# MEDICINAL ESSENTIAL OILS

The Science and Practice of
Evidence-Based Essential Oil Therapy

*Dr. Scott A. Johnson*

Cover design: Scott A. Johnson

Cover Copyright: Scott A. Johnson 2023

Medicinal essential oils: The science and practice of evidence-based essential oil therapy (2ⁿᵈ Edition)/Scott A. Johnson

ISBN-13: 979-8988720607

Discover more books by Scott A. Johnson at www.authorscott.com.

Published by Scott A. Johnson Professional Writing Services, LLC, Orem, Utah

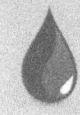

# DISCLAIMERS OF WARRANTY AND LIMITATION OF LIABILITY

The author provides all information on an "as is" and "as available" basis and for informational purposes only. The author makes no representations or warranties of any kind, expressed or implied, as to the information, materials, or products mentioned. Every effort has been made to ensure accuracy and completeness of the information contained; however, it is not intended to replace any medical advice or to halt proper medical treatment, nor diagnose, treat, cure, or prevent any health condition or disease.

Always consult a qualified medical professional before using any dietary supplement or natural product, engaging in physical activity, or modifying your diet; and seek the advice of your physician with any questions you may have regarding any medical condition. Always consult your OB/GYN if you are pregnant or think you may become pregnant before using any dietary supplement or natural product, and to ensure you are healthy enough for exercise or any dietary modifications. The information contained in this book is for educational and informational purposes only, and it is not meant to replace medical advice, diagnosis, or treatment in any manner. Never delay or disregard professional medical advice. Use the information solely at your own risk; the author accepts no responsibility for the use thereof. This book is sold with the understanding that neither the author nor publisher shall be liable for any loss, injury, or harm allegedly arising from any information or suggestion in this book.

The Food and Drug Administration (FDA) has not evaluated the statements contained in this book. The information and materials are not meant to diagnose, prescribe, treat, or cure any disease, condition, illness, or injury.

# ACKNOWLEDGEMENTS

The author gratefully acknowledges the assistance of the following people in the completion and achievement of this book:

My Heavenly Father for blessing me with the talents, knowledge, and wisdom to write this book.

My wife and children, who endured long days (and nights) of writing and research, and offered continual support and encouragement. They are the motivation and inspiration behind my writing. I love them dearly and hope that I will help them achieve health, happiness, and success.

My dedicated fans, who offered encouragement and kind words, and purchased my books, so that I could continue my efforts and contributions to evidence-based natural health and essential oils.

Drs. Prabodh Satyal, Joshua Plant, and Matthew Bernart for providing valuable data during the completion of the book.

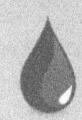

# CONTENTS

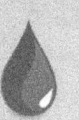

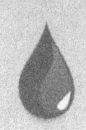

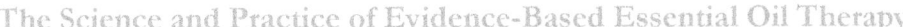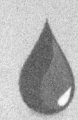

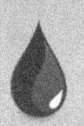

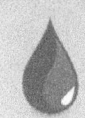

# EVIDENCE-BASED ESSENTIAL OIL THERAPY

Modern medicine, also called allopathic medicine, has ushered in a wonder of scientific advancements and achievements that have greatly benefited humanity. The study of the human body and scientific research have discovered intricate details of human anatomy and physiology, helped us better understand disease cause and progression, revealed our genetic makeup, and much, much more. Organ transplants, medical imaging, and trauma treatment are just a few of the advances of modern medicine that save countless lives each year.

That being said, modern medicine is still largely ineffective in key areas. It emphasizes the treatment of symptoms rather than eradicating the root cause of disease, struggles to adequately address some chronic illnesses, focuses too heavily on invasive treatments, and often causes severe side effects. In addition, modern medicine largely fails when it comes to preventive care, with most doctors lacking the knowledge or time to offer nutritional and lifestyle guidance that could significantly reduce the disease burden facing the world today. Quite frankly, nutrition and lifestyle behaviors are the foundation of health and should be "medical doctor 101," because no amount of drugs (or supplements or essential oils for that matter) can replace eating better and being physically active.

## The Case for Complementary and Integrative Medicine

Where modern medicine fails, alternative—or more appropriately said, complementary or integrative—medicine excels. Complementary medicine relies on gifts provided by Mother Nature as remedies and employs these remedies to support the body's remarkable innate ability to heal. After all, the natural state of man is health, not disease, and the body is well equipped to combat a variety of illnesses and injuries that cause disease, especially when supported in this process. One of the major differences between natural and allopathic medicine is that natural medicine aids processes in the body divinely designed to maintain a state of good health, whereas allopathic medicine thwarts these processes causing the body to go deeper in its repertoire to take corrective actions.

The perception that no evidence exists regarding the safety and efficacy of natural remedies is misguided and entirely incorrect. We have used allopathic interventions with far less evidence than exists for some natural remedies in the modern era. The truth is there are tens of thousands of studies supporting numerous natural remedies as valuable solutions for just as many health conditions and diseases. One need only search PubMed, the U.S. National Library of Medicine's database, to find this evidence. The primary challenge is that much of this research lies in the form of preclinical research that validates decades or centuries of traditional use. In reality, the historical use may be more valuable in some cases because it means the remedy is proven in a "clinical" setting.

The best form of medicine truly is integrative—meaning it combines the best of both modern (Western) and complementary medicine, with pre-ference to the safest, least invasive, and most effective remedy first. Both worlds have something to offer and can improve the lives of men and women if used prudently.

**Essential Oils: The Natural Remedies of the Future**
When it comes to natural remedies, one modality reigns supreme—essential oils. Essential oils offer several key advantages that make them ideal choices as the medicine of the future:

- *They work simultaneously on the emotional, physical, mental, and spiritual levels of health.* Essential oils connect the mind, emotions, body, and spirit to influence all aspects of well-being.
- *A virtually indefinite shelf life for many oils.* When essential oils are unopened and stored in a cool, dark place away from heat and sunlight, their therapeutic value lasts for a very long time. Keep in mind that long-term storage (more than five years) of essential

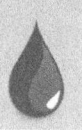 

oils may result in some loss of therapeutic value and potency and increases the risk of oxidation of some of the essential oil constituents. The stability of essential oils depends on several chemical and external (temperature, light, presence of atmospheric oxygen) factors. Citrus oils are more susceptible to degradation because of the high limonene content (very prone to oxidation) and should be discarded if they smell unpleasant or appear cloudy. On the other hand, some essential oils like copaiba, cedarwood, patchouli, myrrh, sandalwood, and vetiver tend to get better with age. Once the bottle is opened, follow the guidelines in the box below.

---

### ESSENTIAL OIL SHELF LIFE*

**1–2 Years**
Citrus oils, lemon verbena, lemongrass, tea tree, melissa, neroli, pine, spruce oils

**2–4 Years**
Virtually all other essential oils

**5–10 Years**
Amyris, cedarwood, copaiba, ginger, myrrh, patchouli, sandalwood, spikenard, vetiver

*Storing essential oils in the refrigerator after opening may extend the shelf life by up to 100%.

---

However, it is noteworthy that modern research suggests essential oils do indeed have a long shelflife when they are left sealed (unopened) and stored in a dark glass bottle and in a cool and dark place. Bulgarian researchers were presented with 5 mL of peppermint essential oil that had been stored for 50 years in dark glass sealed with wax. When they compared this historical peppermint with a fresh sample they concluded that the historical sample's quality met or exceeded the fresh sample in regards to composition, aroma characteristics, and antimicrobial activity.[1] Another study found properly stored 70-year-old lavender had very little oxidation (0.41%).[2]

- *Unmatched versatility.* One essential oil can be used for a variety of purposes and health conditions. This is a remarkable quality that allows a person to store a reasonable quantity of essential oils to use for a variety of ailments and purposes because each essential oil possesses numerous therapeutic properties and uses.

- *Potency.* Essential oils are highly concentrated plant extracts that offer rapid correction, regeneration, protection, and balance, with little or no side effects when used properly. Sometimes one or two drops are all it takes to realize the desired results.

- *Safety.* Essential oils are very safe, with very few contraindications or unintended reactions when used responsibly and prudently.

- *Easy to use.* A complicated materia medica, like used in homeopathy, is not necessary; in fact, many users experience positive results even when the "wrong" essential oil is used.

### The Future of Aromatherapy: The Evidence-based Model

Over the course of recent history, three methodologies, or systems, of aromatherapy have dominated the landscape—dubbed the "British model," the "French model," and to a lesser extent the "German model." While the reality of their existence by the aforementioned names could be argued, the fact that different methodologies exist cannot. Just like divisions and specialties exist in Western Medicine (osteopaths, MDs, neurologists, cardiologists, etc.), some aromatherapists apply different methods or focus on a narrow aspect of essential oils. Each of these methods has contributed to the current knowledge and clinical use of essential oils in different ways.

The "French model" emerged in the early 1900s when French chemists and physicians began experimenting with and investigating the therapeutic properties of essential oils. This model advocates the neat—without diluting in carrier oil—topical application and oral administration of essential oils. A deep understanding of pharmacology, toxicology, anatomy, and physiology is used to determine the therapeutic application of essential oils.

Essential oils are often chosen based on the results of an aromatogram and based on the knowledge of essential oil properties possessed by the clinician. The aromatogram is a laboratory technique and diagnostics method used to guide practitioners to the preferred essential oil for a patient or client. A biological sample from the patient or client (blood, urine, feces, vomit, vaginal discharge, skin, etc.) is cultured in the appropriate medium in a petri dish. Small quantities of essential oils are introduced around the perimeter of the petri dish to determine their antimicrobial activity. The greater the diameter, or zone, of inhibition in the petri

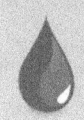

dish, the higher the efficacy of the essential oil. The most efficacious essential oil(s) are then prescribed to be ingested to eliminate what was believed to be the cause of the patient or client's illness. However, the limitation of the aromatogram is that it focuses only on the antimicrobial properties of essential oils and not the fact that they act on many other levels—both biological and psychophysiological—to produce correction.

The therapeutic application of essential oils was introduced to England during the 1950s by Marguerite Maury, who encouraged the heavy dilution of essential oils before applying them to the body and discouraged oral administration because she was not a medical doctor. Her essential oil formulas were individualized based on the receiver's emotional and physical state. The "British model" uses small amounts of essential oils mixed in abundant amounts of carrier oil before topical administration as part of an aromatherapy massage. One of the key contributions of this model to essential oil therapy is a greater knowledge of the safety of essential oils, and possible drug interactions and health contraindications.

The "German model" mainly consists of using essential oils for inhalation purposes. However, Germans greatly advanced the knowledge of distillation procedures during the sixteenth century. Studies suggest that even this simple model, largely relying on the inhalation of essential oils, can have profound psychophysiological effects.

It could be argued that a fourth unrecognized model— the "American model" of aromatherapy—also exists. Each model has its strengths and offers something useful for the essential oil practitioner and layperson alike. The most progressive practitioners will seek to understand each of the methodologies used during essential oil therapy and utilize aspects from each, with a focus on the most evidence-based therapies. The American model recognized this fact and incorporated a bit of each system of thinking.

The future of essential oil therapy, and the one recommended and utilized in this book, is the evidence-based model. This model integrates the best of all models and enriches them with scientific evidence. It combines ancient healing traditions, established protocols, consensus of user testimonials, and scientific evidence to determine therapeutic and safe uses and protocols for countless health conditions.

Evidence-based essential oil therapy is a balanced approach to the therapeutic use of essential oils and suggests a range of dilution—from neat to highly diluted—for topical application. By suggesting a dilution range, each person is able to customize his or her essential oil usage according to his or her knowledge, current state of health, body physiology, propensity toward sensitivity, and level of comfort.

Evidence-based essential oil therapy also supports the oral administration of essential oils, and suggests standardized dosages based on body weight and age. A significant amount of evidence exists to suggest that ingesting reasonable amounts of essential oils is not only safe but offers wide-ranging benefits to human health. In general, only excess or extreme doses are problematic.

Another aspect of the evidence-based model of essential oil therapy is its use of science to determine contraindications and drug interactions. Many essential oils have the potential to interact with drugs if taken concurrently, and so it is important to be knowledgeable of these possible interactions. Indeed, the medical literature and clinical case reports verify that interactions do occur. In addition, some medical conditions require more cautious use of essential oils to prevent the possible aggravation of the condition, and this too is shared as part of this model.

Science and natural remedies are not archenemies and can exist harmoniously with an open-minded practitioner. Truthfully, science is a very welcome member of the evidence-based practitioner's toolbox and can be an influential guide in deciding which oils will work best to restore homeostasis and balance to the body. Those who have used this model have likely realized that its efficacy and safety are unmatched.

The evidence-based practitioners (or average users) of essential oil therapy recognize that essential oils are a big part of a complete integrative approach to human health. This practical approach incorporates all available medical methodologies, with an emphasis on the least invasive remedy that is still effective. They prudently involve their Western physician or modern medical practitioner in their health decisions, inform him or her of their activities, and seek permission to incorporate natural remedies. This book is written with this understood and is in no way meant to replace any advice or care recommended by your primary health practitioner. The reader should always seek physician (or other healthcare practitioner) approval before using any of the recommended protocols.

# SOME ESSENTIAL OIL CONSTITUENTS WITH POSSIBLE
## DRUG INTERACTIONS OR CONTRAINDICATIONS

**Antibiotics, Antifungals:** *Constituents that may increase or decrease the antimicrobial activity of various antibiotics or antifungals when taken together.*

1,8-Cineole (when synergized by other components), Alpha-Terpineol, Bergamottin, Beta-Bisabolene, Cadinenes, Carvacrol, (E)-Cinnamaldehyde, (E)-Cinnamic acid, Citral (Geranial + Neral), Citronellol, Cuminaldehyde, Estragole (Methyl Chavicol), Eugenol, Farnesol, Geraniol, Linalool, Menthol, Methyl Eugenol, (E)-Nerolidol, Piperitenone Oxide, Piperitone, Rosemary (unknown constituents), Terpinen-4-ol, Thymol, Thymoquinone

Note: The synergistic or antagonistic activity of essential oil constituents may be attributed to a combination of the constituents present in the essential oil rather than one single constituent.

**Antidepressants (MAOIs, SSRIs):** *Constituents that may inhibit MAO enzymes or increase serotonin levels in the central nervous system leading to cardiovascular complications, confusion, headache, and convulsions.*

Eugenol, Ethyl-p-Methoxycinnamate, Myristicin

**Antidiabetic Drugs:** *Constituents that may influence blood sugar levels and cause high or low blood sugar.*

1,8-cineole (in synergy with Myrtenyl Acetate, Para-cymene, Beta-Pinene, or Alpha-Pinene), *ar*-Turmerone Carvacrol (weak), Carvone, (E)-Cinnamaldehyde, Citral (Geranial + Neral), Fenugreek (unknown constituents), Geranium (unknown constituents), Thymoquinone, Trans-Anethole, (Z)-Ligustilide, Xanthorrhiozol

**Antiplatelets, Anticoagulants, Blood Pressure Meds, Aspirin:** *Constituents that may increase the blood thinning effects of medications.*

1,8-Cineole (weak), Alpha-Bulnesene, *ar*-turmerone, Ascaridole, Benzoic Acid, Borneol, Carvacrol, Caryophyllene Oxide, Diallyl Trisulfide, (E)-Cinnamaldehyde, (E)-Methylcinnamate, Elemicin (weak), Eugenol, Fenchone, Garlic Sulfides, Isoascaridole, Isoeugenol, Lavandin (synergy of all main components), Menthol, Menthone, Methyl Allyl Trisulfide, Methyl Chavicol (Estragole), Methyl Salicylate, Safrole, Thymol, Thymoquinone, Trans-Anethole, Verbenone, (Z)-Ligustilide

**CYP450 Enzymes:** *Constituents that may interfere with enzymes involved in the metabolism of drugs.*

1,8-Cineole, Alantolactone, Alpha-Bisabolol, Alpha-Humulene, Alpha-Thujone, Beta-Cedrene, Beta-Caryophyllene, Beta-Myrcene, Bergamottin, Bergapten, Borneol, Caryophyllene Oxide, Cedrol, Chalepensin, Chamazulene, Citral (Geranial + Neral), Diallyl Disulfide, Diallyl Trisulfide, (E)-Cinnamaldehyde, (E,E)-Farnesol, Ethyl-p-Methoxycinnamate, Frankincense (lipophilic gum-resin terpene fractions), Garlic Sulfides, Geraniol, Isoimperatorin, Menthofuran, Menthol (weak-moderate), Menthone (very weak), Menthyl Acetate, Methyl Chavicol, Myristicin, Safrole, Spiroether <cis-, trans->, Thujopsene, Thymoquinone, Trans-Anethole, Trans-Carveol

**Diuretic Drugs:** *Constituents that may reduce the passing of urine.*

Trans-Anethole

**Seizures, Epilepsy, Convulsions:** *Constituents that may reduce the seizure threshold—the level at which your brain will have a seizure—of medications or exacerbate or trigger seizures and convulsions.*

1,8-cineole, Camphor, Fenchone, Isopinocamphone, Methyl Salicylate, Pinocamphone, Pulegone, (E)-Sabinyl Acetate, Thujones (Alpha- & Beta-)

Note: The constituents generally need to be present in sufficient quantities to cause an interaction, and some (like 1,8-cineole) require other constituents to be present to create the interaction. Those essential oils considered to have sufficient quantities of the constituent(s) are contraindicated in the individual essential oil monographs.

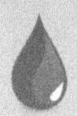

## What Are Essential Oils?

Essential oils are natural aromatic constituents and volatile liquids extracted from the seeds, roots, bark, stems, leaves, flowers, resins, and other parts of plants. These valuable liquids are most commonly obtained from plants through distillation—often by using steam. They can also be expressed mechanically or cold-pressed, as is the case with citrus oils extracted from peels. The chemical makeup of essential oils is highly complex and may consist of hundreds of distinct chemical constituents. Some delicate botanicals (i.e. rose and jasmine) may be extracted with solvents like n-Hexane. When solvent extraction is used, the end product is an absolute that contains both essential oils and other plant constituents (i.e. waxes and coloring constituents). This extract is not a true essential oil, but it is often used by aromatherapists.

## Essential Oil Constituents

A considerable variety of—often structurally related—constituents have been identified in essential oils. Each essential oil can contain from a few to a complex mixture of hundreds of individual constituents. In general, most essential oil constituents can be assigned as lipophilic terpenoids, phenylpropanoids, or short-chain aliphatic hydrocarbon derivatives.[3] Among these, the major constituents found in essential oils can be classified as follows:

*Alcohols*: The name of alcohols start with the parent terpene they were derived from and always end in "-ol." Alcohols often possess good antiseptic, antiviral, and antifungal properties. They are generally nonirritating to the skin and nontoxic. Alcohols can be uplifting and energizing. Some examples of alcohols include linalool, menthol, borneol, cedrol, citronellol, and geraniol.

*Aldehydes*: Aldehydes are responsible for the characteristic fragrance, or aroma, of many essential oils. Some properties of the various aldehydes include: anti-infectious, tonic, immune-stimulating, hypotensive, antiseptic, anti-inflammatory, vasodilating, fever-reducing, and calming properties. Essential oils with high levels of aldehydes, like lemongrass, may irritate the skin and cause sensitization in some individuals. Aldehydes are unstable and susceptible to oxidation when exposed to oxygen and low heat, making it important to store them properly. Aldehydes end in "-al." Common aldehydes include cinnamaldehyde, neral, geranial, and citronellal.

*Alkanes*: Only a few essential oils contain alkanes and usually in very small quantities. Rose essential oil has one of the highest concentrations of alkanes, which may be one reason it possesses such unique properties. The purpose of alkanes in plants is to protect the plant from harmful organisms and predators, as well as decrease water and mineral loss. Examples include tricosane, undecane, nonadecane, eicosane, and dodecane.

*Alkenes*: Abundant in trees and other plants, alkenes influence the characteristic odor of essential oils. These constituents can be identified by their "-ene" ending. They frequently possess anti-inflammatory, relaxant, anticancer, analgesic, antifungal, and antimicrobial properties. Examples include delta-cadinene, alpha-cedrene, chamazulene, alpha-humulene, farnesene, and beta-myrcene.

*Carboxylic Acids*: Carboxylic acids are organic acids formed by the oxidation of aldehydes that usually end in "-ic acid." They are rarely found in essential oils because they are not very volatile. They are anti-inflammatory and antiallergenic. An example of a carboxylic acid in essential oils is cotronellic acid.

*Coumarins*: Coumarin-containing essential oils may be solid at room temperature. Furanocoumarins are typically phototoxic and should not be used immediately prior to sun or UV ray exposure and for twelve hours thereafter. They are not easily extracted during the distillation process because they are not very volatile. Coumarins may be blood thinning, hypotensive, antispasmodic, anticonvulsant, and antimicrobial. They include coumarin, umbelliferone, bergapten, psoralen, angelicin, and citropen.

*Esters*: Essential oils that contain esters are generally very fragrant, often producing a fruity aroma. They can possess antispasmodic, anti-inflammatory, antifungal, relaxant, antimicrobial, and skin-nourishing properties. Essential oils high in esters are good choices for muscle spasms and skin rashes. These constituents are widely found in essential oils and usually end in "-ate." Some examples of esters include linalyl acetate, eugenyl acetate, methyl salicylate, and geranyl acetate.

*Ethers*: Ethers have similar properties and characteristics to esters but are considered much stronger constituents. Because of their powerful effect, essential oils that contain ethers should not be taken in high doses or used for extended periods. They often possess antiseptic, anti-infectious, anti-inflammatory, diuretic, antispasmodic, expectorant, stimulant, and nervine (calms and soothes the nerves) properties. Ethers usually end in "-ole" and include 1,8-cineole and caryophyllene oxide.

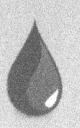 

*Ketones*: These reasonably stable constituents are not easily metabolized by the liver, so those with liver diseases should use very small quantities of essential oils high in ketones and only for short periods. Ketones are extremely powerful and often considered toxic because of their potency. Some do have neurotoxic potential at higher doses, such as pulegone, pinocamphone, and alpha-thujone, but others like carvone and menthone are safer. Some ketones aid the removal of mucous, stimulate cell and tissue regeneration, promote the removal of scar tissue, aid digestion, normalize inflammation, relieve pain, reduce fever, may inhibit coagulation of blood, and encourage relaxation. Other examples of ketones include turmerone and fenchone.

*Lactones*: Lactones are organic esters that commonly possess antimicrobial, antiviral, anti-inflammatory, relaxing, expectorant, analgesic, hypotensive, and fever reducing properties. They are primarily found in expressed oils because of their molecular weight, but are sometimes found in solvent-extracted absolutes as well. Examples include alantolactone and nepetalactone.

*Oxides*: Oxides are formed when an element is oxidized by exposure to the oxygen in the air. Eucalyptol (1,8-cineole) is by far the most common ether oxide found in essential oils. They can be expectorants, mildly anti-infectious, antiseptic, and anesthetic. Examples include eucalyptol, linalyl oxide, and caryophyllene oxide.

*Phenols or Phenolics*: The most common phenols found in essential oils include thymol, carvacrol, eugenol, and chavicol. Their names end in "-ol" or "phenol." Essential oils that contain phenols are highly susceptible to oxidation, may irritate the stomach lining in large quantities, and are very likely to cause skin sensitivity and/or reactions, so essential oils that contain them must always be diluted before topical application. Essential oils with phenols should only be used for short periods and taken in lower doses internally because they are very powerful. They can be stimulating to the nervous and immune systems, act as a tonic within the body, are powerful anti-infectious agents, help rid the body of parasites, may elevate body temperature, help normalize inflammation, useful for rheumatic conditions, help expel excess gas from the intestines, diuretic, antiseptic, and have been shown to clean cell-receptor sites.

*Phenylpropenes (phenylpropanoids)*: A molecule that contains both a phenol molecule and a propyl radical is known as a phenylpropanoid. Examples of phenylpropanoids include eugenol, methyleugenol, elemicin, safrole, estragole (methyl chavicol), and myristicin. These essential oil compounds are very important because they interact with substances attached to cell receptor sites to trigger healing and homeostasis. They can be cleansing, protect against free radicals, aid immune function, and repel insects.

*Terpenes*: Terpenes can be subdivided into monoterpenes, sesquiterpenes, and diterpenes based on the number of carbon atoms they have (mono 10, sesqui 15, di 20). Terpenes can inhibit both the initiation and progression of cancerous cells.[4,5] Another remarkable property of terpenes is their ability to readily cross the blood-brain barrier and to enter brain tissues.[6,7] According to research, terpenes increase cerebral blood flow, thus indirectly enhancing delivery of oxygen to the brain.[5] Given their great diversity, they possesses myriad properties: antiviral, antibacterial, antifungal, antiseptic, analgesic, antioxidant, protective of DNA, antitumoral, anti-inflammatory, antispasmodic, expectorant, antiallergenic, stimulative of organs, encourage proper delivery of oxygen to tissues, supportive of the detoxification processes, and can be both uplifting and relaxing. Monoterpenes are widely found in essential oils. Examples of terpenes include limonene, alpha-pinene, myrcene, camphene, chamazulene, beta-phellandrene, beta-caryophyllene, farnesene, cedrene, delta-cadinene, and sabinene.

### A Brief History of Essential Oils and Aromatics

A collection of ancient texts and historical and archaeological evidence—including Egyptian hieroglyphs, Chinese manuscripts, Greek physicians' records, and biblical references—suggest that aromatic essences and essential oils have been an integral part of health and wellness for centuries. Aromatic extracts have been used extensively throughout recorded history for medicinal and ritual purposes, psychological, social reasons, food preparation, beautification, and even as currency.

The Egyptians were among the first to use aromatic essences and resins as medicines, cosmetics, embalming agents, and as a central component of important rituals. Traces of aromatics have been discovered in jars collected from Egyptian tombs and identified on mummy bandages.[8,9,10] Pots containing frankincense and another aromatic essence were discovered when Tutankhamen's tomb was opened in 1922, and remarkably still offered a hint of aromatic scent after thousands of years being sealed in a tomb. Historical records also suggest that Imhotep, the Grand Vizier of King Djoser (2780–2720 BC) promoted the use of aromatic essences for medicinal purposes.[11,12]

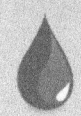

The ancient healing traditions of Chinese and Ayurvedic medicine similarly used aromatic plants to promote well-being. Ancient Buddhists were believed to have used incense for purification and ceremonial purposes. Ancient Chinese texts also refer to the use of aromatic essences for medicinal purposes.[13]

The Greeks incorporated essential oils into therapeutic massages, and the Romans used them for personal hygiene and to promote health. The Persians borrowed from Roman, Greek, Chinese, and Indian teachings as they integrated aromatic plants into their healing system. The Greek physician Hippocrates (460 to c. 375 BC), considered the father of modern medicine, purportedly advocated aromatic baths and fumigation with aromatics for medicinal purposes. According to historical records, he fumigated the city of Athens with an aromatic oil saving the city's inhabitants from a devastating plague.[14] Aromatic botanicals and resins are mentioned throughout the Bible as integral parts of spiritual and ritual ceremonies.

French chemists are credited with discovering the antibacterial properties of essential oils in 1887.[15,16] The modern term aromatherapy was coined by French chemist and perfumer Rene-Maurice Gattefosse. After burning his hand in a laboratory accident in 1910, he treated it with lavender essence, or lavender oil. He explained that after applying lavender, his pain diminished, the gas gangrene ended, and over time, his hand healed without infection. Inspired by the results of Gattefosse's experiments, Dr. Jean Valnet used essential oils to successfully treat the infections and wounds of soldiers during World War II. During the 1950s, Marguerite Maury began diluting essential oils in carrier oil for direct topical application and invented essential oil blends for specific health conditions.

Today, an abundant amount of evidence is building that suggests essential oils possess significant healing properties. Clinical studies in Europe, Australia, Japan, India, Canada, Iran, the United States, and elsewhere have revealed remarkable healing properties of many essential oils. These studies have found that essential oils are effective for a variety of health concerns, including infections, pain, anxiety, depression, nausea, hormone balance, memory, and much more.

## The Importance of Essential Oil Purity and Authenticity

Pure, authentic oils—not the fragrance-grade kind that is often sold for use as perfumes or as scents—are very concentrated constituents, which are far more potent than dried herbs. They are powerful yet gentle remedies that can be used by adults, children, infants, and some pets to restore homeostasis, correct mood disturbances, physical ailments, cognitive difficulties, and even influence spiritual awareness.

The importance of essential oil purity cannot be overstated. Quite frankly, there are many oils on the market that are manipulated for consistency of scent or to pad the company's pockets, rather than produced for clinical use. The majority of essential oils on the market today are used for perfumes—it is estimated that up to 98 percent of essential oils are used in the perfume or food industries or to add scents to candles, soaps, and other household care items. Unfortunately, even those that are intended for therapeutic application are frequently diluted or adulterated by unscrupulous traders to increase profitability, control consistency, and create essential oils with a more appealing aroma.

A significant number of essential oil traders regularly adulterate their oils with cheaper—but similar—oils, isolated synthetic constituents, essential oils of similar species, or less expensive parts of the same plant. This is done to produce a more consistent taste and smell but, ultimately, to generate more profits for the trader. Some common adulterations include reducing the menthol content of cornmint essential oil and passing it off as pure peppermint oil, adding synthetic phenylethyl alcohol to rose otto, adding lavandin to lavender, diluting citronella with lemongrass, or using cinnamon leaf instead of bark.

Synthetic constituents are less expensive and offer greater consistency in constituent profile that cannot be achieved in natural plants. Plants inherently have varying degrees of constituents in them based on harvest time, growing type, geographic region, soil quality, altitude, weather, cultivation practices, and water quality. It is remarkable how significantly an essential oils constituent profile can change based on these factors. In fact, the same species can produce a different chemotype—an essential oil where one constituent is produced more abundantly or an essential oil with unique properties and constituent profile based on growing conditions or location. In order to provide a constant constituent profile, one must use synthetic constituents that are meticulously controlled for consistency through creation in a lab.

If an essential oil smells differently than the natural aroma of the plant, this is not a sign of purity, but rather an indication that the constituents in the oil have been altered from what is found in nature. For example, some

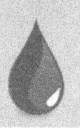 

companies want their lavender to smell better, so after distilling the plant materials, they add a synthetic version of a constituent that is naturally found in lavender, such as linalool or linalyl acetate. They do this because adding more linalool or linalyl acetate improves the fragrance of the oil. This offers no improvement in the therapeutic value of the oil—in fact, quite the opposite. It augments the smell and places the natural constituents found in the oil out of balance.

Another common adulteration seen on the market is with wintergreen oil. Wintergreen plants are naturally high in methyl salicylate—a constituent similar to aspirin. In fact, wintergreen plants usually contain more than 95 percent methyl salicylate. However, many wintergreen oils sold on the market have added synthetic methyl salicylate as either a complete substitution or to dilute the oil. These oils are obviously adulterated and not fit for clinical use.

**The Dangers of Synthetic or Adulterated Essential Oils**

Frankly, using these synthetic and adulterated essential oils can cause significant harm. While even synthetic and adulterated essential oils may produce results in the short term, long-term use may cause allergies, headaches, and chemical sensitivities, and result in body toxicity. We know that toxins—like those synthetically created in a lab—are harmful to the body. Those who are concerned about their health make a concerted effort to avoid toxins, chemicals, and synthetic constituents in personal care products, soaps, and more. Yet, by using an adulterated essential oil, such as those mentioned above, people are inviting these chemicals and toxins to make their bodies their home. This is counterintuitive, that a "health product" would contain harmful ingredients that can be detrimental to your health.

To ensure you are using a pure oil, look for:

- a company that has expertise in the distillation process and innovative distillation equipment—this is generally through their partners, vendors, and suppliers, not the actual retailer of the essential oils;

- a company that utilizes the published essential oils research in scientific journals and takes a clinical approach to essential oil development;

- a company that is personally involved in the farming and cultivation process through the inspection of supplier farms by a qualified expert;

- a company that verifies purity with their own laboratories or third-party testing facilities, and

retains educated scientists experienced in essential oil analysis to read and interpret test results;

- a company that uses advanced testing methods (you need more than a GC-MS test to determine purity and clinical value);

- a company with essential oils that smell like the natural plants and whose single oils vary slightly in aroma from batch to batch due to inherent variations in plants. (Slight variations in the smell of each batch of oil is a good indication that Mother Nature has created the essential oil and not a lab. This trait is desirable and normal; whereas if your lavender oil always smells exactly the same, it could be an indication that the oil is adulterated.); and

- a company that is willing to share results from the tests their essential oils have undergone to ensure purity and authenticity, for the specific batch of oil you have purchased. If a company is not willing to share this information, you are placing blind faith in them and may very well be using a product that doesn't meet the high quality standards required for clinical use.

Many traders (and consumers for that matter) equate purity to organic; however, organic does not always mean pure. Essential oils that are certified organic have been grown according to standards set and verified by approved organizations. The certification process is lengthy and costly, prohibiting some farmers and distillers from receiving certification despite following organic standards. Although essential oils distilled from organically grown plants are greatly preferred, essential oils certified organic are not generally superior to essential oils extracted form organically grown plants. In fact, the chemical constituents in an essential oil certified organic and not certified organic are virtually identical.

In addition, some organic pesticides are known to negatively affect the nervous system and the mitochondria of living cells. This is problematic considering that organic pest control products often require intense applications to be effective (sometimes 20 times the amount of synthetic equivalents). Lastly, the small percentage of certified organic essential oil suppliers (estimated by some to be less than 2% of the market) is not sufficient to meet current demands. Organic essential oils are simply not sustainable and not worth the additional cost to the consumer. Instead, the focus should be on distilling essential oils from organically grown plants, not certified organic.

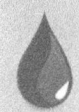

## Usage, Best Practices, and Safety Guidelines

As with any remedy, natural or otherwise, a few guidelines, or best practices, must be followed to maximize effectiveness and foster safety:

- Essential oils should be applied at the first signs of symptoms—when you first start feeling ill—or immediately following an injury. The sooner an essential oil is administered during the onset of illness or after injury, the more rapid and complete your results will be.

- Apply essential oils as often as every five minutes with severe injuries or where illness is progressing, two to four times daily if you catch the illness early, or one to three times daily for chronic conditions.

- Apply oils based on body size—up to 6 to 15 drops per application for a large body (though often 1 to 2 drops is all it takes to obtain the desired results), up to 5 to 10 drops for adolescents and teenagers (but again think less is more, particularly the younger the child), up to 1 to 5 drops for small children, and small amounts of essential oil diluted to a 0.3% to 1.0% dilution ratio for infants and very small children. More is not always better, and this is definitely the case with essential oils, particularly as it relates to children. Children will naturally respond more rapidly and vigorously to natural remedies and so using large amounts of essential oils is unnecessary. Excessive use of essential oils can lead to unintended and undesirable reactions, so start with lower amounts (like 1 to 2 drops) and work up from there if necessary. While these are averages and common doses used, it doesn't hurt to start out with smaller doses (even 1 or 2 drops) and then increase the dosage as necessary. Where specific dosages are recommended, they are generally recommended for the average size adult (154 lb. or 70 kg), so adjust the dosage accordingly.

### ORAL DOSAGE GUIDELINES[+]

| Age/Weight | Total Daily Oral Dosage | Sublingual Dose (Per Dose) |
|---|---|---|
| Birth–12 mos. (Up to 22 lb.) | Not recommended | Not recommended |
| 1–5 yrs. (23–44 lb.) | Not Recommended | Not Recommended |
| 6–11 yrs. (45–77 lb.) | 1–2 drops/4–6 hrs; 8 drops/24 hrs (0.5 mL max.) | 1 drop |
| 12–17 yrs. (78-153 lb.) | 1–3 drops/4–6 hrs; 15 drops/24 hrs (1.0 mL max.) | 1–2 drops |
| 18+ (154+ lb.) | 1–5 drops/4–6 hrs; 25 drops/24 hrs max. (1.65 mL max.) | 1–3 drops (The higher end should be reserved for very mild oils) |

### TOPICAL DOSAGE GUIDELINES[+]

| Age/Weight | Recommended Dilution Ratio | Total Daily Topical Usage |
|---|---|---|
| Birth–12 mos. (Up to 22 lb.) | 0.3% dilution | Up to 1.5 drops EO |
| 1–5 yrs. (23–44 lb.) | 1.5%–3% dilution; neat for some applications | Up to 15 drops EO |
| 6–11 yrs. (45–77 lb.) | 1.5%–5% dilution; neat for rare applications | Up to 17 drops EO |
| 12–17 yrs. (78–153 lb.) | 1.5%–20% dilution; neat for some applications | Up to 25 drops EO |
| 18+ yrs. (154+ lb.) | 1.5%–neat for some applications | Up to 45 drops EO |

[+] Except where otherwise recommended in this book or a published clinical study. Based on a 60 mg drop. The dosage recommendations are offered as a guide and should not be considered perfect and fast rules. The age, height, weight, and current health status of the individual, the essential oil being used, and the health condition being managed must all be considered. Use lower dosages with the elderly, those taking medications, and alcoholics.

- Apply essential oils on the feet, spine, or affected area unless otherwise directed. The feet are one of the best, and preferred, places to apply oils for a few reasons.

  1) The feet are less prone to sensitivity and irritation than other areas of the body. Applying oils on the feet will reduce the probability of causing skin sensitivity and reactions. When in doubt, apply to the feet.

  2) The entire body is represented on the feet. For example, the big toe is your head, the

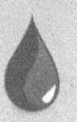 

insides of both feet represent the spine, and so forth. When you apply essential oils to the feet with varied pressure and massage, you can profoundly influence areas of the body far from the feet through reflex responses sent by the nervous system, including vital organs. If you want to affect a specific area, system, or organ of the body through the feet please refer to the chart at the end of this book.

3) Sweat may enhance absorption of essential oils through the skin. The feet are often moist from perspiration, which provides a great location to enhance absorption. Research suggests that warm, wet, and hydrated skin can increase the absorption of some essential oil constituents up to three times.[17]

4) And lastly, decades of aromatic foot massages by savvy clinicians and essential oils users, and emerging clinical research, has demonstrated that remarkable results are obtained by taking care of our feet.

- Use multiple application methods—topical, oral, inhalation, and retention—for specific health concerns or to amplify therapeutic effects. A great example of a time when this is necessary is when treating a respiratory complaint. In this case, it would be best to apply essential oils topically to the chest area, diffuse/inhale to get essential oil molecules into the lungs, and possibly ingest oils to boost immune system activity.

- Combine (blend) multiple essential oils for improved efficacy. Great results can be obtained with one single oil, but an additive or synergistic effect may be achieved when a combination of oils is administered. Essential oil combinations often work on different aspects of a health condition helping to get to the root causes of illness.

- Continue essential oil therapy for a few to several days following relief of symptoms to ensure full and deep healing has occurred. If you don't continue therapy after symptoms cease, the cause of the illness may transfer to other tissues within the body and remain dormant until reactivated (usually by diet, environmental exposures, or inactivity) to cause illness again.

- A general rule of thumb is that for every year you have suffered with a chronic condition, it may take one month of therapy to correct the condition. For example, if you have suffered from migraines for three years, it will likely take at least three months to establish harmony and homeostasis in the body again. However, if you experience an acute condition and don't obtain results within a few hours—often within minutes—try a different oil, or different method of application. You may also have used insufficient or too much essential oil for the therapy to be effective. Each person is biologically unique and will respond differently to different oils; what works for one person may not work for another. Allow your body to "tell" you which oil to use by the way you respond and feel. Not all effective oils are listed for every condition, but rather those essential oils that have proven effective for most people or have the greatest scientific evidence to support usage.

## Essential Oils Cautions with Children

Although children's responses to remedies have much in common with adult responses because of similar basic cellular and physiological processes, the administration of essential oils in children requires adjustment. Differences in body composition, organ function at certain ages of maturity (e.g. liver function in infants), timing of the phases of uptake and distribution, and distinctive skin characteristics each have important implications regarding essential oil effect, loading dose, and dosage interval.

Certain essential oil constituents have a greater toxicity potential in children than adults. Essential oils that contain significant amounts of 1,8-cineole (potentially over 50%), camphor (potentially over 20%), menthol (potentially over 25%), thujone, and methyl salicylate should be avoided at certain ages in children. Commonly available essential oils that contain significant amounts of these constituents include peppermint, cornmint, eucalyptus, bay laurel, rosemary, wintergreen, common sage, and mugwort.

Essential oils rich in menthol or 1,8-cineole or menthol should be avoided in children under 3, particularly around the nose and mouth, due to the potential to decrease respiratory rate. Use each of these oils very cautiously, both topically and diffused, for children up to age 5 (see individual recommendations). In the case of sensitive children, it may be necessary to avoid these essential oils up to age 10, though this is very rare. Blends that contain these individual oils are less likely to pose a risk because the other oils may balance their intensity, but the safest approach is to treat these blends the same way you would an individual oil.

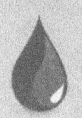

Wintergreen and birch contain methyl salicylate, which is a constituent very similar to aspirin. Ingesting as little as 2.5 mL can be extremely toxic to children, and several well-documented fatalities have resulted after the ingestion of as little as 4 mL in young children.[18,19,20,21,22,23,24] Wintergreen and birch should be avoided by children under age 12 to prevent salicylate poisoning and serious adverse events. This is particularly important with children who are currently experiencing a viral infection, flu-like symptoms, or a fever.

Common sage, mugwort, and other essential oils can contain significant amounts of neurotoxic alpha-thujone or beta-thujone. Given that children's nervous systems are more sensitive to toxicity than adults, it is best to avoid the use of thujone-rich oils with children under age 6, and perhaps longer depending on their individual sensitivity.

It is quite uncommon—thought to affect a very, very small minority of children—but essential oils with the aforementioned constituents may cause adverse reactions in young children, including central nervous system problems,[25,26,27] respiratory distress (difficulty breathing or labored breathing), nystagmus (involuntary eye movement)[28,29] and toxicity,[30,31,32,33,34,35,36] and this reaction can occur from inhalation only. The risk of a reaction depends on the method of administration and amounts exposed to. The greater the level of exposure, the greater the risk of an adverse reaction.

Do not apply any of these essential oils on or near a child's face and avoid diffusing them near young children. This includes applying them on your own body in a place where they would be exposed to them. Use mild oils like copaiba, lavender, German chamomile, lemon, and frankincense instead.

Although the chance of these few essential oils causing harm is extremely remote and largely dependent on exposure amount, it is important to be extra cautious when it comes to the health and safety of children, and no parent wants to see his or her child experience any of these adverse reactions. Very young children, from birth to 24 months, are more likely to experience adverse reactions because their breathing and airway defensive reflexes are still maturing. This is particularly true of premature infants. One study found that when forty-four premature infants were exposed to menthol fumes, they experienced altered airway resistance such as temporary cessation of breathing or a decrease in breathing rate.[37]

Some parents have found that they can use the essential oils associated with respiratory problems on children under 5. If you have used any of the oils mentioned and your child did not experience a reaction, it may be that your child is not sensitive to the constituents associated with problems. However, parents are strongly encouraged to con-sider alternatives (myrtle, balsam fir, etc.) that have proven to be just as effective without the risks of unintended reactions—particularly since there are so many essential oils with similar properties.

Avoid oral administration of essential oils with children under the age of 3. Oral administration in children under the age of 6 should be limited to the mildest of essential oils and very small doses, and when medically deemed necessary—meaning the benefits of doing so far outweigh the risks. Some essential oils may cause acute toxicity in children under the age of 6 if administered orally (almost always very large quantities). Always check the cautions section of this book before using any essential oil with your children.

Please see the specific section titled "ESSENTIAL OILS FOR INFANTS AND CHILDREN" for precise and detailed information about how to use essential oils with children. This chapter also outlines child-specific protocols for the most common health conditions that children experience. Children naturally respond more rapidly and remarkably to small amounts of essential oils, making the use of large amounts unnecessary. As a child matures to adulthood (based on both size and age), he or she may use the adult protocols.

### Do Lavender and Tea Tree Oil Cause Breast Growth in Young Boys?

A number of websites warn parents against using lavender and tea tree oil on their young boys because of a study that claims the topical application of these oils causes prepubertal gynecomastia (enlargement of the breast tissue in males).[38] However, this conclusion is flawed and hotly contested by other scientists and essential oil experts. First, the researchers failed to analyze the commercial products that allegedly caused the breast growth, so we don't even know for sure if the products contained lavender or tea tree oils. Another flaw to the study authors' conclusion is that none of the boys' hormone tests were abnormal except one (case two), who had elevated testosterone levels (not estrogen). In addition, the products that were used in each of the three cases would not allow sufficient absorption of essential oils into the bloodstream to disrupt the endocrine system in such a way to cause

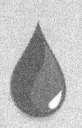 

gynecomastia. Lastly, the study authors conducted *in vitro* testing to determine the estrogenic activity of the oils, which concluded that only extreme levels of the oils produced any estrogenic effects, and these estrogenic effects were one million times less than that of natural estradiol. These extreme levels couldn't have been achieved with the products allegedly causing the breast enlargement, so in reality the researchers' own findings contradict their conclusions.

The first case reports the use of a "healing balm" containing lavender shortly before the breast development occurred in a four-year-old boy. Since the breast enlargement occurred shortly after the topical application of the product, it is unlikely that enough lavender could have entered the bloodstream to cause the breast enlargement.

The second case alleges that a ten-year-old boy experienced breast enlargement after using a styling gel and shampoo with lavender and tea tree oil listed as ingredients. A later report suggests that the hair care products used were analyzed and contained very low concentrations to virtually undetectable amounts of tea tree oil (lavender content was not verified). Based on the low concentrations of tea tree oil and the fact that one of the two products is a wash-off product, it is highly unlikely that either product caused the breast enlargement. Again, not enough of the oils could have entered the bloodstream to cause the condition.

The third report claims that a boy (almost eight) experienced breast enlargement after frequently using a lavender-scented soap and after occasionally applying a lavender-scented lotion. Interestingly, his fraternal twin also used the lavender-scented lotion (but not the soap) and did not experience breast enlargement. Very little essential oil is used in scented soaps, and the product is washed off leaving very little time for absorption. Combining these facts with the point that the twin brother did not experience breast enlargement suggests that something else may have caused the gynecomastia, not the essential oils.

Traditional use and other clinical trials have not reported endocrine-disrupting effects of lavender and tea tree oils. Given the number of young boys regularly exposed to these essential oils, it would be logical that thousands of cases of gynecomastia would be reported if this was a real concern. Based on the evidence, it is highly unlikely that reasonable topical application of lavender and tea tree products will result in any breast development in young boys. Indeed, animal research suggests that not

even the topical application of up to 100 mg/kg (equivalent to over 1.1 mL in a 154-pound adult human) of lavender oil disrupted endocrine system function, nor the subsequent production of develop-mental and reproductive hormones.[39] It is more likely that the personal care products used contained endocrine disrupting chemicals that are frequently found in personal care products than that the essential oil fragrances caused gynecomastia. It is however possible that the essential oils increased the absorption of these chemicals because many essential oils are known to enhance the penetration of substances through the skin. This points to the importance of using more natural personal care products without harmful chemicals.

## Hormone-sensitive Cancers and Phytoestrogen-containing Oils

A great deal of controversy surrounds the role of phytoestrogens among women with a history of or greater risk of hormone-sensitive cancers. Hormone-sensitive cancer cells have receptors that activate when specific hormones bind to them. Once activated these receptors alter gene expression and may stimulate uncontrolled cell growth. If the cancer cells contain estrogen receptors, the cancer is called estrogen receptor-positive, or ER-positive. If the cancer cells contain progesterone receptors, the cancer is considered PR-positive. If the cancer cells lack estrogen and/or progesterone receptors, the cancer is called ER- or PR-negative.

Drugs used for hormone-sensitive cancers block ovarian function (the ovaries are the primary source of estrogen production in premenopausal women), inhibit aromatase activity (an enzyme involved in estrogen production), or bind to estrogen receptors to prevent estrogen from binding. Given our current understanding that phytoestrogens can bind to estrogen cell receptors and either block or mimic the action of estrogen,[40] it is likely that some phytoestrogens have the ability to reduce the risk of estrogen-positive cancers. The current body of scientific evidence seems to support this conclusion. For example, both sclareol and anethole—phytoestrogen essential oil constituents found in clary sage and fennel essential oils respectively—possess anticancer activity against ER-positive breast cancer cells.[41,42]

However, some scientists suggest that the ability of phytoestrogen byproducts to exert mild estrogenic activity may increase the risk of hormone-sensitive cancers.[43,44] One study concluded that late-stage cancer cells (without ERbeta—an estrogen receptor that is associated with a reduction in the spread and metastatic

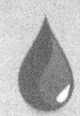

activity of breast cancer cells)[45] increase tumor activity when exposed to phytoestrogens.[46] However, given the important role of ERbeta in breast cancer prevention, it is possible that the lack of ERbeta receptors had more to do with the increased tumor activity than the presence of phytoestrogens.

Limited research has been conducted regarding phytoestrogens found in essential oils and cancer risk. Clary sage contains the phytoestrogen sclareol, which is structurally similar to estradiol. However, the available research does not suggest that clary sage increases the risk of estrogen-dependent cancers.[47,48,49,50,51] In fact, one study determined that the presence of estradiol (originating from natural production within the body) increased the spread of breast cancer cells—with or without the presence of phytoestrogens—but when only the phytoestrogens were present, breast cancer cell apoptosis (destruction) increased.[52] Another study found that the dietary phytoestrogen genistein (from soy) reversed BRCA1 gene deficiency—the dysfunction of which is strongly associated with increased breast cancer risk—and triggered the expression of apoptosis-related genes.[53]

At present, the science surrounding phytoestrogens and whether they increase or decrease hormone-sensitive cancers is inconclusive and debated. However, moderate intake of dietary phyto-estrogens is suspected of reducing cancer risk based on a lower incidence of cancer among populations that consume more dietary phytoestrogens.[54,55]

Overall, essential oil phytoestrogens are considered balancing, with the ability to moderately distinguish body needs and either compete with or mimic estrogen. It is likely that the reasonable use of phytoestrogen-containing essential oils may have a protective effect against some cancers (even among ER-positive populations). Based on the available evidence, it is recommended that women with a history of or higher risk of hormone-sensitive cancers consult their physician for his or her recommendation as to whether to use essential oils that contain phytoestrogens.

### Contraceptives and Essential Oils

Interactions between essential oils—particularly those that contain phytoestrogens or interact with estrogen receptors—and oral contraceptives has not been fully investigated. Essential oils that contain phytoestrogens, like fennel, have demonstrated estrogenic effects, but significantly weaker than estrogens naturally produced by the body or synthetic estrogen.[56] Some essential oil constituents (citral, geraniol, nerol, and eugenol) do not exert estrogenic activity unless present in high concentrations, but they are able to displace 17-beta-estradiol from estrogen cell receptors (ERα and ERβ).[57] However, this displacement was not significant enough to affect the activity or function of estrogen. This research suggests that high concentrations of phytoestrogens are required to interact with estrogen receptors, whereas low concentrations do not interact. Indeed, the weak estrogenic activity of low concentrations of phytoestrogens may provide a range of health benefits, such as prevention of breast, prostate, and hormone-related cancers, reduced risk of cardiovascular disease, improvement of menopausal symptoms, decreased osteoporosis risk, and maintenance of cognitive function, according to our current knowledge.[58,59]

Oral contraceptives contain synthetic progesterone and/or estrogen to suppress ovulation or make the cervical mucous impenetrable to sperm to prevent conception. Whether phytoestrogens amplify or block this effect is not fully known. But it is reasonable to suppose that reports of interactions would be available in populations that consume large amounts of phytoestrogens in their diet if interactions were actually occurring on a regular basis.

While science has yet to fully investigate the relationship between phytoestrogens and contraceptives, it is highly unlikely that the weak estrogenic activity of essential oils containing phytoestrogens will interfere with oral contraceptives that have a much stronger activity. Dietary phytoestrogens appear to pose no risk according to the available research—which is sparse. Researchers reported that soy phytoestrogens do not alter the menstrual cycle or hormone levels, even among those taking an oral contraceptive.[60] Currently, no evidence exists that suggests phytoestrogens found in essential oils will interfere with oral contraceptives because their activity is significantly weaker than that of synthetic hormones.

### Essential Oils Care during Pregnancy and Lactation

Always consult your OBGYN before using any essential oils. Very little information exists regarding the safety of essential oils during pregnancy and lactation. Because of this, caution and common sense is advised, especially during the first trimester, with a sensible approach being to focus on essential oils that are mild (citrus oils, for example) and avoid more than normal dosages. In addition, one should be very cautious with oral administration during pregnancy because it is highly

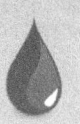

likely that essential oils cross the placenta to the fetus. Knowing this, it is recommended to limit oral consumption of essential oils to a dosage range of 10 to 25 percent of the standard adult dose.

Some essential oils contain constituents that can be toxic and prevent conception, harm the fetus, or result in birth defects—usually when used in significant quantities. The use of the following common oils should be avoided by any method of application throughout pregnancy and while nursing (primarily because these essential oils have a greater toxic potential to infants as well): Anise, applemint (pulegone CTs), auracaria, basil (methyl chavicol and methyl eugenol CTs), bay (West Indies), bay laurel, betony (bicyclogermacrene CT), birch, blue cypress (wood oil), boldo, buchu, calamus (various CTs), carrot seed, cassia, chaste tree, cinnamon bark, cinnamon leaf, clove, dill (with apiol), elecampane, fennel, Formosan cypress (twig oil), genipi, hairy basil (various CTs), hemp, holy basil (various CTs), hyssop (various CTs), juniper (Chinese), kumquat (linalool CT), ledum (*L. palustre*), lovage, mountain savory, mugwort, myrrh, nutmeg, oregano, parsley, pennyroyal, Ponderosa pine, ravensara (various CTs), rosalina (methyl eugenol CT), rue, sage, savin, savory (wild—carvacrol & thymol CTs), spearmint (pulegone-menthone-isomenthone CT), star anise, summer savory, tamala (various CTs), tansy, tarragon, thuja, western red cedar (leaves), white turmeric, wintergreen, wormseed (American), wormwood, and yarrow. Other essential oils should be used cautiously and in lower doses (if needed) during pregnancy and lactation due to the presence of potentially problematic constituents. These include the following essential oils: allspice, black cumin, black pepper (eugenol CT), blue spruce, camphor, citronella, feverfew, fingerroot ((E)-beta-ocimene and camphor CTs), honey myrtle, hops, hyssop (various CTs), Japanese cedarwood (bark), kanuka (37+ weeks), lemon basil, lemon catnip, lemon myrtle (citral CT), lemon tea tree, lemon verbena, lemongrass, manuka (37+ weeks), may chang, melissa, ocotea, ravintsara (camphor CT), rosemary (1,8-cineole, camphor CTs), Spanish sage, spike lavender, sweet wormwood, wild turmeric, verbena, white sage, white spruce, and white verbena (camphor CT).[61,62,63,64,65,66,67,68,69,70,71,72,73,74,75,76]

While this list is comprehensive, it does not include all possible safety issues during pregnancy and nursing. It is strongly advised that lower doses (stronger dilution ratios) of mild oils are used during pregnancy and lactation and to always consult your OBGYN before using essential oils during pregnancy and lactation.

## Essential Oils before and after Surgery or Medical Procedures

Avoid topical and oral essential oil usage for a minimum of forty-eight hours before and up to one week (though usually two to three days is sufficient) after surgery to prevent excess bleeding or interference with anesthesia or other medications administered during the surgery. Inhalation is usually acceptable, but always seek your physician's approval before using essential oils while under medical care or recovering from a medical procedure/surgery.

## Epilepsy Cautions with Essential Oils

Those with epilepsy, prone to convulsions, or who take antiseizure medications should be very cautious with or avoid essential oils containing significant levels of camphor, methyl salicylate, pinocamphone, isopinocamphone, 1,8-cineole (eucalyptol), trans-sabinyl acetate, fenchone, pulegone, and thujone (alpha- and beta-).[77,78,79] Essential oils containing moderate to significant amounts of these constituents could exacerbate or trigger seizures and convulsions or may interact with antiseizure medications, reducing their efficacy. This precaution is predominantly with oral administration, but it may be prudent to limit or avoid topical administration as well. Rarely, seizures have been observed after inhalation. These constituents are found in essential oils like rosemary, eucalyptus, camphor, cardamom, fennel, Spanish sage, common sage, hyssop, pennyroyal, wintergreen, birch, and others.

Not all potentially problematic essential oils have been listed, and those prone to seizures are advised to check GC-MS reports for the problematic constituents in essential oils they desire to use. While peppermint is often recommended as an essential oil to avoid and contains pulegone, it is in diminutive amounts, and the reported convulsions associated with pulegone were with extremely large doses—5 mL to 30 mL—of pennyroyal (up to 87 percent pulegone).[80] Moreover, administration of peppermint oil to animals did not cause seizures, and in fact demonstrated the ability to protect mice from drug-induced seizures.[81]

In younger children, the primary constituent found in eucalyptus essential oil, eucalyptol (1,8-cineole), may cause convulsions, which is another reason why it is not recommended for those under age three, and to use cautiously through age five.[82,83]

In addition to the essential oils mentioned, epileptics are advised to avoid the carrier oils evening primrose oil and borage seed oil as they may lower the seizure threshold

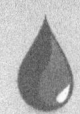

(the balance between forces in the brain that trigger or reduce the risk of seizures in susceptible people).[84] These essential oils should also be avoided by those with Parkinson's disease (PD) because PD is associated with an increased risk of seizures.

**Essential Oils and the Eyes**

Keep essential oils away from the eyes and other sensitive areas. Essential oils should never be placed directly in the eye, and great caution should be exercised when applying near the eye. Always dilute oils before applying near the eye, and apply them widely around the eye. The orbit, or eye socket, can be used as guide by applying oils outside the orbit area, but never inside. Some reports of damaged corneal tissue, corneal abrasions, vision loss, or chemical burns have occurred from applying oils directly into the eye.[85]

If essential oils accidently get into the eye, add a fatty oil (e.g. coconut or olive oil) or milk to the eye and pat the eye with a paper towel. Repeat this process until relief is achieved and then rinse the eyes well with water. Seek medical attention of vision is altered or irritation or pain do not subside.

**Essential Oils and the Ears**

Never put oils directly into the ear canal. Some anecdotal reports suggest that this may result in a ruptured eardrum and, at the very least, may cause severe pain. Add several drops of carrier oil to the ear, and continue to do so, until the pain is relieved if this occurs accidentally. The preferred method for managing conditions of the ear is to place one to two drops of oil, diluted in carrier oil, on a cotton ball and insert the cotton ball into the ear. Replace the cotton ball regularly, at least every four hours, to maintain the therapeutic benefits. Individuals with sensitive skin may experience discomfort of the skin inside the ear with this method, so the essential oil on the cotton ball should be positioned as to not contact the ear and more carrier oil added.

**Photosensitizing Essential Oils**

| PHOTOTOXIC CONSTITUENTS | |
|---|---|
| Constituent | Degree of Phototoxicity |
| Angelicin | Moderate |
| Bergamottin | Negligible |
| Bergapten | Strong |
| Bergaptol | Negligible |
| Citropten | Moderate |
| Isoimperatorin | Weak |
| Isobergapten | Negligible |
| Isopimpinellin | Negligible |
| Imperatorin | Moderate |
| Methoxsalen | Strong |
| Oxypeucedanin | Moderate |
| Psoralen | Strong |

Avoid sun exposure at least twelve hours after topical application of photosensitizing oils. Certain essential oils contain constituents called furanocoumarins that are known to be phototoxic—making the skin more susceptible to damage by UV exposure. The ability of an oil to be phototoxic depends on the concentration of phototoxic furanocoumarin constituent(s) in the essential oil, such as angelicin, bergamottin, bergapten, citropten, imperatorin, psoralen, isobergapten, isoimperatorin, methoxsalen, and oxypeucedanin, and the duration and power of exposure to UV rays or sunlight.[86,87] Linear furanocoumarins are generally more phototoxic than angular furanocoumarins. The phototoxic action of furanocoumarins is due to their ability to enter epithelial (skin) cells and react with nucleobases in DNA when exposed to UV-A radiation. UV-A radiation triggers a chemical reaction that inhibits DNA replication and transcription and initiates the formation of adducts that react to neighboring nucleobases creating crosslinks (bonds) with DNA that initiate inflammation and cell death. The characteristic sign of phytophotodermatitis is acute inflammatory lesions (rash, blisters) or skin discoloration at the site of application.

Aqueous dilutions of essential oils with citral (geranial + neral) were also determined to be phototoxic according to *in vitro* (3T3 Neutral Red Uptake Phototoxicity Test—a first step test as part of a broader phototoxicity testing strategy) and human skin photopatch tests, but this reaction with the actual essential oil has not been observed in humans, nor in phototoxicity studies in animals.[88,89,90]

Another test used to determine the phototoxic potential of essential oil constituents is the photohaemolysis assay (PA). This test is an *in vitro* method used to determine the potential destruction of red blood cells caused by reactions between UV rays and constituents. According to this test, a number of essential oils or essential oil constituents have the potential to cause moderate hemolysis: citronellal, cinnamic alcohol, bergamot, costus root, lime, orange, bay laurel, cinnamaldehyde,

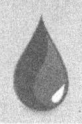

and alpha-amyl cinnamic aldehyde. Oakmoss absolute was determined to be strongly phototoxic based on the PA. However, the PA does not always translate directly to human risk. Essential oils known to be phototoxic in humans or with a relative risk of phototoxicity include: angelica, bay laurel absolute, bergamot, bitter orange, celery, citron, cumin, fennel, grapefruit, khella, Mediterranean mandarin, neroli, lemon (expressed), lime (expressed), petitgrain, rue, and tagetes.

Exposing your skin to UV rays or sunlight after applying a photosensitizing oil could result in pigmentation, blisters, rash, or even serious burns. The preferred place to apply photosensitizing oils is the bottoms of the feet or places that clothing will cover to protect the area from UV exposure.

## Essential Oils with Thymol

Oils with high levels of the phenol thymol should not be taken orally long-term, nor in large doses. Thymol has a longer half-life—the time it takes the body to metabolize or excrete half of the dosage—than most essential oil constituents, meaning it will remain in the body longer.[91] It is recommended to avoid administering more than 16 drops per day and to discontinue use for a minimum of forty-eight hours after seven days of administration. Alternately, use of essential oils high in thymol may be limited to weekdays (Monday – Friday) with a rest period on weekends (Saturday and Sunday). This primarily applies to thyme, ajowan, oregano CT thymol, wild savory CT thymol, mountain savory CT thymol, black cumin CT thymol, monarda CT thymol, hairy basil CT thymol, and summer savory CT thymol, although a number of other essential oils contain small to notable amounts of thymol as well.

| Methyl salicylate[98] | Bath | 2.4–4.0 |
|---|---|---|
| Thymol[99] | Oral | 10.2 |

| HALF-LIVES OF SOME ESSENTIAL OIL CONSTITUENTS IN HUMANS | | |
|---|---|---|
| Constituent | Route | Half-life (hour |
| 1,8-cineole[92] | Inhale | 0.50–2.95 |
| Alpha-pinene[93] | Inhale | 4.8 |
| | Inhale | 5.3 |
| Limonene[95] | Inhale | 1.25 |
| Linalool[96] | Topic | 0.23 |
| Menthol[97] (Menthol | Oral | 0.9 |

## Essential Oils: Kidney Transplants and Compromised Kidneys

Those with kidney disorders are more susceptible to experience nephrotoxicity (kidney toxicity), and therefore, caution is warranted for both oral and topical administration. It would be wise to significantly reduce typical dosages of both methods of administration to reduce the risk of nephrotoxicity, particularly orally. Diffusion is generally acceptable and some physicians have approved the topical use of essential oils as well. Check with your physician to determine his or her recommendation for essential oil use.

## Medical Implants and Essential Oils

Some have expressed concerns about possible interactions between essential oils and plastic or metals implants (hip, knee, etc.). When essential oils are applied topically they will enter the bloodstream via the capillaries before they would come in contact with a medical implant. Oral use is even less of a concern, as the essential oils will be metabolized and a portion will enter the bloodstream to be delivered to cells and tissues, not to a medical implant. There has never been a documented case of essential oils causing a problem with medical implants and so this should not be a concern.

## Breast Implants and Essential Oils

Some women who have undergone breast augmentation have expressed concern about the possible interaction between essential oils and breast implants. Essential oils will only penetrate a few layers deep in the breast tissue before they enter the bloodstream via the capillaries located in the breast tissue over the implant. It is highly unlikely that an essential oil (topically applied) will penetrate the dermal (and potentially muscle tissue depending on the insertion point of the implant—over or under the pectoral muscle) tissue that covers breast implants. Oral use poses even less risk of interacting with or degrading breast implants. There has never been a report of any essential oil degrading breast implants; therefore, oral and topical use of essential oils should not be a concern for those who have had breast augmentation.

## Essential Oils: Immunosuppressive Drugs and Patients

Little is known concerning interactions with immunosuppressive drugs, and the simultaneous use of essential oils, and limited research has been conducted with

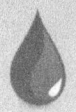

herbs. Some immunostimulating herbs (herbs that may stimulate immune function) have been implicated in interfering (decreasing or enhancing the effectiveness of) immunosuppressive medications.[100,101,102,103,104] In theory, because essential oils are significantly more potent than herbs, they too could enhance or decrease the effectiveness of immunosuppressive medications, especially essential oils that stimulate immune system activity. Many physicians approve the inhalation of essential oils in their patients taking immunosuppressants, and some permit limited topical application as well. Until research suggests otherwise, it is prudent to avoid the use of essential oils orally, and be very cautious with the topical application of essential oils, especially among those who are taking medications to prevent the rejection of transplanted organs and tissues. Seek your physician's approval before using essential oils in this case.

## Essential Oils during Chemotherapy and Cancer Treatment

Another poorly understood potential interaction is the simultaneous use of essential oils with chemotherapy and radiation treatment for cancer. Presently, evidence does not exist as to whether the immune mechanisms and other pharmacological activity of essential oils could potentiate or interfere with conventional cancer treatment. Research suggests that linalool, for example, increases doxorubicin (a chemotherapy drug) permeability in tumor cells, which enhanced the antitumor activity of doxorubicin *in vitro* and *in vivo*.[105] The essential oils of *Inula japonica* (9,12-octadecadienoic acid 9.2%, and 2-pentadecanone,6,10,14-trimethyl 8.8%) and *Angelicae dahuricae* (alpha-pinene 12.5% and 9,12-octadecadienoic acid 9.9%) also enhance the sensitivity of breast cancer cells to doxorubicin and reduce drug resistance via multiple mechanisms *in vitro*.[106] Thymoquinone from black cumin seed essential oil also amplifies the anticancer effect of doxorubicin against certain cancer cell lines *in vitro*.[107] Geraniol reduced colon tumor size by 26% when administered alone, but this reduction increased to 53% when coadministered with 5-fluorouracil (a chemotherapy drug used to treat skin cancer) *in vitro*.[108] Interestingly, 5-fluorouracil was unable to reduce the colon tumor alone. Eucalyptus and peppermint essential oils have shown the ability to increase the absorption of 5-fluorouracil 60- and 46-fold respectively.[109] Similar synergistic activity between chemotherapy drugs and essential oils has been observed with frankincense, chamomile, garlic, tea tree, and other essential oils. The potential of essential oils to increase the

effectiveness of chemotherapy agents and therefore reduce the dose of these agents required is promising and makes it possible to reduce chemotherapy side effects. Based on the available research, it appears that essential oils, or isolated essential oil constituents, may have a positive interaction with chemotherapy agents, but far more research needs to be conducted, including clinical trials, to determine whether essential oils should be considered as an adjunctive therapy for cancer treatment. At the very least, essential oils are becoming more accepted as complementary solutions for the side effects of cancer treatment such as nausea and vomiting, sleep disturbance, anxiety, stress, pain, and quality of life.

When it comes to natural antioxidant constituents, one review of 280 articles concluded that "nonprescription antioxidants and other nutrients do not interfere with therapeutic modalities for cancer."[110] In fact, the study found just the opposite, that antioxidant supplementation enhanced the ability of cancer therapy to kill cancerous cells and increased patient survival rate. A conflicting review determined that high-dose antioxidant supplementation interfered with tumor control by conventional cancer therapies and reduced survival rates of patients.[111]

It is widely known that some essential oils can enhance the penetration of other substances through the skin, but the interaction of essential oils with the range of cancer drugs used is still unanswered. Because of this, it is recommended to avoid the use of essential oils topically and orally for a minimum of forty-eight hours prior to treatment and four to seven days following chemotherapy or radiation treatment. Most chemotherapy drugs will exit the system within three days of use, despite the fact that side effects continue long after this due to associated tissue and organ damage. By limiting the use of essential oils topically and orally, there is minimal risk of interactions with chemotherapy and associated medications and treatments for cancer.

On the other hand, inhalation of essential oils can be a greatly supportive adjunct therapy for those undergoing chemotherapy and radiation therapy. Inhalation of essential oils (such as ginger, spearmint, and peppermint) can greatly benefit the nausea, loss of appetite, and discomfort often associated with cancer treatments.[112,113] In addition, it is widely known that some essential oils can reduce anxiety associated with medical and dental procedures, suggesting that inhalation of calming essential oils (lavender, orange, ylang ylang) may improve the psychological state of the person receiving cancer treatment. It is strongly

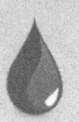 

recommended that you discuss the possibility of inhaling essential oils during your treatments with your doctor. These oils can simply be added to a cotton ball and placed in an oxygen mask, applied to a diffuser necklace or aromastone, or inhaled directly from the cotton ball. Likewise, personal care products that contain essential oils are acceptable when undergoing cancer treatment.

## Drug Tests and Essential Oils

Some individuals have expressed concern about the use of essential oils and whether it will affect a drug test or produce a positive drug test result. This appears to be largely based on the presence of cannabinoids and terpenes found in cannabis present in some essential oils, such as beta-caryophyllene, (E)-beta-caryophyllene, (Z)-beta-caryophyllene, caryophyllene oxide, and alpha-humulene. Several essential oils do contain these constituents, which serve significant roles in their therapeutic benefits.

Beta-caryophyllene is a bicyclic sesquiterpenoid alkene widely distributed in essential oils, but present in high concentrations in black pepper, copaiba, guava leaf (beta-caryophyllene CT), hairy basil (beta-caryophyllene CT), and hemp (myrcene CT) essential oils. It is a natural selective agonist (able to selectively activate a specific cell receptor) of the cannabinoid receptor 2 (CB2R), which when triggered reduces pain associated with inflammation and neuropathy.[114] Both (E)- and (Z)-beta-caryophyllene also selectively bind to CB2R, with the (E) form showing higher binding affinity. Many scientists consider beta-caryophyllene a potential therapeutic target for inflammatory and chronic pain due to its excellent safety and efficacy profile (extremely low toxicity), combined with an absence of the psychoactive effects of the more well-known cannabinoid delta(9)-tetrahydro-cannabinol (THC) found in marijuana.

Caryophyllene oxide is a bicyclic sesquiterpenoid alkene oxide/ether commonly found in melissa essential oil and other essential oils. It is formed when the alkene of beta-caryophyllene becomes an epoxide (an organic molecule that contains a three-membered ring involving an oxygen atom and two carbon atoms). This constituent is responsible for the ability of drug-sniffing dogs to detect cannabis.[115] Caryophyllene oxide does not have binding affinity for CB receptors.

Alpha-humulene, also called alpha-caryophyllene, is a monocyclic sesquiterpene found naturally occurring in some essential oils (guava leaf CT beta-caryophyllene 1.0%–17.2%, catnip CT 1,8-cineole 14.4%, wild sage 4.0%–13.5%, and others). It is commonly present in plants that contain beta-caryophyllene (its isomer),

although typically in lesser quantities. It does not appear to have an affinity for CB receptors. Like beta-caryophyllene it has anti-inflammatory properties, producing similar effects to dexamethasone (a corticosteroid drug used to treat inflammation, severe allergies, adrenal problems, arthritis, skin conditions, and flare-ups of multiple sclerosis).[116]

Marijuana drug tests analyze for the presence of tetrahydrocannabinol carboxylic acid (THC-COOH), which is the major metabolite of THC. THC-COOH has a long half-life and remains in the urine for more than seven days after a single use of marijuana. The most common maximum level for THC-COOH used by drug screening companies is 50 ng/ml, although it ranges from 15 ng/mL to 100 ng/mL. A positive test over 15 ng/mL is a strong indication of marijuana use, while greater than 500 ng/mL suggests chronic and recent use.

Hemp seeds and hemp seed fixed oil are dietary sources of cannabinoids, including trace amounts of THC (seeds: 5 mcg/g; fixed oil: 2 mcg/g).[117] Scientists evaluated the effects of hemp seed fixed oil on drug tests and determined that it required the equivalent of regularly consuming 125 mL (4.4 oz) of hemp seed fixed oil to produce a positive drug test.[118] Based on these findings the study authors concluded the THC concentrations are "sufficiently low to prevent confirmed positives from the extended and extensive consumption of hemp foods." However, another study reports that individuals tested positive for THC-COOH (20 ng/mL and 50 ng/mL) when they ingested three hemp flour cookies or a hemp seed bar.[119] Lack of quality control in the amount of THC present in certain hemp food products could account for this discrepancy.

When it comes to essential oils, there is little concern for producing a positive drug test after their use. First, THC is only present in trace amounts of less than 0.2% in hemp essential oil according to published reports. No other essential oils are known to contain THC. Second, beta-caryophyllene, caryophyllene oxide, and alpha-humulene do not produce the THC-COOH metabolite.[4151,4152] Both of these facts suggest that people using essential oils with cannabinoids have little to worry about in regards to a positive drug test. Whether drug dogs will sniff out these terpenes shared with cannabis is not fully known.

Athletes that are required to submit to performance-enhancing drug tests should be aware that bitter orange is classified by the NCAA as a stimulant and it is on the NCAA banned substances list.[120] It was largely banned because it contains the stimulatory alkaloid P-synephrine—a compound similar in structure to

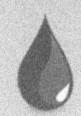

ephedrine—and has been associated with increased blood pressure, heart rate, and cardiac events among some consumers. Although P-synephrine is highly unlikely to be present in bitter orange essential oil (despite being present in the peel of citrus fruits), athletes are encouraged to seek qualified counsel regarding whether bitter orange essential oil can be used in their sport.

**Is It Possible to Build a Tolerance to Essential Oils?**

It is a best practice to limit the use of the exact same oil or oils to twenty-one days before taking a one-week break (or use five days during the week with two days of break). This is recommended for two reasons. One, this reduces the risk of sensitization to the essential oil or oils that you are using. And, two, this reduces the chance that your body will develop a resistance or tolerance to the effectiveness of the essential oils you are using.

Despite resistance being a remote possibility, some users have reported that the long-term use of the same essential oils has reduced its efficacy. While it may be that the person's health condition progressed to cause a decrease in effectiveness, the rotation of essential oils still has merit. For example, one could use one combination of essential oils for one week and then a different combination the next week, continuing this pattern. Alternately, use the same combination for three weeks and switch to another for one week. Herbal remedies have been rotated in a similar manner for centuries to maintain their effectiveness.

Bacteria readily develop resistance against drugs, which expose bacteria to the exact same chemical composition each time permitting microbial adaptation. The bacteria do this to preserve their existence. However, this has not been observed frequently with natural plant extracts, whether from herbs or essential oils. This is because plant extracts, including essential oils, naturally have chemical and structural variance that limits the ability of the bacterium to adapt and become resistant.[121,122,123,124] Very rarely is resistance reported among plant extracts.[125,126]

**Essential Oil Use with Medications**

Essential oils work in harmony with the human body; however, with all potent substances, caution and common sense is required. Some essential oils (as well as blends and supplements that contain them) have the potential to interact with medications and/or are contraindicated with certain health conditions. While possible, drug–essential oil interactions are infrequently observed in clinical practice. Observed interactions in studies typically occur

after administering very high doses of essential oils that far exceed typical amounts used. Clinical experience and practical use suggest that the risk of essential oil–medication interactions is remote and unusual. Nevertheless, individuals should be aware of these potential interactions and use common sense. If you take medications while using essential oils, you should check with your doctor or pharmacist for possible interactions or contraindications before using essential oils at the same time.

Some choose to use medications and essential oils concurrently. If you chose to do so, it is best to use essential oils approximately two to four hours (minimum one hour) following the administration of medications and to reduce the normal (or recommended) essential oil dose by half.

Interaction risk will vary based on method of administration with the risk from greatest to least being: oral > retention > topical > diffusion. Some interactions may only occur when oils are ingested, but interactions are possible with other methods of administration as well (e.g. topical application of wintergreen essential oil).

Although every effort has been made to identify potential drug interactions, known cautions, and contraindications with essential oils, the list may not include every possible caution required. Consequently, always check with your doctor or pharmacist before using medications and essential oils together.

**Reducing Reliance on Medications**

You should never reduce or stop taking any medication without your healthcare professional's approval. Do not do so unless your provider tells you to! Doing so can be dangerous and have serious consequences. However, with physician approval it is possible to reduce reliance on medications in favor of a natural option with reduced risk of side effects.

1. You should discuss the possible effects you might experience as you work toward medication reduction with your healthcare professional.

2. Slowly introduce small doses of the essential oil you wish to use about two to four hours after taking your medication (unless there is an obvious risk and contraindication).

3. You need to reduce your medication gradually over a period of weeks or months. This largely depends on how long you have been taking the medication. As a guide, the Royal College of Psychiatrists recommends the following for antipsychotic medication reduction: treatment for less than eight

weeks—reduce medication over one to two weeks; treatment of six to eight months—taper medication over six to eight weeks; and longer treatment periods, reduce medication by 25 percent every four to six weeks.[127] People who take weeks to months to reduce their medications are more likely to be successful.

4. Follow up regularly with your healthcare professional.

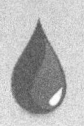 ## TOPICAL APPLICATION

Topical administration of essential oils requires care, and ordinarily dilution, due to the potentially irritating, sensitizing, and photosensitizing constituents contained in essential oils. The evidence-based model allows for neat to highly diluted topical applications according to your comfort level and current state of health; however, dilution is strongly encouraged as a best practice because it also improves absorption of the essential oils through the skin.

Once applied to the skin, essential oil constituents rapidly penetrate the tissues and enter the bloodstream quickly, circulating throughout the body. Scientists suspect that constituents below 500 to 600 Daltons in molecular weight readily cross the skin layers and are absorbed by the body.[128] Since essential oil constituents are well below this threshold (usually less than 300 Daltons except for some heavier diterpenoids), penetration of and entrance into the bloodstream by these constituents is logical.

| Molecular Weight of Common Essential Oil Constituents/Fatty Acids | |
|---|---|
| 1,8-Cineole | 154.3 |
| Alpha-Pinene | 136.2 |
| Alpha-Terpineol | 154.3 |
| Beta-Pinene | 136.2 |
| Beta-Caryophyllene | 204.4 |
| Bisabolol Oxide A | 238.4 |
| Borneol | 154.3 |
| Camphor | 152.2 |
| Carvacrol | 150.2 |
| Cinnamaldehyde | 132.2 |
| Eugenol | 164.2 |
| Gamma-Terpinene | 136.2 |
| Geranial | 152.2 |
| Germacrene D | 204.4 |
| Limonene | 136.2 |
| Linalool | 154.3 |
| Menthol | 156.3 |
| Myrcene | 136.2 |
| Neral | 152.2 |
| Terpinen-4-ol | 154.3 |
| Thymol | 154.3 |
| Arachidic Acid<br>*Jojoba Oil* | 312.5 |
| Lauric Acid<br>*Coconut Oil* | 200.3 |
| Linoleic Acid<br>*Grapeseed Oil, Sesame Oil* | 280.5 |
| Oleic Acid<br>*Olive Oil, Almond Oil* | |

SOURCE: US National Library of Medicine, National Center for Biotechnology Information, PubChem.

**Enhancing Absorption of Essential Oils through the Skin**

There are ways to enhance the absorption, and therefore the effectiveness, of essential oils. Absorption and effectiveness of essential oils may be enhanced by applying a warm wet towel over the area of application and then covering this wet towel with a warm dry towel to retain the heat. Wet skin also helps to improve absorption. Applying essential oils immediately following a warm bath or shower when the pores or more open significantly improve oil absorption. Note, that some find this too intense depending on the oil used. Another way to improve absorption is by directing warm air on the site of application (for example, from a blow dryer).

The 4/10/75 guideline is an easy acronym to remember to improve absorption. One study estimated that 75 percent of various applied oils were absorbed through the skin if the area was covered after application. If the skin was left uncovered, only about 4 percent of the oil was absorbed.[129] Another study found that about 10 percent of lavender oil was absorbed when diluted to a 2 percent dilution ratio, peaking at about twenty minutes after application.[130] Ninety minutes post application, the lavender constituents tested for had reduced to almost zero. This suggests frequent topical application is necessary to maintain a therapeutic effect. In other words, neat (no carrier oil) applications result in about 4 percent absorption, diluted applications about 10 percent, and covered applications (occlusive) 75 percent.

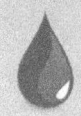

The absorption of essential oils through the skin also depends on the application site (skin thickness, nature of stratum corneum, density). Not all body areas are equally permeable. For example, application to the genitals (scrotum, vulva) may increase absorption of some compounds up to 40-fold.[131,132,133] Clinical experience and current published data suggests permeability can be ranked accordingly (greatest to least): genitals>forehead>armpit>face/scalp>trunk/extremities>palms/soles>nails.[134,135] Other factors that affect essential oil absorption through the skin include: skin age (younger skin is more permeable than aged skin), skin hydration (permeability increases significantly in hydrated skin), skin temperature (permeability increases with higher temperatures), skin pH (higher pH increases permeability), skin pigment (darker skin=superior barrier function) and essential oil concentration applied.[136,137,138]

**Where to Apply Essential Oils**

The application site will depend on the purpose of the application. In general, essential oils should be applied to the area that needs correction. For example, if you have a sore shoulder, you would apply the oil to the shoulder that is sore. If you have diarrhea, you would apply to the lower abdomen in a clockwise motion. However, when in doubt about the location to apply, a common place to apply essential oils is to the feet. This is often a preferred site for the reasons mentioned earlier in this chapter. It is important to note that applying to the feet may reduce the absorption of the essential oils because of the nature of the skin and pores on the bottoms of the feet. In addition, infants will put their feet in their mouths so keep this in mind. Another preferred location to apply essential oils is to the back (along the spine) because this can influence the central nervous system that is located there. The face and near the eyes should usually be avoided, especially in children.

Applying essential oils diluted with a carrier oil is strongly encouraged to avoid sensitization and irritation, especially among those with a chronic skin condition, allergies (food or seasonal), or with an autoimmune or autoinflammatory condition. These people are more likely to experience discomfort, sensitivity, or a reaction to the topical application of essential oils. Dilution is particularly important for "hot" oils like oregano, thyme, and cinnamon (for all populations). The maximum strength recommended should be reserved for serious injuries, infections, wounds, or severe illnesses, and should only be used for short periods by those who are sensitive.

**Carrier Oils**

Carrier oils are an integral part of essential oil therapy and possess their own therapeutic value. They are necessary to reduce the risk of skin sensitivity from topical application and provide soothing comfort if irritation or redness occurs. Moreover, they can extend the therapeutic action of essential oils, prolonging the benefits you receive. This is particularly true if you are administering the essential oils to influence mood and emotions because it lengthens the time the aroma is available to the olfactory system. It is also important when soothing aches and pain, because carrier oils prolong the essential oil contact to areas over distressed muscles and tissues.

Vegetable oils make up the bulk of carrier oils used in essential oil therapy. It is important that you use an unrefined, cold-expeller pressed or cold-pressed vegetable oil. If it doesn't say unrefined, cold-expeller pressed or cold-pressed on the label—even if it says "pure"—it is likely a refined product extracted by high pressure, intense heat, and possibly solvents. Carrier oils extracted from organic plants are also preferred to avoid exposure to toxic fertilizers, pesticides, and fungicides.

Carrier oils contain fatty acids, fat-soluble vitamins, minerals, and other beneficial nutrients. The fatty acids contained in vegetable oils may help reduce cholesterol levels, strengthen cell membranes, and reduce the appearance of fine lines and wrinkles. Olive oil is loaded with vitamins A, K, and omega-3 and -6 fatty acids. Some carrier oils contain gamma linolenic acid (GLA)—borage seed oil and evening primrose oil, which is frequently used for inflammatory and hormone-related conditions. Some studies suggest that GLA may stop cancer progression and angiogenesis (the growth of blood vessels to supply blood to cancerous tumors),[139] and GLA is used to create prostaglandins—hormone-like substances that are involved in many body processes, including immune system function.

Depending on the carrier oil, the average shelf life of a carrier oil is about six months when kept in a cool and dark place. Carrier oils are susceptible to oxidation and rancidity, particularly after opened and used. The empty space in bottles promotes oxidation. When oxidized, carrier oils break down and form free radicals, which, left unchecked, damage cells, accelerate the aging process, and have a detrimental effect on the skin. It is advised to keep carrier oils in the fridge—with the exception of avocado oil—in order to preserve them. This may increase their shelf life to nine months, but be mindful that it may cause them to solidify or turn cloudy, so they will need to be removed to return to room temperature before use. Extra-virgin olive oil will

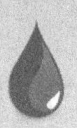 

generally keep well even when stored outside the refrigerator. On the opposite spectrum is wheat germ oil, which becomes rancid after only a few weeks.

## Common Carrier Oils and Bases and Their Properties/Benefits

*Aloe Vera.* While different from aloe vera gel, aloe vera oil has a long history of medicinal and cosmetic use. It is cooling, hydrating, rejuvenating, tonifying, and healing to the skin. It is useful for preventing scars. It has been used medicinally for healing wounds, treating burns, relieving muscle pain, diminishing varicose veins, and restoring damaged tissues. It possesses antifungal, antiseptic, antimicrobial, and anti-inflammatory properties, and the lectins it contains stimulate immune system activity. Aloe vera contains seven of the eight essential amino acids; vitamins A and C; and the minerals magnesium, zinc, copper, and selenium.

*Argan Oil.* Best known for its anti-aging properties, argan oil is rich in fatty acids (oleic, linoleic, palmitic, stearic), vitamin E, and antioxidants. It nourishes and hydrates the skin and is suitable for all skin types, especially sensitive, dry, or damaged skin, or for people prone to breakouts. It is often used for eczema, itching, wound/burn healing, stretch marks, scarring, and healthy hair and nails.

*Avocado Oil.* Rich in monounsaturated fats, lecithin, vitamins A, B, D, E, sterol, lutein, beta-carotene, and essential fatty acids, avocado oil provides significant healing properties for the skin. Look for avocado oils that are dark—the darker the better. Clear or pale green oil is an indication the oil has been refined and highly processed. It has a fruity smell and should be blended with complementary aromas. It is hydrating, nourishing, and easily absorbed into the skin. Indeed, it enhances the penetration of other oils into the skin. It is appropriate for all skin types, but particularly useful for aged, dry, or fragile skin. It may be combined with essential oils to create a natural sunscreen because of its ability to partly block UV rays. Avocado oil encourages cellular regeneration, reduces the appearance of wrinkles, and may improve skin elasticity.

*Beeswax.* Mostly used as an emulsifier and thickening agent to create creams, lotions, and salves, beeswax is an excellent skin softener. It hydrates the skin, promotes a clear complexion, and tightens the pores without clogging them making it an excellent choice for acne. Beeswax may also be used to form a protective barrier on the skin or as a lip balm. Products with beeswax should not be used by those with bee allergies.

*Borage Seed Oil.* Borage seed oil is often taken internally to support skin health, but external application also has therapeutic benefits. Its high levels of gamma linolenic acid (GLA) make it very suitable for damaged and dry skin, stretch marks, eczema, or psoriasis. It is also useful for relieving female reproductive complaints, such as premenstrual syndrome, endometriosis, and menopausal symptoms. Borage seed oil may promote a youthful glow to the skin, and its scent is uplifting. Avoid with epilepsy or convulsions because GLA has been reported (mostly after ingestion) to lower the seizure threshold.

*Caprylic Capric Triglycerides.* Caprylic capric triglycerides are a specialized esterification of coconut oil with a very light, silky, and nongreasy feel. This carrier oil offers several key benefits, including nourishing the skin, helping to extend the shelf life of products due to its antioxidant properties, and provides a noticeable silkiness to the skin. Caprylic capric triglycerides encourage rejuvenation of the skin and form a protective barrier for the skin. In addition, it is nonallergenic making it an excellent choice for those with sensitive and oily skin.

*Castor Oil:* Made by pressing the seeds of the *Ricinus communis* plant, castor oil is an excellent skin moisturizer. It has been used for hundreds of years, and possibly even by the Egyptians thousands of years ago, to encourage healthy skin and hair. It supports scalp circulation and helps hair shafts retain moisture. Castor oil moisturizes dry, flaky skin and soothes irritated skin. It is occasionally used internally after 39 weeks of pregnancy to induce labor, and in packs to help relieve constipation in the elderly. It is reported to possess antimicrobial, immune stimulating, and lymph stimulating properties. In addition, it is anti-inflammatory and helps relieve pain, making it an excellent choice for pain mixtures—particularly sprains. Caution is warranted when using castor oil orally as taking more than the recommended dose or prolonged use (more than one week) can cause fluid and electrolyte disturbances.[140]

*Cocoa Butter.* Obtained from roasted cocoa beans, cocoa butter is solid at room temperature but liquefies easily at about body temperature. Cocoa butter is an excellent choice for creating suppositories, creams, and lotions. It softens and rejuvenates the skin, may help prevent stretch marks, helps reduce the appearance of scars, and forms a protective barrier for the skin. Pure cocoa butters have a very slight chocolate aroma that may not blend well with some oils.

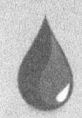

*Coconut oil.* Virtually odorless, coconut oil is a very popular carrier oil because its scent doesn't compete with the essential oils that are added to it. With the exception of fractionated coconut oil, coconut oils remain semisolid at room temperature. It softens the skin and helps to reduce dry, inflamed, and itchy skin. Coconut oil is a useful and beneficial carrier oil when applying essential oil blends to the scalp or hair. Interestingly, inhabitants of the Pacific Isles are less prone to baldness and graying of hair, and some attribute this to their practice of oiling the hair with coconut oil from childhood. It is often used as a base for sunscreens because of its natural ability to block about 20 percent of the sun's UV rays.[141] A significant amount of the fatty acids contained in coconut oil are lauric acid, which can kill bacteria, viruses, and fungi.

*Dimethyl sulfoxide (DMSO).* DMSO is an organosulfur constituent that significantly increases the penetration, effectiveness, and absorption of essential oils and other substances through the skin. It is naturally derived from wood pulp and is also found in spearmint extract, barley, malt, asparagus, and corn.[142] Because of its ability to increase the absorption of some compounds through tissues, including the skin, drug manufacturers have investigated it for use as a transdermal drug-delivery system. It is most often combined with another carrier like aloe vera to calm its scent and reduce the possibility of skin irritation. It possesses antibacterial, analgesic, and anti-inflammatory[143] properties and is often combined with or applied over the top of pain-relieving essential oils. The FDA approved the use of DMSO for the treatment of interstitial cystitis in 1978; however, it is currently available only by prescription or for use as a solvent.[144] DMSO may increase the effect of myriad drugs, so it should not be used in tandem with medications. It has been reported that DMSO dissolves synthetic fibers, so contact with clothing should be avoided. Not for long-term use and should only be a very small percent of the total blend.

*Evening Primrose Oil.* One of the most expensive carrier oils, evening primrose oil is generally added to other carrier oils to reduce the cost of aromatherapy blends. Besides the cost, evening primrose oil is highly unstable and susceptible to oxidation when exposed to air or heat. It is a rich source of GLA, making it helpful for such conditions as dry and scaly skin, eczema, psoriasis, dry skin, and tender breasts. Avoid with epilepsy or convulsions.

*Grapeseed Oil.* Grapeseed oil is suitable for all skin types and is nonallergenic. It is a very gentle moisturizer and leaves the skin feeling smooth. It is odorless, tasteless, and easily absorbed. Grapeseed oil contains proanthocyanidins, which are very potent antioxidants that help protect against cellular and tissue damage. Grapeseed oil contains high levels of vitamin E and helps promote healthy circulation, aids the healing of wounds, speeds up cell regeneration, helps shrink swelling from cysts, reduces the appearance of blemishes and scars, reduces varicose veins, and encourages a youthful glow of the skin. It also has anti-inflammatory properties making it a great choice to add to a soothing aromatherapy blend.

*Hazelnut oil.* Hazelnut oil easily penetrates the skin without drying it. It has appreciable amounts of vitamins A, B, and E, as well as essential fatty acids. Hazelnut stimulates the circulatory system, is a great skin toner, and powerful astringent. It moisturizes and rejuvenates the skin and is a useful carrier oil for acne. The primary drawback to this carrier oil is that it shouldn't be used on those with a nut allergy.

*Jojoba.* Jojoba is a liquid ester similar to the one in our skin and not an oil. It rapidly penetrates the skin, is nonallergenic, and is beneficial to all skin types. It doesn't go rancid and has a very long shelf life. It balances the skin's pH, helps to unclog pores, hydrates the skin, and may prevent stretch marks. Jojoba is popular for acne blends because it helps unclog pores and helps control the buildup of excess sebum. It contains a waxy substance that mimics collagen and is antibacterial to prevent or treat skin infections. It is also a popular carrier oil for the hair, where it increases its luster, reduces the appearance of gray hair, encourages healthy hair growth, and flavonoid oligomeric procyanidin (OPC), decreases scalp dryness.

*Olive oil.* Olive oil contains essential fatty acids, vitamins E and A, minerals, and proteins that are beneficial to the skin. It is revitalizing and moisturizing to dry, chapped, and scaly skin and is known to help wounds heal. It is indicated for sensitive skin and may help soothe eczema and psoriasis. Olive oil contains the anti-inflammatory and antioxidant constituent hydroxytyrosol that prevents free-radical damage to skin cells. In addition, olive oil contains the anti-inflammatory constituent oleocanthal, which inhibits both the COX-1 and COX-2 enzymes responsible for inflammatory conditions within the body.[145] To receive this benefit, one would need to ingest at least two ounces of olive oil daily. Olive oil can leave the skin feeling sticky.

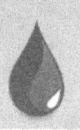

*Sesame Seed Oil.* With a long history of use dating back thousands of years, unrefined sesame oil is highly nutritious. Rich in vitamins A, B-complex, and E, it is protective of the skin, and research suggests it blocks 30 percent of the sun's UV rays.[146] It also contains the minerals calcium, copper, iron, magnesium, and zinc; the latter of which is essential to produce healthy collagen and provides more elasticity to skin. Sesame seed oil contains the constituent sesamol—a constituent that studies suggest protects against DNA damage caused by radiation.[147,148] It is often used as a carrier for blends created to soothe arthritis or rheumatism. Some people suggest sesame seed oil helps protect the body from the negative effects of chlorine in swimming pools. It is naturally moisturizing and useful for conditions like eczema, psoriasis, and dry skin. Some people are allergic to the proteins in cold pressed or expressed sesame oil, but highly refined sesame oil removes most of these proteins making them less allergenic according to allergy experts.

*Shea Butter.* Shea butter leaves the skin feeling oily and waxy and is particularly beneficial to speeding the healing process of skin. It contains high levels of nonsaponifiable fats (keratin, allantoin), vitamins A, E, and F. Shea butter is softening and moisturizing to the skin, and its enhancement of microcirculation aids wound healing, cellular rejuvenation, and scar tissue repair. Its mild properties make it a useful base for baby care products. Shea butter is an excellent choice for chapped or mature skin.

*Sweet Almond Oil.* Sweet almond oil is widely used as an aromatherapy carrier oil and an excellent choice for general aromatherapy applications. It is easily absorbed, slightly viscous, very oily, and carries a delicate, sweet smell. It contains vitamins A, B1, B2, B6, D, and E, as well as trace minerals. It is appropriate for all skin types, but particularly beneficial for sensitive, stressed, dry, or inflamed skin. Sweet almond oil is nourishing and protective of the skin and helps to relieve dry, itchy, and inflamed skin conditions, such as eczema, psoriasis, and dermatitis.

*Vitamin E Oil:* The vitamin E family (tocopherols and tocotrienols) helps prevent cell damage from free radicals, which unchecked can lead to tissue damage, collagen damage, and interfere with the formation of healthy skin cells. It is often added to other carrier oils as a stabilizer, and as little as 0.05% can help protect other carrier oils from oxidation. Vitamin E oil is useful for wound healing, radiation burns, scars, and protection from sun damage. If you are prone to breakouts, vitamin E is thick and greasy, so it may exacerbate this condition.

*Wheat Germ Oil.* A valuable source of vitamin E, wheat germ oil helps relieve dermatitis, enhances circulation, promotes healthy skin cell formation, encourages younger looking skin, and helps reduce scarring. It is a very heavy and sticky oil with a slightly nutty aroma. Wheat germ is beneficial for dry and aged skin and has been used to soothe sore muscles.

**Skin Sensitivity and Reactions to the Topical Application of Essential Oils**

Potent substances like essential oils require respect, particularly as you first introduce your body to these concentrated healing molecules. In some cases, sensitive individuals, or even those without a sensitivity, can become sensitive to essential oils through misuse or the overuse of undiluted (neat) essential oils. It has also been observed that those with compromised immune systems, such as allergies (food or seasonal), chronic skin conditions, or autoimmune and autoinflammatory conditions, are more prone to sensitivity, even pure oils of the highest quality.

When applying topically, first do a skin patch test by applying one drop of oil on the underside of the arm and observing for irritation or redness. If irritation or redness occurs after application, apply a pure carrier oil (olive, coconut, jojoba, etc.), not water. For very sensitive skin, place 1 to 2 drops of oil in a teaspoon of carrier oil before application. When possible, thoroughly cleanse your skin before applying essential oils topically. Essential oils can react with perfumes, deodorants, and other chemicals present on the skin leading to sensitivity. This is because essential oils are likely to carry chemicals within these products across membranes (some of which may be toxic) into the bloodstream.

Contrary to popular belief, skin reactions when using essential oils are not always detoxification reactions, and the continued use of essential oils will not correct this reaction. It is also not entirely accurate to say that essential oils cannot cause allergies because they are devoid of nitrogen compounds—peptides, proteins, and amino acids. While these compounds are typically involved in a true antigen-antibody allergy, other substances devoid of them are known allergens. For example, neither penicillin nor nickel contains these nitrogen compounds, but they are still known to cause allergic reactions.

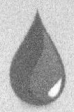

Typically, when an allergy occurs, your body's immune system responds inappropriately to an inert substance by creating antibodies, which are responsible for defending the body against foreign invaders. While it is true—as of this writing—that scientists have not observed antibodies produced in response to essential oil constituents, there are many documented cases of allergic reactions to essential oils, especially topical use.[149,150,151,152,153] The need for essential oils molecules to attach to a carrier protein (peptides at the surface of skin cells) makes skin reactions caused by oral administration extremely rare. Indeed, the majority of people who experience an adverse skin reaction to the topical application of essential oils report that they are not affected by ingesting essential oils.

Multiple studies report that essential oils and fragrance constituents can act as prehaptens and prohaptens, sensitizing constituents, or skin allergens through varying pathways within the body. Haptens are potent sensitizing substances that cause powerful contact allergies by common reactions, such as air oxidation (autoxidation), photoactivation, chemical bonding, or attachment to a carrier protein in the skin after topical application, which forms a complete antigen via enzyme catalysis (bioactivation).[154,155,156,157,158,159,160,161,162,163]

Essential oil constituents such as aldehydes and ketones are electrophilic—molecules attracted to electrons that participate in chemical reactions involving the exchange of electrons. These electrophilic substances can bind to proteins within the skin to trigger an allergic reaction.[164] Research suggests that these adverse skin reactions occur in up to 96 percent of individuals who are more sensitive to aromatic constituents (like people with eczema), depending on the combination of oils used and their chemical structure.[165,166,167]

Moreover, some essential oils or essential oil constituents (especially monoterpenes like limonene) are more prone to oxidation than others.[168,169,170,171] When these oils are exposed to the air they combine with oxygen to form skin allergens known as peroxides or hydroperoxides.[172] This risk is greater as the essential oil ages. Tea tree (*Melaleuca alternifolia*) provides an example of these oxidation reactions. The oxidation of two of its components (terpinen-4-ol and alpha-terpinene) forms small amounts of peroxides, endoperoxides and epoxides, such as ascaridole and 1,2,4-trihydroxymenthane.[173] Ascaridole is a known skin sensitizer and triggers a cascade of events—upregulating costimulatory molecules on antigen-presenting cells (CD86, CD80, and CD4) and stimulating the release of proinflammatory cytokines ((IL)-1ß, TNF-α, IL-6, and IL-8).[174] Ascaridole can also be "activated" by free radical generators like iron, which makes them more highly reactive. In other words, the essential oils are not necessarily allergenic themselves but are activated in the skin or before skin contact to become powerful sensitizers and contact allergens. Furthermore, the journal *Contact Dermatitis* reported in October of 2013 that twenty-eight essential oils and some constituents can be categorized as contact allergens in humans.[175]

Reactions observed on the skin when using essential oils topically—whether at the site of application or not—are best categorized as contact dermatitis. Contact dermatitis is characterized by red, sore, itchy, and inflamed skin after direct contact with a substance that can take from several days to weeks to heal. Two types of contact dermatitis can occur, allergic contact dermatitis and irritant (nonimmunological) contact dermatitis. Contact urticaria (hives) may also occur, which is the immediate—usually within minutes to hours—formation of a rash or hives following exposure to a substance. It will usually fade away after several hours to a few days. It is important to avoid such sensitization because as many essential oils users have discovered the sensitivity is extremely difficult to reverse and may even become permanent in some individuals.

Normally the immune system employs protective mechanisms against harmful substances (antigens) that enter the body, but occasionally the immune system triggers an unfavorable reaction known as hypersensitivity reactions to constituents found in essential oils. These reactions are divided into four categories, but only two are correctly applied to essential oil therapy—type 1 and type 4 reactions.

Type 1 reactions are immediate and typically involve the production of the antibody immunoglobulin E (IgE), which binds to sensitizing substances and activates the release of substances from mast cells (like histamine) that triggers inflammation and an allergic reaction. Although possible, it is extremely rare for a Type 1 reaction to result in anaphylaxis—a serious and potentially life-threatening reaction that occurs within seconds to minutes of exposure to a substance. Type 1 reactions are less common than Type 4 reactions.

# HAPTEN-INDUCED SKIN REACTIONS TO ESSENTIAL OILS

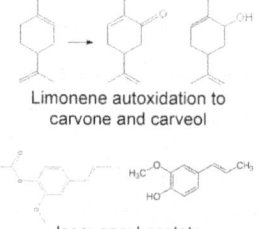

Limonene autoxidation to
carvone and carveol

Isoeuganyl acetate
bioactivation to isoeugenol

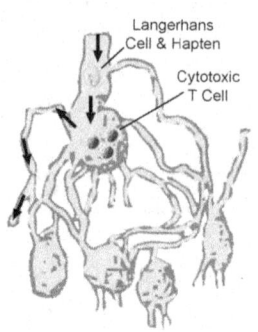

Langerhans
Cell & Hapten

Cytotoxic
T Cell

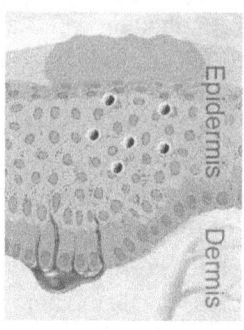

1. Prehapten molecules in essential oils (such as limonene, linalool, and linalyl acetate) undergo chemical reactions like autoxidation (transfer of a hydrogen atom to a free radical in the presence of oxygen) when exposed to the air to become haptens (peroxyl radicals).

Prohapten molecules (certain aldehydes and their corresponding alcohol; i.e. geranial - geraniol) are transformed into haptens by bioactivation through enzymatic reactions.

2. Haptens penetrate the skin and bind to a carrier protein (peptides at the surface of langerhans cells, keratinocytes, or dermal dendritic cells). Normally, the carrier is ignored by the immune system, but the hapten changes its surface structure to to form an antigen (the hapten is too small on its own to form an antigen), which is recognized by the immune system.

3. The langerhans cells migrate to a local lymph node. Helper T cells recognize the modified langerhans cells (peptide-hapten complex) as an antigen and 'prime' cytotoxic T cells (CD8+). Once activated (primed), cytotoxic T cells travel throughout the body to locate and kill the infected 'target' cells.

4. Memory T cells travel to the epidermis to more rapidly respond to subsequent encounters with the peptide-hapten complex.

Subsequent application of the hapten molecules triggers an allergic reaction.

Type 4 reactions involve delayed hypersensitivity reactions caused by T cells rather than antibodies. Contact dermatitis would fall into this category. When an essential oil is applied topically it diffuses through the skin and in the case of a sensitivity reaction interacts with proteins and changes its properties to become an antigen. This modified protein travels through the lymph system where it activates T cells. T cells secrete molecules that trigger inflammation and allergic responses in response to the antigen. It is very difficult to reverse Type 4 reactions once they occur, because memory cells produced from prior exposure to the essential oil remain in the body to respond more rapidly the next time the same constituent is encountered. Type 4 reactions usually occur from one to a few days after exposure to a substance and commonly result in contact dermatitis. This contact dermatitis can persist for days, weeks, or in severe cases months.

Type 4 reactions are generally built up to over prolonged use and exposure to essential oils, particularly if they are applied undiluted too often. In other words, it is not really the single application of one essential oil or a particular essential oil that causes the reaction, but repeated exposure that "primes" the immune system for an allergic reaction. The reaction occurs after applying a single essential oil or blend because sensitivity has been building up due to chronic overexposure to significant quantities of essential oils over the course of months or even years.

Sensitization among aromatherapists and chemists has also been reported. Studies suggest that those who are regularly exposed to significant amounts of essential oils based on their occupation can experience type 4 hypersensitivity reactions to essential oils, and these reactions can result in sensitivities to multiple oils.[176,177,178,179] What we can learn from these studies is that excessive use of essential oils, or perhaps prolonged daily exposure to the same essential oils (particularly undiluted) may increase the risk of hypersensitivity reactions and sensitization.

An anaphylactic reaction to essential oils is extremely rare, but possible. Interestingly an immediate hypersensitive systemic reaction that resulted in anaphylaxis in a thirty-eight-year-old male reportedly caused by tea tree oil did not produce antibodies (IgG or IgE).[180] But a subsequent wheal and flare response (a characteristic irregular red raised bump, or "wheal," surrounded by areas of redness that appears on the skin in response to administration of a substance, usually as part of an allergy test) to an allergy test did determine he was sensitive to tea tree oil.

In the very extraordinary chance that an essential oil does cause an anaphylactic reaction, seek emergency medical help immediately. Anaphylaxis is a severe and potentially life-threatening medical emergency that requires prompt medical attention.

Some tell-tale symptoms of anaphylaxis include hives, flushed or pale skin, airway constriction, swollen tongue or throat, trouble breathing, weak or rapid pulse, very low

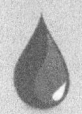

blood pressure, dizziness, anxiety, fainting, headache, confusion, nausea, vomiting, and/or diarrhea. Anaphylaxis usually starts with redness and irritation of the skin, quickly followed by hives, then swelling and inflammation of various areas of the body. The swelling can lead to airway constriction and trouble breathing. Because anaphylaxis is systemic (affecting the whole body), it can lead to the other symptoms mentioned as well.

If these symptoms occur within minutes, or in less common cases half-hour or longer, after the administration of an essential oil contact emergency medical services for help. Time is of the essence if the person is experiencing trouble breathing, loses consciousness, or faints. It is also useful to know that limonene and lavender may reduce anaphylactic reactions, but it would be unwise to apply or administer either of these essential oils in a life-threatening situation.[181,182]

Those with known allergies, food sensitivities, autoinflammatory or autoimmune disorders, and skin conditions (eczema, psoriasis, etc.) are more likely to develop skin sensitivities to essential oils. Essential oils that aromatherapy texts suggest may cause skin sensitivity in those with allergies include basil, cedarwood, German chamomile, clary sage, clove, fennel, ginger, juniper, lemon, lemongrass, orange, peppermint, pine, melaleuca, thyme, and ylang ylang. This is an extensive list and only includes essential oils recommended in the protocols in this book. Many with allergies find they can still use these essential oils as long as they are diluted heavily (less than or equal to 3% dilution). In addition, continuous daily exposure to the same oil(s) increases the risk of skin sensitivities, and clinical observations suggest that a tolerance may be built up with repeated use of the exact same oils without a break. Because of this, it is recommended that you regularly rotate the essential oils you use after continuous use. Another reason for this recommendation is to avoid building up a tolerance to any one, or group, of essential oils. Interestingly, men appear to be more susceptible to adverse skin reactions than women are, and stress and lack of sleep also make skin sensitivities more likely.[183]

To reduce the risk of oxidation and formation of hydroperoxides (1) essential oil caps should be replaced immediately after use, (2) citrus oils are best stored in the refrigerator, (3) keep bottles out of direct sunlight and away from heat sources, and (4) transfer partially used bottles to smaller bottles (e.g. 15 mL to a 10 mL bottle) when the headspace (empty part of the bottle) is near 50 percent.

**Ways to Avoid Sensitization**

One way to avoid sensitization is to dilute essential oils with a pure carrier oil, particularly when first introducing them onto your body. Combining essential oils with a pure carrier oil may help prevent some of the essential oil oxidation that occurs and reduce the risk of skin sensitivity and irritation. This practice may also be desirable when the objective is to keep the essential oil at the site of application for as long as possible (for example, when treating certain skin conditions like eczema or dermatitis). By combining an essential oil with a carrier oil, it helps prevent evaporation and may prolong the time you are able to benefit from both the topical application and the subsequent inhalation of the aroma.

Another strategy is to rotate the site of essential oil application. For instance, you may start with the feet, then move progressively to the ankles, knees, side of the torso, spine, side of the chest, sternum, and wrists. The following table contains dilution recommendations in a range. People with known sensitivities and who are new to essential oils should generally use the essential oils diluted with more carrier oil.

| DILUTION RATIOS *(The number of drops per teaspoon of carrier oil for general use and for individuals with sensitive skin.)* | |
| --- | --- |
| **Dilution %** | **Approximate number of drops of essential oil per teaspoon(s) of carrier oil[a]** |
| 0.3% | 1 drop EO per 2 teaspoons carrier oil |
| 1.5% | 2 drops EO per teaspoon of carrier oil |
| 3.0% | 4 drops of EO per teaspoon of carrier oil |
| 5.0% | 7 drops of EO per teaspoon of carrier oil |

| SIMPLE DILUTION RATIOS *(The number of drops per teaspoon of carrier oil for general use and for those with sensitive skin simplified.)* | |
| --- | --- |
| **Dilution %** | **Approximate number of drops of essential oil per teaspoon(s) of carrier oil[a]** |
| 0.3% | 1 drop EO per 3 teaspoons of carrier oil |
| 1.5% | 3 drops EO per 2 teaspoons of carrier oil |
| 3.0% | 3 drops of EO per teaspoon of carrier oil |
| 5.0% | 5 drops of EO per teaspoon of carrier oil |

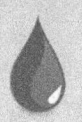 

| MAXIMUM STRENGTH DILUTION RATIOS (*The maximum number of drops per teaspoon of carrier oil for a maximum strength application*) | |
| --- | --- |
| Dilution % | Approximate number of drops of essential oil per teaspoon(s) of carrier oil[a] |
| 20% | 30 drops EO per teaspoon carrier oil |
| 33% | 48 drops EO per teaspoon of carrier oil |
| 50% | 73 drops of EO per teaspoon of carrier oil |
| Neat (NE) | EO only, with no carrier oil added |

[a] Rounded to the nearest whole drop for ease of use. One teaspoon is equivalent to 4.93 mL. On average 1 mL of essential oil contains 30 drops, though this figure can range from 15 to 40 depending on the essential oil and orifice reducer used. If you want to make things simpler for the maximum strength dilution ratios, you can use the following: 20% dilution—1 drop EO per 5 drops carrier, 33% dilution—1 drop EO per 3 drops carrier, and 50% dilution—1 drop EO per 1 drop carrier.

## Reversing Sensitivity

If sensitivity or contact dermatitis occurs, one must stop using the offending—and possibly all—essential oils topically until the skin heals. Immediately after sensitivity occurs apply carrier oil to the area and then wipe off with a dry cloth. Continue adding carrier oil and wiping it off with a dry cloth until the person experiences relief. My experience has been that diffusing and oral consumption do not result in the same reactions, but you may want to eliminate those two methods of application as well to allow your body to reset. The healing process may take several days or even weeks and, in rare cases, may become chronic. In addition to removing contact with one or all essential oils, here are a few other options that may help speed the healing process. Because each person responds differently, many options are recommended to determine which will best help you manage and reverse your skin reaction.

- Apply a natural, thick and creamy, fragrance-free lotion or Shea butter to the area often to keep the skin moist. This is probably the most important, and effective, way to reduce the irritation. It keeps the skin moist and allows it to heal.
- Apply homeopathic cardiospermum cream or gel to the area as directed on the product label.

Cardiospermum is a natural anti-inflammatory and possesses cortisone-like properties.

- Apply a cold washcloth or ice to the area of irritation 2 times daily.
- Take 5,000 to 10,000 IU of vitamin D daily for 30 days. Vitamin D plays a role in allergic diseases and directly modulates immune responses. Vitamin D receptors are located on antigen-presenting dendritic cells and activated T cells.[184] It is also involved in reducing the production of proinflammatory molecules, while simultaneously promoting the production of anti-inflammatory molecules.[185] Lastly, people with low blood levels of vitamin D seem to have a greater risk of atopic dermatitis (eczema), which is also initiated by CD8+ T cells.[186,187]
- The supplement N-acetyl cysteine may reduce the hypersensitivity response by increasing glutathione production in the skin and decreasing the inflammatory response.[188,189] Take 200-400 mg up to 3 times daily.
- Mix together one-quarter cup each of baking soda and water. Massage mixture into the irritated area and leave in place for twenty minutes before rinsing thoroughly. Baking soda helps neutralize acids, makes the skin more alkaline, and helps to remove dead skin.
- Fill a bowl with about half a cup of oatmeal (not the sweetened kind from the store) and then add enough hot water to make a paste-like consistency. Allow to cool until lukewarm and then apply to the irritated skin, leaving it in place for twenty to thirty minutes before rinsing thoroughly with water. Oatmeal will help cleanse and moisturize the skin, and it possesses antioxidants that may help neutralize inflammation.
- Apply aloe vera directly to the irritated skin up to six times daily. The anti-inflammatory and antimicrobial properties of aloe vera will help to soothe irritation and encourage healing.
- Consider taking 2 drops each of lavender, German chamomile, and blue tansy in a capsule one to three times daily to reduce the histamine-reaction and abnormal immune activity related to the reaction.
- Take high doses of a broad-spectrum probiotic (aim for 20 billion or more organisms daily) with a meal. Probiotics support the immune system and may alleviate allergies, particularly in children.
- Consider taking high doses of MSM (methylsulfonylmethane), up to 10 grams daily, which

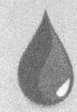

- is useful for allergies and may nourish the skin.
- ⚬ Some people have found cleansing helps relieve this situation. Start with a colon cleanse and then continue cleansing if necessary.
- ⚬ If these natural methods are ineffective in reducing the itching and sensitivity, it may be time to consider an oral antihistamine and/or topical hydrocortisone cream to get the reac- tion under control. Excessive scratching could lead to a worsening of the symptoms and even damaged or scarred skin.

Once sensitivity and the contact dermatitis clears, it is recommended that you slowly reintroduce highly diluted essential oils to your body one single oil at a time. It is possible that the topical application of very concentrated or undiluted (not recommended for those who have experienced sensitivity) essential oils will result in some irritation permanently, so it may be necessary to continually use the lower dilution ratios (0.3% to 5%) to avoid further sensitization and discomfort.

**The Waterfall Technique®**
Essential oil applications to the spine and feet have the potential to dramatically influence multiple body systems and the health of the whole person. With this in mind, the Waterfall Technique® was born. The Waterfall Technique® is an extraordinary essential oil application technique that provides systemic benefits for the whole person by combining ancient healing arts with cutting-edge science. It employs a unique sequence of clinically significant essential oils (six blends and two singles) and proven restorative touch techniques, each of which serves a specific purpose to balance, renew, oxygenate, protect, soothe, quench, synergize, enhance, and rejuvenate. The uniting of ancient healing arts, science, restorative touch, and clinically significant essential oils brings about rejuvenation and optimal wellness.

The three primary purposes of the Waterfall Technique® are: 1) to support and rejuvenate cells at the subcellular level (unblock cell receptors, enhance cellular communication, positively influence cellular behavior and function), 2) optimize key body systems (nervous, circulatory, immune, lymphatic, musculoskeletal, and endocrine) function, and 3) reduce limiting factors in wellness (stress, negative emotions, toxins, and pathogens). Through this technique, a remarkable wide-ranging wellness experience is realized.

## INHALATION

Inhalation is the safest and one of the easiest ways to use essential oils, but still produces remarkable psychophysiological outcomes that should not be underestimated. Inhalation provides several key benefits, including soothing throat infections, overcoming mental fatigue and exhaustion, encouraging the expulsion of mucous, relieving stress, anxiety and nervous tension, and purifying the air (including removing toxins), killing airborne germs to prevent the spread of infections, altering mood, and encouraging restful sleep. It is a must with respiratory concerns because essential oil molecules enter the lungs, bronchi, bronchioles, and alveoli. If your sinuses are congested or affected, you must inhale deeply and hold this breath for as long as possible. This allows the essential oil molecules to travel to the sinuses where they can provide benefit rather than into the lungs, as is the case when you breathe normally. Inhaled essential oils also directly influence the limbic system—the area of the brain associated with memory and emotions—significantly influencing mood, stress, anxiety, and depressive symptoms.

To diffuse essential oils in a diffuser, add 1 to 3 drops of essential oil per 100 mL of water in your diffuser. Diffuse as desired in a well-ventilated area. Place close to an ill person for best results.

If you don't have a diffuser, you can simulate diffusing through a steam inhalation. This can be accomplished by adding 1 to 4 drops of essential oils to three inches of hot water and then cover your head and the container of water with a towel and breathe deeply (depending on the oil used this can be quite intense, so closing your eyes is recommended).

Alternately try palm diffusing by placing 1 to 2 drops of essential oil in one palm, rubbing your palms together and cupping your hands over your nose and mouth to breathe deeply. Another method that can be used for inhalation is to place 1 to 6 drops of essential oil on a cotton ball, tissue, or cloth and inhale as desired.

**The Powerful Influence of Aromas**
The influence of essential oil inhalation and the subsequent psychophysiological actions that follow is quite extraordinary. When an aroma is inhaled, odor molecules travel up the nose and attach to olfactory cell-receptor sites. Once bound to the olfactory nerves, odor molecules travel to the olfactory bulb, where the odor is significantly intensified. The intensified odor stimulates the bipolar receptor to fire, and impulses are transmitted to the limbic system. The limbic system is a complex set of structures—hypothalamus, hippocampus, amygdala, and limbic cortex—that regulates the endocrine and nervous systems and is responsible for controlling memory, learning, emotions, instinct, motivation, and

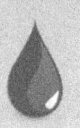

influential to sleep, libido, appetite, thirst, heart rate, blood pressure, breathing, stress levels, and hormone balance. In response to the odor, the limbic system initiates physiological responses in the body by releasing hormones, neurotransmitters, and chemicals that influence myriad body functions, including pain perception, appetite, metabolism, libido, wakefulness, insulin production, body temperature, relaxation level, and sense of well-being. Eventually, this cascade of events modifies emotions and behavior and generates memories that cause profound psychophysiological responses.

## Essential Oil Inhalation: Asthma and Chronic Respiratory Disorders

One concern often raised when inhaling essential oils is the possibility of aggravating asthma or other chronic respiratory condition symptoms. Asthma, particularly, may be triggered by volatile organic compounds like essential oils. Research suggests that terpenes, particularly limonene, may exacerbate bronchial hyperresponsiveness,[190] which is a hallmark symptom of asthma. Because of this, direct inhalation of essential oils very high in limonene—mainly citrus oils, some of which are up to 95 percent limonene—should be limited or avoided by those with asthma or other chronic respiratory conditions. Another essential oil commonly reported to trigger asthma-like symptoms in persons with chronic respiratory disorders is lavender. Those who have chronic respiratory conditions should take care when inhaling essential oils and limit the time that they do so. In addition, those that are sensitive to fragrances or strong odors may need to avoid direct inhalation of essential oils, and use dilutions of less than 3 percent for topical application.

While myrtle contains the terpenes alpha-pinene (up to 56 percent) and limonene (up to 12 percent), it is known to reverse respiratory distress. Myrtle and ginger are known bronchodilators, so they may also be useful in relieving asthma symptoms and bronchial hyperresponsiveness.[191,192] Lavender also has small amounts of terpenes, but anecdotal evidence, preclinical research, and user experience suggests it may be beneficial for relieving asthma symptoms, due to its ability to suppress allergic airway inflammation and the accumulation of mucous in the airways.[193,194] This just goes to show that what may be a trigger for an adverse response in one person, may be beneficial for another person. Ginger is another essential oil with multiple terpenes, such as zingiberene, curcumene, sesquiphellandrene, camphene, beta-bisabolene, beta-

phellandrene, alpha-pinene, and beta-elemene, but is useful in asthma because of its bronchodilatory properties.

While not proven definitively in science, it is possible, and some people report, that essential oils that are known to cause respiratory difficulty in children could exacerbate asthma and bronchial hyperresponsiveness in those who are more susceptible—people with asthma or other chronic respiratory disorders. Based on this assumption, it would be wise to be cautious with or avoid essential oils high in camphor, eucalyptol, and menthol among more sensitive people.

## Sensory Irritation During Essential Oil Inhalation or Diffusion

Sensory irritation, such as nosebleeds, eye, ear, or throat irritation have occasionally been reported among people who have inhaled essential oils. This phenomenon is likely caused by irritation of the mucous membranes among more sensitive populations (younger children, persons with nasal allergies or chemical sensitivities).[195,196,197] When enough of the volatile essential oil compounds are present in the air, sensory pathways within the body are triggered that may lead to irritation, stinging, burning, itching, changes in temperature sensations, nosebleed, and headache.[198]

It appears that terpenes are more likely to cause this type of sensory irritation than other essential oil constituents.[199,200,201] Their structure—comprised of one or more carbon to carbon bonds—makes them extremely susceptible to reactions with atmospheric compounds.[3917,3918] When these reactions occur, toxic oxidation products are produced such as formaldehyde, acetaldehyde, organic acid, and hydrogen peroxide, which are called hydroxyl radicals and secondary organic aerosols (SOAs).[3919–3922] These oxidation products can be harmful to human health if present in sufficient quantities. Children, the elderly, people who are obese, diabetics, and people with chronic respiratory disorders are more likely to experience these adverse health effects.

The risk of reactions between terpenes and atmospheric compounds is dependent on temperature and the amount of ozone present indoors. Reactions are more likely to occur in warm seasons when temperatures are higher as opposed to the colder temperatures of cold seasons.[202] In addition, higher levels of ozone provide more atmospheric compounds for essential oil terpenes to react with. Indoor ozone quantities can increase based on the amount of ozone present outside or through the use

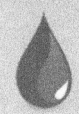

of certain equipment (laser printers, photocopiers, and some air cleaning units).

Limonene (found in two isomeric forms: *d*-limonene—citrusy scent and found in citrus oils; and *l*-limonene—piney scent and found in tree oils) is more susceptible to these reactions than other terpenes like linalool (a monoterpene alcohol). This suggests that essential oils with significant amounts of limonene may require more caution when diffusing, particularly during warm seasons and when the presence of ozone is elevated. In addition, the available evidence suggests that oxidized terpenes[203] and low humidity may exacerbate or trigger sensory irritation. However, studies using synthetic versions of constituents found in essential oils demonstrate that reasonable and normal usage does not result in the production of enough terpene reaction products to be harmful to health.[204] Based on this knowledge, it is sensible for those with known chemical sensitivities, chronic respiratory conditions, or who are prone to headaches and nosebleeds to avoid direct inhalation of essential oils and to limit diffusing. Those without these sensitivities are unlikely to experience adverse effects from diffusing.

### Do Essential Oils Benefit Individuals with a Deficient Sense of Smell?

A common question is whether individuals who have anosmia (loss of sense of smell) or deficient ability to smell (hyposmia) can benefit from essential oil inhalation. Fortunately, the answer is yes. Essential oils are not dependent on the sense of smell to produce beneficial effects. Once essential oil odor molecules are inhaled, they interact with olfactory scent receptors and trigger extraordinary psychophysiological responses. They can also enter the bloodstream through the lungs and produce benefits, the same way nicotine, air pollution, or chemicals can enter the bloodstream and cause damage when they are inhaled. In other words, essential oil molecules will still produce health benefits even if you can't smell the aroma of the essential oil itself because they enter the bloodstream, interact with cells, and trigger a cascade of events through the limbic system.

Indeed, science suggests that those with anosmia still receive benefits from essential oils. Lavender essential oil is well-known for producing a relaxed state and relieving anxiety. When animals with anosmia were exposed to lavender essential oil aroma they still experienced reduced anxiety.[205] This is likely due to lavender's influence on the production of hormones and neurotransmitters like gamma-aminobutyric acid (GABA) and serotonin.

Some practitioners even recommend inhaling essential oils to restore a diminished or lost sense of smell. Thomas Hummel experimented with odors (phenyl ethyl alcohol: rose; eucalyptol: eucalyptus; citronellal: citronella; and eugenol: clove) in an attempt to regain some smell sensation in those with olfactory dysfunction. Constituents found in essential oils were placed on a pad (one constituent at a time) and placed within an inch of the nose to inhale the molecules through the nose. The pad was then removed from the nose and the same oil was inhaled again, repeating this process multiple times. Then the individual was given a five-minute break before repeating the process with the next oil until all constituents were inhaled. The whole process, with all four constituents, was repeated twice daily. A statistically significant number of individuals (30%) reported improvement in their sense of smell at the conclusion of the study.[206]

A more recent study evaluated the effectiveness of the same set of synthetic aromas in people with post-traumatic and post-infectious olfactory dysfunction. This study found that two-thirds of people with post-infectious and one-third with post-traumatic olfactory dysfunction experienced improved olfactory function after inhaling the scents.[207] Those who did not experience positive results in both studies may have had more long-term or extensive damage to olfactory neurons, which prevented positive results. Imagine what may be the results if a genuine essential oil is used in place of the synthetic aromas used in the studies.

These animal and human studies provide evidence that essential oils can still be used effectively despite deficient smell sensation, and may even improve olfaction in some individuals. One caution for those with anosmia is to follow reasonable diffusion and inhalation practices. This is because your senses may not produce the same sensory warnings that a person with a full sense of smell receives when they have "overused" essential oils.

## ORAL ADMINISTRATION

Some essential oils can be administered orally, which allows for greater precision in dosing, increased convenience, and good bioavailability. Oral administration may also increase the risk of drug interactions and stomach discomfort (see below), so it is strongly advised that you check for contraindications, safety precautions, and drug interactions before administering oils orally. The risk of

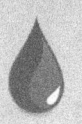

stomach discomfort can be reduced if you take the essential oil in a capsule or softgel with food rather than on an empty stomach and use reasonable doses. It is strongly recommended that you always take essential oils orally with food and a full glass of water.

To administer essential oils orally, add the desired number of drops of essential oil to an empty vegetable capsule, in a beverage (almond or rice milk, herbal tea), in honey, or directly on or under the tongue (sublingual). Adding a carrier oil to the capsule (approximately 50% of the capsule filled with olive oil, MCT, coconut oil, or another edible vegetable oil) will improve bioavailability and reduce disintegration of the capsule, but it is not completely necessary if the capsule will be consumed immediately. The lipid component of food, or carrier oils, influences metabolism, efflux transporter activity, intestinal permeability, length of time present in the digestive tract for absorption, and transport via the lymphatic system to enhance bioavailability and therefore efficacy of orally administered essential oils.[4925] Coconut oil, MCT, black seed oil, and olive oil are each good choices to add to a capsule. Another way to ingest essential oils is to place a drop in your mouth and swish it around to mix it with saliva. This can be very beneficial for oral health, particularly if mixed with coconut oil.

Taking essential oils in capsules is the preferred oral method. Lipophilic molecules, like essential oils, have the high absorption in the intestines. Putting them inside capsules allows greater dispersion of the essential oil to occur in the intestines, and therefore increases absorption into the bloodstream. This is obviously desirable from an efficacy standpoint. Administering essential oils in a capsule will also reduce the likelihood of throat and oral cavity irritation. If oil is added directly to water to ingest, separation will occur, and much of the oil will remain in and be absorbed through the buccal cavity (the portion of the oral cavity enclosed by the lips, cheeks, and gums). Depending on the essential oil, this may result in irritation of the mucous linings in the mouth. This will also reduce essential oil dispersion and bioavailability, allow for the degradation of some of the essential oil molecules in the stomach acid, and likely reduce efficacy.

If desired, multiple essential oil capsules may be prepared prior to administration rather than immediately prior to use. However, many essential oils will cause the capsule to dissolve, making early preparation impractical. This obstacle can be overcome by preparing the capsules with a fatty oil and then immediately placing them in the freezer for future use.

Essential oils can also be taken sublingually (under the tongue) or directly on the tongue, which results in rapid absorption due to the high concentration of capillaries (tiny blood vessels) under the tongue. Essential oils will be absorbed directly into the bloodstream with this method without needing to go through the digestive process. Direct and sublingual administration should be reserved for mild oils that have less potential to irritate the mouth, lips, and tongue.

**Oral Administration and Irritation of the Gastrointestinal System**

Some essential oils users are concerned about the long-term effects that ingesting essential oils may have on the oral cavity, esophagus, stomach, and intestinal mucosa. These linings are more sensitive to irritation, and there have been occasional reports of irritation, inflammation, burp-back, or a burning sensation following oral administration.[208,209,210,211,212] But these effects were usually minor and were reversed when the irritating essential oil was eliminated.

Burp-back of essential oils is common and can be expected when taking them orally. Taking essential oils with food and at least eight ounces of water may reduce this effect. In addition, using enteric coated or delayed release capsules is also beneficial.

It is suspected that larger doses are more likely to cause irritation, particularly if taken directly in a liquid rather than in a capsule. Studies demonstrate that lower doses protect the gastrointestinal system while larger doses of the same oil irritate it.[213,214,215] It is also reasonable to presume that taking essential oils orally on an empty stomach will increase the risk of stomach discomfort. However, the overwhelming body of scientific evidence suggests many essential oils are gastroprotective and even promote healing of irritated and inflamed tissues, even among essential oils commonly reported to irritate the stomach or gastrointestinal tract (thyme, oregano) when administered in smaller doses.[216,217,218,219,220,221,222,223] These studies suggest that the essential oils promote healing of these sensitive linings due to their ability to stimulate stomach mucous lining production, reduce inflammation, destroy harmful bacteria associated with ulcers, and their antioxidant properties. Based on current knowledge, and the available literature, oral administration of essential oils does not pose a long-term risk of damage to the oral cavity, esophagus, stomach, or intestines when taken in reasonable doses and with food.

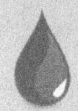

Some research and years of clinical experience supports this theory.

Many traditional aromatherapists argue that oral administration poses a risk of organ toxicity, despite a lack of factual evidence to support this assertion. In essence, they come to this conclusion largely based on assumption and a lack of long-term safety studies for each essential oil used therapeutically. While few controlled safety studies have been conducted regarding the oral administration of essential oils, those that have been completed were favorable for this practice, reporting few if any adverse outcomes, even when liver enzymes were closely monitored. No clinical, blood, kidney, or liver toxicity or abnormalities were reported when turmeric essential oil was administered to healthy individuals (0.6 mL three times daily for one month and 1 mL in three divided doses for three months).[224] No acute side effects were reported during the course of daily administration for up to three months. Another study safely administered 0.45 mL of geranium essential oil daily for two months, reporting positive effects to blood pressure and cortisol levels.[225] Those studies that do report adverse effects in humans are usually case reports of accidental or intentional ingestion of extreme amounts (10 mL+). One study determined that the oral administration of "1–2 mL [of myrtle essential oil] daily is considered to be too low to influence the hepatic [liver] parameters," suggesting that liver toxicity is unlikely at this dosage.[226] A review of multiple published clinical studies reveals that clinical doses for essential oils range from 50 mcL to 3 mL daily depending on the essential oil used and the condition being treated. It is therefore reasonable to conclude that many essential oils have a wide safety profile when taken orally and pose little long-term or short-term (acute) risk when sensible dosing guidelines are followed.

In addition, hundreds of thousands—if not millions—of people have been taking essential oils orally for decades. It is logical that many of these people would experience adverse events if it was a real problem, yet very few reports of adverse reactions exist (most of which are poorly documented and lacking critical information). It is also unlikely that all of these reported adverse side effects are real effects. Adverse events are commonly reported in both active treatment groups and placebo groups in double-blind clinical trials, with some placebos "causing" adverse events so significant that participants discontinue the study.[227] The significant influence of the nocebo effect caused by placebos cannot be ignored. Amazingly, a systematic review of trials in people with fibromyalgia noted that two-thirds of study participants reported adverse reactions to placebos.[228] Similarly, 25 percent of study participants reported allergic symptoms to placebos in a study of allergy treatments.[229] Without adequate documentation and better monitoring, these disorganized and inconclusive online adverse event reports truly provide little real evidence of the adverse effects of essential oils ingestion, especially if you consider the fraction of a percent that the adverse event reports represent compared to global essential oil users. Moreover, it is possible that the adverse reaction was due to another substance the person was consuming or an underlying health condition.

Furthermore, lavender (1–2 drops daily) and peppermint (3–6 drops, three to six times daily) essential oils have significant safety records in clinical studies that administered them orally for anxiety and irritable bowel syndrome.[230,231,232,233,234,235,236,237,238,239,240,241,242] Based on the current knowledge and available research, the assertions that the oral administration of reasonable doses of essential oils is toxic to the liver, or poses long-term health risks, is unwarranted and scientifically inaccurate. Those essential oils that do pose a higher degree of risk are indicated in this reference with appropriate cautions.

**Essential Oils and Gastrointestinal Flora (Probiotics)**

A common question is whether essential oils with antimicrobial properties kill harmful as well as beneficial intestinal flora (probiotics) similarly to antibiotic medications. What published research we have suggests that essential oils are partially selective and do discriminate between healthy and harmful microbes to some degree. Or at least that they are more effective against harmful than beneficial bacteria residing in the gut microbiome.

A study that tested the inhibitory effects of sixty-six essential oils or essential oil constituents against pathogenic bacteria and two probiotic strains determined that essential oils could selectively inhibit harmful bacteria without harming probiotics.[243] Although the essential oils and constituents tested significantly inhibited harmful bacteria, they had little effect on the tested probiotics. Another study found that cinnamon, clove, and mint essential oils demonstrated some antimicrobial activity against the probiotic *L. rhamnosus* in yogurt, but the activity was minimal.[244] In fact, enough probiotics remained in the yogurt product that the product could still meet the minimum requirements to be considered a probiotic food.

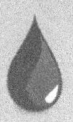 

Other studies have determined that some essential oils may destroy beneficial flora and decrease their ability to reproduce. Cinnamon oil concentrations damaged the cell membrane of *L. rhamnosus* and caused a significant reduction in the number of viable probiotics in one study.[245] Cassia essential oil, which is closely related to cinnamon essential oil, also inhibited some probiotics. Interestingly, the researchers discovered that cassia significantly inhibited some intestinal bacteria (*Bi. bifidum*, *B. fragilis*, and *Cl. perfringens*), but did not inhibit or only weakly inhibited the common probiotics *Bi. longum* and *L. acidophilus*.[246] Another study tested the antimicrobial activity of hairy basil (*O. americanum*) essential oil against two pathogenic organisms and the probiotic *L. casei*. This study also found that the essential oil demonstrated antimicrobial activity against all the organisms, but that *L. casei* was less susceptible to destruction by the essential oil.[247] Two additional studies found similar results with tea tree oil against *Lactobacillus* spp., suggesting probiotics are more resilient to destruction by essential oils than harmful pathogens.[248,249]

Some research even suggests that essential oils may improve the gut microbiome rather than promote imbalance (dysbiosis). Interestingly, cinnamon essential oil enhanced the diversity and richness of intestinal bacteria—reduced harmful *Helicobacter* and bacteroides (bacteria normally found in the mouth, gastrointestinal tract, and female genital tract) and increased bacteroidales and short-chain fatty acids-producing bacteria in an experimental model of colitis.[250] Similarly, orange essential oil and isolated limonene improved the gut microbiome in the caecum and colon in mice.[251] Patchouli essential oil and its isolated constituents also enhanced the gut microbiome and presence of short-chain fatty acids in mice.[252] Even emerging clinical research suggests that ingestion of peppermint essential oil can improve the intestinal microenvironment. Children who consumed peppermint oil experienced improvements in gut microbiome diversity. Specifically, *Collinsella* bacteria increased and the firmicutes/bacteroidetes ratio improved.[253]

Based on the available research, it appears that essential oils are somewhat selective and can distinguish between friendly and harmful bacteria to a certain degree. Nevertheless, considering the far-reaching benefits of probiotics, it is reasonable to supplement more heavily with probiotics four hours after ingesting antimicrobial essential oils. Further clinical research is necessary, but our current understanding of essential oils and probiotics

suggests that they can live in harmony within the human body.

**Liver Toxicity and Essential Oils: Fact or Fabricated Fiction?**

Lipophilic (lipid- or fat-soluble) substances like essential oils swiftly enter the bloodstream and are processed by the liver, unlike hydrophilic (water-soluble) substances that are inclined to stay in the blood or are transported to aqueous compartments within the body. The fastest way to the liver is oral administration, at which point the liver distributes and eliminates the various essential oil constituents. The liver metabolizes essential oil constituents for elimination in two phases through a process called biotransformation. This process converts lipophilic (fat-soluble) substances to hydrophilic (water-soluble) substances, which are more easily excreted by the kidneys. Common phase I reactions include oxidation, reduction, and hydrolysis. The most common phase II reactions include glucuronidation, sulfation, and conjugation. Metabolites of essential oil constituents are identified in the blood of people who consume essential oils, demonstrating that the body and the liver does process them efficiently.

Topical, vaginal, and rectal administration of essential oils bypasses the first phase of biotransformation, but the essential oil constituents are eventually distributed to the liver for processing and elimination through the cytochrome P450 pathway. In addition, dermal (skin) enzymes can catalyze phase I and phase II reactions, though the reactions generally occur with less efficiency than within the liver.

It is important to note that metabolism chemically alters the original constituent, making its metabolite possess different pharmacological and/or toxicological properties. Essential oils are naturally detoxifying; however, toxification is also possible—methyleugenol is an example of a toxic essential oil constituent.[254,255] And if excessive quantities of essential oils are consumed, it is possible to overwhelm the body's detoxification system, potentially causing harm to the liver. It has been reported that the depletion of glutathione levels in the liver is an important mechanism of action for liver injury to occur. The liver contains the highest levels of reduced glutathione (GSH) in the body as a protective mechanism against reactive molecules produced in the liver during the normal detoxification and metabolism processes.

Excessive oral doses of essential oils could potentially deplete liver glutathione stores and overwhelm the liver, creating liver toxicity (hepatotoxicity). This result

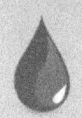

seems to be rare and isolated to megadoses of a few essential oils. Aromatherapy texts often list hepatotoxic essential oils as cassia (coumarin and cinnamaldehyde), cinnamon (cinnamaldehyde), pennyroyal (pulegone), thyme (thymol), oregano (carvacrol), clove (eugenol), and fennel (anethole) because they contain constituents (in parenthesis) reported to reduce glutathione S-transferase activity and/or deplete liver glutathione levels and have been reported as hepatotoxic. Dosages that could potentially produce toxicity are frequently extreme—often exceeding 5 or 10 mL in a single dose for the average-size human adult (154 pounds). For instance, a study found that it required the administration of 67.5 mg/kg/BW/day of coumarin (not cassia essential oil) to produce hepatotoxic effects in male baboons while no adverse effects were observed at a dosage of 22.5 mg/kg/BW/day.[256] In other words, it would require the human equivalent dosage of nearly 2.7 mL of coumarin—not cassia essential oil that has other constituents that may potentially buffer this effect—daily to cause harm in a 154-pound (70 kg) human and this same individual could potentially consume 0.875 mL daily without causing harm.

One study reporting the development of acute liver failure (ALF) in a 15-month-old who ingested 10 mL of clove oil concluded that a single dose of 10 mL of clove could cause hepatotoxicity.[257] The ALF was reversed by administering N-acetyl cysteine. Another young child—2 years old—ingested a single dose of 10 mL of clove oil, which resulted in liver toxicity and excessive clotting of the blood.[258] These results are not surprising, given the amount ingested and the age of the children. So, in other words, the cases of liver toxicity that are sensationalized by those who oppose oral consumption of essential oils are from unreasonably excessive doses, and far greater than recommended amounts.

Oregano is often listed as toxic to the liver because it contains minute amounts of thymol. However, at least one study suggests that thymol protects the liver against toxicity by inhibiting lipid peroxidation—free-radical damage to the lipid cellular membrane, resulting in degradation of lipids[259]—and the major constituent in oregano called carvacrol is hepatoprotective.[260] So, oregano appears to be naturally balanced and buffered by Mother Nature.

Another aspect to consider in the toxicity debate is the fact that many studies on toxicity focus on a single essential oil constituent, not all of the constituents naturally found in the plant. This places the constituents out of balance with what Mother Nature produces and may eliminate many constituents that offer a balancing, buffering, or protective effects when compared to a single constituent. For example, high doses of anethole deplete glutathione,[261] but even though fennel essential oil contains greater than 65 percent trans-anethole the whole oil significantly stimulates glutathione production and may protect the liver from oxidative damage.[262,263] This is because fennel contains buffering and balancing constituents found naturally in the essential oil, rather than just the one isolated constituent.

### Compromised Livers or Liver Damage and Essential Oils Use

If a person has a compromised liver, liver damage, or liver failure, then there is potential for essential oils to exacerbate this condition, particularly essential oils that are known to be hepatotoxic in larger doses.[264,265] The liver is the primary site of essential oil metabolism, and a compromised liver may be overtaxed by the additional responsibility of metabolizing essential oil molecules. Even smaller doses of certain essential oils could potentially be harmful to a person with impaired liver function. Caution is warranted for both oral and topical administration (though topical is low risk considering the amount of essential oil that enters the bloodstream after topical administration) of essential oils among those with liver disorders, particularly oral administration.

### Oral Consumption is Reasonable, Beneficial, and Safe

Based on the available data, it seems reasonable to suggest that essential oils are safe when administered orally in sensible doses (as opposed to the extreme dosages that cause toxicity) for a reasonable amount of time. Those who advise against this practice want to treat essential oils more like drugs where only licensed professionals can dispense or administer them orally. These individuals also ignore the fact that essential oils contain dozens to hundreds of naturally occurring constituents, some of which act as buffers to balance or counteract the toxicity of other constituents. This is likely why, despite being extremely potent remedies, adverse reactions to essential oils are significantly lower and less severe than those of drugs. If reasonable dosages are followed and safety precautions observed, oral administration can be of great benefit.

### RETENTION (RECTAL AND VAGINAL ADMINISTRATION)

Retention is a very efficient method to deliver essential oils to the lower colon and into the vagina, cervix,

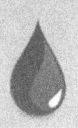

urethra, and ureters. Vaginal pessaries can deliver targeted doses of essential oils to heal the tissues of the vagina, reduce vaginal atrophy and dryness, promote postpartum healing, and fight vaginal and bladder infections. Suppositories may be helpful for hemorrhoids, anal fissures, constipation, cleansing, and inflammation of the colon. Both methods deliver essential oils systemically into the bloodstream for the management of a variety of conditions as well. The retention method may be a viable administration method for people who have difficulty swallowing or are experiencing nausea as well. This method also bypasses the gastrointestinal system, avoiding the breakdown of essential oils during metabolism.

The mucous membranes of the colon and vagina are highly susceptible to irritation, so caution is advised with this method. Dilution ratios of 3% to 5% are recommended. To create a suppository, mix 12 to 21 drops of essential oil with 1 tablespoon of carrier oil and insert through the rectum. Ideal carrier oils include coconut oil, cocoa butter, or shea butter because they are solid at room temperature and melt at body temperature Suppositories should be about 1 gram in total weight, while pessaries should be about 3 to 4 grams each. For vaginal insertion, mix the same essential oil to carrier oil ratio but make them slightly larger and insert through the vagina. Alternately, dip a tampon in the mixture, then insert into vagina and retain up to eight hours, or replace the tampon three to four times daily. Sensitive individuals may need to use dilutions of 1% instead (3 to 4 drops essential oil per tablespoon of carrier oil). Be cautious with "hot" oils (cinnamon, oregano, thyme, lemongrass, etc.) when using this method, and try mild oils first. For a douche, add 3 to 8 drops of oil in one liter of water and douche twice daily.

Essential oils may also be inserted in the rectum or vagina in a capsule. Capsules inserted into the rectum or vagina disintegrate and deliver calibrated doses of essential oils to local tissues and some enters the bloodstream. For the capsule method, add 1 drop of essential oil to a "00" capsule and fill the rest with carrier oil, and then insert as far up the rectum or vagina as possible.

To create an essential oil suppository or pessary, melt your chosen oil or butter over low temperature. Once liquid, remove from heat and slowly add the essential oils (add herbs if desired), stirring gently to mix well. Pour the mixture into an ice cube tray (preferably one that makes small, round cubes) or another mold, then place in the refrigerator or freezer. Once solid, the suppository can be inserted into the rectum or vagina. If frozen, remove and allow to thaw for 20 to 30 minutes nefore insertion.

## Using the Protocols

The method (or methods) of application will depend on the severity of the condition and how accustomed you are to a particular oil or protocol. Using more than one method of application at a time can often exponentially increase the effectiveness of essential oil therapy. However, you can select just one application method to start if desired.

When more than one essential oil is indicated, you may apply them one at a time, waiting a few minutes between each oil for the previous one to absorb—called layering—or create a blend of the suggested oils and apply this blend all at once. It is convenient to create the mixture in a bottle and use the desired or suggested number of drops. Create topical blends in a roller bottle and blends meant to be ingested in a bottle with a dropper. A premade and labeled roller bottle keeps you prepared for those times when you need a specific blend of essential oils.

Unless otherwise recommended in the protocol it is expected that the suggested essential oils will be diluted according to age, current state of health, susceptibility to sensitivity, and body size.

## Recommended Essential Oils

While profiles for more than two hundred essential oils are included in this text, the protocols will adhere to a smaller list of thirty-nine essential oils for convenience. The thirty-nine essential oils are more commonly and usually readily available commercially. In addition, tried and true essential oils often provide the best results. The chosen essential oils for the protocols include balsam fir, basil, blue tansy, cedarwood, cinnamon bark, clary sage, clove, copaiba, cypress, eucalyptus, fennel, frankincense, geranium, German chamomile (or Roman), ginger, grapefruit, helichrysum, juniper, lavender, lemon, lemongrass, lime, marjoram, melissa, myrrh, myrtle, nutmeg, orange, oregano, peppermint, pine, rosemary, sandalwood, spruce (black), tea tree, thyme, vetiver, wintergreen, and ylang ylang. This group of essential oils will allow you to manage most ailments you can expect to experience and still leave the list of essential oils reasonably affordable and easy to carry with you. However, you may substitute essential oils with similar properties or chemical constituents as necessary.

It is critical that you have a supply of essential oils on hand to be prepared before you find yourself in a

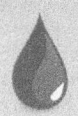

situation where you need it. If you know you have a specific health condition, it is wise to have a reasonable supply of the oil, or oils, recommended for that condition.

## One Final Conversation on Purity, Quality, Testing, and Transparency

The essential oil industry is at a crossroads when it comes to purity, essential oil testing, and transparency. Testing laboratories, consumers, and essential oil wholesalers and retailers are the key players, with varying interests and desires regarding this subject. A shift where consumers demand proof that their essential oil is pure enough for medicinal use is replacing the obsolete practice of blindly buying essential oils without reviewing tests results. While consumers almost universally desire more transparency and access to pertinent test results, retailers and wholesalers fall on one of two sides of this topic: either they refuse to adapt and share the information consumers need, or they do their best to make purity and quality test results available to the consumer.

Savvy health-conscious shoppers read food labels. They want to know if there are any harmful ingredients (artificial sweeteners, high fructose corn syrup, food colors, MSG, trans-fats, to name a few) in the foods they purchase. Equally, they want to be informed of the ingredients a food product contains that may benefit their health (anthocyanins, vitamins, minerals, amino acids, protein, fatty acids, etc.). Dietary supplements similarly provide the consumer an accounting of what is inside the supplements—although proprietary blends often diminish this transparency. Why should essential oil consumers deserve any less?

The inherent variances in essential oil composition, and the sheer number of different chemotypes in some botanicals, makes purity, quality, and quantitative analysis critical to the end consumer, and even more importantly, the clinician. If a health professional uses an essential oil in a clinical setting without having test results to prove purity, they are putting not only their patients or clients, but themselves, at risk. An adulterated or poor quality product may not be effective, and worse, could harm patients or clients. Reliable clinical results require consistent product quality and purity.

What if the supplier is passing spike lavender off for true lavender and this is applied to the burn of a patient or client? The potential for aggravating the burn due to a higher camphor content is possible. What if the bottle of spearmint is the more toxic pulegone chemotype (instead of the more common carvone chemotype) and the patient or client is advised to take it orally on a regular basis? What if a consumer takes a copaiba essential oil rich in beta-caryophyllene to reduce inflammation with good results and then the retailer they purchase copaiba from changes suppliers to a copaiba with far lower beta-caryophyllene content (say 35% versus 80%)? A decline in the efficacy of the product may be experienced. These are just a few of the many examples of why transparency—by providing test results—is so crucial in the industry.

Until recently, essential oil consumers have not had the same privilege as food label readers to review the makeup of their essential oils. Consumers have been forced to purchase essential oils blindly without knowing what is inside their essential oil bottle, nor its chemical makeup. However, as the demand for this information increases by clinicians and consumers, so does the number of companies willing to share this information. The increased demand is driven by several factors: 1) scientific implications regarding replication of scientific research and biological activity; 2) limitations for certain constituents set by governing bodies (i.e. thujone, furanocoumarins, pulegone); 3) the necessity to quality control and ferret out adulterated products; and 4) the need to meet the specifications set by international bodies, committees, pharmacopeias, and the scientific community. This increased demand is a positive driver to elevate transparency and quality in the industry and allows consumers to purchase brands that consistently meet higher standards for clinical use.

Nevertheless, quantitative analysis is a complex task that is not without its difficulties and detractors. Some of the difficulty is that quantitation (the measurement of the amount of each constituent in the essential oil) has generally been considered secondary to the discovery of new constituents. The ambiguity (inconsistency in names of constituents, for example) of several aspects of analysis is also tricky. The complexity of essential oil constituents present in essential oils must also be dealt with. GC/MS analysis of essential oils requires several factors (advanced instruments, a robust library, qualified scientists to interpret results, etc.) to provide quality and relevant results.

The most commonly used approach in essential oil analysis is relative % abundance. Unfortunately, its usefulness is limited to the measurement of constituent percentages in a single sample, not necessarily across a series of samples.[266] Truly comparing a series of samples

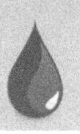 

of the same essential oil (i.e. peppermint, lavender, lemon) requires a more standardized approach like normalized % abundance (the data of essential oil components is normalized against an internal standard to limit performance variations) or true quantitation (specific constituent percentages are determined from the chromatographic area normalized by a standard and calculated using a calibration curve created from a pure constituent reference standard). If the essential oil being tested has limited variance in the number of constituents present and their ratios, normalized % abundance can be applied to make results across the series correctly comparable. On the other hand, true quantitation should be used if an essential oil series produces a significant difference in the number of constituents present and their ratios. True quantitation is limited to certain marker constituents for which a standard is available due to the unacceptably long analysis time of complex essential oils.

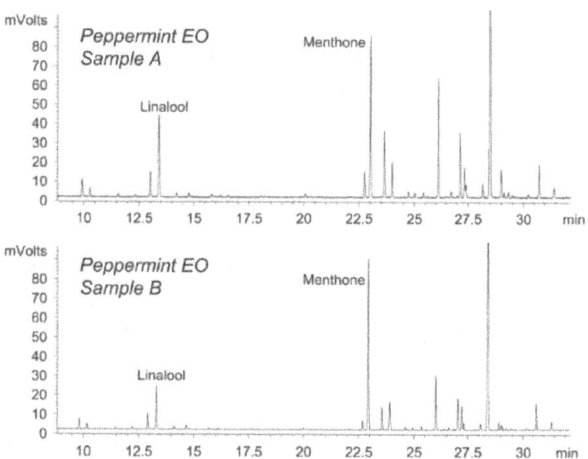

Figure used with permission and courtesy of John Wiley and Sons, *Flavour and Fragrance Journal*.

The above figure demonstrates some of the inherent challenges in determining essential oil constituent percentages. While the menthone peaks appear similar in size on the chromatogram (the absolute area in sample A is about 5% larger than in sample B), the normalized % abundance is contradictory and incorrect (the menthone percentage is calculated as almost double in sample B compared to sample A, 20.7% to 11.2%). Linalool has a similar discrepancy. The absolute areas of the linalool peaks in the chromatogram are significantly different, but the relative % abundance calculates their percentages as very similar—0.39% in sample A and 0.35% in sample B. The results are only fully consistent with the absolute peak areas when a true quantification approach with calibration curves is used.

Detraction against the sharing of test results mostly comes from people affiliated with companies that refuse to provide the data demanded. These individuals grow increasingly vocal about why it is not in the consumer's best interest to provide such data as the shift to make it an industry standard accelerates. Some of these individuals say that the average consumer is incapable of reading essential oil analyses, so the information is useless. This is true to a certain degree. The vast majority of consumers are not trained in organic chemistry or how to interpret GC/MS data. However, this book is the first of its kind to empower consumers to do exactly that—interpret results in a simple and straightforward manner. The key bioactive constituents—including a range of percentages that these constituents should fall within—have been identified in the Preferred Composition for Clinical Use tables included in each essential oil monograph. Empowered with this knowledge and clinical standard, consumers can now simply compare data provided by a laboratory GC/MS to the percentages listed in the table to determine if their essential oil meets these quality standards.

Another argument by companies that choose not to share GC/MS data is that the results of this instrumental analysis are overemphasized. This argument also has merit, because of the inherent, and sizable, margins of error in the data that are generated during a GC/MS analysis. One of the most glaring is that, like all scientific data, the person interpreting the data has the potential to wrongly interpret the data. Mass spectrometry relies on libraries that are challenged when it comes to precisely identifying constituents (particularly complex sesquiterpene mixtures). One only needs to attempt to make sense of a marjoram essential oil analysis to see this (different databases identify the exact same compound—sabinene-hydrate—as different stereoisomers, or use different nomenclature—4-thuyanol or 4-thujanol).[267]

It is true that interpretation—especially computerized interpretation—of GC/MS data is not immune to errors. After all, the reliability of these interpretations is based on the quality of the library that the scientist uses. A scientist who has added specific essential oil components to his private library through years of essential oil analysis will be better equipped to properly identify constituents (not to mention untangle constituents that coelute) based on GC peaks and elution times. Contrarily, a scientist just starting out with a basic library will struggle to provide accurate analysis of essential oil

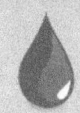

constituents. A robust and customized scientific library reduces the influence of misinterpretation.

Another subject that needs to be discussed before leaving the topic of purity, testing, and transparency is the topic of grades. Several essential oil retailers have adopted terms such as "Therapeutic Grade" to differentiate their essential oils from the competition. It is important to understand that these are all internal standards that have been established by that particular company and that there is not a universally industry recognized standard established by an independent organization. Consumers should ask the company what their established grade means (is it simply purity, or does it also have a quality meaning?) and what methods they use to determine an essential oil meets this internal standard.

Despite the lack of an organizational standard that is universally accepted, one can create a standard from which to compare essential oils through data published in peer-reviewed scientific literature. Studies published in peer-reviewed journals undergo a scrutinizing process by experts before being published. This evaluation of the manuscript includes challenging and dissecting methods, results, and the source of the materials used in the study. Only manuscripts that pass this evaluation and are considered sound science are published. Today, there are thousands of scientific studies on essential oils that have passed this scrutinizing process. The Preferred Composition for Clinical Use has assembled these studies and combined them with reference standards from validated essentials oils used by scientists whenever possible. The results are a standard validated by the scientific community which all essential oils can be compared to. Less common essential oils with few studies, compositional analyses, or the lack of a validated reference standard may require adaptation as these become available. The adoption and acceptance of this validated standard across all essential oil companies could create a universal pharmaceutical- or clinical-grade essential oil standard.

The final word is that while there are challenges in providing GC/MS data to the consumer, they can be overcome. Consumers can be empowered with a comparison database (like the one in this book), scientists can improve their libraries to reduce misinterpretations, and the industry can adopt the standard validated by the scientific community to ensure the industry provides consumers and clinicians what they need to use essential oils safely and effectively.

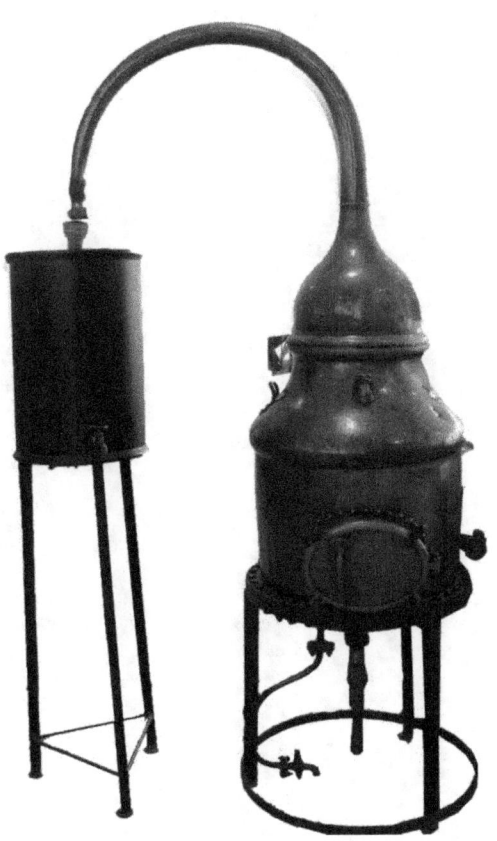

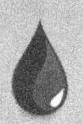

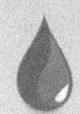

# ESSENTIAL OIL MONOGRAPHS

The following essential oils monographs can be used as a guide to determine the constituent profile of a therapeutic essential oil, the potential therapeutic uses, cautions, recommended dilution ratios, and more. It is always recommended that you ask for a GC/MS analysis of the oils that you purchase to ensure that you are getting a pure and therapeutic oil. In addition, this will help identify chemotypes of essential oils, which can be very different in constituent profile, and are used for different purposes and have different cautions.

The primary constituents generally make up 5% or more of the essential oil, while the other constituents can be found in the essential oil from trace (tr) to 4.9%. When multiple chemotypes or distillation types exist, the constituents that make up less than 5% of the essential oil may be provided to help identify the chemotype or distillation type.

**FAMILY:** Identifies the family the plant belongs to.

**NOTE:** Identifies how volatile the essential oil is and how long the aroma may last.

**AROMA:** Describes the odor characteristics of the essential oil.

**AROMA INTENSITY:** Describes the intensity of the odor.

**COMMON EXTRACTION METHOD:** Identifies the part(s) of the plant commonly used to obtain the essential oil from.

**BLENDS WELL WITH:** Lists blending suggestions or other essential oils that the essential oil is commonly blended with or may blend well with.

**SUBCELLULAR LOCALIZATION | EPIGENETIC INFLUENCE:**[4973] Identifies where within the cell (to what organelle) the essential oil constituents localize after penetration of the plasma membrane when directly exposed to live cells. This helps to create blends that more fully influence complete cellular function and trigger rapid correction without overwhelming a single organelle. Classifies essential oils per their principal influence on the human genome (positive influence on genes in relation to body systems), which reveals how the essential oil affects human genetic health and cellular function and behavior. *Italics indicates a preliminary determination with further analysis in a larger human genome study necessary.*

**POSSIBLE SUBSTITUTE OILS:** Lists essential oils that could possibly be used as a substitute if the recommended oil is not available based on constituent profile and/or reported properties.

**RECOMMENDED DILUTION RANGE:** Suggests a range for diluting the essential oil for topical application.

**PRIMARY CONSTITUENTS:** Identifies the constituents that are commonly reported in the essential oil based on the published research/studies/GC-MS reports.

**OTHER CONSTITUENTS:** Lists constituents that are usually found in the essential oil in the range of 0.5% to 4.9%.

**PREFERRED COMPOSITION FOR CLINICAL USE:** While scientific studies report the range of essential oil composition found in nature, these can lead to extremes that make it difficult to consistently and reliably produce positive human health benefits. A pharmaceutical-grade essential oil destined for clinical use must meet a more narrowly defined range and contain optimal levels of key bioactive and inactive (inactives often act as buffering constituents) constituents to more consistently and reliably produce therapeutic results. The preferred composition lists the desired composition for the key bioactives and markers of the essential oil. This preferred composition was established based on composition published in peer-reviewed journals with preference for studies demonstrating a positive health benefit—particularly human clinical studies, a comprehensive review of commercially available samples, and an emphasis to include optimum levels of key bioactives that possess desirable therapeutic properties. Pharmaceutical-grade essential oils will ideally match all standards for the key bioactive constituents listed, but slight deviations are acceptable. In addition, less common essential oils may require adjustment as greater numbers of analyses are available to further validate the percentages of key bioactives. A "–" means that the essential oil constituent may be present in some chemotypes but doesn't need to be present in the current chemotype to be considered pharmaceutical- or clinical-grade.

**REPORTED THERAPEUTIC PROPERTIES:** Lists the therapeutic properties based on traditional uses, known protocols, empirical evidence, and scientific research. *Properties listed in bold are primary properties of the essential oil or conditions for which the essential oil is often a preferred choice.*

**CAUTIONS:** Identifies known cautions with the essential oil, in regard to drug interactions, and contraindications for children, pregnancy and lactation, and certain health conditions.

**SELECTED EVIDENCE:** Shares and succinctly summarizes published preclinical and clinical studies that suggest a therapeutic or beneficial quality of the oil.

# AFRICAN BLUEGRASS
## (Blue Citronella Grass, Giant Turpentine Grass)

*Cymbopogon validus* (Stapf) Stapf ex Burtt Davy

**FAMILY:** Poaceae (Gramineae)
**NOTE:** Middle
**AROMA INTENSITY:** Medium-Strong
**AROMA:** Lemony, musky, grassy, herbaceous
**COMMON EXTRACTION METHOD:** Steam distilled from the aerial parts
**POSSIBLE SUBSTITUTE OILS:** Hemp, lemon catnip
**BLENDS WELL WITH:** Bergamot, bergamot mint, cedarwood, citronella, hemp, lavandin, lavender, lemon, lemongrass, lime, palmarosa, sandalwood, tangerine
**SUBCELLULAR LOCALIZATION | EPIGENETIC INFLUENCE:** Currently unknown | Currently unknown
**RECOMMENDED DILUTION RANGE:** 3.0%–33.0%; neat for limited conditions

**PRIMARY CONSTITUENTS:**[268,269]

| *Linalool CT* | | *Myrcene CT* | |
|---|---|---|---|
| Linalool | 28.0%–29.6% | Myrcene | 11.6%–35.6% |
| Northujane | 12.3%–16.8% | Geraniol | 1.7%–17.1% |
| Delta-Cadinene | 0.0%–8.1% | Delta-Cadinene | 0.0%–12.8% |
| Hedycaryol | 5.4%–7.6% | Gamma-Cadinene | 0.0%–12.3% |
| Alpha-Eudesmol | 6.5%–6.7% | (Z)-Beta-Ocimene | 6.0%–12.2% |
| Beta-Dihydroagarofuran | 2.4%–6.4% | Borneol | 2.4%–9.5% |
| Gamma-Eudesmol | 4.0%–4.5% | Alpha-Cadinol | 1.0%–9.5% |
| Cubenol | 3.5%–4.1% | Germacrene-D-4-ol | 0.8%–9.4% |
| | | Camphene | 2.6%–7.1% |
| *Artemisia Ketone CT* | | Gamma-Terpinene | 0.0%–5.7% |
| Artemisia Ketone | 37.5% | Alpha-Pinene | 2.3%–5.4% |
| Verbenone | 13.5% | (E)-Beta-Ocimene | 0.1%–5.3% |
| Naphthalene | 9.6% | | |
| Northujane | 4.4% | | |
| Myrcene | 4.2% | | |

Note: The myrcene CT appears to be the most common commercially available.

**OTHER CONSTITUENTS:** *Myrcene CT*—tricyclene, limonene, beta-phellandrene, beta-bourbonene, undecan-4-one, bornyl acetate, elemicine, alpha-humulene, neral, germacrene D, germacrene A, alpha-muurolene, alpha-cadinene, elemol, beta-cadinol, T-muurolol, torreyol, dill apiol (<1.8%), apiol (<1.4%); *Linalool CT*—camphene, myrcene, cis-linalool oxide, naphthalene, alpha-cubebene, alpha-longipinene, cyclosativene, beta-elemene, alpha-muurolene,

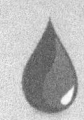

elemol, globulol, caryophyllene oxide, guaiol, beta-eudesmol; *Artemisia Ketone CT*—sabinene, alpha-phellandrene, m-cymene, linalool, alpha-terpineol, carvone, alpha-cubebene, beta-cubebene, beta-caryophyllene, germacrene-D-4-ol, delta-cadinene, caryophyllene oxide

**PREFERRED COMPOSITION FOR CLINICAL USE:**

| Constituent | Linalool CT | Myrcene CT | Artemisia Ketone CT |
|---|---|---|---|
| **Linalool** | 20%–35% | – | – |
| **Northujane** | 10%–20% | – | – |
| **Eudesmol <alpha + gamma>** | 10%–15% | – | – |
| **Hedycaryol** | 5%–10% | – | – |
| **Beta-Dihydroagarofuran** | 0.5%–7% | – | – |
| **Cubenol** | 0.1%–5% | – | – |
| **Myrcene** | – | 20%–40% | – |
| **Geraniol** | – | 4%–18% | – |
| **(Z)-Beta-Ocimene** | – | 5%–15% | – |
| **Borneol** | – | 4%–10% | – |
| **Alpha-Cadinol** | – | 4%–10% | – |
| **Germacrene D-4-ol** | – | 2%–10% | – |
| **Camphene** | – | 3%–8% | – |
| **Alpha Pinene** | – | 2%–6% | – |
| **Artemisia Ketone** | – | – | 30%–40% |
| **Verbenone** | – | – | 10%–20% |
| **Naphthalene** | – | – | 5%–15% |

**REPORTED THERAPEUTIC PROPERTIES:** Antiseptic, antibacterial, antifungal, antiviral, antiparasitic, **analgesic**, anti-inflammatory, antispasmodic, anticancer, astringent, anti-aging, relieves constipation, aids digestion, relieves chronic skin conditions, **antioxidant**, antiallergic, relieves headache/migraine, reduces painful menstruation, eases cough, supports immune function, **soothes sore muscles,** relieves sprains and strains, insecticide, insect repellent, stress management, relieves anxiety, antidepressant

**CAUTIONS:**

■ *Myrcene CT*: May interact with diabetic medications and cause low blood sugar based on geraniol content (low risk).[270,271,272]

■ *Myrcene CT*: Dilution recommended for topical application due to geraniol content. Geraniol is metabolized and autoxidized into metabolites like geranial and neral (citral) and may cause sensitization and irritation when applied topically.[273]

**SELECTED EVIDENCE:**

☐ Animal research concluded that African bluegrass essential oil (Artemisia Ketone or Linalool CT) is significantly anti-inflammatory for up to one hundred twenty minutes.[274] This study compared the results of essential oil obtained from fresh leaves (Artemisia Ketone CT), dry leaves (Linalool CT), and dry flowers (Linalool CT). Interestingly, the study authors noted that the fresh leaves and dry flowers demonstrated significantly greater inflammatory effects than aspirin during the sixty- and one-hundred-twenty-minute test, whereas the dry leaves were similar to aspirin. An *in vitro* study demonstrated that African bluegrass essential oil mildly inhibits the 5-LOX enzyme.[275] The 5-LOX enzyme converts arachidonic acid to leukotrienes, increasing inflammation and allergic reactions, and is associated with chronic degenerative inflammatory diseases.

☐ African bluegrass essential oil exhibits excellent antioxidant activity *in vitro,* scavenging over 80 percent of DPPH free radicals.[276]

☐ African bluegrass essential oil possesses excellent larvicidal (100% mortality) and repellent activity (100%, although only tested for three minutes on rodents), and good insecticidal (53.7% mortality) activity against the *Anopheles arabiensis* mosquito.[277]

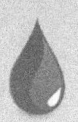 

# AGARWOOD
## (Aloes Wood, Agar, Eaglewood, Oud, Oodh, Gaharu)

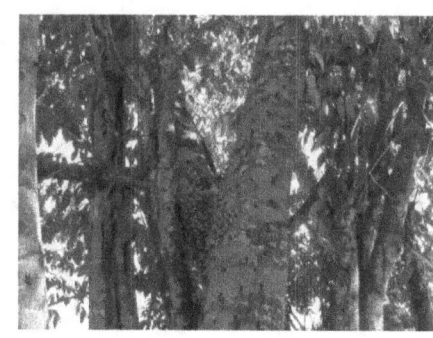

*Aquilaria crassna* Pierre ex Lecomte, *A. agallocha* Roxb., *A. malaccensis* Lamk., *A. beccariana* Tiegh., *A. hirta* Ridl., *A. microcarpa* Baill., *A. sinensis* (Lour.) Gilg; *Gyrinops* spp.

**FAMILY:** Thymelaeaceae
**NOTE:** Base-Middle
**AROMA INTENSITY:** Medium
**AROMA:** Sweet, woody, resinous, earthy, exotic
**COMMON EXTRACTION METHOD:** Hydrodistilled from the fungus-infected wood
**POSSIBLE SUBSTITUTE OILS:** Blue cypress, sandalwood, cedarwood, copaiba
**BLENDS WELL WITH:** Cassia, cedarwood, chamomile (German, Roman), cinnamon, copaiba, cypress, geranium, hinoki, lavender, myrrh, patchouli, pine, rose, sandalwood, spikenard, spruce (black)
**SUBCELLULAR LOCALIZATION | EPIGENETIC INFLUENCE:** Currently unknown | Currently unknown
**RECOMMENDED DILUTION RANGE:** 5%–Neat

**PRIMARY CONSTITUENTS:**[278,279,280,281,282,283,284,285,286,287,288,289,290,291,292,293,294]

*Aquilaria crassna*

| | |
|---|---|
| Selina-3,11-Dien-9-One | 1.1%–17.2% |
| Gamma-Selinene | 0.0%–13.7% |
| Isoamyl Decanoate | 0.0%–13.4% |
| Delta-Selinene | 0.0%–12.4% |
| Beta-Agarofuran | 0.4%–10.3% |
| 1,3,5-Trimethyl-6-methylidene-tricyclo [3.2.1.0(2,7)]oct6-3-en-8-exo-ol | 0.0%–10.3% |
| Spathulenol | 0.0%–9.9% |
| 4a,5-Dimethyl-3-(1-ethylidene)-4,4a,5, 6,7,8-hexahydro-2(3H)-Naphthalenone | 0.0%–9.7% |
| 10-Epi-Gamma-Eudesmol | 0.0%–9.0% |
| Alpha-Guaiene | 0.0%–8.9% |
| Tetradecenal | 0.0%–8.6% |
| Valerianol (Kusunol) | 0.0%–8.2% |
| Guaia-3,9-Diene | 0.0%–7.8% |
| Dehydrojinkoh-Eremol | 0.0%–7.3% |
| 9,1-Eremophiladien-8-One | 0.0%–6.3% |
| Agarospirol | 3.7%–5.8% |
| Epoxybulnesene | 0.0%–5.3% |
| Jinkho-Eremol | 2.3%–4.5% |
| Beta-Guaiene | 0.0%–4.4% |
| Beta-Epi-Eudesmol | 0.0%–4.2% |
| Selina-3,11-Dien-14-al | 0.0%–4.0% |

*Aquilaria malaccensis*

| | |
|---|---|
| Isoamyl Dodecanoate | 0.0%–55.6% |
| 4-Phenyl 2-Butanone | 0.4%–32.1% |
| 2-Hydroxyguaia-1(10),11-Dien-15-oic Acid | 0.0%–14.6% |
| Epoxybulnesene | 0.0%–11.0% |

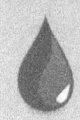

| | |
|---|---|
| 10-Epi-Gamma-Eudesmol | 0.0%–9.2% |
| Norketoagarofuran | 0.0%–8.4% |
| Bulnesol (Guai-1(10)-en-11-ol) | 0.0%–8.1% |
| Guaia-1(10),11-Dien-15-ol | 0.0%–6.5% |
| Jinkho-Eremol | 0.0%–6.5% |
| Selina-3,11-Dien-9-One | 0.0%–6.2% |
| Tetradecanal | 0.0%–6.1% |
| Caryophyllene Oxide | 0.0%–6.1% |
| Alpha-Guaiene | 0.0%–5.8% |
| Selina-4,11-Dien-14-oic Acid | 0.0%–5.2% |
| Selina-3,11-Dien-14-al | 0.0%–4.9% |
| Karanone | 0.0%–4.9% |
| Dehydrojinkoh-Eremol | 0.1%–4.8% |
| Cyclocolorenone | 0.0%–4.7% |
| Valerianol (Kusunol) | 0.0%–4.3% |
| 1,5-Epoxy-Nor-Ketoguaiene | 0.0%–4.1% |

*A. crassna (Thailand)*

| | |
|---|---|
| Allo-Aromadendrene | 10.3% |
| Kusunol | 8.3% |
| 9-Hydroxyselina-4,11-Dien-14-oic Acid | 6.1% |
| Dihydrofukinone | 5.2% |
| Epi-Alpha-Cadinol | 4.9% |
| Epi-Alpha-Bisabolol | 3.5% |
| Agarospirol | 2.6% |

*Malaysian (A. malaccensis, A. beccariana, A. hirta, A. microcarpa)*

| | |
|---|---|
| 10-Epi-Gamma-Eudesmol | 7.1%–30.4% |
| Aromadendrene | 0.0%–25.9% |
| Agarospirol | 0.0%–24.2% |
| Valerianol (Kusunol) | 0.0%–19.4% |
| Alpha-Eudesmol | 0.0%–17.3% |
| Beta-Eudesmol | 0.0%–8.4% |
| Selina-3,11-dien-14-ol | 0.0%–7.1% |
| Hexadecanoic Acid | 0.0%–7.0% |
| Beta-Agarofuran | 1.0%–5.0% |
| Guaia-3,9-Dien-11-ol | 0.0%–4.9% |
| Alpha-Agarofuran | 1.4%–3.5% |

*Thailand (Healthy wood, A. malaccensis, A. subintegra, A. crassna)*

| | |
|---|---|
| Isoamyl Dodecanoate | 13.4%–55.6% |
| Beta-Agorufuran | 0.4%–10.3% |
| Kusunol | 3.9%–8.2% |
| Dehydrojuinkoh-Eremol | 0.5%–7.3% |
| Guaia-1(10),11-Dien-15-ol | 1.9%–6.5% |
| 9,11-Eremophiladien-8-One | 0.1%–6.3% |
| Agarospirol | 0.6%–5.8% |
| Jinkoh-Eremol | 4.2%–5.6% |
| Karanone | 1.5%–4.9% |
| Epoxybulnesene | 1.3%–4.9% |
| Cyclocolorenone | 3.4%–4.7% |

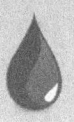
Selina-3,11-Dien-9-Ol                    0.2%–2.8%
Alpha-Bisabolol Acetate                  0.4%–2.5%

*India (A. malaccensis)*
Agarospirol                              11.7%
Epi-Alpha-Cadinol                        9.9%
T-Cadinol                                9.3%
Beta-Eudesmol                            4.1%
9-Hydroxyselina-4,11-Dien-14-oic Acid    3.9%

*Aquilaria sinensis*
Benzylacetone                            1.1%–19.5%
Baimuxinal                               0.0%–14.8%
Guaiol                                   0.0%–14.1%
1,3,5-Trimethyl-2-(2,2,2-Trifluoro-
    Ethoxy)-benzene                      0.0%–13.4%
7-Methyltridecane                        0.0%–11.3%
Guaia-1(10),11-Diene-9-One               0.0%–10.9%
Alpha-Copaen-11-ol                       0.0%–10.8%
Bulnesol (Guai-1(10)-en-11-ol)           0.0%–6.4%
Hinesol                                  0.3%–6.3%
2-Cyclohexylanisole                      0.0%–6.2%
Diepi-Alpha-Cedrene Epoxide              0.0%–6.0%
1,2,5,5,8a-Pentamethyl-1,2,3,5,
    6,7,8,8aoctahydronaphthalene-1-ol    0.0%–5.8%
2,3,4,5-Tetramethyltricyclo[3.2.1.02,7]
    oct-3-ene                            0.0%–5.8%
Selina-3,11-Dien-14-al                   0.0%–5.5%
Eremophila-7(11),9-Dien-8-One            0.0%–5.4%
Aristolene                               0.6%–4.7%
Cis-Z-Alpha-Bisabolene Epoxide           0.0%–4.7%
Eudesm-7(11)-en-4alpha-ol                0.0%–4.4%
Alpha-Selinene                           0.3%–4.1%
Dehydrofukinone                          0.0%–4.1%
Agarospirol                              0.0%–4.0%
6-Isopropyl-4,8-alpha-Dimethyl-1,2,3,7,8,8-
    Hexahydronaphthalene                 0.0%–3.5%
2,3,3,3,4,5-Hexahydro-7-Isopropyl-3-
    Methyl-1H-Cyclopenta[1,3]Cyclopropa-
    [1,2]benzene-3,6 (7H)-dione          0.0%–3.2%
Sandal                                   0.0%–3.0%
1,1,7-Trimethyl-4-Methylenedecahydro-
    1H-Cyclopropa[e]azulene              0.0%–2.9%

*A. sinensis (Artificially induced with fungi)*
6-Hydroxy-2-(2-phenylethyl)Chromone      6.2%–14.8%
6-Methoxy-2-(2-Phenylethyl)Chromone      5.5%–9.4%
6-Methoxy-2-[2-(4-methoxyphenyl)ethyl]
    Chromone                             1.6%–7.3%
6-Hydroxy-2-(4-Methoxyphenethyl)
    Chromone                             0.7%–4.3%

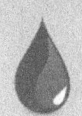
6,7-Dimethoxy-2-[2-(4-Mmethoxyphenyl)
   Ethyl] Chromone                    2.3%–2.7%
[3S-(3.alpha.,4a.alpha.,5.alpha.)]-3,4,4a,5,6,7-
   Hexahydro-4a,5-dimethyl-3-
   (1-methylethenyl)-1(2H)-naphthalenone  0.4%–2.8%

*G. walla (Sri Lanka)*
Gamma-Selinene                        72.5%
3-Phenyl-2-Butanone                   2.0%
3-Pentanone                           2.0%

### Major constituents of *A. crassna from Asia*[295]

| Constituent | India | Indonesia | Laos | Taiwan | Thailand | Vietnam |
|---|---|---|---|---|---|---|
| n-Hexadecanoic acid | 2.6% | 0.4% | 15.0% | 7.8% | 1.7% | – |
| Neopetastone | – | 3.1% | 3.2% | 6.2% | – | 14.4% |
| Dihydroagarofuran-15-al | 3.1% | 4.4% | 2.6% | 5.1% | 5.0% | 9.2% |
| Valerianol (Kusunol) | 4.0% | 6.0% | 6.2% | 9.1% | 6.9% | 4.9% |
| Beta-agarofuran | 7.0% | 5.7% | 2.0% | 3.5% | 8.3% | 8.0% |
| Jinko-Eremol | 3.0% | 4.5% | 4.8% | 7.0% | 5.3% | 5.0% |
| Valenca-1(10),8-dien-11-ol | 4.5% | 5.0% | 4.2% | 6.4% | 4.9% | 6.0% |
| Dihydrokaranone | 6.0% | 6.2% | 4.6% | 2.6% | 4.6% | 3.3% |
| Agarospirol | 2.4% | 4.1% | 3.5% | 5.3% | 5.8% | 5.6% |
| Beta-eudesmol | 4.1% | 3.5% | 2.4% | 3.3% | 3.1% | – |
| Alpha-eudesmol | 2.4% | 3.3% | 1.4% | 2.5% | 1.1% | 2.2% |
| Benzylacetone | 1.6% | 1.6% | 0.4% | 0.3% | 1.1% | 1.5% |
| **Key and minor aroma constituents not included in major constituents** | | | | | | |
| Alpha-agarofuran | – | 0.5% | 0.6% | 1.1% | 0.9% | 0.5% |
| Benzaldehyde | – | – | – | – | – | – |
| Furfural | – | – | – | – | – | – |
| 4-phenyl-2-butanone | – | – | – | – | – | – |
| (E)-alpha-bergamotene | – | – | – | – | – | – |
| Alpha-humulene | – | – | – | – | – | – |
| Alpha-bulnesene | 0.3% | – | – | – | – | – |
| nor-Ketoagarofuran | 0.2% | 0.8% | 0.4% | 0.5% | 0.8% | 0.4% |
| Epoxybulnesene | 1.6% | 3.6% | 0.5% | 0.9% | 0.6% | 1.3% |
| Kusunol | – | – | – | – | – | – |
| Acorenone B | – | – | – | – | – | – |
| Selina-3,11-dien-14-al | 1.8% | 2.6% | – | 1.4% | – | 2.0% |
| 9,11-eremophiladien-8-one | – | – | – | – | – | – |

Note: Agarwood is one of the most expensive woods in the world to procure, making a high-quality agarwood essential oil more difficult to obtain. In addition, agarwood must be infected by mold before it will produce a dark, aromatic resin resulting in dense, dark, embedded heartwood that the essential oil is produced from. Resin production is a defense mechanism that can take many years in the tree's natural habitat. More recently, trees have been induced to produce resin through physical (burning, wounding, chisel drilling) or chemical (solvents that contain ions or microbes) means. They type of fungus that infects the wood can also affect the resulting chemistry and the quality of the oil.[296] Agarwood oil (*A. malaccensis*) artificially inoculated with *Fusarium solani* and extracted by ethyl acetate produced an oil with 8.0% aromadendrene oxide I, 5.4% tridecanoic acid, 5.3% oleic acid, 4.7% beta-elemene, 3.3% alpha-santalol, and 2.7% isoaromadendrene oxide 2.[297] The quality and composition of agarwood will vary greatly, depending on the extent of the infection and how much resin is produced. Other factors that significantly influence the composition of agarwood are the distillation time (long distillation times are required for high-quality agarwood essential oil), fermentation/soaking time of the wood in water before distillation (usually 14–90 days), and the age of the tree. Some scientists suggest the ideal soaking time to maximize oil yield is 14 days. Agarospirol and agarofurans are considered the main constituents responsible for the signature woody notes released from burning agarwood. The major constituents responsible for the characteristic aroma of agarwood are: beta-agarofuran, 4-phenyl-2-butanone, furfural and benzaldehyde; while the minor aroma notes are attributed to (E)-alpha-bergamotene, alpha-humulene, alpha-bulnesene, alpha-agarofuran, nor-ketoagarofuran, epoxybulnesene, agarospirol, jinkoh-eremol, valerianol (kusunol), acorenone B, selina-3,11-dien-14-al and 9,11-eremophiladien-8-one. A review determined that a high-quality agarwood essential oil (*A. agallocha*) should contain alpha-guaiene, (-)-guaia-1(10),11-dien-15-al, (-)-selina-3,11-dien,9-one, (+)-selina-3,11-dien,9-ol, guaiene, eudesmane, beta-agarofuran (the most important constituent), alpha-agarofuran, 10-epi-gamma-eudesmol, and higher abundance of benzaldehyde and anisealdehyde.[298] Three sesquiterpenoid constituents are detected only in the highest quality agarwood: (-)-guaia-1(10),11-dien-15-al, (-)-selina-3,11-dien,9-one, and (+)-selina-3,11-dien,9-ol; while 9-11-eremophiladien-8-one and oxo-agarospirol are typically found in lower quality agarwood oils. Although it should be noted that agarwood oil extracted from different origins and species, as well as the type of wood, will have different marker compounds that predominantly characterize the oil. For example, agarwood extracted from low-quality resin-impregnated wood or leftover wood—Indian *A. malaccensis*—from processing (called extractable wood) usually contains agarospirol in the range of 5%–20%; *A. malaccensis* from Bangladesh similarly contains 5%–10% agarospirol; while white wood (non-infected, India) is primarily composed of fatty acids with only traces of sesquiterpenes. Agarospirol has also been identified as a marker of *A. crassna* grown in Laos (5%–20%) and Vietnam (2%–10%). On the contrary, Vietnamese agarwood oil (*A. crassna*) has the marker compound allo-aromadendrene at 5%–15%, Indonesian *A. beccariana* is characterized by 10%–30% jinkoh-eremol, and *A. malaccensis* from Malaysia is predominantly alpha-eudesmol (5%–15%). Grades of agarwood may also be listed: *khara* (highest grade), *boha*, and *boya* (non-odiferous white wood) grades. Other proposed grading is based upon sesquiterpenoid content: A (70%+), B (30%–69.9%), C (10%–29.9%), and D (0%–9.9%); or infection level: highly infected (Grade 1), moderately infected (Grade 2), less infected (Grade 3), and healthy wood (Grade 4). Isolates or synthetic chemicals may be combined to create a faux agarwood and simulate its composition and aroma, including 3-n-propyl-phenol, 3-ethylphenol, 3-i-butyl-phenol, 3-n-butyl-phenol, castoreum, benzylacetone (naturally present in some agarwood oils), pentanoic acid, 2,6,6-trimethyl-l,Safranal, 4-(4-methoxyphenyl)-2-butanone, 3,3- dimethyl-5-(2,2,3-trimethyl-3-cyclopenten-l-yl)-4-penten-2-ol, β-santalol, and sandalwood oil.

| Natural and Cultivated Agarwood Species and Their Distribution (IUCN, 2018) | |
|---|---|
| **Habitat** | **Species** |
| Bhutan | *A. malaccensis* |
| Brunei | *A. microcarpa* |
| Cambodia | *A. baillonii, A. crassna, A. malaccensis. A. macrocarpa, A. rostrata* |
| China | *A. sinensis* |
| Indonesia | *A. audate, A. beccariana, A. cumingiana, A. filarial, A. hirta, A. malaccensis, A. macrocarpa, Gyrinops decipiens, G. salicifolia, G. versteegii* |
| Laos | *A. crassna* |
| Malaysia | *A. beccariana, A. hirta, A. malaccensis, A. macrocarpa, A. rostrata,* |
| Myanmar | *A. malaccensis* |
| Papua New Guinea | *A. Filarial, G. caudate, G. ledermannii, G. moluccanna, G. salicifolia, G. versteegii* |
| Sri Lanka | *G. walla* |
| Thailand | *A. crassna, A. malaccensis, A. rugosa, A. subintegra,* |
| The Philippines | *A. apiculate, A. brachyantha, A. citrinicarpa, A. decemcostata, A. malaccensis, A. parviflora, A. urdanetensis, A. filarial* |
| Vietnam | *A. baillonii, A. banaensis, A. crassna, A. rugosa* |

**OTHER CONSTITUENTS:** *Aquilaria crassna*—p-methoxyphenol, hexadecanoic acid, alpha-selinene, tridecanal, alpha-bulnesene, dodecanoic acid, norketoagarfuran, guiacol, 1,5-epoxy-nor-ketoguaiene, tridecanoic acid, pentadecanal, rotundone, selina-3,11-dien-9-ol, selina-4,11-dien-14-al, guaia-1(10),11-dien-15-ol, oxo-agarospirol, 2-hydroxyquia-1(10),11-dien-15-oic acid, 5,19-cyclo-5a-androst-6-ene-3,17-dione, benzylacetone; *Aquilaria malaccensis*—gamma-selinene, aromadendrene, humulene, beta-guaiene, gamma-gurjunene, alpha-selinene, alpha-elemol, agarospirol, alpha-bisabolol, rotundone, Selina-3,11-dien-9-ol, 2-hexadecanone, dihydrokaranone, guai-1(10),11-dien-15-al, oxo-agarospirol, pentadecanoic acid, n-hexadecanoic acid; *A. crassna (Thailand)*—4-phenyl-2-butanone, kessane dihydro-aromadendrene, nor-ketogarofuran, caryophyllene oxide, gamma-eudesmol, jonkoh-eremol, bulnesol, alpha-bisabolol, selina-3,11-dien-9-ol, selina-4,11-dien-14-al, selina-3,11-dien-9-al, guaia-1(10),11-dien-9-one, oxo-agarospirol; *Malaysian*—alpha-guaiene, beta-copaene, 4-phenyl-3butanone, benzaldehyde, benzeacetonitrile, gamma-elemene, valencene, ar-curcumene, alpha-muurolene, beta-dihydroagarofuran, elemol, gamma-vetivenene, spathulenol, beta-gurjunene, alloaromadendrene epoxide, beta-costol, alpha-bisabolol, Selina-3,11-diene-9-one, cyperotundone, 10-nor-calamenene, aristolone, thujopsenal, cyclohexa decanolide, dihydrocolumellarin, selina-3,11-dien-9-one; *Thailand (Healthy wood, A. malaccensis, A. subintegra, A. crassna)*—Dihydroagarofuran, nor-ketoagarofuran, beta-epi-eudesmol, Selina-3,11-dien-9-one, acorenone B, cyperotundone, Alpha-(Z)-atlantone, Selina-3,11-dien-14-ol, alpha-(Z)-santalol acetate, beta-eudesmol acetae, oxo-agarospirol, beta-(E)-santalol acetate;

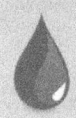

*India (A. malaccensis)*—4-phenyl-2-butanone, gamma-cadinene, dehydro-aromadendrene, caryophyllene oxide, gamma-eudesmol, kusnol, dehydrojonkoh-eremol, epi-alpha-bisabolol, selina-3,11-dien-9-ol, selina-3,11-dien-9-al, selina-4,11-dien-14-al, guaia-1(10),11-dien-15-ol, dehydrofukinone; *Aquilaria sinensis*—Elemol, 5β,7βH,10α-eudesm-11-en-1α-ol, isoaromadendrene epoxide, gamma-eudesmol, cubenol, cis-Z-α-Bisabolene epoxide, aromadendrene oxide, 6-isopropenyl-4,8a-dimethyl-1,2,3,5,6,7,8,8a-octahydronaphthalen-2-ol, eicosane, butylated hydroxytoluene, 4-nitrophthalhydrazide, pyrethone, chamigrene, longifolenaldehyde, 3-ethylpyridine oxide, 1-cycloexeneethanol, 4-methoxycoumarin, perhydropyrene, ortho-tert-butylphenol, isodurol, valencene, trans-N,N'-diferuloylputrescine; *A. sinensis (Artificially induced with fungi)*—Alpa-santalol, agarospirol, 4a,5-dimethyl-3-(prop-1-en-2-yl)-1,2,3,4,4a,5,6,7-octahydronaphthalen-1-ol; *G. walla (Sri Lanka)*—11-isopropylidentricycloundec-3-en-10-one, beta-patchoulene

**PREFERRED COMPOSITION FOR CLINICAL USE:**

| Constituent | Aquilaria crassna |
|---|---|
| **Selina-3,11-Dien-9-One** | 5%–20% |
| **Beta-Agarofuran** | 5%–10% |
| **10-Epi-Gamma-Eudesmol** | 2%–10% |
| **Alpha-Guaiene** | 2%–10% |
| **Agarospirol** | 2%–8% |
| **Eudesmane** | 0.1%–5% |
| **Selina-3,11-Dien-9-ol** | 0.1%–5% |
| **Benzaldehyde** | 0.1%–5% |
| **Alpha-Agarofuran** | 0.1%–5% |
| **(-)-Guaia-1(10),11-Dien-15-al** | 0.1%–5% |
| **Oxo-Agarospirol** | 0% |
| **9-11-Eremophiladien-8-one** | 0% |

**REPORTED THERAPEUTIC PROPERTIES:** Antibacterial, antimicrobial, **antifungal**, antirheumatic, analgesic, anti-inflammatory, anticancer, reduces fever, supports respiratory function, aids digestion, diuretic, expels excess gas, antispasmodic, relieves nausea, aids liver function, supports urinary tract function, **aphrodisiac**, stress management, **calming and relaxing**, relieves anxiety, encourages motivation, aids meditation

**CAUTIONS:**
■ None currently known.

**SELECTED EVIDENCE:**
□ *In vitro* research concluded that Malaysian agarwood essential oil reduced breast-cancer-cell viability and inhibited cancer-cell attachment.[299] Other research demonstrates that *A. crassna* kills colon cancer cells *in vitro*.[300] The same authors conducted oral toxicity studies in mice and found that it took greater than 2,000 mg/kg/day to cause harm and repeated oral dosing of 100 mg/kg and 500 mg/kg for 2 twenty-eight days did not cause significant changes in animal health.

□ Single and repeated administration (injection) of Chinese agarwood essential oil produced a significant sedative and hypnotic effect in mice dosed with pentobarbital. The effects of the oil were attributed to elevated expression of GABA$_A$ receptor subunits and subtypes in the cerebral cortex and by potentiating GABA$_A$ receptor function.[301] Inhalation of agarwood oil (species unknown—one purchased in Hong Kong market, 47.1% benzylacetone; and the other produced in Vietnam, 61.5% alpha-gurjenene and 24.7% calarene) caused a sedative effect in mice.[302] It is possible the second oil is actually spikenard because of the composition.

□ Agarwood essential oil (*A. sinensis*) inhibited *Bacillus subtilis* and *Staphylococcus aureus*.[303] Another study concluded that agarwood essential oil (*A. crassna*) inhibited *S. aureus* and *C. albicans*.[304] A third study concluded that agarwood inhibited the fungi *L. theobromae, Fusarium oxysporum,* and *C. albicans*.[305]

□ Inhaling agarwood essential oil (*A. sinensis*) or benzoylacetone produced sedation in mice.[306]

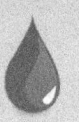 

- ☐ Agarwood essential oil incorporated into silver nanoparticles was toxic to *Aedes albopictus* mosquitoes.[307]
- ☐ An agarwood essential oil (*A. crassna*, 12.3% valerianol, 8.0% gamma-eudesmol, 3.7% epi-cyclocolorenone, 3.7% nootkatone, 3.7% beta-eudesmol, 3.0% methyl phenethyl ketone) nanoemulsion reduced inflammation and increased antioxidant activity in cigarette-smoke-exposed airway cells. It did so by reducing the expression of proinflammatory cytokines (IL-1α, IL-1β, IL-8, and GDF-15), increasing anti-inflammatory mediators (IL-10, IL-18BP, TFF3, GH, VDBP, relaxin-2, IFN-γ, and PDGF), inducing the expression of antioxidant genes (GCLC and GSTP1), and activating prosurvival signaling pathway (PI3K).[308]

# AJOWAN
## (Bishop's Weed, Ajwain, Wild Celery Seed, Sprague)

*Trachyspermum ammi* (L.) Sprague ex Turrill, *T. copticum* L. Link, *Carum copticum* (L.) Benth. & Hook. f. ex C.B. Clarke, *Ammi copticum* L.

**FAMILY:** Apiaceae (Umbelliferae)
**NOTE:** Top
**AROMA INTENSITY:** Strong
**AROMA:** Spicy, herbaceous, medicinal
**COMMON EXTRACTION METHOD:** Steam distilled from the seeds (fruits); may also be steam distilled from the leaves
**POSSIBLE SUBSTITUTE OILS:** Thyme, oregano, mountain savory
**BLENDS WELL WITH:** Bay laurel, bergamot, camphor, clary sage, copaiba, cypress, eucalyptus, geranium, grapefruit, lavender, lemon, juniper, marjoram, tea tree, orange, oregano, petitgrain, pine, ravensara, rose, rosemary, sage, Spanish sage, thyme
**SUBCELLULAR LOCALIZATION | EPIGENETIC INFLUENCE:** Currently unknown | Currently unknown
**RECOMMENDED DILUTION RANGE:** 1.5%–20%; 50% for some conditions

**PRIMARY CONSTITUENTS:**[309,310,311,312,313]

*Thymol CT*

| | |
|---|---|
| Thymol | 39.1%–67.4% |
| Para-Cymene | 17.9%–30.8% |
| Gamma-Terpinene | 11.3%–27.8% |

*Gamma-Terpinene/Para-Cymene CT*

| | |
|---|---|
| Para-Cymene | 33.7%–57.3% |
| Gamma-Terpinene | 21.3%–48.1% |
| Thymol | 1.5%–17.4% |
| Beta-Pinene | 0.0%–3.6% |

*Gamma-Terpinolene CT*

| | |
|---|---|
| Gamma-Terpinolene | 53.6% |
| Thymol | 16.8% |
| Para-Cymene | 13.5% |
| Beta-Pinene | 8.9% |

Note: The thymol CT is most commonly available in commercial samples.

**OTHER CONSTITUENTS:** *Thymol* CT—beta-pinene, terpinen-4-ol, carvacrol, alpha-pinene, limonene, beta-phellandrene, thujene, beta-myrcene; *Gamma-Terpinolene CT*—alpha-pinene, beta-myrcene, alpha-terpinene, limonene, beta-phellandrene; *Gamma-Terpinene/Para-Cymene CT*—thujene, alpha-pinene, myrcene, alpha-terpinene

**PREFERRED COMPOSITION FOR CLINICAL USE:**

| Constituent | Thymol CT |
|---|---|
| Thymol | 45%–65% |
| Para-Cymene | 18%–32% |
| Gamma-Terpinene | 12%–28% |

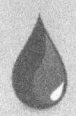

**REPORTED THERAPEUTIC PROPERTIES:** Antibacterial, antifungal, **antiviral**, anti-infectious, antiparasitic, antiseptic, **antispasmodic**, aids circulation, expels excess mucus, supports respiratory function, soothes stomach upset, relieves diarrhea, expels excess gas, regulates menstruation, antioxidant, **analgesic**, anti-inflammatory, **antineuralgic**, supports urinary tract health, eases cough, relieves fever, relieves nausea, encourages restful sleep, immune stimulant, stimulates appetite, **insecticide**, stimulating, combats mental fatigue, antidepressant, instills self-confidence, combats anger

**CAUTIONS:**

■ Oral caution. Thymol has a longer half-life (the time it takes for half of the medication to metabolize or excrete half of the dosage) than most essential oil constituents and should not be administered orally for long periods of time.[314] Thymol is a monoterpene phenol. Reports of fatalities in infants who consumed 50 to 500 mg of phenol have been reported.[315] It is recommended that chemotypes with high levels of thymol be limited to 10 drops per day orally for adults Monday through Friday, with Saturday and Sunday off; or a two to seven-day break monthly.

■ May interact with aspirin, blood pressure, antiplatelet, and anticoagulant medications, and increase the risk of bleeding among people with bleeding disorders due to thymol content.[316,317,318]

■ May interact with anticholinergic (drugs used for asthma, incontinence, gastrointestinal cramps, muscular spasms, depression, and sleep disorders) and cholinergic medications (drugs used to reduce urinary retention, diagnose myasthenia gravis, and for glaucoma) based on thymol content.[319,320,321]

■ May interact with antibiotics and possibly enhance their effects due to thymol content.[322,323,324,325]

■ May irritate mucous membranes (eyes, mouth, nasal passages, vagina, rectum).

**SELECTED EVIDENCE:**

☐ A randomized, double-blind, placebo-controlled study found that a 10% topical ajowan cream significantly reduced feet burning, neuropathic pain, numbness, and tingling among people with neuropathy.[326]

☐ Ajowan essential oil inhibits the Japanese encephalitis virus transmitted by mosquitoes both prior to and after cellular exposure *in vitro*.[327]

☐ *In vitro* research reports that ajowan essential oil inhibits multidrug-resistant *Staphylococcus aureus* (MRSA), *P. vulgaris*, *B. subtilis*, *B. megaterium*, *K. pneumoniae*, and *E. coli*.[328,329] Its antimicrobial activity was stronger when combined with nutmeg essential oil.[330] A gamma-terpinene CT of ajowan essential oil inhibited *E. coli* and *P. aeruginosa* isolated from patients.[331] A fraction of the same oil high in thymol inhibited to a *Salmonella* isolate, in addition to *E. coli* and *P. aeruginosa*, suggesting thymol is the active antimicrobial constituent in ajowan essential oil. Another study reports antimicrobial activity against *Salmonella typhi*, *E. coli*, *S. aureus*, *Bacillus subtilis*, *Aspergillus niger*, and *C. albicans*.[332]

☐ Ajowan essential oil moderately inhibited several oral pathogens *in vitro*, including standard species of *S. mutans*, *S. sanguis*, *S. salivarius*, *S. sobrinus*, *E. faecalis*, *S. aureus*, *C. albicans*, *C. dubliniensis*, *C. tropicalis*, *C. krusei*, *C. glabrata*, and four clinical isolates of *S. mutans*.[333]

☐ Animal research suggests that ajowan essential oil significantly reduces pain (in a mechanism other than by opioid receptors) and inflammation in mice.[334]

☐ *In vitro* research reports that ajowan essential acts as an antagonist for histamine H1 receptors, which is involved in smooth muscle contraction and the release and binding of neurotransmitters in the central nervous system.[335] The study authors also suggest that ajowan essential oil may stimulate beta-adrenergic receptors, which may increase energy production and utilization; and that it may possess anti-cholinergic properties, suggesting it may be useful for gastrointestinal disorders, respiratory disorders, dizziness, and insomnia.

☐ Ajowan essential oil inhibits *C. albicans* isolated from HIV patients.[336] A gamma-terpinene CT and fraction of the essential oil rich in thymol inhibited *C. albicans*, including clinical isolates, better than the antifungal drug fluconazol.[337] Ajowan essential oil (thymol CT) significantly inhibits *Aspergillus niger*, *A. flavus*, *A. parasiticus*, and *A. fumigatus* and their subsequent production of aflatoxin.[338,339,340,341] Ajowan essential oil inhibits *Trichosporon asahii* and *T. cutaneum* (fungi commonly found in the soil that colonize the skin and gastrointestinal tract of humans), *Epidermophyton floccosum*, *Microsporum canis*, and *Trichophyton mentagrophytes*.[342,343]

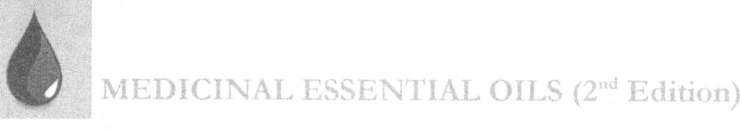

- *In vitro* research demonstrates that ajowan essential oil (thymol CT) significantly inhibits hydatid cyst protoscolices (a cyst caused by a parasitic infection by a tapeworm of the genus *Echinococcus* that affects the liver, lungs, brain, and other organs).[344]

- Ajowan essential oil kills the Indian meal moth (*Plodia interpunctella*), Asian tiger mosquito (*Aedes albopictus*), German cockroach (*Blattella germanica*), water flea (*Daphnia magna*), Japanese termite (*Reticulitermes speratus* Kolbe), pulse beetle (*Callosobruchus chinensis*), and malaria-carrying mosquito (*Anopheles stephensi*)—though thymol was twice as potent against *A. stephensi* as the whole oil.[345,346,347,348,349,350,351]

- *In vitro* research suggests that ajowan essential oil may decrease sperm viability and membrane integrity, therefore acting as a male contraceptive.[352,353]

- Animal research using isolated rat aorta suggests that ajowan essential oil with near equal thymol (38.1%) and gamma-terpinene (33.3%) content triggers vasodilation.[354]

- The thymol CT of ajowan essential oil inhibited *Salmonella typhimurium*.[355]

- Ajowan essential oil potently repelled male and female German cockroaches (*Blatella germanica*).[356]

- Ajowan essential oil (unidentified CT) inhibited *S. aureus, E. coli, L. monocytogenes,* and *P. aeruginosa* and enhanced the antimicrobial activity of the antibiotic vancomycin against *E. coli* and *S. aureus* and improved the efficacy of ciprofloxacin against *S. epidermidis*.[357]

- Laboratory research concluded that the thymol CT of ajowan essential oil possesses significant antioxidant activity, which is comparable to ascorbic acid.[358]

- The thymol CT of ajowan essential oil inhibited over twenty bacteria and seven yeasts and demonstrated anti-quorum-sensing activity against *Chromobacterium violaceum*.[359] The same researchers reported that the oil exhibited antioxidant activity.

- Ajowan CT thymol essential oil demonstrated broad-spectrum antimicrobial activity when tested against three standard strains and six resistant clinical isolates of major respiratory pathogens (*Pseudomonas aeruginosa, Staphylococcus aureus, Streptococcus pneumoniae*).[360] It also synergized the activities of amoxicillin against MRSA (clinical isolates), ciprofloxacin against *P. aeruginosa, S. aureus,* and penicillin-resistant *S. pneumoniae* bacteria. Isolated thymol only synergized ciprofloxacin against *P. aeruginosa* and penicillin-resistant *S. pneumoniae* bacteria.

- Oral administration of ajowan CT para-cymene essential oil (37.2% para-cymene, 35.4% gamma-terpinene, 20.5% thymol)—500, 250, 125, 62.5, 31.25 mg/kg body weight—noticeably reduced the number of peptic ulcers in rats.[361] The scientists found that thymol was more effective than para-cymene. The essential oil reduced peptic ulcers 98.6% at the 500 mg/kg body weight dose and thymol reduced ulcers by 79.4% at 100 mg/kg body weight.

- The thymol CT of ajowan essential oil moderately inhibited *S. aureus, B. cereus, E. coli, S. typhimurium,* and *L. monocytogenes,* and significantly enhanced the antimicrobial activity of propolis extract against the same bacteria.[362]

- Geranium and ajowan CT thymol essential oil demonstrated remarkable antimycobacterial activity against multidrug-resistant *M. tuberculosis, M. kansasii, M. fortuitum,* and a standard strain of *M. tuberculosis* depending on the concentration used.[363]

- Ajowan CT thymol, and two of its constituents—carvacrol and thymol, displayed strong repellent activity against bean bug (*Riptortus clavatus*) nymphs and adults.[364]

- Laboratory research found that ajowan CT thymol essential oil improved the quantity, quality, and viability of spermatogonia cells—undifferentiated male germ cells that mature to spermatozoa in the testis.[365]

- Food products that require refrigeration during transportation must maintain specific temperatures to avoid the growth of microbes. *E. coli* is a common and serious contaminant of meat products due to its ability to grow when temperatures fall outside ideal ranges during transportation. Adding ajowan essential oil (0.75% concentration) to tryptone soy broth media inhibited *E. coli* growth for forty-eight hours with a progressive increase in bacteria until seventy-two hours.[366] The oil also reduced Shiga-toxin gene expression in minced beef during storage.

- The tomato leafminer moth (*Tuta absoluta*) is a major pest of tomato crops. A laboratory study found that ajowan essential oil and thymol were both larvicidal to tomato leafminer moth larvae.[367]

- Laboratory research found that ajowan essential oil (PLGA-based nano-encapsulation) exhibited a cancer-specific cytotoxic effect against colorectal cancer cells.[368]

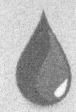

☐ A core-shell nanofiber mat dressing containing ajowan essential oil provided excellent antibacterial and antioxidant activity and wound closure potential in *S. aureus* infected full-thickness rat wounds.[369] A prolonged release of the essential oil was also noted. The findings suggest that the ajowan-loaded dressing has potential to improve wound healing and reduce wound infections that inhibit healing.

☐ A combination of red-light irradiation and ajowan essential oil killed colorectal cancer cells.[370] It was most effective when the cancer cells were first treated with ajowan essential oil and then irradiated.

☐ A tissue conditioner with ajowan CT thymol essential oil possessed antimicrobial properties useful for denture stomatitis.[371]

☐ Dermatophyte infections are caused by a group of filamentous fungi that require keratin (structural proteins found in the hair, nails, and outermost layers of the skin) for growth. It is estimated that up to 25 percent of the world's population is affected by dermatophyte infections, with *Trichophyton rubrum* and *T. mentagrophytes* accounting for 70 percent of infections. Terbinafine is a first-line drug used to treat these infections, but its side effects (liver injury, gastrointestinal disturbances, headache, change in taste, and rash), interactions with other drugs, and the emergence of drug-resistant strains reduce its clinical use and efficacy. An *in vitro* study found that ajowan CT thymol, coriander, caraway CT carvone, and anise weakly to moderately inhibited *T. rubrum* and *T. mentagrophytes*—ajowan was the most effective and anise the least effective.[372] In addition, the essential oils significantly potentiated the activity of terbinafine when used in combination, suggesting essential oils could reduce the amount of the drug needed to be effective and therefore potentially its side effects. None of the essential oils reduced white blood cell (neutrophil) viability at the tested concentrations but did moderately inhibit their release of proinflammatory cytokines (IL-1β, IL-8, and TNF-α). Each oil reduced IL-1β and IL-8 (ajowan most active against IL-1β and coriander most active against IL-8) and only coriander and caraway reduced TNF-α.

☐ Spanish oregano, ajowan, and pennyroyal essential oils (composition not reported) each exhibited good antimicrobial activity against multidrug-resistant *E. coli* strains, producing extended-spectrum β-lactamase (ESBL) enzymes, with Spanish oregano displaying the most important effect.[373]

☐ A comparative study of ajowan essential oil and ajowan essential oil nanoemulsion (thymol CTs) showed that the nanoemulsion had greater antioxidant activity (DPPH assay), and antibacterial and antibiofilm activity against *E. coli* and *L. monocytogenes*.[374]

☐ Nanoemulsions of ajowan essential oil and thymol had better larvicidal activity against *A. aegypti* mosquitoes than free oil and bulk emulsions.[375]

☐ Oral administration of thymol isolated from ajowan essential oil (10 mg/kg and 20 mg/kg BW) reduced blood glucose levels and nerve damage associated with diabetic neuropathy in diabetic rats.[376] The oil demonstrated healing effects in the liver and sciatic nerve, with the higher does being most effective.

☐ Ajowan CT thymol displayed good antioxidant activity in the DPPH, FRAP, and TAC assays and inhibited *E. coli* and *S. aureus*.[377]

☐ Ajowan CT thymol displayed good antioxidant activity in the DPPH and FRAP assays.[378]

*Did you know?*

Essential oils are small enough in size and weight to cross the blood-brain barrier and enter the upper and lower repiratory tract. As such, they are highly valuable remedies for neurological and respiratory health.

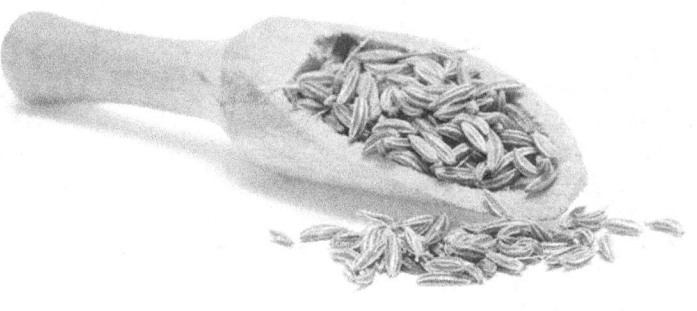

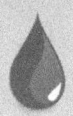 

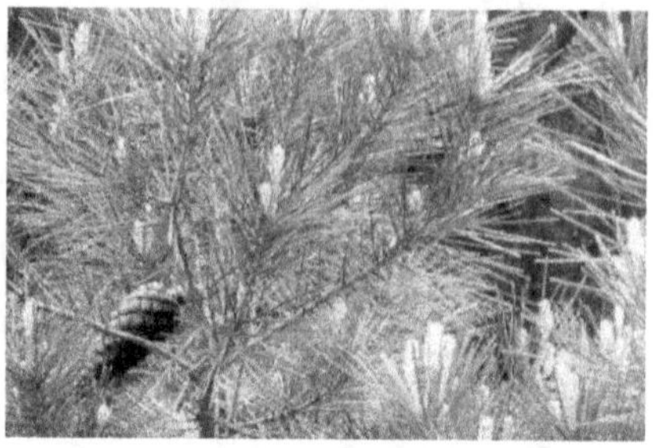

# ALEPPO PINE
*Pinus halepensis* Mill.

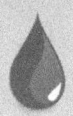

**FAMILY:** Pinaceae
**NOTE:** Top-Middle
**AROMA INTENSITY:** Medium-Strong
**AROMA:** Woody, fresh, balsamic, piney
**COMMON EXTRACTION METHOD:** Steam distilled from the needles (leaves) and twigs; may also be distilled from the cones
**POSSIBLE SUBSTITUTE OILS:** Pine, copaiba, black pepper, white pine, maritime pine, juniper, balsam fir
**BLENDS WELL WITH:** Balsam fir, bergamot, blue spruce, cedarwood, elemi, frankincense, galbanaum, grapefruit, juniper, lavender, lavandin, lemon, orange, pine, peppermint, rosemary, sandalwood, spruce (black), silver fir, tangerine, white fir
**SUBCELLULAR LOCALIZATION | EPIGENETIC INFLUENCE:** Currently unknown | Currently unknown
**RECOMMENDED DILUTION RANGE:** 3%–50%; neat for limited conditions

**PRIMARY CONSTITUENTS:**[379,380,381,382,383,384,385,386]

*Needles*

| | |
|---|---|
| Beta-Caryophyllene | 0.0%–49.7% |
| Beta-Pinene | 0.2%–46.8% |
| Cis-Beta-Caryophyllene | 0.0%–40.3% |
| Beta-Myrcene | 0.3%–27.9% |
| Alpha-Pinene | 1.2%–22.2% |
| Phenylethyl 2-Methylbutanoate | 0.0%–10.3% |
| Alpha-Terpinolene | 0.0%–9.9% |
| Sabinene | 0.1%–9.4% |
| Germacrene D | 0.1%–8.8% |
| Alpha-Humulene | 1.4%–8.0% |
| Aromadendrene | 0.0%–7.1% |
| Phenylethyl 3-Methylbutanoate | 0.0%–6.2% |
| Cembrene | 0.0%–5.4% |

*Twigs*

| | |
|---|---|
| Beta-Pinene | 18.7% |
| Limonene | 18.7% |
| Delta-3-Carene | 16.3% |
| Beta-Caryophyllene | 9.5% |

*Branches*

| | |
|---|---|
| Beta-Myrcene | 42.1% |
| Alpha-Pinene | 27.9% |
| Beta-Caryophyllene | 14.3% |

*Aerial Parts (Needles, Twigs, & Buds)*

| | |
|---|---|
| Caryophyllene Oxide | 0.0%–48.2% |
| Alpha-Pinene | 0.0%–47.1% |
| Beta-Pinene | 0.2%–46.8% |
| Cis-Beta-Caryophyllene | 0.0%–40.3% |
| Myrcene | 0.5%–27.9% |
| Limonene | 0.0%–18.7% |
| Delta-3-Carene | 0.0%–16.3% |
| Para-Cymene | 0.0%–11.4% |
| Beta-Caryophyllene | 0.0%–11.2% |
| Alpha-Humulene | 0.0%–10.5% |
| Alpha-Terpinolene | 0.0%–10.1% |
| Sabinene | 0.0%–9.4% |
| Germacrene D | 0.0%–8.8% |
| Phenylethyl 3-Methylbutanoate | 0.0%–8.4% |
| Thunbergol | 0.0%–8.3% |
| Bulnesol | 0.0%–7.6% |
| Aromadendrene | 0.0%–7.1% |
| Humulene Oxide | 0.0%–6.7% |
| Alpha-Pinene | 0.0%–6.4% |

*Cones*

| | |
|---|---|
| Alpha-Pinene | 47.1%–53.6% |
| Beta-Myrcene | 6.3%–13.7% |
| Beta-Caryophyllene | 6.7%–11.2% |
| Caryophyllene Oxide | 2.3%–7.5% |

Note: Aleppo pine essential oil varies greatly based on location and even trees within the same locale can have significantly different chemical composition. The needles essential oil could be separated into at least five distinct chemotypes (alpha-pinene, beta-pinene, beta-caryophyllene, cis-beta-caryophyllene, and myrcene), but they are combined in this work. The aerial parts essential oil could similarly be separated into at least five distinct chemotypes (alpha-pinene, caryophyllene oxide, myrcene, cis-beta-caryophyllene, and beta-pinene).

**OTHER CONSTITUENTS:** *Needles*—Delta-3-carene, alpha-thujene, tricyclene, beta-phellandrene, alpha-terpinene, gamma-terpinene, (E)-beta-ocimene, (Z)-beta-ocimene, linalool, menthol, cis-caran-2-ol, alpha-terpineol, terpinene-

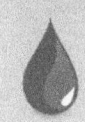

4-ol, alpha-terpinyl acetate, delta-cadinene, limonene, alpha-copaene, hedycaryol, 2-phenyl ethyl tiglate, caryophyllene oxide, guaiol, cubenol, alpha-eudesmol, biformene, cembrene A, alpha-elemene, terpenyl n-butyrate, hexyl acetate, alpha-ylangene, beta-sesquiphellandrene, elemol, 4-epi-isocembrol, isocembrol; *Twigs*—Sabinene, myrcene, beta-phellandrene, terpinolene, menthone, isomenthone, longifolene, bornyl acetate, neomenthol, menthol, alpha-humulene, alpha-terpineol, Germacrene D; *Cones*—Camphene, tricyclene, 2,4(10)-thujadiene, beta-pinene, delta-3-carene, limonene, beta-phellandrene, alpha-campholene aldehyde, trans-pinocarveol, trans-verbenol, cis-verbenol, pinocarvone, p-mentha-1,5-dien-8-ol, myrtenol, myrtenal, bornyl acetate, isobornyl acetate, verbenone, alpha-humulene, humulene epoxide, caryophyllene oxide, isopimaradiene, 18-norabieta-8,11,13-triene, abieta-8,11,13-triene, abieta-7,13-diene, neoabitadiene, cis-abienol; *Branches*—Beta-pinene, delta-3-carene, cyclosativene, alpha-copaene, alpha-humulene, germacrene D, alpha-muurolene, delta-cadinene; *Aerial Parts*—Terpinolene, terpinen-4-ol

### PREFERRED COMPOSITION FOR CLINICAL USE:

| Constituent | Cones |
|---|---|
| Alpha-Pinene | 45%–55% |
| Beta-Caryophyllene | 5%–15% |
| Beta-Myrcene | 5%–15% |
| Caryophyllene Oxide | 2%–8% |
| Beta-Pinene | 1%–4% |
| Alpha-Humulene | 1%–4% |
| Limonene | 0.1%–2% |

**REPORTED THERAPEUTIC PROPERTIES: Wound healing**, analgesic (pain relief), anti-inflammatory, antineuralgic, nervine (calms and soothes the nerves), antirheumatic, antiseptic, antimicrobial, antibacterial, antifungal, soothes chronic skin conditions, expels excess mucus, aids digestion, diuretic, supports respiratory function, eases cough, **aids cognition**, protects the liver and kidneys, insecticide, insect repellent, stimulating, stress management, reduces anxiety, reduces anger, grounding, relieves fatigue

**CAUTIONS:**
■ May interact with anticholinergic (drugs used for asthma, incontinence, gastrointestinal cramps, muscular spasms, depression, and sleep disorders) and cholinergic medications (drugs used to reduce urinary retention, diagnose myasthenia gravis, and for glaucoma) based on AChE inhibitory activity.[387]
■ May decrease the bioavailability of many medications (NSAIDs, proton-pump inhibitors, acetaminophen, antiepileptics, immune modulators, blood-sugar medications, blood pressure medications, antidepressants, antipsychotics, diabetic medications, antihistamines, antibiotics, and anesthetics) due to the ability of caryophyllene oxide, alpha-humulene, and beta-caryophyllene to inhibit CYP3A enzyme activity.[388]
■ *Branches*: May weakly interfere with the enzymes responsible for metabolizing medications (NSAIDs, proton-pump inhibitors, acetaminophen, antiepileptics, immune modulators, blood-sugar medications, blood pressure medications, antidepressants, antipsychotics, diabetic medications, antihistamines, antibiotics, and anesthetics) based on myrcene content.[389,390,391]
■ *Branches*: May interfere with pentobarbital and other barbiturates (medications for anxiety and insomnia) based on beta-myrcene content.[392]

**SELECTED EVIDENCE:**
  □ Animal research demonstrated that an ointment (consisting of glycol stearate, 1,2 propylene glycol, liquid paraffin, and 1% essential oil) with Aleppo cone essential oil encouraged wound healing (closure of the wound was) and increased wound tensile strength (collagen accumulates during the wound healing process to strengthen the ability of the skin to remain closed and withstand injury).[393] Interestingly, the needle essential oil was ineffective, suggesting that the unique composition of the cones is responsible for the wound healing properties.
  □ *In vitro* research demonstrates that Aleppo pine essential oil (aerial parts) exhibits antimicrobial activity against *Listeria monocytogenes, Enterococcus faecalis, Pseudomonas aeruginosa, Acinetobacter baumanii*,

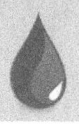

*Citrobacter freundii*, and *Klebsiella pneumoniae*, but was inactive against *S. aureus, B. cereus, E. coli, Salmonella typhimurium,* and *P. miribilis*.[394]

☐ Aleppo essential oil (twig and needle) significantly inhibits AChE (83.9% and 58.5%) and BChE (80.6% and 51.8%) enzyme activity, with the twig oil exhibiting more potent inhibition.[395] The twig oil composition was well-balanced in its primary constituents: beta-pinene (18.7%), limonene (18.7%), alpha-pinene (16.4%), delta-3-carene (16.3%), and beta-caryophyllene (9.5%); whereas the needles essential oil was dominated by beta-pinene (46.8%) and alpha-pinene (18.4%), with beta-caryophyllene (9.2%) the third highest constituent. Inhibition of AChE prevents the breakdown of acetylcholine, which is essential for memory and thinking. People with neurodegenerative diseases make less acetylcholine, and the diseases often break it down at a faster rate, leading to acetylcholine deficits. Selective inhibition of BChE is also desirable in neurodegenerative diseases because it interferes with acetylcholine activity. In addition, BChE is often found in the plaques and tangles in the brains of people with Alzheimer's disease.[396]

☐ Animal research shows that Aleppo essential oil (needle, unidentified composition) protects the liver and kidneys against damage caused by aspirin.[397] Oral administration of 600 mg/kg reversed an increase in lipid peroxidation and reduction in antioxidant activities (superoxide dismutase, catalase, and glutathione peroxidase) in the organs that was caused by administration of aspirin.

☐ Aleppo pine essential oil (needle and twig) exhibited weak antioxidant activity.[398,399]

☐ Aleppo pine essential oil (needle, beta-caryophyllene CT) strongly repelled and killed the larvae of the Asian tiger mosquito (*Ae. albopictus*), which transmits yellow fever.[400] A branch essential oil also killed the stored food mite *Tyrophagus putrescentiae*.[401]

---

# ALLSPICE
## (Pimento Leaf, Jamaica Pepper, Pimento Berry, Myrtle Pepper, Newspice)

*Pimenta dioica* (L.) Merr., *P. officinalis* Lindl.

**FAMILY:** Myrtaceae
**NOTE:** Middle
**AROMA INTENSITY:** Strong
**AROMA:** Spicy, sweet, sharp, hint of clove, black pepper, and cinnamon
**COMMON EXTRACTION METHOD:** Steam distilled from leaves or berries (fruits)
**POSSIBLE SUBSTITUTE OILS:** Clove, black pepper
**BLENDS WELL WITH:** Bay laurel, black pepper, cardamom, cassia, cinnamon, cistus, clove, coriander, geranium, ginger, lavender, neroli, nutmeg, orange, patchouli, petitgrain, spearmint, tangerine, ylang ylang
**SUBCELLULAR LOCALIZATION | EPIGENETIC INFLUENCE:** Currently unknown | Currently unknown
**RECOMMENDED DILUTION RANGE:** 1.5%–20%; 50% for some conditions

**PRIMARY CONSTITUENTS:**[402,403,404,405,406,407,408,409,410,411,412,413]

| *Leaves, Eugenol CT* | | *Berries, Eugenol CT* | |
|---|---|---|---|
| Eugenol | 54.3%–85.3% | Eugenol | 68.8%–86.4% |
| Myrcene | 0.0%–19.3% | Methyl Eugenol | 0.0%–13.1% |
| Beta-Caryophyllene | 1.4%–8.7% | Beta-Caryophyllene | 3.3%–7.7% |
| Methyl Eugenol | 0.0%–7.1% | Beta-Pinene | 0.0%–6.5% |
| Limonene | 0.0%–6.5% | 5-Indanol | 0.0%–5.9% |
| Chavicol | 0.0%–4.8% | | |
| | | | |
| 1,8-Cineole | 0.0%–4.6% | *Berries, Methyl Eugenol CT* | |
| Alpha-Humulene | 0.6%–3.9% | Methyl Eugenol | 43.0%–67.9% |
| Alpha-Cadinol | 0.0%–3.2% | Eugenol | 8.3%–28.8% |
| T-Cadinol | 0.0%–3.1% | Beta-Caryophyllene | 2.7%–6.6% |

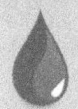

*Leaves, Methyl Eugenol CT*

| | | | |
|---|---|---|---|
| Methyl Eugenol | 62.7% | Alpha-Pinene | 0.1%–6.3% |
| Eugenol | 8.3% | 1,8-Cineole | 1.3%–4.1% |
| 1,8-Cineole | 4.1% | Methyl Chavicol | 0.0%–1.7% |
| Caryophyllene | 2.7% | | |
| Beta-Caryophyllene | 2.5% | | |

Note: The berry essential oil is typically called allspice, whereas the leaf oil is called Pimenta leaf.

**OTHER CONSTITUENTS:** *Leaves, Eugenol CT*—Para-cymene, terpinolene, beta-selinene, linalool, alpha-terpinolene; *Leaves, Methyl Eugenol CT*—Alpha-pinene, beta-pinene, limonene, alpha-copaene, alpha-terpineol, delta-guaiene, terpinen-4-ol, borneol; *Berries, Eugenol CT*—1,8-cineole, alpha-pinene, para-cymene, gamma-terpinene, terpinolene, gamma-cadinene, beta-selinene, terpinen-4-ol, alpha-terpineol; *Berries, Methyl Eugenol CT*—(Z)-beta-ocimene, gamma-terpinene, terpinolene, alpha-humulene, gamma-cadinene, alpha-terpineol, (Z)-pseudoisoeugenyl 2-methyl-butrate, (E)-pseudoisoeugenyl 2-methyl-butrate

**PREFERRED COMPOSITION FOR CLINICAL USE:**

| Constituent | Berries, Eugenol CT | Leaves, Eugenol CT |
|---|---|---|
| **Eugenol** | 60%–82% | 65%–85% |
| **Beta-Caryophyllene** | 5%–15% | 2%–10% |
| **Methyl Eugenol** | 0%–10% | – |
| **Limonene** | 0.5%–7% | 0%–7% |
| **Alpha-Humulene** | 0.5%–4% | 0.1%–5% |
| **Para-Cymene** | 0.5%–4% | 0.01%–3% |

**REPORTED THERAPEUTIC PROPERTIES:** Antibacterial, **antifungal**, antiviral, **antimicrobial**, analgesic, anti-inflammatory, antiarthritic, antirheumatic, anesthetic, relieves stomachache and stomach cramps, **antioxidant**, antiseptic, anti-aging, aids digestion, **stimulates the production of digestive juices**, expels excess gas, anticancer, supports immune function, stimulates localized circulation, relieves headaches, nervine, eases cough, relieves tooth pain, cleanses the urinary tract, relieves insect bites, combats anger, antidepressant

**CAUTIONS:**

■ *Methyl Eugenol CTs*: Avoid in children under age 12 due to the multisite cancerous tumors and DNA mutation caused by methyl eugenol in animal studies.[414,415,416,417]

■ Use very cautiously during pregnancy and lactation due to eugenol, methyl eugenol, and myrcene content. Animal studies suggest that large doses of clove (also with significant eugenol) may negatively impact embryonic development and encourage fetal cell death.[418,419] Another animal study did not detect any negative influence of clove oil.[420] Eugenol is considered strongly toxic to embryos according to animal studies.[421] Very large doses of methyl eugenol may adversely affect the mother's liver and infant body weight according to animal research.[422] Animal research suggests that methyl eugenol may cause changes in embryo form and structure and chromosomal changes in ovary cells, as well as multi-site cancerous tumors.[423,424,425,426] Extremely high doses (500 mg/kg) of beta-myrcene have been toxic to fetuses according to animal research.[427,428] Based on these studies, it is best to limit the use of allspice essential oil during pregnancy and lactation.

■ *Methyl Eugenol CTs*: Avoid oral consumption due to the multisite carcinogenic potential of methyl eugenol.[429,430,431,432]

■ May interact with aspirin, blood pressure, antiplatelet, and anticoagulant medications, and increase the risk of bleeding among people with bleeding disorders based on eugenol content.[433,434,435,436]

■ May interact with MAOI antidepressants. Animal research suggests that eugenol produces antidepressant effects via the monoamine oxidase pathway, which may cause interactions with antidepressants that also interact with this pathway.[437]

■ May interfere with enzymes responsible for metabolizing medications (NSAIDs, proton-pump inhibitors, acetaminophen, antiepileptics, immune modulators, blood-sugar medications, blood pressure medications, antidepressants, antipsychotics, diabetic medications, antihistamines, antibiotics, and anesthetics) based on eugenol content.[438]

■ May interact with anticholinergic (drugs used for asthma, incontinence, gastrointestinal cramps, muscular spasms, depression, and sleep disorders) and cholinergic medications (drugs used to reduce urinary retention, diagnose myasthenia gravis, and for glaucoma) based on AChE inhibitory activity of eugenol and methyl eugenol.[439,440]

■ May interact with antibiotics or antifungal drugs and possibly enhance their effects based on eugenol and methyl eugenol content.[441,442,443]

■ May irritate mucous membranes (eyes, mouth, nasal passages, vagina, rectum).[444,445]

### SELECTED EVIDENCE:

☐ *In vitro* research demonstrates that allspice (berry) essential oil is a potent antioxidant and chelates metals (the process of removing heavy metals from the bloodstream), with some research reporting twice the antioxidant activity of BHT (a synthetic antioxidant and preservative).[446,447,448,449,450] Its antioxidant potency also protects DNA against damage caused by oxidative stress.[451]

☐ Allspice essential oil is toxic to Asian blue tick (*Rhipicephalus microplus*) larvae.[452] It also kills the Japanese termite (*Reticulitermes speratus* Kolbe), pine wood nematode (*Bursaphelenchus xylophilus*), and gall gnat (*Camptomyia corticalis*).[453,454]

☐ Allspice essential oil inhibits *Pseudomonas putida* (a bacterium associated with meat spoilage, and uncommon cause of skin and soft tissue infections).[455] It also moderately inhibits *E. coli, L. monocytogenes, Salmonella typhimurium,* and *Staphylococcus aureus*.[456]

☐ *In vitro* research concluded that allspice essential oil was the most potent antifungal essential oil of twenty-five species tested against *Fusarium oxysporum, Fusarium verticillioides, Penicillium expansum, Penicillium brevicompactum, Aspergillus flavus,* and *Aspergillus fumigatus*, with almost balanced inhibition of all fungi tested.[457] The study also reported that allspice essential oil did not exhibit acute toxicity even at high doses, whereas synthetic drugs used for mycoses caused by the tested fungi do cause toxicity and side effects.

☐ *Borrelia burgdorferi* is a diderm bacterium responsible for Lyme disease in the United States. Of thirty-five essential oils screened, garlic, allspice, cumin, palmarosa, myrrh, ginger lily, amyris, thyme, may chang, and lemon eucalyptus each demonstrated excellent activity against *Borrelia burgdorferi*.[458] Garlic (19% diallyl disulfide), allspice CT eugenol, and myrrh (38% curzerene) were the most active essential oils.

☐ An odd CT of allspice essential oil with alpha-terpineol (30.3%) and beta-linalool (6.8%) as the major constituents completely inhibited the growth of the aflatoxin $B_1$ secreting strain of *A. flavus*.[459]

☐ Allspice CT eugenol essential oil inhibited the growth of *Listeria monocytogenes* and *Salmonella typhimurium in vitro* and on alfalfa seeds (in vapor phase).[460]

☐ Star anise, allspice, and nutmeg all demonstrated larvicidal and adulticidal activity against the *Aedes aegypti* mosquito.[461] Nutmeg essential oil produced the highest mortality.

☐ Allspice essential oil inhibited *A. baumannii*, MRSA, *P. aeruginosa, S. aureus,* and *C. albicans*.[462]

☐ Allspice CT eugenol, bay laurel CT camphene, betle CT safrole, and kaffir lime peel exhibited varying degrees of antioxidant activity in multiple assays (DPPH, XO, NO, ABTS).[463]

☐ *E. coli* is the most common uropathogenic cause of urinary tract infections (UTIs), but the most frequently used antibiotics do not effectively eliminate the organism making recurrent UTIs common. Of 140 essential oils tested, oregano, allspice, cinnamon bark, and clove bud were the most effective against uropathogenic *E. coli*.[464]

☐ *In vitro* research showed that cinnamon bark, oregano, thyme CT thymol, lemongrass (*C. flexuosus*), allspice, palmarosa, and amyris all significantly inhibited *S. aureus* in the stationary phase, which is when the size of a bacterial population remains constant, even though some cells continue to divide, and others begin to die.[465]

☐ Allspice CT eugenol inhibited *B. subtilis, S. enterica, S. aureus,* and *E. coli* in laboratory research.[466]

☐ An odd CT of allspice with myrcene as the primary constituent and basil CT methyl chavicol (estragole) essential oil inhibited *S. aureus, S. enteritidis, P. aeruginosa, L. monocytogenes,* and *E. coli*.[467] Allspice was

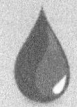

more effective against each bacterium. The researchers then created beta-cyclodextrin inclusion complexes with the oils and found that the antimicrobial activity of allspice was improved in these complexes.

☐ Laboratory research showed that allspice essential oil significantly inhibited *Acinetobacter baumannii*.[468] Topical application of the oil also remarkably reduced *A. baumannii* microbial load in a mice-wound infection model.

☐ The eugenol CT of allspice and bay (West Indies) essential oils were cytotoxic to cervical, liver, and breast cancer cells.[469] Evaluation of the main constituents in the oils found that o-Cymene and eugenol inhibited proteins (human DNA topoisomerase II, human cyclin-dependent kinase 2, and matrix metalloproteinase 13) involved in cancer nearly as well as doxorubicin.

☐ Allspice essential oil exhibited strong antioxidant activity and inhibited *A. flavus*.[470]

☐ *In vitro* research showed that allspice essential oil possesses strong antioxidant activity and antifungal activity against *A. flavus*.[471]

☐ A chitosan nanoemulsion containing allspice essential oil effectively inhibited *A. flavus* and its production of aflatoxin B1.[472] The nanoemulsified oil was more effective than the free oil.

☐ Allspice essential oil was larvicidal to *Aedes, Culex*, and *Armigeres* species insects, repelled pests of stored products from (*Sitophilus, Callosobruchus*, and *Tribolium*), and was toxic to these same stored pests in fumigant test.[473] Contact toxicity was high against *Sitophilus* and *Callosobruchus*. The oil was found to be safe for nontarget organisms (guppy fish) and nongenotoxic in an *Allium cepa* model.

☐ Allspice is considered a viable alternative to conventional insecticides against the litter beetle (*Alphitobius diaperinus*).[474]

☐ Both allspice essential oil and eugenol were active against foodborne pathogens (*L. monocytogenes, S. enterica, B. subtilis, V. vulnificus, S. aureus, Sh. flexneri, E. coli*, and *P. aeruginosa*).[475] Additionally, allspice oil inhibited the production of violacein—a sign of reduced quorum sensing—by *Chromobacterium violaceum* and was active against biofilm potency at low concentrations. Eugenol also inhibited the formation of biofilms by the bacteria on glass and polystyrene.

☐ A combination of cinnamon bark and star allspice essential oil in soybean oil (5% of each oil in 90% soybean oil) was highly larvicidal to and significantly repelled the American cockroach (*Periplaneta americana*).[476]

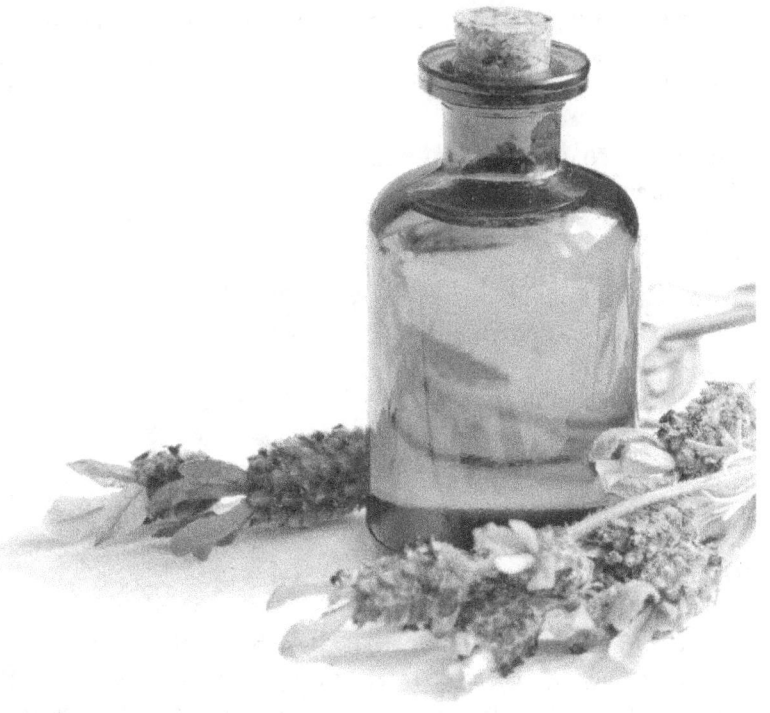

*Did you know?*

Emerging research shows that essential oils influence the expression of genes (epigenetics), which can improve hormone production, metabolism, and many other areas, leading to improved overall health. Learn more about this fascinating information in the book *Synergy, I'ts an Essential Oil Thing: Revealing the Science of Essential Oil Synergy with Cells, Genes, and Human Health.*

# AMYRIS
## (Balsam Torchwood, West Indian Sandalwood)
*Amyris balsamifera* L.

**FAMILY:** Rutaceae
**NOTE:** Base
**AROMA INTENSITY:** Medium
**AROMA:** Woody, balsamic, earthy, musty, slight hint of vanilla
**COMMON EXTRACTION METHOD:** Steam distilled from the seasoned wood
**POSSIBLE SUBSTITUTE OILS:** Sandalwood, spikenard
**BLENDS WELL WITH:** Agarwood, balsam fir, cedarwood, citronella, elemi, frankincense, geranium, ginger, lavandin, lavender, patchouli, Peru balsam, sandalwood, tolu balsam, vetiver, white fir, ylang ylang
**SUBCELLULAR LOCALIZATION | EPIGENETIC INFLUENCE:** Currently unknown | Currently unknown
**RECOMMENDED DILUTION RANGE:** 5.0%–50.0%; neat for limited conditions

**PRIMARY CONSTITUENTS:**[477,478,479,480]

| | |
|---|---|
| Valerianol | 21.5%–26.0% |
| Elemol | 8.7%–10.9% |
| 7-Epi-Alpha-Eudesmol | 9.4%–10.7% |
| Beta-Eudesmol | 7.9%–8.2% |
| Gamma-Eudesmol | 6.6%–8.5% |
| 10-Epi-Gamma-Eudesmol | 6.8%–9.7% |
| Alpha-Eudesmol | 4.8%–9.4% |
| Beta-Sesquiphellandrene | 1.5%–4.7% |
| Alpha-Zingiberene | 1.2%–2.9% |
| ar-Curcumene | 1.5%–2.7% |

**OTHER CONSTITUENTS:** Beta-caryophyllene, alpha-acoradiene, beta-acoradiene, alpha-selinene, beta-santalene, beta-bisabolene, seliol isomer, jinkoh-eremol, nerolidol, gamma-cadinol, alpha-acorenol, cadinol isomer, gamma-curcumene, sesquisabinene hydrate, delta-cadinene, selina-3,7(11)-diene, guaiol, epi-alpha-selinene, guai-9-en-11-ol, drimenol

**PREFERRED COMPOSITION FOR CLINICAL USE:**

| Constituent | |
|---|---|
| **Valerianol** | 20%–35% |
| **Elemol** | 7%–15% |
| **7-Epi-Alpha-Eudesmol** | 5%–15% |
| **10-Epi-Gamma-Eudesmol** | 4%–12% |
| **Beta-Eudesmol** | 5%–10% |
| **Gamma-Eudesmol** | 5%–10% |
| **Alpha-Eudesmol** | 4%–10% |
| **Beta-Sesquiphellandrene** | 1%–5% |
| **Alpha-Zingiberene** | 1%–5% |
| **ar-Curcumene** | 1%–5% |
| **Drimenol** | 0.1%–3% |

**REPORTED THERAPEUTIC PROPERTIES:** Antibacterial, antifungal, antiseptic, analgesic, anti-inflammatory, supports respiratory function, decongestant, eases cough, expels excess mucus, balances blood pressure, support cardiovascular function, **reduces the appearance of wrinkles, scars, and blemishes**, moisturizes skin, soothes irritated skin and

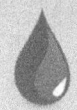

chronic skin conditions, wound healing, supports vaginal health, reduces male impotence, relieves cystitis, **anti-aging**, relieves hemorrhoids, relieves diarrhea, insect repellent, insecticide, **encourages restful sleep**, relaxing/calming, reduces fear (especially about the future), stress management, relieves frustration, aids mental clarity, reduces anxiety, aphrodisiac, antidepressant

**CAUTIONS:**
■ May be photosensitzing due to the presence of psoralen and isoimponellin (low risk).[481] Avoid UV rays for at least twelve hours following topical application.

**SELECTED EVIDENCE:**
- □ *In vitro* research demonstrates that amyris essential oil inhibits *S. aureus, K. pneumoniae,* and *C. albicans.*[482]
- □ Amyris essential oil is a strong inhibitor of the 5-LOX enzyme according to *in vitro* research.[483] The 5-LOX enzyme converts arachidonic acid to leukotrienes, increasing inflammation and allergic reactions, and is associated with chronic degenerative inflammatory diseases and cancer.
- □ Amyris essential oil repels the blacklegged tick (*Ixodes scapularis*) and the lone star tick (*Amblyomma americanun*).[484] It is also larvicidal to three mosquito species: *Aedes aegypti, Anopheles stephensi,* and *Aedes albopictus.* But the *Culex quinquefasciatus* mosquito was more resistant to amyris.[485,486]
- □ *Borrelia burgdorferi* is a diderm bacteria responsible for Lyme disease in the United States. Of thirty-five essential oils screened, garlic, allspice, cumin, palmarosa, myrrh, ginger lily, amyris, thyme, may chang, and lemon eucalyptus each demonstrated excellent activity against *Borrelia burgdorferi.*[487] Garlic (19% diallyl disulfide), allspice CT eugenol, and myrrh (38% curzerene) were the most active essential oils.
- □ *In vitro* research showed that cinnamon bark, oregano, thyme CT thymol, lemongrass (*C. flexuosus*), allspice, palmarosa, and amyris all significantly inhibited *S. aureus* in the stationary phase, which is when the size of a bacterial population remains constant, even though some cells continue to divide and others begin to die.[488]
- □ A study evaluated the chemical composition and antimicrobial (nine respiratory tract pathogens) activity of forty-nine commercial essential oils recommended for respiratory tract infections. Amyris, coriander, and sandalwood (*S. austrocaledonicum*) were identified as having the greatest activity.[489] The oils tested were balsam fir, amyris, frankincense (*B. carterii*), elemi, caraway, camphor, cinnamon leaf, lime, bergamot, lemon, orange, myrrh, coriander, cypress, lemongrass (*C. citratus*), carrot seed, cardamom, eucalyptus (*E. globulus*), fennel, helichrysum, hyssop CT isopinocamphone, star anise, cedarwood (*J. virginiana*), bay laurel, lavender, lavandin (*L. burnati*), spike lavender, tea tree, cajeput, niaouli, peppermint, myrtle, basil CT methyl chavicol, marjoram, oregano CT carvacrol, pimento, pine, black pepper, rose, rosemary CT camphor, sage, clary sage, benzoin, clove bud, tagetes (*T. minuta*), thyme CT para-cymene, and ginger.

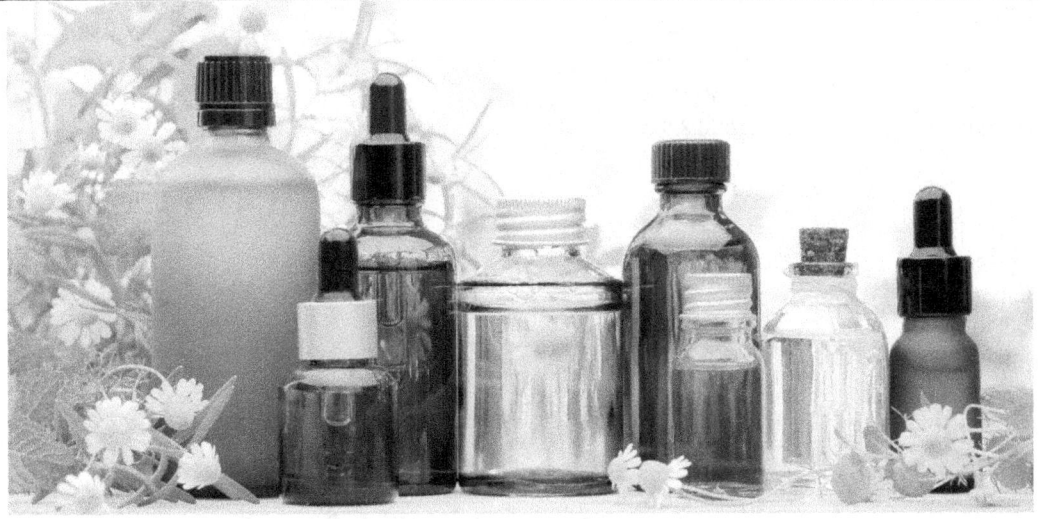

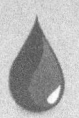 

# ANGELICA ROOT
## (Garden Angelica, Norwegian Angelica, Angelica)

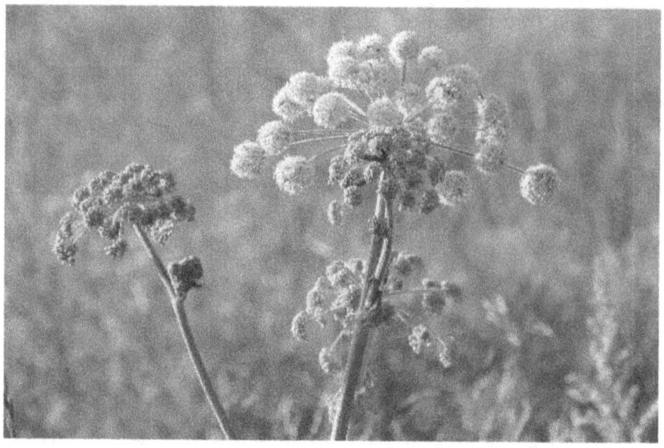

*Angelica archangelica* L., *A. officinalis* (Moench) Hoffm.

**FAMILY:** Apiaceae
**NOTE:** Middle-Base
**AROMA INTENSITY:** Strong
**AROMA:** Rich, peppery, herbaceous, woody
**COMMON EXTRACTION METHOD:** Steam distilled from the roots
**POSSIBLE SUBSTITUTE OILS:** Pine, balsam fir, cypress
**BLENDS WELL WITH:** Basil, cedarwood, chamomile (German, Roman), frankincense, geranium, grapefruit, lavender, myrrh, patchouli, sandalwood, tangerine
**SUBCELLULAR LOCALIZATION | EPIGENETIC INFLUENCE:** Currently unknown | Currently unknown
**RECOMMENDED DILUTION RANGE:** 3%–50%; neat for limited conditions

**PRIMARY CONSTITUENTS:**[490,491,492]

| | |
|---|---|
| Alpha-Pinene | 3.8%–35.7% |
| Delta-3-Carene | 3.4%–17.1% |
| Limonene | 0.0%–16.4% |
| Beta-Phellandrene | 0.1%–15.4% |
| 15-Pentadecanolide | 2.0%–14.9% |
| Alpha-Phellandrene | 0.8%–9.1% |
| Osthol | 1.5%–8.8% |
| Sabinene | 0.4%–7.0% |
| 13-Tridecanolide | 1.5%–6.1% |
| Myrcene | 0.3%–5.9% |
| Terpinen-4-ol | 0.5%–5.9% |
| Trans-Beta-Ocimene | 0.0%–4.8% |
| Para-Cymenene | 0.0%–4.6% |
| Bornyl Acetate | 0.8%–4.2% |
| Longipinanol | 1.3%–4.2% |
| Para-Cymene | 0.6%–3.9% |
| Alpha-Humulene | 0.4%–3.2% |
| Gamma-Terpinene | 0.4%–3.1% |
| Beta-Pinene | 0.2%–3.1% |
| 17-Heptadecanolide | 0.2%–2.9% |
| Octanal | 0.0%–2.8% |
| Trans-Beta-Farnesene | 0.1%–2.7% |
| Mentha-1.5-Dien-8-ol | 0.1%–2.6% |
| Alpha-Copaene-11-ol | 0.1%–2.5% |
| Gamma-Elemene | 0.6%–2.2% |
| Germacrene D | 0.2%–2.1% |
| Alpha-Terpinene | 0.1%–2.0% |
| Alpha-Humulene Epoxide | 0.1%–2.0% |
| Alpha-Terpinolene | 0.5%–1.9% |
| Beta-Eudesmol | 0.4%–1.8% |
| Cis-Beta-Ocimene | 0.0%–1.8% |

*Angelica sinensis*[493,494]
(Provided for comparison purposes only)

| | |
|---|---|
| (Z)-Ligustilide | 18.7%–43.1% |
| (E)-3-Butylidenephthalide | 4.8%–14.5% |
| (Z)-Beta-Ocimene | 0.0%–12.9% |
| Apiole | 0.0%–11.2% |
| Beta-Pinene | 0.0%–5.8% |
| Alpha-Pinene | 4.1%–4.7% |
| Allo-Ocimene | 0.0%–3.8% |
| Carvacrol | 0.0%–3.8% |
| 2-Methoxy-4-Vinylphenol | 0.0%–3.8% |

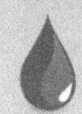

| | |
|---|---|
| Camphene | 0.2%–1.5% |
| Trans-P-Mentha-2.8-Diene | 0.0%–1.5% |
| Beta-Bisabolene | 0.3%–1.3% |
| Trans-Verbenol | 0.1%–1.3% |
| Gamma-Eudesmol | 0.1%–1.2% |
| Trans-Sabinene Hydrate | 0.0%–1.2% |

Note: Some consider angelica root to have two distinct chemotypes—one with beta-phellandrene and one without.

**OTHER CONSTITUENTS:** Cis-menth-2-en-1-ol, cis-verbenol, menthol, para-cymen-8-ol, alpha-terpineol, myrtenal, myrtenol, cis-chrysanthenyl acetate, para-cymen-7-ol, sabinyl acetate, beta-elemene, gamma-caryophyllene, bicyclogermacrene, zingiberene, delta-cadinene, cadinadiene-1.4, spathulenol, tridecanolide.12-methyl, 7-epi-g-eudesmol, 16-hexadecanolide, alpha-thujene, alpha-copaene, alpha-eudesmol, alpha-murrolene, trans-chrysanthenyl acetate

**PREFERRED COMPOSITION FOR CLINICAL USE:**

| Constituent | |
|---|---|
| **Alpha-Pinene** | 20%–40% |
| **Delta-3-Carene** | 10%–20% |
| **Limonene** | 5%–15% |
| **Alpha-Phellandrene** | 4%–12% |
| **Beta-Phellandrene** | 0.1%–12% |
| **Sabinene** | 2%–6% |
| **Myrcene** | 2%–6% |
| **(Z)-Beta-Ocimene** | 1%–6% |
| **Terpinen-4-ol** | 0.1%–5% |
| **Para-Cymene** | 0.1%–4% |
| **(E)-Beta-Ocimene** | 0.5%–3% |
| **Gamma-Terpinene** | 0.5%–3% |
| **Beta-Pinene** | 0.5%–3% |
| **Camphene** | 0.5%–3% |
| **Alpha-Terpinene** | 0.1%–3% |
| **Alpha-Humulene** | 0.1%–3% |

**REPORTED THERAPEUTIC PROPERTIES:** Antispasmodic, expels excess gas, aids digestion, diuretic, nervine, **purification**, purifies the blood, promotes sweating, supports liver function, regulates menstruation, expectorant, reduces fever, supports the immune system, encourages lymph flow and drainage, **encourages restful sleep**, relaxing, stimulating, **reduces anxiety**, stress management

**CAUTIONS:**

■ Photosensitizing due to the presence of angelicin, psoralen, and bergapten.[495,496] Do not expose skin to UV rays for up to twelve hours following topical application.

■ Some aromatherapy texts suggest that angelica root may interact with diabetic medications. However, this appears to be based on studies using *Angelica sinensis*, which lowers blood sugar but is significantly different chemically (predominantly ligustilide) from chaste tree.[497,498,499]

■ Angelica is also frequently listed as an essential oil to avoid during pregnancy and lactation. But again, this seems to be a conclusion drawn from animal studies using *Angelica sinensis*, which is contraindicated during pregnancy.[500,501]

**SELECTED EVIDENCE:**

☐ Angelica oil demonstrated good antimicrobial activity against *C. difficile, C. perfringens, E. faecalis, E. limosum, P. anaerobius*, and *C. albicans*, while only mildly inhibiting the beneficial flora bifidobacteria and lactobacilli.[502]

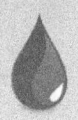

    ☐  *In vitro* research demonstrated that angelica root essential oil reduces inflammation by decreasing proinflammatory cytokine (IL-6) levels and downregulating the expression of miR-126 and miR-146a (microRNAs involved in inflammation).[503]

    ☐  Angelica root, ledum (*R. tomentosum*), and common tansy each showed broad-spectrum antimicrobial activity against tested microbes—*S. aureus, P. aeruginosa, C. albicans, A. niger, Cl. cladosporioides,* and *P. venetum.*[504] Co2 aromatics of each oil were also tested, with ledum Co2 aromatic exhibiting very strong effects against *S. aureus* and a strong effect against *C. albicans.*

Animal research suggests that angelica root oil may protect against seizures and promote a faster recovery during seizure.[505]

---

# ANISE
## (Aniseed, Anise Oil, Burnet Saxifrage)

*Pimpinella anisum* L., *Anisum vulgare* Gaertn.

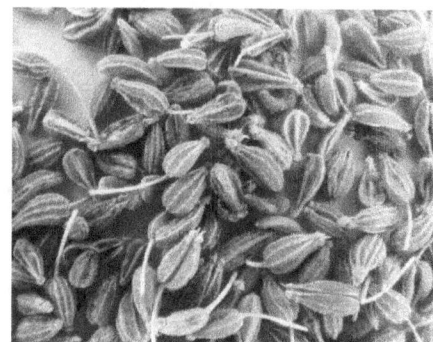

**FAMILY:** Apiaceae (Umbelliferae)
**NOTE:** Top-Middle
**AROMA INTENSITY:** Medium
**AROMA:** Licorice-like, rich, sweet
**COMMON EXTRACTION METHOD:** Steam distilled from the dried/crushed seeds (fruits)
**POSSIBLE SUBSTITUTE OILS:** Fennel, basil, ginger
**BLENDS WELL WITH:** Basil, bay laurel, black pepper, cardamom, coriander, fennel, ginger, lavender, orange, petitgrain, pine, rose, tangerine
**SUBCELLULAR LOCALIZATION | EPIGENETIC INFLUENCE:** Currently unknown | Currently unknown
**RECOMMENDED DILUTION RANGE:** 5%–50%; neat for limited conditions

**PRIMARY CONSTITUENTS:**[506,507,508,509,510,511,512]

| | |
|---|---|
| Trans-Anethole | 76.9%–95.6% |
| Estragole (Methyl Chavicol) | 0.0%–9.1% |
| Gamma-Himachalene | 0.0%–8.2% |
| Trans-Pseudoisoeugenyl 2-Methylbutyrate | 0.0%–6.4% |
| P-Anisaldehyde | 0.0%–5.4% |

**OTHER CONSTITUENTS:** Alpha-pinene, alpha-himachalene, limonene, beta-bisabolene, cis-anethole, linalool, methyl eugenol, and cis-dihydrocarvone

**PREFERRED COMPOSITION FOR CLINICAL USE:**

| *Constituent* | |
|---|---|
| **Trans-Anethole** | 80%–94% |
| **Gamma-Himachalene** | 0.5%–5% |
| **Trans-Pseudoisoeugenyl 2-Methylbutyrate** | 0.1%–5% |
| **Methyl Chavicol** | 0.1%–4% |
| **P-Anisaldehyde** | 0.1%–3% |
| **Cis-Anethole** | 0.1%–1% |

**REPORTED THERAPEUTIC PROPERTIES:** Antiseptic, antibacterial, **antifungal**, analgesic, anti-inflammatory, antiparasitic, antioxidant, antirheumatic, antispasmodic, **supports digestive function**, eases cough, **expels excess gas**, decongestant, **expectorant**, sedative, antiepileptic, aids circulation, balances blood sugar levels, reduces painful menstruation, supports respiratory function, reduces drug withdrawal, insecticide, promotes restful sleep, purification, stimulates the mind, promotes self-confidence, relieves anxiety, antidepressant

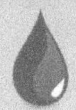

**CAUTIONS:**

■ Use with caution and highly diluted for children under 6 due to methyl chavicol and trans-anethole content.[513]

■ Avoid during pregnancy and lactation due to estrogenic activity.[514,515,516] Large doses of fennel may be toxic to fetal cells based on animal research.[517,518] Nephrotoxicity (kidney toxicity) has been reported in breastfed infants whose mothers drank an herbal tea that contained anise, fennel, licorice, and goat's rue.[519]

■ Long-term oral use of anise is not advised in young girls because of reports that fennel tea (also high in anethole) may cause premature breast development in very young girls when used chronically. Long-term oral use is not recommended for children under age 12.[520]

■ May interact with aspirin, blood pressure, antiplatelet, and anticoagulant medications, and increase the risk of bleeding among people with bleeding disorders.[521,522,523] It is also worth noting that trans-anethole may negatively affect fertility. Animal research suggests it decreases fertility by preventing the implantation of a fertilized egg in the uterus.[524]

■ May interact with diabetes medications and cause low blood sugar because anise oil increases glucose absorption and due to trans-anethole content.[525,526,527]

■ May decrease the effectiveness of diuretic medications due to anise oil's anti-diuretic effects.[528]

■ May interact with acetaminophen and caffeine and reduce their bioavailability and effectiveness.[529]

■ May interact with ibuprofen and enhance its anti-inflammatory activity.[530]

■ May interact with benzodiazepines and increase motor impairment.[531]

■ May interact with barbiturates and reduce sleeping time and effectiveness.[532]

■ May interact with codeine and increase its analgesic effect.[533]

■ May interact with antidepressants (fluoxetine and imipramine) and decrease their effectiveness.[534]

■ Anise oil contains significant amounts of the phytoestrogen anethole. Anethole exhibits weak estrogenic activity,[535] and many aromatherapy texts suggest avoiding anise with endometriosis, oral contraceptives, hormone replacement therapy, and estrogen-dependent cancers because of this. However, research suggests that anethole may promote destruction (apoptosis) of cancer cells—including both estrogen-positive and estrogen-negative breast cancer cells—and phytoestrogens are generally balancing with the ability to either mimic or block the action of estrogen according to current knowledge.[536,537] In addition, anethole reduced painful uterine contractions in the rat uterus.[538] A follow-up clinical study confirmed the animal results, and suggests that anethole-rich fennel essential oil reduces painful menstruation and excess menstrual bleeding, and relaxes the smooth muscles of the uterus.[539] Lastly, anise essential oil reduces the frequency and severity of hot flashes in menopausal women.[540] Theoretically, anise could interact with synthetic hormone therapies by competing for estrogen receptor sites, but reasonable doses pose little risk of interaction or contraindication.

■ May interfere with the enzymes responsible for metabolizing medications based on estragole and trans-anethole content (NSAIDs, proton-pump inhibitors, acetaminophen, antiepileptics, immune modulators, blood-sugar medications, blood pressure medications, antidepressants, antipsychotics, diabetic medications, antihistamines, antibiotics, and anesthetics).[541,542,543,544,545,546]

**SELECTED EVIDENCE:**

☐ Anise essential oil weakly to moderately kills liver, breast, and acute monocytic leukemia cancer cells *in vitro*.[547] It was most active against acute monocytic leukemia cancer cells.

☐ Oral administration of anise essential oil (300 mg/kg) or trans-anethole (100 mg/kg) prevents glucose-6-phosphate-dehydrogenase deficiency (G6PD) associated disorders (elevated bilirubin and serum alkaline phosphatase, and significant decreases in hemoglobin, hematocrit, red and white blood cell counts, serum glucose, blood glutathione, glucose-6-phosphate dehydrogenase, total protein, globulin, alanine and aspartate aminotransferases levels).[548]

☐ *In vitro* research suggests that anise essential oil does not kill the bacterium *C. perfringens* (a bacterium that commonly causes food-borne illness), but it does prevent it from spreading.[549] Additional research concluded that anise oil strongly inhibited several pathogenic bacteria including: *L. innocua, S. aureus, S. typhimurium, P. mirabilis, E. coli* (o157:H7), and *K. oxytoca*.[550]

☐ Anise oil possess good antifungal properties and strongly inhibits five tested Penicillium species, and four *Candida* species (*Candida albicans, C. parapsilosis, C. tropicalis, C. pseudotropicalis, C. glabrata,* and *C.*

*krusei),* and *Alternaria alternata, A. niger,* and *A. parasiticus.*[551,552,553,554] Other research reports that anise oil inhibits *A. niger* better than amphotericin B (an antifungal drug administered for serious systemic fungal infections).[555]

☐ A study concluded that anise essential oil can be used as an expectorant with antibiotics without reducing the effectiveness of the antibiotics against *S. pneumoniae.*[556]

☐ Animal research suggests that anise oil possesses anticonvulsant properties and may reduce tonic convulsions and clonic seizures.[557] Additional research found that anise oil reduced seizure attacks and protected neuron damage caused by the drug pentylenetetrazol (PTZ).[558]

☐ Injection of anise oil may reduce morphine dependence and effect by affecting the GABAergic system (a system of structures that release or bind gamma-aminobutyric acid and regulate anxiety, muscle tension, memory, and convulsive activity).[559]

☐ Anise oil significantly reduces pain comparably to aspirin and morphine in mice.[560] Interestingly, anise carrier oil demonstrated anti-inflammatory properties as strong as the prescription NSAID indomethacin, and analgesic (pain relief) effects comparable to morphine and aspirin in mice.[561] Oral administration of anethole reduces both acute and chronic pain in mice.[562]

☐ A clinical trial concluded that oral administration of 200 mg of anise oil three times daily for four weeks reduced depression in people with irritable bowel syndrome.[563]

☐ Anise essential oil prevents adsorption (attachment of the virus to a susceptible cell) of HSV-1.[564] Other research suggests anise destroys HSV-2.[565]

☐ *In vitro* research suggests anise oil effectively kills head lice.[566,567]

☐ Anise essential oil demonstrates good antioxidant activity *in vitro*, which is improved when the plants are supplemented with zinc fertilizer.[568]

☐ Research demonstrates that anise essential oil and hydroethanolic extract reduces total cholesterol, LDL cholesterol, and biomarkers of oxidative damage (myeloperoxidase, lipid peroxidation, total thiol molecules, and ferric-reducing ability of plasma), accumulation of fat in the liver, and indicators of liver injury (aspartate aminotransferase, alanine aminotransferase) in an animal model of nonalcoholic fatty liver disease.[569]

☐ A double-blind, two-arm, randomized, placebo-controlled pilot clinical study evaluated the effects of anise essential oil against migraine headaches.[570] Men and women aged eighteen to sixty-five (twenty-five in the intervention group and twenty-five in the placebo group) who experienced at least two migraine attacks per month applied 2 mL of anise essential oil (7% dilution in a cold cream base of borax, beeswax, and mineral oil) on the temples and forehead at the onset of migraine. The placebo group applied a cold cream with no essential oil on the same locations of the head at the onset of migraine. The group that applied anise essential oil experienced significant reductions in the frequency and duration of migraine when compared to the placebo group and required fewer analgesic medications.

☐ A double-blind placebo-controlled clinical trial that compared enteric coated anise essential oil capsules (200 mg anise oleogel, three times daily) with Colpermin (peppermint oil capsules) reported that the anise capsules were more effective in reducing symptoms of irritable bowel syndrome. Seventy-five percent of people taking anise capsules experienced significant improvement in IBS symptoms (abdominal discomfort or pain, bloating, diarrhea, constipation severity, difficulty in defecation, gastroesophageal reflux, headache, tiredness, overall satisfaction, and quality of life) compared to 52.5 percent who took Colpermin.[571]

☐ A randomized double-blind placebo-controlled clinical trial concluded that anise essential oil (200 mg anise oleogel, three times daily) effectively relieved mild to moderate depression in people with irritable bowel syndrome.[572]

☐ Human aryl hydrocarbon receptor (AhR: a gene that encodes a protein that helps regulate responses to planar aromatic hydrocarbons and significantly affects the immune activity in the gastrointestinal tract) regulates the circadian rhythm, helps regulate the cell cycle, and plays an important role in tissue development. Cumin, jasmine, vanilla, and bay leaf fully activate AhR; clove, dill, thyme, nutmeg, and oregano partially activate AhR; and tarragon, caraway, turmeric, lovage, fennel, spearmint, star anise, and anise inhibit the AhR activity.[573]

☐ A nanoemulsion of anise essential oil was toxic to the red flour beetle (*Tribolium castaneum*).[574] The nanoemulsion improved the efficacy and stability of the essential oil.

☐ Cumin, fennel, dill, and anise essential oils each demonstrated inhibitory activity against *Candida* species, with cumin being the most active.[575] Fennel and anise were not cytotoxic to mouse fibroblasts at minimum inhibitory concentrations.

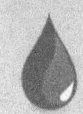

- Anise and encapsulated anise essential oil were both toxic to the Colorado potato beetle (*Leptinotarsa decemlineata*), with the encapsulated form being far more effective.[576]

- Synthetic pesticides are a growing environmental and human health threat and often adversely affect nontarget organisms. The search for safer and natural alternatives has led many scientists to explore essential oils. Anise essential oil was toxic to the red flour beetle (*Tribolium castaneum*) because some of its components—(E)-anethole, limonene, alpha-himachalene, linalool, and trans-verbenol bound to the site for enzymes—aspartate aminotransferase (AST) alanine aminotransferase (ALT)—important for the insects function.[577]

- Nanoencapsulated anise essential oil exhibited improved antifungal activity against *Aspergillus* fungi and reduced fungal production of aflatoxin B1.[578]

- Dermatophyte infections are caused by a group of filamentous fungi that require keratin (structural proteins found in the hair, nails, and outermost layers of the skin) for growth. It is estimated that up to 25 percent of the world's population is affected by dermatophyte infections, with *Trichophyton rubrum* and *T. mentagrophytes* accounting for 70 percent of infections. Terbinafine is a first-line drug used to treat these infections, but its side effects (liver injury, gastrointestinal disturbances, headache, change in taste, and rash), interactions with other drugs, and the emergence of drug-resistant strains reduce its clinical use and efficacy. An *in vitro* study found that ajowan CT thymol, coriander, caraway CT carvone, and anise weakly to moderately inhibited *T. rubrum* and *T. mentagrophytes*—ajowan was the most effective and anise the least effective.[579] In addition, the essential oils significantly potentiated the activity of terbinafine when used in combination, suggesting essential oils could reduce the amount of the drug needed to be effective and therefore potentially its side effects. None of the essential oils reduced white blood cell (neutrophil) viability at the tested concentrations, but did moderately inhibit their release of proinflammatory cytokines (IL-1β, IL-8, and TNF-α). Each oil reduced IL-1β and IL-8 (ajowan most active against IL-1β and coriander most active against IL-8), and only coriander and caraway reduced TNF-α.

- *In vitro* research showed that cumin, anise, and caraway essential oil each inhibited *H. pylori*, with cumin exhibiting the greatest activity and cuminaldehyde the best docking potential to inhibit *H. pylori*.[580] The three oils were also evaluated for their ability to reduce the production of COX-2 (an enzyme responsible for pain and inflammation). Cumin reduced COX-2 expression nearly as well as celecoxib, followed by caraway and anise.

- Anise and tagetes (*T. minuta*) showed strong insecticidal activity against the corn sap beetle (*Carpophilus dimidiatus*) and the merchant grain beetle (*Oryzaephilus mercator*), while cumin was strongly insecticidal against the merchant grain beetle.[581]

- A topical anise essential oil emulgel exhibited greater antibacterial activity against *E. coli* than the free essential oil.[582] The anise emulgel possessed a high affinity for the bacterial adhesin protein FimH in computer-based docking study.

- *In vitro* research demonstrated that anise essential oil inhibits and kills *E. faecalis*, *L. casei*, *A. naeslundii*, and *A. actinomycetemcomitans*, with the greatest activity against *E. faecalis*.[583]

*Did you know?*

Adding a fatty oil (olive, avocado, MCT, coconut) to your essential oil capsule improves bioavailability and helps preserve the capsule from degradation during storage.

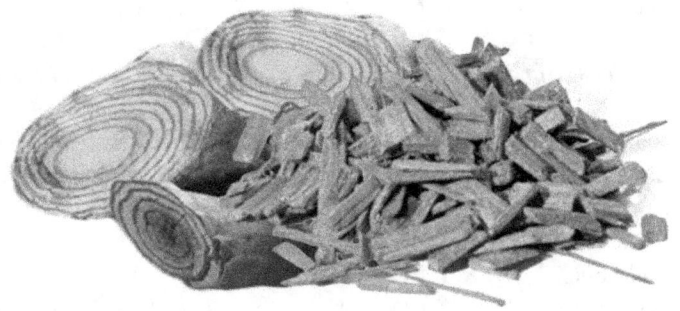

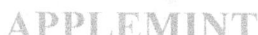 

# APPLEMINT
## (Apple Mint, Hierbabuena)

*Mentha suaveolens* Ehrh., *Mentha rotundifolia* auct. non (L.) Huds.;
*Mentha rotundifolia* auct. (L.) Huds.

**FAMILY:** Lamiaceae (Labiatae)
**NOTE:** Top-Middle
**AROMA INTENSITY:** Medium
**AROMA:** Fruity, sweet, slightly minty (often described as a mixture of apple and spearmint)
**COMMON EXTRACTION METHOD:** Steam distilled from the leaves
**POSSIBLE SUBSTITUTE OILS:** Spearmint, peppermint, pennyroyal, davana
**BLENDS WELL WITH:** Bergamot, copaiba, grapefruit, lavender, lavandin, lemon, lime, neroli, orange, pennyroyal, peppermint, petitgrain, rosemary, spearmint, tangerine
**SUBCELLULAR LOCALIZATION | EPIGENETIC INFLUENCE:** Currently unknown | Currently unknown
**RECOMMENDED DILUTION RANGE:** Piperitenone Oxide, Piperitenone, Pipertone, PO-PEO, and Linalool CTs—5% to neat; Pulegone CT—1.0%–5.0%; Carvone CT—3.0%–50%, neat for limited conditions; Menthol CT—3.0%–33.0%, neat for limited conditions

**PRIMARY CONSTITUENTS:**[584,585,586,587,588,589,590,591,592,593,594,595,596,597,598,599,600 3504–3520]

### *M. suaveolens (Piperitenone Oxide CT)*

| | |
|---|---|
| Piperitenone Oxide | 55.5%–81.7% |
| Carvone | 0.0%–14.0% |
| Piperitenone | 0.0%–10.1% |
| Germacrene D | 0.0%–7.0% |
| Gamma-Muurolene | 0.0%–5.5% |
| Dihydroedulan II | 0.0%–4.1% |
| Alpha-Pinene | 0.0%–3.4% |
| Limonene | 0.6%–3.3% |
| Dihydrocarvone | 0.0%–2.8% |
| Trans-Calamenene | 0.0%–2.7% |
| Pulegone | 0.5%–2.4% |

### *M. suaveolens (Pulegone CT)*

| | |
|---|---|
| Pulegone | 50.0% |
| Para-Cymen-8-ol | 10.4% |
| Borneol | 5.6% |
| 1,8-Cineole+Limonene | 5.5% |
| Cis-8-Menthene | 4.2% |
| Fenchone | 3.6% |

### *M. suaveolens (Carvone CT)*

| | |
|---|---|
| Carvone | 24.7%–55.7% |
| Limonene | 22.6%–29.2% |
| Beta-Caryophyllene | 2.5%–8.5% |
| Germacrene D | 0.0%–8.5% |
| Alpha-Pinene | 0.0%–6.5% |
| Beta-Bourbonene | 1.6%–5.2% |
| Alpha-Humulene | 0.0%–4.0% |
| Sabinene | 0.0%–4.0% |
| Gamma-Muurolene | 0.4%–3.0% |

### *M. rotundifolia (Piperitenone Oxide CT)*

| | |
|---|---|
| Piperitenone Oxide | 23.5%–80.8% |
| Piperitone Oxide | 0.0%–31.4% |
| Borneol | 0.0%–6.4% |
| Carvacrol | 0.0%–6.0% |
| Germacrene D | 0.6%–4.7% |
| Beta-Caryophyllene | 0.4%–4.4% |
| Terpinen-4-ol | 0.3%–4.0% |
| Piperitenone | 0.0%–2.6% |
| Bicyclo-sesquiphellandrene | 0.0%–2.5% |

### *M. rotundifolia (Pulegone CT)*

| | |
|---|---|
| Pulegone | 32.1%–85.5% |
| Piperitenone Oxide | 0.0%–17.3% |
| 5-Acetyl Thiazole | 0.0%–11.3% |
| Germacrene D | 0.0%–6.8% |
| Diosphenol | 0.0%–3.8% |
| Beta-Caryophyllene | 0.0%–3.2% |
| Piperidine | 0.0%–3.0% |

### *M. rotundifolia (Piperitone CT)*

| | |
|---|---|
| Piperitone | 54.9% |
| Piperitenone Oxide | 17.6% |
| Borneol | 5.1% |
| Terpinen-4-ol | 3.0% |

### *M. rotundifolia (Piperitenone CT)*

| | |
|---|---|
| Piperitenone | 35.6% |
| Piperitone | 21.2% |
| Alpha-Terpineol | 10.9% |

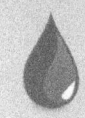

*M. suaveolens (PO-PEO CT)*

| | |
|---|---|
| Piperitenone Oxide | 26.0% |
| Piperitone Oxide | 25.0% |
| Delta-Fenchol | 5.9% |
| Borneol | 3.4% |
| Geraniol | 3.4% |
| Para-Cymen-8-ol | 2.9% |
| Cis-8-Menthene | 2.9% |

*M. suaveolens (Piperitenone CT)*

| | |
|---|---|
| Piperitenone | 33.0% |
| Pulegone | 17.6% |
| Piperitone | 9.2% |
| Menthone | 3.3% |

*M. suaveolens (Menthol CT)*[#]

| | |
|---|---|
| Menthol | 48.3% |
| Pulegone | 20.3% |
| Menthone | 8.9% |
| Neomenthol | 3.8% |
| Menthyl Acetate | 3.4% |
| Piperitone | 3.0% |

*M. suaveolens*
*(Piperitenone Oxide CT—Italian)*

| | |
|---|---|
| Piperitenone Oxide | 35.6%–87.3% |
| Cinerolone | 0.0%–18.8% |
| Alpha-Farnesene | 0.0%–16.5% |
| Beta-Caryophyllene Oxide | 0.3%–14.2% |
| Alpha-Cubebene | 0.0%–10.1% |
| Para-Cymen-8-ol | 0.0%–9.2% |
| Spathulenol | 0.8%–9.0% |
| Limonene | 0.0%–6.2% |
| 3-Octanyl Acetate | 0.0%–4.9% |
| 3-Octanol | 0.0%–4.7% |
| 1,8-Cineole | 0.0%–4.2% |
| Menthone | 0.0%–2.6% |
| Calamenene | 0.4%–2.5% |
| Viridiflorol | 0.0%–2.5% |
| Para-Cymenene | 0.0%–2.5% |
| Bicyclosesquiphellandrene | 0.0%–2.4% |
| Beta-Farnesene | 0.0%–2.3% |
| Demelverine | 0.1%–2.2% |

| | |
|---|---|
| Pulegone | 6.5% |
| Piperitenone Oxide | 4.0% |
| Menthol | 3.3% |
| Menthone | 3.1% |
| Neomenthol | 2.8% |

*M. rotundifolia (β-Caryophyllene CT)*

| | |
|---|---|
| Beta-Caryophyllene | 26.7% |
| Germacrene D | 12.3% |
| Trans-Carveol | 7.3% |
| Bicyclo-sesquiphellandrene | 4.5% |
| Alpha-Humulene | 3.9% |
| Viridiflorol | 3.8% |
| Piperitenone Oxide | 3.4% |
| Bornyl Acetate | 3.3% |
| Gamma-Muurolene | 3.2% |
| Piperidine | 2.7% |
| Pulegone | 2.4% |

*M. suaveolens (Linalool CT)*

| | |
|---|---|
| Linalool | 35.3% |
| Alpha-Terpineol | 11.1% |
| Geranyl Acetate | 10.9% |
| 1,8-Cineole | 8.5% |
| Neryl Acetate | 6.1% |
| Myrcene | 5.3% |
| Geraniol | 2.7% |

Note: *M. suaveolens* composition is very diverse, but the piperitenone oxide CT appears to be the most commonly reported in the literature and, frankly, the preferred CT for safety and efficacy. Some experts and studies consider *M.* x *rotundifolia* auct. (L.) Huds. a synonym for *M. suaveolens*, but it is actually a cross between *M. suaveolens* and *M. longifolia*. However, it is also called applemint and contains similar composition to *M. suaveolens*. In addition, subspecies of *M. suaveolens* can vary greatly in chemical composition. *M. suaveolens* var. *suaveolens* is dominated by piperitenone (73.5%) or piperitenone oxide (72%);[3511] *M. suaveolens* var. *timija* can be dominated by menthone (10.8%–62.6%), pulegone (34.3%–62.3%), piperitenone oxide (19.2%–28.6%), or piperitone (17.7%–35.5%);[3522] whereas *M. suaveolens* var. *insularis* is dominated by pulegone (46.5%) and cis-cis-p-menthenolide (27.3%).[3511,3516] Most studies distill applemint for one to four hours. It is interesting to note that Italian researchers who investigated the influence of distillation times on chemical composition found that distillation times of six to twenty-four hours significantly altered the chemical composition of applemint, reducing piperitenone oxide (0.0%–26.0%) levels while dramatically increasing demelverine (9.5%–43.5%), alpha-cadinol (7.6%–10.7%), verbenone (3.0%–6.6%), and cubenol levels (4.2%–7.5%). In addition, the researchers discovered that the highest content of piperitenone oxide is obtained from plants harvested in July and distilled for one hour.

# The study authors state that the menthol chemotype of *M. suaveolens* is unusual and closely resembles essential oil obtained from *Mentha arvensis* var. *piperascens*, suggesting the plant may have actually been a hybrid (*M. arvensis* var. *piperascens* x *M. suaveolens*).

OTHER CONSTITUENTS: *M. suaveolens (Piperitenone Oxide CT)*—menthone, menthol, cis-jasmone, beta-bourbonene, beta-cis-farnesene, viridiflorol, bet-pinene, cis-sabinene hydrate, terpinen-4-ol, 4a,alpha,-7-beta,7a-alpha-mepetalactone, beta-caryophyllene, khusimene, cis-cadina-1(6),4-diene, spathulenol; *M. suaveolens (Pulegone CT)*—beta-pinene, bornyl acetate, terpine-4-ol, delta-fenchol, geraniol, piperitenone, piperitenone oxide; *M. suaveolens (Carvone CT)*—pulegone (<2.0%), beta-pinene, borneol, cis-dihydrocarvone, trans-carveol, neo-dihydrocarveol acetate, trans-carvyl acetate, cis-carvyl acetate, cis-jasmone, beta-copaene, bicyclogermacrene, trans-calamenene, germacrene D-4-ol, spathulenol, 1,10-di-epi-cubenol, epi-alpha-cadinol, epi-alpha-muurolol, alpha-bisabolene oxide; *M. suaveolens (PO-PEO CT)*—camphene, beta-pinene, 1,8-cineole, limonene, fenchone, bornyl acetate, terpinen-4-ol, piperitenone; *M. suaveolens (Piperitenone CT)*—only traces of other constituents; *M. suaveolens (Menthol CT)*—isomenthone, menthofuran, alpha-terpineol, delta-elemene, alpha-cubebene, alpha-copaene, beta-caryophyllene; *M. suaveolens (Linalool CT)*—nerol, geranial, neral, viridiflorol; *M. rotundifolia (Pulegone CT)*—menthyl acetate, menthol, menthone, limonene, camphor, isomenthone, limonene aldehyde, amyl vinyl carbinol, borneol, terpine-4-ol, para-cymen-8-ol, alpha-terpineol, carvone, bornyl acetate, 2-allyl-4-methylphenol, T-cadinol, calamenene, cis-jasmone, gamma-muurolene, alpha-humulene, bicyclosesquiphellandrene; *M. rotundifolia (Piperitone CT)*—menthofuran, isomenthone, carvone, geranyl acetate, germacrene D, limonene; *M. rotundifolia (Piperitenone CT)*—limonene, 1-octenyl-3-yl acetate, piperitone, bornyl acetate, beta-caryophyllene, bicyclosesquiphellandrene, germacrene D, caryophyllene oxide; *M. rotundifolia (β-Caryophyllene CT)*—1,8-cineole, camphor, borneol, para-cymen-8-ol, carvone, 2-allyl-4-methylphenol, beta-elemene, cis-jasmone, beta-gurjunene, bicyclogermacrene, calamenene, alpha-cadinene, alpha-amorphene, caryophyllene oxide, T-cadinol, alpha-cadinol, naphthalene; *M. suaveolens (Piperitenone Oxide CT—Italian)*—alpha-pinene, beta-myrcene, beta-ocimene, delta-cadinene, alpha-cadinol, cubenol, T-cadinol, T-muurolol, verbenone, ylangene, eugenol, alpha-terpineol, thymol

PREFERRED COMPOSITION FOR CLINICAL USE:

| Constituent | |
| --- | --- |
| **Piperitenone Oxide** | 65%–88% |
| **Spathulenol** | 0.5%–10% |
| **Beta-Caryophyllene Oxide** | 0.1%–10% |
| **Calamenene** | 0.1%–3% |
| **Pulegone** | <2.5% |

Note: One study determined that piperitenone oxide-rich essential oil is obtained from plants harvested in July and maximum therapeutic value may be achieved by distilling for a maximum of three hours.[3520]

REPORTED THERAPEUTIC PROPERTIES: Antibacterial, **antifungal**, **anti-infectious**, antiviral, antiseptic, disinfectant, anti-aging, analgesic, anti-inflammatory, antispasmodic, anticonvulsant, antirheumatic, reduces the appearance of acne, blemishes, and wrinkles, balances blood pressure, aids digestion, expels excess gas, encourages the release of bile from the gallbladder, supports liver function, antioxidant, supports respiratory function, relieves chronic skin conditions, soothes irritated skin, **supports vaginal health**, eases cough, aids immune function, **insecticide**, relaxing/calming, relieves anxiety, stress management, mentally refreshing

CAUTIONS:

■ *Pulegone CTs and CTs with potentially more than 15% pulegone*: Avoid with children under age twelve. Multiple organ failure, liver failure, brain swelling (cerebral edema), severe epileptic encephalopathy (severe brain disorder with seizures), organ cell death (necrosis), and death have been reported in infants who were administered mint tea

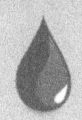

containing pennyroyal essential oil (very high in pulegone).[601] Pulegone and its metabolite menthofuran (or metabolites of menthofuran) are believed to cause the toxic effects of pennyroyal, which include liver and kidney toxicity, bronchiolar cell destruction, depletion of liver glutathione levels (the primary protective antioxidant of the liver), and direct cellular damage.[602,603,604,605] Children are more likely to experience these effects.[606]

■ *Menthol CTs*: Avoid in children under age three and use cautiously in children under six, particularly near the face or nose. Essential oils high in menthol content may cause respiratory distress or breathing problems in very young children.[607,608,609,610]

■ *Pulegone CTs and CTs with potentially more than 15% pulegone*: Avoid during pregnancy and lactation due to significant amounts of pulegone and potential toxicity to multiple organs properties of essential oil rich in pulegone.[611,612]

■ *Pulegone CTs and CTs with potentially more than 15% pulegone*: Avoid oral administration due to pulegone being metabolized to menthofuran via the CYP450 enzyme pathway.[613,614,615,616,617,618] Menthofuran is a known liver toxin and can cause acute liver injury in high doses.[619,620]

■ *Pulegone CTs*: Avoid use with drugs (acetaminophen, barbiturates, carbamazepine, phenobarbital, rifampin, phenytoin, nevirapine, secobarbital, enzalutamide, dexamethasone, modafinil, etc.) that are activated to toxic metabolites by CYP enzymes due to the potentially significant increase in liver toxicity caused by pulegone metabolites.[621,622]

■ *Pulegone CTs and CTs with potentially more than 15% pulegone*: Avoid with epilepsy and Parkinson's disease due to pulegone content.[623]

■ *Menthol CTs*: The menthol content in applemint may negatively impact red blood cells and increase the risk of jaundice in children with glucose-6-phosphate dehydrogenase deficiency (G6PD).[624,625]

■ *Menthol CT*: Avoid use in those with iron deficiency and iron-deficiency anemia. Animal research suggests that mint essential oils with menthol may decrease iron absorption and, therefore, aggravate iron-deficiency symptoms and anemia.[626]

■ *Menthol CTs*: May weakly interfere with enzymes responsible for metabolizing medications (NSAIDs, proton-pump inhibitors, acetaminophen, antiepileptics, immune modulators, blood-sugar medications, blood pressure medications, antidepressants, antipsychotics, diabetic medications, antihistamines, antibiotics, and anesthetics) due to menthol and menthone.[627,628,5059] May also interfere with the anticoagulant effect of warfarin by increasing the expression of CYP4A and CYP2C due to menthol content.[629]

■ *Menthol CT*: May interact with caffeine due to menthol content. Menthol slows the absorption rate of caffeine.[630]

■ *Menthol CTs*: Avoid use in those with ventricular fibrillation (a severely abnormal heart rhythm). The menthol content in this CT of applemint may destabilize the heart rhythm.[631]

■ *Pulegone CTs and CTs with potentially more than 15% pulegone*: Avoid with compromised liver or kidney due to significant potential of pulegone and its metabolite (menthofuran) to cause liver and kidney toxicity (or acute liver/kidney injuries).[632,633,634,635,636]

■ *M. suaveolens (Carvone CT)*: May interact with diabetes medications and cause low blood sugar based on carvone content.[637]

■ *M. suaveolens (Carvone CT)*: May interact with aspirin, blood pressure, antiplatelet, and anticoagulant medications, and increase the risk of bleeding among people with bleeding disorders based on carvone content. Carvone is a potent calcium channel blocker, which may decrease blood pressure.[638,639]

■ *M. suaveolens (Carvone CT)*: May interact with barbiturates (medications for anxiety and insomnia), antihistamines, benzodiazepines, tricyclic antidepressants, or other central nervous system depressant drugs, increasing depressant effects, due to carvone content.[640]

■ May interact with antibiotics, antifungal, or antiviral drugs and increase their effectiveness (applemint essential oils with significant piperitenone oxide, piperitone, or menthol content).[641,642,643,644,645,646,647]

■ May interact with anticholinergic (drugs used for asthma, incontinence, gastrointestinal cramps, muscular spasms, depression, and sleep disorders) and cholinergic medications (drugs used to reduce urinary retention, diagnose myasthenia gravis, and for glaucoma) based on AChE inhibitory activity.[648]

■ *M. rotundifolia (Beta-Caryophyllene CT)*: May decrease the bioavailability of many medications (NSAIDs, proton-pump inhibitors, acetaminophen, antiepileptics, immune modulators, blood-sugar medications, blood pressure medications, antidepressants, antipsychotics, diabetic medications, antihistamines, antibiotics, and anesthetics) due to the ability of caryophyllene oxide, alpha-humulene, and beta-caryophyllene to inhibit CYP3A enzyme activity.[649]

## SELECTED EVIDENCE:

☐ *In vitro* demonstrates that the chemical composition of applemint greatly influences its antimicrobial activity. A pulegone-rich applemint inhibited nineteen bacteria (three strains of *S. aureus*, two strains of *S. simulans*, *S. saprophyticus*, *Enterococcus*, *Bacillus anthracis*, three strains of *Escherichia coli*, two strains of *P. aeruginosa*, *P. fluorescens*, *Citrobacter freundii*, *Enterobacter avium*, and *Proteus mirabilis*) and three fungi (two strains of *C. albicans* and *C. glabrata*); whereas a CT rich in piperitenone oxide exhibited moderate inhibition, and an oil balanced in piperitenone oxide and piperitone oxide was a moderate-to-weak inhibitor of the same microorganisms.[650] A pulegone-rich *M. rotundifolia* also inhibited three bacteria (*Escherichia coli*, *Bacillus subtilis*, *Staphylococcus aureus*), and three fungi (*Trametes pini*, *Aspergillus niger*, *Pénicillium parasiticus*).[651] Both the pulegone and beta-caryophyllene CTs of *M. rotundifolia* strongly inhibited *Escherichia coli*, *Salmonella typhimurium*, *Staphylococcus aureus*, and *Bacillus cereus*.[652]

☐ Italian applemint essential oil effectively inactivated infectious elementary bodies (nonreplicating infectious particles that are released when infected cells rupture, which are responsible for the bacteria's ability to spread from person to person) and inhibited replication of *Chlamydia trachomatis* (the most common cause of sexually transmitted bacterial infection worldwide) *in vitro*.[653] This activity suggests that Italian applemint essential oil may help prevent the transmission of *C. trachomatis* during sexual intercourse, and reduce the number of new chlamydial infections.

☐ *In vitro* research reports piperitenone oxide-rich (65.6%–87.3%) Italian applemint significantly inhibits *C. albicans,* with the amount of piperitenone oxide present directly correlating with antifungal activity (higher PO, greater antifungal activity).[654] The inhibitory action was comparable to the synthetic antifungal drug miconazole. *In vitro* and animal research concluded that a piperitenone oxide CT of applemint potently eradicates *Candida* (*C. albicans*) and prevents its spread, making it a promising candidate for vaginal candidiasis in humans.[655,656] A third study reports that applemint (piperitenone oxide CT—90%) essential oil inhibits *C. albicans* yeast cells and biofilms, and demonstrates synergism with the antifungal drugs fluconazole and micafungin.[657]

☐ Applemint essential oil (piperitenone oxide CT) did not prevent attachment of HSV-1 to cells, but it strongly inhibited HSV-1 replication once attached by reducing the ability of HSV-1 to reduce glutathione levels inside the cell.[658] HSV-1 is known to cause a pro-oxidative state to increase viral replication by reducing glutathione levels inside cells. A synergistic effect against the virus when combined with acyclovir (an antiviral drug) was also observed. The authors attributed the antiviral properties of applemint essential oil to its high composition of piperitenone oxide due to the ability of isolated piperitenone oxide to inhibit HSV-1 to a greater degree than the whole oil.

☐ *In vitro* research reports that applemint essential oil (unidentified CT) inhibits acetylcholinesterase (AChE) enzyme activity greater than 50%.[659] Inhibition of AChE prevents the breakdown of acetylcholine, which is essential for memory and thinking. People with neurodegenerative diseases make less acetylcholine, and the diseases often break it down at a faster rate, leading to acetylcholine deficits and cognitive decline.

☐ *M. suaveolens var. timija* demonstrated weak antioxidant activity (menthone-pulegone CT).[660] However, applemint essential oil rich in piperitenone oxide (88.0%) demonstrated significant antioxidant activity in another study.[661] Another study reports that *M. rotundifolia* (pulegone CT) demonstrated considerable antioxidant properties.[662]

☐ Applemint essential oil (piperitenone CT) is toxic to two species of food storage insects (*Sitophilus oryzae* and *Rhyzopertha dominica*).[663] The piperitenone oxide CT is toxic to the mosquito *Culex quinquefasciatus* (a mosquito that transmits the West Nile virus and St. Louis encephalitis virus) and the *Culex pipiens* mosquito (a transmitter of West Nile virus, Japanese encephalitis, meningitis, and urticaria, and possibly the Zika virus).[664,665] Another study reports that the piperitenone oxide CT is highly toxic to the rice weevil (Sitophilus oryzae).[666] A pulegone-rich applemint essential oil was toxic to two cereal insects (*Rhyzopertha dominica* and *Sitophilus*

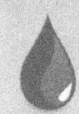

*oryzae*).[667] *M. suaveolens* var. *timija* (menthone-pulegone CT) was highly toxic to the red flour beetle (*Tribolium castaneum*).[668,669]

- ☐ A menthone/pulegone CT of apple mint (*M. suaveolens* subsp. *timja*) demonstrated good antioxidant activity.[670]
- ☐ Apple mint (*M. suaveolens*, CT pulegone) prevented biofilm formation and violacein production by *Chromobacterium violaceum*, which allow it to disrupt bacterial communication (quorum sensing).[671]
- ☐ The pulegone-menthone CT of apple mint (*Mentha suaveolens* var. *timja*) was toxic to the *Hyalomma aegyptium* tick.[672]
- ☐ Of five Moroccan essential oils tested, apple mint CT cinerone (*M. suaveolens*) exhibited the greatest antioxidant activity in the DPPH assay and the highest antibacterial activity against *L. monocytogenes* and *S. enterica* in the microdilution broth method.[673]
- ☐ The carvone CT of apple mint grown in Saudi Arabia displayed moderate antioxidant activity, while its ethanolic extract had high activity and demonstrated food antifungal activity possibly due to its rosmarinic acid content.[674]
- ☐ Researchers analyzed the composition and antimicrobial activity of mint essential oils, including bergamot mint, peppermint, pennyroyal, spearmint, and apple mint (*M. suaveolens*). Bergamot mint inhibited *S. typhi* and *C. albicans*, *peppermint E. coli, B. subtilis*, and *C. albicans*, pennyroyal *K. pneumoniae, B. subtilis*, and *C. albicans*; spearmint significantly inhibited *S. typhi* and *B. subtilis*; and apple mint inhibited *K. pneumoniae*, *C. albicans*, and *S. typhi*.[675]
- ☐ Apple mint (*M. suaveolens*) CT piperitenone oxide, thyme (*T. zygis*) CT carvacrol, and sage CT beta-thujone essential oil each exhibited insecticidal activity against tomato leafminer (*Tuta absoluta*) larvae and medfly (*Ceratitis capitata*) adults.[676]
- ☐ Thyme CT carvacrol, sage CT beta-thujone, and apple mint CT piperitenone oxide were insecticidal to the medfly (*Ceratitis capitata*) and larvicidal to the tomato leafminer (*Tuta absoluta*), with apple mint being the most effective.[677]

---

# ARNICA
## (Mountain Arnica, Leopard's Bane, Wolf's Bane, Mountain Tobacco)

*Arnica montana* L.

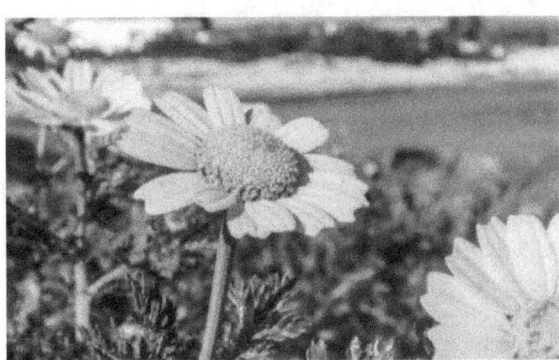

**FAMILY:** Asteraceae (Compositae)
**NOTE:** Middle
**AROMA INTENSITY:** Medium
**AROMA:** Herbaceous, bitter, earthy
**COMMON EXTRACTION METHOD:** Hydrodistilled or steam distilled from the flowers, roots, or rhizomes
**POSSIBLE SUBSTITUTE OILS:** Copaiba, black pepper, hemp, guava leaf, tagetes
**BLENDS WELL WITH:** Bergamot, cardamom, clary sage, coriander, frankincense, geranium, ginger, grapefruit, lavender, lemon, lemon verbena, lemongrass, lime, orange, oregano, palo santo, patchouli, rose, sandalwood, spikenard, tangerine, ylang ylang
**SUBCELLULAR LOCALIZATION | EPIGENETIC INFLUENCE:** Currently unknown | Currently unknown
**RECOMMENDED DILUTION RANGE:** 3%–20%; 50% for some conditions

**PRIMARY CONSTITUENTS:**[678,679,680]

| Flowers | | Roots/Rhizomes (2,5-Dimethoxy-p-Cymene CT) | |
|---|---|---|---|
| Beta-Caryophyllene | 31.6%–34.6% | 2,5-Dimethoxy-p-Cymene | 28.9%–40.6% |
| Germacrene D | 12.5%–16.3% | Thymol Methyl Ether | 9.6%–27.2% |
| Decanal | 2.7%–5.3% | 2,6-Diisopropylanisole | 8.9%–14.1% |
| (E)-Alpha-Ionone | 4.0%–4.3% | p-Methoxyheptanophenone | 6.1%–8.9% |
| Gamma-Muurolene | 2.7%–3.3% | Alpha-Isocomene | 1.3%–7.6% |
| Hexahydrofarnesyl Acetate | 1.8%–3.1% | p-Diisopropyl-Benzene | 1.6%–5.7% |
| | | Pinchotene Acetate | 2.5%–4.7% |

*Hairy Roots/Roots (Thymol Derivatives CT)*

| | |
|---|---|
| 10-Isobutyryloxy-8,9-Didehydrothymol Isobutyrate | 10.3%–12.3% |
| Alpha-Isocomene | 6.9%–9.1% |
| 10-Isobutyryloxy-8,9-Didehydro Thymol Methyl Ether | 6.9%–8.6% |
| 4-Hydroxy-8,9-Didehydrothymol Dimethyl Ether | 4.7%–7.4% |
| Hexadecanoic Acid | 4.1%–7.2% |
| 9-Isobutyryloxy Thymol Isobutyrate | 5.3%–6.7% |
| Para-Cymene | 0.1%–4.9% |
| 4-Hydroxythymol Dimethyl Ether | 3.9%–4.8% |
| 10-Isovaleroxy-8,9-Didehydrothymol Methyl Ether | 3.4%–3.6% |
| Linoleic Acid | 2.9%–3.3% |
| 7-Isobutyryloxy Thymol Isobutyrate | 2.1%–3.1% |
| AETIB | 1.0%–4.2% |
| Beta-Caryophyllene | 0.0%–3.4% |

Note: Arnica root essential oil can be obtained from the hairy roots (roots transformed by the soil bacterium *Agrobacterium rhizogenes*, which produces hairy root disease) or non-transformed roots that have not been infected with the bacterium. One study reports a flower oil with the composition as follows: (Z,Z)-geranyl linalool (14.7%), unknown 2 (13.8%), (2E,6E)-farnesol (4.6%), n-eicosane (4.5%), unknown 1 (4.5%).[4826]

**OTHER CONSTITUENTS:** *Flowers*—Heptanal, thuja-2,3(10)-diene, alpha-terpinene, para-cymene, linalool, nonanal, pinocarvone, (E,E,Z)-1,3,5,8-undecatriene, (E,E)-1,3,5,-undecatriene, dodecane, carvone, bornyl acetate, carvacrol, eugenol, silphin-1-ene, modhephene, trans-alpha-bergamotene, trans-beta-damascone, alpha-humulene, trans-beta-farnesene, trans-beta-ionone, geranyl propionate, alpha-muurolene, caryophyllene oxide, humulene epoxide II, salvia-4(14)-en-1-one, heptadecane, pentadecane, 4,8-dimethyl-7-hydroxycoumarin, (E)-phytol, alpha-linoleic acid, tricosane, pentacosane; *Roots/Rhizomes (2,5-Dimethoxy-p-Cymene CT)*—Alpha-phellandrene, para-cymene, limonene, carvacrol methyl ether, silpherfol-6-ene, modheph-2-ene, beta-isocomene, isobornyl isobutanoate, alpha-trans-bergamotene, germacrene D, beta-sesquiphellandrene, zierone, 3-(3-Hydroxy-4-methyl-phenyl)-3,4,4-trimethyl-cyclopentanone; *Hairy Roots/Roots (Thymol Derivatives CT)*—Gamma-terpinene, methyl thymol, 8,9-didehydrothymol methyl ether, 7aH-silphiperphol-5-ene, silphin-1-ene, modhephene, beta-isocoemene, trans-alpha-bergamotene, beta-sesquiphellandrene, arnicenone, 6-methoxythymol isobutyrate, 6-methoxy-8,9-didehydrothymol isobutyrate, 9-isobutyryloxythymol methyl ether, 7-isobutyryloxythymol methyl ether, 9-(2-methylbutyryloxy)thymol methyl ether, 10-(2-methylbutyryloxy)-8,9-didehydrothymol methyl ether, 9-isovaleroxythymol methyl ether, 7-isobutyryloxy-8,9-didehydrothymol isobutyrate, 9-(2-methylbutyryloxy) thymol isobutyrate, 10-(2-methylbutyryloxy)-8,9-didehydrothymol isobutyrate, 9-isovaleroxythymol isobutyrate, 10-isovaleroxy-8,9-didehydrothymol isobutyrate

**PREFERRED COMPOSITION FOR CLINICAL USE:**

| *Constituent* | *Flowers* |
|---|---|
| **Beta-Caryophyllene** | 30%–40% |
| **Germacrene D** | 10%–18% |
| **Decanal** | 2%–7% |
| **(E)-Alpha-Ionone** | 3%–6% |
| **Gamma-Muurolene** | 2%–5% |
| **Hexahydrofarnesyl Acetone** | 1%–5% |
| **Alpha-Humulene** | 1%–5% |
| **Trans-Beta-Farnesene** | 2%–4% |
| **Pinocarvone** | 0.5%–3% |
| **Linalool** | 0.5%–2% |

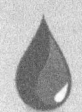

| Trans-Beta-Ionene | 0.5%–2% |
| Alpha-Muurolene | 0.5%–2% |
| Trans-Alpha-Bergamotene | 0.5%–2% |
| Bornyl Acetate | 0.1%–2% |

**REPORTED THERAPEUTIC PROPERTIES:** Antibacterial, antifungal, antimicrobial, **analgesic**, **anti-inflammatory**, antispasmodic, antirheumatic, antiarthritic, **heals bruises**, aids circulation, vasodilator, relieves sports injuries, sprains, and strains, combats negative emotions, encourages feelings of gratitude

**CAUTIONS:**

*Flowers*
■ May decrease the bioavailability of many medications (NSAIDs, proton-pump inhibitors, acetaminophen, antiepileptics, immune modulators, blood-sugar medications, blood pressure medications, antidepressants, antipsychotics, diabetic medications, antihistamines, antibiotics, and anesthetics) due to the ability of beta-caryophyllene to inhibit CYP3A enzyme activity.[681]

*Roots/Rhizomes*
■ The root and rhizome essential oil is not recommended for essential oil therapy due to a lack of safety data surrounding the abundance of phenol (thymol) derivatives it contains. Many references suggest that arnica root essential oil is toxic, but this may be based on severe or fatal poisoning reports caused by oral consumption of the herb.[682,683,684] The herb contains the sesquiterpene lactones helenalin and 1-alpha,13-dihydrohelenalin that inhibit platelet aggregation, but these constituents are not reported in the essential oil.[685]

**SELECTED EVIDENCE:**
☐ None found.

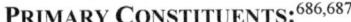

# ARAUCARIA

*Neocallitropsis pancheri* (Carriere) de Laub., *N. araucarioides* (Compton) Florin, *Callitropsis araucarioides* Compton, *C. compton*

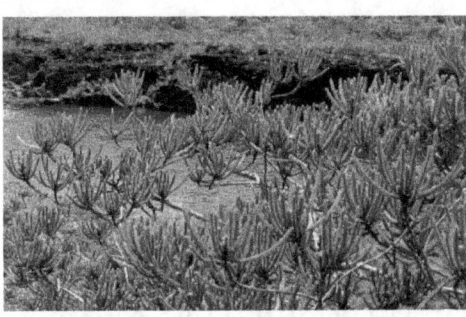

**FAMILY:** Cupressaceae
**NOTE:** Base-Middle
**AROMA INTENSITY:** Medium
**AROMA:** Woody, balsamic, sweet
**COMMON EXTRACTION METHOD:** Steam distilled from the heartwood
**POSSIBLE SUBSTITUTE OILS:** Blue cypress, kumquat (*F. margarita*, leaves), Formosan cypress, balsam poplar, amyris, Japanese cedarwood, elemi, sandalwood
**BLENDS WELL WITH:** Agarwood, balsam fir, cedarwood, copaiba, elemi, frankincense, guaiacwood, lavandin, lavender, muhuhu, Peru balsam, sandalwood, Texas cedarwood, tolu balsam, vetiver, Virginia cedarwood, white fir, ylang ylang
**SUBCELLULAR LOCALIZATION | EPIGENETIC INFLUENCE:** Currently unknown | Currently unknown
**RECOMMENDED DILUTION RANGE:** 5.0%–50.0%; neat for limited conditions

**PRIMARY CONSTITUENTS:**[686,687]

| Beta-Eudesmol | 25.9%–31.1% |
| Gamma-Eudesmol | 19.0%–19.1% |
| Alpha-Eudesmol | 10.8%–13.3% |
| Elemol | 5.0%–7.6% |
| Guaiol | 6.0%–6.9% |

Note: This botanical is native to New Caledonia, only found in small, scattered populations along rivers, and is considered an endangered species. The essential oil may solidify at room temperature.

**OTHER CONSTITUENTS:** Carissone, beta-acoradiene, beta-bisabolene, beta-selinene, beta-bisabolenal, bulnesol, beta-bisabolenol

**PREFERRED COMPOSITION FOR CLINICAL USE:**

| *Constituent* | |
|---|---|
| **Beta-Eudesmol** | 22%–35% |
| **Gamma-Eudesmol** | 15%–22% |
| **Alpha-Eudesmol** | 10%–15% |
| **Elemol** | 4%–8% |
| **Guaiol** | 4%–8% |

**REPORTED THERAPEUTIC PROPERTIES:** Antibacterial, antifungal, analgesic, anti-inflammatory, relieves chronic skin conditions, nourishes and strengthens the hair and skin, **relieves skin itching**, **wound healing**, antiallergic, encourages restful sleep, insecticide, relaxing, combats pessimism

**CAUTIONS:**

■ Avoid during pregnancy and lactation (low risk) due to beta-eudesmol content. Beta-eudesmol strongly inhibits the growth of new blood vessels, which is necessary for implantation, and placental and embryonic development.[688]

■ May interact with aspirin, blood pressure, antiplatelet, and anticoagulant medications, and increase the risk of bleeding among people with bleeding disorders based on beta-eudesmol content (low risk).[689,690]

**SELECTED EVIDENCE:**

☐ *In vitro* research demonstrates that araucaria essential oil kills the cattle tick (*Rhipicephalus* (Boophilus) *microplus*), with an effectiveness similar to synthetic insecticides.[691]

---

# BALSAM FIR
# (Fir Needle)

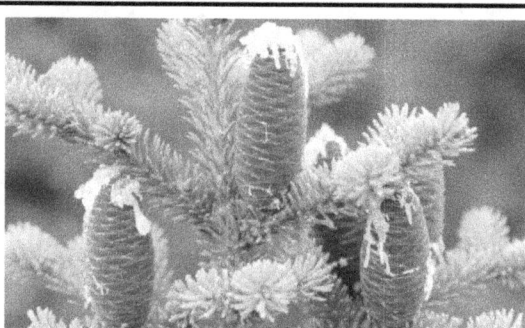

*Abies balsamea* L. (Mill.)

**FAMILY:** Pinaceae
**NOTE:** Middle
**AROMA INTENSITY:** Strong
**AROMA:** Fresh, piney, balsamic, warm, woody
**COMMON EXTRACTION METHOD:** Steam distillation of the needles (leaves)
**POSSIBLE SUBSTITUTE OILS:** Silver fir, white fir, pine, cedarwood, blue spruce, spruce (black)
**BLENDS WELL WITH:** Birch, blue spruce, cassia, cedarwood, cypress, galbanum, German chamomile, frankincense, lavender, lemon, myrtle, palo santo, pine, silver fir, spruce (black), tsuga, white fir
**SUBCELLULAR LOCALIZATION | EPIGENETIC INFLUENCE:** Mitochondria | Circulatory/Respiratory
**RECOMMENDED DILUTION RANGE:** 5%–Neat

**PRIMARY CONSTITUENTS:**[202–207,210 692,693,694,695,696,697,698]

| Beta-Pinene | 27.3%–38.0% |
|---|---|
| Delta-3-Carene | 0.0%–27.7% |
| Alpha-Pinene | 6.2%–25.8% |
| Beta-Phellandrene | 4.4%–23.1% |
| Bornyl Acetate | 4.9%–17.6% |
| Limonene | 1.8%–15.6% |
| Camphene | 3.5%–9.7% |

**OTHER CONSTITUENTS:** Beta-myrcene, terpinolene, alpha-terpineol, santene

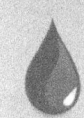

PREFERRED COMPOSITION FOR CLINICAL USE:

| Constituent | Needles | Bark |
|---|---|---|
| **Beta-Pinene** | 20%–37% | 20%–35% |
| **Delta-3-Carene** | 12%–25% | 1%–5% |
| **Alpha-Pinene** | 10%–20% | 15%–30% |
| **Limonene** | 7%–18% | 15%–25% |
| **Bornyl Acetate** | 5%–15% | tr–2% |
| **Beta-Phellandrene** | 3%–15% | 4%–15% |
| **Camphene** | 4%–10% | 0.1%–3% |
| **Beta-Myrcene** | 0.5%–3% | 1%–6% |

REPORTED THERAPEUTIC PROPERTIES: **Anti-inflammatory**, antirheumatic, immune-supportive, **respiratory supportive**, removes excess mucus, **decongestant**, analgesic (pain relief), **relieves bone pain**, antibacterial, anticancer, antioxidant, **antimicrobial**, antifungal, antispasmodic, **supportive of endocrine and thyroid function**, eases cough, wound healing, anxiolytic (reduces anxiety), relaxing, grounding, warming, emotionally stabilizing, uplifting, corrects negative emotions, **aids concentration and meditation**

CAUTIONS:

■ May weakly interfere with the enzymes responsible for metabolizing medications (NSAIDs, proton-pump inhibitors, acetaminophen, antiepileptics, immune modulators, blood-sugar medications, blood pressure medications, antidepressants, antipsychotics, diabetic medications, antihistamines, antibiotics, and anesthetics).[208]

SELECTED EVIDENCE:

☐ *In vitro* research showed that balsam fir essential oil is active against breast, prostate, lung, colon, melanoma, and murine colon cancer cells by depleting cellular glutathione and increasing reactive oxygen species production in cancer cells.[699] All tested isolated constituents from the oil were inactive except of ralph-humulene.

☐ Components of balsam fir essential oil actively inhibit *Staphylococcus aureus*.[700]

☐ Balsam fir essential oil kills some cancer cells (Breast, prostate, lung, colorectal, and melanoma).[210]

☐ Both the whole-needle essential oil of balsam fir and beta-pinene killed overwintering blacklegged ticks (*Ixodes scapularis*).[701] Interestingly, it was found that lower outside temperatures increased its efficacy, while higher temperatures reduced efficacy.

## BALSAM POPLAR
### (Cottonwood, Balm of Gilead, Hackmatack)

*Populus balsamifera* L.

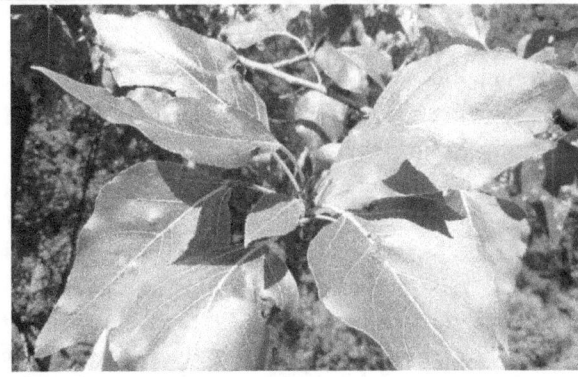

FAMILY: Salicaceae
NOTE: Base
AROMA INTENSITY: Medium
AROMA: Sweet, woody, balsamic, resinous
COMMON EXTRACTION METHOD: Steam distilled from the buds
POSSIBLE SUBSTITUTE OILS: Helichrysum, German chamomile, Roman chamomile
BLENDS WELL WITH: Balsam fir, bergamot, chamomile (German, Roman), frankincense, grapefruit, helichrysum, lavender, lemon, lime, marjoram, palo santo, tangerine, thyme, vetiver, yarrow, ylang ylang
SUBCELLULAR LOCALIZATION | EPIGENETIC INFLUENCE: Currently unknown | Currently unknown
RECOMMENDED DILUTION RANGE: 5%–Neat

**PRIMARY CONSTITUENTS:** [702,703,704]

| | | | | |
|---|---|---|---|---|
| Alpha-Bisabolol | 18.2%–67.7% | *Commercial Samples* | | |
| Delta-Cadinene | 2.2%–10.0% | Alpha-Bisabolol | 23.5%–25.8% |
| (E)-Beta-Farnesene | 1.2%–6.6% | Beta-Eudesmol | 3.4%–11.4% |
| (E)-Nerolidol | 4.2%–6.4% | Gamma-Curcumene | 4.6%–6.4% |
| Delta-Amorphene | 0.8%–5.5% | Delta-Cadinene | 0.0%–5.7% |
| Gamma-Curcumene | 0.2%–5.2% | (E)-Nerolidol | 4.9%–5.4% |
| (E)-Alpha-Bergamotene | 0.7%–5.1% | Beta-Curcumene | 0.0%–3.9% |
| Alpha-Amorphene | 1.2%–4.8% | Alpha-Eudesmol | 0.0%–3.7% |
| Beta-Curcumene | 1.4%–4.5% | | |
| Gamma-Cadinene | 0.0%–4.3% | | |
| Epizonarene | 1.1%–3.0% | | |
| T-Cadinol | 0.4%–2.3% | | |
| Gamma-Amorphene | 0.0%–2.0% | | |

**OTHER CONSTITUENTS:** Limonene, 1,8-cineole, alpha-ylangene, alpha-copaene, alpha-cedrene, beta-caryophyllene, alpha-humulene, trans-cadina-1(6),4-diene, gamma-muurolene, ar-curcumene, alpha-muurolene, beta-guaiene, beta-bisabolene, beta-sesquiphellandrene, zonarene, trans-cadina-1,4-diene, alpha-cadinene, selina-3,7(11)-diene, fokienol, 1,10-di-epi-cubenol, T-muurolol, alpha-bisabolol oxide B, alpha-muurolol, alpha-cadinol, beta-bisabolol oxide B, beta-bisabolol, epi-beta-bisabolol, n-tricosane; *Commercial Samples*—Alpha-trans-bergamotene, alpha-humulene, allo-aromadendrene, alpha-cedrene, calamenene, ylangene, selinadiene isomer, alpha-selinene, germacrene D, alpha-bisabolene, gamma-cadinene, alpha-muurolene, gamma-muurolene, muuroladiene isomer, cedrene isomer, Selina-3,7(11)-diene, (E)-beta-farnesene, cadinol isomer, sesquiterpenol mw+222, t-cadinol, copaenol isomer, gamma-eudesmol, bisabolol epoxide isomer, aromatic component mw=220, 1,8-cineole, epizonarene, amorphene

**PREFERRED COMPOSITION FOR CLINICAL USE:**

*Constituent*

| | |
|---|---|
| **Alpha-Bisabolol** | 20%–28% |
| **Beta-Eudesmol** | 3%–12% |
| **Gamma-Curcumene** | 4%–8% |
| **(E)-Nerolidol** | 4%–8% |
| **Delta-Cadinene** | 4%–8% |
| **Alpha-Eudesmol** | 2%–5% |
| **Beta-Curcumene** | 0.1%–5% |
| **(E)-Beta-Farnesene** | 2%–4% |
| **Gamma-Eudesmol** | 1%–4% |
| **Alpha-Murrolene** | 1%–3% |
| **Gamma-Muurolene** | 1%–3% |
| **Alpha-Curcumene** | 0.5%–3% |

**REPORTED THERAPEUTIC PROPERTIES:** Antibacterial, antifungal, antimicrobial, analgesic, anti-inflammatory, antiseptic, **relieves tendonitis, sprains, and strains**, antiarthritic, antirheumatic, antioxidant, **wound healing**, bruises, antispasmodic, antiallergic, **reduces the appearance of scars and wrinkles**, **deeply skin nourishing**, relieves chronic skin conditions, supports respiratory function, stress management, grounding, aids deep emotional healing

**CAUTIONS:**

■ May interfere with the enzymes responsible for metabolizing medications (NSAIDs, proton-pump inhibitors, acetaminophen, antiepileptics, immune modulators, blood-sugar medications, blood pressure medications, antidepressants, antipsychotics, diabetic medications, antihistamines, antibiotics, and anesthetics) based on alpha-bisabolol content.[895]

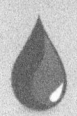

■ May interact with anticholinergic (drugs used for asthma, incontinence, gastrointestinal cramps, muscular spasms, depression, and sleep disorders) and cholinergic medications (drugs used to reduce urinary retention, diagnose myasthenia gravis, and for glaucoma) based on alpha-bisabolol content.[4979]

**SELECTED EVIDENCE:**

☐ Balsam poplar essential oil killed lung carcinoma, colorectal adenocarcinoma, and glioma cancer cells *in vitro*.[705] Isolated alpha-bisabolol was also highly active against lung and colorectal cancer cells. The activity of the whole oil exceeded alpha-bisabolol against glioma.

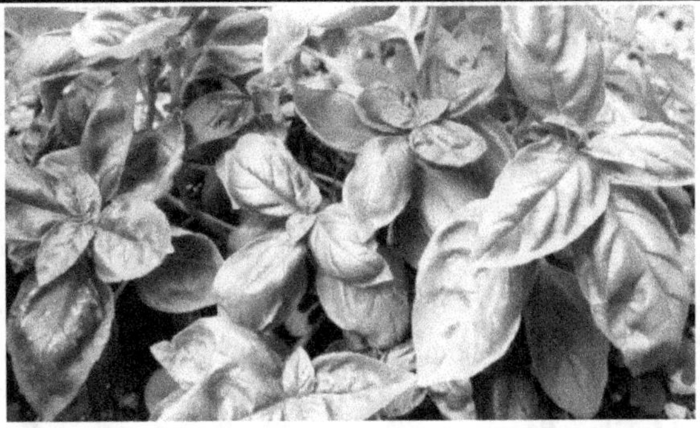

# BASIL (SWEET, LINALOOL CT)
# BASIL (TROPICAL, EXOTIC)

*Ocimum basilicum* L.

**FAMILY:** Lamiaceae (Labiatae)
**NOTE:** Middle-Top
**AROMA INTENSITY:** Strong
**AROMA:** Herbal, spicy, sharp, licorice-like
**COMMON EXTRACTION METHOD:** Steam distillation of the leaves
**POSSIBLE SUBSTITUTE OILS:** Black pepper, thyme (linalool and geraniol CT), marjoram, lavandin, lavender
**BLENDS WELL WITH:** Balsam fir, bergamot, black spruce, blue spruce, camphor, copaiba, cypress, eucalyptus, fennel, geranium, lavender, lemongrass, lime, marjoram, neroli, pine, rosemary
**SUBCELLULAR LOCALIZATION | EPIGENETIC INFLUENCE:** Cytoplasm, Endocytic Vesicles | Lymphatic/Endocrine
**RECOMMENDED DILUTION RANGE:** 3%–20%; neat for limited conditions

**PRIMARY CONSTITUENTS:**[706,707,708,709,710,711]

*Linalool CT*

| | |
|---|---|
| Linalool | 45.3%–69.3% |
| Epi-Alpha-Cadinol | 3.4%–13.1% |
| Eugenol | 4.7%–11.2% |
| Alpha-Bergamotene | 2.6%–11.2% |
| Terpinen-4-ol | 0.0%–5.4% |
| 1,8-Cineole | 0.2%–5.0% |
| Germacrene D | 0.8%–3.3% |

*Methyl Chavicol (estragole) CT*

| | |
|---|---|
| Methyl Chavicol | 78.0%–90.7% |
| Linalool | 0.9%–8.6% |
| Methyl Eugenol | 0.4%–4.0% |

*Methyl Eugenol CT*

| | |
|---|---|
| Methyl Eugenol | 44.6%–78.0% |
| Linalool | 0.1%–37.5% |
| Eugenol | 0.1%–7.6% |
| Linalyl Acetate | 0.2%–7.2% |
| Alpha-Bergamotene | 0.1%–6.8% |
| Alpha-Cubebene | 0.1%–6.2% |
| Limonene | 0.1%–6.2% |
| 1,8-Cineole | 0.0%–6.2% |
| Beta-Cadinene | 0.0%–5.4% |
| Methyl Acetate | 0.0%–5.2% |

Note: Only the linalool CT is considered sweet basil; the methyl chavicol CT of basil is usually called reunion basil, tropical basil, or exotic basil.

**OTHER CONSTITUENTS:** *Linalool CT*—Myrcene, limonene, (E)-beta-ocimene, allo-ocimene, alpha-terpineol, nerol, bornyl acetate, neryl acetate, geranyl acetate, beta-caryophyllene, alpha-amorphene, elemol, viridiflorol, gamma-eudesmol, geraniol, alpha-bulnesene, cubenol, spathulenol, phytol, camphor, borneol; *Methyl Chavicol CT*—limonene, delta-cadinene, geraniol, methyl acetate, germacrene D, eugenol, camphor, (E)-beta-ocimene, 1,8-cineole, 4-terpineol, geranyl formate, trans-alpha-bergamotene, T-cadinol, Germacrene A; *Methyl Eugenol CT*—methyl chavicol, delta-cadinene, germacrene D, trans-caryophyllene, borneol, bornyl acetate, terpinolene, (Z)-beta-ocimene, para-cymene, alpha-pinene, sabinene, myrcene, alpha-muurolene, gamma-cadinene

**PREFERRED COMPOSITION FOR CLINICAL USE:**

| Constituent | Sweet Basil (Preferred) | Tropical/Exotic/ Reunion Basil |
|---|---|---|
| Linalool | 40%–65% | 0.1%–5% |
| Eugenol | 1%–8% | – |
| (E)-Alpha-Bergamotene | tr–10% | – |
| 1,8-Cineole | 2%–12% | 1%–5% |
| Germacrene D | 0.5%–5% | – |
| Epi-Alpha-Cadinol | 0.1%–4% | – |
| Terpinen-4-ol | 0.1%–4% | 0.01%–1% |
| (E)-Beta-Ocimene | 0.1%–2% | 0.5%–3% |
| Camphor | < 2% | 0.1%–1% |
| Methyl Chavicol | < 5% | 75%–90% |
| Methyl Eugenol | < 1% | < 4% |

**REPORTED THERAPEUTIC PROPERTIES: Analgesic (pain relief), antispasmodic,** antibacterial, antiviral, antineuralgic, wound healing, **relieves insect bites and stings,** decongestant, diuretic, anti-inflammatory, antioxidant, anticancer, **muscle relaxer,** nervine (calms and soothes the nerves), improves skin luster, supports adrenal function, **aids digestion, eases cough (especially spasmodic coughs),** supports normal respiration, aids circulation, **headache (migraine),** soothes nausea, expels excess gas, **eases earache,** improves muscle tone, relaxing, warming, **mentally stimulating,** stress management, **relieves anxiety,** encourages self-confidence and motivation, aids mental clarity, reduces burnout and confusion

**CAUTIONS:**

■ *Methyl Chavicol (estragole) and Methyl Eugenol CTs*: Use with great caution for children under age six due to animal reports of liver cancer caused by methyl chavicol (estragole) content.[712] The European Medicines Agency recommends exposure to estragole be limited in young children. Methyl eugenol is associated with multisite cancerous tumors and DNA mutation caused according to animal studies.[713,714,715,716]

■ *Methyl Chavicol (estragole) and Methyl Eugenol CTs*: Avoid during pregnancy and lactation due to high methyl chavicol (estragole) content.[717] Methyl chavicol (estragole) may cause genetic mutations and oxidative DNA damage.[718,719] The European Medicines Agency recommends exposure to estragole be limited in women who are pregnant or nursing.[720] Animal research suggests that methyl eugenol may cause changes in embryo form and structure and chromosomal changes in ovary cells, as well as multi-site cancerous tumors.[721,722,723,724]

■ *Methyl Chavicol (estragole) CT and Methyl Eugenol CTs*: Avoid oral use due to carcinogenic (cancer-causing) or toxic potential of methyl chavicol (estragole) and methyl eugenol.[725,726,727,728] The metabolite of estragole (1'-hydroxyestragole) is considered a stronger carcinogen and humans rapidly metabolize estragole to 1'-hydroxyestragole when ingested.[729] Animal research suggests that methyl eugenol may cause multisite cancerous tumors.[730,731,732,733]

■ May interfere with enzymes responsible for metabolizing medications (NSAIDs, proton-pump inhibitors, acetaminophen, antiepileptics, immune modulators, blood-sugar medications, blood pressure medications, antidepressants, antipsychotics, diabetic medications, antihistamines, antibiotics, and anesthetics).[734,735,736]

■ May interact with aspirin, blood pressure, antiplatelet, and anticoagulant medications, and increase the risk of bleeding among people with bleeding disorders.[737,738,739]

■ May interact with diabetic medications and cause hypoglycemia.[740]

■ *Methyl Eugenol CT*: May interact with anticholinergic (drugs used for asthma, incontinence, gastrointestinal cramps, muscular spasms, depression, and sleep disorders) and cholinergic medications (drugs used to reduce urinary retention, diagnose myasthenia gravis, and for glaucoma) based on the potent AChE inhibitory activity of methyl eugenol.[741]

■ May interact with antibiotics or antifungal drugs and possibly enhance their effects based on eugenol, methyl eugenol, estragole, or linalool content.[637,742,743,744,745,746,747]

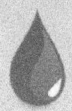

**SELECTED EVIDENCE:**

☐ Sweet basil showed significant activity in preventing the spread of glioblastoma cells.[748] Glioblastomas are tumors that occur in the star-shaped cells in the supportive tissue of the brain called astrocytes.

☐ Sweet basil may help prevent the spread of human oral and mouse leukemia cancer cells.[749]

☐ A twice-per-week thirty-minute aromatherapy massage with orange, geranium, and basil helped relieve depression.[750] The authors speculate that this antidepressant activity was achieved by increasing blood flow to the prefrontal cortex (the front part of the brain responsible for regulating behavior).

☐ A topical mixture of sweet basil (3%) and orange (5%) essential oils and acetic acid was tested against acne in seven volunteers. The antiseptic and keratolytic (the softening and peeling of the horny outer layer of skin) activity of the mixture improved the acne in 75% of the volunteers.[751]

☐ An animal model of fibromyalgia suggests that the oral administration of 25 mg/kg of sweet basil oil or linalool significantly reduces pain and modified FOS protein expression (an indication of modified neuronal activity pathways in the central nervous system, particularly the pain pathway).[752,753] Increased FOS expression from the central nervous system (spinal cord) triggers a cascade of events that produces chronic pain.[754] The studies observed that the pain-relieving effect lasted much longer when the oil or linalool was combined with beta-cyclodextrin (a chemical that causes an enzymatic reaction that makes the oil more water-soluble and bioavailable).

☐ Animal research suggests that sweet basil helps reduce pain by influencing prostaglandins and prostacyclins.[755]

☐ Inhalation of a combination of peppermint, basil, and helichrysum oils reduced mental exhaustion and moderate burnout in a small pilot study.[756]

☐ Sweet basil may protect DNA from damage and mutation due to its antioxidant properties.[757]

☐ Animal research suggests that an ethanolic extract of sweet basil protects the myocardium against damage during a heart attack.[758]

☐ Animal research suggests that sweet basil may significantly alleviate acute ear infections.[759]

☐ Sweet basil actively inhibits gram-negative and gram-positive bacteria, drug-resistant bacteria, fungi, and parasites (including *Giardia lamblia*).[760,761,762,763,764] Basil essential oil inhibits mycotoxin production by *Aspergilus* species *in vitro*.[765] Reunion basil inhibited gram-negative bacteria (multidrug-resistant *Acinetobacter baumannii*, extended-spectrum-beta-lactamase (ESBL) producing *Escherichia coli*, and carbapenemase-producing *Klebsiella pneumoniae*) associated with healthcare-acquired infections.[766]

☐ An animal study concluded that a combination of lavender, monarda, and basil oils reduces cholesterol in the aorta and adverse effects by accumulation of atherosclerotic plaques in the aorta.[767]

☐ Sweet basil is up to 100% effective against dust mites and helps kill the larvae of mosquitos that carry malaria.[768,769]

☐ An increase in fingertip skin temperature and sensory experience has been observed in a clinical study where participants inhaled sweet basil.[770]

☐ Basil essential oil inhibits *T. vaginalis* trophozites, which are responsible for trichomoniasis (a sexually transmitted disease that causes vaginal inflammation, discharge, itching, and pain).[771]

☐ *In vitro* research demonstrated that low doses of marjoram, lemon, basil, clove, thyme, rosemary CT 1,8-cineole, and tea tree essential oils prevented the shortening of telomeres after exposure to hydrogen peroxide.[772] The same research reported that vetiver, black pepper, eucalyptus (*E. globulus*), ginger, clove, and rosemary increased the length of already shortened telomeres. This activity suggests that these essential oils can help maintain the youth and health of cells, or turn back the clock on the cell to make it more youthful depending on the essential oil used. Interestingly, cinnamon and peppermint essential oil decreased the length of telomeres slightly.

☐ A study concluded that oregano (*O. onites*) may be used in combination with basil to preserve meat and control *S. typhimurium* in minced beef.[773]

☐ Basil essential oil may be a viable option to treat *Acanthamoeba* spp. infections due to its ability to kill *A. castellani* cysts and trophozoites.[774]

☐ *In vitro* research demonstrates that sweet basil essential oil is highly effective against *C. albicans*.[775]

- Tropical basil essential oil demonstrated oviposition deterrent activity against the leafminer (*Tuta absoluta*), which is one of the most important pests of the tomato, significantly decimating crop yields.[776]
- Sweet basil, cinnamon bark, sweet fennel, kaffir lime petitgrain, kaffir lime peel, black pepper, peppermint, and spearmint essential oils all demonstrated antimicrobial activity against bacteria linked to cavities (*Streptococcus mutans* and *Lactobacillus casei*).[777] Cinnamon was the most active against both bacteria, kaffir lime petitgrain was the weakest of the tested oils against both bacteria, and black pepper was inactive against *L. casei*.
- Thyme CT gamma-terpinene, lemon CT citral, geranium CT p-menthone, cassia CT cinnamaldehyde, clove CT eugenol, and basil CT 1,8-cineole each demonstrated fungistatic and fungicidal activity toward *C. albicans* and *C. glabrata* isolates with cassia demonstrated the highest activity.[778]
- Marjoram, pink savory (*Satureja thymbra*), spearmint CT piperitenone oxide, melissa, and dittany (*Origanum dictamnus*) demonstrated the greatest repellency toward *Ae. albopictus* mosquitoes of fourteen Lamiaceae species tested.[779] Thyme CT thymol, basil, dittany, marjoram, and oregano CT carvacrol were the most larvicidal.
- Basil essential oil was toxic to stored grain insects and produced a synergistic activity when combined with diatomaceous Earth.[780]
- Algerian basil CT linalool essential oil exhibited moderate antioxidant activity in the DPPH, ABTS, AEAC+FRAP, and AEAC+phosphomolybdenum assays and inhibited *B. subtilis, S. epidermidis, S. aureus, E. coli, K. pneumoniae, C. albicans*, and *C. glabrata,* and was cytotoxic to breast (two types), adenocarcinoma, prostate, and leukemia cancer cells.[781]
- Sage CT alpha-thujone and sweet basil CT linalool both inhibited clinically isolated *P. aeruginosa* biofilm formation and motility suggesting they are highly efficient antipseudomonal agents that could be used in acute and chronic infections.[782]
- Basil CT linalool and oregano CT carvacrol essential oils displayed strong antioxidant activity in the DPPH assay. The same research showed that oregano actively inhibited *S. aureus*.[783]
- Basil CT linalool inhibited *E. coli* isolated from turkeys.[784]
- People with depression exhibit decreased brain serotonin (5-hydroxytryptamine, 5-HT) levels and function and elevated cortisol levels in the bloodstream. Serotonin deficits are often treated by selective serotonin reuptake inhibitors (SSRIs) drugs with significant side effects, such as weight gain, sexual dysfunction, insomnia, anxiety, agitation or restlessness, and stomach disorders. An experimental model of depression evaluated whether basil essential oil (composition not reported) could correct abnormal serotonin and cortisol levels in depressed male mice.[785] Twenty-seven mice were split into three groups: (1) control, nondepressed, (2) depressed, no treatment, and (3) depressed, oral administration of basil essential oil for four weeks. The basil group experienced lower cortisol levels than the depressed and untreated group, but not as low as the normal group. Additionally, serotonin levels were significantly elevated in the basil group, which exceeded that of the depressed (untreated) group and the normal group.
- Thyme, tea tree, tropical basil, rosemary CT 1,8-cineole, eucalyptus, corn mint, and lavender essential oil each inhibited biofilm-forming *S. aureus*, with thyme and rosemary being the most active in liquid phase.[786] Thyme was the most active in vapor phase, with varying degrees of inhibition observed depending on the strain of *S. aureus* with tea tree, rosemary, eucalyptus, corn mint, and lavender. Tea tree and lavender oils displayed the weakest activity in the vapor phase.
- *Fusarium graminearum* is a fungus that contaminates cereals, fruit, and vegetables. Thyme, oregano, basil, nutmeg, hyssop, and clove essential oils inhibited mycelial growth of *F. graminearum*, with oregano performing best, followed by clove and thyme.[787] The composition of the oils was not reported.
- Some experts hypothesize that exposure to chronic stress and altered living conditions may be contributing factors in the development and progression of Alzheimer's disease. Researchers compared the effectiveness of sweet basil CT linalool essential oil and fluoxetine in preventing neurodegenerative changes caused by chronic unpredictable mild stress in mice. Fluoxetine was administered orally, and basil oil was inhaled for fifteen minutes daily from a cotton ball for two weeks. Inhalation of the basil oil alleviated memory impairment, neurodegenerative changes in the hippocampus, and depressed mood caused by chronic stress and also positively altered brain chemicals. Basil's effects frequently exceeded that of fluoxetine.
- Basil (33.3% linalyl acetate and 25.1% citronellal), rosemary CT borneol, and lemongrass (*C. citratus*) were each effective against microbes associated with endometriosis in mares (*S. equi, S. aureus, K. pneumoniae, E. coli*, and *C. albicans*).[788]
- Chronic stress can trigger maladaptive responses in the autonomic nervous system (ANS), which maintains internal homeostasis and controls metabolism. Additionally, chronic stress can interfere with the activation

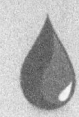

of the sympathetic and parasympathetic nervous systems because the ANS regulates these systems. Dysregulation of the ANS often negatively affects the cardiovascular system (dyslipidemia, high blood pressure, fast heart rate) and contributes to obesity (increased visceral fat, insulin resistance, excess white fat, metabolic syndrome). Inhalation of basil CT linalool essential oil for only twenty minutes reduced total weight gain, total cholesterol, and triglycerides, inhaling it for only five minutes reduced heart rate, while inhalation of isolated linalool reduced white-fat accumulation in rats.[789] Both linalool and basil reduced LDL cholesterol, regardless of inhalation time. Inhaling it for twenty minutes promoted the greatest reduction in LDL cholesterol, and HDL increased in both the five- and two-minute inhalation groups. Moreover, cardiovascular risk and atherogenic index decreased when inhaling basil oil. Overall, this research suggests that inhaling basil and its primary constituent linalool may reduce dyslipidemia and improve cardiovascular health, while contributing to a healthy body weight.

☐ Basil and cumin essential oil exhibited moderate larvicidal activity against mosquitoes *C. pipiens*, with their nanoemulsion forms showing enhanced larvicidal activity.[790]

☐ Investigation of the antifungal and antivirulence activity of basil CT linalool, cinnamon bark, clove, tea tree, oregano CT carvacrol, and thyme CT thymol essential oils (EOs) on five *Candida* species (*C. albicans, C. auris, C. krusei, C. parapsilosis*, and *C. guillermondii*) revealed that clove and cinnamon inhibited all fungal species tested, cinnamon, oregano, and thyme inhibited biofilm formation of *C. albicans, C. guilliermondii*, and *C. parapsilosis*, and each oil except tea tree downregulated virulence genes in *C. albicans*.[791] In addition, thyme synergized the activity of fluconazole against all tested *Candida* species.

☐ Pine, melissa (43.0% citral, 25.0% beta-caryophyllene), ginger, lemon, thyme CT thymol, and basil CT methyl chavicol essential oils each showed activity against MRSA and *E. coli*. Thyme completely inhibited all bacteria at all concentrations tested.[792]

☐ Inhalation of sweet basil essential oil for twenty minutes reduced total weight gain and total cholesterol and triglycerides levels in rats.[793] Inhalation of the whole oil resulted in greater reductions in LDL cholesterol than isolated linalool. Inhaling the oil for five minutes promoted a reduction in heart rate. Inhaling isolated linalool reduced the amount of white fat—less metabolically active fat and the most common type of fat found in humans. The data from this study suggests that simply inhaling sweet basil essential oil may have a positive effect on body composition, cholesterol, and cardiovascular health.

☐ Oregano CT carvacrol, thyme CT thymol, and tropical basil and their postdistillation byproducts—total, spent, and residual-water extracts—were evaluated in enzyme inhibitory and antioxidant assays.[794] The oils and extracts displayed antioxidant activity with the extracts exhibiting greater activity in the DPPH and ABTS assays, but the essential oils had the highest metal-reducing power in the CUPRAC assay. Tropical basil and thyme essential oil also demonstrated good inhibition of acetylcholinesterase, suggesting they may aid cognition. The best butyrylcholinesterase inhibitory activity was observed with tropical basil essential oil. The oils also inhibited tyrosinase and amylase, which indicates they may be useful for skin brightening and glucose management as well.

☐ Odd chemotypes of peppermint (28.0% alloaromadendrene, 18.3% levomenthol) and basil (32.3% alpha-humulene, 27.2% alpha-farnesene, 19.2% estragole) essential oils were lethal to the American tomato moth (*Phthorimaea absoluta*), with peppermint being most effective.[795]

☐ Basil essential oil produced 90 percent mortality in the South American tomato moth (*Phthorimaea absoluta*), which was attributed to alpha-humulene, alpha-farnesene, estragole, and 4-cerene.[796]

# BAY (WEST INDIES)
## (Bayrumtree)

*Pimenta racemosa* (Mill.) J.W. Moore, *P. racemosa* var. *racemosa*

**FAMILY:** Myrtaceae
**NOTE:** Top-Middle
**AROMA INTENSITY:** Medium-Strong
**AROMA:** Spicy, sweet, balsamic, medicinal
**COMMON EXTRACTION METHOD:** Steam distilled from the leaves

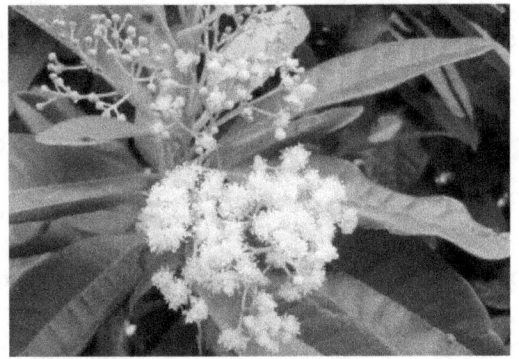

**POSSIBLE SUBSTITUTE OILS:** Clove, allspice, tamala, holy basil (eugenol CT)

**BLENDS WELL WITH:** Bergamot, black pepper, cardamom, cassia, cinnamon, clove, coriander, frankincense, geranium, ginger, lavender, grapefruit, lemon, lime, mandarin, neroli, nutmeg, orange, patchouli, petitgrain, rosemary, sandalwood, tangerine, vetiver, ylang ylang

**SUBCELLULAR LOCALIZATION | EPIGENETIC INFLUENCE:** Currently unknown | Currently unknown

**RECOMMENDED DILUTION RANGE:** 1.5%–20%; 50% for some conditions

**PRIMARY CONSTITUENTS:**[797,798,799]

| | |
|---|---|
| Eugenol | 45.2%–92.9% |
| Myrcene | 0.3%–30.9% |
| Chavicol | 7.1%–9.3% |
| Limonene | 0.1%–4.0% |
| 1,8-Cineole | 0.0%–3.2% |

**OTHER CONSTITUENTS:** Alpha-pinene, 1-octen-3-ol, 3-octanone, alpha-terpinene, para-cymene, (E)-beta-ocimene, linalool, alpha-terpineol, terpinen-4-ol, isoeugenol, beta-caryophyllene, alpha-humulene, (E,E)-alpha-farnesene, delta-cadinene, (E)-nerolidol, methyl chavicol (<0.1%), methyl eugenol (<1.1%)

**PREFERRED COMPOSITION FOR CLINICAL USE:**

| *Constituent* | |
|---|---|
| **Eugenol** | 45%–60% |
| **Myrcene** | 20%–30% |
| **Chavicol** | 7%–10% |
| **Limonene** | 1%–4% |
| **Linalool** | 0.1%–3% |
| **Methyl Eugenol** | < 2% |

**REPORTED THERAPEUTIC PROPERTIES:** Antiseptic, antibacterial, antifungal, **antimicrobial, antioxidant**, analgesic, antineuralgic, antispasmodic, relieves toothache, astringent, balances menstruation, aids digestion, reduces fever, supports liver and gallbladder function, increases sweating, **insecticide**, stimulating, reduces mental fatigue, antidepressant

**CAUTIONS:**

■ Use very cautiously during pregnancy and lactation due to eugenol, methyl eugenol, and myrcene content. Animal studies suggest that large doses of clove (also with significant eugenol) may negatively impact embryonic development and encourage fetal cell death.[800,801] Another animal study did not detect any negative influence of clove oil.[802] Eugenol is considered strongly toxic to embryos according to animal studies.[803] Very large doses of methyl eugenol may adversely affect the mother's liver and infant body weight according to animal research.[804]

■ May interact with aspirin, blood pressure, antiplatelet, and anticoagulant medications, and increase the risk of bleeding among people with bleeding disorders based on eugenol content.[805,806,807,808 632-635]

■ May interact with MAOI antidepressants. Animal research suggests that eugenol produces antidepressant effects via the monoamine oxidase pathway, which may cause interactions with antidepressants that also interact with this pathway.[809]

■ May interfere with enzymes responsible for metabolizing medications (NSAIDs, proton-pump inhibitors, acetaminophen, antiepileptics, immune modulators, blood-sugar medications, blood pressure medications, antidepressants, antipsychotics, diabetic medications, antihistamines, antibiotics, and anesthetics) based on eugenol and beta-myrcene content.[810,811,812]

■ May interfere with pentobarbital and other barbiturates (medications for anxiety and insomnia) based on beta-myrcene content.[813]

■ May interact with anticholinergic (drugs used for asthma, incontinence, gastrointestinal cramps, muscular spasms, depression, and sleep disorders) and cholinergic medications (drugs used to reduce urinary retention, diagnose myasthenia gravis, and for glaucoma) based on AChE inhibitory activity of eugenol.[814,815]

■ May interact with antibiotics or antifungal drugs and possibly enhance their effects based on eugenol content.[816,817,818]

■ May irritate mucous membranes (eyes, mouth, nasal passages, vagina, rectum).[819,820]

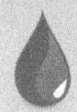

**SELECTED EVIDENCE:**

- *In vitro* research shows that bay (West Indies) inhibits fungi (*C. albicans, Aspergillus ochraceus,* and *Penicillium digitatum,* and bacteria (*S. aureus, E. coli, Salmonella typhi, Strep D – alpha-hemolysate*), with significant activity against *C. albicans* and *S. aureus*.[821,822] It also preserves food products by inhibiting *S. aureus* and *E. coli*, and molds belonging to the Aspergillus, Penicillium, Fusarium and Scopulariopsis genera.[823,824]

- Bay (West Indies) is a potent antioxidant.[825,826]

- Bay (West Indies) kills the tropical bont tick (*Amblyomma variegatum*), cecidomyiid gall midge (*Camptomyia corticalis*), German cockroach (*Blatella germanica*), and the mosquitoes (*Aedes aegypti* and *Culex pipiens pallens*).[827,828,829,830]

- *In vitro* research suggests that bay (West Indies) does not possess anti-inflammatory activity.[831]

- *In vitro* research demonstrated that bay (West Indies) berry essential oil was bactericidal to *Acinetobacter baumannii*.[832]

- Bay (West Indies) leaf and stem oil showed promising inhibitory activity against *H. pylori*, with the stem being most effective and comparable to clarithromycin.[833] Molecular-docking research showed that decanal, eugenol, terpineol, delta-cadinene, and amyl vinyl have potential to inhibit *H. pylori* urease activity due their high binding affinity to active sites.

---

# BAY LAUREL
## (Laurel Leaf, Bay Leaf, Sweet Bay)

*Laurus nobilis* L.

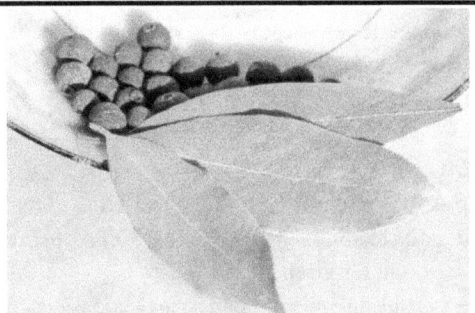

**FAMILY:** Lauraceae
**NOTE:** Middle-Top
**AROMA INTENSITY:** Strong
**AROMA:** Medicinal, herbaceous, spicy
**COMMON EXTRACTION METHOD:** Steam distillation of the leaves
**POSSIBLE SUBSTITUTE OILS:** Eucalyptus, cajeput, cardamom, ravintsara (1,8-cineole CT), ravensara (1,8-cineole CT), niaouli (1,8-cineole CT)
**BLENDS WELL WITH:** Bergamot, cedarwood, clary sage, coriander, cypress, eucalyptus, fennel, frankincense, geranium, ginger, juniper, lavender, lemon, orange, patchouli, pine, neroli, rose, rosemary, thyme, ylang ylang
**SUBCELLULAR LOCALIZATION | EPIGENETIC INFLUENCE:** Currently unknown | Currently unknown
**RECOMMENDED DILUTION RANGE:** 5%–20%; 50% for some conditions

**PRIMARY CONSTITUENTS:**[834,835,836,837,838,839 242–247]

|  |  |
| --- | --- |
| 1,8-Cineole | 18.8%–68.8% |
| Linalool | 0.4%–17.7% |
| Methyl Eugenol | 0.1%–15.8% |
| Alpha-Terpinyl Acetate | 0.0%–14.6% |
| Isovaleraldehyde | 0.0%–10.5% |
| Beta-Phellandrene | 0.0%–10.5% |
| Sabinene | 0.1%–10.2% |
| Camphene | 0.2%–8.9% |
| Alpha-Pinene | 1.9%–7.7% |
| Beta-Pinene | 1.4%–4.7% |

**OTHER CONSTITUENTS:** Terpinen-4-ol, limonene, myrcenol, para-cymene, o-cymene, alpha-terpinene, gamma-terpinene, alpha-terpinolene, endo-bornyl acetate, pinocarvone, 1,4-terpineole, trans-pinocarveol, eugenol, eremophilene, ledene, 2-naphthalenemethanol, linalyl acetate, alpha-terpineol, camphor

**PREFERRED COMPOSITION FOR CLINICAL USE:**

*Constituent*

| | |
|---|---|
| **1,8-Cineole** | 40%–60% |
| **Linalool** | 0.5%–16% |
| **Alpha-Terpinyl Acetate** | 5%–15% |
| **Sabinene** | 5%–12% |
| **Beta-Pinene** | 3%–8% |
| **Alpha-Pinene** | 3%–8% |
| **Camphene** | 0.1%–8% |
| **Alpha-Terpineol** | 1%–5% |
| **Terpinen-4-ol** | 1%–5% |
| **Para-Cymene** | 0.5%–5% |
| **Limonene** | 0.1%–5% |
| **Methyl Eugenol** | < 5% |

**REPORTED THERAPEUTIC PROPERTIES: Analgesic (pain relief)**, anti-inflammatory, anesthetic, antibacterial, **antimicrobial**, antifungal, antirheumatic, antiseptic, anticancer, antispasmodic, antineuralgic, **stimulates lymph flow**, reduces fever, **expels excess mucus**, decongestant, promotes the discharge of bile, reduces inflamed glands, expels excess gas, stimulates the appetite, diuretic, sedating, warming, aids focus and concentration, **enhances confidence**, reduces mental confusion

**CAUTIONS:**

■ Avoid in children under age 12 due to the multisite cancerous tumors and DNA mutation caused by methyl eugenol in animal studies.[840,841,842,843] 1,8-cineole may cause seizures, central nervous system problems, or respiratory distress in young children.[844,845,846,847]

■ Avoid during pregnancy and lactation due to changes in embryo form and structure and chromosomal changes in ovary cells caused by methyl eugenol as well as the carcinogenic (cancer-causing) potential of methyl eugenol.[848,849,850,851] Very large doses of methyl eugenol may adversely affect the mother's liver and infant body weight according to animal research.[852]

■ Avoid oral consumption due to the multisite carcinogenic potential of methyl eugenol.[853,854,855,856]

■ May interact with aspirin, blood pressure, antiplatelet, and anticoagulant medications, and increase the risk of bleeding among people with bleeding disorders (low risk).[857] 1,8-cineole is a weak inhibitor of platelet aggregation.[858]

■ May interact with diabetic medications due to the ability of 1,8-cineole to significantly inhibit alpha-glucosidase activity, particularly when synergized with other constituents (alpha-pinene and beta-pinene).[859,860,861] Alpha-glucosidase is an enzyme that breaks down carbohydrates by chemical reaction with water. Inhibiting its activity postpones glucose absorption and therefore the impact of carbohydrates on blood sugar levels.

■ Avoid with epilepsy and Parkinson's disease due to 1,8-cineole content. May exacerbate or cause seizures or convulsions when inhaled, applied topically, or ingested based on 1,8-cineole content.[862,863,864,865,866,867] One animal study suggests that bay laurel essential oil is anticonvulsive, but the totality of evidence suggests high 1,8-cineole essential oils may be convulsive in people prone to seizures.[868]

■ Bay laurel may cause motor impairment according to animal studies.[869] Do not drive or operate machinery while using.

■ May interfere with pentobarbital and other barbiturates (medications for anxiety/insomnia) based on 1,8-cineole content.[870,871]

■ May interact with antibiotics or antifungal drugs and possibly enhance their effects based on methyl eugenol content.[872]

■ May be mildly photosensitizing (bay laurel absolute only).[873] Avoid sun exposure to area of application for at least twelve hours after topical application.

**SELECTED EVIDENCE:**

☐ Bay laurel may prevent the spread of myeloid leukemia and breast cancer cells according to *in vitro* research.[874,875] Other research has found that it may help destroy leukemia, melanoma, and kidney cancer cells.[876,877]

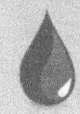

- Animal research suggests that bay laurel provides analgesic and anti-inflammatory effects comparable to the drugs morphine and piroxicam.[878]

- Inhaling bay laurel may improve careful concentration and attention to task performance (something critical to reading, writing, learning, and social behavior).[879]

- Bay laurel significantly inhibits the acetylcholinesterase enzyme from breaking down acetylcholine.[880] This activity may benefit a number of neurological disorders including Alzheimer's disease, myasthenia gravis, Lewy body dementia, and schizophrenia.

- Bay laurel effectively inhibits the common bacteria *S. aureus, Enterococcus faecalis, S. epidermidis, E. coli, L. monocytogenes, S. typhimurium,* and *Pseudomonas aeruginosa*.[881,882] It is also active against the SARS-coronavirus (SARS-CoV).[883]

- *In vitro* research demonstrates that bay laurel berry essential oil (Beta-ocimene – 21.8%, 1,8-cineole – 9.4%, alpha-pinene – 3.7%, and beta-pinene – 2.1%) inhibited the SARS coronavirus (SARS-CoV) and herpes simplex virus (HSV-1).[884]

- An interesting bay laurel essential oil with isoeugenol as the primary constituent inhibits *C. albicans* and prevents its biofilm formation.[885] The 1,8-cineole CT of bay laurel essential oil inhibited thirteen filamentous fungi *in vitro*.[886]

- Bay laurel essential oil killed neuroblastoma cancer cells.[887]

- *In vitro* research demonstrates that bay laurel essential oil inhibits *B. cereus, S. aureus, E. coli,* and *P. aeruginosa* better than 1,8-cineole alone.[888] The same researchers reports that bay laurel essential oil inhibits *A. niger, A. versicolor, P. citrinum,* and *P. expansum*.

- Human aryl hydrocarbon receptor (AhR: a gene that encodes a protein that helps regulate responses to planar aromatic hydrocarbons and significantly affects the immune activity in the gastrointestinal tract) regulates the circadian rhythm, helps regulate the cell cycle, and plays an important role in tissue development. Cumin, jasmine, vanilla, and bay leaf fully activate AhR; clove, dill, thyme, nutmeg, and oregano partially activate AhR; and tarragon, caraway, turmeric, lovage, fennel, spearmint, star anise, and anise inhibit the AhR activity.[889]

- Fractions (FR1: sabinene 37.8%, beta-pinene 13.5%, 1,8-cineole 12.7%, and alpha-pinene 12.6%; FR8: alpha-terpineol 79.2%) efficiently controlled cattle tick (*Rhipicephalus microplus*) adults and larvae.[890]

- Bay laurel leaf, twig, and fruit (1,8-cineole CTs) oils exhibited antimicrobial activity, with the leaf oil demonstrating the best activity.[891] The leaf oil inhibited *S. aureus, B. subtilis, K. rhizophila, S. abony, S. cerevisiae, C. albicans,* and *A. brasiliensis*; fruit oil *S. aureus, K. rhizophila, S. abony, S. cerevisiae,* and *A. brasiliensis*; and the tig-oil-only *S. aureus*.

- Cinnamon leaf CT eugenol, bay laurel CT camphene, guava leaf CT caryophyllene oxide, and Monterey cypress CT alpha-pinene essential oils each inhibited glycation—the nonenzymatic bonding of lipids to sugars creating advanced glycation end products—in laboratory research.[892] Damage caused by glycation can lead to stiffening of the blood vessel walls and high blood pressure, particularly among diabetics.

- Allspice CT eugenol, bay laurel CT camphene, betle CT safrole, and kaffir lime peel, exhibited varying degrees of antioxidant activity in multiple assays (DPPH, XO, NO, ABTS).[893]

- Of five essential oils tested (bay laurel, thyme, peppermint, lemongrass, and *Lippia junelliana*), bay laurel and thyme were the most active against *Candida* species, including species that were drug resistant.[894]

- The 1,8-cineole CT of bay laurel significantly inhibited *M. luteus, S. aureus, B. subtilis, E. coli, P. aeruginosa, K. pneumoniae,* and *Candida* species and improved the antimicrobial effects of fluconazole, ciprofloxacin, and vancomycin.[895]

- A comparison of hydrodistilled and steam-distilled bay laurel essential oil determined that while hydrodistillation increases yield, steam distillation produces a more bioactive oil.[896] The steam-distilled oil exhibited greater antioxidant and antimicrobial activity.

- Type 2 diabetes can be managed by inhibiting the carbohydrate-hydrolyzing enzymes alpha-amylase and alpha-glucosidase, which decreases spikes in blood sugar after a meal. A laboratory study found that eucalyptus (*E. radiata*), bay laurel, and nutmeg (West Indian) essential oils each inhibited alpha-amylase comparably to acarbose (an alpha-amylase and alpha-glucosidase inhibiting drug used to control blood sugar levels in people with type 2 diabetes).[897] Remarkably, eucalyptus and nutmeg essential oils displayed higher activity than acarbose. Another study reported that the 1,8-cineole CT of bay laurel essential oil inhibited both alpha-amylase and alpha-glucosidase, and inhibited lipase (suggesting it may have antiobesity activity by reducing the absorption of fats in the gastrointestinal tract).[898] The same researchers reported that the oil

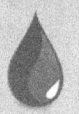

inhibited acetylcholinesterase (antidementia activity), and significantly reduces inflammation (5-LOX and in rats), and possesses antimicrobial activity (*C. albicans, L. monocytogenes, S. aureus, B. subtilis, E. coli, P. mirabilis, A. niger, T. rubrum, S. typhimurium,* and *P. aeruginosa*).

☐ Bay laurel CT 1,8-cineole inhibited *S. faecalis, S. aureus, P. mirabilis, E. coli,* and *P. aeruginosa,* with the greatest activity observed against *S. faecalis* and *S. aureus.*[899]

☐ *In vitro* research showed that bay laurel CT 1,8-cineole essential oil possesses broad-spectrum antifungal activity and remarkable antifungal activity in a food-model study (wheat) as well as good antioxidant activity in the DPPH assay and moderate antioxidant activity in the β-carotene bleaching assay.[900]

☐ Two bay laurel essential oils from Greece and Georgia (both 1,8-cineole CTs) inhibited bacteria (*E. faecalis, S. aureus, B. cereus, E. coli, S. abony, S. flexneri, L. monocytogenes,* and *K. pneumoniae*) and yeasts (*C. albicans, C. glabrata,* and *C. tropicalis*).[901] The oil from Greece exhibited far greater antimicrobial activity, which eclipsed the activity of ciprofloxacin for *E. faecalis, S. aureus,* and *S. abony* and was greater than fluconazole against *C. albicans* and *C. tropicalis.* The oil from Greece had higher levels of alpha-terpineol, terpinen-4-ol, gamma-terpinene, eugenol, and caryophyllene oxide, which may account for the greater antimicrobial activity.

☐ A 10% dilution of bay laurel essential oil caused 80.5 percent mortality among engorged female Asian blue ticks (*Rhipicephalus microplus*) after twenty-four hours, which reached 100 percent on day three.[902]

☐ A bay laurel essential oil (1,8-cineole CT) nanoemulsion was more active against bacteria than the free oil.[903]

☐ The 1,8-cineole CT of bay laurel essential oil was strongly acaricidal to ticks and mites that infest livestock and poultry (*Hyalomma scupense* and *Dermanyssus gallinae*).[904]

☐ Bay laurel essential oil CT 1,8-cineole loaded into polylactic-co-glycolic acid (PLGA) nanoparticles exhibited promise as a natural controlled-release cancer treatment.[905] The nano-bay laurel demonstrated dual inhibition of PI3K/mTOR—the main regulatory pathways of cancer—and antiproliferative activity of its major constituents (in descending order of binding affinity: methyleugenol, sabinene, 1,8-cineole, and alpha-terpinyl acetate) was confirmed in computer-based docking studies. All four constituents indicated very high-absorption and permeability properties in the Caco-2 and MDCK assays, suggesting high human oral absorption.

☐ Oral administration of bay laurel CT 1,8-cineole or myrtle CT 1,8-cineole (0.5 mL mixed in equal parts sunflower oil, for two weeks) was evaluated for their benefits on body weight control, antioxidant status, and lipid control in rats.[906] Both oils promoted weight loss, reduced blood glucose levels, and decreased lipid levels (total cholesterol, LDL, VLDL) and atherogenic indicators, leading to cardiovascular protection. Overall, bay laurel was more effective and considered an excellent candidate to combat obesity caused by medications due to its ability to inhibit enzymes responsible for conversion of carbohydrates into glucose and effects on lipid metabolism in the liver. This activity suggests that ingestion of bay laurel essential oil may result in weight loss. Myrtle exhibited better antioxidant capacity in most tissues, except for the kidneys where it caused a pro-oxidant effect. Myrtle also increased the permeability and instability of red blood cell membranes, which reduced their ability to decrease entry of toxic substances into the cell, and increased intestinal inflammation by reducing probiotic bacteria and increasing *Enterobacter* colonization.

☐ Bay laurel essential oil demonstrated insecticidal activity against the red flour beetle (*Tribolium castaneum*)[907]

☐ Bay laurel essential oil inhibited *A. niger, C. parapsilosis, C. krusei, C. glabrata, C. albicans, E. coli, K. pneumoniae, L. monocytogenes, S. enteritidis, P. aeruginosa, S. aureus, B. cereus, M. luteus, E. faecalis,* with its inhibition zones exceeding fluconazole against *A. niger,* and showing greater inhibition zones than ciprofloxacin against *E. coli, K. pneumoniae, L. monocytogenes, S. aureus,* and *E. faecalis.*[908]

☐ Cinnamon bark, clove bud, and bay laurel essential oils inhibited *L. monocytogenes, L. innocua, L. welshimeri, L. ivanovii, L. grayi,* and *V. parahaemolyticus,* with cinnamon bark being the most effective.[909]

*Did you know?*

Olfactory (smell) receptors have been identified in organs and tissues outside the olfactory system, including sperm cells, the heart, kidney, intestine, and testes. These receptors are involved in chemical reactions that adjust blood pressure, stimulate hormone secretion, trigger release of enzymes, direct the migration of cells in response to chemical stimuli and more.

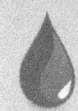

# BENZOIN ABSOLUTE
## (Gum Benjamin, Onycha)

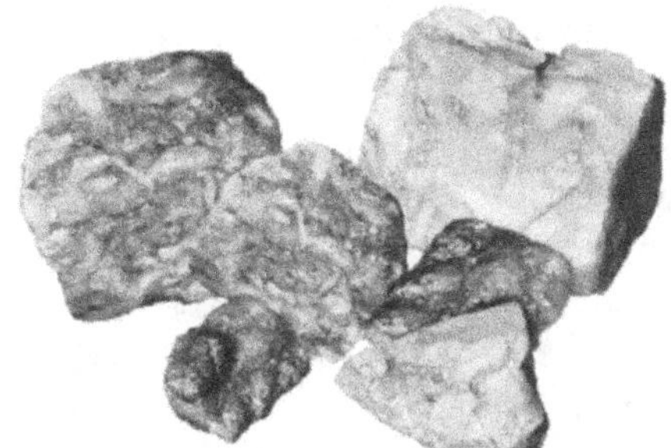

Sumatra Benzoin: *Styrax benzoin* Dryand., *S. paralelloneurus* Perkins;
Siam Benzoin: *S. tonkinensis* Pierre

**FAMILY:** Styracaceae
**NOTE:** Base
**AROMA INTENSITY:** Medium
**AROMA:** Rich, slightly woody, hint of vanilla
**COMMON EXTRACTION METHOD:** Solvent extracted from the oleoresin; also hydrodistilled from the oleoresin
**POSSIBLE SUBSTITUTE OILS:** Copaiba, Peru balsam, tolu balsam, frankincense
**BLENDS WELL WITH:** Bergamot, black pepper, copaiba, coriander, frankincense, ginger, juniper berry, Phoenician juniper, lavender, lemon, lime, myrrh, orange, petitgrain, rose, sandalwood
**SUBCELLULAR LOCALIZATION | EPIGENETIC INFLUENCE:** Currently unknown | Currently unknown
**RECOMMENDED DILUTION RANGE:** 1.0%–3.0%

**PRIMARY CONSTITUENTS:**[910,911,912,913,914]

*Sumatra Benzoin Absolute*

| | |
|---|---|
| Benzyl Benzoate | 50.7% |
| Benzyl Alcohol | 43.4% |

*Siam Benzoin Absolute*

| | |
|---|---|
| Benzyl Benzoate | 39.3% |
| Benzyl Alcohol | 38.8% |
| Benzoic Acid | 18.4% |

*Sumatra Benzoin Absolute (Ethanol)*

| | |
|---|---|
| Undetermined Non-volatiles[#] | 19.0%–40.0% |
| Cinnamic Acid | 16.0%–26.0% |
| P-Coumaryl Acetate[#] | 5.0%–23.0% |
| Undetermined Volatiles | 6.0%–20.0% |
| Cinnamyl Cinnamate[#] | 5.0%–8.0% |
| Benzoic Acid | 2.0%–4.0% |

*Siam Benzoin Absolute (Ethanol)*

| | |
|---|---|
| Coniferyl Benzoate[#] | 29.0%–56.0% |
| Benzoic Acid | 31.0%–36.0% |
| Undetermined Volatiles | 0.0%–20.0% |
| Undetermined Nonvolatiles[#] | 1.0%–10.0% |
| Coniferyl Derivatives[#] | 5.0%–5.0% |

*Siam Benzoin Absolute (S-HS, Grades 3 and 5)*

| | |
|---|---|
| Toluene[#] | 5.2%–79.6% |
| Benzaldehyde | 10.2%–46.8% |
| Methyl Benzoate | 6.2%–17.5% |
| Benzyl Alcohol | 0.9%–6.9% |
| 1,8-Cineole | 0.5%–5.5% |
| Benzyl Formate | 0.5%–3.7% |

*Sumatra Benzoin Hydrodistilled*

| | |
|---|---|
| Benzyl Benzoate | 76.1% |
| Cinnamic Acid | 3.5% |
| Benzyl Cinnamate | 3.3% |

*Siam Benzoin Hydrodistilled*

| | |
|---|---|
| Benzyl Benzoate | 80.1% |
| Benzoic Acid | 12.5% |

*Sumatra Benzoin Absolute (SPME)*

| | |
|---|---|
| Styrene | 72.4%–89.0% |
| Benzoic Acid | 2.1%–6.3% |
| Benzaldehyde | 3.1%–4.5% |

*Siam Benzoin Absolute (SPME, Grades 3 and 5)*

| | |
|---|---|
| Toluene[#] | 1.7%–28.5% |
| Methyl Benzoate | 22.0%–27.7% |
| Benzaldehyde | 17.3%–21.9% |
| Benzoic Acid | 8.5%–15.3% |
| Vanillin | 4.3%–8.0% |
| Benzyl Alcohol | 3.3%–6.7% |
| Alpha-Pinene | 1.8%–6.6% |

*Sumatra Benzoin Absolute (S-HS)*

| | |
|---|---|
| Styrene | 90.0%–93.2% |
| Benzaldehyde | 4.7%–6.6% |

*Sumatra Benzoin Absolute (HSSE)*

| | |
|---|---|
| Styrene | 83.4%–93.1% |
| Benzaldehyde | 3.5%–6.0% |

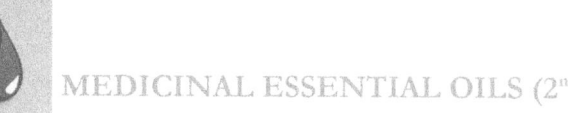

*Siam Benzoin Absolute*
*(HSSE, Grades 3 and 5)*

| | |
|---|---|
| Benzaldehyde | 15.0%–30.2% |
| Methyl Benzoate | 17.7%–21.9% |
| Benzyl Alcohol | 1.8%–12.3% |
| Benzoic Acid | 1.1%–6.8% |
| Vanillin | 2.6%–6.1% |
| Benzyl Benzoate | 0.7%–4.8% |

*S. benzoin Absolute*
*(Dichloromethane Solvent, Grades 1 and 3)*

| | |
|---|---|
| P-Coumaryl Benzoate[#] | 30.5%–52.2% |
| Benzoic Acid | 19.2%–28.2% |
| Coniferyl Benzoate[#] | 15.6%–18.2% |
| Cinnamic Acid | 1.8%–7.5% |

*S. paralleloneurum Absolute (Dichloromethane Solvent, Grades 1 and 3)*

| | |
|---|---|
| P-Coumaryl Cinnamate[#] | 52.5%–74.1% |
| Cinnamic Acid | 5.7%–23.2% |
| Cinnamyl Cinnamate[#] | 4.6%–6.8% |
| P-Coumaryl Benzoate[#] | 1.3%–3.3% |

[#] Non-volatile components.

Note: Differences in extraction method (static-headspace (S-HS), headspace-solid-phase microextraction (SPME), headspace sorptive extraction (HSSE), solvent, and hydrodistillation) can dramatically alter the chemical composition or benzoin absolute. Benzoin is not a true essential oil due to its extraction methods.

**OTHER CONSTITUENTS:** *Sumatra Benzoin Absolute*—cinnamyl cinnamate, cinnamic acid, ethyl cinnamate, benzoic acid; *Siam Benzoin Absolute*—ethyl cinnamate; *Sumatra Benzoin Hydrodistilled*—styrene, benzaldehyde, acetophenone, methyl benzoate, benzoic acid, allyl benzoate, 4-ethylguaiacol, eugenol, allyl cinnamate, cinnamyl benzoate; *Siam Benzoin Hydrodistilled*—methyl benzoate, ethyl benzoate, allyl benzoate, eugenol; *Sumatra Benzoin Absolute (Ethanol)*—N/A; *Siam Benzoin Absolute (Ethanol)*—N/A; *Siam Benzoin Absolute (S-HS, Grades 3 and 5)*—styrene, beta-pinene, nonanol, benzoic acid, propyl benzoate, alpha-copaene, benzyl benzoate; *Sumatra Benzoin Absolute (S-HS)*—para-cymene; *Siam Benzoin Absolute (SPME, Grades 3 and 5)*—formic acid, acetic acid, hexanal, para-cymene, benzyl formate, ethyl benzoate, isobutyl benzoate, benzyl benzoate; *Sumatra Benzoin Absolute (SPME)*—formic acid, para-cymene, 1,8-cineole, acetophenone, (E)-cinnamaldehyde; *Siam Benzoin Absolute (HSSE, Grades 3 and 5)*—limonene, benzyl formate, nonanol, ethyl benzoate, propyl benzoate, eugenol; *Sumatra Benzoin Absolute (HSSE)*—para-cymene, acetophenone, p-ethylphenol; *S. benzoin Absolute (Dichloromethane Solvent, Grade 1 and 3)*—cinnamyl benzoate, p-coumaryl cinnamate, benzoic acid esters; *S. paralleloneurum Absolute (Dichloromethane Solvent, Grade 1 and 3)*—benzoic acid, benzyl cinnamate, coniferyl benzoate, coniferyl cinnamate, cinnamic acid esters

**PREFERRED COMPOSITION FOR CLINICAL USE:**

| *Constituent* | *Sumatra* | *Siam* |
|---|---|---|
| **Benzyl Benzoate** | 45%–55% | 35%–45% |
| **Benzyl Alcohol** | 35%–45% | 35%–45% |
| **Benzoic Acid** | – | 10%–20% |

**REPORTED THERAPEUTIC PROPERTIES:** Antibacterial, antimicrobial, antifungal, antiseptic, disinfectant, antioxidant, anti-inflammatory, analgesic, antirheumatic, stimulates hormone release from various organs, aids immune function, supports respiratory function, eases cough, expels excess mucus, astringent, **wound healing**, diuretic, aids circulation, promotes restful sleep, calming/relaxing, **sedating**, antidepressant, stress management

**CAUTIONS:**

■ Avoid oral consumption. Absolutes contain solvent residue and should not be taken orally. In addition, salicylic acid (the active metabolite of aspirin) is rapidly created (synthesized) from benzoic acid when ingested.[915]

■ May interact with aspirin, blood pressure, antiplatelet, and anticoagulant medications, and increase the risk of bleeding among people with bleeding disorders (low risk) due to due to benzoic acid and 1,8-cineole content.[916,917] *Sumatra Benzoin Absolute*

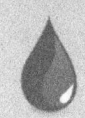

*(Ethanol):* May interact with statins due to significant cinnamic acid content. Cinnamic acid significantly inhibits rosuvastatin transport in to bile and increases the plasma exposure.[918]

■ May interact with antibiotics and possibly enhance their effects based on (E)-cinnamic acid content.[919,920,921]

■ The maximum dilution percentage of 3.0% should not be exceeded during topical application due to presence of solvents and reports of contact dermatitis caused by benzoin extracts.[922,923,924,925,926]

**SELECTED EVIDENCE:**

☐ *In vitro* research demonstrates that Siam benzoin inhibits the fungus *A. niger* and, to a lesser extent, *A. flavus* and *A. parasiticus*.[927,928]

## BERGAMOT

*Citrus bergamia* Risso & Poit., *C.* × *aurantium* subsp. *bergamia* (Risso & Poit) Wight & Arn. ex Engl.

**FAMILY:** Rutaceae (Citrus)
**NOTE:** Top
**AROMA INTENSITY:** Medium
**AROMA:** Citrusy, fruity, fresh, sweet
**COMMON EXTRACTION METHOD:** Cold-pressed/expressed or hydrodistilled from the fruit peel (rind)
**POSSIBLE SUBSTITUTE OILS:** Neroli, lime, lemon, grapefruit
**BLENDS WELL WITH:** Bay leaf, balsam fir, black pepper, cardamom, carrot seed, cassia, coriander, cedarwood, chamomile (Roman, German), camphor, cypress, clary sage, fennel, frankincense, geranium, helichrysum, lavender, lemon, lemon verbena, lime, neroli, niaouli, nutmeg, palmarosa, petitgrain, ravensara, sage, Spanish sage, vetiver, ylang ylang
**SUBCELLULAR LOCALIZATION | EPIGENETIC INFLUENCE:** Cytoplasm | Skeletal/Integumentary
**RECOMMENDED DILUTION RANGE:** 5%–50%; neat for limited conditions

**PRIMARY CONSTITUENTS:**[929,930,931,932]

| *Cold-pressed/expressed* | | *Distilled* | |
|---|---|---|---|
| Limonene | 10.5%–53.2% | Limonene | 31.7%–59.2% |
| Linalyl Acetate | 15.6%–40.5% | Linalool | 9.5%–31.8% |
| Linalool | 1.8%–20.3% | Linalyl Acetate | 10.7%–16.8% |
| Beta-Pinene | 0.1%–12.1% | Gamma-Terpinene | 0.1%–10.3% |
| Gamma-Terpinene | 4.3%–11.4% | Beta-Pinene | 0.8%–4.4% |

**OTHER CONSTITUENTS:** *Cold-pressed/expressed*—Alpha-pinene, beta-myrcene, beta-pinene, sabinene, beta-bisabolene, neryl acetate, alpha-bergamotene, terpinolene, neral, geranial, trans-caryophyllene, valencene, bergamottin; *Distilled*—Alpha-pinene, myrcene, alpha-terpineol, geraniol, geranyl acetate, alpha-bergamotene, beta-bisabolene

**PREFERRED COMPOSITION FOR CLINICAL USE:**

| Constituent | Cold-Pressed | Calabrian* | Distilled |
|---|---|---|---|
| **Limonene** | 30%–45% | 25%–55% | 35%–58% |
| **Linalyl Acetate** | 25%–38% | 15%–41% | 10%–20% |
| **Linalool** | 5%–18% | 2%–20% | 15%–25% |
| **Gamma-Terpinene** | 5%–10% | 5%–12% | 5%–10% |
| **Beta-Pinene** | 4%–10% | 4%–13% | 1%–5% |
| **Alpha-Pinene** | 0.1%–2% | 0.5%–2% | 0.1%–2% |
| **Sabinene** | 0.1%–2% | – | 0%–2% |
| **Beta-Myrcene** | 0.1%–2% | 0.5%–2% | 0.1%–2% |
| **Geranial** | 0.1%–1% | 0.2%–0.5% | – |
| **Beta-Bisabolene** | tr–1% | 0.3%–0.7% | – |

* Some experts consider cold-pressed bergamot essential oil from Calabria, Italy to be the highest quality.[933]

**REPORTED THERAPEUTIC PROPERTIES:** Stimulates hormone release, antibacterial, disinfectant, analgesic (pain relief), anti-inflammatory, **aids digestion**, reduces appearance of blemishes, **supports endothelial and cardiovascular function**, reduces fever, anticancer, antiparasitic, antispasmodic, wound healing, **relieves sore throat**, **antiseptic**, encourages a restful night's sleep, evens skin tone, decongestant, **antidepressant**, relaxing, sedating, uplifting, helps release suppressed negative emotions, **relieves anxiety**, combats aggression, reduces insecurity, despondency, and loneliness, reduces mood swings

**CAUTIONS:**

■ Very photosensitizing due to bergapten, bergamottin, psoralen, and citropten content; do not expose skin to UV rays for up to twenty-four hours following topical application.[934,935]

■ May interfere with the enzymes responsible for drug metabolism (NSAIDs, proton-pump inhibitors, acetaminophen, antiepileptics, immune modulators, blood-sugar medications, blood pressure medications, antidepressants, antipsychotics, diabetic medications, antihistamines, antibiotics, and anesthetics).[936]

■ May interact with anticholinergic (drugs used for asthma, incontinence, gastrointestinal cramps, muscular spasms, depression, and sleep disorders) and cholinergic medications (drugs used to reduce urinary retention, diagnose myasthenia gravis, and for glaucoma) based on AChE inhibitory activity.[937]

**SELECTED EVIDENCE:**

☐ Bergamot may enhance autophagy (the body's housekeeping process to remove cellular waste and pathogens, and maintain balanced sources of energy).[938]

☐ Two of the major components of bergamot, limonene and linalyl acetate, are reported to play leading roles in bergamot's ability to trigger neuroblastoma cancer-cell death.[939] Bergamot may prevent the spread and promote the death of neuroblastomas.[940,941,942]

☐ Bergamot influences calcium ion activity and endothelial inflammation to promote relaxation of the blood vessel walls (vasorelaxation), which may decrease blood pressure.[943,944,945,946] Another study found that inhaling lavender, ylang ylang, and bergamot oils once daily for four weeks reduced cortisol levels, psychological stress, and blood pressure in people with essential hypertension.[947]

☐ Bergamot may help reduce skin inflammation and therefore chronic inflammatory conditions of the skin.[948]

☐ Bergamot may prevent the spread of melanoma cancer cells.[949]

☐ *In vitro* research suggests that bergamot inhibits several mycoplasmas (bacteria that lack a cell wall, which makes them resistant to several common antibiotics) including *M. hominis, M. pneumoniae,* and *M. fermentans.*[950]

☐ Bergamot profoundly influences the nervous system to help reduce anxiety, correct mild mood disorders, protect against brain injury/damage, and reduce pain (including pain caused by something that normally would not cause pain).[951,952,953,954,955,956]

☐ Clinical research shows that inhalation of bergamot may reduce stress, depression, negative emotions, anxiety, and fatigue.[957,958,959,960] [299–302]

☐ Animal research suggests that bergamot essential oil reduces the hypothalamic-pituitary-adrenal axis (HPA) response to stress by reducing corticosterone release, which makes it a valuable remedy for anxiety and stress management.[961]

☐ A hand massage with equal parts of frankincense, bergamot, and lavender (as a 1.5% dilution with sweet almond carrier oil) reduced the pain and depression of hospice patients with terminal cancer.[962]

☐ *In vitro* research suggests that bergamot oil inhibits acetylcholinesterase (AChE) and butyrylcholinesterase (BChE) enzyme activity.[963] Inhibition of AChE prevents the breakdown of acetylcholine, which is essential for memory and thinking. People with neurodegenerative diseases make less acetylcholine, and the diseases often break it down at a faster rate leading to acetylcholine deficits. Selective inhibition of BChE is also desirable in neurodegenerative diseases because it interferes with acetylcholine activity. In addition, BChE is often found in the plaques and tangles in the brains of people with Alzheimer's disease.[964]

☐ *In vitro* research suggests that vapors of a combination of bergamot and orange essential oils inhibit the growth of drug-resistant and drug-sensitive strains of *E. faecalis* and *E. faecium.*[965] Another study determined that bergamot

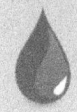

and orange oil kill and inhibit the growth of these bacteria by affecting the cell membrane and cell homeostasis.[966]

☐ Inhalation from personal aromasticks containing either bergamot and sandalwood, or frankincense, tangerine, and lavender essential oils improved sleep quality among cancer patients.[967] Remarkably, 92% of study participants indicated they would continue to use their aromasticks for sleep improvement.

☐ Bergamot essential oil kills the larvae of the mosquito that carries arbovirus (*Aedes albopictus*).[968] Bergamot essential oil demonstrated 84.9%–90.5% efficacy against the *Rhipicephalus microplus* tick depending on the concentration used (1%–10%).[969]

☐ A preclinical model of chronic skin inflammation demonstrates that bergamot essential oil inhibits protein molecules involved in inflammation, immune responses, and tissue remodeling, which suggests that it reduces skin inflammation and promotes wound healing.[970]

☐ Lemon, bergamot, and bitter orange were the most effective of citrus oils (lemon, bitter orange, bergamot, sweet orange, and mandarin) tested in the inhibition of mycelial growth of *A. flavus*.[971] These three oils also were most effective at reducing aflatoxin B1 production.

☐ Researchers found that bergamot exerts an antianxiety effect that works outside of interaction with gamma-aminobutyric acid type A receptors in rats, suggesting it doesn't work on the same pathway as benzodiazepines.[972]

☐ The process of autophagy—a process in the body that removes damaged cells in order to regenerate newer, healthier cells—is impaired in chronic pain conditions, particularly neuropathic pain. Activation of autophagy has been shown to reduce chronic pain in various models. A review study highlighted how bergamot essential oil reduced pain partly by enhancing autophagy and also enhanced the pain-relieving effects of morphine.[973]

☐ Research suggests that bergamot, lemon, and myrtle-leaved orange essential oil may act as green weed control agents. Depending on the oil used, they reduced the germination and radical elongation of *R. sativus, L. sativa, S. lycopersicum, L. sativum, L. multiflorum*, and *P. oleracea*.[974]

☐ Serotonergic (5-HT) neurotransmission plays a significant role in anxiety, particularly the 5-HT1A subtype. Research showed that bergamot essential oil modulates 5-HT1A activity as a selective agonist ((±)8-OH-DPAT) or antagonist (WAY-100635) that may partly explain the anxiety-relieving effects of bergamot oil.

☐ FCF (furanocoumarin free) bergamot essential oil significantly reduced pain and inflammation by reducing proinflammatory chemicals (IL-1β, IL-6, TNF-α, nitrite/nitrate, and PGE2).[975] In addition, bergamot oil displayed good antioxidant activity.

☐ Bergamot essential oil killed oral bacteria (*P. micra, S. intermedius, Veillonella* sp., and *Peptostreptococcus* sp.) without harming gingival cells at lower concentrations.[976] Nutmeg, cajeput, cypress, citronella (*C. winterianus*), myrtle (red), dwarf pine, gully gum, black pepper CT delta-3-carene, pine, eucalyptus (*E. globulus*) peppermint, and rosemary CT 1,8-cineole each exhibited varying degrees of antimicrobial activity against the oral bacteria as well. Dwarf pine, citronella, pine, eucalyptus, and peppermint oils also displayed low toxicity to gingival cells at low concentrations.

☐ Both bergamot and grapefruit essential oil showed anthelmintic activity against *Haemonchus contortus* in laboratory research.[977]

☐ Laboratory research confirmed that bergamottin (BRG) and 5-geranyloxy-7-methoxycoumarin (5G7M) are important constituents in bergamot oil for its anticancer activity against neuroblastoma, and that the natural ratio of these constituents found in bergamot oil creates the highest synergistic activity of BRG and 5G7M against neuroblastoma.[978]

☐ Headaches are common among emergency and critical care nurses, and headaches occur among nurses at a higher rate than in the general population. A study evaluated the benefits of inhaling essential oils on headache occurrence among nurses.[979] Nurses wore a necklace with lavender and bergamot essential oil (0.1 mL of each) for twenty-eight days. Although no reduction in headache was observed, the nurses did show significant improvement in their overall quality of life, especially in relation to their workplace roles and responsibilities.

☐ A placebo-controlled clinical study evaluated the benefits of an abdominal massage with lavender and bergamot essential oil on mood and mental state.[980] One mL of the blend consisting of 9.6% lavender, 0.4% bergamot, and 90% sweet almond carrier oil was self-massaged into the lower abdomen for five minutes, followed by covering the area with a plastic film to prevent evaporation. Compared to the control group (sweet almond oil only), the essential oil group experienced significant reductions in heart rate and blood pressure (systolic and diastolic) and rated themselves as more calm/relaxed.

☐ Prostaglandins play an important role in primary dysmenorrhea (PD: painful menstruation including cramping in the lower abdomen at the onset of menstruation without an identifiable cause). Research suggests that women who experience severe menstrual pain have higher levels of prostaglandin PGF2alpha and PGE2. Administration of bergamot essential oil—via gastric perfusion—reduced symptoms of PD (pain and uterine tissue alterations) in rats by reducing PGF2alpha and PGE2 levels, decreasing the inflammatory response (inhibit the release of inducible nitric oxide), and diminishing oxidative stress in uterine tissues (reduces MDA and increases antioxidant activities—T-AOC, SOD, CAT, and GSH).[981] The essential oil was more effective than bergamot juice and ethanol extract.

☐ Roughly 10–20 percent of new mothers experience postpartum depression. It is believed that postpartum depression stems from dramatic hormone changes that occur during and after childbirth. A randomized controlled clinical study evaluated the benefits of bergamot aromatherapy to improve mood and alleviate sleep challenges in postpartum women.[982] The bergamot group inhaled bergamot essential oil (4 drops in 15 mL of water dispersed from an ultrasonic diffuser) for fifteen minutes daily in the afternoon over the course of four weeks, while the control group inhaled 15 mL of water from a diffuser. What the researchers found was that depression was significantly lower in the bergamot group, but sleep quality did not change. The results of the study suggest that inhaling bergamot essential oil during the critical month after childbirth could reduce the severity of postpartum depression. Another study confirmed these results, showing that bergamot inhalation is effective in reducing postpartum depression.[983]

☐ Researchers investigated the effects of emulsions of bergamot, sweet orange, and clove essential oils in healthy and cancerous cells.[984] Clove essential oil emulsion was toxic to both healthy (keratinocytes and gingival fibroblasts) and cancerous (melanoma and oral squamous carcinoma) cells in a dose-dependent manner. Sweet orange oil emulsion increased healthy (keratinocytes) and cancerous (melanoma) cells but reduced proliferation of gingival fibroblasts and squamous carcinoma cells at the highest concentration. Bergamot oil emulsion decreased viability of squamous carcinoma cells. Combining sweet orange and clove oil emulsions increased their activity against tumor cell lines, and combining bergamot and orange essential oil emulsions also increased their anticancer activity with little effect on skin cells.

☐ Human monoamine oxidases (MAOs) are a family of enzymes that are well-established targets for the management of neurological disorders such as depression, Alzheimer's disease, and Parkinson's disease. Although both MAO forms break down all monoamines, MAO-A preferentially metabolizes noradrenaline, melatonin, and serotonin, while MAO-B preferentially metabolizes dopamine, benzylamine, phenylethylamine, and phenylethanolamine. Inhibition of MAOs allows monoamine brain chemicals to apply their effects for longer and can minimize the symptoms of neurological disorders. Molecular-modeling simulations found that constituents in bergamot inhibit MAOs—one furocoumarin (bergamottin) found in the essential oil and three flavones (nobiletin, sinensetin, and tangeritin) in the fruit and juice.[985] Among the identified constituents, bergamottin significantly and preferentially inhibited MAO-B but also inhibited MAO-A in computer-based models and experimental assays. The researchers concluded that administration of bergamot oil could limit oxidative stress in brain neuronal cells and potentially prevent neurodegenerative conditions. Of particular interest would be Parkinson's disease since MAO-B inhibitors are used in its treatment.

☐ Irritable bowel syndrome (IBS) is a painful condition at least partially caused by neurotransmitter dysfunction in the enteric nervous system (ENS: the nervous system within the gut) leading to weak or strong muscular contractions in the intestines. Strong contractions can make food pass though the digestive system too fast, resulting in diarrhea. On the other hand, if contractions are weak, constipation can occur. A preclinical model found that bergamot essential oil influences ENS activity to reduce intestinal spasms (strong contractions), making it a promising candidate to manage IBS.[986]

☐ Physical fatigue is characterized by a temporary decrease in body functions, which can be caused by strenuous physical work, excessive exercise, or continuous long-term study or physical activity. Exercise-induced fatigue occurs due to energy depletion (exhaustion of glucose and glycogen stores), metabolite accumulation (lactic acid, which impairs muscle contractility and promotes muscle fatigue; blood urea nitrogen, which is associated with fatigue), oxidative stress (can damage cell membranes and trigger muscle injury), and inflammatory responses (aggravate fatigue). A preclinical study evaluated whether inhaling citrus essential oils—sweet orange, lemon, and bergamot—can reduce exercise-induced fatigue and have any effects of exercise performance.[987] Sweet orange and lemon essential oil improved exercise performance (swimming time) by 276 percent and 46.5 percent in rats respectively, but bergamot had no effect of performance. However, bergamot showed the greatest ability to reduce exercise-induced fatigue (increased muscle glycogen levels, regulated blood glucose, decreased blood urea nitrogen, inhibited oxidative stress, and protecting muscles against injury caused by free radicals). The researchers identified constituents in bergamot—limonene, linalyl butyrate, and linalool—that were positively associated with relieving exercise-induced fatigue.

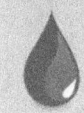

- Alzheimer's disease (AD) is the most prevalent type of dementia, and the number of people living with it is expected to triple by 2050. The progressive memory loss and behavioral changes over years is a painful process for those with AD and their families and caregivers. A randomized controlled clinical trial investigated the effects of aromatherapy (sleep quality, neuropsychiatric behavioral disorders, quality of life, and biochemical measures) for people with AD.[988] Six drops of a blend of lavender, sweet orange, and bergamot essential oils (2 drops of each) were added to 200 mL of water in a diffuser, which was operated every night at 9:00 p.m. for one hour over a twelve-week period. The control group inhaled from a diffuser with water only. Inhaling the essential oil blend improved sleep quality, alleviated psychobehavioral symptoms, and improved overall quality of life. Biochemical evaluation also showed a decrease in oxidative stress (by increasing superoxide dismutase levels) and inflammation (decreased TNF-α and IL-6 levels). The biochemical results are noteworthy because oxidative stress and inflammation are linked to further deterioration of AD.

- Researchers evaluated the activity of bergamot, tea tree, star anise, and eucalyptus (*E. globulus*) against influenza virus type A (H1N1) while in vapor phase.[989] Both bergamot and tea tree essential oils strongly reduced the cytopathic (structural changes to cells after infection) of H1N1 without being toxic to healthy cells. Eucalyptus was moderately effective without being toxic to healthy cells, whereas star anise was inactive. Further evaluation of the mechanism that these essential oils reduced H1N1 infectivity found that the oils interfere with the lipid bilayer of the viral envelope triggering decomposition of membranes. This research suggests that diffusing essential oils, which creates a vapor, may help to reduce viral load and their potential to infect humans.

- A randomized, controlled trial evaluated the effects of mindfulness combined with topical application of an essential oil blend containing 5% lavender and 0.04% bergamot essential oils in an alcohol solution on sexual function, anxiety, and depression in postmenopausal women.[990] Two to three drops of the blend were applied to the forearm three times daily and inhaled from over an eight-week period. The aromatherapy-mindfulness group experienced improvements in sexual function, anxiety, and depression.

- A clinical trial found that inhaling bergamot essential oil from a diffuser reduced work-related stress in nurses (ICU, palliative care, general, and ob-gyn) depending on the department they worked in.[991] Five drops of bergamot oil were added to an ultrasonic diffuser, which was operated at the nursing station, twice daily, from 8:00 a.m. to 12:00 p.m. and 16:00 p.m. to 20:00 p.m. General nurses reported the greatest improvements in psychological perception, while ICU nurses did not experience improvements, and some objective measures were worse in these nurses. Ranking results in the various departments was as follows: general department > ob-gyn department > palliative care department > ICU.

- *In vitro* research showed that bergamot essential oil inhibits *S. typhimurium, B. cereus, S. aureus, E. coli, L. monocytogenes, P. expansum,* and *A. niger.*[992]

- Asthma is a chronic respiratory condition characterized by narrowing of the airways, lung inflammation, and physical changes to the airways (collagen deposition, membrane thickening, smooth muscle enlargement) over time. A laboratory model of asthma found that bergamot essential oil possesses antiasthmatic properties due to its improvement of lung inflammation and reduction of collagen deposition.

# BERGAMOT MINT
## (Water Mint, Bergamot-mint)
*Mentha aquatica* L., *Mentha citrata* Ehrh.

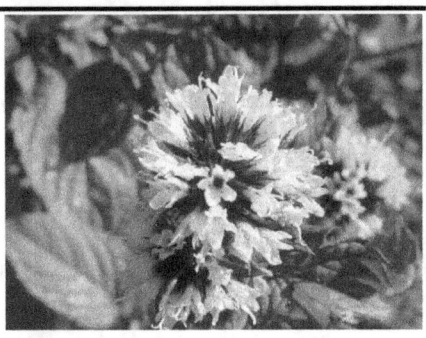

**FAMILY:** Lamiaceae (Labiatae)
**NOTE:** Top-Middle
**AROMA INTENSITY:** Medium
**AROMA:** Citrusy, fresh, minty
**COMMON EXTRACTION METHOD:** Steam or hydrodistilled from the leaves or flowering tops
**POSSIBLE SUBSTITUTE OILS:** Neroli, petitgrain, bergamot, lavender
**BLENDS WELL WITH:** Basil, bergamot, clary sage, geranium, lavender, lemon, lime, marjoram, neroli, orange (sweet), peppermint, petitgrain, rose, sage, spearmint, ylang ylang
**SUBCELLULAR LOCALIZATION | EPIGENETIC INFLUENCE:** Currently unknown | Currently unknown
**RECOMMENDED DILUTION RANGE:** 5%–50%; neat for limited conditions

**PRIMARY CONSTITUENTS:**[993,994,995]

| | |
|---|---|
| Linalool | 23.8%–67.9% |
| Linalyl Acetate | 4.8%–60.9% |
| Alpha-Terpineol | 1.5%–24.9% |

**OTHER CONSTITUENTS:** Alpha-pinene, beta-pinene, myrcene, n-Octanol, limonene, 1,8-cineole, (Z)-beta-ocimene, (E)-beta-ocimene, (Z)-linalool oxide, (E)-linalool oxide, menthol, nerol, neryl acetate, geranyl acetate, beta-caryophyllene, beta-boubonene, gamma-muurolene, elemol, viridiflorol, beta-eudesmol, trans-p-menth-1-en-ol, caryophyllene oxide

**PREFERRED COMPOSITION FOR CLINICAL USE:**

| *Constituent* | |
|---|---|
| **Linalool** | 33%–45% |
| **Linalyl Acetate** | 25%–45% |
| **Beta-Caryophyllene** | 1%–5% |
| **Alpha-Terpineol** | 0.5%–5% |
| **Geranyl Acetate** | 1%–3% |
| **Menthol** | 0.1%–3% |
| **(Z)-Beta-Ocimene** | 0.1%–3% |
| **(E)-Beta-Ocimene** | 0.1%–3% |
| **Beta-Myrcene** | 0.5%–2% |
| **Neryl Acetate** | 0.1%–2% |

**REPORTED THERAPEUTIC PROPERTIES: Antispasmodic**, analgesic, anti-inflammatory, antimicrobial, antifungal, antibacterial, antiviral, antiparasitic, antioxidant, aids immune function, relieves upset stomach, expels excess gas, reduces blood pressure, **wound healing**, relieves painful menstruation, reduces menopausal symptoms, stress management, sedating, **relieves anxiety**, aids mental clarity, antidepressant

**CAUTIONS:**

■ None currently known.

**SELECTED EVIDENCE:**

☐ *In vitro* research demonstrates that bergamot mint essential oil inhibits gram positive (*Staphylococcus aureus, S. epidermidis, Streptococcus mutans*) and gram negative (*Salmonella typhimurium, K. pneumonia*, two strains of *E. coli*, and *P. aeruginosa*) bacteria.[996]

☐ Bergamot mint essential oil is very toxic to the African cotton leafworm (*Spodoptera littoralis*).[997]

☐ Bergamot mint demonstrated promising cytotoxic activity on colon cancer cells in laboratory research.[998] The oil also exhibited antioxidant activity in the DPPH assay.

☐ Researchers analyzed the composition and antimicrobial activity of mint essential oils, including bergamot mint, peppermint, pennyroyal, spearmint, and apple mint. Bergamot mint inhibited *S. typhi* and *C. albicans*; peppermint *E. coli, B. subtilis*, and *C. albicans*; pennyroyal *K. pneumoniae, B. subtilis*, and *C. albicans*; spearmint significantly inhibited *S. typhi* and *B. subtilis*; and apple mint inhibited *K. pneumoniae, C. albicans*, and *S. typhi*.[999]

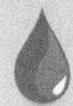

## BETONY
## (Pink Cotton Lamb's Ear, Mountain Tea, Chaye Koohi)

*Stachys lavandulifolia* Vahl.

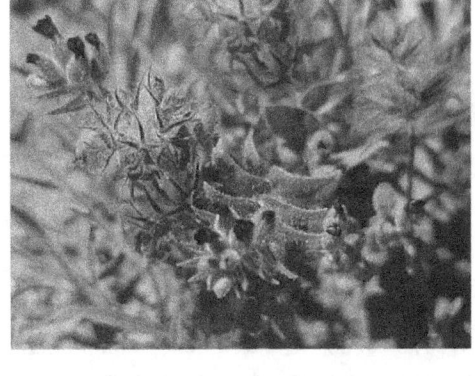

**FAMILY:** Lamiaceae
**NOTE:** Middle
**AROMA INTENSITY:** Medium
**AROMA:** Pungent, herbaceous, slightly floral
**COMMON EXTRACTION METHOD:** Steam distilled from the aerial parts
**POSSIBLE SUBSTITUTE OILS:** Goldenrod, hemp, ylang ylang, ginger
**BLENDS WELL WITH:** Bergamot, copaiba, frankincense, goldenrod, hemp, hyssop, ginger, lavender, lemon, lime, marjoram, orange, patchouli, sage, Spanish sage, vetiver
**SUBCELLULAR LOCALIZATION | EPIGENETIC INFLUENCE:** Currently unknown | Currently unknown
**RECOMMENDED DILUTION RANGE:** 3%–33%; neat for limited conditions

**PRIMARY CONSTITUENTS:**[1000,1001,1002,1003,1004,1005,1006]

*Bicyclogermacrene CT*

| | |
|---|---|
| Bicyclogermacrene | 6.8%–18.0% |
| Pulegone | 0.0%–15.1% |
| Beta-Caryophyllene | 3.1%–13.4% |
| Germacrene D | 4.2%–12.5% |
| Delta-Cadinene | 2.3%–12.2% |
| Spathulenol | 3.3%–12.0% |
| Caryophyllene Oxide | 1.2%–8.5% |
| (Z)-Hex-3-enyl Tiglate | 0.0%–8.4% |
| Limonene | 1.9%–8.2% |
| Alpha-Muurolol | 0.0%–7.7% |
| (2Z,6E)-Farnesol | 0.0%–7.4% |
| Alpha-Copaene | 1.7%–6.5% |
| Myrcene | 1.7%–5.8% |
| Beta-Phellandrene | 0.0%–5.8% |
| Alpha-Pinene | 0.6%–5.1% |

*Beta-Phellandrene/Alpha-Pinene CT*

| | |
|---|---|
| Beta-Phellandrene | 4.6%–37.9% |
| Alpha-Pinene | 8.4%–37.3% |
| Myrcene | 0.7%–23.9% |
| Beta-Caryophyllene | 0.0%–16.9% |
| Germacrene D | 2.5%–13.2% |
| Beta-Pinene | 0.0%–12.1% |
| Spathulenol | 0.0%–7.2% |
| (Z)-Beta-Ocimene | 0.2%–5.8% |
| Alpha-Copaene | 0.0%–4.4% |
| Bicyclogermacrene | 0.0%–4.0% |

*Alpha-Thujene CT*

| | |
|---|---|
| Alpha-Thujene | 13.4%–32.3% |
| Myrcene | 0.5%–15.9% |
| Beta-Phellandrene | 1.1%–14.4% |

*Myrcene/Limonene/Delta-Cadinene CT*

| | |
|---|---|
| Myrcene | 4.3%–26.2% |
| Limonene | 15.3%–24.5% |
| Delta-Cadinene | 9.5%–16.0% |
| Germacrene D | 7.5%–13.5% |
| Alpha-Pinene | 4.9%–8.4% |
| Alpha-Copaene | 4.8%–7.3% |
| Bicyclogermacrene | 3.1%–4.5% |
| Spathulenol | 1.6%–4.3% |
| Cis-m-Mentha-2,8-Diene | 1.4%–4.3% |

*Germacrene D–Spathulenol CT*

| | |
|---|---|
| Germacrene D | 19.3% |
| Spathulenol | 11.1% |
| Bicyclogermacrene | 8.1% |
| Beta-Caryophyllene | 7.8% |
| Delta-Cadinene | 6.5% |

*Alpha-Zingiberene CT*

| | |
|---|---|
| Alpha-Zingiberene | 12.2% |
| Delta-Cadinene | 9.1% |
| Germacrene D | 8.4% |
| Decane | 6.0% |
| Beta-Caryophyllene | 4.6% |
| Spathulenol | 4.1% |

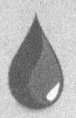 

| | |
|---|---|
| Alpha-Phellandrene | 0.1%–14.0% |
| Delta-Cadinene | 0.1%–11.6% |
| Germacrene D | 0.4%–11.3% |
| Bicyclogermacrene | 0.0%–10.7% |
| Sativene (1,4-methano-1 H-indene) | 0.0%–10.1% |
| Sabinene | 0.0%–4.7% |

**OTHER CONSTITUENTS:** *Bicyclogermacrene CT*—alpha-pinene, cis-m-mentha-2,8-diene, decane, delta-3-carene, (E)-beta-ocimene, delta-elemene, piperitenone, beta-elemene, dihydro-alpha-ionene, beta-copaene, alpha-trans-bergamotene, (E)-beta-farnesene, sesquisabinene, alpha-terpinene, gamma-terpinene, 1,8-cineole, cis-muurola-4(14),5-diene, ar-curcumene, alpha-zingiberene, nootkatene, gamma-cadinene, (E)-gamma-bisabolene, globulol, beta-cedrene epoxide, geranial, neral, alpha-cadinol, intermedeol, guaia-3,10(14)-dien-11-ol, epi-alpha-bisabolol, terpinen-4-ol, mint sulfide; *Myrcene/Limonene/Delta–Cadinene CT*—beta-pinene, alpha-phellandrene, delta-3-carene, alpha-terpinene, gamma-terpinene, delta-elemene, beta-elemene, dihydro-alpha-ionone, (E)-beta-farnesene, sesquisabinene, cis-muurola-4(14),5-diene, ar-curcumene, alpha-zingiberene, nootkatene, (E)-gamma-bisabolene, caryophyllene oxide, alpha-muurolol, alpha-cadinol, guaia-3,10(14)-dien-11-ol, epi-alpha-bisabolol, mint sulfide; *Beta-Phellandrene/Alpha-Pinene CT*—alpha-thujene, alpha-terpinene, (E)-beta-ocimene, gamma-terpinene, linalool, trans-anethole, beta-bourbonene, beta-elemene, trans-alpha-bergamotene, (Z)-beta-farnesene, (E)-beta-farnesene, beta-bisabolene, gamma-cadinene, delta-cadinene, globulol, valeranone, alpha-bisabolol, trans-phytol; *Alpha-Thujene CT*—alpha-pinene, beta-pinene, (Z)-beta-ocimene, linalool, alpha-copaene, beta-bourbonene, naphthalene, cis-alpha-bisabolene; *Germacrene D/Spathulenol CT*—(Z)-hex-3-enyl tiglate, delta-elemene, alpha-copaene, beta-elemene, dihydro-alpha-ionone, alpha-trans-bergamotene, (E)-beta-farnesene, sesquisabinene, cis-muurola-4(14),5-diene, ar-curcumene, alpha-zingiberene, nootkatene, (E)-gamma-bisabolene, caryophyllene oxide, globulol, beta-cedrene epoxide, alpha-muurolol, alpha-cadinol, guaia-3,10(14)-dien-11-ol, epi-alpha-bisabolol; *Alpha-Zingiberene CT*—alpha-thujene, cis-m-mentha-2,8-diene, myrcene, limonene, gamma-terpinene, delta-elemene, beta-elemene, alpha-copaene, dihydro-alpha-ionone, beta-copaene, ar-curcumene, nootkatene, alpha-trans-bergamotene, (E)-beta-farnesene, sesquisabinene, cis-muurola-4(14),5-diene, gamma-cadinene, caryophyllene oxide, globulol, alpha-muurolol, alpha-cadinol, epi-alpha-bisabolol, (2Z,6E)-farnesol, mint sulfide

**PREFERRED COMPOSITION FOR CLINICAL USE:**

| Constituent | Myrcene/Limonene/ Delta-Cadinene CT | Beta-Phellandrene/ Alpha-Pinene CT |
|---|---|---|
| **Myrcene** | 15%–30% | 10%–25% |
| **Limonene** | 15%–30% | – |
| **Delta-Cadinene** | 10%–20% | – |
| **Germacrene D** | 8%–15% | 5%–15% |
| **Alpha-Pinene** | 5%–10% | 20%–40% |
| **Alpha-Copaene** | 5%–10% | – |
| **Bicyclogermacrene** | 2%–5% | – |
| **Spathulenol** | 2%–5% | 1%–8% |
| **Cis-m-Mentha-2,8-Diene** | 2%–5% | – |
| **Beta-Phellandrene** | – | 20%–40% |
| **Beta-Caryophyllene** | – | 10%–20% |
| **Beta-Pinene** | – | 5%–15% |
| **(Z)-Beta-Ocimene** | – | 0.5%–7% |

**REPORTED THERAPEUTIC PROPERTIES:** Antibacterial, antifungal, antimicrobial, analgesic, anti-inflammatory, antirheumatic, anticancer, supports respiratory function, **wound healing**, antioxidant, aids circulation, balances female hormones, reduces painful menstruation, aids digestion, nervine, antineuralgic, relieves headache/migraine, purification, stress management, relieves anxiety, combats nightmares, calming/relaxing

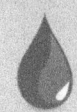

**CAUTIONS:**

■ *Bicyclogermacrene CT*: Caution is warranted in children under age twelve due to the possible presence of pulegone. Multiple organ failure, liver failure, brain swelling (cerebral edema), severe epileptic encephalopathy (severe brain disorder with seizures), organ cell death (necrosis), and death has been reported in infants who were administered mint tea containing pennyroyal essential oil (very high in pulegone).[1007] Pulegone and its metabolite menthofuran (or metabolites of menthofuran) are believed to cause the toxic effects of pennyroyal, which include liver and kidney toxicity, bronchiolar cell destruction, depletion of liver glutathione levels (the primary protective antioxidant of the liver), and direct cellular damage.[1008,1009,1010,1011] Children are more likely to experience these effects.[1012]

■ *Bicyclogermacrene CT*: Avoid during pregnancy and lactation due to potentially high beta-myrcene content and moderate pulegone content. Pulegone-rich essential oils are potentially toxicity to multiple organs, believed to trigger uterine contractions by irritating the genito-urinary system, and commonly used to induce abortions.[1013,1014,1015,1016] Extremely high doses (500 mg/kg) of beta-myrcene have been toxic to fetuses according to animal research.[1017,1018] Pulegone may potentially cause toxicity to multiple organs.[1019,1020]

■ *Bicyclogermacrene CT*: Avoid oral consumption due to the toxic potential of pulegone, which can damage multiple organs. Pulegone is metabolized by human liver cytochrome P-450s (CYP2E1, CYP1A2, and CYP2C19) to its more toxic metabolite menthofuran after administration, which actually increases its toxic effect to the liver.[1021,1022,1023] Animal research suggests oral administration of pulegone is significantly toxic to the liver and causes death at 300 mg/kg body weight per day (over 3.3 mL for a human adult equivalent dose) for two weeks.[1024] Lower doses of 75 and 150 mg/kg body weight per day for three months resulted in liver, kidney, bone marrow, heart, stomach, lung, ovarian, and thymus damage, and one death in animals.[1025] A two-year animal study reported urinary cancer and papillomas, liver cancer, osteosarcoma, and multiple organ damage or enlargement (liver, kidney, olfactory epithelium, lung, bile duct).[1026] Ingestion of essential oils with moderate to significant amounts of pulegone can cause abdominal pain and tenderness, nausea, bloody vomiting, burning of the throat, fever, lethargy alternating with agitation, confusion, delirium, restlessness, seizures, dizziness, auditory and visual hallucinations, increased blood pressure, rapid heartbeat, swollen blood vessels in the lungs and filling of the alveoli with blood, excessive acidity of the blood, blood clots, abortion, liver failure, kidney failure, respiratory failure, shock, coma, and death.[1027]

■ *Bicyclogermacrene CT*: Avoid use with drugs (acetaminophen, barbiturates, carbamazepine, phenobarbital, rifampin, phenytoin, nevirapine, secobarbital, enzalutamide, dexamethasone, modafinil, etc.) that are activated to toxic metabolites by CYP enzymes due to the potentially significant increase in liver toxicity caused by pulegone metabolites.[1028,1029]

■ *Bicyclogermacrene CT*: Avoid with epilepsy and Parkinson's disease due to pulegone content.[1030]

■ *Beta-Phellandrene CT*: May interact with anticholinergic (drugs used for asthma, incontinence, gastrointestinal cramps, muscular spasms, depression, and sleep disorders) and cholinergic medications (drugs used to reduce urinary retention, diagnose myasthenia gravis, and for glaucoma) based on AChE inhibitory activity of beta-phellandrene.[1031]

■ *Bicyclogermacrene CT*: Avoid with compromised liver or kidney due to significant potential of pulegone and its metabolites to cause liver and kidney toxicity (or acute liver/kidney injuries).[1032,1033,1034,1035,1036]

■ *Alpha-Zingiberene CT*: May interfere with the enzymes responsible for metabolizing medications (NSAIDs, proton-pump inhibitors, acetaminophen, antiepileptics, immune modulators, blood-sugar medications, blood pressure medications, antidepressants, antipsychotics, diabetic medications, antihistamines, antibiotics, and anesthetics) due to alpha-zingiberene content.[1037,1038]

**SELECTED EVIDENCE:**

☐ *In vitro* research demonstrates that betony essential oil (alpha-pinene CT, rich in hexadecanoic acid) moderately inhibits *S. aureus* and *E. coli*.[1039] Interestingly, the study authors noted that it exhibited higher activity against gram-negative bacteria than gram-positive bacteria, which is the opposite of most other essential oils.

☐ Oral administration of betony CT alpha-bisabolol significantly reduces orofacial pain (antinociceptive) and inflammation (notably reducing TNF-α and IL-1β) in mice.[1040] Isolated alpha-bisabolol was more effective in reducing pain.

☐ Drying betony plants before essential oil extraction improved their antioxidant activity in the DPPH assay, especially plants that were freeze dried.[1041] Drying techniques (microwave, oven, and sunlight) also reduced monoterpene hydrocarbons (alpha-pinene, beta-pinene, myrcene, and beta-phellandrene) significantly.

# BIG BADJA GUM

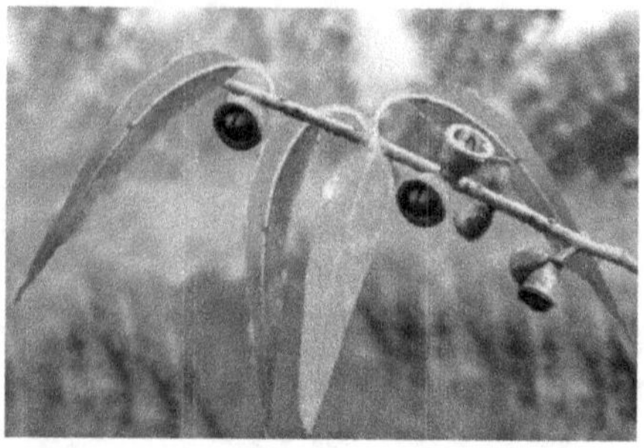

*Eucalyptus badjensis* Beuzev. & M.B. Welch

**FAMILY:** Myrtaceae

**NOTE:** Top

**AROMA INTENSITY:** Medium

**AROMA:** Sweet, camphoraceous, fresh, medicinal

**COMMON EXTRACTION METHOD:** Steam distilled from the leaves

**POSSIBLE SUBSTITUTE OILS:** Eucalyptus, ravintsara (1,8-cineole CT), cajeput, rosemary (1,8-cineole CT), myrtle, cardamom (1,8-cineole CT), Southern blue gum, gully gum, blue mallee

**BLENDS WELL WITH:** Angelica, bay laurel, blue cypress, cajeput, camphor, eucalyptus, lemon, lemon eucalyptus, myrtle, niaouli, peppermint, ravintsara, rosemary, tea tree, thyme

**SUBCELLULAR LOCALIZATION | EPIGENETIC INFLUENCE:** Currently unknown | Currently unknown

**RECOMMENDED DILUTION RANGE:** 3%–33%; neat for limited conditions

**PRIMARY CONSTITUENTS:** [1042,1043,1044]

| | |
|---|---|
| 1,8-Cineole | 71.7%–81.2% |
| Alpha-Pinene | 5.1%–8.4% |
| Beta-Eudesmol | 0.0%–7.8% |
| Limonene | 5.6%–6.0% |

**OTHER CONSTITUENTS:** Para-cymene, alpha-terpineol, gamma-terpinene, viridiflorol

**PREFERRED COMPOSITION FOR CLINICAL USE:**

| Constituent | |
|---|---|
| **1,8-Cineole** | 70%–80% |
| **Alpha-Pinene** | 5%–10% |
| **Limonene** | 5%–10% |

**REPORTED THERAPEUTIC PROPERTIES:** Antibacterial, antifungal, anti-infectious, antiparasitic, antiviral, antiseptic, analgesic, anti-inflammatory, antiarthritic, antirheumatic, wound healing, relieves blisters, **supports respiratory function**, eases cough, relieves headache/migraine, expels excess mucus, decongestant, relieves sinus pressure (sinusitis), relieves sore throat, combats acne, purification, **insecticide**, insect repellent, aids focus/concentration, mentally stimulating

**CAUTIONS:**

■ Avoid with children under age three, particularly around the nose and mouth. Use very cautiously in children under age five due to high 1,8-cineole content. 1,8-cineole may cause seizures, central nervous system problems, or respiratory distress in young children.[1045,1046,1047,1048]

■ Avoid with epilepsy and Parkinson's disease due to 1,8-cineole content. May exacerbate or cause seizures/convulsions or reduce seizure medication efficacy based on 1,8-cineole content.[1049,1050,1051]

■ Caution is warranted orally due to the significant amounts of 1,8-cineole. Limit it to small doses internally (adults—maximum 10 drops daily). One text recommends a maximum daily dose of 6 drops, whereas the European Medicines Agency recommends 2 to 4 drops (100–200 mg) of high 1,8-cineole essential oils orally, 2 to 5 times daily for adolescents, adults, and the elderly.[1052,1053] Additionally, 200 mg of isolated 1,8-cineole has been ingested three times daily for up to six months in clinical research.[1054,1055] Toxicity has been reported when eucalyptus (also high in 1,8-cineole) was ingested in large doses, and as few as 4 to 5 drops may cause problems in very sensitive individuals.[1056,1057,1058,1059,1060,1061] In humans, 3.5 to 5 mL has proven fatal orally.[1062]

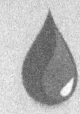

■ May weakly interfere with the enzymes responsible for metabolizing medications (NSAIDs, proton-pump inhibitors, acetaminophen, antiepileptics, immune modulators, blood-sugar medications, blood pressure medications, antidepressants, antipsychotics, diabetic medications, antihistamines, antibiotics, and anesthetics) based on research with an herbal extract of eucalyptus and 1,8-cineole content.[1063,1064,1065]

■ May interact with diabetic medications due to the ability of 1,8-cineole to significantly inhibit alpha-glucosidase activity, particularly when synergized with other constituents (alpha-pinene).[1066,1067,1068] Alpha-glucosidase is an enzyme that breaks down carbohydrates by chemical reaction with water. Inhibiting its activity postpones glucose absorption and therefore the impact of carbohydrates on blood sugar levels.

■ May interact with aspirin, blood pressure, antiplatelet, and anticoagulant medications, and increase the risk of bleeding among people with bleeding disorders (low risk).[1069] 1,8-cineole is a weak inhibitor of platelet aggregation.[1070]

■ May interfere with pentobarbital and other barbiturates (medications for anxiety and insomnia) based on 1,8-cineole content.[1071,1072]

### SELECTED EVIDENCE:

☐ Big badja essential oil possesses fumigant (seventh of fifteen eucalyptus oil tested) and larvicidal properties against the mosquito (*Aedes aegypti*).[1073,1074]

## BIRCH
### (Sweet Birch, Black Birch, Cherry Birch)
*Betula lenta* L.; *Betula carpinifolia* Siebold & Zucc.

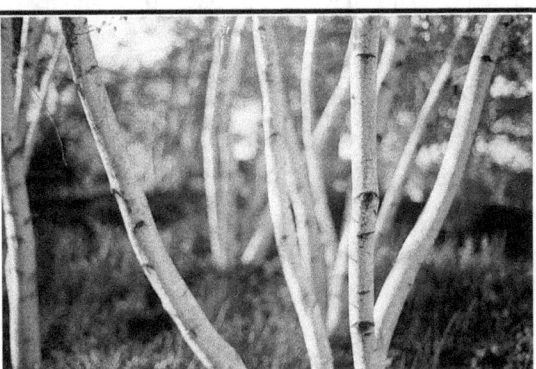

**FAMILY:** Betulaceae
**NOTE:** Top
**AROMA INTENSITY:** Strong
**AROMA:** Intense, balsamic, sweet, woody, smoky, pungent
**COMMON EXTRACTION METHOD:** Steam distillation of the bark
**POSSIBLE SUBSTITUTE OILS:** Wintergreen
**BLENDS WELL WITH:** Balsam fir, basil, bergamot, blue spruce, cajeput, cedarwood, chamomile (German, Roman), copaiba, frankincense, juniper, lavender, lemon, lemongrass, marjoram, myrtle, peppermint, pine, rosemary, sandalwood, silver fir, spruce (black), tsuga, white fir, wintergreen
**SUBCELLULAR LOCALIZATION | EPIGENETIC INFLUENCE:** Currently unknown | Currently unknown
**RECOMMENDED DILUTION RANGE:** 1.5%–20%; 50% for some conditions

**PRIMARY CONSTITUENTS:**[1075,1076]
Methyl Salicylate          97.0%–99.0%

**OTHER CONSTITUENTS:** Ethyl-salicylate, linalyl acetate

**PREFERRED COMPOSITION FOR CLINICAL USE:**

| *Constituent* | |
|---|---|
| **Methyl Salicylate** | 92%–99.9% |
| **Total Other Volatile Constituents:** 2-trans-4-cis-Decadienal, 2-trans-4-trans-Decadienal, ortho-Guaiacol, Veratrole, Ethyl Salicylate, Methyl ortho-Anisate, Etc. | tr–8% |
| **Absent Synthetic Markers:** Methyl 4-Hydroxybenzoate, Dimethyl 4-Hydroxyisophthalate, Dimethyl 2-Hydroxyisophthalate, Methyl Paraben, Dimethyl 2-Hydroxyterephthalate | 0% |

Note: Carbon-14 isotope analysis should be performed as a step to confirm authenticity, but this will only authenticate natural versus synthetic methyl salicylate and not if wintergreen has been used as a substitute for birch. In addition, the presence of beta-dehydroelshotzia ketone and vitispirane are suggestive of the addition of wintergreen oil, while ricenalidic acid would indicate addition of castor oil.

**REPORTED THERAPEUTIC PROPERTIES: Analgesic (pain relief), anti-inflammatory, anti-rheumatic**, antispasmodic, astringent, expels excess gas, **diuretic**, antiseptic, astringent, circulatory stimulant, promotes perspiration, reduces fever, antimicrobial, purifies the blood, aids detoxification, aids digestion, antidepressant, stimulating, encourages focus

### CAUTIONS:

■ Avoid with children under age 12. The high salicylate content in birch may increase the risk of a very serious and life-threatening illness called Reye syndrome in children under 12. Reye syndrome is sudden brain damage and liver dysfunction that most commonly occurs in children ages 4 to 12. It has an unknown cause, but it typically occurs in children who were given aspirin when they are experiencing a fever or recovering from flu-like symptoms or chickenpocks.[1077]

■ Do not use during pregnancy or lactation. May cause congenital abnormalities and fetal malformations.[1078,1079]

■ Oral caution—As little as 2.5 mL can cause toxicity and 4 mL may be fatal in children. As little as 5 mL could result in methyl salicylate poisoning in adults, and more than 5 mL can be fatal.[1080,1081,1082,1083,1084] Methyl salicylate is structurally similar to aspirin (acetylsalicylic acid) and readily metabolized to salicylic acid—the same bioactive intermediate as aspirin—after ingestion. Since authentic bitrch essential oil is 92%+ methyl salicylate, its mode of action is identical to aspirin. One drop of birch essential oil is roughly equivalent to a baby aspirin in salicylate content and four drops is equivalent to a 325 mg aspirin tablet. Do not exceed 5 drops of wintergreen oil per day orally for an adult.

■ Avoid with epilepsy and Parkinson's disease due to methyl salicylate content.[1085,1086]

■ May interact with aspirin, blood pressure, antiplatelet, and anticoagulant medications, and increase the risk of bleeding among people with bleeding disorders both topically and orally.[1087,1088,1089,1090]

■ Toxicity may occur with overuse topically and the absorption of methyl salicylate increases with repeated applications.[1091] Not intended for long-term use.

■ Avoid orally with gastroesophageal reflux disease (GERD). May cause accumulation of fluid in the larynx (laryngeal edema) and lead to airway obstruction in sensitive individuals.[1092]

■ Avoid in individuals allergic to aspirin, methyl salicylate, or other NSAIDs; or those with salicylate sensitivities. Methyl salicylate may be metabolized to the known NSAID, salicylic acid, by the liver.[1093]

### SELECTED EVIDENCE:

□ Birch essential oil (leaf oils of *B. browicziana, B. litwinowii, B.recurvata,* and *B. medwediewii,* with *B. medwediewii* having methyl salicylate as the main constituent and the others 14-Hydroxy-4,5-dihydro-beta-caryophyllene) showed strong antifungal activity against four fungi (*Cephalosporium aphidicola, Drechslera sorokinianse, Fusarium solani,* and *Rhizoctonia cerealis*).[1094]

□ *In vitro* research showed that birch essential oil is active against *B. burgdorferi* and *B. garinii,* causative agents of Lyme disease.[1095]

□ Topical application of methyl salicylate, the primary constituent of birch oil, relieved pain in adults with knee osteoarthritis.[1096] Subjects in the crossover, double-blind, randomized controlled trial applied 400 mg of a methyl salicylate in 20 g of plaster in the morning after a shower or bath and at night, twice daily, for one to two weeks. The methyl salicylate plaster was comparable in efficacy to a plaster with indomethacin.

*Did you know?*

The definition of an essential oil is debated among scientists and aromatherapy organizations. Some organizations choose to use a narrow definition that only includes aromatics extracted via traditionally steam distillation, excluding cold pressed oils. Other scientists want to include a broader range of aromatics extracted by methods such as Co2 and microwave-assited extraction.

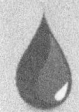

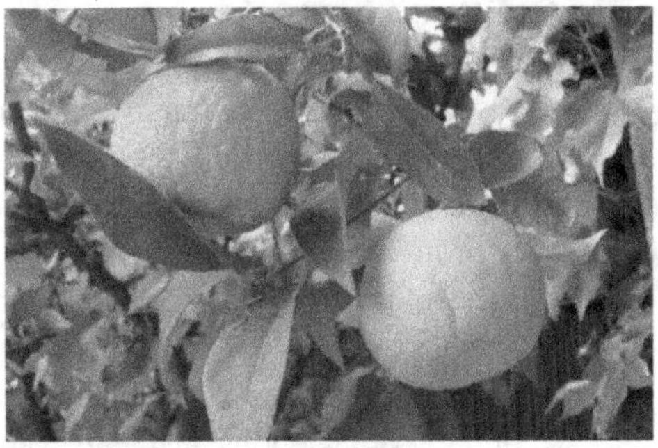

# BITTER ORANGE

*Citrus* × *aurantium* L. (pro sp.) [maxima × reticulata],
*C. aurantium* × L. var. *amara*

**FAMILY:** Rutaceae
**NOTE:** Top
**AROMA INTENSITY:** Medium
**AROMA:** Citrusy, bitter, fresh, slightly woody
**COMMON EXTRACTION METHOD:** Cold-pressed/expressed from the fruit rind (peel)
**POSSIBLE SUBSTITUTE OILS:** Orange (sweet), bergamot, lemon, tangerine, grapefruit, lime
**BLENDS WELL WITH:** Bay laurel, bergamot, black pepper, camphor, cassia, citronella, cinnamon, clary sage, clove, copaiba, coriander, frankincense, geranium, ginger, grapefruit, juniper, lavender, lemon, lemon verbena, lime, marjoram, melissa, myrrh, neroli, nutmeg, patchouli, tangerine, rose, sage, Spanish sage, sandalwood, spikenard, vetiver, ylang ylang
**SUBCELLULAR LOCALIZATION | EPIGENETIC INFLUENCE:** Currently unknown | Currently unknown
**RECOMMENDED DILUTION RANGE:** 3%–50%; Neat for limited conditions

**PRIMARY CONSTITUENTS:**[1097,1098,1099]

| | |
|---|---|
| Limonene | 90.3%–98.7% |
| Myrcene | 0.5%–2.0% |
| Linalool | 0.0%–1.6% |

**OTHER CONSTITUENTS:** Beta-pinene, alpha-pinene, sabinene, 1,8-cineole, alpha-terpineol, (E,Z)-farnesyl acetate, germacrene D, (E)-nerolidol, octanal, decenal, beta-caryophyllene

**PREFERRED COMPOSITION FOR CLINICAL USE:**

| Constituent | |
|---|---|
| Limonene | 90%–95% |
| Myrcene | 1%–3% |
| Linalool | 0.1%–2% |
| Beta-Pinene | 0.1%–2% |
| Alpha-Pinene | 0.1%–1% |
| Linalyl Acetate | 0.1%–1% |
| Geranyl Acetate | < 0.5% |

**REPORTED THERAPEUTIC PROPERTIES:** Anti-inflammatory, antiseptic, astringent, antibacterial, antispasmodic, expels excess gas, deodorant, aids digestion, antifungal, anticancer, helps maintain normal cholesterol levels, relieves diarrhea, **protects the stomach mucosal lining**, reduces the appearance of blemishes and acne, supports cardiovascular function, **soothes sore throat**, weight management, **antidepressant**, **relieves anxiety**, stimulating, combats fatigue, encourages restful sleep

**CAUTIONS:**

■ May cause photosensitivity (low risk). Avoid sun exposure to area of application for at least 12 hours after topical application.[1100,1101]

■ May interact with anticholinergic (drugs used for asthma, incontinence, gastrointestinal cramps, muscular spasms, depression, and sleep disorders) and cholinergic medications (drugs used to reduce urinary retention, diagnose myasthenia gravis, and for glaucoma) based on AChE inhibitory activity.[1102]

■ The NCAA considers bitter orange a stimulant because of its synephrine content and it is on the NCAA banned substances list.[1103] Synephrine is an alkaloid found in the peel and reportedly not present in the essential oil, but athletes are advised to seek professional medical and legal guidance regarding the use of bitter orange essential oil.

**SELECTED RESEARCH**:

- Oral administration of bitter orange (single dose of 5 mg/kg or repeated dose of 1 mg/kg per day for 14 days) reduced anxiety in mice by influencing serotonin levels.[1104] Interestingly the same study found that mice administered bitter orange experienced reduced cholesterol levels.

- Bitter orange may help prevent and treat intestinal dysbiosis (a state of altered intestinal flora to one of harmful bacteria that contributes to a variety of chronic and degenerative diseases) by selectively destroying harmful bacteria while leaving probiotics intact.[1105]

- Animal research suggests that bitter orange heals stomach ulcers and encourages the production of the mucosal lining of the stomach in middle-aged animals.[1106] Another study observed that oral administration of 245 mg/kg of bitter orange prevented 99 percent of stomach ulcers caused by ethanol and NSAIDs in rats.[1107]

- *In vitro* research suggests that bitter orange oil inhibits acetylcholinesterase (AChE) and mildly inhibits butyrylcholinesterase (BChE) enzyme activity.[1108] Inhibition of AChE prevents the breakdown of acetylcholine, which is essential for memory and thinking. People with neurodegenerative diseases make less acetylcholine, and the diseases often break it down at a faster rate leading to acetylcholine deficits. Selective inhibition of BChE is also desirable in neurodegenerative diseases because it interferes with acetylcholine activity. In addition, BChE is often found in the plaques and tangles in the brains of people with Alzheimer's disease.[1109]

- Animal research suggests that the oral administration of 0.5 to 1.0 g/kg of bitter orange oil prevents seizures, reduces anxiety, and is sedating.[2494,2809] Another study concluded that inhaling bitter orange oil for seven minutes reduced anxiety and increased social interaction in rats better than diazepam (a drug used to treat anxiety, spasms, and seizures).[2495]

- Massaging ginger and bitter orange oil to the knees of older adults six times over a three-week period relieved moderate-to-severe knee pain and increased physical function in the short-term.[1110]

- Bitter orange essential oil is larvicidal to the mosquito *An. Stephensi*.[1111]

- Bitter orange essential oil kills the parasitic worm *Schistosoma mansoni*, which is responsible for the acute and chronic disease schistosomiasis (a parasitic disease characterized by rash, itchy skin, fever, chills, cough, muscle aches, and inflammation of the bladder and intestines if the parasites travel to and are lodged in these organs.[1112]

- *In vitro* research demonstrates that bitter orange essential oil exhibits good antioxidant activity (DPPH and beta-carotene bleaching assays) and reduces inflammation (reduces nitric oxide produce by LPS-stimulated macrophages).[1113] The same researchers studied the effects of bitter orange essential oil in rats and found that it protected against liver damage caused by tetrachloride.

- Bitter orange essential oil exhibited good antioxidant activity, which exceeded that of isolated limonene.[1114] In addition, it inhibited *S. aureus, Salmonella* sp. (clinical isolate), *P. aeruginosa, B. subtilis*, and *E. coli*, demonstrating greater activity against gram-positive bacteria.

- Lemon, bergamot, and bitter orange were the most effective of citrus oils (lemon, bitter orange, bergamot, sweet orange, and mandarin) tested in the inhibition of mycelial growth of *A. flavus*.[1115] These three oils also were most effective at reducing aflatoxin B1 production.

- A mixture of bitter orange essential oil in grape (*Vitis vinifera*) hydrolat—1/100 ratio—inhibited yeasts (*Candida, Saccharomyces*, and *Galattomyces* species) isolated from the gut of people with irritable bowel syndrome (IBS).[1116] The final product contained 38.8% linalool, 25.4% geraniol, and 17.7% limonene as major constituents. The mixture reduced inflammatory markers IL-10 and TNF-α in peripheral blood mononuclear cells without harming human gingival fibroblasts. The researchers concluded that the mixture favors an increase in beneficial probiotic bacteria strains while simultaneously reducing pathogenic fungal strains, resulting in microbiome balance and could be useful in the treatment of IBS.

- Anxiety and agitation are common among people admitted to intensive care units (ICU) and this can interfere with treatment and recovery. A randomized parallel placebo-controlled trial evaluated the effects of lavender and bitter orange essential oil on people in the ICU.[1117] Subjects were randomly divided into one of three groups: lavender inhalation, bitter orange inhalation, and saline placebo. Five drops of lavender, bitter orange, or saline were added to gauze and placed 10 cm from the nose. The subjects inhaled from the gauze for thirty minutes. Both the lavender and bitter orange groups experienced significantly reduced anxiety compared to control, but agitation levels were not statistically different among the three groups—all three groups experienced reduced agitation. The conclusion of the study was that "aromatherapy can be used as an effective and safe intervention to reduce anxiety in ICUs."

- Bitter orange essential oil with 35.2% limonene, 18.2% linalool, and 17.6% myrcene weakly inhibited alpha-

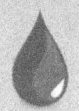

glucosidase and alpha-amylase activity.[1118] Inhibiting either enzyme helps reduce glucose absorption in the intestine and therefore blood sugar spikes after eating.

☐ Yuzu, bitter orange, and citron essential oils each exhibited good antioxidant activity in the ABTS and DPPH assays.[1119]

☐ A study investigated the chemical composition and antioxidant activity of several cultivars ("Canaliculata," "Consolei," "Crispifolia," "Fasciata," "Foetifera," "Listata," and "Bizzaria") of bitter orange in FRAP, DPPH, ABTS, and β-carotene bleaching assays.[1120] Limonene was the main constituent of all cultivars ranging from 33.4%–89.2%. "Crispifolia" was the most dissimilar with only 33.4% limonene and higher levels of linalool, alpha-terpineol, bergamatol, geraniol, geranyl acetate, germacrene D, (E)-nerolidol, and neryl acetate. The "Fasciata" variety (76.0% limonene) had the highest antioxidant potential based on the global antioxidant score.

☐ Anxiety is commonly experienced by men and women before surgery. Men and women respond differently to some interventions due to differences in metabolism (phase 1 and 2 liver enzyme activity), distribution, and excretion of therapeutics, body size, and sex hormones. A randomized, single-blind, placebo-controlled, prospective clinical study compared the effects of lavender, neroli, or control in reducing presurgery anxiety.[1121] Inhalation of lavender and neroli essential oil—2 drops on a napkin and inhaled from for twenty minutes—reduced presurgery severe anxiety in men, but lavender was more effective than neroli in women. Both neroli and lavender essential oil reduced anxiety in male and female subjects.

☐ Bitter orange essential oil showed potent antioxidant activity in the DPPH and FRAP assays and was also active against pathogenic bacteria (*E. coli*, *S. aureus*, *E. faecalis*, *M. luteus*, *S. epidermidis*, *B. cereus*, and *S. typhimurium*).[1122]

☐ Bitter orange essential oil exhibited insecticidal activity against the stable fly (*Stomoxys calcitrans*) in both the contact and fumigant assays.[1123]

☐ Pain and impaired blood pressure are common complaints following surgery. Aromatherapy is a leading solution to help control pain because essential oils trigger endorphin release in the brain, which promotes a general sense of well-being. A human clinical study evaluated the effects of inhaling bitter orange on pain and blood pressure following gastrectomy (partial or total removal of the stomach).[1124] After entering the postoperative recovery room and before receiving analgesic medications, 5 drops of bitter orange (diluted to 30%) were added to a pad placed about five centimeters from the nose, and the participants inhaled for ten breaths. The pad was then attached to the participant's collar for ninety minutes. Participants in the control group inhaled distilled water from a pad. The aromatherapy group experienced significant reductions in blood pressure (systolic and diastolic) and pain intensity when compared to the control group.

☐ Both bitter orange (37.3% diethyl o-phthalate, 10.0% limonene) and grapefruit (60.5% limonene, 11.8% diethyl o-phthalate) essential oil were larvicidal to mosquitoes (*Aedes albopictus*).[1125] Limonene was also reported to be a potent larvicide, with a limonene nanoemulsion providing a longer duration of effect.

☐ Ravintsara, turmeric, petitgrain (*C. aurantium*), and bitter orange essential oil each inhibited *Mycobacterium smegmatis* (a bacterial strain commonly used as a model for inhibition of *M. tuberculosis*), *C. albicans*, and *C. tropicalis*.[1126] The oils also displayed activity against collagenase, indicating an antiaging activity. Petitgrain and turmeric also inhibited elastase, which would preserve skin strength and flexibility.

*Did you know?*

Essential oils enter tissues and the bloodstream rapidly after use. Essential oil compounds can be detected in the blood within five minutes after topical application. Peak blood concentration is achieved around nineteen minutes. Inhaling aromatic constituents—considered the most rapid way to enter the blood and tissues, particularly in the brain and respiratory system—leads to detection in the bloodstream within minutes, peaking about twenty minutes. Ingested essential oils may be more slowly absorbed and are efficiently metabolized by the body. Some constituents act as a prodrug (a substance that is converted into an active form during normal metabolism), such as linalyl acetate, which is readily converted to linalool.

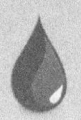

# BLACK CUMIN SEED
## (Black Seed, Black Caraway, Roman Coriander)
*Nigella sativa* L.

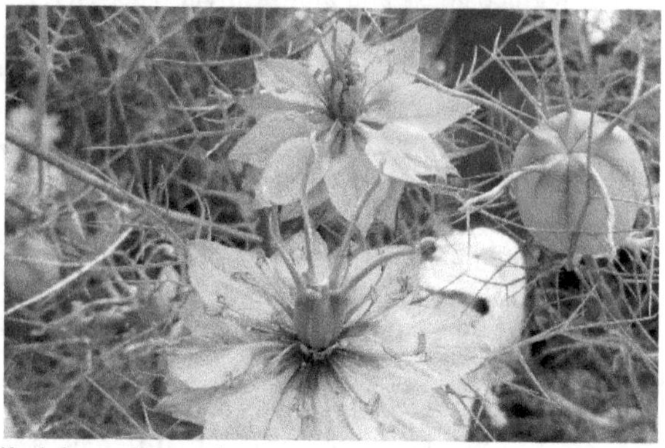

**FAMILY:** Ranunculaceae
**NOTE:** Base
**AROMA INTENSITY:** Medium
**AROMA:** Pungent, spicy, herbaceous, peppery
**COMMON EXTRACTION METHOD:** Hydrodistilled or steam distilled from the seeds
**POSSIBLE SUBSTITUTE OILS:** Thyme, oregano
**BLENDS WELL WITH:** Anise, black pepper, caraway, cardamom, cassia, cinnamon, clove, coriander, fennel, frankincense, hyssop, lavender, marjoram, myrrh, oregano, patchouli, star anise
**SUBCELLULAR LOCALIZATION | EPIGENETIC INFLUENCE:** Currently unknown | Currently unknown
**RECOMMENDED DILUTION RANGE:** 3%–50%; sensitive populations (those with chronic skin conditions, autoimmune/autoinflammatory disorders, allergies, or chronic respiratory ailments should dilute to 0.3%–0.5% due to a higher risk of sensitization when applied topically, including type 4 sensitivity reactions)[3619–3621]

**PRIMARY CONSTITUENTS:**[1127,1128,1129,1130,1131,1132,1133,1134,1135]

*Para-Cymene CT*

| | |
|---|---|
| Para-Cymene | 6.3%–60.2% |
| Thymol | 0.1%–45.0% |
| Alpha-Thujene | 0.0%–15.3% |
| Alpha-Pinene | 0.7%–13.8% |
| Thymoquinone | 0.1%–13.7% |
| Gamma-Terpinene | 0.2%–12.9% |
| Thujol | 0.0%–11.2% |
| Beta-Elemene | 0.0%–11.0% |
| Linalool | 0.0%–9.9% |
| Alpha-Terpinolene | 0.0%–9.1% |
| Ortho-Cymene | 0.0%–7.3% |
| Alpha-Selinene | 0.0%–6.5% |
| Longifolene | 0.0%–6.4% |
| Terpinen-4-ol | 0.0%–4.3% |
| Trans-4-Methoxythujane | 0.0%–4.0% |
| Beta-Pinene | 0.0%–3.7% |
| Myrtenol | 0.0%–3.0% |
| Carvacrol | 0.0%–3.0% |
| Beta-Selinene | 0.0%–2.7% |
| Limonene | 0.0%–2.6% |
| Junipene | 0.0%–2.4% |

*Thymoquinone CT*

| | |
|---|---|
| Thymoquinone | 26.8%–54.8% |
| Para-Cymene | 14.7%–38.0% |
| Alpha-Thujene | 1.3%–10.5% |
| Carvacrol | 0.0%–10.3% |
| Longifolene | 1.2%–10.2% |
| Beta-Pinene | 0.4%–3.0% |
| Alpha-Cubebene | 0.0%–3.0% |
| Limonene | 0.7%–2.3% |

*Trans-Anethole CT*

| | |
|---|---|
| Trans-Anethole | 27.1%–38.3% |
| Para-Cymene | 9.0%–14.8% |
| Thymoquinone | 0.6%–11.8% |
| Longifolene | 0.0%–5.7% |
| Limonene | 4.3%–4.3% |
| Carvone | 2.0%–4.0% |
| Carvacrol | 1.6%–3.7% |
| Naphthalenone | 0.0%–2.6% |
| Alpha-Thujene | 2.4%–2.4% |

Note: Black cumin may also be steam distilled from the fixed oil that has been solvent extracted (produces the thymoquinone CT). Hydrodistillation generally extracts higher thymoquinone content, whereas steam distillation usually only has trace amounts.[1136] Higher thymoquinone content is desirable for greater therapeutic value. A fixed oil from *N. sativa* called black seed oil also exists.

**OTHER CONSTITUENTS:** *Para-Cymene CT*—sabinene, trans-thujan-4-ol, trans-dihydrocarvone, beta-myrcene, trans-sabinene hydrate, 7-epi-selinene, ethyl hexanoate, ethyl heptanoate, alpha-longipinene, estragole (<1.0%), alpha-amorphene, germacrene A, L-carvenol, ethyl octadecanoate, ethyl oleate, ethyl tetradecanoate; *Thymoquinone CT*—

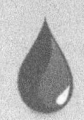

sabinene, gamma-terpinene, bornyl acetate; *Trans-Anethole CT*—n-nonane, 1,2,5,-trimethyl benzene, 1-methyl-3-propyl benzene, alpha-pinene, sabinene, beta-pinene, alpha-phellandrene, myristicin, gamma-terpinene, dihydrocarvone, estragole (<2.0%), anisaldehyde, dill apiol, apiol, longifolene

**PREFERRED COMPOSITION FOR CLINICAL USE:**

| Constituent | Thymoquinone CT | Supercritical (SFE) |
|---|---|---|
| **Thymoquinone** | 30%–55% | 32%–85% |
| **Para-Cymene** | 20%–40% | 0%–20% |
| **Alpha-Thujene** | 2%–12% | 0%–4% |
| **Longifolene** | 2%–10% | – |
| **Beta-Pinene** | 0.5%–5% | – |
| **Limonene** | 0.5%–5% | – |

Note: Greater percentages of thymoquinone are possible, and desirable, with an SFE extract from the crude fixed oil.

**REPORTED THERAPEUTIC PROPERTIES:** Antibacterial, antifungal, antiviral, **antiparasitic**, **antimicrobial**, **antioxidant**, **boosts antioxidant activity**, **analgesic**, anti-inflammatory, antispasmodic, anticonvulsive, antirheumatic, antiseptic, **anticancer**, modulates immune activity, **balances blood sugar levels**, relieves headache/migraine, aids cardiovascular function, antiallergic, expels excess gas, weight management, **protects cognitive function**, aids detoxification, **supports liver and kidney function**, reduces hair loss, combats acne, wound healing, soothes chronic skin conditions, **supports respiratory function**, eases cough, reduces fever, relieves dizziness, supports normal cholesterol levels, reduces blood pressure, insecticide, antidepressant, relieves anxiety, reduces mental exhaustion

**CAUTIONS:**

■ Caution is advised during pregnancy and lactation due to trans-anethole or thymoquinone content. Trans-anethole possesses estrogenic activity that decreases fertility in animals by preventing the implantation of a fertilized egg in the uterus.[1137,1138,1139,1140,1141] Thymoquinone potently prevents the formation of new blood vessels (angiogenesis), which occurs during pregnancy beginning twenty-one days after conception.[1142,1143,1144] The growth of a dense network of blood vessels within the placenta is necessary for the exchange of respiratory gases, nutrients, and wastes between the mother and fetus. If angiogenesis is inhibited during pregnancy it may lead to insufficient blood supply to the placenta and pregnancy complications (fetal growth restriction, preeclampsia, and fetal death). Thymoquinone also negatively effects embryonic development if administered during the second trimester (fetal malformations).[1145]

■ *Trans-Anethole CT*: Use with caution and highly diluted for children under six due to trans-anethole content.[1146]

■ *Trans-Anethole CT*: Long-term oral use of black cumin essential oil is not advised in young girls because of reports that fennel tea (also high in anethole) may cause premature breast development in very young girls when used chronically.[1147] Long-term oral use is not recommended for children under age twelve.

■ *Para-Cymene CT*: Oral caution. Some black cumin essential oils contain up to 45.0% thymol. Thymol has a longer half-life (the time it takes for half of the medication to metabolize or excrete half of the dosage) than most essential oil constituents and should not be administered orally for long periods of time.[1148] Thymol is a monoterpene phenol. Reports of fatalities in children who consumed 50 to 200 mg of phenols have been reported.[1149] It is recommended that the para-cymene CT be limited to 10 drops per day orally for adults with a two- to seven-day break after twenty-one days of use. Alternately, one may take the oil Monday through Friday with a weekly break Saturday and Sunday.

■ May interact with diabetes medications and cause low blood sugar based on thymoquinone and trans-anethole content.[1150,1151,1152,1153,1154,1155,1156] Higher thymoquinone content will increase the effect on blood sugar levels.[1157]

■ May interact with aspirin, blood pressure, antiplatelet, and anticoagulant medications, and increase the risk of bleeding among people with bleeding disorders due to thymol, carvacrol, trans-anethole and thymoquinone content.[1158,1159,1160,1161] Thymoquinone is known to cause platelet apoptosis (cell death).[1162,1163]

■ May interact with anticholinergic (drugs used for asthma, incontinence, gastrointestinal cramps, muscular spasms, depression, and sleep disorders) and cholinergic medications (drugs used to reduce urinary retention, diagnose myasthenia gravis, and for glaucoma) based on thymoquinone, thymol, and carvacrol content.[1164]

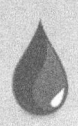

■ May interfere with the enzymes responsible for metabolizing medications based on trans-anethole and thymoquinone content (NSAIDs, proton-pump inhibitors, acetaminophen, antiepileptics, immune modulators, blood-sugar medications, blood pressure medications, antidepressants, antipsychotics, diabetic medications, antihistamines, antibiotics, and anesthetics).[1165,1166,1167,1168,1169,1170,1171,1172,1173,1174]

■ May interact with antibiotics and possibly enhance their effects due to thymol, thymoquinone, or carvacrol content.[1175,1176]

■ May interfere with the antiseizure medication valproate (possibly other antiseizure drugs) and enhance its anticonvulsive activity due to thymoquinone content.[1177]

### SELECTED EVIDENCE:

☐ An ultrasonic nanoemulsion of black cumin essential significantly reduced the viability of breast cancer cells.[1178] Black cumin essential oil kills two rat-leukemia-cell lines, human-gastric-cancer cells, and cancer-associated mouse fibroblasts.[1179] It also prevents colon cancer formation, possibly by inhibiting cancer cell proliferation in the mucosal lining of the colon.[1180] Thymoquinone markedly triggers apoptosis in two cervical cancer cells lines and prevents their proliferation and migration.[1181,1182] Thymoquinone triggers apoptosis of colorectal cancer cells.[1183] Thymoquinone also increases the anticancer activity of doxorubicin (a chemotherapy drug) against promyelocytic leukemia and drug-resistant breast-cancer cells.[1184] A thymoquinone-rich essential oil killed sheep heart cancer cells *in vitro* and prevented cancer metastasis and increased survivability of mice.[1185]

☐ A randomized, placebo-controlled clinical study demonstrated that a boiled extract of black cumin seed (containing volatile oils and 10 g% glucose) reduces the severity and frequency of asthma symptoms (wheezing, cough, chest tightness, and overall pulmonary function) when administered orally at a dose of 15 mL/kg of a 0.1 g% daily for three months.[1186] The longer the participants used the black cumin extract the greater the effects in the study, including a reduced requirement for steroid inhalers, oral corticosteroids, and oral theophylline.

☐ Oral administration (100 or 200 mg of a 0.1 g% volatile extract, twice daily, for eight weeks) of black cumin essential oil (para-cymene CT) significantly reduced blood pressure in healthy adults with mild high blood pressure.[1187] Animal research suggests that oral administration of black cumin essential oil (thymoquinone CT) decreases blood pressure and depresses cardiovascular activity through 5-hydroxytryptaminergic (5-hydroxytryptamine, or serotonin, is a neurotransmitter involved in constriction of the arteries) and muscarinic (muscarinic receptors play an essential oil role in regulation of cardiovascular function) mechanisms.[1188]

☐ Oral administration of black cumin essential oil (para-cymene CT with 13.7% thymoquinone), or thymoquinone, significantly reduced pain but did not reduce inflammation.[1189,1190] Injection of the same oil reduced inflammation and edema.[1191] The study authors suggest that the analgesic activity was not related to opioid receptors because naloxone (a drug used to block or reverse the effects of opioid medications) could not reverse the pain-relieving effect.

☐ *In vitro* research reported that black cumin essential oil inhibits multiple fungi: *Candida albicans, C. zeylanoides, C. dubliniensis, C. glabrata, C. krusei, C. tropicalis, C. parapsilosis, Aspergillus niger, A. flavus, A. fumigatus, Fusarium moniliforme, F. semitectum, F. oxysporum, F. nivale, F. graminearum, F. moniliforme, Penicillium viridicatum, Drechslera hawaiiensis, Alternaria alternata*, and pathogenic dermatophytes (*T. mentagrophytes, M. canis*, and *M. gypseum*).[1192,1193,1194,1195,1196,1197,1198,1199,1200,1201,1202,1203] It also inhibited the production of aflatoxin.[1204] Another study reported that black cumin essential oil prevented the growth of *C. albicans* on dentures.[1205]

☐ Black cumin essential oil (para-cymene CT) completely inhibits the gram-negative and gram-positive bacteria *Penicillium citrinum, Bacillus cereus, Bacillus subtilis, Staphylococcus aureus*, and *Pseudomonas aeruginosa in vitro*.[1206] A microemulsion of black cumin essential oil (thymoquinone CT) is highly effective against *S. aureus, B. cereus* and *S. typhimurium*.[1207] Other research reports thymoquinone-rich black cumin essential oil inhibits *B. cereus, C. subtilis, E. faecalis, S. epidermidis, S. pyogenes, Bacteroides fragilis, E. coli, Salmonella typhi, P. aeruginosa, S. aureus, Micrococcus lysodeikticus*, and *Sarcina lutea*.[1208,1209,1210]

☐ Black cumin essential oil causes vasorelaxation (relaxation of the blood vessels) in isolated rat aorta by influencing calcium channels instead of through influencing nitric oxide production or the endothelium.[1211]

☐ *In vitro* research reports that black cumin essential oil (para-cymene CT) demonstrates stronger antioxidant capacity than the synthetic antioxidants BHA and BHT.[1212,1213,1214,1215] Animal research also reports that black

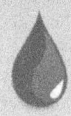

cumin essential oil positively influences the activities of antioxidant enzymes including catalase (CAT), superoxide dismutase (SOD), glutathione transferase (GST), glutathione reductase (GR), and glutathione peroxidase (GPx).[1216] In addition, the study authors reported that black cumin essential oil boosted immunity. Another animal study reports that black cumin essential oil (thymoquinone CT) significantly reduces free radicals and improves antioxidant production and activity to reduce the risk of diabetic complications, including improving cholesterol profile and protecting the integrity of pancreatic beta-cells that produce insulin.[1217,1218,1219]

- Oral administration of black cumin essential oil protects against damage and toxicity of the liver and heart by reducing oxidative stress and balancing cardiac and liver enzymes in rats.[1220]

- Animal research reports that black cumin essential oil protects against lung injury and inflammation caused by mustard gas.[1221]

- A thymoquinone-rich black cumin essential oil killed hydatid cysts, a parasitic tapeworm that affects multiple organs.[1222] The thymoquinone CT also killed *Leishmania tropica* (a parasite that causes cutaneous leishmaniasis) and *Leishmania infantum* (a parasite that causes visceral leishmaniasis in infants) *in vitro*.[1223] Another study reports that black cumin essential oil kills and expels some cestode and nematode parasites.[1224]

- Black cumin essential oil modulates immune activity, including reducing neutrophil chemotaxis (the migration of neutrophils from the bloodstream to tissues in response to infections), which can reduce inflammatory responses.[1225] In addition, excess chemotaxis can result in tissue damage to the area that the neutrophils migrate to. Another study concluded that black cumin essential oil possesses immunosuppressive properties due to its ability to reduce splenocytes and neutrophils, while increasing lymphocytes and monocytes in animals.[1226]

- *In vitro* research demonstrates that black cumin essential oil (para-cymene CT with 13.7% thymoquinone) inhibits human neutrophil elastase (HNE) activity, which may make it useful for chronic obstructive pulmonary disease (COPD) and emphysema.[1227] HNE is a major contributor to lung-tissue damage and reduced lung function in COPD and emphysema.[1228,1229] The authors attributed this effect to the presence of carvacrol (11.8%). Animal research suggests that thymoquinone-rich black cumin essential oil acts as a respiratory stimulant by inhibiting histamine (known to constrict the airways and cause wheezing) and muscarinic acetylcholine receptor (receptors in the airways and blood vessels that cause constriction of airways and mucus secretion) activity.[1230]

- Animal research reports that black cumin essential oil inhibits uterine contractions—even when stimulated by oxytocin—in isolated Guinea pig uterus.[1231]

- Thymoquinone protects neurons against synaptic toxicity (deterioration of synapses that can lead to alterations in nervous system function, damage to nervous system tissue, and neuron cell death), which makes it a promising agent for Parkinson's disease and dementia with Lewy bodies (abnormal groups of proteins that develop in neurons in the brain).[1232] Other research reports that it increases antioxidant activity and production to effectively protect kidney cells from toxicity and premature death, protects cells from toxicity and cancer formation, potently scavenges superoxide anion, and reduces high blood pressure.[1233,1234,1235,3671,1236] It also reduces inflammation and rheumatoid arthritis symptoms in rats when taken orally at doses of 2.5 or 5 mg/kg.[1237]

- Black cumin essential oil (rich in thymol) is larvicidal to *Aedes aegypti, Anopheles stephensi*, and *Culex quinquefasciatus* mosquitoes.[1238]

- Research suggests that microwave-assisted extraction of black cumin essential oil increases the thymoquinone content.[1239] The same research suggests that higher thymoquinone content improves the antioxidant activity of black cumin essential oil.

- Black cumin essential oil demonstrated activity against *E. coli, Citrobacter freundii*, and *C. albicans*.[1240]

- Cancer development is a multistep process wherein normal cells gain the ability to proliferate continuously and migrate to distant sites in the human body. Agents that interfere with these processes are considered potential anticancer therapeutics. Thymoquinone, the major constituent in black cumin essential oil has demonstrated the ability to modulate several major signaling pathways and key oncogenic molecules that play a prominent role in cancer initiation, progression, invasion, metastasis, and angiogenesis, and has proven effective in improving the effectiveness of and reducing the toxicity of other chemotherapy agents.[1241] Thymoquinone has demonstrated inhibition of the growth of breast, prostate, pancreatic, colon, lung, and hematological malignancies in preclinical models of cancer.

- *In vitro* research demonstrated that black cumin essential oil effectively inhibits multi-antibiotic resistant *Salmonella enterica*, which is a major foodborne pathogen and public health problem.[1242]

- Oral administration of 300 mg/kg body weight of fish oil with black cumin essential oil CT Thymoquinone

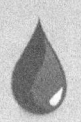 

(68.1%; extracted from the crude fixed/herbal black cumin oil) reduced liver and kidney injury by diminishing oxidative stress and inflammation in rats.[1243] The study included five groups (six rats in each group): a normal control group, a liver-injured control group, and three treatment groups that received either fish oil, black cumin fixed/herbal oil, or fish oil/black cumin essential oil combination. The fish oil/black cumin essential oil was the most effective treatment. Liver enzymes (transaminases (AST and ALT)) were also normalized by the combination. Remarkably liver function was improved in the treatment group pointing to liver regeneration, of which the fish oil/black cumin essential oil was the most effective in regenerating the liver.

☐ Black cumin essential oil and two of its constituents (thymoquinone and carvacrol) significantly inhibited *Listeria monocytogenes* and improved the efficacy of EtBr and ciprofloxacin against *Listeria monocytogenes*.[1244]

☐ Black cumin essential oil demonstrated antimicrobial activity against pathogens (*Staphylococcus aureus, Staphylococcus epidermidis, Streptococcus pneumoniae, Enterococcus faecalis, Klebsiella pneumoniae, Proteus* sp., *Acinetobacter baumannii/calcoaceticus, Porphyromonas* sp., *Veillonella* sp., *Candida* sp., and *Saccharomyces* sp.) isolated from human (periodontal patients') mouths.[1245]

☐ Black cumin essential oil—as well as carvacrol and para-cymene—exhibited antibacterial activity against *S. aureus* and reduced the resistance of MRSA to inhibition.[1246]

☐ *Bacillus* bacteria are widely found in nature and responsible for food poisoning and food spoilage. Black cumin, clove, cinnamon, and marjoram essential oils each reduced *Bacillus* spp. presence in raw and processed meat, with black cumin being the most effective oil.[1247]

☐ Isolated thymoquinone form black cumin seed essential oil protected against brain cell (hippocampal) death in an excitatory model of neurological damage.[1248]

☐ *In vitro* research demonstrated that five different black cumin essential oils—Morocco, Saudi Arabia, Syria, India, and France—inhibited multidrug-resistant pathogenic strains clinically isolated from patients (MRSA, *Escherichia coli, Pseudomonas aeruginosa,* and *Acinetobacter baumannii*).[1249] Interestingly, the five oils did not have thymoquinone and instead were dominated by alpha-phellandrene (Saudi Arabia, Morocco, Syria), 4-caranol (India), and estragole (France).

☐ In rat hypothyroidism and hyperthyroidism models, gavage administration of black cumin essential oil (200 mg/kg BW) balanced thyroid hormone production.[1250] The oil increased triiodothyronine (T3) hormone and decreased nitric oxide (NO)—NO levels are a biomarker for cardiovascular risk in people with hypothyroidism—in hypothyroid rats and decreased T3 in hyperthyroid rats. The oil also increased antioxidant capacity.

☐ Clumping factor B (clfB) is an enzyme in *S. aureus* that plays a key role in its infectivity in humans. Molecular docking research showed that black cumin essential oil inhibited *S. aureus* clfB by docking with the clfB protein and significantly altering intercellular adhesion genes (icaA and icaD).[1251] In addition, isolated para-cymene, thymoquinone, and carvacrol robustly docked to the clfB protein.

☐ CD4+ and CD8+ T lymphocytes are cells involved in cell-mediated immunity. CD4+ cells release cytokines to recruit other cells involved in immune responses, whereas CD8+ cells trigger cell death themselves. Although these cells are important for immune responses, their abnormal function are associated with autoimmune and allergic conditions such as asthma, allergic rhinitis, and rheumatoid arthritis. Black cumin essential oil (49.3% para-cymene, only 2.3% thymoquinone) demonstrated powerful immunomodulatory activity in laboratory research—significantly inhibited the proliferation of CD4+ and CD8+ T lymphocytes, triggered cell death, and reduced the expression of CD28 and CD25 antigens (antigens essential for lymphocyte activation).[1252] Isolated thymoquinone also reduced T lymphocyte proliferation and triggered cell death. The research suggests that black cumin essential oil may contribute to immune balance and alleviate autoimmune and allergic conditions.

☐ Black cumin essential oil with ortho-cymene (37.8%) as the primary constituent displayed significant antioxidant activity and total antioxidant capacity, promising antibacterial activity against antibiotic-resistant bacteria (*B. subtilis, E. coli, P. mirabilis, S. aureus*), and significant antifungal activity against *F. oxysporum* and moderate activity against drug-resistant *C. albicans*.[1253]

☐ A black cumin essential oil with alpha-phellandrene and beta-cymene (0.1% thymoquinone) as the main constituents displayed good antioxidant (DPPH and FRAP assays), alpha-amylase inhibition (reduces the conversion of carbohydrates to sugars), and hemoglobin antiglycation activity (reduces the linking of glucose to sugar, which can result in cell dysfunction and cause diabetic complications like cataracts).[1254] Molecular docking studies showed that thymol, 4-caranol, and alpha-phellandrene had the highest binding affinity to alpha-amylase protein, while alpha-pinene, thymol, alpha-phellandrene, and beta-cymene exhibited good binding potential to human hemoglobin.

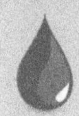

# BLACK PEPPER
*Piper nigrum* L.

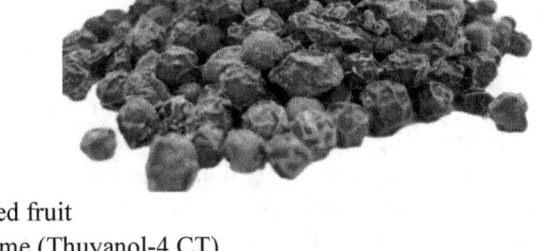

**FAMILY:** Piperaceae
**NOTE:** Top-Middle
**AROMA INTENSITY:** Medium
**AROMA:** Spicy, warming, stimulating
**COMMON EXTRACTION METHOD:** Steam distillation of the dried fruit
**POSSIBLE SUBSTITUTE OILS:** Copaiba, basil (Linalool CT), thyme (Thuyanol-4 CT)
**BLENDS WELL WITH:** Basil, cardamom, cassia, clove, coriander, frankincense, lavender, lemon, marjoram, nutmeg, palo santo, patchouli, pine, ravensara, rosemary, sandalwood, ylang ylang
**SUBCELLULAR LOCALIZATION | EPIGENETIC INFLUENCE:** Endocytic Vesicles | Currently unknown
**RECOMMENDED DILUTION RANGE:** 5%–20%; 50% for some conditions

**PRIMARY CONSTITUENTS:**[1255,1256,1257,1258,1259]

*Beta-Caryophyllene CT*

| | |
|---|---|
| Beta-Caryophyllene | 18.4%–70.4% |
| Limonene | 2.0%–17.4% |
| Alpha-Pinene | 0.3%–16.7% |
| Beta-Pinene | 0.7%–13.6% |
| Sabinene | 0.0%–10.0% |
| Delta-3-Carene | 0.0%–9.2% |
| Beta-Bisabolene | 0.0%–7.1% |
| Alpha-Copaene | 0.2%–5.5% |
| Beta-Elemene | 0.2%–5.1% |
| Bicyclogermacrene | 0.0%–5.1% |
| Alpha-Humulene | 0.0%–4.9% |
| Caryophyllene Oxide | 0.0%–4.9% |
| Alpha-Cadinol | 0.0%–4.9% |
| Alpha-Selinene | 0.0%–4.1% |
| Linalool | 0.5%–4.0% |
| Alpha-Farnesene | 0.0%–3.9% |
| 1,4,7-Cycloundecatrien,1,5,9,9-Tetramethyl-,Z,Z,Z-100 | 0.0%–3.4% |
| Zingiberene | 0.0%–3.4% |

*Limonene CT*

| | |
|---|---|
| Limonene | 10.3%–38.4% |
| Beta-Pinene | 4.7%–25.6% |
| Sabinene | 0.8%–18.1% |
| Beta-Caryophyllene | 1.4%–14.0% |
| Delta-3-Carene | 0.0%–11.3% |
| Germacrene D | 0.0%–11.0% |
| Alpha-Pinene | 4.5%–10.4% |
| Alpha-Phellandrene | 0.5%–8.6% |
| Beta-Biasabolene | 0.2%–8.0% |
| Para-Cymene | 0.0%–5.2% |
| Alpha-Thujene | 0.1%–4.9% |
| Alpha-Copaene | 0.1%–4.8% |

*Delta-3-Carene CT*

| | |
|---|---|
| Delta-3-Carene | 19.0%–32.6% |
| Beta-Pinene | 13.2%–18.3% |
| Limonene | 14.1%–15.2% |
| Beta-Caryophyllene | 2.1%–10.6% |
| Alpha-Pinene | 7.4%–8.3% |
| Beta-Phellandrene | 3.2%–4.5% |
| Alpha-Thujene | 0.0%–4.2% |
| Sabinene | 0.0%–4.1% |
| Para-Cymene | 1.4%–3.5% |
| Alpha-Phellandrene | 2.9%–3.4% |

*Eugenol CT*

| | |
|---|---|
| Eugenol | 12.1%–41.0% |
| Sabinene | 0.0%–12.1% |
| Beta-Eudesmol | 0.9%–9.7% |
| Hedycaryol | 1.3%–9.1% |
| Terpinen-4-ol | 0.0%–8.8% |
| Limonene | 4.9%–7.7% |
| Caryophyllene Oxide | 2.6%–7.2% |
| Delta-3-Carene | 4.2%–6.4% |
| Beta-Pinene | 1.7%–4.7% |
| T-Cadinol | 1.5%–4.7% |
| Beta-Caryophyllene | 3.5%–4.4% |
| T-Muurolol | 2.6%–3.8% |
| Alpha-Pinene | 0.9%–3.8% |

*Beta-Pinene CT*

| | |
|---|---|
| Beta-Pinene | 41.2% |
| 1,8-Cineole | 17.2% |
| Alpha-Pinene | 13.6% |
| Gamma-Terpinene | 5.7% |

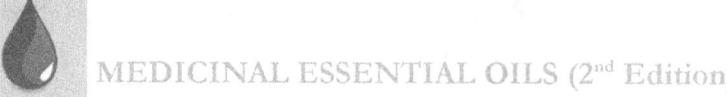
| Linalool | 0.6%–3.9% | Myrcene | 4.4% |
| Myrcene | 1.7%–3.6% | (Z)-Beta-Ocimene | 3.6% |
| Alpha-Terpinene | 0.0%–3.4% | Allo-Ocimene | 3.4% |
| (Z)-Beta-Ocimene | 0.0%–3.2% | | |

Note: The most common CT commercially available is the beta-caryophyllene CT.

**OTHER CONSTITUENTS:** *Beta-Caryophyllene CT*—myrcene, alpha-phellandrene, para-cymene, terpinolene, terpinen-4-ol, eugenol, (E)-beta-farnesene, gamma-muurolene, alpha-selinene, delta-cadinene, hedycaryol, (E)-nerolidol, beta-eudesmol, T-muurolol, alpha-bisabolol, cyclohexene, 1-napthalenol, naphthalene; *Limonene CT*—gamma-terpinene, terpinolene, alpha-terpineol, eugenol, hedycaryol, alpha-cadinol, delta-elemene, alpha-humulene, beta-cubebene, beta-selinene, alpha-selinene, gamma-cadinene, spathulenol, amorphan-3en-9-ol, T-nerolidol, T-muurolol; *Delta-3-Carene CT*—myrcene, alpha-terpinene, para-cymene, gamma-terpinene, linalool, terpinen-4-ol, alpha-terpineol, alpha-copaene, hedycaryolbeta-eudesmol T-cadinol, cyclohexene, (+)-4-carene, beta-humulene, 1,4,7-Cycloundecatrien,1,5,9,9-tetramethylZ,Z,Z-100; *Eugenol CT*—alpha-thujene, myrcene, alpha-phellandrene, beta-phellandrene, gamma-terpinene, terpinolene, linalool, alpha-terpineol, beta-selinene, alpha-farnesene, (E)-nerolidol, ledol, delta-cadinol, alpha-cadinol, alpha-farensol, alpha-bisabolol; *Beta-Pinene CT*—benzyl alcohol, pinene-2-ol, alpha-thujene, neral, geranial, linalool, borneol

**PREFERRED COMPOSITION FOR CLINICAL USE:**

| Constituent | β-Caryophyllene CT | Balanced |
| --- | --- | --- |
| **Beta-Caryophyllene** | 20%–40% | 15%–30% |
| **Limonene** | 10%–22% | 15%–25% |
| **Alpha-Pinene** | 7%–20% | 10%–20% |
| **Beta-Pinene** | 5%–15% | 8%–18% |
| **Delta-3-Carene** | 5%–15% | 8%–18% |
| **Sabinene** | 5%–12% | tr–5% |
| **Alpha-Copaene** | 0.1%–7% | – |
| **Beta-Elemene** | 0.1%–5% | – |
| **Alpha-Phellandrene** | – | 1%–6% |

**REPORTED THERAPEUTIC PROPERTIES: Analgesic (pain relief)**, anti-inflammatory, **aids digestion**, enhances stomach acid production, weight management, protects skin from UV damage, encourages production of skin pigment, **aids circulation**, decongestant, expectorant, antibacterial, **smoking cessation**, antioxidant, antiviral, improves nutrient absorption, aids cognition and memory, increases glutathione and superoxide dismutase production, helps repair gastrointestinal tract damage, respiratory stimulant, helps reduce fear, reduces fatigue and low energy, fosters courage

**CAUTIONS:**

*Limonene, & Delta-3-Carene CTs*
■ None currently known.

*Beta-Caryophyllene CT*
■ May decrease the bioavailability of many medications (NSAIDs, proton-pump inhibitors, acetaminophen, antiepileptics, immune modulators, blood-sugar medications, blood pressure medications, antidepressants, antipsychotics, diabetic medications, antihistamines, antibiotics, and anesthetics) due to the ability of caryophyllene oxide, alpha-humulene, and beta-caryophyllene to inhibit CYP3A enzyme activity.[1260]

*Eugenol CT:*
■ Caution with pregnancy and lactation. Animal studies suggest that large doses of clove (also with significant eugenol content) may negatively impact embryonic development and encourage fetal cell death.[1261,1262] Another animal study did not detect any negative influence of clove oil.[1263] Eugenol is considered strongly toxic to embryos according to animal studies.[1264] Based on these studies it is best to limit clove oil during pregnancy and lactation.
■ May interact with aspirin, blood pressure, antiplatelet, and anticoagulant medications, and increase the risk of bleeding among people with bleeding disorders.[1265,1266,1267,1268]

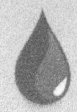

■ May interact with MAOI antidepressants. Animal research suggests that eugenol produces antidepressant effects via the monoamine oxidase pathway, which may cause interactions with antidepressants that also interact with this pathway.[1269]

■ May interfere with enzymes responsible for metabolizing medications (NSAIDs, proton-pump inhibitors, acetaminophen, antiepileptics, immune modulators, blood-sugar medications, blood pressure medications, antidepressants, antipsychotics, diabetic medications, antihistamines, antibiotics, and anesthetics) based on eugenol content.[1270,1271]

■ May interact with antibiotics and possibly enhance their effects due to eugenol content.[1272]

■ May interact with diabetic medications due to inhibition of alpha-glucosidase activity by black pepper essential oil.[1273] Alpha-glucosidase is an enzyme that breaks down carbohydrates by chemical reaction with water. Inhibiting its activity postpones glucose absorption and therefore the impact of carbohydrates on blood sugar levels.

■ May irritate mucous membranes (eyes, mouth, nasal passages, vagina, rectum).[1274,1275]

*Beta-Pinene CT*:

■ Avoid with epilepsy and Parkinson's disease due to 1,8-cineole content (low risk). May exacerbate or cause seizures/convulsions or reduce seizure medication efficacy based on 1,8-cineole content.[1276,1277,1278]

■ May interact with diabetic medications due to inhibition of alpha-glucosidase activity by black pepper essential oil.[1279] This activity may be due to the presence of moderate quantities of 1,8-cineole, which is a known alpha-glucosidase inhibitor when alpha-pinene and beta-pinene are also present.[1280,1281,1282] Alpha-glucosidase is an enzyme that breaks down carbohydrates by chemical reaction with water. Inhibiting its activity postpones glucose absorption and therefore the impact of carbohydrates on blood sugar levels.

**SELECTED EVIDENCE:**

☐ Inhalation of pepper essential oil—20 mcL of a 2% solution added to a cotton pad inhaled for 3 to 7 minutes—increases sympathetic nervous system activity and adrenaline levels, which suggests it may improve alertness.[1283]

☐ Inhalation of black pepper essential oil—1 drop for 2 minutes—significantly decreases nicotine cravings among smokers.[1284,1285,1286]

☐ Topical application of black pepper essential oil—10 to 12 swipes of a 20% dilution (diluted in aloe vera gel) from a roller bottle—prior to intravenous (IV) insertion improves vein visibility and ease of IV insertion.[1287]

☐ A combination of marjoram, black pepper, lavender, and peppermint applied topically decreases neck pain and improves range of motion in people with a history of neck pain.[1288]

☐ Inhalation of black pepper may improve reflexive swallowing movement and may benefit those who have trouble swallowing regardless of consciousness, physical, and mental status.[1289]

☐ Black pepper oil may significantly prevent DNA from bonding to cancer-causing chemicals (DNA adduct formation) and therefore help prevent cancer.[1290]

☐ Animal research suggests oral administration of black pepper essential oil significantly increases superoxide dismutase, glutathione, and glutathione reductase enzyme levels, reduces acute inflammation, and helps relieve pain.[1291]

☐ Black pepper essential oil (composition not reported) helps prevent the growth of *A. calcoacetica, A. faelcais, B. subtilis, B. natriegens, B. linens, F. thermosphacta, C. freundii, C. sporogenes, E. faecalis, E. carotovora, E. coli, F. suaveolens, L. cremoris, M. luteus, Moracella* sp., *P. vulgaris, P. aeruginosa, S. pullorum, S. marcescens, S. aureus,* and *Y. enterocolitica.*[1292]

☐ *In vitro* research demonstrated that low doses of marjoram, lemon, basil, clove, thyme, rosemary CT 1,8-cineole, and tea tree essential oils prevented the shortening of telomeres after exposure to hydrogen peroxide.[1293] The same research reported that vetiver, black pepper, eucalyptus (*E. globulus*), ginger, clove, and rosemary increased the length of already shortened telomeres. This activity suggests that these essential oils can help maintain the youth and health of cells, or turn back the clock on the cell to make it more youthful depending on the essential oil used. Interestingly, cinnamon and peppermint essential oil decreased the length of telomeres slightly.

☐ Black pepper essential oil improves the quality of fresh pork by inhibiting *Pseudomonas* spp. and *Enterobacteriaceae*, and maintaining color quality.[1294]

☐ A small randomized, double-blind, placebo-controlled clinical study with fourteen subjects with back pain found that inhaling black pepper essential oil directly from a vial for fifteen minutes significantly reduced back pain in

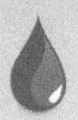 

comparison to placebo (sesame oil).[1295] Subjects were asked to rate their back pain on a scale of one to ten prior to intervention. The average pain rating was 6.07, with a low of three and a high of eight. After intervention the average pain intensity reported reduced to 4.57, demonstrating nearly a 50 percent reduction in back pain.

□ A randomized, double-blind, placebo-controlled study evaluated the benefits of inhaling black pepper essential oil compared to inhaling sesame oil (placebo).[1296] Fifty-four subjects presenting with pain were randomly assigned to two groups and asked to rate their pain from zero to ten, with zero being no pain and ten being maximum pain. Then they inhaled either black pepper or sesame oil for fifteen minutes. The group that inhaled black pepper essential oil experienced significant reduction in pain intensity (a 36.1% reduction) compared to the sesame group, which reported increased pain after inhalation.

□ *In vitro* research demonstrated that black pepper (beta-pinene CT), lemon, and tea tree essential oil possess broad-spectrum antimicrobial activity. Interestingly, of the three essential oils tested, lemon (low limonene content—37.5%) was the most active against bacteria and tea tree was the most active against fungi. The EOs demonstrated synergistic antimicrobial activity when used in combination.[1297]

□ A combination of lemon and black pepper (beta-caryophyllene CT) essential oil demonstrated an additive toxic effect against ticks (*Rhipicephalus microplus*). The individual essential oils also demonstrated varying degrees of efficacy.[1298]

□ Sweet basil, cinnamon bark, sweet fennel, kaffir lime petitgrain, kaffir lime peel, black pepper, peppermint, and spearmint essential oils all demonstrated antimicrobial activity against bacteria linked to cavities (Streptococcus *mutans* and *Lactobacillus casei*).[1299] Cinnamon was the most active against both bacteria, kaffir lime petitgrain was the weakest of the tested oils against both bacteria, and black pepper was inactive against *L. casei*.

□ Black pepper essential oil significantly inhibited the proliferation of cytokine-stimulated skin cells (human dermal fibroblasts) and the production of collagen I, collagen III, and plasminogen activator inhibitor 1, and modulated the expression of genes and signaling pathways related to metabolism, inflammation, tissue remodeling, and cancer signaling.[1300] This data suggests that black pepper essential oil is a promising candidate for wound healing, inflammatory conditions, metabolic diseases, and cancer.

□ *In vitro* research showed that black pepper CT beta-caryophyllene and clove bud essential oils both inhibited *Fusarium oxysporum* and *Aspergillus niger*.[1301]

□ Babesiosis is a rare and life-threatening infection of the red blood cells that occurs when an infected tick bites a human and transmits parasites like *Babesia duncani* or *B. microti*. Current drugs (atovaquone + azithromycin) used to treat babesiosis are ineffective and frequently cause side effects. Both garlic and black pepper essential oil showed good inhibitor activity against *B. duncani* in a hamster red blood cell culture model. Their main constituents, diallyl sulfide and beta-caryophyllene, also exhibited activity. Treatment with atovaquone + azithromycin showed eradication of *B. duncani*, but relapse occurred even at high concentration. On the contrary, garlic oil (or diallyl disulfide) combined with azithromycin killed *B. duncani* parasites at low concentrations without regrowth.

□ Black pepper essential oil displayed good to strong antioxidant activity in the beta-carotene bleaching, FTC, and TBA assays and inhibited the growth of the spoilage fungus *A. flavus* in corn.[1302] The same researchers found that black pepper oil protects against liver and kidney injury caused by carbon tetrachloride in mice. Administration of black pepper essential oil increased catalase (CAT), glutathione (GSH), and total superoxide dismutase (T-SOD) activities present in the liver and kidney, and reversed markers for liver damage such as elevations in total bilirubin (TBIL), glutamate pyruvate transaminase (ALT), aspartate aminotransferase (AST), alkaline phosphatase (AKP), and malondialdehyde (MDA) level.

□ Acute oral and repetitive oral administration of black pepper CT limonene essential oil showed an antidepressant-like and anxiolytic effect in mice, possibly by influencing the serotonin system.[1303] The oil did not alter monoamine levels in mice brains, nor did it impair locomotor activity, cause toxicity, trigger biochemical abnormalities, or change body weight. As a side benefit, total cholesterol level decreased.

□ Black pepper essential oil displayed broad-spectrum antioxidant activity both intracellular and *in vitro*, which was attributed to a synergistic activity of all the constituents.[1304]

□ A randomized controlled clinical study found that topical application of 20% black pepper essential (in a base of aloe vera gel and using a roller bottle) to the forearm ten minutes before vein puncture improved vein selection and successful catheter insertion.[1305] In addition, the application of black pepper oil improved patient and nurse satisfaction.

□ The limonene CT of black pepper essential oil demonstrated moderate anti-*H. pylori* activity.

□ Acetylcholine is a neurotransmitter and neuromodulator that modulates nervous system activity by sending signals between nerves. It is vital for cognitive function, particularly memory and attention. Acetylcholinesterase is an enzyme that breaks down acetylcholine into acetic acid and choline to terminate signaling and transmission

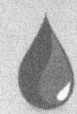

between neurons. Therefore, inhibiting this enzyme can increase the amount of acetylcholine available to neurons and potentially improve cognitive function. Investigating the anticholinesterase activity of spice essential oils (cassia, cardamom, black pepper CT beta-caryophyllene, white pepper CT beta-caryophyllene), researchers found that black pepper (both black and white peppercorns) possess the most potent acetylcholinesterase inhibitory activity.[1306] Molecular docking analysis and *in vitro* validation suggested that delta-3-carene, alpha-pinene, and beta-pinene may be responsible for the anticholinesterase activity of pepper oils.

☐ A black pepper essential oil with 19.6% beta-caryophyllene and 19.1% limonene inhibited the lipolytic activity and type II secretion system P. psychrophile.[1307]

☐ *Clostridioides difficile* (*C. diff*) is a very virulent and multidrug resistant bacterium that causes healthcare-acquired infections that are very difficult to treat and have frequent recurrence. A laboratory study evaluated the anticlostridial potential of three essential oils—wild oregano (*Origanum minutiflorum*), garlic, and black pepper—against C. diff strains isolated from hospitalized people.[1308] Each of the oils inhibited C. diff and its formation of biofilms, with oregano being the most active. The researchers concluded that these oils represent promising candidates for "adjunctive therapeutics in the treatment of CDI [C. diff infections]."

☐ Immunosuppressive steroids like dexamethasone are commonly used to treat rheumatic conditions, skin diseases, sever allergies, lung conditions, brain swelling, and more. Unfortunately, it is associated with a variety of adverse effects such as high blood sugar in people without diabetes, pancreatic cell death due to increased reactive oxygen species, oxidative stress and nitrosative stress—the formation of reactive nitrogen species due to abnormal nitric oxide levels, which plays an important role in cardiovascular and metabolic diseases. A preclinical study evaluated the effects of black pepper CT limonene essential oil against the adverse effects of dexamethasone.[1309] Rats were divided into five groups: (1) dexamethasone treatment alone; (2) dexamethasone with black pepper essential oil (0.5 mL/kg BW); (3) dexamethasone with black pepper essential oil (1 mL/kg BW); (4) dexamethasone with metformin; and (5) a control group that received no interventions. After four consecutive days of intervention, serum insulin, blood glucose, total cholesterol, triglycerides, insulin resistance, pancreatic damage, oxidative stress, and nitrosative stress were all worse in the dexamethasone group compared to the control group. All these parameters were improved in the black pepper oil and metformin groups, suggesting that oral administration of black pepper oil can suppress oxidative/nitrosative stress, protect the pancreas against dexamethasone damage, and alleviate high blood sugar, insulin resistance, hyperinsulinemia, and dyslipidemia caused by dexamethasone treatment.

☐ Black pepper essential oil nanoparticles inhibited proliferation, migration, and invasion of triple negative breast cancer cells.[1310]

☐ Polymeric particles loaded with black pepper essential oil was larvicidal to *Anopheles aquasalis* mosquitoes.[1311]

☐ The sabinene CT of black pepper essential oil demonstrated contact and fumigant toxicity against the stable fly (*Stomoxys calcitrans*).[1312]

---

# BLACK SAGE
## (Cordia, Erva Baleeira)

*Cordia verbenacea* DC, *C. curassavica* (Jacq.) Roem. & Schult., *C. macrostachya* (Jacq.) Roem. & Schult, *Varronia curassavica* Jacq.

**FAMILY:** Boraginaceae
**NOTE:** Middle
**AROMA INTENSITY:** Strong
**AROMA:** Herbaceous, earthy, pungent, slightly sweet
**COMMON EXTRACTION METHOD:** Steam distilled from leaves; may also be distilled from the aerial parts, stems, or roots
**POSSIBLE SUBSTITUTE OILS:** Copaiba, hemp, guava leaf, black pepper, hairy basil (trans-caryophyllene CT), shell ginger
**BLENDS WELL WITH:** Agarwood, cedarwood, chamomile (German, Roman), copaiba, davana, eucalyptus, geranium, hemp, kanuka, kunzea, lavender, manuka, rose, rosewood, sandalwood, tagetes, tea tree, wild chamomile, ylang ylang
**SUBCELLULAR LOCALIZATION | EPIGENETIC INFLUENCE:** Currently unknown | Currently unknown
**RECOMMENDED DILUTION RANGE:** 3.0%–33.0%; neat for limited conditions

**PRIMARY CONSTITUENTS:**[1313,1314,1315,1316,1317,1318,1319]

*Leaves (Caryophyllene Oxide CT)*

| | |
|---|---|
| Caryophyllene Oxide | 15.0%–23.1% |
| Beta-Caryophyllene | 7.7%–14.8% |
| Alpha-Pinene | 1.1%–14.4% |
| Aromadendrene | 0.0%–6.8% |
| 9-Epi-(E)-Caryophyllene | 0.6%–6.0% |
| Humulene Epoxide II | 3.1%–5.0% |
| Delta-Cadinene | 2.5%–4.1% |

*Leaves (Beta-Caryophyllene CT)*

| | |
|---|---|
| Beta-Caryophyllene | 25.4% |
| Bicyclogermacrene | 11.3% |
| Alpha-Pinene | 9.5% |
| Delta-Cadinene | 9.4% |
| Cadina-1,4-Diene | 5.9% |
| Spathulenol | 5.7% |
| Alpha-Humulene | 4.8% |
| Germacrene D | 4.5% |
| Beta-Farnesene | 4.2% |

*Leaves (Alpha-Santalene CT)*

| | |
|---|---|
| Alpha-Santalene | 35.6% |
| Beta-Sinensal | 17.7% |
| Alpha-Trans-Bergamotol | 12.9% |
| (Z)-Beta-Farnesene | 8.8% |
| Alpha-Farnesene | 6.4% |

*Leaves (Alpha-Pinene CT)*

| | |
|---|---|
| Alpha-Pinene | 20.5%–52.3% |
| Beta-Caryophyllene | 11.7%–16.5% |
| Bicyclogermacrene | 0.0%–13.8% |
| Beta-Pinene | 0.1%–13.1% |
| Alpha-Santalene | 0.0%–10.6% |
| Germacrene D | 0.0%–6.7% |
| Sabinene | 0.0%–5.0% |
| Alpha-Humulene | 1.6%–4.8% |
| Allo-Aromadendrene | 0.0%–4.3% |

*Leaves (Beta-Phellandrene CT)*

| | |
|---|---|
| Beta-Phellandrene | 25.3% |
| Cubebol | 23.9% |
| Alpha-Pinene | 10.4% |
| Alpha-Gurjunene | 6.2% |

*Leaves (Tricyclene CT)*

| | |
|---|---|
| Tricyclene | 23.9% |
| Bicyclogermacrene | 11.7% |
| Germacrene D | 9.9% |
| Beta-Caryophyllene | 8.2% |
| Camphene | 7.0% |
| Alpha-Copaene | 6.0% |
| Alpha-Pinene | 5.1% |

Note: Other chemotypes are also reported in the literature (beta-caryophyllene/ar-turmerone, tricyclene/camphene, alpha-zingiberene/beta-sesquiphellandrene, 7-cyclodecen-1-one/7-methyl-3-methylene-10-(1-propyl), sabinene, shyobunol, and shyobunones) but no complete composition data was found for all chemotypes.[1320,1321,1322,1323,1324,1325,1326,1327,1328,1329] The stem oil is primarily composed of spathulenol (27.1%), trans-sesquisabinene hydrate (11.0%), viridiflorol (10.7%), thujopsan-2-alpha-ol (9.6%), and 1,10-di-epi-cubenol (8.3%).[4155] The aerial parts produce an essential oil with 4-Methyl,4-ethenyl-3-(1-methyl ethenyl)-1-(1-methyl methanol)cyclohexane (37.3%), beta-eudesmol (19.2%), spathulenol (11.3%), and cadina 4(5), 10(14) diene (7.9%).[4156]

**OTHER CONSTITUENTS:** *Leaves (Caryophyllene Oxide CT)*—beta-pinene, 1,8-cineole, alpha-thujone (< 2.1%), camphenol, alpha-campholenal, trans-verbenol, cis-beta-terpineol, trans-carveol, isobornyl acetate, cis-4-thujanol acetate, neo-verbenol acetate, neo-iso-verbenol acetate, delta-elemene, verbenol acetate, citronellyl acetate, beta-elemene, 1.7-di-epi-alpha-cedrene, gamma-curcumene, alpha-humulene, germacrene D, germacrene A, epizonarene, spathulenol, ar-turmerone, (Z)-alpha-santalol, acarenone, iso-longifolol, pentadecanol, 14-hydroxy-9-epi-(E)-caryophyllene, beta-bisabolene, 14-hydroxy-alpha-humulene; *Leaves (Alpha-Pinene CT)*—alpha-phellandrene, camphene, myrcene, para-cymene, limonene, gamma-terpinene, linalool, camphor, terpinen-4-ol, alpha-copaene, beta-bourbonene, beta-elemene, alpha-bergamotene, spathulenol, viridiflorol, caryophyllene oxide; *Leaves (Beta-Caryophyllene CT)*—sabinene, beta-myrcene, linalool, camphor, alpha-cubebene, beta-elemene, beta-bisabolene; *Leaves (Beta-Phellandrene CT)*—sabinene, alpha-phellandrene, cis-p-menth-2-en-1-ol, trans-pinocarveol, bornyl acetate, delta-elemene, alpha-copaene, alpha-cubebene, beta-cubebene, beta-bourbonene, valencene, trans-beta-guaiene, cubebol, gamma-cadinene, alpha-cadinene, spathulenol, caryophyllene oxide, globulol, beta-copaene-4alpha-ol, viridiflorol; *Leaves (Alpha-Santalene CT)*—alpha-pinene, alpha-cedrene, alpha-santalene, cis-gamma-bisabolene, (Z)-nerolidol, caratol, caryophyllene oxide, alpha-trans-bergamotol acetate, (Z)-epi-beta-santalol acetate; *Leaves (Tricyclene CT)*—beta-myrcene, limonene, fenchyl acetate, bornyl acetate, beta-bourbonene, beta-cubebene, alpha-humulene, alpha-amorphene, gamma-curcumene, alpha-muurolene, gamma-cadinene, beta-bisabolene, delta-cadinene

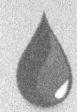

**PREFERRED COMPOSITION FOR CLINICAL USE:**

| Constituent | Alpha-Pinene CT |
|---|---|
| Alpha-Pinene | 20%–40% |
| Beta-Caryophyllene | 10%–25% |
| Bicyclogermacrene | 5%–15% |
| Alpha-Humulene | 2%–10% |
| Beta-Pinene | 0.1%–10% |

**REPORTED THERAPEUTIC PROPERTIES: Analgesic (pain relief), anti-inflammatory**, antirheumatic, antiarthritic, antibacterial, antifungal, antiparasitic, wound healing, stomach protection, aids digestion, astringent, stops excess bleeding, relieves chronic skin conditions, reduces fever, **antiallergic**, supports respiratory function, eases cough, protects the heart, supports oral health, encourages restful sleep, insecticide, stress management, relieves anxiety

**CAUTIONS:**

■ May interact with antibiotics and increase or decrease their effectiveness.[1330]

■ *Beta-Phellandrene CT*: May interact with anticholinergic (drugs used for asthma, incontinence, gastrointestinal cramps, muscular spasms, depression, and sleep disorders) and cholinergic medications (drugs used to reduce urinary retention, diagnose myasthenia gravis, and for glaucoma) based on AChE inhibitory activity of beta-phellandrene.[1331]

■ *Caryophyllene oxide and Beta Caryophyllene CTs*: May decrease the bioavailability of many medications (NSAIDs, proton-pump inhibitors, acetaminophen, antiepileptics, immune modulators, blood-sugar medications, blood pressure medications, antidepressants, antipsychotics, diabetic medications, antihistamines, antibiotics, and anesthetics) due to the ability of caryophyllene oxide and beta-caryophyllene to inhibit CYP3A enzyme activity.[1332]

**SELECTED EVIDENCE:**

☐ Animal research demonstrates that oral administration of black sage essential oil reduces inflammation and allergic responses.[1333] It prevented edema caused by carrageenan, bradykinin, substance P, histamine and platelet-activating factor, myeloperoxidase activity (the most abundant proinflammatory enzyme stored in neutrophils, which is linked to a number of diseases including atherosclerosis, heart attack, atrial fibrillation, multiple sclerosis, Alzheimer's disease, lung cancer, and transplant rejection),[1334] neutrophil migration, edema caused by honey bee (*Apis mellifera*) venom, and significantly decreased TNF-alpha production. Alpha-humulene isolated from black sage essential oil was found to be 18% bioavailable when administered orally to mice, and was distributed to the liver, kidneys, heart, lungs, spleen, and brain thirty minutes following administration. The study authors also observed that alpha-humulene produced a rapid systemic anti-inflammatory and pain relieving effect when administered topically or orally.[4164] Another study reported that oral administration of beta-caryophyllene and alpha-humulene produced anti-inflammatory effects similar to dexamethasone (a corticosteroid drug used to treat inflammation, severe allergies, adrenal problems, arthritis, skin conditions, and flare-ups of multiple sclerosis).[4165] In addition, both constituents reduced edema, prostaglandin production (E(2) (PGE(2)), decreased nitric oxide synthase (iNOS), and COX-2 activity. Alpha-humulene also reduced edema caused by histamine. Other research reports that alpha-humulene and beta-caryophyllene both inhibit inflammation caused by the protein NF-κB and neutrophil migration (neutrophils migrate from the bloodstream to sites of injury to release inflammatory chemicals, and are involved in inflammation, tissue, bone, and cartilage damage associated with rheumatoid arthritis).[4166] Only alpha-humulene prevented the production of proinflammatory cytokines (TNF-alpha and IL-1 beta) when isolated from black sage oil.

☐ Animal research demonstrates that topical application of 5 mg/kg of black sage essential oil three times daily for eleven days reduces bone loss associated with periodontitis, reduced the presence of *Porphyromonas gingivalis* (a pathogenic bacterium involved in the initiation and progression of periodontal disease) in the oral cavity, and encouraged a healthy inflammatory response (balanced the pro/anti-inflammatory system).[1335]

☐ Black sage essential oil (beta-caryophyllene CT) inhibits the growth of fungi (*Candida albicans* and *C. krusei*), and possesses antibacterial activity against gram-positive bacteria (*Staphylococcus aureus* and *Bacillus cereus*), and one multi-resistant gram-negative bacterium (*Escherichia coli*) *in vitro*.[1336] The tricyclene CT is active against gram-positive bacteria (*S. aureus* and *Enterococcus faecalis*).[1337] *In vitro* research demonstrated that black sage CT elemol essential oil inhibited *Artemia salina, Staphylococcus aureus, Staphylococcus epidermidis, Bacillus subtilis,*

*Sarcina lutea, Vibrio cholera, Vibrio cholera, Vibrio cholera (two strains), Escherichia coli, Aspergillus niger, Trichophyton mentagrophytes, Fusarium sporotrichum, Fusarium moniliforme*, and *Rhyzoctonia solani.*[1338]

☐ *In vitro* research shows that a trans-beta-caryophyllene CT of black sage is a more potent antioxidant that vitamin E (alpha-tocopherol) and synthetic BHT.[1339]

☐ Black sage essential oil (alpha-pinene CT) is toxic to the larvae of the *Aedes aegypti* mosquito.[1340]

# BLUE CYPRESS
## (Northern Cypress Pine)
*Callitris intratropica* R. T. Baker & H. G. Smith

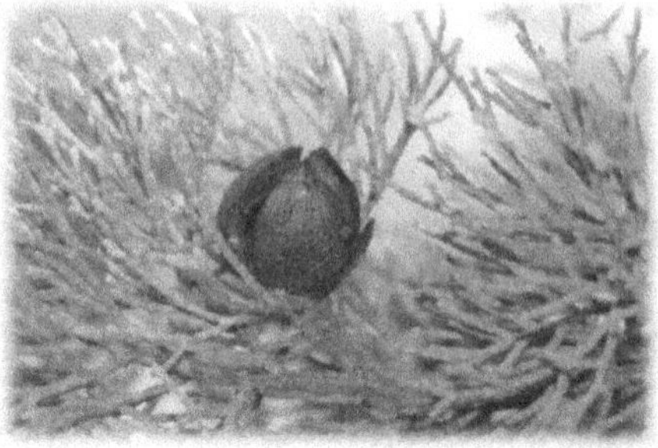

**FAMILY:** Cupressaceae
**NOTE:** Top-Middle
**AROMA INTENSITY:** Medium
**AROMA:** Fresh, balsamic, woody, fruity
**COMMON EXTRACTION METHOD:** Steam distilled from the wood or leaves
**POSSIBLE SUBSTITUTE OILS:** Blue tansy, German chamomile, frankincense
**BLENDS WELL WITH:** Cedarwood, eucalyptus, orange, rosemary, sandalwood
**SUBCELLULAR LOCALIZATION | EPIGENETIC INFLUENCE:** Currently unknown | Currently unknown
**RECOMMENDED DILUTION RANGE:** 5%–Neat

**PRIMARY CONSTITUENTS:**[1341,1342,1343]

*Wood*

| Constituent | Percentage |
|---|---|
| Bulnesol (5-Azulenemethanol) | 13.8%–18.0% |
| Guaiol | 13.7%–15.3% |
| Beta-Eudesmol | 8.5%–14.0% |
| Dihydrocolumellarin | 1.3%–14.0% |
| Alpha-Eudesmol | 7.6%–11.2% |
| Gamma-Eudesmol | 8.0%–9.7% |
| Guaiazulene | 0.1%–6.2% |
| Chamazulene | 0.0%–5.6% |

*Leaves*

| Constituent | Percentage |
|---|---|
| Alpha-pinene | 35.9%–55.6% |
| Limonene | 21.6%–50.5% |
| Myrcene | 6.0%–10.1% |

**OTHER CONSTITUENTS:** Alpha-selinene, beta-chamigrene, beta-elemene, beta-selinene, beta-guaiene, elemol, callitrisin, callitrin, cadalene

**PREFERRED COMPOSITION FOR CLINICAL USE:**

| Constituent | Wood |
|---|---|
| **Guaiol** | 13%–20% |
| **Bulnesol** | 8%–20% |
| **Beta-Eudesmol** | 5%–15% |
| **Gamma-Eudesmol** | 5%–12% |
| **Alpha-Eudesmol** | 2%–12% |
| **Dihydrocolumellarin** | 1%–12% |
| **Beta-Selinene** | 2%–10% |
| **Alpha-Selinene** | 2%–7% |
| **Callitrin** | 0.1%–2% |
| **Callitrisin** | 0.1%–2% |
| **Guaiazulene** | 0.1%–2% |
| **Chamazulene** | 0%–1% |

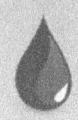

**REPORTED THERAPEUTIC PROPERTIES:** Analgesic, anti-inflammatory, antibacterial, antifungal, antiviral, anti-infectious, antiallergic, relieves itching and skin conditions, **supports respiratory function**, wound healing, calming, helps remove pessimism, grounding, **inspires confidence**

**CAUTIONS:**

■ *Wood oil*: Avoid during pregnancy and lactation (low risk) due to beta-eudesmol content. Beta-eudesmol strongly inhibits the growth of new blood vessels, which is necessary for implantation, and placental and embryonic development.[1344]

■ *Wood oil*: May interact with aspirin, blood pressure, antiplatelet, and anticoagulant medications, and increase the risk of bleeding among people with bleeding disorders based on beta-eudesmol content (low risk).[1345,1346]

**SELECTED EVIDENCE:**

☐ Blue cypress may support a normal inflammatory response by suppressing the production of proinflammatory prostaglandins and moderately inhibiting the 5-lipoxygenase (5-LOX) enzyme that is involved in the inflammation process.[1347,1348]

☐ Blue cypress may mildly inhibit MRSA.[1349]

# BLUE MALLEE
## (Eucalyptus Polybractea, Blue-Leaved Mallee)

*Eucalyptus polybractea* R. Baker

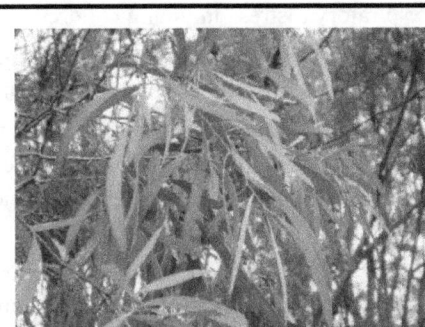

**FAMILY:** Myrtaceae
**NOTE:** Top
**AROMA INTENSITY:** Medium
**AROMA:** Sweet, camphoraceous, fresh, medicinal
**COMMON EXTRACTION METHOD:** Steam distilled from the leaves
**POSSIBLE SUBSTITUTE OILS:** Eucalyptus, ravintsara (1,8-cineole CT), cajeput, rosemary (1,8-cineole CT), myrtle, cardamom (1,8-cineole CT), Southern blue gum, big badja gum, gully gum
**BLENDS WELL WITH:** Angelica, bay laurel, blue cypress, cajeput, camphor, eucalyptus, lemon, lemon eucalyptus, myrtle, niaouli, peppermint, ravintsara, rosemary, tea tree, thyme
**SUBCELLULAR LOCALIZATION | EPIGENETIC INFLUENCE:** Currently unknown | Currently unknown
**RECOMMENDED DILUTION RANGE:** 3%–33%; neat for limited conditions

**PRIMARY CONSTITUENTS:**[1350,1351,1352]

*1,8-Cineole CT*

| | |
|---|---|
| 1,8-Cineole | 85.0%–94.2% |
| Para-Cymene | 1.2%–4.1% |
| Beta-Pinene | 0.0%–2.3% |
| Alpha-Pinene | 0.0%–2.1% |
| Globulol | 0.0%–1.7% |
| Terpinen-4-ol | 0.6%–1.5% |
| Limonene | 0.2%–1.3% |

*Cryptone CT*

| | |
|---|---|
| 1,8-Cineole | 41.0%–58.2% |
| Alpha-Pinene | 5.4%–18.2% |
| Para-Cymene | 3.2%–7.5% |
| Cryptone | 1.3%–4.9% |
| Beta-Pinene | 0.7%–3.8% |
| Spathulenol | 2.0%–3.8% |

**OTHER CONSTITUENTS:** *1,8-Cineole CT*—cryptone (<1.0%), alpha-terpinyl acetate, myrtenal, trans-pinocarveol, aromadendrene; *Cryptone CT*—limonene, terpinen-4-ol, myrtenal, pinocarvone, trans-pinocarveol, carveol, verbenol, verbenone, globulol, para-cymen-8-ol, cuminol, aromadendrene, calamenene, caryophyllene oxide

**PREFERRED COMPOSITION FOR CLINICAL USE:**

| Constituent | Cryptone CT | 1,8-Cineole CT |
|---|---|---|
| **1,8-Cineole** | 45%–60% | 75%–95% |
| **Alpha-Pinene** | 10%–18% | 1–5% |

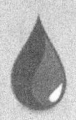
| Para-Cymene | 2%–8% | 0%–7% |
|---|---|---|
| Cryptone | 2%–5% | – |
| Beta-Pinene | 1–5% | 0%–2% |
| Spathulenol | 1–5% | – |
| Limonene | 0.1%–2% | 0%–8% |

**REPORTED THERAPEUTIC PROPERTIES:** Antibacterial, antifungal, anti-infectious, antiparasitic, antiviral, antiseptic, analgesic, anti-inflammatory, antiarthritic, antirheumatic, wound healing, relieves blisters, **supports respiratory function**, eases cough, relieves headache/migraine, expels excess mucus, **decongestant**, relieves sinus pressure (sinusitis), relieves sore throat, combats acne, purification, insect repellent, **insecticide**, aids focus/concentration, mentally stimulating

## CAUTIONS:

■ Avoid with children under age three, particularly around the nose and mouth. Use very cautiously in children under age five due to high 1,8-cineole content. 1,8-cineole may cause seizures, central nervous system problems, or respiratory distress in young children.[1353,1354,1355,1356]

■ Avoid with epilepsy and Parkinson's disease due to 1,8-cineole content. May exacerbate or cause seizures/convulsions or reduce seizure medication efficacy based on 1,8-cineole content.[1357,1358,1359]

■ Caution is warranted orally due to the significant amounts of 1,8-cineole. Limit it to small doses internally (adults— maximum 10 drops daily). One text recommends a maximum daily dose of 6 drops.[1360] Toxicity has been reported when eucalyptus (also high in 1,8-cineole) was ingested in large doses, and as few as 4 to 5 drops may cause problems in very sensitive individuals.[1361,1362,1363,1364,1365,1366] In humans, 3.5 to 5 mL has proven fatal orally.[1367]

■ May weakly interfere with the enzymes responsible for metabolizing medications (NSAIDs, proton-pump inhibitors, acetaminophen, antiepileptics, immune modulators, blood-sugar medications, blood pressure medications, antidepressants, antipsychotics, diabetic medications, antihistamines, antibiotics, and anesthetics) based on research with an herbal extract of eucalyptus and 1,8-cineole content.[1368,1369,1370]

■ May interact with diabetic medications due to the ability of 1,8-cineole to significantly inhibit alpha-glucosidase activity, particularly when synergized with other constituents (alpha-pinene, beta-pinene, and para-cymene).[1371,1372,1373] Alpha-glucosidase is an enzyme that breaks down carbohydrates by chemical reaction with water. Inhibiting its activity postpones glucose absorption and therefore the impact of carbohydrates on blood sugar levels. Studies suggest that eucalyptus oil significantly lowers glucose in animals, which may increase the action of diabetic medications.[1374,1375]

■ May interact with aspirin, blood pressure, antiplatelet, and anticoagulant medications, and increase the risk of bleeding among people with bleeding disorders (low risk).[1376] 1,8-cineole is a weak inhibitor of platelet aggregation.[1377]

■ May interfere with pentobarbital and other barbiturates (medications for anxiety and insomnia) based on 1,8-cineole content.[1378,1379]

## SELECTED EVIDENCE:

☐ Of sixteen eucalyptus species tested, blue mallee essential oil (1,8-cineole CT) was the most effective eucalyptus species tested for mosquito (*Aedes aegypti*) fumigant properties and demonstrated the third strongest larvicidal activity.[1380,1381]

☐ *In vitro* research reported that blue mallee essential oil inhibited *S. aureus, Serratia marcescens, K. pneumoniae, E. coli, Enterococcus faecalis, C. albicans, Aeromonas sobria,* and *Acinetobacter baumanii.*[1382]

☐ Eucalyptus (*E. globulus*) and blue mallee essential oil inhibited *E. coli. S. aureus, E. faecalis, S. typhimurium, A. baumannii, C. albicans, S. epidermidis,* and MRSA, with *E. faecalis* and *C. albicans* being the most susceptible microbes and *A. baumannii* the least susceptible.[1383]

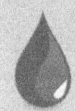

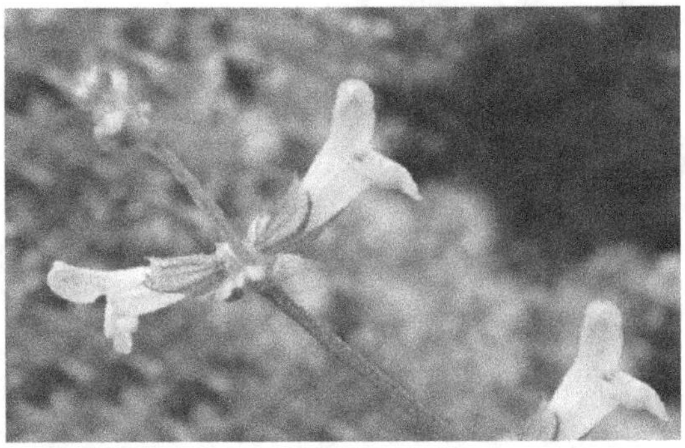

## BLUE MOUNTAIN SAGE
### (African Tea Tree)

*Salvia stenophylla* Burch. ex Benth

**FAMILY:** Lamiaceae (Labiatae)
**NOTE:** Top
**AROMA INTENSITY:** Medium-Strong
**AROMA:** Herbaceous, pungent, fresh, slightly floral
**COMMON EXTRACTION METHOD:** Steam distilled from the flowering aerial parts
**POSSIBLE SUBSTITUTE OILS:** German chamomile, cypress, pine, pink pepper
**BLENDS WELL WITH:** Basil, bergamot, cedarwood, copaiba, cypress, frankincense, geranium, ginger, grapefruit, hyssop, juniper berry, lavender, lemon, lime, marjoram, myrrh, orange, palo santo, rosemary, sage, sandalwood, Spanish sage, vetiver, ylang ylang
**SUBCELLULAR LOCALIZATION | EPIGENETIC INFLUENCE:** Currently unknown | Currently unknown
**RECOMMENDED DILUTION RANGE:** 3%–Neat

### PRIMARY CONSTITUENTS:[1384,1385]

*Delta-3-Carene CT*

| | |
|---|---|
| Delta-3-Carene | 18.4%–25.0% |
| Manool | 0.9%–20.9% |
| Alpha-Bisabolol | 8.2%–19.7% |
| 1,8-Cineole | 0.0%–10.9% |
| Beta-Bisabolene | 0.2%–11.3% |
| Beta-Caryophyllene | 0.0%–7.3% |
| Limonene | 2.8%–6.1% |
| Camphor | 1.0%–6.0% |
| Alpha-Pinene | 2.4%–5.0% |
| Borneol | 1.3%–4.8% |

*(E)-Nerolidol CT*

| | |
|---|---|
| (E)-Nerolidol | 46.7%–53.6% |
| Manool | 12.1%–12.7% |
| Myrcene | 4.4%–12.3% |
| Gamma-Terpinene | 0.1%–11.3% |
| Alpha-Bisabolol | 1.3%–4.7% |

*Gamma-Terpinene CT*

| | |
|---|---|
| Gamma-Terpinene | 20.3% |
| Para-Cymene | 18.4% |
| Alpha-Bisabolol | 17.4% |
| (E)-Nerolidol | 15.1% |
| Manool | 5.6% |

*Alpha-Bisabolol CT*

| | |
|---|---|
| Alpha-Bisabolol | 37.4%–47.6% |
| Delta-3-Carene | 7.0%–19.3% |
| Myrcene | 0.0%–18.8% |
| (Z)-Lanceol | 0.2%–8.7% |
| Manool | 0.0%–8.6% |
| Alpha-Bisabolol Oxide | 0.0%–5.3% |
| Limonene | 2.0%–4.5% |

*Limonene CT*

| | |
|---|---|
| Limonene | 19.3% |
| Delta-3-Carene | 10.2% |
| Beta-Phellandrene | 7.8% |
| Manool | 6.3% |
| Viridiflorol | 5.7% |
| Beta-Caryophyllene | 5.4% |
| Camphor | 4.7% |
| Alpha-Pinene | 4.5% |

**OTHER CONSTITUENTS:** *Alpha-Bisabolol CT*—alpha-pinene, camphene, beta-pinene, sylvestrene, limonene, gamma-terpinene, para-cymene, beta-phellandrene, camphor, linalool, trans-alpha-bergamotene, trans-beta-bergamotene, (Z)-beta-farnesene, bicyclogermacrene, (E)-bisabolene, beta-caryophyllene, borneol, beta-bisabolene, (E)-alpha-bisabolene, alpha-campholenealcohol, caryophyllene oxide; *(E)-Nerolidol CT*—alpha-pinene, camphene, delta-3-carene, limonene, 1,8-cineole, para-cymene, camphor, linalool, terpinen-4-ol, alpha-terpineol, borneol, (Z)-lanceol; *Delta-3-Carene CT*—camphene, beta-pinene, myrcene, sylvestrene, gamma-terpinene, para-cymene, isoterpinolene, terpinolene, linalool, terpinen-4-ol,

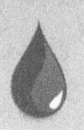

aromadendrene, nonanol, alpha-humulene, alpha-terpineol, delta-cadinene, caryophyllene oxide, trans-alpha-bisabolene, myrtenol, viridiflorol, alpha-eudesmol, beta-eudesmol, caryophyllenol-II; *Limonene CT*—camphene, beta-pinene, alpha-phellandrene, alpha-terpinene, para-cymene, linalool, trans-p-menth-2-en-ol, aromadendrene, cis-p-menth-2-en-ol, alpha-humulene, alpha-terpineol, borneol, delta-cadinene, selina-3-(7)-11-diene, caryophyllene oxide, (E)-nerolidol, humulene epoxide II, spathulenol, alpha-bisabolol, caryophylladienol-I, caryophylladienol-II, caryophyllenol-II, (Z)-lanceol; *Gamma-Terpinene CT*—alpha-pinene, alpha-thujene, camphene, beta-pinene, myrcene, alpha-terpinene, limonene, 1,8-cineole, camphor, terpinen-4-ol, borneol, alpha-bisabolol oxide, isothymol, isocarvacrol, carvacrol, (Z)-lanceol

### PREFERRED COMPOSITION FOR CLINICAL USE:

| Constituent | Delta-3-Carene CT | Alpha-Bisabolol CT |
| --- | --- | --- |
| **Delta-3-Carene** | 18%–30% | 7%–20% |
| **Manool** | 10%–25% | 5%–10% |
| **Alpha-Bisabolol** | 5%–20% | 35%–50% |
| **Beta-Caryophyllene** | 5%–10% | – |
| **Limonene** | 5%–10% | 2%–8% |
| **Beta-Bisabolene** | 0.5%–10% | – |
| **Camphor** | 3%–8% | – |
| **Alpha-Pinene** | 2%–7% | – |
| **Borneol** | 2%–5% | – |
| **Myrcene** | – | 7%–20% |
| **(Z)-Lanceol** | – | 3%–10% |

**REPORTED THERAPEUTIC PROPERTIES:** Antibacterial, **antiviral**, antiseptic, wound healing, eases cough, supports respiratory function, relieves sore throat, aids digestion, expels excess gas, relieves menstrual discomfort, **anti-inflammatory**, antispasmodic, **soothes chronic skin conditions**, moisturizes/softens the skin, insect repellent, relieves insect bites/stings, relieves anxiety, antidepressant, enhances meditation, stress management

### CAUTIONS:

■ *Alpha-Bisabolol CT*: May interfere with the enzymes responsible for metabolizing medications (NSAIDs, proton-pump inhibitors, acetaminophen, antiepileptics, immune modulators, blood-sugar medications, blood pressure medications, antidepressants, antipsychotics, diabetic medications, antihistamines, antibiotics, and anesthetics) due to alpha-bisabolol content.[1386]

■ *Alpha-Bisabolol CT*: May interact with anticholinergic (drugs used for asthma, incontinence, gastrointestinal cramps, muscular spasms, depression, and sleep disorders) and cholinergic medications (drugs used to reduce urinary retention, diagnose myasthenia gravis, and for glaucoma) based on alpha-bisabolol content.[1387]

■ *(E)-Nerolidol CT*: May interfere with antibiotics and increase their effectiveness ((E)-nerolidol sensitizes bacteria to antibiotics).[1388]

### SELECTED EVIDENCE:

☐ *In vitro* research demonstrated that blue mountain sage essential oil (delta-3-carene CT) decreases inflammation by inhibiting both the 5-LOX and COX-2 enzymes.[1389] The 5-LOX enzyme converts arachidonic acid to leukotrienes, increasing inflammation and allergic reactions, and is associated with chronic degenerative inflammatory diseases. The COX-2 enzyme is present and active in cells when inflammation occurs.

☐ Blue mountain sage essential oil (delta-3-carene CT) exhibits good antimalarial activity *in vitro*.[1390]

☐ *In vitro* research reports that blue mountain sage essential oil (alpha-bisabolol CT) exhibits good antimicrobial activity against *S. aureus* and *B. cereus*.[1391]

☐ Blue mountain sage essential oil (delta-3-carene CT) is a poor antioxidant.[1392]

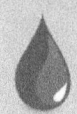

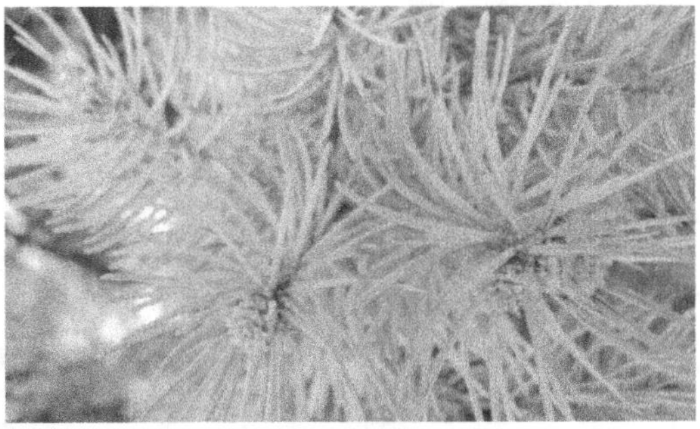

# BLUE SPRUCE
## (Colorado Blue Spruce, Colorado Spruce)

*Picea pungens* Engelm., *P. pungens* Engelm. f. a*rgentea* Beissn.

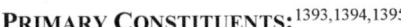

**FAMILY:** Pinaceae
**NOTE:** Middle
**AROMA INTENSITY:** Medium
**AROMA:** Woody, evergreen, earthy
**COMMON EXTRACTION METHOD:** Steam distilled from the needles
**POSSIBLE SUBSTITUTE OILS:** Spruce (black), tsuga, silver fir, rosemary (Bornyl acetate CT), balsam fir, white fir
**BLENDS WELL WITH:** Balsam fir, birch, black spruce, cedarwood, chamomile (German, Roman), copaiba, frankincense, galbanum, lavender, lemon, myrtle, palo santo, pine, silver fir, tsuga, white fir
**SUBCELLULAR LOCALIZATION | EPIGENETIC INFLUENCE:** Currently unknown | Currently unknown
**RECOMMENDED DILUTION RANGE:** 5%–Neat

**PRIMARY CONSTITUENTS:** [1393,1394,1395]

| | |
|---|---|
| Bornyl Acetate | 6.7%–29.4% |
| Camphor | 0.0%–26.4% |
| Limonene | 0.0%–24.8% |
| Alpha-Pinene | 4.1%–23.8% |
| Camphene | 7.1%–18.0% |
| Beta-Pinene | 0.0%–8.8% |
| Myrcene | 5.1%–7.5% |
| Delta-3-Carene | 0.0%–6.4% |

**OTHER CONSTITUENTS:** 1,8-cineole, alpha-terpinolene, beta-elemene, bicyclo[3.1.0]hexan-2-ol, exo-methylcamophenillol, gamma-cadinene, linalool, germacrene D, 3-cyclohexene-1-methanol, borneol, 2-cyclohexene-1-one

**PREFERRED COMPOSITION FOR CLINICAL USE:**

| Constituent | |
|---|---|
| **Bornyl Acetate** | 15%–30% |
| **Limonene** | 15%–25% |
| **Alpha-Pinene** | 10%–25% |
| **Camphene** | 7%–15% |
| **Myrcene** | 5%–10% |
| **Beta-Pinene** | 5%–10% |
| **Delta-3-Carene** | 5%–10% |
| **Camphor** | > 10% |

**REPORTED THERAPEUTIC PROPERTIES:** Antioxidant, **stimulates androgenic hormone production**, analgesic (pain relief), **nervine (calms and soothes the nerves)**, antineuralgic, antiseptic, anti-inflammatory, supports the respiratory system, antibacterial, grounding, relaxing, **releases past trauma and emotional blocks**

**CAUTIONS:**

■ Use very cautiously with children under 6 due to potentially high camphor content. Several cases of camphor poisoning and/or seizures from ingestion and topical application have been reported in children.[1396,1397] Ingestion of camphor-containing products has been lethal in children under age 2 (estimated to be roughly 2,000 mg of camphor for a 20 kg child as the minimum potential fatal dose).[1398,1399] Children 5 years and up may use camphor-containing essential oils topically in dilutions no stronger than 5%.

■ Caution is warranted during pregnancy and while lactating due to potentially high camphor content. Ingestion of essential oils with significant levels of camphor may lead to abortion because fetuses lack the enzymes to process it.[1400] Camphor ingestion by infants and young children may cause cough, vomiting, seizure, burning sensation in the mucous membranes and eyes, or lack of voluntary coordination of muscle movements.[1401]

■ Avoid with epilepsy and Parkinson's due to potentially high camphor content.[1402,1403,1404]

■ Oral caution—Essential oils with significant levels of camphor can be toxic when taken orally. Oral—Camphor can be toxic when taken orally (usually single doses exceeding 2 mL), although the lethal dose for adult humans is estimated to be (more than 5 mL) in a single dose.[1405,1406,1407]

■ The potentially high camphor content in blue spruce may negatively impact red blood cells and increase the risk of jaundice in children with Glucose-6-phosphate dehydrogenase deficiency (G6PD).[1408,1409]

**SELECTED EVIDENCE:**

☐ Topical application of blue spruce—8 drops of neat oil applied to the chest or testicles every day after showering for fourteen days—may increase total and free-testosterone levels an average of 9% and 26.8% respectively.[1410]

☐ Bornyl acetate reduces proinflammatory cytokine levels and may reduce pain and inflammation.[1411,1412]

☐ Blue spruce seed and cone essential oils (consisting primarily of limonene, alpha-pinene, and beta-pinene) exhibited mild antimicrobial activity and demonstrated safety in human skin cells and cardiovascular cells.[1413]

---

# BLUE TANSY
## (Moroccan Tansy, Moroccan Blue Chamomile)
*Tanacetum annuum* L.

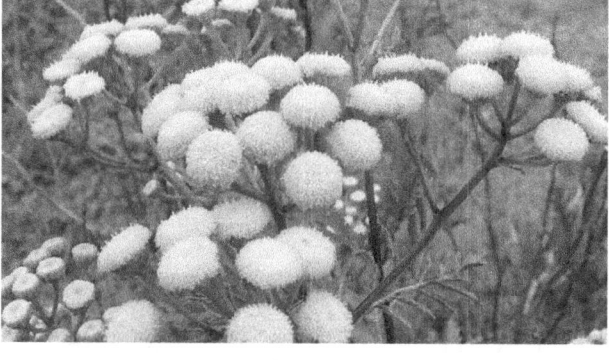

**FAMILY:** Asteraceae (Compositae)
**NOTE:** Middle
**AROMA INTENSITY:** Medium
**AROMA:** Warm, sweet, soft, herbaceous
**COMMON EXTRACTION METHOD:** Steam distilled from the aerial parts of the flowering plants
**POSSIBLE SUBSTITUTE OILS:** Blue cypress, German chamomile, ravensara (sabinene CT), cistus, helichrysum
**BLENDS WELL WITH:** Bergamot, blue cypress, cedarwood, eucalyptus, frankincense, geranium, helichrysum, lavender, neroli, patchouli, pine, rose, spruce (black)
**SUBCELLULAR LOCALIZATION | EPIGENETIC INFLUENCE:** Currently unknown | Currently unknown
**RECOMMENDED DILUTION RANGE:** 5%–Neat

**PRIMARY CONSTITUENTS:**[1414,1415,1416,1417]

| Sabinene CT | | Chamazulene CT | |
|---|---|---|---|
| Sabinene | 13.3%–22.3% | Chamazulene | 17.0%–38.0% |
| Myrcene | 4.4%–18.3% | Beta-Myrcene | 1.0%–18.4% |
| Camphor | 11.7%–13.2% | Camphor | 4.0%–18.0% |
| Beta-Pinene | 5.3%–10.1% | Sabinene | 4.0%–8.6% |
| Alpha-Phellandrene | 7.1%–9.2% | Beta-Eudesmol | 3.0%–7.0% |
| Para-Cymene | 5.9%–8.9% | | |
| Chamazulene | 2.8%–5.0% | | |
| Alpha-Pinene | 2.1%–4.9% | | |

Note: The sabinene CT is the most common CT commercially available.

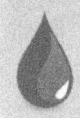

**OTHER CONSTITUENTS:** *Sabinene CT*—Camphene, limonene, alpha-terpinene, beta-phellandrene, gamma-terpinene, thymol, beta-caryophyllene, 1,8-cineole, borneol, 3,6-dihydrochamazulene, borneol, 5,6-dihydrochamazulene, farnesene isomer, germacrene D, terpinen-4-ol, beta-eudesmol; *Chamazulene CT*—Beta-pinene, alpha-bisabolol, borneol, camphene, beta-caryophyllene, caryophyllene oxide, 1,8-cineole, para-cymene, dehydro-5,6,7,8-tetrahydrochazulene, beta-farnesene, 3,6-dihydrochamazulene, 5,6-dihydrochamazulene, beta-elemene, elemol, limonene, terpinen-4-ol, alpha-terpinene, gamma-terpinene, alpha-terpineol, thymol

**PREFERRED COMPOSITION FOR CLINICAL USE:**

| Constituent | Sabinene CT |
| --- | --- |
| Chamazulenes (Chamazulene + 1,9-Dihydrochamazulene + 3,6-Dihydrochamazulene + 5,6-Dihydrochamazulene, 7,8-Dihydrochamazulene) | 8%–36% |
| Sabinene | 10%–28% |
| Myrcene | 2%–18% |
| Camphor | 3%–15% |
| Alpha-Phellandrene | 3%–10% |
| Para-Cymene | 2%–10% |
| Beta-Pinene | 2%–8% |
| Alpha-Pinene | 1.5%–5% |
| Limonene | 1%–4% |
| Borneol | 0.5%–4% |
| Terpinen-4-ol | 0.5%–4% |
| Gamma-Terpinene | 0.5%–4% |
| Beta-Caryophyllene | 1%–3% |
| Germacrene D | 0.1%–3% |
| 1,8-Cineole | 0.1%–3% |

**REPORTED THERAPEUTIC PROPERTIES: Antiallergic, wound healing, anti-inflammatory**, analgesic (pain relief), antibacterial, antifungal, antiviral, antioxidant, antispasmodic, **nourishes skin**, stimulates immune function, reduces excess mucus, **supports tissue regeneration**, reduces anxiety, relaxing, sedating, stress management, reduces anger

**CAUTIONS:**

■ *Chamazulene CT*: May interfere (low risk) with the enzymes responsible for drug metabolism (NSAIDs, proton-pump inhibitors, acetaminophen, antiepileptics, immune modulators, blood-sugar medications, blood pressure medications, antidepressants, antipsychotics, diabetic medications, antihistamines, antibiotics, and anesthetics) due to chamazulene content.[1418]

■ The potentially moderate camphor content in blue tansy may negatively impact red blood cells and increase the risk of jaundice in children with Glucose-6-phosphate dehydrogenase deficiency (G6PD).[1419,1420]

■ Avoid with epilepsy and Parkinson's disease due to camphor content (moderate risk). May exacerbate or cause seizures or convulsions based on camphor content.[1421,1422]

**SELECTED EVIDENCE:**

☐ Blue tansy kills human rhabdomyosarcoma cancer cells *in vitro*.[1423]

☐ Blue tansy helps decrease inflammation by mildly inhibiting the 5-lipoxygenase (5-LOX) enzyme that is involved in the inflammation response according to *in vitro* research.[1424]

☐ Blue tansy inhibits the growth of common food fungi, including *Botrytis cinerea, Helminthosporium oryzae, Alternaria solani, Piricularia oryzae*, and *Verticillium dahliae*.[1425]

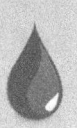

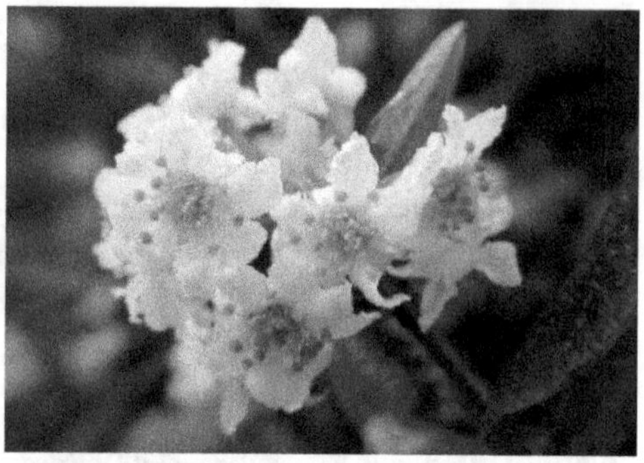

# BOLDO
## (Boldo Leaf, Boldu Boldus, Boldoa Fragrans)
*Peumus boldus* Mol., *Boldus fragrans* Gay

**FAMILY:** Monimiaceae
**NOTE:** Middle
**AROMA INTENSITY:** Strong
**AROMA:** Pungent, spicy, disagreeable
**COMMON EXTRACTION METHOD:** Hydrodistilled from the dried leaves
**POSSIBLE SUBSTITUTE OILS:** Bay laurel, niaouli, rosemary, American wormseed
**BLENDS WELL WITH:** Doesn't blend well with other oils due to its strong disagreeable odor
**SUBCELLULAR LOCALIZATION | EPIGENETIC INFLUENCE:** Currently unknown | Currently unknown
**RECOMMENDED DILUTION RANGE:** < 0.5%

**PRIMARY CONSTITUENTS:**[1426,1427,1428,1429,1430,1431]

*Ascaridole CT*

| | |
|---|---|
| Ascaridole | 21.3%–51.2% |
| 1,8-Cineole | 12.0%–21.1% |
| Para-Cymene | 0.0%–16.3% |
| Limonene | 0.0%–16.1% |
| Alpha-Thujone | 0.0%–14.3% |
| Guaiazulene | 0.0%–8.8% |
| Para-Cymol | 0.0%–7.9% |
| (Z)-Verbenol | 0.0%–7.2% |
| Beta-Thujone | 0.0%–7.2% |
| Beta-Phellandrene | 0.0%–5.4% |
| (E)-Nerolidol | 0.0%–5.0% |

*1,8-Cineole/Para-Cymene/Limonene CT*

| | |
|---|---|
| 1,8-Cineole | 11.8%–36.6% |
| Para-Cymene | 13.6%–29.8% |
| Limonene | 2.7%–17.0% |
| Beta-Phellandrene | 0.0%–8.4% |
| Sabinene | 5.1%–6.3% |
| Ascaridole | 1.0%–6.3% |
| Alpha-Pinene | 4.2%–5.3% |
| Terpinen-4-ol | 4.4%–5.3% |
| Alpha-Terpineol | 1.9%–5.2% |

*Ascaridole CT (no 1,8-cineole)*

| | |
|---|---|
| Ascaridole | 36.5%–46.9% |
| Limonene | 18.5%–23.2% |
| Para-Cymene | 12.9%–19.0% |

**OTHER CONSTITUENTS:** *Ascaridole CT*—delta-3-carene, alpha-phellandrene, alpha-pinene, beta-pinene, 1.3.8-para-menthatriene, cis-sabinene hydrate, trans-sabinene hydrate, trans-pinocarveol, delta-terpineol, terpinen-5-ol, myrtenol, methyl eugenol (< 1.3%), linalool, 1,4-cineole, sabinyl acetate; *Ascaridole CT (no 1,8-cineole)*—alpha-pinene, sabinene, beta-pinene, gamma-terpinene, terpinolene, trans-pinocarveol, pinocarvone, 1-terpinen-4-ol, alpha-terpineol, methyl eugenol (< 1.2%), spathulenol; *1,8-Cineole/Para-Cymene/Limonene CT*—alpha-thujene, camphene, beta-pinene, myrcene, alpha-phellandrene, alpha-terpinene, delta-3-carene, linalool, fenchol, campholenal, bornyl acetate, trans-pinocarveol,

**PREFERRED COMPOSITION FOR CLINICAL USE:**

| Constituent | 1,8-Cineole/ Para-Cymene/ Limonene CT |
|---|---|
| **1,8-Cineole** | 20%–35% |
| **Para-Cymene** | 15%–30% |
| **Limonene** | 5%–15% |
| **Sabinene** | 4%–6% |
| **Alpha-Pinene** | 4%–6% |

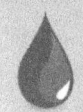

| Terpinen-4-ol | 4%–6% |
|---|---|
| Ascaridole | < 6% |
| Alpha-Terpineol | 2%–5% |

Note: Should only be used clinically when the benefits outweigh the risks as determined by a health professional.

**REPORTED THERAPEUTIC PROPERTIES:** Antibacterial, antimicrobial, antiseptic, antiparasitic, analgesic, anti-inflammatory, antirheumatic, aids digestion, diuretic, aids liver and gallbladder function, helps eliminate gallstones, nervine, insecticide, stimulating

**CAUTIONS:**
*Boldo is not recommended for use in essential oil therapy in any form of administration, but the profile is included for informational purposes and safety information.*

■ Avoid use in children due to toxicity concerns and known poisoning and fatalities with ascaridole-containing essential oils in humans.[1432] Cases of seizure have been reported in young children due to exposure to thujone rich essential oils.[1433,1434]

■ Avoid during pregnancy and lactation. Hydro-alcohol extracts of boldo have reportedly caused abortions, fetal abnormalities, and low birth weight in animal studies when administered at 800 mg/kg/day.[1435,1436] Boldo leaf teas are reportedly used to induce illegal abortions in humans.[1437] Essential oils high in thujone content may cause abortion.[1438,1439]

■ Avoid oral consumption—very toxic due to ascaridole and potential thujones content. Oral use of boldo can cause respiratory depression, overstimulation of the CNS (exaggerated reflexes, lack of coordination, convulsions, paralysis of motor and sensory nerves, and death by respiratory arrest), liver toxicity, and anaphylactic reactions.[1440,1441,1442] Human toxicity and fatal poisoning have been reported in children and adults with chenopodium essential oil (also high in ascaridole).[1443] Thujone is considered significantly neurotoxic and may damage the liver, and it is estimated that as little as 15 mg orally may negatively impact the central nervous system.[1444,1445,1446]

■ Avoid with epilepsy and Parkinson's disease due to thujone and 1,8-cineole content, and reports in animals that boldo essential oil causes convulsions at doses of 70 mg/kg.[1447]

■ May interact with aspirin, blood pressure, antiplatelet, and anticoagulant medications, and increase the risk of bleeding among people with bleeding disorders based on ascaridole and isoascaridole content.[1448,1449]

■ Avoid with those who have a compromised liver or kidneys due to the risk of kidney toxicity, kidney failure, or liver toxicity (ascaridole and thujones content).[1450,1451,1452,1453] Consuming extremely large amounts of thujone rich essential oils (10 mL) has caused kidney failure.[1454] This would also suggest that those taking medications that could cause liver damage should also use boldo very cautiously or avoid it entirely.

■ Topical application, sensitization. Boldo may cause skin sensitization when applied topically due to ascaridole content.[1455,1456,1457]

■ *1,8-cineole and 1,8-Cineole/Para-Cymene/Limonene CTs*: May interfere with pentobarbital and other barbiturates (medications for anxiety and insomnia) based on 1,8-cineole content.[1458,1459]

■ *1,8-cineole and 1,8-Cineole/Para-Cymene/Limonene CTs*: May weakly interfere with the enzymes responsible for metabolizing medications (NSAIDs, proton-pump inhibitors, acetaminophen, antiepileptics, immune modulators, blood-sugar medications, blood pressure medications, antidepressants, antipsychotics, diabetic medications, antihistamines, antibiotics, and anesthetics) due to 1,8-cineole content.[1460,1461,1462]

**SELECTED EVIDENCE:**
☐ *In vitro* research shows that boldo essential oil completely inhibits *Aspergillus niger* and *A. carbonarius*, and prevented the accumulation of ochratoxin A in peanuts.[1463] Other research demonstrates that boldo essential oil inhibits *A. flavus* and *A. parasiticus* and completely prevented their production of aflatoxin AFB(1).[1464,1465] Boldo oil also inhibited *Rhizoctonia solani Phragmidium violaceum*, and *Fusarium oxysporum*.[1466]

☐ Boldo essential oil inhibited several gram-positive (*Streptococcus pyogenes, Micrococcus sp., Staphylococcus aureus, Bacillus subtilis*, and *Enterococcus faecalis*) and gram-negative (*Shigella sonnei, Salmonella Sp., Morganella morganii, Acinetobacter baumannii, Escherichia coli,* and *Pseudomonas aeruginosa*) bacteria, and *C. albicans in vitro*.[1467]

☐ Boldo essential oil showed potent insecticidal activity against the house fly *Musca domestica*.[1468]

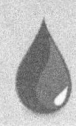 

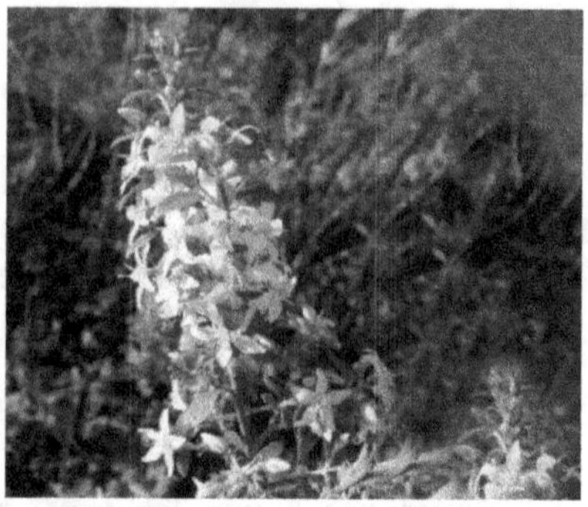

# BUCHU
## (Bucku)

Round Leaf Buchu: *Agathosma betulina* Bergius, *Barosma betulina* Bergius;
Oval Leaf Buchu: *A. crenulata* L., *B. crenulata* L.

**FAMILY:** Rutaceae
**NOTE:** Middle
**AROMA INTENSITY:** Strong
**AROMA:** Medicinal, hints of black currant, slightly sweet to minty, herbaceous, camphoraceous
**COMMON EXTRACTION METHOD:** Steam distilled from the leaves
**POSSIBLE SUBSTITUTE OILS:** Pennyroyal, spearmint, peppermint
**BLENDS WELL WITH:** African bluegrass, cedarwood, frankincense, geranium, ginger, hyssop, jasmine absolute, lavandin, lavender, lemon, may chang, neroli, orange, palmarosa, patchouli, petitgrain, ravintsara, rosewood, sandalwood, Texas cedarwood, Virginia cedarwood, ylang ylang
**SUBCELLULAR LOCALIZATION | EPIGENETIC INFLUENCE:** Currently unknown | Currently unknown
**RECOMMENDED DILUTION RANGE:** 1.0%–5.0%

**PRIMARY CONSTITUENTS:**[1469,1470,1471]

*A. betulina (Isomenthone CT)*

| | |
|---|---|
| Isomenthone | 4.6%–29.1% |
| Limonene | 11.6%–28.2% |
| Diosphenol | 12.0%–26.3% |
| Menthone | 2.5%–25.0% |
| psi-Diosphenol | 10.3%–23.3% |
| 8-Mercapto-p-Menthan-3-one (cis + trans) | 0.7%–6.6% |
| Alpha-Pulegone | 0.4%–4.6% |
| (1S)-(-)-Beta-Pulegone | 0.6%–4.5% |

*A. crenulata*

| | |
|---|---|
| (1R)-(+)-Beta-Pulegone | 31.6%–73.2% |
| Isomenthone | 3.6%–27.6% |
| Limonene | 2.1%–17.2% |
| Menthone | 1.3%–16.6% |
| (E)-8-Acetylthio-p-menthan-3-one | 0.4%–10.4% |
| 8-Hydroxymenthone | 0.0%–4.9% |
| (-)-(E)-Alpha-Pulegone | 0.0%–4.8% |

*A. betulina (Menthone CT)*

| | |
|---|---|
| Menthone | 29.2% |
| Isomenthone | 14.2% |
| Pulegone | 8.4% |
| psi-Diosphenol | 2.9% |

**OTHER CONSTITUENTS:** *A. betulina (Isomenthone CT)*—1,8-cineole, beta-myrcene, sabinene; *A. crenulata*—beta-phellandrene, para-cymene, 3-methylcyclohexanone, linalool, (+)-(Z)-alpha-pulegone, (Z)-8-mercapto-p-menthan-3-one, cis-isopulegole, trans-isopulegole, terpinen-4-ol, (E)-isopulegone beta-myrcene, (Z)-isopulegone, (E)-beta-ocimene, (E)-8-mercapto-p-menthan-3-one, alpha-pinene, beta-pinene, 1,8-cineole, sabinene, (Z)-8-acetylthio-p-menthan-3-one, 8-hydroxy-4-menthen-3-one, cis-piperitone oxide, (E)-8-methylthiomenth-3-one, (E)-p-menthon-8-thioacetate; *A. betulina (Menthone CT)*—alpha-pinene, myrcene, 1,8-cineole, gamma-terpinene, (E)-beta-ocimene, para-cymene, linalool, trans-isopulegole, terpinen-4-ol, 8-hydroxymenthone, 1-hydroxy-pseudo-diosphenol, 4-hydroxy-diosphenol

**PREFERRED COMPOSITION FOR CLINICAL USE:**

| Constituent | Isomenthone CT |
|---|---|
| **Limonene** | 15%–30% |
| **Isomenthone** | 10%–30% |
| **Diosphenol** | 12%–25% |

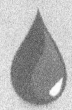

| Psi-Diosphenol | 10%–20% |
| 8-Mercapto-p-Menthan-3-one <cis + trans> | 0.5%–6% |
| Alpha-Pulegone | 0.5%–5% |
| (1S)-(-)-Beta-Pulegone | < 5% |

Note: Should only be used clinically when the benefits outweigh the risks as determined by a health professional.

**REPORTED THERAPEUTIC PROPERTIES:** Antiseptic, anti-infectious, analgesic, antimicrobial, anti-inflammatory, antirheumatic, antiarthritic, antispasmodic, aids immune function, expels excess gas, diuretic, eases cough, aids digestion, supports and protects urinary tract health, aids detoxification, relieves sprains, soothes sore muscles, reduces fever, insecticide, insect repellent, reduces hysteria, reduces jealousy, relaxing/calming

**CAUTIONS:**

*Buchu is not commonly used in essential oil therapy due to the toxicity of pulegone, which is known to be toxic to the liver and deplete glutathione levels. Glutathione is essential to several detoxification processes and its depletion can lead to liver damage. Buchu is not recommended for use in essential oil therapy, but listed here to report composition and safety information.*

■ Avoid with children under age twelve. Multiple organ failure, liver failure, brain swelling (cerebral edema), severe epileptic encephalopathy (severe brain disorder with seizures), organ cell death (necrosis), and death has been reported in infants who were administered mint tea containing pennyroyal essential oil (similar in composition to buchu oil and also high in pulegone).[1472] Pulegone and its metabolite menthofuran (or metabolites of menthofuran) are believed to cause the toxic effects of buchu and other essential oils high in pulegone, which include liver and kidney toxicity, bronchiolar cell destruction, depletion of liver glutathione levels (the primary protective antioxidant of the liver), and direct cellular damage.[1473,1474,1475,1476] Children are more likely to experience these adverse effects.[1477]

■ Avoid during pregnancy and lactation due to significant amounts of pulegone and the potential toxicity of buchu essential oil to multiple organs.[1478,1479] Pennyroyal (similar in composition to buchu oil and also high in pulegone) is believed to trigger uterine contractions by irritating the genito-urinary system. It is commonly used to induce abortions.[1480,1481] Pennyroyal essential oil (similar in composition to buchu oil and also high in pulegone) is commonly used to induce abortion, which generally is unsuccessful but causes serious health consequences to the mother. Carachipita is an abortant sold over the counter in South America that contains pennyroyal, yerba de la perdiz, oregano, and marsh rosemary. The literature reports successful use of Carachipita to induce abortion, but not without serious consequences to the mother (multiple organ failure, vaginal bleeding, destruction of red blood cells, numbness, dizziness, and death).[1482,1483,1484] It is prudent to avoid buchu oil while pregnant or nursing due to its toxicity alone, despite a lack of evidence that it is a direct abortifacient.

■ Avoid oral consumption due to the toxic potential of pulegone, its metabolite menthofuran, and buchu essential oil to multiple organs. Pulegone is metabolized by human liver cytochrome P-450s (CYP2E1, CYP1A2, and CYP2C19) to menthofuran after administration, which actually increases its toxic effect to the liver.[1485,1486] Animal research suggests oral administration of pulegone is significantly toxic to the liver and causes death at 300 mg/kg body weight per day (over 3.3 mL for a human adult equivalent dose) for two weeks.[1487] Lower doses of 75 and 150 mg/kg body weight per day for three months resulted in liver, kidney, bone marrow, heart, stomach, lung, ovarian, and thymus damage, and one death in animals.[1488] A two-year animal study reported urinary cancer and papillomas, liver cancer, osteosarcoma, and multiple organ damage or enlargement (liver, kidney, olfactory epithelium, lung, bile duct).[1489] Ingestion of pennyroyal essential oil (similar in composition to buchu oil and also high in pulegone) can cause abdominal pain and tenderness, nausea, bloody vomiting, burning of the throat, fever, lethargy alternating with agitation, confusion, delirium, restlessness, seizures, dizziness, auditory and visual hallucinations, increased blood pressure, rapid heartbeat, swollen blood vessels in the lungs and filling of the alveoli with blood, excessive acidity of the blood, blood clots, abortion, liver failure, kidney failure, respiratory failure, shock, coma, and death.[1490] Neurological damage has been reported in adults who consumed 2.5 to 5.0 mL of pennyroyal essential oil (similar in composition to buchu oil and also high in pulegone), moderate to severe poisoning with single doses of 10 mL, and deaths occurred at over 15 mL of ingestion.[1491,1492,1493,1494,1495,1496,1497,1498,1499,1500,1501]

■ Avoid with epilepsy and Parkinson's disease due to pulegone and 1,8-cineole content. May exacerbate or cause seizures or convulsions when inhaled, applied topically, or ingested based on 1,8-cineole content.[1502,1503,1504,1505,1506,1507]

■ Avoid with compromised liver or kidney due to the potential of pulegone to cause liver and kidney toxicity and damage.[1508,1509,1510,1511,1512,1513] This would suggest medications that have the potential to damage the liver should also be avoided.

**SELECTED EVIDENCE:**

☐ A double-blind, placebo-controlled study demonstrated that the topical application of a thin layer of buchu essential oil gel three times daily (to the exercised bicep) for four days reduced post-exercise swelling.[1514] However, the researchers also reported that the reduced swelling was accompanied by a reduction in muscle function and did not reduce muscle pain.

☐ Both *A. betulina* and *A. crenulata* essential oil initially increased spasms and then reduced spasms in isolated guinea-pig ileum, possibly by blocking calcium from entering cells (calcium channel blocker).[1515]

☐ Buchu essential oil inhibits the 5-LOX enzyme, which is involved in the initiation and maintenance of a variety of inflammatory diseases.[1516] The study authors attributed the anti-inflammatory activity of buchu oil to the presence of limonene, which also inhibits 5-LOX when used as an isolated constituent.

☐ *In vitro* research suggests that buchu essential oil is a poor antimicrobial, demonstrating insignificant to no inhibition of *E. coli, Enterococcus hirae, P. aeruginosa, Saccharomyces cerevisiae,* and *S. aureus*.[1517] Another study reported that it was inactive against the *Malassezia furfur* fungus.[1518] Interestingly, one study found that buchu (high in menthone content) moderately inhibited *S aureus, B. cereus, K. pneumoniae,* and *C. albicans*.[1519]

☐ *In vitro* research reported that both species of buchu essential oil are weak antioxidants.[1520,1521]

---

## BUDDHA WOOD
### (Desert Rosewood, False Sandalwood)
*Eremophila mitchellii* Benth.

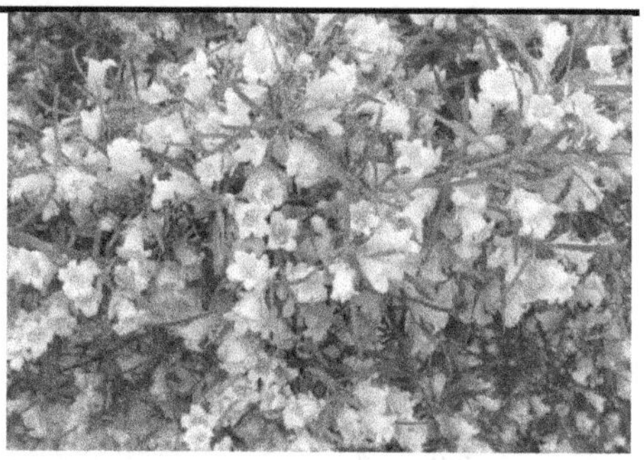

**FAMILY:** Myoporaceae
**NOTE:** Base
**AROMA INTENSITY:** Medium
**AROMA:** Woody, balsamic, resinous, spicy-sweet, slightly smokey
**COMMON EXTRACTION METHOD:** Steam distilled or hydrodistilled from the heartwood
**POSSIBLE SUBSTITUTE OILS:** Frankincense, vetiver
**BLENDS WELL WITH:** Agarwood, allspice, balsam fir, cassia, cedarwood, cinnamon, copaiba, cypress, frankincense, hinoki, myrrh, nutmeg, Peru balsam, sandalwood, tolu balsam, vetiver
**SUBCELLULAR LOCALIZATION | EPIGENETIC INFLUENCE:** Currently unknown | Currently unknown
**RECOMMENDED DILUTION RANGE:** 3%–50%; Neat for limited conditions

**PRIMARY CONSTITUENTS:**[1522,1523]

| | |
|---|---|
| Eremophilone | 40.5%–43.0% |
| 9-Hydroxy-7(11),9-Eremophiladien-8-one | 18.0%–37.0% |
| Santalcamphor | 0.0%–17.5% |
| 9-Hydroxy-1,7,9-Eremophilatrien-8-one | 0.0%–6.7% |
| 8-Hydroxy-10(11), Eremophiladien-9-one | 0.1%–4.1% |

**OTHER CONSTITUENTS:** Beta-selinene, alpha-selinene, 9-hydroxy-1,7(11),9-eremophilatrien-8-one, eremophilenol isomer

**PREFERRED COMPOSITION FOR CLINICAL USE:**

| *Constituent* | |
|---|---|
| **Eremophilone** | 30%–50% |
| 1(10),11-Eremophiladien-9-one* | |
| **9-Hydroxy-7(11),9-Eremophiladien-8-one** | 10%–40% |

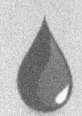

| 2-Hydroxyeremophilone*; 8-Hydroxy Eremophilone* | |
|---|---|
| **8-Hydroxy-10(11), Eremophiladien-9-one** | 10%–30% |
| 2-Hydroxy-2-dihydroeremophilone*; 8-Hydroxy-Dihydro Eremophilone* | |

\* The constituents with a star are not necessarily recognized synonyms but may be what is listed on GC-MS reports for the constituents in bold. There is great confusion and inconsistency in buddha wood constituent nomenclature because the constituents are positional isomers, retention times overlap, and mass spectra are similar.

**REPORTED THERAPEUTIC PROPERTIES:** Analgesic, anti-inflammatory, anticancer, antimicrobial, antiviral, antibacterial, supports cardiovascular system function, aids immune function, insect repellant, insecticide, antidepressant, relieves anxiety, calming, sedating, **enhances meditation**

**CAUTIONS:**
- None currently known.

**SELECTED EVIDENCE:**
- *In vitro* research shows that buddha wood essential oil kills P388D(1) mouse lymphoblast cells.[1524]
- Buddha wood essential oil demonstrated good antioxidant activity.[1525]

# CAJEPUT
## (Cajuput, Swamp Tea Tree)

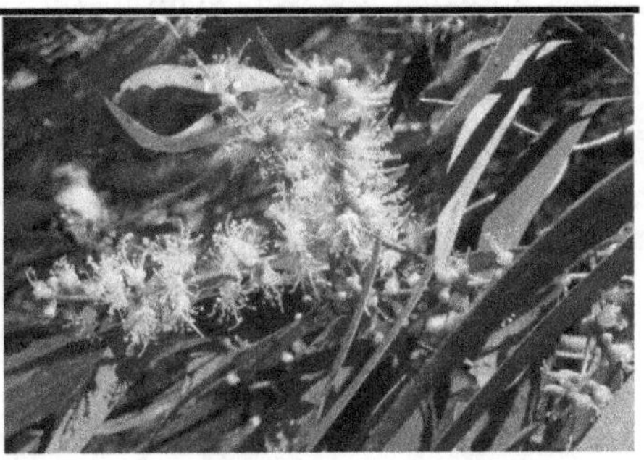

*Melaleuca cajuputi* Powell, *M. leucadendron* var. *cajuputi* Roxb.

**FAMILY:** Myrtaceae
**NOTE:** Middle
**AROMA INTENSITY:** Medium
**AROMA:** Medicinal, penetrating, slightly sweet, slightly woody
**COMMON EXTRACTION METHOD:** Steam distilled from the leaves and twigs
**POSSIBLE SUBSTITUTE OILS:** Eucalyptus, niaouli (1,8-cineole CT), ravintsara (1,8-cineole CT), ravensara (1,8-cineole CT), cardamom, rosemary (1,8-cineole CT)
**BLENDS WELL WITH:** Birch, clove, clary sage, eucalyptus, juniper, lavender, marjoram, tea tree, neroli, patchouli, peppermint, pine, rosemary, spearmint, wintergreen, ylang ylang
**SUBCELLULAR LOCALIZATION | EPIGENETIC INFLUENCE:** Currently unknown | Currently unknown
**RECOMMENDED DILUTION RANGE:** 5%–50%; neat for limited conditions

**PRIMARY CONSTITUENTS:**[1526,1527,1528,1529,1530]

*(Indonesian, Vietnamese)*

| | |
|---|---|
| 1,8-Cineole | 44.8%–70.1% |
| Alpha-Terpineol | 5.9%–12.5% |
| Limonene | 4.5%–8.9% |
| Beta-Caryophyllene | 0.2%–7.6% |

**OTHER CONSTITUENTS:** (Indonesian, Vietnamese)—Alpha-pinene, beta-pinene, beta-myrcene, alpha-thujene, carene, para-cymene, gamma-terpinene, terpinolene, terpinen-4-ol, gamma-terpineol, cedrene, humulene, beta-eudesmene, patchoulene, germacrene D, globulol, cubenol, eugenol, 2-pentanone

**PREFERRED COMPOSITION FOR CLINICAL USE:**

| Constituent | Indonesian/ Vietnamese | Australian |
|---|---|---|
| **1,8-Cineole** | 48%–65% | 65%–73% |
| **Alpha-Terpineol** | 5%–15% | 0.5%–1% |
| **Limonene** | 4%–11% | 8%–15% |

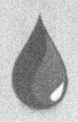

| Alpha-Pinene | 1%–6% | 1%–4% |
|---|---|---|
| Beta-Caryophyllene | 0.5%–6% | 0.1%–1% |
| Linalool | 0.1%–4% | 0.01%–1% |
| Beta-Myrcene | 1%–3% | 0.1%–1% |
| Gamma-Terpinene | 1%–3% | 2%–7% |
| Beta-Pinene | 1%–3% | 0.1%–1% |
| Para Cymene | 0.1%–2% | 5%–10% |

**REPORTED THERAPEUTIC PROPERTIES:** Analgesic (pain relief), anti-inflammatory, antiseptic, antiviral, antifungal, antispasmodic, antibacterial, antimicrobial, antineuralgic, astringent, balances menstruation, aids digestion, supports respiratory health, expels excess gas, reduces fever, brightens skin, reduces the appearance of blemishes, wound healing, protects against radiation, aids circulation, eases cough, decongestant, expels excess mucus, supports liver function, relieves earache, antiparasitic, warming, stimulating, reduces fatigue, combats mental confusion

### CAUTIONS:

■ Avoid with children under age 3, particularly around the nose and mouth. Use very cautiously in children under age 5 due to high 1,8-cineole content. 1,8-cineole may cause seizures, central nervous system problems, or respiratory distress in young children.[1531,1532,1533,1534]

■ Avoid with epilepsy and Parkinson's disease due to 1,8-cineole content. May exacerbate or cause seizures/convulsions or reduce seizure medication efficacy based on 1,8-cineole content.[1535,1536,1537]

■ Caution is warranted orally due to the significant amounts of 1,8-cineole. Limit it to small doses internally (adults—maximum 10 drops daily). Toxicity has been reported when eucalyptus (also high in 1,8-cineole) was ingested in large doses, and as few as 4 to 5 drops may cause problems in very sensitive individuals.[1538,1539,1540,1541,1542,1543] In humans, 3.5 to 5 mL has proven fatal orally.[1544]

■ May weakly interfere with the enzymes responsible for metabolizing medications (NSAIDs, proton-pump inhibitors, acetaminophen, antiepileptics, immune modulators, blood-sugar medications, blood pressure medications, antidepressants, antipsychotics, diabetic medications, antihistamines, antibiotics, and anesthetics) due to 1,8-cineole content.[1545,1546]

■ May interact with aspirin, blood pressure, antiplatelet, and anticoagulant medications, and increase the risk of bleeding among people with bleeding disorders (low risk).[1547] 1,8-cineole is a weak inhibitor of platelet aggregation.[1548]

■ May interfere with pentobarbital and other barbiturates (medications for anxiety and insomnia) based on 1,8-cineole content.[1549,1550]

### SELECTED EVIDENCE:

☐ Cajeput inhibits the herpes simplex virus type 1 (HSV-1).[1551]

☐ Cajeput inhibits several microorganisms, including *A. baumanii, A. veronii, C. albicans, E. faecalis, E. coli, K. pneumoniae, P. aeruginosa, S. enterica, S. marcescens*, and *S. aureus*.[1552] Another study found that cajeput oil inhibits multidrug-resistant *S. aureus* isolated from lower limb wounds.[1553]

☐ *In vitro* research suggests that cajeput essential oil is a potent antioxidant and free-radical scavenger.[1554]

☐ Cajeput repels disease-carrying mosquitoes.[1555,1556]

☐ *In vitro* research demonstrated that cajeput essential oil inhibits mycobacterial species.[1557]

☐ Thyme CT thymol, garlic, tea tree, cajeput, may chang, lemongrass (*C. citratus*), and verbena CT citral exhibited fungistatic activity (100 percent) against *F. culmorum* and *F. graminearum*, and all but garlic (89.4%) were 100% fungistatic against *F. avenaceum* and *F. oxysporum*.[1558]

☐ A study found that cajeput bark essential oil with alpha-eudesmol as the main constituent was larvicidal to *Aedes aegypti, Aedes albopictus*, and *Culex quinquefasciatus* mosquitoes and good antimicrobial activity against *E. faecalis*.[1559]

☐ Cajuputs candy is an Indonesian function food that leverages the bioactivity of cajeput essential oil to maintain oral health. Cajuputs candy inhibited biofilm formation of mixed-biofilm comprising *C. albicans* and *S. mutans*, which interact to cause cavities in children.[1560]

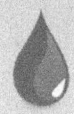

- ☐ Cajeput essential oil inhibited the growth of *Leishmania amazonensis* and *Trypanosoma brucei*, and controlled both lesion size and parasite burden in mice with cutaneous leishmaniasis.[1561] The researchers also reported the oil was cytotoxic to breast, prostate, and ovarian cancer cells (including some drug-resistant cells), with lower toxicity against nonmalignant cells.

---

# CALAMUS
## (Calamus Root, Sweet Flag, Sweet Sedge)

*Acorus calamus* L.; North American (Sweet Flag): *A. calamus* L. var. *americanus* (Raf.) H.D. Wulff., *A. americanus* (Raf.) Raf

**FAMILY:** Acoraceae
**NOTE:** Base/Middle
**AROMA INTENSITY:** Medium
**AROMA:** Refreshing, faintly sweet, woody, slightly fruity
**COMMON EXTRACTION METHOD:** Steam distilled from the dried root (rhizome); also distilled from the leaves
**POSSIBLE SUBSTITUTE OILS:** Cinnamon, catnip, oregano, thyme
**BLENDS WELL WITH:** Cassia, cedarwood, cinnamon, clary sage, geranium, lavender, marjoram, ocotea, oregano, patchouli, rosemary, sandalwood, spikenard, tamala, tea tree, ylang ylang
**SUBCELLULAR LOCALIZATION | EPIGENETIC INFLUENCE:** Currently unknown | Currently unknown
**RECOMMENDED DILUTION RANGE:** 1.5%–20%; 50% for some conditions

**PRIMARY CONSTITUENTS:**[1562,1563,1564,1565,1566,1567,1568,1569,1570,1571,1572]

*Beta-Asarone CT (India, Nepal, Japan, Europe)*

| | |
|---|---|
| Beta-Asarone | 79.4%–95.9% |
| Alpha-Asarone | 0.1%–17.3% |
| Shyobunones | 0.0%–3.3% |
| 1-H-Cyclopropa[a]naphthalene Octahydro Constituent | 0.0%–2.9% |

*Acorenone CT (Europe)*

| | |
|---|---|
| Acorenone | 22.4%–27.5% |
| Shyobunones | 13.1%–19.9% |
| Beta-Asarone | 9.3%–10.2% |
| Preisocalamendiol | 8.1%–8.1% |
| Isoacorone | 0.0%–5.0% |
| Isocalamendiol Isomer | 0.0%–4.7% |
| Dehydroisocalamendiol | 3.5%–4.5% |

*Shyobunones CT (North America)*

| | |
|---|---|
| Shyobunones | 13.0%–45.0% |
| Acorenone | 9.0%–13.0% |
| Preisocalamendiol | 7.0%–12.0% |
| Acorone + Isoacorone | 8.0%–10.0% |
| Isocalamendiol | 2.0%–3.0% |
| Beta-Sesquiphellandrene | 0.0%–3.0% |

*Alpha-Asarone CT (China)*

| | |
|---|---|
| Alpha-Asarone | 50.1% |
| (E)-Methylisoeugenol | 14.0% |
| Methyl Eugenol | 8.6% |
| Beta-Asarone | 3.5% |
| Alpha-Cedrene | 3.1% |

*(E)-Methylisoeugenol CT (Korean)*

| | |
|---|---|
| (E)-Methylisoeugenol | 41.5% |
| Cyclohexanone | 21.3% |
| 1H-3A,7-Methanoazulene | 6.9% |
| Benzenaminium | 4.9% |

Note: The chemical composition of calamus essential oil varies somewhat—although not always—according to ploidy (the number of sets of chromosomes in the plant cells). A diploid variety grows in North America that is devoid of beta-asarone and the preferred variety for essential oil therapy due to its better safety profile. European plants are generally triploid with lower content of beta-asarone, and the tetraploid variety with high content of beta-asarone is found in East Asia, India, and Japan. Hexaploid types grow in the Kashmir Region (the northernmost geographical region of South Asia) and usually contain high beta-asarone content as well.[1573,1574,1575,1576,1577,1578,1579,1580]

OTHER CONSTITUENTS: *Beta-Asarone CT*—cis-ocimene, methylisoeugenol, alpha-farnesol, linalool, dehydroisocalamendiol, caryophyllene oxide, ledene oxide I, geranyl acetone, acorenone, (Z)-isoelimicin, alpha-bisabolol, eurasarone, aristolene, carvacrol, 1,8-cineole, iso-velleral, (1R,5S,E)-2 methyl-4-[2,2,3-trimethyl-6-methylidenecyclohex-2-, elema-1,3,11(13)-trien-12-ol; *Acorenone CT*—camphene, camphor, beta-sedrene, methyl eugenol (<1.5%), alpha-gurjunene, beta-gurjunene, alpha-humulene, (Z)-methylisoeugenol, ar-curcumene, delta-cadinene, alpha-calacorene, (E)-nerolidol, spathulenol, caryophyllene oxide, ledene oxide II, (E)-alpha-cadinol, cis-calamenen-10-ol, alpha-asarone, 1,8-dimethyl -4-isopropyl-spiro[4,5]decan-7-one, cyclocolorenone isomer (NI 2), n-heptadecae, isocalamendiol, cyclocorenone, acorone; *Shyobunones CT*—calamendiol, alpha-cadinol, delta-cadinene; *Alpha-Asarone CT*—camphene, *d*-limonene, linalool, terpinen-4-ol, estragole (<1.0%), alpha-terpineol, copaene, alpha-gurjunene, beta-cedrene, germacrene D, cuparene, beta-calacorene; *(E)-Methylisoeugenol CT*—alpha-asarone (<2.4%), cyclohexanol, calarene, alpha-gurjuene, 2,5-cyclohexadiene, (+)-cuparene

PREFERRED COMPOSITION FOR CLINICAL USE:

| Constituent | North American | Beta-Asarone CT* |
|---|---|---|
| **Shyobunones** | 20%–45% | 0%–5% |
| **Acorenone** | 5%–15% | – |
| **Preisocalamendiol** | 5%–15% | – |
| **Acorone + Isoacorone** | 5%–12% | – |
| **Isocalamendiol** | 1%–5% | – |
| **Beta-Asarone** | – | 80%–95% |
| **Alpha-Asarone** | – | 1%–15% |

* The beta-asarone CT should only be used when recommended by a qualified professional.

REPORTED THERAPEUTIC PROPERTIES: Antibacterial, antifungal, **antiparasitic**, anti-inflammatory, analgesic, antirheumatic, antiarthritic, antispasmodic, supports brain and cognitive function, aids memory, nervine, aids digestion, expels excess gas, relieves diarrhea, supports cardiovascular function, reduces high cholesterol, aids circulation, eases cough, antiallergic, antioxidant, insect repellent, **insecticide**, relaxing, promotes restful sleep, relieves shock, antidepressant, aids mental clarity

CAUTIONS:

*Shyobunones CT*

■ None currently known.

*(E)-Methylisoeugenol CT*

■ May interfere with pentobarbital and other barbiturates (medications for anxiety and insomnia) and increase depressive effect due to (E)-methylisoeugenol content.[4345]

*Beta-Asarone, Alpha-Asarone, and Acorenone CTs:*

***These chemotypes are not generally recommended during essential oil therapy unless the benefits far outweigh the risks as determined by a qualified professional.***

■ Avoid in children under age 12 due to liver toxicity concerns of asarones and methyl eugenol content.[1581,1582,1583,1584,1585,1586,1587,1588]

■ Avoid during pregnancy and lactation due to genotoxicity of beta-asarone, and reduced maternal weight gain, embryo toxicity, abortion, and fetal malformations (hydrocephaly, extra-ribs, clubfeet, and cleft lips) reportedly caused by alpha-asarone in animal studies.[4061] However, one animal study did not report toxicity to embryos or fetuses nor birth defects.[1589] The alpha-asarone CT also contains methyl eugenol. Very large doses of methyl eugenol may adversely affect the mother's liver and infant body weight according to animal research.[1590] Animal research suggests that methyl eugenol may cause changes in embryo form and structure and chromosomal changes in ovary cells, as well as multi-site cancerous tumors.[1591,1592,1593,1594] Based on these studies, it is best to limit the use of calamus essential oil during pregnancy and lactation.

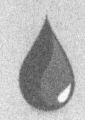

■ Avoid oral consumption due to asarone and methyl eugenol content. Beta-asarone is genotoxic (destructive to a cells genetic material—DNA, RNA—and integrity), and may cause damage to organs (liver, heart, and kidneys), abnormal fluid accumulation in the abdominal (peritoneal cavity), and malignant intestinal tumors at large to extreme doses according to animal research.[1595,1596,1597,1598,1599,1600] Long-term administration increases the damage caused. The exposure limit for total asarones (alpha- and beta-) was set to 115 mcg (or 2 mcg/kg/day) from herbal medicinal products, which would equate to less than one drop of essential oil.[1601] A case report involving a middle-aged woman reports tachycardia, dizziness, tremor, irregular breathing, pallor, anxiety, nausea and vomiting reportedly due to asarone intoxication after consuming an unknown quantity of asarone-containing herbal medicines. Methyl eugenol is considered an animal carcinogen and a possible human carcinogen.[1602]

■ May interact with aspirin, blood pressure, antiplatelet, and anticoagulant medications, and increase the risk of bleeding among people with bleeding disorders based on beta-asarone content.[1603]

■ May interfere with pentobarbital and other barbiturates (medications for anxiety and insomnia) due to asarone content.[1604,1605,1606,1607]

■ Avoid with compromised liver or kidney due to significant potential to cause liver and kidney toxicity.[1608,1609,1610,1611,1612,1613]

■ May interact with anticholinergic (drugs used for asthma, incontinence, gastrointestinal cramps, muscular spasms, depression, and sleep disorders) and cholinergic medications (drugs used to reduce urinary retention, diagnose myasthenia gravis, and for glaucoma) based on AChE inhibitory activity.[1614]

■ Calamus oil is not contraindicated topically because research suggests that it is poorly absorbed.[1615]

## SELECTED EVIDENCE:

☐ Calamus essential oil (beta-asarone and alpha-asarone CTs) inhibited *A. niger* and *A. flavus in vitro*.[1616,1617,1618] *In vitro* research demonstrates that calamus essential oil ((E)-Methylisoeugenol CT) strongly inhibits *Salmonella tryphimurium, S. aureus, B. subtilis, P. acne,* and *C. albicans,* but only weakly inhibits *E. coli*.[1619] Calamus essential oil (beta-asarone CT) also inhibits pathogenic seed borne fungi: *Alternaria solani, Colletotrichum* sp., *Fusarium moniliforme,* and *Rhizoctonia solani*.[1620]

☐ Calamus essential oil (beta-asarone CT) and its major constituents inhibit acetylcholinesterase (AChE) *in vitro*, which may make it useful for Alzheimer's disease.[1621] Inhibition of AChE prevents the breakdown of acetylcholine, which is essential for memory and thinking. People with neurodegenerative diseases make less acetylcholine, and the diseases often break it down at a faster rate leading to acetylcholine deficits.

☐ Beta-asarone and calamus essential oil (beta-asarone CT) demonstrated anthelmintic properties (expel parasitic worms by killing or stunning them without harming the host) against the parasitic roundworm (*Ascaridia galli*).[1622] An unidentified CT of calamus essential oil was also anthelmintic against the small roundworm (*Ascaris lumbricoides*) better than piperazine citrate (a synthetic drug used to expel roundworms).[1623] Interestingly, the essential oil partially paralyzed the parasites within five minutes, but the non-phenolic fractions of the same oil caused complete paralysis within five to twenty-five minutes.

☐ Shyobunones isolated from calamus essential oil repelled and killed the cigar beetle (*Lasioderma serricorne*) and red flour beetle (*Tribolium castaneum*).[1624] The alpha-asarone CT is toxic to the book louse (*Liposcelis bostrychophila* Badonnel) due to its methyl eugenol and (E)-methylisoeugenol content.[1625] An unidentified CT of calamus essential oil killed the tobacco armyworm (*Spodoptera litura*).[1626]

☐ Calamus essential oil exhibited promising fumigant activity against the pulse beetle (*Callosobruchus maculatus*) and bean weevil (*Callosobruchus chinensis*).[1627] Synergistic activity was observed when calamus was combined with lavender essential oil.

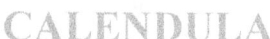 

# CALENDULA
## (Marigold, Pot Marigold)

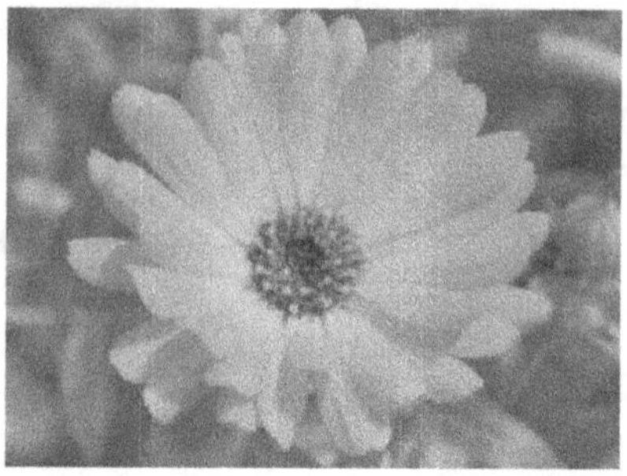

*Calendula officinalis* L., *C. officinalis* L. var. *prolifera* hort.

**FAMILY:** Asteraceae (Compositae)
**NOTE:** Middle
**AROMA INTENSITY:** Medium
**AROMA:** Musky, earthy, pungent, hay-like, slightly floral
**COMMON EXTRACTION METHOD:** Steam distilled from the flowers; may also be solvent extracted or obtained by enfleurage
**POSSIBLE SUBSTITUTE OILS:** Helichrysum, tagetes, lavender, frankincense, betony
**BLENDS WELL WITH:** Bergamot, cypress, frankincense, geranium, kunzea, lavender, lemon, lime, orange, rose, tagetes, tangerine, vetiver, ylang ylang
**SUBCELLULAR LOCALIZATION | EPIGENETIC INFLUENCE:** Currently unknown | Currently unknown
**RECOMMENDED DILUTION RANGE:** 3%–50%; neat for limited conditions

**PRIMARY CONSTITUENTS:**[1628,1629,1630,1631,1632,1633,1634]

*Alpha-Cadinol/Delta-Cadinene CT*

| | |
|---|---|
| Alpha-Cadinol | 2.0%–33.6% |
| Delta-Cadinene | 5.1%–22.5% |
| Beta-Eudesmol | 0.0%–14.5% |
| T-Muurolol | 0.0%–13.0% |
| Gamma-Cadinene | 0.0%–11.9% |
| Aromadendrene | 0.0%–9.4% |
| Borneol | 0.0%–9.1% |
| Bornyl Acetate | 0.0%–8.7% |
| (E)-Nerolidol | 0.0%–8.1% |
| 1-Epi-Cubenol | 0.0%–8.0% |
| Alpha-Cadinene | 0.5%–6.8% |
| Beta-Cubebene | 0.0%–6.5% |
| Alpha-Muurolol | 0.0%–5.7% |
| Alpha-Muurolene | 0.0%–5.6% |
| Caryophyllene Oxide | 0.0%–5.0% |
| T-Cadinol | 0.0%–4.8% |
| Alpha-Patchoulene | 0.0%–4.3% |
| Alpha-Cubebene | 0.0%–3.8% |
| Isoborneol | 0.0%–3.8% |
| Geranyl Acetate | 0.0%–3.8% |
| Beta-Acorenol | 0.0%–3.6% |
| Beta-Patchoulol | 0.0%–3.4% |
| Beta-Ionone | 0.0%–3.2% |
| Alpha-Humulene | 0.0%–3.0% |
| Pentacosane | 0.0%–3.0% |
| Geraniol | 0.0%–3.0% |

*Alpha-Thujene CT*

| | |
|---|---|
| Alpha-Thujene | 26.9% |
| T-Muurolol | 24.9% |
| Delta-Cadinene | 13.1% |

*(E)-Beta-Ocimene CT\**

| | |
|---|---|
| (E)-Beta-Ocimene | 46.2% |
| Dihydrotagetone | 31.7% |
| (Z)-Tagetone | 4.6% |
| Neo-Allo-Ocimene | 3.7% |
| Artemisia Ketone | 3.4% |

*Solvent Extracted*

| | |
|---|---|
| Delta-Cadinene | 10.2% |
| Alpha-Cadinene | 7.2% |
| Alpha-Thujene | 3.9% |
| Alpha-Murolene | 3.1% |

*Enfleurage*

| | |
|---|---|
| Alpha-Cadinene | 6.8% |
| Delta-Cadinene | 4.4% |

\* It is possible that the (E)-Beta-Ocimene CT is not calendula but tagetes essential oil based on the composition reported.

**OTHER CONSTITUENTS:** *Alpha-Cadinol/Delta-Cadinene CT*—alpha-pinene, beta-farnesene, alpha-copaene, beta-fenchene, para-cymene, beta-ylangene, trans-p-mentha-2,8-dienol, neryl acetate, myrtenol, alpha-gurjunene, beta-caryophyllene, calamenene, cubenol, p,a,a-trimethylbenzyl alcohol, alpha-patchoulol, guaiol, beta-acorenol, bulnesol, bisabolol, alpha-ionone, gamma-muurolene, ledene, alpha-calacorene, beta-oplopenone, copaen-4-alpha-ol,

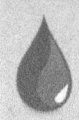

viridiflorol, ledol, 1,10-di-epi -cubenol, cadalene, 3,5-di-tert-butylcatechol, 2,5,6-trimethylbenzimidazole, 2,3,5,6-tetramethyl-p-phenylene; *Alpha-Thujene CT*—alpha-pinene, sabinene, myrcene, 1,8-cineole, gamma-terpinene, terpinen-4-ol, beta-cubebene, alpha-gurjunene, alpha-copaene, beta-caryophyllene, alpha-humulene, alpha-amorphene, germacrene D, gamma-cadinene, (E)-nerolidol, beta-endobourbonene; *(E)-Beta-Ocimene CT*—limonene, verbenone; *Solvent Extracted*—methyl heptanone, (e,e)-2,4-heptadienal, germacrene D, ledol, alpha-cubebene, copaene, [r-(r*,r*)]-2,3-butanediol, beta-cubebene, caryophyllene, gamma-murolene, alpha-cadinol; *Enfleurage*—alpha-murolene, 3-methyl-3-buten-2-one

### PREFERRED COMPOSITION FOR CLINICAL USE:

| Constituent | Alpha-Cadinol/ Delta-Cadinene CT |
|---|---|
| Alpha-Cadinol | 20%–35% |
| Delta-Cadinene | 20%–30% |
| Epi-Alpha-Muurolol | 12%–22% |
| Gamma-Cadinene | 1%–10% |
| Alpha-Cadinene | 0.5%–10% |
| Alpha-Muurolene | 0.1%–7% |

**REPORTED THERAPEUTIC PROPERTIES:** Antioxidant, anti-inflammatory, antispasmodic, analgesic, antifungal, antibacterial, **antiseptic**, antiparasitic, **relieves chronic skin conditions**, **wound healing**, relieves boils and bruises, **aids and strengthens the circulatory system**, soothes burns, relieves insect bites, reduces the appearance of aging, acne, and blemishes, relieves itching, **protects against UV radiation**, supports oral health, relieves painful menstruation, stress management, relieves anxiety, emotionally balancing, encourages compassion

### CAUTIONS:

■ *Alpha-Cadinol/Delta-Cadinene CT*: May moderately interfere (low risk) with the enzymes responsible for metabolizing medications (NSAIDs, proton-pump inhibitors, acetaminophen, antiepileptics, immune modulators, blood-sugar medications, blood-pressure medications, antidepressants, antipsychotics, diabetic medications, antihistamines, antibiotics, and anesthetics) based on cadinene content.[1635]

### SELECTED EVIDENCE:

☐ Animal research suggests that the topical application of a 4% or 5% calendula essential oil cream significantly decreased malondialdehyde (a product of lipid peroxidation—when lipids are degraded by free radicals, resulting in cell damage—that is a marker for oxidative stress) levels and significantly increased antioxidant activity (catalase, glutathione, superoxide dismutase, and ascorbic acid) in the skin after UV-B radiation exposure. This study suggests that calendula essential oil may diminish reductions in antioxidants caused by UV-B exposure.[1636] An *in vitro* study also reported that calendula essential oil ((E)-beta-ocimene CT) protects against UV radiation, providing a remarkable 14.84 SPF (sun protection factor).[1637]

☐ The alpha-cadinol/delta-cadinene CT of calendula essential oil (50% concentration) protected human volunteers against mosquito bites for 2.15 hours, which was significantly lower than DEET (6.23 hours).[1638]

☐ *In vitro* research shows that calendula essential oil inhibits 23 clinical fungal strains (*Candida albicans, C. dubliniensis, C. parapsilosis, C. glabrata*, and *C. krusei*; and the following yeasts clinically isolated from humans: *C. albicans, C. dubliniensis, C. parapsilosis, C. glabrata, C. tropicalis, C. guilliermondii, C. krusei*, and *Rhodotorulla* sp.).[1639]

☐ Scientists determined that geranium and calendula essential oils are useful additions to cosmetics due to their antioxidant (slows skin aging) and SPF (6.45 and 8.36 respectively) properties.[1640]

# CAMPHOR
## (Hon-Sho, True Camphor)

*Cinnamomum camphora* (L.) J. Presl, *Laurus camphora* L.

**FAMILY:** Lauraceae
**NOTE:** Top
**AROMA INTENSITY:** Strong
**AROMA:** Fresh, medicinal, intense, woody
**COMMON EXTRACTION METHOD:** Steam distilled from the wood, branches, leaves, and flowers
**POSSIBLE SUBSTITUTE OILS:** Ravintsara (camphor CT), sage (camphor CT), rosemary (camphor CT), basil (linalool CT), lavandin, Spanish sage
**BLENDS WELL WITH:** Balsam fir, chamomile (German, Roman), copaiba, eucalyptus, frankincense, juniper, lavandin, peppermint, pine, rosemary, spearmint, spruce (black), wintergreen
**SUBCELLULAR LOCALIZATION | EPIGENETIC INFLUENCE:** Currently unknown | Currently unknown
**RECOMMENDED DILUTION RANGE:** 1.5%–20%; 50% for some conditions

**PRIMARY CONSTITUENTS:**[1641,1642,1643,1644,1645,1646,1647]

*Camphor CT*

| | |
|---|---|
| Camphor | 36.5%–98.0% |
| Linalool | 0.6%–22.3% |
| 1,8-Cineole | 1.0%–12.0% |
| Camphene | 0.2%–11.7% |
| Limonene | 0.0%–9.0% |
| Sabinene | 0.2%–6.3% |
| Beta-Pinene | 0.0%–6.3% |
| Terpinen-4-ol | 0.0%–6.3% |
| Alpha-Pinene | 2.0%–4.7% |

*Linalool CT (Leaves, flowers, stems)*

| | |
|---|---|
| Linalool | 40.3%–87.3% |
| Camphor | 0.7%–33.5% |
| Beta-Caryophyllene | 1.5%–5.5% |
| Eugenol | 0.0%–3.6% |
| 1,8-Cineole | 0.1%–3.0% |
| Beta-Selinene | 0.5%–2.9% |

Note: Camphor is separated (fractionated) into different classes of camphor after the crystals are removed by filtration. Technically, none of these classes would be considered a true essential oil, but fractions of an essential oil. The classes are as follows: white camphor (light fraction, contains 1,8-cineole and monoterpenes), yellow camphor (medium fraction), brown camphor (medium fraction, up to 80% safrole), and blue camphor (heavy fraction, contains sesquiterpenes). Only white camphor is typically used for therapeutic purposes. The above composition is for the whole oil and not the fractions.

**OTHER CONSTITUENTS:** Camphor CT—Myrcene, para-cymene, myrtenol, borneol, alpha-terpineol, myrtenal, caryophyllene oxide; Linalool CT—Alpha-pinene, alpha-terpineol, geraniol, safrole, methyl eugenol (< 0.8%), sabinene, beta-myrcene, alpha-terpinolene, gamma-muurolene, germacrene D, delta-cadinene, 1-epi-cubenol, alpha-cadinol, gamma-elemene, alpha-humulene, safrole

**PREFERRED COMPOSITION FOR CLINICAL USE:**

| Constituent | Camphor CT | Balanced CT | Linalool CT, Rectified | Linalool CT |
|---|---|---|---|---|
| **Camphor** | 50%–75% | 25%–35% | 0%–0.2% | 10%–25% |
| **Linalool** | 10%–25% | – | 97%–99% | 50%–75% |
| **1,8-Cineole** | 5%–15% | 25%–38% | 0%–0.2% | 1%–5% |
| **Camphene** | 2%–12% | 0.1%–3% | – | – |
| **Sabinene** | 0.1%–7% | 8%–15% | – | – |
| **Alpha-Pinene** | 1%–5% | 5%–10% | – | 0%–3% |
| **Beta-Pinene** | 0%–6% | 3%–8% | – | – |
| **Beta-Caryophyllene** | – | – | – | 1%–7% |
| **Beta-Selinene** | – | – | – | 0.5%–5% |
| **Linalool Oxide <cis + trans>** | – | – | 0.01%–1% | – |
| **Beta-Myrcene** | – | 1%–5% | 0.01%–0.5% | 0%–3% |
| **Limonene** | 0%–10% | 0.1%–5% | 0%–0.3% | – |

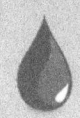

**REPORTED THERAPEUTIC PROPERTIES:** Analgesic (pain relief), anti-inflammatory, antiseptic, antispasmodic, **antiviral**, **antibacterial**, antimicrobial, anticancer, diuretic, expectorant, **stimulates the heart**, antiparasitic, enhances the penetration of other essential oils, increases sweating and redness of the skin, respiratory stimulant, antirheumatic, reduces appearance of skin blemishes, **eases cough**, stimulating

**CAUTIONS:**

■ Avoid with children under 6 due to high camphor content. Several cases of camphor poisoning and/or seizures from ingestion and topical application have been reported in children.[1648,1649] Ingestion of camphor-containing products has been lethal in children under age 2 (estimated to be roughly 2,000 mg of camphor for a 20 kg child as the minimum potential fatal dose).[1650,1651] Children 5 years and up may use camphor topically in dilutions no stronger than 5%. 1,8-cineole may cause seizures, central nervous system problems, or respiratory distress in young children.[1652,1653,1654,1655]

■ Caution is warranted during pregnancy and while lactating. Camphor ingestion may lead to abortion because fetuses lack the enzymes to process it.[1656] Camphor ingestion by infants and young children may cause cough, vomiting, seizure, burning sensation in the mucous membranes and eyes, or lack of voluntary coordination of muscle movements.[1657]

■ Avoid with epilepsy and Parkinson's disease due to camphor content.[1658,1659,1660]

■ Oral—Camphor can be toxic when taken orally (usually single doses exceeding 2 mL), although the lethal dose for adult humans is estimated to be (more than 5 mL) in a single dose.[1661,1662,1663]

■ The potentially high camphor content in camphor may negatively impact red blood cells and increase the risk of jaundice in children with Glucose-6-phosphate dehydrogenase deficiency (G6PD).[1664,1665]

■ Avoid with those who have a compromised liver due to the risk of increased liver enzymes and liver damage.[1666] This would also suggest that those taking medications that could cause liver damage should also use camphor very cautiously or avoid it entirely.

■ *Linalool CT*: May interact with antifungal drugs and enhance their effectiveness based on linalool content.[1667]

■ Caution is warranted for the topical application of camphor on broken or injured skin due to an increased risk of toxicity.[1668]

**SELECTED EVIDENCE:**

☐ Camphor extracts influences cytokine, nitric oxide, and prostaglandin production to exert an anti-inflammatory effect.[1669]

☐ Camphor enhances the penetration of other substances through the skin.[1670]

☐ Camphor essential oil killed and repelled the cotton aphid (*Aphis gossypii* Glover), with linalool being considered a major factor in its insecticidal and repellent properties.[1671] The camphor CT also displayed strong toxicity against stored product pests (*Tribolium castaneum* and *Lasioderma serricorne*).[1672]

☐ Camphor, cinnamon, and ginger essential oils caused significant mortality of *Cephalopina titillator* (a botfly that causes nasopharyngeal myiasis in camels in the Middle East and North Africa), with camphor being the fastest acting and most effective.[1673]

☐ Daily topical application of white camphor essential oil (a light fraction containing monoterpenes like 1,8-cineole and limonene) exhibited cancer preventive (dramatically regressed premalignant skin tumors and two-fold reduction in cutaneous squamous cell carcinomas) properties in a mouse model of keratinocyte-derived skin cancer.[1674]

☐ The linalool CT of camphor oil was significantly bactericidal to *E. coli* in vapor phase.[1675]

☐ Bacterial biofilms allow bacteria to cause localized chronic infections. *E. coli* is one of the most common pathogenic microbes that creates biofilms that can cause diarrhea, endometritis, and mastitis. Camphor CT linalool essential oil inhibited *E. coli* isolated from cows with clinical endometritis and its formation of biofilms.[1676] Bacterial killing was observed during planktonic growth and biofilm formation.

☐ Camphor essential oil—distilled from the wood only—exhibited good antibacterial activity against *Serratia marcescens*, and also inhibited *S. epidermidis, P. acnes, T. mentagrophytes. A. niger, A. fumigatus, C. Albicans, M. canis, M. gypseum*, and *T. rubrum*.[1677] The oil distilled from wood, branches, and leaves was significantly active against *A. niger* and *A. fumigatus*, and also inhibited *B. cereus, P. acnes, S. epidermidis, T. mentagrophytes, C. albicans, M. canis, M. gypseum*, and *T. rubrum*.

☐ Intragastric administration of camphor CT borneol essential oil had a sedative-hypnotic effect in mice.[1678] Further evaluation identified constituents within the oil that interact with proteins (dopamine receptor D2, opioid receptor mu 1, opioid receptor kappa 1) and act on seventeen targets—mainly through response to alkaloid and catecholamine transport, and neuroactive ligand-receptor interaction—to produce these effects.

# CANADIAN FLEABANE
## (Fleabane, Erigeron, Canadian Horseweed, Fleawort)
*Conyza canadensis* (L.) Cronquist, *Erigeron canadensis* L.

**FAMILY:** Asteraceae (Compositae)
**NOTE:** Middle
**AROMA INTENSITY:** Medium
**AROMA:** Herbaceous, complex, earthy, slightly spicy, slightly musky, slightly sweet
**COMMON EXTRACTION METHOD:** Steam distilled from the flowering aerial parts (flowers, stems, and leaves)
**POSSIBLE SUBSTITUTE OILS:** Palo santo, balsam fir, silver fir
**BLENDS WELL WITH:** Balsam fir, basil (sweet), bergamot, blue cypress, cardamom, carrot seed, chamomile (German, Roman), cilantro, clove, copaiba, cypress, davana, Douglas fir, geranium, grapefruit, helichrysum, lavandin, lavender, lemon, lime, melissa, orange, petitgrain, rose, rosewood, Siberian fir, silver fir, tangerine, tsuga, white fir, ylang ylang
**SUBCELLULAR LOCALIZATION | EPIGENETIC INFLUENCE:** Currently unknown | Currently unknown
**RECOMMENDED DILUTION RANGE:** 5%–Neat

**PRIMARY CONSTITUENTS:**[1679,1680,1681,1682,1683,1684,1685]

| | |
|---|---|
| Limonene | 31.2%–81.1% |
| Delta-3-Carene | 0.0%–15.9% |
| Camphene | 0.0%–14.2% |
| Germacrene D | 0.0%–11.3% |
| (Z)-Beta-Farnesene | 0.0%–11.1% |
| Cis-Alpha-Bergamotene | 0.0%–9.9% |
| (E)-Beta-Ocimene | 0.0%–9.1% |
| Trans-Alpha-Bergamotene | 0.0%–8.9% |
| Alpha-Santalene | 0.0%–5.8% |

Note: The best time to harvest Canadian fleabane is the early flower phase for highest oil yield and greatest consistency in chemical composition. Limonene is the abundant constituent, but the other major and minor constituents vary greatly from absent to over 5% of total essential oil composition.

**OTHER CONSTITUENTS:** Beta-pinene, (E)-beta-farnesene, (Z,Z)-matricaria ester (<4.0%), myrcene, thujone (<1.7%), trans-carveol, carvone, beta-caryophyllene, ar-curcumene, (Z)-lachnophyllum ester, caryophyllene oxide

**PREFERRED COMPOSITION FOR CLINICAL USE:**

| Constituent | |
|---|---|
| **Limonene** | 55%–70% |
| **(Z,Z)-Matricaria Ester** | 0.1%–15% |
| **Alpha-Bergamotene <cis + trans>** | 3%–12% |
| **Beta-Pinene** | 2%–10% |
| **(E)-Beta-Ocimene** | 2%–10% |
| **Germacrene D** | 0.1%–7% |
| **Beta-Myrcene** | 0.5%–5% |

**REPORTED THERAPEUTIC PROPERTIES:** Antibacterial, antifungal, analgesic, **anti-inflammatory**, **astringent**, antioxidant, antispasmodic, antirheumatic, supports normal blood pressure, diuretic, aids liver and pancreas function, anti-aging, balances blood sugar, stops excess bleeding, supports respiratory function, **relieves diarrhea**, soothes sore throat, supports kidney function, vasodilating, reduces fever, balances hormones, promotes hGH production, insect repellent, insecticide, uplifting, stress management

**CAUTIONS:**
- None currently known.

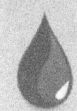

**SELECTED EVIDENCE:**

☐ *In vitro* research concluded that Canadian fleabane moderately to strongly inhibits *Candida albicans* (UK-NEQUAS4661), *Candida glabrata* (ATCC90030), *Candida parapsilosis* (ATCC22019), *Candida tropicalis* (UK-NEQUAS4893), *Cryptococcus neoformans* (INF5855) reference fungal strains, and *Candida kefyr, Rhodotorula glutinis, Trichophyton interdigitale, Aspergillus fumigatus* fungal strains isolated from infected patients.[1686]

☐ An ethanolic extract of Canadian fleabane (which contains the volatile constituent limonene) demonstrated significant anti-inflammatory activity and significantly inhibited brain AChE levels (suggesting it may be useful for memory and cognition) in mice.[1687,1688]

☐ Canadian fleabane essential oil exhibited notable larvicidal activities against *Ae. Aegypti* and *Ae. Albopictus* mosquitoes.[1689]

# CANGERANA
## (Canjerana, Cedro-Cangerana, Canharana, Caierana)

*Cabralea canjerana* Saldanha, *C. cangerana*

**FAMILY:** Meliaceae
**NOTE:** Middle
**AROMA INTENSITY:** Medium
**AROMA:** Woody, spicy-sweet, earthy
**COMMON EXTRACTION METHOD:** Steam distilled or hydrodistilled from the wood; may also be distilled from the leaves, seeds, or fruits
**POSSIBLE SUBSTITUTE OILS:** Copaiba, betony, vilayti tulsi, black pepper
**BLENDS WELL WITH:** Balsam fir, bergamot, cedarwood, copaiba, frankincense, galbanum, hemp, hops, lavender, lemon, orange, palo santo, pine, tangerine, ylang ylang
**SUBCELLULAR LOCALIZATION | EPIGENETIC INFLUENCE:** Currently unknown | Currently unknown
**RECOMMENDED DILUTION RANGE:** 5%–Neat

**PRIMARY CONSTITUENTS:**[1690,1691]

| *Leaves* | | *Wood* | |
|---|---|---|---|
| Spathulenol | 10.8%–16.5% | Beta-Caryophyllene | 28.6% |
| Caryophyllene Oxide | 2.2%–9.8% | Germacrene D | 9.3% |
| Globulol | 0.0%–9.8% | Delta-Cadinene | 7.4% |
| Cubebol | 0.0%–9.3% | Germacrene B | 6.2% |
| Alpha-Cadinol | 0.9%–8.0% | Gamma-Muurolene | 5.0% |
| Dihydroeudesmol | 0.0%–4.0% | | |

**OTHER CONSTITUENTS:** *Wood*—Safrole (0.5%), delta-elemene, alpha-cubebene, alpha-copaene, beta-elemene, 4,8-beta-epoxycaryophyllane, gamma-elelemen, aromadendrene, alpha-muurolene, alpha-humulene, allo-aromadendrene, eudesma-4(15),11-diene, gamma-amorphene, gamma-cadinene, trans-calamenene, alpha-calacorene, eudesma-3,7(11)-diene, caryolan-8-ol, 10-epi-junenol, 1alphaH,5betaH-guaia-6,10(14)-dien-4beta-ol, 10-epi-cubenol, T-cadinol, humulene epoxide III, cubenol, 10beta-hydroxycalamenene, eudesm-7(11)-en-4alpha-ol; *Leaves*—Not reported

**PREFERRED COMPOSITION FOR CLINICAL USE:**

| Constituent | Wood |
|---|---|
| **Beta-Caryophyllene** | 20%–40% |
| **Germacrenes <D + B>** | 8%–25% |
| **Cadinenes <δ + γ>** | 5%–20% |

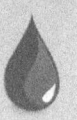 

| | |
|---|---|
| **Muurolenes <γ + α>** | 4%–15% |
| **Elemenes <δ + β + γ>** | 3%–10% |
| **Alpha-Calacorene** | 0.5%–5% |
| **T-Cadinol** | 0.5%–5% |

**REPORTED THERAPEUTIC PROPERTIES:** Analgesic, **anti-inflammatory**, antiarthritic, antirheumatic, aids digestion, reduces chronic skin conditions, wound healing, antibacterial, reduces fever, stress management, relaxing, encourages emotional healing

**CAUTIONS:**

■ May decrease the bioavailability of many medications (NSAIDs, proton-pump inhibitors, acetaminophen, antiepileptics, immune modulators, blood-sugar medications, blood pressure medications, antidepressants, antipsychotics, diabetic medications, antihistamines, antibiotics, and anesthetics) due to the ability of caryophyllene oxide and beta-caryophyllene to inhibit CYP3A enzyme activity.[1692]

**SELECTED EVIDENCE:**

☐ *In vitro* research demonstrates that cangerana leaf essential oil inhibits *S. aureus, S. epidermidis, E. faecalis, E. coli, P. aeruginosa, S. thyphimurium,* and *S. flexneri* with varying activity depending on the harvest time of the leaves and the composition of the essential oil.[1693]

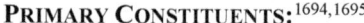

## CAPE CHAMOMILE
### (African Chamomile)

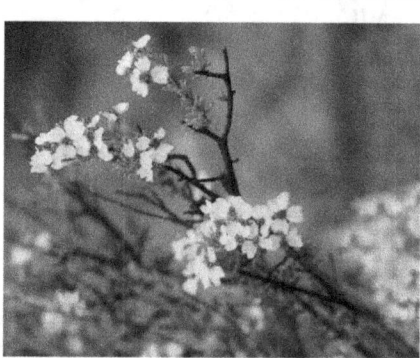

*Eriocephalus punctulatus* DC.

**FAMILY:** Asteraceae (Compositae)
**NOTE:** Middle
**AROMA INTENSITY:** Medium-Strong
**AROMA:** Floral, earthy, herbaceous, fruity, sweet
**COMMON EXTRACTION METHOD:** Steam distilled from the buds/flowers
**POSSIBLE SUBSTITUTE OILS:** Roman chamomile, rose
**BLENDS WELL WITH:** Basil, bergamot, cardamom, cassia, chamomile (Roman), clary sage, coriander, frankincense, geranium, lavender, neroli, orange (sweet), petitgrain, rose, tangerine, ylang ylang, zdravetz
**SUBCELLULAR LOCALIZATION | EPIGENETIC INFLUENCE:** Currently unknown | Currently unknown
**RECOMMENDED DILUTION RANGE:** 5%–Neat

**PRIMARY CONSTITUENTS:**[1694,1695]

| | |
|---|---|
| 2-Methyl Butyl Isobutyrate | 21.2%–27.4% |
| Isobutyl Isobutyrate | 5.3%–14.3% |
| 2-Methylbutyl 2-Methylbutyrate | 5.5%–5.6% |
| 7-Methyl-2-Octyl Acetate | 0.0%–4.5% |
| Linalyl Acetate | 2.9%–4.4% |
| Terpinen-4-ol | 1.7%–3.7% |
| 2-Methylbutyl Angelate | 0.0%–3.5% |

**OTHER CONSTITUENTS:** Alpha-pinene, camphene, dehydroxylinalool oxide A, isobutyl 2-methyl butyrate, 2-methylpropyl 3-methylbutanoate, 3-methylbutyl 2-methylpropanoate, para-cymene, beta-phellandrene, limonene, isobutyl angelate, gamma-terpinene, alpha-terpineol, trans-sabinene hydrate, 7-methyl-2-octanol, butyl angelate, 2-nonanone, para-cymenene, linalool, isoamyl 2-methyl butyrate, 2-methylbutyl isovalerate, camphor, borneol, pentyl tiglate, 2-nonyl acetate, neryl acetate, 2-methylbutyl phenylacetate, artedouglasia oxide A, artedouglasia oxide B, artedouglasia oxide C, artedouglasia oxide D, laciniate furanone H, spathulenol, caryophyllene oxide, beta-copaen-4-alpha-ol, caryophylla-3(15),7(14)-dien-6-ol

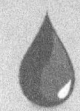

**PREFERRED COMPOSITION FOR CLINICAL USE:**

| *Constituent* | |
|---|---|
| **2-Methyl Butyl Isobutyrate** | 20%–32% |
| **Isobutyl Isobutyrate** | 5%–20% |
| **2-Methylbutyl 2-Methylbutyrate** | 3%–7% |
| **Artedouglasia Oxides** | 2%–6% |
| **Linalyl Acetate** | 1%–6% |
| **7-Methyl-2-Octyl Acetate** | 2%–5% |
| **Borneol** | 1%–4% |
| **Para-Cymene** | 1%–4% |
| **Camphor** | 1%–4% |
| **Terpinen-4-ol** | 0.5%–4% |
| **Isobutyl Angelate** | 0.1%–4% |
| **Isoamyl Angelate** | 1%–3% |
| **Alpha-Pinene** | 0.5%–3% |
| **Gamma-Terpinene** | 0.1%–2% |

**REPORTED THERAPEUTIC PROPERTIES:** Anti-inflammatory, analgesic, antispasmodic, antiparasitic, anti-infectious, antiseptic, relieves boils, **wound healing**, **relieves chronic skin conditions**, skin regenerative, relieves stomachache, **promotes restful sleep**, reduces fear, relieves anxiety, stress management, reduces irritability

**CAUTIONS:**

■ None currently known.

**SELECTED EVIDENCE:**

☐ Several individual constituents within Cape chamomile essential oil were toxic to the Japanese termite (*Reticulitermes speratus*), which led the researchers to conclude the whole essential oil merits further investigation for termite control.[1696]

# CARAWAY
## (Caraway Seed)

*Carum carvi* L., *Carum velenovskyi* Rohlena

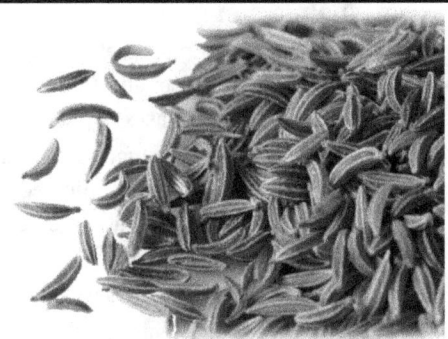

**FAMILY:** Apiaceae (Umbelliferae)
**NOTE:** Middle
**AROMA INTENSITY:** Medium
**AROMA:** Sweet, spicy, herbaceous
**COMMON EXTRACTION METHOD:** Steam distilled from the seeds
**POSSIBLE SUBSTITUTE OILS:** Spearmint, peppermint, fennel, ginger
**BLENDS WELL WITH:** Anise, basil, cardamom, cassia, chamomile (German, Roman), cinnamon, clove, coriander, dill, fennel, frankincense, ginger, lavender, nutmeg, orange, peppermint, spearmint, tangerine
**SUBCELLULAR LOCALIZATION | EPIGENETIC INFLUENCE:** Currently unknown | Currently unknown
**RECOMMENDED DILUTION RANGE:** 1.5%–50%

**PRIMARY CONSTITUENTS:**[1697,1698,1699,1700]

| | |
|---|---|
| Carvone | 38.0%–80.5% |
| Limonene | 13.1%–35.5% |
| Alpha-Pinene | 0.0%–5.2% |
| Cis-Carveol | 0.0%–5.0% |
| Beta-Myrcene | 0.5%–4.7% |

Note: The literature reports other chemotypes of caraway essential oil such as cuminaldehyde, gamma-terpinene, and thymol, but by far the most common chemotype reported in the literature is the carvone chemotype, sometimes with carvone and limonene close to equal in proportion.[1701]

OTHER CONSTITUENTS: Myrcene, trans-limonene oxide, perilla alcohol, carvacrol, beta-caryophyllene, trans-carveol, linalool, menthone, 4-terpineol, cis-dihydrocarvone

PREFERRED COMPOSITION FOR CLINICAL USE:

| Constituent | |
|---|---|
| Carvone | 45%–70% |
| Limonene | 28%–45% |
| Beta-Myrcene | 0.1%–3% |
| Cis-Dihydrocarvone | 0.1%–2% |
| Carveol (cis + trans) | 0.1%–1% |

REPORTED THERAPEUTIC PROPERTIES: Antimicrobial, antibacterial, antiseptic, antispasmodic, **anticonvulsive**, disinfectant, antiallergic, stimulates lactation, **supports cardiac function**, **aids digestion**, expels excess gas, diuretic, supports liver function, relieves congestion, acne, soothes rashes, antiarthritic, **protects the stomach**, reduces painful menstruation, stimulates appetite, supports normal blood pressure, relieves mental fatigue, antidepressant, relieves anxiety, **stress management**

CAUTIONS:

■ May interact with diabetes medications and cause low blood sugar.[1702,1703]

■ May interact with aspirin, blood pressure, antiplatelet, and anticoagulant medications, and increase the risk of bleeding among people with bleeding disorders based on carvone content. Carvone is a potent calcium channel blocker, which may decrease blood pressure.[1704,1705]

■ May interact with barbiturates (medications for anxiety and insomnia), antihistamines, benzodiazepines, tricyclic antidepressants, or other central nervous system depressant drugs, increasing depressant effects, due to carvone content.[1706]

SELECTED EVIDENCE:

☐ *In vitro* and animal research suggests that caraway essential oil may help prevent and treat intestinal dysbiosis (a state of altered intestinal flora to one of harmful bacteria that contributes to a variety of chronic and degenerative diseases) by selectively destroying harmful bacteria while leaving probiotics intact.[1707]

☐ Animal research suggests that caraway essential oil reduces colon lesions and experimental colitis when administered orally or injected into the intraperitoneum.[2833] Another animal study demonstrated that oral administration of caraway essential oil reduces stomach ulcers similarly to the prescription proton-pump inhibitor omeprazole.[1708]

☐ Caraway essential oil is larvacidal to several species of mosquitoes and the German cockroach.[1709,1710,1711,1712]

☐ Animal research suggests that caraway essential oil protects the kidneys from oxidative stress caused by sepsis (a life-threatening complication of an infection that occurs when chemicals released into the bloodstream to fight infections trigger a systemic inflammatory response).[1713]

☐ Caraway essential oil demonstrated strong antioxidant activity and protected the liver against free radicals.[1714]

☐ *In vitro* research concluded that caraway essential oil prevents the reproduction and spread (bacteriostatic) of *E. coli* and moderately inhibited *S. aureus*.[1715,1716]

☐ An enteric-coated capsule containing 90 mg of peppermint and 50 mg of caraway essential oil (about 2 and 1 drops respectively) helped relieve symptoms of non-ulcer dyspepsia as well as the drug cisapride.[1717,1718,1719,1720,1721]

☐ Animal research found that injection of caraway essential oil prevented seizures in mice, which was not due to muscle relaxant activity.[1722] The study concluded that caraway warrants further research to prevent petit mal seizures (a type of seizure that involves brief, sudden lapses in attention) in humans.

☐ Human aryl hydrocarbon receptor (AhR: a gene that encodes a protein that helps regulate responses to planar aromatic hydrocarbons and significantly affects the immune activity in the gastrointestinal tract) regulates the circadian rhythm, helps regulate the cell cycle, and plays an important role in tissue development. Cumin, jasmine,

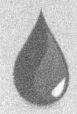

vanilla, and bay leaf fully activate AhR; clove, dill, thyme, nutmeg, and oregano partially activate AhR; and tarragon, caraway, turmeric, lovage, fennel, spearmint, star anise, and anise inhibit the AhR activity.[1723]

☐ A nanoemulsion of caraway essential oil was toxic to and promoted cell death of colon cancer cells.[1724] Another study also reported that caraway essential oil nanoemulsion is selectively cytotoxic to colon cancer cells.[1725]

☐ Caraway essential oil and fractions rich in carvone inhibited food spoilage fungi (*R. oryzae, R. stolonifera, A. penicillioides*).[1726]

☐ Lower concentrations of caraway essential oil repelled the rice weevil (*Sitophilus oryzae*), whereas higher concentrations of the oil or isolated carvone were ineffective.[1727] A 0.5% concentration of caraway and 1% concentration of carvone was insecticidal to the rice weevil.

☐ *In vitro* research demonstrated that caraway essential oil inhibits *C. albicans* and reduces its expression of virulence factors.[1728]

☐ The carvone CT of caraway essential oil inhibited an aflatoxin B1 (AFB1) producing strain of *A. niger*, completely inhibiting its growth and AFB1 secretion at concentrations of 0.7 mcL/mL and 0.6 mcL/mL respectively.[1729] The oil also displayed remarkable antioxidant activity in the DPPH assay.

☐ Dermatophyte infections are caused by a group of filamentous fungi that require keratin (structural proteins found in the hair, nails, and outermost layers of the skin) for growth. It is estimated that up to 25 percent of the world's population is affected by dermatophyte infections, with *Trichophyton rubrum* and *T. mentagrophytes* accounting for 70 percent of infections. Terbinafine is a first-line drug used to treat these infections, but its side effects (liver injury, gastrointestinal disturbances, headache, change in taste, and rash), interactions with other drugs, and the emergence of drug-resistant strains reduce its clinical use and efficacy. An *in vitro* study found that ajowan CT thymol, coriander, caraway CT carvone, and anise weakly to moderately inhibited *T. rubrum* and *T. mentagrophytes*—ajowan was the most effective and anise the least effective.[1730] In addition, the essential oils significantly potentiated the activity of terbinafine when used in combination, suggesting essential oils could reduce the amount of the drug needed to be effective and therefore potentially its side effects. None of the essential oils reduced white blood cell (neutrophil) viability at the tested concentrations, but did moderately inhibit their release of proinflammatory cytokines (IL-1β, IL-8, and TNF-α). Each oil reduced IL-1β and IL-8 (ajowan most active against IL-1β and coriander most active against IL-8) and only coriander and caraway reduced TNF-α.

☐ Caraway was effective against *Vibrio* species bacteria, demonstrating bacteriostatic and inhibitory activity, and inhibited swarming motility and production of elastase and protease in *P. aeruginosa* PAO1, and violacein production in *C. violaceum*.[1731] The oil also exhibited antioxidant capacity in the DPPH, reducing power, beta-carotene, and chelating power assays.

☐ Caraway essential oil exhibited good antioxidant activity in the DPPH and metal chelating assays, antimicrobial activity against *E. coli, S. typhimurium, B. cereus, S. aureus, C. albicans,* and *A. niger* (greatest activity against *S. aureus*), and anticancer activity against colorectal and liver cancer cells.[1732]

☐ *In vitro* research showed that cumin, anise, and caraway essential oil each inhibited *H. pylori*, with cumin exhibiting the greatest activity and cuminaldehyde the best docking potential to inhibit *H. pylori*.[1733] The three oils were also evaluated for their ability to reduce the production of COX-2 (an enzyme responsible for pain and inflammation). Cumin reduced COX-2 expression nearly as well as celecoxib, followed by caraway and anise.

☐ Caraway essential oil was remarkable insecticidal to the cigarette beetle (*L. serricorne*).[1734]

☐ *In vitro* research showed that caraway essential oil significantly inhibited the growth of planktonic bacteria and biofilm in MRSA cells by affecting amino acid metabolism.[1735]

☐ A nanoemulsion gel loaded with caraway essential oil substantially inhibited and reduced the viability of *E. coli* and *S. aureus*.[1736]

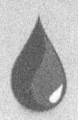 

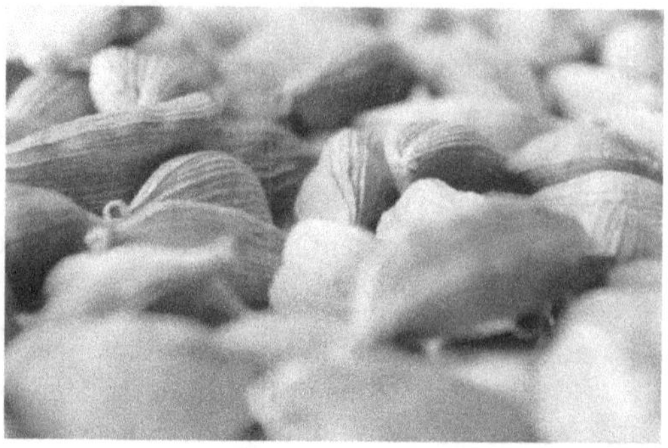

# CARDAMOM

*Elettaria cardamomum* (L.) Maton, *Amomum cardamomum* L.

**FAMILY:** Zingiberaceae
**NOTE:** Middle
**AROMA INTENSITY:** Strong
**AROMA:** Warm, spicy, slightly balsamic
**COMMON EXTRACTION METHOD:** Steam distilled from the seeds
**POSSIBLE SUBSTITUTE OILS:** Eucalyptus, niaouli (1,8-cineole CT), ravintsara (1,8-cineole CT), ravensara (1,8-cineole CT), cajeput, rosemary (1,8-cineole CT), bay laurel, neroli, basil (Linalool CT)
**BLENDS WELL WITH:** Bergamot, black pepper, cinnamon, clove, cedarwood, fennel, ginger, grapefruit, lemon, lemongrass, neroli, orange, patchouli, rose, sandalwood, tangerine, vetiver, ylang ylang
**SUBCELLULAR LOCALIZATION | EPIGENETIC INFLUENCE:** Currently unknown | Currently unknown
**RECOMMENDED DILUTION RANGE:** 3%–33%; neat for limited conditions

**PRIMARY CONSTITUENTS:**[1737,1738,1739,1740,1741]

*Alpha-Terpinyl-Acetate CT*

| | |
|---|---|
| Alpha-Terpinyl Acetate | 10.2%–68.2% |
| 1,8-Cineole | 4.3%–27.2% |
| Linalool | 0.0%–10.2% |
| Nerolidol | 0.3%–8.9% |
| Alpha-Terpineol | 2.1%–7.4% |
| Nerol | 0.0%–6.8% |
| Sabinene | 2.6%–4.3% |

*1,8-Cineole CT*

| | |
|---|---|
| 1,8-Cineole | 15.9%–55.6% |
| Alpha-Terpinyl Acetate | 0.9%–35.3% |
| Linalool | 0.6%–6.4% |

**OTHER CONSTITUENTS:** 1,8-Cineole—Cis-ocimene, alpha-pinene, sabinene, myrcene, gamma-terpinene, terpinolene, fenchyl alcohol, alpha-selinene, farnesol, linalyl acetate, terpinen-4-ol, geranyl acetate, geraniol, nerolidol; Alpha-Terpinyl Acetate CT—Alpha-pinene, alpha-myrcene, 4-terpineol, geranyl acetate

**PREFERRED COMPOSITION FOR CLINICAL USE:**

| Constituent | α-Terpinyl Acetate CT |
|---|---|
| **Alpha-Terpinyl Acetate** | 35%–50% |
| **1,8-Cineole** | 20%–35% |
| **Linalyl Acetate** | 2%–8% |
| **Linalool** | 2%–8% |
| **Alpha-Terpineol** | 1%–7% |
| **Sabinene** | 2%–6% |
| **Limonene** | 1.5%–5% |
| **Myrcene** | 0.1%–3% |
| **Terpinen-4-ol** | 0.1%–3% |
| **Alpha-Pinene** | 0.5%–2% |

**REPORTED THERAPEUTIC PROPERTIES:** Antiseptic, antispasmodic, antimicrobial, **expels excess gas**, **aids digestion**, enhances metabolism, relieves insect bites, stimulates the release of hormones, diuretic, relieves constipation, **stimulates appetite**, anticancer, nervine (calms and soothes the nerves), stimulating, warming, stress management, **aids concentration and focus**, helps relieve overwhelming feelings, aphrodisiac, reduces shame and guilt, combats frustration

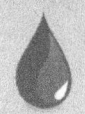

**CAUTIONS:**

■ Avoid with children under age 3 (1,8-cineole CT), particularly around the nose and mouth. Use very cautiously in children under age 5 due to high 1,8-cineole content. 1,8-cineole may cause seizures, central nervous system problems, or respiratory distress in young children.[1742,1743,1744,1745]

■ Avoid with epilepsy and Parkinson's disease due to 1,8-cineole content. May exacerbate or cause seizures/convulsions or reduce seizure medication efficacy based on 1,8-cineole content.[1746,1747,1748]

■ Caution is warranted orally due to the significant amounts of 1,8-cineole (1,8-cineole CT). Limit to small doses internally (adults—maximum 10 drops daily). Toxicity has been reported when eucalyptus (also high in 1,8-cineole) was ingested in large doses, and as few as 4 to 5 drops may cause problems in very sensitive individuals.[1749,1750,1751,1752,1753,1754] In humans, 3.5 to 5 mL has proven fatal orally.[1755]

■ May interfere with enzymes responsible for metabolizing medications (NSAIDs, proton-pump inhibitors, acetaminophen, antiepileptics, immune modulators, blood-sugar medications, blood pressure medications, antidepressants, antipsychotics, diabetic medications, antihistamines, antibiotics, and anesthetics).[1756,1757]

■ May interfere with pentobarbital and other barbiturates (medications for anxiety and insomnia) based on 1,8-cineole content.[1758,1759]

**SELECTED EVIDENCE:**

☐ Cardamom may help prevent tumor formation at the molecular level.[1760,1761]

☐ Extracts of cardamom demonstrated better protection against stomach ulcers than Zantac (ranitidine) in animals.[464] It also protects against aspirin-caused stomach lesions.[1762]

☐ Cardamom oil may significantly prevent DNA from bonding to a cancer-causing chemicals (DNA adduct formation) and therefore help prevent cancer.[1763]

☐ A marked anti-inflammatory and antispasmodic effect has been observed in animals administered cardamom.[1764]

☐ Cardamom demonstrates antimicrobial activity against *Staphylococcus aureus*, *Bacillus cereus*, *Escherichia coli*, and *Salmonella typhi*.[1765]

☐ Extracts of cardamom may help destroy microbes associated with dental cavities.[1766]

☐ Cardamom and dill CT carvone essential oils significantly inhibited *Campylobacter* spp. (*C. jejuni* and *C. coli*) by affecting their membrane integrity.[1767]

☐ *Campylobacter jejuni* is the most commonly reported cause of foodborne infection (food poisoning) in the United States and human infections by this bacterium are increasing worldwide, including multidrug-resistant strains. Oral administration of cardamom essential oil (258 mg/kg body weight daily in drinking water) decreased *C. jejuni* pathogen load and improved clinical outcomes in mice by modulating immune responses.[1768] The treated mice had less gastrointestinal inflammation, but remarkably a decrease in proinflammatory molecule secretion was observed outside the intestinal tract and in systemic organs as well.

☐ *In vitro* research showed that two different cardamom essential oils inhibited *P. aeruginosa* and *E. coli*. The oil also reduced diarrhea caused by castor oil and reduced intestinal contractions when administered orally at 100 and 200 mg/kg body weight in mice.[1769] The oil with higher alpha-terpinyl acetate (24.7% vs. 18.7%) and 1,8-cineole (14.0% vs. 10.6%) content performed best in all tests.

☐ Both cardamom and cinnamon bark essential oils inhibited the growth of *B. subtilis* and *E. coli*, but cardamom was only effective at the highest concentration tested.[1770] The individual oils and their combination inhibited cell attachment for both bacteria, with stronger activity observed against *E. coli*. A combination of both oils was synergistic against *B. subtilis* and reduced biofilm formation by both bacteria.

☐ The incidence of nausea and vomiting during elective cesarean section is estimated to be between 40% and 81%. A randomized placebo-controlled trial evaluated the effects of inhaling cardamom essential oil on nausea and vomiting during and after cesarean section.[1771] Women in the intervention group inhaled from a plastic bag containing sterile gauze pads saturated in 2 mL of saline and 2 drops of cardamom essential oil at the first signs of nausea. They were asked to inhale from the bag three times and repeat the process two minutes later over a five-minute period. Breathing was performed through the nose slowly counting to four and exhalation through the mouth to a slow count of seven. The placebo group followed the same procedure inhaling from a bag with saline saturated gauze pads only. The frequency and severity of nausea and vomiting were significantly lower in the cardamom group than in the placebo group and the need of antiemetic medications was reduced in the cardamom group.

- Cardamom essential oil demonstrated promising adulticidal, larvicidal, and repellent effects against ticks (*Hyalomma anatolicum*) infesting cattle in Saudi Arabia.[1772]

- The hydatid worm (*Echinococcus granulosus*) is a parasite that lives in the small intestine of dogs as an adult, but uses intermediate hosts like livestock and humans, where it causes cystic echinococcosis (hydatid disease). Both cardamom and its main constituent 1,8-cineole reduced hydatid worm protoscoleces viability with 200 mcl/ml being the most effective dose in a laboratory setting.[1773] Combining 1,8-cineole with albendazole at this dose caused 100 percent destruction of protoscoleces. Cardamom and 1,8-cineole, alone and in combination with albendazole, took longer to be effective in the *ex vivo* evaluation.

- Cardamom essential oil inhibited *S. aureus*, *S. epidermidis*, *C. tropicalis*, *P. mirabilis*, and *A. baumannii*, but was inactive against *E. coli*, *K. pneumoniae*, and *P. aeruginosa*.[1774] The oil also displayed weak antioxidant activity in the DPPH and FRAP assays.

- Cardamom essential oil was active against *Candida* strains (clinical and reference) in their planktonic form (resting state concentrated in liquid water) and against exoenzymes and biofilm production.[1775]

- Both cardamom and wild marjoram CT 1,8-cineole essential oils demonstrated antimicrobial activity (*C. glabrata*, *L. monocytogenes*, *C. tropicalis*, *H. influenzae*, *S. pneumoniae*, *S. aureus*, *C. albicans*, *Y. enterocolitica*, *P. fluorescens* biofilm, and *E. coli*), with wild marjoram being the more active against bacteria and cardamom better against fungi.[1776] Cardamom also exhibited mild anticancer activity against breast cancer cells.

- Cardamom exhibited antioxidant activity in the DPPH and TEAC assays.[1777]

# CARROT SEED
## (Queen Anne's Lace, Wild Carrot)
*Daucus carota* L.

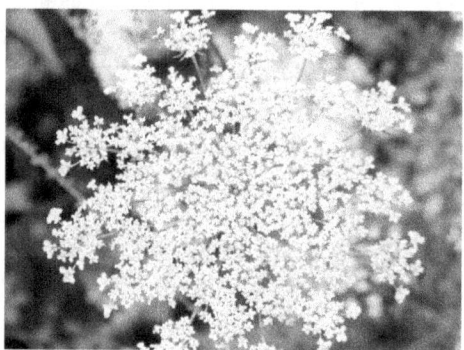

**FAMILY:** Apiaceae (Umbelliferae)
**NOTE:** Middle
**AROMA INTENSITY:** Medium
**AROMA:** Slightly sweet, earthy, woody
**COMMON EXTRACTION METHOD:** Steam distilled from the seeds
**POSSIBLE SUBSTITUTE OILS:** Cistus, rose
**BLENDS WELL WITH:** Bergamot, cedarwood, cinnamon, fennel, geranium, ginger, lavender, lemon, lime, tea tree, orange, neroli, patchouli, tangerine
**SUBCELLULAR LOCALIZATION | EPIGENETIC INFLUENCE:** Currently unknown | Currently unknown
**RECOMMENDED DILUTION RANGE:** 5%–Neat

**PRIMARY CONSTITUENTS:**[1778,1779]

| | |
|---|---|
| Carotol | 38.9%–66.8% |
| Daucol | 2.0%–12.6% |
| Beta-Caryophyllene | 0.0%–10.7% |
| Daucene | 0.0%–8.7% |
| Alpha-Farnesene | 0.2%–5.9% |
| Caryophyllene Oxide | 0.0%–4.3% |
| (E)-Beta-Farnesene | 0.5%–4.0% |

**OTHER CONSTITUENTS:** Camphene, alpha-pinene, sabinene, myrcene, limonene, terpinolene, beta-pinene, linalool, trans-pinocarveol, trans-verbenol, para-cymen-8-ol, alpha-terpineol, verbenone, carvone, cis-alpha-bergamotene, germacrene D, ar-curcumene, beta-selinene, bicyclogermacrene, beta-bisabolene, Z-gamma-bisabolene, beta-sesquiphellandrene, 15-copaenol, alpha-eudesmol, alpha-cadinol

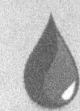

**PREFERRED COMPOSITION FOR CLINICAL USE:**

| Constituent | Carotol Rich | Balanced |
|---|---|---|
| Carotol | 60%–80% | 30%–45% |
| Daucene | 2%–10% | 1%–3% |
| Daucol | 1%–10% | 1%–3% |
| Cedrene Oxide | 0%–6% | – |
| (E)-Beta-Farnesene | 1%–5% | 0.5%–3% |
| Beta-Bisabolene | 1%–5% | 3%–10% |
| Beta-Caryophyllene | 0.1%–5% | 3%–10% |
| Caryophyllene Oxide | 0.1%–5% | 1%–4% |
| Alpha-Pinene | 0.1%–5% | 5%–15% |
| Sabinene | – | 3%–11% |
| (Z)-Beta-Farnesene | – | 0.5%–2% |

**REPORTED THERAPEUTIC PROPERTIES: Promotes cellular regeneration**, antioxidant, aids detoxification, aids circulation, **nourishes skin**, **reduces the appearance of blemishes and wrinkles**, antiparasitic, antiseptic, expels excess gas, diuretic, supports liver function, strengthens nails, supports hair strength, stimulating, antidepressant, reduces anxiety, combats mood swings

**CAUTIONS:**

■ Avoid during pregnancy. Animal studies suggest very large doses of carrot seed oil blocks progesterone synthesis and prevents implantation of the fertilized egg into the uterine wall.[1780,1781,1782]

**SELECTED EVIDENCE:**

☐ The main ingredient in carrot seed essential oil, carotol, inhibits the growth of multidrug-resistant fungi.[1783]

☐ A commercial carrot seed essential oil with 60.7% methyl isoeugenol was significantly more toxic to mosquito larvae (*Cx. Restuans, Cx. Pipiens*, and *Ae. Aegypti*) than essential oil extracted from wild carrot populations (33.0% alpha-pinene, 25.8% beta-pinene).[1784] Three constituents (terpinolene, para cymene, and gamma-terpinene) were more toxic than the whole essential oil.

☐ Laboratory research found that sweet fennel and carrot (leaf and stem; caryophyllene oxide and isospathulenol as primary constituents) inhibited gram-positive (*S. aureus, B. subtilis, B. amyloliquefaciens*) and gram-negative bacteria and the yeast *C. albicans*.[1785] One variety of fennel oil tested was more active against *C. albicans* than gentamicin.

☐ Carrot seed essential oil and its main component carotol significantly repelled *Aedes aegypti* and *Anopheles quadrimaculatus* mosquitoes and enhanced the repellent activity of DEET when mixed together.[1786]

☐ *In vitro* research concluded that carrot seed essential oil was bactericidal against *Campylobacter jejuni*.[1787]

☐ Carrot flower and stem essential oil inhibited *E. coli* and *S. aureus*, and the flower oil improved the activity of superoxide dismutase, catalase, and glutathione peroxidase in polymorphonuclear leukocytes (white blood cells that protect the body against infectious organisms).[1788] The healthy activity of these enzymatic antioxidants is important for the ability of polymorphonuclear leukocytes to protect against bacteria.

# CASSIA
## (Chinese Cinnamon)

*Cinnamomum cassia* Nees ex Blume, *C. aromaticum* Nees

**FAMILY:** Lauraceae
**NOTE:** Middle
**AROMA INTENSITY:** Strong
**AROMA:** Spicy, warm, potent, slightly woody
**COMMON EXTRACTION METHOD:** Steam distilled from the leaves or bark
**POSSIBLE SUBSTITUTE OILS:** Cinnamon

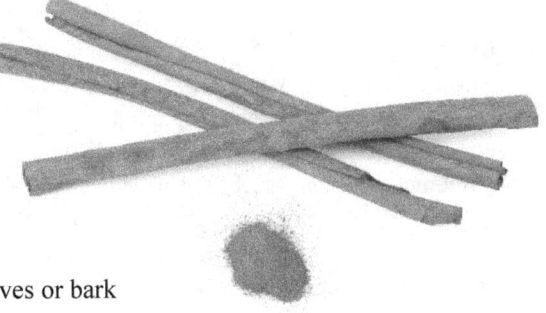

**BLENDS WELL WITH:** Balsam fir, bergamot, black pepper, chamomile (Roman, German), coriander, frankincense, ginger, geranium, grapefruit, lavender, lemon, lime, neroli, nutmeg, orange, petitgrain, rosemary, silver fir, tangerine, white fir

**SUBCELLULAR LOCALIZATION | EPIGENETIC INFLUENCE:** Currently unknown | Currently unknown

**RECOMMENDED DILUTION RANGE:** 1.5%–20%

**PRIMARY CONSTITUENTS:**[1789,1790,1791,1792,1793,1794,1795,1796]

*Cassia Bark*

| | |
|---|---|
| (E)-Cinnamaldehyde | 24.6%–92.3% |
| Cis-2-Methoxy Cinnamic Acid | 0.0%–43.1% |
| 2-Methoxycinnamaldehyde | 0.0%–13.2% |
| (Z)-Cinnamaldehyde | 4.4%–10.5% |
| Acetophenone | 0.0%–6.9% |
| (E)-Cinnamic Acid | 0.0%–5.5% |
| Cinnamyl Acetate | 0.0%–4.2% |

*Cassia Leaves*

| | |
|---|---|
| (E)-Cinnamaldehyde | 57.9%–78.4% |
| Cinnamyl Acetate | 0.0%–9.2% |
| Eugenol | 0.0%–4.5% |
| Alpha-Terpineol | 0.0%–4.2% |

**OTHER CONSTITUENTS:** *Cassia Bark*—Alpha-pinene, benzaldehyde, beta-phellandrene, benzenepropanal, borneol, alpha-terpineol, coumaran, hydrocinnamic alcohol, bornyl acetate, (E)-cinnamyl acetate, (E)-cinnamyl alcohol, citronellol acetate, alpha-ylangene, coumarin, chamigrene, alpha-curcumene, caryophyllene oxide, beta-naphthalenedione, ethanone; *Cassia Leaves*—Beta-terpineol, gamma terpineol, trans-caryophyllene, benzaldehyde, benzyl benzoate, salicylaldehyde, coumarin, alpha-copaene, phenylpropanal, anisaldehyde

**PREFERRED COMPOSITION FOR CLINICAL USE:**

| Constituent | Bark | Leaf |
|---|---|---|
| **(E)-Cinnamaldehyde** | 72%–90% | 60%–92% |
| **(E)-o-Methoxycinnamaldehyde** | 0.5%–15% | — |
| **(E)-Cinnamyl Acetate** | 0%–6% | 0%–6% |
| **Coumarin** | 1%–5% | tr–5% |
| **Benzaldehyde** | 0.1%–2% | — |
| **O-Methoxycinnamyl Acetate** | 0.1%–2% | — |
| **(Z)-Cinnamaldehyde** | | < 1% |
| **Phenylethyl Alcohol** | | < 1% |
| **Eugenol** | | < 1% |
| **Salicylaldehyde** | | < 0.7% |
| **Acetophenone** | | < 0.5% |
| **Stryrene** | | < 0.4% |

**REPORTED THERAPEUTIC PROPERTIES:** Analgesic (pain relief), antirheumatic, antiarthritic, antispasmodic, **antimicrobial**, antibacterial, **antiviral**, astringent, expels excess gas, aids circulation, **antiparasitic**, eases nausea, enhances libido, **relieves diarrhea**, eases cough, aids digestions, **supports normal blood-sugar levels**, energizing, stimulating, antidepressant

**CAUTIONS:**

■ Avoid during pregnancy and lactation. Several studies have tested the major constituents of cinnamon and cassia essential oils with pregnant animals, and the results have been inconsistent. Therefore, it is advised to avoid essential oils with significant quantities of cinnamaldehyde during pregnancy until further research is conclusive.[1797,1798,1799]

■ May interact with aspirin, blood pressure, antiplatelet, and anticoagulant medications, and increase the risk of bleeding among people with bleeding disorders.[1800,1801,1802]

■ May interfere with enzymes responsible for metabolizing medications (NSAIDs, proton-pump inhibitors, acetaminophen, antiepileptics, immune modulators, blood-sugar medications, blood pressure medications, antidepressants, antipsychotics, diabetic medications, antihistamines, antibiotics, and anesthetics).[1803,1804,1805]

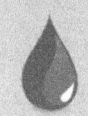

■ May interact with diabetes medications and cause low blood-sugar levels.[1806,1807,1808]
■ May interact with antibiotics and possibly enhance their effects.[1809,1810]
■ May irritate mucous membranes (eyes, mouth, nasal passages, vagina, rectum).[1811]
■ Topical application (significant dilution strongly encouraged). Cinnamon and cassia are very high in cinnamaldehyde, which is very irritating to the skin and prone to cause severe reactions.[1812]

**SELECTED EVIDENCE:**

☐ Cassia inhibits proinflammatory molecules (nitric oxide synthase, COX-2, prostaglandins) and also activates anti-inflammatory molecules (cytokines IL-10, transforming growth factor-beta).[1813] Another study found that oral administration of 15, 30, and 60 mg/kg of cassia twig essential oil significantly inhibited inflammation and reduced pain in mice by decreasing cytokines (TNF-alpha, IL-1 beta, PGE2, COX-2 activity, and iNOS expression).[1814]

☐ Cinnamaldehyde strongly inhibits multidrug-resistant bacteria, molds, and dermatophytes (fungi that require keratin for growth and infect the skin, hair, and nails).[1815,1816] It also inhibits *S. aureus* and prevents the formation of biofilms, which caused the researchers to determine it was a potential surface sanitizer.[1817]

☐ Cassia degrades the integrity of the membranes of pathogenic bacteria to cause their destruction.[1818]

☐ Cassia decreases blood-glucose levels and stimulates pancreas beta-cells to produce insulin in animals (slightly better than true cinnamon bark).[1819] Other research suggests that it reduces fasting blood-sugar levels up to 29%.[1820]

☐ Inhalation of cinnamaldehyde significantly increased survivability among mice infected with the influenza A virus.[1821] Cinnamaldehyde also inhibited virus growth *in vitro*.

☐ Cassia, or its main constituent cinnamaldehyde, may reduce the production of melanin and whiten the skin.[1822] It does so by inhibiting the tyrosinase enzyme.[1823] Tyrosinase is an enzyme involved in the production of melanin (a dark brown to black pigment that is responsible for tanning of skin when exposed to sunlight) by oxidation of tyrosine.

☐ Animal and *in vitro* research concluded that cinnamaldehyde inhibits influenza A/PR/8 growth if administered within three hours after infection.[1824] The same research also found that inhalation of 50 mg and administration of 250 mcg of cinnamaldehyde per day through the nasal passages reduced virus spread and increased survivability in mice.

☐ *In vitro* research suggests cassia oil effectively kills head lice.[1825] Cassia was the second most effective essential oil of six tested.

☐ Cassia essential oil significantly reduces the number of viable *C. albicans* organisms and biofilm formation on dentures.[1826]

☐ Cassia essential oil was toxic to the adult spotted wing drosophila (*Drosophila suzukii*) when in direct contact with the drosophila.[1827]

☐ Cassia essential oil was insecticidal against *Ricania* sp. pests.[1828]

☐ Cassia, bitter ginger, Vietnamese balm, and large cardamom each demonstrated toxicity against *Leishmania Mexicana* (a parasite responsible for cutaneous leishmaniasis), but the most promising oil was clove basil essential oil due to its selectivity.[1829]

☐ Thyme CT gamma-terpinene, lemon CT citral, geranium CT p-menthone, cassia CT cinnamaldehyde, clove CT eugenol, and basil CT 1,8-cineole each demonstrated fungistatic and fungicidal activity toward *C. albicans* and *C. glabrata* isolates with cassia demonstrating the highest activity.[1830]

☐ Both cinnamon and cassia essential oils inhibited and reduced biofilm biomasses of *Streptococcus pyogenes, Pseudomonas aeruginosa,* and *Escherichia coli*.[1831] The same research found that cinnamaldehyde also exhibited antimicrobial and antibiofilm activity.

☐ Cinnamon bark essential oil was the most effective essential oil of seven tested (clove, cinnamon bark, eucalyptus, thyme CT thymol, Scots pine, peppermint, and citronella) against respiratory tract pathogens (*Streptococcus pneumoniae, S. mutans, S. pyogenes, Haemophilus influenzae, H. parainfluenzae,* and *Moraxella catarrhalis*) in vapor phase.[1832] In liquid phase, thyme was most effective against *S. mutans* and cinnamon and clove significantly inhibited *S. pneumoniae* and *S. pyogenes*.

☐ *In vitro* examination of sixty essential oils demonstrated that sandalwood (Indian, Australian, and Hawaiian), melissa, lemongrass (*C. flexuosus*), cilantro, cassia, cinnamon, patchouli, and vetiver essential oils possess

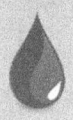

remarkable anticancer (two breast cancer cells) and antifungal (*Aspergillus niger, Candida albicans,* and *Cryptococcus neoformans*) activities.[1833]

☐ Cassia essential oil showed the ability to improve antibiotic effectiveness against three multidrug-resistant bacteria (*Escherichia coli, Staphylococcus aureus,* and *Pseudomonas aeruginosa*). Cassia EO produced synergy against *S. aureus* when combined with ampicillin and chloramphenicol, synergy against *E. coli* when combined with chloramphenicol, and an additive effect against all bacterial strains with streptomycin.[1834]

☐ Cassia essential oil improved erectile function in isolated human corpus cavernosum (CC; from males undergoing penile prosthesis surgery) and CC isolated from diabetic and normal rats.[1835] Erectile dysfunction was noted in the diabetic rats, which was restored after injection of cassia essential oil in to the corpus cavernosum in the *in vivo* arm of the study.

☐ Laboratory research concluded that oregano CT carvacrol, thyme CT thymol, cassia, lemongrass (*C. flexuosus*), and Western red cedar (arborvitae) essential oils exhibit very strong antimicrobial activity against drug-resistant pathogens (*Pseudomonas aeruginosa, Proteus vulgaris, Citrobacter koseri, Klebsiella pneumoniae, Candida albicans,* and *C. parapsilosis*.[1836] Ten essential oils—oregano, thyme, clove, arborvitae, cassia, lemongrass, tea tree, eucalyptus (*E. radiata*), lavender, and clary sage —were tested, and these five were the most effective. The researchers also concluded the essential oils were not genotoxic (cause DNA damage) compared to control cells. In addition, each of the oils exhibited antioxidant activity, with cassia and oregano demonstrating the greatest increase in total antioxidant status, followed by tea tree, thyme, clove, clary sage, eucalyptus, arborvitae, and lavender.

☐ Oral administration of cinnamaldehyde, the main constituent in cassia and cinnamon bark essential oils, significantly inhibited the release of proinflammatory cytokines (IL-6, IL-8, TNF-α) from synoviocyte cells—a specialized type of cells found in joints that play a crucial role in rheumatoid arthritis—in arthritic rats.[1837] Cinnamaldehyde also impaired Jak/Stat signaling pathways—critical pathways in the onset and progression of rheumatoid arthritis—and reduced collagen-induced swollen paws. The anti-inflammatory effects of cinnamaldehyde decreased the severity of arthritis, joint swelling, and reduced bone erosion and destruction.

☐ Both cassia and cinnamon essential oil protected neuron cells against toxicity and cell death caused by 6-hydroxydopamine (a neurotoxic synthetic organic compound used by researchers to destroy neurons that produce dopamine and noradrenaline in the brain) in an *in vitro* model of Parkinson's disease (PD).[1838] The initial research is promising that these essential oils could play a role in reducing a hallmark cause of PD such as the loss of dopamine-producing neurons.

☐ *In vitro* research showed that 8-hydroxyquinoline (a chelating agent) improved the antimicrobial activity of cassia essential oil against *S. aureus*.[1839]

☐ Oregano CT carvacrol, thyme CT thymol, cassia bark, lemongrass, and Western red cedar essential oils each demonstrated significant antibacterial and antifungal activity against several drug-resistant pathogens (*Ps. Aeruginosa, Pr. Vulgaris, C. koseri, K. pneumoniae, C. albicans,* and *C. parapsilosis*) known to infect the skin.[1840] The oils were not toxic to healthy keratinocytes and increased total antioxidant status in the cells as well.

☐ Cassia essential oil improved the antibacterial activity of the antibiotic polymyxin B against carbapenemase-producing *Klebsiella pneumoniae* and *Serratia marcescens*.[1841]

☐ *In vitro* research showed that cassia essential oil inhibited drug-resistant *Klebsiella aerogenes*.[1842]

☐ Cassia essential oil was active against 5 *Listeria monocytogenes* strains *in vitro*.[1843]

☐ A chitin nanofibril stabilized emulsion with cassia essential oil showed prolonged antibacterial activity and enhanced diffusion efficiency, which proved to be a good system for the controlled release of essential oils.[1844]

☐ Cassia essential oil and isolated trans-cinnamaldehyde were acaricidal, larvicidal, and nymphicidal to the Asian longhorned tick (*Haemaphysalis longicornis*).[1845]

☐ Cassia and lemongrass (*C. citratus*) essential oil both exhibited anti-inflammatory (reduced TNF-α, IL-6, COX-2, and NF-κB P65) and antioxidant activities.[1846]

☐ Cassia and ho wood essential oils were the most active fumigants of seven essential oils tested against the poultry ectoparasite *Dermanyssus gallinae*, causing 96 and 61 percent mortality respectively.[1847] Isolated trans-cinnamaldehyde and linalool were less toxic suggesting a synergy of multiple constituents in the oils.

☐ Clove bud essential oil inhibited extended-spectrum β-lactamase bacteria (*E. coli* and *K. pneumoniae*), which are commonly resistant to multiple antibiotics.[1848]

☐ Five essential oils (cassia, oregano CT carvacrol, thyme CT thymol, summer savory CT carvacrol, and clove bud) were evaluated for their ability to reduce colonization of *Salmonella* spp. in an *in vivo* infection model using *Caenorhabditis elegans*.[1849] Both cassia and clove significantly inhibited bacterial colonization in the digestive tract, which the researchers suggested may be related to reduced swimming motility.

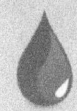

- Clostridioides difficile is a bacterium that produces two exotoxins: toxin A and toxin B. Infections with *C. diff* can be mild to moderate (watery diarrhea three or more times daily for more than one day accompanied by mild abdominal cramping and tenderness) or severe (watery diarrhea up to fifteen times daily, moderate to severe abdominal cramping, rapid heart rate, fever, dehydration, and nausea). Severe cases can cause kidney failure, loss of appetite, blood or pus in the stool, and inflammation of the colon (colitis), which can be life-threatening. Illness caused by *C. diff* typically occurs after antibiotic use and most commonly affects older adults in healthcare facilities. However, because the bacterium is shed in feces it can contaminate any surface, material, or device and spread outside of healthcare settings and in younger people as well. Repeat infections are common among the elderly because the bacterium is resistant to multiple antibiotics, making it very difficult to eradicate. A laboratory study investigated the activity of ten essential oils—cassia bark, cinnamon bark, citronella (*C. nardus*), coriander, clove bud, oregano CT carvacrol, Greek oregano (*O. heracleoticum*) CT carvacrol, marjoram, clary sage, and thyme CT thymol—against *C. diff* isolated from infected patients and contaminated foods.[1850] Isolated constituents within the essential oils were also tested (carvacrol, trans-cinnamaldehyde, eugenol, linalool, and thymol) as well as common antibiotics used to treat *C. diff* infections (chloramphenicol, clindamycin, erythromycin, gentamicin, metronidazole, and vancomycin). Cassia and cinnamon bark were the most effective, with thyme, oregano, Greek oregano, and marjoram also demonstrating high activity. Coriander and clary sage exhibited medium activity, while clove and citronella displayed low activity. Among the isolated constituents, trans-cinnamaldehyde, thymol, and carvacrol showed high activity and eugenol and linalool low activity. Cinnamon and cassia consistently exceeded the activity of all antibiotics, with very few exceptions, and thyme, oregano, and Greek oregano outperformed all antibiotics but metronidazole.
- Cassia, clove, oregano (near equal carvacrol and thymol), ginger, and thyme CT thymol essential oils each showed activity against *L. monocytogenes* in a dry-cured ham-based model.[1851]
- The antioxidant activity of cassia oil nanoemulsion was greater than the free oil alone in the DPPH assay, but lower than free oil in the ABTS assay.[1852] The nanoemulsion also showed a higher antimicrobial activity against gram-positive and gram-negative bacteria.
- Cassia essential oil impregnated chitosan nanoparticles exhibited enhanced antitumor activity against breast cancer cells when compared to free oil.[1853]
- Cassia bark essential oil inhibited *C. auris* better than isolated trans-cinnamaldehyde and nanoencapsulated cassia.[1854]
- A cassia nanoemulsion was more effective than the free oil against *K. pneumoniae* and non-small cell lung cancer cells, and displayed greater antioxidant activity (DPPH and hydrogen peroxide assays).[1855]

# CATNIP
## (Catnep, Catmint)

*Nepeta cataria* L.

**FAMILY:** Lamiaceae (Labiatae)
**NOTE:** Middle
**AROMA INTENSITY:** Medium
**AROMA:** Herbaceous, slightly floral, slightly minty
**COMMON EXTRACTION METHOD:** Steam distilled from the aerial parts
**POSSIBLE SUBSTITUTE OILS:** Applemint, lemon catnip, celery seed
**BLENDS WELL WITH:** Bergamot, big badja gum, cajeput, eucalyptus, grapefruit, gully gum, lavender, lemon, lime, marjoram, myrrh, myrtle, orange, peppermint, rosemary, spearmint
**SUBCELLULAR LOCALIZATION | EPIGENETIC INFLUENCE:** Currently unknown | Currently unknown
**RECOMMENDED DILUTION RANGE:** 3.0%–33.0%; neat for limited conditions

**PRIMARY CONSTITUENTS:**[1856,1857,1858,1859,1860,1861,1862,1863,1864]

| *Nepetalactone CT*[#] | | *1,8-Cineole CT*[*] | |
|---|---|---|---|
| Nepetalactone Isomers | 22.3%–92.2% | 1,8-Cineole | 21.0% |
| Beta-Caryophyllene | 0.2%–24.6% | Alpha-Humulene | 14.4% |
| Caryophyllene Oxide | 0.0%–14.3% | Alpha-Pinene | 10.4% |

| | | | |
|---|---|---|---|
| 1,8-Cineole | 0.0%–13.5% | Geranyl Acetate | 8.2% |
| Citronellyl Acetate | 0.0%–5.2% | Beta-Caryophyllene | 6.4% |
| Dehydronepetalactone | 0.0%–5.0% | (E)-Beta-Ocimene | 5.0% |
| Alpha-Pinene | 0.0%–4.6% | (Z)-Beta-Ocimene | 2.7% |
| Terpinene | 0.0%–4.2% | | |
| Limonene | 0.0%–4.1% | | |
| (Z)-Beta-Farnesene | 0.0%–3.6% | | |
| (Z)-Beta-Ocimene | 0.0%–3.1% | | |
| Beta-Pinene | 0.0%–3.0% | | |

# Other texts and websites (likely reporting what they found in the texts) report catnip essential oil to contain nepetalic acid (a metabolite of nepetalactones formed by condensation interaction of a ketone or aldehyde and semicarbazide—a derivative of urea); however, this is based on two reports from 1941 and 1978 that mention employing fractional distillation to get significant amounts of nepetalic acid (up to 43.0%) from catnip essential oil.[1865,1866] Modern analyses do not report nepetalic acid as a constituent of catnip essential oil unless the oil is combined with other components to react with.

* The 1,8-cineole CT of catnip essential oil doesn't appear to be available commercially. This CT is interesting because it is devoid of the characteristic constituents, nepetalactones, found in catnip essential oil. Other plants of the genus *Nepeta*, such as *N. pogonosperma, N. assurgens, N. binaludensis, N. menthoides, N. crispa,* and *N. parnassica,* do contain significant amounts of 1,8-cineole but they often still contain appreciable amounts of nepetalactone isomers.[1867] It is also important to note that a geranial CT of catnip essential oil is mentioned in the literature consisting of geranial (51.9%–52.0%), nerol (32.2%–34.0%), beta-citronellol (8.0%–9.0%), and geraniol (4.3%–5.5%), but this is solvent extracted, making it an absolute and not a true essential oil.[1868,1869]

**OTHER CONSTITUENTS:** *Nepetalactone CT*—pinocarvone, pulegone (<1.8%), piperitone, thymol, carvacrol, piperitenone, piperitenone oxide, beta-pinene, camphene, thymol, curcumene, farnesol, (E)-beta-ocimene, alpha-humulene, spathulenol, 11-dodecenol, beta-elemene, 3-hexenyl ester, (E)-beta-farnesene, thymol methyl ether, humulene oxide I, Germacrene D, beta-bisabolene, beta-sesquiphellandrene; *1,8-Cineole CT*—alpha-fenchene, beta-pinene, alpha-phellandrene, alpha-terpinene, terpinen-4-acetate, linalool, terpinolene, terpinen-4-ol, caran-3beta-ol, alpha-copaene, Germacrene D, delta-cadinene, beta-caryophyllene oxide, santalol

**PREFERRED COMPOSITION FOR CLINICAL USE:**

| Constituent | Nepetalactone CT |
|---|---|
| **Nepetalactone Isomers** | 70%–90% |
| **Beta-Caryophyllene** | 5%–15% |
| **Caryophyllene Oxide** | 0.5%–10% |
| **Carvone** | 0.1%–3% |
| **Alpha-Pinene** | 0.1%–3% |
| **Beta-Pinene** | 0.1%–3% |

**REPORTED THERAPEUTIC PROPERTIES:** Antibacterial, antifungal, **antimicrobial**, antiseptic, antispasmodic, analgesic, anti-inflammatory, expels excess gas, aids digestion, encourages sweating, nervine, aids the flow of bile and gastric juices, diuretic, astringent, promotes menstrual regularity, encourages the release of hormones, supports respiratory function, balances blood pressure, weight management, reduces headache/migraine, **promotes restful sleep**, disinfectant, insecticide, **insect repellent**, calming/relaxing, stress management, relieves anxiety, uplifting

**CAUTIONS:**

■ May interact with drugs that depress the central nervous system (benzodiazepines, barbiturates, pentobarbital, phenobarbital, secobarbital, fentanyl, morphine, zolpidem, and others). Animal research suggests that catnip extracts or essential oil significantly increases the sleeping time caused by barbiturates, modifies sleep time when administered alone (lower doses increase sleeping time, high doses decrease sleeping time), increases locomotion, amplifies stereotypic behaviors (repetitive and unchanging behaviors without a purpose or goal), and increases susceptibility to seizures.[1870,1871,1872] One case report describes decreased alertness, stomachache, and irritability, followed by prolonged central nervous system depression (lethargy and a hypnotic state) in a nineteen-month-old who ingested raisins soaked in catnip tea and chewing on the tea bag.[1873] The literature also reports altered consciousness similar to marijuana when catnip herb was smoked.[1874]

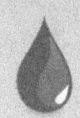

**SELECTED EVIDENCE:**

- *In vitro* research concluded that catnip essential oil (nepetalactone CT) inhibits several common foodborne pathogens, including bacteria: two strains of MRSA, resistant *Escherichia coli*, resistant enterohemorrhagic *E. coli*, *Shigella flexneri*, *Bacillus cereus*, and *P. aeruginosa*; and fungi: *Aspergillus flavus*, two strains of *A. fumigatus*, *A. clavatus*, *A. oryzae*; and clinical isolates of *S. aureus*, *E. coli*, *Shigella spp*, *Salmonella spp*, *Listeria monocytogenes*, and *P. aeruginosa*.[1875] Another study reports that the nepetalactone-rich catnip oil inhibits the fungi: *C. albicans*, *C. tropicalis*, *C. glabrata*, *Aspergillus niger*, *Microsporum canis*, *Microsporum gypseum*, and *Trichophyton tubrum*.[1876] A third study determined that essential oils richer in nepetalactones are more active against pathogens, demonstrating that the essential oil inhibits the fungi: *C. albicans* and *A. niger*; and the bacteria: *E. coli*, *Streptococcus faecalis*, *Staphylococcus aureus*, *P. aeruginosa*, and *Mycobacterium smegmatis*.[1877] A nepetalactone-poor essential oil was ineffective against the same pathogens unless enriched. The nepetalactone CT inhibited the bacteria: *B. subtilis* (two strains), *B. abortus*, *B. macerans*, *Proteus vulgaris*, *S. aureus*, *S. epidermis*, *S. pyogenes* and *E. coli* in another study.[1878]

- The 1,8-cineole CT of catnip essential oil reduced spasms and promoted muscle relaxation in isolated guinea pig trachea, suggesting it may act as a bronchodilator.[1879]

- Animal research found that injection of (0.0005 mL/kg) of catnip essential oil (nepetalactone CT) reduced pain (acted as a central analgesic), inflammation, and edema in mice.[1880]

- Catnip essential oil (nepetalactone CT) potently repels the mosquitoes *Aedes aegypti* (yellow fever vector), *Anopheles gambiae* (malarial vector), *An. Stephensi* (malarial vector), and *Culex quinquefasciatus* (filariasis and encephalitis vector), and *Ae. intrudens* Dyar, house dust mites (*Dermatophagoides pteronyssinus* and *D. farina*), two species of subterranean termite (*Reticulitermes flavipes* Kollar and *R. virginicus*), brown ear tick (*Rhipicephalus appendiculatus*), red poultry mite (*Dermanyssus gallinae*), house fly (*Musca domestica*), black flies (*Simulium decorum* Walker) and stable fly (*Stomoxys calcitrans*).[1881,1882,1883,1884,1885,1886,1887,1888] Its repellency of *Anopheles gambiae* was considered comparable to DEET. Remarkably, a lotion with 15% hydrogenated catnip essential oil completely protected against mosquito bites for greater than eight hours.[1889,1890] Catnip essential oil repels insects when applied topically or dispersed into the air according to more than one study. E,Z,-Nepetalactone was more active than DEET or the whole essential oil in repelling the German cockroach (*Blattella germanica*).[1891]

- Catnip essential oil disrupts neural pathways to repel and prevent female *Aedes aegypti* mosquitoes from biting.[1892]

- *Anopheles* mosquitoes are responsible for transmitting the plasmodium virus and malaria. It is estimated that 212 million people contract malaria annually resulting in more than four hundred thousand deaths. Mosquito nets impregnated with DEET have reduced the mortality rate but have also modified the feeding patterns of mosquitoes. They are now more active in feeding at dusk and early morning rather than after 10:00 p.m. Nepetalactone demonstrates equivalent activity to DEET and its hydrogenated form (dihydronepetalactone) is two times more active. The nepetalactone CT of catnip essential oil effectively reduced mosquito bites when applied by people in the east African country Burundi.[1893]

- Catnip CT nepetalactones (> 86% nepetalactones; different percentages of the Z,E and E,Z isomers) essential oils achieved greater than 95% repellency against *Aedes aegypti* mosquitoes, which lasted from two to four hours.[1894] Remarkably, the lowest concentrations of the oils tested were more effective than DEET at reducing the number of mosquito landings.

- Oral administration of SFE catnip essential oil (composition not reported) protected against liver damage and dysfunction caused by acetaminophen.[1895] The oil was administered for three days after acetaminophen exposure. It did so by increasing the expression of glucuronosyltransferases (a family of liver enzymes that metabolize lipophilic drugs and play a key role in detoxification) and sulfotransferases (a family of phase II enzymes involved in detoxification, drug metabolism, and hormone regulation), as well as by inhibiting CYP2E1 (a member of the cytochrome P450 enzymes that is known to increase liver inflammation and oxidative damage of liver cells). Moreover, the oil significantly increased the expression of Nrf2. Nrf2 is a potent protein found within all cells (but particularly in the liver and kidneys) that acts as the master regulator of the cellular antioxidant system when activated by AREs. Once triggered, Nrf2 activates over 200 genes that metabolize drugs and toxins, protect against oxidative stress, remove damaged proteins, and normalize inflammation. It also interacts with other cells that together determine longevity and protect against age-

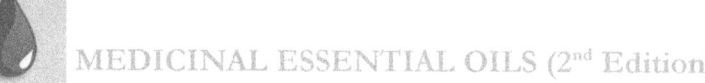

related diseases like cancer and neurological disorders.

- Fumigation of greenhouse plants with pennyroyal, catnip (reduced fertility), and thyme essential oil acted as an effective insecticide against flower thrips (*Frankliniella occidentalis*), which is an insect pest of greenhouse plants.[1896]

- Catnip, oregano, and wild marjoram essential oils each exhibited high antioxidant activity in the DPPH, total reducing power, and β-carotene/linoleic acid assays, anticancer activity against human breast cancer, and broad-spectrum antibacterial activity.[1897]

- Research showed that catnip essential oil was toxic to invertebrate cells but had a protective effect on vertebrate cell lines.[1898]

- The nepetalactones CT of catnip essential oil was strongly larvicidal against *Aedes aegypti* mosquitoes.[1899] The active larvicidal constituents in the oil were determined to be 1,8-cineole, camphor, 4aα,7α,7aβ-Nepetalactone, 4aα,7β,7aα-Nepetalactone, and thymol.

- Catnip essential oil provided over 94 percent repellency against the common bed bug (*Cimex lectularius*) at 10% concentration, which increased to 100 percent at 25% concentration.[1900] Its effectiveness waned at seventy-two hours. In addition, the oil completely prevented bed bug infestation of soiled socks at 20% concentration, which exceeded the effectiveness of DEET.

- Beta-cyclodextrin complexes with essential oils are used to improve the physiochemical and pharmacological effects of essential oils. A study compared the tick repellent activity of free catnip essential oil and a catnip cyclodextrin complex. At 5%, the free oil significantly repelled blacklegged ticks (*Ixodes scapularis*), being comparable to DEET in efficacy.[1901] The cyclodextrin complex oil also exhibited significant tick repellence at a lower concentration (1%), and consistently released the oil for six hours.

- Catnip CT 1,8-cineole, summer savory CT carvacrol, and dill aerial parts essential oil demonstrated promising insecticidal activity against the red spider mite (*Tetranychus urticae*) with some minor potential to decrease populations of insect predators (*Amblyseius swirskii*).[1902]

- The nepetalactone CT of catnip essential oil displayed weak antioxidant activity in the FRAP, ABTS, and DPPH assays and strong anticancer activity against small cell lung cancer cells.[1903]

- A special cultivar (cv. CR9) of catnip essential oil rich in (Z,E)-nepetalactone (84.3%) exhibited moderate antibacterial activity against the plant pathogens *Pseudomonas cichorii*, *P. syringae*, and *Xanthomonas perforans*, and strong insect repellent activity against bed bugs (*Cimex lectularius*).[1904] Mixing it with oregano improved the repellent activity.

# CEDARWOOD

Atlas Cedarwood: *Cedrus atlantica* (Endl.) Manetti ex Carrière;
Himalayan/Indian Cedarwood: *C. deodara* (Roxb.) G. Don f.

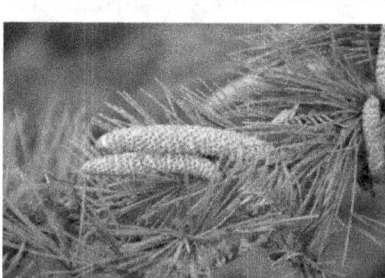

**FAMILY:** Pinaceae
**NOTE:** Base-Middle
**AROMA INTENSITY:** Strong
**AROMA:** Woody, balsamic, rich, earthy
**COMMON EXTRACTION METHOD:** Steam distilled from the wood or needles
**POSSIBLE SUBSTITUTE OILS:** *C. atlantica*—Frankincense, cypress, sandalwood, cistus; *C. deodara*—Sandalwood, frankincense
**SUBCELLULAR LOCALIZATION | EPIGENETIC INFLUENCE:** Currently unknown | Currently unknown
**BLENDS WELL WITH:** Bay laurel, balsam fir, bergamot, blue cypress, blue spruce, carrot seed, cinnamon, copaiba, cypress, myrtle, jasmine, juniper, lemon, neroli, palmarosa, patchouli, petitgrain, pine, rose, rosemary, ravensara, sandalwood, Spanish sage, silver fir, spruce, thyme, tsuga, vetiver, white fir
**RECOMMENDED DILUTION RANGE:** 5.0%–Neat

**PRIMARY CONSTITUENTS:**[1905,1906,1907,1908,1909,1910,1911,1912,1913,1914,1915]

| *Cedrus atlantica*, Wood (Atlas cedarwood) | | *Cedrus deodara*, Wood (Himalayan cedarwood) | |
|---|---|---|---|
| Alpha-Pinene | 14.9%–79.4% | Beta-Himachalene | 12.3%–38.3% |
| Himachalol | 5.3%–66.2% | Alpha-Himachalene | 10.4%–30.8% |
| Beta-Himachalene | 9.9%–40.4% | Himachalol | 12.1%–18.2% |

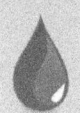

| Cis-Alpha-Atlantone | 5.2%–29.5% | Alpha-Cedrene | 0.0%–15.8% |
| Beta-Pinene | 2.4%–21.4% | Beta-Himachalene Oxide | 0.0%–14.9% |
| Alpha-Himachalene | 4.2%–16.4% | Gamma-Himachalene | 7.0%–12.6% |
| Gamma-Himachalene | 5.1%–11.0% | Gamma-Atlantone | 6.0%–8.6% |

*Cedrus deodara, Needles (Himalayan cedarwood)*

| Alpha-Terpineol | 30.2% |
| Linalool | 24.5% |
| Limonene | 17.0% |
| Anethole | 14.6% |

Note: Heartwood essential oil from *C. atlantica* could be divided into multiple chemotypes including alpha-pinene, himachalenes, himachalol, and atlantones.

**OTHER CONSTITUENTS:** *Cedrus atlantica*—Alpha-terpinene, alpha-cubebene, cis-ocimene, humulene, beta-caryophyllene, delta-himachalene, cadinene, isocaryophyllene, germacrene D, beta-copaene, cymene, 3-carene, verbenol, limonene, ylangene, beta-phellandrene, gamma-amorphane, terpinen-4-ol; *Cedrus deodara*—Himachalene isomer, alpha-bisabolene, sesquiterpenol MW=222, allo-himachalol, epoxy sesquiterpene component, benzocycloheptenone isomer MW=178, alpha-atlantone, atlantone isomer, beta-atlantone, turmerone isomer MW=218, cedrol, ar-himachalene, limona ketone, 5-epi-aristolochene, allo-aromadendra-4(15),10(14)-diene, longifolene

**PREFERRED COMPOSITION FOR CLINICAL USE:**

| Constituent | Atlas, Wood | Himalayan, Wood |
| --- | --- | --- |
| **Beta-Himachalene** | 40%–55% | 32%–45% |
| **Alpha-Himachalene** | 10%–20% | 10%–20% |
| **Gamma-Himachalene** | 7%–15% | 7%–15% |
| **Gamma-Atlantone \<cis- & trans-\>** | 1%–6% | 6%–12% |
| **Alpha-Atlantone \<cis- & trans-\>** | 0.5%–6% | 0.5%–14% |
| **Himachalol \<alpha-, beta-, allo-\>** | 0.1%–5% | 1%–13% |

**REPORTED THERAPEUTIC PROPERTIES:** Antifungal, antiseptic, aphrodisiac, anti-inflammatory, astringent, diuretic, **expectorant**, regenerative, sedating, **encourages a restful night's sleep**, antispasmodic, circulatory stimulant, antirheumatic, calms cough, **reduces the appearance of blemishes**, slows hair loss, **stress management**, grounding, **reduces anxiety**, fear, and insecurity

**CAUTIONS:**
■ None currently known.

**SELECTED EVIDENCE:**
- ☐ Atlas cedarwood prevents the spread of myeloid leukemia cells.[1916]
- ☐ Atlas cedarwood supports a normal inflammatory response by moderately inhibiting the 5-LOX enzyme *in vitro*.[1917]
- ☐ Himalayan cedarwood has demonstrated the ability to reduce stomach acid volume, create a more alkaline stomach environment, reduce stomach lining inflammation, and protect against stomach ulcers in animals.[1918]
- ☐ By balancing mast cell (cells that regulate immune system function through the release of chemical mediators like histamine, interleukins, proteoglycans, and enzymes) activity and inhibiting the production of leukotrienes, Himalayan cedar may reduce inflammation, allergic diseases (asthma, eczema, etc.), autoimmune disorders (rheumatoid arthritis, multiple sclerosis, etc.), and reproductive disorders (endometriosis, decreased sperm motility).[1919]
- ☐ Animal research suggests that oral administration of Himalayan cedarwood helps relieve pain and inflammation.[1920,1921] Himalayan cedarwood is a stronger anti-inflammatory and 5-LOX inhibitor than Atlas cedarwood (strongly inhibits 5-LOX).[1922]
- ☐ Oral administration of Himalayan cedarwood oil may modulate the immune response (both humoral and cell-mediated responses).[1923]
- ☐ A daily scalp massage with thyme, rosemary, lavender, and cedarwood oils in a mixture of carrier oils (jojoba and grapeseed) improved alopecia areata (round patches of hair loss) in 44% of study participants.[1924]

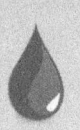
- Inhalation of Atlas cedarwood relieves pain by activating descending pain modulation pathways (opioidergic, serotonergic, noradrenergic, and dopaminergic systems) in mice.[1925]
- Atlas cedarwood essential oil demonstrated 100% efficacy against the *Rhipicephalus microplus* tick even at the lowest concentration tested (1%).[1926]
- Inhalation of Atlas cedarwood essential oil reduced pain possibly by activating the endocannabinoid system in a preclinical model of postoperative pain in mice.[1927] They concluded this because inhibition of the endocannabinoid enzymes that break down cannabinoids prolonged the effects of essential oil inhalation.
- Himalayan cedarwood bark essential oil with a unique composition of 26.3% 2-(tert-Butyl)-6-methyl-3-(2-(trifluoromethyl) benzyl)imidazo[1,2-a]pyridine, 8.0% 9-octadecanoic acid, 5.2% alpha-copaene, and 4.4% 2-(4-Methoxy-2,6-dimethylphenyl)-3-methyl-2Hbenzo[g]indazole was potently cytotoxic to colon cancer cells and reduced cancer cell proliferation *in vitro*.[1928] The researchers discovered that its mechanism of anticancer activity was inhibition of nuclear factor kappa B (NF$_K$B). NF$_K$B plays a role in cancer initiation, development, metastasis, and resistance to treatment because it promotes cancer cell proliferation, suppresses cancer cell destruction (apoptosis), stimulates angiogenesis (the growth of blood vessels to feed the tumor), and causes epithelialmesenchymal transition, which facilitates metastasis.
- Researchers compared the pain-relieving and anti-inflammatory activity of atlas cedarwood essential oil against diclofenac, sodium salicylate, and a control group in mice.[1929] Oral administration of Atlas cedarwood essential oil (three different dosage groups: 12.5, 25, and 50 mg/kg BW) provided excellent pain-relieving effects when compared to diclofenac and excellent anti-inflammatory activity compared to sodium salicylate. Its pain-reliving and anti-inflammatory activity exceeded both diclofenac and sodium salicylate respectively at the 50 mg/kg dose. In addition, the oil demonstrated total safety in the acute toxicity assessment (biochemical markers, organ weight, animal behavior). The study authors concluded that the demonstrated safety and efficacy of Atlas cedarwood essential oil make it a promising replacement for "synthetic and conventional analgesics and anti-inflammatories."

---

# CELERY
## (Celery Seed, Celery Leaf)
*Apium graveolens* L.

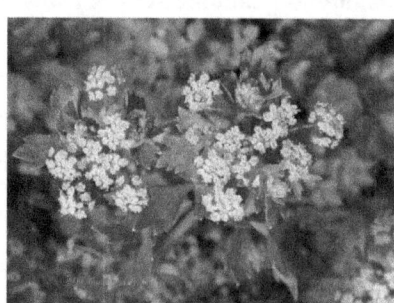

**FAMILY:** Apiaceae (Umbelliferae)
**NOTE:** Middle
**AROMA INTENSITY:** Medium
**AROMA:** Earthy, sweet, slightly spicy, and peppery
**COMMON EXTRACTION METHOD:** Steam distilled from the seeds or leaves and stems
**POSSIBLE SUBSTITUTE OILS:** Helichrysum, grapefruit, dill
**BLENDS WELL WITH:** Black pepper, chamomile (German, Roman), coriander, geranium, ginger, lavender, pine, rose, tea tree
**SUBCELLULAR LOCALIZATION | EPIGENETIC INFLUENCE:** Currently unknown | Currently unknown
**RECOMMENDED DILUTION RANGE:** 3.0%–50.0%; neat for limited conditions

**PRIMARY CONSTITUENTS:**[1930,1931,1932,1933]

| Celery Leaf | | Celery Seed | |
|---|---|---|---|
| Limonene | 16.0%–63.1% | Limonene | 58.4%–63.5% |
| Beta-Selinene | 9.2%–37.4% | Beta-Selinene | 10.1%–27.0% |
| Phellandral | 0.0%–17.2% | Beta-Caryophyllene | 0.9%–5.5% |
| Epiglobulol | 0.0%–7.7% | 3-Butylphthalide | 0.0%–3.5% |
| Beta-Caryophyllene | 3.7%–6.7% | Kessane | 0.0%–3.3% |
| Alpha-Selinene | 1.2%–4.3% | Sedanenolide | 0.0%–2.8% |
| Kessane | 0.0%–3.5% | Alpha-Selinene | 1.3%–2.7% |
| 3-Butylphthalide | 0.0%–3.5% | Beta-Myrcene | 1.2%–2.3% |

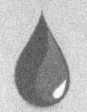

| | |
|---|---|
| Sedanenolide | 0.0%–2.8% |
| Beta-Pinene | 0.0%–2.5% |

Note: Lawrence reports a celery leaf essential oil high in beta-myrcene (33.6%) and limonene (26.3%), but higher beta-myrcene content is typically only found in Chinese celery (*A. graveolens* var. *secalinum* Alef.), which contains limonene (38.5%–58.3%) and beta-myrcene (19.5%–44.6%) as the major constituents.[3459,3460,3461] An odd chemotype obtained from the leaves of celery plants growing in South Korea reports the main constituents as valerophenone (19.9%), 1-dodecanol (16.6%), 9-Octadecen-12-ynoic acid methyl ester (4.9%), ethyl 4,4-D2-n-hexyl ether (4.1%), and 3-(Hydroxymethyl)-1-phenyl-1-heptadecyn-3-ol (3.3%).[3458] Most commercial samples that were identified were celery seed and reported limonene and beta-selinene as major constituents.

**OTHER CONSTITUENTS:** *Celery Seed*—alpha-pinene, sabinene, beta-pinene, L-carvone; *Celery Leaf*—beta-myrcene, alpha-humulene

**PREFERRED COMPOSITION FOR CLINICAL USE:**

| Constituent | Seed |
|---|---|
| **Limonene** | 50%–65% |
| **Beta-Selinene** | 7%–20% |
| **Sedanolide** | 1%–8% |
| **Alpha-Selinene** | 1%–7% |
| **Beta-Caryophyllene** | 0.1%–7% |
| **3-Butylphthalide** | tr–5% |

**REPORTED THERAPEUTIC PROPERTIES:** Antibacterial, antifungal, antispasmodic, antirheumatic, antiarthritic, analgesic, anti-inflammatory, **antioxidant**, decreases uric acid, nervine, aids digestion, **expels excess gas**, reduces appetite, eliminates gallstones and kidney stones, **protects the stomach**, supports respiratory health, balances blood pressure, supports liver function, encourages lymph flow and drainage, relieves painful menstruation, protects the male reproductive system, **diuretic**, insecticide, encourages restful sleep, calming/relaxing, uplifting, aphrodisiac

**CAUTIONS:**

■ Photosensitzing due to the presence of psoralen, bergapten, isoimponellin, and xanthotixin.[1934] Avoid UV rays for at least twelve hours following topical application.

**SELECTED EVIDENCE:**

☐ *In vitro* research reports that celery seed and leaf essential oils act as moderate antioxidants, with the seed demonstrating stronger antioxidant activity.[1935,1936,1937]

☐ Celery seed and leaf essential oil mildly to moderately inhibited several bacterial strains representing gram positive: *Bacillus cereus* and *Staphylococcus aureus*; gram negative: *Escherichia coli*, *Pseudomonas aeruginosa*, and *Salmonella*; in addition to two strains of yeast: *Saccharomyces cerevisiae* and *Candida lipolytica*; and five strains of mold: *Aspergillus niger, Aspergillus flavus, Aspergillus Fumigatus, Aspergillus Parasiticus*, and *Penicillium digitatum*.[1938] The gram-positive bacteria were most susceptible to celery essential oil and the seed essential oil was a stronger inhibitor. Another study reported that celery leaf essential oil demonstrated varying degrees of inhibition against nine bacterial strains: *Ae. hydrophila, Ps. fragi, Ac. denitrificans, S. marcescens, Sh. putrefaciens, Al. faecalis, E. amnigenus, L. innocua*, and *E. gergoviae*; five yeasts: *Y. lipolytica, S. cerevisiae, C. zeylanoides, D. hansenii*, and *Pi. carsonii*; and two molds: *M. racemosus, P. chrysogenum*.[1939] Celery seed essential oil strongly inhibited *E. coli* and moderately inhibited *P. aeruginosa* and *S. aureus*. Another study tested celery essential oil against the same three bacteria, showing similar results but stronger inhibition of all three bacteria when a 700-mg concentration was used.[1940]

☐ Oral administration of celery seed essential oil protected the testes of male rats against damage caused by di-(2-ethylhexyl) phthalate (DEHP), including a reduced production of testosterone.[1941] DEHP is a common phthalate added to plastics to make them flexible and can negatively affect the liver, testes, ovaries, kidneys, thyroid, and blood of animals, with unknown consequences for humans.

- Celery seed essential oil strongly inhibits *C. jejuni* (a gram-negative bacterium that is one of the most common causes of food poisoning in the U.S.).[1942]

- A methanolic (aerial parts) and aqueous extract (seed) of celery—both of which contain volatile oils—prevented gastric lesions caused by a hydrogen chloride-ethanol solution as well as omeprazole (a proton-pump inhibitor used to treat GERD and other conditions caused by excess stomach acid production).[1943] Another study reported that oral administration of 250 to 500 mg/kg celery extract protects against gastric ulcers caused by indomethacin (an NSAID) in rats.[1944] A third study demonstrates that oral administration of celery Co2 aromatic—volatiles extracted by supercritical carbon dioxide—(100, 200, or 300 mg/kg) reduces stomach lesions/ulcers as well as, or better than, the drug omeprazole.[1945]

- Celery leaf essential oil is significantly toxic to the *Aedes aegypti* mosquito, and provides a remarkable 100% repellency protection against bites for 165 minutes, allowing only two bites through 180 minutes.[1946,1947]

- A nanoemulsion of celery seed essential oil exhibited anticancer activity against oral cancer cells by promoting apoptosis and disrupting colony formation.[1948] The oil also inhibited *S. aureus*.

- Celery seed essential oil displayed very weak antioxidant activity in the DPPH assay and inhibited bacteria (*Pseudomonas aeruginosa, Escherichia coli, Bacillus subtilis, Staphylococcus aureus*), yeast (*Candida vini*), and molds (*Aspergillus niger, Penicillium expansum*).[1949]

- Celery leaf essential oil with isocnidilide (40.1%) as the major constituent showed good antimicrobial activity against *C. albicans, B. subtilis, S, aureus, K. pneumoniae,* and *E. coli*, strong anti-inflammatory activity, and weak antioxidant capacity.[1950] Isocnidilide demonstrated high binding activity to COX-2 in a computer model.

# CHASTE TREE
## (Vitex, Monk's Pepper)

*Vitex agnus-castus* L., *Agnus-castus robusta* (Lebas) Carriere, *Agnus-castus vulgaris* Carriere, *Vitex agnus* Stokes

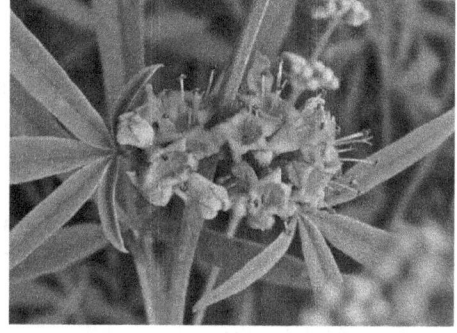

**FAMILY:** Verbenaceae
**NOTE:** Middle
**AROMA INTENSITY:** Medium
**AROMA:** Minty, herbaceous, slightly woody
**COMMON EXTRACTION METHOD:** Steam distilled from the leaves or berries (seeds), or both
**POSSIBLE SUBSTITUTE OILS:** Clary sage, ravensara (sabinene CT), ravintsara (1,8-cineole CT), geranium, bergamot, rose
**BLENDS WELL WITH:** Clary sage, geranium, lavender, melissa, rose
**SUBCELLULAR LOCALIZATION | EPIGENETIC INFLUENCE:** Currently unknown | *Lymphatic/Endocrine*
**RECOMMENDED DILUTION RANGE:** 3%–50%; neat for limited conditions

**PRIMARY CONSTITUENTS:**[1951,1952,1953,1954,1955,1956]

| *Berries (Seeds)* | | *Leaves* | |
|---|---|---|---|
| Sabinene | 3.5%–44.1% | 1,8-Cineole | 15.6%–35.2% |
| Caryophyllene Oxide | 0.0%–24.9% | Sabinene | 2.3%–17.1% |
| Limonene | 0.8%–23.0% | Alpha-Pinene | 1.0%–13.9% |
| Alpha-Pinene | 1.2%–18.9% | Trans-Beta-Farnesene | 0.0%–9.4% |
| 1,8-Cineole | 8.4%–17.5% | Alpha-Terpineol | 1.4%–9.2% |
| Alpha-Terpinyl Acetate | 2.9%–16.8% | Gamma-Elemene | 0.0%–9.1% |
| Beta-Pinene | 0.6%–13.2% | Beta-Selinene | 0.0%–9.0% |
| N-Heptadecane | 0.0%–12.5% | Trans-Beta-Caryophyllene | 1.1%–8.2% |
| N-Hexadecane | 0.0%–12.4% | Terpinen-4-ol | 1.4%–7.8% |
| Trans-Beta-Farnesene | 0.1%–11.7% | Citronellyl Acetate | 0.3%–7.8% |

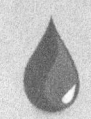

| Beta-Caryophyllene | 2.1%–9.5% | Citronellic Acid | 0.0%–6.6% |
| Bicyclogermacrene | 0.0%–8.4% | Limonene | 0.1%–4.8% |
| Linalool | 0.2%–6.5% | Caryophyllene Oxide | 2.2%–4.8% |
| Spathulenol | 0.1%–4.7% | Beta-Myrcene | 0.0%–3.5% |
| Para-Cymene | 0.0%–4.2% | Sclarene | 0.0%–3.3% |
| Germacrene B | 0.0%–4.2% | Alpha-Terpinyl Acetate | 0.0%–3.1% |
| Terpinen-4-ol | 0.3%–3.3% | Para-Cymene | 0.0%–3.0% |
| N-Tetradecane | 0.0%–3.3% | T-Cadinol | 0.0%–2.7% |
| Manool | 0.0%–3.1% | Alpha-Bisabolol | 0.0%–2.7% |
| T-Cadinol | 0.6%–3.0% | (E)-Nerolidol | 0.0%–2.5% |
| Alpha-Humulene | 0.0%–2.7% | | |
| Alpha-Terpineol | 0.2%–2.6% | | |
| N-Pentadecane | 0.0%–2.6% | | |

**OTHER CONSTITUENTS:** *Berries (seeds)*—Beta-eudesmol, beta-myrcene, sclarene, trans-alpha-bergamotene, n-octadecane, germacrene D, manool oxide, abietatriene, beta-gurjunene, gamma-terpinene, camphor, beta-farnesyl acetate, alpha-thujene, alpha-terpinene, 3-octanone, trans-sabinene-hydrate, cis-sabinene-hydrate, torreyol, citronellyl acetate, ledol, delta-terpineol; *Leaves*—beta-pinene, (Z)-beta-ocimene, (E,Z)-geranyl linalool, alloaromadendrene, trans-isovalencenol, spathulenol, (E)-dihydroterpineol, gamma-terpinene, alpha-gurjunene, guaiol, manool, alpha-guaiene, (3E)-cembrene A, dodecane, thymol, alpha-thujene, linalool, delta-terpineol, beta-citronellol, cis-beta-farnesene, oxacyclotridec-10-en-2-one

**PREFERRED COMPOSITION FOR CLINICAL USE:**

| Constituent | Berries | Leaves | Both |
| --- | --- | --- | --- |
| Sabinene | 15%–32% | 10%–32% | 17%–35% |
| Alpha-Pinene | 5%–15% | 5%–20% | 2%–12% |
| Limonene | 5%–15% | 1%–5% | 1.5%–10% |
| 1,8-Cineole | 5%–15% | 20%–35% | 18%–25% |
| (E)-Beta-Farnesene | 1%–12% | 4%–11% | 3%–9% |
| Beta-Caryophyllene | 2%–10% | 3%–10% | 3%–8% |
| Alpha-Terpinyl Acetate | 1%–10% | 0%–3% | tr–6% |
| Beta-Pinene | 0.5%–8% | 0.5%–3% | 1%–6% |
| Linalool | 0.1%–5% | – | tr–3% |
| Spathulenol | 0.1%–5% | 0.1%–3% | 0.1%–1% |
| Terpinen-4-ol | 0.1%–5% | 1.5%–5% | 1%–6% |
| T-Cadinol | 0.1%–3% | – | 0%–0.5% |
| Alpha-Terpineol | 0.1%–3% | 0.1%–3% | 0.5%–3% |
| Terpinene (Alpha + Gamma) | – | 1%–5% | 1%–5% |
| Caryophyllene Oxide | – | 0.1%–5% | tr–0.5% |
| Citronellyl Acetate | – | 0.1%–5% | – |
| Beta-Myrcene | – | 0%–3% | 1%–3% |
| Para-Cymene | – | 0%–3% | 0.1%–3% |
| Bicyclogermacrene | – | – | 1%–5% |
| Phellandrene < alpha- + beta-> | – | – | 0.1%–4% |

**REPORTED THERAPEUTIC PROPERTIES: Encourages female hormone balance (particularly increasing progesterone), eases premenstrual symptoms,** balances menstruation, eases menopausal symptoms, reduces headache, relieves hair loss, decongestant, reduces libido, antibacterial, antispasmodic, analgesic (pain relief), diuretic, reduces fever, **regulates pituitary function,** reduces enlarged prostate caused by hormone imbalance, **supports endocrine (particularly thyroid) function,** nervine, sedating, relaxing, antidepressant, anaphrodisiac

CAUTIONS:

■ Avoid during pregnancy and lactation. Chaste tree oil may be a uterine stimulant, promote menstrual bleeding, and effect progesterone-estrogen balance.[1957,1958,1959] Oral use of chaste tree may suppress prolactin, the hormone that stimulates breast development and milk production in women, based on studies using the extract.[1960] However, another study found that constituents within chaste tree extract positively affects lactation.[1961]

■ Avoid with hormone replacement therapy medications. Reports of increased menopausal symptoms and breakthrough bleeding have been reported when using chaste tree oil with progesterone drug therapies.[1962,1963] Some aromatherapy texts contraindicate chaste tree with contraceptives, but one study did not find any adverse interactions between chaste tree and contraceptives among thirteen women using both concomitantly.[1964]

■ Avoid with epilepsy and Parkinson's disease (leaf oil) due to 1,8-cineole content. May exacerbate or cause seizures or convulsions when inhaled, applied topically, or ingested based on 1,8-cineole content.[1965,1966,1967,1968,1969,1970]

■ May interfere with pentobarbital and other barbiturates (medications for anxiety and insomnia) based on 1,8-cineole content (leaf oil).[1971,1972]

■ May interact with aspirin, blood pressure, antiplatelet, and anticoagulant medications, and increase the risk of bleeding among people with bleeding disorders due to caryophyllene oxide content.[1973]

■ May interact with antipsychotic (drugs used to treat psychosis, schizophrenia, and bipolar disorder that reduce or increase the effect of neurotransmitters—particularly dopamine—in the brain) and dopamine agonist drugs (pramipexole, ropinirole, rotigotine, and apomorphine: drugs used to treat Parkinson's disease that mimic the effect of dopamine without having to be converted to it) due to the dopaminergic (a substance that increases dopamine-related activity in the brain) activity of chaste tree extracts.[1974,1975] However, this activity is attributed to the diterpenes found in chaste tree extracts not the essential oil.

■ May weakly interfere with the enzymes responsible for metabolizing medications (NSAIDs, proton-pump inhibitors, acetaminophen, antiepileptics, immune modulators, blood-sugar medications, blood pressure medications, antidepressants, antipsychotics, diabetic medications, antihistamines, antibiotics, and anesthetics) based on 1,8-cineole and alpha-bisabolol content (leaf oil).[1976,1977]

SELECTED EVIDENCE:

☐ Animal research suggests that chaste tree oil (injection of 60 mg/kg for three weeks) regulates the hypothalamic-pituitary-thyroid axis, causing functional changes to the thyroid and pituitary glands and increasing thyroid stimulating hormone (TSH) and total thyroxine and triiodothyronine (TH) levels, and decreased adrenocorticotrophic hormone (ACTH). Functional changes to the pituitary included increased pituitary thyrotrophs (endocrine cells in the anterior pituitary that produce TSH) and decreased pituitary corticotrophs (basophilic cells that produce melanocyte-stimulating hormone, TSH, ACTH, and lipotropin) in middle-aged male rats.[1978] Functional changes to the thyroid included increased follicular epithelium (thyroid cells that produce the thyroid hormones thyroxine (T4) and triiodothyronine (T3), reduced luminal colloid size (part of the thyroid gland that contains thyroglobulin from which thyroid hormone is created), and increased expression of sodium-iodide symporter-immunopositivity (a protein involved in the uptake of iodide by follicular cells of the thyroid gland, which is the first step in the creation of thyroid hormone) in the basolateral epithelial membrane.

☐ Injection of 60 mg/kg of chaste tree essential oil once per day for three weeks increased thyroid C cells (parafollicular cells) and serum calcitonin levels, and decreased serum calcium (8%) and osteocalcin (31%) levels in middle-aged male rats.[1979] Thyroid C cells secrete calcitonin, which plays a significant role in calcium homeostasis. The results of this study suggest that vitex essential oil influences thyroid function and subsequently balances bone remodeling to possibly reduce the risk of osteoporosis.

☐ In vitro research concluded that chaste tree oil effectively inhibits S. enteritidis, P. aeruginosa, E. coli, S. aureus, and B. subtilis.[1980]

☐ Vitex agnus-castus extract (not essential oil, although the extract does contain some volatile constituents found in the essential oil) is approved by the German Commission E for the treatment of irregular menstruation, premenstrual symptoms, and premenstrual breast tenderness.[1981]

☐ Chaste tree berry (Vitex agnus-castus) essential oil may help reduce pain by affecting the opioid system according to research.[1982]

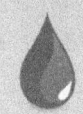

- ☐ Chaste tree may reduce symptoms of menopause in some women, but almost 25% of women who participated in the study also reported that it made symptoms worse.[1983,1984]
- ☐ Chaste tree berry (leaves) effectively inhibited a wide variety of *Candida* species, causing the study authors to conclude that it "may represent alternative therapies for candidiasis" because it is cheaper and has fewer side effects than drugs used for the same purpose.[1985]
- ☐ Chaste tree berry and leaf oil is toxic to the plant-feeding mite (*Tetranychus urticae*).[1986] Interestingly, the leaf oil is more toxic through fumigation, but the fruit oil is more toxic through residual contact.
- ☐ *In vitro* research demonstrates that chaste tree leaf essential oil inhibits the bacteria associated with cavities formation (*Streptococcus mutans*, S. *mitis*, and *Lactobacillus casei*).[1987]
- ☐ The 1,8-cineole CT of chaste tree leaf essential oil displayed anticancer activity against pro-myelocytic leukemia, breast, lung, and cervical cancer cells and was moderately larvicidal to the *Aedes aegypti* mosquito. Pro-myelocytic leukemia were the most sensitive to the oil.
- ☐ Chaste tree essential oil demonstrated strong antioxidant activity and the ability to trigger apoptosis (caspase-dependent) in multidrug-resistant lung cancer cells *in vitro*.[1988]
- ☐ Chaste tree essential oil was insecticidal to the Mexican bean weevil (*Zabrotes subfasciatus*), exhibiting 100 percent mortality at a concentration of 0.004 mcL/L air after twenty-four hours of exposure.[1989]
- ☐ *In vitro* research demonstrated that chaste tree essential oil inhibited S. *abony*, S. *aureus*, and B. *subtilis*, but gram-negative bacteria (*E. coli*, P. *aeruginosa*) were resistant to the oil.[1990]

# CHINESE CEDARWOOD
## (Mourning Cypress, Chinese Weeping Cypress)
*Cupressus funebris* Endl., *Chamaecyparis funebris* (Endl.) Franco

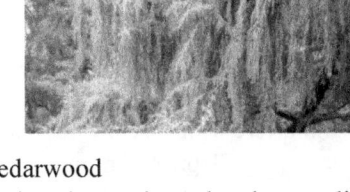

**FAMILY:** Cupressaceae
**NOTE:** Base
**AROMA INTENSITY:** Mild
**AROMA:** Woody, sweet, earthy
**COMMON EXTRACTION METHOD:** Steam distilled from the wood
**POSSIBLE SUBSTITUTE OILS:** Texas cedarwood, Virginia cedarwood, cedarwood
**BLENDS WELL WITH:** Agarwood, bergamot, cedarwood, cypress, juniper berry, lavender, lemon, lime, orange, patchouli, rose, sandalwood, tangerine, Texas cedarwood, vetiver, Virginia cedarwood
**SUBCELLULAR LOCALIZATION | EPIGENETIC INFLUENCE:** Currently unknown | Currently unknown
**RECOMMENDED DILUTION RANGE:** 3%–50%; neat for limited conditions

**PRIMARY CONSTITUENTS:**[1991,1992,1993,1994]

| | |
|---|---|
| Cedrol | 0.0%–54.6% |
| Alpha-Cedrene | 0.7%–44.2% |
| Iso-Alpha-Cedrene | 0.0%–32.0% |
| Thujopsene | 0.0%–37.4% |
| Beta-Cedrene | 0.0%–11.5% |
| Cuparene | 0.0%–10.2% |
| Manool | 0.0%–7.6% |
| Beta-Himachalene | 0.0%–6.4% |
| Cedrenol | 0.0%–6.1% |
| Abietadiene | 0.0%–5.3% |
| Alpha-Alaskene | 0.0%–4.8% |
| Abienol | 0.0%–4.5% |
| Longifolene | 0.0%–4.2% |
| Trans-Calamenene | 0.0%–3.9% |
| Beta-Funebrene | 0.0%–3.4% |

**OTHER CONSTITUENTS:** Alpha-pinene, limonene, terpinolene, methyl chavicol (< 2.4%), 2-epi-alpha-funebrene, alpha-duprezianene, beta-elemene, alpha-chamipinene, longifolene, prezizaene, (E)-beta-farnesene, alpha-acoradiene, beta-acoradiene, alpha-neocallitropscene, beta-chamigrene isomer, beta-chamigrene, gamma-muurolene, ar-curcumene, widdra-2,4(14)-diene, beta-selinene, beta-alaskene, pseudowiddrene, bicyclogermacrene, alpha-chamigrene, germacrene A, delta-cadinene, (E)-gamma-bisabolene, gamma-cuparenene, alpha-cadinene, delta-cuparenene, alpha-calacorene, elemon, eremophilla ketone, caryolan-8-ol, naphthalene. Thujopsan-2alpha-ol, allo-cedrol, widdrol, beta-biotine, beta-biotol, junenol, epi-cedrol, 2-epi-alpha-cedren-3-one, alpha-acorenol isomer, gamma-eudesmol, alpha-acorenol, epi-alpha-muurolol, beta-eudesmol, alpha-eudesmol, alpha-cadinol, 3-thujopsanone, epi-alpha-bisabolol, junicedranol, mayurone, cedryl acetate, cryptomeridol, 11-acetoxyeudesman-4alpha-ol, nootkatin, abietatriene, sclareol (< 0.8%), sandaracopimarinol, torulosol

**PREFERRED COMPOSITION FOR CLINICAL USE:**

| *Constituent* | |
|---|---|
| **Thujopsene** | 18%–39% |
| **Alpha-Cedrene** | 12%–30% |
| **Cedrol** | 10%–22% |
| **Beta-Cedrene** | 4%–12% |
| **Cuparene** | 1%–4% |
| **Widdrol** | 0.1%–3% |
| **Beta-Funebrene** | 0%–3% |

**REPORTED THERAPEUTIC PROPERTIES:** Astringent, relieves chronic skin conditions, **reduces the appearance of acne, wrinkles, and blemishes**, antiseptic, **wound healing**, anti-inflammatory, antiarthritic, antirheumatic, aids immune function, balances menstruation, stops excess bleeding, supports respiratory function, expels excess mucus, insect repellent, insecticide, **encourages restful sleep**, promotes tranquility and peace, combats negative thoughts and emotions, stress management

**CAUTIONS:**

■ May weakly interfere with the enzymes responsible for metabolizing medications (NSAIDs, proton-pump inhibitors, acetaminophen, antiepileptics, immune modulators, blood-sugar medications, blood pressure medications, antidepressants, antipsychotics, diabetic medications, antihistamines, antibiotics, and anesthetics) due to thujopsene, cedrol, and beta-cedrene content.[1995]

**SELECTED EVIDENCE:**

☐ Chinese cedarwood essential oil repels and kills the blacklegged tick (*Amblyomma americanum*), but did not repel the *Ae. aegypti* mosquito.[1996,1997] It also kills and repels the *Liposcelis bostrychophila* booklouse.[4722]

☐ *In vitro* research demonstrated that Chinese cedarwood leaf essential oil inhibited gram-positive (*S. aureus, B. subtilis*) and gram-negative (*E. coli, P. aeruginosa*) bacteria, and fungi (*A. niger, A. flavus, A. fumigatus, C. albicans*).[1998]

*Did you know?*

Essential oils are not actually oils, at least in the sense that they don't contain fatty acids like olive or coconut oil. Instead, essential oils are aromatic and volatile phytoconstituents like terpenes, esters, phenols, ketones, and others. Simple essential oils contain about a dozen of these constituents, while complex essential oils can contain hundreds constituents.

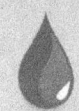

# CHINESE RED PINE
## (Masson's Pine, Horsetail Pine)

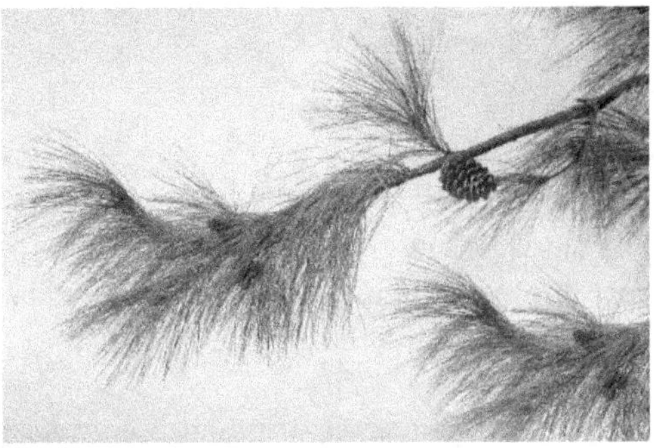

*Pinus massoniana* Lamb.

**FAMILY:** Pinaceae
**NOTE:** Top
**AROMA INTENSITY:** Strong
**AROMA:** Crisp, piney, fresh, resinous
**COMMON EXTRACTION METHOD:** Steam distilled from needles or twigs; may also be distilled from the gum resin
**POSSIBLE SUBSTITUTE OILS:** Pine, juniper berry, white pine, red pine, Maritime pine
**BLENDS WELL WITH:** Agarwood, bergamot, cajeput, camphor, cedarwood, clary sage, coriander, Douglas fir, Engelmann spruce, eucalyptus, frankincense, galbanum, grapefruit, juniper, lavender, lemon, lime, marjoram, tea tree, neroli, niaouli, peppermint, ravensara, ravintsara, rosemary, Spanish sage, spikenard, thyme, Siberian fir, silver fir, white fir, white pine, white spruce
**SUBCELLULAR LOCALIZATION | EPIGENETIC INFLUENCE:** Currently unknown | Currently unknown
**RECOMMENDED DILUTION RANGE:** 3%–50%; neat for limited conditions

**PRIMARY CONSTITUENTS:**[1999,2000,2001]

| *Needles* | | *Twigs* | |
|---|---|---|---|
| Alpha-Pinene | 8.2%–45.5% | Alpha-Pinene | 28.1%–39.1% |
| Beta-Caryophyllene | 0.7%–18.5% | Beta-Pinene | 20.8%–24.3% |
| Beta-Pinene | 3.0%–15.4% | Beta-Phellandrene | 14.9%–25.2% |
| Germacrene D | 0.0%–9.8% | Bornyl Acetate | 8.4%–8.7% |
| Bornyl Acetate | 0.9%–7.8% | Limonene | 1.8%–5.3% |
| 1-Methyl-5-(1-methylethenyl)- | | Alpha-Terpineol | 0.1%–3.3% |
|   Cyclohexene | 0.0%–6.0% | | |
| Limonene | 0.0%–4.7% | | |
| Aristolochene | 0.0%–3.7% | | |
| Alpha-Guaiene | 0.0%–3.7% | | |
| Alpha-Humulene | 1.7%–3.4% | | |
| Beta-Elemene | 0.0%–3.4% | | |
| Alpha-Terpineol | 0.0%–3.3% | | |

Note: The needle essential oil could be divided into at least two distinct chemotypes, one with low alpha-pinene and high beta-caryophyllene content and one with higher alpha-pinene and beta-pinene content. The latter was more commonly reported in the literature.

**OTHER CONSTITUENTS:** *Leaves*—Alpha-thujene, camphene, alpha-terpinolene, santene, acetic acid linalool ester, beta-phellandrene, myrcene, gamma-terpinene, aromadendrene, alpha-amorphene, phenylethyl isovalerate, alpha-selinene, beta-cadinene, cadina-1,4-diene, para-cymene, terpinen-4-ol, myrtenal, 4-isopropyl cyclohexanone, alpha-muurolene, delta-cadinene, alpha-cadinene, alpha-calacorene, caryophyllene oxide, globulol, beta-oplopenone, alpha-eudesmol, beta-bisabolol, pentadecanal, palustradiene, 1-ethyl-1-methyl-2,4-bis(1-methylethyl)-cyclohexane, beta-farnesene, longifolene, gamma-elemene, cadinene, T-muurolol, T-cadinol; *Twigs*—Santene, camphene, para-cymene, myrtenal

**PREFERRED COMPOSITION FOR CLINICAL USE:**

| Constituent | Needles |
|---|---|
| **Alpha-Pinene** | 40%–50% |
| **Beta-Pinene** | 10%–18% |
| **Beta-Caryophyllene** | 0.5%–12% |

| Bornyl Acetate | 0.5%–8% |
|---|---|
| Alpha-Humulene | 1%–4% |
| Camphene | 1%–4% |

**REPORTED THERAPEUTIC PROPERTIES: Antiseptic**, analgesic, anti-inflammatory, **antiarthritic**, antirheumatic, antineuralgic, nervine, antioxidant, supports normal respiratory function, expels excess mucus, eases cough, relieves sore throat, aids immune function, grounding, stress management

**CAUTIONS:**

■ *Twigs*: May interact with anticholinergic (drugs used for asthma, incontinence, gastrointestinal cramps, muscular spasms, depression, and sleep disorders) and cholinergic medications (drugs used to reduce urinary retention, diagnose myasthenia gravis, and for glaucoma) based on AChE inhibitory activity of beta-phellandrene.[2002]

**SELECTED EVIDENCE:**

☐ Chinese red pine leaf essential oil demonstrated moderate antioxidant activity.[2003]

# CILANTRO
## (Coriander Leaf, Santo, Chinese Parsley)

*Coriandrum sativum* L.

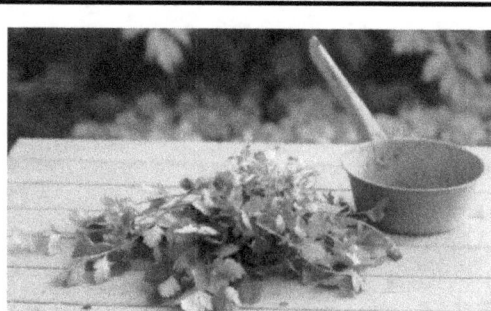

**FAMILY:** Apiaceae
**NOTE:** Top
**AROMA INTENSITY:** Medium
**AROMA:** Fresh, sweet, slightly herbaceous, pleasantly pungent
**COMMON EXTRACTION METHOD:** Steam distilled from the leaves
**POSSIBLE SUBSTITUTE OILS:** Peppermint, fennel, coriander
**BLENDS WELL WITH:** Balsam fir, basil, bergamot, black pepper, carrot, cassia, chamomile (German, Roman), cinnamon, galbanum, ginger, grapefruit, lemon, lime, marjoram, orange, oregano, tangerine
**SUBCELLULAR LOCALIZATION | EPIGENETIC INFLUENCE:** Currently unknown | Currently unknown
**RECOMMENDED DILUTION RANGE:** 5%–50%; neat for limited conditions

**PRIMARY CONSTITUENTS:**[2004,2005]

| | |
|---|---|
| (E)-2-Decen-1-ol | 14.2%–26.0% |
| n-Decanol (1-Decanol) | 13.6%–19.6% |
| (E)-2-Decenal | 9.1%–15.9% |
| Decanal | 6.6%–14.3% |
| (E)-2-Tetradecenal | 0.0%–7.0% |
| (E)-2-Tridecenal | 0.4%–6.8% |
| (E)-2-Dodecenal | 5.4%–6.2% |
| (E)-2-Dodecenol | 0.0%–4.6% |
| Dodecanal | 3.0%–4.4% |

**OTHER CONSTITUENTS:** 2-Undecenal, nonane, (E)-2-hexen-1-ol, (E)-2-undecen-1-ol, (E)-2-tetradecene-pl, (Z)-3-hexen-1-ol, octanal, undecanal, tetradecanal, (E)-2-undecenal, (E)-2-pentadecenal, para-cymene, 1,8-cineole (eucalyptol), nonanal, tridecanal, undecanol

**PREFERRED COMPOSITION FOR CLINICAL USE:**

| Constituent | | Linalool Rich* |
|---|---|---|
| (E)-2-Decen-1-ol | 15%–30% | 5%–25% |
| n-Decanol | 10%–20% | 1%–8% |
| (E)-2-Decenal | 8%–17% | 10%–38% |

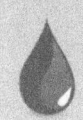

| Decanal | 7%–15% | 3%–10% |
|---|---|---|
| (E)-2-Dodecenal | 5%–10% | 2%–15% |
| (E)-2-Tetradecenal | 1%–7% | 0.1%–5% |
| (E)-2-Tridecenal | 1%–7% | tr–2% |
| Dodecanal | 2%–5% | 2%–8% |
| (E)-2-Dodecenol | 0%–5% | 0.1%–3% |
| Linalool | < 1% | 15%–45% |
| Alpha-Pinene | – | 1%–5% |

\* Commercial samples report linalool as the main component of cilantro essential oil, which is conflicting with published analyses in the literature. These commercial samples may be codistillations of seeds and leaves or distillations of the aerial parts after they have gone to seed.

**REPORTED THERAPEUTIC PROPERTIES:** Analgesic (pain relief), antioxidant, antispasmodic, antibacterial, **aids digestion**, **appetite stimulant**, expels excess gas, antifungal, **aids detoxification**, **antiarthritic**, antirheumatic, antispasmodic, reduces headache (migraine), nervine (calms or soothes nerves) reduces diarrhea, supports normal blood sugar levels, soothes skin irritation, stimulating, revitalizing, stress management, stimulates courage, combats anger, reduces anxiety

**CAUTIONS:**
■ None currently known.

**SELECTED EVIDENCE:**
☐ Cilantro essential oil actively inhibits *Candida* species without harming healthy human cells.[2006]
☐ A review article concluded that cilantro essential oil is a promising antibacterial agent against bacteria that cause cavities.[2007]
☐ Cilantro essential oil is significantly toxic to the larvae of Aedes aegypti (the mosquito that can carry and transmit Dengue fever, yellow fever, and other diseases).[2008]
☐ A preclinical model of chronic skin inflammation demonstrates that cilantro essential oil inhibits protein molecules involved in inflammation, immune responses, and tissue remodeling, which suggests that it reduces skin inflammation and promotes wound healing.[2009]
☐ *In vitro* examination of sixty essential oils demonstrated that sandalwood (Indian, Australian, and Hawaiian), melissa, lemongrass (*C. flexuosus*), cilantro, cassia, cinnamon, patchouli, and vetiver essential oils possess remarkable anticancer (two breast cancer cells) and antifungal (*Aspergillus niger, Candida albicans,* and *Cryptococcus neoformans*) activities.[2010]
☐ Cilantro essential oil demonstrated excellent anti-inflammatory activity, comparable to ibuprofen in the egg albumin assay.[2011] In addition, the oil displayed low antioxidant capacity in the DPPH and ferric chloride scavenging assays but excellent antimicrobial activity, inhibiting *S. subtilis, K. pneumoniae, C. albicans,* and *S, aureus,* but being inactive against *E. coli.*
☐ Laboratory research demonstrated that cilantro CT linalool essential oil possesses significant anti-inflammatory activity and promising antioxidant activity.[2012]

## CINNAMON BARK OR LEAF
### (Ceylon Cinnamon, True Cinnamon)

*Cinnamomum verum* J. Presl, *C. zeylanicum* Garcin ex Blume

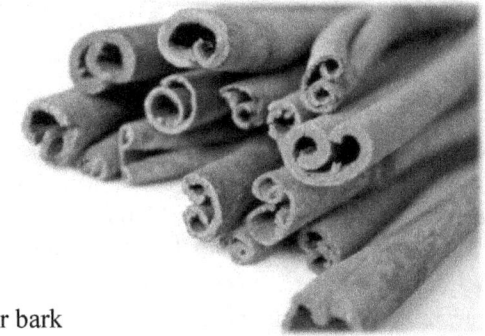

**FAMILY:** Lauraceae
**NOTE:** Middle
**AROMA INTENSITY:** Strong
**AROMA:** Spicy, warm
**COMMON EXTRACTION METHOD:** Steam distilled from the dried inner bark
**POSSIBLE SUBSTITUTE OILS:** Cassia

**BLENDS WELL WITH:** Black pepper, carrot seed, clove, coriander, eucalyptus, geranium, juniper, lavender, pine, tea tree, nutmeg, orange, patchouli, rosemary, Spanish sage, turmeric, vetiver

**SUBCELLULAR LOCALIZATION | EPIGENETIC INFLUENCE:** Actin Cytoskeleton | Circulatory/Respiratory

**RECOMMENDED DILUTION RANGE:** 1.5%–20%

**PRIMARY CONSTITUENTS:**[2013,2014,2015,2016,2017,2018]

| *Cinnamon Bark* | | *Cinnamon Leaves* | |
|---|---|---|---|
| (E)-Cinnamaldehyde | 50.5%–91.0% | Eugenol | 74.9%–81.7% |
| Benzyl Benzoate | 0.3%–15.1% | Linalool | 2.5%–8.5% |
| Beta-Caryophyllene | 0.7%–10.4% | Beta-Caryophyllene | 1.7%–4.1% |
| Eugenol | 1.9%–10.0% | Benzyl Benzoate | 3.0%–4.0% |
| Benzaldehyde | 0.6%–9.9% | Piperitone | 0.0%–3.3% |
| Cinnamyl Acetate | 0.1%–8.8% | (E)-Cinnamaldehyde | 0.8%–2.7% |
| Methyl Isoeugenol | 0.0%–7.8% | | |
| Linalool | 0.0%–6.3% | | |
| 1,8-Cineole | 0.0%–4.6% | | |

**OTHER CONSTITUENTS:** *Cinnamon Bark*—camphene, alpha-phellandrene, para-cymene, limonene, benzyl alcohol, (Z)-cinnamaldehyde, benzenepropanol, carvone, linalyl acetate; *Cinnamon Leaves*—alpha-pinene, myrcene, alpha-terpinene, para-cymene, terpinolene, 1,8-cineole, (Z)-cinnamyl acetate, alpha-humulene

**PREFERRED COMPOSITION FOR CLINICAL USE:**

| Constituent | Bark | Leaf |
|---|---|---|
| **(E)-Cinnamaldehyde** | 55%–80% | 0.5%–3% |
| **Eugenol** | 2%–15% | 70%–85% |
| **Benzyl Benzoate** | 0.01%–10% | 1%–7% |
| **Beta-Caryophyllene** | 1%–8% | 1%–7% |
| **(E)-Cinnamyl Acetate** | 1%–8% | 0.5%–5% |
| **Linalool** | 1%–6% | – |
| **Benzaldehyde** | tr–5% | – |
| **1,8-Cineole** | 0%–3% | – |
| **Eugenyl Acetate** | – | 0.5%–8% |
| **Safrole** | – | 0.5%–5% |
| **Alpha-Pinene** | – | 0.5%–3% |
| **Alpha-Phellandrene** | – | 0.5%–3% |

**REPORTED THERAPEUTIC PROPERTIES:** Aids brain function, **supports balanced blood-sugar levels**, purifies the blood, aids circulation, analgesic (pain relief), **antiviral**, antiseptic, antibacterial, **anti-infectious, antimicrobial, antiparasitic, aids digestion**, relieves PMS and cramps, reduces bruises, helps remove warts, enhances metabolism, relieves sore throat, helps with morale and courage, grounding, uplifting

**CAUTIONS:**

*Cinnamon Bark*:

■ Avoid during pregnancy and lactation. Several studies have tested the major constituents of cinnamon and cassia essential oils with pregnant animals, and the results have been inconsistent. Therefore, it is advised to avoid essential oils with significant quantities of cinnamaldehyde during pregnancy until further research is conclusive.[2019,2020,2021]

■ May interact with aspirin, blood pressure, antiplatelet, and anticoagulant medications, and increase the risk of bleeding among people with bleeding disorders.[2022,2023,2024]

■ May interfere with enzymes responsible for metabolizing medications (NSAIDs, proton-pump inhibitors, acetaminophen, antiepileptics, immune modulators, blood-sugar medications, blood pressure medications, antidepressants, antipsychotics, diabetic medications, antihistamines, antibiotics, and anesthetics).[2025,2026,2027]

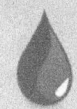

■ May interact with diabetes medications and cause low blood-sugar levels.[2028,2029,2030]

■ May interact with antibiotics and possibly enhance their effects.[2031,2032]

■ May irritate mucous membranes (eyes, mouth, nasal passages, vagina, rectum).[2033]

■ Topical application (significant dilution strongly encouraged). Cinnamon and cassia are very high in cinnamaldehyde, which is very irritating to the skin and prone to cause severe reactions.[2034]

*Cinnamon Leaves*:

■ Caution with pregnancy and lactation. Animal studies suggest that large doses of clove (also with significant eugenol) may negatively impact embryonic development and encourage fetal cell death.[2035,2036] Another animal study did not detect any negative influence of clove oil.[2037] Eugenol is considered strongly toxic to embryos according to animal studies.[2038] Based on these studies it is best to limit clove oil during pregnancy and lactation.

■ May interact with aspirin, blood pressure, antiplatelet, and anticoagulant medications, and increase the risk of bleeding among people with bleeding disorders.[2039,2040,2041,2042]

■ May interact with MAOI antidepressants. Animal research suggests that eugenol produces antidepressant effects via the monoamine oxidase pathway, which may cause interactions with antidepressants that also interact with this pathway.[2043]

■ May interfere with enzymes responsible for metabolizing medications (NSAIDs, proton-pump inhibitors, acetaminophen, antiepileptics, immune modulators, blood-sugar medications, blood pressure medications, antidepressants, antipsychotics, diabetic medications, antihistamines, antibiotics, and anesthetics) based on eugenol content.[2044]

■ May interact with anticholinergic (drugs used for asthma, incontinence, gastrointestinal cramps, muscular spasms, depression, and sleep disorders) and cholinergic medications (drugs used to reduce urinary retention, diagnose myasthenia gravis, and for glaucoma) based on AChE inhibitory activity of eugenol.[2045]

■ May interact with antibiotics and possibly enhance their effects due to eugenol content.[2046]

■ May irritate mucous membranes (eyes, mouth, nasal passages, vagina, rectum).[2047,2048]

**SELECTED EVIDENCE:**

▫ Cinnamaldehyde is a strong inhibitor of multidrug-resistant bacteria, molds, and dermatophytes (fungi that require keratin for growth and infect the skin, hair, and nails).[2049,2050] Cinnamon bark is a potent inhibitor of both gram-positive and gram-negative bacterium that belong to the *Staphylococcus, Enterococcus, Enterobacter,* and *Acinetobacter* families, and the fungi *Candida albicans*.[2051,2052,2053] It also inhibits and prevents the formation of mycotoxins by *Aspergillus* species.[2054] Cinnamon bark essential oil inhibited planktonic and biofilm *E. faecalis* without harming fibroblasts (cells in connective tissue that produce collagen), which caused the researchers to conclude it was a viable antimicrobial agent for use during root canal treatments.[2055] The gaseous phase of cinnamon bark essential oil inhibited *E. coli*.[2056] Cinnamon essential oil strongly inhibited *Pseudomonas aeruginosa, Staphylococcus aureus, Escherichia coli,* and four yeasts: *Torulopsis utilis, Schizosaccharomyces pombe, Candida albicans,* and *Saccharomyces cerevisiae*.[2057]

▫ Researchers concluded that cinnamon oil inhibited several *Candida* species and bacteria known to cause hospital-acquired infections according to *in vitro* research.[2058]

▫ Cinnamon bark decreases blood glucose levels and stimulates pancreas beta-cells to produce insulin in animals.[2059] Other research concluded that cinnamon bark essential oil improves glucose tolerance, stimulates pancreas function, lowers blood-sugar levels, reduces triglycerides, and increases HDL cholesterol.[2060,2061]

▫ Cinnamon bark essential oil effectively killed prostate, head and neck, lung, and breast cancer cells *in vitro*.[2062,2063]

▫ Inhalation of cinnamaldehyde significantly increased survivability among mice infected with influenza A virus.[2064] Cinnamaldehyde also inhibited virus growth *in vitro*.

▫ The main constituent in cinnamon bark, cinnamaldehyde, may reduce the production of melanin and whiten the skin.[2065]

▫ Cinnamon bark may increase sperm motility and quality according to animal research.[2066] Another study concluded that cinnamon essential oil significantly protects against taxanes-induced male reproductive system damage (organ weight, testosterone levels, sperm quality, antioxidant balance, germ cell numbers, sperm DNA and quality, and testicular lesions) in rats.[2067]

▫ A foot bath (107∘ F water) with salts and either oregano, thyme, cinnamon bark, lemongrass, clove, palmarosa, peppermint, lavender, or geranium significantly reduced fungi associated with athlete's foot *in vitro*.[2068]

- Cinnamon oil increased the effectiveness of gentamicin (an antibiotic drug) against multi-drug-resistant *Acinetobacter* species *in vitro*.[2069]

- Animal research suggests that cinnamon bark oil may protect the kidneys from damage associated with diabetes and uncontrolled high blood sugar.[2070]

- Cinnamon bark essential oil enhances the effectiveness of clindamycin (an antibiotic used to treat serious bacterial infections) against *C. difficile* when used together.[2071]

- *In vitro* research suggests that cinnamon oil, whether alone or in combination with peppermint, marjoram, lemon, and nutmeg, strongly inhibits the bacterium *Brucella abortus*, which is a cause of brucellosis (a disease spread from animals to people that causes fever, joint pain, muscle aches, and fatigue).[2072]

- The vapor of cinnamon bark oil inhibited both penicillin-susceptible and penicillin-resistant respiratory pathogens (*H. influenzae, S. pneumoniae, S. pyogenes,* and *S. aureus*) *in vitro*.[2073]

- Of 21 essential oils tested, cinnamon was the most effective inhibitor of *S. aureus, B. subtilis, K. pneumoniae, P. vulgaris, P. aeruginosa,* and *E. coli*.[2074] Cinnamon bark essential oil has the potential to increase the susceptibility of multi-drug-resistant *E. coli* to piperacillin by irreversibly damaging the bacteria's membrane and reducing its surface charge.[2075] Another study reported that cinnamon essential oil effectively inhibited MRSA and the addition of liposomes improves its stability and antimicrobial activity.[2076]

- Peppermint, thyme, cinnamon, and lemongrass oils inhibited the respiratory tract pathogens *S. pyogenes* (a bacterium that causes strep throat, scarlet fever, impetigo, cellulitis, and tonsillitis) and *S. pneumoniae*.[2077]

- Cinnamon bark oil is considered a viable candidate to replace methylparaben in cosmetics to ensure they remain free of harmful microbes.[2078]

- *In vitro* research suggests that a blend of essential oils containing wild orange, clove, cinnamon, eucalyptus, and rosemary reduced influenza (A/PR8/34) infection activity by preventing the virus from hijacking the cell's production of genetic information in favor of producing the virus' genetic information.[2079]

- Animal and *in vitro* research concluded that cinnamaldehyde inhibits influenza A/PR/8 growth if administered within three hours after infection.[2080] The same research also found that inhalation of 50 mg and administration of 250 mcg of cinnamaldehyde through the nasal per day reduced virus spread and increased survivability of mice.

- An *in vitro* study that tested the antimicrobial activity of fifty-one essential oils demonstrated that all fifty-one demonstrated activity against at least one of the seven organisms (13 essential oils—*Ps. aeruginosa,* unidentified number against *S. aureus,* but it was the second most resistant microbe, 20—*E. coli,* 47—*C. albicans,* 49—*S. pombe,* and 50—*S. cerevisiae* and *T. utilis*).[2081] The study authors pointed out that clove, cinnamon, and thyme essential oils demonstrated significant inhibition, inhibiting greater than 50% reduction in all organisms, and greater than 90% reduction in two or more organisms. Thyme inhibited all organisms at greater than 94% except for *E. coli* and *Ps. Aeruginosa.*

- Chewing gum flavored with cinnamon essential oil or inhalation of cinnamon aroma enhanced cognitive function in humans by improving attentional processes, virtual recognition memory, working memory, and visual-motor response speed.[2082]

- Animal research suggests that cinnamon essential oil and cinnamaldehyde may reduce the risk of mastitis in dairy cows by preventing *S. aureus* biofilm formation on surfaces.[2083] *S. aureus* is the most commonly isolated cause of bovine mastitis and inflammation of the mammary glands.

- A rare benzyl benzoate CT (65.4% benzyl benzoate) of cinnamon leaf essential oil was acaricidal to the Asian blue tick (*Rhipicephalus microplus*).[2084]

- Preclinical research demonstrates that cinnamon essential oil modulates the expression of several genes and signaling pathways associated with inflammation, tissue remodeling, and cancer in skin cells. The authors concluded that this activity may be useful to reduce chronic skin inflammation and fibrosis (thickening and scarring of connective tissue).[2085]

- *In vitro* research demonstrates that cinnamon essential oil is highly effective against *C. albicans*.[2086]

- Of ten essential oils tested (galangal, plai, ginger, line, kaffir lime, sweet basil, clove basil (*Ocimum gratissimum*), lemongrass, clove, and cinnamon), cinnamon essential oil displayed the most potent antibacterial activity against human pathogens—*S. aureus, E. coli, P. aeruginosa,* and *A. baumannii*.[2087]

- Cinnamon essential oil was insecticidal against *Ricania* sp. pests.[2088]

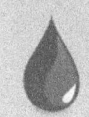

- Cinnamon essential oil may be a viable candidate to reduce bad breath due to its ability to by inhibit growth, kill biofilm, and reduce hydrogen sulfide production by the bacterium *Solobacterium moorei* (a gram-positive bacterium strongly associated with bad breath) without harming oral keratinocytes.[2089]

- Cinnamaldehyde demonstrated the strongest activity against the growth of aflatoxigenic fungi and aflatoxin production when cinnamon, oregano, cinnamaldehyde, and carvacrol were tested as part of bioactive films.[2090]

- A cinnamaldehyde-rich (91.8%) cinnamon bark essential oil killed 100% of hydatid cysts (protoscoleces) after 5 min of exposure at doses of 100 and 50 mcL/mL. The essential oil demonstrated a wide safety margin when injected in mice up to 1.52 mL/kg body weight and no significant toxicity following oral administration of for two weeks.[2091] *Echinococcus granulosus* tapeworms are responsible for cystic echinococcosis (CE)— a zoonotic parasitic disease transmitted in a cycle between dogs, domestic livestock, and humans. CE may develop in humans after the accidental ingestion of tapeworm eggs excreted with the feces of an infected dog, allowing the eggs to hatch in the intestine, penetrate into the intestinal wall, and reach the liver, lungs, or other organs, eventually developing into a hydatid cyst.

- A rare chemotype (65.4% benzyl benzoate) of cinnamon essential oil demonstrated acaricidal activity against the Asian blue tick (*Rhipicephalus microplus*).[2092]

- Laboratory research concluded that cinnamon essential oil inhibits the growth of *E. coli* and its virulence factors (production of Shiga toxin 2).[2093]

- Sweet basil, cinnamon bark, sweet fennel, kaffir lime petitgrain, kaffir lime peel, black pepper, peppermint, and spearmint essential oils all demonstrated antimicrobial activity against bacteria linked to cavities (Streptococcus *mutans* and *Lactobacillus casei*).[2094] Cinnamon was the most active against both bacteria, kaffir lime petitgrain was the weakest of the tested oils against both bacteria, and black pepper was inactive against *L. casei*.

- *In vitro* research demonstrates that both cinnamon bark essential oil and cinnamaldehyde prevent biofilm formation by *Porphyromonas gingivalis*.[2095] *Porphyromonas gingivalis* is a bacterium found in the oral cavity that is associated with periodontal disease, as well as gastrointestinal, respiratory, and vaginal infections. Interestingly, only the oil (not cinnamaldehyde) was able to decrease established biofilms.

- Both vetiver and cinnamon essential oil killed sheep blowfly (*Lucilia sericata*) larvae.[2096] This makes them promising biopesticides to control the spread of myiasis—an infection transmitted to humans when flies transmit their larvae to people, characterized by lumps under the skin.

- Cinnamon bark essential oil inhibits *C. albicans* by disrupting beta tubulin distribution, which caused mitotic spindle defects and compromised the cell wall allowing leakage of cellular components.[2097] Isolated cinnamaldehyde completely inhibited *C. albicans* as well. Another study found that cinnamon essential oil inhibits secreted aspartic protease activity in *C. albicans* (which is a factor in the yeasts virulence) and enhances the activity of fluconazole.[2098]

- Cinnamon, clove, oregano, and red thyme essential oils effectively inhibited multidrug-resistant *Salmonella enterica* (a cause of foodborne illness) and enhanced the activity of antibiotics (enrofloxacin, ceftiofur, and trimethoprim-sulfamethoxazole).[2099] The most effective combination was cinnamon with enrofloxacin reducing the minimum inhibitory concentration (MIC) of cinnamon from 1250 to 312.5 µg/mL and the MIC of ENR from 2 to 0.031 µg/mL.

- Both cinnamon bark and leaf essential oil inhibited *Salmonella Typhimurium* and *Listeria monocytogenes* growth in strawberry shakes.[2100] The cinnamon bark essential oil provided better sensory experience.

- Both cinnamon bark and cassia essential oils inhibited and reduced biofilm biomasses of *Streptococcus pyogenes, Pseudomonas aeruginosa*, and *Escherichia coli*.[2101] The same research found that cinnamaldehyde also exhibited antimicrobial and antibiofilm activity.

- Both cinnamon CT eugenol and clove essential oil were toxic to the wheat weevil (*Sitophilus granarius*).[2102] Eugenol was the most toxic to the weevil of the major constituents tested.

- Cinnamon and its main constituent cinnamaldehyde both inhibited *Aspergillus flavus* and *Aspergillus parasiticus*, which are aflatoxigenic fungi species that cause cancer, DNA mutations, dysregulate immune function, and disrupt fetal development.[2103]

- Both cinnamon and clove essential oils showed significant activity against human pathogens (*S. aureus, S. epidermidis, E. faecalis, S. pyogenes, E. coli, P. aeruginosa, A. hydrophila, P. mirabilis, K. pneumoniae*, and *C. albicans*) and their mature biofilms.[2104]

- *In vitro* examination of sixty essential oils demonstrated that sandalwood (Indian, Australian, and Hawaiian), melissa, lemongrass (*C. flexuosus*), cilantro, cassia, cinnamon, patchouli, and vetiver essential oils possess remarkable anticancer (two breast cancer cells) and antifungal (*Aspergillus niger, Candida albicans*, and

*Cryptococcus neoformans*) activities.[2105]

- Clove and cinnamon bark CT eugenol essential oils each exhibited insecticidal activities against the cowpea weevil (*Callosobruchus maculatus*) by impacting oviposition and offspring emergence.[2106]

- The eugenol CT of cinnamon leaf essential oil prevented the biofilm formation of *Candida* spp. Monospecies and multispecies without showing toxicity to healthy human cells.[2107] This suggests it may be beneficial for reducing oral infections.

- The common green bottle fly (*Lucilia sericata*) is a facultative insect that causes myasis (a skin disease characterized by painful, itchy boil-like lesions that occurs when the flies lay their larvae (maggots) in wounds or on the moist skin) in humans and other warm-blooded vertebrates. Low concentrations (0.2%) of vetiver, cinnamon (leaf and twig oil), lavender, and their blends killed the flies within five minutes.[2108] Vetiver significantly deterred flies from the oviposition medium and reduced adult longevity, while sunflower fixed oil repelled flies, deterred oviposition, and reduced adult fly lifespan. The greatest repellency was achieved with a blend of the four oils (2 mL of each essential oil and 4 mL of sunflower as carrier oil).

- Cinnamon bark, nut grass CT cyperene, and galangal CT beta-bisabolene each synergized the insecticidal activity of permethrin against mosquitoes (*Ae. Aegypti*).[2109]

- Cinnamon (46.3% cinnamaldehyde), oregano (*O. vulgare*; 33.9% cis-p-menth-2-en-1-ol), and turmeric (55.4% ar-turmerone) essential oils each inhibited *S. aureus, E. coli,* and *P. aeruginosa.*[2110]

- Fungal pathogens have caused significant declines in economically and agriculturally important animal species, like bees and bats. Current drug antifungals have limited use due to their toxicity to sensitive animal species. Cinnamon bark, citronella, and lemongrass essential oils each significantly inhibited *Ascosphaera apis* and *Pseudogymnoascus destructans*, the causative agents of chalkbrood disease among honey bee larvae and white-nose syndrome among bats, respectively.[2111]

- Cinnamon bark essential oil protected against kidney and liver toxicity caused by carbon tetrachloride.[2112]

- *In vitro* evidence showed that cinnamon bark essential oil disrupts multiple pathways associated with the ability of *Klebsiella pneumoniae* bacterium survival.[2113]

- Cinnamon bark essential oil enhanced the penetration of ibuprofen through rat skin.[2114]

- Of ten essential oils tested (thyme, pennyroyal, oregano, peppermint, lemongrass, rosemary, cinnamon, mandarin, holy basil, and mint asavi), cinnamon and thyme essential oils demonstrated the greatest efficacy against MRSA.[2115] Each oil demonstrated varying levels of inhibition. Oregano and pennyroyal also showed a strong synergistic activity with penicillin.

- Marjoram CT terpinen-4-ol, cinnamon bark, and thyme CT thymol essential oils each exhibited antibiofilm effects on *L. monocytogenes, P. putida*, and *S. aureus*, but were less effective against biofilms with two species unless higher concentrations were used.[2116] Cinnamon bark and its major constituent trans-cinnamaldehyde showed the greatest inhibitory effects.

- *In vitro* research found that both cinnamon bark and clove essential oil (and their mixtures) inhibited *Salmonella enterica* (Enteritidis and Typhimurium serotypes) isolated from poultry, suggesting they may be useful as farm disinfectants and in poultry diet to avoid *Salmonella* infections.[2117]

- Oral administration of cinnamon bark essential oil significantly improved liver enzymes and liver damage caused by formaldehyde in rats.[2118]

- Cinnamon bark and cinnamaldehyde both produced relaxant responses in isolated human and rat corpus cavernosum, suggesting they may be useful for erectile dysfunction.[2119]

- Both cinnamon bark and vetiver essential oils strongly repelled house flies (*Musca domestica*)—84 percent and 78 percent respectively.[2120] In addition, vetiver, cinnamon, and lavender essential oils were significantly toxic to house flies (100 percent).

- Of sixteen commercial essential oils tested (frankincense sacra, frankincense serrata, fennel, cistus, mountain savory CT carvacrol, oregano CT carvacrol, thyme CT thymol, cinnamon bark, may chang, clove bud, lemongrass—*C. citratus*, bitter orange, lemon, sweet orange, star anise, and lemon verbena), may chang and cinnamon bark essential oil were the most active against tested human cancer cells (breast—three types, chronic myelogenous erythroleukemia, and neuroblastoma).[2121] Other notable activity was observed with frankincense sacra and sweet orange against myelogenous leukemia.

- Cinnamon leaf CT eugenol, bay laurel CT camphene, guava leaf CT caryophyllene oxide, and Monterey cypress CT alpha-pinene essential oils each inhibited glycation—the nonenzymatic bonding of lipids to sugars creating advanced glycation end products—in laboratory research.[2122] Damage caused by glycation can lead to stiffening of the blood vessel walls and high blood pressure, particularly among diabetics.

- Cinnamon bark essential oil exhibited broad-spectrum antimicrobial activity against gram-positive and gram-negative bacteria, with the ability to rapidly kill *P. aeruginosa* at low concentrations.[2123]

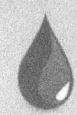

- Preliminary research found that cinnamon bark essential oil inhibits *Klebsiella pneumoniae*—one of the most prevalent pathogens responsible for healthcare-acquired infections—by causing oxidative stress and bacterial membrane disruption.[2124]

- Laboratory research concluded that cinnamon bark essential oil possesses anticancer activity against cervical and lymphoma cancer cells and good antioxidant activity in the phosphomolybdenum and DPPH assays.[2125]

- Immunomodulatory activity of essential oils was assessed by the simultaneous evaluation of phagocytosis, production of iNOS, and secretion of IL-6, induced by contact of RAW 264.7 cells with LPS. What the researchers found was that both clove and cinnamon essential oils modulate immune activity, which suggest they may be helpful for inflammatory and infectious conditions.[2126]

- *E. coli* is the most common uropathogenic cause of urinary tract infections (UTIs), but the most frequently used antibiotics do not effectively eliminate the organism, making recurrent UTIs common. Of 140 essential oils tested, oregano, allspice, cinnamon bark, and clove bud were the most effective against uropathogenic *E. coli*.[2127]

- Tahini is a popular food product in the Middle East, but tahini and its products have been linked to foodborne illness outbreaks and the subjects of worldwide recalls as a result of Salmonella contamination. Of ten essential oils tested, cinnamon bark and thyme essential oils were the most effective against *Salmonella* species bacteria.[2128]

- Oral administration of cinnamaldehyde, the main constituent in cassia and cinnamon bark essential oils, significantly inhibited the release of proinflammatory cytokines (IL-6, IL-8, TNF-α) from synoviocyte cells—a specialized type of cells found in joints that play a crucial role in rheumatoid arthritis—in arthritis rats. Cinnamaldehyde also impaired Jak/Stat signaling pathways—critical pathways in the onset and progression of rheumatoid arthritis—and reduced collagen-induced swollen paws. The anti-inflammatory effects of cinnamaldehyde decreased the severity of arthritis, joint swelling, and reduced bone erosion and destruction.

- Cinnamon bark essential oil inhibited MAO-A (monoamine oxidase A; antidepressant) and MAO-B (anti-Parkinson's), AchE and BchE (anti-Alzheimer's), alpha-amylase (antidiabetic), and tyrosinase (skin whitening), and showed good antioxidant activity.[2129] Its MAO-B inhibiting activity was as high as rasagiline, which is an antidepressant that selectively inhibits MAO-B and is often used to treat Parkinson's disease.

- *In vitro* research showed that cinnamon bark, oregano, thyme CT thymol, lemongrass (*C. flexuosus*), allspice, palmarosa, and amyris all significantly inhibited *S. aureus* in the stationary phase, which is when the size of a bacterial population remains constant, even though some cells continue to divide and others begin to die.[2130]

- Cinnamon bark, thyme, and clove essential oil showed important antibacterial activity against multidrug-resistant bacteria isolated from people (*E. coli, K. pneumoniae, A. baumanii, P. aeruginosa, C. freundii, K. oxytoca, S. enteritidis, S. typhimurium, S. zanzibar, S. Livingstone, S. derby, S. Heidelberg, C. striatum*, and *S. aureus*).[2131] They exhibited a remarkable antibiofilm and anti-quorum-sensing activity and good antioxidant activity. The highest antioxidant activity was observed from clove (90.3% DPPH).

- Inflammatory bowel diseases, like colitis, are associated with poor bacterial balance in the gut, which decreases the barrier function of the intestinal mucosa. Decreased barrier function increases inflammation and allows the growth of harmful bacteria in the intestine. An experimental model of colitis showed that cinnamon essential oil protects against intestinal inflammation and improves bacterial balance in the intestine.[2132] In contrast to antibiotics, which don't improve bacterial balance, cinnamon essential oil enhanced the diversity and richness of intestinal bacteria and reduce inflammation. Simultaneously, it reduced *Helicobacter* and bacteroides—bacteria normally found in the mouth, gastrointestinal tract, and female genital tract—and increased bacteroidales and short-chain fatty acids-producing bacteria. Despite what many believe, this research provides evidence that potent antimicrobial oils improve the gut microflora rather than causing imbalance.

- The human body has a remarkable ability to heal itself. A great example is the wound healing process. Wound healing follows an organized process that involves (1) stopping the flow of blood; (2) inflammation; (3) rebuilding of the wound with new tissue; and (4) remodeling of tissues to fully close the wound. This process works very well as long as no foreign object, infection, or poor circulation (like in diabetics) is present. Cinnamon bark essential oil accelerated the wound healing process in an infected wound model in mice. Mice topically treated with 2% and 4% cinnamon bark essential oil reduced the inflammatory phase of wound healing, increased fibroblast distribution, collagen deposition, and antioxidant power, and accelerated cellular proliferation, reepithelialization, and keratin synthesis, and upregulated the IGF-1, FGF-2, and VEGF expression.[2133]

- Cinnamon bark, lemongrass, and rosemary essential oil each repelled mosquitoes when used as spatial repellents in a laboratory setting.[2134] Synergistic interactions were observed when two or more essential oils

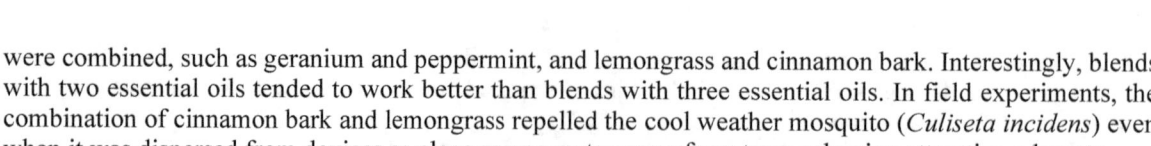

were combined, such as geranium and peppermint, and lemongrass and cinnamon bark. Interestingly, blends with two essential oils tended to work better than blends with three essential oils. In field experiments, the combination of cinnamon bark and lemongrass repelled the cool weather mosquito (*Culiseta incidens*) even when it was dispersed from devices as close as one meter away from traps releasing attractive odorants.

☐ *Listeria monocytogenes* is a pathogenic bacteria that causes listeriosis—a condition characterized by fever, muscle aches, diarrhea, and nausea, which can also spread to the nervous system and cause headache, stiff neck, confusion, and changes in alertness. Onion, garlic, and cinnamon bark essential oils inhibited biofilm formation by *L. monocytogenes in vitro*.[2135]

☐ Cinnamon bark essential oil inhibited food-spoilage bacteria (e.g., *L. innocua*, *S. aureus*, and *B. cereus*) quickly by disrupting the cell envelope and facilitating the leakage of intracellular compounds and also exhibited good antioxidant activity.[2136]

☐ The hydatid worm (*Echinococcus granulosus*) is a tapeworm that inhabits the small intestine of dogs, but can use humans and other livestock as intermediate hosts. It can cause cystic echinococcosis in intermediate hosts. Cinnamon bark essential oil and its main component cinnamaldehyde showed good activity against hydatid worm protoscoleces—larval stage of the tapeworm—but cinnamaldehyde exhibited a more pronounced effect.[2137]

☐ A cinnamon bark essential oil nanoemulsion encapsulated in whey protein concentrate reversed disturbances in biochemical, cytological, and histopathological changes in diabetic rats.[2138] The oil increased antioxidant capacity, reduced oxidative stress, modulated gene expression related to diabetes (downregulated hepatic GLU2, FAS, SREBP-1c, and PEPCK; upregulated IGF-1 mRNA expression), enhanced liver and pancreas histology, and improved glucose, insulin, amylase, and lipid levels.

☐ Of twenty-eight essential oils tested, cinnamon bark essential oil was the most active against the maize weevil (*Sitophilus zeamais*) in both the contact/residual and fumigant bioassays.[2139] However, the oil was primarily effective in empty containers—killing 100 percent of weevils—but ineffective in rice-filled containers—killing only 15 percent of weevils. Testing of individual constituents found that trans-cinnamaldehyde and terpinen-4-ol (in tea tree and marjoram) were the most active constituents.

☐ Thyme CT thymol and cinnamon bark essential oil reduced airway inflammation and hyperresponsiveness—both important features of asthma and chronic obstructive pulmonary disease—in a mouse model of airway inflammation caused by exposure to an endotoxin.[2140] Two drops of oil were placed on filter paper and taped to the bottom of the box mice were placed in during a thirty-minute-long inhalation period. On the contrary, Ceylon citronella essential oil showed an irritating effect on inflamed airways that could exacerbate the airway hyperresponsiveness.

☐ Cinnamon leaf CT eugenol essential oil reduced virulence factors (adhesion ability, germ tube formation, biofilm formation) of *Candida* spp. without causing toxicity.[2141] Another group of researchers evaluated the fungicidal properties of both cinnamon bark and cinnamon leaf CT eugenol essential oils and found that cinnamon bark was more active against *C. albicans* and *C. auris*.[2142]

☐ *Bacillus* bacteria are widely found in nature and responsible for food poisoning and food spoilage. Black cumin, clove, cinnamon, and marjoram essential oils each reduced *Bacillus* spp. presence in raw and processed meat, with black cumin being the most effective oil.[2143]

☐ A randomized, controlled, and blinded clinical trial that included 36 individuals with oral candidiasis compared the benefits of cinnamon leaf essential oil with nystatin (an antifungal medication). Subjects in the cinnamon group used 10 mL of a mouthwash (one minute, three times daily) and applied an oral spray containing 0.5 mg/mL of cinnamon leaf essential oil for fifteen days. The nystatin group followed a similar protocol with a nystatin mouth rinse. The results showed that cinnamon essential oil reduced *Candida* colonies in the mouth and on dentures and improved candidiasis symptoms based on clinical observation.[2144]

☐ *In vitro* research demonstrated that cinnamon bark essential oil is a better antifungal agent than nystatin against *C. albicans*.[2145]

☐ Injection of cinnamon bark essential oil (0.5 mg/kg BW) in male rats protected against neurobehavioral deficits—anxiety-like behavior, significant increase in digging frequency, and a marked decrease in sleeping frequency and duration—caused by the insecticide deltamethrin (DLM).[2146] DLM significantly suppressed acetylcholinesterase (AchE) activity, elevated serotonin and corticosterone concentrations, altered superoxide dismutase (SOD) activity and malondialdehyde (MDA) concentration, and upregulated mRNA expression of brain CYP1A1 and iNOS. Co-treatment with cinnamon oil improved the deleterious activity of DLM on these parameters and reduced its neurotoxicity.

☐ Researchers evaluated the composition and antibacterial activity of six medicinally important essential oils: tarragon CT p-allylanisole, dill CT alpha-phellandrene/para-cymene, lemon, orange, cinnamon bark, and

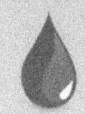

ginger. Interestingly orange essential oil had the greatest antibacterial activity against *S. aureus* and *P. aeruginosa*.[2147] Cinnamon bark and tarragon were most active against *E. coli* and *K. pneumoniae*.

☐ *In vitro* research showed that cinnamon bark essential oil possesses antibacterial activity against multidrug-resistant *Shigella* isolates, most of which were resistant to six antibiotics.[2148]

☐ Cinnamon leaf essential oil inhibited *Pseudomonas aeruginosa, Staphylococcus aureus*, and *Klebsiella pneumoniae* in vapor phase, inhibited biofilm formation, and eradicated existing biofilms without showing toxicity to healthy cells.[2149]

☐ Cinnamon bark, grapefruit, tangerine, and lemon essential oil each inhibited *Bacillus subtilis, Penicillium chrysogenum, Fusarium moniliforme, Aspergillus niger, Aspergillus flavus, Saccharomyces cerevisiae, Escherichia coli, Salmonella abony, Staphylococcus aureus, Pseudomonas aeruginosa*, and *Candida albicans*, with the greatest activity observed from cinnamon bark.[2150] The highest antioxidant activity was found in grapefruit oi, followed by lemon, tangerine, and cinnamon bark.

☐ A cinnamon bark essential oil nanoemulsion showed greater larvicidal activity, with residual effects, against *Anopheles stephensi* mosquito larvae.[2151]

☐ Cinnamon bark, palmarosa, and ginger essential oil each exhibited good antioxidant activity in the DPPH, ABTS, and FRAP assays, with cinnamon being the most effective. Additionally, the oils inhibited the growth of *Fusarium verticillioides* and reduced its production of mycotoxins (fumonisin B1 and B2).[2152] Cinnamon bark and palmarosa were the most effective against *Fusarium verticillioides*.

☐ Cinnamon essential oil-laden bioactive glass/soy protein scaffolds displayed a controlled release over seven days, enhanced antioxidant activity, and improved antibacterial activity against *S. aureus* and *E. coli*.[2153] The oil scaffolds were also nontoxic to osteoblasts, causing the researchers to conclude that the essential oil scaffolds represent promising solutions for bone tissue engineering, bone infections, and to protect against oxidative stress damage.

☐ Cinnamon bark essential oil demonstrated antibiofilm activity against multidrug-resistant *S. agalactiae*.[2154] However, its efficacy was reduced when combined with silver nanoparticles.

☐ Cinnamon bark essential oil was acaricidal to the Asian blue tick (*Rhipicephalus microplus*).[2155]

☐ Both cardamom and cinnamon bark essential oils inhibited the growth of *B. subtilis* and *E. coli*, but cardamom was only effective at the highest concentration tested.[2156] The individual oils and their combination inhibited cell attachment for both bacteria, with stronger activity observed against *E. coli*. A combination of both oils was synergistic against *B. subtilis* and reduced biofilm formation by both bacteria.

☐ Cinnamon leaf essential oil (35.6% I-cinnamaldehyde, 18.9% linalool, 18.7% eugenol) inhibited *E. coli, S. aureus, P. aeruginosa*, and *S. enteritidis*.[2157] The oil was also active against grain pests rice weevil and cowpea weevil (*Sitophilus oryzae* and *Callosobruchus maculatus*) and mosquito (*Ae. aegypti*) larvae without being toxic to guppy fishes or negatively affecting seed germination.

☐ Vapor of cinnamon leaf essential oil (77.2% eugenol) inhibited *C. albicans, C. tropicalis*, and *C. dubliniensis* and was effective against existing biofilms.[2158]

☐ Of fourteen commercial essential oils tested, cinnamon bark, thyme CT thymol, clove bud, geranium, and manuka essential oils were most active against fungi that commonly infect animal and human skin (*Microsporum gypseum, Microsporum canis, Trichophyton mentagrophytes, Trichophyton violaceum, Aspergillus niger, Scopulariopsis brevicaulis*, (IZ 1) dog skin isolate).[2159] (E)-cinnamaldehyde, thymol, and carvacrol displayed the strongest activity of isolated constituents against dermatophyteI(E); cinnamaldehyde, eugenol, carvacrol, geraniol, and thymol were most active against IZ 1.

☐ Terpene/phenol-rich (oregano CT carvacrol, thyme CT carvacrol, and summer savory CT carvacrol) and phenylpropanoid-rich (clove bud and cinnamon leaf) essential oils each showed good absolute antioxidant activity—comparable to BHT—in cumene and squalene during the peroxyl radical trapping assay.[2160]

☐ Cinnamon bark and thyme CT thymol essential oil both inhibited *Streptococcus suis*, which is a zoonotic pathogen that causes disease in pigs and humans and is developing resistance to antibiotics.[2161]

☐ Clove bud and cinnamon bark essential oil each exhibited inhibitory activity against bacteria associated with wound infections (*P. aeruginosa, E. coli*, and *K. pneumoniae*), with cinnamon bark being more effective.[2162] The researchers concluded that these oils may be useful in the prevention of healthcare-acquired infections.

☐ A study investigated a topical nanostructured lipid carrier (NLC) gel loaded cinnamon oil for *Pseudomonas aeruginosa* wound infection. *P. aeruginosa* is an antibiotic-resistant bacterium that commonly infects wounds and complicates wound care and healing. The NLC-cinnamon gel effectively healed burn wounds after six days of application, showing its promise for use in *P. aeruginosa* infected wound treatment.[2163]

☐ *Clostridioides difficile* is a bacterium that produces two exotoxins: toxin A and toxin B. Infections with *C. diff* can be mild to moderate (watery diarrhea three or more times daily for more than one day accompanied

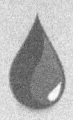

by mild abdominal cramping and tenderness) or severe (watery diarrhea up to fifteen times daily, moderate to severe abdominal cramping, rapid heart rate, fever, dehydration, and nausea). Severe cases can cause kidney failure, loss of appetite, blood or pus in the stool, and inflammation of the colon (colitis), which can be life-threatening. Illness caused by *C. diff* typically occurs after antibiotic use and most commonly affects older adults in healthcare facilities. However, because the bacterium is shed in feces it can contaminate any surface, material, or device and spread outside of healthcare settings and in younger people as well. Repeat infections are common among the elderly because the bacterium is resistant to multiple antibiotics, making it very difficult to eradicate. A laboratory study investigated the activity of ten essential oils—cassia bark, cinnamon bark, citronella (*C. nardus*), coriander, clove bud, oregano CT carvacrol, Greek oregano (*O. heracleoticum*) CT carvacrol, marjoram, clary sage, and thyme CT thymol—against *C. diff* isolated from infected patients and contaminated foods.[2164] Isolated constituents within the essential oils were also tested (carvacrol, trans-cinnamaldehyde, eugenol, linalool, and thymol) as well as common antibiotics used to treat *C. diff* infections (chloramphenicol, clindamycin, erythromycin, gentamicin, metronidazole, and vancomycin). Cassia and cinnamon bark were the most effective, with thyme, oregano, Greek oregano, and marjoram also demonstrating high activity. Coriander and clary sage exhibited medium activity, while clove and citronella displayed low activity. Among the isolated constituents, trans-cinnamaldehyde, thymol, and carvacrol showed high activity and eugenol and linalool low activity. Cinnamon and cassia consistently exceeded the activity of all antibiotics, with very few exceptions, and thyme, oregano, and Greek oregano outperformed all antibiotics but metronidazole.

- The bacterium *H. pylori* can express the cytotoxin-associated gene A (cagA) and vacuolating cytotoxin A (vacA) genes. CagA increases the cancer-causing ability of *H. pylori* in the colon and is associated with cardiovascular disease (inflammation of aortic endothelium and acceleration of atherosclerosis) and vacA is a key toxin secreted by the bacterium to colonize and persist in the human stomach. A recent study found that cagA and vacA were found in 67.7 percent and 93.5 percent of people infected with *H. pylori* respectively. Researchers further evaluated the activity of five essential oils—cinnamon bark, clove bud, thyme, rosemary, and chamomile—against the ability of drug-resistant *H. pylori* to produce cytotoxic genes.[2165] Of the oils tested, cinnamon bark essential oil was the most effective, followed by clove, thyme, rosemary, and chamomile. The activity of both cinnamon and thyme oil exceeded that of levofloxacin (an antibiotic used to treat several bacterial infections, including *H. pylori*).

- The antidiabetic activity of cinnamon essential oil was investigated in molecular docking analysis and by evaluation of activity on enzymes involved in glucose metabolism.[2166] The inhibition of alpha-amylase and alpha-glucosidase enzymes by small molecules like essential oil constituents allows these molecules to bind to active receptor sites and block the subsequent binding of complex carbohydrates to receptor sites therefore slowing increases in blood sugar following eating. Inhibition of PTP1B (protein tyrosine phosphatase 1B) enzyme is also desirable because doing so decreases blood sugar levels by increasing glucose clearance in the blood through cellular uptake. Hexokinases are also enzymatic targets to manage blood glucose because inhibiting their activity helps regulate healthy glucose levels in the human body. Lastly, inducing glucokinase enzymatic activity can increase glucose metabolism. Cinnamaldehyde and eugenol both exhibited high binding potential for the PTP1B active site and alpha-glucosidase active pocket, beta-caryophyllene at the active site for alpha-amylase and hexokinases, beta-caryophyllene and eugenol relatively strong binding affinity to glucokinase sites. Altogether, the research suggests that cinnamon essential oil contains constituents that may positively affect multiple enzymes involved in blood glucose management.

- Cinnamon, eucalyptus (*E. globulus*), and clove bud essential oil effectively inhibited MRSA, with cinnamon producing the greatest zone of inhibition and eucalyptus having the lowest minimum inhibitory concentration.[2167]

- When testing four essential oils (cinnamon bark, clove, oregano, and peppermint) and isolated constituents (allyl isothiocyanate, carvacrol, citral, eugenol, and (+)-limonene), researchers found that allyl isothiocyanate, cinnamon, carvacrol, eugenol, and oregano were active against all microorganisms tested (*E. coli, L. monocytogenes, S. typhimurium, P. fluorescens,* and *En. faecalis*) in vapor phase.[2168] *P. fluorescens* was the most resistant to the oils and isolated.

- A study evaluated the antimicrobial activity of multiple essential oils (cinnamon bark, lavender, tea tree, lemon, oregano CT carvacrol, peppermint, bay laurel and eucalyptus—*E. globulus*) against human pathogens (*S. pyogenes, S. aureus, S. aglactiae*).[2169] Oregano, cinnamon, and tea tree exhibited the strongest antibacterial activity and combinations of tea tree/lavender and cinnamon/lavender displayed synergistic activity.

- Nanofibrous scaffolds with cinnamon bark or nano-cinnamon bark essential oil demonstrated promise for the

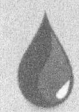

effective management of diabetic wounds *in vitro*.[2170]

☐ A comparison of the activity of ten essential oils against antibiotic-resistant *E. coli* and *L. monocytogenes* showed that clove, thyme, cinnamon, and garlic were highly active against both bacteria, but turmeric, cumin, black pepper, and marjoram were inactive against *L. monocytogenes*.[2171] Ginger and parsley were moderately active against both bacteria. A combination of clove and thyme exhibited the strongest activity against *L. monocytogenes*. Combinations of clove+cinnamon, cinnamon+garlic, and cinnamon+thyme were synergistic against *E. coli*; the same combinations plus clove+thyme, and clove+garlic were synergistic against *L. monocytogenes*. Composition was not reported for the essential oils used in the study.

☐ Nanogels containing clove bud or cinnamon bark essential oil showed significant anti-inflammatory and pain-relieving (antinociceptive) activity in rats.[2172]

☐ *Sarcoptes scabiei* mites are responsible for scabies, an itchy contagious skin infection in humans. More than thirty essential oils used in traditional treatments for dermatological conditions in Madagascar were evaluated against scabies mites. Both cinnamon leaf and holy basil CT eugenol essential oil were most active against *S. scabiei* in a laboratory setting, suggesting they should be further investigated as topical solutions for scabies.[2173]

☐ Investigation of the antifungal and antivirulence activity of basil CT linalool, cinnamon bark, clove, tea tree, oregano CT carvacrol, and thyme CT thymol essential oils (EOs) on five *Candida* species (*C. albicans*, *C. auris*, *C. krusei*, *C. parapsilosis* and *C. guillermondii*) revealed that clove and cinnamon inhibited all fungal species tested, cinnamon, oregano, and thyme inhibited biofilm formation of *C. albicans*, *C. guilliermondii*, and *C. parapsilosis*, and each oil except tea tree downregulate virulence genes in *C. albicans*.[2174] In addition, thyme synergized the activity of fluconazole against all tested *Candida* species.

☐ Cinnamon bark essential oil was acaricidal to unfed adults, nymphs, and larvae of the Asian longhorned tick (*Haemaphysalis longicornis*).[2175] Furthermore, the oil interfered with reproduction.

☐ A combination of cinnamon bark and allspice essential oil in soybean oil (5% of each oil in 90% soybean oil) was highly larvicidal to and significantly repelled the American cockroach (*Periplaneta americana*).[2176]

☐ Colistin (polymyxin E) is an antibiotic used to treat severe infections caused by multidrug-resistant gram-negative bacteria (*E. coli*, *P. mirabilis*). Cinnamon bark essential oil exhibited the highest activity against colistin-resistant bacteria, followed by thyme (composition note reported) and eucalyptus (species not reported) oils.[2177]

☐ Oral administration of cinnamon bark essential oil (50 mg/kg BW) reduced tumor cell count, viability, and proliferation by inhibiting tumor growth rate in a well-established experimental breast cancer cell (Ehrlich ascites carcinoma) in mice.[2178] Moreover, the oil triggered a significant antitumor immune response by elevating splenic T helper (CD3+CD4+) and T cytotoxic (CD3+CD8+) cells, and restored altered kidney and liver functions.

☐ Nanoliposomes containing 2.5% cinnamon bark essential oil provided complete protection against mosquitoes (*Anopheles stephensi*), which lasted significantly longer than DEET.[2179]

☐ *Enterococcus faecalis* is a bacterium that can cause high fever, fatigue, painful urination, gum swelling, breathing difficulties, vomiting, nausea, severe headache, abdominal cramps, and diarrhea depending on the location of the infection. Cinnamon bark, clove bud, and black cumin essential oil each showed strong inhibition of antibiotic-resistant *E. faecalis* strains isolated from children with diarrhea. This research suggests that these oils could be considered for the management of diarrhea caused by *E. faecalis* infection.

☐ Cinnamon, clove, and thyme essential oils demonstrated remarkable antibacterial properties against multidrug-resistant strains of *S. enteritidis*.[2180] Moreover, biofilm formation was reduced by cinnamon, clove, thyme, turmeric, rosemary, and sage essential oils. Clove exhibited the greatest inhibition of violacein production, followed by thyme and cinnamon.

☐ Cinnamon bark essential oil reduced the toxicity of doxorubicin in a brine shrimp assay and improved its effectiveness against leukemia.[2181]

☐ Cinnamon bark, clove bud, and bay laurel essential oils inhibited *L. monocytogenes*, *L. innocua*, *L. welshimeri*, *L. ivanovii*, *L. grayi*, and *V. parahaemolyticus*, with cinnamon bark being the most effective.[2182]

☐ Cinnamon bark essential oil demonstrated antibiofilm activity—initial attachment of microbial cells as well as the eradication of mature biofilm—against *S. aureus* and *K. pneumoniae*.[2183]

☐ Cumin, cinnamon leaf, and oregano CT carvacrol essential oil effectively inhibited *Aspergillus* spp. and *Penicillium* spp., with clove showing the greatest activity.[2184] Electrospun nanofiber films with clove and cinnamon prevented fungal growth on bread samples.

☐ When testing six plants traditionally used to improve memory via inhalation—cinnamon bark, myrtle, rue, saffron, dill, and nutmeg, cinnamon bark essential oil was the most potent inhibitor of acetylcholinesterase

(AChE) and butyrylcholinesterase (BChE) and also inhibited beta-secretase 1, suggesting it may aid healthy cognitive function.[2185] However, the oil did not show neuroprotective activity against toxicity caused by beta-amyloid. Altogether, this laboratory research suggests that cinnamon bark essential oil may be helpful in the management of advanced Alzheimer's disease.

- Inhalation of cinnamon bark essential oil reduced anxiety in two separate mouse models by modifying gene expression in the hippocampus, particularly Dcc, Egr2, and Fos, which are crucial genes involved in anxiety-related biological processes and pathways.[2186] These genes are associated with neuron cell survival and inflammation. Its main constituent, trans-cinnamaldehyde, also reduced anxiety in a zebrafish model.

- Combining cinnamon bark essential oil with sertraline (Zoloft)—a selective serotonin reuptake inhibitor used to treat depression that also shows antibacterial activity—produced a synergistic effect against gram-positive and gram-negative bacteria (B. subtilis, E. faecalis, S, aureus, A. baumannii, C. striatum, and E. coli).[2187]

- When evaluating cinnamon bark, oregano, and thyme essential oils against E. coli and T. pyogenes isolated from dairy cows with clinical endometritis, cinnamon bark was the most effective.[2188]

- Solid lipid nanoparticles (SLN) loaded with cinnamon bark essential oil inhibited ten multidrug-resistant E. coli strains better than free oil.[2189] The SLN cinnamon bark also inhibited biofilm formation better.

- Oral administration of cinnamon essential oil (200 mg/kg BW) significantly reduced total cholesterol, VLDL, and triglycerides in rats with acute hyperlipidemia—high levels of fats (cholesterol and triglycerides) in the blood.[2190] Remarkably, cinnamon oil was more effective than the drug atorvastatin. No liver harm (based on liver enzyme monitoring) was observed.

- Cinnamon leaf essential oil with trans-cinnamaldehyde (73.0%) as the major constituent displayed strong antioxidant activity in the DPPH and ABTS assays and was effective in reducing copper and iron. The oil was also highly effective as an inhibitor of human carbonic anhydrase II (hCA II; plays a prominent role in the regulation of intraocular pressure and its inhibition could help manage glaucoma), AChE (inhibition aids cognition and memory), and alpha-amylase (inhibition helps manage blood glucose).

- Cinnamon bark essential oil and isolated trans-cinnamaldehyde exhibited strong ovicidal activity against mosquitoes (Ae. aegypti and Ae. albopictus) and were not toxic to their aquatic fish predators (Poecilia latipinna and Poecilia reticulata).[2191] The combination of cinnamon bark essential oil with geranial was the most effective.

- Cinnamon (plant part and composition not reported; commercial sample) and lemongrass (species not identified) essential oils both inhibited planktonic C. albicans and eradicated established biofilms when sed at eight times the minimum inhibitory concentration.[2192]

- Kappa-carrageenan hydrogel with cinnamon essential oil and beta-hydroxypropyl cyclodextrin displayed effective antimicrobial activity and prolonged the shelf-life of sliced bread at least two days.[2193]

- Both cinnamon bark essential oil and isolated trans-cinnamaldehyde exhibited significant ovicidal activity against mosquitoes (Ae. aegypti and Ae. albopictus) without being toxic to aquatic mosquito predators (Poecilia latipinna and P. reticulata).[2194] Lemongrass and bitter orange also showed good activity. A combination of cinnamon bark and geranial showed the strongest activity, which was five times more effective than 1% temephos.

- Both cinnamaldehyde and eugenol CTs of cinnamon essential oil inhibited metastatic melanoma cell proliferation by increasing HMOX1, FTH1, SLC7A11, DGKK, and GSR expression but suppressing OXR1, SOD3, Tf, and TfR1 expression.[2195] The eugenol CT was the most active.

- Of fifteen essential oils screened, cinnamon bark was the most effective against C. auris.[2196] The oil also synergized the activity oil fluconazole against C. auris, while its main constituent, trans-cinnamaldehyde, only had an additive effect.

- Cinnamon bark and clove bud essential oils exhibited promising antibacterial activity (E. coli, K. pneumoniae, P. aeruginosa, S. aureus, and E. fecalis) and potent antiviral activity (SARS-CoV-2).[2197]

- Nanofiber mats coated with chitosan microcapsules containing cinnamon essential oil improved wound healing in rats.[2198]

- Cinnamon essential oil encapsulated in silica nanoparticles was insecticidal to the rice moth (Corcyra cephalonica), and its activity exceeded the free oil, silica gel, and peppermint.[2199]

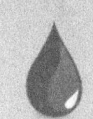

# CISTUS
## (Gum Rockrose)

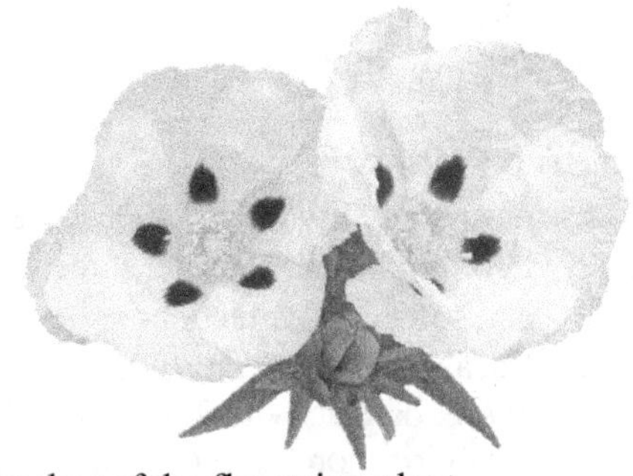

*Cistus ladanifer* L., *Cistus ladaniferus* L., orth. var.

**FAMILY:** Cistaceae
**NOTE:** Middle-Base
**AROMA INTENSITY:** Medium
**AROMA:** Warm, sweet, herbaceous
**COMMON EXTRACTION METHOD:** Steam distilled from the leaves and branches of the flowering plant
**POSSIBLE SUBSTITUTE OILS:** Niaouli (viridiflorol CT), Spanish sage, geranium
**BLENDS WELL WITH:** Bergamot, cedarwood, chamomile (German, Roman), clary sage, copaiba, cypress, frankincense, lavender, juniper, patchouli, pine, sandalwood, spikenard, turmeric, vetiver
**SUBCELLULAR LOCALIZATION | EPIGENETIC INFLUENCE:** Currently unknown | Currently unknown
**RECOMMENDED DILUTION RANGE:** 5%–Neat

**PRIMARY CONSTITUENTS:**[2200,2201,2202,2203,2204,2205,2206]

*Alpha-Pinene CT*

| | |
|---|---|
| Alpha-Pinene | 5.3%–56.0% |
| Ledol | 0.0%–13.8% |
| 2,2,6-Trimethylcyclohexanone | 0.9%–11.9% |
| Viridiflorol | 0.0%–11.8% |
| Camphene | 0.9%–10.0% |
| Para-Cymene | 1.0%–4.8% |
| Bornyl Acetate | 1.9%–3.7% |

*Viridiflorol/Trans-Pinocarveol CT*

| | |
|---|---|
| Viridiflorol | 13.6%–21.3% |
| Trans-Pinocarveol | 1.2%–20.0% |
| Bornyl Acetate | 0.0%–16.7% |
| Ledol | 0.4%–6.6% |
| Terpinen-4-ol | 0.7%–6.4% |
| Globulol | 0.0%–5.0% |
| Alpha-Pinene | 0.1%–4.5% |

**OTHER CONSTITUENTS:** *Alpha-Pinene CT*—Tricyclene, alpha-thujene, sabinene, beta-pinene, alpha-terpinene, para-cymene, *d*-limonene, gamma-terpinene, terpinolene, alpha-campholene aldehyde, camphor, exo-methyl-camphenilol, terpineol-4, para-cymen-8-ol, alpha-terpineol, verbenone, para-mentha-1,4-dien-7-ol, alpha-cubebene, cyclosativen, delta-cadinene, diethyl phthalate, cyercene, pinadiene, borneol; *Viridifloro/Trans-Pinocarveol CT*—Para-cymene, pinocarvone, bornyl acetate, 2,2,6-trimethylcyclohexanone, allo-aromadendrene, (Z)-ocimenone, viridiflorene, delta-cadinene, delta-verbenone, spathulenol, ambrox, sclareol oxide

**PREFERRED COMPOSITION FOR CLINICAL USE:**

| Constituent | *α-Pinene/Viridiflorene CT* | *α-Pinene CT* |
|---|---|---|
| **Alpha-Pinene** | 20%–30% | 30%–55% |
| **Viridiflorene** | 2%–12% | – |
| **2,2,6-Trimethylcyclohexanone** | 0.5%–7% | 0.1%–10% |
| **Bornyl Acetate** | 3%–8% | 3%–6% |
| **Camphene** | 2%–8% | 2%–8% |
| **Para-Cymene** | 2%–7% | 1%–5% |
| **Trans-Pinocarveol** | 2%–6% | 1%–5% |
| **Limonene** | 0.5%–3% | 0.5%–3% |
| **Viridiflorol** | 2%–10% | 0.5%–3% |
| **Gamma-Terpinene** | 0.5%–3% | 0.5%–3% |

**REPORTED THERAPEUTIC PROPERTIES:** Antimicrobial, antiseptic, astringent, expectorant, antiviral, antibacterial, **immune modulator**, anti-inflammatory, antineuralgic, eases cough, nervine (calms and soothes the nerves), **cell regenerating**, reduces appearance of scars, relieves shock, supports normal respiratory function, encourages lymph drainage, stops excess bleeding, helps relieve chronic skin conditions, relieves hemorrhoids and anal fissures, **wound healing**, helps one deal with traumatic events, promotes a peaceful feeling, reduces anxiety

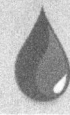
**CAUTIONS:**

■ None currently known.

**SELECTED EVIDENCE:**

- □ Cistus essential oil demonstrates significant activity against multidrug-resistant *Enterobacter aerogenes* EA289.[2207] Enterobacter infections are associated with urinary tract infections, respiratory infections, skin, and soft-tissue infections.
- □ Eucalyptus (*E. globulus*), pine, rosemary, cistus, Maritime pine, and juniper berry each displayed good antioxidant activity in the ORAC assay.[2208]
- □ The viridiflorol CT of cistus essential oil demonstrated powerful antibacterial activity against *E. coli*, *A. baumannii* (fully resistant to antibiotics), *S. aureus*, and *S. typhi*.[2209] The oil also inhibited fungi (*C. albicans*, *C, tropicalis*, *C. glabrata*, *C. dubliniensis*, *Candida* sp., *R. rubra*, *A, niger*, *C. neoformans*, *Penicillium* sp, *Fusarium* sp.), with *C. tropicalis* and *C. neoformans* being the most susceptible strains.
- □ Cistus oils (CT viridiflorol and CT alpha-pinene) demonstrated high antibacterial and cellular antioxidant activity.[2210] Juniper essential oil exhibited cytotoxicity to breast cancer cells, while cypress and cistus essential oils were most effective against lung cancer cells.
- □ Cistus essential oil displayed good anti-inflammatory activity and wound healing potential in laboratory research.[2211]
- □ *In vitro* research showed that cistus essential oil inhibited *L. monocytogenes*, *L. innocua*, *S. aureus*, *E. coli*, *S. choleraesuis*, and *B. cereus*.[2212]

# CITRON
## (Citron Melon)

*Citrus medica* L., *C. medica* L. cv. 'Diamante,' 'Liscia,' and 'Rugosa'; Fingered Citron, Buddha's Hand: *C. medica* L. var. *sarcodactylis* Swingle

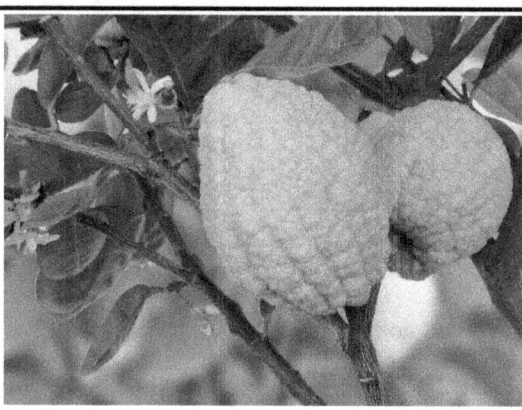

**FAMILY:** Rutaceae
**NOTE:** Top
**AROMA INTENSITY:** Medium
**AROMA:** Citrusy, fruity, sweet, lemon-lime like
**COMMON EXTRACTION METHOD:** Cold pressed/expressed or hydrodistilled from the peel; may also be distilled from the leaves (petitgrain of citron)
**POSSIBLE SUBSTITUTE OILS:** Lime, lemon, bergamot, Persian lime, Mediterranean mandarin
**BLENDS WELL WITH:** African bluegrass, agarwood, amyris, anise, balsam fir, bergamot, bitter orange, cassia, cedarwood, chamomile (German, Roman), cinnamon, citronella, clary sage, clove, copaiba, cypress, davana, frankincense, grapefruit, hinoki, kaffir lime petitgrain, lavandin, lavender, lemon, lime, may chang, melissa, neroli, orange, patchouli, petitgrain, pine, spruce (black), tangerine, ylang ylang
**SUBCELLULAR LOCALIZATION | EPIGENETIC INFLUENCE:** Currently unknown | *Immune/Nervous*
**RECOMMENDED DILUTION RANGE:** 3%–50%; neat for limited conditions

**PRIMARY CONSTITUENTS:**[2213,2214,2215,2216,2217,2218,2219,2220]

| Distilled | | Cold-Pressed/Expressed | |
|---|---|---|---|
| Limonene | 35.4%–67.2% | Limonene | 44.5%–56.6% |
| Gamma-Terpinene | 0.3%–24.5% | Gamma-Terpinene | 21.7%–26.2% |
| Camphene | 0.0%–10.9% | Geranial | 2.9%–6.3% |
| Geranial | 0.1%–8.2% | Neral | 1.1%–3.8% |
| Geraniol | 0.3%–6.6% | | |
| Nerol | 0.0%–5.9% | | |
| Neral | 0.1%–5.7% | | |

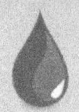

*Fingered Citron, C. medica* L. var. *sarcodactylis (Distilled)*

| | |
|---|---|
| Limonene | 52.4%–59.0% |
| Gamma-Terpinene | 22.5%–28.4% |
| Para-Cymene | 0.0%–5.7% |

**OTHER CONSTITUENTS:** *Hydrodistilled*—Alpha-pinene, beta-pinene, alpha-phellandrene, cis-limonene oxide, alpha-terpineol, neo iso-isopulegol, linalool, endo-fenchyl acetate, neryl acetate, longifolene, alpha-trans-bergamotene, alpha-selinene, eudesm-7(11)-en-4-ol; *Cold-Pressed/Expressed*—Alpha-thujene, alpha-pinene, beta-pinene, myrcene, (Z)-beta-ocimene, (E)-beta-ocimene, terpinolene, alpha-terpineol, beta-bisabolene, neral, citropten; *C. medica* L. var. *sarcodactylis (Distilled)*—Alpha-thujene, alpha-pinene, camphene, beta-pinene, beta-myrcene, alpha-terpinene, benzene, cis-ocimene, beta-ocimene, alpha-terpinolene, alpha-terpinyl acetate, geranial, neral, linalool, trans-p-mentha-2,8-dien-1-ol, terpinen-4-ol, alpha-terpineol

**PREFERRED COMPOSITION FOR CLINICAL USE:**

| Constituent | Distilled | Cold-Pressed/ Expressed | Fingered (var. sarcodactylis) |
|---|---|---|---|
| **Limonene** | 35%–55% | 45%–60% | 50%–60% |
| **Gamma-Terpinene** | 10%–25% | 20%–30% | 22%–32% |
| **Geranial** | 2%–8% | 2%–7% | – |
| **Neral** | 1%–7% | 1%–5% | – |
| **Geraniol** | 1%–7% | – | – |

Note: Higher gamma-terpinene content, like that found in cold-pressed/expressed citron and fingered citron is preferred.

**REPORTED THERAPEUTIC PROPERTIES:** Aids digestion, antifungal, antibacterial, anticancer, expels excess mucus, **anti-inflammatory**, analgesic, antiarthritic, antirheumatic, diuretic, **balances blood sugar levels**, supports cardiovascular function, relieves motion sickness, supports immune function, **aids memory and cognition**, **antidepressant**, stress management, relieves anxiety

**CAUTIONS:**

■ Photosensitizing due to the presence of citropten and bergapten.[2221,2222] Avoid UV rays for at least twelve hours following topical application.

■ May interact with anticholinergic (drugs used for asthma, incontinence, gastrointestinal cramps, muscular spasms, depression, and sleep disorders) and cholinergic medications (drugs used to reduce urinary retention, diagnose myasthenia gravis, and for glaucoma) due to anticholinergic activity of citron essential oil (particularly distilled essential oils).[2223]

■ May interact with diabetic medications and cause hypoglycemia due to insulin secretion and alpha-glucosidase inhibitory properties.[2224,2225]

**SELECTED EVIDENCE:**

☐ Citron essential oil inhibits the growth of neuroblastoma cells better than isolated limonene.[2226] It also selectively kills malignant melanoma cells after 100 minutes of UV radiation exposure, which made the study authors conclude it may be useful for lentigo maligna (an early form of melanoma where the malignant cells are confined to the tissue of origin—the epidermis) and lentigo maligna melanoma (when the malignant cells have invaded the dermis and deeper layers of the skin).[2227]

☐ Citron essential oil significantly increases adenylate cyclase 1 (ADCY1) protein expression (a protein primarily expressed in the brain that is crucial for memory) and, consequently, the intracellular production of cAMP (cyclic adenosine monophosphate).[2228] Increased ADCY1 expression and production of cAMP is associated with improved memory, particularly long-term memory retention. The researchers reported that limonene similarly increased ADCY1 expression and cAMP production.

☐ Animal research demonstrates that fingered citron essential oil increases insulin secretion from the pancreas and, consequently, decreases blood sugar levels.[2229] It also inhibits alpha-glucosidase activity, which was attributed to its high gamma-terpinene content.[2230] Alpha-glucosidase is an enzyme that breaks down carbohydrates by chemical reaction with water. Inhibiting its activity postpones glucose absorption and therefore the impact of carbohydrates on blood sugar levels.

☐ *In vitro* research shows that citron essential oil inhibits *P. aeruginosa*, and moderately inhibits *B. cereus*, *E. coli*, and *S. aureus*.[2231] Fingered citron essential oil inhibits *Enterobacter cloacae*, *E. coli*, *P. aeruginosa*, *K. pneumoniae*, *Proteus mirabilis*, *Bacillus* sp., *Streptococcus* spp., and *S. aureus*.[2232]

☐ Distilled citron essential oil may prevent and manage neurodegenerative diseases caused by oxidative stress by inhibiting acetylcholinesterase (AChE) and butyrylcholinesterase (BChE) enzyme activity.[2233] The cold-pressed essential oil selectively inhibits AChE. Inhibition of AChE prevents the breakdown of acetylcholine, which is essential for memory and thinking. People with neurodegenerative diseases make less acetylcholine, and the diseases often break it down at a faster rate, leading to acetylcholine deficits. Selective inhibition of BChE is also desirable in neurodegenerative diseases because it interferes with acetylcholine activity. In addition, BChE is often found in the plaques and tangles in the brains of people with Alzheimer's disease.[2234]

☐ Citron essential oil (distilled) exerts anti-inflammatory activity by significantly inhibiting excess production of nitric oxide (NO).[2235] Cold-pressed citron moderately inhibits NO production. Excess NO production can cause cellular damage and trigger an abnormal inflammatory response in the joints, gut, and lungs.[2236] Fingered citron also reduces inflammation by inhibiting NO and PGE2 (prostaglandin E2) production, suppressing protein expression of inducible nitric oxide synthase (iNOS) and the COX-2 enzyme, NF-κB activation, and production of TNF-alpha, IL-1 beta, and IL-6.[2237] In addition, it blocked activation of c-Jun N-terminal kinase (JNK) and extracellular signal-regulated kinase (ERK) but not that of p38 mitogen-activated protein kinase in macrophages.

☐ Fingered citron essential oil demonstrated good antioxidant and antimicrobial activity depending on the method of essential oil extraction.[2238] Interestingly, the essential oil obtained by vacuum distillation (47.6% limonene, 29.5% gamma-terpinene) demonstrated the greatest antioxidant activity when compared to hydrodistilled (60.1% limonene, 17.6% para-cymene) and cold-pressed ultrafiltration (64.7% limonene, 26.1% para-cymene) essential oil (descending order of activity: VD > HD > CP). The cold-pressed essential oil was the best antimicrobial, demonstrating notable inhibition of *Staphylococcus aureus*, *Bacillus cereus*, *Pseudomonas aeruginosa*, and *Aspergillus niger*. The vacuum distilled EO was only marginally active against *S. aureus*, *B. cereus*, and *P. aeruginosa*, and strongly active against *A. niger*. The HD oil was the weakest antimicrobial.

☐ Fingered citron essential oil exhibited moderate antibacterial activity against common food-borne bacteria: *Escherichia coli*, *Staphylococcus aureus*, *Bacillus subtilis*, and *Micrococcus luteus*, with better activity against gram-positive than gram-negative bacteria.[2239]

☐ Citron essential oil demonstrated strong antifungal activity against organisms that typically infect ginseng root, which makes it a promising safe and environmentally friendly way to protect ginseng against diseases.

☐ Fingered citron essential oil exhibited strong anti-listerial (*L. monocytogenes*) activity and altered cell morphology and cellular responses.[2240]

☐ Yuzu, bitter orange, and citron essential oils each exhibited good antioxidant activity in the ABTS and DPPH assays.[2241]

☐ Fingered citron essential oil (distilled) exhibited good antioxidant activity in the ABTS assay, buts its activity was weaker in the DPPH assay.[2242] The oil also exhibited antibacterial activity against *B. cereus* but was inactive against *E. coli*. Lastly, the oil was cytotoxic to leukemia cancer cells.

☐ The composition and antioxidant activity of citron essential oil was measured according to ripening stage—green mature (GM), intermediate (INT), yellow ripe (MAT) and overripe stage (OR).[2243] The GM fruit essential oil had the highest limonene content, but the highest antioxidant activity was observed in the OR fruit essential oil.

☐ Thyme CT thymol, cinnamon bark, and tea tree essential oils each inhibited *E. coli* strains isolated from the drinking water of grazing animals in Italy.[2244] Thyme and cinnamon oils showed greater activity than antibiotics used in veterinary and human medicine (repen, macramid, baytril, augmentin, bimixin).

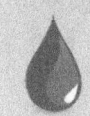

# CITRONELLA
## (Java Citronella, Ceylon Citronella)

Java: *Cymbopogon winterianus* Jowitt ex Bor;
Ceylon: *C. nardus* (L.) Rendle, *Andropogon nardus*

**FAMILY:** Poaceae (Gramineae)
**NOTE:** Top-Middle
**AROMA INTENSITY:** Medium
**AROMA:** Citrusy, slightly fruity, sweet, fresh, clean
**COMMON EXTRACTION METHOD:** Steam distilled from the grass
**POSSIBLE SUBSTITUTE OILS:** Melissa, lemongrass, lemon verbena
**BLENDS WELL WITH:** Bergamot, cedarwood, geranium, grapefruit, lemon, lime, melissa, orange, pine, Spanish sage, tangerine
**SUBCELLULAR LOCALIZATION | EPIGENETIC INFLUENCE:** Currently unknown | Currently unknown
**RECOMMENDED DILUTION RANGE:** 3%–50%; neat for limited conditions

**PRIMARY CONSTITUENTS:**[2245,2246,2247,2248,2249,2250,2251,2252,2253]

| *Ceylon Citronella: C. nardus* | | *Java Citronella: C. winteranius* | |
|---|---|---|---|
| Citronellal | 5.2%–41.3% | Citronellal | 26.5%–42.8% |
| Geraniol | 2.4%–36.5% | Geraniol | 16.2%–40.1% |
| Geranial | 1.2%–22.7% | Elemol | 2.0%–14.5% |
| Neral | 0.0%–14.2% | Citronellol | 5.2%–11.5% |
| Limonene | 0.0%–11.0% | Geranial | 1.5%–8.1% |
| Methyl Isoeugenol | 0.0%–11.0% | Alpha-Cadinol | 0.5%–8.0% |
| Geranyl Acetate | 0.0%–9.7% | Germacrene B | 0.0%–6.8% |
| Citronellol | 4.6%–9.2% | Neral | 0.3%–6.0% |
| Eugenol | 0.0%–8.1% | Geranyl Acetate | 1.8%–4.0% |
| Camphene | 0.0%–8.0% | | |
| Borneol | 0.0%–6.6% | | |
| Beta-Caryophyllene | 0.8%–6.5% | | |
| Elemol | 0.0%–4.8% | | |

**OTHER CONSTITUENTS:** *C. winteranius*—d-limonene, citronellyl acetate, beta-elemene, germacrene A, germacrene D, delta-cadinene, 1,10-di-epi-Cubenol, 1-epi-cubenol, gamma-eudesmol, alpha-muurolol; *C. nardus*—tricyclene, alpha-pinene, cis-ocimene, trans-ocimene, terpinolene, linalyl acetate, nerol, geranyl butyrate, methyl eugenol (<2.0%), linalool, farnesene, naphthalene

**PREFERRED COMPOSITION FOR CLINICAL USE:**

| Constituent | Ceylon | Java/India, Indonesia | Java/Nepal |
|---|---|---|---|
| **Geraniol** | 18%–30% | 17%–25% | 35%–40% |
| **Citronellal** | 3%–15% | 35%–45% | 5%–10% |
| **Limonene** | 5%–12% | 2%–5% | 1%–3% |
| **Camphene** | 5%–10% | – | – |
| **(E)-Methyl Isoeugenol** | 5%–12% | – | – |
| **Citronellol** | 3%–10% | 7%–13% | 7%–12% |
| **Borneol** | 3%–7% | 0%–3% | – |
| **Geranyl Acetate** | 1%–5% | 2%–7% | 1%–4% |
| **Geranial** | 0.1%–5% | 0.1%–8% | 10%–18% |
| **Methyl Eugenol** | < 2% | < 2% | – |

| Citronellyl Acetate | < 2% | 1%–5% | 1%–3% |
|---|---|---|---|
| Elemol | < 2% | 1%–4% | 0.1%–2% |
| Germacrene D | < 2% | 1%–3% | 0.1%–1% |
| Delta-Cadinene | < 2% | 1%–3% | 0.1%–1% |
| Beta-Elemene | < 2% | 0.5%–3% | 0.1%–1% |
| Neral | 0.1%–2% | 0.1%–2% | 7%–12% |
| Beta-Caryophyllene | – | – | 2%–5% |

**REPORTED THERAPEUTIC PROPERTIES:** Antiseptic, aids digestion, **anti-inflammatory**, antibacterial, antifungal, antispasmodic, antioxidant, astringent, anticonvulsive, diuretic, reduces oily skin, **insect repellent**, relieves excess sweating, **deodorant**, nervine (calms and soothes the nerves), analgesic (pain relief), antirheumatic, antiparasitic, calming, clarifying (mentally)

**CAUTIONS:**

■ Caution is advised during pregnancy and lactation due to citral content (low risk). Large doses of citral may negatively affect fetal development according to animal studies.[2254]

■ May interact with diabetes medications and cause low blood sugar based on citronellol, citral, and geraniol content.[2255,2256,2257,2258,2259,2260]

■ There is a low risk that when citronella is taken orally it may interfere with enzymes responsible for metabolizing medications (NSAIDs, proton-pump inhibitors, acetaminophen, antiepileptics, immune modulators, blood-sugar medications, blood pressure medications, antidepressants, antipsychotics, diabetic medications, antihistamines, antibiotics, and anesthetics).[2261,2262,2263,2264,2265,2266]

■ May interfere with medications used to treat high blood pressure (calcium channel blockers) and cause low blood pressure and irregular heart rhythm according to animal research.[2267]

■ May interact with antibiotics and possibly enhance their effects due to citral and geraniol content.[2268]

■ Dilution recommended for topical application due to citral and geraniol content. Geraniol is metabolized and autoxidized into metabolites like geranial and neral (citral) and may cause sensitization and irritation when applied topically.[2269] Citral is a known skin and mucous membrane irritant.[2270,2271]

**SELECTED EVIDENCE:**

☐ *In vitro* research suggests that inhaling the citronellal and citronellol molecules (found in citronella) interacts with cellular receptors, that triggers calcium-signaling pathways in cells, and significantly increases the calcium concentration in liver cancer cells.[2272] Prolonged substantial increases of calcium inside cells triggers apoptosis, reduces the spread of cancer cells, and increases immune cells activity that target and kill cancer cells.[2273]

☐ The primary constituent in citronella, citronellal, increases the pain threshold and relieves pain according to animal research.[2274] Another animal study also concluded that citronella is anti-inflammatory and helps relieve pain.[2275]

☐ Citronella is a potent scavenger of nitric oxide (NO) and superoxide (SO), which helps relieve pain.[2276] Both NO and SO are highly reactive constituents that cause cellular damage that leads to pain and inflammation.

☐ Citronella may promote vasorelaxation and decrease high blood pressure through calcium-channel blocking according to animal research.[2277]

☐ Citronella demonstrates antifungal activity against *Candida albicans* that is similar in action to the antifungal drugs amphotericin B and nystatin.[2278,2279] Another study concluded that *C. winteranius* essential oil significantly reduces the number of viable *C. albicans* organisms and biofilm formation on dentures.[2280]

☐ Animal research suggests that citronella influences central nervous system activity and modulates gamma-aminobutyric acid (GABA) activity to help prevent seizures and convulsions.[2281]

☐ A study determined that a combination of citronella, turmeric, kaffir lime (*C. hystrix*), hairy basil (*O. americanum*), and vanilla could replace DEET (a common chemical insect repellent that is associated with brain cell damage and behavioral changes in animals) as a natural insect repellent.[2282]

☐ *In vitro* research suggests that citronella is a potent antioxidant, and protects against DNA damage caused by hydrogen peroxide and methyl methanesulfonate (an alkylating and cancer-causing agent).[2283]

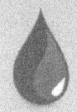

- ☐ Citronellol relieves oral and facial pain by modulating central nervous system activity in mice.[2284]

- ☐ Animal research suggests that citronellol, the primary constituent in citronella essential oil, lowers blood pressure by increasing vasodilation (relaxation of the muscular wall and widening of the blood vessels).[2285]

- ☐ Ceylon citronella repels or kills the larvae of the mosquitos *Anopheles minimus, Aedes aegypti, Culex pipiens, Cx. Quinquefasciatus, Anopheles minimus*, and *An. dirus*, which are mosquitoes that carry and transmit diseases such as malaria, zika virus, dengue fever virus, and West Nile virus.[2286,2287,2288,2289,2290,2291,2292] Another study concluded that mixtures of primary constituents found in Ceylon citronella (citral, myrcene, and citronellal oil) act as a more effective repellent than DEET.[2293]

- ☐ Inhalation of Ceylon citronella decreased appetite and body weight in rats.[2294]

- ☐ Ceylon citronella completely kills lice eggs resistant to the standard drug option (Permethrin) according to *in vitro* research.[2295]

- ☐ *In vitro* research demonstrates that Ceylon citronella significantly inhibits the oral pathogens *Porphyromonas gingivalis* and *Aggregatibacter actinomycetemcomitans* and moderately inhibits *Streptococcus mutans*, which is a causal factor of cavities.[2296] It also markedly prevents *C. albicans* from adhering to dental implants and cover screws, without harming the probiotic l-acidophilus.[2297]

- ☐ Ceylon citronella demonstrated significant antifungal activity against *Pyricularia (Magnaporthe) grisea, Aspergillus* spp., *and Colletotrichum musae*.[3881] Another study found that it inhibits *Aspergillus niger*.[2298]

- ☐ *In vitro* research concluded that Ceylon citronella prevented trypanosomiasis (a disease caused by *T. brucei* and characterized fever, headache, joint pain, itching, confusion, and lack of coordination) by selectively killing cells infected by parasites.[2299]

- ☐ Ceylon citronella kills the ticks *Amblyomma cajennense* and *Anocentor nitens*.[2300]

- ☐ Animal research demonstrates that oral administration of Ceylon citronella relieves pain.[2301]

- ☐ *In vitro* research reports that Ceylon citronella inhibits the bacterium *Pseudomonas putida* (an uncommon bacterial cause of skin and soft tissue infections).[2302]

- ☐ Thyme, clove, and java citronella exhibited toxicity against Turkestan cockroach nymphs.[2303] Thymol was the most toxic essential oil constituent, followed by trans-cinnamaldehyde, eugenol, para-cymene, geraniol, and methyl eugenol.

- ☐ Fungal pathogens have caused significant declines in economically and agriculturally important animal species, like bees and bats. Current drug antifungals have limited use due to their toxicity to sensitive animal species. Cinnamon bark, citronella, and lemongrass essential oils each significantly inhibited *Ascosphaera apis* and *Pseudogymnoascus destructans*, the causative agents of chalkbrood disease among honeybee larvae and white-nose syndrome among bats, respectively.[2304]

- ☐ Lemongrass (*C. citratus*) and citronella (*C. nardus*) essential oils exhibited larvicidal activity against the Asian blue tick (*Rhipicephalus microplus*), while corn mint essential oil was toxic to engorged females.[2305]

- ☐ *Toxoplasma gondii* is a parasite excreted in cat feces. Humans can accidentally ingest the parasites if they come in contact with cat feces and then touch their mouth, causing toxoplasmosis. A laboratory study found that lemongrass (*C. citratus*), marjoram, and citronella (*C. nardus*) inhibited *T. gondii*, with citronella having a high selectivity index.[2306] Based on this, the authors concluded that citronella may be a potential solution for treating toxoplasmosis.

- ☐ Sweet orange, citronella (*C. nardus*), and tea tree essential oils were the most effective nematocidal agents against the southern root-nematode (*Meloidogyne incognita*) of eight essential oils tested.[2307]

- ☐ Pulmonary fibrosis is a lung disease in which the lungs become scarred over time leading to shortness of breath and dry cough. Researchers evaluated the effects of citronella (*C. winterianus*) essential oil in a rat model of pulmonary fibrosis. Oral administration of citronella oil significantly reduced inflammatory markers in bronchoalveolar lavage fluid, reduced signs of oxidative stress (malondialdehyde), and increased antioxidant enzyme (superoxide dismutase) activity.[2308] Additionally, the oil reduced tissue scarring in the lungs. The researchers concluded that the results suggest citronella essential oil "is a potential candidate to be used as a phytotherapeutic in further clinical trials for the treatment of pulmonary fibrosis."

- ☐ Lemongrass (*C. flexuosus*), citronella (*C. winterianus*), and palmarosa essential oil each exhibited activity against MRSA, with the strongest activity observed with lemongrass oil.[2309] Isolated citronellol, citral, and geraniol were also active, with the efficacy of citronellol exceeding whole oils.

- ☐ *Lutzomyia longipalpis* is the most relevant sandfly species for the transmission of visceral leishmaniasis in the

Americas. Researchers investigated the repellent effects of citronella, neem, white verbena CT citral, and *Lippia thymoides* against the sand fly.[2310] Higher concentrations of all oils except neem reduced sand fly biting. Moreover, computer-based molecular docking studies showed that citronellol, citronellyl acetate, citronellal, and geranyl acetate had similar binding interactions with the binding site of DEET (OBP4).

- ☐ Citronella (*C. nardus*) essential oil inhibited the growth and production of mycotoxins by *A. flavus*, *A. carbonarius*, and *F. verticillioides* (aflatoxin B1, ochratoxin A, and fumonisin B1, respectively) in both vapor and liquid phase.[2311]

- ☐ Both lavender and citronella essential oil significantly impaired the feeding activity of the armyworm (*Mythimna separata*) larvae.[2312] Rosemary showed the best repellent activity, while tea tree and lemon essential oil had the best fumigant contact activity.

- ☐ Citronella demonstrated noticeable antimicrobial activity against *S. aureus*, *S. epidermidis*, *S. pyogenes*, *C. albicans*, *M. canis*, and *T. mentagrophytes*.[2313]

# CLARY SAGE
## (Europe Sage)

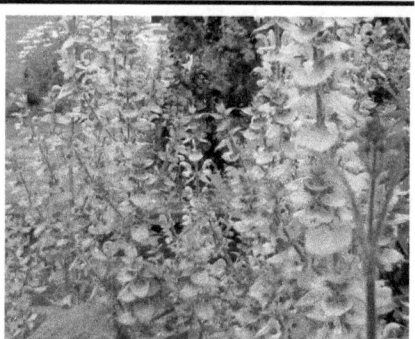

*Salvia sclarea* L., *Salvia sclarea* L. var. *turkestaniana* Mottet

**FAMILY:** Lamiaceae (Labiatae)
**NOTE:** Middle
**AROMA INTENSITY:** Medium
**AROMA:** Musky, herbal, sharp, warm
**COMMON EXTRACTION METHOD:** Steam distilled from the flowers and leaves
**POSSIBLE SUBSTITUTE OILS:** Bergamot, geranium, petitgrain, basil (Linalool CT), chaste tree, equal parts nutmeg and sage
**BLENDS WELL WITH:** Balsam fir, bay laurel, bergamot, black pepper, black spruce, blue spruce, cajeput, cedarwood, chamomile (German Roman), copaiba, coriander, grapefruit, juniper, lemon, lime, lavender, tea tree, neroli, orange, pine, sandalwood, petitgrain, palo santo, ravensara, rose, Spanish sage, spikenard, tangerine, turmeric
**SUBCELLULAR LOCALIZATION | EPIGENETIC INFLUENCE:** Basal Membrane | Currently unknown
**RECOMMENDED DILUTION RANGE:** 3%–20%; 50% for some conditions

**PRIMARY CONSTITUENTS:**[2314,2315,2316,2317,2318,2319,2320]

| | |
|---|---|
| Linalyl Acetate | 16.9%  60.8% |
| Linalool | 12.8%–38.6% |
| Alpha-Terpineol | 1.8%–14.3% |
| Germacrene D | 1.3%–13.3% |
| Geranyl Acetate | 3.8%–12.1% |
| Sclareol | 1.3%–11.5% |
| Epimanoyl oxide | 0.0%–8.6% |
| Beta-Caryophyllene | 3.2%–5.1% |

**OTHER CONSTITUENTS:** Myrcene, (Z)-beta-ocimene, (E)-beta-ocimene, nerol, neryl acetate, alpha-copaene, beta-cubebene, beta-elemene, bicyclogermacrene, delta-cadinene, beta-eudesmol, alpha-eudesmol, sclareol oxide, 1-docosene

**PREFERRED COMPOSITION FOR CLINICAL USE:**

| Constituent | USA/Bulgarian/French | Indian/Russian |
|---|---|---|
| **Linalyl Acetate** | 52%–78% | 45%–55% |
| **Linalool** | 10%–25% | 15%–30% |
| **Germacrene D** | 0.5%–10% | 0%–3% |
| **Sclareol** | 0.1%–10% | 0%–0.5% |
| **Beta-Caryophyllene** | 0.5%–5% | 1%–5% |

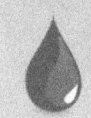

| | | |
|---|---|---|
| Alpha-Terpineol | 0.5%–5% | 1%–5% |
| Geranyl Acetate | 0.5%–5% | 1%–3% |
| Geraniol | 0%–2% | 1%–3% |

Note: plants grown in the USA may yield higher percentages of sclareol.

**REPORTED THERAPEUTIC PROPERTIES:** Antibacterial, **balances estrogenic hormones**, antiseptic, antispasmodic, aphrodisiac, antiviral, **relieves painful menstruation and menstrual cramps**, expels excess gas, astringent, aids digestion, **euphoric**, nervine (calms and soothes the nerves), wound healing, sedating, **encourages a restful night's sleep**, **antidepressant**, reduces anxiety, stress management, promotes inspiration, combats confusion and despondency

**CAUTIONS:**

■ Clary sage contains the phytoestrogen sclareol, which can either block or mimic the action of estrogen according to current knowledge. Some aromatherapists have contraindicated clary sage with estrogen-dependent cancers because of this. However, the available research does not suggest that clary sage increases the risk of estrogen-dependent cancers.[2321,2322,2323,2324,2325] In fact, one study determined that while the presence of estradiol increased breast cancer cell proliferation with or without phytoestrogens, when only phytoestrogens were present breast cancer cell apoptosis increased.[2326] Another study found that the dietary phytoestrogen genistein (from soy) reversed BRCA1 gene deficiency—the dysfunction of which is strongly associated with breast cancer—and triggered the expression of apoptosis-related genes.[2327]

■ Another concern with sclareol is that it may interfere with hormone replacement therapy. Theoretically clary sage could increase estradiol levels and potentiate the action of estrogen-replacement drugs. Because sclareol exerts much weaker estrogenic effects than the hormones administered during hormone replacement therapy, it is highly unlikely that it will interact with hormone-replacement therapy. In general, phytoestrogens are balancing in nature, but women who are undergoing hormone replacement therapy should have their estradiol levels checked regularly and consult with a physician before using clary sage.

■ Avoid with barbiturates. Some evidence suggests that clary sage may increase the sedating effects of barbiturates like hexobarbital.[2328]

**SELECTED EVIDENCE:**

☐ A daily abdominal massage with a combination of lavender, clary sage, and marjoram (2:1:1 ratio) from the end of the last menstruation to the beginning of the next menstruation significantly reduced painful menstruation according to a randomized, double-blind clinical trial.[2329] Another study found that menstrual cramps were alleviated when 2 drops of lavender, and 1 drop each of clary sage, and rose in 5 mL of almond oil was applied to the abdomen.[2330] Menstrual cramps were also reduced in high school girls that received a 10-minute abdominal massage with clary sage, marjoram, cinnamon, ginger, and geranium (1.5:1.5:1:1 ratio) diluted to a 5% concentration in almond carrier oil.[2331]

☐ The topical application of lavender and clary sage oils reduced work-related stress in intensive care unit nurses during three twelve-hour shifts.[2332]

☐ Animal research suggests clary sage influences dopamine activity, which may help relieve depression.[2333]

☐ Clary sage may reduce anxiety, fear, and pain during labor.[2334]

☐ Clary sage moderately reduces inflammation (the whole oil was more effective than individual constituents suspected to be active and responsible for the therapeutic activity of clary sage).[2335]

☐ *In vitro* research suggests that clary sage oil inhibits tetracycline resistant *S. epidermidis* (a gram-positive bacterium that lives on the skin associated with foreign body infections) and increases the effectiveness of tetracycline against the bacterial strain.[2336]

☐ *In vitro* research demonstrates that clary sage essential oil effectively inhibits *L. amazonensis*.[2337]

☐ Oral administration of clary sage essential oil rich in linalool (38.1%) and alpha-terpineol (13.4%) and poor in linalyl acetate (1.0%) demonstrated significant antidiabetic activity at all tested doses (50, 100, and 200 mg/kg BW) in diabetic mice.[2338] The essential oil reduced blood glucose levels by 42.3%, 44.7%, and 51.7% at the respective doses. Interestingly, the scientists compared two clary sage oils, and the second oil with 35.3% linalyl acetate and 10.8% linalool was less effective, reducing blood glucose levels 31.0%, 40.5%,

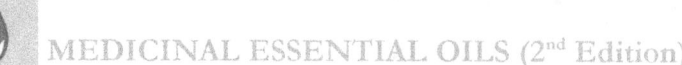

and 42.0% respectively. Further analysis found that isolated linalool reduces blood glucose levels better than isolated linalyl acetate.

- *In vitro* research concluded that clary sage essential oil may be beneficial for wound healing and skin infections due to its antibacterial activity against *Staphylococci* responsible for wound infections.[2339] The study found that clary sage oil was active against *Staphylococcus aureus, S. epidermidis*, and *S. xylosus*.
- Inhalation of clary sage essential oil—0.1 mL on a gauze for 5 minutes—demonstrated an antidepressant-like effect in healthy and depressed menopausal women.[2340] Serotonin levels significantly increased in both healthy women and women with depressive tendencies, but a greater reduction in cortisol was observed in the depressed group (31% versus 16%).
- Topical application of clary sage essential oil diluted in peanut oil to the forearm lead to an increase in heart rate in women, but decreased heart rate in men.[2341] A second experiment by the same group of researchers showed that inhalation of clary sage for thirty minutes decreased pulse rate in both men and women, but the effect was stronger in women than men. The study demonstrates that clary sage essential oil differentially affects men and women.
- Clary sage essential oil was weakly toxic to *Ae. albopictus* mosquitoes, but showed significant repellency.[2342]
- A preclinical model of painful menstruation (dysmenorrhea) and menstrual cramps found that sclareol isolated from clary sage essential oil reduced uterine contractions.[2343] Injection of sclareol inhibited uterine contractions caused by prostaglandin F2α, oxytocin, acetylcholine, carbachol, potassium chloride, and Bay K 8644.
- Clary sage essential oil inhibited clinical and laboratory strains of *S. aureus, E. faecalis, S. pyogenes, E. coli*, and *C. albicans*.[2344]
- Clary sage essential oil with an odd chemistry (6.9% 9-octadecenoic acid, 5.7% n-butyl octadecenoate, 4.7% linalyl acetate, 3.4% octadecanal) demonstrated moderate tyrosinase inhibitory activity *in vitro*, suggesting it may benefit hyperpigmentation of the skin.[2345]
- Clary sage essential oil displayed low antioxidant activity in the DPPH and ABTS assays, moderate antimicrobial activity (*B. subtilis, C. albicans, A. flavus, B. cinerae, P. citrinum, C. glabrata, P. aeruginosa, C. krusei, C. tropicalis, E. faecalis, S. aureus*), good antibiofilm activity (*P. fluorescens*), and good insecticidal activity against the lime seed bug (*Oxycarenus lavatera*).[2346] Isolated beta-caryophyllene was less effective than the whole oil against microbes.

---

# CLOVE BUD

*Syzygium aromaticum* (L.) Merr. & L.M. Perry,
*Eugenia caryophyllata* (Spreng.) Bullock & S. Harrison

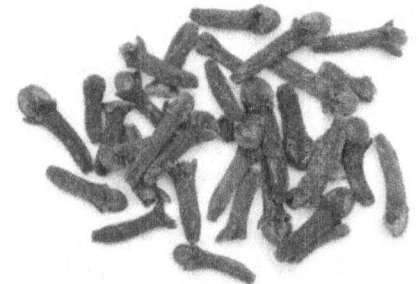

**FAMILY:** Myrtaceae
**NOTE:** Middle
**AROMA INTENSITY:** Medium
**AROMA:** Spicy, warm, slightly fruity
**COMMON EXTRACTION METHOD:** Steam distilled from the flower buds (lesser quality oils also use the flowers, stems, and leaves)
**POSSIBLE SUBSTITUTE OILS:** Black pepper, oregano
**BLENDS WELL WITH:** Black pepper, Cardamom, coriander, cinnamon, cajeput, eucalyptus, ginger, rosemary, Spanish sage, spikenard, turmeric
**SUBCELLULAR LOCALIZATION | EPIGENETIC INFLUENCE:** Cytoplasm, Mitochondria | Muscular/Reproductive
**RECOMMENDED DILUTION RANGE:** 1.5%–20%; 50% for some conditions

**PRIMARY CONSTITUENTS:**[2347,2348,2349,2350,2351,2352]

| Bud | | Leaves | |
|---|---|---|---|
| Eugenol | 69.8%–87.0% | Eugenol | 87.5%–98.8% |
| Eugenyl Acetate | 5.0%–21.3% | Beta-Caryophyllene | 0.5%–9.7% |
| Beta-Caryophyllene | 3.1%–13.0% | Eugenyl Acetate | 0.1%–2.5% |

Note: Clove leaf essential oil is generally only used for industrial purposes due to its very high eugenol content.

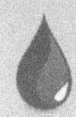

OTHER CONSTITUENTS: *Bud*—Alpha-humulene, beta-caryophyllene oxide, alpha-humulene, epoxide, alpha-pinene, camphene, myrcene, alpha-terpinene, para-cymene, limonene, terpinen-4-ol, thymol, alpha-copaene, terpinolene, beta-phellandrene, methyl salicylate ($< 0.6\%$); *Leaves*—Caryophyllene oxide, humulene, methyl salicylate ($< 0.4\%$), iso-eugenol

## PREFERRED COMPOSITION FOR CLINICAL USE:

| Constituent | Bud |
| --- | --- |
| Eugenol | 72%–85% |
| Eugenyl Acetate | 8%–15% |
| Beta-Caryophyllene | 3%–10% |

**REPORTED THERAPEUTIC PROPERTIES: Analgesic**, anti-aging, antifungal, **aids digestion**, expels excess gas, anti-inflammatory, reduces the appearance of blemishes, **antimicrobial**, **antiviral**, antispasmodic, **antioxidant**, **antiseptic**, stimulates the production of glutathione S-transferase, expectorant, aids circulation, anticancer, stimulates brain function, purifies the blood, helps balance blood-sugar levels, **antiparasitic**, anesthetic, insect repellent, decongestant, stimulating, aphrodisiac, stress management, promotes self-confidence, self-assurance, and courage

## CAUTIONS:

■ Caution with pregnancy and lactation. Animal studies suggest that large doses of clove may negatively impact embryonic development and encourage fetal cell death.[2353,2354] Another animal study did not detect any negative influence of clove oil.[2355] Eugenol is considered strongly toxic to embryos according to animal studies.[2356] Based on these studies it is best to limit clove oil during pregnancy and lactation.

■ May interact with aspirin, blood pressure, antiplatelet, and anticoagulant medications, and increase the risk of bleeding among people with bleeding disorders.[2357,2358,2359,2360]

■ May interact with MAOI antidepressants. Animal research suggests that eugenol produces antidepressant effects via the monoamine oxidase pathway, which may cause interactions with antidepressants that also interact with this pathway.[2361]

■ May interact with antibiotics and possibly enhance their effects due to eugenol content.[2362]

■ May interfere with enzymes responsible for metabolizing medications (NSAIDs, proton-pump inhibitors, acetaminophen, antiepileptics, immune modulators, blood-sugar medications, blood pressure medications, antidepressants, antipsychotics, diabetic medications, antihistamines, antibiotics, and anesthetics) based on eugenol content.[2363]

■ May interact with anticholinergic (drugs used for asthma, incontinence, gastrointestinal cramps, muscular spasms, depression, and sleep disorders) and cholinergic medications (drugs used to reduce urinary retention, diagnose myasthenia gravis, and for glaucoma) based on AChE inhibitory activity of eugenol.[2364]

■ May irritate mucous membranes (eyes, mouth, nasal passages, vagina, rectum).[2365,2366]

■ Extreme oral doses (greater than 5 mL in a single dose) of clove have caused toxicity and serious adverse events (usually liver failure).[2367,2368,2369,2370] Typical doses of clove essential oil should not cause the same problem, nor be a concern.

## SELECTED EVIDENCE:

&#9633; Clove demonstrated excellent activity against breast, colorectal, lung, cervical, ER+ breast, prostate, esophageal, and leukemia cancer cells *in vitro*.[2371,2372,2373,2374 642–644A] Eugenol modulates gene expression and pathways to prevent skin cancer in mice.[2375]

&#9633; Both clove oil and eugenol significantly inhibit the acetylcholinesterase enzyme (AChE) from breaking down acetylcholine.[2376] This activity may be beneficial to a number of neurological disorders including Alzheimer's disease, myasthenia gravis, Lewy body dementia, and schizophrenia.

&#9633; Clove causes the programmed cell death (apoptosis) of *Leishmania donovani* promastigotes (an intracellular parasitic protozoa).[2377,2378]

&#9633; *In vitro* research suggests that clove oil is a strong inhibitor of the bacterium *P. acnes*, which is suspected of being the major bacterium that causes acne.[2379]

&#9633; Eugenol (the main constituent of clove oil) blocks the action of multiple proinflammatory molecules involved

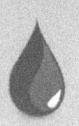

in arthritis according to animal research.[2380] Based on these activities the researchers concluded that clove "could be useful as a beneficial supplement in treating human arthritis." Another study concluded that clove oil provided an equivalent anti-inflammatory effect to the NSAID etodolac.[2381]

- Clove oil modulates and stimulates immune system activity by increasing white blood cell count and reducing inflammation by inhibiting the production and activity of proinflammatory cytokines.[2382,2383,2384] The same research discovered that it also restores cellular and humoral immune responses in animals immunosuppressed by cyclophosphamide (a medication used to treat several types of cancer that suppresses the immune system).

- Clove oil and eugenol stimulate the production of the mucosal lining of the stomach and protect against ulcers according to animal research.[2385]

- *In vitro* research suggests that clove oil can destroy *Candida albicans* (including drug-resistant *C. albicans*) and prevent recurrent infections associated with the growth of *C. albicans*.[2386,2387] It also significantly inhibits *Aspergillus* species and their subsequent production of mycotoxins.[2388] Another study demonstrated that clove essential oil completely inhibited mycelial growth and spore germination of the wilt causing fungus *Fusarium oxysporum* f. sp. *lycopersici* 1322.[2389] Interestingly, clove was more potent than eucalyptus, lemongrass, and peppermint essential oils.

- *In vitro* research concluded that clove oil inhibits the murine norovirus (a norovirus that affects mice but is used in research to study the effects of drugs and other remedies against human norovirus).[2390]

- Low doses of clove oil significantly prevented lipid peroxidation of the membranes and the premature destruction (hemolysis) of red blood cells in mice.[2391]

- Animal research suggests that clove oil may improve cognitive function and enhance memory retention.[2392]

- A case report describes the use of a combination of the essential oil of lemongrass, eucalyptus, tea tree, clove, thyme and BHT, triclosan, and undenatured alcohol to treat a chronic infection of the lower tibia (osteomyelitis) that was not responding to several courses of IV antibiotics. Amputation of the lower leg was being considered when a physician recommended the leg be opened up and the combination inserted directly into the bone (through a drilled hole, 1 mL per day for forty-eight hours). At three months, the wound and bone healed, and symptoms were resolved.[2393]

- Clove oil prevents infection with and kills giardial parasites in a laboratory setting.[2394]

- Animal research suggests that clove oil reduces depression by enhancing hippocampal pathways that modify mood and encourage adaptive behaviors.[2395]

- A foot bath (107°F water) with salts and either oregano, thyme, cinnamon bark, lemongrass, clove, palmarosa, peppermint, lavender, or geranium significantly reduced fungi associated with athlete's foot *in vitro*.[2396]

- Clove oil helps decrease inflammation by mildly inhibiting the 5-lipoxygenase (5-LOX) enzyme that is involved in the inflammation response according to *in vitro* research.[2397]

- Of twenty-one essential oils tested, clove was second only to cinnamon as an inhibitor of *S. aureus, B. subtilis, K. pneumoniae, P. vulgaris, P. aeruginosa,* and *E. coli.*[2398] Clove essential oil strongly inhibited *Pseudomonas aeruginosa, Staphylococcus aureus, Escherichia coli,* and four yeasts: *Torulopsis utilis, Schizosaccharomyces pombe, Candida albicans,* and *Saccharomyces cerevisiae.*[2399] Clove essential oil significantly inhibited clinical and foodborne *Candida* strains (including antibiotic-resistant strains).[2400] Clove essential oil strongly inhibits *C. jejuni* (a gram-negative bacterium that is one of the most common causes of food poisoning in the U.S.) and reduces its virulence (the ability of a microbe to cause disease and damage to a host).[2401]

- Clove and eugenol prevent the production of melanin in melanoma cells.[2402] The presence of melanin may facilitate the development of melanoma if exposed to UV radiation.[2403]

- A combination of clove and thyme oil prevents the degradation of lipids in the skin caused by UV exposure and oxidative damage.[2404]

- Clove oil and its constituents (eugenol, beta-caryophyllene, beta-caryophyllene oxide, alpha-humulene epoxide, and alpha-humulene) found in clove oil may help prevent dental cavities.[2405,2406] The same researchers found that these constituents significantly increased glutathione S-transferase activity.

- Eugenol reduces the growth of cells inside portal tracts of livers and inflammation of the bile ducts in rats with cholestasis (when the flow of bile is slowed or blocked).[2407]

- Eugenol effectively kills scabies mites, which cause an itchy skin rash.[2408]

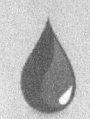

- ☐ An *in vitro* study that tested the antimicrobial activity of fifty-one essential oils showed that all fifty-one demonstrated activity against at least one of the seven organisms (13 essential oils—*Ps. aeruginosa*, unidentified number against *S. aureus*, but it was the second most resistant microbe, 20—*E. coli*, 47—*C. albicans*, 49—*S. pombe*, and 50—*S. cerevisiae* and *T. utilis*).[2409] The study authors pointed out that clove, cinnamon, and thyme essential oils demonstrated significant inhibition, inhibiting greater than 50% reduction in all organisms, and greater than 90% reduction in two or more organisms. Thyme inhibited all organisms at greater than 94% except for *E. coli* and *Ps. Aeruginosa*.

- ☐ Injection of a 0.5% solution (in saline and Tween 80) of clove essential oil, alone or with lidocaine, to the eye significantly reduced acute corneal pain and sensitivity.[2410] Administration of the same solution into the eye also produced a local anesthetic effect.

- ☐ *In vitro* research demonstrated that low doses of marjoram, lemon, basil, clove, thyme, rosemary CT 1,8-cineole, and tea tree essential oils prevented the shortening of telomeres after exposure to hydrogen peroxide.[2411] The same research reported that vetiver, black pepper, eucalyptus (*E. globulus*), ginger, clove, and rosemary increased the length of already shortened telomeres. This activity suggests that these essential oils can help maintain the youth and health of cells, or turn back the clock on the cell to make it more youthful depending on the essential oil used. Interestingly, cinnamon and peppermint essential oil decreased the length of telomeres slightly.

- ☐ *In vitro* research suggests clove oil effectively kills head lice.[2412] Clove was the third most effective essential oil of six tested.

- ☐ An oral gel with clove and thyme essential oils and eugenol and thymol as the primary ingredients demonstrated considerable antifungal activity against *Candida* species, which caused the study authors to conclude that it was a promising product for reduction of oral candidiasis.[2413]

- ☐ An interesting clove bud oil with beta-pinene (45.4%), 1,8-cineole (16.3%), and alpha-pinene (13.1%) as the primary constituents inhibited key enzymes (alpha-amylase, alpha-glucosidase) involved in diabetes in rats, and prevented the oxidation of lipids because it increased the animal's antioxidant defenses.[2414]

- ☐ *In vitro* research demonstrates that clove essential oil is a potent antioxidant and inhibits the excess production of nitric oxide and myeloperoxidase activity (an enzyme that causes oxidation of cholesterol, increases arterial inflammation, and encourages plaque formation in the arteries, all of which increases your risk of heart disease).[2415]

- ☐ Animal research suggests that clove essential oil may restore brain dopamine function by increasing dopamine transporter activity (DAT) in abstinent former drug users.[2416] Drug abuse causes neurobiological changes to the dopamine system, which are linked to relapse and withdrawal symptoms.

- ☐ Clove essential oil significantly inhibited the *C. jejuni* bacterium that is one of the world's most common cases of the stomach flu (gastroenteritis) and *H. pylori* (a pathogen linked to stomach ulcers).[2417]

- ☐ Several essential oils listed in order of efficacy killed the itch mite (*Sarcoptes scabiei*) that burrows into the skin and causes scabies during direct contact (clove > palmarosa > geranium > tea tree > lavender > manuka > petitgrain > eucalyptus > Japanese cedarwood) with the mites and when used as a fumigant (tea tree > clove > eucalyptus > lavender > palmarosa > geranium > Japanese cedarwood > petitgrain > manuka).[2418]

- ☐ Clove essential oil inhibits the gram-positive meat spoilage bacterium *Brochothrix thermosphacta*.[2419]

- ☐ Clove essential oil killed the *Aedes aegypti* and *Anopheles dirus* during immature and larval stages.[2420]

- ☐ Eugenol strongly repelled the body louse (*Pediculus humanus corporis*). Its repellent effects were enhanced when combined with beta-caryophyllene.[2421]

- ☐ Clove essential oil inhibits *S. aureus* by penetrating the bacterial membrane, entering the bacterial cell, destroying its outer cell structure, and then inhibiting the creation of DNA and proteins necessary for bacterial growth.[2422]

- ☐ *In vitro* research demonstrates that clove essential oil is highly antifungal against clinical and foodborne *Candida* strains, including those resistant to antibiotics.[2423]

- ☐ *In vitro* research remonstrates that clove is potently bactericidal against clinical isolates of multidrug-resistant *A. baumannii*.[2424]

- ☐ Clove bud and red thyme essential oil both repelled *Dermacentor reticulatus* ticks at a 3% concentration.[2425] Clove bud was more effective (83% repellency) than red thyme (68% repellency).

- ☐ Spearmint (carvone CT and rich in eugenol), thyme (thymol CT), and clove essential oils all killed head lice, with spearmint being the most effective.[2426]

- Both eugenol and clove essential oil caused 100 percent mortality of cattle tick (*Rhipicephalus microplus*) larvae at low concentrations and 100 percent mortality of adults in higher concentrations.[2427]
- Clove essential oil reduced pain and improved the pain-relieving activity of the NSAID ketorolac.[2428]
- Clove essential oil inhibited *Aspergillus niger* in stored wheat grains without harming the wheat, which made the study authors conclude that clove essential oil could be used as an eco-friendly antifungal product to protect stored wheat.[2429]
- Thyme, clove, and java citronella exhibited toxicity against Turkestan cockroach nymphs.[2430] Thymol was the most toxic essential oil constituent, followed by trans-cinnamaldehyde, eugenol, para-cymene, geraniol, and methyl eugenol.
- Both clove essential oil and eugenol demonstrated activity against the periodontal pathogen *Porphyromonas gingivalis*, which lead the study authors to conclude that it was a viable option to prevent periodontitis.[2431] *Porphyromonas gingivalis* is a major pathogen responsible for the initiation and progression of severe forms of periodontal disease.
- Eugenol obtained from clove essential oil may help prevent the progression of breast cancer by altering cellular energy metabolism pathways according to laboratory research.[2432] Eugenol selectively killed breast cancer cells and reduced ATP (energy) production in breast cancer cells.
- Clove essential oil significantly inhibited the increased production of several proinflammatory molecules (vascular cell adhesion molecule-1 (VCAM-1), interferon γ-induced protein 10 (IP-10), interferon-inducible T-cell α chemoattractant (I-TAC), and monokine induced by γ interferon (MIG)) and tissue remodeling protein molecules (collagen-I, collagen-III, macrophage colony-stimulating factor (M-CSF), and tissue inhibitor of metalloproteinase 2 (TIMP-2)), and significantly modulated gene expression and signaling pathways essential for inflammation, tissue, remodeling, and cancer signaling in a model of chronic inflammation and fibrosis.[2433]
- A review study concluded that clove, tea tree, oregano, thyme, and lemon essential oils have potential to improve indoor air quality by reducing the presence of fungi and molds.[2434]
- Chagas disease is caused by *Trypanosoma cruzi* (a parasite that feeds on blood and lymph) and considered a serious public health concern.[2435] Clove essential oil (CEO), alone or in combination with standard drug treatment (benznidazole, BZ), cured mice of oral chagas disease in the following ascending order: CEO = 12.5%, BZ = 25.0%, and CEO+BZ = 37.5%.
- Oral administration of clove essential oil significantly alleviated histopathological (dilatation in the central vein of the liver, inflammation and binucleation—cells that contain two nuclei commonly found in cancer cells—in the liver, congestion and hemorrhage in the brain, and congestion in the kidney) and biological (blood urea, liver enzymes, total cholesterol, LDL, VLDL, HDL, triglycerides, total protein, and albumin) changes caused by oxidative stress in rats.[2436] The research suggests that the antioxidant properties of clove protect the liver, brain, and kidneys against toxicity. A mixture of clove and argan oil was also very effective.
- *Sarcoptes scabiei* is a mite that causes skin diseases in humans and animals. The few drug treatments available for human infection are poorly effective and the ones used for animals are challenged with increasing development of resistance. Clove essential oil killed all mites within twenty minutes during direct contact of a 1% dilution.[2437] It was also effective in fumigation tests. Other essential oils that performed well in the contact and fumigant bioassays include palmarosa, tea tree, and eucalyptus. Tea tree was the most effective essential oil in the fumigant test.
- Human aryl hydrocarbon receptor (AhR: a gene that encodes a protein that helps regulate responses to planar aromatic hydrocarbons and significantly affects the immune activity in the gastrointestinal tract) regulates the circadian rhythm, helps regulate the cell cycle, and plays an important role in tissue development. Cumin, jasmine, vanilla, and bay leaf fully activate AhR; clove, dill, thyme, nutmeg, and oregano partially activate AhR; and tarragon, caraway, turmeric, lovage, fennel, spearmint, star anise, and anise inhibit the AhR activity.[2438]
- *In vitro* research showed that clove essential oil inhibited bacteria (96.7 percent of which were multidrug resistant) isolated from people with ocular infections, including *S. aureus*, which caused the study authors to conclude it could be helpful in ocular bacterial infections.[2439]
- Thyme CT gamma-terpinene, lemon CT citral, geranium CT p-menthone, cassia CT cinnamaldehyde, clove CT eugenol, and basil CT 1,8-cineole each demonstrated fungistatic and fungicidal activity toward *C. albicans* and *C. glabrata* isolates with cassia demonstrated the highest activity.[2440]
- Cinnamon, clove, oregano, and red thyme essential oils effectively inhibited multidrug-resistant *Salmonella enterica* (a cause of foodborne illness) and enhanced the activity of antibiotics (enrofloxacin, ceftiofur, and trimethoprim-sulfamethoxazole).[2441] The most effective combination was cinnamon with enrofloxacin

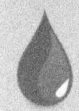

reducing the minimum inhibitory concentration (MIC) of cinnamon from 1250 to 312.5 µg/mL and the MIC of ENR from 2 to 0.031 µg/mL.

- Clove essential oil is significantly active against the bacterial pathogen *S. mutans*, which is associated with dental cavities.[2442]
- Cinnamon bark essential oil was the most effective essential oil of seven tested (clove, cinnamon bark, eucalyptus, thyme CT thymol, Scots pine, peppermint, and citronella) against respiratory tract pathogens (*Streptococcus pneumoniae, S. mutans, S. pyogenes, Haemophilus influenzae, H. parainfluenzae,* and *Moraxella catarrhalis*) in vapor phase.[2443] In liquid phase, thyme was most effective against *S. mutans*, and cinnamon and clove significantly inhibited *S. pneumoniae* and *S. pyogenes*.
- Solid lipid nanoparticles with clove essential oil demonstrated greater inhibition of human pathogens (*Salmonella typhi, Pseudomonas aeruginosa, Staphylococcus aureus,* and *Candida albicans*) than the oil alone in *in vitro* research.[2444]
- Both cinnamon CT eugenol and clove essential oil were toxic to the wheat weevil (*Sitophilus granarius*).[2445] Eugenol was the most toxic to the weevil of the major constituents tested.
- Clove essential oil was moderately toxic to *Culex pipiens* mosquitoes when used as a fumigant.[2446]
- A clove oil-in-water nanoemulsion significantly enhanced the antifungal and mycotoxin inhibitory activity of clove essential oil when compared to nonnanoemulsion oil.[2447]
- Clove bud and thyme CT thymol essential oils significantly reduced biofilm formation by *Candida* species on surfaces, suggesting they can be effectively used in the prevention of *Candida* colonization on abiotic (not derived from living organisms) surfaces.[2448]
- Both cinnamon and clove essential oils showed significant activity against human pathogens (*S. aureus, S. epidermidis, E. faecalis, S. pyogenes, E. coli, P. aeruginosa, A. hydrophila, P. mirabilis, K. pneumoniae,* and *C. albicans*) and their mature biofilms.[2449]
- Clove and cinnamon bark CT eugenol essential oils each exhibited insecticidal activities against the cowpea weevil (*Callosobruchus maculatus*) by impacting oviposition and offspring emergence.[2450]
- Encapsulated (with sodium alginate and emulsifiers) clove essential oil demonstrated *in vitro* inhibition of *S. aureus, E. coli, L. monocytogenes,* and *S. Typhimurium, in situ* antimicrobial against *S. aureus* that was greater than nitrite, but lower antioxidant activity.[2451]
- Clove essential oil demonstrated antifungal activity against *Microsporum* spp., which are dermatophytes that invade the stratum corneum of the skin and hair causing tinea.[2452]
- Rosemary, cinnamon, and grapefruit essential oils each inhibited fungi: *Rhizopus stolonifer* (causes respiratory infections, sinusitis, and otomycosis) and *Trichophyton mentagrophytes* and *Microsporum gypseum* (cause athlete's foot, ringworm, and nail infections).[2453]
- Eucalyptus, clove, mint, oregano, savory, tea tree, and thyme essential oils each inhibited *Venturia inaequalis*, the fungus responsible for apple scab.[2454]
- Clove essential oil was an effective larvicide against the *An. stephensi* mosquito, with the whole oil exceeding the effects of its major component eugenol.[2455]
- Clove essential oil demonstrated the strongest antioxidant activity of five Iranian essential oils tested (oregano CT carvacrol, tarragon CT trans-anethole, lemongrass CT isothymol, cinnamon, and clove) in the DPPH assay.[2456] The same research found that all five essential oils inhibited *Candida*, with lemongrass, cinnamon, and oregano being the most active.
- Clove essential oil was larvicidal to *Aedes aegypti* and *Aedes albopictus* mosquito larvae.[2457]
- Both oregano and clove essential oils prevented the growth of the fungi *Zygosaccharomyces bailii* in salad dressings.[2458]
- Clove essential oil showed significant amoebicidal activity against *Acanthamoeba polyphaga* trophozites, producing effects after only one hour.[2459]
- Glucosyltransferases (GTFs) from *Streptococcus mutans* bacteria play critical roles in the development of virulent dental plaque (ferment carbohydrates that decrease pH of plaque leading to tooth enamel demineralization), which provides an ideal site for colonization by microorganisms and is involved in the development of dental cavities. Laboratory research found that both clove and peppermint essential oils inhibit (allosteric inhibition—bind to a molecule at a site other than its active site so that the enzyme no longer remains able to bind to its specific substrate, making the enzyme inactive) GTFs produced by *S. mutans*.[2460]
- A combination of sweet fennel and clove essential oil killed colon cancer cells without harming normal human cells in laboratory research.[2461]
- Incorporation of clove and tea tree essential oils into chitosan/essential oil wound dressings demonstrated good antimicrobial activity against common wound pathogens.[2462]

- A nanoemulsion of clove bud essential oil was effective against thyroid cancer cells according to the MTT, colony formation, and Annexin V-FITC assays. The nanoemulsion clove oil was also effective against *S. aureus* causing leakage of cytoplasmic contents.[2463]
- *In vitro* research found that both cinnamon bark and clove essential oil (and their mixtures) inhibited *Salmonella enterica* (Enteritidis and Typhimurium serotypes) isolated from poultry, suggesting they may be useful as farm disinfectants and in poultry diet to avoid *Salmonella* infections.[2464]
- *Streptococcus suis* is a bacterial pathogen in pigs that can cause serious human infections like meningitis, septicemia, septicemia, and arthritis. It is becoming increasingly resistant to antibiotics, leading to unsuccessful treatment of *S. suis* infections. Clove oil exhibited significant activity against multidrug-resistant *S. suis* in laboratory research, killing all the bacteria after fifteen minutes of exposure.[2465]
- 1-deoxy-d-xylulose-5-phosphate reductoisomerase (DXR) catalyzes the first step in the nonmevalonate or 2-C-methyl-d-erythritol-4-phosphate (MEP) pathway, which is responsible for generating isoprenoid precursors in bacteria. The MEP pathway is absent in humans and considered a therapeutic target for the development of antibiotics. Oregano and clove essential oil displayed moderate inhibitory activity against DXR, suggesting it plays a role in the antimicrobial activity of the essential oils.[2466] Isolated carvacrol and eugenol also possessed moderate inhibitory activity, whereas thymol, carveol, and linalool exhibited weak activity.
- Immunomodulatory activity of essential oils was assessed by the simultaneous evaluation of phagocytosis, production of iNOS and secretion of IL-6, induced by contact of RAW 264.7 cells with LPS. What the researchers found was that both clove and cinnamon essential oils modulate immune activity, which suggest they may be helpful for inflammatory and infectious conditions.[2467]
- *E. coli* is the most common uropathogenic cause of urinary tract infections (UTIs), but the most frequently used antibiotics do not effectively eliminate the organism, making recurrent UTIs common. Of 140 essential oils tested, oregano, allspice, cinnamon bark, and clove bud were the most effective against uropathogenic *E. coli*.[2468]
- Laboratory research concluded that clove bud and lemongrass (*C. citratus*) essential oil exhibited anticandidal activity and combining the oils or fractions of the oils increased the antifungal activity.[2469]
- Yarrow, clove, and pomelo essential oil (compositions not reported) were active against *Babesia canis*—a parasite transmitted by ticks to dogs that infect and replicate in red blood cells causing a condition called babesiosis.[2470]
- Cinnamon bark, thyme, and clove essential oil showed important antibacterial activity against multidrug-resistant bacteria isolated from people (*E. coli, K. pneumoniae, A. baumanii, P. aeruginosa, C. freunfii, K. oxytica, S. enteridis, S. typhimurium, S. zanizibar, S. livingstone, S. derby, S. heidelberg, C. striatum,* and *S. aureus*).[2471] They exhibited a remarkable antibiofilm and anti-quorum-sensing activity and good antioxidant activity. The highest antioxidant activity was observed from clove (90.3% DPPH).
- Diabetic men are at a higher risk of erectile dysfunction (ED) due to damage to nerves and blood vessels caused by poor long-term blood sugar control. Injection of clove essential oil or eugenol into the base of the penis restored erectile function in male diabetic rats with ED.[2472]
- The cat flea (*Ctenocephalides felis*) is a very common parasitic insect that mainly infects domestic cats. Both clove bud essential oil and eugenol exhibited pediculicidal activity and inhibited the maturation of eggs into adult fleas.[2473]
- *In vitro* research showed that black pepper CT beta-caryophyllene and clove bud essential oils both inhibited *Fusarium oxysporum* and *Aspergillus niger*.[2474]
- Clove exhibited selective insecticidal activity against aphids (*Rhopalosiphum maidis*) while displaying lower toxicity against nontarget ladybugs (*Coleomegilla maculata*).[2475]
- Clove bud essential oil exhibited good antioxidant activity in the DPPH assay.[2476] The greatest antioxidant activity was observed in oil obtained from flowering buds of young trees. The researchers reported that clove bud oil from young trees produced a higher yield and the eugenol content is highest when buds are harvested at the flowering stage in mature trees.
- A nanoemulgel (nanoemulsion of clove essential oil mixed in a hydrogel matrix of chitosan, guar gum, and gum acacia) with clove essential oil and clove oil nanofibers demonstrated the ability to reduce skin inflammation in a mouse model.[2477] Both oil formulas showed the ability to sustain penetration through the skin but the nanofiber oil was more effective as a skin anti-inflammatory. The researchers concluded that the clove nanofibers represented "a promising topical delivery system for effective treatment of inflammatory diseases instead of nonsteroidal anti-inflammatory drugs that possess adverse effects."
- *Vibrio parahaemolyticus* is a gram-negative bacterium that causes gastrointestinal illness in humans

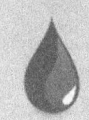

characterized by watery or bloody diarrhea, nausea, vomiting, fever, headache, and abdominal cramps. The bacteria lives in brackish saltwater (like found in the coastal waters of the United States and Canada) and causes symptoms after ingesting contaminated water or food. Clove, thyme CT para-cymene, and garlic (20.0% allyl propyl disulfide, 16.8% diallyl trisulfide, 15.2% allyl sulfide) essential oils reduced bacterial growth, with clove and thyme being the most effective.[2478]

☐ Brain infections like meningitis and encephalitis are difficult to treat due to poor ability of drugs to pass the blood brain barrier (BBB) and reach the brain. Delivery of therapeutic substances through the nose (intranasal) is a way to work around the BBB by delivering those agents through the highly vascularized olfactory region. Clove bud and thyme CT thymol essential oils included in chitosan coated nanoemulsions showed potential to be effective intranasal solutions against multidrug-resistant bacteria such as MRSA, MSSA, *A. baumannii*, and *K. pneumoniae*.[2479]

☐ An animal model (*C. elegans*) of lifespan enhancement discovered that clove bud essential oil extends lifespan and promotes good health.[2480] The oil also exhibited good antioxidant activity, increasing superoxide dismutase-3 and glutathione S-transferase 4 in *C. elegans* nematodes.

☐ *Bacillus* bacteria are widely found in nature and responsible for food poisoning and food spoilage. Black cumin, clove, cinnamon, and marjoram essential oils each reduced *Bacillus* spp. presence in raw and processed meat, with black cumin being the most effective oil.[2481]

☐ Clove bud essential oil encapsulated in a chitosan nanomatrix exhibited enhanced antifungal and anti-aflatoxin B1 inhibitory activity when compared to the free oil.[2482] It also displayed remarkable antioxidant activity. The chitosan encapsulated oil preserved the sensory characteristics of corn seed for up to six months of storage with a considerable safety profile (nontoxic, nonmutagenic, nontumorigenic).

☐ *In vitro* research determined that clove bud essential oil possesses good antioxidant activity, but its primary constituent is more potent. In addition, both clove essential oil and eugenol inhibited *T. cruzi*, with the oil performing better and exhibiting greater selectivity for the parasite than healthy cells.[2483]

☐ Colistin (polymyxin E) is an antibiotic used as a last-resort treatment for multidrug-resistant gram-negative infections. Both clove bud and thyme essential oil (compositions not reported) exhibited good antibacterial activity against *A. baumannii* and *K. pneumoniae*, and enhanced the antibacterial activity of colistin against colistin-resistant and colistin-susceptible strains.[2484]

☐ Clove bud essential oil inhibited *E. coli* isolated from turkeys.[2485]

☐ Clove essential oil moderately inhibited *S. aureus*, *E. faecalis*, *P, aeruginosa*, *K, pneumoniae*, *E. coli*, and *C. albicans*.[2486]

☐ Researchers evaluated the effectiveness of natural gel hand sanitizers with aloe vera gel (90%), glycerin (5%), distilled water (2.45% to 4.95%), vitamin E (0.05%), and the addition of either clove, tea tree, or lavender essential oils (1.25% to 2.5%). The tea tree oil sanitizer exhibited the highest antibacterial activity, the clove sanitizer was effective against all tested microorganisms, and the lavender sanitizer demonstrated the least antimicrobial activity.[2487]

☐ Nanoparticles loaded with clove bud essential oil was toxic to the red flour beetle (*Tribolium castaneum*) and although the nanoparticles did not increase the toxicity of the free oil, it did protect against its degradation and evaporation and allow for a sustained release, as indicated by continued high toxicity for sixteen weeks of storage.[2488]

☐ Comparing ground and unground clove buds, researchers found that grinding the buds before distillation significantly changes its composition. Unground oil contained 87.4% eugenol, 7.2% cyperene, and 3.6% phenethyl isovalerate, whereas the ground oil contained 68.7% eugenol, 20.5% cyperene, and 6.4% phenethyl isovalerate. As far as biological activity, the unground oil displayed greater antioxidant activity in the DPPH and reducing power assays, greater antimicrobial activity (*B. cereus*, *S. aureus*, *L. monocytogenes*, *E. coli*, and *S. enteritidis*), and insecticidal activity against the rice weevil (*S. oryzae*).[2489]

☐ Trypanosoma cruzi is a parasite that causes Chagas disease in humans. This parasite bores into tissue and feeds on blood and lymph increasing the likelihood of disease. It is most commonly spread through contact with feces from an infected kissing bug (a blood-sucking insect that feeds on animals and humans). Clove and ginger essential oil were evaluated against *T. cruzi* II parasite load in mice, alone and in combination with benznidazole.[2490] The mice were inoculated with 10,000 blood trypomastigotes of *T. cruzi* and then orally treated with benznidazole, cinnamon or ginger essential oil, or benznidazole and cinnamon or ginger oil. A control group was untreated. Ginger and the combination of ginger or cinnamon oil with benznidazole each reduced parasitemia, but clove was not effective alone. However, clove did reduce parasite load. Each individual oil and their combinations with benznidazole reduced parasite load. Ginger not only promoted reduced parasite load but also decreased mortality in the mice that received it.

- *Fusarium graminearum* is a fungus that contaminates cereals, fruit, and vegetables. Thyme, oregano, basil, nutmeg, hyssop, and clove essential oils inhibited mycelial growth of *F. graminearum*, with oregano performing best followed by clove and thyme.[2491] The composition of the oils was not reported.

- Of fourteen commercial essential oils tested, cinnamon bark, thyme CT thymol, clove bud, geranium, and manuka essential oils were most active against fungi that commonly infect animal and human skin (*Microsporum gypseum*, *Microsporum canis*, *Trichophyton mentagrophytes*, *Trichophyton violaceum*, *Aspergillus niger*, *Scopulariopsis brevicaulis*, (IZ 1) dog skin isolate).[2492] (E)-cinnamaldehyde, thymol, and carvacrol displayed the strongest activity of isolated constituents against dermatophytes. (E)-cinnamaldehyde, eugenol, carvacrol, geraniol, and thymol were most active against IZ 1.

- *In vitro* research found that clove bud essential oil inhibited a panel of bacteria and fungi with very strong activity observed against *S. aureus*, *P. commune*, *P. expansum*, *P. glabrum*, and *P. chrysogenum*.[2493] Further testing of the oil in vapor phase against yeasts on bread found that it was most effective against *P. glabrum*.

- Clove bud essential oil exhibited antifungal activity against *Candida albicans* and non-*albicans Candida* species and inhibited the growth of a multi-species biofilm isolated from human saliva of people with oral candidiasis.[2494] Its activity was not significantly different than the standard oral antimicrobial chlorhexidine.

- Five essential oils (cassia, oregano CT carvacrol, thyme CT thymol, summer savory CT carvacrol, and clove bud) were evaluated for their ability to reduce colonization of *Salmonella* spp. in an *in vivo* infection model using *Caenorhabditis elegans*.[2495] Both cassia and clove significantly inhibited bacterial colonization in the digestive tract, which the researchers suggested may be related to reduced swimming motility.

- Terpene/phenol-rich (oregano CT carvacrol, thyme CT carvacrol, and summer savory CT carvacrol) and phenylpropanoid-rich (clove bud and cinnamon leaf) essential oils each showed good absolute antioxidant activity—comparable to BHT—in cumene and squalene during the peroxyl radical trapping assay.[2496]

- Both clove essential oil and clove oil in a cream base exhibited moderate antifungal activity against dermatophytes, and the cream also showed good anti-inflammatory activity (similar to the reference drug).[2497]

- Topical application of clove essential oil in a lipid nanocarrier improved the therapeutic activity of free clove oil in *in vitro* and rat models of rheumatoid arthritis.[2498] The nano-clove oil reduced inflammation (inhibited serum lysosomal enzymes and proinflammatory cytokines) and improved joint function slightly better than free oil.

- Clove bud essential oil demonstrated acaricidal activity against the poultry red mite (*Dermanyssus gallinae*) in the contact toxicity test, with toxic effects lasting up to four days post-application.[2499]

- When comparing the contact toxicity and repellent effects of eight essential oils and carrier oils (clove bud, garlic, *Eucalyptus camaldulensis*, lavender, German chamomile, lemon, jojoba, and sweet almond) against the red flour beetle (*Tribolium castaneum*), clove bud essential oil exhibited the highest repellency effect, while garlic, German chamomile, and lemon were the most toxic.[2500]

- Clove bud and cinnamon bark essential oil each exhibited inhibitory activity against bacteria associated with wound infections (*P. aeruginosa*, *E. coli*, and *K. pneumoniae*), with cinnamon bark being more effective.[2501] The researchers concluded that these oils may be useful in the prevention of healthcare-acquired infections.

- Clove and thyme essential oil were evaluated against 36 *Salmonella enterica* (16 *S. typhimurium*, 3 monophasic variant *S. typhimurium*, 8 *S. enteritidis*, 6 *S. rissen*, 1 *S. typhi*, and 2 *S. derby*) strains, isolated from the swine production chain, and for their synergistic potential with antibiotics.[2502] The bacteria were resistant to gentamicin, amikacin, tobramycin, and tetracycline. Both oils showed varying degrees of activity against the tested strains and improved the activity of tetracycline, suggesting the oils restored the susceptibility of *Salmonella* spp. to the antibiotic.

- The human papillomavirus is responsible for more than 90% of all cervical cancer cases. Vaginal gels are designed to deliver targeted agents to the vagina and surrounding tissues. A combination of thyme essential oil and acridine orange derivative (C8) demonstrated promising properties in vaginal fluid stimulant. Combining thyme essential oil with mitoxantrone or acridine orange derivative (C8) resulted in reduced cervical cancer cell viability *in vitro* when compared to the individual agents.[2503]

- Aldose reductase is an enzyme involved in the metabolism of glucose (specifically catalyzing the reduction of glucose to sorbitol) and associated with diabetic complications—cataracts and nerve damage—and inflammatory conditions. Aldose reductase inhibitors are designed to prevent eye and nerve damage in people with diabetes. Researchers investigated the ability of clove essential oil to inhibit aldose reductase in computer docking, laboratory, and rat studies.[2504] The clove oil had an interesting composition of 42.6% 3-allylguaiacol (a eugenol derivative), 15.9% eugenyl acetate, and 15.5% beta-caryophyllene. Computer docking studies showed that 3-allylguaiacol, eugenyl acetate, and beta-caryophyllene each had binding affinity to the alpha reductase receptor, with beta-caryophyllene demonstrating the greatest binding ability.

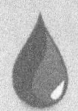

Clove oil inhibited aldose reductase in the laboratory study. Moreover, oral administration of clove (20 mg/kg BW) decreased retinal damage by inhibiting aldose reductase activity in diabetic rats. The study also confirmed the antioxidant capacity of lemongrass oil in the ABTS, hydroxyl, hydrogen peroxide scavenging, DPPH, and phosphomolybdate assays. The research suggests that the oil has a protective effect against diabetic complications due to its antioxidant activity and ability to inhibit aldose reductase activity.

☐ *In vitro* research found that clove bud essential oil nanoemulsion promotes apoptosis in colon cancer cells by upregulating caspase 3 activity (an enzyme responsible for triggering apoptosis in response to increased reactive oxygen species in stressed cells).[2505]

☐ Cinnamon, eucalyptus (*E. globulus*), and clove bud essential oil effectively inhibited MRSA, with cinnamon producing the greatest zone of inhibition and eucalyptus having the lowest minimum inhibitory concentration.[2506]

☐ Cassia, clove bud, oregano (near equal carvacrol and thymol), ginger, and thyme CT thymol essential oils each showed activity against *L. monocytogenes* in a dry-cured ham-based model.[2507]

☐ Clove bud essential oil displayed antioxidant activity in the DPPH assay, inhibited gram-negative and gram-positive bacteria (*B. subtilis, B. cereus, S. aureus, E. coli, P. aeruginosa, E. aerogenes*), and was cytotoxic to breast cancer cells.[2508] However, the oil also showed cytotoxicity to healthy cells.

☐ Nanogels are designed to encapsulate small therapeutic molecules and deliver them across challenging physiological barriers within the body. Topical application of nanogels (100 mg) containing cinnamon bark or clove bud essential oils significantly reduced inflammation and pain in rats.[2509] Cinnamon bark oil was more effective than clove oil. The study authors concluded that the nanogels represent promising therapeutics for the relief of conditions "accompanied by inflammation and pain."

☐ A comparison of the activity of ten essential oils against antibiotic-resistant *E. coli* and *L. monocytogenes* showed that clove, thyme, cinnamon, and garlic were highly active against both bacteria, but turmeric, cumin, black pepper, and marjoram were inactive against *L. monocytogenes*.[2510] Ginger and parsley were moderately active against both bacteria. A combination of clove and thyme exhibited the strongest activity against *L. monocytogenes*. Combinations of clove+cinnamon, cinnamon+garlic, and cinnamon+thyme were synergistic against *E. coli*; the same combinations plus clove+thyme, and clove+garlic were synergistic against *L. monocytogenes*. Composition was not reported for the essential oils used in the study.

☐ Nanogels containing clove bud or cinnamon bark essential oil showed significant anti-inflammatory and pain-relieving (antinociceptive) activity in rats.[2511]

☐ Investigation of the antifungal and antivirulence activity of basil CT linalool, cinnamon bark, clove, tea tree, oregano CT carvacrol, and thyme CT thymol essential oils (EOs) on five *Candida* species (C. albicans, C. auris, C. krusei, C. parapsilosis and C. guillermondii) revealed that clove and cinnamon inhibited all fungal species tested, cinnamon, oregano, and thyme inhibited biofilm formation of *C. albicans, C. guilliermondii,* and *C. parapsilosis*, and each oil except tea tree downregulated virulence genes in *C. albicans*.[2512] In addition, thyme synergized the activity of fluconazole against all tested *Candida* species.

☐ Pneumonitis refers to inflammation in the lungs, which can cause shortness of breath, cough, fatigue, unintentional weight loss, fever, muscle or joint pain, and loss of appetite. Pine (39.4% alpha-pinene, 14.3% limonene, 11.0% beta-pinene) and clove bud essential oils were evaluated for their effects in an acute model of pneumonitis.[2513] Inhalation of pine or clove oils for thirty minutes prior to induction of pneumonitis and four and twenty-three hours afterward significantly reduced airway hyperresponsiveness and respiratory dysfunction (prevented peak expiratory flow, tidal volume increases, and perivascular edema formation), but interestingly increased the inflammatory response (myeloperoxidase activity and cytokine production).

☐ Cadmium is a chemical element chemically similar to zinc and mercury that humans are exposed to primarily through diet (fortunately only about 5 percent of it is absorbed after ingestion) and smoking. It can be toxic in sufficient quantities and cause bone disease accompanied by severe bone pain with kidney failure. It is also associated with brain dysfunction, particularly the prefrontal cortex—the frontal lobe of your brain that regulates behavior, personality, and executive function. A preclinical model of cadmium toxicity found that cadmium significantly reduced glutathione and glutathione S-transferase levels (optimum levels are critical to protect brain cells against damage caused by toxins) and caused neurological deficits. Oral administration of clove bud essential oil significantly protected against these effects by increasing antioxidant activity and preserving neurological function in rats.[2514]

☐ Cinnamon, clove, and thyme essential oils demonstrated remarkable antibacterial properties against multidrug-resistant strains of *S. enteritidis*.[2515] Moreover, biofilm formation was reduced by cinnamon, clove, thyme, turmeric, rosemary, and sage essential oils. Clove exhibited the greatest inhibition of violacein production, followed by thyme and cinnamon.

☐ Clove bud essential oil inhibited *A. niger, C. parapsilosis, C. krusei, C. glabrata, C. albicans, E. coli, K.*

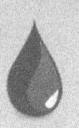
*pneumoniae, L. monocytogenes, S. enteritidis, P. aeruginosa, S. aureus, B. cereus, M. luteus, E. faecalis*, with its inhibition zones exceeding fluconazole against all fungi except *C. albicans*, and showing greater inhibition zones than ciprofloxacin against *E. coli, K. pneumoniae, L. monocytogenes, S. aureus*, and *M. luteus*.[2516]

☐ Isolated eugenol may improve hypopigmentation of the skin due to its ability to enhance melanin production by increasing tyrosinase activity.[2517]

☐ Clove bud essential oil incorporated into bandage-like fibers demonstrated good antimicrobial activity against *C. albicans, E. coli, S. aureus*, and *S. pyogenes*, suggesting the fibers are a promising option for wound care.[2518]

☐ Evaluation of fifteen essential oils found that clove repels the northern yellow spider (*Cheiracanthium mildei*), but caraway attracts it.[2519]

☐ Cinnamon bark, clove bud, and bay laurel essential oils inhibited *L. monocytogenes, L. innocua, L. welshimeri, L. ivanovii, L. grayi*, and *V. parahaemolyticus*, with cinnamon bark being the most effective.[2520]

☐ Clove, lemongrass, and isolated geraniol demonstrated greater than 60 percent repellency against *Ae. aegypti* mosquitoes, eucalyptus greater than 50 percent, and ylang ylang no repellency.[2521]

☐ Clove bud essential oil was effective against multidrug-resistant strains of *P. aeruginosa* isolated from cases of acute and chronic ear infections in dogs.[2522]

☐ *In vitro* research showed that clove bud essential oil inhibited *C. albicans* by decreasing their enzymatic activity, including a strain resistant to fluconazole.[2523]

☐ Topical application of a 5% or 10% concentration of clove essential oil daily improved wound healing of MRSA-infected wounds and reduced bacterial load in the wound in rats.[2524] Combining clove oil with the antibiotic imipenem enhanced the wound-healing process even more.

☐ Both clove and oregano CT carvacrol essential oils were lethal to adult red spider mites (*Tetranychus urticae*), decreased their fertility, and repelled them from two host plants.[2525]

☐ *In vitro* research concluded that clove essential oil and isolated eugenol were effective against *Candida* strains and produced additive or synergistic activity when combined with cetylpyridinium chloride, chlorhexidine, silver nitrate, and triclosan.[2526]

☐ Cinnamon bark and clove bud essential oils exhibited promising antibacterial activity (*E. coli, K. pneumoniae, P. aeruginosa, S. aureus*, and *E. fecalis*) and potent antiviral activity (SARS-CoV-2).[2527]

☐ The ability of *H. pylori* to form biofilms makes it resistant to antibiotics. Clove bud essential oil inhibited drug-resistant clinical and lab strains of *H. pylori*, suppressed its biofilm formation, and demonstrated strong anti-inflammatory activity.[2528]

☐ Clove bud essential oil exhibited powerful antioxidant activity in the DPPH assay, and antiviral activity against herpes simplex virus (HSV-1) and hepatitis A virus (HAV), but was ineffective against an adenovirus. It was most effective against HAV.[2529]

---

# COPAIBA BALSAM
## (Copaiba)

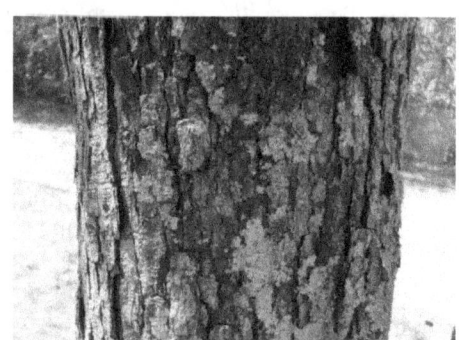

*Copaifera langsdorffii* Desf., *C. langsdorffi* Desf.; *C. officinalis* (Jacq.) L.; *Copaifera reticulata* Ducke, *C. multijuga* Hayne, *C. cearensis* Huber ex Ducke, *C. duckei* Dwyer, *C. paupera* (Herzog) Dwyer, *C. guianensis* Desf., *C. confertiflora* Bth., *C. lucens* Dwyer, *C. coriacea* Mart., *C. martii* Hayne, *C. piresii* Dwyer, *C. pubiflora* Benth.

**FAMILY:** Fabaceae (Leguminosae)
**NOTE:** Base
**AROMA INTENSITY:** Medium
**AROMA:** Woody, mild, slightly balsamic, sweet
**COMMON EXTRACTION METHOD:** Steam distilled from the gum resin; may also be steam distilled from the leaves
**POSSIBLE SUBSTITUTE OILS:** Black pepper, niaouli (1,8-cineole/viridiflorol CT), ginger, frankincense
**BLENDS WELL WITH:** Balsam fir, bergamot, black spruce, blue spruce, cedarwood, clary sage, galbanum, lavender, lemon, lime, orange, palo santo, pine, ravintsara, tangerine, ylang ylang
**SUBCELLULAR LOCALIZATION | EPIGENETIC INFLUENCE:** Lysosomes | Currently unknown
**RECOMMENDED DILUTION RANGE:** 5%–Neat

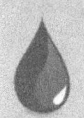

**PRIMARY CONSTITUENTS:**[2530,2531,2532,2533,2534,2535,2536,2537,2538,2539,2540,2541,2542,2543,2544,2545,2546,2547]

*C. langsdorfii or C. officinalis*

| | |
|---|---|
| Beta-Caryophyllene | 36.5%–53.3% |
| Daniellic Acid | 2.6%–33.7% |
| Alpha-Copaene | 1.6%–18.2% |
| Beta-Bisabolene | 1.0%–12.7% |
| Trans-Alpha-Bergamotene | 1.0%–11.8% |
| Caryophyllene Oxide | 0.3%–10.2% |
| Kaurenoic Acid | 0.0%–10.1% |
| Hardwickiic Acid | 0.0%–9.0% |
| Alpha-Humulene | 1.1%–8.6% |
| Copalic Acid | 2.1%–7.6% |
| Delta-Amorphene | 0.0%–5.4% |
| Beta-Selinene | 0.5%–4.7% |
| Germacrene D | 1.2%–4.6% |
| Gamma-Cadinene | 0.8%–4.6% |

*C. langsdorfii (Leaves)*

| | |
|---|---|
| Spathulenol | 12.6%–35.7% |
| Germacrene D | 4.0%–18.0% |
| Caryophyllene Oxide | 7.4%–16.6% |
| Beta-Caryophyllene | 1.1%–9.0% |
| Alpha-Cadinol | 3.2%–7.9% |
| Bicyclogermacrene | 1.5%–5.7% |
| Humulene Epoxy II | 1.7%–3.3% |
| Delta-Cadinene | 1.8%–3.1% |
| Germacrene B | 1.4%–1.8% |
| Alpha-Copaene | 0.1%–1.5% |

*C. reticulata (BC CT)*

| | |
|---|---|
| Beta-Caryophyllene | 27.8%–68.0% |
| Beta-Bisabolene | 0.0%–26.3% |
| (E)-Alpha-Bergamotene | 2.4%–24.0% |
| Beta-Selinene | 0.0%–20.6% |
| Alpha-Selinene | 0.0%–13.2% |
| Alpha-Humulene | 3.9%–9.7% |
| Beta-Elemene | 0.0%–5.6% |
| Germacrene D | 0.0%–5.0% |
| Methyl Kaurenoate | 0.0%–3.9% |
| (Z)-Alpha-Bisabolene | 0.0%–3.6% |
| Methyl Kolavenate | 0.0%–3.4% |
| Alpha-Copaene | 0.0%–3.0% |
| Delta-Cadinene | 0.0%–2.6% |
| Caryophyllene Oxide | 0.0%–2.4% |
| Methyl Copalate | 0.0%–2.4% |
| Methyl Hardwickiate | 0.0%–2.3% |
| Gamma-Amorphene | 0.0%–2.2% |
| Alpha-Bulnesene | 0.0%–2.2% |
| Gamma-Cadinene | 0.0%–2.1% |

*C. multijuga (BC CT)*

| | |
|---|---|
| Beta-Caryophyllene | 16.0%–85.4% |
| Trans-Cadina-1(6),4-Diene | 0.0%–24.6% |
| Germacrene D | 0.0%–18.9% |
| Alpha-Copaene | 0.3%–15.0% |
| Germacrene B | 0.0%–13.6% |
| Caryophyllene Oxide | 0.0%–11.7% |
| Alpha-Humulene | 0.0%–11.3% |
| Copalic Acid | 0.0%–11.0% |
| Copalic Acid Methyl Ester | 0.0%–9.5% |
| (E)-Alpha-Bergamotene | 0.0%–7.5% |
| Delta-Cadinene | 0.0%–6.3% |
| Methyl Copalate | 0.0%–6.2% |
| 3-Acetoxy Copalic Acid | 0.0%–6.2% |
| Beta-Elemene | 0.0%–5.3% |
| Alpha-Amorphene | 0.0%–4.6% |
| Methyl 3-Acetoxy-Copalate | 0.0%–3.4% |
| Alpha-Muurolene | 0.0%–3.4% |
| Delta-Elemene | 0.0%–2.9% |
| Alpha-Cadinol | 0.0%–2.7% |
| Gamma-Muurolene | 0.0%–2.7% |
| Pinifolic Acid | 0.0%–2.6% |
| 3Beta-Hydroxy-Copalic acid | 0.0%–2.2% |
| Dimethyl Agathate | 0.0%–2.1% |

*C. cearensis*

| | |
|---|---|
| Beta-Caryophyllene | 19.7% |
| Methyl Clorechinate | 11.3% |
| Alpha-Copaene | 8.2% |
| Beta-Bisabolol | 8.2% |
| Delta-Cadinene | 7.2% |
| Methyl Hardwickiate | 6.2% |
| Alloaromadendrene | 3.8% |
| Alpha-Humulene | 3.7% |
| Germacrene B | 3.6% |
| Beta-Cubebene | 3.3% |
| Beta-Bisabolene | 2.8% |

*C. pubiflora*

| | |
|---|---|
| Beta-Caryophyllene | 65.9% |
| Beta-Selinene | 10.2% |
| Alpha-Humulene | 7.3% |

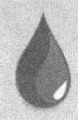

| | |
|---|---|
| (E)-Alpha-Bergamotene | 2.1% |
| Methyl Copalate | 2.1% |

**C. duckei (BC CT)**

| | |
|---|---|
| Beta-Caryophyllene | 31.5%–61.8% |
| Beta-Bisabolene | 5.2%–17.4% |
| (E)-Alpha-Bergamotene | 4.1%–10.3% |
| (E)-Beta-Farnesene | 4.1%–7.6% |
| Beta-Selinene | 0.0%–6.7% |
| Beta-Elemene | 0.4%–4.2% |
| Alpha-Selinene | 0.0%–4.2% |
| (Z)-Alpha-Bisabolene | 1.0%–2.5% |
| Alpha-Bulnesene | 0.0%–2.3% |

**C. reticulata (BB CT)**

| | |
|---|---|
| Beta-Bisabolene | 18.2%–54.0% |
| (E)-Alpha-Bergamotene | 8.1%–36.9% |
| Beta-Caryophyllene | 0.0%–20.1% |
| Beta-Selinene | 0.0%–18.1% |
| Caryophyllene Oxide | 0.0%–15.2% |
| Alpha-Selinene | 0.0%–11.4% |
| Alpha-Guaiene | 0.0%–7.9% |
| (Z)-Alpha-Bisabolene | 0.0%–5.8% |
| (E)-Beta-Guaiene | 0.0%–5.8% |
| Alpha-Humulene | 0.0%–5.3% |
| Beta-Elemene | 0.0%–5.0% |
| (E)-Beta-Farnesene | 0.0%–4.6% |
| Delta-Cadinene | 0.0%–4.4% |
| 7-Epi-Alpha-Selinene | 0.0%–4.0% |
| (Z)-Beta-Farnesene | 0.0%–4.0% |
| (E)-Gamma-Bisabolene | 0.0%–3.8% |
| Viridiflorene | 0.0%–3.4% |
| Cyclosativene | 0.0%–3.3% |
| Cyclosativene | 0.0%–3.2% |
| Cyperene | 0.0%–3.0% |
| Beta-Sesquiphellandrene | 0.0%–2.8% |
| Beta-Chamigrene | 0.0%–2.1% |

**C. pauper (AC CT)**

| | |
|---|---|
| Alpha-Copaene | 42.5% |
| Beta-Caryophyllene | 14.1% |
| Delta-Cadinene | 10.4% |
| Alpha-Cubebene | 5.5% |
| Alloaromadendrene | 3.5% |
| Beta-Cubebene | 3.3% |
| Beta-Bisabolene | 2.6% |

**C. martii (AC CT)**

| | |
|---|---|
| Alpha-Copaene | 36.4%–51.2% |
| Delta-Cadinene | 13.7%–17.2% |

| | |
|---|---|
| Alpha-Selinene | 5.5% |
| Beta-Elemene | 4.7% |

**C. multijuga (TM CT)**

| | |
|---|---|
| Beta-Caryophyllene | 36.2%–60.4% |
| Trans-Muurola-4(14),5-diene | 14.4%–37.0% |
| Alpha-Copaene | 2.4%–18.1% |
| Delta-Elemene | 0.1%–8.5% |
| Alpha-Humulene | 4.2%–6.9% |
| Delta-Cadinene | 0.0%–3.0% |
| Beta-Elemene | 1.1%–2.9% |
| Trans-Cadina-1(6),4-Diene | 0.0%–2.7% |

**C. duckei (B CT)**

| | |
|---|---|
| Beta-Bisabolene | 15.7%–33.6% |
| Beta-Caryophyllene | 13.0%–25.1% |
| Beta-Selinene | 1.8%–15.4% |
| (E)-Alpha-Bergamotene | 8.3%–12.0% |
| Alpha-Selinene | 1.8%–9.9% |
| Beta-Elemene | 3.0%–9.4% |
| Alpha-Guaiene | 0.0%–4.9% |
| (E)-Gamma-Bisabolene | 1.4%–3.3% |
| Alpha-Bulnesene | 1.9%–3.1% |
| Beta-Sesquiphellandrene | 1.1%–2.3% |
| Aromadendrene | 0.8%–3.1% |
| (E)-Beta-Farnesene | 1.4%–2.9% |
| Alpha-Humulene | 1.2%–2.5% |

**C. pauper (BB CT)**

| | |
|---|---|
| Beta-Bisabolene | 20.2% |
| Alpha-Zingiberene | 19.4% |
| Kaurenoic Acid | 13.3% |
| Copalic Acid | 6.1% |

**C. reticu ta (AC CT)**

| | |
|---|---|
| Alpha-Copaene | 25.1% |
| Beta-Caryophyllene | 13.1% |
| Copalic Acid | 7.7% |
| Kaurenoic Acid | 7.5% |
| Hardwickiic Acid | 6.9% |

**C. pires**

| | |
|---|---|
| Alpha-Coapene | 45.5% |
| Delta-Cadinene | 13.7% |
| Beta-Caryophyllene | 10.3% |
| Alpha-Cubebene | 3.5% |
| Beta-Bisabolene | 3.5% |
| Alloaromadendrene | 3.5% |

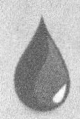

| | | | | |
|---|---|---|---|---|
| Beta-Elemene | 4.1%–6.2% | | Gamma-Muurolene | 2.7% |
| Alloaromadendrene | 4.3%–5.0% | | Alpha-Guaiene | 2.0% |
| Beta-Bisabolene | 2.6%–4.5% | | | |
| Gamma-Muurolene | 2.8%–4.4% | | *C. ltijuga (AB CT)* | |
| Trans-Cadina- | | | (E)-Alpha-Bergamotene | 19.8%–20.9% |
| 1(2),4-Diene | 1.9%–2.5% | | Caryophyllene Oxide | 11.7%–19.9% |
| | | | Beta-Caryophyllene | 7.6%–16.0% |
| *C. reticulata (AB CT)* | | | Beta-Elemene | 5.3%–6.1% |
| (E)-Alpha-Bergamotene | 25.6%–39.3% | | Alpha-Copaene | 5.5%–6.0% |
| Beta-Bisabolene | 24.2%–32.8% | | Ledol | 1.9%–3.5% |
| Beta-Selinene | 0.0%–17.1% | | Alpha-Humulene | 2.0%–3.1% |
| Beta-Caryophyllene | 1.2%–10.8% | | Copalic Acid | 2.5%–2.9% |
| Alpha-Selinene | 0.0%–10.4% | | Germacrene B | 0.5%–2.8% |
| Alpha-Guaiene | 0.0%–9.5% | | 3Beta-Hydroxy- | |
| (E,E)-Alpha-Farnesene | 0.0%–7.6% | | Copalic Acid | 1.2%–2.2% |
| Beta-Elemene | 0.0%–6.0% | | | |
| Valencene | 0.0%–3.1% | | *C. r iculata (BS CT)* | |
| (Z)-Alpha-Bisabolene | 0.0%–2.7% | | Beta-Selinene | 33.0%–35.7% |
| Viridiflorene | 0.0%–2.6% | | Beta-Bisabolene | 8.1%–32.8% |
| (E)-Beta-Farnesene | 0.0%–2.4% | | Alpha-Selinene | 21.2%–23.2% |
| | | | Beta-Elemene | 13.1%–13.4% |
| *C. multijuga (CO CT)* | | | (E)-Alpha-Bergamotene | 10.1%–11.4% |
| Caryophyllene Oxide | 29.2%–44.3% | | Beta-Caryophyllene | 7.5%–10.8% |
| Beta-Caryophyllene | 5.1%–20.8% | | | |
| Alpha-Copaene | 2.0%–15.4% | | *C. rtii (KA CT)* | |
| Beta-Elemene | 0.0%–8.6% | | Kovalenic Acid | 29.0% |
| Copalic Acid | 0.9%–4.9% | | Beta-Bisabolene | 10.7% |
| Pinifolic Acid | 0.8%–4.7% | | Kaurenoic Acid | 7.9% |
| Ledol | 0.0%–4.3% | | Alpha-Zingiberene | 7.2% |
| Alpha-Amorphene | 2.0%–4.1% | | | |
| Alpha-Humulene | 1.0%–4.0% | | *C. luce* | |
| Alpha-Cadinol | 0.3%–2.9% | | Polyathic Acid | 69.8% |
| Spathulenol | 0.0%–2.1% | | Copalic Acid | 11.1% |
| | | | | |
| *C. paupera (AC CT)* | | | | |
| Alpha-Copaene | 34.8% | | | |
| Unidentified | 18.9% | | | |
| Delta-Cadinene | 13.9% | | | |
| Alpha-Cubebene | 9.9% | | | |
| Alloaromadendrene | 7.7% | | | |
| Beta-Caryophyllene | 5.4% | | | |
| Alpha-Humulene | 3.2% | | | |

Note: Higher viscosity oils indicates the presence of greater levels of diterpenes.

**OTHER CONSTITUENTS:** *C. langsdorfii or C. officinalis*—Alpha-elemene, alpha-cubebene, beta-elemene, cyperene, gamma-elemene, gamma-muurolene, alpha-amorphene, alpha-selinene, allo-aromadendrene, bicyclogermacrene, alpha-muurolene, beta-sesquiphellandrene, iso-gamma-bisabolene (E), alpha-muurolol, eperuic acid, kovalenic acid, pinifolic acid, acetoxy-copalic acid; *C. langsdorfii (Leaves)*—beta-elemene, alpha-humulene, gamma-muurolene, alpha-muurolene; *C. reticulata (BC CT)*—Cyclosativene, cyperene, gamma-muurolene, (E,E)-alpha-farnesene, beta-sesquiphellandrene, alpha-gurjunene, aromadendrene, beta-chamigrene, gamma-gurjunene, gamma-curcumene, (E)-gamma-bisabolene, (Z)-beta-farnesene, 7-epi-alpha-selinene, kaurene; *C. reticulata (BB CT)*—Alpha-gurjunene, gamma-muurolene, humulene epoxide II, kaurene, guaia-6,9-diene, gamma-cadinene; *C. reticulata (AC CT)*—Not

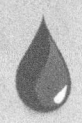 

listed; *C. reticulata (AB CT)*—Guaia-6,9-diene, alpha-humulene, beta-chamigrene, (Z)-gamma-bisabolene, beta-sesquiphellandrene; *C. reticulata (BS CT)*—Cyperene, alpha-humulene, beta-chamigrene, (Z)-alpha-bisabolene, 7-epi-alpha-selinene, delta-cadinene; *C. cearensis*—Alpha-cubebene, longifolene, beta-sesquiphellandrene, aromadendrene, gamma-amorphene, beta-vetivene, ledol, cedrol, alpha-cadinol; *C. multijuga (BC CT)*—Alpha-cubebene, beta-cubebene, bicyclogermacrene, beta-bisabolene, delta-cadinol, (E)-alpha-bergamotene, alloaromadendrene, gamma-cadinene, spathulenol, cis-cadina-1,4-diene, caryophyllene oxide, torreyol, (Z)-beta-ocimene; *C. multijuga (CO CT)*—Alpha-cubebene, gamma-elemene, alloaromadendrene, alpha-muurolene, gamma-cadinene, torreyol, 3beta-hydroxy-copalic acid, 3beta-acetoxy-copalic acid; *C. multijuga (AB CT)*—Delta-elemene, alpha-curcumene, alpha-amorphene, alpha-muurolene, gamma-cadinene, delta-cadinene, torreyol, alpha-cadinol, pinifolic acid; *C. multijuga (TM CT)*—Alpha-cubebene, cyperene, sibirine, alloaromadendrene, gamma-muurolene, gamma-amorphene, gamma-cadinene, germacrene B; *C. duckei (BC CT)*—Alpha-Copaene, alpha-gurjunene, aromadendrene, alpha-humulene, beta-chamigrene, gamma-gurjunene, gamma-curcumene, beta-curcumene, beta-sesquiphellandrene, (E)-gamma-bisabolene; *C. duckei (BB CT)*—(Z)-alpha-bergamotene, beta-chamigrene, gamma-gurjunene, gamma-curcumene, (Z)-alpha-bisabolene, beta-curcumene, epi-alpha-bisabolol, beta-bisabolol; *C. pauper (AC CT)*—(E)-Alpha-bergamotene, alpha-humulene, trans-cadina-1(6),4-diene, epi-cubebol, gamma-cadinene, trans-cadina-1(2),4-diene, T-muurolol; *C. pauper (BB CT)*—Not listed; *C. piresii*—Beta-cubebene, (E)-alpha-bergamotene, alpha-humulene, epi-cubebol, gamma-cadinene, alpha-cadinene, epi-cubenol, cubenol; *C. pubiflora*—(E)-Alpha-bergamotene, germacrene A, caryophyllene oxide; *C. martii (AC CT)*—Alpha-cubebene, (E)-alpha-bergamotene, aromadendrene, beta-selinene, alpha-selinene, alpha-muurolene, gamma-cadinene, alpha-calacorene, gleenol; *C. martii (KA CT)*—Not listed; *C. lucens*—Beta-caryophyllene; *C. paupera (AC CT)*—Isocaryophyllene, beta-bisabolene, caryophyllene oxide

### PREFERRED COMPOSITION FOR CLINICAL USE:

| Constituent | Resin I | Resin II |
|---|---|---|
| **Beta-Caryophyllene** | 50%–83% | 45%–80% |
| **Alpha-Humulene** | 2%–11% | 2%–12% |
| **Trans-Alpha-Bergamotene** | 2%–10% | 2%–12% |
| **Germacrene D** | 0.5%–7% | 0.5%–7% |
| **Alpha-Copaene** | 1%–6% | 2%–12% |
| **Beta-Bisabolene\*** | 0%–5% | — |
| **Delta-Cadinene** | 0.5%–4% | — |
| **Beta-Elemene** | 0.1%–3% | 0.1%–5% |
| **Delta-Elemene** | 0.1%–3% | 0.1%–5% |

Note: Quality copaiba essential oil will usually contain between 1%–4% beta-bisabolene, but it may be absent in some samples.

**REPORTED THERAPEUTIC PROPERTIES:** Analgesic (pain relief), **anti-inflammatory**, **antibacterial**, **antifungal**, antiseptic, **expectorant**, decongestant, supports immune function, **wound healing**, relieves anxiety, aids digestion, stimulates pancreas and liver function, stress management, stimulating, aids concentration and focus, promotes introspection, encourages emotional healing

### CAUTIONS:

■ May decrease the bioavailability of many medications (NSAIDs, proton-pump inhibitors, acetaminophen, antiepileptics, immune modulators, blood-sugar medications, blood pressure medications, antidepressants, antipsychotics, diabetic medications, antihistamines, antibiotics, and anesthetics) due to the ability of caryophyllene oxide, alpha-humulene, and beta-caryophyllene to inhibit CYP3A enzyme activity.[2548]

*C. multijuga (CO CT)*
■ May interact with aspirin, blood pressure, antiplatelet, and anticoagulant medications, and increase the risk of bleeding among people with bleeding disorders, due to caryophyllene-oxide content.[2549]

*C. reticulata (AB CT), C. reticulata (BC CT), C. reticulata (BB CT), C. duckei (BB CT), and C. pauper (BB CT)*
■ May interfere with antibiotics and increase their effectiveness due to significant beta-bisabolene content—beta-bisabolene improves the antimicrobial activity of ampicillin and restores bacterial sensitivity to ampicillin.[2550]

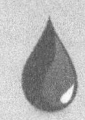

**SELECTED EVIDENCE:**

☐ Animal research suggest copaiba reduces inflammation and both central and peripheral pain.[2551,2552,2553]

☐ Copaiba oil reduces the abnormal growth of endometrial tissue and reduces the severity of endometriosis in animals.[2554]

☐ Topical or oral administration of copaiba oleoresin volatile fraction (48.4% alpha-bergamotene, 11.2% alpha-himachalene, 5.5% beta-caryophyllene, 5% beta-selinene, and diterpene acids) reduces the production of proinflammatory molecules and improves symptoms of psoriasis (skin scaliness, redness, and thickness) in a small clinical trial.[2555] One drop of the fraction was consumed three times daily, increasing the amount to seven drops, three times daily. For topical application, a 5% concentration of the fraction (dissolved in shea butter with 0.1% tea tree oil) was applied twice daily for six weeks.

☐ Copaiba oil is effective against the *S. mutans* bacteria, which is considered the primary organism responsible for dental cavities.[2556,2557]

☐ A 1% copaiba essential oil (47.0% cis-thujopsene, 8.0% seychellene, 7.8% alpha-copaene, 7.3% beta-sesquiphellandrene, and 6.7% beta-caryophyllene) gel significantly decreased the appearance of mild acne in a clinical trial.[2558] The gel was applied twice daily for 21 days and compared to a placebo gel. The copaiba gel was far more effective, which the study authors attributed to the antioxidant, antibacterial, and anti-inflammatory activity of copaiba essential oil.

☐ Copaiba promotes wound healing.[2559] Topical application of copaiba oil increased blood vessel growth (angiogenesis) to and the viability of random skin flaps (skin and tissue that is removed to cover a nearby wound) in rats.[2560] It also reduces inflammation and cellular damage that cause tissue death.[2561]

☐ Copaiba oleo-resin protects the intestines from oxidative damage to tissues and organs caused by a loss of and subsequent return of blood supply (ischemia/reperfusion) according to animal research.[2562] It also protects the stomach from ulcers caused by the NSAID indomethacin.[2563]

☐ Animal research suggests that copaiba oleo-resin protects against colon inflammation and damage caused by colitis.[2564]

☐ Copaiba helps decrease inflammation by strongly inhibiting the 5-lipoxygenase (5-LOX) enzyme that is involved in the inflammation response *in vitro*.[2565]

☐ Beta-caryophyllene selectively inhibits the growth of animal cancer cells without harming normal cells *in vitro*.[2566]

☐ *C. multijuga* essential oil exhibited the strongest anti-inflammatory activity when compared to *C. reticulata* and *C. cearensis*, which isn't surprising since it contained the highest levels of beta-caryophyllene of the three oils (57.5%, 40.9%, and 19.7% respectively) and the lowest diterpenes content (14.5%, 21.85%, and 23.5%).[2567] Some research suggests that the complex mixture of diterpenes and sesquiterpenes may interfere with the active constituents of copaiba oil.[2568] The oil inhibited nitric oxide production *in vitro* and oral administration of 100 mg/kg body weight reduced inflammation in mice (as determined by inhibition of total leukocyte and neutrophil accumulation). Another study found that oral administration (doses of 100 and 200 mg/kg body weight) of *C. multijuga* essential oil reduced lung inflammation *in vitro* and in rats by diminishing leukocyte migration to the pleural cavity.[2569]

☐ Intraperitoneal injection of 400 mg/kg body weight of copaiba resin (*C. reticulata*) protected against damage to the central nervous system caused by the neurotoxin N-Methyl-D-Aspartate in rats.[2570] Its neuroprotective properties were attributed to a reduction in inflammation.

☐ Copaiba oil (*C. multijuga* beta-caryophyllene CT) essential oil promoted healing of the cornea after chemical injury in rats.[2571] Eye drops containing 0.1 and 0.5% of copaiba oil reduced corneal ulcer and improved corneal stroma thickness compared to controls (with similar effectiveness to conventional treatments) without causing any damage to the eye.

☐ Trans-caryophyllene reduces cerebral inflammation (by modulating the production of proinflammatory molecules) and oxidative stress caused by seizures in mice.[2572]

☐ Copaiba oil (*C. reticulata*, beta-bisabolene CT) displayed antimicrobial activity against pathogens that cause periodontitis (*L. casei, E. faecalis, S. salivarius, S. sanguinis, S. mitis, S. sobrinus, P. gingivalis, F. nucleatum, A., naeslundii, P. nigrescens*)—both clinical isolates and cultured strains.[2573]

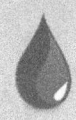 

- Varying species of copaiba essential oils exhibited activity against promastigote forms of *Leishmania amazonensis*, with *C. reticulata* (BC CT; 40.9% beta-caryophyllene) being the most active of the species tested.[2574] Another study reported that copaiba resin (beta-caryophyllene CT) was effective against both promastigotes and amastigotes of *Leishmania chagasi*, without any toxicity to monocytes.[2575]

- Interestingly, copaiba essential oil (*C. multijuga*) promoted anxiety in rats administered 100 and 200 mg/kg body weight (orally), with the higher dose provoking greater effects.[2576]

- Copaiba essential oil inhibits pathogenic oral bacteria, presenting a bacteriostatic or bactericidal effect regardless of the *Copaifera* species it was extracted from.[2577]

- *In vitro* research showed that copaiba CT beta-bisabolene (*C. langsdorfii*) essential oil was most active against *C. tropicalis* and *C. krusei*, but also inhibited *S. aureus*, *P. aeruginosa*, *S. choleraesuis*, and *C. albicans*.[2578] Copaiba oils from other species (*C. pauper* CT alpha-copaene, *C. multifida* CT beta-caryophyllene, and *C. pubiflora* CT beta-caryophyllene) were moderately to weakly active against some of the tested organisms.

- Copaiba essential oil (400 mg/kg body weight by gavage) reduced oxidative stress and cell death signals in rats with pulmonary arterial hypertension, which improved cardiac function.[2579]

- Pulmonary arterial hypertension is high blood pressure that affects the arteries in the lungs and the right side of the heart. It occurs when these blood vessels become narrowed, blocked, or damaged. It is characterized by shortness of breath, chest pressure, and dizziness that worsens over time. Chronically elevated pulmonary arterial pressure can cause right ventricle hypertrophy (abnormal enlargement and thickening of the walls of the right ventricle) and increase pulmonary vascular resistance (resistance against blood flow from the pulmonary artery to the left atrium, which makes the right ventricle work harder to move blood through pulmonary circulation). Oxidative stress in cardiovascular tissue is an early contributing factor to pulmonary hypertension. Oral administration of copaiba essential oil (400 mg/kg BW) daily for one week reduced pulmonary arterial hypertension in rats.[2580] Rats were divided into six groups: (1) control (no treatment or inducement of hypertension); (2) copaiba essential oil; (3) copaiba nanocapsules; (4) medium chain triglycerides (MCT) to trigger oxidative stress, pulmonary vascular resistance, and right ventricle hypertrophy; (5) copaiba oil + MCT; and (6) copaiba nanocapsules + MCT. Echocardiograms were performed to assess cardiovascular effects. The researchers found that both copaiba oil and copaiba nanocapsules significantly reduce right ventricle hypertrophy and oxidative stress, but only copaiba oil reduced pulmonary vascular resistance.

- A 25% dilution of copaiba essential oil improved topical penetration of celecoxib in hairless mice.[2581] The same researchers found that copaiba with celecoxib was up to 3.4 times more effective in reducing inflammation when compared to diethylammonium diclofenac cream gel alone. The study authors concluded that copaiba acts as a penetration enhancer (through the skin) for lipophilic substances. Another study found that a 100% solution increased celecoxib transdermal penetration and retention.[2582]

- An animal model of colitis found that oral administration of large doses of copaiba (*C. reticulata*) oleoresin with a composition very comparable to the essential oil decreased inflammation and oxidative stress.[2583] These large doses (1.15 g/Kg-1 body weight as an acute dose or once daily for seven days) also altered liver enzymes and bilirubin levels, suggesting harm to the liver. However, the doses are extreme and equal to the average adult consuming about five 15mL bottles at once. The oleoresin was composed of 37.6% beta-caryophyllene, 13.9% beta-bisabolene, 9.3% (E)-alpha-bergamotene, 5.3% alpha-humulene + (E)-beta-farnesene, 3.9% beta-selinene, 3.3% beta-elemene, and 3.1% alpha-selinene.

- Copaiba essential oil applied to the suture line improved incision-wound healing of urinary bladders in rats.[2584]

- Preclinical research demonstrated that 25% and 50% concentrations of copaiba oil enhanced the penetration—promotion factors of 4.1 and 3.7 respectively—of kojic acid (a skin-whitening agent from mushrooms) through the skin.[2585]

- An animal model found that topical application of copaiba oil-resin accelerates healing of second intention (also called second healing—when a wound is intentionally left open to heal by granulation, contraction, and epithelialization) wounds by promoting contraction and deposition of type-1 collagen.[2586] Type-1 collagen is essential oil for wound healing to occur. Copaiba oil-resin also promoted better quality scar formation. Copaiba oil-resin outperformed honey and a commercial product containing fibrinolysin, deoxyribonuclease, and chloramphenicol.

- Intragastric administration of copaiba crude oil (oil with volatile components) reduced pain signaling (antinociceptive) in rats, which was reversed by naloxone.[2587]

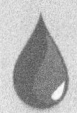

- Proteomic analysis demonstrated that copaiba essential oil influences multiple pathways in brain cells that regulate brain cell metabolism, proliferation, and immunity.[2588] The rapid biological effects of copaiba were fast-acting and suggest it may support healthy cognition and possibly reduce brain inflammation. The same group of researchers reported that copaiba oil positively regulated the pI3K/Akt/mTOR signaling pathway in neuronal and microglial cells where Akt3 is present and negatively regulated the pI3K/Akt/mTOR signaling pathway in liver cells and T lymphocytes where Akt3 is absent.[2589] They also noted that copaiba oil consistently upregulated the MAPK and JAK/STAT signaling pathways in all evaluated cell types, independent of the Akt3 expression level. The findings of this study suggest that the route of administration matters for therapeutic activity. Topical application likely will affect subcutaneous tissues with positive regulation of the pI3K/Akt/mTOR signaling pathway in preadipocytes and adipocytes. Inhalation will likely influence lung and neuronal tissues, with positive regulation of the pI3K/Akt/mTOR signaling pathway. Oral administration of oil in capsules will likely affect intestinal and liver tissues, with negative regulation of the pI3K/Akt/mTOR signaling pathway. The tissue-specific effects of copaiba demonstrate its usefulness in neuroinflammatory pain and possible antidepressant and antianxiety effects because Akt3 is predominantly found in nervous tissues.

- Allergic asthma is a chronic lung inflammatory condition characterized by airflow obstruction caused by a variety of mechanisms. Inflammatory cells infiltrate the lungs and release mediators (e.g., proinflammatory cytokines, induced nitric oxide that make the lining of the lungs [lung epithelium] swell) creating a cycle of chronic inflammation. Oral administration of 50 or 100 mg/kg body weight of copaiba essential oil (62.8% beta-caryophyllene, 9.1% alpha-humulene, 5.1% alpha-copaene, and 4.4% trans-alpha-bergamotene) significantly reduced the number of inflammatory cells infiltrating the lungs, suppressed the production of nitric oxide, and reduced the immune response in a mouse model of allergic asthma.[2590] This preliminary research suggests copaiba oil has a place as a therapy for asthma.

- Chitosan microparticles loaded with essential oils of geranium or copaiba (51.5% beta-caryophyllene)—as well as free oils—inhibited acetylcholinesterase (AChE) activity, indicting potential bioactivity for Alzheimer's disease.[2591] Chitosan-loaded oils also exhibited lower toxicity than the free oils in the brine shrimp assay.

- A 10% dilution of copaiba essential oil caused 84.7 percent mortality among engorged female Asian blue ticks (*Rhipicephalus microplus*) after six days, which reached nearly 100 percent after fifteen days.[2592]

- Spray drying chitosan microparticles (to improve stability) with copaiba (51.5% beta-caryophyllene) or geranium essential oil improved their inhibition of acetylcholinesterase, suggesting they may have potential in the management of Alzheimer's disease.[2593]

- Oral administration of copaiba essential oil (50 mg/kg BW) or its nanoemulsion (50 mg/kg BW) reduced inflammation in mice.[2594] Copaiba essential oil produced a greater effect than diclofenac at three hours, but its activity decreased at six hours, suggesting more frequent dosing is necessary to sustain anti-inflammatory benefits. The nanoemulsion was most effective and produced an anti-inflammatory effect equivalent to diclofenac for the six hours. The nanoemulsion showed no oral acute toxicity at 2,000 mg/kg, and hence is considered a nontoxic product.

- A randomized, controlled clinical trial evaluated the anxiety-relieving effects of inhaling copaiba essential oil in comparison with control (jojoba oil).[2595] Copaiba oil was diffused from an atomizing diffuser (pure oils, no water) placed on the ground in the corner of a room so that the subjects would not easily notice it set to disperse oils for sixty seconds followed by a five-second pause. Subjects then participated in a mental load task involving mental arithmetic. Heart rate, blood pressure, blood oxygen saturation, salivary cortisol, and electroencephalogram were measured as objective gauges of stress and anxiety state. State-Trait Anxiety Inventory (STAI) was used for subjects to self-report perceived stress and anxiety. A significant decrease in heart rate and salivary cortisol, as well as STAI scores, was noted in the copaiba group when compared to the jojoba group. In addition, a remarkable reduction in beta wave activity was observed in the left midfrontal region (F3) of the brain when participants inhaled copaiba oil. The findings of the study show that inhaling copaiba essential oil can reduce anxiety during mentally demanding tasks.

- Polymeric nanocapsules (PNs) are very small shells made from nontoxic polymers that encapsulate liquids like essential oils. PNs containing 1% copaiba essential oil demonstrated antibacterial activity against *S. aureus* and *P. aeruginosa*, which caused the study authors to declare that it represents "a promising candidate for treating skin disorders."[2596]

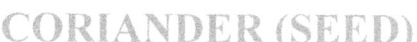 

# CORIANDER (SEED)

*Coriandrum sativum* L.

**FAMILY:** Apiaceae (Umbelliferae)
**NOTE:** Top-Middle
**AROMA INTENSITY:** Medium
**AROMA:** Sweet, spicy, woody, slightly balsamic
**COMMON EXTRACTION METHOD:** Steam distilled from the seeds
**POSSIBLE SUBSTITUTE OILS:** Lavender, petitgrain, basil (Linalool CT), fennel
**BLENDS WELL WITH:** Bergamot, black pepper, cardamom, cinnamon, clary sage, clove, cypress, frankincense, geranium, ginger, grapefruit, lemon, neroli, nutmeg, orange, pine, rosemary, sandalwood, tangerine, vetiver, ylang ylang
**SUBCELLULAR LOCALIZATION | EPIGENETIC INFLUENCE:** Cytoplasm | Currently unknown
**RECOMMENDED DILUTION RANGE:** 5%–50%; neat for limited conditions

**PRIMARY CONSTITUENTS:**[2597,2598,2599]

| | |
|---|---|
| Linalool | 51.0%–79.9% |
| Alpha-Pinene | 1.2%–15.5% |
| Neryl Acetate | 0.0%–14.2% |
| Gamma-Terpinene | 4.6%–13.6% |
| Dodecanal | 0.1%–8.1% |
| Para-Cymene | 0.8%–4.4% |
| Limonene | 0.1%–4.0% |

**OTHER CONSTITUENTS:** Camphene, camphor, beta-pinene, myrcene, camphor, geraniol, geranyl acetate, terpinen-4-ol, alpha-terpineol, sabinene, decanal, nerol, carvacrol, thymol, citronellyl, undecanal, n-tetradecane, beta-caryophyllene, benzyl benzoate, n-hexadecane

**PREFERRED COMPOSITION FOR CLINICAL USE:**

| *Constituent* | |
|---|---|
| **Linalool** | 65%–78% |
| **Alpha-Pinene** | 3%–10% |
| **Gamma-Terpinene** | 3%–10% |
| **Camphor** | 3%–8% |
| **Limonene** | 1%–5% |
| **Geranyl Acetate** | 1%–5% |
| **Geraniol** | 0.5%–3% |
| **Camphene** | 0.5%–3% |
| **Alpha-Terpineol** | 0.1%–2% |
| **Beta-Myrcene** | 0.1%–2% |

**REPORTED THERAPEUTIC PROPERTIES:** Analgesic (pain relief), antibacterial, antirheumatic, antispasmodic, antineuralgic, **antifungal**, aphrodisiac, **expels excess gas**, **aids digestion**, aids weight loss, **encourages blood-sugar balance**, breaks down fats, circulatory stimulant, relieves headache (migraine), purifies the blood, **stimulates appetite**, helps relieve painful menstruation, revitalizing, stimulating, warming, antidepressant, reduces anxiety, reduces irritation (emotional), enhances memory and cognition

**CAUTIONS:**

■ May interact with diabetic medications. Studies suggest that coriander significantly lowers glucose in animals, which may increase the action of diabetic medications.[2600,2601,2602]

■ May interact with antibiotics or antifungals and possibly enhance or reduce their effects.[2603,2604,2605]

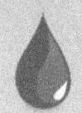

**SELECTED EVIDENCE:**

☐ *In vitro* research demonstrates that linalool from coriander essential oil has potent anti-tumor activity, reducing tumor volume, cancer cell numbers and proliferation, and triggering apoptosis of highly aggressive and metastatic S-180 rodent cancer cells.[2606] Remarkably, linalool did not cause myelosuppression (a decrease in the production of cells responsible for immunity (leukocytes), oxygen carrying (red blood cells), and blood clotting (thrombocytes)) or liver toxicity like the chemotherapy drug (cyclophosphamide) it was compared to. Linalool protected the liver by increasing Nrf2 (a potent protein found within all cells that acts as the master regulator of the cellular antioxidant system when activated by antioxidant response elements) and p21 (cyclin-dependent kinase inhibitor 1, a protein that controls cell cycle arrest—the point in the cell cycle when cell duplication and division is stopped) expression, while simultaneously killing cancer cells.

☐ Coriander moderately inhibits *E. coli*, which is suspected of altering intestinal flora balance.[2607] This disrupted flora balance is suspected as a causal factor in triggering irritable bowel syndrome.

☐ Animal research suggests that the inhalation of coriander oil may improve spatial memory (ability to recall information about one's environment) and reduce oxidative stress of the hippocampus in rats with cognitive impairment.[2608]

☐ Coriander oil possess antifungal activity against *Candida* spp.[2609]

☐ Animal research suggests that coriander selectively kills and prevents the spread of cancer cells while leaving normal cells unharmed.[2610] The researchers concluded that it exerts a pro-oxidant effect to tumor tissue and an antioxidant effect in the liver.

☐ Coriander oil may significantly prevent DNA from bonding to cancer-causing chemicals (DNA adduct formation) and therefore help prevent cancer.[2611]

☐ Coriander oil enhanced the activity of the antibiotics ciprofloxacin, gentamicin, and tetracycline against *A. baumannii* (a bacterium that commonly infects those with a compromised immune system, like those in intensive care units).[2612]

☐ Coriander oil is active against *S. pyogenes* (a bacterium that causes strep throat, scarlet fever, impetigo, cellulitis, and tonsillitis), *S. aureus*, and MRSA, and is tolerated well when applied topically, making it an excellent choice for the prevention and treatment of skin infections by these bacteria.[2613] A synergistic (the sum of the effect is greater than the two individual essential oils combined—i.e. 2 + 2 = 10) antimicrobial activity against *Bacillus cereus, Listeria monocytogenes, Staphylococcus aureus,* and *Escherichia coli,* and an additive (the sum of the effect is equivalent to the sum of the two essential oils separately—i.e. 2 + 2 + 4) effect against *Micrococcus luteus* and *Salmonella typhimurium* and enhanced antioxidant activity was observed when cumin and coriander seed were used in combination.[2614] The researchers concluded that the bioactive compounds responsible for their antimicrobial and antioxidant effects were linalool (coriander) and p-coumaric acid (cumin).

☐ Coriander oil is effective against *C. albicans* alone or in combination with amphotericin B (an antifungal drug used for potentially life-threatening fungal infections).[2615] Another study tested the major constituents of coriander oil and coriander oil against *C. albicans* and found that the oil has stronger activity than any of its major constituents alone.[2616]

☐ Clinical research suggests coriander oil mildly reduces skin inflammation, redness, and rash following UVB exposure at a concentration of 0.5%.[2617]

☐ Extracts of coriander help normalize blood-sugar levels in animals, possibly by inhibiting alpha-glucosidase.[2618,2619]

☐ A review article concluded that coriander essential oil is a leading candidate to use as a natural food preservative due to its ability to inhibit gram-negative and gram-positive bacteria, yeasts, dermatophytes, and filamentous fungi.[4761]

☐ Animal research demonstrates that oral administration of 0.5 mL/kg of coriander seed essential oil alleviated colitis as evidenced by reduced myeloperoxidase activity (an enzyme used as a marker of the extent of inflammation in the colon), colon ulcer severity, and colitis index.[2620]

☐ Coriander CT carvone and thyme CT carvacrol inhibited avian multidrug-resistant strains of *E. coli*, which led the authors to conclude these essential oils have potential to be used as replacements for antibiotics in avian treatment.[2621]

☐ Oral administration of both coriander essential oil and its primary constituent protected against liver harm caused by carbon tetrachloride in rats.[2622] Linalool also improved antioxidant activity (reduced glutathione and catalase).

☐ Aflatoxin B1 (AFB1) is a highly toxic and cancer-causing metabolite produced by *Aspergillus* fungi. These fungi frequently contaminate food and agricultural commodities. Both coriander CT linalool and cumin CT cuminaldehyde essential oils inhibited the growth of *A. flavus* and noticeably reduced its production of AFB1.[2623] Cumin was the most effective essential oil for reducing AFB1.

☐ Leishmaniasis is a neglected tropical disease caused by parasitic protozoa of the *Leishmania* genus. Current treatment options for cutaneous leishmaniasis are limited due to severe side effects, poor efficacy, resistance to first-line drugs, and limited availability to populations who need the medication. A study evaluated the antileishmanial activities of fifty-two essential oils and concluded that frankincense (a combination of *Boswellia carterii, B. sacra, B. papyrifera,* and *B. frereana*), coriander, and wintergreen possesses notable antileishmanial activities that make them promising candidates for the topical treatment of cutaneous leishmaniasis.[2624]

☐ Coriander essential oil exhibited moderate antioxidant activity and strongly inhibited *B. subtilis*, followed by *S. maltophilia* and *Penicillium expansum*.[2625] Moreover, the oil strongly inhibited biofilm formation of *S. maltophilia*.

☐ Coriander (150 µL/L), linaloe (125 µL/L), and lavandin (200 µL/L) essential oil exhibited anesthetic activity in convict cichlid (*Amatitlania nigrofasciata*) fish.[2626]

☐ Aβ1-42 oligomers are toxic to brain cells, causing membrane disruption, and a key molecular factor in the onset and progression of Alzheimer's disease (AD). Laboratory research found that adding lavender or coriander essential oil, or isolated linalool, with brain cells protected against damage caused by Aβ1-42 oligomers.[2627] The research suggests that lavender, coriander, and linalool protect against neurotoxicity and could have potential in AD management.

☐ Caraway (31.0% gamma-terpinene, 18.8% beta-pinene, 17.2% para-cymene, 12.8% bornyl acetate, 12.2% carvone) and coriander essential oils were compared for biological activities alone and in combination.[2628] Caraway had higher antioxidant activity alone, but the combination of the two oils exhibited the highest antioxidant activity. The oils were tested in the DPPH, FRAP, superoxide anion, beta-carotene, and chelating assays. Both oils inhibited a variety of pathogenic organisms (*S. epidermidis, S. aureus, M. luteus, E. faecalis, B. cereus, E. coli, L. monocytogenes, P. aeruginosa, S. typhimurium, Vibrio* spp., *Candida* spp., *S. cerevisiae*) with the combination of the oils more active than the individual oils. Caraway and coriander significantly inhibited acetylcholinesterase (AChE) activity, with the combination enhancing the anti-AChE activity. High antidiabetic activity was also observed for the combination of oils when compared to acarbose. Pharmacokinetic analysis suggests the oils combination has a favorable drug likeness and safety profile.

☐ A study evaluated the chemical composition and antimicrobial (nine respiratory tract pathogens) activity of forty-nine commercial essential oils recommended for respiratory tract infections. Amyris, coriander, and sandalwood (*S. austrocaledonicum*) were identified as having the greatest activity.[2629] The oils tested were balsam fir, amyris, frankincense (*B. carterii*), elemi, caraway, camphor, cinnamon leaf, lime, bergamot, lemon, orange, myrrh, coriander, cypress, lemongrass (*C. citratus*), carrot seed, cardamom, eucalyptus (*E. globulus*), fennel, helichrysum, hyssop CT isopinocamphone, star anise, cedarwood (*J. virginiana*), bay laurel, lavender, lavandin (*L. burnati*), spike lavender, tea tree, cajeput, niaouli, peppermint, myrtle, basil CT methyl chavicol, marjoram, oregano CT carvacrol, pimento, pine, black pepper, rose, rosemary CT camphor, sage, clary sage, benzoin, clove bud, tagetes (*T. minuta*), thyme CT para-cymene, and ginger.

☐ Dermatophyte infections are caused by a group of filamentous fungi that require keratin (structural proteins found in the hair, nails, and outermost layers of the skin) for growth. It is estimated that up to 25 percent of the world's population is affected by dermatophyte infections, with *Trichophyton rubrum* and *T. mentagrophytes* accounting for 70 percent of infections. Terbinafine is a first-line drug used to treat these infections, but its side effects (liver injury, gastrointestinal disturbances, headache, change in taste, and rash), interactions with other drugs, and the emergence of drug-resistant strains reduce its clinical use and efficacy. An *in vitro* study found that ajowan CT thymol, coriander, caraway CT carvone, and anise weakly to moderately inhibited *T. rubrum* and *T. mentagrophytes*—ajowan was the most effective and anise the least effective.[2630] In addition, the essential oils significantly potentiated the activity of terbinafine when used in combination, suggesting essential oils could reduce the amount of the drug needed to be effective and therefore potentially its side effects. None of the essential oils reduced white blood cell (neutrophil) viability at the tested concentrations, but did moderately inhibit their release of proinflammatory cytokines (IL-1β, IL-8, and TNF-α). Each oil reduced IL-1β and IL-8 (ajowan most active against IL-1β and coriander most active against IL-8) and only coriander and caraway reduced TNF-α.

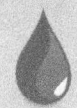

- A nanoemulgel containing coriander essential oil inhibited *P. aeruginosa, K. pneumoniae,* and MRSA and encouraged anticancer activity against breast, liver, and cervical cancer cells.[2631] The bioactivity of the nanoemulgel was greater than the crude oil.

- Transforming growth factor beta (TGFB) is a cytokine that regulates cellular processes, including those related to aging and age-related disorders. TGFB signaling and activity is impaired in certain cell types resulting in age-related changes. Coriander essential oil showed high inhibitory activities against collagenase, elastase, tyrosinase, and hyaluronidase—enzymes that trigger the appearance of skin aging.[2632] Topical application of a cream and nanoparticle formulation with coriander oil diminished UV-induced skin photoaging, increased skin collagen content, and restored healthy TGFB activity, reducing wrinkles and skin aging in mice.

- Comparison of coriander extracted via distillation (61.8% linalool) and SFE (51.3% linalool) showed that the SFE displayed higher antioxidant activity in the DPPH and FRAP assays and stronger antibiofilm activity.[2633] SFE was more effective against *P. multocida* and *A. alternata,* whereas distilled oil was more effective against *E. coli* and *A. niger.*

- Ingestion of coriander essential oil—as part of feed, twice daily for sixty days—improved antioxidant activity, the inflammatory response, and innate immune responses in Nile tilapia.[2634] Hemoglobin, including corpuscular volume and mean cell hemoglobin, increased significantly, and antioxidant activity was enhanced. Survival increased after challenge with *Aeromonas hydrophila,* with the 1.5% and 2% concentrations increasing survival to 100 percent. Expression of anti-inflammatory mediators (IgM and IL-8) significantly increased, with a simultaneous decrease in proinflammatory mediators (TNFα, IL-1β, TGFβ, and HSP 70). The spleen was also protected by coriander.

- Coriander essential oil showed antifungal activity against planktonic and multibiofilm *Candida* spp.[2635]

- Subinhibitory concentrations of coriander, oregano, clove, and thyme essential oils reduce *S. Aureus* biofilm formation by at least 80 percent. Coriander and oregano also demonstrated additive effects when used with cefoperazone.[2636]

- *In vitro* research showed that coriander is antimicrobial against *C. albicans.*[2637]

# CUMIN

*Cuminum cyminum* L., *Cuminum odorum* Salisb.

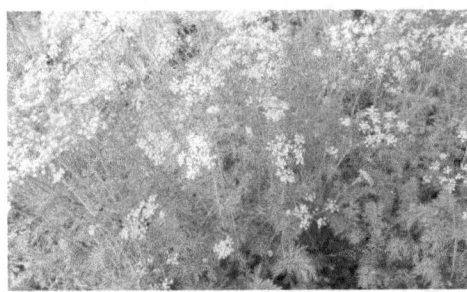

**FAMILY:** Apiaceae (Umbelliferae)
**NOTE:** Middle-Base
**AROMA INTENSITY:** Strong
**AROMA:** Spicy, earthy, musky, slightly nutty
**COMMON EXTRACTION METHOD:** Steam distilled from the seeds; may also be distilled from the roots, stems, leaves, and flowers
**POSSIBLE SUBSTITUTE OILS:** Coriander
**BLENDS WELL WITH:** Angelica root, black pepper, caraway, chamomile (German, Roman), coriander, lavender, rosemary, turmeric
**SUBCELLULAR LOCALIZATION | EPIGENETIC INFLUENCE:** Currently unknown | Currently unknown
**RECOMMENDED DILUTION RANGE:** 5%–50%; neat for limited conditions

**PRIMARY CONSTITUENTS:**[2638,2639,2640,2641]

*Seeds*

| | |
|---|---|
| Cuminaldehyde | 19.9%–39.5% |
| Cuminyl alcohol | 0.2%–30.0% |
| Safranal | 0.0%–26.8% |
| P-Mentha-1,4-Dien-7-al | 0.0%–25.5% |
| P-Mentha-1,3-Dien-7-al | 0.0%–17.5% |
| Beta-Pinene | 6.8%–16.3% |
| Para-Cymene | 4.1%–15.6% |
| Gamma-Terpinene | 0.0%–19.6% |

| | |
|---|---|
| O-Cymene | 0.0%–11.8% |
| 2-Caren-10-al | 0.0%–7.9% |
| Alpha-Terpinene | 0.1%–5.7% |
| Trans-Carveol | 0.0%–4.5% |
| Myrtenal | 0.0%–3.5% |
| 1,8-Cineole | 0.1%–2.2% |
| Alpha-Phellandrene | 0.0%–1.9% |
| Alpha-Pinene Oxide | 0.0%–1.6% |
| Myrcene | 0.0%–1.2% |
| Alpha-Pinene | 0.3%–1.0% |

Note: Cuminaldehyde content will be lower when distilled from unripe fruit. Distilling fully ripe fruit yields greater percentages of cuminaldehyde, gamma-terpinene, and para-cymene but reduces the percentage of beta-phellandrene.

**OTHER CONSTITUENTS:** Perillaldehyde, comphene, sabinene, beta-phellandrene, alpha-cedrene, daucene

**PREFERRED COMPOSITION FOR CLINICAL USE:**

| *Constituent* | |
|---|---|
| **Cuminaldehyde (Cuminal)** | 21%–48% |
| **Gamma-Terpinene** | 5%–20% |
| **P-Mentha-1,3-Dien-7-al (α-Terpinene-7al)** | 5%–20% |
| **Beta-Pinene** | 8%–18% |
| **Para-Cymene** | 4%–16% |
| **P-Mentha-1,4 -Dien-7-al (γ-Terpinene-7al)** | 4%–15% |
| **Alpha-Phellandrene** | 0.1%–5% |
| **Alpha-Pinene** | 0.1%–2% |
| **Myrcene** | 0.1%–2% |

**REPORTED THERAPEUTIC PROPERTIES:** Anti-inflammatory, antibacterial, antifungal, diuretic, antiseptic, antispasmodic, aids circulation, **aids detoxification**, helps relieve colic, eases stomach cramps, expels excess gas, **aids digestion**, nervine, regulates menstruation, reduces fever, encourages normal blood pressure, promotes oral health, tones muscles and skin, purifying, combats fatigue, aphrodisiac, clears past emotional trauma, uplifting

**CAUTIONS:**

■ Cumin is photosensitizing. Avoid UV rays to area of application for at least twelve hours after topical application.[2642]

■ May interact with antibiotics and increase or decrease their effectiveness.[2643]

**SELECTED EVIDENCE:**

☐ *In vitro* research concluded that cumin oil possesses antimicrobial activity similar to penicillin against *Nocardia asterides* (a harmful organism that causes severe pulmonary infections in people whose immune system is compromised), and inhibits *E. coli* and *B. subtilis* similarly to streptomycin.[2644] Another study found that cumin oil was equally or more effective as an antibacterial agent when compared to standard antibiotics.[2645] A synergistic (the sum of the effect is greater than the two individual essential oils combined—i.e. 2 + 2 = 10) antimicrobial activity against *Bacillus cereus, Listeria monocytogenes, Staphylococcus aureus,* and *Escherichia coli,* and an additive (the sum of the effect is equivalent to the sum of the two essential oils separately—i.e. 2 + 2 + 4) effect against *Micrococcus luteus* and *Salmonella typhimurium* and enhanced antioxidant activity was observed when cumin and coriander seed were used in combination.[2646] The researchers concluded that the bioactive compounds responsible for their antimicrobial and antioxidant effects were linalool (coriander) and p-coumaric acid (cumin).

☐ Cumin oil is highly effective against *Vibrio* spp. bacteria (food-borne bacteria that cause diarrhea in healthy individuals and possibly life-threatening bloodstream infections in those who are immunocompromised).[2647] The authors also concluded that cumin oil was antibacterial, antifungal, and antioxidant, which makes it a good option for food preservation and in therapeutic applications.

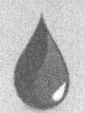

- Cumin inhibits *Candida* species (*C. albicans* and *C. dubliniensis*), which made the authors conclude it may be an effective alternative therapy for candidiasis.[2648] An interesting cumin essential oil with 1,8-cineole (21.1%), cyclopentapyran (18.8%), o-cymene (16.7%), beta-pinene (16.1%), and moslene (16.6%) inhibited *C. albicans* strains isolated from people with recurrent vulvovaginal candidiasis.[2649]
- Cumin oil increases the effectiveness of nisin (an antibacterial peptide used as a food preservative) against the bacteria *B. cereus* and *B. subtilis*.[2650] Researchers concluded that cumin oil decreased bacterial growth by damaging the cell wall.
- *In vitro* research suggests that cumin oil actively inhibits pathogenic yeasts.[2651]
- Cumin oil mildly reduces dental plaque formation, which may help prevent cavities.[2652]
- Research suggests that cumin oil may help reduce the frequency and severity of drug-induced seizures.[2653]
- Cumin exerts significant anti-inflammatory effects by inhibiting nitric oxide synthase, COX-2, IL-1, IL-6, and blocking signaling pathways.[2654]
- Cumin essential oil is active against the parasite *Anisakis Dujardin* (a parasite that causes gastrointestinal and allergic diseases in humans that eat raw or undercooked seafood).[2655]
- A double-blind randomized placebo-controlled clinical trial demonstrated that oral administration of 50 mg and 100 mg of cumin essential oil significantly decreased serum insulin, fasting blood glucose, glycosylated hemoglobin (HgA1c), and inflammatory markers (TNF-α, high-sensitivity C-reactive protein (hsCRP)) and significantly increased insulin sensitivity and adiponectin in people with type II diabetes.[2656] Studies show that TNF-α and hsCRP are increased and adiponectin decreased in type II diabetics. This research suggests that cumin essential oil may help manage diabetes and reduce diabetic-related complications.
- Cumin essential oil demonstrated high (100 percent) acaricidal activity against engorged female cattle ticks (*Rhipicephalus microplus*).[2657]
- Oral administration of cumin (400 mg/kg BW) and German chamomile (250 mg/kg BW) essential oil for two weeks prior to acetaminophen dosing (1 g/kg BW) partially protected against liver toxicity caused by acetaminophen. In rats,[2658] cumin normalized liver enzymes (including alanine aminotransferase and aspartate aminotransferase), preserved liver structure, and ameliorated disruption of the liver antioxidant system. German chamomile slightly reversed the increase in alanine aminotransferase levels and moderately reversed glutathione depletion and decreased superoxide dismutase activity.
- *Borrelia burgdorferi* is a diderm bacteria responsible for Lyme disease in the United States. Of thirty-five essential oils screened, garlic, allspice, cumin, palmarosa, myrrh, ginger lily, amyris, thyme, may chang, and lemon eucalyptus each demonstrated excellent activity against *Borrelia burgdorferi*.[2659] Garlic (19% diallyl disulfide), allspice CT eugenol, and myrrh (38% curzerene) were the most active essential oils.
- Cumin, fennel, dill, and anise essential oils each demonstrated inhibitory activity against *Candida* species, with cumin being the most active.[2660] Fennel and anise were not cytotoxic to mouse fibroblasts at minimum inhibitory concentrations.
- Human aryl hydrocarbon receptor (AhR: a gene that encodes a protein that helps regulate responses to planar aromatic hydrocarbons and significantly affects the immune activity in the gastrointestinal tract) regulates the circadian rhythm, helps regulate the cell cycle, and plays an important role in tissue development. Cumin, jasmine, vanilla, and bay leaf fully activate AhR; clove, dill, thyme, nutmeg, and oregano partially activate AhR; and tarragon, caraway, turmeric, lovage, fennel, spearmint, star anise, and anise inhibit the AhR activity.[2661]
- Cumin essential oil inhibited the germination red-root amaranth (*Amaranthus retroflexus*, an aggressive weed), lettuce (*Lactuca sativa*), and hardheads (*Acroptilon repens*, a significant weed pest), suggesting it has potential as a natural herbicide.[2662]
- The incidence of metabolic syndrome (MetS: a cluster of connected serious disorders) is increasing and a major health problem that increases oxidative stress and inflammation. A randomized, triple blind, placebo-controlled clinical trial found that oral administration of 75 mg of cumin essential oil, three times daily, for eight weeks, reduced markers for MetS in people aged eighteen to sixty years with MetS.[2663] The oil improved antioxidant activity and simultaneously decreased free radicals; therefore reducing oxidative stress. Interestingly, a follow-up clinical (randomized, triple-blind, placebo-controlled) study by the same researchers found that oral administration of 75 mg of cumin essential oil only improved diastolic blood pressure in people with MetS.[2664]
- Both cumin and fennel essential oil showed promise as alternatives to conventional drugs for the treatment of *Candida* infections due to their ability to inhibit *Candida* species isolated from the mouths of edentulous patients.[2665] Cumin was more effective than fennel.

- Aflatoxin B1 (AFB1) is a highly toxic and cancer-causing metabolite produced by *Aspergillus* fungi. These fungi frequently contaminate food and agricultural commodities. Both coriander CT linalool and cumin CT cuminaldehyde essential oils inhibited the growth of *A. flavus* and noticeably reduced its production of AFB1.[2666] Cumin was the most effective essential oil for reducing AFB1.

- Cumin essential oils inhibited *Campylobacter* spp. (*C. jejuni* and *C. coli*) by affecting bacterial cell membrane integrity.[2667]

- Cumin essential oil (28.3% cuminaldehyde) exhibited free radical scavenging activity and a significant inhibitory effect in the beta-carotene bleaching assay (neutralizing hydroperoxides).[2668] The same research reported antimicrobial activity against *C. albicans, S. aureus, L. innocua, E. coli,* and *P. aeruginosa.*

- *Candida* are yeasts present in the gastrointestinal tract and mucous membranes of humans and other mammals associated with localized and systemic illnesses. *Candida* infections are increasingly resistant to first-line drugs causing scientists and health professionals to seek alternative treatment solutions. Laboratory research concluded that cumin, fennel, and Manuka CT leptospermone essential oils each inhibited *Candida* spp. supporting their application as natural solutions for *Candida* infections.[2669]

- A nanoemulsion of cumin seed essential oil exhibited anticancer activity against tongue carcinoma and significant antibacterial activity against *S. aureus* in laboratory research.[2670] The study authors concluded that cumin has potential as a component of cancer therapy and to help overcome antimicrobial resistance.

- Consumption of probiotic soy milk with cumin essential oil for thirty days significantly reduced fasting blood sugar, total cholesterol, and LDL cholesterol, and increased HDL cholesterol in diabetic rats.[2671] The soy-cumin milk also increased weight gain.

- Incorporation of encapsulated cumin essential oil into mayonnaise improved product stability and antioxidant properties.[2672] The same encapsulated cumin oil exhibited slight anticancer effects against breast and brain tumors.

- *In vitro* research demonstrated that cumin essential oil inhibits oral pathogens (*S. mutans* and *S. oralis*).[2673]

- Dill, cumin, and parsley were each toxic to the maize weevil (*Sitophilus zeamais*) in the contact assay.[2674] The same researchers noted that each of the oils and fennel also repelled the insect. Carvone (fumigant and contact) and cuminaldehyde were the most active isolated constituents for toxicity, and cuminaldehyde, carvone, and estragole the most active isolated constituents for repellents.

- Laboratory research found that cumin essential oil was 99 percent effective as an ovicidal (kills the eggs) against the liver fluke (Fasciola hepatica).[2675] The liver fluke is a parasitic trematode that infects the livers of various mammals, including humans.

- *In vitro* research concluded that cumin essential oil inhibited *A. aculeatus*, a fungi responsible for bunch rot in grapes during postharvest.[2676] Isolated cuminaldehyde and alpha-terpinen-7-al were also active. Spraying the grapes with the cumin oil at 1,000 mcg/mL reduced severity and incidence of bunch rot.

- A cumin nanoemulsion enhanced the penetration and pain-relieving effects of diclofenac sodium in mice.[2677]

- Researchers investigated the antibacterial activity of cumin essential oil against ten multidrug-resistant strains of *S. aureus*.[2678] The oil exhibited bacteriostatic and bactericidal properties, which caused the researchers to conclude that cumin is a promising solution to control infections caused by MRSA.

- Immersion tests showed that oregano CT carvacrol and cinnamon bark essential oil are significantly acaricidal against the Asian longhorned tick (*Haemaphysalis longicornis*) larvae and unfed adults.[2679] The fumigant test demonstrated significant acaricidal activity against larvae, unfed and engorged nymphs, and adults.

- Neutrophils serve as the first line of defense against infections and play important roles in initiating inflammatory reactions. An unbalanced response to an infection can trigger uncontrolled inflammation and the progression of neutrophilic inflammatory diseases such as arthritis, psoriasis, asthma, chronic obstructive pulmonary disease, cystic fibrosis, and acute respiratory distress syndrome. Neutrophils are the most abundant innate immune cells and leverage several mechanisms to destroy invading pathogens and activate other immune cells. These activities must maintain a delicate balance to avoid uncontrolled inflammation and destruction of healthy cells. Tropical fennel (methyl chavicol CT) and cumin essential oils significantly suppressed the activation of neutrophils and balanced the mechanisms they use to attack pathogens *in vitro*, suggesting they may be useful for neutrophilic inflammatory diseases.[2680]

- Of four essential oils tested (Zataria CT carvacrol, wild mint CT pulegone, cumin, and *Ferulago angulata*), Zataria essential oil was the most active against drug-resistant *E. coli*. Cumin and wild mint were semi-active.[2681]

- Cumin essential oil was active against fifteen *Vibrio* species, with the highest inhibition recorded against *V. fluvialis, V. parahaemolyticus,* and *V. natrigens*.[2682] Biofilm formation was inhibited by *V. alginolyticus, V. parahaemolyticus, V. cholerae,* and *V. vulnificus.* Both the oil and isolated cuminaldehyde inhibited violacein

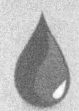

production by *Vibrio* species and elastase and protease production in *P. aeruginosa*. The oil also displayed good antioxidant activity in the DPPH, beta-carotene, FRAP, and chelating power assays.

☐ *In vitro* research showed that cumin, anise, and caraway essential oil each inhibited *H. pylori*, with cumin exhibiting the greatest activity and cuminaldehyde the best docking potential to inhibit *H. pylori*.[2683] The three oils were also evaluated for their ability to reduce the production of COX-2 (an enzyme responsible for pain and inflammation). Cumin reduced COX-2 expression nearly as well as celecoxib, followed by caraway and anise.

☐ Anise and tagetes (*T. minuta*) showed strong insecticidal activity against the corn sap beetle (*Carpophilus dimidiatus*) and the merchant grain beetle (*Oryzaephilus mercator*), while cumin was strongly insecticidal against the merchant grain beetle.[2684]

☐ A nanoemulsion and nanogel loaded with cumin essential oil demonstrated anticancer activity against human melanoma cells, antioxidant activity, antibacterial activity (*P. aeruginosa*, *S. aureus*, and larvicidal activity (*Ae. stephensi*)).[2685]

# CYPRESS
## (Mediterranean Cypress)
*Cupressus sempervirens* L.

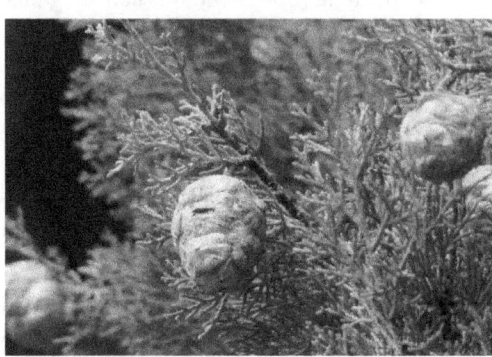

**FAMILY:** Cupressaceae
**NOTE:** Middle
**AROMA INTENSITY:** Medium
**AROMA:** Fresh, slightly woody, evergreen
**COMMON EXTRACTION METHOD:** Steam distilled from the needles and twigs
**POSSIBLE SUBSTITUTE OILS:** Pine, balsam fir, silver fir, cedarwood, juniper berry, helichrysum, frankincense
**BLENDS WELL WITH:** Bay laurel, bergamot, blue cypress, camphor, cedarwood, clary sage, coriander, frankincense, juniper, lavender, lemon, lime, marjoram, orange, palo santo, pine, rosemary, sandalwood, Spanish sage, spikenard
**SUBCELLULAR LOCALIZATION | EPIGENETIC INFLUENCE:** Endocytic Vesicles | Skeletal/Integumentary
**RECOMMENDED DILUTION RANGE:** 3%–Neat

**PRIMARY CONSTITUENTS:**[2686,2687,2688,2689,2690]

| | |
|---|---|
| Alpha-Pinene | 30.0%–64.2% |
| Delta-3-Carene | 11.1%–22.7% |
| Alpha-Terpinolene | 4.5%–6.6% |
| Alpha-Terpinyl Acetate | 0.0%–6.6% |
| Limonene | 2.0%–5.4% |

**OTHER CONSTITUENTS:** Alpha-thujene, alpha-fenchene, camphene, sabinene, beta-pinene, myrcene, 1,3-para-menthadiene, o-cymene, 1,8-cineole, gamma-terpinene, germacrene D, delta-cadinene, alpha-cedrol, 4-terpineol, beta-caryophyllene

**PREFERRED COMPOSITION FOR CLINICAL USE:**

| Constituent | |
|---|---|
| **Alpha-Pinene** | 45%–65% |
| **Delta-3-Carene** | 15%–28% |
| **Alpha-Terpinolene** | 2%–7% |
| **Limonene** | 2%–7% |
| **Myrcene** | 1%–4% |
| **Alpha-Terpinyl Acetate** | 0.5%–4% |
| **Germacrene D** | 0.1%–3% |
| **Beta-Pinene** | 0.1%–3% |

**REPORTED THERAPEUTIC PROPERTIES:** Antibacterial, anti-inflammatory, antiseptic, antispasmodic, **astringent**, relieves painful menstruation, **circulatory stimulant**, **diuretic**, **stops excess bleeding**, supports liver health, helps heal hemorrhoids, deodorant, expectorant, **respiratory stimulant**, eases cough, **helps relieve excess perspiration**, promotes fluid balance and removes excess fluids from the body, relieves oily skin, warming, sedating, combats grief and trauma, aids the emotions during difficult transitions, eases feelings of being overwhelmed, promotes confidence, diminishes guilt and perfectionism, promotes a sense of security

**CAUTIONS:**

■ May interact with aspirin, blood pressure, antiplatelet, and anticoagulant medications, and increase the risk of bleeding among people with bleeding disorders.[2691]

**SELECTED EVIDENCE:**

☐ Cypress oil prevents the spread of melanoma cancer cells *in vitro*.[2692] The study authors also determined that beta-caryophyllene was active against both kidney and melanoma cancer cell lines, as was linalool and alpha-cedrol to a lesser degree.

☐ Cypress oil is an effective nitric oxide free-radical scavenger (antioxidant).[2693] It also prevents the nonenzymatic bonding of lipids to sugars (glycation).[2694] Damage caused by glycation can lead to stiffening of the blood vessel walls and high blood pressure, particularly among diabetics.

☐ Cypress possesses moderate antimicrobial properties against fungi (*A. aspergillus* and *F. oxysporum*) and bacteria (*S. aureus, E. faecalis, B. cereus E. coli*, and *P. aeruginosa*).[2695]

☐ An interesting cedrol CT of the aerial parts of cypress essential oil inhibited the growth of gram-positive (*S. epidermidis, S. pyogenes, S. aureus*) and gram-negative bacteria (*E. coli, K. pneumonia, P. vulgaris, P. aeruginosa, Sh. Boydii*), and the fungi *C. albicans*.[2696]

☐ The essential oils of lemon (fungicidal), cypress (fungicidal), and may chang (fungistatic) each demonstrated anticandidal activity in planktonic (free flowing bacteria in suspension) cells and biofilms (a thin, slimy film of bacteria adhered to a surface) and cypress increased survival of the tested host in the *Caenorhabditis elegans-Candida* model.[2697]

☐ Cypress essential oil and nanoemulsion were toxic to adult and larvae of *C. quinquefasciatus* mosquitoes, with the nanoemulsion demonstrating superior activity.[2698]

☐ Both cypress and pennyroyal essential oil exhibited acaricidal activity and inhibited egg hatching of ticks (*Hyalomma scupense*), with cypress being more active at the concentrations tested.[2699] The highest acaricidal property was observed when the two oils were used in combination. Both oils also acted as a tick repellent.

☐ Cypress essential oil exhibited anticancer activity against lung cancer cells.[2700]

☐ Cypress essential oil displayed strong antioxidant activity in the DPPH and ABTS assays, anticancer activity against two breast cancer cell lines, colon cancer cells, myelogenous leukemia cells (most sensitive cancer cell line), and choriocarcinoma cells (uterine, placental), inhibited *C. albicans, D. subtilis, C. glabrata, P. citrinum, B. cinerae, S. enterica* subsp. *enterica, A. flavus, C. tropicalis, Y. enterocolitica, P. aeuruginosa*, and *C. krusei*, and strong insecticidal activity against the lime seed bug (*Oxycarenus lavaterae*) in a concentration dependent manner.[2701]

---

# DAMIANA
## (Mexican Holly)

*Turnera diffusa* Willd. ex Schult., *T. diffusa* var. *diffusa*, *T. aphrodisiaca*, *T. diffusa* var. *aphrodisiaca*

**FAMILY:** Turneraceae
**NOTE:** Middle
**AROMA INTENSITY:** Medium
**AROMA:** Fruity, bitter-sweet, slightly floral and herbaceous
**COMMON EXTRACTION METHOD:** Steam distilled from the leaves/flowers
**POSSIBLE SUBSTITUTE OILS:** Vilayti tulsi, sage (wild), ylang ylang, kanuka, rosemary, myrtle

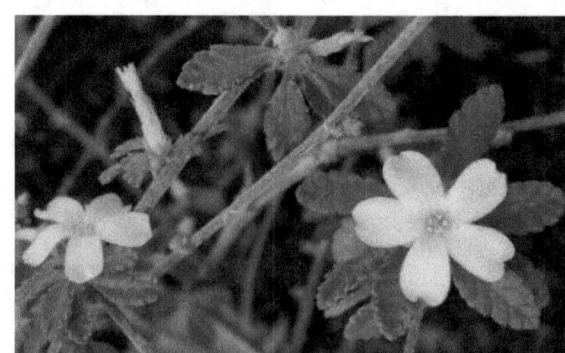

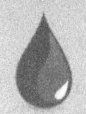

**BLENDS WELL WITH:** Black Pepper, cardamom, cedarwood, chamomile (German, Roman), cinnamon, clary sage, clove, combava, davana, fingerroot, geranium, ginger, jasmine, juniper, lavender, magnolia, neroli, patchouli, petitgrain, rhododendron, rose, sandalwood, ylang ylang, yuzu

**SUBCELLULAR LOCALIZATION | EPIGENETIC INFLUENCE:** Currently unknown | Currently unknown

**RECOMMENDED DILUTION RANGE:** 3%–50%; neat for limited conditions

**PRIMARY CONSTITUENTS:**[2702,2703,2704,2705]

*1,8-Cineole CT*

| | |
|---|---|
| 1,8-Cineole | 11.4%–35.2% |
| Selina-6-en-4-ol <isomer> | 0.0%–12.0% |
| 1,2,3-Trimethyl-2-Cyclopentene -1-carboxylic acid | 0.0%–10.6% |
| Oplopenone | 1.0%–10.3% |
| Guaiol | 0.0%–8.9% |
| Cadalene | 0.0%–5.1% |
| 10-Epi-Gamma-Eudesmol | 0.0%–4.5% |
| 1-Epi-Cubenol | 0.0%–4.1% |
| Caryophyllene Oxide | 0.9%–3.6% |
| Aristolene | 0.0%–3.5% |
| Delta-Cadinene | 1.4%–2.6% |

*Delta-Cadinene CT*

| | |
|---|---|
| Delta-Cadinene | 5.5%–7.7% |
| Caryophyllene Oxide | 2.9%–5.3% |
| 1,8-Cineole | 1.9%–2.8% |
| Beta-Elemene | 2.7%–3.2% |

*Caryophyllene Oxide CT*

| | |
|---|---|
| Caryophyllene Oxide | 9.6%–13.7% |
| Alpha-Cadinene | 0.0%–7.3% |
| Alpha-Cadinol | 0.0%–6.5% |
| Oplopenone | 0.0%–6.0% |
| Beta-Caryophyllene | 0.6%–5.6% |
| Beta-Pinene | 0.0%–3.9% |
| Delta-Cadinene | 1.0%–2.7% |
| Delta-Cadinol | 0.0%–2.6% |

**OTHER CONSTITUENTS:** *1,8-Cineole CT*—alpha-pinene, trans-pinocarveol, p-mentha-1,5-dien-8-ol, alpha-terpineol, damiana<43, 1280>, damiana<149, 1499>, damiana<126, 1502>, damiana<109, 1549>, damiana<135, 1576>, damiana<111, 1590>, damiana<107, 1657>, damiana<177, 1672>, damiana<43, 1701>, alpha-terpinyl acetate, dehydro-isolongifolenene, delta-selinene, (E)-nerolidol, furopelargone B, ledol, humulene epoxide II, uvetiver, 1-epi-cubenol, T-cadinol, T-muurolol, uamyris, velarinol, selin-11-en-4-alpha-ol, lingifolene-8-oxo, juniper camphor, carvacrol dimer, eremophila-7(11),9-dien-8-one, 3-hexen-1-ol, germacrene A, beta-elemene, allyl tiglate, (Z)-3-hexenyl tiglate, alpha-amorphene, alpha-terpineol, gamma-cadinene, globulol, spathulenol, phytol, alpha-copaene, thymol; *Caryophyllene Oxide CT*—alpha-pinene, limonene, 1,8-cineole, delta-3-carene, alpha-copaene, norinone, trans-2-hexenal, 1-hexanol, 3-hexen-1-ol, trans-linalool oxide, cycloisosativen, linalool, pinocarvone, germacrene A, beta-elemene, aristolene, isoledene, allyl tiglate, myrtenal, alloaromadendrene, alpha-terpineol, gamma-cadinene, myrtenol, p-cymen-8-ol, globulol, spathulenol, juniper camphor, phytol, palmitic acid, guaiol, gamma-amorphene; *Delta-cadinene CT*—alpha-pinene, beta-pinene, alpha-cubebene, delta-3-carene, alpha-copaene, linalool, pinocarvone, aristolene, norinone, beta-caryophyllene, alloaromadendrene, myrtenal, gamma-amorphene, germacrene B, gamma-cadinene, spathulenol

**PREFERRED COMPOSITION FOR CLINICAL USE:**

| Constituent | 1,8-Cineole I | 1,8-Cineole CT II |
|---|---|---|
| **1,8-Cineole** | 20%–50% | 18%–38% |
| **Damiana Esters** | – | 3%–12% |
| **Oplopenone** | 0.1%–5% | 1%–10% |
| **Delta-Cadinene** | 2%–7% | 1%–5% |
| **Camphor** | – | 0.1%–5% |
| **Caryophyllene Oxide** | 1%–5% | 0.1%–5% |
| **Selina-6-en-4-ol <isomer>** | 3%–12% | – |
| **Epoxy Drimenene** | 5%–10% | – |
| **Alpha-Pinene** | 2%–5% | – |

**REPORTED THERAPEUTIC PROPERTIES:** Antiseptic, analgesic, antispasmodic, supports respiratory function, astringent, diuretic, relieves headache, immune stimulant, nervine, relieves painful menstruation, balances menstruation, supports kidney function, reduces sexual dysfunction (impotence), eases cough, aids circulation, **aphrodisiac**, relieves anxiety, antidepressant, relieves mental exhaustion

## CAUTIONS:

*Caryophyllene Oxide and Delta-Cadinene CTs*

■ None currently known.

*1,8-Cineole CT*

■ Avoid with epilepsy and Parkinson's due to 1,8-cineole content, which may exacerbate or trigger seizures/convulsions or reduce medication efficacy.[2706,2707,2708]

■ May interfere with pentobarbital and other barbiturates (medications for anxiety and insomnia) if 1,8-cineole content is high.[2709,2710,2711]

■ May weakly interfere with the enzymes responsible for metabolizing medications (NSAIDs, proton-pump inhibitors, acetaminophen, antiepleptics, immune modulators, blood-sugar medications, blood pressure medications, antidepressants, antipsychotics, diabetic medications, antihistamines, antibiotics, and anesthetics) due to 1,8-cineole content.[2712,2713,2714]

## SELECTED EVIDENCE:

☐ *In vitro* research shows that a damiana essential oil with drima-7,9(11)-diene (22.9%) and viridiflorene (6.6%) as the primary constituents inhibits fifteen strains of *Mycobacterium tuberculosis*.[2715] *M. tuberculosis* causes one of the most ancient and opportunistic epidemic diseases in the world—tuberculosis.

☐ May chang CT citral and damiana CT citral demonstrated strong antiviral activity against dengue virus and inhibited viral replication.[2716] Computer docking studies showed that twenty sesquiterpene hydrocarbons, eight oxygenated monoterpenes, and seven monoterpene hydrocarbons had good binding affinity to the DENV-2 E protein with cis-calamenene, delta-cadinene, alpha-cadinene, alpha-guaiene, gamma-cadinene, and viridiflorene having the highest binding affinity.

☐ Damiana demonstrated strong insecticidal and moderate larvicidal activity against *A. aegypti* mosquitoes.[2717]

☐ A 1% concentration of damiana essential oil increased the delivery of a caffeine hydrogel through the skin. Salva-de Marajo (*Lippia origanoides*), eugenol, carvacrol, and limonene were also effective.[2718]

---

*Did you know?*

A special imaging technique called laser scanning confocal microscopy allows scientists to observe essential oils as they interact with live cells. This technique proves that essential oils penetrate the cell membrane and localize within human cells. Interestingly, essential oils tend to localize within certain organelles, such as cypress localizing in the endocytic vesicle. The endocytic vesicle functions to bring large materials from outside the cell inside the cell, which suggests that cypress may facilitate active transport of materials inside the cell.

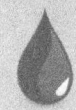

# DAVANA
## (Dhavanam)
*Artemisia pallens* Wall. Ex DC.

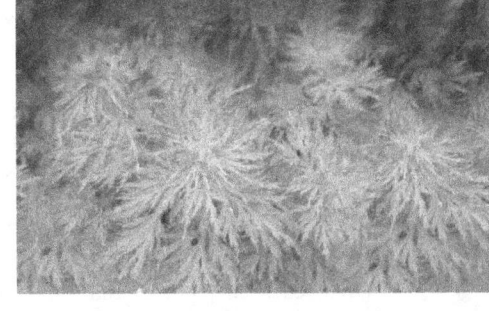

**FAMILY:** Asteraceae (Compositae)
**NOTE:** Base
**AROMA INTENSITY:** Strong
**AROMA:** Rich, fruity, sweet, slightly woody
**COMMON EXTRACTION METHOD:** Steam distilled from the leaves and tops
**POSSIBLE SUBSTITUTE OILS:** Bergamot, geranium, clary sage
**BLENDS WELL WITH:** Bergamot, black pepper, cardamom, cedarwood, chamomile (German, Roman), geranium, grapefruit, lavender, neroli, orange, patchouli, rose, rosewood, sandalwood, spikenard, tangerine, ylang ylang
**SUBCELLULAR LOCALIZATION | EPIGENETIC INFLUENCE:** Currently unknown | Currently unknown
**RECOMMENDED DILUTION RANGE:** 3%–50%; neat for limited conditions

**PRIMARY CONSTITUENTS:**[2719,2720,2721,2722,2723,2724]

| | |
|---|---|
| Davanone | 32.7%–55.0% |
| Caryophyllene | 0.0%–20.7% |
| Beta-Guajene | 0.0%–18.4% |
| Bicyclogermacrene | 0.0%–11.8% |
| Nerol | 0.0%–10.0% |
| (E)-Ethyl Cinnamate | 0.0%–7.8% |
| Davana Ethers | 0.0%–6.0% |
| Geraniol | 0.0%–5.0% |
| (E)-Methyl Cinnamate | 0.0%–4.6% |
| Trans-Isodavanone | 0.0%–3.7% |
| Beta-Eudesmol | 0.0%–3.7% |
| Beta-Davanone-2-ol | 0.0%–3.1% |
| Hydroxy Davanone | 0.0%–3.0% |

Note: The highest quality davana essential oil is produced from plants harvested at full bloom, which increases the davanone and linalool content.[2725]

**OTHER CONSTITUENTS:** Isopropyl butanoate, 2-acetylfuran, unknown esters, o-cymene, linalool, terpinen-4-ol, beta-elemene, aromadendrene, alloaromadendrene, artemone, c-artedouglasia oxide, a-artedouglasia oxide, allo-davanone, beta-artedouglasia oxide, t-cadinol, (Z)-alpha-santalol, hydroxyl dihydrorosefuran, artemone, davana furans, germacrene D, spathulenol, davanone isomer, davana ether isomer, beta-cadinene, beta-selinene, (Z)-methyl cinnamate, geranyl butyrate, trans-arbusculone

**PREFERRED COMPOSITION FOR CLINICAL USE:**

| Constituent | Davanone CT | Nerol/Geraniol CT |
|---|---|---|
| **Davanone** | 40%–60% | 35%–55% |
| **Bicyclogermacrene** | 5%–12% | – |
| **Davana Ether 1** | 0.5%–8% | 0%–3% |
| **Davana Ether 2** | 1%–7% | 0%–3% |
| **(E)-Ethyl Cinnamate** | 1%–6% | – |
| **Davana Ether 4** | 1%–5% | – |
| **Davana Ether 3** | 0.5%–5% | – |
| **Artedouglasia Oxides** | 0%–5% | – |
| **Davanone B** | 0%–3% | – |
| **Germacrene D** | 0%–3% | – |
| **Nerol** | – | 7%–15% |
| **Geraniol** | – | 4%–8% |
| **(E)-Davanone** | 0%–3% | 1%–6% |
| **Isodavanone** | 0%–3% | 1%–5% |
| **(E)-Methyl Cinnamate** | 0.1%–2% | – |

**REPORTED THERAPEUTIC PROPERTIES:** Antibacterial, antimicrobial, antiviral, anti-infectious, antifungal, **antiparasitic**, astringent, analgesic, anti-inflammatory, antioxidant, **antiseptic**, antispasmodic, disinfectant, wound healing, relieves nausea, expels excess gas, vasodilator, relieves headache, relieves cough, supports respiratory function, expels excess mucus, relieves menstrual pain and PMS, **balances menstruation**, nervine, insect repellent, **antidepressant**, combats anger, relaxing and calming, stress management, relieves anxiety

**CAUTIONS:**

■ None currently known.

**SELECTED EVIDENCE:**

☐ *In vitro* research reported that davana essential oil possesses antimicrobial activity against *Staphylococcus aureus*, *Pseudomonas aeruginosa*, *Salmonella enterica* subsp. *enterica*, and *Candida albicans*.[2726]

☐ Davana essential oil exhibits excellent anthelmintic (constituents that have the ability to expel parasitic worms called helminths and other intestinal parasites) activity against earthworms, tapeworms, and roundworms *in vitro*.[2727]

☐ The davanone CT of davana essential oil, and isolated davanone, inhibited the production of proinflammatory cytokines (TNF-α, IL-6) induced by lipopolysaccharide in primary macrophages without causing toxicity to the macrophages.[2728]

---

# DILL SEED
## (Dill, European Dill, Dill Weed)

*Anethum graveolens* L.

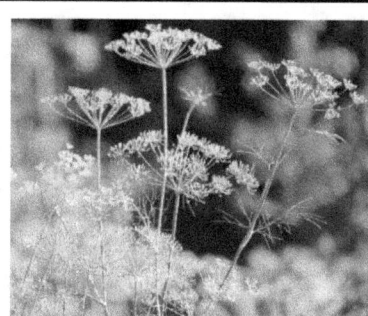

**FAMILY:** Apiaceae (Umbelliferae)
**NOTE:** Middle
**AROMA INTENSITY:** Medium
**AROMA:** Fresh, herbaceous, sweet, slightly earthy
**COMMON EXTRACTION METHOD:** Steam distilled from the seeds; also steam distilled from the aerial parts, leaves, and flowers
**POSSIBLE SUBSTITUTE OILS:** Caraway, spearmint
**BLENDS WELL WITH:** Anise, basil, bergamot, black pepper, caraway, cinnamon, clove, elemi, grapefruit, lemon, lime, nutmeg, orange, peppermint, spearmint, tangerine
**SUBCELLULAR LOCALIZATION | EPIGENETIC INFLUENCE:** Currently unknown | Currently unknown
**RECOMMENDED DILUTION RANGE:** 1.5%–20%

**PRIMARY CONSTITUENTS:**[2729,2730,2731,2732,2733]

*Seeds (fruits)*

| | |
|---|---|
| Carvone | 50.1%–75.9% |
| Limonene | 14.7%–44.1% |
| Cis-Dihydrocarvone | 0.1%–5.9% |
| Trans-Dihydrocarvone | 0.5%–3.0% |

*Leaves*

| | |
|---|---|
| Alpha-Phellandrene | 62.7% |
| Dill Ether | 16.4% |
| Limonene | 13.3% |

*Aerial Parts (Alpha-Phellandrene CT)*

| | |
|---|---|
| Alpha-Phellandrene | 31.8%–63.0% |
| Dill Ether | 0.9%–20.8% |
| Limonene | 3.7%–11.8% |
| Geraniol | 0.0%–10.6% |
| Beta-Phellandrene | 7.4%–7.5% |
| Para-Cymene | 0.7%–5.3% |

*Flowers*

| | |
|---|---|
| Limonene | 33.2% |
| Alpha-Phellandrene | 30.3% |
| Dill Ether | 22.0% |
| Carvone | 10.3% |

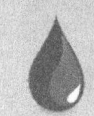

*Aerial Parts (Carvone CT)*

| | |
|---|---|
| Carvone | 36.1%–73.6% |
| Limonene | 6.9%–19.9% |
| Apiole (Apiol) | 0.0%–16.9% |
| Trans-Dihydrocarvone | 0.0%–14.7% |
| Dill Ether | 0.0%–13.2% |
| Alpha-Phellandrene | 0.1%–8.0% |

**OTHER CONSTITUENTS:** *Seeds (fruits)*—alpha-phellandrene, cis-carveol, 1,2-diethoxyethane, diplaniol; *Leaves*—para-cymene, alpha-pinene, neophytadiene; *Aerial parts (alpha-phellandrene CT)*—myristicin, geranial acetate; *Aerial parts (carvone CT)*—linalool, para-cymene, cis-dihydrocarvone, trans-anethole; *Flowers*—alpha-pinene, para-cymene, trans-dihydrocarvone

**PREFERRED COMPOSITION FOR CLINICAL USE:**

| Constituent | Aerial Parts | Seeds |
|---|---|---|
| **Carvone** | 30%–55% | 45%–65% |
| **Limonene** | 15%–35% | 25%–45% |
| **Alpha-Phellandrene** | 10%–25% | 0%–15% |
| **Dill Ether** | 3%–10% | 0%–5% |
| **Trans-Dihydrocarvone** | 1%–5% | 0%–1% |
| **Apiole** | 0% | < 0.5% |

**REPORTED THERAPEUTIC PROPERTIES:** Antibacterial, analgesic, anti-inflammatory, antispasmodic, antiallergic, **antifungal**, antioxidant, expels excess mucous, supports pancreas function, **balances blood sugar levels**, combats food (sugar) addictions, supports respiratory function, **supports normal cholesterol levels**, disinfectant, supports urinary tract function, aids digestion, expels excess gas, encourages normal lactation, wound healing, **insecticide**, relaxing/calming, reduces anxiety, stress management

**CAUTIONS:**

■ *Aerial parts (carvone CT)*: Avoid with children under age twelve. Dill essential oil may contain moderate quantities of apiol, which may cause kidney or liver toxicity, or abnormal quantities of blood components (blood dyscrasias).[2734,2735,2736,2737,2738]

■ *Aerial parts (carvone CT)*: Avoid during pregnancy and lactation due to the abortive properties (parsley apiole causes contractions and necrosis of placental tissue, and has been used for decades to end unwanted pregnancies) and high toxicity (several cases of acute poisoning or death have been reported after ingestion of varying amounts of apiole in single or daily doses) of apiole.[2739,2740,2741,2742,2743,2744,2745]

■ *Aerial parts (carvone CT)*: Avoid oral consumption due to high toxicity of apiol, reported poisonings by apiol, and deaths reported after ingestion of significant amounts of apiol.[2746,2747,2748,2749,2750,2751]

■ *Aerial parts (carvone CT)*: May interact with aspirin, blood pressure, antiplatelet, and anticoagulant medications, and increase the risk of bleeding among people with bleeding disorders based on carvone content. Carvone is a potent calcium channel blocker, which may decrease blood pressure.[2752,2753]

■ *Aerial parts (carvone CT)*: Avoid with compromised liver or kidney due to potential to cause liver and kidney toxicity based on apiole content.[2754,2755,2756,2757,2758]

■ *Aerial parts (carvone CT); Seeds*: May interact with diabetes medications and cause low blood sugar.[2759,2760,2761,2762]

■ *Aerial parts (carvone CT); Seeds*: May interact with barbiturates (medications for anxiety and insomnia), antihistamines, benzodiazepines, tricyclic antidepressants, or other central nervous system depressant drugs, increasing depressant effects, due to carvone content.[2763]

■ May interact with anticholinergic (drugs used for asthma, incontinence, gastrointestinal cramps, muscular spasms, depression, and sleep disorders) and cholinergic medications (drugs used to reduce urinary retention, diagnose myasthenia gravis, and for glaucoma) based on AChE inhibitory activity.[2764]

**SELECTED EVIDENCE:**

☐ *In vitro* research found that dill oil (aerial parts—alpha-phellandrene CT) is a potent antioxidant and inhibits excess nitric oxide production to reduce inflammation.[2765]

☐ Dill essential oil is a potent insecticide and effectively kills several insects.[2766,2767,2768,2769,2770,2771] It also repels mosquitoes for up to half an hour.[2772]

☐ Dill essential oil causes apoptosis (cell death) and metacaspase activation (metacaspases are proteases found in fungi essential for the regulation of cell death) of *C. albicans*.[2773] An additional study found that dill (combined with sage oil and functionalized magnetite nanoparticles) inhibited adherence of *C. albicans* to wound dressings, making it useful to prevent fungal infections of wounds.[2774] Dill oil also disrupts mitochondrial function and increases the production of reactive oxygen species to cause the death of *C. albicans* and other fungi.[2775,2776]

☐ *In vitro* research found that dill oil (seed, carvone CT) strongly inhibits *A. niger, S. cerevisiae,* and *C. albicans*.[2777] Cumin essential oil also is fungicidal to *Fusarium proliferatum* and *F. verticillioides*.[2778]

☐ Animal research found that intravaginal application of dill seed oil is highly effective in clearing candida from the vagina, both as a preventive and as a treatment, making it a potential treatment for vulvovaginal candidiasis.[2779]

☐ Animal research suggests that dill oil reduces triglyceride and blood sugar levels in diabetic mice through PPAR-α activation (a protein normally activated during periods of energy deprivation that promotes the uptake, utilization, and breakdown of fatty acids, is necessary for ketogenesis—a key adaptive response to prolonged fasting, and promotes lipid metabolism in the liver).[2780] The aerial parts (alpha-phellandrene CT) of dill essential oil are used in Iran for high cholesterol. Animal research found that oral administration of dill oil from aerial parts (alpha-phellandrene CT) significantly reduced total cholesterol, triglycerides, and LDL cholesterol, while simultaneously increasing HDL cholesterol levels in rats.[2781]

☐ Dill seed oil is an ingredient in some gripe water products (usually at a dose of 0.005 mL per teaspoon), used to relieve intestinal spasms, excess gas, and colic in babies.[2782]

☐ *In vitro* research suggests that dill oil may prevent and manage neurodegenerative diseases caused by oxidative stress by inhibiting acetylcholinesterase (AchE) and butyrylcholinesterase (BchE) enzyme activity.[2783] Inhibition of AchE prevents the breakdown of acetylcholine, which is essential for memory and thinking. People with neurodegenerative diseases make less acetylcholine, and the diseases often break it down at a faster rate, leading to acetylcholine deficits. Selective inhibition of BchE is also desirable in neurodegenerative diseases because it interferes with acetylcholine activity. In addition, BchE is often found in the plaques and tangles in the brains of people with Alzheimer's disease.[2784]

☐ Dill essential oil potently repelled male and female German cockroaches (*Blattella germanica*).[2785]

☐ A para-cymene/alpha-phellandrene CT effectively killed *An. stephensi* mosquito larvae, with a nanoemulsion form performing significantly better than standard EO.[2786]

☐ Cardamom and dill CT carvone essential oils significantly inhibited *Campylobacter* spp. (*C. jejuni* and *C. coli*) by affecting their membrane integrity.[2787]

☐ Human aryl hydrocarbon receptor (AhR: a gene that encodes a protein that helps regulate responses to planar aromatic hydrocarbons and significantly affects the immune activity in the gastrointestinal tract) regulates the circadian rhythm, helps regulate the cell cycle, and plays an important role in tissue development. Cumin, jasmine, vanilla, and bay leaf fully activate AhR; clove, dill, thyme, nutmeg, and oregano partially activate AhR; and tarragon, caraway, turmeric, lovage, fennel, spearmint, star anise, and anise inhibit the AhR activity.[2788]

☐ Cumin, fennel, dill, and anise essential oils each demonstrated inhibitory activity against *Candida* species, with cumin being the most active.[2789] Fennel and anise were not cytotoxic to mouse fibroblasts at minimum inhibitory concentrations.

☐ Topical application of the alpha-phellandrene CT of dill essential oil (4% in an ointment) promoted wound healing by preventing bacterial growth (MRSA infected wounds), significantly decreasing inflammation, and accelerating re-epithelialization, blood vessel growth to the wound site, and fibroblast and collagen deposition.[2790]

☐ Dill seed essential oil (41.2% carvone, 23.1% limonene) exhibited moderate antioxidant activity, but carvone was highlighted as a potent scavenger of free radicals.[2791]

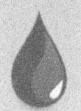

☐ A randomized placebo-controlled trial found that oral administration of dill essential oil solution (40 drops in 30 mL of water, every twenty minutes for a total of three doses) reduced bloating and flatulence in women recovering from a Cesarean section.[2792] The solution was created by dissolving dill essential oil in propylene glycol and water to produce a final dose delivering 10.8–14.8 mg of carvone per 40 drops of solution. The dill group experienced a nearly three-fold greater improvement in symptoms than the placebo group, and no adverse effects were reported.

☐ The carvone CT of dill essential oil killed liver cancer cells by triggering apoptosis.[2793]

☐ Dill, cumin, and parsley were each toxic to the maize weevil (*Sitophilus zeamais*) in the contact assay.[2794] The same researchers noted that each of the oils and fennel also repelled the insect. Carvone (fumigant and contact) and cuminaldehyde were the most active isolated constituents for toxicity, and cuminaldehyde, carvone, and estragole the most active isolated constituents for repellents.

☐ A dill essential oil nanoemulsion displayed antioxidant activity in the FRAP assay and selectively triggered apoptosis in lung cancer cells.[2795]

☐ Vaginal candidiasis (yeast infection) is a fungal infection that causes irritation, discharge, and intense itchiness of the vagina and vulva. This condition affects up to 75 percent of women during their fertility years, most of which have chronic or recurrent episodes. Vaginal suppositories containing 100 mg of cumin essential oil inserted once nightly for six consecutive days significantly relieved symptoms (itching, discharge, painful intercourse) and had a negative culture in 70 percent of women aged eighteen to forty-nine included in the study.[2796] A preliminary evaluation found that the oil suppositories killed *Candida* yeast and was nonirritating to vaginal tissues. This suggests that cumin suppositories may be a viable natural solution for vaginal candidiasis.

☐ Dill essential oils—four separate oils extracted from the flowers (46.9% dill apiole, 22.6% carvone), seeds (33.3% dill apiole, 30.8% limonene), leaves (16.0% dill apiole, 14.1% carvone), and stems (31.9% dill apiole, 14.3% carvone)—exhibited stronger antifungal activity against *A. parasiticus* than the reference drug itraconazole.[2797] The seed oil exhibited the strongest activity, which exceeded gentamicin and tetracycline in efficacy against *S. aureus*.

☐ Catnip CT 1,8-cineole, summer savory CT carvacrol, and dill aerial parts essential oil demonstrated promising insecticidal activity against the red spider mite (*Tetranychus urticae*) with some minor potential to decrease populations of insect predators (*Amblyseius swirskii*).[2798]

# DOUGLAS FIR

*Pseudotsuga menziesii* Mirb. Franco

**FAMILY:** Pinaceae
**NOTE:** Middle-top
**AROMA INTENSITY:** Medium
**AROMA:** Piney, woody, fresh, fruity

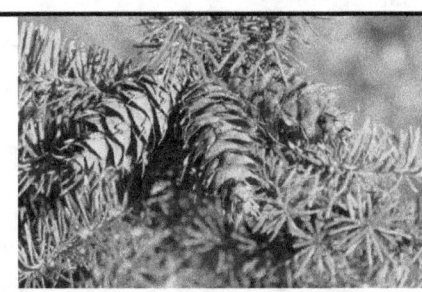

**COMMON EXTRACTION METHOD:** Steam distilled from the needles (leaves); may also be steam distilled from the needles and twigs

**POSSIBLE SUBSTITUTE OILS:** Balsam fir, white fir, pine, spruce (black)

**BLENDS WELL WITH:** Balsam fir, bergamot, cedarwood, frankincense, grapefruit, lavender, lemon, lime, marjoram, neroli, orange, petitgrain, pine, rosemary, sandalwood, silver fir, tangerine, vetiver, white fir

**SUBCELLULAR LOCALIZATION | EPIGENETIC INFLUENCE:** Currently unknown | Currently unknown

**RECOMMENDED DILUTION RANGE:** 5%–Neat

**PRIMARY CONSTITUENTS:**[2799,2800,2801]

| *Needles & Twigs* | | *Needles* | |
|---|---|---|---|
| Bornyl Acetate | 0.0%–34.7% | Beta-Pinene | 21.2%–39.5% |
| Beta-Pinene | 3.7%–31.2% | Sabinene | 11.2%–21.0% |
| Camphene | 0.1%–29.8% | Alpha-Terpinolene | 15.6%–20.2% |
| Sabinene | 0.0%–29.7% | Terpinen-4-ol | 0.0%–12.2% |
| Alpha-Terpinolene | 0.0%–18.8% | Alpha-Pinene | 0.0%–7.6% |

| | | | |
|---|---|---|---|
| Alpha-Pinene | 0.1%–11.7% | Gamma-Terpinene | 1.8%–7.4% |
| Citronellyl Acetate | 0.2%–5.9% | (Z)-Beta Ocimene | 0.0%–7.1% |
| (Z)-Beta Ocimene | 0.0%–5.6% | Alpha-Terpinene | 0.9%–4.3% |
| Santene | 0.0%–5.5% | | |
| Alpha-Terpineol | 0.0%–5.4% | | |
| Limonene | 0.4%–4.5% | | |

Note: The needles and twigs essential oil could be divided into two chemotypes: one with high bornyl acetate and camphene content and another with high beta-pinene and sabinene content.

**OTHER CONSTITUENTS:** *Needles*—alpha-thujene, myrcene, alpha-phellandrene, delta-3-carene, limonene, beta-phellandrene, alpha-terpineol, cis-p-menth-2-en-1-ol, trans-p-menth-en-1-ol, citronellal, citronellol, citronellyl acetate, geranyl acetate, germacrene D; *Needles & Twigs*—tricyclene, citronellol, myrtanol acetate, beta-myrcene, alpha-terpinene, beta-phellandrene, (E)-beta-ocimene, gamma-terpinene, myrcenol, geranyl acetate, alpha-humulene, germacrene D, camphor

**PREFERRED COMPOSITION FOR CLINICAL USE:**

| Constituent | Balanced CT | Beta-Pinene CT | Alpha-Pinene CT | Camphene CT |
|---|---|---|---|---|
| **Bornyl Acetate** | 15%–35% | <5% | 5%–10% | 15%–25% |
| **Camphene** | 15%–35% | — | 5%–10% | 20%–35% |
| **Beta-Pinene** | 10%–25% | 20%–30% | 12%–22% | 5%–20% |
| **Limonene** | 3%–15% | 1%–4% | 3%–9% | 5%–15% |
| **Alpha-Pinene** | 4%–12% | 8%–15% | 18%–30% | 6%–18% |
| **Beta-Phellandrene** | 0.5%–10% | — | — | 0.1%–11% |
| **Beta-Myrcene** | 1%–5% | 1%–4% | 2%–8% | 0.5%–5% |
| **Terpinolene** | — | 8%–15% | 5%–10% | — |
| **Terpinen-4-ol** | — | 4%–10% | 4%–10% | — |
| **Sabinene** | — | 4%–10% | 2%–8% | — |
| **Delta-3-Carene** | — | 3%–10% | 3%–9% | — |
| **Gamma-Terpinene** | — | 3%–8% | 2%–8% | — |
| **Citronellyl Acetate** | — | 2%–6% | 0.1%–4% | — |
| **Alpha-Terpinene** | — | 2%–5% | 1%–5% | — |

**REPORTED THERAPEUTIC PROPERTIES:** Antibacterial, antifungal, antioxidant, antiviral, antimicrobial, antiseptic, antispasmodic, **analgesic**, diuretic, relieves cough, disinfectant, expels excess mucus, supports immune function, **encourages respiratory function**, purification, antirheumatic, nervine, wound healing, enhances focus and concentration, stress management, antidepressant, relieves anxiety, reduces denial

**CAUTIONS:**
■ None currently known.

**SELECTED EVIDENCE:**
- ☐ Douglas fir essential oil demonstrated higher antifungal activity than the antifungal drug bifonazole against several fungi (*Alternaria alternate, Aspergillus niger, Aspergillus ochraceus, Aspergillus versicolor, Aspergillus flavus, Aspergillus terreus, Cladosporium cladosporioides, Fusarium tricinctum, Phomopsis helianthi, Trichoderma viride,* and *Epidermophyton floccosum*).[2802]
- ☐ Douglas fir essential oil exhibited low antimicrobial activity against human respiratory system pathogens (*P. aeruginosa* or *C. albicans*) and weak toxicity against the fruit fly (*Drosophila melanogaster*).[2803]
- ☐ *In vitro* research reported that Douglas fir inhibited *S. aureus, P, aeruginosa, B. subtilis, E. faecalis, E. coli,* and *C. albicans*.[2804] It also potentiated the activity of antibiotics, switching *S. aureus* from resistant to susceptible to oxacillin and tetracycline.

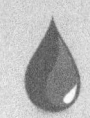

☐ Inhalation of Douglas fir or lavender essential oil via a diffuser promoted relaxation during a leaf-printing activity in older adults, as measured by brainwaves, heart rate, and questionnaires.[2805] The oils modified heart rate variability—low frequency and high frequency heart rate ratio—indicating balanced autonomic nervous system activity. Monitoring of brainwave activity showed a decrease in high beta waves (indicating reduced stress), increased high alpha waves (suggestive of a relaxed but focused state), and decreased gamma waves (corresponding to a more relaxed state). Moreover, participants reported feeling less anxious and more relaxed after inhaling the oils.

# DWARF PINE
## (Mountain Pine)

*Pinus mugo* Turro, *P. montana* Mill., *P. pumilio* Haenke, *P. mughus* Scopoli, *P. mugo* var. *pulilio*, *P. mugo* var. *mugo*

**FAMILY:** Pinaceae
**NOTE:** Top
**AROMA INTENSITY:** Medium-Strong
**AROMA:** Green, resinous, sweet, piney, balsamic
**COMMON EXTRACTION METHOD:** Hydrodistilled from needles (leaves) or twigs; may also be hydrodistilled from the cones
**POSSIBLE SUBSTITUTE OILS:** Pine, cypress, Siberian fir, pink pepper
**BLENDS WELL WITH:** Agarwood, bergamot, cajeput, camphor, cedarwood, clary sage, coriander, Douglas fir, Engelmann spruce, eucalyptus, frankincense, galbanum, grapefruit, juniper, lavender, lemon, lime, marjoram, tea tree, neroli, niaouli, peppermint, ravensara, ravintsara, rosemary, Spanish sage, spikenard, thyme, Siberian fir, silver fir, vetiver, white fir, white pine, white spruce, ylang ylang
**SUBCELLULAR LOCALIZATION | EPIGENETIC INFLUENCE:** Currently unknown | Currently unknown
**RECOMMENDED DILUTION RANGE:** 3%–50%; neat for limited conditions

**PRIMARY CONSTITUENTS:**[2806,2807,2808,2809]

| Needles or Needles/Twigs | | Twigs | |
|---|---|---|---|
| Delta-3-Carene | 13.1%–27.9% | Delta-3-Carene | 24.0%–51.7% |
| Alpha-Pinene | 12.9%–24.5% | Limonene + Beta-Phellandrene | 12.7%–24.3% |
| Limonene + Beta-Phellandrene | 1.6%–18.1% | Beta-Pinene | 2.2%–15.4% |
| Myrcene | 1.4%–12.2% | Trans-Caryophyllene | 4.0%–10.9% |
| Bornyl Acetate | 2.3%–11.6% | Myrcene | 1.6%–10.3% |
| Germacrene D | 0.7%–9.9% | Alpha-Pinene | 5.6%–9.7% |
| Trans-Caryophyllene | 2.4%–9.0% | Germacrene D | 0.1%–6.2% |
| Beta-Pinene | 0.0%–8.7% | Gamma-Terpinolene | 2.5%–4.3% |
| Gamma-Terpinolene | 0.0%–4.3% | Bornyl Acetate | 0.4%–3.0% |
| Camphene | 1.5%–4.0% | | |
| Bicyclogermacrene | 0.0%–3.9% | | |
| Delta-Cadinene | 1.0%–3.6% | | |
| Alpha-Terpinolene | 0.0%–3.4% | | |

**OTHER CONSTITUENTS:** *Needles or Needles/Twigs*—Tricyclene, alpha-thujene, sabinene, alpha-phellandrene, para-cymene, (E)-beta-ocimene, gamma-terpinene, camphor, borneol, thymol methyl ether, alpha-copaene, beta-elemene, longifolene, terpinen-4-ol, cryptone, para-cymen-8-ol, alpha-terpineol, cuminaldehyde, alpha-humulene, aromadendrene, beta-chamigrene, gamma-muurolene, alpha-muurolene, gamma-cadinene, alpha-cadinene, (E)-nerolidol, spathulenol, caryophyllene oxide, epi-alpha-cadinol, piperitenone, alpha-terpinyl acetate, epi-alpha-muurolol, alpha-cadinol; *Twigs*—Camphene, thuja-2,4(10)-diene, sabinene, para-cymene, (E)-beta-ocimene, gamma-terpinene, borneol, myrtenol, beta-elemene, alpha-humulene, aromadendrene, beta-chamigrene, gamma-muurolene, delta-cadinene, caryophyllene oxide, alpha-muurolol

**PREFERRED COMPOSITION FOR CLINICAL USE:**

| Constituent | Needles |
| --- | --- |
| Alpha-Pinene | 20%–25% |
| Delta-3-Carene | 15%–20% |
| Germacrene D | 4%–10% |
| Beta-Caryophyllene | 4%–10% |
| Bornyl Acetate | 3%–10% |
| Limonene + β-Phellandrene | 2%–7% |
| Myrcene | 1%–7% |
| Camphene | 2%–5% |
| Terpinolene <gamma + alpha> | 1%–5% |
| Delta-Cadinene | 1.5%–4% |
| Beta-Pinene | 1%–4% |
| Caryophyllene Oxide | 1%–3% |
| Gamma-Cadinene | 0.5%–3% |
| Beta-Elemene | 0.5%–2% |
| Tricyclene | 0.5%–2% |

**REPORTED THERAPEUTIC PROPERTIES:** Antibacterial, antiparasitic, **antiseptic**, diuretic, analgesic, anti-inflammatory, antiarthritic, supports respiratory function, expels excess mucus, **antioxidant**, aids immune function, aids circulation (localized and systemic), supports/protects cardiovascular health, cleanses and supports urinary tract function, wound healing, relieves blisters/boils, stress management, relieves anxiety

**CAUTIONS:**

■ *Twigs*: May interact with anticholinergic (drugs used for asthma, incontinence, gastrointestinal cramps, muscular spasms, depression, and sleep disorders) and cholinergic medications (drugs used to reduce urinary retention, diagnose myasthenia gravis, and for glaucoma) based on AChE inhibitory activity of delta-3-carene.[2810,2811]

**SELECTED EVIDENCE:**

- ☐ Dwarf pine essential oil exhibits good antioxidant capacity in lipophilic environments, but weak to moderate antioxidant capacity in aqueous environments.[2812] The study also noted that terpinolene exhibited remarkable protection against the oxidation of LDL cholesterol, with gamma-terpinolene producing an even stronger effect. A follow-up study determined that terpinolene, in concert with alpha-tocopherol and beta-carotene, protects against the oxidation of LDL cholesterol by neutralizing free radical damage caused by copper and reducing the oxidation of proteins, as evidenced by delayed tryptophan loss.[2813] Since oxidized LDL cholesterol is a marker for coronary heart disease, this antioxidative protection may reduce the risk of cardiovascular disease. *P. montana* (24% alpha-pinene, 13% camphene, 8% bornyl acetate, 8% alpha-phellandrene, 7% beta-pinene, and 4% limonene) also demonstrated moderate antioxidant activity.[2814]
- ☐ *In vitro* research demonstrates that dwarf pine essential oil (*P. montana*, with very low levels of delta-3-carene) inhibits *Clostridium butyricum, C. hystoliticum, C. perfringens,* and *C. ramnosum.*[2815]
- ☐ Dwarf pine essential oil (needles) kills cervical, breast, and colon cancer cells *in vitro.*[2816] Another laboratory study found that the oil triggers apoptosis in prostate cancer cells.[2817]
- ☐ Dwarf pine essential oil (needles) reduces inflammation by inhibiting the proinflammatory cytokine IL-6.[2818] A more pronounced anti-inflammatory effect was achieved from the twigs' essential oil.
- ☐ Laboratory research found that conifer essential oils are more active antimicrobial agents in vapor phase when compared to liquid phase and tend to have higher concentrations of alpha-pinene in vapor phase.[2819] Dwarf pine inhibited *E. coli, A. bohemicus, K. marina,* and *B. cereus* in liquid phase, which was dramatically improved against all tested organisms (except *E. coli*) in vapor phase. Norway spruce and silver fir inhibited *A. bohemicus, K. marina,* and *B. cereus* in liquid phase, again with significant improvements in vapor phase. Each oil displayed moderate antioxidant activity in the DPPH and ABTS assays.

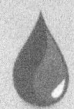

# ELECAMPANE
## (Alantroot, Scabwort)

*Inula helenium* L.

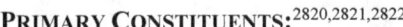

**FAMILY:** Asteraceae (Compositae)
**NOTE:** Middle
**AROMA INTENSITY:** Medium
**AROMA:** Earthy, herbaceous, bitter
**COMMON EXTRACTION METHOD:** Steam distilled or hydrodistilled from the dried roots
**POSSIBLE SUBSTITUTE OILS:** Sweet inula, lovage, camphor
**BLENDS WELL WITH:** Does not blend well with other essential oils.
**SUBCELLULAR LOCALIZATION | EPIGENETIC INFLUENCE:** Currently unknown | Currently unknown
**RECOMMENDED DILUTION RANGE:** < 0.5% (strongly sensitizing)

**PRIMARY CONSTITUENTS:**[2820,2821,2822]

| | |
|---|---|
| Alantolactone | 51.3%–55.8% |
| Isoalantolactone | 26.3%–36.9% |
| Diplophyllin | 0.0%–5.1% |

**OTHER CONSTITUENTS:** Beta-elemene, beta-selinene, caryophyllene oxide, myristic acid, eudesma-5,7(11)-diene-8beta-12 olide, eudesma-4(15),7(11)-diene-8beta-12 olide, oleic acid, dihydroalantolactone

**PREFERRED COMPOSITION FOR CLINICAL USE:**

| Constituent | |
|---|---|
| **Alantolactone** | 50%–56% |
| **Isoalantolactone** | 25%–37% |

**REPORTED THERAPEUTIC PROPERTIES:** Antibacterial, antimicrobial, **antifungal**, antiparasitic, **supports respiratory function**, **expels excess mucus**, ease cough, aids immune function, balances hormones, aids digestion, stimulates metabolism, aids oral health, astringent, reduces the appearance of wrinkles and blemishes, relieves blisters, wound healing, diuretic, releases traumatic memories/emotions

**CAUTIONS:**
*Elecampane is not generally used in essential oil therapy and should be reserved for use by the experienced practitioner. Those who are pregnant or lactating and children under 12 should avoid elecampane until its safety has been fully investigated. If used, it is recommended for inhalation purposes only. Sweet inula (I. graveolens) has largely replaced elecampane in essential oil therapy.*

■ Elecampane should not be used topically because of it is strongly sensitizing and can produce severe allergic reactions. Extremely severe allergic reactions were reported in 23/25 people when elecampane essential oil was applied at a 4% dilution.[2823] A lower concentration of 1% still caused reactions in 4/25 people.

■ May interfere with enzymes that metabolize medications (NSAIDs, proton-pump inhibitors, acetaminophen, antiepileptics, immune modulators, blood-sugar medications, blood pressure medications, antidepressants, antipsychotics, diabetic medications, antihistamines, antibiotics, and anesthetics) due to alantolactone content.[2824,2825]

**SELECTED EVIDENCE:**
◻ *In vitro* research demonstrated that elecampane essential oil, and alantolactone, isoalantolactone, and diplophyllin, significantly inhibited *S. aureus* by damaging its membrane.[2826] Other research reported that it is only active against gram-positive bacteria (*S. aureus, Mycobacterium smegmatis*).[2827] A third study demonstrated that elecampane essential oil strongly inhibits *S. aureus, B. cereus,* and a multi-drug-resistant

strain of *E. faecium*, moderately inhibited a multi-drug-resistant strain of *S. epidermidis*, and weakly inhibited a multi-drug-resistant strain of *A. sobria* and *P. aeruginosa*.[2828]

☐ Elecampane essential oil inhibits the fungi *C. albicans*, *F. oxysporum*, and *C. heteronema*.[2829] Another study shows that elecampane essential oil possesses significant antifungal activities against *C. albicans* (four strains), *C. glabrate* (four strains), *C. parapsilosis* (three strains), and *C. tropicalis* (three strains), which was superior to tea tree and bergamot essential oils.[2830]

☐ Alantolactone and isoalantolcatones kill cancer cells by targeting multiple cellular signaling pathways that are frequently dysregulated in cancers.[2831]

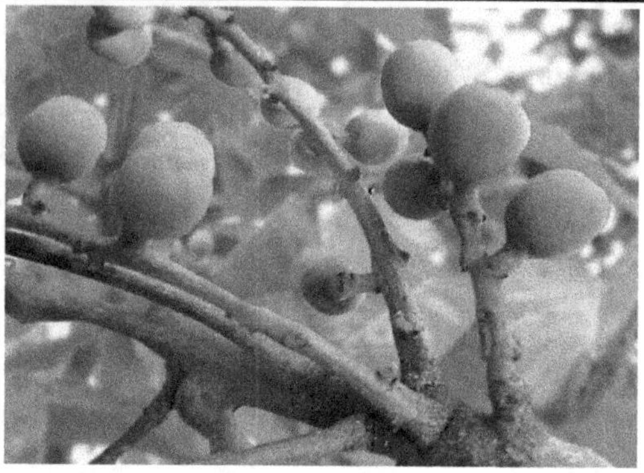

# ELEMI
## (Pisa, Manila Elemi, Java Almond)

*Canarium luzonicum* (Blume) A. Gray; *C. vulgare* Leenh.; *C. commune* L., *C. indicum* L.

**FAMILY:** Burseraceae
**NOTE:** Middle
**AROMA INTENSITY:** Medium
**AROMA:** Fresh, spicy, slightly balsamic, hint of citrus
**COMMON EXTRACTION METHOD:** Steam distilled from the gum/resin
**POSSIBLE SUBSTITUTE OILS:** Frankincense, myrrh, palo santo
**BLENDS WELL WITH:** Cassia, cinnamon, copaiba, frankincense, ginger, lavender, patchouli, rosemary, rosewood, myrrh, sandalwood, sage, Spanish sage, ylang ylang
**SUBCELLULAR LOCALIZATION | EPIGENETIC INFLUENCE:** Currently unknown | *Muscular/Reproductive*
**RECOMMENDED DILUTION RANGE:** 3%–Neat

**PRIMARY CONSTITUENTS:**[2832]

| | |
|---|---|
| Limonene | 54.6%–56.0% |
| Alpha-Phellandrene | 8.8%–17.6% |
| Elemol | 6.3%–13.7% |
| Sabinene | 3.4%–5.7% |
| Elemicin | 2.4%–4.7% |
| Alpha-Terpinolene | 2.5%–2.8% |
| Alpha-Terpineol | 1.1%–2.7% |
| Beta-Phellandrene | 1.8%–2.3% |
| Para-Cymene | 1.1%–1.8% |

**OTHER CONSTITUENTS:** Alpha-pinene, (E)-sabinene hydrate, Terpinene-4-ol, methyl eugenol (< 0.35%)

**PREFERRED COMPOSITION FOR CLINICAL USE:**

| Constituent | Distilled | Co2 (SFE) |
|---|---|---|
| **Limonene** | 45%–65% | 22%–35% |
| **Alpha-Phellandrene** | 10%–22% | 5%–15% |
| **Elemol** | 5%–20% | 15%–30% |
| **Sabinene** | 3%–7% | 0.1%–5% |
| **Elemicin** | 2%–7% | 5%–15% |
| **Para-Cymene** | 1%–5% | — |
| **Alpha-Terpineol** | 1%–3% | — |
| **Beta-Phellandrene** | 1%–3% | — |

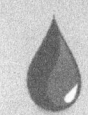

| Alpha-Terpinolene | 0.1%–3% | – |
|---|---|---|
| Beta-Amyrin Acetate | – | 2%–7% |
| Beta-Amyrin | – | 0.1%-4% |

**REPORTED THERAPEUTIC PROPERTIES:** Antiseptic, antibacterial, antiviral, antifungal, antirheumatic, analgesic (pain relief), expels excess mucous, **reduces the appearance of fine lines and wrinkles**, aids circulation, stimulates the endocrine system to release hormones, **boosts the immune system**, soothes sore muscles, **relieves chronic skin conditions**, wound healing, stimulant, calming, reduces anxiety, stress management, beneficial for meditation

**CAUTIONS:**
- None currently known.

**SELECTED EVIDENCE:**
- Elemol, one of the primary constituents in elemi, reduces lesions caused by atopic dermatitis, and reduces serum IgE levels, mast cell infiltration in the dermis and hypodermis, and downregulates the expression of a number of inflammatory cytokines (TNF-α, IL-1β, IL-6 and IκBα) according to animal research.[2833]
- Two separate chemotypes of elemi—para-cymene (Filipino) and limonene (French)—inhibited *B. subtilis*, *B. cereus*, *P. aeruginosa*, and *E. coli*, with the para-cymene CT performing better against all bacteria except for *E. coli*.[2834] The limonene CT exhibited anticancer activity against androgen-positive/dependent and aggressive androgen-negative/independent prostate cancer cells, but the para-cymene CT was only weakly active against androgen-negative/independent prostate cancer cells.

# ENGELMANN SPRUCE
## (Mountain Spruce)

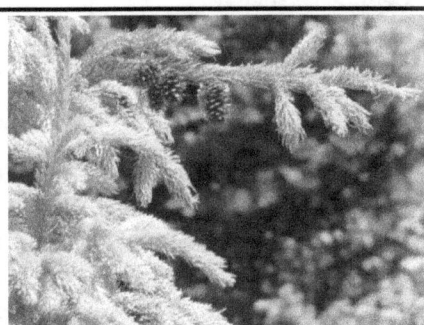

*Picea engelmannii* Parry ex Engelm.

**FAMILY:** Pinaceae
**NOTE:** Middle-Top
**AROMA INTENSITY:** Medium
**AROMA:** Piney, woody, camphoraceous, sweet
**COMMON EXTRACTION METHOD:** Steam distilled from the needles (leaves) and twigs
**POSSIBLE SUBSTITUTE OILS:** Balsam fir, spruce (black), blue spruce, pine, lavandin, spike lavender
**BLENDS WELL WITH:** Balsam fir, blue spruce, camphor, cedarwood, copaiba, cypress, frankincense, lavandin, lavender, palo santo, pine, rosemary, silver fir, spike lavender, spruce (black), white fir
**SUBCELLULAR LOCALIZATION | EPIGENETIC INFLUENCE:** Currently unknown | Currently unknown
**RECOMMENDED DILUTION RANGE:** 3%–50%; neat for limited conditions

**PRIMARY CONSTITUENTS:**[2835,2836,2837,2838]

| | |
|---|---|
| Limonene | 1.6%–30.2% |
| Beta-Pinene | 1.2%–29.7% |
| Alpha-Pinene | 2.3%–24.7% |
| Camphor | 1.0%–14.9% |
| Camphene | 1.7%–14.3% |
| Myrcene | 5.5%–12.2% |
| Delta-3-Carene | 0.2%–9.4% |
| Linalool | 0.1%–6.5% |
| Borneol | 0.3%–5.2% |
| Bornyl Acetate | 1.1%–5.1% |
| Camphene Hydrate | 0.3%–5.0% |
| Piperitone | 0.0%–4.6% |

| | |
|---|---|
| Beta-Phellandrene | 0.6%–3.3% |
| Alpha-Cadinol | 0.0%–3.3% |
| Alpha-Terpineol | 0.3%–3.2% |
| Fenchone | 0.0%–3.0% |

Note: Juvenile foliage tends to have less camphor content and higher alpha-pinene, beta-pinene, and limonene content; whereas older foliage has higher camphor and myrcene content. There are at least two chemotypes of Engelmann spruce, but they are combined in this book.

**OTHER CONSTITUENTS:** Santene, sabinene, gamma-terpinene, terpinolene, endo-fenchol, cis-p-menth-2-en-1-ol, citronellol, trans-cinnamaldehyde, citronellyl acetate, geranyl acetate, beta-caryophyllene, alpha-farnesene, beta-himachalene, cis-gamma-bisabolene, delta-cadinene, alpha-phellandrene, terpinen-4-ol, trans-gamma-bisabolene, 4-beta-hydroxygermaca-1(10),5-diene, T-cadinol, T-muurolol, alpha-bisabolol, methyl chavicol (estragole) <1.0%

**PREFERRED COMPOSITION FOR CLINICAL USE:**

| *Constituent* | |
|---|---|
| **Limonene** | 20%–35% |
| **Alpha-Pinene** | 15%–25% |
| **Camphene** | 10%–15% |
| **Beta-Myrcene** | 6%–12% |
| **Camphor** | 2%–12% |
| **Bornyl Acetate** | 3%–7% |
| **Delta-3-Carene** | 2%–7% |
| **Beta-Pinene** | 1%–5% |
| **Beta-Phellandrene** | 0.1%–3% |
| **Borneol** | 0.1%–3% |
| **Linalool** | 0.1%–3% |
| **Alpha-Terpineol** | 0.1%–3% |

**REPORTED THERAPEUTIC PROPERTIES:** Antibacterial, antimicrobial, antiviral, **analgesic**, anti-inflammatory, antioxidant, antispasmodic, **supports respiratory function**, aids immune function, **relieves coughs**, expels excess mucus, chronic skin conditions, encourages normal endocrine function, increases awareness, grounding, stress management, uplifting, encourages self-acceptance, and forgiveness

**CAUTIONS:**

■ Avoid with epilepsy and Parkinson's disease due to camphor and potential fenchone content.[2839,2840,2841]

■ Caution is warranted in children with glucose-6-phosphate dehydrogenase deficiency (G6PD) due to the camphor content in Engelmann Spruce, which may negatively impact red blood cells and increase the risk of jaundice.[2842,2843]

**SELECTED EVIDENCE:**

☐ None found.

## EUCALYPTUS

Tasmanian Bluegum: *Eucalyptus globulus* Labill.;
Narrow-Leaf Peppermint Gum: *E. radiata* Sieber ex DC.

**FAMILY:** Myrtaceae
**NOTE:** Top
**AROMA INTENSITY:** Strong
**AROMA:** Fresh, clean, medicinal, slightly woody
**COMMON EXTRACTION METHOD:** Steam distilled from the leaves

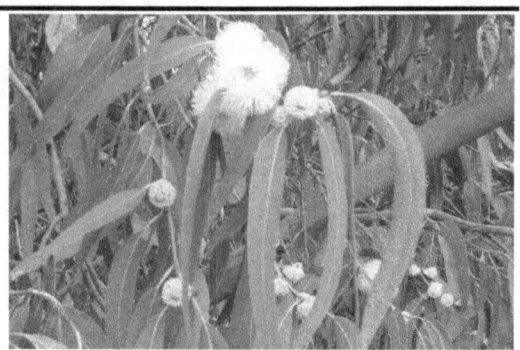

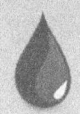

**POSSIBLE SUBSTITUTE OILS:** Niaouli (1,8-cineole CT), bay laurel, cajeput, ravintsara (1,8-cineole CT), ravensara (1,8-cineole CT), cardamom, rosemary (1,8-cineole CT), myrtle, sage (1,8-cineole CT)

**BLENDS WELL WITH:** Bay laurel, bergamot, blue cypress, cajeput, cedarwood, camphor, chamomile (German, Roman), geranium, ginger, grapefruit, peppermint, lavender, lemon, juniper, lemongrass, petitgrain, pine, ravensara, ravintsara, rosemary, sage, tea tree, tangerine, thyme

**SUBCELLULAR LOCALIZATION | EPIGENETIC INFLUENCE:** Endocytic Vesicles | Circulatory/Respiratory (*E. globulus*), Digestive/Excretory (*E. radiata*)

**RECOMMENDED DILUTION RANGE:** 3%–33%; neat for limited conditions

**PRIMARY CONSTITUENTS:**[2844,2845,2846,2847,2848,2849,2850,2851]

| *Eucalyptus globulus* | | *Eucalyptus radiata* | |
|---|---|---|---|
| 1,8-Cineole | 33.6%–83.9% | 1,8-Cineole | 22.4%–74.3% |
| Alpha-Pinene | 4.5%–14.2% | Alpha-Terpineol | 0.0%–15.2% |
| D-Limonene | 0.4%–10.1% | Alpha-Pinene | 0.2%–11.9% |
| Beta-Pinene | 0.3%–5.2% | Trans-Pinocarveol | 0.0%–4.8% |
| Para-Cymene | 0.0%–5.1% | Limonene | 0.5%–4.5% |

Note: *Eucalyptus globulus* essential oil is frequently rectified (redistilled by steam or vacuum to remove impurities or specific constituents) to minimize its odd fruity aroma, which concentrates and increases the 1,8-cineole content from roughly 50%–65% in the crude oil to 70% or higher in the rectified oil.

**OTHER CONSTITUENTS:** *Eucalyptus globulus*—Alpha-phellandrene, alpha-terpinene, alpha-terpineol, alpha-terpineol acetate, beta-myrcene, gamma-terpinene, sabinene, terpinen-4-ol, alloaromadendrene, aromadendrene, globulol, alpha-cadinol; *Eucalyptus radiata*—Beta-pinene, sabinene, alpha-myrcene, isosativene, aristolene, solanone, alpha-myrcene, terpinyl acetate, trans-verbenol, terpinen-4-ol

**PREFERRED COMPOSITION FOR CLINICAL USE:**

| Constituent | *E. globulus* (rectified) | *E. radiata* |
|---|---|---|
| **1,8-Cineole** | 70%–88% | 60%–75% |
| **Limonene** | 3%–12% | 2%–10% |
| **Alpha-Pinene** | 1%–12% | 1%–8% |
| **Gamma-Terpinene** | 0.5%–6% | – |
| **Para-Cymene** | 1%–6% | – |
| **Aromadendrene** | 0%–5% | – |
| **Trans-Pinocarveol** | 0%–5% | – |
| **Alpha-Terpineol** | 0%–5% | 7%–18% |
| **Globulol** | 0%–2% | – |
| **Sabinene** | 0%–2% | 0.1%–4% |
| **Alpha-Terpinyl Acetate** | – | 0.5%–5% |

**REPORTED THERAPEUTIC PROPERTIES: Analgesic**, antibacterial, antifungal, **antirheumatic**, **antiseptic**, antispasmodic, anesthetic, **antiviral**, antineuralgic, **decongestant**, diuretic, **expectorant**, helps balance blood-sugar levels, **supports normal respiration**, reduces fevers, insect repellent, nervine (calms and soothes the nerves), **reduces abnormal bone growth**, promotes oral cleanliness, wound healing, **eases cough**, stimulating, invigorating, refreshing, aids concentration, combats negative emotions, relieves mental exhaustion

**CAUTIONS:**

■ Avoid with children under age 3, particularly around the nose and mouth. Use very cautiously in children under age 5 due to high 1,8-cineole content. 1,8-cineole may cause seizures, central nervous system problems, or respiratory distress in young children.[2852,2853,2854,2855]

■ Avoid with epilepsy and Parkinson's disease due to 1,8-cineole content. May exacerbate or cause seizures/convulsions or reduce seizure medication efficacy based on 1,8-cineole content.[2856,2857,2858] It is also noteworthy that a recent study reports seizures caused by eucalyptus (inhalation (8 cases), intranasal drops (1 case), and massage (1 case)). Most of the

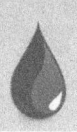

individuals had no previous history or family history of seizures, and each case was the first time the individual was exposed to eucalyptus oil. Although quality and composition of the oil was not tested, this suggests that some individuals may be more prone to seizures when exposed to eucalyptus oil and so caution should be exercised the first time a person is exposed to it.[2859]

■ Caution is warranted orally due to the significant amounts of 1,8-cineole. Limit it to small doses internally (adults—maximum 10 drops daily). One text recommends a maximum daily dose of 6 drops, whereas the European Medicines Agency recommends 2 to 4 drops (100–200 mg) of high 1,8-cineole essential oils orally, 2 to 5 times daily for adolescents, adults, and the elderly. [2860,2861] Additionally, 200 mg of isolated 1,8-cineole has been ingested three times daily for up to six months in clinical research.[2862,2863] Toxicity has been reported when eucalyptus (also high in 1,8-cineole) was ingested in large doses, and as few as 4 to 5 drops may cause problems in very sensitive individuals.[2864,2865,2866,2867,2868,2869] In humans, 3.5 to 5 mL has proven fatal orally.[2870]

■ May weakly interfere with the enzymes responsible for metabolizing medications (NSAIDs, proton-pump inhibitors, acetaminophen, antiepileptics, immune modulators, blood-sugar medications, blood pressure medications, antidepressants, antipsychotics, diabetic medications, antihistamines, antibiotics, and anesthetics) based on research with an herbal extract of eucalyptus and 1,8-cineole content.[2871,2872,2873]

■ May interact with diabetic medications. 1,8-cineole inhibits alpha-glucosidase activity, particularly when synergized with other constituents (alpha-pinene, beta-pinene, para-cymene).[2874,2875,2876] Alpha-glucosidase is an enzyme that breaks down carbohydrates by chemical reaction with water. Inhibiting its activity postpones glucose absorption and therefore the impact of carbohydrates on blood sugar levels. Studies suggest that eucalyptus significantly lowers glucose in animals, which may increase the action of diabetic medications.[2877]

■ May interact with aspirin, blood pressure, antiplatelet, and anticoagulant medications, and increase the risk of bleeding among people with bleeding disorders (low risk).[2878] 1,8-cineole is a weak inhibitor of platelet aggregation.[2879]

■ May interact with antibiotics and increase their antimicrobial activity.[2880,2881,2882,2883]

■ May interfere with pentobarbital and other barbiturates (medications for anxiety and insomnia) based on 1,8-cineole content.[2884,2885]

■ May interact with fluorouracil (a topical medication used for skin cancer and keratosis), and enhance its penetration through the skin.[2886]

### SELECTED EVIDENCE:

◻ The main constituent in eucalyptus, 1,8-cineole, may benefit people with asthma and chronic obstructive pulmonary disease by reducing airway inflammation and excess mucus production (both inflammation and infection caused).[2887]

◻ A study determined that *E. globulus* may be a good candidate for a "natural antibiotic for the treatment of several infections" caused by *S. aureus* and *E. coli*.[2888] It also is an effective treatment for MRSA and *P. aeruginosa*.[2889,2890]

◻ *E. globulus* kills the ectoparasite (*Pediculus humanus*) that cause head lice, including those that are resistant to permethrin (a common drug used to kill head lice).[2891,2892,2893]

◻ A case report describes the use of a combination of the essential oils of lemongrass, eucalyptus, tea tree, clove, thyme and BHT, triclosan, and undenatured alcohol to treat a chronic infection of the lower tibia (osteomyelitis) that was not responding to several courses of IV antibiotics. Amputation of the lower leg was being considered when a physician recommended the leg be opened up and the combination inserted directly into the bone (through a drilled hole, 1 mL per day for forty-eight hours). At three months, the wound and bone healed, and symptoms were resolved.[2894]

◻ An oral spray containing eucalyptus (*E. globulus*), lemon eucalyptus (*E. citriodora*), peppermint (*M. piperita*), Syrian oregano (*O. syriacum*), and rosemary (*R. officinalis*) reduced the severity of the most debilitating symptoms (sore throat, hoarseness, or cough) of upper respiratory tract infections within twenty minutes of application according to a small clinical trial of sixty people.[2895] The spray was continually administered five times a day for three days.

◻ Inhalation of *E. globulus* significantly increased dopamine release (almost a 2.5-fold increase) from rat brain cells.[2896]

◻ *In vitro* research suggests that *E. globulus* is active against six respiratory pathogens: *H. influenzae, H.*

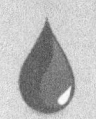

*parainfluenzae, S. maltophilia, S. aureus, S.* pyogenes (a bacterium that causes strep throat, scarlet fever, impetigo, cellulitis, and tonsillitis), and *S. pneumoniae.*[2897,2898]

☐ *E. globulus* essential oil inhibited gram-positive (*S. aureus, B. subtilis*) and gram-negative bacteria (*E. coli*), and fungi (*A. niger, R. solani*).[2899]

☐ *E. globulus* may improve chronic inflammatory airway conditions by reducing toll-like receptor 4 (TLR4) activity in the bronchioles and excess production of airway mucus caused by lipopolysaccharides (LPS) according to animal research.[2900,2901] TLRs are crucial receptors that trigger responses to pathogens. Excess activation of TLRs can lead to allergic and inflammatory responses in the airways.

☐ Topical application of a 1.5% solution containing lavender, marjoram, eucalyptus, rosemary, and peppermint (2:1:2:1:1 ratio), in a carrier oil consisting of 45% apricot, 45% almond, and 10% jojoba carrier oils significantly decreased pain and depression in people with arthritis.[2902]

☐ *In vitro* research suggests that *E. globulus* possesses both central analgesic (act directly on the central nervous system to relieve pain by binding to opioid receptors in the brain and possibly the spinal cord) and peripheral analgesic (inhibit the production of pain-producing substances in the peripheral nervous system) properties.[2903] The peripheral nervous system includes the nerves and ganglia (clusters of nerves and nerve fibers) outside the brain and spinal cord.

☐ Research suggests *E. globulus* possess antimicrobial activity that make it useful as a preservative in the food and pharmaceutical industry.[2904]

☐ *E. globulus* strongly inhibits the fungi *A. fumigatus* (a common fungus that causes respiratory tract infections in people with a suppressed immune system or chronic lung disease) and *A. niger* (a common fungus that can infect humans and produce potent toxins, called mycotoxins).[2905] Eucalyptus essential oil (*E. globulus*) reduced the production of the mycotoxin zearalenone by *Fusarium* species.[2906] Zearalenone is an endocrine-disrupting toxin that attaches to estrogen receptors (ERalpha, ERbeta) in a similar manner to 17beta-estradiol (naturally produced estrogen) and both it and its metabolites (beta-zearalenol, alpha-zearalenol) alter hormone production (progesterone, estradiol, testosterone, and cortisol).[2907,2908,2909]

☐ *E. globulus* scavenges nitric oxide (NO) free radicals and inhibits net NO production to reduce inflammation.[2910] Excess production of NO encourages an abnormal inflammatory response in the joints, gut, and lungs.[2911]

☐ Topical application of a combination of eucalyptus and peppermint oil and ethanol to the forehead and temples of healthy people with a sponge enhanced cognitive performance and produced a muscle-relaxing and mentally relaxing effect.[2912]

☐ *In vitro* research reported that eucalyptus oil provides a sun protection factor (SPF) of 2.625.[2913]

☐ *In vitro* research demonstrated that low doses of marjoram, lemon, basil, clove, thyme, rosemary CT 1,8-cineole, and tea tree essential oils prevented the shortening of telomeres after exposure to hydrogen peroxide.[2914] The same research reported that vetiver, black pepper, eucalyptus (*E. globulus*), ginger, clove, and rosemary increased the length of already shortened telomeres. This activity suggests that these essential oils can help maintain the youth and health of cells, or turn back the clock on the cell to make it more youthful depending on the essential oil used. Interestingly, cinnamon and peppermint essential oil decreased the length of telomeres slightly.

☐ Several essential oils listed in order of efficacy killed the itch mite (*Sarcoptes scabiei*) that burrows into the skin and causes scabies during direct contact (clove > palmarosa > geranium > tea tree > lavender > manuka > petitgrain > eucalyptus > Japanese cedarwood) with the mites and when used as a fumigant (tea tree > clove > eucalyptus (*E. radiata*) > lavender > palmarosa > geranium > Japanese cedarwood > petitgrain > manuka).[2915]

☐ Eucalyptus essential oil is toxic to the brown-banded cockroach (*Supella longipalpa*).[2916] It also repels *Ae. aegypti* mosquitoes for up to 1.5 hours.[2917] A combination of holy basil, peppermint, Indian borage, and eucalyptus (*E. globulus*) provided six hours of mosquito protection, which is comparable to DEET.

☐ Of seven Mediterranean essential oils, eucalyptus and pennyroyal demonstrated the strongest antimicrobial activity.[2918] Rosemary, cistus, and fennel also demonstrated antimicrobial activity. *Eucalyptus globulus* exhibited synergistic activity against *S. aureus* when combined with wild marjoram (*Thymus mastichina*).

☐ *In vitro* and animal research demonstrated that eucalyptus (*E. globulus*) essential oil-loaded lipid nanoparticles produce a synergistic wound healing activity with olive oil.[2919] The wound healing properties of the eucalyptus olive oil mixture were attributed to its antibacterial (*S. aureus, S. pyogenes*) activity and stimulation of cellular migration and proliferation (the phase of wound healing where tissue is rebuilt with tissue composed of collagen and extracellular matrix).

☐ The use of the drug ketamine has been associated with a psychotic state that resembles schizophrenia. Acute and chronic oral administration (500 and 1,000 mg/kg BW) of eucalyptus (*E. globulus*) essential oil protected against ketamine-induced psychosis by facilitating the release of GABA, increasing glutathione (GSH) levels, inhibiting dopamine neurotransmission, and decreasing TNF-α and AChE activity in different regions of the brain.[2920]

☐ *Eucalyptus globulus* essential oil demonstrated consistently strong antimicrobial activity against *L. monocytogenes* and *L. grayi*.[2921]

☐ Eucalyptus (*E. globulus*) essential oil inhibited *Enterococcus faecalis*, whereas *Lactobacillus rhamnosus* presented a higher tolerance to the oil.[2922]

☐ Oral administration of a nanoemulsion formulated with eucalyptus (species not identified; 25 mg/kg BW) essential oil significantly improved wound healing in rats (better than the pure oil alone) by enhancing collagen production at the wound site.[2923]

☐ Eucalyptus (*E. globulus*) essential oil nanoemulsion exhibited antibiofilm and fungicidal activity against *Candida* spp., which was greater than the pure oil.[2924]

☐ Eucalyptus essential oil emulsions exhibited antimicrobial activity against *E. coli, S. aureus,* and *P. aeruginosa* rapidly (less than 1 min).[2925]

☐ *Eucalyptus globulus* essential oil showed insecticidal activity against the housefly (*Musca domestica*) and repelled horn flies (*Haemotobia irritans*) on infested cows.[2926]

☐ Eucalyptus (*E. globulus*) essential oil was toxic to *Culex pipiens* mosquito adults and larvae when used as a fumigant.[2927]

☐ Inhalation of eucalyptus (*E. globulus*) essential oil daily for two to four weeks reduced fatigue during swimming (which was attributed to increased lactate clearance, and reduced creatine kinase, and lactate dehydrogenase concentrations), increased swimming performance and antioxidant capacity, and decreased oxidative damage and inflammatory reactions in tissues in rats.[2928]

☐ Eucalyptus (*E. globulus*) and blue mallee essential oil inhibited *E. coli. S. aureus, E. faecalis, S. typhimurium, A. baumannii, C. albicans, S. epidermidis,* and MRSA, with *E. faecalis* and *C. albicans* being the most susceptible microbes and *A. baumannii* the least susceptible.[2929]

☐ *E. globulus* essential oil showed strong larvicidal activity against mosquitoes (*Anopheles stephensi, Aedes aegypti, Culex quinquefasciatus, Anopheles stephensi, Aedes aegypti, Culex quinquefasciatus*).[2930]

☐ Eucalyptus, clove, mint, oregano, savory, tea tree, and thyme essential oils each inhibited *Venturia inaequalis*, the fungus responsible for apple scab.[2931]

☐ Eucalyptus (*E. globulus*) essential oil demonstrated considerable insecticidal and repellent activity against the *Culex theileri* mosquito.[2932]

☐ A 1% solution of eucalyptus (*E. globulus*) essential oil demonstrated potent scolicidal activity against hydatid cysts obtained from the livers of infected sheep.[2933]

☐ Inhalation or injection of eucalyptus essential oil into mice reduced somatic (skin, tissue, or muscle), inflammatory, and visceral (arising from internal organs) pain by influencing the μ-opioid pain pathway.[2934]

☐ Eucalyptus (*E. globulus*) essential oil was more effective than neem oil in killing mosquito larvae suggesting it is an eco-friendly control measure against *Aedes aegypti* and *Aedes albopictus* mosquitoes.[2935]

☐ Eucalyptus (*E. globulus*) CT 1,8-cineole and fringed lavender CT alpha-thujone were highly acaricidal to ticks (*Hyalomma scupense*).[2936]

☐ Eucalyptus essential oil (*E. globulus*) and ginger, alone and in combination, significantly killed giardial cysts (*Giardia lamblia*) in an experiment that simulated their presence in a human's body.[2937] Eucalyptus killed 73.6 percent of cysts in 480 minutes after exposure.

☐ Male infertility is at least a contributing factor in infertility, about 61 percent of the time due to low quantity (sperm count) or poor quality (decreased mobility, vitality, and sperm morphology) sperm.[2938] Eucalyptus (*E. globulus*) essential oil (composition not reported) significantly improved motility and vitality of human spermatozoa after ten minutes in laboratory research, suggesting it may increase the success of *in vitro* fertilization.[2939]

☐ Both ginger and eucalyptus (*E. globulus*) essential oils effectively repelled the Rhipicephalus bursa tick, which is a transmitter of tick-borne diseases and zoonosis.[2940] The two oils were most effective when used neat (undiluted).

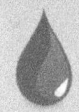

- *In vitro* research demonstrated that eucalyptus (*E. globulus*) completely inhibited *Mycobacterium tuberculosis* subsp. *tuberculosis*, multidrug-resistant *M. tuberculosis*, *M. kansasii,* and *M. gordonae*.[2941]

- Various concentrations of both eucalyptus (*E. globulus*) and lemongrass (*C. citratus*) were effective adulticidal agents against female mosquitoes (*Aedes aegypti* and *Aedes albopictus*) and houseflies (*Musca domestica*).[2942] The highest synergistic activity among the two oils was observed at 2.5% of each oil, which caused a 100 percent knockdown rate and 98.9 percent mortality.

- Nanofibrous membranes with eucalyptus essential oil exhibited good repellent activity against the blood-sucking midge (*Forcipomyia taiwana*).[2943]

- Type 2 diabetes can be managed by inhibiting the carbohydrate-hydrolyzing enzymes alpha-amylase and alpha-glucosidase, which decreases spikes in blood sugar after a meal. A laboratory study found that eucalyptus (*E. radiata*), bay laurel, and nutmeg (West Indian) essential oils each inhibited alpha-amylase comparably to acarbose (an alpha-amylase and alpha-glucosidase inhibiting drug used to control blood sugar levels in people with type 2 diabetes).[2944] Remarkably, eucalyptus and nutmeg essential oils displayed higher activity than acarbose.

- Inhalation of eucalyptus oil with menthol (the primary constituent in peppermint oil; 50:50 ratio) improved pain tolerance, increased blood oxygenation, and increased heart rate variability (as a mechanism to cope with heat stress) during two prospective, randomized, controlled experiments using the Hot Immersion Test Paradigm (HIT).[2945] The oil and menthol were inhaled through an aroma inhaler every thirty seconds by inhaling for three seconds, a two-second hold sequence, and then two-second exhale.

- A 10% concentration of eucalyptus (*E. globulus*) essential oil was acaricidal to the cattle tick (*Rhipicephalus annulatus*), killing 97 percent of ticks.[2946]

- Laboratory research demonstrated that eucalyptus (*E. globulus*) essential oil was toxic to colon cancer cells at lower doses but only toxic to liver cancer cells at high doses (0.5%).[2947] Toxic effects were also observed on human fat cells at higher concentrations (0.5% and 5%), suggesting the oil may not be selective enough for use against cancer cells.

- Eucalyptus (*E. globulus*), pine, rosemary, cistus, Maritime pine, and juniper berry each displayed good antioxidant activity in the ORAC assay.[2948]

- Thyme, tea tree, tropical basil, rosemary CT 1,8-cineole, eucalyptus (*E. globulus*), corn mint, and lavender essential oil each inhibited biofilm-forming *S. aureus*, with thyme and rosemary being the most active in liquid phase.[2949] Thyme was the most active in vapor phase, with varying degrees of inhibition observed depending on the strain of *S. aureus* with tea tree, rosemary, eucalyptus, corn mint, and lavender. Tea tree and lavender oils displayed the weakest activity in the vapor phase.

- Injection of high doses (200 mL/kg BW) of rosemary, Spanish lavender, ravintsara, and eucalyptus (*E. globulus*) essential oil reduced anxiety in rats.[2950]

- Both eucalyptus (*E. globulus*) and clove essential oil repelled mosquitoes (*Anopheles stephensi*), and a combination of the two oils with a ratio of 1:1 of eucalyptus (10%):clove (1%) was more effective.[2951]

- Eucalyptus and cinnamon essential oil reduced inflammation by decreasing superoxide dismutase, TNF-α, and NF-κB levels.[2952]

- Skin barrier integrity is not only important for skin health but also acts as a protective mechanism to limit entry into the body by various substances and microbes. The skin barrier function provided by the *stratum corneum* (SC) is maintained by a delicate balance between water, ions, keratin, natural moisturizing factor, intracellular lipids, skin surface lipids, and the cutaneous microbiome. Substances that possess anti-inflammatory, antimicrobial, and antioxidant activity and trigger adaptive responses in skin characteristics support healthy skin barrier function and improve the appearance of the skin. Preclinical and clinical research evaluated the activity of tea tree, tangerine, eucalyptus (*E. globulus*), and lavender essential oil skin barrier function and characteristics. Two formulas—one with equal parts of tangerine, eucalyptus, and lavender, and one with equal parts of tea tree, tangerine, eucalyptus, and lavender—diluted to 2% in emulsions stabilized with polymers of natural origin were created to investigate their skin benefits. Tangerine showed the deepest penetration through the skin (35% of the oil made it across the SC) in pig ear, while the rest of the oils and combinations of the oils penetrated less than tangerine but were absorbed at higher than 5% through the viable epidermis. In the clinical study, the four essential oil emulsion hydrated the skin better and improved skin barrier function better than the three essential oil emulsion, showing that tea tree oil has a synergistic activity with the other oils. The four-oil group also experienced improvements in skin characteristics compared to a control group and the three-oil emulsion group. The totality of the research suggests that a combination of tea tree, tangerine, eucalyptus, and lavender in an emulsion can improve overall skin barrier function and skin characteristics.[2953]

- Eucalyptus (*E. globulus*) was weakly insecticidal to the three main pests of cotton (*Pectinophora gossypiella*, *Thaumatotibia leucotreta*, and *Helicoverpa armigera*).[2954]

- Cinnamon, eucalyptus (*E. globulus*), and clove bud essential oil effectively inhibited MRSA, with cinnamon producing the greatest zone of inhibition and eucalyptus having the lowest minimum inhibitory concentration.[2955]

- Laboratory research concluded that eucalyptus (*E. globulus*) provides antiaging effects to the skin by decreasing beta-galactosidase and matrix metalloproteinases activation and upregulating collagen type 1.[2956] Moreover, the oil reduced tyrosine activity and melanin production, suggesting it may promote an even skin tone and produced potent anti-inflammatory effects. The oil did not cause irritation or sensitization in cells, revealing the safety of its use topically.

- Combining eucalyptus (*E. globulus*) oil and lovastatin in a nanogel created a synergistic effect against tongue cancer in laboratory research.[2957]

- Interstitial cystitis is a type of bladder pain syndrome characterized by chronic pain in the bladder/pelvic floor area, frequent or urgent need to urinate, and pain during sexual intercourse. Chronic inflammation is a leading trigger of interstitial cystitis because of its damaging effects to bladder tissues and function. Researchers evaluated the activity of lavender and eucalyptus (*E. globulus*) essential oils in a cell culture model (T24 human bladder epithelial cell line on TNF-α-stimulated inflammation) of bladder pain syndrome.[2958] Both oils reduced proinflammatory cytokines (IL-1β, IL-6, IL-8) and NFκB activation (a mediator of proinflammatory gene expression, which when dysregulated contributes to processes that cause multiple inflammatory diseases), but overall lavender was more effective. Both lavender, and its primary constituent linalool, displayed greater effectiveness than the comparative control (ACHP inhibitor). The researchers concluded that this research suggests that lavender oil may be suitable as an adjunct therapy in the treatment of interstitial cystitis.

- *In vitro* (protein denaturation inhibition assay) evidence demonstrated that eucalyptus (*E. globulus*) essential oil possesses anti-inflammatory activity.[2959] Its anti-inflammatory activity was only slightly lower than diclofenac. Further evaluation in rats confirmed this activity when administered orally (250 mcL/kg BW). The anti-inflammatory effect of eucalyptus was superior to ibuprofen for the first four hours but dropped below ibuprofen after hour four suggesting the need for taking the oil every four hours to maintain efficacy.

- Researchers evaluated the activity of bergamot, tea tree, star anise, and eucalyptus (*E. globulus*) against influenza virus type A (H1N1) while in vapor phase.[2960] Both bergamot and tea tree essential oils strongly reduced the cytopathic (structural changes to cells after infection) of H1N1 without being toxic to healthy cells. Eucalyptus was moderately effective without being toxic to healthy cells, whereas star anise was inactive. Further evaluation of the mechanism that these essential oils reduced H1N1 infectivity found that the oils interfere with the lipid bilayer of the viral envelope triggering decomposition of membranes. This research suggests that diffusing essential oils, which creates a vapor, may help to reduce viral load and their potential to infect humans.

- Monocytic/granulocytic cells and macrophages play crucial roles in the recognition of foreign invaders such as bacteria, viruses, and fungi. Phagocytes are immune cells that ingest pathogenic organisms and contribute to tissue homeostasis by eliminating dead cells. A laboratory study found that eucalyptus (*E. globulus*) essential oil stimulated the activation of macrophages (which was attributed to 1,8-cineole), triggers phagocytosis to clear pathogens, and promotes podosome formation (adhesive structures found on the outer surface of cells involved in cell motility and immune responses). These results confirm that eucalyptus oil potently activates innate cell-mediated immunity and may be helpful against infectious illnesses and in people with suppressed immune function.

- Eucalyptus (*E. globulus*) essential oil inhibited *S. aureus*, *B. subtilis*, *P. aeruginosa*, *E. coli*, and *C. albicans*.[2961]

- Of eight essential oils treated, eucalyptus (*E. globulus*) essential oil was the most toxic to the red mite (*Dermanyssus gallinae*) at lower concentrations.[2962] Citronella (*C. winterianus*), pine, clove bud, thyme, rosemary, geranium, and lavender were also effective, with increasing toxicity at higher concentrations.

- Pulmonary fibrosis is a fibrous interstitial pneumonia that damages the lungs, causes accumulation of lymphocytes and monocytes in respiratory fluid, and alters respiratory function. A preclinical model of pulmonary fibrosis evaluated the ingestion of eucalyptus hydrosol (2,000 mg/kg BW) and eucalyptus essential oil (10 mg/kg BW) in rats.[2963] Ingestion of both the hydrosol and oil reversed the harmful effects of pulmonary fibrosis (reduced inflammation, accumulation of lymphocytes and monocytes in respiratory fluid, fibrosis score, and oxidative stress). These preclinical results suggest that ingestion of eucalyptus hydrosol or essential oil could be a natural solution for pulmonary fibrosis.

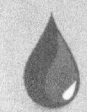

- Humans are exposed to gamma rays (gamma radiation) from cosmic rays in the solar system, medical tests (X-rays, CT scans, etc.), airport scanners, nuclear power plants, some consumer products, and food irradiation, which can alter healthy cells in the body. A preclinical model found that exposure to rosemary, oregano, lavender, or eucalyptus (*E. globulus*) essential oils protected against damage caused by gamma ray exposure.[2964] The best protective effects were observed form lavender and oregano essential oils. Specifically, the oil preserved metabolic enzymes, restored enzymatic antioxidant activity (catalase and superoxide dismutase), and reduced lipid peroxidation.

- Both eucalyptus (*E. globulus*) and rosemary essential oil were insecticidal to and repelled the mill moth (*Ephestia kuehniella*), which is a pest of cereal grains, especially flour.[2965]

- Eucalyptus essential oil was evaluated with and without eucalyptus honey for its antioxidant, antibacterial, and anti-inflammatory activity.[2966] The best antioxidant activity (DPPH, FRAP, and beta-carotene/linoleic acid assays) was observed when eucalyptus was combined with honey, while the best anti-inflammatory activity (5-LOX and tyrosinase inhibition) was noted with eucalyptus only in laboratory tests, but the combination of honey and eucalyptus proved better in rats. The oil also inhibited *E. coli*, *P. mirabilis*, *S. typhimurium*, *B. subtilis*, *S. aureus*, *L. monocytogenes*, *C. albicans*, *T. rubrum*, and *A. niger*, with its activity being reduced when combined with honey.

- Eucalyptus (*E. globulus*) essential oil exhibited good acaricidal activity against camel mites (*Sarcoptes scabiei* var. *cameli*) that cause camel sarcoptic mange in a laboratory setting.[2967]

- Nanoemulsions and nanogels containing eucalyptus (*E. globulus*) essential oil were effective against mosquito (*A. stephensi*) larvae.[2968]

- Post-COVID syndrome, or long haul COVID, involves the persistence of health problems for at least twelve weeks after recovering from COVID-19. A pilot clinical study found that topical application and inhalation of eucalyptus (*E. globulus*) essential oil—application of 2 drops of a 10% dilution to the wrist, inhaled for five minutes, twice daily—reduced post-COVID syndrome symptoms.[2969] All three post-COVID syndrome symptoms measured, specifically difficulty breathing, back pain, and anxiety, significantly improved after four weeks of intervention.

- A preclinical model of dental plaque on teeth showed that both spearmint and eucalyptus essential oils reduced *S. mutans* biofilms at 0.5% concentration.[2970]

- Eucalyptus (*E. globulus*) and tea tree essential oil demonstrated activity against mature biofilms and biofilms in the process of formation, produced by strains belonging to three main categories of antibiotic resistant bacteria (Vancomycin-resistant enterococci, MRSA, and broad-spectrum β-lactamase-producing E. coli), with the greatest activity against biofilm in formation.[2971]

- A eucalyptus nanoemulsion hydrogel inhibited and killed *S. aureus* and effectively promoted wound healing, reduced bacterial load in wounds, decreased inflammation, and accelerated skin tissue recovery.[2972]

- Eucalyptus (*E. globulus*) essential oil inhibited *C. albicans*, *P. citrinum*, *B. cinerae*, *A. flavus*, *C. glabrata*, *B. subtilis*, *S. aureus*, *Y. enterocolitica*, *S. enterica*, *C. tropicalis*, *C. krusei*, and *E. faecalis*, and showed antibiofilm activity against *P. fluorescens*.[2973] Additionally, the oil was insecticidal to the lime seed bug (*Oxycarenus lavaterae*).

# EUCALYPTUS DIVES
## (Peppermint Eucalyptus, Broadleaf Peppermint Gum, Blue Peppermint, Peppermint Gum)

*Eucalyptus dives* Schauer., *E. dives* Schauer. in Walp

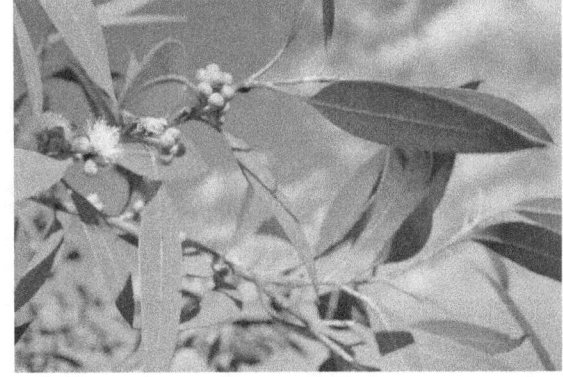

**FAMILY:** Myrtaceae
**NOTE:** Top
**AROMA INTENSITY:** Strong
**AROMA:** Fresh, camphoraceous, sweet, slightly minty
**COMMON EXTRACTION METHOD:** Steam distilled from the leaves
**POSSIBLE SUBSTITUTE OILS:** Peppermint, spearmint, lavandin

**BLENDS WELL WITH:** Basil, bergamot, cajeput, cedarwood, citronella, cypress, eucalyptus, ginger, grapefruit, lavender, lemon, lemon eucalyptus, lime, may chang, myrtle, orange, peppermint, pine, spearmint, tangerine, tea tree

**SUBCELLULAR LOCALIZATION | EPIGENETIC INFLUENCE:** Currently unknown | Currently unknown

**RECOMMENDED DILUTION RANGE:** 3%–50%; neat for limited conditions

**PRIMARY CONSTITUENTS:** [2974,2975,2976,2977,2978]

| | |
|---|---|
| Piperitone | 29.2%–88.4% |
| Alpha-Phellandrene | 0.0%–17.4% (Typically 13.3%–17.4%) |
| Para-Cymene | 0.0%–8.5% |
| Terpinen-4-ol | 0.1%–7.9% |
| Para-Cymen-8-ol | 0.0%–5.1% |
| Para-Mentha-1(7),8-Diene | 0.0%–3.3% |
| Alpha-Thujene | 0.0%–3.1% |
| Beta-Phellandrene | 0.0%–2.8% |

Note: A 1,8-cineole CT is also reported in aromatherapy texts and in the scientific literature, but a review of available commercial samples only found the piperitone CT available.[3031]

**OTHER CONSTITUENTS:** Tricyclene, alpha-pinene, myrcene, alpha-terpinene, 1,8-cineole, gamma-terpinene, terpinolene, linalool, cis-para-menth-2-en-1-ol, trans-para-menth-2-en-1-ol, alpha-terpineol, trans-piperitol, (E)-methyl cinnamate, bicyclogermacrene, terpinen-1-ol

**PREFERRED COMPOSITION FOR CLINICAL USE:**

| *Constituent* | |
|---|---|
| **Piperitone** | 35%–55% |
| **Alpha-Phellandrene** | 15%–30% |
| **Para-Cymene** | 3%–9% |
| **Terpinen-4-ol** | 3%–9% |
| **Alpha-Thujene** | 0.5%–5% |
| **Beta-Phellandrene** | 0.5%–5% |

**REPORTED THERAPEUTIC PROPERTIES:** Antibacterial, antifungal, **antimicrobial**, analgesic, antiseptic, reduces fever, supports respiratory function, **relieves sinusitis**, expels excess mucus, decongestant, **insecticide**, relieves anxiety, mentally stimulating

**CAUTIONS:**

■ May interact with antibiotics and enhance their effectiveness based on piperitone content.[2979,2980]

**SELECTED EVIDENCE:**

☐ The antimicrobial properties of *Eucalyptus dives* against *E. coli. E. faecalis, S. aureus, P. aeruginosa,* and *C. albicans* compare favorably to standard antibiotics.[2981] A piperitone-rich fraction containing 99.2% piperitone inhibited *Pseudomonas fragi, E. coli, Salmonella typhimurium, L. monocytogenes, S. aureus, Saccharomyces cerevisiae.*[2982]

☐ *E. dives* effectively fumigated the plant-feeding mite *Tetranychus urticae.*[2983] It was also effective against *S. oryzae* and *S. zeamais* and the Japanese termite.[2984,2985]

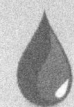

# FENNEL, SWEET OR BITTER

*Foeniculum vulgare* Mill., *F. vulgare dulce*;
Bitter Fennel: *F. vulgare* Mill. ssp. *vulgare* var. *vulgare*,
*F. vulgare* Mill. ssp. *capillaceum* var. *vulgare*

**FAMILY:** Apiaceae (Umbelliferae)
**NOTE:** Middle
**AROMA INTENSITY:** Medium
**AROMA:** Sweet, earthy, licorice-like
**COMMON EXTRACTION METHOD:** Steam distilled from the seeds (fruit)
**POSSIBLE SUBSTITUTE OILS:** Ravensara (methyl chavicol CT), clary sage, basil (linalool CT)
**BLENDS WELL WITH:** Balsam fir, basil, bay laurel, bergamot, black pepper, camphor, cardamom, carrot seed, cinnamon, cypress, eucalyptus, geranium, grapefruit, juniper, lavender, lemon, lemon verbena, marjoram, myrrh, niaouli, orange, patchouli, pine, rose, rosemary, sandalwood, tangerine, ylang ylang
**SUBCELLULAR LOCALIZATION | EPIGENETIC INFLUENCE:** Cell Membrane | Currently unknown
**RECOMMENDED DILUTION RANGE:** 5%–Neat (*trans-anethole CT*); 1.5%–20%, 50% for some conditions (*methyl chavicol (estragole) CT*)

**PRIMARY CONSTITUENTS:**[2986,2987,2988,2989,2990,2991,2992,2993,2994,2995,2996]

*Trans-Anethole CT*

| | |
|---|---|
| Trans-Anethole | 31.0%–94.6% |
| Fenchone | 1.0%–34.7% |
| Limonene | 0.3%–16.5% |
| Carvacrol | 0.0%–12.6% |
| Alpha-Pinene | 0.2%–12.4% |
| Alpha-Phellandrene | 0.1%–10.5% |
| Cis-Anethole | 0.1%–8.6% |
| Methyl Chavicol (Estragole) | 2.6%–8.2% |
| Para-Cymene | 0.0%–6.0% |

*Methyl Chavicol (Estragole) CT*

| | |
|---|---|
| Methyl Chavicol (Estragole) | 57.9%–93.9% |
| Limonene | 0.1%–22.4% |
| Trans-Anethole | 1.4%–19.0% |
| Fenchone | 1.0%–10.4% |
| Alpha-Pinene | 0.2%–3.6% |

*Bitter Fennel, Trans-Anethole CT*

| | |
|---|---|
| Trans-Anethole | 44.2%–71.4% |
| Methyl Chavicol (Estragole) | 1.4%–35.1% |
| Fenchone | 13.2%–24.3% |
| Limonene | 0.9%–1.9% |

*Bitter Fennel, Methyl Chavicol CT*

| | |
|---|---|
| Methyl Chavicol (Estragole) | 47.8%–75% |
| Trans-Anethole | 0.1%–31.5% |
| Fenchone | 12.3%–19.8% |
| Limonene | 0.9%–4.7% |
| 1,8-Cineole | 0.5%–2.0% |

**OTHER CONSTITUENTS:** *Trans-Anethole CT*—Gamma-terpinene, myrcene, para-anisaldehyde, para-acetonylanisole; *Methyl Chavicol (Estragole) CT*—Sabinene, beta-pinene, para-cymene, 1,8-cineole, gamma-terpinene, camphor; *Bitter Fennel, Trans-Anethole CT*—alpha-pinene, beta-myrcene, alpha-phellandrene, gamma-terpinene; *Bitter Fennel, Methyl Chavicol CT*—alpha-pinene, beta-myrcene, gamma-terpinene

**PREFERRED COMPOSITION FOR CLINICAL USE:**

| Constituent | Sweet Fennel (E)-Anethole CT | Bitter Fennel (E)-Anethole CT |
|---|---|---|
| Trans-Anethole | 65%–85% | 55%–72% |
| Fenchone | 3%–17% | 12%–25% |
| Limonene | 0.5%–12% | 1%–4% |
| Alpha-Pinene | 1%–9% | 2%–7% |
| Alpha-Phellandrene | 0.1%–7% | 0.1%–7% |

| | | |
|---|---|---|
| **Methyl Chavicol (Estragole)** | 0.1%–5% | 1%–5% |
| **Gamma-Terpinene** | 0.1%–2% | – |
| **Beta-Myrcene** | 0.1%–2% | 0.1%–2% |
| **Para-Anisaldehyde** | 0%–2% | 0.1%–1% |
| **Cis-Anethole** | < 1% | < 1% |

**REPORTED THERAPEUTIC PROPERTIES: Aids digestion**, expels excess gas, colic, relieves constipation and diarrhea, relieves cough, diuretic, expectorant, helps balance blood-sugar levels, antitumor, antiparasitic, analgesic (pain relief), **antifungal**, enhances metabolism, **helps balance menstruation**, antiseptic, helps reduce the appearance of blemishes, energizing, encourages open communication, promotes self-confidence, reduces anxiety, promotes balanced emotions

**CAUTIONS:**

■ Use with caution and highly diluted for children under 6 due to methyl chavicol (estragole) and trans-anethole content (methyl chavicol and trans-anethole CTs).[2997]

■ Long-term oral use (fennel tea) may cause premature breast development in very young girls—usually under age 2. Long-term oral use is not recommended for children under age 12.[2998]

■ Avoid during pregnancy and lactation. Large doses of fennel may be toxic to fetal cells based on animal research.[2999,3000] Nephrotoxicity (kidney toxicity) has been reported in infants whose mothers drank 2 liters of an herbal tea daily that contained fennel, licorice, anise, and goat's rue. Symptoms improved within 36 hours after the mothers discontinued drinking the tea.[3001] It is also worth noting that trans-anethole may negatively affect fertility. Animal research suggests it decreases fertility by preventing the implantation of a fertilized egg in the uterus.[3002]

■ Oral caution (methyl chavicol CT). Significant amounts of the cancer-causing constituent methyl chavicol (estragole) can be found in fennel (methyl chavicol CT); however, research suggests that other constituents in this CT may inactivate the cancer-causing potential of methyl chavicol. Nevertheless, it would be wise to limit oral consumption of the methyl chavicol CT to no more than 5 drops daily as a precaution.[3003,3004,3005]

■ Photosensitzing due to the presence of psoralen, bergapten, isoimponellin, and xanthotixin.[3006] Avoid UV rays for at least twelve hours following topical application.

■ Avoid with epilepsy and Parkinson's due to fenchone content, which may exacerbate or trigger seizures/convulsions or reduce medication efficacy.[3007,3008]

■ May interact with aspirin, blood pressure, antiplatelet, and anticoagulant medications, and increase the risk of bleeding among people with bleeding disorders based on trans-anethole, fenchone, and methyl chavicol content.[3009,3010,3011,3012,3013]

■ May interact with diabetes medications and cause low blood sugar.[3014]

■ *Trans-Anethole CTs*: May interact with ibuprofen and enhance its anti-inflammatory activity.[3015]

■ Fennel contains significant amounts of the phytoestrogen anethole. Anethole exhibits weak estrogenic activity[3016] and many aromatherapy texts suggest avoiding fennel with endometriosis, oral contraceptives, hormone replacement therapy, and estrogen-dependent cancers because of this. However, research suggests that anethole may promote destruction (apoptosis) of cancer cells—including both estrogen-positive and estrogen-negative breast cancer cells—and phytoestrogens are generally balancing with the ability to either mimic or block the action of estrogen according to current knowledge.[3017,3018] In addition, anethole reduced painful uterine contractions in the rat uterus.[3019] A follow up clinical study confirmed the animal results, and suggests that fennel essential oil reduces painful menstruation and excess menstrual bleeding, and relaxes the smooth muscles of the uterus.[3020] Lastly, another study found that 97.5% of women treated with a traditional Chinese medicine formula containing fennel and cordyceps experienced improvements in their endometrial symptoms.[3021] Based on this, reasonable doses pose little risk of interaction or contraindication.

■ May interfere with fluoroquinolone antibiotics according to research with fennel herb in animals.[3022]

■ May interact with antibiotics or antifungal drugs and possibly enhance or decrease their effectiveness based on trans-anethole and estragole content.[3023,3024,3025,3026]

■ May interfere with the enzymes responsible for metabolizing medications based on research with an herbal extract (NSAIDs, proton-pump inhibitors, acetaminophen, antiepileptics, immune modulators, blood-sugar medications, blood pressure medications, antidepressants, antipsychotics, diabetic medications, antihistamines, antibiotics, and anesthetics).[3027,3028,3029,3030]

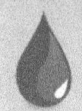

**SELECTED EVIDENCE:**

- *In vitro* research suggests that fennel oil combats fungal infections of the skin, hair, and nails better than standard drug options.[3031]

- Oral administrationof fennel essential oil significantly reduces anxiety in mice.[3032] Lower doses reduced anxiety while higher doses were sedating.

- Fennel oil inhibits the *K. pneumoniae* bacterium that can cause pneumonia, bloodstream infections, wound or surgical site infections, and meningitis.[3033]

- Animal research suggests that fennel oil may protect DNA from damage, reduce bone marrow cell death, and reduce abnormal sperm caused by cyclophosphamide (a drug used to treat leukemia, cancer, and lymphomas).[3034]

- *In vitro* research suggests fennel oil significantly inhibits *C. albicans, S. typhimurium,* and *S. dysenteriae.*[3035] Another study reported that fennel essential oil completely inhibited the mycelial growth of fungi and killed fungi that infect the nails (*Trichophyton rubrum, T. mentagrophytes,* and *Scytalidium dimidiatum*), and demonstrated broad-spectrum antifungal activity against other fungi that infect the nails (*Aspergillus flavus, A. fumigatus, A. niger, A. ustus, Candida albicans, Epidermophyton floccosum, Microporum audouinii, M. canis, M. gypseum, M. nanum, Rhizopus nigricans, Trichophyton tonsurans,* and *T. violaceum*).[3036] The essential oil was non-irritating and caused no adverse reactions when applied to humans at 5% concentration for up to three weeks, which caused the researchers to conclude that fennel essential oil has potential as a therapeutic agent for nail infections.

- Animal research suggests that fennel oil protects against the formation of blood clots by causing vasorelaxation and clot destabilization.[3037]

- Fennel essential oil protects against stomach lesions caused by ethanol according to animal research.[807]

- Inhalation of fennel essential oil increases sympathetic nervous system activity and adrenaline levels, which suggests it may improve alertness.[3038]

- *In vitro* research suggests that anethole may promote destruction (apoptosis) of ovarian and breast cancer cells.[3039,3040]

- Animal research suggests that anethole reduces painful uterine contractions in the rat uterus.[3041] A follow up clinical study confirmed the animal results, and suggests that fennel essential oil (0.3–1.0 mL of a 1% or 2% dilution at onset of pain and then at least every four hours) reduces painful menstruation and excess menstrual bleeding, and relaxes the smooth muscles of the uterus.[3042] Another placebo-controlled clinical study administered 30 mg (about half a drop) of fennel essential oil every four hours beginning from the first day of menstruation reported that fennel oil reduces menstrual pain severity.[3043] The fennel essential oil used in the clinical studies was prepared by Barij Essence, Ltd, Iran, which other studies suggest contains 30% fennel essential oil and 71–90 mg trans-anethole.[3044]

- A clinical study reported that the oral administration of fennel essential oil containing 71–90 mg of trans-anethole resolved amenorrhea (the abnormal absence of menstruation) similarly to a contraceptive known to stimulate menstruation containing 30 mcg ethinylestradiol and 150 mcg levonorgestrel.[3045] The study authors observed that 73 percent of women who took fennel oil resolved amenorrhea (19 percent placebo), whereas 81 percent of those taking both the contraceptive and fennel essential oil experienced amenorrhea resolution. Interestingly, the fennel only group experienced greater menstrual bleeding (20.8 mL) and longer duration of menstrual bleeding/spotting (5.2 days) compared to the contraceptive group (14.4 mL and 4.0 days respectively).

- Fennel oil inhibited multidrug-resistant *A. baumannii* (a bacterium that commonly infects those with a compromised immune system, like those in intensive care units).[3046] It also was active against *E. coli, L. monocytogenes, S. typhimurium,* and *S. aureus* at low concentrations.[3047,3048]

- Animal research suggests that fennel oil possesses bronchodilatory properties, possibly by influencing the potassium channel.[3049]

- Fennel oil protected rats against liver damage caused by carbon tetrachloride (an inorganic constituent associated with liver and kidney damage).[3050]

- Both fennel essential oil and trans-anethole significantly increased extracellular $Ca^{2+}$ (free/unbound calcium ions) entry into endothelial cells when extracellular $Ca^{2+}$ was present, but strongly prevented increased activity of store-operated $Ca^{2+}$ entry (SOCE), which is activated when intracellular calcium stores are depleted.[3051] This activity suggests that fennel and trans-anethole may regulate vasodilation and influence blood pressure.

- Fennel essential oil increases the antioxidant activity of yogurt and acts as a food preservative.[3052]
- A clinical study demonstrated that oral administration of two capsules containing 17.5 mg of fennel essential oil and 42 mg of curcumin, twice daily, relieves irritable bowel symptoms.[3053] Remarkably, the fennel EO-curcumin supplement resulted in complete resolution of IBS symptoms among 25.9% of study participants.
- A unique CT of fennel essential oil (o-cymene) inhibited *Candida* sp.[3054]
- *In vitro* research showed that fennel essential oil (low trans-anethole content—36.8%) was a moderate antioxidant and mildly toxic to cervical, colorectal, breast, T lymphoblast leukemia, and Adriamycin-resistant leukemia cancer cells (in comparison to reference drugs).[3055]
- Oral administration of fennel essential oil (200, 400 mg/kg BW) to rats decreased colon inflammation (via inhibition of NF-KB pathway) in an animal model of colitis.[3056]
- Sweet basil, cinnamon bark, sweet fennel, kaffir lime petitgrain, kaffir lime peel, black pepper, peppermint, and spearmint essential oils all demonstrated antimicrobial activity against bacteria linked to cavities (Streptococcus *mutans* and *Lactobacillus casei*).[3057] Cinnamon was the most active against both bacteria, kaffir lime petitgrain was the weakest of the tested oils against both bacteria, and black pepper was inactive against *L. casei*.
- Sweet fennel essential oil demonstrated good efficacy against the insect pest *Myzus persicae* without harming its natural predator (*Harmonia axyridis*) or the soil organism *Eisenia fetida*.[3058]
- The trans-anethole CT of fennel essential oil, frequently called sweet fennel, exhibited remarkable dose-dependent apoptotic effects against liver cancer cells without causing damage to genetic material.[3059]
- Sweet fennel essential oil demonstrated potent anticancer activity against breast and cervical cancer cells *in vitro*.[3060] The same study noted antibacterial activity against three Gram-negative strains (*Pseudomonas aeruginosa*, *Escherichia coli*, and *Shigella dysenteriae*).
- Human aryl hydrocarbon receptor (AhR: a gene that encodes a protein that helps regulate responses to planar aromatic hydrocarbons and significantly affects the immune activity in the gastrointestinal tract) regulates the circadian rhythm, helps regulate the cell cycle, and plays an important role in tissue development. Cumin, jasmine, vanilla, and bay leaf fully activate AhR; clove, dill, thyme, nutmeg, and oregano partially activate AhR; and tarragon, caraway, turmeric, lovage, fennel, spearmint, star anise, and anise inhibit the AhR activity.[3061]
- *In vitro* research demonstrates that fennel CT trans-anethole essential oil enhances the antimicrobial activity of antibiotics (cefoxitin, mupirocin, co-trimoxazole, and ciprofloxacin) against *S. aureus* isolated from humans, with the greatest enhancement of mupirocin.[3062]
- A triple-blind, placebo-controlled trial of ninety postmenopausal women showed that oral administration of fennel essential oil 100 mg softgels (for eight weeks) significantly reduced postmenopausal symptoms.[3063] Symptoms assessed included total symptoms; somatic/vegetative: hot flashes, heart discomfort, sleep problems, joint or muscular discomfort; psychological symptoms: depression, irritability, anxiety, and physical or mental exhaustion; and urogenital symptoms: sexual dysfunction, bladder problems, and vaginal dryness. Each 100 mg softgel contained 30% fennel essential oil (standardized to 21–27mg of trans-anethole) with sunflower oil.
- Cumin, fennel, dill, and anise essential oils each demonstrated inhibitory activity against *Candida* species, with cumin being the most active.[3064] Fennel and anise were not cytotoxic to mouse fibroblasts at minimum inhibitory concentrations.
- *In vitro* research showed that peppermint and fennel essential oil inhibit *Alternaria* sp.[3065]
- Topical application of a transdermal nanoemulsion (a mixture of oil, water, and a stabilizer that improves systemic and controlled delivery of substances through the skin) of fennel essential oil CT trans-anethole reduced liver dysfunction and toxicity in rats as indicated by improved ALT, AST, ALP, bilirubin, albumin, malondialdehyde, and ammonia plasma levels.[3066]
- Laboratory research found that sweet fennel and carrot (leaf and stem; caryophyllene oxide and isospathulenol as primary constituents) essential oil inhibited gram-positive (*S. aureus, B. subtilis, B. amyloliquefaciens*) and gram-negative bacteria and the yeast *C. albicans*.[3067] One variety of fennel oil tested was more active against *C. albicans* than gentamicin.
- Sweet fennel CT trans-anethole essential oil killed breast cancer cells by altering gene expression—increasing BAX (a gene that contributes to apoptosis) and decreasing Bcl2 (a gene that blocks apoptosis).[3068] The same researchers reported that fennel essential oil demonstrated remarkable antimicrobial activity against *E. coli, S. aureus, S. epidermidis, P. aeruginosa*, and *C. albicans*.
- A combination of sweet fennel and clove essential oil killed colon cancer cells without harming normal human cells in laboratory research.[3069]

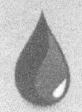

- Both cumin and fennel essential oil showed promise as alternatives to conventional drugs for the treatment of *Candida* infections due to their ability to inhibit *Candida* species isolated from the mouths of edentulous patients.[3070] Cumin was more effective than fennel.
- Tunisian (trans-anethole CT) and French (methyl chavicol CT) fennel exhibited low antioxidant capacity in the DPPH assay, with Tunisian performing better than French.[3071]
- Oral administration of fennel or rosemary oils (or their respective nanoforms) in dyslipidemic rats improved biochemical parameters (reduced cardiovascular disease risk, decreased inflammation and oxidative stress, preserved liver function, and lowered blood sugar levels).[3072]
- Laboratory research demonstrated that fennel essential oil and trans-anethole exhibited moderate antitrichomonal properties against *Trichomonas vaginalis*, which is a parasite that is transmitted via sexual intercourse and infects the vagina, urethra, and foreskin of the penis.[3073]
- Sweet fennel essential oil exhibited good antioxidant (DPPH assay) and antifungal (*C. gloeosporioides, P. capsici, S. sclerotiorum, F. fujikuroi*) activity and inhibited cancer cells (human gastric cancer, human cervical cancer, human lung cancer).[3074]
- Both the trans-anethole and the estragole CTs of fennel exhibited good antioxidant activity in the DPPH, ABTS, and reducing power assays.[3075]
- The widespread use of pesticides is a concern for humans and the environment. Researchers found that fennel essential oil protects against pesticide (triflumuron) toxicity in laboratory research.[3076] The oil increased cell viability and antioxidant (SOD and CAT) activity, reduced reactive oxygen species generation, and significantly decreased DNA damage and malondialdehyde levels.
- Fennel essential oil protected carp (*Cyprinus carpio*) against chlorpyrifos (an organophosphate pesticide) toxicity as measured by significant improvements in impaired antioxidant activity and hematological parameters.[3077]
- Researchers compared sweet fennel essential oil, fluoxetine, and imipramine in a preclinical model of depression. The fennel essential oil produced a dose-dependent antidepressant effect in albino mice without altering animal movement, partly by influencing dopaminergic and serotonergic systems.[3078] Administration of noneffective doses of fennel oil with noneffective doses of fluoxetine or imipramine caused a synergistic antidepressant-like effect in mice.
- Neutrophils serve as the first line of defense against infections and play important roles in initiating inflammatory reactions. An unbalanced response to an infection can trigger uncontrolled inflammation and the progression of neutrophilic inflammatory diseases such as arthritis, psoriasis, asthma, chronic obstructive pulmonary disease, cystic fibrosis, and acute respiratory distress syndrome. Neutrophils are the most abundant innate immune cells and leverage several mechanisms to destroy invading pathogens and activate other immune cells. These activities must maintain a delicate balance to avoid uncontrolled inflammation and destruction of healthy cells. Tropical fennel (methyl chavicol CT) and cumin essential oils significantly suppressed the activation of neutrophils and balanced the mechanisms they use to attack pathogens *in vitro*, suggesting they may be useful for neutrophilic inflammatory diseases.[3079]
- Of twenty-three essential oils tested, fennel exhibited the greatest insecticidal activity against the red flour beetle (*Tribolium castaneum*).[3080] Other essential oils that showed good fumigant activity were tarragon, cardamom, lavender, and black pepper. The researchers reported that the most effective oils contained a diversity of constituents while the least effective consisted mainly of monoterpenes.
- Fennel essential oil was acaricidal to the cattle tick (Rhipicephalus annulatus), which was largely attributed to its main constituent trans-anethole.[3081] Lethal concentrations against adults and larvae were significantly lower when isolated trans-anethole was used compared to whole fennel oil.
- When ten essential oils—lesser calamint CT piperitone oxide, bergamot, lemon petitgrain, tangerine petitgrain, fennel CT methyl chavicol, bay laurel, myrtle CT 1,8-cineole, oregano CT, sage CT alpha-thujone, and rosemary CT 1,8-cineole—were tested against antibiotic-resistant *E. coli*, oregano, lesser calamint, and fennel were the most active at inhibiting bacterial growth.[3082] Further evaluation found that the oils triggered methylation both at adenine and cytosine residues in the genomes of most cell lines, suggesting that the oils can induce epigenetic remodeling.
- Of 11 essential oils tested, oregano CT carvacrol, fennel, winter savory CT para-cymene, and summer savory CT carvacrol were the most effective against gastrointestinal nematodes (*Haemonchus, Trichostrongylus, Teladorsagia,* and *Chabertia*) in the *in vitro* egg hatch test.[3083] Oral administration of the oils diluted in sunflower oil to animals showed that thyme CT para-cymene essential oil was the most effective, even more effective than thyme CT thymol.
- Researchers investigated the benefits of inhaling fennel essential oil in a high-fat diet-induced obesity model.[3084] Rats were divided into four groups: normal diet control, high-fat diet no intervention, high-fat diet

plus inhalation of 0.3% fennel oil, and high-fat diet plus inhalation of 1.0% fennel oil. Inhalation of fennel essential oil—0.3% or 1.0% fennel oil for thirty minutes daily over the course of twelve weeks—resulted in decreased body weight, body fat, and visceral fat in rats fed a high-fat diet. Improvement in lipid metabolism (improved cholesterol profiles and reduced insulin) and reduced systolic blood pressure and heart rate was also observed after inhaling fennel oil. Inhaling the higher concentration (1.0%) of fennel essential oil had the greatest impact on body weight. Interestingly, a decrease in LDL cholesterol and triglycerides and an increase in HDL cholesterol was observed in the 0.3% fennel oil group, but the 1.0% group experienced increases in triglycerides, HDL and LDL cholesterol. Insulin levels decreased in both fennel oil groups, while cortisol only decreased in the 1.0% fennel group. A marked increase in testosterone in male rats was noted in the 0.3% fennel group. Overall, this study suggests that inhaling fennel essential oil protects against metabolic dysfunction associated with obesity and could promote healthy body weight despite a high-fat diet. The study also reported that p-anisaldehyde, limonene, estragole, anethole, and trans-anethole are major contributors to the odor of fennel, with trans-anethole showing the highest odor intensity.

☐ Fennel essential oil produced a synergistic action against *E. faecalis* and *E. coli* when combined with amoxicillin.[3085]

☐ Fennel essential oil (*Foeniculum vulgare* subsp. *piperitum* fruits; CT estragole) showed antitumor effects against triple-negative breast cancer cells.[3086]

☐ A synergistic effect was observed when fennel essential oil was combined with amoxicillin or lavender against *E. faecalis* and *E. coli*.[3087] A blend of lavender and fennel in combination with amoxicillin also showed synergy.

☐ An odd fennel essential oil with para-anisaldehyde (86.6%) as the major constituent demonstrated good anti-inflammatory activity in the mouse ear edema model.[3088]

☐ An unusual fennel essential oil with alpha-pinene (33.8%) and estragole (25.1%) as the main constituents showed excellent antimicrobial activity (*E. coli, S. aureus, B. cereus*), antibiofilm activity, and antioxidant capacity in the BATS assay (increasing SOD, CAT, GPx, and decreasing ROS).[3089]

☐ Fennel essential oil (near equal fenchone and trans-anethole) displayed good antioxidant activity in the beta-carotene bleaching assay but not in the DPPH assay, and inhibited *K. pneumoniae, E. coli, C. albicans, L. monocytogenes, B. cereus, C. tropicalis, S. aureus,* and *P. aeruginosa*.[3090]

☐ Fennel essential oil was pediculicidal against the head louse (*Pediculus capitis*) under laboratory conditions at 15% and 20% concentrations.[3091]

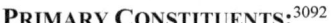

# FENUGREEK
## (Sicklefruit)

*Trigonella foenum-graecum* L.

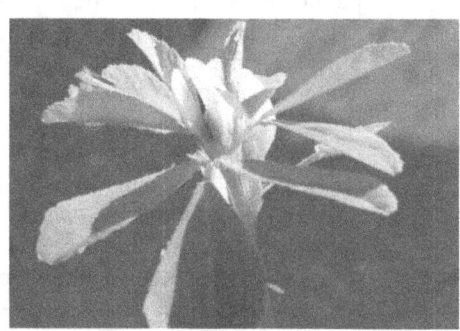

**FAMILY:** Fabaceae (Leguminosae)
**NOTE:** Middle
**AROMA INTENSITY:** Medium
**AROMA:** Green, slightly nutty, somewhat bitter
**COMMON EXTRACTION METHOD:** Steam distilled from seeds; may also be distilled from the aerial parts
**POSSIBLE SUBSTITUTE OILS:** Helichrysum, coriander, fennel
**BLENDS WELL WITH:** Balsam fir, cassia, cinnamon, copaiba, frankincense, lavender, myrrh, palo santo, patchouli, Peru balsam, sandalwood, tolu balsam
**SUBCELLULAR LOCALIZATION | EPIGENETIC INFLUENCE:** Currently unknown | Currently unknown
**RECOMMENDED DILUTION RANGE:** 3%–20%; neat for limited conditions

**PRIMARY CONSTITUENTS:**[3092]

| Constituent | Percent |
|---|---|
| Neryl Acetate | 17.3% |
| Camphor | 16.3% |
| Beta-Pinene | 15.1% |
| Beta-Caryophyllene | 14.6% |
| 2,5-Dimethylpyrazine | 6.1% |

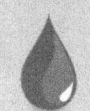

| Geranial | 4.8% |
| 6-Methyl-5-Hepten-2-One | 4.5% |

Note: Fenugreek is more commonly solvent extracted.

**OTHER CONSTITUENTS:** Alpha-pinene, gamma-terpinene, alpha-selinene, 3-octen-2-one, alpha-terpineol, alpha-campholenal

### PREFERRED COMPOSITION FOR CLINICAL USE:

| *Constituent* | |
|---|---|
| **Neryl Acetate** | 15%–25% |
| **Beta-Caryophyllene** | 5%–15% |
| **Beta-Pinene** | 5%–15% |
| **Camphor** | 5%–15% |
| **2,5-Dimethylpyrazine** | 2%–10% |
| **Geranial** | 1%–5% |
| **6-Methyl-5-Hepten-2-One** | 1%–5% |

**REPORTED THERAPEUTIC PROPERTIES:** Antimicrobial, antiviral, antioxidant, anticancer, **balances blood sugar**, antispasmodic, anti-inflammatory, aids immune function, supports respiratory function, expels excess mucus, aids cognitive function, balances blood pressure, supports immune function, encourages lactation, **reduces the appearance of acne and blemishes**, relieves boils and blisters, stomach protective, soothes irritated skin, supports kidney function, liver protective, aids circulation, **relieves painful menstruation**, stress management, aids concentration

### CAUTIONS:

■ May interact with diabetic medications and cause hypoglycemia.[3093]

■ Avoid with epilepsy and Parkinson's due to camphor content. May exacerbate or cause seizures/convulsions or reduce seizure medication efficacy based on 1,8-cineole content.[3094,3095,3096]

■ Fenugreek may negatively impact red blood cells and increase the risk of jaundice in children with Glucose-6-phosphate dehydrogenase deficiency (G6PD) due to camphor content.[3097,3098]

### SELECTED EVIDENCE:

☐ Animal research reports that when fenugreek essential oil terpenes and omega-3 fatty acids reduced alpha-amylase and maltase activities in blood and the pancreas when fed to diabetic rats, which resulted in a 51-percent reduction in blood sugar levels.[3099]

## FERULA
### (Wild Asafoetida)

*Ferula jaeschkeana* Vatke, *Peucedanum jaeschkeanum* (Vatke)
Baill., *F. jaeschkeana* var. *parkeriana* O. E. Schulz, *F. foetidissima*
Regel & Schmalh., *F. parkeriana* H. Wolff ex O. E. Schulz

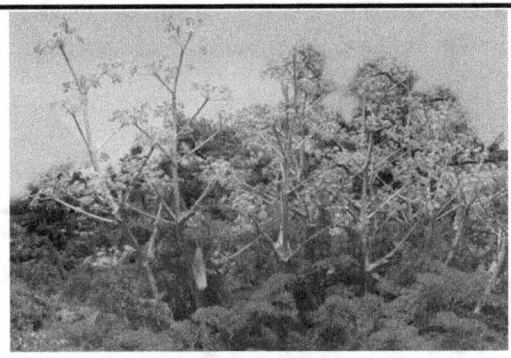

**FAMILY:** Apiaceae (Umbelliferae)
**NOTE:** Middle
**AROMA INTENSITY:** Medium
**AROMA:** Balsamic, earthy, woody
**COMMON EXTRACTION METHOD:** Hydrodistilled from the rhizomes
**POSSIBLE SUBSTITUTE OILS:** Palo santo, pine, frankincense, juniper berry

**BLENDS WELL WITH:** Basil, bay laurel, bergamot, black pepper, camphor, cassia, cinnamon, coriander, cypress, geranium, grapefruit, lavender, lemon, myrrh, neroli, orange, pine, petitgrain, palo santo, ravensara, ravintsara, rose, sandalwood, spikenard, tangerine, vetiver, ylang ylang

**SUBCELLULAR LOCALIZATION | EPIGENETIC INFLUENCE:** Currently unknown | Currently unknown

**RECOMMENDED DILUTION RANGE:** 3%–50%; neat for limited conditions

**PRIMARY CONSTITUENTS:**[3100,3101]

| *Limonene CT* | | *Alpha-Pinene CT* | |
|---|---|---|---|
| Limonene | 26.0% | Alpha-Pinene | 79.5% |
| Para-Cymene | 14.3% | Beta-Pinene | 12.7% |
| Alpha-Pinene | 8.3% | | |
| Terpinen-4-ol | 5.8% | | |
| Cubenol | 3.8% | | |
| Delta-Selinene | 3.5% | | |
| Terpinen-4-yl Acetate | 3.4% | | |
| Epi-Cubenol | 3.2% | | |
| Alpha-Gurjunene | 3.1% | | |

**OTHER CONSTITUENTS:** *Limonene CT*—Alpha-thujene, delta-3-carene, cis-ocimene, alpha-thujone (< 0.9%), alpha-terpineol, para-cymen-7-ol, alpha-terpinyl acetate, 2beta-hydroxy-1,4-cineole, p-menth-1beta,4alpha-diol, p-menth-1beta,2alpha-diol, p-menth-3-en-1,2,-diol, p-menth-4-en-1,2,-diol, p-menth-8-en-1,2,-diol, carvacrol, germacrene D, iso-longifolene; *Alpha-Pinene CT*—camphene

**PREFERRED COMPOSITION FOR CLINICAL USE:**

| Constituent | Limonene CT |
|---|---|
| **Limonene** | 20%–35% |
| **Para-Cymene** | 10%–20% |
| **Alpha-Pinene** | 5%–12% |
| **Terpinen-4-ol** | 3%–8% |

**REPORTED THERAPEUTIC PROPERTIES:** Antibacterial, antifungal, antiparasitic, antispasmodic, diuretic, **supports respiratory function**, expels excess mucus, relieves stomachache, nervine, antioxidant, analgesic, anti-inflammatory, stress management, relieves mental fatigue

**CAUTIONS:**

■ None currently known. The herb is often used as an herbal contraceptive, but research suggests that any anti-fertility activity is due to the presence of compounds only found in hexane and ethanol extracts, not the essential oil.

**SELECTED EVIDENCE:**

☐ None found.

---

*Did you know?*

Essential oil yield—the amount of essential oil that can be extracted from plant materials—is usually quite low. In fact, it takes more than 10,000 freshly picked rose blossoms to produce one 5 mL bottle of rose essential oil.

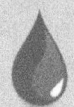

# FEVERFEW
## (Featherleaf Tansy)

*Tanacetum parthenium* (L.) Sch. Bip., *Chrysanthemum parthenium* (L.) Bernh., *Matricaria parthenium* L.

**FAMILY:** Asteraceae (Compositae)
**NOTE:** Top-Middle
**AROMA INTENSITY:** Medium-Strong
**AROMA:** Green, musty, camphoraceous, bitter
**COMMON EXTRACTION METHOD:** Steam distilled from the whole plant (aerial parts, stem, and leaves) or the leaves
**POSSIBLE SUBSTITUTE OILS:** Camphor (camphor CT), rosemary (camphor CT), Spanish sage, ravintsara (camphor CT), fingerroot (camphor CT), white verbena (camphor CT), hairy basil (camphor CT), sweet wormwood (camphor CT), mugwort (camphor CT), sage (camphor CT)
**BLENDS WELL WITH:** Blue tansy, blue spruce, camphor, copaiba, frankincense, lavender, myrrh, peppermint, spearmint, spruce (black), rose
**SUBCELLULAR LOCALIZATION | EPIGENETIC INFLUENCE:** Currently unknown | Currently unknown
**RECOMMENDED DILUTION RANGE:** 1.5%–20%; 50% for some conditions

**PRIMARY CONSTITUENTS:**[3102,3103,3104,3105,3106,3107,3108]

| | |
|---|---|
| Camphor | 42.7%–94.0% |
| (E)-Chrysanthenyl Acetate | 0.0%–25.1% |
| Camphene | 1.6%–12.2% |
| Germacrene D | 0.0%–9.2% |
| Bornyl Acetate | 0.0%–8.7% |
| Chrysanthenol | 0.0%–8.4% |
| (E)-Sesquilavandulol | 0.0%–4.8% |
| (E)-Myrtanol | 0.0%–4.7% |
| Para-Cymene | 0.0%–4.2% |
| 1,3-Cyclopentadiene, 5,5-dimethyl-1-ethyl- | 0.0%–4.2% |

Note: The camphor CT could be divided further into additional chemotypes primarily based on the presence of (E)-chrysanthenyl acetate, although other components vary greatly in these two different chemotypes as well. Feverfew may also be distilled from the inflorescence (valencene 34.3%–43.0, camphor 11.5%–11.6%, chrysanthenyl acetate 7.6%–8.9%, camphene 5.1%–5.5%), seeds (myrcene 36.0%–51.0%, camphor 10.4%–12.4%, camphene 4.2%–6.5%, chrysanthenyl acetate 4.3%–6.3%), or roots (camphor 30.2%, (Z)-chrysanthenyl acetate 26.5%, beta-farnesene 11.1%, spathulenol 8.2%).[4121,4127]

**OTHER CONSTITUENTS:** Alpha-pinene, alpha-thujene, limonene, alpha-terpinene, gamma-terpinene, terpinen-4-ol, (E)-beta-farnesene, borneol, beta-caryophyllene, alpha-phellandrene, para-cymen-8-ol, myrtenal, eugenol, (Z)-chrysanthenyl acetate, ortho-cymene, p-menth-1,5-dien-9-ol, 1,2,3-trimethyl benzene, filifolene, chrysanthenone, cis-carveol, decanoic acid, intermedol, hexadecanoic acid

**PREFERRED COMPOSITION FOR CLINICAL USE:**

| Constituent | |
|---|---|
| Camphor | 45%–65% |
| (E)-Chrysanthenyl Acetate | 10%–25% |
| Camphene | 5%–15% |
| Bornyl Acetate | 2%–10% |
| Limonene | 1%–5% |
| Para-Cymene | 1%–5% |
| (E)-Beta-Farnesene | 0.5%–5% |
| Gamma-Terpinene | 0.5%–4% |

**REPORTED THERAPEUTIC PROPERTIES:** Antibacterial, antifungal, **antimicrobial**, antiarthritic, antirheumatic, **analgesic**, anti-inflammatory, antispasmodic, **relieves headache/migraine**, balances menstruation, relieves chronic skin conditions, supports respiratory function, eases cough, expels excess mucus, reduces nausea/vomiting, insect repellent, stress management, relieves anxiety

## CAUTIONS:

■ Avoid with children under six due to significant camphor content. Several cases of camphor poisoning and/or seizures from ingestion and topical application have been reported in children.[3109,3110] Ingestion of camphor-containing products has been lethal in children under age two.[3111] Children five years and up may use camphor-containing essential oils topically in dilutions no stronger than 5%. Camphor ingestion by infants and young children may cause cough, vomiting, seizure, burning sensation in the mucous membranes and eyes, or lack of voluntary coordination of muscle movements.[3112]

■ Caution is warranted during pregnancy and while lactating due to significant camphor content. Ingestion of essential oils with significant levels of camphor may lead to abortion because fetuses lack the enzymes to process it.[3113] Camphor ingestion by infants and young children may cause cough, vomiting, seizure, burning sensation in the mucous membranes and eyes, or lack of voluntary coordination of muscle movements.[3114]

■ Avoid with epilepsy and Parkinson's due to significant camphor content.[3115,3116,3117]

■ Avoid with those who have a compromised liver due to the risk of increased liver enzymes and liver damage.[3118] This would also suggest that those taking medications that could cause liver damage should also use feverfew very cautiously or avoid it entirely.

■ The significant camphor content in feverfew may negatively impact red blood cells and increase the risk of jaundice in children with glucose-6-phosphate dehydrogenase deficiency (G6PD).[3119,3120]

■ Oral caution—Essential oils with significant levels of camphor can be toxic when taken orally, usually single doses exceeding 2 mL, although the lethal dose for humans is estimated to be more than 5 mL in a single dose.[3121,3122,3123]

■ Caution is warranted for the topical application of camphor-containing essential oils on broken or injured skin due to an increased risk of toxicity.[3124]

## SELECTED EVIDENCE:

☐ Feverfew essential oil kills cervical, lymphoblastic leukemia, and drug-resistant lymphobalstic leukemia cancer cells with a medium cytotoxic activity compared to the chemotherapy drug doxorubicin.[3125]

☐ *In vitro* research demonstrates that feverfew essential oil weakly to moderately inhibits sixteen pathogenic bacterial strains (*Streptococcus pneumoniae, Streptococcus pyogenes* (2), *Enterococcus faecalis, Acinetobacter* sp., *Pseudomonas aeruginosa* (3), *S. aureus* (2), *Klebsiella* sp. (2), *Proteus mirabilis,* and *Escherichia coli* (3).[3126] Research suggests that gram-positive bacteria or more sensitive to feverfew essential oil than gram-negative bacteria, with inhibition of *P. aeruginosa, Yersina enterocolitica, B. cereus, Micrococcus luteus, S. aureus,* and the fungi *C. albicans* notes.[3127] Another study reported that feverfew essential oil only mildly inhibited *S. aureus* and *B. subtilis.*[3128] The leaf, stem, and root essential oils (devoid of (E)-chrysanthenyl acetate) were active against *E. coli* and *Salmonella typhi,* but inactive against *S. aureus.*[3129] An essential oil with camphor and (E)-chrysanthenyl acetate demonstrated considerable antimicrobial effect on gram-positive bacteria (*Staphylococcus aureus* and *S. epidermidis*), gram-negative bacteria (*S. flexneri, Klebsiella pneumonia,* and *E. coli*), and fungi (*A. niger, C. albicans,* and *C. cruise*), suggesting the presence of (E)-chrysanthenyl acetate may improve antimicrobial activity.[3130]

☐ Feverfew essential oil mildly inhibits the 5-LOX enzyme indicating low anti-inflammatory activity.[3131]

☐ Feverfew essential oil is considered a weak antioxidant.[3132,3133]

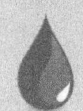

# FINGERROOT
## (Finger Root, Thai Ginger, Chinese Keys)

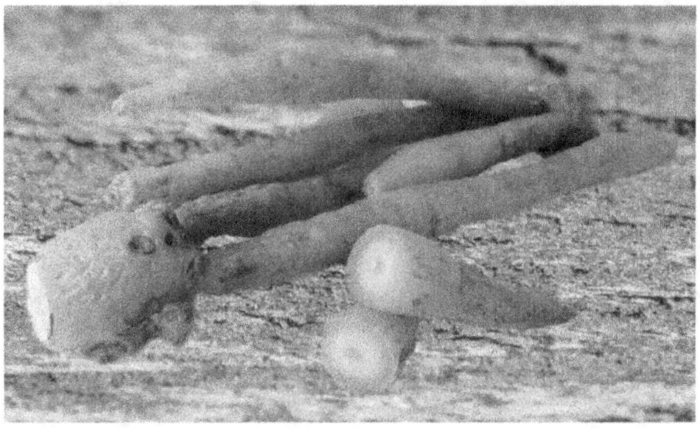

*Boesenbergia pandurata* (Roxb.) Schlecht, *B. rotunda,*
*Kaempferia pandurata, Gastrochilus panduratus* (Roxb.)
Ridl., *Curcuma rotunda* L.

**FAMILY:** Zingiberaceae
**NOTE:** Middle-Base
**AROMA INTENSITY:** Medium
**AROMA:** Earthy, herbaceous, warm, slightly camphoraceous
**COMMON EXTRACTION METHOD:** Steam distilled or hydrodistilled from the rhizomes
**POSSIBLE SUBSTITUTE OILS:** Ginger, turmeric
**BLENDS WELL WITH:** Bay laurel, bergamot, camphor, cardamom, carrot seed, cassia, cedarwood, cinnamon, clove, eucalyptus, fennel, frankincense, geranium, nutmeg, oregano, patchouli, peppermint, sandalwood, spearmint, turmeric, vetiver
**SUBCELLULAR LOCALIZATION | EPIGENETIC INFLUENCE:** Currently unknown | Currently unknown
**RECOMMENDED DILUTION RANGE:** 3%–20%, neat for limited conditions; Camphor and Nerol-Camphor CTs—1.5%–20%; 50% for some conditions

**PRIMARY CONSTITUENTS:**[3134,3135,3136,3137,3138]

*(E)-Beta-Ocimene CT*

| | |
|---|---|
| (E)-Beta-Ocimene | 19.0%–27.0% |
| Geraniol | 11.0%–26.0% |
| Camphor | 16.1%–24.0% |
| 1,8-Cineole | 7.5%–17.0% |
| Camphene | 5.4%–8.0% |

*Camphor CT*

| | |
|---|---|
| Camphor | 32.1%–58.0% |
| Geraniol | 6.2%–16.2% |
| 1,8-Cineole | 2.6%–13.9% |
| Camphene | 0.0%–5.8% |
| Methyl Cinnamate | 0.0%–5.8% |

*Gamma-Terpinene CT*

| | |
|---|---|
| Gamma-Terpinene | 44.0% |
| Geraniol | 20.6% |
| 6-Camphenenone | 18.7% |
| 1,8-Cineole | 12.8% |

*B. rotunda (Nerol-Camphor CT)*

| | |
|---|---|
| Nerol | 39.6% |
| Camphor | 36.0% |
| 1,8-Cineole | 9.5% |
| Methyl Cinnamate | 6.9% |

*B. rotunda (1,8-cineole CT)*

| | |
|---|---|
| 1,8-Cineole | 41.0% |
| Camphor | 13.0% |
| Borneol | 9.2% |
| Alpha-Pinene | 4.1% |

**OTHER CONSTITUENTS:** *(E)-Beta-Ocimene CT*—alpha-pinene, beta-pinene, 3-carene, alpha-terpinolene, isoborneol, borneol, alpha-terpineol, neral, geranial, methyl cinnamate; *Camphor CT*—alpha-pinene, 3-carene, alpha-terpinolene, linalool, borneol, alpha-terpineol, neral, geranial, geranyl formate, neryl acetate, gamma-elemene, delta-elemene; *Gamma-Terpinene CT*—methyl cinnamate, limonene, linalool; *B. rotunda (Nerol-Camphor CT)*—fenchene, cis-p-mentha-2,8-dien-1-ol, cyclohexene; *B. rotunda (1,8-cineole CT)*—alpha-zingiberene, curcumin, zedoarine

**REPORTED THERAPEUTIC PROPERTIES:** Antibacterial, antifungal, **analgesic**, anti-inflammatory, antispasmodic, antiarthritic, antirheumatic, anticancer, antioxidant, antiseptic, **aids digestion**, increases appetite, relieves constipation, expels excess gas, relieves nausea/vomiting, supports respiratory function, eases cough, antiallergic, expels excess mucus, supports liver function, aids detoxification, promotes restful sleep, insecticide, insect repellent, uplifting, stress management, aphrodisiac

## PREFERRED COMPOSITION FOR CLINICAL USE:

| Constituent | 1,8-Cineole CT | Nerol/Camphor CT | (E)-Beta-Ocimene CT |
|---|---|---|---|
| **1,8-Cineole** | 25%–45% | 5%–15% | 10%–20% |
| **Camphor** | 10%–20% | 25%–40% | 15%–25% |
| **Borneol** | 7%–15% | – | – |
| **Alpha-Pinene** | 2%–8% | – | 0.5%–5% |
| **Nerol** | – | 25%–40% | – |
| **(E)-Methyl Cinnamate** | 0%–5% | 2%–10% | 0.5%–5% |
| **(E)-Beta-Ocimene** | – | – | 15%–30% |
| **Geraniol** | – | – | 10%–25% |
| **Camphene** | – | – | 4%–10% |

## CAUTIONS:

■ *(E)-Beta-Ocimene and Camphor CTs; B. rotunda*: Use very cautiously with children under six due to camphor and 1,8-cineole content. Several cases of camphor poisoning and/or seizures from ingestion and topical application have been reported in children.[3139,3140] Ingestion of camphor-containing products has been lethal in children under age two.[3141] 1,8-cineole may cause seizures, central nervous system problems, or respiratory distress in young children.[3142,3143,3144,3145] Children five years and up may use camphor-containing essential oils topically in dilutions no stronger than 5%. Camphor ingestion by infants and young children may cause cough, vomiting, seizure, burning sensation in the mucous membranes and eyes, or lack of voluntary coordination of muscle movements.[3146]

■ *(E)-Beta-Ocimene and Camphor CTs; B. rotunda*: Caution is warranted during pregnancy and while lactating due to potentially high camphor content. Ingestion of essential oils with significant levels of camphor may lead to abortion because fetuses lack the enzymes to process it.[3147]

■ *All CTs*: Avoid with epilepsy and Parkinson's due to potentially high camphor and 1,8-cineole content, which may exacerbate or trigger seizures/convulsions or reduce medication efficacy.[3148]

■ Avoid with those who have a compromised liver due to the risk of increased liver enzymes and liver damage.[3149] This would also suggest that those taking medications that could cause liver damage should also use fingerroot very cautiously or avoid it entirely.

■ *(E)-Beta-Ocimene and Camphor CTs; B. rotunda*: The potentially high camphor content in fingerroot may negatively impact red blood cells and increase the risk of jaundice in children with glucose-6-phosphate dehydrogenase deficiency (G6PD).[3150,3151]

■ *(E)-Beta-Ocimene and Camphor CTs; B. rotunda*: Oral caution—Essential oils with significant levels of camphor and 1,8-cineole can be toxic when taken orally. As few as 4 to 5 drops of high 1,8-cineole oils may be problematic in very sensitive individuals. Oral—Camphor can be toxic when taken orally (usually single doses exceeding 2 mL), although the lethal dose for adult humans is estimated to be (more than 5 mL) in a single dose.[3152,3153,3154]

■ *1,8-Cineole CT*: May interfere with pentobarbital and other barbiturates (medications for anxiety and insomnia) based on 1,8-cineole content.[3155,3156]

■ *(E)-Beta-Ocimene CT*: May weakly to moderately interfere with enzymes responsible for metabolizing medications (NSAIDs, proton-pump inhibitors, acetaminophen, antiepileptics, immune modulators, blood-sugar medications, blood pressure medications, antidepressants, antipsychotics, diabetic medications, antihistamines, antibiotics, and anesthetics) due to geraniol and 1,8-cineole content.[3157,3158,3159,3160]

■ *(E)-Beta-Ocimene CT*: May interact with diabetes medications and cause low blood sugar based on moderate geraniol content.[3161,3162]

■ *(E)-Beta-Ocimene CT*: May interact with antibiotics and/or antifungals and possibly increase their effectiveness based on moderate geraniol content.[3163]

■ *CTs with Geraniol*: May interact with diabetes medications and cause low blood sugar based on geraniol content (low risk).[3164,3165,3166]

■ *CTs with Geraniol*: Dilution recommended for topical application. Geraniol is metabolized and autoxidized into metabolites like geranial and neral, and may cause sensitization and irritation when applied topically.[3167]

■ *Camphor CT*: Caution is warranted for the topical application of camphor-containing essential oils on broken or injured skin due to an increased risk of toxicity.[3168]

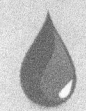

**SELECTED EVIDENCE:**

☐ *In vitro* research demonstrates that fingerroot essential oil moderately inhibits foodborne pathogens (*E. coli, S. enteritidis, S. typhimurium, B. cereus, S. aureus, S. flexneri, S. Typhi,* and *L. monocytogenes*).[3169,3170] *B. rotunda* essential oil inhibited gram-positive (*Staphylococcus aureus* and *Bacillus cereus*) and gram-negative bacteria (*Pseudomonas aeruginosa* and *Escherichia coli*) *in vitro*.[3171] Another study reported that *B. rotunda* actively inhibits *E. coli, Clostridium perfringens, Salmonella typhimurium, S. aureus,* and *B. cereus*.[3172] *In vitro* research demonstrates that fingerroot essential oil inhibits *A. flavus* and *A. parasiticus* and their production of aflatoxin B1.[3173]

☐ Fingerroot essential oil provided equivalent protection against mosquito (*Culex quinquefasciatus* (Say)) bites when compared to DEET—4.3 hours.[3174] It also kills the larvae of *Aedes aegypti* (Linn.) and *Culex quinquefasciatus* (Say) mosquitoes.[3175]

# FORMOSAN CYPRESS
## (Taiwan Red Cypress, Hong Kuai, Meniki, Benihi)

*Chamaecyparis formosensis* Matsum, *Cupressus formosensis* (Matsum.) A. Henry

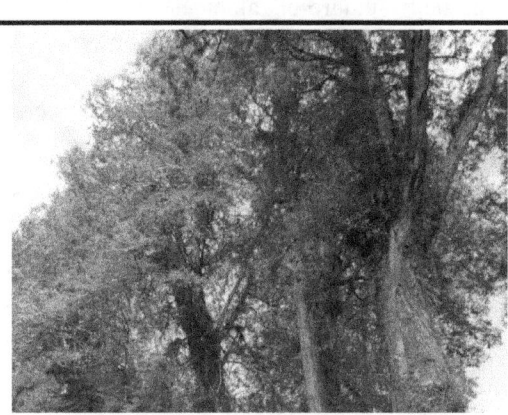

**FAMILY:** Cupressaceae
**NOTE:** Top-Middle
**AROMA INTENSITY:** Medium
**AROMA:** Woody, balsamic, fresh, sweet, slightly citrusy
**COMMON EXTRACTION METHOD:** Steam distilled from the heartwood; may also be distilled from the needles (leaves) or twigs
**POSSIBLE SUBSTITUTE OILS:** Hinoki, blue cypress, sandalwood, cedarwood (atlas), frankincense, juniper berry, agarwood
**BLENDS WELL WITH:** Balsam fir, bergamot, blue cypress, cedarwood, cypress, Douglas fir, grapefruit, Japanese cedarwood, juniper, lavender, lemon, lime, myrrh, orange, pine, rose, sandalwood, spruce (black), tangerine, tsuga, white fir
**SUBCELLULAR LOCALIZATION | EPIGENETIC INFLUENCE:** Currently unknown | Currently unknown
**RECOMMENDED DILUTION RANGE:** 3%–Neat

**PRIMARY CONSTITUENTS:** [3176,3177,3178,3179,3180,3181,3182,3183,3184]

| *Wood (Myrtenol CT)* | | *Wood (Alpha-Eudesmol CT)* | |
|---|---|---|---|
| Myrtenol | 20.3%–48.9% | Alpha-Eudesmol | 18.1% |
| (E)-Myrtanol | 13.1%–19.2% | Beta-Guaiene | 8.0% |
| Alpha-Pinene | 1.3%–15.1% | Beta-Cadinene | 7.9% |
| Delta-Cadinene | 0.6%–11.9% | Gamma-Costal | 7.0% |
| Gamma-Cadinene | 0.0%–11.4% | Alpha-Muurolol | 6.5% |
| Alpha-Amorphene | 0.0%–6.3% | 4a-Hydroxy-4b- | |
| Alpha-Muurolene | 1.3%–5.3% | Methyldihydrocostol | 5.5% |
| Beta-Selinene | 0.0%–4.1% | Alpha-Selinene | 4.8% |
| Alpha-Cadinol | 0.4%–4.1% | Santolina Triene | 4.6% |
| Beta-Elemene | 1.1%–3.6% | Eremophilene | 4.3% |
| | | Cis-Myrtanol | 4.1% |
| *Needles (Leaves)—Germacrene D CT* | | Alpha-Humulene | 4.1% |
| Germacrene D | 35.1%–41.2% | | |
| Alpha-Pinene | 8.1%–13.3% | *Twig* | |
| Delta-Cadinene | 6.3%–10.3% | Beta-Eudesmol | 25.1% |
| Gamma-Muurolene | 5.8%–9.1% | T-Muurolol | 21.6% |

| | | | |
|---|---|---|---|
| Alpha-Humulene | 4.4%–8.7% | Elemol | 15.0% |
| Gamma-Cadinene | 2.3%–5.3% | Totarol | 14.9% |
| | | Alpha-Cadinol | 12.4% |

*Needles (Leaves)—Alpha-Pinene CT*

| | |
|---|---|
| Alpha-Pinene | 89.3%–96.9% |
| Beta-Myrcene | 0.8%–4.7% |
| Beta-Pinene | 1.9%–3.4% |

**OTHER CONSTITUENTS:** *Wood (Myrtenol CT)*—nopinone, beta-elemene, siberene, trans-cadina-1,(6),4-diene, gamma-muurolene, alpha-selinene, alpha-cadinene, alpha-calacorene, elemol, 1-epi-cubenol, valerenol, alpha-copaene, T-muurolol, alpha-cubebene; *Wood (Alpha-Eudesmol CT)*—myrtenal, beta-elemene, isoledene, alpha-gurjunene, T-muurolene, alpha-cubebene, calarene, chamaecynone, 7-(5-hexynyl)-tricyclo(4,2,2,0(2,5))dec-7-ene, epi-cubenol, 2alpha-hydroxycostol, 12-hydroxy-isointermedeol; *Needles (Leaves) Germacrene D CT*—beta-myrcene, delta-3-carene, alpha-cubebene, beta-caryophyllene, gamma-amorphene, alpha-muurolene, alpha-cadinene, ent-16-kaurene; *Needles (Leaves)—Alpha-Pinene CT*—limonene, beta-phellandrene; *Twigs*—not listed

**PREFERRED COMPOSITION FOR CLINICAL USE:**

| Constituent | Wood (Myrtenol CT) |
|---|---|
| **Myrtenol** | 15%–45% |
| **(E)-Myrtanol** | 10%–20% |
| **Delta-Cadinene** | 5%–15% |
| **Alpha-Pinene** | 4%–15% |
| **Gamma-Cadinene** | 3%–12% |
| **Selinene <alpha + beta>** | 2%–8% |
| **Alpha-Cadinol** | 0.1%–6% |
| **Beta-Elemene** | 1%–5% |
| **Alpha-Muurolene** | 1%–5% |

**REPORTED THERAPEUTIC PROPERTIES:** Antibacterial, antifungal, analgesic, anti-inflammatory, antioxidant, antiallergic, supports respiratory function, wound healing, eases cough, aids cardiovascular function, supports immune function, nourishes the skin, insect repellent, insecticide, **stress management**, relieves anxiety, calming/relaxing, encourages confidence, **uplifting to mood**, promotes inspiration

**CAUTIONS:**

■ *Twig oil:* Avoid during pregnancy and lactation due to beta-eudesmol content. Beta-eudesmol strongly inhibits the growth of new blood vessels, which is necessary for implantation, and placental and embryonic development.[3185]

■ *Twig oil:* May interact with aspirin, blood pressure, antiplatelet, and anticoagulant medications, and increase the risk of bleeding among people with bleeding disorders due to beta-eudesmol content (low risk).[3186,3187]

■ *Myrtenol CT (Wood):* May interact with barbiturates and other sedative drugs and increase sleeping time based on myrtenol content.[3188]

**SELECTED EVIDENCE:**

☐ *In vitro* research reported that Formosan cypress moderately kills two liver-cancer cells, adenocarcinoma (lung alveolar) cells, and breast cancer cells (including an invasice—metastatic—breast cancer cell line).[3189]

☐ Inhalation of Formosan cypress essential oil decreased systolic blood pressure, heart rate, and sympathetic nervous system activity; whereas diastolic blood pressure and parasympathetic nervous system activity increased.[3190] This activity stimulated a more pleasant mood.

☐ Formosan cypress essential oil approached 100% termite mortality at a dose of 1.25mg/g after seven days. The study authors determined that of the main components in Formosan cypress, T-cadinol and T-muurolol displayed the most powerful antitermitic activities.[3191]

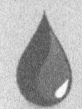

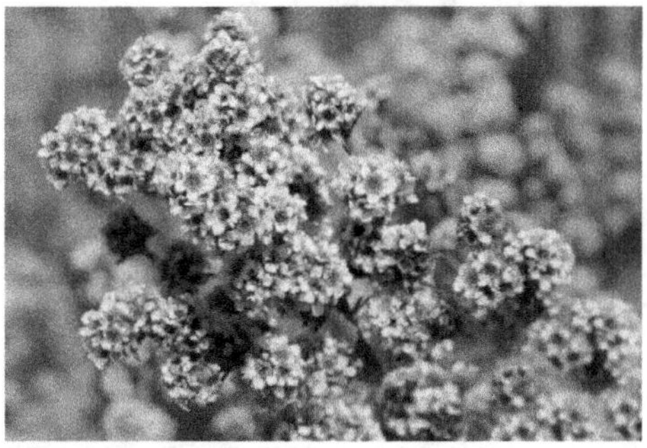

# FRAGONIA
## (Coarse Tea Tree, Agonis)
*Agonis fragrans* J.R. Wheeler & N.G. Marchant

**FAMILY:** Myrtaceae
**NOTE:** Middle
**AROMA INTENSITY:** Medium
**AROMA:** Camphoraceous, medicinal, slightly sweet, floral, and fruity
**COMMON EXTRACTION METHOD:** Steam distilled from the leaves and branches/stems
**POSSIBLE SUBSTITUTE OILS:** Tea tree, rosalina, lavender, myrtle
**BLENDS WELL WITH:** Bergamot, cajeput, copaiba, geranium, grapefruit, frankincense, lavender, lemon, lemon myrtle, myrrh, orange, palmarosa, rhododendron, rosalina, rose, tangerine, tea tree
**SUBCELLULAR LOCALIZATION | EPIGENETIC INFLUENCE:** Currently unknown | Currently unknown
**RECOMMENDED DILUTION RANGE:** 3%–Neat

**PRIMARY CONSTITUENTS:**[3192,3193]

*Balanced CT*

| | |
|---|---|
| 1,8-Cineole | 12.4%–34.2% |
| Alpha-Pinene | 11.6%–28.0% |
| Linalool | 1.7%–14.7% |
| Beta-Pinene | 0.9%–8.3% |
| Beta-Caryophyllene | 0.2%–6.8% |
| Bicyclogermacrene | 0.5%–6.7% |
| Cryptomeridiol | 0.0%–6.6% |
| Alpha-Terpineol | 3.0%–6.3% |
| Myrtenol | 1.7%–5.5% |
| Beta-Eudesmol | 0.0%–5.5% |
| Alpha-Eudesmol | 0.0%–5.1% |

*Alpha-Pinene CT*

| | |
|---|---|
| Alpha-Pinene | 21.5%–38.5% |
| Linalool | 18.3%–25.3% |
| Myrtenol | 12.1%–20.0% |
| Bicyclogermacrene | 2.9%–4.5% |

Note: Interestingly, a well-balanced (oxides: 1,8-cineole; monoterpenes: alpha-pinene, beta-pinene, etc.; and monoterpenols: linalool, alpha-terpineol, myrtenol, etc.; in close to a 1:1:1 ratio) essential oil grown on a plantation in Australia is trademarked (Fragonia™) by The Paperback Co. Pty. Ltd.[4716]

**OTHER CONSTITUENTS:** *Balanced CT*—Alpha-thujene, sabinene, myrcene, alpha-terpinene, para-cymene, limonene, gamma-terpinene, terpinolene, delta-terpineol, terpinen-5-ol, nerol, geraniol, alpha-humulene, cis-calamenen, globulol, caryophyllene oxide, elemol, hedycaryol, gamma-eudesmol, epi-cryptomeridiol, neophytadiene; *Alpha-Pinene* CT—Limonene, 1,8-cineole, delta-terpineol, terpinen-4-ol, alpha-terpineol, nerol, geranol, beta-caryophyllene, delta-cadinene, cis-calamenene, globulol, viridiflorol, humulene oxide, guaia-5-en-11-ol, beta-eudesmol, alpha-eudesmol, cryptomeridiol, trans-myrtanol, (E)-beta-ocimene

**PREFERRED COMPOSITION FOR CLINICAL USE:**

| Constituent | Balanced |
|---|---|
| **1,8-Cineole** | 25%–35% |
| **Alpha-Pinene** | 20%–30% |
| **Linalool** | 7%–12% |
| **Alpha-Terpineol** | 4%–8% |
| **Myrtenol** | 2%–7% |
| **Terpinen-4-ol** | 2%–5% |
| **Para-Cymene** | 1%–4% |
| **Limonene** | 1%–4% |

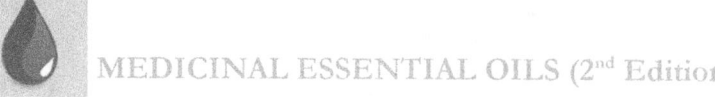

| | |
|---|---|
| **Gamma-Terpinene** | 1%–3% |
| **Beta-Pinene** | 1%–3% |
| **Myrcene** | 1%–3% |
| **Geraniol** | 0.5%–2% |
| **Citronellol** | 0.5%–2% |
| **Beta-Caryophyllene** | 0.1%–1% |
| **Alpha-Humulene** | 0.1%–1% |
| **Bicyclogermacrene** | 0.1%–1% |

**REPORTED THERAPEUTIC PROPERTIES: Antibacterial**, antifungal, anti-infectious, antiviral, antimicrobial, analgesic, **anti-inflammatory**, antispasmodic, antioxidant, aids/modulates immune function, supports respiratory function, expels excess mucus, balances hormones, reduces jet lag, **antiallergic**, encourages restful sleep, encourages self-esteem, relieves past emotional trauma, deeply relaxing, relieves anxiety

**CAUTIONS:**

*Alpha-Pinene CT*

■ None currently known.

*1,8-Cineole CT*

■ Avoid with epilepsy and Parkinson's due to 1,8-cineole content, which may exacerbate or trigger seizures/convulsions or reduce medication efficacy.[3194,3195,3196]

■ May interfere with pentobarbital and other barbiturates (medications for anxiety and insomnia) based on 1,8-cineole content.[3197,3198,3199]

■ May weakly interfere with the enzymes responsible for metabolizing medications (NSAIDs, proton-pump inhibitors, acetaminophen, antiepleptics, immune modulators, blood-sugar medications, blood pressure medications, antidepressants, antipsychotics, diabetic medications, antihistamines, antibiotics, and anesthetics) due to 1,8-cineole content.[3200,3201,3202]

**SELECTED EVIDENCE:**

☐ *In vitro* research shows that Fragonia essential oil (balanced CT) possesses broad-spectrum antimicrobial activity against several bacteria (*S. aureus, E. coli, Acinetobacter* spp., *Klebsiella* spp., *S. marcescens, S. epidermidis,* and *P. aeruginosa*).[3203] *P. aeruginosa* was the least susceptible organism.

☐ Fragonia essential oil (balanced CT) inhibits several aspects immune activity involved in inflammation, autoimmune disease, and atopic dermatitis (eczema), including cytokine IFNγ production by mononuclear cells (MC), Mitogen-induced Th2 cytokine IL-13, and T cell regulatory cytokine IL-10 responses.[3204]

---

# FRANKINCENSE

*Boswellia carterii* Birdw. *(B. carteri)*; *B. sacra* Flueckiger, *B. bhaw-dajiana* Birdw.; *B. frereana* Birdw.; *B. papyrifera* (Delile ex Caill.) Hochst.; *B. serrata* Roxb. ex Colebr., *B. Thurifera* Roxb, ex Flem

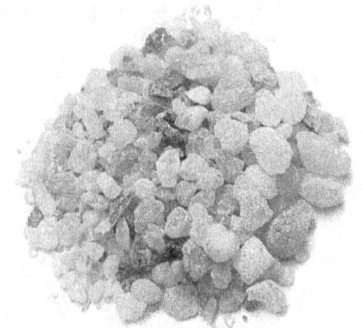

**FAMILY:** Burseraceae
**NOTE:** Base
**AROMA INTENSITY:** Medium
**AROMA:** Balsamic, rich, warm, slightly spicy, sweet, woody
**COMMON EXTRACTION METHOD:** Steam distilled from the resin
**POSSIBLE SUBSTITUTE OILS:** Palo santo, niaouli (viridiflorol/para-cymene/1,8-cineole CT), equal parts petitgrain (mandarin) and cedarwood, equal parts cistus and white fir

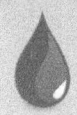

**BLENDS WELL WITH:** Basil, bay laurel, bergamot, black pepper, camphor, cassia, cinnamon, coriander, cypress, geranium, grapefruit, lavender, lemon, myrrh, neroli, orange, pine, petitgrain, palo santo, ravensara, ravintsara, rose, sandalwood, spikenard, tangerine, vetiver, ylang ylang

**SUBCELLULAR LOCALIZATION | EPIGENETIC INFLUENCE:** Lysosomes | Digestive/Excretory

**RECOMMENDED DILUTION RANGE:** 3%–50%; neat for limited conditions

**PRIMARY CONSTITUENTS:**[3205,3206,3207,3208,3209,3210,3211,3212,3213,3214,3215,3216,3217,3218]

*Boswellia carterii*

| | |
|---|---|
| Alpha-Pinene | 2.0%–64.0% |
| Alpha-Thujene | 1.0%–52.4% |
| Octyl Acetate | 0.0%–39.3% |
| Limonene | 1.0%–20.4% |
| Para-Cymene | 3.0%–17.0% |
| 1-Octanol | 0.0%–11.9% |
| Myrcene | 0.5%–8.2% |
| Alpha-Cedrene | 0.0%–6.1% |
| Alpha-Copaene | 0.0%–5.5% |
| Sabinene | 0.0%–4.9% |
| Delta-Cadinene | 0.0%–2.6% |
| Incensole Acetate | 0.0%–2.3% |
| Camphene | 0.0%–2.1% |
| Beta-Pinene | 0.0%–2.1% |

*Boswellia serrata*

| | |
|---|---|
| Alpha-Thujene | 22.5%–69.8% |
| Eudesmol | 0.2%–11.5% |
| Alpha-Pinene | 0.0%–11.2% |
| Tetra-Dihydrolinalool | 0.0%–10.6% |
| Epi-Cubenol | 0.0%–9.1% |
| Delta-3-Carene | 0.5%–9.6% |
| Myrcene | 0.0%–8.9% |
| Limonene | 0.7%–8.5% |
| Alpha-Terpineol | 1.0%–7.8% |
| Sabinene | 0.4%–5.9% |
| Benzyl Tigliate | 0.0%–5.5% |
| 10-Epi-γ-Eudesmol | 0.0%–5.3% |
| Terpinyl Isobutyrate | 0.0%–5.1% |
| Para-Cymene | 1.6%–3.5% |
| Methyl Isoeugenol | 0.0%–3.1% |

*Boswellia sacra*

| | |
|---|---|
| Alpha-Pinene | 5.3%–78.5% |
| Limonene | 5.6%–33.5% |
| (E)-Beta-Ocimene | 0.0%–32.3% |
| Myrcene | 1.0%–8.9% |
| Alpha-Thujene | 0.9%–6.6% |
| Sabinene | 1.1%–5.2% |
| Para-Cymene | 1.6%–2.7% |
| Beta-Elemene | 0.9%–2.6% |

*Boswellia papyrifera*

| | |
|---|---|
| Octyl Acetate | 57.1%–65.7% |
| N-Octanol | 3.4%–8.8% |
| Limonene | 1.4%–3.8% |

*Boswellia frereana*

| | |
|---|---|
| Alpha-Pinene | 2.0%–64.7% |
| Alpha-Thujene | 0.0%–33.1% |
| Para-Cymene | 5.4%–16.9% |
| Trans-Verbenol | 0.0%–4.2% |
| Bornyl Acetate | 0.0%–2.8% |
| Beta-Elemene | 0.0%–2.7% |
| Sabinene | 0.0%–2.6% |
| Limonene | 0.0%–2.4% |

| Frankincense Species Origins | |
|---|---|
| *B. carterii* | Somalia, Ethiopia |
| *B. frereana* | Somalia (primarily), Oman |
| *B. papyrifera* | Eritrea, Ethiopia, Sudan |
| *B. sacra* | Oman, Yemen |
| *B. serrata* | India |

**OTHER CONSTITUENTS:** *B. carterii*—Alpha-phellandrene, hexyl acetate, Z-beta-ocimene, E-beta-ocimene 1,8-cineole, linalool, α-pinene epoxide, trans-verbenol, terpinen-4-ol, bornyl acetate, geranyl acetate, cembrene A, cembrene, incensole; *B. frereana*—Camphene, beta-pinene, alpha-phellandrene, m-cymene, 1,8-cineole, gamma-terpinene, trans-sabinene-hydrate, trans-linalool oxide, cis-linalool oxide, linalool, viridiflorol, verbenone, thujanol, carvone, delta-3-carene, alpha-pinocarveol, octyl acetate, alpha-copaene, terpinen-4-ol, myrtenal; *B. sacra*—Beta-pinene, alpha-phellandrene, camphene, beta-myrcene, beta-caryophyllene, terpinen-4-ol, 2-carene, gamma-terpinene, terpinolene, verbenone, linalool, bornyl acetate, delta-3-carene, delta-cadinene, alpha-caryophyllene, campholene aldehyde, octyl acetate, thujol, calamenene, beta-selinene, alpha-selinene, alpha-humulene, 1,8-cineole; *B. papyrifera*—alpha-pinene, linalool, geraniol; *B. serrata*—trycyclene, dehydrosabinene, beta-pinene, p-1,3,8-menthatriene, ment-2-en-1-ol, trans-sabinol, p-mentha-1,5-diene-8-ol, terpinen-4-ol, trans-anethole, beta-bourbonene, trans-methyl eugenol, (E)-nerolidol, alpha-terpinene, beta-phellandrene, terpinolene, citronellol, cadinene, undecenol

## PREFERRED COMPOSITION FOR CLINICAL USE:

| Constituent | Carterii Balanced | Carterii α-pinene | Frereana | Sacra | Serrata | Papyrifera |
|---|---|---|---|---|---|---|
| Alpha-Pinene | 30%–55% | 50%–75% | 2%–22% | 60%–82% | 0.5%–10% | 0.5%–5% |
| Limonene | 6%–22% | 2%–8% | 0.5%–5% | 1%–10% | 2%–8% | 1%–5% |
| Alpha-Thujene | 5%–20% | 0%–2% | 25%–55% | <5% | 50%–75% | – |
| Sabinene | 3%–10% | 2%–8% | 3%–10% | 1%–5% | 1%–10% | – |
| Myrcene | 2%–10% | 2%–6% | <1% | 0%–5% | 0%–5% | 0.1%–5% |
| Para-Cymene | 2%–6% | 0.5%–3% | 10%–22% | 0%–5% | 1%–10% | – |
| Delta-3-Carene | 0.5%–5% | 0.1%–2% | – | 0.1%–5% | 2%–10% | – |
| Incensoles | 0%–5% | <0.5% | – | – | – | >0.1% |
| Beta-Pinene | 0.5%–4% | 3%–8% | <1% | 1%–5% | 0.5%–5% | <1% |
| Beta-Elemene | 0.1%–3% | <0.5% | – | <1% | – | – |
| Alpha-Terpineol | 0%–2% | <1% | <2% | <1% | 0%–2% | – |
| Octyl Acetate | 0%–3% | 0.5%–3% | – | – | – | 45%–70% |
| N-Octanol | <0.5% | <0.5% | – | – | – | 3%–15% |
| Terpinen-4-ol | tr–2% | <0.5% | 0.5%–6% | <0.5% | <0.6% | <0.5% |
| α-Phellandrene Dimers | – | – | 0%–3% | – | – | – |

Note: Different species of frankincense trees grow together. Resin from more than one species may be mixed together during harvesting or when separated into grades, which means that commercial frankincense essential oil may be a mixture of two or more species and produce a composition profile comprising characteristics of more than one species.

**REPORTED THERAPEUTIC PROPERTIES: Analgesic (pain relief), anticancer**, antitumoral, supports reproductive health, **anti-inflammatory, anti-aging**, antioxidant, antiseptic, astringent, expels excess gas, **antirheumatic**, aids digestion, encourages cellular rejuvenation and a healthy cell cycle, diuretic, expectorant, immune modulating, **soothes cough**, promotes oral cleanliness, antiarthritic, **aids normal respiration, reduces the appearance of scars and blemishes**, wound healing, supports eye health, sedating, **antidepressant**, reduces anxiety, stress management, encourages emotional healing, **supports meditation and focus**, reduces loneliness, grief, and fear, focuses attention

## CAUTIONS:

■ May interfere with the enzymes responsible for metabolizing medications (NSAIDs, proton-pump inhibitors, acetaminophen, antiepileptics, immune modulators, blood-sugar medications, blood pressure medications, antidepressants, antipsychotics, diabetic medications, antihistamines, antibiotics, and anesthetics).[3219]

## SELECTED EVIDENCE:

☐ *In vitro* research suggests that *B. carterii* kills bladder (selectively, via oxidative stress) cancer cells.[3220,3221]

☐ *In vitro* and animal research suggests that *B. sacra* causes pancreas cancer cell death.[3222]

☐ *B. sacra* effectively killed three breast cancer cell lines while normal breast cells were more resistant to cellular death caused by frankincense oil *in vitro*.[3223]

☐ Animal research suggests that oral administration of *B. sacra* essential oil relieves pain.[3224]

☐ A hand massage with equal parts of frankincense, bergamot, and lavender (as a 1.5 percent dilution in sweet almond carrier oil) reduced the pain and depression of hospice patients with terminal cancer.[3225]

☐ Inhalation from personal aromasticks containing either bergamot and sandalwood, or frankincense, tangerine, and lavender improved sleep quality among cancer patients.[3226] Remarkably, 92% of study participants indicated they would continue to use their aromasticks for sleep improvement.

☐ *B. frereana* prevents the production of proinflammatory molecules that may cause cartilage damage, making it a promising natural remedy for inflammation associated with arthritis.[3227]

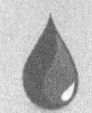

- *B. sacra* inhibits several gram-positive and gram-negative bacteria including *B. subtilis, M. luteus, S. aureus, P. aeruginosa, K. pneumoniae, E. aerogenes*, and *E. coli*.[3228] *B. serrata* exhibited good antimicrobial activity against *K. pneumoniae, Salmonella typhi, S. aureus, P. aeruginosa, C. albicans*, and *C. kefyr*.[3229] Interestingly, the antimicrobial activity greatly varied depending on the specific composition of the five samples tested.

- Animal research suggests that frankincense oil can reduce the appearance of wrinkles and aging of the skin.[3230]

- *In vitro* research suggests that *B. carterii* is an immune modulator and stimulates the transformation (activation of small, resting lymphocytes into large and functional lymphocytes) of lymphocytes.[3231]

- A Chinese mixture of four herbs including *B. carteri* promoted wound healing and the prevention of scar formation in rabbits.[3232]

- The Korean remedy Hyunamdan (made of heat-processed ginseng) and Hangamdan S (made of *Cordyceps militaris, Panax ginseng radix, Commiphora myrrha*, calculus bovis, margarita, *Boswellia carteri, Panax notoginseng* radix and *Cremastra appendiculata* tuber) reduced cancerous nodules in the lungs that had metastasized from the bladder in a seventy-four-year-old man.[3233]

- Alpha-pinene inhibits the production of interleukins (IL-1), nitric oxide, and proteins (NF-kappa-B) that promote inflammation and protects the breakdown of chondrocytes (cells that make up the healthy cartilage in the body).[3234,3235]

- *B. carterii* resin (which contains volatile molecules found in the essential oil) provided mild cardiovascular protection during a heart attack in animal research.[3236]

- *B. papyrifera* essential oil inhibited *Cryptococcus neoformans, S. aureus, P. aeurginosa, Candida albicans*, and *B. cereus in vitro*.[3237] Another study reported that it demonstrated significant activity against *S. aureus* and *S epidermidis*.[3238] *In vitro* research demonstrates that *B. papyrifera* essential oil good antibacterial activity against *E. coli, Bacillus subtilis*, and *S. aureus*.[3239]

- *B. serrata* essential oil demonstrated significant broad spectrum antimicrobial activity against organisms associated with skin, scalp, and nail infections (*Propionibacterium acnes, Malassezia* spp., *Candida albicans*, and *Trichophyton* spp.).[3240]

- Frankincense essential oil (*B. carterii*) inhibits *C. albicans, C. krusei*, and *C. glabrata* isolated from the oral cavity.[3241] Interestingly, the researchers reported that *B. carterii* was more effective than myrrh essential oil, and of the two *B. carterii* samples tested, a sample with lower alpha-thujene content (1.8% versus 12.0%) and higher cadinenes content was more effective.

- An alpha-thujene CT of frankincense essential oil (*B. carterii*) demonstrated strong insecticidal activity against the pulse beetle *Callosobruchus chinensis* and *C. maculatus*.[3242]

- Frankincense (species not identified), geranium, and Japanese red pine (*Pinus densiflora*) exhibited anticancer activity against breast cancer cells, reducing cell viability, proliferation, migration, and invasion *in vitro*.[3243] Moreover, all three oils modulated AMPK/mTOR signaling activity. Further evaluation in mice showed that frankincense oil reduced tumor growth and triggered apoptosis.

- Topical application of 1–2 drops of a 5% dilution (5 drops frankincense in 5 mL of coconut oil) of frankincense essential oil to the soles of the feet, twice daily, the day before chemo, the day of chemo, and continued seven days after chemo reduced cancer-related fatigue.[3244] Interestingly, the case study reported that a reduction in blood sugar levels was also observed, requiring an adjustment in insulin requirements.

- Frankincense (species not identified) nanoemulsion essential oil enhanced the activity of mitomycin C against cervical cancer cells.[3245] Mitomycin C is an antitumoral chemotherapy drug used to treat gastrointestinal, anal, bladder, and breast cancers.

- Pretreatment with frankincense (*B. sacra*) essential oil significantly reduced the viability of melanoma cancer cells (mouse and human) without harming healthy skin cells *in vitro*.[3246] The study authors also reported that administering doses of 1,200 mg/kg body weight of frankincense essential oil did not cause harm over the course of twelve weeks. The *in vivo* study showed that doses of 300 and 600 mg/kg body weight of frankincense oil significantly reduced melanoma tumor burden in mice. Lastly, the researchers reported that frankincense reversed liver damage caused by acetaminophen.

- Topical application of frankincense (*B. carterii*) essential oil significantly diluted in jojoba oil (1/1,000) reduced stress—as observed by reduced corticosterone levels—in sleep-deprived rats.[3247] The oil countered the effects of stress by relieving sleep debt and maintaining antioxidant capacity. Rapid eye movement (REM) sleep deprivation disrupts antioxidant capacity and increases oxidative damage and causes psychological stress. Interestingly, the major constituents of frankincense (alpha-pinene and limonene) increased corticosterone stress hormone levels.

☐ Leishmaniasis is a neglected tropical disease caused by parasitic protozoa of the *Leishmania* genus. Current treatment options for cutaneous leishmaniasis are limited due to severe side effects, poor efficacy, resistance to first-line drugs, and limited availability to populations who need the medication. A study evaluated the antileishmanial activities of fifty-two essential oils and concluded that frankincense (a combination of *Boswellia carterii*, *B. sacra*, *B. papyrifera*, and *B. frereana*), coriander, and wintergreen possesses notable antileishmanial activities that make them promising candidates for the topical treatment of cutaneous leishmaniasis.[3248]

☐ Frankincense essential oil (*B. sacra*) inhibited *S. aureus*, *P. aeruginosa*, *P. acnes*, *C. albicans*, and *M. furfur*.[3249]

☐ Status epilepticus is a single seizure lasting longer than five minutes or when two or more seizures occur close together without the person recovering between. It is a medical emergency that could lead to permanent brain damage or even death. Oral pretreatment of 1,000 mg/kg of frankincense (*B. serrata*) essential oil for five days decreased the severity of seizures caused by pilocarpine in rats.[3250] The oil prevented an increase in malondialdehyde, nitric oxide, IL-1β, IL-6 and acetylcholinesterase and a reduction in reduced glutathione induced by pilocarpine in the studied brain regions (cortex and striatum). Frankincense oil failed to restore decreased levels of serotonin and dopamine in the cortex, but improved serotonin and norepinephrine levels in the striatum. The primary composition of the oil was 67.4% octyl acetate, 16.7% thymol, 10.1% octanol, and 3.0% carvone.

☐ Dendritic cells (DCs) are specialized antigen-presenting cells and sentinel cells (first responder cells of the immune system found in body tissues) involved in regulating the immune response. They act as messengers between the innate and adaptive immune systems, processing and presenting antigen materials to T cells. Immature (undifferentiated) DCs are maintained in the tissues and facilitate immune tolerance—a mechanism whereby the immune system learns to discriminate self-antigens from foreign substances and a key to avoiding a hyperimmune response to environmental substances. Frankincense essential oil (*B. sacra*; 20.6% beta-caryophyllene, 9.5% delta-cadinene, 6.4% beta-cubebene, 5.3% beta-elemene, 5.2% elemol) deviated the differentiation of monocytes into immature DCs without stimulating immature DCs to mature.[3251] This suggests that frankincense may be able to produce DCs that promote immune tolerance in conditions such as autoimmune disorders, allergies, hypersensitivity reactions, and after organ transplantation.

☐ A randomized, double-blinded, placebo-controlled study evaluated the effects of massage with frankincense and myrrh essential oils in people with chronic low back pain. A total of ninety-one individuals who had experienced back pain for at least the past three months were randomly divided into three groups: essential oil (two fifteen-minute sessions of lower lumbar massage with frankincense and myrrh diluted in jojoba oil, twice weekly, for a total of three weeks), placebo (massage with jojoba oil only), and control (standard treatment only). The essential oil group had an average of 3 mL of a 4% dilution (2% each of frankincense and myrrh diluted in jojoba oil) applied. The aromatic massage group experienced improvements in back function and pain by the end of the study.[3252]

☐ Frankincense (*B. serrata*) essential oil was inactive against bacteria (*S. aureus*, *E. faecalis*, *P, aeruginosa*, *K, pneumoniae*, *E. coli*) but strongly inhibited *C. albicans*.[3253]

☐ *In vitro* research found that frankincense (*B. sacra*) essential oil reduces the proliferation of and kills colon cancer cells by decreasing delta-catenin signaling molecules, which play a critical role in cancer cell proliferation.[3254]

☐ Frankincense (*B. serrata*; 76.5%–89.1% alpha-pinene) essential oil extracted by superheated steam inhibited *F. solani*, *P. multocida*, *E. coli*, *A. alternata*, *S. aureus*, *A. flavus*, *B. subtilis*, and *A. niger*.[3255]

☐ A case study reports the ingestion of frankincense (*B. sacra*) essential oil for bladder cancer.[3256] A fifty-two-year-old Hispanic male diagnosed with a large invasive high-grade urothelial cell carcinoma of the urinary bladder declined standard treatment of tumor removal and chemotherapy with or without radiotherapy. Instead, he consumed 3 mL of frankincense oil daily (1 mL under the tongue, three times daily after meals) and made lifestyle changes (regular exercise, practicing religious beliefs, consuming more white meats versus red meats, taking vitamin C, organic multivitamins, broccoli sprout extract, and daily juicing), continuing this regimen for twenty-five months. His first recurrence was detected about two months after beginning the regimen and twenty tumors ranging from 0.2 to 3.0 cm were removed (no tumor was present in the original site). A second recurrence was experienced nearly one year after beginning the regimen and six lesions were removed. Regular surveillance continued (urinalysis and cystoscopy) and no detectible cancer in the bladder was noted for fourteen months. Correspondence with an author of the study on June 6, 2022, confirmed that he is still cancer free. The subject's liver and kidney function were monitored during the regimen, and all parameters remained normal. He reported no adverse effects from ingestion of frankincense.

☐ A case study reports the benefits of topical application of frankincense (*B. sacra*) essential oil for skin cancer

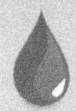

(basal cell carcinoma).[3257] A fifty-six-year-old male diagnosed with nodular basal cell carcinoma on the upper arm and superficial, nodular, and infiltrative basal cell carcinoma on the chest applied neat frankincense oil to the areas several times daily for four months. Examination at the end of four months demonstrated the total resolution of the basal cell carcinoma on the arm and substantial reduction of the basal cell carcinoma on the chest, without causing any adverse effects locally or systemically. Significant increase in apoptotic cells was noted in the residual carcinoma of the chest.

☐ Frankincense essential oil (*B. sacra*) was not very potent against MRSA or multidrug resistant-*P. aeruginosa* (MDR-P), nor did it improve the activity of imipenem or gentamicin against the bacteria.[3258] Further evaluation in a rat model of bacterial pneumonia showed that oral administration of frankincense essential oil—500 mg/kg and 1,000 mg/kg BW—reduced MRSA in rats' lungs after four days of treatment, but it was less effective than the tested antibiotics that were administered intraperitoneally. The lower dose was ineffective against MDR-P, but the higher dose mildly reduced MDR-P in rats' lungs. Moreover, frankincense oil reduced lung inflammation in both MRSA and MDR-P infections.

☐ Both peppermint and frankincense (*B. serrata*; 29.8% beta-thujene, 11.7% alpha-thujene) essential oil inhibited pathogens frequently isolated from the vagina (*P. aeruginosa, P. mirabilis, S. aureus, E. coli, C. albicans*), with the greatest activity observed from peppermint against *P. aeruginosa*.[3259] There activity exceeded that of the tested antibiotics (streptomycin, ampicillin, tetracycline, cefuroxime, and nystatin). Only peppermint showed bactericidal activity against *P. aeruginosa* and *P. mirabilis*, while both were fungicidal to *C. albicans*, which was strain specific.

☐ Nanoparticles loaded with frankincense (*B. sacra*) essential oil improved its anticancer activity against breast cancer cells, doubling its apoptotic activity.[3260]

☐ Frankincense (*B. carterii*) essential oil demonstrated strong antioxidant activity in the DPPH and ABTS assays (exceeding the reference compound Trolox), good antimicrobial activity (*C. glabrata, C. tropicalis, C. albicans, B. subtilis, A. flavus, Y. enterocolitica, S. enterica* biofilm, *P. aeruginosa, S. enterica* ser. Enteritidis, *P. citrinum, B. cinerea, C. krusei*, and *E. faecalis*), which often exceeded controls (cefoxitin, fluconazole), and moderate insecticidal activity against the lime seed bug (*Oxycarenus lavaterae*).[3261]

☐ Two commercial samples of frankincense purchased in Turkey (*B. carterii/B. serrata*; alpha-pinene CT and alpha-thujene CT) demonstrated anticancer activity against androgen-positive/dependent and aggressive androgen-negative/independent prostate cancer cells, with the alpha-thujene CT being more active against aggressive androgen-negative/independent prostate cancer cells.[3262] The oils also inhibited *B. subtilis, B. cereus, P. aeruginosa*, and *E. coli*, but this time the alpha-pinene CT was more active.

# GALANGAL
## (Galanga)

Greater Galangal, Siamese Ginger: *Alpinia galanga* L., *Languas galanga*; Lesser Galangal, Chinese Ginger: *A. officinarum* Hance., *L. officinarum* (Hance) Farwell; False Galangal, Kencur, Galanga: *Kaempferia galanga* L.

**FAMILY:** Zingiberaceae
**NOTE:** Middle
**AROMA INTENSITY:** Medium
**AROMA:** Sweet, woody, camphoraceous, spicy
**COMMON EXTRACTION METHOD:** Steam distilled from the rhizomes
**POSSIBLE SUBSTITUTE OILS:** Ginger, fingerroot, hairy basil, ocotea, lavandin, Spanish sage
**BLENDS WELL WITH:** Black pepper, cardamom, cassia, chamomile (German, Roman), cinnamon, cistus, cypress, elemi, eucalyptus, frankincense, geranium, ginger, hinoki, juniper berry, juniper (Phoenician), lavender, lavandin, lemon myrtle, marjoram, may chang, opoponax, palmarosa, patchouli, pine, rose, rosemary, rosewood, sage, Spanish sage, spike lavender, spikenard, tarragon, turmeric, vetiver, ylang ylang
**SUBCELLULAR LOCALIZATION | EPIGENETIC INFLUENCE:** Currently unknown | Currently unknown
**RECOMMENDED DILUTION RANGE:** 3%–20%; neat for limited conditions

**PRIMARY CONSTITUENTS:**[3263,3264,3265,3266,3267,3268,3269,3270,3271,3272,3273,3274,3275,3276,3277]

*Greater Galangal (1,8-Cineole CT)*

| | |
|---|---|
| 1,8-Cineole | 22.6%–61.9% |
| Alpha-Fenchyl Acetate | 0.0%–18.4% |
| Beta-Pinene | 0.9%–14.4% |
| Camphor | 0.0%–14.0% |
| Alpha-Terpineol | 2.1%–12.7% |
| Alpha-Pinene | 0.5%–10.9% |
| Cis-Sabinene Hydrate | 0.0%–8.8% |
| Borneol | 0.0%–8.4% |
| (Z)-Beta-Ocimene | 0.0%–6.4% |
| Germacrene D | 0.0%–6.1% |
| Chavicol Acetate | 0.0%–5.9% |
| (E)-Methyl Cinnamate | 0.0%–5.3% |
| Beta-Sesquiphellandrene | 0.0%–5.0% |
| Camphene | 0.5%–4.1% |

*Greater Galangal (Piperitenone CT)*

| | |
|---|---|
| Piperitenone | 33.3% |
| Limonene | 29.6% |
| N-Pentadecane | 5.6% |

*False Galangal (Ethyl-p-Methoxycinnamate CT)*

| | |
|---|---|
| Ethyl-p-Methoxycinnamate | 18.4%–51.6% |
| (E)-Ethyl Cinnamate | 13.1%–29.5% |
| 1,8-Cineole | 5.7%–13.6% |
| Carvone | 0.0%–11.1% |
| Gamma-Cadinene | 0.0%–9.8% |
| N-Pentadecane | 0.0%–9.0% |
| Germacrene D-4-ol | 0.0%–8.0% |
| Delta-3-Carene | 0.0%–7.9% |
| (E)-Cinnamaldehyde | 0.0%–5.3% |
| Borneol | 2.6%–5.2% |
| Camphor | 0.0%–4.3% |

*Lesser Galangal*

| | |
|---|---|
| 1,8-Cineole | 28.1%–55.4% |
| Alpha-Fenchyl Acetate | 0.5%–15.2% |
| Carotol | 0.0%–8.9% |
| Delta-3-Carene | 0.0%–8.9% |
| Alpha-Terpineol | 6.4%–9.2% |
| Gamma-Muurolene | 0.0%–7.9% |
| Beta-Pinene | 1.0%–5.7% |
| Alpha-Farnesene | 0.0%–5.7% |
| Beta-Caryophyllene | 0.3%–4.7% |
| Trans-Alpha-Bergamotene | 0.1%–4.2% |
| Alpha-Eudesmol | 0.0%–4.5% |
| (E)-Methyl Cinnamate | 0.0%–4.0% |

*False Galangal (2-Propeonic Acid CT)*

| | |
|---|---|
| 2-Propeonic Acid | 35.5% |
| N-Pentadecane | 26.1% |
| Ethyl-p-Methoxycinnamate | 26.0% |

Note: An unusual CT of greater galangal—grown in a subtropical climate—is also reported in the literature (alpha-fenchyl acetate 54.3%, 1,8-cineole 6.1%, viridiflorol 4.5%), but doesn't appear to be available commercially. It is possible that this was a mistakenly identified snap ginger (*A. calcarata*), which is typically high in alpha-fenchyl acetate (12.9%–40.3%). False galangal may crystallize when standing and left at room temperature.

**OTHER CONSTITUENTS:** *Greater Galangal (1,8-Cineole CT)*—alpha-phellandrene, limonene, farnesol, bornyl acetate, terpinene-4-ol, beta-eudesmol, geraniol, n-pentadecane, (E)-beta-ocimene, gamma-terpinene, alpha-terpinene, carvacrol methyl ether, (E)-nerolidol, viridiflorol, alpha-cadinol, 2,4(8)-p-menthadiene, 2-isopropyltoluene, camphene hydrate, 4-carvomenthenol, benzylacetone, 3,5-Dimethyl-4-octanone, (Z)-geraniol, eugenol, 2-(1,1-Dimethylethyl)-6-(1-methylethyl)phenol, trans-p-menth-2,8-dien-1-ol, chavicol, geranyl acetate, farnesyl acetate, 7-epi-selinene, eugenyl acetate, zingiberenol, T-muurolol, methyl eugenol (< 3.2%), trans-beta-farnesene; *Greater Galangal (Piperitenone CT)*—gamma-terpinene, borneol, para-cymen-8-ol, neral, decanoic acid, beta-elemene, trans-beta-caryophyllene, alpha-amorphene, 7-epi-alpha-selinene, alpha-cadinol, beta-bisabolene, apiole (< 0.7%); *Lesser Galangal*—camphor (< 2.6%), alpha-pinene, camphene, limonene, isoborneol, (E)-cinnamaldehyde, alpha-guaiene, 2-phenylethyl 2-bromopropanoate, (E)-beta-farnesene, alpha-caryophyllene, guaiene, phenethyl 2-methylbutyrate, gamma-gurjunene, r-himachalene, delta-cadinene, alpha-gurjunene, beta-panasinsene, gamma-elemene, epiglobulol, cubenol; *False Galangal (Ethyl-p-Methoxycinnamate CT)*—alpha-pinene, camphene, m-cymene, d-limonene, alpha-

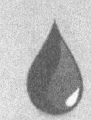

phellandren-8-ol, terpinen-4-ol, para-cymen-8-ol, eucaevone, delta-cadinene, hexylbenzoate, davanone, isoborneol, butyl ethyl ether, beta-pinene, para-cymene, p-Menth-1-en-4-ol, alpha-terpineol, benzenemethanol,α,α, 4-trimethyl-, azulene, octadecyl chloride, linoleoyl chloride, ethyl-m-methoxycinnamate; *False Galangal (2-Propeonic Acid CT)*— borneol, delta-3-carene, 1,8-cineole, heptadecane, 3-4-methoxyphenyl, 1-methyl-2-(1-methylethyl)

## PREFERRED COMPOSITION FOR CLINICAL USE:

| Constituent | Greater | Lesser |
|---|---|---|
| 1,8-Cineole | 35%–60% | 30%–55% |
| Beta-Pinene | 5%–15% | 1%–7% |
| Alpha-Terpineol | 2%–10% | 5%–12% |
| Alpha-Pinene | 2%–10% | 0.5%–3% |
| Borneol | 0%–8% | – |
| Camphene | 0.5%–5% | 0.5%–3% |
| Alpha-Fenchyl Acetate | 0.1%–5% | 2%–15% |
| Beta-Caryophyllene | 0.1%–3% | 1%–5% |
| Trans-Alpha-Bergamotene | – | 0.1%–5% |

**REPORTED THERAPEUTIC PROPERTIES: Antibacterial**, antifungal, antimicrobial, antiseptic, anticancer, disinfectant, anti-inflammatory, antiarthritic, antirheumatic, analgesic, antispasmodic, diuretic, balances menstruation, reduces high blood pressure, relieves upset stomach, expels excess gas, relieves diarrhea, relieves motion sickness, aids digestion, relieves nausea and vomiting, eases cough, **supports respiratory function**, relieves chronic skin conditions, insecticide, aphrodisiac, reduces pessimism, relieves anxiety, reduces mental fatigue, antidepressant

## CAUTIONS:

*Greater (1,8-cineole CT) and Lesser Galangal*

■ Avoid with children under age 3, particularly around the nose and mouth. Use very cautiously in children under age 5 due to high 1,8-cineole and camphor content. 1,8-cineole may cause seizures, central nervous system problems, or respiratory distress in young children.[3278,3279,3280,3281] Several cases of camphor poisoning and/or seizures from ingestion and topical application have been reported in children.[3282,3283] Ingestion of camphor-containing products has been lethal in children under age two.[3284] Camphor ingestion by infants and young children may cause cough, vomiting, seizure, burning sensation in the mucous membranes and eyes, or lack of voluntary coordination of muscle movements.[3285]

■ Avoid with epilepsy and Parkinson's disease due to 1,8-cineole content and camphor. May exacerbate or cause seizures/convulsions or reduce seizure medication efficacy based on 1,8-cineole content.[3286,3287,3288]

■ Caution is warranted orally due to the significant amounts of 1,8-cineole and potential moderate camphor content. Limit it to small doses internally (adults—maximum 10 drops daily). One text recommends a maximum daily dose of 6 drops, whereas the European Medicines Agency recommends 2 to 4 drops (100–200 mg) of high 1,8-cineole essential oils orally, 2 to 5 times daily for adolescents, adults, and the elderly.[3289,3290] Additionally, 200 mg of isolated 1,8-cineole has been ingested three times daily for up to six months in clinical research.[3291,3292] Toxicity has been reported when eucalyptus (also high in 1,8-cineole) was ingested in large doses, and as few as 4 to 5 drops may cause problems in very sensitive individuals.[3293,3294,3295,3296,3297,3298] In humans, 3.5 to 5 mL has proven fatal orally.[3299] Essential oils with significant levels of camphor can be toxic when taken orally, usually single doses exceeding 2 mL, although the lethal dose for humans is estimated to be more than 5 mL in a single dose.[3300,3301,3302]

■ The potential moderate camphor content in galangal may negatively impact red blood cells and increase the risk of jaundice in children with glucose-6-phosphate dehydrogenase deficiency (G6PD).[3303,3304]

■ May weakly interfere with the enzymes responsible for metabolizing medications (NSAIDs, proton-pump inhibitors, acetaminophen, antiepileptics, immune modulators, blood-sugar medications, blood pressure medications, antidepressants, antipsychotics, diabetic medications, antihistamines, antibiotics, and anesthetics) based on 1,8-cineole content.[3305,3306,3307]

■ May interact with diabetic medications. 1,8-cineole inhibits alpha-glucosidase activity, particularly when synergized with other constituents (alpha-pinene, beta-pinene, para-cymene).[3308,3309,3310] Alpha-glucosidase is an enzyme that breaks down carbohydrates by chemical reaction with water. Inhibiting its activity postpones glucose absorption and therefore the impact of carbohydrates on blood sugar levels.

■ May interfere with pentobarbital and other barbiturates (medications for anxiety and insomnia) based on 1,8-cineole content.[3311,3312]

*Greater Galangal (Piperitenone CT)*
■ None currently known.

*False Galangal (Ethyl-p-Methoxycinnamate CT)*
■ May interact with aspirin, blood pressure, antiplatelet, and anticoagulant medications, and increase the risk of bleeding among people with bleeding disorders due to (E)-methyl cinnamate content (low risk as (E)-methyl cinnamate only moderately inhibits platelet aggregation).[3313,3314]
■ May interact with MAOI antidepressants due to Ethyl-p-Methoxycinnamate content. Research suggests that Ethyl-p-Methoxycinnamate inhibits MAO activity.[3315]

*False Galangal (2-Propeonic Acid CT)*
■ May interact with MAOI antidepressants due to Ethyl-p-Methoxycinnamate content. Research suggests that Ethyl-p-Methoxycinnamate inhibits MAO activity.[3316]

**SELECTED EVIDENCE:**

☐ *In vitro* research shows that lesser galangal essential oil inhibits gram positive (*Staphylococcus aureus, Streptococcus bovis,* and *Bacillus subtilis*) and gram-negative (*Escherichia coli, Klebsiella pneumoniae, Pseudomonas aeruginosa* (weakly), and *Salmonella typhi*) bacteria, and the fungus *Candida albicans*.[3317,3318] Greater galangal synergizes the antimicrobial activity of lemongrass essential oil when used in a 3:7 (greater galangal:lemongrass) ratio.[3319] Greater galangal (piperitenone CT) rapidly and strongly inhibited foodborne bacteria (*E. coli, S. typhimurium, S. sonnei, L. monocytogenes,* and *S. aureus*), demonstrating particularly significant activity against *E. coli*, which greatly exceeded that of gentamicin.[3320] False galangal essential oil demonstrated marked antimicrobial activity against gram-positive (*S. aureus, Streptococcus faecalis,* and *B. subtilis*), gram-negative (*Salmonella typhi, Shigella flexneri,* and *E. coli*), and the fungi *C. albicans*.[3321] The antifungal activity of false galangal exceeded that of the antifungal drug clotramazole.[3322]

☐ Lesser galangal essential oil is considered a moderate antioxidant.[3323] False galangal essential oil was inactive for antioxidant activity.[3324]

☐ Greater galangal essential oil is significantly toxic to the cigarette beetle (*Lasioderma serricorne*).[3325] It also repels and is toxic to two species of termites: *Coptotermes gestroi* and *Coptotermes curvignathus*.[3326] False galangal essential oil was toxic to and repelled the booklouse, *Liposcelis bostrychophila*.[3327] The same researchers reported that (E)-ethyl cinnamate was also toxic to and (E)-cinnamaldehyde repelled the booklouse. False galangal (2-propeonic acid CT) was toxic to the larvae of pyrethroid-susceptible and resistant *Ae. aegypti* mosquitoes.[3328] Greater galangal provided protection against mosquito (*Ae. aegypti*) bites comparable to DEET.[3329]

☐ Cinnamon bark, nut grass CT cyperene, and galangal CT beta-bisabolene each synergized the insecticidal activity of permethrin against mosquitoes (*Ae. aegypti*).[3330]

---

*Did you know?*

Essential oils are volatile, meaning they readily evaporate at normal temperatures and pressures. Their volatility indicates it is better to apply them more frequently rather than a large amount all at once. In addition, most essential oil constituents are quickly metabolized when ingested, demonstrating the need to take smaller, more frequent oral doses to maintain efficacy.

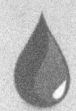

# GALBANUM

*Ferula galbaniflua* Boiss., *F. gummosa* Boiss. & Buhse

**FAMILY:** Apiaceae (Umbelliferae)
**NOTE:** Top-Middle
**AROMA INTENSITY:** Medium
**AROMA:** Woody, spicy, balsamic
**COMMON EXTRACTION METHOD:** Steam distilled from the resin; also distilled from the fruit and seed
**POSSIBLE SUBSTITUTE OILS:** Balsam fir, copaiba, white fir
**BLENDS WELL WITH:** Balsam fir, black spruce, blue spruce, carrot seed, copaiba, geranium, ginger, lavender, pine, rose, silver fir, white fir
**SUBCELLULAR LOCALIZATION | EPIGENETIC INFLUENCE:** Currently unknown | Currently unknown
**RECOMMENDED DILUTION RANGE:** 5%–Neat

**PRIMARY CONSTITUENTS:**[3331,3332,3333]

| | |
|---|---|
| Beta-Pinene | 45.5%–66.3% |
| Alpha-Pinene | 5.4%–36.6% |
| Beta-Phellandrene | 0.1%–22.7% |
| Delta-3-Carene | 0.6%–12.1% |
| Delta-Cadinene | 1.5%–7.2% |
| Beta-Cubebene | 0.0%–4.9% |
| Epi-Bicyclosesquiphellandrene | 0.0%–4.4% |
| Terpinen-4-ol | 0.0%–4.1% |

**OTHER CONSTITUENTS:** Alpha-terpinene, alpha-thuyene, beta-myrcene, d-limonene, beta-elemene, (E)-caryophyllene, Germacrene D, alpha-muurolene, para-cymene, guaiol, gamma-cadinene, methyl carvacrol, terpinyl acetate, alpha-amorphene, spathulenol, viridiflorol

**PREFERRED COMPOSITION FOR CLINICAL USE:**

| *Constituent* | |
|---|---|
| **Beta-Pinene** | 45%–68% |
| **Alpha-Pinene** | 7%–25% |
| **Delta-3-Carene** | 2%–15% |
| **Limonene** | 0.5%–10% |
| **Delta-Cadinene** | 0.1%–7% |
| **Myrcene** | 0.1%–4% |
| **Beta-Phellandrene** | 0.1%–3% |

**REPORTED THERAPEUTIC PROPERTIES:** Analgesic (pain relief), anti-inflammatory, antiarthritic, **antirheumatic**, antispasmodic, antimicrobial, **aids immune function**, **anti-aging**, antiseptic, **aids circulation**, decongestant, aids detoxification, softens skin, **reduces the appearance of scars and blemishes**, aids the absorption of nutrients, **balances menstruation**, stimulates lymph flow, antiparasitic, wound healing, calming, aids concentration and focus, antidepressant, relieves shock, combats emotional rigidity

**CAUTIONS:**
■ None currently known.

**SELECTED EVIDENCE:**
☐ Animal research suggests that galbanum oil reduces intestinal spasms.[3334]

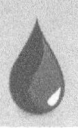

- Galbanum seed oil inhibited *E. coli in vitro*.[3335]
- Galbanum fruit oil remarkably inhibits *S. aureus, S. epidermis, and B. subtilis, E. coli, S. typhi, P. aeruginosa, C. kefyr, and C. albicans*.[3336] The resin oil also inhibits *S. aureus, P. aeruginosa, E. coli, S. enteritidis*, and *L. monocytogenes*.[3337] Other research concluded that galbanum essential oil inhibits multidrug-resistant clinical isolates of *Acinetobacter*, although the alcohol extract demonstrated far greater antimicrobial activity.[3338]
- *In vitro* research demonstrates that galbanum essential oil effectively inhibits *L. amazonensis*.[3339]
- Galbanum essential oil inhibited multidrug-resistant *P. aeruginosa*.[3340]
- A combination of galbanum and bourbon geranium (*Pelargoneum roseum*) essential oil was scolicidal to *Echinococcus granulosus*, with beta-pinene demonstrating the greatest activity followed by citronellol.[3341]
- *In vitro* research showed that galbanum essential oil inhibited *E. coli* and this antibacterial activity was improved when the oil was used in liposomal form.[3342]
- Galbanum essential oil was weakly insecticidal to adult Khapra beetles (*Trogoderma granarium*) and adult large grain borer (*Prostephanus truncatus*), weakly larvicidal to Khapra beetle and Egyptian cotton leafworm (*Spodoptera littoralis*) larvae, moderately larvicidal to mosquito (*Culex quinquefasciatus*) larvae, and displayed good activity against houseflies (*Musca domestica*).[3343] However, the toxicity was not selective and also resulted in cytotoxicity in human cells (fibroblasts) and nontarget aquatic microcrustaceans (*Daphnia magna*).
- Oral administration of galbanum essential oil increased survival in mice experiencing an epileptic seizure without causing toxicity.[3344] Sabinene was able to bind to the GABA$_A$ receptor, which is the same binding site of benzodiazepines.

# GARLIC

*Allium sativum* L.

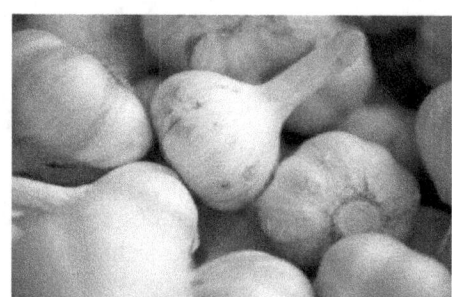

**FAMILY:** Liliaceae
**NOTE:** Top
**AROMA INTENSITY:** Strong
**AROMA:** Pungent, sulfur-like, garlicky
**COMMON EXTRACTION METHOD:** Steam distilled from bulbs
**POSSIBLE SUBSTITUTE OILS:** Bergamot, cinnamon bark, lemongrass, marjoram, ylang ylang
**BLENDS WELL WITH:** Basil (sweet), cumin, lavender, peppermint, rosemary
**SUBCELLULAR LOCALIZATION | EPIGENETIC INFLUENCE:** Currently unknown | Currently unknown
**RECOMMENDED DILUTION RANGE:** 1.5%–5.0%

**PRIMARY CONSTITUENTS:**[3345,3346,3347,3348,3349]

| *Sulfides CT* | | *Vinyldithiins CT* | |
|---|---|---|---|
| Diallyl Trisulfide | 19.9%–45.9% | 2-Vinyl-4H-1,3-Dithiin | 17.7%–38.1% |
| Diallyl Disulfide | 17.5%–44.6% | 3-Vinyl-4H-1,2-Dithiin | 14.5%–32.7% |
| Allyl Methyl Trisulfide | 7.3%–18.2% | Diallyl Sulfide | 6.0%–17.6% |
| Ethyl Vinyl Sulfide | 0.0%–9.7% | Methyl Allyl Trisulfide | 0.1%–14.9% |
| Allyl Methyl Disulfide | 0.0%–9.1% | Diallyl Trisulfide | 0.2%–14.1% |
| 2-Vinyl-4H-1,3-Dithiin | 0.0%–8.7% | Unidentified | 4.2%–11.7% |
| Propyl Allyl Disulfide | 0.0%–7.2% | Ethyl Vinyl Sulfide | 0.0%–9.7% |
| Gamma-Cadinene | 0.0%–6.8% | Methyl Allyl Disulfide | 0.6%–9.0% |
| Diallyl Sulfide | 0.0%–6.6% | 3-(2,3,4-Trithia-5-Heptenyl)-1- | |
| 3-Vinyl-4H-1,2-Dithiin | 0.0%–4.5% | Thia-Cyclohex-5-ene | 2.0%–6.7% |
| Diallyl Tetrasulfide | 0.0%–4.1% | | |

**OTHER CONSTITUENTS:** *Sulfides CT*—dimethyl disulfide, 1.4-dimethyl tetrasulfide, allyl methyl sulfide, eugenol, alpha-humulene, alpha-guaiene, aromadendrene, alpha-bisabolene, elemicin, 3-methoxyoctane; *Vinyldithiins CT*—dimethyl disulfide, diallyl sulfide, dimethyl trisulfide, 3,5-diethyl 1,2,4-trithiolane, pentadecene, heptadecene

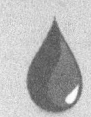

**PREFERRED COMPOSITION FOR CLINICAL USE:**

| Constituent | Sulfides CT |
|---|---|
| **Diallyl Disulfide** | 20%–47% |
| **Diallyl Trisulfide** | 20%–42% |
| **Allyl Methyl Trisulfide** | 10%–20% |
| **Diallyl Sulfide** | 1%–10% |
| **Allyl Methyl Disulfide** | 1%–10% |
| **Diallyl Tetrasulfide** | 0.5%–5% |

**REPORTED THERAPEUTIC PROPERTIES:** Antibacterial, antimicrobial, antifungal, **antiviral**, antiparasitic, analgesic, antirheumatic, anti-inflammatory, **anticancer**, antioxidant, **supports cardiovascular function**, **supports normal blood pressure**, **reduces high cholesterol**, relieves diarrhea, aids respiratory function, expels excess mucus, boosts immune function, removes warts and corns, relieves chronic skin conditions, wound healing (especially deep), reduces the appearance of acne and blemishes, promotes hair growth, aids circulation, relieves male impotence, weight management, insect repellent, **insecticide**, combats anger and rage, releases traumatic memories and emotions, increases awareness, mentally stimulating

**CAUTIONS:**

■ Caution is advised during pregnancy and nursing. Garlic odor was detected in the amniotic fluid of women who consumed a single capsule of ginger herb and a review concluded that garlic herb has the potential to cause abortion, trigger menstruation, or stimulate the uterus.[3350,3351] However, no adverse outcomes were reported in pregnant women who took 800 mg of garlic herb daily during the third trimester of pregnancy, and diallyl sulfide prevents embryo-feto toxicity.[3352,3353,3354] Animal research also reports that garlic herbal oil—containing diallyl trisulfide—reduces pregnancy complications (decreased newborn body weight, abortion, and musculoskeletal abnormalities) due to its ability to reduce cholesterol in pregnant rats with high cholesterol.[3355] Based on conflicting information it is best to use garlic cautiously during pregnancy until definitive research determines its safety. In addition, ingestion of garlic by lactating mothers reportedly altered the flavor of breast milk because garlic constituents are secreted in the breast milk and made infants prone to extended nursing.[3356,3357]

■ May interact with aspirin, blood pressure, antiplatelet, and anticoagulant medications, and increase the risk of bleeding among people with bleeding disorders. Garlic herbal oil, essential oil, and volatile components inhibit platelet aggregation.[3358,3359,3360,3361,3362,3363,3364,3365,3366,3367,3368] The study authors attributed this effect to the presence of essential oil or volatile organosulfur constituents (diallyl trisulfide, methyl allyl trisulfide).

■ May interfere with enzymes responsible for metabolizing medications (NSAIDs, proton-pump inhibitors, acetaminophen, antiepileptics, immune modulators, blood-sugar medications, blood pressure medications, antidepressants, antipsychotics, diabetic medications, antihistamines, antibiotics, and anesthetics) due to diallyl disulfide, diallyl trisulfide, allyl methyl sulfide, and allyl diallyl sulfide content.[3369,3370,3371,3372,3373] Diallyl disulfide and diallyl trisulfide also interfere with protein transporters that move drugs across cell membranes, which can increase or decrease drug effectiveness.[3374]

■ May interact with antifungal medications (ketoconazole) and increase their effectiveness.[3375]

■ May be photosensitizing due to reports that diallyl disulfide causes photo contact dermatitis.[3376,3377] Avoid UV exposure to area of application for at least twelve hours after topical application.

■ Topical application may cause skin irritation or skin sensitivity reactions. Cases of contact dermatitis or irritation have been reported after using garlic herbal oil, with diallyl disulfide being a major cause of this irritation.[3378,3379] Dilutions under 3% are strongly recommended.

**SELECTED EVIDENCE:**

☐ Diallyl trisulfide causes an increase in cystolic free calcium concentration ($[Ca^{2+}]_i$).[3380] $[Ca^{2+}]_i$ acts as a major signaling method that controls cellular proliferation, migration, metabolism, gene transcription, and death, and in some cases kills cancer cells.[3381] Cancer cells may dysregulate $[Ca^{2+}]_i$ homeostasis in order to enhance their survivability, invasiveness, and ability to spread (proliferate); therefore, increases in $[Ca^{2+}]_i$ may contribute to the destruction of cancer cells. Diallyl trisulfide also contributes to the destruction of liver tumor cells possibly by affecting cell viability, triggering structural changes in cancer cells, and controlling cyclin B1 (a regularity protein involved in cellular division that is overexpressed in premalignant and malignant tumors) and Cdk7 (a transcriptional cyclin-dependent kinase that cancer cells are dependent on to survive and spread—inhibition of Cdk7 causes apoptosis) expression.[3382]

☐ *In vitro* research shows that garlic essential oil (sulfides CT) inhibits the gram-negative bacteria *Salmonella typhi*, *E. coli*, *Campylobacter jejuni*, and *Yersinia enterocolitica* and gram-positive bacteria *S. aureus*, *L monocytogenes*, and *B. cereus*.[3383,3384,3385] The sulfides CT of garlic essential oil inhibited both bacteria (*S. aureus*, *S. typhimurium*, *L. monocytogenes*) and fungi (*A. flavus*, *A. niger*).[3386]

☐ Garlic essential oil (sulfides CT) completely inhibited the growth of *Aspergillus versicolor* and production of sterigmatocystin (a mycotoxin produced by *Aspergillus* sp. that is associated with cancer and DNA damage).[3387] Garlic essential oil vapor also strongly inhibits the fungal cause of honey bee larval disease chalkbrood (*Ascosphaera apis*).[3388] Other research reports that garlic essential oil strongly inhibits *Trichophyton rubrum*, *T. erinacei*, and *T. soudanense*, and increases the effectiveness of ketoconazole.[3389]

☐ Garlic essential oil demonstrated stronger anti-inflammatory activity than diclofenac sodium (an NSAID used to treat arthritis and migraines) when used in concentrations higher than 25 mcg/mL *in vitro*.[3390]

☐ Oral administration of 18 mg/day of garlic herbal oil for 4 weeks reduced blood pressure and cholesterol levels in healthy individuals, which was attributed to the herbal oil's volatile components.[3391] Another study administered 120 mg of garlic herbal oil daily for up to 30 days in people with high blood pressure and reported that the dosage moderately to significantly reduced blood pressure in 67% of study participants.[3392] A third study reported that oral administration of the essential oil (0.25 mg/kg in two divided doses daily for ten months) reduced cholesterol and triglyceride levels, while increasing HDL levels.[3393] Another study reported reduced cholesterol and triglyceride levels and increased HDL levels after administering two capsules of garlic ethyl acetate extract (equivalent to 1 g raw garlic per capsule) divided in two doses for three months.[3394]

☐ Animal research shows that oral administration of 2.0 to 4.0 mg/kg of garlic essential oil with 2.0 to 4.0 mL/kg of garlic juice protects rats from heart cell death and damage (necrosis) caused by isoprenaline (a heart medication used to treat slow heart rhythms and associated with myocardial necrosis) and improved animal survivability.[3395] Garlic essential oil added to the diet also reduced total cholesterol and increased HDL levels in rabbits.[3396]

☐ Garlic essential oil completely and irreversible caused paralysis of the liver fluke (*Fasciola gigantica*) after 15 minutes of administration of 3 mg/mL concentration.[3397] The liver fluke is a parasitic flatworm that is regarded as one of the single most important parasitic infections in Asia and Africa and causes fascioliasis (an infection characterized by abdominal pain, enlarged liver, fever, vomiting, diarrhea, hives, and eosinophilia, which can last for months, finally leading to bile duct obstruction and inflammation).

☐ Animal research shows that oral administration of garlic essential oil (50 or 100 mg/kg) or diallyl sulfide (20 mg/kg) protects against nonalcoholic fatty liver diseases by significantly decreasing the release of proinflammatory cytokines in the liver, positively modulating enzyme activity (down-regulating: sterol regulatory element binding protein-1c, acetyl-CoA carboxylase, fatty acid synthase, and 3-hydroxy-3-methylglutaryl-coenzyme A reductase; and stimulating: peroxisome proliferator-activated receptor α, and carnitine palmitoyltransferase-1), and increasing antioxidant capacity.[3398]

☐ Animal research demonstrates that oral administration of (10 mL/kg) garlic essential oil improves memory recognition by increasing the number of neurons (cell proliferation) and neuroblast (neural cells that are in development between a stem cell and fully developed neuron) differentiation, modulating BDNF protein (a protein that promotes neuron cell survival by influencing their growth, maturation, and maintenance) levels, and inhibiting AChE enzyme activity.[3399] Inhibition of AChE prevents the breakdown of acetylcholine, which is essential for memory and thinking. People with neurodegenerative diseases make less acetylcholine, and the diseases often break it down at a faster rate leading to acetylcholine deficits.

☐ Garlic essential oil is a moderate to strong antioxidant.[3400,3401,3402,3403,3404]

☐ Garlic essential oil was toxic to and repelled the darkling beetle (*Alphitobius diaperinus*) for 12 hours (90.4% efficacy).[4359] It was also toxic to the Japanese termite (*Reticulitermes speratus* Kolbe), pear psyllid (*Cacopsylla chinensis*), tick (*Rhipicephalus microplus*), cabbage looper (*Trichoplusia ni Hübner*), Sciarid fly (*Lycoriella*

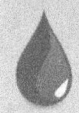

*ingénue*), Japanese beetle (*Popillia japonica* Newman), European chafer (*Rhizotrogus majalis*), oriental beetle (*Anomala orientalis*), mosquito (*Culex pipiens L.*), and northern masked chafer (*Cyclocephala borealis* Arrow).[3405,3406,3407,3408,3409,3410,3411]

☐ Garlic essential oil—and diallyl sulfide and diallyl disulfide—demonstrated significant insecticidal activity against the mealworm beetle (*Tenebrio molitor*).[3412]

☐ *In vitro* research demonstrates that garlic essential oil actively inhibits *Candida* sp. isolated from dental prostheses (dentures), with effects on both biofilms and planktonic cells (bacteria that float in their environment).[3413]

☐ The sulfides CT of garlic essential oil nanoemulsion showed high acaricidal activity against eriophyid olive mites *Aceria oleae* and *Tegolophus hassani* without any toxicity in rats.[3414]

☐ Both garlic (49.1% allyl disulfide and 31.1% diallyl trisulfide) and asafetida (30.0% (E)-sec-butyl propenyl disulfide and 24.3% (Z)-sec-butyl propenyl disulfide) essential oils were toxic to West Nile Virus vector mosquitoes (*Culex pipiens Linnaeus, Culex restuans*).[3415] Garlic was the most effective essential oil, which was attributed to its rich allyl disulfide content. Isolated allyl disulfide also exhibited strong ovicidal and larvicidal activity. Interestingly, an antagonistic effect was observed when garlic and asafetida were used in combination.

☐ Diallyl sulfide from garlic essential oil hinders the virulence of *Pseudomonas aeruginosa* by inactivating key quorum-sensing genes across three difference quorum-sensing systems.[3416]

☐ Oral administration of garlic essential oil demonstrated antiobesity (reduced body weight gain, decreases adipose tissue) and antihyperlipidemic (reduced triglycerides, total cholesterol, and LDL cholesterol) properties that counteract the effects of a high sugar diet in rats.[3417]

☐ *Borrelia burgdorferi* is a diderm bacteria responsible for Lyme disease in the United States. Of thirty-five essential oils screened, garlic, allspice, cumin, palmarosa, myrrh, ginger lily, amyris, thyme, may chang, and lemon eucalyptus each demonstrated excellent activity against *Borrelia burgdorferi*.[3418] Garlic (19% diallyl disulfide), allspice CT eugenol, and myrrh (38% curzerene) were the most active essential oils.

☐ Both garlic and chamomile (species not identified) essential oil combined with the chemotherapy drug mitomycin as nanoparticles improved the anticancer activity of mitomycin against cervical cancer cells.[3419] Garlic essential oil worked by damaging the cell membrane, whereas chamomile passed through the cell membrane and directly affected the cell nucleus.

☐ Oral administration of garlic essential oil (25 and 50 mg/kg BW) for twenty-eight consecutive days significantly reduced depression caused by persistent stress in rats.[3420] The 25 mg dose also effectively decreased the frontal cortex turnover ratio of serotonin (5-HT) and dopamine (DA), which increased levels of both 5-HT and DA. In addition, garlic oil increased brain-derived neurotrophic factor (reduced levels are noted in stressed and depressed animals), c-AMP response element binding protein (involved in the regulation of multiple genes related to the pathophysiology of depression), and protein kinase B (regulates molecular mechanisms that are dysregulated in mood disorders and depression) expression in the hippocampus.

☐ Thyme CT thymol, garlic, tea tree, cajeput, may chang, lemongrass (*C. citratus*), and verbena CT citral exhibited fungistatic activity (100 percent) against *F. culmorum* and *F. graminearum*, and all but garlic (89.4%) were 100% fungistatic against *F. avenaceum* and *F. oxysporum*.[3421]

☐ A garlic essential oil-charged mist sprayed at the entryway of a meat processing room significantly repelled blowflies.[3422] Sage CT alpha-thujone, garlic, and rosemary CT 1,8-cineole essential oil were also toxic to adults blowflies (*C. vomitoria*) by direct topical and fumigant activity. The same oils exerted antimicrobial activity against *B. subtilis, S. aureus, E. coli, C. albicans, P. aeruginosa,* and *S. enterica*.

☐ Collection of COVID-19 research. Angiotensin-converting enzyme 2 (ACE2) is a protease enzyme that regulates cardiovascular function. It does so by controlling angiotensin II levels, which acts on the central nervous system to regulate kidney activity and function and, therefore, blood pressure. ACE2 is found significantly in the gastrointestinal system, heart, and kidneys, and also found in alveolar cells in the lungs. ACE2 has been shown to be a co-receptor for the severe acute respiratory syndrome coronavirus 2 (SARS-CoV-2) to infect cells and increase virulence. Coronaviruses are RNA viruses that trigger the creation of two long polyproteins after infecting a cell. These proteins provide the instructions (replication/transcription complex) that makes more RNA, viral particles (virons), structural proteins, and two proteases that allow the virus to infect more cells and cause illness. Inhibition of the ACE2 protein could potentially prevent and treat SARS-CoV-2 infection.[3423] In addition, SARS-CoV-2 infects cells through its spike proteins, of which the main protein is PDB6LU7.[3424,3425] A study investigated the ability of garlic essential oil and its compounds to inhibit ACE2 and PDB6LU7 via molecular docking technique. What the researchers observed was that sulfur compounds in garlic essential oil interacted with amino acids in and inhibited the ACE2 protein and inhibited PDB6LU7.[3426] The most active compounds were allyl disulfide and allyl trisulfide. The researchers concluded that garlic essential oil is a promising natural antiviral substance with anticoronavirus activity that contributes to the prevention of coronavirus invading the human body. Another study reported that thymoquinone (black cumin essential oil), citral (lemongrass, lemon myrtle, lemon tea tree, may chang, melissa, lemon verbena, and other essential oils), menthol (peppermint), and beta-selinene (celery, ledum, and helichrysum essential oils) also inhibit the PDB6LU7 protein.[3427] A third study reported that 1,8-cineole from eucalyptus essential oil bonds to Mpro/3CLpro (the main viral proteinase of SARS-CoV-2), making it a "potential treatment . . . to act as a COVID-19 mpro inhibitor."[3428] Similarly, a study of cajeput essential oil found that ten of its twenty-four constituents strongly inhibited ACE2 and PDB6LU7 proteins.[3429] The most powerful anticoronavirus activity was observed from: alpha-terpineol = guaiol = linalool > 1,8-cineole > beta-selinenol > alpha-eudesmol > gamma-eudesmol. Excellent inhibition of both proteins was observed when the ten constituents were used in combination, creating significant synergy. Geranium and lemon essential oils and their major constituents citronellol and limonene downregulated ACE2 receptor expression in epithelial cells, suggesting they are valuable natural antiviral agents that may help prevent the invasion of SARS-CoV-2 into the human body.[3430] Coronavirus replication takes place by converting the polypeptide into a functional protein, which is controlled by main protease. A computerized model (molecular docking study) found that eucalyptus (*E. globulus*), lemon eucalyptus (*C. citriodora*), and isolated 1,8-cineole may act as potent inhibitors of SARS-CoV-2 replication and transcription processed by inhibiting Main protease activity.[3431] Rosemary CT 1,8-cineole demonstrated inhibition of ACE2 with anti-inflammatory (5LOX) activity, suggesting it may have potential against coronavirus.[3432] A review article reported that cinnamon essential oil, and isolated trans-cinnamaldehyde, may be useful to "decrease oxidative stress and inflammation in COVID-19 patients."[3433] Evaluating essential oils and essential oil constituents for activity against SARS-CoV-2 based on their physicochemical, pharmacokinetic, and toxicity properties identified 41 essential oil compounds suitable for use because of their drug-likeness and bioactivity.[3434] Essential oils that were considered most promising and contained many of the identified constituents include melissa, Zataria, Surinam cherry (*Eugenia brasiliensis*), shell ginger, Taurus cedar, and vetiver. Fifteen constituents were considered the most promising against SARS-CoV-2: alpha-vetispirene, cadin-4-em-10-ol, caryophyllene oxide, eudesmol, himachalol, (E)-isovalencenol, khusene, khusimol, khusimone, khusol, epi-zizanone, salutarisolide, zerumbone, curione, and spathulenol. Vetiver essential oil contains many of these compounds such as alpha-vetispirene, (E)-isovalencenol, khusene, khusimol, khusimone, khusol, and epi-zizanone, with particularly high levels of khusimol and (E)-isovalencenol. Constituents with anti-SARS-CoV-2 action because of activity against the spike protein or main protease (MPRO—a cysteine protease in the virus that restricts antiviral signaling and is involved in the neuropathology of the virus; inhibiting its activity blocks replication and transcription of the virus) include alpha-eudesmol (katafray, Japanese cedarwood, Formosan cypress, Serrata frankincense, blue cypress, amyris), himachalol (Atlas cedarwood, Himalayan cedarwood), and spathulenol (kunzea, betony, pink pepper) for MPRO; alpha-eudesmol and zerumbone (bitter ginger, *Zingiber zerumbet*) for ACE2; caryophyllene oxide (melissa, black sage, cangerana) for spike protein, replicase polyprotein 1a (RP1a—protein involved in the transcription and replication of viral RNAs), and nonstructural protein 9 RNA binding protein (NSP9—involved in replicating and transcribing the viral genome after a virus infects a host cell); and zerumbone for the spike protein. Thymoquinone, the main ingredient of black cumin essential oil, has a chemical structure indicative of antiviral activity against multiple viruses. Molecular docking research suggests that thymoquinone may prevent COVID-19 by binding to the receptor site on the transmembrane serine proteinase 2 (the activator enzyme that attaches the virus to the cell).[3435] Molecular docking analysis of sesquiterpenes from copaiba essential oil showed that beta-selinene displayed the best binding energy for the SARS-CoV-2 MPRO, while spathulenol strongly interacted with the human ACE2 receptor.[3436] Other sesquiterpenes demonstrating good binding energy for SARS-CoV-2 proteins included alpha-selinene, alpha-humulene, beta-bisabolene (spike protein). A review article concluded that based on the scientific evidence and properties of peppermint essential oil, peppermint may be "effective in prevention of infection as well as symptom treatment of COVID-19."[3437] A laboratory study found that clove bud, lemongrass (*C. citratus*), lemon, geranium, oregano CT carvacrol, star anise, and German chamomile CT (E)-beta-farnesene each blocked entry of the SARS-CoV-2 virus delta variant into cells.[3438] Evaluation of toxicity potential of the oils to healthy cells demonstrated that star anise, lemon, geranium, and clove essential oils are promising candidates to inhibit viral entry due to their high therapeutic index.

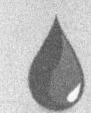

- A multi-center controlled clinical trial evaluated the effects of oral administration of garlic essential oil among ninety-seven people with COVID-19.[3439] People in the experimental group took five capsules with 10 mg of garlic essential oil before breakfast and dinner (total of 100 mg of garlic essential oil) along with conventional treatment (nutritional support, symptomatic treatment, antiviral therapy, and antimicrobial therapy) for up to ten days. A control group of one hundred people received conventional therapy only. Compared to the control group, the garlic group experienced a shorter duration of symptoms, shorter time to a negative COVID test, and shorter time to improvement in lung characteristics (as determined by computed tomography).

- *Listeria monocytogenes* is a pathogenic bacterium that causes listeriosis—a condition characterized by fever, muscle aches, diarrhea, and nausea, which can also spread to the nervous system and cause headache, stiff neck, confusion, and changes in alertness. Onion, garlic, and cinnamon bark essential oils inhibited biofilm formation by *L. monocytogenes in vitro*.[3440]

- Babesiosis is a rare and life-threatening infection of the red blood cells that occurs when an infected tick bites a human and transmits parasites like *Babesia duncani* or *B. microti*. Current drugs (atovaquone + azithromycin) used to treat babesiosis are ineffective and frequently cause side effects. Both garlic and black pepper essential oil showed good inhibitor activity against *B. duncani* in a hamster red blood cell culture model. Their main constituents diallyl sulfide and beta-caryophyllene also exhibited activity. Treatment with atovaquone + azithromycin showed eradication of *B. ducani*, but relapse occurred even at high concentration. On the contrary, garlic oil (or diallyl disulfide) combined with azithromycin killed *B. duncani* parasites at low concentrations without regrowth.

- *Vibrio parahaemolyticus* is a gram-negative bacterium that causes gastrointestinal illness in humans characterized by watery or bloody diarrhea, nausea, vomiting, fever, headache, and abdominal cramps. The bacteria lives in brackish saltwater (like found in the coastal waters of the United States and Canada) and causes symptoms after ingesting contaminated water or food. Clove, thyme CT para-cymene, and garlic (20.0% allyl propyl disulfide, 16.8% diallyl trisulfide, 15.2% allyl sulfide) essential oils reduced bacterial growth, with clove and thyme being the most effective.[3441]

- Garlic essential oil with diallyl disulfide as the major constituent (80%) killed human promyelocytic leukemia cells by inducing apoptosis and significantly increasing the production of intracellular reactive oxygen species.[3442] Isolated diallyl disulfide was also active against leukemia cells.

- Garlic essential oil was the most toxic to the granary weevil (*Sitophilus granarius*) of twenty-five essential oils tested. Other oils that were effective and had a lower cost included wintergreen, cornmint, and eucalyptus dives.[3443]

- A model of acute infection with *Campylobacter jejuni* investigated the benefits of garlic essential oil.[3444] Mice were infected with *C. jejuni* and then given garlic essential oil in their water two days after infection. The mice treated with garlic essential oil experienced less severe clinical symptoms of the infection and had a lower bacterial load when compared to placebo. The essential oil also reduced intestinal cell death in the colon, decreased secretion of proinflammatory molecules, and limited relocation of *C. jejuni* from the intestines to distant organs.

- Several sulfur compounds in garlic essential oil inhibited enzymes—AChE, BChE, and beta-secretase (involved in the amyloid creation pathway)—related to Alzheimer's disease in mice.[3445] In addition, sulfur compounds were detected in the blood and brain six hours after administration, with high levels of allyl mercaptan and allyl methyl sulfide present in the brain. This suggests that other sulfur compounds—such as dimethyl trisulfide, allyl methyl trisulfide, and diallyl trisulfide—are converted to allyl mercaptan or allyl methyl sulfide in the body.

- Garlic essential oil (44.2% diallyl trisulfide, 22.1% diallyl disulfide) exhibited good antioxidant activity in the DPPH and beta-carotene bleaching assays.[3446]

- Chitosan nanoparticles with garlic essential oil showed antifungal activity against *A. versicolor, A. niger,* and *F. oxysporum,* and promoted the growth of wheat, barley, and oats.[3447]

- Toxoplasmosis is an infection caused by the intracellular protozoan parasite *Toxoplasma gondii*. Toxoplasmosis is a significant infection in immunocompromised people and also affects pregnant women. Prophylactic treatment is often recommended in these people to reduce likelihood of infection. Administration of garlic essential oil prior to being challenged with *Toxoplasma gondii* parasites significantly protected mice against toxoplasmosis and increased survival rates without negatively effecting the kidneys or liver.[3448]

- A high-fat diet during pregnancy can trigger high blood pressure in adult offspring. Oral administration of garlic essential oil during pregnancy and lactation protected against high blood pressure by increasing mRNA expression and activity of $H_2S$-generating enzymes in the kidneys, nitric oxide bioavailability, and plasma short chain fatty acid levels, and improved the gut microbiome.[3449]

- Comparing the contact toxicity and repellent effects of eight essential oils and carrier oils (clove bud, garlic, *Eucalyptus camaldulensis*, lavender, German chamomile, lemon, jojoba, and sweet almond) against the red flour beetle (*Tribolium castaneum*), clove bud essential oil exhibited the highest repellency effect, while garlic, German chamomile, and lemon were the most toxic.[3450]

- Both garlic and thyme CT para-cymene essential oil effectively inhibited biofilm formation by *S. typhimurium*, with garlic being most active.[3451]

- Garlic leaf and bulb essential oil with allicin as the main constituent inhibited *A. baumannii*, *E. coli*, *L. monocytogenes*, and *S. aureus*, and their ability to form biofilms.[3452]

- A comparison of the activity of ten essential oils against antibiotic-resistant *E. coli* and *L. monocytogenes* showed that clove, thyme, cinnamon, and garlic were highly active against both bacteria, but turmeric, cumin, black pepper, and marjoram were inactive against *L. monocytogenes*.[3453] Ginger and parsley were moderately active against both bacteria. A combination of clove and thyme exhibited the strongest activity against *L. monocytogenes*. Combinations of clove+cinnamon, cinnamon+garlic, and cinnamon+thyme were synergistic against *E. coli*; the same combinations plus clove+thyme, and clove+garlic were synergistic against *L. monocytogenes*. Composition was not reported for the essential oils used in the study.

- *In vitro* and *in vivo* bioassays showed that garlic essential, its hydrolate, and an organic fraction of garlic essential oil caused high mortality rates of juvenile root-knot nematode (*Meloidogyne javanica*), suppressed egg hatching, and reduced nematode infection and reproduction in tomato plants.[3454]

- *Clostridioides difficile* (C. diff) is a very virulent and multidrug resistant bacterium that causes healthcare-acquired infections that are very difficult to treat and have frequent recurrence. A laboratory study evaluated the anticlostridial potential of three essential oils—wild oregano (*Origanum minutiflorum*), garlic, and black pepper—against C. diff strains isolated from hospitalized people.[3455] Each of the oils inhibited C. diff and its formation of biofilms, with oregano being the most active. The researchers concluded that these oils represent promising candidates for "adjunctive therapeutics in the treatment of CDI [C. diff infections]."

- Nanoemulsions (NEs) with 0.1% ginger or garlic essential oil and varying ratios of neomycin sulphate (0.001%, 0.005%, 0.01%) were prepared and evaluated for their antimicrobial activity against pathogens that commonly infect skin wounds (*B. spizizenii*, *S. aureus*, *E. coli*, and *S. enterica*).[3456] A NE with a blend of 0.05% of each oil was also evaluated. The garlic NE with 0.005% neomycin sulphate was the most active against the pathogens except for against *S. aureus*, which was most susceptible to ginger NE with 0.001% neomycin sulfate. The NEs were evaluated for their wound healing properties in a rabbit-skin excision-wound model and demonstrated that they accelerated wound healing better than a neomycin sulfate NE. The combination of garlic and ginger worked the best for wound healing.

# GENIPI

## (Génépi, Génépy)

*Artemisia genipi* Weber ex. Poljakov, *A. spicata* Wulfen,
*A. mutellina* Vill.; White Genepi: *A. umbelliformis* L.

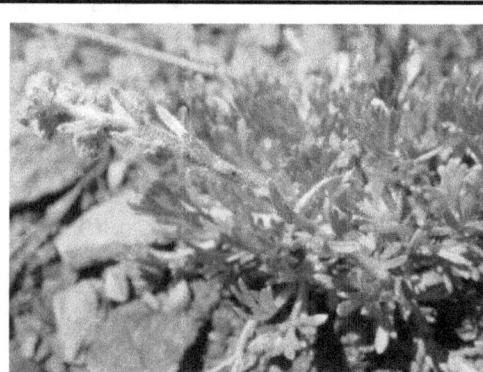

**FAMILY:** Asteraceae (Compositae)
**NOTE:** Top
**AROMA INTENSITY:** Medium
**AROMA:** Herbaceous, medicinal, spicy
**COMMON EXTRACTION METHOD:** Steam distilled from the aerial parts
**POSSIBLE SUBSTITUTE OILS:** Sage, thuja, mugwort
**BLENDS WELL WITH:** Bay laurel, bergamot, cajeput, camphor, chamomile (German, Roman), coriander, eucalyptus, lavender, lemon, lime, orange, neroli, palo santo, peppermint, petitgrain, ravensara, rosemary, Spanish sage, spikenard, tangerine, thyme, turmeric
**SUBCELLULAR LOCALIZATION | EPIGENETIC INFLUENCE:** Currently unknown | Currently unknown **RECOMMENDED DILUTION RANGE:** 1.5%–20%

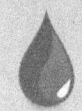

**PRIMARY CONSTITUENTS:**[3457,3458,3459]

*A. genipi*

| | |
|---|---|
| Alpha-Thujone | 26.0%–79.8% |
| Beta-Pinene | 1.3%–17.9% |
| Terpinen-4-ol | 1.0%–12.2% |
| Beta-Thujone | 6.8%–10.4% |

*A. umbelliformis (Alpha-Thujone CT)*

| | |
|---|---|
| Alpha-Thujone | 29.7%–67.5% |
| Beta-Thujone | 4.6%–19.5% |
| 1,8-Cineole | 0.3%–9.5% |
| Sabinyl Valerianate | 0.0%–7.3% |
| Sabinyl Isovalerianate | 0.0%–7.1% |
| Neryl Isovalerianate | 0.0%–6.9% |
| Sabinol | 0.0%–4.1% |
| Borneol | 0.1%–3.9% |

*A. umbelliformis (Cis-Sabinene Hydrate/Borneol CT)*

| | |
|---|---|
| Cis-Sabinene Hydrate | 2.7%–20.1% |
| Borneol | 0.1%–19.4% |
| 1,8-Cineole | 4.1%–14.0% |
| Beta-Pinene | 1.8%–11.5% |
| Neryl Isovalerianate | 1.4%–10.0% |
| Terpinen-4-ol | 3.3%–8.2% |
| Caryophyllene Oxide | 2.2%–5.4% |
| Beta-Caryophyllene | 1.0%–4.6% |
| Alpha-Terpinyl Acetate | 0.7%–4.2% |

**OTHER CONSTITUENTS:** *A. genipi*—alpha-pinene, sabinyl isobutyrate, alpha-thujene, gamma-terpinene, para-cymene, cuminaldehyde, 1,8-cineole, (E)-nerolidol, spathulenol, sabinyl isovalerate, sabinyl n-valerate, valeranone; *A. umbelliformis (Alpha-Thujone CT)*—sabinene, beta-pinene, gamma-terpinene, cis-sabinene hydrate, trans-sabinene hydrate, camphor, terpinen-4-ol, alpha-terpineol, sabinyl isobutyrate, beta-caryophyllene, caryophyllene oxide; *A. umbelliformis (Cis-Sabinene Hydrate/Borneol CT)*—alpha-thujene, alpha-pinene, camphene, beta-myrcene, alpha-terpinene, trans-sabinene hydrate, para-cymene, gamma-terpinene, alpha-thujone (< 2.0%), beta-thujone (< 0.7%), sabinol, camphor, alpha-terpineol, bornyl acetate, sabinyl isovalerianate, sabinyl valerianate

**PREFERRED COMPOSITION FOR CLINICAL USE:**

| Constituent | A. genepi |
|---|---|
| **Alpha-Thujone** | 40%–60% |
| **Beta-Pinene** | 5%–15% |
| **Beta-Thujone** | 5%–12% |
| **Terpinen-4-ol** | 3%–8% |

Note: Should only be used clinically when the benefits outweigh the risks as determined by a health professional experienced with essential oils.

**REPORTED THERAPEUTIC PROPERTIES:** Antimicrobial, antibacterial, antifungal, anti-infectious, antispasmodic, decongestant, expectorant, aids immune function, supports respiratory function, aids digestion, accelerates fat utilization, stimulates appetite, wound healing, relieves bruises, diuretic, reduces fever, insect repellent, **combats mental fatigue**, promotes alertness and concentration

**CAUTIONS:**

*Genipi essential oil is not commonly used in essential oil therapy and should be reserved for use by the very experienced user who can properly weigh the risks-to-benefits ratio of using it.*

■ Avoid with children under six due to thujone content. Cases of seizure have been reported in young children due to exposure to essential oils high in thujones.[3460,3461,3462]

■ Avoid during pregnancy and while lactating. Essential oils high in thujone content may cause abortion.[3463,3464]

■ Avoid oral consumption. Ingesting plants or products high in thujones can cause vomiting, stomachache, diarrhea, and gastroenteritis followed by absorption disorders, headache, nervous agitation, and chronic convulsions, and symptoms of liver and kidney toxicity extending to yellow liver atrophy (extensive and rapid death of liver cells—parenchymal, possibly accompanied by fatty degeneration), arrhythmia and myocardial bleeding.[2852] Thujone is considered significantly neurotoxic and may damage the liver, and it is estimated that as little as 15 mg orally may negatively impact the central nervous system.[3465,3466,3467] Taking 20 drops of thuja oil (also high in thujones) twice daily for five days caused an adult woman to have a tonic seizure and then fall and fracture her skull.[2033] Case reports involving serious adverse health outcomes (seizure, convulsions, and acute kidney failure) have been reported in adults who consumed high thujone essential oils (sage, thuja, wormwood) in doses of one "swallow," 12 drops, and 20 drops twice daily for five days.[3468,3469,3470,3471]

■ Avoid with epilepsy and Parkinson's disease due to thujone, 1,8-cineole, and camphor content.[3472,3473,3474,3475,3476,3477,3478]

■ May weakly interfere with the enzymes responsible for metabolizing medications (NSAIDs, proton-pump inhibitors, acetaminophen, antiepileptics, immune modulators, blood-sugar medications, blood pressure medications, antidepressants, antipsychotics, diabetic medications, antihistamines, antibiotics, and anesthetics) due to alpha-thujone content.[3479]

■ Avoid with those who have a compromised liver or kidneys due to the risk of kidney toxicity, kidney failure, or liver toxicity.[3480,3481] Consuming extremely large amounts of thujone rich essential oils (10 mL) has caused kidney failure.[3482] This would also suggest that those taking medications that could cause liver damage should also use genipi very cautiously or avoid it entirely.

**SELECTED EVIDENCE:**

  ☐   None found.

---

# GERANIUM
## (Rose Geranium, Sweet Scented Geranium)

*Pelargonium graveolens* L'Hér. ex Aiton; *P. capitatum* (L.) L'Hér. ex Aiton; *P. × aspermum*; *P. radens* H.E. Moore, *P. radula* (Cav.) L'Her

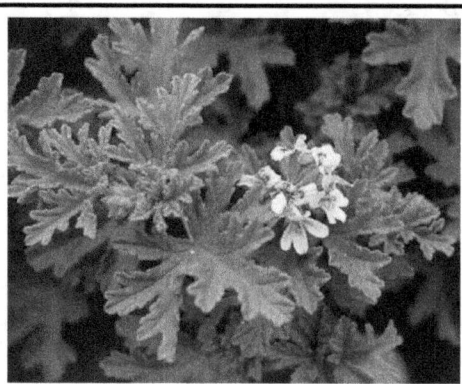

**FAMILY:** Geraniaceae
**NOTE:** Middle
**AROMA INTENSITY:** Strong
**AROMA:** Floral, sweet, fresh, rose-like
**COMMON EXTRACTION METHOD:** Steam distilled from the leaves and flowers
**POSSIBLE SUBSTITUTE OILS:** Rose, melissa, vetiver, cistus
**BLENDS WELL WITH:** Basil, bay laurel, bergamot, carrot seed, cassia, coriander, chamomile (German, Roman), citronella, clary sage, cypress, fennel, galbanum, ginger, grapefruit, juniper, lavandin, lavender, lemon, lemongrass, lime, melissa, neroli, orange, palmarosa, patchouli, peppermint, tangerine, ravensara, rose, rosemary, spikenard, ylang ylang
**SUBCELLULAR LOCALIZATION | EPIGENETIC INFLUENCE:** Mitochondria | Currently unknown
**RECOMMENDED DILUTION RANGE:** 3%–50%; neat for limited conditions

**PRIMARY CONSTITUENTS:**[3483,3484,3485,3486,3487,3488]

| Constituent | Percentage |
| --- | --- |
| Citronellol | 2.4%–45.7% |
| Geraniol | 1.1%–38.4% |
| Citronellyl Formate | 0.0%–18.1% |
| Linalool | 0.3%–16.0% |
| Menthone | 0.3%–16.0% |
| Trans-Caryophyllene | 0.0%–11.0% |
| Isomenthone | 0.0%–7.9% |
| Thymol | 0.0%–7.8% |
| 10-Epi-Gamma-Eudesmol | 0.0%–5.6% |
| Guaia-6,9-Diene | 0.0%–5.4% |
| Cyclohexanone | 0.0%–5.2% |

**OTHER CONSTITUENTS:** Alpha-pinene, beta-pinene, trans rose oxide, alpha-copaene, beta-bourbonene, beta-cubebene, geranyl formate, geranyl tiglate, germacrene, octadiene, butanoic acid, alpha-terpineol, nerol, citral

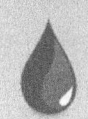

**PREFERRED COMPOSITION FOR CLINICAL USE:**

| Constituent | South African | Bourbon (Reunion Island) | Madagascan | Egyptian | Chinese |
|---|---|---|---|---|---|
| Citronellol | 20%–30% | 18%–28% | 18%–26% | 25%–40% | 30%–43% |
| Geraniol | 9%–18% | 12%–20% | 12%–20% | 12%–16% | 4%–12% |
| Citronellyl Formate | 5%–14% | 6%–15% | 6%–12% | 6%–10% | 7%–14% |
| Guaia-6,9-Diene | 5%–10% | 3%–8% | 5%–10% | 0.1%–0.5% | 5%–12% |
| Isomenthone | 3%–8% | 5%–10% | 5%–10% | 4%–7% | 3%–12% |
| Geranyl Formate | 3%–8% | 4%–8% | 3%–7% | 2%–4% | 1%–8% |
| Linalool | 1%–6% | 4%–11% | 4%–10% | 4%–5% | 1%–5% |
| Beta-Caryophyllene | 1%–3% | 1%–3% | 1%–3% | 1%–2% | 1%–3% |
| Germacrene D | 1%–3% | 0.5%–2% | 0.5%–2% | 1%–2% | 0.1%–3% |
| Geranyl Tiglate | 0.5%–3% | 0.5%–3% | 0.5%–2% | 0.5%–2% | 0.5%–2% |
| Geranyl Butyrate | 0.5%–2% | 0%–2% | 0.5%–2% | 0.5%–2% | 0.1%–1% |
| Cis-Rose Oxide | 0.5%–2% | 0.1%–1.5% | 0.5%–1.5% | 0.5%–1.5% | 1%–4% |
| Bourbonene <α or β> | 0.5%–2% | 0.5%–2% | 0.5%–2% | 0%–1.5% | 1%–3% |
| Geranyl Propionate | 0%–2% | 0%–2% | 0%–2% | 0%–2% | 0.01%–2% |
| Phenylethyl Tiglate | 0.1%–2% | 0.1%–1% | 0.1%–1% | 0.5%–1% | 0.1%–1% |
| Geranial | 0.1%–2% | 0.2%–1% | 0.1%–1% | 0.5%–1% | – |
| Trans Rose Oxide | 0.1%–1% | 0.1%–0.5% | 0.1%–1% | 0.1%–1% | 0.5%–2% |
| Menthone | 0.1%–1% | 0.1%–2% | 0.1%–2% | 1%–2% | 0.1%–5% |
| Nerol | 0.1%–1% | 0.1%–1% | 0.5%–1% | 0.1%–1% | – |
| Alpha-Terpineol | 0.1%–0.5% | 0.1%–1% | 0.1%–1% | 0.1%–0.5% | 0.01%–0.5% |
| 10-Epi-γ-Eudesmol | 0%–0.5% | – | – | 4%–6% | – |
| Beta-Myrcene | 0%–0.2% | 0%–2% | 0.1%–0.2% | 0%–0.2% | 0%–0.3% |

**REPORTED THERAPEUTIC PROPERTIES:** Analgesic (pain relief), antibacterial, antidepressant, supports blood-sugar balance, **stimulates lymph flow and drainage**, anti-inflammatory, antiseptic, astringent, **antineuralgic**, antioxidant, diuretic, **cell regeneration**, aids liver function, **balances menstruation**, stops excess bleeding, regenerative, helps bruises heal, **nervine (calms and soothes the nerves)**, wound healing, **reduces the appearance of scars and blemishes**, sedating, antidepressant, promotes a sense of security, stimulates imagination, promotes balanced emotions

**CAUTIONS:**
■ May interfere with the enzymes responsible for metabolizing medications (NSAIDs, proton-pump inhibitors, acetaminophen, antiepileptics, immune modulators, blood-sugar medications, blood pressure medications, antidepressants, antipsychotics, diabetic medications, antihistamines, antibiotics, and anesthetics).[3489]
■ May interact with diabetes medications and cause low blood sugar.[3490]
■ May interact with antibiotics and/or antifungals and possibly increase their effectiveness.[3491,3492,3493,3494,3495,3496]
■ Dilution recommended for topical application. Geraniol is metabolized and autoxidized into metabolites like geranial and neral and may cause sensitization and irritation when applied topically.[3497]

**SELECTED EVIDENCE:**
☐ Geranium oil reduced the viability of two leukemia cancer cell lines *in vitro*.[3498]
☐ Animal research suggests that geranium oil protects against oxidative testicular damage caused by the xenobiotic insecticide deltamethrin.[3499]
☐ *In vitro* research suggests that geranium oil inhibits *S. enteritidis, P. aeruginosa, E. coli, S. aureus*, and *B. subtilis*.[3500] Other research demonstrates that geranium essential oil inhibits *S. typhimurium* and *E. coli*.[3501]
☐ *In vitro* research suggests that geranium oil inhibits common pathogens that infect the urinary tract and improves the effectiveness of treating UTIs with ciprofloxacin.[3502] It also improves the effectiveness of

norfloxacin (a quinolone antibiotic used to treat urinary tract infections),[3503] ketoconazole (an antifungal drug used to treat seborrheic dermatitis),[3504] and amphotericin B (an antifungal drug used to treat systemic fungal infections).[3505] Geranium increases the antibacterial activity of gentamicin (an antibiotic used to treat eye infections) and may reduce the dose of gentamicin required, and therefore its side effects, according to *in vitro* research.[3506,3507]

☐ Animal research suggests that geranium oil decreases high blood sugar better than glibenclamide (an antidiabetic medication that increases insulin production by the pancreas).[3508] The researchers also reported that geranium oil reduces complications of diabetes associated with oxidative stress. Trans-caryophyllene in geranium stimulates the production of insulin by pancreatic beta-cells in response to glucose according to *in vitro* research.[3509]

☐ A 1% geranium oil topical gel improved dental stomatitis (an oral infection of *Candida* or thrush that causes inflammation of oral mucous membranes that primarily affects denture wearers or those who don't practice appropriate oral care) in 90% of study volunteers.[3510]

☐ Topical application of a combination of lavender, geranium, tea tree, and peppermint oils improved the oral health of hospice patients with terminal cancer.[3511]

☐ Animal research concluded that vaginal washing with geranium oil reduces inflammation and vaginal candidiasis (yeast infection) in mice.[3512]

☐ A foot bath (107∘F water) with salts and either oregano, thyme, cinnamon bark, lemongrass, clove, palmarosa, peppermint, lavender, or geranium significantly reduced fungi associated with athlete's foot *in vitro*.[3513]

☐ Geranium oil reduces inflammation by suppressing neutrophil accumulation of fluid retention in the area of inflammation.[3514,3515]

☐ Geranium oil possesses good antioxidant properties.[3516,3517]

☐ Citronellol relieves oral and facial pain by modulating central nervous system activity in mice.[3518]

☐ Animal research suggests that citronellol, the primary constituent in geranium essential oil, lowers blood pressure by increasing vasodilation (relaxation of the muscular wall and widening of the blood vessels).[3519] A small clinical study reported that oral administration of geranium essential oil (0.15 mL initial load, followed by 0.45 mL daily) for two months significantly reduced blood pressure, platelet aggregation, and cortisol levels.[3520]

☐ Geranium essential oil protected against hypothalamic neuron toxicity caused by zinc.[3521]

☐ Geranium oil contains the constituent 10-epi-gamma-eudesmol, which is considered a natural tick repellent.[3522]

☐ A twenty-minute massage with a 0.5% concentration of lavender and geranium essential oil (diluted in a neutral gel) to the shoulders and back, three times per week, reduced anxiety among people with personality disorders during psychiatric hospitalization, as evidenced by reduced heart and respiratory rates.[3523]

☐ Geranium essential oil demonstrated 85.9%–97.0% efficacy against the *Rhipicephalus microplus* tick depending on the concentration used (1%–10%).[3524]

☐ Several essential oils listed in order of efficacy killed the itch mite (*Sarcoptes scabiei*) that burrows into the skin and causes scabies during direct contact (clove > palmarosa > geranium > tea tree > lavender > manuka > petitgrain > eucalyptus > Japanese cedarwood) with the mites and when used as a fumigant (tea tree > clove > eucalyptus > lavender > palmarosa > geranium > Japanese cedarwood > petitgrain > manuka).[3525]

☐ Animal research demonstrates that oral (100 mg/kg) and topical (5 or 10 mcL) administration of geranium essential oil significantly reduces inflammation.[3526]

☐ Inhalation of rose or geranium essential oil increased salivary estrogen levels in premenopausal women.[3527] Ten different essential oils and absolutes (geranium, rose, orange, lavender, neroli, frankincense, jasmine absolute, ylang ylang, Roman chamomile, and clary sage) were tested among women with an average age of forty-four. Air was pumped through an apparatus containing 15 mL of each of the essential oils and delivered to the participant by a tube and glass funnel. Salivary estrogen levels loosely approximate serum estrogen levels,[3528] suggesting that simply inhaling rose or geranium essential oil could influence estrogen levels in women and promote hormone balance.

☐ Geranium essential oil inhibits *S. aureus* and produces a synergistic effect against the bacteria when used with wild chamomile.[3529]

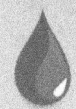

- ☐ Of six essential oil microemulsions tested (marjoram, turmeric, sweet basil, clove bud, geranium, and black cumin), geranium was the most active against the cancer cell lines tested.[3530]
- ☐ *In vitro* research demonstrates that geranium essential oil inhibits secreted aspartic protease activity in *C. albicans* (which is a factor in the yeasts virulence) and enhances the activity of fluconazole.[3531]
- ☐ Diabetic foot ulcers are caused by poor circulation and kidney disease and frequently result in amputation due to improper healing. An herbal cream with geranium and denak essential oils (1% of each oil) promoted wound healing of diabetic foot ulcers by reducing inflammation and triggering tissue regeneration.[3532]
- ☐ A laboratory and clinical study demonstrated that vaginal pessaries with cocoa butter, calendula extract and either geranium and palmarosa or lavender and Roman chamomile essential oils reduced symptoms of vaginal atrophy (muscle weakness/wasting) in breast cancer survivors.[3533]
- ☐ Thyme CT gamma-terpinene, lemon CT citral, geranium CT p-menthone, cassia CT cinnamaldehyde, clove CT eugenol, and basil CT 1,8-cineole each demonstrated fungistatic and fungicidal activity toward *C. albicans* and *C. glabrata* isolates with cassia demonstrated the highest activity.[3534]
- ☐ Lemongrass (*C. citratus*) and geranium essential oil significantly reduced viral replication and viral infectivity and reduced the cytopathic (damage to living cells) effect of the Ross River virus when introduced prior to, during, or after viral adsorption (the first step in the viral life cycle where the virus attaches to the cell).[3535]
- ☐ Scientists determined that geranium and calendula essential oils are useful additions to cosmetics due to their antioxidant (slows skin aging) and SPF (6.45 and 8.36 respectively) properties.[3536]
- ☐ A pilot study found that a back massage with lavender and geranium essential oils—diluted to a concentration of 1% of each oil (2% essential oil total) in a neutral cream—significantly reduced stress in members of a surgical nursing team.[3537] Healthcare professionals received six effleurage massages for ten to fifteen minutes with an average of 42 hours between sessions. Reduction in both blood pressure and heart rate were observed after the massage.
- ☐ Geranium and ajowan CT thymol essential oil demonstrated remarkable antimycobacterial activity against multidrug-resistant *M. tuberculosis*, *M. kansasii*, *M. fortuitum*, and a standard strain of *M. tuberculosis* depending on the concentration used.[3538]
- ☐ Geranium essential oil demonstrated anticandida activity against *C. albicans* and synergized the effects of fluconazole against candida.[3539]
- ☐ Methomyl is a highly toxic pesticide known to impair central nervous system function. Researchers assessed the protective effects of oral administration of geranium essential oil against neurotoxicity caused by methomyl. Specifically, whether it could ameliorate deficits in special working memory in rats. The control group that received oral methomyl only experienced declines in spatial working memory, elevated liver enzymes (a sign of liver harm), and oxidative stress (increased malondialdehyde and decreased glutathione S-transferase and catalase antioxidant enzyme activities). In addition, the CA1 region of the hippocampus was damaged. Rats treated with geranium essential oil showed improvements in special working memory, partial restoration of antioxidant activity, and prevention of neuronal damage in the hippocampus.[3540]
- ☐ Toxoplasmosis is a zoonotic infection caused by *T. gondii* parasites and estimated to affect one-third of the human population chronically. Exiting drugs are not very effective and associated with significant side effects. Geranium was the only oil of five tested (cypress, eucalyptus, tea tree, bergamot, and geranium) that exhibited antiparasitic activity against *T. gondii*, causing the researchers to conclude it represented a potential antiparasitic drug for toxoplasmosis.[3541]
- ☐ Geranium essential oil inhibited *S. aureus*, *E. faecalis*, *P, aeruginosa*, *K, pneumoniae*, *E. coli*, and *C. albicans*.[3542]
- ☐ Researchers evaluated the synergistic activity of rosemary, geranium, and peppermint essential oils in combination with colistin antibiotics against extreme drug-resistant and susceptible *Acinetobacter baumannii* clinical isolates. The highest inhibitory activity was observed with peppermint essential oil, followed by geranium and rosemary essential oils.[3543] Both rosemary and geranium produced strong synergistic activity when combined with colistin, but peppermint was indifferent when combined with colistin.
- ☐ Geranium essential oil demonstrated good anti-inflammatory activity and stabilization of erythrocyte membrane, antioxidant activity, and anticancer activity against gastric, metastatic breast, and melanoma cancer cells.[3544] Gastric cancer was the most susceptible to geranium. Isolated citronellol exhibited stronger anti-inflammatory and antioxidant activity.
- ☐ *Helicobacter pylori* is the main pathogen responsible for peptic ulcer formation. Left untreated, peptic ulcers can cause chronic gastric cancer and lymphoma. Laboratory research showed that geranium essential oil inhibits *H. pylori* and significantly enhances the antibacterial activity of the antibiotic clarithromycin.[3545]
- ☐ Of fourteen commercial essential oils tested, cinnamon bark, thyme CT thymol, clove bud, geranium, and manuka essential oils were most active against fungi that commonly infect animal and human skin

(*Microsporum gypseum, Microsporum canis, Trichophyton mentagrophytes, Trichophyton violaceum, Aspergillus niger, Scopulariopsis brevicaulis,* (IZ 1) dog skin isolate).[3546] (E)-cinnamaldehyde, thymol, and carvacrol displayed the strongest activity of isolated constituents against dermatophytes. (E)-cinnamaldehyde, eugenol, carvacrol, geraniol, and thymol were most active against IZ 1.

☐ Spray drying chitosan microparticles (to improve stability) with copaiba (51.5% beta-caryophyllene) or geranium essential oil improved their inhibition of acetylcholinesterase, suggesting they may have potential in the management of Alzheimer's disease.[3547]

☐ A study found that laser light and mycorrhizal co-treatment improved the essential oil production and antimicrobial activity of geranium plants when compared to controls.[3548] Both geraniol and citronellol content were significantly increased in co-treated plants. Other key marker constituents that increased after co-treatment include linalool, nerol, citronellyl formate, and geraniol formate. Moreover, the essential oil from co-treated plants exhibited significantly higher activity against *E. coli, S. salivarius, Sa. lutea, B. subtilis, P. aeruginosa,* and *S. aureus.*

☐ Although nanoparticles increase bioavailability of therapeutics, emerging evidence suggests that some nanomaterials have the potential to cause deleterious effects on human health. Women are particularly vulnerable to nanoparticle toxicity. A study evaluated the effects of titanium dioxide nanoparticles on reproductive organs in male rats and whether geranium essential oil is protective against nanotoxicity.[3549] Injection of titanium dioxide nanoparticles triggered sperm abnormalities, decreased sperm motility and total sperm count, decreased sex hormone levels, altered testicular antioxidant/oxidant status, interfered with mRNA expression of steroid-related genes, and caused deleterious changes to testicular, epididymal, and prostate gland tissues. Oral administration of geranium essential oil (75 mg/kg body weight per day for sixty days) significantly restored sperm health, sex hormones, antioxidant capacity, steroid-related gene expression, and protected reproductive tissues.

☐ Anxiety following an operation or other invasive procedure is common and can delay postoperative healing and recovery and interfere with pain management. A placebo-controlled randomize human clinical study compared the effects of geranium and lemon essential oil for anxiety following coronary artery bypass.[3550] One hundred and fifty participants were randomly assigned to inhale geranium, lemon, or sweet almond oil (control group). Three drops of the various oils were placed onto a cloth pinned to the subject's shirts approximately 20 cm from their nose. Subjects inhaled from the cloth for twenty minutes after surgery and state anxiety and physiological indices measured. Both the lemon and geranium oil groups experienced increased arterial blood oxygen saturation levels, but other indices (state anxiety scores, heart rate, and blood pressure) showed that geranium was superior to both lemon and control for decreasing overall anxiety state.

☐ Dysautonomia is a condition characterized by imbalance between sympathetic and parasympathetic nervous system function. It may adversely affect organ/gland function (heart, bladder, pupils, blood vessels, sweat glands, and intestines) and cause mental and physical discomfort. A preclinical model of dysautonomia found that inhaling geranium essential oil balanced sympathetic and parasympathetic nervous system function (enhancing parasympathetic activity, which is associated with recovery and recharging from stress).[3551]

☐ Geranium essential oil was active against acaricide-resistant cattle ticks (*Rhipicephalus annulatus*), while its nanoemulsion and combination with sesame oil were effective at lower concentrations.[3552]

☐ Palestinian geranium essential oil (24.4% citronellol, 15.6% citronellyl formate, 7.7% isomenthone, 7.6% gamma-eudesmol) displayed strong antioxidant activity in the DPPH assay and inhibition of alpha-glucosidase (when compared to Acarbose; a desirable activity to reduce blood sugar spikes after eating a carbohydrate-rich meal), but weak suppression of COX-2 and weak inhibition of lipase and alpha-amylase.[3553] Additionally, the oil strongly inhibited MRSA (more than Ampicillin and Ciprofloxacin) and *C. albicans* (compared with Fluconazole), and exhibited anticancer activity against breast, liver, and cervical cancer cells.

☐ The chemistry and biological activities of Moroccan geranium essential oil were evaluated at three different growing stages—vegetative stage, beginning flowering stage, and full flowering stage.[3554] Interestingly, all stages had menthol (15.8%–20.6%), isogeraniol (9.1%–15.5%), p-menthene (6.7%–10%), and eremophilene (8.2%–9.0%) as the major constituents. The best antioxidant activity was observed from the full flowering stage oil (highest menthol and lowest isogeraniol) in the DPPH, FRAP, ABTS, and H2O2 assays, which was moderate compared to ascorbic acid. The full flowering stage oil also showed the greatest antibacterial activity against *L. monocytogenes, S. aureus, B. subtilis, P. mirabilis, E. coli,* and *S. typhimurium.* Significant inhibition of alpha-amylase, alpha-glucosidase, lipase, 5-LOX, and tyrosinase were also observed.

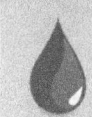

# GERMAN CHAMOMILE
## (German Camomile, Blue Chamomile)

*Matricaria recutita* L., *M. chamomilla* L., *Chamomilla recutita* (L.) Rauschert, *M. suaveolens* L.

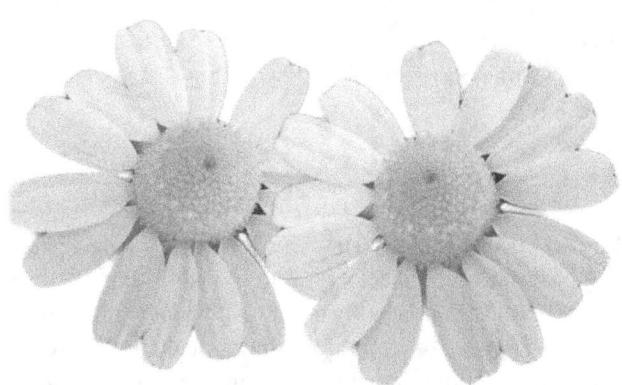

**FAMILY:** Asteraceae (Compositae)
**NOTE:** Middle
**AROMA INTENSITY:** Strong
**AROMA:** Warm, sweet, herbaceous
**COMMON EXTRACTION METHOD:** Steam distilled from the flowers
**POSSIBLE SUBSTITUTE OILS:** Roman chamomile, blue tansy, blue cypress, basil (linalool CT), lavender
**BLENDS WELL WITH:** Bergamot, cassia, cedarwood, eucalyptus, geranium, lavender, neroli, patchouli, pine, ravintsara, rose, silver fir, white fir
**SUBCELLULAR LOCALIZATION | EPIGENETIC INFLUENCE:** Currently unknown | Currently unknown
**RECOMMENDED DILUTION RANGE:** 5%–Neat

**PRIMARY CONSTITUENTS**[3555,3556,3557,3558,3559]

| | |
|---|---|
| Chamazulene | 0.7%–61.3% |
| Bisabolol Oxide A | 3.1%–56.0% |
| Alpha-Bisabolol | 0.1%–44.2% |
| Bisabolol Oxide B | 3.9%–27.2% |
| Cis-Enyne-Bicycloether | 8.8%–26.1% |
| Bisabolone Oxide A | 0.5%–24.8% |
| (Z)-Beta-Farnesene | 0.0%–15.9% |
| (E)-Beta-Farnesene | 2.3%–14.0% |
| Isopropyl Hexadecanoate | 0.0%–12.7% |
| (E,E)-Farnesol | 0.0%–6.9% |
| (E)-Beta-Farnesol | 0.0%–5.2% |
| Decanoic Acid | 0.1%–5.1% |
| Spathulenol | 1.7%–4.8% |

Note: German chamomile composition varies widely based on growing environment. Estonian samples are predominant in bisabolol oxide A; Moldovan, Russian, and Czech Republic samples are predominant in bisabolol oxide A and chamazulene; Armenian samples are predominant in bisabolol oxide B and chamazulene; German samples are predominant in alpha-bisabolol, and Himalayan samples are predominant in bisabolol oxide A and (E)-beta-farnesene. The alpha-bisabolol CT with high trans-beta-farnesene content may be called the Hungarian type and the bisabolol oxide A CT may be called the Egyptian type.

**OTHER CONSTITUENTS:** Artemisia ketone, alpha-eudesmol, geranyl tiglate, gamma-muurolene, germacrene D

**PREFERRED COMPOSITION FOR CLINICAL USE:**

| Constituent | Bisabolol Oxide A CT | Alpha-Bisabolol CT | (E)-Beta-Farnesene CT |
|---|---|---|---|
| **Bisabolol Oxide A** | 35%–55% | see below | 5%–20% |
| **(E)-Beta-Farnesene** | 10%–25% | 15%–40% | 40%–57% |
| **Bisabolol Oxide B** | 3%–15% | see below | 2%–8% |
| **Cis-Enyne-Bicycloether (Cis-Spiroether)** | 3%–10% | > 0.1% | – |
| **Alpha-Bisabolol** | 0.1%–10% | 30%–60% | 0.5%–2% |
| **Bisabolone Oxide A** | 2%–8% | – | 0%–5% |
| **Chamazulene** | 2%–7% | 1%–15% | 0.5%–5% |

| Spathulenol | 0.1%–5% | – | 0.1%–3% |
|---|---|---|---|
| Decanoic Acid | 0%–5% | – | – |
| (E,E)-Alpha-Farnesene | < 3% | 0.1%–7% | 5%–15% |
| Germacrene D | < 3% | 0.5%–5% | 2%–6% |
| Bicyclogermacrene | < 3% | 0.1%–5% | 0%–9% |
| Bisabolol Oxide A + B | – | 5%–25% | – |

**REPORTED THERAPEUTIC PROPERTIES:** Analgesic (pain relief), **anti-inflammatory**, **muscle relaxant**, **antispasmodic**, antibacterial, antioxidant, **expels excess gas**, reduces fever, **antirheumatic**, antiallergenic, **antiarthritic**, stimulates liver and gallbladder function, **antineuralgic**, antiseptic, antidepressant, **antifungal**, eases nausea, **relieves colic**, **reduces the appearance of scars and blemishes**, **reduces painful menstruation**, nervine (calms and soothes the nerves), **aids digestion**, wound healing, calming, sedating, helps eliminate anger and frustration, **stress management**, reduces anxiety, **reduces tantrums**

**CAUTIONS:**

■ May interfere with the enzymes responsible for metabolizing medications (NSAIDs, proton-pump inhibitors, acetaminophen, antiepileptics, immune modulators, blood-sugar medications, blood pressure medications, antidepressants, antipsychotics, diabetic medications, antihistamines, antibiotics, and anesthetics).[3560]

■ May interact with aspirin, blood pressure, antiplatelet, and anticoagulant medications, and increase the risk of bleeding among people with bleeding disorders.[3561,3562,3563]

■ May interact with anticholinergic (drugs used for asthma, incontinence, gastrointestinal cramps, muscular spasms, depression, and sleep disorders) and cholinergic medications (drugs used to reduce urinary retention, diagnose myasthenia gravis, and for glaucoma) based on alpha-bisabolol content.[3564]

**SELECTED EVIDENCE:**

□ *In vitro* research suggests that German chamomile strongly inhibits the growth of colon carcinoma cells through disrupting DNA replication (inhibits DNA polymerase alpha and beta).[3565]

□ German chamomile oil killed two myeloid leukemia cell lines *in vitro*.[3566]

□ A medical hypothesis concluded that German chamomile was an effective natural option for migraine headache relief based on its neuroprotective and anti-inflammatory effects.[3567]

□ A very small observational study concluded that German chamomile is slightly effective for some symptoms (hyperactivity, inattention, and immaturity) of attention-deficit hyperactivity disorder (ADHD).[3568] Two 14- to 16-year-old males with ADHD for at least 6 years consumed tablets—containing 190 mg of German chamomile and 100 mg of alpha-bisabolol—three times daily for four weeks, and then placebo for four weeks, or vice versa. Improvements in symptoms were not equivalent to stimulant drugs but similar to non-stimulants.

□ German chamomile inhibits mast cell degranulation (when mast cells degranulate they rapidly release proinflammatory molecules like histamine and TNF-alpha), which is beneficial to a number of allergic responses and conditions.[3569]

□ Animal research suggests that German chamomile kills the parasitic worm anisakis that infects the stomach and intestines and causes abdominal pain, nausea, intestinal obstruction, and intestinal tract damage.[3570]

□ German chamomile has stronger antioxidant activity than vitamin C, vitamin E, and the synthetic antioxidant butylated hydroxytoluene (BHT).[3571] It also acts as a food preservative an increases antioxidant activity when added to yogurt.[3572]

□ Animal research suggests that German chamomile calms an increased sensitivity to pain (hyperalgesia) and reduces edema caused by inflammatory conditions (through reduced histamine response).[3573]

□ Alpha-bisabolol decreases pain and excess inflammation by decreasing leukocyte activity, TNF-alpha production, and neutrophil degranulation (a common feature of inflammatory disorders) in rodents.[3574]

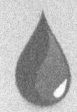

- German chamomile helps decrease inflammation by moderately inhibiting the 5-lipoxygenase (5-LOX) enzyme that is involved in the inflammation response according to *in vitro* research.[3575]

- *In vitro* research suggests that German chamomile prevents oxidative DNA damage to reproductive cells in mice.[3576]

- Animal research suggests that alpha-bisabolol protects the gastrointestinal system against ulcers caused by ethanol and indomethacin (an NSAID).[3577]

- German chamomile prevented the mutagenic (the ability to cause changes in genetic material) action of daunorubicin (a chemotherapeutic drug used to treat lymphocytic and myelocytic leukemias) and methyl methanesulfonate (an alkylating and cancer-causing agent) in mouse bone marrow.[3578]

- Alpha-bisabolol inhibits *L. infantum*, which makes it a promising natural remedy for leishmaniasis (a disease caused by protozoan parasites characterized by skin sores (cutaneous) or organ dysfunction (visceral)).[3579]

- *In vitro* research suggests that German chamomile is highly active against herpes simplex virus type 1 (HSV-1) and prevents the virus from attaching to cells.[3580]

- *In vitro* research suggests that German chamomile inhibits herpes simplex virus type 2 (HSV-2) by interacting with the viral envelope (a lipid bilayer that surrounds the virus and contains proteins that allow the virus to bind to healthy cells).[3581] This activity makes it a promising natural remedy for the treatment for genital herpes.

- Oral administration of German chamomile essential oil or ethyl acetate extract demonstrated that it possesses antipruritic properties (itching caused by sunburn, allergic reactions, chronic skin conditions, insect bites, and microorganism infection) in mice.[3582]

- *In vitro* research suggests that German chamomile oil inhibits various streptococci strains (*S. mutans, S. salivarius, S. faecalis,* and *S. sanguis*) at low concentrations.[3583] Other research suggests that German chamomile essential oil supports oral health by inhibiting *P. gingivalis*, which is a periopathogen associated with periodontitis (a serious gum infection that causes inflammation of the oral cavity and damages or destroys the soft tissue and bone that support the teeth).[3584]

- *In vitro* research discovered that German chamomile oil inhibited *H. pylori* growth (a bacterium strongly associated with stomach ulcers) at extraordinarily low concentrations.[3585]

- German chamomile oil reduces excess inflammation by modulating leukocyte chemotaxis (the movement of leukocytes from the blood to tissues, which causes increased inflammation).[3586] Leukocytes travel to the site of damaged tissue to encourage tissue repair; however, when they migrate excessively to the area it causes an abnormal inflammatory response.

- *In vitro* and animal research suggests that German chamomile accelerated the wound-healing process.[3587]

- Alpha-bisabolol triggers the internal apoptotic (self-destruction) process of glioma (a tumor that begins in the supportive tissue of the brain) cancer cells *in vitro*.[3588]

- *In vitro* research demonstrates that German chamomile essential oil is effective against *L. amazonensis*.[3589]

- A randomized double-blind placebo-controlled clinical trial evaluated the benefits of topical German chamomile CT bisabolene oxide essential oil in people with mild to moderate carpal tunnel syndrome.[3590] Eighty-six subjects were randomly divided into the intervention group or a placebo group that used 10% sesame oil in paraffin with 0.1% chamomile oil to simulate the aroma. Five drops of German chamomile oil (diluted in sesame oil) or placebo were applied to the palmar area of the wrist every morning and evening for four weeks and both groups used a standard wrist splint at night. At the end of the four weeks the German chamomile group experienced significant improvements in symptom severity and functionality when compared to placebo. In addition, the German chamomile oil improved median nerve activity and function.

- German chamomile (bisabolol oxides CT) was cytotoxic to colon cancer cells *in vitro*.[3591]

- Oral administration of German chamomile essential oil reduced systolic and diastolic blood pressure in rats with normal blood pressure levels.[3592]

- A randomized, double-blind, placebo-controlled, crossover clinical trial of 100 people reported that a German chamomile oleogel (standardized to chamazulene content) significantly reduced migraine symptoms (pain, nausea, vomiting, and light and sound sensitivity) in people that experience migraine without aura.[3593] When a migraine attack started, 2mL of the oleogel (10% chamomile oil; 57.4% bisabolene oxide A 14.3% bisabolol oxide A, 9.8% chamazulene) was rubbed into the temples, forehead, and behind the ears, twice.

- German chamomile essential oil (composition not reported) demonstrated the ability to prevent root canal

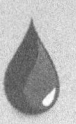 

infections by inhibiting *Enterococcus faecalis*.[3594] The activity was sustained for fourteen days and comparable to chlorhexidine. Vetiver essential oil was the most effective after day one, but its activity was not sustained.

☐ An interesting CT of German chamomile from Iran (42.8% and 40.1% (E)- and (Z)-gamma-bisabolene respectively) demonstrated more potent antioxidant activity than alpha-bisabalone oxide A CTs in the DPPH assay.[3595]

☐ Nanoencapsulated German chamomile essential oil was active against *L. amazonensis* promastigotes and intracellular amastigotes while the nanoecapsulation reduced the oil's toxicity to healthy cells.[3596] Based on the results, the researchers concluded that German chamomile in nanocapsules using an alkylated chitosan biosurfactant represents "a promising therapeutic strategy to treat leishmaniasis."

☐ Approximately 12 percent of the population (children and adults) experience painful and debilitating migraines. Migraines are complex and their exact cause and trigger are not known. Inflammation in the nervous system (neurogenic inflammation), dilation of blood vessels on the surface of the brain, and alterations in neurochemicals and neuropeptides (serotonin, nitric oxide, endothelin, CGRP) are some of the abnormal brain activities associated with migraines. A recent review article concluded that lavender, peppermint, German chamomile, anise, basil CT estragole, rose, and garlic essential oils were useful for migraines.[3597] They further identified constituents in these oils that contribute to relief of factors that contribute to migraines: menthol (pain relief, reduces neurogenic inflammation), borneol (relaxes blood vessels, reduces neurogenic inflammation), 1,8-cineole (dilates blood vessels, reduces neurogenic inflammation, inhibits CNS pain), linalool/linalyl acetate (reduces neurogenic inflammation, inhibits CNS pain), menthone (reduces neurogenic inflammation), limonene (pain relief, reduces neurogenic inflammation, balances vasomotor abnormalities), alpha-pinene (reduces neurogenic inflammation), beta-elemene (reduces neurogenic inflammation), beta-caryophyllene (reduces neurogenic inflammation, balances vasomotor abnormalities), trans-anethole (reduces neurogenic inflammation, balances vasomotor abnormalities), diallyl trisulfide (reduces neurogenic inflammation), estragole (reduces neurogenic inflammation, balances vasomotor abnormalities), and citronellol (relaxes blood vessels, reduces neurogenic inflammation, reduces excess pain response).

☐ Important life changes that occur as we get older—retirement, loneliness, serious illness or chronic health condition, death of a loved one—can increase feelings of sadness, nervousness, and stress. This can reduce overall health and quality of life. Inhalation of Spanish lavender or German chamomile essential oil improved depression, anxiety, and stress in older community-dwelling adults.[3598] As part of the randomized controlled trial, 3 drops of a 1.5% dilution were applied to a cotton ball and pinned to the participant's pillowcase every night at bedtime for thirty consecutive nights. Depression, anxiety, and stress scores improved immediately following inhalation of the oils and continued for the thirty days after the intervention. This suggests that inhaling Spanish lavender or German chamomile may improve the quality of life and health of older adults.

☐ Chitosan nanocapsules with German chamomile essential oil was active against *L. amazonensis* promastigotes and intracellular amastigotes, and the nanocapsules reduced the oils toxicity toward healthy cells.[3599]

☐ Urinary tract infections (UTIs) are among the most common bacterial infections. They occur when bacteria present on the skin or rectum enter the urethra, infecting the urinary tract and triggering inflammation. Common bacteria that cause UTIs include *Escherichia coli, Pseudomonas aeruginosa, Staphylococcus epidermidis, Staphylococcus saprophyticus*, and *Enterococcus faecalis*, with *E. coli* being the most common. Of five essential oils tested (German chamomile, thyme, juniper, Spanish sage, and sage) the best inhibitory activity in vapor phase was observed for German chamomile.[3600] Thyme was also active against all tested bacteria. Interestingly, mixtures of sage or Spanish sage with German chamomile decreased the activity of the individual oils.

☐ Comparing the contact toxicity and repellent effects of eight essential oils and carrier oils (clove bud, garlic, *Eucalyptus camaldulensis*, lavender, German chamomile, lemon, jojoba, and sweet almond) against the red flour beetle (*Tribolium castaneum*), clove bud essential oil exhibited the highest repellency effect, while garlic, German chamomile, and lemon were the most toxic.[3601]

☐ German chamomile essential oil (16.4% camphor, 10.0% delta-3-carene, 8.0% myrcene, 6.5% chamazulene) grown in Morocco displayed antioxidant activity in the DPPH assay, which was improved by combining with honey.[3602] A high anti-inflammatory activity was also observed when the oil was combined with honey (exceeding the reference drug indomethacin). The oil alone showed high antimicrobial activity against *S. aureus, A. niger,* and *C. albicans,* and inhibited *E. coli, P. mirabilis, S. enterica* Typhimurium, *P. aeruginosa, L. monocytogenes,* and *T. rubrum*. The oil also inhibited alpha-glucosidase and alpha-amylase suggesting antidiabetic activity—mixing with honey reduced this activity.

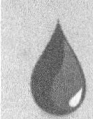

□ A randomized controlled clinical trial found that inhalation of German chamomile essential oil—1 drop of a 5% dilution at four, eight, and twelve hours post-cesarean surgery—for fifteen to twenty minutes significantly reduced pain intensity compared to control (which inhaled a similar smelling and colored placebo).[3603]

□ Investigation of essential oils from the Apiaceae, Asteraceae, Cupressaceae, and Lamiaceae families grown in Serbia showed that German chamomile CT bisabolol oxide essential oil was the most effective DPPH radical scavenger, followed by thyme CT thymol, summer savory CT carvacrol, and sweet basil.[3604] Peppermint CT carvone oil was the strongest in the ABTS assay.

□ Three separate German chamomile CT bisabolol oxide B essential oils samples significantly reduced inflammation by inhibiting inducible nitric oxide, TNF-α, and IL-6 production in macrophages and decreasing activation of CD4+ T cells (these cells are involved in the pathogenesis of inflammatory conditions).[3605] The oils also increased glutamate-cysteine ligase and heme oxygenase-1 antioxidant enzymes expression leading to the rapid scavenging of reactive oxygen species (oxidative stress can trigger macrophages activation and elicit strong immune and inflammatory responses).

□ Diffusion of 3 drops of lavender or German chamomile essential oil beginning twenty minutes before bedtime for two weeks improved sleep quality of pregnant women during their third trimester.[3606] Lavender was the most effective.

# GHANDI ROOT
## (Sugandh Mantri)

*Homalomena aromatica* Schott.

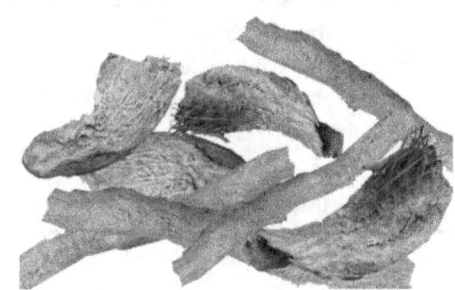

**FAMILY:** Araceae (Compositae)
**NOTE:** Base
**AROMA INTENSITY:** Medium
**AROMA:** Earthy, woody, spicy, balsamic, slightly floral
**COMMON EXTRACTION METHOD:** Steam distilled or hydrodistilled from the rhizomes
**POSSIBLE SUBSTITUTE OILS:** Rosewood, saro, magnolia (flowers), lavender, coriander
**BLENDS WELL WITH:** Agarwood, cedarwood, copaiba, frankincense, lavandin, lavender, patchouli, rosewood, sandalwood, spikenard
**SUBCELLULAR LOCALIZATION | EPIGENETIC INFLUENCE:** Currently unknown | Currently unknown
**RECOMMENDED DILUTION RANGE:** 5%–Neat

**PRIMARY CONSTITUENTS:**[3607,3608,3609,3610,3611]

| | |
|---|---|
| Linalool | 32.4%–71.2% |
| Terpinen-4-ol | 4.6%–16.7% |
| Sabinene | 0.0%–8.3% |
| Delta-Cadinene | 0.1%–5.6% |
| T-Muurolol | 0.0%–5.3% |
| Alpha-Cadinol | 0.0%–3.7% |
| Viridiflorol | 0.0%–3.7% |
| Linalyl Acetate | 0.0%–3.3% |

**OTHER CONSTITUENTS:** Delta-3-carene, beta-pinene, limonene, gamma-terpinene, alpha-phellandrene, beta-caryophyllene, beta-elemene, alpha-selinene, m-cymene, gamma-muurolene, alpha-muurolene, beta-copaene, alpha-terpineol, cedrenol, geraniol, nerol, spathulenol, T-cadinol, cis-linalool oxide, trans-linalool oxide, cryptone, humulene epoxide II, oplopanone

**PREFERRED COMPOSITION FOR CLINICAL USE:**

| Constituent | |
|---|---|
| **Linalool** | 40%–65% |
| **Terpinen-4-ol** | 5%–15% |
| **Cadinene <delta + gamma>** | 0.5%–6% |
| **Para-Cymene** | 1%–5% |

| Alpha-Terpineol | 0.5%–5% |
|---|---|
| Sabinene | 0.5%–3% |
| Geraniol | 0.1%–2% |

**REPORTED THERAPEUTIC PROPERTIES:** Analgesic, anti-inflammatory, antirheumatic, antispasmodic, nervine, anticancer, antibacterial, **antifungal**, anti-infectious, aids immune function, relieves hemorrhoids, relieves chronic skin conditions, insecticide, insect repellent, encourages restful sleep, relieves anxiety, antidepressant, aids meditation, **stress management**, aphrodisiac

**CAUTIONS:**

■ May interact with antifungal drugs and enhance their effectiveness based on linalool content.[3612]

**SELECTED EVIDENCE:**

☐ *In vitro* research demonstrated that Ghandi root essential oil strongly inhibits the dermatophytes and fungi *Trichophyton rubrum, Trichophyton mentagrophytes, Microsporum fulvum, Microsporum gypseum, Trichosporon beigelii,* and *Candida albicans.*[3613] Another study found that it is highly effective against *C. pallescens* and significantly prevented mycelial growth of *A. niger* and *F. graminearum*, but only weakly inhibited *F. solani.*[3614]

☐ Ghandi root essential oil kills the white termite (*Odontotermes obesus* Rhamb.).[3615] It also repelled the blackfly (100% repellency at 5% concentration for two hours; 100% at 7.5% concentration for three hours; 90% at 10% concentration for six hours).[3616]

☐ Nanoencapsulated Ghandi root essential oil (68.5% linalool) inhibited fungal infestation (*A. flavus*), aflatoxin B1 production, lipid peroxidation, and mineral loss *in situ* and was safe in mice.[3617]

# GINGER

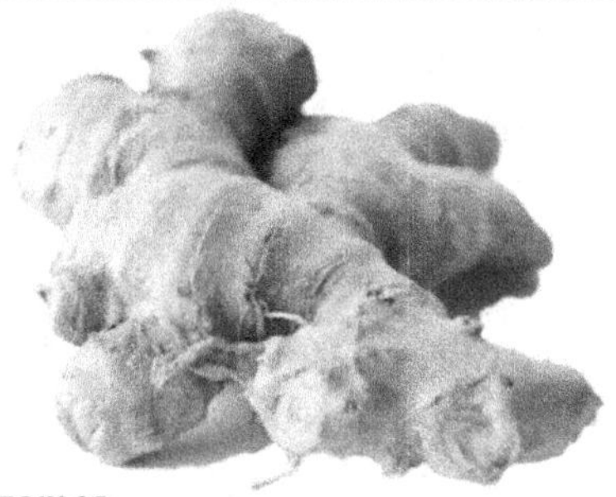

*Zingiber officinale* Roscoe, *Amomum zingiber* L.

**FAMILY:** Zingiberaceae
**NOTE:** Middle-Base
**AROMA INTENSITY:** Medium
**AROMA:** Earthy, woody, sweet, warm
**COMMON EXTRACTION METHOD:** Steam distilled or hydrodistilled from the rhizomes
**POSSIBLE SUBSTITUTE OILS:** Turmeric, melissa
**BLENDS WELL WITH:** Bay laurel, bergamot, camphor, cardamom, carrot seed, cassia, cedarwood, clove, coriander, eucalyptus, fennel, frankincense, galbanum, geranium, grapefruit, lemon, lime, neroli, nutmeg, orange, oregano, patchouli, ravensara, rose, sandalwood, tangerine, turmeric, vetiver
**SUBCELLULAR LOCALIZATION | EPIGENETIC INFLUENCE:** Endocytic Vesicles | Lymphatic/Endocrine
**RECOMMENDED DILUTION RANGE:** 3%–50%; neat for limited conditions

**PRIMARY CONSTITUENTS:**[3618,3619,3620,3621,3622,3623,3624,3625]

| *Alpha-Zingiberene CT* | | *Citral CT (Australian)* * | |
|---|---|---|---|
| Alpha-Zingiberene | 5.7%–32.2% | Geranial | 17.5%–44.3% |
| Geranial | 1.2%–20.1% | Neral | 10.6%–26.5% |
| Geranyl Acetate | 0.0%–18.8% | Alpha-Zingiberene | 1.9%–11.2% |
| Beta-Sesquiphellandrene | 1.9%–18.4% | Beta-Sesquiphellandrene | 2.9%–9.4% |
| ar-Curcumene | 1.9%–16.7% | Geraniol | 1.5%–7.3% |
| (E)-Beta-Farnesene | 0.0%–14.7% | ar-Curcumene | 2.4%–5.7% |
| Geraniol | 0.0%–14.5% | (E,E)-Alpha-Farnesene | 2.1%–4.4% |
| ar-Turmerone | 0.0%–12.8% | Beta-Bisabolene | 1.0%–4.1% |
| Camphene | 0.6%–12.7% | * Not commonly available. Follow cautions for | |
| 1,8-Cineole | 0.2%–10.9% | lemongrass for this CT. | |

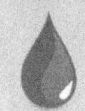

| | |
|---|---|
| Neral | 2.6%–9.4% |
| Beta-Bisabolene | 0.0%–7.8% |
| (E,E)-Alpha-Farnesene | 0.0%–7.0% |
| Borneol | 0.0%–5.6% |
| Linalool | 0.0%–4.8% |
| Beta-Phellandrene | 0.2%–4.3% |

**OTHER CONSTITUENTS:** *Alpha-Zingiberene CT*—Alpha-pinene, sabinene, octenal, alpha-phellandrene, delta-3-carene, alpha-terpinene, para-cymene, d-limonene, gamma-terpinene, alpha-copaene, citronellal, camphor, alpha-terpineol, nerol, carveol, 2-undecanone, neryl acetate, delta-elemene, alpha-bergamotene, germacrene D, alpha muurolene, delta-cadinene, (Z)-nerolidol, elemol, eudesma-3,7(11)-diene, (E)-nerolidol, cubenol, beta-guaiacol, sesquisabinene hydrate, zingerone, alpha-curcumene, beta-curcumene, alpha-muurolol, beta-bisabolol, eudesma-7(11)-en-4-ol, (Z)-alpha-bergamotol, (Z,Z)-farnesol, (Z,E)-farnesol, (E,E)-farnesol, (Z)-lanceol; *Citral CT*—6-Methyl-5-hepten-2-one, myrcene, beta-phellandrene, 1,8-cineole, linalool, borneol, alpha-terpineol, citronellol, 2-undecanone, citronellyl acetate, geranyl acetate, germacrene D, (E)-nerolidol, elemol

**PREFERRED COMPOSITION FOR CLINICAL USE:**

| *Constituent* | |
|---|---|
| **Alpha-Zingiberene** | 25%–45% |
| **Beta-Sesquiphellandrene** | 5%–15% |
| **ar-Curcumene** | 4%–15% |
| **Camphene** | 5%–13% |
| **(E,E)-Alpha-Farnesene** | 3%–11% |
| **1,8-Cineole** | 0.1%–10% |
| **Beta-Bisabolene** | 4%–9% |
| **Beta-Phellandrene** | 3%–8% |
| **Geranial** | tr–7% |
| **Neral** | tr–7% |

Note: Citral (geranial/neral) is not present in all samples. Lower or no citral may be preferred to reduce a strong lemony aroma. Distillation of fresh roots will often produce greater percentages of alpha-zingiberene.

**REPORTED THERAPEUTIC PROPERTIES:** **Analgesic (pain relief)**, **bronchodilator**, anticancer, **anti-inflammatory**, antispasmodic, antineuralgic, antibacterial, antioxidant, antiseptic, aphrodisiac, astringent, **expels excess gas**, relieves menstrual cramps, **eases nausea and vomiting**, aids normal respiration, **aids digestion**, diuretic, expectorant, **relieves constipation and diarrhea**, eases sports injuries, aids circulation, stimulating, promotes courage and motivation, encourages feelings of balance and stability, reduces mental fatigue

**CAUTIONS:**
■ May interact with aspirin, blood pressure, antiplatelet, and anticoagulant medications, and increase the risk of bleeding among people with bleeding disorders.[3626,3627]
■ May interfere with the enzymes responsible for metabolizing medications (NSAIDs, proton-pump inhibitors, acetaminophen, antiepileptics, immune modulators, blood-sugar medications, blood pressure medications, antidepressants, antipsychotics, diabetic medications, antihistamines, antibiotics, and anesthetics).[3628]

**SELECTED EVIDENCE:**
☐ A twice weekly, thirty-minute ginger oil massage (for five weeks total) significantly reduced low back pain and disability (both long- and short-term effectiveness) among 140 study participants.[3629]
☐ Massaging ginger and orange oil to the knees of older adults six times over a three-week period relieved moderate-to-severe knee pain and increased physical function in the short-term.[3630]
☐ Ginger oil modulates enzymatic activity to prevent genetic damage and cancer caused by carcinogens in rats.[3631]

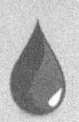 

- Ginger oil triggers bronchodilation (dilates the bronchi and bronchioles to improve airflow to the lungs) possibly by stimulating the beta-adrenergic receptor, which improves breathing in people with chronic respiratory diseases.[3632]
- Ginger oil reduced the production of proinflammatory constituents released during respiratory infections *in vitro*.[3633] An *in vitro* study reported that ginger essential oil exerted anti-inflammatory effects by inhibiting lipoxygenase enzymes as well as quercetin.[3634] Lipoxygenase enzymes are involved in the development of breast, prostate, and colorectal cancers when overexpressed.[3635]
- *In vitro* and animal research discovered that ginger oil reduces inflammation by preventing the migration of excess leukocytes from the blood to tissues.[3636] Leukocytes travel to the site of damaged tissue to encourage tissue repair; however, when they migrate excessively to the area it causes an abnormal inflammatory response.
- Animal research demonstrates that ginger essential oil (injection of 28 mg/kg) prevents chronic joint inflammation in a model of rheumatoid arthritis, but does not affect acute joint swelling.[3637]
- Animal research suggests ginger oil modulates the immune system, influences cell-mediated immune responses, enhances T lymphocyte production, and restores humoral immune responses after drug-induced immunosuppression.[3638,3639,3640] Another study concluded that ginger oil improves immune system activity (lymphocyte numbers) among people who are receiving chemotherapy.[3641]
- An aromatic bath with ginger oil may shorten the second stage of maternal labor by accelerating contractions, increasing cervical dilation, and decreasing pain.[3642]
- Ginger oil may significantly prevent DNA from bonding to cancer-causing chemicals (DNA adduct formation) and therefore help prevent cancer.[3643]
- Inhalation of ginger oil may reduce the frequency and severity of nausea and vomiting, and the need for drugs used to treat nausea and vomiting.[3644] Another study concluded that inhalation of ginger alone or in combination with spearmint, peppermint, and cardamom (three deep inhalations) from a gauze pad following surgery reduced nausea and requirements for medications to reduce nausea and vomiting.[3645]
- Low doses of ginger and lemon oil prevented lipid peroxidation of the membranes and the premature destruction (hemolysis) of red blood cells in mice.[3646] The same researchers discovered that ginger and lemon oil prevent lipid peroxidation of the lipids within the brain and liver. *In vitro* research demonstrates that ginger essential oil is a strong antioxidant and inhibits the excess production of nitric oxide.[3647]
- *In vitro* research discovered that ginger oil prevents HSV-2 infection of healthy cells at an effective rate greater than 90%, and it was highly selective (kill bacteria without harming host cells).[3648] Another study determined that ginger oil possesses high levels of activity against both drug-resistant and non-drug-resistant HSV-1.[3649]
- Ginger oil significantly reduces stomach ulcers (up to 85.1%) caused by ethanol in rodents (rats).[3650]
- Animal research suggests that oral administration of ginger oil protects the liver and reverses fatty liver caused by alcohol.[3651]
- Ginger oil significantly reduces both spontaneous and PGF2alpha-induced uterine contractions in rats.[3652] PGF2-alpha is a natural prostaglandin that stimulates uterine contractions, and as a pharmaceutical (dinoprost) is used to induce abortions in animals.
- *In vitro* research discovered that ginger oil inhibited *H. pylori* growth (a bacterium strongly associated with stomach ulcers) in extraordinarily low concentrations.[3653]
- Ginger essential oil and some of its constituents (beta-pinene, terpinolene, alpha-phellandrene, and alpha-copaene) inhibit the 5-HT3 receptor channel system and reduce intestinal spasms in rats.[3654] Drugs that inhibit this receptor channel system help reduce nausea and vomiting, and treat irritable bowel syndrome, fibromyalgia, anxiety, substance abuse, eating disorders, and neurological disorders.
- Animal research suggests that acetone extracts of ginger, which contain volatile oils, increases the speed at which food moves from the gastrointestinal system (gastrointestinal motility) similar to a drug used to treat gastroesophageal reflux disease (metoclopramide) and domperidone (a drug used to increase peristalsis).[956]
- A mixture of honokiol, magnolol, and ginger oil reduced depressive symptoms in rats by regulating serotonin production.[3655,3656]
- *In vitro* research demonstrated that low doses of marjoram, lemon, basil, clove, thyme, rosemary CT 1,8-cineole, and tea tree essential oils prevented the shortening of telomeres after exposure to hydrogen

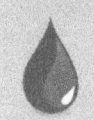

peroxide.[3657] The same research reported that vetiver, black pepper, eucalyptus (*E. globulus*), ginger, clove, and rosemary increased the length of already shortened telomeres. This activity suggests that these essential oils can help maintain the youth and health of cells, or turn back the clock on the cell to make it more youthful depending on the essential oil used. Interestingly, cinnamon and peppermint essential oil decreased the length of telomeres slightly.

☐ Ginger essential oil inhibits *Aspergillus* species and their subsequent production of mycotoxins.[3658]

☐ A review study of nurse-delivered aromatherapy in acute care settings reported that the use of essential oils generally resulted in significant clinical improvements based on their intended use. Marjoram and tangerine essential oils reduced pain, lavender and marjoram essential oil reduced anxiety, and ginger alleviated nausea.[3659]

☐ Patients in the post-anesthesia recovery unit who inhaled ginger essential oil from an aromatherapy necklace

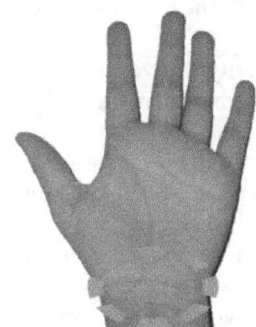

they wore for 24 hours (containing 0.3 mL of ginger essential oil) experienced reduced nausea and vomiting after major abdominal surgery. The intervention caused no side effects and the average person inhaled 0.15 mL of the oil over 24 hours.[3660] Another clinical investigation reported that a topical application of 5% solution (diluted in grapeseed carrier oil and added to a roller bottle) of ginger essential oil to the volar side (the portion of the wrist below the palm; 4x4 cm$^2$ area of application) of the wrist prior to anesthesia reduced postoperative nausea and vomiting (PONV) in people at high risk for PONV.[3661]

☐ Ginger essential oil demonstrated 85.7%–94.0% efficacy against the *Rhipicephalus microplus* tick depending on the concentration used (1%–10%).[3662]

☐ A randomized controlled trial demonstrated that an aromatic bath with a blend of 1.0 mL of lemon and 0.5 mL ginger essential oils (10 minutes before each meal for two weeks) prevented salivary gland damage and dysfunction caused by radioactive iodine therapy for thyroid cancer.[3663]

☐ Injection of ginger essential oil (2.5 g/kg of BW) or rosemary essential oil (2.5 g/kg of BW)—or 5 mg/kg of body weight combined ginger and rosemary—in rats reversed reductions in HDL cholesterol, and elevations in blood glucose, total cholesterol, and triglycerides caused by a high-fat diet.[3664]

☐ Both lemon and ginger essential oils prevented the formation of biofilms by *Klebsiella* species (*K. ornithinolytica, K. oxytoca* and *K. terrigena*).[3665]

☐ A ginger essential oil with higher citral content (19%) was cytotoxic to colon cancer cells *in vitro*.[3666]

☐ Ginger essential oil (gingerol CT) demonstrated strong activity against *Shigella, E. hirae, E. coli, Citrobacter freundii, A. flavus,* and *C. albicans* when compared to tetracycline and clotrimazole.[3667] Interestingly, this gingerol CT of ginger was more active against microbes than oregano (15.9% carvacrol) and black cumin (6.9%) essential oil.

☐ Ginger essential oil CT camphene killed cervical cancer cells *in vitro* even at the lowest concentration tested (32.12 mcg/mL).[3668]

☐ Ginger essential oil (methyl lineolate as the major constituent) inhibits drug-resistant *P. aeruginosa* isolated from burn wound infections according to *in vitro* research.[3669]

☐ Oral administration of 50, 100, or 150 mcL/kg of ginger essential oil reduced lipid peroxidation in reproductive tissues and improved fertility traits in Japanese quail.[3670]

☐ Ginger essential oil may lighten the skin due to its suppression of melanin production, inhibition of tyrosinase and melanogenesis-related proteins, and antioxidant properties (improve the activities of GSH, SOD and CAT).[3671] Tyrosinase is an enzyme involved in the production of melanin (a dark brown to black pigment that is responsible for tanning of skin when exposed to sunlight) by oxidation of tyrosine.

☐ A nanoemulsion ginger essential oil enhanced the cytotoxic activity of mitomycin C against breast cancer cells; similarly, a frankincense (species not identified) nanoemulsion essential oil enhanced the activity of mitomycin C against cervical cancer cells.[3672]

☐ Both ginger and turmeric (76.5% 1,8-cineole) essential oil protected against kidney damage caused by cadmium by reducing inflammation (reduced cytokines: IL-6, IL-10 and TNF-α) and renal adenosine deaminase (ADA) activity.[3673]

☐ Ginger essential oil exhibited antifungal and antimycotoxigenic activities against *F. graminearum*.[3674]

☐ Growing evidence suggest that inflammation plays a role in the pathogenesis of neurological diseases such as Alzheimer's disease, Parkinson's disease, depression, Huntington's disease, amyotrophic lateral sclerosis, stroke and traumatic brain injuries.[3675,3676] Ginger and turmeric CT 1,8-cineole essential oils reduced cadmium-induced neuroinflammation by preventing alterations in cytokines and inflammatory biomarkers (IL-6, IL-10 and TNF-α) and inhibiting both hippocampus and prefrontal cortex acetylcholinesterase (AChE) and adenosine deaminase (ADA) activities (important enzymes relevant in the management/prevention of neurodegenerative diseases).[3677] Both ginger and turmeric were administered to rats orally at a dose of 50 mg/kg body weight daily for fourteen days.

☐ A randomized placebo-controlled study found that inhalation of lavender or ginger essential oil reduced postoperative nausea.[3678] Interestingly, lavender was more effective (82.6% reduction) than ginger (65.2% reduction), while rose oil was similar to placebo (47.8%, 43.5% respectively).

☐ Both ginger and eucalyptus (*E. globulus*) essential oils demonstrated considerable insecticidal and repellent activity against the *Culex theileri* mosquito, with eucalyptus being the most effective.[3679]

☐ Ginger essential oil exhibited virucidal activity against the caprine alphaherpesvirus 1 (CpHV-1) as demonstrated by inactivation of up to 100% of virus before it infected cells.[3680] The CpHV-1 virus is used in animal research to study HSV-2 infection and genital herpes.

☐ Ginger essential oil (15.2% curcumene and 13.5% linalool) reduced the severity of liver toxicity caused by diethylnitrosamine (a toxic and carcinogenic chemical found in tobacco smoke) in rats.[3681] The same researchers reported that the oil displayed anticancer activity against liver cancer.

☐ A controlled clinical trial found that massaging the knee with a combination of ginger and rosemary essential oils diluted in black cumin seed carrier oil reduced osteoarthritis knee pain and improved knee function and quality of life in elderly individuals.[3682] Ten drops each of ginger and rosemary essential oils were added to 20 mL of black cumin seed carrier oil and massaged into the knee using effleurage and petrissage techniques in the direction of lymph drainage for fifteen to twenty minutes. The massage was repeated three times.

☐ Laboratory research concluded that ginger essential oil possesses antimycobacterial activity against *Mycobacterium* spp. (bacteria that cause series diseases like tuberculosis and leprosy in humans).[3683]

☐ Oral administration of the citral CT of ginger essential oil (300 mg/kg BW) exhibited good antitumor and antioxidant activity in the colorectal region of rats.[3684] The study authors concluded that the cancer preventive properties of ginger essential oil were comparable to the drug 5-Florouracil.

☐ *In vitro* research showed that ginger essential oil possesses antibacterial activity against *S. aureus* and *E. coli* most likely by disrupting the bacterial cell membrane.[3685]

☐ Fixed dental appliances significantly hinder tooth brushing and oral hygiene and contribute to bacterial adhesion and biofilm formation. The formation of biofilms around dental appliances can cause a host of adverse effects including white spot lesions, gingivitis, gingival bleeding, and tooth decay. A clinical study found that use of a mouthwash with 0.5% ginger essential oil for seven days inhibited *S. mutans* (a bacterium that forms biofilms in the mouth and contributes to tooth decay), controlled dental biofilms, and reduced gingival bleeding in people with a fixed orthodontic appliance.[3686]

☐ An interesting verbenol CT of ginger essential oil showed that it inhibits *A. flavus* and its production of aflatoxin B1 by targeting the cell membrane, mitochondria, and carbohydrate catabolism.[3687] Verbenol inhibited structural gene products (Nor-1, Omt-1, and Vbs) of aflatoxin biosynthesis.

☐ The citral CT of ginger essential oil—17.3% geranial, 10.3% neral, 9.6% camphene, 7.6% alpha-zingiberene, 6.8% beta-phellandrene, 6.4% nerol—displayed good antioxidant activity and protected against colon cancer in rats.[3688] The oil presented similar results to the standard drug (5-Florouracil) in slowing cell proliferation.

☐ Cinnamon bark, palmarosa, and ginger essential oil each exhibited good antioxidant activity in the DPPH, ABTS and FRAP assays, with cinnamon being the most effective. Additionally, the oils inhibited the growth of *Fusarium verticillioides* and reduced its production of mycotoxins (fumonisin B1 and B2).[3689] Cinnamon bark and palmarosa were the most effective against *Fusarium verticillioides*.

☐ Trypanosoma cruzi is a parasite that causes Chagas disease in humans. This parasite bores into tissue and feeds on blood and lymph increasing the likelihood of disease. It is most commonly spread through contact with feces from an infected kissing bug (a blood-sucking insect that feeds on animals and humans). Clove and ginger essential oil were evaluated against *T. cruzi* II parasite load in mice, alone and in combination with benznidazole.[3690] The mice were inoculated with 10,000 blood trypomastigotes of *T. cruzi* and then orally treated with benznidazole, cinnamon or ginger essential oil, or benznidazole and cinnamon or ginger oil. A control group was untreated. Ginger and the combination of ginger or cinnamon oil with benznidazole each reduced parasitemia, but clove was not effective alone. However, clove did reduce parasite load. Each individual oil and their combinations with benznidazole reduced parasite load. Ginger not only promoted reduced parasite load but also decreased mortality in the mice that received it.

☐ A clinical study compared the effect of oral ginger herb with topical ginger essential oil in reducing pain and

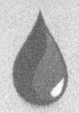

severity of primary dysmenorrhea—menstrual pain in the absence of pelvic disease. Seventy women with moderate to severe primary dysmenorrhea were randomly assigned to receive 250 mg of powdered ginger herb or apply 5 drops of ginger oil to the lower abdomen without massage every six hours from two days before the start of menstruation through the first three days of menstruation. The intervention continued for three menstrual cycles. Both groups experienced reductions in pain severity and duration and need for oral pain relievers (mefenamic acid).[3691] The group that applied the essential oil reported greater reductions in pain severity and the same reduction in pain duration, but a slightly higher need for oral pain-relieving medication, when compared to oral ginger powder.

□ Four varieties of ginger essential oil (high citral content: 12.9%–18.1%) from Malaysia strongly inhibited human cervical cancer cells *in vitro*.[3692]

□ More than half of chemotherapy patients experience nausea and vomiting. A case study of two subjects showed that inhaling ginger (5 to 10 drops from an inhaler stick for five to ten minutes, repeated every thirty minutes for four times) decreased nausea and vomiting scores.[3693]

□ Ginger essential oil inhibited *S. aureus, S. epidermidis, C. tropicalis, P. mirabilis,* and *A. baumannii,* but was inactive against *E. coli, K. pneumoniae,* and *P. aeruginosa*.[3694] The oil also displayed weak antioxidant activity in the DPPH and FRAP assays.

□ Loss of appetite, fatigue, anxiety, and nausea are common complaints of individuals receiving chemotherapy. A controlled clinical trial evaluated the benefits of inhaling a ginger, German chamomile, and bergamot on these common complaints that effect quality of life.[3695] Inhalation of ginger essential oil—7 drops placed on a cotton ball and placed in a bottle to smell from morning, noon, and evening—significant reduced fatigue and anxiety. Surprisingly, bergamot and German chamomile did not have a measurable effect.

□ It is estimated that 40% of individuals aged sixty-five and older experience constipation, which increases to 74% if they live in a nursing home. Left untreated, constipation can cause fecal incontinence, anal fissures, bowel perforation, gas, and bloating. An abdominal massage with lavender and ginger essential oils (diluted to 2% in sweet almond oil) decreased constipation severity, softened stool consistency, and reduced symptoms associated with constipation.[3696] Five mL of the oil blend were massaged into the abdomen for fifteen minutes between 9:30 and 12:00 on five weekdays over the course of four weeks. A control group received no massage.

□ Of sixty-two essential oils tested, ginger essential oil was among the most potent alpha-glucosidase inhibitors (reversible and uncompetitive-type inhibitor).[3697] Inhibition of alpha-glucosidase reduces spikes in blood sugar after consuming carbohydrates suggesting it may be helpful for diabetes.

□ Topical application of ginger essential oil reduced inflammation and swelling better than ibuprofen in mice.[3698] The oil decreased COX-2, IL-6, and NF-$_{\kappa}$B expression and downregulated mRNA expression of IL-6, and NF-$_{\kappa}$B. Additionally, antibacterial activity against *E. coli, P. aeruginosa,* and *S. aureus,* good antioxidant potential in the DPPH assay, and antitumor (lung cancer) properties were observed.

□ Topiramate is a drug used to treat epilepsy and prevent migraines; however, research suggests it may have toxic effects in the brain. A preclinical study found that it triggers neuropathological altercations that increase inflammation and oxidative stress.[3699] Both topiramate and ginger increased mRNA expression of GABA receptors 1 and 3, but interestingly their combination downregulated them. Taking ginger essential oil at the same time with topiramate reduced its potential neurotoxicity.

*Did you know?*

Essential oils are lipophilic, meaning they are attracted to and dissolve in fats. As volatile extracts they contain no fats themselves and do not leave an oil residue. Combining essential oils with a carrier oil improves absorption by reducing volatility.

# GINGERGRASS

*Cymbopogon martinii* Roxb. var. *sofia* Gupta,
*Andropogon martinii* Roxb. var. *sofia* Gupta

**FAMILY:** Poaceae (Gramineae)
**NOTE:** Middle
**AROMA INTENSITY:** Medium
**AROMA:** Spicy, herbaceous, grassy, slightly fruity and floral
**COMMON EXTRACTION METHOD:** Steam distilled from the leaves (grass blades)
**POSSIBLE SUBSTITUTE OILS:** Palmarosa, tsauri grass, lemongrass
**BLENDS WELL WITH:** Agarwood, bergamot, black pepper, cedarwood, elemi, frankincense, geranium, ginger, grapefruit, Japanese cedarwood, lavender, lavandin, lemon, lime, may chang, orange, palmarosa, patchouli, peppermint, rosemary, rosewood, sandalwood, spearmint, vetiver, ylang ylang
**SUBCELLULAR LOCALIZATION | EPIGENETIC INFLUENCE:** Currently unknown | Currently unknown
**RECOMMENDED DILUTION RANGE:** 3%–50%; neat for limited conditions

**PRIMARY CONSTITUENTS:**[3700,3701,3702]

| | |
|---|---|
| (Z)-p-Mentha-1(7),8-Dien-2-ol | 13.0%–31.1% |
| Limonene | 6.0%–30.1% |
| (Z)-p-Mentha-2,8-Dien-1-ol | 9.1%–27.0% |
| (E)-p-Mentha-1(7),8-Dien-2-ol | 8.6%–20.5% |
| Isopiperitenol | 0.0%–13.4% |
| (Z)-Piperitol | 0.0%–11.3% |
| (E)-p-Mentha-2,8-Dien-1-ol | 2.4%–9.8% |
| Carvone | 1.1%–8.5% |
| P-Menthadienol | 0.0%–5.3% |
| (E)-Carveol | 2.1%–4.8% |
| (E)-Limonene Oxide | 0.6%–3.8% |
| (E)-Piperitol | 0.0%–3.6% |
| (Z)-Carveol | 1.0%–3.5% |

**OTHER CONSTITUENTS:** P-mentha-1(7),2,8-triene, p-mentha-1,5,8-triene, dihydrocarvone, cis-limonene oxide, unidentified constituents

**PREFERRED COMPOSITION FOR CLINICAL USE:**

| Constituent | Dienols/Limonene CT | Balanced CT | Geraniol CT |
|---|---|---|---|
| **(Z)-p-Mentha-1(7),8-Dien-2-ol** | 15%–32% | – | – |
| **Limonene** | 10%–30% | 10%–17% | – |
| **(Z)-p-Mentha-2,8-Dien-1-ol** | 10%–25% | – | – |
| **(E)-p-Mentha-1(7),8-Dien-2-ol** | 8%–20% | – | – |
| **(E)-p-Mentha-2,8-Dien-1-ol** | 2%–10% | – | – |
| **Carvone** | 2%–8% | – | – |
| **(E)-Carveol** | 2%–5% | – | – |
| **(E)-Limonene Oxide** | 1%–5% | – | – |
| **(Z)-Carveol** | 1%–5% | – | – |
| **Elemicin** | – | 10%–20% | 8%–15% |
| **Camphene** | – | 10%–15% | 4%–9% |
| **Borneol** | – | 5%–12% | 3%–7% |
| **Beta-Caryophyllene** | – | 3%–9% | 2%–5% |

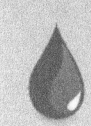

| | | | |
|---|---|---|---|
| Alpha-Pinene | – | 3%–7% | 1%–3% |
| Tricyclene | – | 2%–5% | 1%–3% |
| (Z)-Beta-Ocimene | – | 2%–5% | 0.5%–1% |
| Alpha-Terpineol | – | 1%–3% | 0.5%–2% |
| (E)-Beta-Ocimene | – | 1%–3% | 0.5%–1% |
| Geraniol | – | 0%–2% | 20%–32% |
| Linalool | – | 0%–2% | 1%–3% |
| Geranyl Acetate | – | 0%–0.5% | 1%–4% |
| Geranial | – | 0%–0.2% | 2%–5% |

**REPORTED THERAPEUTIC PROPERTIES:** Antibacterial, antifungal, antiviral, antiseptic, antiparasitic, **analgesic**, anti-inflammatory, antiarthritic, antirheumatic, eases cough, antiallergic, aids circulation, supports immune function, expels excess mucus, supports respiratory function, nourishes the skin, relieves chronic skin conditions, **reduces the appearance of acne, wrinkles, scars, and blemishes**, soothes sore throat, **insect repellent**, relieves anxiety, relaxing/calming, aphrodisiac, antidepressant, improves mental clarity, euphoric

**CAUTIONS:**

■ None currently known.

**SELECTED EVIDENCE:**

☐ Application of 1 mL of neat gingergrass essential oil to exposed body parts (face, arms, and legs) provided 98.7% and 96.5% protection (indoor and outdoor respectively) from mosquito (*An. sundaicus*) bites over a twelve-hour period when tested on 10 different nights.[3703] Other research reports that gingergrass provides 100% protection for twelve hours against mosquito bites from *An. culicifacies,* and 96.3% protection from *An. annularis,* and *An. subpictus* mosquitoes.[3704]

☐ Adding gingergrass essential oil rich in p-Menthadienols to human skin cells protected against inflammation in laboratory research. Further study in mice found that topical application of the oil reduced skin inflammation caused by TPA (12-O-tetradecanoylphorbol-13-acetate)—a chemical used to promote a range of effects in cells including inflammation. Specifically, the oil reduced proinflammatory mediators (IL-6, TNF-α), oxidative stress markers (malondialdehyde and nitric-oxide), and tissue modification in ears. The oil did not cause irritation on rabbit skin. Altogether, the research findings suggest that gingergrass essential oil may be a valuable natural solution for the treatment of skin inflammation.

☐ Ginger essential oil inhibited multiple fungi (*A. alternata, A. flavus, A. niger, A. ochraceus, C. albicans, G. candidum, M. circinelloides,* and *P. roqueforti*) and weakly inhibited one bacterium (*E. faecalis*) but was inactive against *L. innocua* and *S. aureus.*[3705]

☐ Ginger, lemongrass (*C. citratus*), and turmeric each displayed antioxidant activity in the DPPH and ABTS assays, inhibited gram-negative (*K. oxytoca, P. vulgaris, E. coli, P. aeruginosa*) and gram-positive (*S. aureus, E. faecalis, L. grayi, M. luteus*) bacteria and yeasts (*C. albicans, S. cerevisiae*), and mutagen-protecting effects.[3706]

☐ Nanoemulsions (NEs) with 0.1% ginger or garlic essential oil and varying ratios of neomycin sulphate (0.001%, 0.005%, 0.01%) were prepared and evaluated for their antimicrobial activity against pathogens that commonly infect skin wounds (*B. spizizenii, S. aureus, E. coli,* and *S. enterica*).[3707] A NE with a blend of 0.05% of each oil was also evaluated. The garlic NE with 0.005% neomycin sulphate was the most active against the pathogens except for against *S. aureus*, which was most susceptible to ginger NE with 0.001% neomycin sulfate. The NEs were evaluated for their wound healing properties in a rabbit skin excision wound model and demonstrated that they accelerated wound healing better than a neomycin sulfate NE. The combination of garlic and ginger worked the best for wound healing.

# GOBRE SALLA
## (Blue Pine, Bhutan Pine, Himalayan Blue Pine)
*Pinus wallichiana* A.B. Jacks, *P. griffithii McClell.*

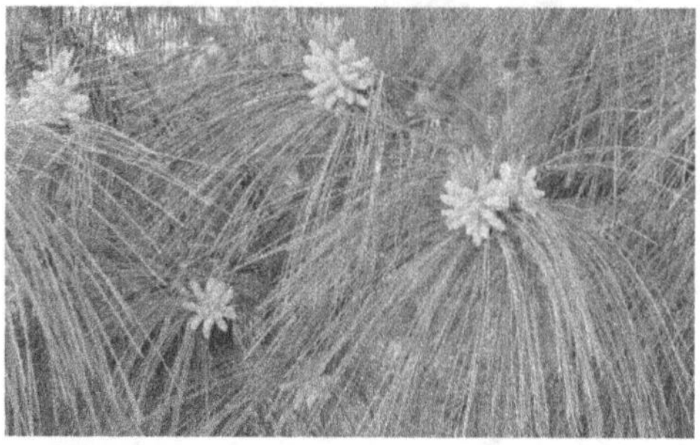

**FAMILY:** Pinaceae
**NOTE:** Top
**AROMA INTENSITY:** Medium
**AROMA:** Fresh, woody, rich, piney, balsamic
**COMMON EXTRACTION METHOD:** Hydrodistilled from needles (leaves)
**POSSIBLE SUBSTITUTE OILS:** White fir, pine, red pine, frankincense, Douglas fir
**BLENDS WELL WITH:** Agarwood, bergamot, cajeput, camphor, cedarwood, clary sage, coriander, Douglas fir, eucalyptus, Engelmann spruce, frankincense, galbanum, grapefruit, juniper, lavender, lemon, lime, tea tree, marjoram, neroli, niaouli, peppermint, ravensara, ravintsara, rosemary, Spanish sage, spikenard, thyme, Siberian fir, silver fir, white fir, white pine, white spruce
**SUBCELLULAR LOCALIZATION | EPIGENETIC INFLUENCE:** Currently unknown | Currently unknown
**RECOMMENDED DILUTION RANGE:** 5%–Neat

**PRIMARY CONSTITUENTS:**[3708,3709]

| | |
|---|---|
| Beta-Pinene | 18.1%–46.8% |
| Alpha-Pinene | 13.8%–25.2% |
| Germacrene D | 0.0%–10.3% |
| Myrcene | 1.2%–9.5% |
| Beta-Caryophyllene | 1.8%–7.2% |
| Germacrene D-4-ol | 0.0%–6.7% |
| Delta-Cadinene | 0.4%–4.6% |
| Alpha-Cadinol | 0.9%–4.3% |

**OTHER CONSTITUENTS:** Camphene, delta-3-carene, limonene, terpinolene, alpha-terpineol, alpha-terpinyl acetate, alpha-humulene, caryophyllene oxide, alpha-bisabolol, bornyl acetate, bicyclogermacrene, alpha-muurolene, gamma-cadinene, cubenol, epi-alpha-cadinol, epi-alpha-muurolol, alpha-muurolol, hexadecanal, 4-epi-isocembrol, methyl daniellate

**PREFERRED COMPOSITION FOR CLINICAL USE:**

| *Constituent* | |
|---|---|
| **Beta-Pinene** | 20%–45% |
| **Alpha-Pinene** | 15%–35% |
| **Bornyl Acetate** | 0%–12% |
| **Myrcene** | 2%–10% |
| **Beta-Caryophyllene** | 0.5%–7% |
| **Delta-Cadinene** | 0%–5% |
| **Alpha-Cadinol** | 0%–5% |

**REPORTED THERAPEUTIC PROPERTIES:** Antibacterial, antifungal, **anticancer**, **antiseptic**, anti-inflammatory, antirheumatic, antiarthritic, antioxidant, supports respiratory function, expels excess mucus, **decongestant**, eases cough, wound healing, aids digestion, stress management, antidepressant

**CAUTIONS:**
■ None currently known

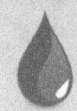

**SELECTED EVIDENCE:**

☐ *In vitro* research demonstrates that gobre salla essential oil prevents the spread of monocytic leukemia (THP-1), lung carcinoma (A-549), liver adenocarcinoma (HEP-2), prostate (PC-3), and ovarian (1GR-OV-1) cancer cells.[3710] Remarkably, gobre salla essential oil inhibited leukemia, lung, liver, and prostate cancer growth better than the chemotherapy drug paclitaxel, and leukemia, lung, ovarian, and prostate cancer better than the chemotherapy drug mitomycin.

☐ Gobre salla is a mild antioxidant, neutralizing free radicals to a lesser degree than ascorbic acid.[3711]

# GOLDENROD

*Solidago canadensis* L.

**FAMILY:** Asteraceae (Compositae)
**NOTE:** Middle
**AROMA INTENSITY:** Medium
**AROMA:** Herbaceous, floral, slightly sweet, green
**COMMON EXTRACTION METHOD:** Steam distilled from the leaves or flowering tops
**POSSIBLE SUBSTITUTE OILS:** Ylang ylang, marjoram
**BLENDS WELL WITH:** Black spruce, blue spruce, copaiba, ginger
**SUBCELLULAR LOCALIZATION | EPIGENETIC INFLUENCE:** Currently unknown | Currently unknown
**RECOMMENDED DILUTION RANGE:** 3%–33%; 50% for some conditions

**PRIMARY CONSTITUENTS:**[3712,3713,3714,3715,3716,3717,3718,3719]

|  |  |
|---|---|
| Germacrene D | 28.4%–69.7% |
| Beta-Cubebene | 0.0%–26.9% |
| Alpha-Pinene | 0.0%–29.2% |
| Delta-Cadinene | 0.0%–20.4% |
| Myrcene | 0.0%–13.7% |
| D-Limonene | 0.2%–12.5% |
| Beta-Copaene | 0.0%–9.8% |
| Beta-Pinene | 0.0%–9.3% |
| Bornyl Acetate | 0.3%–9.2% |
| Delta-Elemene | 0.0%–7.4% |

Note: A chemotype grown in Egypt and obtained from the leaves with beta-myrcene (25.6%), limonene (16.5%), and beta-phellandrene (11.5%) is also reported in the literature.[3720] Plants growing in Canada will generally have higher myrcene content and very little to any beta-cubebene. Summer crops will be higher in alpha-pinene (25.8%–29.2%) and lower in germacrene D (9.9%–10.3%), whereas spring, fall, and winter crops will be characteristically higher in germacrene D.

**OTHER CONSTITUENTS:** Sabinene, alpha-phellandrene, benzene acetaldehyde, beta-elemene, beta-caryophyllene, beta-gurjunene, alpha-humulene, elemol, 1-epi-cubenol, epi-alpha-cadinol, beta-eudesmol, selin-11-en-4-alpha-ol

**PREFERRED COMPOSITION FOR CLINICAL USE:**

| Constituent | |
|---|---|
| **Germacrene D** | 20%–40% |
| **Alpha-Pinene** | 8%–20% |
| **Limonene** | 5%–16% |
| **Myrcene** | 3%–14% |
| **Beta-Cubebene** | 0.1%–12% |
| **Sabinene** | 0.1%–10% |
| **Bornyl Acetate** | 3%–9% |
| **Beta-Pinene** | 1%–5% |

**REPORTED THERAPEUTIC PROPERTIES:** Diuretic, anti-inflammatory, **aids circulation**, **vasodilator**, supports liver function, **anti-infectious**, antiallergenic, antiseptic, expectorant, decongestant, supports lymph circulation, helps prevent kidney stones, **supports cardiovascular and urinary tract health**, soothes cough, wound healing, relaxing, calming

**CAUTIONS:**
■ None currently known.

**SELECTED EVIDENCE:**
- □ Goldenrod prevented the growth and promoted the destruction of liver carcinoma, stomach, and cervical cancer cells, and mildly inhibited skin, breast, and a second liver cancer cell line *in vitro*.[3721,3722]
- □ *In vitro* research concluded that goldenrod oil significantly inhibits *E. faecalis* (formerly known as *S. faecalis*) and *E. coli*, and moderately inhibits *C. albicans*.[3723,3724] Another study reported that it inhibits *Bortrytus cinerea* and prevents decay of strawberries caused by gray mold when in vapor stage.[3725]
- □ Goldenrod oil is considered a natural pesticide.[3726,3727,3728]
- □ *In vitro* research demonstrated that goldenrod essential oil inhibits phytopathogens (*P. fluorescens, C. michiganensis, B. megaterium*).[3729]

# GRAPEFRUIT
## (Pink Grapefruit, White Grapefruit)

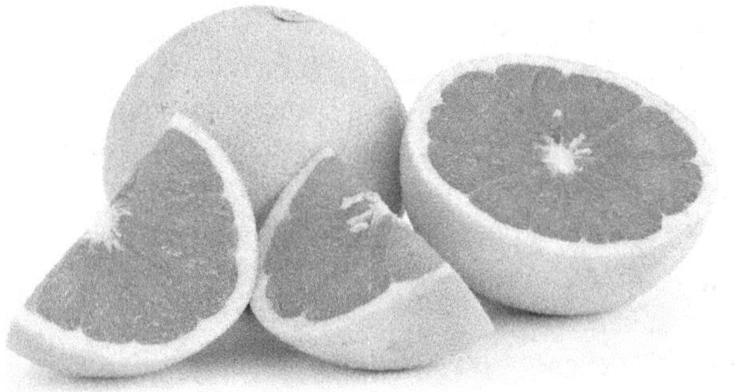

*Citrus × paradisi* Macfad. (pro sp.) [maxima × sinensis],
*C. × paradisii* Macfad. (pro sp.) [maxima × sinensis]

**FAMILY:** Rutaceae
**NOTE:** Top
**AROMA INTENSITY:** Medium
**AROMA:** Citrusy, fresh, clean, slightly bitter
**COMMON EXTRACTION METHOD:** Cold-pressed/expressed or hydrodistilled from the fruit peel (rind)
**POSSIBLE SUBSTITUTE OILS:** Lemon, orange, bergamot, tangerine, lime
**BLENDS WELL WITH:** Bergamot, black pepper, cardamom, cassia, chamomile (German, Roman), citronella, clary sage, clove, coriander, cypress, eucalyptus, fennel, frankincense, geranium, ginger, juniper, lavender, lemon, lemon verbena, lime, orange, neroli, patchouli, peppermint, petitgrain, ravensara, rosemary, Spanish sage, tangerine, thyme, ylang ylang
**SUBCELLULAR LOCALIZATION | EPIGENETIC INFLUENCE:** Endocytic Vesicles | Immune/Nervous
**RECOMMENDED DILUTION RANGE:** 3%–50%; neat for limited conditions

**PRIMARY CONSTITUENTS:**[3730,3731,3732,3733,3734,3735,3736 972–978]

| Cold-pressed/expressed | | Distilled | |
|---|---|---|---|
| Limonene | 86.3%–95.3% | Limonene | 70.9%–88.6% |
| Beta-Myrcene | 1.6%–6.3% | Nootkatone | 0.0%–8.5% |
| | | Beta-Myrcene | 3.5%–7.3% |

**OTHER CONSTITUENTS:** *Cold pressed/expressed*—Beta-caryophyllene, alpha-pinene, beta-pinene, linalool, alpha-terpinene, alpha-cubebene, n-octanal, n-decanal, n-nonanal, beta-phellandrene, tetradecane, citronellol, delta-cadinene; *Distilled*—Alpha-pinene, beta-phellandrene, n-octanal, linalool, n-decanal, copaene, tetradecane, caryophyllene, delta-cadinene, phthalate

**PREFERRED COMPOSITION FOR CLINICAL USE:**

| Constituent | Cold-Pressed |
|---|---|
| **Limonene** | 91%–97% |
| **Beta-Myrcene** | 1%–5% |
| **Alpha-Pinene** | 0.1%–1% |

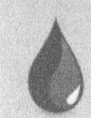

| Sabinene | 0.1%–1% |
|---|---|
| n-Octanal | tr–1% |
| n-Decanal | tr–1% |
| n-Nonanal | tr–1%* |
| Nootkatone | tr–1%* |

Note: Nootkatone and n-Nonanal may be absent in white grapefruit essential oil but are normally present in red/pink/ruby/rose grapefruit essential oil. Growing region may also affect the presence of nootkatone.

**REPORTED THERAPEUTIC PROPERTIES:** Antibacterial, antiseptic, antioxidant, **reduces excess fluid retention**, appetite balancer, supports healthy lymphatic function, astringent, aids digestion, decongestant, diuretic, **weight management**, strengthens nails, immune supportive, **aids detoxification**, reduces the appearance of blemishes, restorative, stimulating, stress management, antidepressant, energizing, reduces fear

**CAUTIONS:**

■ May be mildly photosensitizing. Avoid sun exposure to area of application for at least twelve hours after topical application. Grapefruit essential oil contains very small amounts of the photosensitizing constituents bergapten, bergamottin, and epoxy-bergamottin.[3737,3738,3739,3740,3741]

■ A very common question is whether grapefruit essential oil interferes with medications like grapefruit juice can. The juice contains considerable amounts of furanocoumarin derivatives (bergamottin, bergapten, and dihydroxybergamottin) and flavonoids, which significantly interfere with enzymes that metabolize medications.[3742,3743] While grapefruit essential oil contains bergapten, bergamottin, and epoxybergamottin (flavonoids are not present in the oil), they are present in very small amounts and are weak inhibitors of enzymes. It is highly unlikely, though remotely possible, that grapefruit oil will interfere with the CYP enzymes responsible for metabolizing medications (NSAIDs, proton-pump inhibitors, acetaminophen, antiepileptics, immune modulators, blood-sugar medications, blood pressure medications, antidepressants, antipsychotics, diabetic medications, antihistamines, antibiotics, and anesthetics).[3744,3745,3746,3747] This risk increases with oral administration, as opposed to topical application.

**SELECTED EVIDENCE:**

☐ Grapefruit oil causes the destruction of leukemia cancer cells (apoptosis) *in vitro*.[3748]

☐ A sitz bath with or a soap application with lavender, myrrh, neroli, rose, grapefruit, mandarin, orange, and Roman chamomile improves healing of the perineum following delivery and episiotomy.[3749]

☐ *In vitro* research suggests that grapefruit oil may be useful for weight management because it reduces a process called adipogenesis, whereby adipocytes (fat-laden cells that specialize in the storage of fats) develop and accumulate as body fat at various sites in the body.[3750] Animal research also suggests that inhalation of grapefruit oil decreases appetite and causes an increase in plasma glycerol levels, which indicates that fats have been mobilized from stores for use as energy (adipocyte lipolysis).[3751,3752] Decreased adipocyte lipolysis (the release of fatty acids and glycerol from adipose tissue for use as energy by other organs) is associated with obesity. Adipocytes will release glycerol and fatty acids when triggered by enzymes or proteins.

☐ Grapefruit oil reduces elastase activity (an enzyme involved in the breakdown of elastin) *in vitro*, which may help prevent wrinkles and aging of the skin.[3753] Elastin helps keep skin tight, supple, and flexible.

☐ *In vitro* research concluded that grapefruit oil inhibits *S. aureus, E. faecalis, S. epidermis, E. coli, S. typhimurium, S. marcescens*, and *P. vulgaris*.[3754]

☐ Inhaling the aroma of grapefruit oil for ten minutes increased blood pressure in rats.[3755]

☐ Grapefruit essential oil reduced the production of the mycotoxin zearalenone by *Fusarium* species.[3756] Zearalenone is an endocrine-disrupting toxin that attaches to estrogen receptors (ERalpha, ERbeta) in a similar manner to 17beta-estradiol (naturally produced estrogen) and both it and its metabolites (beta-zearalenol, alpha-zearalenol) alter hormone production (progesterone, estradiol, testosterone, and cortisol).[3757,3758,3759]

☐ A randomized controlled study demonstrated that inhalation of grapefruit essential oil (0.30 mL added to a diffuser with 70 mL of water) significantly reduced abdominal pain exacerbated by severe anxiety during a colonoscopy procedure.[3760] Osmanthus was also effective.

- Rosemary, cinnamon, and grapefruit essential oils each inhibited fungi: *Rhizopus stolonifer* (causes respiratory infections, sinusitis, and otomycosis) and *Trichophyton mentagrophytes* and *Microsporum gypseum* (cause athlete's foot, ringworm, and nail infections).[3761]
- Rosemary CT 1,8-cineole and grapefruit essential oils reduced hepatitis A virus infection in berries.[3762]
- Cold-pressed grapefruit essential oil inhibited the quorum-sensing activity—a virulence factor—of *Pseudomonas aeruginosa*.[3763] Its major constituent, limonene, was less effective than the whole essential oil suggesting synergy between limonene and other minor constituents.
- Molecularly distilled grapefruit essential oil inhibited *B. subtilis*, *E. coli*, *S. aureus*, and *S. phimurium*, exhibited good antioxidant activity in the DPPH and ABTS assays, and displayed anticancer activity against liver and colon cancer cells.[3764]
- Both bergamot and grapefruit essential oil showed anthelmintic activity against *Haemonchus contortus* in laboratory research.[3765]
- Cinnamon bark, grapefruit, tangerine, and lemon essential oil each inhibited *Bacillus subtilis*, *Penicillium chrysogenum*, *Fusarium moniliforme*, *Aspergillus niger*, *Aspergillus flavus*, *Saccharomyces cerevisiae*, *Escherichia coli*, *Salmonella abony*, *Staphylococcus aureus*, *Pseudomonas aeruginosa*, and *Candida albicans*, with the greatest activity observed from cinnamon bark.[3766] The highest antioxidant activity was found in grapefruit oil, followed by lemon, tangerine, and cinnamon bark.
- Oral administration of grapefruit peel or leaf (90.0%–91.0% beta-phellandrene) essential oil significantly reduced inflammation in rats and did not cause any mortality at doses of 5,000 mg/kg body weight.[3767]
- Grapefruit essential oil showed that it is a promising, eco-friendly safe solution to control red imported fire ants (*Solenopsis invicta*). The oil and some of its isolated constituents—alpha-pinene, alpha-terpineol, beta-phellandrene, octanal, and d-carvone—exhibited strong lethal effects against ant workers.[3768]
- A study investigated the chemical composition and biological properties of citrus oils: lemon, sweet orange, grapefruit, and mandarin. All four oils displayed remarkable radical scavenging capacity with grapefruit exhibiting excellent antioxidant activity.[3769] Topical application of the oils showed significant antiedema activity comparable to ibuprofen and reduced the expression of inflammatory cytokines (IL-6, COX-2, NF-κB) to varying degrees. Lemon, grapefruit, and tangerine oil also inhibited lung cancer cells.
- When infected by the bacterium *S. aureus*, skin cells produce proinflammatory molecules and metabolites that irritate the skin. A laboratory study developed to simulate cell damage and inflammation stimulated by *S. aureus* infection evaluated the benefits of grapefruit essential oil.[3770] The researchers found that grapefruit essential oil reduced free radical production by *S. aureus* metabolites, inhibited inflammatory pathways (IL-1 and COX-2), and promoted skin cell proliferation (a sign of tissue healing). This study suggests that grapefruit essential oil has potential to repair the skin and alleviate inflammation and irritation.
- Both bitter orange (37.3% diethyl o-phthalate, 10.0% limonene) and grapefruit (60.5% limonene, 11.8% diethyl o-phthalate) essential oil were larvicidal to mosquitoes (*Aedes albopictus*).[3771] Limonene was also reported to be a potent larvicide, with a limonene nanoemulsion providing a longer duration of effect.
- Laboratory research showed that distilled sweet orange, grapefruit, lemon, and tangerine essential oil each have excellent antioxidant activity in the DPPH assay.[3772] Additionally, all four oils reduced inflammation (remarkably increased G1 phase of the cell cycle, which hinders proinflammatory factor expression) and the expression of proinflammatory molecules (COX-2 and TNF-α). Evaluation in a rat model of rheumatoid arthritis demonstrated that the oils reduce inflammation similarly to the NSAID ibuprofen.
- Chronic inflammation is accompanied by intensified cytokine secretion, which increases the risk of many conditions and leads to premature aging. Macrophages play a critical role in regulating the inflammatory process, and if they don't perform their functions well, inflammation is not resolved, leading to chronic inflammation. Laboratory research found that fractions of grapefruit essential oil rich in aldehydes reduced gene expression and levels of the proinflammatory cytokines IL-6 and TNF-α. The research suggests that grapefruit essential oil fractions may be helpful for a variety of chronic inflammatory conditions.

*Did you know?*

If your sense of smell isn't working properly, essential oils can still produce biological effects. This is because your olfactory receptors will still respond to the aromatic molecules and respond despite your sense of smell being deficient or absent.

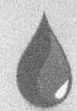

# GRINDELIA
## (Curlycup Gumweed, Curly-Top Gumweed, Gum Plant)

*Grindelia squarrosa* (Pursh) Dunal

**FAMILY:** Asteraceae (Compositae)
**NOTE:** Middle
**AROMA INTENSITY:** Strong
**AROMA:** Herbaceous, earthy, medicinal, slightly camphoraceous
**COMMON EXTRACTION METHOD:** Steam distilled or hydrodistilled from the aerial parts
**POSSIBLE SUBSTITUTE OILS:** Balsam fir, tsuga (Hemlock spruce)
**BLENDS WELL WITH:** Agarwood, balsam fir, blue spruce, cedarwood, copaiba, cypress, frankincense, lavender, palo santo, pine, sandalwood, silver fir, spruce (black), tsuga (Hemlock spruce), white fir, white pine, white spruce
**SUBCELLULAR LOCALIZATION | EPIGENETIC INFLUENCE:** Currently unknown | Currently unknown
**RECOMMENDED DILUTION RANGE:** 5%–Neat

**PRIMARY CONSTITUENTS:**[3773,3774,3775,3776]

|  |  |
|---|---|
| Alpha-Pinene | 8.3%–25.5% |
| Limonene | 3.6%–16.8% |
| Bornyl Acetate | 1.3%–10.8% |
| Germacrene D | 0.0%–6.8% |
| Caryophyllene Oxide | 0.0%–5.9% |
| Spathulenol | 0.0%–5.4% |
| Beta-Pinene | 1.5%–5.2% |
| Borneol | 1.5%–4.5% |
| Camphene | 1.9%–4.2% |

**OTHER CONSTITUENTS:** Thuja-2,4(10)-diene, myrcene, para-cymene, alpha-humulene, beta-caryophyllene, (E)-beta-ocimene, bornyl formate, 2,2,6-trimethylcyclohexanone, camphor, alpha-terpinolene, alpha-campholenol, trans-pinocarveol, trans-sabinol, para-methyl-acetophenone, myrtenal, verbenone, trans-carveol, carvone, trans-chrysanthemyl acetate, alpha-copaene

**PREFERRED COMPOSITION FOR CLINICAL USE:**

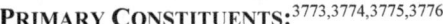

| *Constituent* | |
|---|---|
| **Alpha-Pinene** | 8%–25% |
| **Limonene** | 8%–18% |
| **Bornyl Acetate** | 4%–12% |
| **Beta-Pinene** | 1%–5% |
| **Borneol** | 1%–5% |
| **Camphene** | 1%–5% |

**REPORTED THERAPEUTIC PROPERTIES:** Antibacterial, antifungal, antimicrobial, antispasmodic, anti-inflammatory, aids digestion, **supports respiratory function**, eases cough, decongestant, expels excess mucus, antiallergic, **soothes chronic skin conditions**, relieves hives, astringent, aids immune function, promotes mental clarity, antidepressant

**CAUTIONS:**
■ None currently known.

**SELÉCTED EVIDENCE:**
□   None found.

# GUAIACWOOD
## (Guaiac Wood)

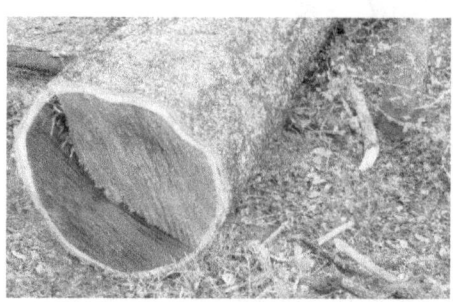

*Bulnesia sarmientoi* Lorentz ex Griseb.

**FAMILY:** Zygophyllaceae
**NOTE:** Base
**AROMA INTENSITY:** Medium
**AROMA:** Balsamic, woody, resinous, sweet, slightly smoky, hint of rose floral
**COMMON EXTRACTION METHOD:** Steam distilled from the wood
**POSSIBLE SUBSTITUTE OILS:** Palo santo, agarwood, Formosan cypress, sandalwood
**BLENDS WELL WITH:** Agarwood, anise, bergamot, chamomile (German, Roman), cassia, cinnamon, clove, cypress, davana, elemi, fennel, Formosan cypress, frankincense, geranium, grapefruit, hinoki, Japanese cedarwood, juniper, lavender, myrrh, neroli, orange, palmarosa, patchouli, petitgrain, rose, sandalwood, vetiver, ylang ylang
**SUBCELLULAR LOCALIZATION | EPIGENETIC INFLUENCE:** Currently unknown | Currently unknown
**RECOMMENDED DILUTION RANGE:** 5%–Neat

**PRIMARY CONSTITUENTS:**[3777,3778]

| | |
|---|---|
| Bulnesol | 34.7%–40.5% |
| Guaiol | 20.3%–26.8% |
| Alpha-Eudesmol | 0.0%–3.7% |
| 7-Epi-Alpha-Eudesmol | 0.0%–3.3% |
| Gamma-Eudesmol | 0.0%–2.6% |
| (-)-Hanamyol | 0.0%–2.5% |
| 10-Epi-Gamma-Eudesmol | 0.0%–2.2% |

**OTHER CONSTITUENTS:** Sesquiterpene oxides, guaioxide, alpha-bulnesene, beta-eudesmol, elemol, eudesm-5-en-11-ol, hannamyol, bulnesol isomer, hanamyol isomer, guaiol isomer

**PREFERRED COMPOSITION FOR CLINICAL USE:**

| *Constituent* | |
|---|---|
| **Bulnesol** | 30%–45% |
| **Guaiol** | 20%–35% |

**REPORTED THERAPEUTIC PROPERTIES:** Anti-inflammatory, **antirheumatic**, relieves gout, antifungal, antiseptic, nervine, diuretic, antioxidant, encourages lymph flow and drainage, balances menstruation, relieves stomachache, **wound healing**, relieves chronic skin conditions, nourishes the skin, supports respiratory function, insect repellent, stress management, relieves anxiety, grounding, aids meditation

**CAUTIONS:**
■ None currently known.

**SELECTED EVIDENCE:**
- ☐ *In vitro* research shows that guaiacwood essential oil inhibited *Fusarium* spp. fungi.[3779]
- ☐ Guaiacwood essential oil was insecticidal to *Myzus persicae, Rhopalosiphum padi*, and *Spodoptera littoralis* aphids.[3780]
- ☐ An ethanolic extract with similar composition to the essential oil (45.0% bulnesol, 27.3% guaiol) demonstrated antibacterial activity against *Mycobacterium tuberculosis* (a virulent bacterium that causes

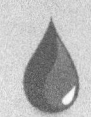

tuberculosis and is associated with increased incidence of disease and mortality among infected individuals).[3781]

☐ *In vitro* research demonstrates that guaiacwood essential oil effectively inhibits *L. amazonensis*.[3782]

☐ Guaiacwood and its two primary constituents—guaiol and bulnesol were acaricidal to *Rhipicephalus evertsi, Rhipicephalus appendiculatus,* and *Rhipicephalus pulchelus* ticks.[3783]

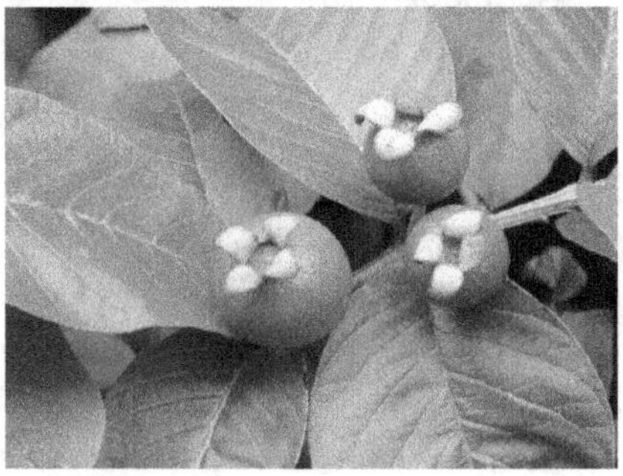

# GUAVA LEAF

*Psidium guajava* L.

**FAMILY:** Myrtaceae
**NOTE:** Top-Middle
**AROMA INTENSITY:** Medium
**AROMA:** Woody, earthy, citrusy, hint of mint
**COMMON EXTRACTION METHOD:** Steam distilled from the leaves
**POSSIBLE SUBSTITUTE OILS:** Copaiba, hemp, black pepper
**BLENDS WELL WITH:** Balsam fir, cedarwood, copaiba, cypress, eucalyptus, geranium, hemp, hinoki, lavender, peppermint, peppermint, rose, sandalwood, spruce (black)
**SUBCELLULAR LOCALIZATION | EPIGENETIC INFLUENCE:** Currently unknown | Currently unknown
**RECOMMENDED DILUTION RANGE:** 5%–Neat

**PRIMARY CONSTITUENTS:**[3784,3785,3786,3787,3788,3789,3790,3791,3792,3793,3794,3795,3796,3797,3798,3799,3800,3801,3802]

*Beta-Caryophyllene CT*

| | |
|---|---|
| Beta-Caryophyllene | 12.0%–46.0% |
| Alpha-Humulene | 1.0%–17.2% |
| Alpha-Pinene | 0.0%–14.7% |
| 1,8-Cineole | 1.8%–12.4% |
| Beta-Selinene | 0.0%–11.0% |
| Alpha-Selinene | 0.0%–10.0% |
| Selin-11-en-4-Alpha-ol | 0.0%–8.3% |
| Humulene Epoxide | 0.0%–6.9% |
| Aromadendrene | 0.2%–6.6% |
| Caryophyllene Oxide | 3.0%–6.5% |
| Alpha-Muurolol | 0.0%–5.6% |
| Alpha-Cadinene | 0.0%–5.3% |
| Daucol | 0.0%–4.8% |
| (E)-Nerolidol | 0.0%–4.7% |
| Phytol | 0.0%–4.8% |
| Cubenol | 0.0%–4.4% |
| Globulol | 0.0%–4.0% |
| Limonene | 0.0%–4.0% |

*Selin-11-en-4-Alpha-ol CT*

| | |
|---|---|
| Selin-11-en-4-Alpha-ol | 21.0%–22.2% |
| 1,8-Cineole | 12.8%–18.8% |
| Beta-Caryophyllene | 8.2%–12.1% |
| Caryophyllene Oxide | 6.9%–9.3% |
| (E)-Nerolidol | 3.3%–8.2% |
| T-Cadinol | 1.2%–8.2% |
| Beta-Guaiene | 3.9%–6.7% |
| Alpha-Selinene | 3.6%–5.8% |

*Limonene CT*

| | |
|---|---|
| Limonene | 27.1%–42.1% |
| Alpha-Pinene | 0.0%–29.5% |
| Alpha-Farnesene | 0.0%–23.3% |
| Beta-Caryophyllene | 6.2%–21.3% |
| Viridiflorol | 0.0%–11.3% |
| Caryophyllene Oxide | 1.6%–9.3% |
| 4,7,10-Cycloundecatriene | 0.0%–4.4% |

*Viridiflorol CT*

| | |
|---|---|
| Viridiflorol | 36.4%–36.4% |
| Germacrene D | 2.7%–16.8% |
| Alpha-Humulene | 0.1%–10.9% |
| Valerenol | 0.1%–10.6% |
| Beta-Caryophyllene | 5.9%–5.9% |

*Beta-Caryophyllene/(E)-Nerolidol CT*

| | |
|---|---|
| Beta-Caryophyllene | 21.6% |
| (E)-Nerolidol | 19.2% |
| Selin-11-en-4-Alpha-ol | 13.4% |
| Viridiflorene | 8.8% |
| Alpha-Selinene | 8.3% |
| Caryophyllene Oxide | 8.2% |
| Cedr-8(15)-en-9-ol | 7.9% |
| Beta-Bisabolol | 3.2% |
| Alpha-Bisabolol | 3.2% |
| Alpha-Humulene | 3.1% |

*Alpha-Pinene CT*

| | |
|---|---|
| Alpha-Pinene | 23.9%–65.4% |
| 1,8-Cineole | 7.6%–21.4% |
| Beta-Caryophyllene | 5.2%–17.4% |
| Beta-Bisabolol | 0.0%–9.2% |
| (E)-Nerolidol | 0.0%–5.0% |
| Beta-Bisabolene | 0.0%–4.8% |

*Beta-Bisabolene/Beta-Sesquiphellandrene CT*

| | |
|---|---|
| Beta-Bisabolene | 19.2% |
| Beta-Sesquiphellandrene | 14.8% |
| Beta-Caryophyllene | 6.0% |
| Trans-Gamma-Bisabolene | 5.3% |
| Alpha-Curcumene | 5.1% |
| (E)-Beta-Farnesene | 4.0% |

*1,8-Cineole CT*

| | |
|---|---|
| 1,8-Cineole | 42.7% |
| Alpha-Terpineol | 38.7% |
| Terpinen-4-ol | 3.9% |

*(E)-Nerolidol CT*

| | |
|---|---|
| (E)-Nerolidol | 35.6% |
| Beta-Caryophyllene | 15.8% |
| (2Z,6E)-Farnesol | 6.7% |
| Ledol | 5.5% |
| Delta-Cadinene | 4.0% |
| Cubenol | 4.0% |
| Alpha-Muurolol | 3.1% |

*(2E)-Hexenal CT*

| | |
|---|---|
| (2E)-Hexenal | 28.4% |
| 1,8-Cineole | 15.9% |
| Globulol | 10.3% |
| Benzaldehyde | 8.2% |
| (E)-Nerolidol | 6.9% |

Note: Based on the diverse composition of guava leaf essential oil, there are at least nine different chemotypes reported in the literature. Some of the nine chemotypes listed here could be further divided into additional chemotypes, but for simplification purposes some chemotypes have been combined when the composition was similar enough. The beta-caryophyllene CT is the most commonly reported in the literature; however, both the limonene and beta-caryophyllene CTs are available commercially.

**OTHER CONSTITUENTS:** *Beta-Caryophyllene CT*—cis-beta-ocimene, alpha-copaene, beta-copaene, allo-aromadendrene, gamma-selinene, alpha-bisabolene, beta-bisabolene, gamma-gurjunene, chamigrene, muuroladiene, valencene, alpha-calamene, alpha-calacorene, beta-oplopenone, viridiflorol, spathulenol, cedr-8(15)-en-9-ol, alpha-terpineol, ledol, delta-cadinol, alpha-santalol, cis-alpha-copaen-8-ol, caryophylla-4(12),8(13)-dien-5-beta-ol, caryophyllenyl alcohol, caryophyll-5-en-12-al; *Limonene CT*—alpha-copaene, myrcene, (E)-beta-ocimene, alpha-humulene, allo-aromadendrene, beta-selinene, alpha-selinene, alpha-copaene, trans-calamenene, delta-cadinene, cadina-1,4-diene, T-cadinol, alpha-cadinol, alpha-terpineol, geranial, methyl cinnamate; *Viridiflorol CT*—aromadendrene, beta-humulene; *Selin-11-en-4-Alpha-ol CT*—benzaldehyde, cis-ocimene, alpha-terpineol, alpha-humulene, humulene epoxide, 14-hydroxy-9-epi-(E)-caryophyllene, beta-bisabolol; *Alpha-Pinene CT*—benzaldehyde, myrcene, alpha-humulene, alpha-acoradiene, gamma-curcumene, ar-curcumene, limonene, alpha-copaene, (E)-gamma-bisabolene, alpha-muurolol, alpha-bisabolol, cis-alpha-bisabolol; *Beta-Caryophyllene/(E)-Nerolidol CT*—ar-curcumene, zingiberene, alpha-muurolol; *Beta-Bisabolene/Beta-Sesquiphellandrene CT*—alpha-ylangene, benzaldehyde, trans-alpha-bergamotene, cis-alpha-bergamotene, (Z)-beta-farnesene, cis-gamma-bisabolene, caryophyllene oxide, (Z)-nerolidol; *(E)-Nerolidol CT*—alpha-terpineol, nerol, geraniol, epi-cubebol, cubebol, trans-cadina-1,4-diene, caryophyllene oxide, alpha-copaene, alpha-humulene, alpha-cadinol; *(2E)-Hexenal CT*—N/A; *1,8-Cineole CT*—trans-sabinene hydrate, borneol, caryophyllene oxide

**PREFERRED COMPOSITION FOR CLINICAL USE:**

| Constituent | B-Caryophyllene CT | Alpha-Pinene CT |
|---|---|---|
| **Beta-Caryophyllene** | 15%–30% | 8%–18% |
| **Alpha-Pinene** | 1%–10% | 25%–45% |
| **Alpha-Humulene** | 1%–10% | 0%–4% |
| **1,8-Cineole** | 1%–8% | 5%–20% |
| **Aromadendrene** | 2%–7% | – |
| **Caryophyllene Oxide** | 2%–7% | – |
| **Alpha-Selinene** | 0.5%–7% | – |

**REPORTED THERAPEUTIC PROPERTIES:** Antibacterial, antifungal, antimicrobial, antispasmodic, **analgesic, anti-inflammatory**, antioxidant, antiseptic, anticancer, aids digestion, **relieves diarrhea**, supports liver function, anti-seizure, balances blood sugar levels, astringent, expels excess gas, aids immune function, relieves painful menstruation, insect repellent, encourages restful sleep, relieves anxiety, stress management

**CAUTIONS:**

■ May decrease the bioavailability of many medications (NSAIDs, proton-pump inhibitors, acetaminophen, antiepileptics, immune modulators, blood-sugar medications, blood pressure medications, antidepressants, antipsychotics, diabetic medications, antihistamines, antibiotics, and anesthetics) due to the ability of caryophyllene oxide, alpha-humulene, and beta-caryophyllene to inhibit CYP3A enzyme activity.[3803]

■ *1,8-Cineole and Alpha-Pinene CTs*: Avoid with epilepsy and Parkinson's due to 1,8-cineole content.[3804,3805,3806] May exacerbate or cause seizures or convulsions when inhaled, applied topically, or ingested based on 1,8-cineole content.[3807,3808,3809,3810,3811,3812]

■ *1,8-Cineole CT*: May interfere with pentobarbital and other barbiturates (medications for anxiety and insomnia) based on 1,8-cineole content.[3813,3814]

■ *1,8-Cineole CT*: May weakly interfere with the enzymes responsible for metabolizing medications (NSAIDs, proton-pump inhibitors, acetaminophen, antiepileptics, immune modulators, blood-sugar medications, blood pressure medications, antidepressants, antipsychotics, diabetic medications, antihistamines, antibiotics, and anesthetics) due to 1,8-cineole content.[3815,3816,3817]

■ *(E)-Nerolidol CT*: May interfere with antibiotics and increase their effectiveness because (E)-nerolidol sensitizes bacteria to antibiotics).[3818]

**SELECTED EVIDENCE:**

☐ *In vitro* research reports that guava leaf essential oil (beta-caryophyllene CT) kills liver cancer cells, mouth cancer cells, murine (common rats and mice) leukemia cells, and mildly kills breast-cancer cells.[3819,3820]

☐ Guava leaf essential oil (beta-caryophyllene CT) reduces inflammation by inhibiting the 5-LOX enzyme (a key enzyme involved in autoimmune and airway related inflammation).[3821] The study authors reported that beta-caryophyllene oxide had the greatest affinity for binding to 5-LOX receptors followed closely by beta-caryophyllene. The beta-caryophyllene CT also reduces inflammation by significantly inhibiting eosinophil migration when administered orally at 100 mg/kg in mice. Eosinophils (white blood cells that release granules in response to allergic diseases, infections, and other medical conditions) are recruited to the lungs and increase inflammation in the respiratory system.[3822]

☐ An unidentified CT of guava leaf essential oil reversed heat-induced infertility (abnormal sperm) in male guinea pigs.[3823]

☐ *In vitro* research concluded that guava leaf essential oil (beta-caryophyllene CT) is a good antioxidant.[3824]

☐ Oral administration of 200 and 400 mg/kg of guava leaf essential oil (alpha-pinene CT) relieved pain caused by chemicals but not heat in mice, likely by activating adenosine receptors.[3825] Activation of adenosine receptors is associated with a reduction of chronic nerve, bone, and chemical-related pain, without building up a tolerance like opioids.[3826]

☐ *In vitro* research demonstrates that guava leaf essential oil (unknown CT) inhibits bacteria that can cause diarrhea (*S. aureus* and *Salmonella* spp.).[3827] Other research reports an undisclosed CT of guava leaf essential oil inhibits *Bacillus cereus, Enterobactor aerogenes,* and *Pseudomonas fluorescens*.[3828]

☐ Animal research reports that guava leaf essential oil reduces the severity of seizures when administered orally at doses of 100, 200, and 400 mg/kg, likely by influencing adenosine receptors and selectively blocking muscle contractions caused by acetylcholine.[3829]

☐ Guava leaf essential oil ((E)-nerolidol CT) was marginally effective in killing *Caenorhabditis elegans* (a non-parasitic nematode that lives in the soil), but proved ineffective as an antimicrobial agent, antioxidant, and against breast-cancer cells.[3830]

☐ A six percent concentration of guava leaf essential oil (beta-caryophyllene CT) repelled the *Anopheles stephensi* mosquito (malarial vector) for up to one hundred and fifty minutes.[3831]

☐ The beta-caryophyllene CT of guava leaf essential oil demonstrated significant antimicrobial activity against gram-positive bacteria (*Bacillus aryabhattai, B. subtilis, B. megaterium, Arthrobacter creatinolyticus*), gram-negative bacteria (*Escherichia coli, Alcaligenes faecalis*) and fungi (*Saccharomyces cervisiae, Rhodotorula* sp.).[3832] The same researchers reported that the beta-caryophyllene CT exhibits poor antioxidant activity.

- The beta-caryophyllene CT of guava leaf essential oil moderately inhibited oral bacteria (*S. mutans, S. mitis, S. sanguinis, S. sobrinus,* and *S. salivarius*).[3833]

- Guava leaf CT beta-caryophyllene essential oil demonstrated significant selectivity against cancer cells, killing breast, cervical, and glioblastoma cancer cells with a lower effect on normal human cells.[3834]

- The limonene CT of guava leaf essential oil significantly inhibited human pathogenic bacteria (MRSA, *S. aureus, S. epidermidis, M. smegmatis*) and plant pathogenic fungi (*Curvularia lunata* and *Fusarium chlamydosporum*), and moderately inhibited *C. krusei*.[3835]

- Guava CT limonene essential oil (51.3% limonene, 21.3% 1,8-cineole, 6.2% caryophyllene oxide, 5.6% beta-caryophyllene, and 4.5% trans-nerolidol) exhibited potent antioxidant activity in the DPPH assay and had nearly the same efficacy against breast and liver cancer cells.[3836] Additionally, molecular docking studies show that constituents of the oil—beta-caryophyllene, caryophyllene oxide, alpha-humulene, 4-hydroxy-9-epi-trans-hydroxycaryophyllene, and trans-calamenene—have potential to inhibit tumor growth due to their resemblance to 4-hydroxytamoxifen (a selective estrogen receptor modulator used to prevent and treat breast cancer), suggesting their possibility as selective estrogen receptor modulators.

- Cinnamon leaf CT eugenol, bay laurel CT camphene, guava leaf CT caryophyllene oxide, and Monterey cypress CT alpha-pinene essential oils each inhibited glycation—the nonenzymatic bonding of lipids to sugars creating advanced glycation end products—in laboratory research.[3837] Damage caused by glycation can lead to stiffening of the blood vessel walls and high blood pressure, particularly among diabetics.

- Guava flower essential oil (37.8% alpha-cadinol, 12.2% beta-caryophyllene, 9.1% (E)-nerolidol, 8.8% alpha-selinene, 7.4% beta-selinene, and 7.2% caryophyllene oxide) exhibited strong trypanocidal activity against trypomastigote forms of *T. cruzi* and promising antibacterial activity against *X. fastidiosa* and *P. carotovorum*.[3838]

- Guava leaf essential oil (13.8% beta-selinene, 10.9% alpha-humulene, 7.6% beta-caryophyllene) demonstrated antioxidant activity in the ABTS, DPPH, and FRAP assays, and inhibited foodborne pathogens (*S. enteritidis, L. monocytogenes, P. aeruginosa*).[3839]

- The limonene CT of guava leaf essential oil was insecticidal to and promoted varying avoidance behaviors in *An. minimus, An. epiroticus,* and *C. quinquefasciatus* mosquitoes.[3840]

- Guava leaf CT beta-caryophyllene essential oil displayed good antioxidant activity in the DPPH, ABTS, and β-carotene bleaching assays, inhibited *S. acidiscabies, E. solanacearum,* and *E. carotovora,* and exhibited remarkable alpha-amylase and alpha-glucosidase inhibitory activity (suggestive of antidiabetic activity).[3841]

- Guava leaf essential oil exhibited weak antioxidant activity in the DPPH assay and inhibited bacteria (*E. coli, Psuedomonas* sp., *C. freundii, E. faecalis,* and *S. aureus*) and fungi (*C. albicans, C. tropicalis, Cr. Neoformans*).[3842]

- Evaluation of seventeen *Myrtaceae* species essential oils for antitrypanosomal activity against *T. cruzi* found that eight of them were promising, including guava leaf essential oil.[3843] Beta-caryophyllene, alpha-humulene, limonene, caryophyllene oxide, and alpha-copaene were identified as important constituents that contribute to the antitryposomal activity.

- Guava leaf CT limonene essential oil displayed weak antioxidant activity in the CUPRAC, FRAP, PM, and MCA assays, potent BChE (cognitive supporting activity) and tyrosinase (skin-whitening activity) inhibitory ability, and also inhibited alpha-amylase and alpha-glucosidase (showing blood glucose control potential).[3844] Several constituents demonstrated good binding potential with the target enzymes, including selin-11-en-4-alpha-ol (AChE, tyrosinase, alpha-amylase) and viridiflorol (BChE, alpha-glucosidase), with limonene, beta-caryophyllene, beta-selinene, 1-epi-cubenol, and caryophylla-4(12),8(13)-dien-5alpha-ol also exhibiting binding potential.

- The limonene CT of guava leaf essential oil (38.0% limonene, 28.0% beta-caryophyllene) inhibited the oral pathogens *C. albicans* and *S. mutans,* and showed significant anticancer activity against oral cancer cells.

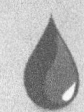

# GUGGUL
## (Gugul, Gugal, Mukul Myrrh, Indian Bdellium, False Myrrh)

*Commiphora mukul* (Hook. ex Stocks) Engl., *C. wightii* (Arn.) Bhandari, *Balsamodendrum wightii* Arn.

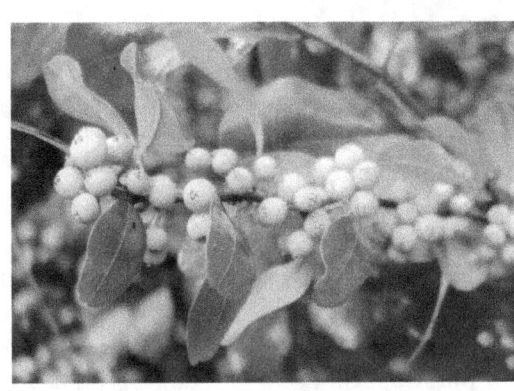

**FAMILY:** Burseraceae
**NOTE:** Base
**AROMA INTENSITY:** Medium
**AROMA:** Balsamic, herbaceous, peppery, slightly sweet, hint of vanilla
**COMMON EXTRACTION METHOD:** Hydrodistilled from the gum resin
**POSSIBLE SUBSTITUTE OILS:** Myrrh, frankincense, copaiba, katafray
**BLENDS WELL WITH:** Agarwood, camphor, cedarwood, copaiba, Formosan cypress, frankincense, guaiacwood, hemp, hinoki, hops, juniper, lavender, myrtle, palo santo, sandalwood, spikenard
**SUBCELLULAR LOCALIZATION | EPIGENETIC INFLUENCE:** Currently unknown | Currently unknown
**RECOMMENDED DILUTION RANGE:** 5%–Neat

**PRIMARY CONSTITUENTS:** [3845]

| | |
|---|---|
| Beta-Caryophyllene | 2.7%–20.8% |
| Alpha-Cadinol | 7.3%–14.5% |
| Delta-Cadinene | 0.0%–11.4% |
| Alpha-Copaene | 0.0%–10.1% |
| Alpha-Selinene | 0.1%–9.3% |
| Alpha-Humulene | 0.0%–8.9% |
| Thunbergol | 0.0%–8.7% |
| Gamma-Cadinene | 0.0%–8.6% |
| Cembrene A | 0.0%–8.2% |
| Alpha-Muurolene | 0.0%–8.1% |
| Alpha-Amorphene | 0.0%–7.6% |
| Alpha-Gurjunene | 0.5%–5.5% |
| Cembrene | 0.0%–5.3% |
| Alpha-Pinene | 2.0%–5.0% |
| Beta-Gurjunene | 0.0%–4.6% |

Note: An analysis from the 1950s reports guggul essential oil composition as 64% myrcene and 11% dimyrcene. [3846]

**OTHER CONSTITUENTS:** Alpha-thujene, sabinene, beta-myrcene, beta-pinene, delta-3-carene, beta-phellandrene, menthol, cyclosativene, delta-elemene, beta-elemene, neo-alloicumene, aromadendrene, germacrene D, beta-selinene, alpha-cadinene, germacrene B, carotol, selin-4,7(11)-diene, caryophyllene oxide

**PREFERRED COMPOSITION FOR CLINICAL USE:**

| Constituent | |
|---|---|
| Beta-Caryophyllene | 12%–22% |
| Alpha-Cadinol | 10%–18% |
| Alpha-Amorphene | 5%–10% |
| Alpha-Selinene | 0.1%–10% |
| Alpha-Muurolene | 0.5%–8% |
| Alpha-Cubebene | 3%–7% |
| Beta-Gurjunene | 3%–7% |

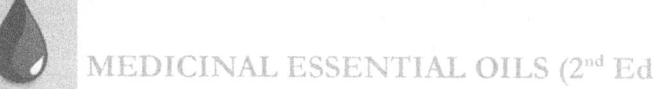

| | |
|---|---|
| Alpha-Humulene | 3%–7% |
| Beta-Elemene | 2%–5% |
| Alpha-Pinene | 1.5%–5% |
| Aromadendrene | 1%–3% |
| Germacrene D | 1%–3% |
| Delta-Elemene | 1%–3% |
| Beta-Phellandrene | 0%–3% |
| Alpha-Gurjunene | 0.5%–2% |
| Selin-4,7(11)-diene | 0.5%–2% |
| Germacrene B | 0.1%–2% |
| Alpha-Copaene | 0.1%–2% |
| Cycloisosativene | 0.1%–2% |

**REPORTED THERAPEUTIC PROPERTIES:** Anti-inflammatory, analgesic, **antiarthritic**, antirheumatic, antioxidant, antibacterial, supports immune function, anticancer, aids digestion, balances blood sugar levels, reduces high cholesterol, weight management, aids detoxification, soothes chronic skin conditions, nourishes and heals the skin, astringent, antiseptic, **wound healing**, balances menstruation, aids meditation, stress management

**CAUTIONS:**

- None currently known.

**SELECTED EVIDENCE:**

- *In vitro* research demonstrates that a guggul ethanol extract exhibits broad-spectrum antifungal activity against *R. stolonifera, A. flavus, A. fumigatus, A. sulphureus*, and *M. fragilis*.[3847] One study reports that guggul essential oil inhibits several gram-positive and gram-negative bacteria, but the composition of the essential oil listed in the study suggests that the essential oil was a misidentified myrrh essential oil sample.[3848]
- Evaluation of the antioxidant capacity of four guggul essential oil samples determined that guggul essential oil is a weak to good antioxidant, with one sample producing comparable activity to vitamin C (ascorbic acid).[3849]

# GULLY GUM
## (Smith's Eucalyptus)
*Eucalyptus smithii* R.T. Baker

**FAMILY:** Myrtaceae
**NOTE:** Top
**AROMA INTENSITY:** Medium
**AROMA:** Sweet, camphoraceous, fresh, woody
**COMMON EXTRACTION METHOD:** Steam distilled from the leaves
**POSSIBLE SUBSTITUTE OILS:** Eucalyptus, ravintsara (1,8-cineole CT), cajeput, rosemary (1,8-cineole CT), myrtle, cardamom (1,8-cineole CT), Southern blue gum, big badja gum, blue mallee
**BLENDS WELL WITH:** Angelica, basil (sweet), bay laurel, blue cypress, camphor, cajeput, eucalyptus, lavender, lemon, lemon eucalyptus, lemon myrtle, myrtle, niaouli, peppermint, ravintsara, rosemary, spearmint, tea tree, thyme
**SUBCELLULAR LOCALIZATION | EPIGENETIC INFLUENCE:** Currently unknown | Currently unknown
**RECOMMENDED DILUTION RANGE:** 3%–33%; neat for limited conditions

**PRIMARY CONSTITUENTS:**[3850,3851,3852,3853]

| | |
|---|---|
| 1,8-Cineole | 72.2%–86.4% |
| Alpha-Terpineol | 0.0%–7.5% |
| Beta-Eudesmol | 0.0%–6.3% |

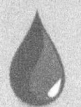

| Limonene | 0.0%–5.9% |
| Alpha-Pinene | 0.4%–4.6% |

**OTHER CONSTITUENTS:** Gamma-terpinene, terpinen-4-ol, para-cymene, linalool, myrcene, pinocarvone, trans-pinocarveol, trans-p-mentha-1(7),8-dien-2-ol, cis-p-mentha-1(7),8-dien-2-ol

**PREFERRED COMPOSITION FOR CLINICAL USE:**

| *Constituent* | |
| --- | --- |
| **1,8-Cineole** | 70%–84% |
| **Alpha-Pinene** | 2%–12% |
| **Limonene** | 2%–8% |
| **Alpha-Terpineol** | 1%–7% |
| **Para-Cymene** | 0.5%–5% |

**REPORTED THERAPEUTIC PROPERTIES:** Antibacterial, antifungal, anti-infectious, antiparasitic, antiviral, antiseptic, analgesic, anti-inflammatory, antiarthritic, antirheumatic, wound healing, relieves blisters, **supports respiratory function**, eases cough, relieves headache/migraine, expels excess mucus, **decongestant**, relieves sinus pressure (sinusitis), relieves sore throat, combats acne, reduces fever, purification, insect repellent, aids focus/concentration, mentally stimulating

**CAUTIONS:**

■ Avoid with children under age three, particularly around the nose and mouth. Use very cautiously in children under age five due to high 1,8-cineole content. 1,8-cineole may cause seizures, central nervous system problems, or respiratory distress in young children.[3854,3855,3856,3857]

■ Avoid with epilepsy and Parkinson's disease due to 1,8-cineole content. May exacerbate or cause seizures or convulsions when inhaled, applied topically, or ingested based on 1,8-cineole content.[3858,3859,3860,3861,3862,3863]

■ Caution is warranted orally due to the significant amounts of 1,8-cineole. Limit it to small doses internally (adults—maximum 10 drops daily). One text recommends a maximum daily dose of 6 drops, whereas the European Medicines Agency recommends 2 to 4 drops (100–200 mg) of high 1,8-cineole essential oils orally, 2 to 5 times daily for adolescents, adults, and the elderly. [3864,3865] Additionally, 200 mg of isolated 1,8-cineole has been ingested three times daily for up to six months in clinical research.[3866,3867] Additionally, 200 mg of isolated 1,8-cineole has been ingested three times daily for up to six months in clinical research.[3868,3869] Toxicity has been reported when eucalyptus (also high in 1,8-cineole) was ingested in large doses, and as few as 4 to 5 drops may cause problems in very sensitive individuals.[3870,3871,3872,3873,3874,3875] In humans, 3.5 to 5 mL has proven fatal orally.[3876]

■ May weakly interfere with the enzymes responsible for metabolizing medications based on research with an herbal extract (NSAIDs, proton-pump inhibitors, acetaminophen, antiepileptics, immune modulators, blood-sugar medications, blood pressure medications, antidepressants, antipsychotics, diabetic medications, antihistamines, antibiotics, and anesthetics) due to 1,8-cineole content.[3877,3878]

■ May interact with diabetic medications due to the ability of 1,8-cineole to significantly inhibit alpha-glucosidase activity, particularly when synergized with other constituents (alpha-pinene).[3879,3880,3881] Alpha-glucosidase is an enzyme that breaks down carbohydrates by chemical reaction with water. Inhibiting its activity postpones glucose absorption and therefore the impact of carbohydrates on blood sugar levels.

■ May interact with aspirin, blood pressure, antiplatelet, and anticoagulant medications, and increase the risk of bleeding among people with bleeding disorders (low risk).[3882] 1,8-cineole is a weak inhibitor of platelet aggregation.[3883]

■ May interfere with pentobarbital and other barbiturates (medications for anxiety and insomnia) based on 1,8-cineole content.[3884,3885]

**SELECTED EVIDENCE:**

☐ *In vitro* research demonstrates that gully gum essential oil inhibits the growth of the dermatophytes *Microsporum canis, M. gypseum, Trichophyton mentagrophytes,* and *T. rubrum.*[3886]

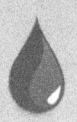

- ☐ Gully gum essential oil inhibits *S. aureus* and *P. aeruginosa*, interfering with biofilm formation and also acting on existing biofilms.[3887] The study author concluded that gully gum is a viable candidate for complementary inhalation therapy for chronic or recurrent upper respiratory infections based on the findings.
- ☐ Gully gum essential oil possesses fumigant and larvicidal properties against the mosquito (*Aedes aegypti*).[3888,3889]

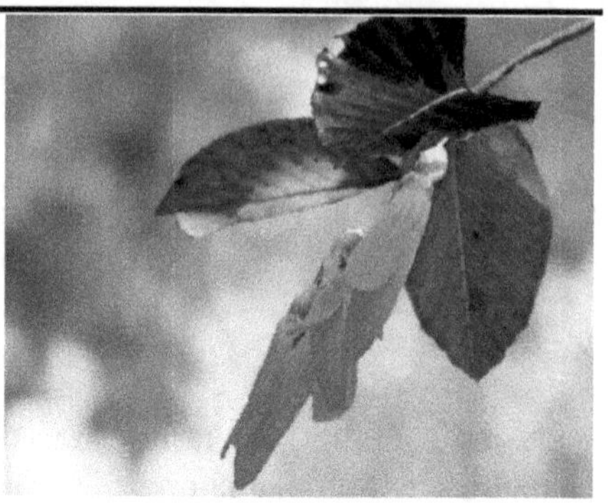

# GURJUN BALSAM
## (Indian Gurjan, Gurgina)

*Dipterocarpus turbinatus* C.F. Gaertn.; *D. tuberculatus* Roxb.; *D. jourdanii* Pierre ex Laness; *D. alatus* Roxb.; *D. kerrii* King

**FAMILY:** Dipterocarpaceae
**NOTE:** Base
**AROMA INTENSITY:** Strong
**AROMA:** Sweet, balsamic, woody
**COMMON EXTRACTION METHOD:** Steam distilled from the balsam resin
**POSSIBLE SUBSTITUTE OILS:** Balsam fir, Peru Balsam, tolu balsam, frankincense
**BLENDS WELL WITH:** Bergamot, cedarwood, copaiba, frankincense, geranium, grapefruit, lavender, myrrh, neroli, palmarosa, patchouli, Peru balsam, rose, sandalwood, tolu balsam, ylang ylang
**SUBCELLULAR LOCALIZATION | EPIGENETIC INFLUENCE:** Currently unknown | Currently unknown
**RECOMMENDED DILUTION RANGE:** 5%–Neat

**PRIMARY CONSTITUENTS:**[3890,3891,3892,3893]

*D. turbinatus*

| Constituent | % |
|---|---|
| Alpha-Gurjunene | 20.0%–75.0% |
| Calarene (Beta-Gurjunene) | 15.0% |
| Allo-Aromadendrene | 4.0%–6.0% |
| Alpha-Copaene | 5.0% |

*D. tuberculatus*

| Constituent | % |
|---|---|
| Alpha-Gurjunene | 90.0% |
| Allo-aromadendrene | 4.0%–6.0% |
| Beta-Caryophyllene | 2.0%–4.0% |

*D. kerrii*

| Constituent | % |
|---|---|
| Alpha-Gurjunene | 79.2% |
| Allo-Aromadendrene | 5.3% |
| Alpha-Copaene | 3.1% |
| Beta-Caryophyllene | 1.1% |
| Calarene (Beta-Gurjunene) | 0.8% |

*D. turbinatus (Commercial Sample)*

| Constituent | % |
|---|---|
| Alpha-Copaene | 47.7% |
| Beta-Caryophyllene | 18.6% |
| Delta-Cadinene | 7.2% |
| Alpha-Humulene | 3.8% |
| Caryophyllene Epoxide | 2.0% |
| Alpha-Gurjunene | 1.4% |
| Gamma-Muurolene | 1.4% |

Note: No complete composition information was found for *D. jourdanii* or *D. alatus*.

**OTHER CONSTITUENTS:** N/A

**PREFERRED COMPOSITION FOR CLINICAL USE:**

| Constituent | Dipterocarpaceae spp. |
|---|---|
| **Alpha-Gurjunene** | 60%–90% |
| **Calarene (Beta-Gurjunene)** | 1%–15% |
| **Allo-Aromadendrene** | 2%–8% |
| **Alpha-Copaene** | 2%–8% |

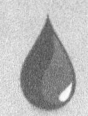

**REPORTED THERAPEUTIC PROPERTIES:** Antibacterial, antifungal, antiseptic, analgesic, anti-inflammatory, antirheumatic, antispasmodic, nervine, aids liver function, **soothes chronic skin conditions**, wound healing, relieves boils, bruises, and blisters, antiallergic, aids immune function, supports respiratory function, expels excess mucus, **eases stomach upset**, relieves anxiety, stress management, reduces hysteria, stimulates creativity, grounding

**CAUTIONS:**
■ None currently known.

**SELECTED EVIDENCE:**
☐ None found.

---

# HAIRY BASIL
## (Hoary Basil)

*Ocimum americanum* auct., *O. americanum* L., *O. canum* Sims; *O. americanum* var. *pilosum*

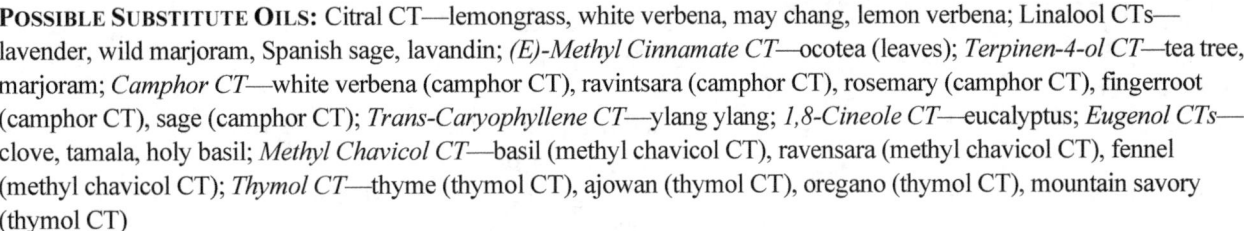

**FAMILY:** Lamiaceae (Labiatae)
**NOTE:** Middle-Top
**AROMA INTENSITY:** Strong
**AROMA:** Herbaceous, spicy, sharp
**COMMON EXTRACTION METHOD:** Steam distillation of the leaves or inflorescences
**POSSIBLE SUBSTITUTE OILS:** Citral CT—lemongrass, white verbena, may chang, lemon verbena; Linalool CTs—lavender, wild marjoram, Spanish sage, lavandin; *(E)-Methyl Cinnamate CT*—ocotea (leaves); *Terpinen-4-ol CT*—tea tree, marjoram; *Camphor CT*—white verbena (camphor CT), ravintsara (camphor CT), rosemary (camphor CT), fingerroot (camphor CT), sage (camphor CT); *Trans-Caryophyllene CT*—ylang ylang; *1,8-Cineole CT*—eucalyptus; *Eugenol CTs*—clove, tamala, holy basil; *Methyl Chavicol CT*—basil (methyl chavicol CT), ravensara (methyl chavicol CT), fennel (methyl chavicol CT); *Thymol CT*—thyme (thymol CT), ajowan (thymol CT), oregano (thymol CT), mountain savory (thymol CT)
**BLENDS WELL WITH:** Balsam fir, bergamot, black spruce, blue spruce, camphor, copaiba, cypress, eucalyptus, fennel, geranium, lavender, lemongrass, lime, marjoram, neroli, pine, rosemary
**SUBCELLULAR LOCALIZATION | EPIGENETIC INFLUENCE:** Currently unknown | Currently unknown
**RECOMMENDED DILUTION RANGE:** 3%–20%; neat for limited conditions

**PRIMARY CONSTITUENTS:**[3894,3895,3896,3897,3898,3899,3900,3901,3902,3903,3904,3905,3906,3907,3908,3909,3910,3911,3912,3913,3914,3915]

*Citral CT (Leaves or Inflorescences)*

| | |
|---|---|
| Geranial | 28.6%–47.2% |
| Neral | 20.2%–36.6% |
| Linalool | 2.0%–12.2% |
| Nerol | 0.0%–7.2% |
| Caryophyllene Oxide | 0.0%–7.1% |

*(E)-Methyl Cinnamate CT (Leaves)*

| | |
|---|---|
| (E)-Methyl Cinnamate | 45.6%–86.6% |
| (Z)-Methyl Cinnamate | 5.8%–11.0% |
| 1,8-Cineole | 0.0%–7.0% |
| (E)-Alpha-Bergamotene | 0.0%–6.8% |
| Linalool | 0.0%–6.6% |
| T-Cadinol | 0.0%–5.3% |
| Beta-Caryophyllene | 0.0%–4.6% |

*Linalool CT\* (var. pilosum, Inflorescences)*

| | |
|---|---|
| Linalool | 29.7%–50.1% |
| Terpinen-4-ol | 0.5%–26.8% |
| (Z)-Cinnamic Acid Methyl Ester | 0.0%–21.5% |
| Beta-Caryophyllene | 1.0%–10.0% |
| (E)-Alpha-Bergamotene | 0.0%–7.6% |
| Sabinene Hydrate& | 0.0%–6.1% |
| Gamma-Terpinene | 0.0%–4.8% |
| Cyclohexanone | 0.0%–4.4% |
| Alpha-Cadinol | 0.0%–4.0% |

*Terpinen-4-ol CT (var. pilosum, Inflorescences)*

| | |
|---|---|
| Terpinen-4-ol | 25.0%–52.8% |
| Linalool | 0.1%–18.5% |
| (E)-Alpha-Bergamotene | 2.7%–11.4% |

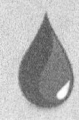 

*Camphor CT (Leaves or Inflorescences)*

| | |
|---|---|
| Camphor | 38.6%–48.2% |
| Limonene | 6.8%–10.6% |
| Beta-Selinene | 3.3%–7.0% |
| Longipinanol | 0.0%–6.2% |
| Alpha-Selinene | 2.9%–5.3% |
| Alpha-Pinene | 3.4%–4.9% |
| Alpha-Thujene | 0.0%–4.9% |
| Camphene | 0.1%–3.7% |
| Trans-Caryophyllene | 3.1%–4.3% |
| Globulol | 0.0%–3.8% |
| Beta-Copaene | 0.0%–3.7% |

*Trans-Caryophyllene CT (Inflorescences)*

| | |
|---|---|
| Trans-Caryophyllene | 43.0% |
| Methyl Eugenol | 26.0% |
| Caryophyllene Oxide | 13.9% |
| (E)-Methyl Cinnamate | 8.3% |

*Eugenol CT (var. pilosum, Inflorescences)*

| | |
|---|---|
| Eugenol | 28.5% |
| Methyl Chavicol (Estragole) | 17.3% |
| Alpha-Terpineol | 15.0% |
| Beta-Farnesene | 9.2% |
| Limonene | 7.5% |
| 1,8-Cineole | 7.4% |
| Beta-Bisabolene | 4.5% |

*1,8-Cineole/Linalool CT (Leaves)*

| | |
|---|---|
| 1,8-Cineole | 17.3%–29.0% |
| Linalool | 19.1%–19.6% |
| Eugenol | 8.0%–14.7% |
| Camphor | 0.0%–14.1% |
| Terpinen-4-ol | 0.7%–7.5% |
| Germacrene D | 0.0%–6.9% |
| Gamma-Cadinene | 0.0%–4.6% |
| (E)-Alpha-Bergamotene | 2.0%–3.5% |

*Linalool CT (Leaves)*

| | |
|---|---|
| Linalool | 20.2% |
| Eugenol | 17.2% |
| Camphor | 12.0% |
| Germacrene D | 3.5% |

| | |
|---|---|
| Gamma-Terpinene | 0.1%–9.2% |
| Beta-Caryophyllene | 2.1%–9.0% |
| Sabinene Hydrate& | 0.3%–7.7% |
| Methyl Chavicol (Estragole) | 0.2%–7.2% |
| Germacrene D | 0.5%–5.0% |
| Limonene | 0.1%–4.3% |

*1,8-Cineole CT (Inflorescences)*

| | |
|---|---|
| 1,8-Cineole | 21.8%–78.3% |
| Beta-Bisabolene | 0.0%–15.9% |
| (E)-Alpha-Bisabolene | 0.0%–13.7% |
| Methyl Chavicol (Estragole) | 0.0%–13.4% |
| Camphor | 0.0%–12.7% |
| (Z)-Beta-Ocimene | 0.0%–11.4% |
| Beta-Pinene | 1.9%–5.8% |
| Germacrene D | 0.0%–3.9% |
| Eugenol | 0.0%–3.6% |

*Eugenol CT (Leaves)*

| | |
|---|---|
| Eugenol | 66.4% |
| Delta-Cadinene + UI# | 9.8% |
| Beta-Elemene | 4.3% |

*Methyl Chavicol (Estragole) CT (Leaves)*

| | |
|---|---|
| Methyl chavicol (Estragole) | 46.4%–56.8% |
| Linalool | 23.9%–33.1% |
| 1,8-Cineole | 2.5%–3.5% |

*Linalool CT (Inflorescences)*

| | |
|---|---|
| Linalool | 61.0%–88.1% |
| Camphor | 0.0%–9.5% |
| (E)-Alpha-Bergamotene | 0.0%–8.2% |
| Beta-Caryophyllene | 2.8%–5.3% |
| Germacrene D | 0.1%–4.8% |

*Thymol CT (Inflorescences)*

| | |
|---|---|
| Thymol | 43.5% |
| Eugenol | 8.1% |

Note: Hairy basil composition is very diverse with at least fourteen chemotypes reported in the literature.

* The linalool CT could be further divided into additional chemotypes, but it is listed as one in this work for simplification purposes.

# Unidentified sesquiterpene hydrocarbon.

& Correct isomer not identified.

**OTHER CONSTITUENTS:** *Citral CT*—limonene, geraniol, neryl acetate, geranyl acetate, trans-alpha-bergamotene, trans-alpha-bisabolene, 6-methyl-5-heptan-2-one, fenchone, cis-linalool oxide, trans-linalool oxide, alpha-farnesene, beta-

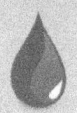

caryophyllene, eugenol, estragole (< 0.7%), alpha-terpineol, methyl crotonate, vivylcyclooctane, vinylcyclohexane, cis-alpha-bisabolol, cyclopentane, methylene, humulene, Germacrene D, bicyclogermacrene, alpha-bulnesene; *(E)-Methyl Cinnamate CT*—alpha-pinene, (E)-beta-farnesene, zingiberene, delta-cadinene; *Camphor CT*—beta-pinene, oct-3-en-1-ol, myrcene, para-cymene, beta-elemene, gamma-terpinene, borneol, terpinen-4-ol, myrtenol, alpha-humulene, delta-cadinene, caryophyllene oxide, epi-alpha-bisabolol, cubebol, beta-cubebene, para-cymen-8-ol, trans-sabinene hydrate, cis-sabinene hydrate, (E)-beta-ocimene, (3E)-Hexenyl acetate, myrcene; *Trans-Caryophyllene CT*—linalool, methyl chavicol (< 2.0%), eugenol, (Z)-methyl cinnamate, beta-selinene, elemol; *Eugenol CT*—alpha-pinene, beta-pinene, myrcene, camphor, linalool, linalyl acetate, isoeugenol, farnesol; *Linalool CT*—2-pentanone,4-hydroxy-4-methyl, (E)-cinnamic acid methyl ester, cyclohexane,2,4-diisopropenyl-1-methyl vinyl, beta-guaiene, 1,4,7-cycloundecatriene,1,5,9,9-tetramethyl, beta-cubebene, germacrene D, limonene, methyl chavicol (< 0.5%), guaia-1(10),11-diene, cadinene, 3,5-pridinedicarboxylic acid,2,6-dimethyldiethyl ester; *Terpinen-4-ol CT*—camphor, alpha-terpineol; *1,8-Cineole CT*—2-methylbutanoic acid ethyl ester, 3-methylbutanoic acid ethyl ester, alpha-pinene, myrcene, sabinene, gamma-terpinene, terpinen-4-ol, alpha-terpineol, linalool, trans-caryophyllene, alpha-caryophyllene, trans-alpha-bergamotene, trans-beta-farnesene, alpha-bisabolol, biccylogermacrene, gamma-cadinene; *Eugenol (Leaves)*—beta-caryophyllene, borneol, beta-selinene, alpha-selinene; *1,8-Cineole/Linalool CT*—alpha-pinene, camphene, limonene, sabinene, beta-pinene, myrcene, para-cymene, (E)-beta-ocimene, gamma-terpinene, linalool oxide, borneol, beta-caryophyllene, bicyclogermacrene, (E)-beta-epoxyximene, fenchone, delta-terpineol, 5-Isopropyl-2-methylbicyclo[3.1.0]hexan-2-ol, alpha-terpineol, beta-elemene, alpha-humulene, (E)-alpha-bisabolene, beta-bisabolene, gamma-muurolene; *Methyl Chavicol (Estragole) CT*—trans-alpha-bergamotene, terpinen-4-ol, alpha-terpineol, bornyl acetate, eugenol, trans-caryophyllene, germacrene D, bicyclogermacrene, germacrene A, gamma-cadinene, delta-cadinene, cadinol; *Linalool CT (Inflorescences)*—3-octanol, oct-1-en-3-ol, alpha-humulene, alpha-terpineol, eugenol, fenchone, beta-elemene, beta-caryophyllene, T-elemene, delta-guaiene, T-cadinol; *Thymol CT*—alpha-pinene, beta-pinene, limonene, 1,8-cineole, gamma-terpinene, para-cymene, terpinen-4-ol, beta-elemene; *Linalool CT (Leaves)*—fenchone, 1-terpinen-4-ol, alpha-terpineol, beta-caryophyllene, alpha-bergamotene, alpha-caryophyllene, T-cadinene, 1,10-di-epi-cubenol, T-cadinol

## PREFERRED COMPOSITION FOR CLINICAL USE:

| Constituent | var. pilosum |
| --- | --- |
| Linalool | 30%–50% |
| Terpinen-4-ol | 10%–25% |
| Beta-Caryophyllene | 4%–10% |
| (E)-Alpha-Bergamotene | 3%–8% |
| Sabinene Hydrate | 2%–6% |
| Gamma-Terpinene | 0.5%–5% |
| Methyl Chavicol (Estragole) | <2% |

REPORTED THERAPEUTIC PROPERTIES: Analgesic (pain relief), antispasmodic, antibacterial, antiviral, **antifungal**, antineuralgic, decongestant, diuretic, anti-inflammatory, antioxidant, antiarthritic, muscle relaxer, nervine (calms and soothes the nerves), aids digestion, eases cough, supports respiratory function, aids circulation, relieves headache (migraine), soothes nausea, expels excess gas, supports oral health, improves muscle tone, **insect repellent**, **insecticide**, mentally stimulating, stress management, relieves anxiety, aids mental clarity, reduces burnout and confusion

## CAUTIONS:
*Linalool var. pilosum (Inflorescences), Linalool (Inflorescences) CTs*
■ May interact with antifungal drugs and enhance their effectiveness based on linalool content.[3916]

*Linalool CT (Leaves)*
■ Avoid during pregnancy and lactation due to eugenol content. Animal studies suggest that large doses of clove (also high in eugenol) may negatively impact embryonic development and encourage fetal cell death.[3917,3918] Another animal

study did not detect any negative influence of clove oil.[3919] Based on these studies it is best to limit clove oil during pregnancy and lactation.

■ May interact with aspirin, blood pressure, antiplatelet, and anticoagulant medications, and increase the risk of bleeding among people with bleeding disorders due to eugenol content.[3920,3921,3922,3923]

■ May interact with MAOI antidepressants due to eugenol content. Animal research suggests that eugenol produces antidepressant effects via the monoamine oxidase pathway, which may cause interactions with antidepressants that also interact with this pathway.[3924,3925]

■ The camphor content in hairy basil (Camphor CT) may negatively impact red blood cells and increase the risk of jaundice in children with glucose-6-phosphate dehydrogenase deficiency (G6PD).[3926,3927]

■ May interact with antibiotics and possibly enhance their effects due to eugenol content.[3928]

## Citral CT

■ Caution is advised during pregnancy and lactation due to high citral content. Large doses of citral may negatively affect fetal development according to animal studies.[3929]

■ May mildly interfere with enzymes responsible for metabolizing medications (NSAIDs, proton-pump inhibitors, acetaminophen, antiepileptics, immune modulators, blood-sugar medications, blood pressure medications, antidepressants, antipsychotics, diabetic medications, antihistamines, antibiotics, and anesthetics).[3930,3931]

■ May interfere with pentobarbital and other barbiturates (medications for anxiety and insomnia) and increase their sleeping effect.[3932]

■ Use cautiously with diabetic medications. Large oral doses of citral may improve insulin sensitivity and lower blood-glucose levels according to animal research.[3933,3934]

■ May interact with antibiotics and possibly enhance their effects due to citral content.[3935,3936]

■ Dilution is recommended for topical application due to high citral content and a study that suggests concentrations of 9.6% or higher may cause skin sensitivity.[3937] Sensitivity occurred at a concentration of 6.3% with isolated citral.

## (E)-Methyl Cinnamate CT

■ May interact with aspirin, blood pressure, antiplatelet, and anticoagulant medications, and increase the risk of bleeding among people with bleeding disorders due to (E)-methyl cinnamate content (low risk as (E)-methyl cinnamate is only moderately inhibits platelet aggregation).[3938,3939]

## Terpinen-4-ol CT

■ Use cautiously for children under six due to methyl chavicol (estragole) content.[3940]

■ Avoid during pregnancy and lactation due to methyl chavicol (estragole) content.[3941] Estragole may cause genetic mutations and oxidative DNA damage.[3942]

■ Avoid oral use due to the toxic and carcinogenic (cancer-causing) potential of methyl chavicol (estragole).[3943,3944]

■ May interact with antifungal drugs and increase their effectiveness due to terpinen-4-ol content.[3945]

## Camphor CT

■ Use very cautiously with children under six due to camphor content. Several cases of camphor poisoning and/or seizures from ingestion and topical application have been reported in children.[3946,3947] Ingestion of camphor-containing products has been lethal in children under age two.[3948] Children five years and up may use camphor-containing essential oils topically in dilutions no stronger than 5%. Camphor ingestion by infants and young children may cause cough, vomiting, seizure, burning sensation in the mucous membranes and eyes, and lack of voluntary coordination of muscle movements.[3949]

■ Caution is warranted during pregnancy and while lactating due to potentially high camphor content. Ingestion of essential oils with significant levels of camphor may lead to abortion because fetuses lack the enzymes to process it.[3950]

■ Avoid with epilepsy and Parkinson's due to camphor content.[3951,3952]

■ Avoid with those who have a compromised liver due to the risk of increased liver enzymes and liver damage (camphor content).[3953] This would also suggest that those taking medications that could cause liver damage should also use hairy basil very cautiously or avoid it entirely.

■ The camphor content in hairy basil (Camphor CT) may negatively impact red blood cells and increase the risk of jaundice in children with glucose-6-phosphate dehydrogenase deficiency (G6PD).[3954,3955]

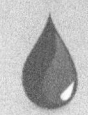

■ Oral caution—Essential oils with significant levels of camphor can be toxic when taken orally. Oral—Camphor can be toxic when taken orally (usually single doses exceeding 2 mL), although the lethal dose for adult humans is estimated to be (more than 5 mL) in a single dose.[3956,3957,3958]

■ Caution is warranted for the topical application of camphor-containing essential oils on broken or injured skin due to an increased risk of toxicity.[3959]

*Trans-Caryophyllene CT*

■ Avoid in children under age 12 due to the multisite cancerous tumors and DNA mutation caused by methyl eugenol in animal studies.[3960,3961,3962,3963]

■ Avoid during pregnancy and lactation due to changes in embryo form and structure and chromosomal changes in ovary cells caused by methyl eugenol as well as the carcinogenic (cancer-causing) potential of methyl eugenol.[3964,3965,3966,3967]

■ Avoid oral consumption due to the multisite carcinogenic potential of methyl eugenol.[3968,3969,3970,3971]

■ May interfere with antibiotics and antifungals and increase their effectiveness due to methyl eugenol content.[3972]

■ May decrease the bioavailability of many medications (NSAIDs, proton-pump inhibitors, acetaminophen, antiepileptics, immune modulators, blood-sugar medications, blood pressure medications, antidepressants, antipsychotics, diabetic medications, antihistamines, antibiotics, and anesthetics) due to the ability of caryophyllene oxide, alpha-humulene, and beta-caryophyllene to inhibit CYP3A enzyme activity.[3973]

*1,8-Cineole CT & 1,8-Cineole/Linalool CT*

■ Avoid with children under age 3, particularly around the nose and mouth (*1,8-Cineole CT*). Use very cautiously in children under age 5 due to high 1,8-cineole content. 1,8-cineole may cause seizures, central nervous system problems, or respiratory distress in young children.[3974,3975,3976,3977] Use cautiously for children under six due to methyl chavicol (estragole) content.[3978]

■ Avoid during pregnancy and lactation due to methyl chavicol (estragole) content.[3979] Estragole may cause genetic mutations and oxidative DNA damage.[3980]

■ Avoid with epilepsy and Parkinson's disease due to 1,8-cineole content. May exacerbate or cause seizures or convulsions when inhaled, applied topically, or ingested based on 1,8-cineole content.[3981,3982,3983,3984,3985,3986]

■ Caution is warranted orally due to the significant amounts of 1,8-cineole and moderate methyl chavicol (estragole content). Limit it to small doses internally (adults—maximum 10 drops daily). One text recommends a maximum daily dose of 6 drops, whereas the European Medicines Agency recommends 2 to 4 drops (100–200 mg) of high 1,8-cineole essential oils orally, 2 to 5 times daily for adolescents, adults, and the elderly.[3987,3988] Additionally, 200 mg of isolated 1,8-cineole has been ingested three times daily for up to six months in clinical research.[3989,3990] Toxicity has been reported when eucalyptus (also high in 1,8-cineole) was ingested in large doses, and as few as 4 to 5 drops may cause problems in very sensitive individuals.[3991,3992,3993,3994,3995,3996] In humans, 3.5 to 5 mL has proven fatal orally.[3997] Methyl chavicol is a possible human carcinogen.[3998,3999]

■ May interact with diabetic medications due to the ability of 1,8-cineole to inhibit alpha-glucosidase activity, particularly when synergized with other constituents (beta-pinene).[4000,4001,4002] Alpha-glucosidase is an enzyme that breaks down carbohydrates by chemical reaction with water. Inhibiting its activity postpones glucose absorption and therefore the impact of carbohydrates on blood sugar levels.

■ May interfere with pentobarbital and other barbiturates (medications for anxiety and insomnia) based on 1,8-cineole content.[4003,4004]

■ May interact with aspirin, blood pressure, antiplatelet, and anticoagulant medications, and increase the risk of bleeding among people with bleeding disorders (low risk).[4005] 1,8-cineole is a weak inhibitor of platelet aggregation.[4006]

■ The camphor content in hairy basil (Camphor CT) may negatively impact red blood cells and increase the risk of jaundice in children with glucose-6-phosphate dehydrogenase deficiency (G6PD).[4007,4008]

■ May weakly interfere with the enzymes responsible for metabolizing medications (NSAIDs, proton-pump inhibitors, acetaminophen, antiepileptics, immune modulators, blood-sugar medications, blood pressure medications, antidepressants, antipsychotics, diabetic medications, antihistamines, antibiotics, and anesthetics) based on 1,8-cineole content.[4009,4010]

*Eugenol CTs*

■ Use with great caution for children under age six due to animal reports of liver cancer caused by methyl chavicol (estragole) content.[4011] The European Medicines Agency recommends exposure to estragole be limited in young children.

■ Avoid during pregnancy and lactation due to methyl chavicol (estragole) and eugenol content. Estragole may cause genetic mutations and oxidative DNA damage.[4012,4013] Animal studies suggest that large doses of clove (also high in eugenol) may negatively impact embryonic development and encourage fetal cell death.[4014,4015] Another animal study did not detect any negative influence of clove oil.[4016] Based on these studies it is best to limit clove oil during pregnancy and lactation. Methyl chavicol (estragole) may cause genetic mutations and oxidative DNA damage.[4017,4018,4019] The European Medicines Agency recommends exposure to estragole be limited in women who are pregnant or nursing.[4020]

■ Avoid oral use due to carcinogenic (cancer-causing) potential of methyl chavicol (estragole).[4021,4022,4023] The metabolite of estragole (1'-hydroxyestragole) is considered a stronger carcinogen and humans rapidly metabolize estragole to 1'-hydroxyestragole when ingested.[4024]

■ May interact with aspirin, blood pressure, antiplatelet, and anticoagulant medications, and increase the risk of bleeding among people with bleeding disorders due to eugenol and methyl chavicol content. [4025,4026,4027,4028,4029]

■ May interact with MAOI antidepressants due to eugenol content. Animal research suggests that eugenol produces antidepressant effects via the monoamine oxidase pathway, which may cause interactions with antidepressants that also interact with this pathway.[4030,4031]

■ May interfere with enzymes responsible for metabolizing medications (NSAIDs, proton-pump inhibitors, acetaminophen, antiepileptics, immune modulators, blood-sugar medications, blood pressure medications, antidepressants, antipsychotics, diabetic medications, antihistamines, antibiotics, and anesthetics) based on eugenol content.[4032]

■ *Leaves, Eugenol CT*: May interact with anticholinergic (drugs used for asthma, incontinence, gastrointestinal cramps, muscular spasms, depression, and sleep disorders) and cholinergic medications (drugs used to reduce urinary retention, diagnose myasthenia gravis, and for glaucoma) based on AChE inhibitory activity of eugenol.[4033]

■ May interact with antibiotics and possibly enhance their effects due to eugenol content.[4034]

■ May irritate mucous membranes (eyes, mouth, nasal passages, vagina, rectum).[4035,4036]

*Methyl Chavicol (Estragole) CT*

■ Use with great caution for children under age six due to animal reports of liver cancer caused by methyl chavicol (estragole) content.[4037] The European Medicines Agency recommends exposure to estragole be limited in young children.

■ Avoid during pregnancy and lactation due to high methyl chavicol (estragole) content.[4038] Methyl chavicol (estragole) may cause genetic mutations and oxidative DNA damage.[4039,4040] The European Medicines Agency recommends exposure to estragole be limited in women who are pregnant or nursing.[4041]

■ Avoid oral use due to carcinogenic (cancer-causing) potential of methyl chavicol (estragole).[4042,4043, 4044] The metabolite of estragole (1'-hydroxyestragole) is considered a stronger carcinogen and humans rapidly metabolize estragole to 1'-hydroxyestragole when ingested.[4045]

■ May interact with aspirin, blood pressure, antiplatelet, and anticoagulant medications, and increase the risk of bleeding among people with bleeding disorders based on methyl chavicol content.[4046]

*Thymol CT*

■ Oral caution. Thymol has a longer half-life (the time it takes for half of the medication to metabolize or excrete half of the dosage) than most essential oil constituents and should not be administered orally for long periods of time.[4047] Thymol is a monoterpene phenol. Reports of fatalities in infants who consumed 50 to 500 mg of phenol have been reported.[4048] It is recommended that chemotypes with high levels of thymol be limited to 10 drops per day orally for adults Monday through Friday, with Saturday and Sunday off; or a two to seven-day break monthly.

■ May interact with aspirin, blood pressure, antiplatelet, and anticoagulant medications, and increase the risk of bleeding among people with bleeding disorders.[4049,4050,4051]

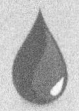

■ May interact with anticholinergic (drugs used for asthma, incontinence, gastrointestinal cramps, muscular spasms, depression, and sleep disorders) and cholinergic medications (drugs used to reduce urinary retention, diagnose myasthenia gravis, and for glaucoma) based on thymol content.[4052,4053,4054]

■ May interact with antibiotics and possibly enhance their effects due to thymol content.[4055,4056,4057,4058]

■ May irritate mucous membranes (eyes, mouth, nasal passages, vagina, rectum).

## SELECTED EVIDENCE:

☐ Animal research demonstrates that hairy basil essential oil (1,8-Cineole/Linalool CT) demonstrated significant anti-inflammatory effects and reduced cartilage destruction in knee joints of arthritic mice.[4059] The authors reported that hairy basil oil protected against leucocyte migration into the synovial membrane of joints and edema. An *in vitro* study reported that hairy basil essential oil (1,8-cineole CT) exerts mild anti-inflammatory effects by inhibiting lipoxygenase enzymes.[4060] Lipoxygenase enzymes are involved in the development of breast, prostate, and colorectal cancers when overexpressed.[4061]

☐ *In vitro* research demonstrates that hairy basil essential oil (citral CT) possesses comparable antioxidant activity to vitamin C.[4062] The 1,8-cineole CT demonstrated significant antioxidant power, especially against hydroxyl radicals in one study, whereas another study noted that it was a weak antioxidant.[4063,4064]

☐ Hairy basil essential oil (citral CT) inhibits fungi (*R. oryzae, A. flavus, C. albicans,* and *F. oxysporum*) and bacteria (*P. aeruginosa, S. mutans, S. aureus, S. epidermis, L. monocytogenes, L. ivanovii, E. faecalis, E. faecium, P. vulgaris,* and *E. coli*), with greater inhibition of fungi than bacteria according to *in vitro* research.[4065,4066] The linalool CT inhibits plant pathogenic fungi (*F. fulva, G. cingulata, A. alternate,* and *F. solani*).[4067] The 1,8-cineole CT of hairy basil essential oil was inactive against five fungi (*M. gypseum, A. pullulans, C. albicans, A. flavus,* and *T. viride*).[4068] The linalool CT possesses broad-spectrum antimicrobial activity against food spoilage bacteria.[4069] A methyl chavicol (estragole) CT inhibits *S. aureus* and *E. coli*.[4070] Hairy basil (unidentified CT) essential oil inhibits the oral pathogens *S. mutans* (a bacterium associated with cavities) and *C. albicans* (a fungus that can cause oral thrush) comparably to the synthetic oral antiseptic chlorhexidine *in vitro*.[4071,4072] The same researchers also reported that it inhibits the probiotics *L. lactis* and *L. casei,* although with a lesser degree of sensitivity than pathogenic organisms. The thymol CT of hairy basil essential oil inhibited several bacteria, including some clinical isolates (two strains of *B. subtilis, Citrobacter* sp., *C. diversus, E. coli, K. oxytoca, K. pneumoniae,* two strains of *P. mirabilis,* two strains *P. vulgaris, S. aureus, S. typhimurium,* and two strains *S. flexneri*.[4073]

☐ Animal research demonstrates that hairy basil essential oil (linalool CT—both leaves and inflorescences varieties) acts as a rapid anesthetic in fish and reduces stress caused by handling.[4074]

☐ Hairy basil essential oil (eugenol CT) repelled and killed the *Agrotis ipsilon* moth.[4075] The 1,8-cineole CT kills the malarial vector mosquito *Anopheles funestus* and inhibits the growth of *Plasmodium falciparum* (a protozoan parasite that causes malaria transmitted by mosquitos).[4076] An unidentified CT of hairy basil essential oil repelled and irritated (caused excitation) the *Anopheles minimus* mosquito (a malarial vector), whereas an unidentified CT of hairy basil only irritated the *Ae. aegypti* mosquito.[4077,4078] Another unidentified CT of hairy basil essential oil repelled, irritated, and killed the *Ae.* aegypti mosquito.[4079] The (E)-methyl cinnamate CT of hairy basil essential oil kill the larvae of *Ae. aegypti*.[4080] An unidentified CT of hairy basil essential oil combined with 5% vanillin repelled *Ae. aegypti, An. dirus* and *C. quinquefasciatus* mosquitoes for up to eight hours in a caged environment.[4081] The camphor CT of hairy basil essential oil repelled and killed the larvae of *Ae. aegypti*.[4082] A study determined that a combination of citronella, turmeric, kaffir lime (*C. hystrix*), hairy basil (*O. americanum*), and vanilla could replace DEET (a common chemical insect repellent that is associated with brain cell damage and behavioral changes in animals) as a natural insect repellent.[4083]

# HELICHRYSUM
## (Immortelle, Everlasting)

*Helichrysum italicum* (Roth) G. Don, *H. angustifolium* (Lam.) DC

**FAMILY:** Asteraceae (Compositae)
**NOTE:** Middle-Base | Peta: Middle
**AROMA INTENSITY:** Medium
**AROMA:** Rich, sweet, floral, earthy | Peta: Herbaceous, fresh, sweet
**COMMON EXTRACTION METHOD:** Steam distilled from the flowering plant
**POSSIBLE SUBSTITUTE OILS:** Cypress, cistus, frankincense, calendula
**BLENDS WELL WITH:** Bergamot, chamomile (German, Roman), clary sage, clove, cypress, geranium, grapefruit, lavender, lemon, lime, tea tree, neroli, orange, oregano, rosemary, tangerine, vetiver, ylang ylang
**SUBCELLULAR LOCALIZATION | EPIGENETIC INFLUENCE:** Endocytic Vesicles | Skeletal/Integumentary
**RECOMMENDED DILUTION RANGE:** 3%–50%; neat for limited conditions

**PRIMARY CONSTITUENTS:**[4084,4085,4086,4087,4088,4089,4090,4091,4092,4093,4094,4095,4096,4097]

*Helichrysum italicum*

| | |
|---|---|
| Gamma-Curcumene | 2.3%–22.5% |
| Alpha-Pinene | 9.3%–21.7% |
| Neryl Acetate | 1.4%–11.5% |
| 2-Methyl-Cyclohexyl Pentanoate | 0.0%–11.1% |
| Alpha-Cedrene | 0.0%–9.6% |
| Italicene | 0.0%–7.1% |
| Beta-Selinene | 2.0%–6.9% |
| 1,7-Di-Epi-Alpha-Cedrene | 0.0%–6.8% |
| Thymol | 0.0%–5.4% |
| Italidione | 0.0%–5.1% |
| Beta-Caryophyllene | 2.0%–5.0% |
| Alpha-Selinene | 0.0%–4.8% |

*Helichrysum italicum* ssp. *italicum*
*(Neryl acetate CT)*

| | |
|---|---|
| Neryl Acetate | 5.6%–45.9% |
| 4,6,9-Trimethyldec-8- en-3,5-dione | 0.3%–19.8% |
| Neryl Propionate | 3.0%–16.4% |
| Gamma-Curcumene | 0.8%–12.9% |
| Nerol | 1.4%–12.8% |
| 4,6-Dimethyloctan-3,5-dione | 0.0%–11.3% |
| 4-Methylhexan-3-one | 0.0%–10.5% |
| Limonene | 0.2%–10.4% |
| Alpha-Pinene | 0.1%–8.6% |
| 2-Methylpentan-3-one | 0.0%–8.2% |
| 2,4,6,9-Tetramethyldec- 8-en-3,5-dione | 0.0%–8.0% |
| Eudesmen-5-en-11-ol | 1.1%–5.8% |
| Ar-Curcumene | 0.9%–4.6% |

*Helichrysum italicum* G. Don ssp. *microphyllum*

| | |
|---|---|
| Neryl Acetate | 16.9%–56.1% |
| Eudesmen-5-en-11-ol | 3.7%–23.5% |
| Rosifoliol | 0.0%–20.2% |
| Gamma-Curcumene | 0.8%–18.2% |
| Beta-Selinene | 6.6%–17.1% |
| Neryl Propionate | 1.5%–16.4% |
| Linalool | 0.0%–14.9% |
| Nerol | 3.7%–14.4% |
| Dihydro-Occidentalol | 7.6%–12.2% |
| Alpha-Selinene | 3.8%–5.4% |
| Italicene | 1.4%–5.1% |

*Helichrusm Italicum (Croatian)*

| | |
|---|---|
| Alpha-Pinene | 12.8%–21.7% |
| Gamma-Curcumene | 0.0%–16.9% |
| 2-Methylcyclohexyl Pentanoate | 0.0%–11.2% |
| Neryl Acetate | 8.2%–10.5% |
| Beta-Selinene | 2.0%–7.9% |
| 1,7-di-epi-Alpha-Cedrene | 0.0%–7.1% |
| Thymol | 0.0%–5.5% |
| Beta-Caryophyllene | 2.0%–4.9% |
| Italicine | 0.0%–4.5% |
| Eremophilene | 0.0%–4.5% |

Note: *H. italicum* samples from Corsica are typically rich in neryl acetate, whereas samples from Croatia (Balkan region) are rich in gamma-curcumene and alpha-pinene. The neryl acetate CT of *H. italicum* (Corsican) appears to be the most common CT commercially available. Corsican helichrysum is rich in esters that make it a good choice for muscle spasms, pain, and

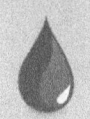

inflammation, whereas Croatian (Balkan) helichrysum is rich in skin/wound healing sesquiterpenes and ketones and is also useful for pain and inflammation.

**OTHER CONSTITUENTS:** *Helichrysum italicum*—Caryophyllene oxide, limonene, selina-4,11-diene, alpha-copaene, (Z)-alpha-bergamotene, (E)-alpha-bergamotene; *Helichrysum italicum* ssp. *Italicum*—Alpha-fenchene, beta-pinene, 1,8-cineole, gamma-terpinene, linalool, nerol oxide, terpinen-4-ol, alpha-terpineol; *Helichrysum italicum* G. Don ssp. *microphyllum*—4,6-Dimethyloctan-3,5-dione, alpha-terpineol, lavandulyl acetate, carvacrol, (Z)-alpha-bergamotene, (E)-alpha-bergamotene, ar-curcumene, geranyl butanoate, guaiol, beta-eudesmol, alpha eudesmol, arzanol; *Helichrusm Italicum (Croatian)*—Limonene, ar-curcumene, (E)-2-methyl-2-butenoic acid, alpha-copaene, italidiones, 2,3,4,7,8,8a-hexahydro-1H-3a,7-methanoazulene, fenchol, linalool, 3,4-octadion, cis-alpha-bergamotene, trans-alpha-bergamotene, gamma-gurjunene, alpha-humulene, alpha-terpineol, alpha-selinene, gamma-selinene, alpha-fenchene, delta-cadinene, neryl propionate, nerol, 2-methylcyclohexyl octanoate, geranyl propionate, guaiol, viridiflorol, phenylethyl tiglate, alpha-copaene, italidiones

**PREFERRED COMPOSITION FOR CLINICAL USE:**

| Constituent | Corsican | Croatian | Balanced |
|---|---|---|---|
| **Neryl Acetate** | 30%–45% | 5%–12% | 17%–30% |
| **Italidiones** | 3%–18% | 3%–15% | 1%–10% |
| **Gamma-Curcumene** | 5%–15% | 8%–23% | 5%–18% |
| **Neryl Propionate** (Neryl Propanoate) | 3%–10% | 0.1%–3% | 0.5%–4% |
| **Limonene** | 2%–8% | 1%–5% | 1%–5% |
| **Nerol** | 2%–8% | 0.1%–3% | 0%–2% |
| **Alpha-Pinene** | 1%–8% | 15%–35% | 15%–35% |
| **Linalool** | 1%–5% | 0.1%–3% | 0.1%–2% |
| **Italicene** | 1%–5% | 3%–7% | 0.1%–5% |
| **ar-Curcumene** (Alpha-Curcumene) | 0.5%–5% | 1%–5% | 1%–3% |
| **Beta-Caryophyllene** | 0%–3% | 2%–6% | 2%–4% |
| **Isoitalicine** | 0.1%–2% | 0.5%–2% | 0.5%–5% |
| **Beta-Selinene** | – | 2%–8% | 1%–5% |
| **Alpha-Selinene** | – | 1%–5% | 1%–5% |
| **Alpha-Copaene** | – | 0%–5% | 0%–2% |
| **Terpinolene** | – | – | 0.1%–3% |
| **Alpha-Terpineol** | – | – | 0.1%–3% |
| **Delta-Cadinene** | – | 0.1%–3% | – |
| **Beta-Pinene** | – | – | 0.1%–3% |

**REPORTED THERAPEUTIC PROPERTIES (Helichrysum):** Antibacterial, **reduces the appearance of scars**, anti-inflammatory, **analgesic (pain relief)**, antimicrobial, antioxidant, antispasmodic, antiallergenic, antifungal, astringent, diuretic, aids detoxification, **supports liver function**, moisturizes the skin, **helps relieve chronic skin conditions**, expectorant, supports spleen function, aids red blood cell production, encourages cell health, **strengthens the circulatory system**, **wound healing**, **nervine (calms and soothes the nerves)**, reduces fever, helps bruises heal, **helps clear blood clots**, stress management, antidepressant, emotionally balancing, stimulating, promotes creativity, helps relieve emotional trauma, fosters forgiveness

**CAUTIONS:**
■ None currently known.

**SELECTED EVIDENCE:**
□ Helichrysum oil significantly reverses multi-drug-resistance of *E. aerogenes, E. coli, P. aeruginosa*, and *A. baumannii in vitro.*[4098]

□ *In vitro* research suggests that arzanol from helichrysum (ssp. *microphyllum*) reduces inflammation (through inhibiting the production of proinflammatory cytokines) and prevents HIV-1 replication.[4099]

- Helichrysum reduces inflammation through multiple pathways (reduced proinflammatory enzyme activity, enhanced free-radical-scavenging activity, and corticoid steroid-like properties) according to *in vitro* research.[4100] Another study determined that helichrysum moderately inhibits 5-LOX activity (an proinflammatory enzyme).[4101]

- Inhalation of a combination of peppermint, basil, and helichrysum oils reduced mental exhaustion and moderate burnout in a small pilot study.[4102]

- *In vitro* research demonstrates that an odd CT of helichrysum essential oil (alpha-cedrene 13.6%, alpha-curcumene 11.4%, geranyl acetate 10.1%, nerol 5.0%, neryl acetate 4.9%, and alpha-pinene 3.8%) inhibited bacteria (*Staphylococcus aureus*, *Micrococcus luteus*, *Enterococcus cereus*, *Bacillus cereus*, *Staphylococcus epidermidis*, *Bacillus subtilis*, *Pseudomonas aeruginosa*, *Enterococcus faecalis*, *Proteus mirabilis*), yeasts (*Candida albicans*, *Saccharomyces cerevisiae*), and fungi (*Fusarium solani var. coeruleum*, *Aspergillus niger*, *Alternaria alternata*, *Ascochyta rabiei*), although the fungi were more resistant to its antimicrobial effects.[4103]

- A preclinical model of chronic skin inflammation demonstrates that helichrysum (Corsican type) essential oil inhibits protein molecules involved in tissue remodeling, which suggests that it promotes wound healing.[4104]

- Helichrysum from Montenegro (21.7% beta-eudesmene, 19.9% beta-bisabolene, 16.9% alpha-pinene, 10.7% neryl acetate) inhibited *C. albicans* and *A. baumannii*.[4105]

- Helichrysum (15.8% neryl acetate, 8.2% alpha-pinene, 7.3% italidione I) inhibited both collagenase and elastase activities *in vitro*.[4106] Collagenases are enzymes that break down the peptide bonds in collagen, which both helps to remove damaged tissues within the skin and participates in tissue degradation in tissue conditions. Elastase is an enzyme that breaks down proteins (elastin) and may reduce the stretchability of skin, causing skin aging (e.g., wrinkles). When some of the major constituents (neryl acetate, nerol, linalool, alpha-pinene, and limonene) were tested alone or in combinations, only alpha-pinene and limonene showed inhibitory activity of both enzymes.

- *Acanthamoeba castellanii* is an opportunistic protozoon found in aquatic environments where it can form symbiotic relationships with over thirty different pathogenic bacteria, including nontuberculous mycobacteria (NTM). Protozoa play an important role in the ability of nontuberculous mycobacteria to infect hosts. Addition of juniper or helichrysum essential oil to tap water infested with *Acanthamoeba castellanii* and NTM (*Mycobacterium avium*, *M. intracellulare*, and *M. gordonae*) essential oil prevented the adhesion of the protozoa to NTM.[4107] This suggests that the essential oils and their combinations weaken the contact of environmental NTMs and free-living amoebae and therefore indirectly reduce their ability to infect hosts.

- Helichrysum (Corsican type), mastic CT myrcene, and myrtle CT tricyclene essential oils demonstrated strong anticancer activity against human ovarian cancer cells.[4108] Rosemary CT alpha-pinene, thyme CT thymol, and yarrow CT 1,8-cineole exhibited weaker activity against cancer cells. All of the oils showed weak or no estrogenic activity in yeast strains expressing the human estrogen receptor alpha, while helichrysum and yarrow essential oils were antiestrogenic. All of the oils affected the proliferation and viability of human peripheral lymphocytes in a dose-dependent manner.

- A laboratory study exploring the anti-inflammatory and antimicrobial potential of various chemotypes of helichrysum essential oil found that its bioactivity is likely a synergistic activation of all constituents, and/or the presence of minor constituents, rather than simply the presence of neryl esters (neryl acetate), alpha-pinene, curcumene (alpha and gamma), and italidiones (diketones).[4109] However, curcumenes and alpha-pinene did correlate with anti-inflammatory activity and overall higher mono- and sesquiterpene hydrocarbon content had the most positive impact on anti-inflammatory activity.

- A helichrysum essential oil with gamma-curcumene (21.5%) as the major constituent and no italidiones displayed weak antioxidant activity in the DPPH and ABTS assays.[4110]

- Wound healing activity is diminished in diabetic subjects—due to several factors: elevated blood sugar narrows blood vessels limiting blood supply and cell migration to the wound area, neuropathy that reduces the ability to detect wounds, immune system deficiency, and infection—making wound care crucial. An ointment with 0.5% helichrysum essential oil improved wound healing in diabetic rats.[4111] Rats were divided into four groups: (1) no treatment; (2) treatment with silver sulfadiazine; (3) treatment with 0.5% ointment base; and (4) treatment with 0.5% helichrysum ointment. Ointments were applied topically once daily for twenty-one days, and wound healing measured regularly. The helichrysum ointment group experienced the greatest wound healing and increased levels of hydroxyproline (reduced levels are a marker for poor wound healing). The helichrysum ointment promoted significant wound contraction from day seven to twenty-one, which was higher than ointment base (81.3%) and no treatment (71.4%) at day 21 (99.3%). In addition, the

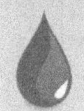

- helichrysum ointment promoted scar fading and increased collagen fiber density.

☐ *In vitro* research demonstrated that helichrysum essential oils from Bosnia (13.7% alpha-pinene, 10.8% beta-himachalene), France (14.9% neryl acetate, 9.9% beta-himachalene), and Corsica (12.4% neryl acetate, 11.0% beta-himachalene) each inhibited *S. aureus, E. faevalis, S. pneumoniae, P. aeruginosa, Y. enterocolitica, S. enterica* subsp. *enterica, C. albicans, C. krusei,* and *C. tropicalis*, with the French oil exhibiting the highest activity overall.[4112]

☐ Helichrysum essential oil from the herb (20.3% neryl acetate, 10.4% alpha-pinene, 9.1% alpha-selinene, 8.2% beta-selinene) exhibited greater antioxidant activity than the inflorescences oil (16.4% neryl acetate, 15.7% nerol) in the ABTS and DPPH assays.[4113] However, the inflorescences oil showed stronger bacteriostatic power against *S. aureus* and MRSA, with both oils showing weaker activity against gram-negative bacteria (*E. coli, P. aeruginosa*).

☐ Helichrysum essential oil (21.2% neryl acetate, 15.9% ar-curcumene, 8.8% beta-longipinene, 7.2% beta-selinene, 6.7% alpha-pinene) exhibited stronger antibacterial activity against respiratory pathogens—*P. aeruginosa, S. pneumoniae, H. influenzae, H. parainfluenzae*—than the reference antibiotics (gentamicin, imipenem, amikacin) *in vitro*.[4114] The oil also inhibited biofilm formation by all the bacteria with *Haemophilus* spp. being the most susceptible and *P. aeruginosa* and *S. pneumoniae* the least susceptible.

☐ Corsican helichrysum essential oil and isolated neryl acetate modulate genes involved in epidermal differentiation (a process to maintain healthy cells in the outermost layer of the skin), skin barrier formation (protects the body from the external environment), and lipid and ceramide synthesis (crucial for skin structure and function and maintain youthful-looking skin) in a skin explant model.[4115]

# HEMP
## (Cannabis)

*Cannabis sativa* L.

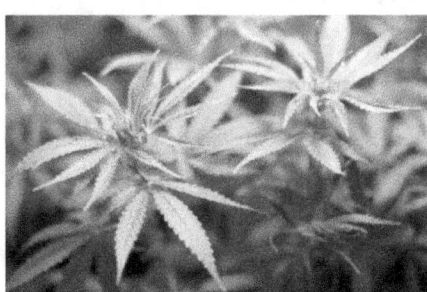

**FAMILY:** Cannabaceae
**NOTE:** Middle-Top
**AROMA INTENSITY:** Strong
**AROMA:** Earthy, herbaceous, pungent, slightly sweet
**COMMON EXTRACTION METHOD:** Steam distilled from the leaves and flowers
**POSSIBLE SUBSTITUTE OILS:** Copaiba, anise
**BLENDS WELL WITH:** Bergamot, copaiba, frankincense, hyssop, lavender, lemon, lime, marjoram, orange, patchouli, vetiver, ylang ylang
**SUBCELLULAR LOCALIZATION | EPIGENETIC INFLUENCE:** Currently unknown | Currently unknown
**RECOMMENDED DILUTION RANGE:** 3.0%–33.0%; neat for limited conditions

**PRIMARY CONSTITUENTS:**[4116,4117,4118,4119,4120]

| *Beta-Caryophyllene CT* | | *Myrcene CT* | |
|---|---|---|---|
| Beta-Caryophyllene | 19.6%–26.1% | Myrcene | 12.5%–67.1% |
| Limonene | 4.1%–15.8% | Beta-Caryophyllene | 11.0%–37.5% |
| Caryophyllene Oxide | 2.0%–10.7% | Alpha-Pinene | 2.3%–31.0% |
| (E)-Beta-Farnesene | 4.8%–8.5% | Alpha-Terpinolene | 0.1%–23.8% |
| Alpha-Humulene | 5.4%–7.8% | Limonene | 0.2%–17.2% |
| Alpha-Pinene | 0.7%–7.7% | Caryophyllene Oxide | 0.1%–11.3% |
| Myrcene | 0.8%–6.0% | (E)-Beta-Ocimene | 0.4%–10.2% |
| Alpha-Terpinolene | 0.2%–6.0% | Beta-Pinene | 0.9%–9.3% |
| Beta-Selinene | 1.8%–5.4% | Alpha-Humulene | 0.7%–8.7% |
| Beta-Sesquiphellandrene | 2.0%–4.6% | | |
| (E)-Beta-Ocimene | 0.4%–4.1% | | |
| Alpha-Selinene | 1.6%–4.0% | | |
| Trans-Alpha-Bergamotene | 2.1%–3.9% | | |

Note: THC (delta(9)-tetrahydrocannabinol), the psychoactive constituent in the plant, is generally only present in trace amounts of less than 0.2% in the essential oil according to published reports. Regulations require extremely low THC levels in commercially produced essential oils. Do not confuse hemp essential oil with hemp seed vegetable/fixed oil (also called hemp oil), which is obtained by pressing the seeds of the plant.

**OTHER CONSTITUENTS:** *Myrcene CT*—alpha-phellandrene, delta-3-carene, cis-beta-ocimene, trans-alpha-bergamotene, cis-beta-guaiene, alpha-selinene, beta-selinene, alpha-zingiberene, alpha-terpinene, beta-bisabolene, germacrene B, 1,8-cineole, gamma-elemene, trans-alpha-farnesene, cis-beta-farnesene, alloaromadendrene, Selina-3,7 (11)-diene; *Beta-Caryophyllene CT*—beta-pinene, gamma-terpinene, cis-sabinene hydrate, linalool, terpinen-4-ol, p-cymen-8-ol, alpha-terpineol, alpha-caryophyllene, gamma-curcumene, germacrene D, beta-bisabolene, (E)-nerolidol, humulene epoxide II

**PREFERRED COMPOSITION FOR CLINICAL USE:**

| Constituent | Beta-Caryophyllene CT | Beta-Myrcene CT |
|---|---|---|
| **Beta-Caryophyllene** | 20%–30% | 20%–35% |
| **Limonene** | 7%–15% | 0.1%–5% |
| **Alpha-Humulene** | 5%–15% | 0.5%–7% |
| **(E)-Beta-Farnesene** | 3%–8% | – |
| **Caryophyllene Oxide** | 2%–8% | 0.1%–5% |
| **Alpha-Pinene** | 2%–8% | 3%–10% |
| **Myrcene** | 2%–8% | 35%–50% |
| **Beta-Selinene** | 2%–7% | – |
| **Beta-Sesquiphellandrene** | 2%–7% | – |
| **(E)-Alpha-Bergamotene** | 2%–5% | – |
| **(E)-Beta-Ocimene** | 1%–5% | 0.5%–5% |
| **Alpha-Selinene** | 1%–5% | – |
| **Alpha-Terpinolene** | 0.1%–5% | 3%–10% |
| **Beta-Pinene** | – | 1%–5% |

**REPORTED THERAPEUTIC PROPERTIES:** Antibacterial, antifungal, anticancer, **analgesic**, **anti-inflammatory**, antispasmodic, antineuralgic, nervine, soothes chronic skin conditions, supports cardiovascular function, aids digestion, increases appetite, protects eye health, relieves headache/migraine, antiallergic, reduces nausea, supports respiratory function, eases cough, balances female hormones, reduces painful menstruation, reduces fever, insect repellent, encourages restful sleep, calming/relaxing, **stress management**, relieves anxiety, antidepressant, promotes creativity, enhances confidence

**CAUTIONS:**

■ Caution is advised during pregnancy and lactation due to high beta-myrcene content. Extremely high doses (500 mg/kg) of beta-myrcene have been toxic to fetuses according to animal research.[4121,4122]

■ May interact with barbiturates (medications for anxiety and insomnia), antihistamines, benzodiazepines, tricyclic antidepressants, or other central nervous system depressant drugs, increasing their depressant effects.[4123,4124,4125]

■ *Myrcene CT*: May weakly interfere with the enzymes responsible for metabolizing medications (NSAIDs, proton-pump inhibitors, acetaminophen, antiepileptics, immune modulators, blood-sugar medications, blood pressure medications, antidepressants, antipsychotics, diabetic medications, antihistamines, antibiotics, and anesthetics) based on myrcene content.[4126,4127,4128]

**SELECTED EVIDENCE:**

☐ *In vitro* research reports that the myrcene CT of hemp essential oil inhibits gram-positive bacteria widely known to cause infections of the human gastrointestinal tract, such as *Enterococcus hirae*, *Enterococcus faecium*, and *S. salivarius* subsp. *thermophiles*.[4129] Another study concluded that hemp essential oil (beta-caryophyllene CT) moderately inhibited two *S. aureus* strains, mildly to moderately inhibited *B. subtilis* and *Streptococcus mutans*, and moderately inhibited *Salmonella typhimurium*.[4130]

☐ Animal research suggests that oral administration of 5 or 10 mg/kg of beta-caryophyllene (an abundant cannabinoid in hemp essential oil) reduces acute and chronic pain by influencing opioid (a group of receptors that

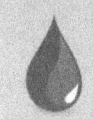

produce opioids—beta-endorphin, met-enkephalins, leu-enkephalins, and dynorphins—that act on cell receptors to reduce pain and modulate rewarding stimuli) and endocannabinoid (a group of receptors located throughout the brain and central nervous system that modulates pain and inflammation) systems, and inhibits proinflammatory molecules.[4131,4132]

☐ Hemp essential oil (19.2% alpha-pinene, 17.2% myrcene, and 15.3% beta-caryophyllene) reduced the virulence (motility) of *L. monocytogenes* isolated from people diagnosed with listeriosis and improved survivability of moth (*Galleria mellonella*) larvae infected with *L. monocytogenes* grown in the presence of the essential oil.[4133]

☐ The beta-caryophyllene CT of hemp essential oil exhibited antioxidant activity (DPPH, CUPRAC, FRAP, phosphomolybdenum, and metal chelating assays), inhibited *S. aureus* (four clinical isolates) and its biofilms, demonstrated antimicrobial activity against *H. pylori* (significantly greater than MNZ and CLR), and significantly inhibited breast (two cell lines: estrogen dependent and triple-negative), colorectal, and bile duct cancer cells with good selectivity.[4134]

☐ Hemp (both the beta-caryophyllene and myrcene CTs) essential oil demonstrated good antimicrobial activity against pathogenic and food spoilage microbes (*S. aureus, L. monocytogenes, E. faecalis, E. hirae, E. faecium, B. subtillis, B. cereus,* and *Bacillus* species).[4135]

☐ Hemp CT beta-caryophyllene essential oil (two types: Chinese accession and var. *fibrante*) exhibited strong antioxidant activity and significantly inhibited acetylcholinesterase (a key enzyme involved in neurodegenerative disorders) activity in mouse and human neurons.[4136] The Chinese accession type with 16.5% beta-caryophyllene and 14.9% alpha-bisabolol exhibited greater antiacetylcholinesterase activity. Furthermore, the hemp oils inhibited spontaneous electrical activity in mouse and human neuronal networks. Interestingly, the hydrodistilled hemp oil contained trace to significant amounts of cannabinoids: Chinese accession—delta9-tetrahydrocannabivarin (8.2%), cannabidiol (3.3%), delta9-tetrahydrocannabinol (0.7%), cannabivarin (0.2%), and cannabigerol (trace); var. *fibrante*—cannabidiol (20.1%), delta⁹-tetrahydrocannabinol (0.5%), cannabigerol (trace), delta⁸-tetrahydrocannabinol (trace), cannabinol (trace).

☐ Hemp essential oil CT beta-caryophyllene displayed significant antioxidant activity in the DPPH assay and good antibacterial activity against gram-positive bacteria such as *S. aureus* and *L. monocytogenes* (three strains of each bacteria).[4137]

☐ The beta-caryophyllene and myrcene CTs of hemp essential oil reduced the expression of proinflammatory genes and proteins and were larvicidal to *An. stephensi* and *An. Gambiae* mosquitoes.[4138]

☐ Hemp CT beta-caryophyllene essential oils extracted from wild-grown plants showed greater antimicrobial activity against *S. aureus, E. faecalis,* and *S. pneumoniae* than hemp CT beta-caryophyllene essential oils extracted from cultivated plants.[4139] Interestingly, the hydrodistilled wild-grown hemp oils had high concentrations of CBD (up to 52.4%) and THC (up to 3.4%).

☐ Three separate cultivars of hemp essential oil (one myrcene CT and two beta-caryophyllene CTs) protected tissues and promoted wound healing after infection with *Leishmania tropica* in mice.[4140] It was observed that the myrcene CT provided the best protection against *L. tropica* parasitic infection. In addition, the oils displayed antioxidant activity in the DPPH, ABTS, CUPRAC, FRAP, metal chelating, and phosphomolybdenum assays, with the myrcene CT and one beta-caryophyllene CT showing the greatest activity. Based on this the researchers identified a minor constituent (0.5%–2.5%) of the oils, selina-3,7(11)-diene, as a significant contributor the bioactivity of hemp essential oil. Further study found that selina-3,7(11)-diene binds to CB2 and PPAR-alpha receptors—suggesting it acts as a cannabinoid—and inhibits acetylcholinesterase activity.

☐ An analysis of the composition of essential oils from commercial varieties of *C. sativa* showed that white shark, lemon conti kush new, lemon conti kush, fresh mountain, and amnesia cookies produce the myrcene CT; while venom OG, pablito, 24 K, and gorilla glue produce the beta-caryophyllene CT.[4141] CBD and THC yield were as follows from hydrodistilled oils: white shark (5.5%, 0.1%), lemon conti kush new (2.9%, 0.1%), lemon konti kush (4.3%, 0.1%), venom OG (5.3%, 0.1%), pablito (3.1%, 0.1%), 24 K (4.0%, 0.1%), fresh mountain (3.9%, 0.1%), amnesia cookies (2.3%, 0.2%), and gorilla glue (3.1%, 0.2%).

☐ Hemp essential oil with near equal beta-caryophyllene and limonene and the alpha-humulene CT of hops essential oil exhibited anticancer activity against acute promyelocytic leukemia, neuroblastoma, metastatic breast, and breast cancer cells, with the greatest activity against acute promyelocytic leukemia.[4142] Good selectivity was observed for hemp and hops against leukemia and neuroblastoma.

☐ Hemp essential oil (16.2% gamma-elemene, 14.2% caryophyllene oxide) was insecticidal to fleas (*Ctenocephalides felis*), demonstrating 100 percent mortality at the highest concentrations for egg, larvae, pupal, and adults.[4143]

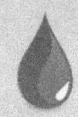 

# HINOKI
## (Japanese Cypress, Hinoki Cypress, Falsecypress)

*Chamaecyparis obtusa* (Siebold & Zucc.) Endl., *Cupressus obtusa* (Siebold & Zucc.) Silba; Taiwan Cypress, Formosan Hinoki Cypress: *Ch. obtusa var. formosana* (Hayata) Hayata

**FAMILY:** Cupressaceae
**NOTE:** Top-Middle
**AROMA INTENSITY:** Medium
**AROMA:** Sweet, woody, balsamic, slightly citrusy
**COMMON EXTRACTION METHOD:** Steam distilled from the wood, or leaves and twigs
**POSSIBLE SUBSTITUTE OILS:** Wood—Pine; *Chamaecyparis obtusa* var. *formosana* wood—Cedarwood, Palo Santo; Leaves—Cardamom, frankincense, juniper; Leaves and Twigs—Turmeric, juniper needles
**BLENDS WELL WITH:** Bergamot, blue cypress, cedarwood, cypress, grapefruit, juniper, lavender, lemon, lime, myrrh, orange, rose, sandalwood, spruce (black), tangerine
**SUBCELLULAR LOCALIZATION | EPIGENETIC INFLUENCE:** Currently unknown | *Skeletal/Integumentary*
**RECOMMENDED DILUTION RANGE:** 3%–neat

**PRIMARY CONSTITUENTS:**[4144,4145,4146,4147,4148,4149,4150]

### Wood

| | |
|---|---|
| Alpha-Cadinol | 20.5% |
| T-Muurolol | 18.5% |
| Gamma-Cadinene | 12.5% |
| Delta-Cadinene | 10.8% |
| T-Cadinol | 10.6% |
| Cadin-1(10)-en-4,beta-ol | 6.8% |
| Alpha-Muurolene | 5.8% |

### Needles and Twigs (Bicyclo [2.2.1] heptan-2-ol CT)

| | |
|---|---|
| Bicyclo [2.2.1] heptan-2-ol | 18.8% |
| 2-Carene | 17.4% |
| Sabinene | 12.8% |
| Limonene | 7.6% |
| Beta-Myrcene | 6.1% |
| Camphene | 5.1% |
| Beyerene | 4.7% |

### Leaves (needles)

| | |
|---|---|
| Beta-Myrcene | 0.0%–26.4% |
| Alpha-Terpinyl Acetate | 0.0%–12.6% |
| Limonene | 2.6%–11.2% |
| 1,7,7-Trimethylbicyclo | 0.0%–10.2% |
| Terpinyl Acetate | 0.0%–10.1% |
| Alpha-Pinene | 0.1%–7.8% |
| Gamma-Terpinene | 0.1%–6.8% |
| Beta-Pinene | 0.0%–6.4% |
| Alpha-Pinene Isomer | 0.0%–5.9% |
| Isobornyl Acetate | 0.0%–5.7% |

### Formosan Hinoki Cypress
*Chamaecyparis obtusa var. formosana wood*

| | |
|---|---|
| Alpha-Terpineol | 2.2%–19.4% |
| T-Muurolol | 0.5%–16.9% |
| Borneol | 3.0%–16.0% |
| Beta-Elemene | 0.2%–15.8% |
| Gamma-Cadinene | 1.4%–12.1% |
| Alpha-Pinene | 0.0%–11.1% |
| Alpha-Cadinol | 0.3%–10.9% |
| Limonene | 0.1%–10.8% |
| Alpha-Amorphene | 0.0%–9.4% |
| Delta-Cadinene | 2.1%–9.0% |
| Beta-Selinene | 0.4%–5.0% |

### Needles and Twigs (Alpha-Terpinene CT)

| | |
|---|---|
| Alpha-Terpinene | 40.6% |
| Bornyl Acetate | 12.5% |
| Alpha-Pinene | 11.4% |
| Beta-Pinene | 7.2% |
| Beta-Phellandrene | 3.5% |
| Alpha-Terpinolene | 3.4% |

### Leaves (Alpha-Terpinolene CT)

| | |
|---|---|
| Alpha-Terpinolene | 19.5% |
| (+)-3-Carene | 15.2% |
| Alpha-Pinene | 10.1% |
| Sabinene | 6.3% |
| Gamma-Terpinene | 4.8% |

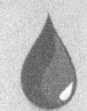

| Terpinene-4-ol | 2.1%–5.3% |
|---|---|
| Elemol | 0.0%–4.2% |
| Epizonarene | 0.0%–4.1% |

Note: One study reports the composition of Japanese hinoki branches essential oil as 58.6% alpha-pinene, 5.7% limonene, 5.3% myrcene, 3.5% terpinolene, and 3.4% beta-pinene.[4151] Another study evaluated the composition of the fruit oil (wildcrafted in Sudan) and reported it as 69.1% alpha-pinene, 12.1% delta-3-carene, 11.6% trans-sabinene hydrate, and 3.1% beta-pinene.[4152]

**OTHER CONSTITUENTS:** *Wood*—beta-caryophyllene alcohol, cadin-1(10)-en-4alpha-ol; *Chamaecyparis obtusa var. formosana* wood—camphene, terpinolene, endo-fenchol, camphor, alpha-terpinyl acetate, alpha-copaene, alpha-selinene, alpha-muurolene, T-muurolol; *leaves*—alpha-thujene, camphene, alpha-terpinolene, delta-cadinene, borneol, delta-himachalene, alpha-bisabolol, beta-phellandrene, alpha-terpineol, epi-bicyclosesquiphellandrene, widdrene; *needles and twigs (Bicyclo [2.2.1] heptan-2-ol CT)*—thujene, alpha-terpinene, alpha-terpinolene, 3-cyclohexen-1-ol, widdrene, germacrene D, beta-cubebene, 2-naphthalenemethanol, beta-eudesmol, alpha-eudesmol, rimuene; *Needles and Twigs (Alpha-Terpinene CT)*—tricyclene, camphene, sabinene, limonene, dehydro-p-cymene, alpha-terpinyl acetate, alpha-cedrene, cedrol, gamma-eudesmol, T-cadinol, hibaene, 13-isopimaradiene; *Leaves (Alpha-Terpinolene CT)*—camphene, beta-pinene, beta-myrcene, alpha-terpinene, o-cymene, bornyl acetate

**PREFERRED COMPOSITION FOR CLINICAL USE:**

| Constituent | Wood | Wood (var. formosana) |
|---|---|---|
| **Alpha-Terpineol** | tr–2% | 12%–25% |
| **Alpha-Pinene** | 25%–60% | 5%–15% |
| **Borneol** | tr–2% | 5%–15% |
| **Alpha-Cadinol** | 5%–15% | 4%–12% |
| **Limonene** | 0.1%–4% | 4%–10% |
| **Gamma-Cadinene** | 3%–10% | 2%–10% |
| **Delta-Cadinene** | 7%–15% | 2%–10% |
| **T-Muurolol** | 3%–12% | 1%–10% |
| **Alpha-Terpinolene** | tr–2% | 2%–8% |
| **Beta-Elemene** | – | 0.1%–8% |
| **Beta-Selinene** | tr–2% | 0.1%–5% |
| **Cadinol <T-, delta->** | 2%–15% | – |

**REPORTED THERAPEUTIC PROPERTIES:** Analgesic, antibacterial, antioxidant, **anti-inflammatory**, antifungal, deters insects, decongestant, antiallergenic, **relieves sinus pressure**, supports lymphatic system, aids normal respiration, nervine, reduces hair loss, calming, sedating, stress management, relieves anxiety, **relaxing**

**CAUTIONS:**

■ May moderately interfere (low risk) with the enzymes responsible for metabolizing medications based on cadinene content (NSAIDs, proton-pump inhibitors, acetaminophen, antiepileptics, immune modulators, blood-sugar medications, blood-pressure medications, antidepressants, antipsychotics, diabetic medications, antihistamines, antibiotics, and anesthetics) based on cadinene content.[4153]

■ May interact with anticholinergic (drugs used for asthma, incontinence, gastrointestinal cramps, muscular spasms, depression, and sleep disorders) and cholinergic medications (drugs used to reduce urinary retention, diagnose myasthenia gravis, and for glaucoma) based on AChE inhibitory activity.[4154]

**SELECTED EVIDENCE:**

☐ Injection of 5 or 10 mg/kg of hinoki essential oil (leaves, beta-myrcene CT) reduced inflammation by inhibiting COX-2 enzyme, TNF-α, IL-1β, and nitric oxide synthase activity, and relieved pain as well as aspirin in mice.[4155] Another study found that injection of a 10% hinoki essential oil (leaves, beta-myrcene CT) diluted in mineral oil significantly reduced arthritic pain and inflammation in rats by inhibiting the proinflammatory molecules COX-2, TNF-α, IL-6, and IL-1β.[4156] A third study determined that hinoki's (*var. formosana*, alpha-

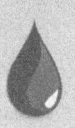 

terpineol CT) anti-inflammatory activity was the result of inhibition of TNF-α, IL-6, and IL-1, pro-IL-1β, nitric oxide (NO), inducible nitric oxide synthase (iNOS), NLRP3 (an inflammasome involved in the inflammatory process).[4157] Another study reported that oral administration of 5 and 10 mg/kg of hinoki essential oil (unidentified CT) reduced peritonitis (inflammation of the membrane lining the abdominal wall and covering abdominal organs).[4158] The study authors reported that the anti-inflammatory activity of hinoki essential oil was achieved through inhibition of TNF-α, IL-1β, IL-6, NO, iNOS, and COX-2. Oral administration o hinoki (leaf and twig) essential oil for two weeks protected against prostaglandin E2 (PGE2)-induced inflammation by reducing TNA-alpha and COX-2 and regulatin g PGE-2 expression in rats.[4159]

☐ Hinoki essential oil fractions promoted the early phase of hair growth in mice by positively influencing hair growth regulating genes and enzymatic activity.[4160] Hinoki oil positively increased alkaline phosphatase (ALP) enzyme activity, gamma-glutamyl transpeptidase (γ-GT) enzyme activity, and insulin-like growth factor-1 (IGF-1), vascular endothelial growth factor (VEGF), and epidermal growth factor (EGF) gene expression. The activity of these enzymes and genes is increased during anagen (hair growth) phase and decreased when hair loss occurs and during the catagen (regression—when the hair follicle shrinks and detaches) and telogen phases (resting—when the old hair is resting and a new hair begins the growth phase), suggesting they play important roles in hair growth and thickness.

☐ Inhalation of hinoki essential oil reduced anxiety in mice by distributing alpha-pinene to each region of the brain (particularly concentrating outside the hippocampus and striatum).[4161]

☐ Inhalation of hinoki essential oil decreased systolic blood pressure and parasympathetic nervous system activity while increasing sympathetic nervous system activity and promoting a more positive mood.[4162]

☐ Hinoki essential oil possesses broad-spectrum antimicrobial activity against general infectious bacteria, MRSA, and vancomycin-resistant enterococci (VRE) strains *in vitro*.[4163,4164] It also inhibits *S. mutans* by inhibiting the expression of some genes (*brpA, gbpB, gtfC,* and *gtfD*) involved in bacterial virulence.[4165]

☐ Application of a 5% hinoki essential oil solution reduced the appearance of acne better than a 5% tea tree essential oil solution by decreasing the size of sebaceous glands and the production of sebum, and reducing inflammatory factors associated with acne.[4166]

☐ One to two hours of inhalation of hinoki essential oil daily for seven days reduced separation anxiety in rats.[4167] Interestingly, hinoki reduced the anxiety by modulating genes that upregulated during anxiety states such as Ccl2, Il6, Cxcl10, Ccl19, and Il1rl in the hippocampus. Another study reported similar results that hinoki inhalation reduces anxiety and stress by regulating cytoskeletal-associated protein (Arc) gene expression, brain-derived neurotrophic factor (a protein that plays a role in anxiety, memory, post-traumatic stress, depression, and aging), and galactokinase 1 protein expression, and increasing nerve growth factor receptor (plays a role in behavioral changes caused by stress).[4168]

☐ Inhaling hinoki essential oil (leaves, alpha-terpinyl acetate CT) protected cognitive function (spatial learning and memory) from impairment caused by beta-amyloid induced Alzheimer's disease in rats.[4169] The essential oil protected neurons from premature death and decreased (AChE) acetylcholinesterase activity (inhibition of AChE prevents the breakdown of acetylcholine, which is essential for memory and thinking).

☐ Hinoki possesses antibacterial properties against *S. aureus, L. monocytogenes,* and *L. anisa,* and antifungal properties against *C. albicans*.[4170]

☐ Exposure to hinoki essential oil reduces the lifespan and activity of flies, and strongly repels them for about five hours.[4171]

☐ An *in vitro* study demonstrated that hinoki essential oil may be effective against inflammatory airway diseases (COPD, asthma, chronic bronchitis, etc.) due to its ability to inhibit proinflammatory molecules (IL-6, IL-5, IL-10, and TNF-α) involved in airway inflammation.[4172] A low concentration of the essential oil (0.05%) inhibited the production of these molecules by CD4+ T cells in response to airborne fungus (*Alternaria alternata*). CD4+ T cells are involved in triggering airway inflammation when they become activated by a substance and infiltrate the airways. Once there they release molecules that increase inflammation of the lungs.

☐ Inhalation of hinoki leaf essential oil (18.9% alpha-terpinyl acetate, 17.5% elemol, 10.4% sabinene) protected the lungs against LPS-induced inflammation (inhibited nitric oxide synthase, COX-2, and degradation of cytostolic p65) and improved alveolar capacity in rats, suggesting hinoki has potential for use in inflammatory respiratory conditions.[4173]

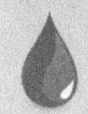

- A hinoki-infused fabric applied six hours per day for fourteen days, significantly improved eczema (lesion severity, water loss in the skin, and inflammation) in mice.[4174]
- Hay fever (allergic rhinitis) is an allergic inflammatory response to pollen characterized by red, itchy, and watery eyes, sneezing, and stuffy nose. Intranasal administration of hinoki leaf (19.5% myrcene, 16.7% sabinene, 15.7% alpha-terpinyl acetate, 9.5% bornyl acetate, 6.0% alpha-pinene) essential oil significantly suppressed hay fever symptoms, such as allergic response, inflammation of the sinuses, and mucus production in mice.[4175] The oil reduced the expression of inflammatory cytokines (L-4, IL-10, and TNF-α) and Th2 and Treg cytokines and their transcription factors. The research suggests that hinoki essential oil is antiallergic and anti-inflammatory.
- Innate immune responses to environmental triggers—pollen, cigarette smoke, viruses, and house dust mite—by the mucosal linings of airways play an important role in airway inflammation and asthma. House dust mites are microscopic, insect-like pests that feed on dead human skin cells found in dust. They are the most abundant allergens that cohabitate with humans, being found on mattresses, bedsheets, carpet, furniture, and surfaces within the home. Pretreating nasal epithelial cells with hinoki essential oil prior to stimulation with house dust mites (*Dermatophagoides pteronyssinus* and *D. farina*) suppressed the expression of multiple inflammatory mediators: NF-κB, AP-1, IL-25, IL-33, and TSLP.[4176] In addition, the essential oil was evaluated in peripheral blood mononuclear cells cultured in epithelial cells. The essential oil was less active in this culture media, only inhibiting TNF-α production.
- Hinoki fruit (seed-bearing cones) essential oil (69.1% alpha-pinene) displayed significant antioxidant activity in the ABTS and PBD assays, good activity in the CUPRAC, FRAP, and MCA assays, and was inactive in the DPPH assay.[4177] The oil also showed significant antiacetylcholinesterase and antibutyrylcholinesterase activity.

# HOLY BASIL
## (Sacred Basil, Tulsi, Rama, Tulasi, Indian Basil, Hot Basil)
*Ocimum tenuiflorum* L., *O. sanctum* L.

**FAMILY:** Lamiaceae
**NOTE:** Top-middle
**AROMA INTENSITY:** Strong
**AROMA:** Warm, spicy, balsamic, clove/basil-like
**COMMON EXTRACTION METHOD:** Steam distilled from the leaves and flower buds
**POSSIBLE SUBSTITUTE OILS:** Clove, sweet basil
**BLENDS WELL WITH:** Bergamot, cedarwood, chamomile (German, Roman), clary sage, grapefruit, hyssop, lavender, lemon, lime, orange, rose, Spanish sage, spikenard, tangerine, turmeric, ylang ylang
**SUBCELLULAR LOCALIZATION | EPIGENETIC INFLUENCE:** Currently unknown | Currently unknown
**RECOMMENDED DILUTION RANGE:** 1.5%–20%; 50% for some conditions

**PRIMARY CONSTITUENTS:**[4178,4179,4180,4181,4182,4183,4184]

*Aerial Parts—Eugenol CT*

| | |
|---|---|
| Eugenol | 15.7%–51.5% |
| Beta-Caryophyllene | 0.1%–25.4% |
| Beta-Bisabolene | 0.0%–21.0% |
| 1,8-Cineole | 2.2%–20.8% |
| Trans-Beta-Guaiene | 0.0%–19.2% |
| Beta-Elemene | 0.0%–18.0% |
| Methyl Chavicol (estragole) | 10.6%–11.5% |
| Gamma-Elemene | 7.7%–10.5% |
| E-Methyl Cinnamate | 0.0%–8.7% |
| (Z)-3-Hexanol | 0.0%–8.1% |
| Bicyclogermacrene | 0.0%–6.3% |
| Beta-Selinene | 0.0%–5.0% |

*Aerial Parts—Beta-Bisabolene CT*

| | |
|---|---|
| Beta-Bisabolene | 24.6%–52.0% |
| 1,8-Cineole | 5.1%–24.9% |
| Methyl Chavicol (estragole) | 3.4%–21.6% |
| Eugenol | 2.9%–7.6% |
| Alpha-Bergamotene | 2.9%–6.6% |
| Caryophyllene Oxide | 2.8%–4.2% |

*Aerial Parts—Methyl Chavicol (Estragole) CT*

| | |
|---|---|
| Methyl Chavicol (estragole) | 25.1%–75.1% |
| 1,8-Cineole | 1.1%–23.4% |
| Linalool | 0.0%–21.8% |
| Eugenol | 0.0%–17.0% |

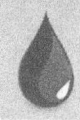

| | | | |
|---|---|---|---|
| Trans-Beta-Farnesene | 0.0%–4.1% | Carvone | 0.0%–6.3% |
| Caryophyllene Oxide | 0.0%–3.9% | Alpha-Humulene | 0.0%–5.5% |
| Alpha-Cis-Bergamotene | 1.3%–3.1% | D-Limonene | 0.0%–4.4% |
| Germacrene D | 0.1%–2.6% | | |
| 1,10 Di-Epi-Cubenol | 0.0%–2.6% | *Aerial Parts or Seeds—Methyl Eugenol CT* | |
| Alpha-Humulene | 1.3%–2.3% | Methyl Eugenol | 82.9%–92.4% |
| | | Beta-Caryophyllene | 1.3%–13.7% |
| *Leaves* | | Eugenol | 0.1%–2.4% |
| Eugenol | 71.3%–75.1% | Borneol | 0.0%–2.4% |
| Beta-Caryophyllene | 10.9%–12.9% | Germacrene D | 0.1%–2.3% |
| Germacrene D | 9.1%–10.2% | | |

Note: Plants harvested at the vegetative stage (as opposed to the budding or full flowering stage) will produce a holy basil essential oil higher in beta-bisabolene and 1,8-cineole than eugenol.

**OTHER CONSTITUENTS:** *Aerial parts—Eugenol CT:* Alpha-pinene, sabinene, myrcene, alpha-terpineol, (E)-beta-ocimene, linalool, delta-cadinene; *Aerial Parts—Beta-Bisabolene CT*: neral, (Z)-methyl cinnamate; *Aerial Parts—Methyl Chavicol (estragole) CT*: humulene epoxide II, (-)-trans-caryophyllene, beta-hydroxylauric acid, beta-pinene, alpha-pinene, isomenthone, alpha-farnesene, menthol, caryophyllene, alpha-citral, p-methoxycinnamate, alpha-caryophyllene; *Aerial Parts—Methyl Eugenol CT*: Linalool, beta-elemene, alpha-copaene, germacrene A, delta-cadinene; *Leaves:* Beta-elemene, beta-bourbonene, camphenol, ethyl linoleate, beta-selinene, elema-1,311(13)-triene-ol

**PREFERRED COMPOSITION FOR CLINICAL USE:**

| Constituent | Eugenol, Aerial Parts 1 | Eugenol, Aerial Parts 2 |
|---|---|---|
| **Eugenol** | 35%–58% | 25%–55% |
| **Beta-Caryophyllene** | 20%–40% | 15%–37% |
| **Alpha-Humulene** | 3%–8% | 0.5%–5% |
| **Elemol** | 1%–5% | – |
| **1,8-Cineole** | 0.5%–3% | tr–3% |
| **Delta-Cadinene** | 0.1%–3% | 0.1%–3% |
| **Methyl Chavicol (Estragole)** | < 3% | < 3% |
| **Trans-Beta-Elemene** | – | 15%–27% |
| **Germacrene D** | – | 1%–5% |

**REPORTED THERAPEUTIC PROPERTIES:** Anti-infectious, **antimicrobial**, **antifungal**, **antibacterial**, antiviral, antiparasitic, analgesic (pain relief), **antioxidant**, high cholesterol, headache/migraine, expectorant, fever, **heart protection**, digestive aid, kidney stones, encourages restful sleep, fatigue, acne, nervine, oral health, respiratory disorders, boosts testosterone, antidepressant, **stress management**, relieves anxiety

**CAUTIONS:**

*Aerial Parts or Leaves—Eugenol CT*

■ Caution with pregnancy and lactation. Animal studies suggest that large doses of clove may negatively impact embryonic development and encourage fetal cell death.[4185,4186] Another animal study did not detect any negative influence of clove oil.[4187] Eugenol is considered strongly toxic to embryos according to animal studies.[4188] Based on these studies it is best to limit clove oil during pregnancy and lactation.

■ May interact with MAOI antidepressants. Animal research suggests that eugenol produces antidepressant effects via the monoamine oxidase pathway, which may cause interactions with antidepressants that also interact with this pathway.[4189]

■ May interact with aspirin, blood pressure, antiplatelet, and anticoagulant medications, and increase the risk of bleeding among people with bleeding disorders due to eugenol content.[4190,4191,4192,4193]

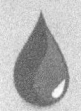

■ May interact with antibiotics or antifungal medications (fluconazole, ketoconazole) and increase their effectiveness due to eugenol content.[4194,4195,4196]

■ May interact with barbiturates and increase their sedative effects based on research using extracts of holy basil.[4197,4198,4199,4200]

■ May interact with anticholinergic (drugs used for asthma, incontinence, gastrointestinal cramps, muscular spasms, depression, and sleep disorders) and cholinergic medications (drugs used to reduce urinary retention, diagnose myasthenia gravis, and for glaucoma) based on AChE inhibitory activity of eugenol and the whole essential oil.[4201]

■ May decrease the bioavailability of many medications (NSAIDs, proton-pump inhibitors, acetaminophen, antiepileptics, immune modulators, blood-sugar medications, blood pressure medications, antidepressants, antipsychotics, diabetic medications, antihistamines, antibiotics, and anesthetics) due to the ability of beta-caryophyllene to inhibit CYP3A enzyme activity.[4202]

*Aerial Parts—Methyl Chavicol (Estragole) CT, Aerial Parts—Beta-Bisabolene CT*

■ Use with great caution for children under age 6 due to animal reports of liver cancer caused by methyl chavicol (estragole) content.[4203,4204,4205] The European Medicines Agency recommends exposure to estragole and methyl eugenol be limited in young children.

■ Avoid during pregnancy and lactation due to high methyl chavicol (estragole) content.[4206] Methyl chavicol (estragole) may cause genetic mutations and oxidative DNA damage.[4207,4208] The European Medicines Agency recommends exposure to estragole and methyl eugenol be limited in women who are pregnant or nursing.[4209]

■ Avoid oral use due to carcinogenic (cancer-causing) or toxic potential of methyl chavicol (estragole).[4210,4211,4212] The metabolite of estragole (1'-hydroxyestragole) is considered a stronger carcinogen and humans rapidly metabolize estragole to 1'-hydroxyestragole when ingested.[4213]

■ May interact with aspirin, blood pressure, antiplatelet, and anticoagulant medications, and increase the risk of bleeding among people with bleeding disorders.[4214,4215,4216,4217]

■ Avoid with epilepsy and Parkinson's disease due to 1,8-cineole content. May exacerbate or cause seizures or convulsions when inhaled, applied topically, or ingested based on 1,8-cineole content.[4218,4219,4220,4221,4222,4223]

■ May interfere with enzymes responsible for metabolizing medications (NSAIDs, proton-pump inhibitors, acetaminophen, antiepileptics, immune modulators, blood-sugar medications, blood pressure medications, antidepressants, antipsychotics, diabetic medications, antihistamines, antibiotics, and anesthetics) due to methyl chavicol (estragole) and 1,8-cineole content.[4224,4225,4226]

■ May irritate mucous membranes (eyes, mouth, nasal passages, vagina, rectum).[4227,4228]

■ May interfere with antibiotics and antifungals and increase or decrease their effectiveness due to methyl eugenol and estragole (methyl chavicol) content.[4229,4230,4231,4232]

*Aerial Parts or Seeds—Methyl Eugenol CT*:

■ Avoid in children under age 12 due to the multisite cancerous tumors and DNA mutation caused by methyl eugenol in animal studies.[4233,4234,4235,4236]

■ Avoid during pregnancy and lactation due to changes in embryo form and structure and chromosomal changes in ovary cells caused by methyl eugenol as well as the carcinogenic (cancer-causing) potential of methyl eugenol.[4237,4238,4239,4240]

■ Avoid oral consumption due to the multisite carcinogenic potential of methyl eugenol.[4241,4242,4243,4244]

■ May interfere with antibiotics and antifungals and increase their effectiveness due to methyl eugenol content.[4245]

■ May interact with anticholinergic (drugs used for asthma, incontinence, gastrointestinal cramps, muscular spasms, depression, and sleep disorders) and cholinergic medications (drugs used to reduce urinary retention, diagnose myasthenia gravis, and for glaucoma) based on the potent AChE inhibitory activity of methyl eugenol.[4246]

**SELECTED EVIDENCE:**

☐ *In vitro* research demonstrates that holy basil essential oil upregulates genes that trigger apoptosis of breast cancer cells.[4247]

☐ Holy basil essential oil demonstrated moderate antimicrobial activity against several common oral pathogens (*S. mutants, S. sanguis, S. salivarius, S. sobrinus, E. faecalis, S. aureus, C. albicans, C. dubliniensis, C. tropicalis, C. krusei,* and *C. glabrata,* and four clinical isolates of *S. mutans*) *in vitro*.[4248] Two additional *in*

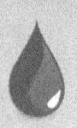

*vitro* studies suggests that holy basil is active against the fungi *Epidermophyton floccosum*, *Microsporum gypseum*, *A. flavus*, *A. fumigatus*, *A. clavatus*, *A. oryzae*, and *Sporothrix schenckii* and the bacteria *Bacillus subtilis*, *Staphylococcus aureus*, *Streptococcus mutans*, *Enterococcus coli*, *P. aeruginosa*, *S. flexneri*, and *Enterococcus faecalis*.[4249,4250] Another study demonstrated that holy basil essential oil completely inhibited *S. aureus* (including MRSA) and *E. coli*, but only partially inhibited the growth of *P. aeruginosa*, which the study authors attributed to the presence of eugenol, camphor, and 1,8-cineole.[4251]

☐ Holy basil essential oil exhibited strong antimicrobial activity against foodborne pathogens (Fungi: *Aspergillus flavus*, *A. fumigatus*, *A. clavatus*, and *A. oryzae*; Bacteria: *Staphylococcus aureus*, *Enterococcus faecalis*, *E. coli*, enterohemorrhagic *E. coli*, *Pseudomonas aeruginosa*, and a clinical isolate of *Shigella flexneri*) in vitro.[4252] Other research suggests holy basil essential oil inhibits *A. flavus* and 12 commonly occurring fungi superior to common synthetic antifungals, and completely inhibits aflatoxin B production.[4253]

☐ *In vitro* research concluded holy basil essential oil possesses antifungal activity and causes apoptosis of *C. albicans* by triggering oxidative damage, and damages cell membrane integrity.[4254,4255] Holy basil is also active against *C. tropicalis*.[2637] Another *in vitro* study found that holy basil decreases enzyme activity and down regulates genes to prevent the spread (virulence) of *C. albicans*.[4256]

☐ Holy basil essential oil is active against drug-sensitive and drug-resistant fungi and improves the antifungal activity of the antifungal drugs fluconazole and ketoconazole.[4257]

☐ Animal and *in vitro* research suggests holy basil essential oil possesses both anti-inflammatory and antibacterial properties.[4258]

☐ Holy basil essential oil demonstrated weak antioxidant activity, but significant antimicrobial activity against *A. niger* and *S. faecalis*.[4259] Interestingly, other *in vitro* research concluded that holy basil has the highest antioxidant activity of 18 essential oils tested and the strongest antioxidant activity of Ocimum species.[4260,4261]

☐ Animal research suggests that holy basil leaf essential oil decreases cholesterol levels and protects heart tissues against damage caused by high cholesterol through its antioxidant properties.[4262]

☐ *In vitro* research suggests that holy basil essential oil (eugenol was found to be a potent AChE inhibitor as well) inhibits acetylcholinesterase (AChE) enzyme activity.[4263] Inhibition of AChE prevents the breakdown of acetylcholine, which is essential for memory and thinking. People with neurodegenerative diseases make less acetylcholine, and the diseases often break it down at a faster rate leading to acetylcholine deficits.

☐ Animal research found that holy basil essential oil increases the penetration and bioavailability of the NSAID flurbiprofen through the skin.[4264]

☐ An *in vitro* study concluded that holy basil essential oil is suitable for acne skin care because of its ability to inhibit *P. acnes*.[4265]

☐ *In vitro* research suggests holy basil essential oil inhibits the Leishmania protozoa.[4266]

☐ Both holy basil essential oil and eugenol demonstrate potent anti-parasitic (anthelmintic) activity.[4267]

☐ Animal research suggests that holy basil essential oil decreased blood pressure by triggering vasodilation and inhibiting platelet aggregation.[4268]

☐ A combination of holy basil, peppermint, Indian borage, and eucalyptus (*E. globulus*)—diluted to 5%—provided six hours of mosquito protection, which is comparable to DEET.[4269]

☐ Holy basil essential oil (CT not reported) significantly reduced bacterial colony-forming units (CFUs) obtained from children aged four to nine after a root canal.[4270]

☐ The eugenol CT of holy basil essential oil was significantly toxic to the coleopteran beetle (*Callosobruchus maculatus*) in fumigant form.[4271] Eugenol was slightly more effective when used alone.

☐ *In vitro* research showed that holy basil essential oil possesses anticancer activity against human gastric cancer.[4272] The oil triggered apoptosis by significantly upregulating pro-apoptotic genes (TP53, BAX, and BAK) and significantly downregulating antiapoptotic genes (BCL-2 and BCL-xL). The oil also markedly increased the expression of CASP8, CASP9, and CASP3 (genes that increase overall survivability of gastric cancer when increased) genes.

☐ *In vitro* research showed that holy basil inhibited *Fusarium verticillioides*, *Penicillium expansum*, and *Aspergillus flavus*, with the greatest activity observed against *A. niger*.[4273] The oil also was insecticidal/larvicidal to house flies, the African cotton leafworm larvae (most susceptible), and *C. quinquefasciatus* mosquito larvae.

☐ *Mycobacterium tuberculosis* is a pathogenic bacterium that cause tuberculosis. Unfortunately, this bacterium

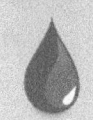

has developed resistance to most available antimicrobials making it difficult to treat and cure. Laboratory research found that holy basil essential oil inhibits both drug-resistant and drug-sensitive strains (nine clinical and one lab strain) of *M. tuberculosis*.[4274] The study authors concluded that research emphasize "the potential use of essential oils from plants as a new source of anti-*M. tuberculosis* drug" and further research including human clinical trials are needed.

☐ *Sarcoptes scabiei* mites are responsible for scabies, an itchy contagious skin infection in humans. More than thirty essential oils used in traditional treatments for dermatological conditions in Madagascar were evaluated against scabies mites. Both cinnamon leaf and holy basil CT eugenol essential oil were most active against *S. scabiei* in a laboratory setting, suggesting they should be further investigated as topical solutions for scabies.[4275]

# HONEY MYRTLE
## (Marsh Honey Myrtle)

*Melaleuca teretifolia* Endl., *Gymnagathis teretifolia* (Endl.) Schauer

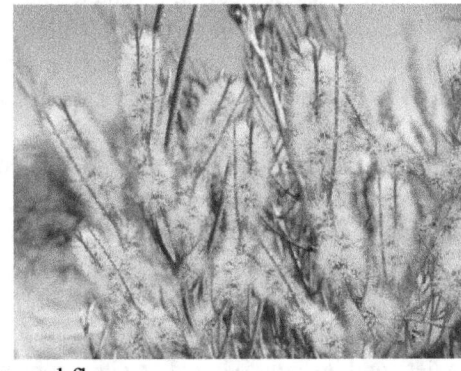

**FAMILY:** Myrtaceae
**NOTE:** Top-Middle
**AROMA INTENSITY:** Strong
**AROMA:** Fresh, lemony, herbaceous
**COMMON EXTRACTION METHOD:** Steam distilled from the leaves, twigs, and flowers
**POSSIBLE SUBSTITUTE OILS:** Lemongrass, melissa, lemon verbena, lemon myrtle (geranial CT), may chang (geranial CT)
**BLENDS WELL WITH:** Bergamot, blue cypress, cedarwood, citronellal, copaiba, cypress, Douglas fir, grapefruit, hyssop, lavender, lemon, lemongrass, lemon eucalyptus, lime, melissa, myrtle, niaouli, orange, ravintsara, rosalina, sandalwood, tangerine, tea tree, vetiver
**SUBCELLULAR LOCALIZATION | EPIGENETIC INFLUENCE:** Currently unknown | Currently unknown
**RECOMMENDED DILUTION RANGE:** 1.5%–20%; neat for limited conditions

**PRIMARY CONSTITUENTS:**[4276,4277,4278]
*Citral CT*

| | |
|---|---|
| Geranial | 38.0%–40.3% |
| Neral | 27.7%–32.3% |
| Beta-Myrcene | 9.8%–11.2% |
| Geraniol | 2.1%–5.3% |
| Nerol | 0.0%–3.6% |
| Terpinen-4-ol | 0.0%–3.4% |
| (E)-Isocitral | 0.0%–2.4% |
| 1,8-Cineole | 0.5%–1.6% |
| (Z)-Isocitral | 0.0%–1.6% |
| Limonene | 0.6%–1.0% |
| Citronellal | 0.2%–1.0% |

Note: A 1,8-cineole CT is produced when only the leaves are distilled and consists of: 1,8-Cineole (84.0%), Alpha-Terpineol (3.3%), Limonene (3.1%), Terpinen-4-ol (1.8%), Alpha-Pinene (1.8%), Beta-Pinene (1.2%).

**OTHER CONSTITUENTS:** Alpha-pinene, alpha-terpineol, geranyl acetate, citronellyl acetate

**PREFERRED COMPOSITION FOR CLINICAL USE:**

| *Constituent* | |
|---|---|
| **Geranial** | 35%–45% |
| **Neral** | 25%–35% |
| **Beta-Myrcene** | 8%–13% |

| Geraniol | 2%–7% |
|---|---|
| Nerol | 1%–5% |

**REPORTED THERAPEUTIC PROPERTIES:** Antibacterial, antifungal, **antimicrobial**, antiviral, antispasmodic, analgesic, anti-infectious, antioxidant, anti-inflammatory, anti-convulsant, balances blood pressure, supports cardiovascular function, aids respiratory function, insect repellent, deodorant, relaxing/calming, antidepressant, relieves anxiety, enhances clarity and focus, stress management

**CAUTIONS:**

■ Caution is advised during pregnancy and lactation due to high citral content. Large doses of citral may negatively affect fetal development according to animal studies.[4279]

■ There is a moderate risk that honey myrtle may interfere with enzymes responsible for metabolizing medications (NSAIDs, proton-pump inhibitors, acetaminophen, antiepileptics, immune modulators, blood-sugar medications, blood pressure medications, antidepressants, antipsychotics, diabetic medications, antihistamines, antibiotics, and anesthetics) due to citral and geraniol content.[4280,4281,4282,4283 1232–1235]

■ Use cautiously with diabetic medications. Large oral doses of citral may improve insulin sensitivity and lower blood-glucose levels according to animal research.[4284,4285]

■ May interact with antibiotics and possibly enhance their effects due to similar composition to lemongrass essential oil.[4286]

■ There is a moderate risk that honey myrtle may interfere with pentobarbital and other barbiturates (medications for anxiety and insomnia) based on citral content.[4287]

■ Dilution is recommended for topical application due to high citral content and the risk for skin irritation or sensitivity.[4288,4289] May also irritate mucous membranes.

**SELECTED EVIDENCE:**

☐ Honey myrtle essential oil repels the fruit fly *B. tryoni,* but only for short periods of time.[4290]

☐ Honey myrtle essential oil demonstrated strong fumigant properties against the spotted-wing drosophila (*D. suzukii*).[4291]

# HOPS
## (Hop, Aroma Hops, Hops Flower)
*Humulus lupulus L.*

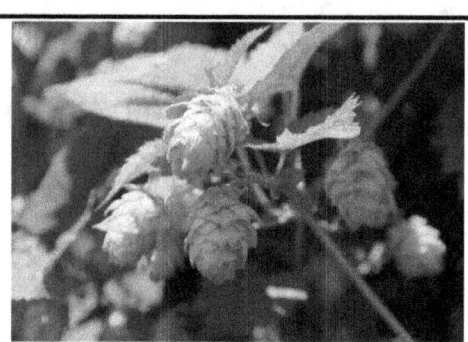

**FAMILY:** Moraceae
**NOTE:** Middle
**AROMA INTENSITY:** Medium
**AROMA:** Rich, earthy/herbaceous, spicy, slightly sweet
**COMMON EXTRACTION METHOD:** Steam distilled from the flowers (hops, or cones)
**POSSIBLE SUBSTITUTE OILS:** Hemp, copaiba, mastic (beta-myrcene CT), verbena (myrcene CT), guava leaf, black sage, black pepper, ginger
**BLENDS WELL WITH:** Bergamot, cassia, cinnamon, clary sage, clove, copaiba, grapefruit, hemp, lavender, lemon, lime, Mediterranean mandarin, nutmeg, orange, patchouli, pine, tangerine, valerian, yuzu
**SUBCELLULAR LOCALIZATION | EPIGENETIC INFLUENCE:** Currently unknown | Currently unknown
**RECOMMENDED DILUTION RANGE:** 3.0%–33.0%; neat for limited conditions

**PRIMARY CONSTITUENTS:**[4292,4293,4294]

| Beta-Myrcene | 5.1%–52.4% |
|---|---|
| Alpha-Humulene | 1.9%–51.2% |
| Beta-Bisabolol | 0.0%–15.0% |

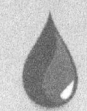

| | |
|---|---|
| Beta-Caryophyllene | 4.1%–14.5% |
| Gamma-Elemene | 0.0%–14.0% |
| (E)-Beta-Farnesene | 0.0%–9.5% |
| Humulene Epoxide II | 0.0%–7.9% |
| Alpha-Zingiberene | 0.0%–5.6% |

Note: Hops essential oil is very complex with more than 400 volatile constituents registering on analyses. Of those 400 constituents about 200 have been identified. Alpha-humulene, myrcene, and beta-caryophyllene typically make up more than half of its total composition, and sometimes reaches 98% of its total composition. 'Olympic,' 'Hallertau mittelfrüh,' 'Hugo de Groot,' 'Hallertauer,' 'Sterling,' 'Vanguard,' and wild-growing hops varieties typically have higher alpha-humulene content, whereas 'Cascade,' 'Saaz,' 'Willamette,' 'Brewers Gold,' 'Hersbrücker spät,' 'Wye Challenger,' 'Wye Northdown,' 'Wye Target,' 'Yeoman,' and 'Northern Brewer' hops varieties are normally dominated by beta-myrcene. The 'Hallertau mittelfrüh' variety is considered by some to be the most desirable for essential oil extraction (alpha-humulene 41.3%, beta-myrcene 27.3%, beta-caryophyllene 11.3%).

**OTHER CONSTITUENTS:** 4-methyl-2-pentanone, 3-methyl-2-pentanone, 3-methyl-2-buten-1-ol, hexanal, 3-methyl-2-butenal, isovaleric acid, 2-methylbutanoic acid, 4-methyl-2-pentenolide, beta-pinene, isoamyl isobutyrate, methyl heptanoate, limonene, beta-phellandrene, heptanoic acid, 2-nonane, linalool, n-nonanal, 2-decanone, methyl nonanoate, 2-undecanone, methyl (4Z)-decenoate, methyl geranate, methyl decanoate, 9-decanoic acid, alpha-copaene, geranyl acetate, alpha-trans-bergamotene, geranyl propionate, gamma-muurolene, beta-selinene, delta-selinene, alpha-selinene, 2-tridecanone, terpinolene, alpha-muurolene, (E,E)-alpha-farnesene, delta-cadinene, geranyl isobutyrate, caryophyllene oxide, alpha-humulene hydrate, T-cadinol, 1-epi-cubenol, caryophylla-4(12),8(13)-dien-5-o, alpha-cadinol, 14-hydroxy-(E)-caryophyllene, (2Z,6E)-farneso, (6Z)-pentadecen-2-one, 2-pentadecanone, alpha-guaiene, beta-gurjunene, ar-curcumene, aromadendrene, alloaromadendrene, Selina-3,7(11)-diene, elemol, germacrene B, guaiol, globulol, viridiflorol, alpha-epi-7-epi-5-eudesmol, 1,10-di-epi-cubenol, bisabolene-11-ol, (Z)-nerolidol acetate

**PREFERRED COMPOSITION FOR CLINICAL USE:**

| *Constituent* | |
|---|---|
| **Alpha-Humulene** | 30%–50% |
| **Beta-Myrcene** | 10%–32% |
| **Beta-Caryophyllene** | 8%–18% |

**REPORTED THERAPEUTIC PROPERTIES: Analgesic, anti-inflammatory,** antispasmodic, antineuralgic, relieves headache/migraine, eases cough (especially spasmodic), supports respiratory function, relieves chronic skin conditions, aids digestion, relieves painful menstruation, nervine, **antiallergic,** encourages restful sleep, relieves anxiety, **sedating,** antidepressant, stress management

**CAUTIONS:**

■ Caution is advised during pregnancy and lactation due to high beta-myrcene content. Extremely high doses (500 mg/kg) of beta-myrcene have been toxic to fetuses according to animal research.[4295,4296]

■ May interact with barbiturates (medications for anxiety and insomnia), antihistamines, benzodiazepines, tricyclic antidepressants, or other central nervous system depressant drugs, increasing their depressant effects due to similar composition to hemp essential oil and beta-myrcene content.[4297,4298,4299]

■ May weakly interfere with the enzymes responsible for metabolizing medications (NSAIDs, proton-pump inhibitors, acetaminophen, antiepileptics, immune modulators, blood-sugar medications, blood pressure medications, antidepressants, antipsychotics, diabetic medications, antihistamines, antibiotics, and anesthetics) based on myrcene content.[4300,4301,4302]

**SELECTED EVIDENCE:**

☐ *In vitro* research demonstrates that hops essential oil (alpha-humulene CT) inhibits gram-positive bacteria (*L. innocua* and *S. aureus*) and gram-negative bacterium *Y. enterocolitica.*[4303] Another study reported that hops essential oil inhibits gram-positive bacteria (*Bacillus subtilis* and *S. aureus*) and the fungus *Trichophyton mentagrophytes* var. *interdigitale*, but almost no activity against the gram-negative bacterium *E. coli* and the yeast *C. albicans*.[4304]

☐ Hops essential oil (alpha-humulene CT) is a moderate antioxidant.[4305]

# HYSSOP (LINALOOL CT)

*Hyssopus officinalis* L. var. *decumbens* Briq.;
*H. officinalis* L., *H. angustifolius* M. Bieb

**FAMILY:** Lamiaceae (Labiatae)
**NOTE:** Middle
**AROMA INTENSITY:** Medium
**AROMA:** Sweet, herbaceous, woody, earthy
**COMMON EXTRACTION METHOD:** Steam distilled from the leaves and flowering tops
**POSSIBLE SUBSTITUTE OILS:** Lavandin, lavender, spike lavender
**BLENDS WELL WITH:** Angelica, bay laurel, clary sage, geranium, grapefruit, lavandin, lavender, lemon, melissa, myrtle, orange, rosemary, sage, tangerine
**SUBCELLULAR LOCALIZATION | EPIGENETIC INFLUENCE:** Currently unknown | Currently unknown
**RECOMMENDED DILUTION RANGE:** 3%–50%, neat for limited conditions; Pinocamphone CT: 1.5%–20%

**PRIMARY CONSTITUENTS:**[4306,4307,4308,4309,4310,4311]

| *Linalool CT (H. officinalis* var. *decumbens)* | | *Pinocamphone CT (H. officinalis, H. angustifolius)* | |
|---|---|---|---|
| Linalool | 48.0%–51.7% | Pinocamphone | 34.0%–53.0% |
| 1,8-Cineole | 12.3%–14.9% | Isopinocamphone | 3.2%–27.5% |
| Limonene | 5.0%–6.0% | Beta-Pinene | 9.9%–18.4% |
| Beta-Pinene | 2.9%–3.0% | Beta-Phellandrene | 3.4%–7.5% |
| Beta-Caryophyllene | 2.4%–2.8% | Germacrene D | 0.7%–6.2% |
| Caryophyllene Oxide | 0.0%–3.2% | Elemol | 0.0%–5.7% |
| Alpha-Pinene | 2.2%–2.5% | Limonene | 0.0%–5.6% |
| Camphene | 0.0%–2.0% | Myrtenol | 0.7%–2.8% |
| Isopinocamphone | 0.1%–1.5% | Beta-Caryophyllene | 0.3%–2.5% |
| Myrcene | 0.0%–1.7% | Myrcene | 0.0%–2.4% |
| Beta-Bourbonene | 0.0%–1.2% | Bicyclogermacrene | 0.0%–2.0% |
| Pinocamphone | 0.1%–1.0% | Sabinene | 1.3%–1.9% |
| Sabinene | 0.8%–1.0% | Alpha-Pinene | 0.1%–1.8% |
| | | Pinocarvone | 0.0%–1.4% |
| *Alpha-Pinene CT* | | Alpha-Thujene | 0.0%–1.0% |
| Alpha-Pinene | 70.9% | Alloaromadendrene | 0.0%–1.0% |
| Beta-Pinene | 10.9% | | |
| Limonene | 2.7% | | |
| Beta-Caryophyllene | 2.7% | | |
| Caryophyllene Oxide | 2.1% | | |
| Alpha-Campholenal | 1.1% | | |
| Viridiflorene | 1.1% | | |
| Guaiol | 1.0% | | |
| Alpha-Guaiene | 1.0% | | |

Note: The linalool CT is the preferred variation of hyssop essential oil for safety and efficacy reasons. Multiple CTs are available commercially, most with moderate to significant amounts of pinocamphones. Other chemotypes include pinocarvone (pinocarvone 36.3%, pinocamphone 19.6%, beta-pinene 10.6%, 1,8-cineole 7.2%), isopinocamphone (isopinocamphone 38.1%, pinocamphone 20.3%, 1,8-cineole 12.2%, beta-pinene 10.2%) myrtenyl acetate (myrtenyl acetate 74.1%, camphor 6.8%), and 1,8-cineole (1,8-

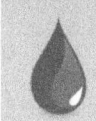

cineole 52.9%–70.0%, beta-pinene 1.0%–16.8%, terpinen-4-ol 4.0%–10.0%, pinocarvone 2.0%–6.0%).[4144,4346] Pinocamphone CTs are typically obtained when the plant material is distilled in the vegetative state, whereas isopinocamphone CTs are obtained during the beginning and full flowering stage. The pinocamphone CT appears to be the most common CT available in commercial samples.

**OTHER CONSTITUENTS:** *Linalool CT*—N/A; *Pinocamphone CT*—Alpha-terpineol, sabinyl acetate, delta-cadinene, beta-bourbonene, camphor, linalool; *Alpha-Pinene CT*—Alpha-thujene, spathulenol, trans-pinocamphone (trace), cis-pinocamhone (trace)

**PREFERRED COMPOSITION FOR CLINICAL USE:**

| Constituent | var. decumbens |
|---|---|
| Linalool | 45%–55% |
| 1,8-Cineole | 10%–18% |
| Limonene | 3%–8% |
| Beta-Pinene | 2%–6% |
| Beta-Caryophyllene | 2%–6% |
| Alpha-Pinene | 1%–6% |
| Sabinene | 0.5%–3% |
| Isopinocamphone | ≤ 1.5%* |
| Pinocamphone | ≤ 1%* |

\* The closer to 0% the better for pinocamphones.

**REPORTED THERAPEUTIC PROPERTIES:** Antiseptic, **antimicrobial**, astringent, antirheumatic, anti-inflammatory, antispasmodic, expels excess gas, aids digestion, diuretic, **decongestant**, promotes normal menstruation, purifying, nervine, reduces fever, wound healing, reduces the appearance of scars and blemishes, relieves sore throat, **supports immune system activity**, encourages sweating, stimulating, aids concentration, combats mental fatigue, stress management, relieves anxiety

**CAUTIONS:**
*Linalool CT & Alpha-Pinene CT:*
■ None currently known.

*All Other CTs:*
**These CTs are not recommended for use during essential oil therapy unless the benefits far outweigh the risks as determined by a qualified professional.**
■ The pinocamphone, isopinocamphone, and all other CTs with high levels of pinocamphones should be avoided with children, during pregnancy/lactation, orally, and by those with epilepsy and Parkinson's disease due to their neurotoxic, uterine/menstrual stimulant, and convulsive properties.[4312,4313,4314,4315] They should also not be used long-term by any administration method, nor applied in concentrations greater than 0.5% topically. Animal research suggests that as little 0.08 g/kg body weight of hyssop oil may negatively affect the central nervous system and cause convulsions, and 1.25 g/kg is lethal. In addition, the daily repeated use of hyssop (injection) produced toxic effects and caused convulsions. Moreover, short-term oral use (several days) of only 2–3 drops of hyssop in children caused tonic-clonic convulsions (a seizure when all the muscles stiffen, air is forced past the vocal cords to cause a groan, the person loses consciousness, followed by jerking of the arms and legs that generally last from one to three minutes).[4316,4317] The linalool CT has very low concentrations of pinocamphones that should not adversely affect the central nervous system, and any minute toxicity is likely countered by linalool.

**SELECTED EVIDENCE:**
  ☐ The linalool CT of hyssop oil possesses stronger antimicrobial activity than other CTs according to *in vitro* research, inhibiting the bacteria *Enterococcus* spp. and *E. coli*, and seven strains of *C. albicans, C. krusei,* and *C. tropicalis*.[4318] The isopinocamphone CT strongly inhibited *Staphylococcus pyogenes, S. aureus, C. albicans,* and *E. coli*; whereas the pinocamphone CT demonstrated weak antimicrobial activity.[4319,4320] An unidentified CT of hyssop essential oil completely inhibited *A. niger*.[4321]

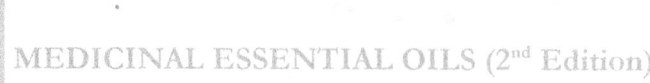

- ☐ Linalool-rich hyssop reduces intestinal spasms according to animal research.[4322] The isopinocamphone CT also prevented intestinal spasms in isolated guinea-pig ileum and rabbit jejunum.[4323]
- ☐ Hyssop CT isopinocamphone essential oil significantly kills adult rice weevils (*S. oryzae*).[4324]
- ☐ Hyssop essential oil (1,8-cineole CT) was strongly active against the African cotton leafworm (*Spodoptera littoralis*).[4325]
- ☐ The isopinocamphone content of hyssop essential oil exhibited strong antioxidant activity in the DPPH assay.[4326]
- ☐ *Fusarium graminearum* is a fungus that contaminates cereals, fruit, and vegetables. Thyme, oregano, basil, nutmeg, hyssop, and clove essential oils inhibited mycelial growth of *F. graminearum*, with oregano performing best followed by clove and thyme.[4327] The composition of the oils was not reported.
- ☐ Hyssop (subsp. *aristatus*) CT 1,8-cineole essential oil exhibited anti-inflammatory activity by inhibiting COX-2 enzyme activity similarly to celecoxib (hyssop: 20 µg/mL 43.7%–52.4%; celecoxib: 8.8 µg/mL 61.6%) *in vitro*.[4328] Further evaluation in rats showed that injection of the oil significantly reduced edema comparably to indomethacin.
- ☐ The pinocamphone CT of hyssop essential oil (grown intercropped with fenugreek) showed good antioxidant activity.[4329]
- ☐ Hyssop CT pinocamphone essential oil produced a synergistic effect against clinical isolates and a reference strain of *C. albicans* when combined with itraconazole and enhanced (additive) the activity of itraconazole and fluconazole against clinical isolates and a reference strain of *C. albicans*.[4330]
- ☐ The antioxidant activity of hyssop CT pinocamphones essential oil was improved when the oil was distilled from plants intercropped with fenugreek.[4331]

# INDIAN BORAGE
## (Mexican Mint, Plectranthus Oregano)

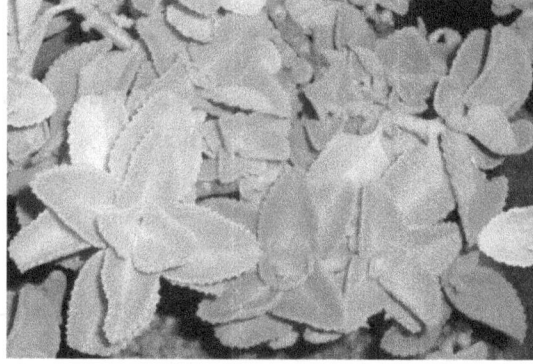

*Plectranthus amboinicus* (Lour.) Spreng., *Coleus amboinicus* Lour., *C. aromaticus* Benth.

**FAMILY:** Lamiaceae
**NOTE:** Middle
**AROMA INTENSITY:** Strong
**AROMA:** Herbaceous, spicy, medicinal
**COMMON EXTRACTION METHOD:** Hydrodistilled or steam distilled from the leaves; may also be distilled from the stems or aerial parts
**POSSIBLE SUBSTITUTE OILS:** Oregano, summer savory, mountain savory, savory (wild)
**BLENDS WELL WITH:** Bergamot, grapefruit, lavender, lemon, lime, mountain savory, orange, oregano, pine, rosemary, savory (wild), tangerine, thyme
**SUBCELLULAR LOCALIZATION | EPIGENETIC INFLUENCE:** Currently unknown | Currently unknown
**RECOMMENDED DILUTION RANGE:** Carvacrol & Thymol CTs—1.5%–20%; 50% for some conditions; Beta-caryophyllene and Delta-Cadinene CTs—3%–50%; neat for limited conditions

**PRIMARY CONSTITUENTS:**[4332,4333,4334,4335,4336,4337,4338,4339,4340]

*Leaves (Carvacrol CT)*

| | | | |
|---|---|---|---|
| Carvacrol | 21.7%–98.0% | *Leaves (Thymol CT)* | |
| Camphor | 0.0%–22.2% | Thymol | 8.8%–58.8% |
| Thymol | 0.0%–21.7% | Eugenol | 0.0%–14.6% |
| Delta-3-Carene | 0.0%–15.0% | (E)-Cycloisolongifol-5-ol | 0.0%–8.0% |
| Gamma-Terpinene | 0.0%–14.7% | Himachalene Epoxide | 0.0%–7.9% |
| Beta-Caryophyllene | 0.0%–14.1% | 1(5),3-Aromadendradiene | 0.0%–7.1% |
| Para-Cymene | 0.0%–12.0% | Germacrene D-4-ol | 0.0%–5.7% |
| Alpha-Humulene | 0.0%–9.7% | Gamma-Gurjunene Epoxide | 0.0%–5.2% |
| Undecanal | 0.0%–8.3% | Alpha-Amorphene | 0.0%–4.2% |

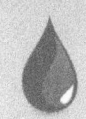

| | | | |
|---|---|---|---|
| Trans-Alpha-Bergamotene | 0.0%–8.2% | (E)-Cadinene Ether | 0.0%–3.9% |
| O-cymene | 0.0%–7.7% | Gamma-Terpinene | 3.2%–3.5% |
| Caryophyllene Oxide | 0.0%–5.9% | | |
| Alpha-Terpinene | 0.0%–4.8% | | |
| Germacrene D | 0.0%–3.9% | *Leaves (Beta-Caryophyllene CT)* | |
| Alpha-Terpineol | 0.0%–3.3% | Beta-Caryophyllene | 12.6% |
| | | Delta-Cadinene | 9.8% |
| | | Eudesm-4(15),7-diene-1-β-1-ol | 9.0% |
| *Leaves (Delta-Cadinene CT)* | | Himachalene Epoxide | 8.6% |
| Delta-Cadinene | 12.5%–18.7% | Alpha-Humulene | 8.0% |
| Alpha-Cadinol | 5.7%–12.5% | Alpha-Copaene | 6.9% |
| Beta-Caryophyllene | 5.3%–9.8% | 1(5),3-Aromadendradiene | 3.2% |
| Alpha-Humulene | 6.3%–8.2% | Thymol | 3.0% |
| Epi-Alpha-Muurolol | 4.4%–7.3% | Alpha-Amorphene | 3.0% |
| Thymol | 2.9%–6.0% | Isospathulenol | 3.0% |
| Carvacrol | 0.1%–6.0% | | |
| Spathulenol | 4.9%–5.7% | | |
| (E)-Cycloisolongifol-5-ol | 0.0%–5.3% | | |
| Alpha-Copaene | 2.6%–5.0% | | |
| Himachalene Epoxide | 1.6%–4.9% | | |
| Alpha-Amorphene | 0.0%–4.8% | | |
| Germacrene D | 0.0%–3.9% | | |

**OTHER CONSTITUENTS:** *Carvacrol CT*—Beta-myrcene, delta-3-carene, limonene, terpinene-4-ol, 2Z-octenol acetate, beta-selinene, 2-phenyl ethyl tiglate, beta-copaen-4-alpha-ol, caryophyllene oxide; *Thymol CT*—octen-3-ol, alpha-terpinene, para-cymene, fenchone, carvacrol, alpha-ylangene, isocaryophyllene, valencene, delta-cadinene, 1,10-di-epi cubenol, epoxy-allo-aromadendrene, epi-alpha-muurolol, alpha-cadinol, cis-alpha-copaene-8-ol, 9-epi-trans-caryophyllene-14-hydroxy, 10-nor-calamenene-10-one, alpha-muurolene-14-hydroxy, phytol, 3E-cembrene A, kaurene; *Delta-Cadinene CT*—octen-3-ol, para-cymene, gamma-terpinene, terpinene-4-ol, thymol acetate, beta-elemene, alpha-gurjunene, trans-alpha-bergamotene, beta-selinene, alpha-muurolene, gamma-gurjunene epoxide, 1(5),3-aromadendradiene, isospathulenol, caryophyllene oxide, humulene epoxide II, 1,10-di-epi cubenol, epi-alpha-cadinol, Eudesm-4(15),7-diene-1-β-1-ol, 10-nor-calamenene-10-one, cembrene; *Beta-Caryophyllene CT*—para-cymene, gamma-terpinene, carvacrol, thymol acetate, alpha-ylangene, beta-bourbonene, trans-alpha-bergamotene, alpha-cuprenene, caryophyllene oxide, humulene epoxide II, beta-copaene-4-alpha-ol, epi-alpha-cadinol, epi-alpha-muurolol, cis-alpha-copaene-8-ol, shyobunol, 10-nor-calamenene-10-one, alpha-muurolene-14-hydroxy, cubitene, phytol

**PREFERRED COMPOSITION FOR CLINICAL USE:**

| Constituent | Carvacrol CT |
|---|---|
| **Carvacrol** | 25%–35% |
| **Thymol** | 20%–28% |
| **Alpha-Humulene** | 7%–12% |
| **Gamma-Terpinene** | 7%–12% |
| **Undecanal** | 5%–10% |
| **Para-Cymene** | 5%–10% |
| **Caryophyllene Oxide** | 3%–7% |
| **Beta-Selinene** | 1%–5% |
| **Alpha-Terpineol** | 1%–5% |

**REPORTED THERAPEUTIC PROPERTIES:** Anti-infectious, antibacterial, antifungal, antiviral, diuretic, **antimicrobial**, antiseptic, analgesic, **anti-inflammatory**, relieves menstrual discomfort, soothes sore throat, relieves diarrhea, supports respiratory function, eases cough, relieves headache, wound healing, relieves insect bites/stings, promotes restful sleep, reduces insecurity, encourages motivation, reduces ego

CAUTIONS:

*Delta-Cadinene CT*
■ None currently known.

*Beta-Caryophyllene CT*
■ May interact with diuretic medications and increase diuretic action.[4341]

*Carvacrol and Thymol CTs*
■ *Carvacrol CT only*: Use very cautiously with children under 6 due to potentially moderate camphor content. Several cases of camphor poisoning and/or seizures from ingestion and topical application have been reported in children.[4342,4343] Ingestion of camphor-containing products has been lethal in children under age 2 (estimated to be roughly 2,000 mg of camphor for a 20 kg child as the minimum potential fatal dose).[4344,4345] Children 5 years and up may use camphor-containing essential oils topically in dilutions no stronger than 5%.

■ Avoid during pregnancy and lactation due to similar composition to oregano essential oil and possible camphor or eugenol content. Oils rich in carvacrol may negatively affect embryonic development and encourage fetal cell death according to animal research.[4346] Camphor ingestion may lead to abortion because fetuses lack the enzymes to process it.[4347] Camphor ingestion by infants and young children may cause cough, vomiting, seizure, burning sensation in the mucous membranes and eyes, or lack of voluntary coordination of muscle movements.[4348] Eugenol is considered strongly toxic to embryos according to animal studies.[4349]

■ Oral caution due to thymol and camphor content. Thymol has a longer half-life (the time it takes for half of the medication to metabolize or excrete half of the dosage) than most essential oil constituents and should not be administered orally for long periods of time.[4350] Thymol is a monoterpene phenol. Reports of fatalities in children who consumed 50 to 200 mg of phenols has been reported.[4351] It is recommended that chemotypes with high levels of thymol be limited to 10 drops per day orally for adults with a two- to seven-day break after twenty-one days of use. Essential oils with significant levels of camphor can be toxic when taken orally. Oral—Camphor can be toxic when taken orally (usually single doses exceeding 2 mL), although the lethal dose for adult humans is estimated to be (more than 5 mL) in a single dose.[4352,4353,4354]

■ May interact with diabetic medications and cause low blood-sugar levels based on carvacrol content.[4355,4356,4357]

■ May interact with aspirin, blood pressure, antiplatelet, and anticoagulant medications, and increase the risk of bleeding among people with bleeding disorders due to thymol, carvacrol, or eugenol content.[4358,4359,4360,4361,4362,4363]

■ *Carvacrol CT only*: Avoid with epilepsy and Parkinson's due to potentially high camphor content.[4364,4365,4366]

■ *Carvacrol CT only*: The potentially moderate camphor content in Indian borage may negatively impact red blood cells and increase the risk of jaundice in children with Glucose-6-phosphate dehydrogenase deficiency (G6PD).[4367,4368]

■ May interact with antibiotics and possibly enhance their effects due to thymol, carvacrol, or eugenol content.[4369,4370]

■ May interact with anticholinergic (drugs used for asthma, incontinence, gastrointestinal cramps, muscular spasms, depression, and sleep disorders) and cholinergic medications (drugs used to reduce urinary retention, diagnose myasthenia gravis, and for glaucoma) based on thymol, carvacrol, or eugenol content.[4371,4372]

■ May irritate mucous membranes (eyes, mouth, nasal passages, vagina, rectum).

SELECTED EVIDENCE:
    ☐   Indian borage essential oil (beta-caryophyllene CT) only weakly killed liver and breast cancer cells when compared to the chemotherapy drug doxorubicin.[4373] Injection of Indian borage essential oil into mice exhibited potent anticancer activity against metastatic lung cancer.[4374]

    ☐   *In vitro* research shows that Indian borage essential oil (carvacrol CT) inhibits the pathogenic yeasts *S. epidermidis, C. albicans, C. gattii* (two strains), *C. neoformans,* and *S. cerevisiae*.[4375] The beta-caryophyllene CT of Indian borage essential oil inhibited *C. albicans, C. parapsilosis, A. flavus,* and *A. niger*.[4376] The carvacrol CT with camphor present inhibited *C. albicans* and *C. tropicalis*, with stronger inhibition noted for *C. tropicalis*.[4377]

    ☐   The carvacrol CT with camphor present inhibited *E. coli* and *S. aureus*, with stronger antimicrobial activity observed against gram-positive bacteria (*S. aureus*).[4378] Indian borage essential oil without camphor inhibited intestinal bacteria: *Salmonella* sp., *Shigella* sp., *E. coli,* and *Vibrio* sp.[4379] An Indian borage essential oil with

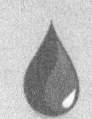

significant carvacrol content completely inhibited *K. pneumoniae*. Interestingly, the researchers noted that its antimicrobial activity increased in higher pH ranges.[4380] The beta-caryophyllene CT of Indian borage essential oil inhibited *S. mutans, E. coli, B. subtilis, S. aureus,* and MRSA, but was ineffective against *K. pneumoniae* and *Ps. Aeruginosa.*[4381] The carvacrol CT with camphor present inhibited *Staphylococcus epidermis, S. aureus, Serratia marcencens, Proteus vulgaris,* MRSA, *E. coli, and B. subtilis*, with the greatest inhibition noted against *E. coli* and *S. aureus.*[4382]

☐ An unidentified CT of Indian borage essential oil inhibited two bacteria commonly associated with swimmer's ear (acute otitis externa): *S. aureus* and *C. krusei.*[4383]

☐ Oral administration of 0.01 mL of Indian borage essential oil (beta-caryophyllene CT) significantly reduces inflammation and pain in animals.[4384]

☐ Indian borage essential oil (beta-caryophyllene CT) significantly increased urine and sodium excretion in animals.[4385]

☐ *In vitro* research demonstrates that the beta-caryophyllene CT of Indian borage essential oil is a powerful antioxidant.[4386]

☐ Indian borage essential oil (close to equal portions of carvacrol and thymol) killed the larvae of malarial vector mosquito *Anopheles stephensi* and African malaria vector mosquito *(Anopheles gambiae).*[4387,4388] The thymol CT of Indian borage essential oil repelled the cat flea *(Ctenocephalides felis).*[4389] A combination of holy basil, peppermint, Indian borage, and eucalyptus *(E. globulus)*—diluted to 5%—provided six hours of mosquito protection, which is comparable to DEET.[4390]

☐ Indian borage CT carvacrol essential oil was larvicidal to *Culex quinquefasciatus* and *Aedes Aegypti* mosquitoes.[4391] The study authors determined that gamma-terpinene and para-cymene were the most larvicidal constituents in the oil, which may have been synergized by beta-caryophyllene.

☐ *In vitro* research showed that Indian borage CT carvacrol essential oil inhibits *F. oxysporum.*[4392]

# JAPANESE CEDARWOOD
## (Sugi)

*Cryptomeria japonica* D. Don

**FAMILY:** Cupressaceae
**NOTE:** Middle-Base
**AROMA INTENSITY:** Medium
**AROMA:** Leaves—fresh, woody, balsamic; Roots—woody, cedar-like, slightly peppery; Wood/Bark—woody, cedar-like, balsamic
**COMMON EXTRACTION METHOD:** Steam distilled from the leaves (needles), roots, wood, or bark
**POSSIBLE SUBSTITUTE OILS:** Hinoki, betony, calendula, Formosan cypress, agarwood, helichrysum
**BLENDS WELL WITH:** Bergamot, blue cypress, cedarwood, cypress, grapefruit, juniper, lavender, lemon, lime, myrrh, orange, rose, sandalwood, spruce (black), tangerine
**SUBCELLULAR LOCALIZATION | EPIGENETIC INFLUENCE:** Currently unknown | Currently unknown
**RECOMMENDED DILUTION RANGE:** 3.0%–Neat

**PRIMARY CONSTITUENTS:**[4393,4394,4395,4396,4397,4398,4399,4400,4401,4402,4403,4404,4405,4406]

| Leaves (16-Kaurene CT) | | Leaves (Alpha-Pinene CT) | |
|---|---|---|---|
| 16-Kaurene | 11.6%–42.1% | Alpha-Pinene | 6.1%–29.5% |
| Elemol | 8.6%–20.5% | (+)-Phyllocladene | 0.0%–24.1% |
| Alpha-Pinene | 3.1%–16.8% | Sabinene | 0.5%–19.9% |
| Alpha-Eudesmol | 0.0%–12.2% | Elemol | 0.2%–12.7% |
| Sabinene | 1.2%–11.1% | Terpinen-4-ol | 0.1%–9.8% |
| Gamma-Eudesmol | 0.0%–10.6% | Gamma-Eudesmol | 0.0%–9.1% |
| Delta-3-Carene | 0.1%–9.9% | 10(15)-Cadinene-4-ol | 0.0%–7.2% |
| Terpinen-4-ol | 0.0%–9.1% | Alpha-Eudesmol | 2.6%–7.1% |

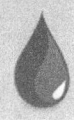

| | |
|---|---|
| Limonene | 1.1%–6.8% |
| Beta-Eudesmol | 0.0%–5.7% |
| Gamma-Selinene | 0.0%–4.4% |
| Biformen | 0.0%–3.9% |
| Lendene | 0.0%–3.8% |
| Epi-Cedrol | 0.0%–3.8% |
| Camphene | 0.1%–3.4% |
| Delta-Cadinene | 0.5%–3.3% |
| Gamma-Terpinene | 0.5%–3.1% |

*Heartwood*

| | |
|---|---|
| Cubebol | 0.0%–39.9% |
| Epi-Cubebol | 0.0%–26.9% |
| 1-Epi-Cubenol | 0.0%–18.9% |
| Alpha-Cadinene | 0.0%–18.6% |
| Cubenol | 0.0%–18.4% |
| Delta-Cadinene | 0.0%–17.3% |
| Elemol | 0.0%–14.1% |
| Isoledene | 0.0%–12.4% |
| Gamma-Muurolene | 0.0%–11.8% |
| Alpha-Eudesmol | 0.0%–10.7% |
| Alpha-Humulene | 0.7%–9.4% |
| Alpha-Muurolene | 1.5%–9.3% |
| Alpha-Cubebene | 0.2%–9.3% |
| T-Muurolol | 0.0%–6.9% |
| 1,1,3a-trimethyl-7-methyl-ene-decahydrocyclo-propa[a]-naphthalene | 0.0%–6.8% |
| Beta-Eudesmol | 0.0%–6.1% |
| Hedycariol | 0.0%–5.7% |
| Trans-Calamenene | 0.0%–5.3% |
| Alpha-Cadinol | 0.0%–5.2% |
| T-Cadinol | 0.0%–3.9% |
| Gamma-Cadinene | 0.0%–3.7% |

*Bark*

| | |
|---|---|
| Camphor | 0.0%–48.4% |
| Delta-3-Carene | 0.0%–18.6% |
| Alpha-Pinene | 0.0%–17.1% |
| Delta-Cadinene | 0.0%–15.9% |
| Cubenol | 0.0%–14.0% |
| Ferruginol | 0.0%–11.5% |
| T-Muurolol | 0.0%–10.7% |
| Cadina-1,3,5-Triene | .0%–10.5% |
| Beta-Eudesmol | 0.0%–9.9% |
| Limonene | 0.1%–9.7% |
| Gamma-Eudesmol | 0.0%–7.0% |
| Hedycariol | 0.0%–6.2% |
| Alpha-Muurolene | 1.3%–5.4% |
| Dehydroferruginol | 0.0%–5.1% |

| | |
|---|---|
| Delta-Cadinene | 0.8%–6.5% |
| Alpha-Terpineol | 0.1%–6.1% |
| Limonene | 0.0%–5.0% |
| Beta-Eudesmol | 0.0%–4.8% |
| T-Cadinol | 0.3%–4.7% |
| Myrcene | 0.0%–3.9% |
| 8Beta-Hydroxysandara-copimarene | 0.0%–3.6% |
| Gamma-Terpinene | 0.0%–3.5% |

*Leaves (16-Kaurene/Valencene CT)*

| | |
|---|---|
| 16-Kaurene | 40.6% |
| Valencene | 19.9% |
| Eudesma-3,7(11)-Diene | .4% |
| Alpha-Gurjunene | 7.9% |
| Beta-Eudesmol | 5.9% |
| Para-Cymene | 3.7% |
| Alpha-Pinene | 3.1% |

*Sapwood*

| | |
|---|---|
| Sclarene | 0.0%–27.6% |
| Cubebol | 0.0%–20.5% |
| Cubenol | 0.0%–13.3% |
| Cupressene | 0.0%–12.6% |
| 1-Epi-Cubenol | 0.0%–12.5% |
| Ferruginol | 0.0%–10.8% |
| Valencene | 0.0%–9.9% |
| Beta-Eudesmol | 0.0%–9.3% |
| 1,1,3a-trimethyl-7-methyl-ene-decahydrocyclo-propa[a]-naphthalene | 0.0%–7.6% |
| 2-methylene-5-(1-methylvinyl)-8-methyl-bicyclo[5.3.0]decane | 0.0%–5.6% |
| Isoledene | 0.0%–5.0% |
| Trans-Calamenene | 0.0%–4.6% |
| Trans-Cadina-1(6),4-Diene | 0.0%–4.1% |
| Alpha-Muurolene | 3.4%–4.0% |
| Alpha-Eudesmol | 0.0%–3.8% |
| Epi-Cubebol | 0.0%–3.7% |
| Sandaracopimarinal | 0.0%–3.7% |
| Verticiol | 0.0%–3.5% |
| Tremetone | 0.0%–3.1% |

*Twig*

| | |
|---|---|
| Alpha-Eudesmol | 10.9%–25.6% |
| Gamma-Eudesmol | 6.1%–11.8% |
| Delta-Cadinene | 0.0%–10.4% |
| Isopimarol | 0.0%–10.9% |
| Elemol | 6.8%–8.7% |

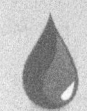

| | | | |
|---|---|---|---|
| Epi-Zonarene | 0.0%–5.0% | Cryptomerione | 7.5%–7.6% |
| Valencene | 0.0%–3.9% | Bisabolatrien-1-ol-4-one | 5.7%–5.8% |
| Alpha-Terpineol | 0.0%–3.7% | Ferruginol | 4.3%–4.8% |
| Alpha-Eudesmol | 0.0%–3.4% | Cubebol | 4.3%–4.5% |
| Sabinene | 0.0%–3.3% | Cubenol | 0.1%–4.0% |
| | | Sandaracopimarinal | 3.2%–3.4% |
| | | Kauran-16-ol | 0.0%–3.4% |
| | | 1-Epi-Cubenol | 3.2%–3.3% |

Note: The leaf alpha-pinene CT generally has less than 0.5% 16-kaurene or none at all. Heartwood, sapwood, and bark essential oils could be divided into additional CTs based on the presence or absence of various constituents, but they are combined in this work for simplification purposes.

**OTHER CONSTITUENTS:** *Leaves (16-Kaurene CT)*—camphene, beta-myrcene, alpha-terpinene, linalool, bornyl acetate, isobornyl acetate, T-muurolol, 5-neo-cedranol, alpha-terpinolene, widdrene, germacrene D, beta-himachalene, alpha-muurolene, alpha-cedrol, 10-epi-gamma-eudesmol, alpha-cadinol, nezukol; *Leaves (Alpha-Pinene CT)*—alpha-thujene, beta-pinene, alpha-phellandrene, alpha-terpinene, beta-phellandrene, para-cymene, terpinolene, thymol, thujopsene, trans-beta-farnesene, germacrene D, camphene, delta-3-carene, bornyl acetate, alpha-muurolene, caryophyllene oxide, cupressene, pimara-8,15-diene; *Leaves (16-Kaurene/Valencene CT)*—beta-pinene, delta-3-carene, terpinen-4-ol, bornyl acetate, cadina-3,9-diene, isoledene, sclareol (< 1.5%); *Heartwood*—germacrene D, beta-cubebene, gamma-elemene, epi-bicyclosesquiphellandrene, beta-maaiene, longiverbenone, verticiol, camphor, cis-muurola-3,5-diene, trans-cadina-1(6),4-diene, trans-muurola-4(14),5-diene, trans-cadina-1(2),4-diene, alpha-calacorene, cis-muurol-5-en-4-α-ol, gleenol, humulene epoxide II, cryptomerione, abietadiene, sandaracopimarinal, phyllocladanol, ferruginol, selin-11-en-4-α-ol; *Sapwood*—camphor, cis-muurola-3,5-diene, alpha-humulene, trans-muurola-4(14),5-diene, trans-cadina-1(2),4-diene, alpha-calacorene, elemol, gleenol, gamma-eudesmol, selin-11-en-4-α-ol, cryptomerione, bisabolatrien-1-ol-4-one, abietadiene, sandaracopimarinal, phyllocladanol, cadala-1(10),3,8-triene, azulene, spathulenol, longiverbenone, pimarinal, abieta-8,11,13-triene; *Bark*—camphene, limonene, terpinen-4-ol, alpha-terpineol, gamma-gurjunene, cubebol, trans-calamenene, trans-cadina-1(2),4-diene, elemol, isophyllocladene; *Twig*—alpha-muurolene, trans-calamenene, trans-cadina-1(2),4-diene, epi-cedrol, alpha-calacorene, eudesm-7(11)-en-4-ol, sandaracopimarinal

**PREFERRED COMPOSITION FOR CLINICAL USE:**

| Constituent | 16-Kaurene CT |
|---|---|
| **16-Kaurene** | 20%–42% |
| **Elemol** | 7%–22% |
| **Alpha-Pinene** | 4%–16% |
| **Sabinene** | 4%–11% |
| **Limonene** | 1%–7% |
| **Delta-Cadinene** | 0.5%–5% |
| **Gamma-Terpinene** | 0.5%–5% |
| **Camphene** | 0.1%–5% |
| **Delta-3-Carene** | 0.1%–5% |

**REPORTED THERAPEUTIC PROPERTIES:** Antibacterial, antifungal, anti-infectious, anticancer, anti-inflammatory, analgesic, antiarthritic, antioxidant, aids detoxification, protects the stomach, **reduces the appearance of acne and blemishes, soothes chronic skin conditions**, supports respiratory function, protects the liver, supports oral health, **insecticide**, insect repellent, relieves anxiety, antidepressant, relaxing, stress management

**CAUTIONS:**

■ May moderately interfere (low risk) with the enzymes responsible for metabolizing medications based on cadinene content (NSAIDs, proton-pump inhibitors, acetaminophen, antiepileptics, immune modulators, blood-sugar medications, blood-pressure medications, antidepressants, antipsychotics, diabetic medications, antihistamines, antibiotics, and anesthetics) based on cadinene content.[4407]

*Bark*

■ Avoid with children under six due to potentially significant camphor content. Several cases of camphor poisoning and/or seizures from ingestion and topical application have been reported in children.[4408,4409] Ingestion of camphor-containing products has been lethal in children under age two.[4410] Children five years and up may use camphor-containing essential oils topically in dilutions no stronger than 5%. Camphor ingestion by infants and young children may cause cough, vomiting, seizure, burning sensation in the mucous membranes and eyes, or lack of voluntary coordination of muscle movements.[4411]

■ Caution is warranted during pregnancy and while lactating due to potentially significant camphor content. Ingestion of essential oils with significant levels of camphor may lead to abortion because fetuses lack the enzymes to process it.[4412] Camphor ingestion by infants and young children may cause cough, vomiting, seizure, burning sensation in the mucous membranes and eyes, or lack of voluntary coordination of muscle movements.[4413]

■ Avoid with epilepsy and Parkinson's due to potentially significant camphor content.[4414,4415]

■ Avoid with those who have a compromised liver due to the risk of increased liver enzymes and liver damage.[4416] This would also suggest that those taking medications that could cause liver damage should also use Japanese cedarwood (bark) essential oil very cautiously or avoid it entirely.

■ The potentially significant camphor content in Japanese cedarwood bark essential oil may negatively impact red blood cells and increase the risk of jaundice in children with glucose-6-phosphate dehydrogenase deficiency (G6PD).[4417,4418]

■ Oral caution—Essential oils with significant levels of camphor can be toxic when taken orally, usually single doses exceeding 2 mL, although the lethal dose for humans is estimated to be more than 5 mL in a single dose.[4419,4420,4421]

■ Caution is warranted for the topical application of camphor-containing essential oils on broken or injured skin due to an increased risk of toxicity.[4422]

## SELECTED EVIDENCE:

☐ *In vitro* research shows that Japanese cedarwood essential oil (elemol CT) killed human oral epidermoid carcinoma (squamous cell carcinoma) by rapidly triggering capsase-3 (a thiol protease that regulates cell death by dismantling intracellular components while avoiding inflammation and damage to surrounding cells) activity and the cleavage of PARP (a family of proteins that are involved in routine repair of DNA damage, and also participate in cell death and survival) and cancer cells.[4423] It also caused mitochondrial stress within cancer cells (triggered changes to Bcl-2 proteins), which leads to apoptosis.

☐ Japanese cedarwood essential oil (16-kaurene CT) may be a good candidate to reduce acne due to its ability to inhibit drug-susceptible and drug resistant skin pathogens (*P. acnes* and *S. epidermidis*) associated with acne and the production of proinflammatory cytokines (PGE2, TNF-alpha, IL-1Beta, IL-6) and nitric oxide production.[4424]

☐ *In vitro* research shows that Japanese cedarwood essential oil (elemol CT) significantly inhibits several oral bacterial strains: *Streptococcus sanguinis, S. mutans, S. ratti, S. criceti, S. anginosus, S. gordonii, S. sobrinus, Actinobacillus actinomycetemcomitans, Fusobacterium nucleatum, Prevotella intermedia,* and *Porphylomonas gingivalis,* and reference strains: *Staphylococcus aureus, S. puogenes, E. coli,* and *Streptococcus pyogenes.*[4425] The weakest activity was observed against *E. coli.* The study authors also reported that individual components within Japanese cedarwood essential oil (alpha-pinene, sabinene, alpha-terpineol, and terpinen-4-ol) all demonstrated antimicrobial activity against all strains tested. The 16-kaurene CT of Japanese cedarwood essential oil only weakly inhibited *E. coli* and *Klebsiella oxytoca,* but effectively inhibited *B. subtilis, Citrobacter freundii, Enterobacter aerogenes, E. Cloacae, Klebsiella pneumoniae, Pseudomonas aeruginosa, Serratia maracescens,* and two strains of *S. aureus.*[4426] The leaf (alpha-pinene CT), heartwood (cubebol and epi-cubebol rich), and bark (cubenol and delta-cadinene rich) oils of Japanese cedarwood essential oil moderately inhibited *Mycobacterium tuberculosis.*[4427]

☐ Essential oil from different parts of Japanese cedarwood demonstrated antifungal activities against wood decay and tree pathogenic fungi: heartwood—*Laetiporus sulphureus, Trametes versicolor, Rhizoctonia solani, Collectotrichum gloeosporioides, Fusarium solani,* and *Ganoderma australe;* sapwood—*T. Versicolor, L. sulphureus,* and *G. trabeum;* and leaf—*T. Versicolor, L. sulphureus,* and *G. trabeum;* but the bark oil was largely inactive.[4428] The 16-kaurene CT of Japanese cedarwood essential oil inhibited several fungi: *Candida albicans, C.*

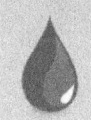

*krusei, C. glabrata, C. tropicalis, C. pseudotropicalis, C. parapsilosis, Cryptococcus neoformans,* and *Aspergillus fumigatus.*[4429] Elemol and eudesmol from Japanese cedarwood essential oil were determined to possess antifungal activity in another study.[4430] The leaf (alpha-pinene CT), heartwood (cubebol and epi-cubebol rich), and bark (cubenol and delta-cadinene rich) oils of Japanese cedarwood essential oil inhibited four phytopathogenic fungi: *B cinera, T. harzianum, C. cladosporioides,* and *Cladosporium sp.*; but were inactive against seven human pathogenic fungi (*Aspergillus fumigatus, Trichophyton rubrum, T. mentagrophytes, Microsporum gypseum, Candida albicans, C. tropicalis,* and *Saccharomyces cerevisiae*), and moderately inhibited *Cryptococcus neoformans.*[4431] Essential oil obtained from waste wood chips of Japanese cedar (25.9% delta-cadinene, 11.6% epi-cubenol) inhibited the activity of DNA polymerase (enzymes that create DNA molecules that are essential for fungal replication) of a fungus responsible for fungal skin infections (*Trichophyton rubrum*).[4432]

- The sapwood, twig, heartwood, bark, and leaf essential oil of Japanese cedarwood demonstrated moderate antioxidant activity, with sapwood being the strongest antioxidant.[4433] Ferruginol possessed the highest antioxidant activity among the constituents in the sapwood essential oil. Other research reported that terpinen-4-ol and delta-cadinene demonstrated high DPPH antioxidant activity, and bornyl acetate and nezukol demonstrated extremely high SOD-like antioxidant activity.[4434]

- Japanese cedarwood essential oil (16-kaurene CT with 18.2% elemol) killed and significantly repelled the silverfish insect (*Lepisma saccharina*).[4435] Japanese cedarwood essential oil also kills the larvae of the *Anopheles gambiae* mosquito, the *Ae. aegypti* mosquito, the *Coptotermes formosanus* Shiraki termite, and the pinewood nematode (*Bursaphelenchus xylophilus*).[4436,4437,4438,4439,4440] Beta-elemol and alpha-terpineol isolated from the essential oil also caused 100% *Coptotermes formosanus* Shiraki termite mortality.[4441] The leaf essential oil was considered the best mosquito repellent (*Aedes aegypti* and *Ae. albopictus*) of four different Japanese cedarwood plant parts tested.[4442] The age of the tree that Japanese cedarwood essential oil is extracted from may also affect its insecticidal activity against mosquitoes (*Aedes aegypti* and *Ae. albopictus*), with older trees being more effective.[4443]

- 16-kaurene, bornyl acetate, and nezukol from Japanese cedarwood essential oil may whiten the skin by inhibiting tyrosinase activity.[4444] Tyrosinase is an enzyme involved in the production of melanin (a dark brown to black pigment that is responsible for tanning of skin when exposed to sunlight) by oxidation of tyrosine.

- Terpinen-4-ol and elemol isolated from Japanese cedarwood essential oil prevented ulcers caused by HCI/ethanol, HCI/aspirin, water-immersion stress, and pylorus-ligation (closing off the blood vessel that supplies blood to the opening from the stomach into the duodenum) in animals.[4445] The most pronounced effect was observed with terpinen-4-ol, which reduced stomach acid output and pepsin activity. Excess stomach acid and pepsin may overcome the defenses of the gastrointestinal tract and erode the mucosal wall, producing ulcers.

- Several essential oils listed in order of efficacy killed the itch mite (*Sarcoptes scabiei*) that burrows into the skin and causes scabies during direct contact (clove > palmarosa > geranium > tea tree > lavender > manuka > petitgrain > eucalyptus > Japanese cedarwood (16-kaurene CT)) with the mites and when used as a fumigant (tea tree > clove > eucalyptus > lavender > palmarosa > geranium > Japanese cedarwood > petitgrain > manuka).[4446]

- Inhalation of Japanese cedarwood essential oil promoted mental relaxation (improved mood and balanced nervous system activity) after performing a monotonous mathematical task.[4447] Women inhaled 0.4 mL of essential oil (mixed with 3.6 mL of a dilute solution) from a diffuser while performing the task.

- Japanese cedarwood essential oil showed high antioxidant activity in the DPPH, ORAC, and ROS reduction assays, but was inactive against *S. aureus, B. subtilis, P. aeruginosa, E. coli, C. albicans,* and *A. brasiliensis.*[4448]

*Did you know?*

Clinical research proves that simply inhaling essential oils can positively influence hormone production. This is likely due to their influence on both the nervous and endocrine systems.

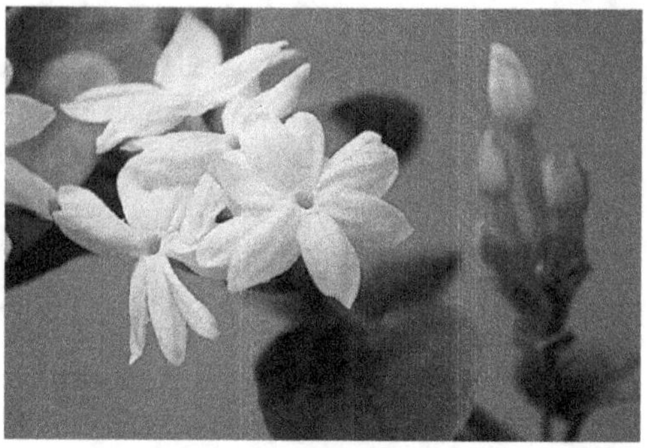

# JASMINE ABSOLUTE
## (Poet's Jasmine)

*Jasminum grandiflorum* L., *J. officinale* L., *J. officinale* L. var. *grandiflorum* (L.) L.H. Bailey; **Jasmine Sambac:** *J. sambac* (L.) Ait

**FAMILY:** Oleaceae
**NOTE:** Middle-Base
**AROMA INTENSITY:** Strong
**AROMA:** Intensely floral, rich, sweet
**COMMON EXTRACTION METHOD:** Solvent extracted from the flowers; may also be hydrodistilled from the flowers
**POSSIBLE SUBSTITUTE OILS:** Rose, ylang ylang, chamomile (German, Roman)
**BLENDS WELL WITH:** Bergamot, chamomile (German, Roman), clary sage, clove, coriander, frankincense, geranium, ginger, grapefruit, lavender, lemon, lime, Mediterranean mandarin, neroli, orange, palmarosa, patchouli, petitgrain, rose, rosewood, sandalwood, tangerine, vetiver, ylang ylang
**SUBCELLULAR LOCALIZATION | EPIGENETIC INFLUENCE:** Currently unknown | Currently unknown
**RECOMMENDED DILUTION RANGE:** Absolute—1.0%–3.0%; Essential oil—3%–25%

**PRIMARY CONSTITUENTS:**[4449,4450,4451,4452,4453,4454]

*Jasmine Absolute (Benzyl Acetate CT)*

| | |
|---|---|
| Benzyl Acetate | 15.0%–31.0% |
| Benzyl Benzoate | 2.5%–20.0% |
| Linalool | 3.0%–12.7% |
| Phytol | 0.0%–12.5% |
| Squalene 2,3-Oxide | 0.0%–12.0% |
| Isophytol | 0.0%–8.0% |
| Phytyl Acetate | 0.0%–7.0% |
| Methyl Benzoate | 0.2%–6.9% |
| Indole | 0.7%–6.5% |
| Phenylethyl Acetate | 0.0%–6.5% |
| M-Cresol | 0.0%–6.1% |
| Squalene | 0.0%–6.0% |
| (3E,6E)-Alpha-Farnesene | 0.0%–5.8% |
| Geranyl Linalool | 0.0%–5.0% |

*Jasmine Absolute (Benzyl Benzoate CT)*

| | |
|---|---|
| Benzyl Benzoate + Phytol | 20.1%–26.6% |
| Jasmine Lactone | 3.1%–8.5% |
| Trans-Methyl Jasmonates | 5.0%–7.8% |
| Benzyl Acetate | 4.8%–7.7% |
| (Z)-Jasmone | 1.8%–7.1% |
| Eugenol | 2.0%–4.0% |
| Methyl Anthranilate | 1.2%–3.6% |

*Hydrodistilled (Essential Oil)*

| | |
|---|---|
| Phytol | 25.8% |
| 3,7,11-trimethyl-1,6,10-Dodecatrien-3-ol | 12.5% |
| 3,7,11,15-tetramethyl-Hexadecen-3-ol | 12.4% |
| Hexadecanoic Acid | 9.2% |
| Perhydrofarnesyl Acetone | 4.9% |
| Benzyl Benzoate | 4.9% |
| 9,12,15-Octadecatrienoic Acid | 4.8% |

*Jasmine Sambac Absolute*

| | |
|---|---|
| (Z)-3-Hexenyl Benzoate | 9.4%–20.7% |
| (E,E)-Alpha-Farnesene | 2.2%–19.7% |
| Benzyl Acetate | 7.5%–14.2% |
| Linalool | 6.3%–14.1% |
| Benzyl Alcohol | 0.3%–8.4% |
| Methyl Anthranilate | 2.8%–6.5% |
| (Z)-3-Hexenyl Acetate | 0.7%–6.4% |
| Methyl Linoleate | 1.4%–3.9% |
| Methyl Stearate | 0.3%–3.8% |
| (Z)-11-Tricosene | 0.0%–3.5% |
| Cis-Linalool Oxide | 0.2%–3.2% |
| Anti-Phenylacetaldoximine | 0.0%–2.6% |
| 5-Methyltricosane | 0.0%–2.0% |
| Palmitic Acid | 0.0%–2.0% |
| Tetracosane | 0.0%–2.0% |

Note: Jasmine sambac and jasmine grandiflorum have a simlar aroma and therapeutic use. Jasmine sambac tends to have a more exotic and youthful aroma, while grandiflorum is often described as greener and more animalic. Grandiflorum blossoms early in the morning and sambac late in the evening.

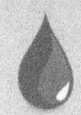

**OTHER CONSTITUENTS:** *Jasmine Absolute (Benzyl Acetate CT)*—octanal, nonanal, naphthalene, methyl salicylate (<3.4%), decanal, (Z)-jasmone, tetradecane, geranyl acetate, eugenol, (Z)-methyl jasmonate, jasmolactone, pentadecane, 3-hexenyl benzoate, 5,10,14-trimethyl-2-pentadecanone; *Jasmine Absolute (Benzyl Benzoate CT)*— benzyl alcohol, n-acetyl; *Hydrodistilled*—methyl myristate, methyl palmitate, 3,7,11,15-tetramethylhexadecanoic acid methyl ester, 9,12,15-octadecatrienoic acid methyl ester, heneicosane, octadecanoic acid methyl ester, tetracosane, pentacosane, hexacosane, heptacosane, octacosane, nonacosane; *Jasmine Sambac Absolute*—Trans-linalool oxide, terpinolene, methyl salicylate (<1.0%), indole, (E)-beta-farnesene, germacrene D, (Z,Z)-alpha-farnesene, delta-cadinene, (E)-nerolidol, alpha-cadinol, (E,E)-farnesol, (E,Z)-farnesol, benzyl benzoate, (E,E)-farnesyl acetate, methyl palmitate, heptadecanoic acid, 9,12-octadecadienol, oleic acid, mixed hydrocarbons

**PREFERRED COMPOSITION FOR CLINICAL USE:**

| Constituent | *J. grandiflorum* Benzyl Acetate CT | *J. grandiflorum* Squalenes CT | *J. Sambac* |
|---|---|---|---|
| Benzyl Acetate | 15%–35% | 5%–17% | 5%–15% |
| Benzyl Benzoate | 7%–25% | 3%–13% | – |
| Phytol | 5%–12% | 5%–12% | – |
| Linalool | 3%–12% | 1%–5% | 4%–14% |
| Phytyl Acetate | 5%–11% | 3%–8% | – |
| Isophytol | 3%–10% | 3%–9% | – |
| Epoxysqualenes | 2%–10% | incl. below | – |
| Squalene | 2%–6% | 22%–38%* | < 5% |
| Indole | 0.1%–6% | 0.1%–4% | tr–8% |
| Jasmone <cis + trans> | 1%–5% | 0.5%–3% | – |
| Geranyl Linalool | 2%–5% | 1%–4% | – |
| Methyl Linolenate | 1%–3% | – | 0.1%–5% |
| Eugenol | 0.5%–3% | 0.5%–3% | – |
| (E,E)-Alpha-Farnesene | 0%–3% | 0.1%–3% | 10%–20% |
| (Z)-3-Hexenyl Benzoate | – | – | 3%–15% |
| Benzyl Alcohol | – | – | 1%–9% |
| Germacrene D-4-ol | – | – | 2%–8% |
| Methyl Anthranilate | – | – | 2%–8% |
| (Z)-3-Hexenyl Acetate | – | – | tr–7% |
| Methyl Linoleate | – | – | 0.5%–5% |
| Linalool Oxide <cis- + trans-> (fur) | – | | tr–5% |

* Total squalenes (trans-trans-trans-Squalene, 2,3-Epoxy dihydro squalene A, 2,3-Epoxy dihydro squalene B, Oxirane squalene, Oxirane squalene 2, Oxirane squalene 3, Hydroxy squalene)

**REPORTED THERAPEUTIC PROPERTIES:** Antibacterial, antimicrobial, antifungal, antiseptic, analgesic, antiarthritic, **antispasmodic**, aids circulation, reduces the appearance of scars and blemishes, nourishes the skin, wound healing, supports respiratory function, expels excess mucus, balances female hormones, reduces painful menstruation, relieves addictions, encourages restful sleep, **sedating**, antidepressant, **stress management**, **relieves anxiety**, reduces hysteria, aphrodisiac

**CAUTIONS:**

■ Avoid oral consumption. Absolutes contain solvent residue and should not be taken orally. In addition, ingestion of benzoic acids, benzoic salts (calcium, potassium, and sodium), benzaldehyde, benzyl acetate, benzyl benzoate, and benzyl alcohol may cause gastrointestinal irritation, vomiting, and diarrhea.[4455]

■ Jasmine absolute and distilled oil should be avoided by individuals with Refsum disease (a neurological disorder caused by the overaccumulation of phytanic acid in cells and tissues) or who are AMACR-deficient (alpha-methylacyl-CoA racemase-deficient) due to phytol content. It is believed that humans can convert phytol to phytanic acid.[4456] Animal research suggests that phytol can cause liver inflammation, liver failure, and death in AMACR-deficient mice.[4457,4458] AMACR is an enzyme found in the mitochondria that plays a role in the breakdown of fatty acids.

AMACR deficiency causes neurological problems (seizures, cognitive decline, migraines, encephalopathy, loss of sensation due to nerve damage, muscle stiffness, lack of coordination, and vision problems) that begin in adulthood and progressively get worse.[4459] Phytol may also weakly promote tumor formation according to animal research.[4460]

■ Do not exceed maximum dilution percentage during topical application due to solvent content and possibility of skin irritation.[4461,4462,4463,4464,4465,4466,4467,4468,4469] Jasmine absolute is a common cause of contact dermatitis, particularly among people who have sensitive skin, chronic skin conditions, or allergies to fragrances.

### SELECTED EVIDENCE:

□ Jasmine absolute reduced spasms in isolated guinea pig small intestine (ileum) by inhibiting cAMP-phosphodiesterase (an enzyme that plays a role in muscle contraction of the airways and cardiovascular tissues).[4470,4471] It also reduces uterine contractions and decreases the tone of isolated phrenic nerve (a nerve that originates at the neck—C3-C5—and passes between the lung and heart to reach the diaphragm) skeletal muscle.[4472,4473]

□ Inhalation of 2 mcL/mL of propylene glycol and diethyl phthalate from a plastic squeeze bottle held 5 cm under the nose for 15 minutes improved mood and increased calmness in thirty-two healthy individuals aged seventeen to thirty-six.[4474]

□ Jasmine absolute demonstrated varying degrees of antimicrobial activity against several human pathogenic bacteria (*E. coli, Bacillus sp., Streptococcus* sp., *Salmonella* sp., *Pseudomonas* sp., *Serratia marcescens, Klebsiella pneumonia,* and *Staphylococcus aureus*).[4475]

□ Jasmine absolute inhibited the fungi *A. flavus* and *A. parasiticus*.[4476]

□ Human aryl hydrocarbon receptor (AhR: a gene that encodes a protein that helps regulate responses to planar aromatic hydrocarbons and significantly affects the immune activity in the gastrointestinal tract) regulates the circadian rhythm, helps regulate the cell cycle, and plays an important role in tissue development. Cumin, jasmine, vanilla, and bay leaf fully activate AhR; clove, dill, thyme, nutmeg, and oregano partially activate AhR; and tarragon, caraway, turmeric, lovage, fennel, spearmint, star anise, and anise inhibit the AhR activity.[4477]

□ Jasmine essential oil was significantly acaricidal against the two-spotted spider mite and improved eggplant growth (height, number of leaves, branches per plant, leaf area, and leaf mass), yield, and quality in a greenhouse investigation.[4478] Moreover, spraying eggplants with the jasmine oil improved photosynthetic pigment, chlorophyll ratio, nitrogen, phosphorus, potassium, ascorbic acid, and phenols.

□ Jasmine essential oil displayed weak anticancer (liver, breast, and leukemia) and antiviral (HSV-1, hepatitis A) effects, but a jasmine essential oil nanoemulsion showed strong anticancer (exceeding doxorubicin efficacy against liver and breast cancer cells) and antiviral activity.[4479]

□ Medical schools are stressful environments and depression is reported among almost one-third of medical students globally.[4480] Despite this, very few medical students seek treatment. A clinical study compared the effects of inhaling lavender essential oil or jasmine (*J. sambac*) absolute to a control (water only) on depression among first- and second-year medical students.[4481] Participants in each group inhaled lavender, jasmine, or water for fifteen to twenty minutes before going to bed for seven consecutive nights. Questionnaires were completed before and after intervention to determine the effects on depressive state. The average depressive state decreased from 19.73 (moderate depression) to 14.73 (mild depression) in the lavender group and from 19.33 (moderate depression) to 14.06 (mild depression) in the jasmine group. Statistical analysis and normalization of the data showed that lavender decreased depression 24% and jasmine 28.9%. This suggests both lavender and jasmine have potential to decrease depression among stressed and depressed medical students.

□ Depot-medroxyprogesterone acetate is an injectable three-month contraceptive used to prevent pregnancy. One of its side effects is impaired sexual function (vaginal drying, pain during sexual intercourse, decreased sexual desire). A clinical trial evaluated the effects of inhaling jasmine sambac—via diffuser for 2.5 hours at night—essential oil with loving yoga (exercises focused on pelvic muscles to increase blood flow and libido).[4482] The combination significantly improved libido and sexual function.

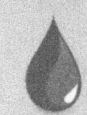

# JUNIPER BERRY

*Juniperus communis* L.; *J. communis* L. ssp. *alpina* (Suter) Celak., *J. alpina* (Sm.) Gray; *J. canadensis* Lodd. Ex Burgsd.; Utah Juniper: *J. osteosperma* (Torr.) Little

**FAMILY:** Cupressaceae (Coniferae)
**NOTE:** Middle
**AROMA INTENSITY:** Medium
**AROMA:** Fresh, slightly balsamic, sweet, woody
**COMMON EXTRACTION METHOD:** Steam distilled from the berries or needles (leaves)
**POSSIBLE SUBSTITUTE OILS:** Frankincense, blue cypress (leaves), pine, blue spruce
**BLENDS WELL WITH:** Balsam fir, bay laurel, cajeput, cedarwood, clary sage, copaiba, cypress (Phoenician), grapefruit, lavender, lemon, lime, niaouli, orange, petitgrain, pine, ravintsara, rosemary, spikenard, tangerine, turmeric, silver fir, white fir
**SUBCELLULAR LOCALIZATION | EPIGENETIC INFLUENCE:** Microtubule Cytoskeleton | Currently unknown
**RECOMMENDED DILUTION RANGE:** 3%–33%; 50% for some conditions

**PRIMARY CONSTITUENTS:**[4483,4484,4485,4486,4487,4488,4489]

| *Berries* | | *Needles (Leaves)* | |
|---|---|---|---|
| Alpha-Pinene | 18.3%–62.3% | Limonene | 2.8%–53.9% |
| Beta-Myrcene | 2.9%–26.5% | Alpha-Pinene | 1.4%–45.6% |
| Sabinene | 2.8%–11.8% | Sabinene | 0.2%–33.6% |
| Germacrene D | 1.1%–9.6% | Beta-Phellandrene | 3.7%–25.2% |
| Gamma-Elemene | 0.1%–6.4% | Beta-Caryophyllene | 0.8%–10.3% |
| Terpinen-4-ol | 0.1%–6.3% | Germacrene D | 3.0%–7.8% |
| Beta-Pinene | 1.7%–5.4% | Beta-Myrcene | 6.5%–6.9% |
| Limonene | 2.9%–5.1% | Alpha-Humulene | 0.8%–6.2% |
| Alpha-Humulene | 1.3%–4.6% | | |
| Germacrene D-4-ol | 0.0%–4.4% | | |

| *J. osteosperma (Needles/Twigs)* * | | *J. osteosperma (Needles/Berries)* * | |
|---|---|---|---|
| Camphor | 5.9%–31.3% | Bornyl Acetate | 14.9% |
| Alpha-Pinene | 10.2%–29.2% | Alpha-Pinene | 14.2% |
| Bornyl Acetate | 9.3%–18.5% | Camphor | 11.4% |
| Limonene | 7.5%–10.2% | Sabinene | 8.9% |
| Sabinene | 1.7%–5.6% | Limonene | 8.9% |
| Gamma-Terpinene | 1.0%–5.2% | Gamma-Terpinene | 5.3% |
| Terpinen-4-ol | 1.7%–5.2% | Terpinen-4-ol | 4.8% |

* Not a true substitute for juniper (*J. communis*) but it is occasionally listed as simply juniper by retailers.

**OTHER CONSTITUENTS:** *Berries*—Alpha-thujene, camphene, para-cymene, beta-phellandrene, cis-verbenol; *Needles*—Alpha-thujene, beta-pinene, myrcene, delta-2-carene, delta-3-carene, alpha-terpinene, para-cymene, 1,8-cineole, gamma-terpinene, terpinolene, terpinen-4-ol, alpha-terpineol, citronellyl acetate, gamma-cadinene, delta-cadinene, (E)-nerolidol, beta-caryophyllene oxide, humulene oxide, T-cadinol, alpha-cadinol; *J. osteosperma (Needles/Twigs)*—Alpha-terpinene, beta-myrcene, camphene, para-cymene, terpinolene, tricyclene, delta-cadinene, elemol, borneol, isobornyl acetate, pinadiene, beta-phellandrene, alpha-phellandrene, beta-caryophyllene, carvone, camphene hydrate, trans-carveol, alpha-thujene; *J. osteosperma (Needles/Berries)*—Para-cymene, terpinolene, pinadiene, alpha-terpinene, camphene, beta-phellandrene, myrcene, tricyclene, alpha-phellandrene, isobornyl acetate

## PREFERRED COMPOSITION FOR CLINICAL USE:

| Constituent | Berries |
|---|---|
| Alpha-Pinene | 28%–48% |
| Beta-Myrcene | 7%–20% |
| Sabinene | 3%–15% |
| Beta-Pinene | 2%–13% |
| Terpinen-4-ol | 1%–9% |
| Limonene | 2%–8% |
| Beta-Caryophyllene | 1%–5% |
| Alpha-Humulene | 1%–5% |
| Germacrene D | 1%–5% |
| Delta-Cadinene | 0.5%–4% |

Note: Essential oils obtained from juniper trees growing in Canada may contain alpha-pinene percentages that reach over 70% with decreased amounts of the other constituents. *Juniperus osteosperma* (Utah Juniper; needles and berries) produces a dissimilar essential oil often poor in alpha-pinene, but rich in camphor and bornyl acetate. The Rocky Mountain juniper (*J. scopulorum*; unidentified plant materials) also produces a dissimilar essential oil with sabinene (49.9%), alpha-terpinene (10.0%), and terpinen-4-ol (6.8%) as the major compounds.[5151]

**REPORTED THERAPEUTIC PROPERTIES:** Analgesic (pain relief), antimicrobial, **antiarthritic**, antiseptic, antispasmodic, antirheumatic, **reduces excess fluid retention**, antioxidant, astringent, **supports urinary tract health**, helps relieve chronic skin conditions, aids digestion, diuretic, **helps reduce kidney stones**, helps relieve painful menstruation, **supports pancreas function**, reduces the appearance of blemishes, **clears the body of uric acid**, **stimulates liver and gallbladder function**, sedating, encourages feelings of love, relieves feelings of being overwhelmed, combats worrisome thoughts and negative thinking, diminishes guilt

## CAUTIONS:

*J. communis, J. alpina, J. canadensis*

■ Some aromatherapy texts suggest that juniper should be avoided with serious kidney disorders because it may irritate the kidneys. However, scientific research to support this assertion is unconvincing, and in fact suggests that juniper protects the kidneys and supports kidney function.[4490,4491,4492]

■ May interact with diuretic drugs and promote increased production of urine due to significant alpha-pinene content according to animal research.[4493]

■ May interact with diabetic medications and promote low blood sugar according to animal research that used ethanolic extracts.[4494] In addition, the diuretic action mentioned above would contraindicate juniper oil in diabetics because diuretics are known to cause short-term disruption in blood sugar control among people with diabetes.

■ *Needles*: May interact with anticholinergic (drugs used for asthma, incontinence, gastrointestinal cramps, muscular spasms, depression, and sleep disorders) and cholinergic medications (drugs used to reduce urinary retention, diagnose myasthenia gravis, and for glaucoma) based on AChE inhibitory activity of beta-phellandrene.[4495]

*Utah Juniper: J. osteosperma*

■ Avoid with children under six due to significant camphor content. Several cases of camphor poisoning and/or seizures from ingestion and topical application have been reported in children.[4496,4497] Ingestion of camphor-containing products has been lethal in children under age two.[4498] Children six years and up may use camphor-containing essential oils topically in dilutions no stronger than 5%. Camphor ingestion by infants and young children may cause cough, vomiting, seizure, burning sensation in the mucous membranes and eyes, or lack of voluntary coordination of muscle movements.[4499]

■ Caution is warranted during pregnancy and while lactating due to significant camphor content. Ingestion of essential oils with significant levels of camphor may lead to abortion because fetuses lack the enzymes to process it.[4500] Camphor ingestion by infants and young children may cause cough, vomiting, seizure, burning sensation in the mucous membranes and eyes, or lack of voluntary coordination of muscle movements.[4501]

■ Avoid with epilepsy and Parkinson's due to significant camphor content.[4502,4503,4504]

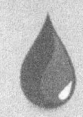

■ The significant camphor content in Utah juniper may negatively impact red blood cells and increase the risk of jaundice in children with glucose-6-phosphate dehydrogenase deficiency (G6PD).[4505,4506]

■ Oral caution—Essential oils with significant levels of camphor can be toxic when taken orally, usually single doses exceeding 2 mL, although the lethal dose for humans is estimated to be more than 5 mL in a single dose.[4507,4508,4509]

**SELECTED EVIDENCE:**

☐ Juniper oil reduces elastase activity (an enzyme involved in the breakdown of elastin) *in vitro*, which may help prevent wrinkles and aging of the skin.[4510] Elastin helps keep skin tight, supple, and flexible.

☐ Juniper oil prevents protein glycation, which plays a key role in diabetes and its cardiovascular complications.[4511]

☐ *In vitro* research suggests that juniper oil inhibits *S. aureus* and *P. aeruginosa*.[4512] The authors concluded that inhalation of juniper oil may be useful for chronic and/or recurrent upper respiratory tract infections.

☐ Juniper essential oil significantly inhibited foodborne pathogens (*E. coli*, *S. paratyphi* A, *K. pneumoniae,* and *Y. enterocolitica*).[4513] Other essential oils that exhibited antibacterial activity against one or more organisms in the study include Turkish pine, myrtle, orange, thyme, lavender, sage, lemon, rosemary, lavender, eucalyptus, and bay laurel.

☐ Juniper oil inhibits several dermatophytes (fungi that require keratin for growth and typically infect the skin, hair, and nails) and *Candida* species *in vitro*.[4514,4515]

☐ Juniper berry oil helps decrease inflammation by moderately inhibiting the 5-lipoxygenase (5-LOX) enzyme that is involved in the inflammation response according to *in vitro* research.[4516]

☐ *In vitro* research suggests that juniper oil prevents lipid peroxidation and possess antioxidant properties.[4517]

☐ An interesting chemotype of juniper essential oil (linalool 18.1%, para-cymene 9.1%) demonstrated 73.8%–96.3% efficacy against the *Rhipicephalus microplus* tick depending on the concentration used (1%–10%).[4518]

☐ Of eleven essential oils tested, lemongrass (*C. citratus*: citronellal formate 42.8%, isobornyl formate 33.5%) essential oil demonstrated the greatest antioxidant activity in the DPPH test and the best overall antimicrobial activity.[4519] Lemon eucalyptus (78.2% citronellal), lemon scented iron bark (1,8-cineole 29.2%, bornyl formate 12.3%, isobornyl formate 12.1%), lavender (French: cuminaldehyde 41.3%, linalool 37.3%; and French high altitude: linalyl formate 41.7%, linalool 23.5%), and juniper (*J communis*: p-mentha-1(7),8 diene 32.3%, delta-cadinene 11.3%) demonstrated very strong antioxidant activity, lavender (Croatian: linalool 47.9%, linalyl formate 22.1%) and rosemary (limonene CT) strong activity, lavender (Croatian, linalool rich 66.8%) moderate activity, and gully gum poor activity (81.7% 1,8-cineole). The other essential oils demonstrated various degrees of antimicrobial activity against the tested bacteria (*E. faecalis, B. cereus, L. monocytogenes, S. aureus*, MRSA, *Salmonella typhimurium, P. aeruginosa, E. coli, K. pneumonia, A. baumannii,* and *Ch. violaceum*.

☐ Juniper essential oil (*J. communis* var. saxatilis, CT alpha-pinene) demonstrated strong antioxidant activity in the DPPH assay and moderate activity in the TBA and FRAP assays, was toxic to human lung cancer cells (exhibiting greater toxicity to cancer cells than normal lung fibroblast cells), and improved the cytotoxicity of doxorubicin against lung cancer cells.[4520]

☐ Juniper berry essential oil prevented the adhesion of *C. jejuni* (a bacterium that is one of the world's most common cases of the stomach flu—gastroenteritis) to surfaces.[4521] *C. jejuni* can adhere to surfaces and form biofilms that increase the risk of human infection by improving its persistence in food processing environments and therefore its spread.

☐ A juniper essential oil from wild harvested plants was toxic to human cervical, lung, and skin cancer cells.[4522] The same researchers reported that it exhibited antimicrobial activity, with better activity against gram-positive bacteria than gram-negative bacteria and the greatest inhibition against *Staphylococcus aureus*.

☐ When bacteria form biofilms, it allows them to survive in adverse environments. Nontuberculosis mycobacteria are found extensively in aqueous environments, where they adhere to surfaces and create biofilms. Their presence in healthcare settings has led to healthcare-associated infections. Juniper essential oil significantly reduced the formation of biofilms by *Mycobacterium avium* and *Mycobacterium intracellulare* at subinhibitory concentrations, suggesting it could be used as a disinfectant of sterilized tap water.[4523] The oil combined with increasing ambient temperature showed a significant effect in reducing biofilm formation of mycobacteria on polystyrene surfaces.

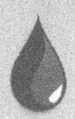

- Juniper, Rocky Mountain juniper, and creeping juniper essential oils each demonstrated antioxidant (via DPPH assay), antifungal (*M. fructicola* and *P. expansum*) and antibacterial (*P. syringae* pv. *phaseolicola* and *B. megaterium*) activity.[4524] Juniper (*J. communis*) also exhibited promising activity against human neuroblastoma cancer cells.

- The leaf and branches essential oil of juniper (11.8% bornyl acetate, 11.6% alpha-cadinol, 8.6% methyleugenol, 7.9% alpha-pinene, 7.6% 4-terpinen-ol) inhibited *S. aureus* and *E. coli* and also reduced the production of proinflammatory cytokines in human white blood cells.[4525]

- *Acanthamoeba castellanii* is an opportunistic protozoa found in aquatic environments where it can form symbiotic relationships with over thirty different pathogenic bacteria, including nontuberculous mycobacteria (NTM). Protozoa play an important role in the ability of nontuberculous mycobacteria to infect hosts. Addition of juniper or helichrysum essential oil to tap water infested with *Acanthamoeba castellanii* and NTM (*Mycobacterium avium*, *M. intracellulare*, and *M. gordonae*) essential oil prevented the adhesion of the protozoa to NTM.[4526] This suggests that the essential oils and their combinations weaken the contact of environmental NTMs and free-living amoebae and therefore indirectly reduce their ability to infect hosts.

- Juniper berry, eucalyptus (*E. globulus*), and helichrysum essential oil exhibited anti-H1N1 influenza virus activity *in vitro*.[4527] The researchers observed a correlation between anti-influenza activity and both limonene and o-cymene and inhibitory activity.

- Juniper and cade essential oil exhibited good antioxidant activity, moderate antimicrobial activity (*Fusarium* spp., *Botrytis cinerea*, *Colletotrichum* spp., *Rhizoctonia solani*, and *Cylindrocarpon pauciseptatum*), and significant repellent and insecticidal activity against two aphid species (*Rhopalosiphum padi* and *Sitobion avenae*).[4528]

- Juniper berry essential oil exhibited cytotoxicity to breast cancer cells.[4529]

- Juniper needle CT sabinene essential oil moderately inhibited alpha-glucosidase activity, suggesting it may be valuable for the management of diabetes.[4530]

- *Mycobacterium avium* complex is a group of mycobacteria—*M. avium*, *M. intracellulare*, and *M. gordonae*—commonly found in food, water, and soil that infect humans. Nearly all humans have these bacteria in their bodies, but those with a strong immune system don't experience symptoms. However, those with weak or compromised immune systems can become very sick and experience respiratory diseases, high fever, abdominal pain, weight loss, diarrhea, fatigue, swollen glands, night sweats, and fewer red blood cells, or more serious symptoms like hepatitis, pneumonia, and blood infections. Of six essential oils tested (juniper berry, ylang ylang, sage, lavandin, bay laurel, and white cedar), juniper berry essential oil was the most active, significantly reducing cell viability of *M. avium*, *M. intracellulare*, and *M. gordonae* in laboratory research.[4531] The researchers concluded that juniper berry essential oil represents a promising alternative water disinfectant in hot water systems such as baths, swimming pools, spa pools, hot tubs, or even foot baths/whirlpools.

---

# JUNIPER (CHINESE)

*Juniperus chinensis* L.

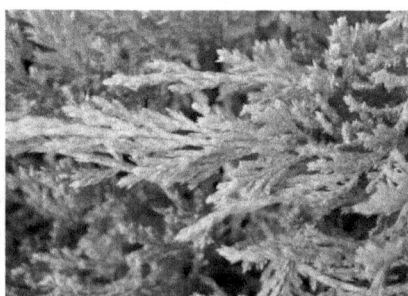

**FAMILY:** Cupressaceae (Coniferae)
**NOTE:** Middle
**AROMA INTENSITY:** Medium
**AROMA:** Fresh, woody, piney, slightly balsamic, sweet
**COMMON EXTRACTION METHOD:** Steam distilled from the needles (leaves); may also be distilled from the heartwood or berries
**POSSIBLE SUBSTITUTE OILS:** Spruce (black), tsuga, balsam fir, Siberian fir
**BLENDS WELL WITH:** Balsam fir, birch, cajeput, cedarwood, clary sage, copaiba, cypress, grapefruit, lavender, lemon, lime, niaouli, orange, petitgrain, pine, ravintsara, rosemary, spikenard, tangerine, turmeric, silver fir, white fir, wintergreen
**SUBCELLULAR LOCALIZATION | EPIGENETIC INFLUENCE:** Currently unknown | Currently unknown
**RECOMMENDED DILUTION RANGE:** 5%–neat

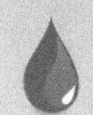

**PRIMARY CONSTITUENTS:**[4532,4533,4534]

*Leaves*

| | |
|---|---|
| Bornyl Acetate | 12.3%–30.4% |
| Sabinene | 15.6%–19.8% |
| Elemol | 0.0%–18.6% |
| Limonene | 3.9%–14.2% |
| Carotol | 0.0%–11.4% |
| Trans-Sabinyl Acetate | 0.0%–11.1% |
| Myrcene | 2.8%–9.2% |
| Alpha-Pinene | 1.3%–6.4% |
| T-Muurolol | 0.0%–5.0% |
| Alpha-Cadinol | 0.0%–4.8% |

**OTHER CONSTITUENTS:** *Leaves*—alpha-thujene, camphene, gamma-terpinene, linalool, terpinene-4-ol, beta-caryophyllene, beta-humulene, germacrene D, delta-cadinene, alpha-muurolol, manool, alpha-muurolene, tricyclene, linalool, delta-3-carene, alpha-terpinene, beta-thujone (<1.7%), gamma-terpinene, terpinolene, gamma-eudesmol

**PREFERRED COMPOSITION FOR CLINICAL USE:**

| Constituent | |
|---|---|
| **Bornyl Acetate** | 16%–30% |
| **Sabinene** | 16%–22% |
| **Limonene** | 7%–15% |
| **Myrcene** | 4%–10% |
| **Elemol** | 1%–10% |
| **Alpha-Pinene** | 2%–7% |
| **Trans-Sabinyl Acetate** | < 5% |

**REPORTED THERAPEUTIC PROPERTIES: Analgesic (pain relief)**, antimicrobial, antiparasitic, antiarthritic, antiseptic, **anti-inflammatory**, antispasmodic, antirheumatic, nervine, antiallergic, relieves diarrhea, astringent, aids digestion, helps relieve painful menstruation, **supports respiratory function**, increases localized circulation, stimulates liver and gallbladder function, insecticide, sedating, stress management, relieves feelings of being overwhelmed, combats worrisome thoughts and negative thinking, diminishes guilt, aphrodisiac

**CAUTIONS:**

■ Avoid in children under age 12 due to the toxic potential of trans-sabinyl acetate.[4535,4536,4537]

■ Avoid during pregnancy. Trans-sabinyl acetate is toxic to developing embryos and prevents implantation during days 0–4 of gestation according to animal research.[4538,4539] Trans-sabinyl acetate can cause abortions and maternal toxicity (which indicated a greater susceptibility to trans-sabinyl acetate toxicity during pregnancy) in animals.[4540] The researchers concluded that trans-sabinyl acetate possesses significant antifertility activity during the pre-implantation period, and attribute the fetotoxic and abortifacient activity to trans-sabinyl acetate.

■ Avoid oral consumption due to trans-sabinyl acetate content. Essential oils with moderate to significant amounts of trans-sabinyl acetate may irritate the mucosal lining of the gastrointestinal tract, damage the kidneys, cause blood in the urine, obstruct blood flow in the abdominal organs, and cause abnormally heavy menstrual bleeding.[4541]

■ Avoid with epilepsy and Parkinson's disease due to thujone and trans-sabinyl acetate content.[4542]

■ Avoid in those who have a compromised liver or kidneys due to the increased risk of liver toxicity, liver damage, and kidney damage.[4543,4544,4545] This would also suggest that those taking medications that could cause liver damage should also use Chinese juniper very cautiously or avoid it entirely.

**SELECTED EVIDENCE:**

☐ Chinese juniper essential oil kills house dust and stored food mites.[4546]

# JUNIPER (HIMALAYAN)

Drooping Juniper: *Juniperus recurva* Buch.-Ham. ex D. Don;
Black Juniper: *J. wallichiana* Hook. f. & Thomson ex E. Brandis,
*J. indica* Bertol., *Sabina wallichiana* (Hook. f. & Thomson ex E.
Brandis) W.C. Cheng & L.K. Fu

**FAMILY:** Cupressaceae (Coniferae)
**NOTE:** Middle
**AROMA INTENSITY:** Medium
**AROMA:** Fresh, woody, piney, slightly balsamic, sweet
**COMMON EXTRACTION METHOD:** Steam distilled from the berries or needles (leaves)
**POSSIBLE SUBSTITUTE OILS:** Pine, balsam fir, juniper (needles), Douglas fir (needles)
**BLENDS WELL WITH:** Balsam fir, bay laurel, cajeput, cedarwood, clary sage, copaiba, cypress, grapefruit, lavender, lemon, lime, niaouli, orange, petitgrain, pine, ravintsara, rosemary, spikenard, tangerine, turmeric, silver fir, white fir
**SUBCELLULAR LOCALIZATION | EPIGENETIC INFLUENCE:** Currently unknown | Currently unknown
**RECOMMENDED DILUTION RANGE:** 3%–33%; 50% for some conditions

**PRIMARY CONSTITUENTS:**[4547,4548,4549,4550,4551,4552,4553]

| *J. recurva, Berries* | | *J. recurva, Needles (Leaves)* | |
|---|---|---|---|
| Delta-3-Carene | 46.1% | Delta-3-Carene | 13.6%–23.7% |
| Alpha-Pinene | 8.3% | Limonene | 0.2%–18.4% |
| Limonene | 5.9% | Sabinene | 0.4%–13.4% |
| Delta-Cadinene | 5.7% | Alpha-Cadinol | 0.8%–13.1% |
| (E)-Muurola-4(14), | | Delta-Cadinene | 0.8%–10.2% |
| 5-Diene | 4.3% | Alpha-Pinene | 0.5%–6.9% |
| (Z)-Cadina-1(6), 4-Diene | 4.0% | Epi-Alpha-Muurolol | 0.5%–5.5% |
| Myrcene | 3.7% | Epi-Alpha-Cadinol | 0.3%–5.5% |
| Terpinolene | 3.6% | Elemol | 3.9%–5.1% |

| *J. wallichiana/J. indica, Leaves* | | *J. wallichiana/J. indica, Berries* | |
|---|---|---|---|
| Sabinene | 27.8%–51.0% | Sabinene | 23.2%–50.2% |
| Terpinen-4-ol | 4.5%–16.1% | Terpinen-4-ol | 2.2%–23.6% |
| Alpha-Pinene | 1.8%–12.2% | Alpha-Pinene | 8.1%–8.8% |
| Gamma-Terpinene | 3.9%–6.4% | Gamma-Terpinene | 0.1%–6.6% |
| Beta-Myrcene | 3.2%–4.7% | Alpha-Terpinene | 0.1%–4.3% |
| Alpha-Terpinene | 1.5%–4.5% | | |
| Delta-Cadinene | 0.6%–4.5% | | |

**OTHER CONSTITUENTS:** *J. recurva, Berries*—alpha-fenchene, sabinene, sylvestrene, (E)-muurola-3,5-diene, alpha-muurolene, delta-amorphene, zonarene, 1-epi-cubenol; *J. recurva, Needles (Leaves)*—Alpha-thujene, alpha-fenchene, myrcene, alpha-terpinene, gamma-terpinene, cis-sabinene hydrate, terpineolene, germacrene d-4-ol, p-menth-1,5-dien-8-ol, terpinen-4-ol, hexyl 3-methylbutyrate, beta-caryophyllene, terpene alcohol, alpha-cadinene, beta-cadinene, gamma-muurolene, trans-muurola-4(14),5-diene, epi-cubenol, gamma-cadinene, beta-oplopenone, cubenol, alpha-muurolol, beta-eudesmol, alpha-eudesmol, selen-11-en-4alpha-ol, bulnesol, 8-alpha-acetoxyelemon, 4-epi-abietal, trans-totarol; *J. Wallichiana/J. indica, Leaves*—alpha-thujene, para-cymene, limonene, 1,8-cineole, cis-sabinene-hydrate, terpinolene, linalool, p-menth-2-en-1-ol, alpha-terpineol, beta-cubebene, alpha-muurolene, gamma-cadinene, alpha-cadinol, beta-eudesmol, nezukol, abietatriene, manool, epi-alpha-cadinol, epi-alpha-muurolol, germacrene D-4-ol; *J. Wallichiana/J. indica, Berries*—alpha-thujene, beta-pinene, myrcene, para-cyemene, limonene, cis-sabinene hydrate, trans-sabinene hydrate, terpinolene, alpha-terpineol, trans-piperitol, gamma-gurjunene, gamma-cadinene, elemol, alpha-cadinol, 6-camphenol, cis-p-menth-2-en-1-ol, trans-verbenol, p-menth-1,5-dien-8-ol, para-cymene-8-ol, myrtenol, bornyl acetate, thymol, delta-elemene, geranyl acetate, oplopanone, khusinol acetate, nexukol

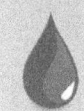

**PREFERRED COMPOSITION FOR CLINICAL USE:**

| Constituent | J. recurva, Needles (Leaves) | J. wallichiana/ J. indica, Berries |
|---|---|---|
| Delta-3-Carene | 15%–25% | – |
| Limonene | 5%–15% | 1%–5% |
| Sabinene | 4%–12% | 28%–50% |
| Alpha-Cadinol | 2%–10% | 0.5%–3% |
| Delta-Cadinene | 2%–10% | 0.1%–4% |
| Elemol | 3%–7% | 0%–3% |
| Alpha-Pinene | 2%–7% | 8%–15% |
| Epi-Alpha-Cadinol | 1%–5% | – |
| Epi-Alpha-Muurolol | 0.5%–5% | – |
| Gamma-Terpinene | 0%–5% | 2%–7% |
| Alpha-Terpinene | 0%–5% | 1%–5% |
| Terpinen-4-ol | 0%–3% | 7%–22% |

**REPORTED THERAPEUTIC PROPERTIES: Analgesic (pain relief)**, antimicrobial, antiparasitic, antiarthritic, antiseptic, **antispasmodic**, anti-inflammatory, antirheumatic, nervine, astringent, aids digestion, helps relieve painful menstruation, protects stomach, supports respiratory function, increases localized circulation, purification, encourages sweating, stimulates liver and gallbladder function, sedating, encourages feelings of love, relieves feelings of being overwhelmed, combats worrisome thoughts and negative thinking, diminishes guilt, aphrodisiac

**CAUTIONS:**

■ *J. recurva, Berries*: May interact with anticholinergic (drugs used for asthma, incontinence, gastrointestinal cramps, muscular spasms, depression, and sleep disorders) and cholinergic medications (drugs used to reduce urinary retention, diagnose myasthenia gravis, and for glaucoma) based on AChE inhibitory activity of δ-3-carene.[4554,4555]

**SELECTED EVIDENCE:**

☐ None found.

---

# JUNIPER (PHOENICIAN)

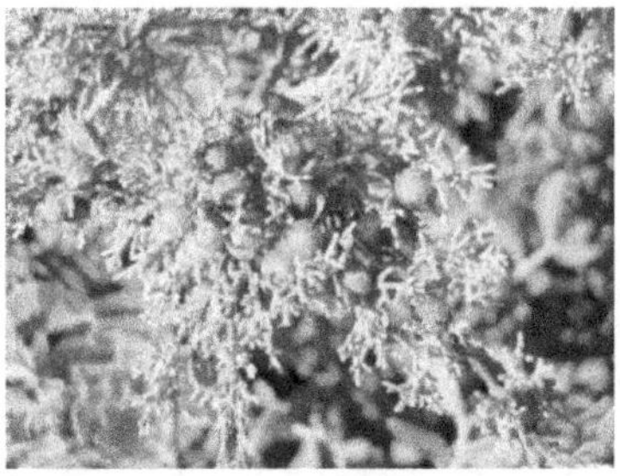

*Juniperus phoenicea* L.

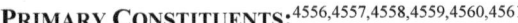

**FAMILY:** Cupressaceae (Coniferae)
**NOTE:** Middle
**AROMA INTENSITY:** Medium
**AROMA:** Fresh, slightly balsamic, sweet, woody
**COMMON EXTRACTION METHOD:** Steam distilled from the berries or needles (leaves)
**POSSIBLE SUBSTITUTE OILS:** Cypress, frankincense, blue cypress (leaves), pine
**BLENDS WELL WITH:** Balsam fir, bay laurel, cajeput, cedarwood, clary sage, copaiba, cypress, Douglas fir, grapefruit, lavender, lemon, lime, niaouli, orange, petitgrain, pine, ravintsara, rosemary, spikenard, tangerine, turmeric, Siberian fir, silver fir, white fir
**SUBCELLULAR LOCALIZATION | EPIGENETIC INFLUENCE:** Currently unknown | Currently unknown
**RECOMMENDED DILUTION RANGE:** 3%–33%; 50% for some conditions

**PRIMARY CONSTITUENTS:**[4556,4557,4558,4559,4560,4561]

| Berries | | Needles (Leaves)—Alpha-Pinene CT | |
|---|---|---|---|
| Alpha-Pinene | 26.9%–86.4% | Alpha-Pinene | 20.3%–65.7% |
| Sabinene | 0.0%–24.3% | Para-Cymene | 0.0%–25.7% |
| Camphor | 0.0%–14.9% | Beta-Phellandrene | 0.1%–24.4% |

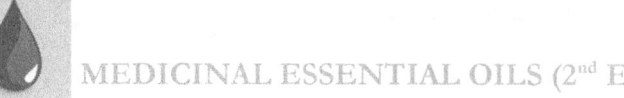
| | | | |
|---|---|---|---|
| Alpha-Terpineol | 0.0%–10.8% | Alpha-Terpineol | 0.0%–19.8% |
| Gamma-Cadinene | 0.0%–10.2% | Alpha-Terpinyl Acetate | 0.0%–12.9% |
| Germacrene B | 0.0%–7.3% | Beta-Bourbonene | 0.0%–12.9% |
| Beta-Selinene | 0.0%–6.9% | Delta-3-Carene | 0.4%–10.7% |
| β-Caryophyllene Oxide | 0.0%–6.3% | Alpha-Phelladrene | 0.0%–6.1% |
| Cubenol | 0.0%–4.9% | Limonene | 0.0%–5.0% |
| Delta-Cadinene | 0.0%–4.9% | Gamma-Cadinene | 0.0%–4.4% |
| Delta-3-Carene | 0.0%–4.5% | | |

*Needles (Leaves)—Isoborneol CT*

| | |
|---|---|
| Isoborneol | 20.9% |
| Alpha-Pinene | 18.3% |
| Beta-Phellandrene | 8.1% |
| Alpha-Camphenal | 7.9% |
| Alpha-Phellandrene | 7.6% |
| Cedrol | 3.7% |
| *d*-Limonene | 3.5% |
| Alpha-Terpinyl Acetate | 3.5% |

Note: There are at least four chemotypes of leaf essential oil depending on the presence or absence of beta-phellandrene, para-cymene, and isoborneol. Likewise, the berry essential oil could be divided into several chemotypes based on the presence or absence of camphor, sabinene, alpha-terpineol, and other constituents.

**OTHER CONSTITUENTS:** *Berries*—alpha-fenchene, camphene, beta-pinene, beta-myrcene, limonene, alpha-phellandrene, beta-phellandrene, beta-elemene, gamma-terpinene, alpha-terpinolene, 6-camphenone, bornyl acetate, alpha-cubebene, beta-caryophyllene, beta-gurjunene, alpha-himachalene, alpha-humulene, allo-aromadendrene, alpha-chamigrene, elemol, (E)-nerolidol, alpha-cedrol, T-muurolol, alpha-cadinol, bulnesol, 13-isopimaradiene, abietatriene, trans-ferruginol; *Needles (Leaves), Alpha-Pinene CT*—alpha-fenchene, beta-pinene, sabinene, beta-myrcene, gamma-terpinene, alpha-terpinolene, alpha-cubebene, beta-bourbonene, beta-caryophyllene oxide, beta-elemene, 6-camphenone, gamma-elemene, beta-gurjunene, camphenol, trans-pinocarveol, camphor, isopulegol, pinocarvone, myrtenal, verbenone, cubenol, delta-cadinene, elemol, cuminaldehyde, carvone, isopulegol acetate, beta-caryophyllene, alpha-himachalene, alpha-humulene, allo-aromadendrene, gamma-muurolene, alpha-chamigrene, trans-ferruginol, heptane 2,4-dimethyl; *Needles (Leaves), Isoborneol CT*—camphene, beta-myrcene, gamma-terpinene, cis-limonene oxide, pinocamphone (< 1.0%), fenchyl acetate, linalyl acetate, myrtenyl acetate, delta-elemene, alpha-cubebene, trans-carvyl acetate, alpha-terpinyl acetate, gamma-cadinene

**PREFERRED COMPOSITION FOR CLINICAL USE:**

| *Constituent* | *Berries* |
|---|---|
| **Alpha-Pinene** | 38%–60% |
| **Sabinene** | 15%–25% |
| **Beta-Phellandrene** | 1%–5% |
| **Trans-Pinocarveol** | 1%–5% |
| **Delta-3-Carene** | 1%–5% |
| **Camphor** | 1%–5% |

**REPORTED THERAPEUTIC PROPERTIES:** Analgesic (pain relief), antimicrobial, antiarthritic, antiseptic, antispasmodic, antirheumatic, **anticancer**, reduces excess fluid retention, **antioxidant**, astringent, **supports urinary tract health**, helps relieve chronic skin conditions, aids digestion, diuretic, helps reduce kidney stones, helps relieve painful menstruation, protects stomach, supports pancreas function, reduces the appearance of blemishes, clears the body of uric acid, stimulates liver and gallbladder function, insecticide, sedating, encourages feelings of love, relieves feelings of being overwhelmed, combats worrisome thoughts and negative thinking, diminishes guilt

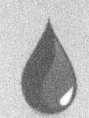

## CAUTIONS:

■ Some aromatherapy texts suggest that juniper should be avoided with serious kidney disorders because it may irritate the kidneys. However, scientific research to support this assertion is unconvincing, and in fact suggests that juniper protects the kidneys and supports kidney function.[4562,4563,4564]

■ The moderate camphor content in Phoenician juniper may negatively impact red blood cells and increase the risk of jaundice in children with Glucose-6-phosphate dehydrogenase deficiency (G6PD).[4565,4566]

■ May interact with diuretic drugs and promote increased production of urine due to significant alpha-pinene content according to animal research.[4567]

■ Avoid with epilepsy and Parkinson's disease due to camphor content.[4568,4569,4570]

■ May interact with diabetic medications and promote low blood sugar according to animal research that used ethanolic extracts.[4571] In addition, the diuretic action mentioned above would contraindicate juniper oil in diabetics because diuretics are known to cause short-term disruption in blood sugar control among people with diabetes.

## SELECTED EVIDENCE:

☐ *In vitro* research demonstrated that Phoenician juniper essential oil is highly toxic to brain (glioma), lung (large cell), liver, and breast cancer cells, and moderately toxic to cervical cancer cells.[4572] The study authors reported that the berry oil demonstrated greater activity against lung, liver, and breast cancer cells than the leaf oil.

☐ Phoenician juniper essential oil moderately inhibits fungi (*A. aspergillus* and *F. oxysporum*) and bacteria (*S. aureus, E. faecalis, B. cereus, E. coli,* and *P. aeruginosa*).[4573] Other research demonstrated that it moderately inhibited only gram-positive bacteria (*S. aureus, E. faecium, L. monocytogenes* 4b, and *L. monocytogenes* EGD-e) but had no activity against gram-negative bacteria (*Salmonella enteritidis, E. coli,* and *P. aeruginosa*), and inhibited the fungus *M. ramamnianus*.[4574,4575] Interestingly, other research reports that Phoenician juniper essential oil demonstrates reasonable antimicrobial activity against gram-positive bacteria (*B. subtillis, S. aureus,* and *L. monocytogenes*), gram-negative bacteria (*P. aeruginosa, E. coli,* and *K. pneumoniae*), and fungi (*M. ramamnianus* and *A. westerdijkiae*).[4576,4577] The leaf essential oil appears to be a more active antimicrobial, inhibiting pathogens responsible for healthcare-associated infections (four gram-negative bacteria, *C. albicans, B. subtilis, S. aureus, B. cereus, Candida* species, and *A. niger*).[4578,4579] In fact, the leaf oil was more effective against *C. albicans* than standard antifungal substances.

☐ An interesting chemotype of Phoenician juniper with isoborneol and alpha-pinene as the primary constituents inhibited the gram-negative bacterium *Legionella pneumophila*, which causes the respiratory disease legionellosis.[4580]

☐ *In vitro* research demonstrates that Phoenician juniper is a good antioxidant.[4581,4582,4583] One study reports that essential oil distilled from ripe berries exhibits stronger antioxidant activity than essential oil obtained from unripe berries.[4584]

☐ Animal research demonstrates that Phoenician juniper essential oil (leaves) protects against stomach ulcers caused by ethanol and excess stomach acid, possibly by reducing stomach acid production and increasing antioxidant activity (superoxide dismutase (SOD), catalase (CAT), and glutathione peroxidase (GPx)).[4585]

☐ Phoenician juniper was moderately toxic to the *Ae. albopictus* mosquito (a vector that carries at least twenty-two arboviruses, including Dengue virus).[4586] It also significantly repels the *ixodes ricinus* L. tick, but only for short periods of time.[4587]

*Did you know?*

Some medical doctors in Europe prescribe essential oils as an adjunct to or replacemt for pharmaceuticals. Essential oil capules are even available as over-the-counter remedies.

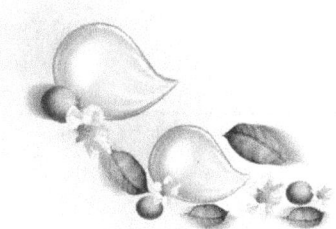

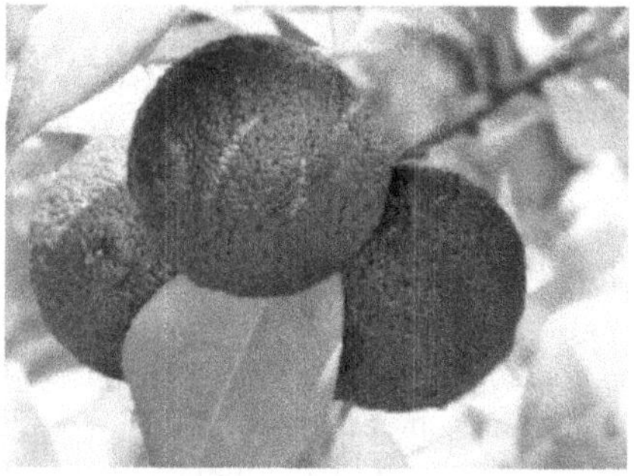

# KABOSU

*Citrus sphaerocarpa* Tanaka

**FAMILY:** Rutaceae
**NOTE:** Top
**AROMA INTENSITY:** Medium
**AROMA:** Citrusy, fruity, sweet
**COMMON EXTRACTION METHOD:** Cold pressed from the fruit rind (peel)
**POSSIBLE SUBSTITUTE OILS:** Grapefruit, lime, lemon, orange, tangerine

**BLENDS WELL WITH:** Allspice, applemint, bergamot, cassia, cedarwood, cinnamon, clove, frankincense, grapefruit, kaffir lime, lavender, lemon, lime, Mediterranean mandarin, patchouli, peppermint, orange, sandalwood, spearmint, tangerine

**SUBCELLULAR LOCALIZATION | EPIGENETIC INFLUENCE:** Currently unknown | Currently unknown

**RECOMMENDED DILUTION RANGE:** 3%–50%; Neat for limited conditions

**PRIMARY CONSTITUENTS:**[4588,4589]

| | |
|---|---|
| Limonene | 70.5%–75.5% |
| Myrcene | 18.5%–20.2% |

**OTHER CONSTITUENTS:** Alpha-pinene, gamma-terpinene, beta-farnesene, decanal, octanal

**PREFERRED COMPOSITION FOR CLINICAL USE:**

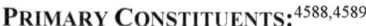

| Constituent | |
|---|---|
| Limonene | 68%–78% |
| Myrcene | 15%–22% |
| Gamma-Terpinene | 2%–5% |
| Beta-Caryophyllene | 0.1%–1% |
| Alpha-Pinene | 0.1%–1% |
| Beta-Pinene | 0.1%–1% |
| Decanal | 0.01%–1% |

**REPORTED THERAPEUTIC PROPERTIES:** Antibacterial, antiseptic, analgesic, anti-inflammatory, **antispasmodic**, anticancer, reduces the appearance of scars and blemishes, relieves acne, aids digestion, diuretic, relieves constipation, promotes restful sleep, reduces restlessness, combats anger, reduces irritability, **antidepressant**, stress management, relieves anxiety

**CAUTIONS:**

■ Thought to be a cross between bitter orange and Ichang papeda (*Citrus ichangensis*), kabosu is likely photosensitizing. Avoid UV exposure to area of application for at least twelve hours after topical application.[4590]

**SELECTED EVIDENCE:**

☐ None found.

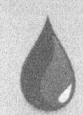

# KAFFIR LIME PETITGRAIN
## (Combava, Thai Lime, Makrut Lime, Swangi, Leech-Lime)

*Citrus hystrix* DC (Swangi)

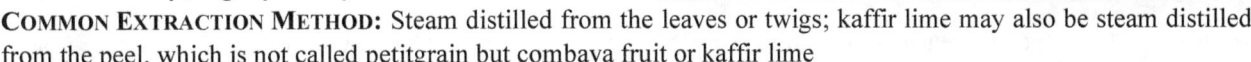

**FAMILY:** Rutaceae
**NOTE:** Top-Middle
**AROMA INTENSITY:** Strong
**AROMA:** Citrusy, slightly woody
**COMMON EXTRACTION METHOD:** Steam distilled from the leaves or twigs; kaffir lime may also be steam distilled from the peel, which is not called petitgrain but combava fruit or kaffir lime
**POSSIBLE SUBSTITUTE OILS:** *Kaffir Lime Petitgrain*—Citronella, melissa; *Peel*—bergamot (cold pressed), lime (cold pressed)
**BLENDS WELL WITH:** Agarwood, balsam fir, bergamot, blue cypress, blue spruce, cedarwood, clary sage, cypress, Douglas fir, frankincense, geranium, grapefruit, lavender, lemon, lime, myrrh, neroli, orange, petitgrain, pine, red pine, rose, sandalwood, Siberian fir, silver fir, spruce (black), tangerine, tsuga, white fir, white pine
**SUBCELLULAR LOCALIZATION | EPIGENETIC INFLUENCE:** Currently unknown | Currently unknown
**RECOMMENDED DILUTION RANGE:** *Petitgrain*—3%–50%, neat for limited conditions; *Peel*—5%–50%; neat for limited conditions

**PRIMARY CONSTITUENTS:**[4591,4592,4593,4594,4595,4596]

*Kaffir Lime Petitgrain (Combava)—leaves or twigs*

| | |
|---|---|
| Citronellal | 65.4%–81.5% |
| Citronellol | 0.0%–6.6% |
| Linalool | 2.9%–6.4% |
| 5,9-Dimethyl-1-Decanol | 0.0%–5.0% |

*Kaffir Lime Peel (distilled)*

| | |
|---|---|
| Sabinene | 1.7%–45.6% |
| Limonene | 5.3%–30.7% |
| Beta-Pinene | 13.5%–30.5% |
| Terpinen-4-ol | 0.0%–17.4% |
| Citronellal | 0.1%–16.8% |
| Alpha-Terpineol | 0.4%–8.4% |
| Citronellol | 0.2%–7.8% |
| Gamma-Terpinene | 0.9%–6.2% |
| Alpha-Terpinene | 0.4%–5.1% |
| Alpha-Terpinolene | 0.3%–4.3% |
| Alpha-Pinene | 2.0%–3.2% |

**OTHER CONSTITUENTS:** *Petitgrain of Kaffir Lime (Combava)*—sabinene, isoprenol, 3-undecanol, methyl citronellate, geranyl acetate, 2-(2-Hydroxy-2-propyl)-5-methyl-cyclohexanol, 4,8-dimethyl-1,7-nonadien-4-ol; *Peel*—camphene, alpha-phellandrene, cis-linalool oxide, linalool, neo-isopulegol, iso-isopulegol, alpha-cubebene, gamma-cadinene, myrcene, delta-2-carene

**PREFERRED COMPOSITION FOR CLINICAL USE:**

| Constituent | Leaves | Peel |
|---|---|---|
| **Citronellal** | 60%–80% | < 1% |
| **Linalool** | 3%–8% | < 2% |

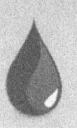
| | | |
|---|---|---|
| **Citronellol** | 0.5%–6% | < 1% |
| **Sabinene** | 0.1%–5% | 1%–5% |
| **Alpha-Pinene** | 0.1%–3% | 2%–5% |
| **Beta-Pinene** | 0.1%–3% | 15%–25% |
| **Limonene** | – | 20%–35% |
| **Terpinen-4-ol** | – | 7%–15% |
| **Alpha-Terpineol** | – | 7%–15% |
| **Gamma-Terpinene** | – | 5%–12% |
| **Alpha-Terpinene** | – | 3%–8% |
| **Terpinolene** | – | 1%–5% |

**REPORTED THERAPEUTIC PROPERTIES: Antibacterial**, antifungal, antiviral, antiseptic, antioxidant, analgesic, anti-inflammatory, antiarthritic, **aids oral health**, detoxification, reduces the appearance of scars, fine lines, and wrinkles, supports immune function, aids digestion, relieves headache/migraine, supports respiratory function, reduces hair loss, insect repellent, **insecticide**, antidepressant, relieves anxiety, stress management, **mentally stimulating**

**CAUTIONS:**

■ Kaffir lime petitgrain may interact with anticholinergic (drugs used for asthma, incontinence, gastrointestinal cramps, muscular spasms, depression, and sleep disorders) and cholinergic medications (drugs used to reduce urinary retention, diagnose myasthenia gravis, and for glaucoma) likely due to a synergistic activity of citronellal, citronellol, and beta-phellandrene (reported as a main ingredient in the study).[4597,4598,4599]

■ Kaffir lime petitgrain may be photosensitizing due to the presence of bergapten, bergamottin, and oxypeucedanin.[4600] It is reasonable to conclude that kaffir lime peel oil may also contain photosensitizing furanocoumarins. Avoid UV rays for at least twelve hours following topical application. Hexanes and extracts of kaffir lime also contain furanocoumarins.

**SELECTED EVIDENCE:**

☐ Massaging 1 mL of a 20% kaffir lime (peel) dilution to the lower abdomen for five minutes, followed by covering with plastic film, increased alertness, attention, cheerfulness, vigor, and blood pressure in forty healthy adults.[4601] Interestingly these benefits were achieved without olfactory stimulation because all participants wore a mask supplying pure air during the study.

☐ *In vitro* research demonstrated that kaffir lime petitgrain killed bacteria associated with periodontal disease (*P. gingivalis, S. sanguinis,* and *S. mutans*) and enhanced the antimicrobial activity of chlorhexidine.[4602]

☐ Both kaffir lime petitgrain and kaffir lime (peel) essential oils inhibited multiple respiratory tract pathogens: 411 isolates of groups A, B, C, F, G *streptococci, Streptococcus pneumoniae, Haemophilus influenzae, Staphylococcus aureus (methicillin-resistant* and *-sensitive S. aureus),* and *Acinetobacter baumannii,* obtained from patients with respiratory tract infections.[4603] However, the petitgrain oil was far more effective.

☐ *In vitro* research shows that a kaffir lime petitgrain essential oil inhibits both AChE and BChE activity, with stronger inhibition of BChE.[4604] Inhibition of AChE prevents the breakdown of acetylcholine, which is essential for memory and thinking. People with neurodegenerative diseases make less acetylcholine, and the diseases often break it down at a faster rate leading to acetylcholine deficits. Selective inhibition of BChE is also desirable in neurodegenerative diseases because it interferes with acetylcholine activity. In addition, BChE is often found in the plaques and tangles in the brains of people with Alzheimer's disease.[4605]

☐ Kaffir lime (peel) essential oil is lethal to mosquito larvae and the leafworm moth.[4606,4607] Kaffir lime essential oil petitgrain repels cockroaches up to 86% when mixed with ethanol and formulated with 20% of kaffir lime essential oil.[4608] Both kaffir lime petitgrain and peel essential oil repelled the *Aedes aegypti* and *Anopheles minimus* mosquito vectors, with the leaf oil being more active against *An. minimus.*[4609] Another study reported that hairy basil was a promising mosquito repellent against *An. minimus.*[4610] A study determined that a combination of citronella, turmeric, kaffir lime (*C. hystrix*), hairy basil (*O. americanum*), and vanilla could

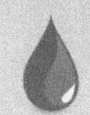

replace DEET (a common chemical insect repellent that is associated with brain cell damage and behavioral changes in animals) as a natural insect repellent.[4611]

☐ Sweet basil, cinnamon bark, sweet fennel, kaffir lime petitgrain, kaffir lime peel, black pepper, peppermint, and spearmint essential oils all demonstrated antimicrobial activity against bacteria linked to cavities (Streptococcus *mutans* and *Lactobacillus casei*).[4612] Cinnamon was the most active against both bacteria, kaffir lime petitgrain was the weakest of the tested oils against both bacteria, and black pepper was inactive against *L. casei*.

☐ Tangerine and kaffir lime peel essential oil both presented antimelanogenic (prevents hyperpigmentation) and antiacetylcholinesterase (a key enzyme involved in neurodegenerative disorders) activity. Kaffir lime peel oil also inhibited collagenase and elastase (enzymes involved in skin aging).[4613] The study authors also reported that cinnamon, kaffir lime, tangerine, and pomelo essential oils inhibited α-glucosidase activity, which is an enzyme linked to diabetes.

☐ Allspice CT eugenol, bay laurel CT camphene, betel CT safrole, and kaffir lime peel, exhibited varying degrees of antioxidant activity in multiple assays (DPPH, XO, NO, ABTS).[4614]

☐ Kaffir lime peel essential oil was evaluated for its skin benefits in various laboratory studies.[4615] The oil and its major constituents were not toxic to healthy human skin cells representing various skin layers (keratinocytes, melanocytes, and fibroblasts) even after prolonged exposure of seventy-two hours. It also demonstrated good anti-inflammatory activity (half the potency of the drug diclofenac) and minimal proinflammatory activity. Kaffir lime oil also exhibited high inhibition of tyrosinase activity, suggesting it may brighten the skin. Lastly, the oil displayed antimelanoma effects in three human melanoma cells of varying degrees of malignancy.

☐ Comparison of citrus leaf essential oils—lemon, calamondin, kaffir lime petitgrain, and ponderosa lemon (*C. pyriformis*)—showed that lemon displayed the greatest antioxidant capacity in the DPPH assay, while kaffir lime was the lowest.[4616] Each oil exhibited potent antiproliferative activity against cervical cancer cells, with lemon leaf oil being the most active at the higher concentrations.

# KANUKA
## (White Tea Tree, Burgan)

*Kunzea ericoides* (A. Rich.) J. Thomp., *K. peduncularis* F. Muell., *Leptospermum ericoides* A. Rich.

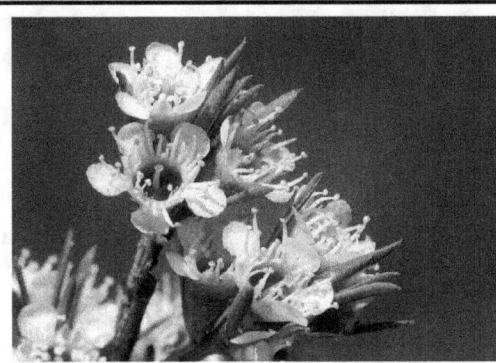

**FAMILY:** Myrtaceae
**NOTE:** Top
**AROMA INTENSITY:** Medium
**AROMA:** Herbaceous, earthy, sweet
**COMMON EXTRACTION METHOD:** Steam distilled from the leaves and twigs
**POSSIBLE SUBSTITUTE OILS:** Tea tree, Kunzea, Manuka
**BLENDS WELL WITH:** Balsam fir, bergamot, cedarwood, copaiba, cypress, Douglas fir, frankincense, honey myrtle, grapefruit, hyssop, juniper, juniper (Phoenician), lavender, lemon, lime, neroli, orange, palo santo, pine, rose, sandalwood, silver fir, spruce (black), tsuga, vetiver, white fir
**SUBCELLULAR LOCALIZATION | EPIGENETIC INFLUENCE:** Currently unknown | Currently unknown
**RECOMMENDED DILUTION RANGE:** 5%–Neat

**PRIMARY CONSTITUENTS:**[4617,4618,4619,4620]

|  |  |
| --- | --- |
| Alpha-Pinene | 54.5%–72.4% |
| 1,8-Cineole | 3.5%–16.4% |
| Viridiflorol | 0.0%–7.2% |
| Alpha-Terpineol | 0.0%–5.7% |
| Para-Cymene | 0.0%–5.1% |
| Gamma-Terpinene | 0.0%–4.1% |
| Limonene | 0.0%–3.9% |
| Calamenene | 0.0%–3.0% |

**OTHER CONSTITUENTS:** Alpha-thujene, beta-pinene, terpinolene, linalool, alpha-copaene, alpha-gurjunene, beta-caryophyllene, delta-cadinene, aromadendrene, cadina-3,5-diene, delta-amorphene, alpha-selinene, alpha-terpinene, (E)-beta-ocimene, viridiflorene, spathulenol

**PREFERRED COMPOSITION FOR CLINICAL USE:**

| Constituent | |
|---|---|
| Alpha-Pinene | 50%–73% |
| 1,8-Cineole | 3%–10% |
| Viridiflorol | 1%–8% |
| Para-Cymene | 2%–5% |
| Trans-Calamenene | 0.5%–5% |
| Limonene | 0.5%–3% |
| Linalool | 0.1%–3% |
| Alpha-Terpineol | 0.1%–3% |

**REPORTED THERAPEUTIC PROPERTIES:** Antibacterial, antifungal, antiviral, analgesic, anti-inflammatory, combats acne, relieves insect bites, enhances the penetration of other constituents through the skin, relieves headache/migraines, supports respiratory function, **wound healing**, removes warts and corns, eases cough, **reduces the appearance of blemishes**, moisturizes the skin, **relieves itching and rashes**, cellular regeneration, antiallergic, relieves insect bites, deodorant, calming/relaxing, stress management, relieves anxiety, uplifting, antidepressant, combats anger

**CAUTIONS:**

■ Caution is sensible after the thirty-seventh week of pregnancy. There is a very small risk that Kanuka essential oil could decrease uterine contractions during active labor based on animal research.[4621]

**SELECTED EVIDENCE:**

□ A small clinical study (nineteen people) found that a gargle with equal parts of Kanuka and Manuka essential oil in water delayed mucositis (painful inflammation of the mucous membranes of the digestive tract—mouth to anus—after chemotherapy or radiation treatment), reduced pain, and reduced weight loss better than a placebo.[4622]

□ *In vitro* research suggests the antibacterial activity of kanuka essential oil against 25 bacterial strains and 20 *Listeria* strains varies from absent to moderate inhibition, and it possessed moderate antioxidant activity.[4623] Other research reports that kanuka essential oil significantly inhibits four infectious and inflammatory fungi (*Trichosporon mucoides, Malassezia furfur, Candida albicans,* and *Candida tropicalis*) and bacteria (*Staphylococcus aureus, Streptococcus sobrinus, Streptococcus mutans,* and *Escherichia coli*).[4624] The study authors determined that the antifungal activity of kanuka essential oil was superior to manuka essential oil.

□ Animal research suggests that Kanuka essential oil relieves muscles spasms by a currently unknown mechanism.[4625] Interestingly, another study found that Kanuka essential oil temporarily increases muscle spasms.[4626]

□ Kanuka essential oil strongly inhibited LPS-induced (bacterial lipopolysaccharide, which is well-known for initiating inflammatory responses) release of the inflammatory cytokine tumor necrosis factor alpha (TNF-$\alpha$) without adversely affecting the immune system.[4627] TNF-$\alpha$ plays a key role in the initiation of systemic inflammation and is associated with chronic inflammatory conditions.

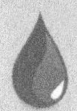

# KATRAFAY
## (Kathrafay, Katafray)
*Cedrelopsis grevei* H. Baillon

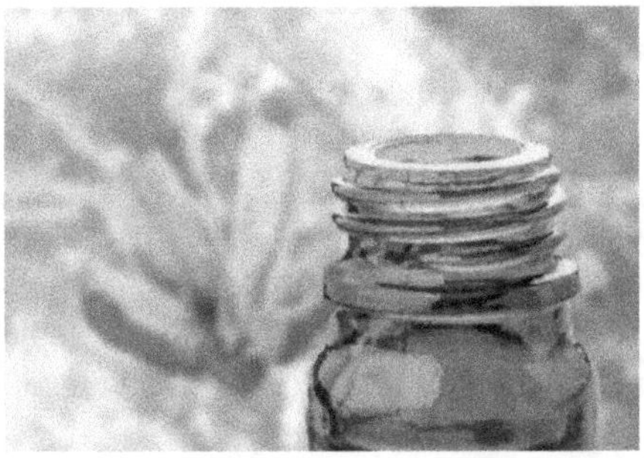

**FAMILY:** Ptaeroxylaceae
**NOTE:** Middle
**AROMA INTENSITY:** Medium
**AROMA:** Woody, earthy, crisp, slightly sweet
**COMMON EXTRACTION METHOD:** Steam distilled from the bark; may also be distilled from the leaves and branches
**POSSIBLE SUBSTITUTE OILS:** Copaiba, Japanese cedarwood, Formosan cypress, helichrysum, calendula, hinoki, ginger
**BLENDS WELL WITH:** Agarwood, cedarwood, lavender, lemon, marjoram, sandalwood, tea tree
**SUBCELLULAR LOCALIZATION | EPIGENETIC INFLUENCE:** Currently unknown | Currently unknown
**RECOMMENDED DILUTION RANGE:** 3%–50%; neat for limited conditions

**PRIMARY CONSTITUENTS:**[4628,4629,4630,4631]

*Ishwarane CT*

| | |
|---|---|
| Ishwarane | 5.8%–22.1% |
| Alpha-Copaene | 5.9%–15.6% |
| (α,β,δ)-Selinene | 0.7%–13.0% |
| Beta-Caryophyllene | 0.8%–10.5% |
| (γ,δ)-Cadinene | 0.6%–9.6% |
| Alpha-Humulene | 0.0%–9.5% |
| Beta-Elemene | 0.0%–8.9% |
| Gamma-Murrolene | 0.0%–8.2% |
| (α,β)-Eudesmol | 0.0%–8.1% |
| Alpha-Muurolene | 0.0%–6.7% |
| Alpha-Bisabolol | 0.0%–5.8% |
| Copaborneol | 0.0%–5.2% |
| Isoledene | 0.9%–4.8% |

*Alpha-Pinene CT*

| | |
|---|---|
| Alpha-Pinene | 2.1%–30.0% |
| Copaborneol | 4.7%–20.0% |
| Alpha-Bisabolol | 0.0%–16.9% |
| Alpha-Eudesmol | 3.9%–11.3% |
| (γ,δ)-Cadinene | 1.1%–7.4% |
| Caryophyllene Oxide | 1.6%–7.1% |
| Gamma-Eudesmol | 0.0%–6.2% |
| Alpha-Copaene | 1.1%–5.1% |
| (α,β,δ)-Selinene | 1.1%–4.5% |

*Leaves*

| | |
|---|---|
| (E)-Beta-Farnesene | 27.7%–35.6% |
| Delta-Cadinene | 0.4%–14.5% |
| Beta-Pinene | 0.2%–12.8% |
| Cis-Sesquisabinene Hydrate | 0.0%–9.8% |
| ar-Curcumene | 0.1%–8.6% |
| Alpha-Copaene | 0.1%–7.7% |
| Beta-Elemene | 1.1%–7.0% |

*Alpha-Eudesmol CT*

| | |
|---|---|
| Alpha-Eudesmol | 9.9%–37.5% |
| Alpha-Pinene | 0.0%–18.1% |
| (α,β,δ)-Selinene | 3.4%–17.2% |
| T-Muurolol | 0.0%–13.7% |
| Ishwarane | 0.0%–13.1% |
| Gamma-Eudesmol | 0.0%–11.1% |
| Copaborneol | 0.0%–9.6% |
| Alpha-Bisabolol | 0.0%–7.1% |

*(γ,δ)-Cadinene CT*

| | |
|---|---|
| (γ,δ)-Cadinene | 0.5%–35.2% |
| Alpha-Cadinol | 0.0%–15.3% |
| Alpha-Copaene | 0.1%–13.8% |
| T-Muurolol | 0.0%–11.8% |
| (α,β,δ)-Selinene | 0.0%–5.6% |
| Caryophyllene Oxide | 0.6%–4.8% |

*Beta-Pinene CT*

| | |
|---|---|
| Beta-Pinene | 17.1% |
| Cis-Sesquisabinene Hydrate | 12.8% |
| Caryophyllene Oxide | 7.0% |

OTHER CONSTITUENTS: *Ishwarane CT*—alpha-pinene, caryophyllene oxide, T-muurolol, gamma-eudesmol; *Alpha-Eudesmol CT*—alpha-copaene, beta-caryophyllene, cadinenens, caryophyllene oxide, alpha-cadinol; *Alpha-Pinene CT*—beta-caryophyllene, ishwarane; *(γ,δ)-Cadinene CT*—alpha-pinene, beta-caryophyllene; *Beta-Pinene CT*—alpha-pinene, beta-myrcene, delta-3-carene, o-cymene, para-cymene, limonene, (Z)-beta-ocimene, linalool, trans-pinocarveol, terpinen-4-ol, alpha-terpineol, myrtenal, myrtenol, alpha-copaene, beta-elemene, alpha-cedrene, beta-caryophyllene, trans-beta-farnesene, alpha-humulene, gamma-curcumene, ar-curcumene, beta-curcumene, gamma-cadinene, delta-cadinene, gamma-eudesmol, alpha-eudesmol, alpha-bisabolol; *Leaves*—alpha-pinene, beta-myrcene, delta-3-carene, limonene, (Z)-beta-ocimene, linalool, alpha-cedrene, alpha-cis-bergamotene, beta-caryophyllene, (Z)-beta-farnesene, alpha-humulene, beta-curcumene, gamma-cadinene, trans-calamenene, trans-sesquisabinene hydrate, caryophyllene oxide

## PREFERRED COMPOSITION FOR CLINICAL USE:

| Constituent | Balanced CT | Ishwarane CT |
|---|---|---|
| Alpha-Copaene | 10%–20% | 5%–11% |
| Selinene <α- + β- + δ-> | 10%–20% | 4%–10% |
| Ishwarane | 5%–15% | 10%–25% |
| Beta-Caryophyllene | 5%–15% | 0.5%–10% |
| (γ,δ)-Cadinene | 5%–10% | 3%–9% |
| Alpha-Humulene | 3%–10% | – |
| (α,β)-Eudesmol | 3%–8% | – |
| Gamma-Muurolene | 2%–7% | – |
| Isoledene | 3%–6% | – |
| Copaborneol | 0.1%–5% | – |
| Allo-Aromadendrene | | 7%–14% |
| Beta-Elemene | – | 5%–12% |
| Ar-Curcumene | – | 0.5%–5% |
| Rotundene | – | 1%–4% |

Note: The preferred composition (balanced CT) is usually obtained from plants growing in southern Madagascar in the Salary and Intampolo regions.

REPORTED THERAPEUTIC PROPERTIES: **Analgesic**, anti-inflammatory, **soothes sore muscles and joints**, relieves sciatica, **nervine**, antineuralgic, antirheumatic, antiarthritic, antiviral, antibacterial, supports respiratory function, reduces fever, moisturizes the skin, relieves headache, aids lymph flow, supports intestinal function, reduces mental fatigue, energizing

CAUTIONS:
■ None currently known.

SELECTED EVIDENCE:

☐ *In vitro* research demonstrates that the leaf essential oil kills breast cancer cells, which was attributed to the synergy of all the terpenes contained in the essential oil.[4632] The study authors also noted a strong correlation with the minor constituent (Z)-beta-farnesene and anticancer activity.

☐ Katrafay leaf essential oil inhibited chloroquine-resistant *P. falciparum* (a protozoan parasite that is one of the causes of malaria in humans).[4633]

☐ Katrafay leaf essential oil reduces inflammation by inhibiting the 5-LOX enzyme.[4634] The 5-LOX enzyme converts arachidonic acid to leukotrienes, increasing inflammation and allergic reactions, and is associated with chronic degenerative inflammatory diseases and cancer.

☐ Katafray leaf essential oil exhibited poor antioxidant activity.[4635]

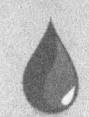

# KHELLA
## (Chellah, Toothpick Weed)
*Ammi visnaga* L., *Visnaga daucoides* Gaertn.

**FAMILY:** Apiaceae (Umbelliferae)
**NOTE:** Middle
**AROMA INTENSITY:** Strong
**AROMA:** Earthy, pungent, herbaceous, medicinal
**COMMON EXTRACTION METHOD:** Steam distilled from the seeds or aerial parts
**POSSIBLE SUBSTITUTE OILS:** Carrot seed, Roman chamomile, balsam fir
**BLENDS WELL WITH:** Carrot seed, clary sage, eucalyptus, lavender, marjoram, oregano, peppermint, sage, spearmint, thyme, turmeric
**SUBCELLULAR LOCALIZATION | EPIGENETIC INFLUENCE:** Currently unknown | Currently unknown
**RECOMMENDED DILUTION RANGE:** 3%–20%; 50% for some applications

**PRIMARY CONSTITUENTS:**[4636,4637,4638,4639,4640,4641]

*Seeds*

| | |
|---|---|
| Linalool | 22.0%–35.0% |
| Isoamyl 2-Methylbutyrate | 23.4%–27.7% |
| Amyl Isobutyrate | 13.2%–16.0% |
| Amyl Valerate | 10.0%–13.2% |
| Alpha-Terpinene | 0.1%–4.0% |

*Aerial Parts (2,2-Dimethylbutanoic Acid CT)*

| | |
|---|---|
| 2,2-Dimethylbutanoic Acid | 30.1% |
| Isobutyl Isobutyrate | 14.0% |
| Croweacin | 12.2% |
| Linalool | 12.1% |
| Bornyl Acetate | 7.3% |
| Thymol | 6.0% |

*Aerial Parts (Isoamyl 2-Methylbutyrate CT)*

| | |
|---|---|
| Isoamyl 2-Methylbutyrate | 10.3%–36.0% |
| Linalool | 4.9%–32.0% |
| Isoamyl Isovalerate | 0.0%–10.0% |
| Verticiol | 0.0%–9.9% |
| Isoamyl Isobutyrate | 0.0%–6.8% |
| Octane-3,3-dimethyl-2-(1-buten-3-on-1-yl) | 0.0%–6.4% |

*Aerial Parts (2-Methylbutyl Butyrate CT)*

| | |
|---|---|
| 2-Methylbutyl Butyrate | 41.8% |
| Linalool | 23.5% |
| Isoamyl 2-Methylbutyrate | 10.0% |
| Amyl Isovalerate | 3.9% |

**OTHER CONSTITUENTS:** *Seeds*—pentyl propanoate, alpha-pinene, limonene, beta-bourbonene, dodecanal, lavandulyl 2-methyl propanoate, germacrene D, lavandulyl 3-methylbutanoate, lavandulyl 2-methylbutanoate, beta-sesquiphellandrene (E)-nerolidol, (Z,E)-farnesyl acetate, alpha-thujene, para-cymene, cis-linalool oxide, trans-linalool oxide, beta-terpineol, alpha-farnesene; *Aerial Parts (Isoamyl 2-Methylbutyrate CT)*—spiro, iso-valerate acid, 2-methyl butyl ester, sabinene, alpha-pinene, butyl isobutyrate, isobutyl isovalerate, alpha-terpinene, limonene, 2-methylbutyl 2-methylbutyrate, amyl isovalerate, gamma-terpinene, beta-bourbonene, alpha-humulene, germacrene D, linalyl valerate, lavandulyl 2-methyl-butyrate, beta-sesquiphellandrene, alpha-bisabolol, (Z)-farnesyl acetate; *Aerial Parts (2,2-Dimethylbutanoic Acid CT)*—alpha-thujene, 3-methylpentenol, methylbutyl 2-methylbutanoate, 2-nonyne, hexenyl isobutanoate, geranyl acetate, lavandulyl acetate, citronellyl propionate; *Aerial Parts (2-Methylbutyl Butyrate CT)*—N/A

**PREFERRED COMPOSITION FOR CLINICAL USE:**

| Constituent | Aerial Parts |
|---|---|
| Linalool | 25%–40% |
| Isoamyl 2-Methylbutyrate | 15%–25% |
| Verticiol | 0%–7% |
| Isoamyl Isobutyrate | 0%–7% |
| Isoamyl Isovalerate | 0%–5% |
| Octane-3,3-Dimethyl -2-(1-buten-3-on-1-yl) | 0%–5% |

**REPORTED THERAPEUTIC PROPERTIES:** Antibacterial, antifungal, antimicrobial, antiallergic, antispasmodic, **supports respiratory function**, **relieves asthma**, eases cough, bronchodilator, decongestant, balances blood pressure, reduces kidney stones, relieves chronic skin conditions, balances menstruation, balancing, grounding, relieves anxiety, stress management

**CAUTIONS:**

■ May be photosensitizing based on possible presence of the furanocoumarins marmesine (marmesine is a precursor to the production of psoralen) and 8-hydroxybergapten (a psoralen).[4642,4643] Avoid sun exposure to area of application for at least twelve hours after topical application.

■ Some texts and websites report that khella essential oil contains the toxic constituent khellin, which is an active and toxic constituent found in the plant at less than 2%.[4644,4645,4646] However, none of the studies in the literature report this constituent in the SD/HD essential oils, only those extracted by carbon dioxide. If it is present, it would contraindicate the essential oil in children, during pregnancy and while nursing, and the oral administration of the essential oil.

**SELECTED EVIDENCE:**

☐ *In vitro* research demonstrates that khella essential oil inhibits *E. coli*, *P. aeruginosa*, *B. subtilis*, and *K. pneumoniae*.[4647,4648,4649,4650]

☐ Khella essential oil inhibits the fungi *Trametes pini*, *Penicillium parasiticus*, and *Aspergillus niger in vitro*.[4651]

☐ The linalool CT of khella essential oil displayed moderate to low antioxidant activity in the DPPH and reducing power assays, but oral administration of the oil in mice showed high antioxidant capacity that protected against acetaminophen toxicity (increased reduced glutathione, superoxide dismutase, and catalase levels, and significantly reduced lipid peroxidation).[4652]

# KUMQUAT
## (Cumquat, Nagami, Oval Kumquat, Round Kumquat)

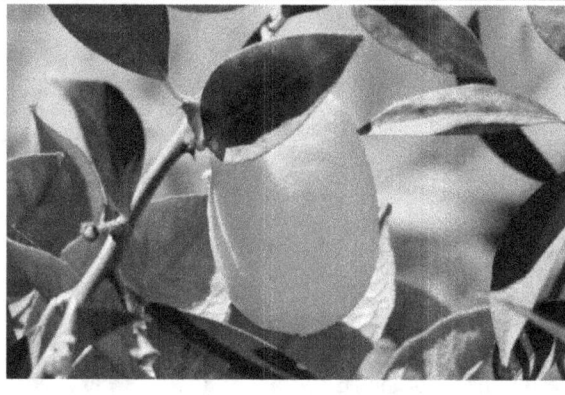

Oval Kumquat: *Fortunella margarita* (Lour.) Swingle, *Fortunella japonica* (Thunb.) Swingle var. *margarita*; Kumquat, Round Kumquat: *Citrus japonica* Thunb., *F. japonica* (Thunb.) Swingle

**FAMILY:** Rutaceae
**NOTE:** Top
**AROMA INTENSITY:** Medium
**AROMA:** Citrusy, fruity, sharp
**COMMON EXTRACTION METHOD:** Steam distilled from the peel (rind) or leaves; may also be hydrodistilled from the whole fruit or cold-pressed from the rind
**POSSIBLE SUBSTITUTE OILS:** Tangerine, orange, lemon, neroli, petitgrain
**BLENDS WELL WITH:** Allspice, bergamot, cassia, cedarwood, cinnamon, clove, frankincense, grapefruit, lavender, lemon, lime, patchouli, peppermint, orange, sandalwood, spearmint, tangerine
**SUBCELLULAR LOCALIZATION | EPIGENETIC INFLUENCE:** Currently unknown | Currently unknown
**RECOMMENDED DILUTION RANGE:** 3%–50%; neat for limited conditions

**PRIMARY CONSTITUENTS:**[4653,4654,4655,4656,4657,4658,4659,4660,4661]

| *F. margarita*, Peel (Steam Distilled) | | *C. japonica*, Leaves (Linalool CT) | |
|---|---|---|---|
| Limonene | 41.6%–94.9% | Linalool | 35.1% |
| Myrcene | 1.8%–16.5% | Eugenol | 14.8% |
| Linalyl Propionate | 0.0%–9.6% | Geraniol | 12.7% |
| Germacrene D | 0.0%–5.9% | Geranial | 7.9% |
| | | Nerol | 5.3% |
| | | (Z)-Asarone | 5.0% |

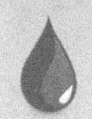

*F. margarita, Peel (Cold-pressed)*

| | |
|---|---|
| Limonene | 95.1% |
| Myrcene | 2.0% |

*F. margarita, Leaves*

| | |
|---|---|
| Beta-Eudesmol | 12.4%–28.3% |
| Gamma-Eudesmol | 8.4%–19.0% |
| Elemol | 0.0%–18.8% |
| Alpha-Muurolene | 0.1%–10.3% |
| Beta-Gurjunene | 0.0%–10.0% |
| Germacrene D | 0.0%–8.9% |
| Beta-Pinene | 0.0%–8.3% |
| Linalool | 1.0%–8.2% |
| Gamma-Muurolene | 0.0%–6.5% |
| Delta-Elemene | 2.3%–5.3% |

*F. margarita, Fruit (Limonene CT)*

| | |
|---|---|
| Limonene | 94.4%–94.6% |
| Myrcene | 1.9%–2.0% |

*F. margarita, Fruit (Alpha-Terpineol CT)*

| | |
|---|---|
| Alpha-Terpineol | 55.5% |
| Carvone | 5.7% |
| Carveol | 5.5% |
| Gamma-Murrolene | 5.5% |
| Citronellal | 5.0% |

*C. japonica, Leaves (Beta-Pinene CT)*

| | |
|---|---|
| Beta-Pinene | 47.4% |
| Limonene | 10.2% |
| Linalool | 9.8% |
| Trans-Ocimene | 7.6% |
| Alpha-Pinene | 7.4% |
| Camphene | 3.6% |
| Myrcene | 3.2% |

*C. japonica, Peel (Cold-pressed)*

| | |
|---|---|
| Limonene | 93.4% |
| Myrcene | 1.9% |

*C. japonica, Peel (Distilled)*

| | |
|---|---|
| Limonene | 51.0% |
| Germacrene D | 12.1% |
| Beta-Myrcene | 8.5% |
| Hexadecene-3(Z) | 3.5% |
| Linoleic Acid | 3.2% |
| Delta-Cadinene | 2.5% |
| Beta-Phellandrene | 2.5% |
| Geranyl Acetate | 2.4% |
| Dodecene-1 | 2.0% |

**OTHER CONSTITUENTS:** *F. margarita, Peel (Steam Distilled)*—camphene, alpha-pinene, p-menta-2,8-dien-1-ol, p-mentha-1,5-dien-8-ol, carvone, octyl acetate; *F. margarita, Peel (Cold-pressed)*—germacrene D, alpha-pinene; *F. margarita, Leaves*—alpha-pinene, limonene, terpinen-4-ol, alpha-terpineol, delta-cadinene, (E)-nerolidol, beta-elemene, alpha-humulene, beta-selinene, bicyclogermacrene, alpha-amorphene, spathulenol; *F. margarita, Fruit (Limonene CT)*—N/A; *F. margarita, Fruit (Alpha-Terpineol CT)*—linalool, limonene, delta-cadinene, trans-gamma-bisabolene, germacrene B, alpha-cadinene, diethylphthalate, cedrol; *C. japonica, Leaves (Linalool CT)*—citronellol, terpinen-4-ol, (E)-isocitral, alpha-terpineol, citronellol, bornyl acetate, T-cadinol, beta-eudesmol, alpha-eudesmol, gamma-cadinene, alpha-trans-bergamotene, elemol, geranyl acetate, beta-elemene, methyl eugenol (<0.2%); *C. japonica, Leaves (Beta-Pinene CT)*—alpha-thujene, alpha-phellandrene, delta-3-carene, terpinolene, alpha-terpineol, 4-terpineol; *C. japonica, Peel (Cold-pressed)*—ethyl acetate; *C. japonica, Peel (Distilled)*—alpha-pinene, nonene-4-methyl-5, decene-2-(Z), 1,6-Octadien-3-ol,3,7,dimethyl, acetic acid (methyl ester), carvone, gamma-elemene, gamma-cadinene, myristicin, germacrene B, heptadecyl 2,2-dichloroacetate

**PREFERRED COMPOSITION FOR CLINICAL USE:**

| Constituent | *F. margarita, Peel, Distilled* | *F. margarita, Peel, Cold-pressed* | *C. japonica, Peel, Cold-pressed* |
|---|---|---|---|
| **Limonene** | 40%–70% | 85%–97% | 83%–95% |
| **Myrcene** | 5%–18% | 1%–5% | 1%–5% |
| **Linalyl Propionate** | 5%–12% | – | – |
| **Germacrene D** | 3%–8% | 0.1%–5% | – |
| **Alpha-Pinene** | 0.1%–5% | 0.1%–5% | 0.1%–3% |
| **Ethyl Acetate** | – | – | 0%–5% |
| **Beta-Pinene** | – | – | 0.5%–3% |

**REPORTED THERAPEUTIC PROPERTIES:** Antibacterial, **antifungal**, antiviral, anticancer, antioxidant, anti-aging, **anti-inflammatory**, reduces the appearance of wrinkles and blemishes, relieves chronic skin conditions, aids digestion, balances blood sugar, weight management, mentally stimulating, antidepressant, relieves anxiety

**CAUTIONS:**

■ May be photosensitizing due to the possible presence of furanocoumarins. Avoid sun exposure to area of application for at least twelve hours after topical application.[4662]

■ *C. japonica, Leaves (Linalool CT)*: Avoid in children under age 12 due to liver toxicity concerns of beta-asarone.[4663,4664,4665,4666,4667]

■ *C. japonica, Leaves (Linalool CT)*: Avoid during pregnancy and lactation due to genotoxicity of beta-asarone, and reduced maternal weight gain, embryo toxicity, abortion, and fetal malformations (hydrocephaly, extra-ribs, clubfeet, and cleft lips) reportedly caused by alpha-asarone in animal studies.[4668] However, one animal study did not report toxicity to embryos or fetuses nor birth defects.[4669]

■ *C. japonica, Leaves (Linalool CT)*: Avoid oral consumption due to asarone content. Beta-asarone is genotoxic (destructive to a cells genetic material—DNA, RNA—and integrity), and may cause damage to organs (liver, heart, and kidneys), abnormal fluid accumulation in the abdominal (peritoneal cavity), and malignant intestinal tumors at large to extreme doses according to animal research.[4670,4671,4672,4673,4674,4675] Long-term administration increases the damage caused. The exposure limit for total asarones (alpha- and beta-) was set to 115 mcg (or 2 mcg/kg/day) from herbal medicinal products, which would equate to less than one drop of essential oil.[4676] A case report involving a middle-aged woman reports tachycardia, dizziness, tremor, irregular breathing, pallor, anxiety, nausea and vomiting reportedly due to asarone intoxication after consuming an unknown quantity of asarone-containing herbal medicines.

■ *C. japonica, Leaves (Linalool CT)*: Avoid with compromised liver or kidney due to significant potential to cause liver and kidney toxicity due to asarone content.[4677,4678,4679,4680,4681]

■ *C. japonica, Leaves (Linalool CT)*: May interfere with pentobarbital and other barbiturates (medications for anxiety and insomnia) due to asarone content.[4682,4683,4684,4685]

**SELECTED EVIDENCE:**

□ *In vitro* research shows that kumquat essential oil (limonene CT) triggered apoptosis of prostate cancer cells.[4686]

□ Kumquat essential oil reduces inflammation by inhibiting the COX-2 enzyme and NF-κB according to *in vitro* research. NF-κB is a protein complex that plays a key role in inflammation by modulating pro- and anti-inflammatory molecules.[4687] Another study reported that kumquat essential oil (limonene CT) reduces inflammation by reducing the secretion of nitric oxide by liposaccharides.[4688]

□ *In vitro* research demonstrates that kumquat essential oil (limonene CT) strongly inhibited four human skin pathogens (*Staphylococcus epidermidis*, *Propionibacterium acnes*, *Malassezia furfur*, and *Candida albicans*) and antibiotic-resistant *S. epidermis*.[4689] The leaf essential oil (beta-eudesmol CT) moderately to strongly inhibited several bacteria: *Bacillus subtilis*, *Staphylococcus aureus*, *Sarcina luta*, *Streptococcus faecalis*, *Escherichia coli*, *Klebsilla pneumonia*, and *Pseudomonas aeruginosa*, whereas the whole fruit oil (alpha-terpineol CT) demonstrated stronger activity against fungi: *A. niger* and *C. albicans*.[4690] The peel oil (limonene CT) demonstrated potent antimicrobial activity against both gram-negative (*E. coli* and *S. typhimurium*) and gram-positive (*S. aureus*, *B. cereus*, *B. subtilis*, *L. bulgaricus*, and *B. laterosporus*) bacteria, and a remarkable antifungal activity against *C. albicans*.[4691] The leaf oil (beta-pinene CT) demonstrated antibacterial activity against *B. subtilis* and *S. aureus* comparable to gentamacin.[4692]

□ The whole fruit oil (alpha-terpineol CT) inhibited the Avian influenza virus (H5N1) almost 80% and the leaf oil (beta-eudesmol CT) inhibited the H5N1 virus by almost 44%.[4693]

□ *In vitro* research suggests kumquat essential oil (limonene and beta-pinene CTs) possesses good to significant antioxidant activity, which is comparable to synthetic vitamin E and BHT.[4694,4695,4696]

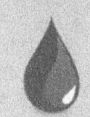

# KUNZEA
## (White Kunzea, White Cloud, Southern Spring Flower, Tick Bush)

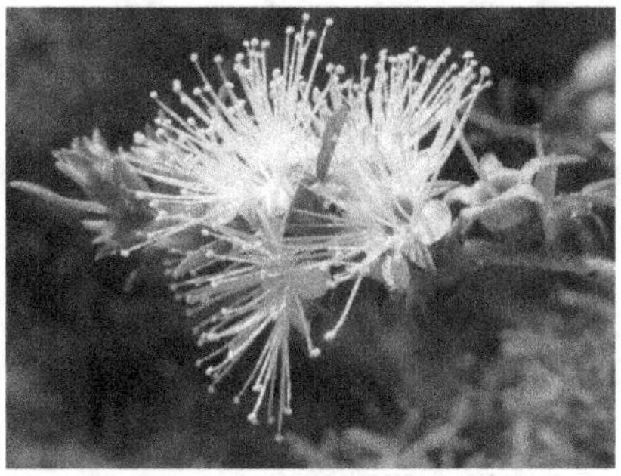

*Kunzea ambigua* (Sm.) Druce

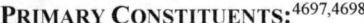

**FAMILY:** Myrtaceae
**NOTE:** Middle
**AROMA INTENSITY:** Medium
**AROMA:** Herbaceous, medicinal, earthy, slightly camphoraceous, slightly sweet
**COMMON EXTRACTION METHOD:** Steam distilled from the flowers, leaves, and twigs
**POSSIBLE SUBSTITUTE OILS:** Kanuka, manuka, tea tree
**BLENDS WELL WITH:** Angelica, cajeput, eucalyptus dives, helichrysum, honey myrtle, Kanuka, lavender, lemon, lemongrass, lemon eucalyptus, lemon myrtle, manuka, niaouli, rosalina, sandalwood, tea tree
**SUBCELLULAR LOCALIZATION | EPIGENETIC INFLUENCE:** Currently unknown | Currently unknown
**RECOMMENDED DILUTION RANGE:** 5%–Neat

**PRIMARY CONSTITUENTS:**[4697,4698]

*Spathulenol/Globulol CT*

|  |  |
|---|---|
| Spathulenol | 12.2%–34.8% |
| Globulol | 15.3%–22.6% |
| Bicyclogermacrene | 7.6%–14.0% |
| Alpha-Pinene | 0.6%–7.3% |
| Viridiflorol | 3.9%–6.4% |
| Ledol | 4.8%–6.3% |
| Viridiflorene | 3.0%–5.1% |
| Alpha-Gurjunene | 1.1%–4.5% |
| Linalool | 0.8%–4.3% |
| Beta-Caryophyllene | 2.9%–4.1% |
| Allo-Aromadendrene | 1.2%–2.9% |
| Isospathulenol | 0.0%–2.8% |
| Palustrol | 2.5%–2.7% |
| Rosifoliol | 0.0%–2.0% |

*Alpha-Pinene CT*

|  |  |
|---|---|
| Alpha-Pinene | 28.3%–62.5% |
| Viridiflorol | 0.3%–38.0% |
| Globulol | 0.5%–16.6% |
| 1,8-Cineole | 3.6%–14.5% |
| Calamenene | 0.6%–4.6% |
| Viridiflorene | 0.3%–4.0% |
| Alpha-Terpineol | 0.0%–4.0% |
| Bicyclogermacrene | 0.4%–3.8% |
| Leptospermone | 0.1%–2.1% |
| Myrtenal | 0.0%–2.1% |

**OTHER CONSTITUENTS:** *Alpha-Pinene CT*—beta-pinene, limonene, isoamyl isovalerate, citronellol, alpha-cubebene, beta-caryophyllene, aromadendrene, alloaromadendrene, delta-cadinene, palustrol, ledol, spathulenol, caryophyllene oxide; *Spathulenol/Globulol CT*—linalool, beta-elemene, aromadendrene, citronellol, caryophyllene oxide

**PREFERRED COMPOSITION FOR CLINICAL USE:**

| Constituent | Alpha-Pinene CT |
|---|---|
| **Alpha-Pinene** | 30%–50% |
| **Viridiflorol** | 5%–20% |
| **1,8-Cineole** | 5%–20% |
| **Globulol** | 2%–15% |
| **Bicyclogermacrene** | 2%–7% |
| **Trans-Calamenene** | 0.5%–5% |
| **Ledol** | 1%–3% |
| **Alpha-Terpineol** | 1%–3% |
| **Ledene (Viridiflorene)** | 0%–3% |
| **Leptospermone** | 0%–3% |

**REPORTED THERAPEUTIC PROPERTIES:** Antibacterial, antifungal, antiviral, **analgesic**, anti-inflammatory, antispasmodic, **antiarthritic**, antirheumatic, anti-infectious, antimicrobial, antioxidant, wound healing, supports respiratory function, expels excess mucus, **relieves sports injuries**, soothes sprains and strains, aids immune function, relieves bruises, relieves headache/migraines (particularly recurrent), soothes chronic skin conditions, vasodilator, insect repellent, stress management, relieves anxiety, releases emotional trauma

**CAUTIONS:**
■ None currently known.

**SELECTED EVIDENCE:**
☐ Kunzea essential oil (30%–40%) completely repelled mosquitoes for a mean protection time of 49 minutes, but its repellency was significantly less than that of DEET or citronella.[4699]

## LAVANDIN

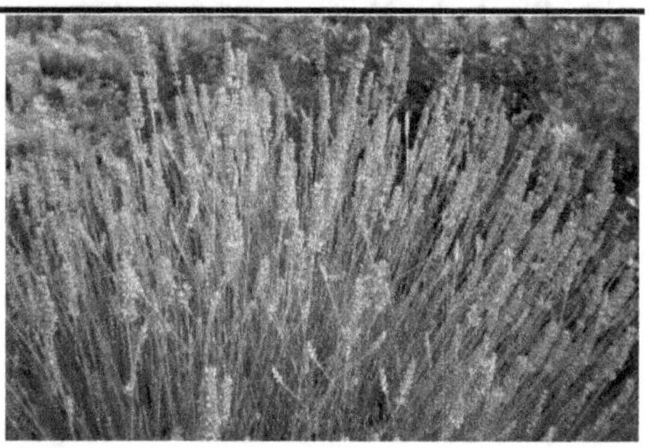

*Lavandula × intermedia* Emeric ex Loisel.,
*L. hybrida* Reverchon, *L. hortensis* Hy

**FAMILY:** Lamiaceae (Labiatae)
**NOTE:** Middle-Top
**AROMA INTENSITY:** Strong
**AROMA:** Fresh, floral, strongly herbaceous
**COMMON EXTRACTION METHOD:** Steam distilled from the fresh flowering tops
**POSSIBLE SUBSTITUTE OILS:** Lavender, spike lavender, neroli, basil (linalool CT)
**BLENDS WELL WITH:** Bergamot, camphor, cedarwood, clary sage, clove, cinnamon, citronella, cypress, grapefruit, lavender, lemon, lime, niaouli, orange, patchouli, pine, ravensara, sandalwood, Spanish sage, tangerine, thyme
**SUBCELLULAR LOCALIZATION | EPIGENETIC INFLUENCE:** Currently unknown | Currently unknown
**RECOMMENDED DILUTION RANGE:** 3%–50%; neat for limited conditions

**PRIMARY CONSTITUENTS:**[4700,4701,4702,4703,4704,4705]

*Lavandin Abrialis*

| | |
|---|---|
| Linalool | 19.6%–39.6% |
| Linalyl Acetate | 18.6%–28.0% |
| Camphor | 8.2%–12.2% |
| 1,8-Cineole | 6.7%–10.4% |
| (E)-Beta-Ocimene | 4.0%–5.5% |
| Borneol | 2.4%–3.7% |

*Lavandin Giant*

| | |
|---|---|
| Linalool | 34.9%–45.7% |
| 1,8-Cineole | 0.0%–26.1% |
| Sabinene | 0.0%–16.9% |
| Borneol | 7.6%–10.1% |
| Camphor | 5.3%–8.4% |
| Linalyl Acetate | 3.8%–4.4% |

*Lavandin Grosso*

| | |
|---|---|
| Linalyl Acetate | 26.2%–36.7% |
| Linalool | 25.7%–35.5% |
| 1,8-Cineole | 4.0%–10.2% |
| Camphor | 5.9%–8.8% |

*Lavandin Dutch*

| | |
|---|---|
| Linalool | 42.5%–47.0% |
| Sabinene | 0.0%–16.7% |
| 1,8-Cineole | 0.0%–15.6% |
| Camphor | 10.0%–12.5% |
| Linalyl Acetate | 4.5%–11.7% |
| Borneol | 3.3%–6.0% |

*Lavandin Super*

| | |
|---|---|
| Linalyl Acetate | 20.4%–45.0% |
| Linalool | 23.0%–41.8% |
| 1,8-Cineole | 0.0%–15.9% |
| Camphor | 0.0%–11.4% |
| Terpinen-4-ol | 1.0%–6.7% |

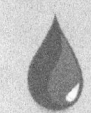

| | | | |
|---|---|---|---|
| Terpinen-4-ol | 1.5%–3.9% | Sabinene | 0.0%–6.5% |
| Borneol | 1.6%–3.6% | Borneol | 1.3%–5.5% |
| Lavandulyl Acetate | 1.6%–2.9% | Sabinene Hydrate | 0.0%–4.6% |

**OTHER CONSTITUENTS:** Myrcene, limonene, butanoic acid hexyl ester, neryl acetate, farnesene, nerol, crypton, alpha-terpineol, geraniol, nonadecane, heneicosane, beta-pinene, 1-octen-4-ol, geranyl acetate, benzaldehyde, cadinol, alpha-pinene, caryophyllene, bisabolol, trans-beta-ocimene, cis-beta-ocimene

**PREFERRED COMPOSITION FOR CLINICAL USE:**

| Constituent | Lavandin Abrialis | Lavandin Grosso | Lavandin Super |
|---|---|---|---|
| Linalool | 25%–40% | 25%–40% | 25%–40% |
| Linalyl Acetate | 20%–32% | 25%–40% | 30%–50% |
| 1,8-Cineole | 5%–15% | 4%–10% | 3%–7% |
| Camphor | 6%–12% | 4%–10% | 3%–7% |
| (E)-Beta-Ocimene | 2%–7% | 0%–2% | 2%–5% |
| Borneol | 1%–5% | 1%–5% | 1%–3% |
| Lavandulyl Acetate | 1%–3% | 1%–5% | 0.5%–3% |
| Beta-Caryophyllene | 1%–3% | 1%–3% | 1%–3% |
| Limonene | 0.5%–2% | 0.5%–2% | 0.5%–2% |
| Terpinen-4-ol | 0.1%–2% | 1%–5% | 0.01%–1% |
| Alpha-Terpineol | 0.1%–2% | 0.1%–2% | 0.5%–2% |
| (E)-Beta-Farnesene | 0.1%–2% | 0%–2% | 0%–2% |
| (Z)-Beta-Ocimene | 0%–2% | 0.5%–2% | 1%–3% |
| Lavandulol | 0.3%–1.5% | 0.1%–1% | 0.01%–1% |
| Myrcene | 0.1%–1% | 0.1%–1% | 0.1%–1% |
| Hexyl Butyrate | 0.1%–0.5% | 0.1%–1% | 0.1%–1.5% |
| 3-Octanone | – | – | 0.1%–2% |

**REPORTED THERAPEUTIC PROPERTIES:** Analgesic (pain relief), wound healing, supports normal menstruation, **antiseptic**, expectorant, **antispasmodic**, antifungal, antiviral, antibacterial, insect repellent, aids normal respiration, reduces the appearance of scars and blemishes, antidepressant, stress management, **reduces anxiety**, helps one overcome shock, calming, relaxing

**CAUTIONS:**
■ Avoid with epilepsy and Parkinson's due to moderate camphor and 1,8-cineole content.[4706,4707,4708]
■ The camphor content in lavandin may negatively impact red blood cells and increase the risk of jaundice in children with Glucose-6-phosphate dehydrogenase deficiency (G6PD).[4709,4710]
■ May interact with aspirin, blood pressure, antiplatelet, and anticoagulant medications, and increase the risk of bleeding among people with bleeding disorders.[4711]
■ May interfere with pentobarbital and other barbiturates (medications for anxiety and insomnia) based on 1,8-cineole content (Lavandin (Giant)).[4712,4713]
■ May weakly interfere with the enzymes responsible for metabolizing medications (NSAIDs, proton-pump inhibitors, acetaminophen, antiepileptics, immune modulators, blood-sugar medications, blood pressure medications, antidepressants, antipsychotics, diabetic medications, antihistamines, antibiotics, and anesthetics) based on 1,8-cineole content (Lavandin (Giant)).[4714,4715]

**SELECTED EVIDENCE:**
☐ Regular inhalation of lavandin oil protects neurons from degeneration or injury by increasing antioxidant enzyme activities (superoxide dismutase and reduced glutathione) and reducing lipid peroxidation in rats with dementia.[4716]
☐ Animal research suggests that lavandin oil inhalation (sixty minutes a day for seven days) reduces anxiety

and improves spatial memory in rats with dementia.[4717]

- Both orally administered (100 mg/kg) or inhaled lavandin (60 minutes) "Grosso" essential oil significantly reduced pain in rodents.[4718] The authors concluded the analgesic activity of lavandin involved opioidergic and cholinergic pathways. Oral administration of lavandin also protected against gastric ulcers caused by ethanol (but not ulcers caused by the NSAID indomethacin) in the same research.
- Lavandin oil inhibits *S. aureus* and Pseudomonas *in vitro*.[4719,4720] It also completely eliminates the parasites *T. vaginalis, G. duodenalis*, and *H. inflata in vitro*.[4721]
- Inhaling lavandin oil reduced test-taking anxiety among graduate nursing students.[4722]
- Topical application of lavandin oil before surgery reduced anxiety.[4723]
- A study concluded that lavandin has potential as a natural "ingredient to fight several skin diseases" due to its antioxidant and anti-inflammatory (mild lipoxygenase inhibitor) properties.[4724]
- An interesting lavandin CT (1,8-cineole rich in borneol) significantly inhibited *E. coli* and *S. agalactiae,* and moderately to significantly inhibited *K. pneumoniae* and *S. aureus*.[4725]
- Lavandin Super essential oil was strongly active against the African cotton leafworm (*Spodoptera littoralis*) and toxic to the hard-bodied tick (*Hyalomma lusitanicum*).[4726]
- The abrialis and RC varieties of lavandin exhibited significant activity against *L. monocytogenes*, especially clinical strains, and *Salmonella enterica*.[4727]
- Aromatherapy massage with 5% lavandin essential oil—to the back for ten minutes prior to surgery—reduced anxiety and improved sleep quality in people undergoing colorectal surgery.[4728]
- Lavandin Grosso essential oil inhibited gram-negative bacteria (*Escherichia coli, Acinetobacter bohemicus*, and *Pseudomonas fluorescens*; bactericidal) and gram-positive bacteria (*Bacillus cereus* and *Kocuria marina*; bacteriostatic) in both liquid and vapor phase.[4729]
- Coriander (150 µL/L), linaloe (125 µL/L), and lavandin (200 µL/L) essential oil exhibited anesthetic activity in convict cichlid (*Amatitlania nigrofasciata*) fish.[4730]
- *Streptococcus agalactiae* (also known as Group B Streptococcus) is the most common cause of neonatal sepsis and frequently a cause of postpartum infections. *Candida albicans* is the primary cause of vulvovaginal yeast infections. Lavandin and cornmint essential oil both exhibited good antimicrobial and antibiofilm activity against *S. agalactiae* and *C. albicans* in laboratory research.[4731] The oils also demonstrated synergistic activity when used with erythromycin and fluconazole.
- Lavandin essential oil triggered apoptosis in leukemia cells, as did isolated terpinen-4-ol and linalyl acetate.[4732]
- Three cultivars of lavandin essential oil were larvicidal to the root-knot nematode (*Meloidogyne incognita*) and toxic to juveniles, with the Sumiens variety (48% linalool, 14.9% linalyl acetate, 12.1% 1,8-cineole) being the most effective against juveniles.[4733] The oils were also active against the lesion nematode (*Pratylenchus vulnus*) and again the Sumiens variety displayed the greatest activity.
- *In vitro* research demonstrated that lavandin essential oil possesses antimicrobial activity against *Candida* spp.[4734]

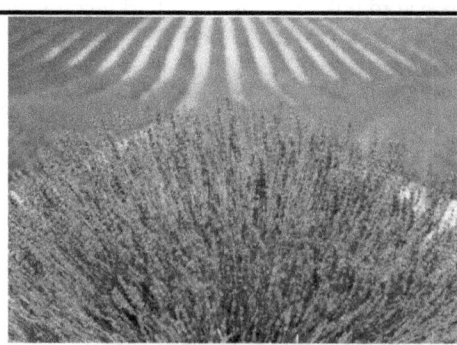

# LAVENDER
## (True Lavender)

*Lavandula angustifolia* Mill., *L. officinalis* Chaix., *L. vera* DC.

**FAMILY:** Lamiaceae (Labiatae)
**NOTE:** Top-Middle
**AROMA INTENSITY:** Medium
**AROMA:** Floral, herbaceous, sweet, woody
**COMMON EXTRACTION METHOD:** Steam distilled from the flowers
**POSSIBLE SUBSTITUTE OILS:** Lavandin, spike lavender, neroli, bergamot, basil (Linalool CT), cistus, frankincense, rosewood
**BLENDS WELL WITH:** All oils
**SUBCELLULAR LOCALIZATION | EPIGENETIC INFLUENCE:** Cytoplasm | Digestive/Excretory
**RECOMMENDED DILUTION RANGE:** 5%–Neat

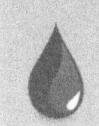

**PRIMARY CONSTITUENTS:**[4735,4736,4737]

*True English Lavender*
*(Lavandula angustifolia Vera,*
*Lavandula angustifolia Mill.)*

| | |
|---|---|
| Linalool | 24.5%–50.6% |
| Linalyl Acetate | 3.7%–45.0% |
| Caryophyllene | 0.0%–24.1% |
| 1,8 Cineole | 0.0%–19.8%* |
| Beta-Phellandrene | 0.0%–16.0% |
| Sabinene | 0.1%–11.0% |
| Terpinen-4-ol | 7.8%–9.6% |
| (Z)-Beta-Ocimene | 0.0%–7.8% |
| Lavandulyl Acetate | 2.7%–6.4% |
| Beta-Caryophyllene | 2.0%–6.1% |
| Alpha-Terpineol | 1.5%–6.0% |
| Borneol | 0.4%–5.1% |
| Germacrene D | 0.2%–4.7% |
| Santalene | 0.4%–4.5% |
| Naphthalene | 0.0%–4.2% |
| Beta-Farnesene | 0.1%–4.2% |

*Lavandula angustifolia* 'Munstead'

| | |
|---|---|
| Linalool | 37.8%–46.1% |
| Alpha-Terpineol | 19.2%–20.6% |
| Terpinen-4-ol | 0.3%–19.5% |
| Linalyl Acetate | 6.1%–12.2% |
| Cymene | 4.8%–8.3% |
| Neryl Acetate | 0.7%–4.4% |

*Indian*

| | |
|---|---|
| Linalyl Acetate | 35.4%–49.5% |
| Linalool | 26.7%–37.1% |
| Lavandulyl Acetate | 0.6%–4.5% |
| Beta-Caryophyllene | 0.9%–4.0% |
| Alpha-Terpineol | 1.2%–3.8% |

*Brazilian*

| | |
|---|---|
| Borneol | 22.4% |
| Epi-Alpha-Muurolol | 13.4% |
| Alpha-Bisabolol | 13.1% |
| Precocene I | 13.0% |
| 1,8-Cineole | 7.9% |
| Caryophyllene Oxide | 4.5% |
| Camphor | 3.5% |

*Bulgarian*

| | |
|---|---|
| Linalool | 25.4%–47.3% |
| Linalyl Acetate | 19.9%–37.6% |
| Terpinen-4-ol | 0.1%–7.4% |
| (Z)-Beta-Ocimene | 1.7%–7.7% |
| Beta-Caryophyllene | 1.7%–5.2% |
| Beta-Farnesene | 1.0%–4.7% |
| Lavandulyl Acetate | 2.5%–4.4% |
| Trans-Beta-Ocimene | 1.0%–4.2% |
| 1,8-Cineole | 0.4%–4.2% |

*French*

| | |
|---|---|
| Linalool | 9.3%–68.8% |
| Linalyl Acetate | 1.2%–59.4% |
| Lavandulyl Acetate | 0.3%–21.6% |
| Ocimene | 0.2%–18.1% |
| Terpinen-4-ol | 0.1%–13.5% |
| Lavandulol | 0.0%–4.3% |
| 1,8-Cineole | 0.0%–3.4% |

*Polish*

| | |
|---|---|
| Linalool | 27.3%–34.7% |
| Linalyl Acetate | 19.7%–22.4% |
| Lavandulyl Acetate | 4.5%–5.7% |
| Ocimene | 1.9%–2.9% |
| Terpinen-4-ol | 1.1%–2.0% |

*Italian*

| | |
|---|---|
| Linalool | 33.3%–45.0% |
| Linalyl Acetate | 31.7%–41.2% |
| Terpinen-4-ol | 1.1%–3.6% |

Note: Some reports suggest lavender contains significant amounts of 1,8-cineole (eucalyptol); however, these may be misidentified lavandin or spike lavender (*Lavandula spica*) samples, or adulterated samples. Lavender essential oil is often adulterated with lavandin. Shorter distillation times also increase the 1,8-cineole content of lavender essential oils.[1081] The lavender essential oil composition reported from Brazil is very odd and unlike any other lavender composition reported.

**OTHER CONSTITUENTS:** Limonene, alpha-pinene, camphene, cymene, butanoic acid hexyl ester, 1-octen-3-ol, 3-octanone, hexyl acetate, neryl acetate, beta-farnesene, alpha-terpineol, borneol, geranyl acetate, geraniol, camphor, caryophyllene, bisabolol, octene-3-yl-acetate, p-cymene-1-ol-8, beta-caryophyllene

**PREFERRED COMPOSITION FOR CLINICAL USE:**

| Constituent | Bulgarian | French | Chinese (Blue/White) | Lavender Blend |
|---|---|---|---|---|
| Linalyl Acetate | 26%–46% | 24%–46% | 26%–40% | 28%–40% |
| Linalool | 25%–45% | 25%–45% | 25%–40% | 28%–40% |
| (Z)-Beta-Ocimene | 2%–8% | 1%–6% | 2%–10% | 2%–6% |
| Beta-Caryophyllene | 2%–6% | 2%–7% | 1%–6% | 1%–5% |
| Lavandulyl Acetate | 2%–6% | 0.5%–5% | 2%–9% | 3%–7% |
| Terpinen-4-ol | 1%–6% | 0.1%–6% | 0.5%–6% | 2%–6% |
| (E)-Beta-Ocimene | 1%–5% | 0.5%–10% | 0.5%–5% | 1%–5% |
| 1,8-Cineole | < 4% | < 4% | < 4% | < 4% |
| Alpha-Terpineol | 0.5%–3% | 0.1%–3% | 0.5%–3% | 0.5%–3% |
| Borneol | 0.1%–3% | 0.1%–3% | 0.1%–3% | 0.1%–3% |
| 3-Octanone | 0.1%–3% | tr–3% | 0.1%–3% | 0.1%–3% |
| Camphor | < 1.5% | < 1.5% | < 1.5% | < 1.5% |
| Limonene | < 1% | < 1% | < 1% | < 1% |
| Lavandulol | > 0.1% | > 0.1% | > 0.1% | > 0.1% |
| Furano-Linalool Oxide Acetates <cis-, trans-> | Absent* | Absent* | Absent* | Absent* |

Note: The best lavender essential oils typically come from Bulgaria and France.
* Marker of synthetic adulteration.

**REPORTED THERAPEUTIC PROPERTIES: Skin healing**, analgesic (pain relief), antibacterial, anti-inflammatory, **relives burns and sunburn**, immune supportive, anticancer, antimicrobial, antiseptic, **antifungal, antispasmodic**, diuretic, nervine (calms and soothes the nerves), sedating, **reduces the appearance of scars and blemishes**, aids digestion, reduces fever, **helps bruises and boils heal**, helps relieve colic, helps relieve painful menstruation, **encourages restful sleep**, eases cough, **helps relieve headache**, balances blood pressure, stimulating, relaxing, combats irritability, **adaptogenic**, antidepressant, **reduces anxiety**, **stress management**, reduces fear, **calms shock and panic attacks,** encourages feelings of love

**CAUTIONS:**

■ May interact with antifungal drugs and enhance their effectiveness based on linalool content.[4738]
■ May interact with antibiotics and enhance their effectiveness (terpinen-4-ol rich, like Munstead).[4739]

**SELECTED EVIDENCE:**

☐ *In vitro* research concluded that lavender oil promoted the destruction (apoptosis) of breast cancer cells, but had little effect on normal healthy cells.[4740] Another study demonstrated that lavender essential oil and its two primary constituents (linalool and linalyl acetate) triggered apoptosis and prevented the spread of highly metastatic prostate cancer cells (PC-3 cells), but demonstrated weaker activity against another prostate cancer cell line (DU-145).[4741] Other research demonstrates that lavender essential oil (about a 3:1 ratio of linalool: linalyl acetate) prevents the spread of acute lymphoblastic leukemia, breast, and lung (large cell) cancers, with best activity against the leukemia line.[4742] Lavender essential oil is also cytotoxic to colorectal cancer cells.[4743]

☐ A daily abdominal massage with a combination of lavender, clary sage, and marjoram (2:1:1 ratio) from the end of the last menstruation to the beginning of the next menstruation significantly reduced painful menstruation according to a randomized, double-blind clinical trial.[4744]

☐ A sitz bath with or soap application of lavender, myrrh, neroli, rose, grapefruit, mandarin, orange, and Roman chamomile improves healing of the perineum following delivery and episiotomy.[4745] Another study observed that a lavender oil sitz bath (five to seven drops of lavender oil in four liters of water) twice daily for ten days reduced inflammation and redness of the episiotomy area better than the standard treatment option (Povidone-iodine).[4746] Pain relief was equivalent in the two groups. Two additional studies concluded that lavender essential oil may be preferable to Betadine and povidone-iodine for episiotomy wound care.[4747,4748]

☐ A daily abdominal massage with a combination of rose, cinnamon, clove, and lavender oils in an almond carrier

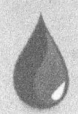

oil for seven days prior to menstruation significantly reduced painful menstruation and excess menstrual bleeding in women suffering from painful menstruation.[4749] A second study found that painful menstrual cramps were relieved in women by massaging the abdomen with two drops of lavender, and one drop each of rose and clary sage in 5 mL of almond oil.[4750]

☐ Regular inhalation of lavender oil protects neurons from degeneration or injury by increasing antioxidant enzyme activities (superoxide dismutase and reduced glutathione) and reducing lipid peroxidation in rats with dementia.[4751]

☐ A lavender massage between the hours of 3:00 and 4:00 p.m. decreased the agitated behavior in people with dementia better than inhalation of lavender alone.[4752]

☐ Animal research suggests that lavender oil inhalation (sixty minutes a day for seven days) reduces anxiety and improves spatial memory in rats with dementia.[4753]

☐ *In vitro* and animal research suggests that lavender oil may help prevent and treat intestinal dysbiosis (a state of altered intestinal flora to one of harmful bacteria that contributes to a variety of chronic and degenerative diseases) by selectively destroying harmful bacteria while leaving probiotics intact.[4754,4755]

☐ Multiple clinical studies suggest that the oral administration of 80 mg of lavender essential oil in softgels or capsules (Silexan, standardized to 20%–45% linalool and 25%–46% linalyl acetate) significantly reduces anxiety (comparable to standard drug options), improves depressive symptoms, relieves post-traumatic stress disorder, and enhances overall mental health.[4756,4757,4758,4759,4760,4761,4762,4763,4764,4765] Taking two doses daily seems to be most effective.

☐ A hand massage with equal parts of frankincense, bergamot, and lavender (as a 1.5 dilution with sweet almond carrier oil) reduced the pain and depression of hospice patients with terminal cancer.[4766]

☐ Bathing with a solution containing 20% lavender oil and 80% grapeseed oil for fourteen days positively affected mood, and reduced negative thoughts about the future in forty women being treated for psychological disorders.[4767]

☐ A lavender oil hand massage enhances emotions and reduces aggressive behavior in elderly people with dementia.[4768]

☐ A foot bath (107∘F water) with salts and either oregano, thyme, cinnamon bark, lemongrass, clove, palmarosa, peppermint, lavender, or geranium significantly reduced fungi associated with athlete's foot *in vitro*.[4769]

☐ Postpartum women who received a thirty-minute massage on the second postpartum day with 7 drops of lavender and 3 drops of neroli in 100 mL of carrier oil experienced significantly lower postpartum depression, reduced anxiety, and were more interactive with their infant.[4770]

☐ Animal research suggests that lavender can protect the myocardium (the muscular tissue of the heart) against damage during a heart attack.[4771] Another animal study concluded that a combination of lavender, monarda, and basil oils reduces cholesterol in the aorta and adverse effects by accumulation of atherosclerotic plaques in the aorta.[4772]

☐ Injection of lavender essential oil in mice reduced anxiety-induced conflict as well as the drug diazepam (a psychoactive drug used to treat psychological disorders like anxiety and panic attacks).[4773,4774]

☐ Inhalation of lavender oil influenced serotonin production and prevented serotonin syndrome caused by a combination of fluoxetine (an SSRI antidepressant drug) and 5-HTP in mice.[4775]

☐ Lavender oil helps reverse drug-resistance by *E. coli* by disrupting bacterial cell membrane integrity.[4776]

☐ Lavender oil completely eliminates the parasites *T. vaginalis, G. duodenalis,* and *H. inflata in vitro*.[4777]

☐ *In vitro* research discovered that lavender oil prevented the formation of germ tubes by *C. albicans* and killed all *C. albicans* cells within fifteen minutes of exposure.[4778] Germ tubes are used by the spores to reproduce and spread. Other research shows that lavender essential oil inhibits the growth and activity of *C. albicans* isolated from vaginal swabs better than the antifungal drug clotrimazole.[4779]

☐ Topical application of a spray with tea tree and lavender oils twice daily for three months decreased unwanted, male-pattern hair growth in women (hirsutism).[4780]

☐ Massaging the hands with lavender and rose oil (2% dilution) for fifteen minutes twice weekly for four consecutive weeks reduced depression and anxiety in postpartum women.[4781]

☐ Inhalation of lavender oil improves parasympathetic nervous system activity and relieves emotional symptoms related to PMS (premenstrual syndrome).[4782]

☐ The oral administration of 0.2 mL of lavender essential oil decreased anxiety of volunteers watching anxiety-provoking movies.[4783]

☐ Animal research suggests that lavender oil significantly reduces excess accumulation of fluid in the brain (cerebral edema) and protects neurons and tissue from oxidative damage caused by a loss of and subsequent return of blood supply (ischemia/reperfusion, like during a stroke) by enhancing the body's production of key antioxidants (reduced glutathione, superoxide dismutase, and catalase) according to animal research.[4784,4785]

- *In vitro* research reported that lavender oil provides a sun protection factor (SPF) of 5.624.[4786]

- Topical application of lavender essential oil reduced painful menstruation in a study that included forty-four female college students.[4787]

- Inhalation of lavender oil reduces the need for oral pain relievers but not the intensity of pain or frequency of nighttime awakening in children following tonsillectomy.[4788]

- Lavender inhalation directly from a glass bottle from 10:00 p.m. to 6:00 a.m. improved sleep quality of hospital patients in an intermediate care unit.[1124] Inhalation from personal aromasticks containing either bergamot and sandalwood, or frankincense, tangerine, and lavender improved sleep quality among cancer patients.[4789] Remarkably, 92% of study participants indicated they would continue to use their aromasticks for sleep improvement.

- Inhaling lavender, lemon, and ylang ylang oil (2:2:1 ratio) reduced systolic blood pressure, and influenced heart rate and sympathetic nervous system activity in people with essential hypertension (high blood pressure without an identifiable cause).[4790] Another study found that inhaling lavender, ylang ylang, and bergamot oils once daily for four weeks reduced cortisol levels, psychological stress, and blood pressure in people with essential hypertension.[4791]

- A clinical study concluded that both cortisol and systolic blood pressure declines after inhalation of a combination of lavender, ylang ylang, marjoram, and neroli oil in those with high blood pressure or pre-high blood pressure.[4792]

- Healthy volunteers experienced an increase in chromogranin A (CgA)—an indication of psychological stress—after performing an arithmetic task for ten minutes. The CgA levels of the volunteers significantly decreased after ten minutes of lavender oil inhalation.[4793]

- Inhalation of lavender oil moderates the stress response by decreasing blood pressure, heart rate, and skin temperature. In addition, the researchers observed that those who inhaled lavender oil reported mood improvements (more active, fresher, and more relaxed).[4794]

- *In vitro* research suggests that lavender oil may reduce agitation by reducing the release of neurotransmitters, and therefore reducing arousal and stimulation of the brain.[4795]

- Women who inhaled lavender oil after a cesarean section experienced decreased pain when compared to those who inhaled a placebo.[4796]

- Topical application of lavender oil significantly reduced inflammation, pain, ulcer size, and healing time (from two to four days) of canker sores (aphthous ulcers) in humans and animals.[4797]

- The topical application of lavender and clary sage oils reduced work-related stress in intensive care unit nurses during three twelve-hour shifts.[4798] Another study found similar results among nurses who inhaled lavender oil from small bottles pinned to their clothes on the right chest.[4799]

- Inhaling lavender oil for fifteen minutes relieved the pain and other symptoms associated with acute migraines in a small clinical trial.[4800]

- A small clinical study observed that inhalation of lavender decreased alpha-amylase levels in the saliva of fifteen young, healthy adults.[4801] Elevated alpha-amylase is an indication of stress and stress-related activity.

- Gerbils exposed to the aroma of lavender oil experienced decreased anxiety similar to diazepam (a drug used to treat anxiety disorders), and were more willing to explore.[4802]

- Inhaling a combination of peppermint, artemisia, sage, lavender, and monarda improved the symptoms of people with chronic bronchitis being treated with standard options concurrently.[4803]

- Lavender oil prevented the mutagenic (the ability to cause changes in genetic material) action of the toxins 1-nitropyrene and 2-nitrofluorene in *S. typhumurin*.[4804]

- Animal research suggests that inhalation of lavender oil suppresses respiratory inflammation caused by inhaled allergens (antigens), and may be useful for asthma.[4805] Another study determined that lavender may decrease inflammation by increasing the cell's protective mechanism against stress-induced damage.[4806]

- When mice were administered 200 mg/kg of lavender essential oil they experienced reduced pain and inflammation, including both phases of the formalin test, and the essential oil also prevented edema caused by carrageenan (a chemical irritant that is commonly used to produce inflammation in rodents).[4807] The formalin test involves administration of the chemical irritant formalin to determine both the immediate pain relieving effect (phase I) and the anti-inflammatory effect of another constituent (phase II), which in this case is lavender oil.

- Both spike lavender and true lavender reduce inflammation by inhibiting lipoxygenase (LOX) activity, which activity was attributed to the presence of linalool, camphor, para-cymene, and limonene.[4808]

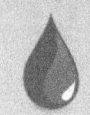

- Diffusion of lavender oil nightly reduced insomnia and anxiety among residents with dementia and disturbed sleep patterns in four different nursing homes.[4809]
- Lavender oil reduces intestinal spasms in rats.[4810]
- Inhalation of lavender oil reversed hyperactivity caused by an injection of caffeine in animals.[4811]
- Animal research suggests that lavender oil can produce a local anesthetic effect.[4812] Another study observed a sedative effect in mice administered lavender oil orally and enhanced the sleep-inducing effect of pentobarbital (a drug used to treat anxiety, sleeplessness, and nervousness).[4813]
- Animal research suggests that lavender oil is adaptogenic. Mice that inhaled lavender negated the impact of stress or experienced increased stress activity depending on their current state of stress.[4814]
- Lavender oil inhalation via a face mask for five minutes reduced the stress and pain associated with needle insertion among healthy volunteers.[4815]
- A preliminary study found that medical staff who worked night shifts experienced endothelial dysfunction (a risk factor that often precedes atherosclerosis), which was alleviated by inhaling lavender for thirty minutes.[4816]
- Topical application of a combination of lavender, geranium, tea tree, and peppermint oils improved the oral health of hospice patients with terminal cancer.[4817]
- Inhalation of humidified lavender oil positively improved blood pressure, heart rate, pain, anxiety, depression, and sense of well-being in seventeen cancer hospice patients.[4818]
- Topical application of a product containing 1% lavender and 10% tea tree oils worked better than the chemical alternative of pyrethrins and piperonyl butoxide, and as well as a suffocation product to eliminate head lice (louse).[4819] Another study concluded that the same combination of oils was slightly less effective than the suffocation method (44.4% versus 68.3%).[4820]
- Inhaling lavender oil in the waiting room prior to dental visits reduces anxiety in dental patients.[4821,4822]
- Both lavender and vetiver oil decreased inhalation and increased exhalation in healthy sleepers when the oils were diffused for nine to fifteen minutes up to thirty-seven times per night.[4823]
- A lavender oil bath decreased stress and cortisol levels in both the mothers and the infants, reduced infant crying, and improved deep-sleep time for the infants following the bath.[4824]
- A clinical study determined that inhalation of lavender oil in an oxygen face mask following laparoscopic gastric banding surgery reduced the patient's demand for opioid pain relievers.[4825]
- Healthy men experienced decreased cortisol and improved coronary flow velocity reserve (a test used to determine the effectiveness of a remedy to dilate the arteries and improve blood flow through the blood vessels) after inhaling four drops of lavender oil in 20 mL of hot water for thirty minutes.[4826]
- Intermittent inhalation of lavender oil while sleeping increases deep sleep in healthy young men and women.[4827] Another study determined that inhalation of lavender oil improved mild insomnia in ten volunteers.[4828]
- Topical application of a 1.5% solution containing lavender, marjoram, eucalyptus, rosemary, and peppermint (2:1:2:1:1 ratio) in a carrier oil consisting of 45% apricot, 45% almond, and 10% jojoba carrier oils significantly decreased pain and depression in people with arthritis.[4829]
- Inhalation of a 2% lavender oil preparation reduced agitated behavior in nine people with severe dementia.[4830]
- *In vitro* and animal research suggests that topical application and injection of lavender oil prevents immediate allergic reactions by inhibiting mast cell degranulation (when mast cells degranulate they rapidly release proinflammatory molecules like histamine and tumor necrosis factor-alpha).[4831]
- A daily scalp massage with thyme, rosemary, lavender, and cedarwood oils in a mixture of carrier oils (jojoba and grapeseed) improved alopecia areata (round patches of hair loss) in 44% of study participants.[4832]
- A 10% or 20% solution of lavender provided equivalent tick repellency as DEET over a two-hour period.[4833]
- Lavender essential oil stimulates innate macrophage responses to bacteria by the immune system to prevent hospital-acquired infections and balances the inflammatory response to these bacteria.[4834]
- A massage to the shoulders and back with a 0.5% dilution of lavender and geranium essential oils reduced anxiety in people with personality disorders.[4835]
- Oral administration of lavender essential oil to mice with cognitive deficits similar to Alzheimer's disease protected cognition by significantly reducing AChE activity and malondialdehyde (MDA) levels and increasing antioxidant activity (superoxide dismutase (SOD) and glutathione peroxidase (GPX)). AChE inhibition prevents the breakdown of acetylcholine, which is a neurotransmitter critical for memory and cognition. People with neurodegenerative

diseases make less acetylcholine, and they often break it down more rapidly leading to acetylcholine deficits.[4836] Higher malondialdehyde levels indicate a state of oxidative stress and are associated with cognitive dysfunction and memory impairment.

☐ True lavender essential oil is considered a good antioxidant due to its high concentration of oxygenated terpenes.[4837,4838] A study in mice determined that its antioxidative properties combined with rose essential oil, vitamin C, and water-soluble vitamin E (Trolox) used during levodopa (L-dopa is a chemical naturally produced in the body by biosynthesis of the amino acid L-tyrosine, but it is also used as a drug treatment for Parkinson's disease) therapy reduces neuron toxicity caused by L-dopa.[4839]

☐ Lavender essential oil inhibits *Aspergillus* species and their subsequent production of mycotoxins.[4840]

☐ A twenty-minute massage with a 0.5% concentration of lavender and geranium essential oil (diluted in a neutral gel) to the shoulders and back, three times per week, reduced anxiety among people with personality disorders during psychiatric hospitalization, as evidenced by reduced heart and respiratory rates.[4841]

☐ Inhalation of lavender essential oil (one to two drops of lavender on a cotton ball placed 10 cm from the person's nose) for twenty minutes prior to removal of a chest tube after surgery reduced anxiety and pain during the procedure.[4842]

☐ A review study of nurse-delivered aromatherapy in acute care settings reported that the use of essential oils generally resulted in significant clinical improvements based on their intended use. Marjoram and tangerine essential oils reduced pain, lavender and marjoram essential oil reduced anxiety, and ginger alleviated nausea.[4843]

☐ Animal research concluded that lavender and thyme essential oil alone or blended together (2:1 ratio) decreased atopic dermatitis symptoms (decreased free radical activity, mast cell degranulation, and epidermal thickness).[4844]

☐ A 20-minute effleurage massage to the knees, three times weekly for three weeks, with 5 mL of a 3% dilution of lavender essential oil (diluted in sweet almond oil) reduced pain severity in people with knee osteoarthritis after the first application and one week after intervention. However, no significant difference in pain relief was observed between the lavender and control group (almond oil only) at the end of the three-week study.[4845]

☐ Animal research demonstrates that topical application of 1% lavender essential oil promoted accelerated wound healing by triggering the expression of type I and II collagen, increasing fibroblasts (which create collagen), and increasing myofibroblasts (necessary for wound closure) at the wound site.[4846]

☐ Several essential oils listed in order of efficacy killed the itch mite (*Sarcoptes scabiei*) that burrows into the skin and causes scabies during direct contact (clove > palmarosa > geranium > tea tree > lavender > manuka > petitgrain > eucalyptus > Japanese cedarwood) with the mites and when used as a fumigant (tea tree > clove > eucalyptus > lavender > palmarosa > geranium > Japanese cedarwood > petitgrain > manuka).[4847]

☐ Lavender essential oil with high terpinene-4-ol content (14.9%) created a synergistic or additive antimicrobial effect against *C. albicans (CA), S. aureus (SA),* and *P. aeruginosa (PA)* when used with antibiotics (chloramphenicol: *CA*—additive, *SA*—additive, *PA*—synergistic; nystatin: *CA*—no interaction noted; ciprofloxacin: *SA*—synergistic, *PA*—additive; fusidic acid: *SA*—additive, *PA*—no interaction noted). The most prominent interaction of synergism was with lavender and chloramphenicol.[4848]

☐ *In vitro* research demonstrated that lavender essential oil inhibits *Listeria innocua*.[4849]

☐ Inhalation of 3 drops of lavender essential oil (placed on an aroma stone 10 cm from the nose) for three minutes after working a night shift, followed by placing the aroma stone next to the bed while sleeping, improved sleep quality of nurses working night shifts.[4850]

☐ Oral administration of lavender essential oil (100 mg/kg BW) significantly protected mice against cognitive deficits caused by D-galactose and aluminum trichloride in a model of Alzheimer's disease.[4851] Lavender, or linalool at the same dose, protected against decreased activity of superoxide dismutase (SOD), glutathione peroxidase (GPX), and inhibited acetylcholinesterase activity and increased malondialdehyde levels. In addition, they prevented decreased expression of nuclear factor-erythroid 2-related factor 2 (Nrf2) and heme oxygenase-1 (HO-1) expression significantly, and improved expression of synapse plasticity-related proteins, calcium-calmodulin-dependent protein kinase II (CaMKII), p-CaMKII, brain-derived neurotrophic factor (BDNF), and TrkB in the hippocampus.

☐ Laboratory research demonstrates that lavender essential oil protects against DNA damage caused by hydrogen

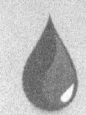

peroxide and tert-butyl hydroperoxide through its own antioxidant activity and improvement of the levels of enzymatic and nonenzymatic antioxidants (SOD-superoxide dismutase, GPx-glutathione peroxidase, GSH-glutathione).[4852]

☐ Inhalation of lavender essential oil reduced labor pain but did not affect labor duration.[4853]

☐ A twenty-minute self-massage with 5 mL of a 3% dilution of lavender essential oil (diluted in sweet almond carrier oil) nine times over the course of three weeks effectively reduced knee pain in people with knee osteoarthritis.[4854]

☐ The use of 0.01%, 0.001%, and 0.0001% lavender essential oil stimulated skin cells (HSF) to produce procollagen.[4855] The production of procollagen is a marker for the healing of wounds, which suggests that lavender promotes healing of skin wounds.

☐ Of eleven essential oils tested, lemongrass (*C. citratus*: citronellal formate 42.8%, isobornyl formate 33.5%) essential oil demonstrated the greatest antioxidant activity in the DPPH test and the best overall antimicrobial activity.[4856] Lemon eucalyptus (78.2% citronellal), lemon scented iron bark (1,8-cineole 29.2%, bornyl formate 12.3%, isobornyl formate 12.1%), lavender (French: cuminaldehyde 41.3%, linalool 37.3%; and French high altitude: linalyl formate 41.7%, linalool 23.5%), and juniper (*J. communis*: p-mentha-1(7),8 diene 32.3%, delta-cadinene 11.3%) demonstrated very strong antioxidant activity, lavender (Croatian: linalool 47.9%, linalyl formate 22.1%) and rosemary (limonene CT) strong activity, lavender (Croatian, linalool rich 66.8%) moderate activity, and gully gum poor activity (81.7% 1,8-cineole). The other essential oils demonstrated various degrees of antimicrobial activity against the tested bacteria (*E. faecalis, B. cereus, L. monocytogenes, S. aureus,* MRSA, *Salmonella typhimurium, P. aeruginosa, E. coli, K. pneumonia, A. baumannii,* and *Ch. violaceum.*

☐ Lavender essential oil was toxic to colon cancer cells. [4857]

☐ Inhalation of lavender essential (3 drops for three minutes prior to insertion) reduced pain related to needle insertion into an implantable central venous port catheter during chemotherapy.[4858] The same research reported that eucalyptus was no better than the control group that received no intervention prior to needle insertion.

☐ The common green bottle fly (*Lucilia sericata*) is a facultative insect that causes myasis (a skin disease characterized by painful, itchy boil-like lesions that occurs when the flies lay their larvae [maggots] in wounds or on the moist skin) in humans and other warm-blooded vertebrates. Low concentrations (0.2%) of vetiver, cinnamon, lavender, and their blends killed the flies within five minutes.[4859] Vetiver significantly deterred flies from the oviposition medium and reduced adult longevity, while sunflower fixed oil repelled flies, deterred oviposition, and reduced adult fly lifespan. The greatest repellency was achieved with a blend of the four oils (2 mL of each essential oil and 4 mL of sunflower as carrier oil).

☐ Lavender essential oil (or linalool) reduced neuronal excitability through modulation of T-type calcium channels (TTCCs).[4860] Inhibition of TTCCs are involved in the antianxiety and neuroprotective effects of lavender essential oil.

☐ Animal research demonstrates that inhalation of lavender essential oil prevents a viscous cycle of anticipatory anxiety that causes anxious and fearful feelings.[4861]

☐ Nanoemulsions of both lavender and rosemary essential oils demonstrated antileishmanial activity against *L. major* without any toxicity to normal cells.[4862] The lavender nanoemulsion was more effective than the standard drug treatment (meglumine antimoniate).

☐ A laboratory and clinical study demonstrated that vaginal pessaries with cocoa butter, calendula extract, and either geranium and palmarosa or lavender and Roman chamomile essential oils reduced symptoms of vaginal atrophy (muscle weakness/wasting) in breast cancer survivors.[4863]

☐ Lavender essential oil demonstrated antimicrobial activity *in vitro* and improved production performance of broiler chickens when added to their water at 0.2 mL/L or 0.4 mL/L.[4864] The higher concentration was the most effective.

☐ Roman chamomile (isobutyl angelate as the primary constituent), lime, and lavender (an interesting CT with 36.0% linalyl acetate and 29.2% trans-sabinene hydrate as the major constituents) essential oils effectively inhibited the parasite *Haemonchus contortus*, hindering adult worm motility completely within the first eight to twelve hours.[4865]

☐ Oral administration of 75 and 100 mg/kg body weight of lavender essential oil (Brazilian; 39.8% 1,8-cineole, 22.6% borneol, and 22.1% camphor) reduced acute inflammation, at least in part by modulating prostanoids, nitric oxide, proinflammatory cytokines, and histamine, in mice.[4866]

☐ A topical massage with a 3% dilution of lavender (5 mL for twenty minutes) essential oil reduced disability in people with osteoarthritis of the knee.[4867]

☐ Lavender, lemongrass (*C. citratus*), marjoram, peppermint, tea tree, and rosewood essential oils all exhibited significant activity against clinical isolates of multidrug-resistant *Burkholderia cepacia* complex (a group of bacteria commonly resistant to antibiotics that cause health problems in people with weakened immune systems and are known to cause healthcare related infections).[4868]

- Inhalation of 2 drops of lavender essential oil (5% dilution) decreased fatigue in people undergoing hemodialysis better than relaxation techniques in a controlled clinical study.[4869]
- Injection of lavender (200 mg/kg BW) essential oil blocked stress-induced anxiety after being exposed to a social defeat encounter.[4870] Stressed mice displayed heightened anxiety and social avoidance after the social defeat, but both linalool and lavender reversed social aversion and depression when administered. Interestingly, linalool (100 mg/kg) did not reduce stress-induced anxiety suggesting a synergy of other components is necessary for this effect.
- Application of a lavender essential oil plaster to the right shoulder relaxed ten healthy females and increased their arousal level.[4871] Heart rate variable (HRV; measurement of variations in the time interval between heartbeats and a standard to measure the state of the body and mind in humans) was monitored and a significant increase in HF (high-frequency heart rate band) and reduction in LF/HF (low-frequency to high-frequency heart rate band) ratios was observed during lavender use. These results suggest that lavender oil increased parasympathetic nervous system activity and reduced sympathetic activity, resulting in a more relaxed but alert state. Interestingly, the authors found through brain positron emission tomography (PET) scan that the response did not involve the olfactory regions but the orbitofrontal cortex, thalamus, and cerebellum.
- Inhalation of 5 drops of lavender essential oil (2% dilution from a patch placed on the shirt) for twenty minutes, thirty minutes prior to intravenous catheter insertion reduced pain severity during insertion in preschool children.[4872]
- Fear and anxiety surrounding gynecological examinations may deter women from having regular important physical exams. A randomized controlled trial of 156 women concluded that inhalation of a 10% lavender solution from a heat lamp (placed 15 cm from the exam table) for ten to fifteen minutes significantly reduced anxiety during the exam.[4873] The control group experienced increased anxiety following the exam, but women who inhaled lavender oil experienced reduced anxiety from the initial time of the appointment. The lavender group also reported less pain and discomfort during the exam.
- A randomized placebo-controlled study found that inhalation of lavender or ginger essential oil reduced postoperative nausea.[4874] Interestingly, lavender was more effective (82.6% reduction) than ginger (65.2% reduction), while rose oil was similar to placebo (47.8%, 43.5%, respectively).
- The current body of evidence suggests that lavender has a positive effect on mood and anxiety state. Daily inhalation of lavender essential oil for fourteen days reduced depressive-like behavior caused by chronic administration of corticosterone in rats.[4875] Brain examination found that lavender essential oil improved neurogenesis (growth and development of new brain cells) and neuroplasticity (the ability of the brain to form new connections to optimize brain function, behavior, thinking, and emotions).
- Lavender essential oil (35.2% linalool, 33.4% linalyl acetate) was toxic to eggs and larvae of the common green bottle fly (*Lucilia sericata*) and completely deterred oviposition up to three hours.[4876] The same researchers reported that the oil demonstrated antifungal and antibacterial activity against *E. coli, B. subtilis, S. aureus, C. albicans,* and *S. abaetetuba.*
- Clinical research found that inhalation of lavender essential oil (2% concentration, twenty minutes before bedtime every night for a month) improved quality of life and reduced both physical and psychological symptoms in postmenopausal women.[4877]
- Kidney injury and loss of kidney function can occur following kidney transplant due to an acute inflammatory response and a return of blood supply after a period of lack of oxygen (ischemia-reperfusion). Intraperitoneal administration of lavender essential oil preserved normal kidney function and reduced kidney damage by improving antioxidant enzyme activity and significantly decreasing inflammatory cytokines.[4878]
- Oral administration of lavender essential oil (100 mg/kg) alleviated mechanical allodynia (neuropathic pain caused by harmless stimuli like light touch) through multiple mechanisms, including involvement of the endocannabinoid system.[4879] Lavender oil mildly inhibited the enzymes (FAAH—fatty acid amide hydrolase; MAGL—monoacylglycerol lipase) that regulate the production of endocannabinoids (cannabinoids produced by the body), particularly FAAH. FAAH and MAGL can synthesize or degrade endocannabinoids. If they degrade endocannabinoids, there may be insufficient endocannabinoids to minimize the occurrence and progression of multiple health conditions. Inhibition of these enzymes is considered a therapeutic target for neuropathic pain, anxiety, inflammatory bowel diseases, and cancer metastasis.[4880]
- Inhalation of lavender essential oil with 30.6% linalool and 20.4% linalyl acetate reduced mechanical hyperalgesia—increased sensitivity to pain from stimuli that is usually not painful—in both a chronic inflammatory and neuropathic pain model in mice.[4881] Further investigation determined that the oil reduced pain through modulation of peripheral and central opioid and cannabinoid 2 receptors.
- Lavender essential oil improved memory in a mouse model of Alzheimer's disease by decreasing oxidative stress in neurons (increased glutathione peroxidase, catalase, and superoxide dismutase).[4882]

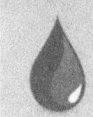

- An animal model of corticosterone-induced depression and anxiety found that inhalation of lavender—rich in linalool—daily for fourteen days reduced depression and the production of neurons from stem cells (neurogenesis).[4883] Remarkably, the oil increased dendritic complexity of immature neurons, demonstrating a clear restorative effect of neurological function. In addition, the lavender group experienced increased BDNF (a protein that promotes neuron cell survival by influencing their growth, maturation, and maintenance) and oxytocin (an important hormone for pair bonds and social behaviors) two to three days after treatment.
- Oral administration of lavender essential oil (100 mg/kg) reduced oxidative stress associated with psychological stress and reduced behavioral and biochemical changes caused by stress better than ibuprofen in rats.[4884]
- A randomized clinical trial found that inhalation of lavender essential oil reduced anxiety related to oral surgery (wisdom teeth removal) as evidenced by decreased blood pressure and subject satisfaction.[4885] Subjects aged eighteen to thirty-seven years old inhaled 100% lavender for three minutes prior to surgery from a medical patch, avoiding skin contact. Almost 90% of subjects were satisfied with their experience and 97.6% stated they would prefer the same protocol be followed during subsequent oral procedures.
- A pilot study found that a back massage with lavender and geranium essential oils—diluted to a concentration of 1% of each oil (2% essential oil total) in a neutral cream—significantly reduced stress in members of a surgical nursing team.[4886] Healthcare professionals received six effleurage massages for ten to fifteen minutes with an average of forty-two hours between sessions. Reduction in both blood pressure and heart rate were observed after the massage.
- A double-blind crossover clinical trial of one hundred menopausal women—fifty in the lavender group and fifty in the placebo group—found that lavender essential oil inhalation (twenty minutes, twice weekly for twelve weeks) significantly reduced hot flashes during menopause.[4887]
- Difficulty sleeping is commonly reported among women transitioning to menopause, affecting 39%–47% of perimenopausal women and 35%–60% of postmenopausal women. A controlled clinical trial found that inhalation of lavender essential oil modulated parasympathetic nervous system activity and significantly improved sleep quality in women aged forty-five to fifty-five years old.[4888] Women relaxed in a chair with arm support for ten minutes before inhaling 0.25 mL of lavender oil from an ultrasonic diffuser (10 to 15 cm from the women) for twenty minutes, twice weekly in the evening, over the course of twelve weeks (twenty-four total times).
- Both cinnamon bark and vetiver essential oils strongly repelled house flies (*Musca domestica*)—84% and 78% respectively.[4889] In addition, vetiver, cinnamon, and lavender essential oils were significantly toxic to house fly larvae (100 percent).
- Melatonin is known as the "sleep hormone" because it regulates the circadian rhythm and directly affects sleep. The production of melatonin changes throughout life, peaking in humans in newborns and children up to puberty, after which production declines. Inhalation of Bulgarian lavender essential oil from an ultrasonic diffuser (5 drops in 80 mL of water) significantly increased serum melatonin in older adults (aged sixty-plus).[4890] The subjects inhaled the lavender for thirty minutes in a room where the diffuser was operating for fifteen minutes prior to entry, twice weekly for four weeks.
- Having type 2 diabetes can lead to disorders that reduce sleep quality and quantity, which in turn reduces the control of diabetes. A randomized, placebo-controlled, crossover clinical trial found that inhalation of lavender essential oil improved sleep quantity and quality, as well as quality of life and mood in people with diabetes.[4891] The lavender oil was inhaled by placing 3 drops in a linen cloth and inhaling slowly and rhythmically for five minutes before bedtime. Each participant in the study inhaled lavender and then placebo (sweet almond oil) for two periods of four weeks separated by one week as a washout period.
- *In vitro* research found that lavender essential oil inhibited bacteria (gram-positive bacilli) in mixed facial skin microbiota, suggesting it is cleansing to the face.[4892]
- Lavender essential oil added to an ostomy bag—10 drops added to a clean bag at each colostomy bag exchange, spreading the oil around the entire inner surface of the bag—reduced odor and improved quality of life in a small clinical study.[4893]
- Lavender essential oil reduced cardiac injury after myocardial infarction (heart attack) in rats.[4894] Intraperitoneal administration of the oil immediately after ischemia (inadequate blood supply to an organ) reduced inflammation and oxidative stress to protect the heart against damage.
- Awake craniotomy is a type of surgery where a piece of the skull is removed to access the brain and the patient is woken during the surgery to provide feedback. As you can imagine, this can cause anxiety. A preliminary feasibility study of thirty-one people undergoing awake craniotomy found that inhaling lavender essential oil during the procedure mildly reduced anxiety (considered not statistically significant).[4895] Patients inhaled lavender from a nasal essential oil inhaler with 15 drops of lavender and 4 drops of grapeseed oil. Lavender was inhaled for up to five minutes at designated time points prior to surgery, every thirty minutes during surgery, and anytime

the patient requested it. Although the study didn't show good efficacy of the intervention, it did prove that essential oils can be used in the operating room during surgeries.

- Tooth extractions can be stressful and trigger anxiety in children. A recent clinical trial found that inhalation of lavender (2 drops on medical patches) for three minutes prior to tooth extraction significantly reduced both pain and anxiety in children at the conclusion of the procedure.[4896]

- Inhalation of lavender essential oil (150 mcL on filter paper) significantly reduced stress in healthy female college students (measured by decreased chromogranin A levels) while watching a stressful video for ten minutes.[4897] Chromogranin A is a glycoprotein that is released along with other chemicals from the adrenal glands and sympathetic nerve endings during stress.

- Bone marrow biopsy is a common procedure used to identify and diagnose disorders of the blood and blood-forming organs. Anxiety and tension prior to biopsy can increase pain intensity during the procedure. Inhalation of lavender essential oil (3 drops of 10% dilution on a cotton ball in a closed container and placed 7 to 10 cm from the nose) for fifteen minutes prior to bone marrow biopsy significantly reduced anxiety in people undergoing this procedure.[4898]

- Ferulic acid is an organic plant compound used as an antioxidant that helps protect overall skin integrity and improves the appearance of skin when used in skin care products. Lavender essential oil-ferulic acid nanoparticles promoted skin cell proliferation and migration *in vitro* suggesting that the combination represents a promising strategy for wound healing.[4899]

- Lavender essential oil increased the susceptibility of MRSA to the antiseptic octenidine dihydrochloride.[4900] Lavender represents a promising solution to improve the antimicrobial activity of conventional antiseptics.

- Th-1 and Th-17 cells release inflammatory cytokines that are involved in both the initiation and continuation of psoriasis. Th-17 cytokines, especially IL-17A plays a pivotal role in sustaining inflammation in psoriatic lesions. Topical application of 10% lavender essential oil effectively reduced psoriasis like skin inflammation in mice as determined by reduced psoriatic lesions and reduced Th-17 cell expressing cytokines.[4901] The major constituents of lavender essential oil, linalool and linalyl acetate, were also effective at a 2% concentration. Both linalool and linalyl acetate significantly reduced Th-1 cytokine release, but only linalool reduced TH-17 cytokine release.

- Lavender essential oil synergized the activity of piperacillin against multidrug-resistant *E. coli* by modifying expression of genes related to microbial metabolism.[4902]

- Learning and memory play a crucial role in anxiety because cues related to negative situations trigger high arousal and great anticipation. Researchers suggest that obstructing memory reconsolidation—the process of recalling previously consolidated memories and actively consolidating them to maintain, modify, or strengthen memories—or improving memory extinction—detaching a learned response from a stimulus—may minimize cognitive cues that initiate anxiety. Exposure to 1% vaporized lavender essential oil reduced fear memory in mice by enhancing memory extinction.[4903] Interestingly, concentrations of 2.5% and 5% were ineffective.

- Lavender essential oil deterred the spotted-wing drosophila (*Drosophila suzukii*) from infesting raspberries but was ineffective on blueberries in a two-choice laboratory bioassay.[4904]

- Sleeping difficulties is commonly experienced by menopausal women. A nonrandomized placebo-controlled clinical trial found that inhalation of lavender and lemon essential oils improved sleep quality and quality of life in menopausal women with sleep difficulty.[4905] Two drops of each oil were added to a bowl of 200 mL of boiling water, and the participants inhaled the steam through the nose and exhaled through the mouth for five minutes. This procedure was repeated daily for thirty consecutive days.

- Up to 50 percent of infants over the age of six months continue to awaken during the night, which can also negatively affect the sleep of the parents. Massaging infants with 2 drops of lavender essential oil in 50 mL of carrier oil for thirty minutes during three consecutive days reduced sleep disturbances in infants aged six to twelve months.[4906] The lavender oil massage helped infants fall asleep and stay asleep and reduced overall disturbances in sleep patterns. The control group inhaled steam from boiling water only. At the end of the study, the control group experienced no change is sleep quality, but significant improvements were noted in the aromatherapy group.

- Individuals who require hemodialysis may experience a reduced quality of life, such as sleep disturbances, distress, and compromised physical and social well-being. A randomized clinical trial of 105 hemodialysis patients evaluated the effects of aromatherapy massage on their quality of life.[4907] Participants were randomized into three groups: a lavender massage group, a bitter orange massage group, and a control group (massage only). Aromatherapy massage was performed for about one hour after hemodialysis began with approximately 10 to 15 mL of a 1.5% dilution of the oils. The aromatherapy massage groups had a significant increase in quality-of-life scores after the intervention when compared to the control group. Another study found that massage with 5% lavender essential oil (diluted in sesame oil) reduced the severity of restless leg syndrome in people undergoing hemodialysis.[4908]

- Lavender essential oil displayed significant antioxidant activity in the DPPH assay. Based on these findings, the

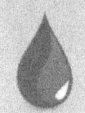

researchers evaluated the organ (liver and kidney) protective effects of lavender in a mouse model. Intraperitoneal injection of lavender essential oil corrected the harmful effects caused by hydrogen peroxide in both organs.[4909]

☐ Myogenous temporomandibular disorders (MTD, also called masticatory myalgia) are characterized by pain and dysfunction of the muscles of the jaw (masticatory muscles). Researchers set out to determine the benefits of massage with lavender essential oil for MTD. Ninety-one people with MTD were divided into three different groups: 1) massage with lavender, 2) massage with sweet almond oil, and 3) control (no intervention). The lavender group received a massage with 100 mL of a 3% dilution of lavender essential oil (ten minutes to the intraoral area, twenty minutes to the myofascial area, and thirteen minutes to the remaining areas), twice weekly, for eight weeks. Both massage groups experienced improvements in maximal mouth opening, with the lavender group experiencing the most improvement.[4910] In addition, the lavender group had the largest decrease in pain levels.

☐ Oral administration of lavender essential oil (Silexan at 30 mg/kg BW) reduced depression comparably to the tricyclic antidepressant imipramine (20 mg/kg BW) after nine days of treatment in rats. Further investigation found that the lavender preparation triggered neurite outgrowth (the process whereby developing neurons produce new projections as they grow in response to cues from the cell's environment) and synaptogenesis (the formation of new synapses between neurons) in two different neuronal cell models, leading to a significant increase in synaptogenesis in primary hippocampal neurons.

☐ A post-dural-puncture headache (PDPH) occurs as a complication of neuraxial anesthesia (such as an epidural) when the dural is inadvertently punctured. Following the puncture, cerebrospinal fluid leaks causing reduced fluid levels in the brain and spinal cord and a severe headache involving the back and front of the head that is exacerbated by movement, sitting, and standing. The pain may radiate down the neck and shoulders and sometimes cause neck stiffness. A small randomized placebo-controlled study found that inhalation of lavender essential oil for fifteen minutes reduced the severity of PDPH, but only immediately following the intervention, while only minimal effects were observed during successive time intervals.[4911]

☐ Premature infants are more sensitive to pain and stress than full-term infants. A double-blind randomized clinical study found that inhalation of lavender essential oil significantly reduced pain after heel-stick sampling for metabolic screening in premature infants.[4912] The pain was determined by recording facial expressions three minutes before and after heel-stick sampling.

☐ Pain, stress, and anxiety can reduce the likelihood that children will receive proper dental care and represents a major obstacle to regular dental visits. Previous research has shown that lavender essential oil can reduce dental-visit-related anxiety, but much of the research relied upon questionnaires from study participants rather than biometric measures. A randomized, crossover clinical trial evaluated the effect of lavender essential oil on salivary cortisol and heart rate (to determine anxiety/stress level) and face rating scale (FRS; to assess pain) during injections at a dental visit. Two drops of pure lavender essential oil were added to 100 mL of water and diffused for thirty minutes prior to the child's arrival. Plain water was diffused on the days the child was not included in the intervention group. The researchers found that inhalation of lavender reduced both dental anxiety/stress and pain as evidenced by significant reductions in salivary cortisol, heart rate, and FRS.[4913]

☐ White wormwood CT alpha-thujone, pennyroyal CT pulegone, Phoenician juniper, lavender, and cade essential oils each displayed varying degrees of antioxidant activity in the DPPH, FRAP, and ABTS assays.[4914] The same researchers reported that the oils exhibited moderate to good acetylcholinesterase (AChE) inhibition activity (in descending order): lavender, pennyroyal, cade, white wormwood, Phoenician juniper; moderate to weak butyrylcholinesterase (BChE) inhibition activity (in descending order): pennyroyal, white wormwood, lavender, cade, and Phoenician juniper; and moderate to weak tyrosinase inhibition activity (in descending order): cade, lavender, white wormwood, pennyroyal, and Phoenician juniper. Each of the oils was toxic to two types of breast cancer cells as well, with white wormwood being the most effective, followed by Phoenician juniper, pennyroyal, lavender, and cade.

☐ A randomized clinical trial that included 147 participants found that lavender essential oil aided in the control of pain following abdominal surgery but only in individuals who received a regional nerve block.[4915] One drop of undiluted lavender oil was applied topically to the back of the neck, temple, ear, wrist, or other area of preference at each episode of reported surgical pain. Pain medication was administered at typical intervals but before lavender oil application. The improvement in pain scores was a remarkable fivefold after aromatherapy in this subgroup of participants.

☐ A parallel randomized placebo-controlled clinical trial evaluated the benefits of lavender or neroli essential oil inhalation against a placebo (saline) on the pain of people admitted to an intensive care unit. Five drops of either oil or saline were added to a gauze strip, which was placed about 10 cm from the person's nose and inhaled for thirty

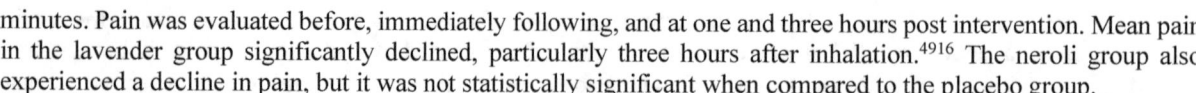

minutes. Pain was evaluated before, immediately following, and at one and three hours post intervention. Mean pain in the lavender group significantly declined, particularly three hours after inhalation.[4916] The neroli group also experienced a decline in pain, but it was not statistically significant when compared to the placebo group.

☐ Chemotherapy drugs can cause daytime sleepiness, which can make sleep more difficult at night. A randomized, placebo-controlled study evaluated the benefits of lavender essential oil for sleep among people receiving cancer chemotherapy. Three drops of lavender or tea tree oil were added to cotton that was placed on the subject's neck or shoulder about ten inches below the nose nightly before going to sleep. The control group did not inhale any essential oils. Inhalation of the lavender oil reduced the participant's anxiety and improved sleep quality.[4917]

☐ A lavender essential oil with low linalool (23.2%) and high lavandulyl acetate (40.6%) induced IL-6, which suggests it may promote wound healing.[4918] Interestingly, the lab-distilled oil poor in linalool performed better than a commercial sample with a composition more consistent with quality lavender oil (44.0% linalyl acetate, 40.2% linalool, 5.5% lavandulyl acetate). The oil also increased the production of vascular endothelial growth factor (VEGF)—an important factor in the formation of new blood vessels to accelerate wound healing. Further research by the same researchers found that a lavender-loaded nanoemulsion promotes regeneration of skin after wound without irritation, sensitization, or damage to the skin.[4919]

☐ Physical, psychological, and hormonal changes during menopause can cause sleep problems such as insomnia, sleep-disordered breathing, and hot flashes. A double-blind, randomized controlled clinical trial compared the sleep benefits of inhaled lavender essential oil to placebo (sunflower oil) in postmenopausal women.[4920] A 6% dilution of lavender oil was inhaled directly from the bottle for two minutes followed by a ten-minute rest and another two minutes of inhalation before bedtime. Both groups were instructed on good sleep hygiene, which improved sleep outcomes for both groups. However, women who inhaled lavender experienced improved overall sleep patterns, quality, and sleep efficiency.

☐ Researchers compared the pharmacological effects—via EEG (electroencephalogram) fingerprint and sleep-wake profiles—of inhaling lavender essential oil and intraperitoneal injection of diazepam in male rats. EEG is a test that records the electrical activity of the brain.[4921] EEG signals were recorded for 180 minutes after injection of diazepam and for the whole duration of lavender inhalation. Both diazepam and lavender essential oil increased parietal powers with lower magnitudes of significant change, with some frequency increases lasting for sixty to ninety minutes. Diazepam significantly reduced time spent awake, increased time spent in nonrapid eye movement (NREM), increased duration of NREM, reduced waking episodes, and decreased rapid eye movement (REM) sleep latency. On the contrary, lavender oil only significantly decreased awake episodes and latency to REM sleep. Importantly, lavender oil reduced wake episode but maintained the normal time spent in wake, NREM, and REM sleep. The findings suggest lavender is beneficial for its distinct anxiety-reducing effects to improve sleep.

☐ A lavender essential oil from Morocco with an odd composition (39.1% 1,8-cineole, 24.2% camphor, and 8.3% borneol) inhibited foodborne bacteria and synergized the activity of ciprofloxacin.[4922]

☐ A systemic review and network meta-analysis of forty studies concluded that inhalation of lavender essential oil is most effective for relieving anxiety acutely, but oral administration of lavender is better for long-term relief of anxiety.[4923]

☐ Poorly controlled diabetes can lead to damage of nerves, particularly in the legs and feet—a condition called diabetic neuropathy. Diabetic neuropathy can range from pain, numbness, and tingling in the legs and feet to problems with digestion, urination, and the cardiovascular system. A single-blind, randomized, and controlled clinical trial evaluated the benefits of lavender essential oil for diabetic neuropathy.[4924] Participants were randomly assigned to three groups: lavender essential oil massage, sunflower oil massage, and control (no intervention). Participants in the lavender group received a gentle foot massage with 2.5 mL of 3% lavender (mixed in sunflower oil) from the knee down ten minutes every night before bed. The placebo group applied 2.5 mL of sunflower oil in the same manner each night. The lavender group experienced significant pain reductions in the short- and long-term compared to placebo and control. Additionally, the lavender group had an improved quality of life after four weeks of intervention. No side effects were reported.

☐ An odd lavender essential oil with 13.1% carbitol, 10.9% alpha-terpinyl acetate, 10.7% linalool, and 9.6% linalyl acetate inhibited S. aureus (two strains) in laboratory research.[4925]

☐ Pain control after a burn is a major challenge and difficult to accomplish with medications. Increased pain levels are associated with delayed burn healing, and uncontrolled pain can lead to chronic pain and psychological and mood disturbances such as depression, anxiety, and acute stress. A randomized controlled study of 108 children (aged two months to seven years) with second-degree superficial burns evaluated the benefits of inhaling lavender essential oil before burn dressing application.[4926] The children were divided into three groups randomly: 1) inhalation of jojoba oil fifteen minutes prior to dressing, 2) inhalation of lavender EO fifteen minutes prior to

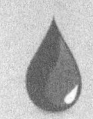

dressing, and 3) inhalation of lavender EO sixty minutes prior to dressing. The jojoba or lavender EO (0.5 mL) was applied to gauze and placed about 20 cm from the child's nose for inhalation. Both groups that inhaled lavender EO experienced lower pain than the jojoba group as evidenced by lower heart rate, blood pressure, respiratory rate, and reported pain levels.

☐ *In vitro* research demonstrated that lavender essential oil (36.1% 1,8-cineole and 15.8% linalool) inhibits *C. jejuni*, reduces its motility, degrades its biofilms, and downregulates genes important for biofilm formation.[4927] Its reduction of *C. jejuni* adhesion conforms to European Food Safety Authority recommendations.

☐ Nanostructured lipid carriers (NLCs) are emerging as a novel way to deliver essential oils intranasally for the management of neurodegenerative diseases. NLCs containing rosemary or lavender essential oil showed the formation of more ordered structures and high cytocompatibility on two cell lines (murine and human fibroblasts) when compared to Tegosoft CT and neem oil.[4928]

☐ Rosemary CT 1,8-cineole and lavender essential oils exhibited anticancer activity against neuroblastoma cells.[4929] Both oils also demonstrated good antibacterial activity against *E. coli*, *P. fluorescens*, *A. bohemicus*, *K. marina*, and *B. cereus*. Furthermore, the oils exhibited good antioxidant activity in the ABTS and DPPH assays.

☐ Lavender essential oil showed good antibacterial activity against *B. subtilis*, *P. fluorescens*, *X. campestris*, and *E. carotovara* at higher concentrations and *E. amylovora and C. utilis* at lower concentrations.[4930] The residual water (floral water) and an extract from the leftover plant material after distillation also showed high antimicrobial activity against *A. alternata*, *P. chrysogenum*, *Bacillus* sp., and *P. aeruginosa*.

☐ Headaches are common among emergency and critical care nurses and headaches occur among nurses at a higher rate than in the general population. A study evaluated the benefits of inhaling essential oils on headache occurrence among nurses.[4931] Nurses wore a necklace with lavender and bergamot essential oil (0.1 mL of each) for twenty-eight days. Although no reduction in headache was observed, the nurses did show significant improvement in their overall quality of life, especially in relation to their workplace roles and responsibilities.

☐ Both dried and fresh flower essential oil from lavender grown in Italy (poor in linalyl acetate and higher in borneol) inhibited *B. subtilis* and *E. coli* and exhibited antioxidant activity.[4932]

☐ Poor cardiac function can lead to fatigue, and fatigue is among the most common complaints among cardiac patients. A randomized placebo-controlled trial evaluated the effects of inhaling peppermint or lavender essential oil in subjects in a cardiac care unit.[4933] Three drops of peppermint, lavender, or placebo were added to a cotton ball and attached to the subject's shirt collar for twenty minutes at 9:00 p.m. The intervention continued for seven nights. Interestingly, both lavender and peppermint oil inhalation reduced reported fatigue better than placebo.

☐ A poor night's sleep interferes with restorative body processes that can alter your mood, performance, energy levels, cognitive function, and overall well-being. Researchers evaluated the benefits of diffused lavender essential oil—30 mcL lavender oil in 500 mL of water—after a short sleep cycle.[4934] The first night of the study, subjects slept without any intervention to determine their normal sleep pattern and state via pure sleep waveform. On the second and third days, subjects were randomly divided into groups to receive aromatherapy with lavender oil or distilled water only and allowed to sleep only ninety minutes. Sleep state was confirmed via electroencephalograph (EEG), and a saliva sample taken to evaluate for cortisol, α-amylase, and chromogranin A—objective measures of stress response. Mood was evaluated subjectively by the Japanese version of the UWIST Mood Adjective Checklist. The lavender group did not experience decreases in cortisol or mood improvements, but alpha-amylase and chromogranin A significantly decreased, suggesting lavender suppressed the stress response to interrupted and insufficient sleep.

☐ Oregano CT carvacrol, lemon, lavender, mastic, and mandarin essential oil each inhibited *S. aureus*.[4935]

☐ Lavender essential oil exhibited antitoxoplasma activity against *T. gondii*.[4936]

☐ Anxiety and agitation are common among people admitted to intensive care units (ICU), and this can interfere with treatment and recovery. A randomized parallel placebo-controlled trial evaluated the effects of lavender and bitter orange essential oil on people in the ICU.[4937] Subjects were randomly divided into one of three groups: lavender inhalation, bitter orange inhalation, and saline placebo. Five drops of lavender, bitter orange, or saline were added to gauze and placed 10 cm from the nose. The subjects inhaled from the gauze for thirty minutes. Both the lavender and bitter orange groups experienced significantly reduced anxiety compared to control, but agitation levels were not statistically different among the three groups—all three groups experienced reduced agitation. The conclusion of the study was that "aromatherapy can be used as an effective and safe intervention to reduce anxiety in ICUs."

☐ Being overweight or obese may increase the risk of several conditions, including pain-related conditions. The excess accumulation of fat can increase biochemical tension in the joints and keep that person in a chronic inflammatory state. A placebo-controlled clinical trial evaluated the benefits of lavender essential oil for spinal pain in obese women.[4938] The treatment group received a thirty-five-minute massage with 3% lavender essential oil (diluted in sweet almond oil) and heated stones. One drop of the oil was also placed on their pillows at night for the duration of the study—thirty days. The placebo group received the same procedure substituting sweet almond with lavender fragrance. A control group received no intervention. The lavender group experienced significant decreases in total spinal pain—cervical and lumbar regions—when compared to the placebo and control groups.

□ Artificial intrauterine insemination can be associated with significant anxiety, which could potentially decrease the effectiveness of the procedure. A randomized controlled trial found that inhaling lavender—smelling from a pouch containing a cotton ball with 1 drop of lavender essential oil during the procedure—essential oil significantly reduced anxiety during intrauterine insemination procedure.[4939]

□ Both lavender essential oil and linalool effectively decreased proinflammatory cytokines—IL-8, IL-1β, NFkB—in THP-1 human monocyte/macrophage cells. Lavender exhibited stronger activity in reducing IL-8 and IL-1β.[4940] Lavender oil distilled preflowering stage (36.3% linalool, 21.5% linalyl acetate, 95% terpinen-4-ol) and postflowering stage (41.6% linalool, 16.7% terpinen-4-ol, 14.8% linalyl acetate) behaved differently, with the preflowering oil inhibiting cytokine release but the postflowering oil only decreased IL-6, IL-1β and IL-8 mRNA expression.

□ A fistula is an abnormal connection or passageway between two organs that do not normally connect. They can develop in the intestines, skin, vagina, rectum, and other places. An arteriovenous fistula (AVF) connects a vein and an artery in a person's arm who is undergoing hemodialysis to allow blood to flow from the body into a dialysis machine and back into the same place. AVF cannulation—inserting a flexible catheter into the AVF—is challenging for nurses and painful for the patient. Researchers evaluated the benefits of inhaling lavender essential oil during AVF cannulation.[4941] Subjects inhaled 5 drops of pure lavender essential oil for five minutes as part of a steam inhalation. The lavender was added to 200 mL of boiled water and placed approximately 30 cm (11.8 inches) away and then the subject completely covered with a cloth. Inhaling the lavender oil significantly reduced AVF puncture-related pain and anxiety.

□ Restless leg syndrome (RLS) is a condition that causes an uncomfortable sensation that creates an uncontrollable urge to move your legs. RLS frequently occurs in people undergoing hemodialysis. A randomized placebo-controlled clinical trial compared the effectiveness of lavender essential oil massage with reflexology to reduce RLS in people undergoing hemodialysis.[4942] Lavender essential oil diluted in carrier oil (10 drops) was massaged to the subject's feet for fifteen minutes on each foot using mild pressure and the therapist's fist to stimulate reflex points (thyroid, parathyroid, pancreas, adrenal glands, and solar plexus). The lavender massage was repeated three times per week for eight consecutive weeks. The reflexology group received a general foot massage with 6 drops of sweet almond oil on each foot similar to the lavender group, followed by fifteen minutes of reflexology on each foot to stimulate the same reflex points. Placebo massage was performed using only sweet almond oil and without specifically stimulating the reflex points. According to the RLS scale, the lavender massage group experienced reduced RLS severity, but placebo and reflexology had no effect.

□ Over 50 percent of women experience some sort of menstrual pain with their period, and up to 10 percent of women experience pain severe enough to disrupt their lifestyle. A randomized controlled human trial evaluated the benefits of abdominal massage with lavender and clary sage essential oil for menstrual pain. Clary sage and lavender were diluted in sweet almond oil and massaged to the lower abdomen during the first three days of menses for two consecutive cyles. Compared to the control group of sweet almond oil only, lavender/clary sage massage significantly reduced menstrual pain during the first two days of menses, but the pain reduction was not maintained through day three.[4943]

□ Chronic nicotine exposure is known to exacerbate rheumatoid arthritis by causing muscle wasting. Rats were chronically exposed to nicotine after inducing rheumatoid arthritis. Increased hind paw thickness and inflammatory cytokines (IL-6), loss of gastrocnemius muscle mass, as well as decreased body weight and serum insulin-like growth factor were noted in rats with arthritis. Injection of lavender essential oil or isolated linalyl acetate, twice weekly for twenty-one days, prevented these alterations, suggesting they can counteract muscle wasting associated with chronic nicotine exposure.[4944] Isolated linalyl acetate was more effective than the whole oil.

□ High blood pressure (hypertension) is a global health concern with nearly one-third of adults affected (2010). Lifestyle factors are the leading cause of hypertension, including excess sodium intake, low potassium intake, obesity, alcohol consumption, physical inactivity, and unhealthy diet. In addition to making positive lifestyle changes, essential oils may be helpful to support healthy blood pressure. A foot massage with lavender essential oil decreased blood pressure in people with hypertension.[4945] Subjects received a fifteen- to twenty-minute foot massage with lavender essential oil, twice daily, and after three days of massage with lavender blood pressure was reduced from 150/90 to 120/80 and 170/100 to 150/90 in a small pilot clinical study.

□ The pathogenic fungus *C. auris* is considered a major threat to public health because of its intrinsic resistance to conventional antifungals and its biofilm characteristics that promote prolonged survival (persister cells) after

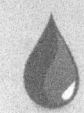

disinfection and antifungal treatments. Lavender essential oil, free or encapsulated in liposomes, was able to eradicate primary *C. auris* and persister cells in biofilms.[4946]

☐ Electroconvulsive therapy is used to treat depression, often among people who have not responded to conventional drug therapies. Unfortunately, this invasive therapy causes significant anxiety related to the procedure. A randomized controlled clinical trial compared the benefits of lavender essential oil inhalation, breathing exercises, or routine care among people receiving electroconvulsive therapy. The lavender group inhaled 2 drops of lavender oil added to a sterile gauze pad for three to five minutes prior to electroconvulsive therapy. The breathing exercise group performed slow breathing exercises in a quiet environment for ten minutes before electroconvulsive therapy, and the routine care group received no intervention before electroconvulsive therapy. Anxiety state was measured twenty minutes before and thirty minutes after electroconvulsive therapy. Both the lavender oil group and the breathing exercise group reported decreased anxiety scores after electroconvulsive therapy, with lavender oil providing the greatest benefits.[4947]

☐ Essential hypertension is high blood pressure (systolic blood pressure >120 mmHg and diastolic blood pressure >80 mmHg) without an identifiable secondary cause like renal failure, renovascular disease, aldosteronism (excess production of the hormone aldosterone), thyroid dysfunction, obesity, pregnancy, or other causes. Essential hypertension accounts for approximately 85 percent of high blood pressure cases with the rest being secondary hypertension caused by another health condition. A clinical study evaluated the benefits of inhaling lavender essential oil among people with essential hypertension. Subjects inhaled 5 to 6 drops of lavender essential oil from an ultrasonic diffuser for fifteen minutes over the course of six days. Blood pressure was measured before and after lavender inhalation on the first and sixth days of the study. Mean systolic blood pressure declined from 145.60 mmHg to 136.93 mmHg and mean diastolic blood pressure declined from 92.00 mmHg to 83.87 mmHg at the end of the six days.[4948] This suggests that inhaling lavender essential oil daily for short periods can help reduce high blood pressure in people with essential hypertension.

☐ Skin barrier integrity is not only important for skin health but also acts as a protective mechanism to limit entry into the body by various substances and microbes. The skin barrier function provided by the *stratum corneum* (SC) is maintained by a delicate balance between water, ions, keratin, natural moisturizing factor, intracellular lipids, skin surface lipids, and the cutaneous microbiome. Substances that possess anti-inflammatory, antimicrobial, and antioxidant activity and trigger adaptive responses in skin characteristics support healthy skin barrier function and improve the appearance of the skin. Preclinical and clinical research evaluated the activity of tea tree, tangerine, eucalyptus (*E. globulus*), and lavender essential oil skin barrier function and characteristics. Two formulas—one with equal parts of tangerine, eucalyptus, and lavender, and one with equal parts of tea tree, tangerine, eucalyptus, and lavender—diluted to 2% in emulsions stabilized with polymers of natural origin were created to investigate their skin benefits. Tangerine showed the deepest penetration through the skin (35% of the oil made it across the SC) in pig ear, while the rest of the oils and combinations of the oils penetrated less than tangerine but were absorbed at higher than 5% through the viable epidermis. In the clinical study, the four essential oil emulsion hydrated the skin better and improved skin barrier function better than the three essential oil emulsion, showing that tea tree oil has a synergistic activity with the other oils. The four-oil group also experienced improvements in skin characteristics compared to a control group and the three-oil emulsion group. The totality of the research suggests that a combination of tea tree, tangerine, eucalyptus, and lavender in an emulsion can improve overall skin barrier function and skin characteristics.[4949]

☐ Impairment of working memory is frequently reported in people with multiple sclerosis (MS) because of lesions in the brain or spinal cord. A randomized clinical study evaluated the benefits of inhaling lavender essential oil on working memory in women with MS.[4950] Women in the aromatherapy group inhaled 2 drops of lavender essential oil from a cotton ball for ten minutes, twice daily, for two weeks. The placebo group inhaled distilled water. At the end of two weeks, the aromatherapy groups showed improved working memory (5.9% average improvement) that exceeded the improvements experienced in the placebo group (2.2%).

☐ Inhalation of lavender essential oil (as aromatabs attached to subject's clothing) improved the comfort of women following cesarean birth but did not affect anxiety state.[4951]

☐ Fatigue is the most commonly reported symptom experienced by people undergoing hemodialysis, which can significantly decrease quality of life. A clinical study compared the effectiveness of lavender essential oil or orange essential oil with distilled water (so subjects in each group). For fourteen days, the participants inhaled 5 drops of lavender, orange, or water from a cotton ball pinned to the subject's collar. Both sweet orange and lavender essential oil significantly reduced fatigue in people receiving hemodialysis.[4952] Another study found that inhaling lavender essential oil reduced fatigue in people undergoing hemodialysis.[4953]

☐ Researchers evaluated the efficacy of auricular acupuncture with lavender essential oil on anxiety state prior to cardiovascular intervention during a randomized blinded and placebo-controlled trial. Eighty subjects undergoing

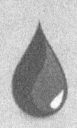

coronary angiography (with or without percutaneous coronary intervention) and right heart catheterization, transcatheter aortic valve replacement, and percutaneous mitral valve repair were included in the study. The intervention group received auricular acupuncture at the "relaxation point" and had lavender oil (5% dilution) applied above the sternum. The acupuncture/lavender group experienced significant declines in anxiety state when compared to the control group (sham acupuncture and application of a placebo). Decreased anxiety during catheter placement and fifteen minutes after the procedure was observed in the lavender group when compared to control.

- Multichannel urodynamics (urodynamic evaluation) is an office procedure that measures the pressure on the bladder to evaluate bladder function during filling and emptying. A randomized controlled pilot trial evaluated the benefits of lavender essential oil to reduce anxiety and pain during multichannel urodynamics.[4954] Two drops of lavender or placebo (distilled water) were placed on a paper towel, and the participants breathed with this three inches from their face prior to procedure and were told to hold the paper towel over their mouths when asked to cough during the procedure. Inhalation of the lavender oil significantly reduced anxiety during and after the procedure but did not affect pain levels.

- Pain and discomfort following orthopedic surgery is unavoidable and sometimes long-lasting. Effective pain management is a vital part of the healing process after these surgeries. A placebo-controlled clinical study found that inhalation of lavender essential oil (2 drops of lavender oil on the pillow cover and top bed sheet each evening for three consecutive days) significantly reduced pain and discomfort following orthopedic surgery—total knee replacement, total hip replacement, insertion of metal to repair a broken bone, or external fixation of broken bones after fracture—when compared to control (distilled water).[4955]

- Laboratory research showed that lavender essential oil significantly kills liver and lung cancer cells and also reduces genotoxicity (damage resulting in mutations to genetic information within a cell) and liver tissue damage.[4956]

- Menstrual pain (dysmenorrhea) is estimated to affect nearly 80% of adolescent girls, with 38% reporting suffering regularly from severe dysmenorrhea. This shows there is a great need to find safe and effective solutions to relieve dysmenorrhea.[4957] Indonesian researchers evaluated the dysmenorrhea relieving effects of inhaling lavender essential oil in adolescent girls. Inhalation of lavender essential oil significantly reduced average menstrual pain from 5.44 (prior to inhalation) to 2.97 (after inhalation).

- Researchers evaluated the psychophysiological responses of women to nine essential oils and one absolute (lavender, rosemary, rose, eucalyptus, jasmine, geranium, chamomile, clary sage, thyme, and peppermint).[4958] Participants inhaled each essential oil for ninety seconds through a glass funnel, and electroencephalography, blood pressure, and pulse rate were measured before and during inhalation of the oils. The study showed that inhaling lavender, rosemary, eucalyptus, jasmine, chamomile, clary sage, and thyme oils reduced relative alpha brainpower, indicating relaxation and a resting state. The ratio of alpha to high beta brainpower—an indication of brain stability and relaxation—significantly increased when rosemary, jasmine, clary sage, and peppermint were inhaled. The relative low beta power—an indicator of brain activity in the absence of stress—significantly increased with lavender, rosemary, rose, and geranium. In addition, systolic blood pressure decreased after inhaling all ten aromatics, suggesting a decline in stress state. The research suggests that inhaling one or a combination of the oils can promote a relaxed state and increase resilience to stress.

- Lavender essential oil grown in Tuscany (19.3%–34.2% linalool, 19.4%–26.3% linalyl acetate, 5.4%–19.4% terpinen-4-ol) inhibited *S. aureus, E. faecalis. L. monocytogenes, P. aeruginosa, E. coli,* and *S. enterica,* with four-year-old plants (highest linalool and terpinen-4-ol content) showing the highest activity.[4959]

- Sepsis is a systemic inflammatory response caused by a severe infection that frequently causes multi-organ dysfunction/failure and has high mortality rates. The lungs are one of the most vulnerable organs during sepsis, and almost half of people with severe sepsis develop acute lung injury. An experimental model of sepsis-induced acute lung injury found that ingestion of lavender essential oil protected rats against sepsis-induced acute lung injury.[4960] Specifically, the oil reduced inflammation and oxidative stress (which triggers cell death) and reduced overexpression of genes linked to lung injury.

- Collagen is the main structural protein in the skin and a basic building block of tissues (connective, tendons, bones, muscles, and cartilage). It is constantly being repaired and regenerated to heal and strengthen tissues and make them resilient to stretching. Evaluation of the biological activities of four lavender essential oil varieties (*L. angustifolia* 'Xinxun-1'-'Xinxun-4') showed that each variety possesses significant antioxidant activity and increased collagen regeneration activity.[4961] Xinxun-2 displayed the highest ferrous ion chelating activity and reducing power, and the greatest collagen regeneration activity.

- An investigation of three essential oils from the *Lamiaceae* family (peppermint, rosemary, and lavender) found that rosemary CT camphor was the most effective larvicidal agent against third instar larvae mosquitoes (*Culex*

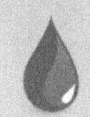

*pipiens*).[4962] Lavender essential oil was the least effective larvicide but demonstrated the highest knockdown rate, followed by peppermint. In addition, lavender and peppermint essential oils showed the highest adult mosquito mortality rates.

☐ Menopause marks the end of a woman's reproductive years and may be accompanied with undesirable symptoms such as hot flashes, vertigo, fatigue, muscle pain, headache, heart palpitations, and abnormal skin sensations. A comparative quasi-experimental human clinical study evaluated the effects of aromatic massage on relieving menopausal symptoms.[4963] Participants of the study were divided into an intervention group (aromatic massage with clary sage, lavender, rose, and jasmine in a base of sweet almond oil) and control group (massage only). Both groups received two twenty-minute massages—back and arms—twice weekly over a five-week period. At the end of the study, the aromatic massage group experienced significant improvement in hot flashes, vertigo, fatigue, muscle pain, headache, heart palpitations, and abnormal skin sensations when compared to the massage only group.

☐ Stroke is a multifaceted disabling neurodegenerative condition that causes the degeneration of neurons leading to cognitive and muscular problems. Researchers found that oral administration of lavender essential oil (200 mg/kg BW) with gallic acid (100 mg/kg BW) prior to stroke preserved cognitive—including memory—and muscular function and reduced anxiousness in rats.[4964] This preclinical research suggests that ingestion of lavender essential oil with gallic acid may be beneficial in people with a higher risk of stroke to preserve cognitive and muscular function if a stroke occurs, but more confirmatory human clinical research is necessary.

☐ Vitamin C (ascorbate) is a vital antioxidant in the brain where it acts as a key signaling molecule and regulator of oxidative stress. Under certain circumstances ascorbate produces hydroxyl radicals and hydrogen peroxide. A laboratory study evaluated how essential oils either enhance (pro-oxidant) or suppress (antioxidant) the production of hydrogen peroxide in the brain.[4965] The researchers reported that lavender, tea tree, and rosemary essential oil suppress the production of hydrogen peroxide by brain ascorbate and produce an overall antioxidant effect, which can reduce anxiety. Isolated beta-pinene was also effective. On the contrary, juniper berry, elecampane, and alpha-pinene had pro-oxidant effects that may be useful for antimicrobial, anti-inflammatory, and anticancer effects.

☐ Low back pain is one of the most common complaints during pregnancy, affecting up to 70 percent of pregnant mothers. This is especially true during the third trimester because production of the hormone relaxin increases, which causes the joints of the pelvic bones to stretch to facilitate the delivery process. A clinical study evaluated the benefits of massage with lavender essential oil to reduce lower back pain the third trimester of pregnancy.[4966] Participants received an effleurage massage with 3 to 10 mL of diluted lavender (diluted to a concentration of 1.5%–3%) essential oil for fifteen to twenty minutes a total of four times. The lavender massage significantly reduced lower back pain when compared to the control group.

☐ Endoscopic retrograde cholangiopancreatography (DRC) is a procedure that combines upper gastrointestinal endoscopy with X-ray used to diagnose and treat problems in the liver, gallbladder, bile duct, and pancreas. A randomized and controlled study evaluated the benefits of lavender oil inhalation with people undergoing DRC. Ninety subjects were randomly divided into a control group and lavender inhalation group. The lavender group inhaled 4 drops of lavender oil added to sterile gauze and placed on the person's chest for thirty minutes. Decreases in heart rate, blood pressure, pain, and anxiety levels, and increased oxygen saturation levels were observed in the lavender group when compared to control. This study suggests that inhaling lavender essential oil can improve patient satisfaction during medical procedures by reducing anxiety and pain and increasing oxygen saturation.[4967]

☐ For decades, physicians wrongly believed that newborns experienced little to no pain due to the immaturity of their nervous systems. However, evidence shows that they not only feel pain, but they may be more sensitive to it and its long-term negative effects. Few viable options exist to relieve pain in newborns, with oral sucrose, swaddling, breastfeeding, and pacifiers most commonly used. A frenotomy is a common procedure performed in newborns for "tongue-tie"—when the lingual frenulum is abnormally short or tight, which may impair the infant's ability to breastfeed. A randomized clinical trial evaluated the ability of inhaling lavender essential oil to reduce pain in newborns during frenotomy.[4968] One drop of lavender was placed on a gauze pad and the pad placed under the newborn's nose for two minutes prior to procedure. In addition, the newborns were given oral sucrose, swaddled, and allowed to suck for two minutes. The control group received the same care without inhaling any lavender essential oil. Researchers reported that inhaling lavender essential oil significantly reduced signs of pain (crying and neonatal infant pain scale score) when compared to the control group. This research suggests that inhalation of lavender essential oil may be a safe, noninvasive, and effective way to reduce pain in newborns during painful procedures.

☐ Interstitial cystitis is a type of bladder pain syndrome characterized by chronic pain in the bladder/pelvic floor area, frequent or urgent need to urinate, and pain during sexual intercourse. Chronic inflammation is a leading trigger of interstitial cystitis because of its damaging effects to bladder tissues and function. Researchers evaluated the activity of lavender and eucalyptus (*E. globulus*) essential oils in a cell culture model (T24 human bladder epithelial cell line on TNF-α stimulated inflammation) of bladder pain syndrome.[4969] Both oils reduced proinflammatory cytokines (IL-1 β, IL-6, IL-8) and NFκB activation (a mediator of proinflammatory gene expression, which when dysregulated contributes to processes that cause multiple inflammatory diseases), but overall, lavender was more effective. Both lavender and its primary constituent linalool displayed greater effectiveness than the comparative control (ACHP inhibitor). The researchers concluded that this research suggests that lavender oil may be suitable as an adjunct therapy in the treatment of interstitial cystitis.

☐ Lavender plants sprayed with paclobutrazol—an organic compound that is used as a plant growth retardant and triazole fungicide—reduced essential oil yield and altered its chemical composition.[4970] The interesting lavender oil with camphor and 1,8-cineole as primary constituents exhibited higher antioxidant activity (DPPH assay) and antimicrobial activity (*S. aureus, B. cereus, S. enteritidis, E. coli, C. albicans,* and *A. niger*) than the essential oil extracted from plants not sprayed with paclobutrazol.

☐ Children treated in pediatric intensive care units (PICUs) often experience distress and pain both from the illness or injury that required hospitalization and the frequency of painful or distressful procedures performed daily. Moreover, children are in an unfamiliar environment with noises and people they are unaccustomed to. A clinical observational study evaluated the effects of massage with lavender, German chamomile, and neroli in 111 children aged less than six months to six years old in the PICU.[4971] A mixture of 1% of the above oils was added to grapeseed carrier oil and massaged to the body (from the feet up to the legs, arms, hands, back, shoulders, abdomen, and the head) using the "M" technique for as long as the child was comfortable or when the therapist deemed the massage had been performed sufficiently. Each child participating in the study received one aromatherapy massage. Heart rate and anxiety were significantly lower and overall comfort improved after the intervention. The study suggests that an essential oil massage could improve the comfort and experience of children when admitted to a PICU.

☐ A foot massage with lavender essential oil reduced blood pressure, heart rate, serum cortisol, and subjective anxiety in people with essential hypertension.[4972]

☐ Behavioral (delusions, hallucinations, agitation, depression, anxiety, euphoria, apathy, disinhibition, irritability, wandering, sleep disorders and appetite problems) and psychological symptoms of dementia can significantly reduce quality of life and make interactions with loved ones difficult. Irritability is among the most common and distressing behavioral changes noted among people with dementia and contributes to caregivers' burden. Researchers investigated nonpharmacological interventions for the reduction of irritability related to dementia in a randomized crossover clinical trial.[4973] Sixty individuals with dementia and irritability were randomly assigned to six different groups, and each group received a series of nonpharmacological interventions—validation therapy and psychoeducational program; aromatherapy and massage therapy; and music therapy—in different sequences. All family caregivers participated in validation therapy and a psychoeducational program that lasted two weeks and included twenty-four two-hour seminars. The lavender aromatherapy massage was administered to the lower back and lower limbs for twenty minutes every morning before breakfast. Music preferred by each person with dementia was chosen and listened to for forty-five minutes per session, once per day, every morning after breakfast. The most effective combination for reducing irritability was aromatherapy massage, followed by validation therapy/psychoeducational program, and music therapy.

☐ Pain and fatigue are commonly reported by mothers after giving birth. A clinical study found that inhaling lavender essential oil—2 drops placed on a cotton ball situated close to the nose and inhaled for fifteen to twenty minutes—significantly reduced fatigue and moderately reduced after pain when compared to the control group (standard treatment and medications only).[4974]

☐ Diffusion of lavender in a hospital (2.4 mL of the oil every twenty-four hours in an area 45 m²) reduced the number of bacteria in all hospital areas the oil was diffused in.[4975] The research suggests that essential oils have potential for sanitizing hospital environments.

☐ Lavender essential oils from three varieties (Moldoveanca 4, Vis magic, and Alba) displayed antioxidant activity in the ABTS and DPPH assays, with the highest activity observed for the Alba variety.[4976] The oils also inhibited *S. aureus, E. coli,* and *C. albicans*. Synergy in antibacterial activity was observed against *P. aeruginosa* when lavender oil was combined with geranium or tea tree essential oils.

☐ Students tend to experience poor sleep quality due to various lifestyle factors such as caffeine intake, poor nutrition, stress, being away from home, and irregular sleep-wake patterns. A randomized clinical trial evaluated the effects of lavender essential oil on sleep and fatigue among college students.[4977] Inhalation of lavender was done by decorative stones (20 g of stone powder, 30 mL of water, 7 drops of lavender oil mixed together and poured into a decorative mold) that contained 7 drops of lavender essential oil. The stones were kept in lidded

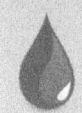

glass jars to maintain the aroma. Students in the lavender group removed the stones from the jar every night and placed it by the bed twenty to twenty-five minutes before retiring every night for a week. No intervention was involved in the control group. Sleep quality and perception of fatigue was improved in the lavender group.

☐ Symptoms—vertigo, dizziness, imbalance—caused by vestibular dysfunction are observed in roughly half of people with multiple sclerosis (MS). Vestibular rehabilitation (VR) involving progressive exercises including eye, head, and body movements with sitting, standing, and walking is used to manage vestibular dysfunction. A controlled clinical trial evaluated the effects of inhaling lavender (0.3 mL of a 2% concentration added to paper that was worn over the nose) in conjunction with VR on balance, fear of falling, and activities of daily living of people with MS.[4978] Both groups performed 45 minutes of VR exercises with one group inhaling lavender essential oil during them. The lavender group performed significantly better on scales measuring balance, fall risk, and MS impact.

☐ Medical schools are stressful environments and depression is reported among almost one-third of medical students globally.[4979] Despite this, very few medical students seek treatment. A clinical study compared the effects of inhaling lavender essential oil or jasmine (*J. sambac*) absolute to a control (water only) on depression among first- and second-year medical students.[4980] Participants in each group inhaled lavender, jasmine, or water for fifteen to twenty minutes before going to bed for seven consecutive nights. Questionnaires were completed before and after intervention to determine the effects on depressive state. The average depressive state decreased from 19.73 (moderate depression) to 14.73 (mild depression) in the lavender group and from 19.33 (moderate depression) to 14.06 (mild depression) in the jasmine group. Statistical analysis and normalization of the data showed that lavender decreased depression 24 percent and jasmine 28.9 percent. This suggests both lavender and jasmine have potential to decrease depression among stressed and depressed medical students.

☐ Acute coronary syndrome (ACS) describes a range of conditions caused by reduced blood flow in the coronary arteries to the heart. The decreased blood flow makes part of the heart muscle unable to function properly and may even cause permanent heart tissue damage. Anxiety while experiencing ACS contributes to poor recovery outcomes and increases the risk of mortality making managing stress and anxiety during ACS critical. A randomized, controlled clinical trial investigated the effects of inhaling lavender essential oil on anxiety and depression during among people with ACS.[4981] In the intervention group, 2 drops of lavender essential oil were placed on an absorbent pad attached to the participant's collar for twenty minutes, morning and evening, for three total days. The control group inhaled sweet almond oil in the same manner. Anxiety and depression levels were measured seven times during the three days. Remarkably, the lavender group experienced significant reductions in anxiety and depression during the first day of intervention at one and nine hours postintervention. Improvements were maintained through the three days of the study, suggesting that lavender could improve ACS patient outcomes because of its effects on anxiety and depression.

☐ Approximately 55 percent of women experience painful menstruation (dysmenorrhea) with rates among adolescent women in Africa higher than 85 percent, Germany 52.1 percent, and the United States nearly 60 percent. A clinical study evaluated the effects of inhaling lavender essential oil while receiving a massage among adolescent women with dysmenorrhea.[4982] Three drops of lavender essential oil were added to 40 mL of water in a diffuser that was operated during the ten-minute massage. Average menstrual pain declined from a rating of eight to three after the massage and aromatherapy demonstrating their effectiveness.

☐ It is estimated that 40 percent of individuals aged sixty-five and older experience constipation, which increases to 74 percent if they live in a nursing home. Left untreated, constipation can cause fecal incontinence, anal fissures, bowel perforation, gas, and bloating. An abdominal massage with lavender and ginger essential oils (diluted to 2% in sweet almond oil) decreased constipation severity, softened stool consistency, and reduced symptoms associated with constipation.[4983] Five mL of the oil blend were massaged into the abdomen for fifteen minutes between 9:30 and 12:00 on five weekdays over the course of four weeks. A control group received no massage.

☐ Lavender essential oil exhibited promising anticancer activity against prostate cancer cells *in vitro*.[4984] The oil also displayed moderate antioxidant activity in the DPPH assay and anti-inflammatory activity in a rat model of arthritis.

☐ The cyclic adenosine monophosphate (cAMP) signaling pathway is involved in the regulation of nausea and vomiting due to its role in relaying information about extracellular stimuli to targets inside cells. A preclinical model found that inhalation of lavender essential oil reduced serotonin, substance P, and dopamine levels, thus regulating downstream the cAMP signaling pathway to reduce nausea and vomiting.[4985]

☐ Humans are exposed to gamma rays (gamma radiation) from cosmic rays in the solar system, medical tests (X-rays, CT scans, etc.), airport scanners, nuclear power plants, some consumer products, and food irradiation, which can alter healthy cells in the body. A preclinical model found that exposure to rosemary, oregano, lavender, or eucalyptus (*E. globulus*) essential oils protected against damage caused by gamma ray exposure.[4986] The best protective effects were observed form lavender and oregano essential oils. Specifically, the oil preserved

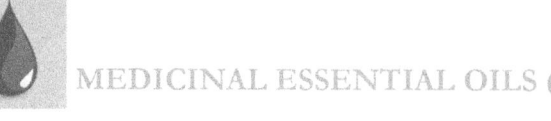

metabolic enzymes, restored enzymatic antioxidant activity (catalase and superoxide dismutase), and reduced lipid peroxidation.

☐ Both lavender (22.4% linalool, 19.2% linalyl acetate, 17.9% camphor) and Spanish lavender (54.7% camphor, 19.2% alpha-fenchone) essential oil inhibited ACE2 and LOX, suggesting they may have potential for the management of cognitive and inflammatory disorders.[4987] Spanish lavender inhibited LOX better, but lavender was significantly more active against ACE2. Isolated camphor and linalool were also active, with camphor being the most effective against ACE2 and linalool against LOX.

☐ Inhalation of Douglas fir or lavender essential oil via a diffuser promoted relaxation during a leaf-printing activity in older adults, as measured by brainwaves, heart rate, and questionnaires.[4988] The oils modified heart rate variability—low frequency and high frequency heart rate ratio—indicating balanced autonomic nervous system activity. Monitoring of brainwave activity showed a decrease in high beta waves (indicating reduced stress), increased high alpha waves (suggestive of a relaxed but focused state), and decreased gamma waves (corresponding to a more relaxed state). Moreover, participants reported feeling less anxious and more relaxed after inhaling the oils.

☐ A randomized, controlled trial evaluated the effects of lavender essential oil and Sujok therapy—a healing therapy based on acupressure that focuses on active points on the palm and foot that correspond to all organs or parts of the human body—for relieving pain after cesarean section.[4989] Participants were divided into four groups: 1) lavender, rose, and eucalyptus aromatherapy, 2) Sujok therapy, 3) aromatherapy with Sujok therapy, and 4) a control group that received only routine pain management. The participants selected among the three oils based on scent preference with twenty-six choosing lavender, seventeen choosing rose, and seventeen preferring eucalyptus. Essential oils were inhaled for thirty minutes. All three intervention groups experienced significant pain reductions. Interestingly, the Sujok-only group experienced the greatest relief.

☐ Absorption of naproxen through the skin is low, so researchers investigated the effects of adding 0.5% lavender essential oil to a topical gel with naproxen sodium.[4990] The addition of the essential oil not only improved the absorption into and across skin layers, but it also enhanced the pain-relieving properties of the gel in mice.

☐ Taikong blue lavender is a cultivar of lavender used to produce an essential oil in Xinjiang Province, China. Taikong blue lavender (41.0% linalyl acetate, 29.5% linalool) reduced oxidative stress indicators (NO, ROS, MDA, and iNOS at the mRNA and protein levels) and preserved antioxidant (SOD, CAT) activities in inflamed cells.[4991] The oil reduced inflammation by inhibiting the expression of TNF-$\alpha$, IL-1$\beta$, IL-6, and key proteins (I$\kappa$B$\alpha$, NF-$\kappa$B p65, p50, JNK, and p38 MAPK). Molecular docking analysis showed that multiple constituents of lavender have high binding affinity to target proteins, particularly beta-caryophyllene, lavandulyl acetate, and geranyl acetate.

☐ Coronary artery bypass graft surgery (CABG) is a procedure used to treat narrowing coronary arteries by bypassing the blocked/narrowed arteries with a piece of healthy blood vessel obtained from elsewhere in the body. Although a primary treatment option for coronary artery disease and usually successful, the procedure may cause undesirable complications—irregular heartbeat, abnormal vital signs, cardiogenic shock (a life-threatening condition where insufficient blood and oxygen is supplied to tissues or organs), delirium, pain (especially chest pain), stress, and gastrointestinal bleeding. A randomized clinical trial found that inhalation of lavender essential oil—5 drops of 20% lavender EO applied to gauze and worn as a necklace for three consecutive days—reduced pain and blood pressure, and the lavender group required less pain meds following CABG.[4992]

☐ Tarragon, lemongrass (C. citratus), and lavender essential oil were each insecticidal against the bean weevil (Acanthoscelides obtectus).[4993]

☐ Inhalation of lavender essential oil—20 drops in an aromatherapy vaporizer placed next to the subject and refreshed every twenty minutes until the dental visit was completed—minimized dental anxiety, pain, and fear related to dental procedures.[4994]

☐ Septorhinoplasty is a procedure used to improve nasal breathing, correct a deviated septum, or improve the appearance of the nose. Rhinoplasty can be cosmetic or function and changes the shape and appearance of the nose. A parallel randomized controlled clinical trial evaluated the effects of inhaling lavender—3 drops of diluted lavender were applied to cotton and attached near the subject's nose for nearly twenty minutes—essential oil to control anxiety before and after septorhinoplasty or rhinoplasty. Lavender inhalation significantly decreased anxiety, blood pressure, and heart rate when compared to the control group.

☐ Inhalation of a 3% dilution of lavender essential oil and its fractions—light fraction (linalool and trans-beta-ocimene) and heavy fraction (linalyl acetate, lavandulyl acetate, beta-caryophyllene)—for thirty minutes relieved sleep disturbances caused by caffeine and anxiety in mice.[4995] Interestingly, the light fraction was more effective for improving sleep maintenance and the heavy fraction for sleep initiation. The effects were achieved through multiple mechanisms involving the GABA, acetylcholine, histamine, and dopamine systems.

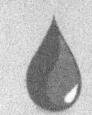

- Lavender essential oil effectively inhibited *C. albicans* isolated from the saliva of children at low concentrations (0.5%–2%).[4996]
- Laboratory research found that lavender essential oil modulates cholesterol metabolism—increases intracellular cholesterol and alters proteins involved cholesterol uptake, biosynthesis, and trafficking—in hepatic cells.[4997] The researchers attributed the effects primarily to terpinen-4-ol.
- Inhalation of a 5% dilution of lavender essential oil for thirty minutes reduced orofacial pain sensation and anxiety in mice.[4998]
- Four varieties of lavender essential oil displayed good antioxidant activity in the DPPH assay.[4999] Varieties with near equal linalool and linalyl acetate produced greater activity than varieties with moderate borneol and camphor content.
- Perineal massage with lavender essential oil starting at thirty-four weeks of pregnancy—ten minutes daily for five consecutive days in one week—significantly reduced perineal tearing during delivery compared to the control group (just normal delivery care). Only one individual (3.8%) had no perineal tears in the control group, while 30.8% of the women in the lavender perineal massage group had no tears.[5000]
- Lavender essential oil enhanced (synergistic) the antifungal effects of fluconazole against *C. albicans*.[5001]
- A randomized, controlled clinical trial found that inhalation of lavender essential oil—20 drops in 50 mL of water diffused in a diffuser near the person's chair in the waiting room for twenty minutes—reduced pain and anxiety related to a dental visit in women. Heart rate, systolic blood pressure, respiratory rate, and oxygen saturation were also improved.
- More than half of people with diabetes have a phobia to needles due to the pain caused by the frequency of insulin injections. A double-blind randomized controlled clinical trial found that topical application of 0.3 mL of lavender essential oil on the arms reduced pain after insulin injection when compared to placebo (distilled water).[5002]
- Diffusion of 3 drops of lavender or German chamomile essential oil beginning twenty minutes before bedtime for two weeks improved sleep quality of pregnant women during their third trimester.[5003] Lavender was the most effective.
- Massage with diluted lavender essential oil to the hands and feet of people with diabetic neuropathy—twenty massage sessions during four weeks; twenty minutes to the feet and ten minutes to the hands—significantly reduced pain.[5004]

# LEDUM
## (Labrador Tea, Marsh Tea, Greenland Moss)

*Rhododendron groenlandicum* Oeder, *Ledum groenlandicum, L. palustre* var. *latifolium* (Jacq.) Michx.; *L. palustre* L., *R. tomentosum* Harmaja

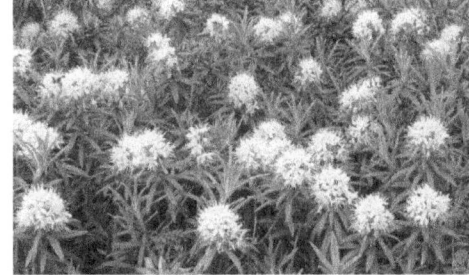

**FAMILY:** Ericaceae
**NOTE:** Middle
**AROMA INTENSITY:** Medium
**AROMA:** Herbaceous, warm, slightly sweet
**COMMON EXTRACTION METHOD:** Steam distilled from the leaves and flowering tops
**POSSIBLE SUBSTITUTE OILS:** Helichrysum, elemi, ylang ylang
**BLENDS WELL WITH:** Bergamot, fennel, grapefruit, lemon, lime, orange, petitgrain, neroli, tangerine
**SUBCELLULAR LOCALIZATION | EPIGENETIC INFLUENCE:** Currently unknown | Currently unknown
**RECOMMENDED DILUTION RANGE:** 3%–Neat

**PRIMARY CONSTITUENTS:**[5005,5006,5007]

| *Rhododendron groenlandicum*# | | *Ledum palustre** | |
|---|---|---|---|
| Limonene | 0.3%–67.2% | Palustrol | 26.2%–43.4% |
| Beta-Selinene | 2.3%–35.4% | Ledol | 21.0%–32.2% |
| Sabinene | 0.1%–35.0% | Ascaridole | 0.1%–14.2% |
| (E,E)-Germacrone | 0.0%–29.3% | Myrcene | 0.9%–11.4% |
| Beta-Bisabolene | 0.0%–12.6% | 5-(3-furyl)-2-methyl-1 -penten-3-ol=lepalol | 0.0%–7.9% |
| Gamma-Terpinene | 0.0%–12.2% | | |
| Alpha-Humulene | 0.0%–12.1% | Cyclocolorenone | 2.7%–6.5% |

| | | | |
|---|---|---|---|
| Alpha-Selinene | 0.3%–9.9% | Para-Cymene | 0.0%–5.0% |
| Germacrene B | 0.0%–9.4% | Alpha-Terpinene | 0.1%–4.5% |
| Eudesma-3,11-Dien-2-One | 0.0%–8.9% | 2-methyl-6-methylene | |
| Beta-Pinene | 1.0%–8.4% | -3,7-octadien-2-ol | 0.0%–4.1% |
| Bornyl Acetate | 0.3%–8.4% | 5-(3-furyl)-2-methyl-1 | |
| Alpha-Pinene | 0.0%–8.0% | -penten-3-one=lepalone | 0.0%–3.5% |
| Trans-p-Mentha-1(7), 8-Dien-2-ol | 0.0%–7.0% | Bornyl Acetate | 0.0%–3.3% |
| Cis-p-Mentha-1(7),8-dien-2-ol | 0.0%–6.2% | Allo-Aromadendrene | 0.8%–3.2% |
| Terpinen-4-ol | 0.1%–5.1% | Carvone | 0.0%–2.4% |
| Myrtenal | 0.3%–4.3% | Beta-Oplopenone | 0.0%–1.7% |
| Rosifoliol | 0.0%–4.3% | Geranyl Acetate | 0.2%–1.7% |
| Menthatriene | 0.0%–4.0% | | |
| Para-Cymene | 0.2%–3.4% | | |
| Isopiperitenol A | 0.0%–3.1% | | |
| Beta-Caryophyllene | 0.0%–3.1% | | |

\# Commercial samples vary widely in composition based on growing conditions and vegetation period. There are at least six ledum chemotypes (limonene, sabinene, beta-selinene, para-cymene, beta-bisabolene, and limonene/beta-selinene) reported in the literature.
\* Essential oils richest in ledol and palustrol are typically harvested in April and October.

**OTHER CONSTITUENTS:** *Rhododendron groenlandicum*—Alpha-terpinene, curzerene, cis-p-mentha-2,3-dien-1-ol, trans-pinocarveol, p-menth-1,5,8-triene, delta-cadinene, cyclocolorenone, nootkatol, trans-sabinol, carvone, pinocarvone, isopiperitenol B, beta-elemene, terpinolene, germacrene D, trans-p-mentha-2,3-dien-1-ol, camphene, (E)-beta-farnesene, beta-phellandrene, germacrene A, beta-myrcene, para-cymene, dehydrosabina ketone, myrtenol, cis-4-caranone, cis carveol, cumin aldehyde, alpha-copaene, alpha-gurjunene, gamma-elemene, trans-alpha-bergamotene, eudesma-2,4,11-triene, gamma-cadinene, zonarene, selina-4(15),7(11)-diene, isozierene, palustrol, humulene epoxide II, beta-Costol; *Ledum palustre*—Ortho-cymene, limonene, iso-citral, beta-pinene-oxide, menthyl acetate, viridiflorene, delta-cadinene, viridiflorol, alpha-cadinol, gamma-terpinene, 2-methyl-6-methylene-1,7-octadien-3-one, 2-methyl-6-methylene-1,7-octadien-3-ol, terpinen-4-ol, myrtenal, gamma-terpineol, 2-methyl-5-(3-furyl)-3-penten-2-ol, epi-alpha-muurolol

**PREFERRED COMPOSITION FOR CLINICAL USE:**

| Constituent | *R. groenlandicum* CT Limonene | *R. groenlandicum* CT Sabinene |
|---|---|---|
| **Limonene** | 20%–35% | 0.5%–5 |
| **Beta-Selinene** | 5%–15% | 7%–15% |
| **Sabinene** | 2%–13% | 15%–25% |
| **Alpha-Selinene** | 2%–10% | 1%–5% |
| **Trans-p-Mentha-1(7),8-dien-2-ol** | 2%–10% | – |
| **Alpha-Pinene** | 2%–8% | 3%–8% |
| **Beta-Pinene** | 1%–7% | 3%–10% |
| **Bornyl Acetate** | 1%–7% | 2%–5% |
| **Cis-p-Mentha-1(7),8-dien-2-ol** | 1%–7% | – |
| **Menthatriene** | 0.1%–5% | – |
| **Para-Cymene** | 0.2%–4% | 1%–5% |
| **Gamma-Terpinene** | – | 5%–10% |
| **Terpinen-4-ol** | – | 3%–10% |
| **Alpha-Terpinene** | – | 1%–5% |
| **Myrtenal** | – | 2%–5% |

**REPORTED THERAPEUTIC PROPERTIES:** Antibacterial, anti-inflammatory, analgesic (pain relief), antirheumatic, soothes cough, antitumoral, antiallergenic, diuretic, **aids detoxification, supports kidney and liver function**, stimulates immune system activity, encourages lymph flow and drainage, reduces nausea, weight management, expels excess gas, reduces chronic skin conditions, encourages normal thyroid function, aids addictive tendencies, eases jealousy, combats rage and anger

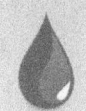
**CAUTIONS:**

■ *L. palustre*: Avoid use in children due to toxicity concerns and known poisoning and fatalities with ascaridole-containing essential oils in humans due to ascaridole content.[5008]

■ *L. palustre*: Avoid during pregnancy and lactation due to ascaridole content. Hydro-alcohol extracts of boldo (containing ascaridole) have reportedly caused abortions, fetal abnormalities, and low birth weight in animal studies when administered at 800 mg/kg/day.[5009,5010] Boldo leaf teas (containing ascaridole) are reportedly used to induce illegal abortions in humans.[5011]

■ *L. palustre:* Avoid oral consumption due to ascaridole content. Oral use of essential oils with significant ascaridole content can cause respiratory depression, overstimulation of the CNS (exaggerated reflexes, lack of coordination, convulsions, paralysis of motor and sensory nerves, and death by respiratory arrest), liver toxicity, and anaphylactic reactions.[5012,5013,5014] Human toxicity and fatal poisoning have been reported in children and adults with chenopodium essential oil (also high in ascaridole).[5015]

■ *L. palustre*: Topical application, sensitization. Ledum may cause skin sensitization when applied topically due to ascaridole content.[5016,5017,5018]

■ *L. groenlandicum*: May interfere with the enzymes responsible for metabolizing medications (NSAIDs, proton-pump inhibitors, acetaminophen, antiepileptics, immune modulators, blood-sugar medications, blood pressure medications, antidepressants, antipsychotics, diabetic medications, antihistamines, antibiotics, and anesthetics) due to possible significant germacrone content.[5019]

**SELECTED EVIDENCE:**

☐ Animal research suggests that ledum oil significantly reduces edema and inflammation similar to the drugs piroxicam and ketoprofen.[5020]

☐ Ledum oil is considered a strong tick repellent. A 10% concentration diluted in acetone provided 95.1% repellency, which is comparable to synthetic DEET (100% repellency).[5021]

☐ Intermediate inhibition of MRSA was found with ledum essential oil *in vitro*.[5022]

☐ A review concluded that ledum essential oil possesses analgesic, anti-inflammatory, antimicrobial, antiviral, antifungal, and insecticidal potential.[5023]

☐ Laboratory research found that ledum essential oils (gamma-terpineol, palustrol/ledol, and ledene oxide CTs) caused apoptosis of blood lymphocytes—cells connected to joint inflammation and damage—and rheumatoid arthritis (RA) synoviocytes—cells in cartilage junctions that contribute to joint destruction—from RA synovia.[5024]

☐ Ledum (*L. palustre*) essential oil rich in ascaridole was insecticidal to mosquitoes (*Culex quinquefasciatus*), moths (*Spodoptera littoralis*), and flies (*Musca domestica*) without causing serious harm to nontarget organisms.[5025]

☐ *Fusobacterium nucleatum* is the main bacterium linked to bad breath. The bacterium aggregates with other bacteria in the mouth to form plaque biofilms that cause bad breath. Ledum (*R. groenlandicum*) CT sabinene, peppermint, and mountain savory CT carvacrol essential oil each inhibited *F. nucleatum* without harming human oral cells in a laboratory study.[5026]

☐ Angelica root, ledum (*R. tomentosum*), and common tansy each showed broad-spectrum antimicrobial activity against tested microbes—*S. aureus, P. aeruginosa, C. albicans, A. niger, Cl. Cladosporioides,* and *P. venetum*.[5027] Co2 aromatics of each oil were also tested, with ledum Co2 aromatic exhibiting very strong effects against *S. aureus* and a strong effect against *C. albicans*.

# LELESHWA
## (African Wild Sage, Camphor Bush)

*Tarchonanthus camphoratus* L.

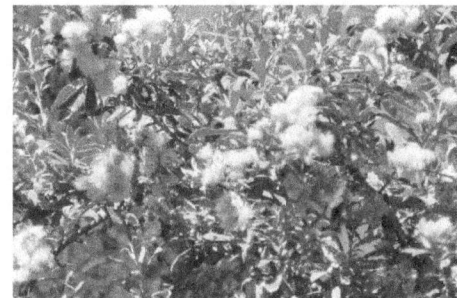

**FAMILY:** Asteraceae
**NOTE:** Top-Middle
**AROMA INTENSITY:** Strong
**AROMA:** Camphoraceous, medicinal, herbaceous
**COMMON EXTRACTION METHOD:** Steam distilled from the leaves and aerial parts

**POSSIBLE SUBSTITUTE OILS:** Vilayti tulsi, white sage, rosemary, tea tree
**BLENDS WELL WITH:** Angelica root, African bluegrass, balsam fir, cardamom, cassia, cedarwood, cinnamon, clary sage, clove, eucalyptus, frankincense, geranium, ginger, lavender, lavandin, palmarosa, patchouli, ravensara, ravintsara, sandalwood, spike lavender, tamala, white fir, white sage
**SUBCELLULAR LOCALIZATION | EPIGENETIC INFLUENCE:** Currently unknown | Currently unknown
**RECOMMENDED DILUTION RANGE:** 3%–Neat

**PRIMARY CONSTITUENTS:**[5028,5029,5030,5031,5032,5033,5034,5035,5036,5037]

| | |
|---|---|
| Alpha-Fenchol | 10.9%–29.1% |
| Alpha-Pinene | 6.9%–16.9% |
| 1,8-Cineole | 13.1%–16.5% |
| Alpha-Terpineol | 0.9%–13.2% |
| (E)-Pinene Hydrate | 3.2%–6.5% |
| Camphene | 3.8%–6.3% |
| Beta-Eudesmol | 0.3%–5.8% |
| Terpinen-4-ol | 2.0%–4.7% |

Note: The leaf oil produces a wide variety of chemotypes that include, but are not limited to: 1,8-cineole, beta-caryophyllene, beta-guaiene, and endo-fenchol.

**OTHER CONSTITUENTS:** Beta-pinene, delta-2-carene, alpha-terpinene, para-cymene, limonene, gamma-terpinene, trans-sabinene hydrate, alpha-terpinolene, nonanal, exo-methyl camphenilol, borneol, beta-caryophyllene, aromadendrene, gamma-curcumene, ar-curcumene, delta-cadinene, caryophyllene oxide, alpha-cadinol, alpha-phellandrene, delta-3-carene, fenchone, isocaryophyllene

**PREFERRED COMPOSITION FOR CLINICAL USE:**

| Constituent | |
|---|---|
| **Alpha-Fenchol** | 15%–30% |
| **1,8-Cineole** | 10%–20% |
| **Alpha-Pinene** | 10%–20% |
| **Alpha-Terpineol** | 6%–15% |
| **(E)-Pinene Hydrate** | 2%–10% |
| **Camphene** | 2%–7% |
| **Terpinen-4-ol** | 2%–7% |
| **Beta-Eudesmol** | 0.1%–5% |

**REPORTED THERAPEUTIC PROPERTIES:** Antiseptic, antifungal, antiviral, antibacterial, soothes chronic skin conditions, astringent, **supports urinary tract and reproductive health**, relieves headaches, analgesic, supports respiratory function, eases cough, reduces the appearance of wrinkles, blemishes, and acne, purification, disinfectant, insect repellent, insecticide, encourages restful sleep, relieves past trauma and negative emotions, mentally stimulating

**CAUTIONS:**
■ None currently known.

**SELECTED EVIDENCE:**
☐ *In vitro* research demonstrated that the endo-fenchol CT of leleshwa kills colon cancer cells.[5038]
☐ The alpha-fenchol CT of leleshwa essential oil exhibited broad-spectrum antifungal (*C. albicans*) and antibacterial (gram-negative: *E. coli*, *K. pneumoniae*, *Proteus mirabilis*, *Salmonella typhi*; gram-positive: *S. aureus*, *Bacillus* spp.) activity.[5039,5040] *In vitro* research reports that the leaf essential oil of leleshwa (1,8-cineole and beta-guaiene CTs) inhibits gram-positive (*S. aureus*, *S. epidermidis*, and *B. cereus*) and gram-negative (*E. coli*, *K. pneumonia*, and *Salmonella* sp.) bacteria, with a broader spectrum of antimicrobial activity than the antibiotic chloramphenicol.[5041] The endo-fenchol CT of leleshwa essential oil moderately inhibited MRSA, *S. aureus*, and *C. albicans* according to *in vitro* research.[5042]
☐ In a study that investigated the effectiveness of plant extracts and essential oils against pathogens that cause

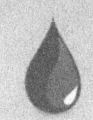

urinary or sexually transmitted infections, leleshwa essential oil (unidentified composition) was significantly active against *Oligella ureolytica* (a gram-negative bacterium associated with urinary tract and cervical infections), and moderately active against *Garderella vaginalis* (a gram-variable bacterium that causes genital tract infections and vaginitis), *Ureaplasma urealyticum* (a bacterium and commonly sexually transmitted infection that causes urogenital tract infections and may lead to fertility issues), and *C. albicans* (a common cause of vaginal yeast infections), *Neisseria gonorrhoeae* (a gram-negative bacteria responsible for the sexually transmitted infection gonorrhea), and mild activity against *Trichomonas vaginalis* (a protozoan parasite that causes trichomoniasis—a very common STD that can cause mild irritation to severe inflammation).[5043]

- Leleshwa leaf essential oil (1,8-cineole, beta-guaiene, and endo-fenchol CTs) is considered a weak antioxidant according to *in vitro* research.[5044,5045]
- Leleshwa leaf essential oil (near equal portions of alpha-pinene, camphene, and alpha-fenchol) repelled the *Anopheles gambiae* mosquito, but was less effective than DEET.[5046]
- Leleshwa essential oil exhibited good anticancer activity against breast cancer cells, and killed liver and lung cancer cells to a lesser degree.[5047] The oil was less toxic to healthy human cells.

# LEMON

*Citrus × limon* (L.) Burm. f. (pro sp.) [medica × aurantifolia]

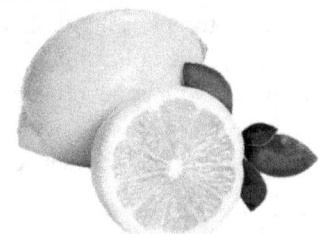

**FAMILY:** Rutaceae
**NOTE:** Top
**AROMA INTENSITY:** Medium
**AROMA:** Clean, fresh, citrusy, fruity
**COMMON EXTRACTION METHOD:** Cold-pressed/expressed or hydrodistilled from the fruit peel (rind)
**POSSIBLE SUBSTITUTE OILS:** Lime, orange, grapefruit, bergamot, tangerine, neroli, petitgrain
**BLENDS WELL WITH:** Bay laurel, bergamot, camphor, cajeput, cardamom, carrot seed, cassia, chamomile (German, Roman), cinnamon, cistus, citronella, copaiba, coriander, eucalyptus, fennel, frankincense, geranium, grapefruit, lavender, lemongrass, lemon verbena, lime, melissa, tea tree, neroli, niaouli, orange, petitgrain, pine, patchouli, ravensara, rose, sage, sandalwood, silver fir, Spanish sage, tangerine, vetiver, white fir
**SUBCELLULAR LOCALIZATION | EPIGENETIC INFLUENCE:** Endocytic vesicles, Mitochondria, Lysosome | Lymphatic/Endocrine
**RECOMMENDED DILUTION RANGE:** 3%–50%; neat for limited conditions

**PRIMARY CONSTITUENTS:**[5048,5049,5050]

| Cold-pressed/expressed | | Distilled | |
|---|---|---|---|
| Limonene | 38.1%–95.8% | Limonene | 61.8%–73.8% |
| Gamma-Terpinene | 0.1%–18.0% | Gamma-Terpinene | 9.8%–10.4% |
| Beta-Pinene | 0.1%–15.8% | Beta-Pinene | 0.0%–6.9% |
| Para-Cymene | 0.0%–7.8% | Sabinene | 0.0%–5.8% |
| Sabinene | 0.1%–6.3% | Citral | 0.0%–5.4% |

Note: Higher limonene content is usually found in essential oils obtained from lemons grown in America.

**OTHER CONSTITUENTS:** *Cold-pressed/expressed*—Alpha-thujene, alpha-pinene, camphene, myrcene, beta-phellandrene, terpinolene, trans-limonene-1,2-oxide, linalool, terpinen-4-ol, alpha-terpineol, nerol, linalyl acetate, terpinyl acetate, neryl acetate, geranyl acetate, beta-bisabolene, trans-R-bergamotene, beta-elemene, neral, geranial, germacrene D, thymol; *Distilled*—Alpha-thujene, alpha-pinene, camphene, myrcene, alpha-terpinene, 1,8-cineole, linalool, terpinen-4-ol, alpha-terpineol, nerol, linalyl acetate, germacrene D, beta-bisabolene

**PREFERRED COMPOSITION FOR CLINICAL USE:**

| Constituent | Cold-Pressed | Distilled |
|---|---|---|
| Limonene | 60%–78% | 60%–75% |
| Beta-Pinene | 8%–17% | 5%–13% |
| Gamma-Terpinene | 7%–14% | 5%–13% |

| Sabinene | 1%–3% | 0.1%–3% |
|---|---|---|
| Neryl Acetate + Geranyl Acetate | 0.1%–4% | 0.5%–3% |
| Geranial | 0.1%–3% | 1%–5% |
| Alpha-Pinene | 0.1%–3% | 0.1%–3% |
| Neral | 0.1%–2% | 0%–3% |

REPORTED THERAPEUTIC PROPERTIES: Antibacterial, analgesic (pain relief), antifungal, **antiseptic**, anti-inflammatory, **immune supportive**, antimicrobial, antineuralgic, **diuretic**, improves skin luster, nourishes the skin, **reduces the appearance of wrinkles and blemishes**, disinfectant, strengthens nails, **weight management**, reduces fever, nourishes hair, antirheumatic, soothes mouth sores, antiseptic, astringent, **helps boils heal**, expels excess gas, aids digestion, encourages a restful night's sleep, relieves constipation, helps lower high blood pressure, soothes swollen glands, **relieves nausea and vomiting**, aids detoxification, antiparasitic, **adaptogenic**, combats frustration, stress management, sedating, **antidepressant**, uplifting, aids concentration, **combats nightmares**

CAUTIONS:

■ May be photosensitizing (cold-pressed/expressed). Avoid sun exposure to area of application for at least twelve hours after topical application.[5051,5052,5053]

■ May interact with anticholinergic (drugs used for asthma, incontinence, gastrointestinal cramps, muscular spasms, depression, and sleep disorders) and cholinergic medications (drugs used to reduce urinary retention, diagnose myasthenia gravis, and for glaucoma) based on AChE inhibitory activity.[5054]

SELECTED EVIDENCE:

☐ *In vitro* research suggests that lemon oil activates enzyme activity (like caspases) that promotes apoptosis of astrocytoma cells (cancerous astrocyte cells that make up the supportive tissue of the brain and form brain tumors).[5055]

☐ Lemon oil reduces elastase activity (an enzyme involved in the breakdown of elastin) *in vitro*, which may help prevent wrinkles and aging of the skin.[5056] Elastin helps keep skin tight, supple, and flexible.

☐ Inhaling lavender, lemon, and ylang ylang oil (2:2:1 ratio) reduced systolic blood pressure, and influenced heart rate and sympathetic nervous system activity in people with essential hypertension (also called primary hypertension, it is high blood pressure without an identifiable cause).[5057]

☐ Animal research suggests that inhalation of lemon oil reduces anxiety and depression by influencing dopamine and serotonin activity.[5058]

☐ Pregnant women who inhaled 1 to 2 drops of lemon oil on a cotton ball placed directly under their nose experienced improvements in pregnancy-associated nausea and vomiting.[5059]

☐ After seventeen days of soaking a plantar wart followed by the topical application of lavender, wintergreen, lemongrass, peppermint, and two blends of oils (containing wintergreen, helichrysum, clove, peppermint, coconut oil, grape seed oil, almond oil, olive oil, oregano, eucalyptus, elemi, vetiver, lemongrass, and thyme), the wart fell off in a immunosuppressed (from chemotherapy) fifty-three-year-old female.[5060] This is significant considering that a plantar wart can take a few weeks to fall off after cryotherapy.

☐ Constituents found in lemon (limonene and perillyl alcohol) improved dementia caused by the drug scopolamine in animals.[5061]

☐ A nasal spray with lemon, ravensara, and niaouli oils (0.14 mL consisting of 0.014 mL lemon, 0.042 mL aloe vera juice, 0.0007 mL ravensara, 0.0007 g propolis and 0.00042 mL niaouli oil) decreased the symptoms of allergic and nonallergic rhinopathy (nasal congestion, drainage, and obstruction of the nasal passages) in a clinical trial.[5062]

☐ *In vitro* research concluded that lemon oil enhanced the penetration of vitamins A, C, E, and B6 through the skin.[5063]

☐ An abdominal massage with lemon, rosemary, and peppermint oil relieved constipation in the elderly.[5064] Interestingly, the effect of the massage lasted for two weeks after treatment.

☐ Three minutes of oral cleansing daily with a combination of tea tree, peppermint, and lemon oils helped reduce bad breath and production of volatile sulfur compounds (compounds excreted by oral bacteria that cause bad breath) in intensive care patients.[5065] Another study combined alpha-bisabolol with tea tree oil and found that this combination killed the bacteria associated with bad breath (*S. moorei*).[5066]

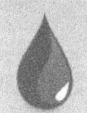

- *In vitro* research suggests that lemon oil may prevent and manage neurodegenerative diseases caused by oxidative stress by inhibiting acetylcholinesterase (AChE) and butyrylcholinesterase (BChE) enzyme activity, and preventing lipid peroxidation.[5067] Inhibition of AChE prevents the breakdown of acetylcholine, which is essential for memory and thinking. People with neurodegenerative diseases make less acetylcholine, and the diseases often break it down at a faster rate leading to acetylcholine deficits. Selective inhibition of BChE is also desirable in neurodegenerative diseases because it interferes with acetylcholine activity. In addition, BChE is often found in the plaques and tangles in the brains of people with Alzheimer's disease.[5068]

- Direct infusions of 20–30 mL of limonene dissolved gallstones in people in as few as three days.[5069,5070] While these are extreme doses and were administered through injection, anecdotal evidence from user testimonials suggest that smaller amounts of lemon oil may also be effective.

- Oral administration of 1,000 mg of d-limonene every day or every other day relieved heartburn and GERD symptoms in 89% of people after fourteen days of use.[5071,5072]

- Lemon oil increased the effectiveness of gentamicin (an antibiotic drug) against multi-drug-resistant *Acinetobacter* species *in vitro*.[5073]

- *In vitro* research concluded that lemon oil is effective against the bacteria *B. subtilis, S. capitis, M. luteus,* and *P. fluorescens,* and the *yeasts S. cerevisiae* and *C. parapsilosis.*[5074]

- Animal research suggests that lemon oil prevents damage to the hippocampus (the part of the brain involved in the storage of long-term memory, knowledge, experiences, and the related emotions) caused by oxidative stress associated with neurodegenerative diseases.[5075]

- Lemon oil helps decrease inflammation by strongly inhibiting the 5-lipoxygenase (5-LOX) enzyme that is involved in the inflammation response according to *in vitro* research.[5076] Other research reports that oral administration of hydrodistilled lemon essential oil (100 mg/kg) reduces inflammation by decreasing cell migration (white blood cell movement to tissues), cytokine production, and protein extravasation (the movement of proteins excreted by white blood cells from capillaries to surrounding tissues, which plays a key role in inflammation).[5077]

- Oral administration of 50–100 mg/kg of lemon oil relieves pain by binding to and activating opioid receptors in mice.[5078]

- Lemon essential oil protects the gastrointestinal tract from damage caused by aspirin.[5079]

- Animal research suggests that lemon oil reduced anxiety and depression by interacting with GABA receptors (GABA binds to receptors to reduce the excitatory activity of the brain that causes anxiety, panic, and fear) and possibly by modulating serotonin and noradrenaline levels.[5080] Another study concluded that inhalation of lemon oil reliably elevated mood and increased norepinephrine levels (low norepinephrine levels are associated with depression).[5081]

- Inhalation of lemon oil balances the autonomic nervous system (ANS)—adaptogenic. It differentially influenced ANS activity in healthy and depressed persons. Healthy subjects experienced increased sympathetic and parasympathetic activity after inhalation, whereas depressed persons experienced increased parasympathetic activity.[5082] Sympathetic nervous system activity is often elevated and parasympathetic activity decreased in people who are depressed.

- *In vitro* research reported that lemon oil provides a sun protection factor (SPF) of 2.81.[5083]

- Lemon oil demonstrated better anticandidal activity than the anticandidal drugs miconazole and clotrimazole *in vitro*.[5084]

- Oral administration of d-limonene reduced metabolic disorders (reduced high blood-sugar levels and improved cholesterol profiles) in high-fat diet caused obese mice.[5085] The researchers concluded this effect was caused by activation of peroxisome proliferator-activated receptors, PPARs for short, (receptor proteins that regulate gene expression, cellular differentiation, metabolism, and tumor growth) and liver X receptor-beta signaling (receptors that detect cholesterol and activate pathways that lower cholesterol levels).

- Lemon oil may help prevent cavities by preventing glucosyltransferase (GST) and lactate dehydrogenase activity, and reducing acid production and water insoluble glucans in the mouth. All of these factors work together to increase the risk of cavities and other oral conditions.[5086] The existence of streptococci in the mouth is strongly associated with cavities; however, they require the presence of both sugar and the enzyme GST to cause cavities. GST enhances the formation of sticky water insoluble glucans from sugar, which adhere Streptococci bacteria to the teeth and form plaque. In addition, streptococci in the plaque use sugar to create acid that attacks the teeth and creates the holes in them known as cavities.

☐ Animal research suggests that lemon oil may enhance the learning ability of rats.[5087] Rats who inhaled lemon oil were able to find a target faster than the control group.

☐ Researchers concluded that lemon oil inhibited several *Candida* species and bacteria known to cause hospital-acquired infections according to *in vitro* research.[5088]

☐ Rats exposed to the aroma of lemon oil (3 drops added to the cage every three days for eleven to twelve days) experienced changes in corticosterone levels and neuronal responses that decreased anxiety and pain.[5089,5090,5091]

☐ Preclinical research demonstrates that oral administration of lemon essential oil prevented liver and kidney damage caused by aspirin.[5092]

☐ *In vitro* research demonstrated that low doses of marjoram, lemon, basil, clove, thyme, rosemary CT 1,8-cineole, and tea tree essential oils prevented the shortening of telomeres after exposure to hydrogen peroxide.[5093] The same research reported that vetiver, black pepper, eucalyptus (*E. globulus*), ginger, clove, and rosemary increased the length of already shortened telomeres. This activity suggests that these essential oils can help maintain the youth and health of cells, or turn back the clock on the cell to make it more youthful depending on the essential oil used. Interestingly, cinnamon and peppermint essential oil decreased the length of telomeres slightly.

☐ Lemon essential oil inhibits *Aspergillus* species and their subsequent production of mycotoxins.[5094] It also reduced the production of the mycotoxin zearalenone by *Fusarium* species.[5095] Zearalenone is an endocrine-disrupting toxin that attaches to estrogen receptors (ERalpha, ERbeta) in a similar manner to 17beta-estradiol (naturally produced estrogen) and both it and its metabolites (beta-zearalenol, alpha-zearalenol) alter hormone production (progesterone, estradiol, testosterone, and cortisol).[5096,5097,5098]

☐ *In vitro* research demonstrated that hydrodistilled lemon peel essential oil is a potent antioxidant.[5099]

☐ Lemon essential oil kills the larvae of the mosquito that carries arbovirus (*Aedes albopictus*).[5100]

☐ A randomized controlled trial demonstrated that an aromatic bath with a blend of 1.0 mL of lemon and 0.5 mL ginger essential oils (10-minutes before each meal for two weeks) prevented salivary gland damage and dysfunction caused by radioactive iodine therapy for thyroid cancer.[5101]

☐ *In vitro* research demonstrated that black pepper (beta-pinene CT), lemon, and tea tree essential oil possess broad-spectrum antimicrobial activity. Interestingly, of the three essential oils tested, lemon (low limonene content—37.5%) was the most active against bacteria and tea tree was the most active against fungi. The Eos demonstrated synergistic antimicrobial activity when used in combination.[5102]

☐ Both lemon and ginger essential oils prevented the formation of biofilms by *Klebsiella* species (*K. ornithinolytica* [now *Raoultella ornithinolytica*], *K. oxytoca*, and *K. terrigena*).[5103]

☐ A combination of lemon and black pepper (beta-caryophyllene CT) essential oil demonstrated an additive toxic effect against ticks (*Rhipicephalus microplus*). The individual essential oils also demonstrated varying degrees of efficacy.[5104]

☐ Animal research shows that oral administration of lemon essential oil improved high-density lipoprotein levels and significantly decreased total cholesterol, triglycerides, and very low-density lipoprotein concentrations.[5105] Additionally, the oil improved antioxidant status, which is important because oxidation of low-density lipoprotein is a contributing factor in atherosclerosis and cardiovascular disease.

☐ Thyme CT gamma-terpinene, lemon CT citral, geranium CT p-menthone, cassia CT cinnamaldehyde, clove CT eugenol, and basil CT 1,8-cineole each demonstrated fungistatic and fungicidal activity toward *C. albicans* and *C. glabrata* isolates with cassia demonstrated the highest activity.[5106]

☐ Oral administration of lemon leaf essential oil (composition not reported) protected against damage to the brain, lung, and intestines caused by aspirin when given before aspirin administration in rats.[5107]

☐ Dispersion of lemon and silver fir essential oils together in a hospital significantly reduced the concentration of airborne bacteria and fungi (40 percent and 60 percent, respectively).[5108]

☐ Lemon, bergamot, and bitter orange were the most effective of citrus oils (lemon, bitter orange, bergamot, sweet orange, and mandarin) tested in the inhibition of mycelial growth of *A. flavus*.[5109] These three oils also were most effective at reducing aflatoxin B1 production.

☐ The essential oils of lemon (fungicidal), cypress (fungicidal), and may chang (fungistatic) each demonstrated anticandidal activity in planktonic (free flowing bacteria in suspension) cells and biofilms (a thin, slimy film

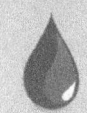

of bacteria adhered to a surface) and cypress increased survival of the tested host in the *Caenorhabditis elegans-Candida* model.[5110]

☐ Loss of synaptic density is found in many brain disorders and associated with cognitive impairment in Alzheimer's disease (AD). A preclinical model of AD found that inhalation of lemon essential oil for one hour daily over a period of thirty days reduced cognitive dysfunction and improved memory in mice with AD.[5111] The researchers discovered that inhalation of lemon oil increased synaptic density and reduced acetylcholinesterase activity. The oil also increased brain-derived neurotrophic factor and enhanced synaptic plasticity.

☐ A heart attack can produce significant anxiety and can cause complications like high blood pressure, which results in a poor prognosis. A randomized, multi-centered, blinded clinical trial found that inhalation of lemon essential oil—5 drops of lemon on a cotton ball placed 20 cm from the individuals for at least two hours—reduced systolic blood pressure and anxiety and improved electrocardiogram results in people diagnosed with a heart attack.[5112] Lemon was inhaled from day one of admittance to a care center and for three consecutive days thereafter.

☐ Estimates suggest that 50 to 90 percent of pregnant women experience nausea and vomiting during their first trimester. This usually occurs between the fourth and sixth week of gestational age and peaks between week eight and twelve. A double-blind, randomized clinical trial found that inhalation of a combination of lemon and peppermint essential oils reduced the time and intensity of nausea and vomiting in pregnant women experiencing mild to moderate nausea and vomiting during six to sixteen weeks of gestational age.[5113] Ten mL of the oil blend (5 percent lemon and 5 percent peppermint oil in a carrier) were provided to the women with instructions to place 3 drops of the blend onto a cotton ball and inhale from the cotton ball kept 3 cm from the nose (three deep breaths through the nose) whenever feeling nausea, and repeat every five minutes as necessary. Another study confirmed this combination is effective for pregnancy-associated nausea. A clinical trial found that inhalation of a combination of lemon and peppermint essential oil significantly reduced the intensity of nausea and vomiting among women during their first trimester of pregnancy.[5114]

☐ Lemon leaf essential oil (29.5% neryl acetate, 13.8% nerol, 12.9% limonene) exhibited antileishmanial activity against intracellular *Leishmania major* amastigotes.[5115] The activity of lemon leaf essential oil was close to Miltefosine, and the oil demonstrated low toxicity to healthy cells and good selectivity toward infected cells. Mastic essential oil also showed moderate activity.

☐ Cinnamon bark, grapefruit, tangerine, and lemon essential oil each inhibited *Bacillus subtilis, Penicillium chrysogenum, Fusarium moniliforme, Aspergillus niger, Aspergillus flavus, Saccharomyces cerevisiae, Escherichia coli, Salmonella abony, Staphylococcus aureus, Pseudomonas aeruginosa,* and *Candida albicans,* with the greatest activity observed from cinnamon bark.[5116] The highest antioxidant activity was found in grapefruit oil, followed by lemon, tangerine, and cinnamon bark.

☐ Textiles treated with may chang and lemon essential oil microemulsion displayed strong antimicrobial activity against skin-associated microorganisms—*E. coli, S. aureus, S. epidermidis,* and *T. rubrum*—and repelled *Ae. aegypti* mosquitoes.[5117]

☐ Distilled lemon peel and lemon leaf essential oil inhibited gram-positive bacteria (*S. aureus* and *S. epidermidis*) but were weakly active against gram-negative bacteria (*S. typhimurium* and *E. coli*); however, isolated limonene was effective against both gram-positive and gram-negative bacteria.[5118] Both oils were also active against larvae and adult mosquitoes (*Ae. albopictus*).

☐ *In vitro* research showed that cold-pressed lemon peel essential oil reduced virulence factors (production and motility) of two *P. aeruginosa* strains.[5119]

☐ Nanogels are commonly used for topical drug delivery due to their ease of use, high loading capacity, and stability. Nanogels with peppermint, dill, and lemon essential oil were evaluated against *Leishmania tropica* and *L. major,* causes of cutaneous leishmaniasis. Of the three oils tested, lemon was the most active, reducing the viability of both species to zero percent at a concentration of 80 mcg/mL.[5120]

☐ Ingestion of distilled lemon or tangerine (35.0% limonene, 18.8% xanthotoxin, 10.0% n-methyl-D3-Aziridine) essential oil produced improvements in a Harwish fruit fly model of Alzheimer's disease. Fruit flies are considered an acceptable organism to investigate neurodegenerative disorders because of their similarities to humans—share several basic biological, biochemical, neurological, and physiological similarities with mammals and have 75 percent of human disease-causing genes. Adding the oils to the diet of fruit flies significantly improved behavioral patterns, protected neurons (reduced cholinesterase and monoamine activities), and reduced oxidative stress, which suggests they may be helpful for the management of Alzheimer's disease.[5121]

☐ Thyme, tea tree, tropical basil, rosemary CT 1,8-cineole, eucalyptus, corn mint, and lavender essential oil each inhibited biofilm-forming *S. aureus*, with thyme and rosemary being the most active in liquid phase.[5122] Thyme was the most active in vapor phase, with varying degrees of inhibition observed depending on the strain of *S. aureus* with tea tree, rosemary, eucalyptus, corn mint, and lavender. Tea tree and lavender oils displayed the weakest activity in the vapor phase.

☐ Oregano CT carvacrol, lemon, lavender, mastic, and mandarin essential oil each inhibited *S. aureus*.[5123]

☐ Comparing the contact toxicity and repellent effects of eight essential oils and carrier oils (clove bud, garlic, *Eucalyptus camaldulensis*, lavender, German chamomile, lemon, jojoba, and sweet almond) against the red flour beetle (*Tribolium castaneum*), clove bud essential oil exhibited the highest repellency effect, while garlic, German chamomile, and lemon were the most toxic.[5124]

☐ A study investigated the chemical composition and biological properties of citrus oils: lemon, sweet orange, grapefruit, and tangerine. All four oils displayed remarkable radical scavenging capacity with grapefruit exhibiting excellent antioxidant activity.[5125] Topical application of the oils showed significant antiedema activity comparable to ibuprofen and reduced the expression of inflammatory cytokines (IL-6, COX-2, NF-κB) to varying degrees. Lemon, grapefruit, and tangerine oil also inhibited lung cancer cells.

☐ Excessive fat accumulation in the thighs (cellulite) is associated with a greater risk of cardiovascular complications and poor glucose management. Plaster therapy is a beauty treatment used to reduce cellulite that involves cleansing and exfoliation of the skin followed by the application of an active agent and plaster. The plaster absorbs heat released by the body, increasing circulation and also improves the penetration of active agents through the skin. Green clay is often used as the plaster due to its mineral content, which facilitates lipolysis (the breakdown of fats in the body). A pilot controlled clinical study evaluated the effects of using lemon essential oil as part of plaster therapy to reduce cellulite.[5126] Six women with a BMI of 18.5 to 29.9 (normal to pre-obese BMI) were evenly divided into an active treatment group and control. Body fat and thigh fat accumulation were tracked for five weeks, with treatments occurring twice weekly. A five-minute dynamic massage was performed with 20 mL of sweet almond oil and 12 drops of lemon essential oil. Then green clay combined with magnesium sulfate in 30 mL of water was applied to the thighs followed by a plaster bandage impregnated with 10 g of magnesium sulfate in 0.5 L of water. Finally, a plastic film was applied on top of the plaster bandage. While wearing the plaster bandage, the participants performed thirty minutes of moderate-intensity aerobic exercise on an exercise bike. The control group performed aerobic exercise only. At the end of the ten sessions, both groups experienced decreased thigh fat, but the participants in the treatment group experienced a significant decrease in cellulite when compared to control.

☐ Test-taking can provoke anxious feelings due to the cognitive, emotional, and physiological strain it involves. Inhalation of lemon essential oil reduced test-taking anxiety in nursing students in a randomized clinical trial.[5127] Five drops of lemon essential oil were added to 100 mL of water in a diffuser and operated for fifteen to twenty minutes prior to the subjects entering the room to take the test. In addition, subjects inhaled 3 drops of lemon essential oil added to a cloth attached to their collar for fifteen minutes prior to the test. Based on all measures, it was determined that inhaling lemon essential oil reduced test-taking anxiety by 43.3 percent.

☐ Pine, melissa (43.0% citral, 25.0% beta-caryophyllene), ginger, lemon, thyme CT thymol, and basil CT methyl chavicol essential oils each showed activity against MRSA and *E. coli*. Thyme completely inhibited all bacteria at all concentrations tested.[5128]

☐ Laboratory research showed that distilled sweet orange, grapefruit, lemon, and tangerine essential oil each have excellent antioxidant activity in the DPPH assay.[5129] Additionally, all four oils reduced inflammation (remarkably increased G1 phase of the cell cycle, which hinders proinflammatory factor expression) and the expression of proinflammatory molecules (COX-2 and TNF-α). Evaluation in a rat model of rheumatoid arthritis demonstrated that the oils reduce inflammation similarly to the NSAID ibuprofen.

☐ Pregnancy-associated nausea can become severe and persistent and lead to dehydration, electrolyte imbalance, and nutritional deficiencies if not managed properly. A case study reports that inhalation of lemon essential oil (2 to 3 drops on a tissue) for five to ten minutes anytime nausea was experienced significantly improved nausea and vomiting among two women during their first trimester.[5130]

☐ Distilled lemon leaf essential oil (30.1% geranial, 27.1% limonene, 22.9% neral) showed high antileishmanial activity against *L. major* with good selectivity.[5131] The same research reported that clementine leaf essential oil was most effective against *L. infantum*.

☐ Oral application of lemon essential oil in gel form (1.56%) twice daily for two days inhibited *C. albicans* in an immunosuppressed rat model of oral candidiasis. Based on the results, the researchers concluded that lemon essential oil could be used to manage oral candidiasis.

☐ Lemon leaf essential oil (60.5% limonene) exhibited significant antioxidant potential in the DPPH (compared to BHT) and linoleic acid peroxidation assays.[5132]

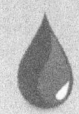

□ Free tea tree and lemon essential oil displayed higher acaricidal activity against phenotypically resistant cattle ticks (*Rhipicephalus annulatus*) when compared to their nanoemulsions.[5133] The combination of the oils was also highly larvicidal, while lemon oil exhibited the most effective ovicidal effects.

□ Researchers evaluated the effects of inhaling lemon, sandalwood (*S. album*), and camphor essential oils on brain activity related to emotions and memory processing via electroencephalography (EEG).[5134] Participants engaged in a working memory task for two minutes and inhaled essential oils for two minutes. Task performance significantly improved after inhaling lemon essential oil and delta and theta band activation in the prefrontal cortex (anterior cingulate gyrus and orbitofrontal cortex, superior temporal gyrus, parahippocampal gyrus, and insula). Sandalwood inhalation resulted in beta and gamma band activation in the prefrontal cortex (cingulate gyrus), which suggests it may help maintain memory. While camphor oil did not significantly alter brain activity, participants rated the task difficulty as easier when they inhaled it.

□ Comparison of citrus leaf essential oils—lemon, calamondin, kaffir lime, and ponderosa lemon (*C. pyriformis*)—showed that lemon displayed the greatest antioxidant capacity in the DPPH assay, while kaffir lime was the lowest.[5135] Each oil exhibited potent antiproliferative activity against cervical cancer cells, with lemon leaf oil being the most active at the higher concentrations.

□ Noroviruses are a group of highly contagious viruses that cause severe vomiting, diarrhea, and stomach pain. They are commonly spread through contaminated food and water or through contaminated surfaces. The murine norovirus is a human norovirus surrogate used in research to assess the potential effects of agents against human norovirus. A preclinical study found that lemon essential oil exerted an immediate reduction in viral infectivity, followed by further reduction twenty-four hours later.[5136] This suggests that lemon essential oil is a promising candidate to reduce norovirus infections.

# LEMON BASIL
## (Pesto Perpetuo)
*Ocimum* × *citriodorum* Vis.

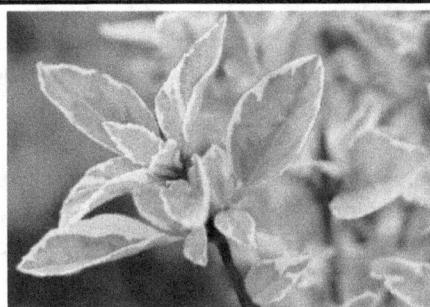

**FAMILY:** Lamiaceae
**NOTE:** Top
**AROMA INTENSITY:** Medium-Strong
**AROMA:** Lemony, citrusy, spicy, herbaceous
**COMMON EXTRACTION METHOD:** Steam distilled from the aerial parts
**POSSIBLE SUBSTITUTE OILS:** Melissa, lemon verbena, lemon myrtle, lemon tea tree, may chang, lemongrass
**BLENDS WELL WITH:** Angelica, bergamot, clary sage, citronella, cumin, geranium, galbanum, kaffir lime, lavender, lemon, lemon eucalyptus, lemon myrtle, lemongrass, lime, may chang, neroli, orange, petitgrain, tangerine, ylang ylang
**SUBCELLULAR LOCALIZATION | EPIGENETIC INFLUENCE:** Currently unknown | Currently unknown
**RECOMMENDED DILUTION RANGE:** 3%–50%; neat for limited conditions

**PRIMARY CONSTITUENTS:**[5137,5138]

| | |
|---|---|
| Geranial | 31.2%–50.9% |
| Neral | 21.8%–39.8% |
| Nerol | 0.0%–14.6% |
| Linalool | 4.5%–7.2% |
| Geraniol | 0.0%–5.1% |
| Caryophyllene Oxide | 0.0%–3.7% |
| Beta-Caryophyllene | 2.1%–3.2% |

**OTHER CONSTITUENTS:** 1,8-cineole, octyl acetate, alpha-terpinolene, alpha-farnesene, estragole (<1.2%), alpha-terpineol, geranyl acetate, alpha-bisabolene, eugenol, benzoic acid, terpinen-4-ol, (E)-alpha-bisabolene

**PREFERRED COMPOSITION FOR CLINICAL USE:**

| Constituent | |
|---|---|
| Geranial | 23%–35% |
| Neral | 18%–28% |
| Nerol | 5%–15% |
| Linalool | 5%–10% |
| Beta-Caryophyllene | 2%–5% |
| Geraniol | 0.5%–5% |

**REPORTED THERAPEUTIC PROPERTIES: Antibacterial**, antifungal, antimicrobial, antiviral, analgesic, relieves headache/migraine, reduces high blood pressure, supports normal cholesterol levels, balances blood sugar levels, supports respiratory function, reduces fever, balances menstruation, reduces mental fatigue, relieves anxiety, **antidepressant**, combats grief, relieves nightmares

**CAUTIONS:**

■ Caution is advised during pregnancy and lactation due to potentially significant citral content. Large doses of citral may negatively affect fetal development according to animal studies.[5139]

■ May mildly interfere with enzymes responsible for metabolizing medications (NSAIDs, proton-pump inhibitors, acetaminophen, antiepileptics, immune modulators, blood sugar medications, blood pressure medications, antidepressants, antipsychotics, diabetic medications, antihistamines, antibiotics, and anesthetics).[5140,5141,5142]

■ Use cautiously with diabetic medications. Large oral doses of citral may improve insulin sensitivity and lower blood-glucose levels according to animal research.[5143,5144]

■ May interact with antibiotics and possibly enhance their effects due to citral content. [5145,5146]

■ There is a moderate risk that lemon basil may interfere with pentobarbital and other barbiturates (medications for anxiety and insomnia) based on citral content.[5147]

■ Dilution is recommended for topical application due to high citral content and the risk for skin irritation or sensitivity.[5148,5149] May also irritate mucous membranes.

**SELECTED EVIDENCE:**

☐ *In vitro* research demonstrates that lemon basil possesses broad-spectrum antimicrobial properties and inhibits *L. monocytogenes, L. ivanovii, E. faecalis. E. faecium, P. vulgaris, S. aureus, S. epidermis,* and *E. coli*.[5150] It was particularly effective against *E. faecalis, E. faecium, P. vulgaris, S. aureus,* and *S. epidermis.*

---

## LEMON CATNIP
### (Lemon Catmint)

*Nepeta cataria* L. var. *citriodora*

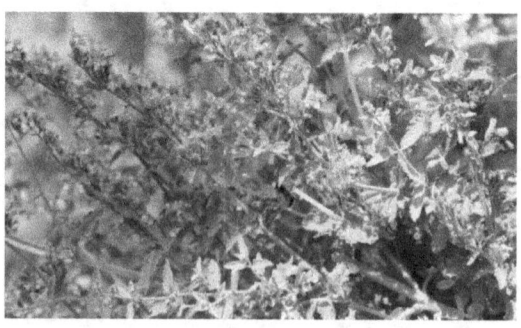

**FAMILY:** Lamiaceae (Labiatae)
**NOTE:** Top-Middle
**AROMA INTENSITY:** Strong
**AROMA:** Lemony, herbaceous, slightly floral
**COMMON EXTRACTION METHOD:** Steam distilled from the aerial parts
**POSSIBLE SUBSTITUTE OILS:** Geranium, rose, palmarosa, citronella, catnip
**BLENDS WELL WITH:** Bergamot, cedarwood, grapefruit, lavender, lemon, lemongrass, lemon eucalyptus, lemon myrtle, lime, marjoram, myrrh, orange, palmarosa, peppermint, rosemary, sandalwood, spearmint
**SUBCELLULAR LOCALIZATION | EPIGENETIC INFLUENCE:** Currently unknown | Currently unknown
**RECOMMENDED DILUTION RANGE:** 3.0%–33.0%; neat for limited conditions

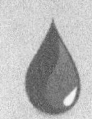

**PRIMARY CONSTITUENTS:**[5151,5152,5153,5154]

| Citronellol CT | | Geraniol/Nerol CT | |
|---|---|---|---|
| Citronellol | 25.2%–39.3% | Geraniol | 23.5%–31.0% |
| Geraniol | 19.6%–32.9% | Nerol | 24.4%–30.7% |
| Nepetalactone Isomers | 0.0%–25.4% | Citronellol | 11.4%–14.0% |
| Geranial | 4.9%–22.3% | Geranial | 4.9%–9.9% |
| Neral | 3.7%–15.4% | Neral | 0.4%–7.1% |
| Beta-Caryophyllene | 0.0%–3.7% | Isoborneol | 0.0%–5.0% |

**OTHER CONSTITUENTS:** *Citronellol CT*—alpha-pinene, sabinene, citronellal, caryophyllene oxide, rhodinol, geranic acid, 11,13-dimethyl-12-tetradecen-1-ol-acetate; *Geraniol/Nerol Ct*—p-cymen-3-ol, linalool citronellal, beta-caryophyllene, beta-caryophyllene oxide, rose oxide, nerol oxide, alpha-pinene, alpha-thujene, trans,trans-photocitral, linalool, linalyl acetate, alpha-humulene, estragole (<0.6%), p-ment-3-en-9-ol

**PREFERRED COMPOSITION FOR CLINICAL USE:**

| Constituent | Citronellol CT |
|---|---|
| **Citronellol** | 25%–35% |
| **Geraniol** | 18%–28% |
| **Nepetalactone Isomers** | 17%–26% |
| **Geranial** | 5%–15% |
| **Neral** | 4%–13% |
| **Beta-Caryophyllene** | 0%–4% |

**REPORTED THERAPEUTIC PROPERTIES:** Antibacterial, antifungal, **antimicrobial**, antiseptic, antispasmodic, analgesic, anti-inflammatory, expels excess gas, aids digestion, encourages sweating, nervine, aids the flow of bile and gastric juices, diuretic, astringent, promotes menstrual regularity, encourages the release of hormones, **supports respiratory function**, balances blood pressure, weight management, reduces headache/migraine, reduces erectile dysfunction, vasodilator, promotes restful sleep, disinfectant, insecticide, **insect repellent**, calming/relaxing, stress management, relieves anxiety, uplifting

**CAUTIONS:**

■ Caution is advised during pregnancy and lactation due to moderate to significant citral content (low risk). Large doses of citral may negatively affect fetal development according to animal studies.[5155]

■ May interact with diabetes medications and cause low blood sugar based on beta-citronellol, citral, and geraniol content.[5156,5157,5158,5159,5160,5161]

■ May interfere with the enzymes responsible for metabolizing medications (NSAIDs, proton-pump inhibitors, acetaminophen, antiepileptics, immune modulators, blood-sugar medications, blood pressure medications, antidepressants, antipsychotics, diabetic medications, antihistamines, antibiotics, and anesthetics).[5162,5163,5164,5165,5166,5167]

■ *Citronellol CT*: May interact with drugs that depress the central nervous system (benzodiazepines, barbiturates, pentobarbital, phenobarbital, secobarbital, fentanyl, morphine, zolpidem, and others). Animal research suggests that catnip extracts or essential oil significantly increases the sleeping time caused by barbiturates, modifies sleep time when administered alone (lower doses increase sleeping time, high doses decrease sleeping time), increases locomotion, amplifies stereotypic behaviors (repetitive and unchanging behaviors without a purpose or goal), and increases susceptibility to seizures based on nepetalactone and citral content.[5168,5169,5170,5171] One case report describes decreased alertness, stomachache, and irritability, followed by prolonged central nervous system depression (lethargy and a hypnotic state) in a nineteen-month-old who ingested raisins soaked in catnip tea and chewing on the tea bag.[5172] The literature also reports altered consciousness similar to marijuana when catnip herb was smoked.[5173]

■ May interact with antibiotics and possibly enhance their effects due to citral content.[5174,5175]

■ Dilution recommended for topical application due to citral and geraniol content. Geraniol is metabolized and autoxidized into metabolites like geranial and neral (citral) and may cause sensitization and irritation when applied topically.[5176] Citral is a known skin and mucous membrane irritant.[5177,5178]

**SELECTED EVIDENCE:**

☐ *In vitro* research demonstrates that lemon catnip essential oil inhibits several gram-positive and gram-negative bacteria, including some common respiratory tract pathogens (*Streptococcus pneumoniae, H. influenza, M. catarrhalis,* and clinical isolates of clinical isolates of *S. aureus*, MRSA, *S. pyogenes, S. pneumoniae, H. influenzae,* and *M. catarrhalis*).[5179] It weakly inhibited *K. pneumoniae* and *E. coli.*

# LEMON EUCALYPTUS
## (Lemon-Scented Gum, Lemon-Scented Iron Gum, Spotted Gum)

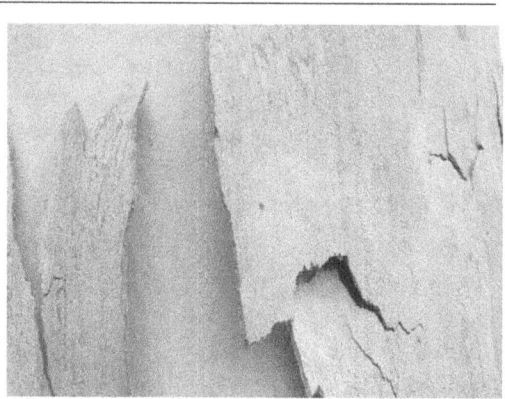

*Corymbia citriodora* (Hook.) K.D. Hill & L.A.S. Johnson, *Eucalyptus citriodora* Hook, *E. maculata* Hook

**FAMILY:** Myrtaceae
**NOTE:** Middle
**AROMA INTENSITY:** Strong
**AROMA:** Fresh, clean, medicinal, lemony
**COMMON EXTRACTION METHOD:** Steam distilled from the leaves and branches
**POSSIBLE SUBSTITUTE OILS:** Citronella, melissa, lemongrass
**BLENDS WELL WITH:** Bay laurel, basil, bergamot, black pepper, blue cypress, cajeput, camphor, cedarwood, chamomile (German, Roman), clary sage, clove, cypress, eucalyptus, frankincense, geranium, ginger, grapefruit, juniper, lavender, lemon myrtle, tea tree, melissa, marjoram, orange, peppermint, pine, ravensara, ravintsara, rosemary, sage, thyme, vetiver, ylang ylang
**SUBCELLULAR LOCALIZATION | EPIGENETIC INFLUENCE:** Currently unknown | Currently unknown
**RECOMMENDED DILUTION RANGE:** 3%–50%; neat for limited conditions

**PRIMARY CONSTITUENTS:**[5180,5181,5182]

| | |
|---|---|
| Citronellal | 40.0%–83.5% |
| Isopulegol | 8.2%–14.6% |
| Beta-Citronellol | 12.6%–13.0% |
| 5-Methyl-2-(2-Hydroxy-2-Propyl) -Cyclohexanol | 0.0%–4.7% |
| 1,8-Cineole | 1.8%–3.4% |
| Beta-Caryophyllene | 1.8%–2.9% |
| Para-Menthane-3,8-diol | 0.0%–2.9% |
| Citronellyl Acetate | 0.0%–2.4% |
| Beta-Pinene | 0.9%–2.2% |
| Linalool | 0.1%–2.2% |
| Methyl Citronellate | 0.0%–2.0% |
| Citronellic Acid(3,7-Dimethyl-6-Octenoic Acid) | 0.0%–1.9% |
| Gamma-Terpinene | 0.3%–1.5% |
| Limonene | 0.5%–1.1% |
| Para-Cymene | 0.6%–1.0% |
| Alpha-Terpineol | 0.1%–1.0% |
| Terpinen-4-ol | 0.0%–1.0% |

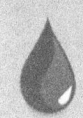

**OTHER CONSTITUENTS:** Alpha-pinene, isoisopulegol, para-mentha-3,8-diene

**PREFERRED COMPOSITION FOR CLINICAL USE:**

| *Constituent* | |
|---|---|
| Citronellal | 65%–80% |
| Beta-Citronellol | 4%–15% |
| Isopulegol | 1%–7% |
| Citronellyl Acetate | 0.5%–4% |
| Beta-Caryophyllene | 0.1%–3% |
| 1,8-Cineole | 0.1%–3% |
| Beta-Pinene | 0.1%–3% |
| Limonene | 0.1%–3% |

**REPORTED THERAPEUTIC PROPERTIES: Antiseptic, antifungal,** antibacterial, antiviral, antioxidant, anti-inflammatory, analgesic (pain relief), expels excess mucous, fever reducer, **insect repellent**, insecticidal, supports respiration, wound healing, calming, uplifting

**CAUTIONS:**
■ None currently known.

**SELECTED EVIDENCE:**
- ☐ Animal research suggests that lemon eucalyptus is anti-inflammatory (possibly through its antioxidant properties), significantly reduced edema, and strongly relieved pain and fever similarly to Aspirin DL-lysine.[5183]
- ☐ Components of lemon eucalyptus and lemon eucalyptus itself mildly inhibited airborne tuberculosis when diffused.[5184] Citronellol, linalool, isopulegol, alpha-terpineol, beta-eudesmol, spathulenol, and T-cadinol were considered the active terpenes in the oil.
- ☐ Animal research suggests that lemon eucalyptus may reduce intestinal contractions associated with diarrhea triggered by acetylcholine.[5185]
- ☐ *In vitro* research suggests that lemon eucalyptus possesses both central analgesic (act directly on the central nervous system to relieve pain by binding to opioid receptors in the brain and possibly the spinal cord) and peripheral analgesic (inhibit the production of pain-producing substances in the peripheral nervous system) properties.[5186]
- ☐ An oral spray containing *E. globulus*, *E. citriodora*, *M. piperita*, *O. syriacum*, and *R. officinalis* (applied five times a day for three days) reduced the severity of the most debilitating symptoms (sore throat, hoarseness, or cough) of upper respiratory tract infections within twenty minutes of application according to a small clinical trial of sixty people.[5187]
- ☐ Lemon eucalyptus exhibited higher inhibition of *Candida* species than two synthetic antifungals (miconazole and clotrimazole) according to *in vitro* research.[5188] Another study found that lemon eucalyptus possesses a wide spectrum of antifungal activity.[5189]
- ☐ Lemon eucalyptus inhibited *T. rubrum*, *H. capsulatum*, *C. albicans* (including drug-resistant), *Cryptococcus neoformans*, and gram-positive bacteria.[5190] *In vitro* research reported that lemon eucalyptus essential oil inhibits gram-negative and gram-positive bacteria and fungi (*Staphylococcus aureus*, *Bacillus subtilis*, *Escherichia coli*, *Aspergillus niger*, and *Rhizopus solani*).[5191]
- ☐ Lemon eucalyptus essential oil repelled the red flour beetle (*Tribolium castaneum* Herbst) for approximately four hours.[5192] It also kills disease-carrying mosquitos: *Anopheles stephensi* Liston, *Culex quinquefasciatus* Say, *Aedes aegypti* Linn, and *Anopheles gambiae* (Giles), which the CDC considers one of the most efficient human malarial vectors in the Afrotropical region.[5193,5194,5195] Another study reports that lemon eucalyptus extracts effectively repel mosquitoes.[5196]
- ☐ *In vitro* research demonstrates that lemon eucalyptus essential oil significantly inhibits *P. gingivalis*, which is a periopathogen associated with periodontitis (a serious gum infection that causes inflammation of the oral cavity and damages or destroys the soft tissue and bone that support the teeth).[5197]
- ☐ Of eleven essential oils tested, lemongrass (*C. citratus*: citronellal formate 42.8%, isobornyl formate 33.5%) essential oil demonstrated the greatest antioxidant activity in the DPPH test and the best overall antimicrobial

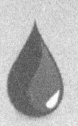
activity.[5198] Lemon eucalyptus (78.2% citronellal), lemon scented iron bark (1,8-cineole 29.2%, bornyl formate 12.3%, isobornyl formate 12.1%), lavender (French: cuminaldehyde 41.3%, linalool 37.3%; and French high altitude: linalyl formate 41.7%, linalool 23.5%), and juniper (*J. communis*: p-mentha-1(7),8 diene 32.3%, delta-cadinene 11.3%) demonstrated very strong antioxidant activity, lavender (Croatian: linalool 47.9%, linalyl formate 22.1%) and rosemary (limonene CT) strong activity, lavender (Croatian, linalool rich 66.8%) moderate activity, and gully gum poor activity (81.7% 1,8-cineole). The other essential oils demonstrated various degrees of antimicrobial activity against the tested bacteria (*E. faecalis, B. cereus, L. monocytogenes, S. aureus*, MRSA, *Salmonella typhimurium, P. aeruginosa, E. coli, K. pneumonia, A. baumannii*, and *Ch. Violaceum*).

☐ Lemon eucalyptus essential oil and salva de marajó (*Lippia origanoides*) essential oils provides good repellency against *Ae. aegypti* mosquitoes when applied at 1,000 PPM.[5199] Salva de marajó was also insecticidal to adults and pupils of the mosquito, while lemon eucalyptus exhibited oviposition-deterrent activity.

☐ Research suggests that lemon eucalyptus has potential to be used as a natural herbicide for weeds. When tested against some of the most noxious weeds in Algeria (*Sinapis arvensis, Sonchus oleraceus, Xanthium strumarium*, and *Avena fatua*), lemon eucalyptus drastically reduced seed germination and seedling growth and completely killed *S. arvensis, S. oleraceus*, and *A. fatua* and severely injured *X. strumarium*.[5200]

☐ *Borrelia burgdorferi* is a diderm bacteria responsible for Lyme disease in the United States. Of thirty-five essential oils screened, garlic, allspice, cumin, palmarosa, myrrh, ginger lily, amyris, thyme, may chang, and lemon eucalyptus each demonstrated excellent activity against *Borrelia burgdorferi*.[5201] Garlic (19% diallyl disulfide), allspice CT eugenol, and myrrh (38% curzerene) were the most active essential oils.

☐ Lemon eucalyptus essential oil demonstrated strong fumigant properties against the spotted-wing drosophila (*D. suzukii*).[5202]

☐ *In vitro* research concluded that lemon eucalyptus essential oil possesses strong antimicrobial activity against *Escherichia coli, Bacillus cereus, Agrobacterium tumefaciens, Pectobacterium atrosepticum, Dickeya solani, Pectobacterium carotovorum*, and *S. aureus*.[5203]

☐ Both lemon eucalyptus and its primary constituent citronellol inhibited sheep gastrointestinal nematodes (*Haemonchus contortus*), with the whole oil showing less toxicity in mice.[5204]

☐ Lemon eucalyptus essential oil improved the antimicrobial activity of multiple antibiotics against drug-resistant *S. aureus* and *E. coli*, despite not showing antimicrobial activity against the two strains alone.[5205]

☐ Lemon eucalyptus essential oil significantly decreased inflammation as evidenced by inhibition of nitric oxide activity in LPS-activated macrophages.[5206] Its fractions also decreased the production of proinflammatory molecules and the expression of COX-2.

☐ Lemon eucalyptus displayed remarkable antioxidant activity in the TAC, DPPH, and ABTS assays, fungitoxic activity, and herbicidal activity (weeds: *Sinapis arvensis, Phalaris canariensis*) that exceeded glyphosate.[5207]

---

# LEMON MYRTLE
## (Lemon Ironwood, Sweet Verbena, Lemon-Scented Myrtle)

*Backhousia citriodora* F. Muell.

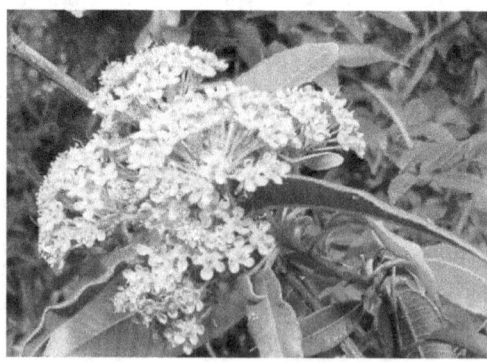

**FAMILY:** Myrtaceae
**NOTE:** Top
**AROMA INTENSITY:** Strong
**AROMA:** Intensely lemon, crisp, fresh, citrusy
**COMMON EXTRACTION METHOD:** Steam distilled from the leaves
**POSSIBLE SUBSTITUTE OILS:** Lemon eucalyptus, citronella, lemon verbena, melissa
**BLENDS WELL WITH:** Bergamot, citronella, grapefruit, lavender, lemon, lemongrass, lime, orange, rosemary, thyme
**SUBCELLULAR LOCALIZATION | EPIGENETIC INFLUENCE:** Currently unknown | Currently unknown
**RECOMMENDED DILUTION RANGE:** 3%–50%; neat for limited conditions

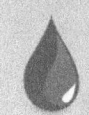

**PRIMARY CONSTITUENTS:**[5208,5209]

| *Citral CT* | | *Citronellal CT* | |
|---|---|---|---|
| Geranial | 46.1%–60.7% | Citronellal | 85.0%–89.2% |
| Neral | 32.0%–40.9% | Isopulegol Isomer (1577) | 4.0%–6.6% |
| Isogeraniol | 1.0%–4.2% | Citronellol | 2.6%–3.4% |
| Isoneral | 0.6%–2.7% | Isopulegol Isomer (1568) | 1.6%–2.5% |
| 6-Methyl-5-Hepten-2-one | 0.1%–2.5% | | |
| Linalool | 0.1%–1.0% | | |

Note: The citral CT appears to be the most common CT available commercially.

**OTHER CONSTITUENTS:** *Citronellal CT*—isopulegol isomer (1631), neral, germacrene D, geraniol, myrcene; *Citral CT*—Citronellal, myrcene, geraniol, nerol

**PREFERRED COMPOSITION FOR CLINICAL USE:**

| Constituent | Citral CT |
|---|---|
| **Geranial** | 43%–55% |
| **Neral** | 35%–45% |
| **Isocitral <Z- + E->** | 0.1%–7% |
| **Geraniol** | 0%–5% |
| **Linalool** | 0%–1% |

* Total citral (geranial + neral) should be ≥ 80%.

**REPORTED THERAPEUTIC PROPERTIES:** Antimicrobial, antiseptic, antibacterial, **antiviral**, antioxidant, disinfectant, **supports immune system function**, decongestant, soothes sore throat, relieves allergies, soothes headache, reduces fever, antispasmodic, relieves stomach discomfort, relaxing, **uplifting**, encourages restful sleep, corrects negative emotions

**CAUTIONS:**

■ *Citral CT*: Caution is advised during pregnancy and lactation due to citral content in the Citral CT (low risk). Large doses of citral may negatively affect fetal development according to animal studies.[5210]

■ *Citral CT*: Use cautiously with diabetic medications. Large oral doses of citral may improve insulin sensitivity and lower blood-glucose levels according to animal research.[5211,5212]

■ *Citral CT*: There is a moderate risk that when lemon myrtle is taken orally it may interfere with enzymes responsible for metabolizing medications (NSAIDs, proton-pump inhibitors, acetaminophen, antiepileptics, immune modulators, blood-sugar medications, blood-pressure medications, antidepressants, antipsychotics, diabetic medications, antihistamines, antibiotics, and anesthetics) due to citral content.[5213,5214,5215,5216]

■ *Citral CT*: May interact with antibiotics and possibly enhance their effects due to citral content.[5217,5218]

■ There is a moderate risk that lemon myrtle may interfere with pentobarbital and other barbiturates (medications for anxiety and insomnia) based on citral content.[5219]

■ *Citral CT*: Dilution is recommended for topical application due to high citral content and the risk for skin irritation or sensitivity.[5220,5221] May also irritate mucous membranes.

**SELECTED EVIDENCE:**

☐ A 10% solution of lemon myrtle oil applied once daily significantly reduced the number of lesions in children with molluscum contagiosum (90% reduction in 9 of 16 children).[5222]

☐ Researchers reported that lemon myrtle oil possesses antibacterial and antifungal properties that were often superior to *Melaleuca alternifolia* (tea tree), which made the study authors conclude that lemon myrtle has potential as an antiseptic and surface disinfectant.[5223]

☐ Lemon myrtle possesses significant antimicrobial activity against *S. aureus, E. coli, P. aeruginosa, C. albicans*, methicillin-resistant *S. aureus* (MRSA), *A. niger, K. pneumoniae*, and P. acnes according to *in vitro* research.[5224]

☐ Lemon myrtle exhibited significant inhibition of MRSA *in vitro*.[5225]

☐ Lemon myrtle essential oil was toxic to engorged female ticks (*Rhipicephalus microplus*) and demonstrated good repellent activity against adult ticks (*Rhipicephalus sanguineus*) up to three hours after application.[5226]

☐ Lemon myrtle displayed strong antioxidant activity in the DPPH and FRAP assays, good antibacterial activity (*S. aureus, S. epidermidis, E. coli, K. pneumoniae*, and *S. epidermidis*), and acted as a potent antibiofilm agent (inhibiting growth and eradicating existing biofilms).[5227]

# LEMON TEA TREE
## (Lemon-Scented Tea Tree)

*Leptospermum petersonii* L.H. Bailey, *L. flavercens* Sm., *L. citratum* Chall. Cheel & Penf.; *L. liversidgei* R.T. Baker & H. G. Smith

**FAMILY:** Myrtaceae
**NOTE:** Middle-Top
**AROMA INTENSITY:** Medium-Strong
**AROMA:** Lemony, citrusy, sweet
**COMMON EXTRACTION METHOD:** Steam distilled from the aerial parts
**POSSIBLE SUBSTITUTE OILS:** White verbena, lemongrass, may chang (citral CT), melissa
**BLENDS WELL WITH:** Big badja gum, cajeput, clove, cypress, eucalyptus, geranium, ginger, gully gum, lavender, lemon, lemongrass, lemon eucalyptus, lime, manuka, niaouli, orange, peppermint, pine, rosemary, spearmint, tangerine, thyme, white verbena
**SUBCELLULAR LOCALIZATION | EPIGENETIC INFLUENCE:** Currently unknown | Currently unknown
**RECOMMENDED DILUTION RANGE:** 1.5%–20%; neat for limited conditions

**PRIMARY CONSTITUENTS:**[5228,5229,5230,5231]

| *L. petersonii—Citral CT* | | *L. liversidgei—Citral CT* | |
|---|---|---|---|
| Geranial | 29.8%–40.7% | Geranial | 31.0%–34.6% |
| Citronellal | 4.3%–33.9% | Neral | 19.7%–21.0% |
| Citronellol | 0.1%–26.8% | Alpha-Pinene | 0.8%–11.0% |
| Neral | 17.9%–23.5% | Linalool | 2.0%–8.5% |
| (E)-Isopulegol | 0.0%–5.2% | Beta-Caryophyllene | 3.0%–3.5% |
| Geraniol | 1.2%–3.9% | | |

Note: A citronella chemotype of lemon tea tree (both *L. petersonii* and *L. liversidgei*) is reported in the literature, but doesn't appear to be available commercially.

**OTHER CONSTITUENTS:** *L. petersonii*—Linalool, alpha-pinene, beta-myrcene, 6-methyl-5-hepten-2-one, citronellyl acetate, geranyl acetate, (E)-caryophyllene, alpha-humulene, beta-chamigrene, alpha-selinene, delta-cadinene, (Z)-isopulegol, bicyclogermacrene, nerol, eugenol; *L. liversidgei*—camphene, beta-selinene, 1,8-cineole, isopulegol, alpha-terpineol, geraniol, caryophyllene epoxide, globulol, karahanaenone, myrtenol, geranyl acetate, germacrene B, spathulenol, cubeban-11-ol, beta-cedrene epoxide, iso-menthol, carvone, eugenol

**PREFERRED COMPOSITION FOR CLINICAL USE:**

| Constituent | *L. petersonii* |
|---|---|
| **Geranial** | 30%–42% |
| **Neral** | 18%–27% |
| **Citronellal** | 12%–25% |
| **Geraniol** | 1%–5% |
| **Citronellol** | 0.1%–5% |
| **(E)-Isopulegol** | 0.1%–5% |
| **Linalool** | 0.1%–3% |

**REPORTED THERAPEUTIC PROPERTIES:** Antibacterial, **antifungal**, antiviral, antimicrobial, antioxidant, anti-infectious, antiseptic, anti-inflammatory, analgesic, wound healing, relieves headache, helps bruises and blisters heal, reduces fever, aids digestion, **weight management**, balances blood sugar levels, encourages restful sleep, nervine, purification, insect repellent, insecticide, relaxing/calming, antidepressant, relieves anxiety, stress management, **antidepressant**

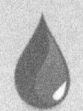

**CAUTIONS:**

■ Caution is advised during pregnancy and lactation due to high citral content. Large doses of citral may negatively affect fetal development according to animal studies.[5232]

■ There is a moderate risk that when lemon tea tree is taken orally it may interfere with enzymes responsible for metabolizing medications (NSAIDs, proton-pump inhibitors, acetaminophen, antiepileptics, immune modulators, blood-sugar medications, blood pressure medications, antidepressants, antipsychotics, diabetic medications, antihistamines, antibiotics, and anesthetics) due to citral content.[5233,5234,5235,5236]

■ Use cautiously with diabetic medications. Large oral doses of citral may improve insulin sensitivity and lower blood-glucose levels according to animal research.[5237,5238]

■ May interfere with pentobarbital and other barbiturates (medications for anxiety and insomnia) based on citral content.[5239]

■ May interact with antibiotics and possibly enhance their effects based on citral content.[5240,5241]

■ Dilution is recommended for topical application due to high citral content and the risk for skin irritation or sensitivity.[5242,5243] May also irritate mucous membranes.

**SELECTED EVIDENCE:**

□ *In vitro* research shows that lemon tea tree essential oil (*L. petersonii*) inhibits *C. albicans*, *Aspergillus niger* and *A. flavus*, largely due to its high citral content.[5244,5245] Animal research confirms the antifungal activity of lemon tea tree essential oil against *Aspergillus* species. No viable fungi were detected in the lungs of animals that inhaled lemon tea tree for three days one to five days after being infected with *A. fumigatus*.[5246]

□ *In vitro* research reports that lemon tea tree essential oil (*L. petersonii*) strongly inhibits the dermatophytes: *Microsporum canis*, *Trichophyton mentagrophytes*, *Trichophyton rubrum*, *Epidermophyton floccosum*, and *Microsporum gypseum*.[5247] The study authors attributed this inhibition effect to geranial content.

□ Lemon tea tree essential oil (*L. liversidgei*) inhibits *S. aureus*, *S. typhi*, and *Myco. Phlei in vitro*.[5248]

□ Lemon tea tree essential oil (*L. petersonii*) is insecticidal against the diamondback moth.[5249] It also provided limited and short-term protection against mosquito bites.[5250]

□ *In vitro* research demonstrated that lemon tea tree CT geranyl acetate essential oil has good antibacterial activity against *Staphylococcus aureus* and *Pectobacterium carotovorum* and reduced *S. aureus* biofilm formation.[5251]

# LEMON VERBENA
## (Lemon Beebrush)

*Lippia citriodora* Kunth, *Aloysia triphylla* (L'Her.) Britton, *A. citriodora* Paláu, *Verbena citriodora* (L'Her.), *V. triphylla* L'Hér.

**FAMILY:** Verbenaceae
**NOTE:** Top
**AROMA INTENSITY:** Medium-Strong
**AROMA:** Fresh, lemony, citrusy, sweet, slightly floral
**COMMON EXTRACTION METHOD:** Steam distilled from the flowering stocks or leaves
**POSSIBLE SUBSTITUTE OILS:** Lemongrass, melissa, lime, rose
**BLENDS WELL WITH:** Bergamot, fennel, grapefruit, lemon, lime, lemongrass, may chang, neroli, niaouli, orange, tangerine
**SUBCELLULAR LOCALIZATION | EPIGENETIC INFLUENCE:** Currently unknown | Currently unknown
**RECOMMENDED DILUTION RANGE:** 3%–20%; neat for limited conditions

**PRIMARY CONSTITUENTS:**[5252,5253,5254]

| Leaves | | Leaves and Stems | |
|---|---|---|---|
| Geranial | 29.5%–38.5% | Geranial | 9.9%–26.0% |
| Neral | 25.7%–27.4% | Limonene | 3.7%–18.6% |

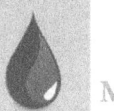

| | | | | |
|---|---|---|---|---|
| Limonene | 5.6%–15.9% | Neral | 6.0%–12.0% |
| Alpha-Zingiberene | 2.8%–5.7% | Methyl Heptenone | 1.4%–7.4% |
| Methyl Heptenone | 0.3%–4.0% | Geraniol | 0.1%–6.0% |
| Geraniol | 0.0%–4.0% | ar-Curcumene | 3.0%–5.7% |
| Geranyl Acetate | 0.9%–4.0% | Spathulenol | 2.5%–5.2% |
| Caryophyllene Oxide | 0.8%–2.5% | Nerol | 0.0%–5.2% |
| ar-Curcumene | 0.6%–1.7% | Caryophyllene Oxide | 3.1%–4.9% |
| | | Beta-Caryophyllene | 0.4%–4.3% |
| *Stems* | | Neryl Acetate | 0.0%–4.0% |
| Geranial | 29.5%–39.6% | | |
| Neral | 23.0%–27.4% | | |
| ar-Curcumene | 1.3%–6.1% | | |
| Limonene | 3.2%–5.4% | | |
| Caryophyllene Oxide | 1.3%–5.1% | | |
| Alpha-Zingiberene | 1.9%–3.7% | | |

**OTHER CONSTITUENTS:** Alpha-pinene, sabinene, beta-pinene, 6-methyl-5-hepten-2-one, myrcene, (E)-beta-ocimene, gamma-terpinene, cis-sabinene hydrate, linalool, beta-thujone, cis-limonene oxide, trans-limonene oxide, citronellal, alpha-terpineol, methyl citronellate, delta-elemene, eugenol, geranyl acetate, trans-caryophyllene, (E)-beta-farnesene, Germacrene D, gamma-cadinene, delta-cadinene, 4-beta-hydroxygermacra-1(10),5-diene, alpha-cadinol, n-nonadecane, n-pentacosane, n-hexacosane, n-octacosane

**PREFERRED COMPOSITION FOR CLINICAL USE:**

| Constituent | Leaves/Stems |
|---|---|
| **Geranial** | 14%–25% |
| **Limonene** | 8%–23% |
| **Neral** | 10%–20% |
| **ar-curcumene** | 3%–10% |
| **1,8-Cineole** | 2%–9% |
| **Beta-Caryophyllene** | 2%–8% |
| **6-Methyl-5-Hepten-2-one** | 1%–7% |
| **Spathulenol** | 1%–7% |
| **Caryophyllene Oxide** | 2%–5% |
| **Geraniol** | 0.1%–5% |
| **Nerol** | 0.1%–5% |
| **Geranyl Acetate** | 0.1%–3% |

**REPORTED THERAPEUTIC PROPERTIES:** Analgesic (pain relief), **anti-inflammatory (especially gastrointestinal)**, antibacterial, antiparasitic, antiseptic, **antiviral**, antispasmodic, stimulates organ (gallbladder, liver, pancreas, thyroid) function, **nourishes the skin,** decreases the appearance of blemishes, reduces fever, aids digestion, increases hair luster, **combats anxiety**, stress management, antidepressant

**CAUTIONS:**

■ Caution is advised during pregnancy and lactation due to high citral content. Large doses of citral may negatively affect fetal development according to animal studies.[5255]

■ May mildly interfere with enzymes responsible for metabolizing medications (NSAIDs, proton-pump inhibitors, acetaminophen, antiepileptics, immune modulators, blood-sugar medications, blood pressure medications, antidepressants, antipsychotics, diabetic medications, antihistamines, antibiotics, and anesthetics).[5256,5257,5258]

■ Use cautiously with diabetic medications. Large oral doses of citral may improve insulin sensitivity and lower blood-glucose levels according to animal research.[5259,5260]

■ May interact with antibiotics and possibly enhance their effects due to citral content.[5261,5262]

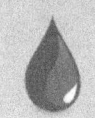

■ There is a moderate risk that lemon verbena may interfere with pentobarbital and other barbiturates (medications for anxiety and insomnia) based on citral content.[5263]

■ Dilution is recommended for topical application due to high citral content and the risk for skin irritation or sensitivity.[5264,5265] May also irritate mucous membranes.

SELECTED EVIDENCE:

□ Lemon verbena essential oil kills murine mastocytoma cancer cells *in vitro*.[5266]

□ Oral administration of 250 mg/kg of lemon verbena oil significantly reduces (85.4%) the protozoan parasite *T. cruzi* in mice.[5267] *T. cruzi* causes the potentially life-threatening illness Chagas disease, also known as American trypanosomiasis. An *in vitro* study found that lemon verbena actively inhibits the parasites *L. chagasi* and *T. cruzi*.[5268]

□ Lemon verbena destroyed *H. pylori* (a pathogen responsible for sores in the stomach and upper part of the small intestine) in mice without promoting resistance (as is often the case with antibiotics).[5269]

□ *In vitro* research concluded that citral and lemon verbena oil prevented yellow fever virus replication before and after attachment to a cell (adsorption).[5270]

□ Lemon verbena oil inactivates and prevents the replication of four dengue viruses before attachment to a cell (adsorption) *in vitro*.[5271]

□ Lemon verbena is considered a promising treatment for candidiasis due to its ability to inhibit several drug-resistant *Candida* species (*C. albicans*, *C. dubliniensis*, *C. glabrata*, *C. krusei*, *C. guilliermondii*, *C. parapsilosis*, and *C. tropicalis*) *in vitro*.[5272,5273]

□ *In vitro* research suggests that lemon verbena inhibits several pathogens including *S. aureus*, *S. epidermidis*, *B. cereus*, *M. luteus*, *Klebsiella* sp., and *P. mirabilis*.[5274]

□ Oral administration of an aqueous lemon verbena extract relieved intestinal spasms in rats.[5275]

□ Lemon verbena essential oil is larvicidal to the *Cx. quinquefasciatus* mosquito.[5276]

□ *In vitro* research demonstrated that lemon eucalyptus essential oil inhibited *Listeria monocytogenes*, *Staphylococcus epidermidis*, *Staphylococcus aureus*, *Saccharomyces cerevisiae*, and *Aspergillus niger*, but not *Escherichia coli*, *Salmonella enteritidis*, *Salmonella typhimurium*, and *Pseudomonas fragi*.[5277] Its primary constituent citral effectively inhibited all microbes. The same study reported lemon verbena is a weak antioxidant, but both the oil and citral were able to protect cells against oxidative damage caused by hydrogen peroxide. When the oil and citral was tested against cancer cells, the oil was active against melanoma, liver, breast, colon, and leukemia cancer cells, whereas citral was very active against breast, colon, and liver cancer cells.

□ Lemon verbena demonstrated good antioxidant properties and prevented lipid peroxidation of sunflower oil better than synthetic BHT.[5278]

□ Lemon verbena and white verbena CT linalool inhibited *Aeromonas* spp., interfered with their biofilm formation, and enhanced the activity of florfenicol against the bacteria.[5279]

□ Oral administration of 10 mL of a syrup containing 1.66 mg/10 mL lemon verbena essential oil and 3.22 mg/10mL quercetin an hour before bedtime for four weeks improved sleep quality in people with insomnia as determined by improvements in Pittsburgh sleep quality index (PSQI) and insomnia severity index (ISI) scores.[5280]

□ Mexican oregano thymol CT, salva de marajó CT carvacrol, salva de marajó CT thymol, white verbena CT citral, and lemon verbena CT citral (in order of highest activity to lowest)—and the isolated constituents para-cymene, geraniol, carvacrol, thymol, citral, and 1,8-cineole—exhibited antigenotoxic activity against ultraviolet radiation (UV)-induced DNA damage that was not related to their antioxidant capacity.[5281]

□ Lemon verbena essential (beta-spathulenol 15.6%, ar-curcumene 14.2%, trans-caryophyllene oxide 14.1%, neral 10.0%) oil killed mouse mast cell neoplasm and human invasive ductal cell carcinoma cancer cells.[5282]

□ *In vitro* research demonstrates that an odd CT of lemon verbena essential oil (beta-spathulenol 15.6%, ar-curcumene 14.2%, trans-caryophyllene oxide 14.1%, neral 10.0%) is significantly active against *Escherichia coli*, *Staphylococcus aureus*, and *Pseudomonas aeruginosa*.[5283]

□ Lemon verbena and peppermint essential oil completely prevented the growth of pathogenic fungi of cultivated button mushroom *in vitro*.[5284]

□ Lemon verbena essential oil extracted from plants grown in two Palestinian regions exhibited good antioxidant activity in the DPPH assay, more potent antibacterial activity against MRSA than ciprofloxacin and ampicillin antibiotics, and greater activity against *C. albicans* than fluconazole.[5285] The oils also inhibited *S. aureus*, *P. vulgaris*, and *K. pneumoniae*, but *E. coli* and *P. aeruginosa* were resistant to the oils. Both oils were cytotoxic to cervical cancer cells, with one oil exhibiting anticancer activity similar to doxorubicin. Lastly, one oil showed potent anti-inflammatory activity (COX-1 and COX-2 inhibition).

- Lemon verbena essential oil inhibited the growth of rodent breast cancer cells *in vitro*, and its oral administration in mice significantly reduced breast tumor size in mice.[5286]
- Lemon verbena, eucalyptus (*E. globulus*), and citronella (*C. winterianus*) showed repellent activity against *Ae. aegypti* mosquitoes.[5287] The researchers further analyzed active constituents within the oils and determined that citronellal, citronellol, citronellyl acetate, and geranyl acetate exhibited synergistic or individual activity in citronella and lemon verbena, while the repellent activity of eucalypts was related to ledol.
- The persistence of parasites (*Trypanosoma cruzi*) combined with a sustained immune response and oxidative stress contributes to the development of cardiac disorders (arrhythmias, ventricular aneurysm, congestive heart failure, thromboembolism, and sudden cardiac death) years or decades after infection. Limonene-enriched and citral/caryophyllene oxide-enriched fractions from lemon verbena essential oil were trypanocidal to *T. cruzi* amastigotes (with comparable efficacy to benznidazole) and improved the efficacy of benznidazole.[5288] The limonene-enriched fraction also decreased oxidative stress, mitochondrial metabolism, and the genotoxicity of benznidazole. Combining the two fractions or combining the limonene-enriched fraction with benznidazole decreased proinflammatory cytokines (IFN-gamma, IL-2, and TNF-α) and increased the anti-inflammatory cytokines (IL-4 and IL-10). Overall, the research suggests that fractions of lemon verbena can modulate immune activity, reduce parasitic load, and help control Chagas disease progression and cardiac symptoms.
- Laboratory research showed that lemon verbena essential oil possesses trypanocidal properties. Further *in vivo* research demonstrated that injection of lemon verbena for twenty days slightly reduced parasitemia by *T. cruzi* on day seven (4.74%), increasing parasitemia reduction significantly by day nine (27.96%) in mice.[5289]

# LEMONGRASS
## (Cochin Grass, Malabar Grass)

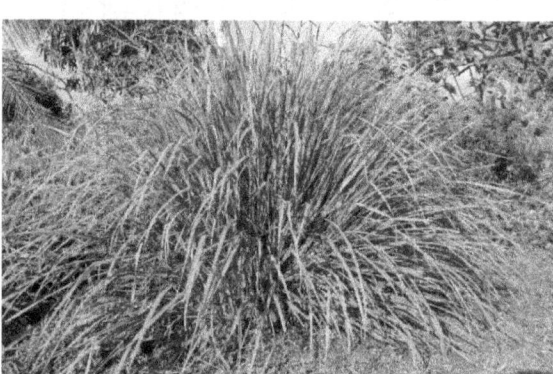

Cochin Grass, Malabar Grass: *Cymbopogon flexuosus* (Nees ex Steud.) J.F. Watson, *Andropogon flexuosus* Nees ex Steud.; *C. citratus* (DC. ex Nees) Stapf, *A. citratus* DC. ex Nees

**FAMILY:** Poaceae (Gramineae)
**NOTE:** Top-Middle
**AROMA INTENSITY:** Strong
**AROMA:** Fresh, lemony, grassy, earthy
**COMMON EXTRACTION METHOD:** Steam distilled from the grass
**POSSIBLE SUBSTITUTE OILS:** Melissa, lemon verbena, lime (distilled), tangerine (distilled), citronella, palmarosa
**BLENDS WELL WITH:** Basil, bergamot, black pepper, camphor, cardamom, cedarwood, citronella, clary sage, copaiba, cypress, fennel, geranium, ginger, grapefruit, lavender, lavandin, lemon, lemon verbena, lime, tea tree, myrrh, neroli, orange, pine, tangerine, thyme, vetiver, ylang ylang
**SUBCELLULAR LOCALIZATION | EPIGENETIC INFLUENCE:** Cytoplasm | *Muscular/Reproductive*
**RECOMMENDED DILUTION RANGE:** 1.5%–20%; neat for limited conditions

**PRIMARY CONSTITUENTS:**[5290,5291,5292,5293,5294,5295]

| *East Indian (Cymbopogon flexuosus)* | | *West Indian (Cymbopogon citratus)* | |
|---|---|---|---|
| Geranial | 25.0%–53.8% | Geranial | 27.0%–48.1% |
| Neral | 19.0%–45.0% | Neral | 19.3%–34.6% |
| Geranyl Acetate | 0.6%–24.0% | Beta-Myrcene | 3.2%–27.0% |
| Caryophyllene Oxide | 1.1%–7.2% | 3-Undecyne | 1.5%–6.1% |
| Geraniol | 0.1%–7.0% | Nerol | 3.1%–3.7% |
| Dodecanoic Acid | 0.0%–5.3% | | |
| Nerol | 0.0%–2.9% | | |

Note: Younger grass (*C. citratus*) will generally produce an essential oil with higher beta-myrcene content.

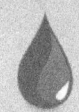

**OTHER CONSTITUENTS:** *East Indian (Cymbopogon flexuosus)*—Neroplomacrol, isamyl acetate, linalool, isogeraniol, alpha-bergamotene, geranic acid, triacontane, beta-caryophyllene, myristoleic acid, 6-Methyl-5-heptene-2-one; *West Indian (Cymbopogon citratus)*—Alpha-pinene oxide, beta-ocimene, linalool, citronellal, geranyl acetate, alpha-bergamotene, gamma-muurolene, isocaryophyllene, delta-cadinene, alpha-cadinol, juniper camphor, di-n-octyl phthalate

**PREFERRED COMPOSITION FOR CLINICAL USE:**

| Constituent | East Indian | West Indian |
|---|---|---|
| Geranial | 35%–50% | 32%–50% |
| Neral | 25%–40% | 24%–40% |
| Geraniol | 3%–10% | 1%–8% |
| Geranyl Acetate | 1.5%–8% | 0.1%–3% |
| Caryophyllene Oxide | 0.1%–5% | 0.1%–2% |
| Limonene | 0.1%–4% | 0%–3% |
| Beta-Caryophyllene | 0.1%–4% | 0%–3% |
| 6-Methyl-5-Hepten-2-one | 0.1%–3% | 1%–3% |
| Nerol | < 0.7% | < 5% |
| Citronellal | < 0.7% | < 5% |
| Beta-Myrcene | < 0.5% | 0%–15% |

Note: Total citral (geranial + neral) should be ≥ 65%.

**REPORTED THERAPEUTIC PROPERTIES:** Analgesic (pain relief), **antifungal**, nervine (calms and soothes the nerves), anti-inflammatory, diuretic, **helps relieve headache**, aids detoxification, supports eye health, anticancer, anticonvulsive, **antimicrobial**, antioxidant, antiallergenic, antiparasitic, antiseptic, antiviral, **astringent**, antibacterial, **antineuralgic**, helps expel excess gas, relieves diarrhea, **insect repellent**, eases sports injuries, aids digestion, helps bruises heal, circulatory aid, reduces fever, deodorant, soothes swollen glands, balances blood sugar levels, sedating, antidepressant, helps ease difficult emotional transitions, energizing, reduces mental fatigue, **stress management**

**CAUTIONS:**

■ Caution is advised during pregnancy and lactation due to high citral and beta-myrcene content. Large doses of citral may negatively affect fetal development according to animal studies.[5296] Extremely high doses of beta-myrcene have been toxic to fetuses according to animal research.[5297]

■ There is a moderate risk that when lemongrass is taken orally it may interfere with enzymes responsible for metabolizing medications (NSAIDs, proton-pump inhibitors, acetaminophen, antiepileptics, immune modulators, blood-sugar medications, blood-pressure medications, antidepressants, antipsychotics, diabetic medications, antihistamines, antibiotics, and anesthetics).[5298,5299,5300,5301]

■ Use cautiously with diabetic medications. Large oral doses of citral may improve insulin sensitivity and lower blood-glucose levels according to animal research.[5302,5303]

■ May interact with antibiotics and possibly enhance their effects.[5304]

■ There is a moderate risk that lemongrass may interfere with pentobarbital and other barbiturates (medications for anxiety and insomnia) based on citral content.[5305]

■ Dilution is recommended for topical application due to high citral content and the risk for skin irritation or sensitivity.[5306,5307] May also irritate mucous membranes.

**SELECTED EVIDENCE:**

☐ Animal research suggests that injection of 200 mg/kg of lemongrass oil into the peritoneal cavity (the fluid-filled gap between the abdominal wall and abdominal organs) promotes destruction of lung sarcoma cells by triggering apoptosis.[5308] The same study concluded that lemongrass oil kills colon and neuroblastoma cancer cells.

☐ Oral administration of lemongrass protected mice from DNA damage and breast cancer caused by the known cancer-causing agent N-methyl-N-nitrosourea.[5309]

☐ Lemongrass oil caused destruction of promyelocytic leukemia cells through activation of both internal and external pathways of apoptosis.[5310]

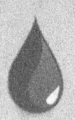 

- A case report describes the use of a combination of the essential oil of lemongrass, eucalyptus, tea tree, clove, thyme and BHT, triclosan, and undenatured alcohol to treat a chronic infection of the lower tibia (osteomyelitis) that was not responding to several courses of IV antibiotics. Amputation of the lower leg was being considered when a physician recommended the leg be opened up and the combination inserted directly into the bone (through a drilled hole, 1 mL per day for forty-eight hours). At three months, the wound and bone healed, and symptoms were resolved.[5311]

- Lemongrass completely inhibits the growth of *H. pylori* (a bacterium involved in the cause of peptic ulcers) without causing bacterial resistance in mice.[5312]

- Animal research suggests that lemongrass influences central nervous system activity and modulates gamma-aminobutyric acid (GABA) activity to help prevent seizures and convulsions.[5313]

- Lemongrass prevented anaphylactic reactions and allergic responses in mice by suppressing immunoglobulin E (IgE) (an antibody that binds to allergens and releases substances from mast cells that cause inflammation and a cascade of events that plays a major role in allergic diseases) activity.[5314]

- *In vitro* research suggests that lemongrass oil can destroy *C. albicans* (including drug-resistant *C. albicans*) and prevent recurrent infections associated with the growth of *C. albicans*.[5315,5316,5317] Another study found that lemongrass oil inhibited oral *C. albicans* infections when it was added to a tissue conditioner typically applied following dental prosthesis insertion *in vitro*.[5318] The same researchers completed a follow up study confirming their previous results, which caused a review article to suggest it is a viable option for dental stomatitis.[5319,5320] One study determined that lemongrass was a valuable remedy for oral and vaginal candidiasis after concluding that it inhibits both mycelial and yeast-form growth of *C. albicans*.[5321] A nanoemulsion of *C. citratus* essential oil demonstrated improved antimicrobial activity against nine bacteria and ten fungal strains of clinical relevance.[5322]

- Animal research concluded that lemongrass protected brain neurons from death due to glutamate toxicity.[5323]

- Lemongrass oil demonstrated better anticandidal activity than the anticandidal drugs miconazole and clotrimazole *in vitro*.[5324]

- Researchers concluded that lemongrass oil inhibited several *Candida* species and bacteria known to cause hospital-acquired infections according to *in vitro* research.[5325]

- The vapor of lemongrass oil inhibited both penicillin-susceptible and penicillin-resistant respiratory pathogens (*H. influenzae, S. pneumoniae, S. pyogenes*, and *S. aureus*) *in vitro*.[5326]

- *In vitro* research concluded that lemongrass oil inhibits *C. albicans, S. aureus, P. aeruginosa*, and *S. bovis*.[5327] Other research demonstrates that lemongrass essential oil inhibits multi-drug-resistant *A. baumannii* (a gram-negative and opportunistic bacterial pathogen that causes healthcare-acquired infections).[5328]

- Lemongrass strongly inhibits the growth and survival of several fungi (*A. alternata, A. niger, F. oxysporum*, and *P. roquefortii*) and yeasts (*C. albicans, C. oleophila, H. anomala, S. cerevisiae, S. pombe, S. uvarum*, and *M. fructicola*) *in vitro*.[5329] Lemongrass essential oil also inhibits dermatophytes (*Trichophyton rubrum* and *Trichophyton mentagrophytes*) linked to athlete's foot without harming healthy cells.[5330]

- *In vitro* research suggests that lemongrass inhibits elastase activity (an enzyme involved in the breakdown of elastin and a causal factor in lung connective tissue diseases, disruption of the body's ability to kill pathogens, and delayed wound healing).[5331] The researchers concluded that topical administration may be beneficial for bullous pemphigoid (a skin condition that causes the formation of large blisters) and pulmonary emphysema (a chronic lung condition characterized by enlargement of the air sacs in the lungs).

- Lemongrass can prevent mosquito bites (up to 98.9%) for up to eighty-eight minutes, which is better than two chemical repellents, but not as effective as DEET (98.5%, for up to 182 minutes).[5332]

- Topical application of a shampoo and cream with lemongrass cleared pityriasis versicolor (a chronic yeast infection of the skin that causes scaling and discoloration) in 60% of people receiving the treatment.[5333]

- A topical gel containing 2% lemongrass oil improved gum health and effectively treated periodontitis (inflammation and infection of the gums that damages the tissue and bone that supports your teeth) in the fifteen people included in the study.[5334]

- Oral administration of lemongrass protected the stomach against ulcers caused by ethanol and the NSAID indomethacin by modulating prostaglandin production in mice.[5335]

- *In vitro* research reported that lemongrass oil provides a sun protection factor (SPF) of 6.282.[5336]

- Animal research suggests that lemongrass prevents edema (swelling caused by excess fluid trapped in body

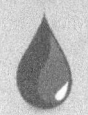

tissues), and strongly relieves pain, decreases inflammation, and reduces fever as well as lysine acetylsalicylate (a NSAID drug that reduces fever, inflammation, and pain).[5337]

☐ Lemongrass decreases pain at doses of 25 to 200 mg/kg in mice.[5338] The researchers found that lemongrass influences both the central and peripheral nervous systems to reduce pain, which makes it a useful natural pain reliever for neuropathy.

☐ Lemongrass may help control leishmaniasis (a disease caused by the bite of the sand-fly parasite characterized by skin sores or organ dysfunction) by promoting apoptosis of Leishmania species.[5339,5340,5341]

☐ *In vitro* research suggests lemongrass oil inhibits *Entamoeba histolytica* (an anaerobic parasitic protozoan that may cause intestinal disorders and bloodstream, liver, brain, and lung infections).[5342]

☐ Lemongrass protects against tissue alteration caused by N-methyl-N-nitrosourea (a cancer-causing alkylating agent) in mice by triggering apoptosis and reducing cellular reproduction.[5343]

☐ Animal research suggests that lemongrass oil reduces anxiety by influencing the GABAergic system (a system of structures that release or bind gamma-aminobutyric acid and regulate anxiety, muscle tension, memory, and convulsive activity).[5344]

☐ *In vitro* research suggests that a 2% lemongrass oil shampoo inhibits Malassezia furfur (a yeast associated with dandruff).[5345]

☐ Oral administration of 100 mg/kg lemongrass oil daily for twenty-one days reduced total blood cholesterol in mice.[5346]

☐ Lemongrass oil reduces inflammation by inhibiting the production of the proinflammatory cytokines (IL-1 beta and IL-6).[5347] Citral triggered PPARa and PPARy gene expression to suppress the COX-2 enzyme (an enzyme present in cells when inflammation occurs, like arthritis).[5348]

☐ *In vitro* research concluded that lemongrass effectively inhibits *T. cruzi* trypomastigotes and amastigotes (a parasite that can cause fever, anorexia, myocarditis, swollen lymph nodes, and the simultaneous enlargement of the spleen and liver).[5349]

☐ Animal research concluded that lemongrass oil relieves anxiety, is sedating, and prevents convulsions.[5350]

☐ Administration of 400 or 800 mg of lemongrass essential oil per kg reduced blood sugar levels in diabetic rats.[5351] Another study found that oral administration of lemongrass essential oil (400 mg/kg) reduced blood sugar levels in diabetic rats with the whole oil or constituents interacting with three key targets—PTP-1B (myrcenol, linalool, α-elemol and β-Eudesmol), PPAR-γ (myrcenol, linalool, α-elemol and β-Eudesmol), and DPP-IV ((E,E)-farnesyl primethyl dihydrazide)—involved in diabetes.[5352] Lemongrass increases PPAR-γ activation, which regulates gene transcription involved in glucose metabolism and glucose disposal (the rate of glucose uptake from the blood and peripheral tissues). Lemongrass improves insulin sensitivity by inhibiting PTP-1B activity, which plays an important role in regulating insulin signaling. DPP-IV activity is blocked by lemongrass essential oil. DPP-IV is an enzyme that remove incretin (a hormone that stimulates insulin secretion after meals) from your body. Inhibiting DPP-IV allows incretin to stay in the body longer and triggers the release of insulin to reduce blood sugar levels.

☐ *In vitro* research suggests that peppermint, thyme, cinnamon, and lemongrass oils inhibited the respiratory tract pathogens *S. pyogenes* (a bacterium that causes strep throat, scarlet fever, impetigo, cellulitis, and tonsillitis) and *S. pneumoniae*.[5353]

☐ Oral administration of lemongrass oil (500 mg/kg) prevented malaria (86.6%) caused by a parasitic infection in mice, which is slightly less effective than the antimalarial drug chloroquine (100%).[5354]

☐ *In vitro* research found that lemongrass oil inhibits several microorganisms responsible for urinary tract infections (85.7% efficiency against *K. pneumoniae*, 50% against *E. aerogenes*, 89.9% against *E. coli*, 16.6% against *P. mirabilis*, and 50% against *M. morganii*).[5355]

☐ Lemongrass oil has better antimicrobial properties against clinically significant oral pathogens than standard oral antiseptics (chlorhexidine digluconate) according to *in vitro* research.[5356]

☐ Application of oregano and lemongrass oil to ground beef controls the growth of *S. enteritidis* (a very common foodborne pathogen that may cause stomach flu, fever with rash, serious bacterial infections of the blood, and systemic bacterial infection) during refrigerated storage.[5357]

☐ Lemongrass oil increases the effectiveness of phenoxyethanol (a chemical preservative often used in cosmetics).[5358]

☐ A hair tonic with a 10% lemongrass essential oil solution (applied twice daily) significantly reduced dandruff by day 7 of use and provided even greater results after 14 days of use.[5359]

□ A 0.25% lemongrass mouthwash reduced plaque and improved gingival index (a measurement of periodontal disease based on severity and location of lesions) better than the standard drug treatment of chlorhexidine.[5360] Another clinical study found that swishing with an essential oil mouthwash containing lemongrass (0.5%), thyme (0.5%), rosemary (0.5%), PEG-40-hydrogenated-castor-oils-emulsifier (6%), and water (92.5%) for twenty minutes following scaling and root planing significantly reduced microbe populations in the mouth and prevented subgingival biofilm formation.[5361]

□ Inhalation of 3 to 6 drops of lemongrass essential oil reduces anxiety and tension immediately following inhalation.[5362]

□ *In vitro* research demonstrated that lemongrass essential oil kills and inhibits multi-drug-resistant *Acinetobacter baumannii* strains (an opportunistic gram-negative bacterium that commonly infects those with a compromised immune system).[5363]

□ Lemongrass essential oil demonstrated 100% efficacy against the *Rhipicephalus microplus* tick even at the lowest concentration tested (1%).[4932] *C. citratus* essential oil killed the *Aedes aegypti* and *Anopheles dirus* during immature stages.[5364] It also kills the *An. gambiae* mosquito.[5365]

□ *In vitro* research demonstrates that lemongrass essential oil prevents the formation of *S. mutans* biofilms, suggesting it may be useful in the prevention of dental cavities.[5366]

□ Lemongrass essential oil (*C. citratus*) was insecticidal to the housefly (*Musca domestica*).[5367]

□ *In vitro* research demonstrates that lemongrass essential oil (*C. citratus*) inhibits bacteria isolated from pet turtles (*E. tarda, A. hydrophila, C. freundii, P. mirabilis, S. enterica*), many of which were resistant to multiple antibiotics.[5368]

□ Of eleven essential oils tested, lemongrass (*C. citratus*: citronellal formate 42.8%, isobornyl formate 33.5%) essential oil demonstrated the greatest antioxidant activity in the DPPH test and the best overall antimicrobial activity.[5369] Lemon eucalyptus (78.2% citronellal), lemon scented iron bark (1,8-cineole 29.2%, bornyl formate 12.3%, isobornyl formate 12.1%), lavender (French: cuminaldehyde 41.3%, linalool 37.3%; and French high altitude: linalyl formate 41.7%, linalool 23.5%), and juniper (*J communis*: p-mentha-1(7),8 diene 32.3%, delta-cadinene 11.3%) demonstrated very strong antioxidant activity, lavender (Croatian: linalool 47.9%, linalyl formate 22.1%) and rosemary (limonene CT) strong activity, lavender (Croatian, linalool rich 66.8%) moderate activity, and gully gum poor activity (81.7% 1,8-cineole). The other essential oils demonstrated various degrees of antimicrobial activity against the tested bacteria (*E. faecalis, B. cereus, L. monocytogenes, S. aureus*, MRSA, *Salmonella typhimurium, P. aeruginosa, E. coli, K. pneumonia, A. baumannii*, and *Ch. Violaceum*).

□ Lemongrass essential oil (*C. flexuosus*) demonstrated significant antimicrobial activity against rapidly growing mycobacteria (*Mycobacterium fortuitum, M. massiliense*, and *M. abscessus*) when the essential oil was used in its nanoemulsion form.[5370]

□ Lemongrass (*C. citratus*) and cade juniper (*J. oxycedrus*) essential oil each demonstrated significant activity against *Trypanosoma brucei brucei*, which was attributed to citral and alpha-pinene respectively.[5371] The oils were also nontoxic to macrophage cells.

□ Lemongrass (*Cymbopogon citratus*) essential oil and its main compound (citral) demonstrated antimicrobial activity against primary dental colonizers and bacteria associated with cavities (*Actinomyces naeslundii, Lactobacillus acidophilus, S. gordonii, S. mitis, S. mutans, S. sanguinis*, and *S. sobrinus*).[5372] The researchers concluded that lemongrass should be incorporated into dental products like mouthwash due to its low toxicity to human cells.

□ *In vitro* research demonstrated that lemongrass (*C. citratus*; 59.2% neral, 22.5% beta-pinene) essential oil actively interfered with HIV-1 Tat protein function. The Tat protein plays a central role in and drastically enhances HIV transcription (resulting in the production of multiple copies of the viral RNA and improved infectivity).[5373]

□ Both lemongrass (*C. citratus*) and geraniol accelerated the gastric healing process by 34.5% (10mg/kg body weight EO) and 80.57% (3mg/kg body weight geraniol) in mice.[5374] They promoted stomach ulcer healing following an ethanol-induced ulcer. Interestingly, citral was not effective.

□ Lemongrass (*C. flexuosus*) and citral both prevented oxidative stress in the liver caused by acetaminophen at an oral dose of 400 mg/kg body weight.[5375] The study determined that lemongrass and citral modify drug metabolizing enzymes but do not affect the detoxification of acetaminophen.

□ Lemongrass (*C. citratus*) essential oil killed prostate (two cell lines: one highly metastatic, one low) and

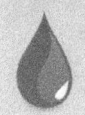

glioblastoma cancer cells.[5376] Its primary constituent, citral, was equally effective against cancer cell lines. Interestingly, when lemongrass and tsauri grass were combined, antagonism (prostate LNCaP, highly metastatic), additive (prostate PC-3, lowly metastatic), indifferent (glioblastoma SF-767), and synergistic (glioblastoma SF-763) interactions were observed. The same research reported that lemongrass oil acted as a good antioxidant.

☐ Lemongrass (*C. citratus*) essential oil prevented the growth of *Penicillium expansum* (blue mold) on bread when used in the vapor phase.[5377]

☐ Lemongrass (*C. citratus*) and geranium essential oil significantly reduced viral replication and viral infectivity and reduced the cytopathic (damage to living cells) effect of the Ross River virus when introduced prior to, during, or after viral adsorption (the first step in the viral life cycle where the virus attaches to the cell).[5378]

☐ A tea tree and lemongrass (*C. flexuosus*) essential oil solution reduced *Candida* biofilms form dentures.[5379]

☐ Lemongrass (*C. flexuosus*) exhibited anticancer activity against breast cancer cells. The oil was cytotoxic to the cells and suppressed the expression of the HSP90 gene (a chaperone protein involved in tumor growth).[5380] New cancer drugs target the inhibition of HSP90 to improve cancer therapy.

☐ Rosemary CT 1,8-cineole, lemongrass (*C. citratus*), and wintergreen essential oils each repelled, knocked down, and were lethal to moths (*Anarsia lineatella*).[5381] Rosemary was the most effective repellent and most lethal.

☐ Lavender, lemongrass (*C. citratus*), marjoram, peppermint, tea tree, and rosewood essential oils all exhibited significant activity against clinical isolates of multidrug-resistant *Burkholderia cepacia* complex (a group of bacteria commonly resistant to antibiotics that cause health problems in people with weakened immune systems and are known to cause healthcare related infections).[5382]

☐ Both lemongrass (*C. flexuosus*) and thyme essential oils were active against foodborne pathogens (multidrug-resistant *Enterococcus* spp. and *Aeromonas* spp.) and eradicated preformed biofilms from *Aeromonas* spp.[5383]

☐ *In vitro* examination of sixty essential oils demonstrated that sandalwood (Indian, Australian, and Hawaiian), melissa, lemongrass (*C. flexuosus*), cilantro, cassia, cinnamon, patchouli, and vetiver essential oils possess remarkable anticancer (two breast cancer cells) and antifungal (*Aspergillus niger, Candida albicans,* and *Cryptococcus neoformans*) activities.[5384]

☐ Fungal pathogens have caused significant declines in economically and agriculturally important animal species, like bees and bats. Current drug antifungals have limited use due to their toxicity to sensitive animal species. Cinnamon bark, citronella, and lemongrass essential oils each significantly inhibited *Ascosphaera apis* and *Pseudogymnoascus destructans*, the causative agents of chalkbrood disease among honeybee larvae and white-nose syndrome among bats, respectively.[5385]

☐ Lemongrass essential oil demonstrated remarkable 100% inhibition of MRSA *in vitro*.[5386] Lemon myrtle, mountain savory, cinnamon bark, and melissa also exhibited significant activity against MRSA.

☐ Lemongrass (*C. citratus*) essential oil repelled, irritated, and was toxic to nymphs of the spined soldier bug (*Podisus nigrispinus*; a predatory bug of gypsy moth caterpillars and the larvae of beetles).[5387]

☐ Lemongrass (*C. citratus*) inhibited *Staphylococcus* strains isolated from newborns in laboratory and animal (rat) research.[5388] The oil has the same therapeutic effect as vancomycin in *S. aureus* when tested in rats.

☐ A lemongrass (*C. citratus*) essential oil nanoemulsion effectively killed gastrointestinal nematodes (*H. contortus*) in sheep with greater efficacy and less toxicity than the free essential oil.[5389]

☐ Laboratory research concluded that oregano CT carvacrol, thyme CT thymol, cassia, lemongrass (*C. flexuosus*), and Western red cedar (arborvitae) essential oils exhibit very strong antimicrobial activity against drug resistant pathogens (*Pseudomonas aeruginosa, Proteus vulgaris, Citrobacter koseri, Klebsiella pneumoniae, Candida albicans,* and *C. parapsilosis*).[5390] Ten essential oils—oregano, thyme, clove, arborvitae, cassia, lemongrass, tea tree, eucalyptus (*E. radiata*), lavender, and clary sage —were tested, and these five were the most effective. The researchers also concluded the essential oils were not genotoxic (cause DNA damage) compared to control cells. In addition, each of the oils exhibited antioxidant activity, with cassia and oregano demonstrating the greatest increase in total antioxidant status, followed by tea tree, thyme, clove, clary sage, eucalyptus, arborvitae, and lavender.

☐ Thyme CT thymol, garlic, tea tree, cajeput, may chang, lemongrass (*C. citratus*), and verbena CT citral exhibited fungistatic activity (100%) against *F. culmorum* and *F. graminearum*, and all but garlic (89.4%) were 100% fungistatic against *F. avenaceum* and *F. oxysporum*.[5391]

☐ Lemongrass (*C. citratus*) essential oil with 60% citral exhibited moderate inhibitory activity of acetylcholinesterase (AChE), while isolated citral (geranial + neral) exhibited potent activity. By inhibiting AChE, the oil or citral can increase both the level and duration of action of the neurotransmitter acetylcholine. Acetylcholine is important for memory, learning ability, alertness, and attention.

- *Helicobacter pylori* is a bacterium that lives in the digestive tract that can cause sores and ulcers in the lining of the stomach or upper part of the small intestine. Thyme, lemongrass, Virginia cedarwood, and melissa essential oils were the most active of 26 commercial essential oils examined against *H. pylori*.[5392] Oregano, tea tree, pine, and silver fir were also bactericidal.

- Lemongrass (*C. citratus*) and its constituents citral (geranial + neral) and geraniol inhibited biofilm formation by *E. coli* through inhibition of glucosyltransferase activity and glucans production.[5393]

- *In vitro* research showed that cinnamon bark, oregano, thyme CT thymol, lemongrass (*C. flexuosus*), allspice, palmarosa, and amyris all significantly inhibited *S. aureus* in the stationary phase, which is when the size of a bacterial population remains constant, even though some cells continue to divide and others begin to die.[5394]

- Various concentrations of both eucalyptus (*E. globulus*) and lemongrass (*C. citratus*) were effective adulticidal agents against female mosquitoes (*Aedes aegypti* and *Aedes albopictus*) and houseflies (*Musca domestica*).[5395] The highest synergistic activity among the two oils was observed at 2.5% of each oil, which caused a 100 percent knockdown rate and 98.9 percent mortality.

- The itch mite (*Sarcoptes scabiei*) is a parasitic mite that burrows into the skin and causes the condition known as scabies. Lemongrass concentrations of 5% and 10% killed itch mites within twenty-five and ten minutes respectively and concentrations ranging from 0.1%–10% significantly decreased hatching rate of itch mite eggs.[5396]

- Lemongrass (*C. citratus*) essential oil killed adult and nymph Asian longhorned ticks (*Haemaphysalis longicornis*)—mortality rate of 98 percent and 100 percent respectively.[5397]

- Oregano CT carvacrol, thyme CT thymol, cassia, lemongrass (*C. flexuosus*), and Western red cedar essential oils each demonstrated significant antibacterial and antifungal activity against several drug-resistant pathogens (*Ps. aeruginosa, Pr. vulgaris, C. koseri, K. pneumoniae, C. albicans,* and *C. parapsilosis*) known to infect the skin.[5398] The oils were not toxic to healthy keratinocytes and increased total antioxidant status in the cells as well.

- Lemongrass (*C. citratus*) essential oil demonstrated insecticidal and repellent activity against the granary weevil (*Sitophilus granarius*).[5399] Isolated geranyl acetate and geranial were more effective insecticides than the whole oil.

- Laboratory research concluded that clove bud and lemongrass (*C. citratus*) essential oil exhibited anticandidal activity and combining the oils or fractions of the oils increased the antifungal activity.[5400]

- *Candida tropicalis* forms biofilms on prosthetics and other medical devices, posing a risk of serious skin infection and shortened lifespan of the prosthesis. Lemongrass (*C. citratus*) essential oil inhibited *C. tropicalis* and prevented its formation of biofilms on silicone rubber prosthesis.[5401]

- Lemongrass (*C. citratus*) essential oil relieved anxiety in zebra fish possibly through influencing $GABA_A$ receptors.[5402] Its main constituents citral and geraniol also exhibited a synergistic anxiolytic activity.

- *In vitro* research demonstrated that lemongrass (*C. citratus*) essential oil possesses anticancer activity against lung cancer cells by triggering apoptosis and cell cycle arrest.[5403]

- Repeated oral administration of lemongrass (*C. citratus*) essential oil (50, 100, and 200 mg/kg body weight per day for 14 weeks) reduced breast cancer tumors in mice without showing signs of toxicity.[5404] In addition the oil reduced tumor necrosis (a sign of more aggressive breast cancer) and mitosis (cellular division where the cell makes an exact copy of the original cell's chromosomes during growth and repair). Cancer is a disease of mitosis where genes inside cells that control mitosis are overrun and the cell replicates itself in an out-of-control manner creating cancer cells. The essential oil was primarily comprised of 40.5% geranial, 31.8% neral, and 13.6% myrcene.

- Oral administration of lemongrass (*C. citratus*) essential oil—50 or 100 mg/kg body weight for fifteen days—substantially protected the brains of rats against aluminum chloride toxicity.[5405] The oil markedly reduced abnormal behaviors caused by the aluminum and normalized antioxidant to free radical ratios.

- Lemongrass (*C. citratus*) essential oil was toxic to *Dolops discoidalis* (a marine parasite) and *Argulus* sp. (a marine parasite).[5406]

- Lemongrass (*C. citratus*) and citronella (*C. nardus*) essential oils exhibited larvicidal activity against the Asian blue tick (*Rhipicephalus microplus*), while corn mint essential oil was toxic to engorged females.[5407]

- *Toxoplasma gondii* is a parasite excreted in cat feces. Humans can accidentally ingest the parasites if they come in contact with cat feces and then touch their mouth causing toxoplasmosis. A laboratory study found that lemongrass (*C. citratus*), marjoram, and citronella (*C. nardus*) inhibited *T. gondii*, with citronella having a high selectivity index.[5408] Based on this, the authors concluded that citronella may be a potential solution for treating toxoplasmosis.

- Knowing that lemongrass possesses strong antimicrobial activity, researchers investigated its effects on polymicrobial (more than one species of microbe) biofilms. What the researchers found was that both

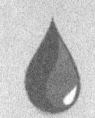

lemongrass (*C. flexuosus*) and isolated citral reduced polymicrobial (*S. aureus* and *C. albicans*) biofilm biomass and cell viability.[5409] Lemongrass and citral interfered with the ability of the microbes to adhere to surfaces by counteracting nucleic acids, proteins, and carbohydrates in the biofilm.

☐ Microencapsulation—in maltodextrin or gelatin—of lemongrass (*C. citratus*) essential oil improved the oil's thermal and oxidative stability.[5410]

☐ Cinnamon (plant part and composition not reported; commercial sample) and lemongrass (species not identified) essential oils both inhibited planktonic *C. albicans* and eradicated established biofilms when used at eight times the minimum inhibitory concentration.[5411]

☐ Medical professionals and researchers are searching for alternatives to control epilepsy because the current drugs used often have undesirable effects. Exposure—by immersion—to lemongrass (*C. citratus*) essential oil prior to a seizure-inducing chemical (pentylenetetrazole) increased time to the first seizure in zebrafish.[5412] The researchers found that the efficacy of lemongrass oil partially involved $GABA_A$ receptors, and the oil decreased malondialdehyde and nitric oxide levels, while increasing glutathione and catalase in the brain. Isolated geranium and citral in combination exhibited a synergistic anticonvulsant activity. Altogether, the research suggests that lemongrass, geraniol, and citral have anticonvulsant and neuroprotective activity that may be beneficial for epilepsy treatment.

☐ Lemongrass (*C. citratus*) was toxic to fish ectoparasites (*Dolops discoidalis* and *Argulus* sp.).[5413]

☐ Lemongrass, ginger, black pepper, turmeric, and kaffir lime, as well as isolated constituents (citral, camphene, camphor, delta-3-carene, limonene, myrcene, alpha-pinene, beta-pinene, and terpinen-4-ol), reduced adipogenesis and triggered lipolysis (the breakdown of fats in the body) in a laboratory model of cellulite control that investigated the use of botanicals as part of an herbal compress.[5414] Adipogenesis is the process that adipocytes are created, and more adipocytes as we age makes cellulite more visible.

☐ A clinical study found that topical application of lemongrass essential oil every day for thirty days significantly decreased pain associated with rheumatoid arthritis.[5415] Pain levels gradually decreased over the course of thirty days, decreasing from an average of eight (on a scale of one to ten) to five at the end of the study.

☐ A lemongrass (*C. citratus*) essential oil nanoemulsion showed notable antibacterial and antibiofilm (forming and preformed) activity against *Enterococcus faecalis* and some antioxidant activity.[5416] Based on the results, the researchers recommended further exploration of the nanoemulsion in dental practice for infected teeth during root canal.

☐ Application of clove basil (para-cymene and thymol as major constituents) or lemongrass (*C. citratus*) essential oil to cotton were insecticidal to pests of cotton.[5417]

☐ Lemongrass (*C. citratus*) essential oil was insecticidal to the black cutworm (*Agrotis ipsilon*).[5418]

☐ Red blood cells (erythrocytes) exposed to high blood sugar (glucose) levels are constantly subjected to assault from reactive oxygens species, which oxidizes their membranes and damages red blood cells. Lemongrass (*C. citratus*) essential oil improved antioxidant activity and prevented the oxidation of red blood cell membranes in laboratory research.[5419] The research suggests that lemongrass essential oil may protect red blood cells against oxidation caused by high blood sugar levels.

☐ Mountain savory, nutmeg, and lemongrass (*C. flexuosus*) were each fungicidal to *A. niger* and *A. ochraceus*.[5420] The oils also inhibited the production of ochratoxin A by the fungus *A. ochraceus* and the production of aflatoxin B1 and aflatoxin B2.

☐ Thyme (near equal thymol and para-cymene) and lemongrass (*C. citratus*) significantly inhibited *B. cinerea* and their vapors reduced gray mold, with thyme being more effective.[5421]

☐ Lemongrass (*C. citratus*) essential oil was acaricidal to cattle tick (*Rhipicephalus microplus*) larvae.[5422] Interestingly, combining lemongrass with kaffir lime reduced the efficacy of lemongrass oil.

☐ Lemongrass (*C. citratus*) essential oil was cytotoxic and neurotoxic to the Asian longhorned tick (*Haemaphysalis longicornis*), triggering mitochondrial calcium overload and depolarization. Isolated citronellal was also effective.[5423]

☐ Lemongrass (*C. citratus*) displayed significant antioxidant activity in the DPPH, FRAP, and ABTS assays and significant anti-inflammatory activity as compared to Diclofenac sodium.[5424] Computer modeled (*in silico*) molecular docking revealed that beta-caryophyllene possesses considerable binding potential with human peroxiredoxin 5 (PB5) and cyclooxygenase 2 receptor (COX-2) proteins with significant stable interactions. PB5 is a protein and enzyme found in various tissues that responds to oxidative stress and is involved in the initiation of inflammatory processes. Higher levels of PB5 are noted in people with chronic inflammatory conditions like osteoarthritis, tendonitis, and myasthenia gravis.[5425,5426,5427] It has even been implicated in neuroinflammation in people with autism.[5428] COX-2 plays a major role in inflammatory reactions and regulated pain responses. Reducing its activity is associated with decreased pain and inflammation. The researchers concluded that beta-caryophyllene possesses drug likeness and "can be used as a potential candidate to replace the synthetic anti-inflammatory drugs."

- Maxillofacial silicone prosthetics are used by dentists to restore or replace structures of the mouth, jaw, or face. Adherence of fungi to these prosthetics is an important medical risk. *In vitro* research concluded that lemongrass (*C. citratus*) essential oil is fungicidal to *Candida albicans* biofilms established on the surface of maxillofacial silicone prosthetics in a dose-dependent manner.[5429] Concentrations of 2.5% were as effective as 20% nystatin.

- Adipocytes are fat cells that specialize in storing energy as fat. They also play a role in appetite regulation (secrete adipokines), and control thermogenesis (the production of heat in the human body by physiological processes). Adipogenesis is the process whereby adipocytes develop and accumulate as adipose tissue. Enlargement of existing adipocytes (hypertrophy) increases the risk of obesity and cardiovascular disease. There are three general types of adipocytes: white adipocytes that store energy as a single large lipid (fat) droplet and are important for endocrine system function; brown adipocytes, which store energy as multiple lipid droplets specifically for use as fuel to create body heat; and brite (inducible brown, beige, or brown-in-white) adipocytes that may form by conversion of white adipocytes to brown adipocytes and are important for obesity control because of their activity in metabolism and fatty acid utilization. White adipocytes may adopt characteristics of brown adipocytes and vice versa depending on diet and temperature. Laboratory research found that lemongrass (*C. flexuosus*) and isolated citral reduced lipid accumulation by decreasing lipid uptake, increasing the breakdown of triglycerides into glycerol and free fatty acids to use for energy (lipolysis), reducing the production of adipocytes (differentiation), and downregulating the creation of lipids.[5430] This suggests that lemongrass oil may reduce fat accumulation and therefore combat weight gain and obesity.

- Lemongrass (*C. flexuosus*), citronella (*C. winterianus*), and palmarosa essential oil each exhibited activity against MRSA, with the strongest activity observed with lemongrass oil.[5431] Isolated citronellol, citral, and geraniol were also active, with the efficacy of citronellol exceeding whole oils.

- Lemongrass essential oil was larvicidal to *Ae. aegypti* mosquitoes, showing similar activity to the commercial growth inhibitor diflubenzuron.[5432]

- Chitosan nanomatrix incorporated with lemongrass (*C. citratus*) essential oil significantly protected the deterioration of pear millet (*Pennisetum glaucum*) seeds by *A. flavus*, aflatoxin B1 contamination, and lipid peroxidation.[5433] The findings suggest the oil can be used to control foodborne molds and aflatoxin B1 contamination in foods.

- *Trichophyton* is a genus of fungi that infect humans and cause conditions such as athlete's foot, ringworm, jock itch, and similar infections of the nail, beard, skin, and scalp. Japanese researchers investigated the benefits of lemongrass (*C. citratus*) essential oil applied in shoes to prevent athlete's foot. A combination of citral and perillaldehyde produced antimicrobial activity against *Trichophyton mentagrophytes*, *Bacillus subtilis*, and *Candida albicans*, which was superior to citronellal, cinnamaldehyde, cuminaldehyde, hydroxycitronellal, and vanillin.[5434] The researchers concluded that the combination is a sage and useful way to disinfect shoes.

- Lemongrass (*C. citratus*) essential oil showed antifungal activity against yeasts commonly found in the oral cavity (*Candida* spp., *Cl. lusitaniae*, *I. orientalis*, *M. guillermondii*, *P. norvegensis*, *Cy. Jadinii*, *K. marxianus*, and *S. cerevisiae*) that cause oral thrush (oral candidiasis).[5435] The oil also improved the antifungal activity of nystatin (additive).

- A computer-based molecular docking and *in vitro* study found that lemongrass (*C. citratus*) essential oil inhibits the growth of a fungal strain associated with aspergillosis (*Aspergillus fumigatum*).[5436] Citral (geranial + neral) effectively bound to UDP-glycosyltransferase, Glucosamine-6-phosphate synthase, and chitin synthase and displayed drug likeness.

- Nanoencapsulated lemongrass (*C. flexuosus*) essential oil with nearly 98% citral and incorporated into nanofibers demonstrated antifungal activity against *Aspergillus* fungi, reducing mycelial growths and the production of ochratoxin A.[5437]

- Microencapsulated lemongrass (*C. citratus*) essential oil had antibacterial activity against *S. aureus* and *E. coli* and displayed antioxidant activity in the DPPH assay.[5438]

- Lemongrass (*C. citratus*) essential oil exhibited insecticidal and repellent activity against the maize weevil (*Sitophilus zeamais*).[5439]

- Thyme, oregano, lemongrass (*C. citratus*), spearmint, and rosemary essential oils were each inhibited multidrug-resistant foodborne pathogens isolated from raw milk (*Escherichia, Enterobacter, Citrobacter,*

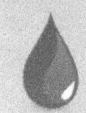

*Proteus, Klebsiella*, and *Staphylococcus*) but were ineffective against *Pseudomonas*.[5440] Thyme was the most active followed by oregano.

☐ Of five essential oils tested (lemon verbena, two morphotypes of *Croton cajucara*, lemongrass, and *Lippia gracilis*), *L. gracilis* and lemongrass (*C. citratus*) showed the best antimicrobial activity against *Aeromonas* strains, interfering with biofilm formation and consolidated biofilm.[5441] Lemon verbena, lemongrass, and *L. gracilis* each exhibited synergistic activity when combined with florfenicol.

☐ Lemongrass (*C. citratus*) essential oil inhibited MRSA and strongly potentiated the activity of tetracycline, streptomycin, and amoxicillin against MRSA.[5442]

☐ Both lemongrass (*C. citratus*) and isolated citral were toxic to the eastern subterranean termite (*Reticulitermes flaviceps*) in vapor phase, with citral being more toxic.[5443]

☐ *In vitro* research concluded that lemongrass (*C. citratus*) essential oil improved the antibiofilm activity of chlorhexidine against microcosms (polymicrobial) biofilms in human saliva and exposed to sucrose.[5444]

☐ Essential oils are susceptible to volatilization and oxidation when added to food matrices, making a barrier material necessary to preserve their activity. The bioactivity of microencapsulated (as a protective barrier) and free lemongrass essential oil was compared.[5445] The microencapsulated oil showed good antioxidant activity in the DPPH, ABTS, and FRAP assays, and was bactericidal to gram-positive (*B. cereus, C. perfringens, L. innocua, S. aureus*) and gram-negative bacteria (*C. jejuni, E. coli. S. typhimurium*). However, the antibacterial activity of lemongrass decreased after microencapsulation.

☐ Lemongrass (*C. citratus*), basil, and turmeric essential oils were toxic to the red flour beetle (*Tribolium castaneum*), which was improved when combined with diatomaceous earth in emulsion form.[5446]

☐ Tarragon, lemongrass (*C. citratus*), and lavender essential oil were each insecticidal against the bean weevil (*Acanthoscelides obtectus*).[5447]

☐ Ginger, lemongrass (*C. citratus*), and turmeric each displayed antioxidant activity in the DPPH and ABTS assays, inhibited gram-negative (*K. oxytoca, P. vulgaris, E. coli, P. aeruginosa*) and gram-positive (*S. aureus, E. faecalis, L. grayi, M. luteus*) bacteria and yeasts (*C. albicans, S. cervisiae*), and mutagen-protecting effects.[5448]

☐ Lemongrass (*C. flexuosus*) essential oil inhibited the growth of *A. hydrophila* of fish origin, with greater activity against oxytetracycline-resistant strains than oxytetracycline-sensitive strains.[5449] Computer-based molecular docking study showed that some of the constituents of the oil strongly bonded to DNA gyrase-B—a vital macromolecule in bacterial cell—comparably to oxytetracycline, inhibiting the enzyme's efficacy.

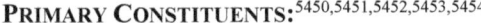

# LIME
## (Key Lime)

*Citrus × aurantifolia* (Christm.) Swingle (pro sp.)
[medica × sp.], *Limonia aurantifolia* Christm.

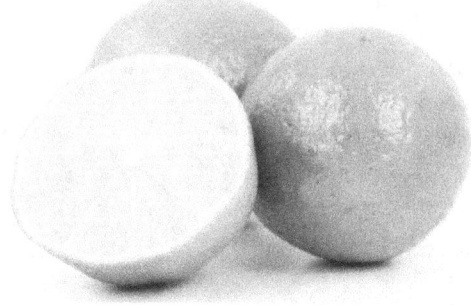

**FAMILY:** Rutaceae
**NOTE:** Top
**AROMA INTENSITY:** Medium
**AROMA:** Sharp, citrusy, fruity, tart
**COMMON EXTRACTION METHOD:** Cold-pressed/expressed or hydrodistilled from the fruit peel (rind)
**POSSIBLE SUBSTITUTE OILS:** Orange, lemon, tangerine, bergamot, grapefruit, neroli, petitgrain
**BLENDS WELL WITH:** Bergamot, camphor, carrot seed, cassia, chamomile (German, Roman), cinnamon, citronella, geranium, grapefruit, lavender, lemon, lemon verbena, lemongrass, tea tree, neroli, nutmeg, orange, palmarosa, patchouli, petitgrain, pine, ravensara, rose, rosemary, sage, Spanish sage, tangerine, vetiver, ylang ylang
**SUBCELLULAR LOCALIZATION | EPIGENETIC INFLUENCE:** Currently unknown | Currently unknown
**RECOMMENDED DILUTION RANGE:** 3%–50%; neat for limited conditions

**PRIMARY CONSTITUENTS:**[5450,5451,5452,5453,5454]
*Cold-pressed/expressed*

| | |
|---|---|
| Limonene | 39.9%–94.4% |
| Gamma-Terpinene | 0.1%–20.6% |

| | |
|---|---|
| Sabinene | 0.1%–19.6% |
| Beta-pinene | 0.1%–19.2% |
| Geranial | 0.0%–6.1% |
| Para-Cymene | 0.0%–5.6% |

*Distilled*

| | |
|---|---|
| Limonene | 49.7%–53.8% |
| Gamma-Terpinene | 0.0%–16.5% |
| Beta-Pinene | 0.9%–12.6% |
| Alpha-Terpineol | 0.4%–7.4% |
| Alpha-Terpinene | 0.4%–3.0% |

*Commercial Samples (Distilled)*

| | |
|---|---|
| Limonene | 45.9%–55.0% |
| Gamma-Terpinene | 12.4%–12.8% |
| Terpinolene | 7.0%–9.6% |
| Alpha-Terpineol | 3.7%–6.7% |
| Para-Cymene | 2.6%–2.8% |
| Beta-Pinene | 2.6%–2.7% |
| Alpha-Terpinene | 2.5%–2.7% |

**OTHER CONSTITUENTS:** *Cold-pressed/expressed*—Alpha-thujene, alpha-pinene, myrcene, beta-caryophyllene, (Z)-beta-ocimene, (E)-beta-ocimene, terpinolene, citronellal, linalool, trans-alpha-bergamotene, thymol methyl oxide, terpinen-4-ol, neral, alpha-terpineol, germacrene D, beta-bisabolene, neryl acetate, (E,E)-alpha-farnesene, citronellol; *Distilled*—Alpha-thujene, alpha-pinene, myrcene, beta-caryophyllene, trans-alpha-bergamotene, beta-bisabolene, gamma-terpineol

**PREFERRED COMPOSITION FOR CLINICAL USE:**

| Constituent | Distilled | Cold-pressed |
|---|---|---|
| **Limonene** | 40%–60% | 40%–58% |
| **Gamma-Terpinene** | 5%–15% | 7%–15% |
| **Terpinolene** | 5%–12% | < 1% |
| **Alpha-Terpineol** | 4%–10% | 0.1%–2% |
| **Beta-Pinene** | 1%–10% | 8%–20% |
| **Alpha-Terpinene** | 2%–5% | – |
| **Para-Cymene** | 2%–5% | < 1.5% |
| **Alpha-Pinene** | 0.5%–3% | 1%–3% |
| **Myrcene** | 0.5%–3% | 0.5%–2% |
| **Geranial** | 0%–3% | 1%–4% |
| **Neral** | 0%–3% | 1%–3% |
| **Beta-Bisabolene** | 0.1%–2% | 1%–5% |
| **Trans-Alpha-Bergamotene** | 0.1%–2% | 0.5%–2% |
| **Neryl Acetate** | 0%–2% | 0.1%–2% |
| **(E,E)-Alpha-Farnesene** | 0.1%–2% | 0%–2% |
| **Terpinen-4-ol** | 0%–2% | 0.1%–1% |
| **Geranyl Acetate** | 0%–2% | 0.1%–1% |
| **Sabinene** | 0.1%–2% | 1%–5% |

**REPORTED THERAPEUTIC PROPERTIES:** Antiseptic, antiviral, astringent, anti-bacterial, **anti-inflammatory**, appetite stimulant, antispasmodic, disinfectant, **reduces fever**, stops excess bleeding, **aids immune function**, regenerative, circulatory aid, reduces appearance of blemishes, encourages restful sleep, **weight management**, antidepressant, reduces anxiety, **stress management**, uplifting

**CAUTIONS:**

■ Very photosensitizing (cold-pressed/expressed). Avoid sun exposure to area of application for at least twelve hours after topical application.[5455]

■ May interfere with enzymes responsible for metabolizing medications (NSAIDs, proton-pump inhibitors, acetaminophen, antiepileptics, immune modulators, blood-sugar medications, blood pressure medications, antidepressants, antipsychotics, diabetic medications, antihistamines, antibiotics, and anesthetics).[5456]

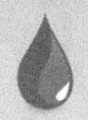

■ May interact with anticholinergic (drugs used for asthma, incontinence, gastrointestinal cramps, muscular spasms, depression, and sleep disorders) and cholinergic medications (drugs used to reduce urinary retention, diagnose myasthenia gravis, and for glaucoma) based on AChE inhibitory activity.[5457,5458]

**SELECTED EVIDENCE:**

☐ Oral administration of lime oil promoted weight loss, and prevented obesity caused by ketotifen (a drug associated with weight gain) in mice.[5459]

☐ *In vitro* research suggests that lime oil significantly inhibits the pathogenic fungi *M. hiemalis* and *F. proliferatum*.[5460]

☐ Distilled lime oil prevented the spread of colon cancer cells by triggering apoptosis *in vitro*.[5461]

☐ *In vitro* research suggests that lime oil inhibits acetylcholinesterase (AChE) and mildly inhibits butyrylcholinesterase (BChE) enzyme activity.[5462,5463] Lime oil also had the highest free-radical-scavenging (antioxidant) activity of three citrus oils tested. Inhibition of AChE prevents the breakdown of acetylcholine, which is essential for memory and thinking. People with neurodegenerative diseases make less acetylcholine, and the diseases often break it down at a faster rate leading to acetylcholine deficits. Selective inhibition of BChE is also desirable in neurodegenerative diseases because it interferes with acetylcholine activity. In addition, BChE is often found in the plaques and tangles in the brains of people with Alzheimer's disease.[5464]

☐ *In vitro* research found that lime oil inhibits both gram-negative and gram-positive bacteria including *S. aureus, B. subtilis, K. pneumoniae, P. vulgaris, P. aeruginosa*, and *E. coli*.[5465]

☐ Oral administration of hydrodistilled lime essential oil (100 mg/kg) reduces inflammation by decreasing cell migration (white blood cell movement to tissues), cytokine production, and protein extravasation (the movement of proteins excreted by white blood cells from capillaries to surrounding tissues, which plays a key role in inflammation).[5466]

☐ Laboratory research demonstrates that lime leaf essential oil inhibits the phytopathogen *Xanthomonas citri* subsp. *citri* (Xcc)—one of the most devastating phytopathogens of citrus fruits worldwide. The same researchers reported that constituents (alpha-terpineol and citral; citral and citronellal; citral and geraniol; and citronellal and geraniol) within essential oils produce a synergistic antimicrobial effect.[5467]

☐ Roman chamomile (isobutyl angelate as the primary constituent), lime, and lavender essential oils effectively inhibited the parasite *Haemonchus contortus*, hindering adult worm motility completely within the first eight to twelve hours.[5468]

☐ Distilled lime peel and leaf essential oil inhibited bacteria associated with cavities, with promising activity against *Streptococcus mutans* and *Lactobacillus casei*.[5469]

☐ Intraperitoneal administration of lime essential oil (100 mg/kg BW) in diabetic rats resulted in significant reductions in fasting blood and liver glucose levels while simultaneously increasing liver glycogen levels.[5470] Improvements in lipid levels (significant LDL decrease and HDL increase) was also observed suggesting amelioration of diabetic-related cardiovascular problems.

☐ Steam-distilled lime essential oil exhibited good antioxidant activity in the DPPH and ABTS assays.[5471] Based on the findings, the study authors examined the protective effects of lime essential oil against high cholesterol in rats. Oral administration of 0.74 g/100 g and 2.23 g/100 g in their diets improved total serum cholesterol, triglycerides, LDL cholesterol, and liver enzymes. Lime oil also improved overall health of the rats in terms of obesity, atherogenic index, and fatty liver.

☐ Oral administration of distilled unripe lime essential oil (49.0% germacrene A, 14.3% alpha-pinene, 12.2% germacrene B, and 11.3% bornane) reduced benign prostatic hyperplasia (BPH; enlarged prostate)—less thickened glandular epithelium, smaller acini, fewer prostatic secretions, and more fibromuscular stroma—and significantly reduced prostate-specific antigen (PSA) in rats.[5472] Improved histomorphological characteristics were also observed in the testis, kidneys, and liver of the lime-treated group.

☐ Lime peel and leaf essential oil exhibited ovicidal (capable of killing eggs) activity against *Aedes aegypti* mosquitoes.[5473] Citral from the leaf oil also exhibited significant ovicidal activity (higher than the whole oil).

☐ A study tested the ability of five essential oils to act as herbal pesticides by inhibiting native and recombinant acetylcholinesterases (AChE) from the Asian blue tick (Rhipicephalus microplus).[5474] Lime, eucalyptus (*E. globulus*), sweet orange, and peppermint essential oils inhibited susceptible AChE extract (S.AChE) and native resistant AChE extract (R.AChE). Eucalyptus also inhibited recombinant enzyme (rBmAChE1), exhibiting significant inhibition at the highest concentration tested. Citronella (*C. winterianus*) did not inhibit AChE, but displays acaricidal activity via another mechanism making it a viable option for ticks resistant to organophosphates.

- ☐ The abnormal proliferation of vascular smooth muscle cells (VSMCs) plays a major role in cardiovascular diseases like atherosclerosis. VSMCs are found in the vascular wall and responsible for the tone and contractions of arteries, which regulates blood pressure and flow in response to specific metabolic demands. Cold-pressed lime essential oil inhibited the proliferation of VSMCs, suggesting lime oil may be helpful for abnormal proliferation of VSMCs associated with cardiovascular diseases.[5475] The researchers concluded that lime oil represents a promising "nature-based therapeutic agent for obstructive vascular disease."

- ☐ Delayed onset muscle soreness (DOMS) is muscle pain that occurs a day or two—at least twelve hours and up to six days—after physical exertion. A controlled clinical study evaluated the effects of massage with lime essential oil to massage with normal lotion and no massage after exercise (three times weekly for four weeks) for DOMS. Massage was performed for thirty minutes following the exercise and lactic acid and pain levels monitored. The lime massage group experienced the greatest reductions in lactic acid levels and pain intensity when compared to lotion massage and no massage.

# LOVAGE
## (Lovage Leaf, Garden Lovage)

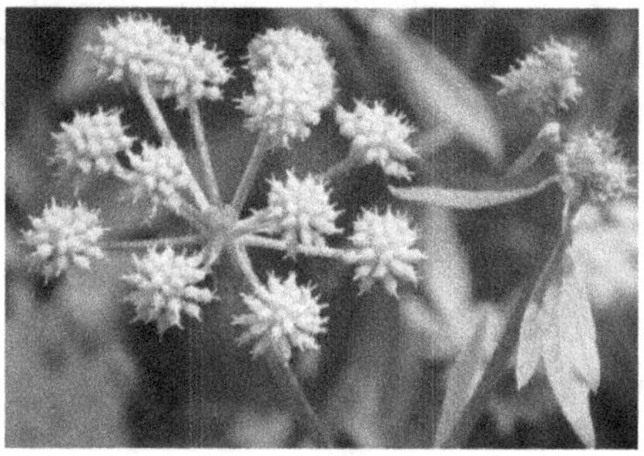

*Levisticum officinale* W.D.J. Koch, *L. paludapifolium* Asch.,
*Hipposelinum levisticum* (L.) Britton & Rose

**FAMILY:** Apiaceae (Umbelliferae)
**NOTE:** Middle
**AROMA INTENSITY:** Medium
**AROMA:** Fresh, sweet, green, spicy
**COMMON EXTRACTION METHOD:** Steam distilled from the leaves; may also be distilled from the aerial parts, seeds, roots, flowers, fruits, or stems
**POSSIBLE SUBSTITUTE OILS:** Cardamom, betony, juniper (needles), balsam fir, clary sage
**BLENDS WELL WITH:** Basil (sweet), bay laurel, cassia, cinnamon, clove, frankincense, hairy basil, holy basil, lavender, myrrh, oakmoss, ocotea, patchouli, opoponax, rose, tamala
**SUBCELLULAR LOCALIZATION | EPIGENETIC INFLUENCE:** Currently unknown | Currently unknown
**RECOMMENDED DILUTION RANGE:** 3%–20%; 50% for some conditions

**PRIMARY CONSTITUENTS:**[5476,5477,5478,5479,5480,5481,5482]

*Leaves*

| | |
|---|---|
| Alpha-Terpinyl Acetate | 26.1%–70.0% |
| Beta-Phellandrene | 9.6%–44.0% |
| (Z)-Ligustilide | 3.9%–32.1% |
| Myrcene | 1.3%–6.2% |
| (Z)-Beta-Ocimene | 0.0%–6.2% |

*Roots*

| | |
|---|---|
| (Z)-Ligustilide | 9.4%–79.7% |
| Beta-Phellandrene | 0.4%–62.5% |
| Alpha-Terpinyl Acetate | 0.0%–46.4% |
| Phenylacetaldehyde | 0.0%–29.0% |
| (Z)-3-Butylidene Phthalide | 0.0%–28.6% |
| Pentylcyclohexa-1,5-diene | 0.0%–12.3% |
| Trans-Sabinyl Acetate | 0.0%–12.1% |
| P-Allylanisole | 0.0%–7.0% |
| Methyl Hexadevenoate | 0.0%–6.1% |

*Aerial Parts*

| | |
|---|---|
| Alpha-Terpinyl Acetate | 1.6%–52.4% |
| Beta-Phellandrene | 12.9%–42.5% |
| (Z)-Ligustilide | 0.0%–29.7% |
| Alpha-Terpineol | 0.8%–27.9% |
| (Z)-Beta-Ocimene | 0.0%–7.5% |
| Dehydro-1,8-Cineole | 0.0%–6.8% |
| Gamma-Terpinene | 0.0%–4.9% |

*Seeds*

| | |
|---|---|
| Beta-Phellandrene | 63.2%–79.3% |
| (Z)-Beta-Ocimene | 0.1%–9.2% |
| (Z)-Ligustilide | 0.0%–5.6% |

*Flowers*

| | |
|---|---|
| (Z)-Ligustilide | 53.4% |
| Beta-Phellandrene | 26.6% |
| Alpha-Terpinyl Acetate | 10.4% |

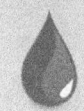

*Fruits*

Beta-Phellandrene          34.4%–47.8%

(Z)-Ligustilide          35.1%–38.5%

OTHER CONSTITUENTS: *Leaves*—alpha-pinene, sabinene, camphene, alpha-phellandrene, (E)-beta-ocimene, gamma-terpinene, p-menth-2,4(8)-diene, (4E,6Z)-allo-ocimene, alpha-terpineol, geranyl acetate, (E)-ligustilide; *Roots*—nonane, alpha-pinene, camphene, sabinene, beta-pinene, 2,3-dihydro-1,8-cineole, myrcene, 2-methyl-6-methylene, alpha-phellandrene, terpinolene, linalool, pentylbenzene, 2-methylene-6,6-dimethyl, alpha-terpineol, geraniol, bornyl acetate, perrillyl alcohol, beta-elemene, germacrene D, beta-selinene, bornyl 2-methylbutyrate, (E)-ligustilide, methyl pentadecanoate, methyl hexadecadienoate; *Seeds*—alpha-pinene, limonene, alpha-terpinyl acetate, alpha-phellandrene, myrcene; *Aerial Parts*—alpha-thujene, alpha-pinene, camphene, beta-pinene, alpha-terpinene, o-cymene, trans-verbenol, neryl acetate, dibutyl phthalate, myrcene; *Fruits*—alpha-pinene, sabinene, beta-pinene, myrcene, alpha-phellandrene, (E)-ligustilide, linalool, alpha-terpinyl acetate, alpha-humulene, E-Butylidene phthalide, Z-Butylidene phthalide; *Flowers*—myrcene, alpha-phellandrene, (E)-beta-ocimene, (E)-ligustilide

PREFERRED COMPOSITION FOR CLINICAL USE:

| *Constituent* | |
|---|---|
| **Alpha-Terpinyl Acetate** | 45%–60% |
| **Beta-Phellandrene** | 10%–20% |
| **Beta-Myrcene** | 2%–7% |
| **(Z)-Ligustilide** | 3%–8% |
| **Alpha-Pinene** | 1%–5% |

REPORTED THERAPEUTIC PROPERTIES: Antibacterial, antifungal, antiseptic, antiparasitic, antispasmodic, analgesic, antirheumatic, anti-inflammatory, aids circulation, balances menstruation, relieves painful menstruation, expels excess mucus, supports respiratory function, eases cough, supports liver and kidney function, soothes chronic skin conditions, aids detoxification, relieves gout, nervine, **diuretic**, relieves fever, soothes stomachache, expels excess gas, soothes sore throat, aphrodisiac, releases traumatic memories

CAUTIONS:

■ Avoid during pregnancy and lactation due to the estrogenic activity of (Z)-ligustilide and *A. sinensis* (also with significant ligustilide content) and potential trans-sabinyl acetate content (root oil). (Z)-ligustilide may prolong menstruation and stimulate or relax the uterus.[5483,5484,5485] Trans-sabinyl acetate is toxic to developing embryos and prevents implantation during days 0–4 of gestation according to animal research.[5486,5487] Trans-sabinyl acetate can cause abortions and maternal toxicity (which indicated a greater susceptibility to trans-sabinyl acetate toxicity during pregnancy) in animals.[5488] The researchers concluded that trans-sabinyl acetate possesses significant antifertility activity during the pre-implantation period, and attribute the fetotoxic and abortifacient activity to trans-sabinyl acetate.

■ *Root oil*: Avoid oral consumption due to trans-sabinyl acetate content. Essential oils with moderate to significant amounts of trans-sabinyl acetate may irritate the mucosal lining of the gastrointestinal tract, damage the kidneys, cause blood in the urine, obstruct blood flow in the abdominal organs, and cause abnormally heavy menstrual bleeding.[5489]

■ May interact with diabetic medications and cause low blood-sugar levels based on ligustilide or (Z)-3-butylidene phthalide content.[5490]

■ May interact with aspirin, blood pressure, antiplatelet, and anticoagulant medications, and increase the risk of bleeding among people with bleeding disorders due to ligustilide content. (Z)-ligustilide inhibits platelet aggregation without affecting coagulation time of peripheral blood.[5491]

■ May interact with levodopa (L-dopa) and increase its cytotoxic effects (causes neuronal cell death).[5492]

■ May interfere with pentobarbital and other barbiturates (medications for anxiety and insomnia) based on (Z)-Ligustilide content.[5493]

■ May interact with anticholinergic (drugs used for asthma, incontinence, gastrointestinal cramps, muscular spasms, depression, and sleep disorders) and cholinergic medications (drugs used to reduce urinary retention, diagnose myasthenia gravis, and for glaucoma) based on AChE inhibitory activity.[5494,5495]

■ May interact with diuretic drugs and promote increased production of urine due to diuretic effects of lovage essential oil.[5496]

■ *Root oil*: Use very cautiously with epilepsy and Parkinson's disease due to trans-sabinyl acetate content.[5497]

**SELECTED EVIDENCE:**

- *In vitro* research shows that lovage essential oil (leaves, alpha-terpinyl acetate rich) kills head and neck squamous cancer cells by positively influencing genes involved in apoptosis, cancer, cellular growth, and cell cycle regulation.[5498]

- Oral administration of (Z)-ligustilide reduced cognitive decline and brain damage caused by inadequate blood supply to the brain in rats.[5499] The authors attributed this affect to the ability of (Z)-ligustilide to reduce malondialdehyde, increase super oxide dismutase (SOD) activity, and significantly inhibit AChE activity. Inhibition of AChE prevents the breakdown of acetylcholine, which is essential for memory and thinking. People with neurodegenerative diseases make less acetylcholine, and the diseases often break it down at a faster rate leading to acetylcholine deficits.

- Human aryl hydrocarbon receptor (AhR: a gene that encodes a protein that helps regulate responses to planar aromatic hydrocarbons and significantly affects the immune activity in the gastrointestinal tract) regulates the circadian rhythm, helps regulate the cell cycle, and plays an important role in tissue development. Cumin, jasmine, vanilla, and bay leaf fully activate AhR; clove, dill, thyme, nutmeg, and oregano partially activate AhR; and tarragon, caraway, turmeric, lovage, fennel, spearmint, star anise, and anise inhibit the AhR activity.[5500]

---

# MAGNOLIA
## (Magnolia Leaf, Magnolia Flower, White Champaca)
*Michelia* x *alba* DC

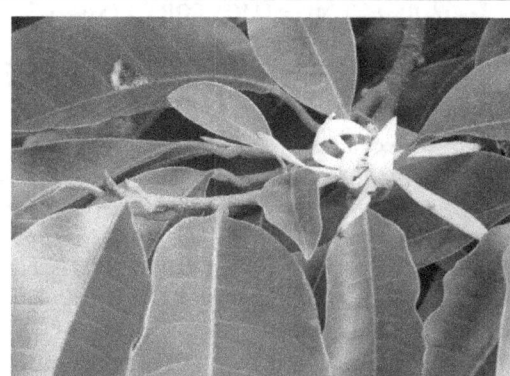

**FAMILY:** Magnoliaceae
**NOTE:** Top/Middle
**AROMA INTENSITY:** Strong
**AROMA:** Fruity, floral, balsamic
**COMMON EXTRACTION METHOD:** Steam distilled from the leaves or flowers; the flowers may also be solvent extracted or obtained by enfleurage
**POSSIBLE SUBSTITUTE OILS:** Lavender, ylang ylang
**BLENDS WELL WITH:** Basil, bergamot, cedarwood, combava, eucalyptus, lavender, lemon, lime, Mediterranean mandarin, neroli, orange, petitgrain, sandalwood, tangerine, ylang ylang
**SUBCELLULAR LOCALIZATION | EPIGENETIC INFLUENCE:** Currently unknown | Currently unknown
**RECOMMENDED DILUTION RANGE:** 5%–neat

**PRIMARY CONSTITUENTS:**[5501,5502,5503,5504]

| *Flowers* | | *Leaves* | |
|---|---|---|---|
| Linalool | 66.9%–91.7% | Linalool | 76.6%–80.1% |
| Methyl-2-Methylbutyrate | 1.3%–7.8% | Farnesol | 0.0%–5.5% |
| Ethyl-2-Methylbutyrate | 1.5%–6.8% | Beta-Elemene | 1.7%–3.7% |
| Beta-Elemene | 1.3%–3.8% | Beta-Caryophyllene | 0.0%–3.0% |
| Methyl Eugenol | 0.0%–3.6% | | |

Note: The flower oil may also produce a chemotype with beta-caryophyllene and bicyclogermacrene as the primary compounds.

**OTHER CONSTITUENTS:** *Leaves*—Caryophyllene oxide, (E)-nerolidol; *Flowers*—(Z)-beta-ocimene, (E)-beta-ocimene, delta-cadinene

**PREFERRED COMPOSITION FOR CLINICAL USE:**

| Constituent | Flowers | Leaves |
|---|---|---|
| **Linalool** | 58%–75% | 70%–82% |
| **Beta-Elemene, Trans-Beta-Elemene** | 1.5%–7% | 1%–5% |
| **Methyl-2-Methylbutyrate** | 1%–7% | – |

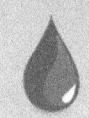

| | | |
|---|---|---|
| (Methyl Alpha-Methyl Butyrate) | | |
| **Beta-Caryophyllene** | 1%–7% | 0.1%–7% |
| **Ethyl-2-Methylbutyrate** | tr–5% | – |
| **Methyl Eugenol** | < 4% | – |
| **(E)-Beta-Ocimene** | 1%–4% | – |
| **(Z)-Beta-Ocimene** | 0.5%–3% | – |
| **Delta-Cadinene** | 0.1%–3% | – |
| **(E)-Nerolidol** | 0.1%–1% | 0.1%–3% |
| **Farnesol** | – | 0%–5% |

**REPORTED THERAPEUTIC PROPERTIES:** Antibacterial, aids digestion, deodorant, eases cough, supports respiratory function, decongestant, promotes healthy circulation, soothes chronic skin conditions, **encourages restful sleep**, relieves anxiety, stress management, **deeply relaxing**

**CAUTIONS:**

■ *Linalool CT*: May interact with antifungal drugs and enhance their effectiveness based on linalool content.[5505]

**SELECTED EVIDENCE:**

☐ Inhalation of magnolia leaf essential oil (50 mcL on filter paper attached to the nose) promoted relaxation and decreased alertness in a small clinical study.[5506] Thirty-two-channel electroencephalography was used to record brainwave activity among the twenty-five participants (ten male, fifteen female; ten men and women received the oil and five inhaled from filter paper with no oil as a control group). The oil caused decreased beta brainwaves and increased fast alpha wave activity, which indicates the oil may trigger relaxation and sleep. Inhalation of isolated linalool showed virtually identical results, suggesting that linalool may be the main driver of brainwave changes and relaxation activity.

☐ A randomized, controlled study reported that inhaling fragrant brown rice (with magnolia essential oil) increases alpha and beta brainwave activity, promoting reduced stress and a relaxed mood.[5507] Vapor of the oil also inhibited *A. flavus*, which is a causative fungi of brown rice mold.

# MANUKA
## (New Zealand Tea Tree, Broom Tea Tree)

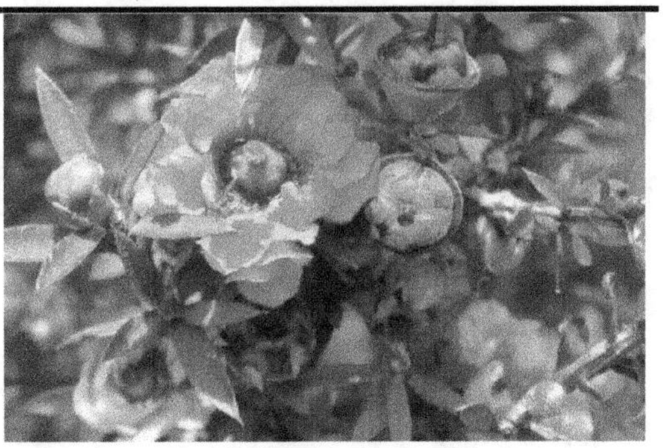

*Leptospermum scoparium* J.R. Forst. & G. Forst., *L. scoparium* J.R. Forst. & G. Forst. var. *martinii* hort and var. *nichollsii* (Dorr. Sm.) Turrill

**FAMILY:** Myrtaceae
**NOTE:** Middle
**AROMA INTENSITY:** Medium
**AROMA:** Herbaceous, earthy, sweet, rich
**COMMON EXTRACTION METHOD:** Steam distilled from the leaves and twigs
**POSSIBLE SUBSTITUTE OILS:** Helichrysum, tea tree, kanuka, niaouli, palmarosa, geranium
**BLENDS WELL WITH:** Basil, bergamot, black pepper, cajeput, chamomile (German, Roman), clary sage, cypress, eucalyptus, geranium, grapefruit, kanuka, lavender, lemon, lime, marjoram, may chang, neroli, orange, patchouli, petitgrain, peppermint, pine, ravensara, rosemary, sage, Spanish sage, sandalwood, tangerine, tea tree, thyme
**SUBCELLULAR LOCALIZATION | EPIGENETIC INFLUENCE:** Currently unknown | Currently unknown
**RECOMMENDED DILUTION RANGE:** 5%–Neat

**PRIMARY CONSTITUENTS:**[5508,5509,5510,5511]

| *Leptospermone CT* | | *Selinene/Beta-Elemene CT* | |
|---|---|---|---|
| *(Also called Triketone CT or East Cape CT)* | | Alpha-Selinene/Viridiflorene | 13.5% |
| Leptospermone | 8.7%–29.4% | Beta-Elemene | 10.8% |

| | | | |
|---|---|---|---|
| Trans-Calamenene* | 3.1%–22.7% | (E)-Methyl Cinnamate/ | |
| Flavesone | 0.0%–12.3% | Alpha-Cubebene | 10.6% |
| Isoleptospermone | 1.4%–11.5% | Beta-Selinene | 10.0% |
| Alpha-Pinene | 1.0%–11.0% | Gamma-Ylangene + | |
| Delta-Cadinene | 4.8%–8.6% | Alpha-Copaene | 6.0% |
| Cadina-3,5-Diene | 0.0%–8.0% | Trans-Calamenene | 3.3% |
| Alpha-Copaene | 0.6%–6.6% | Beta-Caryophyllene | 3.2% |
| Alpha-Selinene | 2.7%–6.1% | Linalool | 3.2% |
| Beta-Selinene | 0.3%–5.8% | Alpha-Muurolene | 3.1% |
| Cadina-1.4-Diene | 0.0%–5.3% | Alpha-Amorphene | 2.8% |
| Viridiflorene | 0.7%–4.4% | Alpha-Humulene | 2.6% |
| Alpha-Cubebene | 3.0%–4.4% | Citronellyl Formate | 2.3% |
| Delta-Amorphene | 0.0%–4.2% | | |
| Beta-Caryophyllene | 2.0%–3.2% | | |
| Aromadendrene | 1.6%–2.2% | | |

Note: Ten chemotypes of Manuka essential oil are described in the literature including a-pinene; sesquiterpene-rich with high myrcene; sesquiterpene-rich with elevated caryophyllene and humulene; sesquiterpene-rich with an unidentified sesquiterpene hydrocarbon; high geranyl acetate; sesquiterpene-rich with high gamma-ylangene+a-copaene and elevated triketones; sesquiterpene-rich with no distinctive components; sesquiterpene-rich with high trans-methyl cinnamate; high linalool; and sesquiterpene-rich with elevated elemene and selinene. The leptospermone and elemene-selinene were identified in commercially available samples, with leptospermone being the most common sample.

**OTHER CONSTITUENTS:** *Leptospermone CT*—Myrcene, 1,8-cineole, para-cymene, alpha-gurjunene, beta-elemene, allo-aromadendrene, gamma-muurolene, germacrene D, bicyclogermacrene, (E,E)-alpha-farnesene, alpha-calacorene, gamma-calacorene, caryophyllene oxide, cubenol, globulol, viridiflorol, spathulenol; *Selinene/Beta-Elemene CT*—Alpha-pinene, myrcene, 1,8-cineole, alpha-terpineol, citronellol, methyl geranate, citronellyl acetate, geranyl acetate, alpha-gurjunene, aromadendrene, gamma-cadinene, flavesone, delta-cadinene, leptospermone, beta-eudesmol, alpha-eudesmol

**PREFERRED COMPOSITION FOR CLINICAL USE:**

| Constituent | Leptospermone CT |
|---|---|
| **Leptospermone** | 10%–25% |
| **Calamenene\* <cis- + trans->** | 5%–20% |
| **Isoleptospermone** | 2%–12% |
| **Delta-Cadinene** | 2%–10% |
| **Alpha-Copaene** | 2%–8% |
| **Flavesone** | 2%–8% |
| **Alpha-Selinene** | 3%–7% |
| **Alpha-Cubebene** | 2%–7% |
| **Cadina-3,5-diene** or **Trans-Muurola-3,5-diene** | 1%–7% |
| **Trans-Cadina-1,4-diene** | 3%–6% |
| **Beta-Selinene** | 0.5%–6% |
| **Beta-Caryophyllene** | 1%–5% |
| **Alpha-Pinene** | 0.5%–5% |
| **Aromadendrene** | 0.5%–3% |

\* Calamenene is identified as both cis- and trans- in GC/MS reports, suggesting there may be confusion in identifying the correct isomer. Trans-calamenene is the constituent present in manuka essential oil.

**REPORTED THERAPEUTIC PROPERTIES: Antibacterial**, antifungal, antimicrobial, **antiviral**, analgesic, anti-inflammatory, antiallergic, antispasmodic, supports respiratory function, expels excess mucous, decongestant,

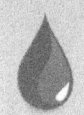

combats acne, eases cough, relieves cold sores, **supports oral health**, removes warts, **reduces the appearance of scars and blemishes**, relieves chronic skin conditions, relieves insect bites, supports immune function, relieves headache/migraine, relaxing/calming, stress management, combats disappointment, encourages motivation

## CAUTIONS:

■ Caution is sensible after the thirty-seventh week of pregnancy. There is a very small risk that Manuka essential oil could decrease uterine contractions during active labor based on animal research.[5512]

## SELECTED EVIDENCE:

☐ A small clinical study (nineteen people) found that a gargle with equal parts of Kanuka and Manuka essential oil in water delayed mucositis (painful inflammation of the mucous membranes of the digestive tract—mouth to anus—after chemotherapy or radiation treatment), reduced pain, and reduced weight loss better than placebo.[5513]

☐ Manuka essential oil significantly inhibits cariogenic bacteria (bacteria associated with cavities) and periodontopathic bacteria, completely killing the bacteria at a concentration of 0.2% *in vitro*.[5514] A mouth rinse with Manuka, cinnamon, tea tree, *Leptospermum morrisonii*, arnica, eucalyptus, grapefruit, the essential oil mouth rinse Cool Mint Listerine and two of its components, menthol and thymol inhibited *S. mutans* and *L. plantarum*, which are oral pathogens associated with cavities. The essential oils also reduced the amount of chlorhexidine required to inhibit the oral pathogens up to ten-fold.[5515] Another study reported that a mouthwash (GingiNat) containing Manuka essential oil, avocado oil, propolis oil, grapeseed extract, *Aloe vera*, green tea, and coenzyme Q10 is a viable natural extract to support oral health (reduce plaque and gingivitis) due to its antiseptic, antioxidant, and immunoregulatory properties on oral tissues.[5516] A small clinical study (twenty participants with significant gingivitis) demonstrated that swishing with a 6% solution of GingiNat two to three times daily for twenty-one days significantly decreased the periodontal index (plaque, gingivitis, and bad breath) 30% by day 4, 49% by day seven and 78% by day twenty-one.[5517]

☐ *In vitro* research concluded that oregano and manuka essential oils, alone and in combination, inhibit *S. aureus* strains, making them an "effective alternative to chemotherapic [sic] drugs in staphylococcal infections and useful tools to enhance food security." Synergistic and additive effects were seen almost half of the time when oregano and manuka were used together.[4989]

☐ Animal and *in vitro* research suggests that Manuka essential oil relieved muscles spasms and delayed an increase in the resting tone of the diaphragm (suggesting it may increase blood supply to the respiratory system).[3072,3073]

☐ Manuka essential oil possesses moderate antioxidant properties.[3073]

☐ *In vitro* research suggests the antibacterial activity of Manuka essential oil against twenty-five bacterial strains and twenty *Listeria* strains varies from absent to moderate inhibition.[3073] Additional research concluded that Manuka essential oil (or its polar triketones) actively inhibits gram-positive bacteria, *S. aureus*, MRSA, *E. coli*, *P. aeruginosa*, *B. subtilis*, *T. mentagrophytes*, dermatophytes, and *C. albicans*.[3064,3071,3082] Research suggests the antimicrobial activity of Manuka essential oil is directly related to its triketone (leptospermone, isoleptospermone, and flavesone) content, and that chemotypes other than leptospermone have little to no antimicrobial activity. Another study reports that manuka essential oil significantly inhibits four infectious and inflammatory fungi (*Trichosporon mucoides, Malassezia furfur, Candida albicans,* and *Candida tropicalis*) and bacteria (*Staphylococcus aureus, Streptococcus sobrinus, Streptococcus mutans,* and *Escherichia coli*).[4785] The study authors determined that the antifungal activity of kanuka essential oil was superior to manuka essential oil.

☐ Manuka essential oil strongly kills and prevents the replication of HSV-1 and drug-resistant HSV-1.[5518] Another study reported that Manuka essential oil (leptospermone CT) significantly inhibits HSV-1 and prevents plaque formation (plaque formation in cell cultures is indicative of virus replication and spread) of HSV-1 and HSV-2.[5519]

☐ Animal research suggests that a 10% Manuka essential oil prevented skin inflammation and aging (reduced the appearance of wrinkles and protected against collagen fiber loss and epidermal hyperplasia—the enlargement of the outer layer of skin caused by an increased rate of cell reproduction often as an initial stage in the development of skin cancer,) caused by UV-B rays.[5520]

- *In vitro* research found that Manuka essential oil (leptospermone CT) inhibits *Staphylococcus pseudintermedius* and meticillin-resistant *S. pseudintermedius*, which is a common pathogen of skin and ear infections in dogs.[5521]

- Manuka essential oil strongly inhibited LPS-induced (bacterial lipopolysaccharide, which is well-known for initiating inflammatory responses) release of the inflammatory cytokine tumor necrosis factor alpha (TNF-α) without adversely affecting the immune system.[5522] TNF-α plays a key role in the initiation of systemic inflammation and is associated with chronic inflammatory conditions.

- Several essential oils listed in order of efficacy killed the itch mite (*Sarcoptes scabiei*) that burrows into the skin and causes scabies during direct contact (clove > palmarosa > geranium > tea tree > lavender > manuka > petitgrain > eucalyptus > Japanese cedarwood) with the mites and when used as a fumigant (tea tree > clove > eucalyptus > lavender > palmarosa > geranium > Japanese cedarwood > petitgrain > manuka (leptospermone CT)).[5523]

- Manuka essential oil prevented the production of enterotoxins by *S. aureus*.[5524]

- Manuka essential oil (East Cape CT) was toxic to *Aedes aegypti* mosquito larvae, which was improved when combined with bio-based amylose-N-1-hexadecylammonium chloride inclusion complexes.[5525] Alpha-pinene, ledene, and aromadendrene were two to seven times less toxic than the whole essential suggesting that the toxicity of Manuka is likely due to synergistic interactions among all the chemical constituents or possibly a constituent not tested.

- Manuka essential oil has been traditionally used for wound care and as an antimicrobial. However, the essential oil is not well retained in mucosal sites, limiting its benefits for oral care. Manuka essential oil in a semisolid emulsion displayed greater bactericidal penetrative effects against *Streptococci gordonii* biofilms when compared to the oil alone.[5526] The oil emulsion was also less toxic to human gingival fibroblasts when compared to chlorhexidine. Altogether, the research suggests that manuka essential oil has potential for use in oral care when used as an emulsion.

- Of fourteen commercial essential oils tested, cinnamon bark, thyme CT thymol, clove bud, geranium, and manuka essential oils were most active against fungi that commonly infect animal and human skin (*Microsporum gypseum, Microsporum canis, Trichophyton mentagrophytes, Trichophyton violaceum, Aspergillus niger, Scopulariopsis brevicaulis,* (IZ 1) dog skin isolate).[5527] (E)-cinnamaldehyde, thymol, and carvacrol displayed the strongest activity of isolated constituents against dermatophytes. (E)-cinnamaldehyde, eugenol, carvacrol, geraniol, and thymol were most active against IZ 1.

- Oregano CT carvacrol, may chang, and manuka each displayed acaricidal activity against the Asian blue tick (*Rhipicephalus microplus*).[5528] Beta-triketone fractions from manuka caused significant larval mortality, while its sesquiterpene fraction was far less effective. Interestingly, the sesquiterpene fractions were more effective on adults than the beta-triketone fractions.

- Manuka essential oil (24.0% (Z)-calamenene, 18.3% leptospermone) demonstrated good antimicrobial activity against *L. monocytogenes* and *S. aureus*.[5529]

- Tea tree and manuka essential oils inhibited *S. aureus* and *P. aeruginosa*.[5530]

- Manuka inhibited *C. albicans, C. glabrata,* and *C. krusei*.[5531]

# MARITIME PINE
## (Terebinth)

*Pinus pinaster* Aiton

**FAMILY:** Pinaceae
**NOTE:** *Gum Resin*—Middle-Base;
*Needles*—Top-Middle
**AROMA INTENSITY:** Medium
**AROMA:** Coniferous, balsamic, piney, woody
**COMMON EXTRACTION METHOD:** Steam distilled from the gum resin; also steam distilled from the needles (leaves)
**POSSIBLE SUBSTITUTE OILS:** Pine, red pine, white pine, cedarwood (Atlas)

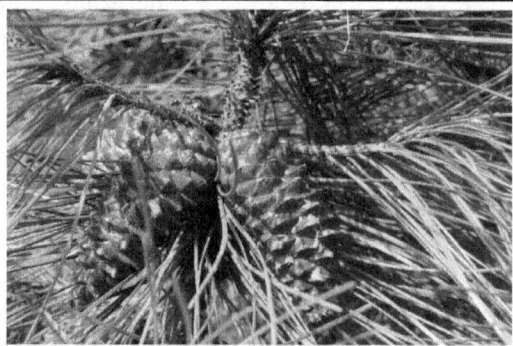

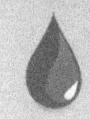
**BLENDS WELL WITH:** Angelica, balsam fir, camphor, cedarwood, copaiba, cypress, eucalyptus, frankincense, ginger, juniper berry, lavender, myrtle, oregano, palo santo, pine, ponderosa pine, red pine, rosemary, sandalwood, silver fir, thyme, white fir

**SUBCELLULAR LOCALIZATION | EPIGENETIC INFLUENCE:** Currently unknown | Currently unknown

**RECOMMENDED DILUTION RANGE:** 3%–50%; neat for limited conditions

**PRIMARY CONSTITUENTS:**[5532,5533,5534,5535,5536,5537,5538,5539]

*Gum Resin*

| Alpha-Pinene | 44.1%–78.0% |
|---|---|
| Beta-Pinene | 17.0%–29.5% |
| Beta-Myrcene | 0.0%–4.7% |
| Beta-Caryophyllene | 0.1%–3.5% |
| Delta-3-Carene | 0.0%–3.3% |
| Limonene | 1.4%–3.2% |

*Needles (Alpha-Pinene CT)*

| Alpha-Pinene | 10.2%–28.9% |
|---|---|
| Beta-Pinene | 0.9%–21.7% |
| Germacrene D | 2.9%–19.2% |
| Beta-Caryophyllene | 0.2%–14.8% |
| Limonene | 0.8%–7.5% |
| Beta-Myrcene | 0.4%–6.1% |
| Phenylethyl 2-Methylbutyrate | 0.0%–6.1% |
| Delta-Cadinene | 1.4%–5.0% |
| Alpha-Terpinene | 0.0%–3.8% |
| Delta-3-Carene | 0.0%–3.5% |
| Alpha-Cadinol | 0.0%–3.5% |

*Needles (Beta-Caryophyllene CT)*

| Beta-Caryophyllene | 26.6%–30.9% |
|---|---|
| Beta-Selinene | 0.0%–13.5% |
| Allo-Aromadendrene | 0.0%–12.5% |
| Delta-Cadinene | 0.0%–7.8% |
| Alpha-Humulene | 4.3%–6.9% |
| Alpha-Copaene | 0.0%–5.1% |
| Gamma-Cadinene | 0.0%–3.9% |
| Germacrene D | 0.0%–3.8% |
| Alpha-Selinene | 0.0%–3.5% |

Note: Generally, only the gum resin essential oil is called terebinth.

**OTHER CONSTITUENTS:** *Gum Resin*—camphene, beta-phellandrene, terpinolene, longifolene, alpha-humulene, alpha-terpineol, germacrene D, delta-cadinene, gamma-cadinene; *Needles (Alpha-Pinene CT)*—delta-elemene, geranyl acetate, alpha-gurjunene, alpha-humulene, aristolene, butanoic acid, longifolene, gamma-cadinene, 3-methyl, 2-phenyl ethyl ester, (E)-2-hexen-1-ol, phenyl-3-methyl butanoate, beta-phellandrene, alpha-muurolene, gamma-murolene, guaiol, cembrene, alpha-terpineol, cis-hexenol, linalool, copaene, methyl eugenol (<0.6%); *Needles (Beta-Caryophyllene CT)*—alpha-thujene, alpha-pinene, tricyclene, beta-myrcene, methyl acetate, alpha-terpinyl acetate, alpha-murolene, beta-copaene, humulene epoxide II, beta-bisabolol, phenyl ethyl anthanilate, cis-ferruginol, benzyl acetate, cyclosativene, longicyclene, geranyl acetate, phenylethyl 3-methyl butanoate, epi-cubebol, alpha-methyl-ionone, beta-sesquiphellandrene-8-ol, trans-sesquisabinene hydrate

**PREFERRED COMPOSITION FOR CLINICAL USE:**

| Constituent | Gum Resin |
|---|---|
| **Alpha-Pinene** | 65%–80% |
| **Beta-Pinene** | 12%–25% |
| **Limonene** | 1%–5% |
| **Beta-Caryophyllene** | 0.1%–4% |
| **Longifolene** | 0.1%–3% |
| **Beta-Myrcene** | 0.1%–5% |
| **Camphene** | 0.5%–2% |
| **Delta-3-Carene** | 0%–2% |

**REPORTED THERAPEUTIC PROPERTIES:** Antibacterial, antifungal, **antimicrobial**, antiviral, antiparasitic, antioxidant, antiseptic, analgesic, anti-inflammatory, antirheumatic, relieves gout, nervine, antineuralgic, diuretic, astringent, aids circulation, supports kidney and urinary tract function, helps dissolve gallstones, aids digestion, **supports respiratory function**, expels excess mucus, eases cough, stops excess bleeding, supports immune function, insect repellent, grounding, stress management, relieves mental fatigue, combats fear, relieves anxiety, enhances mental clarity

**CAUTIONS:**

■ *Needles (Beta-Caryophyllene CT)*: May decrease the bioavailability of many medications (NSAIDs, proton-pump inhibitors, acetaminophen, antiepileptics, immune modulators, blood-sugar medications, blood pressure medications, antidepressants, antipsychotics, diabetic medications, antihistamines, antibiotics, and anesthetics) due to the ability of caryophyllene oxide, alpha-humulene, and beta-caryophyllene to inhibit CYP3A enzyme activity.[5540]

**SELECTED EVIDENCE:**

☐ *In vitro* research demonstrates that maritime pine essential oil (needles—alpha-pinene CT) actively inhibits *Sarcina lutea, Streptococcus faecalis, Staphylococcus aureus (two strains), Salmonella typhi, Salmonella typhimurium, Salmonella arizona, Salmonella enteritidis, Klebsiella pneumoniae, Klebsiella ozonae, Klebsiella oxytoca, Enterobacter cloaca, Serratia marescens, Aeromonas* sp., *Escherichia coli (two strains), Pseudomonas fluorescens, Pseudomonas aeruginosa, Proteus vulgaris, Proteus mirabilis,* and *Morganella morganeii.*[3813] Interestingly, the main component in the essential oil (alpha-pinene), as well as minor components (beta-myrcene and beta-caryophyllene), exhibited very little inhibition, suggesting minor components in the essential oil, or a synergistic effect of all essential oil constituents, may be responsible for the broad antimicrobial activity. On the contrary, research is conflicting against *Aspergillus* fungi. One study concluded that maritime pine essential oil (needles—beta-caryophyllene CT) was not active against the fungi *A. flavus* and *A. niger,* while another observed inhibition of *A. parasiticus* and *A. flavus* and their production of aflatoxin B1.[5541,5542]

☐ Maritime pinecone essential oil (alpha-pinene CT) demonstrated remarkable anti-inflammatory and wound healing activities.[5543]

☐ Maritime pine essential oil inhibited *S. aureus, B. subtilis, P. aeruginosa, E. coli,* and *C. albicans* but displayed only weak antioxidant activity in the DPPH, ORAC, and ROS reduction assays.[5544]

☐ Maritime pine essential oil displayed good antioxidant activity in the beta-carotene bleaching assay but not in the DPPH assay, and inhibited *K. pneumoniae, E. coli, C. albicans, L. monocytogenes, B. cereus, C. tropicalis, S. aureus,* and *P. aeruginosa.*[5545]

# MARJORAM, SWEET

*Origanum majorana* L., *O. dubium* Boiss., *Majorana hortensis* Moench

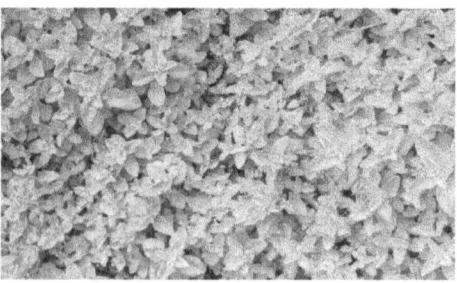

**FAMILY:** Lamiaceae (Labiatae)
**NOTE:** Middle
**AROMA INTENSITY:** Medium
**AROMA:** Herbaceous, warm, medicinal
**COMMON EXTRACTION METHOD:** Steam distilled from the flowers and leaves
**POSSIBLE SUBSTITUTE OILS:** Oregano (terpinen-4-ol CT), tea tree, thyme (thuyanol-4 CT), basil (linalool CT), lavender
**BLENDS WELL WITH:** Basil, bergamot, cajeput, camphor, chamomile (German, Roman), cypress, eucalyptus, fennel, ginger, juniper, lavender, tea tree, orange, oregano, patchouli, petitgrain, pine, ravensara, rosemary, thyme
**SUBCELLULAR LOCALIZATION | EPIGENETIC INFLUENCE:** Cell Membrane | Circulatory/Respiratory
**RECOMMENDED DILUTION RANGE:** 3%–20%; neat for limited conditions

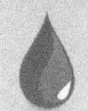

**PRIMARY CONSTITUENTS:**[5546,5547,5548,5549,5550,5551,5552]

| | | | |
|---|---|---|---|
| Terpinen-4-ol | 28.9%–38.4% | *Turkish Marjoram** | |
| Cis-Sabinene Hydrate | 3.0%–30.2% | Carvacrol | 56.4%–83.5% |
| Linalyl-Acetate | 0.3%–26.1% | Linalool | 0.0%–31.7% |
| Gamma-Terpinene | 6.9%–14.3% | O-Cymene | 0.0%–8.1% |
| Sabinene | 4.9%–12.0% | Gamma-Terpinene | 2.0%–6.9% |
| Alpha-Terpinene | 2.8%–8.2% | Para-Cymene | 0.0%–4.7% |
| Para-Cymene | 3.5%–7.0% | * Follow cautions for oregano. | |
| Alpha-Terpineol | 4.9%–6.9% | | |
| Trans-Sabinene Hydrate | 3.5%–4.4% | | |

Note: Marjoram composition varies widely depending on the season it is harvested, with spikes in certain constituents: winter—cis-sabinene hydrate (up to 54.4%); spring—thymol (up to 38.4%) and cis-sabinene hydrate (up to 25.3%); fall/autumn—terpinolene (43.1%).

**OTHER CONSTITUENTS:** *Terpinen-4-ol CT*—Alpha-phellandrene, alpha-pinene, beta-phellandrene, d-limonene, terpinolene, thujene, beta-caryophyllene, bicyclogermacrene, linalool, piperitol, thymol; *Turkish Marjoram*—Alpha-pinene, alpha-thujene, myrcene, alpha-terpinene, delta-2-carene, beta-phellandrene, cis-sabinene hydrate, trans-sabinene hydrate, terpinen-4-ol, trans-caryophyllene, alpha-terpineol, boorneol, thymol

**PREFERRED COMPOSITION FOR CLINICAL USE:**

| Constituent | |
|---|---|
| **Terpinen-4-ol** | 20%–32% |
| **Sabinene Hydrate <cis- + trans->** (4-Thujanol <cis-, trans->, 4-Thuyanol <cis-, trans->) | 8%–28% |
| **Gamma-Terpinene** | 10%–20% |
| **Alpha-Terpinene** | 5%–12% |
| **Sabinene** | 4%–10% |
| **Alpha-Terpineol** | 2%–10% |
| **Linalool** | 0.1%–8% |
| **Linalyl Acetate** | 1%–5% |
| **Para-Cymene** | 0.5%–5% |
| **Beta-Caryophyllene** | 1%–4% |
| **Limonene** | 1%–4% |
| **Trans-p-Menth-2-en-1-ol** | 0.1%–2% |
| **Cis-p-Menth-2-en-1-ol** | 0.1%–2% |

**REPORTED THERAPEUTIC PROPERTIES: Analgesic (pain relief)**, antibacterial, antifungal, anti-inflammatory, helps expel excess gas, antiviral, antiseptic, **antispasmodic**, **antiarthritic**, **antirheumatic**, supports heart muscle function, decongestant, expectorant, **nervine (calms and soothes the nerves)**, supports brain health, relieves constipation, **strengthens muscle tone**, relieves painful menstruation, wound healing, **antineuralgic**, circulatory stimulant, vasodilator, encourages restful sleep, lowers blood pressure, warming, relieves anxiety, stress management, sedating, **decreases overactive sex drive**, reduces obsessive thinking, helps relieve trauma and grief, combats mood swings

**CAUTIONS:**
■ May interact with anticholinergic (drugs used for asthma, incontinence, gastrointestinal cramps, muscular spasms, depression, and sleep disorders) and cholinergic medications (drugs used to reduce urinary retention, diagnose myasthenia gravis, and for glaucoma) based on AChE inhibitory activity.[5553]
■ May interact with antifungals and increase their effectiveness due to terpinen-4-ol content.[5554]

**SELECTED EVIDENCE:**
   □ Sweet marjoram oil kills two myeloid leukemia cells lines according to *in vitro* research.[5555] Other research reports that marjoram essential oil kills breast and prostate cancer cells.[5556]

- A clinical study concluded that both cortisol and systolic blood pressure declines after inhalation of a combination of lavender, ylang ylang, marjoram, and neroli oil in those with high blood pressure or pre-high blood pressure.[5557]
- A daily abdominal massage with a combination of lavender, clary sage, and marjoram (2:1:1 ratio) from the end of the last menstruation to the beginning of the next menstruation significantly reduced painful menstruation according to a randomized, double-blind clinical trial.[5558]
- Topical application of a 1.5% solution containing lavender, marjoram, eucalyptus, rosemary, and peppermint (2:1:2:1:1 ratio) in a carrier oil consisting of 45% apricot, 45% almond, and 10% jojoba carrier oils significantly decreased pain and depression in people with arthritis.[5559]
- *In vitro* research concluded that marjoram essential oil inhibited *P. insidiosum* (a pathogenic oomycete that infects mammals and causes gangrenous ulcers on the skin and may restrict blood flow in the surrounding arteries).[5560]
- Rats administered 160 µL/kg of marjoram oil twice daily for twenty-eight days were protected against oxidative damage of the kidneys caused by prallethrin (an insecticide known to cause oxidative damage and toxicity in the kidneys of animals).[5561] The same amount of oral administration also prevented prallethrin-induced oxidative stress and liver toxicity and injury in rats.[5562]
- Marjoram essential oil protected bone marrow cells from DNA and chromosomal damage caused by prallethrin (an insecticide that causes damage to DNA and chromosomes in animals).[5563]
- Animal research suggests that oral administration of marjoram oil (0.16 mL/kg) prevented damage to reproductive, liver, and brain tissues caused by ethanol in male rats.[5564]
- *In vitro* research suggests that marjoram oil inhibits acetylcholinesterase (AChE) and is a weak to potent antioxidant (depending on its composition, with essential oils containing terpinen-4-ol, trans-sabinene hydrate, gamma-terpinene, and alpha-terpinene as major constituents demonstrating greater antioxidant activity).[5565,5566,5567] Inhibition of AChE prevents the breakdown of acetylcholine, which is essential for memory and thinking. People with neurodegenerative diseases make less acetylcholine, and the diseases often break it down at a faster rate leading to acetylcholine deficits.
- An ethanolic extract of marjoram prevented ulcers caused by ethanol and indomethacin (an NSAID), and replenished lost stomach mucous in animals.[5568]
- Oral administration of 0.16 mL/kg of marjoram oil protected liver and kidney cells against DNA damage caused by lead and improved liver and kidney function in mice.[5569]
- *In vitro* research suggests that marjoram oil significantly inhibits *A. niger, B. natriegens, E. carotovora, E. coli, Streptococcus A, S. dysenteriae, S. enteritidis,* and *Moraxella* sp.[5570,1312] Another study demonstrated that marjoram essential oil possesses antimicrobial activity against *S. aureus, B. cereus, B. subtilis, B. pumilis, P. aeruginosa, Salmonella poona, E. coli,* and drug-resistant *E. coli.*[4872]
- *In vitro* research demonstrated that low doses of marjoram, lemon, basil, clove, thyme, rosemary CT 1,8-cineole, and tea tree essential oils prevented the shortening of telomeres after exposure to hydrogen peroxide.[4779] The same research reported that vetiver, black pepper, eucalyptus (*E. globulus*), ginger, clove, and rosemary increased the length of already shortened telomeres. This activity suggests that these essential oils can help maintain the youth and health of cells, or turn back the clock on the cell to make it more youthful depending on the essential oil used. Interestingly, cinnamon and peppermint essential oil decreased the length of telomeres slightly.
- A review study of nurse-delivered aromatherapy in acute care settings reported that the use of essential oils generally resulted in significant clinical improvements based on their intended use. Marjoram and tangerine essential oils reduced pain, lavender and marjoram essential oil reduced anxiety, and ginger alleviated nausea.[4857]
- *In vitro* research demonstrates that marjoram essential oil inhibits 18 fungal isolates of *Sporothrix brasiliensis* (n: 17) from humans, dogs and cats, and a standard strain of *Sporothrix schenckii* (n: 1).[4871] It also inhibits dermatophytes (*T. rubrum, T. tonsurans, T. mentagrophyte, M. gypseum, M. canis, E. floccosum*) and bacteria (*S. aureus, Strep. pyogens*).[4873]
- Marjoram SFE essential oil exerts anti-inflammatory effects by inhibiting the production of proinflammatory cytokines (TNF-α, IL-1β, IL-6 and IL-10), COX-2 enzyme activity, and NH$_K$B gene expression in an

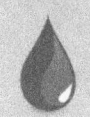

atherosclerotic environment.[4874] The study authors further tested individual constituents and found that terpinen-4-ol and trans-sabinene hydrate were responsible for the anti-inflammatory activity.

- Marjoram essential oil significantly kills adult rice weevils (*S. oryzae*).[5571]

- *In vitro* research demonstrates that marjoram essential oil inhibits several bacteria (*Escherichia coli, Salmonella enteritidis, Listeria ivanovii, Listeria inocula,* and *Listeria monocytogenes*)—with gram-negative bacteria being more sensitive than gram-positive bacteria. The same research reported that marjoram essential oil possesses significant antioxidant activity.[5572]

- Marjoram oil demonstrated the greatest activity of five essential oils tested against *Prototheca zopfii* strains that cause inflammation of the udder (mastitis) in cows.[5573]

- Lavender, lemongrass (*C. citratus*), marjoram, peppermint, tea tree, and rosewood essential oils all exhibited significant activity against clinical isolates of multidrug-resistant *Burkholderia cepacia* complex (a group of bacteria commonly resistant to antibiotics that cause health problems in people with weakened immune systems and are known to cause healthcare related infections).[5574]

- Marjoram, pink savory (*Satureja thymbra*), spearmint CT piperitenone oxide, melissa, and dittany (*Origanum dictamnus*) demonstrated the greatest repellency toward *Ae. albopictus* mosquitoes of fourteen Lamiaceae species tested.[5575] Thyme CT thymol, basil, dittany, marjoram, and oregano CT carvacrol were the most larvicidal.

- Marjoram essential oil demonstrated a relaxant effect on isolated rat and rabbit intestines.[5576]

- Bruxism is excessive teeth grinding or jaw clenching that can reduce sleep quality. Inhalation of marjoram essential oil combined with neurofeedback training modified brain activity as well as myeloperoxidase activity to reduce stress and anxiety in people diagnosed with bruxism.[5577] The marjoram essential oil was inhaled via nasal filters impregnated with 1% marjoram essential oil (23.6% terpinen-4-ol, 15.3% cis-sabinene hydrate, 14.1% alpha-terpinene, 14.1% gamma-terpinene, 8.3% sabinene, 3.4% trans-sabinene hydrate, 3.2% terpinolene, and 3.1% alpha-terpineol).

- *E. coli* causes up to 85 percent of urinary tract infections (UTIs). Thyme CT linalool, marjoram, and rosemary CT 1,8-cineole essential oils each inhibited *E. coli* isolated from the urinary tract of people with a UTI.[5578] Thyme was the most effective.

- Marjoram CT terpinen-4-ol, cinnamon bark, and thyme CT thymol essential oils each exhibited antibiofilm effects on *L. monocytogenes, P. putida,* and *S. aureus,* but were less effective against biofilms with two species unless higher concentrations were used.[5579]

- Oral administration of marjoram essential oil (80 mg/kg BW) for thirty days significantly improved cutaneous sporotichosis—a skin infection caused by fungi like *Sporothrix brasiliensis*—in rats.[5580] Marjoram oil resolved cutaneous lesions and decreased the fungal burden in systemic organs better than itraconazole. The oil's composition was: 34.1% terpinen-4-ol, 14.3% gamma-terpinene, and 9.6% alpha-terpinene.

- Marjoram essential oil and fractions rich in terpinen-4-ol inhibited food spoilage fungi (*R. oryzae, R. stolonifera, A. penicilioides*).[5581]

- Nursing students frequently experience a high level of stress and anxiety while completing their education and learning fundamental skills, particularly while taking tests. A double-blind, randomized, and controlled trial demonstrated that inhalation of marjoram and sweet orange (3 drops of a 1:1 blend of the oils) essential oil from an aroma lamp combined with music therapy for twenty minutes significantly reduced test anxiety, general anxiety, and stress.[5582] The intervention also improved performance of fundamental nursing skills.

- Rosemary CT 1,8-cineole, oregano (*Th. capitatus*) CT carvacrol, marjoram, and sage CT alpha-thujone demonstrated promising antibacterial activity against bacteria (*P. aeruginosa, E. coli, S. enterica, B. subtilis,* and *S. aureus*) responsible for healthcare-associated infections and foodborne illnesses.[5583] Oregano exhibited the strongest activity, which exceeded gentamicin in effectiveness.

- Colorectal cancer is a leading cause of mortality worldwide, ranking third for incidence and mortality. Marjoram essential oil significantly reduced colon cancer cell growth and viability by inducing autophagy, downregulating genes, and triggering apoptosis (considered the main anticancer mechanism of the oil).[5584]

- Both marjoram and white wormwood inhibited several microorganisms isolated from spoiled butter in a concentration-dependent manner.[5585]

- Marjoram CT pulegone essential oil exhibited high larvicidal activity against *Aedes aegypti* mosquito larvae.[5586] The same research concluded that the oil inhibited *E. coli* and *P. aeruginosa,* but did not display antioxidant activity in the DPPH assay.

- Nanoencapsulation of marjoram essential oil significantly improved its antifungal activity against *A. flavus* and its production of aflatoxin B1.[5587] The nanoencapsulated oil also exhibited better antioxidant activity than the free oil.

- Marjoram essential oil reduced parasite load and increased the lifespan of mice infected with *Plasmodium* parasites (the cause of malaria), without causing healthy cell death in mouse fibroblasts (in a separate laboratory study).[5588]
- Inhalation of marjoram essential oil (five days after inducement of Alzheimer's disease and for fifteen minutes daily over the course of twenty-one days) increased antioxidant activity and enhanced brain-derived neurotrophic factor (BDNF) expression, which together improved memory and cognitive function in rats.[5589] BDNF is a protein found in the brain and spinal cord that promotes the survival of neurons by influencing growth, maturation, and maintenance of these cells.
- *Toxoplasma gondii* is a parasite excreted in cat feces. Humans can accidentally ingest the parasites if they come in contact with cat feces and then touch their mouth causing toxoplasmosis. A laboratory study found that lemongrass (*C. citratus*), marjoram, and citronella (*C. nardus*) inhibited *T. gondii*, with citronella having a high selectivity index.[5590] Based on this, the authors concluded that citronella may be a potential solution for treating toxoplasmosis.
- *Bacillus* bacteria are widely found in nature and responsible for food poisoning and food spoilage. Black cumin, clove, cinnamon, and marjoram essential oils each reduced *Bacillus* spp. presence in raw and processed meat, with black cumin being the most effective oil.[5591]
- Bisphenol A (BPA) is an industrial chemical used to make some plastics, which is an endocrine disruptor and known to increase estrogen load in the body and contribute to estrogen-related cancers. A preclinical study employed isobaric tags to determine the relative and absolute effects of ginger essential oil on the proliferation of breast cancer cells induced by BPA. What the researchers found was that ginger essential oil reduced the proliferation of breast cancer cells by altering the expression of multiple proteins and possibly via oxidative phosphorylation.[5592]
- Marjoram essential oil demonstrated promise as a biofungicide because of its ability to inhibit *F. verticilliodies*, which is a rice seed-born fungus.[5593]
- Marjoram essential oil caused 100 percent mortality by the third day after exposure against castor bean tick (*Ixodes Ricinus*) nymphs and caused paralysis or less movement after two hours of exposure.[5594]
- *In vitro* research showed that marjoram, rosemary CT 1,8-cineole, sage CT camphor, and pennyroyal CT limonene/piperitone inhibited *L. monocytogenes* and *Salmonella enterica* and displayed antioxidant activity in the DPPH assay.[5595]
- Marjoram (*O. dubium* and *O. majorana*), Greek sage, and bay laurel essential oils each inhibited promastigotes of *L. tropica*, with marjoram (*O. dubium*; 81.8% carvacrol) being the most active.[5596]
- Of three essential oils tested (marjoram, spearmint, and wild mint), marjoram exhibited the highest antioxidant capacity in the DPPH free radical-scavenging and ABTS assays, followed by spearmint and wild mint CT pulegone.[5597]
- The carvacrol CT of marjoram essential oil showed high antifungal activity against clinically relevant *Candida* spp., inhibition of biofilm formation, and reduction of virulence factors (germ-tube formation and its length) and on cell surface hydrophobicity.[5598]
- Marjoram CT carvacrol, oregano CT carvacrol, Turkish oregano CT carvacrol, as well as isolated carvacrol each inhibited angiotensin-converting enzyme 2 (ACE2) activity, with marjoram being the most effective. Blockade of ACE2 reduces the production of angiotensin II, which is a substance that narrows blood vessels and releases hormones (aldosterone, norepinephrine) to increase blood pressure and urine production. ACE inhibitors are primarily used to treat heart and kidney conditions. All of the oils also inhibited lipoxygenase (LOX) enzyme activity, with marjoram being the most active again. Stopping LOX activity reduces the production of inflammatory leukotrienes, which is a major cause of inflammation in conditions such as asthma, osteoarthritis, and allergic rhinitis. Additionally, computer-based protein docking confirmed the docking potential of the carvacrol and agreed with the significant enzyme inhibition activity observed in the laboratory studies.
- Marjoram essential oil inhibited drug-sensitive and drug-resistant *S. aureus* and *E. coli* strains.[5599] In addition, isolated gamma-terpinene, terpinen-4-ol, sabinene, sabinene hydrate, and linalool were effective inhibitors of biofilm formation by both bacteria.
- Marjoram essential oil significantly decreased the viability of two non-small cell lung cancer (NSCLC) cells *in vitro* and further slowed the growth, migration, invasion, and lymph nodes metastasis in xenografted mice.[5600]
- Nepalese marjoram essential oil with poor sabinene hydrate and higher linalool exhibited weak to moderate antioxidant activity in the FRAP and DPPH assays and good antifungal activity against *A. niger* and *C. albicans*.[5601]
- Researchers evaluated the ability of marjoram essential oil to preserve testicular function and sexual behavior in male rats after exposure to the insecticide imidacloprid (IMI).[5602] Twenty-eight rats were divided into four

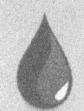

groups: 1) control group, 2) oral marjoram essential oil only, 3) oral IMI only, and 4) IMI and marjoram essential oil. The rats received the oil or IMI daily for sixty days. Notable abnormalities in territorial aggressive and sexual behaviors were observed in the IMI treated rats. Moreover, these rats experienced elevated follicle-stimulating hormone and luteinizing hormone, altered testicular antioxidant status, abnormal sperm, degeneration of testicular cells, and decreased testosterone. Co-administration of marjoram improved all the above-mentioned parameters and restored sexual behavior, supporting marjoram as a male fertility enhancer and reproductive organ protector.

- Marjoram was acaricidal to the cattle tick (*Rhipicephalus annulatus*).[5603] Addition of vitamins E and C increased its efficacy, but hydrogen peroxide decreased its effectiveness, suggesting that its antioxidant activity plays a role in its acaricidal activity.

- Administration of marjoram essential oil (30 mg and 45 mg) protected rats against kidney damage caused by ciprofloxacin possibly because marjoram activated the antioxidant defenses pathway.[5604]

- Marjoram CT terpinen-4-ol, oregano CT thymol, inhibited *B. subtilis, M. luteus, S. aureus, E, coli, K. pneumoniae,* and *P. aeruginosa*, while citronella (*C. winterianus*), geranium, and catnip CT nepetalactones were only active against some gram-positive bacteria.[5605]

# MASTIC
## (Lentisk)

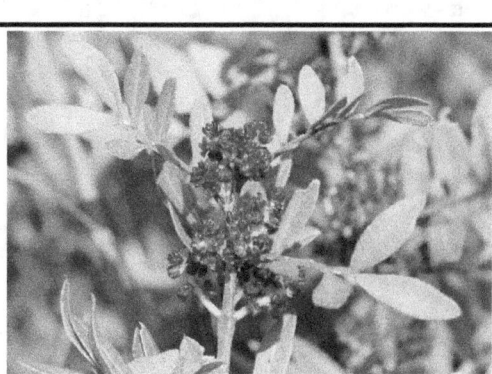

*Pistacia lentiscus* L., *Lentiscus massiliensis, L. vulgaris, Terebinthus lentiscus; P. lentiscus* L. var. *latifolius* Coss, *P. lentiscus* var. Chia

**FAMILY:** Anacardiaceae
**NOTE:** Base-Middle
**AROMA INTENSITY:** Strong
**AROMA:** Balsamic, herbaceous, earthy, resinous
**COMMON EXTRACTION METHOD:** Steam distilled from the gum resin; may also be steam distilled from the leaves and twigs/branches (aerial parts)
**POSSIBLE SUBSTITUTE OILS:** Cedarwood (Atlas), frankincense, tea tree, hemp, pine, palo santo
**BLENDS WELL WITH:** Allspice, balsam fir, bay laurel, bergamot, carrot seed, cassia, cedarwood, cistus, cinnamon, clary sage, clove, coriander, frankincense, galbanum, grapefruit, lavender, lavandin, lemon, lime, Mediterranean mandarin, myrrh, nutmeg, orange, palo santo, rose, rosewood, sandalwood, silver fir, sweet inula, tangerine, vetiver, ylang ylang, white fir
**SUBCELLULAR LOCALIZATION | EPIGENETIC INFLUENCE:** Currently unknown | Currently unknown
**RECOMMENDED DILUTION RANGE:** Beta-Myrcene CTs—3%–20%, 50% for some conditions; Terpinen-4-ol CT—3%–50%, neat for limited conditions; All other CTs—5%–Neat

**PRIMARY CONSTITUENTS:**[5606,5607,5608,5609,5610,5611,5612,5613,5614,5615,5616,5617,5618,5619]

| *Gum Resin* | | *Leaves & Twigs/Branches (Alpha-Pinene CT)* | |
|---|---|---|---|
| Alpha-Pinene | 21.7%–82.3% | Alpha-Pinene | 16.5%–40.2% |
| Beta-Pinene | 3.0%–38.7% | Limonene | 5.2%–17.8% |
| Pinocarvone | 0.0%–5.3% | Terpinen-4-ol | 6.8%–14.8% |
| Alpha-Ylangene | 0.0%–4.0% | Alpha-Phellandrene | 1.2%–13.4% |
| Limonene | 0.2%–3.8% | Beta-Pinene | 2.0%–12.8% |
| N-Nonanal | 0.0%–3.5% | Beta-Myrcene | 1.3%–11.5% |
| Beta-Myrcene | 1.9%–3.2% | Sabinene | 1.0%–6.8% |
| | | Beta-Phellandrene | 0.0%–5.8% |
| *Leaves & Twigs/Branches (Terpinen-4-ol CT)* | | Camphene | 1.1%–5.1% |
| Terpinen-4-ol | 25.1%–43.8% | Alpha-Terpineol | 2.5%–5.0% |
| Alpha-Pinene | 7.1%–22.4% | Gamma-Terpinene | 2.2%–4.2% |
| Sabinene | 4.2%–10.5% | Alpha-Thujene | 0.8%–4.2% |
| Bornyl Acetate | 0.5%–10.3% | | |

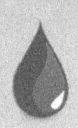

| | |
|---|---|
| Para-Cymene | 4.8%–10.2% |
| Alpha-Phellandrene | 4.3%–10.0% |
| Gamma-Terpinene | 4.9%–7.8% |
| Limonene | 4.0%–5.2% |
| Beta-Caryophyllene | 1.1%–5.2% |
| Beta-Pinene | 2.3%–5.1% |
| Alpha-Terpineol | 3.7%–5.0% |
| Alpha-Terpinene | 3.6%–5.0% |
| Beta-Phellandrene | 3.7%–4.8% |
| Germacrene D | 2.2%–4.1% |
| Camphene | 2.2%–4.0% |

*Leaves & Twigs/Branches (Beta-Myrcene CT)*

| | |
|---|---|
| Beta-Myrcene | 75.5%–89.5% |
| Alpha-Pinene | 2.5%–5.5% |
| Alpha-Phellandrene | 1.5%–3.5% |
| Germacrene D | 0.8%–2.1% |
| Terpinen-4-ol | 0.5%–2.0% |

*Leaves & Twigs/Branches (Germacrene D CT)*

| | |
|---|---|
| Germacrene D | 13.5% |
| Terpinen-4-ol | 10.0% |
| Alpha-Pinene | 9.4% |
| Limonene | 9.0% |
| Sabinene | 6.7% |
| Beta-Caryophyllene | 4.1% |
| Alpha-Terpineol | 4.0% |
| Alpha-Cadinol | 3.8% |
| Delta-Cadinene | 3.4% |
| Gamma-Terpinene | 3.1% |
| Beta-Pinene | 2.9% |

*Twigs (Alpha-Pinene CT)*

| | |
|---|---|
| Alpha-Pinene | 19.2% |
| Tricyclene | 8.2% |
| Beta-Caryophyllene | 6.2% |
| (E)-Beta-Ocimene | 6.9% |
| Germacrene D | 5.2% |
| Delta-3-Carene | 5.2% |
| Delta-Cadinene | 4.0% |
| Aromadendrene Oxide | 3.8% |
| Para-Cymene | 3.5% |
| Alpha-Phellandrene | 3.4% |

*Aerial Parts (Beta-Eudesmol CT)*

| | |
|---|---|
| Beta-Eudesmol | 16.3% |
| Alpha-Pinene | 8.6% |
| (–)-Cedreanol | 7.7% |
| Beta-Caryophyllene | 6.6% |
| Delta-Cadinene | 5.6% |
| Sabinene | 5.5% |

*Leaves & Twigs/Branches (Limonene CT)*

| | |
|---|---|
| Limonene | 46.2%–51.8% |
| Terpinen-4-ol | 10.2%–15.3% |
| Alpha-Pinene | 4.9%–6.5% |
| Beta-Myrcene | 3.0%–4.5% |
| Sabinene | 2.3%–3.2% |
| Germacrene D | 1.8%–3.1% |
| Gamma-Terpinene | 1.9%–2.5% |
| Camphene | 0.9%–2.3% |
| Beta-Caryophyllene | 0.7%–2.3% |

*Leaves*

| | |
|---|---|
| Beta-Myrcene | 0.2%–39.2% |
| Terpinen-4-ol | 1.6%–29.9% |
| Alpha-Pinene | 0.0%–24.3% |
| Germacrene D | 0.0%–14.3% |
| Beta-Caryophyllene | 0.0%–12.8% |
| Beta-Pinene | 0.0%–12.6% |
| Alpha-Terpineol | 0.1%–11.6% |
| Limonene | 0.0%–10.6% |
| Epi-Alpha-Muurolol | 0.0%–9.1% |
| Para-Cymene | 0.0%–8.5% |
| Beta-Gurjunene | 0.0%–7.8% |
| Tricyclene | 0.0%–7.7% |
| Delta-3-Carene | 0.0%–7.2% |
| Sabinene | 0.0%–7.0% |
| (Z)-3-Hex-1-Enyl Benzoate | 0.0%–6.7% |
| Caryophyllene Oxide | 0.0%–6.1% |
| Delta-Cadinene | 0.4%–5.2% |
| Beta-Phellandrene | 0.0%–5.0% |
| Epi-Alpha-Cadinol | 0.0%–4.9% |
| Gamma-Terpinene | 0.0%–4.5% |
| (E)-Beta-Ocimene | 0.0%–3.9% |
| Alpha-Phellandrene | 0.0%–3.5% |
| Bornyl Acetate | 0.1%–3.3% |
| Alpha-Humulene | 0.0%–3.3% |
| Verbenol | 0.0%–3.1% |
| Alpha-Cadinol | 0.0%–3.0% |

*Twigs (Beta-Myrcene CT)*

| | |
|---|---|
| Beta-Myrcene | 34.1% |
| Limonene | 9.6% |
| Beta-Gurjunene | 6.5% |
| Terpinen-4-ol | 6.3% |
| Germacrene D | 4.1% |
| Alpha-Pinene | 3.8% |
| Alpha-Terpinene | 3.6% |

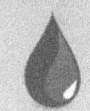

| Myrcene | 5.3% |
| Gamma-Cadinene | 5.0% |
| Terpinen-4-ol | 4.1% |

Note: Mastic leaf essential oil could be split into at least four different chemotypes (beta-myrcene, terpinen-4-ol, alpha-pinene, and limonene) but they are combined for simplification. Many experts consider the essential oil obtained from the gum resin to be the most therapeutic.

**OTHER CONSTITUENTS:** *Gum Resin*—camphene, dimyrcene I-a, dimyrcene II-b, n-undecane, pinocarveol, borneol, alpha-terpineol, myrtenol, verbenone, (Z)-carveol, bornyl acetate, thymol, carvacrol, n-tridecane, alpha-guianene, germacrene D; *Leaves & Twigs/Branches (Terpinen-4-ol CT)*—tricyclene, beta-myrcene, alpha-thujene, terpinolene, (E)-beta-ocimene, nonan-2-one, endecan-2-one, delta-cadinene, T-muurolol, alpha-cadinol; *Leaves & Twigs/Branches (Alpha-Pinene CT)*—tricyclene, beta-myrcene, alpha-terpinene, (E)-beta-ocimene, terpinolene, para-cymene, nonan-2-one, bornyl acetate, beta-caryophyllene, undecan-2-one, delta-cadinene, T-muurolol, alpha-cadinol; *Leaves & Twigs/Branches (Limonene CT)*—tricyclene, beta-pinene, alpha-phellandrene, alpha-terpinene, beta-phellandrene, (E)-beta-ocimene, para-cymene, terpinolene, nonan-2-one, bornyl acetate, undecan-2-one, alpha-terpineol, delta-cadinene, alpha-cadinol; *Leaves & Twigs/Branches (Beta-Myrcene CT)*—beta-pinene, limonene, beta-phellandrene, gamma-terpinene, beta-caryophyllene, alpha-terpineol, delta-cadinene, alpha-cadinol; *Leaves & Twigs/Branches (Germacrene D CT)*— camphene, beta-myrcene, alpha-phellandrene, alpha-terpinene, copaene, alpha-humulene, gamma-cadinene, alpha-muurolene, gamma-cadinene, 1-epi-cubenol, caryophyllene oxide, epi-alpha-cadinol, cadinol isomer; *Leaves*—camphene, para-cymenene, geraniol, beta-elemene, alpha-caryophyllene, benzoic acid, pentyl ester, aromadendrene, 3-methyl butyl hexanoate, alpha-copaene, beta-cubebene, 2-undecanone, alloaromadendrene, trans-p-meth-2-en-ol, gamma-muurolene, alpha-terpinyl acetate, alpha-muurolene, bicyclogermacrene, gamma-cadinene, caryophyllene oxide, (E)-geranyl acetate, cis-calamenene, para-cymen-8-ol, (E)-geranyl acetone, isoamylbenzene, humulene epoxide I, 1-epi-cubenol, T-muurolol, delta-cadinol, alpha-amorphene, linalool, 1,8-cineole; *Twigs (Alpha-Pinene CT)*—camphene, terpinene-4-ol, alpha-terpineol, trans-carveol, bornyl acetate, undecanone, alpha-cubebene, beta-elemene, alpha-caryophyllene, aromadendrene, alpha-muurolene, gamma-cadinene, spathulenol, caryophyllene oxide; *Twigs (Beta-Myrcene CT)*—beta-pinene, alpha-phellandrene, para-cymene, 1,8-cineole, linalool, camphor, para-cymene-8-ol, 2-undecanone, alpha-copaene, epi-cicyclosesquiphellandrene, alpha-humulene, alla-aromadendrene, delta-muurolene, caryophyllene oxide, humulene epoxide, T-cadinol; *Aerial Parts (Beta-Eudesmol CT)*—Gamma-terpinene, para-cymene, 2-carene terpinolene, trans-2-caren-4-ol, alpha-copaene, calamenene, n-methylbenzenamide, 1-endo-bourbonanol, phenylethyl isovalerate, caryophyllene oxide, cumin alcohol, carvacrol, ε-cadinene, allo-aromadendrene, 2-naphthoic acid, patchoulane, 1-naphthalenepropanol

**PREFERRED COMPOSITION FOR CLINICAL USE:**

| Constituent | Balanced CT | α-Pinene CT | Gum Chios Mastiha | Gum Resin |
|---|---|---|---|---|
| **Alpha-Pinene** | 14%–30% | 15%–30% | 55%–88% | 45%–60% |
| **Beta-Myrcene** | 12%–30% | 0.1%–6% | 4%–28% | 2%–7% |
| **Limonene** | 3%–15% | 5%–20% | 0.1%–5% | 1%–5% |
| **Terpinen-4-ol** | 3%–10% | 5%–15% | – | – |
| **Alpha-Phellandrene** | 3%–10% | 1%–7% | – | – |
| **Gamma-Terpinene** | 2%–10% | 2%–5% | – | – |
| **Alpha-Terpinene** | 1%–6% | – | – | – |
| **Sabinene** | 0.1%–6% | 2%–7% | – | – |
| **Beta-Pinene** | 2%–5% | 2%–10% | 0.5%–5% | 10%–25% |
| **Beta-Phellandrene** | 1%–5% | – | – | – |
| **Beta-Caryophyllene** | 0.5%–5% | – | tr–5% | – |
| **Germacrene D** | 0.5%–5% | – | – | – |
| **Camphene** | 1%–3% | 2%–5% | tr–3% | 0.1%–3% |
| **Alpha-Terpinolene** | 0.5%–3% | – | – | – |
| **Alpha-Terpineol** | 0.1%–2% | 2%–5% | – | 0.1%–3% |
| **Alpha-Thujene** | 0%–2% | 2%–5% | – | – |

**REPORTED THERAPEUTIC PROPERTIES:** Antibacterial, antifungal, antimicrobial, antiviral, antiparasitic, antiseptic, **analgesic**, anti-inflammatory, antispasmodic, aids lymph flow, **supports respiratory function**, expels excess mucus, supports oral health, wound healing, relieves boils and bruises, reduces edema, aids circulation, reduces varicose veins, astringent, supports prostate and urinary tract health, aids digestion, supports cognitive function, grounding, stress management, relieves anxiety

## CAUTIONS:

*Beta-Eudesmol CT*

■ May interact with antibiotics and possibly enhance their effects.[5620]

*Beat-Myrcene CTs*

■ May weakly interfere with the enzymes responsible for metabolizing medications (NSAIDs, proton-pump inhibitors, acetaminophen, antiepileptics, immune modulators, blood-sugar medications, blood pressure medications, antidepressants, antipsychotics, diabetic medications, antihistamines, antibiotics, and anesthetics) based on myrcene content.[5621,5622,5623]

■ May interfere with pentobarbital and other barbiturates (medications for anxiety and insomnia) based on beta-myrcene content.[5624]

*All other CTs*

■ None currently known.

■ Two case reports of acute generalized exanthematous pustulosis (an uncommon skin eruption characterized by pustules that is generally caused by taking a drug) are reported in the literature following the ingestion of mastic essential oil.[5625] However, the authors do not report the amount of the oil ingested or the duration it was taken, nor did they analyze the essential oil to determine its authenticity and chemical composition. Insufficient information is available currently from these case studies to warrant cautions for oral administration particularly since this type of reaction has not been reported from ingesting essential oils of similar composition.

## SELECTED EVIDENCE:

☐ Animal research demonstrates that injection of mastic gum essential oil (45–625 mg/kg) every other day for up to 20 days significantly inhibited the growth of Lewis lung carcinoma by increasing apoptosis, reducing neovascularization (the formation of functional microvascular networks to supply blood to tumors), and inhibiting chemokine expression (regulate the migration of leukocytes into tumors, which can have protumor and antitumor effects).[5626] A complex/balanced beta-myrcene CT of mastic (aerial parts: myrcene 25.3%, alpha-pinene 18.6%, limonene + beta-phellandrene 9.8%, alpha-phellandrene 7.3%, terpinen-4-ol 7.1%) was cytotoxic to thyroid cancer cells without harming healthy cells, and potentiated the cytotoxic effects of cisplatin, 5-fluorouracil, and etoposide.[5627]

☐ *In vitro* research demonstrates that mastic essential oil actively inhibits *S. aureus, E. coli, B. subtilis Salmonella sp., Bacillus sp., Enterococcus faecalis, Mycobacterium aurum, M. smegmatis, K. pneumonia,* and *P. aeruginosa.*[5628,5629,5630] The beta-eudesmol CT of mastic essential oil significantly inhibited three clinical isolates of MRSA, and moderately inhibited multidrug-resistant *E. coli* and *A. baumannii.*[5631] It also created a synergistic antimicrobial activity with some synthetic antibiotics and helped reverse bacterial resistance to some bacterial strains (tetracycline and pipercillin with *E.coli*, ofloxacin with *A. baumannii*, and pipercillin, ofloxacin, amoxicillin, and tetracycline against MRSA).

☐ Mastic essential oil inhibits the fungus *R. solani.*[5632] Another study reported that two chemotypes were weakly active against *A. flavus.*[5633]

☐ Mastic essential oil kills *Trichomonas vaginalis* (an anaerobic, flagellated protozoan parasite that causes the sexually transmitted disease trichomoniasis).[5634]

☐ Animal research demonstrates that mastic essential oil protects the liver against oxidative damage and dysfunction caused by arsenic.[5635] Another animal study demonstrates that mastic essential oil protects the liver against injury caused by a loss of and return of blood supply (ischemia-reperfusion) due to its antioxidant and anti-inflammatory effects.[5636]

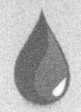

- Oral administration of mastic essential oil (supercritical $CO_2$ extraction, high in Germacrene D) prevented the loss of DHA in the frontal cortex and decreased COX-2 enzyme levels after loss of blood, oxygen, and nutrient supply to the brain due to a blocked artery in rats.[5637]

- Topical application of mastic essential oil reduced inflammation (decreasing the proinflammatory molecules IL-6 and TNF-alpha, leukocyte migration, and mast cell degranulation) in rats.[5638] Mast cell degranulation increases inflammation in allergic diseases.

- Mastic essential oil demonstrates good antioxidant activity.[5639]

- Mastic essential oil is insecticidal to the *Culex pipiens* mosquito (a carrier of West Nile and Rift Valley fever viruses).[5640]

- Constituents extracted in mastic essential oil (alpha-terpineol and (E)-methyl isoeugenol) inhibit the bacterium *H. pylori*, which is associated with an increased risk of peptic ulcers.[5641]

- Various chemotypes of mastic essential oil demonstrated varying cytotoxicity to breast, ovarian, and colorectal cancer cells.[5642] The activity of the mastic essential oil samples of various composition ranged from high activity on some cancer cells to being inactive, leading the study authors to conclude that it is likely the phytocomplexes of the whole essential oil determined its anticancer activity rather than a single compound.

- *In vitro* research demonstrates that mastic essential oil inhibits the fungus *Cryptococcus neoformans*.[5643]

- Oral administration (0.58 g/kg body weight/day for 13 days) of essential oil extracted from mastic resin (67.7% alpha-pinene and 18.8% myrcene) significantly suppressed the growth of colon cancer cells in mice.[5644]

- Mastic leaf essential oil (11.5% terpinen-4-ol, 8.6% germacrene D, 6% alpha-pinene, 5.1% caryophyllene) exhibited potent antioxidant activity (improved cell viability, ROS scavenging, and overall antioxidant activity) and protected lung epithelial cells against cytotoxicity caused by nickel oxide nanoparticles.[5645]

- Mastic essential oil exhibited good antioxidant activity at higher concentrations in the DPPH and ABTS assays and inhibited *E. coli, S. enteritidis, S. aureus,* and *L. monocytogenes*.[5646]

- Pistacia leaf essential oil exhibited broad-spectrum activity against periodontal bacteria and *Candida* and also showed a dual inhibitory action against COX-2 and LOX inflammatory enzymes without adverse effects against healthy oral cells.[5647]

- Helichrysum (Corsican type), mastic CT myrcene, and myrtle CT tricyclene essential oils demonstrated strong anticancer activity against human ovarian cancer cells.[5648] Rosemary CT alpha-pinene, thyme CT thymol, and yarrow CT 1,8-cineole exhibited weaker activity against cancer cells. All of the oils showed weak or no estrogenic activity in yeast strains expressing the human estrogen receptor alpha, while helichrysum and yarrow essential oils were antiestrogenic. All of the oils affected the proliferation and viability of human peripheral lymphocytes in a dose-dependent manner.

- Mastic resin CT myrcene essential oil increased the mRNA levels of genes involved in antioxidant activity but did not show any direct antioxidant activity in the performed tests.[5649] The oil also demonstrated the ability to protect human skin (keratinocyte) cells against UVB irradiation when added before exposure. One of its main constituents, myrcene was able to protect against UVB damage when added to skin cells after exposure. Additionally, the oil protected cells against damage caused by hydrogen peroxide and myrcene favorably influenced wound healing (increased cell migration and wound closure).

- Three separate mastic resin essential oils (alpha-pinene CTs)—two wild and one cultivated—exhibited anti-inflammatory activity based on inhibition of iNOS, with the wild types being more active. The oils also exhibited cytotoxicity toward various cancer cells: pancreatic, breast (two types), prostate, colorectal, cervical, bladder, non-small cell lung, macrophage-like, melanoma, primary glioblastoma, liver, and kidney. Remarkably, the wild types exceeded the anticancer activity of doxorubicin against pancreatic and glioblastoma cancer cells. The cultivated type was more active than the wild types against ER/PR negative breast, cervical and macrophage-like cancer cells. The wild types had higher percentages of myrcene (20.1% and 18.6% compared to 2.5%) and less alpha-pinene (56.2% and 51.9% compared to 70.8%) when compared to the cultivated type. Lastly, the researchers found that the oils were weak antimicrobials against *E. coli, S. aureus, L. monocytogenes, K. pneumoniae, S. typhimurium,* and *C. albicans*.

- Oregano CT carvacrol, lemon, lavender, mastic, and mandarin essential oil each inhibited *S. aureus*.[5650]

- Mastic CT alpha-pinene essential oil displayed weak to moderate antioxidant activity in the DPPH, beta-carotene bleaching, and ferrous ion chelating assays.[5651]

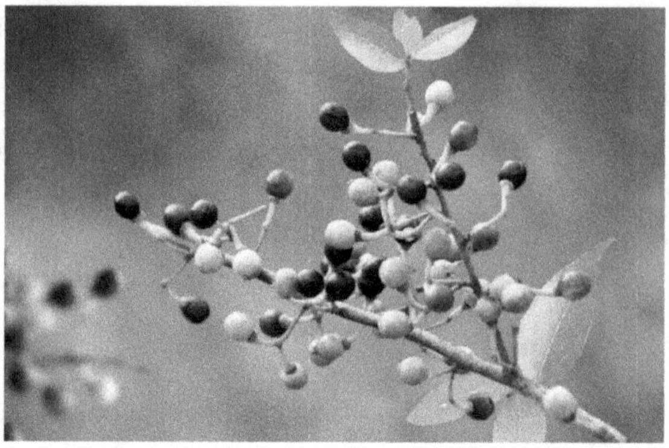

## MAY CHANG
### (Litsea, Pheasant Pepper Tree, Mountain Pepper, Cubeba, Chinese Pepper)

*Litsea cubeba* (Lour.) Pers.

**FAMILY:** Lauraceae
**NOTE:** Top-Middle
**AROMA INTENSITY:** Strong
**AROMA:** Lemony, fresh, grassy, sharp
**COMMON EXTRACTION METHOD:** Steam distilled from the fruits
**POSSIBLE SUBSTITUTE OILS:** Lemongrass, lemon verbena, Melissa, palmarosa, citronella
**BLENDS WELL WITH:** Basil, bay laurel, black pepper, cardamom, cedarwood, chamomile (German, Roman), clary sage, coriander, cypress, eucalyptus, frankincense, geranium, ginger, grapefruit, juniper, lavender, lemon, marjoram, neroli, orange, palmarosa, patchouli, petitgrain, rosemary, sandalwood, tea tree, thyme, vetiver, ylang ylang
**SUBCELLULAR LOCALIZATION | EPIGENETIC INFLUENCE:** Currently unknown | Currently unknown
**RECOMMENDED DILUTION RANGE:** 1.5%–20%; neat for limited conditions

**PRIMARY CONSTITUENTS:**[5652,5653,5654,5655,5656,5657]

*Citral CT*

| | |
|---|---|
| Geranial | 33.2%–50.0% |
| Neral | 26.1%–36.3% |
| D-Limonene | 0.7%–22.9% |
| Citronellal | 0.0%–6.2% |
| Bornyl Acetate | 0.0%–4.0% |
| Beta-Caryophyllene | 0.1%–3.5% |
| Geraniol | 0.4%–2.6% |

*Neral CT*

| | |
|---|---|
| Neral | 63.6% |
| Limonene | 7.4% |
| Camphene | 3.1% |
| Methyl heptenone | 3.5% |
| Alpha-Pinene | 2.9% |
| Para-Cymene | 2.1% |

*Citronellal CT*

| | |
|---|---|
| Citronellal | 44.8%–77.2% |
| Citronellol | 10.9%–14.0% |
| Limonene | 2.2%–6.1% |
| Geraniol | 1.1%–4.6% |
| Sabinene | 0.8%–2.4% |

Note: The citral CT is more commonly reported in the literature and seems to be more commonly available commercially. The leaf oil is primarily 1,8-cineole, gamma-elemene, beta-caryophyllene, linalool, and limonene; the flower oil is predominantly beta-terpinene, 1,8-cineole, alpha-pinene, and beta-pinene; and the stem oil is primarily beta-phellandrene, terpinen-4-ol, limonene, alpha-thujanol, and beta-pinene.

**OTHER CONSTITUENTS:** *Citral CT*—Methyl heptene, beta-myrcene, 1,8-cineole, linalool, verbenol, isopulegone, alpha-terpineol, nerol, beta-farnesene, thujanol, para-cymene, camphene, gamma-terpinene, sabinene, alpha-terpineol, eugenol, geranyl acetate; *Citronellal CT*—Alpha-pinene, beta-pinene, 1,8-cineole, linalool, isopulegol, iso(iso)pulegol, terpinen-4-ol, alpha-terpineol; *Neral CT*—beta-phellandrene, beta-pinene, beta-myrcene, 1,8-cineole, linalool, citronellal, terpinen-4-ol, geraniol, safrole (<1.2%), geranyl acetate, n-(E)-nerolidol

**PREFERRED COMPOSITION FOR CLINICAL USE:**

| Constituent | Citral CT (China) | Citral CT (India) |
|---|---|---|
| Geranial | 35%–50% | 35%–45% |
| Neral | 28%–40% | 24%–35% |

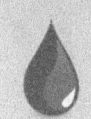

| | | |
|---|---|---|
| Limonene | 9%–18% | 9%–18% |
| Linalool | 1%–4% | 0.01%–3% |
| 5-Heptan-2-One, 6-Methyl | 0.1%–3% | 1%–3% |
| Beta-Caryophyllene | 0.1%–3% | < 1% |
| Citronellal | < 3% | 0.1%–8% |
| Geraniol | 0.5%–2% | 0.5%–2% |
| Citronellol | 0.5%–2% | < 0.5% |
| Nerol | 0.1%–2% | < 0.5% |
| Alpha-Pinene | < 2% | < 2% |
| Camphene | < 1% | 0.1%–4% |
| Alpha-Humulene | < 0.5% | 0%–2% |

Note: Citral (geranial + neral) content should be ≥ 65%.

**REPORTED THERAPEUTIC PROPERTIES:** Analgesic, antimicrobial, antifungal, astringent, antiseptic, antispasmodic, anti-inflammatory, anticancer, antirheumatic, **antiallergic**, antioxidant, anti-infectious, digestive aid, nervine, cardiovascular support, acne, headache, fever reducing, relieves dermatitis, **nourishes the skin**, supports respiratory function, expels excess gas, relieves excess sweating, encourages restful sleep, lowers blood pressure, deodorant, **insecticide**, uplifting to the emotions, relaxing, stress management, **relieves anxiety**, **antidepressant**

**CAUTIONS:**

■ Caution is advised during pregnancy and lactation due to high citral content. Large doses of citral may negatively affect fetal development according to animal studies.[5658]

■ May mildly interfere with enzymes responsible for metabolizing medications (NSAIDs, proton-pump inhibitors, acetaminophen, antiepileptics, immune modulators, blood-sugar medications, blood pressure medications, antidepressants, antipsychotics, diabetic medications, antihistamines, antibiotics, and anesthetics).[5659,5660]

■ May interfere with pentobarbital and other barbiturates (medications for anxiety and insomnia) and increase their sleeping effect.[5661]

■ Use cautiously with diabetic medications. Large oral doses of citral may improve insulin sensitivity and lower blood-glucose levels according to animal research.[5662,5663]

■ May interact with antibiotics and possibly enhance their effects due to citral content.[5664,5665]

■ Dilution is recommended for topical application due to high citral content and a study that suggests concentrations of 9.6% or higher may cause skin sensitivity.[5666] Sensitivity occurred at a concentration of 6.3% with isolated citral, and citral is a known skin and mucous membrane irritant.[5667,5668]

**SELECTED EVIDENCE:**

☐ *In vitro* research reported that the vapors of May Chang essential oil triggered apoptosis and cell cycle arrest (reducing cancer proliferation) of non-small cell lung cancer.[5669] Other research found that May Chang fruit oil is cytotoxic to human lung, liver, and oral cancer cells.[5670]

☐ May Chang essential oil actively inhibits a number of dermatophytes and was considered among the most effective of twenty essential oils tested.[5671]

☐ Animal research suggests that May Chang regulates central nervous system activity (modulating GABA receptor subtypes) to reduce anxiety.[5672]

☐ May Chang (citronellol CT) demonstrated wide spectrum inhibition against gram-positive bacteria, yeast, and fungi, but not against gram-negative bacteria.[5673] Another study found that it demonstrated antimicrobial activity against *E. coli* by destroying the outer and inner membrane of infected cells.[5674]

☐ May Chang essential oil moderately inhibits *B. subtilis, E. coli, E. faecalis, M. albicans, P. aeruginosa,* and S. aureus.[5675] Other research reports it is bactericidal against *Aer. hydrophila, Edwarsiella tarda, Vibrio furnissii, Vibrio parahaemolyticus, Streptococcus garvieae, Escherichia coli,* and *Salmonella Typhimurium.*[5676]

☐ *In vitro* research concluded that May Chang essential oil inhibits the fungus *Microsporum canis* (a fungus that infects the outer layer of skin on cats that can cause ringworm in humans).[5677]

☐ A review paper concluded that May Chang demonstrates anticancer, anti-rheumatic, antiallergic, and antioxidant effects, and positively benefits the cardiovascular and respiratory systems.[5678] Some of the review's conclusions were based on Chinese studies of May Chang where no abstract or English translation is available.[5679,5680,5681]

☐ May Chang essential oil (often leaf oil) repels and/or kills mosquitoes, termites, cabbage looper, beetles, and mealworms (*Tenebrio molitor*).[5682,5683,5684,5685,5686]

☐ Animal research shows that may chang essential oil reduces contact hypersensitivity by suppressing the immune response of infiltrative T cells (T cells that have migrated to allergen-exposed sites and initiate skin reactions), which may make it helpful for hypersensitivity reactions, autoimmune disorders, and inflammatory diseases.[5687]

☐ Citral (geranial + neral), alleviates an animal model of lupus nephrititis (inflammation of the kidneys caused by lupus) by inhibiting inflammasome activation (a pathway responsible for activating the inflammatory response) and levels of reactive oxygen species, IL-1beta, and COX-2, and enhancing Nrf2 activation.[5688] Nrf2 is a potent protein found within all cells (but particularly in the liver and kidneys) that acts as the master regulator of the cellular antioxidant system when activated by AREs (antioxidant response elements). Once triggered, Nrf2 activates over 200 genes that metabolize drugs and toxins, protect against oxidative stress, remove damaged proteins, and normalize inflammation. It also interacts with other cells that together determine longevity and protect against age-related diseases like cancer and neurological disorders.[5689] The same researchers discovered that citral reduces abnormal quantities of protein in the urine, kidney function impairment, and kidney disease.

☐ *In vitro* research concluded that the 1,8-cineole and linalool CTs of may chang essential oil possess antibacterial activity against eight bacterial strains.[5690] The linalool CT was more effective and damaged bacterial (*E. coli*) cell integrity leading to cell permeabilization (providing the ability to detect intracellular or extracellular antigens and access for antibodies) and altered nucleoid morphology (changes to the form of the part of the cell that houses primary DNA). The 1,8-cineole CT also damaged cell morphology, caused DNA loss, and modified cell integrity and permeability.

☐ Clove (diluted in coconut or sunflower oil) and may chang (diluted in coconut oil) essential oil showed significant efficacy against head lice (*Pediculus humanus capitis*).[5691] Clove demonstrated the best adulticidal activity at > 90 percent mortality within two hours after 30-minutes of contact.

☐ *Borrelia burgdorferi* is a diderm bacteria responsible for Lyme disease in the United States. Of thirty-five essential oils screened, garlic, allspice, cumin, palmarosa, myrrh, ginger lily, amyris, thyme, may chang, and lemon eucalyptus each demonstrated excellent activity against *Borrelia burgdorferi*.[5692] Garlic (19% diallyl disulfide), allspice CT eugenol, and myrrh (38% curzerene) were the most active essential oils.

☐ The citral CT of may chang essential oil exhibited good antimicrobial (*Staphylococcus aureus, Escherichia coli*, and *Salmonella typhimurium*) and antioxidant activity in the OH, DPPH, and FRAP assays.[5693]

☐ May chang CT citral essential oil synergized the activity of another antimicrobial agent against *E. coli* by increasing bacterial cell membrane permeability, which allows more uptake and diffusion of antimicrobial substances inside the cell.[5694]

☐ The essential oils of lemon (fungicidal), cypress (fungicidal), and may chang (fungistatic) each demonstrated anticandidal activity in planktonic (free flowing bacteria in suspension) cells and biofilms (a thin, slimy film of bacteria adhered to a surface) and cypress increased survival of the tested host in the *Caenorhabditis elegans-Candida* model.[5695]

☐ Of sixteen commercial essential oils tested (frankincense sacra, frankincense serrata, fennel, cistus, mountain savory CT carvacrol, oregano CT carvacrol, thyme CT thymol, cinnamon bark, may chang, clove bud, lemongrass—*C. citratus*, bitter orange, lemon, sweet orange, star anise, and lemon verbena), may chang and cinnamon bark essential oil were the most active against tested human cancer cells (breast—three types, chronic myelogenous erythroleukemia, and neuroblastoma).[5696] Other notable activity was observed with frankincense sacra and sweet orange against myelogenous leukemia.

☐ Thyme CT thymol, garlic, tea tree, cajeput, may chang, lemongrass (*C. citratus*), and verbena CT citral exhibited fungistatic activity (100 percent) against *F. culmorum* and *F. graminearum*, and all but garlic (89.4%) were 100% fungistatic against *F. avenaceum* and *F. oxyporum*.[5697]

☐ Inhalation of diffused may chang essential oil for thirty minutes improved total mood state and reduced confusion in 15 healthy adults. Salivary cortisol levels were reduced, suggesting reduced stress.[5698]

☐ *In vitro* research showed that may chang essential oil inhibits *S. aureus* by modifying its gene expression.[5699]

☐ An unidentified CT of may chang essential oil alleviated pain associated with irritation or injury in mice.[5700]

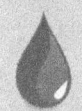

The oil was injected at 150, 300, and 600 mg/kg body weight reduced pain by 17 percent, 30 percent, and 54 percent respectively. The same study showed the oil decreased fever and inhibited (in descending order of inhibition) *C. albicans, A. fumigatus*, MRSA, *S. aureus, E. faecalis, E. coli, S. enteritidis*, and *P. aeruginosa*.

☐ *In vitro* research demonstrated that may chang essential oil inhibits *E. coli* and its addition to different vegetable juices at the minimum inhibitory concentration maintained antibacterial activity above 99.9 percent for four days without significantly influencing food sensory quality.[5701]

☐ May chang essential oil inactivated *S. aureus* and *E. coli* when added to packaging material at 20% concentrations.[5702] Isolated citral was bactericidal to *S. aureus* and *E. coli* at 20% concentrations and inactivated *S. cerevisiae* and *A. niger* at 3% and 5% concentrations.

☐ The citral CT of may chang essential oil displayed good antioxidant activity in the DPPH and ABTS assays, killed colorectal and cervical cancer cells, and inhibited *F. verticillioides*.[5703]

☐ May chang, Virginia cedarwood, spearmint, and tea tree essential oils each demonstrated contact toxicity against third instar larvae of the cotton leafworm (*Alabama argillacea*).[5704] Each oil changed the histochemistry of the testicles, while tea tree, Virginia cedarwood, and spearmint altered morphology. In addition, the histochemistry of the ovarioles was altered by Virginia cedarwood, tea tree, and may chang.

☐ Deep eutectic solvent-homogenate based microwave-assisted hydrodistillation (DES-HMAHD) extraction of may chang essential oil produced an EO with lower citral and higher alpha-terpineol.[5705] The biological activity of the oil showed it had higher antioxidant (DPPH and ABTS) activity but lower antifungal activity than traditionally distilled oil.

☐ Textiles treated with may chang and lemon essential oil microemulsion displayed strong antimicrobial activity against skin-associated microorganisms—*E. coli, S. aureus, S. epidermidis*, and *T. rubrum*—and repelled *Ae. aegypti* mosquitoes.[5706]

☐ A clinical study evaluated the effects of inhaling may chang, turmeric, and garlic essential oils on mood.[5707] Electroencephalography was used to measure brainwave activity during a non-task resting state, and mood state was self-reported. Fifty microliters of three different dilution ratios of each oil were dropped onto filter paper, which was attached to the subject's nose. May chang reduced alpha and beta brainwave power, promoting sedation. Garlic oil increased alpha power at lower concentrations but decreased alpha power at higher concentrations. Both may chang and turmeric essential oils improved subjective mood, whereas garlic produced more negative moods.

☐ Oregano CT carvacrol, may chang, and manuka each displayed acaricidal activity against the Asian blue tick (Rhipicephalus microplus).[5708] Beta-triketone fractions from manuka caused significant larval mortality, while its sesquiterpene fraction was far less effective. Interestingly, the sesquiterpene fractions were more effective on adults than the beta-triketone fractions.

☐ *Cutibacterium acnes* is a bacterium normally found on the skin associated with acne and surgical infections. May chang essential oil exhibited promising antibacterial activity against *C. acnes* by altering eighty-six metabolites and thirty-four metabolic pathways in the bacterium.[5709]

☐ May chang essential oil demonstrated synergistic and additive antibacterial activity against *V. parahaemolyticus* when used with tetracycline or oxytetracycline hydrochloride.[5710] The essential oil alone also inhibited growth and promoted removal of biofilms.

☐ May chang essential oil inhibited *C. albicans* with molecular docking studies showing that geranial, neral, and limonene bound to cellular targets to inhibit its growth.[5711]

☐ Incorporation of may chang essential oil into three soft lining materials (GC soft liner, Viscogel and Coe-Comfort) inhibited common oral pathogens (*C. albicans* and *S. mutans*).[5712]

☐ May chang CT citral and damiana CT citral demonstrated strong antiviral activity against dengue virus and inhibited viral replication.[5713] Computer docking studies showed that twenty sesquiterpene hydrocarbons, eight oxygenated monoterpenes, and seven monoterpene hydrocarbons had good binding affinity to the DENV-2 E protein with cis-calamenene, delta-cadinene, alpha-cadinene, alpha-guiene, gamma-cadinene, and viridiflorene having the highest binding affinity.

☐ Inhalation of may chang CT citral essential oil promoted relaxation and alertness in healthy men and women according to EEG (electroencephalogram) readings.[5714] Twenty-five men and women aged twenty to twenty-five years old first inhaled sweet almond oil (control) via a face mask. After a seven-day washout period, they inhaled a 10% dilution of may chang essential oil via face mask. Inhalation of the oil increased absolute powers of alpha and beta brainwaves, suggesting calmness and alertness, respectively, when compared to sweet almond oil.

☐ May chang essential oil extracted by solvent-free microwave (SFME) extraction significantly increased limonene content and yield compared to hydrodistillation.[5715] The SFME oil also exhibited enhanced inhibition of tyrosinase and melanogenesis, indicating a skin-whitening effect.

□ *Cronobacter sakazakii* is a foodborne bacterium able to survive in very dry places (xerotolerance) that can causer neonatal meningitis, necrotizing enterocolitis, and bacteremia, with an alarming mortality rate. Infected people that do survive may have lasting complications such as ventriculitis (inflammation of the ventricles in the brain) and cerebral abscess (a pus-filled pocket of infected material in the brain). May chang essential oil inhibited clinical and foodborne isolates of *C. sakazakii* in laboratory research and inhibited the bacteria in reconstructed infant formula. Moreover, the oil inactivated *C. sakazakii* biofilms on stainless steel surfaces, suggesting it has potential to cleanse surfaces and prevent and control *C. sakazakii* in industry and healthcare settings.

□ May chang essential oil strongly inhibited *S. sonnei* without negatively affecting the sensory quality of lettuce.[5716]

# MEDITERRANEAN MANDARIN
## (Sicilian Mandarin, Willowleaf Mandarin)
*Citrus* × *deliciosa* Ten.; *C.* × *deliciosa* Ten. var. *tangerina*

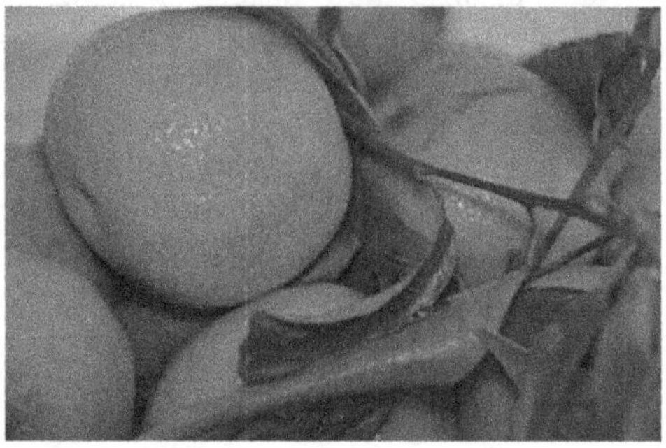

**FAMILY:** Rutaceae
**NOTE:** Top
**AROMA INTENSITY:** Medium
**AROMA:** Citrusy, sweet, fruity
**COMMON EXTRACTION METHOD:** Cold pressed/expressed or hydrodistilled from the peel (rind)
**POSSIBLE SUBSTITUTE OILS:** Lime, lemon, tangerine
**BLENDS WELL WITH:** Allspice, bergamot, cassia, cedarwood, cinnamon, clove, frankincense, grapefruit, lavender, lemon, lime, patchouli, peppermint, orange, sandalwood, spearmint, tangerine
**SUBCELLULAR LOCALIZATION | EPIGENETIC INFLUENCE:** Currently unknown | Currently unknown
**RECOMMENDED DILUTION RANGE:** 3.0%–50%; neat for limited conditions

**PRIMARY CONSTITUENTS:** [5717,5718,5719,5720,5721,5722]

| Hydrodistilled | | Cold Pressed | |
|---|---|---|---|
| Limonene | 70.5%–90.0% | Limonene | 65.3%–77.6% |
| Gamma-Terpinene | 0.1%–15.8% | Gamma-Terpinene | 13.1%–20.7% |
| Beta-Myrcene | 1.5%–3.5% | Alpha-Pinene | 0.3%–5.2% |
| N-Dodecanal | 0.0%–3.0% | Beta-Pinene | 0.5%–2.4% |
| Terpinen-4-ol | 0.0%–2.4% | Beta-Myrcene | 0.0%–1.8% |
| Alpha-Terpineol | 0.0%–2.2% | Alpha-Terpinolene | 0.0%–1.6% |
| Alpha-Pinene | 0.6%–1.5% | | |
| Methyl N-Methylanthranilate | 0.0%–1.5% | | |
| Sabinene | 0.2%–1.4% | | |

**OTHER CONSTITUENTS:** *Cold Pressed*—alpha-thujene, para-cymene, methyl n-methylanthranilate, alpha-sinesal, (E,E)-alpha-farnesene; *Hydrodistilled*—delta-3-carene, trans-beta-ocimene, decanal, linalool, alpha-terpinolene, thymol

**PREFERRED COMPOSITION FOR CLINICAL USE:**

| Constituent | Distilled | Cold-pressed |
|---|---|---|
| **Limonene** | 75%–90% | 65%–78% |
| **Myrcene** | 1%–5% | < 2% |
| **Alpha-Pinene** | 0.5%–2% | 0.1%–5% |
| **Sabinene** | 0.5%–2% | – |

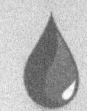

| | | |
|---|---|---|
| **Gamma-Terpinene** | 0.1%–2% | 12%–22% |
| **Alpha-Terpinolene** | 0.1%–2% | < 2% |
| **Beta-Pinene** | – | 0.5%–3% |

**REPORTED THERAPEUTIC PROPERTIES:** Antibacterial, antifungal, antiviral, antiseptic, antispasmodic, anticancer, aids lymph circulation, **promotes even skin tone**, reduces the appearance of scars and blemishes, relieves acne, **aids digestion**, supports gallbladder function and encourages the release of bile, diuretic, relieves constipation, promotes restful sleep, **reduces restlessness**, combats anger, reduces irritability, antidepressant, stress management, **relieves anxiety**

**CAUTIONS:**

■ May be photosensitizing (cold-pressed/expressed). Avoid sun exposure to area of application for at least twelve hours after topical application.[5723] The Mediterranean mandarin is a cross between the tangerine and pummelo. Reports suggest that tangerines are almost completely devoid of furanocoumarins that cause photosensitivity. However, the pummelo can contain significant amounts of these photosensitizing constituents.

**SELECTED EVIDENCE:**

☐ *In vitro* research reports that Mediterranean mandarin peel essential oil selectively kills liver, cervix, and breast-cancer cells, with some varieties demonstrating efficacy similar to doxorubicin (a chemotherapy drug used to treat multiple types of cancer).[5724]

☐ Mediterranean mandarin peel essential oil is a potent antioxidant when high levels of limonene are present.[5725]

☐ *In vitro* research demonstrates that Mediterranean mandarin peel essential oil inhibits the bacteria *S. aureus, Micrococcus luteus, E. coli, Proteus vulgarus,* and *Saccharomyces cervaceae* to varying degrees.[5726]

☐ Mediterranean mandarin peel essential oil inactivates the Avian bird flu virus (H5N1).[5727]

# MELISSA
## (Lemon Balm)
*Melissa officinalis* L.

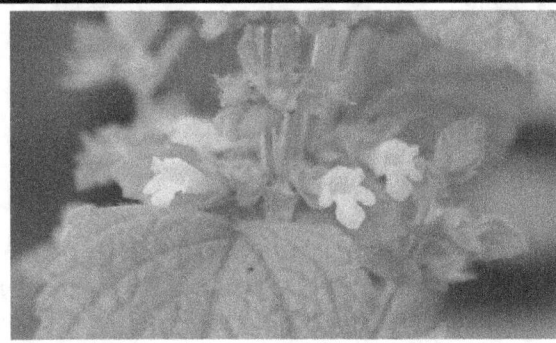

**FAMILY:** Lamiaceae (Labiatae)
**NOTE:** Middle
**AROMA INTENSITY:** Medium
**AROMA:** Fresh, herbaceous, lemony
**COMMON EXTRACTION METHOD:** Steam distilled from the flowers and leaves
**POSSIBLE SUBSTITUTE OILS:** Lemongrass, lemon verbena, lime (distilled)
**BLENDS WELL WITH:** Citronella, geranium, lavender, lemon, lemon verbena, myrtle, orange, neroli, palo santo, rose, ylang ylang
**SUBCELLULAR LOCALIZATION | EPIGENETIC INFLUENCE:** Currently unknown | Currently unknown
**RECOMMENDED DILUTION RANGE:** 3%–50%; neat for limited conditions

**PRIMARY CONSTITUENTS:**[5728,5729,5730,5731,5732]

| | |
|---|---|
| Geranial | 6.6%–45.2% |
| Neral | 4.6%–33.8% |
| Caryophyllene Oxide | 1.3%–31.7% |
| Citronellal | 0.4%–20.3% |
| Beta-Caryophyllene | 0.1%–15.3% |
| Geraniol | 0.1%–11.8% |

| | |
|---|---|
| Germacrene D | 0.1%–8.3% |
| Nerol | 0.0%–7.9% |
| Citronellol | 0.1%–7.7% |
| Geranyl Acetate | 0.1%–7.1% |
| Delta-3-Carene | 0.0%–5.0% |
| Citronellyl Acetate | 0.0%–3.7% |

Note: Multiple chemotypes of melissa essential oil are reported in the literature including citral, citronellal, citronellal/geranyl acetate, geraniol, alpha-muurolene, beta-caryophyllene, beta-pinene, terpinen-4-ol, caryophyllene oxide, limonene, and germacrene D (subsp. *altissima*).

**OTHER CONSTITUENTS:** (E)-beta-ocimene, neryl acetate, 6-methyl-5-hepten-2-ol, delta-cadinene, 6-methyl-5-hepten-2-one, alpha-copaene, methyl citronellate, alpha-terpineol, alpha caryophyllene, 1-octen-3-ol

**PREFERRED COMPOSITION FOR CLINICAL USE:**

| Constituent | Citral CT I | Citral CT II |
|---|---|---|
| **Geranial** | 25%–48% | 7%–28% |
| **Neral** | 15%–32% | 5%–20% |
| **Beta-Caryophyllene** | 5%–15% | 10%–30% |
| **Citronellal** | 5%–15% | 1%–10% |
| **Geraniol** | 2%–6% | 0.5%–2% |
| **Geranyl Acetate** | 1%–5% | 0.1%–3% |
| **Caryophyllene Oxide** | 0.5%–5% | 0.1%–2% |
| **6-Methyl-5-Hepten-2-one** | ≤ 5% | ≤ 3% |
| **Nerol** | ≤ 2.5% | ≤ 1.5% |
| **Alpha-Humulene** | ≤ 2% | 1%–5% |
| **Linalool** | 0.5%–2% | ≤ 2% |
| **Citronellol** | ≤ 1.5% | 0.1%–2% |
| **Delta-Cadinene** | ≤ 1% | 0.1%–4% |
| **Germacrene D** | ≤ 1% | 5%–24% |
| **Linalyl Acetate** | ≤ 0.5% | ≤ 2% |
| **(E)-Beta-Ocimene** | ≤ 0.5% | 0.5%–6% |

**REPORTED THERAPEUTIC PROPERTIES: Antiseptic, antiviral**, antibacterial, antifungal, **antispasmodic**, antitumor, **strengthens the heart**, expels excess gas, balances hormones, helps lower high blood pressure, **reduces the appearance of blemishes**, encourages the flow of bile, reduces fever, aids digestion, regulates menstruation, nervine (calms and soothes the nerves), relieves skin conditions, **regulates breathing**, encourages restful sleep, **antidepressant**, relieves vertigo, **heals cold sores and cankers**, warming, relaxing, reduces anxiety, comforts during grief, sedating, eases agitation, uplifting, combats anger and rage, relieves nightmares, calms hysteria

**CAUTIONS:**

■ Caution is advised during pregnancy and lactation due to high citral content. Large doses of citral may negatively affect fetal development according to animal studies.[5733]

■ May mildly interfere with enzymes responsible for metabolizing medications (NSAIDs, proton-pump inhibitors, acetaminophen, antiepileptics, immune modulators, blood sugar medications, blood pressure medications, antidepressants, antipsychotics, diabetic medications, antihistamines, antibiotics, and anesthetics).[5734,5735,5736,5737]

■ Use cautiously with diabetic medications. Large oral doses of citral may improve insulin sensitivity and lower blood-glucose levels according to animal research.[5738,5739] Also, low doses of melissa essential oil may decrease blood-sugar levels through enhanced glucose uptake and metabolism according to animal research.[5740]

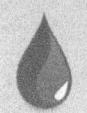

■ May interact with aspirin, blood pressure, antiplatelet, and anticoagulant medications, and increase the risk of bleeding among people with bleeding disorders due to caryophyllene oxide content.[5741]

■ May interact with anticholinergic (drugs used for asthma, incontinence, gastrointestinal cramps, muscular spasms, depression, and sleep disorders) and cholinergic medications (drugs used to reduce urinary retention, diagnose myasthenia gravis, and for glaucoma) based on AChE inhibitory activity.[5742,5743]

■ May interact with antibiotics and possibly enhance their effects due to citral content.[5744,5745]

■ There is a moderate risk that melissa may interfere with pentobarbital and other barbiturates (medications for anxiety and insomnia) based on citral content.[5746]

■ Dilution is recommended for topical application due to high citral content and the risk for skin irritation or sensitivity.[5747,5748] May also irritate mucous membranes.

**SELECTED EVIDENCE:**

☐ Melissa oil may prevent the formation of tumors and destroys lung carcinoma, breast, colorectal adenocarcinoma, promyelocytic leukemia, and myeloid leukemia cancer cells *in vitro*.[5749]

☐ Melissa oil causes apoptosis of glioblastoma multiforme cells (GBM). GBM is a common and aggressive tumor that begin in astrocytes (star-shaped cells that make up the supportive tissue of the brain) *in vitro*.[5750]

☐ Topical application of a lotion with melissa oil to the faces and arms of people with severe dementia reduced agitation in 35% of study participants.[5751]

☐ *In vitro* and animal research suggests that melissa oil may reduce agitation by reducing the release of neurotransmitters and interacting with brain cell receptors (nicotinic, muscarinic), and therefore reducing arousal, anxiety, and stimulation of the brain.[5752,5753,5754]

☐ Animal research suggests that melissa essential oil reduces pain associated with diabetic neuropathy in mice.[5755]

☐ *In vitro* research suggests that melissa oil may prevent and manage neurodegenerative diseases caused by oxidative stress by inhibiting acetylcholinesterase (AChE) and butyrylcholinesterase (BChE) enzyme activity, and preventing lipid peroxidation.[5756,5757] Inhibition of AChE prevents the breakdown of acetylcholine, which is essential for memory and thinking. People with neurodegenerative diseases make less acetylcholine, and the diseases often break it down at a faster rate leading to acetylcholine deficits. Selective inhibition of BChE is also desirable in neurodegenerative diseases because it interferes with acetylcholine activity. In addition, BChE is often found in the plaques and tangles in the brains of people with Alzheimer's disease.[5758]

☐ Melissa oil enhances glucose uptake and metabolism and prevents the production of sugar from noncarbohydrate sources within the body (gluconeogenesis) in type 2 diabetic mice.[5759]

☐ *In vitro* research suggests that melissa oil prevents the infection of healthy cells by the herpes virus.[5760] Other research concluded that melissa oil prevented the attachment of HSV-1 to host cells (adsorption) and killed HSV-1 at low concentrations.[5761,5762] Melissa also prevented HSV-2 replication (the duplication of genetic material to divide and produce to identical cells called daughter cells).[5763]

☐ Melissa oil helps decrease inflammation by inhibiting the 5-lipoxygenase (5-LOX) enzyme that is involved in the inflammation response according to *in vitro* research.[5764]

☐ A clinical study concluded that a twice-daily massage with a melissa oil cream (containing a total of 200 mg of oil; roughly four drops) reduced agitation and improved the quality of life in people with severe dementia.[5765]

☐ Melissa oil reduces inflammation, pain, and edema (swelling caused by excess fluid trapped in body tissues) in mice at a dose of 200 to 400 mg/kg.[5766]

☐ Melissa essential oil inhibits avian influenza A virus (H9N2) replication *in vitro*, with significant antiviral activity observed when cells were incubated with melissa essential oil before infection.[5767]

☐ Animal research suggests that oral administration of melissa oil reduces blood triglycerides by preventing the creation of fatty acids.[5768]

☐ Melissa oil significantly inhibits *C. albicans* and *T. brucei in vitro*.[5769,5770]

☐ *In vitro* research concluded that melissa is a potent free-radical scavenger (antioxidant), prevents lipid peroxidation (free-radical deterioration of lipids, which can disrupt cellular communication, destroy cells, and damage proteins or DNA), and inhibits *S. sonnei* and *Trichophyton* species.[5771]

☐ Animal research suggests that both melissa oil and citral reduce intestinal spasms in rats.[5772]

☐ A review recommended the topical application of diluted tea tree, peppermint, or melissa oil three to four times daily for recurrent herpetic infections (cold sores and genital herpes).[5773]

- *In vitro* research demonstrates that melissa essential oil effectively inhibits *L. amazonensis*.[5774]

- Melissa essential oil may be a viable option to treat *Acanthamoeba* spp. infections due to its ability to kill *A. castellani* cysts and trophozoites.[5775]

- Marjoram, pink savory (*Satureja thymbra*), spearmint CT piperitenone oxide, melissa, and dittany (*Origanum dictamnus*) demonstrated the greatest repellency toward *Ae. albopictus* mosquitoes of fourteen Lamiaceae species tested.[5776] Thyme CT thymol, basil, dittany, marjoram, and oregano CT carvacrol were the most larvicidal.

- *In vitro* examination of sixty essential oils demonstrated that sandalwood (Indian, Australian, and Hawaiian), melissa, lemongrass (*C. flexuosus*), cilantro, cassia, cinnamon, patchouli, and vetiver essential oils possess remarkable anticancer (two breast cancer cells) and antifungal (*Aspergillus niger, Candida albicans,* and *Cryptococcus neoformans*) activities.[5777]

- A randomized clinical trial found that melissa and lavender essential oils differently affect agitated behavior in elderly people with and without dementia. Melissa essential oil was more effective in reducing agitation (irritability, nonphysical aggressive behavior) in people without dementia, whereas lavender reduced agitation (physical nonaggressive behavior) in people with dementia.[5778] Two drops of the oils were applied to a cotton patch, and the pad was attached to the clothes of participants for fourteen days. The reduction in agitation were assessed by the Neuropsychiatric Inventory (NPI; a test used to detect, quantify, and track changes in psychiatric symptoms in people with dementia) and Cohen-Mansfield Agitation Inventory (CMAI; a scale used to address agitation in elderly persons) tests.

- *Candida* species are the most prevalent fungi in the human microbiome and opportunistic pathogens that can cause various illnesses. Management of these infections is difficult because of a limited number of antifungal drugs, their relatively high toxicity and side effects, and increasing fungal resistance. Hydrogels with 2% melissa essential oil successfully inhibited the growth of *C. albicans*, which suggests it may be helpful for the treatment of oral candidiasis.[5779]

- *Helicobacter pylori* is a bacterium that lives in the digestive tract that can cause sores and ulcers in the lining of the stomach or upper part of the small intestine. Thyme, lemongrass, Virginia cedarwood, and melissa essential oils were the most active of 26 commercial essential oils examined against *H. pylori*.[5780] Oregano, tea tree, pine, and silver fir were also bactericidal.

- Loading essential oils inside nanocarriers is a strategy to increase the stability and effectiveness. Glycerosomes are fluid-filled pouches that act as nanocarriers composed of phospholipids in a high amount of glycerol. Melissa essential oil (36.7% geranial, 27.3% neral, 14.9% beta-caryophyllene) glycerosomes were highly effective in inhibiting herpes simplex virus type 1 infection *in vitro*, without causing harm to healthy cells.[5781]

- Acute coronary syndrome (ACS) describes a range of conditions caused by reduced blood flow in the coronary arteries to the heart. The decreased blood flow makes part of the heart muscle unable to function properly and may even cause permanent heart tissue damage. A double-blind placebo-controlled clinical trial of 72 subjects evaluated the effects of inhaling melissa essential oil after admission to the emergency department for ACS.[5782] Subjects who inhaled 2 drops of melissa for ten minutes at ninety-minute intervals experienced a significant decrease in stress, heart rate, and mean arterial pressure, suggesting that melissa can reduce the stress response and improve cardiovascular function during ACS. The composition of the melissa essential oil was reported as 24.4% beta-caryophyllene, 8.6% geranial, 6.9% 1,8-cineole, 6.7% neral, 5.8% dehydroaromadendrene, and 4.8% thymol.

- An interesting melissa essential oil with beta-cubebene (27.7%) as the main constituent displayed good antioxidant activity in the DPPH and ABTS assays and a strong antioxidant activity in the beta-carotene bleaching assay.[5783] Molecular docking study showed that the oil may exert *in vitro* antioxidant activity by inhibiting xanthine oxidoreductase.

- Of nine commercial essential oils tested (fennel, geranium, lavender, melissa, oregano CT carvacrol, thyme CT thymol, and sage), pine essential oil was strongly antifungal against non-*albicans Candida* isolates and uncommon yeasts that are growingly associated with yeast infections. Melissa and isolated alpha-pinene also exhibited strong activity against non-*albicans Candida* isolates, and isolated thymol inhibited all uncommon yeasts.

- A 4-aminopyridine (4-AP)-brain slice *in vitro* model of epilepsy demonstrated the anticonvulsant activity of melissa essential oil. Furthermore, injection of melissa essential oil (25.6% geranial, 19.5% neral, 13.2% caryophyllene oxide, 11.6% beta-caryophyllene, 4.8% citronellal) protected mice from maximal electroshock

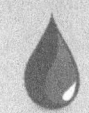

(MES)- and pentylenetetrazole (PTZ)-induced seizures and mortality.[5784] In addition, the oil ameliorated seizure severity, combated fear avoidance, reduced depressive-like behavior and cognitive deficits, and diminished neuron loss and oxidative stress.

☐ The citral/citronellal CT of melissa essential oil (23.8% geranial, 22.2% citronellal, 17.9% neral) exhibited antianxiety activity in both *in vitro* and *in vivo* models.[5785] Melissa oil reduced anxiety by inhibiting the activity of acetylcholinesterase and also influenced isolated intestinal and cardiac tissues, suggesting possible modification of voltage-gated calcium channels or muscarinic receptors. The whole oil did not negatively affect muscle balance or strength, but isolated citronellal did slightly interfere with muscle function.

☐ *Vibrio parahaemolyticus* is a bacterium found in the sea that causes gastrointestinal illness when ingested by humans. It can also cause wound infections and in severe cases, sepsis. Melissa essential oil (38.3% geraniol, 27.9% citronellal, 11.4% citronellol, 7.4% geranyl acetate) inhibited *V. parahaemolyticus* biofilm formation, biofilm motility, extracellular polysaccharide production, and genes associated with its infection abilities *in vitro*.[5786]

☐ Pine, melissa (43.0% citral, 25.0% beta-caryophyllene), ginger, lemon, thyme CT thymol, and basil CT methyl chavicol essential oils each showed activity against MRSA and *E. coli*. Thyme completely inhibited all bacteria at all concentrations tested.[5787]

☐ Melissa essential oil exhibited good antibacterial activity against pathogens (*S. aureus, E. coli*) isolated from dairy cows with subclinical mastitis.[5788]

☐ Evaluation of *Lamiaceae* family essential oils (melissa, oregano CT carvacrol, thyme CT para-cymene, Spanish lavender, sage, rosemary CT 1,8-cineole, and peppermint) showed that melissa and oregano exhibit the best anticandidal activity (*C. albicans, C. glabrata, C. guilliermondii, C. krusei, C. parapsilosis*, and *C. tropicalis*), with Spanish lavender, peppermint, rosemary, and thyme also being very active.[5789] Oregano and thyme demonstrated the strongest antibiofilm activity, followed by Spanish lavender, peppermint, and rosemary.

# MONARDA
## (Wild Bergamot, Bee Balm, Horsemint, Mintleaf Bergamot)

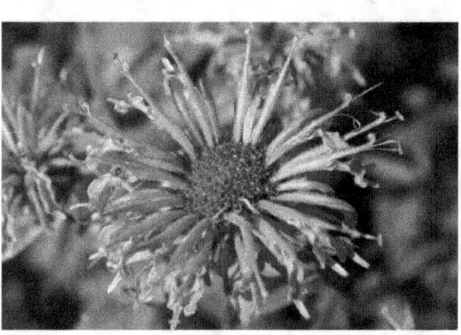

*Monarda fistulosa* L. var. *menthaefolia (or menthifolia)* (Graham) Fernald, *M. menthifolia* L.; *M. fistulosa* L.; Cambridge Scarlet: *M. didyma* L.

**FAMILY:** Lamiaceae (Labiatae)
**NOTE:** Middle
**AROMA INTENSITY:** Medium
**AROMA:** Citrusy (somewhat like bergamot), herbaceous, slightly sweet and floral
**COMMON EXTRACTION METHOD:** Steam distilled from the flowering plant
**POSSIBLE SUBSTITUTE OILS:** Palmarosa, thyme (geraniol CT), geranium, thyme, oregano, summer savory, mountain savory, mountain savory, savory (wild)
**BLENDS WELL WITH:** Chamomile (German, Roman), citronella, frankincense, geranium, lavender, lemon, lemon verbena, magnolia, myrtle, neroli, orange, neroli, palo santo, petitgrain, rosalina, rose, sandalwood, tangerine, ylang ylang, yuzu
**SUBCELLULAR LOCALIZATION | EPIGENETIC INFLUENCE:** Currently unknown | Currently unknown
**RECOMMENDED DILUTION RANGE:** Geraniol CT—3%–50%, neat for limited conditions; All other CTs—1.5%–20%, 50% for some conditions

**PRIMARY CONSTITUENTS:**[5790,5791,5792,5793,5794,5795 4580–4585]

| *M. fistulosa* var. *menthaefolia (Geraniol CT)* | | *Linalool CT* | |
|---|---|---|---|
| Geraniol | 86.8%–93.2% | Linalool | 45.7%–67.0% |
| | | Carvacrol | 17.8%–33.3% |
| *Thymol CT* | | Beta-Pinene | 0.8%–7.6% |
| Thymol | 20.8%–43.6% | (Z)-Beta-Ocimene | 2.3%–6.9% |
| Beta-Phellandrene | 0.0%–17.0% | 1,8-Cineole | 0.4%–4.8% |
| Para-Cymene | 6.0%–14.9% | | |

| | | | |
|---|---|---|---|
| 1,8-Cineole | 0.0%–14.1% | *Carvacrol/Para-Cymene CT* | |
| Alpha-Phellandrene | 0.4%–13.7% | Carvacrol | 23.9%–39.1% |
| Beta-Pinene | 1.6%–10.9% | Para-Cymene | 32.5%–35.4% |
| Carvacrol Methyl Ether | 0.0%–9.8% | Thymol | 0.2%–12.6% |
| Beta-Myrcene | 2.4%–8.1% | 1-Octen-3-ol | 0.0%–10.3% |
| Alpha-Terpineol | 0.6%–7.8% | Aliphatic Aldehyde | 0.0%–6.3% |
| (Z)-Beta-Ocimene | 0.0%–5.9% | Carvacrol Methyl Ether | 0.2%–5.5% |

*Carvacrol CT*

| | |
|---|---|
| Carvacrol | 22.3%–73.5% |
| (Z)-Beta-Ocimene | 6.2%–27.1% |
| 1,8-Cineole | 1.0%–22.2% |
| Alpha-Terpineol | 0.1%–12.0% |
| Para-Cymene + Limonene | 1.7%–6.0% |

Note: *M. fistulosa* L. var. *menthaefolia* rich in geraniol is the most common commercially available sample.

OTHER CONSTITUENTS: *M. fistulosa* L. var. *menthaefolia (Geraniol CT)*—linalool, neral, gamma-terpinene, geranial, nerol, beta-myrcene, ocimene, Germacrene D, 1-octen-3-ol; *Linalool CT*—alpha-thujene, alpha-pinene, 1-heptan-3-ol, beta-myrcene, alpha-terpinene, bornyl acetate, terpinen-4-ol, geraniol, thymol, germacrene D; *Carvacrol CT*—alpha-thujene, alpha-pinene, camphene, 1-heptan-3-ol, beta-myrcene, alpha-terpinene, bornyl acetate, borneol, terpinen-4-ol, nerol, thymol, geranial, beta-caryophyllene, germacrene D; *Thymol CT*—alpha-thujene, alpha-pinene, camphene, 1-hepten-3-ol, delta-3-carene, beta-terpineol, alpha-caryophyllene, beta-caryophyllene, epibicyclosesquiphellandrene, delta-cadinene, gamma-cadinene, alpha-terpinene, limonene, bornyl acetate, linalool, borneol, terpinen-4-ol, germacrene D; *Carvacrol/Para-Cymene CT*—alpha-thujene, alpha-pinene, beta-pinene, alpha-terpinene, limonene, gamma-terpinene, beta-phellandrene, sabinene hydrate, menthone, beta-caryophyllene, citronellyl acetate, terpinen-4-ol, para-cymen-8-ol

PREFERRED COMPOSITION FOR CLINICAL USE:

| Constituent | var. *menthaefolia* (Geraniol CT) |
|---|---|
| **Geraniol** | 85%–95% |
| **Linalool** | 1%–5% |
| **Neral** | 0.1%–3% |
| **Geranial** | 0.1%–3% |

REPORTED THERAPEUTIC PROPERTIES: Analgesic, antispasmodic, anti-inflammatory, nervine, relieves headache, aids digestion, supports liver and gallbladder function, **antibacterial**, antifungal, antimicrobial, antiviral, anti-infectious, antiparasitic, antioxidant, supports respiratory function, expels excess mucus, wound healing, relieves fever, **relieves chronic skin conditions**, encourages restful sleep, relaxing, antidepressant, relieves anxiety

CAUTIONS:

*Geraniol CTs*

■ May moderately interfere with enzymes responsible for metabolizing medications (NSAIDs, proton-pump inhibitors, acetaminophen, antiepileptics, immune modulators, blood-sugar medications, blood pressure medications, antidepressants, antipsychotics, diabetic medications, antihistamines, antibiotics, and anesthetics) due to significant geraniol content.[5796]

■ May interact with aspirin, blood pressure, antiplatelet, and anticoagulant medications, and increase the risk of bleeding among people with bleeding disorders based on antiplatelet activity.[5797]

■ May interact with diabetic medications and cause low blood sugar based on significant geraniol content.[5798,5799]

■ May interact with antibiotics and/or antifungals and possibly increase their effectiveness based on significant geraniol content.[5800]

■ Dilution recommended for topical application. Geraniol is metabolized and autoxidized into metabolites like geranial and neral, and may cause sensitization and irritation when applied topically.[5801]

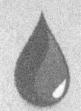

### Linalool, Carvacrol, Carvacrol/Para-Cymene CTs

■ May interact with diabetic medications and cause low blood-sugar levels based on carvacrol/thymol content.[5802,5803,5804]

■ May interact with aspirin, blood pressure, antiplatelet, and anticoagulant medications, and increase the risk of bleeding among people with bleeding disorders due to carvacrol and thymol content.[5805,5806,5807]

■ May interact with antibiotics and possibly enhance their effects due to carvacrol and thymol content.[5808]

■ May interact with anticholinergic (drugs used for asthma, incontinence, gastrointestinal cramps, muscular spasms, depression, and sleep disorders) and cholinergic medications (drugs used to reduce urinary retention, diagnose myasthenia gravis, and for glaucoma) based carvacrol and thymol content.[5809]

■ May irritate mucous membranes (eyes, mouth, nasal passages, vagina, rectum).

### Thymol CT

■ Oral caution. Thymol has a longer half-life (the time it takes for half of the medication to metabolize or excrete half of the dosage) than most essential oil constituents and should not be administered orally for long periods of time.[5810] Thymol is a monoterpene phenol. Reports of fatalities in infants who consumed 50 to 500 mg of phenol have been reported.[5811] It is recommended that chemotypes with high levels of thymol be limited to 10 drops per day orally for adults Monday through Friday, with Saturday and Sunday off; or a two to seven-day break monthly.

■ May interact with aspirin, blood pressure, antiplatelet, and anticoagulant medications, and increase the risk of bleeding among people with bleeding disorders due to thymol content.[5812,5813,5814]

■ May interact with anticholinergic (drugs used for asthma, incontinence, gastrointestinal cramps, muscular spasms, depression, and sleep disorders) and cholinergic medications (drugs used to reduce urinary retention, diagnose myasthenia gravis, and for glaucoma) based on thymol content.[5815,5816,5817]

■ May interact with antibiotics and possibly enhance their effects due to thymol content.[5818,5819,5820,5821]

■ May irritate mucous membranes (eyes, mouth, nasal passages, vagina, rectum).

### SELECTED EVIDENCE:

☐ *In vitro* research shows that monarda essential oil inhibits *P. aeruginosa, E. coli, Proteus vulgaris, Staphylococcus* sp., *B. subtilis, Penicillium* sp., and *C. albicans*.[5822]

☐ Inhaling a combination of peppermint, artemisia, sage, lavender, and monarda improved the symptoms of people with chronic bronchitis being treated with standard options concurrently.[5823]

☐ An animal study concluded that a combination of lavender, monarda, and basil oils reduces cholesterol in the aorta and adverse effects by accumulation of atherosclerotic plaques in the aorta.[5824]

☐ Monarda essential oil is a mild inhibitor of the 5-LOX enzyme according to *in vitro* research.[5825] The 5-LOX enzyme converts arachidonic acid to leukotrienes, increasing inflammation and allergic reactions, and is associated with chronic degenerative inflammatory diseases and cancer.

☐ Animal research reported that monarda essential oil reduced inflammation and hypersensitivity skin reactions superior to hydrocortisone when injected with vitamin B6.[5826]

☐ Monarda essential oil with thymol, carvacrol, eugenol, and carvacrol methyl ether repelled the *Aedes aegypti* just slightly less effectively than DEET.[5827]

☐ Leaf and flower monarda essential oils (both with carvacrol as the major constituent) transiently activated TRPA1 but not TRPV1 or TRPV4 channels, with the leaf oil being the most effective.[5828] The isolated monoterpenes myrcene, carvacrol, and thymol also activated TRPA1 channels.

☐ Monarda (*M. didyma*) CT thymol essential oil inhibited *E. coli, S. aureus,* and *C. perfringens* and increased the body weight of mice and chickens when supplemented in the diet, suggesting it can be a natural substitute for antibiotic growth promoters.[5829] Another study concluded that monarda (*M. didyma*) CT thymol essential oil inhibited clinical and laboratory strains of *S. aureus, E. faecalis, S. pyogenes, E. coli,* and *C. albicans*.[5830]

☐ The carvacrol CT of monarda (*M. didyma*) essential oil decreased the expression of the proinflammatory cytokine IL-6 and increased the expression of the anti-inflammatory micro-RNA miR-146a, showing an anti-inflammatory effect via toll-like receptor signaling pathway.[5831] The oil also showed moderate antioxidant activity in the DPPH assay.

# MORINGA
## (Miracle Tree, Drumstick Tree, Horseradish Tree)

*Moringa oleifera* L., *M. pterygosperma* Gaertn.

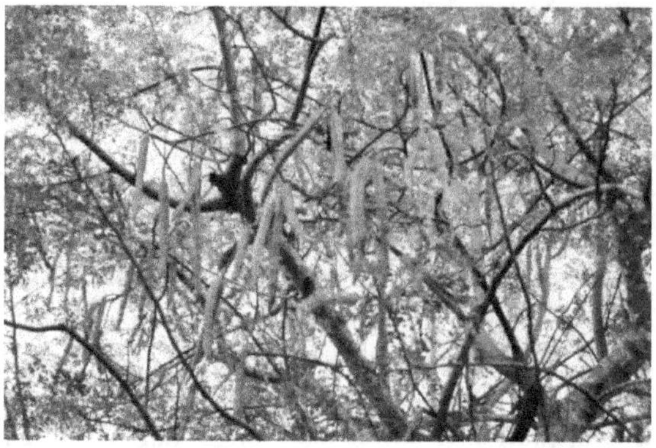

**FAMILY:** Moringaceae
**NOTE:** Middle
**AROMA INTENSITY:** Strong
**AROMA:** Herbaceous, earthy, slightly floral, hay-like
**COMMON EXTRACTION METHOD:** Hydrodistilled from the leaves; may also be hydrodistilled from the flowers, fruits, or seeds; the seeds may also be solvent extracted
**POSSIBLE SUBSTITUTE OILS:** Rose, geranium, palmarosa
**BLENDS WELL WITH:** Bay laurel, bergamot, black pepper, cardamom, cedarwood, chamomile (German, Roman), citronella, clary sage, copaiba, eucalyptus, geranium, helichrysum, jasmine, kunzea, lavender, lemongrass, manuka, melissa, neroli, palo santo, patchouli, pine, sandalwood, spikenard, vetiver, ylang ylang
**SUBCELLULAR LOCALIZATION | EPIGENETIC INFLUENCE:** Currently unknown | Currently unknown
**RECOMMENDED DILUTION RANGE:** 3%–50%; neat for limited conditions

**PRIMARY CONSTITUENTS:**[5832,5833,5834,5835,5836]

*Pentacosane CT (Leaves)*

| | |
|---|---|
| Pentacosane | 13.3%–17.4% |
| Hexacosane | 11.2%–13.9% |
| Heptacosane | 0.0%–11.4% |
| Nonacosane | 0.0%–10.5% |
| Octacosane | 0.0%–10.0% |
| Tetracosane | 1.5%–9.7% |
| Tricosane | 0.0%–8.1% |
| (E)-Phytol | 0.0%–7.7% |
| Docosane | 0.3%–6.8% |

*Flowers*

| | |
|---|---|
| Tetracosane | 27.4% |
| Hexadecyl Acetate | 21.0% |
| n-Hexadecanoic Acid | 18.4% |
| 9,12-Octadeca dienoic acid | 12.2% |
| Nonacosane | 10.5% |
| n-Pentadecanol | 10.5% |

*Fruits*

| | |
|---|---|
| Docosane | 32.7% |
| Tetracosane | 24.0% |
| Octacosane | 19.1% |
| Octadecane | 13.1% |
| Eiocosane | 5.2% |

*(E)-Phytol CT (Brazilian)*

| | |
|---|---|
| (E)-Phytol | 21.9% |
| n-Hexadecanoic Acid | 13.8% |
| Thymol | 9.7% |
| Hexahydrofarnesyl acetone | 8.5% |
| 9,12-Octadeca dienoic acid | 7.8% |
| Nonadecane | 3.7% |

*Seeds (Naphthalene CT)*

| | |
|---|---|
| Naphthalene | 35.6% |
| Benzene Isothio-cyanatomethyl | 34.9% |
| Butylated Hydroxytoluene | 6.1% |
| Methyl Chavicol (Estragole) | 4.5% |

*Seeds (Cyclopentane CT)*

| | |
|---|---|
| Cyclopentane | 51.5% |
| n-Hexadecanoic Acid | 11.1% |
| 1,2-Dimethyl-4-(2-propenyl)benzene | 8.7% |
| 2-(E)-Decenal | 4.4% |

Note: The Pentacosane CT of Moringa essential oil could be divided into additional chemotypes, but they are combined in this work for simplification purposes. The flowers may also produce an essential oil with (E)-nerolidol (13.3%), alpha-terpineol (7.8%), and isothiocyanate (6.4%) as the primary constituents.[3983] A fixed oil is also obtained from moringa seeds and called moringa oil, which should not be confused with the essential oil. One study mistakenly identifies moringa fixed oil as moringa essential oil.[3986]

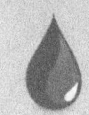

**PREFERRED COMPOSITION FOR CLINICAL USE:**

| Constituent | Pentacosane CT |
|---|---|
| Pentacosane | 12%–20% |
| Hexacosane | 9%–17% |
| Heptacosane | 0%–12% |
| Nonacosane | 0%–11% |
| Octacosane | 0%–10% |
| Tetracosane | 2%–10% |
| Tricosane | 0%–8% |
| Docosane | 2%–7% |
| (E)-Phytol | 0%–3% |

**OTHER CONSTITUENTS:** *Pentacosane CT*—benzeneacetaldehyde, benzylnitrile, indole, ledene oxide, dihydro-actiridioide, megastigmatrienone, 1-[2,3,6-Trimethyl-phenyl]-2-butanone, 1-[2,3,6-Trimethyl-phenyl]-3-buten-2-one, isolongifolene, hexahydrofarnesylactone, n-hexadecanoic acid, eiocosane, heneicosane, triacontane, pseudo phytol; *(E)-Phytol CT*—linalool, alpha-terpineol, geraniol, methyl eugenol (< 2.3%), (Z)-isoelimicin, spathulenol, caryophyllene oxide, octadecane, docosane, nonacosane; *Flowers*—N/A; *Fruits*—N/A; *Seeds (Cyclopentane CT)*—nonanal, 1-nonanol, tridecane, 1,6-dibromo-silane, heptadecane, propanoic acid, butanoic acid, 2,4-diphenyl-4-methyl-2-(E)-pentene, docosane, nonadecane, isamoxole, 8-dimethyl-2-isopropylphenanthrene, 2,2-bipyridine-3,3-diol, phthalic acid, propanenitrile, 1,5-dimethyl-2-pyrrolecarbonitrile, phenol, eicosane; *Seeds (Naphthalene CT)*—tetratriacontyl heptafluorobutyrate, hexadecane, caryophyllene, (-)-aristolene, benzene, 1-(1,5-dimethyl-4-hexenyl-4-methyl, anethole, 1-methyl-5-(1-methylethyl)-1H-pyrrol-3-ol, thymol, 2-pentadecanone, hexadecanoic acid methyl ester, methyl stearate, 11-octadecenoic acid methyl ester, trans-13-octadecenoic acid methyl ester, 9,12-octadecadienoic acid methyl ester

**REPORTED THERAPEUTIC PROPERTIES:** Anticancer, antibacterial, antimicrobial, antifungal, antioxidant, antiseptic, analgesic, anti-inflammatory, antispasmodic, diuretic, relieves diarrhea, relieves stomachache and ulcers, supports respiratory function, supports normal cholesterol levels, balances blood pressure, aids/protects liver function, wound healing, **relieves chronic skin conditions**, relieves boils and abscesses, **reduces the appearance of acne, blemishes, scars, and wrinkles**, deeply nourishes and softens skin, anti-aging, antiallergic, aids immune function, balances blood sugar levels, reduces anxiety, encourages restful sleep, antidepressant, **aphrodisiac**

**CAUTIONS:**
*Pentacosane CT (Leaves), Seeds, Fruits, Flowers*
■ None currently known.

*(E)-Phytol CT*
■ Moringa CT (E)-Phytol should be avoided by individuals with Refsum disease (a neurological disorder caused by the overaccumulation of phytanic acid in cells and tissues) or who are AMACR-deficient (alpha-methylacyl-CoA racemase-deficient) due to phytol content. It is believed that humans can convert phytol to phytanic acid. .[5837] Animal research suggests that phytol can cause liver inflammation, liver failure, and death in AMACR-deficient mice.[5838,5839] AMACR is an enzyme found in the mitochondria that plays a role in the breakdown of fatty acids. AMACR deficiency causes neurological problems (seizures, cognitive decline, migraines, encephalopathy, loss of sensation due to nerve damage, muscle stiffness, lack of coordination, and vision problems) that begin in adulthood and progressively get worse.[5840] Phytol may also weakly promote tumor formation according to animal research.[5841]

**SELECTED EVIDENCE:**
☐ Moringa seed essential oil (naphthalene CT) kills breast, colon, liver, larynx, and cervical cancer cells *in vitro*.[5842]
☐ *In vitro* research reports that moringa essential oil (leaf, pentacosane CT) inhibits the fungi *Trichophyton*

*rubrum, T. mentagrophytes, E. floccosum,* and *M. canis,* but had little effect on dermatophytes.[5843] Moringa leaf essential oil (pentacosane CT) inhibits two gram-positive bacteria (*B. cereus* and *Pseudomonas aeruginosa*) and five fungi (*Penicillium aurantiogriseum, P. expansum, P. citrinum, P. digitatum,* and *Aspergillus niger* spp.).[5844]

☐ Moringa seed essential oil (naphthalene CT) possesses stronger antioxidant properties than vitamin C or water-soluble vitamin E (Trolox) according to *in vitro* research.[3985] The leaf essential oil (pentacosane CT) was only mildly antioxidant.[5845]

---

# MOUNTAIN SAVORY
## (Winter Savory)

*Satureja montana* L.

**FAMILY:** Lamiaceae (Labiatae)
**NOTE:** Middle
**AROMA INTENSITY:** Strong
**AROMA:** Herbaceous, mildly sweet, sharp, medicinal
**COMMON EXTRACTION METHOD:** Steam distilled from the dried aerial parts
**POSSIBLE SUBSTITUTE OILS:** Oregano, thyme (carvacrol CT)
**BLENDS WELL WITH:** Ajowan, bergamot, grapefruit, lavender, lemon, lime, marjoram, orange, oregano, pine, rosemary, tangerine, thyme
**SUBCELLULAR LOCALIZATION | EPIGENETIC INFLUENCE:** Currently unknown | Currently unknown
**RECOMMENDED DILUTION RANGE:** 1.5%–20%; 50% for some conditions

**PRIMARY CONSTITUENTS:**[5846,5847,5848,5849,5850,5851]

| *Thymol CT* | | *Carvacrol CT* | |
|---|---|---|---|
| Thymol | 30.9%–46.0% | Carvacrol | 16.1%–63.4% |
| Para-Cymene | 6.4%–13.5% | Para-Cymene | 3.0%–28.9% |
| Gamma-Terpinene | 5.9%–9.8% | Linalool | 0.5%–24.8% |
| Carvacrol | 3.8%–6.9% | Thymol | 0.0%–20.6% |
| Geraniol | 0.0%–6.4% | Gamma-Terpinene | 0.0%–13.5% |
| Carvacrol Methyl Ether | 4.0%–5.1% | Thymol Methyl Ether | 0.0%–12.8% |
| Thymol Methyl Ether | 3.9%–5.1% | Borneol | 0.0%–11.5% |
| Borneol | 2.4%–4.1% | Carvacrol Methyl Ether | 0.0%–11.0% |
| Alpha-Terpinene | 1.7%–3.9% | Geraniol | 0.0%–10.2% |
| Beta-Caryophyllene | 1.7%–3.8% | Geranyl Acetate | 0.0%–6.7% |
| Linalool | 0.4%–3.2% | | |

Note: The carvacrol CT is the most common CT reported in the literature, with the thymol CT the second most common reported. Other CTs are also infrequently reported.

**OTHER CONSTITUENTS:** *Carvacrol CT*—Alpha-terpinene, beta-caryophyllene, alpha-thujene, alpha-pinene, myrcene, alpha-terpinene, limonene, cis-beta-ocimene, allo-ocimene, 1-octen-3-ol, trans-sabinene hydrate, camphor, beta-bourbonene, aromadendrene, neral, alpha-terpineol, beta-cubebene, geranial, beta-bisabolene, nerol, caryophyllene oxide, spathulenol; *Thymol CT*—Alpha-thujene, alpha-pinene, myrcene, limonene, allocimene, 1-octen-3-ol, ledene, geranial, beta-bisabolene, nerol

**PREFERRED COMPOSITION FOR CLINICAL USE:**

| Constituent | |
|---|---|
| **Carvacrol** | 25%–50% |
| **Thymol** | 5%–25% |
| **Para-Cymene** | 8%–20% |

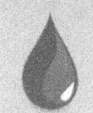

| Gamma-Terpinene | 5%–15% |
|---|---|
| Carvacrol Methyl Ether | 4%–12% |
| Linalool | 0.5%–10% |
| Thymol Methyl Ether | 0%–5% |

**REPORTED THERAPEUTIC PROPERTIES: Antibacterial**, antifungal, antiviral, anti-infectious, **antimicrobial**, antioxidant, abscesses and bruises, coughs, cold/flu, aids digestion, expels excess gas, immune stimulant, supports circulatory function, antiarthritic, relieves diarrhea, muscle soreness, intestinal cramps, expels excess mucus, sore throat, reduces the appearance of scars, insect bites/stings, **insect repellent**, reduces excess ego, combats fear, motivating

## CAUTIONS:

■ *Carvacrol and Thymol CTs*: Avoid during pregnancy and lactation due to similar composition to oregano essential oil. Oils rich in carvacrol may negatively affect embryonic development and encourage fetal cell death according to animal research.[5852]

■ *Thymol CT*: Oral caution. Some thyme chemotypes contain up to 46.0% thymol. Thymol has a longer half-life (the time it takes for half of the medication to metabolize or excrete half of the dosage) than most essential oil constituents and should not be administered orally for long periods of time.[5853] Thymol is a monoterpene phenol. Reports of fatalities in children who consumed 50 to 200 mg of phenols has been reported.[5854] It is recommended that chemotypes with high levels of thymol be limited to 10 drops per day orally for adults with a two- to seven-day break after twenty-one days of use.

■ *Carvacrol CT*: May interact with diabetic medications and cause low blood-sugar levels based on carvacrol content.[5855,5856,5857]

■ May interact with aspirin, blood pressure, antiplatelet, and anticoagulant medications, and increase the risk of bleeding among people with bleeding disorders due to thymol and carvacrol content.[5858,5859,5860]

■ May interact with antibiotics and possibly enhance their effects due to thymol and carvacrol content.[5861]

■ May interact with anticholinergic (drugs used for asthma, incontinence, gastrointestinal cramps, muscular spasms, depression, and sleep disorders) and cholinergic medications (drugs used to reduce urinary retention, diagnose myasthenia gravis, and for glaucoma) based on thymol and carvacrol content.[5862]

■ May irritate mucous membranes (eyes, mouth, nasal passages, vagina, rectum).

## SELECTED EVIDENCE:

☐ *In vitro* research suggests that mountain savory (*Satureja montana* subsp. *pisidica*, with primary constituents of carvacrol, thymol, and carvacrol methyl ether) oil is cytotoxic to cervical and metastatic breast-cancer cells.[5863] The same research reported that mountain savory oil was highly antimicrobial. Another study found that mountain savory oil (alpha-terpineol/linalool CT) prevents growth of erythroleukemic cells.[5864]

☐ Mountain savory oil strongly inhibited six bacteria strains responsible for mastitis in animals: *Staphylococcus aureus, S. chromogenes, S. sciuri, S. warneri, S. xylosus,* and *E. coli.*[5865] It effectively inhibited eight common food-borne pathogenic bacteria as well: *B. thermosphacta, E. coli, L. innocua, L. monocytogenes, P. putida, Salmonella typhimurium, S. enteritidis,* and *Shewanella putrefaciens.*[5866,5867,5868,5869,5870,5871] Mountain savory actively inhibits MRSA.[5872]

☐ Mountain savory essential oil inhibits the gram-positive meat spoilage bacterium *Brochothrix thermosphacta.*[5873]

☐ *In vitro* research demonstrates that mountain savory essential oil possesses remarkable antibiofilm, anti-adhesive, and bactericidal properties against two reference strains of *Salmonella typhimurium* and twelve *Salmonella* spp. isolated from food.[5874]

☐ Mountain savory oil significantly repels and kills the larvae of the *Culex pipiens* mosquito.[5875]

☐ *In vitro* research demonstrated that mountain savory essential oil possesses maximum inhibitory activity against *C. albicans.*[5876,5877] Another study shows that mountain savory oil inhibits the growth and activity of *C. albicans* isolated from vaginal swabs better than the antifungal drug clotrimazole.[5878]

☐ Mountain savory demonstrated strong antioxidant properties in *in vitro* testing.[5879]

☐ Mountain savory essential oil is larvicidal to the *Cx. quinquefasciatus* mosquito.[5880]

□ Laboratory research demonstrated that mountain savory CT carvacrol possesses good antioxidant capacity and inhibited bacteria involved in food spoilage (*P. fluorescens*, *B. thermosphacta*, and *E. faecium*) and pathogenic bacteria (*Salmonella enterica* serotype Enteritidis, *Salmonella enterica* serotype Typhimurium, *L. monocytogenes*, and *S. aureus*).[5881]

□ *Fusobacterium nucleatum* is the main bacterium linked to bad breath. The bacterium aggregates with other bacteria in the mouth to form plaque biofilms that cause bad breath. Ledum (*R. groenlandicum*) CT sabinene, peppermint, and mountain savory CT carvacrol essential oil each inhibited *F. nucleatum* without harming human oral cells in a laboratory study.[5882]

□ Two subspecies of winter savory (subsp. *variegata*, carvacrol CT; subsp. *montana*, carvacrol CT) both exhibited noteworthy antioxidant activity in the DPPH, ABTS, and FRAP assays.[5883]

□ *In vitro* research demonstrated that winter savory CT carvacrol exerted antimicrobial activity against *S. aureus* (three strains), *E. coli* (three strains), and *L. monocytogenes* (three strains) and synergized the activity of gentamicin against many of the microbes (an additive effect was seen against some strains).[5884]

□ The carvacrol CT of winter savory essential oil inhibited clinical isolates of *L. monocytogenes*, *S. aureus*, *S. haemolyticus*, *E. coli*, *K. pneumoniae*, *P. aeruginosa*, and *S. marcescens*.[5885]

□ *In vitro* research showed that winter savory CT carvacrol essential oil inhibited the food pathogen *Campylobacter jejuni*, which is the most common cause of food poisoning in the United States and Europe.[5886] Carvacrol, thymol, and thymoquinone were each more potent inhibitors than the whole oil, and a synergistic activity between thymol and carvacrol was observed against the pathogen.

□ A nanoemulsion of winter savory essential oil exhibited greater inhibitory effects against planktonic *E. coli* than the free oil and reduced its biofilm production.[5887]

□ Winter savory showed the ability to damage the reproductive system of the Asian blue tick (*Rhipicephalus microplus*), suggesting it could be used as a natural solution to control tick populations.[5888]

□ The carvacrol CT of winter savory inhibited *A. flavus* growth and its production of aflatoxin.[5889]

□ Winter savory, nutmeg, and lemongrass (*C. flexuosus*) were each fungicidal to *A. niger* and *A. ochraceus*.[5890] The oils also inhibited the production of ochratoxin A by the fungus *A. ochraceus* and the production of aflatoxin B1 and aflatoxin B2.

□ Both Greek oregano CT carvacrol (80.4% carvacrol) and winter savory CT carvacrol (55.0% carvacrol) essential oils exhibited good activity against pathogens associated with bovine mastitis.[5891]

□ The thymol CT of Greek oregano essential oil reduced anxiety-like behavior and improved cognitive deficits caused by scopolamine in a zebra fish model of cognitive impairment.[5892] The oil reduced brain oxidative stress and inhibited acetylcholinesterase activity that were both increased by scopolamine.

□ Toxoplasmosis is an illness caused by infection with the *Toxoplasma gondii* parasite characterized by muscle aches, fever, and headache. Infection usually occurs after exposure to infected cat feces or by eating undercooked contaminated meat. A laboratory study found that both oregano CT carvacrol essential oil and isolated carvacrol inhibited the growth of *T. gondii*, with carvacrol being most effective.[5893] Carvacrol prevented proliferation of and invasion by the parasite, suggesting it may be an "effective drug for treating toxoplasmosis."

□ Oregano CT carvacrol, may chang, and manuka each displayed acaricidal activity against the Asian blue tick (Rhipicephalus microplus).[5894] Beta-triketone fractions from manuka caused significant larval mortality, while its sesquiterpene fraction was far less effective. Interestingly, the sesquiterpene fractions were more effective on adults than the beta-triketone fractions.

□ Terpene/phenol-rich (oregano CT carvacrol, thyme CT carvacrol, and summer savory CT carvacrol) and phenylpropanoid-rich (clove and cinnamon leaf) essential oils each showed good absolute antioxidant activity—comparable to BHT—in cumene and squalene during the peroxyl radical trapping assay.[5895]

□ Of 11 essential oils tested, oregano CT carvacrol, fennel, winter savory CT para-cymene, and summer savory CT carvacrol were the most effective against gastrointestinal nematodes (*Haemonchus*, *Trichostrongylus*, *Teladorsagia*, and *Chabertia*) in the *in vitro* egg hatch test.[5896] Oral administration of the oils diluted in sunflower oil to animals showed that thyme CT para-cymene essential oil was the most effective, even more effective than thyme CT thymol.

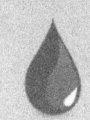

- Winter savory CT borneol, lemongrass (*C. flexuosus*), and nutmeg exhibited antioxidant (DPPH, beta-carotene bleaching assays) and antimicrobial activity in laboratory research. Winter savory was active against *E. coli*, while nutmeg was bactericidal against *E. coli* and *S. aureus*.[5897]

- The carvacrol CT (near equal carvacrol and para-cymene) of winter savory inhibited *B. cereus, S. aureus, E. faecalis, E. coli, S. typhimurium, S, cerevisiae, C. albicans, A. brasiliensis,* and *P. aeruginosa,* and exhibited good antioxidant activity in the ABTS assay, while weak activity in the DPPH, SOA, and reducing power assays.[5898]

- Oregano CT carvacrol, thyme CT thymol, and winter savory CT carvacrol essential oils and there mixtures were effective against clinical bacterial strains—*Staphylococcus* sp., *Streptococcus* sp., *P. aeruginosa, E. coli, K. pneumoniae, S. marcescens,* and *M. pachydermatis* strains—cultured from the ears of dogs affected by otitis externa (ear infection).[5899] The mixture contained equal parts of each oil and was the most active against the tested strains.

# MUGWORT
## (Common Mugwort, Indian Wormwood)

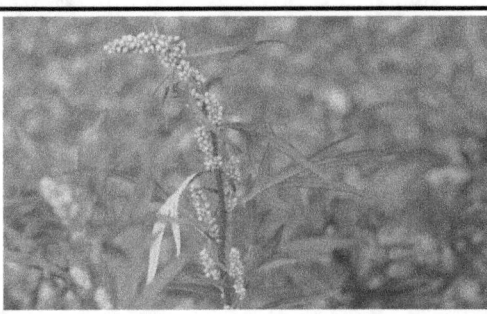

*Artemisia vulgaris* L.; Great Mugwort: *A. aborescens* L.

**FAMILY:** Asteraceae (Compositae)
**NOTE:** Middle
**AROMA INTENSITY:** Strong
**AROMA:** Fresh, camphorous, earthy, bittersweet
**COMMON EXTRACTION METHOD:** Steam distilled from the aerial parts
**POSSIBLE SUBSTITUTE OILS:** Sage, Western red cedar (Leaves), thuja, wormwood, tansy, white sage, Spanish sage
**BLENDS WELL WITH:** Cedarwood, clary sage, lavandin, lavender, patchouli, pine, rosemary, sage, sandalwood, Spanish sage
**SUBCELLULAR LOCALIZATION | EPIGENETIC INFLUENCE:** Currently unknown | Currently unknown
**RECOMMENDED DILUTION RANGE:** 1,8-cineole, alpha-thujone, beta-thujone, camphor CTs—1.5%–20%; Alpha-phellandrene, beta-caryophyllene, chrysanthenyl acetate, germacrene D, isobornyl isobutyrate CTs—3%–50%, Neat for limited conditions

**PRIMARY CONSTITUENTS:**[5900,5901,5902,5903,5904,5905,5906,5907,5908]

| *1,8-Cineole CT* | | *Alpha-Thujone CT* | |
|---|---|---|---|
| 1,8-Cineole | 24.9%–32.2% | Alpha-Thujone | 14.4%–48.5% |
| Camphor | 1.4%–16.3% | Fenchone | 0.0%–16.6% |
| Sabinene | 0.0%–13.7% | Beta-Caryophyllene | 6.3%–16.5% |
| Beta-Thujone | 0.0%–13.5% | 1,8-Cineole | 1.0%–13.2% |
| Borneol | 0.0%–9.0% | Camphor | 0.0%–10.9% |
| Terpinen-4-ol | 2.2%–7.6% | Para-Cymene | 2.7%–10.6% |
| Para-Cymene | 0.1%–7.5% | Beta-Thujone | 5.2%–8.7% |
| Caryophyllene Oxide | 3.6%–6.5% | (Z)-Beta-Farnesene | 0.0%–8.1% |
| Alpha-Pinene | 0.8%–5.9% | Alpha-Pinene | 1.8%–5.7% |
| Caryophyllene | 1.2%–5.3% | Beta-Myrcene | 4.9%–5.0% |
| Gamma-Terpinene | 0.0%–5.1% | Germacrene D | 4.5%–4.5% |
| Beta-Selinene | 2.1%–4.7% | Camphene | 0.0%–4.0% |
| Alpha-Terpinene | 0.0%–4.6% | Beta-Phellandrene | 2.9%–3.7% |
| Santolinatriene | 2.2%–4.0% | Alpha-Humulene | 2.6%–3.1% |
| Germacrene D | 0.0%–3.2% | Trans-2-Hexenal | 0.4%–3.1% |
| Artemisia Ketone | 0.0%–3.2% | Limonene | 0.0%–2.7% |
| Gamma-Gurjunene | 0.0%–2.8% | Borneol | 0.0%–2.2% |
| Trans-Sabinene Hydrate Acetate | 0.0%–2.5% | Beta-Pinene | 0.7%–1.9% |
| Alpha-Thujone | 0.0%–2.5% | 1-Octen-3-ol | 1.4%–1.7% |
| Anethole | 0.0%–2.2% | Bornyl Acetate | 0.0%–1.0% |

| | | |
|---|---|---|
| Beta-Phellandrene | 0.0%–2.2% | |
| 1-Octen-3-ol | 0.0%–1.8% | |
| Alpha-Terpineol | 0.0%–1.8% | |
| Alpha-Humulene | 0.5%–1.6% | |
| Beta-Elemene | 0.0%–1.4% | |
| Alpha-Copaene | 0.6%–1.3% | |
| Beta-Myrcene | 0.0%–1.3% | |
| Delta-Cadinene | 0.0%–1.3% | |
| Humulene Oxide | 0.0%–1.2% | |
| Gamma-Humulene | 0.0%–1.1% | |
| 2-Hexenal | 0.0%–1.1% | |
| Cis-Sabinol | 0.0%–1.1% | |
| Alpha-Zingiberene | 0.0%–1.0% | |
| Alpha-Thujene | 0.0%–1.0% | |
| Menthol | 0.0%–1.0% | |

*Beta-Caryophyllene CT*

| | |
|---|---|
| Beta-Caryophyllene | 17.5% |
| Santolinatriene | 10.0% |
| 1,8-Cineole | 9.5% |
| (Z)-Beta-Farnesene | 7.1% |
| Para-Cymene | 6.8% |
| Germacrene D | 6.7% |
| Beta-Myrcene | 5.9% |
| Borneol | 5.4% |
| Alpha-Humulene | 4.4% |
| Beta-Pinene | 3.8% |
| Camphene | 3.3% |
| Trans-2-Hexenal | 2.3% |
| Alpha-Pinene | 2.1% |

*Camphor CT*

| | |
|---|---|
| Camphor | 17.3%–47.7% |
| Camphene | 3.9%–17.4% |
| 1,8-Cineole | 3.9%–14.1% |
| Alpha-Thujone | 10.2%–10.7% |
| Gamma-Muurolene | 0.0%–9.0% |
| Borneol | 0.8%–8.9% |
| Para-Cymene | 0.0%–8.9% |
| Isoborneol | 0.0%–8.2% |
| Trans-Verbenol | 0.0%–7.0% |
| Beta-Thujone | 2.8%–5.8% |
| Beta-Caryophyllene | 0.0%–5.8% |
| Isobornyl 2-Methylbutyrate | 0.0%–5.3% |
| Artemisia Alcohol | 0.0%–4.5% |
| Alpha-Fenchene | 0.0%–3.9% |
| Delta-Cadinene | 0.0%–2.5% |
| Cis-Davanone | 0.0%–2.5% |
| Sabinene | 0.0%–2.4% |
| Caryophyllene Oxide | 1.2%–2.3% |
| Alpha-Thujene | 0.0%–2.2% |
| Beta-Pinene | 0.0%–2.1% |
| Alpha-Pinene | 0.1%–2.0% |

*Alpha-Phellandrene CT*

| | |
|---|---|
| Alpha-Phellandrene | 17.3% |
| Lyratol | 15.1% |
| Trans-Isoelemicin | 15.1% |
| Alpha-Humulene | 8.8% |
| Gamma-Elemene | 8.8% |
| Camphene | 4.2% |
| 1,8-Cineole | 3.6% |
| Beta-Pinene | 1.8% |
| Alpha-Pinene | 1.3% |
| Beta-Myrcene | 1.3% |

*Beta-Thujone CT*

| | |
|---|---|
| Beta-Thujone | 20.8% |
| Alpha-Pinene | 15.1% |
| 1,8-Cineole | 11.7% |
| Camphor | 8.7% |
| Artemisia Alcohol | 8.5% |
| Alpha-Phellandrene | 6.3% |
| Borneol | 2.4% |

*Chrysanthenyl Acetate CT*

| | |
|---|---|
| Chrysanthenyl Acetate | 39.6% |
| Para-Cymene | 17.2% |
| Beta-Phellandrene | 11.4% |
| Trans-2-Hexenal | 5.0% |
| Santolinatriene | 3.6% |
| Limonene | 3.5% |
| Beta-Myrcene | 2.7% |
| Beta-Caryophyllene | 1.6% |
| Ocimene | 1.2% |
| 1-Octen-3yl Acetate | 1.1% |
| 1-Octene | 1.0% |
| Beta-Selinene | 1.0% |

*Germacrene D CT*

| | |
|---|---|
| Germacrene D | 25.3% |
| Caryophyllene | 19.6% |
| Alpha-Zingiberene | 14.9% |
| Borneol | 10.8% |
| ar-Curcumene | 6.0% |
| Alpha-Humulene | 5.0% |
| Delta-Cadinene | 3.9% |
| 1,8-Cineole | 1.8% |
| Beta-Selinene | 1.2% |
| Caryophyllene Oxide | 1.1% |
| Trans-2-Hexenal | 1.0% |
| Bornyl Acetate | 1.0% |

*Isobornyl Isobutyrate CT*

| | |
|---|---|
| Isobornyl Isobutyrate | 38.1% |
| Beta-Pinene | 30.1% |
| Limonene | 6.2% |

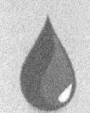

| | | |
|---|---|---|
| Alpha-Humulene | 0.0%–1.9% | |
| Gamma-Terpinene | 0.0%–1.8% | |
| Bicyclogermacrene | 0.0%–1.6% | |
| Alpha-Gurjunene | 0.0%–1.3% | |
| Beta-Thujone | 0.0%–1.2% | |
| Spathulenol | 0.0%–1.1% | |
| 2-Hexenal | 0.0%–1.1% | |
| Alpha-Thujone | 0.0%–1.3% | |

| Limonene | 6.2% |
|---|---|
| Delta-3-Carene | 4.8% |
| Alpha-Pinene | 4.0% |
| Gamma-Terpinene | 2.8% |
| Trans-Rose-Oxide | 2.0% |
| Spathulenol | 1.5% |
| Alpha-Humulene | 1.3% |

*Artemisia Ketone CT*

| Artemisia Ketone | 18.8%–29.4% |
|---|---|
| 1,8-Cineole | 3.4%–13.2% |
| Para-Cymene | 1.7%–7.6% |
| Yomogi Alcohol | 4.4%–5.5% |
| Limonene | 0.9%–4.8% |
| Beta-Caryophyllene | 0.0%–4.8% |
| Germacrene D | 0.2%–4.4% |
| Beta-Pinene | 1.8%–4.3% |
| Artemisia Alcohol | 1.3%–4.1% |
| Santolina Triene | 4.0%–4.0% |
| Caryophyllene Oxide | 0.6%–3.7% |
| Camphene | 1.4%–3.6% |
| Camphor | 3.4%–3.5% |
| Alpha-Pinene | 3.5%–4.5% |
| Alpha-Thujone | 0.2%–3.1% |

*A. aborescens (Great Mugwort)*[#]

| Beta-Thujone | 19.6%–71.3% |
|---|---|
| Chamzulene | 3.6%–49.4% |
| Camphor | 1.1%–25.7% |
| Terpinen-4-ol | 1.0%–7.7% |
| Myrcene | 0.5%–6.8% |
| Alpha-Thujone | 0.5%–4.4% |
| Germacrene D | 0.6%–4.3% |
| Chrysanthenyl Acetate | 0.0%–3.2% |
| Sabinene | 0.1%–3.0% |

Note: The alpha-thujone CT was the most common CT found commercially among four samples. Three were alpha-thujone CT and one was 1,8-cineole CT. The isobornyl isobutyrate, germacrene D, alpha-phellandrene, beta-caryophyllene, and chrysanthenyl acetate CTs are preferred for safety reasons. Some companies report a beta-myrcene chemotype of mugwort, but this CT is not found in the scientific literature and more likely *Artemisia absinthium* (Absinthe, Wormwood), which has a beta-myrcene CT.[5909]

[#] Great mugwort has at least three distinct chemotypes (likely more), one with chamazulene and one without, and another with almost equal portions of chamazulene and beta-thujone and devoid of camphor. They are combined in this text.

OTHER CONSTITUENTS: *1,8-Cineole* CT—Camphene, bornyl acetate, ar-curcumene; *Alpha-Thujone CT*—Limonene; *Alpha-Phellandrene CT*—Alpha-thujene, alpha-terpineol; *Beta-Caryophyllene CT*—Beta-phellandrene, 1-Octen-3-ol, limonene; *Beta-Thujone CT*—Caryophyllene oxide; *Camphor CT*—Artemisiatriene, beta-pinene, 3-thujanol, myrtenal, para-cymene, bornyl acetate, alpha-copaene, beta-cubebene, alpha-muurolene, gamma-cadinene, alpha-cadinol; *Chrysanthenyl Acetate CT*—Alpha-phellandrene, 1,8-cineole, gamma-terpinene, camphor, terpinolene; *Germacrene D CT*—Alpha-pinene, terpinen-4-ol; *Isobornyl Isobutyrate CT*—Cis-beta-ocimene, caryophyllene alcohol; *A. aborescens (Great Mugwort)*—alpha-pinene, camphene, alpha-copaene, beta-pinene, alpha-terpinene, para-cymene, gamma-terpinene, cis-sabinene hydrate, linalool, nerol, beta-bourbonene, beta-caryophyllene, caryophyllene oxide, alpha-terpineol, carvacrol, geranyl isovalerate, methyl butyl-2-methyl butyrate; *Artemisia Ketone CT*—Artemisia triene, davanone, alpha-fenchene, sabinene, alpha-terpinene, bergamal, cis-thujone, (Z)-p-mentha-2,8-dien-1-ol, trans-chrysanthenol, trans-pinocarveol, terpinen-4-ol, alpha-terpineol, borneol, bornyl acetate, alpha-copaene, alpha-humulene, gamma-curcumene, delta-cadinene

PREFERRED COMPOSITION FOR CLINICAL USE:

| Constituent | Artemisia Ketone CT | Great Mugwort |
|---|---|---|
| **Artemisia Ketone** | 15%–30% | – |
| **1,8-Cineole** | 5%–15% | < 1% |
| **Yomogi Alcohol** | 3%–6% | – |
| **Para-Cymene** | 1%–7% | 0%–2% |
| **Santolina Triene** | 3%–7% | – |
| **Alpha-Pinene** | 3%–7% | – |

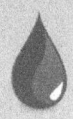

| Camphor | 3%–6% | – |
|---|---|---|
| Beta-Pinene | 2%–6% | – |
| Artemisia Alcohol | 2%–5% | – |
| Beta-Caryophyllene | 1%–5% | 0.1%–3% |
| Germacrene D | 1%–5% | 2%–7% |
| Camphene | 1%–5% | – |
| Limonene | 0.5%–5% | – |
| Caryophyllene Oxide | 0.5%–5% | 0%–2% |
| Chamazulene | – | 34%–52% |
| Beta-Thujone | < 2% | 28%–38% |
| Terpinen-4-ol | 0.1%–3% | 0.5%–5% |
| Alpha-Thujone | < 2% | < 2% |

**REPORTED THERAPEUTIC PROPERTIES:** Antibacterial, antifungal, antiviral, **antispasmodic**, aids digestion, diuretic, **promotes normal menstruation**, nervine, antiparasitic, antiviral, warming, anti-infectious, promotes healthy uterine function, stimulates the release of hormones, **relieves chronic skin conditions (especially inflammatory conditions)**, stimulant, combats feelings of hysteria, relieves anxiety, stress management, aids concentration and memory, promotes valor and courage

**CAUTIONS:**

*Mugwort essential oil is not commonly used in essential oil therapy unless the exact composition of the bottle (batch) being used is known. It should be reserved for use by the very experienced user who can properly weigh the risks-to-benefits ratio of using it.*

■ Avoid with children under 6 due to thujone, 1,8-cineole, and camphor content. Essential oils high in thujones, camphor, and 1,8-cineole (all of which can be found in many chemotypes of mugwort) are powerful convulsants and may adversely affect the nervous system and/or cause toxicity/ neurotoxicity.[5910,5911,5912,5913,5914,5915,5916,5917,5918,5919,5920] Ingestion of camphor-containing products has been lethal in children under age 2 (estimated to be roughly 2,000 mg of camphor for a 20 kg child as the minimum potential fatal dose).[5921,5922] In addition, thujone may cause altered visual perception.[5923] Camphor ingestion by infants and young children may cause cough, vomiting, seizure, burning sensation in the mucous membranes and eyes, or lack of voluntary coordination of muscle movements.[5924]

■ Avoid during pregnancy and while lactating due to thujone and camphor. Camphor ingestion may lead to abortion because fetuses lack the enzymes to process it.[5925] Essential oils high in thujone content may cause abortion.[5926,5927,5928]

■ Avoid oral consumption. Thujone is considered significantly neurotoxic and may damage the liver, and it is estimated that as little as 15 mg orally may negatively impact the central nervous system.[5929,5930,5931] Oral—Camphor can be toxic when taken orally (usually single doses exceeding 2 mL), although the lethal dose for adult humans is estimated to be (more than 5 mL) in a single dose.[5932,5933,5934]

■ Avoid with epilepsy and Parkinson's disease due to camphor, thujone, fenchone, and 1,8-cineole content.[5935,5936,5937,5938,5939]

■ The potentially high camphor content in various mugwort CTs may negatively impact red blood cells and increase the risk of jaundice in children with Glucose-6-phosphate dehydrogenase deficiency (G6PD).[5940,5941]

■ Avoid with those who have a compromised liver or kidneys due to the risk of kidney toxicity, kidney failure, or liver toxicity.[5942,5943,5944] Consuming extremely large amounts of thujone rich essential oils (10 mL) has caused kidney failure.[5945] This would also suggest that those taking medications that could cause liver damage should also use mugwort very cautiously or avoid it entirely.

■ *1,8-cineole CT*: May interfere with pentobarbital and other barbiturates (medications for anxiety and insomnia) based on 1,8-cineole content.[5946,5947]

■ *1,8-cineole and Alpha-Thujone CTs and A. aborescens (Great Mugwort)*: May weakly interfere with the enzymes responsible for metabolizing medications (NSAIDs, proton-pump inhibitors, acetaminophen, antiepileptics, immune modulators, blood-sugar medications, blood pressure medications, antidepressants, antipsychotics, diabetic medications, antihistamines, antibiotics, and anesthetics) due to 1,8-cineole, alpha-thujone, or chamazulene content.[5948,5949,5950]

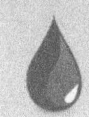
**SELECTED EVIDENCE:**

- *In vitro* research concluded that mugwort oil from both the leaves (Germacrene D CT) and the buds (1,8-cineole CT) effectively killed leukemia cells by selectively inducing apoptosis (mediated by caspase-dependent pathways).[5951]

- Mugwort oil is a mild antioxidant and possesses antimicrobial activity against *S. pyogenes* and *P. acnes*.[5952]

- Great mugwort essential oil inhibits several strains of the common foodborne pathogen *L. monocytogenes in vitro*.[5953,5954]

- Animal research demonstrated that great mugwort essential oil protected the liver from toxicity caused by synthetic estrogen/progestrogen hormone therapy and restored normal liver activity.[5955] Synthetic hormone replacement therapy has been associated with an increased risk of liver problems in some women.

- A chamazulene-rich great mugwort essential oil inhibited tumor cell growth of malignant melanoma and colorectal cancer cells *in vitro*.[5956] The same research reported that great mugwort essential oil potently scavenged the ABTS radical cation, which is a free radical associated with skin inflammation.

- Great mugwort essential oil kills the German cockroach (*Blattella germanica*) and the grain borer (Rhyzopertha dominica).[5957,5958]

- *In vitro* research reports that great mugwort essential oil (chamazulene CT) inhibits the plant fungus *R. solani*.[5959]

- Great mugwort essential oil rich in chamazulene inhibits both HSV-1 and HSV-2 *in vitro* by killing the virus.[5960,5961,5962]

- *In vitro* research demonstrates that great mugwort essential oil moderately prevent lipid peroxidation (the attack of and oxidation of lipids by free radicals, which causes cell and tissue damage).[5963]

- The beta-thujone CT of mugwort essential oil demonstrated good antioxidant and antibacterial (*Enterococcus* sp., *Staphylococcus aureus, Bacillus subtilis*, and *Klebsiella pneumonia*) activity.[5964]

- Mugwort essential oil CT 1,8-cineole (no thujones) was larvicidal to and repelled the *Ae. aegypti* mosquito (a vector that spreads dengue and yellow fever).[5965]

- The beta-caryophyllene CT of mugwort essential oil was bactericidal and fungicidal to *S. aureus* and *C. albicans*.[5966]

- Oral administration of mugwort of 1,8-cineole for three days prevented acetaminophen-induced liver injury by activating the Nrf2 pathway (a major intracellular antioxidant pathway) and increasing clearance of the drug through nontoxic metabolic pathway.[5967]

- Mugwort essential oil was insecticidal to the red flour beetle (*Tribolium castaneum*).[5968]

- The 1,8-cineole CT of mugwort essential oil exhibited strong antimicrobial activity against *S. oryzae, F. oxysporum, B. cereus*, and *S. aureus*.[5969]

---

# MUHUHU
## (African Sandalwood, Mkarambaki, Silver Oak, Muhugu)

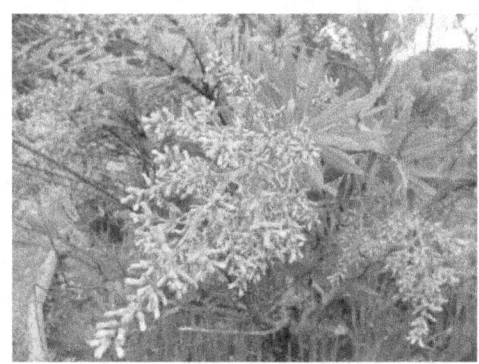

*Brachylaena hutchinsii* Hutch., *B. huillensis* O. Hoffm.

**FAMILY:** Asteraceae (Compositae)
**NOTE:** Base
**AROMA INTENSITY:** Strong
**AROMA:** Woody, earthy, balsamic, slightly musky, smoky-sweet
**COMMON EXTRACTION METHOD:** Steam distilled from the wood; may also be steam distilled from the leaves
**POSSIBLE SUBSTITUTE OILS:** Cedarwood, sandalwood
**BLENDS WELL WITH:** Bergamot, cedarwood, copaiba, frankincense, geranium, grapefruit, lavender, lemon, lime, mastic, Mediterranean mandarin, myrrh, neroli, orange, petitgrain, rose, rosewood, sandalwood, tangerine, vetiver, ylang ylang
**SUBCELLULAR LOCALIZATION | EPIGENETIC INFLUENCE:** Currently unknown | Currently unknown
**RECOMMENDED DILUTION RANGE:** 5%–Neat

**PRIMARY CONSTITUENTS:**[5970,5971,5972]

| *Wood* | | *Leaves* | |
|---|---|---|---|
| Alpha-Amorphene | 11.9%–16.5% | Beta-Caryophyllene | 19.1% |
| Brachyl Oxide | 10.0%–10.6% | Beta-Cubebene | 15.5% |
| Copaenal | 7.2%–7.5% | Cis-Calamenene | 10.5% |
| Copaenol | 6.3%–7.5% | Alpha-Copaene | 9.0% |
| Delta-Cadinene | 3.3%–6.5% | Delta-Cadinene | 8.5% |
| Alpha-Calacorene | 4.4%–5.0% | Alpha-Muurolene | 8.0% |
| Ylangenal | 0.5%–4.0% | Alpha-Calacorene | 6.0% |
| Oplopenone | 0.0%–3.5% | Alpha-Ylangene | 5.2% |
| Cadalene | 3.0%–3.2% | Gamma-Cadinene | 3.5% |
| Alpha-Copaene | 1.2%–3.0% | | |
| Alpha-Muurolene | 0.9%–3.0% | | |
| (E)-Muurola-4(14),5-Diene | 0.0%–2.9% | | |
| Viridiflorol | 0.0%–2.9% | | |
| Delta-Amorphene | 0.0%–2.7% | | |
| 1-Epi-Cubenol | 0.0%–2.6% | | |

**OTHER CONSTITUENTS:** *Wood*—Alpha-ylangene, albicanol, delta-selinene, gamma-cadinene, cis-calamenene, trans-calamenene, zonarene, ylangenol, alpha-dehydro-ar-himachalenene, naphthalenedione, juniper camphor, T-cadinol, delta-cadinol, 8-oxy-neoisolongifolene, muhuhu sesquiterpenols, muhuhu sesquiterpenes, muhuhu ester; *Leaves*—alpha-thujene, beta-calacorene, spathulenol, beta-oplopenone, beta-eudesmol, cadalene

**PREFERRED COMPOSITION FOR CLINICAL USE:**

| *Constituent* | *Wood* |
|---|---|
| **Alpha-Amorphene** | 8%–20% |
| **15-Copaenol** | 5%–15% |
| **Brachyl Oxide** | 5%–12% |
| **Copaenal** | 5%–10% |
| **Delta-Cadinene** | 3%–7% |
| **Alpha-Calacorene** | 3%–6% |
| **Cadalene** | 0.1%–5% |
| **Ylangenal** | 0.1%–5% |
| **Alpha-Copaene** | 1%–4% |
| **Alpha-Muurolene** | 0.5%–4% |

**REPORTED THERAPEUTIC PROPERTIES:** Antibacterial, antimicrobial, antiseptic, analgesic, anti-inflammatory, soothes chronic skin conditions, combats acne, supports respiratory function, eases cough, antidepressant, encourages acceptance of and adaptation to change, grounding, **relieves anxiety**, **stress management**, aphrodisiac, enhances meditation

**CAUTIONS:**

■ None currently known.

**SELECTED EVIDENCE:**

☐ *In vitro* research reports that muhuhu (leaf) essential oil inhibits *Proteus mirabilis* with effectiveness similar to the antibiotic gentamycin.[5973] In addition, it inhibited *E. faecalis, M. luteus, B. cereus, S. aureus,* and *S. epidermidis.* It was inactive against *E. coli, Klebsiella* spp., and *C. albicans.*

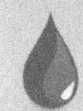

# MYRRH

*Commiphora myrrha* (Nees) Engl., *C. molmol* Engl.

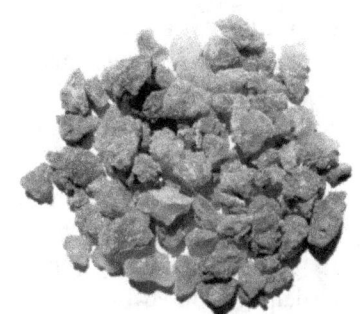

**FAMILY:** Burseraceae
**NOTE:** Base
**AROMA INTENSITY:** Medium
**AROMA:** Rich, balsamic, warm, earthy
**COMMON EXTRACTION METHOD:** Steam distilled from the resin
**POSSIBLE SUBSTITUTE OILS:** Cistus, frankincense, lavender
**BLENDS WELL WITH:** Camphor, cedarwood, frankincense, juniper, lavender, myrtle, palo santo, sandalwood, spikenard
**SUBCELLULAR LOCALIZATION | EPIGENETIC INFLUENCE:** Endocytic Vesicles | Currently unknown
**RECOMMENDED DILUTION RANGE:** 5%–Neat

**PRIMARY CONSTITUENTS**[5974,5975,5976,5977]

| Constituent | |
|---|---|
| Furanoeudesma-1,3-Diene | 15.0%–49.1% |
| Curzerene | 8.5%–40.1% |
| Furanodiene* | 0.0%–19.7% |
| Lindestrene | 3.6%–12.9% |
| Beta-Elemene | 4.4%–10.9% |
| Germacrene Isomer I | 0.4%–6.5% |
| Germacrone | 0.0%–5.8% |
| Alpha-Copaene | 0.0%–5.5% |
| Germacrene B | 0.9%–4.3% |

\* Furanodiene is often mistakenly identified as curzerene in GC/MS analyses.

**OTHER CONSTITUENTS:** Delta-elemene, beta-bourbonene, trans-caryophyllene, alpha-humulene, germacrene D, beta-selinene, gamma-cadinene, furanoeudesma-1,4-diene, t-cadinol, 2-methoxyfuranodiene

**PREFERRED COMPOSITION FOR CLINICAL USE:**

| Constituent | |
|---|---|
| **Furanoeudesma-1,3-Diene** | 25%–45% |
| **Curzerene** | 15%–35% |
| **Lindestrene** | 5%–15% |
| **Furanodiene*** | 0%–15% |
| **Beta-Elemene <cis + trans>** | 2%–8% |
| **2-Methoxyfurano-1(10),4-Diene** | 0%–5% |
| **Germacrene B** | 1%–5% |
| **Gamma-Elemene** | 0.1%–3% |
| **Germacrene D** | 0.5%–2% |

Note: Furanodiene converts to curzerene when exposed to heat (e.g. steam distillation), which is why it may not be found in some myrrh essential oils, or only in very small quantities.[5087]

**REPORTED THERAPEUTIC PROPERTIES: Anti-inflammatory**, antimicrobial, antitumor, **antiseptic**, antispasmodic, **antifungal**, antiviral, astringent, expels excess gas, **cell rejuvenator**, expectorant, decongestant, aids digestion, strengthens nails, circulatory stimulant, wound healing, **helps relieve chronic skin conditions**, sedating, calms the mind, encourages feelings of peace, reduces mental distractions, enhances meditation and focus, promotes creativity, reduces irritability

**CAUTIONS:**

■ Avoid during pregnancy and lactation (very low risk). Myrrh may contain moderate amounts of furanodiene and beta-elemene, which may prevent the formation of blood vessels necessary for fetal development according to animal research.[5978,5979,5980]

**SELECTED EVIDENCE:**

- Myrrh essential oil triggered apoptosis of breast and skin cancer cells at a greater rate than frankincense oil (*B. carterii*) *in vitro*.[5981]

- A sitz bath with or soap application of lavender, myrrh, neroli, rose, grapefruit, mandarin, orange, and Roman chamomile improves healing of the perineum following delivery and episiotomy.[5982]

- When combined with frankincense, myrrh inhibits *C. neoformans*, *P. aeruginosa*, and *B. cereus*.[5983]

- Myrrh oil prevents sebum squalene peroxidation by singlet oxygen (the main trigger of sebum squalene peroxidation during sun exposure, and a cause of DNA damage), which plays an important role in skin damage caused by sunburn and UV exposure.[5984] Another study found that myrrh oil neutralizes singlet oxygen better than vitamin E.[5985]

- Oral administration of myrrh oil and resin (12 mg/kg daily for six days) reduced Fasciola egg count and all signs and symptoms of fascioliasis—a parasitic infection that causes abdominal pain, fever, vomiting, diarrhea, swelling of the liver, hives, and eosinophilia (abnormally high number of the disease-fighting white blood cells called eosinophils) in a small clinical study.[5986]

- *In vitro* research concluded that myrrh oil modulates the pathways involved in inflammation of the gums.[5987]

- Myrrh oil helps decrease inflammation by inhibiting the 5-lipoxygenase (5-LOX) enzyme that is involved in the inflammation response according to *in vitro* research.[5988]

- *In vitro* research suggests that myrrh oil inhibits *T. vaginalis* (a protozoan parasite that is spread by sexual intercourse and causes a foul-smelling discharge from the vagina, painful urination, and vaginal itching in women; men typically have no symptoms).[5989]

- Myrrh essential oil significantly inhibited dermatophytes responsible for fungal infections of the skin, and inhibited elastase activity.[5990]

- Lyme disease is the most common vector-borne illness in the United States. It is transmitted to humans through the bite of a blacklegged tick infected with the bacterium *Borrelia burgdorferi*, and rarely *B. mayonii*. Symptoms of infection include fever, skin rash, headache, and fatigue. Left untreated, symptoms can become systematic and affect the heart, joints, and nervous system. Of thirty-five essential oils screened, garlic, allspice, cumin, palmarosa, myrrh, ginger lily, amyris, thyme, may chang, and lemon eucalyptus each demonstrated excellent activity against *Borrelia burgdorferi*.[5991] Garlic (19% diallyl disulfide), allspice CT eugenol, and myrrh (38% curzerene) were the most active essential oils.

- A combination of sandalwood and myrrh essential oil displayed noteworthy antimicrobial activity against wound pathogens.[5992] This suggests the combination may be a good option for preventing wound infections and promoting healing.

- *In vitro* research showed that myrrh essential oil inhibits *S. aureus* and *P. aeruginosa* better than its methanolic extract.[5993] The researchers further tested the antibacterial activity and found that it inhibited MRSA, multidrug-resistant *E. coli*, multidrug-resistant *P. aeruginosa*, and multidrug-resistant *K. pneumoniae*. The weakest activity was observed against *K. pneumoniae* and best activity against *P. aeruginosa*. Myrrh essential oil also demonstrated anticancer activity against human liver, breast (highest activity), and colon cancer cells *in vitro*.

- Oral administration of myrrh essential oil (50 and 100 mg/kg BW) to rats for thirty days prior to inducing heart attack by isoproterenol protected against cardiovascular deviations and injury.[5994] Specifically, the oil prevented elevations in blood pressure, heart to body weight ratio, and biochemical markers such as myocytes (CK-MB, CPK, LDH, cTnT, cTnI), lipid peroxidation, protein expression of Nrf2 and HO-1, apoptotic markers (Caspase 3,9), and inflammatory indicators.

- A double-blind, randomized clinical trial assessed the antiplaque, anti-inflammatory, and antimicrobial activity of myrrh essential oil as an adjunctive treatment during scaling and root planning in people with gingival inflammation. People aged eighteen to thirty-five with moderate to severe gingivitis applied 2 drops of a product containing myrrh oil along the gums twice daily after brushing teeth. The myrrh oil did not reduce plaque but significantly reduced gingival inflammation after forty-eight hours and reduced bacterial counts in the mouth.[5995]

- Gastritis is a general term used for inflammation of the stomach characterized by abdominal pain, indigestion, nausea, or bloating. Oral administration of myrrh essential oil reduced stomach ulcers caused by alcohol in rats.[5996] The extract was more effective than the oil.

- Myrrh essential oil protected plasmid DNA against damage caused by hydrogen peroxide and ultraviolet light and was only cytogenic to human peripheral lymphocytes at higher concentrations.[5997]

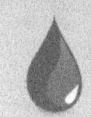

- Myrrh essential oil added to yogurt improved the yogurt's physical characteristics and inhibited the growth of bacteria, particularly *L. monocytogenes*.[5998]
- *In vitro* evaluation of essential oils and extracts from *Commiphora* oleoresins found that myrrh essential oil (29.7% curzerene, 17.4% furanoeudesma-1,3-diene, 9.1% beta-elemene) was highly toxic to skin cancer cells (epidermoid carcinoma and malignant melanoma), but less toxic to healthy skin cells.[5999]
- Oral administration of myrrh essential oil (100 mg/kg BW, for three weeks) protected against ischemia/reperfusion (I/R)-induced renal injury in rats.[6000] The oil restored antioxidant (SOD, CAT, and GPx) activity, reduced lipid peroxidation, reduced TLR4 and NFκB gene expression, leading to decreased inflammation and destruction of renal cells.

# MYRTLE
## (Red Myrtle, Green Myrtle)

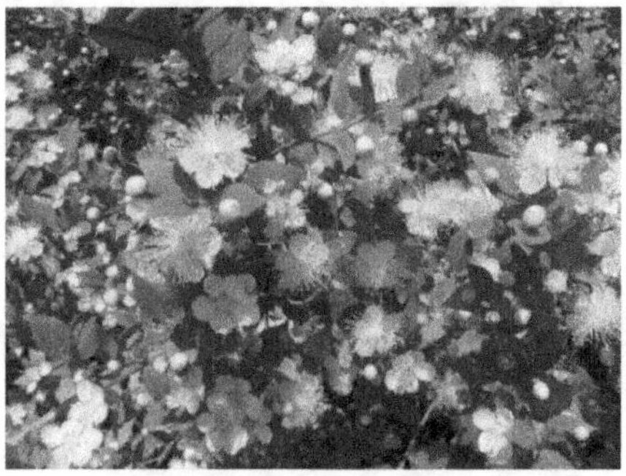

*Myrtus communis* L.

**FAMILY:** Myrtaceae
**NOTE:** Top-Middle
**AROMA INTENSITY:** Medium
**AROMA:** Sweet, slightly medicinal, fresh
**COMMON EXTRACTION METHOD:** Steam distilled from the leaves
**POSSIBLE SUBSTITUTE OILS:** Cypress, rosemary (alpha-pinene CT), niaouli (viridiflorol CT), balsam fir
**BLENDS WELL WITH:** Bergamot, black pepper, cedarwood, clary sage, clove, eucalyptus, frankincense, ginger, lavender, lemon, lemongrass, lime, melissa, myrrh, neroli, peppermint, rosemary, silver fir, white fir, ylang ylang
**SUBCELLULAR LOCALIZATION | EPIGENETIC INFLUENCE:** Endoplasmic Reticulum | Circulatory/Respiratory
**RECOMMENDED DILUTION RANGE:** 3%–Neat

**PRIMARY CONSTITUENTS:**[6001,6002,6003,6004,6005,6006,6007,6008,6009,6010]

*Alpha-Pinene CT (Green Myrtle)*

| | |
|---|---|
| Alpha-Pinene | 26.4%–64.0% |
| 1,8-Cineole | 6.5%–30.4% |
| Limonene | 0.3%–23.9% |
| Linalool | 0.7%–18.4% |
| Delta-3-Carene | 0.0%–6.1% |
| Myrtenyl Acetate | 0.0%–5.4% |
| Alpha-Terpinyl Acetate | 0.0%–4.9% |

*1,8-Cineole CT (Red Myrtle)*

| | |
|---|---|
| 1,8-Cineole | 25.7%–40.4% |
| Alpha-Pinene | 14.7%–22.5% |
| Linalool | 3.2%–17.6% |
| Alpha-Terpineol | 0.0%–8.4% |
| Myrtenyl Acetate | 0.0%–7.4% |
| Geranyl Acetate | 1.9%–6.3% |
| Linalyl Acetate | 0.0%–5.3% |
| Bornyl Acetate | 0.0%–5.2% |
| Methyl Eugenol | 0.0%–4.8% |

*Myrtenyl Acetate CT*

| | |
|---|---|
| 1,8-Cineole | 16.6%–25.7% |
| Myrtenyl Acetate | 20.8%–21.6% |
| Alpha-Pinene | 14.7%–15.6% |
| Linalool | 10.1%–13.3% |
| Limonene | 4.1%–8.9% |

*Limonene CT*

| | |
|---|---|
| Limonene | 23.4%–44.2% |
| Alpha-Pinene | 10.7%–18.9% |
| Linalool | 1.0%–15.4% |
| Geranyl Acetate | 0.9%–10.9% |
| 1,8-Cineole | 6.6%–8.7% |
| Linalyl Acetate | 0.5%–8.2% |
| Para-Cymene | 0.0%–5.1% |

Note: The 1,8-cineole CT, also called red myrtle, is the most common commercially available sample, with green myrtle (alpha-pinene CT) the second most common. The myrtenyl acetate CT may also be found commercially.

**OTHER CONSTITUENTS:** *Alpha-Pinene CT*—Alpha-thujene, beta-pinene, myrcene, alpha-phellandrene, gamma-terpinene, alpha-terpinolene, linalyl acetate, beta-caryophyllene, alpha-humulene, caryophyllene oxide methyl eugenol (<2.2%); *1,8-Cineole CT*—Beta-pinene, terpinolene, terpinen-4-ol, cinerolone, isobutyl isobutyrate, alpha-terpinyl acetate, neral acetate, eugenol, beta-caryophyllene, alpha-humulene, 4-isopropyl-2,5-dimethoxybenzyl acetate, caryophyllene oxide, beta-bisabolene, 5,8-tri decadiene, methyl eugenol (<4.8%); *Myrtenyl Acetate CT—* Alpha-thujene, alpha-terpineol, myrtenol, linalyl acetate, terpinyl acetate, alpha-humulene, beta-caryophyllene, methyl eugenol (<1.2%); *Limonene CT—*Alpha-thujene, beta-pinene, myrcene, alpha-phellandrene, delta-3-carene, gamma-terpinene, alpha-terpinolene, alpha-terpineol, methyl eugenol (<3.1%), caryophyllene oxide

### PREFERRED COMPOSITION FOR CLINICAL USE:

| Constituent | Green Myrtle | Red Myrtle |
|---|---|---|
| **Alpha-Pinene** | 40%–65% | 15%–25% |
| **1,8-Cineole** | 15%–30% | 25%–40% |
| **Limonene** | 5%–15% | 5%–15% |
| **Linalool** | 1.5%–8% | 2%–8% |
| **Geranyl Acetate** | 0.5%–3% | 2%–7% |
| **Myrtenyl Acetate** | < 3% | 5%–22% |
| **Methyl Eugenol** | < 2% | < 5% |
| **Alpha-Terpineol** | < 2% | 1%–6% |

### REPORTED THERAPEUTIC PROPERTIES:

Antiseptic, astringent, antibacterial, antimicrobial, **bronchodilator**, expectorant, decongestant, **eases cough**, nervine (calms and soothes the nerves), reduces the appearance of blemishes, **balances respiratory function**, **stimulates thyroid function and the release of thyroid hormones**, supports urinary tract health, aphrodisiac, **encourages restful sleep**, invigorating, enhances mental clarity, sedating, reduces self-destructive behavior

### CAUTIONS:

■ Some aromatherapy texts suggest being cautious with the oral administration of myrtle because it may contain methyl chavicol (estragole) and methyl eugenol. These constituents or their metabolites may potentially cause cancer in very large amounts.[6011,6012] However, animal research suggests that it takes extreme amounts (6.6 mL/kg) for ten to twenty-one days to cause liver toxicity.[6013] The same study concluded that daily intake of 1 to 2 mL of myrtle by humans is too low to cause liver problems. Based on the available evidence reasonable oral doses of myrtle pose very little risk.

■ Avoid with epilepsy and Parkinson's due to 1,8-cineole content (*all CTs except limonene*), which may exacerbate or trigger seizures/convulsions or reduce medication efficacy.[6014,6015,6016]

■ May interfere with pentobarbital and other barbiturates (medications for anxiety and insomnia) if 1,8-cineole content is high.[6017,6018,6019]

■ May interact with diabetes medications and cause low blood sugar.[6020] Myrtle is known to reduce blood glucose levels in animals and 1,8-cineole inhibits alpha-glucosidase activity, particularly when synergized with other constituents (myrtenyl acetate and alpha-pinene).[6021,6022,6023] Alpha-glucosidase is an enzyme that breaks down carbohydrates by chemical reaction with water. Inhibiting its activity postpones glucose absorption and therefore the impact of carbohydrates on blood sugar levels.

■ May weakly interfere with the enzymes responsible for metabolizing medications (NSAIDs, proton-pump inhibitors, acetaminophen, antiepileptics, immune modulators, blood-sugar medications, blood pressure medications, antidepressants, antipsychotics, diabetic medications, antihistamines, antibiotics, and anesthetics) due to 1,8-cineole content.[6024,6025,6026]

■ May interact with antibiotics or antifungals and increase their effectiveness.[6027]

■ While myrtle can contain up to 40% 1,8-cineole, it has not been associated with the same respiratory distress problems in young children as eucalyptus has. This makes it a preferred choice for respiratory support for younger children.

### SELECTED EVIDENCE:

☐ A linalool CT of myrtle (linalool 29.1%, 1,8-cineole 18.4%, alpha-terpineol 10.8%) exhibited moderate antitumor activity against colon cancer.[6028]

☐ *In vitro* research suggests that myrtle oil enhances the antimicrobial activity of conventional antibiotics and resensitizes multi-drug-resistant pathogens to traditional antibiotics and improves the effectiveness of antifungal drugs.[6029,6030]

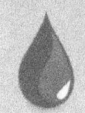

- Myrtle oil inhibited both drug-resistant and nonresistant strains of *M. tuberculosis* (the cause of tuberculosis) *in vitro*.[6031]

- Animal research suggests that topical application of myrtle oil reduces inflammation by inhibiting excess leukocyte migration to damaged tissue, and inhibiting the proinflammatory molecules TNF-alpha and IL-6.[6032] Leukocytes travel to the site of damaged tissue to encourage tissue repair; however, when they migrate excessively to the area it causes an abnormal inflammatory response. An *in vitro* study suggests that it also inhibits excess nitric oxide production.[6033]

- Myrtle oil inhibits *E. rhusiopathiae* (a pathogenic bacterium that causes minor to serious skin infections and systemic infections) *in vitro*.[6034]

- *In vitro* research concluded that myrtle oil inhibits *P. gingivalis* (a pathogenic bacterium associated with periodontal disease) *in vitro*.[6035]

- Myrtle oil inhibits *C. albicans*, *C. tropicalis*, *C. glabrata*, and *C. parapsilosis* according to *in vitro* research.[6036,6037]

- An animal study found that 150 mg/kg of myrtle oil significantly reduced blood-sugar levels, decreased inflammation about as well as the NSAID indomethacin, and relieved pain in mice.[6038]

- Oral administration of 50 mg/kg of myrtle essential oil reduced blood-sugar levels and blood triglyceride levels in diabetic and normal rabbits. The study attributed this affect to myrtle's ability to inhibit the enzyme responsible for breaking down starch and disaccharides to glucose (alpha-glucosidase), enhance glycolysis (the metabolic pathway used to convert glucose to pyruvate, which is typically conserved for glucose production in diabetes), and improve glycogenesis (the formation of glycogen from glucose, which is the storage form of glucose in humans).[6039]

- *In vitro* research concluded that myrtle oil prevents both oxidative damage and genetic mutation.[6040,6041,6042]

- Myrtle oil eradicates *H. pylori* (a bacterium associated with peptic ulcers, stomach cancer, and stomach inflammation) *in vitro*.[6043]

- *In vitro* research suggests that myrtle oil is active against *P. falciparum* (a protozoan parasite that causes malaria in humans).[6044]

- Myrtle essential oil CT linalool demonstrates moderate to potent antimicrobial activity against *B. subtilis*, *S. aureus*, and *C. albicans*.[6045]

- Myrtle oil significantly inhibits *T. vaginalis* (a protozoan parasite that is spread by sexual intercourse and causes a foul-smelling discharge from the vagina, painful urination, and vaginal itching in women; men typically have no symptoms) *in vitro*.[6046]

- A mixture of myrtle, eucalyptus, sweet orange, and lemon increased mucus, bacterial, and inflammatory molecule clearance from the respiratory system *in vitro*.[6047]

- A methanolic extract of myrtle (which contains volatile constituents ground within the essential oil) reduced intestinal and aorta spasms, enhanced bronchodilation (relaxation of the bronchi and bronchioles to increase airflow in the lungs) and vasodilation (relaxation of the blood vessel walls, which causes decreased blood pressure) in rabbit intestines and hearts, possibly by blocking calcium channels.[6048] Agents that block calcium channels prevent calcium from entering heart and blood vessel cells, which results in relaxed blood vessels and greater supply of blood and oxygen to the heart. They are useful for such conditions as high blood pressure, migraines, chest pain, cardiomyopathy, and Raynaud's syndrome.

- Topical application of a 5% solution (10 drops on a cotton ball and applied to the lesion for 20–30 seconds, three to six times daily for seven days or until complete improvement) of myrtle essential oil decreased the average healing time and size of canker sores (Aphthous stomatitis) and reduced pain without any reported significant side effects.[6049,6050,6051,6052,6053] One of the studies demonstrated comparable efficacy to topical triamcinolone (a long acting corticosteroid). Interestingly, a 10% solution of myrtle essential oil was less effective than placebo and the 5% solution (oral or paste).

- *In vitro* research demonstrates that myrtle CT linalool is a moderate antioxidant.[6054]

- Myrtle essential oil (myrtenyl acetate and alpha-pinene CTs) inhibited the *Biscogniauxia mediterranea* fungus, which causes charcoal canker in trees.[6055]

- A review of three clinical trials concluded that myrtle essential oil significantly improves bleeding, permanent pain, pain during defecation, anal irritation, anal itching and anal heaviness in patients with hemorrhoids types I (mild: rare presence of bleeding) and II (symptoms interfere with work and average bleeding), including people who did not respond to drug treatments.[6056,6057,6058,6059] The oil was incorporated in a lotion or ointment and standardized to 1,8-cineole content.

☐ An increasing resistance to antifungal medications has prompted a search for novel alternative antifungal agents. Myrtle essential oil (CT geranyl acetate; 16.4% geranyl acetate, 10.3% 1,8-cineole, 7.1% alpha-terpineol, 7.0% myrtenyl acetate, and 6.0% nerol) demonstrated broad-spectrum antimicrobial activities against *Malassezia* sp. isolated from the skin of people with pityriasis versicolor.[6060]

☐ Niosomal (formed by nonionic surfactants and cholesterol) myrtle essential oil inhibited *Staphylococcus aureus, Staphylococcus epidermidis, Serratia marcescens,* and *Bacillus subtilis* better than traditional myrtle essential oil.[6061]

☐ Both an odd CT (with methyleugenol as the major constituent) and the 1,8-cineole CT of myrtle essential oil were effective against breast cancer cells.[6062]

☐ Sepsis (a potentially life-threatening condition that occurs when chemicals released in the bloodstream to fight infection trigger systemic inflammation and damage to multiple organs) is associated with severe endothelial cell damage and dysfunction leading to poor vascular function and tissue swelling. Myrtle essential oil was unable to reduce cellular damage caused by sepsis, but isolated 1,8-cineole and alpha-pinene from the oil were effective.[6063]

☐ Helichrysum (Corsican type), mastic CT myrcene, and myrtle CT tricyclene essential oils demonstrated strong anticancer activity against human ovarian cancer cells.[6064] Rosemary CT alpha-pinene, thyme CT thymol, and yarrow CT 1,8-cineole exhibited weaker activity against cancer cells. All of the oils showed weak or no estrogenic activity in yeast strains expressing the human estrogen receptor alpha, while helichrysum and yarrow essential oils were antiestrogenic. All of the oils affected the proliferation and viability of human peripheral lymphocytes in a dose-dependent manner.

☐ Hypothyroidism can cause oxidative stress (where more free radicals are present than the body has capacity to neutralize), which can damage tissues throughout the body. Administration of myrtle essential oil improved antioxidant capacity in rats with hypothyroidism.[6065]

☐ Commonly found in cat feces and raw or undercooked meat, *Toxoplasma gondii* is a parasite that infects warm-blooded mammals, including humans. While many people are infected and display no symptoms, toxoplasmosis can be dangerous in pregnant women (can cause birth abnormalities and even fatalities in unborn babies) and people with a compromised immune system. Oral administration of myrtle CT alpha-pinene essential oil for fifteen days prior to infection with *T. gondii* and continuing for six days after infection significantly reduced total *T. gondii* cysts in the brain of mice. The most effective doses were 200 and 300 mg/kg body weight. The oil improved the immune system's response to the infection and displayed low toxicity.

☐ Gastric (or stomach) ulcers are common in modern society and caused by a variety of factors including *H. pylori* infection, NSAIDs, psychological stress, heavy alcohol consumption, and smoking. Evidence suggests that oxidative stress plays a significant role in the damage of the stomach lining. The protective effect of myrtle CT myrtenyl acetate essential oil was evaluated in rats with ulcers caused by ethanol/hydrogen chloride.[6066] Rats were divided into six groups: 1) normal control, 2) ulcer control, 3) 250 mg/kg body weight myrtle oil, 4) 500 mg/kg BW myrtle oil, 5) 1,000 mg/kg BW myrtle oil, and 6) famotidine (brand name Pepcid—a stomach acid lowering medication used to treat ulcers and GERD). Oral administration of microencapsulated myrtle essential oil before exposure to ethanol/hydrogen chloride significantly protected against gastric ulcers, with the 500 and 1,000 mg dosage groups performing better than famotidine. The protective benefits of the oil were attributed to a reduction in overall stomach acidity, potent anti-inflammatory effects, prevention of depletion of antioxidant enzyme activity (SOD, CAT, GPx), and reduced gastric lipoperoxidation. Overall, the research suggests that oral use of myrtle essential oil reduces oxidative stress and inflammation that contribute to gastric ulcers.

☐ Human papillomaviruses (HPV) are a group of over one hundred related viruses that affect the genitals and skin. HPV is spread through intimate skin to skin contact and most sexually active men and women are carriers of the virus by their early twenties. Side effects of current medications and a high recurrence rate make finding new solutions important for global health. A double-blind, randomized controlled trial investigated the benefits of vaginal suppositories containing myrtle extract (10%; aqueous) and essential oil (0.5%).[6067] Women between the ages of eighteen and fifteen years in the active treatment group used twenty myrtle suppositories each month (one suppository at bedtime daily except during menstruation) for up to three months. The control group used placebo vaginal suppositories without any herbal extract or essential oil. At the end of the study, an HPV test was negative in 92.6 percent of the myrtle group and 62.6 percent of the placebo group (the body can often clear HPV without any intervention). In addition, a cervical exam

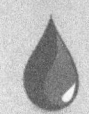

showed that lesion reduction was 71.4 percent in the myrtle group and 30.4 percent in the placebo group. The study demonstrates that myrtle suppositories can speed HPV clearance and improve cervical tissue state.

- ☐ Oral administration of bay laurel CT 1,8-cineole or myrtle CT 1,8-cineole (0.5 mL mixed in equal parts sunflower oil, for two weeks) was evaluated for their benefits on body weight control, antioxidant status, and lipid control in rats.[6068] Both oils promoted weight loss, reduced blood glucose levels, and decreased lipid levels (total cholesterol, LDL, VLDL) and atherogenic indicators, leading to cardiovascular protection. Overall, bay laurel was more effective and considered an excellent candidate to combat obesity caused by medications due to its ability to inhibit enzymes responsible for conversion of carbohydrates into glucose and effects on lipid metabolism in the liver. This activity suggests that ingestion of bay laurel essential oil may result in weight loss. Myrtle exhibited better antioxidant capacity in most tissues, except for the kidneys where it caused a pro-oxidant effect. Myrtle also increased the permeability and instability of red blood cell membranes, which reduced their ability to decrease entry of toxic substances into the cell, and increased intestinal inflammation by reducing probiotic bacteria and increasing *Enterobacter* colonization.

- ☐ *Toxoplasma gondii* is a parasite excreted in cat feces. Humans can accidentally ingest the parasites if they come in contact with cat feces and then touch their mouth causing toxoplasmosis. Oral administration of myrtle CT alpha-pinene (green myrtle) essential oil reduced the number of brain tissues cysts in a dose-dependent manner in mice.[6069] The oil improved innate immunity and exhibited low toxicity.

- ☐ Myrtle CT myrtenyl acetate essential oil inhibited *L. monocytogenes, P. aeruginosa, P. carotovorum, S. aureus,* and *E. coli,* inhibited *S. aureus* biofilm formation, was cytotoxic to neuroblastoma cancer cells, and exhibited good antiacetylcholinesterase activity (suggesting it may benefit memory and thinking). Myrtenyl acetate, alpha-pinene, and linalool were also active against all tested strains. 1,8-cineole and alpha-pinene displayed greater antiacetylcholinesterase activity than the whole oil.

- ☐ The alpha-pinene CT of myrtle essential oil was anthelmintic to the gastrointestinal parasites *Haemonchus contortus* and *Heligosomoides polygyrus in vitro* and in a rodent model.[6070]

- ☐ Myrtle (subsp. *tarentina*; 17.7% alpha-pinene, 12.4% alpha-humulene) reduced the viability of prostate cancer cells (triggered apoptosis) and decreased the capacity of these cancer cells to migrate to other areas of the body.[6071]

---

# NEROLI

*Citrus × aurantium* L. (flowers), *C. × aurantium* L. var. *amara,*
*C. × aurantium* L. var. *bigaradia*; *C. × sinensis* (L.) Osbeck (flower)

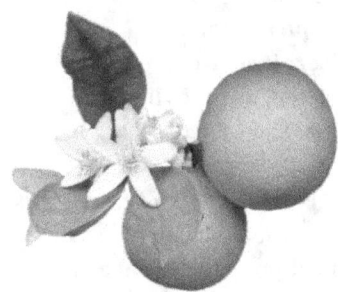

**FAMILY:** Rutaceae
**NOTE:** Middle
**AROMA INTENSITY:** Strong
**AROMA:** Sweet, floral, citrusy, fresh
**COMMON EXTRACTION METHOD:** Steam distilled from the flowers; may also be solvent extracted
**POSSIBLE SUBSTITUTE OILS:** Petitgrain (bergamot), bergamot, petitgrain (mandarin)
**BLENDS WELL WITH:** Bay laurel, cajeput, cardamom, carrot seed, cassia, chamomile (German, Roman), clary sage, coriander, geranium, grapefruit, lavender, lemon, lemon verbena, lime, melissa, orange, petitgrain, pine, rose, rosemary, sage, spikenard, tangerine, ylang ylang
**SUBCELLULAR LOCALIZATION | EPIGENETIC INFLUENCE:** Currently unknown | Currently unknown
**RECOMMENDED DILUTION RANGE:** 3%–50%; neat for limited conditions

**PRIMARY CONSTITUENTS:**[6072,6073,6074,6075,6076]

| *C. aurantium* | | *C. sinensis* | |
|---|---|---|---|
| Linalool | 26.6%–34.4% | Sabinene | 31.4%–41.4% |
| Limonene | 9.2%–27.5% | Linalool | 16.4%–31.8% |
| Beta-Pinene | 3.5%–19.1% | Limonene | 4.0%–10.0% |
| (E)-Nerolidol | 1.8%–17.5% | (E)-Nerolidol | 2.9%–10.0% |
| Alpha-Terpineol | 4.6%–14.0% | Terpinen-4-ol | 2.3%–5.6% |
| Alpha-Terpinyl Acetate | 0.2%–11.7% | Beta-Caryophyllene | 0.1%–4.9% |

| Linalyl Acetate | 3.3%–11.3% | (E)-Beta-Ocimene | 0.1%–4.8% |
| (E,E)-Farnesol | 0.0%–8.0% | (E,Z)-Farnesol | 0.1%–4.6% |
| Trans-Beta-Ocimene | 0.0%–6.6% | Beta-Caryophyllene Oxide | 0.0%–3.9% |
| Geranyl Acetate | 2.6%–4.9% | Myrcene | 2.1%–3.7% |
| Geraniol | 0.4%–4.3% | | |

**OTHER CONSTITUENTS:** *C. aurantium*—Alpha-pinene, sabinene, myrcene, cis-beta-ocimene, terpinen-4-ol, nerol, alpha-terpinolene, neryl acetate, beta-caryophyllene; *C. sinensis*—Alpha-pinene, beta-pinene, delta-3-carene, benzene acetaldehyde, para-cymene, beta-phellandrene, gamma-terpinene, terpinolene, alpha-terpineol, indole, methyl anthranilate, beta-elemene, (E)-beta-farnesene

**PREFERRED COMPOSITION FOR CLINICAL USE:**

| Constituent | C. aurantium | C. sinensis |
| --- | --- | --- |
| Linalool | 28%–50% | 15%–35% |
| Limonene | 8%–22% | 4%–12% |
| Beta-Pinene | 4%–18% | 1%–3% |
| Linalyl Acetate | 1%–16% | – |
| Trans-Beta-Ocimene | 2%–9% | 0.1%–5% |
| Alpha-Terpineol | 3%–8% | 0.1%–1% |
| (E)-Nerolidol | 1.5%–7% | 3%–10% |
| Geranyl Acetate | 2%–5% | – |
| Geraniol | 1%–5% | < 0.5% |
| Neryl Acetate | 0.1%–5% | – |
| Farnesol (E,Z; Z,E; or E,E) | 0.5%–4% | 0.1%–5% |
| Myrcene | 0.1%–4% | 2%–5% |
| Sabinene | 0.1%–3% | 30%–45% |
| Alpha-Pinene | 0.1%–2% | 0.1%–2% |
| Terpinen-4-ol | 0.1%–2% | 2%–6% |
| Beta-Caryophyllene | 0.1%–2% | 0.1%–5% |

Note: Moroccan neroli (*C. aurantium*) will have lower percentages of linalyl acetate than Egyptian neroli.

**REPORTED THERAPEUTIC PROPERTIES:** Antibacterial, **analgesic (pain relief)**, anti-inflammatory, antiseptic, antispasmodic, aphrodisiac, expels excess gas, aids digestion, **cell regenerator**, antifungal, anti-infectious, balances blood pressure, **reduces the appearance of scars, blemishes, and spots**, anticonvulsive, helps hemorrhoids heal, deodorant, regenerative, sedating, **antidepressant**, **reduces anxiety**, combats shock, encourages a restful night's sleep, **stress management**, encourages creativity

**CAUTIONS:**

■ May be mildly photosensitizing (very low risk) due to the presence of psoralen, bergapten, isopompinellin, and xanthotoxin.[6077,6078] Avoid UV rays for at least twelve hours following topical application.

**SELECTED EVIDENCE:**

☐ A sitz bath with or soap application of lavender, myrrh, neroli, rose, grapefruit, mandarin, orange, and Roman chamomile improves healing of the perineum following delivery and episiotomy.[6079]

☐ Applying a gauze pad with 4 mL of a neroli oil distillate (hydrosol) and changed every thirty minutes significantly reduced anxiety during the first stage of labor among pregnant women aged 18 to 35 years.[6080]

☐ Inhalation of neroli oil from a pad for five minutes several times daily helps relieve menopausal symptoms, increase libido, reduce blood pressure, and balance the endocrine system according to clinical research.[6081]

☐ Administering 20–40 mg/kg of neroli to animals prevented drug-induced convulsions by balancing the GABAergic system (a system of structures that release or bind gamma-aminobutyric acid and regulate

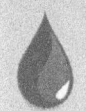

anxiety, muscle tension, memory, and convulsive activity).[6082]

- ☐ A clinical study concluded that both cortisol and systolic blood pressure declines after inhalation of a combination of lavender, ylang ylang, marjoram, and neroli oil in those with high blood pressure or pre-high blood pressure.[6083]

- ☐ *In vitro* research discovered that neroli oil inhibited *H. pylori* growth (a bacterium strongly associated with stomach ulcers) in extraordinarily low concentrations.[6084]

- ☐ Postpartum women who received a thirty-minute massage on the second postpartum day with 7 drops of lavender and 3 drops of neroli in 100 mL of carrier oil experienced significantly lower postpartum depression, reduced anxiety, and were more interactive with their infant.[6085]

- ☐ Inhalation (ten deep breaths from aromatherapy stones with two drops of the blend) of lavender, Roman chamomile, and neroli reduced the anxiety and stress of patients undergoing coronary angioplasty (the insertion of a catheter to open blocked coronary arteries).[6086]

- ☐ Neroli oil helps decrease inflammation by mildly inhibiting the 5-lipoxygenase (5-LOX) enzyme that is involved in the inflammation response *in vitro*.[6087]

- ☐ *In vitro* research found that neroli oil is a potent antioxidant and that it moderately to strongly inhibits thirteen bacteria and eight fungal strains.[6088,6089]

- ☐ A twenty-minute foot massage with neroli oil one day after heart surgery significantly improved the mental and emotional state of the heart patients, and improved respiratory rate in people who had heart surgery.[6090]

- ☐ Inhalation of neroli oil encourages a relaxed state in mice. The researchers also found that neroli oil constituents were detected in the blood of mice one hour after inhalation.[6091,6092]

- ☐ Inhalation of spearmint or *C. sinensis* flower essential oils (0.02 mL/kg mixed with 2 mL of saline) through a nebulizer five minutes prior to a 1500 meter running test increased athletic performance in male college students (mean age 19.1 to 19.8, 50% to 10% smokers for the spearmint and orange groups respectively).[6093] Lung function was increased 20% in the spearmint group and 75% in the orange flower group, and the mean time to run the 1500 m was significantly decreased after inhaling both essential oils. Interestingly, a significant increase in Forced Expiratory Volume 1 (FEV1, the maximal amount of air that can be forcefully exhaled in one second, and a test used to measure airway obstruction, bronchoconstriction, or bronchodilation) and Forced Vital Capacity (FVC, the maximum amount of air that can be exhaled from the lungs) was observed after essential oil inhalation.

- ☐ Neroli (*C. aurantium* L. var. *amara*) essential oil triggers vasodilation by influencing the NO-sGC pathway (a pathway involved in vascular tone, platelet aggregation, and vasorelaxation) and modulating calcium entry into endothelial cells (prevention of calcium entry into cells reduces heart contraction force and opens the blood vessels).[6094]

- ☐ Animal research demonstrates that neroli (*C. aurantium* L.) significantly reduces acute and chronic inflammation and reduces pain (centrally and peripherally).[6095]

- ☐ A linalool rich neroli essential oil (64.6% linalool, 7.6% alpha-terpineol, 6.2% limonene, 5.0% linalyl acetate) demonstrated good anti-inflammatory activity by markedly decreasing COX-2, and inhibited nitric oxide production, IL-6, TNF-α, and IL-1β, as well as their gene expression level.[6096]

- ☐ A clinical trial found that inhalation of a 0.5% concentration of neroli (*C. aurantium*) essential oil improved premenstrual syndrome symptoms in college students.[6097] Participants inhaled neroli for five minutes from a cotton pad placed about 30cm from their nose, twice daily, from about one week prior to menstruation (for five days) during two consecutive menstrual cycles.

- ☐ Another randomized, controlled clinical study by the same research team concluded that inhalation of 4% rose or 0.5% neroli essential oil decreased symptoms (mental, physical, social) associated with premenstrual symptoms.[6098] Participants inhaled the oils (10 drops on an eye pad, which was placed 30 cm from the nose) for five minutes, twice daily, for five days one week prior to menstruation. Rose was far more effective than neroli and the control (sweet almond oil).

- ☐ A double-blind placebo-controlled clinical trial found that inhalation of neroli essential oil (30% solution, three times daily, two days after hospitalization) significantly reduced anxiety in people who had acute coronary syndrome (ACS).[6099] ACS is the term used for conditions associated with a sudden, reduced flow of blood to the heart. Anxiety occurs at higher rates among people with ACS and anxiety adversely affects cardiovascular outcomes in people with ACS.[6100]

- Neroli essential oil inhibited *E. coli, S. typhimurium S. aureus, B. cereus*, and *L. monocytogenes*, and demonstrated good antioxidant activity in the DPPH assay.[6101] Interestingly, the hydrosol exhibited nearly identical antioxidant activity.

- A nanoemulsion of neroli (*C. aurantium*) with 22.9% linalyl acetate, 14.2% linalool, and 13.6% farnesol killed human lung cancer cells.[6102] The same research found that gavage administration of the oil (10 to 20 mg/kg BW) daily for thirty days did not cause harm to the liver and kidneys, but instead improved intestinal structure and liver antioxidant potential. Based on the results the study authors concluded that the oil represents a promising solution to prevent lung cancer progression.

- Inhalation of aurantium acid isolated from *C. aurantium*—fifteen to twenty minutes about 60 minutes prior to angiography (a procedure to examine your blood vessels)—alleviated anxiety about the procedure as measured by Spielberger's state-trait anxiety inventory, blood pressure, and respiratory and pulse rate.[6103]

- Neroli (*C. aurantium*) essential oil exhibited strong antifungal activity against two strains of *C. albicans* and synergized the effects of fluconazole and amphotericin B against the fungi.[6104] The major compounds in the oil were beta-pinene, delta-3-carene, and limonene.

- Postmenopausal sleep problems are common occurrences for many women due to both psychological (stress, overwork) and physical (hormone imbalances—decreased estrogen, progesterone, serotonin, and melatonin) disturbances. A randomized controlled trial evaluated the sleep benefits of topical application of neroli essential oil in postmenopausal women.[6105] Participants in the neroli group applied 2 drops of the oil (diluted to 10% in sweet almond oil) to the forearm twice daily (10:00 a.m. and 10:00 p.m.), for four consecutive days per week, continuing this pattern for four weeks. The women were instructed to lie comfortable and inhale the aroma from their forearm for five minutes after application. The control group applied and inhaled sweet almond oil only. At the end of the four-week study, all dimensions of the Pittsburgh Sleep Quality Index were significantly improved in the neroli group compared to the sweet almond oil only group. The findings suggest that inhaling neroli essential oil can significantly improve sleep quality of postmenopausal women.

- Sleep quality diminishes during pregnancy, especially during the last trimester. Sleep troubles during pregnancy reportedly affects about 50 percent of women. A neroli essential oil extracted using enfleurage was investigated for its effects on sleep quality among pregnant women in a clinical study.[6106] Five drops of the oil were placed inside a face mask and the masks were inhaled from morning and before going to bed for twenty minutes over a one-month period. A placebo group inhaled from masks saturated with 5 drops of sweet almond oil instead. At the end of a month, sleep quality significantly improved in the neroli group when compared to placebo.

- A decrease of sex hormones during menopause can cause many changes such as hot flashes, heart palpitations, sleep disturbance, mood disorders, and sexual dysfunction. Sexual dysfunction is among the most common issues experienced during menopause because a decline in circulating estrogen and androgen hormones can decrease blood flow to the vagina causing dryness and vaginal atrophy, painful sexual intercourse, and reduced libido. A randomized, placebo-controlled human clinical trial investigated the benefits of inhaling neroli essential oil in menopausal women reporting sexual dysfunction.[6107] Women in the neroli group applied 2 drops of neroli essential oil (10% dilution) to the forearm twice daily (10:00 a.m. and 10:00 p.m.), while sitting in a comfortable position and inhaled from their forearm for five minutes, for four consecutive days per week, continuing for four weeks. The placebo group applied odorless sweet almond oil only and inhaled from their forearm in the same manner. The results of the study demonstrated that inhaling neroli oil significantly improved sexual function—increased libido, sexual satisfaction, reduced pain during intercourse, and vaginal dryness—compared to the control group.

- Breastfeeding can affect sex drive due to hormonal changes after delivery—decrease in estrogen and progesterone and increased prolactin and oxytocin. A randomized controlled trial found that applying 10% bitter orange or lavender essential oil to the forearm (2 drops, twice daily, for forty days) and inhaling it for five minutes improved sexual satisfaction in breastfeeding women.[6108]

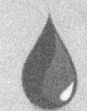

# NIAOULI

*Melaleuca quinquenervia* (Cav.) S.T. Blake;
*M. viridiflora* Sol. ex Gaertn

**FAMILY:** Myrtaceae
**NOTE:** Middle
**AROMA INTENSITY:** Medium
**AROMA:** Sharp, medicinal, slightly sweet, citrusy
**COMMON EXTRACTION METHOD:** Steam distilled from the leaves and twigs
**POSSIBLE SUBSTITUTE OILS:** Eucalyptus, Spanish sage, sage (1,8-cineole CT)
**BLENDS WELL WITH:** Bergamot, coriander, eucalyptus, fennel, juniper, lavandin, lavender, lemon, lime, tea tree, myrtle, orange, peppermint, pine, spearmint, tangerine
**SUBCELLULAR LOCALIZATION | EPIGENETIC INFLUENCE:** Currently unknown | Currently unknown
**RECOMMENDED DILUTION RANGE:** 3%–50%; neat for limited conditions

**PRIMARY CONSTITUENTS:**[6109,6110,6111,6112,6113,6114,6115,6116]

### *M. quinquenervia (1,8-Cineole CT)*

| | |
|---|---|
| 1,8-Cineole | 19.1%–76.3% |
| Viridiflorol | 0.0%–47.9% |
| Alpha-Pinene | 0.8%–25.0% |
| Limonene | 0.5%–15.0% |
| Alpha-Terpineol | 0.0%–15.0% |
| Alpha-Terpinyl Acetate | 0.0%–11.4% |
| Para-Cymene | 0.0%–10.0% |
| Beta-Pinene | 0.5%–5.0% |
| (E,E)-Farnesol | 0.0%–5.0% |
| Terpinen-4-ol | 0.0%–3.0% |

### *M. quinquenervia (1,8-Cineole & Viridiflorol CT)*

| | |
|---|---|
| 1,8-Cineole | 0.4%–75.0% |
| Viridiflorol | 8.4%–66.0% |
| Beta-Caryophyllene | 0.5%–28.0% |
| Alpha-Terpineol | 0.0%–14.0% |
| Terpinolene | 1.4%–8.3% |
| Alpha-Pinene | 1.3%–7.9% |
| (E)-Nerolidol | 0.1%–2.3% |
| Gamma-Terpinene | 0.1%–2.0% |

### *M. quinquenervia (Viridiflorol/Para-Cymene/1,8-Cineole CT)*

| | |
|---|---|
| Viridiflorol | 4.0%–50.0% |
| 1,8-Cineole | 0.4%–47.0% |
| Para-Cymene | 0.4%–40.0% |
| Gamma-Terpinene | 0.0%–32.4% |
| Alpha-Terpineol | 0.5%–24.5% |
| Terpinolene | 0.1%–19.2% |
| Alpha-Pinene | 0.0%–17.0% |
| (E,E)-Farnesol | 0.0%–10.8% |
| Limonene | 1.0%–6.0% |
| Terpinen-4-ol | 0.5%–5.0% |

### *M. quinquenervia ((E)-Nerolidol CT)*

| | |
|---|---|
| (E)-Nerolidol | 56.0%–95.0% |
| Linalool | 0.0%–30.0% |
| Beta-Caryophyllene | 0.5%–8.7% |
| 1,8-Cineole | 0.1%–6.6% |
| Alpha-Pinene | 0.0%–4.5% |

### *M. quinquenervia (Viridiflorol CT)*

| | |
|---|---|
| Viridiflorol | 10.0%–67.4% |
| 1,8-Cineole | 0.1%–40.0% |
| Alpha-Pinene | 0.2%–27.7% |
| Beta-Caryophyllene | 1.3%–24.6% |
| Alpha-Terpineol | 1.5%–13.6% |
| Limonene | 1.0%–10.0% |
| (E,E)-Farnesol | 0.0%–10.0% |
| (E)-Nerolidol | 0.1%–8.3% |
| Beta-Pinene | 0.4%–5.0% |

### *M. viridiflora (1,8-cineole CT)*

| | |
|---|---|
| 1,8-Cineole | 67.0%–72.9% |
| Alpha-Terpineol | 8.2%–8.4% |
| Alpha-Pinene | 5.8%–7.2% |

### *M. viridiflora (Terpinen-4-ol CT)*

| | |
|---|---|
| Terpinen-4-ol | 29.1% |
| Alpha-Pinene | 21.6% |
| Limonene | 17.4% |
| Alpha-Terpineol | 8.1% |
| Beta-Pinene | 7.3% |

| | |
|---|---|
| Alpha-Terpinyl Acetate | 0.0%–5.0% |
| Beta-Pinene | 0.1%–2.0% |

Note: Niaouli essential oil is obtained from *M. quinquenervia*, but often mistakenly identified as *M. viridiflora*.[6117] Both species may be available commercially and called niaouli. The 1,8-cineole CT is the most common CT of *M. quinquenervia* and estimated to make up more than 90% of commercially available niaouli essential oils. The (E)-Nerolidol/Linalool CT may be called nerolina.

**OTHER CONSTITUENTS:** *M. quinquenervia (1,8-Cineole CT)*—Myrcene, linalool, benzaldehyde, terpinolene, beta-caryophyllene, viridiflorene, delta-cadinene, gamma-cadinene, ledol, caryophyllene oxide, alpha-muurolol; *M. quinquenervia (1,8-Cineole & Viridiflorol CT)*—Myrcene, alpha-phellandrene, alpha-thujene, gamma-cadinene, delta-cadinene, ledol, alpha-gurjunene, caryophyllene oxide; *M. quinquenervia ((E)-Nerolidol CT)*—Alpha-thujene, alpha-humulene, alpha-terpineol, viridiflorene, ledol, viridiflorol, delta-cadinol, caryophyllene oxide, camphor, benzaldehyde; *M. quinquenervia (Viridiflorol/ Para-Cymene/1,8-Cineole CT)*—Alpha-thujene, alpha-gurjunene, linalool, gamma-cadinene, delta-cadinene, (E)-nerolidol; *M. quinquenervia (Viridiflorol CT)*—Myrcene; *M. viridiflora (1,8-cineole CT)*—Beta-myrcene, alpha-terpinene, gamma-terpinene, terpinolene, 1,8-cineole; *M. viridiflora (Terpinen-4-ol CT)*—Beta-pinene, myrcene, para-cymene, beta-caryophyllene, estragole (< 0.6%), neral

**PREFERRED COMPOSITION FOR CLINICAL USE:**

| Constituent | 1,8-Cineole CT | Nerolina CT | (E)-Nerolidol CT |
|---|---|---|---|
| **1,8-Cineole** | 48%–68% | 2%–10% | 0.1%–5% |
| **Alpha-Pinene** | 5%–15% | 0.5%–3% | – |
| **Limonene** | 4%–12% | < 2% | – |
| **Alpha-Terpineol** | 3%–10% | < 2% | – |
| **Viridiflorol** | 2%–10% | < 2% | – |
| **Beta-Caryophyllene** | 0.1%–7% | < 2% | 0.5%–10% |
| **Linalool** | 0.1%–6% | 25%–50% | 0%–10% |
| **(E)-Nerolidol** | 0%–6% | 35%–60% | 65%–85% |
| **Beta-Pinene** | 1%–5% | < 0.5% | |
| | | | |
| **Caryophyllene Oxide** | 0%–3% | – | 0.1%–5% |
| **Ledol** | 0%–3% | < 0.5% | 0.1%–3% |

**REPORTED THERAPEUTIC PROPERTIES:** Analgesic (relieves pain), antispasmodic, **antibacterial**, antirheumatic, **antiseptic**, aids nutrient absorption, decongestant, **expectorant**, removes excess mucus, aids circulation, **relieves burns (including radiation burns), helps boils and abscesses heal**, relieves insect bites and stings, **supports respiratory health**, reduces the appearance of scars and blemishes, antiparasitic, reduces fever, **wound healing**, stimulating, uplifting, reduces fear, encourages confidence, aids concentration

**CAUTIONS:**

■ Avoid with children under age 3, particularly around the nose and mouth (1,8-cineole and 1,8-cineole & viridiflorol CT). Use very cautiously in children under age 5 due to high 1,8-cineole content. 1,8-cineole may cause seizures, central nervous system problems, or respiratory distress in young children.[6118,6119,6120,6121]

■ Avoid with epilepsy and Parkinson's disease due to 1,8-cineole content (*all CTs except (E)-Nerolidol and Terpinen-4-ol*). May exacerbate or cause seizures or convulsions when inhaled, applied topically, or ingested based on 1,8-cineole content.[6122,6123,6124,6125,6126,6127]

■ Caution is warranted orally due to the significant amounts of 1,8-cineole. Limit it to small doses internally (adults—maximum 10 drops daily). Toxicity has been reported when eucalyptus (also high in 1,8-cineole) was ingested in large doses, and as few as 4 to 5 drops may cause problems in very sensitive individuals.[6128,6129,6130,6131,6132,6133] In humans, 3.5 to 5 mL has proven fatal orally.[6134]

■ May interact with diabetic medications due to the ability of 1,8-cineole to inhibit alpha-glucosidase activity, particularly when synergized with other constituents (alpha-pinene, para-cymene, and beta-pinene).[6135,6136,6137] Alpha-

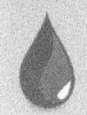

glucosidase is an enzyme that breaks down carbohydrates by chemical reaction with water. Inhibiting its activity postpones glucose absorption and therefore the impact of carbohydrates on blood sugar levels.

■ Chemotypes rich in 1,8-cineole may interact with aspirin, blood pressure, antiplatelet, and anticoagulant medications, and increase the risk of bleeding among people with bleeding disorders.[6138] 1,8-cineole is a weak inhibitor of platelet aggregation.[6139]

■ May weakly interfere with the enzymes responsible for metabolizing medications (NSAIDs, proton-pump inhibitors, acetaminophen, antiepileptics, immune modulators, blood-sugar medications, blood pressure medications, antidepressants, antipsychotics, diabetic medications, antihistamines, antibiotics, and anesthetics) based on 1,8-cineole content.[6140,6141,6142]

■ May interfere with pentobarbital and other barbiturates (medications for anxiety and insomnia) based on 1,8-cineole content.[6143,6144]

■ *(E)-Nerolidol CT*: May interfere with antibiotics and increase their effectiveness because (E)-nerolidol sensitizes bacteria to antibiotics).[6145]

### SELECTED EVIDENCE:

☐ A nasal spray with lemon, ravensara, and niaouli oils (0.14 mL consisting of 0.014 mL lemon, 0.042 mL aloe vera juice, 0.0007 mL ravensara, 0.0007 g Propolis, and 0.00042 mL niaouli oil) decreased the symptoms of allergic and nonallergic rhinopathy (nasal congestion, drainage, and obstruction of the nasal passages) in a clinical trial.[6146]

☐ Animal research suggests that niaouli oil enhances cellular immunity by upregulating T-cell (lymphocytes that respond to specific pathogens) and macrophage (a type of white blood cell that ingest foreign materials) activity.[6147]

☐ Niaouli oil is considered a safe and natural way to control the mosquito population by killing mosquito larvae.[6148]

☐ *In vitro* research suggests that niaouli oil may increase the skin penetration of estradiol, diclofenac sodium (a drug used to relieve pain, inflammation, and joint stiffness caused by arthritis), and other substances.[6149,6150,6151]

☐ Niaouli essential oil kills adults and larvae of three mosquito vectors (*Aedes aegypti, Aedes albopictus*, and *Culex quinquefasciatus*) known to carry and transmit disease.[6152]

☐ The 1,8-cineole CT (21.6% 1,8-cineole) balanced well with alpha-pinene (15.9%), viridiflorol (14.6%), and alpha-terpineol (13.7%) brightened the skin by inhibiting tyrosine activity and melanin production.[6153] The essential oil, 1,8-cineole, alpha-pinene, and alpha-terpineol all inhibited tyrosinase activity and reduced melanin production. Tyrosinase is an enzyme involved in the production of melanin (a dark brown to black pigment that is responsible for tanning of skin when exposed to sunlight) by oxidation of tyrosine.

☐ Ingestion of niaouli CT 1,8-cineole essential oil protected against peptic ulcers caused by alcohol in rats due to its antioxidant properties.[6154]

☐ A nanoemulsion of niaouli essential oil (10% niaouli, 9.25% Kolliphor EL, 27.75% Carbitol, and 53% water) improved skin permeation and exhibited a marked effect on acne pathogens (*P. acnes* and *S. epidermidis*).[6155]

☐ Silver fir and niaouli CT 1,8-cineole essential oils inhibited *P. expansum, P. citrinum*, and *P. crustosum* in a dose-dependent manner (in vapor phase), with *P. citrinum* being the most sensitive and *P. crustosum* the least sensitive.[6156]

# NUTMEG

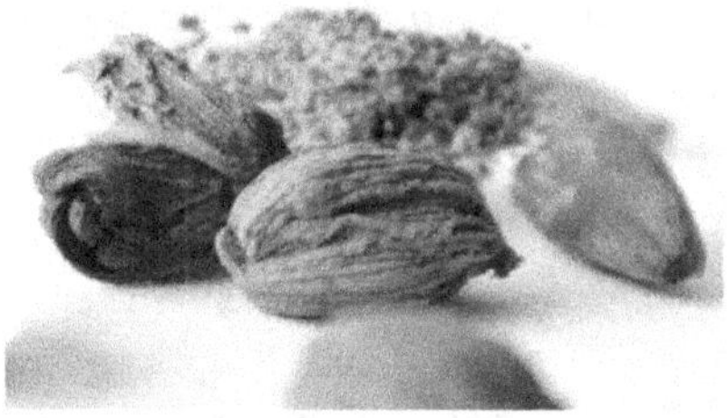

*Myristica fragrans* Houtt., *M. officinalis* L. f.

**FAMILY:** Myristicaceae
**NOTE:** Middle
**AROMA INTENSITY:** Medium
**AROMA:** Spicy, warm, nutty
**COMMON EXTRACTION METHOD:** Steam distilled from the seeds
**POSSIBLE SUBSTITUTE OILS:** Ravensara (Sabinene CT), ravintsara (Camphor CT)
**BLENDS WELL WITH:** Camphor, cassia, cinnamon, clary sage, copaiba, coriander, clove, eucalyptus, fennel, geranium, ginger, lavender, lime, orange, oregano, patchouli, pine, rosemary, turmeric, vetiver, ylang ylang
**SUBCELLULAR LOCALIZATION | EPIGENETIC INFLUENCE:** Nuclear Membrane | Currently unknown
**RECOMMENDED DILUTION RANGE:** 3%–33%; 50% for some conditions

**PRIMARY CONSTITUENTS:**[6157,6158,6159,6160,6161,6162,6163]

*East Indian*

| | |
|---|---|
| Myristicin | 0.3%–45.6% |
| Sabinene | 6.3%–44.8% |
| Elemicin | 0.6%–30.9% |
| Alpha-Pinene | 10.2%–26.5% |
| Safrole | 0.0%–22.1% |
| Beta-Pinene | 0.0%–17.7% |
| Terpinen-4-ol | 1.0%–10.9% |
| Linalool | 0.2%–7.4% |
| Limonene | 2.0%–7.0% |
| Alpha-Phellandrene | 0.0%–5.8% |
| Gamma-Terpinene | 0.1%–5.2% |
| Alpha-Terpinene | 0.1%–5.2% |

*West Indian (Indonesian)*

| | |
|---|---|
| Sabinene | 33.0%–57.0% |
| Alpha-Pinene | 9.4%–19.9% |
| Beta-Pinene | 7.3%–18.8% |
| Terpinen-4-ol | 5.8%–17.8% |
| Elemicin | 0.4%–6.1% |
| Gamma-Terpinene | 1.7%–4.7% |
| Limonene | 2.9%–4.4% |
| Myristicin | 0.2%–3.9% |
| Safrole | 0.1%–1.4% |

**OTHER CONSTITUENTS:** Alpha-thujene, alpha-myrcene, terpinolene, linalool, alpha-terpineol, citronellol, eugenol, methyl eugenol

**PREFERRED COMPOSITION FOR CLINICAL USE:**

| Constituent | Indonesian |
|---|---|
| **Alpha-Pinene** | 15%–30% |
| **Sabinene** | 15%–30% |
| **Myristicin** | 5%–20% |
| **Beta-Pinene** | 10%–18% |
| **Terpinen-4-ol** | 4%–10% |
| **Limonene** | 2%–6% |
| **Gamma-Terpinene** | 2%–6% |
| **Alpha-Terpinene** | 1%–5% |
| **Safrole** | 1%–3% |
| **Elemicin** | 0.1%–3% |
| **Delta-3-Carene** | 0.1%–3% |

**REPORTED THERAPEUTIC PROPERTIES: Analgesic (pain relief)**, antioxidant, antiseptic, antirheumatic, antispasmodic, **relieves menstrual cramps and painful menstruation, aids digestion**, expels excess gas, supports cardiovascular health, relieves constipation, eases cough, deodorant, increases redness and circulation of a localized area, supports brain health, aids detoxification, supports liver and adrenal function, stimulating, **reduces anxiety**,

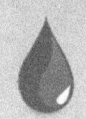

**stress management**, reduces feelings of being overwhelmed, combats worrisome and negative thoughts, aphrodisiac, reduces mental fatigue

### CAUTIONS:

■ Avoid nutmeg use in children under 6, and use cautiously with children through age 12. Children are more susceptible to nutmeg toxicity, which can produce dry mouth, flushing, irregular heart rhythm, tremors, agitation, and delirium.[6164,6165,6166]

■ Avoid oral use and use cautiously topically during pregnancy and lactation due to myristicin and safrole content, particularly East Indian nutmeg, that has higher levels of myristicin and safrole. Animal research suggests that higher doses of safrole or myristicin (0.01 mL/kg every two days while nursing, and 0.001 to 10 mg while pregnant) taken orally during pregnancy and while nursing may cause liver toxicity in offspring born to the mother and increase the offspring's risk of liver cancer.[6167,6168]

■ Long-term oral use of small doses (1 to 6 drops) for more than twenty-one days without at least a seven-day break and single large doses (5 g or more of the whole herb) should be avoided due to the psychotropic activity of nutmeg, as well as its constituents methyl eugenol and safrole. Safrole and methyl eugenol can be toxic in large doses.[6169,6170,6171] Myristicin is believed to be at least partially responsible for the psychotropic (a substance capable of affecting the mind, emotions, and behavior) effects of nutmeg; although it is likely a combination of more than one component of nutmeg oil that produces this effect. Large doses of nutmeg with high myristicin content (5 g in a single dose), and long-term use of as few as 120 mg of the whole herb daily may produce a psychotropic (hallucinations, anxiety, fear, and delusions) effect in adults.[6172,6173] In addition, scientists suspect nutmeg may be chemically modified once ingested to amphetamine-like constituents, though this has not been proven conclusively.[6174]

■ There is a moderate risk that East Indian nutmeg may interact with aspirin, blood pressure, antiplatelet, and anticoagulant medications, and increase the risk of bleeding among people with bleeding disorders (low risk) based on safrole content.[6175]

■ May interact with psychotropic medications—medications prescribed for anxiety, depression, schizophrenia, mania, obsessive-compulsive disorder, ADHD, and bipolar disorder.[6176,6177]

■ May interact with monoamine oxidase inhibitors (MAOIs)—medications prescribed for the treatment of depression.[6178]

■ May interfere with enzymes responsible for metabolizing medications (NSAIDs, proton-pump inhibitors, acetaminophen, antiepileptics, immune modulators, blood-sugar medications, blood pressure medications, antidepressants, antipsychotics, diabetic medications, antihistamines, antibiotics, and anesthetics).[6179,6180,6181,6182,6183,6184,6185]

### SELECTED EVIDENCE:

☐ Nutmeg oil significantly prevented DNA from bonding to cancer-causing chemicals (DNA adduct formation) *in vitro* and therefore may help prevent cancer.[6186] It also prevents the formation of blood vessels (angiogenesis) by cancerous tumors *in vitro*.[6187]

☐ A study concluded that nutmeg inhibited the growth and survival of the food-borne pathogens *Y. enterocolitica* (a bacterium that can cause right-sided abdominal pain, fever, and bloody diarrhea) and *L. monocytogenes* (a bacterium that causes a serious infection that causes muscle aches, sometimes preceded by gastrointestinal symptoms like diarrhea) on barbecued chicken.[6188]

☐ *In vitro* research demonstrates that nutmeg essential oil inhibits *S. aureus, B. subtilis, B. megaterium, K. pneumoniae, P. vulgaris*, and *E. coli*, with greater antimicrobial activity when combined with ajowan essential oil.[6189]

☐ Nutmeg oil significantly prevented convulsions of grand mal and partial seizures in mice, but the researchers concluded it was not preferred for myoclonic and absence seizures.[6190]

☐ *In vitro* research suggests that nutmeg inhibits twenty-five microorganisms of significant importance.[6191]

☐ Animal research suggests that oral administration of myristicin provides extraordinary protection against liver damage.[6192]

☐ *In vitro* research demonstrates that nutmeg essential oil is a potent antioxidant.[6193]

☐ Human aryl hydrocarbon receptor (AhR: a gene that encodes a protein that helps regulate responses to planar aromatic hydrocarbons and significantly affects the immune activity in the gastrointestinal tract, regulates the circadian rhythm, helps regulate the cell cycle, and plays an important role in tissue development). Cumin, jasmine, vanilla, and bay leaf fully activate AhR; clove, dill, thyme, nutmeg, and oregano partially activate AhR; and tarragon, caraway, turmeric, lovage, fennel, spearmint, star anise, and anise inhibit the AhR activity.[6194]

☐ East Indian nutmeg essential oil exhibited broad-spectrum inhibition of food deteriorating fungi and disrupted cellular methylglyoxal content, which produces aflatoxin.[6195]

☐ Star anise, allspice, and nutmeg all demonstrated larvicidal and adulticidal activity against the *Aedes aegypti* mosquito.[6196] Nutmeg essential oil produced the highest mortality.

☐ Elderly individuals may experience a loss of appetite or a decrease in eating behaviors, particularly those with dementia, which leads to frailty. Inhalation of nutmeg essential oil—or myristicin or methyl eugenol—enhanced appetite in mice.[6197]

☐ Inclusion of nutmeg essential oil in beta-cyclodextrin complexes improved its antimicrobial activity against *Staphylococcus aureus, Staphylococcus epidermidis, Escherichia coli, Klebsiella pneumoniae, Saccharomyces cerevisiae*, and *Bacillus subtilis*.[6198]

☐ Nutmeg hydrodistilled with aluminometasilicate as an excipient significantly increased levels of key compounds (sabinene, alpha-pinene, and limonene), which improved some of its biological activities when compared to a traditionally distilled oil.[6199] Antimicrobial activity was observed in the aluminometasilicate oil against *E. faecalis, S. mutans* (referent), and *P. multocida*, whereas the traditional oil was only active against *P. multocida*. The antioxidant was comparable for both oils, but the anti-inflammatory activity was better with the aluminometasilicate oil.

☐ A study found that longer distillation times decreased alpha-thujene, alpha-pinene, camphene, sabinene, beta-pinene, alpha-phellandrene, delta-3-carene, para-cymene, and limonene amounts and increased alpha-terpinene, gamma-terpinene, terpinolene, and myristicin levels.[6200] The fraction removed at 120 to 240 minutes was slightly active against *C. neoformans*, while another fraction removed at 1 to 2.5 minutes had higher inhibitory activity against *P. falciparum*. The antimalarial activity against *P. falciparum* was attributed to the higher levels of sabinene in this fraction.

☐ Complete elimination of microorganisms during a root canal is vital to successful endodontic treatment but increasing resistance to antibiotics and adverse effects of these drugs limits their use. West Indian nutmeg essential oil inhibited common endodontic pathogens (*Escherichia coli, Staphylococcus aureus, Enterococcus faecalis, Streptococcus mutans, Candida albicans, Lactobacillus casei, Actinomyces viscosus, Prevotella intermedia*, and *Porphyromonas gingivalis*) making it a promising alternative to synthetic drugs.[6201]

☐ Type 2 diabetes can be managed by inhibiting the carbohydrate-hydrolyzing enzymes alpha-amylase and alpha-glucosidase, which decreases spikes in blood sugar after a meal. A laboratory study found that eucalyptus (*E. radiata*), bay laurel, and nutmeg (West Indian) essential oils each inhibited alpha-amylase comparably to acarbose (an alpha-amylase and alpha-glucosidase inhibiting drug used to control blood sugar levels in people with type 2 diabetes).[6202] Remarkably, eucalyptus and nutmeg essential oils displayed higher activity than acarbose.

☐ Isolated constituents from nutmeg (myristicin and safrole) and rosemary (terpinolene) essential oil repelled ticks (*Dermacentor variabilis*) better than DEET in a no-human horizontal Petri dish assay.[6203] 2-undecanone also performed well.

☐ Nutmeg was found to be very effective against housefly (*Musca domestica*) larvae—at 5% using the immersion method.[6204] Topical application was more toxic to blow fly (*Chrysomya albiceps*) adults and paper impregnated with the oil was equally effective against both fly species.

☐ A study found that nutmeg essential oil acts as efflux pump inhibitor for MRSA and synergizes the activity of ciprofloxacin against MRSA.[6205] In addition, the isolated constituents were active efflux pump inhibitors, in descending order: elemicin, myristicin, methoxyeugenol, myristicin, and asarone.

☐ *Fusarium graminearum* is a fungus that contaminates cereals, fruit, and vegetables. Thyme, oregano, basil, nutmeg, hyssop, and clove essential oils inhibited mycelial growth of *F. graminearum*, with oregano performing best followed by clove and thyme.[6206] The composition of the oils was not reported.

☐ Mountain savory, nutmeg, and lemongrass (*C. flexuosus*) were each fungicidal to *A. niger* and *A. ochraceus*.[6207] The oils also inhibited the production of ochratoxin A by the fungus *A. ochraceus* and the production of aflatoxin B1 and aflatoxin B2.

☐ Of ten essential oils tested, massoia and nutmeg essential oils were the most active larvicides to Asian tiger mosquito (*Ae. albopictus*).[6208] Cellulose nanocrystal-stabilized Pickering emulsions of massoia and nutmeg

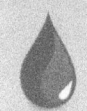

EOs were stable for at least ten days and more active than the free oil. Isolated benzyl salicylate, terpinolene, C12 massoia lactone, sabinene, benzyl benzoate, methyl eugenol, and C10 massoia lactone were also highly active.

☐ Mountain CT borneol, lemongrass (*C. flexuosus*), and nutmeg exhibited antioxidant (DPPH, beta-carotene bleaching assays) and antimicrobial activity in laboratory research. Mountain savory was active against *E. coli*, while nutmeg was bactericidal against *E. coli* and *S. aureus*.[6209]

# OAKMOSS ABSOLUTE

*Evernia prunastri* L.

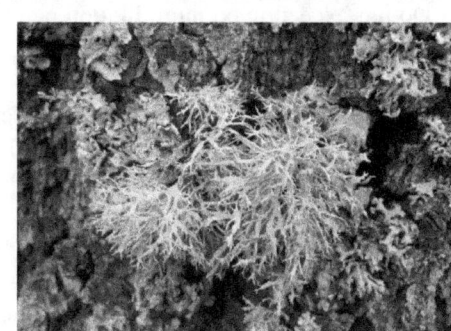

**FAMILY:** Usneaceae
**NOTE:** Base
**AROMA INTENSITY:** Strong
**AROMA:** Earthy, slightly woody, and piney
**COMMON EXTRACTION METHOD:** Solvent extracted from the lichen
**POSSIBLE SUBSTITUTE OILS:** Blue spruce, benzoin, copaiba, vetiver

**BLENDS WELL WITH:** Anise, bay laurel, clary sage, cypress, eucalyptus, geranium, ginger, jasmine, lavender, lemon, lime, neroli, orange, palmarosa, patchouli, petitgrain, rose, tea tree, vetiver, ylang ylang

**SUBCELLULAR LOCALIZATION | EPIGENETIC INFLUENCE:** Currently unknown | Currently unknown

**RECOMMENDED DILUTION RANGE:** 0.1%–1.0%

**PRIMARY CONSTITUENTS:**[6210,6211,6212,6213,6214,6215,6216,6217]

*Oakmoss Absolute*

| | |
|---|---|
| Methyl Beta-Orcinolcarboxylate | 18.6%–30.1% |
| Ethyl Everninate | 0.0%–3.7% |
| Ethyl Hematommate | 1.4%–3.4% |

*Hydrodistilled and Dissolved in Hexane*

| | |
|---|---|
| Veramoss | 11.5% |
| 1-Tricosene | 10.1% |
| (E)-Citronellyl Tiglate | 7.8% |
| Alpha-Pinene | 6.6% |
| Diisobutyl Phthalate | 6.5% |
| Beta-Pinene | 6.3% |
| Tricosane | 4.3% |

Note: Two Swiss studies from the 1970s report oakmoss absolute contained alpha-pinene, beta-pinene, limonene, gamma-terpinene, trans-pinocarveol, and alpha-copaene as major constituents, but no complete composition data with percentages is available. Oakmoss is typically rectified to reduce levels of the major allergens atranol and chloroatranol (to meet IFRA cosmetic usage guidelines) and may be labeled "low atranol".

**OTHER CONSTITUENTS:** *Absolute*—ethyl chlorohematommate; *Hydrodistilled*—tricyclene, camphene, alpha-phellandrene, limonene, gamma-terpinene, trans-pinocarveol, alpha-terpinen-7-al, alpha-copaene, alpha-humulene, alpha-muurolene, caryophyllene oxide, abietatriene, epi-13-manoyl oxide, bornyl acetate, heptadecane, eicosane, heneicosane, 1-docosane, pentacosane, 2-pentyl furan

**PREFERRED COMPOSITION FOR CLINICAL USE:**

| Constituent | |
|---|---|
| **Methyl Beta-Orcinolcarboxylate** | 15%–35% |
| **Ethyl Everninate** | 1%–5% |
| **Ethyl Hematommate** | 0%–5% |

**REPORTED THERAPEUTIC PROPERTIES:** Antibacterial, antimicrobial, antifungal, antiseptic, analgesic, anti-inflammatory, antioxidant, soothes skin irritation, wound healing, supports respiratory function, expels excess mucus, eases cough, grounding, **releases traumatic emotions**

**CAUTIONS:**

■ Avoid oral consumption. Absolutes contain solvent residue and should not be taken orally.

■ Do not exceed maximum dilution percentage during topical application due to solvent content and possibility of skin irritation.[6218,6219,6220,6221,6222] Oakmoss absolute is a very common cause of contact dermatitis, particularly among people who have sensitive skin, chronic skin conditions, or allergies to fragrances. Atranol and chloroatranol are considered the most potent sensitizing constituents of oakmoss absolute, but the mixture of all the allergenic constituents in oakmoss absolute are more potent than atranol or chloratranol alone.[6223,6224,6225,6226] "Hypoallergenic" oakmoss absolutes with low content of ethyl hematommate, ethyl chlorohematommate, atranorin, and chloratranorin may also be available.

**SELECTED EVIDENCE:**

☐ *In vitro* research suggests that oakmoss absolute inhibits *C. albicans*, but it is inactive against gram-negative and gram-positive bacteria.[6227]

---

# OCOTEA
## (American Cinnamon, Ishpingo)

*Ocotea quixos* (Lam.) Kosterm., *Laurus quixos* Lam.

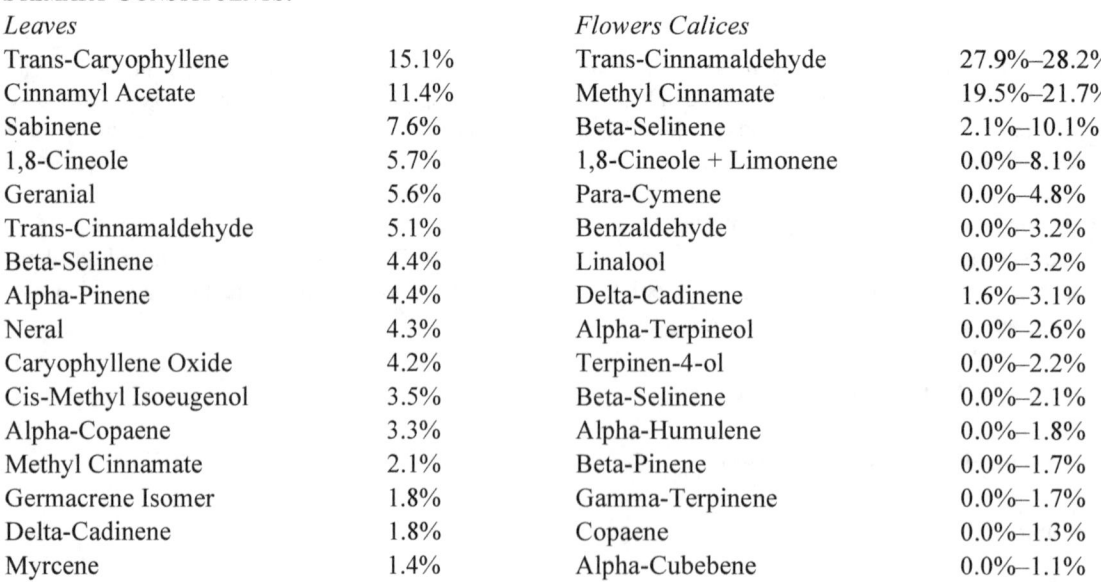

**FAMILY:** Lauraceae
**NOTE:** Middle
**AROMA INTENSITY:** Medium
**AROMA:** Mildly cinnamon, warm, herbaceous, sweet, spicy
**COMMON EXTRACTION METHOD:** Steam distilled from the leaves or flowers calices
**POSSIBLE SUBSTITUTE OILS:** Cinnamon, cassia, tamala, copaiba
**BLENDS WELL WITH:** Bergamot, black pepper, cassia, cinnamon, frankincense, ginger, grapefruit, lavender, lemon, lime, nutmeg, orange, patchouli, tangerine
**SUBCELLULAR LOCALIZATION | EPIGENETIC INFLUENCE:** Currently unknown | Currently unknown
**RECOMMENDED DILUTION RANGE:** 3%–33%; 50% for some conditions

**PRIMARY CONSTITUENTS:**[6228,6229,6230]

| Leaves | | Flowers Calices | |
|---|---|---|---|
| Trans-Caryophyllene | 15.1% | Trans-Cinnamaldehyde | 27.9%–28.2% |
| Cinnamyl Acetate | 11.4% | Methyl Cinnamate | 19.5%–21.7% |
| Sabinene | 7.6% | Beta-Selinene | 2.1%–10.1% |
| 1,8-Cineole | 5.7% | 1,8-Cineole + Limonene | 0.0%–8.1% |
| Geranial | 5.6% | Para-Cymene | 0.0%–4.8% |
| Trans-Cinnamaldehyde | 5.1% | Benzaldehyde | 0.0%–3.2% |
| Beta-Selinene | 4.4% | Linalool | 0.0%–3.2% |
| Alpha-Pinene | 4.4% | Delta-Cadinene | 1.6%–3.1% |
| Neral | 4.3% | Alpha-Terpineol | 0.0%–2.6% |
| Caryophyllene Oxide | 4.2% | Terpinen-4-ol | 0.0%–2.2% |
| Cis-Methyl Isoeugenol | 3.5% | Beta-Selinene | 0.0%–2.1% |
| Alpha-Copaene | 3.3% | Alpha-Humulene | 0.0%–1.8% |
| Methyl Cinnamate | 2.1% | Beta-Pinene | 0.0%–1.7% |
| Germacrene Isomer | 1.8% | Gamma-Terpinene | 0.0%–1.7% |
| Delta-Cadinene | 1.8% | Copaene | 0.0%–1.3% |
| Myrcene | 1.4% | Alpha-Cubebene | 0.0%–1.1% |

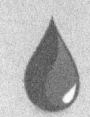

**OTHER CONSTITUENTS:** *Flowers Calices*–Styrene, alpha-thujene, alpha-phellandrene, 3-carene, hydrocinnamic aldehyde, alpha-bergamotene, alpha-selinene, gamma-cadinene, beta-bisabolene, beta-caryophyllene; *Leaves*–Camphene, benzaldehyde, para-cymene, gamma-terpinene, linalool, terpinen-4-ol, alpha-terpineol, cis-cinnamaldehyde, gamma-elemene, beta-elemene, 7-epi-alpha-selinene, cis-gamma-bisabolene

**PREFERRED COMPOSITION FOR CLINICAL USE:**

| Constituent | Calices |
|---|---|
| (E)-Cinnamaldehyde | 25%–35% |
| Methyl Cinnamate | 15%–25% |
| Beta-Selinene | 2%–12% |
| Limonene | 3%–9% |
| Para-Cymene | 3%–8% |
| Benzaldehyde | 2%–5% |
| Linalool | 1%–4% |
| Alpha-Pinene | 1%–4% |
| Delta-Cadinene | 1%–4% |
| Alpha-Terpineol | 1%–3% |
| Terpinen-4-ol | 1%–3% |

**REPORTED THERAPEUTIC PROPERTIES:** Antibacterial, antioxidant, **anti-inflammatory**, antiparasitic, **antifungal**, disinfectant, balances the body's response to irritation and injury, balances blood sugar, **supports normal blood pressure**, aids digestion, aids liver function, relieves diarrhea, reduces appetite, balances mood, stimulating, energizing, antidepressant

**CAUTIONS:**

■ Use very cautiously during pregnancy and lactation due to cinnamaldehyde content. Several studies have tested the major constituents of ocotea's cousins cinnamon and cassia essential oils with pregnant animals, and the results have been inconsistent. Therefore, it is advised to be very cautious with ocotea during pregnancy because it can contain nearly 30% cinnamaldehyde.[6231,6232,6233]

■ May interact with aspirin, blood pressure, antiplatelet, and anticoagulant medications, and increase the risk of bleeding among people with bleeding disorders.[6234,6235]

■ May interfere with enzymes responsible for metabolizing medications (NSAIDs, proton-pump inhibitors, acetaminophen, antiepileptics, immune modulators, blood-sugar medications, blood pressure medications, antidepressants, antipsychotics, diabetic medications, antihistamines, antibiotics, and anesthetics).[6236,6237,6238]

■ Ocotea may interact with diabetes medications and decrease blood sugar based on cinnamaldehyde content.[6239] However, research is conflicting and some scientists don't believe cinnamaldehyde is the primary constituent in cinnamon and cassia that decreases blood sugar.[6240]

■ May interact with antibiotics and possibly enhance their effects.[6241]

■ May irritate mucous membranes (eyes, mouth, nasal passages, vagina, rectum).[6242]

**SELECTED EVIDENCE:**

☐ Ocotea oil protects the stomach and potently inhibits inflammation by strongly inhibiting the lipopolysaccharide-induced release of nitric oxide by macrophages and inhibiting the COX-2 enzyme *in vitro*.[6243]

☐ Animal research suggests that ocotea oil helps prevent and shrink blood clots and relaxes blood vessels without causing unfavorable bleeding.[6244]

☐ A review study concluded that ocotea possesses good antioxidant, antibacterial (gram negative bacteria), and antifungal properties.[6245]

☐ Ocotea CT 1,8-cineole essential oil produced rapid toxicity against *Aedes aegypti* mosquitoes.[6246]

# OPOPONAX
## (Opopanax, Sweet Myrrh, Scented Myrrh, Bisabol Myrrh)

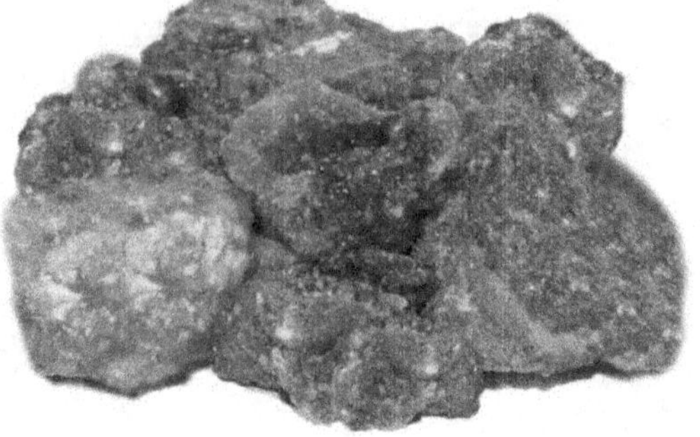

*Commiphora guidotti* Chiov.; *C. holtziana* Engl., *C. erythraea* (Ehrenb.) Engl., *C. erythraea* (Ehrenb.) Engl. var. *glabrescens, C. kataf* (Forssk.) Engl., *C. pseudopaoli* J.B. Gillet

**FAMILY:** Burseraceae
**NOTE:** Base-Middle
**AROMA INTENSITY:** Medium
**AROMA:** Earthy, rich, resinous, sweet, slightly woody
**COMMON EXTRACTION METHOD:** Steam distilled from the resin
**POSSIBLE SUBSTITUTE OILS:** Myrrh, frankincense
**BLENDS WELL WITH:** Bergamot, cedarwood, frankincense, grapefruit, lavender, lemon, lime, Mediterranean mandarin, myrrh, neroli, orange, patchouli, peppermint, petitgrain, pine, sandalwood, tangerine, vetiver, yuzu
**SUBCELLULAR LOCALIZATION | EPIGENETIC INFLUENCE:** Currently unknown | Currently unknown
**RECOMMENDED DILUTION RANGE:** 5%–Neat

**PRIMARY CONSTITUENTS:**[6247,6248,6249,6250,6251,6252,6253,6254]

| *C. erythraea* | | *C. guidotti* | |
|---|---|---|---|
| 1(10),4-Furanodien-6-one | 9.0%–20.6% | (E)-Beta-Ocimene | 6.7%–52.6% |
| 1,10(15)-Furanogermacra-Dien-6-one | 4.3%–10.4% | Cis-Alpha-Bisabolene | 2.3%–27.0% |
| Beta-Elemene | 5.4%–8.2% | Alpha-Santalene | 11.1%–21.9% |
| Camphene | 0.0%–8.2% | Furanoeudesma-1,3-diene | 0.0%–18.6% |
| Alpha-Copaene | 4.4%–6.6% | Curzerene | 0.0%–11.4% |
| Alpha-Gurjunene | 4.3%–6.0% | Trans-Alpha-Bergamotene | 0.0%–9.3% |
| Alpha-Pinene | 3.4%–4.5% | Trans-Beta-Bergamotene | 0.0%–9.0% |
| Aromadendrene | 3.5%–4.4% | Isofuranodiene | 0.0%–6.8% |
| Dihydropyrocurzerenone | 1.1%–4.2% | Beta-Bisabolene | 0.0%–5.1% |
| Alpha-Selinene | 3.2%–3.8% | Alpha-Santalol | 0.0%–4.0% |
| Beta-Selinene | 3.3%–3.6% | Gamma-Bisabolene | 0.0%–3.9% |
| Alloaromadendrene | 2.0%–3.6% | Alpha-Bergamotene | 0.0%–3.0% |
| rel-3R-Methoxy-4S-Furanogermacra-1E,10(15)-dien-6-one | 0.9%–3.9% | | |
| rel-2R-Methoxy-4R-Furanogermacra-1(10)E-en-6-one | 0.9%–3.1% | | |
| Delta-3-Carene | 0.4%–3.0% | | |

Note: No reliable or complete composition analysis was found for *C. kataf, C. holtziana*, and *C. pseudopaoli. Opopanax chironium* is believed to be the original source of opoponax.

**OTHER CONSTITUENTS:** *C. guidotti*—(Z)-beta-ocimene, 1-methyl-4-acetylcyclohex-1-ene, epi-beta-santalene, (Z)-beta-farnesene, (E)-beta-farnesene, germacrene D, decanol, 2,6-dimethyl-3(E),5(E),7-octatriene-2-ol, cis-alpha-ocimene, cis-alpha-bergamotene, beta-caryophyllene; *C. erythraea*—alpha-thujene, sabinene, beta-pinene, para-cymene, limonene, 4-terpineol, delta-elemene, alpha-cubebene, beta-bourbonene, beta-caryophyllene, alpha-guaiene, alpha-humulene, germacrene D, curzerene, gamma-cadinene, delta-cadinene, germacrene B, curzerenone, alismol, beta-eudesmol, alpha-eudesmol, germacrone

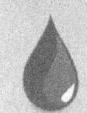

**PREFERRED COMPOSITION FOR CLINICAL USE:**

| Constituent | C. guidotti |
|---|---|
| (E)-Beta-Ocimene | 15%–50% |
| Cis-Alpha-Bisabolene | 10%–30% |
| Alpha-Santalene | 10%–25% |
| Trans-Beta-Bergamotene | 3%–10% |
| Cis-Alpha-Santalol | 0.5%–5% |
| Cis-Alpha-Bergamotene | 0.1%–5% |
| Germacrene D | 0.1%–3% |
| Cis-Alpha-Bisabolol | 0.1%–3% |

**REPORTED THERAPEUTIC PROPERTIES: Antibacterial, antifungal,** antiparasitic, antiseptic, analgesic, anti-inflammatory, antispasmodic, aids digestion, **wound healing,** reduces the appearance of scars, wrinkles, and blemishes, supports respiratory function, expels excess mucus, eases cough, aids circulation, soothes sore throat, purification, stress management, relieves anxiety, stimulates creativity, increases intuition

**CAUTIONS:**

■ None currently known. Opoponax is often listed as photosensitizing, but this appears to be based on the original source of the essential oil (*Opopanax chironium*), which contains furanocoumarins, particularly in the roots.[6255] Photosensitizing constituents are not reported in the current species used to produce opoponax essential oil.

**SELECTED EVIDENCE:**

☐ *In vitro* research reported that *C. guidotti* inhibits the bacteria: *S. aureus, B. cereus,* and *P. aeruginosa,* and the yeasts: *C. albicans* and *Crypto neoformans.*[6256] Another study found that *C. guidotti* (an interesting composition with alpha-santalene (19.5%), furanoeudesma-1,3-diene (18.6%), and curzerene (11.4%), possibly distilled from a mixture of myrrh and opoponax resins) demonstrates broad spectrum antibacterial action, significantly inhibiting gram-negative bacteria (*E. coli, V. cholera,* and *S. typhi* Ty2), moderately inhibiting other gram-negative bacteria (*Shigella* spp.), moderately inhibiting gram-positive bacteria (*B. pumilus* and *B. subtilis*), and inhibiting the fungi *A. niger, C. albicans, P. funiculosum,* and *P. notatum* as effectively as the antifungal drug griseofulvin.[6257] Both the steam distilled and hydrodistilled essential oils of *C. erythraea* completely inhibited the plant fungus *A. solani,* significantly inhibited *F. culmorum,* and moderately inhibited *P. cryptogea.*[6258]

☐ Animal research demonstrates that an ointment with 4% *C. guidotti* essential oil (an interesting composition with alpha-santalene (19.5%), furanoeudesma-1,3-diene (18.6%), and curzerene (11.4%), possibly distilled from a mixture of myrrh and opoponax resins) encourages healing of incisions.[6259] An ointment with resin instead of essential oil added to the ointment also demonstrated anti-inflammatory effects.

☐ *C. erythraea* essential oil demonstrated moderate antioxidant activity.[6260] Interestingly, the hydrodistilled essential oil was a stronger antioxidant than the steam distilled essential oil, with afractionated essential oil rich in 1(10),4-Furanodien-6-one (24.7%) and 1, 10(15)-Furanogermacra-Dien-6-one (10.4%) being the most potent antioxidant.

☐ *C. erythraea* essential oil is a strong inhibitor of the 5-LOX enzyme according to *in vitro* research.[6261] The 5-LOX enzyme converts arachidonic acid to leukotrienes, increasing inflammation and allergic reactions, and is associated with chronic degenerative inflammatory diseases and cancer.

☐ Opoponax essential oil was active against *Cx. restuans, Cx. pipiens,* and *Ae. aegypti* mosquito larvae, but its fractions with 62.5% (fraction 2) or 23.8% (fraction 4) bisabolene, curzerene (fraction 1), and alpha-santalene (fraction 3) were inactive suggesting synergy among all components is responsible for its larvicidal activity.[6262]

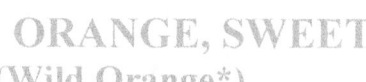 

# ORANGE, SWEET
## (Wild Orange*)

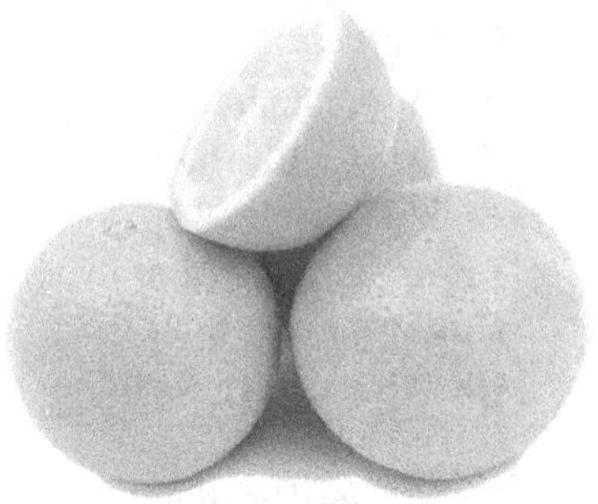

*Citrus* × *sinensis* (L.) Osbeck (pro sp.) [maxima × reticulata],
*C. aurantium* L. var. *sinensis* L., *C. aurantium dulcis*

**FAMILY:** Rutaceae
**NOTE:** Top
**AROMA INTENSITY:** Medium
**AROMA:** Citrusy, sweet, fruity
**COMMON EXTRACTION METHOD:** Cold-pressed/expressed or hydrodistilled from the fruit peel (rind)
**POSSIBLE SUBSTITUTE OILS:** Lemon, grapefruit, tangerine, lime, bergamot
**BLENDS WELL WITH:** Bergamot, black pepper, camphor, cassia, cinnamon, citronella, clove, copaiba, coriander, frankincense, geranium, ginger, grapefruit, juniper, lavender, lemon, lemon verbena, lime, marjoram, melissa, myrrh, neroli, niaouli, nutmeg, vetiver, patchouli, tangerine, rose, sage, Spanish sage, sandalwood, spikenard, ylang ylang
**SUBCELLULAR LOCALIZATION | EPIGENETIC INFLUENCE:** Cytoplasm | Muscular/Reproductive
**RECOMMENDED DILUTION RANGE:** 3%–50%; neat for limited conditions

**PRIMARY CONSTITUENTS:**[6263,6264,6265,6266,6267]

*Cold-pressed/expressed*

| | |
|---|---|
| Limonene | 85.4%–95.4% |
| Bornyl Acetate | 0.0%–4.2% |
| Beta-Myrcene | 0.7%–2.4% |
| Alpha-Pinene | 0.5%–2.4% |

*Distilled*

| | |
|---|---|
| Limonene | 81.5%–93.7% |
| Beta-Myrcene | 0.9%–2.1% |
| Linalool | 0.1%–1.4% |

**OTHER CONSTITUENTS:** *Cold-pressed/expressed*—Beta-pinene, octanal, decanal; *Distilled*—Camphene, alpha-pinene, beta-pinene, alpha-terpinene, cis-linalool oxide, terpinolene, camphor, borneol, alpha-terpineol, linalyl acetate, bornyl acetate, carvacrol, decanal

**PREFERRED COMPOSITION FOR CLINICAL USE:**

| Constituent | Cold-pressed | Distilled |
|---|---|---|
| **Limonene** | 93%–97% | 80%–95% |
| **Beta-Myrcene** | 1%–4% | 1%–5% |
| **Alpha-Pinene** | 0.5%–2% | 1%–3% |
| **Linalool** | 0.1%–1% | 0.1%–2% |
| **Sabinene** | 0.1%–1% | 0%–1% |
| **n-Octanal** | tr–1% | – |
| **Beta-Pinene** | tr–1% | 0.1%–1% |
| **n-Decanal** | tr–1% | 0%–2% |
| **Valencene** | tr–0.5% | 0.1%–2% |
| **Geranial + Neral** | tr–0.5% | – |
| **Sinensal <beta + alpha>** | 0%–0.5% | < 2% |
| **Alpha-Terpineol** | – | 0%–3% |

\* Wild orange essential oil is customarily cold-pressed from the ripe peel of oranges from trees growing wild in Italy.

**REPORTED THERAPEUTIC PROPERTIES:** Anti-inflammatory, **antiseptic**, antispasmodic, antibacterial, expels excess gas, disinfectant, **aids digestion**, diuretic, expectorant, supports lymph drainage, antifungal, **anticancer**, stimulating, uplifting, **supports glutathione production**, **antidepressant**, aphrodisiac, helps reduce perfectionism, **reduces anxiety**, combats pessimism, **stress management**

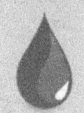

**CAUTIONS:**

■ None currently known. Sweet orange has generally been considered nonphotosensitizing and devoid of photosensitizing constituents; however, recent findings suggest it may be mildly photosensitizing due to the presence of furanocoumarins depending on growing location and type (navel, Valencia, etc.).[6268,6269,6270] Avoid UV rays (sun and artificial) for at least 12 hours after topical application.

**SELECTED EVIDENCE:**

- □ *In vitro* and animal research suggests that d-limonene or orange essential oil may prevent cancer by stimulating enzymes that metabolize and detoxify cancer-causing molecules and by triggering apoptosis.[6271,6272,6273]

- □ Orange oil prevents the spread and causes the death of colon cancer cells, and inhibits angiogenesis (the formation of new blood vessels, which allows a tumor to become malignant) *in vitro*.[6274]

- □ Topical application of 10 drops, 3 times per day, of a 2% concentrated solution of orange oil reduced depressive symptoms better than Prozac (fluoxetine) according to a clinical trial that included 150 adults with major depressive disorder.[6275] Interestingly, the study authors observed that 20 drops of the same solution decreased its effectiveness, suggesting more is not always better when it comes to essential oils.

- □ A topical mixture of sweet basil (3%) and orange (5%) essential oils and acetic acid was tested against acne in seven volunteers. The antiseptic and keratolytic activity of the mixture improved the acne in 75% of the volunteers.[6276]

- □ Massaging ginger and orange oil to the knees of older adults six times over a three-week period relieved moderate-to-severe knee pain and increased physical function in the short-term.[6277]

- □ A sitz bath with or soap application of lavender, myrrh, neroli, rose, grapefruit, mandarin, orange, and Roman chamomile improves healing of the perineum following delivery and episiotomy.[6278]

- □ *In vitro* research reported that orange oil provides a sun protection factor (SPF) of 3.975.[6279]

- □ An *in vitro* dressing model concluded that orange oil prevents infections caused by *S. aureus* without harming skin cells (keratinocytes).[6280]

- □ Inhaling orange oil in the waiting room prior to dental visits reduces anxiety in dental patients, including children.[6281,6282,6283]

- □ Animal research suggests that inhalation of orange oil has a calming effect and reduces anxiety.[6284]

- □ Inhalation of 2.5 to 10 drops of orange oil increased tranquility, reduced anxiety, and decreased tension in healthy males.[6285]

- □ *In vitro* research suggests that the vapors of a combination of bergamot and orange oils inhibits the growth of drug-resistant and drug-sensitive strains of *E. faecalis* and *E. faecium*.[6286] Another study determined that bergamot and orange oil kill and inhibit the growth of these bacteria by affecting the cell membrane and cell homeostasis.[6287]

- □ Orange oil inhibits several *Salmonella* species *in vitro*.[6288]

- □ *In vitro* research concluded that orange oil inhibits *A. niger* (a common fungus that can infect humans and produce potent toxins, called mycotoxins and causes black mold in produce), *Aspergillus* species, and their subsequent production of mycotoxins.[6289,6290]

- □ Orange oil helps decrease inflammation by strongly inhibiting the 5-lipoxygenase (5-LOX) enzyme that is involved in the inflammation response according to *in vitro* research.[6291]

- □ Animal research concluded that oral administration of orange oil protected rats against oxidative injury during an acute middle-ear infection.[6292]

- □ *In vitro* research suggests that orange oil is a potent free-radical scavenger and inhibits aflatoxin B1 (a common mycotoxin found in foods that can damage DNA and cause cancer) production and food contaminating molds.[6293]

- □ Injection of 40 mg/kg of D-limonene prevents lipid peroxidation (free-radical deterioration of lipids, which can disrupt cellular communication, destroy cells, and damage proteins or DNA) and the depletion of reduced glutathione (GSH), vitamins C and E, and increases liver GSH in diabetic rats.[6294] Another study observed that d-limonene effectively restored GSH levels in mice.[6295]

- □ Orange essential oil inhibited toxic fungi (two strains of *A. parasiticus* and *A. flavus*) *in vitro*.[6296]

- Orange essential oil kills the larvae of the mosquito that carries arbovirus (*Aedes albopictus*).[6297]

- *In vitro* research demonstrated that distilled orange essential oil inhibits *S. aureus, L. monocytogens,* and *P. aeruginosa.*[6298]

- Post-traumatic stress disorder (PTSD) is a disorder characterized by intense fear, flashbacks, and anxiety after a traumatic experience. Over the last several years, researchers have performed various experiments to better understand what leads to PTSD. Leading theories include alterations in fear memory circuits within the brain, neurohormonal changes (catecholamine, serotonin, epinephrine, norepinephrine), exacerbation of inflammation in the peripheral immune system, and mitochondrial dysfunction. Inhalation of 25% orange essential oil prior to and after fear conditioning showed that orange oil helped mice extinguish fear memory forty-eight hours after fearful experience.[6299] Further evaluation found that orange oil balanced the neuroimmune response during recollection of a fearful event previously experienced. The research suggests that inhaling orange oil helps reduce inflammation associated with chronic stress and fear and may be valuable in the management of PTSD.

- Orange essential oil demonstrated mosquitocidal activity against *Culex pipiens*, with the greatest effect against larvae.[6300]

- Russian scientists determined that inhalation of orange essential oil reduces stress related to student exams based on its ability to regulate heart rate.[6301]

- Inhalation of sweet orange essential oil reduced anxiety and caused mild sedation in mice without affecting melatonin and corticosterone hormone levels.[6302]

- Orange peel essential oil protected against food spoilage mold growth and provided about 74 percent, 74 percent, 73 percent, and 69 percent protection against *Aspergillus niger, Mucor wutungkiao, Penicillium funiculosum,* and *Rhizopus oryzae.*[6303]

- Both cold-pressed and molecularly distilled sweet orange (Gannan variety; *Citrus sinensis* Osbeck cv. Newhall) peel essential oils exhibited antimicrobial activity against *Saccharomyces cerevisiae, Escherichia coli, Bacillus subtilis,* and *Staphylococcus aureus,* with the distilled oil displaying greater antimicrobial activity.[6304]

- Hydrodistilled sweet orange essential oil inhibited proliferation of human lung and prostate cancer cells in laboratory research.[6305] Its major constituents also displayed anticancer activity in a concentration-dependent manner in decreasing order as follows: linalool, 3-carene, alpha-terpineol, decanal, citral, d-limonene, and alpha-pinene.

- Recently scientists discovered that nitric oxide (NO), which can act as a neurotransmitter, helps regulate anxiety. Orange essential oil reduced anxiety by modulating NO neurotransmission in mice.[6306]

- Oral administration of orange essential oil, limonene, linalool, and citral (geranial + neral) each increased the abundance of *Lactobacillus* in the caecum and colon of mice.[6307] Limonene produced the greatest improvements in gut microbiome in both the caecum and colon, which will also result in improvements in blood immune index and short-chain fatty acids.

- Inhalation of orange essential oil alleviated depressive-like behavior caused by chronic unpredictable mild stress in mice by modulating neuroendocrine, neurotrophic, and monoaminergic systems.[6308] Inhalation of isolated limonene balanced the hypothalamic-pituitary-adrenal axis and improved the release of monoamine brain neurotransmitters. The antidepressant effects were attributed to limonene, suggesting other citrus essential oils might have similar effects.

- Hydrodistilled orange cv. Gannanzao essential oil significantly reduced the migration of colorectal and liver cancer cells.[6309]

- Both orange and Persian lime essential oils prevented DNA mutations caused by MNNG and demonstrated good antioxidant activity in the β-carotene bleaching assay.[6310] Persian lime also prevented DNA mutation caused by ENNG.

- Oral administration of sweet orange essential oil microcapsules reduced body weight gain by 41.4 percent in obese rats fed a high-fat diet.[6311] The oil also decreased total cholesterol and alleviated pathological alteration of liver and adipose tissue. The oil did so through multiple mechanisms: decreasing the expression of peroxisome proliferators-activated receptor-γ (PPAR-γ; decreased expression reduces fat storage), upregulating of uncoupling protein 2 (protects against obesity and improves glucose control), hormone sensitive lipase (regulates storage and release of fats), and carnitine palmitoyltransferase I (an important enzyme involved in the regulation of mitochondrial fatty acid oxidation), inhibiting the expression of acetyl-CoA carboxylase (involved in the energy metabolism of fatty acids).

- Nursing students frequently experience a high level of stress and anxiety while completing their education and learning fundamental skills, particularly while taking tests. A double-blind, randomized, and controlled

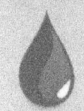

trial demonstrated that inhalation of marjoram and sweet orange (3 drops of a 1:1 blend of the oils) essential oil from an aroma lamp combined with music therapy for 20 minutes significantly reduced test anxiety, general anxiety, and stress.[6312] The intervention also improved performance of fundamental nursing skills.

□ Hydrodistilled orange essential oil was insecticidal to the cowpea weevil (*Callosobruchus maculatus*) and maize weevil (Sitophilus zeamais).[6313] Of its constituents, alpha-terpineol exhibited the highest contact toxicity against the cowpea weevil, which delta-3-carene was the most toxic against the maize weevil. Citral showed the highest toxicity against both insects in the fumigant test.

□ Cold-pressed orange essential oil incorporated into chitosan nanoemulsions demonstrated promise as a fruit juice preservative due to its improved bactericidal effect compared to the free oil.[6314]

□ Sweet orange, citronella (*C. nardus*), and tea tree essential oils were the most effective nematocidal agents against the southern root-nematode (*Meloidogyne incognita*) of 8 essential oils tested.[6315]

□ Researchers evaluated the composition and antibacterial activity of six medicinally important essential oils: tarragon CT p-allylanisole, dill CT alpha-phellandrene/para-cymene, lemon, orange, cinnamon bark, and ginger. Interestingly, orange essential oil had the greatest antibacterial activity against *S. aureus* and *P. aeruginosa*.[6316] Cinnamon bark and tarragon were most active against *E. coli* and *K. pneumoniae*.

□ Yeast-encapsulated sweet orange oil was highly active against *Ae. aegypti* mosquito larvae, including deltamethrin- and temephos-resistant strains, in both laboratory and environmental conditions.[6317]

□ Distilled tangerine, Nanfeng mandarin (*Citrus reticulata* Blanco cv. *Kinokuni*), kumquat, and sweet orange essential oil inhibited *Bacillus subtilis, Staphylococcus aureus, Escherichia coli, Pseudomonas aeruginosa*, and *Salmonella typhimurium*, with kumquat being the most active against three (*B. subtilis, E. coli*, and *S. typhimurium*) of the five microorganisms.[6318] Each of the essential oils also exhibited antioxidant activities in the DPPH and ABTS assays, with Nanfeng mandarin oil presenting the best activity.

□ Laboratory research reported that sweet orange leaf essential oil—sabinene (8.25%–28.81%), delta-2-carene (11.25%–16.72%) and cis-beta-ocimene (10.22%–13.93%)—was cytotoxic to cervical, liver, and breast cancer cells, with the cervical cancer cells being most sensitive.[6319]

□ Distilled sweet orange essential oil exhibited good antioxidant activity.[6320]

□ A randomized double-blinded, and parallel-group controlled clinical trial evaluated the benefits of inhaling sweet orange, rose, or placebo (distilled water) to reduce abdominal pain after open abdominal surgeries.[6321] The 120 participants were randomly assigned to groups that inhaled the various substances via adding 4 drops to a clean gauze pad that was attached to the subject's collar. Subjects were asked to inhale the aroma through normal breathing for thirty minutes. Abdominal pain severity significantly decreased in the sweet orange groups at eight and twelve hours after intervention and rose 12 hours after intervention. Sweet orange was therefore the most effective intervention in reducing postoperative abdominal pain.

□ Fatigue is the most commonly reported symptom experienced by people undergoing hemodialysis, which can significantly decrease quality of life. A clinical study compared the effectiveness of lavender essential oil or orange essential oil with distilled water (so, subjects in each group). For fourteen days, the participants inhaled 5 drops of lavender, orange, or water from a cotton ball pinned to the subject's collar. Both sweet orange and lavender essential oil significantly reduced fatigue in people receiving hemodialysis.[6322]

□ Distilled tangerine and sweet orange essential oil exhibited stronger antioxidant activity than the positive control of quercetin in the DPPH assay.[6323]

□ Methyl tertbutyl ether (MTBE) is used to dissolve (litholytic activity) cholesterol gallstones. Researchers compared the ability of citrus essential oils—clementine, bitter orange, sweet orange, and grapefruit, and their main constituents, to dissolve gallstones against MTBE in a laboratory study.[6324] All citrus oils deteriorated the gallstones, with sweet orange demonstrating remarkable litholytic activity after one day. Sweet orange reached a dissolution capacity of 95.8%, followed by clementine 94.8%, and bitter orange 93.0%, all of which were more effective than MBTE. Grapefruit was less effective than MBTE and other oils at 87.7% dissolution capacity. Isolated limonene and linalool also showed good litholytic activity, exceeding that of MBTE. Taken together, the research suggests that citrus essential oils may be an effective natural solution for cholesterol gallstones.

□ Junior high school (middle school) is a critical time of growth and development for children full of varying emotions that they may not understand how to express or cope with. Academic emotions refer to the emotional experiences of students in relation to education, the learning process, and academic failure or success. A clinical study investigated the inhalation of five essential oils (rosemary, lavender, mint, lemon, and sweet orange) among middle school students in a classroom setting.[6325] Classes were randomly assigned to one of three groups: no aromatherapy, daily aromatherapy, or aromatherapy every other day. Students randomly smelled the five different oils directly from the bottle, smelling their own skin to neutralize the previous smell between each oil, and rated their pleasantness and relaxation ability. The results showed that sweet orange was superior to the other oils in promoting positive emotions. Emotional questionnaires before intervention and eight weeks later showed that sweet orange essential oil significantly promoted greater feelings of joy, hope, positive academic emotion, and relaxation and reduced anger and negative academic emotions. The results suggest that inhaling sweet orange essential oil may improve emotional states among middle school students in an academic setting.

☐ Nonalcoholic fatty liver disease (NAFLD) is a liver conditions characterized by fat inside the liver among people who drink little to no alcohol. Over time, these fat deposits can affect liver function and cause liver damage. Although the cause of NAFLD is not fully understood, it has been linked to overweight/obesity, insulin resistance, diabetes, high blood pressure, high fats (particularly triglycerides) in the blood, and a high-fat diet. Inhaling sweet orange essential oil protected against NAFLD caused by a high-fat diet in mice.[6326] The oil reduced obesity, high triglycerides, total cholesterol, LDL cholesterol, and the accumulation of fats in liver cells.

☐ A study investigated the chemical composition and biological properties of citrus oils: lemon, sweet orange, grapefruit, and tangerine. All four oils displayed remarkable radical scavenging capacity with grapefruit exhibiting excellent antioxidant activity.[6327] Topical application of the oils showed significant antiedema activity comparable to ibuprofen and reduced the expression of inflammatory cytokines (IL-6, COX-2, NF-κB) to varying degrees. Lemon, grapefruit, and tangerine oil also inhibited lung cancer cells.

☐ Researchers evaluated the effects of inhaling sweet orange or pine essential oils on stress based on their visual-motor reaction to the aromas.[6328] Twenty-one young adults aged eighteen to twenty-one years participated in a visual-motor assessment where they had to push the down arrow key as quickly as possible in response to different colored shapes. Fifteen of the participants inhaled orange essential oil for twenty-five minutes, while six inhaled pine essential oil before participating in the assessment. Reaction times and error rates were recorded for each group. Reaction times increased after inhaling both oils, but error rate increased in the orange group and decreased in the pine group. The results suggest that orange essential oil promoted relaxation and alleviated psychoemotional arousal, while pine oil reduced fatigue and promoted greater vigilance.

☐ A study evaluated the effects of various administration methods (inhalation, gavage, and food additive) of orange essential oil on the gut microbiome and immunity in mice.[6329] Remarkably, both inhalation and medium concentration feeding altered the gut microbiome, increasing diversity of intestinal microflora (increased the abundance of Bacteroidetes and *Lactobacillus*). Inhalation of orange oil improved immunoglobulins better than feeding and gavage. Low concentration feeding improved the spleen index, while high and medium concentrations increased interleukin-2 (IL-2) levels—a cytokine signaling molecule that regulated white blood cell responses. Gavage administration significantly increased H+ K+ -ATPase activity.

☐ Laboratory research showed that distilled sweet orange, grapefruit, lemon, and tangerine essential oil each have excellent antioxidant activity in the DPPH assay.[6330] Additionally, all four oils reduced inflammation (remarkably increased G1 phase of the cell cycle, which hinders proinflammatory factor expression) and the expression of proinflammatory molecules (COX-2 and TNF-α). Evaluation in a rat model of rheumatoid arthritis demonstrated that the oils reduce inflammation similarly to the NSAID ibuprofen.

☐ Of nine essential oils tested (cumin, ajowan, neem, clove, moringa, spearmint, rose gum, garlic, and sweet orange), orange essential oil showed the largest zone of inhibition against *F. oxysporum*, which was also confirmed in field testing.[6331] A computer-aided docking study showed that nootkatone had the best docking ability to *F. oxysporum* polyketide synthase beta-ketoacyl synthase.

☐ A sweet orange essential oil based nanoformulation showed good aphicidal activity against aphids (*Aphis gossypii*) in both laboratory and field trials at moderate concentrations, but high concentrations were toxic to citrus plants.[6332]

☐ Comparison of steam-distilled and cold-pressed sweet orange essential oil found that the cold-pressed oil possessed greater antioxidant activity (phosphomolybdenum, CUPRAC, NO radical, and ABTS radical assays).[6333] Both oils also inhibited *S. aureus* and *P. aeruginosa* biofilms and the production of elastase, pyocyanin, and quorum-sensing autoinducers. The whole oil was more effective than isolated limonene on the bacteria.

☐ Inhalation of orange essential oil—2 drops on sterile gauze, three times daily (at 10:00 a.m., 4:00 p.m., and before bedtime) for three days—significantly improved sleep quality in hospitalized children.[6334] The intervention improved time to fall asleep, waking up during the night, and sleep disturbances.

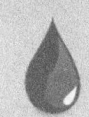

# OREGANO
## (Origanum)

*Origanum vulgare* L., *O. compactum* Benth., *O. hirtum* Link; Turkish Oregano: *O. onites* L., *Majorana onites* L.; **Syrian Oregano, Bible Hyssop**: *Origanum syriacum* L., *Majorana syriaca* (L.) Raf.; Spanish/ **Greek Oregano**: *Thymus capitatus* L. Hoffsgg. & Link, *Thymbra capitata* (L.) Cav.; *O. vulgare* subsp. *hirtum*

**FAMILY:** Lamiaceae (Labiatae)
**NOTE:** Middle
**AROMA INTENSITY:** Strong
**AROMA:** Herbaceous, warm, spicy, medicinal
**COMMON EXTRACTION METHOD:** Steam distilled from the leaves
**POSSIBLE SUBSTITUTE OILS:** Marjoram, thyme (carvacrol CT)
**BLENDS WELL WITH:** Bergamot, camphor, cedarwood, cinnamon, chamomile (German, Roman), clove, cypress, eucalyptus, frankincense, ginger, lavender, lemon, marjoram, tea tree, myrrh, orange, pine, rosemary, thyme
**SUBCELLULAR LOCALIZATION | EPIGENETIC INFLUENCE:** Endoplasmic Reticulum | Circulatory/Respiratory
**RECOMMENDED DILUTION RANGE:** 1.5%–20%; 50% for some conditions

**PRIMARY CONSTITUENTS:** [6335,6336,6337,6338,6339,6340,6341,6342,6343,6344,6345,6346,6347,6348,6349,6350,6351,6352,6353]

*Origanum vulgare (Carvacrol CT)*

| | |
|---|---|
| Carvacrol | 48.5%–83.4% |
| Para-Cymene | 3.0%–12.6% |
| Gamma-Terpinene | 0.0%–6.3% |
| Thymol | 0.9%–5.9% |
| Caryophyllene Oxide | 0.0%–4.9% |
| Borneol | 0.9%–2.4% |

*T. capitatus (Carvacrol CT)* [+]

| | |
|---|---|
| Carvacrol | 51.1%–81.5% |
| Para-Cymene | 3.2%–24.0% |
| Gamma-Terpinene | 1.4%–16.4% |
| Thymol | 0.1%–12.3% |
| Beta-Caryophyllene | 2.9%–9.3% |

*O. vulgare (Terpinen-4-ol CT)*

| | |
|---|---|
| Terpinen-4-ol | 41.2%–48.0% |
| Thymol | 8.4%–22.0% |
| Linalool | 2.1%–15.2% |
| Carvacrol | 4.7%–9.4% |
| Alpha-Terpineol | 5.0%–7.6% |
| Alpha-Terpinene | 2.8%–5.9% |
| Gamma-Terpinene | 0.0%–5.0% |

*Origanum onites (Turkish)* [*]

| | |
|---|---|
| Carvacrol | 65.5%–79.4% |
| Linalool | 0.0%–12.5%* |
| Gamma-Terpinene | 1.7%–5.2% |
| Para-Cymene | 2.5%–4.9% |
| Borneol | 0.5%–4.6% |
| Thymol | 0.2%–2.8% |

*Origanum syriacum (Syrian) Carvacrol CT* [#]

| | |
|---|---|
| Carvacrol | 47.1%–57.7% |
| Thymol | 19.2%–21.0% |
| Para-Cymene | 3.7%–5.2% |
| Gamma-Terpinene | 3.4%–4.8% |

*O. syriacum (Syrian) Thymol CT* [#]

| | |
|---|---|
| Thymol | 36.3%–65.6% |
| Carvacrol | 3.4%–33.8% |
| Para-Cymene | 7.0%–8.4% |
| Gamma-Terpinene | 6.5%–8.0% |

*O. vulgare subsp. hirtum (Carvacrol CT)*

| | |
|---|---|
| Carvacrol | 63.3%–89.7% |
| Gamma-Terpinene | 2.7%–9.9% |
| Para-Cymene | 4.5%–8.7% |
| Myrcene | 1.9%–2.6% |
| Alpha-Pinene | 0.5%–2.2% |
| Beta-Caryophyllene | 0.4%–2.1% |

*O. vulgare subsp. hirtum (Linalool CT)*

| | |
|---|---|
| Linalool | 28.3%–96.3% |
| Carvacrol | 0.3%–51.4% |
| Gamma-Terpinene | 0.0%–6.0% |
| Para-Cymene | 0.0%–4.8% |

Alpha-Terpinene     1.3%–2.0%
Alpha-Thujene     0.0%–2.0%

*O. vulgare subsp. hirtum (Thymol CT)*

| | |
|---|---|
| Thymol | 38.8% |
| Para-Cymene | 20.3% |
| Gamma-Terpinene | 19.6% |
| Alpha-Terpinene | 3.5% |
| Carvacrol Methyl Ether | 3.1% |
| Myrcene | 2.1% |

\* Most *O. onites* samples have very little to any linalool based on the available research.

\# *O. syriacum* composition varies widely based on the season harvested: summer/spring—thymol and carvacrol CTs; autumn/fall—thymol CT; winter—sabinene hydrate and thymol CTs.[6354]

\+ Linalool and thymol chemotypes of *T. capitatus* (*Thymbra capitata*) are also reported in the literature, but the most common CT (and the one that most closely matches other oreganos) is the carvacrol CT.[6355]

**OTHER CONSTITUENTS:** *O. vulgare (Carvacrol CT)*—Alpha-thujene, alpha-pinene, beta-myrcene, alpha-terpinene, trans-alpha-ocimene, sabinene hydrate, terpinen-4-ol, carvacrol acetate, beta-caryophyllene, beta-bisabolene, delta-cadinene, alpha-cadinol; *O. vulgare (Terpinen-4-ol CT)*—Alpha-phellandrene, para-cymene, limonene, terpinolene, methyl thymol ester, methyl carvacrol ester, geraniol/neral, beta-caryophyllene, spathulenol, 1,8-cineole; *O. onites (Turkish)*— Alpha-thujene, alpha-pinene, beta-myrcene, alpha-terpinene, trans sabinene hydrate, thymoquinone, beta-caryophyllene, beta-bisabolene, 4-terpineol, beta-caryophyllene, limonene, camphor; *Origanum syriacum*—Alpha-thujene, alpha-pinene, myrcene, alpha-terpinene, 1,8-cineole, trans-sabinene-hydrate, carvone, beta-caryophyllene, aromadendrene, cis-sabinene hydrate; *T. capitatus (Carvacrol CT)*—alpha-terpinene, beta-myrcene, linalool, terpinen-4-ol, alpha-pinene, borneol, 4-terpineol, caryophyllene oxide ; *O. vulgare subsp. hirtum (Carvacrol CT)*—Octen-3-ol, limonene, thymol methyl ether, 1,8-cineole, terpinen-4-ol, alpha-terpineol, trans-sabinene hydrate, beta-bisabolene, delta-cadinene; *O. vulgare subsp. hirtum (Linalool CT)*—Alpha-thujene, alpha-pinene, myrcene, alpha-terpinene, 1,8-cineole, beta-caryophyllene, alpha-terpineol; *O. vulgare subsp. hirtum (Thymol CT)*—Alpha-thujene, alpha-pinene, limonene, terpinen-4-ol, thymol methyl ether, carvacrol, beta-caryophyllene, beta-bisabolene, delta-cadinene

**PREFERRED COMPOSITION FOR CLINICAL USE:**

| Constituent | *O. vulgare* | *T. capitatus* | *O. onites* |
|---|---|---|---|
| **Carvacrol** | 60%–75% | 60%–75% | 65%–80% |
| **Para-Cymene** | 3%–15% | 5%–15% | 2%–7% |
| **Gamma-Terpinene** | 2%–10% | 3%–10% | 2%–6% |
| **Thymol** | 0.5%–7% | 0.1%–7% | 0.1%–4% |
| **Linalool** | 0.1%–7% | 0.1%–3% | 0%–5% |
| **Beta-Caryophyllene** | 0.5%–5% | 3%–7% | 0%–3% |
| **Myrcene** | 0.5%–3% | 0.5%–3% | 1%–5% |
| **Borneol** | 0%–2% | 0%–2% | 0.5%–5% |

**REPORTED THERAPEUTIC PROPERTIES:** Analgesic (pain relief), anti-inflammatory, **antibacterial**, **antifungal**, antioxidant, **antimicrobial** (particularly systemic infection), **antiviral**, anti-infectious, anticancer, antispasmodic, antiallergenic, diuretic, **immune stimulant**, expels excess gas, expectorant, bronchodilator, **helps relieve menstrual discomfort**, **removes warts**, warming, antidepressant, encourages a general feeling of well-being, promotes a sense of security

**CAUTIONS:**

■ Avoid during pregnancy and lactation. Oregano may negatively affect embryonic development and encourage fetal cell death according to animal research.[6356]

■ May interact with diabetic medications and cause low blood-sugar levels.[6357]

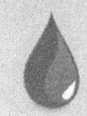

■ May interact with aspirin, blood pressure, antiplatelet, and anticoagulant medications, and increase the risk of bleeding among people with bleeding disorders.[6358,6359,6360]

■ May interact with antibiotics or antifungals and possibly enhance or decrease their effects due to carvacrol or thymol content, and based on research with the whole essential oil.[6361,6362,6363,6364]

■ *Terpinen-4-ol CT*: May interact with antifungals and increase their effectiveness due to terpinene-4-ol content.[6365]

■ May irritate mucous membranes (eyes, mouth, nasal passages, vagina, rectum).

■ *O. syriacum (Syrian) Thymol CT*: Oral caution. The thymol CT of Syrian oregano can contain up to 65.6% thymol. Thymol has a longer half-life (the time it takes for half of the medication to metabolize or excrete half of the dosage) than most essential oil constituents and should not be administered orally for long periods of time.[6366] Thymol is a monoterpene phenol. Reports of fatalities in children who consumed 50 to 200 mg of phenols has been reported.[6367] It is recommended that chemotypes with high levels of thymol be limited to 10 drops per day orally for adults with a two- to seven-day break after twenty-one days of use.

■ May interact with anticholinergic (drugs used for asthma, incontinence, gastrointestinal cramps, muscular spasms, depression, and sleep disorders) and cholinergic medications (drugs used to reduce urinary retention, diagnose myasthenia gravis, and for glaucoma) based on thymol and carvacrol content.[6368]

SELECTED EVIDENCE:

☐ *O. onites* oil significantly inhibited cell viability, angiogenesis (the formation of new blood vessels, which allows a tumor to become malignant), and triggered apoptosis (destruction) of cancerous connective tissue cells from rat embryos *in vitro*.[6369]

☐ *In vitro* research concluded that carvacrol from *O. onites* may be useful in cancer therapy after they found that it inhibited the growth of mouse myoblast cells (an embryonic cell that becomes a muscle cell or fiber) after activation of a human oncogene (activated oncogenes have the potential to cause cancer by allowing the cell to proliferate instead of self-destruct when they are supposed to).[6370]

☐ Carvacrol effectively inhibits glioblastomas *in vitro*, which are cancerous tumors that arise from astrocytes (brain cells that make up the supportive tissue of the brain).[6371]

☐ Oregano with high carvacrol content may cause bronchodilation according to animal research.[6372]

☐ A 4-terpineol-rich oregano oil kills colon adenocarcinoma cells *in vitro*.[6373]

☐ Oregano oil increased antioxidant enzyme activity (up to three times) and decreased lung carcinoma tumor size in mice after three months of administration.[6374]

☐ *O. vulgare* inactivates the yellow fever virus *in vitro*, which is a disease transmitted by mosquitos characterized by fever, muscle pain, backache, headache, loss of appetite, and nausea or vomiting.[6375]

☐ Administration of 200 mg (about four drops) of an emulsified (sustained release form) of *O. vulgare* oil three times daily for six weeks completely eradicated parasites (*Entamoeba hartmanni*, *Endolimax nana*, and *Blastocystis hominis*) in the majority of people included in the study (77%).[6376]

☐ Oregano essential oil is strongly active against the parasite *Anisakis Dujardin* (a parasite that causes gastrointestinal and allergic diseases in humans that eat raw or undercooked seafood).[6377]

☐ Animal research concluded that administration of 0.1 to 1 mg/kg daily of *O. onites* in the rectum or injected into the peritoneal cavity (the fluid-filled gap between the abdominal wall and abdominal organs) protects the colon from injury in rats.[6378] The study observed a significant reduction in ulcers, mucous cell depletion, inflammation, abscesses characteristic of chronic bowel disorders, and mucosal atrophy.

☐ *In vitro* research concluded that oregano and carvacrol effectively inhibit the murine norovirus (a norovirus that affects mice but is used in research to study the effects of drugs and other remedies against human norovirus).[6379,6380]

☐ Oregano oil strongly inhibits *C. albicans*, *S. aureus*, *E. coli*, *L. monocytogenes*, and *S. mutans in vitro*.[6381,6382,6383,6384] Remarkably, a study found that oregano oil inhibits 111 gram-positive bacteria from twenty-three species related to three genre of bacteria.[6385] One study concluded that oregano's strong antimicrobial activity against *C. albicans* make it a possible alternative treatment for candidiasis.[6386] Oregano essential oil inhibits *Aspergillus* species and their subsequent production of mycotoxins.[6387] The gaseous phase of oregano essential oil inhibited *E. coli*.[6388] Oregano essential oil inhibited a number of bacteria (methicillin-sensitive *S. aureus*, *Streptococcus*, *E. coli*, *K. pneumoniae*, *K. pneumoniae*, *Salmonella enterica* serovar Enteritidis, *S. enterica* serovar Typhimurium UK-1, and MRSA) and several clinical isolates (ESBL-producing *E. coli* and two isolates of carbapenemase-producing *E. coli* from urinary tract infections, one isolate of carbapenem-resistant *A. baumannii* from inguinal-rectal swabs, and two isolates of MRSA strains from secretions-general discharges), with greater potency than silver particles.[6389] Bacterial resistance to silver particles by genetic alterations has been reported, making it more challenging to treat infections with them. Oregano essential oil synergized or created an additive antimicrobial effect when used with silver particles against *S. aureus* and *E. coli*. Oregano essential oil inhibited gram-negative bacteria (multidrug-resistant *Acinetobacter baumannii*, extended-spectrum-beta-lactamase (ESBL) producing *Escherichia coli*, and carbapenemase-producing *Klebsiella pneumoniae*) and weakly inhibited *P. aeruginosa*, which are associated with healthcare-acquired infections.[6390]

☐ Oregano essential oil inhibits fifty-nine strains (most of which were resistant to multiple antibiotics) of the major human opportunistic pathogens responsible for respiratory infections in people with cystic fibrosis: methicillin-resistant *Staphylococcus aureus*, *Stenotrophomonas maltophilia*, and *Achromobacter xylosoxidans*.[6391]

☐ *In vitro* research concluded that oregano and manuka essential oils, alone and in combination, inhibit *S. aureus* strains, making them an "effective alternative to chemotherapic [sic] drugs in staphylococcal infections and useful tools to enhance food security." Synergistic and additive effects were seen almost half of the time when oregano and manuka were used together.[6392]

☐ Oregano essential oil may reduce the risk of denture stomatitis (an oral infection of Candida or thrush that causes inflammation of oral mucous membranes that primarily affects denture wearers or those who don't practice appropriate oral care) because it kills *C. albicans* and inhibits its adhesion and colonization to tissue conditioners.[6393,6394]

☐ *In vitro* research suggests that oregano oil is active against *T. cruzi*.[6395] *T. cruzi* causes the potentially life-threatening illness Chagas disease, also known as American trypanosomiasis.

☐ According to *in vitro* research oregano oil prevents the formation of enterotoxins (toxins produced by pathogens that target the intestines) by *S. aureus*.[6396]

☐ *In vitro* research concluded that oregano essential oil strongly inhibited *P. insidiosum* (a pathogenic oomycete that infects mammals and causes gangrenous ulcers on the skin and may restrict blood flow in the surrounding arteries).[6397]

☐ Oregano inhibited the growth and survival of the food-associated pathogens *Y. enterocolitica* (a bacterium that can cause right-sided abdominal pain, fever, and bloody diarrhea) and *L. monocytogenes* (a bacterium that causes a serious infection that causes muscle aches, sometimes preceded by gastrointestinal symptoms like diarrhea) on barbecued chicken.[6398] The carvacrol CT of oregano (*O. onites*) essential oil significantly inhibited the foodborne pathogens *E. coli*, *Salmonella paratyphi* A, *K. pneumoniae*, *Y. enterocolitica*, *P. aeruginosa*, *A. hydrophila,* and *C. jejuni*.[6399]

☐ Oregano oil (Terpinen-4-ol CT) controls the production of aflatoxin B1 (a common mycotoxin found in foods that can damage DNA and cause cancer) by *A. flavus* in corn, grapes, and soybeans *in vitro*.[6400,6401]

☐ *In vitro* research concluded that oregano oil possesses strong antioxidant properties.[6402,6403,6404]

☐ Oregano oil prevents oxidation of LDL cholesterol *in vitro*.[6405] Higher oxidized LDL levels are associated with a significantly increased risk of heart disease.[6406] Spanish oregano essential oil also inhibits the activity of myeloperoxidase (an enzyme that causes oxidation of cholesterol, increases arterial inflammation, and encourages plaque formation in the arteries, all of which increases your risk of heart disease).[6407]

☐ Oregano oil inhibited *Listeria* strains (*L. monocytogenes* and *L. innocua*), whereas its hot water extract was ineffective *in vitro*.[6408]

☐ Application of oregano and lemongrass oil to ground beef controls the growth of *S. enteritidis* (a very common foodborne pathogen that may cause stomach flu, fever with rash, serious bacterial infections of the blood, and systemic bacterial infection) during refrigerated storage.[6409] Additional studies reported that oregano oil is a promising natural food preservative that could possibly replace chemical preservatives currently used by the food industry.[6410,6411,6412,6413]

☐ *In vitro* research concluded that oregano oil inhibits MRSA, as do its components carvacrol and thymol.[6414]

☐ A foot bath (107°F water) with salts and either oregano, thyme, cinnamon bark, lemongrass, clove, palmarosa,

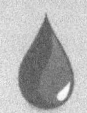

peppermint, lavender, or geranium significantly reduced fungi associated with athlete's foot *in vitro*.[6415]

☐ Animal research found that oral administration of (12 mg per 100 dl) of *O. onites* for twelve weeks protected against toxicity and diabetic-related tissue injury caused by streptozotocin (a chemical that is highly toxic to insulin-producing beta-cells and is used to induce experimental diabetes in animals) in rats.[6416]

☐ *O. syriacum* inhibits 13 bacteria (*C. xerosis, B. brevis, B. megaterium, B. subtilis, M. smegmatis, P. aeruginosa, S. aureus, K. pneumoniae, K. oxytoca, E. faecalis, M. luteus, E. coli,* and *Y. enterocolitica*), and two fungi (*S. cerevisiae* and *S. sclerotiorum*) *in vitro*.[6417,6418]

☐ *Th. capitata* prevented the growth of leukemia cells.[6419]

☐ Spanish/Greek oregano essential oil demonstrated significant broad-spectrum antibacterial (*B. cereus, M. flavus, S. aureus, L. monocytogenes, E. coli, P. aeruginosa, Proteus mirabilis,* and *Salmonella enterica* Typhimurium) and antifungal (*Penicillium funiculosum, P ochrochloron, A. fumigatus, A. niger, A. flavus, A. orchraceus, C. albicans,* and *T. viride*) activity *in vitro*, and reduced the adhesion to and colonization of *E. coli* and *L. monocytogenes* in colon cells.[6420,6421,6422,6423,6424] *Th. Capitata* essential oil inhibits miltdrug-resistant *Enterococcus faecalis* in both planktonic and biofilm state.[6425] Planktonic bacteria are more susceptible to antimicrobial agents. Most infections in humans are caused by bacteria in a biofilm state, making antimicrobial testing of bacteria in a biofilm state more relevant to human health.

☐ Research suggests that the carvacrol chemotype of *T. capitatus* essential oil possesses stronger antifungal activity than the thymol CT.[6426] *Th. capitata* essential oil reduced biofilm formation by *C. albicans*, which made the study authors conclude that it has potential to manage resistant mucocutaneous candidiasis (a group of disorders characterized by infections of the skin, mucous membranes, and nails with *Candida* organisms).[6427] *In vitro* research shows that oregano (*Th. capitatus*) essential oil inhibits the growth and activity of *C. albicans* isolated from vaginal swabs better than the antifungal drug clotrimazole.[6428] Another study reports that *Th. capitata* essential oil inhibits three strains of *C. albicans*, two strains of *C. tropicalis*, two strains of *C. glabrata, C. krusei, C. guilermondii, C. parapsilosis, M. gypseum, M. canis*, three strains of *A. niger, A. flavus,* and five strains of *A. fumigatus* and the dermatophytes *E. floccosum, T. rubrum,* and *T. mentagrophytes*.[6429] Another study reported that *Th. capitata* inhibited *Candida* (7 clinical isolates and 3 ATCC type strains), *Aspergillus* (5 clinical isolates, 2 CECT and 2 ATCC type strains) and 5 dermatophyte clinical strains, with significant activity against dermatophytes.[6430]

☐ *In vitro* research demonstrates that *Th. capitata* is active against the protozoan parasite responsible for giardia (*Giardia lamblia*).[6431,6432]

☐ Research reports that Spanish/Greek oregano possesses strong antioxidant activity.[6433,6434,6435] Another study concluded that *T. capitatus* essential oil is a strong antioxidant, and that its antioxidant activity directly correlates with its ability to decreased blood pressure.[6436]

☐ *T. capitatus* essential oil kills fresh water snails (*Biomphalaria alexandrina*), mosquitoes (*Culex pipiens*), and the pinewood nematode (*Bursaphelenchus xylophilus*).[6437,6438]

☐ Preclinical research suggests that *Th. Capitata* essential oil prevented the death of heart cells *in vitro* when used in small doses, but causes damage when used in higher doses (> 440 PPM).[6439]

☐ A 2:1 mixture of summer savory essential oil and oregano reduced *H. pylori* colonization and eradicated the pathogen in 70% of mice.[6440] Oregano oil significantly inhibited the *C. jejuni* bacterium that is one of the world's most common cases of the stomach flu (gastroenteritis) and *H. pylori* (a pathogen linked to stomach ulcers).[6441]

☐ Oregano essential oil demonstrated potent antioxidant activity when tested via several methods, good anti-inflammatory activity (LOX inhibition), and inhibited acetylcholinesterase (AChE).[6442] Inhibition of AChE prevents the breakdown of acetylcholine, which is essential for memory and thinking. People with neurodegenerative diseases make less acetylcholine, and the diseases often break it down at a faster rate leading to acetylcholine deficits.

☐ Oregano essential oil (*O. vulgare*) was fungicidal to *R. stolonifer* and *A. niger* and reduced black mold formation and soft rot caused by these fungi in cherry tomatoes.[6443] It similarly reduced microbe populations in Brussels sprouts.[6444] Another study concluded that oregano (*O. onites*) may be used in combination with basil to preserve meat and control *S. typhimurium* in minced beef.[6445]

☐ *In vitro* research demonstrates that oregano essential oil *(O. vulgare)* inhibited clinical strains of *C. albicans* isolated from women experiencing symptoms of vaginal infection.[6446]

☐ Oregano essential oil kills and repels the brown-banded cockroach (*Supella longipalpa*).[6447]

☐ Oral administration of 3, 6, 12 mg/kg of oregano essential oil (*Th. capitatus*) relieved pain in rodents by blocking peripheral nervous excitability.[6448]

☐ *In vitro* research demonstrates that oregano essential oil is antimicrobial to *P. insidiosum*.[6449]

☐ Oregano (*O. vulgare* subsp. *hirtum*, CT linalool) demonstrated significant metal chelating and anti-tyrosinase activity and moderate antimicrobial activity.[6450]

☐ Exposure to oregano (*O. vulgare* subsp. *hirtum*, CT thymol) reduced anxiety-like behavior and improved cognition and brain oxidative stress, and decreased acetylcholinesterase activity in a zebra fish model.[6451]

☐ Oregano essential oil exhibited the highest antimicrobial activity of five essential oils tested (manuka, thyme, marjoram, oregano, and mountain savory) against *S. aureus*.[6452]

☐ Greek oregano essential oil (*O. vulgare* ssp. *hirtum*) rich in carvacrol effectively inhibited the lesser mealworm (*Alphitobius diaperinus*) when used as a feed additive (1%) in poultry, as well as its transmission of bacterial and fungal pathogens.[6453]

☐ Both thyme and oregano (*T. capitatus*) essential oils demonstrated good antioxidant and antimicrobial activity against all tested bacteria (*Listeria innocua, Serratia marcescens, Pseudomonas fragi, P. fluorescens, Aeromonas hydrophila, Shewanella putrefaciens, Achromobacter denitrificans, Enterobacter amnigenus, E. gergoviae,* and *Alcaligenes faecalis*), making them good options as meat preservatives.[6454]

☐ Oregano essential oil demonstrated activity against *Shigella, E. hirae,* and *S. typhi*.[6455]

☐ Spanish oregano (*Th. capitatus* CT carvacrol; 81.5% carvacrol) effectively inhibited *Acanthamoeba* species, which are amoebas that cause serious human infections that are difficult to treat with current drugs.[6456] Two isolated constituents—thymol and 2,3-dihydroxy-para-cymene—of the essential oil demonstrated effectiveness against the trophozoite stage.

☐ Turkish oregano demonstrated antimicrobial activity against *E. coli* (both standard and extended spectrum beta lactamase (ESBL) positive strains isolated from patients).[6457]

☐ Oregano essential oil inhibited *Prototheca zopfii* strains that cause inflammation of the udder (mastitis) in cows.[6458]

☐ Laboratory research demonstrated that oregano CT thymol possesses good antioxidant capacity and inhibited bacteria involved in food spoilage (*P. fluorescens, B. thermosphacta,* and *E. faecium*) and pathogenic bacteria (*Salmonella enterica* serotype Enteritidis, *Salmonella enterica* serotype Typhimurium, *L. monocytogenes,* and *S. aureus*).[6459] The same researchers reported that rosemary, sage CT alpha-thujone, peppermint, and garlic CT diallyl disulfide essential oils demonstrated limited spectrum of activity against gram-positive and gram-negative bacteria.

☐ *In vitro* research concluded that oregano CT carvacrol (78%) essential oil is beneficial for wound healing, skin care, and to possibly prevent skin cancer due to its anti-inflammatory, tissue remodeling, and immunomodulatory activities.[6460] The oregano oil inhibited inflammatory markers (MVP-1, VCAM-1, ICAM-1, IP-10, I-TAC, and MIG), tissue remodeling markers (collagen I, collagen III, EGFR, MMP-1, PAI-1, TIMP-1, and TIMP-2), and the immunomodulatory biomarker M-CSF. It also significantly modulated global gene expression and signaling pathways involved in inflammation, tissue remodeling, and cancer signaling processes.

☐ An oregano essential oil with terpinen-4-ol as the primary constituent inhibited phospholipase enzyme activity produced by *C. albicans* strains isolated from dentures.[6461]

☐ Rosemary, clove, oregano (*T. capitatus*), thyme, manuka, sage, eucalyptus (*E. globulus*), lavandin, myrtle, tea tree, peppermint, sage, and corn mint essential oils all showed antimicrobial activity against oral pathogens (*S. mutans, Lactobacillus* spp.) isolated from dental surgery patients.[6462] The essential oils also improved the antimicrobial effects of chlorhexidine, particularly rosemary, thyme, and oregano oils.

☐ *In vitro* research demonstrates that oregano (or isolated carvacrol) essential oil enhances the activity of itraconazole against *Cryptococcus neoformans* (a difficult to treat encapsulated yeast that few molecules actively inhibit and a serious problem for people with a compromised immune system).[6463] This suggests that oregano essential oil could reduce drug resistance, drug requirement, and drug side effects.

☐ Human aryl hydrocarbon receptor (AhR: a gene that encodes a protein that helps regulate responses to planar aromatic hydrocarbons and significantly effects the immune activity in the gastrointestinal tract, regulates the circadian rhythm, helps regulate the cell cycle, and plays an important role in tissue development). Cumin, jasmine, vanilla, and bay leaf fully activate AhR; clove, dill, thyme, nutmeg, and oregano partially activate AhR; and tarragon, caraway, turmeric, lovage, fennel, spearmint, star anise, and anise inhibit the AhR activity.[6464]

☐ Oregano CT carvacrol inhibited *Malassezia furfur* (a fungus associated with skin disorders) isolates.[6465]

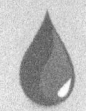

- Cinnamon, clove, oregano, and red thyme essential oils effectively inhibited multidrug-resistant *Salmonella enterica* (a cause of foodborne illness) and enhanced the activity of antibiotics (enrofloxacin, ceftiofur, and trimethoprim-sulfamethoxazole).[6466] The most effective combination was cinnamon with enrofloxacin reducing the minimum inhibitory concentration (MIC) of cinnamon from 1250 to 312.5 μg/mL and the MIC of ENR from 2 to 0.031 μg/mL.

- Oregano essential oil inhibited the foodborne molds *Penicillium verrucosum* and *Aspergillus westerdijkiae*.[6467] The study authors also tested isolated essential oil constituents and reported their antifungal activity in decreasing effectiveness as: trans-cinnamaldehyde > carvacrol = thymol > eugenol > 1,8-cineole.

- Combining oregano essential oil with honey improved the antimicrobial activity of the honey.[6468]

- Oregano essential oil, and carvacrol and thymol, killed liver cancer cells.[6469] Interestingly this study also reported that citral was equally toxic to cancer cells and healthy cells.

- Both oregano CT carvacrol and thyme CT thymol essential oil inhibited multidrug-resistant strains of pathogens (*Escherichia coli*, *Enterococcus* spp., *Candida albicans*, and *Candida famata*) responsible for urinary tract infections that had been isolated from cats and dogs.[6470]

- An odd CT of oregano with pulegone as the major constituent demonstrated the best antioxidant (better than BHT), antibacterial (*B. cereus*, *D. solani*, *E. coli*, *L. monocytogenes*, *M. flavus*, *P. aeruginosa*, *S. aureus*), and anticancer (breast, cervical, colon—better than vinblastine sulfate, T cell leukemia, bladder) activities of twelve essential oils tested.[6471] The same researchers reported that rosemary CT camphor was the best antifungal (*A. flavus*, *A. ochraceus*, *A. niger*, *P. funiculosum*, *P. ochrochloron*, *C. albicans*).

- Oregano CT thymol ad thyme CT thymol essential oils exhibited strong antimicrobial activity against bacteria (*Propionibacterium acnes* and *Staphylococcus epidermidis*) associated with acne that are becoming increasing resistant to first-line antibiotics.[6472] Oregano essential oil was further tested in mice as a topical nanoemulsion, which demonstrated superior healing and antimicrobial effects against acne.

- Marjoram, pink savory (*Satureja thymbra*), spearmint CT piperitenone oxide, melissa, and dittany (*Origanum dictamnus*) demonstrated the greatest repellency toward *Ae. albopictus* mosquitoes of fourteen Lamiaceae species tested.[6473] Thyme CT thymol, basil, dittany, marjoram, and oregano CT carvacrol were the most larvicidal.

- Oregano CT carvacrol and sage CT alpha-thujone inhibited the growth and biofilm formation of *S. pyogenes*, which caused the study authors to conclude that they are potential "plant-derived antimicrobial agents in the management of streptococcal pharyngitis [strep throat]."[6474]

- Oregano and its main constituent carvacrol both inhibited *Aspergillus flavus* and *Aspergillus parasiticus*, which are aflatoxigenic fungi species that cause cancer, DNA mutations, dysregulate immune function, and disrupt fetal development.[6475]

- Syrian oregano rich in carvacrol demonstrated significant antityrosinase activity, which was attributed to its high carvacrol content.[6476] This activity suggests a possible whitening effect on the skin. Interestingly, the researchers found that the presence of thymoquinone reduced the antityrosinase efficacy of carvacrol.

- Oregano essential oil killed human stomach cancer cells by triggering mitochondrial mediated apoptosis and influencing gene pathways and lipogenesis.[6477]

- Oregano (*Th. capitatus*) essential oil exhibited antiviral activity against herpes simplex virus Type 2 (HSV-2), with carvacrol exhibiting moderate antiviral activity.[6478]

- Both oregano (*Th. capitatus*) and mountain savory essential oil (unidentified compositions) were the most effective of twelve essential oils (tea tree, bay laurel, anise, basil, bergamot, lavender, mint, oregano, grapefruit, rosemary, mountain savory, and ginger) tested against vaginal azole-sensitive (clotrimazole, fluconazole, itraconazole) and -resistant *Candida glabrata* strains isolated from women.[6479] Spike lavender and grapefruit essential oils also demonstrated moderate activity.

- Summer savory CT thymol and oregano CT pulegone essential oils prevented biofilm formation and subsequent colonization of *S. pneumoniae* at subminimum inhibitory concentrations.[6480] Summer savory also downregulated genes (LuxS, pfs) involved in quorum sensing.

- Oregano essential oil was the most effective of five essential oils tested (oregano, red thyme, thyme, cinnamon, and clove) antimicrobial against eighty-five *Salmonella* strains belonging to twenty-three serotypes of animal origin.[6481] The researchers also reported that the Typhimurium serotypes were more susceptible to clove and Enteritidis to cinnamon.

- Eucalyptus, clove, mint, oregano, savory, tea tree, and thyme essential oils each inhibited *Venturia inaequalis*, the fungus responsible for apple scab.[6482]

- Cinnamon (46.3% cinnamaldehyde), oregano (*O. vulgare*; 33.9% cis-p-menth-2-en-1-ol), and turmeric (55.4% ar-turmerone) essential oils each inhibited *S. aureus*, *E. coli*, and *P. aeruginosa*.[6483]

- An alpha-terpineol CT of oregano essential oil showed better repellency against bed bugs (*Cimex lectularius*) than DEET when used at 40% concentration.[6484]
- The terpinen-4-ol CT of oregano essential oil inhibited S. aureus (most sensitive pathogen), *Br. bronchiseptica, S. cerevisiae, B. subtilis*, and *S. epidermidis*.[6485] An emulsion of the essential oil demonstrated rapid inhibition of *E. coli, B. subtilis, S. epidermidis*, and *S. cerevisiae*.
- Spanish oregano (*Th. capitatus*) essential oil CT carvacrol demonstrated significant activity against *Echinococcus multilocularis* tapeworms.[6486]
- Oregano, thyme, and creeping thyme (*Thymus serpyllum*) each inhibited biofilm formation by *Salmonella Enteritidis*.[6487]
- Oregano CT beta-terpineol and sweet basil CT linalool essential oils inhibited pathogenic bacterial isolates (*Staphylococcus aureus, Streptococcus pyogenes, Escherichia coli*, and *Streptococcus typhimurium*) and one fungal isolate (*Candida albicans*).[6488]
- Both oregano and clove essential oils prevented the growth of the fungi *Zygosaccharomyces bailii* in salad dressings.[6489]
- The carvacrol CT of oregano essential oil demonstrated significant toxicity against the house fly (*Musca domestica*).[6490]
- Syrian oregano CT thymol reduced the excessive activation of AMPA (a subtype of the excitatory glutamate receptor) receptors.[6491] Specifically, the oil triggered a decrease in desensitization rate of GluA1 and GluA2 homomers. Excessive activation of glutamate receptors can cause brain damage and neurological disorders like seizures, ALS, and stroke.
- Oral administration (370 mg/kg body weight daily for thirteen days) of Turkish oregano CT carvacrol as a preventative measure reduced the formation of colon cancer tumors in mice.[6492]
- Syrian oregano CT carvacrol (82.6%) was effective against the gastrointestinal parasite *Anisakiasis simplex* and insecticidal to the *Culex quinquefasciatus* mosquito.[6493] Carvacrol was also effective against mosquito larvae and adult mosquitoes.
- Oregano essential oil CT carvacrol inhibited antibiotic-resistant *Staphylococcus aureus* strains isolated from pigs.[6494] Another study reported that oregano oil CT carvacrol (71.0%) rapidly and consistently inhibited carbapenem-resistant gram-negative bacteria.[6495]
- An interesting oregano oil with 13.3% caryophyllene oxide, 8.2% beta-caryophyllene, and 5.2% ortho-cymene as major constituents exhibited significant antioxidant activity, moderate antimicrobial activity, metal-chelating, and tyrosinase inhibitory activity.
- Thyme and oregano essential oils demonstrated the ability to increase the stability of minced pork and prevent the oxidation of lipids after two weeks of storage.[6496]
- Of ten essential oils tested (thyme, pennyroyal, oregano, peppermint, lemongrass, rosemary, cinnamon, mandarin, holy basil, and mint asavi), cinnamon and thyme essential oils demonstrated the greatest efficacy against MRSA.[6497] Each oil demonstrated varying levels of inhibition. Oregano and pennyroyal also showed a strong synergistic activity with penicillin.
- A comparative study of the antimicrobial activity of oregano grown in Saudi Arabia (CT carvacrol) and Jordan (CT thymol) found that they effectively inhibited various gram-positive and gram-negative microorganisms.[6498] Of the individual constituents, thymol was superior to carvacrol in this study.
- Male infertility is at least a contributing factor in infertility about 61 percent of the time due to low quantity (sperm count) or poor quality (decreased mobility, vitality, and sperm morphology) sperm.[6499] Oregano essential oil (composition not reported) significantly improved motility and vitality of human spermatozoa in laboratory research, suggesting it may increase the success of *in vitro* fertilization.[6500]
- Laboratory research concluded that oregano CT carvacrol, thyme CT thymol, cassia, lemongrass (*C. flexuosus*), and Western red cedar (arborvitae) essential oils exhibit very strong antimicrobial activity against drug resistant pathogens (*Pseudomonas aeruginosa, Proteus vulgaris, Citrobacter koseri, Klebsiella pneumoniae, Candida albicans*, and *C. parapsilosis*).[6501] Ten essential oils—oregano, thyme, clove, arborvitae, cassia, lemongrass, tea tree, eucalyptus (*E. radiata*), lavender, and clary sage —were tested, and these five were the most effective. The researchers also concluded the essential oils were not genotoxic (cause DNA damage) compared to control cells. In addition, each of the oils exhibited antioxidant activity, with cassia and oregano demonstrating the greatest increase in total antioxidant status, followed by tea tree, thyme, clove, clary sage, eucalyptus, arborvitae, and lavender.
- *Bartonella henselae* is a gram-negative bacteria transmitted to humans by arthropod vectors (fleas, sheep keds, lice, sandflies, ticks, mites, and spiders) and causing acute and chronic infections, including endocarditis—an infection of the inner lining of the heart chambers and valves, bacteremia, and central

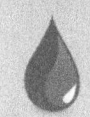

nervous system disorders. *In vitro* research showed that oregano CT thymol, cinnamon bark, mountain savory CT carvacrol, cinnamon leaf, geranium (*P. graveolens* and *P. asperum*), clove bud, allspice, geranium (bourbon), ylang ylang, citronella (*C. winterianus*), elemi, and vetiver eradicated stationary phase *Bartonella henselae* cells within seven days at a concentration of 0.032% (v/v).[6502] Isolated carvacrol and cinnamaldehyde also exhibited significant activity against the bacterium.

☐ Hyperpigmentation of the skin occurs when excess melanin is produced in melanocytes. This can lead to premature skin aging and blotchy appearance of the skin. Most ingredients that are effective against hyperpigmentation block the activity of tyrosinase—an oxidase enzyme that limits the production of melanin. Syrian oregano significantly reduced melanin levels in melanocytes (14 percent reduction) without affecting intracellular tyrosinase, suggesting the oil inhibits oxidation of tyrosinase to reduce the production of melanin.[6503] Carvacrol also reduced melanin by 30 percent without effects on tyrosinase.

☐ Syrian oregano CT carvacrol essential oil was significantly active against *Trypanosoma brucei rhodesiense* (a parasite transmitted to humans by tsetse fly bites that causes African sleeping sickness), moderately active against *Leishmania donovani* (a parasite that is responsible for the most severe form of leishmaniasis—visceral leishmaniasis) and *Plasmodium falciparum* (the deadliest species of *Plasmodium* that causes malaria in humans), and inactive against *T. cruzi* (the parasite responsible for American trypanosomiasis).[6504] The oil was not harmful to the normal cells tested.

☐ Spanish oregano CT carvacrol exhibited excellent antioxidant activity and inhibited bacteria (*S. typhimurium, S. aureus, S. epidermidis,* and *E. coli*) and fungi (*A. niger* and *A. flavus*), with greater activity against bacteria.[6505]

☐ 1-deoxy-d-xylulose-5-phosphate reductoisomerase (DXR) catalyzes the first step in the nonmevalonate or 2-C-methyl-d-erythritol-4-phosphate (MEP) pathway, which is responsible for generating isoprenoid precursors in bacteria. The MEP pathway is absent in humans and considered a therapeutic target for the development of antibiotics. Oregano and clove essential oil displayed moderate inhibitory activity against DXR, suggesting it plays a role in the antimicrobial activity of the essential oils.[6506] Isolated carvacrol and eugenol also possessed moderate inhibitory activity, whereas thymol, carveol, and linalool exhibited weak activity.

☐ Catnip, oregano, and wild marjoram essential oils each exhibited high antioxidant activity in the DPPH, total reducing power, and β-carotene/linoleic acid assays, anticancer activity against human breast cancer, and broad-spectrum antibacterial activity.[6507]

☐ *E. coli* is the most common uropathogenic cause of urinary tract infections (UTIs), but the most frequently used antibiotics do not effectively eliminate the organism making recurrent UTIs common. Oregano essential oil exhibited higher antibacterial activity against uropathogenic *E. coli* than tosufloxacin—a fluoroquinolone antibiotic used for chronic UTIs associated with severe side effects like thrombocytopenia and liver and kidney toxicity.[6508]Allspice, cinnamon bark, and clove bud were also highly effective. Thirty-nine additional oils inhibited *E. coli* at 0.5% concentration, and eight more essential oils at 0.25%.

☐ A study found that a combination of oregano and thyme CT thymol, in gaseous form, essential oil produced a synergistic effect against *L. monocytogenes* on surfaces and radishes.[6509] Oregano with cinnamon and thyme with cinnamon also displayed synergistic activity against the bacteria.

☐ *Helicobacter pylori* is a bacterium that lives in the digestive tract that can cause sores and ulcers in the lining of the stomach or upper part of the small intestine. Thyme, lemongrass, Virginia cedarwood, and melissa essential oils were the most active of 26 commercial essential oils examined against *H. pylori*.[6510] Oregano, tea tree, pine, and silver fir were also bactericidal.

☐ Experimental research showed that oregano CT carvacrol essential oil possesses skin antiaging properties, which exceeded the anti-skin-aging properties of vitamin C.[6511] Two oils were compared—one with 79.5% carvacrol and one with 64.6% carvacrol. The higher carvacrol oil showed good antioxidant activity and significantly higher reductions in lipid peroxidation compared to the lower carvacrol oil. Both oils exhibited comparable antihyaluronidase activity, but the high carvacrol oil had superior anticollagenase and antielastase activity. By inhibiting hyaluronidase the oil could make more hyaluronic acid available to the skin, which retains skin moisture. Inhibiting collagenase and elastase reduces the visible signs of aging by maintaining the firmness and flexibility of the skin.

☐ *In vitro* research showed that cinnamon bark, oregano, thyme CT thymol, lemongrass (*C. flexuosus*), allspice, palmarosa, and amyris all significantly inhibited *S. aureus* in the stationary phase, which is when the size of a bacterial population remains constant, even though some cells continue to divide and others begin to die.[6512]

☐ The carvacrol CT of oregano essential oil inhibited *Aggregatibacter actinomycetemcomitans*, which is a bacterium associated with aggressive periodontitis.[6513] Periodontitis is a severe infection of the specialized tissues that both surround and support the teeth. The antibacterial effect of oregano essential oil was comparable or superior to amoxicillin, amoxicillin and clavulanic acid, and doxycycline. This suggests that oregano could be incorporated into an oral care system to prevent or treat periodontal diseases.

☐ Oregano CT carvacrol essential oil was larvicidal and ovicidal to the cotton bollworm (*Helicoverpa armigera*), making it a promising eco-friendly insecticide against the cotton bollworm,.[6514] Carvacrol, para-cymene, and gamma-terpinene were also effective larvicides when tested individually.

☐ Rosemary CT 1,8-cineole, oregano (*Th. capitatus*) CT carvacrol, marjoram, and sage CT alpha-thujone demonstrated promising antibacterial activity against bacteria (*P. aeruginosa, E. coli, S. enterica, B. subtilis,* and *S. aureus*) responsible for healthcare-associated infections and foodborne illnesses.[6515] Oregano exhibited the strongest activity, which exceeded gentamicin in effectiveness.

☐ Oregano CT carvacrol essential oil exhibited significant antimicrobial activity against thirty-nine bacteria, sixteen fungi, and two yeast species.[6516]

☐ Oregano CT carvacrol, thyme CT thymol, cassia, lemongrass, and Western red cedar essential oils each demonstrated significant antibacterial and antifungal activity against several drug-resistant pathogens (*Ps. aeruginosa, Pr. vulgaris, C. koseri, K. pneumoniae, C. albicans,* and *C. parapsilosis*) known to infect the skin.[6517] The oils were not toxic to healthy keratinocytes and increased total antioxidant status in the cells as well.

☐ Laboratory research demonstrated that oregano essential oil significantly enhances the integrity of human sperm DNA collected from twenty-five male infertile volunteers during incubation.[6518] The oil improved the sperm parameters of mobility—curvilinear velocity (VCL), linear velocity (VSL), the mean velocity of the path (VAP), and the amplitude of the displacement (ALH).

☐ Evaluation of 13 medicinal aromatic plants of Greece found that essential oils rich in carvacrol, para-cymene, and gamma-terpinene, like Greek oregano CT carvacrol, Spanish oregano CT carvacrol, and pink savory CT carvacrol, exhibited the strongest inhibitory activity against bacterial pathogens and the greatest total antioxidant activity.[6519]

☐ Oregano essential oil reduced the expression of proinflammatory mediators (reactive oxygen species, inter-cellular adhesion molecule, inducible nitric oxide synthase, and cyclooxygenase, a marker of DNA damage (formation of 8-oxo-7,8-dihydro-2'-deoxyguanosine), and abnormal modification of extracellular matrix components (metalloproteinase-1 and metalloproteinase-2).[6520] This preliminary research suggests that oregano may be helpful to reduce inflammation to facilitate wound healing.

☐ Excess pigmentation (hyperpigmentation; when patches of skin are darker than normal surrounding skin) of the skin due to disorders that cause excessive melanin production is considered a sign of aging and unattractive to some.[6521] Syrian oregano CT carvacrol essential oil significantly reduced the production of melanin by inhibiting the oxidation of tyrosinase and deregulating the production of melanin. Isolated carvacrol reduced melanin production by 30%. Neither the oil or isolated carvacrol significantly affected intracellular tyrosinate levels.

☐ Syrian oregano CT carvacrol showed superior antimicrobial activity against *S. aureus, S. mutans,* and *C. albicans,* which are microbes commonly associated with denture stomatitis.[6522]

☐ Basil CT linalool and oregano CT carvacrol essential oils displayed strong antioxidant activity in the DPPH assay. The same research showed that oregano actively inhibited *S. aureus*.[6523]

☐ The thymol CT of oregano essential oil inhibited pathogenic bacteria (*S. aureus, B. subtilis, S. enterica, E. coli,* and *P. aeruginosa*) and displayed antioxidant activity in the DPPH, ABTS, FRAP, and TPC assays.[6524]

☐ An interesting CT of oregano essential oil with germacrene D as the main constituent moderately inhibited *E. coli* and *S. aureus*.[6525]

☐ A carvacrol rich (71.0%) oregano essential oil inhibited reference and multidrug-resistant clinical isolates of *Acinetobacter baumannii* and significantly enhanced the antibacterial activity of polymyxin B.[6526]

☐ A nanoemulsion of oregano essential oil with alpha-terpinolene as the main constituent displayed antimicrobial activity and novel quorum-sensing inhibition activity against *P. aeruginosa, S. aureus, E. coli,* and *L. monocytogenes*.[6527] The free oil was ineffective against *P. aeruginosa* and *S. aureus*.

☐ Goldenrod (*Solidago canadensis*) is considered an invasive and dangerous plant invader in Europe because it suppresses the growth of indigenous flora. Researchers tested the effects of sage CT beta-thujone, peppermint, oregano CT carvacrol, fennel (near equal estragole and trans-anethole), and dill essential oils. Oregano essential oil significantly inhibited goldenrod germination, suggesting it may be a natural herbicide.[6528] In addition, the researchers noted that isolated trans-anethole and estragole exhibited high phytotoxicity.

☐ A study comparing the effects of three CTs of oregano essential oil —carvacrol CT, thymol/para-cymene CT, and thymol/gamma-terpinene CT—found that although each CT was toxic to blowfly (*Calliphora*

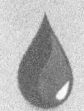

*vomitoria*) adults and eggs and could deter oviposition, the thymol CTs were more active and effective than the carvacrol CT.[6529]

☐ Metabolic syndrome (a cluster of conditions—increased blood pressure, excess body fat, high cholesterol and triglycerides, low HDL, high blood sugar) that increase the risk of type 2 diabetes and cardiovascular disease) promotes acute and chronic infections because of increased inflammation, which impairs immune function. In addition, metabolic syndrome alters the gut microbiome (dysbiosis), creating a more favorable environment for opportunistic pathogens. This is problematic because antibiotics are commonly administered to treat infections, exacerbating dysbiosis. A clinical study reported that oral administration of oregano CT carvacrol essential oil (0.8 mL of oregano essential oil) twice daily, for ten days, reduced minor infections with *Staphylococcus aureus, Streptococcus pyogenes,* and *Escherichia coli* without increasing dysbiosis.[6530] The participants were divided into four groups: 1) *Staphylococcal* infection group, 2) *Escherichia coli* infection group, 3) *Streptococcal* infection group, and 4) control group (no infection or treatment). Moreover, the oil reduced diarrhea, gastrointestinal pain, and flatulence, and improved the subject's health and cellular function.

☐ Oral administration of the carvacrol CT of oregano essential oil protected against liver and kidney damage caused by carbon tetrachloride in rats.[6531] The protective effect was improved when the oil was added to thyme honey.

☐ Oregano (near equal carvacrol and thymol) and Zataria CT thymol essential oils exhibited good antioxidant activity in the DPPH and ferric reducing assays, and they strongly inhibited *E. coli*.[6532] They also inhibited *L. monocytogenes, S. putrefaciens,* and *P. fluorescens*.

☐ Both oregano CT carvacrol and thyme CT thymol essential oil inhibited *S. aureus* in vapor and liquid phase, with thyme generally showing greater activity.[6533] Combining oregano and thyme essential oils showed a synergistic and strong antibacterial activity against *S. aureus* in both liquid and vapor phases.

☐ A comparison of Greek oregano CT carvacrol and oregano (*O. vulgare*) essential oil CT sabinene/terpinen-4-ol revealed that Greek oregano possess stronger antibacterial activity (*E. coli, S. enteritidis, B. cereus, L. monocytogenes,* and *S. aureus*) but the antioxidant activity was near equal in the DPPH, ABTS, and FRAP assays.[6534]

☐ Nanovesicles loaded with Turkish oregano CT carvacrol or pink savory CT carvacrol inhibited foodborne pathogens and spoilage organisms.[6535]

☐ *Candida* spp. can form biofilms on mucosal surfaces, the skin, and medical implants, which contribute to infections that respond poorly to medications. Turkish oregano essential oil inhibited biofilm formation by *Candida* spp. and reduced existing biofilms and acted as a dual inhibitor of *C. albicans* + *S. aureus*.[6536]

☐ Spanish oregano (*Th. capitatus*) CT carvacrol essential oil was significantly effective against *Ascosphaera apis*, the etiological agent of chalkbrood, an invasive honeybee mycosis.[6537] Other oils that showed activity include myrtle, rosemary, eucalyptus (*E. globulus*), cinnamon bark, and helichrysum.

☐ Oregano CT thymol essential oil showed high antibacterial activity against extended-spectrum β-lactamases (ESBL-) and non-ESBL-producing *Enterobacteriaceae* isolates, with the ESBL-producing isolates being more susceptible to the oil.[6538]

☐ An odd CT of oregano essential oil with 16.5% methyleugenol, 15.6% myristicin, and 15.1% carvacrol, strongly inhibited *Botrytis cinerea* mycelial growth and spore germination.[6539] Isolated carvacrol and thymol were also significantly active, completely suppressing grey mold at 125 mg/L.

☐ Both oregano CT carvacrol and thyme CT para-cymene (40.0% para-cymene, 32.0% thymol) essential oils demonstrated good antifungal activity against *C. albicans*, showing high activity during the adherence phase and during biofilm formation.[6540] The pinocamphone CT of hyssop, rosemary CT 1,8-cineole, and sage CT 1,8-cineole were active as well but to lesser degrees.

☐ Immersion tests showed that oregano CT carvacrol and cinnamon bark essential oil are significantly acaricidal against the Asian longhorned tick (*Haemaphysalis longicornis*) larvae and unfed adults.[6541] The fumigant test demonstrated significant acaricidal activity against larvae, unfed and engorged nymphs, and adults.

☐ Oregano CT carvacrol and marjoram CT carvacrol significantly increased HDL cholesterol in trained athletes, but only marjoram decreased LDL cholesterol.[6542] Participants ingested 2 mL of oil in 150 mL of warm water after each meal for 14 consecutive days. There was no change in total cholesterol, triglycerides, or liver biomarkers.

☐ *Fusarium graminearum* is a fungus that contaminates cereals, fruit, and vegetables. Thyme, oregano, basil, nutmeg, hyssop, and clove essential oils inhibited mycelial growth of *F. graminearum*, with oregano performing best followed by clove and thyme.[6543] The composition of the oils was not reported.

- Oregano CT carvacrol, lemon, lavender, mastic, and mandarin essential oil each inhibited *S. aureus*.[6544]

- Oregano CT carvacrol essential oil was insecticidal to the mealworm beetle (*Tenebrio molitor*) at varying developmental stages, affected their behavior, and displayed repellency effects.[6545]

- An oregano essential oil with 84.4% carvacrol exhibited potent antimicrobial activity against *S. aureus*.[6546]

- The carvacrol CT of oregano essential oil inhibited the growth of cariogenic bacteria, which was improved by the addition of isolated carvacrol.[6547]

- When ten essential oils—lesser calamint CT piperitone oxide, bergamot, lemon petitgrain, tangerine petitgrain, fennel CT methyl chavicol, bay laurel, myrtle CT 1,8-cineole, oregano CT, sage CT alpha-thujone, and rosemary CT 1,8-cineole—were tested against antibiotic-resistant *E. coli*, oregano, lesser calamint, and fennel were the most active at inhibiting bacterial growth.[6548] Further evaluation found that the oils triggered methylation both at adenine and cytosine residues in the genomes of most cell lines, suggesting that the oils can induce epigenetic remodeling.

- Honey has been used medicinal since ancient times for a variety of ailments. Medical-grade honey (not the raw honey you purchase at a grocery store) is particularly useful for wound healing because of its antibacterial and anti-inflammatory activity, which speeds the healing of wounds. An experimental study evaluated the healing effects of a mixture of honey with selected essential oils—oregano CT ethanone, rosemary CT camphor, and thyme CT 1,3-Cyclopentadiene—in burn and chemical wound models in rabbits.[6549] The oils were added to honey in a concentration of 0.5% per 100g of honey. The honey/essential oil groups were compared versus a control (no treatment) and standard treatment with madecassol ointment. All of the honey/essential oil groups experienced faster healing times than the control group and standard treatment group. The best healing effect for burns was observed with honey and thyme essential oil for burns. The oils were not irritating when used at 0.5% in the honey, but showed irritation at 5%.

- *Clostridioides difficile* is a bacterium that produces two exotoxins: toxin A and toxin B. Infections with *C. diff* can be mild to moderate (watery diarrhea three or more times daily for more than one day accompanied by mild abdominal cramping and tenderness) or severe (watery diarrhea up to fifteen times daily, moderate to severe abdominal cramping, rapid heart rate, fever, dehydration, and nausea). Severe cases can cause kidney failure, loss of appetite, blood or pus in the stool, and inflammation of the colon (colitis), which can be life-threatening. Illness caused by *C. diff* typically occurs after antibiotic use and most commonly affects older adults in healthcare facilities. However, because the bacterium is shed in feces it can contaminate any surface, material, or device and spread outside of healthcare settings and in younger people as well. Repeat infections are common among the elderly because the bacterium is resistant to multiple antibiotics, making it very difficult to eradicate. A laboratory study investigated the activity of ten essential oils—cassia bark, cinnamon bark, citronella (*C. nardus*), coriander, clove bud, oregano CT carvacrol, Greek oregano (*O. heracleoticum*) CT carvacrol, marjoram, clary sage, and thyme CT thymol—against *C. diff* isolated from infected patients and contaminated foods.[6550] Isolated constituents within the essential oils were also tested (carvacrol, trans-cinnamaldehyde, eugenol, linalool, and thymol) as well as common antibiotics used to treat *C. diff* infections (chloramphenicol, clindamycin, erythromycin, gentamicin, metronidazole, and vancomycin). Cassia and cinnamon bark were the most effective, with thyme, oregano, Greek oregano, and marjoram also demonstrating high activity. Coriander and clary sage exhibited medium activity, while clove and citronella displayed low activity. Among the isolated constituents, trans-cinnamaldehyde, thymol, and carvacrol showed high activity and eugenol and linalool low activity. Cinnamon and cassia consistently exceeded the activity of all antibiotics, with very few exceptions, and thyme, oregano, and Greek oregano outperformed all antibiotics but metronidazole.

- Of eleven essential oils tested, oregano CT carvacrol, fennel, mountain savory CT para-cymene, and summer savory CT carvacrol were the most effective against gastrointestinal nematodes (*Haemonchus, Trichostrongylus, Teladorsagia*, and *Chabertia*) in the *in vitro* egg hatch test.[6551] Oral administration of the oils diluted in sunflower oil to animals showed that thyme CT para-cymene essential oil was the most effective, even more effective than thyme CT thymol.

- *In vitro* research showed that oregano essential oil inhibits *Candida* spp. (in descending order of inhibition—*C. albicans, C. dubliniensis, C. krusei*) and synergistically improved the activity of fluconazole and nystatin.[6552]

- Oral administration of Turkish oregano essential oil CT carvacrol (0.25 mL/kg of BW) significantly protected against neurological deficits—memory and learning impairments—in a scopolamine-induced amnesia/Alzheimer's disease model in rats.[6553] The researchers suggested that the oil's activity was possibly due to inhibition of acetylcholinesterase, reduction of oxidative stress, and prevention of brain cell loss in the hippocampus and frontal cortex. Computer-based models also predicted that the oil may reduce

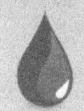

proinflammatory enzyme (COX-2, inducible nitric oxide synthase, and myeloperoxidase) activity.

☐ When testing four essential oils (cinnamon bark, clove, oregano, and peppermint) and isolated constituents (allyl isothiocyanate, carvacrol, citral, eugenol, and (+)-limonene), researchers found that allyl isothiocyanate, cinnamon, carvacrol, eugenol, and oregano were active against all microorganisms tested (*E. coli, L. monocytogenes, S. typhimurium, P. fluorescens*, and *En. faecalis*) in vapor phase.[6554] *P. fluorescens* was the most resistant to the oils and isolated.

☐ A study evaluated the antimicrobial activity of multiple essential oils (cinnamon bark, lavender, tea tree, lemon, oregano CT carvacrol, peppermint, bay laurel, and eucalyptus—*E. globulus*) against human pathogens (*S. pyogenes, S. aureus, S. agalactiae*).[6555] Oregano, cinnamon, and tea tree exhibited the strongest antibacterial activity and combinations of tea tree/lavender and cinnamon/lavender displayed synergistic activity.

☐ An oregano essential oil rich in beta-caryophyllene (6.4%–8.2%) and caryophyllene oxide (11.2%–13.4%) produced significant antinociceptive and anti-inflammatory activity when injected in mice.[6556]

☐ Cassia, clove, oregano (near equal carvacrol and thymol), ginger, and thyme CT thymol essential oils each showed activity against *L. monocytogenes* in a dry-cured ham-based model.[6557]

☐ Spanish oregano, ajowan, and pennyroyal essential oils (composition not reported) each exhibited good antimicrobial activity against multidrug-resistant *E. coli* strains, producing extended-spectrum β-lactamase (ESBL) enzymes, with Spanish oregano displaying the most important effect.[6558]

☐ Marjoram CT carvacrol, oregano CT carvacrol, Turkish oregano CT carvacrol, as well as isolated carvacrol each inhibited angiotensin-converting enzyme 2 (ACE2) activity, with marjoram being the most effective. Blockade of ACE2 reduces the production of angiotensin II, which is a substance that narrows blood vessels and releases hormones (aldosterone, norepinephrine) to increase blood pressure and urine production. ACE inhibitors are primarily used to treat heart and kidney conditions. All of the oils also inhibited lipoxygenase (LOX) enzyme activity, with marjoram being the most active again. Stopping LOX activity reduces the production of inflammatory leukotrienes, which is a major cause of inflammation in conditions such as asthma, osteoarthritis, and allergic rhinitis. Additionally, computer-based protein docking confirmed the docking potential of the carvacrol and agreed with the significant enzyme inhibition activity observed in the laboratory studies.

☐ Oregano (*Th. capitatus*) CT carvacrol displayed significant antioxidant capacity based on ORAC score, did not promote mutagenic activity, and inhibited fungi (*C. albicans, A. fumigatus, T. rubrum, E. floccosum, M. canis*) at low concentrations.[6559]

☐ Investigation of the antifungal and antivirulence activity of basil CT linalool, cinnamon bark, clove, tea tree, oregano CT carvacrol, and thyme CT thymol essential oils (EOs) on five *Candida* species (*C. albicans, C. auris, C. krusei, C. parapsilosis*, and *C. guillermondii*) revealed that clove and cinnamon inhibited all fungal species tested, cinnamon, oregano, and thyme inhibited biofilm formation of *C. albicans, C. guilliermondii*, and *C. parapsilosis*, and each oil except tea tree downregulated virulence genes in *C. albicans*.[6560] In addition, thyme synergized the activity of fluconazole against all tested *Candida* species.

☐ Oregano CT carvacrol essential oil nanoemulsion was strongly active against prostate cancer cells.[6561]

☐ Acetylcholine is an important cholinergic neurotransmitter and neuromodulator involved in various functions throughout the body, but particularly in the nervous system. It works by attaching to receptors and sending signals between nerves. Acetylcholine has multiple functions in the body including motor neuron function (muscular movement), dilation of blood vessels, motivation, attention, learning, and memory. The activity and function of the cholinergic system is controlled by the enzymes acetylcholinesterase (AChE) and butyrylcholinesterase (BChE). People with neurodegenerative conditions make less acetylcholine and experience excessive BChE activity. Inhibition of AChE and BChE are targets for the treatment of neurodegenerative conditions. The outgrowth of neurites (called neuritogenesis—the formation of any projection from neurons) occurs during brain development and when neurons are regenerated. These outgrowths of dendrites or axons allow neurons to form networks and connections and communicate with other cells and ultimately maintain youthful brain function. A preclinical model of Alzheimer's disease evaluated essential oils from the *Lamiaceae* family for their effects on brain function and brain cell protection.[6562] Oregano CT alpha-terpineol, peppermint, rosemary CT 1,8-cineole, and sage essential oils each inhibited BChE activity. The carvacrol CT of oregano inhibited both BChE and AChE activity. Isolated linalool from lavender significantly reduced reactive oxygen species (ROS) inside neurons, suggesting it can protect against oxidative stress and death of neurons. In addition, oregano CT alpha-terpineol, peppermint, rosemary, and sage triggered neurite outgrowth, with the greatest activity observed from oregano. The researchers concluded that these oils have properties that could potentially prevent or delay dementia-related diseases.

☐ Nanoencapsulation of oregano essential oil into liposomes (Phospholipon 90H)—to help maintain and improve its biological activity—significantly increased its cytotoxicity against breast cancer cells.[6563]

- Turkish oregano CT carvacrol and marjoram CT carvacrol essential oils were larvicidal to and repelled the cattle tick (*Rhipicephalus annulatus*).[6564]
- Humans are exposed to gamma rays (gamma radiation) from cosmic rays in the solar system, medical tests (X-rays, CT scans, etc.), airport scanners, nuclear power plants, some consumer products, and food irradiation, which can alter healthy cells in the body. A preclinical model found that exposure to rosemary, oregano, lavender, or eucalyptus (*E. globulus*) essential oils protected against damage caused by gamma ray exposure.[6565] The best protective effects were observed form lavender and oregano essential oils. Specifically, the oil preserved metabolic enzymes, restored enzymatic antioxidant activity (catalase and superoxide dismutase), and reduced lipid peroxidation.
- Pennyroyal, Spanish lavender CT camphor, rosemary CT camphor, and oregano CT thymol essential oil were each acaricidal to two spider mites (*Tetranychus urticae* and *Eutetranychus orientalis*) in the fumigant toxicity test, with pennyroyal displaying the highest activity.[6566] A combination of oregano with acequinocyl exhibited the greatest results of mixtures tried.
- An odd oregano essential oil with p-Vinylguaiacol as the primary constituent was active against *S. aureus, L. monocytogenes, V. vulnificus, S. flexeneri, B. subtilis, S. enterica, E. coli,* and *P. aeruginosa*.[6567] Its activity frequently exceeded isolated terpinen-4-ol and gentamicin against the tested pathogens.
- Four essential oils—*Lepidium pinnatifidum*, wild mint CT piperitone oxide, oregano CT carvacrol, and *Agrimonia eupatoria*—were evaluated for their repellent activity against *Ae. aegypti* mosquitoes.[6568] Each oil provided repellent effects with wild mint and oregano preventing bites for ninety and seventy-five minutes respectively.
- The antimicrobial, antioxidant (DPPH, ABTS, and FRAP assays), and anti-inflammatory (LOX inhibition) activity of thyme CT carvacrol (80.7%), oregano CT carvacrol (68.0%), and sage CT 1,8-cineole (55.8%) essential oils were evaluated in laboratory research.[6569] Oregano displayed the highest antioxidant activity, followed by thyme and sage. The greatest anti-inflammatory activity was observed with thyme. Oregano and thyme had higher antimicrobial activity against *S. aureus, E. coli,* and *L. fermentum*. Additionally, oregano and thyme essential oils inhibited intracellular invasion of sporozoites from the poultry parasite (*E. tenella*).
- Oregano essential oil formulated as polymeric micelles demonstrated promise against skin tags due to its ability to decrease human keratinocyte (a major component of skin tags) cell migration and trigger keratinocyte cell death without harming dendritic cells.[6570] The oil formulation also decreased inflammation and exhibited antimicrobial activity.
- Both oregano and thyme essential oils inhibited *S. epidermidis* and *E. coli* in pure and diluted forms (50% and 75%), with a higher inhibition observed when the antimicrobial effect was due to both liquid and vapor phase components.[6571]
- Both clove and oregano CT carvacrol essential oils were lethal to adult red spider mites (*Tetranychus urticae*), decreased their fertility, and repelled them from two host plants.[6572]
- Oregano CT carvacrol, thyme CT thymol, and mountain savory CT carvacrol essential oils and there mixtures were effective against clinical bacterial strains—*Staphylococcus* sp., *Streptococcus* sp., *P. aeruginosa, E. coli, K. pneumoniae, S. marcescens,* and *M. pachydermatis* strains—cultured from the ears of dogs affected by otitis externa (ear infection).[6573] The mixture contained equal parts of each oil and was the most active against the tested strains.
- Oregano CT carvacrol, thyme CT thymol, and tropical basil and their post-distillation byproducts—total, spent, and residual water extracts—were evaluated in enzyme inhibitory and antioxidant assays.[6574] The oils and extracts displayed antioxidant activity with the extracts exhibiting greater activity in the DPPH and ABTS assays, but the essential oils had the highest metal-reducing power in the CUPRAC assay. Tropical basil and thyme essential oil also demonstrated good inhibition of acetylcholinesterase, suggesting they may aid cognition. The best butyrylcholinesterase inhibitory activity was observed with tropical basil essential oil. The oils also inhibited tyrosinase and amylase, which indicates they may be useful for skin brightening and glucose management as well.
- Oregano CT carvacrol essential oil displayed antimicrobial and bactericidal activity against *K. pneumoniae* and a synergistic activity when combined with ampicillin and gentamicin.[6575]
- Mycotoxins, aflatoxin B1 (AFB1), produced by *Aspergillus* spp. fungi is found in one-quarter of feed components and can harm animals that eat the feed (liver or kidney damage and cancer, malnutrition, growth impairment, and suppressed immune function). Oregano CT oleic acid essential oil (1 g/kg diet) added to feed decreased the toxic effects of AFB1, oxidative stress, lipid peroxidation levels, DNA damage, and inflammation, and protected the kidneys in rabbits.[6576]
- Evaluation of *Lamiaceae* family essential oils (melissa, oregano CT carvacrol, thyme CT para-cymene, Spanish

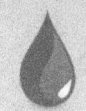

lavender, sage, rosemary CT 1,8-cineole, and peppermint) showed that melissa and oregano exhibit the best anticandidal activity (*C. albicans, C. glabrata, C. guilliermondii, C. krusei, C. parapsilosis,* and *C. tropicalis*), with Spanish lavender, peppermint, rosemary, and thyme also being very active.[6577] Oregano and thyme demonstrated the strongest antibiofilm activity, followed by Spanish lavender, peppermint, and rosemary.

☐ Oregano essential oil strongly inhibited *S. aureus* and displayed strong antibiofilm activity even at half its minimum inhibitory concentration.[6578] None of the MRSA strains were resistant to its activity.

☐ *In vitro* research demonstrated that oregano essential oil inhibits the acid production and reduced the hydrophobicity and biofilm formation of *S. mutans*, suggesting it may help prevent dental cavities.[6579]

☐ The thymol CT of oregano (*Th. capitatus*) displayed high antioxidant activity (AA and TPC assays), good antibacterial activity (*S. enterica* ser. *Typhimurium, L. monocytogenes,* and *Y. enterocolitica*), and completely destroyed mature biofilms of all three bacteria.[6580]

☐ Marjoram CT terpinen-4-ol, oregano CT thymol, inhibited *B. subtilis, M. luteus, S. aureus, E, coli, K. pneumoniae,* and *P. aeruginosa*, while citronella (*C. winterianus*), geranium, and catnip CT nepetalactones were only active against some gram-positive bacteria.[6581]

☐ Comparison of the thymol (> 47%) and carvacrol (> 80%) CTs of oregano essential oil, showed that both exhibit high antimicrobial activity *in vitro* and in a food matrix challenge test and did not alter the epithelial layer of intestinal cells to reduce the adhesion of selected pathogens at low concentrations.[6582]

☐ Oregano and carvacrol both inhibited *Malassezia sympodialis* and *M. furfur*, which are opportunistic fungi associated with skin and systemic infections.[6583]

☐ A special cultivar (cv. Pierre; 61.9% carvacrol, 25.2% para-cymene) of oregano essential oil exhibited strong antibacterial activity against the plant pathogens *Pseudomonas cichorii, P. syringae,* and *Xanthomonas perforans*, and strong insect repellent activity against bed bugs (*Cimex lectularius*).[6584] Mixing it with catnip improved the repellent activity.

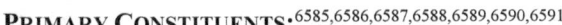

# ORIENTAL ARBORVITAE
## (Chinese Thuja, Oriental Thuja, Chinese Arborvitae, Biota)

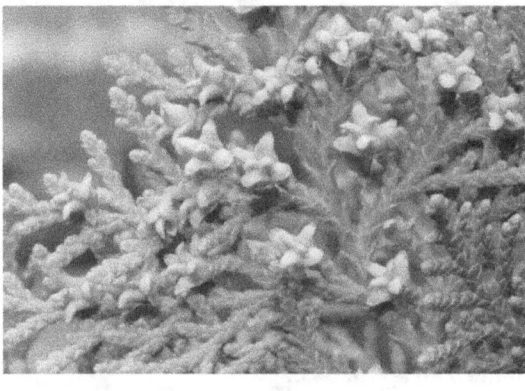

*Platycladus orientalis* (L.) Franco, *Thuja orientalis* L., *Biota orientalis* (L.) Endl.

**FAMILY:** Cupressaceae
**NOTE:** Top
**AROMA INTENSITY:** Strong
**AROMA:** Piney, woody, fresh, balsamic
**COMMON EXTRACTION METHOD:** Steam distilled from the needles (leaves); may also be steam distilled from the berries or wood
**POSSIBLE SUBSTITUTE OILS:** Virginia cedarwood, Texas cedarwood, cypress, pine, balsam fir
**BLENDS WELL WITH:** Balsam fir, birch, blue spruce, cassia, cedarwood, Chinese cedarwood, Chinese red pine, cypress, galbanum, German chamomile, frankincense, lavender, lemon, myrtle, palo santo, pine, sandalwood, silver fir, spruce (black), tsuga, white fir
**SUBCELLULAR LOCALIZATION | EPIGENETIC INFLUENCE:** Currently unknown | Currently unknown
**RECOMMENDED DILUTION RANGE:** 3%–50%; Neat for limited conditions

**PRIMARY CONSTITUENTS:**[6585,6586,6587,6588,6589,6590,6591]

| Needles | | Berries | |
|---|---|---|---|
| Alpha-Pinene | 15.0%–35.7% | Alpha-Pinene | 23.5%–52.4% |
| Alpha-Cedrol | 9.8%–20.3% | Delta-3-Carene | 9.5%–23.8% |
| Delta-3-Carene | 6.3%–20.1% | Sabinene | 2.1%–11.1% |
| Sabinene | 0.5%–10.0% | Alpha-Cedrol | 6.5%–9.6% |
| Limonene | 3.6%–8.2% | Beta-Phellandrene | 0.0%–5.5% |
| Beta-Caryophyllene | 3.0%–7.5% | Thujopsene | 0.0%–5.0% |

| | | | |
|---|---|---|---|
| Alpha-Humulene | 0.0%–5.6% | Myrcene | 1.6%–4.7% |
| Alpha-Terpinolene | 2.1%–5.3% | Limonene | 0.0%–4.7% |
| Myrcene | 1.6%–5.0% | Beta-Caryophyllene | 1.9%–4.1% |
| Thujopsene | 0.0%–5.0% | Alpha-Terpinolene | 1.7%–4.0% |
| Terpinyl Acetate | 0.0%–4.7% | | |

Note: The wood oil reportedly contains 45% thujopsene and 21% cedrol as the primary constituents.[6592]

**OTHER CONSTITUENTS:** *Needles*—Para-cymene, alpha-thujene, beta-pinene, gamma-terpinene, alpha-fenchene, alpha-phellandrene, delta-terpinene, terpinen-4-ol, beta-cedrene, germacrene D, trans-pinocarveol, camphor, bornyl acetate, alpha-ylangene, beta-elemene, beta-acoradiene, elemol, beta-bisabolene, bicyclo[4.4.0]dec-1-en-2-isopropyl-5-methyl-9-methylene, delta-cadinene, plaustrol; *Berries*—Alpha-thujene, alpha-phellandrene, alpha-fenchene, sabinene, terpinen-4-ol, beta-cedrene, gamma-terpinene, trans-pinocarveol, camphor, pinocamphone ($< 0.4\%$), isopinocamphone ($< 0.5\%$), bornyl acetate, alpha-copaene, (E)-beta-farnesene, beta-acoradiene, beta-bisabolene, beta-pinene, terpinyl acetate

**PREFERRED COMPOSITION FOR CLINICAL USE:**

| Constituent | Needles | Berries |
|---|---|---|
| **Alpha-Pinene** | 25%–38% | 35%–55% |
| **Alpha-Cedrol** | 10%–20% | 5%–10% |
| **Delta-3-Carene** | 6%–15% | 9%–15% |
| **Limonene** | 3%–8% | 1%–5% |
| **Beta-Caryophyllene** | 3%–8% | 2%–5% |
| **Alpha-Terpinolene** | 2%–5% | 2%–5% |
| **Myrcene** | 2%–5% | 2%–5% |
| **Sabinene** | 0.5%–5% | 2%–12% |

**REPORTED THERAPEUTIC PROPERTIES:** Anticancer, antibacterial, antifungal, antiviral, **antiseptic**, diuretic, **supports respiratory function**, ease cough, astringent, moisturizes the skin, relieves chronic skin conditions, aids digestion, balances menstruation, stops excess bleeding, reduces constipation, insecticide, sedating, stress management

**CAUTIONS:**
■ None currently known.

**SELECTED EVIDENCE:**
☐ *In vitro* research demonstrates that Oriental arborvitae prevents the spread of melanoma and kidney cancer cells.[6593] Eleven sesquiterpenes and sesquiterpenoid constituents (3α-methoxy-4α-epoxythujopsane; δ3,15-4β-epoxythujopsene; δ3,4-thujopsen-2,15-diol; thujopsadiene; 3α-hydroxy-4-thujopsene; 3β-hydroxy-4-thujopsene; mayurone oxide; thujopsen-12-ol; mayurone; thujopsan-2α-ol; and dihydromayurone) isolated from Oriental arborvitae leaf essential oil (methanol extracted) prevented the spread of melanoma cancer cells.[6594] Seven of the eleven constituents prevented the spread of drug-resistant and TNF-resistant ovarian cancer cells. Two constituents (3β-hydroxy-4-thujopsene and mayurone oxide) prevented the spread of lung and colon cancer cells.

☐ Oriental arborvitae leaf essential oil inhibited the plant fungus *Alternaria alternata*, with the study authors determining that alpha-cedrol was the active antifungal constituent.[6595] Oriental arborvitae berry essential oil moderately inhibits *Aspergillus niger, A. fumigatus, Rhizopus oryzae, Fusarium psidi,* and *Curvularia lunate*.[6596]

☐ *In vitro* research demonstrates that Oriental arborvitae berry essential oil remarkably inhibits *S. typhi* and demonstrates moderate to good antibacterial activity against *B. subtilis, Corynaebacterium diphtheriae, S. aureus, Shigella* sp., and *E. coli*.[6597]

☐ The berry essential oil of Oriental arborvitae potently inhibited the SARS coronavirus (SARS-CoV) with a wide safety margin but was inactive against HSV-1 according to *in vitro* research. The SARS-CoV causes severe acute respiratory syndrome (SARS).[6598]

☐ *In vitro* research shows that Oriental arborvitae essential oil is a strong antioxidant.[6599]

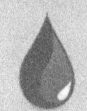

- Oriental arborvitae leaf essential oil is toxic to the cigarette beetle (*Lasioderma serricorne*). The fruit oil was also toxic to the cigarette beetle, but to a lesser degree.[6600] It was also toxic to three stored-product pests: cowpea weevil (*Callosobruchus maculatus* Fab.), rice weevil (*Sitophilus oryzae* L.), and red flour beetle (*Tribolium castaneum* Herbst).[6601]
- Oriental arborvitae leaf essential oil was larvicidal to two mosquito species (*Anopheles stephensi* and *Culex pipiens*).[6602]
- Topical application of Oriental arborvitae essential oil promoted the proliferation of dermal papilla cells (cells that regulate hair follicle development and growth) and hair growth in mice.[6603] At times during the twenty-eight-day study, the hair growth exceeded that of minoxidil.
- Oriental arborvitae leaf essential oil significantly reduced inflammation in multiple rodent models of inflammation.[6604] The oil reduced ear swelling and peritoneal (the membrane that lines the walls of the abdominal cavity) capillary permeability in mice, and granuloma (small area of inflammation) swelling and paw swelling in rats. Furthermore, decreased inflammatory markers (IL-1$\beta$, TNF-$\alpha$) and lung damage was observed, with a simultaneous increase in anti-inflammatory markers (IL-10).
- Thyme, oregano, lemongrass, spearmint, and rosemary essential oils were each inhibited multidrug-resistant foodborne pathogens isolated from raw milk (*Escherichia, Enterobacter, Citrobacter, Proteus, Klebsiella,* and *Staphylococcus*) but were ineffective against *Pseudomonas*.[6605] Thyme was the most active, followed by oregano.
- Evaluation of eight varieties of oregano essential oil—thymol CT, spathulenol CT, gamma-terpinene CT, and para-cymene/gamma-terpinene CT—showed that the thymol CT was the most effective against *Cronobacter sakazakii* (a bacterium frequently found in infant formula).[6606]

# PALMAROSA
## (East Indian Geranium, Rosha Grass)

*Cymbopogon martinii* (Roxb.) J.F. Watson,
*Andropogon martinii* Roxb.

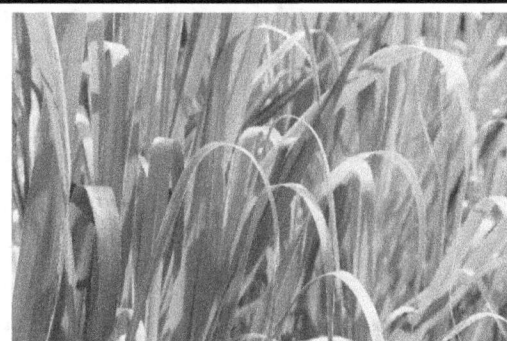

**FAMILY:** Poaceae (Gramineae)
**NOTE:** Middle
**AROMA INTENSITY:** Medium
**AROMA:** Floral, sweet, slightly rose-like
**COMMON EXTRACTION METHOD:** Steam distilled from the leaves
**POSSIBLE SUBSTITUTE OILS:** Thyme (Geraniol CT), citronella, lemongrass, rose, geranium
**BLENDS WELL WITH:** Bergamot, cedarwood, chamomile (Roman), coriander, frankincense, geranium, juniper, lavandin, lavender, lemon, lemongrass, lime, magnolia, neroli, orange, patchouli, petitgrain, rose, rosemary, sandalwood, spikenard, ylang ylang
**SUBCELLULAR LOCALIZATION | EPIGENETIC INFLUENCE:** Currently unknown | Currently unknown
**RECOMMENDED DILUTION RANGE:** 3%–50%; neat for limited conditions

**PRIMARY CONSTITUENTS:**[6607,6608,6609,6610,6611]

|  |  |
| --- | --- |
| Geraniol | 63.5%–83.8% |
| Geranyl Acetate | 2.3%–14.8% |
| (E)-Beta-Ocimene | 1.2%–4.3% |
| (E,Z)-Farnesol | 1.6%–3.4% |
| Linalool | 0.8%–2.6% |
| Geranial | 0.0%–2.1% |

**OTHER CONSTITUENTS:** Limonene, beta-caryophyllene, geranyl hexanoate

**PREFERRED COMPOSITION FOR CLINICAL USE:**

| Constituent | |
| --- | --- |
| **Geraniol** | 70%–85% |
| **Geranyl Acetate** | 5%–18% |
| **Linalool** | 1%–5% |
| **(E)-Beta-Ocimene** | 1%–4% |

| Beta-Caryophyllene | 0.5%–3% |
|---|---|
| Geranial | 0.1%–3% |
| Farnesol (E,Z) or (E,E) | 0.1%–2% |
| Limonene | tr–2% |
| Neral | 0%–2% |

**REPORTED THERAPEUTIC PROPERTIES:** Antiseptic, antibacterial, antiviral, aids digestion, reduces fever, **moisturizes and tones skin**, aids circulation, **promotes cellular growth and regeneration**, relieves skin conditions, wound healing (especially cracks), relaxes muscles, helps reduce the appearance of blemishes, uplifting, reduces anxiety, antidepressant, stress management, supports one through change, calms the mind, combats jealous and possessive feelings

**CAUTIONS:**

■ May moderately interfere with enzymes responsible for metabolizing medications (NSAIDs, proton-pump inhibitors, acetaminophen, antiepileptics, immune modulators, blood-sugar medications, blood pressure medications, antidepressants, antipsychotics, diabetic medications, antihistamines, antibiotics, and anesthetics).[6612]

■ May interact with diabetes medications and cause low blood sugar based on significant geraniol content.[6613,6614]

■ May interact with antibiotics and/or antifungals and possibly increase their effectiveness based on significant geraniol content.[6615]

■ Dilution recommended for topical application. Geraniol is metabolized and autoxidized into metabolites like geranial and neral, and may cause sensitization and irritation when applied topically.[6616]

**SELECTED EVIDENCE:**

☐ Inhalation of palmarosa increases glutathione peroxides levels (enzymes responsible for protecting the body from damage caused by hydroperoxide free radicals) and catalase (an enzyme responsible for breaking down hydrogen peroxide produced by cells into oxygen and water) in rats, which reduces oxidative stress.[6617] This activity protects the liver against toxicity. Interestingly, the same researchers found that if geraniol is isolated from palmarosa it increases creatinine and alanine aminotransferase levels in the blood, which suggests that geraniol may cause liver toxicity if not buffered by the other constituents in palmarosa.

☐ *In vitro* research suggests that palmarosa reduces inflammation by modulating the immune response and increases the production of interleukin-10 (an anti-inflammatory cytokine).[6618]

☐ Palmarosa oil relieves pain by activating the TRPV1 receptor (a molecular sensor that detects painful sensations, and when activated triggers pathways that reduce pain caused by heat and inflammation) *in vitro*.[6619]

☐ Palmarosa reduces the production of proinflammatory cytokines (TNF-alpha, IL-1 Beta, and IL-8), and is a potent antioxidant according to *in vitro* research.[6620,6621]

☐ *In silico* research suggests that palmarosa inhibits elastase activity (an enzyme involved in the breakdown of elastin and a causal factor in lung connective tissue diseases, disruption of the body's ability to kill pathogens, and delayed wound healing).[6622] The researchers concluded that topical administration may be beneficial for bullous pemphigoid (a skin condition that causes the formation of large blisters) and pulmonary emphysema (a chronic lung condition characterized by enlargement of the air sacs in the lungs).

☐ Animal research concluded that the oral administration of palmarosa (50 to 100 mg/kg) significantly prevented damage to neurons caused by a loss of and subsequent return of blood supply (ischemia/reperfusion) to the brain.[6623] Palmarosa decreased lipid peroxidation and returned superoxide dismutase, catalase, total thiols (organic constituents that contain a sulfur and hydrogen atom that play a significant role in the body's defense mechanisms against reactive oxygen species), and reduced glutathione levels to normal.

☐ Animal and *in vitro* research suggests that the topical application of palmarosa may be an effective alternative treatment to synthetic drugs for the topical treatment of dermatophytes (fungi that require keratin for growth and infect the skin, hair, and nails).[6624]

☐ Geraniol, the main constituent in palmarosa, may reverse diabetic neuropathy by balancing biochemicals involved in neuropathy (like dopamine levels).[6625]

☐ A foot bath (107°F water) with salts and either oregano, thyme, cinnamon bark, lemongrass, clove, palmarosa, peppermint, lavender, or geranium significantly reduced fungi associated with athlete's foot *in vitro*.[6626]

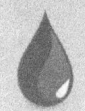

- Palmarosa oil demonstrated significant activity against *E. coli in vitro*.[6627]

- *In vitro* research suggests that palmarosa oil inhibits *E. coli, S. aureus, P. acnes, C. albicans, P. putida,* and *P. ovale*.[6628,6629,6630,6631] One *in vitro* study concluded that palmarosa was more effective than amphotericin B (a drug used to treat fungal infections) at inhibiting *C. albicans*.[6632]

- Palmarosa prevents the spread, growth of, and production of mycotoxins by Aspergillus spores better than synthetic preservatives created for the same purpose *in vitro*.[6633] It also reduced the production of the mycotoxin zearalenone by *Fusarium* species.[6634] Zearalenone is an endocrine-disrupting toxin that attaches to estrogen receptors (ERalpha, ERbeta) in a similar manner to 17beta-estradiol (naturally produced estrogen) and both it and its metabolites (beta-zearalenol, alpha-zearalenol) alter hormone production (progesterone, estradiol, testosterone, and cortisol).[6635,6636,6637]

- The main constituent in palmarosa, geraniol, blocks both calcium and potassium channels of the heart, which may make it useful for arrhythmia.[6638]

- *In vitro* research demonstrates that palmarosa essential oil is a potent antioxidant.[6639]

- Palmarosa essential oil demonstrated 99%–100% efficacy against the *Rhipicephalus microplus* tick at concentrations ranging from 1% to 10%.[6640]

- Several essential oils listed in order of efficacy killed the itch mite (*Sarcoptes scabiei*) that burrows into the skin and causes scabies during direct contact (clove > palmarosa > geranium > tea tree > lavender > manuka > petitgrain > eucalyptus > Japanese cedarwood) with the mites and when used as a fumigant (tea tree > clove > eucalyptus > lavender > palmarosa > geranium > Japanese cedarwood > petitgrain > manuka).[6641]

- A laboratory and clinical study demonstrated that vaginal pessaries with cocoa butter, calendula extract and either geranium and palmarosa or lavender and Roman chamomile essential oils reduced symptoms of vaginal atrophy (muscle weakness/wasting) in breast cancer survivors.[6642]

- *Borrelia burgdorferi* is a diderm bacteria responsible for Lyme disease in the United States. Of thirty-five essential oils screened, garlic, allspice, cumin, palmarosa, myrrh, ginger lily, amyris, thyme, may chang, and lemon eucalyptus each demonstrated excellent activity against *Borrelia burgdorferi*.[6643] Garlic (19% diallyl disulfide), allspice CT eugenol, and myrrh (38% curzerene) were the most active essential oils.

- Although the human skin contains bacteria belonging to *Staphylococcus, Cutibacterium, Micrococcus,* and *Corynebacterium* families, the skin of the face is about 50% *Cutibacterium* (formerly *Propionibacterium*) *acnes*, which is associated with acne. Palmarosa essential oil inhibited *C. acnes* without cytotoxic effects to keratinocytes (epidermal cells that produce keratin).[6644]

- Palmarosa essential oil demonstrated broad-spectrum antimicrobial activity against pathogens associated with skin infections, with complete inhibition of *Trichophyton mentagrophytes* and *Trichophyton rubrum* at concentrations above 1% of oil and *Microsporum canis* and *Trichophyton verrucosum* at a concentration of 4% oil.[6645] Neither a hydrophilic nor macrogol blend ointment containing 5% palmarosa oil caused skin sensitization in guinea pigs.

- *In vitro* research showed that cinnamon bark, oregano, thyme CT thymol, lemongrass (*C. flexuosus*), allspice, palmarosa, and amyris all significantly inhibited *S. aureus* in the stationary phase, which is when the size of a bacterial population remains constant, even though some cells continue to divide and others begin to die.[6646]

- Palmarosa essential oil demonstrated the ability to disrupt biofilm formation by oral pathogens (*S. mitis, S. sanguinis,* and *E. faecalis*) in an experimental model of root canals.[6647] Thyme essential oil also showed antibiofilm activity, which was 2-fold higher than the control (1.5% sodium hypochlorite). Successive irrigations with palmarosa was more efficient than the control as well.

- Palmarosa essential oil demonstrated anticandida activity against *C. albicans* and synergized the effects of fluconazole against candida.[6648]

- Cinnamon bark, palmarosa, and ginger essential oil each exhibited good antioxidant activity in the DPPH, ABTS and FRAP assays, with cinnamon being the most effective. Additionally, the oils inhibited the growth of *Fusarium verticillioides* and reduced its production of mycotoxins (fumonisin B1 and B2).[6649] Cinnamon bark and palmarosa were the most effective against *Fusarium verticillioides*.

- Lemongrass (*C. flexuosus*), citronella (*C. winterianus*), and palmarosa essential oil each exhibited activity against MRSA, with the strongest activity observed with lemongrass oil.[6650] Isolated citronellol, citral, and geraniol were also active, with the efficacy of citronellol exceeding whole oils.

# PALO SANTO
## (Holy Wood, Sacred Wood, Anthony's Wood)

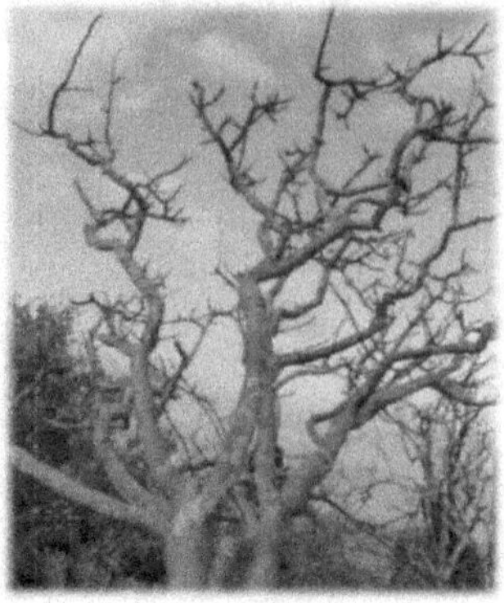

*Bursera graveolens* (Kunth) Triana & Planch.

**FAMILY:** Burseraceae
**NOTE:** Middle
**AROMA INTENSITY:** Strong
**AROMA:** Woody, sharp, citrusy, slightly sweet
**COMMON EXTRACTION METHOD:** Steam distilled from the wood or leaves
**POSSIBLE SUBSTITUTE OILS:** Frankincense
**BLENDS WELL WITH:** Balsam fir, black pepper, blue spruce, clary sage, copaiba, cypress, frankincense, lavender, melissa, myrrh, rose, sandalwood, spruce (black), vetiver, silver fir, white fir
**SUBCELLULAR LOCALIZATION | EPIGENETIC INFLUENCE:** Currently unknown | Currently unknown
**RECOMMENDED DILUTION RANGE:** 5%–Neat

**PRIMARY CONSTITUENTS:**[6651,6652,6653,6654]

| *Wood* | | *Leaves, Aerial Parts* | |
|---|---|---|---|
| Limonene | 60.7%–68.7% | Limonene | 26.5%–30.7% |
| Menthofuran | 0.0%–13.4% | (E)-Beta-Ocimene | 13.0%–20.8% |
| Alpha-Terpineol | 5.8%–10.9% | Beta-Elemene | 11.3%–14.1% |
| Gamma-Terpineol | 0.0%–8.7% | Menthofuran | 0.0%–5.1% |
| Germacrene D | 0.0%–2.1% | Germacrene A | 0.0%–3.9% |

**OTHER CONSTITUENTS:** Beta-cymene, para-cymene, alpha-farnesene, trans-pinocarveol, carvone, pulegone, gamma-muurolene, piperitol, trans-carveol

**PREFERRED COMPOSITION FOR CLINICAL USE:**

| *Constituent* | *Wood* |
|---|---|
| **Limonene** | 60%–72% |
| **Alpha-Terpineol** | 7%–15% |
| **Menthofuran** | 5%–15% |
| **Para-Cymene** | 0.1%–2% |
| **Carvone** | 0.1%–2% |
| **Germacrene D** | 0.1%–2% |

**REPORTED THERAPEUTIC PROPERTIES: Analgesic, anti-inflammatory**, antispasmodic, antibacterial, antiseptic, **anticancer**, antioxidant, immune stimulant, eases cough, relieves menstrual pain, antiallergenic, **decongestant**, expectorant, **supports respiratory function**, encourages calm, **relieves anxiety, stress management**, relaxing, promotes focus, enhances creativity, grounding, enhances meditation

**CAUTIONS:**

■ Oral caution for long-term use (palo santo wood). Large doses of menthofuran (greater than 5 mL) and pulegone can be toxic to the liver.[6655,6656,6657,6658] However, limonene is considered nontoxic (even at high doses—a single acute dose of 20 g) and no animal or human toxicity studies for palo santo oil have been reported as of this writing.[6659] Based on this information it is recommended that palo santo be used cautiously orally until safety studies are completed. Limit oral consumption to no more than 5 drops of palo santo per day for up to twenty-one days with a seven-day break afterwards, or no more than 3 drops daily for long-term use.

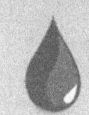

**SELECTED EVIDENCE:**

☐ Animal and *in vitro* research concluded that palo santo oil prevents the growth of breast tumor cells.[6660,6661]

☐ A topical gel with amphotericin B and palo santo essential oil inhibited *C. albicans*, *C. glabrata*, and *C. parapsilosis* and performed well in the *ex vivo* permeation study in human skin.[6662] The incorporation of palo santo oil into the gel proved to improve permeation and retention suggesting the gel is a promising candidate for cutaneous candidiasis.

---

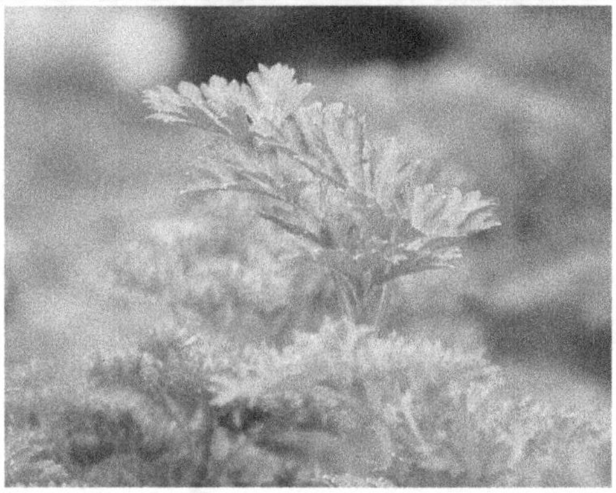

# PARSLEY
## (Garden Parsley)

*Petroselinum crispum* (Mill.) Nyman ex A.W. Hill, *P. sativum* Hoffm., *P. hortense* Hoffm., *P. vulgare* Lagasca, *Apium petroselinum* L., *Carum petroselinum* (L.) Benth. & Hook. f.

**FAMILY:** Apiaceae (Umbilliferae)
**NOTE:** Middle
**AROMA INTENSITY:** Medium
**AROMA:** Herbaceous, spicy, slightly woody
**COMMON EXTRACTION METHOD:** Steam distilled from the seeds or leaves (most commercial oil samples are obtained from the seeds or the whole herb harvested at seed formation)
**POSSIBLE SUBSTITUTE OILS:** Nutmeg, dill seed
**BLENDS WELL WITH:** Anise, bay laurel, black pepper, clary sage, coriander, dill seed, ginger, neroli, orange, petitgrain, rose, tangerine, tea tree, ylang ylang
**SUBCELLULAR LOCALIZATION | EPIGENETIC INFLUENCE:** Currently unknown | Currently unknown
**RECOMMENDED DILUTION RANGE:** 1.5%–20%

**PRIMARY CONSTITUENTS:**[6663,6664,6665,6666,6667,6668,6669,6670]

*Seeds*

| | |
|---|---|
| Myristicin | 12.4%–42.2% |
| Alpha-Pinene | 26.0%–40.6% |
| Beta-Pinene | 18.6%–27.2% |
| 1-Allyl-2,3,4,5-Tetramethoxybenzene | 2.0%–12.8% |
| Parsley Apiol | 0.1%–10.2% |
| Beta-Phellandrene | 4.4%–8.8% |

*Leaves—1,3,8-Para-Menthatriene CT*

| | |
|---|---|
| 1,3,8-Para-Menthatriene | 29.3%–64.7% |
| Beta-Phellandrene | 3.1%–29.8% |
| Parsley Apiol | 0.0%–22.1% |
| Beta-Myrcene | 2.9%–16.3% |
| Alpha-Terpinolene | 2.1%–13.9% |
| Alpha-Para-Dimethylstyrene | 2.1%–13.9% |
| Myristicin | 0.0%–12.2% |

*Leaves—Myristicin CT*

| | |
|---|---|
| Myristicin | 12.6%–60.5% |
| Beta-Phellandrene | 6.2%–35.9% |
| 1,3,8-Para-Menthatriene | 5.4%–24.2% |
| Para-Cymene | 0.4%–18.9% |
| Parsley Apiol | 0.1%–13.5% |
| Alpha-Terpinolene | 0.8%–10.3% |
| Tricyclene | 0.0%–8.8% |
| Beta-Myrcene | 2.8%–8.7% |
| Alpha-Phellandrene | 0.3%–8.7% |

*Whole Plant*

| | |
|---|---|
| Myristicin | 32.8%–36.2% |
| Parsley Apiol | 17.5%–21.0% |
| Alpha-Pinene | 15.5%–16.6% |
| Beta-Pinene | 10.4%–11.6% |
| 1-Allyl-2,3,4,5-Tetramethoxybenzene | 6.5%–10.0% |
| Limonene | 0.6%–4.8% |
| Beta-Phellandrene | 0.0%–4.2% |
| Elemicin | 2.7%–4.1% |

**OTHER CONSTITUENTS:** *Seeds*—beta-myrcene, myrtenal, elemicin; *Leaves, Myristicin CT*—alpha-pinene, limonene, para-cymenene, alpha-terpineol, (E,E)-decadienal, 2,5-dimethoxy-p-cymene, 2,5-dimethyl-p-cymene, germacrene D, alpha-bergaptene, alpha-muurolene, elemicin; *Leaves, 1,3,8-Para-Menthatriene CT*—alpha-pinene, beta-pinene, alpha-phellandrene, alpha-terpinene, thymol; *Whole plant*—sabinene, carotol, beta-myrcene

**PREFERRED COMPOSITION FOR CLINICAL USE:**

| Constituent | Seed | Whole Plant |
|---|---|---|
| **Myristicin** | 25%–55% | 25%–45% |
| **Alpha-Pinene** | 10%–35% | 10%–20% |
| **Beta-Pinene** | 5%–20% | 10%–20% |
| **Apiole** | 4%–10% | 15%–35% |
| **1-Allyl-2,3,4,5-Tetramethoxybenzene** (6-Methoxyelemicin) | 1%–12% | 1%–12% |
| **Elemecin** | 1%–12% | 1%–12% |
| **Limonene** | – | 1%–7% |

**REPORTED THERAPEUTIC PROPERTIES:** Antibacterial, antifungal, antimicrobial, antiseptic, antioxidant, antiallergic, astringent, analgesic, anti-inflammatory, antiarthritic, antirheumatic, anticancer, aids digestion, expels excess gas, **diuretic**, reduces fever, aids detoxification, balances blood pressure, reduces constipation, eases cough, **balances blood sugar levels**, wound healing, soothes hemorrhoids, relieves swollen breasts, soothes blisters, stimulates uterus function and menstruation, relieves painful menstruation, cleanses the urinary tract, **strengthens blood vessels**, reduces cellulitis, **immune modulator**, increases libido, insecticide, combats paranoia, reduces fear, encourages self-esteem and self-love

**CAUTIONS:**

■ Avoid with children under age twelve. Parsley seed essential oil may contain large quantities of apiol or myristicin, which may cause kidney or liver toxicity, abnormal quantities of blood components (blood dyscrasias), dizziness, or hallucinations.[6671,6672,6673,6674,6675]

■ Avoid during pregnancy and lactation due to the abortive properties (parsley apiol causes contractions and necrosis of placental tissue and has been used for decades to end unwanted pregnancies) and high toxicity (several cases of acute poisoning or death have been reported after ingestion of varying amounts of apiol in single or daily doses) of apiol.[6676,6677,6678,6679,6680,6681,6682] Essential oils with high myristicin content should also be used cautiously during pregnancy due to decreased male fertility and chromosomal damage reported in animal studies using extremely high doses of nutmeg (also high in myristicin content).[6683] Animal research suggests that higher doses of myristicin (0.01 mL/kg every two days while nursing, and 0.001 to 10 mg while pregnant) taken orally during pregnancy and while nursing may cause liver toxicity in offspring born to the mother and increase the offspring's risk of liver cancer.[6684]

■ Avoid oral consumption due to high toxicity of apiol, reported poisonings by apiol, and deaths reported after ingestion of significant amounts of apiol.[6685,6686,6687,6688,6689,6690] Also, myristicin is believed to be at least partially responsible for the psychotropic (a substance capable of affecting the mind, emotions, and behavior) effects of nutmeg, although it is likely a combination of more than one component of nutmeg oil that produces this effect. Large doses of nutmeg with high myristicin content (5 g in a single dose), and long-term use of as few as 120 mg of the whole herb daily may produce a psychotropic (hallucinations, anxiety, fear, and delusions) effect in adults.[6691,6692] In addition, scientists suspect nutmeg may be chemically modified once ingested to amphetamine-like constituents, though this has not been proven conclusively.[6693]

■ May interact with psychotropic medications—medications prescribed for anxiety, depression, schizophrenia, mania, obsessive-compulsive disorder, ADHD, and bipolar disorder.[6694,6695]

■ May interact with monoamine oxidase inhibitors (MAOIs)—medications prescribed for the treatment of depression.[6696]

■ May interact with diabetic medications and produce an additive effect that may cause low blood sugar levels based on animal research using herbal extracts (herbal extracts contain volatile components like apiol and myristicin).[6697,6698,6699]

■ *Leaves (both CTs)*: May interact with anticholinergic (drugs used for asthma, incontinence, gastrointestinal cramps, muscular spasms, depression, and sleep disorders) and cholinergic medications (drugs used to reduce urinary retention, diagnose myasthenia gravis, and for glaucoma) based on AChE inhibitory activity of beta-phellandrene.[6700]

■ May interact with diuretic medications and increase their diuretic effects based on animal and *in vitro* research that suggests that the herbal extract influences electrolyte (sodium and potassium) balance and increases the production and excretion of urine.[6701,6702]

■ May interfere with enzymes responsible for metabolizing medications (NSAIDs, proton-pump inhibitors, acetaminophen, antiepileptics, immune modulators, blood-sugar medications, blood pressure medications,

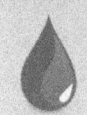

antidepressants, antipsychotics, diabetic medications, antihistamines, antibiotics, and anesthetics).[6703,6704,6705,6706,6707,6708,6709]

■ Avoid in those with a compromised liver and kidneys due to potential of apiol or myristicin to cause kidney or liver damage and toxicity.[6710,6711,6712,6713,6714]

■ Photosensitzing due to the presence of psoralen, bergapten, oxypeucedanin, isoimponellin, and xanthotixin.[6715] Avoid UV rays for at least twelve hours following topical application. Interestingly, no phototoxic effects were reported when parsley essential oil was tested undiluted (neat) on animals.[6716]

### SELECTED EVIDENCE:

☐ Parsley seed essential oil inhibits the production of malondialdehyde (MDA) from squalene (a common lipid produced by skin cells) after exposure to UV radiation by 67%, which was greater than rose (46%) and celery seed (23%).[6717] MDA may damage and alter DNA, contributing to cancer and other genetic diseases.[6718]

☐ Parsley leaf essential oil inhibits and eradicates Vibrio strains (gram-negative bacteria *in vitro*, some of which are pathogenic—like *V. cholerae* serotype 01 El Tor N16961 that causes pandemic cholera, and several species that cause gastroenteritis).[6719] The whole plant essential oil moderately inhibits *Listeria innocua* (a harmless gram-positive bacterium).[6720] The leaf essential oil (1,3,8-Para-Menthatriene CT) strongly inhibited *Staphylococcus aureus* and *Salmonella tryphimurium*, and moderately inhibited *E. coli*.[6721] Parsley essential oil also inhibited *Alcaligenes faecalis, Providencia rettgeri, Serratia marcescens, Klebsiella oxytoca, Staphylococcus aureus, Shigella dysenteriae*, and *Listeria monocytogenes*, with greater antimicrobial activity against gram-positive bacteria versus gram-negative bacteria.[6722] Another study found that parsley seed essential oil mildly inhibits several bacteria that cause foodborne illness and food spoilage (*Listeria* spp., *Staphylococcus aureus, Lactobacillus* spp., *Bacillus cereus, Salmonella, Enterobacter* spp., *Escherichia coli*, and *Pseudomonas* spp.) again with greater activity on gram-positive bacteria.[6723] Parsley oil (aerial parts) inhibited the bacteria (*S. aureus, L. monocytogenes*, and *Salmonella enterica*) and fungi (*Penicillium ochrochloron* and *Trichoderma viride*) as efficiently or more efficiently than antibiotic and antifungal drugs.[6724] Parsley essential oil (whole plant) inhibits *Listeria innocua*.[6725]

☐ *In vitro* research concluded that parsley essential oil (whole plant) possesses moderate antioxidant properties, whereas apiol demonstrates stronger antioxidant properties alone.[6726,6727,6728] The seed essential oil also demonstrates antioxidant activity.[6729]

☐ Parsley essential oil suppresses humoral and cellular immune responses by inhibiting the function of splenocytes and macrophages and reduces the production of nitric oxide, which suggests it may be beneficial for unwanted immune responses (allergies, autoimmune diseases, autoinflammatory, and transplant rejections).[6730,6731]

☐ Parsley essential oil is a mild inhibitor of the 5-LOX enzyme according to *in vitro* research.[6732] The 5-LOX enzyme converts arachidonic acid to leukotrienes, increasing inflammation and allergic reactions, and is associated with chronic degenerative inflammatory diseases and cancer.

☐ Parsley essential oil is larvicidal to the Asian tiger mosquito (*Aedes albopictus*) and kills adults and larvae of pyrethroid-resistant and pyrethroid-susceptible *Ae. aegytpi* mosquitoes.[6733,6734]

☐ A study concluded that parsley seed essential oil is an attractive alternative option for control of mosquitoes due to its larvicidal activity against pyrethroid-resistant *Ae. aegypti* mosquitoes and activity against mosquito acetylcholinesterase (AChE) and mixed-function oxidases (MFO).[6735]

☐ Parsley Co2 aromatic extract (82.1% apiole and 11.4% myristicin) exhibited activity on acetylcholinesterase (AChE), tyrosinase, and alpha-glucosidase, suggesting it may be helpful for cognition, skin brightening, and diabetes.[6736] It was inactive in the ABTS antioxidant assay.

☐ Dill, cumin, and parsley were each toxic to the maize weevil (*Sitophilus zeamais*) in the contact assay.[6737] The same researchers noted that each of the oils and fennel also repelled the insect. Carvone (fumigant and contact) and cuminaldehyde were the most active isolated constituents for toxicity and cuminaldehyde, carvone, and estragole the most active isolated constituents for repellents.

☐ A parsley essential oil with thymol as its main constituent (74.6%) was larvicidal to *Ae. aegypti* mosquitoes—both pyrethroid-susceptible and resistant strains.[6738] In addition, the researchers found that parsley oil (as well as thymol, para-cymene, and gamma-terpinene) significantly improved the efficacy of the pesticides temephos and deltamethrin.

☐ Researchers evaluated the activities of essential oils from three exotic and two endemic plants from Mauritius. Parsley essential oil exhibited antiamylase (prevents starch from being absorbed and influences

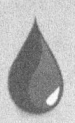

blood sugar levels) and antityrosinase (skin brightening) activity in laboratory research.[6739] The oil also displayed good antioxidant activity in the DPPH and ABTS assays. Analysis of isolated constituents from the five oils tested showed that 1,8-cineole had the strongest affinity with butyrylcholinesterase, amylase, and tyrosinase; myristicin and beta-pinene with acetylcholinesterase; and beta-pinene with glucosidase(antidiabetic).

☐ Ravintsara CT 1,8-cineole selectively inhibited AChE (anti-Alzheimer's activity) and inhibited tyrosinase (skin brightening activity). The oil also showed moderate antioxidant activity in the DPPH and ABTS assays.[6740]

☐ Carbon tetrachloride is an organic compound that was previously used in refrigerants, cleaning products, and fire extinguishers that has since been discontinued because of safety and environmental concerns. Exposure to high concentration of carbon tetrachloride can harm the central nervous system, liver, kidneys, thyroid, and reproductive organs. Administration of carbon tetrachloride to male mice caused decreased antioxidant enzyme activity (catalase, superoxide dismutase), increased lipid peroxidation and malondialdehyde levels, significantly reduced hormone levels (testosterone, follicle-stimulating hormone, luteinizing hormone, thyroid-stimulating hormone, and thyroid hormones—T3, fT3, T4, fT4), altered sperm health, and caused irregular-shaped seminiferous tubules with prominent swelling. Intragastric administration of parsley essential oil (0.5 mL/kg body weight for four weeks) significantly reduced testicular and thyroid harm caused by oxidative stress and improved testosterone, FSH, LH, T3, fT3, T4, and fT4 levels.[6741] The research suggests that parsley oil may protect against hypogonadism by protecting against oxidative stress and preserving healthy thyroid function.

☐ Parsley essential oil with myristicin as the major constituent inhibited *C. albicans, S. aureus,* and *B. subtilis* at lower concentrations, and *E. coli* and *K. pneumoniae* at higher concentrations.[6742] The oil also showed excellent anti-inflammatory activity in the albumin and trypsin assays, which was comparable in efficacy to ibuprofen. Parsley oil exhibited weak antioxidant activity in the DPPH and FeCl3 assays when compared to ascorbic acid. Computer-based molecular docking studies showed that myristicin has binding affinity for target proteins involved in antimicrobial, antioxidant, and anti-inflammatory (COX-2 and COX-1) activity.

☐ Parsley herb essential oil inhibited multiple fungi (*A. flavus, A. ochraceus, G. candidum, M. circinelloides,* and *P. roqueforti*) but was inactive against bacteria (*E. faecalis, L. innocua,* and *S. aureus*).[6743]

☐ Dysbiosis can lead to elevated levels of trimethylamine-N-oxide (TMAO)—a compound associated with chronic disease, including cardiovascular disease and diabetes. Ingestion of summer savory, parsley, or rosemary essential oil emulsions with L-carnitine improved the gut microbiome (primarily *Lactobacillus* genus bacteria), decreased TMAO levels, and increased short-chain fatty acids in mouse models of ischemic heart disease and type 2 diabetes.[6744] Additionally, rosemary and parsley decreased proinflammatory cytokines, while savory increased chemokines (signaling proteins crucial for the migration of white blood cells during normal inflammatory processes to maintain homeostasis). The essential oil emulsions acted as prebiotics to improve gut microbiome and reduce the risk of cardiovascular and metabolic disorders.

# PATCHOULI

*Pogostemon cablin* (Blanco) Benth., *P. patchouli* Pellet

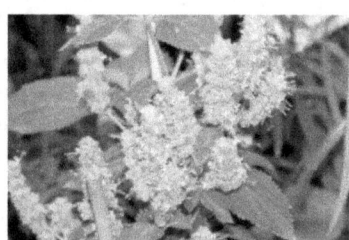

**FAMILY:** Lamiaceae (Labiatae)
**NOTE:** Middle
**AROMA INTENSITY:** Medium
**AROMA:** Rich, herbaceous, musky, earthy, spicy
**COMMON EXTRACTION METHOD:** Steam distilled from the leaves; may be distilled from the stems also (usually high in pogostone)
**POSSIBLE SUBSTITUTE OILS:** Spikenard, vetiver
**BLENDS WELL WITH:** Bay laurel, bergamot, black pepper, cajeput, camphor, cardamom, carrot seed, cedarwood, chamomile (German, Roman), cinnamon, clary sage, clove, eucalyptus, frankincense, geranium, ginger, lavender, lemongrass, myrrh, neroli, pine, orange, rose, sandalwood, Spanish sage, spikenard, vetiver
**SUBCELLULAR LOCALIZATION | EPIGENETIC INFLUENCE:** Cytoplasm | Currently unknown
**RECOMMENDED DILUTION RANGE:** 5%–Neat

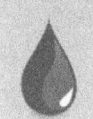

**PRIMARY CONSTITUENTS:**[6745,6746,6747,6748,6749,6750,6751,6752]

*Indonesian, Malaysian, Vietnamese*

| | |
|---|---|
| Patchoulol | 37.8%–68.0% |
| Alpha-Bulnesene (Delta-Guaiene) | 6.8%–14.7% |
| Alpha-Guaiene | 4.3%–13.4% |
| Alpha-Patchoulene | 1.8%–8.0% |
| Seychellene | 3.7%–7.5% |
| Pogostol | 3.7%–5.5% |

*Chinese*

| | |
|---|---|
| Patchoulol | 22.9%–78.2% |
| Alpha-Guaiene | 1.7%–21.5% |
| Pogostone | 6.0%–32.7% |
| Alpha-Bulnesene (Delta-Guaiene) | 0.9%–11.8% |
| Seychellene | 0.0%–9.6% |
| Alpha-Patchoulene | 0.0%–9.1% |
| Caryophyllene | 0.5%–6.8% |
| Beta-Patchoulene | 0.0%–5.8% |

*Brazilian*

| | |
|---|---|
| Patchoulol | 36.6%–70.7% |
| Alpha-Bulnesene (Delta-Guaiene) | 6.9%–55.1% |
| Alpha-Guaiene | 2.9%–12.0% |
| Alpha-Patchoulene | 5.2%–6.7% |

Note: Patchouli essential oil may be labeled as light or dark. Although both are steam distilled from the *Pogostemon cablin* plant, the container in which the patchouli plant is distilled determines the type of oil produced. Use of a stainless steel container produces a light patchouli oil that is thin and golden brown. Distillation in cast iron containers (more traditional) produces an oil that is thick and a rich brown in color with more depth of aroma. It should be noted that some suppliers do not distinguish light and dark patchouli oils based on the contianer it is distilled in but rather based on aroma or color alone.

**OTHER CONSTITUENTS:** 1-octen-3-ol, beta-patchoulene, trans-caryophyllene, gamma-patchoulene, dihydro-aromadendrene, trans-beta-guaiene, beta-copaen-4-alpha-ol

**PREFERRED COMPOSITION FOR CLINICAL USE:**

| Constituent | Ind/Mal/Viet. | Chinese |
|---|---|---|
| **Patchoulol** | 30%–40% | 45%–65% |
| **Alpha-Bulnesene** | 10%–20% | 5%–15% |
| **Alpha-Guaiene** | 8%–18% | 4%–12% |
| **Seychellene** | 4%–10% | 2%–5% |
| **Alpha-Patchoulene** | 3%–9% | 0%–5% |
| **Beta-Caryophyllene** | 2%–5% | 0.1%–3% |
| **Aciphyllene (Guaia-4,11-diene)** | 1%–5% | – |
| **Pogostol** | 0.1%–5% | – |
| **Beta-Patchoulene** | 1%–4% | 0.1%–5% |
| **nor-Patchulenol** | 0.1%–2% | – |
| **Pogostone** | < 2% | 8%–25% |
| **Spathulenol** | – | 0.1%–3% |

**REPORTED THERAPEUTIC PROPERTIES:** Antibacterial, anti-inflammatory, **antiseptic**, antiviral, **antifungal**, expels excess gas, decongestant, eases nausea and vomiting, reduces constipation, nervine (calms and soothes the nerves), **circulatory aid**, aids digestion, reduces fever, protects skin from UV-radiation damage, reduces the appearance of blemishes, **nourishes and moisturizes the skin**, regenerative, **soothes skin conditions**, wound healing, stimulating, **antidepressant**, aphrodisiac, promotes clarity of thought, **stress management**, balances overactive minds

**CAUTIONS:**

■ May interact with aspirin, blood pressure, antiplatelet, and anticoagulant medications, and increase the risk of bleeding among people with bleeding disorders based on alpha-bulnesene content.[6753,6754]

**SELECTED EVIDENCE:**

☐ *In vitro* research suggests that patchouli oil exerts anticancer activity by decreasing cell growth and triggering apoptosis in human colorectal cancer cells.[6755]

☐ Patchouli oil prevented the spread of cervical cancer cells *in vitro*.[6756]

☐ Patchouli oil helps decrease inflammation by moderately inhibiting the 5-lipoxygenase (5-LOX) enzyme that is involved in the inflammation response according to *in vitro* research.[6757] Both *in vitro* and animal (oral administration of 100, 200, or 300 mg/kg) research suggests that patchouli essential oil reduces inflammation by decreasing leukocyte recruitment (a key immunological process that allows leukocytes to leave the smallest system of blood vessels and migrate to tissues, which influences inflammation), nitric oxide (NO) production (NO is anti-inflammatory under normal circumstances, but proinflammatory when it is produced in excess), and the number of leukocytes in the microcirculation (a reduced number of leukocytes in microcirculation reduces the inflammatory response by reducing the number of leukocytes available to migrate to tissues).[6758]

☐ Animal research concluded that patchouli oil helps maintain the structural integrity of the skin and prevents damage to the skin caused by UV exposure by enhancing the activity of glutathione peroxidase, superoxide dismutase, and catalase.[6759]

☐ Inhalation of patchouli oil is sedating, particularly if combined with other oils based on animal research.[6760]

☐ Oral administration of patchoulol, a primary constituent in patchouli essential oil, bolsters the body's defenses against the flu by improving the immune response and reducing whole-body and respiratory inflammatory responses according to research with mice.[6761]

☐ Animal research suggests that pogostone (found in Chinese patchouli oil) inhibits *C. albicans* and is a promising candidate for the treatment of *Candida* infections, especially vulvovaginal candidiasis.[6762,6763]

☐ Patchouli essential oil slowed biofilm formation by *S. aureus* and reduced the number of biofilm cells at higher concentrations.[6764]

☐ Oral administration of patchouli oil has a significant immunomodulatory effect in mice and enhances leukocyte and macrophage (key immune cells) activity.[6765,6766]

☐ *In vitro* research concluded that patchouli oil inhibits sixteen strains of common skin bacteria that are associated with foot and armpit odor.[6767]

☐ Patchouli oil helps repel and kill, moths, and dust mites.[6768,6769,6770]

☐ Patchouli essential oil incorporated into silver nanoparticles was toxic to *Aedes albopictus* mosquitoes.[6771]

☐ Animal research demonstrates that rectal administration of 270 mg/kg of body weight of patchouli essential oil relieves the symptoms of inflammatory bowel disease.[6772]

☐ Pogostone from patchouli essential oil demonstrated immunomodulatory activity that may be beneficial for autoimmune and inflammatory disorders due to its ability to regulate inflammatory cytokines and suppress T cell responses. It reduced the release of anti-inflammatory interleukin 10 (IL-10) and pro-inflammatory IL-6 from the stimulated lymphocytes in laboratory research and alleviated T-cell mediated delayed type hypersensitivity responses when administered orally (10, 20, and 40 mg/kg BW) to mice.[6773]

☐ Patchouli essential oil and its nanoformulation demonstrated efficient insecticidal activity and irritability to three species of leaf-cutting ants from the genus Atta.[6774]

☐ *In vitro* examination of sixty essential oils demonstrated that sandalwood (Indian, Australian, and Hawaiian), melissa, lemongrass (*C. flexuosus*), cilantro, cassia, cinnamon, patchouli, and vetiver essential oils possess remarkable anticancer (two breast cancer cells) and antifungal (*Aspergillus niger, Candida albicans,* and *Cryptococcus neoformans*) activities.[6775]

☐ Pogostone, a major constituent of Chinese patchouli essential oil, showed promising anti-inflammatory activity in an acute lung injury model in mice. Pogostone activated nuclear factor erythroid 2-related factor 2 (Nrf2), inhibited nuclear factor-kappa B (NF-κB), suppressed the levels of inflammatory cytokines [interleukin (IL)-6, IL-1β, and IL-8], and enhanced the expression of antioxidant genes (quinine oxidoreductase 1, glutamate cysteine ligase catalytic subunit, heme oxygenase-1).[6776]

☐ *In vitro* research concluded that patchouli essential oil inhibits *S. aureus, P. aeruginosa,* and *E. coli.*[6777] The same researchers found that the oil was toxic to *Aedes aegypti* mosquito larvae.

☐ Oral administration of patchouli essential oil (40 mg/kg BW) or three of its main components (patchoulol—20 mg/kg; pogostone—20 mg/kg; and beta-patchoulene—20 mg/kg) for fifteen consecutive days positively altered the gut microbiome in mice.[6778] A significant increase in gut microflora diversity and short chain fatty acids-producing bacteria (*Anaerostipes butyraticus, Butyrivibrio fibrisolvens, Clostridium jejuense, Eubacterium uniforme,* and *Lactobacillus lactis*) and simultaneous reduction in abundance of pathogens was observed.

☐ Inhalation of patchouli essential oil reduced food intake, decreased body weight, reduced blood pressure, and improved cholesterol profiles (increased HDL and decreased LDL) in obese rats.[6779]

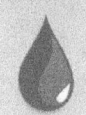

- Patchouli essential oil displayed good antioxidant activity in the DPPH assay and inhibited *Chromobacterium violaceum* and *P. aeruginosa*.[6780] Another study concluded that patchouli essential oil possesses antioxidant activity according to free radical sequestration experiments and inhibits (fungistatic) *F. graminearum*.[6781]

- 5-Fluorouracil is an anticancer drug that can cause intestinal mucositis—ulcers in the lining of the intestines that cause pain and upset stomach. Researchers investigated the ability of oral administration of patchouli essential oil to protect against intestinal mucositis caused by 5-fluorouracil. Oral administration of patchouli significantly reduced the expression of inflammatory cytokines and increased the mRNA expression of ZO-1 and Occludin, which stabilizes the intestinal barrier to protect against ulcers in rats.[6782] The oil also prevented the loss of intestinal mucosal cells by modulating the activity of proteins (reduced: caspase-8, caspase-3, and Bax; increased: Bcl-2). Furthermore, the oil restored water absorption from the gastrointestinal tract, thus alleviating diarrhea.

- Inhalation of patchouli essential oil (0.3%–1%, inhaled for thirty minutes for six to twelve weeks) reduced food intake and body weight in a preclinical model of obesity.[6783] Moreover, HDL increased and LDL and leptin decreased in the rats that inhaled patchouli. Lastly, the patchouli oil reduced systolic blood pressure.

- Three separate patchouli essential oils grown in different regions of India—Northern (alpha-guaiene CT), Southern (patchoulol CT), and North Eastern (patchoulol CT)—each showed significant nematocidal activity against the southern root nematode (*Meloidogyne incognita*).[6784] Molecular docking study revealed that alpha-bulnesene and alpha-guaiene had the highest affinity for three target proteins: acetyl cholinesterase (AChE), odorant response gene-1 (ODR1), and odorant response gene-3 (ODR3). Furthermore, the researchers concluded that the presence of a hydroxyl group is not essential for nematocidal activity, rather this activity depends on a synergistic activity of sesquiterpene hydrocarbons.

- Oral administration of patchouli essential oil, or its isolated constituents patchoulol and pogostone, reduced colon cancer tumor burden in mice. The oil also strengthened the intestinal epithelial barrier (improved intestinal integrity) by increasing Paneth (intestinal cells that secrete peptides and proteins to protect against pathogenic microbes and facilitate probiotic colonization) and goblet cells (intestinal cells that secrete mucus to protect mucous membranes), enhancing tight junctions in the intestine (critical to maintain optimum permeability of the intestines, which is important to prevent allergies), and increasing adhesion molecules (surface proteins that regulate cellular interactions and play an important role in inflammation).[6785] Additionally, improvements in the gut microbiome and presence of short-chain fatty acids and receptors and alterations in immune-inflammatory pathways was observed. Altogether, the research suggests that patchouli oil, patchoulol, or pogostone possesses potent anticancer effects by improving the intestinal microenvironment and positively altering the gut microbiome.

- Patchouli essential oil, and its emulsion, were toxic to the coffee berry borer (*Hypothenemus hampei*) and sublethal exposure of females to the oil reduced reproduction and feeding and modified their behavior.[6786] Based on this, patchouli oil may be an eco-friendly insecticide.

- Patchouli essential oil with a high amount of patchoulol (60.7%) was evaluated in a preclinical model of depression. Five drops of patchouli essential oil were added to 40 mL of distilled water and diffused for five minutes inside a cage before the rats were introduced to the cage.[6787] The results showed that inhaling patchouli oil reduced depressive-like behaviors by increasing dopamine levels in the brain.

- Patchouli essential oil exhibited moderate antimelanoma (murine melanoma) and antioxidant (DPPH assay) properties in laboratory research, and anti-inflammatory activity in a rodent model of arthritis.[6788]

- Patchouli essential oil demonstrated insecticidal activity against cat fleas (*Ctenocephalides felis*).[6789]

*Did you know?*

Due to their complexity, essential oils share many of the same constituents. Limonene is found in high percentage in most citrus oils. Alpha- and beta-pinene are common constituents in needle oils. Some of the most common constituents shared across essential oils are limonene, alpha-pinene, beta-pinene, and gamma-terpinene.

# PENNYROYAL

European: *Mentha pulegium* L.; North American: *M. pulegioides* L.;
Turkish: *Micromeria fruticosa* L., *Satureja fruticosa* (L.) Béguinot

**FAMILY:** Lamiaceae (Labiatae)
**NOTE:** Middle
**AROMA INTENSITY:** Strong
**AROMA:** Minty, fresh, herbaceous
**COMMON EXTRACTION METHOD:** Steam distilled from the flowering plant (aerial parts)
**POSSIBLE SUBSTITUTE OILS:** Spearmint, peppermint, applemint (pulegone CT)
**BLENDS WELL WITH:** Citronella, geranium, lavender, peppermint, rosemary, sage, Spanish sage, spearmint
**SUBCELLULAR LOCALIZATION | EPIGENETIC INFLUENCE:** Currently unknown | Currently unknown
**RECOMMENDED DILUTION RANGE:** 1.0%–5.0%

**PRIMARY CONSTITUENTS:**[6790,6791,6792,6793,6794,6795,6796,6797]

*M. pulegium* (European)

| | |
|---|---|
| (1R)-(+)-Beta-Pulegone | 38.8%–73.4% |
| Menthone | 0.0%–19.2% |
| Piperitenone | 0.0%–16.5% |
| Menthol | 0.0%–13.0% |
| Isomenthone | 0.0%–12.9% |
| 1,8-Cineole | 0.1%–11.1% |
| Piperitone | 0.0%–6.4% |
| Limonene | 0.9%–4.3% |
| Isopulegone | 1.4%–2.5% |
| Beta-Pinene | 0.4%–2.5% |

*M. pulegioides* (North American)

| | |
|---|---|
| (1R)-(+)-Beta-Pulegone | 67.6%–86.7% |
| Menthone | 1.5%–16.0% |
| Isomenthone | 0.8%–8.6% |
| Piperitenone | 0.5%–2.5% |

*Micromeria fruticosa* (Turkish) CT Pulegone

| | |
|---|---|
| (1R)-(+)-Beta-Pulegone | 56.6%–62.9% |
| Isomenthone | 15.2%–19.3% |
| Piperitenone | 7.1%–10.3% |
| Beta-Pinene | 1.2%–3.6% |
| Limonene | 1.2%–3.0% |

*Micromeria fruticosa* (Turkish) CT Isomenthol

| | |
|---|---|
| Isomenthol | 48.1%–67.1% |
| (1R)-(+)-Beta-Pulegone | 0.0%–22.5% |
| Pulegol | 11.1%–15.3% |
| Neoisomenthol | 4.5%–10.0% |
| Beta-Caryophyllene | 5.1%–6.6% |
| Isomenthone | 0.0%–4.9% |

Note: *M. fruticosa* composition varies greatly based on season and developmental stage at time of harvest.[6798] Plants harvested in June have very high pulegone content, declining to about 5% by December. In addition, isomenthol content is low in summer months, steadily increasing to 60% during the fall and winter. *M. fruticosa* also has multiple subspecies that varies greatly in chemical composition. *M. frutitcosa* ssp. *giresunica* contains pulegone (39.6%), menthol (23.3%), and menthone (24.2%) as major constituents. *M. fruticosa* ssp. *serpyllifolia* CT Linalool contains linalool (30.3%), Pulegone (16.7%), p-menthone (10.3%), menthone (7.8%), and 1,8-cineole (6.7%) as major constituents. *M. fruticosa* ssp. *serpyllifolia* CT Piperitenone contains piperitenone (50.6%) and pulegone (29.2%) as major constituents. *M. fruticosa* ssp. *brachycalyx* contains linalool (39.9%), piperitenone (31.9%), pulegone (9.5%), and 1,8-cineole (7.1%) as major constituents. European pennyroyal composition also varies greatly.

**OTHER CONSTITUENTS:** *M. pulegium*—alpha-pinene, sabinene, octan-3-one, octan-3-ol, isopulegole, alpha-humulene, neo-isomenthol, trans-ocimene, camphene, menthofuran; *M. pulegioides*—limonene, 3-octyl-acetate, menthofuran, neoisoomenthol, 3-octanol, alpha-caryophyllene, (-)-(E)-alpha-pulegone; *Micromeria fruticosa CT Pulegone*—sabinene, beta-myrcene, 1,8-cineole, cis-isopulegone, trans-isopulegone, beta-caryophyllene, 2-cyclohexen-1-ol, piperitone, 5-hexen-2-one, 2-cyclohexen-one, 4-nitro-o-cresol, caryophyllene oxide, patchulane; *Micromeria fruticosa CT Isomenthol*—neoiso-isopulegol, isopulegone, isopulegol, germacrene D, bicyclogermacrene

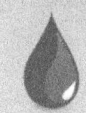

**PREFERRED COMPOSITION FOR CLINICAL USE:**

| Constituent | European |
|---|---|
| Piperitone | 30%–40% |
| Piperitenone | 20%–35% |
| Alpha-Terpineol | 4%–11% |
| (1R)-(+)-Beta-Pulegone | 2%–8% |
| Piperitone Oxide | 2%–6% |
| Menthone | 2%–4% |

Note: Should only be used clinically when the benefits outweigh the risks as determined by a health professional.

**REPORTED THERAPEUTIC PROPERTIES:** Antibacterial, antifungal, antimicrobial, antiarthritic, antirheumatic, anti-inflammatory, antiseptic, antispasmodic, antiparasitic, aids liver and gallbladder function, purifies the blood, aids digestion, relieves stomachache, expels excess gas, relieves headache, encourages menstruation (especially if delayed or stagnant), relieves painful menstruation, stimulates the release of female hormones, soothes boils and blisters, astringent, aids circulation, decongestant, eases cough, insect repellent, insecticide, reduces hysteria, reduces jealousy, relaxing/calming

**CAUTIONS:**

*Pennyroyal is rarely used in essential oil therapy due to the potential to cause serious adverse effects and damage multiple organs. Some texts and resellers of pennyroyal essential oil suggest that North American pennyroyal essential oil is less toxic than European pennyroyal because it has less pulegone. However, North American pennyroyal essential oil can have higher levels of pulegone according to the literature; therefore, this assumption is incorrect.* **Pennyroyal is not recommended for use in essential oil therapy, but listed here to report composition and safety information.**

■ Avoid with children under age twelve. Multiple organ failure, liver failure, brain swelling (cerebral edema), severe epileptic encephalopathy (severe brain disorder with seizures), organ cell death (necrosis), and death has been reported in infants who were administered mint tea containing pennyroyal essential oil.[6799] Pulegone and its metabolite menthofuran (or metabolites of menthofuran) are believed to cause the toxic effects of pennyroyal, which include liver and kidney toxicity, bronchiolar cell destruction, depletion of liver glutathione levels (the primary protective antioxidant of the liver), and direct cellular damage.[6800,6801,6802,6803] Children are more likely to experience these effects.[6804]

■ Avoid during pregnancy and lactation due to significant amounts of pulegone and potential toxicity to multiple organs properties of pennyroyal.[6805,6806] Pennyroyal is believed to trigger uterine contractions by irritating the genito-urinary system. It is commonly used to induce abortions.[6807,6808] While pennyroyal herb is considered abortifacient, the essential oil is not.[6809] When pennyroyal essential oil is used alone to induce abortion, it generally is unsuccessful but causes serious health consequences to the mother. Carachipita is an abortant sold over the counter in South America that contains pennyroyal, yerba de la perdiz, oregano, and marsh rosemary. The literature reports successful use of Carachipita to induce abortion, but not without serious consequences to the mother (multiple organ failure, vaginal bleeding, destruction of red blood cells, numbness, dizziness, and death).[6810,6811,6812] It is prudent to avoid pennyroyal oil while pregnant or nursing due to its toxicity alone, despite a lack of evidence that it is a direct abortifacient.

■ Avoid oral consumption due to the toxic potential of pulegone, menthofuran, and pennyroyal essential oil to multiple organs. Menthofuran is generally a very minor constituent of pennyroyal essential oil, but it is considered more toxic than pulegone.[6813] In addition, pulegone is metabolized by human liver cytochrome P-450s (CYP2E1, CYP1A2, and CYP2C19) to menthofuran after administration, which actually increases its toxic effect to the liver.[6814,6815] Animal research suggests oral administration of pulegone is significantly toxic to the liver and causes death at 300 mg/kg (over 3.3 mL for a human adult equivalent dose) for two weeks.[6816] Lower doses of 75 and 150 mg/kg for three months resulted in liver, kidney, bone marrow, heart, stomach, lung, ovarian, and thymus damage, and one death in animals.[6817] A two-year animal study reported urinary cancer and papillomas, liver cancer, osteosarcoma, and multiple organ damage or enlargement (liver, kidney, olfactory epithelium, lung, bile duct).[6818] Ingestion of pennyroyal essential oil can cause abdominal pain and tenderness, nausea, bloody vomiting, burning of the throat, fever, lethargy alternating with agitation, confusion, delirium, restlessness, seizures, dizziness, auditory and visual hallucinations, increased blood pressure, rapid heartbeat, swollen blood vessels in the lungs and filling of the alveoli with blood, excessive acidity of the blood, blood clots, abortion, liver failure, kidney failure, respiratory failure, shock, coma, and death.[6819] Neurological damage has been reported in adults who consumed 2.5 to 5.0 mL of pennyroyal essential oil, moderate to severe poisoning with single doses of 10 mL, and deaths occurred at over 15 mL of ingestion.[6820,6821,6822,6823,6824,6825,6826,6827,6828,6829,6830]

■ Avoid with epilepsy and Parkinson's disease due to pulegone and 1,8-cineole content. May exacerbate or cause seizures or convulsions when inhaled, applied topically, or ingested based on 1,8-cineole content.[6831,6832,6833,6834,6835,6836]

■ Avoid with compromised liver or kidney due to significant potential to cause liver and kidney toxicity.[6837,6838,6839,6840,6841,6842]

■ May interact with antibiotics and antifungals and increase or decrease their effectiveness.[6843]

**SELECTED EVIDENCE:**

☐ *In vitro* research reports that European pennyroyal essential oil inhibits *Streptococcus pyogenes, S. aureus, L. monocytogenes, E. faecium, S. enteritidis,* gram-positive bacteria, and *Klebsiella* sp. (including antibiotic resistant strains of *Klebsiella*).[6844,6845,6846,6847] Turkish pennyroyal essential oil inhibited the bacteria *Micrococcus luteus, Bacillus megaterium, Bacillus brevis, Enterococcus faecalis, Pseudomonas pyocyaneus, Mycobacterium smegmatis, Escherichia coli, Aeromonas hydrophila, Yersinia enterocolitica, Staphylococcus aureus, Streptococcus faecalis,* and the fungi *Saccharomyces cerevisiae, Kluvyeromyces fragilis.*[6848] The researchers also reported that Turkish pennyroyal increased the effectiveness of three antibiotics (gentamicin, cephalothin, and ceftriaxone). Pennyroyal essential oil also inhibits several foodborne and spoilage bacteria: gram-positive—*Listeria monocytogenes, Clostridium perfringens, Bacillus cereus, Staphylococcus aureus, Enterococcus faecium, Enterococcus faecalis,* and *Staphylococcus epidermidis,* and gram-negative—*Salmonella enterica,* and *Escherichia coli* strains.[6849]

☐ Turkish pennyroyal essential oil was ineffective against *C. albicans,* but European pennyroyal exhibited moderate antifungal activity against *Botrytis cinerea* (a plant pathogen that causes gray mold disease).[6850,6851]

☐ Interestingly, injection of European pennyroyal essential oil reduced the occurrence of seizure and increased the survivability of animals when administered pentylenetetrazol (PTZ) to cause seizures.[6852]

☐ European pennyroyal essential oil reduced muscle spasms in isolated animal trachea and bladder, likely by inhibiting calcium entrance into cells.[6853] The authors attributed this effect to pulegone. Another study found that it reduces uterine contractions in isolated rat uterus through calcium channel blocking properties.[6854]

☐ Research demonstrates that pennyroyal essential oil repels and kills the head louse (*Pediculus humanus capitis*) that causes head lice, particularly during the vapor phase.[6855,6856]

☐ A piperitone-oxide rich European pennyroyal essential oil demonstrated marked toxicity and expelling ability against the hydatid worm (*Echinococcus granulosus*), also called the hyper tape-worm, which is a parasite that infests the small intestines of canines, but also lives in the liver, lungs, or other organs of humans.[6857] Pennyroyal essential oil significantly repelled wasps (*Polistes dominulus*) and yellowjackets (*Vespula pensylvanica*), moderately repelled fleas (*Diamanus montanus*), and kills gall midge (*Camptomyia corticalis*) larvae, the twospotted spider mite (*Tetranychus urticae* Koch), melon thrip (*Thrips palmi* Karny), and greenhouse whitefly (*Trialeurodes vaporariorum* Westwood).[6858,6859,6860,6861,6862,6863,6864] It also kills the house dust mites *Dermatophagoides farinae* and *D. pteronyssinus.*[6865]

☐ Components of spearmint and pennyroyal essential oils (piperitenone and piperitone oxide) were biocidal (destroy, deter, render harmless, or control insects and harmful organisms by chemical or biological means) to the Colorado potato beetle (*Leptinotarsa decemlineata*); piperitone oxide and pulegone was biocidal to the African cotton leafworm (*Spodoptera littoralis*); and piperitenone oxide strongly inhibited the plant root-knot nematode (*Meloydogine javanica*), followed by piperitone oxide, piperitenone, and carvone.[6866] Based on these properties, scientists concluded that these compounds may be useful as natural crop protectants.

☐ Of seven Mediterranean essential oils, eucalyptus and pennyroyal demonstrated the strongest antimicrobial activity.[6867]

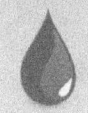

- Pennyroyal essential oil (41% pulegone and 21.2% menthone) showed remarkable antioxidant capacity in comparison to vitamin C, demonstrated leishmanicidal activity against *L. major*, and strongly inhibited *Bacillus subtilis* and *Proteus mirabilis*.[6868]

- Peppermint and pennyroyal essential oils demonstrated good toxicity against the *Aphis gossypii* aphid.[6869] The toxicity was improved when the two oils were combined with the fungus *Lecanicillium muscarium*.

- Encapsulation of pennyroyal essential oil in yeast cell microcarriers prolonged the insecticidal activity of the oil against the green peach aphid (*Myzus persicae*) by three days.[6870]

- Pennyroyal essential oil (86.2% pulegone) inhibited *C. albicans* germ tube formation at amounts well below its minimum inhibitory concentration (MIC).[6871]

- Of ten essential oils tested (thyme, pennyroyal, oregano, peppermint, lemongrass, rosemary, cinnamon, mandarin, holy basil, and mint asavi), cinnamon and thyme essential oils demonstrated the greatest efficacy against MRSA.[6872] Each oil demonstrated varying levels of inhibition. Oregano and pennyroyal also showed a strong synergistic activity with penicillin.

- Fumigation of greenhouse plants with pennyroyal, catnip (reduced fertility), and thyme essential oil acted as an effective insecticide against flower thrips (*Frankliniella occidentalis*), which is an insect pest of greenhouse plants.[6873]

- White wormwood CT alpha-thujone, pennyroyal CT pulegone, Phoenician juniper, lavender, and cade essential oils each displayed varying degrees of antioxidant activity in the DPPH, FRAP, and ABTS assays.[6874] The same researchers reported that the oils exhibited moderate to good acetylcholinesterase (AChE) inhibition activity (in descending order): lavender, pennyroyal, cade, white wormwood, Phoenician juniper; moderate to weak butyrylcholinesterase (BChE) inhibition activity (in descending order): pennyroyal, white wormwood, lavender, cade, and Phoenician juniper; and moderate to weak tyrosinase inhibition activity (in descending order): Cade, lavender, white wormwood, pennyroyal, and Phoenician juniper. Each of the oils was toxic to two types of breast cancer cells as well, with white wormwood being the most effective, followed by Phoenician juniper, pennyroyal, lavender, and cade.

- A rodent model of parasite infection found that administration of pennyroyal essential oil once daily for six consecutive days completely paralyzed *Heligosomoides polygyrus* worms six hours after treatment.[6875] In addition, the researchers reported that the oil displayed good antioxidant activity in the DPPH, ABTS, and FRAP assays, as well as increased endogenous antioxidants (superoxide dismutase, catalase, glutathione) after the parasite infection.

- *In vitro* research showed that marjoram, rosemary CT 1,8-cineole, sage CT camphor, and pulegone CT limonene/piperitone inhibited *L. monocytogenes* and *Salmonella enterica* and displayed antioxidant activity in the DPPH assay.[6876]

- A 1,8-cineole CT of pennyroyal essential oil (70.0% 1,8-cineole) was termiticidal to *Nasutitermes corniger* termites and insecticidal to the maize weevil (*Sitophilus zeamais*).[6877]

- Pennyroyal essential oil inhibited *S. aureus, B. subtilis, P. aeruginosa, E. coli*, and *C. albicans*, but very weak antioxidant activity in the DPPH and ABTS assays.[6878]

- Both cypress and pennyroyal CT pulegone essential oil exhibited acaricidal activity and inhibited egg hatching of ticks (*Hyalomma scupense*), with cypress being more active at the concentrations tested.[6879] The highest acaricidal property was observed when the two oils were used in combination. Both oils also acted as a tick repellent.

- Spanish oregano, ajowan, and pennyroyal essential oils (composition not reported) each exhibited good antimicrobial activity against multidrug-resistant *E. coli* strains, producing extended-spectrum β-lactamase (ESBL) enzymes, with Spanish oregano displaying the most important effect.[6880]

- Pennyroyal CT pulegone, rosemary CT camphor, and their main constituents (carvone, pulegone, 1,8-cineole, camphor, and alpha-pinene) showed insecticidal activity against *C. pipiens* mosquitoes.[6881]

- Researchers analyzed the composition and antimicrobial activity of mint essential oils, including bergamot mint, peppermint, pennyroyal, spearmint, and apple mint. Bergamot mint inhibited *S. typhi* and *C. albicans*; *peppermint E. coli, B. subtilis*, and *C. albicans*; pennyroyal *K. pneumoniae, B. subtilis*, and *C. albicans*; spearmint significantly inhibited *S. typhi* and *B. subtilis*; and apple mint inhibited *K. pneumoniae, C. albicans*, and *S. typhi*.[6882]

- Pennyroyal, Spanish lavender CT camphor, rosemary CT camphor, and oregano CT thymol essential oil were each acaricidal to two spider mites (*Tetranychus urticae* and *Eutetranychus orientalis*) in the fumigant toxicity test, with pennyroyal displaying the highest activity.[6883] A combination of oregano with acequinocyl exhibited the greatest results of mixtures tried.

□ Pennyroyal essential oil displayed good antioxidant activity in the beta-carotene bleaching assay and very strong activity in the DPPH assay, and inhibited *K. pneumoniae, E. coli, C. albicans, L. monocytogenes, B. cereus, C. tropicalis, S. aureus,* and *P. aeruginosa.*[6884]

□ A nanogel and nano-scaled emulsion showed anticancer activity against melanoma cells, with the nanogel being more effective.[6885] Additionally, the Bax gene (a pro-apoptotic and tumor suppressor protein that plays a crucial role in cell death regulation) was upregulated and Bcl-2 (an antiapoptotic protein) was downregulatred.

# PEPPERMINT
## (Mint)

*Mentha × piperita* L. (pro sp.) [aquatica × spicata]

**FAMILY:** Lamiaceae (Labiatae)
**NOTE:** Top
**AROMA INTENSITY:** Strong
**AROMA:** Minty, cool, invigorating, sharp
**COMMON EXTRACTION METHOD:** Steam distilled from the leaves
**POSSIBLE SUBSTITUTE OILS:** Spearmint, rosemary
**BLENDS WELL WITH:** Basil, bergamot, cajeput, cypress, eucalyptus, ginger, grapefruit, lavender, lemon, lemongrass, lime, marjoram, tea tree, niaouli, petitgrain, pine, ravintsara, rosemary, sage, spearmint, tangerine, thyme
**SUBCELLULAR LOCALIZATION | EPIGENETIC INFLUENCE:** Mitochondria, Cytoplasm, Endoplasmic Reticulum | Skeletal/Integumentary
**RECOMMENDED DILUTION RANGE:** 3%–33%; neat for limited conditions

**PRIMARY CONSTITUENTS:**[6886,6887,6888,6889,6890,6891]

| *Peppermint (M. piperita)* | | Cornmint (*M. arvensis*)* |
|---|---|---|
| Menthol | 25.2%–76.7% | 61.9%–82.2% |
| Menthone | 2.5%–30.6% | 3.4%–19.3% |
| Menthol Acetate (Menthyl Acetate) | 0.4%–17.4% | 0.6%–4.4% |
| Menthofuran | 0.1%–11.2% | Not reported |
| Limonene | 0.2%–10.8% | 0.6%–4.7% |
| Beta-Phellandrene | 0.1%–9.2% | Not reported |
| 1,8-Cineole | 4.1%–6.7% | 0.0%–0.1% |
| Isomenthone | 0.0%–5.3% | 2.4%–6.1% |
| Pulegone | 0.3%–4.4% | 0.0%–0.8% |

\* The composition of cornmint (also known as menthol mint) essential oil is provided to help identify a common adulteration of peppermint essential oil. One possible indicator of adulteration of peppermint essential oil with cheaper cornmint is low menthofuran levels. True peppermint oil typically contains between 0.4% and 14.6% menthofuran, while it is not typically detected in cornmint. The odor of cornmint also tends to be slightly harsher.[6892]

**OTHER CONSTITUENTS:** Cis-sabinene hydrate, neomenthone, isomenthone, neomenthyl acetate, isomenthyl acetate, beta-caryophyllene, germacrene D

**PREFERRED COMPOSITION FOR CLINICAL USE:**

| *Constituent* | |
|---|---|
| **Menthol** | 30%–55% |
| **Menthone** | 14%–30% |
| **Menthyl Acetate** | 3%–8% |
| **1,8-Cineole** | 3%–8% |

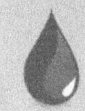

| Isomenthone | 0.5%–6% |
| Menthofuran | 0.5%–6% |
| Neomenthol | 2%–5% |
| Limonene | 1%–5% |
| Beta-Caryophyllene | 1%–4% |
| Pulegone | 0.1%–3.5% |
| Isopulegol | < 0.2% |

REPORTED THERAPEUTIC PROPERTIES: **Analgesic (pain relief)**, antibacterial, anti-inflammatory, antifungal, immune supportive, **relieves headache**, bronchodilator, antimicrobial, antiseptic, antispasmodic, **antineuralgic**, astringent, expels excess gas, **aids digestion**, anticancer, expectorant, decongestant, **reduces fever**, nervine (calms and soothes the nerves), **eases nausea and vomiting**, promotes oral cleanliness, stimulates liver and gallbladder function and encourages the release of bile, **stimulates pancreas function**, stimulating, anesthetic, aids concentration, **promotes alertness**, invigorating, **combats fatigue**, encourages self-confidence, enhances creativity, calms anger, encourages a fresh perspective

CAUTIONS:
■ Avoid in children under age 3 and use cautiously in children under 6, particularly near the face or nose. Essential oils high in menthol and 1,8-cineole content may cause respiratory distress or breathing problems in very young children.[6893,6894,6895,6896 1715–1718]

■ The menthol content in peppermint may negatively impact red blood cells and increase the risk of jaundice in children with glucose-6-phosphate dehydrogenase deficiency (G6PD).[6897,6898]

■ Avoid use in those with ventricular fibrillation (a severely abnormal heart rhythm). Oral use of peppermint may destabilize the heart rhythm based on menthol content.[6899]

■ Avoid use in those with iron-deficiency and iron-deficiency anemia. Animal research suggests that peppermint may decrease iron absorption and therefore aggravate iron-deficiency symptoms and anemia.[6900]

■ May interact with cyclosporine (a medication used to suppress the immune system and avoid transplant rejection) and possibly other immunosuppressants. Very large doses of peppermint may enhance the bioavailability of cyclosporine, increase blood levels of the drug, and intensify its immune-suppressing activity.[6901,6902]

■ Extremely large doses of peppermint (greater than 5 mL daily) may interact with codeine and significantly reduce its pain relieving effect based on animal research.[6903]

■ Extremely large doses of peppermint (greater than 5 mL daily) may interact with pentobarbital (a medication for anxiety, insomnia, and epilepsy) and midazolam (a drug used before surgery to encourage relaxation and sleepiness) and prolong the sleeping effect based on animal research.[6904]

■ May interact with fluorouracil (a topical medication used for skin cancer and keratosis), and enhance its penetration through the skin.[6905]

■ May possibly interact with the antibiotics or antifungals and enhance or decrease their effectiveness.[6906,6907,6908]

■ May weakly interfere with enzymes responsible for metabolizing medications (NSAIDs, proton-pump inhibitors, acetaminophen, antiepileptics, immune modulators, blood-sugar medications, blood pressure medications, antidepressants, antipsychotics, diabetic medications, antihistamines, antibiotics, and anesthetics).[6909,6910,6911,6912] May also interfere with the anticoagulant effect of warfarin by increasing the expression of CYP4A and CYP2C due to menthol content.[6913]

■ May interact with caffeine due to menthol content. Menthol slows the absorption rate of caffeine.[6914]

■ May irritate mucous membranes (eyes, mouth, nasal passages, vagina, rectum).

■ Use with caution with gastroesophageal reflux disease (low risk). Peppermint relaxes smooth muscles and may relax the lower esophageal sphincter muscle. Relaxation of this sphincter may increase heartburn and acid reflux symptoms. This appears to be isolated to sensitive individuals.[6915,6916]

■ Some have suggested that peppermint oil should be limited orally because very large doses of menthofuran, pulegone, menthone, and menthol can be toxic to the liver.[6917,6918,6919,6920,6921] But it takes a very extreme amount of peppermint oil ingestion to cause fatalities in animals, and the equivalent of about 6 to 14 drops daily has been used in studies for irritable bowel syndrome, and up to 8 mL per liter of water has been administered through the rectum during a colonoscopy.[6922,6923,6924,6925] Based on this information it can be concluded that reasonable doses of peppermint pose little risk of actual toxicity.

**SELECTED EVIDENCE:**

- *In vitro* research suggests that peppermint oil is significantly active against lung carcinoma, leukemia, and stomach cancer cells.[6926] The same research concluded that peppermint is a mild antioxidant, and inhibits proinflammatory production of nitric oxide and prostaglandin E2.

- Peppermint potently inhibits *E. coli*, which is suspected of altering intestinal flora balance.[6927] This disrupted flora balance is suspected as a causal factor in triggering irritable bowel syndrome. Other research concluded that peppermint oil inhibits *E. coli, S, aureus, P. aeruginosa, S. faecalis*, and *K. pneumoniae*.[6928] The gaseous phase of peppermint essential oil inhibited *E. coli*.[6929]

- Multiple clinical studies suggest that the oral administration of peppermint oil (0.1 to 0.2 mL, three times daily) is associated with relief of irritable bowel syndrome symptoms and associated pain, largely through preventing gastrointestinal spasms.[6930,6931,6932,6933,6934,6935]

- Inhalation of peppermint oil may reduce the frequency and severity of nausea and vomiting, and the need for drugs used to treat nausea and vomiting.[6936,6937] Another study concluded that inhalation of ginger, spearmint, peppermint, and cardamom (three deep inhalations) from a gauze pad following surgery reduced nausea and requirements for medications to reduce nausea and vomiting.[6938]

- Animal research suggests that inhalation of menthol causes bronchodilation.[6939]

- Oral administration of 0.05 mL of peppermint oil in 500 mL of water daily for ten days resulted in improved exercise performance, blood pressure, and respiratory performance in young males.[6940]

- Peppermint significantly kills HSV-1 and HSV-2, prevents healthy cells from being infected with both viruses, and is active against acyclovir (commonly known as Zovirax, it is an antiviral drug used to treat herpes virus infections) resistant HSV-1.[6941] A review recommended the topical application of diluted tea tree, peppermint, or melissa oil three to four times daily for recurrent herpetic infections (cold sores and genital herpes).[6942]

- Animal and *in vitro* research suggests that peppermint oil kills the parasitic worm Anisakis that infects the stomach and intestines and causes abdominal pain, nausea, intestinal obstruction, and intestinal tract damage.[6943] Peppermint oil effectively prevented gastrointestinal lesions caused by the Anisakis parasite, whereas 46.7% of animals treated with albendazole (a drug used to treat worm infections, including Anisakis) experienced gastrointestinal lesions.

- Inhalation of a combination of peppermint, basil, and helichrysum oils reduced mental exhaustion and moderate burnout in a small pilot study.[6944]

- Topical application of a combination of lavender, geranium, tea tree, and peppermint oils improved the oral health of hospice patients with terminal cancer.[6945]

- Inhalation of peppermint oil enhances attention, speed, and accuracy while performing clerical tasks, which increased task performance.[6946]

- Topical application of a 1.5% solution containing lavender, marjoram, eucalyptus, rosemary, and peppermint (2:1:2:1:1 ratio), in a carrier oil consisting of 45% apricot, 45% almond, and 10% jojoba carrier oils significantly decreased pain and depression in people with arthritis.[6947]

- An abdominal massage with lemon, rosemary, and peppermint oil relieved constipation in the elderly.[6948] Interestingly, the effect of the massage lasted for two weeks after treatment.

- *In vitro* research suggests that peppermint essential oil inhibits *C. albicans*.[6949,6950] Other research demonstrates that peppermint essential oil inhibits *Fusarium sporotrichioides*, a plant fungus that is responsible for crop damage.[6951]

- Peppermint oil completely inhibits the yeasts *T. asahii* and *T. cutaneum* that are known to cause potentially life-threatening infections (urinary tract, skin, and bloodstream) in those with a compromised immune system.[6952]

- *In vitro* research concluded that peppermint essential oil inhibited *P. insidiosum* (a pathogenic oomycete that infects mammals and causes gangrenous ulcers on the skin and may restrict blood flow in the surrounding arteries).[6953]

- *In vitro* research suggests that peppermint inhibits elastase activity (an enzyme involved in the breakdown of elastin and a causal factor in lung connective tissue diseases, disruption of the body's ability to kill pathogens, and delayed wound healing).[6954] The researchers concluded that topical administration may be beneficial for bullous pemphigoid (a skin condition that causes the formation of large blisters) and pulmonary emphysema (a chronic lung condition characterized by enlargement of the air sacs in the lungs).

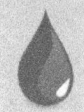

- Injection of peppermint oil into animals prior to pentylenetetrazol (a drug used to experimentally study seizures in animals) protected mice from seizures and increased survival rate to 100%.[6955]
- Peppermint oil effectively kills the larvae of and repels the mosquito responsible for dengue fever.[6956,6957]
- Oral administration of 2 drops each of peppermint and spearmint oils (the rest of the capsule was filled with sugar) in addition to traditional drugs (granisetron, dexamethasone, or metoclopramide) significantly reduced the number and severity of nausea and vomiting episodes in chemotherapy patients within the first twenty-four hours of taking the oils.[6958]
- Peppermint has been used to reduce itching caused by allergies, drugs, kidney, or liver disease, and other health conditions.[6959]
- *In vitro* and animal research suggests that peppermint oil is a good free-radical scavenger, significantly decreases uric acid levels in the blood (higher uric acid levels are associated with increased gout risk), and significantly killed cervical cancer cells.[6960,6961,6962] The same research found that peppermint extract reduced lung tumors.
- Animal research suggests that peppermint oil relaxes tracheal spasms caused by carbachol (a drug used to induce spasms in animals).[6963]
- Researchers evaluated the effectiveness of a spray (administered as four sprays, five times daily) containing 30% *Origanum syriacum* (Syrian oregano), 20% peppermint, rosemary, and *Eucalyptus globulus*, and 10% *E. citriodora* in people with upper respiratory tract infections (URTI). The researchers concluded that people who used the spray experienced significant reductions in their most debilitating URTI symptoms within twenty minutes of application.[6964] Another study concluded that peppermint, thyme, cinnamon, and lemongrass oils inhibited the respiratory tract pathogens *S. pyogenes* (a bacterium that causes scarlet fever) and *S. pneumoniae*.[6965]
- *In vitro* and clinical research concluded that peppermint was more effective than chlorhexidine (a drug used to treat diseases of the teeth and gums) in preventing the bacteria *S. mutans* and *S. pyogenes* from sticking together and forming plaque (biofilm), possibly leading to the prevention of cavities.[6966,6967] Another study determined that peppermint oil kills pathogenic oral bacteria.[6968]
- Inhalation of peppermint oil enhanced cognitive performance and memory in people.[6969]
- Oral administration of peppermint oil in capsules prior to colonoscopy decreased the time required to perform the entire procedure, reduced colon spasm and pain, and improved patient satisfaction with the procedure in thirty-three adults.[6970] Another study found that spraying the stomach chamber directly with 20 mL of a 0.8% menthol solution prior to upper gastrointestinal endoscopy reduced peristalsis before and after the procedure.[6971] A third study concluded that when peppermint oil was mixed with the barium enema solution, residual spasms were significantly reduced during a barium enema examination.[6972]
- Three minutes of oral cleansing daily with a combination of tea tree, peppermint, and lemon oils helped reduce bad breath and production of volatile sulfur compounds (compounds excreted by oral bacteria that cause bad breath) in intensive care patients.[6973]
- Russian scientists found that inhaling peppermint oil (twenty minutes daily for two months) improved symptoms of pulmonary (lung) tuberculosis and prevented its recurrence in people.[6974,6975]
- *In vitro* research reported that peppermint oil provides a sun protection factor (SPF) of almost 7.[6976]
- Clinical research suggests that peppermint oil slows gastrointestinal motility (the time required for food to travel through the digestive system), which may make it beneficial for diarrhea.[6977]
- Peppermint enhanced the absorption of aminophylline (a drug used to treat asthma and lung conditions) by 28% in healthy people.[6978] Interestingly, peppermint reduced the absorption of benzoic acid through the skin in low concentrations.[6979]
- A foot bath (107°F water) with salts and either oregano, thyme, cinnamon bark, lemongrass, clove, palmarosa, peppermint, lavender, or geranium significantly reduced fungi associated with athlete's foot *in vitro*.[6980]
- *In vitro* research concluded that peppermint oil enhances the effectiveness of oxytetracycline (a broad-spectrum antibiotic used to treat bacterial infections like acne, rosacea, and chest infections).[6981]
- The combination of peppermint and caraway oils reduces internal organ pain after inflammation has ceased in rats.[6982]
- Inhalation of peppermint oil reduced daytime sleepiness in people when they were subjected to conditions that normally increase daytime sleepiness.[6983]

- Headache was relieved when a combination of peppermint oil and ethanol was applied to the forehead and temples of healthy people with a sponge.[6984] When eucalyptus was added to the mixture the pain relieving effect was diminished, but cognitive performance was enhanced, as was the muscle-relaxing and mentally relaxing effect.

- Animal research shows that topical application of peppermint essential oil encouraged hair growth (significantly increased dermal thickness, follicle number, and follicle depth) by increasing alkaline phosphatase (ALP) enzymatic activity and insulin-like growth factor-1 gene expression (IGF-1).[6985] Both ALP and IGF-1 levels are significantly diminished in areas experiencing hair loss, suggesting they play an important role in hair growth and thickness. Increased ALP activity is also associated with hair staying in the anagen (hair growth) stage longer. Interestingly, peppermint oil increased ALP and IGF-1 levels more rapidly and to a greater extent than minoxidil (a hair loss drug that targets ALP and IGF-1).

- Peppermint essential oil may be a viable option to treat *Acanthamoeba* spp. infections due to its ability to kill *A. castellani* cysts and trophozoites.[6986]

- Peppermint essential oil reduced counts of *E. coli, Salmonella enteritidis,* and *L. monocytogenes* in cashew, guava, mango, and pineapple juices at concentrations of 10 mcl/mL.[6987]

- Peppermint essential oil moderately inhibited the *C. jejuni* bacterium that is one of the world's most common cases of the stomach flu (gastroenteritis) and *H. pylori* (a pathogen linked to stomach ulcers).[6988]

- Peppermint essential oil is toxic to the brown-banded cockroach (*Supella longipalpa*).[6989]

- A combination of holy basil, peppermint, Indian borage, and eucalyptus (*E. globulus*)—diluted to 5%—provided six hours of mosquito protection, which is comparable to DEET.[6990]

- A double-blinded randomized crossover study demonstrated that oral administration of a sustained release capsule containing 0.2 mL (187 mg; roughly four drops) of peppermint essential oil (once daily for three days beginning when menstruation starts) significantly reduced pain duration and severity of painful menstruation in young women.[6991] The peppermint capsules also reduced nausea and diarrhea.

- *In vitro* research demonstrates that peppermint essential oil is antimicrobial to *P. insidiosum*.[6992]

- Peppermint essential oil inhibited multiple bacteria (*Escherichia coli, Pseudomonas aeruginosa, Micrococcus luteus, Staphylococcus aureus, Bacillus subtilis, Salmonella typhimurium,* and *Bacillus cereus*), with *P. aeruginosa* being the least sensitive.[6993]

- Peppermint essential oil inhibited *E. faecalis, E. coli,* and *S. epidermidis in vitro*.[6994]

- Peppermint and pennyroyal essential oils demonstrated good toxicity against the *Aphis gossypii* aphid.[6995] The toxicity was improved when the two oils were combined with the fungus *Lecanicillium muscarium*.

- Research suggests that peppermint essential oil is a safe fumigant to control the rice weevil (*Sitophilus oryzae*) due to its effectiveness and nonharmful effects.[6996]

- Peppermint essential oil demonstrated superior repellency against the house fly (*M. domestica*) when used alone or in conjunction with lemongrass (*C. citratus*)—70% peppermint and 30% lemongrass. Isolated menthol also demonstrated excellent repellency in the research.[6997]

- Sweet basil, cinnamon bark, sweet fennel, kaffir lime petitgrain, kaffir lime peel, black pepper, peppermint, and spearmint essential oils all demonstrated antimicrobial activity against bacteria linked to cavities (*Streptococcus mutans* and *Lactobacillus casei*).[6998] Cinnamon was the most active against both bacteria, kaffir lime petitgrain was the weakest of the tested oils against both bacteria, and black pepper was inactive against *L. casei*.

- Oral administration of 15 or 40mg/kg body weight of peppermint essential oil protected rats against liver and kidney toxicity caused by tetrachloride.[6999] The protective effect was attributed to a decrease in stress parameters (alanine aminotransferase, aspartate aminotransferase, alkaline phosphatase), creatinine, urea, lactate dehydrogenase, and γ-glutamyl transpeptidase) and liver and kidney lipid peroxidation, and an increase in liver and kidney antioxidant activity (superoxide dismutase, catalase, and glutathione peroxidase).

- Injection of peppermint essential oil significantly improved liver fibrosis in rats as evidenced by improved liver injury markers, reduced lipid peroxidation, enhanced antioxidant activity, and alteration of gene expression.[7000] In addition, the scientists observed that peppermint essential oil improved redox status (the balance of antioxidants, free radicals, and several sets of metabolites), regulated tumor suppressor p53 (a gene involved in liver fibrosis and injury), and modulated desmin (a marker for elevated fat-storing cells—hepatic stellate cells), α-smooth muscle actin (α-SMA; a marker for elevated fat-storing cells linked to liver fibrosis and chronic liver disease), transforming growth factor-β (TGF-β1; a regulator of liver disease

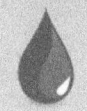

involved in all stages from initiation to fibrosis and cirrhosis), and SMAD3 (an intracellular regulator of TGF-β1 and protein that stimulated fibrosis) protein expression.

- Peppermint essential oil (rich in menthol—68.0%) improved the antimicrobial activity of gentamicin against all bacteria tested in a large panel of gram-positive and gram-negative bacteria.[7001] Its synergistic effect with antifungals was less pronounced.

- Topical application of peppermint essential oil accelerated wound healing in mice despite wounds being infected by *Staphylococcus aureus* and *Pseudomonas aeruginosa*.[7002] The oil reduced bacterial count in the wound, edema, and inflammation, while simultaneously increasing migration of fibroblasts to wound site, collagen production, and re-epithelization (the process that covers a wound with epithelial tissue).

- Lavender, lemongrass (*C. citratus*), marjoram, peppermint, tea tree, and rosewood essential oils all exhibited significant activity against clinical isolates of multidrug-resistant *Burkholderia cepacia* complex (a group of bacteria commonly resistant to antibiotics that cause health problems in people with weakened immune systems and are known to cause healthcare related infections).[7003]

- A double-blind, placebo-controlled, balanced crossover study demonstrated that ingestion of 1.0 mL (two 0.5 mL capsules with 0.1 mL peppermint and the rest filled with vegetable oil, about 2 to 3 drops) of peppermint essential oil reduced fatigue and improved performance during a cognitively demanding task (one and three hours after taking it).[7004] The same researchers reported that peppermint essential oil (36.7% menthol and 24.9% menthone) demonstrated high $GABA_A$ and nicotinic receptor binding activity, as well as inhibited AChE (acetylcholinesterase).

- Peppermint essential oil inactivated *E. coli, L. monocytogenes*, and *S. enteritidis* when added to pineapple and mango juice through multi mechanisms (cytoplasmic membranes disruption, increased permeability, potential depolarization, and inhibition of efflux pump and respiratory activity).[7005]

- The addition of 0.2% peppermint or thyme essential oil to a yogurt-based drink inhibited *S. aureus*.[7006]

- SENLAT (also called TRIBOLA/DEBONEL) is an illness caused by the tick-borne bacterium *Rickettsia slovaca* characterized by necrosis of the scalp and painfully enlarged cervical lymph nodes. Peppermint and cornmint essential oils both significantly inhibited the growth of *R. slovaca* in laboratory research.[7007]

- *In vitro* research showed that peppermint and fennel essential oil inhibit *Alternaria* sp.[7008]

- Peppermint essential oil (in vapor form) prevented the growth of *C. albicans* comparably to amphotericin-B and strongly reduced its biofilm formation and transition (change from blastospore to hyphae forms).[7009] The scientists also observed that peppermint disrupted existing *c. albicans* biofilms and reduced expression of genes related to its virulence.

- Peppermint essential oil exhibited noteworthy insecticidal properties against stored grain pests (*Sitophilus oryzae* and *Tribolium castaneum*).[7010]

- Peppermint essential oil reduced virulence factors of *Campylobacter jejuni* (a cause of food poisoning) by influencing expression go genes related to virulence.[7011]

- Peppermint essential oil chitosan nanogel showed potential as an antibiofilm agent in toothpaste or mouthwash based on its ability to inhibit biofilm formation by *S. mutans*.[7012] *S. mutans* metabolizes sugar to initiate the formation of biofilms on the surface of teeth and consequently produces lactic acid to degrade the tooth's enamel and cause cavities (caries). By preventing this process from occurring peppermint essential oil may help reduce the risk of cavities and help maintain strong tooth enamel.

- Glucosyltransferases (GTFs) from *Streptococcus mutans* bacteria play critical roles in the development of virulent dental plaque (ferment carbohydrates that decrease pH of plaque leading to tooth enamel demineralization), which provides an ideal site for colonization by microorganisms and is involved in the development of dental cavities. Laboratory research found that both clove and peppermint essential oils inhibit (allosteric inhibition—bind to a molecule at a site other than its active site so that the enzyme no longer remains able to bind to its specific substrate, making the enzyme inactive) GTFs produced by *S. mutans*.[7013]

- The ability of essential oils to enhance the antimicrobial activity of antibiotics has led researchers to combine them with antimicrobial drugs to use less drug toxicity, side effects, and resistance. Peppermint essential oil (41.7% menthol, 21.8% menthone) was fungistatic to dermatophytes and fungicidal to yeasts. In addition, peppermint improved the efficacy of itraconazole against *Candida* spp., *C. neoformans*, and *T. mentagrophytes*.[7014]

- A double-blind clinical trial compared the effects of 4% lidocaine, 1.5% peppermint, and placebo for migraine headaches. Study participants administered 2 drops of the peppermint oil (or placebo or lidocaine) into the nose at the first signs of migraine attack while laying down with their head hanging over a table edge and turned thirty degrees toward the site of the pain. They remained laying down for at least thirty seconds after administration of the remedy. A significant decrease in headache intensity and frequency was experienced by both the peppermint and lidocaine groups.[7015] Peppermint was considered similar in its efficacy to lidocaine.

☐ Peppermint essential oil showed significant fumigation and contact toxicity against three stored product insects (*Tribolium castaneum, Lasioderma serricorne,* and *Liposcelis bostrychophila*).[7016] Peppermint oil also exhibited comparable repellent efficacy to the control at the highest concentration. Isolated menthone showed good insecticidal activity, while menthol exhibited the most notable repellent effects.

☐ Peppermint essential oil nanoemulsion demonstrated significant insecticidal activity against the cotton aphid (*Aphis gossypii*).[7017]

☐ A single-blind randomized controlled trial showed that inhalation of peppermint essential oil—2 drops of a 10% or 30% concentration added to 2 mL of distilled water placed on a gauze pads— for five minutes significantly reduced nausea after abdominal surgery.[7018]

☐ Both hydrodistilled and microwave-assisted hydrodistilled peppermint essential oils displayed weak antioxidant activity in the DPPH and ABTS assays.[7019]

☐ Nanoencapsulation of peppermint essential oil was significantly toxic to stored-grain pests (*T. castaneum* and *S. oryzae*).[7020]

☐ *Fusobacterium nucleatum* is the main bacterium linked to bad breath. The bacterium aggregates with other bacteria in the mouth to form plaque biofilms that cause bad breath. Ledum (*R. groenlandicum*) CT sabinene, peppermint, and mountain savory CT carvacrol essential oil each inhibited *F. nucleatum* without harming human oral cells in a laboratory study.[7021]

☐ Exposure to fine particulate matter (PM) can exacerbate airway remodeling, fibrosis, and pulmonary destruction in people with asthma. Small particles in the air—pollution, smoke, airborne dust, haze, etc.— pass through the nose or mouth and enter the lungs to trigger asthma symptoms. Inhalation of nebulized peppermint essential oil reduced respiratory epithelium hyperplasia (thickening of the lining of the lung due to excessive proliferation of lung epithelial cells), collagen deposition (part of the tissue healing process after injury of epithelial cells, which can enhance inflammation of the lungs and worsen fibrosis), and goblet cell activation (increased activation of goblet cells negatively changes the tissue structure of the lungs) in asthmatic mice exposed to PM with particles of a diameter generally 10 micrometers and smaller.[7022] To identify the mechanism by which peppermint oil exerts its antiasthmatic effects, the researchers performed a network pharmacological analysis and determined the oil reduces inflammation (reduced IL-6 and proinflammatory and T helper 2-specific cytokines through modulating the cytokine-cytokine receptor interaction and JAK/STAT pathway).

☐ Laboratory research found that the anticancer activity of peppermint essential oil against three human breast cancer cell lines was improved when it was prepared as a nanoemulsion.[7023]

☐ Shigella infection (shigellosis) is a very contagious intestinal infection caused by a family of bacteria known as shigella. The infection is characterized by diarrhea, which is often bloody (dysentery). It is most commonly acquired in poor and crowded communities, certain occupations (agriculture, animal husbandry, tanning) and in hospitals. Researchers identified the ideal concentration (0.6%) of peppermint essential oil to inhibit the bacterium *Shigella dysenteriae* in the lab. Then, as part of a preclinical model of Shigella infection, they administered 0.1 mL of the ideal concentration to rats with shigellosis for seven days. Remarkably, the peppermint oil reduced the *S. dysenteriae* infection to nearly zero.[7024]

☐ Peppermint showed good fumigant toxicity against eggs, second instar larvae, fourth instar larvae, and adults of the Khapra Beetle (*Trogoderma granarium*; a stored grain pest) and repelled the beetles from infesting wheat sprayed with the oil.[7025]

☐ Researchers evaluated the synergistic activity of rosemary, geranium, and peppermint essential oils in combination with colistin antibiotics against extreme drug-resistant and susceptible *Acinetobacter baumannii* clinical isolates. The highest inhibitory activity was observed with peppermint essential oil, followed by geranium and rosemary essential oils.[7026] Both rosemary and geranium produced strong synergistic activity when combined with colistin, but peppermint was indifferent when combined with colistin.

☐ A placebo-controlled clinical trial found that prolonged exposure—via inhalation from a patch—to peppermint essential oil enhances cognition and mood in healthy adults.[7027] Participants wore an aroma patch infused with peppermint or without any oil at all for six hours, and cognitive and mood parameters were assessed. Those in the peppermint group experienced improved word recall, memory, alertness, and subjective mood.

☐ The Kristinka variety of peppermint oil, which was rich in menthol (70.1%), demonstrated promising antifungal activity against *Botrytis cinerea, Monilinia fructicola, Penicillium expansum,* and *Aspergillus*

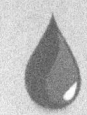

*niger*, but only moderate antibacterial activity against *C. michiganensis* and *P. syringae* pv. *Phaseolicola* and weak activity against *P. savastanoi*.[7028]

- Poor cardiac function can lead to fatigue and fatigue is among the most common complaints among cardiac patients. A randomized placebo-controlled trial evaluated the effects of inhaling peppermint or lavender essential oil in subjects in a cardiac care unit.[7029] Three drops of peppermint, lavender, or placebo were added to a cotton ball and attached to the subject's shirt collar for twenty minutes at 9:00 p.m. The intervention continued for seven nights. Interestingly, both lavender and peppermint oil inhalation reduced reported fatigue better than placebo.

- A preclinical model of kidney stones evaluated the ability of peppermint essential oil to block and manage the development of oxalate kidney stones (urolithiasis) and compared against the standard antiurolithic drug. Kidney stones are frequently accompanied by abnormal urinary conditions such as crystalluria (the presence of crystals in the urine, which may impair kidney function), polyuria (excessive production or passage of urine), and acidic urine (abnormally acid urine promotes uric acid or cystine stones, whereas overly alkaline urine promotes calcium- and phosphate-containing stones). Administration of peppermint essential oil protected against crystalluria, polyuria, and acidic urine, and neutralized altered urinary or blood levels of uric acid, magnesium, total protein, creatinine, and blood urea nitrogen.[7030]

- *In vitro* research concluded that peppermint essential oil inhibited *S. aureus* and *L. monocytogenes*, was toxic to rat glioma cancer cells, and displayed potent antioxidant activity in the ABTS assay while maintaining a good safety profile based on 90% viability of human keratinocyte cells.[7031]

- A significant number of people experience anxiety after developing acute coronary syndrome (ACS; a condition characterized by reduced blood flow in the coronary arteries that makes part of the heart muscle unable to function properly and becomes damaged)—up to 60 percent. A randomized, controlled clinical study evaluated the benefits of inhaling peppermint in sixty-four people experiencing ACS.[7032] In the peppermint group, 3 drops of peppermint essential oil (diluted 1 drop of peppermint per 20 drops of sweet almond oil) were added to a cotton ball and placed on the participant's collar, and the participant inhaled gently for one hour. The placebo group had 3 drops of water added to the cotton ball instead. The peppermint group experienced significant reductions in anxiety levels after inhaling peppermint compared to control.

- A healthy gut microbiome is vital for overall health, influencing gastrointestinal health, immunity, mood, cognition, cardiovascular function, pain, and more. The gut microbiome changes throughout life from intrinsic (e.g., stress) and extrinsic factors (e.g., diet and drugs). Research suggests that early colonization of *Bifidobacterium* and *Collinsella* populations in children during the first months of life supports healthy childhood development and growth. Low populations of Collinsella bacteria are observed in adults with irritable bowel syndrome. In addition, low Collinsella colonization in the microbiome is associated with higher morbidity and mortality after infections, suggesting that these bacteria may mitigate infection and reduce symptom severity. A clinical study investigated the effects of ingesting peppermint essential oil on the gut microbiome in children aged seven to twelve with functional abdominal pain.[7033] Children were assigned to three different dosage groups—180 mg once daily, 180 mg twice daily (360 mg/day), and 180 mg three times daily (540 mg/day)—and the assigned dosage was taken in capsules for one week. At the end of one week, there was no significant difference in alpha diversity (a measurement of the richness and balance of the microbial community) from pre- and post-intervention; however, a marked increase in Collinsella bacteria was observed in all groups. In addition, the firmicutes/Bacteroidetes ratio was lower in children who received the highest dose of peppermint oil. Firmicutes/Bacteroidetes ratio is considered a health biomarker that is disrupted in obesity, metabolic disorders, and inflammatory conditions. While more research is necessary, especially of longer duration, it suggests that peppermint oil ingestion can improve populations of important microbiota in the gut.

- A study evaluated the antimicrobial activity of multiple essential oils (cinnamon bark, lavender, tea tree, lemon, oregano CT carvacrol, peppermint, bay laurel, and eucalyptus—*E. globulus*) against human pathogens (*S. pyogenes, S. aureus, S. agalactiae*).[7034] Oregano, cinnamon, and tea tree exhibited the strongest antibacterial activity and combinations of tea tree/lavender and cinnamon/lavender displayed synergistic activity.

- The effects of peppermint essential oil inhalation was evaluated in an APP/PS1 mouse model of Alzheimer's disease (a model that involves elevated beta-amyloid production associated with behavioral modifications and age-related deterioration of learning and memory).[7035] Mice were split into three groups: 1) normal mice without AD, 2) mice with AD that inhaled peppermint oil, one hour, twice daily, for twenty-one days, 3) mice with AD that inhaled rosemary oil, one hour, twice daily, for twenty-one days. Inhaling peppermint improved memory and the health of neurons in the hippocampus (returned to normal), and the deposition of amyloid reduced. In addition, markers of brain oxidative stress reduced and enzymatic antioxidant activity

(SOD, GSH-PX) increased significantly to normal levels. Models were used to identify the mechanism of action and the researchers reported that peppermint improves cognitive function by improving amino acid metabolism (arginine, proline, cysteine, and methionine) and energy production, and reducing brain oxidative damage, and protecting brain cells.

☐ Activities involving standing or walking for extended periods of time can cause swelling, pain, and fatigue in the feet and legs. A clinical study investigated the benefits of an aromatic foot bath or aromatic spray on lower extremity swelling and pain in nurses.[7036] For the foot bath, 0.5 mL of a blend of peppermint and grapefruit were added to 9 L of water heated to 40° C (104° F) and the participants soaked their feet for thirty minutes. The spray was created by combining 6 mL of grapefruit and peppermint oils (1:1 ratio) in 94 mL of distilled water. About 4 mL of the spray was sprayed to participant's lower limbs three separate times at ten-minute intervals while sitting in chairs, shaking the bottle before each use. A control group sat in a chair for thirty minutes without any intervention. Swelling significantly reduced in the foot bath and spray groups (as measured by calf circumference) and reported lower extremity pain and fatigue was remarkably reduced when compared to control group.

☐ Saliva is important for chewing, swallowing, tasting, and talking. Dry mouth occurs when insufficient saliva is produced to keep the mouth moist, which can be caused by salivary gland dysfunction, medications, radiation therapy to the head or neck, chemotherapy, Sjogren syndrome, diabetes, sarcoidosis, viral infection, and smoking. A clinical trial evaluated an oral spray with peppermint essential oil (1 mL), propolis (1.5 mL), xylitol (700 mg), and water (50 mL) for dry mouth.[7037] A control group used an alcohol-based spray with pineapple-flavored water and xylitol. Both groups used the spray—two to three sprays from the bottle directly onto the tongue and teeth—four times daily after consuming food for four weeks. At the conclusion of the study, the peppermint oil spray improved dry mouth and oral health (dental hypersensitivity and plaque accumulation on the teeth). The subjects in the peppermint group also used the spray with greater compliance because they reported it made their mouth feel fresh.

☐ Acetylcholine is an important cholinergic neurotransmitter and neuromodulator involved in various functions throughout the body, but particularly in the nervous system. It works by attaching to receptors and sending signals between nerves. Acetylcholine has multiple functions in the body including motor neuron function (muscular movement), dilation of blood vessels, motivation, attention, learning, and memory. The activity and function of the cholinergic system is controlled by the enzymes acetylcholinesterase (AChE) and butyrylcholinesterase (BChE). People with neurodegenerative conditions make less acetylcholine and experience excessive BChE activity. Inhibition of AChE and BChE are targets for the treatment of neurodegenerative conditions. The outgrowth of neurites (called neuritogenesis—the formation of any projection from neurons) occurs during brain development and when neurons are regenerated. These outgrowths of dendrites or axons allow neurons to form networks and connections and communicate with other cells and ultimately maintain youthful brain function. A preclinical model of Alzheimer's disease evaluated essential oils from the *Lamiaceae* family for their effects on brain function and brain cell protection.[7038] Oregano CT alpha-terpineol, peppermint, rosemary CT 1,8-cineole, and sage essential oils each inhibited BChE activity. The carvacrol CT of oregano inhibited both BChE and AChE activity. Isolated linalool from lavender significantly reduced reactive oxygen species (ROS) inside neurons, suggesting it can protect against oxidative stress and death of neurons. In addition, oregano CT alpha-terpineol, peppermint, rosemary, and sage triggered neurite outgrowth, with the greatest activity observed from oregano. The researchers concluded that these oils have properties that could potentially prevent or delay dementia-related diseases.

☐ Menstrual pain is one of the most common complaints of women during their reproductive years. A survey of more than four hundred young women found that 84.1 percent report menstrual pain, with 43.1 percent of them reporting pain during every period.[7039] Researchers found that applying a warm compress with peppermint essential oil significantly reduced menstrual pain in young women.[7040] The compress was made by adding 4 to 5 drops of peppermint essential oil to 500 mL of warm water and then soaking a cotton, wool, or flannel cloth in the bowl. The cloth was wrung out and then placed over the supra pubic area, repeating the process when the cloth cooled down.

☐ An investigation of three essential oils from the *Lamiaceae* family (peppermint, rosemary, and lavender) found that rosemary CT camphor was the most effective larvicidal agent against third instar larvae mosquitoes (*Culex pipiens*).[7041] Lavender essential oil was the least effective larvicide, but demonstrated the highest knockdown rate, followed by peppermint. In addition, lavender and peppermint essential oils showed the highest adult mosquito mortality rates.

☐ Peppermint essential oil (29.2% menthone, 38.7% levomenthol) inhibited *S. aureus, B. cereus, L.*

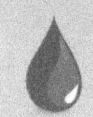

*monocytogenes, E. coli, P. aeruginosa,* and *S. typhimurium,* of which its activity against *S. aureus, B. cereus, P. aeruginosa,* and *S. typhimurium* was considered significant when compared against chloramphenicol.[7042]

☐ A clinical trial assessed the effects of peppermint essential oil (20.1% menthone, 16.0% limonene, 11.6% menthol) inhalation while under white, red, and blue color lights.[7043] Approximately 0.1 g of oil was added to scented wood placed close to the subject's nose at the beginning of the experiment and electroencephalographic (EEG) activity response recorded. Both alpha and beta brainwave activity increased after the inhalation of peppermint essential oil. Alpha waves increased in the prefrontal areas of the brain with white light and peppermint, which enhanced learning and thinking. The blue light/peppermint group had a less pronounced effect and the alpha wave activity was more controlled in the occipital area of the brain, suggesting an increase in visual function. Beta waves increased in the red light/peppermint group, which is indicative of greater alertness.

☐ Researchers analyzed the composition and antimicrobial activity of mint essential oils, including bergamot mint, peppermint, pennyroyal, spearmint, and apple mint. Bergamot mint inhibited *S. typhi* and *C. albicans*; *peppermint E. coli, B. subtilis,* and *C. albicans*; pennyroyal *K. pneumoniae, B. subtilis,* and *C. albicans*; spearmint significantly inhibited *S. typhi* and *B. subtilis*; and apple mint inhibited *K. pneumoniae, C. albicans,* and *S. typhi.*[7044]

☐ Peppermint (29.0% menthone, 22.4% menthol, 12.6% 1,8-cineole) and rosemary CT 1,8-cineole essential oil were evaluated for their biological effects (antimicrobial, antioxidant, anti-inflammatory and cytotoxic in different cancer cells) with an emphasis on their use as a complementary treatment for colorectal cancer.[7045] Peppermint exhibited potent antimicrobial activity (*S. mutans, S. pyogenes, S. aureus, E. coli, P. aeruginosa, C. albicans,* and *C. parapsilosis*), moderate antioxidant activity, and low cytotoxicity to colorectal cancer cells. Rosemary was significantly cytotoxic to colorectal cancer cells but presented a low antimicrobial and antioxidant activity.

☐ A nanogels containing peppermint essential oil (31.1% menthol, 22.1% menthone) completely protected against mosquitoes (*A. stephensi*) and inhibited *E. coli* and *S. aureus.*[7046]

☐ Injection of peppermint essential oil significantly reduced seizure occurrence, severity, and death in two mouse models of epilepsy.[7047]

☐ Both peppermint and frankincense (*B. serrata*; 29.8% beta-thujene, 11.7% alpha-thujene) essential oil inhibited pathogens frequently isolated from the vagina (*P. aeruginosa, P. mirabilis, S. aureus, E. coli,* and *C. albicans*), with the greatest activity observed from peppermint against *P. aeruginosa.*[7048] There activity exceeded that of the tested antibiotics (streptomycin, ampicillin, tetracycline, cefuroxime, and nystatin). Only peppermint showed bactericidal activity against *P. aeruginosa* and *P. mirabilis*, while both were fungicidal to *C. albicans*, which was strain specific.

☐ Peppermint and isolated menthol were toxic to the red spider mite (*Tetranychus urticae*) when used in fumigant form.[7049]

☐ Odd chemotypes of peppermint (28.0% alloaromadendrene, 18.3% levomenthol) and basil (32.3% alpha-humulene, 27.2% alpha-farnesene, 19.2% estragole) essential oils were lethal to the American tomato moth (*Phthorimaea absoluta*), with peppermint being most effective.[7050]

☐ Laboratory research showed that peppermint CT isomenthone essential oil inhibited both AChE and BChE (comparable to the standard drug galantamine in AChE and more active in BChE), which suggests that peppermint essential oil may help preserve memory and cognition.[7051]

☐ Inhalation—5 drops on a diffuser pad dispersed via unheated fan thirty minutes prior to participating in a driving simulator that included emergency situations, heavy traffic, and pedestrian encounters—of peppermint essential oil reduced aggressive driving behaviors in healthy adults.[7052]

☐ Peppermint essential oil produced 100 percent mortality in the South American tomato moth (*Phthorimaea absoluta*), which was attributed to alloaromadendrene, levomenthol, and santolina triene.[7053]

☐ Oral administration of rosemary (30.7% 1,8-cineole, 19.9% camphor, 8.0% alpha-pinene) or peppermint essential oil—equivalent to between 5 and 10 drops in humans—improved cognition (working memory, reference memory, and long-term memory) in a rat model of amnesia-like Alzheimer's disease.[7054] The oils significantly elevated BDNF—a protein in the central nervous system that promotes the survival of neurons by influencing growth, maturation, and maintenance of these cells—and increased hippocampal neurogenesis—the generation of new functional neurons (dentate granule cells) to improve neural plasticity. The combination of the oils produced even better enhancements in cognition.

☐ Adding 2% peppermint essential oil to ozone increased the efficacy against oral pathogens common in dental plaque (*C. albicans > E. coli > P. aeruginosa > S. aureus > S. mutans*).[7055]

# PERSIAN LIME
## (Tahiti Lime)

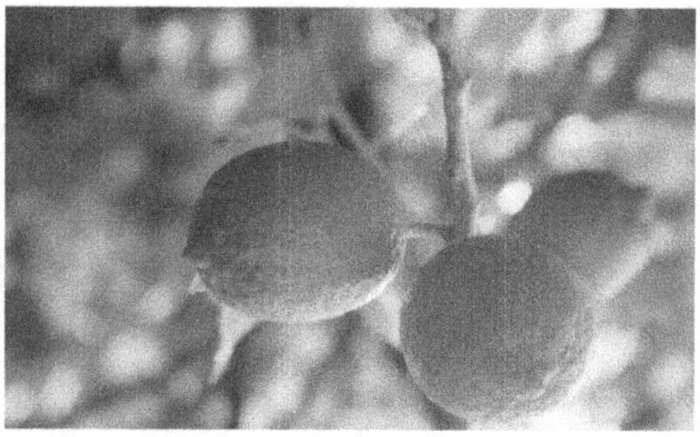

*Citrus × latifolia* Tanaka ex Q. Jiménez

**FAMILY:** Rutaceae
**NOTE:** Top
**AROMA INTENSITY:** Medium
**AROMA:** Citrusy, fruity, sharp
**COMMON EXTRACTION METHOD:** Cold-pressed/expressed or hydrodistilled from the fruit rind (peel)
**POSSIBLE SUBSTITUTE OILS:** Lime, bergamot, tangerine, orange
**BLENDS WELL WITH:** Bergamot, camphor, carrot seed, cassia, chamomile (German, Roman), cinnamon, citronella, geranium, grapefruit, lavender, lemon, lemon verbena, lemongrass, lime, Mediterranean mandarin, tea tree, neroli, nutmeg, orange, palmarosa, patchouli, petitgrain, pine, ravensara, rose, rosemary, sage, Spanish sage, tangerine, vetiver, ylang ylang
**SUBCELLULAR LOCALIZATION | EPIGENETIC INFLUENCE:** Currently unknown | Currently unknown
**RECOMMENDED DILUTION RANGE:** 3.0%–50.0%; neat for limited conditions

**PRIMARY CONSTITUENTS:**[7056,7057,7058,7059,7060,7061,7062,7063]

*Distilled*

| | |
|---|---|
| *d*-Limonene | 47.5%–62.0% |
| Gamma-Terpinene | 11.8%–17.0% |
| Beta-Thujene | 0.0%–14.9% |
| Beta-Pinene | 1.8%–13.0% |
| Alpha-Terpineol | 1.4%–6.6% |
| Geranial | 0.0%–6.4% |
| Para-Cymene | 0.1%–5.3% |
| Alpha-Terpinolene | 0.0%–5.2% |
| Neral | 0.0%–4.7% |
| Alpha-Pinene | 1.8%–2.8% |

*Cold-Pressed/Expressed*

| | |
|---|---|
| *d*-Limonene | 40.3%–59.8% |
| Gamma-Terpinene | 12.5%–21.5% |
| Beta-Pinene | 7.9%–15.3% |
| Geranial | 1.0%–4.0% |
| Beta-Bisabolene | 0.8%–2.4% |
| Geranyl Acetate | 0.2%–2.4% |
| Alpha-Pinene | 1.9%–2.3% |
| Neral | 1.1%–2.3% |

**OTHER CONSTITUENTS:** *Cold-Pressed/Expressed*—Sabinene, alpha-thujene, myrcene, 1,8-cineole, alpha-terpineolene, linalool, trans-alpha-bergamotene, beta-caryophyllene, alpha-terpineol, neryl acetate; *Distilled*—Camphene, alpha-thujene, sabinene, myrcene, linalool, 2,2,6-trimethyl-2-vinyl-tetrahydropyran, 1,4-cineole, p-cymene, alpha-fenchol, terpinen-1-ol, cis-beta-terpineol, terpinen-4-ol, neryl acetate, beta-bisabolene

**PREFERRED COMPOSITION FOR CLINICAL USE:**

| Constituent | Cold-pressed | Distilled |
|---|---|---|
| **Limonene** | 45%–60% | 40%–60% |
| **Gamma-Terpinene** | 10%–15% | 10%–20% |
| **Beta-Pinene** | 8%–15% | 8%–17% |
| **Alpha-Terpineol** | 1%–5% | 0%–5% |
| **Alpha-Pinene** | 1.5%–3% | 1.5%–3% |
| **Geranial** | 1%–3% | 0%–2% |
| **Neral** | 1%–3% | 1%–3% |
| **Myrcene** | 1%–2% | 1%–3% |
| **Neryl Acetate + Geranyl Acetate** | 0.5%–2% | 0.2%–2% |

**REPORTED THERAPEUTIC PROPERTIES:** Antiseptic, **antifungal**, antiviral, astringent, antibacterial, anti-inflammatory, appetite stimulant, antispasmodic, disinfectant, **antioxidant**, reduces fever, stops excess bleeding, aids immune function, regenerative, circulatory aid, reduces appearance of blemishes, tones the skin, reduces cellulite, encourages restful sleep, weight management, antidepressant, **reduces anxiety**, stress management, uplifting

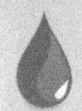

**CAUTIONS:**

■ May be photosensitizing (cold-pressed/expressed). Avoid sun exposure to area of application for at least twelve hours after topical application.[7064]

■ May interfere with enzymes responsible for metabolizing medications (NSAIDs, proton-pump inhibitors, acetaminophen, antiepileptics, immune modulators, blood-sugar medications, blood pressure medications, antidepressants, antipsychotics, diabetic medications, antihistamines, antibiotics, and anesthetics).[7065]

**SELECTED EVIDENCE:**

☐ *In vitro* research concluded that Persian lime essential oil (distilled) reduces inflammation by inhibiting proinflammatory mediators (TNF-alpha and neutrophil migration).[7066] Neutrophils migrate from circulation to the site of inflammation and into inflamed tissue and produce reactive oxygen species (ROS) to kill pathogens. However, this release of ROS can also damage normal tissues when inappropriately activated, like in autoimmune disease.

☐ Oral administration of 0.5 g/kg of Persian lime essential oil (distilled) reduced anxiety (interestingly 1.0 g/kg did not reduce anxiety) and oral administration of 1.0 and 1.5 g/kg significantly reduced obsessive-compulsive disorder (marble-burying) in experimental animal models.[7067]

☐ *In vitro* research concluded that Persian lime essential oil (distilled) inhibits several fungi (*C. albicans, C. tropicalis, C. glabrata, C. lusitaniae,* and *C. guilliermondii*), including some antimycotic activity greater than amphotericin B (a drug used for serious, usually potentially life-threatening, systemic fungal infections).[7068]

☐ Persian lime essential oil demonstrates strong antioxidant properties.[7069]

☐ Both orange and Persian lime essential oils prevented DNA mutations caused by MNNG (N-methyl-N′-nitro-N-nitrosoguanidine) and demonstrated good antioxidant activity in the β-carotene bleaching assay.[7070] Persian lime also prevented DNA mutation caused by ENNG.

# PERU BALSAM
## (Balsam of Peru)

*Myroxylon pereirae* (Royle) Klotzsch, *M. balsamum* (L.) Harms var. *pereirae* (Royle) Harms, *Myrospermum sonsonatense* Per.

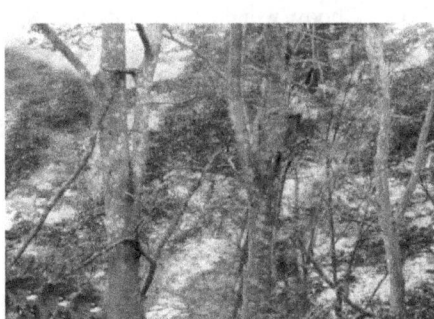

**FAMILY:** Fabaceae
**NOTE:** Base
**AROMA INTENSITY:** Medium
**AROMA:** Balsamic, rich, sweet, earthy, soft hint of vanilla and cinnamon
**COMMON EXTRACTION METHOD:** Steam distilled from the resin
**POSSIBLE SUBSTITUTE OILS:** Tolu balsam, ylang ylang, copaiba, frankincense
**BLENDS WELL WITH:** Balsam fir, black pepper, cardamom, cedarwood, cinnamon, clove, copaiba, frankincense, ginger, lemon, lime, neroli, orange, patchouli, petitgrain, rose, sandalwood, tangerine, ylang ylang
**SUBCELLULAR LOCALIZATION | EPIGENETIC INFLUENCE:** Currently unknown | Currently unknown
**RECOMMENDED DILUTION RANGE:** 1.5%–5.0%

**PRIMARY CONSTITUENTS:**[7071,7072,7073]

| *Essential Oil* | | *Resinoid Absolute* | |
|---|---|---|---|
| Benzyl Benzoate | 56.6%–66.2% | Benzyl Benzoate | 25.0%–40.0% |
| Benzyl Cinnamate | 15.9%–22.1% | Benzyl Cinnamate | 10.0%–25.0% |
| Benzoic Acid | 8.1%–8.9% | (E)-Nerolidol | 0.0%–5.0% |
| (E)-Cinnamic Acid | 3.0%–5.1% | (Z)-Nerolidol | 0.0%–5.0% |
| (E)-Nerolidol | 3.4%–4.8% | | |

**OTHER CONSTITUENTS:** *Essential* oil—Benzyl alcohol, vanillin, benzyl cinnamate isomer; *Resinoid Absolute—*vanillin, (E)-cinnamic acid, benzoic acid

**PREFERRED COMPOSITION FOR CLINICAL USE:**

| *Constituent* | *EO* |
|---|---|
| **Benzyl Benzoate** | 43%–67% |
| **(E)-Benzyl Cinnamate** | 10%–30% |
| **(E)-Cinnamic Acid** | 3%–12% |
| **Benzoic Acid** | 2%–10% |
| **(E)-Nerolidol** | 3%–6% |
| **Vanillin** | 0.2%–1% |
| **Benzyl Alcohol** | 0.1%–1% |

**REPORTED THERAPEUTIC PROPERTIES:** Antibacterial, antifungal, antiseptic, antiparasitic, anti-inflammatory, antiarthritic, antirheumatic, diuretic, astringent, nourishes the hair and skin, relieves chronic skin conditions, aids circulation, antioxidant, supports respiratory function, expels excess mucus, **combats lice**, relieves painful menstruation, aids detoxification, eases cough, supports oral health, relieves diarrhea, insecticide, relieves anxiety, stress management, combats anger, **relieves emotional trauma**

**CAUTIONS:**

■ Oral caution. Ingestion of benzoic acids, benzoic salts (calcium, potassium, and sodium), benzaldehyde, benzyl acetate, benzyl benzoate, and benzyl alcohol may cause gastrointestinal irritation, vomiting, and diarrhea.[7074] The Joint Expert Committee for Food Additives (JECFA) has established an acceptable daily limit for the aforementioned constituents of 0–5mg/kg body weight for adults to avoid GI discomfort.[7075] Based on this limit, it is suggested to limit the oral consumption to no more than 4 drops daily.

■ Dilutions of less than 1.0% are strongly recommended for people with chronic skin conditions, allergies, compromised immune systems, or chronic respiratory conditions based on reports of sensitization among individuals with and without a compromised immune system.[7076,7077,7078]

**SELECTED EVIDENCE:**

☐ Peru balsam essential oil is larvacidal to the mosquito *A. aegypti* and the water flea *Daphnia magna*.[7079]

☐ Peru balsam essential oil demonstrated potent antioxidant activity.[7080]

---

# PETA

*Helichrysum splendidum* (Thunb.) Less

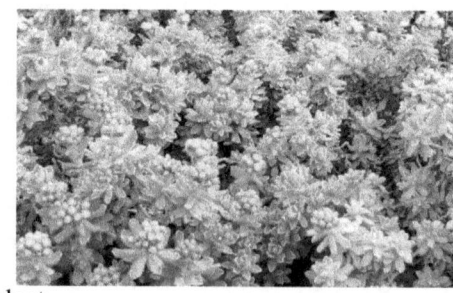

**FAMILY:** Asteraceae (Compositae)
**NOTE:** Middle-Base | Peta: Middle
**AROMA INTENSITY:** Medium
**AROMA:** Herbaceous, fresh, sweet
**COMMON EXTRACTION METHOD:** Steam distilled from the flowering plant
**POSSIBLE SUBSTITUTE OILS:** Cypress, cistus, frankincense, calendula
**BLENDS WELL WITH:** Bergamot, chamomile (German, Roman), clary sage, clove, cypress, geranium, grapefruit, lavender, lemon, lime, tea tree, neroli, orange, oregano, rosemary, tangerine, vetiver, ylang ylang
**SUBCELLULAR LOCALIZATION | EPIGENETIC INFLUENCE:** Currently Unknown
**RECOMMENDED DILUTION RANGE:** 3%–50%; neat for limited conditions

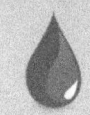

**PRIMARY CONSTITUENTS:**[7081,7082,7083,7084,7085,7086,7087,7088,7089,7090,7091,7092,7093,7094]

*Delta-Cadinene CT*

| | |
|---|---|
| Delta-Cadinene | 9.3%–16.9% |
| Alpha-Cadinol | 5.8%–16.8% |
| Germacrene D | 3.4%–10.1% |
| T-Cadinol | 0.0%–9.0% |
| Alpha-Cadinene | 1.1%–7.6% |
| Alpha-Muurolol | 3.4%–7.5% |
| Bicyclogermacrene | 0.8%–6.3% |
| Spathulenol | 0.0%–6.1% |

*Spathulenol CT*

| | |
|---|---|
| Spathulenol | 12.2%–30.7% |
| Bicyclogermacrene | 7.4%–20.5% |
| Delta-Cadinene | 1.4%–6.9% |
| Alpha-Cadinol | 0.5%–6.5% |
| T-Cadinol | 0.4%–3.4% |
| Alpha-Muurolol | 0.4%–2.9% |

*Alpha-Terpinene CT*

| | |
|---|---|
| Alpha-Terpinene | 14.9% |
| Beta-Pinene | 10.2% |
| 1,8-Cineole | 8.6% |
| Bicyclogermacrene | 7.9% |
| Delta-Cadinene | 7.4% |
| Cubebol | 7.3% |
| Alpha-Phellandrene | 5.5% |
| Para-Cymene | 3.0% |
| Germacrene D-4-ol | 2.5% |
| Sabinene | 2.4% |
| Alpha-Thujene | 1.6% |
| Alpha-Cadinol | 1.6% |
| Camphor | 1.2% |

**OTHER CONSTITUENTS:** *Delta-Cadinene CT*—beta-phellandrene, beta-pinene, borneol, alpha-cubebene, alpha-copaene, beta-bourbonene, beta-cubebene, beta-elemene, trans-caryophyllene, allo-aromadendrene, germacrene D-isomer, gamma-muurolene, beta-selinene, cadina-1,4-diene, viridiflorol, 1,10-di-epi-cubenol, 1-epi-cubenol, guaiazulene; *Sapthulenol CT*—not reported in study; *Alpha-Terpinene CT*—limonene, terpinolene, beta-caryophyllene, terpinen-4-ol, germacrene D, alpha-cadinene, T-muurolol, T-cadinol

**PREFERRED COMPOSITION FOR CLINICAL USE:**

| Constituent | |
|---|---|
| **Beta-Phellandrene** | 15%–25% |
| **Delta-Cadinene** | 10%–15% |
| **Beta-Pinene** | 7%–15% |
| **Germacrene D** | 1%–8% |
| **Gamma-Cadinene** | 3%–7% |
| **Alpha-Pinene** | 2%–5% |
| **Bicyclogermacrene** | 2%–5% |
| **Alpha Muurolene** | 2%–5% |
| **Beta-Bourbonene** | 2%–5% |
| **Beta-Elemene** | 2%–5% |
| **Epi-Cubebol** | 1%–3% |
| **Germacrene D-4-ol** | 1%–3% |
| **Sabinene** | 1%–3% |
| **Borneol** | 0.1%–2% |
| **Cubebol** | 0.1%–2% |
| **Alpha-Copaene** | 0.0%–2.0% |

**REPORTED THERAPEUTIC PROPERTIES (Peta):** Antibacterial, antifungal, antiviral, **anti-inflammatory**, antirheumatic, antiarthritic, analgesic, antioxidant, relieves burns/chronic skin conditions, wound healing, antiseptic, antispasmodic, **supports respiratory function**, aids mental clarity, combats anger, stress management

**CAUTIONS:**
■ None currently known.

**SELECTED EVIDENCE:**
☐ None found.

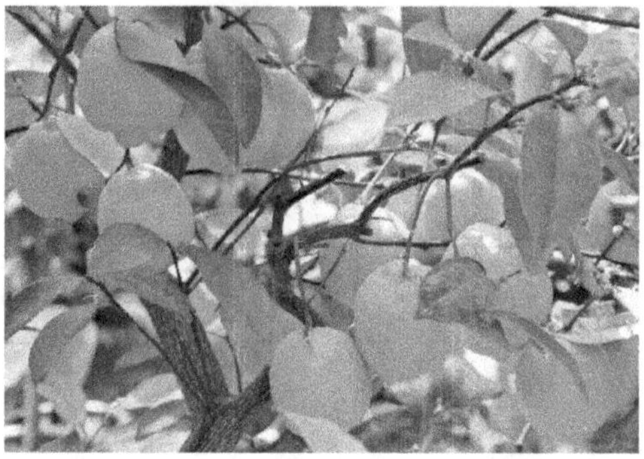

# PETITGRAIN

Petitgrain of Bergamot: *Citrus bergamia* Risso & Poit., *C. bigaradia* Risso & Poit.; Petitgrain of Bitter Orange: *C. × aurantium* L., *C. × aurantium* subsp. *amara*; Petitgrain of Mandarin: *C. reticulata* Blanco; Petitgrain of Lemon: *C. limon* (L.) Burm. f.; Petitgrain of Lime: *C. × aurantiifolia* (Christm.) Swingle, *C. latifolia* Tanaka ex Q. Jiménez

**FAMILY:** Rutaceae
**NOTE:** Top-Middle
**AROMA INTENSITY:** Strong
**AROMA:** Citrusy, fresh, floral, slightly woody and herbaceous
**COMMON EXTRACTION METHOD:** Steam distilled from the leaves and twigs
**POSSIBLE SUBSTITUTE OILS:** Neroli, combava, lavender, bergamot, niaouli (viridiflorol/para-cymene/1,8-cineole CT), lemon, lime, Persian lime
**BLENDS WELL WITH:** Bergamot, cassia, cinnamon, citronella, geranium, lemon, lemongrass, lime, lemon verbena, neroli, sage, spikenard, tangerine
**SUBCELLULAR LOCALIZATION | EPIGENETIC INFLUENCE:** Currently unknown | Currently unknown
**RECOMMENDED DILUTION RANGE:** 3%–50%; neat for limited conditions

**PRIMARY CONSTITUENTS:**[7095,7096,7097,7098,7099,7100,7101,7102,]

*Pettigrain of Bergamot*
*Petitgrain of Bitter Orange*

| | |
|---|---|
| Linalool | 18.6%–66.0% |
| Linalyl Acetate | 12.4%–50.0% |
| Alpha-Terpineol | 7.1%–12.9% |
| Trans-Carveol | 0.0%–11.9% |
| Geranyl Acetate | 0.0%–8.7% |
| Cis-Linalool Oxide | 0.0%–8.1% |
| Gamma-Terpinene | 0.0%–7.0% |
| Carvone | 0.0%–5.8% |
| Neryl Acetate | 2.2%–4.5% |
| Trans-Beta-Ocimene | 3.1%–4.1% |
| Beta-Pinene | 1.6%–3.6% |

*Petitgrain of Mandarin*

| | |
|---|---|
| Dimethyl Anthranilate | 13.2%–65.3% |
| Gamma-Terpinene | 19.8%–47.9% |
| Para-Cymene | 0.1%–16.3% |
| Limonene | 0.0%–12.6% |
| Linalool | 0.0%–9.6% |
| Alpha-Terpinene | 0.0%–7.4% |
| Terpinen-4-ol | 0.1%–7.1% |
| Beta-Phellandrene | 0.0%–6.3% |
| Trans-Isolimonene | 0.0%–5.9% |
| Alpha-Terpinolene | 0.6%–4.6% |
| Myrcene | 0.0%–3.2% |
| Alpha-Pinene | 1.7%–2.8% |
| Beta-Pinene | 0.0%–2.3% |

*Petitgrain of Lemon*

| | |
|---|---|
| Limonene | 17.8%–33.5% |
| Beta-Pinene | 10.5%–25.1% |
| Geranial | 14.3%–22.6% |
| Neral | 10.4%–16.1% |
| 1,8-Cineole | 0.0%–5.2% |
| Sabinene | 1.9%–5.1% |
| Neryl Acetate | 0.7%–5.1% |
| Nerol | 1.2%–3.4% |
| Geranyl Acetate | 0.8%–3.2% |
| 6-Methylhept-5-en-2-one | 0.7%–3.2% |
| Geraniol | 0.8%–2.4% |
| Trans-Beta-Ocimene | 1.5%–2.2% |
| Linalool | 1.4%–2.1% |

*Petitgrain of Lime*

| | |
|---|---|
| Limonene | 22.1%–53.4% |
| Geranial | 11.8%–26.9% |
| Neral | 8.3%–20.5% |
| Santal-10-en-2-ol | 0.0%–8.5% |
| Geranyl Acetate | 1.7%–8.3% |
| Linalool | 0.9%–8.1% |
| Neryl Acetate | 0.6%–6.1% |
| Geraniol | 1.3%–3.8% |
| Nerol | 1.1%–3.1% |
| 6-Methylhept-5-en-2-one | 1.1%–2.5% |

Note: Petitgrain of lemon can also have other chemotypes including one with linalool and linalyl acetate, but the limonene CT is more common.

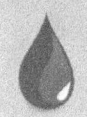

**OTHER CONSTITUENTS:** *Petitgrain of Bergamot/Bitter Orange*—Sabinene, myrcene, limonene, cis-beta-ocimene, trans-beta-ocimene, nerol, neryl acetate, geranyl acetate; *Petitgrain of Mandarin*—Alloocimene, limonene oxide, linalyl propionate, cuminic aldehyde, linalool oxide, caryophyllene oxide, alpha-thujene, sabinene, trans-ocimene; *Petitgrain of Lemon*—Alpha-pinene, delta-3-carene, myrcene, gamma-terpinene, (Z)-beta-ocimene, citronellal, terpinen-4-ol, alpha-terpineol, citronellol; *Petitgrain of Lime*—sabinene, myrcene, 1,8-cineole, beta-phellandrene, trans-beta-ocimene, alpha-terpineol, citronellol

**PREFERRED COMPOSITION FOR CLINICAL USE:**

| Constituent | Petitgrain of Bergamot | Petitgrain of Bitter Orange | Petitgrain of Mandarin | Petitgrain of Lemon | Petitgrain of Lime |
|---|---|---|---|---|---|
| Linalyl Acetate | 55%–70% | 45%–60% | – | – | – |
| Linalool | 8%–15% | 18%–35% | – | 1%–4% | 1%–3% |
| Alpha-Terpineol | 2%–5% | 2%–7% | – | – | – |
| Geranyl Acetate | 2%–5% | 2%–5% | – | 1%–4% | 2%–6% |
| Neryl Acetate | 2%–5% | 1%–5% | – | 1.5%–6% | 1%–6% |
| Trans-Beta-Ocimene | 2%–4% | 2%–4% | – | 1.5%–3% | |
| Limonene | 1%–3% | 1%–5% | 7%–12% | 20%–35% | 30%–42% |
| Beta-Pinene | 1%–3% | 0.1%–3% | 1%–3% | 12%–25% | – |
| Myrcene | 1%–3% | 0.1%–4% | – | – | – |
| Beta-Caryophyllene | 1%–2% | 0%–2% | – | – | – |
| Nerol | 0.1%–1% | 0%–1% | – | 1%–4% | 1%–3% |
| Geraniol | < 1% | 1%–4% | – | 0.5%–3% | 1%–3% |
| Dimethyl Anthranilate | – | – | 40%–60% | – | – |
| Gamma-Terpinene | – | – | 20%–27% | – | – |
| Para-Cymene | – | – | 4%–8% | – | – |
| Alpha-Pinene | – | – | 1.5%–3% | – | – |
| Alpha-Terpinolene | – | – | 0.1%–3% | – | – |
| Terpinen-4-ol | – | – | 0.1%–3% | – | – |
| Geranial | – | – | – | 12%–22% | 11%–28% |
| Neral | – | – | – | 10%–16% | 8%–20% |
| 1,8-Cineole | – | – | – | 0.5%–5% | – |
| Sabinene | – | – | – | 2%–6% | – |
| 6-Methyl Hept-5-en-2-one | – | – | – | 0.5%–3% | 0.5%–3% |

**REPORTED THERAPEUTIC PROPERTIES: Antiseptic**, **anti-inflammatory**, **antifungal**, antispasmodic, **antibacterial**, expels excess gas, deodorant, nervine (calms and soothes the nerves), supports liver function, eases nausea, encourages restful sleep, reduces excess sweating, helps reduce the appearance of blemishes, aids digestion, relaxing, uplifting, **antidepressant**, **reduces anxiety**, calms anger, stimulates creativity, encourages a fresh perspective

**CAUTIONS:**

■ May be mildly photosensitizing (low risk). Avoid sun exposure to area of application for at least twelve hours after topical application.[7103,7104]

**SELECTED EVIDENCE:**

- ☐ *C. reticulata* was effective against two leukemia cell lines *in vitro*.[7105]
- ☐ Oral administration of 0.5 to 1.0 g/kg of *C. aurantium* (leaf and peel) oil reduced anxiety and increased sleeping times of barbiturate drugs in mice.[7106]
- ☐ Inhalation of petitgrain essential oil improved workplace performance by balance the autonomic nervous system, which led to an improved mental and emotional state, reduced stress level, and increased attentiveness and alertness.[7107]
- ☐ *C. aurantium* petitgrain essential oil acts as an antioxidant, and is more effective as a free radical scavenger

than the peel or flower (particularly old leaves as opposed to young leaves).[7108]

☐ *C. aurantium* petitgrain essential oil inhibited gram-positive (*B. subtilis and S. aureus*) bacteria and moderately inhibited yeasts (*S. cerecisiae*) and fungi (*M. ramannianus*).[7109]

☐ Petitgrain of bitter orange repelled the *Ae. aegypti* mosquito.[7110]

☐ Several essential oils listed in order of efficacy killed the itch mite (*Sarcoptes scabiei*) that burrows into the skin and causes scabies during direct contact clove > palmarosa > geranium > tea tree > lavender > manuka > petitgrain of bitter orange > eucalyptus > Japanese cedarwood) with the mites and when used as a fumigant (tea tree > clove > eucalyptus > lavender > palmarosa > geranium > Japanese cedarwood > petitgrain > manuka).[7111]

☐ Petitgrain of bitter orange inhibited *B. subtilis* on carrots and weakly inhibited fungi (*Penicillium crustosum, P. citrinum*, and *P. expansum*) on bread.[7112]

☐ Ravintsara, turmeric, petitgrain (*C. aurantium*), and bitter orange essential oil each inhibited *Mycobacterium smegmatis* (a bacterial strain commonly used as a model for inhibition of *M. tuberculosis*), *C. albicans*, and *C. tropicalis*.[7113] The oils also displayed activity against collagenase, indicating an antiaging activity. Petitgrain and turmeric also inhibited elastase, which would preserve skin strength and flexibility.

☐ Three cultivars of petitgrain of mandarin—Kishu, Cara, and Willow leaf—demonstrated antiaging potential due to their ability to inhibit hyaluronidase, collagenase, and elastase *in vitro*.[7114] Computer docking analysis revealed that thymol, dimethyl anthranilate, and linalool were the most active constituents with strong docking potential to the enzyme binding sites.

☐ Petitgrain (*C. sinensis*) essential oil extracted from fresh spring leaves and nanoemulsified was effective against third instar larvae *Culex pipiens* (common house mosquito).[7115]

# PINE
## (Scots Pine, Scotch Pine)
*Pinus sylvestris* L.

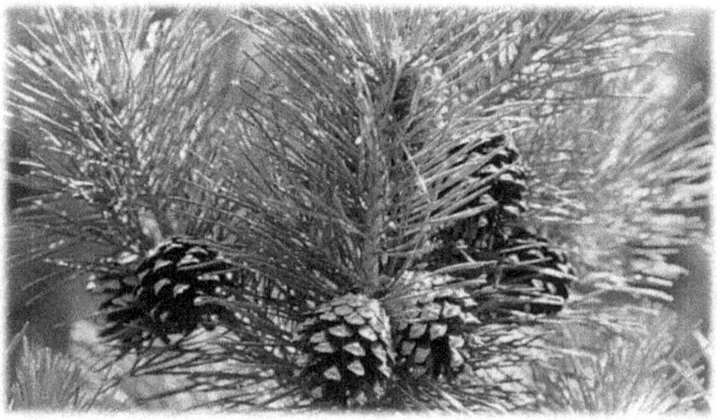

**FAMILY:** Pinaceae
**NOTE:** Top
**AROMA INTENSITY:** Strong
**AROMA:** Fresh, woody, balsamic, clean
**COMMON EXTRACTION METHOD:** Steam distilled from the needles and twigs
**POSSIBLE SUBSTITUTE OILS:** Balsam fir, cypress, silver fir, galbanum, blue spruce
**BLENDS WELL WITH:** Bergamot, cajeput, camphor, cedarwood, clary sage, coriander, eucalyptus, frankincense, galbanum, grapefruit, juniper, lavender, lemon, lime, tea tree, marjoram, neroli, niaouli, peppermint, ravensara, ravintsara, rosemary, Spanish sage, spikenard, thyme, silver fir, white fir
**SUBCELLULAR LOCALIZATION | EPIGENETIC INFLUENCE:** Currently unknown | Currently unknown
**RECOMMENDED DILUTION RANGE:** 3%–50%; neat for limited conditions

**PRIMARY CONSTITUENTS:**[7116,7117,7118,7119,7120,7121]

| | |
|---|---|
| Alpha-Pinene | 14.8%–51.1% |
| Delta-3-Carene | 0.1%–33.7% |
| Beta-Pinene | 1.8%–29.4% |
| Camphene | 0.4%–16.8% |
| Caryophyllene Oxide | 0.0%–12.6% |
| Delta-Cadinene | 0.0%–11.6% |
| Gamma-Cadinene | 0.0%–11.1% |
| Alpha-Longifolene | 0.0%–9.6% |
| Alpha-Cadinol | 0.0%–7.7% |
| Germacrene D | 0.2%–6.5% |

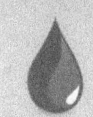

| | |
|---|---|
| Bicyclogermacrene | 0.0%–6.2% |
| Cubenol | 0.0%–5.1% |
| Beta-Caryophyllene | 0.6%–4.9% |
| Tricyclene | 0.1%–4.3% |
| Bornyl Acetate | 0.1%–3.9% |
| Trans-Verbenol | 0.1%–3.5% |
| Beta-Myrcene | 0.2%–3.4 % |

**OTHER CONSTITUENTS:** Para-cymene, limonene, beta-phellandrene, alpha-campholene aldehyde, trans-pinocarveol, alpha-humulene, humulene epoxide, alpha-cadinene, alpha-muurolene, beta-bisabolene, alpha-terpinene, terpinolene, sabinene, (Z)-beta-ocimene, (E)-beta-ocimene, gamma-terpinene, borneol, p-mentha-1,5-dien-8-ol, terpinen-4-ol, alpha-terpineol, thymol, undecanone-2, delta-elemene, terpinyl acetate, alpha-cubebene, alpha-copaene, beta-elemene, aromadendrene, alpha-humulene, alpha-cadinene, germacrene-d-4-ol, spathulenol, gleenol, 1-epi-cubenol, 1,10-di-epi-cubenol

**PREFERRED COMPOSITION FOR CLINICAL USE:**

| Constituent | Scots | Scots 2 | Pinion* |
|---|---|---|---|
| **Alpha-Pinene** | 45%–62% | 30%–50% | 45%–60% |
| **Beta-Pinene** | 5%–25% | 10%–25% | 5%–15% |
| **Delta-3-Carene** | 5%–15% | 10%–25% | 2%–7% |
| **Limonene** | 3%–10% | 3%–20% | 1%–3% |
| **Myrcene** | 4%–7% | 0.5%–7% | 3%–6% |
| **Camphene** | 1%–4% | 0.5%–7% | 1%–3% |
| **Beta-Caryophyllene** | 1%–3% | 0.5%–3% | – |
| **Bornyl Acetate** | 0.1%–3% | 0.5%–5% | 1%–5% |
| **Beta-Phellandrene** | 0.1%–3% | 0.1%–3% | 5%–15% |

\* Pinion pine (*Pinus edulis*) is included because of its similar composition to Scots pine. Some retailers carry pinion pine instead of Scots pine. It can be used similarly because of its comparable composition.

**REPORTED THERAPEUTIC PROPERTIES:** Analgesic (pain relief), antibacterial, **antifungal**, anti-inflammatory, **antineuralgic**, antimicrobial, **antioxidant**, **nervine (calms and soothes the nerves)**, antirheumatic, aids detoxification, **antiseptic**, antiviral, anti-infectious, soothes various skin conditions, **decongestant**, clears excess mucus, disinfectant, diuretic, expectorant, antiparasitic, encourages normal bone turnover (remodeling), helps eliminate uric acid, **eases cough**, enhances metabolism, **balances respiratory function**, improves eye health and protects eyes from oxidative damage, reduces gallbladder inflammation and helps eliminate gallstones, stimulating, **stress management**, reduces anxiety, reduces anger, grounding, **relieves fatigue**

**CAUTIONS:**
■ None currently known.

**SELECTED EVIDENCE:**
- □ Pine essential oil demonstrated the ability to inhibit both estrogen positive and estrogen negative breast cancer cells.[7122]
- □ Animal research suggests that Siberian pine essential oil (*Pinus sibirica*) may protect against osteoporosis by inhibiting osteoclast (cells that break down bone tissue to release minerals into the circulatory system) activity and normalizing bone turnover.[7123] Alpha-pinene, beta-pinene, and bornyl acetate from this pine oil were all potent inhibitors of bone resorption, suggesting Scots pine may also be effective.
- □ Pine oil inhibits *C. hystoliticum* (a bacterium that can cause acute infection, fever, pain, edema, organ failure, and gas gangrene) and *C. ramosum* (a bacterium associated with obesity in animals).[7124]
- □ Animal research suggests that pine oil enhances the production of airway surface liquid (liquid found in the airways that is important in normal respiration, traps inhaled particles, and is involved in mucous secretion) in the trachea and salivary glands.[7125]

- *In vitro* research concluded that pine oil improves air quality by inhibiting several fungi, yeast, bacteria, and toxins associated with difficulty breathing, allergic rhinitis, watery eyes, headaches, and flu-like symptoms.[7126]
- Pine essential oil demonstrated significant antifungal activity against clinical isolates of *Candida* spp. in both liquid and vapor phases.[7127]
- *In vitro* research demonstrates that pine essential oil inhibits *Cryptococcus neoformans* (a difficult to treat encapsulated yeast that few molecules actively inhibit and a serious problem for people with a compromised immune system).[7128]
- *Helicobacter pylori* is a bacterium that lives in the digestive tract that can cause sores and ulcers in the lining of the stomach or upper part of the small intestine. Thyme, lemongrass, Virginia cedarwood, and melissa essential oils were the most active of 26 commercial essential oils examined against *H. pylori*.[7129] Oregano, tea tree, pine, and silver fir were also bactericidal.
- Eucalyptus (*E. globulus*), pine, rosemary, cistus, Maritime pine, and juniper berry each displayed good antioxidant activity in the ORAC assay.[7130]
- Of nine commercial essential oils tested (fennel, geranium, lavender, melissa, oregano CT carvacrol, thyme CT thymol, and sage), pine essential oil was strongly antifungal against non-*albicans Candida* isolates and uncommon yeasts that are growingly associated with yeast infections. Melissa and isolated alpha-pinene also exhibited strong activity against non-*albicans Candida* isolates, and isolated thymol inhibited all uncommon yeasts.
- Pneumonitis refers to inflammation in the lungs, which can cause shortness of breath, cough, fatigue, unintentional weight loss, fever, muscle or joint pain, and loss of appetite. Pine (39.4% alpha-pinene, 14.3% limonene, 11.0% beta-pinene) and clove bud essential oils were evaluated for their effects in an acute model of pneumonitis.[7131] Inhalation of pine or clove oils for thirty minutes prior to induction of pneumonitis and four and twenty-three hours afterward significantly reduced airway hyperresponsiveness and respiratory dysfunction (prevented peak expiratory flow, tidal volume increases, and perivascular edema formation), but interestingly increased the inflammatory response (myeloperoxidase activity and cytokine production).
- Researchers evaluated the effects of inhaling sweet orange or pine essential oils on stress based on their visual-motor reaction to the aromas.[7132] Twenty-one young adults aged eighteen to twenty-one years participated in a visual-motor assessment where they had to push the down arrow key as quickly as possible in response to different colored shapes. Fifteen of the participants inhaled orange essential oil for twenty-five minutes, while six inhaled pine essential oil before participating in the assessment. Reaction times and error rates were recorded for each group. Reaction times increased after inhaling both oils, but error rate increased in the orange group and decreased in the pine group. The results suggest that orange essential oil promoted relaxation and alleviated psychoemotional arousal, while pine oil reduced fatigue and promoted greater vigilance.
- Pine, melissa (43.0% citral, 25.0% beta-caryophyllene), ginger, lemon, thyme CT thymol, and basil CT methyl chavicol essential oils each showed activity against MRSA and *E. coli*. Thyme completely inhibited all bacteria at all concentrations tested.[7133]

---

# PINK PEPPER
(California Pepper, Peruvian Pepper/ Mastic, Aguaribay, Aroeira, Baies Roses, Brazilian Pepper)

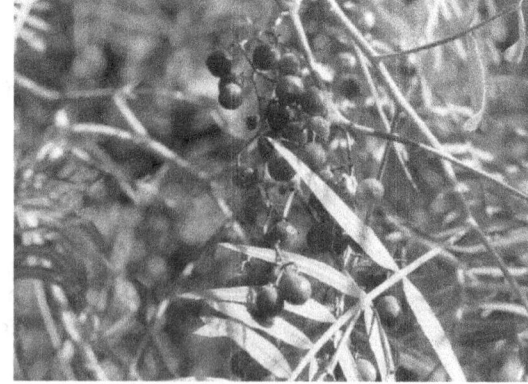

Peruvian/California Pepper: *Schinus molle* L.;
Brazilian Pepper: *S. terebinthifolius* Raddi

**FAMILY:** Anacardiaceae
**NOTE:** Middle
**AROMA INTENSITY:** Medium
**AROMA:** Spicy, sweet, peppery, slightly fruity
**COMMON EXTRACTION METHOD:** Steam distilled from the dried fruits; may also be distilled from the dried leaves, stems/branches, flowers, or aerial parts

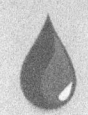

**POSSIBLE SUBSTITUTE OILS:** Elemi, *Eucalyptus dives*, pine, balsam fir, hemp, dill, helichrysum (*H. slendidum*), black pepper, copaiba

**BLENDS WELL WITH:** Amyris, bergamot, black pepper, cedarwood, cardamom, carrot, clary sage, clove, frankincense, geranium, ginger, grapefruit, lavandin, lavender, lemon, lime, marjoram, may chang, myrrh, neroli, nutmeg, orange, palo santo, patchouli, rosemary, sage, sandalwood, Spanish sage, tangerine, tea tree, vetiver, yarrow, ylang ylang

**SUBCELLULAR LOCALIZATION | EPIGENETIC INFLUENCE:** Currently unknown | Currently unknown

**RECOMMENDED DILUTION RANGE:** 3%–Neat

**PRIMARY CONSTITUENTS:**[7134,7135,7136,7137,7138,7139,7140,7141,7142,7143,7144,7145,7146,7147,7148,7149,7150,7151,7152]

*S. molle (Fruits—Alpha-Phellandrene CT)*

| | |
|---|---|
| Alpha-Phellandrene | 22.1%–46.5% |
| Limonene | 0.0%–20.9% |
| Beta-Phellandrene | 0.0%–20.8% |
| Myrcene | 0.0%–16.8% |
| Alpha-Terpineol | 0.0%–8.4% |
| Alpha-Cadinol | 0.1%–7.2% |
| Para-Cymene | 1.8%–6.4% |
| Methyl Octanoate | 0.6%–5.2% |
| Beta-Pinene | 0.0%–5.0% |
| Octanoic Acid | 0.0%–4.4% |
| Alpha-Pinene | 1.1%–4.3% |
| Delta-Cadinene | 0.3%–4.0% |

*S. molle (Fruits/Leaves—Alpha-Phellandrene/Sylvestrene CT)*

| | |
|---|---|
| Alpha-Phellandrene | 32.8%–45.0% |
| Sylvestrene | 22.3%–38.5% |
| O-Cymene | 0.0%–8.5% |
| Para-Cymene | 0.0%–8.1% |
| Delta-Cadinene | 1.1%–7.6% |
| Myrcene | 1.0%–5.1% |
| Sabinene | 0.9%–5.1% |
| Beta-Caryophyllene | 0.0%–4.5% |
| Elemol | 0.8%–4.3% |

*S. molle (Leaves—Alpha-Phellandrene CT)*

| | |
|---|---|
| Alpha-Phellandrene | 26.5%–45.7% |
| Beta-Phellandrene | 9.6%–13.6% |
| Limonene | 0.0%–13.4% |
| Elemol | 0.1%–13.3% |
| Para-Cymene | 0.0%–7.3% |
| Alpha-Pinene | 0.2%–6.5% |
| Alpha-Eudesmol | 0.0%–6.1% |
| Alpha-Terpineol | 0.0%–5.6% |
| Germacrene D | 0.0%–5.2% |
| Gamma-Cadinol | 0.0%–4.7% |
| Beta-Eudesmol | 0.0%–4.2% |
| Myrcene | 0.0%–4.1% |
| Bicyclogermacrene | 0.0%–4.1% |

*S. molle (Leaves—Beta-Pinene CT)*

| | |
|---|---|
| Beta-Pinene | 31.1% |
| Alpha-Pinene | 22.7% |

*S. terebinthifolius (Fruits—Delta-3-Carene CT)*

| | |
|---|---|
| Delta-3-Carene | 5.8%–55.4% |
| Beta-Phellandrene | 0.0%–18.5% |
| Limonene | 0.0%–17.4% |
| Alpha-Pinene | 1.8%–16.3% |
| Alpha-Cadinol | 0.0%–16.3% |
| Elemol | 0.0%–13.6% |
| Alpha-Phellandrene | 2.9%–12.9% |
| Sylvestrene | 0.0%–10.7% |
| Germacrene D | 0.0%–8.7% |
| Delta-Cadinene | 0.3%–7.1% |
| Myrcene | 1.0%–5.8% |
| Germacrene D-4-ol | 0.0%–5.3% |
| Epi-Alpha-Cadinol | 0.1%–4.6% |

*S. terebinthifolius (Fruits—Alpha-Phellandrene CT)*

| | |
|---|---|
| Alpha-Phellandrene | 34.4% |
| Gamma-Cadinene | 18.0% |
| Beta-Phellandrene | 10.6% |
| Para-Cymene | 7.3% |
| Alpha-Pinene | 6.5% |
| Alpha-Terpineol | 5.6% |

*S. terebinthifolius (Fruits or Leaves—Bicyclogermacrene CT)*

| | |
|---|---|
| Bicyclogermacrene | 23.6%–35.6% |
| Alpha-Phellandrene | 11.7%–22.2% |
| Germacrene B | 0.0%–13.7% |
| Alpha-Pinene | 5.2%–9.6% |
| Spathulenol | 0.6%–8.3% |
| Germacrene D | 0.0%–7.4% |
| Beta-Elemene | 0.0%–7.3% |
| Beta-Phellandrene | 0.0%–6.5% |
| Elemol | 0.0%–4.0% |

*S. terebinthifolius (Fruits—Limonene CT)*

| | |
|---|---|
| Limonene | 31.8%–44.1% |
| Alpha-Thujene | 3.0%–21.7% |
| Sabinene | 0.0%–15.8% |
| Alpha-Phellandrene | 11.9%–15.7% |

*S. terebinthifolius (Leaves—Sabinene CT)*

| | |
|---|---|
| Sabinene | 40.7% |
| Alpha-Pinene | 30.3% |

| | |
|---|---|
| Gamma-Cadinene | 6.0% |
| Epi-Alpha-Cadinol | 5.6% |
| Beta-Caryophyllene | 4.7% |
| Allo-Aromadendrene | 4.0% |

*S. molle Leaves (Bicyclogermacrene CT)*

| | |
|---|---|
| Bicyclogermacrene | 20.5%–29.2% |
| Beta-Caryophyllene | 7.7%–19.7% |
| Spathulenol | 0.0%–19.2% |
| Beta-Pinene | 1.1%–14.0% |
| Sabinene | 0.0%–12.9% |
| Germacrene D | 7.4%–12.1% |
| Terpinen-4-ol | 1.2%–10.6% |
| Globulol | 0.0%–9.5% |
| Myrcene | 0.2%–5.5% |
| Caryophyllene Oxide | 0.5%–5.3% |

*S. molle (Leaves—Elemol/Beta-Eudesmol CT)*

| | |
|---|---|
| Elemol | 10.3% |
| Beta-Eudesmol | 10.3% |
| Para-Cymene | 9.4% |
| Beta-Bisabolenol | 5.1% |
| Alpha-Pinene | 4.5% |
| Myrcene | 4.5% |
| Limonene | 4.4% |
| 10-Epi-Gamma-Eudesmol | 4.3% |

*S. molle*
*(Leaves—Epi-Bicyclosesquiphellandrene CT)*

| | |
|---|---|
| Epi-Bicyclosesqui-Phellandrene | 18.6% |
| Beta-Pinene | 14.7% |
| Alpha-Pinene | 11.5% |
| Limonene | 9.2% |
| Gamma-Cadinene | 6.9% |
| Delta-Cadinene | 4.9% |

*S. molle (Leaves or Fruits—Sabinene CT)*

| | |
|---|---|
| Sabinene | 34.7%–51.7% |
| Limonene | 3.8%–17.0% |
| Beta-Pinene | 0.6%–12.7% |
| Alpha-Pinene | 0.7%–11.7% |
| Germacrene D | 0.0%–7.1% |
| Beta-Caryophyllene | 1.2%–6.1% |
| Terpinen-4-ol | 0.8%–5.5% |

| | |
|---|---|
| Alpha-Phellandrene | 9.9% |
| Beta-Pinene | 8.0% |
| Myrcene | 6.6% |

*S. terebinthifolius*
*(Fruits—Myrcene/Limonene CT)*

| | |
|---|---|
| Myrcene | 1.6%–20.4% |
| Limonene | 14.2%–17.0% |
| Germacrene D | 10.9%–11.5% |
| Alpha-Copaene | 3.5%–8.0% |
| Alpha-Pinene | 6.0%–7.9% |

*S. terebinthifolius (Leaves—Para-Cymen-7-ol CT)*

| | |
|---|---|
| Para-Cymen-7-ol | 22.5% |
| 9-Epi-(E)-Caryophyllene | 10.1% |
| Carvone | 7.5% |
| Verbenone | 7.4% |
| Caryophyllene Oxide | 5.2% |
| Beta-Dehydroelsholtzione | 4.6% |
| m-Cymen-8-ol | 4.1% |

*S. molle (Leaves—Limonene CT)*

| | |
|---|---|
| Limonene | 41.9% |
| Beta-Caryophyllene | 15.6% |
| Bicyclogermacrene | 11.6% |
| Germacrene D | 8.9% |
| Sabinene | 5.9% |

*S. molle (Fruits or Leaves—Para-Cymene CT)*

| | |
|---|---|
| Para-Cymene | 32.8%–69.4% |
| Beta-Pinene | 1.8%–19.0% |
| Alpha-Terpinene | 2.2%–18.3% |

*S. molle (Aerial Parts)*

| | |
|---|---|
| Alpha-Phellandrene | 35.9% |
| Beta-Phellandrene | 29.3% |
| Beta-Pinene | 15.7% |
| Para-Cymene | 5.4% |
| Alpha-Pinene | 5.2% |

Note: Pink pepper essential oil composition varies greatly and multiple chemotypes exist in both fruit and leaf essential oils from both species (*S. molle* and *S. terebinthifolius*). Other chemotypes not listed in this work are also reported in the literature.

**OTHER CONSTITUENTS:** *S. molle (Fruits—Alpha-Phellandrene CT)*—linalool, carveol, 10-undecenal, aromadendrene, beta-selinene, trans-piperitol, cubenol, terpinen-4-ol, beta-caryophyllene, Germacrene D, alpha-muurolene, alpha-humulene, elemol, bicyclogermacrene, cis-piperitol, geranyl acetate, p-mentha-1(7),5-dien-2-ol, 1,6-germacradien-5-ol, neryl hexanoate, T-cadinol, dodecanoic acid, epi-alpha-muurolol, gamma-eudesmol, shyobunol; *S. molle*

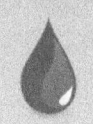

*(Fruits/Leaves—Alpha-Phellandrene/Sylvestrene CT)*—alpha-pinene, camphene, alpha-gurjunene, alpha-humulene, germacrene D, epi-bicyclosesquiphellandrene, delta-amorphene, alpha-cadinol, T-cadinol; *S. molle (Leaves—Alpha-Phellandrene CT)*— methyl octanoate, terpinen-4-ol, alpha-muurolene, beta-caryophyllene, delta-cadinene, linalool, camphor, borneol, thymol, alpha-terpinyl acetate, 1,10-di-epi-cubenol, 1,6-germacradien-5-ol, octanoic acid, T-muurolol, alpha-cadinol; *S. molle (Leaves—Beta-Pinene CT)*—camphene, beta-phellandrene, alpha-humulene, germacrene D, bicyclogermacrene, alpha-muurolene, delta-cadinene, alpha-cadinene, spathulenol, globulol, 1,10-di-epi-cubenol, alpha-cadinol; *S. molle (Leaves—Elemol/Beta-Eudesmol CT)*—alpha-phellandrene, cryptone, cis-pulegol, trans-piperitone epoxide, perilla aldehyde, (3Z,6Z,9Z)-tetradecatriene, gamma-terpinene-7-al, trans-(E)-jasmonol, beta-elemene, alpha-humulene, gamma-muurolene, alpha-muurolene, gamma-cadinene, delta-cadinene, elemol, epi-alpha-muurolol, trans-calamenen-10-ol, guaia-3,10(14)-dien-11-ol, elemol acetate, trien-1-alpha-ol, oplopanone, alpha-costol, 8-alpha-acetoxyelemol, alpha-chenopodiol, kudtdiol, 11,12dihydrocy-valencene; *S. molle Leaves (Bicyclogermacrene CT)*—limonene, gamma-terpinene, linalool, beta-elemene, alpha-humulene, delta-cadinene, germacrone, epiglobulol, aromadendrene, isospathulenol, cubenol; *(Leaves—Epi-Bicyclosesquiphellandrene CT)*—camphene, myrcene, alpha-ocimene, beta-caryophyllene, azulene derivative, germacrene D, isoledene, spathulenol, eudol, alpha-cadinol; *S. molle (Leaves or Fruits—Sabinene CT)*—myrcene, gamma-terpinene, alpha-thujene, para-cymene, alpha-terpinene, alpha-terpinolene, alpha-terpineol, beta-elemene, alpha-humulene, alloaromadendrene, beta-selinene, germacrene B, germacrene A, gamma-cadinene, delta-cadinene, spathulenol, caryophyllene oxide, delta-cadinol; *S. molle (Leaves—Limonene CT)*—alpha-pinene, myrcene; *S. molle (Fruits or Leaves—Para-Cymene CT)*—3-penten-1-ol, alpha-pinene, alpha-phellandrene, 1,8-cineole, methyl caprylate, borneol, 4-thujanol, cis-p-menth-2,8-dienol, alpha-terpineol, (E)-3-caren-2-ol, alpha-terpinyl acetate, carvotanacetone, pulegone (< 0.9%), perillaldehyde, bornyl acetate, (E)-2,3-epoxycarane, 1,5,7-octatrien-3-ol,2,6-dimethyl, 4-isopropenyl-1-methyl-1,2-cyclohexanediol, limonene-1,2-epoxide, calamenene, alpha-calacorene, beta-vatrienene, eudesma-4(14),11-diene, epi-bicyclosesquiphellandrene; *S. molle (Aerial Parts)*—alpha-terpinolene, terpinen-4-ol; *S. terebinthifolius (Fruits—Delta-3-Carene CT)*—sabinene, beta-pinene, o-cymene, isoterpinolene, para-cymene, terpinen-4-ol, alpha-terpinenolene, delta-elemene, beta-elemene, beta-caryophyllene, alpha-humulene, alpha-muurolene, gamma-cadinene, germacrene B, caryophyllene oxide, alpha-bisabolol, T-cadinol; *S. terebinthifolius (Fruits—Alpha-Phellandrene CT)*—beta-pinene, alpha-terpinolene, delta-elemene, beta-gurjunene, gamma-elemene, alpha-chamigrene, germacrene B, caryophyllene oxide, alpha-eudesmol, alpha-cadinol, syringaldehyde, grandisol, lineatin; *S. terebinthifolius (Fruits or Leaves—Bicyclogermacrene CT)*—alpha-thujene, sabinene, beta-pinene, m-cymene, para-cymene, carvacrol, beta-chamigrene, viridiflorol, gamma-cadinol, alpha-eudesmol, 4-carene, o-cymene, cis-ocimene, gamma-terpinene, gamma-elemene, aromadendrene, allo-aromadendrene, delta-cadinene, myrcene, gamma-(E)-bisabolene, globulol, o-menth-8-ene, spathulenol; *S. terebinthifolius (Fruits—Limonene CT)*—alpha-thujene, beta-pinene, iso-sylvestrene, o-cymene, alpha-terpinolene, alpha-terpineol, viridene, cis-4-caranone, carvone, neo-menthyl acetate, alpha-terpinen-7-al, para-cymen-7-ol, trans-pinocarvyl acetate, verbanyl acetate, mertenyl acetate, alpha-cubebene, allo-aromadendrene, delta-cadinene, beta-copaen-4-alpha-ol, guaiol, 10-epi-gamma-eudesmol; *S. terebinthifolius (Leaves—Sabinene CT)*—camphene, myrcene, alpha-terpinene, gamma-terpinene, 3-cyclohexen-1-ol; *S. terebinthifolius (Fruits—Myrcene/Limonene CT)*—alpha-thujene, beta-pinene, sabinene, alpha-phellandrene, alpha-terpinene, para-cymene, alpha-cubebene, beta-caryophyllene, terpinen-4-ol, aromadendrene, alpha-humulene, (E)-beta-farnesene, bicyclogermacrene, gamma-cadinene, alpha-amorphene; *S. terebinthifolius (Leaves—Para-Cymen-7-ol CT)*—o-cymene, m-cymenene, 2,5-dimethyl styrene, perillinen, myrcenol, alpha-campholenal, trans-limonene oxide, trans-verbenol, p-cymen-8-ol, alpha-terpineol, alpha-terpien-7-al, neo-dihydro carveol acetate, iso-longifolene, cis-muurola-4(14),5-diene, beta-chamigrene, gamm-muurolene, alpha-bulnesene, spathulenol, beta-eudesmol, alpha-cadinol, aristolene

### PREFERRED COMPOSITION FOR CLINICAL USE:

| Constituent | S. molle, Fruits (Alpha-Phellandrene CT) | S. molle, Fruits/ Leaves (Sabinene CT) | S. terebinthifolius, Fruits (Limonene CT) | S. terebinthifolius, Fruits (δ-3-Carene CT) |
|---|---|---|---|---|
| **Alpha-Phellandrene** | 20%–40% | – | 10%–20% | 5%–15% |
| **Limonene** | 10%–20% | 4%–15% | 30%–45% | 5%–20% |
| **Myrcene** | 10%–20% | – | – | 1%–7% |
| **Alpha-Pinene** | 2%–15% | 2%–12% | – | 5%–20% |
| **Beta-Phellandrene** | 1%–11% | – | – | – |
| **Para-Cymene** | 2%–8% | – | – | – |

| | | | | |
|---|---|---|---|---|
| Alpha-Cadinol | 0.1%–8% | – | – | – |
| Methyl Octanoate | 0.5%–5% | – | – | – |
| Delta-Cadinene | 0.5%–5% | – | – | – |
| Sabinene | – | 35%–55% | 5%–15% | – |
| Beta-Pinene | – | 5%–20% | – | – |
| Terpinen-4-ol | – | 3%–13% | – | – |
| Delta-3-Carene | – | – | – | 35%–55% |
| Alpha-Thujene | – | – | 5%–20% | – |

**REPORTED THERAPEUTIC PROPERTIES:** Antibacterial, antifungal, antiviral, **antimicrobial**, **anticancer**, antioxidant, antiseptic, astringent, **wound healing**, diuretic, aids digestion, stops excess bleeding, aids circulation, supports respiratory function, removes warts, analgesic, anti-inflammatory, antirheumatic, antiarthritic, relieves gout, soothes sprains/strains, nervine, antineuralgic, relieves toothache, balances menstruation, reduces high blood pressure, balances cardiovascular function, **insecticide**, insect repellent, antidepressant, relieves anxiety, calming

**CAUTIONS:**

■ *S. molle, Aerial Parts, Alpha-Phellandrene CT*: May interact with anticholinergic (drugs used for asthma, incontinence, gastrointestinal cramps, muscular spasms, depression, and sleep disorders) and cholinergic medications (drugs used to reduce urinary retention, diagnose myasthenia gravis, and for glaucoma) based on AChE inhibitory activity of beta-phellandrene.[7153]

■ *S. terebinthifolius, Fruits, δ-3-carene CT*: May interact with anticholinergic (drugs used for asthma, incontinence, gastrointestinal cramps, muscular spasms, depression, and sleep disorders) and cholinergic medications (drugs used to reduce urinary retention, diagnose myasthenia gravis, and for glaucoma) based on AChE inhibitory activity of δ-3-carene.[7154,7155]

**SELECTED EVIDENCE:**

☐ *In vitro* research shows that pink pepper essential oil (*S. molle*, alpha-phellandrene CT) kills colon, liver, and breast cancer cells, with the fruit oil being more active against colon and liver cancer and the flower oil (para-cymene 25.6%, beta-eudesmol 10.1%, myrcene 6.1%, and alpha-pinene 5.4%) being more active against breast cancer.[7156] The researchers also reported that alpha-phellandrene, myrcene (myrcene was most active against all cancer cells), and limonene were highly toxic to all three cancer cell lines, while para-cymene was only moderately toxic. The beta-pinene CT of *S. molle* triggered apoptosis of mouse breast and myelogenous leukemia (erythroleukemic) cancer cells, and moderately caused apoptosis in liver (HepG2) and bladder cancer cells, while leaving healthy cells intact.[7157] *S. terebinthifolius* essential oil (berries, alpha-phellandrene CT rich in gamma-cadinene) killed breast cancer cells more effectively than an *S. molle* essential oil (alpha-phellandrene CT devoid of myrcene).[7158] A germacrene D CT (germacrene D 23.7%, bicyclogermacrene 15.0%, beta-pinene 9.1%, beta-longipinene 8.1%) of *S. terebinthifolius* killed leukemia and cervical cancer cells.[7159] The same researchers reported that alpha-pinene and beta-pinene demonstrated activity against melanoma, breast, leukemia, and cervical cancer cells, either alone or in combination.

☐ Pink pepper essential oil (*S. molle*, alpha-phellandrene CT) inhibited gram-positive bacteria (*S. aureus* and *St. pyogenes*) and gram-negative bacteria (*E. coli*) according to *in vitro* research.[7160] Pink pepper essential oil (*S. molle*, alpha-phellandrene CT) preserved minced beef meet against gram-positive and gram-negative bacteria: *S. aureus, P. aeruginosa* (two strains), *E. coli,* and *En. faecalis,* and one fungus (*C. albicans*): and against clinical, foodborne and waterborne isolated pathogens: *L. monocytogenes, P. morgani, K. pneumoniae, S. enteritidis* (2 strains), *Salmonella anatum,* and *E. coli,* (2 strains).[7161] *S. molle* (alpha-phellandrene/sylvestrene CT) inhibited *S. aureus* and *S. pyogenes*, which cause skin infections that potentially may lead to sepsis, but was not antifungal in nature.[7162] *S. terebinthifolius* (para-cymen-7-ol CT) was only mildly bactericidal to *S. intermedius* isolated from dogs with ear infections, even though it demonstrated inhibitory activity against nine isolates of coagulase-positive *Staphylococci* obtained from diseased dogs, some resistant to several antibiotics typically used for treatment.[7163] *S. terebinthifolius* (sabinene CT) demonstrated potent antibacterial activity against *Yersinia enterocolitica, Pseudomonas aeruginosa, E. coli, A. calcoaceticus, B. subtilis, and K. pneumoniae,* and moderate antifungal activity against

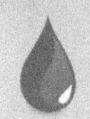

*Aspergillus flavus, A. niger,* and *C. albicans.*[7164] *S. terebinthifolius* essential oil (delta-3-carene CT) inhibited bacteria acquired from a public hospital in Brazil, including gram-negative bacteria: *E. coli, Klebsiella oxytoca, Pseudomonas* sp., *Enterobacter* sp., and *En. agglomerans,* and gram-positive bacteria: *Streptococcus* group D, *S. aureus, Corynebacterium* sp., *Bacillus* sp., and *Nocardia* sp.[7165] The essential oil was more effective against gram-positive bacteria than gram-negative bacteria. *S. molle* essential oil (alpha-phellandrene CT with myrcene) exhibited antimicrobial activity against gram-negative, gram-positive, and food spoilage bacteria.[7166] The sabinene CT demonstrates potent antibacterial activity on *S. aureus,* strong/moderate effect on *E. coli,* and moderate/weak effect on *P. aeruginosa.*[7167] An unidentified CT of *S. molle* inhibited *A. parasiticus* and *F. moniliforme* growth and the production of mycotoxin by *F. moniliforme.*[7168] Pink pepper essential oil (*S. molle,* unidentified CT) exhibited significant antimicrobial activity against bacteria (*K. pneumoniae, Al. faecalis, P. aeruginosa, L. cremoris, En. aerogenes, P. vulgaris, C. sporogenes, Ac. calcoacetica, E. coli, Be. natriegens, C. freundii, Se. marcescens, B. subtilis,* and *Br. thermosphacata*) and fungi (*A. ochraceus, A. parasiticus, F. culmorum,* and *Al. alternata*). A Germacrene D CT of *S. terebinthifolius* (Germacrene D 21%, alpha-phellandrene 18.2%, limonene 16.7%) inhibited *E. coli, S. aureus,* and *B. cereus,* with a July crop outperforming a spring crop.[7169] *S. terebinthifolius* leaf essential oil inhibited three strains of gram-positive bacteria (*B. megaterium, B. mojavensis,* and *Cl. michiganensis*) and four strains of gram-negative bacteria (*E. coli, X. campestris, Ps. savastanoi,* and *Ps. syringae* pv. *phaseolicola*), and was fungicidal to and prevented mycelial growth of *C. acutatum* and *B. cinereal.*[7170]

- Both *S. molle* (alpha-phellandrene CT devoid of myrcene) and *S. terebinthifolius* (berries, alpha-phellandrene CT rich in gamma-cadinene) demonstrated antioxidant properties, with *S. terebinthifolius* being the stronger antioxidant of the two essential oils.[7171] Another study reported that the alpha-phellandrene/sylvestrene CT of *S. molle* (leaf oil) was a weak antioxidant.[7172] *S. terebinthifolius* (sabinene CT) demonstrated moderate antioxidant activity.[7173] The bicyclogermacrene CT of *S. terebinthifolius* showed moderate antioxidant activity, with the fruit oil being more potent than the leaf oil.[7174] *S. molle* (alpha-phellandrene CT with myrcene) exhibited low to moderate antioxidant activity.[7175]

- Pink pepper essential oil (unidentified CT) demonstrates significant activity against the protozoan parasite *Trypanosoma evansi,* which causes a form of surra (fever, weakness, lethargy, anemia, and possibly death) in animals.[7176]

- Topical application of an ointment containing 5% pink pepper essential oil (*S. terebinthifolius,* unidentified composition), 30% lanolin, 70% vasoline, and 0.5% vitamin E promoted wound closure in rats by increasing mast cell concentration in the wound area.[7177] Mast cells are essential for complete wound healing because they stimulate endothelial and epithelial cell growth and participate in collagen remodeling.

- Animal research demonstrated that oral administration of pink pepper essential oil (*S. terebinthifolius,* fruit oil, unidentified composition, but with limonene and alpha-phellandrene present) at a dose of 100 mg/kg reduced pain caused by mechanical stimulation in a model that simulates peripheral neuropathic pain.[7178] The same researchers reported that alpha-phellandrene (10 mg/kg) reduced pain caused by mechanical stimulation and pain caused by cold stimulus. The study authors also reported that the essential oil, alpha-phellandrene, and limonene all reduced depressive-like behavior. Limonene also reduced pain associated with mechanical stimulation.

- Pink pepper essential oil (*S. molle,* para-cymene CT) fruit and leaf essential oil repelled and killed the khapra beetle (*Trogoderma granarium*) and the red flour beetle (*Tribolium castaneum*). The fruit essential oil (with lower concentration of para-cymene) more effectively repelled and killed both beetles.[7179] Both ripe and unripe fruit essential oil (*S. terebinthifolius,* limonene CT) exhibited significant repellent activity against the spider mite (*Tetranychus urticae*), and was also toxic to the spider mite.[7180] An *S. molle* essential oil with major constituents of myrtenal, terpineol, spathulenol, and cubenol killed adult fleas (*Ctenocephalides felis*) that commonly infect cats and dogs with a 100% efficacy, but had no effect against flea eggs.[7181]

- Pink pepper essential oil (*S. molle*) inhibits *Paenibacillus* larvae (the bacterium responsible for American foulbrood in honeybees).[7182]

- A pink pepper (*S. terebinthifolius*) fruit essential oil with alpha-pinene and alpha-phellandrene as the major constituents actively inhibited *S. aureus* and *P. aeruginosa* and exhibited good antioxidant activity.[7183]

- Pink pepper (*S. molle*) essential oil demonstrated an acaricidal effect against larvae and reproductive parameters of engorged female brown dog ticks (*Rhipicephalus sanguineus*).[7184]

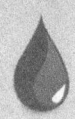

- *In vitro* research found that pink pepper (*S. molle*, 25.2% beta-pinene, 21.3% T-cadinol) significantly inhibited *Paracoccidioides brasiliensis*, but only weakly inhibited *C. neoformans* and *T. quinckeanum*, and was inactive against *Candida* species.[7185] Paracoccidioidomycosis is a systemic fungal infection of the lungs, skin, mucous membranes, lymph nodes, and internal organs of great clinical importance in Latin America. Symptoms include lesions in the mouth or throat, swollen lymph nodes, weight loss, fever, fatigue, cough, shortness of breath, skin lesions, enlarged liver or spleen, and less commonly premature death.

- The alpha-pinene CT of pink pepper (*S. molle*) essential oil activates the immune system by modulating the production of interleukin-10 and tumor necrosis factor alpha.[7186]

- Pink pepper essential oil CT terpinen-4-ol exhibited good moderate antioxidant activity in the DPPH and ABTS assays.[7187] The same researchers reported that it displayed antigout activity by inhibiting xanthine oxidase activity.

- Pink pepper (*S. molle*) CT alpha-phellandrene essential oil exhibited antiproliferative activity against breast and colon cancer cells.[7188]

- Pink pepper (*S. terebinthifolius*) essential oil reduced memory impairment caused by scopolamine by improving acetylcholine (via inhibition of acetylcholinesterase) levels in the brain and reducing oxidative stress in an animal model.[7189]

- Experimental research demonstrates that oral administration of pink pepper (*S. terebinthifolius*) essential oil reduced eye pain in zebrafish.[7190] The effects were slightly similar to morphine, which was used as a positive control. The oil reduced pain by modulating the opioid system, NMDA receptors, transient receptor potential ankyrin 1 (TRPA1), transient receptor potential vanilloid 1 (TRPV1), and acid-sensing ion channels. It also exhibited moderate to good antioxidant activity in the ferrous ion-chelating capacity and beta-carotene tests.

- Both pink pepper (*S. terebinthifolius*) essential oil and its nanoemulsion were larvicidal and insecticidal to Culex pipiens mosquitoes and exhibited repellent activity.[7191] Isolated limonene and alpha-phellandrene were also larvicidal.

- *Culex quinquefasciatus* are filarial vector mosquitoes with resistance to common insecticides. Pink pepper (*S. molle*) CT sabinene essential oil was larvicidal against *C. quinquefasciatus* mosquitoes.[7192]

- Pink pepper fruit and leaf essential oil from *S. molle* and *S. terebinthifolius* (limonene as the major constituent of all oils) displayed weak to moderate antioxidant activity with the fruits and *S. terebinthifolius* being most active.[7193] The oils were also insecticidal to the rice weevil (*Sitophilus oryzae*), *S. molle* fruit oil being the strongest insecticide.

- Pink pepper (*S. molle*) berries were insecticidal to the carob moth (*Ectomyelois ceratoniae*) and the Mediterranean flour moth (*Ephestia kuehniella*) and larvicidal to Mediterranean flour moth larvae.[7194]

---

# PLAI
## (Thai Ginger, Cassumnar Ginger)

*Zingiber cassumunar* Roxb., *Z. montanum* (J. Koenig)
Link ex A. Dietr., *Z. purpureum* Roscoe

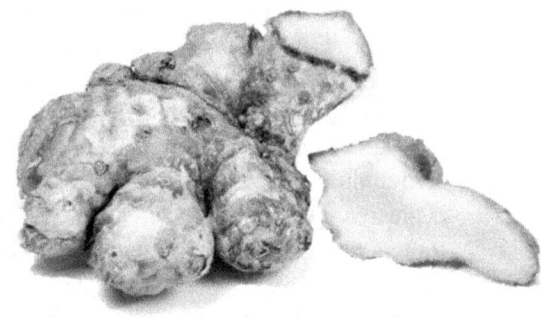

**FAMILY:** Zingiberaceae
**NOTE:** Middle
**AROMA INTENSITY:** Medium
**AROMA:** Peppery, spicy, medicinal, herbaceous, earthy
**COMMON EXTRACTION METHOD:** Steam distilled or hydrodistilled from the rhizomes; may also be distilled from the leaves
**POSSIBLE SUBSTITUTE OILS:** Tea tree, ginger, black pepper, pink pepper, Himalayan juniper (leaves), shell ginger, marjoram, nutmeg
**BLENDS WELL WITH:** Bergamot, black pepper, cassia, cinnamon, cypress, ginger, helichrysum, lavender, lemon, marjoram, nutmeg, orange, rosemary, sage, Spanish sage, tangerine
**SUBCELLULAR LOCALIZATION | EPIGENETIC INFLUENCE:** Currently unknown | *Muscular/Reproductive*
**RECOMMENDED DILUTION RANGE:** 3%–50%; Neat for limited conditions

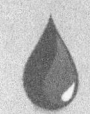

**PRIMARY CONSTITUENTS:**[7195,7196,7197,7198,7199,7200,7201,7202,7203,7204]

*Terpinen-4-ol CT*

| | |
|---|---|
| Terpinen-4-ol | 10.2%–50.5% |
| (E)-1-(3,4-Dimethoxyphenyl) Butadiene | 9.8%–19.1% |
| Sabinene | 3.7%–10.1% |
| (E)-1-(3,4-Dimethoxyphenyl) But-1-ene | 6.0%–7.4% |
| Beta-Sesquiphellandrene | 5.9%–7.0% |
| Para-Cymene | 0.0%–5.2% |
| Curzerenone | 0.1%–3.7% |
| (Z)-1-(3,4-Dimethoxyphenyl) Butadiene | 0.0%–3.7% |
| Gamma-Terpinene | 1.8%–3.6% |
| Terpinolene | 0.4%–3.4% |

*2,6,9,9-Tetramethyl-2,6,10-Cycloundecatrien-1-one CT*

| | |
|---|---|
| 2,6,9,9-Tetramethyl-2,6,10-Cycloundecatrien-1-one | 60.8% |
| Alpha-Caryophyllene | 23.9% |
| Caryophyllene Oxide | 4.8% |
| 1,5,5,8-Tetramethyl-12-Oxabic-yclo[9.1.0]dodeca-3,7-diene | 3.3% |

*Sabinene CT*

| | |
|---|---|
| Sabinene | 34.0%–53.5% |
| Terpinen-4-ol | 11.5%–30.0% |
| (E)-1-(3,4-Dimethoxyphenyl) Butadiene | 1.0%–27.5% |
| Gamma-Terpinene | 5.3%–9.0% |
| Alpha-Terpinene | 2.0%–6.0% |
| Beta-Pinene | 2.3%–3.8% |

*Terpinen-4-ol (No Phenylbutanoids) CT*

| | |
|---|---|
| Terpinen-4-ol | 40.5%–67.1% |
| Sabinene | 0.0%–17.4% |
| Gamma-Terpinene | 5.8%–13.3% |
| Alpha-Terpinene | 0.4%–6.4% |
| Alpha-Terpinolene | 2.2%–3.0% |

*Triquinacene,1,4-Bis(Methoxy)- CT*

| | |
|---|---|
| Triquinacene,1,4-Bis(Methoxy)- | 26.5% |
| (Z)-Ocimene | 22.0% |
| Terpinen-4-ol | 18.5% |
| Gamma-Terpinene | 3.9% |
| Beta-Phellandrene | 3.5% |
| Cis-Sabinene Hydrate | 3.0% |

Note: The fresh rhizomes (as opposed to dried rhizomes) produce a higher yield and an essential oil that is reportedly a stronger anti-inflammatory and analgesic.

**OTHER CONSTITUENTS:** *Sabinene CT [fresh rhizomes]*—Alpha-thujene, alpha-pinene, beta-myrcene, para-cymene, beta-phellandrene, terpinolene, trans-sabinene hydrate, beta-sesquiphellandrene, (E)-1-(3,4-dimethoxyphenyl)but-1-ene; *Terpinen-4-ol CT [fresh rhizomes]*—Alpha-thujene, alpha-pinene, camphene, beta-pinene, beta-phellandrene, zingiberene, alpha-phellandrene, beta-myrcene, alpha-terpinene, limonene, delta-3-carene, trans-sabinene hydrate, cis-sabinene hydrate, trans-menth-2-en-ol, cis-menth-2-en-ol, alpha-terpineol, trans-piperitol, p-mentha-2,4(8)diene, cis-1(3,4-dimethoxyphenyl)but-1-ene, beta-bisabolene, 1-(2,4,5-trimethoxyphenyl)but-1-ene, cis-1-(2,4,5-trimethoxyphenyl)butadiene; *Terpinen-4-ol (No Phenylbutanoids) CT [fresh rhizomes]*—Alpha-thujene, alpha-pinene, beta-pinene, alpha-phellandrene, para-cymene, cis-sabinene hydrate, trans-linalool oxide, neo-alloocimene, p-cymen-8-ol, dill ether, cis-piperitol, trans-piperitol, all-ocimene, caryophyllene oxide, 1-terpineol, gamma-terpineol, beta-sesquiphellandrene; *Triquinacene,1,4-Bis(Methoxy) CT [dried rhizomes]*—Alpha-thujene, alpha-pinene, beta-pinene, beta-myrcene, 4-terpinyl acetate, m-cymene, 2-carene, terpinyl acetate, beta-sesquiphellandrene, methyleugenol (<2.1%), lachnophyllum ester, 2-Allyl-1,4-dimethoxy-3-methyl benzene; *2,6,9,9-Tetramethyl-2,6,10-Cycloundecatrien-1-one CT [fresh rhizomes]*—Beta-caryophyllene, gamma-gurjunene epoxide I, 1-Oxaspiro[2.5]octane, 5,5-dimethyl-4-(3-methyl-1,3-butadienyl), 4,6,6-Trimethyl-2-(3-methylbuta-1,3-dienyl)-3-oxatricyclo[5.1.0.0(2,4)]octane

**PREFERRED COMPOSITION FOR CLINICAL USE:**

| Constituent | Balanced CT | Sabinene CT |
|---|---|---|
| Terpinen-4-ol | 28%–40% | 10%–25% |
| Sabinene | 25%–40% | 45%–60% |
| Gamma-Terpinene | 5%–10% | 4%–8% |
| Alpha-Terpinene | 2%–7% | 1%–4% |
| Para-Cymene | 1%–6% | 0.1%–2% |
| Beta-Pinene | 2%–5% | 2%–5% |

| | | |
|---|---|---|
| Beta-Sesquiphellandrene | 0.5%–4% | 0.5%–2% |
| Terpinolene | 0.5%–3% | 0.5%–2% |
| Alpha-Pinene | 0.5%–2% | 1%–3% |
| (E)-1-(3,4-Dimethoxyphenyl)Butadiene | 0.5%–2% | 2%–7% |
| (E)-1-(3,4-Dimethoxyphenyl)But-1-ene | – | 0.1%–1% |

**REPORTED THERAPEUTIC PROPERTIES: Analgesic, anti-inflammatory**, antirheumatic, antiarthritic, antispasmodic, **relieves sports injuries, sprains, and strains**, antiseptic, antiallergic, antiviral, antibacterial, **antifungal**, antimicrobial, aids immune function, astringent, supports respiratory function, expels excess gas, aids digestion, relieves stomachache, relieves diarrhea and constipation, heals bruises, insect repellent, insecticide, energizing, relieves anxiety, combats anger

## CAUTIONS:

■ *Terpinen-4-ol, Sabinene, and Terpinen-4-ol (No Phenylbutanoids) CTs*: May interact with anticholinergic (drugs used for asthma, incontinence, gastrointestinal cramps, muscular spasms, depression, and sleep disorders) and cholinergic medications (drugs used to reduce urinary retention, diagnose myasthenia gravis, and for glaucoma) likely due to a synergistic activity of terpinen-4-ol and sabinene or gamma-terpinene.[7205,7206,7207,7208]

■ *Terpinen-4-ol, Sabinene, and Terpinen-4-ol (No Phenylbutanoids) CTs*: May interact with antifungal/antibiotic drugs and increase their effectiveness.[7209,7210]

## SELECTED EVIDENCE:

☐ *In vitro* research shows that plai essential oil (terpinen-4-ol CT) and a 5% plai gel potently inhibits yeasts (*C. albicans, Cryptococcus neoformans*) and dermatophytes (*Epidermophyton floccisum, Microsporum gypseum, Trichophyton mentagrophytes, T. rubrum*), but bacteria were less susceptible.[7211] The study reported that plai essential oil inhibited gram-positive bacteria (*B. subtilis, P. acnes*) and gram-negative bacteria (*E. coli, Salmonella typhi*), but only weakly inhibited *S. aureus, St. pyogenes, St. epidermidis, P. aeruginosa, K. pneumonia*, and *Pr. vulgaris*. The gel was far less effective against bacteria. Studies suggest that the antimicrobial activity of plai essential oil is primarily due to terpinen-4-ol, with sabinene also contributing.[7212,7213] The sabinene CT inhibited *A. baumanniii*, including multidrug-resistant strains, and potentiated antibiotics.[7214] The 2,6,9,9-Tetramethyl-2,6,10-Cycloundecatrien-1-one CT of plai essential oil only weakly inhibited *B. cereus* and *E. coli*, and was inactive against *S. aureus, P. aeruginosa, C. albicans*, and *C. neoformans*.[7215]

☐ Animal research demonstrated that topical application of plai essential oil (sabinene CT) exhibited a significant anti-inflammatory effect, which was attributed to the (E)-1-(3,4-dimethoxyphenyl)butadiene (DMPBD), terpinen-4-ol, and alpha-terpinene content.[7216] Remarkably, (E)-1-(3,4-dimethoxyphenyl)butadiene demonstrated an anti-inflammatory effect that was twice that of the NSAID diclofenac. Another study attributed the significant anti-inflammatory activity of plai essential oil to (E)-1-(3,4-dimethoxyphenyl)but-1-ene.[7217] A fraction of plai essential oil enriched with phenylbutanoids ((E)-4-(3,4-dimethoxyphenyl)but-3-en-l-ol, (E)-4-(3,4-dimethoxyphenyl)but-3-en-l-yl acetate, (E)-1-(3,4-dimethoxyphenyl)butadiene, and (E)-3-(3,4-dimethoxyphenyl)-4-[(E)-3,4-dimethoxystyryl]cyclohex-1-ene) significantly inhibited the production of nitric oxide and was more potent than the essential oil or any of the individual components in the phenylbutanoids fraction.[7218] A microemulsion of plai essential oil enhanced the anti-inflammatory activity of plai essential oil without harming human cells.[7219] Sabinene and terpinen-4-ol significantly balanced the inflammatory response by inhibiting interleukin-6 (IL-6) secretion and nuclear factor-kappa B (NF-kB) expression. NF-kB plays a key role in the inflammatory signaling pathways (cytokines, genes, chemokines, and adhesion molecules) and IL-6 modulates (pro- or anti-inflammatory) the inflammation response.

☐ *In vitro* research shows that a microemulsion of plai essential oil (Terpinen-4-ol—No Phenylbutanoids CT) inhibits both AChE (28.4%) and BChE (47.5%) activity, with stronger inhibition of BChE.[4810] The microemulsion is a much stronger inhibitor than the essential oil.[7220,7221] Inhibition of AChE prevents the breakdown of acetylcholine, which is essential for memory and thinking. People with neurodegenerative diseases make less acetylcholine, and the diseases often break it down at a faster rate leading to acetylcholine deficits. Selective inhibition of BChE is also desirable in neurodegenerative diseases because it interferes with

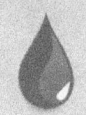

acetylcholine activity. In addition, BChE is often accumulates in plaques and tangles inside the brains of people with Alzheimer's disease.[7222]

☐ Plai essential oil from Thailand exhibits varying antioxidant capacity depending on its composition: north (80.9%), east (76.5%), south (72.5%), northeast (67.4%), west (66.7%), and central (57.6%).[7223] Based on the composition of these essential oils, it appears that a relatively balanced amount of sabinene (33.4%–38.2%), terpinen-4-ol (11.5%–24.4%), and DMPBD (20.4%–27.5%) produces the greatest antioxidant activity.

☐ Plai essential oil effectively kills brown dog ticks (*Rhipicephalus sanguineus*).[7224] It also repels three mosquito vectors (*Aedes aegypti, Anopheles minimus*, and *Culex quinquefasciatus*), providing a protection time of 205 minutes (0.9% biting rate), 165 minutes (0.9% biting rate), and 90 minutes (0.8% biting rate) respectively.[7225,7226] Undiluted plai oil repelled *Leptotrombidium chiggers* (the vector of scrub typhus) 100%.[7227]

☐ *In vitro* research demonstrates that plai essential oil exhibits low to good antibacterial activity and moderate antifungal activity.[7228]

☐ Plai CT terpinen-4-ol essential oil showed moderate repellent activity against *Ae. albopictus* mosquitoes in an in-cage experiment, moderate larvicidal activity against first instar larvae, and moderate adulticidal activity in fumigant bioassays.[7229] Isolated terpinen-4-ol demonstrated significant adulticidal activity, suggesting that it is primarily responsible for the activity of plai oil.

# PONDEROSA PINE
## (Western Yellow Pine)

*Pinus ponderosa* Lawson & C. Lawson

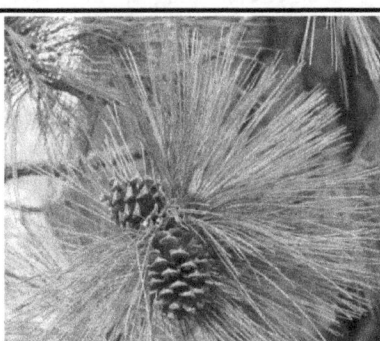

**FAMILY:** Pinaceae
**NOTE:** Top
**AROMA INTENSITY:** Medium
**AROMA:** Piney, woody, fresh, balsamic, earthy
**COMMON EXTRACTION METHOD:** Steam distilled from the needles (leaves)
**POSSIBLE SUBSTITUTE OILS:** Pine, red pine, white pine, balsam fir, cypress
**BLENDS WELL WITH:** Agarwood, bergamot, cajeput, camphor, cedarwood, clary sage, coriander, Douglas fir, eucalyptus, Engelmann spruce, frankincense, galbanum, grapefruit, juniper, lavandin, lavender, lemon, lime, tea tree, marjoram, neroli, niaouli, peppermint, ravensara, ravintsara, rosemary, Spanish sage, spikenard, thyme, Siberian fir, silver fir, white fir, white pine, white spruce, ylang ylang
**SUBCELLULAR LOCALIZATION | EPIGENETIC INFLUENCE:** Currently unknown | Currently unknown
**RECOMMENDED DILUTION RANGE:** 1.5%–5%

**PRIMARY CONSTITUENTS:**[7230,7231,7232,7233,7234]

| | |
|---|---|
| Beta-Pinene | 17.0%–66.0% |
| Alpha-Pinene | 9.1%–37.2% |
| Methyl Chavicol (Estragole) | 0.0%–20.4% |
| Delta-3-Carene | 0.2%–19.3% |
| Germacrene D | 0.1%–19.0% |
| Alpha-Terpineol | 0.0%–10.0% |
| Linalyl Anthranilate | 0.0%–9.0% |
| Beta-Myrcene | 0.9%–7.4% |
| Delta-Cadinene | 0.0%–4.6% |
| Limonene | 0.1%–3.7% |

**OTHER CONSTITUENTS:** Camphene, terpinolene, cis-ocimene, beta-phellandrene, beta-elemene, methyleugenol (<0.6%)

**PREFERRED COMPOSITION FOR CLINICAL USE:**

*Constituent*

| | |
|---|---|
| **Alpha-Pinene** | 25%–40% |
| **Beta-Pinene** | 20%–30% |
| **Delta-3-Carene** | 10%–20% |
| **Bornyl Acetate** | 3%–6% |
| **Limonene** | 2%–6% |
| **Myrcene** | 2%–5% |
| **Camphene** | 1%–3% |
| **Beta-Phellandrene** | 0.5%–3% |
| **Beta-Caryophyllene** | 0.5%–3% |
| **Delta-Cadinene** | 0.1%–1% |
| **Methyl Chavicol** | < 5% |

**REPORTED THERAPEUTIC PROPERTIES:** Antibacterial, antifungal, anti-infectious, **analgesic**, anti-inflammatory, antiarthritic, antispasmodic, supports respiratory function, expels excess mucus, decongestant, eases cough, antiparasitic, antiseptic, wound healing, antioxidant, **relieves chronic skin conditions**, immune stimulant, increases localized circulation, relaxing/calming, stress management

**CAUTIONS:**

■ Use with great caution for children under age six due to animal reports of liver cancer caused by methyl chavicol (estragole).[7235] The European Medicines Agency recommends exposure to estragole be limited in young children.

■ Avoid during pregnancy and lactation due to high methyl chavicol (estragole) content.[7236] Methyl chavicol (estragole) may cause genetic mutations and oxidative DNA damage.[7237,7238] The European Medicines Agency recommends exposure to estragole be limited in women who are pregnant or nursing.[7239] Pregnant cattle who ate ponderosa pine needles have experienced abortions, endometriosis, and kidney and nervous system toxicity.[7240,7241] Although these adverse effects are suspected to be caused by isocupressic acid (not found in the essential oil), it is wise to avoid ponderosa pine until further research rules out the volatile constituents as contributors to the adverse outcomes.

■ Avoid oral use due to carcinogenic (cancer-causing) potential of methyl chavicol (estragole). [7242,7243,7244] The metabolite of estragole (1'-hydroxyestragole) is considered a stronger carcinogen and humans rapidly metabolize estragole to 1'-hydroxyestragole when ingested.[7245]

**SELECTED EVIDENCE:**

☐ Ponderosa pine demonstrated strong antifungal activity against *F. culmorum, F. poae,* and *F. solani.*[7246]

---

# RABBITBRUSH
## (Rubber Rabbitbrush, Chamisa, Gray Rabbitbrush, Golden Hare)

*Ericameria nauseosa* (Pall. Ex Pursh) G.L. Nesom & G.I. Baird,
*Chrysothamnus nauseosus* (Pall. ex Pursh) Britton

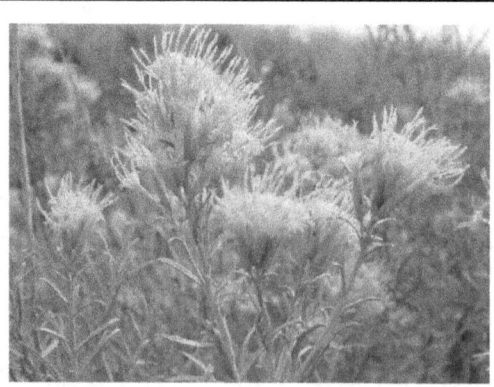

**FAMILY:** Asteraceae (Compositae)
**NOTE:** Middle
**AROMA INTENSITY:** Strong
**AROMA:** Herbaceous, green, piney
**COMMON EXTRACTION METHOD:** Hydrodistilled from the flowering aerial parts
**POSSIBLE SUBSTITUTE OILS:** Balsam fir, galbanum
**BLENDS WELL WITH:** Cedarwood, copaiba, cypress, Douglas fir, juniper berry, lavender, Phoenician juniper, sage, sandalwood, Spanish sage, Texas cedarwood, vetiver

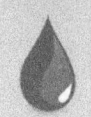

**SUBCELLULAR LOCALIZATION | EPIGENETIC INFLUENCE:** Currently unknown | Currently unknown
**RECOMMENDED DILUTION RANGE:** 5%–Neat

**PRIMARY CONSTITUENTS:**[7247,7248]

*E. nauseosa* var. *nauseosa*

| | |
|---|---|
| Beta-Phellandrene | 22.8% |
| Beta-Pinene | 19.8% |
| Beta-Eudesmol | 7.7% |
| Sabinene | 5.7% |
| Limonene | 4.7% |
| Gamma-Terpinene | 2.6% |
| Cryptone | 2.6% |
| Carvacrol | 2.5% |
| Terpinen-4-ol | 2.4% |

*C. nauseosa* var. *consimilis*

| | |
|---|---|
| Limonene | 33.2% |
| Beta-Phellandrene | 18.0% |
| (Z)-Beta-Ocimene | 14.6% |
| Beta-Myrcene | 3.2% |
| Terpinen-4-ol | 3.0% |

*C. nauseosa* var. *albicaulis*

| | |
|---|---|
| Beta-Phellandrene | 26.0% |
| Limonene | 18.6% |
| Beta-Pinene | 16.8% |
| Beta-Myrcene | 6.9% |
| (Z)-Beta-Ocimene | 4.8% |
| Terpinen-4-ol | 4.3% |
| (E)-Beta-Ocimene | 3.3% |
| Sabinene | 3.4% |

*C. nauseosa* var. *glabratus*

| | |
|---|---|
| Beta-Pinene | 30.3% |
| Limonene | 16.5% |
| Beta-Phellandrene | 10.9% |
| Beta-Myrcene | 10.5% |
| (E)-Beta-Ocimene | 9.1% |
| Terpinen-4-ol | 2.3% |

**OTHER CONSTITUENTS:** *E. nauseosa* var. *nauseosa*—alpha-pinene, alpha-thujene, beta-myrcene, alpha-terpinene, dehydro-1,8-cineole, trans-sabinene hydrate, cis-sabinene hydrate, para-cymene, trans-p-menth-2-en-1-ol, cis-p-menth-2-en-ol, trans-pinocarveol, delta-cadinene, ar-curcumene, cuminaldehyde, elemol; *C. nauseosa* var. *albicaulis*—alpha-pinene, alpha-terpinene, gamma-terpinene, terpinolene, alpha-terpineol, geranyl acetate; *C. nauseosa* var. *consimilis*—alpha-pinene, sabinene, alpha-phellandrene, alpha-terpinene, (E)-beta-ocimene, gamma-terpinene, terpinolene, geranyl acetate; *C. nauseosa* var. *glabratus*—alpha-pinene, alpha-terpinene, (Z)-beta-ocimene, gamma-terpinene, citronellyl acetate, alpha-terpineol, geranyl acetate, delta-cadinene

**PREFERRED COMPOSITION FOR CLINICAL USE:**

| Constituent | Limonene CT |
|---|---|
| **Limonene** | 30%–45% |
| **Beta-Phellandrene** | 10%–25% |
| **(Z)-Beta-Ocimene** | 5%–20% |
| **Beta-Myrcene** | 2%–6% |
| **Terpinen-4-ol** | 2%–5% |

**REPORTED THERAPEUTIC PROPERTIES:** Antibacterial, antifungal, antiparasitic, antiseptic, analgesic, anti-inflammatory, antirheumatic, antiarthritic, antispasmodic, expels excess gas, **eases cough**, supports respiratory function, expels excess mucus, aids digestion, relieves diarrhea, eases stomachache, relieves headache/migraine, balances blood pressure, **soothes chronic skin conditions**, soothes blisters and boils, wound healing, relieves anxiety, stress management, promotes alertness, aids mental clarity

**CAUTIONS:**

■ *var. albicaulis*: May interact with anticholinergic (drugs used for asthma, incontinence, gastrointestinal cramps, muscular spasms, depression, and sleep disorders) and cholinergic medications (drugs used to reduce urinary retention, diagnose myasthenia gravis, and for glaucoma) based on AChE inhibitory activity of beta-phellandrene.[7249]

**SELECTED EVIDENCE:**

☐ Rabbitbrush was found to be ineffective against malaria and human pathogens (*C. albicans, Cr. neoformans, A. fumigatus, S. aureus*, MRSA, *P. aeruginosa*, and *M. intracellulare*).[7250]

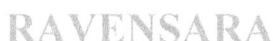 

# RAVENSARA
## (Clove Nutmeg, Ravensare)

*Ravensara aromatica* Sonn., *R. anisata* Danguy et Choux,
*Agathophyllum aromatica* Willd.

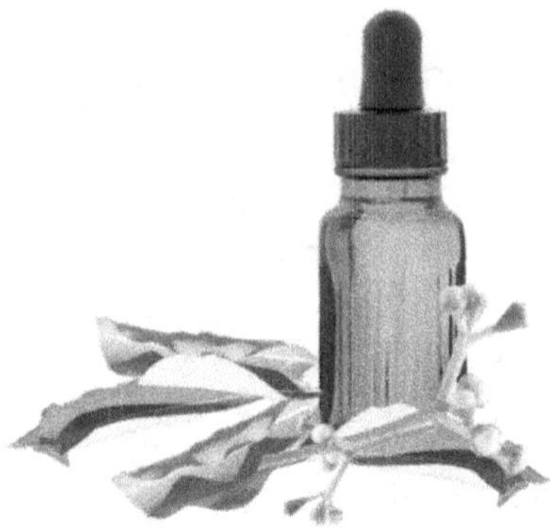

**FAMILY:** Lauraceae
**NOTE:** Top-Middle
**AROMA INTENSITY:** Medium
**AROMA:** Medicinal, woody, herbaceous, slightly spicy
**COMMON EXTRACTION METHOD:** Steam distilled from the leaves; also extracted from the bark (which is characterized by high levels of methyl chavicol (estragole)—83.0%–98.0%[1823]
**POSSIBLE SUBSTITUTE OILS:** Ravintsara (1,8-cineole CT), eucalyptus, myrtle, cajeput, cardamom, bay laurel, niaouli (1,8-cineole CT), petitgrain (mandarin), fennel (methyl chavicol CT), bay laurel
**BLENDS WELL WITH:** Bergamot, black pepper, cardamom, clary sage, cedarwood, eucalyptus, frankincense, geranium, ginger, grapefruit, lavender, lavandin, lemon, lime, marjoram, tea tree, pine, rosemary, sandalwood, thyme
**SUBCELLULAR LOCALIZATION | EPIGENETIC INFLUENCE:** Currently unknown | Currently unknown
**RECOMMENDED DILUTION RANGE:** Methyl chavicol and Methyl eugenol CT 1.5%–5%; 3%–20%; Alpha-terpinene, Sabinene, and Limonene CT 3%–50%; neat for limited conditions

**PRIMARY CONSTITUENTS:**[7251,7252,7253,7254,7255,7256]

*Methyl Chavicol (Estragole) CT\**

| | |
|---|---|
| Methyl Chavicol (Estragole) | 61.6%–94.5% |
| Trans-Anethole | 0.0%–20.1% |
| Methyl Eugenol | 0.1%–8.5% |
| Limonene | 0.1%–4.2% |
| Sabinene | 0.1%–3.4% |
| Terpinen-4-ol | 0.0%–2.2% |
| Linalool | 0.7%–1.9% |
| Alpha-Copaene | 0.0%–1.9% |
| Beta-Caryophyllene | 0.4%–1.8% |
| Germacrene D | 0.1%–1.6% |
| Alpha-Terpinene | 0.1%–0.8% |

*1,8-Cineole CT\#*

| | |
|---|---|
| 1,8-Cineole | 31.0%–60.8% |
| Sabinene | 11.0%–17.2% |
| Alpha-Terpineol | 0.0%–12.4% |
| Limonene | 0.0%–0.8% |
| Methyl-Chavicol (Estragole) | 0.0%–0.7% |

*Alpha-Terpinene CT*

| | |
|---|---|
| Alpha-Terpinene | 25.3%–27.7% |
| Limonene | 14.8%–21.8% |
| Sabinene | 16.8%–19.4% |
| Terpinen-4-ol | 7.0%–7.2% |
| Gamma-Terpinene | 5.7%–5.9% |
| Alpha-Pinene | 3.9%–4.5% |
| Linalool | 3.3%–4.5% |

*Limonene CT*

| | |
|---|---|
| Limonene | 13.9%–22.5% |
| Sabinene | 3.9%–16.4% |
| Isoledene | 0.0%–14.2% |
| Methyl Chavicol (Estragole) | 0.1%–11.9% |
| Beta-Caryophyllene | 1.5%–8.4% |
| Beta-Myrcene | 5.0%–7.3% |
| Alpha-Terpinene | 1.8%–7.1% |
| Alpha-Pinene | 3.0%–6.4% |
| Linalool | 3.0%–5.7% |
| Methyl Eugenol | 0.0%–5.2% |
| Terpinen-4-ol | 1.7%–4.8% |
| Gamma-Terpinene | 1.8%–4.1% |
| 1,8-Cineole | 0.1%–3.9% |
| Beta-Pinene | 2.2%–2.9% |
| Beta-Phellandrene | 1.0%–2.9% |
| Alpha-Thujene | 0.4%–2.1% |

*Sabinene CT*

| | |
|---|---|
| Sabinene | 25.0%–34.4% |
| Linalool | 6.5%–21.4% |
| Terpinen-4-ol | 6.2%–12.0% |
| Limonene | 7.2%–8.5% |
| Alpha-Pinene | 5.6%–8.1% |
| Beta-Pinene | 3.9%–7.7% |
| Methyl Chavicol (Estragole) | 1.8%–5.0% |
| Gamma-Terpinene | 1.9%–4.4% |
| Myrcene | 2.5%–3.4% |

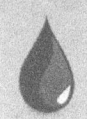

| | | | |
|---|---|---|---|
| Myrcene | 2.8%–3.2% | Para-Cymene | 1.4%–3.0% |
| Beta-Pinene | 2.7%–2.9% | Alpha-Phellandrene | 1.1%–2.8% |
| Methyl Chavicol (Estragole) | 0.0%–1.4% | Germacrene D | 1.5%–2.2% |
| Alpha-Thujene | 1.2%–1.3% | Alpha-Thujene | 1.2%–1.6% |
| Alpha-Phellandrene | 1.2%–1.3% | Methyl Eugenol | 0.3%–1.3% |
| Germacrene D | 0.5%–1.1% | | |
| Methyl Eugenol | 0.1%–1.1% | | |

*Methyl Eugenol CT*

| | |
|---|---|
| Methyl Eugenol | 74.0%–81.6% |
| Alpha-Terpinene | 0.6%–7.8% |
| Linalool | 0.4%–4.7% |
| Methyl Chavicol (Estragole) | 2.5%–4.5% |
| Limonene | 0.7%–4.5% |
| Elemicin | 0.6%–1.7% |
| Gamma-Terpinene | 0.7%–1.6% |
| 1,8-Cineole | 0.0%–1.4% |
| Para-Cymene | 0.5%–1.2% |
| Alpha-Pinene | 0.2%–1.2% |
| Beta-Caryophyllene | 0.1%–0.9% |
| Terpinen-4-ol | 0.6%–0.7% |
| Eugenol | 0.0%–0.6% |
| Sabinene | 0.4%–0.5% |

*The methyl chavicol (estragole) CT is the most commonly reported in the literature.

#Given the great confusion between ravintsara (*Cinnamomum camphora*, leaves) and ravensara, it is possible that the 1,8-cineole CT is a misidentified sample from ravintsara.

**OTHER CONSTITUENTS:** Delta-3-carene, camphene, gamma-cadinene, beta-elemene, (Z)-beta-ocimene

**PREFERRED COMPOSITION FOR CLINICAL USE:**

| Constituent | Limonene CT |
|---|---|
| Limonene | 12%–25% |
| Sabinene | 5%–18% |
| Beta-Caryophyllene | 4%–10% |
| Alpha-Pinene | 3%–7% |
| Methyl Eugenol | 2%–7% |
| Linalool | 3%–6% |
| Delta-3-Carene | 3%–6% |
| Beta-Myrcene | 2%–6% |
| Methyl Chavicol | 1%–6% |
| Alpha-Terpinene | 1%–4% |
| Gamma-Terpinene | 1%–4% |
| Beta-Pinene | 2%–3% |
| Alpha-Phellandrene | 1%–3% |
| 1,8-Cineole | 0.5%–3% |
| Beta-Phellandrene | 0.5%–3% |
| Alpha-Copaene | 15%–2% |
| Camphene | 0.5%–2% |
| Cis-Beta-Ocimene | 0.5%–2% |
| Delta-Cadinene | 0.5%–2% |
| Alpha-Humulene | 0.5%–2% |
| Alpha-Thujene | 0.1%–2% |

**REPORTED THERAPEUTIC PROPERTIES:** Analgesic (pain relief), antiallergenic, antibacterial, **antimicrobial, anti-infectious**, antiseptic, **antiviral**, antispasmodic, diuretic, eases cough, expectorant, **antifungal**, expels excess gas, **supports respiratory function**, aids lymph circulation, wound healing, strengthens nails, simulating, antidepressant, reduces anxiety, stress management, energizing, encourages creativity, aphrodisiac

**CAUTIONS:**

■ Avoid with children under age 3 (1,8-cineole CT), particularly around the nose and mouth. Use very cautiously in children under age 5 due to high 1,8-cineole content. 1,8-cineole may cause seizures, central nervous system problems, or respiratory distress in young children.[7257,7258,7259,7260] Use with great caution for children under age six due to animal reports of liver cancer caused by methyl chavicol (estragole) content.[7261] The European Medicines Agency recommends exposure to estragole be limited in young children. Avoid the *Methyl Eugenol CT* in children under age 12 due to the multisite cancerous tumors and DNA mutation caused by methyl eugenol in animal studies.[7262,7263,7264,7265]

■ Avoid during pregnancy and lactation due to potentially high estragole and/or methyl eugenol content.[7266] Estragole may cause genetic mutations and oxidative DNA damage.[7267] The European Medicines Agency recommends exposure to estragole be limited in women who are pregnant or nursing.[7268] Animal research suggests that methyl eugenol may cause changes in embryo form and structure and chromosomal changes in ovary cells, as well as multi-site cancerous tumors.[7269,7270,7271,7272]

■ Avoid oral use (limonene, methyl chavicol, methyl eugenol CTs) due to toxic and carcinogenic (cancer-causing) potential of methyl eugenol and methyl chavicol.[7273,7274,7275,7276] The metabolite of estragole (1'-hydroxyestragole) is considered a stronger carcinogen and humans rapidly metabolize estragole to 1'-hydroxyestragole when ingested.[7277] Caution is warranted orally for the 1,8-cineole CT due to the significant amounts of 1,8-cineole. Limit to small doses internally (adults—maximum 10 drops daily) for 1,8-cineole CT. Toxicity has been reported when eucalyptus (also high in 1,8-cineole) was ingested in large doses, and as few as 4 to 5 drops may cause problems in very sensitive individuals.[7278,7279,7280,7281,7282,7283] In humans, 3.5 to 5 mL has proven fatal orally.[7284] Methyl eugenol may cause multisite cancerous tumors according to animal research.[7285,7286,7287,7288]

■ Avoid with epilepsy and Parkinson's disease due to 1,8-cineole content. May exacerbate or cause seizures or convulsions when inhaled, applied topically, or ingested based on 1,8-cineole content.[7289,7290,7291,7292,7293,7294]

■ May interact with antibiotics or antifungal drugs and possibly enhance or decrease their effectiveness based on methyl eugenol or estragole content.[7295,7296,7297,7298]

■ May interact with aspirin, blood pressure, antiplatelet, and anticoagulant medications, and increase the risk of bleeding among people with bleeding disorders based on methyl chavicol content.[7299,7300,7301,7302] Methyl chavicol is a more potent inhibitor of platelet aggregation than aspirin (*methyl chavicol CT*).[7303]

■ *Methyl Eugenol CT*: May interact with anticholinergic (drugs used for asthma, incontinence, gastrointestinal cramps, muscular spasms, depression, and sleep disorders) and cholinergic medications (drugs used to reduce urinary retention, diagnose myasthenia gravis, and for glaucoma) based on the potent AChE inhibitory activity of methyl eugenol.[7304]

■ *1,8-Cineole CT*: May interfere with enzymes responsible for metabolizing medications (NSAIDs, proton-pump inhibitors, acetaminophen, antiepileptics, immune modulators, blood-sugar medications, blood pressure medications, antidepressants, antipsychotics, diabetic medications, antihistamines, antibiotics, and anesthetics) due to methyl chavicol (estragole) and 1,8-cineole content.[7305]

■ *1,8-Cineole, Methyl Chavicol CTs*: May weakly interfere with the enzymes responsible for metabolizing medications (NSAIDs, proton-pump inhibitors, acetaminophen, antiepileptics, immune modulators, blood-sugar medications, blood pressure medications, antidepressants, antipsychotics, diabetic medications, antihistamines, antibiotics, and anesthetics) due to 1,8-cineole content.[7306,7307,7308]

■ *1,8-Cineole CT*: May interfere with pentobarbital and other barbiturates (medications for anxiety and insomnia) based on 1,8-cineole content.[7309,7310]

**SELECTED EVIDENCE:**

☐ A nasal spray with lemon, ravensara, and niaouli oils (0.14 mL consisting of 0.014 mL lemon, 0.042 mL aloe vera juice, 0.0007 mL ravensara, 0.0007 g propolis, and 0.00042 mL niaouli oil) decreased the symptoms of allergic and nonallergic rhinopathy (nasal congestion, drainage, and obstruction of the nasal passages) in a clinical trial.[7311]

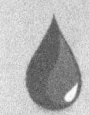

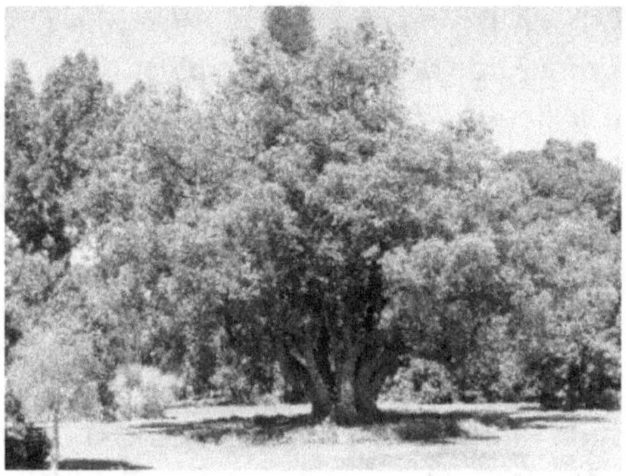

# RAVINTSARA
## (Ho Leaf, Ho Sho)

*Cinnamomum camphora* (L.) J. Presl, *Laurus camphora* L.; *C. camphora* chvar. Borneol

**FAMILY:** Lauraceae
**NOTE:** Middle
**AROMA INTENSITY:** Strong
**AROMA:** Medicinal, penetrating, woody
**COMMON EXTRACTION METHOD:** Steam distilled from the leaves
**POSSIBLE SUBSTITUTE OILS:** Eucalyptus, niaouli (1,8-cineole CT), bay laurel, cajeput, cardamom, rosemary (1,8-cineole CT), ravensara (1,8-cineole CT), camphor (camphor CT), sage (camphor CT), rosemary (camphor CT), thyme (linalool CT), camphor (linalool CT)
**BLENDS WELL WITH:** Chamomile (German, Roman), copaiba, eucalyptus, frankincense, juniper, peppermint, pine, rosemary, wintergreen,
**SUBCELLULAR LOCALIZATION | EPIGENETIC INFLUENCE:** Currently unknown | Currently unknown
**RECOMMENDED DILUTION RANGE:** 3%–33%; neat for limited conditions

**PRIMARY CONSTITUENTS:**[7312,7313,7314,7315,7316,7317,7318,7319,7320,7321,7322,7323,7324]

| *1,8-Cineole CT* | | *Camphor CT* | |
|---|---|---|---|
| 1,8-Cineole | 53.8%–63.0% | Camphor | 40.5%–72.5% |
| Sabinene | 14.1%–16.8% | Linalool | 0.5%–22.9% |
| Alpha-Terpineol | 3.8%–10.3% | 1,8-Cineole | 1.0%–11.3% |
| Alpha-Pinene | 3.7%–5.0% | Alpha-Pinene | 2.1%–5.0% |
| Beta-Pinene | 0.0%–3.5% | Safrole | 0.1%–5.0% |
| Alpha-Myrcene | 0.0%–3.2% | Bicyclogermacrene | 0.0%–5.0% |
| | | Limonene | 0.0%–4.5% |
| *Linalool CT* | | Allo-Aromadendrene | 0.0%–4.4% |
| Linalool | 87.2%–95.3% | Camphene | 0.0%–2.8% |
| Beta-Caryophyllene | 0.5%–2.2% | Alpha-Terpineol | 0.0%–2.3% |
| Camphene Hydrate | 0.0%–1.5% | Caryophyllene | 0.0%–2.2% |

| *chvar. Borneol* | |
|---|---|
| Borneol | 10.7%–81.6% |
| Alpha-Pinene | 0.0%–21.9% |
| Alpha-Phellandrene | 0.0%–15.2% |
| Limonene | 0.0%–12.0% |
| Camphor | 0.0%–11.7% |
| Beta-Pinene | 0.0%–10.0% |
| (3E)-2,7-Dimethyl-3-Octen-5-yne | 0.0%–8.2% |
| Alpha-Humulene | 0.1%–8.1% |
| Camphene | 0.0%–6.1% |
| Beta-Caryophyllene | 0.0%–5.0% |
| Para-Cymene | 0.0%–4.7% |
| 1,8-Cineole | 1.8%–4.1% |
| Germacrene D | 0.0%–4.1% |

Note: *C. camphora* chvar. Borneol is a byproduct of steam distillation to produce natural crystalline borneol. The branches and flowers can also produce a borneol CT.

**OTHER CONSTITUENTS:** *1,8-Cineole CT*—Alpha-thujene, myrcene, para-cymene, gamma-terpinene, cis-sabinene hydrate, delta-terpineol, terpinen-4-ol, alpha-humulene, beta-caryophyllene, Germacrene D, bicyclogermacrene; *Camphor CT*—2-Thujene, sabinene, p-mentha-1-en-4-ol, p-menth-1-en-8-ol, dihydro-cis-alpha-copaene-8-ol, gamma-elemene, germacrene D; *Linalool CT*—Beta-ocimene, camphor, alpha-terpineol, elemol, germacrene D, bicyclogermacrene; *chvar. Borneol*—Alpha-thujene, sabinene, delta-3-carene, myrcene, alpha-terpinene, gamma-terpinene, beta-ocimene, linalool, terpinen-4-ol, caryophyllene oxide, beta-bisabolene, spathulenol, bicyclogermacrene, beta-cadinene, alpha-copaene, terpinolene, selina-3,11-diene, beta-elemene, germacrene B, alpha-cadinol, neointermedeol, 1,2-dimethoxy-4-(1-propenyl)-benzene

**PREFERRED COMPOSITION FOR CLINICAL USE:**

| Constituent | 1,8-Cineole CT |
|---|---|
| **1,8-Cineole** | 50%–62% |
| **Sabinene** | 10%–20% |
| **Alpha-Terpineol** | 4%–10% |
| **Alpha-Pinene** | 3%–6% |
| **Beta-Pinene** | 1%–6% |
| **Terpinen-4-ol** | 1%–4% |
| **Beta-Caryophyllene** | 0.5%–3% |
| **Beta-Myrcene** | 0.1%–2% |
| **Gamma-Terpinene** | 0.1%–2% |

**REPORTED THERAPEUTIC PROPERTIES:** Analgesic (pain relief), anti-inflammatory, antirheumatic, antiarthritic, **antibacterial**, **antiviral**, **antifungal**, **anti-infectious**, antiseptic, reduces the appearance of blemishes, eases cough, relieves skin conditions, **supports respiratory system**, **relieves sinusitis**, reduces fever, antidepressant, reduces anxiety, stress management, combats fear, encourages self-confidence

**CAUTIONS:**

■ Avoid with children under age 3 (camphor and 1,8-cineole CT), particularly around the nose and mouth. Use very cautiously in children under age 5 due to high 1,8-cineole content. 1,8-cineole may cause seizures, central nervous system problems, or respiratory distress in young children.[7325,7326,7327,7328] Ingestion of camphor-containing products has been lethal in children under age 2 (estimated to be roughly 2,000 mg of camphor for a 20 kg child as the minimum potential fatal dose).[7329,7330] Children 5 years and up may use camphor topically in dilutions no stronger than 5%.

■ Caution is warranted during pregnancy and while lactating due to significant camphor content (camphor CT). Ingestion of essential oils with significant levels of camphor may lead to abortion because fetuses lack the enzymes to process it.[7331] Camphor ingestion by infants and young children may cause cough, vomiting, seizure, burning sensation in the mucous membranes and eyes, or lack of voluntary coordination of muscle movements.[7332]

■ Avoid with epilepsy and Parkinson's disease due to 1,8-cineole and camphor content. May exacerbate or cause seizures/convulsions or reduce seizure medication efficacy based on 1,8-cineole and camphor content.[7333,7334,7335]

■ Caution is warranted orally due to the significant amounts of 1,8-cineole content (1,8-cineole CT) and the camphor CT should be avoided orally. Limit to small doses internally (adults—maximum 10 drops daily). Toxicity has been reported when eucalyptus (also high in 1,8-cineole) was ingested in large doses, and as few as 4 to 5 drops may cause problems in very sensitive individuals.[7336,7337,7338,7339,7340,7341] In humans, 3.5 to 5 mL has proven fatal orally.[7342] Oral—Camphor can be toxic when taken orally (usually single doses exceeding 2 mL), although the lethal dose for adult humans is estimated to be (more than 5 mL) in a single dose.[7343,7344,7345]

■ The significant camphor content in ravintsara (camphor CT) may negatively impact red blood cells and increase the risk of jaundice in children with Glucose-6-phosphate dehydrogenase deficiency (G6PD).[7346,7347]

■ May weakly interfere with the enzymes responsible for metabolizing medications (NSAIDs, proton-pump inhibitors, acetaminophen, antiepileptics, immune modulators, blood-sugar medications, blood pressure medications, antidepressants, antipsychotics, diabetic medications, antihistamines, antibiotics, and anesthetics) due to 1,8-cineole content.[7348,7349,7350]

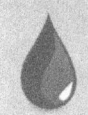

■ *Linalool CT*: May interact with antifungal drugs and enhance their effectiveness based on linalool content.[7351]

■ May interfere with pentobarbital and other barbiturates (medications for anxiety and insomnia) based on 1,8-cineole content.[7352,7353]

■ Avoid with those who have a compromised liver due to the risk of increased liver enzymes and liver damage (camphor CT).[7354] This would also suggest that those taking medications that could cause liver damage should also use ravintsara very cautiously or avoid it entirely.

■ Caution is warranted for the topical application of camphor-containing essential oils on broken or injured skin due to an increased risk of toxicity.[7355]

**SELECTED EVIDENCE:**

☐ Research shows that amino acid neurotransmitter levels—like glycine, aspartate, and D-serine—as well as serine racemase (the enzyme responsible for producing D-serine) are altered in subjects with learning and memory impairment. Multiple metabolites in the blood and brain tissue play important roles in cognitive function. Inhalation of ravintsara essential oil CT borneol (one hour, twice daily, for 21 days) modified 11 differential blood metabolites—including glycine, azelaic acid, citraconic acid, adenine, methionine, isoleucine, cholesterol, tyrosine, proline, phenylalanine and leucine—and 26 different brain tissue metabolites—including adenine, aspartic acid, D-serine, valine, glucose, ornithine, glutamic acid, lysine, isoleucine, lactic acid, citric acid, gluconic acid, α-alanine, β-alanine, cholesterol, citrulline, glycine, leucine, methionine, myo-inositol, myristic acid, oleic acid, phenylalanine, proline, tyrosine and uracil in mice.[7356] These metabolites are involved in metabolic pathways important for healthy cognition, comprising phenylalanine, tyrosine and tryptophan biosynthesis, phenylalanine metabolism, alanine, aspartate and glutamate metabolism, arginine biosynthesis, and beta-alanine metabolism, glyoxylate and dicarboxylate metabolism and aminoacyl-tRNA biosynthesis. Based on the activity of ravintsara essential oil on these metabolic pathways, the researchers concluded that the oil may improve learning and memory impairment by regulating amino acid metabolism and improving neurotransmitter balance.

☐ Repeated topical application of ravintsara (chvar. Borneol) to the abdomen for six days, significantly reduce pain in mice, with higher concentrations producing greater effects.[7357] Blood markers for pain and inflammation (prostaglandin E2 and TPRM8 were significantly reduced. The oil was virtually nontoxic when ingested by male mice (LD50 5081 mg/kg BW) and showed low toxicity in female mice (LD50 2749 mg/kg BW), and was not irritating to the skin or eye when applied topically up to 50%.

☐ Ravintsara essential oil inhibits *A. niger* (a common fungus that can infect humans and produce potent toxins, called mycotoxins) *in vitro*.[7358] Another study found that ravintsara inhibits *A. flavus* and its subsequent production of the toxin aflatoxin B1.[7359] Ravintsara (chvar. Borneol) inhibited *C. globosum, E. coli, P. aeruginosa, S. aureus, B. subtilis, H. anomala, A. niger,* and *cerevisiae*.[7360] Another study showed the borneol CT inhibited *B. subtilis, S. typhimurium, E. coli, S. aureus, A. niger,* and *P. aurantiogriseum*.[7361]

☐ Ravintsara (chvar. Borneol) exhibited good antioxidant activity in the beta-carotene/linoleic acid and moderate activity in the reducing power assays.[7362]

☐ *In vitro* research concluded that ravintsara is a natural insecticide for fire ants, butterflies, and fruit flies.[7363] The camphor CT of ravintsara essential oil killed and repelled the cotton aphid (*Aphis gossypii* Glover).[7364] Ravintsara (chvar. borneol) repelled and was miticidal against the dust mite.[7365]

☐ Ravintsara's ability to inhibit *Candida* is superior to the antifungals miconazole and clotrimazole.[7366]

☐ *In vitro* research suggests that ravintsara oil inhibits *S. pyogenes* (a bacterium that causes strep throat, scarlet fever, impetigo, cellulitis, and tonsillitis).[7367]

☐ The camphor CT of ravintsara displayed strong toxicity against stored product pests (*Tribolium castaneum* and *Lasioderma serricorne*).[7368]

☐ The linalool CT of ravintsara essential oil inhibited *P. aeruginosa, S. aureus, C. violaceum,* and *E. coli* and exhibited antiquorum-sensing activity, which reduces virulence factors in bacteria.[7369]

☐ Ravintsara CT 1,8-cineole essential oil displayed larvicidal activity against the *Anopheles stephensi* mosquito, which is the main malaria vector in Southeast Asia.[7370]

☐ The linalool CT of ravintsara essential oil inhibited MRSA, *S. aureus, E. faecalis, B. subtilis, S. gallinarum,* and *E. coli*.[7371]

- Topical application of a borneol CT of ravintsara essential oil significantly reduced swelling and expression of inflammatory mediators (IL-1β and tumor necrosis factor α) in mice.[7372] Another study from a different group of researchers found that ravintsara CT linalool essential oil decreases the release of nitric oxide and the mRNA expression of inducible NO synthase (iNOS) and inflammatory cytokines (IL-6, IL-8, IL-1β, and TNF-α).[7373]

- The 1,8-cineole CT of camphor essential oil moderately inhibited *L. monocytogenes, S. aureus, E. faecalis, S. typhimurium, E. coli,* and *P. aeruginosa* and high antibacterial activity against the same microorganisms.[7374]

- Ravintsara CT camphor essential oil inhibited *T. rubrum, S. epidermidis, T. mentagrophytes, P. acnes, A. niger, A. fumigatus, C. albicans, M. canis,* and *M. gypseum.*[7375]

- Injection of high doses (200 mL/kg BW) of rosemary, Spanish lavender, ravintsara, and eucalyptus (*E. globulus*) essential oil reduced anxiety in rats.[7376]

- Research shows that amino acid neurotransmitter levels—like glycine, aspartate, and D-serine—as well as serine racemase (the enzyme responsible for producing D-serine) are altered in subjects with learning and memory impairment. Multiple metabolites in the blood and brain tissue play important roles in cognitive function. Inhalation of ravintsara essential oil CT borneol (one hour, twice daily, for twenty-one days) modified eleven differential blood metabolites—including glycine, azelaic acid, citraconic acid, adenine, methionine, isoleucine, cholesterol, tyrosine, proline, phenylalanine and leucine—and twenty-six different brain tissue metabolites—including adenine, aspartic acid, D-serine, valine, glucose, ornithine, glutamic acid, lysine, isoleucine, lactic acid, citric acid, gluconic acid, α-alanine, β-alanine, cholesterol, citrulline, glycine, leucine, methionine, myo-inositol, myristic acid, oleic acid, phenylalanine, proline, tyrosine, and uracil in mice.[7377] These metabolites are involved in metabolic pathways important for healthy cognition, comprising phenylalanine, tyrosine and tryptophan biosynthesis, phenylalanine metabolism, alanine, aspartate and glutamate metabolism, arginine biosynthesis, and beta-alanine metabolism, glyoxylate and dicarboxylate metabolism, and aminoacyl-tRNA biosynthesis. Based on the activity of ravintsara essential oil on these metabolic pathways, the researchers concluded that the oil may improve learning and memory impairment by regulating amino acid metabolism and improving neurotransmitter balance.

- Ravintsara inhibited multidrug-resistant bacteria (*S. aureus, A. baumannii, K. pneumonia, E. coli*) obtained from clinical samples.[7378]

- An interesting chemotype of ravintsara with geranial and neral as the primary constituents, displayed good antioxidant activity in the DPPH, ABTS, and FRAP assays.[7379]

- Ravintsara CT 1,8-cineole selectively inhibited AChE (anti-Alzheimer's activity) and inhibited tyrosinase (skin brightening activity). The oil also showed moderate antioxidant activity in the DPPH and ABTS assays.[7380]

- Topical application of a ravintsara CT of borneol essential oil for six days significantly reduced pain in mice.[7381] The oil significantly reduced mediators of pain: serum prostaglandin E2 (PGE2) and transient receptor potential melastatin-8 (TRPM8). No acute skin or eye irritation was observed when the oil was used at less than 50% dilution.

- Ravintsara, turmeric, petitgrain (*C. aurantium*), and bitter orange essential oil each inhibited *Mycobacterium smegmatis* (a bacterial strain commonly used as a model for inhibition of *M. tuberculosis*), *C. albicans,* and *C. tropicalis.*[7382] The oils also displayed activity against collagenase, indicating an antiaging activity. Petitgrain and turmeric also inhibited elastase, which would preserve skin strength and flexibility.

---

# RED PINE
## (Norway Pine)

*Pinus resinosa* Aiton

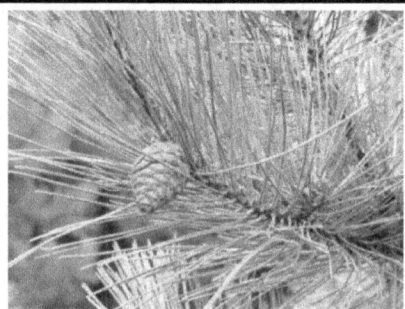

**FAMILY:** Pinaceae
**NOTE:** Top
**AROMA INTENSITY:** Medium
**AROMA:** Piney, woody, fresh, balsamic, earthy
**COMMON EXTRACTION METHOD:** Steam distilled from the needles and twigs
**POSSIBLE SUBSTITUTE OILS:** Pine, balsam fir, cypress, white pine

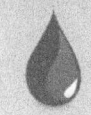

**BLENDS WELL WITH:** Agarwood, bergamot, cajeput, camphor, cedarwood, clary sage, coriander, Douglas fir, eucalyptus, Engelmann spruce, frankincense, galbanum, grapefruit, juniper, lavender, lemon, lime, tea tree, marjoram, neroli, niaouli, peppermint, ravensara, ravintsara, rosemary, Spanish sage, spikenard, thyme, Siberian fir, silver fir, white fir, white pine, white spruce

**SUBCELLULAR LOCALIZATION | EPIGENETIC INFLUENCE:** Currently unknown | Currently unknown

**RECOMMENDED DILUTION RANGE:** 5%–Neat

**PRIMARY CONSTITUENTS:**[7383,7384,7385,7386]

| | |
|---|---|
| Alpha-Pinene | 13.0%–50.1% |
| Beta-Pinene | 1.9%–42.4% |
| Beta-Caryophyllene | 0.7%–27.6% |
| Beta-Myrcene | 3.5%–14.5% |
| Delta-3-Carene | 0.5%–12.9% |
| Naphthalene | 0.0%–9.4% |
| Germacrene D | 0.1%–4.9% |
| Borneol | 0.0%–3.5% |

**OTHER CONSTITUENTS:** Terpinolene, limonene, camphene, beta-phellandrene, alpha-terpinolene, alpha-fenchene, longifolene, 1,3,5-cycloheptatriene, limonene oxide, beta-bisabolene, alpha-amorphene, isoborneol, alpha-terpineol

**PREFERRED COMPOSITION FOR CLINICAL USE:**

| *Constituent* | |
|---|---|
| **Alpha-Pinene** | 35%–55% |
| **Beta-Pinene** | 25%–45% |
| **Beta-Myrcene** | 3%–12% |
| **Delta-3-Carene** | 3%–8% |
| **Beta-Caryophyllene** | 0.5%–5% |
| **Germacrene D** | 0.1%–4% |
| **Limonene** | 1%–3% |
| **Camphene** | 0%–3% |
| **Beta-Phellandrene** | 1%–2% |

**REPORTED THERAPEUTIC PROPERTIES:** Antibacterial, antifungal, anti-infectious, **analgesic**, anti-inflammatory, antiarthritic, antispasmodic, **supports respiratory function**, expels excess mucus, eases cough, relieves sore throat, aids immune function, stimulates localized circulation, supports endocrine and adrenal function, grounding, stress management, relieves anxiety, encourages self-esteem

**CAUTIONS:**

■ May decrease the bioavailability of many medications (NSAIDs, proton-pump inhibitors, acetaminophen, antiepileptics, immune modulators, blood-sugar medications, blood pressure medications, antidepressants, antipsychotics, diabetic medications, antihistamines, antibiotics, and anesthetics) due to the ability of beta-caryophyllene to inhibit CYP3A enzyme activity.[7387]

**SELECTED EVIDENCE:**

☐ *In vitro* research demonstrates that red pine essential oil is active against the fungi *Fusarium culmorum, F. poae,* and *F. solani.*[7388]

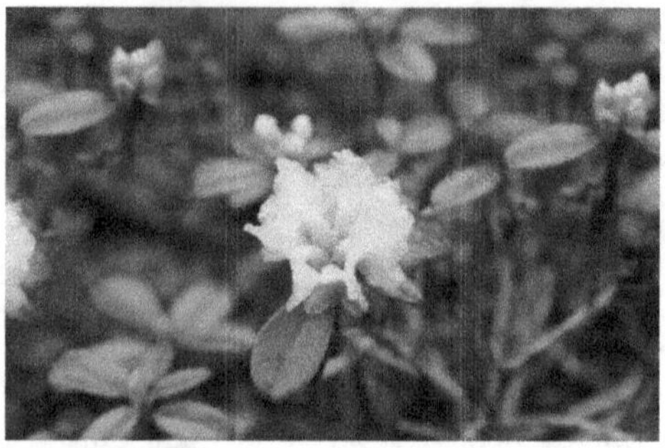

# RHODODENDRON
## (Anthropogon, Sunpati)
*Rhododendron anthopogon* D. Don

**FAMILY:** Ericaceae
**NOTE:** Middle
**AROMA INTENSITY:** Medium
**AROMA:** Floral, sweet, fruity, slightly balsamic and herbaceous
**COMMON EXTRACTION METHOD:** Steam distilled from the aerial parts (flowers and leaves)
**POSSIBLE SUBSTITUTE OILS:** Grindelia, frankincense
**BLENDS WELL WITH:** Balsam fir, cedarwood, clary sage, davana, Douglas fir, frankincense, geranium, ginger, lavender, orange, palmarosa, sandalwood, spruce (black), white fir, ylang ylang
**SUBCELLULAR LOCALIZATION | EPIGENETIC INFLUENCE:** Currently unknown | Currently unknown
**RECOMMENDED DILUTION RANGE:** 5%–Neat

**PRIMARY CONSTITUENTS:**[7389,7390,7391,7392,7393]

*Aerial Parts*

| | |
|---|---|
| Alpha Pinene | 8.3%–37.4% |
| Beta-Pinene | 6.2%–16.0% |
| Limonene | 7.1%–13.3% |
| Delta-Cadinene | 9.1%–11.4% |
| Beta-Caryophyllene | 2.3%–6.5% |
| Alpha-Muurolene | 2.7%–5.9% |
| (Z)-Beta-Ocimene | 3.7%–5.3% |
| Alpha-Amorphene | 3.2%–5.3% |

*Flowers*

| | |
|---|---|
| N-Acetyl-1,2,3,4-Tetrahydro -Isoquinoline | 29.2% |
| 2-Ethoxypropane | 12.5% |
| 3-Methyl-6-Tert-Butylphenol | 10.8% |
| 3-Methyl-5-Phenyl-Isothiazole | 6.4% |
| Diphenylamine | 4.2% |

*Leaves*

| | |
|---|---|
| Beta-Caryophyllene | 11.6% |
| Limonene | 11.3% |
| Alpha-Humulene | 7.2% |
| Aromadendrene | 6.3% |
| Gamma-Terpinene | 6.1% |
| (E)-Nerolidol | 5.8% |
| Citronellyl Formate | 5.5% |

**OTHER CONSTITUENTS:** *Aerial Parts*—Beta-myrcene, para-cymene, gamma-terpinene, alpha-copaene, (E)-beta-farnesene, alpha-humulene, alpha-selinene, ar-curcumene, cis-calamenene, alpha-cadinol, T-cadinol, germacrene D; *Leaves*—Alpha-terpinene, beta-phellandrene, (E)-beta-ocimene, para-cymene, alpha-terpinolene, linalool, calarene, bornyl acetate, terpinen-4-ol, gamma-gurjunene, (E)-beta-farnesene, alpha-terpineol, ledene, alpha-muurolene, E,E-alpha-farnesene, citronellol, globulol, spathulenol, alpha-eudesmol, beta-eudesmol, tetracosane, 2-furan carboxylic acid; *Flowers*—N-ethyl-1,2,3,4-tetrahydro-naphthalenamine, pentacosane, tricosane

**PREFERRED COMPOSITION FOR CLINICAL USE:**

| *Constituent* | *Aerial Parts* |
|---|---|
| **Alpha-Pinene** | 23%–38% |
| **Beta-Pinene** | 10%–17% |
| **Limonene** | 8%–15% |
| **Delta-Cadinene** | 4%–14% |
| **(Z)-Beta-Ocimene** | 1%–8% |

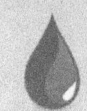

| | |
|---|---|
| **Beta-Caryophyllene** | 2%–6% |
| **Alpha-Amorphene** | 0%–5% |
| **Gamma-Cadinene** | 2%–5% |
| **Alpha-Muurolene** | 0.5%–5% |
| **Gamma-Muurolene** | 1%–4% |
| **Gamma-Terpinene** | 1%–4% |
| **Para-Cymene** | 0.1%–4% |

**REPORTED THERAPEUTIC PROPERTIES:** Antibacterial, antifungal, anti-inflammatory, analgesic, antispasmodic, nervine, **supports respiratory function**, eases cough, aids cardiovascular function, detoxification, aids circulation, encourages lymph flow, aids digestion, reduces the appearance of blemishes, **aids kidney and adrenal function**, encourages restful sleep, increases clarity, **aids meditation**, encourages feelings of love, antidepressant, stress management, relieves grief

**CAUTIONS:**
- None currently known.

**SELECTED EVIDENCE:**
- *In vitro* research demonstrates that rhododendron essential oil kills ovarian, cervical, and colon cancer cells.[7394]
- Rhododendron essential oil strongly inhibits *B. subtilis* and *E. faecalis*, moderately inhibits *S. aureus, C. amycolatum, C. albicans,* and *A. ochraceus*, and weakly inhibits *E. coli* according to *in vitro* research.[7395,7396]

---

# ROMAN CHAMOMILE
## (Roman Camomile)

*Chamaemelum nobile* (L.) All., *Anthemis nobilis* L.

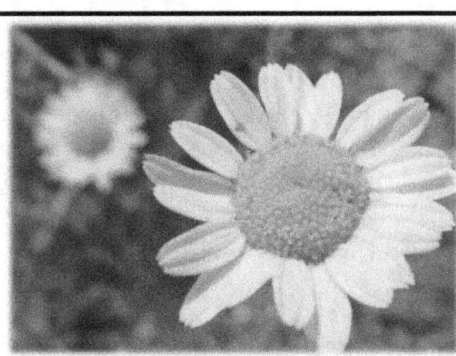

**FAMILY:** Asteraceae (Compositae)
**NOTE:** Middle
**AROMA INTENSITY:** Medium
**AROMA:** Fresh, sweet, fruity, herbaceous
**COMMON EXTRACTION METHOD:** Steam distilled from the flowers
**POSSIBLE SUBSTITUTE OILS:** German chamomile, lavender
**BLENDS WELL WITH:** Bergamot, cassia, chamomile (German), clary sage, eucalyptus, geranium, grapefruit, lavender, lemon, lime, tea tree, neroli, ravintsara, rose, tangerine, silver fir, white fir, ylang ylang
**SUBCELLULAR LOCALIZATION | EPIGENETIC INFLUENCE:** Endocytic Vesicles | Lymphatic/Endocrine
**RECOMMENDED DILUTION RANGE:** 5%–Neat

**PRIMARY CONSTITUENTS:**[7397,7398,7399,7400]

| | |
|---|---|
| Isobutyl Angelate | 24.5%–36.0% |
| Isoamyl Isobutyrate | 5.3%–23.7% |
| 2-Methylbutyl Angelate | 13.0%–20.3% |
| Isoamyl Tigliate | 11.7%–19.9% |
| Isoamyl Angelate | 3.7%–17.9% |
| Propyl Tigliate | 10.8%–13.1% |
| 3-Methylbutyl Isobutyrate | 5.2%–6.3% |
| Isobutyl Isobutyrate | 1.4%–5.3% |
| Isoamyl 2-Methylbutyrate | 3.9%–4.5% |
| Trans-Pinocarveol | 0.1%–4.5% |

**OTHER CONSTITUENTS:** Methyl 2-methylbutyrate, prenyl acetate, 2-methylbutyl acetate, 2-methylbutyl isobutyrate, alpha-pinene, camphene, pinocarvone, 2-methylbutyl methacrylate, isobutyl methacrylate, isopropyl angelate, methyl allyl angelate

**PREFERRED COMPOSITION FOR CLINICAL USE:**

| Constituent | Bulgarian/ Italian | English | French |
|---|---|---|---|
| **Isobutyl Angelate** | 28%–42% | 3%–12% | 28%–38% |
| **2-Methylbutyl Angelate** | 10%–25% | 3%–10% | 5%–21% |
| **Methyallyl Angelate** | 5%–10% | 8%–18% | 7%–17% |
| **Isoamyl Angelate** (Isoamyl Tiglate) | 3%–10% | 4%–12% | 4%–23% |
| **Isobutyl Isobutyrate** | 2%–8% | 0.1%–2% | 1%–8% |
| **Trans-Pinocarveol** | 0.5%–8% | 4%–10% | 2%–8% |
| **Isoamyl Isobutyrate** | 0.1%–5% | 0.5%–2% | 0.1%–4% |
| **Pinocarvone** | 1%–5% | 2%–5% | 1%–5% |
| **Alpha-Pinene** | 1%–5% | 1.5%–8% | 1%–5% |
| **Isobutyl Methacrylate** | tr–3% | 0.1%–2% | tr–4% |
| **2-Methylbutyl Methacrylate** | 0.1%–5% | 1%–3% | tr–3% |
| **3-Methylpentyl Angelate** (3-Methylamyl Angelate, Methylamyl Angelate) | 0.01%–1% | 10%–25% | tr–2% |

**REPORTED THERAPEUTIC PROPERTIES: Analgesic (pain relief)**, anti-inflammatory, antibacterial, antimicrobial, antiparasitic, **relieves headache**, nervine (calms and soothes the nerves), reduces fever, **relieves colic**, antiseptic, antirheumatic, **antineuralgic, antispasmodic**, expels excess gas, aids digestion, disinfectant, diuretic, **helps boils heal**, diminishes the appearance of scars and blemishes, **relieves skin conditions**, aids detoxification, supports liver function, **helps relieve painful menstruation**, wound healing, **relieves sunburn**, calming, relaxing, **reduces anxiety**, antidepressant, combats worrisome thoughts, helps eliminate sensitivity, stress management, **calms tantrums**, reduces anger, combats loneliness, reduces insecurity

**CAUTIONS:**

■ None currently known.

**SELECTED EVIDENCE:**

    □  Roman chamomile helps decrease inflammation by mildly inhibiting the 5-lipoxygenase (5-LOX) enzyme that is involved in the inflammation response according to *in vitro* research.[7401]

    □  Inhalation (ten deep breaths from aromatherapy stones with 2 drops of the blend) of lavender, Roman chamomile, and neroli reduced the anxiety and stress of patients undergoing coronary angioplasty (the insertion of a catheter to open blocked coronary arteries).[7402]

    □  A sitz bath with, or soap application of, lavender, myrrh, neroli, rose, grapefruit, mandarin, orange, and Roman chamomile improves healing of the perineum following delivery and episiotomy.[7403]

    □  Animal research suggests that Roman chamomile is anti-inflammatory, relaxing, and sedating.[7404]

    □  Topical application of Roman chamomile extracts soothes a variety of inflammatory skin conditions in animals.[7405]

    □  Inhalation of a combination of essential oils (anise, fennel, Roman chamomile, and peppermint) relieved the nausea of people suffering from nausea in a hospice or palliative care program.[7406]

    □  Clinical and *in vitro* studies found that Roman chamomile extracts and essential oils penetrate into the deeper skin layers where it reduces the production and activity of proinflammatory molecules (prostaglandins, and COX-2 enzyme, without affecting the COX-1 enzyme) to reduce inflammatory skin conditions.[7407,7408]

    □  Massage with Roman chamomile essential oil diluted in carrier oil reduced anxiety, improved mood/stress, and enhanced quality of life in people receiving palliative care.[7409] Participants in the study received three

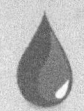

full-body massages over three consecutive weeks with either Roman chamomile/carrier oil or sweet almond carrier oil only. The Roman chamomile group experienced greater improvements than the carrier oil group.

☐ A laboratory and clinical study demonstrated that vaginal pessaries with cocoa butter, calendula extract and either geranium and palmarosa or lavender and Roman chamomile essential oils reduced symptoms of vaginal atrophy (muscle weakness/wasting) in breast cancer survivors.[7410]

☐ Roman chamomile (isobutyl angelate as the primary constituent), lime, and lavender essential oils effectively inhibited the parasite *Haemonchus contortus*, hindering adult worm motility completely within the first eight to twelve hours.[7411]

☐ A model of treatment-resistance depressive-like behavior found that inhalation of Roman chamomile essential oil improved the antidepressant effects of the tricyclic antidepressant clomipramine.[7412] The researchers observed that nerve growth factor (NGF)—a factor involved in neuron growth, maintenance, proliferation, and survival—was significantly decreased in the hippocampus of stressed mice exhibiting depressive-like behavior and that clomipramine did not correct this deficiency. The mice also had fewer doublecortin (DCX)-positive cells in the subgranular zone of the dentate gyrus, which suggests poor production of new neurons. Reduced neuron production in the dentate gyrus region of the hippocampus is also linked to depression. Roman chamomile significantly improved NGF levels. It also increased DCX-positive cells in the dentate gyrus when combined with clomipramine. The combination treatment also reduced corticosterone levels in the blood.

☐ A preclinical model of anxiety in zebrafish found that exposure to Roman chamomile reduces anxiety without interfering with typical behaviors, while tangerine essential oil had a minimal effect.[7413]

# ROSALINA
## (Lavender Tea Tree, Swamp Paperback)

*Melaleuca ericifolia* Smith

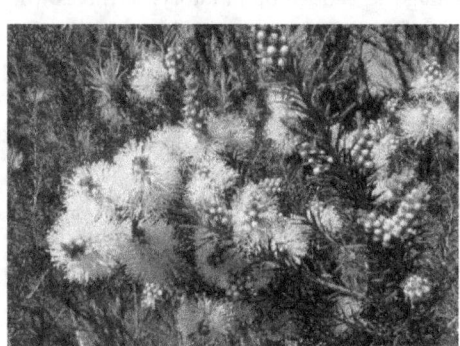

**FAMILY:** Myrtaceae
**NOTE:** Base-Middle
**AROMA INTENSITY:** Medium
**AROMA:** Herbaceous, spicy, earthy, slightly floral, slightly citrusy
**COMMON EXTRACTION METHOD:** Steam distilled from the leaves
**POSSIBLE SUBSTITUTE OILS:** Lavandin, spike lavender, tea tree
**BLENDS WELL WITH:** Balsam fir, bergamot, blue cypress, blue spruce, blue tansy, cajeput, citronella, cypress, Douglas fir, geranium, grapefruit, lavender, lavandin, lemon, lime, Manuka, niaouli, orange, palmarosa, palo santo, Siberian fir, silver fir, spike lavender, spruce (black), sweet inula, tangerine, tea tree, thyme, white fir
**SUBCELLULAR LOCALIZATION | EPIGENETIC INFLUENCE:** Currently unknown | Currently unknown
**RECOMMENDED DILUTION RANGE:** 5%–Neat

**PRIMARY CONSTITUENTS:**[7414]

| *Linalool CT (Northern)* | | *1,8-Cineole CT (Southern)* | |
|---|---|---|---|
| Linalool | 36.3%–56.2% | 1,8-Cineole | 43.6%–79.5% |
| 1,8-Cineole | 13.3%–29.4% | Alpha-Pinene | 0.0%–13.1% |
| Alpha-Pinene | 6.3%–13.1% | Alpha-Terpineol | 6.5%–8.0% |
| Para-Cymene | 0.0%–4.3% | Limonene | 0.0%–7.1% |
| Aromadendrene | 2.0%–4.1% | Alpha-Thujene | 0.0%–5.9% |
| Alpha-Terpineol | 0.0%–3.6% | Linalool | 0.0%–5.1% |
| Terpinen-4-ol | 0.0%–3.6% | | |
| Alpha-Terpinolene | 0.0%–3.6% | *Methyl Eugenol CT* | |
| Limonene | 0.0%–3.4% | Methyl Eugenol | 96.8% |
| Gamma-Terpinene | 0.0%–3.2% | | |

Note: The methyl eugenol and 1,8-cineole CTs were not found in commercial samples. All retailers that identified the constituents of their rosalina essential oil reported carrying the linalool CT (nine of nine). Rosalina oils from the northern part of Australia are the linalool CT, whereas oils from the southern part of Australia are the 1,8-cineole CT.

**OTHER CONSTITUENTS:** *Linalool CT*—linalool oxide, alpha-cubebene, beta-caryophyllene, allo-aromadendrene, viridiflorene, geranial, globulol, spathulenol; *1,8-Cineole CT*—gamma-terpinene, beta-pinene, para-cymene, aromadendrene, delta-cadinene, ledol, globulol, viridiflorol, alpha-eudesmol, beta-eudesmol; *Methyl Eugenol CT* (other components <0.5% each)—alpha-pinene, beta-pinene, estragol, gamma-elemene, eugenol, elemecin

**PREFERRED COMPOSITION FOR CLINICAL USE:**

| Constituent | Linalool CT | 1,8-Cineole CT |
|---|---|---|
| **Linalool** | 35%–50% | 0.1%–10% |
| **1,8-Cineole** | 15%–30% | 35%–75% |
| **Alpha-Pinene** | 5%–15% | 7%–25% |
| **Aromadendrene** | 1%–6% | – |
| **Alpha-Terpineol** | 1.5%–5% | 3%–12% |
| **Para-Cymene** | 1%–5% | 0.1%–5% |
| **Limonene** | 1%–5% | 2%–10% |
| **Gamma-Terpinene** | 0.5%–5% | 0.1%–5% |
| **Terpinen-4-ol** | 0.5%–5% | 0.1%–5% |

**REPORTED THERAPEUTIC PROPERTIES:** Antibacterial, antifungal, antiviral, anti-infectious, antimicrobial, antiallergic, analgesic, anti-inflammatory, **reduces the appearance of scars and blemishes**, cellular regeneration, anti-aging, disinfectant, **supports respiratory function (especially for children's respiratory complaints)**, expels excess mucous, decongestant, combats acne, **soothes chronic skin conditions**, relieves boils and blisters, aids immune function, removes warts, encourages restful sleep, relaxing/calming, stress management, antidepressant, relieves anxiety, boosts self-esteem, instills confidence

**CAUTIONS:**

*Linalool CT*

■ Avoid with epilepsy and Parkinson's disease due to 1,8-cineole content. May exacerbate or cause seizures or convulsions when inhaled, applied topically, or ingested based on 1,8-cineole content.[7415,7416,7417,7418,7419,7420]

■ There is a low risk that oral administration of rosalina may interfere with enzymes responsible for metabolizing medications (NSAIDs, proton-pump inhibitors, acetaminophen, antiepileptics, immune modulators, blood-sugar medications, blood pressure medications, antidepressants, antipsychotics, diabetic medications, antihistamines, antibiotics, and anesthetics) due to 1,8-cineole content.[7421,7422]

■ There is a low risk that rosalina May interfere with pentobarbital and other barbiturates (medications for anxiety and insomnia) based on 1,8-cineole content.[7423,7424]

*1,8-Cineole CT*

■ Avoid with children under age three, particularly around the nose and mouth. Use very cautiously in children under age five due to high 1,8-cineole content. 1,8-cineole may cause seizures, central nervous system problems, or respiratory distress in young children.[7425,7426,7427,7428]

■ Avoid with epilepsy and Parkinson's disease due to 1,8-cineole content. May exacerbate or cause seizures/convulsions or reduce seizure medication efficacy based on 1,8-cineole content.[7429,7430,7431]

■ Caution is warranted orally due to the significant amounts of 1,8-cineole. Limit it to small doses internally (adults—maximum 10 drops daily). One text recommends a maximum daily dose of 6 drops, whereas the European Medicines Agency recommends 2 to 4 drops (100–200 mg) of high 1,8-cineole essential oils orally, 2 to 5 times daily for adolescents, adults, and the elderly.[7432,7433] Additionally, 200 mg of isolated 1,8-cineole has been ingested three times daily for up to six months in clinical research.[7434,7435] Toxicity has been reported when eucalyptus (also high in 1,8-cineole) was ingested in large doses, and as few as 4 to 5 drops may cause problems in very sensitive individuals.[7436,7437,7438,7439,7440,7441] In humans, 3.5 to 5 mL has proven fatal orally.[7442]

■ May interact with diabetic medications due to the ability of 1,8-cineole to inhibit alpha-glucosidase activity, particularly when synergized with other constituents (alpha-pinene).[7443,7444,7445] Alpha-glucosidase is an enzyme that

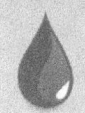

breaks down carbohydrates by chemical reaction with water. Inhibiting its activity postpones glucose absorption and therefore the impact of carbohydrates on blood sugar levels.

■ May weakly interfere with the enzymes responsible for metabolizing medications (NSAIDs, proton-pump inhibitors, acetaminophen, antiepileptics, immune modulators, blood-sugar medications, blood pressure medications, antidepressants, antipsychotics, diabetic medications, antihistamines, antibiotics, and anesthetics) based on 1,8-cineole content.[7446,7447]

■ May interact with aspirin, blood pressure, antiplatelet, and anticoagulant medications, and increase the risk of bleeding among people with bleeding disorders (low risk).[7448] 1,8-cineole is a weak inhibitor of platelet aggregation.[7449]

■ May interfere with pentobarbital and other barbiturates (medications for anxiety and insomnia) based on 1,8-cineole content.[7450,7451]

### Methyl Eugenol CT

***The methyl eugenol CT of rosalina is very rare, not found in commercial samples, and not recommended for essential oil therapy.***

■ Avoid in children under age 12 due to the multisite cancerous tumors and DNA mutation caused by methyl eugenol in animal studies.[7452,7453,7454,7455]

■ Avoid during pregnancy and lactation due to changes in embryo form and structure and chromosomal changes in ovary cells caused by methyl eugenol as well as the carcinogenic (cancer-causing) potential of methyl eugenol.[7456,7457,7458,7459]

■ Avoid oral consumption due to the multisite carcinogenic potential of methyl eugenol.[7460,7461,7462,7463]

■ May interfere with antibiotics and antifungal medications and increase their effectiveness due to methyl eugenol content.[7464]

■ May interact with anticholinergic (drugs used for asthma, incontinence, gastrointestinal cramps, muscular spasms, depression, and sleep disorders) and cholinergic medications (drugs used to reduce urinary retention, diagnose myasthenia gravis, and for glaucoma) based on the potent AChE inhibitory activity of methyl eugenol.[7465]

### SELECTED EVIDENCE:

☐ *In vitro* evidence suggests that rosalina (methyl eugenol CT) is antiviral and inhibits the HSV-1 virus 91.5%.[3105] The same research reported that rosalina is a potent inhibitor of the gram-positive bacterium *B. subtiles* and the fungus *A. niger*.[7466]

## ROSE OTTO
### (Rose, Damask Rose)

*Rosa × damascena* Mill. (pro sp.) [gallica × moschata]

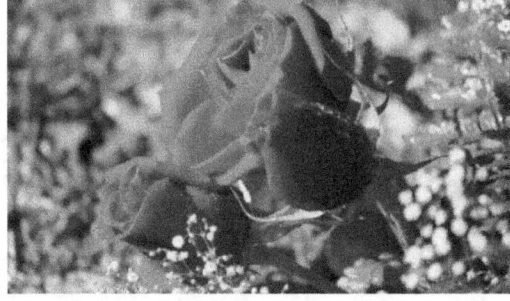

**FAMILY:** Anacardiaceae
**NOTE:** Middle
**AROMA INTENSITY:** Strong
**AROMA:** Strong floral, sweet
**COMMON EXTRACTION METHOD:** Steam distilled from the flowers
**POSSIBLE SUBSTITUTE OILS:** Geranium, citronella
**BLENDS WELL WITH:** Bay laurel, bergamot, black pepper, cardamom, cedarwood, chamomile (German, Roman), citronella, clary sage, copaiba, eucalyptus, geranium, helichrysum, jasmine, lavender, lemongrass, melissa, neroli, palo santo, patchouli, pine, sandalwood, spikenard, vetiver, ylang ylang
**SUBCELLULAR LOCALIZATION | EPIGENETIC INFLUENCE:** Currently unknown | Currently unknown
**RECOMMENDED DILUTION RANGE:** 3%–50%; neat for limited conditions

**PRIMARY CONSTITUENTS:**[7467,7468,7469,7470,7471,7472,7473,7474]

| Bulgarian | | Turkish | |
|---|---|---|---|
| Citronellol + Nerol | 21.6%–31.9% | Citronellol | 24.5%–43.0% |
| Geraniol | 4.8%–25.3% | Geraniol | 2.1%–18.0% |

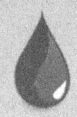

| | | | |
|---|---|---|---|
| Nonadecane | 8.1%–19.2% | Nonadecane | 8.2%–18.9% |
| Heneicosane | 1.1%–8.6% | Ethanol | 0.0%–13.4% |
| Heptadecane | 2.7%–5.1% | Heneicosane | 2.9%–8.9% |
| 2-Phenylethanol | 0.2%–1.2% | Nerol | 0.8%–7.6% |
| Ethanol | 0.0%–0.9% | 2-Phenylethanol | 0.5%–1.2% |
| | | Heptadecane | 0.2%–0.5% |

*Iranian\**

| | | | |
|---|---|---|---|
| Citronellol | 12.6%–53.4% | *Indian#* | |
| Nonadecane | 0.0%–51.2% | Citronellol + Nerol | 2.2%–44.9% |
| Neral | 0.0%–44.8% | Geraniol | 2.5%–26.5% |
| Dihydrolinalool | 0.0%–39.2% | Nonadecane | 7.3%–24.7% |
| Geraniol | 0.0%–22.7% | Heneicosane | 0.0%–19.7% |
| Eicosane | 0.7%–20.5% | Tricosane | 0.0%–11.3% |
| Docosane | 0.0%–19.5% | 2-Phenylethanol | 0.4%–9.6%# |
| Heneicosane | 0.0%–18.0% | Heptadecane | 0.5%–6.0% |
| Disiloxane | 0.0%–17.6% | Farnesol | 0.3%–5.4% |
| Citronellyl Formate | 0.0%–14.6% | Eicosane | 0.1%–5.0% |
| Geranial | 0.0%–12.3% | Geranyl Acetate | 0.1%–4.1% |
| Linalyl Formate | 0.0%–11.9% | Eugenol | 0.0%–3.3% |
| Hexadecanol | 0.0%–7.8% | Alpha-Terpineol | 0.1%–2.7% |
| Octadecane | 0.0%–6.1% | | |
| Undecanol | 0.0%–5.5% | | |
| Occidentalol Acetate | 0.0%–4.0% | | |

\* Iranian rose oil has five distinct chemotypes: Citronellol—40.3%–42.2% (nonadecane 15.9%–26.3%, geranial 0.0%–12.3%); Dihydrolinalool—30.8%–39.2% (nonadecane 10.7%–26.5%, linalyl formate 0.0%–11.9%); Geraniol—37.5% (citronellyl formate 14.6%, nonadecane 13.9%); Neral—31.7%–44.8% (nonadecane 20.0%–20.5%, citronellyl formate 7.5%–7.8%); and Nonadecane—22.4%–51.2% (heneicosane 18.0%, eicosane 6.2%).[7475]

# Indian rose oil should not contain more than 7% 2-phenylethyl alcohol according to the Bureau of Indian standard for rose essential oil. Essential oils reporting more than this are generally fraudulent and adulterated with synthetic 2-phenylethyl alcohol.

**OTHER CONSTITUENTS:** *Bulgarian*—Gamma-muurolene, methyl eugenol (up to 3.3%), linalool, citronellyl acetate, farnesol, beta-caryophyllene, eugenol, geranyl acetate, alpha-guaiene, alpha-caryophyllene, octadecane; *Indian*—Para-cymene, alpha-pinene, linalool, octadecane, 1-docosene, tetracosane, pentacosane, methyl eugenol (less than 1.2%), beta-bourbonene, beta-elemene, beta-caryophyllene, alpha-humulene, alpha-cadinene; *Iranian*—Nerol, kaempferol, methyl eugenol (up to 2.6%), cis-farnesol, heptadecane, pentacosane; *Turkish*—Alpha-pinene, gamma-muurolene, myrcene, methyl eugenol (up to 2.5%), cis-rose oxide, pentadecane, alpha-guaiene, linalool, citronellyl acetate, alpha-humulene, neral, delta-guaiene, heptadecene, geranyl acetate, beta-caryophyllene, eugenol, alpha-guaiene, heptadecane, alpha-caryophyllene, octadecane, tricosane, eicosane, 2-phenylethyl acetate

**PREFERRED COMPOSITION FOR CLINICAL USE:**

| Constituent | Bulgarian | Turkish | Moroccan | Indian | Iranian |
|---|---|---|---|---|---|
| **Citronellol** | 20%–32% | 30%–45% | 28%–45% | 22%–32% | 23%–35% |
| **Geraniol** | 12%–23% | 8%–24% | 8%–22% | 22%–32% | 6%–18% |
| **Nonadecane** | 8%–17% | 7%–15% | 7%–15% | 8%–18% | 22%–40% |
| **Nerol** | 5%–14% | 3%–11% | 3%–11% | 10%–14% | – |
| **Heneicosane** | 3%–8% | 3%–6% | 2%–6% | 0%–10% | 0%–10% |
| **Heptadecane** | 1%–4% | 0.5%–2% | 0.5%–5% | 0.5%–4% | 1%–3% |
| **2-Phenylethanol** | ≤ 4% | ≤ 3% | ≤ 3% | ≤ 3% | ≤ 5% |
| **Ethanol** | < 2% | < 7% | < 3% | < 7% | < 7% |

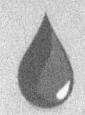

**REPORTED THERAPEUTIC PROPERTIES:** Anti-inflammatory, **antiseptic**, antispasmodic, astringent, antiviral, reduces fever, antibacterial, anticonvulsive, **balances heart function**, reduces the appearance of blemishes, stretch marks, and scars, **nourishes and moistens skin**, **balances female hormones and helps regulate menstruation**, supports liver function, eases cough, relieves constipation, **nervine (calms and soothes the nerves)**, purifies the blood, encourages restful sleep, **stress management**, **antidepressant**, **aphrodisiac**, combats anger, relieves deep despair and grief, encourages feelings of love, **releases traumatic memories**, reduces loneliness

**CAUTIONS:**
- Use cautiously with diabetic medications (low risk). Large oral doses of citronellol and geraniol may lower blood-glucose levels.[7476,7477]
- May interact with antibiotics and possibly enhance their effects due to citronellol and geraniol content.[7478,7479]
- Dilution recommended for topical application of rose oil with high levels of geraniol. Geraniol is metabolized via the CYP450 pathway into metabolites such as geranial and neral and may cause sensitization and irritation when applied topically.[7480]

**SELECTED EVIDENCE:**
- A sitz bath with (or soap application) of lavender, myrrh, neroli, rose, grapefruit, mandarin, orange, and Roman chamomile improves healing of the perineum following delivery and episiotomy.[7481]
- A daily abdominal massage with a combination of rose, cinnamon, clove, and lavender oils in an almond carrier oil for seven days prior to menstruation significantly reduced painful menstruation and excess menstrual bleeding in women suffering from painful menstruation.[7482] A second study found that painful menstrual cramps were relieved in women by massaging the abdomen with two drops of lavender, and one drop each of rose and clary sage in 5 mL of almond oil.[7483]
- Massaging the hands with lavender and rose oil (2% dilution) for fifteen minutes twice weekly for four consecutive weeks reduced depression and anxiety in postpartum women.[7484]
- Citronellol, a primary constituent in rose oil, relieves oral and facial pain by modulating central nervous system activity in mice.[7485]
- Animal research suggests that citronellol, a primary constituent in rose oil, lowers blood pressure by increasing, (relaxation of the muscular wall and widening of the blood vessels).[7486]
- Rose oil helps decrease inflammation by mildly inhibiting the 5-lipoxygenase (5-LOX) enzyme that is involved in the inflammation response according to *in vitro* research.[7487]
- Animal research suggests that rose oil prevents intestinal spasms.[7488]
- Rose oil relieves pain by activating the TRPV1 receptor (a molecular sensor that detects painful sensations, and when activated triggers pathways that reduce pain caused by heat and inflammation) *in vitro*.[7489]
- Animal research suggests that injection of rose oil influences neurotransmitter production pathways and reduces morphine withdrawal symptoms.[7490]
- Rose oil reduces the number and severity of seizures caused by PTZ in rats.[7491,7492]
- Oral administration of rose oil (5 mg/kg three times daily; 10% rose essential oil solution in vegetable oil) significantly reduced the frequency of seizures in children (aged 3 to 13 years old) that were not controlled by standard drug options.[7493]
- Animal research concluded that rose oil significantly relaxes the smooth muscle of the trachea, with comparable effectiveness to the drug theophylline.[7494]
- Rose oil possesses strong antimicrobial activity against *E. coli, P. aeruginosa, B. subtilis, S. aureus, C. violaceum*, and *E. carotovora in vitro*.[7495]
- Inhalation of rose oil significantly reduced the pain associated with kidney stones in emergency room patients when combined with conventional medications.[7496]
- Inhalation of rose oil reverses disruption in the function of the skin barrier (protection against harmful organisms, encouraging hydration, and gatekeeper for nutrient absorption) caused by chronic stress in rats and humans.[7497]
- Animal research suggests that inhalation of rose oil reduces anxiety and conflict in mice and rats.[7498,7499,7500]
- Rose essential oil protected hypothalamic neurons against toxicity caused by aluminum.[7501] Another study

found that the combination of rose and lavender essential oils with vitamin C, and water-soluble vitamin E (Trolox) used during levodopa (L-dopa is a chemical naturally produced in the body by biosynthesis of the amino acid L-tyrosine, but it is also used as a drug treatment for Parkinson's disease) therapy reduces neuron toxicity caused by L-dopa.[7502] *In vitro* studies suggest that L-dopa may be toxic to dopaminergic neurons and prolonged use can cause motor complications and limitations. The study authors concluded that the essential oils and vitamins act as antioxidants to reduce the production of reactive oxygen species (ROS) and reactive nitrogen species (RNS), therefore limiting neuron toxicity.

☐ Rose essential oil was toxic to the adult spotted wing drosophila (*Drosophila suzukii*) when in direct contact with the drosophila.[7503]

☐ Inhalation of a 2% dilution of rose essential oil reduced painful menstruation when combined with diclofenac sodium better than diclofenac sodium alone.[7504]

☐ Inhalation of rose or geranium essential oil increased salivary estrogen levels in premenopausal women.[7505] Salivary estrogen levels loosely approximate serum estrogen levels,[7506] suggesting that simply inhaling rose or geranium essential oil could influence estrogen levels in women and promote hormone balance.

☐ Topical application of rose essential oil (7 drops of diluted rose oil—unspecified dilution ratio in sweet almond oil, twice daily for four weeks) to the lower back reduced pregnancy-related lower back pain.[7507]

☐ Oral administration of rose essential oil (50, 100, 200, and 400 mcg/kg body weight daily, for twenty-eight days) protected against testicular damage in diabetic rats without affecting testosterone levels, body weight, or blood glucose levels.[7508] The rats treated with rose essential oil—especially at the two higher doses—had higher sperm counts and healthier seminiferous tubules.

☐ A triple blind randomized clinical trial concluded that rose essential oil improved premenstrual syndrome symptoms (psychological, physical, social, and total). Women inhaled 10 drops of a 4% concentration of rose essential oil for five minutes (placed on a pad and held 30 cm from their nose), twice daily during the luteal phase (total of five days).[7509]

☐ Many children experience sleep disorders, interrupted sleep, or nightmares. Side effects associated with sleep aids make it difficult for parents to improve the sleep quality of their children. A clinical study found that inhaling rose essential oil (5 drops of a 10% dilution on a cotton ball for twenty minutes after going to bed) improved sleep quality in children aged five to twelve diagnosed with sleep disorders.[7510] The rose oil significantly reduced resistance going to sleep, difficulty waking in the morning, nightmares, and waking during the night.

☐ Topical application of 2 mL of a macerated rose essential oil to the forehead and temporal zones at the onset of migraine reduced pain in people experiencing a "hot" type (eye redness, aggravation by light or heat, pulsing or throbbing, find certain odors disagreeable, and a hot sensation in the face during headache attacks) migraine.[7511]

☐ A randomized clinical trial of 110 nulliparous (women who has never given birth) women found that inhaling 0.08 mL of rose essential oil every thirty minutes reduced severity of pain and anxiety at each level of cervical dilation (4–5, 6–7, and 8–10 cm; and 4–7 and 8–10 cm).[7512]

☐ L-dopa is one of the most common treatment options for people with Parkinson's disease, but it is limited by frequent side effects and toxicity. Intraperitoneal administration of (400mg/kg BW) of rose essential oil reduced L-dopa toxicity due to its antioxidant activity.[7513]

☐ Methadone maintenance therapy (MMT) is frequently used as a treatment for heroin and narcotic (like opioids) addiction. However, the therapy is not without side effects. One such side effect in men is sexual dysfunction, including erectile dysfunction. A double-blind, placebo-controlled clinical trial found that oral administration of a 2 mL rose essential oil oral drops (containing 17 mg of citronellol; roughly just about one drop of rose oil in the solution) in water daily reduced sexual dysfunction in men on MMT.[7514] The scientists observed improvements in sexual drive, erectile function, sexual satisfaction, and testosterone levels. Another study evaluated the effects of the same dose of rose oil in male sexual function in men with depression and taking a selective serotonin-reuptake inhibitor (SSRI). One of the side effects of SSRI medications is sexual dysfunction. The double-blind, randomized, and placebo-controlled clinical trial showed that the administration of rose oil solution reduces sexual dysfunction in men taking an SSRI. In addition, improvements in depressive symptoms were observed as sexual function improved. Interestingly, the same researchers reported that the rose oil solution also mildly improves sexual function (sexual desire, orgasms, and sexual satisfaction) in women taking SSRIs in another study.[7515]

☐ Sepsis is a potentially life-threatening condition that occurs when the body releases excess chemicals in response to an infection, which can damage multiple organ systems. Oral administration of deuterium-depleted water with rose essential oil (100 mg/kg body weight plus 15 to 30 PPM deuterium-depleted water)

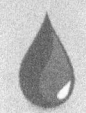

for two weeks reduced sepsis by regulating oxidative stress.[7516] The natural solution reduced lipid peroxidation and inflammation, increased antioxidant activity, and healed liver tissue injuries caused by sepsis. Further research by the same authors concluded that rose essential oil alone (50 and 100 mg/kg BW) reduces oxidative injury caused by sepsis by reducing inflammation, increasing antioxidant activity, and protecting the liver.[7517]

☐ Patients in a cardiac unit frequently experience disrupted sleep and anxiety. A randomized controlled clinical trial evaluated the effects of rose essential oil on sleep quality and anxiety in people in a cardiac unit. Five drops of a 40% (diluted in distilled water) rose essential oil was added to an absorbent cloth napkin and attached to the collar of the participant's shirt approximately 20 cm from the nose. The rose napkin was left on for eight hours. The intervention significantly reduced anxiety and improved sleep quality.[7518]

☐ A comparison of multiple Iranian rose essential oil samples found that samples higher in alkenes/alkanes (29.7% nonadecene, 16.9% heneicosane, 16.3% citronellol, 7.1% 1-nonadecene, 4.7% eicosane) inhibited bacteria with efficacy similar to that of rifampin (an antibiotic used to treat several types of bacterial infections), and inhibited *C. albicans* four times better than nystatin (an antifungal medication to treat *Candida* infections).[7519]

☐ An Iranian rose essential oil with 24.7% nonadecane, 19.3% heneicosane, 17.6% oleic acid, and 12.6% citronellol inhibited *S. aureus, S. pyogenes, K. pneumoniae,* and *A. basiliensis.*[7520]

☐ Rose essential oil reduced herpes simplex virus type 1 (HSV-1) viral adsorption (attachment of the virus to a susceptible cell) and extracellular virons and protected healthy cells from subsequent infection in a laboratory study, but failed to prevent HSV-1 replication.[7521] The oil also synergized low doses of acyclovir, increasing its ability to inhibit viral replication.

☐ Having an infant in the neonatal intensive care unit (NICU) can cause significant stress and anxiety in mothers and fathers. A placebo-controlled clinical study evaluated the effects of inhaling rose essential oil in mothers of premature infants in the NICU.[7522] Mothers inhaled rose essential oil (diluted to 10%) for five to ten minutes over ten consecutive nights. Anxiety significant reduced in the rose group when compared to the control (standard care only) suggesting that inhaling rose essential oil is an effective and noninvasive way to decrease stress/anxiety in mothers with children in the NICU.

☐ Nurses are the cornerstone of healthcare because they are on the frontlines of patient care. Operating room nurses are frequently exposed to high-stress situations that can increase stress and anxiety and potentially reduce job accuracy. A clinical study investigated the effects of inhaling rose essential oil on job stress/anxiety and accuracy among operating room nurses.[7523] Two drops of rose essential oil (40% dilution) were added to cotton and the nurses placed the cotton on their upper lip and inhaled for ten minutes. The placebo group inhaled normal saline from cotton. Mean anxiety and stress scores significantly decreased and job accuracy significantly increased after inhaling the rose oil, when compared to the placebo group. The results suggest that inhalation of rose essential oil could significantly improve nurse job satisfaction and performance. Another randomized, controlled, nonblinded, parallel-group clinical study evaluated the effects of inhaling rose essential oil among operating room nurses during the COVID-19 pandemic.[7524] Five drops of either rose essential oil or paraffin (placebo group) were placed on an absorbent cloth and pinned to the side of their pillow before a night's sleep for thirty consecutive nights. The rose oil group experienced significant improvements in anxiety state and sleep quality.

☐ Rose essential oil relaxed contracted rat thoracic aorta with or without endothelium through the NO-cGMP-dependent pathway, showing that rose oil has a vasorelaxant effect.[7525] Additional research from the same author reported that geraniol and citronellol participate in the vasodilatory effects of rose essential oil.[7526]

☐ Nursing involves high levels of stress, which can cause a cascade of events that increase oxidative stress, inflammation, and the risk of several adverse health conditions (diabetes, high cholesterol, hypertension, premature aging, and cardiovascular events). A study evaluated the benefits of an aromatic massage with rose essential oil among nurses after finishing a night shift at the hospital.[7527] Forty-two nurses were randomly assigned to receive an aromatic rose massage (rose essential oil diluted to 1% in grapeseed oil) or the control group that received a massage with grapeseed only. The neck and shoulder massage lasted fifteen minutes in each group. Sleep and anxiety surveys were completed, modified visual analog scale evaluated, and saliva collected and analyzed for chromogranin A (a marker for psychological stress) and biological antioxidant potential levels. Biological antioxidant potentials, sleep quality, and anxiety all improved after receiving the rose massage when compared to massage with grapeseed only.

☐ Preclinical research demonstrated that rose essential oil relaxes contracted rat trachea, which shows that the oil triggers bronchodilation and may be useful for asthma, emphysema, and COPD.[7528]

☐ Coronary angiography is a diagnostic procedure that helps diagnose cardiovascular disease by injecting dye into your arteries through a catheter while evaluating how blood flows through your heart via X-ray. Since the procedure is done while you are awake, anxiety and stress during the procedure are common and a sedative is often given. A randomized clinical trial evaluated whether inhalation of rose essential oil can reduce stress, anxiety, and how blood flows through blood vessels.[7529] Subjects in the intervention group inhaled 5 drops of a 40% dilution of rose essential oil for 20 minutes, while the control group inhaled distilled water. Significant changes in anxiety, stress, and hemodynamics (heart rate, mean arterial pressure, blood pressure, and blood oxygen saturation) were observed in the rose group when compared to controls.

☐ A double-blind randomized clinical trial compared the effects of lavender and rose essential oil inhalation on anxiety and pain severity after C-section. Ninety women were randomized to one of three groups: 1) control, 2) lavender inhalation, and 3) rose inhalation following C-section. Three drops of the respective oils were added to a cotton ball and then inhaled from for thirty minutes followed by assessment of pain and anxiety five minutes after intervention. Pain severity significantly declined in both the lavender and rose groups, with rose being the most effective, while overall anxiety slightly improved compared to control.

☐ Women have higher rates of high blood pressure (hypertension) rates than men as they age, suggesting hormones may have a prominent role in hypertension. Hypertension is a silent killer and can cause damage to the arteries, heart, brain, kidneys, and eyes for years before being detected. It is also associated with higher heart attack, stroke, and sexual dysfunction risk. Inhalation of rose essential oil decreased blood pressure in menopausal women.[7530,]

☐ A randomized controlled clinical trial found that inhaling rose essential oil—10 mL of a 2% dilution added to a paper handkerchief for fifteen minutes—reduced menstrual pain and the need for oral analgesics (diclofenac) in women with primary dysmenorrhea.[7531]

---

# ROSEMARY

*Salvia rosmarinus* Spenn., *Rosmarinus officinalis* L.,
*R. officinalis* L. var. *prostratus* hort.

**FAMILY:** Lamiaceae (Labiatae)
**NOTE:** Top-Middle
**AROMA INTENSITY:** Strong
**AROMA:** Strongly herbaceous, slightly woody and balsamic, medicinal
**COMMON EXTRACTION METHOD:** Steam distilled from the flowers and leaves
**POSSIBLE SUBSTITUTE OILS:** Sage (1,8-cineole CT), spike lavender, lavandin, myrtle, niaouli (viridiflorol CT), Spanish sage, spike lavender, spruce (black), blue spruce, sage (camphor CT), Spanish sage, balsam fir, silver fir
**BLENDS WELL WITH:** Bay laurel, basil, bergamot, black pepper, blue cypress, cajeput, camphor, cassia, cedarwood, cinnamon, citronella, clary sage, clove, coriander, eucalyptus, frankincense, geranium, grapefruit, lavender, lemon, lime, marjoram, tea tree, orange, oregano, palmarosa, patchouli, peppermint, pine, petitgrain, ravensara, ravintsara, sage, tangerine, thyme, vetiver
**SUBCELLULAR LOCALIZATION | EPIGENETIC INFLUENCE:** Endocytic Vesicles | Skeletal/Integumentary
**RECOMMENDED DILUTION RANGE:** 3%–20%; neat for limited conditions

**PRIMARY CONSTITUENTS:**[7532,7533,7534,7535,7536,7537,7538,7539,7540,7541,7542,7543,7544,7545]

| *1,8-Cineole CT* | | *Beta-Myrcene CT* | |
|---|---|---|---|
| 1,8-Cineole | 41.6%–52.4% | Beta-Myrcene | 17.9%–30.0% |
| Camphor | 7.9%–18.9% | Alpha-Pinene | 8.8%–16.5% |
| Alpha-Pinene | 5.2%–15.8% | 1,8-Cineole | 8.0%–14.5% |
| Camphene | 3.0%–11.1% | Limonene | 2.9%–10.6% |
| Beta-Pinene | 4.8%–7.5% | Camphor | 2.1%–9.0% |
| Alpha-Terpineol | 0.0%–4.9% | Caryophyllene | 0.0%–8.3% |
| Borneol | 2.6%–4.8% | Camphene | 1.3%–5.1% |
| Caryophyllene | 0.1%–4.2% | | |

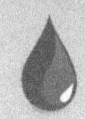

*Alpha-Pinene CT*

| | |
|---|---|
| Alpha-Pinene | 14.1%–62.2% |
| 1,8-Cineole | 5.3%–26.5% |
| Camphor | 2.4%–18.9% |
| Verbenone | 2.3%–15.3% |
| Bornyl Acetate | 0.0%–14.3% |
| Borneol | 3.4%–13.7% |
| Beta-Pinene | 1.1%–12.0% |
| Camphene | 5.5%–11.5% |
| Alpha-Phellandrene | 0.1%–7.9% |
| Myrcene | 0.6%–4.9% |
| Sabinene | 0.0%–4.6% |

*Borneol CT*

| | |
|---|---|
| 1,8-Cineole | 20.0% |
| Borneol | 15.6% |
| Camphor | 15.3% |
| Verbenone | 8.4% |
| Alpha-Pinene | 8.3% |
| Bornyl Acetate | 5.0% |

*Bornyl Acetate CT*

| | |
|---|---|
| Alpha-Pinene | 7.7%–35.8% |
| Bornyl Acetate | 14.3%–20.3% |
| Verbenone | 0.0%–20.3% |
| Caryophyllene | 0.0%–13.6% |
| 1,8-Cineole | 5.3%–12.8% |
| Camphor | 6.4%–10.4% |
| Borneol | 3.6%–8.4% |
| Camphene | 4.2%–7.0% |
| Verbenone | 0.0%–5.7% |
| Limonene | 0.1%–4.6% |

*Camphor CT*

| | |
|---|---|
| Camphor | 14.9%–35.8% |
| 1,8-Cineole | 9.0%–31.6% |
| Alpha-Pinene | 6.7%–24.7% |
| Borneol | 0.0%–11.6% |
| Camphene | 5.2%–11.2% |
| Sabinene | 0.0%–5.1% |
| Myrcene | 2.3%–4.9% |
| Para-Cymene | 0.0%–3.8% |
| Beta-Pinene | 2.5%–3.4% |
| Limonene | 2.8%–3.1% |
| Linalool | 0.0%–3.1% |
| Borneol | 2.9%–3.0% |

*Verbenone CT*

| | |
|---|---|
| Verbenone | 7.6%–24.9% |
| Bornyl Acetate | 2.0%–17.0% |
| Camphor | 2.9%–14.9% |
| Alpha-Pinene | 2.5%–14.7% |
| 1,8-Cineole | 3.4%–9.0% |
| Borneol | 0.3%–7.3% |
| Limonene | 0.0%–7.1% |
| Linalool | 1.0%–6.6% |
| Para-Cymene | 1.1%–6.3% |
| Myrcene | 0.5%–5.4% |
| Alpha-Terpineol | 2.4%–4.9% |

**OTHER CONSTITUENTS:** Linalool, alpha-terpineol, para-cymene, ar-curcumene, 1-nonalol, terpinen-4-ol, limonene, 1-octen-3-ol, alpha-phellandrene, sabinene, (E)-pinocarveol, (E)-myrtanol, carvone, (Z)-myrtanol

**PREFERRED COMPOSITION FOR CLINICAL USE:**

| Constituent | 1,8-Cineole CT (CT2) | Balanced CT (CT1) | Verbenone CT (CT3) |
|---|---|---|---|
| **1,8-Cineole** | 40%–55% | 15%–25% | 5%–11% |
| **Camphor** | 8%–18% | 14%–25% | 3%–16% |
| **Alpha-Pinene** | 7%–16% | 15%–27% | 15%–40% |
| **Camphene** | 3%–10% | 6%–13% | 4%–11% |
| **Beta-Pinene** | 3%–9% | 1.5%–6% | 0.5%–4% |
| **Borneol** | 2%–5% | 1%–4% | 2%–8% |
| **Limonene** | 1%–5% | 3%–6% | 3%–7% |
| **Beta-Caryophyllene** | 0.5%–5% | 1%–5% | 0.5%–3% |
| **Alpha-Terpineol** | 0.5%–3% | 1%–3% | 0.5%–3% |
| **Para-Cymene** | 0.5%–3% | 0.5%–2% | 0.5%–3% |
| **Myrcene** | 0.5%–2% | 2%–6% | 0.5%–3% |
| **Bornyl Acetate** | 0.1%–2% | 0.5%–2% | 6%–13% |
| **Verbenone** | – | – | 3%–15% |
| **Isopinocamphone** | – | – | ≤1.7% |

**REPORTED THERAPEUTIC PROPERTIES:** Analgesic, antiarthritic, **antibacterial**, antioxidant, antirheumatic, **antispasmodic**, antineuralgic, aphrodisiac, **antiseptic**, astringent, anticancer, expels excess gas, decongestant, stops excess bleeding, strengthens and nourishes hair, **stimulates hair growth**, oral cleanliness, **relieves painful menstruation**, stimulates and strengthens cardiovascular function, **aids digestion**, diuretic, helps normalize bone remodeling, expectorant, antifungal, **helps reduce the appearance of blemishes**, supports liver function, nervine (calms and soothes the nerves), regenerative, **relieves headache (migraine)**, increases redness and circulation to a localized area, stimulates gallbladder function and the release of bile, **relieves skin conditions**, wound healing, immune support, increases sweating, insect repellent, **aids memory**, **boosts mental activity**, mentally stimulating, stress management, reduces fatigue and burnout, energizing, promotes confidence, antidepressant, reduces confusion

## CAUTIONS:

■ Avoid with children under age 3, particularly around the nose and mouth (1,8-cineole CT and camphor CT). Use very cautiously in children under age 5 due to high 1,8-cineole and camphor content. 1,8-cineole may cause seizures, central nervous system problems, or respiratory distress in young children.[7546,7547,7548,7549] Several cases of camphor poisoning and/or seizures from ingestion and topical application have been reported in children.[7550,7551] Ingestion of camphor-containing products has been lethal in children under age 2 (estimated to be roughly 2,000 mg of camphor for a 20 kg child as the minimum potential fatal dose).[7552,7553] Children 5 years and up may use camphor-containing essential oils topically in dilutions no stronger than 5%.

■ Caution is warranted during pregnancy and while lactating due to potentially high camphor content (1,8-cineole CT and camphor CT). Ingestion of essential oils with significant levels of camphor may lead to abortion because fetuses lack the enzymes to process it.[7554] Camphor ingestion by infants and young children may cause cough, vomiting, seizure, burning sensation in the mucous membranes and eyes, or lack of voluntary coordination of muscle movements.[7555]

■ Caution is warranted orally due to the significant amounts of 1,8-cineole and camphor present in some CTs. Limit it to small doses internally (adults—maximum 10 drops daily). Toxicity has been reported when eucalyptus (also high in 1,8-cineole) was ingested in large doses, and as few as 4 to 5 drops may cause problems in very sensitive individuals.[7556,7557,7558,7559,7560,7561] In humans, 3.5 to 5 mL has proven fatal orally.[7562] Doses between 0.1 and 1.0 mL (3 to 30 drops) have been used in studies.[1959] Essential oils that contain significant amounts of camphor can be toxic when taken orally (usually single doses exceeding 2 mL), although the lethal dose for adult humans is estimated to be more than 5 mL in a single dose.[7563,7564,7565]

■ Avoid with epilepsy and Parkinson's disease due to 1,8-cineole and camphor content. May exacerbate or cause seizures or convulsions when inhaled, applied topically, or ingested based on 1,8-cineole content.[7566,7567,7568,7569,7570,7571]

■ The potentially high camphor content in various rosemary CTs may negatively impact red blood cells and increase the risk of jaundice in children with Glucose-6-phosphate dehydrogenase deficiency (G6PD).[7572,7573]

■ May interfere with enzymes that metabolize medications (NSAIDs, proton-pump inhibitors, acetaminophen, antiepileptics, immune modulators, blood-sugar medications, blood pressure medications, antidepressants, antipsychotics, diabetic medications, antihistamines, antibiotics, and anesthetics).[7574,7575,7576,7577]

■ May interfere with pentobarbital and other barbiturates (medications for anxiety and insomnia) based on 1,8-cineole or beta-myrcene content.[7578,7579,7580]

■ May interact with diabetic medications (1,8-cineole CT) due to the ability of 1,8-cineole to significantly inhibit alpha-glucosidase activity when synergized by other components (alpha-pinene and beta-pinene).[7581,7582,7583] Alpha-glucosidase is an enzyme that breaks down carbohydrates by chemical reaction with water. Inhibiting its activity postpones glucose absorption and therefore the impact of carbohydrates on blood sugar levels.

■ May interact with antibiotics and decrease their effectiveness by competing for primary target sites on cells.[7584]

■ Very large oral doses (1.54 mL) may interact with the pain-relievers codeine and paracetamol and increase their analgesic effects.[7585]

■ Avoid with those who have a compromised liver due to the risk of increased liver enzymes and liver damage (camphor CT).[7586] This would also suggest that those taking medications that could cause liver damage should also use rosemary very cautiously or avoid it entirely.

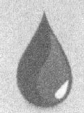

**SELECTED EVIDENCE:**

- Rosemary oil killed two ovarian cancer cell lines and one liver cancer cell line *in vitro*.[7587] A preclinical perspective review suggested that rosemary is a good candidate for clinical cancer studies because of its ability to suppress tumor development in several organs/tissues including the colon, breast, liver, stomach, and melanoma and leukemia cells.[7588]

- *In vitro* research concluded that rosemary prevents the spread of breast and androgen-sensitive prostate cancer cells.[7589] Another *in vitro* study concluded that rosemary oil protects DNA from damage and kills and promotes apoptosis of liver cancer cells.[7590]

- Rosemary oil causes destruction of liver cancer cells by modulating BCL2 and BAX genes expression *in vitro*.[7591] The BCL2 and BAX genes work together to weaken cell membranes and promote apoptosis.

- Topical application of a 1.5% solution containing lavender, marjoram, eucalyptus, rosemary, and peppermint (2:1:2:1:1 ratio), in a carrier oil consisting of 45% apricot, 45% almond, and 10% jojoba carrier oils significantly decreased pain and depression in people with arthritis.[7592]

- Oral administration of 1 mL of rosemary oil (1,8-cineole CT) every eight hours for forty-four weeks increased the blood pressure of people with low blood pressure without affecting heart rate.[7593]

- A daily scalp massage with thyme, rosemary, lavender, and cedarwood oils in a mixture of carrier oils (jojoba and grapeseed) improved alopecia areata (round patches of hair loss) in 44% of study participants.[7594]

- An abdominal massage with lemon, rosemary, and peppermint oil relieved constipation in the elderly.[7595] Interestingly, the effect of the massage lasted for two weeks after treatment.

- *In vitro* research concluded that rosemary essential oil inhibited *P. insidiosum* (a pathogenic oomycete that infects mammals and causes gangrenous ulcers on the skin and may restrict blood flow in the surrounding arteries).[7596]

- Animal research concluded that rosemary oil relieves pain by influencing opioid and serotonin receptor activity.[7597] Opioids are molecules naturally produced by the body that work similarly to morphine.

- *In vitro* research suggests that rosemary inhibits elastase activity (an enzyme involved in the breakdown of elastin and a causal factor in lung connective tissue diseases, disruption of the body's ability to kill pathogens, and delayed wound healing).[7598] The researchers concluded that topical administration may be beneficial for bullous pemphigoid (a skin condition that causes the formation of large blisters) and pulmonary emphysema (a chronic lung condition characterized by enlargement of the air sacs in the lungs).

- Rosemary oil helps decrease inflammation by mildly inhibiting the 5-lipoxygenase (5-LOX) enzyme that is involved in the inflammation response according to *in vitro* research.[7599] Another study concluded that rosemary oil stimulates nerve cell receptor function of alpha(1) and alpha(2) adrenergic receptors, which improves local blood circulation and relieves pain.[7600]

- *In vitro* research suggests that rosemary oil inhibits *P. falciparum* (a protozoan parasite that causes malaria in humans).[7601]

- Animal research concluded that rosemary oil protects the male reproductive system against oxidative stress and functional damage in diabetic rats.[7602]

- Rosemary oil completely inhibits germ tube formation (used by the spores to reproduce and spread) of *C. albicans* isolated from the mouths of denture wearers.[7603]

- Inhalation of rosemary oil increases feelings of alertness and affects brain wave activity (decreases alpha waves and increases beta waves) to a state of greater alertness.[7604] Increased alpha waves are associated with an awake but relaxed state (i.e. daydreaming), whereas elevated beta waves are associated with normal consciousness and a state of elevated alertness, logic, and critical reasoning.

- Oral administration of 100 to 400 μl/kg of rosemary reduced colon lesions and inflammation in rats with colitis.[7605]

- Animal research suggests that rosemary oil may protect against osteoporosis by inhibiting osteoclast (cells that breakdown bone tissue to release minerals into the circulatory system) activity and normalizing bone turnover.[7606]

- *In vitro* and animal research suggests that rosemary oil reduces inflammation by inhibiting excessive leukocyte migration and adhesion to damaged tissue.[7607,7608] Leukocytes travel to the site of damaged tissue to encourage tissue repair; however, when they migrate excessively to the area it causes an abnormal inflammatory response.

☐ Rosemary oil increases intracellular reduced glutathione (GSH) levels and Nrf2-antioxidant responsive element (ARE)-reporter activity, which protects liver cells from damage and enhances liver cell survival *in vitro*.[7609] Nrf2 is a potent protein found within all cells (but particularly in the liver and kidneys) that acts as the master regulator of the cellular antioxidant system when activated by AREs. Once triggered, Nrf2 activates over 200 genes that metabolize drugs and toxins, protect against oxidative stress, remove damaged proteins, and normalize inflammation. It also interacts with other cells that together determine longevity and protect against age-related diseases like cancer and neurological disorders.[7610]

☐ Animal research suggests that rosemary oil is useful for diabetic wounds. Topical application of rosemary oil accelerated the healing of wounds that had cut through all the layers of skin in diabetic mice.[7611]

☐ Exposing people with dementia to 0.04 mL of lemon and 0.08 mL of rosemary oils on a gauze pad with an electric fan in the morning (9:00 a.m. to 11:00 a.m.) and 0.08 mL of lavender and 0.04 mL of orange oils in the evening (7:30 p.m. to 9:00 p. m.) significantly improved personal orientation related to cognitive function without any side effects.[7612]

☐ Inhalation of rosemary and lavender oils reduced test-taking stress of graduate nursing students.[7613]

☐ *In vitro* research suggests that rosemary oil inhibits gram-positive and drug-resistant bacteria (*E. faecalis, E. coli*) and fungi (*C. albicans*).[7614] Another *in vitro* study concluded that rosemary oil significantly inhibits *E. coli, S. typhi, S. enteritidis, S. sonnei*, and *C. albicans*, and reduced lipid peroxidation.[7615] A third study concluded that rosemary oil provides broad-spectrum antimicrobial activity against several bacteria and yeast strains that are associated with food spoilage, food poisoning, and human disease.[7616] Rosemary essential oil inhibits *Aspergillus* species and their subsequent production of mycotoxins.[7617] The alpha-pinene CT of rosemary essential oil weakly inhibited *Candida neoformans*.[7618]

☐ Rosemary oil caused *P. acnes* (the bacterium associated with acne) cell death by causing them to shed their lining, lose their normal shape, and leak their fluid *in vitro*.[7619]

☐ Smelling rosemary or lavender for five minutes decreased cortisol levels and increased free-radical-scavenging activity in twenty-two healthy people.[7620]

☐ *In vitro* research suggests that rosemary oil partially inhibits HSV-1.[7621]

☐ Inhalation of rosemary oil improves overall memory quality and secondary memory (the ability to recall stored memories after a distraction and some time has passed) in healthy adults.[7622] A subsequent study attributed the cognitive and memory benefits of oral and inhaled rosemary oil to its 1,8-cineole content, which researchers concluded triggers neurochemical pathways involved in memory.[7623]

☐ Oral administration of rosemary oil protected the liver from damage and prevented genetic mutation in rats.[7624]

☐ Animal research concluded that rosemary oil prevents tracheal contractions.[7625]

☐ A 1,8-cineole rich rosemary oil provided 68.3% repellency against ticks.[7626]

☐ Rosemary essential oil protected against hypothalamic neuron toxicity caused by excessive zinc.[7627]

☐ *In vitro* research demonstrated that low doses of marjoram, lemon, basil, clove, thyme, rosemary CT 1,8-cineole, and tea tree essential oils prevented the shortening of telomeres after exposure to hydrogen peroxide.[7628] The same research reported that vetiver, black pepper, eucalyptus (*E. globulus*), ginger, clove, and rosemary increased the length of already shortened telomeres. This activity suggests that these essential oils can help maintain the youth and health of cells, or turn back the clock on the cell to make it more youthful depending on the essential oil used. Interestingly, cinnamon and peppermint essential oil decreased the length of telomeres slightly.

☐ A clinical study found that swishing with an essential oil mouthwash containing lemongrass (0.5%), thyme (0.5%), rosemary (0.5%), PEG-40-hydrogenated-castor-oils-emulsifier (6%), and water (92.5%) for twenty minutes following scaling and root planing significantly reduced microbe populations in the mouth and prevented subgingival biofilm formation.[7629]

☐ Rosemary essential oil is toxic to the brown-banded cockroach (*Supella longipalpa*).[7630] It was the most toxic of five essential oils tested (eucalyptus, peppermint, oregano, yarrow, and rosemary).

☐ Rosemary essential oil demonstrates meat preservation properties by reducing psychrotrophics, *Brochothrix thermosphacta, Pseudomonas* spp., and *Enterobacteriaceae* counts in meat.[7631]

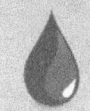

- The alpha-pinene CT of rosemary essential oil weakly inhibited tyrosinase activity, suggesting it may mildly whiten the skin.[7632]
- Animal research suggests that rosemary essential oil (1,8-cineole CT) inhibits *Candida albicans* strains isolated from bovine clinical mastitis.[7633]
- A controlled clinical trial found that inhalation of rosemary essential oil improved short-term image and number memory in students aged thirteen to fifteen years old when compared to the control group.[7634]
- Oral administration of a nanoemulsion of rosemary essential oil CT 1,8-cineole/camphor (830 mcg/kg effective dose—46% inhibition; 100 mg/kg—55% inhibition) reduced inflammation and pain in rats.[7635]
- Injection of ginger essential oil (2.5 g/kg BW) or rosemary essential oil CT alpha-pinene (2.5 g/kg BW)—or 5 mg/kg of body weight combined ginger and rosemary—in rats reversed reductions in HDL cholesterol, and elevations in blood glucose, total cholesterol, and triglycerides caused by a high-fat diet.[7636]
- The 1,8-cineole CT of rosemary essential oil showed significant antioxidant activity compared to vitamin C and inhibited *Listeria monocytogenes*, *Bacillus subtilis*, and *Escherichia coli*.[7637]
- Of eleven essential oils tested, lemongrass (*C. citratus*: citronellal formate 42.8%, isobornyl formate 33.5%) essential oil demonstrated the greatest antioxidant activity in the DPPH test and the best overall antimicrobial activity.[7638] Lemon eucalyptus (78.2% citronellal), lemon scented iron bark (1,8-cineole 29.2%, bornyl formate 12.3%, isobornyl formate 12.1%), lavender (French: cuminaldehyde 41.3%, linalool 37.3%; and French high altitude: linalyl formate 41.7%, linalool 23.5%), and juniper (*J communis*: p-mentha-1(7),8 diene 32.3%, delta-cadinene 11.3%) demonstrated very strong antioxidant activity, lavender (Croatian: linalool 47.9%, linalyl formate 22.1%) and rosemary (limonene CT) strong activity, lavender (Croatian, linalool rich 66.8%) moderate activity, and gully gum poor activity (81.7% 1,8-cineole). The other essential oils demonstrated various degrees of antimicrobial activity against the tested bacteria (*E. faecalis*, *B. cereus*, *L. monocytogenes*, *S. aureus*, MRSA, *Salmonella typhimurium*, *P. aeruginosa*, *E. coli*, *K. pneumonia*, *A. baumannii*, And *Ch. violaceum*).
- Rosemary essential oil (1,8-cineole CT) corrected depletions in antioxidant enzyme activities, oxidative stress, kidney and liver dysfunction, abnormal lipid profiles, and hyperglycemia in an experimental model of diabetes.[7639]
- The 1,8-cineole CT of rosemary essential oil inhibited and killed *S. aureus* and *S. epidermidis* and prevented eradicated existing biofilm and prevented new biofilm formation.[7640] The same researchers found that rosemary essential oil strongly inhibited the proliferation of breast and cervical cancer cells.
- *In vitro* research demonstrated that rosemary CT 1,8-cineole essential oil actively interfered with HIV-1 Tat protein function. The Tat protein plays a central role in and drastically enhances HIV transcription (resulting in the production of multiple copies of the viral RNA and improved infectivity).[7641]
- Inhalation of the camphor CT of rosemary essential oil increased brain dopamine levels in mice by activating the stress response system through the nerve growth factor (NGF) and hypothalamus-pituitary-adrenal axis.[5332] Further investigation concluded that rosemary essential oil caused the differentiation (the process whereby a cell becomes specialized to perform a specific function) of neurons by modulating intracellular acetylcholine, choline, and Gap43 gene expression levels.
- Rosemary essential oil reduced neuronal excitability through modulation of T-type calcium channels (TTCCs).[7642] Inhibition of TTCCs are involved in the antianxiety and neuroprotective effects of rosemary essential oil.
- Two different chemotypes of rosemary essential oil demonstrated the ability to kill head lice.[7643]
- Nanoemulsions of both lavender and rosemary essential oils demonstrated antileishmanial activity against *L. major* without any toxicity to normal cells.[7644] The lavender nanoemulsion was more effective than the standard drug treatment (meglumine antimoniate).
- Laboratory research demonstrated that rosemary CT camphor possesses good antioxidant capacity and inhibited bacteria involved in food spoilage (*P. fluorescens*) and pathogenic bacteria (*Salmonella enterica serotype Typhimurium*, *L. monocytogenes*, and *S. aureus*).[7645]
- *In vitro* and animal research demonstrate that rosemary essential oil nanoemulsion is a more potent anti-inflammatory than the oil alone and demonstrates good antioxidant activity (comparable to quercetin).[7646] Rosemary reduced inflammation by modulating immune activity (inhibiting nitric oxide production). The anti-inflammatory properties of rosemary were attributed to the presence of alpha-pinene, 1,8-cineole, and camphor, which targeted cell receptor sites involved in inflammation.
- Rosemary, clove, oregano (*T. capitatus*), thyme, manuka, sage, eucalyptus (*E. globulus*), lavandin, myrtle, tea tree, peppermint, sage, and corn mint essential oils all showed antimicrobial activity against oral pathogens (*S. mutans*, *Lactobacillus* spp.) isolated from dental surgery patients.[7647] The essential oils also

improved the antimicrobial effects of chlorhexidine, particularly rosemary, thyme, and oregano oils.

□ Rosemary CT 1,8-cineole, lemongrass (*C. citratus*), and wintergreen essential oils each repelled, knocked down, and were lethal to moths (*Anarsia lineatella*).[7648] Rosemary was the most effective repellent and most lethal.

□ An odd CT of oregano with pulegone as the major constituent demonstrated the best antioxidant (better than BHT), antibacterial (*B. cereus, D. solani, E. coli, L. monocytogenes, M. flavus, P. aeruginosa, S. aureus*), and anticancer (breast, cervical, colon—better than vinblastine sulfate, T cell leukemia, bladder) activities of twelve essential oils tested.[7649] The same researchers reported that rosemary CT camphor was the best antifungal (*A. flavus, A. ochraceus, A. niger, P. funiculosum, P. ochrochloron, C. albicans*).

□ Raynaud's disease, also known as Raynaud or Raynaud's phenomenon or syndrome, is an early manifestation of systemic sclerosis characterized by a numb and cool feeling in some areas of the body—such as the fingers and toes—during periods of stress or during temperature changes. This is caused by narrowing of the small arteries that supply blood to the skin. A case study reported that topical application of 10 drops of rosemary CT 1,8-cineole essential oil once daily for three days reduced Raynaud's disease symptoms (significantly warmed the right hand, minimally warmed the left hand, and produced an increased feeling of warmth through the entire body—particularly the face after thirty minutes) in a fifty-three-year-old female.[7650] A 10% dilution (mixed in olive oil) was applied to both the back of the hand and the palm of the hand from the wrist to the finger for thirty seconds.

□ Rosemary, cinnamon, and grapefruit essential oils each inhibited fungi: *Rhizopus stolonifer* (causes respiratory infections, sinusitis, and otomycosis) and *Trichophyton mentagrophytes* and *Microsporum gypseum* (cause athlete's foot, ringworm, and nail infections).[7651]

□ Rosemary (27.4% alpha-pinene, 20.9% 1,8-cineole, 20.6% camphor) essential oil inhibited the growth of *Listeria monocytogenes* and *Salmonella Typhimurium in vitro* and on alfalfa seeds (in vapor phase).[7652]

□ *E. coli* causes up to 85 percent of urinary tract infections (UTIs). Thyme CT linalool, marjoram, and rosemary CT 1,8-cineole essential oils each inhibited *E. coli* isolated from the urinary tract of people with a UTI.[7653] Thyme was the most effective.

□ Rosemary CT 1,8-cineole essential oil killed castor bean tick (*Ixodes ricinus*) nymphs.[7654]

□ A controlled clinical trial found that massaging the knee with a combination of ginger and rosemary essential oils diluted in black cumin seed carrier oil reduced osteoarthritis knee pain and improved knee function and quality of life in elderly individuals.[7655] Ten drops each of ginger and rosemary essential oils were added to 20 mL of black cumin seed carrier oil and massaged into the knee using effleurage and petrissage techniques in the direction of lymph drainage for fifteen to twenty minutes. The massage was repeated three times.

□ Rosemary essential oil (27.0% alpha-pinene, 21.0% camphor, 21.0% 1,8-cineole) inhibited *A. baumannii* and *C. albicans* and demonstrated a significant anti-inflammatory activity.[7656]

□ Rosemary CT 1,8-cineole and grapefruit essential oils reduced hepatitis A virus infection in berries.[7657]

□ Rosemary essential oil preloaded in β-Cyclodextrin protected ram sperm against damage caused by cryopreservation.[7658] The β-Cyclodextrin oil was more effective than the oil alone.

□ Oral administration of fennel or rosemary oils (or their respective nanoforms) in dyslipidemic rats improved biochemical parameters (reduced cardiovascular disease risk, decreased inflammation and oxidative stress, preserved liver function, and lowered blood sugar levels).[7659]

□ A chitosan-based topical formulation with either rosemary or tea tree essential oil or a combination of both demonstrated significant wound healing benefits. The blend of both oils significantly increased wound contraction in comparison to the placebo and the individual essential oil groups and promoted complete re-epithelialization with active hair follicles.[7660]

□ Rosemary essential oil CT 1,8-cineole significantly inhibited egg hatching and larval migration—demonstrating both ovicidal and larvicidal activity—against gastrointestinal nematodes isolated from sheep.[7661]

□ Laboratory research reported that rosemary essential oil inhibited *A. flavus* and its production of aflatoxins B1 and B2.[7662]

□ Rosemary CT 1,8-cineole and thyme CT para-cymene essential oils, alone or in combination, reduced viable counts of food-borne and spoilage bacteria (*Listeria monocytogenes, Salmonella enteritidis, Yersinia enterocolitica, Escherichia coli,* and *Pseudomonas* spp.) in ready-to-eat vegetables.[7663]

□ Tea tree and rosemary essential oil exhibited good antibacterial activity against multidrug-resistant bacteria (*Staphylococcus aureus, S. epidermidis,* and *Cutibacterium acnes*) associated with acne.[7664]

□ Rosemary essential oil (balanced CT) reversed anxiety, depression, memory impairment, and brain oxidative stress caused by scopolamine in zebrafish by reducing acetylcholinesterase (AChE) activity.[7665]

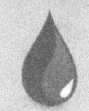

- Sage CT alpha-thujone, garlic, and rosemary CT 1,8-cineole essential oil were also toxic to adults blowflies (*C. vomitoria*) by direct topical and fumigant activity.[7666] The same oils exerted antimicrobial activity against *B. subtilis, S. aureus, E. coli, C. albicans, P. aeruginosa,* and *S. enterica.*

- The kidney plays an important role in detoxification and excretion of toxic substances. Because of this, it is susceptible to toxicity when excess toxins are present. Rosemary CT camphor essential oil reduced or prevented the severity of kidney damage caused by diethylnitrosamine in rats.[7667] Rats that received rosemary oil showed a significant increase in HDL cholesterol and glutathione peroxidase (GSH-Px) activity accompanied by a reduction in LDL cholesterol.

- Rosemary CT 1,8-cineole, oregano (*Th. capitatus*) CT carvacrol, marjoram, and sage CT alpha-thujone demonstrated promising antibacterial activity against bacteria (*P. aeruginosa, E. coli, S. enterica, B. subtilis,* and *S. aureus*) responsible for healthcare-associated infections and foodborne illnesses.[7668] Oregano exhibited the strongest activity, which exceeded gentamicin in effectiveness.

- Moroccan rosemary essential oil (33.9% 1,8-cineole, 14.7% camphor, 12.8% alpha-pinene) inhibited *M. luteus, B. cereus, B. subtilis, C. tropicalis, E. coli, C. albicans, M. aurum, M. smegmatis,* and *P. aeruginosa.*[7669] The oil also showed a remarkable synergistic activity when combined with isolated carvacrol.

- Rosemary CT 1,8-cineole and rosemary with calcium hydroxide inhibited *E. faecalis,* which is an important pathogen during root canal therapy that is resistant to calcium hydroxide (the gold standard antimicrobial used during root canals) alone.[7670] Ginger, neroli, and copaiba essential oils also demonstrated moderate antibacterial activity.

- The 1,8-cineole CT of rosemary essential oil demonstrated neuroprotective properties (AChE inhibition) and antioxidant activity in various assays.[7671] Inhibition of AChE preserves acetylcholine levels in the brain, which is important for memory and brain function. Severe depletion of acetylcholine is associated with Alzheimer's disease.

- Used as a fumigant, rosemary CT camphor essential oil was insecticidal to the cowpea weevil (*Callosobruchus maculatus*).[7672]

- Rosemary and tea tree essential oils significantly inhibited the formation of biofilms and destroyed mature biofilms produced by *S. aureus* and *E. coli.*[7673] Tea tree was more active than rosemary.

- Rosemary CT 1,8-cineole essential oil demonstrated good antioxidant activity in the DPPH, ABTS, beta-carotene bleaching, and FRAP assays.[7674] The same research reported that the oil effectively inhibited acetylcholinesterase activity, showing promising activity for Alzheimer's disease.

- Hexavalent chromium (HC) is a known carcinogen and has the potential to cause liver toxicity and harm. Administration of rosemary essential oil (0.5 mL/kg body weight prior to or after injection of HC) restored deleterious changes in liver and antioxidant function caused by HC in rats.[7675] The oil improved glutathione content, enzymatic antioxidant activity, liver enzymes, and serum liver function biomarkers. Rats pretreated with rosemary oil experienced greater improvements than rats administered the oil after HC administration.

- A nanoemulsion with rosemary and peppermint essential oils reduced osteoarthritis pain in rats.[7676] Thirty-six rats were randomly assigned to six different groups: control (no osteoarthritis), osteoarthritis, osteoarthritis treated with EO nanoemulsion gel, osteoarthritis treated with EO nanoemulsion, osteoarthritis treated with rosemary and peppermint EO gel, and osteoarthritis treated with diclofenac sodium. The treatments were administered topically at an amount of 1 mL daily. The EO nanoemulsion reduced osteoarthritis pain by increasing antioxidant capacity and improving joint structure and function.

- Sleepiness is a common complaint of those required to work night shifts. Sleepiness during a shift among nurses could lead to accidents and medical errors. A randomized, controlled trial evaluated the effects of inhaling rosemary essential oil during a night shift. Eighty night-shift nurses in a critical care unit (CCU) were randomly assigned to two groups: forty in the control group (distilled water) and forty in the essential oil group. Participants completed sleep surveys at the beginning and end of the study. One drop of rosemary essential oil was added to gauze and placed inside a mask, which was used to inhale the oil for ten to fifteen minutes while working. At the end of the study, the nurses who received the essential oil reported significantly less sleepiness and improved alertness during their shifts when compared to control groups.[7677]

- Potassium dichromate (PD) is a common inorganic chemical reagent that primarily affects the respiratory tract causing ulcerations, shortness of breath, and respiratory conditions (bronchitis, asthma, pneumonia). It is also known to cause oxidative stress and kidney toxicity in animals and humans. Rats injected with PD experienced increased oxidative stress and notable declines in glutathione (GSH), total protein content, and enzymatic antioxidants (SOD, CAT GPX, and GST). In addition, signs of kidney damage (serum urea, creatinine, and uric acid) increased significantly. Oral administration of rosemary CT 1,8-cineole essential oil (0.5 mL/kg BW) before or after administration of PD restored most of the biochemical parameters, diminished oxidative stress markers, and improved kidney tissue architecture.[7678]

- *In vitro* research showed that marjoram, rosemary CT 1,8-cineole, sage CT camphor, and pulegone CT limonene/piperitone inhibited *L. monocytogenes* and *Salmonella enterica* and displayed antioxidant activity in the DPPH assay.[7679]
- Rosemary CT 1,8-cineole essential oil inhibited *S. aureus* (two strains) in laboratory research.[7680]
- Researchers evaluated the synergistic activity of rosemary, geranium, and peppermint essential oils in combination with colistin antibiotics against extreme drug-resistant and susceptible *Acinetobacter baumannii* clinical isolates. The highest inhibitory activity was observed with peppermint essential oil, followed by geranium and rosemary essential oils.[7681] Both rosemary and geranium produced strong synergistic activity when combined with colistin, but peppermint was indifferent when combined with colistin.
- Eucalyptus (*E. globulus*), pine, rosemary CT camphor, cistus, Maritime pine, and juniper berry each displayed good antioxidant activity in the ORAC assay.[7682]
- Nanostructured lipid carriers (NLCs) are emerging as a novel way to deliver essential oils intranasally for the management of neurodegenerative diseases. NLCs containing rosemary or lavender essential oil showed the formation of more ordered structures and high cytocompatibility on two cell lines (murine and human fibroblasts) when compared to Tegosoft CT and neem oil.[7683]
- Rosemary CT 1,8-cineole and lavender essential oils exhibited anticancer activity against neuroblastoma cells.[7684] Both oils also demonstrated good antibacterial activity against *E. coli*, *P. fluorescens*, *A. bohemicus*, *K. marina*, and *B. cereus*. Furthermore, the oils exhibited good antioxidant activity in the ABTS and DPPH assays.
- *Sporothrix brasiliensis* is a fungus that causes human and animal sporotrichosis—an infection that affects the skin, lungs, bones, and joints, causing firm, painless modules that later become ulcers. Itraconazole is the first-line drug treatment option, but the emergence of itraconazole-resistant strains makes treating sporotrichosis more difficult. Oral administration of rosemary CT 1,8-cineole essential oil for thirty days delayed fungal spread, reduced fungal load (better than itraconazole), and protected systemic organs—primarily the liver and spleen—in rats.[7685]
- Thyme, tea tree, tropical basil, rosemary CT 1,8-cineole, eucalyptus, corn mint, and lavender essential oil each inhibited biofilm-forming *S. aureus*, with thyme and rosemary being the most active in liquid phase.[7686] Thyme was the most active in vapor phase, with varying degrees of inhibition observed depending on the strain of *S. aureus* with tea tree, rosemary, eucalyptus, corn mint, and lavender. Tea tree and lavender oils displayed the weakest activity in the vapor phase.
- Injection of high doses (200 mL/kg BW) of rosemary, Spanish lavender, ravintsara, and eucalyptus (*E. globulus*) essential oil reduced anxiety in rats.[7687]
- The 1,8-cineole CT of rosemary essential oil was active against *A. niger*, *S. aureus*, and Adenovirus 35, and good antioxidant activity in the DPPH, ferric-reducing, and ABTS assays.[7688] The oil was not genotoxic in the Ames test at dilutions of 5% and 90% respectively.
- Dyslipidemias (increased levels of serum lipoprotein, cholesterol, and triglycerides) are associated with a higher incidence of cardiovascular diseases. Rats fed a saturated fat diet experienced abdominal fat gain, high cholesterol and triglycerides, increased LDL cholesterol, and atherogenesis in the aorta. Similarly, rats administered Triton experienced significantly increased total cholesterol, LDL, and triglycerides levels. Oral administration of rosemary (33.7% 1,8-cineole, 27.7% camphor, 22.0% limonene, and 8.1% alpha-pinene) essential oil or its nanoemulsion significantly reduced total cholesterol, LDL, and triglycerides in rats with dyslipidemia.[7689] The group that received rosemary essential oil reversed dyslipidemia and abdominal fat accumulation in the Triton-induced dyslipidemia model, which was superior to simvastatin. The oil also reduced dyslipidemia in the saturated fat model.
- Emergency personnel work in an environment where they are exposed to factors that increase occupational stress. Indeed, rates of posttraumatic stress disorder among emergency personnel rival, and occasionally, surpass those of combat veterans. A randomized controlled trial evaluated the benefits of rose essential oil inhalation among emergency department nurses.[7690] Nurses inhaled from cotton swabs containing 2 drops of 40% rose essential oil for ten minutes, while the control group inhaled cotton swabs with 2 drops of distilled water instead. The rose group experienced a significant decrease in reported stress, but the control group experienced a slight increase in stress. Inhalation of rose essential oil therefore may be a viable natural way to reduce stress among emergency personnel.
- Honey has been used medicinal since ancient times for a variety of ailments. Medical-grade honey (not the raw honey you purchase at a grocery store) is particularly useful for wound healing because of its antibacterial and anti-inflammatory activity, which speeds the healing of wounds. An experimental study evaluated the healing effects of a mixture of honey with selected essential oils—oregano CT ethanone, rosemary CT

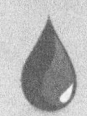

camphor, and thyme CT 1,3-Cyclopentadiene—in burn and chemical wound models in rabbits.[7691] The oils were added to honey in a concentration of 0.5% per 100g of honey. The honey/essential oil groups were compared versus a control (no treatment) and standard treatment with madecassol ointment. All of the honey/essential oil groups experienced faster healing times than the control group and standard treatment group. The best healing effect for burns was observed with honey and thyme essential oil for burns. The oils were not irritating when used at 0.5% in the honey, but showed irritation at 5%.

☐ Raynaud's phenomenon (Raynaud's syndrome) is a condition characterized by spasms of the small arteries resulting in reduced blood flow to the end arterioles of the fingers. It may also occur in the ears, toes, nipples, knees, or nose. Spasms generally occur in response to cold, stress, or emotional upset, causing the extremity to turn pale or white then blue. Warming the hands brings red color back but may also cause swelling and pain. An open-label pilot study investigated the benefits of topical rosemary essential oil for Raynaud's phenomenon.[7692] Twelve subjects with progressive systemic sclerosis and Raynaud's phenomenon received an application of olive oil as a control and then a 10% dilution of rosemary essential oil three hours later. Skin temperature increased significantly after both the olive oil and rosemary oil massage, but self-reported warmth perception increased only after the rosemary oil application.

☐ Vitamin C (ascorbate) is a vital antioxidant in the brain where it acts as a key signaling molecule and regulator of oxidative stress. Under certain circumstances ascorbate produces hydroxyl radicals and hydrogen peroxide. A laboratory study evaluated how essential oils either enhance (pro-oxidant) or suppress (antioxidant) the production of hydrogen peroxide in the brain.[7693] The researchers reported that lavender, tea tree, and rosemary essential oil suppress the production of hydrogen peroxide by brain ascorbate and produce an overall antioxidant effect, which can reduce anxiety. Isolated beta-pinene was also effective. On the contrary, juniper berry, elecampane, and alpha-pinene had pro-oxidant effects that may be useful for antimicrobial, anti-inflammatory, and anticancer effects.

☐ Currently, the accumulation of amyloid-beta peptide as aging plaque, the deposition of neurofibrillary tangles in brain cells (due to hyperphosphorylation of tau protein), massive cholinergic brain cell death, oxidative stress, and brain inflammation are considered the major causes of Alzheimer's disease. The hippocampus—the area of the brain associated with memory, feelings, thoughts, personality, and behavior—is most vulnerable to these alterations. Stem cell-based therapy has emerged as a potential solution for AD in the past few years due to positive results in preclinical trials. Researchers evaluated the benefits of ingesting rosemary CT 1,8-cineole essential oil in conjunction with stem cell therapy in a rat model of AD.[7694] Human olfactory bulb neuronal stem cells (hOBNSCs) were injected into the hippocampus twenty-two days after inducement of AD via ibotenic acid injection. Rosemary essential oil was administered (30 mg/kg BW) once daily before or with hOBNSC transplant. Combined stem cell therapy and rosemary oil significantly enhanced learning and memory, reduced brain inflammation, improved antioxidant activity (CAT, GSH, and SOD), and reduced the expression of genes associated with the deposition of amyloid-beta plaque and the death of brain cells. In addition, the oil promoted fast differentiation and integration of stem cells.

☐ Moroccan grown rosemary essential oil (28.6%–47.3% 1,8-cineole, 5.8%–18.8% camphor, and 9.9%–15.4% alpha-pinene) inhibited *M. smegmatis*, *E. coli*, and *B. subtilis* in a concentration-dependent manner.[7695] Samples collected during summer were characterized by high 1,8-cineole and a higher yield, whereas samples collected during the winter has higher alpha-pinene and a lower yield.

☐ Thyme, oregano, lemongrass, spearmint, and rosemary essential oils each inhibited multidrug-resistant foodborne pathogens isolated from raw milk (*Escherichia, Enterobacter, Citrobacter, Proteus, Klebsiella,* and *Staphylococcus*) but were ineffective against *Pseudomonas*.[7696] Thyme was the most active followed by oregano.

☐ Acetylcholine is an important cholinergic neurotransmitter and neuromodulator involved in various functions throughout the body, but particularly in the nervous system. It works by attaching to receptors and sending signals between nerves. Acetylcholine has multiple functions in the body including motor neuron function (muscular movement), dilation of blood vessels, motivation, attention, learning, and memory. The activity and function of the cholinergic system is controlled by the enzymes acetylcholinesterase (AChE) and butyrylcholinesterase (BChE). People with neurodegenerative conditions make less acetylcholine and experience excessive BChE activity. Inhibition of AChE and BChE are targets for the treatment of neurodegenerative conditions. The outgrowth of neurites (called neuritogenesis—the formation of any projection from neurons) occurs during brain development and when neurons are regenerated. These outgrowths of dendrites or axons allow neurons to form networks and connections and communicate with other cells and ultimately maintain youthful brain function. A preclinical model of Alzheimer's disease evaluated essential oils from the *Lamiaceae* family for their effects on brain function and brain cell protection.[7697] Oregano CT alpha-terpineol, peppermint, rosemary CT 1,8-cineole, and sage essential oils each inhibited BChE activity. The carvacrol CT of oregano inhibited both BChE and AChE activity. Isolated linalool from lavender significantly reduced reactive oxygen species (ROS) inside neurons, suggesting it can protect against oxidative stress and death of neurons. In addition, oregano CT alpha-terpineol, peppermint, rosemary, and sage triggered neurite outgrowth, with the greatest activity observed from oregano. The researchers concluded that these oils have properties that could potentially prevent or delay dementia-related diseases.

☐ An investigation of three essential oils from the *Lamiaceae* family (peppermint, rosemary, and lavender) found that rosemary CT camphor was the most effective larvicidal agent against third instar larvae mosquitoes (*Culex pipiens*).[7698] Lavender essential oil was the least effective larvicide, but demonstrated the highest knockdown rate, followed by peppermint. In addition, lavender and peppermint essential oils showed the highest adult mosquito mortality rates.

☐ Exposure to ionizing radiation (depending on the type, amount absorbed, exposure time, distance, and tissue sensitivity) can harm humans by destroying cells or causing them to mutate. Exposure to radiation with rosemary essential oil (composition not reported) present significantly increased the survival and reduced damage and death to human peripheral blood mononuclear cells (PBMCs).[7699]

☐ Both rosemary (30.1% 1,8-cineole, 22.0% camphor) and tea tree essential oil displayed significant antibiofilm effectiveness against *P. aeruginosa* in liquid and vapor forms.[7700]

☐ The camphor CT of rosemary essential oil was toxic to the lesser grain weevil (*Sitophilus oryzae*) and red flour beetle (*Tribolium castaneum*).[7701]

☐ Rosemary CT levo-verbenone essential oil exhibited moderate anticancer (murine melanoma and human prostate) and antioxidant (DPPH assay) properties in laboratory research, and anti-inflammatory activity in a rodent model of arthritis.[7702]

☐ Humans are exposed to gamma rays (gamma radiation) from cosmic rays in the solar system, medical tests (X-rays, CT scans, etc.), airport scanners, nuclear power plants, some consumer products, and food irradiation, which can alter healthy cells in the body. A preclinical model found that exposure to rosemary, oregano, lavender, or eucalyptus (*E. globulus*) essential oils protected against damage caused by gamma ray exposure.[7703] The best protective effects were observed form lavender and oregano essential oils. Specifically, the oil preserved metabolic enzymes, restored enzymatic antioxidant activity (catalase and superoxide dismutase), and reduced lipid peroxidation.

☐ Both eucalyptus (*E. globulus*) and rosemary essential oil were insecticidal to and repelled the mill moth (*Ephestia kuehniella*), which is a pest of cereal grains, especially flour.[7704]

☐ The 1,8-cineole CT of rosemary essential oil demonstrated good antioxidant activity in the DPPH, FRAP, and beta-carotene bleaching assays.[7705]

☐ Peppermint (29.0% menthone, 22.4% menthol, 12.6% 1,8-cineole) and rosemary CT 1,8-cineole essential oil were evaluated for their biological effects (antimicrobial, antioxidant, anti-inflammatory and cytotoxic in different cancer cells) with an emphasis on their use as a complementary treatment for colorectal cancer.[7706] Peppermint exhibited potent antimicrobial activity (*S. mutans, S. pyogenes, S. aureus, E. coli, P. aeruginosa, C. albicans,* and *C. parapsilosis*), moderate antioxidant activity, and low cytotoxicity to colorectal cancer cells. Rosemary was significantly cytotoxic to colorectal cancer cells but presented a low antimicrobial and antioxidant activity.

☐ Pennyroyal, Spanish lavender CT camphor, rosemary CT camphor, and oregano CT thymol essential oil were each acaricidal to two spider mites (*Tetranychus urticae* and *Eutetranychus orientalis*) in the fumigant toxicity test, with pennyroyal displaying the highest activity.[7707] A combination of oregano with acequinocyl exhibited the greatest results of mixtures tried.

☐ Rosemary CT alpha-pinene essential oil showed moderate acaricidal activity against the two-spotted spider mite (*Tetranychus urticae*), but isolated alpha-pinene showed more toxicity than the whole oil.[7708]

☐ Dysbiosis can lead to elevated levels of trimethylamine-N-oxide (TMAO)—a compound associated with chronic disease, including cardiovascular disease and diabetes. Ingestion of summer savory, parsley, or rosemary essential oil emulsions with L-carnitine improved the gut microbiome (primarily *Lactobacillus* genus bacteria), decreased TMAO levels, and increased short-chain fatty acids in mouse models of ischemic heart disease and type 2 diabetes.[7709] Additionally, rosemary and parsley decreased proinflammatory cytokines, while savory increased chemokines (signaling proteins crucial for the migration of white blood cells during normal inflammatory processes to maintain homeostasis). The essential oil emulsions acted as prebiotics to improve gut microbiome and reduce the risk of cardiovascular and metabolic disorders.

☐ Rosemary essential oil inhibited virulence factors of *C. albicans*, with a mixture of 1,8-cineole and alpha-pinene showing partial synergy against the fungus.[7710]

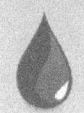

- Co-administration of rosemary essential oil CT 1,8-cineole with curcumin protected against livery injury in mice caused by acetaminophen better than either rosemary of curcumin alone.[7711] Rosemary also enhanced the bioavailability of curcumin. Further investigation found that the liver protection was produced by the combination triggering the overexpression of MEK and ERK proteins.
- Etoposide is a chemotherapy drug used to treat a variety of cancers. Its use is restricted due to significant toxicity to healthy tissues and organs, particularly the liver. A preclinical model evaluated the protective effects of rosemary CT alpha-pinene essential oil against etoposide toxicity.[7712] Etoposide damaged the liver (elevated liver enzymes) and testis of male rats, which was diminished by ingestion of rosemary essential oil. Additionally, rosemary essential oil improved lipid profile (decreased total cholesterol and triglycerides and raised HDL cholesterol) and increased testosterone levels. This research suggests that ingestion of rosemary oil may alleviate some of the toxic effects and damage caused by etoposide.
- Researchers concluded that the NO/cGMP/KATP pathway may be important for the pain-relieving effects of rosemary essential oil.[7713]
- Evaluation of rosemary essential oil from six cultivars showed that they displayed good antioxidant activity, with verbenone content being closely related to antioxidant capacity.[7714] The researchers also reported that rosemary CT alpha-pinene are more toxic to human keratinocytes. Additionally, all the oils demonstrated better activity against pancreatic and epithelial cell cancer cells when tested against six cell types.
- Myrtle CT alpha-pinene and rosemary CT 1,8-cineole exhibited antioxidant activity (DPPH and ferrous chelating assays), with rosemary being more effective.[7715] Similar antibacterial (*E. coli*, *S. enterica*, *P. aeruginosa*, *E. aerogenes*, *L. monocytogenes*, *S. aureus*, *B. cereus*, *M. luteus*) activities were reported from both oils with rosemary being more active against *M. luteus* and myrtle against *S. enterica*. Another group of researchers also investigated myrtle CT alpha-pinene and rosemary CT 1,8-cineole essential oils against *S. aureus* and found that the oils possess antibacterial activity (bactericidal and inhibitory), reduce virulence factors, and remove preformed biofilms.[7716]
- Co-administration of insulin and rosemary essential oil (nasogastric) restored normal blood glucose levels, renal function, and antioxidant activity in diabetic rats better than insulin alone.[7717] Rosemary alone also improved these parameters but not to the degree insulin and insulin plus rosemary did.
- Oral administration of rosemary (30.7% 1,8-cineole, 19.9% camphor, 8.0% alpha-pinene) or peppermint essential oil—equivalent to between 5 and 10 drops in humans—improved cognition (working memory, reference memory, and long-term memory) in a rat model of amnesia-like Alzheimer's disease.[7718] The oils significantly elevated BDNF—a protein in the central nervous system that promotes the survival of neurons by influencing growth, maturation, and maintenance of these cells—and increased hippocampal neurogenesis—the generation of new functional neurons (dentate granule cells) to improve neural plasticity. The combination of the oils produced even better enhancements in cognition.
- Clary sage, rosemary CT 1,8-cineole, creeping thyme (*Thymus serpyllum*), spearmint, melissa CT citronellal, marjoram CT 1,8-cineole, peppermint, basil, and lavender were each toxic to termites (*Reticulitermes dabieshanensis*).[7719]

# ROSEWOOD

*Aniba rosaeodora* Ducke, *A. amazonica* Ducke, *A. parviflora* Meissner Mez.

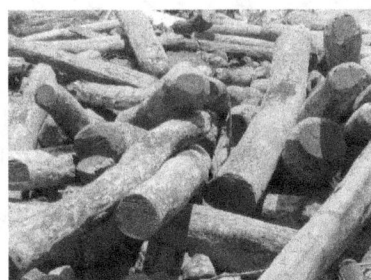

**FAMILY:** Lauraceae
**NOTE:** Middle
**AROMA INTENSITY:** Medium
**AROMA:** Sweet, woody, slightly fruity, floral
**COMMON EXTRACTION METHOD:** Steam distilled from the wood; also distilled from the leaves
**POSSIBLE SUBSTITUTE OILS:** Ravintsara (linalool CT), rose
**BLENDS WELL WITH:** Bergamot, chamomile (German, Roman), geranium, grapefruit, lavender, lemon, lime, neroli, orange, petitgrain, rose
**SUBCELLULAR LOCALIZATION | EPIGENETIC INFLUENCE:** Currently unknown | Currently unknown
**RECOMMENDED DILUTION RANGE:** 5%–neat

**PRIMARY CONSTITUENTS:**[7720,7721,7722]

| *Wood* | | *Leaves* | |
|---|---|---|---|
| Linalool | 73.0%–99.0% | Linalool | 82.5% |
| Alpha-Terpineol | 0.1%–18.8% | Alpha-Terpineol | 3.6% |
| Alpha-Cubebene | 0.0%–2.8% | Geraniol | 1.3% |
| Trans-Linalool Oxide | 1.2%–2.1% | Alpha-Selinene | 1.1% |
| Cis-Linalool Oxide | 1.3%–2.1% | Trans-Linalool Oxide | 0.8% |
| Nerol | 0.2%–1.7% | Cis-Linalool Oxide | 0.8% |
| Delta-Cadinene | 0.1%–1.4% | | |
| Alpha-Selinene | 0.7%–1.3% | | |
| Geraniol | 0.7%–1.3% | | |
| 1,8-Cineole | 0.6%–1.2% | | |

**OTHER CONSTITUENTS:** Sabinene, limonene, alpha-pinene, alpha-copaene, beta-selinene, delta-guaiene, hotrienol, benzyl benzoate, caryophyllene oxide, gamma-selinene, germacrene D, cyperene, spathulenol

**PREFERRED COMPOSITION FOR CLINICAL USE:**

| Constituent | Wood |
|---|---|
| **Linalool** | 72%–90% |
| **Alpha-Terpineol** | 0.1%–8% |
| **1,8-Cineole** | 0.5%–3% |
| **Cis-Linalool Oxide** | 1%–3% |
| **Trans-Linalool Oxide** | 1%–3% |
| **Alpha-Copaene** | 0.1%–3% |
| **Geraniol** | 0.1%–3% |
| **Benzyl Benzoate** | 0.1%–2% |
| **Limonene** | 0.1%–2% |
| **Alpha-Pinene** | 0.01%–1% |

**REPORTED THERAPEUTIC PROPERTIES:** Analgesic (pain relief), antiseptic, antibacterial, deodorant, skin disorders, encourages the secretion of hormones, fever reducer, tissue regenerative, **helps reduce the appearance of wrinkles and blemishes**, wound healing, stimulating, relaxing, strengthening, **stress management**, antidepressant, relieves anxiety, aphrodisiac

**CAUTIONS:**
- May interact with antibiotics or antifungals and possibly enhance their effects.[7723,7724]
- Large doses (100 mg/kg) may interact with pentobarbital (a barbiturate) and increase sleeping time caused by the drug.[7725]

**SELECTED EVIDENCE:**
- *In vitro* research suggests that rosewood oil selectively causes apoptosis of cancerous and precancerous skin cells through mechanisms inside and outside the cell.[7726]
- Rosewood oil interacts with the central nervous system (adenosine receptors) to promote relaxation according to animal research.[7727]
- Scientists observed that rosewood oil synergistically enhances the antibacterial activity of Gentamicin, which may allow a reduced dose of Gentamicin and reduced side effects.[7728]
- Animal research suggests that rosewood oil encourages a relaxed and calm state by reducing neuronal excitability.[7729]
- Animal research demonstrates that rosewood essential oil produces rapid (within 1 to 3 seconds) cardiovascular effects (reduced blood pressure, vasodilation, and lowered heart rate) via a vago-vagal reflex response.[7730]
- *In vitro* research demonstrates that rosewood essential oil inhibits *A. flavus* and *A. parasiticus* and their production of aflatoxin B1.[7731]

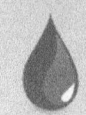

- Intraperitoneal injection of rosewood essential oil exhibited antidepressant activity in rats without causing sedation or memory impairment in rodents.[7732] The study authors attributed this effect to the presence of linalool, which is synergized by the other minor constituents in the oil.
- Lavender, lemongrass (*C. citratus*), marjoram, peppermint, tea tree, and rosewood essential oils all exhibited significant activity against clinical isolates of multidrug-resistant *Burkholderia cepacia* complex (a group of bacteria commonly resistant to antibiotics that cause health problems in people with weakened immune systems and are known to cause healthcare related infections).[7733]
- The benefits of inhaling essential oils was evaluated in a mouse model of Alzheimer's disease.[7734] The mice were exposed to a blend of lemon and rosemary essential oils at nighttime and a blend of lavender and orange oil in the daytime over a period of two months. The cognitive function of the mice improved after the intervention based on improved performance in the Y-maze test. Moreover, brain amyloid beta and abnormally phosphorylated tau proteins were both considerably reduced, while brain-derived neurotrophic factor marginally increased.
- Rosewood essential oil displayed efficient antioxidant activity in the ABTS assay, exhibited antitrypanosomal activity against epimastigote forms and intracellular amastigotes of *T. cruzi* at higher concentrations, reduced nitric oxide production in unstimulated macrophages, and was not toxic to BALB/c peritoneal macrophages.[7735] The oil and linalool were also antibacterial against bacteria isolated from marine environments (*A. caviae, E. faecalis, A. hydrophila, K. pneumoniae, P. stuartii*) and pathogenic bacterial cultures (*S. aureus, E. coli, S. choleraesuis, P. aeruginosa*). In addition, the oil was not toxic to mice peritoneal macrophages and reduced nitrite levels in unstimulated cells, suggesting a potential to modulate nitric oxide production. Linalool also exhibited antimicrobial activity, although it was generally less effective than the whole oil. Linalool displayed greater antioxidant activity than the whole oil, weaker activity against epimastigotes and greater activity against intracellular amastigotes.
- Rosewood chitosan nanoemulsion essential oil completely inhibited the growth and production of aflatoxin B1 by *A. flavus*, which exceeded the activity of the free oil.[7736]

# RUE
## (Common Rue, Arruda, Garden Rue)

*Ruta graveolens* L., *Ruta montana* Mill.

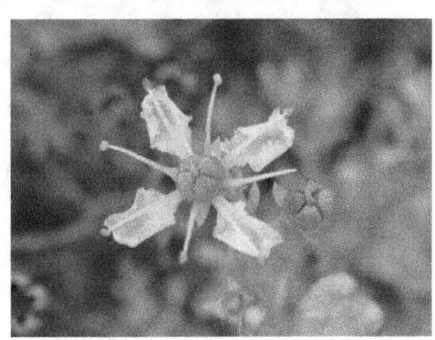

**FAMILY:** Rutaceae
**NOTE:** Top
**AROMA INTENSITY:** Strong
**AROMA:** Bitter, herbaceous, acrid
**COMMON EXTRACTION METHOD:** Steam distilled from the aerial parts
**POSSIBLE SUBSTITUTE OILS:** Vetiver, spikenard
**BLENDS WELL WITH:** Bay laurel, chamomile (German, Roman), fennel, frankincense, lavender, myrrh, thyme, wormwood
**SUBCELLULAR LOCALIZATION | EPIGENETIC INFLUENCE:** Currently unknown | Currently unknown
**RECOMMENDED DILUTION RANGE:** 1.5%–20% (a dilution of under 1.5% is recommended to avoid photosensitivity)

**PRIMARY CONSTITUENTS:**[7737,7738,7739,7740,7741,7742,7743,7744]

| *2-Undecanone CT* | | *n-Hex-4-en-3-one CT* | |
|---|---|---|---|
| 2-Undecanone | 30.7%–73.2% | n-Hex-4-en-3-one | 53.6%–55.1% |
| 2-Nonanone | 4.9%–41.7% | n-Pent-3-one | 28.2%–37.8% |
| 2-Heptanol Acetate | 0.0%–17.5% | n-Hex-3-en-2-one | 7.2%–14.1% |
| 2-Acetoxy Tetradecanone | 0.0%–14.5% | | |
| 2-Acetyltridecane | 0.0%–12.7% | | |
| 2-Nonylacetate | 0.0%–11.1% | | |
| 1-Dodecanol | 0.0%–11.0% | | |
| Geyrene | 0.0%–10.4% | | |

| Nonyl Cyclopropane- | |
|---|---|
| carboxylate | 0.0%–9.2% |
| Xanthotoxine | 0.0%–7.2% |
| 1-Nonene | 0.0%–4.4% |
| Limonene | 0.0%–4.3% |
| Tridecanol | 0.0%–4.2% |
| Undecane | 0.0%–3.5% |
| 5,6-Diethenyl-1-Methyl- | |
| Cyclohexene | 0.0%–3.4% |
| 2-Nonene | 0.0%–3.1% |

Note: Undecanone content will increase in rue essential oil (undecanone CT) when harvested at wax ripeness stage instead of full blossoming stage.[7745] Drying the plant materials also increases essential oil yield.

**OTHER CONSTITUENTS:** *2-Undecanone CT*—2-octanone, anthracene, 3,4-dihydrobenzo [b] fluoranthene, tetradecanal, dodecanal, 2-decanone, 2-dodecanone, elemol, 12-methyl-oxa-cyclododec-6-en-2-one, myrtenol, 1,3-benodioxide; *n-Hex-4-en-3-one CT*—n-hex-3-one, n-pent-3-en-2-one, n-hex-5-en-2-one, n-hex-5-en-3-one, n-hept-4,6-dien-3-one

**PREFERRED COMPOSITION FOR CLINICAL USE:**

| Constituent | Wood |
|---|---|
| **2-Undecanone** | 42%–62% |
| **2-Nonanone** | 10%–22% |

Note: The rest of the compounds will vary greatly.

**REPORTED THERAPEUTIC PROPERTIES: Antibacterial**, antifungal, antiviral, analgesic, antiarthritic, antirheumatic, nervine, anticonvulsive, antispasmodic, aids digestion, remove warts, helps boils heal, relieves insect bites/stings, **encourages restful sleep**, counters poisoning, antidote to snake bites, insecticide, calming/relaxing, combats regret and grief, relieves anxiety, antidepressant, stress management

**CAUTIONS:**

*Rue is not commonly used in essential oil therapy largely because of the toxic history of the herb. Ingesting 120 grams of the leaves can cause severe kidney and liver damage. It takes ingesting about 100 mL of the essential oil to cause the same damage.[7746] Toxic hepatitis has also been reported due to ingestion of rue herb.[7747] These adverse effects are caused by excessive amounts, which far exceed recommended doses of the herb and essential oil, suggesting that its reputation as a highly toxic plant may be exaggerated based on misuse. Rue generally should not be used alone, and only be a small part of a blend.*

■ Avoid during pregnancy and lactation. Rue herb (*Ruta graveolens* or *R. chalepensis,* called fringed rue and also high in 2-undecanone) is one of the most common plants used to induce abortion.[7748,7749,7750] This practice often leads to abortion, but has severe consequences for the mother as well, including gastrointestinal disturbances, genital hemorrhaging, anemia, jaundice, liver enlargement, respiratory distress, acute kidney failure, multiple organ system failure, and even death.[7751] Constituents in the plant (pilocarpine and chalepensin) are used to prevent conception in animals.[7752,7753,7754] One animal study reports antifertility properties of rue herb (chloroform extract, with chalepensin as the constituent with antifertility properties) at a human equivalent dose of only 2.5 grams.[7755] However, this is all based on the herb, not the essential oil, which is chemically different. Scientists believe that pilocarpine (present in the herb) may be responsible for its abortifacient effects.[7756,7757] It required extreme acute doses of rue essential oil to cause abortions and harm animals (both mother and fetus).[7758,7759] Lower acute doses of up to 75 mL did not disrupt embryo or fetal development.[7760] Repeated (chronic) doses of 1 mL/kg (equivalent to giving the average adult 59 mL regularly) led to abortions in guinea pigs.[7761] One study reports that the volatile oil (even the smell) can induce abortion, but it appears to be based on traditional usage rather than actual case reports.[7762] In the end, caution is the most reasonable approach and the use of rue should be avoided during pregnancy.

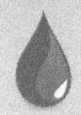

■ Caution is advised orally. Unknown amounts of rue essential oil ingestion (when trying to induce abortion) have led to death in humans. Animal studies report toxicity, multiple organ system failure, and death at acute doses ranging from 2.54 g/kg to over 5 g/kg.[7763,7764] The European Union allows from 630 to 9000 mcg/kg (human equivalent dose approximately 0.05 to 0.7 mL) in beverages and food products; whereas, the United States allows 2,000 to 10,000 mcg/kg (human equivalent dose approximately 0.15 to 0.75 mL).[7765] The 1999 edition of the British Herbal Pharmacopoeia recommends 0.5 to 1 g of dried herb, or 0.5 to 1 mL of herbal extract, but makes no recommendation for the essential oil.[7766] Another text reports 65 mg (just over one drop) of essential oil is the traditional dosage used.[7767]

■ Rue essential oil may be photosensitizing (moderate risk) due to the possible presence of furanocoumarins (bergapten, methoxsalen, psoralen, and xanthotoxine).[7768,7769,7770,7771] Avoid exposing the area of application to UV rays for at least twelve hours after application. Dilution of 1.5% is strongly recommended topically to avoid local irritation and photodermatitis.

SELECTED EVIDENCE:

☐ *In vitro* research demonstrates that rue essential oil strongly inhibits several strains of *Legionella pneumophila* (a bacterium that causes a respiratory disease called legionellosis in humans).[7772]

☐ Rue essential oil (rich in 2-nonanone and undecanal) inhibits six clinical isolates of bacteria (MRSA, *S. epidermidis, B. subtilis, Escherichia coli, Enterobacter aerogenes,* and *P. aeruginosa*), demonstrating more effective against gram-positive bacterial strains.[7773]

☐ *In vitro* research demonstrates that rue essential oil significantly inhibits the fungi *A. fumigatus* and *C. herbarum*.[7774]

☐ Rue essential oil repels the weevil *Aegorhinus superciliosus*, which is a significant pest of fruit crops in some countries.[7775] It is also lethal to the pinewood nematode (*Bursaphelenchus xylophilus*) and repels and kills the *Aedes egypti* mosquito.[7776,7777]

☐ *In vitro* research demonstrated that rue essential oil inhibits *Candida* spp. (hospital-acquired, antifungal resistant) and synergized the efficacy of amphotericin B.[7778] *C. albicans* and *C. tropicalis* were the most sensitive strains.

☐ Rue weakly inhibited fungi (*A. flavus* and *F. oxysporum*), exhibited repellent activity against insect pests (*Rhizopus stolonifera, Mucor racemosus,* and *Trichoderma viride*) comparable to DEET, and was weakly insecticidal.[7779]

☐ Rue essential oil displayed good antioxidant activity in the beta-carotene bleaching assay but not in the DPPH assay, and inhibited *K. pneumoniae, E. coli, C. albicans, L. monocytogenes, B. cereus, C. tropicalis, S. aureus,* and *P. aeruginosa*.[7780]

☐ Rue was larvicidal to fruit flies (*Drosophila melanogaster*) and mosquitoes (*Culex pipiens, Culiseta longiareolata*).[7781]

# SAGE
## (Common Sage, Dalmatian Sage)

*Salvia officinalis* L.

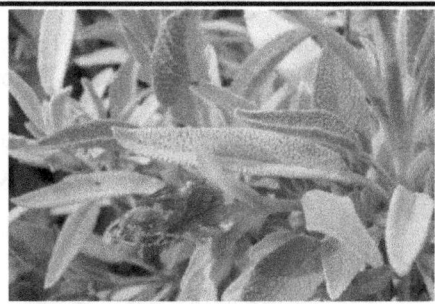

**FAMILY:** Lamiaceae (Labiatae)
**NOTE:** Top
**AROMA INTENSITY:** Medium
**AROMA:** Fresh, warm, spicy, herbaceous, slightly medicinal
**COMMON EXTRACTION METHOD:** Steam distilled from the dried leaves
**POSSIBLE SUBSTITUTE OILS:** Rosemary (1,8-cineole CT), cajeput, cardamom, Spanish sage, camphor (camphor CT), ravintsara (camphor CT)
**BLENDS WELL WITH:** Bay laurel, bergamot, cajeput, camphor, chamomile (German, Roman), coriander, eucalyptus, lavender, lemon, lime, orange, neroli, palo santo, peppermint, petitgrain, ravensara, rosemary, Spanish sage, spikenard, tangerine, thyme, turmeric
**SUBCELLULAR LOCALIZATION | EPIGENETIC INFLUENCE:** Currently unknown | Currently unknown
**RECOMMENDED DILUTION RANGE:** Alpha-thujone, beta-thujone, and camphor CT, Wild—1.5%–20%; Cineole CT—3%–20%; 50% for some conditions

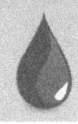
**PRIMARY CONSTITUENTS:**[7782,7783,7784,7785,7786,7787,7788,7789,7790,7791]

*1,8-Cineole CT*

| | |
|---|---|
| 1,8-Cineole | 39.5%–50.3% |
| Camphor | 8.8%–25.0% |
| Alpha-Thujone | 0.1%–9.9% |
| Beta-Pinene | 3.3%–7.3% |
| Beta-Caryophyllene | 1.4%–5.5% |
| Camphene | 0.2%–3.9% |
| Beta-Thujone | 0.1%–3.7% |
| Alpha-Terpineol | 2.6%–3.1% |
| Alpha-Terpinyl Acetate | 1.4%–2.9% |
| Viridiflorol | 0.5%–2.9% |
| Borneol | 1.5%–2.4% |

*Camphor CT*

| | |
|---|---|
| Camphor | 19.8%–36.5% |
| Beta-Thujone | 2.1%–28.6% |
| Alpha-Thujone | 1.5%–28.3% |
| 1,8-Cineole | 3.6%–24.7% |
| Beta-Pinene | 1.4%–14.5% |
| Camphene | 2.1%–9.7% |
| Borneol | 0.3%–6.2% |
| Limonene | 1.8%–6.2% |
| Alpha-Pinene | 0.1%–5.3% |

*Wild*

| | |
|---|---|
| Alpha-Thujone | 14.1%–29.8% |
| Beta-Caryophyllene | 5.2%–19.8% |
| 1,8-Cineole | 5.1%–16.8% |
| Viridiflorol | 9.9%–16.4% |
| Alpha-Humulene | 4.0%–13.5% |

*Alpha-Thujone CT*

| | |
|---|---|
| Alpha-Thujone | 24.5%–52.9% |
| Camphor | 5.5%–26.1% |
| Beta-Thujone | 3.5%–17.9% |
| 1,8-Cineole | 1.9%–15.9% |
| Camphene | 4.8%–8.5% |
| Alpha-Pinene | 0.1%–5.9% |
| Alpha-Humulene | 0.0%–5.6% |
| Beta-Pinene | 0.7%–4.8% |
| Beta-Caryophyllene | 0.0%–4.7% |
| Bornyl Acetate | 0.0%–4.5% |
| Limonene | 1.1%–2.4% |
| Borneol | 0.8%–2.3% |

*Beta-Thujone CT*

| | |
|---|---|
| Beta-Thujone | 20.4%–49.7% |
| Camphor | 5.2%–29.5% |
| Alpha-Thujone | 2.2%–18.4% |
| 1,8–Cineole | 5.0%–15.7% |
| Camphene | 1.0%–9.9% |
| Beta-Pinene | 1.0%–7.7% |
| Borneol | 1.1%–8.8% |
| Limonene | 1.3%–6.5% |
| Alpha-Pinene | 0.1%–5.5% |

Note: Camphor and alpha-thujone were the most common chemotypes identified among commercial samples reviewed.

**OTHER CONSTITUENTS:** Alpha-pinene, camphene, alpha-humulene, borneol, myrcene, beta-pinene, limonene, tricyclene, alpha-terpinolene, endo bornyl acetate, gamma-terpinene, terpinen-4-ol, (Z)-salvene, para-cymene, alpha-thujene, thymol, alpha-terpineol, alpha-phellandrene, (E)-beta-ocimene, myrtenol, (Z)-beta-ocimene, viridiflorol

**PREFERRED COMPOSITION FOR CLINICAL USE:**

| Constituent | *1,8-Cineole CT* | *Alpha-Thujone CT* |
|---|---|---|
| **1,8-Cineole** | 35%–50% | 5%–12% |
| **Camphor** | 8%–20% | 6%–23% |
| **Beta-Pinene** | 3%–8% | 0.5%–4% |
| **Alpha-Thujone** | 0.1%–7% | 23%–45% |
| **Beta-Caryophyllene** | 2%–6% | 2%–6% |
| **Alpha-Terpineol** | 2%–4% | – |
| **Camphene** | 1%–4% | 4%–9% |
| **Alpha-Terpinyl Acetate** | 1%–4% | – |
| **Borneol** | 1.5%–3% | 0.1%–3% |
| **Alpha-Pinene** | 0.5%–3% | 1%–5% |
| **Viridiflorol** | 0.5%–3% | – |
| **Beta-Thujone** | 0.1%–3% | 3%–10% |

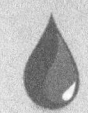

| | | |
|---|---|---|
| **Alpha-Humulene** | – | 0%–7% |
| **Limonene** | – | 1%–3% |
| **Bornyl Acetate** | – | < 3% |
| **Linalool** | – | < 1% |
| **Linalool Esters** | – | < 1% |

**REPORTED THERAPEUTIC PROPERTIES: Antiseptic, antibacterial, antiviral,** antifungal, anti-inflammatory, antispasmodic, astringent, decongestant, expectorant, expels excess mucus, reduces excess sweating, **immune booster,** helps balance hormones, diuretic, wound healing, promotes fat utilization, nervine (calms and soothes the nerves), muscle relaxant, helps normalize bone remodeling, **aids memory,** mentally stimulating

**CAUTIONS:**

■ Avoid with children under 6 due to thujone, 1,8-cineole, and camphor content. Cases of seizure have been reported in young children due to sage essential oil exposure or other oils rich on thujones. [7792,7793,7794] Several cases of camphor poisoning and/or seizures from ingestion and topical application have been reported in children.[7795,7796] Ingestion of camphor-containing products has been lethal in children under age 2 (estimated to be roughly 2,000 mg of camphor for a 20 kg child as the minimum potential fatal dose).[7797,7798] 1,8-cineole may cause seizures, central nervous system problems, or respiratory distress in young children.[7799,7800,7801,7802] Children 6 years and up may use sage essential oil topically in dilutions no stronger than 5%.

■ Avoid during pregnancy and while lactating. Camphor ingestion may lead to abortion because fetuses lack the enzymes to process it.[7803] Essential oils high in thujone content may cause abortion.[7804,7805,7806] Camphor ingestion by infants and young children may cause cough, vomiting, seizure, burning sensation in the mucous membranes and eyes, or lack of voluntary coordination of muscle movements.[7807]

■ Avoid oral consumption. Thujone is considered significantly neurotoxic and may damage the liver, and it is estimated that as little as 15 mg orally may negatively impact the central nervous system.[7808,7809,7810] As few as 12 drops of sage oil (high in thujones) orally have reportedly caused a seizure and short coma in an adult.[7811] Camphor can be toxic when taken orally (usually single doses exceeding 2 mL), although the lethal dose for adult humans is estimated to be more than 5 mL in a single dose.[7812,7813,7814]

■ Avoid with epilepsy and Parkinson's disease due to camphor, thujone, and 1,8-cineole content.[7815,7816,7817,7818,7819]

■ The potentially high camphor content in various sage CTs may negatively impact red blood cells and increase the risk of jaundice in children with Glucose-6-phosphate dehydrogenase deficiency (G6PD).[7820,7821]

■ Avoid with those who have a compromised liver or kidneys due to the risk of kidney toxicity, kidney failure, or liver toxicity.[7822,7823,7824] Consuming extremely large amounts of thujone-rich essential oils (10 mL) has caused kidney failure.[7825] This would also suggest that those taking medications that could cause liver damage should also use sage very cautiously or avoid it entirely.

■ Chemotypes high in 1,8-cineole may interfere with pentobarbital and other barbiturates (medications for anxiety and insomnia).[7826,7827]

■ May interact with diabetes medications and cause low blood-sugar levels.[2049]

■ May weakly interfere with the enzymes responsible for metabolizing medications (NSAIDs, proton-pump inhibitors, acetaminophen, antiepileptics, immune modulators, blood-sugar medications, blood pressure medications, antidepressants, antipsychotics, diabetic medications, antihistamines, antibiotics, and anesthetics) due to 1,8-cineole and alpha-thujone content.[7828,7829,7830,7831]

**SELECTED EVIDENCE:**

☐ Sage essential oil enhances cognitive performance in both healthy individuals and people with dementia or cognitive impairments according to a review of eight clinical studies.[7832,7833]

☐ An *in vitro* study concluded that sage promotes the destruction (apoptosis) of three melanoma cancer cell lines.[7834] Other research has found that it destroys leukemia, melanoma, and kidney cancer cells *in vitro*.[7835]

☐ Sage oil inhibits oral squamous cancer cell growth *in vitro*.[7836]

☐ *In vitro* research found that sage oil inhibits several microorganisms responsible for urinary tract infections (100% efficiency against *Klebsiella* and *Enterobacter* species, 96% against *E. coli*, 83% against *P. mirabilis*, and 75% against *M. morganii*).[7837]

- A topical cream that contains St. John's wort, olive oil, *Origanum tourn*, and sage oil stimulated the various stages of the wound healing process and demonstrated remarkable wound healing properties in mice and rats.[7838]
- An *in vitro* study concluded that sage oil significantly inhibits *E. coli*, *S. typhi*, *S. enteritidis*, and *S. sonnei*, and reduced lipid peroxidation.[2472] Other research reports it effectively inhibits *P. aeruginosa in vitro*.[7839]
- Sage oil reduces inflammation by inhibiting the excess production of nitric oxide without harming cells *in vitro*.[7840]
- Animal research suggests that sage oil may protect against osteoporosis by inhibiting osteoclast (cells that break down bone tissue to release minerals into the circulatory system) activity and normalizing bone turnover.[7841]
- *In vitro* research concluded that sage oil significantly inhibited *T. rubrum*, *E. floccosum*, and *C. neoformans*.[7842] Sage oil disrupts the cytoplasmic membrane integrity of MRSA epidermidis, and enhances the effectiveness of oxacillin (a penicillin antibiotic that treats bacterial infections) against MRSA.[7843] It inhibits *S. aureus* and prevents the formation of biofilms, which caused the researchers to determine it was a potential surface sanitizer.[7844]
- Sage oil may reduce the risk of denture stomatitis (an oral infection of *Candida* or thrush that causes inflammation of oral mucous membranes that primarily affects denture wearers or those who don't practice appropriate oral care) because it kills *C. albicans* and inhibits its adhesion to resinous surfaces *in vitro*.[7845]
- Diffusion of 0.25 mL of sage oil in a room (for one, six, and twenty-four hours) disinfected the room of total airborne microbes (up to 73%) and yeasts and molds (up to 55%).[7846]
- Sage oil increased cell sensitivity to insulin and prevented the production of sugar from noncarbohydrate sources within the body (gluconeogenesis) similar to the diabetes drug metformin in animals and *in vitro*.[7847] The researchers concluded that sage is a promising option to reduce the risk of type 2 diabetes.
- Inhaling a combination of peppermint, artemisia, sage, lavender, and monarda improved the symptoms of people with chronic bronchitis being treated with standard options concurrently.[7848]
- Sage essential oil inhibited *C. albicans*, *C. parapsilosis*, *C. krusei* (standard species), and *C. albicans* and *C. glabrata* (isolated from patients) with comparable efficacy to synthetic antifungal drugs *in vitro*.[7849]
- Sage essential oil protected (1,8-cineole CT) rats against liver toxicity caused by Co-amoxiclav (an antibiotic associated with liver toxicity).[7850]
- The addition of plant growth-promoting rhizobacteria (PGPR) during growing stages enhances the production of essential oils in sage and leads to improved antioxidant and antimicrobial activity.[7851]
- Sage essential oil CT camphor demonstrated significant insecticidal activity against *Spodoptera littoralis* larvae and *Tribolium castaneum* adults.[7852]
- *In vitro* research demonstrates that sage essential oil CT camphor inhibits gram-positive bacteria (*S. aureus*, *M. luteus*, *B. cereus*, and *B. subtilis*), and fungi (*A. niger*, *A. flavus*, and *A. alternata*), and mildly inhibits gram-negative bacteria (*E. coli*, *S. enteritidis*, and *A. tumefaciens*).[7853] Another study concluded that sage essential oil CT alpha-thujone inhibited *E. coli*, *S. aureus*, and *C. albicans*.[7854]
- Oral administration of 15 mg/kg body weight of the alpha-thujone CT of sage essential oil significantly reduced kidney toxicity (restored biochemical markers and reduced pathological lesions) caused by vanadium in rats.[7855]
- An unidentified CT of sage effectively killed *Varroa destructor*, an external parasitic mite that attacks honeybees.[7856]
- Sage essential oil CT camphor or alpha-thujone demonstrated good antioxidant activity but lower than the synthetic antioxidant BHT.[7857,7858]
- Individual constituents of sage essential oil inhibit lipoxygenase and acetylcholinesterase activity (enzymes associated with inflammation and Alzheimer's disease).[7859]
- The alpha-thujone chemotype of sage essential oil (four separate samples) demonstrated moderate antioxidant, insecticidal, anti-inflammatory (inhibit LOX, bornyl acetate and limonene demonstrated the highest inhibition of the individual constituents tested), and anti-Alzheimer activity (inhibit AChE, with essential oils higher in 1,8-cineole demonstrating the greatest inhibition). The same researchers reported that the four sage essential oils tested inhibited *E. coli*, *S. aureus*, and *C. albicans*.[7860]
- Injection of sage essential oil (acute: 1.2 mL/kg body weight; subacute: 0.8 mL/kg; three days per week, for two weeks) in mice prevented modulate testicular genetic (DNA) damage and histological (distortion of testis) alteration caused by carbon tetrachloride.[7861]
- The 1,8-cineole CT of sage essential oil significantly inhibited *S. aureus* biofilm formation when used at its minimum inhibitory concentration (MIC).[7862]
- Sage essential oil demonstrated greater antioxidant activity than clary sage in laboratory research.[7863]
- Thyme CT gamma-terpinene and sage CT beta-caryophyllene both inhibited *Fusarium graminearum* and

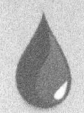

demonstrated a synergistic antifungal activity when used together.[7864] The same study found that both oils exhibited antiproliferative activity against two melanoma lines (A375 human melanoma and B164A5 mouse melanoma) alone and in combination, with sage being the most effective.

☐ Oral administration of sage essential oil (0.1, 0.2, and 0.4 mL/kg body weight, for two weeks, five times per week) protected the liver and kidneys against damage (lowered liver enzymes, bilirubin, urea, creatinine, lipid peroxidation, DNA breakage levels; increased total protein, albumin, globulin, prothrombin, and glutathione S transferase; and repaired the histo-architectural distortions) caused by carbon tetrachloride.[7865] The composition of the sage essential oil obtained from Egyptian sage leaves was not reported.

☐ Oregano CT carvacrol and sage CT alpha-thujone inhibited the growth and biofilm formation of *S. pyogenes*, which caused the study authors to conclude that they are potential "plant-derived antimicrobial agents in the management of streptococcal pharyngitis [strep throat]."[7866]

☐ Sage essential oil showed larvicidal activity against the *Ae. aegypti* mosquito.[7867]

☐ Oral administration of sage CT alpha-thujone reduced hyperglycemia by 60 percent, stored glycogen in the liver by 43.7 percent, and alleviated metabolic and tissue impairments caused by diabetes (protected liver and kidney function and reduced obesity) in rats.[7868]

☐ Male infertility is at least a contributing factor in infertility about 61 percent of the time due to low quantity (sperm count) or poor quality (decreased mobility, vitality, and sperm morphology) sperm.[7869] Sage essential oil (composition not reported) improved motility of human spermatozoa in laboratory research, suggesting it may increase the success of *in vitro* fertilization.[7870]

☐ Sage CT alpha-thujone, garlic, and rosemary CT 1,8-cineole essential oil were toxic to adults blowflies (*C. vomitoria*) by direct topical and fumigant activity.[7871] The same oils exerted antimicrobial activity against *B. subtilis, S. aureus, E. coli, C. albicans, P. aeruginosa,* and *S. enterica.*

☐ Oral administration of sage CT 1,8-cineole essential oil (4 mg/kg body weight dissolved in 100 mcL of corn oil by gavage) reduced high cholesterol, weight gain, disruption of liver and kidney functions, and production of free radicals (reactive oxygen species) in mice fed a high-fat diet.[7872] Remarkably, sage oil reduced high cholesterol better than simvastatin.

☐ Rosemary CT 1,8-cineole, oregano (*Th. capitatus*) CT carvacrol, marjoram, and sage CT alpha-thujone demonstrated promising antibacterial activity against bacteria (*P. aeruginosa, E. coli, S. enterica, B. subtilis,* and *S. aureus*) responsible for healthcare-associated infections and foodborne illnesses.[7873] Oregano exhibited the strongest activity, which exceeded gentamicin in effectiveness.

☐ Topical application of the alpha-thujone CT of sage essential oil accelerated the wound healing process by reducing the expression of proinflammatory cytokines (IL-6, IL-1β and TNF-α), accelerating growth factors (cellular proliferation, revascularization, collagen deposition, and re-epithelialization), and enhancing total antioxidant capacity.[7874]

☐ Sage CT alpha-thujone and sweet basil CT linalool both inhibited clinically isolated *P. aeruginosa* biofilm formation and motility suggesting they are highly efficient antipseudomonal agents that could be used in acute and chronic infections.[7875]

☐ Sage essential oil exhibited antiproliferative effects against three human colon cancer cell lines.[7876]

☐ Oral administration of sage essential oil (15 mg/kg body weight by gavage) significantly protected rats against oxidative damage and histological changes in the liver caused by vanadium (a metal linked to liver damage).[7877] The protective effect of the oil was attributed to its ability to modulate the activity of detoxification enzymes and scavenge free radicals.

☐ The camphor CT of sage essential oil exhibited good antioxidant activity in the ABTS and lipid peroxidation assays and inhibited BChE (butyrylcholinesterase) activity, suggesting it may have antidementia properties.[7878]

☐ Sage essential oil exhibited moderate activity against bovine viral diarrhea virus (BVDV), an enveloped RNA virus that causes significant disease in cattle.[7879] Of sage's major constituents, alpha-humulene was the most active—and more potent than the whole oil—followed by beta-caryophyllene.

☐ Three separate sage CT camphor essential oils exhibited good antioxidant activity in the DPPH, ABTS, beta-carotene bleaching, and FRAP assays, with the oil having the highest beta-pinene content being the most effective.[7880] In addition, the oils inhibited AChE and BChE.

☐ *In vitro* research showed that marjoram, rosemary CT 1,8-cineole, sage CT camphor, and pulegone CT limonene/piperitone inhibited *L. monocytogenes* and *Salmonella enterica* and displayed antioxidant activity in the DPPH assay.[7881]

☐ The 1,8-cineole CT of sage essential oil (less than 4% thujones) exhibited liver protective properties (reduced liver enzymes and significantly increased protein levels) in rats compared to rats that received acetaminophen only.[7882] Sage essential oil's effects were similar to that of silymarin. The oil also reduced creatinine,

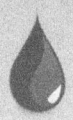 

cholesterol, and triglycerides in rats. *In vitro* experiments showed an increase in total antioxidant capacity, reduced malondialdehyde, and improved cell viability.

☐ The spotted wing drosophila (*Drosophila suzukii*) is a significant fruit fly pest of thin-skinned fruit crops. Rosemary essential oil exhibited high toxicity against fruit fly adults, larvicidal activity, and isolated dry residues of alpha-pinene, 1,8-cineole, and camphor provided poor repellent activity.[7883]

☐ Comparison of Serbian CT alpha-pinene and Russian CT 1,8-cineole rosemary essential oil found that the Serbian oil possessed significantly higher antimicrobial activity, but the Russian oil was a better antioxidant in sunflower oil during frying.[7884]

☐ Sage essential oil (composition not reported) inhibited oral cariogenic (*S. mutans*) and periodontopathic bacteria (*P. gingivalis*).[7885]

☐ Viridiflorol CTs of sage essential oil (17.7%–33.1% viridiflorol, 8.6%–19.5% camphor, 6.7%–10.4% borneol, 3.5%–12.2% alpha-thujone, 3.7%–4.6% beta-thujone) displayed antioxidant activity in the DPPH, CUPRAC, FRAP, ABTS, HRSA and, TBARS assays, was toxic to cervical, lung, and colorectal cancer cells, and inhibited *S. aureus, E. coli, B. subtilis, P. aeruginosa, C. albicans*, and *A. niger*.[7886]

☐ The 1,8-cineole CT of sage essential oil (39.2% 1,8-cineole, 12.8% beta-caryophyllene, 10.3% alpha-terpineol) remarkably inhibited antibiotic-resistant *S. enterica*.[7887]

☐ After screening thirty-two essential oils for larvicidal activity against the early fourth larvae of *Culex pipiens* mosquitoes, researchers found that garlic CT (Z)-9-octadecenamide, dill, fennel CT estragole, black cumin, sage CT terpinen-4-ol, thyme CT 2-ethynyl-3-hydroxypyridine, and violet leaf were highly effective, and frankincense (*B. serrata*), cumin, and wild turmeric were moderately effective.[7888]

☐ A lab hydrodistilled sage essential oil with 1,8-cineole (18.0%), borneol (15.9%), beta-pinene (10.5%), alpha-thujone (8.7%), camphene (8.7%), and alpha-humulene (8.6%) as major constituents was evaluated for its biological activity in laboratory and humans.[7889] It exhibited a moderate antioxidant capacity in the DPPH and ABTS assays. As part of the human study, 174 hospitalized subjects aged twenty-three to eighty-five years diagnosed with a chronic condition who had been previously hospitalized at least once were randomized to inhale sage oil or to the control group (only routine care). Two drops of sage oil were added to a cotton ball that was kept on the subject's pillow for a minimum of thirty minutes. Subjects' perception of the quality of in-hospital services and their overall well-being were evaluated via questionnaire. More people in the aromatherapy group rated the services as excellent or very good when compared to the control group (76 percent and 64 percent, respectively), but the results were not considered statistically significant.

☐ Acetylcholine is an important cholinergic neurotransmitter and neuromodulator involved in various functions throughout the body, but particularly in the nervous system. It works by attaching to receptors and sending signals between nerves. Acetylcholine has multiple functions in the body including motor neuron function (muscular movement), dilation of blood vessels, motivation, attention, learning, and memory. The activity and function of the cholinergic system is controlled by the enzymes acetylcholinesterase (AChE) and butyrylcholinesterase (BChE). People with neurodegenerative conditions make less acetylcholine and experience excessive BChE activity. Inhibition of AChE and BChE are targets for the treatment of neurodegenerative conditions. The outgrowth of neurites (called neuritogenesis—the formation of any projection from neurons) occurs during brain development and when neurons are regenerated. These outgrowths of dendrites or axons allow neurons to form networks and connections and communicate with other cells and ultimately maintain youthful brain function. A preclinical model of Alzheimer's disease evaluated essential oils from the *Lamiaceae* family for their effects on brain function and brain cell protection.[7890] Oregano CT alpha-terpineol, peppermint, rosemary CT 1,8-cineole, and sage essential oils each inhibited BChE activity. The carvacrol CT of oregano inhibited both BChE and AChE activity. Isolated linalool from lavender significantly reduced reactive oxygen species (ROS) inside neurons, suggesting it can protect against oxidative stress and death of neurons. In addition, oregano CT alpha-terpineol, peppermint, rosemary, and sage triggered neurite outgrowth, with the greatest activity observed from oregano. The researchers concluded that these oils have properties that could potentially prevent or delay dementia-related diseases.

☐ The chemical element vanadium has been shown to accelerate the production of reactive oxygen species, which may result in testicular dysfunction or damage. A rat model showed that vanadium significantly reduced the weight of reproductive organs, serum testosterone levels, and sperm health (number and motility).[7891] In addition, vanadium increased the oxidation of lipids and proteins as well as the activities of antioxidant enzymes in the testes and seminal vesicles, demonstrating vanadium toxicity. However, oral administration of sage essential oil improved all these parameters, suggesting it can reduce damage to the male reproductive system caused by vanadium.

☐ Sage essential oil extracted from plants harvested at different stages——was evaluated for their antioxidant,

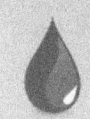

antidiabetic, and anti-inflammatory activity.[7892] Sage (20.8% naphthalenone, 14.4% camphor, 10.8% 1,8-cineole, 9.6% beta-caryophyllene) extracted from plants harvested at the full flowering stage showed the best antioxidant activity. It also demonstrated important antidiabetic (based on inhibition of alpha-amylase, alpha-glucosidase, and lipase) and anti-inflammatory (5-LOX inhibition) activity. All three oils exhibited strong antibacterial activity against *L. monocytogenes, S. aureus, B. subtilis, P. mirabilis, E. coli*, and *S. typhimurium*.

◻ Sage CT alpha-thujone essential oil demonstrated acetylcholinesterase, tyrosinase, inhibitory activity *in vitro*, suggesting it may benefit Alzheimer's disease and hyperpigmentation of the skin.[7893]

◻ Thyme CT carvacrol, sage CT beta-thujone, and apple mint CT piperitenone oxide were insecticidal to the medfly (*Ceratitis capitata*) and larvicidal to the tomato leafminer (*Tuta absoluta*), with apple mint being the most effective.[7894]

# SANDALWOOD

*Santalum album* L.; *S. paniculatum* Hook. & Arn.;
*S. spicatum* A. DC. (syn. *Fusanus spicatus* R.Br.);
*S. austrocaledonicum* Vieill.

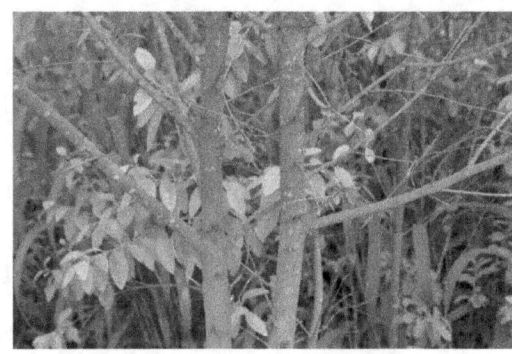

**FAMILY:** Santalaceae
**NOTE:** Base
**AROMA INTENSITY:** Medium
**AROMA:** Woody, earthy, slightly balsamic
**COMMON EXTRACTION METHOD:** Steam distilled from the wood
**POSSIBLE SUBSTITUTE OILS:** Cedarwood, lavender
**BLENDS WELL WITH:** Basil, bergamot, black pepper, blue cypress, cardamom, cedarwood, chamomile (German, Roman), coriander, cypress, frankincense, juniper, lavender, myrrh, neroli, palo santo, palmarosa, patchouli, petitgrain, ravensara, rose, Spanish sage, vetiver, ylang ylang
**SUBCELLULAR LOCALIZATION | EPIGENETIC INFLUENCE:** Endocytic Vesicles | Circulatory/Respiratory
**RECOMMENDED DILUTION RANGE:** 3%–33%; neat for limited conditions

**PRIMARY CONSTITUENTS:**[7895,7896,7897,7898,7899,7900,7901,7902,7903,7904,7905,7906]

| *S. album (East Indian)* | | *S. paniculatum (Hawaiian)* | |
|---|---|---|---|
| (Z)-Alpha-Santalol | 40.4%–57.1% | (Z)-Alpha-Santalol | 39.8%–42.6% |
| (Z)-Beta-Santalol | 20.3%–30.5% | (Z)-Beta-Santalol | 13.7%–16.2% |
| (Z)-Alpha-Trans-Bergamotol | 2.2%–17.2% | (Z)-Alpha-Trans-Bergamotol | 4.2%–5.1% |
| (Z)-Epi-Beta-Santalol | 4.9%–11.2% | (Z)-Epi-Beta-Santalol | 3.1%–4.2% |
| Beta-Santalene | 0.9%–5.9% | (Z)-Nuciferol | 3.2%–4.8% |
| (Z)-Nuciferol | 1.8%–5.2% | | |

| *S. austrocaledonicum (New Caledonian, Pacific Island)*[#] | | *Santalum spicatum (West Australian)* | |
|---|---|---|---|
| (Z)-Alpha-Santalol | 28.9%–48.4% | (E,E)-Farnesol | 9.3%–38.7% |
| (Z)-Beta-Santalol | 13.5%–22.0% | (Z)-Alpha-Santalol | 5.5%–27.3% |
| (Z)-Lanceol | 0.0%–9.1% | Alpha-Bisabolol | 4.9%–10.7% |
| (Z)-Alpha-Trans-Bergamotol | 0.2%–9.0% | (Z)-Beta-Santalol | 2.1%–10.5% |
| (Z)-Nuciferol | 1.6%–8.7% | Beta-Curcumene-12-ol | 0.0%–7.2% |
| (Z)-Epi-Beta-Santalol | 1.9%–5.4% | (Z)-Nuciferol | 5.6%–6.5% |

[#] Chemotypes high in (Z)-Nuciferol (7-25%) and (Z)-Lanceol (15-41%) may also be found among New Caledonian sandalwood essential oil samples. Some scientists consider *S. austrocaledonicum* var. *glabrum* (Loyalty Sandalwood) essential oil a true substitute for East Indian sandalwood essential oil because it meets the ISO 3518 standards for *S. album* santalol content ((Z)-alpha-santalol—44.3%–47.4% and (Z)-beta-santalol—19.4%–21.3%), but it also has higher (Z)-lanceol content like Australian sandalwood. New Caledonian is more likley to have a constiuent profile that more closely matches East Indian sandlwood quality, followed by Hawaiian sandalwood.

**OTHER CONSTITUENTS:** *Santalum album (East Indian)*—Para-benzoquinone, alpha-santalene, teresantalol, epi-beta-santalene, 2-carene, alpha-curcumene, (E)-beta-santalol, cis lanceol; *Santalum paniculatum (Hawaiian)*—E-nerolidol, beta-bisabolol, alpha-bisabolol, (Z)-lanceol, (Z)-gamma-curcumen-12-ol, z-beta-curcumene-12-ol, alpha-santalene, beta-santalene, epi-beta-santalene, alpha-santalol; *Santalum austrocaledonicum (New Caledonian, Pacific Island Sandalwood)*—Beta-santalene, epi-beta-santalene, alpha-curcumene, epi-beta-santalol, alpha-santalol, alpha-bisabolol, dihydro-alpha-santalol, (E,E)-farnesol, campherenol, epi-alpha-santalol, (Z)-gamma-curcumene-12-ol, (Z)-gamma-bisabolen-12-ol, spirosantalol, beta-bisabolol, epi-beta-bisabolol; *Santalum spicatum (West Australian)*—(Z)-beta-curcumene-12-ol, (Z)-alpha-trans-bergamotol, (Z)-gamma-curcumen-12-ol, bisabola-2,10-dien-6,13-diol, dendrolasin, (Z)-lanceol, beta-bisabolol, epi-beta-bisabolol, (Z)-12-hydroxy-sesquicineole, alpha-santalene, beta-curcumene, beta-santalene, guaiol

## PREFERRED COMPOSITION FOR CLINICAL USE:

| Constituent | East Indian | New Caledonian | Loyalty | Hawaiian | West Australian |
|---|---|---|---|---|---|
| **(Z)-Alpha-Santalol** | 40%–55% | 40%–50% | 40%–50% | 35%–50% | 14%–32% |
| **(Z)-Beta-Santalol** | 15%–30% | 15%–25% | 15%–25% | 12%–20% | 5%–20% |
| **(Z)-Epi-Beta-Santalol** | 3%–11% | 2%–6% | 2%–6% | 2%–6% | 0.5%–4% |
| **(Z)-Alpha-Trans-Bergamotol** | 3%–11% | 3%–10% | 3%–10% | 0.5%–10% | 0.1%–10% |
| **(Z)-Nuciferol** | 0.5%–6% | 2%–10% | 2%–10% | 2%–13% | 5%–22% |
| **Farnesol <E,E + E,Z>** | – | – | – | – | 2%–22%* |
| **α-Bisabolol + epi-α-Bisabolol** | – | – | – | – | 4%–15% |
| **(Z)-Lanceol** | 0.5%–5% | 5%–12% | 5%–15% | 1%–10% | 0.5%–10% |

* Lower (E,E)-Farnesol/(E,Z)-Farnesol content is preferred because it typically indicates higher alpha- and beta-santalol content. In addition, (E,E)-Farnesol is considered a skin irritant that may promote sensitization.

**REPORTED THERAPEUTIC PROPERTIES:** Analgesic (pain relief), antiseptic, antispasmodic, astringent, antibacterial, anti-inflammatory, antitumor, stimulates lymph drainage, expels excess gas, antineuralgic, reduces fever, **tones and strengthens the cardiovascular system**, disinfectant, reduces the appearance of scars and blemishes, **relieves skin conditions** (especially those that involve inflammation), decongestant, **eases cough**, diuretic, **nourishes and softens skin**, helps lower high blood pressure, **antifungal**, sedating, aids concentration and memory, **aphrodisiac**, grounding, reduces aggressive behavior, encourages acceptance, stress management, reduces irritability and despondency, diminishes guilt

## CAUTIONS:

■ West Australian sandalwood may interfere (very low risk) with enzymes responsible for metabolizing medications based on alpha-bisabolol content (NSAIDs, proton-pump inhibitors, acetaminophen, antiepileptics, immune modulators, blood-sugar medications, blood pressure medications, antidepressants, antipsychotics, diabetic medications, antihistamines, antibiotics, and anesthetics).[2076] This difference from other sandalwood species is likely due to the presence of farnesol, which weakly induces CYP enzymes, and alpha-bisabolol (inhibits CYP enzymes).[7907]
■ West Australian sandalwood may interact with antibiotics and/or antifungals and possibly increase their effectiveness based on farnesol content.[7908]

## SELECTED EVIDENCE:

- ☐ Sandalwood kills bladder cancer cells according to *in vitro* research.[7909]
- ☐ *In vitro* research suggests that East Indian sandalwood essential oil may prevent skin cancer by reducing the progression of pre-cancerous cells to skin cancer cells and inhibition of UV-induced AP-1 activity (two major cellular mechanisms known to trigger skin cancer).[7910]
- ☐ *In vitro* research concluded that *S. album* oil prevented the replication of HSV-1 and HSV-2, with a stronger activity against HSV-1.[7911,7912] Another study determined that sandalwood oil possesses high levels of virucidal activity against both drug-resistant and non-drug-resistant HSV-1.[7913]
- ☐ Sandalwood helps decrease inflammation by strongly inhibiting the 5-lipoxygenase (5-LOX) enzyme that is involved in the inflammation response according to *in vitro* research.[7914]
- ☐ Topical application of S. album reduced the number and spread of skin papillomas (benign skin growths caused by the human papilloma virus, HPV, which may be a precursor to squamous cell skin cancer) in

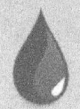

mice.[7915] Another study concluded that topical application of sandalwood oil prevented skin cancer caused by chemicals in mice.[7916]

☐ *In vitro* research suggests that sandalwood prevents the formation of proinflammatory molecules (cytokines, chemokines, prostaglandins, and COX enzymes) in skin cells in a similar manner to ibuprofen.[7917]

☐ Sandalwood oil inhibits P. falciparum (the parasite that causes malaria in humans) *in vitro*.[7918]

☐ Inhalation of sandalwood oil increased arousal, alertness, attentiveness, pulse rate, and blood pressure in humans.[7919]

☐ Massaging a 20% sandalwood oil to the lower abdomen of healthy people balanced autonomic nervous system function and created more harmonized states and moods (adaptogenic).[7920]

☐ Inhalation from personal aromasticks containing either bergamot and sandalwood, or frankincense, tangerine, and lavender improved sleep quality among cancer patients.[7921] Remarkably, 92% of study participants indicated they would continue to use their aromasticks for sleep improvement.

☐ Sandalwood (*S. album*) essential oil was toxic to the adult spotted wing drosophila (*Drosophila suzukii*) when in direct contact with the drosophila.[7922]

☐ A review concluded that East Indian sandalwood essential oil is useful in dermatology, and it shows promise in clinical trials for the treatment of acne, psoriasis, eczema, common warts, and molluscum contagiosum.[7923]

☐ *In vitro* examination of sixty essential oils demonstrated that sandalwood (Indian, Australian, and Hawaiian), melissa, lemongrass (*C. flexuosus*), cilantro, cassia, cinnamon, patchouli, and vetiver essential oils possess remarkable anticancer (two breast cancer cells) and antifungal (*Aspergillus niger, Candida albicans,* and *Cryptococcus neoformans*) activities.[7924]

☐ A combination of sandalwood and myrrh essential oil displayed noteworthy antimicrobial activity against wound pathogens.[7925] This suggests the combination may be a good option for preventing wound infections and promoting healing.

☐ Doxorubicin is a chemotherapy drug associated with cardiotoxicity (which can occur within two to three days of its administration), limiting its usefulness as a cancer treatment. Administration of sandalwood with the doxorubicin protected rats against cardiotoxicity as determined by reduced cardiac injury biomarkers, heart rate anomalies, and inflammation, improved antioxidant activity, and reversing ECG changes and blood pressure.[7926]

☐ Gas gangrene is a potentially deadly condition that occurs when bacteria—usually *Clostridium perfringens* or *C. septicum*—gather in a wound that has no blood supply and produce toxins that release gas causing tissue death. Of the fifty-six essential oils tested, sandalwood (*S. austrocaledonicum*) essential oil exhibited the highest inhibition of *C. perfringens* or *C. septicum*, which was improved when combined with palmarosa oil.[7927] Other oils that demonstrated high activity—exceeding inhibition of one or more of the reference drugs (clindamycin, penicillin, ciprofloxacin, and a combination of clindamycin and penicillin)—include cinnamon leaf, patchouli, oregano CT carvacrol, lemongrass (*C. citratus*), palmarosa, Virginia cedarwood, thyme CT para-cymene, vetiver, and coriander.

☐ A study evaluated the chemical composition and antimicrobial (nine respiratory tract pathogens) activity of forty-nine commercial essential oils recommended for respiratory tract infections. Amyris, coriander, and sandalwood (*S. austrocaledonicum*) were identified as having the greatest activity.[7928] The oils tested were balsam fir, amyris, frankincense (*B. carterii*), elemi, caraway, camphor, cinnamon leaf, lime, bergamot, lemon, orange, myrrh, coriander, cypress, lemongrass (*C. citratus*), carrot seed, cardamom, eucalyptus (*E. globulus*), fennel, helichrysum, hyssop CT isopinocamphone, star anise, cedarwood (*J. virginiana*), bay laurel, lavender, lavandin (*L. burnati*), spike lavender, tea tree, cajeput, niaouli, peppermint, myrtle, basil CT methyl chavicol, marjoram, oregano CT carvacrol, pimento, pine, black pepper, rose, rosemary CT camphor, sage, clary sage, benzoin, clove bud, tagetes (*T. minuta*), thyme CT para-cymene, and ginger.

☐ Researchers evaluated the effects of inhaling lemon, sandalwood (*S. album*), and camphor essential oils on brain activity related to emotions and memory processing via electroencephalography (EEG).[7929] Participants engaged in a working memory task for two minutes and inhaled essential oils for two minutes. Task performance significantly improved after inhaling lemon essential oil and delta and theta band activation in the prefrontal cortex (anterior cingulate gyrus and orbitofrontal cortex, superior temporal gyrus, parahippocampal gyrus, and insula). Sandalwood inhalation resulted in beta and gamma band activation in the prefrontal cortex (cingulate gyrus), which suggests it may help maintain memory. While camphor oil did not significantly alter brain activity, participants rated the task difficulty as easier when they inhaled it.

# SARO
## (Mandravasarotra)

*Cinnamosma fragrans* Baillon

**FAMILY:** Canaellaceae
**NOTE:** Top
**AROMA INTENSITY:** Medium-Strong
**AROMA:** Medicinal, camphoraceous, fresh, slightly fruity/floral
**COMMON EXTRACTION METHOD:** Steam distilled from the leaves
**POSSIBLE SUBSTITUTE OILS:** Myrtle, eucalyptus, cajeput, white sage, rosewood, magnolia, lavender
**BLENDS WELL WITH:** Bay laurel, blue mallee, cypress, cajeput, camphor, eucalyptus, ginger, lavender, lemon, orange, peppermint, ravintsara, rosemary, spearmint, tangerine, tea tree
**SUBCELLULAR LOCALIZATION | EPIGENETIC INFLUENCE:** Currently unknown | Currently unknown
**RECOMMENDED DILUTION RANGE:** 3%–Neat

**PRIMARY CONSTITUENTS:**[7930]

| *1,8-Cineole CT* | | *Linalool CT* | |
|---|---|---|---|
| 1,8-Cineole | 47.3%–71.6% | Linalool | 72.5%–95.8% |
| Beta-Pinene | 2.1%–8.0% | | |
| Camphene | 1.2%–4.8% | | |
| 1-Terpineol | 2.1%–4.2% | | |
| Alpha-Pinene | 1.1%–3.5% | | |
| Sabinene | 1.8%–3.2% | | |

**OTHER CONSTITUENTS:** *1,8-Cineole CT*—delta-3-carene, myrcene, alpha-phellandrene, alpha-terpinene, limonene, beta-phellandrene, (Z)-beta-ocimene, (E)-beta-ocimene, para-cymene, terpinolene, cis-linalool oxide, linalool, bornyl acetate, (E)-2,6 dimethyl-3,7-octadien-2,6-diol, nerol, geraniol, alpha-copaene, beta-caryophyllene, alpha-humulene, germacrene D, delta-cadinene, cis-calamenene, caryophyllene oxide; *Linalool CT*—alpha-pinene, camphene, beta-pinene, sabinene, delta-3-carene, alpha-terpinene, limonene, (Z)-beta-ocimene, terpinolene, 1,8-cineole, cis-linalool oxide, trans-linalool oxide, camphor, terpinen-4-ol, 1-terpineol, nerol, geraniol, alpha-copaene, beta-cubebene, beta-caryophyllene, germacrene D, delta-cadinene, cadina-1,4-diene, cis-calamenene, caryophyllene oxide, 6-methyl-5-heptan-2-one

**PREFERRED COMPOSITION FOR CLINICAL USE:**

| Constituent | 1,8-Cineole CT | Linalool CT |
|---|---|---|
| **1,8-Cineole** | 40%–60% | 0.1%–2% |
| **Sabinene** | 5%–12% | 0.1%–2% |
| **Linalool** | 3%–12% | 70%–96% |
| **Limonene** | 3%–11% | 0.1%–2% |
| **Beta-Pinene** | 4%–10% | 0.1%–2% |
| **Alpha-Pinene** | 3%–7% | 0.1%–3% |
| **Alpha-Terpineol** | 2%–5% | – |
| **Terpinen-4-ol** | 1%–5% | 0.1%–3% |
| **Myrcene** | 0.5%–3% | – |

**THERAPEUTIC PROPERTIES:** Antibacterial, antifungal, antimicrobial, antiviral, antiparasitic, antiseptic, anti-inflammatory, analgesic, **soothes sore muscles**, supports immune function, eases cough, supports respiratory function, expels excess mucus, energizing, relieves anxiety, antidepressant

**CAUTIONS:**
*Linalool CT*
■ May interact with antifungal drugs and enhance their effectiveness based on linalool content.[7931]

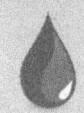

*1,8-Cineole CT*

■ Avoid with epilepsy and Parkinson's due to 1,8-cineole content, which may exacerbate or trigger seizures/convulsions or reduce medication efficacy.[7932,7933,7934]

■ Caution is warranted orally due to the significant amounts of 1,8-cineole. Limit it to small doses internally (adults—maximum 10 drops daily). One text recommends a maximum daily dose of 6 drops, whereas the European Medicines Agency recommends 2 to 4 drops (100–200 mg) of high 1,8-cineole essential oils orally, 2 to 5 times daily for adolescents, adults, and the elderly.[7935,7936] Additionally, 200 mg of isolated 1,8-cineole has been ingested three times daily for up to six months in clinical research.[7937,7938] Toxicity has been reported when eucalyptus (also high in 1,8-cineole) was ingested in large doses, and as few as 4 to 5 drops may cause problems in very sensitive individuals.[7939,7940,7941,7942,7943,7944] In humans, 3.5 to 5 mL has proven fatal orally.[7945]

■ May interfere with pentobarbital and other barbiturates (medications for anxiety and insomnia) based on 1,8-cineole content.[7946,7947]

■ May interact with diabetes medications and cause low blood sugar.[7948] Essential oils with significant 1,8-cineole content may reduce blood glucose levels by inhibiting alpha-glucosidase activity, particularly when synergized with other constituents (beta-pinene and alpha-pinene).[7949,7950,7951] Alpha-glucosidase is an enzyme that breaks down carbohydrates by chemical reaction with water. Inhibiting its activity postpones glucose absorption and therefore the impact of carbohydrates on blood sugar levels.

■ May weakly interfere with the enzymes responsible for metabolizing medications (NSAIDs, proton-pump inhibitors, acetaminophen, antiepileptics, immune modulators, blood-sugar medications, blood pressure medications, antidepressants, antipsychotics, diabetic medications, antihistamines, antibiotics, and anesthetics) due to 1,8-cineole content.[7952,7953,7954]

■ May interact with aspirin, blood pressure, antiplatelet, and anticoagulant medications, and increase the risk of bleeding among people with bleeding disorders (low risk).[7955] 1,8-cineole is a weak inhibitor of platelet aggregation.[7956]

**SELECTED EVIDENCE:**

☐ *In vitro* research demonstrates that both the 1,8-cineole and linalool CTs of saro essential oil singnificantly inhibit gram-positive (*S. aureus*, *B. subtilis*) bacteria, and moderately inhibit gram-negative bacteria (*S. typhimurium, E. coli, V. fisheri, C. anguillarum, V. harveyi, V. alinolyticus*) and fungi (*F. oxysporum*).[7957] Interestingly, the researchers reported that when they compared the antimicrobial activity of the whole essential oils against their primary constituents a synergistic and antagonistic effect was observed among the primary components (1,8-cineole and linalool respectively) and the minor components against gram-negative bacteria and fungi. Other research reports the 1,8-cineole CT of saro essential oil strongly inhibits a number of human pathogens (*B. cereus, C. neoformans, E. cloacae, K. pneumoniae, N, gonorrhoe, P. multicida, Sh. Sonnei, S. aureus, St. pneumoniae, T. rubrum, T. mucoides*), and moderately inhibits others (*A. dispar, C. albicans, E. coli, G. vaginalis, L. seeligeri, S. typhi*).[4701]

## SAVIN
### (Sabina, Savin Juniper)

*Juniperus sabina* L.

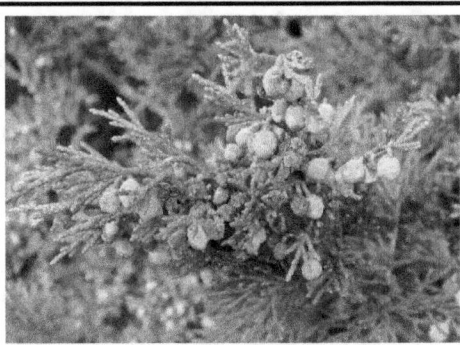

**FAMILY:** Coniferae (Cupressaceae)
**NOTE:** Middle
**AROMA INTENSITY:** Strong
**AROMA:** Unpleasant, pungent, herbaceous, piney
**COMMON EXTRACTION METHOD:** Steam distilled from the needles (leaves) and terminal branches or berries
**POSSIBLE SUBSTITUTE OILS:** Himalayan juniper, juniper berry, Phoenician juniper, Douglas fir, blue tansy, vilayti tulsi
**SUBCELLULAR LOCALIZATION | EPIGENETIC INFLUENCE:** Currently unknown | Currently unknown
**BLENDS WELL WITH:** Doesn't blend well with other essential oils due to its very unpleasant odor
**RECOMMENDED DILUTION RANGE:** < 0.5%

**PRIMARY CONSTITUENTS:**[7958,7959,7960,7961,7962]

| Needles & Branches | | Berries | |
|---|---|---|---|
| Sabinene | 18.3%–56.7% | Sabinene | 48.6%–82.9% |
| (E)-Sabinyl Acetate | 0.0%–54.4% | Myrcene | 5.8%–10.8% |
| Cedrol | 0.0%–15.9% | Alpha-Pinene | 5.0%–8.1% |
| Alpha-Pinene | 1.2%–15.8% | Alpha-Thujene | 0.0%–5.4% |
| Terpinen-4-ol | 1.1%–14.4% | Gamma-Terpinene | 0.6%–4.3% |
| Methyl Eugenol | 0.0%–12.1% | Terpinen-4-ol | 1.1%–4.3% |
| Beta-Thujone | 0.0%–8.7% | | |
| Elemol | 0.0%–8.3% | | |
| Safrole | 0.0%–6.6% | | |
| Citronellol | 0.1%–6.4% | | |
| Alpha-Terpinene | 0.3%–5.4% | | |
| Delta-Cadinene | 0.1%–5.4% | | |
| Alpha-Thujene | 0.6%–4.8% | | |
| Limonene | 0.6%–4.3% | | |
| Myrcene | 3.0%–4.2% | | |

Note: Savin essential oil is banned in the European Union and Canada as a cosmetic ingredient and can only be sold in a pharmacy (under the supervision of a licensed pharmacist) in the U.K.

**OTHER CONSTITUENTS:** Beta-pinene, beta-phellandrene, gamma-terpinene, cis-sabinene hydrate, alpha-thujone (< 0.5%), terpinolene, trans-sabinene hydrate, linalool, cis-p-menth-2-en-ol, trans-sabinol, methyl citronellate, methyl geranate, gamma-cadinene, elemicin, germacrene D-4-ol, alpha-cadinol, cis-ocimene, beta-elemene, trans-caryophyllene, germacrene D, cis-beta-elemone, T-cadinol, beta-oplopenone, linalyl acetate, pregeijerene, terpinyl acetate, geranyl acetate, caryophyllene oxide, gamma-eudesmol, alpha-eudesmol, sandaracopimara-8(14),15-diene, 2,6-Dimethyl-1,5-heptadien-4-ol acetate; *Berries*—limonene, alpha-terpinolene, beta-elemene, methyl eugenol (<2.7%)

**PREFERRED COMPOSITION FOR CLINICAL USE:**

| Constituent | Berries |
|---|---|
| **Sabinene** | 55%–70% |
| **Myrcene** | 5%–15% |
| **Alpha-Pinene** | 4%–10% |
| **Gamma-Terpinene** | 0.5%–5% |
| **Terpinen-4-ol** | 1%–4% |
| **Methyl Eugenol** | < 2.5% |

**REPORTED THERAPEUTIC PROPERTIES:** Antimicrobial, antiparasitic, anticancer, analgesic, antirheumatic, relieves blisters, wound healing, encourages menstruation, diuretic, removes warts, relieves headache, grounding, relaxing

**CAUTIONS:**

*Savin is not recommended for use in essential oil therapy in any form of administration, but the profile is included for informational purposes and safety information. The berries essential oil is much safer than the needles and branches essential oil.*

■ Avoid in children due to toxicity or cancer concerns from trans-sabinyl acetate, thujone, and methyl eugenol content.[7963,7964,7965,7966,7967,7968] Cases of seizure have been reported in young children due to exposure to essential oils high in thujones.[7969,7970,7971]

■ Avoid during pregnancy. Savin essential oil (containing 50% sabinyl acetate) is toxic to developing embryos and prevents implantation during days 0–4 of gestation according to animal research.[7972,7973] Other research using a Spanish Sage essential oil (containing 50% trans-sabinyl acetate) demonstrated trans-sabinyl acetate can cause abortions and maternal toxicity (which indicated a greater susceptibility to trans-sabinyl acetate toxicity during pregnancy) in animals.[7974] The researchers concluded that trans-sabinyl acetate possesses significant antifertility

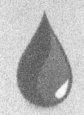

activity during the pre-implantation period, and attribute the fetotoxic and abortifacient activity of savin essential oil to this constituent. Very large doses of methyl eugenol may adversely affect the mother's liver and infant body weight according to animal research.[7975] Animal research suggests that methyl eugenol may cause changes in embryo form and structure and chromosomal changes in ovary cells, as well as multi-site cancerous tumors.[7976,7977,7978,7979] Essential oils high in thujone content may cause abortion.[7980,7981,7982] Animal research suggests that higher doses of safrole or myristicin (0.01 mL/kg every two days while nursing, and 0.001 to 10 mg while pregnant) taken orally during pregnancy and while nursing may cause liver toxicity in offspring born to the mother and increase the offspring's risk of liver cancer.[7983,7984]

■ Avoid oral consumption. Savin essential oil irritates the mucosal lining of the gastrointestinal tract, damages the kidneys, causes blood in the urine, obstructs blood flow in the abdominal organs, and causes abnormally heavy menstrual bleeding, which the study authors attributed to the combined effects of sabinene, sabinol, and trans-sabinyl acetate.[7985] However, more recent research suggests it is the trans-sabinyl acetate content of savin essential oil that causes toxicity and other adverse effects. Ingesting essential oils high in thujones can cause vomiting, stomachache, diarrhea, and gastroenteritis followed by absorption disorders, headache, nervous agitation, and chronic convulsions, and symptoms of liver and kidney toxicity extending to yellow liver atrophy (extensive and rapid death of liver cells—parenchymal, possibly accompanied by fatty degeneration), arrhythmia, and myocardial bleeding.[7986] Thujone is considered significantly neurotoxic and may damage the liver, and it is estimated that as little as 15 mg orally may negatively impact the central nervous system.[7987,7988,7989] Case reports involving serious adverse health outcomes (seizure, convulsions, and acute kidney failure) have been reported in adults who consumed high thujone essential oils (sage, thuja, wormwood) in doses of one "swallow," 12 drops, and 20 drops twice daily for five days.[7990,7991,7992,7993] Safrole and methyl eugenol can be toxic in large doses.[7994,7995,7996] Methyl eugenol may cause multisite cancerous tumors according to animal research.[7997,7998,7999,8000]

■ Avoid with epilepsy and Parkinson's disease due to thujone and trans-sabinyl acetate content.[8001,8002]

■ Avoid in those who have a compromised liver due to the increased risk of liver toxicity and liver damage.[8003,8004] This would also suggest that those taking medications that could cause liver damage should also use savin very cautiously or avoid it entirely.

■ Avoid with those who have compromised kidneys due to the risk of kidney toxicity or kidney failure.[8005]

■ May interact with antibiotics or antifungal drugs and possibly enhance their effects based on methyl eugenol content.[8006]

### SELECTED EVIDENCE:

☐ *In vitro* research shows that savin essential oil possesses weak antimicrobial activity against *Bacillus subtilis*, *Candida albicans*, *Escherichia coli*, and *Staphylococcus aureus*, which was significantly lower than gentamycin.[8007] Another study reported that savin essential oil prevented the growth (bacteriostatic activity of >12 mm) of *E. coli*, *Salmonella para*, *S. spomb*, *S. aureus* ATCC 25923, MRSA, and a clinical isolate of *S. aureus*.[8008]

☐ *In vitro* research demonstrates that savin essential oil weakly to moderately inhibits *Fusarium verticillioides* and *Fusarium graminearum*.[8009]

☐ Savin CT sabinene and low (E)-sabinyl acetate protected against liver damage—based on tissue study and liver enzymes levels—caused by carbon tetrachloride in rats.[8010] Its protective effects were similar to silymarin at the highest dose of 200 mg/kg body weight.

☐ The sabinene CT of savin essential oil inhibited *S. aureus*, *H. influenzae*, *Sh. sonnei*, *E. coli*, *S. pneumoniae*, and *Y. enterocolitica*.[8011] The oil was also insecticidal to two aphid species (Sitobion avenae and Rhopalosiphum padi) and exhibited antioxidant activity.

# SAVORY (WILD)
## (Acegrea)

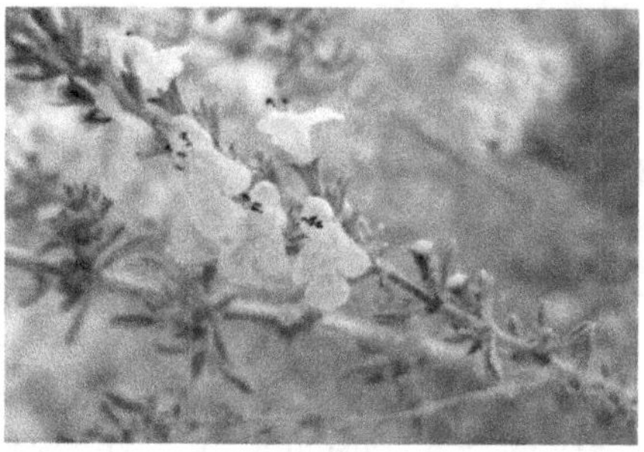

*Satureja cuneifolia* Ten., *Clinopodium cuneifolium* (Ten.) Kuntze

**FAMILY:** Lamiaceae (Labiatae)
**NOTE:** Middle
**AROMA INTENSITY:** Strong
**AROMA:** Herbaceous, medicinal, spicy
**COMMON EXTRACTION METHOD:** Steam distilled from the flowering aerial parts
**POSSIBLE SUBSTITUTE OILS:** Oregano, thyme (carvacrol CT), mountain savory
**BLENDS WELL WITH:** Ajowan, bergamot, grapefruit, lavender, lemon, lime, mountain savory, orange, oregano, pine, rosemary, tangerine, thyme
**SUBCELLULAR LOCALIZATION | EPIGENETIC INFLUENCE:** Currently unknown | Currently unknown
**RECOMMENDED DILUTION RANGE:** 1.5%–20%; 50% for some conditions

**PRIMARY CONSTITUENTS:**[8012,8013,8014,8015,8016,8017,8018]

*Carvacrol CT*

| | |
|---|---|
| Carvacrol | 17.7%–71.6% |
| Para-Cymene | 8.1%–31.2% |
| Thymol | 0.1%–15.7% |
| Gamma-Terpinene | 0.8%–14.8% |
| Linalool | 0.1%–6.6% |
| Limonene | 0.0%–6.2% |
| Borneol | 0.0%–4.2% |

*Thymol CT*

| | |
|---|---|
| Thymol | 22.0%–57.9% |
| Para-Cymene | 7.1%–24.3% |
| Carvacrol | 2.4%–19.0% |
| Gamma-Terpinene | 2.2%–18.7% |
| Thymoquinone | 0.0%–4.5% |

*Linalool CT*

| | |
|---|---|
| Linalool | 17.2%–18.2% |
| Carvacrol | 5.0%–16.3% |
| Para-Cymene | 1.8%–14.8% |
| Alpha-Pinene | 5.8%–12.0% |
| Limonene | 1.8%–11.0% |
| Beta-Caryophyllene | 2.8%–9.3% |
| Beta-Cubebene | 1.7%–9.1% |
| Borneol | 2.8%–7.6% |
| Terpinen-4-ol | 2.8%–6.4% |
| (Z)-Beta-Ocimene | 0.0%–4.2% |
| Gamma-Terpinene | 0.0%–4.1% |

Note: Other uncommon CTs of wild savory are also reported in the literature including alpha-pinene, borneol, alpha-pinene/borneol, beta-cubebene/limonene, ortho-cymene, and carvacrol/spathulenol.

**OTHER CONSTITUENTS:** *Carvacrol CT*—1-octene-3-ol, n-octanol, allo-ocimene, isoborneol, terpinen-4-ol, alpha-terpineol, myrtenol, geraniol, linalyl acetate, alpha-copaene, geranyl acetate, delta-cadinene, carvacrol methyl ether, beta-caryophyllene, 2,6-octadenal, alpha-phellandrene, alpha-pinene, beta-bisabolene, myrcene; *Thymol CT*—alpha-pinene, camphene, myrcene, alpha-terpinene, limonene, 1,8-cineole, (Z)-beta-ocimene, linalool, terpinen-4-ol, borneol, beta-bisabolene, caryophyllene oxide; *Linalool CT*—beta-pinene, myrcene, allo-ocimene, 1-octen-3-ol, sabinene hydrate, alpha-copaene, camphor, calarene, neral, alpha-terpineol, beta-bisabolene, delta-cadinene, nerol, geraniol, caryophyllene oxide, spathulenol, thymol

**PREFERRED COMPOSITION FOR CLINICAL USE:**

| Constituent | Carvacrol CT | Linalool CT |
|---|---|---|
| **Carvacrol** | 45%–60% | 5%–20% |
| **Para-Cymene** | 9%–22% | 5%–15% |
| **Thymol** | 5%–16% | 0.5%–3% |
| **Gamma-Terpinene** | 3%–9% | – |
| **Linalool** | 0.5%–5% | 15%–20% |

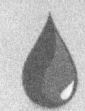

| Borneol | 1%–4% | 3%–10% |
|---|---|---|
| Alpha-Pinene | – | 5%–15% |
| Limonene | – | 2%–10% |
| Beta-Caryophyllene | – | 2%–10% |
| Terpinen-4-ol | – | 3%–8% |
| Beta-Cubebene | – | 1%–4% |

REPORTED THERAPEUTIC PROPERTIES: **Antibacterial**, antifungal, antiviral, **antimicrobial**, antioxidant, heals abscesses and bruises, eases cough, aids digestion, expels excess gas, immune stimulant, supports circulatory function, anti-inflammatory, analgesic, antiarthritic, relieves diarrhea, **aids cognition**, relieves intestinal cramps, expels excess mucus, soothes sore throat, reduces the appearance of scars, soothes insect bites/stings, insect repellent, reduces excess ego, combats fear, motivating

CAUTIONS:

■ *Carvacrol and Thymol CTs*: Avoid during pregnancy and lactation due to similar composition to oregano essential oil. Oils rich in carvacrol may negatively affect embryonic development and encourage fetal cell death according to animal research.[8019]

■ *Thymol CTs*: Oral caution. May contain up to 45.2% thymol. Thymol has a longer half-life (the time it takes for half of the medication to metabolize or excrete half of the dosage) than most essential oil constituents and should not be administered orally for long periods of time.[8020] Thymol is a monoterpene phenol. Reports of fatalities in children who consumed 50 to 200 mg of phenols has been reported.[8021] It is recommended that chemotypes with high levels of thymol be limited to 10 drops per day orally for adults with a two- to seven-day break after twenty-one days of use.

■ *Carvacrol CT*: May interact with diabetic medications and cause low blood-sugar levels based on carvacrol content.[8022,8023,8024]

■ *Carvacrol and Thymol CTs*: May interact with aspirin, blood pressure, antiplatelet, and anticoagulant medications, and increase the risk of bleeding among people with bleeding disorders due to thymol and carvacrol content.[8025,8026,8027]

■ *Carvacrol and Thymol CTs*: May interact with antibiotics and possibly enhance their effects due to thymol and carvacrol content.[8028]

■ *Carvacrol and Thymol CTs*: May interact with anticholinergic (drugs used for asthma, incontinence, gastrointestinal cramps, muscular spasms, depression, and sleep disorders) and cholinergic medications (drugs used to reduce urinary retention, diagnose myasthenia gravis, and for glaucoma) based on thymol content and research using the whole essential oil.[8029,8030]

■ *Carvacrol and Thymol CTs*: May irritate mucous membranes (eyes, mouth, nasal passages, vagina, rectum).

SELECTED EVIDENCE:

☐ *In vitro* research shows that wild savory essential oil (linalool CT) possesses broad-spectrum antimicrobial activity with maximum activity observed against *C. albicans, E. coli, Salmonella typhimurium, P. mirabilis, S. aureus,* and *B. cereus.*[8031] The carvacrol CT demonstrates antimicrobial activity against gram-positive (*S. aureus, B. cereus, S. lutea, L. monocytogenes*) and gram-negative (*P. aeruginosa, E. coli, C. jejuni, S. sonnei, S. enteritidis*) bacteria.[8032,8033] Wild savory essential oil (thymol CT) demonstrated moderate antimicrobial activity against *C. albicans.*[8034] An interesting ortho-cymene CT of wild savory inhibited the gram-negative bacteria *K. pneumoniae* that is associated with healthcare-acquired infections, including pneumonia, bloodstream infections, wound or surgical site infections, and meningitis.[8035] An odd beta-cubebene/limonene CT of wild savory essential oil (low in thymol and carvacrol) inhibited bacteria (*S. aureus, E. coli*, MRSA, *B. subtilis*) and fungi (*A. niger, C. albicans*).[8036]

☐ Wild savory essential oil (carvacrol CT) demonstrates remarkable antioxidant activity *in vitro.*[8037] The thymol CT of wild savory essential oil demonstrated good antioxidant activity and inhibited lipid peroxidation at almost the same effectiveness level as synthetic BHT.[8038]

☐ The carvacrol CT of wild savory essential oil kills *Legionella pneumophila*, which is responsible for Legionellosis infections (a bacterial disease of the respiratory system that could lead to pneumonia).[8039]

□ Wild savory essential oil strongly inhibited AChE and BChE enzyme activity (86.5% and 98.4% respectively), whereas thymol and carvacrol were less effective than the whole essential oil (28.4% and 70.3% respectively).[8040] Inhibition of AChE prevents the breakdown of acetylcholine, which is essential for memory and thinking. People with neurodegenerative diseases make less acetylcholine, and the diseases often break it down at a faster rate leading to acetylcholine deficits. Selective inhibition of BChE is also desirable in neurodegenerative diseases because it interferes with acetylcholine activity. In addition, BChE is often found in the plaques and tangles in the brains of people with Alzheimer's disease.[8041]

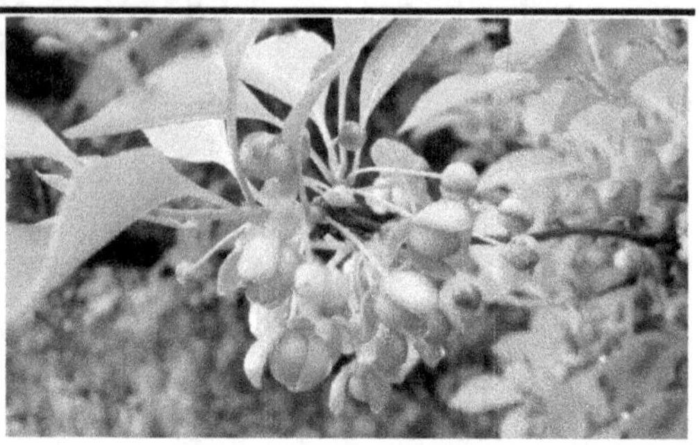

# SCHISANDRA FRUIT
## (Nan Wu-wei-zi, Wu Wei Zi)

*Schisandra sphenanthera* Rehd. et Wils.; *S. chinensis* (Turcz.) Baill.

**FAMILY:** Schisandraceae
**NOTE:** Middle
**AROMA INTENSITY:** Medium
**AROMA:** Sweet, fruity, slightly bitter-sour
**COMMON EXTRACTION METHOD:** Steam distilled from the fruits (berries); commonly CO2 extracted
**POSSIBLE SUBSTITUTE OILS:** Helichrysum, betony, hinoki, Formosan cypress, manuka, cedarwood
**BLENDS WELL WITH:** Bergamot, cassia, cinnamon, clove, geranium, ginger, grapefruit, lavender, lemon, lime, may chang, Mediterranean mandarin, orange, palmarosa, Persian lime, rose, tangerine, ylang ylang
**SUBCELLULAR LOCALIZATION | EPIGENETIC INFLUENCE:** Currently unknown | Currently unknown
**RECOMMENDED DILUTION RANGE:** 5%–Neat

**PRIMARY CONSTITUENTS:**[8042,8043,8044,8045,8046]

*S. sphenanthera, Delta-Cadinene CT*

| | |
|---|---|
| Delta-Cadinene | 25.6% |
| Beta-Himachalene | 19.8% |
| Alpha-Santalene | 10.1% |
| Unknown Cadinene Compound | 7.7% |
| Isocaryophyllene | 5.6% |
| Beta-Longifolene | 4.8% |

*S. chinensis*

| | |
|---|---|
| Ylangene | 37.7%–50.4% |
| Alpha-Himachalene | 8.8%–11.4% |
| Alpha-Bergamotene | 8.6%–10.5% |
| Beta-Chamigrene | 4.9%–6.6% |
| Calamenene | 2.1%–5.3% |
| Acoradiene | 1.8%–3.0% |

*S. sphenanthera, Alpha-Cadinene CT*

| | |
|---|---|
| Alpha-Cadinene | 18.3% |
| Alpha-Santalene | 13.0% |
| Beta-Himachalene | 11.4% |
| Cuparene | 8.7% |
| 3-Methylenecyclohexene | 4.4% |
| Alpha-Selinene | 3.8% |
| 15-Copaenol | 3.0% |
| Beta-Chamigrene | 3.0% |

**OTHER CONSTITUENTS:** *S. sphenanthera, Delta-Cadinene CT*—alpha-copaene, beta-chamigrene, gamma-muurolene, beta-bisabolene, gamma-elemene; *S. sphenanthera, Alpha-Cadinene CT*—alpha-copaene, isoledene, gamma-cadinene, alpha-caryophyllene, 2-isopropyl-5-methyl-9-methylene-bicyclo[4.4.0]dec-1-ene, delta-cadinene, beta-ionene, 3,7,11-trimethyl-3-hydroxy-6,10-dodecadien-1-yl acetate, epi-beta-santalene; *S. chinensis*—para-cymene, gamma-terpinene, thymol methyl ether, bornyl acetate, alpha-gurjunene, beta-farnesene, alpha-cedrene, bicyclogermacrene, alpha-muurolene, 2-tert-butyl-1,4-dimethoxybenzene, alpha-chamigrene, gamma-muurolene, cyclosativene, bicyclo[4.4.0]dec-1-ene,2-isopropyl-5-methyl-9-methylene-, isoledene, cuparene, delta-cadinene, gamma-himachalene, tricyclo[4.4.0.0(2,7)]dec-3-ene-3-methanol,1-methyl-8-(1,methylethyl)-

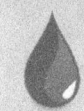

**PREFERRED COMPOSITION FOR CLINICAL USE:**

| Constituent | S. sphenanthera | S. chinensis |
|---|---|---|
| Delta-Cadinene | 20%–35% | – |
| Beta-Himachalene | 15%–25% | – |
| Alpha-Santalene | 10%–20% | – |
| Isocaryophyllene | 3%–9% | – |
| Beta-Longifolene | 2%–7% | – |
| Ylangene | – | 35%–50% |
| Alpha-Himachalene | – | 7%–15% |
| Alpha-Bergamotene | – | 7%–14% |
| Beta-Chamigrene | – | 3%–9% |
| Calamenene | – | 2%–7% |
| Acoradiene | – | 1%–5% |

**THERAPEUTIC PROPERTIES:** Anti-aging, antioxidant, antibacterial, antifungal, supports respiratory function, anti-inflammatory, liver protective/supportive, antiallergic, aids digestion, antidepressant, relieves mental fatigue, **stress management**, relieves anxiety

**CAUTIONS:**

■ None currently known.

**SELECTED EVIDENCE:**

□ *S. sphenanthera* essential oil (delta-cadinene CT) significantly killed liver cancer cells.[8047]

□ *In vitro* research demonstrates that schisandra fruit essential oil (*S. chinensis*) inhibits gram-positive (*S. epidermidis, S. aureus, B. subtilis*) and gram-negative (*E. coli, Ps. aeruginosa, Proteus vulgaris*) bacteria.[8048] Schisandra fruit essential oil (*S. sphenanthera*, delta-cadinene CT) strongly inhibtied gram-positive bacteria (*S. aureus, B. subtilis*) and the fungi (*S. cerevisiae*), but was ineffective against gram-positive bacteria (*E.coli, E. aerogenes*).[8049]

□ Schisandra fruit essential oil (*S. chinensis*) is a good antioxidant, demonstrating equivalent or greater antioxidant activity than the synthetic antioxidant BHT.[8050,8051,8052] On the contrary, *S. sphenanthera* (alpha-cadinene CT) essential oil displayed no antioxidant activity.[8053] Another study reported that *S. sphenanthera* (delta-cadinene CT) remarkably inhibited the production of malondialdehyde.[8054]

□ A schisandra fruit essential oil with Longiverbenone as the primary constituent exhibited good antioxidant activity in the DPPH, superoxide anion, and hydroxyl radical assays.[8055]

□ Schisandra (*S. chinensis*) essential oil exhibited antidepressant-like activity in a behavioral despair mouse model.[8056] Mice were randomly divided into four groups: control, oral fluoxetine, oral schisandra (250 mg/kg BW), and oral schisandra (750 mg/kg BW). Oral administration of schisandra oil improved oxidative stress (upregulated the PI3K/AKT/GSK3β signaling, and then promoted Nrf2/HO-1 pathway) and exerted antidepressant-like effects.

# SHELL GINGER
## (Shell Flower, Butterfly Ginger, Shellplant)

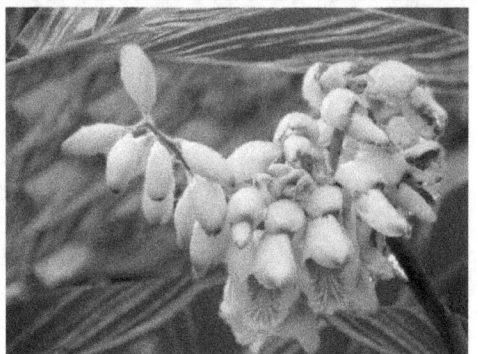

*Alpinia zerumbet* (Pers.) B.L. Burtt & R.M. Sm., *A. speciosa* (Wendl.) K. Schum., *A. nutans* (L.) Roscoe, *Catimbium speciosum* (Wendl.) Holttum, *Languas speciosa* (Wendl.) Merr.

**FAMILY:** Zingiberaceae
**NOTE:** Middle
**AROMA INTENSITY:** Medium
**AROMA:** Herbaceous, medicinal, fresh
**COMMON EXTRACTION METHOD:** Hydrodistilled from the leaves or aerial parts

**POSSIBLE SUBSTITUTE OILS:** Tea tree, marjoram, niaouli

**BLENDS WELL WITH:** Agarwood, cedarwood, chamomile (German, Roman), copaiba, davana, eucalyptus, geranium, kanuka, kunzea, lavender, manuka, rose, rosewood, sandalwood, tagetes, tea tree, wild chamomile, ylang ylang

**SUBCELLULAR LOCALIZATION | EPIGENETIC INFLUENCE:** Currently unknown | Currently unknown

**RECOMMENDED DILUTION RANGE:** 3%–50%; neat for limited conditions

**PRIMARY CONSTITUENTS:**[8057,8058,8059,8060,8061,8062]

*Terpinen-4-ol CT*

| | |
|---|---|
| Terpinen-4-ol | 17.3%–55.7% |
| 1,8-Cineole | 10.8%–23.1% |
| Gamma-Terpinene | 5.7%–16.1% |
| Sabinene | 1.4%–10.1% |
| Para-Cymene | 4.1%–5.9% |
| Alpha-Terpinene | 0.7%–4.7% |
| Alpha-Terpineol | 0.0%–4.2% |
| Beta-Pinene | 0.3%–4.3% |
| Alpha-Pinene | 0.0%–4.1% |

*p-Mentha-1,3-Dien-7-al CT*

| | |
|---|---|
| p-Mentha-1,3-Dien-7-al | 40.5% |
| Trans-Sabinene Hydrate | 15.4% |
| p-Mentha-4,8-Diene | 10.0% |
| Gamma-Terpinene | 4.1% |

*1,8-Cineole CT*

| | |
|---|---|
| 1,8-Cineole | 13.8%–37.8% |
| Para-Cymene | 0.0%–22.6% |
| Terpinen-4-ol | 0.0%–17.4% |
| Linalool | 0.0%–17.1% |
| Gamma-Terpinene | 0.0%–14.5% |
| Sabinene | 0.0%–12.5% |
| Caryophyllene Oxide | 5.0%–10.4% |
| 4-Carene | 0.0%–7.3% |
| Methyl Cinnamate | 4.2%–6.3% |
| Silvestrene | 0.0%–4.6% |
| Benzylacetone | 0.1%–4.2% |
| Alpha-Thujene | 0.0%–4.1% |

*Para-Cymene CT*

| | |
|---|---|
| Para-Cymene | 33.1% |
| 1,8-Cineole | 18.9% |
| Terpinen-4-ol | 18.8% |

Note: Spring crops will generally produce essential oil rich in p-Mentha-1,3-dien-7-al, whereas summer crops are rich in terpinen-4-ol. The 1,8-cineole CT may be obtained from the aerial parts of the plant, rather than just the leaves, and its composition varies greatly. An alpha-pinene chemotype is also reported in the literature, but no complete information on its full composition was available.

**OTHER CONSTITUENTS:** *Terpinen-4-ol CT*—limonene, myrcene, beta-caryophyllene, alpha-phellandrene, caryophyllene oxide, cis-sabinene hydrate, trans-sabinene hydrate, trans-p-menth-2-en-ol, linalool, camphor, trans-piperitol, ethyl isoborneol, alpha-eudesmol; *1,8-Cineole CT*—alpha-pinene, beta-pinene, myrcene, cis-beta-terpineol, 2,5-norbornadiene, cis-p-menth-2-en-ol, gamma-terpineol, 2-tert-butylphenyl pivalate, carvacrol, caryophyllene, 2,6-diethylnitrosobenzene, p-cymen-7-ol; *p-Mentha-1,3-Dien-7-al CT*—(Z)-3-hexenol, sabinene, myrcene, delta-2-carene, p-2menth-4,8-diene, p-cymenene, cis-beta-terpineol, thujyl alcohol, trans-beta-terpineol, neomenthol, cis-sabinene hydrate acetate, germacrene A, caryophyllene oxide; *Para-cymene CT*—alpha-thujene, sabinene, alpha-terpineol, beta-pinene, alpha-terpinolene, linalool, undecanone-2, beta-caryophyllene

**PREFERRED COMPOSITION FOR CLINICAL USE:**

| Constituent | Terpinen-4-ol CT |
|---|---|
| **Terpinen-4-ol** | 25%–45% |
| **1,8-Cineole** | 10%–25% |
| **Gamma-Terpinene** | 5%–20% |
| **Sabinene** | 3%–8% |
| **Para-Cymene** | 3%–7% |
| **Alpha-Terpinene** | 0.5%–5% |
| **Beta-Pinene** | 1%–6% |
| **Alpha-Pinene** | 0.5%–4% |
| **Alpha-Terpineol** | 0.5%–4% |
| **Limonene** | 0.1%–3% |
| **Beta-Caryophyllene** | 0.1%–3% |

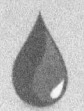

**REPORTED THERAPEUTIC PROPERTIES:** Antibacterial, antifungal, antiviral, antimicrobial, **antioxidant**, antiseptic, **anti-aging**, analgesic, anti-inflammatory, **antispasmodic**, diuretic, relieves diarrhea, aids digestion, expels excess gas, reduces fever, **supports cardiovascular function**, balances blood pressure, reduces cholesterol levels, relieves headache/migraine, aids liver function, eases cough, expels excess mucus, antiallergic, relieves dizziness or motions sickness, combats mental fatigue, stress management, **relieves anxiety**, antidepressant

## CAUTIONS:

■ *1,8-cineole, Terpinen-4-ol CTs*: Avoid with epilepsy and Parkinson's disease due to 1,8-cineole content, which may exacerbate or cause seizures or convulsions when inhaled, applied topically, or ingested based on 1,8-cineole content.[8063,8064,8065,8066,8067,8068]

■ *1,8-cineole, Terpinen-4-ol CTs*: May weakly interfere with the enzymes responsible for metabolizing medications (NSAIDs, proton-pump inhibitors, acetaminophen, antiepileptics, immune modulators, blood-sugar medications, blood pressure medications, antidepressants, antipsychotics, diabetic medications, antihistamines, antibiotics, and anesthetics) based on 1,8-cineole content.[8069,8070]

■ May interact with antibiotics or antifungals and increase their effectiveness.[8071,8072]

■ *1,8-cineole, Terpinen-4-ol CTs*: May interfere with pentobarbital and other barbiturates (medications for anxiety and insomnia) based on 1,8-cineole content.[8073,8074]

## SELECTED EVIDENCE:

☐ *In vitro* research demonstrates that shell ginger essential oil (terpinen-4-ol CT) inhibits multi-drug-resistant clinical isolates of *S. aureus* and *E. coli*, and moderately inhibits *Aeromonas caviae, Klebsiella pneumonia,* and *Listeria monocytogenes.*[8075] The same research reports that shell ginger essential oil increases the effectiveness of aminoglycoside antibiotics against bacterial strains. Other research reports that it significantly inhibits the bacteria *S. aureus, P. aeruginosa, E. coli,* and *B. subtilis,* moderately inhibits *Mycobacterium phlei* and *Sarcina lutea,* and significantly inhibits the fungi *C. albicans.*[8076] Other research reports that shell ginger essential oil (1,8-cineole CT) effectively inhibits a number of clinically isolated dermatophytes (fungi that require keratin for growth and typically infect the skin, hair, and nails): *T. rubrum, T. mentagraphytes, M. canis,* and *Epidermophyton floccosum.*[8077] Shell ginger flower essential oil with near equal percentages of 1,8-cineole and terpinene-4-ol was significantly active against *B. cereus, E. coli, A. niger, S. aureus, C. albicans, L. innocua,* and *S. enteritidis.*[8078]

☐ Animal research shows that inhalation of shell ginger essential oil (multiple CTs) reduces anxiety without affecting the GABA system (a group of receptors that respond to the neurotransmitter gamma-aminobutyric acid and encourage relaxation when more GABA is present).[8079,8080,8081]

☐ A 1,8-cineole-rich shell ginger essential oil demonstrated good antioxidant properties.[8082] Shell ginger essential oil also protects against DNA damage caused by free radicals and increases glutathione (GSH) levels.[8083,8084]

☐ Shell ginger essential oil (1,8-cineole CT) possesses anti-aging properties based on its ability to significantly inhibit collagenase and elastase activities (these enzymes break down collagen and elastase, which reduces the flexibility of the skin and can increase the appearance of aging).[8085]

☐ *In vitro* research reports that shell ginger essential oil (1,8-cineole CT) reduces the production of melanin in melanoma cells. Reducing melanin production in melanoma cells is desirable because it may reduce the progression of skin cancer caused by UV exposure.[8086] The study authors also suggest that shell ginger essential oil may be able to whiten the skin.[8087]

☐ Topical application of 0.05 mL of shell ginger essential oil (terpinen-4-ol CT) to each calf once daily for ten days reduced muscle spasms and improved muscle performance in individuals suffering from post-stroke spasticity.[8088] Injury to the brain following a stroke may cause involuntary muscle contractions (like a serious Charlie horse), which further aggravates the muscle by tightening the surrounding ligaments and tendons, and can result in permanently frozen muscles if left untreated. Animal research also suggests that shell ginger essential oil (para-cymene CT) relaxes intestinal muscles and prevent muscle spasms.[8089]

☐ *In vitro* research concluded that shell ginger essential oil (terpinen-4-ol CT) protects against endothelial dysfunction caused by oxidation of LDL cholesterol by acting as an antioxidant and modulating nitric oxide pathways.[8090,8091] Animal research also reports that shell ginger essential oil (terpinen-4-ol CT) decreases left atrial force of contraction in the heart by regulating the amount of calcium that enters cells and heart tissue, causing cardiodepression.[8092] Both the 1,8-cineole CT and the terpinene-4-ol CT reduce blood pressure through vasorelaxation (relaxing and widening of the blood vessels).[8093,8094] Injection of the terpinen-4-ol CT produced an immediate and significant decrease in blood pressure in rats.[8095] All of the study authors acknowledged the vasorelaxant and blood pressure lowering effects of terpinene-4-ol, and that it was at least partially responsible for the results.

☐ Shell ginger essential oil (1,8-cineole CT) prevents larval development of *Haemonchus contortus* (a very common parasitic gastrointestinal nematode that attaches to the stomach mucosa and feeds on blood) *in vitro*.[8096] Shell ginger flower essential oil demonstrates significant repellent and toxicity against the *Ae. aegypti* mosquito.[8097]

☐ Animal research demonstrates that injection of shell ginger essential oil possesses antipsychotic properties and reduces incessant movement due to overstimulation of the nervous system.[8098,8099]

☐ Oral administration of 100 or 300 mg/kg of shell ginger essential oil (terpinen-4-ol CT) relieves pain in mice, likely by interacting with opiate receptors.[8100]

☐ Animal research suggests that shell ginger essential oil can reduce the excitability of tissues (sciatic nerve) by calming the nervous system.[8101]

☐ Animal research demonstrated that topical application of 0.3 mL/kg body weight of shell ginger essential oil (unidentified CT, diluted to 33%) to severed Achilles tendons promoted healing and tissue repair by reducing inflammation and increasing fibroblasts and type I collagen fibers.[8102] Fibroblasts are cells in connective tissue that produce collagen and other fibers, which are critical to wound closure and healing.

☐ Oral administration of shell ginger essential oil (0.135 g/kg BW) significantly decreased pain and inflammation in mice.[8103] The researchers concluded that alpha-pinene, beta-pinene, and camphor were at least partially responsible for the analgesic and anti-inflammatory activity of shell ginger essential oil.

☐ The terpinen-4-ol CT of shell ginger essential oil were toxic to *Rhodnius nasutus* (a large blood-sucking insect and carrier of *T. cruzi* that causes Chagas disease).[8104] Terpinen-4-ol was even more effective and caused 100 percent mortality, compared to 73.3% with the whole oil.

☐ High blood glucose levels and diabetes are associated with damage to the cardiovascular system. Shell ginger essential oil protected endothelial cells against damage caused by high glucose levels (reduced IL-8, TNF-$\alpha$, ICAM-1, and VCAM-1 and translocation of the p65 subunit of NF-$\kappa$B triggered by high glucose).[8105]

☐ Shell ginger essential oil demonstrated cardioprotective properties by preventing aortic endothelial cell injury and inflammation in preclinical research.[8106]

☐ Endothelial to mesenchymal transition is a biological process whereby endothelial cells undergo a cascade of molecular events that cause the cells to adopt a mesenchymal phenotype—a group of cellular processes that involve gene and protein expression and affect the cell's structure and function. This process is associated with cardiovascular diseases such as pulmonary hypertension and atherosclerosis and the development of cancer, inflammatory disorders, and fibrotic disorders. Shell ginger essential oil impeded TGF-$\beta$1-induced endothelial to mesenchymal transition *in vitro* through the downregulation of Krüppel-like factor 4 (KLF4).[8107] KLF4 plays an important role in phenotype transitions and its inhibition is associated with reduced development of human diseases associated with phenotype transition.

☐ Schizophrenia is a serious mental disorder characterized by an altered interpretation of reality (hallucinations, delusions, and extremely discorded thinking and behaviors). Current drugs for schizophrenia only partly treat its symptoms—reduce acute psychosis and its recurrence but poorly controls cognitive deficits and negative symptoms (normal behaviors and functions related to motivation and interest, or verbal/emotional expression). In addition, these drugs are associated with negative side effects, such as weight gain and catalepsy (diminished responsiveness and rigidity or posture). Shell ginger essential oil prevented and reversed most schizophrenia-like behavioral alterations like the drug olanzapine and modestly improved working memory in mice.[8108] The oil also efficiently protected against oxidative stress and inflammation in the hippocampus, and impaired BDNF (a protein that promotes neuron cell survival by influencing their growth, maturation, and maintenance). Moreover, shell ginger essential oil showed a far more favorable side effect profile, including less catalepsy and weight gain. The findings of this study suggest that shell ginger essential oil may have therapeutic potential to reduce symptoms of schizophrenia without significant side effects.

☐ Muscular fibrosis involves the excessive formation of fibrous bands of scar tissue, especially excessive collagen, between muscle fibers. Skeletal muscle fibrosis occurs in disorders like Duchenne or Becker muscular dystrophy and amyotrophic lateral sclerosis. Muscular fibrosis can occur in musculoskeletal or cardiac tissue and may cause

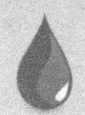

muscle weakness, fatigue, or the inability to perform regular daily activities. Caveolin-1 (CAV-1) is a protein that regulates numerous signaling pathways and biological processes, including processes that cause fibrosis. Reduction in the expression of CAV-1 has been observed in people with fibrotic conditions. Topical application of shell ginger essential oil at three different concentrations to the gastrocnemius muscle regulated the quality of collagen and therefore reducing fibrosis in rats.[8109] Only the lowest concentration of the oil restored healthy expression of CAV-1 gene expression to a level similar to healthy animals. Overall, the findings of this study suggests that topical application of shell ginger oil may be a low-cost, noninvasive, and effective solution to manage muscular fibrosis.

☐ Muscle fibrosis impairs muscle function, negatively affects muscle recovery and regeneration after injury, and increases susceptibility to re-injury. Topical application of shell ginger essential oil (31.0% para-cymene, 23.3% 1,8-cineole, 22.7% terpinen-4-ol) for thirty days improved muscle function and movement in a preclinical model of muscular fibrosis.[8110]

☐ Shell ginger essential oil protected against vascular endothelial cell injury in laboratory research, which suggests it may reduce the development of cardiovascular diseases.[8111]

# SIAM WOOD
## (Coffin Wood, Fujian Cypress, Fokienia, Po Mu, Peimou, Pemou)

*Fokienia hodginsii* (Dunn) Henry et Thomas, *Chamaecyparis hodginsii* (Dunn) Rushforth, *Cupressus hodginsii* Dunn

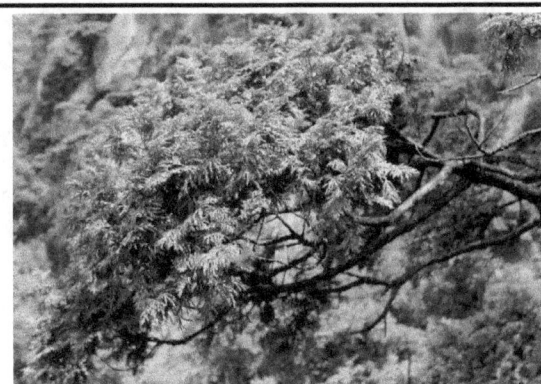

**FAMILY:** Cupressaceae
**NOTE:** Base
**AROMA INTENSITY:** Medium
**AROMA:** Woody, balsamic, rich, sweet
**COMMON EXTRACTION METHOD:** Hydrodistilled or steam distilled from the root bark/wood; may also be distilled from the leaves
**POSSIBLE SUBSTITUTE OILS:** Niaouli, guava leaf, hinoki, neroli, helichrysum, lemon eucalyptus
**BLENDS WELL WITH:** Agarwood, balsam fir, cassia, cedarwood, cinnamon, davana, elemi, frankincense, gobre salla, geranium, jasmine, lavender, lemon, neroli, orange, palmarosa, sandalwood, Siberian fir, silver fir, spruce (black), tangerine, white fir, ylang ylang
**SUBCELLULAR LOCALIZATION | EPIGENETIC INFLUENCE:** Currently unknown | Currently unknown
**RECOMMENDED DILUTION RANGE:** 3%–50%; Neat for limited conditions

**PRIMARY CONSTITUENTS:**[8112,8113,8114]

| *Root Bark* | | *Leaves* | |
|---|---|---|---|
| (E)-Nerolidol | 24.0%–35.5% | Alpha-Pinene | 24.9% |
| Delta-Cadinene | 4.2%–32.6% | Limonene | 8.5% |
| Fokienol | 24.0%–26.4% | Caryophyllene Oxide | 4.0% |
| Gamma-Cadinene | 2.3%–15.6% | Rimuene | 3.3% |
| Alpha-Muurolene | 1.8%–10.4% | | |
| Gamma-Muurolene | 0.0%–7.1% | | |
| Beta-Eudesmol | 3.2%–4.5% | | |
| Beta-Elemol | 3.2%–4.5% | | |
| Dauc-6(14),11-dien-5-ol | 1.8%–3.9% | | |
| Alpha-Muurolol | 0.0%–3.3% | | |
| Gamma-Eudesmol | 2.0%–3.0% | | |

**OTHER CONSTITUENTS:** *Root Bark*—Alpha-copaene, beta-elemene, beta-cedrene, beta-caryophyllene, beta-copaene, (E)-beta-farnesene, alpha-humulene, alpha-curcumene, alpha-neocallitropsene, capartriene, (Z)-alpha-bisabolene, beta-bisabolene, zonarene, alpha-cadinene, alpha-calacorene, beta-calacorene, eremoligenol, T-cadinol, T-muurolol, alpha-cadinol, alpha-eudesmol; *Leaves*—Beta-pinene, alpha-campholene aldehyde, trans-pinocarveol, terpinen-4-ol, borneol, alpha-terpineol, bornyl acetate, myrtenal, myrtenol, trans-carveol, terpinyl acetate, carvone, verbenone, geranyl acetate, isopiperitenone, calamenene, (E)-nerolidol, elemol, beta-eudesmol

**PREFERRED COMPOSITION FOR CLINICAL USE:**

| Constituent | Root Bark |
| --- | --- |
| **(E)-Nerolidol** | 25%–40% |
| **Fokienol** | 20%–30% |
| **Delta-Cadinene** | 5%–20% |
| **Gamma-Cadinene** | 2%–10% |
| **Beta-Eudesmol** | 3%–7% |
| **Beta-Elemol** | 3%–7% |
| **Alpha-Muurolene** | 1%–6% |
| **Gamma-Eudesmol** | 2%–5% |
| **Alpha-Eudesmol** | 1%–5% |
| **Alpha-Cadinol** | 1%–5% |
| **Dauc-6(14),11-dien-5-ol** | 1%–5% |
| **Beta-Elemene** | 0.1%–1% |

**THERAPEUTIC PROPERTIES:** Antioxidant, anti-aging, analgesic, **anti-inflammatory**, anti-rheumatic, antifungal, protects the stomach, supports endocrine, adrenal, and pituitary function, relieves chronic skin conditions, insecticide, **insect repellent**, reduces confusion, increases confidence, aphrodisiac, sedating, combats feelings of grief and abandonment, mentally stimulating

**CAUTIONS:**

■ *Root Bark*: May interfere with antibiotics and increase their effectiveness because (E)-nerolidol sensitizes bacteria to antibiotics).[8115]

**SELECTED EVIDENCE:**

☐ Siam wood essential oil (root bark) repels and kills the *Aedes aegypti* mosquito and its primary compounds ((E)-nerolidol and fokienol) are significantly toxic to house flies (*Musca domestica* L.).[8116]

## SIBERIAN FIR
### (Russian Fir)

*Abies sibirica* L.

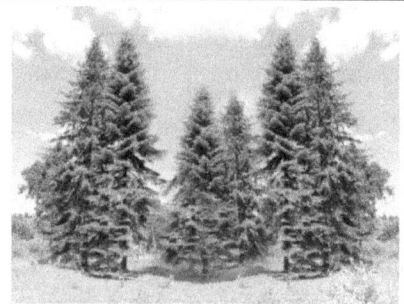

**FAMILY:** Pinaceae
**NOTE:** Top-Middle
**AROMA INTENSITY:** Medium
**AROMA:** Piney, woody, fresh, balsamic
**COMMON EXTRACTION METHOD:** Steam distilled from the needles (leaves) and twigs
**POSSIBLE SUBSTITUTE OILS:** Spruce (black), tsuga, silver fir, balsam fir, Douglas fir, white fir
**BLENDS WELL WITH:** Balsam fir, bergamot, cedarwood, Douglas fir, frankincense, grapefruit, lavender, lemon, lime, orange, palo santo, rosemary, sandalwood, silver fir, spruce (black), tangerine, tsuga, vetiver, white fir
**SUBCELLULAR LOCALIZATION | EPIGENETIC INFLUENCE:** Currently unknown | Currently unknown
**RECOMMENDED DILUTION RANGE:** 3%–Neat

**PRIMARY CONSTITUENTS:**[8117,8118,8119,8120]

| | |
| --- | --- |
| Bornyl Acetate | 31.0%–37.6% |
| Camphene | 17.5%–28.4% |

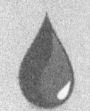
| | |
|---|---|
| Alpha-Pinene | 6.7%–13.7% |
| Delta-3-Carene | 6.2%–12.2% |
| Beta-Phellandrene | 2.4%–9.3% |
| Borneol | 0.0%–6.1% |
| Limonene | 0.0%–5.5% |
| Tricyclene | 2.3%–3.1% |

**OTHER CONSTITUENTS:** Beta-pinene, alpha-terpinolene, santene, myrcene, calarene, cis-alpha-bisabolol, trans-alpha-bisabolol, beta-bisabolene

**PREFERRED COMPOSITION FOR CLINICAL USE:**

| *Constituent* | |
|---|---|
| **Bornyl Acetate** | 25%–40% |
| **Camphene** | 15%–30% |
| **Alpha-Pinene** | 10%–20% |
| **Delta-3-Carene** | 10%–18% |
| **Limonene** | 3%–9% |
| **Beta-Phellandrene** | 2%–6% |
| **Tricyclene** | 1%–5% |
| **Beta-Pinene** | 1%–4% |
| **Santene** | 0.5%–4% |
| **Borneol** | 1%–3% |
| **Beta-Caryophyllene** | 0.5%–3% |
| **Alpha-Phellandrene** | tr–3% |
| **Alpha-Humulene** | 0.5%–2% |

**REPORTED THERAPEUTIC PROPERTIES:** Antibacterial, antifungal, antiseptic, anti-infectious, **analgesic**, anti-inflammatory, antispasmodic, antirheumatic, aids circulation, supports respiratory function, expels excess mucous, eases cough, reduces fever, **boosts antioxidant activity**, protects cognition and memory, increases localized circulation, supports oral health, stress management, **relieves anxiety**

**CAUTIONS:**
- None currently known.

**SELECTED EVIDENCE:**
- ☐ Inhalation of Siberian fir essential oil (132 mcg) via olfactometer for 40 minutes (5 minutes before, 30 minutes during, and 5 minutes after a task) promoted a relaxed state (slower heart rate and increased theta brainwaves—suggesting meditative thought and decreased arousal) after performing a visual discrimination task (tasks involving the ability to detect differences in variables such as features, patterns, and shapes).[8121]
- ☐ Siberian fir essential oil inhibits AChE (acetylcholinesterase), which suggests it may preserve cognitive abilities and memory.[8122] The same research reported that Siberian fir essential oil increases antioxidant activity (catalase and glutathione reductase) 2.5 and 8 times, respectively.
- ☐ *In vitro* research demonstrates that Siberian fir essential oil inhibits *C. albicans* when incorporated into a dental gel.[8123]

---

## Did you know?

Some constituents found in essential oils are not present in the plant. These constituents, like methyl salicylate and chamazulene, are byproducts of the distillation process that converts constituents (galtherin, matricine) present in the plant to other constituents.

# SILVER FIR
## (Silver Spruce)

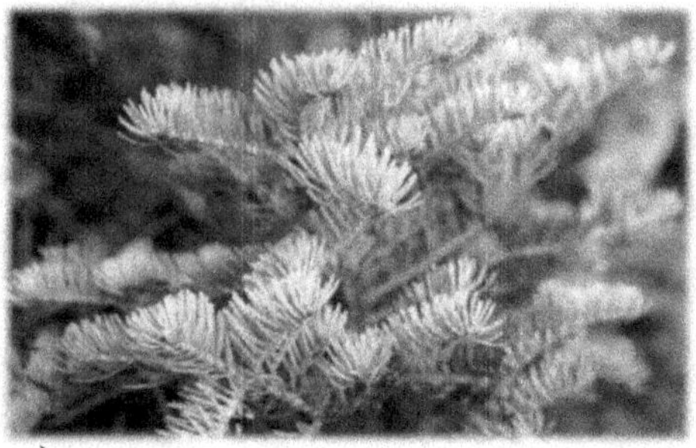

*Abies alba* Mill.

**FAMILY:** Pinaceae
**NOTE:** Top-Middle
**AROMA INTENSITY:** Medium
**AROMA:** Fresh, piney, clean, woody
**COMMON EXTRACTION METHOD:** Steam distilled from the needles (leaves)
**POSSIBLE SUBSTITUTE OILS:** White fir, balsam fir, blue spruce, spruce (black), palo santo, blue cypress, juniper (needles)
**BLENDS WELL WITH:** Balsam fir, birch, cassia, blue spruce, cedarwood, chamomile (German, Roman), cypress, frankincense, galbanum, lavender, lemon, myrtle, palo santo, pine, sandalwood, spruce (black), tsuga, white fir, wintergreen
**SUBCELLULAR LOCALIZATION | EPIGENETIC INFLUENCE:** Currently unknown | Currently unknown
**RECOMMENDED DILUTION RANGE:** 5%–Neat

**PRIMARY CONSTITUENTS:**[8124,8125,8126]

| | |
|---|---|
| Limonene | 7.5%–54.7% |
| Alpha-Pinene | 2.9%–31.7% |
| Bornyl Acetate | 1.0%–30.3% |
| Camphene | 5.6%–19.8% |
| Beta-Pinene | 0.5%–15.5% |
| Delta-3-Carene | 0.0%–13.9% |
| Tricyclene | 0.8%–12.9% |
| Beta-Caryophyllene | 2.2%–8.4% |
| Santene | 0.0%–5.0% |
| Alpha-Humulene | 0.8%–4.6% |
| Sabinene | 0.0%–4.3% |

Note: Silver fir could be split into at least two distinct chemotypes—one with significant limonene content and the other with higher bornyl acetate. Both *Abies alba* and *Abies concolor* are referred to as white fir, and both are available on the essential oil market. *A. alba* is more commonly called silver fir or silver spruce, whereas *A. concolor* is called white fir according to the United States Department of Agriculture.[8127] They are two distinct species, and the chemical constituents are very different.[8128] *A. concolor* is the true white fir essential oil.

**OTHER CONSTITUENTS:** Myrcene, beta-phellandrene, alpha-terpinolene, linalool, alpha-campholenic aldehyde, endoborneol, alpha-terpineol, alpha-longipinene, delta-3-carene, alpha-cedrene, alpha-himachalene, cis-caryophyllene, gamma-himachalene, widdrene, beta-selinene, alpha-selinene, beta-himachalene, alpha-amorphene, delta-cadinene, caryophyllene oxide, longiborneol, beta-paciulan, alpha-cadinol, t-muurolol

**PREFERRED COMPOSITION FOR CLINICAL USE:**

| Constituent | Bornyl Acetate CT | Limonene CT | Beta-Pinene CT |
|---|---|---|---|
| **Bornyl Acetate** | 12%–32% | 1.5%–12% | 5%–15% |
| **Limonene** | 6%–25% | 30%–55% | 15%–25% |
| **Camphene** | 6%–20% | 5%–15% | 10%–20% |
| **Alpha-Pinene** | 3%–15% | 7%–30% | 10%–20% |
| **Delta-3-Carene** | 0.5%–14% | < 1% | – |
| **Tricyclene** | 1.5%–13% | < 2% | 1%–2% |
| **Beta-Pinene** | 0.5%–12% | 2%–8% | 22%–35% |
| **Beta-Caryophyllene** | 0.5%–7% | 1%–3% | < 1% |

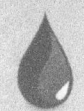

| Alpha-Humulene | 0.1%–5% | 0.1%–2% | < 0.5% |
| Santene | < 4% | 0.1%–2% | 1%–3% |
| Beta-Phellandrene | < 4% | < 1% | 2%–5% |

**THERAPEUTIC PROPERTIES: Analgesic (pain relief), anti-inflammatory**, antiarthritic, antirheumatic, antimicrobial, anticancer, antiseptic, **antioxidant**, **aids circulation**, increases redness and circulation of a localized area, **antispasmodic**, expectorant, disinfectant, removes excess mucus, relieves cough, **supports respiratory function**, reduces fever, stimulating, energizing, **encourages feelings of stability and empowerment**

**CAUTIONS:**
- None currently known.

**SELECTED EVIDENCE:**
- Silver fir seed and cone essential oil only weakly killed two breast cancer cells lines.[8129]
- Silver fir essential oil inhibits organisms (*C. butyricum, C. intestinale*, and *C. ramosum*) that commonly infect the gastrointestinal system, cervix, and vagina and cause a variety of human diseases.[8130]
- *In vitro* research reports that silver fir essential oil mildly inhibits *S. aureus*.[8131] The seed and cone essential oil was only weakly antimicrobial (*S. aureus, E. faecalis, E. faecium, E, coli, K, pneumoniae*, and *A. baumannii*).[8132]
- Silver fir essential oil is a potent free-radical scavenger according to *in vitro* research.[8133,8134]
- Dispersion of lemon and silver fir essential oils together in a hospital significantly reduced the concentration of airborne bacteria and fungi (40% and 30%–60%) respectively.[8135]
- *Helicobacter pylori* is a bacterium that lives in the digestive tract that can cause sores and ulcers in the lining of the stomach or upper part of the small intestine. Thyme, lemongrass, Virginia cedarwood, and melissa essential oils were the most active of 26 commercial essential oils examined against *H. pylori*.[8136] Oregano, tea tree, pine, and silver fir were also bactericidal.
- Laboratory research found that conifer essential oils are more active antimicrobial agents in vapor phase when compared to liquid phase and tend to have higher concentrations of alpha-pinene in vapor phase.[8137] Dwarf pine inhibited *E. coli, A. bohemicus, K. marina*, and *B. cereus* in liquid phase, which was dramatically improved against all tested organisms (except *E. coli*) in vapor phase. Norway spruce and silver fir inhibited *A. bohemicus, K. marina*, and *B. cereus* in liquid phase, again with significant improvements in vapor phase. Each oil displayed moderate antioxidant activity in the DPPH and ABTS assays.
- Silver fir and niaouli essential oils inhibited *P. expansum, P. citrinum*, and *P. crustosum* in a dose-dependent manner (in vapor phase), with *P. citrinum* being the most sensitive and *P. crustosum* the least sensitive.[8138]

## SOUTHERN BLUE GUM
### (Eurabbie, Victorian Blue Gum, Blue Eucalyptus)

*Eucalyptus bicostata* Maiden, Blakely & Simmons.,
*E. globulus* Labill. subsp. *bicostata*

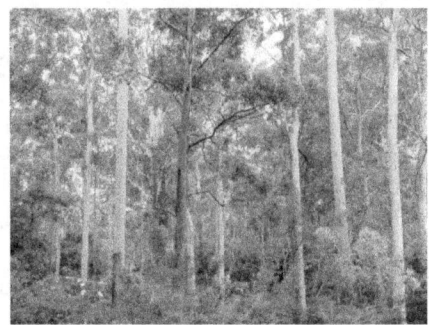

**FAMILY:** Myrtaceae
**NOTE:** Top
**AROMA INTENSITY:** Strong
**AROMA:** Fresh, clean, medicinal, slightly woody
**COMMON EXTRACTION METHOD:** Steam distilled from the leaves
**POSSIBLE SUBSTITUTE OILS:** Eucalyptus, niaouli (1,8-cineole CT), bay laurel, cajeput, ravintsara (1,8-cineole CT), ravensara (1,8-cineole CT), cardamom, rosemary (1,8-cineole CT), myrtle, sage (1,8-cineole CT)
**BLENDS WELL WITH:** Bay laurel, bergamot, blue cypress, cajeput, camphor, cedarwood, chamomile (German, Roman), geranium, ginger, grapefruit, juniper, lavender, lemon, lemongrass, tea tree, peppermint, petitgrain, pine, ravensara, ravintsara, rosemary, sage, tangerine, thyme
**SUBCELLULAR LOCALIZATION | EPIGENETIC INFLUENCE:** Currently unknown | Currently unknown
**RECOMMENDED DILUTION RANGE:** 3%–33%; neat for limited conditions

[611]

**PRIMARY CONSTITUENTS:**[8139,8140,8141]

| | |
|---|---|
| 1,8-cineole | 44.0%–81.3% |
| Aromadendrene | 2.0%–16.9% |
| Alpha-Pinene | 1.2%–12.2% |
| Globulol | 1.8%–5.5% |
| Trans-Pinocarveol | 0.2%–4.6% |
| Limonene | 0.0%–4.4% |
| Pinocarvone | 0.1%–3.9% |
| Alloaromadendrene | 0.0%–3.0% |
| Alpha-Terpineol | 0.3%–2.4% |
| Para-Cymene | 0.2%–1.4% |
| Viridiflorol | 0.2%–1.4% |
| Epiglobulol | 0.0%–1.2% |
| Trans-p-Mentha-1.7.8 dien-2-ol | 0.0%–1.1% |
| Cis-p-Mentha-1.7.8 dien-2-ol | 0.0%–1.1% |
| Beta-Caryophyllene | 0.1%–1.0% |

**OTHER CONSTITUENTS:** Beta-elemene, spathulenol, alpha-eudesmol, beta-eudesmol, torquatone

**PREFERRED COMPOSITION FOR CLINICAL USE:**

| Constituent | |
|---|---|
| **1,8-Cineole** | 60%–82% |
| **Alpha-Pinene** | 2%–10% |
| **Globulol** | 0.5%–7% |
| **Trans-Pinocarveol** | 2%–6% |
| **Pinocarvone** | 1%–5% |
| **Aromadendrene** | 0.1%–3% |

**REPORTED THERAPEUTIC PROPERTIES: Analgesic**, antibacterial, antifungal, **antirheumatic**, **antiseptic**, antispasmodic, anesthetic, **antiviral**, antineuralgic, **decongestant**, diuretic, **expectorant**, helps balance blood-sugar levels, **supports normal respiration**, reduces fevers, insect repellent, nervine (calms and soothes the nerves), **reduces abnormal bone growth**, promotes oral cleanliness, wound healing, **eases cough**, stimulating, invigorating, refreshing, aids concentration, combats negative emotions, relieves mental exhaustion

**CAUTIONS:**

■ Avoid with children under age 3, particularly around the nose and mouth. Use very cautiously in children under age 5 due to high 1,8-cineole content. 1,8-cineole may cause seizures, central nervous system problems, or respiratory distress in young children.[8142,8143,8144,8145]

■ Avoid with epilepsy and Parkinson's disease due to 1,8-cineole content. May exacerbate or cause seizures/convulsions or reduce seizure medication efficacy based on 1,8-cineole content.[8146,8147,8148]

■ Caution is warranted orally due to the significant amounts of 1,8-cineole. Limit it to small doses internally (adults—maximum 10 drops daily). One text recommends a maximum daily dose of 6 drops, whereas the European Medicines Agency recommends 2 to 4 drops (100–200 mg) of high 1,8-cineole essential oils orally, 2 to 5 times daily for adolescents, adults, and the elderly.[8149,8150] Additionally, 200 mg of isolated 1,8-cineole has been ingested three times daily for up to six months in clinical research.[8151,8152] Toxicity has been reported when eucalyptus (also high in 1,8-cineole) was ingested in large doses, and as few as 4 to 5 drops may cause problems in very sensitive individuals.[8153,8154,8155,8156,8157,8158] In humans, 3.5 to 5 mL has proven fatal orally.[8159]

■ May weakly interfere with the enzymes responsible for metabolizing medications (NSAIDs, proton-pump inhibitors, acetaminophen, antiepileptics, immune modulators, blood-sugar medications, blood pressure medications, antidepressants, antipsychotics, diabetic medications, antihistamines, antibiotics, and anesthetics) based on 1,8-cineole content.[8160,8161]

■ May interact with diabetic medications due to the ability of 1,8-cineole to significantly inhibit alpha-glucosidase activity, particularly when synergized with other constituents (alpha-pinene and para-cymene).[8162,8163,8164] Alpha-

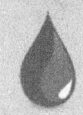

glucosidase is an enzyme that breaks down carbohydrates by chemical reaction with water. Inhibiting its activity postpones glucose absorption and therefore the impact of carbohydrates on blood sugar levels.

■ May interact with aspirin, blood pressure, antiplatelet, and anticoagulant medications, and increase the risk of bleeding among people with bleeding disorders (low risk).[8165] 1,8-cineole is a weak inhibitor of platelet aggregation.[8166]

■ May interfere with pentobarbital and other barbiturates (medications for anxiety and insomnia) based on 1,8-cineole content.[8167,8168]

**SELECTED EVIDENCE:**

☐ *In vitro* research concluded that *E. bicostata* inhibited *S. pneumoniae*, *S. aureus*, *C. albicans*, and *M. canis*, and possessed the greatest antiviral activity of the eight Eucalyptus species tested.[2773] Another study concluded that it had the highest antibacterial activity of seven Eucalyptus species against *L. ivanovii* and *B. cereus*.[8169]

---

# SPANISH SAGE
## (Lavender Sage)

*Salvia lavandulifolia* Vahl., *S. lavandulaefolia*, *S. hispanorum* Lag.

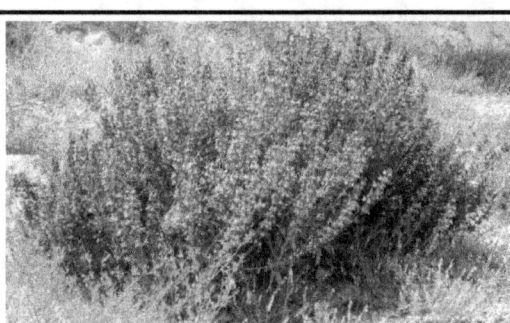

**FAMILY:** Lamiaceae (Labiatae)
**NOTE:** Middle
**AROMA INTENSITY:** Medium
**AROMA:** Herbaceous, medicinal, slightly woody and balsamic
**COMMON EXTRACTION METHOD:** Steam distilled from the flowers, buds, and leaves
**POSSIBLE SUBSTITUTE OILS:** Sage (1,8-cineole CT), rosemary (1,8-cineole CT), niaouli (viridiflorol CT), spike lavender, lavandin
**BLENDS WELL WITH:** Bergamot, camphor, cedarwood, cinnamon, citronella, clary sage, clove, cypress, grapefruit, lavandin, lavender, lemon, lime, orange, patchouli, pine, sandalwood, tangerine, thyme
**SUBCELLULAR LOCALIZATION | EPIGENETIC INFLUENCE:** Currently unknown | Currently unknown
**RECOMMENDED DILUTION RANGE:** 3%–20%; neat for limited conditions

**PRIMARY CONSTITUENTS:**[8170,8171,8172,8173]

| | |
|---|---|
| 1,8-Cineole | 13.0%–33.8% |
| Camphor | 6.1%–31.0% |
| Alpha-Pinene | 4.9%–17.5% |
| Beta-Pinene | 4.6%–17.3% |
| Viridiflorol | 0.0%–12.0% |
| Delta-Terpineol | 0.3%–12.0% |
| Camphene | 5.6%–11.0% |
| Limonene | 0.0%–10.4% |
| Ledol | 0.0%–10.8% |
| Myrcene | 0.1%–10.0% |
| Beta-Phellandrene | 0.1%–9.3% |
| Beta-Caryophyllene | 1.2%–8.5% |
| Camphene | 5.2%–7.1% |
| Geranyl Acetate | 0.0%–4.9% |
| Linalyl Acetate | 0.0%–4.2% |

**OTHER CONSTITUENTS:** Sabinene, linalool, trans-sabinol, borneol, terpinen-4-ol, alpha-terpineol, linalyl acetate, sabinyl acetate, bornyl acetate, terpinyl acetate, geranyl propionate

**PREFERRED COMPOSITION FOR CLINICAL USE:**

*Constituent*

| | |
|---|---|
| **Camphor** | 18%–36% |
| **1,8-Cineole** | 12%–30% |
| **Alpha-Pinene** | 4%–10% |
| **Borneol** | 1%–10% |
| **Alpha-Terpinyl Acetate** | 0.5%–9% |
| **Limonene** | 2%–8% |
| **Camphene** | 3%–7% |
| **Beta-Pinene** | 2%–7% |
| **Beta-Caryophyllene** | 1%–6% |
| **Linalyl Acetate** | 0.1%–6% |
| **Myrcene** | 0.1%–5% |
| **Trans-Sabinyl Acetate** | < 5% |
| **Linalool** | 0.1%–4% |
| **Sabinene** | 0.1%–4% |
| **Terpinen-4-ol** | 0%–2% |

**THERAPEUTIC PROPERTIES: Analgesic (pain relief)**, anti-inflammatory, antispasmodic, antirheumatic, **antimicrobial**, decongestant, eases cough, balances menstruation, balances hormones, **relieves skin disorders**, reduces excess sweating, aids circulation, reduces fever, wound healing, **aids memory**, reduces anxiety, revitalizing, aids concentration, stress management, antidepressant, **aids cognition**, combats grief and fear

**CAUTIONS:**

■ Use very cautiously with children under 6 due to potentially high camphor and 1,8-cineole content. Several cases of camphor poisoning and/or seizures from ingestion and topical application have been reported in children.[8174,8175] Ingestion of camphor-containing products has been lethal in children under age 2 (estimated to be roughly 2,000 mg of camphor for a 20 kg child as the minimum potential fatal dose).[8176,8177] 1,8-cineole may cause seizures, central nervous system problems, or respiratory distress in young children.[8178,8179,8180,8181] Children 5 years and up may use camphor-containing essential oils topically in dilutions no stronger than 5%. Camphor ingestion by infants and young children may cause cough, vomiting, seizure, burning sensation in the mucous membranes and eyes, or lack of voluntary coordination of muscle movements.[8182]

■ Caution is warranted during pregnancy and while lactating due to potentially high camphor and small sabinyl acetate content. Ingestion of essential oils with significant levels of camphor may lead to abortion because fetuses lack the enzymes to process it.[8183] Sabinyl acetate is also considered an abortifacient based on large doses administered to animals that prevented implantation and impaired fertility.[8184,8185] However, Spanish sage usually has less than 5% sabinyl acetate, and the studies that considered it an abortifacient injected large doses of sabinyl acetate directly into pregnant mice. When the camphor and sabinyl acetate content of Spanish sage are both considered, it is reasonable to limit topical application and avoid oral administration during pregnancy and lactation.

■ Avoid with epilepsy and Parkinson's due to potentially high camphor and 1,8-cineole content.[8186,8187,8188,8189,8190]

■ The potentially high camphor content in Spanish sage may negatively impact red blood cells and increase the risk of jaundice in children with Glucose-6-phosphate dehydrogenase deficiency (G6PD).[8191,8192]

■ Oral caution—Essential oils with significant levels of camphor and 1,8-cineole can be toxic when taken orally. As few as 4 to 5 drops of high 1,8-cineole oils may be problematic in very sensitive individuals. Camphor can be toxic when taken orally (usually single doses exceeding 2 mL), although the lethal dose for adult humans is estimated to be (more than 5 mL) in a single dose.[8193,8194,8195]

■ May interfere with pentobarbital and other barbiturates (medications for anxiety and insomnia) based on 1,8-cineole content.[8196,8197]

■ May weakly interfere with the enzymes responsible for metabolizing medications (NSAIDs, proton-pump inhibitors, acetaminophen, antiepileptics, immune modulators, blood-sugar medications, blood pressure medications,

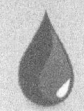

antidepressants, antipsychotics, diabetic medications, antihistamines, antibiotics, and anesthetics) due to 1,8-cineole content.[8198,8199,8200]

■ May interact with anticholinergic (drugs used for asthma, incontinence, gastrointestinal cramps, muscular spasms, depression, and sleep disorders) and cholinergic medications (drugs used to reduce urinary retention, diagnose myasthenia gravis, and for glaucoma) based on AChE inhibitory activity.[8201,8202,8203]

### SELECTED EVIDENCE:

☐ Spanish sage essential oil enhances cognitive performance in both healthy people and people with dementia or cognitive impairments according to a review of eight clinical studies.[8204,8205] Another study found that speed of memory, secondary memory, alertness, and mood were all enhanced by the administration of about one drop of Spanish sage oil daily for seven days in young healthy individuals.[8206]

☐ Oral administration of about one drop of Spanish sage in a capsule (one capsule daily week one, two capsules daily week two, three capsules daily week three) moderately improved memory and attention in people with Alzheimer's disease with good tolerability and no adverse effects directly attributable to the Spanish sage.[8207]

☐ *In vitro* research discovered that Spanish sage protects neurons from oxidative stress-induced damage by preventing morphological changes associated with Alzheimer's disease (plaques, neurofibrillary tangles, etc.), protecting cell viability, improving glutathione to oxidized glutathione levels, and reducing the production of damaging reactive oxygen species.[8208]

☐ The monoterpenes alpha-pinene and 1,8-cineole in Spanish sage balance the production of reactive oxygen species to reactive oxygen scavengers (cellular redox balance), which prevents injury to and death of astrocytes (glial cells of the central nervous system).[8209] Astrocytes degeneration or destruction is associated with dementia.

☐ *In vitro* research suggests that Spanish sage oil and its major constituents inhibits acetylcholinesterase (AChE).[8210,8211,8212] Inhibition of AChE prevents the break-down of acetylcholine, which is essential for memory and thinking. People with neurodegenerative diseases make less acetylcholine, and the diseases often break it down at a faster rate leading to acetylcholine deficits.

☐ Spanish sage possesses mild estrogenic activity (a substance that can activate or inhibit endocrine system and estrogen activity).[8213]

☐ The camphor CT of Spanish sage demonstrated antioxidant and antimicrobial (*Escherichia coli*, *Staphylococcus aureus*, and *Candida albicans*) activity, and inhibited acetylcholinesterase and lipoxygenase (an enzyme that catalyzes the addition of oxygen to fatty acids and is involved in inflammation, cancer, and chronic conditions) activity.[8214] Inhibition of AChE prevents the break-down of acetylcholine, which is essential for memory and thinking. People with neurodegenerative diseases make less acetylcholine, and the diseases often break it down at a faster rate leading to acetylcholine deficits. In addition, 1,8-cineole demonstrated the greatest inhibition of AChE, while bornyl acetate and limonene were most active against lipoxygenase.

☐ Spanish sage CT camphor essential oil showed acaricidal activity against synanthropic mites (*D. farinae, D. pteronyssinus*, and *T. putrescentiae*).[8215]

☐ Chronic oral administration of Spanish sage CT 1,8-cineole essential oil (essential oil encapsulated with acacia gum; 83.3 mg/kg/day) improved memory and learning in normal adult mice.[8216] The activity of the oil was improved when combined with an aqueous extract of sage (*S. officinalis*). Interestingly, memory improvements were observed after only one administration of the oil.

*Did you know?*

Essential oils are frequently used to reduce the side effects of medical interventions and a growing number of integrative hospitals and healthcare facilities are using them to improve patient satisfaction and quality of care.

# SPEARMINT
## (Spear Mint)

*Mentha spicata* L., *M. viridis* (L.) L., *M. crispa* L.;
**Scotch Spearmint**: *M. cardiaca* L., *M.* x *gracilis* Sole

**FAMILY:** Lamiaceae (Labiatae)
**NOTE:** Top
**AROMA INTENSITY:** Medium
**AROMA:** Minty, warm, herbaceous
**COMMON EXTRACTION METHOD:** Steam distilled from the leaves
**POSSIBLE SUBSTITUTE OILS:** Peppermint
**BLENDS WELL WITH:** Basil, bergamot, cajeput, eucalyptus, ginger, grapefruit, lavender, lemon, lemongrass, marjoram, niaouli, orange, peppermint, petitgrain, pine, rosemary, tangerine, thyme
**SUBCELLULAR LOCALIZATION | EPIGENETIC INFLUENCE:** Currently unknown | Currently unknown
**RECOMMENDED DILUTION RANGE:** 3%–50%; neat for limited conditions; Pulegone-Menthone-Isomenthone CT—1.5%–20%

**PRIMARY CONSTITUENTS:**[8217,8218,8219,8220,8221,8222,8223,8224,8225,8226,8227,8228,8229,8230,8231]

*Mentha spicata (Carvone CT)\**

| | |
|---|---|
| Carvone | 48.6%–76.5% |
| Limonene | 5.8%–25.2% |
| Menthone | 0.9%–21.9% |
| Dihydrocarvone | 0.0%–21.5% |
| Cis-Carveol | 14.0%–21.3% |
| Trans-Carveol | 0.2%–14.0% |
| Linalool | 0.3%–11.3% |
| 1,8-Cineole | 1.0%–6.8% |
| Germacrene D | 0.0%–4.7% |

*Mentha spicata (Piperitenone Oxide CT)*

| | |
|---|---|
| Piperitenone Oxide | 63.5%–70.3% |
| Germacrene D | 4.2%–7. 2% |
| 1,8-Cineole | 0.4%–3.5% |
| Piperitenone | 1.0%–2.8% |
| Carhydranol | 1.5%–2.0% |
| Beta-Pinene | 0.4%–2.0% |
| Limonene | 1.1%–1.8% |
| Delta-Cadinene | 0.1%–1.6% |

*Mentha spicata (Menthone CT)*

| | |
|---|---|
| Menthone | 44.5% |
| Neoisomenthyl Acetate | 8.4% |
| Menthol | 5.4% |
| 1,8-Cineole | 5.2% |
| Caryophyllene | 2.9% |
| Isomenthone | 2.6% |

*Mentha spicata (Piperitone Oxide CT)*

| | |
|---|---|
| Piperitone Oxide | 54.2%–72.3% |
| Germacrene D | 2.0%–7.5% |

*Mentha spicata (Pulegone/Menthone/Isomenthone CT)*

| | |
|---|---|
| Pulegone | 26.7%–72.1% |
| Menthone | 15.6%–31.4% |
| Isomenthone | 2.6%–31.4% |
| Piperitone | 0.0%–28.2% |
| Octadecanol | 0.0%–15.0% |
| Trans-Beta-Caryophyllene | 0.0%–8.0% |
| 1,8-Cineole | 1.6%–7.8% |
| Germacrene D | 0.0%–5.3% |
| Limonene | 0.7%–5.2% |
| Phytene-2 | 0.0%–3.5% |
| Beta-Phellandrene | 0.0%–3.0% |
| Caryophyllene Oxide | 0.0%–3.0% |
| Sabinene Hydrate | 0.0%–2.8% |
| Phytol | 0.0%–2.5% |

*Mentha spicata (Linalool CT)*

| | |
|---|---|
| Linalool | 65.2%–75.3% |
| Beta-Caryophyllene | 4.4%–6.3% |
| Myrcene | 4.7%–5.9% |
| 1,8-Cineole | 4.7%–4.9% |
| Germacrene D | 1.9%–3.0% |
| Beta-Terpineol | 1.0%–3.0% |
| Alpha-Terpineol | 0.9%–3.0% |

*Mentha spicata var. viridis (Cis-Ocimenone CT)*

| | |
|---|---|
| Cis-Ocimenone | 61.7% |
| Limonene | 10.5% |
| Trans-Carveol | 5.0% |
| Alpha-Selinene | 1.7% |
| Neo-Isodihydrocarveol Acetate | 1.5% |

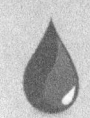

| | | | |
|---|---|---|---|
| 1,8-Cineole | 0.4%–5.8% | (Z)-Jasmone | 1.3% |
| Limonene | 0.4%–4.8% | 1,8-Cineole | 1.2% |
| Piperitenone Oxide | 0.1%–4.8% | | |
| Beta-Pinene | 0.4%–2.0% | *M. cri a (Rotundifolone, syn. Piperitenone Oxide CT)* | |
| Carhydranol | 0.2%–2.0% | Rotundifolone | 58.1% |
| Delta-Cadinene | 0.1%–1.9% | Limonene | 10.6% |
| Piperitone | 0.1%–1.8% | Myrcene | 7.8% |
| Piperitenone | 0.1%–1.3% | Germacrene D | 6.6% |
| | | Beta-Pinene | 4.4% |

*M. cardiaca* (Scotch Spearmint)

| | |
|---|---|
| Carvone | 60.9%–74.1% |
| Limonene | 6.8%–21.6% |

\* The carvone CT is the most commonly reported in the literature and the most common commercially available chemotype.

**OTHER CONSTITUENTS:** *Carvone CT*—Sabinene, beta-myrcene, para-cymene, gamma-terpinene, menthol, terpinene-4-ol, piperitone, trans-anethole, alpha-bourbonene, carvyl acetate, beta-bourbonene, beta-caryophyllene, germacrene A, diisobutyl carbinol, 4-hydroxy-3,5,5-trimethylcyclohex-2-enone, jasmine, ledol, 2-napthol,1,2,3,4,4a,5,6,7-octahydro-4a-methyl, trans-sabinene hydrate, 13-tetradeca-11-yn-1-ol; *Pulegone/Menthone/Isomenthone CT*—Myrcene, camphene, beta-pinene, alpha-pinene, 3-octanol, 3-thujanol, (Z)-beta-ocimene, terpinene-4-ol, carvone, elixene, delta-cadinene, caryophyllene oxide, alpha-cadinol; *Piperitenone Oxide CT*—Sabinene, myrcene, beta-bourbonene, bornyl acetate, piperitenone, piperitone, pulegone (< 2.3%), piperitone, dehydroedulan II, trans-caryophyllene, cis-Muurola-4(14),5-diene, alpha-cadinene, alpha-cadinol; *Linalool CT*—gamma-terpinene, 1-octen-3-ol, beta-elemene, neodihydrocarveol; *Menthone CT*—Dodecatriene, n-decanoic acid, 3,7,11,15-tetramethyl-2-hexadecenol, phytol, 1,2-benzenedicarboxylic acid, n-decanoic acid, octadecanol, tetradecanol; *Cis-Ocimenone CT*—Myrcene, alpha-terpinene, (E)-beta-ocimene, (Z)-beta-ocimene, cis-dihydrocarveol, cis-carveol, beta-gurjunene, beta-caryophyllene, alpha-cadinol; *Piperitone Oxide CT*—Sabinene, myrcene, isomenthone, alpha-copaene, beta-bourbonene, bornyl acetate; *M. crispa*—Alpha-pinene, sabinene, trans-caryophyllene; *M. cardiaca*—alpha-bourbonene, 1,8-cineole, cis-carveol, dihydrocarvone, jasmine, germacrene D, piperitone, menthone, beta-pinene, sabinene, 6-undecanol, alpha-pinene

**PREFERRED COMPOSITION FOR CLINICAL USE:**

| *Constituent* | |
|---|---|
| **Carvone** | 55%–70% |
| **Limonene** | 10%–23% |
| **Cis-Dihydrocarvone** | 0.5%–4% |
| **Beta-Bourbonene** | 1%–3% |
| **3-Octanol** | 0.4%–2% |
| **Trans-Dihydrocarvyl Acetate** | 0.1%–2% |
| **Cis-Sabinene Hydrate** | 0.1%–1.5% |
| **Cis-Carvyl Acetate** | 0.1%–1% |
| **Cis-Jasmone** | 0.1%–1% |
| **Viridiflorol** | 0%–1% |
| **Menthone** | < 0.5% |

**REPORTED THERAPEUTIC PROPERTIES:** Analgesic (pain relief), anesthetic, antibacterial, anti-inflammatory, antiseptic, **antispasmodic**, antifungal, anticonvulsive, antineuralgic, expels excess gas, **decongestant**, **aids digestion**, **relieves headache**, expectorant, diuretic, reduces fever, nervine (calms and soothes the nerves), supports and protects the liver, stimulating, energizing, reduces anxiety, stress management, **antidepressant**, combats fatigue

**CAUTIONS:**

*Rotundifolone, Menthone, and Linalool CTs*

■ Avoid use in those with iron-deficiency and iron-deficiency anemia. Animal research suggests that spearmint may decrease iron absorption and therefore aggravate iron-deficiency symptoms and anemia.[8232]

*Pulegone/menthone/isomenthone CT*

■ Avoid with children under age 12. Multiple organ failure, liver failure, brain swelling (cerebral edema), severe epileptic encephalopathy (severe brain disorder with seizures), organ cell death (necrosis), and death has been reported in infants who were administered mint tea containing pennyroyal essential oil.[8233] Pulegone and its metabolite menthofuran (or metabolites of menthofuran) are believed to cause the toxic effects of pennyroyal, which include liver and kidney toxicity, bronchiolar cell destruction, depletion of liver glutathione levels (the primary protective antioxidant of the liver), and direct cellular damage.[8234,8235,8236,8237] Children are more likely to experience these effects.[8238]

■ Avoid during pregnancy and lactation due to significant amounts of pulegone and potential toxicity to multiple organs properties of essential oil rich in pulegone.[8239,8240,8241]

■ Avoid oral administration due to the metabolism of pulegone to menthofuran via the CYP450 enzyme pathway.[8242,8243,8244,8245,8246,8247] Menthofuran is a known liver toxin and can cause acute liver injury in high doses.[8248,8249]

■ Avoid use with drugs (acetaminophen, barbiturates, carbamazepine, phenobarbital, rifampin, phenytoin, nevirapine, secobarbital, enzalutamide, dexamethasone, modafinil, etc.) that are activated to toxic metabolites by CYP enzymes due to the potentially significant increase in liver toxicity caused by pulegone metabolites.[8250,8251]

■ Avoid with compromised liver or kidney due to significant potential of pulegone and its metabolites to cause liver and kidney toxicity (or acute liver/kidney injuries).[8252,8253,8254,8255,8256]

■ Avoid with epilepsy and Parkinson's disease due to pulegone content.[8257]

■ Avoid use in those with iron-deficiency and iron-deficiency anemia. Animal research suggests that spearmint may decrease iron absorption and therefore aggravate iron-deficiency symptoms and anemia.[8258]

*Carvone CT*

■ May interact with diabetes medications and cause low blood sugar based on carvone content.[8259]

■ May interact with aspirin, blood pressure, antiplatelet, and anticoagulant medications, and increase the risk of bleeding among people with bleeding disorders based on carvone content. Carvone is a potent calcium channel blocker, which may decrease blood pressure.[8260,8261]

■ May interact with barbiturates (medications for anxiety and insomnia), antihistamines, benzodiazepines, tricyclic antidepressants, or other central nervous system depressant drugs, increasing depressant effects, due to carvone content.[8262]

■ Avoid use in those with iron-deficiency and iron-deficiency anemia. Animal research suggests that spearmint may decrease iron absorption and therefore aggravate iron-deficiency symptoms and anemia.[8263]

*Piperitenone Oxide CTs*

■ May interact with antibiotics, antifungal, or antiviral drugs and increase their effectiveness.[8264,8265,8266]

■ Avoid use in those with iron-deficiency and iron-deficiency anemia. Animal research suggests that spearmint may decrease iron absorption and therefore aggravate iron-deficiency symptoms and anemia.[8267]

*Linalool CT*

■ *Linalool CT*: May interact with antifungal drugs and enhance their effectiveness based on linalool content.[8268]

**SELECTED EVIDENCE:**

☐ The oral administration of two drops each of peppermint and spearmint in a capsule every four hours in conjunction with normal antiemetic medications significantly reduced the number and severity of nausea/vomiting associated with chemotherapy treatment when compared to antiemetic drugs alone.[8269] Another study concluded that inhalation of ginger, spearmint, peppermint, and cardamom (three deep inhalations) from a gauze pad following surgery reduced nausea and requirements for medications to reduce nausea and vomiting.[8270]

☐ Spearmint oil, or carvone, reduces intestinal spasms according to animal research.[2154] Interestingly, the researchers concluded that carvone was a 100 times more potent calcium channel blocker than verapamil (a drug calcium channel blocker used to treat high blood pressure chest pain, and irregular heart rhythm). Agents that block calcium channels prevent calcium from entering heart and blood vessel cells, which results in

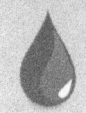

relaxed blood vessels and greater supply of blood and oxygen to the heart. Other research shows that oral administration of carvone reduces blood pressure by acting as a calcium channel blocker, reduces total cholesterol and triglycerides, and increases antioxidant (Vitamins C and E, reduced glutathione—GSH) activity.[8271]

- *In vitro* research suggest that spearmint oil inhibits *C. albicans*, *A. flavus*, *A. parasiticus*, *A. ochraceus*, and *F. moniliforme*, and drug-resistant and -susceptible *H. pylori*, and *S. aureus*.[8272,8273,8274] Another study determined that spearmint oil is a stronger antifungal than bifonazole (an antifungal drug).[8275] The carvone CT of spearmint essential oil inhibited three of thirteen filamentous (*Fusarium graminearum*, *F. moniliforme*, and *Penicillium expansum*) fungi *in vitro*.[8276]

- Spearmint oil prevents *S. mutans* from sticking together and forming plaque (biofilm) *in vitro*, possibly leading to the prevention of cavities.[8277]

- Animal research concluded that spearmint oil significantly reduces lung injury and inflammation in rats with chronic obstructive pulmonary disease (COPD).[8278]

- *In vitro* research suggests that spearmint oil increases the antibacterial effect of nitrofurantoin (an antibiotic used to treat bacterial urinary tract infections).[8279]

- Inhalation of spearmint or orange flower essential oils (0.02 mL/kg mixed with 2 mL of saline) through a nebulizer five minutes prior to a 1500 meter running test increased athletic performance in male college students (mean age 19.1 to 19.8, 50% to 10% smokers for the spearmint and orange groups respectively).[8280] Lung function was increased 20% in the spearmint group and 75% in the orange group, and the mean time to run the 1500 m was significantly decreased after inhaling both essential oils. Interestingly, a significant increase in Forced Expiratory Volume 1 (FEV1, the maximal amount of air that can be forcefully exhaled in one second, and a test used to measure airway obstruction, bronchoconstriction, or bronchodilation) and Forced Vital Capacity (FVC, the maximum amount of air that can be exhaled from the lungs) was observed after essential oil inhalation.

- Components of spearmint and pennyroyal essential oils (piperitenone and piperitone oxide) were biocidal (destroy, deter, render harmless, or control insects and harmful organisms by chemical or biological means) to the Colorado potato beetle (*Leptinotarsa decemlineata*); piperitone oxide and pulegone was biocidal to the African cotton leafworm (*Spodoptera littoralis*); and piperitenone oxide strongly inhibited the plant root-knot nematode (*Meloydogine javanica*), followed by piperitone oxide, piperitenone, and carvone.[8281] Based on these properties scientists concluded that these compounds may be useful as natural crop protectants.

- Rotundifolone and perillyl aldehyde from spearmint essential oil killed and inhibited the parasitic protozoan *T. brucei*, which is a cause of sleeping sickness (African trypanosomiasis) in humans and Nagana disease in animals.[8282]

- A review concluded that preclinical research demonstrates a beneficial effect of spearmint essential oil on osteoarthritic pain.[8283]

- The carvone CT of spearmint essential oil demonstrated significant anti-inflammatory and antinociceptive activity in animal research.[8284]

- Spearmint (carvone CT and rich in eugenol), thyme (thymol CT), and clove essential oils all killed head lice, with spearmint being the most effective.[8285]

- Sweet basil, cinnamon bark, sweet fennel, kaffir lime petitgrain, kaffir lime peel, black pepper, peppermint, and spearmint essential oils all demonstrated antimicrobial activity against bacteria linked to cavities (*Streptococcus mutans* and *Lactobacillus casei*).[8286] Cinnamon was the most active against both bacteria, kaffir lime petitgrain was the weakest of the tested oils against both bacteria, and black pepper was inactive against *L. casei*.

- Spearmint (carvone CT) essential oil significantly inhibited *S. aureus* biofilm formation when used at its minimum inhibitory concentration (MIC) and was still able to inhibit biofilm formation at half of its MIC.[8287]

- An animal model of polycystic ovarian syndrome demonstrates that oral administration of spearmint essential oil (150 or 300mg/kg BW) has treatment potential for PCOS by reducing testosterone production and restoring normal follicular development in ovarian tissue.[8288]

- Human aryl hydrocarbon receptor (AhR: a gene that encodes a protein that helps regulate responses to planar aromatic hydrocarbons and significantly affects the immune activity in the gastrointestinal tract, regulates the circadian rhythm, helps regulate the cell cycle, and plays an important role in tissue development). Cumin, jasmine, vanilla, and bay leaf fully activate AhR; clove, dill, thyme, nutmeg, and oregano partially activate AhR; and tarragon, caraway, turmeric, lovage, fennel, spearmint, star anise, and anise inhibit the AhR activity.[8289]

- Spearmint CT carvone and mojito mint CT piperitenone oxide essential oils both inactivated spoilage yeasts (*C. albicans, P. anomala*, and *S. cerevisiae*) in nut and fruit juices.[8290]
- The carvone CT of spearmint essential oil exhibited moderate antioxidant activity and weak to moderate antimicrobial activities against *Candida glabrata, Escherichia coli*, and *Staphylococcus epidermidis*.[8291]
- Spearmint CT rotundifoliae essential oil was toxic to glioblastoma (the most common and aggressive brain tumor) cancer cells and increased expression of genes associated with antioxidant activity without causing genetic damage in blood cells.[8292]
- Marjoram, pink savory (*Satureja thymbra*), spearmint CT piperitenone oxide, melissa, and dittany (*Origanum dictamnus*) demonstrated the greatest repellency toward *Ae. albopictus* mosquitoes of fourteen Lamiaceae species tested.[8293] Thyme CT thymol, basil, dittany, marjoram, and oregano CT carvacrol were the most larvicidal.
- The carvone (69.2%) CT of spearmint essential oil was antifungal to *Cryptococcus neoformans* and the dermatophytes *Trichophyton rubrum* and *T. verrucosum*, and inhibited *C. albicans* germ tube formation at amounts well below its minimum inhibitory concentration (MIC).[8294]
- Both native and Scotch spearmint with carvone as the major constituent of both oils exhibited good antioxidant activity in the DPPH and TEAC assays and increased natural production of glutathione.[8295]
- Spanish lavender CT camphor and spearmint CT carvone essential oils both exhibited mild antibacterial activity against pathogens that cause sinusitis (*Streptococcus pneumoniae, Streptococcus pyogenes, Staphylococcus aureus, Haemophilus influenzae, Moraxella catarrhalis*, and *Pseudomonas aeruginosa*).[8296]
- Rewiring mice to have cellular sensitivity to spearmint (mice-bearing designer cells) permitted the inhalation or ingestion of spearmint CT carvone essential oil to reduce chronic inflammatory and neuropathic pain without any adverse cardiovascular, immune, or behavioral side effects.[8297]
- Spearmint CT carvone exhibited strong inhibitory activities against the principal enzymes associated with Alzheimer's disease and obesity (cholinesterase and porcine pancreatic lipase), including synergism with standard drugs used for obesity and overweight.[8298] The same study showed that it possesses strong antidermatophytic activity against *Microsporum canis, Trichophyton rubrum, T. mentagrophytes*, and *Epidermophyton floccosum*, and inhibited biofilm formation by MRSA.
- Pants treated with 5% spearmint or thyme essential oil caused ticks to significantly drop off the pants within three minutes. Blankets treated with 5% spearmint or oregano essential oil significantly repelled ticks.[8299] The results showed that oregano and spearmint essential oils are promising natural clothing repellents, with an effective equivalence to 20% DEET.
- Spearmint essential oil inhibited MRSA and *Y. enterocolitica* and increased the antimicrobial activity of sodium benzoate.[8300]
- May chang, Virginia cedarwood, spearmint, and tea tree essential oils each demonstrated contact toxicity against third instar larvae of the cotton leafworm (*Alabama argillacea*).[8301] Each oil changed the histochemistry of the testicles, while tea tree, Virginia cedarwood, and spearmint altered morphology. In addition, the histochemistry of the ovarioles was altered by Virginia cedarwood, tea tree, and may chang.
- Spearmint essential oil exhibited promising fumigant toxicity against pulse beetles (*Callosobruchus chinensis*), followed by peppermint (pulse beetles: *Callosobruchus maculatus*).[8302] Combining peppermint with tagetes (*T. minuta*) increased the toxicity against *C. chinensis*. The essential oils also repelled the beetles and interfered with reproduction.
- Thyme, oregano, lemongrass, spearmint, and rosemary essential oils were each inhibited multidrug-resistant foodborne pathogens isolated from raw milk (*Escherichia, Enterobacter, Citrobacter, Proteus, Klebsiella*, and *Staphylococcus*) but were ineffective against *Pseudomonas*.[8303] Thyme was the most active followed by oregano.
- Researchers analyzed the composition and antimicrobial activity of mint essential oils, including bergamot mint, peppermint, pennyroyal, spearmint, and apple mint. Bergamot mint inhibited *S. typhi* and *C. albicans*, peppermint *E. coli, B. subtilis*, and *C. albicans*; pennyroyal *K. pneumoniae, B. subtilis*, and *C. albicans*; spearmint significantly inhibited *S. typhi* and *B. subtilis*; and apple mint inhibited *K. pneumoniae, C. albicans*, and *S. typhi*.[8304]
- A nanogel with spearmint CT carvone essential oil was significantly more potent as an antioxidant than the free essential oil.[8305] The nanogel also exhibited antibacterial activity against *S. aureus* and *E. coli*.
- A preclinical model of dental plaque on teeth showed that both spearmint and eucalyptus essential oils reduced *S. mutans* biofilms at 0.5% concentration.[8306]

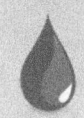

# SPIKE LAVENDER

*Lavandula latifolia* Medikus, *Lavandula spica* DC

**FAMILY:** Lamiaceae
**NOTE:** Middle
**AROMA INTENSITY:** Strong
**AROMA:** Spicy, medicinal, fresh, floral
**COMMON EXTRACTION METHOD:** Steam distilled from the flowers
**POSSIBLE SUBSTITUTE OILS:** Spanish sage, lavender, lavandin
**BLENDS WELL WITH:** Cedarwood, cinnamon, clary sage, clove, eucalyptus, lavender, patchouli, neroli, nutmeg, pine, rosemary, sage
**SUBCELLULAR LOCALIZATION | EPIGENETIC INFLUENCE:** Currently unknown | Currently unknown
**RECOMMENDED DILUTION RANGE:** 3%–50%; neat for limited conditions

**PRIMARY CONSTITUENTS:**[8307,8308,8309]

| | |
|---|---|
| Linalool | 27.2%–43.1% |
| 1,8-Cineole | 28.0%–34.9% |
| Camphor | 10.8%–23.2% |
| Borneol | 0.9%–10.1% |
| Beta-Pinene | 0.8%–2.6% |
| (E)-Alpha-Bisabolene | 0.2%–2.3% |
| Beta-Caryophyllene | 0.5%–1.9% |
| Alpha-Terpineol | 0.8%–1.6% |
| Trans-Caryophyllene Oxide | 0.0%–1.6% |

**OTHER CONSTITUENTS:** Alpha-pinene, beta-myrcene, camphene, cis-beta-ocimene, d-limonene, sabinene, beta-farnesene, gamma-terpineol, caryophyllene oxide, linalyl acetate

**PREFERRED COMPOSITION FOR CLINICAL USE:**

| *Constituent* | |
|---|---|
| **Linalool** | 34%–50% |
| **1,8-Cineole** | 20%–35% |
| **Camphor** | 10%–20% |
| **Beta-Pinene** | 1%–3% |
| **Trans-Alpha-Bisabolene** | 1%–3% |
| **Alpha-Pinene** | 1%–3% |
| **Limonene** | 0.5%–3.0% |
| **Linalyl Acetate** | 0.1%–3% |
| **Alpha-Terpineol** | 0.5%–2.0% |

**REPORTED THERAPEUTIC PROPERTIES: Analgesic (pain relief)**, anti-inflammatory, antifungal, antimicrobial, **antiseptic**, antispasmodic, expels excess gas, relieves insect bites, promotes the flow of bile, diuretic, **expectorant**, nervine (calms and soothes the nerves), aids digestion, increases redness and circulation of a localized area, **relieves skin conditions**, increases sweating, **wound healing**, stimulating, antidepressant, combats shock, relieves anxiety, **stress management**

**CAUTIONS:**

■ Avoid with children under 6 due to high camphor content. Several cases of camphor poisoning and/or seizures from ingestion and topical application have been reported in children.[8310,8311] Ingestion of camphor-containing products has been lethal in children under age 2 (estimated to be roughly 2,000 mg of camphor for a 20 kg child as the minimum potential fatal dose).[8312,8313] Children 5 years and up may use camphor topically in dilutions no stronger than 5%. 1,8-cineole may cause seizures, central nervous system problems, or respiratory distress in young children.[8314,8315,8316,8317]

■ Caution is warranted during pregnancy and while lactating due to potentially high camphor content. Ingestion of essential oils with significant levels of camphor may lead to abortion because fetuses lack the enzymes to process it.[8318] Camphor ingestion by infants and young children may cause cough, vomiting, seizure, burning sensation in the mucous membranes and eyes, or lack of voluntary coordination of muscle movements.[8319]

■ Caution is warranted orally due to the significant amounts of 1,8-cineole and camphor content. Limit it to small doses internally (adults—maximum 10 drops daily). Toxicity has been reported when eucalyptus (also high in 1,8-cineole) was ingested in large doses, and as few as 4 to 5 drops may cause problems in very sensitive individuals.[8320,8321,8322,8323,8324,8325] In humans, 3.5 to 5 mL has proven fatal orally.[8326] Essential oils that contain significant amounts of camphor can be toxic when taken orally (usually single doses exceeding 2 mL), although the lethal dose for adult humans is estimated to be more than 5 mL in a single dose.[8327,8328,8329]

■ Avoid with epilepsy and Parkinson's disease due to 1,8-cineole and camphor content. May exacerbate or cause seizures or convulsions when inhaled, applied topically, or ingested based on 1,8-cineole content.[8330,8331,8332,8333,8334,8335]

■ The camphor content in spike lavender may negatively impact red blood cells and increase the risk of jaundice in children with Glucose-6-phosphate dehydrogenase deficiency (G6PD).[8336,8337]

■ May interfere with pentobarbital and other barbiturates (medications for anxiety and insomnia) based on 1,8-cineole content.[8338,8339]

■ May weakly interfere with the enzymes responsible for metabolizing medications (NSAIDs, proton-pump inhibitors, acetaminophen, antiepileptics, immune modulators, blood-sugar medications, blood pressure medications, antidepressants, antipsychotics, diabetic medications, antihistamines, antibiotics, and anesthetics) due to 1,8-cineole content.[8340,8341,8342]

■ Avoid with those who have a compromised liver due to the risk of increased liver enzymes and liver damage.[8343] This would also suggest that those taking medications that could cause liver damage should also use spike lavender very cautiously or avoid it entirely.

**SELECTED EVIDENCE:**

□ Spike lavender inhibits the growth of *S. aureus* and MRSA *in vitro*.[8344]

□ *In vitro* research concluded that spike lavender inhibits several foodborne pathogens (*S. Enteritidis, S. Typhimurium, E. coli, Y. enterocolitica, S. flexneri, L. monocytogenes serovar*, and *S. aureus*).[8345]

□ Inhalation of spike lavender helped clear the sinuses and increased the expectoration of mucus from the bronchi and lungs (lasting from twenty minutes to two hours) in 40 people with sinus or nasal congestion.[8346]

□ Both spike lavender and true lavender reduce inflammation by inhibiting lipoxygenase (LOX) activity, which activity was attributed to the presence of linalool, camphor, para-cymene, and limonene.[8347]

□ Spike lavender is considered a good antioxidant due to its high concentration of oxygenated terpenes.[8348]

□ *In vitro* research found that spike lavender inhibits *S. aureus* and *L. monocytogenes* and this activity is improved when the oil is combined with isolated camphor.[8349]

# SPIKENARD
## (Green Spikenard)

*Nardostachys grandiflora* DC, *N. jatamansi* (D.Don) DC.

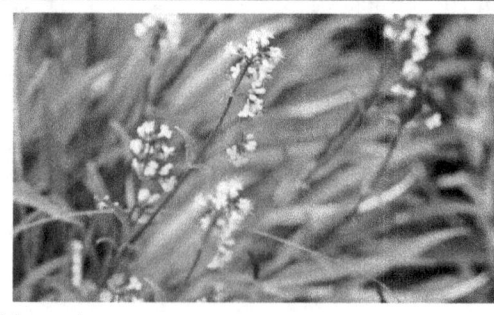

**FAMILY:** Valerianaceae
**NOTE:** Base
**AROMA INTENSITY:** Strong
**AROMA:** Woody, spicy, musty
**COMMON EXTRACTION METHOD:** Steam distilled from the roots (rhizome)
**POSSIBLE SUBSTITUTE OILS:** Patchouli, vetiver
**BLENDS WELL WITH:** Cistus, clary sage, clove, cypress, frankincense, geranium, juniper, lavender, myrrh, neroli, orange, palmarosa, patchouli, petitgrain, pine, rose, sage, vetiver

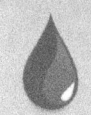

**SUBCELLULAR LOCALIZATION | EPIGENETIC INFLUENCE:** Currently unknown | *Immune/Nervous*
**RECOMMENDED DILUTION RANGE:** 5%–Neat

**PRIMARY CONSTITUENTS:**[8350,8351,8352,8353,8354,8355,8356 2196–2201A]

*Calarene CT*

| | |
|---|---|
| Calarene (Beta-Gurjunene) | 25.9%–35.4% |
| Aristolone | 6.3%–15.6% |
| Patchoulol | 0.0%–10.6% |
| Beta-Maaliene | 5.6%–10.2% |
| Valeranone (Jatamansone) | 3.7%–9.7% |
| Alpha-Gurjunene | 0.1%–9.1% |
| Valerena-4,7-Diene | 0.0%–6.6% |
| Spathulenol | 0.0%–4.3% |

*Calarene CT (Nepal)*

| | |
|---|---|
| Calarene (Beta-Gurjunene) | 9.4%–29.1% |
| 1(10)-Aristolen-9beta-ol | 0.0%–11.6% |
| Valeranone (Jatamansone) | 7.9%–9.7% |
| Valerena-4,7(11)-diene | 0.0%–7.1% |
| Aristolenone | 0.0%–6.5% |
| Nardol A | 0.0%–6.0% |
| Cis-Valerinic Acid | 0.0%–5.7% |
| Valerenal | 0.0%–5.6% |
| Beta-Maaliene | 0.0%–5.6% |

*Ledene Oxide CT (Pakistani)*

| | |
|---|---|
| Ledene Oxide | 13.0% |
| Patchoulol | 9.6% |
| Spathulenol | 2.7% |
| Globulol | 1.9% |

*Valeranone CT (Indian)*

| | |
|---|---|
| Valeranone (Jatamansone) | 36.7% |
| Epi-Alpha-Cadinol | 22.7% |
| Alpha-Eudesmol | 3.0% |

*Nardol CT (Indian)*

| | |
|---|---|
| Nardol | 10.1% |
| Formic Acid | 9.4% |
| Alpha-Selinene | 9.2% |
| Dihydro-Beta-Ionene | 7.9% |

**OTHER CONSTITUENTS:** Isovaleric acid, 3-methylvaleric acid, alpha-pinene, camphene, beta-pinene, 1,8-cineole, gamma-terpinene, linalool, 4-terpineol, alpha-terpineol, beta-patchoulene, beta-gurjunene, beta-maaliene, aromadendrene, beta-Ionone, alpha-selinene, alpha-bulnesene, alloaromadendrene, delta-cadinene, spathulenol, viridiflorol, 3,7 guaiadiene, alpha-bulnesene, beta-elemene, cis-4,5-muuroladiene, epi-alpha-selinene, seychellene, daucol, spirojatamol isomer, valerenal MW=218; *Calarene CT Nepal*—beta-patchoulene, gamma-cadinene, delta-cadinene, carotol, alpha-cadinol, 4-methoxy-7H-furo3,2-g-1-benzopyran-7-one, alpha-panasinsen, aristolene, aristolone, 1,2,3,4,5,6,7,8a-octahydro-3,6,8,8-tetramethyl-1H-3a,methazulene, 1,2,3,4,5,6,7,8,8a-decahydro-1,4a-dimethyl-7-(1-methylethylidene)-1-napthalenol

**PREFERRED COMPOSITION FOR CLINICAL USE:**

| Constituent | Calarene CT | Green | Nepal I | Nepal II |
|---|---|---|---|---|
| **Calarene (Beta-Gurjunene)** | 25%–40% | 5%–15% | 5%–10% | 2%–7% |
| **Aristolone** | 6%–15% | – | – | – |
| **Beta-Maaliene** | 5%–11% | – | – | 0.5%–3% |
| **Valeranone (Jatamansone)** | 4%–10% | 2%–10% | 3%–10% | 5%–28% |
| **Alpha-Gurjunene** | 0.1%–5% | 1%–3% | 0.5%–3% | 0.1%–1% |
| **Valencene** | – | 5%–15% | 0%–3% | – |
| **6,9-Guaiadiene** | – | 5%–15% | 0%–10% | – |
| **Nardol Isomers** | | 0%–10% | 0%–10% | – |
| **Valerena-4,7(11)-diene** | – | 3%–8% | 0%–7% | – |
| **3,7-Guaiadiene** | – | – | 0%–7% | 0%–7% |
| **Beta-Pinene** | – | 1%–8% | 0%–3% | 0%–3% |
| **Valerenal** | – | – | 4%–9% | 2%–9% |
| **Seychellene** | – | 2%–6% | 0%–4% | 0.5%–5% |
| **Alpha-Patchoulene** | – | 2%–5% | 0.5%–6% | 0%–3% |

| | | | | |
|---|---|---|---|---|
| Beta-Patchoulene | – | 1%–4% | 1%–3% | 0%–2% |
| Alpha-Guaiene | – | 1%–4% | 0.5%–4% | 0%–2% |
| (E)-Beta-Guaiene | – | 1%–3% | – | – |
| Patchoulol | | 1%–3% | 0%–2% | 0%–2% |
| Spirojatamol | – | 0%–3% | 0%–6% | 3%–25% |
| Alpha-Pinene | – | 0%–3% | 0.5%–2% | 0%–2% |

Note: There is very little consistency in spikenard samples from batch to batch even when sourced from the same location. In addition, some reports list both beta-gurjunene and calarene even though they are considered synonyms by some experts, though it is not accepted by all chemists/experts/databases as a synonym.

**REPORTED THERAPEUTIC PROPERTIES:** Antibacterial, antifungal, anti-infectious, antispasmodic, anti-inflammatory, antiseptic, **antiallergic**, relieves constipation, promotes cellular regeneration, **relieves headache (migraine)**, stimulates production of female hormones, **balances heart function**, promotes lymph circulation, aids circulation, **wound healing**, **sedating**, encourages calm and peace, stress management, **relieves anxiety**

**CAUTIONS:**

■ None currently known.

**SELECTED EVIDENCE:**

□ Spikenard essential oil (Nepal) killed breast cancer cells *in vitro*.[8357]

□ *In vitro* research concluded that spikenard oil (root and rhizome) protected heart muscle cells from oxidative stress and death, which is a major cause of heart disorders.[8358]

□ Spikenard oil prevents the growth of *A. flavus, A. fumigatus, A. sulphureus, M. fragilis, R. stolonifer, A. niger,* and *F. oxysporum in vitro*.[2203,2204] Other research demonstrates that spikenard essential oil (Nepal) possesses antimicrobial activity against *Bacillus cereus, Escherichia coli*, and *Candida albicans*.[8359]

□ Spikenard essential oil triggers vasodilation through multiple channels: rapidly activating the release of nitric oxide, increasing phosphorylation of eNOS, enhancing intracellular Ca2+ and BAPTA-AM levels, and markedly decreasing phosphorylation of Akt kinase.[8360]

□ Spikenard essential oil protected heart muscle cells (cardiomyocytes) from oxidative stress-induced cell death by reducing reactive oxygen species (ROS) inside cells, activating Akt phosphorylation, and enhancing gene expression of antioxidant enzymes (glutathione S-transferase, NAD(P)H quinone oxidoreductase, glutamate-cysteine ligase catalytic and modulatory subunits).[8361]

□ A preclinical model of chronic skin inflammation demonstrates that spikenard essential oil inhibits protein molecules involved in inflammation, immune responses, and tissue remodeling, which suggests that it reduces skin inflammation and promotes wound healing.[8362]

□ Spikenard essential oil was significantly toxic to the cigarette beetle (*Lasioderma serricorne*).[8363]

□ Of three essential oils tested (spikenard, valerian, and *Valeriana jatamansi*), spikenard essential oil exhibited the highest acetylcholinesterase (AChE) inhibitory activity, followed by valerian.[8364] Spikenard and valerian also inhibited neuron activity—inhibited spontaneous electrical activity—based on microelectrode arrays analyses on rat cortical neurons. The researchers noted that the presence of oxygenated compounds, such as aldehydes and ketones, was a major factor in the potency and effects of the oils. The results suggest that the traditional use of these two oils for neurological disorders, like anxiety, depression, and dementia, warrants further investigation in humans.

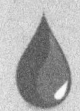

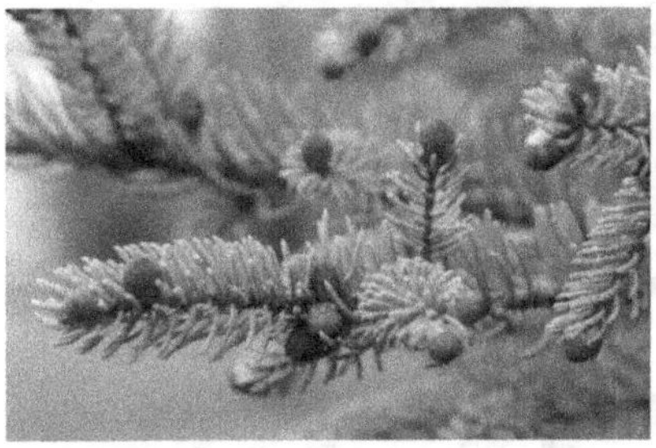

# SPRUCE (BLACK)

*Picea mariana* (Mill.) Britton, Sterns & Poggenb.

**FAMILY:** Pinaceae
**NOTE:** Top-Middle
**AROMA INTENSITY:** Medium
**AROMA:** Woody, earthy, evergreen
**COMMON EXTRACTION METHOD:** Steam distilled from the needles
**POSSIBLE SUBSTITUTE OILS:** Blue spruce, tsuga, silver fir, rosemary (bornyl acetate CT), balsam fir, white fir, pine
**BLENDS WELL WITH:** Birch, blue spruce, cedarwood, eucalyptus, frankincense, galbanum, helichrysum, lavender, palo santo, pine, rosemary, silver fir, white fir, wintergreen
**SUBCELLULAR LOCALIZATION | EPIGENETIC INFLUENCE:** Nuclear Membrane | Circulatory/Respiratory
**RECOMMENDED DILUTION RANGE:** 5%–50%; neat for limited conditions

**PRIMARY CONSTITUENTS:**[8365,8366,8367,8368,8369]

| | |
|---|---|
| Bornyl acetate | 21.6%–52.0% |
| Camphene | 14.0%–22.0% |
| Alpha-pinene | 7.4%–16.6% |
| Borneol | 0.0%–7.8% |
| Limonene | 2.6%–5.5% |
| Tricyclene | 0.0%–4.6% |

**OTHER CONSTITUENTS:** Beta-myrcene, beta-pinene, fenchyl acetate, beta-elemene, caryophyllene, beta-phellandrene, isobornyl acetate, camphor, delta-cadinene, alpha-amorphene, germacrene D, 1,3-cyclohexadiene, longifolene, santene

**PREFERRED COMPOSITION FOR CLINICAL USE:**

| *Constituent* | |
|---|---|
| **Bornyl Acetate** | 22%–40% |
| **Camphene** | 12%–25% |
| **Alpha-Pinene** | 12%–22% |
| **Delta-3-Carene** | 6%–12% |
| **Beta-Pinene** | 3%–12% |
| **Limonene** | 2%–6% |
| **Beta-Myrcene** | 2%–6% |
| **Santene** | 1%–5% |
| **Tricyclene** | 1%–5% |

**REPORTED THERAPEUTIC PROPERTIES: Analgesic (pain relief)**, antimicrobial, antiseptic, eases cough, anti-inflammatory, antispasmodic, astringent, diuretic, expectorant, **nervine (calms and soothes the nerves)**, stimulates thyroid function, **supports adrenal gland function**, increases redness and circulation of a localized area, warming, **relieves exhaustion**, grounding, calming, reduces mood swings, encourages self-confidence, self-acceptance, and forgiveness, **relieves anxiety**, stress management, promotes a sense of security

**CAUTIONS:**
■ None currently known.

**SELECTED EVIDENCE:**
□ Black spruce oil inhibits MRSA *in vitro*.[8370]
□ Inhalation of bornyl acetate, the main constituent in black spruce, for 40 minutes influenced autonomic nervous system activity and provided a calming effect in healthy males without influencing task performance.[8371] This study suggests that black spruce may be beneficial for those who are anxious while performing tasks.

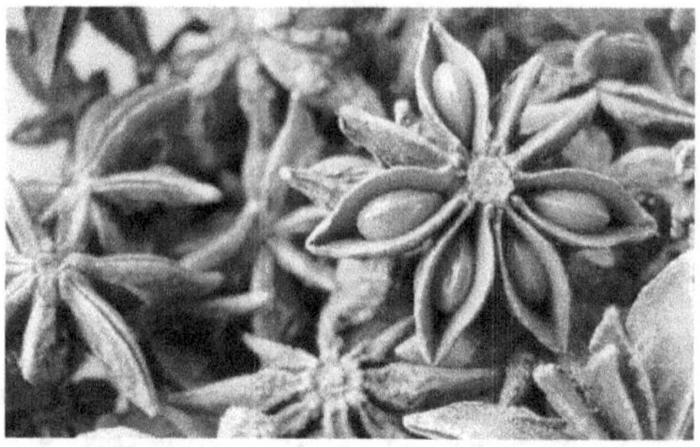

# STAR ANISE
## (Chinese Anise)

*Illicium verum* Hook. f.

**FAMILY:** Illiciaceae

**NOTE:** Middle

**AROMA INTENSITY:** Strong

**AROMA:** Licorice-like, sharp, fresh, sweet, spicy

**COMMON EXTRACTION METHOD:** Steam distilled from the fresh and partly dried seeds

**POSSIBLE SUBSTITUTE OILS:** Anise, fennel (trans-anethole CT)

**BLENDS WELL WITH:** Anise, bay laurel, cardamom, caraway, cedarwood, coriander, dill, fennel, lavender, lemon, neroli, orange, petitgrain, rosewood, tangerine

**SUBCELLULAR LOCALIZATION | EPIGENETIC INFLUENCE:** Currently unknown | Currently unknown

**RECOMMENDED DILUTION RANGE:** 3%–50%; sensitive populations (those with chronic skin conditions, autoimmune/autoinflammatory disorders, allergies, or chronic respiratory ailments should dilute star anise to 0.3%–0.5% due to a higher risk of sensitization when applied topically).[2867]

**PRIMARY CONSTITUENTS:**[8372,8373,8374,8375]

| | |
|---|---|
| Trans-Anethole | 87.4%–94.1% |
| Limonene | 0.4%–6.5% |
| Methyl Chavicol (Estragole) | 0.0%–5.2% |
| Chavicol | 0.0%–2.7% |
| Anisaldehyde | 0.0%–1.8% |

**OTHER CONSTITUENTS:** Cis-anethole, alpha-pinene, 2-(1-cyclopentenyl)-furan, cinnamyl acetate, foeniculin, anisketone, linalool, alpha-phellandrene, beta-caryophyllene, trans-alpha-bergamotene

**PREFERRED COMPOSITION FOR CLINICAL USE:**

| *Constituent* | |
|---|---|
| **Trans-Anethole** | 85%–95% |
| **Limonene** | 0.1%–6% |
| **Methyl Chavicol (Estragole)** | < 5% |
| **Foeniculin ((E)-Foeniculin)** | 0.1%–3% |
| **Linalool** | 0.1%–3% |
| **Alpha-Pinene** | 0.1%–2% |
| **Para-Anisaldehyde** | < 2% |
| **Trans- + Cis-Alpha-Bergamotene** | tr–1% |
| **Cis-Anethole** | tr–1% |

**REPORTED THERAPEUTIC PROPERTIES:** Antiseptic, antibacterial, antifungal, **analgesic** (especially chronic), **antiviral**, anti-inflammatory, antiparasitic, antioxidant, antirheumatic, antispasmodic, supports digestive function, eases cough, expels excess gas, decongestant, expectorant, supports respiratory function, anti-epileptic, aids circulation, balances blood sugar levels, reduces painful menstruation, **insecticide**, **insect repellent**, promotes restful sleep, purification, promotes self-confidence, relieves anxiety, antidepressant

**CAUTIONS:**

■ Use with caution and highly diluted for children under six due to methyl chavicol (estragole) and trans-anethole content.[8376]

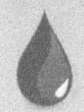

■ Long-term oral use of star anise is not advised in young girls because of reports that fennel tea (also high in anethole) may cause premature breast development in very young girls when used chronically.[8377] Long-term oral use is not recommended for children under age twelve.

■ Avoid during pregnancy and lactation due to estrogenic activity of trans-anethole.[8378,8379,8380,8381] It is also worth noting that trans-anethole may negatively affect fertility. Animal research suggests it decreases fertility by preventing the implantation of a fertilized egg in the uterus.[8382] Large doses of fennel (also high in anethole) may be toxic to fetal cells based on animal research.[8383,8384] Nephrotoxicity (kidney toxicity) has been reported in breastfed infants whose mothers drank an herbal tea that contained anise, fennel, licorice, and goat's rue.[8385]

■ May interact with aspirin, blood pressure, antiplatelet, and anticoagulant medications, and increase the risk of bleeding among people with bleeding disorders based on its similar consistency to fennel oil.[8386,8387,8388]

■ May interact with diabetes medications and cause low blood sugar due to trans-anethole content.[8389,8390,8391]

■ May decrease the effectiveness of diuretic medications due to anise oil's antidiuretic effects and star anise has a very similar constituency profile.[8392]

■ May interact with acetaminophen and caffeine and reduce their bioavailability and effectiveness based on a very similar constituency profile to anise oil.[8393]

■ May interact with benzodiazepines and increase motor impairment based on a very similar constituency profile to anise oil.[8394]

■ May interact with barbiturates and reduce sleeping time and effectiveness based on a very similar constituency profile to anise oil.[8395]

■ May interact with ibuprofen and enhance its anti-inflammatory activity.[8396]

■ May interact with codeine and increase its analgesic effect based on a very similar constituency profile to anise oil.[8397]

■ May interact with antidepressants (fluoxetine and imipramine) and decrease their effectiveness based on a very similar constituency profile to anise oil.[8398]

■ Star anise oil contains significant amounts of the phytoestrogen anethole. Anethole exhibits weak estrogenic activity[8399] and many aromatherapy texts suggest avoiding star anise with endometriosis, oral contraceptives, hormone replacement therapy, and estrogen-dependent cancers because of this. However, research suggests that anethole may promote destruction (apoptosis) of cancer cells—including both estrogen-positive and estrogen-negative breast cancer cells— and phytoestrogens are generally balancing with the ability to either mimic or block the action of estrogen according to current knowledge.[8400,8401] In addition, anethole reduced painful uterine contractions in the rat uterus.[8402] A follow up clinical study confirmed the animal results, and suggests that fennel essential oil reduces painful menstruation and excess menstrual bleeding, and relaxes the smooth muscles of the uterus.[8403] Lastly, another study found that 97.5% of women treated with a traditional Chinese medicine formula containing fennel and cordyceps experienced improvements in their endometrial symptoms.[8404] Based on this, reasonable doses pose little risk of interaction or contraindication.

■ May interfere with the enzymes responsible for metabolizing medications based on estragole and trans-anethole content (NSAIDs, proton-pump inhibitors, acetaminophen, antiepileptics, immune modulators, blood-sugar medications, blood pressure medications, antidepressants, antipsychotics, diabetic medications, antihistamines, antibiotics, and anesthetics).[8405,8406,8407,8408,8409,8410]

### SELECTED EVIDENCE:

☐ *In vitro* research concluded that star anise oil is antimicrobial against *S. pneumoniae, B. cereus, A. lwoffii, E. coli, K. pneumoniae, C. perfingens, C. albicans* and *C. krusei.*[8411] Another study reported that fennel essential oil inhibits *Listeria innocua.*[8412]

☐ Star anise essential oil proved more potent than DEET in repelling the mites *Leptotrombidium pallidum.*[8413] Another study found that it strongly inhibited egg laying by female house flies.[8414] A third study reported that star anise kills the *Aedes aegypti* mosquito.[8415]

☐ *In vitro* research discovered that star anise reduces HSV-1 (herpes simplex virus type 1) infection of cells by greater than 99%.[8416]

☐ Anethole reduces pain sensation, acute lung inflammation, nonimmune acute inflammation (an inflammatory response mediated by white cell count, plasma lactoferrin, C-reactive protein, ferritin, iron, and iron-binding capacity), and acute and chronic inflammatory pain in animals.[8417,8418,8419,8420]

- ☐ Star anise essential oil was toxic to the adult spotted wing drosophila (*Drosophila suzukii*) when used as a fumigant.[8421]

- ☐ Nanoencapsulated star anise essential oil may prolong the shelf-life of food items due to its antifungal activity and ability to inhibit the production of aflatoxin B1.[8422]

- ☐ Human aryl hydrocarbon receptor (AhR: a gene that encodes a protein that helps regulate responses to planar aromatic hydrocarbons and significantly affects the immune activity in the gastrointestinal tract, regulates the circadian rhythm, helps regulate the cell cycle, and plays an important role in tissue development). Cumin, jasmine, vanilla, and bay leaf fully activate AhR; clove, dill, thyme, nutmeg, and oregano partially activate AhR; and tarragon, caraway, turmeric, lovage, fennel, spearmint, star anise, and anise inhibit the AhR activity.[8423]

- ☐ Encapsulation of star anise essential oil in hydroxypropyl and beta-cyclodextrin (HPCD) improved its antibacterial activity against *Rhizopus stolonifer, Saccharomyces cerevisiae*, and *E. coli*.[8424]

- ☐ Ylang ylang and star anise essential oil exhibited strong acaricidal activity against the castor bean tick (*Ixodes ricinus*)—a tick that can transmit both bacterial and viral pathogens such as the causative agents of Lyme disease and tick-borne encephalitis.[8425]

- ☐ Star anise CT methyleugenol, allspice, and nutmeg all demonstrated larvicidal and adulticidal activity against the *Aedes aegypti* mosquito.[8426] Nutmeg essential oil produced the highest mortality.

- ☐ Both star anise and geranium essential oils showed insecticidal activity against cat fleas (*Ctenocephalides felis felis*), with star anise being more effective.[8427]

- ☐ Complexes of beta-cyclodextrin and vaporized star anise essential oil demonstrated stronger antibacterial activity against *E. coli, B. subtilis, S. epidermidis*, and *S. aureus* than the free oil and good antioxidant activity.[8428]

# SUMMER SAVORY
## (Garden Savory)

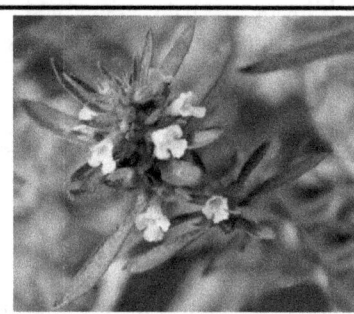

*Satureja hortensis* L., *Calamintha hortensis* Hort.

**FAMILY:** Lamiaceae (Labiatae)
**NOTE:** Middle
**AROMA INTENSITY:** Strong
**AROMA:** Herbaceous, medicinal, spicy, slightly sweet
**COMMON EXTRACTION METHOD:** Steam distilled or hydrodistilled from the flowering aerial parts
**POSSIBLE SUBSTITUTE OILS:** Oregano, thyme (carvacrol CT), mountain savory
**BLENDS WELL WITH:** Bergamot, grapefruit, lavender, lemon, lime, orange, oregano, pine, rosemary, tangerine, thyme
**SUBCELLULAR LOCALIZATION | EPIGENETIC INFLUENCE:** Currently unknown | Currently unknown
**RECOMMENDED DILUTION RANGE:** 1.5%–20%; 50% for some conditions

**PRIMARY CONSTITUENTS:**[8429,8430,8431,8432,8433,8434,8435,8436]

*Carvacrol CT*

| | |
|---|---|
| Carvacrol | 44.0%–79.2% |
| Gamma-Terpinene | 9.1%–41.8% |
| Para-Cymene | 3.1%–6.7% |

*Gamma-Terpinene CT*

| | |
|---|---|
| Gamma-Terpinene | 27.4%–70.4% |
| Carvacrol | 12.3%–40.2% |
| Para-Cymene | 1.7%–11.1% |
| Alpha-Terpinene | 0.0%–10.2% |
| Alpha-Pinene | 0.0%–5.1% |
| Myrcene | 0.0%–5.1% |

*Thymol CT*

| | |
|---|---|
| Thymol | 28.2%–40.5% |
| Para-Cymene | 9.0%–19.6% |
| Gamma-Terpinene | 16.0%–18.6% |
| Carvacrol | 11.0%–14.0% |
| Beta-Pinene | 1.2%–4.5% |
| Sabinene | 1.3%–4.4% |

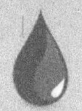

**OTHER CONSTITUENTS:** *Carvacrol CT*—alpha-thujene, alpha-pinene, myrcene, limonene, alpha-terpinene, beta-caryophyllene, beta-bisabolene, bicyclogermacrene; *Thymol CT*—alpha-thujene, myrcene, alpha-terpinene, camphor, pinocarvone, terpinen-4-ol, alpha-phellandrene, cuminal, trans-anethole, gamma-cadinene, caryophyllene oxide, T-cadinol; *Gamma-Terpinene CT*—alpha-thujene, camphene, beta-pinene, alpha-phellandrene, beta-thujene, sylvestrene, terpinen-4-ol, para-thymol, d-carvone, carvacrol acetate, beta-caryophyllene, beta-bisabolene

**PREFERRED COMPOSITION FOR CLINICAL USE:**

| Constituent | Carvacrol CT | Thymol CT |
| --- | --- | --- |
| **Carvacrol** | 45%–70% | 10%–15% |
| **Gamma-Terpinene** | 18%–38% | 15%–20% |
| **Para-Cymene** | 3%–7% | 8%–15% |
| **Alpha-Terpinene** | 2%–7% | – |
| **Thymol** | – | 28%–42% |
| **Beta-Pinene** | – | 1%–5% |
| **Sabinene** | – | 1%–5% |
| **Myrcene** | – | 0.5%–2% |

**REPORTED THERAPEUTIC PROPERTIES:** Antibacterial, antifungal, antiviral, **antimicrobial**, antiparasitic, **antioxidant**, **antiseptic**, eases cough, aids digestion, expels excess gas, immune stimulant, supports circulatory function, analgesic, antispasmodic, anti-inflammatory, antiarthritic, **supports oral health**, relieves diarrhea, aids respiratory function, relieves intestinal cramps, balances menstruation, expels excess mucus, soothes sore throat, reduces shock, combats fear, stress management

**CAUTIONS:**

■ Avoid during pregnancy and lactation due to similar composition to oregano essential oil. Oils rich in carvacrol may negatively affect embryonic development and encourage fetal cell death according to animal research.[8437]

■ *Thymol CT*: Oral caution. May contain up to 45.2% thymol. Thymol has a longer half-life (the time it takes for half of the medication to metabolize or excrete half of the dosage) than most essential oil constituents and should not be administered orally for long periods of time.[8438] Thymol is a monoterpene phenol. Reports of fatalities in children who consumed 50 to 200 mg of phenols has been reported.[8439] It is recommended that chemotypes with high levels of thymol be limited to 10 drops per day orally for adults with a two- to seven-day break after twenty-one days of use.

■ *Carvacrol CT*: May interact with diabetic medications and cause low blood-sugar levels based on carvacrol content.[8440,8441,8442]

■ *Carvacrol and Thymol CTs*: May interact with aspirin, blood pressure, antiplatelet, and anticoagulant medications, and increase the risk of bleeding among people with bleeding disorders due to thymol and carvacrol content.[8443,8444,8445]

■ *Carvacrol and Thymol CTs*: May interact with antibiotics and possibly enhance their effects due to thymol and carvacrol content.[8446]

■ May interact with anticholinergic (drugs used for asthma, incontinence, gastrointestinal cramps, muscular spasms, depression, and sleep disorders) and cholinergic medications (drugs used to reduce urinary retention, diagnose myasthenia gravis, and for glaucoma) based on thymol and carvacrol content.[8447]

■ May irritate mucous membranes (eyes, mouth, nasal passages, vagina, rectum).

**SELECTED EVIDENCE:**

☐ Summer savory essential oil (thymol CT) moderately to strongly inhibits both foodborne bacteria (*Acinetobacter lwof, A. baumanii, Bacillus macerans, B. megaterium, Burkholderia cepracia, Cedecea davisae, Enterobacter cloacae, Klebsiella pneumoniae* (two strains), *Pseudomonas aeruginosa* (two strains), *P. pseudoalkaligenes, Salmonella cholerasuis arizonae, S. enteritidis, Serratia plymuthica, Staphylococcus aureus, S. epidermis, S. hominis, Streptococcus pyogenes, Shigella sonnei,* and *Yersinia enterocolitica*) and fungi (*Aspergillus flavus, Fusarium Solani,* and *Penicillum* spp.).[8448] Another study reported that the thymol CT was bactericidal and fungicidal to a variety of bacteria (*Staphylococcus aureus, S. saprophyticus, S.*

*epidermidis, Enterococcus faecalis, E. faecium, E. coli, Streptococcus sanguis, S. salivarius, Pseudomonas aeruginosa Klebsiella pneumoniae, Salmonella typhimurium, Proteus vulgaris, Enterobacter aerogenes, Shigella dysantri, Sh. flexeneri, Serratia marcescens*) and fungi (*Candida albicans, C. glabrata, Aspergillus flavus, A. niger, A. parasiticus*), with *S. sanguis, S. salivarius, S. aureus, Sh. flexeneri, Sh. dysantri*, and *K. pneumoniae* being the most sensitive pathogens,[8449] while a third study reports the thymol CT possesses antimicrobial activity against 23 bacteria and 15 fungi.[8450] Interestingly, scientists have discovered that higher para-cymene content reduces the antimicrobial activity of high phenol essential oils.[8451] The carvacrol CT also demonstrates significant antimicrobial activity against a wide spectrum of pathogenic gram-negative (*E. coli, Salmonella enteritidis, P. aeruginosa, Erwinia amylovora*) and gram-positive (*B. subtilis, S. aureus* (two strains), *C. perfringens, S. lutea, M. flavus*) bacteria and fungi (*A. niger, C. cerevisiae, C. albicans*), with its activity against gram-positive bacteria higher than that of the antibiotic streptomycin.[8452,8453,8454] *In vitro* research also concluded that the carvacrol CT of summer savory essential oil preserves food products that are highly oxidative and microbial sensitive due to its antioxidant and antimicrobial properties against *S. aureus, B. cereus, P. aeruginosa, Salmonella typhimurium*, and *E. coli*.[8455] The gamma-terpinene CT of summer savory also demonstrates strong antibacterial and antifungal activity.[8456] Unidentified CTs of summer savory oil strongly inhibited *A. flavus* and the production of aflatoxin by *A. parasiticus*.[8457,8458]

☐ The carvacrol CT of summer savory essential oil prevented the colonization of *C. albicans* on wound dressings when combined with biohybrid nanostructured iron oxide nanoparticles, which suggests it may be useful in reducing local infections that prevent wound healing.[8459]

☐ A 2:1 mixture of summer savory essential oil and oregano reduced *H. pylori* colonization and eradicated the pathogen in 70% of mice.[8460]

☐ Summer savory was considered a poor antioxidant in one study.[8461] The study authors concluded that para-cymene, carvacrol, and beta-bisabolene are possibly the antioxidant constituents present in summer savory essential oil. Interestingly, another study found that summer savory essential oil (rich in carvacrol—79.2%) is a strong antioxidant and prevents DNA damage, which may protect against cell mutations and cancer.[8462] An unidentified CT of summer savory essential oil prevented oxidative DNA damage caused by hydrogen peroxide.[8463] The gamma-terpinene CT of summer savory essential oil also demonstrated significant antioxidant activity, with the researchers reporting that using a sulfur fertilizer during plant growth can enhance the antioxidant activity by increasing the alpha-terpinene, para-cymene, myrcene, thujene, and alpha-pinene content.[8464] However, other research suggests that the antioxidant activity of essential oils is not dependent on the main components, but rather an interaction of various components, which can produce synergism, antagonism, or additivity (a substance that can improve, strengthen or otherwise alter another substance).[8465]

☐ *In vitro* research shows that summer savory essential oil helps prevent periodontal diseases by inhibiting the periodontopathogen *Fusobacterium nucleatum*, matrix metalloproteinase (MMP-2 and MMP-9) activities (MMPs are enzymes responsible for tissue growth and turnover, but their overexpression can cause acute and chronic inflammation and undesirable tissue destruction, particularly when triggered by bacterial infection), and gelatinolytic activity (the release of enzymes by neutrophils that are associated with destruction of the periodontium), as well as preventing cell death caused by free radical attack.[8466,8467,8468] A randomized, controlled clinical study shows that a 1% topical gel of summer savory essential oil (carvacrol CT) significantly reduced lesions and Candida colonies associated with denture stomatitis in denture wearers.[8469]

☐ Animal research demonstrates that summer savory seed essential oil (gamma-terpinene 50.5%, thymol 32.7%, para-cymene 9.2%) reduces inflammation and pain.[8470]

☐ Summer savory essential oil reduced diarrhea caused by castor oil in mice.[8471]

☐ An *in vitro* study concluded that reduces spasms and relaxes isolated rat intestines.[8472]

☐ *In vitro* research shows that summer savory essential oil (carvacrol CT) inhibits the growth and spore formation of *Alternaria citri* (a plant pathogen that causes black rot in citrus fruits).[8473] It also inhibits a wide variety of phytopathogenic organisms: *Agrobacterium tumefaciens, Bacillus pumilus, Clavibacter michiganensis* ssp. *michiganensis, Enterobacter intermedius, Erwinia caratovora* ssp. *caratovora, E. chrysanthemi, Pseudomonas corrugate, P. fluorescens, P. syringae* pv. *Syringae, P. syringae* pv. *tomato, Ralstonia solanacearum*, and *Xanthomonas vesicatoria*.[8474]

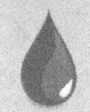

- Summer savory essential oil is toxic to the gall midge (*Camptomyia corticalis*).[8475]

- Summer savory (carvacrol CT) essential oil inhibited *S. aureus* isolates and disrupted its formation of biofilms.[8476]

- Summer savory CT thymol and oregano CT pulegone essential oils prevented biofilm formation and subsequent colonization of *S. pneumoniae* at subminimum inhibitory concentrations.[8477] Summer savory also downregulated genes (LuxS, pfs) involved in quorum sensing.

- Terpene/phenol-rich (oregano CT carvacrol, thyme CT carvacrol, and summer savory CT carvacrol) and phenylpropanoid-rich (clove bud and cinnamon leaf) essential oils each showed good absolute antioxidant activity—comparable to BHT—in cumene and squalene during the peroxyl radical trapping assay.[8478]

- Of eleven essential oils tested, oregano CT carvacrol, fennel, mountain savory CT para-cymene, and summer savory CT carvacrol were the most effective against gastrointestinal nematodes (*Haemonchus*, *Trichostrongylus*, *Teladorsagia*, and *Chabertia*) in the *in vitro* egg hatch test.[8479] Oral administration of the oils diluted in sunflower oil to animals showed that thyme CT para-cymene essential oil was the most effective, even more effective than thyme CT thymol.

- Catnip CT 1,8-cineole, summer savory CT carvacrol, and dill aerial parts essential oil demonstrated promising insecticidal activity against the red spider mite (*Tetranychus urticae*) with some minor potential to decrease populations of insect predators (*Amblyseius swirskii*).[8480]

- Dysbiosis can lead to elevated levels of trimethylamine-N-oxide (TMAO)—a compound associated with chronic disease, including cardiovascular disease and diabetes. Ingestion of summer savory, parsley, or rosemary essential oil emulsions with L-carnitine improved the gut microbiome (primarily *Lactobacillus* genus bacteria), decreased TMAO levels, and increased short-chain fatty acids in mouse models of ischemic heart disease and type 2 diabetes.[8481] Additionally, rosemary and parsley decreased proinflammatory cytokines, while savory increased chemokines (signaling proteins crucial for the migration of white blood cells during normal inflammatory processes to maintain homeostasis). The essential oil emulsions acted as prebiotics to improve gut microbiome and reduce the risk of cardiovascular and metabolic disorders.

## SWEET INULA
### (Stinkwort, Camphor Inula)

*Dittrichia graveolens* L. Greuter, *Inula graveolens* L. Desf.

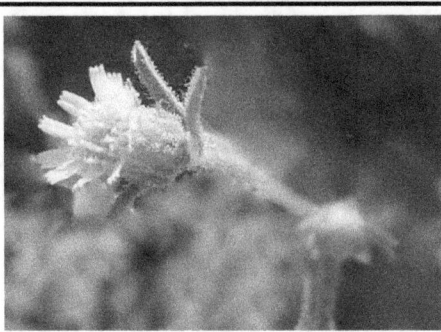

**FAMILY:** Asteraceae (Compositae)
**NOTE:** Middle
**AROMA INTENSITY:** Medium
**AROMA:** Fresh, earthy, camphoraceous, medicinal, slightly sweet/floral
**COMMON EXTRACTION METHOD:** Steam distilled from the aerial parts (stem, leaves, and flowers)
**POSSIBLE SUBSTITUTE OILS:** *Bornyl acetate CT*—rosemary (bronyl acetate CT), spruce (black), tsuga; *Borneol CT*—rosemary, lavandin; *1,8-cineole CT*—rosemary (1,8-cineole CT), spike lavender, Spanish sage; *T-cadinol CT*—spikenard, basil (linalool CT)
**BLENDS WELL WITH:** Bay laurel, bergamot, cajeput, eucalyptus, frankincense, geranium, grapefruit, helichrysum, hyssop, lavender, lemon, lemon myrtle, lime, orange, rosalina, rose, rosemary, thyme
**SUBCELLULAR LOCALIZATION | EPIGENETIC INFLUENCE:** Currently unknown | Currently unknown
**RECOMMENDED DILUTION RANGE:** 3%–33%; neat for limited conditions

**PRIMARY CONSTITUENTS:**[8482,8483,8484,8485,8486,8487,8488,8489]

| Bornyl Acetate CT | | Borneol CT | |
|---|---|---|---|
| Bornyl Acetate | 43.1%–72.3% | Borneol | 34.5%–43.6% |
| Borneol | 2.7%–32.2% | Bornyl Acetate | 0.6%–38.3% |
| T-Cadinol | 0.0%–13.4% | T-Cadinol | 0.0%–23.8% |
| Camphene | 0.6%–7.1% | 3,4-Decadienal | 0.0%–7.5% |
| Caryophyllene Oxide | 1.1%–5.7% | Beta-Cubebene | 0.0%–7.1% |
| Alpha-Chamigrene | 0.0%–2.9% | Camphene | 0.0%–5.7% |
| 1[7]2-Mentha-Diene-8-ol | 0.0%–2.1% | Caryophyllene Oxide | 2.5%–4.2% |

| | | | |
|---|---|---|---|
| Caryophyllene | 0.5%–2.1% | Caryophyllene | 0.5%–2.8% |
| Gamma-Cadinene | 0.1%–2.0% | Caryophylla-4(14),8(15)- | |
| | | Dien-5α-ol | 0.0%–2.7% |
| *1,8-Cineole CT* | | Hexafarnesyl Acetone | 0.0%–2.5% |
| 1,8-Cineole | 22.4%–54.9% | Trans-P-Mentha-1(7),8- | |
| Borneol | 5.4%–20.4% | Dien-2-ol | 2.2%–2.2% |
| Para-Cymene | 3.5%–16.2% | Alpha-Terpineol | 0.0%–2.2% |
| Alpha-Cadinol | 0.0%–11.8% | P-Mentha-1,5-Dien-8-ol | 0.0%–2.1% |
| Beta-Pinene | 3.6%–6.9% | Isovaleric Acid 3- | |
| Bornyl Acetate | 0.2%–5.3% | Phenylpropyl Ester | 0.0%–2.1% |
| Beta-Caryophyllene | 1.6%–4.8% | Geranyl Butyrate | 0.0%–2.0% |
| Camphene | 0.0%–4.6% | | |
| Alpha-Pinene | 2.3%–3.2% | | |
| Alpha-Humulene | 1.9%–2.0% | | |

*T-Cadinol (Epi-Alpha-Cadinol) CT*

| | |
|---|---|
| T-Cadinol (Epi-Alpha-Cadinol) | 30.2% |
| Bornyl Acetate | 25.4% |
| Borneol | 12.8% |
| Caryophyllene | 6.3% |
| Beta-Caryophyllene | 4.4% |
| Camphene | 4.3% |
| Gamma-Cadinene | 3.3% |
| T-Muurolol | 3.0% |
| 1,8-Cineole | 2.6% |

Note: The bornyl acetate CT appears to be the most commercially available CT.

**OTHER CONSTITUENTS:** *Bornyl Acetate CT*—para-cymene-8-ol, beta-caryophyllene, ocimenone, occidentallo acetate, epi-cadinol, nerolidol, alpha-eudesmol, beta-selinene, germacrene B; *Borneol CT*—beta-pinene, limonene, gamma-cadinene, alcanfor, para-cymen-8-ol, beta-methyl-benzenepropanal, geranyl propionate, cyercene, 5-epi-paradisiol, geranyl hexanoate; *1,8-Cineole CT*—sabinene, limonene, gamma-terpinene, alpha-terpineol, thymol, beta-elemene, terpinen-4-ol, delta-cadinene, beta-selinene, spathulenol, ledol, linalool, trans-pinocarveol, pinocarvone; *T-Cadinol CT*—beta-pinene, delta-cadinene, 14-hydroxy-9-epi-beta-caryophyllene

**PREFERRED COMPOSITION FOR CLINICAL USE:**

| *Constituent* | *Bornyl Acetate CT* |
|---|---|
| **Bornyl Acetate** | 40%–65% |
| **Borneol** | 8%–30% |
| **Camphene** | 4%–10% |
| **T-Cadinol** | 0.5%–5% |
| **Beta-Caryophyllene** | 0.5%–5% |
| **Caryophyllene Oxide** | 0.1%–5% |
| **Cadinene <gamma + delta>** | 0.1%–3% |

**REPORTED THERAPEUTIC PROPERTIES:** Antibacterial, antifungal, antiviral, analgesic, anti-inflammatory, reduces the appearance of scars and blemishes, antiallergic, wound healing, antioxidant, expels excess mucus, supports immune function, decongestant, **supports respiratory function**, diuretic, combats acne, relieves insect bites, soothes chronic skin conditions, **antioxidant**, supports cardiovascular function, balances blood pressure, **relieves sinusitis**, aids meditation, relieves anxiety, antidepressant

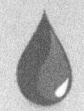

**CAUTIONS:**

■ Avoid with children under age three (1,8-cineole CT), particularly around the nose and mouth. Use very cautiously in children under age five due to high 1,8-cineole content. 1,8-cineole may cause seizures, central nervous system problems, or respiratory distress in young children.[8490,8491,8492,8493]

■ May interact with aspirin, blood pressure, antiplatelet, and anticoagulant medications, and increase the risk of bleeding among people with bleeding disorders based on high borneol percentages in some CTs.[8494] Borneol possesses anticoagulant properties.

■ Avoid with epilepsy and Parkinson's disease due to 1,8-cineole content. May exacerbate or cause seizures or convulsions when inhaled, applied topically, or ingested based on 1,8-cineole content.[8495,8496,8497,8498,8499,8500]

■ Caution is warranted orally due to the significant amounts of 1,8-cineole (1,8-cineole CT). Limit to small doses internally (adults—maximum 10 drops daily). Toxicity has been reported when eucalyptus (also high in 1,8-cineole) was ingested in large doses, and as few as 4 to 5 drops may cause problems in very sensitive individuals.[8501,8502,8503,8504,8505,8506] In humans, 3.5 to 5 mL has proven fatal orally.[8507]

■ May interfere with enzymes responsible for metabolizing medications (NSAIDs, proton-pump inhibitors, acetaminophen, antiepileptics, immune modulators, blood-sugar medications, blood pressure medications, antidepressants, antipsychotics, diabetic medications, antihistamines, antibiotics, and anesthetics) based on high borneol content in some CTs.[8508,8509,8510,8511,8512]

■ May interact with diabetic medications (1,8-cineole CT) due to the ability of 1,8-cineole to inhibit alpha-glucosidase activity when synergized by other components (alpha-pinene, beta-pinene, and para-cymene).[8513,8514] Alpha-glucosidase is an enzyme that breaks down carbohydrates by chemical reaction with water. Inhibiting its activity postpones glucose absorption and therefore the impact of carbohydrates on blood sugar levels.

■ May interact with antibiotics and increase or decrease their effectiveness.[8515]

■ May interfere with pentobarbital and other barbiturates (medications for anxiety and insomnia) based on 1,8-cineole content (1,8-cineole CT).[8516,8517]

**SELECTED EVIDENCE:**

☐ *In vitro* research demonstrates that sweet inula (borneol CT) is active against gram-positive bacteria (*S. aureus* and *B. subtilis*) but was ineffective against gram-negative bacteria (*P. aeruginosa, S. typhimurium,* and *E. coli*) and the fungi *C. albicans*.[8518] Sweet inula essential oil (bornyl acetate CT) kills *S. aureus* by folding the cell membrane back on itself (invaginations) and damaging (thickening) the cell wall.[8519] Other research found that sweet inula (1,8-cineole CT) was effective against *C. albicans*.[8520] Another study confirmed the strong activity of the borneol CT against the gram-positive bacterium *E. faecalis*, even antibiotic resistant strains.[8521] Interestingly this research also reported varying degrees of activity against gram-positive (*S. aureus, E. faecalis, B. subtilis*), gram-negative bacteria (*E. coli, P. aeruginosa*), yeast (*C. albicans, C. glabrata*), and fungi (*A. niger, A. parasiticus*). The most susceptible microbes were *E. faecalis, C. glabrata,* and *C. albicans*.

☐ The bornyl acetate CT of sweet inula increases the effectiveness of antibiotics (chloramphenicol and tetracycline) against five bacterial strains, but reduced the effectiveness of streptomycin against *S. aureus, E. coli,* and *P. aeruginosa*.[8522]

☐ Sweet inula demonstrated stronger antioxidant properties than trolox (a water-soluble form of vitamin E).[8523]

☐ *In vitro* research suggests that sweet inula essential oil (bornyl acetate CT) inhibits acetylcholinesterase (AChE) enzyme activity.[8524] Inhibition of AChE prevents the breakdown of acetylcholine, which is essential for memory and thinking. People with neurodegenerative diseases make less acetylcholine, and the diseases often break it down at a faster rate, leading to acetylcholine deficits.

☐ The bornyl acetate CT of sweet inula essential oil exhibited slight antibacterial activity against thirteen bacterial strains—*E. coli, S. enteritidis,* K. pneumoniae (two strains), *P. mirabilis, P. aeruginosa* (two strains), *E. aerogenes, E. faecalis, B. cereus, S. aureus* (two strains), and *L. monocytogenes*—and improved the activity of chloramphenicol and tetracycline.[8525] A borneol CT was only active against gram-positive bacteria.[8526]

☐ Both roots and aerial parts of sweet inula essential oil repelled and were toxic to the red flour beetle (*Tribolium castaneum*) with the aerial parts oil being more effective.[8527] Fractions of the oil were more effective than the whole oil.

# SWEET NANCY
## (English Mace, Yellow Flowered Yarrow)
*Achillea ageratum* L.

**FAMILY:** Asteraceae (Compositae)
**NOTE:** Top-Middle
**AROMA INTENSITY:** Medium
**AROMA:** Herbaceous, floral, slightly sweet
**COMMON EXTRACTION METHOD:** Steam distilled from the flowering aerial parts
**POSSIBLE SUBSTITUTE OILS:** Sweet wormwood, yarrow, geranium, copaiba, cistus
**BLENDS WELL WITH:** Bay laurel, black pepper, bergamot, cedarwood, chamomile (German, Roman), clary sage, copaiba, cypress, grapefruit, lavender, lemon, lime, neroli, orange, pine, sandalwood, tangerine, vetiver, ylang ylang
**SUBCELLULAR LOCALIZATION | EPIGENETIC INFLUENCE:** Currently unknown | Currently unknown
**RECOMMENDED DILUTION RANGE:** 5%–Neat

**PRIMARY CONSTITUENTS:**[8528, 8529,8530]

| *Artemisyl Acetate CT* | | *Yomogi Alcohol/1,8-Cineole CT* | |
|---|---|---|---|
| Artemisyl Acetate | 62.3%–78.8% | Yomogi Alcohol | 22.3%–44.1% |
| Yomogi Alcohol | 4.9%–12.4% | 1,8-Cineole | 20.2%–41.0% |
| Santolina Alcohol | 4.9%–11.8% | Santolina Alcohol | 0.0%–10.0% |
| Cis-Alpha-Copaene-8-ol | 0.0%–7.4% | Artemisia Alcohol | 4.1%–8.6% |
| Artemisia Alcohol | 3.4%–7.1% | Artemisia Triene | 0.0%–8.3% |
| | | Artemisia Acetate | 0.0%–7.6% |

| *Artemisia Ketone CT* | |
|---|---|
| Artemisia Ketone | 55.7% |
| 1,8-Cineole | 10.6% |
| Beta-Caryophyllene Oxide | 3.8% |
| Artemisia Alcohol | 2.7% |

**OTHER CONSTITUENTS:** *Artemisyl Acetate CT*—cis-p-mentha-1(7),8-dien-2-ol, silphiperfol-6-ene, beta-elemene, verbenyl propionate, presilphiperfolan-8-ol; *Yomogi Alcohol/1,8-Cineole CT*—alpha-pinocarvone, trans-pinocarveol, myrtenal, terpinen-4-ol, para-cymene, dehydrosabina ketone, sabina ketone, delta-terpineol, cuminaldehyde; *Artemisia Ketone CT*—3-buten-2-ol,2-methyl, butanoic acid,2-methyl-ethyl ester, butanoic acid,3-methyl-ethyl ester, butanoic acid,2-methyl-2-methylbutyl, 5,6 epoxy,3,3,6-trimethyl-1-hepten-4-on, 2(5H) furanone,5-hexyldihydro, carvone, piperitone, terpinen-4-ol, beta-elemene, beta-humulene, borenol, thymol, carvacrol

**PREFERRED COMPOSITION FOR CLINICAL USE:**

| *Constituent* | *Artemisyl Acetate CT* |
|---|---|
| **Artemisyl Acetate** | 60%–78% |
| **Yomogi Alcohol** | 5%–12% |
| **Santolina Alcohol** | 5%–12% |
| **Artemisia Alcohol** | 2%–7% |

**REPORTED THERAPEUTIC PROPERTIES:** Antibacterial, antifungal, analgesic, anti-inflammatory, antirheumatic, antispasmodic, antioxidant, antiseptic, aids digestion, expels excess gas, **relieves chronic skin conditions, wound healing**, astringent, supports respiratory function, expels excess mucus, balances blood pressure, stops excess bleeding, insect repellent, insecticide, releases emotional trauma, combats anger and irritability, stress management, calming/relaxing

**CAUTIONS:**

■ *Yomogi Alcohol/1,8-Cineole CT*: Avoid with epilepsy and Parkinson's due to 1,8-cineole content, which may exacerbate or trigger seizures/convulsions or reduce medication efficacy.[8531,8532,8533]

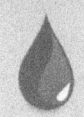

■ *Yomogi Alcohol/1,8-Cineole CT*: May interfere with pentobarbital and other barbiturates (medications for anxiety and insomnia) based on 1,8-cineole content.[8534,8535]

■ *Yomogi Alcohol/1,8-Cineole CT*: May weakly interfere with the enzymes responsible for metabolizing medications (NSAIDs, proton-pump inhibitors, acetaminophen, antiepileptics, immune modulators, blood-sugar medications, blood pressure medications, antidepressants, antipsychotics, diabetic medications, antihistamines, antibiotics, and anesthetics) due to 1,8-cineole content.[8536,8537,8538]

**SELECTED EVIDENCE:**

☐ *In vitro* research demonstrates that sweet nancy essential oil (Artemisyl acetate CT) significantly inhibited gram-positive bacteria (*S. aureus, M. luteus, B. subtilis*, and *B cereus*), mildly inhibited gram-negative bacteria (*E. coli, E. cloacae, Salmonella* sp.), and inhibited five yeasts (two strains of *C. albicans, C. krusei, C. glabrata, C. parapsilosis*).[8539] Another study reports that the Artemisia ketone CT of sweet nancy inhibited *S. aureus, B. subtilis, C. cereus, B. megaterium*, and moderately inhibited *E. coli*.[8540]

☐ Sweet nancy essential oil (Yomogi alcohol/1,8-cineole CT) moderately inhibited *C. albicans*, preventing its virulence by inhibiting germ tube formation and biofilm formation.[8541]

☐ Animal research reported that sweet nancy essential oil relieves intestinal spasms in isolated duodenum.[8542]

☐ Sweet nancy essential oil (Artemisyl acetate CT) possesses only a mild antioxidant properties according to *in vitro* research.[8543]

# SWEET WORMWOOD
## (Annual Wormwood, Sweet Annie, Sweet Sagewort)
*Artemisia annua* L.

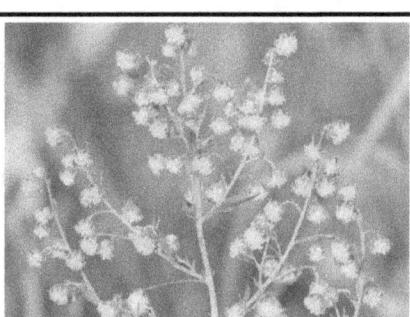

**FAMILY:** Asteraceae (Compositae)
**NOTE:** Top-Middle
**AROMA INTENSITY:** Medium
**AROMA:** Herbaceous, floral, slightly sweet
**COMMON EXTRACTION METHOD:** Steam distilled from the flowering aerial parts
**POSSIBLE SUBSTITUTE OILS:** Sweet nancy, yarrow, camphor
**BLENDS WELL WITH:** Bay laurel, black pepper, bergamot, cedarwood, chamomile (German, Roman), clary sage, copaiba, cypress, grapefruit, lavender, lemon, lime, neroli, orange, pine, sandalwood, tangerine, vetiver, ylang ylang
**SUBCELLULAR LOCALIZATION | EPIGENETIC INFLUENCE:** Currently unknown | Currently unknown
**RECOMMENDED DILUTION RANGE:** 1.5%–20%; neat for limited conditions
**PRIMARY CONSTITUENTS:**[8544,8545,8546,8547,8548,8549,8550,8551,8552,8553]

| Artemisia Ketone CT | | Camphor CT | |
|---|---|---|---|
| Artemisia Ketone | 28.3%–75.5% | Camphor | 17.7%–48.0% |
| Artemisia Alcohol | 3.7%–56.0% | Germacrene D | 0.0%–15.6% |
| Camphor | 0.0%–23.8% | 1,8-Cineole | 1.2%–13.9% |
| Alpha-Pinene | 0.0%–16.5% | Trans-Pinocarveol | 0.0%–10.9% |
| 1,8-Cineole | 0.0%–10.4% | Alpha-Pinene | 0.0%–9.7% |
| Yomogi Alcohol | 0.0%–6.1% | Beta-Selinene | 0.0%–9.4% |
| Beta-Pinene | 0.0%–6.0% | Beta-Caryophyllene | 0.3%–8.9% |
| Camphene | 0.0%–5.0% | Camphene | 0.0%–7.0% |
| Trans-Pinocarveol | 0.0%–4.8% | Artemisia Ketone | 2.7%–6.3% |
| Beta-Selinene | 0.0%–4.6% | Spathulenol | 0.0%–4.9% |
| Pinocarvone | 0.0%–4.0% | Gamma-Gurjunene | 0.0%–4.3% |
| Beta-Cubebene | 0.0%–3.9% | Terpinolene | 0.0%–3.7% |
| Caryophyllene Oxide | 0.0%–3.9% | | |

Note: An uncommon chemotype of *A. annua* from Bulgaria was also reported in the literature that was rich in alpha-humulene (24.7%), alpha-cubebene (13.5%), artemisia ketone (8.5%), and alpha-selinene (8.2%).

**OTHER CONSTITUENTS:** *Artemisia Ketone CT*—sabinene, myrcene, 4-carvomenthenol, copaene, beta-caryophyllene, Santolina alcohol, cis-sabinene hydrate, borneol, cis-pinocamphone, terpinen-4-ol, alpha-terpineol, myrtenol, eugenol, isobutyl phenylacetate, 4-methylpentylcyclohexane, 9-epi-(E)-caryophyllene, humulene epoxide II, 1,10-di-epi-cubenol, allo-aromadendrene epoxide, himachalol, bulnesol, arteannuic acid; *Camphor CT*—tricyclene, delta-3-carene, alpha-terpinene, cymol, cis-sabinene hydrate, trans-sabinene hydrate, pinocarvone, borneol, terpinen-4-ol, trans-carveol, myrtenal, myrtenol, cis-carveol, germacrene A, epi-cubenol, ledene oxide, alpha-copaene, verbenone, artemisia alcohol, gamma-muurolene

**PREFERRED COMPOSITION FOR CLINICAL USE:**

| Constituent | Artemisia Ketone CT |
|---|---|
| Artemisia Ketone | 30%–65% |
| Camphor | 4%–20% |
| Artemisia Alcohol | 3%–10% |
| 1,8-Cineole | 0%–6% |
| Myrcene | 0.5%–5% |
| Beta-Caryophyllene | 0.5%–3% |
| Alpha-Pinene | 0.1%–1% |
| Camphene | 0.1%–1% |

**REPORTED THERAPEUTIC PROPERTIES:** Antibacterial, antifungal, antiviral, **antimicrobial**, analgesic, anti-inflammatory, antirheumatic, antispasmodic, antioxidant, antiseptic, anticancer, aids digestion, expels excess gas, **relieves chronic skin conditions**, **wound healing**, astringent, supports respiratory function, expels excess mucus, balances blood pressure, stops excess bleeding, insect repellent, **insecticide**, releases emotional trauma, combats anger and irritability, stress management, calming/relaxing

**CAUTIONS:**

■ Avoid with children under six due to high camphor content. Several cases of camphor poisoning and/or seizures from ingestion and topical application have been reported in children.[8554,8555] Ingestion of camphor-containing products has been lethal in children under age two.[8556] Children five years and up may use camphor topically in dilutions no stronger than 5%. 1,8-cineole may cause seizures, central nervous system problems, or respiratory distress in young children.[8557,8558,8559,8560]

■ Caution is warranted during pregnancy and while lactating. Camphor ingestion may lead to abortion because fetuses lack the enzymes to process it.[8561] Camphor ingestion by infants and young children may cause cough, vomiting, seizure, burning sensation in the mucous membranes and eyes, or lack of voluntary coordination of muscle movements.[8562]

■ Avoid with epilepsy and Parkinson's disease due to camphor and 1,8-cineole content.[8563,8564,8565]

■ Oral caution—Camphor can be toxic when taken orally (usually single doses exceeding 2 mL), although the lethal dose for adult humans is estimated to be (more than 5 mL) in a single dose.[8566,8567,8568] To date, toxicity studies have only been completed with the artemisia ketone CT of sweet wormwood, with little to no camphor content. Artemisia ketone and Artemisia alcohol are considered non-toxic and therefore this does not adequately determine the toxicity of high camphor sweet wormwood essential oils. While the acute toxicity of the artemisia ketone CT in mice is 1500 mg/kg after injection, one study reports i.p. administration of 790 mg/kg of the camphor CT was lethal to 50 percent of rats, which the study authors considered a high acute toxicity.[8569] A sesquiterpene endoperoxide lactone called artemisinin is semi-synthesized from artemisinic acid in *A. annua* plants and used orally to treat malaria, particularly chloroquine-resistant and cerebral malaria. However, the plant must be harvested far before flowering stage to obtain appreciable amounts of this constituent, which reduces essential oil yield.

■ The potentially high camphor content in sweet wormwoodor may negatively impact red blood cells and increase the risk of jaundice in children with glucose-6-phosphate dehydrogenase deficiency (G6PD).[8570,8571]

■ Avoid with those who have a compromised liver due to the risk of increased liver enzymes and liver damage from high camphor content.[8572] This would also suggest that those taking medications that could cause liver damage should also use camphor-containing essential oils very cautiously or avoid them.

■ May interact with anticholinergic (drugs used for asthma, incontinence, gastrointestinal cramps, muscular spasms, depression, and sleep disorders) and cholinergic medications (drugs used to reduce urinary retention, diagnose

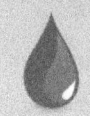

myasthenia gravis, and for glaucoma) due to its strong depressant activity on the CNS, cholinergic action, and AChE inhibitory activity.[8573,8574]

■ Caution is warranted for the topical application of camphor-containing essential oils on broken or injured skin due to an increased risk of toxicity.[8575]

## SELECTED EVIDENCE:

☐ *In vitro* research reports that sweet wormwood essential oil induces apoptosis of liver cancer cells.[8576]

☐ *In vitro* research demonstrates that sweet wormwood possesses broad antimicrobial activity against gram-positive bacteria (*S. aureus, E. hirae, E. faecalis, S. pneumoniae, B. cereus, B. subtilis, B. thuringensis, Sarcina lutea*), gram-negative bacteria (*E. coli*, EPEC, *Shigella* sp., *S. enteritidis, K. pneumoniae, H. influenza, P. aeruginosa*), and fungi (*C. albicans, C. krusei, S. cervisiae, A. fumigatus*).[8577,8578,8579,8580,8581,8582,8583] Another report suggests that the Artemisia ketone chemotype (main constituents artemisia ketone—14.0% and 1,8-cineole—8.1%) of sweet wormwood essential oil is ineffective against *L. innocua*.[8584] The camphor CT demonstrated varying degrees of inhibition of gram-positive bacteria (*S. aureus*, MRSA, *B. subtilis, E. faecalis*), gram-negative bacteria (*K. pneumoniae, P. aeruginosa, A. baumannii),* and yeasts (*C. famata, C. albicans, C. utilis, C. famata*).[8585]

☐ *In vitro* research demonstrates that sweet wormwood essential oil (*Artemisia Ketone CT*) inhibits ten clinical isolates of *Candida* spp.[8586] Interestingly, the antifungal activity was greater in vapor phase than liquid phase.

☐ Animal research reports that sweet wormwood essential oil (Artemisia ketone CT) mildly reduced pain, but was not as effective as aspirin.[8587]

☐ Sweet wormwood essential oil (Artemisia ketone CT) moderately protected the liver and kidneys against damage caused by carbon tetrachloride in rats.[8588] The authors noted that because sweet wormwood essential oil is a weak antioxidant, this protection was likely produced through another mechanism.

☐ Sweet wormwood is considered a weak antioxidant.[8589,8590] Interestingly, one study reports that sweet wormwood essential oil (Artemisia ketone CT) showed a pro-oxidant effect.[8591]

☐ A camphor-rich sweet wormwood essential oil significantly inhibited *L. donovani* both *in vitro* and *in vivo*, demonstrating the ability to reduce visceral leishmaniasis without causing liver or kidney toxicity.[8592]

☐ *In vitro* research suggests that sweet wormwood essential oil (camphor CT) inhibits acetylcholinesterase (AChE) enzyme activity.[8593] Inhibition of AChE prevents the breakdown of acetylcholine, which is essential for memory and thinking. People with neurodegenerative diseases make less acetylcholine, and the diseases often break it down at a faster rate, leading to acetylcholine deficits.

☐ The camphor CT of sweet wormwood essential oil was toxic to red fire ants.[8594] An unidentified chemotype of sweet wormwood essential oil was toxic to cattle ticks (*Rhipicephalus* (Boophilus) *annulatus*) and prevented female ticks from laying eggs.[8595] The Artemisia ketone CT of sweet wormwood moderately killed the house fly (*Musca domestica*).[8596] An unidentified CT of sweet wormwood essential oil was toxic to and repelled two types of beetles: *Tribolium castaneum* (Herbst) and *Callosobruchus maculatus* (L.).[3502] Sweet wormwood essential oil (artemisia ketone CT) was insecticidal to the disease-carrying blowfly (*Calliphora vomitoria*), which spread pathogenic microorganisms.[8597]

☐ The camphor CT of sweet wormwood essential oil demonstrated strong antimicrobial activity against most of twenty tested strains of *Malassezia* spp. in both the liquid and vapor phase.[8598]

☐ Sweet wormwood CT artemisia ketone essential oil demonstrated good antioxidant activity.[8599]

☐ The artemisia ketone CT of sweet wormwood essential oil demonstrated considerable ability to repel two storage pests (*Lasioderma serricorne* and *Tribolium castaneum* adults).[8600]

☐ Sweet wormwood essential oil nanoemulsion inhibited *Candida* biofilms better than Tween 80 stabilized emulsion and an ethanolic solution of sweet wormwood.[8601]

☐ *In vitro* research demonstrated that sweet wormwood essential oil inhibited multidrug-resistant *E. coli*, which caused the researchers to conclude that it could be used as a substitute for thirteen antibiotics (oxacillin, amoxicillin, ampicillin, amoxicillin-clavulanic acid, tetracycline, streptomycin, ciprofloxacin, ceftriaxone, cefazolin, cefuroxime, cefotaxime, ceftazidime and cefixime).[8602]

☐ Bones are living tissue that continually change throughout life through a process called bone remodeling.

During this process, new bone cells replace older and damaged ones. This is accomplished through a delicate balance of two types of bones cells: osteoclasts (break down bone and remove older bone matrix; called resorption) and osteoblasts that (build new bone matrix). It is estimated that the human skeleton is completely remodeled every ten years through this process. An increase in the number or function of osteoclasts can lead to brittle bones and conditions like osteoporosis. Cell differentiation is the process through which a cell undergoes changes to become a more specific type of cell, like an osteoclast. Increased osteoclast differentiation can increase their activity and removal of bone so that osteoblasts can't replace removed bone at the necessary pace to keep bones healthy. Sweet wormwood CT essential oil (main constituents: camphor, borneol, eucalyptol, and piperitone) inhibited mouse osteoclast differentiation in laboratory research, suggesting it may reduce bone resorption and play a role in bone health and metabolic bone diseases.

☐ Sweet wormwood and isolated camphor and 1,8-cineole were toxic to the fall webworm (*Hyphantria cunea*).[8603]

☐ Sweet wormwood essential oil displayed remarkable antioxidant activity in the DPPH and FRAP assays. The oil also showed antimicrobial activity against *E. coli*, *F. oxysporum*, and *C. albicans*.[8604]

# TAGETES
## (Taget, Wild Marigold, Muster John Henry, Aztec Marigold, African Marigold)

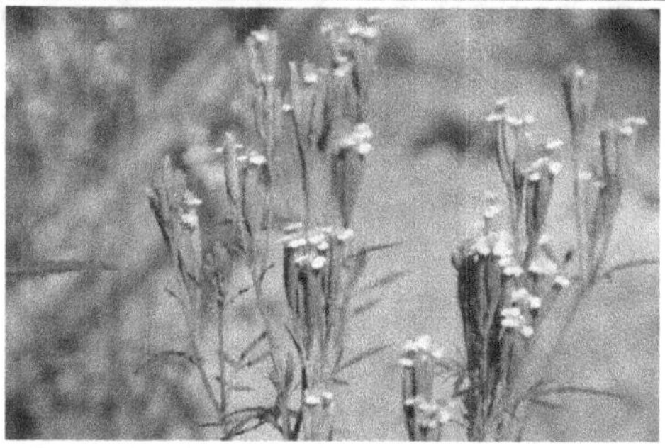

*Tagetes minuta* L., *T. bonariensis* Pers., *T. porophylla* Vell, *T. glandulifera* Schrank; French Marigold: *T. patula* L.; Aztec Marigold: *T. erecta* L.

**FAMILY:** Asteraceae (Compositae)
**NOTE:** Top-Middle
**AROMA INTENSITY:** Medium
**AROMA:** Herbaceous, green, slightly floral and fruity
**COMMON EXTRACTION METHOD:** Steam distilled from the aerial parts; may also be distilled from the flowers or leaves
**POSSIBLE SUBSTITUTE OILS:** Palo santo, neroli, spearmint, sweet basil
**BLENDS WELL WITH:** Bergamot, clary sage, frankincense, geranium, grapefruit, juniper berry, juniper (Phoenician), lavender, lemon, lime, myrrh, orange, rose, sandalwood, tangerine, tea tree, ylang ylang
**SUBCELLULAR LOCALIZATION | EPIGENETIC INFLUENCE:** Currently unknown | Currently unknown
**RECOMMENDED DILUTION RANGE:** 5%–50%; neat for limited conditions

**PRIMARY CONSTITUENTS:**[8605,8606,8607,8608,8609,8610,8611,8612,8613,8614,8615,8616,8617,8618,8619,8620,8621,8622,8623,8624]

*T. minuta ((Z)-Beta-Ocimene CT)*

| | |
|---|---|
| (Z)-Beta-Ocimene | 8.3%–51.7% |
| (E)-Ocimenone | 5.8%–34.8% |
| (Z)-Tagetone | 1.8%–17.7% |
| Dihydrotagetone | 3.0%–16.4% |
| (Z)-Ocimenone | 4.0%–15.9% |
| Limonene | 0.0%–7.1% |

*T. minuta (Limonene CT)*

| | |
|---|---|
| Limonene | 13.0%–66.3% |
| (E)-Ocimenone | 0.0%–19.1% |
| Piperitenone | 0.0%–12.2% |
| Alpha-Pinene | 0.5%–11.8% |
| Alpha-Terpinolene | 0.0%–11.0% |
| Piperitone | 0.0%–6.0% |
| (E)-Tagetone | 0.0%–5.7% |
| (Z)-Ocimenone | 2.7%–5.1% |
| Docosane | 0.0%–5.0% |
| Tricosane | 0.0%–4.2% |

*T. minuta (Dihydrotagetone CT)*

| | |
|---|---|
| Dihydrotagetone | 33.8%–54.2% |
| (Z)-Tagetone | 0.2%–23.0% |
| (E)-Tagetone | 6.2%–17.1% |
| Limonene | 5.4%–12.3% |
| (Z)-Beta-Ocimene | 0.0%–7.9% |

*T. minuta (Alpha-Terpineol CT)*

| | |
|---|---|
| Alpha-Terpineol | 20.8% |
| (Z)-Beta-Ocimene | 17.7% |
| Dihydrotagetone | 13.7% |
| (E)-Ocimenone | 13.3% |
| (Z)-Tagetone | 8.4% |
| (Z)-Ocimenone | 6.1% |
| Cis-Dihydrocarvone | 5.0% |

*T. minuta (Piperitone CT)*

| | |
|---|---|
| Piperitone | 86.3% |
| Limonene | 13.7% |

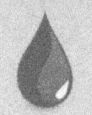

*T. patula (Limonene CT)*

| | |
|---|---|
| Limonene | 13.6%–19.2% |
| Caryophyllene | 11.9%–17.7% |
| (Z)-Ocimenone | 10.9%–13.4% |
| (E)-Ocimenone | 10.8%–13.4% |
| Alpha-Terpinolene | 0.0%–11.2% |
| Unknown | 7.6%–9.5% |
| (Z)-Beta-Ocimene | 0.0%–8.3% |
| Beta-Caryophyllene | 0.0%–8.0% |
| (Z)-Tagetone | 4.3%–7.0% |
| Piperitone | 0.0%–6.1% |
| Para-Cymen-8-ol | 0.0%–5.4% |
| Piperitenone | 0.0%–4.9% |
| Dihydrotagetone | 0.0%–4.5% |

*T. patula (Aerial parts, 4-Vinyl-Guaiacol/Gamma Terpinene CT)*

| | |
|---|---|
| 4-Vinyl-Guaiacol | 8.6% |
| Gamma-Terpinene | 8.4% |
| Limonene | 6.3% |
| 3,9-Epoxy-p-Mentha-1,8(10)-Diene | 6.2% |
| (E)-Tagetone | 5.3% |
| Rotundifolene | 4.6% |
| 1,3,8-p-Menthatriene | 3.9% |
| Trans-Carveol | 3.7% |
| Caryophyllene Oxide | 3.7% |
| Alpha-Ocimene | 3.4% |
| (Z)-Nerolidol | 3.2% |
| Cis-Epoxy-Ocimene | 2.7% |
| (Z)-Beta-Ocimene | 2.3% |
| Dihydrotagetone | 2.3% |

*T. erecta (Aerial Parts)*

| | |
|---|---|
| Piperitone | 3.4%–45.7% |
| (Z)-Beta-Ocimene | 5.0%–18.5% |
| (E)-Beta-Ocimene | 8.7%–14.8% |
| Alpha-Terpinolene | 0.1%–13.9% |
| (E)-Tagetone | 0.1%–10.6% |
| Limonene | 7.8%–8.6% |
| Beta-Caryophyllene | 1.7%–8.6% |
| Piperitenone | 0.0%–5.9% |

*T. patula (Flowers, Piperitone CT)*

| | |
|---|---|
| Piperitone | 24.7% |
| Piperitenone | 22.9% |
| Alpha-Terpinolene | 7.8% |
| Dihydrotagetone | 4.9% |
| (Z)-Tagetone | 4.6% |
| Limonene | 4.5% |
| Allo-Ocimene | 3.7% |

*T. erecta (Leaves)*

| | |
|---|---|
| Piperitone | 8.9%–52.4% |
| Alpha-Terpinolene | 11.2%–22.2% |
| Limonene | 1.4%–10.4% |
| Piperitenone | 5.0%–9.7% |
| (Z)-Beta-Ocimene | 0.3%–7.0% |
| (E)-Beta-Ocimene | 0.6%–7.0% |
| (Z)-Myroxide | 0.0%–4.2% |

*T. erecta (Flowers)*

| | |
|---|---|
| Beta-caryophyllene | 7.1%–35.2% |
| Piperitone | 0.6%–28.5% |
| (Z)-Beta-Ocimene | 2.8%–13.7% |
| Piperitenone | 2.6%–11.0% |
| (E)-Ocimenone | 0.0%–9.8% |
| (Z)-Myroxide | 0.0%–7.9% |
| (Z)-Ocimenone | 0.0%–7.7% |
| Piperitenone Oxide | 0.0%–7.2% |
| Limonene | 2.5%–6.9% |
| Terpinolene | 4.7%–6.3% |
| Germacrene D | 1.5%–4.1% |

Note: Leaf oils generally contain more dihydrotagetone, whereas the flower oils contain more (Z)-beta-ocimene.[3237] In addition, dihydrotagetone content sharply declines and (Z)-beta-ocimene content simultaneously increases from flower bud stage to seed shedding stage. Most commercial samples of tagetes essential oil are *T. minuta* and report the (Z)-beta-ocimene CT, although other CTs may also be available.

**OTHER CONSTITUENTS:** *T. minuta ((Z)-Beta-Ocimene CT)*—sabinene, trans-linalool oxide, neo-alloocimene, (E)-tagetone, elsholtzia ketone, alpha-gurjunene, beta-caryophyllene, alpha-humulene, germacrene D, gamma-elemene; *T. minuta (Dihydrotagetone CT)*—sabinene, trans-linalool oxide, trans-p-menth-2-en-ol, linalool, borneol, terpinen-4-ol, (Z)-ocimenone, alpha-gurjunene, spathulenol; *T. minuta (Limonene CT)*—sabinene, dihydrotagetone, 1-methyl-4-isopropenylbenzene, cis-epoxy-ocimene, trans-epoxy-ocimene, (Z)-tagetone, p-cymene-8-ol, linalyl propionate, verbenone, piperitone oxide, beta-caryophyllene, spathulenol, caryophyllene oxide, heptadecane, neophytadiene, nonadecane, heneicosane; *T. minuta (Alpha-Terpineol CT)*—limonene, terpinen-1-ol, (E)-tagetone, trans-beta-terpineol, borneol, terpinen-4-ol, (Z)-jasmone, beta-caryophyllene, bicyclogermacrene, spathulenol; *T. minuta (Piperitone CT)*—N/A; *T patula (Limonene CT)*—alpha-pinene, beta-pinene, (E)-beta-ocimene, linalool, isopinocampheol, isobornyl acetate, alpha-gurjunene, (E)-beta-farnesene, spathulenol, trans-sesquisabinene hydrate; *T. patula (Aerial parts, 4-Vinyl-Guaiacol/Gamma Terpinene CT)*—borneol, (E)-beta-farnesene, spathulenol, Artemisia ketone, alpha-terpineolene; *T. patula (Flowers, Piperitone CT)*—(Z)-ocimene, (E)-ocimene, linalool, 4-terpineol, (E)-tagetone, alpha-terpinolene, 2-phenyl ethyl acetate, caryophyllene, caryophyllene oxide; *T. erecta (Leaves)*—sabinene, (E)-beta-ocimene, dihydrotagetone, linalool, alpha-terpineol, (E)-tagetenone, linalyl acetate, indole, beta-caryophyllene, (E)-epoxyocimene; *T. erecta (Flowers)*—sabinene, gamma-terpinene, allo-ocimene, bicyclogermacrene, caryophyllene oxide; *T. erecta (Aerial Parts)*—sabinene, allo-oscimine, piperitone, bicyclogermacrene

## PREFERRED COMPOSITION FOR CLINICAL USE:

| Constituent | (Z)-Beta-Ocimene CT | (E)-Ocimenone-Rich | Dihydrotagetone CT |
|---|---|---|---|
| **(Z)-Beta-Ocimene** | 30%–55% | 8%–33% | 0.5%–10% |
| **(E)-Ocimenone ((E)-Tagetenone)** | 5%–20% | 30%–45% | 0%–1% |
| **Dihydrotagetone** | 3%–18% | 1%–5% | 30%–55% |
| **(Z)-Tagetone** | 5%–15% | 5%–15% | 10%–25% |
| **(Z)-Ocimenone ((Z)-Tagetenone)** | 4%–10% | 5%–20% | 0%–1% |
| **Limonene** | 4%–10% | 0.5%–3% | 5%–15% |
| **(E)-Tagetone** | 1%–3% | 1%–3% | 10%–20% |
| **Linalool** | < 3% | < 3% | 0.5%–3% |

**REPORTED THERAPEUTIC PROPERTIES: Antibacterial**, antifungal, antiparasitic, antimicrobial, anti-infectious, antiseptic, antispasmodic, analgesic, anti-inflammatory, **anticancer**, disinfectant, supports normal blood pressure, soothes chronic skin conditions, wound healing, supports respiratory function, expels excess mucus, diuretic, relieves burns, **insect repellent**, **insecticide**, sedating, calming/relaxing, combats anger, **combats negative thoughts**, combats mental fatigue, antidepressant

## CAUTIONS:

■ May be photosensitizing due to possible presence of psoralen.[8625] Avoid sun exposure to the area of application for at least twelve hours after topical application.

■ May interact with benzodiazepine medications based on animal research.[8626,8627]

■ *T. minuta (Piperitone CT), T. erecta (Aerial parts, leaves, flowers); T. patula (Flowers)*: May interact with antibiotics and enhance their effectiveness based on piperitone content.[8628,8629]

■ *T. erecta (Flowers)*: May decrease the bioavailability of many medications (NSAIDs, proton-pump inhibitors, acetaminophen, antiepileptics, immune modulators, blood-sugar medications, blood pressure medications, antidepressants, antipsychotics, diabetic medications, antihistamines, antibiotics, and anesthetics) due to the ability of caryophyllene oxide, alpha-humulene, and beta-caryophyllene to inhibit CYP3A enzyme activity.[8630]

## SELECTED EVIDENCE:

☐ The dihydrotagetone CT of *T. minuta* killed nasopharyngeal and liver hepatocellular carcinoma cancer cells at higher concentrations (50 to 200 mcg/mL) but had no effect under 50 mcg/mL *in vitro*.[8631] Another study reported that the (E)-ocimenone CT of *T. minuta* moderately killed breast-cancer cells.[8632] *T. erecta* essential oil rich in alpha-terpinolene and (E)-ocimenone prevented the spread of six cancer cell lines (colon adenocarcinoma, two glioblastoma cells lines, human cervical adenocarcinoma, breast adenocarcinoma, and hepatocellular carcinoma) *in vitro*.[8633]

☐ *T. minuta* (dihydrotagetone and beta-ocimene CTs) demonstrates potent antioxidant and free radical scavenging activity, inhibiting reactive oxygen species (ROS) and reactive nitrogen species (RNS).[8634,8635] A (E)-ocimenone-rich *T. minuta* also demonstrated potent antioxidant activity.[8636]

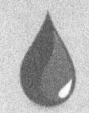

- *In vitro* research reported that tagetes essential oil (*T. minuta*, (Z)-Beta-Ocimene CT) completely inhibited thirteen gram-positive and nineteen gram-negative bacteria and seven fungi, and partially inhibited an additional gram-negative bacterium.[8637] Another study compared the antimicrobial activity of the dihydrotagetone and (Z)-beta-ocimene CTs of *T. minuta* against gram-positive and gram-negative bacteria, reporting that the dihydrotagetone CT more actively inhibited *Bacillus cereus, B. subtilis, Staphylococcus aureus, Streptococcus faecalis, E. coli, Proteus mirabilis, Pseudomonas aeruginosa,* and *Salmonella typhi.*[8638] The (Z)-beta-ocimene CT also inhibited all organisms but required higher concentrations to produce inhibition, particularly a CT with 32% beta-ocimene and 16.4% dihydrotagetone. Overall the researchers reported that both CTs were more effective against gram-negative bacteria. More research tested the antimicrobial activity of the dihydrotagetone CT of *T. minuta* and found that it inhibited *S. typhi, E. coli, S. aureus,* and *B. subtilis,* with greater activity against the gram-positive bacteria (*S. aureus* and *B. subtilis*).[8639] *T. erecta* ((Z)-beta-ocimene CT) inhibited four bacteria: gram-positive bacteria—*Staphylococcus aureus,* and gram-negative bacteria—*Klebsiella pneumonia, Pseudomonas aeruginosa,* and *Xanthomonas oryzae in vitro,* with greater activity against gram-positive bacteria.[8640]

- The beta-ocimene CT demonstrated remarkable antifungal activity against *C. albicans* and significantly inhibited MRSA *in vitro.*[8641] Additional research reported that the beta-ocimene CT demonstrated moderate antifungal activity (partially preventing mycelial growth) against seven pathogenic fungi: *Fusarium moniliforme, F. oxysporum, Colletotrichum falcatum, Trichothecium roseum, Curvularia pallescens, Aspergillus niger,* and *A. terreus.*[8642] Another study reported moderate antifungal activity of *T. erecta* (beta-ocimene CT) against three phytopathogenic fungi: *R. solani, S. rolfsii,* and *M. phaseolina.*[8643] An unknown CT of *T. minuta* essential oil inhibited the fungi: *Trichophyton mentagrophytes, Microsporum gypsum, Candida albicans ATCC 10231, Cryptococcus neoformans, Aspergillus niger,* and *Penicillium* species. Its ability to inhibit filamentous fungi was greater than that of standard antifungal drugs, but less active on yeast.[8644] *T. patula* (piperitone CT) completely inhibits the phytopathogenic fungi *Botrytis cinerea* and *Penicillium digitatum.*[8645]

- *T. minuta* (dihydrotagetone CT) significantly inhibited proinflammatory processes (NADH oxidase, inducible nitric oxide synthase, and TNF-alpha) and potently scavenged ROS and RNS, suggesting it could potentially modulate the immune-inflammatory response and reduce the associated oxidative damage.[8646]

- *In vitro* research demonstrates that *T. minuta* (piperitone CT) inhibits the gastrointestinal nematode *Haemonchus contortus* (a common and highly pathogenic parasite that attaches to mucous membranes in the stomach—of both animals and humans—and feeds on the blood of its host).[8647]

- A 20% concentration of *T. minuta* essential oil (dihydrotagetone CT) effectively killed—over 95% efficacy—four species of ticks: *Rhipicephalus (B.) microplus, Rhipicephalus sanguineus, Amblyomma cajennense,* and *Argas miniatus* Koch.[8648,8649] *T. minuta* (rich in (E)-ocimenone) killed *Aedes aegypti* mosquito larvae.[8650] A 25% concentration of *T. minuta* (unknown CT) prevented *A. aegypti* from biting for ninety minutes.[8651] Interestingly, a 50% concentration only protected against bites for sixty-three minutes. The beta-ocimene CT also kills the *Odontotermes obesus* Rhamb. Termite, demonstrating 100% mortality at higher doses (6 mcL/Petri-plate).[8652] *T. minuta* (beta-ocimene CT) also significantly repels the brown ear tick (*Rhipicephalus appendiculatus*), *Hyalomma rufipes* tick, and *Triatoma infestans* (a nocturnal insect that feeds on the blood of mammals while they sleep).[8653,8654,8655] Interestingly, *T. minuta* (beta-ocimene CT) attracts male Mediterranean fruit flies but repels females.[8656] *T. patula* (rich in 4-vinyl-guaiacol and gamma-terpinene) is larvicidal against the tick *Rhipicephalus sanguineus.*[8657] *T. patula* (limonene CT) was larvicidal to three mosquitoes (*Aedes aegypti, Anopheles stephensi,* and *Culex quinquefasciatus*), with the greatest activity against *A. aegypti.*[8658] *T. erecta* (piperitone CT) effectively killed the larvae of the mosquito *A. aegypti.*[8659] Tagetes (*T. minuta*) essential oil demonstrated 100% efficacy against tick (*Rhipicephalus sanguineus*) larvae, nymphs and adults.[8660] *T. patula* essential oil is toxic to bed bugs (*Cimex lectularius* L.) without harming human cells.[8661] An unidentified CT of *T. minuta* repelled sandflies (*Phlebotomus duboscqi*), which is a vector of zoonotic cutaneous leishmaniasis.[8662]

- Animal research reported that oral administration of *T. minuta* (unidentified CT) increases anxiety in chicks during maze tests by negatively modulating GABAergic function (the GABAergic system is a system of structures that release or bind gamma-aminobutyric acid and regulate anxiety, muscle tension, memory, and convulsive activity).[8663] Another study reports that *T. minuta* essential oil (unknown CT) interacts with brain membranes and disrupts the binding of benzodiazepine in the brain at benzodiazepine sites, which suggests it may reduce depressive symptoms.[8664]

☐ *Tagetes patula* essential oil CT piperitenone/piperitone demonstrated 100 percent inhibition of multidrug-resistant *Haemonchus contortus* (a very common parasitic gastrointestinal nematode of ruminant animals—cattle, sheep, goats, etc.—that attaches to the stomach mucosa and feeds on blood).[8665]

☐ The beta-ocimene CT of tagetes essential oil exhibited good antioxidant activity and demonstrated antimicrobial activity against *S. aureus, M. smegmatis, S. uberis, L. ivanovii, Vibrio* spp., *E. cloacae,* and *E. coli.*[8666]

☐ *Tagetes minuta* CT dihydrotagetone was strongly insecticidal to the blowfly (*Lucilia cuprina*).[8667]

☐ Tagetes (*T. patula*) acted as a natural and safe method to control cattle ticks (*Rhipicephalus microplus*), both repelling and killing the tick.[8668]

☐ Tagetes (*T. minuta*) essential oil was larvicidal to the Australian sheep blowfly (*Lucilia cuprina*).[8669]

☐ Administration of tagetes (*T. erecta*) essential oil in rats upregulated antioxidant and immune system activity in an experimental model of gastric cancer caused by methylnitronitrosoguanidine (a biochemical used to trigger cancer and mutations in research).[8670] The oil also reduced release of inflammatory cytokines and changed the expression of multiple proteins involved in cancer initiation and progression. Overall, the results suggest that tagetes essential oil may shield against gastric cancer.

☐ Tagetes (*T. patula*) and lavender cotton essential oil were toxic to aphids.[8671]

☐ Stress and inflammation are contributing factors in depression. Intragastric administration of tagetes (*T. minuta*) essential oil reversed depressive-like behavior caused by stress and inflammation in mice.[8672] The researchers hypothesized that the antidepressant activity of tagetes essential oil was due to its ability to reverse oxidative stress in the hippocampus, reduce corticosterone levels, and restore levels of brain-derived neurotrophic factor (BDNF), phosphatidylinositol-3-kinase (P3K), protein kinase B (PKB), and extracellular signal-regulated kinase 2 (ESRK-2). BDNF is a neurotrophic factor vital for neuronal plasticity and associated with antidepressant activity. Dysregulation of P3K and ESRK-2 has been linked to major depressive episodes. PKB is the receptor for BDNF and has been implicated as a causative factor in major depressive disorder and response to antidepressant therapies.

☐ Tagetes (*T. patula*) essential oil with trans-beta-caryophyllene as the major constituent displayed potent antioxidant activity in the DPPH, NO, and FRAP assays.[8673] Oral administration of the oil in rats relieved all of the toxic effects of carbon tetrachloride—significantly increased oxidative stress markers (malonaldehyde, total protein, and non-protein sulfhydryl), elevated liver markers (aminotransferase, gamma-glutamyl transferase, alkaline phosphatase, and bilirubin), and disrupted lipid profiles.

☐ Anise and tagetes (*T. minuta*) showed strong insecticidal activity against the corn sap beetle (*Carpophilus dimidiatus*) and the merchant grain beetle (*Oryzaephilus mercator*), while cumin was strongly insecticidal against the merchant grain beetle.[8674]

---

# TAMALA
## (Indian Bay Leaf, Indian Cassia, Tejpat)

*Cinnamomum tamala* (Buch.-Ham) T. Nees & Eberm.

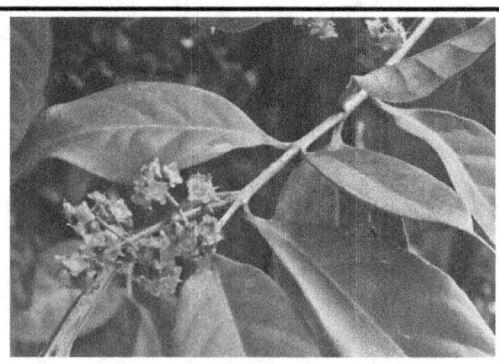

**FAMILY:** Lauraceae
**NOTE:** Middle
**AROMA INTENSITY:** Medium
**AROMA:** Spicy, warm, peppery, clove-cinnamon like
**COMMON EXTRACTION METHOD:** Hydrodistilled from the leaves
**POSSIBLE SUBSTITUTE OILS:** Clove, cinnamon, cassia
**BLENDS WELL WITH:** Bergamot, cassia, cinnamon, clove, grapefruit, lavender, lemon, lime, orange, Mediterranean mandarin, patchouli, tangerine
**SUBCELLULAR LOCALIZATION | EPIGENETIC INFLUENCE:** Currently unknown | Currently unknown

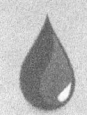

**RECOMMENDED DILUTION RANGE:** Eugenol, Eugenol/Eugenyl Acetate, (E)Cinnamaldehyde, Linalool/(E)Cinnamaldehyde CT, (E)-Cinnamaldehyde/Cinnamyl Acetate CTs—1.5%–20%; Linalool, Beta-Caryophyllene, Trans-Sabinene Hydrate CT—5%–Neat

**PRIMARY CONSTITUENTS:**[8675,8676,8677,8678,8679,8680,8681,8682,8683,8684]

*Eugenol CT*

| | |
|---|---|
| Eugenol | 66.1%–91.4% |
| Spathulenol | 0.6%–12.7% |
| Beta-Pinene | 0.1%–10.0% |
| Eugenyl Acetate | 0.0%–9.8% |
| Beta-Myrcene | 0.0%–9.7% |
| Methyl Eugenol | 0.0%–6.4% |
| (Z)-Beta-Ocimene | 0.0%–4.5% |
| Beta-Humulene | 0.0%–4.4% |
| Beta-Costol | 0.0%–3.9% |
| Beta-Caryophyllene | 0.1%–3.6% |

*(E)-Cinnamaldehyde CT*

| | |
|---|---|
| (E)-Cinnamaldehyde | 60.1%–82.0% |
| Linalool | 2.9%–18.5% |
| Cinnamyl Acetate | 1.3%–11.1% |
| Benzaldehyde | 2.0%–3.2% |

*Linalool CT*

| | |
|---|---|
| Linalool | 60.7% |
| Alpha-Pinene | 10.5% |
| Beta-Pinene | 10.4% |
| Limonene | 3.2% |
| Camphene | 3.0% |

*Beta-Caryophyllene CT*

| | |
|---|---|
| Beta-Caryophyllene | 25.3% |
| Linalool | 13.4% |
| Caryophyllene Oxide | 10.3% |
| Alpha-Humulene | 6.2% |
| Alpha-Terpinyl Acetate | 3.2% |
| Spathulenol | 2.8% |

*Eugenol/Eugenyl Acetate CT*

| | |
|---|---|
| Eugenol | 41.8%–77.8% |
| Eugenyl Acetate | 12.3%–47.1% |
| Bicyclogermacrene | 1.5%–4.9% |

*Linalool/(E)Cinnamaldehyde CT*

| | |
|---|---|
| Linalool | 22.7%–62.0% |
| (E)-Cinnamaldehyde | 7.7%–61.7% |
| Cinnamyl Acetate | 0.6%–13.7% |
| 1,8-Cineole | 0.2%–3.7% |

*(E)-Cinnamaldehyde/Cinnamyl Acetate CT*

| | |
|---|---|
| (E)-Cinnamaldehyde | 28.2%–55.0% |
| Cinnamyl Acetate | 18.4%–42.3% |
| Benzyl Benzoate | 0.0%–15.3% |
| Linalool | 0.3%–13.5% |
| 1,8-Cineole | 0.1%–4.4% |
| Benzaldehyde | 1.3%–4.1% |

*Trans-Sabinene Hydrate CT*

| | |
|---|---|
| Trans-Sabinene Hydrate | 29.8% |
| (Z)-Beta-Ocimene | 17.9% |
| Germacrene A | 11.3% |
| Alpha-Gurjunene | 4.7% |
| Beta-Myrcene | 4.6% |
| Alpha-Pinene | 3.1% |

**OTHER CONSTITUENTS:** *Eugenol CT*—para-cymene, 1,8-cineole, thujyl alcohol isomer, cis-sabinene, alpha-phellandrene, beta-elemene, delta-cadinene, germacrene B, germacrene D, globulol, viridiflorol, guaiol, alpha-cadinol, alpha-terpineol, (E)-cinnamaldehyde, aromadendrene, gamma-muurolene, bicyclogermacrene; *Eugenol/Eugenyl Acetate CT*—alpha-pinene, alpha-phellandrene, para-cymene, 1,8-cineole, beta-caryophyllene, germacrene D, spathulenol, globulol; *Linalool/(E)-Cinnamaldehyde CT*—beta-pinene, benzaldehyde, caryophyllene oxide; *(E)-Cinnamaldehyde CT*—beta-pinene, 1,8-cineole; *(E)-Cinnamaldehyde/Cinnamyl Acetate CT*—beta-pinene, caryophyllene oxide; *Linalool CT*—benzaldehyde, geraniol, eugenol; *Beta-Caryophyllene CT*—alpha-pinene, para-cymene, alpha-ylangene, alpha-copaene, beta-elemene, terpinen-4-ol, gamma-muurolene, alpha-terpineol, germacrene D, alpha-muurolene, delta-cadinene, cuminaldehyde, cis-calamenene, (E)-geranyl acetate, isocaryophyllene oxide, 1-epi-cubenol, globulol, T-cadinol, T-muurolol, alpha-cadinol, caryophylladienol II, dodecanoic acid, hexadecanoic acid; *Trans-Sabinene Hydrate CT*—camphene, sabinene, beta-pinene, trans-verbenol, citronellal, terpinen-4-ol, alpha-terpineol, carvone, 2,6-dimethyl-2(3), 7-octadiene, alpha-guaiene, aromadendrene, beta-selinene, beta-bisabolene, gamma-cadinene, ledol, spathulenol, epi-globulol, caryophyllene oxide, hexadecanoic acid

PREFERRED COMPOSITION FOR CLINICAL USE:

| Constituent | Eugenol CT | (E)-Cinnamaldehyde/ Cinnamyl Acetate CT |
|---|---|---|
| Eugenol | 45%–70% | – |
| Beta-Pinene | 0.1%–10% | – |
| Beta-Myrcene | 0.1%–10% | – |
| Spathulenol | 0.1%–5% | – |
| Eugenyl Acetate | 0.1%–5% | – |
| Beta-Caryophyllene | 0.1%–5% | – |
| Methyl Eugenol | < 5% | – |
| (E)-Cinnamaldehyde | – | 45%–55% |
| Cinnamyl Acetate | – | 20%–35% |
| Benzyl Benzoate | – | 0.1%–10% |
| Benzaldehyde | – | 1%–5% |
| Linalool | – | 0.1%–5% |
| 1,8-Cineole | – | 0.1%–5% |
| Linalool | – | 0.1%–5% |

REPORTED THERAPEUTIC PROPERTIES: Antibacterial, **antifungal**, antimicrobial, anti-infectious, anticancer, liver supportive, analgesic, anti-inflammatory, antiarthritic, antirheumatic, antispasmodic, **antioxidant**, soothes sprains and sports injuries, aids circulation, reduces cholesterol levels, relieves painful menstruation, aids digestion, relieves diarrhea, increases appetite, **balances blood sugar levels**, uplifting, relieves anxiety, stress management, relieves mental fatigue, eases difficult emotional transitions

CAUTIONS:

■ *Eugenol, Eugenol/Eugenyl Acetate, (E)Cinnamaldehyde, Linalool/(E)Cinnamaldehyde CT, (E)-Cinnamaldehyde/Cinnamyl Acetate CTs*: Avoid during pregnancy and lactation due to eugenol and cinnamaldehyde content. Several animal studies have tested cinnamaldehyde with pregnant animals, and the results have been inconsistent. Therefore, it is advised to avoid essential oils with significant quantities of cinnamaldehyde during pregnancy until further research is conclusive.[8685,8686,8687] Animal studies suggest that large doses of clove (also with significant eugenol) may negatively impact embryonic development and encourage fetal cell death.[8688,8689] Another animal study did not detect any negative influence of clove oil.[8690] Eugenol is considered strongly toxic to embryos according to animal studies.[8691] Based on these studies it is best to limit clove oil during pregnancy and lactation.

■ *Eugenol, Eugenol/Eugenyl Acetate, (E)Cinnamaldehyde, Linalool/(E)Cinnamaldehyde CT, (E)-Cinnamaldehyde/Cinnamyl Acetate CTs*: May interact with aspirin, blood pressure, antiplatelet, and anticoagulant medications, and increase the risk of bleeding among people with bleeding disorders based on cinnamaldehyde and eugenol content.[8692,8693,8694,8695,8696,8697,8698]

■ *Eugenol, Eugenol/Eugenyl Acetate CTs*: May interact with MAOI antidepressants based on eugenol content. Animal research suggests that eugenol produces antidepressant effects via the monoamine oxidase pathway, which may cause interactions with antidepressants that also interact with this pathway.[8699,8700]

■ *Eugenol, Eugenol/Eugenyl Acetate, (E)Cinnamaldehyde, Linalool/(E)Cinnamaldehyde CT, (E)-Cinnamaldehyde/Cinnamyl Acetate CTs*: May interfere with enzymes responsible for metabolizing medications (NSAIDs, proton-pump inhibitors, acetaminophen, antiepileptics, immune modulators, blood-sugar medications, blood pressure medications, antidepressants, antipsychotics, diabetic medications, antihistamines, antibiotics, and anesthetics) based on eugenol or cinnamaldehyde content.[8701,8702,8703]

■ *(E)Cinnamaldehyde, Linalool/(E)Cinnamaldehyde CT, (E)-Cinnamaldehyde/Cinnamyl Acetate CTs*: May interact with diabetes medications and cause low blood-sugar levels based on cinnamaldehyde content and similar composition to cassia and cinnamon essential oils.[8704,8705,8706,8707]

■ *Eugenol, Eugenol/Eugenyl Acetate, (E)Cinnamaldehyde, Linalool/(E)Cinnamaldehyde CT, (E)-Cinnamaldehyde/Cinnamyl Acetate CTs*: May interact with antibiotics and possibly enhance their effects based on cinnamaldehyde and eugenol content.[8708,8709,8710]

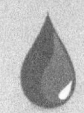

■ *Eugenol, Eugenol/Eugenyl Acetate CTs*: May interact with anticholinergic (drugs used for asthma, incontinence, gastrointestinal cramps, muscular spasms, depression, and sleep disorders) and cholinergic medications (drugs used to reduce urinary retention, diagnose myasthenia gravis, and for glaucoma) based on AChE inhibitory activity of eugenol.[8711]

■ *CTs with cinnamaldehyde and eugenol*: May irritate mucous membranes (eyes, mouth, nasal passages, vagina, rectum).[8712,8713,8714]

■ *(E)Cinnamaldehyde, Linalool/(E)Cinnamaldehyde CT, (E)-Cinnamaldehyde/Cinnamyl Acetate CTs*: Topical application (significant dilution strongly encouraged). Some CTs of tamala are very high in cinnamaldehyde, which is very irritating to the skin and prone to cause severe reactions.[8715]

**SELECTED EVIDENCE:**

☐ *In vitro* research demonstrated that tamala essential oil (eugenol CT) significantly inhibits the pathogenic plant fungi *Aspergillus fumigatus, A. niger, Cladosporium cladosporioides, Curvularia lunata, Fusarium oxysporum, Helminthosporium oryzae, Macrophomina phaseolina, Mucor racemosus, Penicillium italicum, Rhizoctonia solani,* and *Sclerotium rolfsii.*[8716] Remarkably, tamala essential oil inhibited nine of the eleven fungi completely (all but *A. niger* (49.6%) and *A. fumigatus* (91.9%)), which was more potent than some common synthetic fungicides. The study authors also reported that it reduced the production of aflatoxin. Another study concluded that tamala essential oil (eugenol CT) completely inhibited *F. moniliforme, A. niger, A. oryzae,* and *A. solani.*[8717] The (E)-cinnamaldehyde CT of tamala essential oil inhibited *A. niger* and *A. falvus.*[8718]

☐ Tamala essential oil (eugenol CT) strongly inhibits the bacteria *P. aeruginosa, K. pneumoniae, S. aureus, Proteus vulgaris, B. cereus,* and *E. coli.*[8719] The study authors attributed the antimicrobial activity predominantly to the presence of the phenolic constituents eugenol and spathulenol.

☐ Animal research demonstrates that oral administration of the cinnamaldehyde/cinnamyl acetate CT of tamala essential oil (100 or 200 mg/kg) reduces blood glucose, plasma insulin levels, and total cholesterol as well as the antidiabetic drug glibenclamide.[8720]

☐ *In vitro* research reports that tamala essential oil (eugenol CT) possesses considerable antioxidant capacity and increases reduced glutathione (GSH) levels.[8721,8722]

☐ Tamala essential oil is toxic to mosquitoes and fire ants.[8723]

☐ *In vitro* research demonstrates that tamala essential oil (linalool/(E)-cinnamaldehyde CT) inhibits *Pseudomonas aeruginosa* through inhibition of its quorum-sensing ability.[8724] The same research reported that tamala essential oil works in synergy with DNase (DNaseI)—a bovine pancreatic enzyme—and a DNase (MBD)—an enzyme isolated from the marine bacterium *Vibrio alginolyticus.*

☐ Tamala essential oil prevented biofilm formation and reduced virulence factors like staphyloxanthin and hemolysin in MRSA.[8725] Another study reported that tamala essential oil disrupted *Candida* biofilm formation.[8726]

☐ Both tamala CT eugenol and cinnamon leaf essential oil exhibited antispasmodic activity in isolated rat intestine (ileum), with tamala being the most effective.[8727]

# TANGERINE
## (Mandarin*)

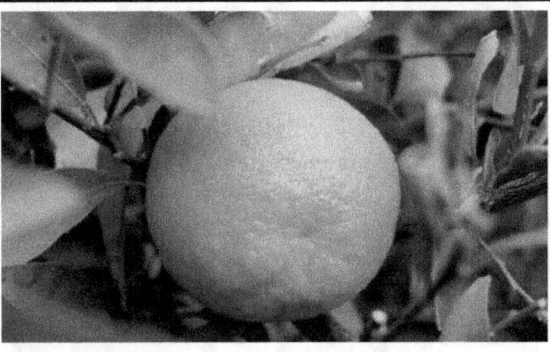

Tangerine: *Citrus reticulata* Blanco;
Mandarin/Green Mandarin: *C. nobilis* Andrews, *C. reticulata*

**FAMILY:** Rutaceae
**NOTE:** Top
**AROMA INTENSITY:** Medium
**AROMA:** Fresh, citrusy, sweet, fruity, orange-like
**COMMON EXTRACTION METHOD:** Cold-pressed/expressed or hydrodistilled from the fruit peel (rind)
**POSSIBLE SUBSTITUTE OILS:** Orange, lemon, grapefruit, lime, bergamot
**BLENDS WELL WITH:** Basil, bergamot, cardamom, carrot seed, cassia, chamomile (German, Roman), cinnamon, clary sage, clove, coriander, frankincense, grapefruit, juniper, lavender, lemon, lemon verbena, lime, nutmeg, neroli, niaouli, orange, patchouli, petitgrain, rose, sage, sandalwood, Spanish sage, ylang ylang

**SUBCELLULAR LOCALIZATION | EPIGENETIC INFLUENCE:** Golgi Apparatus | Muscular/Reproductive
**RECOMMENDED DILUTION RANGE:** 3%–50%; neat for limited conditions

**PRIMARY CONSTITUENTS:**[8728,8729,8730,8731,8732,8733]

| *Distilled* | | *Cold-pressed/expressed* | |
|---|---|---|---|
| Limonene | 45.7%–92.4% | Limonene | 87.1%–94.7% |
| Geranial | 0.1%–19.0% | Gamma-Terpinene | 0.1%–5.4% |
| Neral | 0.1%–14.5% | Myrcene | 0.7%–2.2% |
| Octanol | 0.0%–6.9% | | |
| Alpha-Myrcene | 0.0%–4.2% | | |
| Geranyl Acetate | 0.0%–3.9% | | |
| Geraniol | 0.0%–3.5% | | |

\* There is a great deal of confusion regarding mandarin and tangerine essential oil. They are frequently used synonymously in the essential oil industry, but technically are two different species of mandarin. Tangerine *(C. reticulata* Blanco; also *C. nobilis)* is a subtype of mandarin *(C. reticulata)*. Tangerine has a sweeter citrus aroma when compared to the light citrus aroma of mandarin. Tangerine essential oil typically has higher limonene levels and lower gamma-terpinene levels than mandarin essential oil. In addition, mandarin is further subdivided into green (from unripened fruits; soft, tangy, and less sweet aroma; light yellow appearance), and yellow (partially ripened fruits; slightly sweeter aroma; yellow appearance), and red (mature fruit; sweetest aroma; yellowish-orange appearance).

**OTHER CONSTITUENTS:** *Cold-pressed/expressed*—Linalool, alpha-pinene, (E)-beta-ocimene; *Distilled*—Linalool, alpha-pinene, beta-myrcene, (E)-beta-ocimene, gamma-terpinene

**PREFERRED COMPOSITION FOR CLINICAL USE:**

| Constituent | Tangerine Cold-pressed | Mandarin Cold-pressed | Green Mandarin | Yellow Mandarin | Red Mandarin |
|---|---|---|---|---|---|
| **Limonene** | 80%–95% | 60%–75% | 60%–72% | 62%–72% | 65%–80% |
| **Gamma-Terpinene** | 0.5%–5% | 15%–23% | 15%–25% | 15%–23% | 13%–21% |
| **Para-Cymene** | tr–5% | 0%–2.5% | 0.1%–2% | 0.1%–2% | 0.5%–3% |
| **Myrcene** | 1%–3% | 1%–3% | 1%–3% | 1%–3% | 1%–3% |
| **Alpha-Pinene** | 0.1%–3% | 1%–4% | 1%–4% | 1%–4% | 1%–4% |
| **Beta-Pinene** | tr–2% | 0.5%–2% | 1%-3% | 1%–3% | 1%–3% |
| **Linalool** | 0.1%–1% | tr–1% | tr–1% | tr–0.5% | tr–0.5% |
| **Octanal** | tr–1% | 0%–1% | < 0.5% | < 0.5% | < 0.5% |
| **Decanal** | 0%–1% | tr–1% | < 0.5% | < 0.5% | < 0.5% |
| **Methyl N-Methylanthranilate** | < 0.2% | 0.3%–1% | 0.5%–1% | 0.5%–1% | 0.5%–1% |
| **Alpha-Sinensal** | < 0.5% | tr–1% | 0.1%–1% | 0.1%–1% | 0.1%–1% |

**REPORTED THERAPEUTIC PROPERTIES:** Antimicrobial, antiseptic, **antispasmodic**, anti-inflammatory, expels excess gas, aids digestion, diuretic, relieves constipation, regenerative, **reduces the appearance of blemishes**, stimulates healthy cell cycle, promotes fluid balance and removes excess fluids from the body, purifies the blood, **encourages restful sleep**, stimulating, **stress management**, **antidepressant**, **relieves anxiety**

**CAUTIONS:**

■ Tangerine is considered nonphotosensitizing according to the available research.[8734] However, the International Fragrance Association (IFRA) considers tangerine a possible mild photosensitizer.[8735] Mandarin essential oil contains higher percentages of 5-methoxypsoralen (250 ppm) than tangerine (50 ppm), and is photosensitizing. Avoid sun exposure for twelve hours following topical application of mandarin essential oil. Based on IFRAs determination, it may be best to avoid UV exposure for twelve hours following application of tangerine essential oil.

■ May interfere with enzymes responsible for metabolizing medications (NSAIDs, proton-pump inhibitors, acetaminophen, antiepileptics, immune modulators, blood-sugar medications, blood pressure medications, antidepressants antipsychotics, diabetic medications, antihistamines, antibiotics, and anesthetics).[8736,8737,8738,8739,8740]

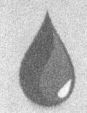

■ *Distilled Tangerine*: Use cautiously with diabetic medications. Large oral doses of citral may improve insulin sensitivity and lower blood-glucose levels according to animal research.[8741,8742]

■ *Distilled Tangerine*: May interact with antibiotics and possibly enhance their effects due to citral content (low risk).[8743]

■ *Distilled Tangerine*: Dilution is recommended for topical application due to moderate citral content and the risk for skin irritation or sensitivity.[8744,8745] May also irritate mucous membranes.

SELECTED EVIDENCE:

- Tangerine oil helps decrease inflammation by strongly inhibiting the 5-lipoxygenase (5-LOX) enzyme that is involved in the inflammation response according to *in vitro* research.[8746]

- Tangerine oil completely prevents the production of aflatoxin B(1) by *A. flavus in vitro*.[8747]

- *In vitro* research suggests that tangerine oil kills mosquito larvae and is a potential natural option to control mosquito-borne disease.[8748]

- Tangerine essential oil prevents pulmonary fibrosis in rats possibly by preventing oxidation, reducing collagen deposition and fibrosis (the formation of excess connective tissue) in the lungs, and down-regulating CTGF protein and mRNA expression (CTGF and mRNA activity are involved triggering of fibrosis).[8749]

- Inhalation from personal aromasticks containing either bergamot and sandalwood, or frankincense, tangerine, and lavender improved sleep quality among cancer patients.[8750] Remarkably, 92% of study participants indicated they would continue to use their aromasticks for sleep improvement.

- A review study of nurse-delivered aromatherapy in acute care settings reported that the use of essential oils generally resulted in significant clinical improvements based on their intended use. Marjoram and tangerine essential oils reduced pain, lavender and marjoram essential oil reduced anxiety, and ginger alleviated nausea.[8751]

- Tangerine essential oil kills the larvae of the mosquito that carries arbovirus (*Aedes albopictus*).[8752]

- Both mandarin and tangerine essential oil demonstrated mosquitocidal activity against *Culex pipiens*, with mandarin demonstrating greater effectiveness against adults.[8753]

- Tangerine essential oil showed potent contact, repellent, and fumigant activity against the rusty grain beetle (*Cryptolestes ferrugineus*), which is a major insect pest of stored products.[8754]

- Mandarin essential oil was active against tumor cells, which caused the scientists to state that citrus peels prevent cancer and act as anticancer agents.[8755]

- Tangerine and kaffir lime peel essential oil both presented antimelanogenic (prevents hyperpigmentation) and antiacetylcholinesterase (a key enzyme involved in neurodegenerative disorders) activity. Kaffir lime peel oil also inhibited collagenase and elastase (enzymes involved in skin aging).[8756] The study authors also reported that cinnamon, kaffir lime, tangerine, and pomelo essential oils inhibited α-glucosidase activity, which is an enzyme linked to diabetes.

- Application of distilled tangerine and tea tree essential oils deterred fruit flies (*Drosophila suzukii*) from infesting small fruits (strawberries, cherries, and blueberries) without negatively impacting their taste.[8757]

- Distilled tangerine essential oil exhibited good antioxidant activity in the DPPH assay and antibacterial activity against *E. coli*.[8758] Topical application of the oil on rabbits also improved the wound healing process without causing skin irritation.

- Oral administration (0.5 to 0.75% of the diet) of tangerine peel extracted by subcritical extraction (76.6% limonene, 12.9% gamma-terpinene, 2.5% myrcene) significantly reduced high cholesterol—decreased total cholesterol, triglycerides, and LDL cholesterol—and fatty liver in rats fed a high-fat diet.[8759] Moreover, genes related to the production of cholesterol (SREBP-1c, ACC, and FAS) were downregulated and genes related to bile acid production (LXRα, CYP7A1, and CYP27A1) upregulated.

- *In vitro* research showed that mandarin essential oil inhibited *S. aureus* by depolarizing and increasing the cell permeability of the bacterial cell membrane, which allowed the cellular contents to leak out.[8760]

- Inhalation of diluted tangerine essential oil (50 mcL placed on filter paper attached to the subject's nose approximately 3 cm away) improved the time it took healthy people aged nineteen to twenty-five years old to fall asleep.[8761] The researchers also measured how tangerine essential oil affected the brainwave activity of the subjects. Inhalation of undiluted essential oil reduced alpha brainwave powers (slow and fast) and elevated beta powers (low and mid). Diluted tangerine oil produced an opposite effect, decreasing both alpha and beta powers while increasing theta power. The diluted oil's effects on brainwave activity suggest a relaxing and sedating effect, whereas the undiluted oil produces a fresh and alert state based on brainwaves.

- Hydrodistilled tangerine essential oil with an interesting composition (7.2% 1,8-cineole, 3.8% methyl palmitate, 3.7% alpha-terpineol, 2.6% methyl octadecanoate) inhibited *E. coli* and *S. aureus*, while its inhibitory capabilities were slightly reduced when incorporated into a gelatin-based film.[8762]

- Cinnamon bark, grapefruit, tangerine, and lemon essential oil each inhibited *Bacillus subtilis, Penicillium chrysogenum, Fusarium moniliforme, Aspergillus niger, Aspergillus flavus, Saccharomyces cerevisiae, Escherichia coli, Salmonella abony, Staphylococcus aureus, Pseudomonas aeruginosa,* and *Candida albicans*, with the greatest activity observed from cinnamon bark.[8763] The highest antioxidant activity was found in grapefruit oil, followed by lemon, tangerine, and cinnamon bark.

- Distilled tangerine, Nanfeng mandarin (*Citrus reticulata* Blanco cv. *Kinokuni*), kumquat, and sweet orange essential oil inhibited *Bacillus subtilis, Staphylococcus aureus, Escherichia coli, Pseudomonas aeruginosa,* and *Salmonella typhimurium*, with kumquat being the most active against three (*B. subtilis, E. coli,* and *S. typhimurium*) of the five microorganisms.[8764] Each of the essential oils also exhibited antioxidant activities in the DPPH and ABTS assays, with Nanfeng mandarin oil presenting the best activity.

- Distilled tangerine essential oil was significantly active against promastigote forms of *Leishmania amazonensis* and larvicidal to *Ae. aegypti* mosquitoes.[8765]

- Oregano CT carvacrol, lemon, lavender, mastic, and mandarin essential oil each inhibited *S. aureus*.[8766]

- Distilled tangerine and sweet orange essential oil exhibited stronger antioxidant activity than the positive control of quercetin in the DPPH assay.[8767]

- Reserpine was a drug formerly used to treat high blood pressure, often in combination with a thiazide diuretic, that works by slowing down the nervous system. Unfortunately, it was associated with significant side effects such as mood disorders, lack of energy, sleep problems, and weight gain or loss. A preclinical model evaluated the benefits of inhaling mandarin essential oil in reserpine-induced depressive mice.[8768] Reserpine resulted in weight loss, lack of energy, significantly reduced serotonin and glucocorticoid receptors (GR) and Nissl bodies (NB) in brain tissue, and elevated brain-derived neurotrophic factor (BDNF). Inhalation of mandarin essential oil for one hour daily prevented weight loss, lack of energy, and reversed changes in serotonin, GR, NB, and BDNF. Limonene was considered the most active constituent of the oil. Taken together, the research suggests that inhalation of mandarin essential oil balances hypothalamic-pituitary-adrenal (HPA) axis function resulting in increased neurotransmitter production and brain cell restoration to reduce depression caused by reserpine. Impressively, mandarin oil was more effective than fluoxetine.

- Skin barrier integrity is not only important for skin health but also acts as a protective mechanism to limit entry into the body by various substances and microbes. The skin barrier function provided by the *stratum corneum* (SC) is maintained by a delicate balance between water, ions, keratin, natural moisturizing factor, intracellular lipids, skin surface lipids, and the cutaneous microbiome. Substances that possess anti-inflammatory, antimicrobial, and antioxidant activity and trigger adaptive responses in skin characteristics support healthy skin barrier function and improve the appearance of the skin. Preclinical and clinical research evaluated the activity of tea tree, tangerine, eucalyptus (*E. globulus*), and lavender essential oil skin barrier function and characteristics. Two formulas—one with equal parts of tangerine, eucalyptus, and lavender, and one with equal parts of tea tree, tangerine, eucalyptus, and lavender—diluted to 2% in emulsions stabilized with polymers of natural origin were created to investigate their skin benefits. Tangerine showed the deepest penetration through the skin (35 percent of the oil made it across the SC) in pig ear, while the rest of the oils and combinations of the oils penetrated less than tangerine but were absorbed at higher than 5% through the viable epidermis. In the clinical study, the four essential oil emulsion hydrated the skin better and improved skin barrier function better than the three essential oil emulsion, showing that tea tree oil has a synergistic activity with the other oils. The four-oil group also experienced improvements in skin characteristics compared to a control group and the three-oil emulsion group. The totality of the research suggests that a combination of tea tree, tangerine, eucalyptus, and lavender in an emulsion can improve overall skin barrier function and skin characteristics.[8769]

- A study investigated the chemical composition and biological properties of citrus oils: lemon, sweet orange, grapefruit, and tangerine. All four oils displayed remarkable radical scavenging capacity with grapefruit exhibiting excellent antioxidant activity.[8770] Topical application of the oils showed significant antiedema activity comparable to ibuprofen and reduced the expression of inflammatory cytokines (IL-6, COX-2, NF-κB) to varying degrees. Lemon, grapefruit, and tangerine oil also inhibited lung cancer cells.

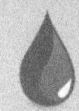

- Inhaling (200 mcL on cotton wool) Sai-Nam-Paung tangerine Co2 aromatic produced electroencephalographic (EEG) patterns similar to that of diazepam in male rats.[8771] However, diazepam increased episode number of awake and non-rapid eye movement (REM) sleep and reduced episode duration, while tangerine significantly decreased REM sleep latency and increased total time and episode numbers of REM sleep. The findings suggest that inhaling tangerine could improve sleep quality in some neurodegenerative conditions.

- Laboratory research showed that distilled sweet orange, grapefruit, lemon, and tangerine essential oil each have excellent antioxidant activity in the DPPH assay.[8772] Additionally, all four oils reduced inflammation (remarkably increased G1 phase of the cell cycle, which hinders proinflammatory factor expression) and the expression of proinflammatory molecules (COX-2 and TNF-$\alpha$). Evaluation in a rat model of rheumatoid arthritis demonstrated that the oils reduce inflammation similarly to the NSAID ibuprofen.

- Free and nanoencapsulated tangerine essential oil were compared against chlorhexidine against *S. mutans*, one of the main bacteria responsible for the development of dental cavities.[8773] The nanoencapsulated essential oil had a lower minimum inhibitory concentration (only slightly higher than chlorhexidine) and exhibited the greatest antibiofilm activity of the three agents tested. The nanoencapsulated oil was also less toxic to healthy cells.

- Tangerine displayed good repellent activity against *Ae. aegypti* mosquitoes.[8774]

# TANSY
## (Common Tansy, Bitter Buttons)

*Tanacetum vulgare* L., *Chrysanthemum tanacetum* Karsch,
*Ch. Vulgare* (L.) Bernh.

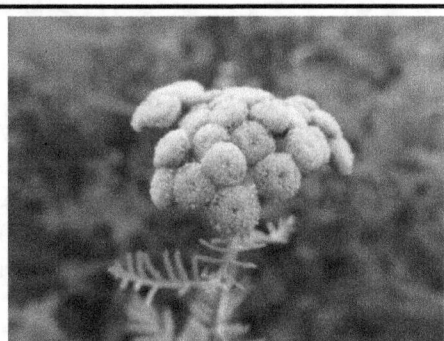

**FAMILY:** Asteraceae (Compositae)
**NOTE:** Middle-Base
**AROMA INTENSITY:** Strong
**AROMA:** Pungent, herbaceous
**COMMON EXTRACTION METHOD:** Steam distilled from the aerial parts
**POSSIBLE SUBSTITUTE OILS:** Sage
**BLENDS WELL WITH:** Chamomile (German, Roman), citronella, cypress, eucalyptus, lemongrass, lemon verbena, tea tree, peppermint, spearmint
**SUBCELLULAR LOCALIZATION | EPIGENETIC INFLUENCE:** Currently unknown | Currently unknown
**RECOMMENDED DILUTION RANGE:** $\leq 0.5\%$

**PRIMARY CONSTITUENTS:**[8775,8776,8777,8778,8779,8780,8781,8782,8783,8784,8785,8786,8787]

*Beta-Thujone CT*

| | |
|---|---|
| Beta-Thujone | 28.1%–97.9% |
| Artemisia Ketone | 0.0%–23.5% |
| Camphor | 0.0%–23.0% |
| Trans-Chrysanthenyl Acetate | 0.0%–20.0% |
| 1,8-Cineole | 0.5%–11.8% |
| Alpha-Thujone | 0.0%–11.0% |
| Thujyl Alcohol | 0.0%–8.7% |
| Carvone | 0.0%–6.6% |
| Germacrene D | 0.0%–5.0% |
| Sabinene | 0.0%–2.1% |
| Para-Cymene | 0.0%–1.6% |
| Borneol | 0.0%–1.0% |
| Camphene | 0.0%–1.0% |

Note: Several chemotypes of tansy exist, including alpha-thujone, thujyl alcohol, myrtenol, bornyl acetate, borneol, piperitone, camphor, chrysanthenyl/chrysanthenol, trans-carvyl acetate, chrysanthenone, artemisia ketone/artemisia alcohol, trans-dihydrocarvone, and 1,8-

cineole; and the beta-thujone CT could be divided into further CTs. One study found that 55% of samples obtained were the beta-thujone variety, with camphor the next most common CT noted (20%).[8788]

**OTHER CONSTITUENTS:** *Beta-thujone CT*—Alpha-pinene, para-cymene, terpinen-4-ol, eugenol, gamma-terpinene, terpinolene, beta-caryophyllene, davadone D

**PREFERRED COMPOSITION FOR CLINICAL USE:**

| Constituent | |
|---|---|
| **Beta-Thujone** | 60%–80% |
| **Camphor** | 2%–10% |
| **Germacrene D** | 1%–5% |
| **Sabinene** | 0.5%–4% |
| **1,8-Cineole** | 0.5%–4% |

**REPORTED THERAPEUTIC PROPERTIES:** Antibacterial, antimicrobial, antiviral, antifungal, antiallergenic, analgesic (pain relief), antiparasitic, anti-inflammatory, antirheumatic, anti-infectious, stimulates hormone release from the endocrine system, immune stimulant, insect repellent, stimulating, stress management, relieves anxiety, antidepressant

**CAUTIONS:**
*It is best to avoid the use of tansy in essential oil therapy—particularly by children, women who are pregnant/nursing, people with epilepsy or prone to convulsion, and people with compromised liver or kidney function— unless you absolutely know the chemotype and exact composition of the bottle (batch) you are using.*
■ Avoid with children under six due to thujone and camphor content. Cases of seizure have been reported in young children due to exposure to thujone rich essential oils.[8789,8790,8791] Several cases of camphor poisoning and/or seizures from ingestion and topical application have been reported in children.[8792,8793] Ingestion of camphor-containing products has been lethal in children under age 2 (estimated to be roughly 2,000 mg of camphor for a 20 kg child as the minimum potential fatal dose).[8794,8795]
■ Avoid during pregnancy and while lactating. Essential oils rich in thujone content may cause abortion.[8796,8797,8798] Camphor ingestion may lead to abortion because fetuses lack the enzymes to process it.[8799] Camphor ingestion by infants and young children may cause cough, vomiting, seizure, burning sensation in the mucous membranes and eyes, or lack of voluntary coordination of muscle movements.[8800]
■ Avoid oral consumption. Ingesting plants or products high in thujones can cause vomiting, stomachache, diarrhea, and gastroenteritis followed by absorption disorders, headache, nervous agitation, and chronic convulsions, and symptoms of liver and kidney toxicity extending to yellow liver atrophy (extensive and rapid death of liver cells— parenchymal, possibly accompanied by fatty degeneration), arrhythmia, and myocardial bleeding.[8801] Thujone is considered significantly neurotoxic and may damage the liver, and it is estimated that as little as 15 mg orally may negatively impact the central nervous system.[8802,8803,8804] Taking 20 drops of thuja oil (also with significant thujones content) twice daily for five days caused an adult woman to have a tonic seizure.[2033] As few as 12 drops of sage oil (also with significant thujones content) orally have reportedly caused a seizure and short coma in an adult.[8805]
■ Avoid with epilepsy and Parkinson's disease due to thujone, 1,8-cineole, and camphor content.[8806,8807,8808,8809,8810,8811,8812]
■ The potentially high camphor content in tansy may negatively impact red blood cells and increase the risk of jaundice in children with Glucose-6-phosphate dehydrogenase deficiency (G6PD).[8813,8814]
■ Avoid with those who have a compromised liver or kidneys due to the risk of kidney toxicity, kidney failure, or liver toxicity.[8815,8816,8817] Consuming extremely large amounts of thujone rich essential oils (10 mL) has caused kidney failure.[8818] This would also suggest that those taking medications that could cause liver damage should also use tansy very cautiously or avoid it entirely.
■ May heighten and alter the effect of alcohol.[8819]

**SELECTED EVIDENCE:**
  □ Doses of 200 µg/mL of tansy decreased motor activity and killed 100% of adult *Schistosoma mansoni* (parasitic worms that infect the intestinal tract and cause itchy skin, fever, chills, cough, muscle aches, abdominal pain, enlarged liver, blood stool or urine, and an increased risk of bladder cancer).[8820]

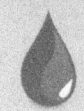

- Three of the primary constituents in tansy (beta-thujone, alpha-thujone, 1,8-cineole) possess tick repellency properties (64%–72%).[8821]

- The camphor CT of tansy essential oil demonstrated anti-inflammatory (inhibited nitric oxide production) and antioxidant activity.[8822] The anti-inflammatory activity was attributed to alpha-humulene, while the antioxidant activity was driven by alpha-pinene and caryophyllene oxide. The essential oil also inhibited *Escherichia coli* and *Staphylococcus aureus* (attributed to camphor and caryophyllene oxide) and was slightly toxic to lung cancer cells and moderately toxic to colon cancer cells.

- Tansy essential oil reduced gypsy moth (*Lymantria dispar*) larval survival, development, and nutritional physiology, suggesting it could be considered as a green pesticide.[8823]

- The Colorado potato beetle (Leptinotarsa decemlineata) is a significantly destructive pest of potato crops, which has developed resistance to most chemical pesticides. Tansy essential oil was an effective insecticide against adult beetles.[8824]

- Angelica root, ledum (*R. tomentosum*), and common tansy each showed broad-spectrum antimicrobial activity against tested microbes—*S. aureus, P. aeruginosa, C. albicans, A. niger, Cl. cladosporioides,* and *P. venetum.*[8825] Co2 aromatics of each oil were also tested, with ledum Co2 aromatic exhibiting very strong effects against *S. aureus* and a strong effect against *C. albicans.*

---

# TARRAGON
## (French Tarragon, Estragon)

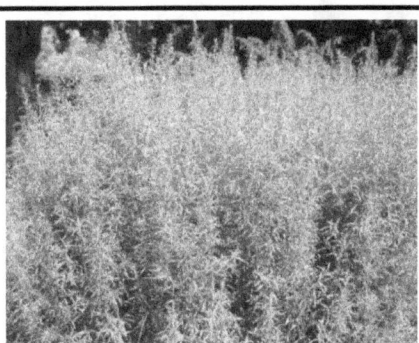

*Artemisia dracunculus* L., *A. dracunculoides* Pursh, *A. dracunculus* L. subsp. *glauca* (Pall. ex Willd.) H.M. Hall & Clem., *A. glauca* Pall. ex Willd., *Oligosporus dracunculus* (L.) Poljakov

**FAMILY:** Asteraceae (Compositae)

**NOTE:** Middle

**AROMA INTENSITY:** Medium

**AROMA:** Sweet, spicy, herbaceous, somewhat licorice-like

**COMMON EXTRACTION METHOD:** Steam distilled from the aerial parts

**POSSIBLE SUBSTITUTE OILS:** Ravensara (methyl chavicol CT), fennel (methyl chavicol CT), ginger, anise

**BLENDS WELL WITH:** Basil, carrot seed, cistus, fennel, galbanum, holy basil, lavender, lemon, lime, orange, pine, ravensara, rosewood

**SUBCELLULAR LOCALIZATION | EPIGENETIC INFLUENCE:** Currently unknown | Currently unknown

**RECOMMENDED DILUTION RANGE:** 1.5%–5%

**PRIMARY CONSTITUENTS:**[8826,8827,8828,8829]

*Methyl Chavicol (Estragole) CT*

| Methyl Chavicol (Estragole) | 71.3%–84.1% |
| --- | --- |
| (Z)-Beta-Ocimene | 1.3%–8.3% |
| (E)-Beta-Ocimene | 1.0%–7.8% |
| Carvacrol | 0.0%–7.7% |
| Limonene | 2.8%–5.4% |
| Herniarin | 0.0%–4.3% |
| Beta-Pinene | 0.0%–3.4% |
| Alpha-Copaene | 0.0%–2.2% |
| Methyl Eugenol | 0.0%–2.2% |

Note: Tarragon has a wide variety of chemotypes depending on growing conditions and locations. The French (predominantly methyl chavicol—estragole CT) and Russian (methyleugenol, elemicin, sabinene, and terpinene-4-ol CTs) varieties are considered the two most common types.[8830] A review of samples available commercially reveals that virtually all tarragon essential oil samples are the methyl chavicol CT. For this reason, the composition of this chemotype will be the only one reported and safety and caution information will also be related to the methyl chavicol chemotype.

**OTHER CONSTITUENTS:** *Methyl Chavicol (estragole) CT*—Alpha-pinene, bornyl acetate, eugenol, hexyl hexanoate, cis-davanone, anethole

**PREFERRED COMPOSITION FOR CLINICAL USE:**

| *Constituent* | |
|---|---|
| **Methyl Chavicol (Estragole)** | 70%–84% |
| **(Z)-Beta-Ocimene** | 3%–12% |
| **(E)-Beta-Ocimene** | 3%–10% |
| **Limonene** | 2%–8% |
| **Alpha-Pinene** | 0.1%–2% |
| **Methyl Eugenol** | < 1% |

**REPORTED THERAPEUTIC PROPERTIES: Antibacterial**, antioxidant, antiparasitic, **antirheumatic**, antiarthritic, analgesic, aids digestion, expels excess gas, circulatory stimulant, promotes normal menstruation, aids detoxification, improves appetite, cough, muscle aches, **relieves painful menstruation and PMS**, supports normal blood sugar levels, mentally stimulating, **uplifting**, stress management, antidepressant, combats fear

**CAUTIONS:**

■ Use with great caution for children under age six due to animal reports of liver cancer caused by methyl chavicol (estragole) content.[8831] The European Medicines Agency recommends exposure to estragole be limited in young children.

■ Avoid during pregnancy and lactation due to high methyl chavicol (estragole) content.[8832] Methyl chavicol (estragole) may cause genetic mutations and oxidative DNA damage.[8833,8834] The European Medicines Agency recommends exposure to estragole be limited in women who are pregnant or nursing.[8835]

■ Avoid oral use due to the carcinogenic (cancer-causing) potential of methyl chavicol (estragole).[8836,8837,8838,8839] The metabolite of estragole (1'-hydroxyestragole) is considered a stronger carcinogen and humans rapidly metabolize estragole to 1'-hydroxyestragole when ingested.[8840]

■ May interact with aspirin, blood pressure, antiplatelet, and anticoagulant medications, and increase the risk of bleeding among people with bleeding disorders based on methyl chavicol content.[8841,8842,8843,8844] Methyl chavicol is a more potent inhibitor of platelet aggregation than aspirin.[8845]

■ May interfere with enzymes responsible for metabolizing medications (NSAIDs, proton-pump inhibitors, acetaminophen, antiepileptics, immune modulators, blood-sugar medications, blood pressure medications, antidepressants, antipsychotics, diabetic medications, antihistamines, antibiotics, and anesthetics) due to methyl chavicol (estragole) content.[8846]

■ May interact with anticholinergic (drugs used for asthma, incontinence, gastrointestinal cramps, muscular spasms, depression, and sleep disorders) and cholinergic medications (drugs used to reduce urinary retention, diagnose myasthenia gravis, and for glaucoma) based on AChE inhibitory activity.[8847]

■ May interact with barbiturates (medications for anxiety and insomnia), antihistamines, benzodiazepines, tricyclic antidepressants, or other central nervous system depressant drugs.[8848]

■ May interact with antibiotics or antifungal drugs and possibly enhance or decrease their effectiveness based on estragole content.[8849,8850,8851]

**SELECTED EVIDENCE:**

☐ Tarragon oil relieves pain both centrally and peripherally using mechanisms other than interacting with opioid receptors.[8852]

☐ *In vitro* research suggests that tarragon essential oil possesses antimicrobial activity against *C. albicans, E. coli, B. subtilis,* and *S. aureus.*[8853,8854,8855]

☐ Tarragon oil inhibits acetylcholinesterase (AChE) activity, which may make it beneficial for neurodegenerative diseases.[8856] Inhibition of AChE prevents the break-down of acetylcholine, which is essential for memory and thinking. People with neurodegenerative diseases make less acetylcholine, and the diseases often break it down at a faster rate, leading to acetylcholine deficits.

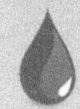

- Research suggests that tarragon oil (trans-anethole CT) reduces convulsions and experimental seizures in animals.[8857]

- Tarragon essential oil was insecticidal to the disease-carrying blowfly (*Calliphora vomitoria*), which spread pathogenic microorganisms.[8858]

- Human aryl hydrocarbon receptor (AhR: a gene that encodes a protein that helps regulate responses to planar aromatic hydrocarbons and significantly effects the immune activity in the gastrointestinal tract, regulates the circadian rhythm, helps regulate the cell cycle, and plays an important role in tissue development). Cumin, jasmine, vanilla, and bay leaf fully activate AhR; clove, dill, thyme, nutmeg, and oregano partially activate AhR; and tarragon, caraway, turmeric, lovage, fennel, spearmint, star anise, and anise inhibit the AhR activity.[8859]

- *In vitro* research demonstrated that tarragon essential oil inhibited *Salmonella enterica* serovar Typhimurium and *S. aureus*, exhibited anti-quorum-sensing properties, and disrupted biofilm formation at subminimum inhibitory concentrations.[8860]

- Researchers evaluated the composition and antibacterial activity of six medicinally important essential oils: tarragon CT p-allylanisole, dill CT alpha-phellandrene/para-cymene, lemon, orange, cinnamon bark, and ginger. Interestingly orange essential oil had the greatest antibacterial activity against *S. aureus* and *P. aeruginosa*.[8861] Cinnamon bark and tarragon were most active against *E. coli* and *K. pneumoniae*.

- Comparison of free tarragon essential oil versus nanoemulsion tarragon essential oil (NEO) showed that NEO displays better antioxidant activity in the DPPH assay because of a greater hydrogen donation capacity, but the ferric reducing potential was very similar.[8862] Furthermore, the NEO exhibited greater antibacterial activity against *S. aureus, Sh. dysenteriae,* and *L. monocytogenes.*

- *In vitro* research demonstrated that tarragon essential oil activates cellular antioxidant enzymes—catalase and superoxide dismutase—to increase cell survival in BV-2 microglial wild type and acyl-CoA oxidase (ACOX) type 1 deficient cells.[8863] ACOX cells were used as a cellular model of oxidative damage and 3-(4, 5-dimethylthiazol-2-yl)-2,5-diphenyltetrazolium bromide used to challenge the cells.

- Tarragon essential oil inhibited the lipolytic activity and type II secretion system P. psychrophile.[8864]

- Both a nanogel and nanoemulsion with tarragon essential oil were larvicidal to mosquitoes (*Anopheles stephensi*), inhibited *S. aureus*, and weakly inhibited *P. aeruginosa*.[8865]

- Tarragon, lemongrass (*C. citratus*), and lavender essential oil were each insecticidal against the bean weevil (*Acanthoscelides obtectus*).[8866]

---

# TEA TREE
## (Melaleuca)

*Melaleuca alternifolia* (Maiden & Betche) Cheel.,
*M. linariifolia* var. *alternifolia* Maiden & Betche

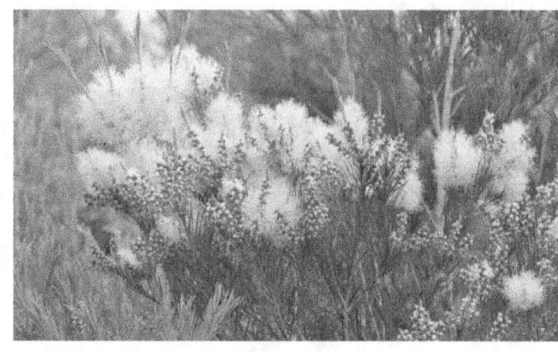

**FAMILY:** Myrtaceae
**NOTE:** Middle
**AROMA INTENSITY:** Medium
**AROMA:** Fresh, medicinal, earthy, herbaceous
**COMMON EXTRACTION METHOD:** Steam distilled from the leaves
**POSSIBLE SUBSTITUTE OILS:** Marjoram, equal parts oregano (terpinen-4-ol CT) and petitgrain (Mandarin)
**BLENDS WELL WITH:** Bergamot, cajeput, carrot seed, chamomile (German, Roman), cedarwood, clary sage, clove, cypress, eucalyptus, fennel, grapefruit, lavender, lemon, lime, myrrh, orange, patchouli, petitgrain, pine, ravensara, rosemary, sandalwood, tangerine, thyme
**SUBCELLULAR LOCALIZATION | EPIGENETIC INFLUENCE:** Endocytic Vesicles | Skeletal/Integumentary
**RECOMMENDED DILUTION RANGE:** 3%–50%; Neat for limited conditions

**PRIMARY CONSTITUENTS:**[8867,8868,8869,8870,8871 1313–1317]

| | |
|---|---|
| Terpinen-4-ol | 37.0%–46.9% |
| Gamma-Terpinene | 10.0%–28.0% |
| 1,8-Cineole | 0.1%–16.5%* |
| Para-Cymene | 0.5%–12.0% |
| Alpha-Terpinene | 7.9%–10.4% |

* Most studies report 1,8-cineole ranges of 3.0%–3.6%, and the ISO 4730 standard is ≤15.0%.

**OTHER CONSTITUENTS:** Alpha-pinene, d-limonene, terpinolene, delta-cadinene, aromadendrene, ledene, alpha-terpineol, viridiflorol, globulol

**PREFERRED COMPOSITION FOR CLINICAL USE:**

| *Constituent* | |
|---|---|
| **Terpinen-4-ol** | 35%–48% |
| **Gamma-Terpinene** | 10%–28% |
| **Alpha-Terpinene** | 5%–13% |
| **1,8-Cineole** | 0.1%–10% (Best 1%–5%) |
| **Alpha-Terpineol** | 2%–8% |
| **Alpha-Pinene** | 1%–6% |
| **Terpinolene** | 1%–5% |
| **Para-Cymene** | 0.5%–5% |
| **Delta-Cadinene** | 0.1%–5% |
| **Aromadendrene** | 0.1%–3% |
| **Ledene (Viridiflorene)** | 0.1–3% |

**REPORTED THERAPEUTIC PROPERTIES:** Analgesic (pain relief), **antibacterial**, sports injury recovery, anti-inflammatory, **anti-infectious**, **anticancer**, **antifungal**, improves nutrient absorption, **antiviral**, **antimicrobial**, expectorant, reduces hair loss, antiseptic, **helps reduce the appearance of blemishes**, helps burns heal, stimulates secretion of hormones, aids detoxification, **helps boils, blisters, and abscesses heal**, helps remove warts, relieves insect bites, helps hemorrhoids heal, **relieves inflammation of the gums**, stimulates immune function, **relieves diarrhea caused by pathogens**, protects against radiation damage and helps radiation burns heal, eases cough, relieves shock, builds confidence, reduces feelings of oppression

**CAUTIONS:**

■ May interact with antibiotics or antifungal drugs and increase or decrease their effectiveness due to terpinen-4-ol content, and based on research using the whole essential oil.[8872,8873,8874]

■ Several medical references and aromatherapy texts suggest oral administration of tea tree oil is contraindicated. Large doses, usually more than 10 mL (and up to 70 mL) in a single dose, have caused toxicity, and one case of toxicity was reported with an unidentified "small quantity" of tea tree oil in a 4-year old boy. Two cases of toxicity in adults are also reported in the literature. One adult ingested half a teacup of tea tree essential oil and the other half a teaspoon full (2.5 mL; which he had ingested previously without problems).[8875,8876] Both of these are extreme doses—one acute and one chronic—and far beyond reasonable oral use of tea tree essential oil. Most cases of toxicity have involved the ingestion of 10 to 25 mL of tea tree oil.[8877] Based on the amounts ingested, and the fact that ingestion of oils is not recommended for children under age 6, it is unlikely that tea tree oil will cause problems orally except in the case of very small children who ingest significant quantities.[8878,8879,8880,8881] Toxicity appears to occur at extreme doses; therefore it is best to limit tea tree essential oil consumption to 300 mg (about 6 drops based on an average of 45 mg per drop) daily, and avoid long-term use orally.

**SELECTED EVIDENCE:**

☐ A tea tree gel proved more effective at preventing dental plaque and inhibiting oral bacteria than Colgate Total in a small clinical trial of thirty-four volunteers.[8882] Another study concluded the tea tree oil gel improves overall gum health, but has little effect on plaque accumulation.[8883] Other research suggests tea tree essential oil supports oral health by inhibiting *P. gingivalis*, which is a periopathogen associated with

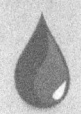

periodontitis (a serious gum infection that causes inflammation of the oral cavity and damages or destroys the soft tissue and bone that support the teeth).[8884] Tea tree essential oil reduces the amount of bacteria in the mouth and their production of volatile Sulphur compounds, which can help reduce bad breath.[8885]

☐ A tissue conditioner combined with a 20% solution of tea tree oil completely inhibited *C. albicans* and reduced inflammation in nine patients with dental stomatitis (an oral infection of *Candida* or thrush that causes inflammation of oral mucous membranes that primarily affects denture wearers or those who don't practice appropriate oral care).[8886] An *in vitro* study reported that a tissue conditioner with tea tree essential oil was superior to a tissue conditioner with 5% fluconazole against *C. albicans*, retaining its antifungal action through seven days, whereas the fluconazole formula completely lost its antifungal activity after 24 hours.[8887] These studies caused a review study to conclude that tea tree essential oil conditioners are a viable option for dental stomatitis.[8888]

☐ *In vitro* research concluded that tea tree oil significantly reduced influenza virus A/PR/8 (H1N1) replication if administered within two hours of the infection; however, it did not prevent attachment of the virus to healthy cells (adsorption).[8889,8890]

☐ Application of tea tree oil to the mouth with a cotton swab reduced oral candidiasis caused by drug-resistant *C. albicans* in mice.[8891]

☐ Tea tree oil may relieve psoriasis because of its ability to inhibit proinflammatory molecules, pathways, and cellular mechanisms involved in the cause of psoriasis.[8892]

☐ A small clinical study reported that topical application of tea tree oil significantly reduced histamine-induced allergic skin eruptions characterized by swelling, redness, and the appearance of an irregular wheal within ten minutes of application.[8893] Another study also concluded that tea tree oil prevents the histamine reaction involved in some skin eruptions.[8894]

☐ *In vitro* research discovered that tea tree oil causes transcriptional alteration of *S. aureus* and *Candida* sp. that damages the pathogens protein structure, membrane, and alters its membrane functions for destruction.[8895,8896] Another *in vitro* study observed that tea tree oil efficiently kills *S. aureus* during the stationary phase (when the size of the bacterial population remains relatively constant after a period of growth).[8897] *In vitro* studies concluded that tea tree oil inhibits *S. aureus* and *E. coli* by damaging their plasma membrane and emptying their cytoplasmic (the fluid that fills a cell) contents, and by inhibiting the pathogens ability to participate in cellular respiration (the process that cells use to release energy from food molecules for use by the living organism they inhabit).[8898,8899,8900] Tea tree essential oil significantly inhibited clinical and foodborne *Candida* strains (including antibiotic-resistant strains).[8901] Tea tree essential oil demonstrated antimicrobial activity against bacteria (*E. coli*, *S. aureus*) and *C. albicans*.[8902] Tea tree essential oil inhibits *B. cinerea* and *P. expansum*.[8903]

☐ A case report indicates that tea tree oil may help remove warts caused by the human papilloma virus (HPV) in children. When tea tree oil was applied on hand warts once daily for twelve days the wart was removed.[8904]

☐ Washing hands with soap and tea tree was as effective as washing hands with soap that contains triclosan (an antibacterial agent) in removing hand germs according to clinical research.[8905,8906] Rubbing alcohol with soap was more effective than tea tree and soap.

☐ A small clinical trial found that tea tree oil significantly increased the healing of wounds infected with *S. aureus*.[8907] Other research suggests that tea tree essential oil is a viable alternative antimicrobial agent for the treatment of chronic, infected wounds because of its ability to interact with multiple intracellular components to cause disruption of pathogen cellular function and kill pathogens.[8908]

☐ A case report describes the use of a combination of the essential oil of lemongrass, eucalyptus, tea tree, clove, thyme and BHT, triclosan, and undenatured alcohol to treat a chronic infection of the lower tibia (osteomyelitis) that was not responding to several courses of IV antibiotics. Amputation of the lower leg was being considered when a physician recommended the leg be opened up and the combination inserted directly into the bone (through a drilled hole, 1 mL per day for forty-eight hours). At three months, the wound and bone healed, and symptoms were resolved.[8909]

☐ *In vitro* research concluded that tea tree concentrate protects mice against Group A *Streptococcus pyogenes* infection (a bacteria that causes strep throat, scarlet fever, impetigo, cellulitis, and tonsillitis), and prevented skin damage caused by the bacteria called necrotizing fasciitis (commonly referred to as flesh-eating bacteria, which causes rapid destruction of the body's soft tissue).[8910]

- ☐ Tea tree oil reduces acne lesions in people with mild-to-moderate acne with good tolerability.[8911] One study found that tea tree oil was as effective as benzoyl peroxide with fewer side effects, but the results were achieved more slowly.[8912] A third study concluded that a 5% tea tree oil gel reduced both the number and severity of acne in thirty people.[8913]

- ☐ An *in vitro* study concluded that tea tree oil enhances the effectiveness of the antibiotic tobramycin against *E. coli* and *S. aureus*, which makes it a possible natural agent for the treatment of skin lesions, and infections of the conjunctiva (the membrane that covers the inside of the eyelids and the white part of the eyeball) and respiratory tract via inhalation.[8914]

- ☐ Topical application of tea tree oil is useful for the control of staphylococcal infections, including antibiotic-resistant infections according to in vitro research.[8915]

- ☐ *In vitro* research concluded that tea tree oil had broad antimicrobial activity against *M. hominis* (twenty-five vaginal, urethral, and cervical strains, and one reference strain), *M. pneumoniae* (one clinical and one reference strain), and *M. fermentans* (four vaginal strains and two reference strains).[8916] Another study found that tea tree essential oil inhibits *Aeromonas hydrophila* (a gram-negative bacterium that is present in fresh water environments and brackish water that can cause infections in animals and humans) in Silver catfish and reduced the anatomical alterations in the gills that the bacterium can cause.[8917]

- ☐ Topical application of a product containing 1% lavender and 10% tea tree oils worked better than the chemical alternative of pyrethrins and piperonyl butoxide, and as well as a suffocation product to eliminate head lice (louse).[8918] Another study concluded that the same combination of oils was slightly less effective than the suffocation method (44.4% versus 68.3%).[8919]

- ☐ A 1% solution of tea tree killed 100% of head lice in thirty minutes. When it was combined with nerolidol in a 1:2 ratio (tea tree 0.5% plus 1% nerolidol) the solution killed 100% of the head lice in thirty minutes and the louse eggs after five days.[8920]

- ☐ Topical application of a spray with tea tree and lavender oils twice daily for three months decreased unwanted, male-pattern hair growth in women (hirsutism).[8921]

- ☐ *In vitro* research reported that tea tree oil provides a sun protection factor (SPF) of 1.702.[8922]

- ☐ Animal research suggests that the topical application of 10% tea tree and DMSO solution triggers the accumulation of dendritic cells and T cells in tumors directly beneath the skin (subcutaneous), and kills tumor cells, resulting in rapid destruction of the tumor.[8923] Another study found that the combination of tea tree oil and DMSO significantly inhibited the growth of an aggressive subcutaneous tumor that was resistant to chemotherapy in mice.[8924]

- ☐ Tea tree oil prevents the growth of melanoma cells, interferes with the migration and invasion process of melanoma cells, and decreases drug resistance by melanoma cells *in vitro*.[8925,8926]

- ☐ *In vitro* research suggests that tea tree oil significantly prevents the spread of and kills aggressive mesothelioma and melanoma tumor cancer cells.[8927] The research concluded that tea tree oil triggers cell cycle arrest (a natural process in the cell cycle where the cell stops self-duplication and division).

- ☐ Topical application of a combination of lavender, geranium, tea tree, and peppermint oils improved the oral health of hospice patients with terminal cancer.[8928]

- ☐ *In vitro* research concluded that a 12.5% tea tree solution inhibits *C. albicans* and the microscopic lesions of candidiasis.[8929,8930] Another study found that tea tree oil prevents *C. albicans* from forming germ tubes, which are used by the spores to reproduce and spread.[8931]

- ☐ Tea tree oil, or terpinen-4-ol, reduces the production of the proinflammatory molecules IL-1β, IL-6, and IL-10 according to *in vitro* research.[8932,8933]

- ☐ A review of the dermatological uses of tea tree oil concluded that tea tree oil may be useful for acne, seborrheic dermatitis (a chronic inflammatory skin condition that causes scaly, red patches on the skin and dandruff), chronic gingivitis, wound healing, and skin cancer.[8934]

- ☐ Tea tree oil is a mild inhibitor of HSV-1, HSV-2, and *Pseudomonas* sp. *in vitro*.[8935,8936]

- ☐ Tea tree oil reduces inflammation by preventing oxidation and the release of proinflammatory molecules by cells without affecting the cells ability to release anti-inflammatory molecules.[8937,8938,8939]

- ☐ *In vitro* research concluded that tea tree oil effectively inhibited both drug-resistant and nonresistant fungal infections obtained from people with compromised immune system due to cancer treatment.[8940,8941] The study

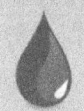

authors recommended that tea tree oil be considered for use as a natural remedy to prevent and treat oral fungal infections in immunocompromised people.

☐ Tea tree oil effectively inhibits a large range of oral bacteria, suggesting that tea tree oil may promote oral hygiene.[8942,8943] Another study found that a mouthwash with tea tree oil reduced plaque formation and gum inflammation.[8944]

☐ An *in vitro* study suggests that tea tree oil may be an effective treatment for inflammation of the ear canal (otitis externa) caused by allergies, infection, or swimmer's ear.[8945]

☐ Multiple components within tea tree oil, or tea tree oil itself, possess antifungal activity against a range of fungi (both drug-resistant and drug-susceptible) and dermatophytes according to *in vitro* studies.[8946,8947,8948,8949,8950,8951]

☐ *In vitro* research suggests that tea tree oil inhibits some Malassezia species (fungi that inhabit the skin and may cause or exacerbate many skin conditions like tinea versicolor, Pityrosporum folliculitis, and seborrheic dermatitis).[8952,8953]

☐ Tea tree oil was more effective than zinc oxide and clobetasone butyrate (a topical corticosteroid used to treat inflammatory skin conditions) in relieving allergic contact dermatitis.[8954]

☐ Tea tree oil inhibited three bacteria that are commonly associated with hospital-acquired infections *S. marcescens*, *P. aeruginosa*, and *K. pneumoniae*.[8955] Other research reported that tea tree essential oil inhibited gram-negative bacteria (multidrug-resistant *Acinetobacter baumannii*, extended-spectrum-beta-lactamase (ESBL) producing *Escherichia coli*, carbapenemase-producing *Klebsiella pneumoniae, and P. aeruginosa*), which are associated with healthcare-acquired infections.[8956] Remarkably, this study reported that tea tree essential oil demonstrated greater antimicrobial activity than oregano, thyme, and reunion basil. A study that tested the antimicrobial activity of tea tree essential oil against 193 strains of anaerobic bacteria isolated from people with oral and respiratory infections reported that tea tree essential oil was most effective against gram negative (*Veillonella* and *Porphyromonas* species) and gram-positive (*Anaerococcus, Ruminococcus, Eubacterium*, and *Eggerthella* species) bacteria.[8957] Tea tree essential oil also prevents *P. aeruginosa* biofilm formation.[8958]

☐ After sixteen weeks of treatment with a cream containing 5% tea tree oil and 2% butenafine hydrochloride (an antifungal drug used to treat athlete's foot and other fungal infections) 80% of people experienced complete remission of toenail onychomycosis (a fungal infection of the nail) without relapse.[8959] Another study reported similar findings that neat topical application of tea tree oil (twice daily for six months) was as effective as the standard treatment option of clotrimazole.[8960]

☐ Topical application of a 25% or 50% tea tree oil solution improved the symptoms of tinea pedis (commonly called athlete's foot, a fungal infection of the feet) in up to 72% of people.[8961]

☐ *In vitro* and clinical research suggests that tea tree oil inhibits methicillin-resistant *Staphylococcus aureus* (MRSA).[8962,8963,8964,8965,8966,8967]

☐ *In vitro* and animal research suggests that terpinen-4-ol and tea tree oil can control *C. albicans* vaginal infections, even infections by pathogens resistant to fluconazole and itraconazole (antifungal drugs used for the treatment of vaginal candidiasis).[8968,8969,8970] *In vitro* research shows that tea tree essential oil inhibits the growth and activity of *C. albicans* isolated from vaginal swabs better than the antifungal drug clotrimazole.[4232] Tea tree essential oil (in both liquid and vapor form) reduces fungal contamination in residential and occupational buildings better than industrial disinfectants (Carvicide, Virkon), 70% ethanol, and vinegar.[4907]

☐ A gel with tea tree oil, hyaluronic acid, and methyl-sulfonyl-methane effectively reduced hemorrhoid symptoms (anal pain, pain during a bowel movement, irritation, and inflammation) in eighteen people with hemorrhoids.[8971]

☐ Topical application of tea tree oil with organically bound iodine (twice daily) cleared molluscum contagiosum (a viral skin infection that causes round bumps on the skin) in 90% of children included in the study.[8972]

☐ A daily eyelid massage with a 5% solution of tea tree oil relieved ocular itching in all twenty-four patients receiving treatment, and completely cleared the itching in 67% of patients.[8973] ***Never place oils directly in your eye, and it is advised not to apply them on the eyelid to avoid damage to the eye.*** Contrarily, the standard treatment of chlortetracycline hydrochloride (a topical antibiotic ointment that reduces inflammation) provided little relief after four weeks of use.

- A review recommended the topical application of diluted tea tree, peppermint, or melissa oil three to four times daily for recurrent herpetic infections (cold sores and genital herpes).[8974]
- Topical application of neat tea tree oil prevented hypersensitive reactions to nickel in humans.[8975]
- A 5% tea tree oil solution effectively eliminated sarcoptes scabiei var hominis (commonly called scabies—a contagious skin infection caused by the mite burrowing into the skin and laying its eggs, which leads to intense itching and secondary infection).[8976,8977]
- Clinical research suggests that a shampoo with 5% tea tree oil is an effective treatment for dandruff.[8978]
- Swishing with an oral solution containing tea tree oil four times daily for two to four weeks cured or improved oropharyngeal thrush in 60% of people with AIDS.[8979]
- *In vitro* research concluded that tea tree exerts its antiseptic properties partially through activation of white blood cells, which help fight infections.[8980]
- An extract of tea tree oil composed predominantly of monoterpenes and sesquiterpenes modulated immune system activity by inhibiting NF-KB (a protein complex that is involved in cellular responses to stimuli, stress, and free radicals and plays a critical role in immune system activity) and IKB phosphorylation (a process that activates the IKB enzyme complex, which is a hallmark of chronic inflammatory diseases and cancer).[8981]
- Terpinen-4-ol triggers autophagic (the cell partially digests itself for programmed cell death) and apoptosis of leukemia cancer cells.[8982]
- Tea tree essential oil, and terpinen-4-ol, both decreased parasitic worm infections by *Haemonchus contortus* in gerbils and protected the liver against damage cause by the infection based on a reduction in alanine aminotransferase (ALT) and aspartate aminotransferase (AST) levels.[8983] Increased ALT and AAST levels are a blood test used to identify organ damage and severity.
- *In vitro* research demonstrated that low doses of marjoram, lemon, basil, clove, thyme, rosemary CT 1,8-cineole, and tea tree essential oils prevented the shortening of telomeres after exposure to hydrogen peroxide.[8984] The same research reported that vetiver, black pepper, eucalyptus (*E. globulus*), ginger, clove, and rosemary increased the length of already shortened telomeres. This activity suggests that these essential oils can help maintain the youth and health of cells, or turn back the clock on the cell to make it more youthful depending on the essential oil used. Interestingly, cinnamon and peppermint essential oil decreased the length of telomeres slightly.
- Several essential oils listed in order of efficacy killed the itch mite (*Sarcoptes scabiei*) that burrows into the skin and causes scabies during direct contact (clove > palmarosa > geranium > tea tree > lavender > manuka > petitgrain > eucalyptus > Japanese cedarwood) with the mites and when used as a fumigant (tea tree > clove > eucalyptus > lavender > palmarosa > geranium > Japanese cedarwood > petitgrain > manuka).[8985]
- Tea tree essential oil is insecticidal to the cereal weevil (*Sitophilus zeamais*).[4980] It also effectively repels and kills the cattle tick (*Rh. australis*).[8986,8987]
- *In vitro* research demonstrates that tea tree essential oil is antimicrobial to *P. insidiosum*.[8988]
- *In vitro* research demonstrates that tea tree essential oil is highly antifungal against clinical and foodborne *Candida* strains, including those resistant to antibiotics.[8989]
- A semi *in vivo* study determined that tea tree essential oil is 100 percent effective against *Acanthamoeba* trophozoites and cysts.[8990] Acanthamoeba keratitis is a sight-threatening parasitic disease that currently has no completely effective drug treatment.
- *In vitro* research demonstrated that black pepper (beta-pinene CT), lemon, and tea tree essential oil possess broad-spectrum antimicrobial activity. Interestingly, of the three essential oils tested, lemon (low limonene content—37.5%) was the most active against bacteria and tea tree was the most active against fungi. The EOs demonstrated synergistic antimicrobial activity when used in combination.[8991]
- Clinical research demonstrates that a tea tree essential oil (1.5%) mouthwash reduces gingivitis and mouth bleeding better than chlorhexidine, but was not quite as effective in controlling bacterial plaque.[8992]
- A study found that the antifungal activity of tea tree essential oil against *Botrytis cinerea* involves the following molecular mechanisms: destruction of cell membranes, decreasing the activity of three enzymes related to the tricarboxylic acid cycle, inhibiting glycolysis, and inducing mitochondrial dysfunction, thereby disrupting energy metabolism.[8993]

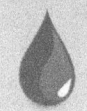

☐ Cystic echinococcosis is a disease that affects the liver, lungs, brain, and other organs spread by contact with animal feces contaminated with tapeworm eggs. Tea tree essential oil (20 mg mL-1 concentration) killed 90 percent of tapeworm cysts in five minutes, suggesting it may be a viable option for the treatment of cystic echinococcosis.[8994]

☐ Tea tree essential oil demonstrated anti-inflammatory activity by inducing the p38 MAPK and JNK pathways.[8995] The p38 MAPK and JNK pathways are key regulators of proinflammatory cytokines involved in inflammatory diseases, such as inflammatory bowel disease.

☐ Synthetic pediculicides (agents that kill lice) have suffered considerable loss of efficacy worldwide, creating a need for a natural alternative for head lice. Clove (diluted in coco or sunflower oil) demonstrated good activity against *Pediculus humanus* capitis *in vitro*, while bergamot, lavender, and tea tree showed lower activity.[8996]

☐ *In vitro* research demonstrates that tea tree possesses antioxidant activity (reduces DPPH, inhibits lipid peroxidation, and eliminates hydroxyl radicals) and strongly inhibits the growth of *E. coli, S. aureus, P. aeruginosa, P. italicum.* and *P. digitatum.*[8997]

☐ A tea tree and lemongrass (*C. flexuosus*) essential oil solution reduced *Candida* biofilms from dentures.[8998]

☐ Administration of tea tree beta-cyclodextrin powder in the lungs (inhalation) demonstrated activity against fungal and bacterial pneumonia in rats.[8999] Its antipneumonic effect mechanism involved blocking the recruitment of leucocytes and neutrophils, eliminating the microbes, downregulating proinflammatory cytokines (including tumor necrosis factor-α, IL-1β and IL-6), suppressing cyclooxygenase 2 expression, and further reducing lung injury in rats. Its efficacy was greater than fluconazole and similar to penicillin. The powder also showed good pulmonary delivery, high-stability, high lung deposition, and was portable, making it an excellent option for the treatment of fungal and bacterial pneumonia.

☐ A clinical study found that a toothpaste with tea tree essential oil and polish propolis improved overall oral hygiene as evidenced by significant reduction in the plaque index, modified sulcus bleeding index (a measurement of gingival/gum bleeding), and improvements in the simplified oral hygiene index and oral microbiome balance after seven and twenty-eight days.[9000]

☐ *S. aureus* biofilms exposed to tea tree oil significantly changed 304 genes (glycine, serine and threonine metabolism pathway, purine metabolism pathway, pyrimidine metabolism pathway and amino acid biosynthesis pathway were dramatically changed) in the biofilms.[9001]

☐ Tea tree essential oil demonstrated excellent (greater than chlorhexidine) antimicrobial activity against multibacterial dental biofilms.[9002]

☐ A nanoemulsion with tea tree essential oil and silver particles eradicated gram-negative and gram-positive bacteria, with synergistic activity observed against *E. coli* and an additive effect against *S. aureus*.[9003]

☐ Lavender, lemongrass (*C. citratus*), marjoram, peppermint, tea tree, and rosewood essential oils all exhibited significant activity against clinical isolates of multidrug-resistant *Burkholderia cepacia* complex (a group of bacteria commonly resistant to antibiotics that cause health problems in people with weakened immune systems and are known to cause healthcare-related infections).[9004]

☐ Tea tree essential oil exhibited repellent effects and pronounced contact mortality against the green peach aphid (*Myzus persicae*).[9005] Additionally, tea tree bound to proteins to disrupt the reproduction and development of the aphid.

☐ *In vitro* research revealed that tea tree essential oil has anti-quorum-sensing and antibiofilm activities at very low concentrations against *Chromobacterium violaceum* and *Pseudomonas aeruginosa*.[9006]

☐ Tea tree essential oil showed potent bactericidal activity against methicillin-sensitive *S. aureus, E. coli,* and clinical strains of methicillin-resistant *S. aureus*, extended-spectrum beta lactamases producer carbapenem-sensitive *K. pneumoniae*, carbapenem-resistant *K. pneumoniae, A. baumannii,* and *P. aeruginosa*.[9007] The oil also showed a high level of synergism with reference drugs (amikacin, oxacillin, cefazolin, vancomycin, rifampin, meropenem, and colistin).

☐ Tea tree essential oil exhibited antitumor activity against human and mouse breast cancer cells without cytotoxic effects on normal cells (fibroblasts or peripheral blood mononuclear) in laboratory research. The study authors concluded that tea tree oil has potential for "the development of new alternative therapies to treat topically locally advanced breast cancer."[9008]

☐ Tea tree essential oil exhibited insecticidal activity against the red flour beetle (*Tribolium confusum*) by targeting intracellular NAD+/NADH dehydrogenase, which blocked the mitochondrial respiratory chain.[9009]

☐ The biological properties of tea tree essential oil are often attributed to terpinen-4-ol content. One study found that its antimicrobial (MRSA, *C. glabrata*) and anti-infectious (HSV-1) properties resulted from a complex interaction among different constituents.[9010]

☐ Eucalyptus, clove, mint, oregano, savory, tea tree, and thyme essential oils each inhibited *Venturia inaequalis*, the fungus responsible for apple scab.[9011]

☐ Tea tree essential oil effectively killed malignant melanoma and squamous cell carcinoma skin cancer cells, indicating it may be a promising solution for the prevention and treatment of cancer in topical formulations.[9012] Tea tree oil triggered apoptosis, upregulated pro-apoptotic genes (P53 and BAX), downregulated antiapoptotic genes (BCL-2), and caused cell cycle arrest.

☐ Tea tree essential oil exhibited good antimicrobial activity against foodborne pathogens (*L. monocytogenes* and *E. coli*) when added to fresh cucumber juice.[9013]

☐ Toothbrushes can get heavily contaminated by bacteria, yeasts, viruses, and fungi that originates from the mouth or the environment where they are stored. A review concluded that tea tree essential oil may be an effective toothbrush cleaner. Immersion of a toothbrush in a 0.2% tea tree essential oil solution for twelve hours effectively reduced bacterial loads (71.9% reduction in *S. mutans*) on toothbrushes, making it a good option to sanitize toothbrushes.[9014]

☐ Incorporation of clove and tea tree essential oils into chitosan/essential oil wound dressings demonstrated good antimicrobial activity against common wound pathogens.[9015]

☐ Blepharitis is inflammation of the eyelid that occurs when tiny oil glands at the base of the eyelashes become inflamed. Chronic blepharitis is difficult to treat and causes irritated and red eyes. A double-blind, randomized clinical trial found that topical application of a gel with 3% tea tree oil reduced symptoms of chronic blepharitis.[9016] Another study found that a 7.5% tea tree eyelash shampoo reduced Demodex mite infection in people with demodectic blepharitis and relieved their eye symptoms.[9017]

☐ A chitosan-based topical formulation with either rosemary or tea tree essential oil or a combination of both demonstrated significant wound-healing benefits. The blend of both oils significantly increased wound contraction in comparison to the placebo and the individual essential oil groups and promoted complete re-epithelialization with active hair follicles.[9018]

☐ *In vitro* research demonstrated that tea tree essential oil enhanced the ability of polymorphonuclear leucocytes to kill *Candida krusei*—a yeast that primarily infects people with a compromised immune system and is naturally resistant to fluconazole.[9019]

☐ Both *in vitro* and *in vivo* research demonstrated that tea tree essential oil inhibits the dermatophyte *Trichophyton interdigitale*, with the capacity to reduce fungal burden and to preserve tissue architecture.[9020] Interestingly, the combination of tea tree oil and ketoconazole produced an antagonistic reaction and caused tissue damage.

☐ Tea tree and rosemary essential oil exhibited good antibacterial activity against multidrug-resistant bacteria (*Staphylococcus aureus*, *S. epidermidis*, and *Cutibacterium acnes*) associated with acne.[9021]

☐ Thyme CT thymol, garlic, tea tree, cajeput, may chang, lemongrass (*C. citratus*), and verbena CT citral exhibited fungistatic activity (100 percent) against *F. culmorum* and *F. graminearum*, and all but garlic (89.4%) were 100 percent fungistatic against *F. avenaceum* and *F. oxysporum*.[9022]

☐ *Helicobacter pylori* is a bacterium that lives in the digestive tract that can cause sores and ulcers in the lining of the stomach or upper part of the small intestine. Thyme, lemongrass, Virginia cedarwood, and melissa essential oils were the most active of 26 commercial essential oils examined against *H. pylori*.[9023] Oregano, tea tree, pine, and silver fir were also bactericidal.

☐ Use of a tea tree mouthwash for four weeks reduced plaque, gingivitis, and *S. mutans* in the oral cavity in children with a similar efficacy to chlorhexidine.[9024]

☐ Tea tree and thyme CT geraniol essential oils were active against sixteen multidrug-resistant *P. aeruginosa* strains isolated from infected hip implants.[9025] Tea tree was more effective than thyme.

☐ Tea tree essential oil demonstrated insecticidal activity against stable fly (*Stomoxys calcitrans*) adults at a 5% concentration.[9026]

☐ Both terpinen-4-ol and tea tree essential oil interfered with biofilm formation by *Candida albicans* strains (genotypes A and B), making it a promising natural solution for oral candidiasis.[9027]

☐ Rosemary and tea tree essential oils significantly inhibited the formation of biofilms and destroyed mature biofilms produced by *S. aureus* and *E. coli*.[9028] Tea tree was more active than rosemary.

☐ Tea tree and thyme CT linalool essential oils were active against seven antibiotic-resistant and antibiotic-sensitive bacteria that cause urinary tract infections (*E. coli*, *K. pneumoniae*, *En. cloacae*, *P. mirabilis*, *Ps. aeruginosa*, *En. faecalis*, *S. saprophyticus*). A synergistic activity of the two oils was observed when they were combined. In addition, the oils increased the activity of fosfomycin and pivmecillinam, but not nitrofurantoin, against *E. coli*.

☐ Application of distilled tangerine and tea tree essential oils deterred fruit flies (*Drosophila suzukii*) from infesting small fruits (strawberries, cherries, and blueberries) without negatively impacting their taste.[9029]

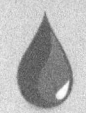

- A microemulsion (consisting of 31.05% Kolliphor HS 15, 3.45% Span 80, 34.5% isopropyl myristate, and 31% distilled water) containing 3.45% tea tree oil demonstrated good antibacterial activity and contributed to the wound healing process in mice when applied topically once per day.[9030]

- Tea tree essential oil inhibited two fungi (*Trichophyton rubrum* and *T. mentagrophytes*) responsible for onychomycosis (a fungal infection of the nail that manifests as white or yellow nail discoloration, thickening of the nail, and nail separation from the nail bed).[9031] The oil inhibited *T. rubrum* growth at 0.04% and *T. mentagrophytes* at 0.02%, with complete inhibition of *T. mentagrophytes* at 0.07%.

- *In vitro* research confirmed that tea tree essential oil effectively inhibits *S. mutans* and reduced bacterial aggregation, biofilm formation, and biofilm thickness, suggesting it may help prevent dental caries (cavities).[9032]

- Onychomycosis is a fungal infection of the nails that is treated with oral and topical medications with little success. A Pickering nanoemulsion with tea tree essential oil and tioconazole exhibited significant synergistic activity against *Candida albicans* and *Trichophyton rubrum*, suggesting that the combination may be useful as a topical solution for onychomycosis.[9033]

- A 2% concentration of tea tree essential oil displayed antimicrobial activity against *Cutibacterium acnes* (formerly *Propionibacterium acnes*), suggesting it may be helpful for acne.[9034]

- Sweet orange, citronella (*C. nardus*), and tea tree essential oils were the most effective nematocidal agents against the southern root-nematode (*Meloidogyne incognita*) of eight essential oils tested.[9035]

- *Trichophyton rubrum* accounts for about 70 percent of ringworm—a fungal infection of the skin that causes a red, itchy, scaly, circular rash—cases, for which imidazoles (ketoconazole) and triazoles (itraconazole) are the primary treatment options. Unfortunately, *T. rubrum* can develop resistance to azole medications resulting in failure to clear the infection and chronic infections. Tea tree essential oil was fungicidal to *T. rubrum* and created a synergistic effect when used in combination with azoles.[9036]

- A prospective triple-blinded randomized clinical trial evaluated the benefits of an eye shampoo containing tea tree oil on dry eyes following cataract surgery. Scrubbing the eyelid with the shampoo decreased *Demodex* numbers and improved other aspects of dry eyes after cataract surgery.[9037]

- Researchers compared four soaps for handwashing among healthcare workers: tea tree oil, triclosan, chlorhexidine, and a reference soap. What the researchers found was that the triclosan soap was the most effective for reducing *E. coli* colony-forming units (but it isn't ideal because it is irritating to the skin and contributes to superbugs) followed by the tea tree soap, chlorhexidine, and reference soap.[9038] However, the test subjects enjoyed the aroma of the tea tree soap and remarked that it didn't dry their hands.

- May chang, Virginia cedarwood, spearmint, and tea tree essential oils each demonstrated contact toxicity against third instar larvae of the cotton leafworm (*Alabama argillacea*).[9039] Each oil changed the histochemistry of the testicles, while tea tree, Virginia cedarwood, and spearmint altered morphology. In addition, the histochemistry of the ovarioles was altered by Virginia cedarwood, tea tree, and may chang.

- After identifying a high prevalence of bacteria (*S. aureus* and *Enterobacteriaceae* spp.) on keyboards in an intensive care unit (ICU), researchers found that a 3M Tegaderm film with tea tree oil over the keyboard significantly reduced bacterial presence.[9040]

- Tea tree essential oil strongly inhibited *S. aureus, E. faecalis, P, aeruginosa, K, pneumoniae, E. coli*, and *C. albicans*.[9041]

- Hand hygiene is vital in preventing healthcare-associated infections in medical centers and to reduce the spread of infectious illnesses in community settings. A randomized controlled clinical trial compared the effectiveness of a tea tree oil disinfectant handwash (mixed in a ratio of 2:2:1:15 of tea tree oil, solubilizer, glycerin, and sterile distilled water) with an alcohol-based hand sanitizer gel (83% ethanol), a foam-type hand sanitizer containing benzalkonium chloride, and no hand sanitizing.[9042] The study proved that the tea tree handwash was effective in reducing bacterial count on the hands and could be used to reduce the spread of infections in healthcare and community settings. No significant difference was observed for skin moistness, dryness, or exfoliation.

- Diabetic foot ulcers are a common complication of poorly managed diabetes. Ulcers form when skin tissue breaks down exposing the layers underneath. A clinical study compared the impact of honey and a natural ointment with honey and tea tree oil (TTO) on the healing of diabetic foot ulcers.[9043] Twenty-seven participants were divided into two groups: thirteen in the control group (honey only) and fourteen in the intervention group (honey-TTO ointment). Wounds were cleansed with antiseptic soap and debrided and then the honey or honey-TTO ointment applied with absorbent dressing followed by an occlusive dressing. Wound care was performed every two days and wound healing evaluated on days one, seven, and fourteen. Both honey and honey-TTO ointment significantly improved wound healing, with the honey-TTO ointment being the most effective.

- Among four essential oils tested (rosemary CT 1,8-cineole, tea tree, *Eucalyptus obliqua*, and lavender with carbitol as the main constituent), tea tree essential oil exhibited the strongest antimicrobial activity against pathogenic bacteria (*Escherichia coli*, *Staphylococcus aureus*, *Salmonella typhi*, and *Citrobacter koseri*).[9044] Tea tree oil inhibited *E. coli* (two strains), *S. typhi*, and *C. koseri*; rosemary and lavender inhibited *S. aureus* (two strains); and *Eucalyptus obliqua* inhibited *S. aureus* (two strains) and *S. typhi*.

- Tea tree and black pepper essential oils were insecticidal to the green peach aphid (*Myzus persicae*), producing 80 percent mortality.[9045] A combination of black pepper, tea tree, and rosemary essential oils produced a synergistic insecticidal effect that caused 98.33 percent mortality.

- *In vitro* testing of sixty-one essential oils against melanoma and lung cancer cells found that tea tree, pine, lavender, grapefruit, and cypress were the most effective in reducing tumor cell viability/proliferation, without harming normal healthy cells (fibroblasts).[9046] Further evaluation of the oils in a preclinical melanoma model found that topical application of tea tree oil—and isolated terpinen-4-ol—reduced melanoma tumors by recruiting immune cells to the site and reducing the growth of melanoma on the skin. Combining tea tree oil with dabrafenib and/or trametinib synergistically enhanced the activity of the anticancer drugs.

- Periodontitis is a type of gum disease involving a serious gum infection that damages the soft tissue, and without proper treatment, can also damage bone that supports the teeth. Periodontitis is categorized by stage, from Stage 1 to Stage 4, with Stage 4 being the worst. A randomized, controlled clinical trial with thirty subjects with Stage 2 periodontitis evaluated the benefits of tea tree oil gel along with scaling and toot planning (the standard treatment for periodontitis).[9047] Intrapocket application of the 5% tea tree oil gel improved all clinical and biochemical parameters, proving it to be an effective adjunctive treatment in Stage 2 periodontitis.

- Fungal infection of the nails (onychomycosis) is a common cause of nail alteration, but the available drugs are associated with significant side effects. Tea tree essential oil maintained inhibition of two fungi associated with onychomycosis at low concentrations: *Trichophyton rubrum* (0.04%) and *Trichophyton mentagrophytes* (0.02%; complete inhibition 0.07%).[9048]

- A toothpaste containing tea tree essential oil and propolis extract was evaluated in fifty subjects using removable acrylic partial dentures. The effects of the toothpaste on microflora and overall oral health (plaque, gum bleeding, oral hygiene) was evaluated during the study. Significant improvements in all evaluated indexes were observed after seven and twenty-eight days of using the toothpaste, including stabilization of oral microflora.[9049]

- Tea tree essential oil inhibited *E. faecalis* and its formation of biofilms.[9050] The researchers concluded it has the potential to be further developed into an antibacterial agent because it destroys cell membrane, inhibits biofilm formation, and eliminates mature formed biofilms.

- The comparison of 0.2% chlorhexidine, 2% lemongrass essential oil, and 2% tea tree essential oil mouth rinse found that tea tree oil mouth rinse gives a greater increase in salivary pH, suggesting it may be helpful for oral health and to produce an environment unfavorable to bacterial growth.[9051]

- Tungiasis is an inflammatory skin disease characterized by pain, itching, and lesions that occurs when female sand fleas embed themselves into the skin. Itching and scratching of the lesions can promote bacterial superinfection and abscesses. Long-term, the infection may result in deformation and loss of nails, tissue necrosis, disfigurement, disability, and changes in the way a person walks. An ongoing randomized controlled trial of school children aged 6 to 15 years is evaluating the effectiveness of 5% tea tree oil gel (with 0.05% potassium permanganate) in the treatment of tungiasis.[9052] The gel is applied twice daily for three days and observation of effects continued for ten days. If the tea tree oil gel proves effective, the trial will provide compelling evidence for the use of tea tree oil gel as a simple, affordable, and effective treatment for tungiasis.

- A laboratory study found that tea tree essential oil containing product (*Melaleuca alternifolia* concentrate) triggered the apoptotic pathway in prostate and breast cancer cells.[9053] Follow up in mice showed that injecting the concentrate significantly suppressed tumor progression with greater levels of tumor infiltrating neutrophils exhibiting anticancer cytotoxic activity in mice with spontaneously arising breast cancer.

- Thyme, tea tree, tropical basil, rosemary CT 1,8-cineole, eucalyptus, corn mint, and lavender essential oil each inhibited biofilm-forming *S. aureus*, with thyme and rosemary being the most active in liquid phase.[9054] Thyme was the most active in vapor phase, with varying degrees of inhibition observed depending on the strain of *S. aureus* with tea tree, rosemary, eucalyptus, corn mint, and lavender. Tea tree and lavender oils displayed the weakest activity in the vapor phase.

- *Pseudomonas aeruginosa* is an opportunistic pathogen that commonly infects the lungs of people with cystic

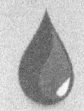

fibrosis, accelerating declines in lung function. Unfortunately, *P. aeruginosa* is significantly resistant to antibiotics and undergoes adaptive mutations during chronic infections, making it difficult for the innate immune system to eradicate. Laboratory research found that tea tree essential oil inhibits biofilm formation by multidrug-resistant *P. aeruginosa* isolated from people with cystic fibrosis.[9055] The researchers concluded that tea tree oil is "a promising candidate as a potential therapeutic agent" for cystic fibrosis *P. aeruginosa* infections.

- ☐ Tea tree essential oil inhibited *Fusarium* spp., *Alternaria* spp., *B. cereus, B. subtilis, A. niger, P. putida, C. albicans, A. flavus,* and *E. coli.*[9056]

- ☐ A double-blind randomized clinical trial compared the effectiveness of swabs containing tea tree and chamomile essential oils against a baby shampoo for seborrheic blepharitis.[9057] The subjects were treated for eight weeks followed by four weeks of no treatment and changes in symptoms, demodex count, and other index measures evaluated to determine efficacy. Overall, the subjects using swabs showed greater relief of symptoms and index improvements after treatment.

- ☐ Keyboards in the intensive care unit coated with a film containing tea tree essential oil significantly reduced pathogen presence on the keyboards.[9058]

- ☐ Tungiasis is a neglected tropical disease most prevalent in Latin America, the Caribbean, and sub-Saharan Africa without a standard drug treatment. It occurs when sand fleas (*Tunga penetrans*) burrow into a person's skin—usually the feet—causing immense pain. Because there is no standard treatment, affected people extract the fleas with non-sterile instruments increasing the risk of secondary infections. A review concluded that tea tree oil has a potential role to manage tungiasis because of its antiparasitic and antiseptic properties and extensive safety and efficacy data.[9059]

- ☐ Adding tea tree essential oil to gel formulations of ketoconazole improved the penetration and retention of ketoconazole through artificial skin membrane, particularly the hydrogel formulation.[9060]

- ☐ Repeated oral administration of a tea tree nanoemulsion for twenty-eight days in mice revealed no significant adverse effects on growth, behavior, blood, biochemistry, or tissues.[9061] The study suggests that nano-tea tree oil can be considered a potential oral antimicrobial agent.

- ☐ Skin barrier integrity is not only important for skin health but also acts as a protective mechanism to limit entry into the body by various substances and microbes. The skin barrier function provided by the *stratum corneum* (SC) is maintained by a delicate balance between water, ions, keratin, natural moisturizing factor, intracellular lipids, skin surface lipids, and the cutaneous microbiome. Substances that possess anti-inflammatory, antimicrobial, and antioxidant activity and trigger adaptive responses in skin characteristics support healthy skin barrier function and improve the appearance of the skin. Preclinical and clinical research evaluated the activity of tea tree, tangerine, eucalyptus (*E. globulus*), and lavender essential oil skin barrier function and characteristics. Two formulas—one with equal parts of tangerine, eucalyptus, and lavender, and one with equal parts of tea tree, tangerine, eucalyptus, and lavender—diluted to 2% in emulsions stabilized with polymers of natural origin were created to investigate their skin benefits. Tangerine showed the deepest penetration through the skin (35 percent of the oil made it across the SC) in pig ear, while the rest of the oils and combinations of the oils penetrated less than tangerine but were absorbed at higher than 5 percent through the viable epidermis. In the clinical study, the four essential oil emulsion hydrated the skin better and improved skin barrier function better than the three essential oil emulsion, showing that tea tree oil has a synergistic activity with the other oils. The four-oil group also experienced improvements in skin characteristics compared to a control group and the three-oil emulsion group. The totality of the research suggests that a combination of tea tree, tangerine, eucalyptus, and lavender in an emulsion can improve overall skin barrier function and skin characteristics.[9062]

- ☐ Crotamiton is a prescription lotion-based drug used to treat scabies—a noncontagious skin infestation by *Sarcoptes scabiei* mites—and general itching. However, it is not very bioavailable and has side effects that limit its use. To overcome these issues, researchers developed a microemulsion hydrogel formula containing tea tree essential oil and crotamiton. The gel was nonirritant and penetrated and distributed better in the skin of mice, suggesting that it would be more effective and safer in the treatment of scabies.[9063]

- ☐ Meibomian gland dysfunction (MGD) is a common condition characterized by insufficient oil (meibum) or poor-quality oil production from the meibomian glands in the eyelids. These glands can become clogged resulting in dry eyes and blepharitis (inflammation, redness, scaling, and crusting of the eyelid). A double-masked randomized clinical trial compared the effectiveness of a tea tree oil shampoo (1% tea tree) with regular eyelid shampoo for the treatment of MGD. The forty-three subjects were randomly assigned to gently apply either tea tree oil shampoo or standard eyelid shampoo for sixty to ninety seconds, then rinse thoroughly, each day for three months. At the end of the study, the tea tree oil shampoo was found to be more effective in controlling symptoms of MGD, but it also resulted in more ocular surface irritation.[9064]

- Glioblastoma multiforme (GBM) is the most common primary malignant brain tumor in humans, exhibiting aggressive proliferation and invasion of healthy brain tissue. Standard treatment involves surgical removal of the tumor followed by radiotherapy and chemotherapy with temozolomide, but despite this, 95 percent of people with GBM die within five years of diagnosis. Tea tree essential oil showed inhibited GBM proliferation and displayed synergistic activity with temozolomide in cell culture and rodents.[9065]

- Tea tree essential oil exhibited weak antioxidant activity but was active against a series of gram-positive and gram-negative bacteria and yeasts, with the best antimicrobial activity observed against *E. faecalis* and *C. albicans*.[9066] It also demonstrated antibiofilm activity against *P. fluorescens* and *S. enterica*.

- Vitamin C (ascorbate) is a vital antioxidant in the brain where it acts as a key signaling molecule and regulator of oxidative stress. Under certain circumstances ascorbate produces hydroxyl radicals and hydrogen peroxide. A laboratory study evaluated how essential oils either enhance (pro-oxidant) or suppress (antioxidant) the production of hydrogen peroxide in the brain.[9067] The researchers reported that lavender, tea tree, and rosemary essential oil suppress the production of hydrogen peroxide by brain ascorbate and produce an overall antioxidant effect, which can reduce anxiety. Isolated beta-pinene was also effective. On the contrary, juniper berry, elecampane, and alpha-pinene had pro-oxidant effects that may be useful for antimicrobial, anti-inflammatory, and anticancer effects.

- A study evaluated the antimicrobial activity of multiple essential oils (cinnamon bark, lavender, tea tree, lemon, oregano CT carvacrol, peppermint, bay laurel and eucalyptus—*E. globulus*) against human pathogens (*S. pyogenes, S. aureus, S. agalactiae*).[9068] Oregano, cinnamon, and tea tree exhibited the strongest antibacterial activity and combinations of tea tree/lavender and cinnamon/lavender displayed synergistic activity.

- Investigation of the antifungal and antivirulence activity of basil CT linalool, cinnamon bark, clove, tea tree, oregano CT carvacrol, and thyme CT thymol essential oils (EOs) on five *Candida* species (*C. albicans, C. auris, C. krusei, C. parapsilosis*, and *C. guillermondii*) revealed that clove and cinnamon inhibited all fungal species tested; cinnamon, oregano, and thyme inhibited biofilm formation of *C. albicans, C. guilliermondii*, and *C. parapsilosis*; and each oil except tea tree downregulated virulence genes in *C. albicans*.[9069] In addition, thyme synergized the activity of fluconazole against all tested *Candida* species.

- Pythiosis is a skin condition caused by invasion of *Pythium insidiosum* (a fungus-like oomycete) that most commonly affects dogs, horses, and humans. Intralesional administration of tea tree nanoemulsion reduced lesions in rabbits but topical application did not.[9070] The nanoemulsion was nontoxic to the skin.

- Demodex mites are associated with several skin disorders. They typically live on the skin or hair follicles without causing problems, but *Demodex folliculorum* mites have the potential to trigger an inflammatory response in people with rosacea. Researchers evaluated the effects of tea tree essential oil in skin biopsy samples taken from people with rosacea and *D. folliculorum* mites and compared its effectiveness against permethrin and a negative control group (no treatment).[9071] Tea tree oil (25%) had comparable efficacy to permethrin and reduced mite survival times significantly when compared to the negative control group.

- Researchers evaluated the activity of bergamot, tea tree, star anise, and eucalyptus (*E. globulus*) against influenza virus type A (H1N1) while in vapor phase.[9072] Both bergamot and tea tree essential oils strongly reduced the cytopathic (structural changes to cells after infection) of H1N1 without being toxic to healthy cells. Eucalyptus was moderately effective without being toxic to healthy cells, whereas star anise was inactive. Further evaluation of the mechanism that these essential oils reduced H1N1 infectivity found that the oils interfere with the lipid bilayer of the viral envelope triggering decomposition of membranes. This research suggests that diffusing essential oils, which creates a vapor, may help to reduce viral load and their potential to infect humans.

- Laboratory research demonstrated that tea tree essential oil is virucidal against feline coronavirus (FCoVII) and the human coronavirus OC43 (HCoV-OC43), which are used as surrogates for SARS-CoV-2 in research.[9073] The research suggests that tea tree oil may be a natural disinfectant for SARS-CoV-2.

- Both rosemary and tea tree essential oil displayed significant antibiofilm effectiveness against *P. aeruginosa* in liquid and vapor forms.[9074]

- A tea tree nanoemulsion potentiated the activity of antibiotics against multidrug-resistant *E. coli* and showed efficacy in the *Galleria mellonella* infection model and mouse peritonitis model.[9075]

- Tea tree essential oil inhibited *E. faecalis, S. mutans*, and *P. gingivalis*.[9076]

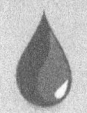

- Adapalene is a topical retinoid primarily used to treat mild to moderate acne and other skin conditions. A twelve-week clinical study evaluated the effects of a tea tree essential oil nanogel with adapalene (TTNE+ADA) compared to adapalene (ADA) alone.[9077] A total of one hundred subjects were randomized to groups that applied TTNE+ADA or ADA once daily at night. The subject's acne was evaluated at four, eight, and twelve weeks. Significantly better reduction in total, inflammatory, and noninflammatory acne lesions was achieved with TTNE+ADA than ADA alone and safety was similar in both groups.

- Tea tree and manuka essential oils inhibited *S. aureus* and *P. aeruginosa*.[9078]

- The vapor phase of tea tree essential oil exhibited promising activity against *Candida* biofilm formation and against existing biofilms.[9079]

- A laboratory model of intestinal integrity assessed the benefits of tea tree, ginger, and thyme essential oils. Each oil showed antioxidant benefits and the reduction of reactive oxygen species (ROS)—elevated ROS can increase inflammation and damage intestinal tissues leading to poor intestinal integrity.[9080] In addition, ginger and thyme oils improved barrier integrity and reduced levels of claudin 2 and claudin 15 (key biomarkers for leaky gut). The findings suggest that thyme and ginger essential oil could support gut barrier function and intestinal integrity.

- Topical application of a nanolipogel containing tea tree essential oil daily for seven days significantly accelerated the healing of second-degree burns in rats.[9081]

- Hydrogels containing tea tree essential oil displayed good antioxidant activity in the OH and DPPH assays, reduced intracellular reactive oxygen species (ROS), protected cells against injury and death caused by ROS, and inhibited *S. aureus* and *E. coli* (better effects against *S. aureus*).[9082] Based on the laboratory findings the tea tree hydrogel was evaluated in an anal fistula model and showed the ability to improve wound healing time.

- Due to an increased prevalence of scabies and their growing resistance to permethrin and ivermectin, researchers are seeking new solutions to manage scabies cases. Comparison of permethrin, 5% tea tree oil, and 25% tea tree oil to control found that tea tree oil was more effective in killing live scabies mites collected from people.[9083] The 25% tea tree oil was the most effective and far superior to permethrin, killing mites in nearly one-third the time of permethrin.

- Free tea tree and lemon essential oil displayed higher acaricidal activity against phenotypically resistant cattle ticks (*Rhipicephalus annulatus*) when compared to their nanoemulsions.[9084] The combination of the oils was also highly larvicidal, while lemon oil exhibited the most effective ovicidal effects.

- Thyme CT thymol, cinnamon bark, and tea tree essential oils each inhibited *E. coli* strains isolated from the drinking water of grazing animals in Italy.[9085] Thyme and cinnamon oils showed greater activity than antibiotics used in veterinary and human medicine (repen, macramid, baytril, augmentin, bimixin).

- Tea tree, thyme CT thymol, and peppermint essential oil demonstrated the ability to enhance human polymorphonuclear leukocytes' capacity to kill *C. albicans* and *C. krusei* even at concentrations lower than the oils' ability to inhibit the yeasts.[9086] Their activity was comparable or superior to the comparative drug (anidulafungin).

- Tea tree essential oil nanoliposomes improved the antibacterial activity of the oil against *E. coli* when compared to the free oil *in vitro*.[9087] Further evaluation in chickens found that the tea tree nanoliposome remarkably reduced colibacillosis caused by *E. coli* infection.

- Eucalyptus (*E. globulus*) and tea tree essential oil demonstrated activity against mature biofilms and biofilms in the process of formation, produced by strains belonging to three main categories of antibiotic resistant bacteria (Vancomycin-resistant enterococci, MRSA, and broad-spectrum β-lactamase-producing E. coli), with the greatest activity against biofilm in formation.[9088]

- The microencapsulation of tea tree essential oil in chitosan-sodium alginate microspheres improved its antioxidant activity in the DPPH and ABTS assays and inhibited bacterial pathogens while maintaining negligible cytotoxicity to healthy cells.[9089] Altogether, the research suggests this product could be used as a wound dressing.

- Topical application of 10% tea tree essential oil in glycerin twice daily suppressed local inflammation and cell death and increased collagen synthesis in a rat pressure ulcer model better than glycerin alone.[9090]

- Topical application of tea tree essential oil to the nipples on the third, seventh, and tenth days postpartum, significantly reduced nipple crack formation and pain.[9091]

# TEXAS CEDARWOOD
## (Alligator Juniper, Ashe's Juniper, Mountain Cedar)

*Juniperus deppeana* Steud., *J. deppeana* Steud. var. *pachyphlaea* (Torr.) Martinez, *J. deppeana* Steud. var. *sperryi* Correll, *J. mexicana* Schltdl. & Cham., *J. pachyderma* Sitgr., *J. ashei* Buckholz

**FAMILY:** Cupressaceae (Coniferae)
**NOTE:** Base
**AROMA INTENSITY:** Medium
**AROMA:** Woody, sweet, rich, balsamic
**COMMON EXTRACTION METHOD:** Steam distilled from the wood (trunk and limbs); often rectified or fractionated to reduce crystallization
**POSSIBLE SUBSTITUTE OILS:** Virginia cedarwood, atlas cedarwood, Himalayan cedarwood, sandalwood
**BLENDS WELL WITH:** Balsam fir, bay laurel, bergamot, blue cypress, blue spruce, carrot seed, cinnamon, copaiba, cypress, myrtle, jasmine, juniper, lemon, neroli, palmarosa, patchouli, petitgrain, pine, rose, rosemary, ravensara, sandalwood, Spanish sage, silver fir, spruce, thyme, tsuga, vetiver, white fir
**SUBCELLULAR LOCALIZATION | EPIGENETIC INFLUENCE:** Currently unknown | Currently unknown
**RECOMMENDED DILUTION RANGE:** 5%–Neat

**PRIMARY CONSTITUENTS:**[9092,9093,9094]

| | |
|---|---|
| Thujopsene | 25.0%–60.4% |
| Alpha-Cedrene | 1.8%–30.7% |
| Cedrol | 12.2%–29.5% |
| Beta-Cedrene | 0.1%–5.5% |

**OTHER CONSTITUENTS:** Alpha-copaene, cuparene, widdrol, alpha-chamigrene, alpha-selinene, alpha-acorneol, beta-himachalene, gamma-himachalene, beta-chamigrene, himachala-2,4-diene, alpha-acoradiene, beta-acoradiene

**PREFERRED COMPOSITION FOR CLINICAL USE:**

| Constituent | Co2 (SFE) | Distilled |
|---|---|---|
| **Thujopsene** | 25%–45% | 25%–40% |
| **Cedrol** | 25%–45% | 20%–35% |
| **Widdrol** | 2%–7% | 2%–7% |
| **Beta-Cedrene** | 0.5%–7% | 2%–7% |
| **Alpha-Cedrene** | 0.1%–7% | 10%–25% |
| **Cuparene** | – | 0.1%–5% |

**REPORTED THERAPEUTIC PROPERTIES:** Antibacterial, antifungal, analgesic, anti-inflammatory, antiarthritic, antirheumatic, eases cough, expels excess mucus, combats acne, **reduces the appearance of blemishes**, soothes chronic skin conditions, nourishes the hair, relieves hemorrhoids, insect repellent, **encourages restful sleep**, stress management, relieves anxiety, **relaxing/calming**, promotes clarity of thought, balances emotions, reduces fear

**CAUTIONS:**
■ May weakly interfere with the enzymes responsible for metabolizing medications (NSAIDs, proton-pump inhibitors, acetaminophen, antiepileptics, immune modulators, blood-sugar medications, blood pressure medications, antidepressants, antipsychotics, diabetic medications, antihistamines, antibiotics, and anesthetics) due to thujopsene, cedrol, and beta-cedrene content.[9095]

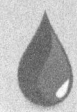

**SELECTED EVIDENCE:**

☐ Topical application of Texas cedarwood essential oil (supercritical carbon dioxide oil (SC-CO₂) with very similar composition to steam distilled oil) to incisions moderately improved wound healing time in rats.[9096]

☐ *In vitro* research reports that Texas cedarwood inhibits ten different strains of gram-positive and gram-negative bacteria associated with food poisoning and spoilage and plant disease.[9097]

# THUJA
## (American Arborvitae, Eastern Arborvitae, White Cedar, Cedar Leaf, Eastern White Cedar, Northern White Cedar)

*Thuja occidentalis* L.

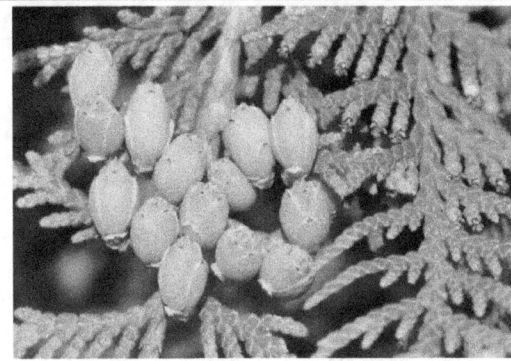

**FAMILY:** Cupressaceae
**NOTE:** Top
**AROMA INTENSITY:** Medium
**AROMA:** Woody, earthy, sharp, spicy, camphoraceous
**COMMON EXTRACTION METHOD:** Steam distilled from the leaves and branches
**POSSIBLE SUBSTITUTE OILS:** Sage (alpha-thujone CT), mugwort (alpha-thujone CT), western red cedar
**BLENDS WELL WITH:** Cedarwood, copaiba, geranium, lavender, lemon, neroli, petitgrain, pine, sage, tangerine
**SUBCELLULAR LOCALIZATION | EPIGENETIC INFLUENCE:** Currently unknown | Currently unknown
**RECOMMENDED DILUTION RANGE:** 1.5%–20%

**PRIMARY CONSTITUENTS:**[9098,9099,9100]

| | |
|---|---|
| Alpha-Thujone | 42.6%–69.8% |
| Fenchone | 0.4%–14.5% |
| Beyerene | 1.1%–13.2% |
| Camphor | 0.7%–13.0% |
| Beta-Thujone | 3.1%–10.0% |
| Sabinene | 1.4%–7.6% |
| Rimuene | 0.3%–5.0% |
| Bornyl Acetate | 0.8%–4.5% |
| Terpinen-4-ol | 2.0%–3.1% |
| Para-Cymene-8-ol | 0.0%–2.7% |

Note: *T. occidentalis* is sometimes called Arborvitae and sold as an essential oil under this name; however, it shouldn't be confused with *T. plicata*, which is also called Arborvitae in the essential oil market. *T. occidentalis* is more appropriately referred to as thuja or white cedar essential oil, whereas *T. plicata* is more appropriately called giant arborvitae or western red cedar.

**OTHER CONSTITUENTS:** Para-cymene, camphene, fenchyl acetate, isobornyl acetate, alpha-humulene, limonene, alpha-terpinene, myrcene, alpha-fenchene, alpha-pinene, beyerene-19-ol, trans-totarol

**PREFERRED COMPOSITION FOR CLINICAL USE:**

| Constituent | |
|---|---|
| **Alpha-Thujone** | 55%–70% |
| **Fenchone** | 5%–15% |
| **Beta-Thujone** | 3%–10% |
| **Beyerene** | 1%–7% |
| **Camphor** | 0.5%–7% |
| **Sabinene** | 1%–5% |

| Terpinen-4-ol | 2%–4% |
|---|---|
| Bornyl Acetate | 0.5%–4% |
| Rimuene | 0.1%–3% |

**REPORTED THERAPEUTIC PROPERTIES:** Antimicrobial, antibacterial, antiviral, antifungal, **antiparasitic,** anticancer, antirheumatic, astringent, diuretic, promotes menstruation, removes excess mucus, stimulates localized circulation, cough, warts, aids detoxification, stress management, relieves worrisome thoughts

**CAUTIONS:**

*Thuja essential oil is not commonly used in essential oil therapy and should be reserved for use by the very experienced user who can properly weigh the risks-to-benefits ratio of using it.*

■ Avoid with children under six due to thujone and camphor content. Cases of seizure have been reported in young children due to sage essential oil (also high in thujones) exposure.[9101,9102,9103] A seven-month-old child experienced eight generalized tonic-clonic seizures after being administered a 30C homeopathic preparation made from thuja essential oil daily.[2851] This case is very interesting considering the fact that a 30C homeopathic dilution would have less than one molecule of thuja left in it. It is possible that the preparation was not diluted properly therefore providing a more potent strength of the essential oil. Several cases of camphor poisoning and/or seizures from ingestion and topical application have been reported in children.[9104,9105] Ingestion of camphor-containing products has been lethal in children under age two.[9106]

■ Avoid during pregnancy and while lactating. Camphor ingestion may lead to abortion because fetuses lack the enzymes to process it.[9107] Essential oils high in thujone content may cause abortion.[9108,9109] Camphor ingestion by infants and young children may cause cough, vomiting, seizure, burning sensation in the mucous membranes and eyes, or lack of voluntary coordination of muscle movements.[9110]

■ Avoid oral consumption. Ingesting thuja essential oil can cause vomiting, stomachache, diarrhea, and gastroenteritis followed by absorption disorders, headache, nervous agitation, and chronic convulsions, and symptoms of liver and kidney toxicity extending to yellow liver atrophy (extensive and rapid death of liver cells—parenchymal, possibly accompanied by fatty degeneration), arrhythmia, and myocardial bleeding.[9111] Thujone is considered significantly neurotoxic and may damage the liver, and it is estimated that as little as 15 mg orally may negatively impact the central nervous system.[9112,9113,9114] Taking 20 drops of thuja oil twice daily for five days caused an adult woman to have a tonic seizure and then fall and fracture her skull.[2033] Case reports involving serious adverse health outcomes (seizure, convulsions, and acute kidney failure) have been reported in adults who consumed high thujone essential oils (sage, thuja, wormwood) in doses of one "swallow," 12 drops, and 20 drops twice daily for five days.[9115,9116,9117,9118] Camphor can be toxic when taken orally (usually single doses exceeding 2 mL), although the lethal dose for adult humans is estimated to be more than 5 mL in a single dose.[9119,9120,9121]

■ Avoid with epilepsy and Parkinson's disease due to camphor, fenchone, and thujone content.[9122,9123,9124,9125,9126]

■ May weakly interfere with the enzymes responsible for metabolizing medications (NSAIDs, proton-pump inhibitors, acetaminophen, antiepileptics, immune modulators, blood-sugar medications, blood pressure medications, antidepressants, antipsychotics, diabetic medications, antihistamines, antibiotics, and anesthetics) due to alpha-thujone content.[9127]

■ The small amounts of camphor in thuja essential oil may negatively impact red blood cells and increase the risk of jaundice in children with glucose-6-phosphate dehydrogenase deficiency (G6PD).[9128,9129]

■ Avoid with those who have a compromised liver or kidneys due to the risk of increased liver enzymes, liver damage, kidney toxicity, and kidney failure.[9130,9131] This would also suggest that those taking medications that could cause liver damage should also use thuja very cautiously or avoid it entirely.

**SELECTED EVIDENCE:**

☐ Animal research suggests that thuja oil and alpha-thujone significantly increases estradiol and progesterone levels while decreasing luteinizing hormone and testosterone, which made it beneficial for polycystic ovary syndrome (PCOS).[9132]

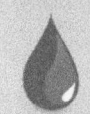

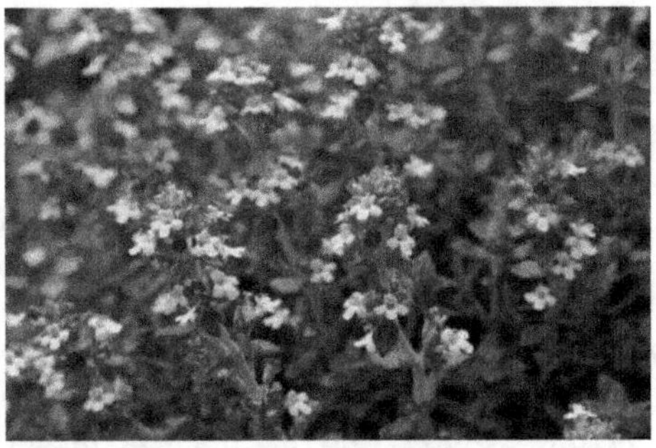

# THYME
## (Red Thyme, Garden Thyme)
*Thymus vulgaris* L.; *Thymus zygis* L.

**FAMILY:** Lamiaceae (Labiatae)
**NOTE:** Top-Middle
**AROMA INTENSITY:** Strong
**AROMA:** Fresh, herbaceous, medicinal
**COMMON EXTRACTION METHOD:** Steam distilled from the flowers and leaves
**POSSIBLE SUBSTITUTE OILS:** Oregano, ajowan, niaouli, geranium, marjoram, palmarosa
**BLENDS WELL WITH:** Bay laurel, bergamot, camphor, clary sage, copaiba, cypress, eucalyptus, geranium, grapefruit, lavender, lemon, juniper, tea tree, marjoram, orange, oregano, petitgrain, pine, ravensara, rose, rosemary, sage, Spanish sage
**SUBCELLULAR LOCALIZATION | EPIGENETIC INFLUENCE:** Endocytic Vesicles | Skeletal/Integumentary
**RECOMMENDED DILUTION RANGE:** 1.5%–20%; 50% for some conditions

## PRIMARY CONSTITUENTS:[9133,9134]

*Thymol CT*

| | |
|---|---|
| Thymol | 21.4%–72.9% |
| Para-Cymene | 0.0%–29.0% |
| Carvacrol | 0.8%–26.8% |
| Gamma-Terpinene | 0.0%–23.5% |
| Linalool | 1.1%–13.4% |
| Geraniol | 0.0%–8.9% |
| Beta-Caryophyllene | 0.0%–7.8% |
| Alpha-Terpineol | 0.0%–6.1% |
| Terpinen-4-ol | 0.0%–5.0% |
| 1,8-Cineole | 0.0%–3.8% |
| Thuyanol-4 | 0.0%–3.3% |

*Alpha-Terpineol CT*

| | |
|---|---|
| Alpha-Terpineol | 40.9%–90.4% |
| Thymol | 0.0%–27.4% |
| Linalool | 0.4%–19.2% |
| Thuyanol-4 | 0.0%–13.9% |
| 1,8-Cineole | 0.1%–13.2% |
| Terpinen-4-ol | 0.0%–6.2% |
| Gamma-Terpinene | 0.0%–3.3% |
| Carvacrol | 0.0%–3.0% |

*Thuyanol-4 CT*

| | |
|---|---|
| Thuyanol-4 | 1.6%–52.2% |
| Linalool | 2.4%–32.5% |
| Terpinen-4-ol | 2.2%–29.6% |
| Carvacrol | 0.0%–21.4% |
| 1,8-Cineole | 0.0%–21.2% |
| Beta-Caryophyllene | 0.8%–20.3% |
| Myrcenol-8 | 0.0%–18.7% |
| Alpha-Terpineol | 2.0%–13.9% |

*Linalool CT*

| | |
|---|---|
| Linalool | 32.2%–93.8% |
| Geraniol | 0.0%–30.0% |
| Thymol | 0.0%–23.6% |
| Thuyanol-4 | 0.0%–20.6% |
| Alpha-Terpineol | 0.0%–14.2% |
| Beta-Caryophyllene | 0.5%–12.3% |
| 1,8-Cineole | 0.0%–10.7% |
| Terpinen-4-ol | 0.0%–8.5% |
| Myrcenol-8 | 0.0%–7.1% |
| Carvacrol | 0.0%–6.8% |

*Carvacrol CT*

| | |
|---|---|
| Carvacrol | 21.5%–84.1% |
| Para-Cymene | 0.0%–34.6% |
| Linalool | 1.1%–29.9% |
| Thymol | 0.0%–27.2% |
| Gamma-Terpinene | 0.0%–26.8% |
| Thuyanol-4 | 0.0%–12.2% |
| Beta-Caryophyllene | 0.0%–10.3% |
| Geraniol | 0.0%–10.3% |
| Alpha-Terpineol | 0.0%–8.2% |
| Terpinen-4-ol | 0.0%–7.1% |
| 1,8-Cineole | 0.0%–3.1% |

*Geraniol CT*

| | |
|---|---|
| Geraniol | 23.5%–72.7% |
| Linalool | 0.4%–40.8% |
| Beta-Caryophyllene | 0.3%–9.6% |
| Thymol | 0.0%–7.9% |
| Carvacrol | 0.0%–6.9% |
| Gamma-Terpinene | 0.0%–5.3% |

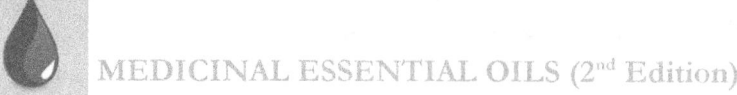

| | |
|---|---|
| Thymol | 0.0%–9.3% |
| Gamma-Terpinene | 0.0%–5.0% |
| Para-Cymene | 0.0%–5.0% |

Note: The thymol CT, often called red thyme, is the most common chemotype commercially available. White thyme may also be available, which is red thyme that has been redistilled (rectified) to remove some of the phenols (thymol and carvacrol); often making it rich in linalool. White thyme is technically an essential oil fraction and not a true essential oil. Adding to the confusion, some distinguish *T. vulgaris* and *T. zygis* by calling them red and white thyme respectively. White thyme can be extracted from either *T. vulgaris* or *T. zygis*.

**OTHER CONSTITUENTS:** *Alpha-Terpineol CT*—Para-cymene, thymol, myrcenol-8, beta-caryophyllene; *Carvacrol CT*—N/A; *Geraniol CT*—Alpha-terpineol, para-cymene; *Linalool CT*—Gamma-terpinene, para-cymene; *Thuyanol-4 CT*—NA; *Thymol CT*—N/A

**PREFERRED COMPOSITION FOR CLINICAL USE:**

| Constituent | Thymol CT (Red Thyme) | Linalool CT (France) | Linalool CT (Spain) |
|---|---|---|---|
| **Thymol** | 40%–60% | 8%–18% | < 1.5% |
| **Para-Cymene** | 14%–28% | 2%–7% | 1%–3% |
| **Gamma-Terpinene** | 5%–12% | 1%–3% | 3%–9% |
| **Linalool** | 3%–7% | 45%–65% | 30%–65% |
| **Carvacrol** | 0.5%–7% | 7%–15% | – |
| **Terpinen-4-ol** | 0.1%–4% | 2%–4% | 5%–15% |
| **Myrcene** | 0.5%–3% | 0.5%–1% | 2%–10% |
| **Alpha-Terpinene** | 0.5%–3% | 0.5%–2% | 1%–5% |
| **Alpha-Pinene** | 0.5%–3% | 0.1%–1% | 2%–5% |
| **Beta-Caryophyllene** | 0.1%–3% | 1%–3% | 0.1%–2% |
| **Alpha-Thujene** | 0.1%–2% | < 0.5% | < 1% |
| **Carvacrol Methyl Ether** | tr–2% | tr–1% | – |
| **Geraniol** | – | 1%–5% | < 0.5% |
| **4-Thuyanol <cis- + trans->** | < 2% | < 5% | 1.5%–8% |
| **Limonene** | < 1% | < 1% | 2%–5% |

**REPORTED THERAPEUTIC PROPERTIES:** Analgesic (pain relief), antiparasitic, **antibacterial**, antifungal, antiviral, anti-inflammatory, **antiarthritic**, anesthetic, antimicrobial, antirheumatic, **antiseptic**, supports cardiac function, antitumor, antioxidant, antispasmodic, **antiviral**, expels excess gas, supports healthy cell division, **encourages normal bone turnover (remodeling)**, diuretic, **reduces the appearance of scars and blemishes, eases chronic and deep-set cough**, relieves sports injuries, **reduces hair loss**, expectorant, **wound healing**, increases redness and circulation of a localized area, **reduces headache**, stimulating, antidepressant, boosts memory and concentration, promotes self-confidence and self-assurance, combats despondency, **relieves fatigue,** diminishes guilt

**CAUTIONS:**

■ Oral caution. Some thyme chemotypes contain up to 72.9% thymol. Thymol has a longer half-life (the time it takes for half of the medication to metabolize or excrete half of the dosage) than most essential oil constituents and should not be administered orally for long periods of time.[9135] Thymol is a monoterpene phenol. Reports of fatalities in children who consumed 50 to 200 mg of phenols has been reported.[9136] It is recommended that chemotypes with high levels of thymol be limited to 10 drops per day orally for adults with a two- to seven-day break after twenty-one days of use.

■ Avoid with epilepsy or Parkinson's disease due to 1,8-cineole content (alpha-terpineol, linalool, and thuyanol CTs). May exacerbate or cause seizures or convulsions when inhaled, applied topically, or ingested based on 1,8-cineole content.[9137,9138,9139,9140,9141,9142]

■ May interact with aspirin, blood pressure, antiplatelet, and anticoagulant medications, and increase the risk of bleeding among people with bleeding disorders.[9143,9144,9145]

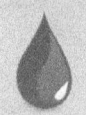

■ May interfere with enzymes that metabolize medications (NSAIDs, proton-pump inhibitors, acetaminophen, antiepileptics, immune modulators, blood-sugar medications, blood pressure medications, antidepressants, antipsychotics, diabetic medications, antihistamines, antibiotics, and anesthetics).[9146,9147,9148,9149]

■ May interact with anticholinergic (drugs used for asthma, incontinence, gastrointestinal cramps, muscular spasms, depression, and sleep disorders) and cholinergic medications (drugs used to reduce urinary retention, diagnose myasthenia gravis, and for glaucoma) based on thymol and carvacrol content.[9150,9151]

■ May interact with antibiotics or antifungals and possibly enhance their effects based on thymol, carvacrol, or linalool content.[9152,9153,9154,9155,9156,9157,9158,9159]

■ May irritate mucous membranes (eyes, mouth, nasal passages, vagina, rectum).

■ Dilution recommended for topical application with the geraniol, linalool, and carvacrol chemotypes due to geraniol content. Geraniol is metabolized via the CYP450 pathway into metabolites such as geranial and neral and may cause sensitization and irritation when applied topically.[9160]

■ May interact with diabetes medications and cause low blood sugar based on significant geraniol content (geraniol and linalool CTs).[9161,9162]

**SELECTED EVIDENCE:**

☐ *In vitro* research suggests that thyme essential oil is highly toxic to breast, prostate, oral, and lung cancer cells.[9163,9164] Another study concluded that carvacrol from thyme oil prevents tumor formation and triggers apoptosis of liver cancer cells through the mitochondrial pathway.[9165] Thymol causes cell death among cells that are responsible for causing glioblastomas (tumors that arise from astrocyte cells that make up the connective tissue of the brain).[9166]

☐ Thyme potently inhibits several common pathogenic organisms (*S. pyogenes*, *S. agalactiae*, *S. pneumoniae and K. pneumoniae*, *H. influenzae*, *S. aureus*, and *S. maltophilia*) that cause respiratory tract infections.[9167,9168] Another study found that thyme oil inhibited 120 drug-resistant bacterial strains from people with oral, abdominal cavity, respiratory, skin, and genitourinary infections from hospitals.[9169] One study reported that thyme oil reduced biofilm formation by *S. aureus*, but some cellular adaptation to thyme oil was observed, suggesting rotation of antimicrobial essential oils is important to increase effectiveness and reduce the risk of bacterial resistance.[9170] It also effectively inhibits clinical isolates of *P. aeruginosa*.[9171] Both the thymol and the linalool CTs of thyme essential oil inhibited *E. coli* in the gaseous phase, with the thymol CT being more potent.[9172] Thyme essential oil slowed biofilm formation by *S. aureus* and significantly reduced the number of biofilm cells in high concentrations.[9173] Interestingly, the study authors reported that some cellular adaptation to thyme essential oil was observed, suggesting a resistance was building. Thyme essential oil significantly inhibits *L. monocytogenes* (a bacterium that infects food and is associated with serious infections).[9174] Thyme essential oil reduced yeast film formation in meat.[9175] Thyme essential oil inactivates *Salmonella enteritidis* on turkey products.[9176]

☐ *In vitro* research concluded that thyme essential oil inhibits MRSA and *E. coli*.[9177,9178] Thyme essential oil strongly inhibited *Pseudomonas aeruginosa*, *Staphylococcus aureus*, *Escherichia coli*, and four yeasts: *Torulopsis utilis*, *Schizosaccharomyces pombe*, *Candida albicans*, and *Saccharomyces cerevisiae*.[9179] Thyme essential oil significantly inhibited clinical and foodborne *Candida* strains (including antibiotic-resistant strains).[9180] Thyme essential oil demonstrated significant antifungal activity against clinical isolates of *Candida* spp. in both liquid and vapor phases.[9181]

☐ Thyme essential oil CT linalool inhibits *Clostridium perfringens* and three microaerophilic *Campylobacter jejuni* strains.[9182]

☐ *In vitro* research demonstrates that thyme essential oil possesses remarkable antibiofilm, anti-adhesive, and bactericidal properties against two reference strains of *Salmonella typhimurium* and twelve *Salmonella* spp. isolated from food.[9183]

☐ Thyme essential oil inhibited gram-negative bacteria (multidrug-resistant *A. baumannii*, extended-spectrum-beta-lactamase (ESBL) producing *E. coli*, and carbapenemase-producing *K. pneumoniae*) and weakly inhibited *P. aeruginosa*, which are associated with healthcare-acquired infections.[9184]

☐ Thyme oil prevents oxidation of LDL cholesterol *in vitro*.[9185] Higher oxidized LDL levels are associated with a significantly increased risk of heart disease.[9186] Thyme essential oil also inhibits the activity of myeloperoxidase (an enzyme that causes oxidation of cholesterol, increases arterial inflammation, and encourages plaque formation

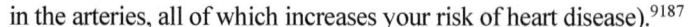

in the arteries, all of which increases your risk of heart disease).[9187]

- *In vitro* research suggests that thyme is a strong inhibitor of the bacterium *P. acnes*, which is suspected of being a major bacterial cause of acne.[9188]

- Oral administration of 25 drops of a 2% thyme oil solution every six hours for two consecutive menstrual cycles significantly reduced the pain and severity of painful menstruation (dysmenorrhea) in young women.[9189]

- A foot bath (107∘F water) with salts and either oregano, thyme, cinnamon bark, lemongrass, clove, palmarosa, peppermint, lavender, or geranium significantly reduced fungi associated with athlete's foot *in vitro*.[9190]

- Researchers concluded that thyme oil inhibited several *Candida* species and bacteria known to cause hospital-acquired infections according to *in vitro* research.[9191] Thyme also inhibited drug-resistant *C. albicans* and enhances the effect of antifungal drugs.[9192,9193,9194] Thyme essential oil demonstrated significant antifungal activity against antibiotic-resistant clinical isolates and foodborne strains of *Candida*.[9195] The linalool CT of thyme essential oil inhibited the filamentous fungal strain *Aspergillus ochraceus*.[9196] Thyme essential oil inhibits *Aspergillus* species and their subsequent production of mycotoxins.[9197] Thyme essential oil is fungicidal to *Fusarium proliferatum, F. verticillioides,* and *F. oxysporum* strains.[9198,9199]

- *In vitro* research discovered that thyme oil prevents HSV-2 infection of healthy cells at an effective rate greater than 90%.[9200] Another study determined that thyme oil possesses high levels of virucidal activity against both drug-resistant and non-drug-resistant HSV-1.[9201]

- A daily scalp massage with thyme, rosemary, lavender, and cedarwood oils in a mixture of carrier oils (jojoba and grapeseed) improved alopecia areata (round patches of hair loss) in 44% of study participants.[9202]

- Animal research suggests that thyme oil may protect against osteoporosis by inhibiting osteoclast (cells that breakdown bone tissue to release minerals into the circulatory system) activity and normalizing bone turnover.[9203]

- The vapor of thyme oil inhibited both penicillin-susceptible and penicillin-resistant respiratory pathogens (*H. influenzae, S. pneumoniae, S. pyogenes,* and *S. aureus*) *in vitro*.[9204]

- A case report describes the use of a combination of the essential oils of lemongrass, eucalyptus, tea tree, clove, thyme and BHT, triclosan, and undenatured alcohol to treat a chronic infection of the lower tibia (osteomyelitis) that was not responding to several courses of IV antibiotics. Amputation of the lower leg was being considered when a physician recommended the leg be opened up and the combination inserted directly into the bone (through a drilled hole, 1 mL per day for forty-eight hours). At three months, the wound and bone healed, and symptoms were resolved.[9205]

- *In vitro* research concluded that thyme oil possesses strong antioxidant properties.[9206,9207,9208,9209]

- *In vitro* research suggests that thyme oil inhibits the parasitic protozoan *T. cruzi*.[9210] *T. cruzi* causes the potentially life-threatening illness Chagas disease, also known as American trypanosomiasis.

- A combination of clove and thyme oil prevents the degradation of lipids in the skin caused by UV exposure and oxidative damage.[9211]

- Thyme oil prevents the growth of *A. flavus* and *A. parasiticus,* and the subsequent production of aflatoxin.[9212,9213] Another study concluded that thyme oil prevents the growth of *T. rubrum* and *Aspergillus* species.[9214]

- Animal research found that oral administration of thyme oil (250 to 500 mg/kg) prevented liver damage caused by acetaminophen comparable to the herbal remedy silymarin.[9215]

- Both oral and topical administration of thyme oil and/or carvacrol (alpha-terpineol CT) reduced inflammation, edema (swelling caused by excess fluid trapped in body tissues), and leukocyte migration (the movement of leukocytes from the blood to tissues, which causes increased inflammation) in rats.[9216] Another study concluded that thyme inhibits a number of proinflammatory molecules.[9217]

- *In vitro* research suggests that thyme oil inhibits *R. oryzae* (a fungus that causes mucormycosis, which is an infection characterized by sinus infection, sinus pain, fever, headache, and lung infection).[9218]

- Thyme oil inhibits multi-drug-resistant clinical strains of *E. coli in vitro*.[9219,9220]

- *In vitro* research suggests thyme oil inhibits *Entamoeba histolytica* (an anaerobic parasitic protozoan that may cause intestinal disorders, and bloodstream, liver, brain, and lung infections).[9221]

- Animal research suggests that the topical application of a 1% thyme oil solution cures dermatomycoses (a fungal skin disease that causes scaling and redness) in rats.[9222]

- Both carvacrol and thymol inhibit acetylcholinesterase (AChE). Inhibition of AChE prevents the breakdown of acetylcholine, which is essential for memory and thinking.[9223] People with neurodegenerative diseases

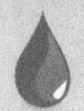

make less acetylcholine, and the diseases often break it down at a faster rate leading to acetylcholine deficits.

- *In vitro* research concluded that thyme oil inhibits nitric oxide (NO) production and scavenges NO, which reduces inflammation.[9224]

- Thyme oil inhibits the growth of the protozoan *G. lamblia*, which colonizes the small intestine and causes giardia (an intestinal infection characterized by abdominal cramps, bloating, nausea, and diarrhea).[9225,9226]

- Thymol (the primary constituent in thyme CT thymol) balances mast cell production with cell death, which may make it beneficial for skin inflammation.[9227]

- Alpha-terpineol prevents the growth of tumor cells by inhibiting NF-kappaB (a protein that helps regulates a variety of cellular and organism processes including inflammation, immune activity, developmental factors, cellular growth, and apoptosis).[9228]

- Thyme essential (carvacrol chemotype) oil proved very effective against 11 bacterial species (6 gram-positive, 5 gram-negative) and 7 fungi.[9229]

- Thyme essential oil kills head lice (*Pediculus humanus capitis*) *in vitro*.[9230] Another study reported that thyme essential oil kills the eggs of *Pediculus humanus capitis* in the fumigant test and killed adults without causing skin irritation.[9231]

- A study concluded that the addition of thyme and clove essential oils to Orabase formulations demonstrated considerable antifungal activity against *Candida* species that are associated with mild to severe oral infections.[9232] Another study reported that an essential oil mouthrinse containing lemongrass, thyme, and rosemary essential oils positively affected oral health and clinical variables of moderate chronic periodontitis after scaling and root planing.[9233] The study participants rinsed with the five drops of the mouthwash for sixty seconds, twice daily, for a total of fourteen days.

- An oral gel with clove and thyme essential oils and eugenol and thymol as the primary ingredients demonstrated considerable antifungal activity against *Candida* species, which caused the study authors to conclude that it was a promising product for reduction of oral candidiasis.[9234]

- Thyme essential oil and its components are highly active against foodborne pathogens.[9235] Research demonstrates that thyme essential oil inhibits and prevents meat spoilage (20 mg/mL) caused by *Brochothrix thermosphacta*.[9236]

- Animal research reports that thyme essential oil improves intestinal integrity without creating dysbiosis (a state of altered intestinal flora to one of harmful bacteria that contributes to a variety of chronic and degenerative diseases).[9237] The same research reported that thyme oil increases total antioxidant status and glutathione peroxidase (GPX) activity in the liver.

- Topical application of a blend of lavender and thyme essential oils (2:1 ratio) for twenty-one days reduced atopic dermatitis (eczema) by decreasing superoxide radical, mast cell degranulation, IgE production, and epidermal thickness in mice.[9238]

- An *in vitro* study that tested the antimicrobial activity of fifty-one essential oils demonstrated that all fifty-one demonstrated activity against at least one of the seven organisms (13 essential oils—*Ps. aeruginosa*, unidentified number against *S. aureus*, but it was the second most resistant microbe, 20—*E. coli*, 47—*C. albicans*, 49—*S. pombe*, and 50—*S. cerevisiae* and *T. utilis*).[9239] The study authors pointed out that clove, cinnamon, and thyme essential oils demonstrated significant inhibition, inhibiting greater than 50% reduction in all organisms, and greater than 90% reduction in two or more organisms. Thyme inhibited all organisms at greater than 94% except for *E. coli* and *P. Aeruginosa*.

- Thyme essential oil completely inhibited the three main stages, egg hatching, larval development, and motility of *Haemonchus contortus* (a common and highly pathogenic parasite that attaches to mucous membranes in the stomach—of both animals and humans—and feeds on the blood of its host).[9240] The effectiveness was comparable to levamisole (a drug used to treat parasitic worm infections). Thymol was equally effective, causing the study authors to conclude that the antiparasitic activity of thyme oil is due to thymol.

- *In vitro* research demonstrated that low doses of marjoram, lemon, basil, clove, thyme, rosemary CT 1,8-cineole, and tea tree essential oils prevented the shortening of telomeres after exposure to hydrogen peroxide.[9241] The same research reported that vetiver, black pepper, eucalyptus (*E. globulus*), ginger, clove, and rosemary increased the length of already shortened telomeres. This activity suggests that these essential oils can help maintain the youth and health of cells, or turn back the clock on the cell to make it more youthful depending on the essential oil used. Interestingly, cinnamon and peppermint essential oil decreased the length of telomeres slightly.

☐ Animal research concluded that lavender and thyme essential oil alone or blended together (2:1 ratio) decreased atopic dermatitis symptoms (decreased free radical activity, mast cell degranulation, and epidermal thickness).[9242]

☐ Adding thyme essential oil to the food of rabbits resulted in significant increases in total antioxidant status in the blood plasma, glutathione peroxidase (GPX) activity in the liver, and decreased malondialdehyde in the duodenal (the first part of the small intestine) tissue. In addition, thyme oil strengthened the intestinal integrity while maintaining a balanced gut microbiome (increasing beneficial microbes in the gut).[9243]

☐ Thyme essential oil (linalool CT) significantly kills adult rice weevils (*S. oryzae*).[9244]

☐ Thyme essential oil strongly inhibited several oral pathogens (*Streptococcus pyogenes, Streptococcus mutans, Candida albicans, Porphyromonas gingivalis*, and *Aggregatibacter actinomycetemcomitans*) with *Streptococcus pyogenes* and *Streptococcus mutans* being the most sensitive.[9245]

☐ *In vitro* research demonstrates that thyme essential oil is highly antifungal against clinical and foodborne *Candida* strains, including those resistant to antibiotics.[9246]

☐ Clove bud and red thyme essential oil both repelled *Dermacentor reticulatus* ticks at a 3% concentration.[9247] Clove bud was more effective (83 percent repellency) than red thyme (68 percent repellency).

☐ *In vitro* research demonstrates that thyme essential oil inhibits *S. aureus*.[9248]

☐ Spearmint (carvone CT and rich in eugenol), thyme (thymol CT), and clove essential oils all killed head lice, with spearmint being the most effective.[9249]

☐ Thyme essential oil inhibits *S. mutans* and reduces its colonization on dental enamel.[9250]

☐ Both thyme and oregano (*T. capitatus*) essential oils demonstrated good antioxidant and antimicrobial activity against all tested bacteria (*Listeria innocua, Serratia marcescens, Pseudomonas fragi, Pseudomonas fluorescens, Aeromonas hydrophila, Shewanella putrefaciens, Achromobacter denitrificans, Enterobacter amnigenus, Enterobacter gergoviae*, and *Alcaligenes faecalis*), making them good options as meat preservatives.[5243] Another study concluded that thyme and thymol and carvacrol inhibited *Salmonella* in minced pork meat, but also modified its sensory attributes (texture, flavor, or aroma).[9251]

☐ Thyme, clove, and java citronella exhibited toxicity against Turkestan cockroach nymphs.[9252] Thymol was the most toxic essential oil constituent, followed by trans-cinnamaldehyde, eugenol, para-cymene, geraniol, and methyl eugenol.

☐ *In vitro* research demonstrated that thyme CT thymol essential oil actively interfered with HIV-1 Tat protein function. The Tat protein plays a central role in and drastically enhances HIV transcription (resulting in the production of multiple copies of the viral RNA and improved infectivity).[9253]

☐ Thyme essential oil inhibited *Prototheca zopfii* strains that cause inflammation of the udder (mastitis) in cows.[9254]

☐ Thyme-oil-loaded hydrogel membranes (carrageenan/polyethylene glycol) significantly inhibited both gram-positive and gram-negative bacteria, suggesting the potential to use these membranes as part of a wound care system.[9255]

☐ Laboratory research demonstrated that thyme CT thymol possesses good antioxidant capacity and inhibited bacteria involved in food spoilage (*P. fluorescens, B. thermosphacta*, and *E. faecium*) and pathogenic bacteria (*Salmonella enterica* serotype *Enteritidis, Salmonella enterica* serotype *Typhimurium, L. monocytogenes*, and *S. aureus*).[9256]

☐ Rosemary, clove, oregano (*T. capitatus*), thyme, manuka, sage, eucalyptus (*E. globulus*), lavandin, myrtle, tea tree, peppermint, sage, and corn mint essential oils all showed antimicrobial activity against oral pathogens (*S. mutans, Lactobacillus* spp.) isolated from dental surgery patients.[9257] The essential oils also improved the antimicrobial effects of chlorhexidine, particularly rosemary, thyme, and oregano oils.

☐ *In vitro* research demonstrates that thyme essential oil enhances the activity of itraconazole against *Cryptococcus neoformans* (a difficult to treat encapsulated yeast that few molecules actively inhibit and a serious problem for people with a compromised immune system).[9258]

☐ Human aryl hydrocarbon receptor (AhR: a gene that encodes a protein that helps regulate responses to planar aromatic hydrocarbons and significantly effects the immune activity in the gastrointestinal tract, regulates the circadian rhythm, helps regulate the cell cycle, and plays an important role in tissue development). Cumin, jasmine, vanilla, and bay leaf fully activate AhR; clove, dill, thyme, nutmeg, and oregano partially activate AhR; and tarragon, caraway, turmeric, lovage, fennel, spearmint, star anise, and anise inhibit the AhR activity.[9259]

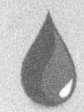

- Thyme CT gamma-terpinene, lemon CT citral, geranium CT p-menthone, cassia CT cinnamaldehyde, clove CT eugenol, and basil CT 1,8-cineole each demonstrated fungistatic and fungicidal activity toward *C. albicans* and *C. glabrata* isolates with cassia demonstrated the highest activity.[9260]
- The carvacrol CT of thyme essential oil reduces neutrophil infiltration during an inflammatory response.[9261]
- Thyme CT carvacrol inhibited *Malassezia furfur* (a fungus associated with skin disorders) isolates.[9262]
- The thymol (34.5%) CT of thyme essential oil was highly active against blaESBL-producing multidrug-resistant *Enterobacteriaceae* isolates and synergized the activity of cefotaxime against blaSHV-12 producing *E. coli* and an additive effect against ESBL producing *Enterobacter cloacae*.[9263]
- Cinnamon, clove, oregano, and red thyme essential oils effectively inhibited multidrug-resistant *Salmonella enterica* (a cause of foodborne illness) and enhanced the activity of antibiotics (enrofloxacin, ceftiofur, and trimethoprim-sulfamethoxazole).[9264] The most effective combination was cinnamon with enrofloxacin reducing the minimum inhibitory concentration (MIC) of cinnamon from 1250 to 312.5 µg/mL and the MIC of ENR from 2 to 0.031 µg/mL.
- Thyme essential oil inhibited MRSA biofilm formation up to 88.7 percent after forty-eight hours of exposure to a 0.1% concentration.[9265]
- Thyme, oregano, and clove essential oils each inhibited *Burkholderia cepacia* complex (a bacterium that affects people with a compromised immune system that is highly resistant to antibiotics), with improved efficacy when combined with an efflux inhibitor.[9266]
- The thymol CT of thyme demonstrated acaricidal activity against the Carmine Spider Mite (*Tetranychus Cinnabarinus*).[5536] The researchers also tested individual constituents and found thymol to be the strongest acting, with the greatest effect when all of the putatively active and inactive constituents were present.
- Cinnamon bark essential oil was the most effective essential oil of seven tested (clove, cinnamon bark, eucalyptus, thyme CT thymol, Scots pine, peppermint, and citronella) against respiratory tract pathogens (*Streptococcus pneumoniae*, *S. mutans*, *S. pyogenes*, *Haemophilus influenzae*, *H. parainfluenzae*, and *Moraxella catarrhalis*) in vapor phase.[9267] In liquid phase, thyme was most effective against *S. mutans*, and cinnamon and clove significantly inhibited *S. pneumoniae* and *S. pyogenes*.
- Thyme CT gamma-terpinene and sage CT beta-caryophyllene both inhibited *Fusarium graminearum* and demonstrated a synergistic antifungal activity when used together.[5565] The same study found that both oils exhibited antiproliferative activity against two melanoma lines (A375 human melanoma and B164A5 mouse melanoma) alone and in combination, with sage being the most effective.
- Oregano CT thymol and thyme CT thymol essential oils exhibited strong antimicrobial activity against bacteria (*Propionibacterium acnes* and *Staphylococcus epidermidis*) associated with acne that are becoming increasing resistant to first-line antibiotics.[5594]
- Marjoram, pink savory (*Satureja thymbra*), spearmint CT piperitenone oxide, melissa, and dittany (*Origanum dictamnus*) demonstrated the greatest repellency toward *Ae. albopictus* mosquitoes of fourteen Lamiaceae species tested.[5595] Thyme CT thymol, basil, dittany, marjoram, and oregano CT carvacrol were the most larvicidal.
- Thyme CT thymol essential oil exhibited higher efficacy against *S. aureus* biofilms than peracetic acid and sodium hypochlorite formed on polystyrene and stainless-steel surfaces.[5598] An even greater effect was observed when thyme was combined with *Lippia sidoides* essential oil or peracetic acid.
- Both lemongrass (*C. flexuosus*) and thyme essential oils were active against foodborne pathogens (multidrug-resistant *Enterococcus* spp. and *Aeromonas* spp.) and eradicated preformed biofilms from *Aeromonas* spp.[5604]
- The thymol CT of thyme essential oil inhibited *Vibrio alginolyticus* and *V. parahaemolyticus*, which are important bacteria that live in water and cause ear, gastrointestinal, and wound infections.[5605]
- *Borrelia burgdorferi* is a diderm bacteria responsible for Lyme disease in the United States. Of thirty-five essential oils screened, garlic, allspice, cumin, palmarosa, myrrh, ginger lily, amyris, thyme, may chang, and lemon eucalyptus each demonstrated excellent activity against *Borrelia burgdorferi*.[9268] Garlic (19% diallyl disulfide), allspice CT eugenol, and myrrh (38% curzerene) were the most active essential oils.
- The addition of 0.2% peppermint or thyme essential oil to a yogurt-based drink inhibited *S. aureus*.[9269]
- Coriander CT carvone and thyme CT carvacrol inhibited avian multidrug-resistant strains of *E. coli*, which led the authors to conclude these essential oils have potential to be used as replacements for antibiotics in avian treatment.[9270]
- Formulations of the carvacrol CT of thyme essential oil demonstrated good antioxidant activity and antibacterial activity against bacteria associated with cavities (S. mutans, L. acidophilus), suggesting the oil may be useful for the treatment of oral cavity diseases.[9271]
- Eucalyptus, clove, mint, oregano, savory, tea tree, and thyme essential oils each inhibited *Venturia*

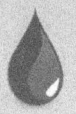

*inaequalis*, the fungus responsible for apple scab.[9272]

☐ Thyme (composition not reported) essential oil inhibited the foodborne pathogen *L. monocytogenes*.[9273]

☐ The m-cymene CT of thyme essential oil potently inhibited the growth of planktonic *B. cereus* by damaging its cell membrane.[9274] It also inhibited *B. cereus* biofilm formation.

☐ Thyme essential oil significantly inhibited the growth of *Listeria monocytogenes* and *Salmonella Typhimurium in vitro* and on alfalfa seeds (in vapor phase).[9275]

☐ *E. coli* causes up to 85% of urinary tract infections (UTIs). Thyme CT linalool, marjoram, and rosemary CT 1,8-cineole essential oils each inhibited *E. coli* isolated from the urinary tract of people with a UTI.[9276] Thyme was the most effective.

☐ Thyme CT thymol exhibited good antioxidant activity and inhibited *B. cereus, S. aureus, S. epidermidis, E. coli, S. enteritidis, S. typhimurium.*[9277]

☐ An *in vitro* study found that thyme essential oil denture cleanser was more effective than a commercially available denture cleanser in preserving surface toughness and flexural strength of denture base resins.[9278]

☐ Thyme and oregano essential oils demonstrated the ability to increase the stability of minced pork and prevent the oxidation of lipids after two weeks of storage.[9279]

☐ Thyme essential oil with nearly equal para-cymene (43.1%) and thymol (39.8%) significantly reduced tumor volumes in a mouse and rat model of breast cancer, reducing tumor frequency by 84 percent and 53 percent, respectively.[9280] The oil was added to the rodent's diet at a concentration of 1% to be effective.

☐ Of ten essential oils tested (thyme, pennyroyal, oregano, peppermint, lemongrass, rosemary, cinnamon, mandarin, holy basil, and mint asavi), cinnamon and thyme essential oils demonstrated the greatest efficacy against MRSA.[9281] Each oil demonstrated varying levels of inhibition. Oregano and pennyroyal also showed a strong synergistic activity with penicillin.

☐ Marjoram CT terpinen-4-ol, cinnamon bark, and thyme CT thymol essential oils each exhibited antibiofilm effects on *L. monocytogenes, P. putida*, and *S. aureus*, but were less effective against biofilms with two species unless higher concentrations were used.[9282]

☐ Thyme essential oil inhibited *A. flavus* and its production of aflatoxins in both the liquid- and vapor-phase, with greater inhibition in vapor-phase.[9283] The oil substantially reduced aflatoxin production in brown rice (72.7%) and white rice (18.0%) as well.

☐ *In vitro* research found that of five Lamiaceae family essential oils (lavender, peppermint, marjoram, sage, and thyme) thyme CT thymol was the most effective against eighteen strains of multidrug-resistant *S. aureus* isolated from humans.[9284] Peppermint also exhibited inhibition, followed by sage, marjoram, and lavender in efficacy.

☐ Laboratory research concluded that oregano CT carvacrol, thyme CT thymol, cassia, lemongrass (*C. flexuosus*), and Western red cedar (arborvitae) essential oils exhibit very strong antimicrobial activity against drug resistant pathogens (*Pseudomonas aeruginosa, Proteus vulgaris, Citrobacter koseri, Klebsiella pneumoniae, Candida albicans*, and *C. parapsilosis*).[9285] Ten essential oils—oregano, thyme, clove, arborvitae, cassia, lemongrass, tea tree, eucalyptus (*E. radiata*), lavender, and clary sage —were tested and these five were the most effective. The researchers also concluded the essential oils were not genotoxic (cause DNA damage) compared to control cells. In addition, each of the oils exhibited antioxidant activity, with cassia and oregano demonstrating the greatest increase in total antioxidant status, followed by tea tree, thyme, clove, clary sage, eucalyptus, arborvitae, and lavender.

☐ Rosemary CT 1,8-cineole and thyme CT para-cymene essential oils, alone or in combination, reduced viable counts of food-borne and spoilage bacteria (*Listeria monocytogenes, Salmonella enteritidis, Yersinia enterocolitica, Escherichia coli*, and *Pseudomonas* spp.) in ready-to-eat vegetables.[9286]

☐ Clove bud and thyme CT thymol essential oils significantly reduced biofilm formation by *Candida* species on surfaces, suggesting they can be effectively used in the prevention of *Candida* colonization on abiotic (not derived from living organisms) surfaces.[9287]

☐ Thyme CT thymol, garlic, tea tree, cajeput, may chang, lemongrass (*C. citratus*), and verbena CT citral exhibited fungistatic activity (100 percent) against *F. culmorum* and *F. graminearum*, and all but garlic (89.4 percent) were 100 percent fungistatic against *F. avenaceum* and *F. oxysporum*.[9288]

☐ Fumigation of greenhouse plants with pennyroyal, catnip (reduced fertility), and thyme essential oil acted as an effective insecticide against flower thrips (*Frankliniella occidentalis*), which is an insect pest of greenhouse plants.[9289]

☐ Tahini is a popular food product in the Middle East, but tahini and its products have been linked to foodborne illness outbreaks and the subjects of worldwide recalls as a result of Salmonella contamination. Of ten essential oils tested, cinnamon bark and thyme essential oils were the most effective against *Salmonella* species bacteria.[9290]

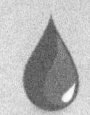

- A study found that a combination of oregano and thyme CT thymol, in gaseous form, essential oil produced a synergistic effect against *L. monocytogenes* on surfaces and radishes.[9291] Oregano with cinnamon and thyme with cinnamon also displayed synergistic activity against the bacteria.

- *Helicobacter pylori* is a bacterium that lives in the digestive tract that can cause sores and ulcers in the lining of the stomach or upper part of the small intestine. Thyme, lemongrass, Virginia cedarwood, and melissa essential oils were the most active of twenty-six commercial essential oils examined against *H. pylori*.[9292] Oregano, tea tree, pine, and silver fir were also bactericidal.

- Thyme CT thymol essential oil inhibited the formation of biofilms by *Candida* species and produced a synergistic activity of fluconazole against *C. albicans* and *C. tropicalis*.[9293]

- Of five essential oils tested (bay laurel, thyme, peppermint, lemongrass, and *Lippia junelliana*), bay laurel and thyme were the most active against *Candida* species including species that were drug resistant.[9294]

- *In vitro* research showed that cinnamon bark, oregano, thyme CT thymol, lemongrass (*C. flexuosus*), allspice, palmarosa, and amyris all significantly inhibited *S. aureus* in the stationary phase, which is when the size of a bacterial population remains constant, even though some cells continue to divide and others begin to die.[9295]

- Tea tree and thyme CT geraniol essential oils were active against sixteen multidrug-resistant P. aeruginosa strains isolated from infected hip implants.[9296] Tea tree was more effective than thyme.

- Cinnamon bark, thyme, and clove essential oil showed important antibacterial activity against multidrug-resistant bacteria isolated from people (*E. coli, K. pneumoniae, A. baumanii, P. aeruginosa, C. freundii, K. oxytoca, S. enteritidis, S. typhimurium, S. zanizibar, S. Livingstone, S. derby, S. Heidelberg, C. striatum*, and *S. aureus*).[9297] They exhibited a remarkable antibiofilm and anti-quorum-sensing activity and good antioxidant activity. The highest antioxidant activity was observed from clove (90.3% DPPH).

- Adding thyme essential oil (composition not reported) to the diet of African catfish (*Clarias gariepinus*) partly reduced liver and kidney toxicity caused by thiamethoxam due to its anti-inflammatory, antioxidant, antiapoptotic, and immune-stimulant effects.[9298]

- Thyme essential oil was active—caused apoptotic-like cell death—against *A. flavus* and significantly reduced its production of aflatoxin $B_1$.[9299]

- Oregano, thyme, and their major constituents carvacrol and thymol showed good *in vitro* bactericidal and fungicidal activity against 100 bacterial and fungal isolates from dogs with external ear infections, some of which were highly drug-resistant.[9300]

- Oregano CT carvacrol, thyme CT thymol, cassia, lemongrass, and Western red cedar essential oils each demonstrated significant antibacterial and antifungal activity against several drug-resistant pathogens (*Ps. aeruginosa, Pr. vulgaris, C. koseri, K. pneumoniae, C. albicans,* and *C. parapsilosis*) known to infect the skin.[9301] The oils were not toxic to healthy keratinocytes and increased total antioxidant status in the cells as well.

- *Vibrio parahaemolyticus* is a gram-negative bacterium that causes gastrointestinal illness in humans characterized by watery or bloody diarrhea, nausea, vomiting, fever, headache, and abdominal cramps. The bacteria lives in brackish saltwater (like found in the coastal waters of the United States and Canada) and causes symptoms after ingesting contaminated water or food. Clove, thyme CT para-cymene, and garlic (20.0% allyl propyl disulfide, 16.8% diallyl trisulfide, 15.2% allyl sulfide) essential oils reduced bacterial growth, with clove and thyme being the most effective.[9302]

- A specially formulated thyme CT thymol essential oil with the oil linked to solid excipients and the free oil (not linked to excipients) inhibited *Staphylococcus aureus, Streptococcus pyogenes, Pseudomonas aeruginosa, Escherichia coli, Salmonella typhimurium,* and *Candida albicans* without harming good bacteria involved in intestinal homeostasis (*Bifidobacterium breve, Lactobacillus fermentum*).[9303] The free oil was most effective in reducing intestinal spasms in isolated Guinea-pig ileum and colon but the special formulated oil also exhibited antispasmodic activity.

- Palmarosa essential oil demonstrated the ability to disrupt biofilm formation by oral pathogens (*S. mitis, S. sanguinis,* and *E. faecalis*) in an experimental model of root canals.[9304] Thyme essential oil also showed antibiofilm activity, which was 2-fold higher than the control (1.5% sodium hypochlorite). Successive irrigations with palmarosa was more efficient than the control as well.

- Thyme CT thymol essential oil exerted good antimicrobial activity against clinical and foodborne strains of the bacterium *L. monocytogenes*.[9305] Oils obtained from plants using three mulching methods were compared, with the grass cover mulch oil (36.9% thymol, 21.7% para-cymene, 18.4% gamma-terpinene) being the most effective.

- Brain infections like meningitis and encephalitis are difficult to treat due to poor ability of drugs to pass the blood brain barrier (BBB) and reach the brain. Delivery of therapeutic substances through the nose (intranasal) is a way to work around the BBB by delivering those agents through the highly vascularized olfactory region. Clove bud and thyme CT thymol essential oils included in chitosan-coated nanoemulsions showed potential to be effective intranasal solutions against multidrug-resistant bacteria such as MRSA, MSSA, *A. baumannii*, and *K. pneumoniae*.[9306]

☐ Tea tree and thyme CT linalool essential oils were active against seven antibiotic-resistant and antibiotic-sensitive bacteria that cause urinary tract infections (*E. coli, K. pneumoniae, En. cloacae, P. mirabilis, Ps. aeruginosa, En. faecalis, S. saprophyticus*). A synergistic activity of the two oils was observed when they were combined. In addition, the oils increased the activity of fosfomycin and pivmecillinam, but not nitrofurantoin, against *E. coli*.

☐ Application of thyme CT thymol essential oil to beans significantly reduced the survival and longevity of the bean weevil (*Acanthoscelides obtectus*).[9307]

☐ Thyme CT thymol and cinnamon bark essential oil reduced airway inflammation and hyperresponsiveness—both important features of asthma and chronic obstructive pulmonary disease—in a mouse model of airway inflammation caused by exposure to an endotoxin.[9308] Two drops of oil were placed on filter paper and taped to the bottom of the box mice were placed in during a thirty-minute-long inhalation period. On the contrary, Ceylon citronella essential oil showed an irritating effect on inflamed airways that could exacerbate the airway hyperresponsiveness.

☐ Nitrates are chemicals added to processed meats as a preservative and to improve the color. Concern over the association of nitrates to cancer has led experts to seek alternatives. Thyme essential oil inhibited *L. innocua* (a foodborne pathogen that infests meat products) in both a laboratory setting and in salami.[9309]

☐ Evaluation of the isolated constituents from thyme CT thymol essential oil found that thymol, gamma-terpinene, and para-cymene (in order of effectiveness) inhibited fungal species associated with postharvest spoilage—*Botrytis, Penicillium, Alternaria*, and *Monilinia*—in vapor phase.[9310]

☐ MRSA poses a major threat to human health because of its ability to develop biofilms, which are complex biological systems that are difficult to treat with antibiotics, and infect humans. Thyme CT linalool, marjoram, and rosemary CT alpha-pinene essential oils each exhibited antibacterial activity against MRSA, inhibited its formation of biofilms, and eradicated existing biofilms.[9311] Thyme had the highest antibacterial activity followed by marjoram and rosemary. Interestingly, marjoram demonstrated the highest biofilm inhibition and eradication activity.

☐ The thymol CT of thyme essential oil ameliorated memory impairment caused by scopolamine in zebrafish. The oil was administered by immersion once daily for thirteen days.[9312] Thyme oil reduced scopolamine-induced increases in acetylcholinesterase (AChE) activity and the oxidative stress response, restoring brain antioxidant capacity.

☐ Laboratory research found that thyme essential oil inhibits the formation of biofilms by bacteria associated with cavities (*Streptococcus mutans, Streptococcus gordonii, Streptococcus sanguinis, Streptococcus mitis, Streptococcus sobrinus, Lactobacillus acidophilus*, and *Actinomyces naeslundii*).[9313]

☐ Both oregano CT carvacrol and thyme CT thymol essential oil inhibited *S. aureus* in vapor and liquid phase, with thyme generally showing greater activity.[9314] Combining oregano and thyme essential oils showed a synergistic and strong antibacterial activity against *S. aureus* in both liquid and vapor phases.

☐ Thyme CT thymol and creeping thyme CT thymol were both active against bovine mastitis-associated bacteria, with thyme being more effective against the fourteen bacteria tested.[9315]

☐ Feline infectious peritonitis is an infection of cats caused by coronavirus. Thyme (composition not reported) essential oil inhibited coronavirus replication and reduced viral load.[9316]

☐ Thyme CT thymol essential oil inhibited *E. coli* isolated from turkeys.[9317]

☐ A solid thyme CT thymol essential oil formulation (liquid essential oil linked to solid excipients) exerted relaxant (antispasmodic) activity in isolated intestines (ileum and colon).[9318] The free oil was effective as well. The solid oil also displayed antimicrobial activity against *Staphylococcus aureus, Streptococcus pyogenes, Pseudomonas aeruginosa, Escherichia coli, Salmonella typhimurium*, and *Candida albicans* similarly to the free oil.

☐ Researchers compared three different chemotypes of thyme (*Thymus vulgaris*) essential oil (geraniol, linalool, and thuyanol-4) and their main constituents in a model of neuroinflammation. Pretreatment of microglia with the essential oils or their main constituents reduced inflammation by modulating the expression of inflammatory cytokines (IL-6 and TNFα).[9319] The main constituents were more active than the whole oil, with geraniol and linalool being very effective.

☐ Researchers evaluated the correlation of chemical constituents with antimicrobial activity and concluded that phenols and aldehydes had the strongest positive effects on the antimicrobial properties of essential oils.[9320]

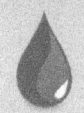

Thyme CT thymol, cinnamon bark, garlic, and oregano CT carvacrol essential oils were the most active oils of thirty-eight tested against foodborne pathogens—*E. coli* (three types), *Listeria* (two types), *Bacillus* (two types), *S. enterica* (two types), *S. aureus* (three types), *C. tyrobutyricum*, *P. aeruginosa*, *B. thermosphacta*, *C. jejuni*, *C. divergens*, *Aspergillus* (four types), and *Penicillium* (four types).

☐ Oxidative stress—an imbalance in free radicals to antioxidants to neutralize them—has been associated with a variety of conditions such as Parkinson's, Alzheimer's, diabetes, cardiovascular disease, and cancer formation and progression. Thyme CT thymol and summer savory CT carvacrol demonstrated potent antioxidant capacity in the DPPH and ABTS assays, which is related to their high phenol (thymol and carvacrol) content.[9321]

☐ Thyme CT thymol essential oil was toxic to breast, lung carcinoma, and acute lymphoblastic leukemia cancer cells, but was also toxic to brine shrimp.[9322]

☐ The thymol CT of thyme essential oil exhibited high efficacy in interfering with *Candida* biofilm formation.[9323]

☐ Both oregano CT carvacrol and thyme CT para-cymene (40.0% para-cymene, 32.0% thymol) essential oils demonstrated good antifungal activity against *C. albicans*, showing high activity during the adherence phase and during biofilm formation.[9324] The pinocamphone CT of hyssop, rosemary CT 1,8-cineole, and sage CT 1,8-cineole were active as well but to lesser degrees.

☐ Cassia, clove, oregano (near equal carvacrol and thymol), ginger, and thyme CT thymol essential oils each showed activity against *L. monocytogenes* in a dry-cured ham-based model.[9325]

☐ Thyme, tea tree, tropical basil, rosemary CT 1,8-cineole, eucalyptus, corn mint, and lavender essential oil each inhibited biofilm-forming *S. aureus*, with thyme and rosemary being the most active in liquid phase.[9326] Thyme was the most active in vapor phase, with varying degrees of inhibition observed depending on the strain of *S. aureus* with tea tree, rosemary, eucalyptus, corn mint, and lavender. Tea tree and lavender oils displayed the weakest activity in the vapor phase.

☐ Thyme CT thymol essential oil exhibited good antioxidant activity, moderate to very strong antimicrobial activity (in order of greatest to least zone of inhibition: *P. fluorescens* biofilm, *S. marcescens*, *S. enterica*, *C. glabrata*, *C. krusei*, *S. enteritidis* biofilm, *B. subtilis*, *S. aureus*, *P. aeruginosa*, *C. albicans*, *E. faecalis*, and *C. tropicalis*), and antifungal (*Penicillium*) activity when used in vapor phase on bread.[9327]

☐ The thymol CT of thyme essential oil demonstrated antimicrobial activity against gram-positive and gram-negative bacteria and fungal pathogens, with the greatest activity observed against *S. pyogenes*, *S. flexneri*, *S. typhimurium*, and *C. parapsilosis*.[9328]

☐ Comparing thyme and oregano essential oils against their nanoencapsulated versions showed that both oils exhibited enhanced bactericidal activity against foodborne pathogens (*S. aureus*, *E. coli*, and *L. monocytogenes*) than the free essential oils.[9329]

☐ *Fusarium graminearum* is a fungus that contaminates cereals, fruit, and vegetables. Thyme, oregano, basil, nutmeg, hyssop, and clove essential oils inhibited mycelial growth of *F. graminearum*, with oregano performing best followed by clove and thyme.[9330] The composition of the oils was not reported.

☐ *In vitro* research showed that thyme CT thymol essential oil strongly inhibited *Fusarium oxysporum* sp. *lactucae*.[9331]

☐ Thyme (near equal thymol and para-cymene) and lemongrass (*C. citratus*) significantly inhibited *B. cinerea*, and their vapors reduced gray mold, with thyme being more effective.[9332]

☐ Of fourteen commercial essential oils tested, cinnamon bark, thyme CT thymol, clove bud, geranium, and manuka essential oils were most active against fungi that commonly infect animal and human skin (*Microsporum gypseum*, *Microsporum canis*, *Trichophyton mentagrophytes*, *Trichophyton violaceum*, *Aspergillus niger*, *Scopulariopsis brevicaulis*, (IZ 1) dog skin isolate).[9333] (E)-cinnamaldehyde, thymol, and carvacrol displayed the strongest activity of isolated constituents against dermatophytes. (E)-cinnamaldehyde, eugenol, carvacrol, geraniol, and thymol were most active against IZ 1.

☐ When thyme CT thymol, marjoram, and oregano (caryophyllene oxide as the major constituent) were tested for antioxidant activity, thyme showed the greatest activity.[9334]

☐ The thymol CT of thyme essential oil inhibited *H. influenzae*, *S. aureus*, and *St. pyogenes*.[9335]

☐ Terpene/phenol-rich (oregano CT carvacrol, thyme CT carvacrol, and summer savory CT carvacrol) and phenylpropanoid-rich (clove bud and cinnamon leaf) essential oils each showed good absolute antioxidant activity—comparable to BHT—in cumene and squalene during the peroxyl radical trapping assay.[9336]

☐ Thyme CT thymol successfully reduced the growth of drug-resistant clinical *C. albicans* isolates, exhibiting fungistatic and fungicidal activity at very low doses.[9337] The oil was more effective than fluconazole.

☐ Microbes can form biofilms, which allows microbial populations to survive and resist drug treatment. Researchers investigated the activity of 15 essential oils against *E. coli* and *S. aureus*. Thyme CT thymol essential oil exhibited significant antibacterial activity and reduced biofilm formation.[9338]

- Cinnamon bark and thyme CT thymol essential oil both inhibited *Streptococcus suis*, which is a zoonotic pathogen that causes disease in pigs and humans and is developing resistance to antibiotics.[9339]

- Researchers evaluated the benefits of using thyme essential oil for people hospitalized with COVID-19 for one week.[9340] Eighty-three subjects were randomly assigned to receive thyme essential oil with conventional treatment (forty subjects) or conventional treatment only (forty-three subjects). Five mL of thyme essential oil (dilution and carrier not reported, but essential oils are frequently mixed into a liquid syrup in Iran and then standardized to active—thymol—content) was administered orally every eight hours for seven days. Subjects who received thyme essential oil experienced significantly greater reductions in their symptoms (fever, cough, difficulty breathing, dizziness, muscular pain, headache, sore throat, vomiting, weakness/lethargy, fatigue, and chest pain) when compared to standard treatment alone.

- The carvacrol CT of thyme essential oil displayed excellent antioxidant activity in the DPPH and FRAP assays and showed strong antimicrobial activities against multidrug-resistant *A. baumannii* at low concentrations, also exhibiting antimicrobial activity against *E. cloacae, S. aureus, S. typhi, S. dysenteriae, C. glabrata, C. albicans, Candida* spp., *F, solani,* and *A. fischeri.*[9341]

- Honey has been used medicinal since ancient times for a variety of ailments. Medical-grade honey (not the raw honey you purchase at a grocery store) is particularly useful for wound healing because of its antibacterial and anti-inflammatory activity, which speeds the healing of wounds. An experimental study evaluated the healing effects of a mixture of honey with selected essential oils—oregano CT ethanone, rosemary CT camphor, and thyme CT 1,3-Cyclopentadiene—in burn and chemical wound models in rabbits.[9342] The oils were added to honey in a concentration of 0.5% per 100g of honey. The honey/essential oil groups were compared versus a control (no treatment) and standard treatment with madecassol ointment. All of the honey/essential oil groups experienced faster healing times than the control group and standard treatment group. The best healing effect for burns was observed with honey and thyme essential oil for burns. The oils were not irritating when used at 0.5% in the honey, but showed irritation at 5%.

- Infection with the bacterium *E. coli* can have deleterious effects on hormone production, blood parameters, immune system activity, and organ (liver, kidney, pancreas, and small intestine) damage. Oral administration of thyme essential oil partially improved blood parameters, protected against organ damage, and restored immune-inflammatory dysfunction.[9343]

- *Clostridioides difficile* is a bacterium that produces two exotoxins: toxin A and toxin B. Infections with *C. diff* can be mild to moderate (watery diarrhea three or more times daily for more than one day accompanied by mild abdominal cramping and tenderness) or severe (watery diarrhea up to fifteen times daily, moderate to severe abdominal cramping, rapid heart rate, fever, dehydration, and nausea). Severe cases can cause kidney failure, loss of appetite, blood or pus in the stool, and inflammation of the colon (colitis), which can be life-threatening. Illness caused by *C. diff* typically occurs after antibiotic use and most commonly affects older adults in healthcare facilities. However, because the bacterium is shed in feces it can contaminate any surface, material, or device and spread outside of healthcare settings and in younger people as well. Repeat infections are common among the elderly because the bacterium is resistant to multiple antibiotics, making it very difficult to eradicate. A laboratory study investigated the activity of ten essential oils—cassia bark, cinnamon bark, citronella (*C. nardus*), coriander, clove bud, oregano CT carvacrol, Greek oregano (*O. heracleoticum*) CT carvacrol, marjoram, clary sage, and thyme CT thymol—against *C. diff* isolated from infected patients and contaminated foods.[9344] Isolated constituents within the essential oils were also tested (carvacrol, trans-cinnamaldehyde, eugenol, linalool, and thymol) as well as common antibiotics used to treat *C. diff* infections (chloramphenicol, clindamycin, erythromycin, gentamicin, metronidazole, and vancomycin). Cassia and cinnamon bark were the most effective, with thyme, oregano, Greek oregano, and marjoram also demonstrating high activity. Coriander and clary sage exhibited medium activity, while clove and citronella displayed low activity. Among the isolated constituents, trans-cinnamaldehyde, thymol, and carvacrol showed high activity and eugenol and linalool low activity. Cinnamon and cassia consistently exceeded the activity of all antibiotics, with very few exceptions, and thyme, oregano, and Greek oregano outperformed all antibiotics but metronidazole.

- Of 11 essential oils tested, oregano CT carvacrol, fennel, mountain savory CT para-cymene, and summer savory CT carvacrol were the most effective against gastrointestinal nematodes (*Haemonchus, Trichostrongylus, Teladorsagia,* and *Chabertia*) in the *in vitro* egg hatch test.[9345] Oral administration of the oils diluted in sunflower oil to animals showed that thyme CT para-cymene essential oil was the most effective, even more effective than thyme CT thymol.

- Thyme CT thymol displayed antioxidant activity in the DPPH and beta-carotene-bleaching assays and was antibacterial to *S. aureus.*[9346] Its inhibitory activity exceeded that of tetracycline against all three strains of *S.*

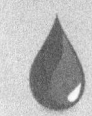

*aureus* tested. Moreover, the oil exhibited antibiofilm and antihemolytic properties and a synergistic and additive activity in combination with ampicillin, ciprofloxacin, or vancomycin against *S. aureus*.

☐ The fungus *Fusarium graminearum* can produce mycotoxins—deoxynivalenol (DON) and zearalenone (ZEA)—that are seriously toxic to animal reproductive systems. The essential oils of thyme, ginger, and rosemary were fungicidal to *F. graminearum*, and both thyme and ginger exhibited the most potent antimycotoxigenic activity against DON and ZEA.[9347]

☐ Doxorubicin is an anticancer drug associated with many adverse effects on various organs, including the liver. Oral administration (via gavage) of thyme oil, or thymol, at 250 and 100 mg/kg body weight respectively, four time per week reversed markers of liver damage—high AST, ALT, and ALP and total bilirubin, AFP, and CA19.9 levels —in rats.[9348] Both the oil and thymol also reduced inflammation, reduced lipid peroxidation caused by reduced enzymatic antioxidant activity, augmented mRNA expression of antiapoptotic protein Bcl-2 and significantly downregulated nuclear and cytoplasmic levels of the hepatic apoptotic mediator p53. Overall, the research results suggest that thyme, or thymol, can reduce liver toxicity and damage caused by doxorubicin.

☐ A comparison of the activity of ten essential oils against antibiotic-resistant *E. coli* and *L. monocytogenes* showed that clove, thyme, cinnamon, and garlic were highly active against both bacteria, but turmeric, cumin, black pepper, and marjoram were inactive against *L. monocytogenes*.[9349] Ginger and parsley were moderately active against both bacteria. A combination of clove and thyme exhibited the strongest activity against *L. monocytogenes*. Combinations of clove + cinnamon, cinnamon + garlic, and cinnamon + thyme were synergistic against *E. coli*; the same combinations plus clove + thyme, and clove + garlic were synergistic against *L. monocytogenes*. Composition was not reported for the essential oils used in the study.

☐ Thyme, oregano, lemongrass, spearmint, and rosemary essential oils each inhibited multidrug-resistant foodborne pathogens isolated from raw milk (*Escherichia, Enterobacter, Citrobacter, Proteus, Klebsiella*, and *Staphylococcus*) but were ineffective against *Pseudomonas*.[9350] Thyme was the most active followed by oregano.

☐ Investigation of the antifungal and antivirulence activity of basil CT linalool, cinnamon bark, clove, tea tree, oregano CT carvacrol, and thyme CT thymol essential oils (EOs) on five *Candida* species (*C. albicans, C. auris, C. krusei, C. parapsilosis*, and *C. guillermondii*) revealed that clove and cinnamon inhibited all fungal species tested; cinnamon, oregano, and thyme inhibited biofilm formation of *C. albicans, C. guilliermondii*, and *C. parapsilosis;* and each oil except tea tree downregulated virulence genes in *C. albicans*.[9351] In addition, thyme synergized the activity of fluconazole against all tested *Candida* species.

☐ Thyme CT geraniol was insecticidal to the lesser grain borer (*Rhyzopertha dominica*).[9352]

☐ Comparison of *Thymus* genus essential oils—*T. vulgaris* (thyme; 63.1% thymol), *T. zygis* (thyme; 26.5% thymol, 22.7% carvacrol), *T. satureioides* (thyme borneol; 29.3% borneol), and *T. mastichina* (wild marjoram; 31.9% linalool)—showed that *T. vulgaris* had the greatest antifungal effect on preformed biofilms in vapor phase and *T. mastichina* the lowest.[9353] Direct contact of *T. vulgaris* and *T. zygis* oils demonstrated higher antifungal activity when compared to vapor phase.

☐ The thymol CT of thyme essential oil inhibited *S. enterica, S. aureus,* and *L. monocytogenes*.[9354] Further research into its mechanism of action found that thymol and beta-sesquiphellandrene possibly target multiple bacterial pathways (topoisomerase II and DNA and RNA polymerases) that impair bacterial cell replication and transcription processes.

☐ Thyme essential oil enhanced (additive) the activity of itraconazole and fluconazole against clinical isolates and a reference strain of *C. albicans*.[9355]

☐ Cinnamon, clove, and thyme essential oils demonstrated remarkable antibacterial properties against multidrug-resistant strains of *S. enteritidis*.[9356] Moreover, biofilm formation was reduced by cinnamon, clove, thyme, turmeric, rosemary, and sage essential oils. Clove exhibited the greatest inhibition of violacein production, followed by thyme and cinnamon.

☐ Of five essential oils tested (tea tree, clove, thyme, spearmint, basil), thyme CT thymol essential oil exhibited the greatest activity against bacteria associated with acne (*C. acnes* and *S. epidermidis*).[9357] Moreover, thyme EO nanoemulsion suppressed the inflammatory response and reduced bacterial loads in acne animal models.

☐ A laboratory model of intestinal integrity assessed the benefits of tea tree, ginger, and thyme essential oils. Each oil showed antioxidant benefits and the reduction of reactive oxygen species (ROS)—elevated ROS can increase inflammation and damage intestinal tissues leading to poor intestinal integrity.[9358] In addition, ginger and thyme oils improved barrier integrity and reduced levels of claudin 2 and claudin 15 (key biomarkers for leaky gut). The findings suggest that thyme and ginger essential oil could support gut barrier function and intestinal integrity.

☐ Eight essential oils—thyme CT 1,8-cineole, spearmint, horsemint, rosemary, fringed lavender, marjoram, lemongrass (*C. citratus*), and eucalyptus (*E. globulus*)—were evaluated for their antimicrobial (*E. coli, S. aureus, C. albicans*) and beverage preservation (apple juice) properties.[9359] Thyme essential oil was the most effective, and the other oils showed a concentration-dependent inhibition.

☐ Thyme (26.0% para-cymene, 22.6% thymol, 21.3% carvacrol) was potently larvicidal against *Anisakis* larvae—killing all larvae within four hours—and displayed high activity against *L. monocytogenes* on smoked fish.[9360]

☐ Incorporation of thyme into a nanocomposite hydrogel (NCHG) improved the sustained release of the oil and significantly higher antibacterial effects in comparison to free oil. Moreover, the NCHG remarkably promoted wound healing.[9361]

☐ The thymol CT of thyme essential oil (26.9% thymol, 14.5% para-cymene, 13.4% linalool, 5.7% carvacrol) was toxic to the mulberry pyralid (*Glyphodes pyloalis*), with the whole oil being more effective than isolated thymol and carvacrol.[9362]

☐ Thyme CT carvacrol, sage CT beta-thujone, and apple mint CT piperitenone oxide were insecticidal to the medfly (*Ceratitis capitata*) and larvicidal to the tomato leafminer (*Tuta absoluta*), with apple mint being the most effective.[9363]

☐ A clinical study found that 2% thyme essential oil—spraying the internal surface every night after washing and then rinse after fifteen minutes—significantly decreased colony count of *C. albicans* on removable orthodontic appliances, exerting efficacy similar to chlorhexidine.[9364]

☐ The antimicrobial, antioxidant (DPPH, ABTS, and FRAP assays), and anti-inflammatory (LOX inhibition) activity of thyme CT carvacrol (80.7%), oregano CT carvacrol (68.0%), and sage CT 1,8-cineole (55.8%) essential oils were evaluated in laboratory research.[9365] Oregano displayed the highest antioxidant activity, followed by thyme and sage. The greatest anti-inflammatory activity was observed with thyme. Oregano and thyme had higher antimicrobial activity against *S. aureus, E. coli,* and *L. fermentum*. Additionally, oregano and thyme essential oils inhibited intracellular invasion of sporozoites from the poultry parasite (*E. tenella*).

☐ Ischemia-reperfusion injuries (IRI) involve the loss of blood supply to tissues or an organ followed by the reestablishment of blood flow to the area. Loss of blood supply causes metabolic dysfunction leading to cellular damage and death. While restoration of blood flow is essential to rescue ischemic tissues, this process ironically causes further damage that threatens the function and viability of the tissue/organ. Oral administration of thyme essential oil as a preventive measure showed that it protects the liver during renal IRI by decreasing inflammation and oxidative stress.[9366]

☐ Thyme CT thymol, cinnamon bark, and tea tree essential oils each inhibited *E. coli* strains isolated from the drinking water of grazing animals in Italy.[9367] Thyme and cinnamon oils showed greater activity than antibiotics used in veterinary and human medicine (repen, macramid, baytril, augmentin, bimixin).

☐ Encapsulation of thyme CT thymol in the natural biosurfactant mannosylerythritol lipid enhanced its antimicrobial activity against *E. coli, S. aureus, B. subtilis, P. aeruginosa, Penicillium* sp., *A. flavus, F. oxysporum,* and *C. albicans*.[9368] It also increased its antioxidant capacity (ORAC and TEAC).

☐ Oregano CT carvacrol, thyme CT thymol, and mountain savory CT carvacrol essential oils and there mixtures were effective against clinical bacterial strains—*Staphylococcus* sp., *Streptococcus* sp., *P. aeruginosa, E. coli, K. pneumoniae, S. marcescens,* and *M. pachydermatis* strains—cultured from the ears of dogs affected by otitis externa (ear infection).[9369] The mixture contained equal parts of each oil and was the most active against the tested strains.

☐ Oregano CT carvacrol, thyme CT thymol, and tropical basil and their post-distillation byproducts—total, spent, and residual water extracts—were evaluated in enzyme inhibitory and antioxidant assays.[9370] The oils and extracts displayed antioxidant activity with the extracts exhibiting greater activity in the DPPH and ABTS assays, but the essential oils had the highest metal reducing power in the CUPRAC assay. Tropical basil and thyme essential oil also demonstrated good inhibition of acetylcholinesterase, suggesting they may aid cognition. The best butyrylcholinesterase inhibitory activity was observed with tropical basil essential oil. The oils also inhibited tyrosinase and amylase, which indicates they may be useful for skin brightening and glucose management as well.

☐ Encapsulating thyme essential oil with a natural biosurfactant (mannosylerythritol lipid) improved its antioxidant capacity and antimicrobial activity against *E. coli, S. aureus, Penicillium* sp., *A, flavus, F. oxysporum,* and *C. albicans*.[9371]

☐ Evaluation of *Lamiaceae* family essential oils (melissa, oregano CT carvacrol, thyme CT para-cymene, Spanish lavender, sage, rosemary CT 1,8-cineole, and peppermint) showed that melissa and oregano exhibit the best anticandidal activity (*C. albicans, C. glabrata, C. guilliermondii, C. krusei, C. parapsilosis,* and *C. tropicalis*), with Spanish lavender, peppermint, rosemary, and thyme also being very active.[9372] Oregano and thyme

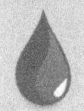

demonstrated the strongest antibiofilm activity, followed by Spanish lavender, peppermint, and rosemary.

☐ Thyme CT thymol essential oil helped protect against *E. coli* infection in the intestines by effectively maintaining epithelial integrity and tight junctions and reducing inflammation in a laboratory setting.[9373]

☐ Thyme essential oil with 44.4% thymol and 69.4% limonene demonstrated bacteriostatic and bactericidal activity against widespread foodborne pathogens (*S. enterica* subsp. *enterica* serovar Typhimurium and *B. cereus*).[9374] It also exhibited antibiofilm activity.

☐ Sodium hypochlorite (used to purify pools) can wreak havoc on the skin, lungs, and eyes. Inhaling thyme essential oil reduced the harmful effects of sodium hypochlorite in rats.[9375]

☐ Pine, melissa (43.0% citral, 25.0% beta-caryophyllene), ginger, lemon, thyme CT thymol, and basil CT methyl chavicol essential oils each showed activity against MRSA and *E. coli*. Thyme completely inhibited all bacteria at all concentrations tested.[9376]

☐ Thyme CT thymol essential from plants harvested at the beginning of the flowering phase acted as a potent inhibitor of cytokine production (IL-6, IL-8, IL-beta, and TNF-α) in *P. aeruginosa*–induced macrophages, showing an anti-inflammatory effect.[9377] Both the oil and isolated thymol also increased CAT and SOD antioxidant activity.

---

# TOLU BALSAM
## (Balsam of Tolu, Thomas Balsam, Opobalsam)

*Myroxylon balsamum* (L.) Harms. var. *balsamum*, *M. balsamum* (L.) Harms. var. *genuinum*, *Toluifera balsamum* L., *M. toluiferum* H.B. et K.

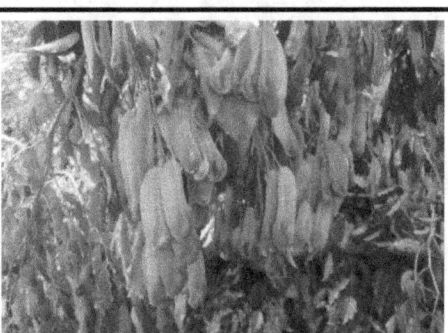

**FAMILY:** Fabaceae

**NOTE:** Base

**AROMA INTENSITY:** Medium

**AROMA:** Balsamic, rich, sweet, soft hint of vanilla

**COMMON EXTRACTION METHOD:** Steam distilled from the resin

**POSSIBLE SUBSTITUTE OILS:** Peru balsam, ylang ylang, copaiba, frankincense

**BLENDS WELL WITH:** Balsam fir, black pepper, cardamom, cassia, cedarwood, cinnamon, clove, copaiba, frankincense, ginger, lemon, lime, neroli, orange, palo santo, patchouli, Peru balsam, petitgrain, rose, sandalwood, tangerine, ylang ylang

**SUBCELLULAR LOCALIZATION | EPIGENETIC INFLUENCE:** Currently unknown | Currently unknown

**RECOMMENDED DILUTION RANGE:** 1.5%–5.0%

**PRIMARY CONSTITUENTS:**[9378]

| Constituent | Percent |
|---|---|
| Benzyl Benzoate | 46.6% |
| Benzyl Alcohol | 41.8% |
| (E)-Cinnamic Acid | 2.7% |
| Benzoic Acid | 2.5% |

Note: Tolu balsam essential oil is very difficult to extract through hydrodistillation or steam distillation so it is often extracted with alcohol (ethanol), which is actually a resinoid absolute and not an essential oil.

**OTHER CONSTITUENTS:** (Z,E)-cinnamyl acetate, vanillin, ethyl cinnamate

**PREFERRED COMPOSITION FOR CLINICAL USE:**

| Constituent | |
|---|---|
| Benzyl Benzoate | 35%–55% |
| Benzyl Alcohol | 30%–50% |
| (E)-Cinnamic Acid | 1%–5% |
| Benzoic Acid | 1%–5% |

**REPORTED THERAPEUTIC PROPERTIES:** Antibacterial, antifungal, antiseptic, antiparasitic, **analgesic**, anti-inflammatory, antiarthritic, **antirheumatic**, eases cough, relieves sprains and strains, diuretic, astringent, relieves headache, UV protection, wound healing, nourishes the hair and skin, relieves chronic skin conditions, relieves dandruff, aids circulation, antioxidant, **supports respiratory function**, expels excess mucus, relieves painful menstruation, aids detoxification, eases cough, supports oral health, relieves diarrhea, insecticide, relieves anxiety, stress management, combats anger, relieves emotional trauma, antidepressant

**CAUTIONS:**

■ Oral caution. Ingestion of benzoic acids, benzoic salts (calcium, potassium, and sodium), benzaldehyde, benzyl acetate, benzyl benzoate, and benzyl alcohol may cause gastrointestinal irritation, vomiting, and diarrhea.[9379] The Joint Expert Committee for Food Additives (JECFA) has established an acceptable daily limit for the aforementioned constituents of 0–5mg/kg body weight for adults to avoid GI discomfort.[9380] Based on this limit, it is suggested to limit the oral consumption to no more than 4 drops daily.

■ Dilutions of less than 1.0% are strongly recommended for people with chronic skin conditions, allergies, compromised immune systems, or chronic respiratory conditions based on reports of sensitization among those with a compromised immune system and people without a compromised immune system using Peru balsam (similar composition to tolu balsam).[9381,9382,9383] Contact dermatitis has also been reported with tolu balsam.[9384]

■ Resinoids and absolutes should not be taken orally due to the presence of solvent residue. If the oil is extracted with a solvent, avoid oral administration.

**SELECTED EVIDENCE:**

  □ *In vitro* research suggests that the hexane extract of tolu balsam (that contains volatile constituents found in the essential oil) demonstrated good activity against twenty-one multiresistant strains of *P. aeruginosa*, sixteen multi drug-resistant MRSA strains, and eight drug-sensitive *Staphylococcus aureus* strains isolated from patients in three Brazilian hospitals.[9385]

  □ Tolu balsam is considered a natural sun-block agent based on *in vitro* research.[9386]

---

# TSAURI GRASS
## (Beignefata, Ahibero)

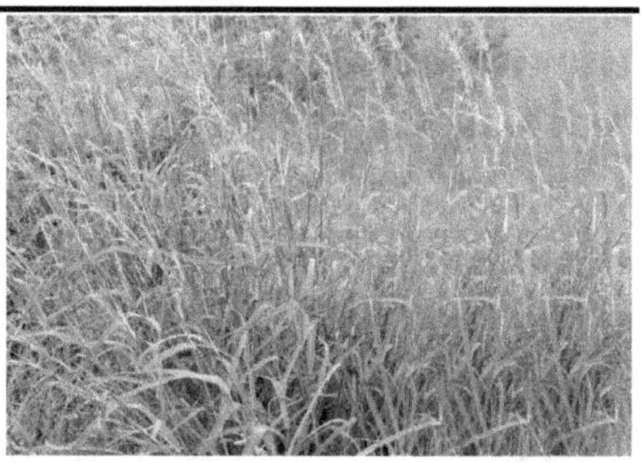

*Cymbopogon giganteus* (Hochst.) Chiov., *Andropogon giganteus* Hochst.; **Citronella of Madagascar, Ahibero**: *Cymbopogon giganteus* (Hochst.) Chiov. var. *madagascariensis*

**FAMILY:** Poaceae (Gramineae)
**NOTE:** Middle-Top
**AROMA INTENSITY:** Medium
**AROMA:** Fresh, spicy, earthy, musky, grassy, weakly fruity-floral
**COMMON EXTRACTION METHOD:** Steam distilled from the leaves (grass blades)
**POSSIBLE SUBSTITUTE OILS:** Gingergrass, palmarosa, lemongrass
**BLENDS WELL WITH:** Agarwood, bergamot, black pepper, cedarwood, elemi, frankincense, geranium, ginger, gingergrass, grapefruit, Japanese cedarwood, lavender, lavandin, lemon, lime, may chang, orange, palmarosa, patchouli, peppermint, rosemary, rosewood, sandalwood, spearmint, vetiver, ylang ylang
**SUBCELLULAR LOCALIZATION | EPIGENETIC INFLUENCE:** Currently unknown | Currently unknown
**RECOMMENDED DILUTION RANGE:** 3%–50%; neat for limited conditions

**PRIMARY CONSTITUENTS:**[9387,9388,9389,9390,9391,9392,9393]

| *Cymbopogon giganteus* | | *Cymbopogon giganteus* var. *madagascariensis* | |
|---|---|---|---|
| Limonene | 7.7%–42.0% | Limonene | 5.1%–24.0% |
| (Z)-p-Mentha-1(7),8-Dien-2-ol | 0.0%–27.7% | (E)-p-Mentha-1(7),8-Dien-2-ol | 14.7%–22.4% |
| (E)-p-Mentha-2,8-Dien-1-ol | 0.0%–26.2% | (Z)-p-Mentha-1(7),8-Dien-2-ol | 12.3%–19.0% |

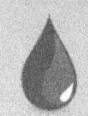

| | | | |
|---|---|---|---|
| (E)-p-Mentha-1(7),8-Dien-2-ol | 0.0%–22.3% | (E)-p-Mentha-2,8-Dien-1-ol | 11.2%–19.0% |
| Carvotanacetone | 0.0%–19.9% | (Z)-p-Mentha-2,8-Dien-1-ol | 8.3%–9.8% |
| (Z)-Limonene Oxide | 0.0%–19.2% | Carvone | 3.1%–3.9% |
| Cis-DihydroCarvone | 0.0%–17.2% | (E)-Isopiperitenol | 2.3%–3.9% |
| (Z)-p-Mentha-2,8-Dien-1-ol | 0.0%–16.3% | | |
| (Z)-Verbenol | 0.0%–9.6% | | |
| 2-Pinen-4-ol | 0.0%–8.9% | | |
| (E)-Isopiperitenol | 0.0%–7.1% | | |
| (Z)-Carveol | 0.0%–6.4% | | |
| (E)-Piperitol | 0.0%–5.4% | | |
| Myrtenol | 0.0%–5.3% | | |
| (Z)-Ocimenone | 0.0%–5.2% | | |
| (E)-Carveol | 0.0%–5.1% | | |
| (Z)-Isopiperitenol | 0.0%–4.2% | | |
| Dihydrocarvylacetate | 0.0%–4.2% | | |
| Neo-Dihydrocarvylacetate | 0.0%–4.2% | | |
| Alpha-Pinene | 0.0%–4.1% | | |
| (Z)-Piperitol | 0.0%–3.9% | | |

Note: Tsauri grass essential oil composition varies greatly and could be divided into at least four chemotypes. Most samples are predominantly p-menthadienols and limonene.

**OTHER CONSTITUENTS:** *Cymbopogon giganteus*—para-cymene, isoamyl hexanoate, (E)-beta-terpineol, p-methyl-acetophenone, 4-methylene-isophorone, dien-2-ol, nerol, (E)-carvone, geranial, gamma-terpin-7-al, citronellyl acetate, 1,3,8-p-menthatriene; *Cymbopogon giganteus* var. *madagascariensis*—para-cymene, para-cymenene, (E)-limonene-1,2-oxide, (Z)-limonene-1,2-oxide, (Z)-isopiperitenol, 3,9-oxy-mentha-1,8(10)-diene, (Z)-dihydroperillaldehyde, (E)-dihydroperillaldehyde, (E)-carveol, (Z)-carveol, phenylethyl hexanoate, ascaridole (<0.4%)

**PREFERRED COMPOSITION FOR CLINICAL USE:**

| Constituent | var. *madagascariensis* |
|---|---|
| **Limonene** | 8%–30% |
| **(E)-p-Mentha-1(7),8-Dien-2-ol** | 15%–25% |
| **(Z)-p-Mentha-1(7),8-Dien-2-ol** | 10%–20% |
| **(E)-p-Mentha-2,8-Dien-1-ol** | 10%–20% |
| **(Z)-p-Mentha-2,8-Dien-1-ol** | 5%–10% |
| **Carvone** | 2%–5% |
| **(E)-Isopiperitenol** | 2%–5% |

**REPORTED THERAPEUTIC PROPERTIES: Antibacterial**, antifungal, antiviral, antiseptic, antiparasitic, anticancer, analgesic, anti-inflammatory, relieves toothache, antiarthritic, antirheumatic, reduces high blood pressure, aids circulation, supports immune function, expels excess mucus, supports respiratory function, eases cough, nourishes the skin, **relieves chronic skin conditions**, astringent, reduces the appearance of acne, wrinkles, scars, and blemishes, soothes sore throat, insect repellent, relieves anxiety, relaxing/calming, improves focus/concentration, aids mental clarity

**CAUTIONS:**
- None currently known.

**SELECTED EVIDENCE:**
- □ Tsauri grass essential oil produces its anti-inflammatory activity partly by inhibiting the 5-LOX enzyme, COX enzymes, and weakly inhibiting the LOX-1 enzyme.[9394,9395]
- □ *In vitro* research shows that tsauri grass essential oil moderately to significantly inhibits gram-positive bacteria (*S. aureus* and a clinical isolate of *Enterococcus faecalis*), gram-negative bacteria (*E. coli, Pseudomonas aeruginosa,* and clinical isolates of *Klebsiella pneumoniae, Proteus vulgaris,* and *Salmonella*

sp.), and the fungus *C. albicans*.[9396] The study authors suggested that the antimicrobial activity of tsauri grass essential oil may be attributed to the presence of limonene and the p-menthadienols. Another study reported that tsauri grass essential oil inhibited gram-positive bacteria (*S. aureus, E. faecalis,* and *L. monocytogenes*), and gram-negative bacteria (*E. coli, P. aeruginosa, Salmonella enterica, S. typhimurium, Enterobacter aerogenes* and *Shigella dysenteriae*).[9397] The essential oil was more active than standard antibiotics (tetracycline and erythromycin) against *E. faecalis, L. monocytogenes, S. typhimurium, S. dysenteria,* and *P. aeruginosa,* and produced a synergistic or additive antimicrobial effect with lemongrass essential oil against *S. aureus, L. monocytogenes, E. coli, E. aerogenes, S. typhimurium,* and *S. dysenteria*.

- ☐ Tsauri grass essential oil demonstrated weak antioxidant activity compared to BHT.[9398]
- ☐ Lemongrass (*C. citratus*) and tsauri grass both demonstrated good antioxidant activity with lemongrass performing better in DPPH test and tsauri grass performing better in the ABTS test.[9399]

# TSUGA
## (Hemlock Spruce, Eastern Hemlock)

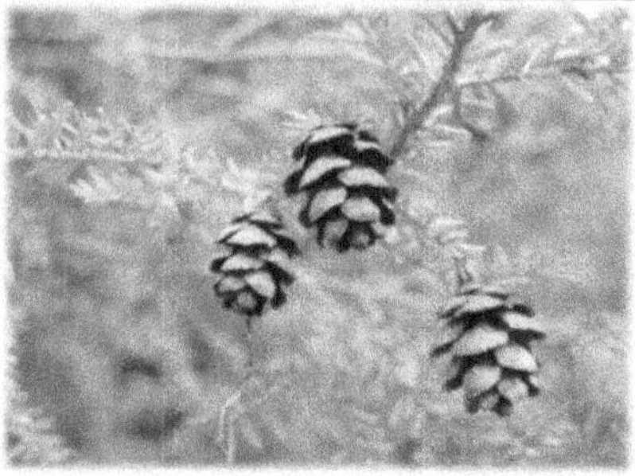

*Tsuga canadensis* (L.) Carrière, *Pinus canadensis* L.

**FAMILY:** Pinaceae
**NOTE:** Top-Middle
**AROMA INTENSITY:** Medium
**AROMA:** Woody, balsamic, slightly fruity
**COMMON EXTRACTION METHOD:** Steam distilled from the needles and twigs
**POSSIBLE SUBSTITUTE OILS:** Blue spruce, spruce (black), silver fir, rosemary (bornyl acetate CT), balsam fir, white fir, pine
**BLENDS WELL WITH:** Balsam fir, blue spruce, cedarwood, clary sage, lavender, pine, rosemary, sandalwood, spruce (black), silver fir, white fir
**SUBCELLULAR LOCALIZATION | EPIGENETIC INFLUENCE:** Currently unknown | Currently unknown
**RECOMMENDED DILUTION RANGE:** 3%–33%; neat for limited conditions

**PRIMARY CONSTITUENTS:**[9400,9401]

| | |
|---|---|
| Bornyl Acetate* | 26.8%–39.6% |
| Alpha-Pinene | 16.4%–23.7% |
| Camphene | 11.9%–14.5% |
| Limonene | 3.4%–6.2% |
| Tricyclene | 0.0%–6.2% |
| Beta-Phellandrene | 0.0%–4.4% |

**OTHER CONSTITUENTS:** Beta-pinene, alpha-phellandrene, beta-myrcene, alpha-terpinolene, para-cymene, beta-caryophyllene, alpha-humulene, alpha-terpineol, terpinen-4-ol, camphor, cycloheptane, piperitone, 1,3-cyclopentadiene, 2-cyclohexene-1-one, 1,3-benzenediamine, borneol

**PREFERRED COMPOSITION FOR CLINICAL USE:**

| Constituent | CT 1 | CT 2 |
|---|---|---|
| **Isobornyl Acetate/Bornyl Acetate*** | 20%–40% | 30%–40% |
| **Alpha-Pinene** | 15%–25% | 10%–20% |
| **Camphene** | 5%–20% | 3%–10% |
| **Limonene** | 3%–10% | 3%–10% |
| **Beta-Pinene** | 1%–6% | 10%–25% |
| **Tricyclene** | 1%–5% | – |
| **Myrcene** | 1%–5% | 0.5%–4% |
| **Isobornyl Acetate/Bornyl Acetate*** | 0.1%–4% | 0%–5% |
| **Beta-Phellandrene** | 0.1%–4% | 1%–4% |

\* GC/MS reports identify the primary constituent in *T. canadensis* as bornyl acetate, but a recent study suggests that this may

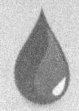

actually be isobornyl acetate.[9402] This misidentification is understandable considering they share the same Kovats Retention Indices (1285) and their close elution. Interpretation of the Adams GC/MS database and identification of electron impact conditions is required to properly identify the correct constituent.

**REPORTED THERAPEUTIC PROPERTIES: Analgesic (pain relief), anti-inflammatory**, anti-infectious, antimicrobial, antiseptic, antioxidant, astringent, diuretic, expectorant, removes excess mucus, **aids endocrine system function**, nervine (calms and soothes the nerves), increases redness and circulation of a localized area, aids circulation, **supports normal respiration, eases cough**, antifungal, grounding, uplifting, encourages a sense of calm, helps remove emotional blocks

**CAUTIONS:**
■ None currently known.

**SELECTED EVIDENCE:**
☐ Tsuga essential oil kills bladder cancer cells *in vitro*.[9403]

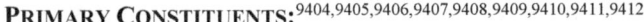

# TURKISH PINE
## (Calabrian Pine, Brutia Pine)
*Pinus brutia* Ten.

**FAMILY:** Pinaceae
**NOTE:** Top-Middle
**AROMA INTENSITY:** Medium-Strong
**AROMA:** Woody, fresh, balsamic, piney
**COMMON EXTRACTION METHOD:** Steam distilled from the

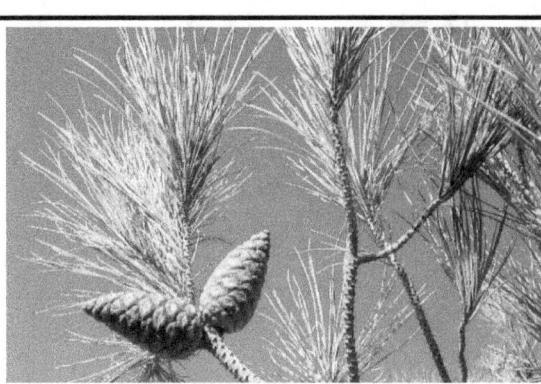

needles (leaves); may also be distilled from the resin, twigs, cones, needles/twigs, or bark
**POSSIBLE SUBSTITUTE OILS:** Pine, white pine, maritime pine, juniper, balsam fir, dwarf pine
**BLENDS WELL WITH:** Balsam fir, bergamot, blue spruce, cedarwood, frankincense, galbanaum, grapefruit, juniper, lavender, lavandin, lemon, orange, pine, peppermint, rosemary, sandalwood, spruce (black), silver fir, tangerine, white fir
**SUBCELLULAR LOCALIZATION | EPIGENETIC INFLUENCE:** Currently unknown | Currently unknown
**RECOMMENDED DILUTION RANGE:** 3%–50%; neat for limited conditions

**PRIMARY CONSTITUENTS:**[9404,9405,9406,9407,9408,9409,9410,9411,9412]

| Needles/Twigs | | Twigs | |
|---|---|---|---|
| Beta-Pinene | 20.0%–26.8% | Delta-3-Carene | 14.2%–25.1% |
| Delta-3-Carene | 11.3%–21.2% | Beta-Pinene | 17.5%–19.2% |
| Alpha-Pinene | 18.1%–19.0% | Alpha-Pinene | 14.5%–18.2% |
| Germacrene D | 3.3%–8.1% | Limonene | 1.5%–13.4% |
| Myrcene | 4.9%–7.6% | Myrcene | 5.5%–11.0% |
| Beta-Caryophyllene | 5.6%–6.2% | Beta-Caryophyllene | 6.8%–9.7% |
| | | Germacrene D | 1.4%–5.5% |
| *Needles* | | | |
| Alpha-Pinene | 14.4%–90.2% | *Resin* | |
| Beta-Pinene | 0.0%–47.5% | Alpha-Pinene | 21.4% |
| Germacrene D | 0.0%–17.9% | Beta-Pinene | 9.7% |
| Beta-Caryophyllene | 0.0%–14.5% | Beta-Caryophyllene | 9.1% |
| Alpha-Terpinyl Acetate | 0.0%–5.3% | Longifolene | 8.6% |
| | | Limonene | 5.8% |

*Bark*

| | | | | |
|---|---|---|---|---|
| Alpha-Pinene | 14.9% | *Cones* | | |
| Beta-Caryophyllene | 11.2% | Alpha-Pinene | 30.9%–40.7% |
| Delta-3-Carene | 9.6% | Beta-Pinene | 28.3%–39.6% |
| Caryophyllene Oxide | 6.9% | Delta-3-Carene | 7.8%–13.4% |
| Alpha-Terpineol | 6.7% | Beta-Caryophyllene | 0.0%–5.1% |
| Neryl Acetate | 5.9% | | |
| Beta-Pinene | 5.7% | | |

**OTHER CONSTITUENTS:** *Needles/Twigs*—Camphene, (E)-beta-ocimene, gamma-terpinene, terpinolene, linalyl acetate, longifolene, alpha-humulene, (E)-methyl isoeugenol, gamma-cadinene; *Needles*—Limonene, sabinene, myrcene, alpha-terpineol, camphene, beta-phellandrene, 1,3,6-octatriene, linalyl acetate, alpha-humulene, butanoic acid, delta-cadinene, alpha-bisabolene, caryophyllene oxide; *Twigs*—Camphene, gamma-terpinene, limonene, beta-phellandrene, terpinolene, alpha-terpineol, trans-anethole, longifolene, alpha-humulene, delta-cadinene, caryophyllene oxide, alpha-acorenol, thymol; *Bark*—Camphene, benzene,1-methyl-2, limonene, gamma-terpinolene, trans-pinocarveol, borneol, terpinene-4-ol, benzene,1-methoxy-4, 2-4,decadienal, alpha-longipinene, alpha-humulene, alpha-cadinol, benzyl benzoate, n-hexadecanoic acid, 9,12-octadecanoic acid, abietal, stilbene, dehydroabietal, dehydroabietic acid, rosin acids; *Resin*—Camphene, myrcene, alpha-phellandrene, beta-phellandrene, 1,3,8-o-menthatriene, 4-carene, verbenene, camphanone, trans-verbenol, alpha-phellandren-8-ol, alpha-humulene, caryophyllene oxide, aromadendrene oxide, seychellene; *Cones*—Camphene, myrcene, limonene, beta-phellandrene, alpha-terpinolene, trans-pinocarveol, alpha-terpineol, myrtenal, myrtenol, alpha-humulene, caryophyllene oxide

**PREFERRED COMPOSITION FOR CLINICAL USE:**

| Constituent | Needles/Twigs |
|---|---|
| **Beta-Pinene** | 20%–30% |
| **Alpha-Pinene** | 15%–25% |
| **Delta-3-Carene** | 11%–22% |
| **Myrcene** | 5%–10% |
| **Beta-Caryophyllene** | 5%–10% |
| **Germacrene D** | 3%–10% |
| **Terpinolene** | 1%–5% |
| **Alpha-Humulene** | 1%–4% |
| **Gamma-Cadinene** | 0.1%–3% |

**REPORTED THERAPEUTIC PROPERTIES:** Analgesic (pain relief), anti-inflammatory, antineuralgic, nervine (calms and soothes the nerves), antirheumatic, antiseptic, **antimicrobial**, antibacterial, antifungal, antioxidant, soothes chronic skin conditions, expels excess mucus, aids digestion, diuretic, **supports respiratory function**, eases cough, aids cognition, insecticide, stimulating, stress management, reduces anxiety, reduces anger, grounding, relieves fatigue

**CAUTIONS:**

■ None currently known.

**SELECTED EVIDENCE:**

◻ *In vitro* research demonstrates that Turkish pine essential oil (needles) inhibits the foodborne pathogens *E. coli, Salmonella paratyphi* A, *K. pneumoniae,* and *Y. enterocolitica.*[9413] Other research suggests that Turkish pine essential oil (resin) inhibits several bacteria (*B. cereus, S. aureus, E. faecalis, E. casseliflavus,* and *E. hormaechei*) and *C. albicans*, with greatest activity observed against *Micrococcus luteus* and *Bacillus subtilis.*[9414] Interestingly, the cone essential oil inhibited gram-negative bacteria (*E. coli*) better than gram-positive bacteria (*S. aureus, B, subtilis*) and fungi (*C. albicans*).[9415]

◻ Turkish pine essential oil (resin) kills the phytopathogens *Lactuca sativa, Lepidium sativum,* and *Portulaca oleracea.*[9416]

◻ *In vitro* research demonstrates that Turkish pine (needles, twigs, or resin) is a moderate antioxidant.[9417,9418] An

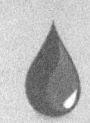

interesting chemotype of Turkish pine essential oil (aerial parts) with alpha-terpinolene (35.5%), terpinen-4-ol (11.9%), and beta-phellandrene (8.4%) as primary constituents demonstrated weak antioxidant activity.[9419]

◻ Turkish pine essential oil (needle) weakly inhibited AChE and BChE enzyme activity, which was attributed to its alpha-pinene, beta-pinene, and limonene content.[9420] The twig oil was a very weak (almost inactive) inhibitor. Inhibition of AChE prevents the breakdown of acetylcholine, which is essential for memory and thinking. People with neurodegenerative diseases make less acetylcholine, and the diseases often break it down at a faster rate, leading to acetylcholine deficits. Selective inhibition of BChE is also desirable in neurodegenerative diseases because it interferes with acetylcholine activity. In addition, BChE is often found in the plaques and tangles in the brains of people with Alzheimer's disease.[9421]

◻ Turkish pine essential oil (resin) kills Mediterranean flour moth (*Ephestia kuehniella*) eggs.[9422] The needle essential oil effectively killed and significantly repelled the *Ae. albopictus* mosquito.[9423]

# TURMERIC
## (Curcuma Oil, Indian Saffron)

*Curcuma longa* L., *C. domestica* Valeton; **White Turmeric, Zedoary**: *C. zedoaria* (Berg.) Rosc.; **Wild Turmeric**: *C. aromatica* Salisb.

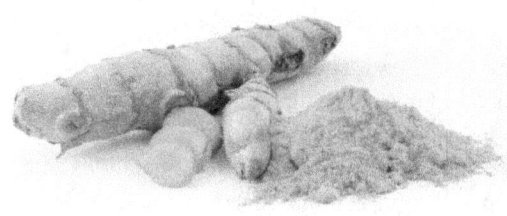

**FAMILY:** Zingiberaceae
**NOTE:** Base
**AROMA INTENSITY:** Medium
**AROMA:** Earthy, warm, slightly spicy and woody
**COMMON EXTRACTION METHOD:** Steam distilled from the rhizomes or leaves; may also be solvent extracted from the rhizomes
**POSSIBLE SUBSTITUTE OILS:** Ginger, sandalwood
**BLENDS WELL WITH:** Cistus, clary sage, clove, copaiba, cinnamon, frankincense, ginger, helichrysum, juniper, lavender, nutmeg, vetiver, wintergreen, ylang ylang
**SUBCELLULAR LOCALIZATION | EPIGENETIC INFLUENCE:** Currently unknown | *Musculoskeletal/Reproductive*
**RECOMMENDED DILUTION RANGE:** 5%–50%; neat for limited conditions

**PRIMARY CONSTITUENTS:**[9424,9425,9426,9427,9428,9429,9430,9431,9432,9433,9434,9435,9436,9437,9438,9439]

| *C. longa, Rhizome (Distilled)* | | *C. longa, Rhizome (Solvent Extracted)* | |
|---|---|---|---|
| ar-Turmerone | 5.4%–61.8% | ar-Turmerone | 5.4%–33.2% |
| Alpha-Turmerone | 0.0%–44.1% | Alpha-Turmerone | 6.5%–53.4% |
| Beta-Turmerone (Curlone) | 10.6%–18.5% | Beta-Turmerone (Curlone) | 18.1%–22.7% |
| Alpha-Phellandrene | 0.5%–9.4% | 3,5-Ditert-Butyl Phenol | 0.0%–5.4% |
| Alpha-Santalene | 0.8%–6.6% | | |
| ar-Curcumene | 0.5%–6.6% | *C. longa, Leaves* | |
| Beta-Sesquiphellandrene | 0.0%–5.6% | Alpha-Phellandrene | 8.0%–57.8% |
| 2-Carene | 0.0%–4.8% | Alpha-Terpinolene | 11.5%–26.4% |
| Zingiberene | 0.0%–4.4% | Para-Cymene | 4.8%–11.1% |
| | | 1,8-Cineole | 0.0%–10.5% |
| *C. zedoaria, Rhizomes (Distilled)* | | Beta-Pinene | 0.1%–4.7% |
| Curzerenone | 0.0%–31.6% | Limonene | 0.0%–4.6% |
| Curzerene | 0.0%–29.4% | | |
| Curdione | 0.0%–19.6% | *C. aromatica (Distilled)* | |
| Epi-Curzerenone | 0.0%–19.0% | Beta-Curcumene | 0.0%–29.9% |
| 1,8-Cineole | 0.0%–15.9% | Camphor | 2.4%–26.9% |
| ar-Curcumene | 0.0%–12.1% | Xanthorrhizol | 4.8%–25.7% |
| Alpha-Zingiberene | 0.0%–12.0% | ar-Curcumene | 0.0%–23.2% |
| Germacrone | 0.0%–10.8% | Camphene | 0.0%–10.2% |
| Camphor | 2.9%–10.3% | 1,8-Cineole | 0.1%–10.1% |
| Beta-Sesquiphellandrene | 0.0%–9.8% | Borneol | 0.0%–8.2% |

| | | | |
|---|---|---|---|
| Beta-Elemene | 0.0%–8.3% | Beta-Elemene | 0.4%–7.5% |
| Germacrene B | 0.6%–6.0% | Germacrone | 0.0%–4.9% |
| | | Curdione | 0.0%–4.8% |

*C. zedoaria, Rhizomes (Solvent Extracted)*

| | |
|---|---|
| Epi-Curzerenone | 24.1%–44.6% |
| Curzerene | 0.0%–10.4% |
| Curdione | 7.0%–13.8% |
| 5-Isopropylidene-3,8-Dimethyl-1(5H)-azulenone | 4.3%–9.2% |

*C. aromatica (Solvent Extracted)*

| | |
|---|---|
| Curcumol | 35.8% |
| ar-Turmerone | 7.0% |
| Linalool | 6.4% |
| Humulene Oxide | 6.4% |
| Caryophyllene Oxide | 5.9% |

Note: The rhizome essential oil is more commonly used in aromatherapy. However, essential oils distilled from the rhizome and the herb are both available commercially. Consumers should also be aware that solvent extracted turmeric absolutes are available commercially. As can be seen above, the composition of white turmeric and wild turmeric varies widely. Other chemotypes (1,8-cineole, curdione, etc.) are also reported in the literature.

**OTHER CONSTITUENTS:** *C. longa, Leaves*—Terpinen-4-ol, 2-octanol, alpha-pinene, gamma-terpinene, delta-3-carene, undecanol, alpha-terpinene, linalool, neral, ar-turmerone; *C. longa, Rhizome (Distilled)*—Alpha-bisabolene, beta-bisabolene, trans-ocimene, 1,8-cineole, benzene, 1-ethyl-4-isobutylbenzene, benzaldehyde, silane, 1,2,3,4,-tetramethyl-benzene, phenol, 2-octanol, delta-3-carene, terpinolene, viridiflorol, T-cadinol, (E)-alpha-atlantone, heptyl salicylate, humulene epoxide II; *C. longa, Rhizome (Solvent Extracted)*—Alpha-pinene, vinyl propionate, para-cymene, 1,8-cineole, gamma-curcumene, ar-curcumene, zingiberene, beta-sesquiphellandrene, ar-turmerol, alpha-cadinol, bisabolene, (E)-alpha-atlantone; *C. zedoaria, Rhizomes (Distilled)*—camphene, 1,8-cineole, iso-borneol, borneol, beta-bourbonene, beta-selinene, caryophyllene oxide, alpha-cadinol, T-cadinol, ar-turmerone (<1.5%), gamma-trans-atlantone, curcumenol, beta-turmerone, borneol, alpha-terpineol, beta-elemene, gamma-elemene, alpha-farnesene; *C. zedoaria, Rhizomes (Solvent Extracted)*—1,8-cineole, camphor, beta-elemene, alpha-terpineol, ar-curcumene, curcumol, isocucumenol; *C. aromatica (Distilled)*—alpha-piene, beta-myrcene, linalool, iso-borneol, caryophyllene, germacrene D, germacrene B, neo-curdione, curzerenone, curzerene, gamma-curcumene, beta-farnesene, ar-turmerol, alpha-bergamotene, alpha-terpineol, alpha-zingiberene; *C. aromatica (Solvent Extracted)*—2-nonanol, beta-elemene, terpinen-4-ol, caryophyllene, alpha-humulene, alpha-terpineol, alpha-selinene, beta-selinene, delta-cadinene, dodecanoic acid

**PREFERRED COMPOSITION FOR CLINICAL USE:**

| Constituent | CO2 C. longa | C. longa |
|---|---|---|
| **ar-Turmerone** | 30%–55% | 25%–42% |
| **Alpha-Turmerone** | 7%–25% | 5%–25% |
| **Beta-Turmerone** | 10%–20% | 1%–11% |
| **Alpha-Curcumene (ar-Curcumene)** | 3%–10% | 3%–8% |
| **Alpha-Zingiberene** | 0%–5% | 2%–7% |
| **Beta-Sesquiphellandrene** | 2%–7% | 2%–7% |

**REPORTED THERAPEUTIC PROPERTIES:** Antimicrobial, antibacterial, antimicrobial, antifungal, antiparasitic, antiviral, **antioxidant**, antiseptic, antispasmodic, relieves insect and snake bites, **anticancer**, antiarthritic, antitumor, **analgesic (pain relief)**, **anti-inflammatory**, **antirheumatic**, diuretic, **nervine (calms and soothes the nerves)**, **regenerates brain neurons**, supports liver function, nourishes and protects the skin, weight management, expels excess gas, **aids digestion**, eases cough, warming, **aids cognition**, relieves anxiety, promotes stability, stress management, improves mental clarity

**CAUTIONS:**

*Turmeric, C. longa*

■ May interact with aspirin, blood pressure, antiplatelet, and anticoagulant medications, and increase the risk of bleeding among people with bleeding disorders based on ar-turmerone content.[9440]

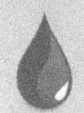

■ May interact with diabetes medications and cause low blood-sugar levels due to ar-turmerone content.[9441,9442] The primary constituent in the rhizome oil, ar-turmerone, inhibits alpha-glucosidase activity. Alpha-glucosidase is an enzyme that breaks down carbohydrates by chemical reaction with water. Inhibiting its activity postpones glucose absorption and therefore the impact of carbohydrates on blood sugar levels.

■ May interfere with enzymes that metabolize medications (NSAIDs, proton-pump inhibitors, acetaminophen, antiepileptics, immune modulators, blood-sugar medications, blood pressure medications, antidepressants, antipsychotics, diabetic medications, antihistamines, antibiotics, and anesthetics).[9443]

*White Turmeric, C. zedoaria*

■ Avoid during pregnancy and lactation. Animal research suggests that white turmeric essential oil (curzerene 29.4%, curdione 19.6%, 1,8-cineole 9.7%, germacrone 9.2%, beta-elemene 8.1%, camphor 2.9%, gamma-elemene 2.8%) is toxic to embryos and pregnant mothers (weight loss, abnormal blood results, and detrimental biochemical affects), and inhibits blood vessel growth for the placenta, which may cause placental calcification.[9444] The study authors attributed this effect to a combination of terpenoids present in the essential oil (1,8-cineole, camphor, beta-elemene, and germacrone, and possibly curzerene, curdione, and neocurdione), which were present in the blood of the animals.

*Wild Turmeric, C. aromatica*

■ Avoid with children under six due to potential moderate camphor content. Several cases of camphor poisoning and/or seizures from ingestion and topical application have been reported in children.[9445,9446] Ingestion of camphor-containing products has been lethal in children under age two.[9447] Children five years and up may use camphor-containing essential oils topically in dilutions no stronger than 5%. Camphor ingestion by infants and young children may cause cough, vomiting, seizure, burning sensation in the mucous membranes and eyes, or lack of voluntary coordination of muscle movements.[9448]

■ Caution is warranted during pregnancy and while lactating due to potential moderate camphor content. Ingestion of essential oils with significant levels of camphor may lead to abortion because fetuses lack the enzymes to process it.[9449] Camphor ingestion by infants and young children may cause cough, vomiting, seizure, burning sensation in the mucous membranes and eyes, or lack of voluntary coordination of muscle movements.[9450]

■ Avoid with epilepsy and Parkinson's due to potential moderate camphor content.[9451,9452]

■ The potential moderate camphor content in wild turmeric may negatively impact red blood cells and increase the risk of jaundice in children with glucose-6-phosphate dehydrogenase deficiency (G6PD).[9453,9454]

■ Oral caution—Essential oils with significant levels of camphor can be toxic when taken orally, usually single doses exceeding 2 mL, although the lethal dose for humans is estimated to be more than 5 mL in a single dose.[9455,9456,9457]

■ *Distilled*: Avoid with tamoxifen. Animal research suggests chronic administration of xanthorrhizol with tamoxifen increases cancer progression and tumor size.[9458]

■ *Distilled*: May interact with diabetic medications and cause low blood sugar due to xanthorrhizol content.[9459]

SELECTED EVIDENCE:

   □ White turmeric essential oil (primary components neocurdione, curdione, germacrone, curzerene, furanodiene, gamma-elemene, and 8,9-dehydro-9-formyl-cycloisolongifolene) kills and prevents the growth of ovarian cancer cells and increases the effectiveness of paclitaxel (a first-line chemotherapy drug for ovarian cancer).[9460] A white turmeric essential oil with major constituents of 8,9-dehydro-9-formyl-cycloisolongifolene, 6-ethenyl-4,5,6,7-tetrahydro-3,6-dimethyl-5-isopropenyl-trans-benzofuran, eucalyptol, and gamma-elemene triggered apoptosis in non-small cells lung carcinoma cells by altering various signaling pathways.[9461] White turmeric absolute suppressed melanoma growth and lung cancer metastasis by inhibiting angiogenesis (a process used by cancer cells to create their own blood vessel network).[9462] Another study concluded that white turmeric essential oil could inhibit promyelocytic leukemia cell proliferation.[9463]

   □ Injection of 100 mg/kg of wild turmeric every three days preserved manganese superoxide dismutase (MnSOD) in esophageal epithelium, which prevented the formation of Barrett's esophagus (a serious complication of acid reflux that causes tissue similar to the lining of the stomach to line the esophagus) and esophageal cancer in rats.[9464]

   □ A study determined that a combination of citronella, turmeric, kaffir lime (*C. hystrix*), hairy basil (*O.*

*americanum*), and vanilla could replace DEET (a common chemical insect repellent that is associated with brain cell damage and behavioral changes in animals) as a natural insect repellent.[9465]

☐ Turmeric oil significantly reduces stomach ulcers (up to 84.7%) caused by ethanol in rats.[9466]

☐ *In vitro* research concluded that turmeric oil inhibits alpha-glucosidase and alpha-amylase activity more effectively than acarbose (a drug used to control blood-sugar levels and treat diabetes).[9467] Inhibition of these enzymes is valuable in the treatment of diabetes because it slows the digestion of starches and therefore reduces blood-sugar spikes following the consumption of carbohydrates. Another study concluded that turmeric oil or oleoresin modulated gene expression related to glycolysis (cellular production of energy from glucose), which led to better glucose and lipid metabolism in mice.[9468]

☐ Oral administration of turmeric oil was mildly joint protective and antiarthritic when administered to rats.[9469]

☐ Animal research suggests that oral administration of 250 to 500 mg/kg of turmeric oil protects neurons and the brain from damage caused during a stroke.[9470,9471,9472]

☐ Turmeric oil helps decrease inflammation by strongly inhibiting the 5-lipoxygenase (5-LOX) enzyme that is involved in the inflammation response according to *in vitro* research.[9473] An animal study found that when turmeric oil was administered orally, with or without fish oil, it provided equivalent or better anti-inflammatory activity than aspirin.[9474] Interestingly, turmeric oil relieved pain better alone, as opposed to with fish oil.

☐ A 0.5% turmeric oil solution completely inhibited the growth of *A. flavus* (a fungus that produces aflatoxin), and prevented aflatoxin production by the fungus by more than 96%.[9475,9476,9477]

☐ Oral administration of 300 mg/kg of turmeric oil reduced high cholesterol as effectively as the drug Ezetimibe (a drug used to lower cholesterol) by modulating genes (PPARa and LXRa) involved in lipid metabolism and transport in hamsters.[9478] Interestingly, the researchers also noted that turmeric oil reduced oxidative stress, platelet activation, and blood-vessel dysfunction.

☐ Turmeric oil prevents *S. mutans* from sticking together and forming plaque (biofilm) *in vitro*, possibly leading to the prevention of cavities.[9479]

☐ *In vitro* research demonstrates that turmeric (*C. longa*) essential oil rich in beta-sesquiphellandrene (38.7%) and alpha-curcumene (18.4%) inhibits gram-positive bacteria (*B. subtilis, B. atrophaeus, S. aureus*), gram-negative bacteria (*E. coli, K. pneumonia, S, typhimurium, P. aeruginosa, E. carotovora, A. tumefaciens*), and *C. albicans*.[9480]

☐ A cream containing 6% turmeric oil inhibited the growth of dermatophytes (fungi that require keratin for growth and typically affect the skin, hair, and nails) on the skin.[9481]

☐ Clinical research suggests that 600 mg of turmeric oil (about 10 drops) mixed with 3 g of turmeric herb protected, in three equal doses, and reversed DNA damage and prevented cancer caused by oral submucous fibrosis (a precancerous condition of the oral mucosa that causes the formation of excess connective tissue of the oral mucosa, recurrent ulceration, ear pain and deafness, and decreased mouth opening).[9482] Participants in the trial consumed the oil/herb mixture orally in capsules for three months.

☐ Turmeric (*C. longa*) essential oil supports oral health by inhibiting *P. gingivalis*, which is a periopathogen associated with periodontitis (a serious gum infection that causes inflammation of the oral cavity and damages or destroys the soft tissue and bone that support the teeth).[9483]

☐ Turmerones prevent the growth of cancer cells *in vitro*.[9484,9485,9486] Research concluded that turmerones prevent migration of and trigger apoptosis in breast cancer cells, leukemia cells, and liver cancer cells, and stimulate the production of normal blood lymphocytes.[9487,9488,9489,9490,9491]

☐ Research suggests that ar-turmerone may slow or reverse neurodegenerative disorders like dementia, Alzheimer's disease, Parkinson's disease, and Huntington's disease. Researchers discovered that ar-turmerone significantly increased the production of neural stem cells (brain stem cells that are essential for the repair and recovery of brain function) *in vitro* and in rats.[9492] Another *in vitro* study found that ar-turmerone inhibited pathways involved in inflammation and protected hippocampal cells from toxicity.[9493]

☐ *In vitro* research shows that white turmeric absolute inhibits gram-positive (*S. aureus and B. cereus*) and gram-negative (*P. aeruginosa, V. parahaemolyticus, and S. typhimurium*) bacteria.[9494]

☐ White turmeric essential oil rich in curzerenone exhibited potent antioxidant activities.[9495] Another study concluded that white turmeric rich in epicurzerenone absolute is a moderate to good antioxidant—good in

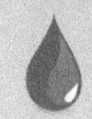

reducing power and excellent in the scavenging of 1,1-diphenyl-2-picrylhydrazyl radicals, but weak in chelating ferrous iron.[9496] Turmeric and wild turmeric absolutes were moderate to weak antioxidants when compared to BHA, vitamin E, and ascorbic acid.[9497] Wild turmeric exhibited potent antioxidant activity (greater than BHA) in another study.[9498]

☐ A 10% white turmeric essential oil protected against mosquito (*Aedes aegypti* and *Culex quinquefasciatus*) bites for 2.6 hours and caused 100% mortality of the larvae of both mosquito vectors.[9499,9500] Other research reports that white turmeric essential oil is significantly toxic to *Anopheles dirus* and *Ae. aegypti* mosquitoes.[9501,9502,9503] White turmeric essential oil was toxic to the maize weevil (*Sitophilus zeamais*) and red flour beetle (*Tribolium castaneum*).[9504] Wild turmeric absolute was a stronger repellent of the *Ae. aegypti* mosquito than the distilled oil (providing 1–1.5 hours of protection versus 0.5 hours).[9505]

☐ Turmeric essential oil (*C. longa*) promoted angiogenesis (the formation of new blood vessels, which is important for wound healing) in fertilized chicken eggs.[9506]

☐ Oral administration of ar-turmerone from turmeric essential oil prevented brain damage and memory impairment caused by neuroinflammation by normalizing brain glucose intake and metabolism and inhibiting the activation of microglia (nerve cells that act as key mediators of neuroinflammation and are important to triggering the brain degeneration process) and the production of inflammatory chemicals (cytokines).[9507] These properties suggest that ar-turmerone may be useful for multiple sclerosis and Alzheimer's disease, among many other neurological disorders.

☐ Turmeric essential oil killed prostate and liver cancer cells.[9508]

☐ Turmeric essential oil (*C. longa*, 35.9% ar-turmerone) demonstrated anxiolytic (relieves anxiety), sedative, and anticonvulsive activity in mice when injected.[9509] The essential oil was considered slightly toxic orally (LD50 2154 mg/kg) and moderately toxic when injected (LD50 693 mg/kg).

☐ Turmeric essential oil killed cervical cancer cells *in vitro* even at the lowest concentration tested (32.81 mcg/mL).[9510]

☐ *In vitro* research demonstrates that turmeric leaf essential oil (52.9% alpha-terpinolene, 21.1% alpha-phellandrene) alleviates skin inflammation by inhibiting proinflammatory cytokines (TNF-α, IL-6, IL-1β).[9511] Topical application of the oil reduced ear thickness and weight and reduced proinflammatory cytokines in a mouse model of inflammation.

☐ Human aryl hydrocarbon receptor (AhR: a gene that encodes a protein that helps regulate responses to planar aromatic hydrocarbons and significantly affects the immune activity in the gastrointestinal tract) regulates the circadian rhythm, helps regulate the cell cycle, and plays an important role in tissue development. Cumin, jasmine, vanilla, and bay leaf fully activate AhR; clove, dill, thyme, nutmeg, and oregano partially activate AhR; and tarragon, caraway, turmeric, lovage, fennel, spearmint, star anise, and anise inhibit the AhR activity.[9512]

☐ Aromatic-turmerone (*ar*-Turmerone) from turmeric essential oil reduced skin inflammation and ameliorated psoriasis in mice by inhibiting transfer of CD8+ T cells in epidermis and reducing expression of NF-κB and COX-2 as well as phosphorylation of p38 MAPK.[9513]

☐ Both ginger and turmeric (76.5% 1,8-cineole) essential oil protected against kidney damage caused by cadmium by reducing inflammation (reduced cytokines: IL-6, IL-10 and TNF-α) and renal adenosine deaminase (ADA) activity.[9514]

☐ Cinnamon (46.3% cinnamaldehyde), oregano (*O. vulgare*; 33.9% cis-p-menth-2-en-1-ol), and turmeric (55.4% ar-turmerone) essential oils each inhibited *S. aureus*, *E. coli*, and *P. aeruginosa*.[9515] Turmeric essential oil also exhibited potent antileishmanial activity against *L. amazonensis*.

☐ Turmeric leaf CT alpha-phellandrene essential oil was toxic to Australian sheep blowfly (*Lucilia cuprina*) larvae.[9516] Female flies lay their eggs in the open wounds of sheep, which cause large lesions on the sheep when they emerge.

☐ Turmeric (21.8% beta-turmerone, 14.7% ar-turmerone, 12.4% alpha-turmerone) essential oil demonstrated promising scolicidal effects against hydatid cysts protoscoleces *in vitro* and *in vivo*—killing 100% of protoscoleces at the dose of 100 μL/mL.[9517]

☐ Trypanosomiasis (also called sleeping sickness) is caused by *Trypanosoma brucei* (a parasite spread by tsetse flies in sub-Saharan Africa). Turmeric, white turmeric, and ginger essential oils all demonstrated antitrypanosomal activity against *Trypanosoma brucei* without harming human cells.[9518] The most promising oil was turmeric CT alpha-zingiberene.

☐ Topical application of turmeric essential oil reduced skin aging caused by UVB rays in a nude mouse model.[9519]

☐ A laboratory and rat model of benign prostatic hyperplasia (BPH; enlarged prostate) found that turmeric essential oil effectively triggered cell death (apoptosis) of BPH-1 cells and significantly reduced prostate weight and hyperplasia by modulating inflammatory pathways and suppressing the expression of 5alpha-reductase and the subsequent production of dihydrotestosterone (DHT).[9520] The suppression of 5alpha-reductase and the production of dihydrotestosterone is essential to reduce an enlarge prostate.

- An interesting turmeric essential oil with neral as the primary constituent and turmerones absent inhibited various fungi—sometimes better than the antimicrobial drugs clotrimazole, fluconazole, ketoconazole, and terbinafine—and displayed a synergistic or indifferent activity when combined with these drugs.[9521]

- Turmeric essential oil extracted from roots harvested from four separate provinces in China demonstrated good antioxidant activity in the DPPH assay.[9522] The turmeric oil with the highest ar-curcumene exhibited the highest antioxidant capacity.

- Ingestion of ar-turmerone, a primary constituent of turmeric essential oil, improved ulcerative colitis (prevented colon shortening, reduced colon tissue damage, and decreased inflammation (lowering COX-2 and TNF-$\alpha$) in mice.[9523] In addition, ar-turmerone improved the gut microbiome (abundance of flora, beneficial flora, and reducing harmful bacteria), which is known to improve colitis symptoms.

- Molecular docking studies of the major constituents found in turmeric leaf essential oil found that 3,7-cyclodecadien-1-one has strong binding potential to antifungal proteins (cytochrome P450 14 alpha-sterol demethylase, PDB ID: 1EA1, and N-myristoyl transferase, PDB ID: 1IYL), antioxidant (human peroxiredoxin 5, PDB ID: 1HD2), and antidiabetic proteins (human pancreatic alpha-amylase, PDB ID: 1HNY).[9524]

- Preclinical research found that turmeric oil and its terpenoids (beta-elemene, curcumol, furanodiene, and germacrone) have potential to stop the growth of gynecological cancers (cervical, endometrial, ovarian), limit the formation of tumors, and improve effectiveness of chemotherapy drugs.[9525]

- Turmeric leaf essential oil (31.3% alpha-phellandrene, 21.7% delta-2-carene, 13.5% 1,8-cineole, 5.5% o-Cymene)

- exhibited good antioxidant potential in the DPPH, ABTS, and hydrogen peroxide assays and was active against two breast cancer cell lines.[9526] It also demonstrated antibacterial activity against *E. coli, P. aeruginosa, S. aureus,* and *S. enterica.* Wild turmeric leaf essential oil (19.8% camphor, 15.3% curdione, 12.3% 2-bornanone) displayed weaker antioxidant, anticancer, and antimicrobial activity

- Ravintsara, turmeric, petitgrain (*C. aurantium*), and bitter orange essential oil each inhibited *Mycobacterium smegmatis* (a bacterial strain commonly used as a model for inhibition of *M. tuberculosis*), *C. albicans,* and *C. tropicalis.*[9527] The oils also displayed activity against collagenase, indicating an antiaging activity. Petitgrain and turmeric also inhibited elastase, which would preserve skin strength and flexibility.

- Lemongrass (*C. citratus*), basil, and turmeric essential oils were toxic to the red flour beetle (*Tribolium castaneum*), which was improved when combined with diatomaceous earth in emulsion form.[9528]

- Ginger, lemongrass (*C. citratus*), and turmeric each displayed antioxidant activity in the DPPH and ABTS assays, inhibited gram-negative (*K. oxytoca, P. vulgaris, E. coli, P. aeruginosa*) and gram-positive (*S. aureus, E. faecalis, L. grayi, M. luteus*) bacteria and yeasts (*C. albicans, S. cervisiae*), and mutagen-protecting effects.[9529]

- Immersion in white turmeric and eucalyptus (*E. globulus*) essential oils prevented hatching of head lice (*Pediculus humanus capitis*) eggs for seven to fourteen days, which significantly exceeded the efficacy of permethrin.[9530] Bitter ginger and temulawak essential oils also demonstrated a synergistic effect against head lice eggs when combined with eucalyptus (*E. globulus*).

# VALERIAN
## (European Valerian, Garden Valerian, Valerian Root)
*Valeriana officinalis* L.

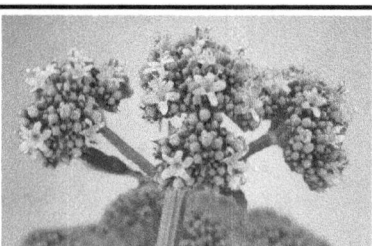

**FAMILY:** Valerianaceae
**NOTE:** Base
**AROMA INTENSITY:** Medium
**AROMA:** Musky, pungent, smoky, warm-woody, balsamic
**COMMON EXTRACTION METHOD:** Steam distilled from the roots
**POSSIBLE SUBSTITUTE OILS:** Spikenard, vetiver, lavender, spruce (black)
**BLENDS WELL WITH:** Basil, bay laurel, cassia, cedarwood, cinnamon, geranium, lavender, nutmeg, patchouli, petitgrain, pine, rosemary, sage, Spanish sage, spikenard, tangerine, vetiver
**SUBCELLULAR LOCALIZATION | EPIGENETIC INFLUENCE:** Currently unknown | Currently unknown
**RECOMMENDED DILUTION RANGE:** 5%–50%; neat for limited conditions

**PRIMARY CONSTITUENTS:**[9531,9532,9533]

| | |
|---|---|
| Bornyl Acetate | 2.9%–35.5% |
| Valerianol | 0.2%–33.9% |
| Alpha-Fenchene | 0.0%–28.3% |
| Valerenal | 0.1%–15.6% |
| Alpha-Pinene | 0.0%–14.8% |
| Nonyl Phenylacetate | 0.0%–13.8% |
| Isovaleric Acid | 0.0%–13.1% |
| Ledol | 0.0%–12.0% |
| Camphene | 0.0%–11.0% |
| Valeranone | 0.5%–10.9% |
| Myrtenyl Isovalerate | 0.3%–10.5% |
| Valerenic Acid | 0.0%–9.8% |
| Myrtenyl Acetate | 0.1%–9.1% |
| Beta-Eudesmol | 0.0%–8.3% |
| Kessane | 0.0%–8.2% |
| Butylated Hydroxytoluene | 0.0%–8.0% |
| Farnesal | 0.0%–8.0% |
| Eudesma-2,6,8-Triene | 0.0%–7.6% |
| Spathulenol | 0.0%–7.3% |
| Farnesyl Acetate | 0.0%–7.1% |
| Alloaromadendrene | 0.0%–6.9% |
| Borneol | 0.0%–6.6% |
| Trans-Pinocarveol Acetate | 0.0%–6.2% |
| Alpha-Bisabolol | 0.0%–5.4% |
| Hexadecanoic Acid | 0.0%–5.0% |
| Eugenyl Hexanoate | 0.0%–4.9% |
| Kessyl Alcohol | 0.0%–4.7% |
| Delta-Elemene | 0.0%–4.4% |
| Drimenol | 0.0%–4.4% |
| Epi-Bicyclosesquiphellandrene | 0.0%–4.2% |
| Limonene | 0.0%–4.0% |
| Aromadendrene | 0.0%–4.0% |

Note: Other chemotypes are also reported (maaliol, isovaleric acid, alpha-fenchene, valerenol, valeranone, and valerianol) but this is the most common chemotype reported in the literature.[9534] Valerenic acid (one of the constituents in valerian credited for its sedative effects—along with isovaleric acid) generally reaches its maximum concentration in plants harvested February to March.[9535]

**OTHER CONSTITUENTS:** Tricyclene, alpha-thujene, beta-pinene, para-cymene, gamma-terpinene, isoamyl isovalerate, menthone, terpinen-4-ol, alpha-terpineol, myrtenol, (E)-carveol, n-hexyl isovalerate, isomenthyl acetate, alpha-gurjunene, alpha-terpinyl acetate, caryophyllene, 2,6-dimethoxy-p-cymene, dehydroisolongifolene, beta-caryophyllene, sabinene, alpha-guaiene, alpha-humulene, linalyl isovalerate, germacrene B, germacrene D, ar-curcumene, beta-cedrene, beta-ionone, zingiberene, alpha-farnesene, bornyl isovalerate, bicyclogermacrene, valencene, gamma-cadinene, delta-cadinene, valencene ketone, caryophyllene oxide, neryl isovalerate, epi-globulol, t-muurolol, geranyl valerate, (Z,E)-farnesol, valerenol, cis-valerenyl acetate, kessyl acetate, trans-valerenyl isovalerate, pulegone (<1.5%), pacifigrgiol isomer

**PREFERRED COMPOSITION FOR CLINICAL USE:**

| Constituent | Bornyl Acetate CT | Balanced CT | Isovaleric Acid CT |
|---|---|---|---|
| **Bornyl Acetate** | 35%–55% | 8%–20% | 0.1%–3% |
| **Valerenal** | 4%–15% | 5%–15% | 0.1%–5% |

| | | | |
|---|---|---|---|
| Valerenic Acid | – | 5%–10% | 0.1%–3% |
| Isovaleric Acid | – | 1%–13% | 10%–22% |
| Vetiverol (Sesquiterpene Alcohol C) | – | 4%–8% | – |
| Spathulenol | 0.1%–3% | 3%–8% | 0.1%–3% |
| Allo-Aromadendrene | – | 1%–5% | 0.1%–3% |
| Valeranone | – | 0.6%–4% | – |
| Valerianol | – | 0.5%–3% | – |
| Camphene | 10%–25% | 0%–3% | 0.1%–3% |
| Alpha-Fenchene | 0.5%–5% | 0%–3% | 0.1%–3% |
| Maaliol | – | – | 5%–15% |
| Alpha-Copaene | – | – | 5%–15% |
| Patchoulol | – | – | 4%–10% |
| Beta-Caryophyllene | 0.5%–5% | – | 2%–8% |
| Alpha-Bulnesene | – | – | 2%–8% |
| Delta-Cadinene | – | – | 2%–8% |
| Beta-Gurjunene (Calarene) | – | – | 2%–8% |
| Valerana7,11-diene | – | – | 2%–8% |
| Valeric Acid | – | – | 2%–6% |
| Seychellene | – | – | 1%–5% |
| Jatamansone | – | – | 1%–5% |
| Alpha-Pinene | 4%–10% | – | – |
| Beta-Pinene | 3%–8% | – | – |
| Myrtenyl Acetate | 1%–5% | – | – |

Note: Essential oils with the bornyl acetate preferred composition may be found among plants grown in Belgium, the Czech Republic, and Germany.

**REPORTED THERAPEUTIC PROPERTIES:** Antimicrobial, antibacterial, anti-inflammatory, **antispasmodic**, supports cardiovascular balance, antineuralgic, nervine, anesthetic, headache/migraine, relieves digestive upset, **relieves menstrual cramps**, high blood pressure, relieves chronic skin conditions, reduces fever, expels excess gas, weight management, **promotes restful sleep**, aids cognitive function, sedating, stress management, **deeply relaxing**, relieves anxiety, antidepressant

**CAUTIONS:**

■ Volatile constituents in valerian are known to produce pronounced sedative effects. Theoretically, valerian could increase the sedating effects of alcohol, although this has not been proven in humans.[9536,9537] Nevertheless, caution is still warranted.

■ May interact with benzodiazepines, barbiturates (medications for anxiety and insomnia), antihistamines, tricyclic antidepressants, and other central nervous system depressants based on information from valerian root herb, which contains volatile constituents credited for some of the sedative effects of valerian.[9538,9539]

**SELECTED EVIDENCE:**

☐ *In vitro* research reported that a valerian essential oil rich in bornyl acetate, valeranone, and valerenic acid had a strong antimicrobial effect against *A. niger, E. coli, S. aureus,* and *Saccharomyces cerevisiae*.[9540] Interestingly, another variety rich in bornyl acetate, alpha-humulene, camphene, valerenone, and valerenic acid demonstrated low or no antimicrobial activity against the tested microbes. The study authors concluded that the antimicrobial activity of valerian depends on the plant variety and its developmental stage.

☐ The quality and quantity of sleep was improved in ICU patients by applying a 2.5% dilution of valerian essential oil to three acupressure points (Neiguan, Shenmen, and Yongquan—see image below for acupressure point locations) on each wrist and foot, followed by acupressure stimulation of the six points (five seconds of pressure and then released for one second) continuously for three minutes at each point.[9541]

☐ The volatile components of valerian directly act on the amygdaloid body (the amygdala serves to alert the body of danger and can go into overdrive and release noradrenaline in sleep-deprived individuals) of the

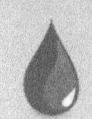

brain and valerenic acid inhibits the breakdown of GABA (gamma-aminobutyric acid) by enzymes, which causes a deeply relaxed and sedated state.[9542]

☐ Valerian essential oil was significantly toxic to the red flour beetle (*Tribolium castaneum*) and moderately toxic to the cigarette beetle (*Lasioderma serricorne*) and the booklouse (*Liposcelis bostrychophila*).[9543]

☐ Valerian exhibited contact toxicity against three stored-product insects (cigarette beetle booklouse, and red flour beetle), with the strongest activity observed against the red flour beetle.[9544]

☐ A preclinical model of insomnia found that ingestion of valerian essential oil relieves insomnia and increases sleep duration.[9545] Further evaluation of its mechanism determined that beta-caryophyllene attaches to serotonin receptors and activates pathways that increase serotonin and GABA, which could relieve anxiety and insomnia.

☐ Secondary insomnia is a condition caused by an underlying medical, neurological, or psychiatric condition, such as neuropathy, depression, anxiety, and Alzheimer's disease. A clinical study evaluated the effects of valerian, lavender, and Roman chamomile essential oil (25.9% 3-methylpentyl angelate) on neurotransmitter levels in people with dementia.[9546] Each oil was massaged on the participants diluted to 3% in jojoba oil. Lavender significantly decreased urinary free cortisol (a sign of decreased stress), valerian significantly increased serum serotonin (supports mood and healthy sleep patterns), and Roman chamomile significantly increased urinary norepinephrine (involved in healthy sleep-wake cycles). Valerian also promoted better quality sleep. Based on the results, the researchers evaluated three separate blends of the three oils (also at 3% in jojoba). The highest levels of serotonin were achieved with a 2:2:1 blend of valerian, lavender, and Roman chamomile.

Neiguan

Shenmen

Yongquan

---

## VERBENA
### (Honey Verbena, Wild Verbena, Lippia Oil, Zinziba)
*Lippia javanica* Spreng.

**FAMILY:** Verbenacea
**NOTE:** Middle
**AROMA INTENSITY:** Medium
**AROMA:** Sweet, fruity, intense, green, slightly minty and floral
**COMMON EXTRACTION METHOD:** Steam distilled from the leaves and flowering tops
**POSSIBLE SUBSTITUTE OILS:** Frankincense, silver fir, balsam fir, lemon verbena, lavender
**BLENDS WELL WITH:** Basil, black pepper, cinnamon, clary sage, clove, geranium, lavender, lemon, lemon verbena, neroli, nutmeg, orange, palmarosa, sage, Spanish sage
**SUBCELLULAR LOCALIZATION | EPIGENETIC INFLUENCE:** Currently unknown | Currently unknown
**RECOMMENDED DILUTION RANGE:** *Myrcenone and myrcene CTs*: 3%–33%, 50% for some conditions; *Linalool and Limonene-Piperitenone CTs*: 5%–Neat

**PRIMARY CONSTITUENTS:** [9547,9548,9549]

| Myrcenone CT | | Limonene/Piperitenone CT | |
|---|---|---|---|
| Myrcenone | 36.2%–71.6% | Limonene | 27.5%–51.7% |
| Myrcene | 0.1%–28.8% | Piperitenone | 32.5%–47.3% |
| Limonene | 0.0%–16.0% | Beta-Caryophyllene | 1.8%–4.5% |

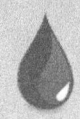 

| | | | |
|---|---|---|---|
| Eugenol | 0.0%–15.3% | 1,8-Cineole | 0.0%–4.0% |
| (E)-Ocimenone | 0.0%–11.2% | Germacrene D | 0.0%–2.3% |
| Geranial | 0.0%–9.5% | | |
| Carvone | 0.0%–5.9% | *Linalool CT* | |
| Beta-Caryophyllene | 0.0%–5.5% | Linalool | 27.3%–65.2% |
| Cis-Tagetenone | 0.0%–4.9% | Limonene | 0.5%–26.2% |
| Alpha-Terpineol | 0.0%–4.6% | (Z)-Beta-Ocimene | 0.0%–13.0% |
| Germacrene D | 0.0%–4.3% | Alpha-Pinene | 0.2%–10.3% |
| | | Beta-Caryophyllene | 1.6%–9.8% |
| *Myrcene CT* | | Myrcene | 2.6%–9.1% |
| Myrcene | 33.1%–53.2% | 1,8-Cineole | 0.0%–7.0% |
| Linalool | 1.7%–19.1% | (E)-Beta-Ocimene | 1.6%–6.2% |
| Beta-Caryophyllene | 0.1%–8.4% | Isomyrcenol | 0.0%–6.2% |
| Limonene | 5.3%–7.7% | Myrtenal | 0.0%–6.0% |
| 2.6-Dimethylstyrene | 1.0%–7.2% | Germacrene D | 0.2%–3.8% |
| Camphor | 0.1%–5.0% | 2.6-Dimethylstyrene | 0.0%–3.8% |
| 1,8-Cineole | 0.1%–4.5% | | |
| Perillene | 0.0%–4.3% | | |
| (Z)-Beta-Ocimene | 1.9%–3.8% | | |
| Alpha-Pinene | 0.4%–3.1% | | |

Note: A number of chemotypes of verbena essential oil exist, including some not listed in this work; however, the most commercially available chemotype appears to be the myrcenone CT. The myrcenone CT may be the least therapeutic based on the current research.

**OTHER CONSTITUENTS:** *Myrcenone CT*—1,8-cineole, isomyrcenol, dihydrotagetone, 1-octen-3-ol, ipsdienol, verbenone, trans-tagetenone, caryophyllene oxide, 2-methyl-6-methylene-3,7-octadien-2-ol, linalool, 6,7-epoxymyrcene, alloaromadendrene, alpha-humulene, (E)-beta-farnesene, ar-curcumene; *Limonene/Piperitenone CT*—sabinene, para-cymene, trans-1,2-Limonene epoxide, linalool, trans-p-mentha-2,8-dien-1-ol, carvone, trans-carvyl acetate, trans-carveol, isopiperitone, caryophyllene oxide; *Myrcene CT*—sabinene, gamma-terpinene, (E)-beta-ocimene, para-cymene, dihydrotagetenone, 6-methyl-5-hepten-2-one, 2-octanone, perillene, trans-sabinene hydrate, citronellal, beta-bourbonene, myrtenal, tagetenone, geranial, nerol, p-cymen-8-ol, caryophyllene oxide; *Linalool CT*—sabinene, myrcene, gamma-terpinene, (E)-beta-ocimene, para-cymene, camphor, beta-bourbonene, (E)-tagetone, nerol, geraniol, caryophyllene oxide, ipsenone

**PREFERRED COMPOSITION FOR CLINICAL USE:**

| Constituent | Limonene/ Piperitenone CT | Linalool CT |
|---|---|---|
| **Piperitenone** | 35%–50% | – |
| **Limonene** | 25%–35% | – |
| **Beta-Caryophyllene** | 1.5%–4% | 2%–8% |
| **Linalool** | < 3% | 50%–65% |
| **(Z)-Beta-Ocimene** | – | 1%–13% |
| **Myrcene** | – | 2.5%–9% |
| **(E)-Beta-Ocimene** | – | 2%–7% |
| **Germacrene D** | – | 0.1%–5% |

**REPORTED THERAPEUTIC PROPERTIES:** Antibacterial, analgesic, reduces fever, **reduces cough (especially chronic)**, antispasmodic, anti-inflammatory, supports respiratory function, **chronic respiratory ailments**, decongestant, relieves insect bites/stings, soothes sore muscles, antiarthritic, antirheumatic, relieves painful menstruation and PMS, **antiparasitic**, relieves sore throat, **relieves diarrhea and associated diseases (malaria, dysentery)**, abscesses, wound healing, aids circulation, relaxing, stress management, antidepressant

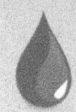

**CAUTIONS:**

■ Caution is advised during pregnancy and lactation due to potentially high myrcene content (myrcenone and myrcene CTs). Extremely high doses of myrcene have been toxic to fetuses according to animal research.[9550]

■ There is a moderate risk that when verbena is taken orally it may interfere with enzymes responsible for metabolizing medications (NSAIDs, proton-pump inhibitors, acetaminophen, antiepileptics, immune modulators, blood-sugar medications, blood pressure medications, antidepressants, antipsychotics, diabetic medications, antihistamines, antibiotics, and anesthetics) due to myrcene content (myrcenone and myrcene CTs).[9551,9552]

■ *Myrcene and Myrcenone CTs*: May interfere with pentobarbital and other barbiturates (medications for anxiety and insomnia) based on beta-myrcene content.[9553]

**SELECTED EVIDENCE:**

☐ *In vitro* research demonstrated that a linalool CT of verbena essential oil prevented three common respiratory tract pathogens (*K. pneumoniae, C. neoformans,* and *B. cereus*) from reproducing.[9554]

☐ Verbena essential oil protected against mosquito bites for 2.5 hours.[9555,9556]

☐ Piperitonone isolated from verbena essential oil demonstrated marked activity against *Entamoeba histolytica* (an anaerobic parasitic protozoan that may cause intestinal disorders and bloodstream, liver, brain, and lung infections).[9557]

☐ *In vitro* research demonstrated that a piperitenone-rich CT (74.4%) of verbena essential oil inhibited *Plasmodium falciparum* (a protozoan parasite that causes the most dangerous form of malaria—malignant malaria—in humans) in micromolar concentrations (8 mcg/ml).[9558]

☐ Thyme CT thymol, garlic, tea tree, cajeput, may chang, lemongrass (*C. citratus*), and verbena CT citral exhibited fungistatic activity (100 percent) against *F. culmorum* and *F. graminearum*, and all but garlic (89.4%) were 100% fungistatic against *F. avenaceum* and *F. oxysporum.*[9559]

# VETIVER
## (Khus)

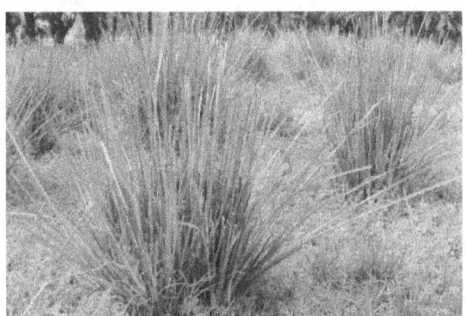

*Vetiveria zizanioides* (L.) Nash, *Anatherum zizanioides* (L.) Hitchc. & Chase, *Chrysopogon zizanioides* (L.) Roberty, *Phalaris zizanioides* L.

**FAMILY:** Poaceae (Gramineae)
**NOTE:** Base
**AROMA INTENSITY:** Strong
**AROMA:** Earthy, balsamic, slightly sweet and spicy
**COMMON EXTRACTION METHOD:** Steam distilled from the roots
**POSSIBLE SUBSTITUTE OILS:** Patchouli, spikenard, geranium
**BLENDS WELL WITH:** Bergamot, cardamom, clary sage, coriander, frankincense, geranium, ginger, grapefruit, lavender, lemon, lemon verbena, lemongrass, lime, orange, oregano, palo santo, patchouli, rose, sandalwood, spikenard, tangerine, ylang ylang
**SUBCELLULAR LOCALIZATION | EPIGENETIC INFLUENCE:** Endocytic Vesicles | Immune/Nervous
**RECOMMENDED DILUTION RANGE:** 5%–50%; neat for limited conditions

**PRIMARY CONSTITUENTS:**[9560,9561,9562,9563,9564,9565,9566]

|  |  |
|---|---|
| Khusimol | 3.4%–24.6% |
| (E)-Isovalencenol | 0.0%–15.6% |
| Calarene (Beta-Gurjunene) | 0.5%–9.9% |
| Beta-Vetivenene | 0.0%–9.8% |
| Dehydro-Aromadendrene | 0.0%–7.3% |
| Alpha-Vetivone | 2.0%–6.3% |

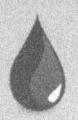
| Cycloisolongifolene | 0.0%–5.9% |
|---|---|
| Vetiselinenol | 0.0%–5.6% |
| Beta-Bisabolol | 0.0%–4.7% |
| Alpha-Longipinene | 0.0%–4.2% |
| Nootkatone | 0.0%–4.1% |
| Gamma-Selinene | 0.0%–4.1% |
| Delta-Cadinene | 0.0%–4.0% |
| Valerenol | 0.0%–3.9% |

**OTHER CONSTITUENTS:** Beta-vetispirene, terpinen-4-ol, 5-epiprezizane, khusimene, alpha-muurolene, calacorene, beta-humulene, delta-selinene, valencene, gamma-vetivene, alpha-amorphene, epizizanal, 3-epi-zizanol, delta-amorphene, iso-khusimol, beta-vetivone, (E)-isoeugenol, elemol, alpha-cadinol, eudesm-7(11)-en-4-ol, nootkatol, (E)-isovalencenol, 14-hydroxy-delta-cadinene, khusimone, epi-zizanone

**PREFERRED COMPOSITION FOR CLINICAL USE:**

| Constituent | Reunion Island (Bourbon) | Haitian | Indonesian | Indian |
|---|---|---|---|---|
| **Khusimol** | 12%–20% | 10%–16% | 4%–13% | 5%–20% |
| **(E)-Isovalencenol** | 5%–15% | 10%–20% | 0.5%–7% | 5%–11% |
| **Alpha-Vetivone** | 3%–6% | 2%–7% | 2%–5% | 2%–9% |
| **Beta-Vetivenene** | 3%–6% | 0.5%–5% | 4%–10% | 5%–7% |
| **Beta-Vetivone** | 2%–5% | 2%–6% | 2%–5% | 1%–4% |
| **Vetiselinenol** | 1%–5% | 3%–6% | 0.5%–2% | 0.5%–6% |
| **Cadinol <alpha + T>** | 0.5%–5% | 0.5%–6% | < 1% | < 3% |
| **Zizanol** | 0%–3% | 1%–6% | 1%–2% | 0.1%–2% |
| **Zizanoic Acid** | < 2% | < 2% | 3%–5% | 0%–6% |
| **Selina-6-en-4-ol Isomer** | – | 0%–5% | < 1% | – |
| **Beta-Vetispirene** | 0.1%–3% | 0.1%–3% | 1%–4% | 0.5%–5% |

**REPORTED THERAPEUTIC PROPERTIES:** Analgesic (pain relief), antibacterial, antifungal, anti-inflammatory, antimicrobial, antioxidant, antiseptic, antispasmodic, **antirheumatic**, **antiarthritic**, supports healthy cell division, insect repellent, increases redness and circulation of a localized area, wound healing, **nervine (calms and soothes the nerves)**, aids detoxification, antiparasitic, reduces the appearance of scars, aphrodisiac, **encourages restful sleep**, antidepressant, **relieves anxiety**, **encourages focus and concentration**, reduces anger, grounding, **stress management**, combats grief, reduces fear

**CAUTIONS:**

■ None currently known.

**SELECTED EVIDENCE:**

☐ Vetiver essential oil provides potent antioxidant protection, reduces lipid peroxidation, and prevents the formation of melanin by melanoma cancer cells.[9567] Other research confirmed that vetiver essential oil is a potent free-radical scavenger.[9568]

☐ Inhalation of low doses of vetiver oil enhances reaction time and improves attention while performing visual discrimination tasks (something critical to reading, writing, learning, and social behavior).[9569]

☐ *In vitro* research suggests that vetiver essential oil inhibits *S. aureus*.[9570]

☐ Animal research concluded that vetiver essential oil reduces anxiety by altering central amygdaloid nucleus (part of the amygdala that is involved in the expression of conditioned fear and processes pain) activity.[9571]

☐ Vetiver root extract inhibited two *M. tuberculosis* strains, making it a useful natural remedy for tuberculosis.[9572]

☐ Vetiver essential oil repelled two mosquito vectors (*Aedes aegypti* and *Anopheles minimus*).[9573] Interestingly, vetiver essential oil only weakly repelled and did not kill any *Aedes aegypti* mosquitoes, but significantly repelled and killed (91% to 100% mortality) the *An. minimus* mosquito. Another study also found that vetiver essential oil kills and repels the *An. minimus* mosquito.[9574]

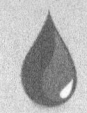

- *In vitro* research demonstrated that low doses of marjoram, lemon, basil, clove, thyme, rosemary CT 1,8-cineole, and tea tree essential oils prevented the shortening of telomeres after exposure to hydrogen peroxide.[9575] The same research reported that vetiver, black pepper, eucalyptus (*E. globulus*), ginger, clove, and rosemary increased the length of already shortened telomeres. This activity suggests that these essential oils can help maintain the youth and health of cells, or turn back the clock on the cell to make it more youthful depending on the essential oil used.

- Inhalation of 20 mcL of vetiver in 200 mcL of water modified sleep-waking patterns in rats by modifying brainwave activity (decreased alpha and beta1 activity, and increased gamma activity), increasing alertness, and decreasing slow wave sleep time almost from the start of inhalation.[9576]

- Vetiver essential oil demonstrated antimicrobial activity against *S. aureus* (both susceptible and resistant to methicillin), *Corynebacterium striatum*, *Bacillus* sp., *B. subtilis*, and *Candida glabrata*.[9577]

- Both vetiver and cinnamon essential oil killed sheep blowfly (*Lucilia sericata*) larvae.[9578] This makes them promising biopesticides to control the spread of myiasis—an infection transmitted to humans when flies transmit their larvae to people, characterized by lumps under the skin.

- *In vitro* examination of sixty essential oils demonstrated that sandalwood (Indian, Australian, and Hawaiian), melissa, lemongrass (*C. flexuosus*), cilantro, cassia, cinnamon, patchouli, and vetiver essential oils possess remarkable anticancer (two types of breast cancer cells) and antifungal (*Aspergillus niger, Candida albicans,* and *Cryptococcus neoformans*) activities.[9579]

- The common green bottle fly (*Lucilia sericata*) is a facultative insect that causes myasis (a skin disease characterized by painful, itchy boil-like lesions that occurs when the flies lay their larvae (maggots) in wounds or on the moist skin) in humans and other warm-blooded vertebrates. Low concentrations (0.2%) of vetiver, cinnamon, lavender, and their blends killed the flies within five minutes.[9580] Vetiver significantly deterred flies from the oviposition medium and reduced adult longevity, while sunflower fixed oil repelled flies, deterred oviposition, and reduced adult fly lifespan. The greatest repellency was achieved with a blend of the four oils (2 mL of each essential oil and 4 mL of sunflower as carrier oil).

- Vetiver essential oil inhibited *E. faecalis* and MRSA *in vitro*.[9581] A fraction of the oil rich in cedren-8-en-13-ol was found to be the most active against MRSA.

- Both cinnamon bark and vetiver essential oils strongly repelled houseflies (*Musca domestica*)—84% and 78% respectively.[9582] In addition, vetiver, cinnamon, and lavender essential oils were significantly toxic to house flies (100 percent).

- Vetiver essential oil relaxed precontracted isolated rat aortic rings through the muscarinic pathway and by acting as calcium channel blocker.[9583] This suggests that vetiver may help maintain healthy blood pressure levels, which is very important for cardiovascular health.

- After demonstrating that vetiver essential oil possesses noteworthy antimicrobial activity against pathogens—*Cutibacterium acnes, Staphylococcus aureus, Staphylococcus epidermidis*, and *Streptococcus pyogenes*—associated with acne *in vitro*, researchers created an oil-in-water emulsified lotion. The lotion also completely inhibited the growth of *C. acnes* and killed *S. aureus, S. epidermidis*, and *S. pyogenes* within twenty-four hours.[9584] Moreover, the lotion retained antimicrobial activity against the tested microorganisms during an 84-day stability study.

- An interesting vetiver essential oil (Indonesian: 15.4% beta-caryophyllene, 8.9% cuminone, 8.5% myrcenol, 8.1% alpha-humulene) arrested the growth of colon and murine breast cancer cells, while the oil increased apoptosis of progesterone receptor-positive breast cancer and colon cancer cells.[9585] CB2 receptors were highly expressed in the murine breast cancer cells and beta-caryophyllene bound to these receptors, which might have contributed to its cytotoxicity against the cancer cells. The researchers concluded that the molecular interaction of vetiver oil and CB2 receptors make it better suited for use as an anticancer agent against triple negative breast cancer.

- Vetiver essential oil (30.0% khusimol, 10.8% beta-eudesmol, 6.0% alpha-muurolene, 5.6% patchoulol) exhibited good antibacterial activity against antibacterial activity against *P. nigrescens, F. nucleatum, P. melaninogenica*, and *A. actinomycetemcomitans*, and was highly active against *L. amazonensis* promastigote and amastigote forms and *T. cruzi* trypomastigote form (with good selectivity).

- Vetiver and two of its constituents, valencene and vetiverol, demonstrated mosquito repellency (*Ae. aegypti* and *Ae. albopictus*) without genotoxicity.[9586]

# VILAYTI TULSI
## (Dorado Azul, Pignut, Chan, Wild Spikenard)
*Hyptis suaveolens* (L.) Poit., *Mesosphaerum suaveolens* (L.) Kuntze

**FAMILY:** Lamiaceae (Labiatae)
**NOTE:** Top-Middle
**AROMA INTENSITY:** Medium
**AROMA:** Herbaceous, camphoraceous, medicinal
**COMMON EXTRACTION METHOD:** Steam distilled from the aerial parts (stems, leaves, and flowers)
**POSSIBLE SUBSTITUTE OILS:** *1,8-Cineole CT*—myrtle, cardamom, niaouli; *Sabinene CT*—nutmeg (West Indian); *Fenchone CT*—fennel
**BLENDS WELL WITH:** Bergamot, cajeput, cedarwood, clary sage, eucalyptus, grapefruit, hyssop, lavender, lemon, lime, niaouli, orange, palo santo, peppermint, sage, sandalwood, Spanish sage, tangerine
**SUBCELLULAR LOCALIZATION | EPIGENETIC INFLUENCE:** Currently unknown | Currently unknown
**RECOMMENDED DILUTION RANGE:** 3%–50%; neat for limited conditions

**PRIMARY CONSTITUENTS:**[9587,9588,9589,9590,9591,9592,9593,9594,9595,9596]

| *1,8-Cineole CT* | | *Sabinene CT* | |
|---|---|---|---|
| 1,8-Cineole | 32.0%–47.6% | Sabinene | 7.3%–31.3% |
| Beta-Caryophyllene | 4.7%–29.0% | 1,8-Cineole | 5.2%–24.6% |
| Gamma-Elemene | 0.0%–8.2% | Alpha-Terpinolene | 5.6%–13.8% |
| Beta-Pinene | 4.2%–6.6% | Beta-Caryophyllene | 0.0%–11.7% |
| Germacrene | 0.0%–4.9% | Terpinen-4-ol | 2.9%–11.4% |
| Sabinene | 2.5%–3.9% | Alpha-Phellandrene | 0.0%–10.2% |
| (Z)-Beta-Ocimene | 0.0%–3.6% | Fenchone | 0.0%–8.1% |
| | | P-Mentha-2(7),8-Diene | 0.0%–7.9% |
| *Fenchone CT* | | Bicyclogermacrene | 0.6%–7.5% |
| Fenchone | 8.1%–42.3% | Alpha-Pinene | 2.0%–7.4% |
| Sabinene | 10.3%–18.0% | (Z)-Beta-Ocimene | 0.0%–6.9% |
| Limonene | 0.8%–13.5% | Beta-Pinene | 0.0%–6.7% |
| 1,8-Cineole | 0.0%–11.5% | Limonene | 0.0%–5.9% |
| Beta-Caryophyllene | 7.0%–9.7% | | |
| Fenchol | 0.7%–8.6% | | |
| Gamma-Terpinene | 1.6%–7.0% | | |
| Beta-Pinene | 3.2%–4.9% | | |
| Para-Cymene | 2.7%–4.5% | | |
| P-Mentha-2,4,(8)-Diene | 0.0%–4.5% | | |
| Alpha-Pinene | 0.0%–3.1% | | |

Note: A number of chemotypes of vilayti tulsi are reported in the literature including 1,8-cineole, sabinene, fenchone/fenchol, beta-caryophyllene, alpha-pinene/sabinene, bicyclogermacrene, citronellyl acetate/beta-caryophyllene, spathulenol, beta-phellandrene, and p-mentha-2,4(8)-diene. The 1,8-cineole is reported to be the most frequently observed CT, followed by sabinene, beta-caryophyllene, and the fenchone CTs. This essential oil is rarely commercially available.

**OTHER CONSTITUENTS:** *1,8-cineole*—beta-myrcene, alpha-pinene, alpha-phellandrene, gamma-terpinene, terpinolene, citronellol, alpha-terpineol, 4-terpineol, citronellal, geraniol, beta-bourbonene, beta-elemene, bicyclogermacrene, delta-cadinene, elemol, spathulenol, eugenol, aromadendrene, alpha-humulene; *Sabinene CT*—1-octen-3-ol, alpha-terpinene, para-cymene, fenchol, alpha-bergamotene, alpha-humulene, beta-selinene, spathulenol, bergamotol, naphthalene, phenanthrene; *Fenchone CT*—alpha-thujene, alpha-phellandrene, myrcene, alpha-terpinene, alpha-terpinolene, camphor, borneol, alpha-terpineol, alpha-copaene, beta-elemene, alpha-selinene, alpha-bergamotene, alpha-humulene, beta-bourbonene, germacrene D, bicyclogermacrene, spathulenol, caryophyllene oxide

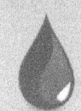

**PREFERRED COMPOSITION FOR CLINICAL USE:**

| Constituent | 1,8-Cineole CT |
|---|---|
| **1,8-Cineole** | 30%–50% |
| **Beta-Caryophyllene** | 5%–20% |
| **Beta-Pinene** | 3%–10% |
| **Sabinene** | 2%–5% |
| **Bicyclogermacrene** | 0.1%–4% |

**REPORTED THERAPEUTIC PROPERTIES:** Antibacterial, **antifungal**, antiseptic, analgesic, anti-inflammatory, antiarthritic, antirheumatic, antiallergic, **supports respiratory function**, aids circulation, relieves cough, supports digestive function, stimulates appetite, expels excess gas, relieves headache/migraine, balances hormones, supports oral health, reduces fever, **insect repellent**, **insecticide**, uplifting, boosts self-confidence, increases mindfulness and meditation

**CAUTIONS:**

■ Caution is warranted orally due to the significant amounts of 1,8-cineole. Limit it to small doses internally (adults—maximum 10 drops daily). One text recommends a maximum daily dose of 6 drops, whereas the European Medicines Agency recommends 2 to 4 drops (100–200 mg) of high 1,8-cineole essential oils orally, 2 to 5 times daily for adolescents, adults, and the elderly.[9597,9598] Additionally, 200 mg of isolated 1,8-cineole has been ingested three times daily for up to six months in clinical research.[9599,9600] Toxicity has been reported when eucalyptus (also high in 1,8-cineole) was ingested in large doses, and as few as 4 to 5 drops may cause problems in very sensitive individuals.[9601,9602,9603,9604,9605,9606] In humans, 3.5 to 5 mL has proven fatal orally.[9607]

■ Avoid with epilepsy and Parkinson's due to 1,8-cineole or fenchone content (*all CTs*). May exacerbate or cause seizures/convulsions or reduce seizure medication efficacy based on 1,8-cineole content.[9608,9609,9610,9611,9612]

■ May weakly interfere with the enzymes responsible for metabolizing medications (NSAIDs, proton-pump inhibitors, acetaminophen, antiepileptics, immune modulators, blood-sugar medications, blood pressure medications, antidepressants, antipsychotics, diabetic medications, antihistamines, antibiotics, and anesthetics) due to 1,8-cineole content.[9613,9614,9615,9616]

■ May interact with aspirin, blood pressure, antiplatelet, and anticoagulant medications, and increase the risk of bleeding among people with bleeding disorders due to fenchone content.[9617]

■ May interfere with pentobarbital and other barbiturates (medications for anxiety and insomnia) if 1,8-cineole content is high (*1,8-cineole CT*).[9618,9619]

**SELECTED EVIDENCE:**

☐ *In vitro* research concluded that vilayti tulsi (caryophyllene CT) inhibits *Staphylococcus aureus, Bacillus subtilis, Escherichia coli, Pseudomonas aeruginosa, Fusarium graminearum, Botrytis cinerea, Exserohilum turcicum, T. mentagrophytes,* and *Lagonosticta acicula.*[9620,9621]

☐ Vilayti tulsi essential oil (most studies used the sabinene CT) repels ticks (*Ixodes ricinus*), repels or kills three mosquito species (*Aedes albopictus, Armigeres,* and *Culex*), repels *Amblyomma cajennense* nymphs for short periods, repel the adult granary weevil *Sitophilus granaries,* and kills the storage grain insect (*Tribolium castaneum* Herbst).[9622,9623,9624,9625,9626,9627,9628]

☐ *In vitro* research demonstrates that vilayti tulsi essential oil (1,8-cineole CT) inhibits the fungi *A. fumigatus* and *A. parasiticus.*[9629]

☐ The 1,8-cineole CT of vilayti tulsi, shell ginger, and clove basil essential oils showed marked efficacy against engorged female ticks (*Rhipicephalus microplus*). Clove basil was the most potent followed by shell ginger and vilayti tulsi.[9630]

☐ Vilayti tulsi CT sabinene displayed antioxidant activity and slowed the proliferation of prostate and cervical cancer cells *in vitro.*[9631]

☐ A nanoemulsion containing vilayti tulsi essential oil was larvicidal against *Cx. quinquefasciatus* mosquitoes.[9632]

# VIRGINIAN CEDARWOOD
## (Eastern Red Cedar, Red Cedar, Virginia Juniper, Red Juniper, Pencil Cedar)
*Juniperus virginiana* L.

**FAMILY:** Cupressaceae (Coniferae)
**NOTE:** Base
**AROMA INTENSITY:** Medium
**AROMA:** Woody, sweet, slightly balsamic
**COMMON EXTRACTION METHOD:** Steam distilled from the wood
**POSSIBLE SUBSTITUTE OILS:** Texas cedarwood, atlas cedarwood, Himalayan cedarwood, sandalwood
**BLENDS WELL WITH:** Balsam fir, bay laurel, bergamot, blue cypress, blue spruce, carrot seed, cinnamon, copaiba, cypress, myrtle, jasmine, juniper, lemon, neroli, palmarosa, patchouli, petitgrain, pine, ravensara, rose, rosemary, sandalwood, silver fir, Spanish sage, spruce, thyme, tsuga, vetiver, white fir
**SUBCELLULAR LOCALIZATION | EPIGENETIC INFLUENCE:** Currently unknown | Currently unknown
**RECOMMENDED DILUTION RANGE:** 5%–Neat

**PRIMARY CONSTITUENTS:**[9633,9634,9635]

| | |
|---|---|
| Alpha-Cedrene | 21.1%–35.0% |
| Thujopsene | 21.3%–30.0% |
| Cedrol | 4.0%–22.2% |
| Beta-Cedrene | 0.0%–9.2% |
| Alpha-Copaene | 0.0%–6.3% |
| Alpha-Selinene | 0.0%–3.0% |
| Widdrol | 1.0%–2.3% |

Note: Older heartwood will have higher levels of alpha-cedrene and cedrol compared to sapwood, which has higher thujopsene.[9636] Virginian cedarwood essential oil may also be rectified, which produces various fractions (light: mainly cedrene; #1025: high-boiling materials).

**OTHER CONSTITUENTS:** Beta-chamigrene, alpha-chamigrene, beta-himachalene, cuparene

**PREFERRED COMPOSITION FOR CLINICAL USE:**

| Constituent | CO2 | Distilled |
|---|---|---|
| Cedrol | 30%–45% | 12%–25% |
| Thujopsene | 25%–45% | 15%–35% |
| Widdrol | 3%–10% | 2%–12% |
| Alpha-Cedrene | 2%–7% | 20%–36% |
| Beta-Cedrene | 1%–7% | 4%–8% |
| Cuparene | – | 0.5%–7% |
| Cedrene Isomer or Beta-Funebrene | – | 0.1%–6% |
| Beta-Himachalene | – | 0.1%–3% |
| Beta-Caryophyllene | – | 0%–3% |

**REPORTED THERAPEUTIC PROPERTIES:** Antibacterial, antifungal, anti-infectious, analgesic, anti-inflammatory, antiarthritic, antirheumatic, eases cough, expels excess mucus, combats acne, **reduces the appearance of blemishes**, astringent, soothes chronic skin conditions, nourishes the hair, relieves dandruff, relieves hemorrhoids, strengthens the cardiovascular system, insect repellent, **encourages restful sleep**, stress management, relieves anxiety, **relaxing/calming**, promotes clarity of thought, balances emotions, reduces fear, grounding

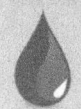

**CAUTIONS:**

■ May weakly interfere with the enzymes responsible for metabolizing medications (NSAIDs, proton-pump inhibitors, acetaminophen, antiepileptics, immune modulators, blood-sugar medications, blood pressure medications, antidepressants, antipsychotics, diabetic medications, antihistamines, antibiotics, and anesthetics) due to thujopsene, cedrol, and beta-cedrene content.[9637]

**SELECTED EVIDENCE:**

☐ Topical application of Virginia cedarwood essential oil (supercritical carbon dioxide oil , SC-CO$_2$) with very similar composition to steam distilled oil) to incisions moderately improved wound healing time in rats.[9638]

☐ Virginia cedarwood essential oil repels the red bud borer (*Resseliella oculiperda*).[9639] A CO$_2$ Virginian cedarwood essential oil effectively repels fire ants and kills ticks, making it a possible natural insect repellent.[9640]

☐ A CO$_2$ aromatic Virginian cedarwood (high in cedrol and thujopsene) was highly anti-inflammatory in an animal study.[9641] An *in vitro* study reported that it is a strong inhibitor of the 5-LOX enzyme.[9642] The 5-LOX enzyme converts arachidonic acid to leukotrienes, increasing inflammation and allergic reactions, and is associated with chronic degenerative inflammatory diseases and cancer.

☐ Oral administration of Virginia cedarwood essential oil (400–800 mg/kg BW) relieved anxiety in mice.[9643] The researchers further investigated the primary constituents in Virginia cedarwood oil and found that cedrol (400–1600 mg/kg boy weight) reduced anxiety but alpha-cedrene had no effect. Furthermore, Virginia cedarwood essential oil increased 5-hydroxytryptamine (5-HT) at 800 mg/kg, whereas cedrol increased 5-HT at 1200–1600mg/kg and reduced dopamine levels at 100–200 mg/kg.

☐ Cedrol, predominantly obtained from Virginia cedarwood essential oil, has demonstrated relaxing and anxiety-relieving effects. A recent preclinical study found that cedrol produces relaxation and relieves anxiety by altering neurotransmitter levels in the brain.[9644] Specifically, cedrol reduced dopamine and norepinephrine levels in the hippocampus, striatum, and hypothalamus.

☐ *Helicobacter pylori* is a bacterium that lives in the digestive tract that can cause sores and ulcers in the lining of the stomach or upper part of the small intestine. *H. pylori* produces urease in the stomach, which reduces stomach acidity allowing the bacteria to colonize the acidic environment of the stomach and trigger gastritis, peptic ulcer, and even gastric cancer. Thyme, lemongrass, Virginia cedarwood, and melissa essential oils were the most active of 26 commercial essential oils examined against *H. pylori*.[9645] Oregano, tea tree, pine, and silver fir were also bactericidal. Virginia cedarwood was the most active inhibitor of urease production at subinhibitory concentrations. Based on its ability to inhibit the bacteria and its production of urease, Virginia cedarwood represents a promising essential oil to eradicate *H. pylori* from the stomach and reduce ulcers and gastric cancer.

☐ May chang, Virginia cedarwood, spearmint, and tea tree essential oils each demonstrated contact toxicity against third instar larvae of the cotton leafworm (*Alabama argillacea*).[9646] Each oil changed the histochemistry of the testicles, while tea tree, Virginia cedarwood, and spearmint altered morphology. In addition, the histochemistry of the ovarioles was altered by Virginia cedarwood, tea tree, and may chang.

☐ Virginia cedarwood essential oil weakly inhibited *S. aureus, E. faecalis, P. aeruginosa, K. pneumoniae, E. coli,* and *C. albicans*.[9647]

☐ Virginia cedarwood needle essential oil (sabinene, limonene, beta-myrcene, bornyl acetate, and terpinen-4-ol as major constituents) was moderately larvicidal to, knocked down, and caused mortality in mosquitoes (*An. gambiae, An. arabiensis*).[9648]

## WESTERN RED CEDAR
### (Western Arborvitae, Pacific Thuja, Arborvitae, Giant Arborvitae)

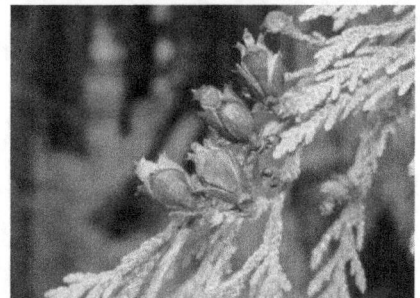

*Thuja plicata* Donn ex D. Don

**FAMILY:** Cupressaceae
**NOTE:** *Wood*—base; *Needles*—top
**AROMA INTENSITY:** Medium
**AROMA:** *Wood*—Woody, earthy, warm; *Needles*—sharp, camphoraceous, fresh

**COMMON EXTRACTION METHOD:** Steam distilled from wood (most commercially available, likely because it is devoid of thujones); may also be steam distilled from the needles (leaves)

**POSSIBLE SUBSTITUTE OILS:** *Wood*—hinoki, agarwood, cedarwood, sandalwood; *Needles*—Thuja, sage (alpha-thujone CT), mugwort (alpha-thujone CT)

**BLENDS WELL WITH:** Bergamot, black pepper, cedarwood, cinnamon, cistus, copaiba, cypress, frankincense, ginger, lavender, lemon, lime, neroli, petitgrain, rose, rosemary, sandalwood, tangerine, thuja

**SUBCELLULAR LOCALIZATION | EPIGENETIC INFLUENCE:** Currently unknown | Currently unknown

**RECOMMENDED DILUTION RANGE:** *Wood*—3%–33%; *Needles*—1.5%–20%

**PRIMARY CONSTITUENTS:** [9649,9650,9651,9652,9653]

| *Wood* | | *Needles (Leaves)* | |
|---|---|---|---|
| Methyl Thujate | 55.8%–59.1% | Alpha-Thujone | 54.1%–77.5% |
| Thujic Acid | 1.8%–25.0% | Fenchone | 0.0%–15.2% |
| Methyl Myrtenate | 4.1%–4.5% | Beta-Thujone | 6.8%–8.3% |
| Unknown Ester | 0.0%–3.8% | Sabinene | 4.2%–6.4% |
| Unknown Ester | 0.0%–3.2% | Terpinen-4-ol | 1.6%–4.7% |
| Unknown Ester | 0.0%–2.7% | | |
| Hinokitiol | 0.0%–2.0% | | |
| Alpha-Terpineol | 1.8%–1.9% | | |
| Thujic Acid Isomer | 0.0%–1.9% | | |
| Terpinen-4-ol | 1.4%–1.7% | | |
| 1,4-Cineole | 1.1%–1.3% | | |
| Para-Cymenene | 1.1%–1.2% | | |

**OTHER CONSTITUENTS:** *Wood*—para-cymene, meta-cymene, myrtanol, methyl thujate isomer, carvacrol, methyl thujate isomer3, benzoic acid, methyl cinnamate, sesquiterpineol, gamma-eudesmol, abietadiene; *Needles (leaves)*—alpha-pinene, alpha-terpinene, limonene, gamma-terpinene, rimuene, myrcene, camphor, camphene, fenchyl acetate, bornyl acetate, thymol, beta-caryophyllene

**PREFERRED COMPOSITION FOR CLINICAL USE:**

| Constituent | Wood |
|---|---|
| **Methyl Thujate** | 48%–65% |
| **Thujic Acid** | 0.1%–12% |
| **Methyl Myrtenate** | 3%–8% |
| **Alpha-Terpineol** | 1%–5% |
| **Terpinen-4-ol** | 1%–5% |
| **1,4-Cineole** | 1%–3% |
| **Para-Cymenene** | 0.5%–3% |
| **Nootkatene** | 0.1%–3% |

**REPORTED THERAPEUTIC PROPERTIES:** Antibacterial, antiseptic, antiparasitic, antifungal, antirheumatic, antispasmodic, eases cough, reduces fever, purification, insecticide, **insect repellent**, supports respiratory function, warts, nourishes the skin, astringent, balances menstruation, expels excess mucus, **calming**, encourages deep meditation, grounding, stress management

**CAUTIONS:**

*Wood*

■ None currently known.

*Needles (leaves) essential oil*

■ Avoid with children under six due to thujone content. Cases of seizure have been reported in young children due to exposure to thujone rich essential oils.[9654,9655,9656]

■ Avoid during pregnancy and while lactating. Essential oils rich in thujone content may cause abortion.[9657,9658]

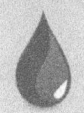

■ Avoid oral consumption. Ingesting plants or products high in thujons like western red cedar leaf can cause vomiting, stomachache, diarrhea, and gastroenteritis followed by absorption disorders, headache, nervous agitation, and chronic convulsions, and symptoms of liver and kidney toxicity extending to yellow liver atrophy (extensive and rapid death of liver cells—parenchymal, possibly accompanied by fatty degeneration), arrhythmia, and myocardial bleeding.[2852] Thujone is considered significantly neurotoxic and may damage the liver, and it is estimated that as little as 15 mg orally may negatively impact the central nervous system.[9659,9660,9661] Taking 20 drops of thuja oil (also with significant thujones content) twice daily for five days caused an adult woman to have a tonic seizure.[9662] As few as 12 drops of sage oil (also with significant thujones content) orally have reportedly caused a seizure and short coma in an adult.[9663]

■ Avoid with epilepsy and Parkinson's disease due to thujone and fenchone content.[9664,9665,9666,9667,9668]

■ May weakly interfere with the enzymes responsible for metabolizing medications (NSAIDs, proton-pump inhibitors, acetaminophen, antiepileptics, immune modulators, blood-sugar medications, blood pressure medications, antidepressants, antipsychotics, diabetic medications, antihistamines, antibiotics, and anesthetics) due to alpha-thujone content.[9669]

■ Avoid with those who have a compromised liver or kidneys due to the risk of kidney toxicity, kidney failure, or liver toxicity.[9670,9671,9672] Consuming extremely large amounts of thujone rich essential oils (10 mL) has caused kidney failure.[9673] This would also suggest that those taking medications that could cause liver damage should also use western red cedar leaf essential oil very cautiously or avoid it entirely.

### SELECTED EVIDENCE:

☐ *In vitro* research reported that western red cedar leaf essential oil inhibited ten pathogenic bacteria, bacterial spores, and two fungi: *Bacillus subtilis, Streptococcus pyogenes, Staphylococcus aureus, Enterococcus fecalis, Pseudomonas aeruginosa. Klebsiella pneumoniae, Acinetobacter baumannii, Haemophilus influenzae, Salmonella enteritidis,* and *Escherichia coli;* and *Candida albicans* and *Aspergillus niger.*[9674,9675]

☐ Western red cedar wood essential oil significantly reduced inflammation by modulating global gene expression (inhibited both the protein and gene expression levels of VCAM-1, IP-10, and I-TAC), immune responses, and signaling pathways involved in inflammatory and tissue remodeling processes (decreased ICAM-1 and MIG).[9676] When vascular cell adhesion molecule-1 (VCAM-1) is inhibited, it blocks leukocyte recruitment and therefore tissue inflammation. Interferon gamma-induced protein 10 (IP-10) is a chemokine involved in systemic inflammation. Elevated interferon-inducible T-cell alpha chemoattractant (I-TAC) expression is involved in triggering inflammatory responses. ICAM-1 is an inflammatory molecule that also negatively affects vascular permeability. Also called CXCL9, monokine induced by gamma interferon (MIG) regulates T cell recruitment to the site of inflammation and is associated with increased cardiovascular inflammation.

☐ *In vitro* research found that western red cedar wood essential oil completely killed *E. coli* and significantly inhibited *S. aureus*, but was inactive against *P. aeruginosa.*[9677]

☐ Laboratory research concluded that oregano CT carvacrol, thyme CT thymol, cassia, lemongrass (*C. flexuosus*), and Western red cedar (arborvitae) essential oils exhibit very strong antimicrobial activity against drug-resistant pathogens (*Pseudomonas aeruginosa, Proteus vulgaris, Citrobacter koseri, Klebsiella pneumoniae, Candida albicans,* and *C. parapsilosis.*[9678] Ten essential oils—oregano, thyme, clove, arborvitae, cassia, lemongrass, tea tree, eucalyptus (*E. radiata*), lavender, and clary sage —were tested and these five were the most effective. The researchers also concluded the essential oils were not genotoxic (cause DNA damage) compared to control cells. In addition, each of the oils exhibited antioxidant activity, with cassia and oregano demonstrating the greatest increase in total antioxidant status, followed by tea tree, thyme, clove, clary sage, eucalyptus, arborvitae, and lavender.

# WHITE FIR

*Abies concolor* (Gord. & Glend.) Lindl. ex Hildebr., *Picea concolor, Pinus concolor*; Sierra White Fir: *Abies iowiana* (Gordon & Glend.), *A. murray* bis

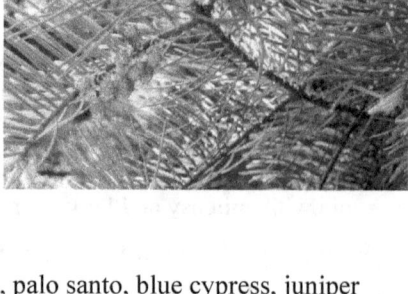

**FAMILY:** Pinaceae
**NOTE:** Top-Middle
**AROMA INTENSITY:** Medium
**AROMA:** Fresh, piney, clean, woody
**COMMON EXTRACTION METHOD:** Steam distilled from the needles (leaves)
**POSSIBLE SUBSTITUTE OILS:** Silver fir, balsam fir, blue spruce, spruce (black), palo santo, blue cypress, juniper (needles)
**BLENDS WELL WITH:** Balsam fir, birch, blue spruce, cassia, cedarwood, cypress, chamomile (German, Roman), frankincense, galbanum, lavender, lemon, myrtle, palo santo, pine, sandalwood, silver fir, spruce (black), tsuga, wintergreen
**SUBCELLULAR LOCALIZATION | EPIGENETIC INFLUENCE:** Currently unknown | Currently unknown
**RECOMMENDED DILUTION RANGE:** 5%–Neat

## PRIMARY CONSTITUENTS:[9679]

| | |
|---|---|
| Beta-Pinene | 41.5%–52.2% |
| Limonene | 1.6%–23.0% |
| Bornyl Acetate | 0.6%–20.2% |
| Camphene | 0.5%–9.0% |
| Alpha-Pinene | 4.4%–7.9% |
| Alpha-Terpineol | 1.2%–6.9% |
| Beta-Phellandrene | 1.1%–6.5% |
| Naphthalenol | 0.0%–6.4% |
| Camphene Hydrate | 0.1%–4.1% |

Note: Both *Abies alba* and *Abies concolor* are referred to as white fir, and both are available on the essential oil market. *A. alba* is more commonly called silver fir or silver spruce, whereas *A. concolor* is called white fir according to the United States Department of Agriculture.[9680] They are two distinct species, and the chemical constituents are very different.[9681] *A. concolor* is the true white fir essential oil. High levels of bornyl acetate and camphene are usually only found in trees growing in the Wasatch Mountains of Utah and New Mexico, U.S.A.

**OTHER CONSTITUENTS:** Tricyclene, myrcene, alpha-phellandrene, delta-3-carene, terpinolene, 2-nonanone, linalool, endo-fenchol, citronellal, borneol, terpinen-4-ol

## PREFERRED COMPOSITION FOR CLINICAL USE:

| *Constituent* | |
|---|---|
| **Beta-Pinene** | 35%–55% |
| **Alpha-Pinene** | 10%–20% |
| **Bornyl Acetate** | 4%–12% |
| **Camphene** | 3%–9% |
| **Limonene** | 3%–8% |
| **Beta-Phellandrene** | 2%–8% |
| **Alpha-Terpineol** | 0.5%–8% |
| **Delta-3-Carene** | 1%–5% |
| **Beta-Myrcene** | 1%–3% |
| **Camphene Hydrate** | 0.1%–2% |

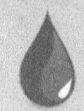

**Reported Therapeutic Properties: Analgesic (pain relief), anti-inflammatory,** antiarthritic, antirheumatic, antimicrobial, antiseptic, **antioxidant, aids circulation,** increases redness and circulation of a localized area, **antispasmodic,** expectorant, decongestant, supports immune system function, disinfectant, removes excess mucus, relieves cough, **supports respiratory function,** reduces fever, stimulating, energizing, **encourages feelings of stability and empowerment**

**Cautions:**
■ None currently known.

**Selected Evidence:**
☐ An ethanolic extract of white fir rich in terpenes reduced adenocarcinoma tumors of the duodenum.[9682]

---

## WHITE PINE
## (Eastern White Pine)

*Pinus strobus* L.

**Family:** Pinaceae
**Note:** Top
**Aroma Intensity:** Medium
**Aroma:** Piney, woody, fresh
**Common Extraction Method:** Steam distilled from the needles (leaves)
**Possible Substitute Oils:** Pine, red pine, balsam fir, cypress
**Blends Well With:** Agarwood, bergamot, cajeput, camphor, cedarwood, clary sage, coriander, Douglas fir, Engelmann spruce, eucalyptus, frankincense, galbanum, grapefruit, juniper, lavender, lemon, lime, marjoram, tea tree, neroli, niaouli, peppermint, ravensara, ravintsara, rosemary, Spanish sage, spikenard, thyme, Siberian fir, silver fir, white fir, white pine, white spruce
**Subcellular Localization | Epigenetic Influence:** Currently unknown | Currently unknown
**Recommended Dilution Range:** 5%–Neat

**Primary Constituents:**[9683,9684,9685,9686]

| | |
|---|---|
| Alpha-Pinene | 17.7%–57.8% |
| Beta-Pinene | 7.9%–35.5% |
| Beta-Myrcene | 1.7%–27.7% |
| Germacrene D | 2.3%–19.6% |
| Beta-Caryophyllene | 3.3%–8.2% |
| Delta-Cadinene | 0.1%–7.5% |
| Alpha-Cadinol | 0.0%–5.7% |
| Beta-Phellandrene | 1.1%–5.3% |
| Camphene | 1.7%–4.6% |
| T-Cadinol | 0.0%–4.0% |
| Limonene | 1.2%–3.0% |
| Delta-3-Carene | 0.0%–3.0% |
| Alpha-Selinene | 0.0%–3.0% |

**Other Constituents:** Tricyclene, terpinolene, beta-bourbonene, beta-elemene, alpha-humulene, gamma-muurolene, beta-selinene, alpha-muurolene, gamma-cadinene, beta-selinene, beta-calacorene, caryophyllene oxide, delta-cadinol, alpha-terpineol, bornyl acetate, humulene, kauranol isomer, manoyloxide

**PREFERRED COMPOSITION FOR CLINICAL USE:**

*Constituent*

| | |
|---|---|
| Alpha-Pinene | 25%–45% |
| Beta-Pinene | 20%–35% |
| Myrcene | 5%–15% |
| Limonene | 2%–10% |
| Camphene | 3%–6% |
| Delta-3-Carene | 2%–6% |
| Beta-Phellandrene | 2%–6% |
| Germacrene D | 0.1%–5% |
| Beta-Caryophyllene | 0.1%–5% |
| Bornyl Acetate | 1%–3% |
| Delta-Cadinene | 0.1%–2% |

**REPORTED THERAPEUTIC PROPERTIES:** Antibacterial, antifungal, antiviral, anti-infectious, **analgesic**, anti-inflammatory, **antiarthritic**, antirheumatic, antispasmodic, aids circulation, supports respiratory function, expels excess mucus, **eases cough**, decongestant, antioxidant, antiallergic, aids immune function, supports kidney function, grounding, stress management, relieves anxiety

**CAUTIONS:**
■ None currently known.

**SELECTED EVIDENCE:**
☐ White pine essential oil mildly repelled mosquitoes.[9687]
☐ *In vitro* research demonstrates that red pine essential oil is mildly active against the fungi *Fusarium culmorum, F. poae,* and *F. solani.*[9688]

---

# WHITE SAGE
## (Bee Sage, Sacred Sage)

*Salvia apiana* Jeps.

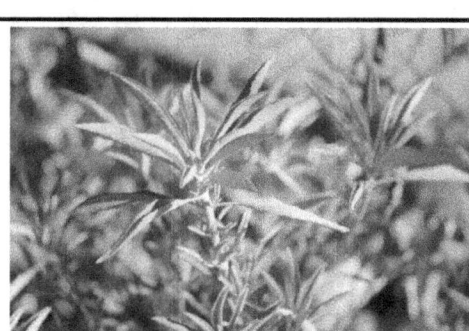

**FAMILY:** Lamiaceae (Labiatae)
**NOTE:** Middle
**AROMA INTENSITY:** Medium
**AROMA:** Herbaceous, earthy, pungent, fresh, camphoraceous
**COMMON EXTRACTION METHOD:** Steam distilled from the aerial parts
**POSSIBLE SUBSTITUTE OILS:** Spanish sage, spike lavender, rosemary (1,8-cineole or camphor CT), eucalyptus, mugwort
**BLENDS WELL WITH:** Bergamot, bitter orange, cedarwood, chamomile (German, Roman), frankincense, geranium, juniper berry, juniper (Phoenician), lavender, lemon, lime, marjoram, neroli, orange, oregano, petitgrain, pine, sandalwood, spruce (black), tangerine, vetiver, white spruce, white pine, yuzu
**SUBCELLULAR LOCALIZATION | EPIGENETIC INFLUENCE:** Currently unknown | Currently unknown
**RECOMMENDED DILUTION RANGE:** 3%–20%; neat for limited conditions

**PRIMARY CONSTITUENTS:**[9689,9690,9691]

| | |
|---|---|
| 1,8-Cineole | 34.5%–71.7% |
| Camphor | 2.1%–21.7% |
| Beta-Pinene | 3.8%–9.1% |

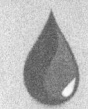

| Alpha-Pinene | 5.1%–9.0% |
| Delta-3-Carene | 1.3%–6.3% |
| Camphene | 0.4%–3.9% |
| Limonene | 1.5%–3.5% |
| Myrcene | 0.5%–3.2% |

**OTHER CONSTITUENTS:** (Z)-beta-ocimene, gamma-terpinene, para-cymene, terpinolene, beta-caryophyllene, terpinen-4-ol, beta-caryophyllene oxide

**PREFERRED COMPOSITION FOR CLINICAL USE:**

| Constituent | |
| --- | --- |
| **1,8-Cineole** | 45%–70% |
| **Camphor** | 3%–15% |
| **Alpha-Pinene** | 5%–10% |
| **Beta-Pinene** | 4%–10% |
| **Delta-3-Carene** | 1%–6% |
| **Limonene** | 1%–5% |
| **Camphene** | 0.1%–4% |
| **Myrcene** | 0.5%–3% |

**REPORTED THERAPEUTIC PROPERTIES:** Antibacterial, antifungal, antimicrobial, anti-infectious, antiviral, antiseptic, astringent, supports respiratory function, **decongestant**, expels excess mucus, **eases cough**, soothes irritated skin, relieves sore throat, purification, aids mental clarity, **stimulating/energizing**, stimulates creativity, dispels negativity, stress management

**CAUTIONS:**

■ Avoid with children under age three, particularly around the nose and mouth due to significant 1,8-cineole content. Use very cautiously in children under age five due to high 1,8-cineole content. 1,8-cineole may cause seizures, central nervous system problems, or respiratory distress in young children.[9692,9693,9694,9695] Ingestion of camphor-containing products has been lethal in children under age two.[9696] Children five years and up may use camphor-containing essential oils topically in dilutions no stronger than 5%. Camphor ingestion by infants and young children may cause cough, vomiting, seizure, burning sensation in the mucous membranes and eyes, or lack of voluntary coordination of muscle movements.[9697]

■ Caution is warranted during pregnancy and while lactating due to potentially high camphor content. Ingestion of essential oils with significant levels of camphor may lead to abortion because fetuses lack the enzymes to process it.[9698]

■ Avoid with epilepsy and Parkinson's disease due to 1,8-cineole content. May exacerbate or cause seizures/convulsions or reduce seizure medication efficacy based on 1,8-cineole content.[9699,9700,9701]

■ The potentially high camphor content in white sage may negatively impact red blood cells and increase the risk of jaundice in children with glucose-6-phosphate dehydrogenase deficiency (G6PD).[9702,9703]

■ Caution is warranted orally due to the significant amounts of 1,8-cineole and camphor. Limit it to small doses internally (adults—maximum 10 drops daily). One text recommends a maximum daily dose of 6 drops, whereas the European Medicines Agency recommends 2 to 4 drops (100–200 mg) of high 1,8-cineole essential oils orally, 2 to 5 times daily for adolescents, adults, and the elderly.[9704,9705] Additionally, 200 mg of isolated 1,8-cineole has been ingested three times daily for up to six months in clinical research.[9706,9707] Toxicity has been reported when eucalyptus (also high in 1,8-cineole) was ingested in large doses, and as few as 4 to 5 drops may cause problems in very sensitive individuals.[9708,9709,9710,9711,9712,9713] In humans, 3.5 to 5 mL has proven fatal orally.[9714] Camphor can be toxic when taken orally (usually single doses exceeding 2 mL), although the lethal dose for adult humans is estimated to be (more than 5 mL) in a single dose.[9715,9716,9717]

■ May weakly interfere with the enzymes responsible for metabolizing medications (NSAIDs, proton-pump inhibitors, acetaminophen, antiepileptics, immune modulators, blood-sugar medications, blood pressure medications, antidepressants, antipsychotics, diabetic medications, antihistamines, antibiotics, and anesthetics) and to 1,8-cineole content.[9718,9719,9720]

■ May interact with diabetic medications due to the ability of 1,8-cineole to significantly inhibit alpha-glucosidase activity, particularly when synergized with other constituents (alpha-pinene and beta-pinene).[9721,9722,9723] Alpha-glucosidase is an enzyme that breaks down carbohydrates by chemical reaction with water. Inhibiting its activity postpones glucose absorption and therefore the impact of carbohydrates on blood sugar levels.

■ May interact with aspirin, blood pressure, antiplatelet, and anticoagulant medications, and increase the risk of bleeding among people with bleeding disorders (low risk).[9724] 1,8-cineole is a weak inhibitor of platelet aggregation.[9725]

■ May interfere with pentobarbital and other barbiturates (medications for anxiety and insomnia) based on 1,8-cineole content.[9726,9727]

**SELECTED EVIDENCE:**

□   None found.

---

# WHITE SPRUCE
## (Canadian Spruce, Black Hills Spruce, Cat Spruce)

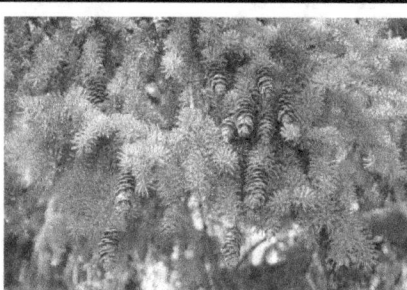

*Picea glauca* (Moench) Voss, *P. alba* (Aiton) Link,
*P. Canadensis* (Mill.) Britton, Sterns & Poggenb

**FAMILY:** Pinaceae
**NOTE:** Middle-Top
**AROMA INTENSITY:** Medium
**AROMA:** Woody, piney, fresh, slightly camphoraceous
**COMMON EXTRACTION METHOD:** Steam distilled from the needles (leaves); may also be steam distilled from the needles (leaves) and twigs, branches, or oleoresin
**POSSIBLE SUBSTITUTE OILS:** Spruce (black), pine, balsam fir, tsuga, silver fir, cedarwood, white fir, Douglas fir, blue spruce
**BLENDS WELL WITH:** Balsam fir, bergamot, cedarwood, copaiba, cypress, Douglas fir, frankincense, honey myrtle, grapefruit, hyssop, juniper, juniper (Phoenician), lavender, lemon, lime, neroli, orange, palo santo, pine, rose, sandalwood, silver fir, spruce (black), tsuga, vetiver, white fir
**SUBCELLULAR LOCALIZATION | EPIGENETIC INFLUENCE:** Currently unknown | Currently unknown
**RECOMMENDED DILUTION RANGE:** 5%–Neat

**PRIMARY CONSTITUENTS:**[9728,9729,9730,9731,9732,9733,9734,9735,9736,9737]

| *Needles* | | *Commercial Samples—Needles* | |
|---|---|---|---|
| Camphor | 0.0%–49.6% | 3.3%–14.4% | |
| Bornyl Acetate | 0.0%–31.3% | 9.7%–19.3% | |
| Limonene | 8.2%–26.5% | 8.0%–13.7% | |
| Alpha-Pinene | 4.1%–24.0% | 12.7%–18.7% | |
| Camphene | 6.2%–18.1% | 5.7%–12.5% | |
| Beta-Pinene | 0.0%–11.3% | 13.9%–26.5% | |
| Beta-Myrcene | 0.0%–8.4% | 4.4%–6.3% | |
| Beta-Phellandrene | 0.0%–5.5% | 0.0%–3.9% | |
| Delta-3-Carene | 0.0%–5.4% | 1.9%–5.8% | |
| Borneol | 0.0%–4.3% | 0.4%–2.2% | |
| | | | |
| *Branches* | | *Oleoresin* | |
| Beta-Pinene | 20.4%–20.5% | Beta-Pinene | 4.7%–23.8% |
| Camphor | 20.2%–20.4% | Limonene | 3.6%–17.8% |
| Alpha-Pinene | 12.0%–12.1% | Alpha-Pinene | 7.5%–11.8% |
| Bornyl Acetate | 11.7%–11.9% | Beta-Myrcene | 3.2%–10.5% |

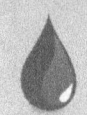

| | | | |
|---|---|---|---|
| Limonene | 8.0%–10.2% | Beta-Phellandrene | 0.1%–4.1% |
| Myrcene | 4.2%–4.3% | | |
| Borneol | 2.7%–3.9% | | |

*Needles and Twigs*

| | |
|---|---|
| Limonene | 9.8%–25.1% |
| Camphor | 8.5%–24.5% |
| Bornyl Acetate | 11.3%–19.6% |
| Beta-Myrcene | 4.8%–16.5% |
| Beta-Pinene | 3.4%–15.1% |
| Alpha-Pinene | 4.8%–13.7% |
| Camphene | 8.0%–12.6% |
| Borneol | 0.2%–5.6% |
| Delta-3-Carene | 1.1%–4.9% |
| Beta-Eudesmol | 0.9%–4.0% |

Note: Many studies report the needle oil is predominantly camphor (26.8%–49.6%), bornyl acetate (7.1%–16.5%), camphene, and limonene; however, commercially available samples are more typically predominant in beta-pinene (13.9%–26.5%), bornyl acetate (9.7%–19.3%), alpha-pinene, camphor, limonene, and camphene.

**PREFERRED COMPOSITION FOR CLINICAL USE:**

| *Constituent* | |
|---|---|
| **Beta-Pinene** | 15%–30% |
| **Alpha-Pinene** | 10%–20% |
| **Bornyl Acetate** | 10%–20% |
| **Limonene** | 8%–15% |
| **Camphene** | 5%–15% |
| **Camphor** | 7%–15% |
| **Myrcene** | 4%–7% |
| **Delta-3-Carene** | 2%–6% |
| **Borneol** | 0.1%–3% |

**OTHER CONSTITUENTS:** *Needles*—santene, alpha-terpinolene, alpha-terpineol, piperitone, delta-cadinene, tricyclene, alpha-phellandrene, gamma-cadinene; *Needles & Twigs*—tricyclene, beta-phellandrene, terpinolene, 1,8-cineole, alpha-terpineol, delta-cadinene; *Branches*—tricyclene, 1,8-cineole, terpinolene, camphene hydrate, alpha-terpineol, piperitone; *Oleoresin*—delta-3-carene

**REPORTED THERAPEUTIC PROPERTIES:** Antibacterial, antifungal, antiviral, antimicrobial, antioxidant, antiseptic, analgesic, **anti-inflammatory**, antirheumatic, antispasmodic, reduces the appearance of scarring and blemishes, aids endocrine system function, circulatory stimulant, **supports respiratory function**, expels excess mucus, supports immune function, decongestant, **calming/relaxing**, uplifting, aids mental clarification, stress management, relieves anxiety, antidepressant

**CAUTIONS:**

■ Avoid with children under 6 due to high camphor content. Several cases of camphor poisoning and/or seizures from ingestion and topical application have been reported in children.[9738,9739] Ingestion of camphor-containing products has been lethal in children under age 2 (estimated to be roughly 2,000 mg of camphor for a 20 kg child as the minimum potential fatal dose).[9740,9741] Children 5 years and up may use camphor topically in dilutions no stronger than 5%.

■ Caution is warranted during pregnancy and while lactating due to moderate to potentially high camphor content. Ingestion of essential oils with significant levels of camphor may lead to abortion because fetuses lack the enzymes to process it.[9742] Camphor ingestion by infants and young children may cause cough, vomiting, seizure, burning sensation in the mucous membranes and eyes, or lack of voluntary coordination of muscle movements.[9743]

■ Oral caution—Essential oils with significant levels of camphor can be toxic when taken orally. Camphor can be toxic when taken orally (usually single doses exceeding 2 mL), although the lethal dose for adult humans is estimated to be more than 5 mL in a single dose.[9744,9745,9746]

■ Avoid with those who have a compromised liver due to the risk of increased liver enzymes and liver damage due to camphor content.[9747] This would also suggest that those taking medications that could cause liver damage should also use white spruce very cautiously or avoid it entirely.

■ Avoid with epilepsy and Parkinson's disease due to camphor content.[9748,9749,9750]

■ Caution is warranted in children with glucose-6-phosphate dehydrogenase deficiency (G6PD) due to the camphor content in White Spruce, which may negatively impact red blood cells and increase the risk of jaundice.[9751,9752]

■ Caution is warranted for the topical application of camphor-containing essential oils on broken or injured skin due to an increased risk of toxicity.[9753]

**SELECTED EVIDENCE:**

☐ *In vitro* research concluded that white spruce demonstrated varying degrees of antimicrobial activity against the bacteria: *E. coli, S. aureus, S. enteritidis,* and *S. typhimurium* and fungi: *A. pullulans* and *A. niger.*[9754]

# WHITE VERBENA
## (Bushy Lippia, White Lippia, Juanilama)

*Lippia alba* (Mill.) N.E. Br. ex Britton & P. Wilson,
*Lantana alba* Mill., *L. germinate* Kunth

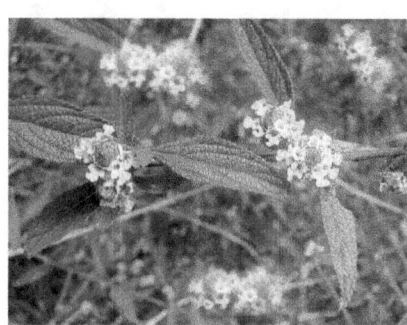

**FAMILY:** Verbenacea
**NOTE:** Middle
**AROMA INTENSITY:** Medium
**AROMA:** Varies from lemony-earthy-grassy to sweet-spicy-herbaceous to herbaceous-earthy-slightly floral depending on CT
**COMMON EXTRACTION METHOD:** Steam distilled from the leaves, flowers, and stems
**POSSIBLE SUBSTITUTE OILS:** *Citral CT*—lemongrass, melissa, may chang, citronella; *Carvone-Limonene CT*—spearmint, caraway; *Linalool CT*—lavender, rosalina
**BLENDS WELL WITH:** Basil, bergamot, black pepper, camphor, cardamom, cedarwood, citronella, clary sage, copaiba, cypress, fennel, geranium, ginger, grapefruit, lavender, lavandin, lemon, lemon eucalyptus, lemon verbena, lime, may chang, tea tree, myrrh, neroli, orange, pine, tangerine, thyme, vetiver, ylang ylang
**SUBCELLULAR LOCALIZATION | EPIGENETIC INFLUENCE:** Currently unknown | Currently unknown
**RECOMMENDED DILUTION RANGE:** *Citral CT*—1.5%–20%, neat for limited conditions; *Carvone-Limonene CT*—3%–50%, neat for limited conditions; *Linalool CT*—5%–Neat

**PRIMARY CONSTITUENTS:**[9755,9756,9757,9758,9759,9760]

| Citral CT | | Carvone/Limonene CT | |
|---|---|---|---|
| Geranial | 30.5%–54.6% | Carvone | 25.3%–77.2% |
| Neral | 23.6%–36.1% | Limonene | 18.5%–33.2% |
| Caryophyllene Oxide | 0.0%–20.5% | Geranial | 0.0%–10.4% |
| Ortho-Cymene | 0.0%–12.4% | Neral | 0.0%–10.4% |
| Limonene | 0.0%–10.2% | Bicyclosesquiphellandrene | 0.0%–7.7% |
| Beta-Myrcene | 0.0%–8.5% | Piperitone | 0.0%–4.4% |
| Geraniol | 0.0%–7.1% | Piperitenone | 2.2%–4.3% |
| Beta-Caryophyllene | 0.0%–6.6% | | |
| 6-Methyl-5-Hepten-2-ol | 0.0%–6.0% | | |

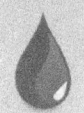

| *Linalool CT* | | *Camphor CT* | |
|---|---|---|---|
| 1,8-Cineole | 0.0%–23.0% | Camphor | 30.7%–52.0% |
| Linalool | 53.4%–84.7% | 1,6-Germacadien-5-ol | 0.0%–8.2% |
| 1,8-Cineole | 4.2%–9.2% | Linalool | 0.0%–4.1% |
| Caryophyllene Oxide | 2.9%–3.6% | | |

Note: Ten chemotypes are reported in the literature: 1) citral, 2) carvone-limonene, 3) linalool, 4) geranial-carvenone, 5) tagetenone, 6) beta-myrcene, 7) gamma-terpinene, 8) camphor-1,8-cineole, 9) camphor, and 10) estragole. However, commercial samples appear to be either citral or carvone-limonene, with the other chemotypes not found in commercial samples.

**OTHER CONSTITUENTS:** *Citral CT*—1-octen-3-al, sabinene, beta-elemene, 6-methyl-5-hepten-2-one, gamma-terpinene, linalool, (E)-isocitral, myrtenal, carvone, myrtanyl acetate, elemol, farnesol, (E)-nerolidol, geranic acid; *Carvone/Limonene CT*—beta-myrcene, gamma-muurolene, 6-methyl-5-hepten-2-ol, alpha-phellandrene, linalool, borneol, trans-carveol, nerol, beta-elemene, beta-caryophyllene, beta-guaiane; *Linalool CT*—neral, geranial, cis-linalool oxide, trans-linalool oxide, myrtenal, trans-beta-caryophyllene, germacrene B, germacrene D, nerolidol, spathulenol, humulene epoxide, beta-caryophyllene, gamma-muurolene, sabinene, beta-elemene, trans-beta-farnesene; *Camphor CT*—verbenone, pinocarvone, borneol, beta-caryophyllene, p-cymen-8-ol, trans-beta-caryophyllene, germacrene B, caryophyllene oxide

**PREFERRED COMPOSITION FOR CLINICAL USE:**

| Constituent | Citral CT | Carvone CT |
|---|---|---|
| **Geranial** | 30%–55% | – |
| **Neral** | 20%–40% | – |
| **Carvone** | – | 40%–65% |
| **Limonene** | – | 10%–25% |
| **Piperitenone** | – | 0%–5% |
| **Piperitone** | – | 0%–5% |

**REPORTED THERAPEUTIC PROPERTIES: Antibacterial**, **antifungal**, antimicrobial, **antiviral**, antioxidant, analgesic, anti-inflammatory, **antispasmodic**, antiseptic, antiallergic, eases sports injuries, helps bruises and blisters heal, reduces fever, aids digestive function, reduces intestinal spasms, anticancer, **anticonvulsant**, reduces nausea/vomiting, relieves diarrhea, **weight management**, soothes chronic skin conditions, brightens skin, aids cardiovascular function, aids normal blood pressure, balances blood sugar levels, supports eye health, encourages restful sleep, aids oral health, nervine, **antineuralgic**, relieves headache/migraine, insecticide, **insect repellent**, calming/relaxing, stress management, antidepressant, **relieves anxiety**, grounding

**CAUTIONS:**
*Citral CT*

■ Caution is advised during pregnancy and lactation due to high citral and beta-myrcene content. Large doses of citral may negatively affect fetal development according to animal studies.[9761] Extremely high doses of beta-myrcene have been toxic to fetuses according to animal research.[9762]

■ There is a moderate risk that when white verbena is taken orally it may interfere with enzymes responsible for metabolizing medications (NSAIDs, proton-pump inhibitors, acetaminophen, antiepileptics, immune modulators, blood-sugar medications, blood pressure medications, antidepressants, antipsychotics, diabetic medications, antihistamines, antibiotics, and anesthetics) due to citral content.[9763,9764,9765,9766]

■ Use cautiously with diabetic medications. Large oral doses of citral may improve insulin sensitivity and lower blood-glucose levels according to animal research.[9767,9768]

■ There is a moderate risk that white verbena may interfere with pentobarbital and other barbiturates (medications for anxiety and insomnia) based on citral, 1,8-cineole, and beta-myrcene content.[9769,9770,9771]

■ May interact with antibiotics and possibly enhance their effects.[9772,9773]

■ Dilution is recommended for topical application due to high citral content and the risk for skin irritation or sensitivity.[9774,9775] May also irritate mucous membranes.

*Carvone-Limonene CT*

■ May interact with aspirin, blood pressure, antiplatelet, and anticoagulant medications, and increase the risk of bleeding among people with bleeding disorders based on carvone content. Carvone is a potent calcium channel blocker, which may decrease blood pressure.[9776,9777]

■ May interact with barbiturates (medications for anxiety and insomnia), antihistamines, benzodiazepines, tricyclic antidepressants, or other central nervous system depressant drugs, increasing depressant effects, due to carvone content.[9778]

■ May interact with diabetes medications and cause low blood sugar based on carvone content.[9779]

*Linalool CT*

■ *Linalool CT*: May interact with antifungal drugs and enhance their effectiveness based on linalool content.[9780]

*Camphor CT*

■ Use very cautiously with children under six due to significant camphor and potentially moderate 1,8-cineole content. Several cases of camphor poisoning and/or seizures from ingestion and topical application have been reported in children.[9781,9782] Ingestion of camphor-containing products has been lethal in children under age two.[9783] 1,8-cineole may cause seizures, central nervous system problems, or respiratory distress in young children.[9784,9785,9786,9787] Children five years and up may use camphor-containing essential oils topically in dilutions no stronger than 5%. Camphor ingestion by infants and young children may cause cough, vomiting, seizure, burning sensation in the mucous membranes and eyes, or lack of voluntary coordination of muscle movements.[9788]

■ Caution is warranted during pregnancy and while lactating due to significant high camphor content. Ingestion of essential oils with significant levels of camphor may lead to abortion because fetuses lack the enzymes to process it.[9789]

■ Avoid with epilepsy and Parkinson's due to significant camphor and potentially moderate 1,8-cineole content.[9790,9791,9792,9793,9794]

■ Avoid with those who have a compromised liver due to the risk of increased liver enzymes and liver damage due to camphor content.[9795] This would also suggest that those taking medications that could cause liver damage should also use white verbena CT camphor very cautiously or avoid it entirely.

■ The significant camphor content in white verbena may negatively impact red blood cells and increase the risk of jaundice in children with glucose-6-phosphate dehydrogenase deficiency (G6PD).[9796,9797]

■ Avoid oral use. Essential oils with significant levels of camphor and 1,8-cineole can be toxic when taken orally. As few as 4 to 5 drops of high 1,8-cineole oils may be problematic in very sensitive individuals. Camphor can be toxic when taken orally (usually single doses exceeding 2 mL), although the lethal dose for adult humans is estimated to be more than 5 mL in a single dose.[9798,9799,9800]

■ May interfere with pentobarbital and other barbiturates (medications for anxiety and insomnia) based on 1,8-cineole content.[9801,9802]

■ Caution is warranted for the topical application of white verbena (camphor CT) on broken or injured skin due to an increased risk of toxicity.[9803]

**SELECTED EVIDENCE:**

☐ Citral-rich white verbena essential oil kills cervical cancer cells *in vitro*.[9804]

☐ *In vitro* research demonstrates that white verbena essential oil (citral CT) potently prevents the growth of and kills fungi (*A. fumigatus* and *C. krusei*), and inhibits the production of aflatoxin B1.[9805,9806,9807] A citral-rich CT also effectively inhibited green molds.[9808] Most research concludes that the citral CT possesses greater antifungal activity than the carvone-limonene CT.

☐ Animal research reports that white verbena (citral CT) reduces gastrointestinal and respiratory spasms by inhibiting the 5-HT3 receptor.[9809] The study also reported that citral, 1,8-cineole, and linalool all inhibit 5-HT3 as well. Compounds that inhibit 5-HT3 are effective in reducing nausea and vomiting and used to relieve symptoms of irritable bowel syndrome. Another study reported that white verbena essential oil (citral and linalool CTs) reduced spasms in isolated rat intestines by inhibiting calcium from enter cells and tissues.[9810] Interestingly the citral CT was five times more potent than the linalool CT, and twenty-eight times more potent than verapamil (a calcium channel blocker used to treat high blood pressure, chest pain, and abnormal

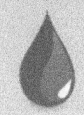

heart rhythms). Calcium channel blockers are also used to treat irritable bowel syndrome, esophageal spasms, and anal fissures due to their smooth muscle relaxant properties. The citral CT also increased nitric oxide production, which signals smooth muscle to relax.

☐ White verbena essential oil (citral CT) reduced sciatic nerve pain and excitability in isolated rat sciatic nerves.[9811]

☐ White verbena effectively killed the cattle tick *Rhipicephalus microplus*.[9812] The carvone CT repelled the same tick.[9813] Interestingly two samples of carvone CTs were used in the tick repellency study, which demonstrated that a more balanced essential oil with 26.6% limonene and 52.6% carvone exhibited greater repellency than a sample with 26.5% and 62.8% (limonene, carvone) respectively. Another study found that while the carvone-limonene CT killed cattle ticks, the citral CT was more effective.[9814]

☐ White verbena essential oil (carvone CT) killed amoebic parasites from the Acanthamoeba genus that cause amoebic keratitis and granulomatous amoebic encephalitis.[9815] Amoebic keratitis is a rare infection of the cornea by amoebae that may result in permanent vision impairment or blindness. Granulomatous amoebic encephalitis is a rare disease of the central nervous system characterized by confusion, headaches, one-sided paralysis, vision problems, low-grade fever, and seizures caused by amoebae that are generally fatal and affects people with a weakened immune system.

☐ *In vitro* research demonstrated that white verbena essential oil (citral and carvone-limonene CTs) inhibited *S. aureus* by inhibiting bacterial cell quorum sensing (the process of bacterial cell-to-cell communication that allows bacteria to share information about cell density and adjust genetic expression accordingly and is involved in its ability to cause disease).[9816] White verbena (citral CT) also inhibited quorum sensing of *E.coli*.[9817] The carvone-limonene CT actively inhibits *B. subtilis, S. aureus, S. epidermidis, Enterococcus faecalis, Enterobacter aerogenes, Escherichia coli, K. pneumoniae, P. aeruginosa,* and *Serratia maracescens*.[9818,9819] Other research reports that the citral CT inhibits *Enterococcus faecalis, S. aureus,* MRSA, *Streptococcus mutans, Candida albicans* (including serotype B), *C. parapsilosis, Cryptococcus neoformans* (serotype A), *Fonsecaea pedrosoi,* and *Trichophyton rubrum*.[9820,9821,9822,9823]

☐ White verbena essential oil (citral and carvone-limonene CTs) inhibit a number of periodontal pathogens and caused osteoclasts (bone cells that break down bone tissue during bone resorption) to die.[9824] Dental abnormalities such as root resorption and loss of permanent teeth can result if osteoclast formation or activity is increased, or if excess osteoclasts exist in relation to osteoblasts.

☐ White verbena essential oil (carvone-limonene CT) moderately killed mosquito larvae.[9825] A citral-rich white verbena essential oil effectively kills and repels the pulse beetle, whereas the carvone-rich chemotype repels the red flour beetle.[9826,9827]

☐ *In vitro* research reports that white verbena essential oil (citral CT) inhibits the adsorption (attachment of the virus to the cells surface) and replication of the yellow fever virus.[9828] Another study determined that white verbena (carvone-limonene CT) inactivates the yellow fever virus.[9829] Another study found that white verbena essential oil (carvone-limonene CT) inactivated the dengue fever virus before attaching to a cell (adsorption).[9830]

☐ A linalool-rich white verbena inhibited the activity of enzymes proteases and keratinases secreted from dermatophytes (fungi that require keratin for growth and usually infect the skin, hair and nails) allowing it to inhibit *Trichophyton rubrum, Epidermophyton floccosum* and *Microsporum gypseum*.[9831] Dermatophytes increase the secretion and activity of proteases and keratinases during infection.

☐ Animal research suggests that white verbena essential oil (carvone-limonene CT) reduces anxiety similarly to the drug diazepam.[9832] The study authors attributed the anxiolytic affect to its carvone content.

☐ White verbena essential oil (citral CT) enhances the antibiotic activity of erythromycin against *S. aureus* and was considered a valid additional treatment option against respiratory tract pathogens by the study authors.[9833]

☐ A citral-rich white verbena essential oil caused vasorelaxation (relaxing and widening of the blood vessels) in isolated rat arteries.[9834]

☐ Both the citral and carvone-limonene CTs prevented genetic damage that is a precursor to cancer initiation.[9835]

☐ *In vitro* research concluded that white verbena essential oil (citral CT) actively inhibits *T. cruzi*—a protozoan parasite that causes Chagas disease.[9836]

- White verbena essential oil (carvone-limonene) exhibited antioxidant activity similar to vitamin E.[9837]

- Animal research suggests that injection of white verbena essential oil (citral, carvone-limonene CTs) reduce anxiety-related behaviors in mice, with the carvone-limonene CT being slightly more effective.[9838] Both CTs also reduced rectal temperature.

- Ethanolic extracts of white verbena (citral and linalool CTs) with a chemical make-up similar to the essential oils prevented convulsions in mice that had clonic seizure induced by pentylenetetrazole.[9839] A citral-rich ethanolic extract also prevented the uptake of GABA, suggesting it makes more GABA available to the brain to promote relaxation. Injection of white verbena essential oil (citral, limonene-citral, and carvone-limonene CTs) reduced seizures caused by pentylenetetrazole in mice and increased survivability after seizure.[9840]

- Oral administration of 1 to 1.5 drops/kg, twice daily, of an alcoholic white verbena tincture (geranial-carvenone CT)—200 grams of leaves in 1 liter of 70% alcohol macerated for ten days and then filtered with filter paper reduced the pain intensity of migraines in frequent migraine sufferers.[9841] This was not the essential oil, but the alcoholic extract contained volatile components.

- The citral CT of white verbena essential oil was the most efficient inhibitor of the phytopathogen *Alternaria solani* Sorauer, which causes early blight on tomatoes and is responsible for great economic loss of crops.[9842] The linalool CT was also active against the phytopathogen, but the camphor CT was inactive.

- Four chemotypes of white verbena essential oil influenced biochemical pathways to lower cholesterol levels, with the tagetenone CT demonstrating greatest efficacy.[9843]

- *In vitro* research demonstrates that white verbena essential oil prevents the formation of *S. mutans* biofilms, suggesting it may be useful in the prevention of dental cavities.[9844]

- Thyme (thymol CT) essential oil inhibited *Aspergillus niger* in stored wheat grains without harming the wheat, which made the study authors conclude that thyme essential oil could be used as an eco-friendly antifungal product to protect stored wheat.[9845]

- Various chemotypes of white verbena essential oil showed antibacterial and antibiofilm activity against *S. aureus*, with the citral chemotype with 9.8% para-cymene demonstrating the greatest efficacy, followed by a citral CT with 24.9% geranic acid and the carvone CT.[9846] Isolated citral was also significantly effective.

- A white verbena CT with closely balanced citral (21.9%) and geraniol/nerol (27.1%) content displayed greater cytotoxic activity against murine melanoma and human lung cancer cells than the chemotherapy drugs cisplatin and paclitaxel.[9847] The same research observed that it inhibited yeasts (*C. albicans, C. dubliniensis, C. tropicalis, C. glabrata, C. parapsilosis, C. krusei, C. grubii, C. gattii, C. neoformans, S. cerevisiae*) better than bacteria (*E. coli, S. marcescens, E. faecalis, S. epidermidis*).

- Both the citral CT of white verbena essential oil and isolated citral reduced tracheal spasms in rats.[9848]

- White verbena essential oil CT citral demonstrated significant trypanocidal activity on three forms of *T. cruzi* (epimastigotes, trypomastigotes, amastigotes), which was greater than the activity of the carvone CT.[9849] In addition, the study authors reported that isolated limonene exhibited synergistic interaction with citral, caryophyllene oxide, and Benznidazole (decreasing its IC50 17 times) and was the most effective and selective treatment.

- The citral CT of white verbena essential oil relaxed isolated rat aortic muscle, suggesting it may dilate blood vessels and reduce blood pressure.[9850]

- White verbena CT citral essential oil — and limonene and citral — relaxed isolated rat uterus demonstrating a tocolytic (anticontraction; suppression of premature labor) effect.[9851]

- Mexican oregano thymol CT, salva-de marajó CT carvacrol, salva-de marajó CT thymol, white verbena CT citral, and lemon verbena CT citral (in order of highest activity to lowest)—and the isolated constituents para-cymene, geraniol, carvacrol, thymol, citral, and 1,8-cineole—exhibited antigenotoxic activity against ultraviolet radiation (UV)-induced DNA damage that was not related to their antioxidant capacity.[9852]

- *Schistosoma mansoni* is a water-borne parasite found in fresh water in subtropical and tropical regions that most commonly infects humans by piercing the skin and entering the bloodstream. The resulting infections, called schistosomiasis, is characterized by abdominal pain (liver and spleen), diarrhea, blood in the urine or stool, and liver enlargement in advanced cases. Schistosomiasis is second only to malaria as the most devastating parasitic infection. *Lippia gracilis* essential oil and its major constituent, carvacrol, reduced adult worm viability by 100 percent, while white verbena essential oil reduced viability by 60 percent, and its major constituent, citral, reduced viability by 75 percent. Immature parasite (schistosomula) viability was reduced by *Lippia gracilis* and white verbena 80 percent and 16 percent respectively.

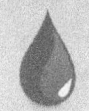

- Obesity is characterized by the increased size of adipocytes (fat-storing cells) caused by the excessive accumulation of fats, which alters their function and promotes chronic inflammation. The carvone CT of white verbena essential oil reduced adipocyte size by increasing the use of stored fats (triglycerides) for energy production in laboratory research.[9853]
- The citral CT of white verbena essential oil promoted vasorelaxation on isolated human umbilical arteries by blocking voltage-operated calcium channels.[9854]
- *Vibrio parahaemolyticus* is a bacterium found in the sea and on raw and undercooked seafood that can cause gastrointestinal illness when ingested by humans. White verbena essential oil demonstrated antibacterial activity against *V. parahaemolyticus*.[9855] The same researchers noted that it possesses antioxidant (DPPH) activity.

# WILD CHAMOMILE
## (Moroccan Chamomile, Weedy Dogfennel)

*Ormenis mixta* (L.) Dumort, *O. mixta* (L.) Dumort. ssp. *multicaulis, Chamaemelum mixtum* (L.) All., *Anthemis mixta* L.; *O. multicaulis* Braun-Blanquet & Maire; *Cladanthus mixtus* (L.) Chevall

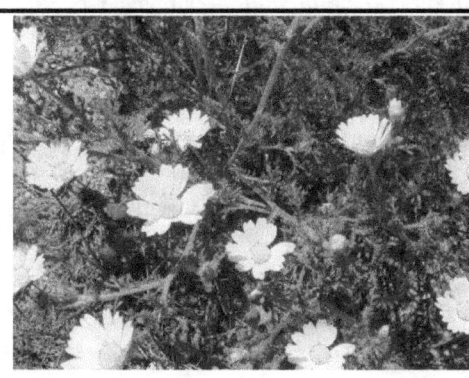

**FAMILY:** Asteraceae (Compositae)
**NOTE:** Top-Middle
**AROMA INTENSITY:** Medium
**AROMA:** Herbaceous, fresh, balsamic
**COMMON EXTRACTION METHOD:** Steam distilled from the aerial parts (flowering plant)
**POSSIBLE SUBSTITUTE OILS:** Chamomile (German, Roman), sandalwood
**BLENDS WELL WITH:** Balsam fir, basil (sweet), blue cypress, chamomile (German, Roman), clove, copaiba, cypress, davana, geranium, helichrysum, lavandin, lavender, melissa, neroli, Peru balsam, sandalwood, tolu balsam, yarrow
**SUBCELLULAR LOCALIZATION | EPIGENETIC INFLUENCE:** Currently unknown | Currently unknown
**RECOMMENDED DILUTION RANGE:** 5%–Neat

**PRIMARY CONSTITUENTS:**[9856,9857,9858,9859,9860,9861]

*O. mixta | O. mixta* (L.) Dumort. ssp. *multicaulis | Chamaemelum mixtum*

| | |
|---|---|
| Santolina alcohol | 12.5%–55.1% |
| Germacrene D | 0.5%–28.6% |
| Yomogi Alcohol | 0.7%–16.2% |
| Alpha-Pinene | 0.6%–16.0% |
| Artemisia Alcohol | 1.2%–13.2% |
| (Z)-Heptadeca-9,16-Dien-7-One | 0.0%–12.7% |
| Bornyl Acetate | 0.1%–12.2% |
| (E)-Beta-Farnesene | 1.5%–11.3% |
| Alpha-Cadinol | 0.1%–8.9% |
| Limonene | 0.1%–8.0% |
| Epi-Alpha-Muurolol | 0.2%–6.6% |
| Epi-Alpha-Cadinol | 0.2%–4.4% |
| Pinocarvone | 0.1%–4.1% |
| (E)-Pinocarveol | 0.1%–3.7% |
| Delta-Cadinene | 0.1%–3.4% |
| Caryophylladienol | 0.0%–3.1% |

*Cladanthus mixtus—Santolina Alcohol CT*

| | |
|---|---|
| Santolina Alcohol | 17.4%–37.7% |
| 1,8-Cineole | 3.2%–11.6% |
| (E)-Nerolidol | 0.7%–9.0% |
| Beta-Elemene | 0.0%–5.0% |
| Alpha-Pinene | 2.7%–4.8% |
| Camphenilone | 0.0%–4.8% |
| Yomogi Alcohol | 0.4%–4.5% |
| Sabinene | 0.3%–3.9% |
| Germacrene D | 1.5%–3.3% |
| Cubenol | 0.0%–3.2% |

*O. multicaulis*

| | |
|---|---|
| Alpha-Pinene | 11.6%–24.9% |
| Santolina Alcohol | 10.2%–15.2% |
| (E)-Beta-Farnesene | 0.0%–8.6% |
| 1,8-Cineole | 7.2%–7.4% |
| Beta-Elemene | 0.0%–6.7% |
| Germacrene D | 0.0%–6.3% |
| Limonene | 0.1%–6.0% |
| Alpha-Humulene | 0.0%–4.1% |

| | |
|---|---|
| Myrcene | 0.1%–3.7% |
| Sabinene | 0.1%–3.4% |

Note: Blue tansy (*Tanacetum annuum*) is sometimes called Moroccan chamomile as well, but it is more appropriately called blue tansy or true Moroccan chamomile. *Cladanthus mixtus* also has camphor/beta-myrcene, trans-beta-farnesene, ar-curcumene, and 2-methyl-2-trans-butenyl methacrylate chemotypes reported in the literature, but none of its chemotypes are commercially available as of this writing.

**OTHER CONSTITUENTS:** *O. mixta/O. mixta* (L.) Dumort. ssp. *multicaulis/Chamaemelum mixtum*—1,8-cineole, camphor, borneol, santolina acetate, myrcene, delta-elemene, beta-maaliene, beta-elemene, beta-caryophyllene, alpha-humulene, bicyclogermacrene, alpha-muurolene, (Z)-nerolidol, germacrene-d-4-ol, caryophyllene oxide, alpha-murolol; *O. multicaulis*—camphene, beta-pinene, gamma-terpinene, trans-pinocarveol, borneol, terpinen-4-ol, alpha-terpineol, bornyl acetate, beta-caryophyllene, (E)-nerolidol; *Cladanthus mixtus*—santolinatriene, alpha-thujene, alpha-terpinene, para-cymene, gamma-terpinene, Artemisia alcohol, isobutyl tiglate, trans-pinocarveol, pinocarvone, terpinen-4-ol, alpha-terpineol, beta-caryophyllene, trans-beta-farnesene, alpha-muurolene, elemol, beta-caryophyllene oxide, ledol, T-cadinol, beta-eudesmol, alpha-bisabolol

**PREFERRED COMPOSITION FOR CLINICAL USE:**

| Constituent | CT 1 | CT2 |
|---|---|---|
| Santolina Alcohol | 30%–47% | 3%–10% |
| (Z)-Heptadeca-9,16-dien-7-one | 0%–13% | – |
| (E)-Beta-Farnesene | 2%–6% | 8%–18% |
| Artemisia Alcohol | 2%–5% | tr–5% |
| Yomogi Alcohol | 2%–5% | tr–5% |
| Alpha-Pinene | 0.5%–5% | 8%–18% |
| Caryophyllene Oxide | 0.5%–3% | 0.1%–5% |
| Limonene | 0.1%–2% | 2%–8% |
| Pinocarvone | 0.1%–2% | – |
| Germacrene D | – | 8%–18% |
| 1,8-Cineole | – | 2%–8% |
| Myrcene | – | 2%–8% |
| Delta-Elemene | – | 2%–8% |
| (E,E)-Alpha-Farnesene | – | 0.1%–6% |

**REPORTED THERAPEUTIC PROPERTIES:** Antibacterial, antifungal, **antimicrobial**, analgesic, antiparasitic, anti-inflammatory, soothes sprains and strains, antiarthritic, antirheumatic, antiallergic, relieves sunburn, **relieves chronic skin conditions**, nourishing to the skin, relieves headache/migraine, antispasmodic, combats acne, supports liver, gallbladder, and pancreas function, aids digestion, balances menstruation, relieves painful menstruation, relaxing/calming, **promotes restful sleep**, stress management, helps one adapt to change, combats irritability

**CAUTIONS:**
■ None currently known.

**SELECTED EVIDENCE:**
☐ *In vitro* research demonstrates that wild chamomile essential oil strongly inhibits *S. aureus, E. coli, C. freundii, E. faecalis, L. monocytogenes,* and *K. pneumoniae,* and a fraction of the oil rich in alcohols (santolina and yomogi) also inhibits *C. albicans* by disc diffusion method.[9862] Minimum-inhibitory concentration method demonstrated that the essential oil strongly inhibited *S. aureus, E. coli, C. freundii, E. faecalis, L. monocytogenes,* and *K. pneumoniae,* whereas the alcohol-rich fraction possessed stronger antimicrobial activity, inhibiting seven bacteria: three gram-positive bacteria, *B. cereus, S. aureus,* and *L. monocytogenes,* and four gram-negative bacteria, *E. coli, C. freundii, E. faecalis,* and *K. pneumoniae,* and

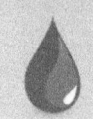

one strain of *C. albicans*.[9863] Another study found that wild chamomile inhibits *B. subtilis, E. coli, Micrococcus luteus, S. aureus, A. niger, Penicillium parasiticus,* and *Trametes pini*.[9864]

☐ Wild chamomile essential oil is insecticidal to the Japanese termite.[9865]

☐ Wild chamomile essential oil inhibits *S. aureus* and produces a synergistic effect against the bacteria when used with geranium.[9866] The same research demonstrates that wild chamomile possesses important antioxidant activity.

# WILD MARJORAM
## (Mastic Thyme, Spanish Marjoram)
*Thymus mastichina* L., *Th. mastichina* L. ssp. *mastichina*

**FAMILY:** Lamiaceae (Labiatae)
**NOTE:** Middle
**AROMA INTENSITY:** Medium
**AROMA:** Herbaceous, medicinal, camphoraceous, spicy
**COMMON EXTRACTION METHOD:** Steam distilled from the aerial parts (flowering plant)
**POSSIBLE SUBSTITUTE OILS:** *1,8-Cineole CT*—eucalyptus, ravintsara (1,8-cineole CT), niaouli (1,8-cineole CT), big badja gum, Southern blue gum, gully gum; *Linalool CT*—Lavandin, ravintsara (linalool CT), lavender, spike lavender
**BLENDS WELL WITH:** Basil, big badja gum, blue cypress, cajeput, chamomile (German, Roman), clary sage, cypress, eucalyptus, elemi, frankincense, grapefruit, gully gum, lavender, lemon, lemongrass, lime, orange, rosemary, rosewood, Southern blue gum, tea tree, tangerine, thyme
**SUBCELLULAR LOCALIZATION | EPIGENETIC INFLUENCE:** Currently unknown | Currently unknown
**RECOMMENDED DILUTION RANGE:** *1,8-Cineole CT*—3%–33%, neat for limited conditions; *Linalool CT*—5%–Neat

**PRIMARY CONSTITUENTS:**[9867,9868,9869,9870,9871]

| *1,8-Cineole CT* | | *Linalool CT* | |
|---|---|---|---|
| 1,8-Cineole | 56.8%–69.6% | Linalool | 59.3%–69.0% |
| Linalool | 1.8%–15.7% | 1,8-Cineole | 1.1%–10.8% |
| Limonene | 1.1%–10.8% | Elemol | 0.9%–6.6% |
| Alpha-Terpineol | 1.7%–6.0% | Gamma-Terpinene | 0.2%–5.8% |
| Beta-Pinene | 1.7%–5.6% | Camphor | 2.4%–5.3% |
| Alpha-Terpinyl Acetate | 0.0%–4.5% | T-Cadinol | 1.2%–4.6% |
| Alpha-Phellandrene | 0.1%–3.8% | Borneol | 0.1%–4.4% |
| Alpha-Pinene | 0.5%–3.6% | Delta-Terpineol | 0.1%–4.4% |
| | | Camphene | 0.9%–3.3% |

Note: Wild marjoram is not related to sweet marjoram chemically or botanically, but is actually a species of wild thyme that grows in Spain.

**OTHER CONSTITUENTS:** *1,8-Cineole CT*—camphene, myrcene, sabinene, para-cymene, (E)-beta-ocimene, gamma-terpinene, trans-sabinene hydrate, borneol, isoborneol, terpinen-4-ol, myrtenol, bornyl acetate, allo-aromadendrene, elemol; *Linalool CT*—alpha-pinene, beta-pinene, para-cymene, (E)-beta-ocimene, beta-caryophyllene, bicyclogermacrene, gamma-cadinene

**PREFERRED COMPOSITION FOR CLINICAL USE:**

| Constituent | *1,8-Cineole CT* |
|---|---|
| **1,8-Cineole** | 50%–70% |
| **Linalool** | 3%–16% |
| **Limonene** | 1.5%–8% |
| **Beta-Pinene** | 2%–6% |

| Alpha-Terpineol | 1.5%–5% |
| Alpha-Pinene | 1%–5% |
| Linalyl Acetate | 0.1%–4% |
| Camphor | 0.1%–2% |
| Borneol | 0.1%–2% |
| Terpinen-4-ol | 0.1%–2% |
| Beta-Caryophyllene | 0.1%–2% |

**REPORTED THERAPEUTIC PROPERTIES:** Antibacterial, antifungal, antioxidant, antiseptic, analgesic, relieves sprains and strains, anti-inflammatory, antirheumatic, antiarthritic, **supports respiratory function**, decongestant, expels excess mucus, eases cough, aids circulation, helps bruises heal, relieves menstrual pain, aids digestion, relieves headache (particularly sinus related), insecticide, mentally stimulating, promotes alertness, **aids concentration**, supports memory function

**CAUTIONS:**

*1,8-Cineole CT*

■ Avoid with children under age three, particularly around the nose and mouth. Use very cautiously in children under age five due to high 1,8-cineole content. 1,8-cineole may cause seizures, central nervous system problems, or respiratory distress in young children.[9872,9873,9874,9875]

■ Avoid with epilepsy and Parkinson's disease due to 1,8-cineole content. May exacerbate or cause seizures/convulsions or reduce seizure medication efficacy based on 1,8-cineole content.[9876,9877,9878]

■ Caution is warranted orally due to the significant amounts of 1,8-cineole. Limit it to small doses internally (adults—maximum 10 drops daily). Toxicity has been reported when eucalyptus (also high in 1,8-cineole) was ingested in large doses, and as few as 4 to 5 drops may cause problems in very sensitive individuals.[9879,9880,9881,9882,9883,9884] In humans, 3.5 to 5 mL has proven fatal orally.[9885]

■ May weakly interfere with the enzymes responsible for metabolizing medications (NSAIDs, proton-pump inhibitors, acetaminophen, antiepileptics, immune modulators, blood-sugar medications, blood pressure medications, antidepressants, antipsychotics, diabetic medications, antihistamines, antibiotics, and anesthetics) based on 1,8-cineole content.[9886,9887]

■ May interact with diabetic medications due to the ability of 1,8-cineole to significantly inhibit alpha-glucosidase activity, particularly when synergized with other constituents (alpha-pinene, beta-pinene, and para-cymene).[9888,9889,9890] Alpha-glucosidase is an enzyme that breaks down carbohydrates by chemical reaction with water. Inhibiting its activity postpones glucose absorption and therefore the impact of carbohydrates on blood sugar levels.

■ May interfere with pentobarbital and other barbiturates (medications for anxiety and insomnia) based on 1,8-cineole content.[9891,9892]

■ May interact with anticholinergic (drugs used for asthma, incontinence, gastrointestinal cramps, muscular spasms, depression, and sleep disorders) and cholinergic medications (drugs used to reduce urinary retention, diagnose myasthenia gravis, and for glaucoma) based on AChE inhibitory activity.[9893]

*Linalool CT*

■ May interact with antifungal drugs and enhance their effectiveness based on significant linalool content.[5053]

■ May interact with anticholinergic (drugs used for asthma, incontinence, gastrointestinal cramps, muscular spasms, depression, and sleep disorders) and cholinergic medications (drugs used to reduce urinary retention, diagnose myasthenia gravis, and for glaucoma) based on AChE inhibitory activity.[9894]

**SELECTED EVIDENCE:**

☐ Wild marjoram essential oil demonstrated mild antioxidant properties *in vitro*.[9895,9896]

☐ Both the 1,8-cineole and linalool CTs of wild marjoram essential oil inhibited both lipoxygenase and acetylcholinesterase (AChE) enzyme activity.[9897] The study authors reported that bornyl acetate and limonene were the strongest inhibitors of lipoxygenase and 1,8-cineole was the best AChE inhibitor. These findings suggest that wild marjoram essential oil may be useful for a variety of inflammatory conditions and dementia

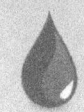

and Alzheimer's disease. The same research reported that the oils exhibited antioxidant and antimicrobial (*Escherichia coli, Staphylococcus aureus*, and *Candida albicans*) activities.

□ *In vitro* research demonstrates that wild marjoram essential oil inhibits poultry origin strains of *Escherichia coli, Salmonella enteritidis*, and *S. essen*, and pig origin strains of enterotoxigenic *E. coli, S. choleraesuis* and *S. typhimurium* at high concentrations.[9898] Another study reported antimicrobial activity against *Salmonella* subsp., *Staphylococcus aureus, Candida albicans, Escherichia coli, Proteus mirabilis*, and *Listeria monocytogenes*, with the linalool CT being more effective than the 1,8-cineole CT.[9899] The 1,8-cineole CT of the oil moderately inhibited several *Candida* species.[9900]

□ Wild marjoram essential oil is highly insecticidal against the Egyptian cotton leafworm.[9901]

□ Laboratory research suggests that wild marjoram essential oil CT 1,8-cineole might be useful for Alzheimer's disease and inflammatory conditions due to its ability to inhibit lipoxygenase and acetylcholinesterase activities.[9902] When individual constituents in wild marjoram were tested, bornyl acetate and limonene demonstrated the highest lipoxygenase inhibition and 1,8-cineole the best inhibition of acetylcholinesterase activities. The same research showed that wild marjoram essential oil inhibits *Escherichia coli, Staphylococcus aureus*, and *Candida albicans*, and is a good antioxidant. Linalool, linalyl acetate, α-terpinene and γ-terpinene also demonstrated antioxidant activities.

□ Catnip, oregano, and wild marjoram essential oils each exhibited high antioxidant activity in the DPPH, total reducing power, and β-carotene/linoleic acid assays, anticancer activity against human breast cancer, and broad-spectrum antibacterial activity.[9903]

□ Wild marjoram CT 1,8-cineole showed antibacterial activity against several bacteria such as *E. coli, P. mirabilis, Salmonella* subsp., methicillin-resistant and methicillin-sensitive *S. aureus, L. monocytogenes* EGD, *B. cereus*, and *Pseudomonas*, and antifungal activity against *Candida* spp. and *Fusarium* spp.[9904]

□ Wild marjoram essential oil CT 1,8-cineole extracted via steam distillation, hydrodistillation, or solvent-free microwave extraction produced a similar composition and possessed similar antioxidant (DPPH assay) and antimicrobial activity.[9905] The oils inhibited MRSA, *S. aureus, E. faecalis, E. coli, P. aeruginosa*, and *C. albicans*.

□ Both cardamom and wild marjoram CT 1,8-cineole essential oils demonstrated antimicrobial activity (*C. glabrata, L. monocytogenes, C. tropicalis, H. influenzae, S. pneumoniae, S. aureus, C. albicans, Y. enterocolitica, P. fluorescens* biofilm, and *E. coli*), with wild marjoram being the more active against bacteria and cardamom better against fungi.[9906] Cardamom also exhibited mild anticancer activity against breast cancer cells.

□ Wild marjoram CT 1,8-cineole essential oil displayed good antioxidant activity in the beta-carotene bleaching assay but not in the DPPH assay, and inhibited *K. pneumoniae, E. coli, C. albicans, L. monocytogenes, B. cereus, C. tropicalis, S. aureus*, and *P. aeruginosa*.[9907]

---

# WINTERGREEN

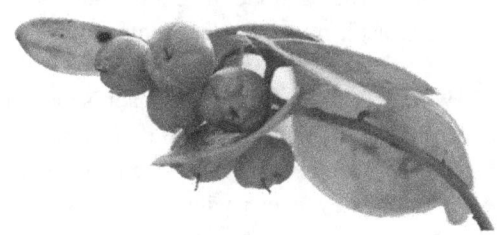

*Gaultheria procumbens* L.; *G. fragrantissima* Wall.;
*G. yunnanensis* (Franch.) Rehd, *G. leucocarpa* var. *yunnanensis*;
*G. semi-infera* (C.B.Clarke) Uiry Shaw; *G. leucocarpa* Blume;
*G. griffithiana* Wight; *G. longibracteolata* R.C.Fang.; *Gaultheria* spp.

**FAMILY:** Ericaceae
**NOTE:** Top-Middle
**AROMA INTENSITY:** Strong
**AROMA:** Sharp, sweet, woody, slightly minty
**COMMON EXTRACTION METHOD:** Steam distilled from the leaves
**POSSIBLE SUBSTITUTE OILS:** Birch
**BLENDS WELL WITH:** Birch, cajeput, oregano, peppermint, ravintsara, spearmint, thyme, ylang ylang
**SUBCELLULAR LOCALIZATION | EPIGENETIC INFLUENCE:** Cell Membrane, Endoplasmic Reticulum, Mitochondria | Immune/Nervous
**RECOMMENDED DILUTION RANGE:** 1.5%–20%; 50% for some conditions

**PRIMARY CONSTITUENTS:**[9908,9909,9910]

Methyl Salicylate          96.9%–99.6%

**OTHER CONSTITUENTS:** Alpha-pinene, delta-3-carene, d-limonene, myrcene, delta-cadinene

**PREFERRED COMPOSITION FOR CLINICAL USE:**

*Constituent*

| | |
|---|---|
| **Methyl Salicylate** | 97%–99.9% |
| **Total Other Volatile Constituents:** Linalool, Ethyl Salicylate, (3Z)-Hexenol, Benzyl Alcohol, Alpha-Pinene, Beta-Pinene, Limonene, Eugenol, etc. | tr–3% |
| **Absent Synthetic Markers:** Methyl 4-Hydroxybenzoate, Dimethyl 4-Hydroxyisophthalate, Dimethyl 2-Hydroxyisophthalate, Methyl Paraben, Dimethyl 2-Hydroxyterephthalate | 0% |

Note: Carbon-14 isotope analysis should be performed as a step to confirm authenticity. Moreover, production of American wintergreen (*G. procumbens*) essential oil is now nearly non-existent, especially at commercial scale. Some markers of American wintergreen may be tuberolactone and massoia lactone.

**REPORTED THERAPEUTIC PROPERTIES: Analgesic (pain relief), anti-inflammatory, antirheumatic,** antiarthritic, antiseptic, antispasmodic, astringent, relieves bone pain, deodorant, expels excess gas, eases sports injuries, **stimulates liver function,** eases cough, supports normal menstruation, diuretic, stimulates gallbladder function, **increases redness and circulation of a localized area,** relaxing, warming, stimulating, promotes mental alertness, promotes a positive self-image and self-acceptance, encourages forgiveness

**CAUTIONS:**

■ Avoid with children under age 12. The high salicylate content in wintergreen may increase the risk of a very serious and life-threatening illness called Reye syndrome in children under 12. Reye syndrome is sudden brain damage and liver dysfunction that most commonly occurs in children ages 4 to 12. It has an unknown cause, but it typically occurs in children who were given aspirin when they were experiencing a fever or recovering from flu-like symptoms or chickenpocks.[9911]

■ Do not use during pregnancy or lactation. May cause congenital abnormalities and fetal malformations.[9912,9913]

■ Oral caution—As little as 2.5 mL can cause toxicity and 4 mL may be fatal in children. As little as 5 mL could result in methyl salicylate poisoning in adults and more than 5 mL can be fatal.[9914,9915,9916,9917,9918] Methyl salicylate is structurally similar to aspirin (acetylsalicylic acid) and readily metabolized to salicylic acid—the same bioactive intermediate as aspirin—after ingestion. Since quality wintergreen essential oil is 97%+ methyl salicylate, this means that wintergreen's mode of action is identical to aspirin. One drop of wintergreen essential oil is roughly equivalent to a baby aspirin in salicylate content and four drops is equivalent to a 325 mg aspirin tablet. Do not exceed 5 drops of wintergreen oil per day orally for an adult.

■ Avoid with epilepsy and Parkinson's disease due to methyl salicylate content.[9919,9920]

■ May interact with aspirin, blood pressure, antiplatelet, and anticoagulant medications, and increase the risk of bleeding among people with bleeding disorders both topically and orally.[9921,9922,9923,9924]

■ Toxicity may occur with overuse topically and the absorption of methyl salicylate increases with repeated applications.[9925] Not intended for long-term use.

■ Avoid orally with gastroesophageal reflux disease (GERD). May cause accumulation of fluid in the larynx (laryngeal edema) and lead to airway obstruction in sensitive individuals.[9926]

■ Avoid in individuals allergic to aspirin, methyl salicylate, or other NSAIDs; or those with salicylate sensitivities. Methyl salicylate may be metabolized to the known NSAID, salicylic acid, by the liver.[9927]

**SELECTED EVIDENCE:**

☐ Oral administration of salicylate glucoside from wintergreen oil (200 to 800 mg/kg) prevented abdominal contractions, and reduced pain and inflammation, in mice similarly to aspirin but without causing stomach ulcers because it released the salicylates slowly in the intestine rather than in the stomach.[9928,9929]

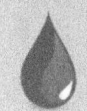

- Salicylate glucoside obtained from wintergreen oil inhibited the production of proinflammatory molecules and the excess production of nitric oxide *in vitro*.[9930,9931,9932]

- A methyl salicylate ointment applied to the temples and jaw relieved a headache caused by electroconvulsive treatment (a procedure used to treat mental illness where electrical currents are passed through the brain to cause a trigger a brief seizure).[9933]

- Wintergreen essential oil was toxic to the adult spotted wing drosophila (*Drosophila suzukii*) when used as a fumigant.[9934]

- Wintergreen essential oil demonstrated good antioxidant and antibacterial (*Enterococcus* sp, *Staphylococcus aureus, Bacillus subtilis*, and *Klebsiella pneumonia*) activity *in vitro*.[9935]

- Rosemary CT 1,8-cineole, lemongrass (*C. citratus*), and wintergreen essential oils each repelled, knocked down, and were lethal to moths (*Anarsia lineatella*).[9936] Rosemary was the most effective repellent and most lethal.

- Leishmaniasis is a neglected tropical disease caused by parasitic protozoa of the *Leishmania* genus. Current treatment options for cutaneous leishmaniasis are limited due to severe side effects, poor efficacy, resistance to first-line drugs, and limited availability to populations who need the medication. A study evaluated the antileishmanial activities of fifty-two essential oils and concluded that frankincense (a combination of *Boswellia carterii, B. sacra, B. papyrifera*, and *B. frereana*), coriander, and wintergreen possesses notable antileishmanial activities that make them promising candidates for the topical treatment of cutaneous leishmaniasis.[9937]

- *In vitro* evidence showed that wintergreen essential oil inhibits *Aeromonas caviae, Candida albicans*, and *Mycobacterium fortuitum*.[9938] The researchers also showed that the oil was not cytogenotoxic.

- Wintergreen essential oil was the toxic to the granary weevil (*Sitophilus granarius*) and considered a potential biocide because of its cost to effectiveness ratio.

---

# WORMSEED, AMERICAN
## (Chenopodium, Mexican Tea, Jesuits' Tea, Epazote)

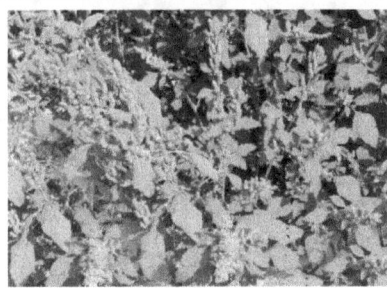

*Dysphania ambrosioides* (L.) Mosyakin & Clemants, *Chenopodium ambrosioides, Ch. obovatum* Moq., *Ch. retusum* Juss. ex Moq., *Teloxys ambrosioides* (L.) W.A. Weber, *T. vagans* (Standl.) W.A. Weber, *Ambrina ambrosioides* (L.) Spach

**FAMILY:** Chenopodiaceae
**NOTE:** Middle
**AROMA INTENSITY:** Strong
**AROMA:** Pungent, medicinal, herbaceous
**COMMON EXTRACTION METHOD:** Hydrodistilled or steam distilled from the whole herb, leaves, or seeds
**POSSIBLE SUBSTITUTE OILS:** Boldo, oregano
**BLENDS WELL WITH:** Doesn't blend well with other oils due to its strong, disagreeable odor
**SUBCELLULAR LOCALIZATION | EPIGENETIC INFLUENCE:** Currently unknown | Currently unknown
**RECOMMENDED DILUTION RANGE:** < 0.5%

**PRIMARY CONSTITUENTS:**[9939,9940,9941,9942,9943,9944,9945,9946,9947,9948,9949,9950,9951]

| *Ascaridole CT* | | *Alpha-Terpinene CT* | |
|---|---|---|---|
| (Z)-Ascaridole | 29.7%–61.4% | Alpha-Terpinene | 40.7%–64.0% |
| Isoascaridole | 0.5%–27.7% | Alpha-Terpinyl Acetate | 0.0%–31.6% |
| Para-Cymene | 2.0%–27.2% | Para-Cymene | 7.3%–26.4% |
| Alpha-Terpinene | 0.7%–20.7% | (Z)-Ascaridole | 0.9%–17.9% |
| Piperitone | 0.0%–5.0% | Thymol | 0.0%–7.9% |
| Carvacrol | 0.0%–4.9% | Carvacrol | 0.0%–4.3% |
| Trans-Ascaridole Glycol | 0.0%–4.5% | | |
| 3,4-Epoxy-ρ-Menthan-2-One | 0.0%–4.1% | | |

*Carvacrol CT*

| | |
|---|---|
| Carvacrol | 62.4% |
| (Z)-Ascaridole | 22.5% |
| Caryophyllene Oxide | 5.6% |

Note: There are at least ten chemotypes of American wormseed essential oil, including ascaridole, alpha-terpinene, alpha-pinene, para-cymene, carvacrol, alpha-terpinyl acetate, sabinene hydrate acetate, ascaridole epoxide, terpinolene, and limonene. The most common CTs reported in the literature are ascaridole, alpha-terpinene, and carvacrol, which are reported above.

**OTHER CONSTITUENTS:** *Ascaridole CT*—para-cymen-8-ol, alpha-terpineol, limonene, (E)-piperitol acetate, trans-p-mentha-2,8-dien-1-ol, cis-p-menth-2-en-1-ol, delta-4-carene, alpha-pinene, ρ,α-dimenthylstyrene, gamma-terpinene, terpinen-1-ol, geraniol, cis-piperitone epoxide, caryophyllene oxide, trans-piperitone epoxide, 2-ethylcyclohexanone, thymol, precocene II, dihydroisojasmone, cis-p-mentha-1(7),8-diene-2-ol, geranyl tigliate, phytol, hexahydrofarnesyl acetone; *Alpha-Terpinene CT*—isoascaridole (< 2.6%), limonene, gamma-terpinene, cis-p-mentha-1(7),8-diene-2-ol, phytol; *Carvacrol CT*—delta-4-carene, para-cymene, isoascaridole (< 1.9%), neomenthyl acetate, hexyl tigliate, apiole (< 2.0%)

**PREFERRED COMPOSITION FOR CLINICAL USE:**

| Constituent | Carvacrol CT |
|---|---|
| **Carvacrol** | 50%–65% |
| **(Z)-Ascaridole** | < 20% |
| **Caryophyllene Oxide** | 2%–8% |

Note: Should only be used clinically when the benefits outweigh the risks as determined by a health professional.

**REPORTED THERAPEUTIC PROPERTIES:** Antibacterial, antifungal, antiparasitic, aids respiratory function, expels excess mucus, stimulates menstruation, diuretic, wound healing, anti-inflammatory, analgesic, antirheumatic, relieves snake bites, soothes hemorrhoids, insect repellent, insecticide, relieves hysteria, relieves anxiety

**CAUTIONS:**

*Wormseed is not recommended for use in essential oil therapy in any form of administration, but the profile is included for informational purposes and safety information. Its anti-leishmanial activity may be useful (and less toxic than standard drugs) if done under the care of a physician, and preferably with the carvacrol CT, which seems to mitigate some of the toxicity of ascaridole, or American wormseed herbal infusions. Infusions contain a hydrophilic component that produces a significant nematocidal effect, while proving to be much safer than the essential oil.[9952]*

■ Avoid use in children due to toxicity concerns and known poisoning and fatalities with ascaridole-containing essential oils in humans.[4111] American wormseed essential oil is considered genotoxic (damages genetic information within a cell resulting in mutations and possibly cancer) and cytotoxic (toxic to living cells).[9953]

■ Avoid during pregnancy and lactation. Hydro-alcohol extracts containing ascaridole have reportedly caused abortions, fetal abnormalities, and low birth weight in animal studies when administered at 800 mg/kg/day.[9954,4113] American wormseed is commonly used to cause abortions.[9955,9956]

■ Avoid oral consumption—very toxic due to ascaridole content. Oral use of essential oils with significant ascaridole can cause respiratory depression, overstimulation of the CNS (exaggerated reflexes, lack of coordination, convulsions, paralysis of motor and sensory nerves, and death by respiratory arrest), liver toxicity, and anaphylactic reactions.[9957,9958,9959] Human toxicity and fatal poisoning have been reported in children and adults with wormseed essential oil.[4111] Ingestion of as little as 10 mg of American wormseed is known to cause cardiac disturbances, convulsions, respiratory disturbances, sleepiness, vomiting, weakness, and even death.[4312]

■ Avoid with epilepsy and Parkinson's disease due to ascaridole content. Ingestion of as little as 10 mg of American wormseed is known to cause convulsions.[4312]

■ May interact with aspirin, blood pressure, antiplatelet, and anticoagulant medications, and increase the risk of bleeding among people with bleeding disorders due to ascaridole, isoascaridole, and carvacrol content.[1610,1611,1612,4115,4313]

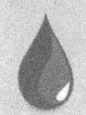

■ Avoid with those who have a compromised liver or kidneys due to the risk of kidney toxicity, kidney failure, or liver toxicity (ascaridole content).[3979,4109,4312] This would suggest that those taking medications that could cause liver damage should also use American wormseed essential oil very cautiously or avoid it entirely.

■ May interact with the antifungal and antiparasitic medication pentamidine and increase its effectiveness.[4325]

■ May interact with antibiotics and possibly enhance their effects due to carvacrol content.[1612,1613]

■ *Carvacrol CT*: May interact with diabetic medications and cause low blood-sugar levels due to carvacrol content.[1609]

■ *Carvacrol CT*: May irritate mucous membranes (eyes, mouth, nasal passages, vagina, rectum).

■ *Carvacrol CT*: May interact with anticholinergic (drugs used for asthma, incontinence, gastrointestinal cramps, muscular spasms, depression, and sleep disorders) and cholinergic medications (drugs used to reduce urinary retention, diagnose myasthenia gravis, and for glaucoma) based on research with the whole essential oil and carvacrol and ascaridole content.[2236,4305]

■ Topical application may promote skin sensitization or irritation. Ascaridole and essential oils with significant amounts of ascaridole are known to cause skin sensitivity.[4248,4249,4250]

### SELECTED EVIDENCE:

☐ *In vitro* research shows that American wormseed essential oil (Ascaridole CT) kills colon adenocarcinoma cells.[4305]

☐ Both ascaridole and the ascaridole CT of American wormseed essential oil inhibits acetylcholinesterase activity.[4305] Inhibition of AChE prevents the breakdown of acetylcholine, which is essential for memory and thinking. People with neurodegenerative diseases make less acetylcholine, and the diseases often break it down at a faster rate, leading to acetylcholine deficits and cognitive decline.

☐ *In vitro* research reports that American wormseed essential oil (ascaridole CT) is a potent antioxidant—more potent than ascorbic acid.[4305] An unknown CT of American wormseed also exhibited potent antioxidant activity.[4329]

☐ Animal research shows that American wormseed essential oil (ascaridole CT) cleared an *Entamoeba histolytica* (a parasite that causes amoebiasis and is estimated to infect 50 million people worldwide) infection.[4307] Another study found that it inhibited parasite growth and reduced intracellular *Leishmania amazonensis* (a parasite that causes leishmaniasis).[4300] The combination of ascaridole and carvacrol (1:4 ratio) demonstrated anti-protozoal activity on Leishmania promastigotes, lower cytotoxicity, and synergistic activity on intracellular amastigotes, which reduced lesion size and parasite burden in mice.[4317] Other research found that the whole essential oil (carvacrol CT with 62.4% carvacrol and 22.5% ascaridole) was superior to both glucantime (a drug considered a first-line agent in the treatment of leishmaniasis) and isolated essential oil constituents (a mix of ascaridole, carvacrol, and caryophyllene oxide) in reversing cutaneous leishmaniasis caused by *L. amazonensis* in mice.[4319,4328] Oral administration of the carvacrol CT (150 mg/kg) demonstrated better anti-leishmanial activity against *L. amazonensis* and resolution of cutaneous leishmaniasis than glucantime, amphotericin B, and pentamidine.[4323] The carvacrol CT also demonstrated antiprotozoal activity against *Plasmodium falciparum* (one of the protozoan parasites that causes malaria in humans) and *Trypanosoma brucei* (a protozoan parasite that causes African trypanosomiasis in humans and other animals).[4320] American wormseed (terpinolene CT; 69.9% terpinolene and 17.1% ascaridole) prevented *T. cruzi* parasite growth and survival—demonstrating activity at the epimastigote, trypomastigote, and amastigote phases—by interacting with the microbe's membrane and drastically reducing membrane permeability without harming healthy cells (mice macrophages).[4322] Another study reported that American wormseed essential oil (carvacrol CT) potently inhibited promastigote and amastigote phases, but was also moderately toxic to mice macrophages.[4330] An unidentified CT of American wormseed essential oil significantly killed *L. donovani* promastigotes and amastigotes *in vitro*.[4326]

☐ *In vitro* research demonstrates that American wormseed essential oil (ascaridole CT) completely inhibits the fungi *Aspergillus flavus*, *A. glaucus*, *A. niger*, *A. ochraceous*, *Colletotrichum gloesporioides*, *C. musae*, *Fusarium oxysporum*, and *F. semitectum*.[4298] An unknown CT of American wormseed essential oil demonstrated broad-spectrum antifungal activity against *Aspergillus niger*, *A. fumigatus*, *Botryodiplodia theobromae, Fusarium oxysporum, Sclerotium rolfsii, Macrophomina phaseolina, Cladosporium cladosporioides, Helminthosporium oryzae,* and *Pythium debaryanum,* and inhibited aflatoxin B1 production by the aflatoxigenic strain of *A. flavus.*[4329]

☐ Topical application of an ointment containing American wormseed or American wormseed in combination with palmarosa strongly inhibited ringworm (a common fungal infection of the skin caused by a dematophyte) in guinea pigs.[4234] Other research reported similar results and concluded that American wormseed essential oil inhibits *Aspergillus fumigatus, Cladosporium trichoides,* and eight dermatophytes, including *Trichophyton rubrum* and *Microsporum gypseum.*[4336,4338]

☐ Interestingly, the ascaridole CT of American wormseed essential oil displayed no antibacterial activity against gram-positive bacteria (*Bacillus cereus* or *Staphylococcus aureus*) or the gram-negative bacterium *Escherichia coli.*[4301]

☐ American wormseed essential oil (various CTs) is toxic to or repels the Cucurbit Beetle (*Diabrotica speciosa*), mosquitoes, maize weevil (*Sitophilus zeamais* (Motsch.)), ticks (*Rhipicephalus lunulatus*), citrus mealybug (*Planococcus citri* (Risso)), longtailed mealybug (*Pseudococcus longispinus* (Targioni Tozzetti)), western flower thrips (*Frankliniella occidentalis* (Pergande)), fungus gnats (*Bradysia* spp.), German cockroach (*Blattella germanica*), twospotted spider mite (*Tetranychus urticae* Koch), European red mite (*Panonychus ulmi* (Koch), common green bottle fly (*Lucilia sericata*), pulse bruchids (*Callosobruchus chinensis* L. and *C. maculatus* F.).[3937A,4303,4309,4314,4315,4316,4318,4321,4327,4332,4333,4335]

# WORMWOOD
## (Absinthe, Artemisia)

*Artemisia absinthium* L., *A. absinthium* L. var. *insipida* Stechmann

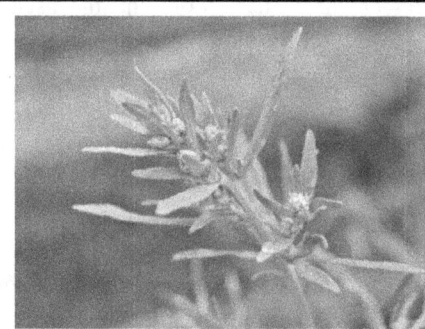

**FAMILY:** Asteraceae (Compositae)
**NOTE:** Base
**AROMA INTENSITY:** Medium
**AROMA:** Bitter, earthy, medicinal, herbaceous
**COMMON EXTRACTION METHOD:** Steam distilled from leaves and flowering tops; may also be steam distilled from the roots or leaves
**POSSIBLE SUBSTITUTE OILS:** Thuja, sage (alpha-thujone CT), mugwort (alpha-thujone CT), western red cedar (leaves)
**BLENDS WELL WITH:** Anise, bergamot, lavender, lemon, lime, neroli, orange, petitgrain, rose, tangerine
**SUBCELLULAR LOCALIZATION | EPIGENETIC INFLUENCE:** Currently unknown | Currently unknown
**RECOMMENDED DILUTION RANGE:** 1.5%–20%

**PRIMARY CONSTITUENTS:**[9960,9961,9962,9963,9964,9965,9966,9967,9968,9969]

| Beta-Thujone CT | | Myrcene CT | |
|---|---|---|---|
| Beta-Thujone | 12.3%–64.6% | Myrcene | 8.6%–44.3% |
| (Z)-Epoxy Ocimene | 0.2%–23.1% | Sabinene | 0.0%–21.1% |
| Trans-Sabinyl Acetate | 0.9%–18.2% | Cis-Chrysanthenyl Acetate | 7.7%–17.9% |
| Linalool | 0.4%–7.3% | Beta-Pinene | 0.1%–11.8% |
| Sabinene | 0.0%–6.3% | Dihydrochamazulene Isomer | 5.5%–11.6% |
| Cis-Chrysanthenyl Acetate | 0.0%–5.2% | Germacrene D | 0.6%–8.0% |
| Alpha-Phellandrene | 0.0%–4.9% | Beta-Thujone | 0.4%–7.3% |
| | | Linalool | 5.3%–7.0% |
| *Chamazulene CT* | | Linalyl Acetate | 0.0%–7.0% |
| Chamazulene | 25.3%–39.9% | Chamazulene | 0.0%–6.8% |
| Beta-Thujone | 17.2%–22.1% | Alpha-Phellandrene | 0.0%–5.3% |
| Trans-Sabinene Hydrate | 5.3%–12.6% | | |

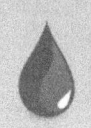

| | |
|---|---|
| Trans-Linalool Oxide | 0.1%–6.0% |
| Beta-Selinene | 4.5%–5.3% |
| Sabinyl Acetate | 0.1%–5.0% |

*Alpha-Thujone CT*

| | |
|---|---|
| Alpha-Thujone | 17.7%–30.7% |
| Trans-Sabinyl Acetate | 9.8%–22.1% |
| Beta-Thujone | 5.6%–13.4% |
| Beta-Pinene | 1.3%–9.0% |
| Trans-Sabinol | 0.1%–6.4% |
| Myrcene | 0.1%–5.1% |
| Linalool | 0.1%–4.7% |

*(Z)-Epoxy Ocimene CT*

| | |
|---|---|
| (Z)-Epoxy Ocimene | 20.6%–59.7% |
| Beta-Thujone | 0.0%–27.8% |
| Cis-Chrysanthenyl Acetate | 0.0%–26.4% |
| Trans-Sabinyl Acetate | 0.0%–23.6% |
| Bicyclo[2.2.1]Hept-2-en-7-ol | 0.0%–18.9% |
| Sabinene | 0.0%–9.3% |
| (E)-Epoxy Ocimene | 0.0%–8.4% |
| 2-Ethyl-4-Methyl-1,3-Pentadienyl Benzene | 0.0%–7.4% |
| Alpha-Phellandrene | 0.0%–6.0% |
| Linalool | 0.0%–5.9% |
| Neryl-3-Methyl Butanoate | 0.0%–5.5% |
| Benzeneacetaldehyde | 0.0%–5.5% |
| Neryl Butanoate | 0.0%–4.9% |

*Trans-Sabinyl Acetate CT*

| | |
|---|---|
| Trans-Sabinyl Acetate | 13.7%–84.5% |
| Alpha-Thujone | 0.0%–15.9% |
| Beta-Pinene | 0.2%–10.4% |
| Myrcene | 0.2%–9.2% |
| Neryl-3-Methyl Butanoate | 0.0%–9.1% |
| Neryl Butanoate | 0.0%–7.9% |
| Sabinene | 1.0%–6.9% |
| 1,8-Cineole | 1.0%–5.2% |
| Linalool | 0.3%–4.8% |
| Alpha-Pinene | 0.2%–4.3% |

*Cis-Chrysanthenyl Acetate CT*

| | |
|---|---|
| Cis-Chrysanthenyl Acetate | 3.6%–36.7% |
| (Z)-Epoxy Ocimene | 24.2%–25.6% |
| Bicyclo[2.2.1]Hept-2-en-7-ol | 3.2%–5.3% |
| (Z)-3-Hexenyl Butyrate | 1.5%–4.8% |
| Benzeneacetaldehyde | 1.6%–3.3% |

*Trans-Sabinene Hydrate CT*

| | |
|---|---|
| Trans-Sabinene Hydrate | 11.0%–21.8% |
| Trans-Sabinyl Acetate | 0.0%–8.8% |
| Alpha-Thujone | 0.1%–8.0% |
| Beta-Thujone | 3.7%–6.7% |
| Beta-Selinene | 0.0%–6.7% |
| Lavandulol | 0.0%–5.5% |
| Myrcene | 0.0%–4.4% |
| Sabinene | 0.0%–4.0% |
| Linalool | 0.0%–4.0% |

*Myrcene/Sabinene CT*

| | |
|---|---|
| Sabinene | 18.0%–30.1% |
| Myrcene | 17.7%–29.9% |
| Beta-Thujone | 0.1%–4.5% |

*Sabinene CT*

| | |
|---|---|
| Sabinene | 17.6%–24.5% |
| Trans-Sabinyl Acetate | 7.8%–13.6% |
| Myrcene | 3.1%–11.0% |
| Cis-Chrysanthenyl Acetate | 0.0%–11.0% |
| Alpha-Phellandrene | 5.4%–10.3% |
| Para-Cymene | 4.7%–6.2% |
| (Z)-Myroxide | 0.0%–5.8% |
| Linalool | 3.9%–4.9% |
| Terpinen-4-ol | 1.4%–4.5% |
| Chamazulene | 0.0%–4.3% |

*Beta-Pinene CT (Pre-flowering Aerial Parts)*

| | |
|---|---|
| Beta-Pinene | 12.3%–31.9% |
| Alpha-Phellandrene | 9.8%–16.4% |
| Chamazulene | 4.2%–13.9% |
| Sabinene | 0.0%–8.8% |
| Para-Cymene | 7.1%–8.2% |
| Alpha-Pinene | 3.2%–5.9% |

*(E)-Beta-Farnesene CT*

| | |
|---|---|
| (E)-Beta-Farnesene | 31.6% |
| (Z)-Beta-Ocimene | 27.8% |
| (Z)-En-yn-Dicycloether | 11.1% |
| Santolina Triene | 4.9% |

**OTHER CONSTITUENTS:** *Beta-Thujone CT*—myrcene, alpha-thujene, beta-phellandrene, para-cymene, allocimene, phellandrene oxide, alpha-thujone (<3.0%), terpinen-4-ol, benzeneacetaldehyde, thujol, nerol, fragranol, geraniol, neryl propionate, linalyl 3-methyl butanoate, caryophyllene oxide, chamazulene, eugenol, neral, alpha-terpineol, diepi-alpha-cedrene, (Z)-3-hexenyl butyrate, (E)-3-hexenyl butyrate geranyl acetate, neryl butanoate, neryl-3-methyl butanoate; *Myrcene*

*CT*—alpha-pinene, para-cymene, 1,8-cineole, santolina alcohol, gamma-terpinene, alpha-thujone (<3.0%), menthone, pulegone (<1.2%), carvone, cis-piperitone epoxide, carvacrol, carvone, thymol, lavandulyl acetate, piperitenone oxide, lavandulyl isobutanoate, neryl isobutanoate, bicyclogermacrene, lavandulyl 2-methylbutyrate, neryl 2-methylbutanoate, neryl isovalerate, 9-geranyl-para-cymene, (E)-nuciferol isobutyrate, (Z)-nuciferol isobutyrate; *Chamazulene CT*—tricyclene, alpha-thujene, alpha-pinene, camphene, sabinene, myrcene, limonene, (Z)-beta-ocimene, (E)-beta-ocimene, alpha-copaene, linalool, cis-sabinene hydrate, linalyl acetate, terpinene-4-ol, cis-dihydrocarvone, cis-verbenol, lavandulol, alpha-humulene, neral, gamma-curcumene, gamma-muurolene, borneol, germacrene D, carvone, geranyl acetate, gamma-cadinene, geraniol, para-cymene-8-ol, eugenol; *Trans-Sabinene Hydrate CT*—beta-pinene, alpha-phellandrene, 1,8-cineole, trans-sabinol, terpinen-4-ol, alpha-acoradiene, lavandulyl 2-methyl butyrate, beta-calacorene, chamazulene, 9-geranyl-para-cymene; *(Z)-Epoxy Ocimene CT*—myrcene, alpha-thujene, gamma-terpinene, 1,8-cineole, neral, alpha-humulene, alpha-terpineol, ar-curcumene, linalyl 3-methyl-butanoate, geranyl pentanoate, (Z)-jasmone, (E)-nerolidol, spathulenol, eugenol, vulgarol B, carvacrol, beta-bisabolol, chamazulene, beta-selinene, gamma-cadinene, thujol, alpha-thujone (<1.2%); *Trans-Sabinyl Acetate CT*—alpha-phellandrene, para-cymene, trans-sabinol, cis-chrysanthenol, terpinen-4-ol, trans-caryophyllene, alpha-humulene, geranyl propionate, germacrene D, gamma-curcumene, lavandulyl isovalerate, lavandulyl 2-methyl butyrate, cis-nerolidol, neryl 2-methyl butyrate, beta-calacorene, chamazulene, 9-geranyl-para-cymene, 9-geranyl-alpha-terpinene; *Myrcene/Sabinene CT*—1,8-cineole, linalool, alpha-thujone, (Z)-epoxy ocimene, neryl butanoate, neryl-3-methyl butanoate; *Cis-Chrysanthenyl Acetate CT*—allocimene, 3-octanol, (E)-epoxy ocimene, linalool, neral, alpha-humulene, alpha-terpineol, gamma-cadinene, ar-curcumene, neryl propionate, geranyl propionate, (Z)-jasmone, spathulenol, bisabolol oxide, alpha-bisabolol, vulgarol B, gamma-gurjunene, eugenol; *Alpha-Thujone CT*—alpha-pinene, sabinene, 1,8-cineole, gamma-terpinene, terpinen-4-ol, alpha-acoradiene, gamma-curcumene, neryl 2-methyl butyrate, beta-calacorene, chamazulene, 9-geranyl-para-cymene; *Sabinene CT*—alpha-pinene, allo-ocimene, beta-thujone (<3.0%), alpha-thujone (<0.6%), beta-caryophyllene, gamma-terpinene, 1,8-cineole, geranyl isovalerate, lavandulyl acetate, lavandulol, cis-sabinol; *Beta-Pinene CT*—alpha-thujene, beta-myrcene, limonene, beta-thujone (<2.4%), linalool, beta-bourbonene, humulene, germacrene D, beta-selinene, delta-cadinene, phytane; *(E)-Beta-Farnesene CT*—hexanal, alpha-pinene, benzaldehyde, para-cymene, (E)-beta-ocimene, gamma-terpinene, allo-ocimene, alpha-terpineol, terpinen-4-ol, cis-verbenyl acetate, beta-caryophyllene, (2Z,6E)-farnesyl acetate, (E)-en-yn-dicycloether

**PREFERRED COMPOSITION FOR CLINICAL USE:**

| Constituent | *(Z)-Epoxy Ocimene CT* |
|---|---|
| **(Z)-Epoxy Ocimene** | 20%–55% |
| **(Z)-Chrysanthenyl Acetate** | 10%–25% |
| **Bicyclo[2.2.1]Hept-2-en-ol** | 5%–15% |
| **Benzeneacetaldehyde** | 1%–6% |
| **(E)-Ocimene Oxide** | 2%–5% |
| **Neryl Propionate** | 0.5%–5% |
| **Linalool** | 1%–4% |
| **Caryophyllene Oxide** | 1%–3% |
| **Gamma-Gurjunene** | 1%–3% |
| **Alpha-Copaene** | 0.5%–3% |
| **Linalyl-3-Methyl Butanoate** | 0.1%–3% |
| **ar-Curcumene** | 0.1%–3% |
| **Eugenol** | 0.5%–3% |
| **Alpha-Bisabolol** | 0.5%–3% |
| **Spathulenol** | 0.1%–2% |

Note: The (Z)-Epoxy Ocimene CT is typically found among plants grown in France.

**REPORTED THERAPEUTIC PROPERTIES: Antibacterial**, antifungal, antimicrobial, **antiparasitic**, anticancer, aids digestion, immune stimulant, **antioxidant**, supports cardiovascular function, balances menstruation, relieves menstrual cramps and PMS, aids liver function, reduces fever, supports endocrine function and the release of hormones, insect repellent, insecticide, promotes restful sleep, antidepressant, relieves anxiety, stress management

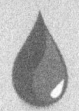

CAUTIONS:

*Wormwood essential oil composition is very complex and diverse with many chemotypes having the potential to have high thujone content. Wormwood is an essential oil best avoided in essential oil therapy unless you know the exact composition of the oil that you are using.*

■ Avoid with children under six due to thujone and trans-sabinyl acetate content. Cases of seizure have been reported in young children who were exposed to essential oils with significant amounts of thujones.[9970,9971,9972] Trans-sabinyl acetate is highly toxic, particularly when thujones are present.[9973,9974,9975]

■ Avoid during pregnancy and while lactating. Essential oils high in thujone content may stimulate menstruation and the uterus resulting in abortion.[9976,9977] Sabinyl acetate containing oils are toxic to developing embryos and prevent implantation during days 0–4 of gestation, can cause abortions, and maternal toxicity (which indicated a greater susceptibility to sabinyl acetate toxicity during pregnancy) according to animal research.[9978,9979,9980] Extremely high doses (500 mg/kg) of beta-myrcene have been toxic to fetuses according to animal research.[9981,9982]

■ Avoid oral consumption. Ingesting high thujone essential oils like wormwood can cause vomiting, stomachache, diarrhea, and gastroenteritis followed by absorption disorders, headache, nervous agitation and chronic convulsions, and symptoms of liver and kidney toxicity extending to yellow liver atrophy (extensive and rapid death of liver cells— parenchymal, possibly accompanied by fatty degeneration), arrhythmia, and myocardial bleeding.[9983] Thujone is considered significantly neurotoxic and may damage the liver, and it is estimated that as little as 15 mg orally may negatively impact the central nervous system.[9984,9985,9986] A thirty-one-year-old man experienced tonic/clonic seizures and acute kidney failure after mistakenly drinking 10 mL of wormwood oil high in thujones.[9987] Case reports involving serious adverse health outcomes (seizure, convulsions, and acute kidney failure) have been reported in adults who consumed high thujone essential oils (sage, thuja, wormwood) in doses of one "swallow," 12 drops, and 20 drops twice daily for five days.[9988,9989,9990,9991] Savin essential oil (also high in sabinyl acetate) irritates the mucosal lining of the gastrointestinal tract, damages the kidneys, causes blood in the urine, obstructs blood flow in the abdominal organs, and causes abnormally heavy menstrual bleeding, which the study authors attributed to the combined effects of sabinene, sabinol, and sabinyl acetate.[9992] However, more recent research suggests it is the sabinyl acetate content of savin essential oil that causes toxicity and other adverse effects.

■ *Alpha-Thujone, Myrcene CT*: May weakly interfere with the enzymes responsible for metabolizing medications (NSAIDs, proton-pump inhibitors, acetaminophen, antiepileptics, immune modulators, blood-sugar medications, blood pressure medications, antidepressants, antipsychotics, diabetic medications, antihistamines, antibiotics, and anesthetics) due to alpha-thujone or beta-myrcene content.[9993,9994]

■ Avoid with epilepsy and Parkinson's disease due to thujone and sabinyl acetate content.[9995,9996,9997,9998,9999]

■ Avoid with those who have a compromised liver or kidneys because of increased risk of kidney toxicity, kidney failure, or liver toxicity due to sabinyl acetate and thujones content.[10000,10001,10002,10003,4135] Consuming extremely large amounts of thujone rich essential oils (10 mL) has caused kidney failure.[10004] Trans-sabinyl acetate is highly toxic to the liver when thujones are also present.[10005,10006,10007,10008] This would also suggest that those taking medications that could cause liver damage should also use wormwood essential oil very cautiously or avoid it entirely.

■ *Myrcene CT*: May interfere with pentobarbital and other barbiturates (medications for anxiety and insomnia) based on beta-myrcene content.[10009]

SELECTED EVIDENCE:

☐ Wormwood essential oil ((Z)-epoxy ocimene CT) killed several cancer cells (adenocarcinoma, squamous non-small cell lung cancer, colorectal carcinoma, breast, melanoma, and bone marrow) *in vitro*.[10010]

☐ *In vitro* research reported that wormwood essential oil (sabinene CT) inhibited three multi-drug-resistant pathogenic bacteria (*Acinetobacter* sp. from wound swabs, *P. aeruginosa* from sputum, and *S. aureus* from nasal swabs).[10011]

☐ High concentrations of wormwood essential oil ((Z)-epoxy ocimene CT) killed the parasites *T. cruzi* and *T. vaginalis*.[10012]

☐ Animal and *in vitro* research concluded that wormwood essential oil (trans-sabinyl acetate CT) killed the parasite *L. amazonensis*, which is one of the parasite responsible for leishmania, better than the drug glucantime (a drug used as the first line of defense to treat cutaneous leishmania).[10013] Another study found that a camphor-rich wormwood essential oil killed two *Leishmanial* strains: *L. aethiopica* and *L. donovani* better than amphotericin B (an antifungal drug administered intravenously for systemic fungal infections and first-line drug for cutaneous leishmania).[10014]

☐ Research suggests wormwood essential oil (sabinene CT) is a potent antioxidant, insecticide, ant antibacterial.[10015,10016] A beta-pinene CT also demonstrated antioxidant activity.[10017] The same research reported that the sabinene CT of wormwood was not irritating to the skin of 30 volunteers when applied neat.

☐ *In vitro* research concluded that wormwood leaf oil (rich in borneol) inhibited *Micrococcus luteus, M. flavus, Bacillus subtilis, Penicillium chrysogenum,* and *Aspergillus fumigatus.*[10018]

☐ Wormwood essential oil (beta-thujone CT and an alpha-fenchene CT from long-term stored aerial parts) inhibited the common human pathogens *E. coli, S. enteritidis, P. aeruginosa, K. pneumoniae, S. aureus, C. albicans,* and *A. niger.*[10019]

☐ Wormwood essential oil (sabinene CT) provided 70% tick repellency.[10020]

☐ *In vitro* research found that wormwood essential oil (chamazulene CT) completely inhibited several plant fungi and weakly inhibited a limited number of sixty-four tested bacteria (plant, food, and clinical).[10021] Another study found that the chamazulene CT of wormwood inhibited the growth of several species of plant fungi.[10022]

☐ Wormwood essential oil ((Z)-epoxy ocimene CT) inhibited *Candida albicans* and *Saccharomyces cerevisiae* var. *chevalieri.*[10023]

☐ Wormwood essential oil (beta-thujone CT) killed the spider mite (*tetranychus urticae* Koch).[10024] The study authors reported that the steam distilled oil was more potent than either the hydrodistilled (direct distillation in contact with water) or microwave-assisted process oils. Other research reports that wormwood essential oil ((E)-beta-farnesene CT) is toxic to six mosquito vectors: *An. stephensi, An. subpictus, Ae. aegypti, Ae. albopictus, Cx. quinquefasciatus,* and *Cx. Tritaeniorhynchus,* without harming other insects (*Chironomous circumdatus, Anisops bouvieri,* and *Gambusia affinis*).[10025] The study authors concluded that (E)-beta-farnesene, (Z)-en-yn-dicycloether, and (Z)-beta-ocimene from wormwood essential oil represent promising eco-friendly larvicides.

☐ Intralesional (direct injection into a lesion) injection of an encochleated (lipid-crystal nanoparticle form that improves bioavailability, targeted delivery, and safety) wormwood essential oil proved to be stable, tolerable, and effective, and improved the systemic delivery of the essential oil in animals with cutaneous leishmaniasis.[10026]

☐ Wormwood CT alpha-fenchene essential oil inhibited *C. parapsilosis, S. aureus* (three strains), *P. aeruginosa, E. coli* (two strains), and *E. faercium,* with the greatest activity observed against *C. parapsilosis.*[10027] It was also found that the oil maintained antimicrobial activity when combined with hydroxyapatite—a combination developed to prevent postoperative infections.

☐ Wormwood CT chamazulene and white wormwood (*A. herba alba*) CT alpha-thujone essential oil reduced the ability of *E. coli* to form a biofilm.[10028]

☐ A cis-davanone CT of wormwood essential oil displayed antioxidant activity in the TAC, FRAP, and DPPH-SA assays and metal chelating activity, with minimal cytotoxicity against cell lines (an indicator of safety).[10029]

☐ Wormwood essential oil displayed strong antioxidant activity in the DPPH and ABTS assays and potently inhibited the growth of *B. subtilis, S. aureus,* and *Aspergillus* sp.[10030] The oil also inhibited acetylcholinesterase and butyrylcholinesterase.

# XANTHOXYLUM
## (Zanthoxylum, Winged Prickly Ash, Tomar Seed)

*Zanthoxylum armatum* DC.

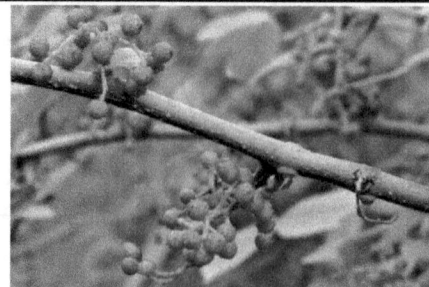

**FAMILY:** Rutaceae
**NOTE:** Middle
**AROMA INTENSITY:** Medium
**AROMA:** Floral, fruity, fresh
**COMMON EXTRACTION METHOD:** Steam distilled from the dried seeds (fruits/berries); may also be distilled from the leaves

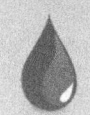

**POSSIBLE SUBSTITUTE OILS:** Neroli, lavender, rosewood, petitgrain
**BLENDS WELL WITH:** Black pepper, buddha wood, cedarwood, copaiba, coriander, elemi, geranium, jasmine, lavender, neroli, orange (sweet), Peru balsam, petitgrain, sandalwood, siam wood, spruce (black)
**SUBCELLULAR LOCALIZATION | EPIGENETIC INFLUENCE:** Currently unknown | Currently unknown
**RECOMMENDED DILUTION RANGE:** 3%–50%; neat for limited conditions

**PRIMARY CONSTITUENTS:**[10031,10032]

| | |
|---|---|
| Linalool | 57.0%–70.6% |
| Limonene | 8.2%–19.8% |
| Beta-Phellandrene | 0.0%–5.7% |
| (E)-Methyl Cinnamate | 0.0%–5.7% |
| (Z)-Methyl Cinnamate | 0.0%–4.9% |

**OTHER CONSTITUENTS:** Myrcene, gamma-terpinene, (Z)-linalool oxide, (E)-linalool oxide, (Z)-pinene oxide, phellandral, (E)-nerolidol, otrienol, terpinene-4-ol, geraniol, (E)-beta-caryophyllene

**PREFERRED COMPOSITION FOR CLINICAL USE:**

| Constituent | Linalool CT | Balanced |
|---|---|---|
| **Linalool** | 45%–65% | 25%–45% |
| **Limonene** | 10%–25% | 25%–45% |
| **Beta-Phellandrene** | 5%–15% | – |
| **(E)-Methyl Cinnamate** | 5%–13% | 5%–20% |
| **Beta-Myrcene** | 2%–6% | 2%–8% |

**REPORTED THERAPEUTIC PROPERTIES:** Analgesic, anti-inflammatory, antirheumatic, antiarthritic, **antispasmodic**, antibacterial, antiviral, antimicrobial, antioxidant, antiallergic, aids immune function, **relieves painful menstruation and PMS**, nervine, relieves strained/sore throat, supports respiratory function, relieves upset stomach, relieves toothache, promotes restful sleep, **stress management**, relieves anxiety, **antidepressant**

**CAUTIONS:**

■ May interact with antifungals and possibly enhance their effects due to significant linalool content.[10033]

**SELECTED EVIDENCE:**

☐ Xanthoxylum essential oil kills the larvae of three mosquito species (*Cx. quinquefasciatus, Ae. aegypti,* and *An. stephensi*).[10034] An interesting CT of xanthoxylum essential oil with trans-anethole and 1,8-cineole as the primary constituents was strongly toxic to two stored-product insects (*Lasioderma serricorne* and *Tribolium castaneum*).[10035]

# YARROW
## (Blue Yarrow, Common Yarrow)
*Achillea millefolium* L.

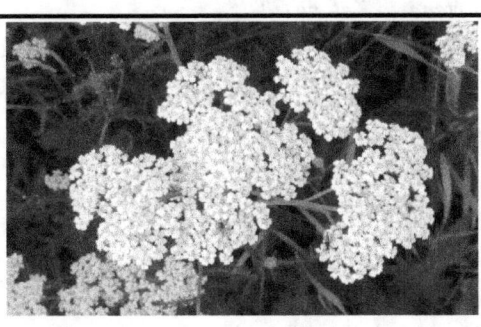

**FAMILY:** Asteraceae (Compositae)
**NOTE:** Middle
**AROMA INTENSITY:** Strong
**AROMA:** Herbaceous, sharp, floral, slightly sweet
**COMMON EXTRACTION METHOD:** Steam distilled from the aerial parts (leaves and tops) of the flowering plant; yarrow may also be steam distilled from the leaves or flowers separately
**POSSIBLE SUBSTITUTE OILS:** German chamomile, blue tansy, cistus, geranium, copaiba

**BLENDS WELL WITH:** Bay laurel, black pepper, bergamot, cedarwood, chamomile (German, Roman), clary sage, copaiba, cypress, grapefruit, lavender, lemon, lime, neroli, orange, pine, sandalwood, tangerine, vetiver, ylang ylang

**SUBCELLULAR LOCALIZATION | EPIGENETIC INFLUENCE:** Currently unknown | Currently unknown

**RECOMMENDED DILUTION RANGE:** 5%–20%, neat for limited conditions; *Beta-Thujone CT*—1.5%–20%; *1,8-Cineole/Camphor CT*—3%–33%, 50% for some conditions

**PRIMARY CONSTITUENTS:**[10036,10037,10038,10039,10040,10041]

*Sabinene CT*

| | |
|---|---|
| Sabinene | 6.7%–41.3% |
| 1,8-Cineole | 4.7%–16.0% |
| Borneol | 0.0%–12.4% |
| Beta-Pinene | 2.3%–12.3% |
| (E)-Nerolidol | 0.0%–9.6% |
| Bornyl Acetate | 0.0%–8.0% |
| Beta-Caryophyllene | 2.3%–7.5% |
| Germacrene D | 1.0%–6.8% |
| (E,E)-Farnesol | 0.0%–6.5% |
| Alpha-Pinene | 2.8%–6.3% |
| Terpinen-4-ol | 0.4%–6.2% |
| Caryophyllene Oxide | 0.0%–6.0% |
| Chamazulene | 0.0%–5.3% |

*1,8-Cineole/Camphor CT*

| | |
|---|---|
| 1,8-Cineole | 8.7%–28.8% |
| Camphor | 11.0%–28.4% |
| Germacrene D | 0.7%–11.5% |
| Borneol | 2.9%–6.2% |
| Beta-Eudesmol | 0.0%–6.1% |
| Alpha-Terpineol | 0.9%–5.9% |
| Alpha-Bisabolol | 0.0%–5.5% |
| Beta-Pinene | 0.5%–5.4% |
| Caryophyllene Oxide | 0.2%–3.3% |
| Terpinen-4-ol | 1.9%–3.1% |
| Beta-Caryophyllene | 1.1%–3.1% |
| Alpha-Elemol | 0.0%–3.0% |
| Alpha-Pinene | 0.6%–2.5% |
| Kongol | 0.0%–2.3% |
| Sabinene | 0.1%–2.0% |

*Artemisia Ketone CT*

| | |
|---|---|
| Artemisia Ketone | 14.9% |
| Camphor | 11.5% |
| Linalyl Acetate | 11.5% |
| 1,8-cineole | 10.2% |
| Limonene | 7.4% |
| Linalool | 6.6% |
| Yomogi Alcohol | 6.4% |
| Borneol | 5.4% |
| O-Cymene | 5.3% |

*Chamazulene CT*

| | |
|---|---|
| Chamazulene | 15.7%–44.3% |
| Beta-Caryophyllene | 2.5%–22.2% |
| Beta-Pinene | 0.1%–19.4% |
| Bornyl Acetate | 0.1%–15.8% |
| Sabinene | 0.0%–15.2% |
| Germacrene D | 0.0%–11.2% |
| 1,8-Cineole | 0.1%–9.6% |
| (E)-Nerolidol | 0.1%–9.6% |
| Piperitone | 0.0%–5.1% |
| Spathulenol | 0.0%–5.1% |
| Caryophyllene Oxide | 0.5%–4.8% |
| Gamma-Muurolene | 0.1%–4.6% |
| Camphor | 0.1%–4.3% |
| Alpha-Pinene | 0.0%–4.1% |
| Terpinen-4-ol | 0.2%–3.1% |
| Isophytol | 0.0%–2.9% |
| Delta-Cadinene | 0.5%–2.8% |
| T-Muurolol | 0.0%–2.7% |
| Isocaryophyllene Oxide | 0.0%–2.6% |
| Phytol | 0.0%–2.6% |
| Delta-Cadinol | 0.0%–2.3% |
| Trans-Sabinyl Acetate | 0.0%–2.1% |
| Alpha-Thujone | 0.0%–2.1% |
| Pentadecanoic Acid | 0.0%–2.1% |
| Alpha-Guaiene | 0.1%–2.0% |
| Alpha-Terpineol | 0.3%–1.9% |
| Humulene Epoxide | 0.1%–1.9% |
| Borneol | 0.0%–1.8% |
| Alpha-Cadinol | 0.0%–1.8% |

*Beta-Thujone CT*

| | |
|---|---|
| Beta-Thujone | 8.3%–96.2% |
| 1,8-Cineole | 0.4%–15.2% |
| Camphor | 0.0%–11.7% |
| Sabinene | 0.0%–8.9% |
| Beta-Pinene | 0.0%–7.8% |
| Terpinen-4-ol | 0.0%–5.8% |

Note: Myriad chemotypes of yarrow essential oil are reported in the literature and its chemical composition varies widely based on growing environment and location: Yugoslavia (1,8-cineole/camphor CT), Canada (beta-thujone CT), Greece (ascaridole CT), Cuba (caryophyllene oxide CT), Germany (chamazulene, linalool, and sabinene CTs), Estonia (chamazulene CT), Czech Republic (chamazulene CT), Romania (1,8-cineole-camphor CT), Latvia (chamazulene CT), Ukraine (chamazulene CT), Austria

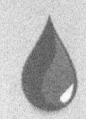

(chamazulene CT), Norway (sabinene CT), Portugal (sabinene, 1,8-cineole-camphor, and beta-thujone CTs), Algeria (chrysanthenone CT), Italy (alpha-asarone CT), India (sabinene, beta-pinene, and 1,8-cineole-camphor CTs), Chile (beta-thujone CT), Greece (ascaridole CT), Australia and Kazakhstan (artemisia ketone CT), and Iran (alpha-bisabolol CT).[2936,2937,2941,2943,2943A,2943B,2944,2950,2951] Changes in composition of yarrow are associated with environmental factors and plant maturity at time of harvest, with increasing amounts of monoterpenes in relation to sesquiterpenes (increased alpha-pinene, beta-pinene, and alpha-thujone and decreased sabinene, borneol, and bornyl acetate) from vegetative state to full bloom.[2953] Much of Europe produces chamazulene CTs, but the sabinene CT appears to be the most common CT available commercially.

**OTHER CONSTITUENTS:** *Sabinene CT*—myrcene, alpha-terpinene, para-cymene, limonene, gamma-terpinene, gamma-muurolene, alloaromadendrene, terpinolene, alpha-thujone (<1.0%), thujanol, camphor (<2.2%), alpha-terpineol, azulen, gamma-cadinene, alpha-cadinol, epiglobulol, beta-bisabolol, t-muurolol; *1,8-Cineole/Camphor CT*—camphene, myrcene, alpha-terpinene, gamma-terpinene, para-cymene, trans-sabinene hydrate, cis-sabinene hydrate, cis-chrysanthenyl acetate, cis-chrysanthenol, delta-cadinene, bornyl acetate, eugenol, spathulenol, caryophylladienol 2, germacrene-D isomer; *Chamazulene CT*—alpha-terpinene, camphene, myrcene, artemesia ketone, linalool, cis-verbenol, trans-verbenol, myrtenal, fenchyl acetate, carvone, geranyl acetate, aromadendrene, ar-curcumene, beta-Ionone, gamma-cadinene, viridiflorol, guaiol, beta-bisabolol, alpha-bisabolol, (E,E)-farnesyl acetate, hexadecane-1-ol; *Beta-thujone CT*—carvotanacetone, camphene, myrcene, alpha-phellandrene, alpha-terpinene, limonene, gamma-terpinene, para-cymene, terpinolene, chamazulene, alpha-cadinol, T-cadinol, gamma-cadinene, beta-caryophyllene, borneol, terpineol, caryohyllenol-1, alpha-thujone (<1.4%), bornyl acetate, caryophyllene oxide; *Artemisia Ketone CT*—camphene, alpha-pinene, beta-pinene, artemisia alcohol, beta-thujone (<1.7%), terpinen-4-ol, (Z)-chrysanthenyl acetate, caryophyllene, germacrene D, viridiflorol

## PREFERRED COMPOSITION FOR CLINICAL USE:

| Constituent | Sabinene CT |
|---|---|
| Sabinene | 15%–30% |
| Beta-Pinene | 5%–20% |
| Germacrene D | 5%–18% |
| Beta-Caryophyllene | 5%–15% |
| Chamazulene | 2%–12% |
| Artemisia Ketone | 4%–10% |
| 1,8-Cineole | 3%–5% |
| Terpinen-4-ol | 1.5%–5% |
| Alpha-Pinene | 2%–4% |
| Alpha-Humulene | 1%–3% |
| Caryophyllene Oxide | 1%–3% |
| (E)-Nerolidol | 0%–3% |
| Bornyl Acetate | 0.1%–2% |
| Camphor | < 1% |

**REPORTED THERAPEUTIC PROPERTIES:** Analgesic, **anti-inflammatory**, antiseptic, astringent, antirheumatic, **antispasmodic**, stops excess bleeding, **wound healing**, nourishes and softens the skin, reduces the appearance of scars and other blemishes, chronic skin conditions, relieves burns, acne, circulatory aid, insecticide, **aids digestion**, encourages secretion of digestive juices, supports liver and intestinal function, **increases bile release from the liver**, reduces varicose veins, migraine/headaches, hemorrhoids, antiallergic, relieves sore muscles, nourishes hair, lowers high blood pressure, **anti-aging (skin)**, reduces fever, increases sweating, expels excess mucus, promotes restful sleep, stress management

## CAUTIONS:

■ Avoid in children (Beta-thujone CT). Cases of seizure have been reported in young children exposed to thujone-rich essential oils.[10042,10043,10044] Use very cautiously with children under six due to potentially high camphor and thujone content, moderate 1,8-cineole content, and small trans-sabinyl acetate content (1,8-cineole/camphor, chamazulene CTs). Trans-sabinyl acetate has a high risk of toxicity.[10045,10046,10047] Several cases of camphor poisoning and/or seizures from ingestion and topical application have been reported in children.[10048,10049] Ingestion of camphor-containing products has been lethal in children under age two.[10050] Thujone is a powerful convulsant and neurotoxin, which has cumulative adverse effects.[10051,10052,10053,10054,10055,10056,10057,10058,10059,10060,10061] Children five years and up may use camphor-containing essential oils topically in dilutions no stronger than 5%. Camphor ingestion by infants and young children may cause cough, vomiting, seizure, burning sensation in the mucous membranes and eyes, or lack of voluntary coordination of muscle movements.[10062]

■ Avoid during pregnancy and lactation (Beta-thujone CT). Essential oils high in thujone content may cause abortion.[10063,10064,10065] Caution is warranted during pregnancy and while lactating due to potentially moderate to high camphor content or small trans-sabinyl acetate content (1,8-cineole/camphor, Chamazulene, Artemisia ketone CTs). Ingestion of essential oils with significant levels of camphor may lead to abortion because fetuses lack the enzymes to process it.[10066] Sabinyl acetate is also considered an abortifacient based on large doses administered to animals that prevented implantation and impaired fertility.[10067,10068] However, blue yarrow usually has less than 2.5% sabinyl acetate, and the studies that considered it an abortifacient injected large doses of sabinyl acetate directly into pregnant mice.

■ Avoid oral consumption (beta-thujone CT, 1,8-cineole/camphor CTs) and use the camphor and chamazulene CTs cautiously orally. Thujone is considered significantly neurotoxic and may damage the liver, and it is estimated that as little as 15 mg orally may negatively impact the central nervous system.[10069,10070,10071] Essential oils with moderate to significant amounts of trans-sabinyl acetate may irritate the mucosal lining of the gastrointestinal tract, damage the kidneys, cause blood in the urine, obstruct blood flow in the abdominal organs, and cause abnormally heavy menstrual bleeding.[10072] Camphor can be toxic when taken orally (usually single doses exceeding 2 mL), although the lethal dose for adult humans is estimated to be more than 5 mL in a single dose.[10073,10074,10075] Case reports involving serious adverse health outcomes (seizure, convulsions, and acute kidney failure) have been reported in adults who consumed high thujone essential oils (sage, thuja, wormwood) in doses of one "swallow," 12 drops, and 20 drops twice daily for five days.[10076,10077,10078,10079]

■ Avoid with epilepsy and Parkinson's disease due to camphor, thujone, 1,8-cineole, and trans-sabinyl acetate content (all CTs).[10080,10081,10082,10083,10084]

■ The potentially high camphor content in yarrow (1,8-cineole/camphor, artemisia ketone CTs) may negatively impact red blood cells and increase the risk of jaundice in children with glucose-6-phosphate dehydrogenase deficiency (G6PD).[10085,10086]

■ May interfere with pentobarbital and other barbiturates (medications for anxiety and insomnia) based on 1,8-cineole content (1,8-cineole/camphor CT).[10087,10088]

■ May interfere with the enzymes responsible for metabolizing medications (NSAIDs, proton-pump inhibitors, acetaminophen, antiepileptics, immune modulators, blood-sugar medications, blood pressure medications, antidepressants, antipsychotics, diabetic medications, antihistamines, antibiotics, and anesthetics) due to chamazulene or 1,8-cineole content (chamazulene and 1,8-cineole/camphor CTs).[10089,10090]

■ May interact with aspirin, blood pressure, antiplatelet, and anticoagulant medications, and increase the risk of bleeding among people with bleeding disorders due to similar constituent profile as German chamomile (chamazulene CT).[10091,10092,10093]

■ Avoid with those who have a compromised liver or kidneys due to the risk of kidney toxicity, kidney failure, or liver toxicity.[10094,10095,10096] Consuming extremely large amounts of thujone rich essential oils (10 mL) has caused kidney failure.[10097] This would also suggest that those taking medications that could cause liver damage should also use yarrow very cautiously or avoid it entirely

**SELECTED EVIDENCE:**

☐ *In vitro* research found that yarrow essential oil prevents hyperpigmentation and suppresses the production of melanin in melanoma cells.[10098] Malignant melanoma cells generally exhibit increased formation of melanin and hyperpigmentation defects.[10099]

☐ Yarrow essential is considered a potent insecticide and repellent against a number of insects, including mosquitoes and ticks.[10100,10101,10102,10103,10104]

☐ Yarrow essential oil (Artemisia ketone CT) reduces inflammation through a number of mechanisms, including suppressing the inflammatory responses of LPS macrophages, decreasing cellular levels of nitric oxide, and downregulating the COX-2 enzyme, TNF-alpha, IL-6, and heme oxygenase 1 (HO-1).[10105]

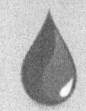

- *In vitro* research demonstrated that yarrow essential oil possesses antifungal properties, particularly against dermatophytes (fungi that require keratin for growth and typically affect the skin, hair, and nails).[10106]

- Yarrow essential oil inhibits *Leishmania* protozoan parasites that cause leishmaniasis (a disease of tropical and subtropical climates characterized by skin lesions and ulcers, damage to mucous membranes, or in rare cases enlargement of the spleen and liver—vascular leishmaniasis).[10107]

- A chamazulene CT of yarrow essential oil was antifungal against *Aspergillus nidulans* (a fungus with low pathogenicity seen almost exclusively in people with chronic granulomatous disease).[10108]

- *In vitro* research reported that yarrow essential oil inhibits the growth of the parasite *T. cruzi*.[10109] *T. cruzi* causes the potentially life-threatening illness Chagas disease, also known as American trypanosomiasis.

- Yarrow essential oil demonstrated strong antioxidant properties and prevented lipid peroxidation.[10110] The same research reported that yarrow actively inhibited *S. pneumoniae*, *C. perfringens*, *C. albicans*, *Mycobacterium smegmatis*, *Acinetobacter lwoffii*, and *C. krusei*.

- Yarrow essential oil is toxic to the brown-banded cockroach (*Supella longipalpa*).[10111]

- Yarrow essential oil (12.8% camphor, 12.0% germacrene D, 7.3% (E)-nerolidol, 6.7% sabinene) demonstrated strong antioxidant activity (better than BHT at the highest concentration) and inhibited *B. cereus*, *S. typhimurium*, and *S. Agona*, with remarkable activity against plant fungi (*R. stolonifera*, *V. dahliae*, *C. gloeosporioides*, *Botrytis cinerea*, and *Aspergillus niger*).[10112]

- Yarrow, clove, and pomelo essential oil (compositions not reported) were active against *Babesia canis*—a parasite transmitted by ticks to dogs that infect and replicate in red blood cells causing a condition called babesiosis.[10113]

- Oral administration of 100 mg/kg body weight of yarrow essential oil (26.2% germacrene D, 14.3% sabinene, 11.4% beta-pinene, 10.4% beta-caryophyllene, and 10.0% chamazulene) markedly reduced the severity of ulcerative colitis in mice.[10114] Inflammation markers (downregulated NF-κB, normalized TNF-α expression, restored normal serum IL-10, reduced serum IL-6, upregulated PPAR-γ, and enhanced the expression of transforming growth factor-β) and colon length were improved and the inner lining of the colon was protected against lesions.

- Yarrow CT camphor essential oil inhibited *E. coli* and *S. aureus*, with significant activity observed against *S. aureus*.[10115]

- *Babesia canis* is a parasite transmitted by certain ticks. The parasite invades mammalian red blood cells and can cause anemia. Yarrow CT chamazulene essential oil was active against *B. canis*, suggesting it may be useful in the prevention and treatment of *Babesia* infections.[10116] Previous research by the same group identified yarrow, clove, and pomelo as active against the parasite.[10117]

- Ulcerative colitis is a condition characterized by inflammation of and sores in the inner lining of the colon. The length of the colon also appears to shorten in people with ulcerative colitis. It can occur due to infection, lifestyle factors, autoimmune attack, or poor blood supply to the colon. Oral administration of yarrow essential oil CT germacrene D decreased ulcerative colitis severity by significantly reducing inflammation—normalized TNF-α expression (an inflammatory cytokine), reduced IL-6 (an inflammatory cytokine), and balanced IL-10 (an anti-inflammatory cytokine and a major regulator of immune responses to infection)—and restoring colon length in mice.[10118] The oil downregulated nuclear factor kappa light chain enhancer of activated B cells (NF-κB), upregulated peroxisome proliferator-activated receptor gamma (PPAR-γ), and enhanced transforming growth factor-β expression.

- Nanoliposomes and nanoniosomes loaded with yarrow essential oil showed greater antimicrobial and anticancer activity than the free essential oil in laboratory research.[10119]

- Oral administration of yarrow essential oil protected against stomach ulcers by recovering antioxidant enzyme activities, balancing gastrointestinal pH, increasing pepsin activity, reducing inflammation, and preserving gastrointestinal cells.[10120] These benefits were mediated through the Nrf2/HO-1 pathway. Another study found that oral administration of yarrow essential oil reduced ulcers in a rat model of ulcerative colitis.[10121] The hydroalcoholic extract was more effective, especially in reducing malonaldehyde content and inflammation.

- Yarrow flower and leaf essential oils (both rich in germacrene D, but flower oil higher in camphor) demonstrated significant acaricidal and repellent activity against the blacklegged tick (*Ixodes scapularis*), with the flower oil being more effective.[10122]

# YLANG YLANG
## (Ylang-Ylang, Ilang-Ilang; Cananga)

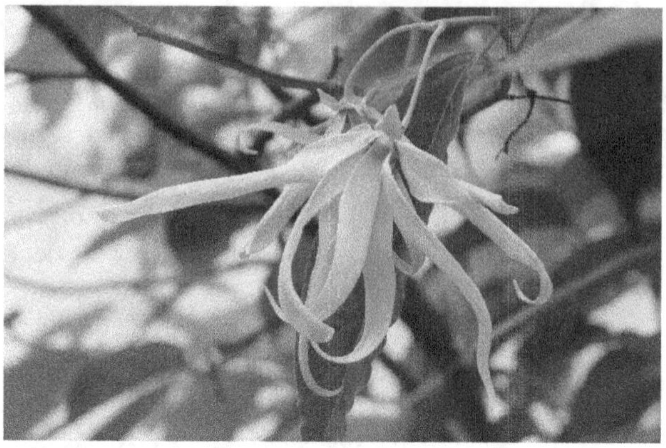

*Cananga odorata* (Lam.) Hook. f. & Thomson, *Uvaria odorata* Lam.; **Cananga**: *C. odorata* Hook fil. et Thompson forma *macrophylla* Koolhaas, *Cangarium odoratum* f. *macrophylla*

**FAMILY:** Annonaceae
**NOTE:** Middle-Base
**AROMA INTENSITY:** Medium
**AROMA:** Intensely sweet, floral, rich
**COMMON EXTRACTION METHOD:** Steam distilled from the flowers; also solvent extracted (particularly for the perfume industry)
**POSSIBLE SUBSTITUTE OILS:** Goldenrod, petitgrain, neroli, helichrysum, jasmine
**BLENDS WELL WITH:** Bay laurel, bergamot, cajeput, cardamom, chamomile (German, Roman), clary sage, clove, copaiba, coriander, cypress, eucalyptus, geranium, ginger, juniper, lavender, melissa, neroli, orange, palmarosa, patchouli, rose, sandalwood, turmeric, vetiver
**SUBCELLULAR LOCALIZATION | EPIGENETIC INFLUENCE:** Endoplasmic Reticulum | Skeletal/Integumentary
**RECOMMENDED DILUTION RANGE:** 3%–33%; neat for limited conditions

**PRIMARY CONSTITUENTS:**[10123,10124,10125,10126,10127,10128,10129,10130]

*Ylang Ylang Complete*

|  |  |
|---|---|
| Germacrene D | 18.8%–24.4% |
| Beta-Caryophyllene | 1.5%–18.8% |
| Alpha-Farnesene | 3.9%–12.9% |
| Geranyl Acetate | 7.6%–12.6% |
| Linalool | 1.3%–10.6% |
| Benzyl Benzoate | 0.0%–7.6% |

*Ylang Ylang I French*

|  |  |
|---|---|
| Benzyl Acetate | 27.5% |
| Para-Cresyl Methyl Ether | 9.7% |
| Linalool | 9.0% |
| Methyl Benzoate | 6.1% |
| 3-Methyl-2-Butenyl Acetate | 4.2% |
| Neryl Acetate | 2.7% |
| 3-Methyl-3-Buten-1-ol Acetate | 2.2% |
| Alpha-Farnesene | 1.6% |

*Ylang Ylang IV French*

|  |  |
|---|---|
| (E,E)-Alpha-Farnesene | 10.1% |
| Sesquiterpene (MW 204) | 7.5% |
| Methyl Caprylate | 7.2% |
| Alpha-Humulene | 6.2% |
| T-Muurolol | 4.4% |
| Benzyl Salicylate | 4.1% |
| Beta-Curcumene | 2.7% |
| Gamma-Cadinene | 2.1% |

*Ylang Ylang I Madagascan*

|  |  |
|---|---|
| Linalool | 11.7%–30.0% |
| Benzyl Benzoate | 4.3%–14.9% |
| Germacrene D | 0.1%–13.5% |
| Beta-Caryophyllene | 1.1%–11.2% |
| Geranyl Acetate | 6.2%–11.0% |
| Methyl Salicylate | 1.7%–10.4% |
| Para-Cresyl Methyl Ether | 1.1%–10.4% |
| Benzyl Acetate | 3.3%–8.0% |
| (E,E)-Farnesyl Acetate | 0.5%–7.8% |
| Methyl Benzoate | 1.7%–5.6% |

*Ylang Ylang II Madagascan*

|  |  |
|---|---|
| Beta-Caryophyllene | 1.7%–19.6% |
| Germacrene D | 1.5%–19.3% |
| Gamma-Cadinene + Alpha-Farnesene | 1.7%–12.7% |
| Benzyl Benzoate | 5.3%–12.3% |
| Linalool | 3.9%–12.2% |
| Geranyl Acetate | 2.6%–7.2% |
| (E,E)-Farnesyl Acetate | 0.7%–6.2% |
| Alpha-Caryophyllene + (E)-Cadinene | 3.4%–5.8% |
| Para-Cresyl Methyl Ether | 0.6%–5.3% |
| Methyl Salicylate | 0.6%–5.3% |
| Delta-Cadinene | 2.1%–5.2% |

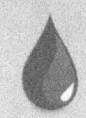

| | | |
|---|---|---|
| (2E,6E)-Farnesyl Acetate | 2.1% | |
| Isogermacrene-D | 1.8% | |
| Para-Cresyl Methyl Ether | 1.6% | |
| Cinnamyl Acetate | 1.6% | |
| Aromadendrene | 1.5% | |
| Alpha-Cadinol | 1.5% | |
| (2Z,6Z)-Farnesol | 1.4% | |

*Ylang Ylang III Madagascan*

| | |
|---|---|
| Germacrene D | 15.1%–25.1% |
| Beta-Caryophyllene | 14.8%–21.5% |
| Gamma-Cadinene + Alpha-Farnesene | 6.5%–17.4% |
| Benzyl Benzoate | 5.9%–12.8% |
| Alpha-Caryophyllene + (E)-Cadinene | 3.9%–5.8% |

*Cananga*

| | |
|---|---|
| Beta-Caryophyllene | 11.0%–38.2% |
| Caryophyllene Oxide | 0.0%–17.6% |
| Alpha-Humulene | 4.2%–9.2% |
| Germacrene D | 1.3%–8.3% |
| Benzyl Alcohol | 0.0%–7.8% |
| Benzyl Benzoate | 2.0%–7.6% |
| Delta-Cadinene | 0.5%–6.0% |
| Linalool | 1.0%–5.6% |
| (Z,Z)-Alpha-Farnesene | 0.4%–4.4% |
| (E,E)-Farnesol | 0.0%–3.9% |
| Trans-Beta-Guaiene | 0.0%–4.2% |
| (E,E)-Alpha-Farnesene | 0.1%–3.8% |

*Solvent Extracted (Absolute)*

| | |
|---|---|
| Trans-Caryophyllene | 25.0%–26.1% |
| Germacrene D | 10.3%–12.0% |
| Alpha-Humulene | 10.7%–10.8% |
| Linalool | 6.8%–7.4% |
| Delta-Cadinene | 5.4%–7.6% |
| Alpha-Longipinene | 6.8%–6.9% |
| Alpha-Farnesene | 6.2%–6.8% |

**OTHER CONSTITUENTS:** 3-methyl-3-buten-1-ol acetate, 3-methyl-2-butenyl acetate, n-hexyl acetate, benzyl alcohol, methyl caprylate, alpha-cadinene, alpha-bergamotene, alpha-caryophyllene, copaene, geraniol, farnesol, muurolol, benzyl salicylate, eugenol, 2-phenylethyl acetate, neryl acetate, alpha-copaene, beta-cubebene, beta-ylangene, beta-copaene, cinnamyl acetate, isoeugenol, beta-curcumene, guaiol; *Cananga*—Gamma-muurolene, p-cresyl methyl ether, alpha-copaene, geraniol, geranyl acetate, alpha-muurolene, bicyclosesquiphellandrene, alpha-cadinol, benzaldehyde, eugenol, beta-cubebene, beta-cadinene, cis-calamenene, (Z)-nerolidol, dihydro-eugenol acetate, globulol, humulene epoxide II, epi-alpha-cadinol, alpha-muurolol, beta-eudesmol, alpha-eudesmol, 7-epi-alpha-eudesmol, beta-bisabolol, aromadendrene oxide-(1), aromadendrene oxide-(2), (Z)-alpha-santalol, 8-cedren-13-ol, (E,E)-farnesyl acetate, benzyl salicylate, geranyl benzoate, methyl eugenol ( < 0.6%)

**PREFERRED COMPOSITION FOR CLINICAL USE:**

## Ylang Ylang

| Constituent | Complete | I | II | III | Extra | Extra Super |
|---|---|---|---|---|---|---|
| | *Madagascar* | | | | *Comoros/Mayotte/Indonesia* | |
| **Germacrene D** | 15%–25% | 9%–18% | 12%–28% | 15%–34% | 10%–20% | 10%–15% |
| **Beta-Caryophyllene** | 10%–18% | 5%–12% | 10%–18% | 14%–20% | 3%–9% | 2%–7% |
| **(E,E)-Alpha-Farnesene** | 3%–14% | 3%–8% | 5%–12% | 8%–25% | 3%–15% | 2%–7% |
| **Geranyl Acetate** | 4%–12% | 7%–15% | 5%–12% | 1%–6% | 5%–15% | 2%–7% |
| **Benzyl Benzoate** | 5%–10% | 5%–10% | 6%–11% | 5%–10% | 4%–16% | 3%–6% |
| **Linalool** | 2%–9% | 5%–20% | 4%–11% | 0.5%–4% | 6%–12% | 8%–14% |
| **Alpha-Humulene** | 2%–6% | 0.1%–5% | 0.5%–6% | 1%–6% | 1%–4% | 2%–8% |
| **Delta-Cadinene** | 2%–6% | 0.1%–5% | 1%–6% | 2%–7% | 0.1%–3% | 0.5%–5% |
| **4-Methylanisole** (p-Methyl Anisole, p-Cresyl Methyl Ether, Methyl-p-Cresol) | 0.5%–4% | 4%–10% | 0.5%–5% | 0.1%–2% | 3%–15% | 7%–13% |
| **Farnesol <E,E- or E,Z->** | 1%–3% | 0.1%–3% | 1%–4% | 1%–4% | 0.5%–4% | 0.5%–2% |
| **(E,E)-Farnesyl Acetate** | 1%–3% | 0.5%–3% | 0.5%–5% | 1%–5% | 1.5%–15% | 1%–4% |
| **Benzyl Acetate** | 1%–3% | 2%–10% | 0.1%–5% | 0.1%–3% | 5%–15% | 12%–20% |

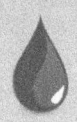 

| Benzyl Salicylate | 0.5%–3% | 1%–4% | 1.5%–4% | 2%–5% | 2%–5% | 1%–4% |
|---|---|---|---|---|---|---|
| Geraniol | 0.1%–2% | 0.1%–3% | 0.5%–3% | 0.1%–1% | 0.1%–1.5% | 0.1%–1% |
| Methyl Benzoate | 0.5%–2% | 2%–6% | 1%–3% | 0.1%–1% | 2%–7% | 4%–9% |
| (E)-Cinnamyl Acetate | 0.1%–2% | 0.5%–2% | 0.1%–3% | 0.1%–2% | 1%–7% | 4%–7% |
| Prenyl Acetate | < 0.5% | 0.1%–1% | 0.1%–0.5% | tr–0.5% | 1%–3% | 1.5%–4% |

## Cananga

| Constituent | |
|---|---|
| Beta-Caryophyllene | 28%–40% |
| Alpha-Humulene | 6%–11% |
| Germacrene D | 5%–10% |
| Delta-Cadinene | 2%–7% |
| (E,E)-Alpha-Farnesene | 3%–9% |
| (Z,E)-Alpha-Farnesene | 2%–9% |
| Benzyl Benzoate | 3%–6% |
| Linalool | 1%–4% |
| Geranyl Acetate | 1%–3% |
| Alpha-Cadinol | 1%–3% |
| 4-Methylanisole | 0.5%–3% |
| Farnesol <E,E- or E,Z-> | tr–3% |
| Geraniol | 0.5%–2% |
| Benzyl Salicylate | 0.1%–1% |

## Comoros Complete

| Constituent | |
|---|---|
| Germacrene D | 15%–25% |
| (E,E)-Alpha-Farnesene | 7%–22% |
| Beta-Caryophyllene | 5%–15% |
| Benzyl Benzoate | 4%–10% |
| (E,E)-Farnesyl Acetate | 1%–6% |
| Benzyl Salicylate | 1%–5% |
| Linalool | 2%–8% |
| Delta-Cadinene | 2%–6% |
| Benzyl Acetate | 1%–5% |
| Geranyl Acetate | 3%–10% |
| 4-Methylanisole | 0.5%–3% |
| (E,E)-Farnesol | 1%–3% |
| Alpha-Humulene | 1%–5% |
| (E)-Cinnamyl Acetate | 0.1%–3% |
| Methyl Benzoate | 0.5%–3% |
| Geraniol | 0.1%–2% |

**REPORTED THERAPEUTIC PROPERTIES:** Antibacterial, antifungal, anti-inflammatory, antiseptic, antispasmodic, **balances breathing rate**, supports healthy cell division, benefits oily skin, encourages hair growth, **balances and regulates heart function**, **helps lower high blood pressure**, disinfectant, expectorant, nervine (calms and soothes the nerves), wound healing, sedating, **stress management**, **reduces anxiety**, **aphrodisiac**, promotes euphoria, stress management, increases feelings of love, pleasure, and joy, **antidepressant**, reduces fear, anger, despondency, and frustration, reduces mood swings

**CAUTIONS:**

■ Dilution is recommended as ylang ylang is commonly reported to cause skin sensitization or irritation.

■ May decrease the bioavailability of many medications (NSAIDs, proton-pump inhibitors, acetaminophen, antiepileptics, immune modulators, blood-sugar medications, blood pressure medications, antidepressants, antipsychotics, diabetic medications, antihistamines, antibiotics, and anesthetics) due to the ability of caryophyllene oxide and beta-caryophyllene to inhibit CYP3A enzyme activity.[10131]

■ *Ylang Ylang I Fractions*: Oral caution. Oral caution. Ingestion of benzoic acids, benzoic salts (calcium, potassium, and sodium), benzaldehyde, benzyl acetate, benzyl benzoate, and benzyl alcohol may cause gastrointestinal irritation, vomiting, and diarrhea.[10132] The Joint Expert Committee for Food Additives (JECFA) has established an acceptable daily limit for the aforementioned constituents of 0–5mg/kg body weight for adults to avoid GI discomfort.[10133] Based on this limit, it is suggested to limit the oral consumption to no more than 10 drops daily.

**SELECTED EVIDENCE:**

□ Inhaling lavender, lemon, and ylang ylang oil (2:2:1 ratio) reduced systolic blood pressure, and influenced heart rate and sympathetic nervous system activity in people with essential hypertension (high blood pressure without an identifiable cause).[10134] Another study found that inhaling lavender, ylang ylang, and bergamot oils once daily for four weeks reduced cortisol levels, psychological stress, and blood pressure in people with essential hypertension.[10135]

□ Animal research demonstrates that ylang ylang essential oil and its major constituents (benzyl benzoate,

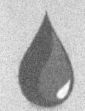

linalool, and benzyl alcohol) reduces anxiety in male mice, and modifies neurotransmitter levels (decreases dopamine in the striatum and increase serotonin in the hippocampus) more dramatically in male than female mice.[10136] Isolated benzyl benzoate also modified neurotransmitters in accordance with the whole essential oil.

- A clinical study concluded that both cortisol and systolic blood pressure declines after inhalation of a combination of lavender, ylang ylang, marjoram, and neroli oil in those with high blood pressure or pre-high blood pressure.[10137]

- Ylang ylang can prevent mosquito bites (up to 98.9%) for up to eighty-eight minutes, which is better than two chemical repellents, but not as effective as DEET (98.5%, for up to 182 minutes).[10138,10139]

- *In vitro* research concluded that ylang ylang oil prevented the adherence of *K. pneumonia* and *S. aureus* to catheters, which could help prevent hospital-acquired infections.[10140]

- Both the topical application and inhalation of ylang ylang increased the perceived self-esteem among healthy individuals.[10141]

- Topical application of ylang ylang oil (1 mL of a 20% solution in sweet almond oil) to the lower abdomen increased skin temperature and reduced blood pressure, which promoted a calmer and more relaxed state among healthy individuals.[10142]

- Animal (intravenous injection of 0.01 to 0.005 mL) and *in vitro* research suggests that ylang ylang oil relaxes an overactive bladder.[10143]

- *In vitro* research demonstrates that ylang ylang essential oil inhibits *A. flavus* and *A. parasiticus* and their production of aflatoxin B1.[10144]

- A preclinical model of chronic skin inflammation demonstrates that ylang ylang essential oil inhibits protein molecules involved in tissue remodeling, which suggests that it promotes wound healing.[10145]

- Ylang ylang and star anise essential oil exhibited strong acaricidal activity against the castor bean tick (*Ixodes ricinus*)—a tick that can transmit both bacterial and viral pathogens such as the causative agents of Lyme disease and tick-borne encephalitis.[10146]

- A 50-minute massage, received from one to five times during treatment, with ylang ylang oil—10% ylang ylang in *monoi* oil (an infused perfume-oil made by soaking flower petals in coconut oil)—reduced suicide attempts and suicide among individuals admitted to the hospital who had contacted a suicide crisis line after suicidal ideation or attempts.[10147]

- *In vitro* research showed that nanoencapsulated ylang ylang essential oil (24.6% linalool, 22.4% benzyl benzoate) completely inhibited the growth and aflatoxin-B1 production of a toxigenic strain of *A. flavus*. Additionally, the nanoencapsulated oil showed improved antioxidant activity when compared to the free oil.[10148]

- Loading ylang ylang essential oil into a chitosan nanoemulsion improved its antioxidant activity and completely inhibited *A. flavus*.[10149] The oil also suppressed fungal growth, aflatoxin B1 secretion, and lipid peroxidation in peanuts (*Arachis hypogea*) without harming seed germination.

- An *in vitro* study found that the antioxidant (radical scavenging activity) of ylang ylang is related to its distillation time, with germacrene D, alpha-farnesene, eugenol, and linalool contributing to its antioxidant capacity.[10150] Ylang ylang complete oils were more effective than fractions.

- Ylang ylang essential oil repelled mosquitoes (*A. dirus, Ae. aegypti*) when used at 2.5% and produced a knockdown effect on *Anopheles* mosquitoes at 5.0% concentration.[10151]

- Ylang ylang and frankincense (*Boswellia* spp.) CT alpha-thujene demonstrated insecticidal activity against mosquito larvae (*C. quinquefasciatus*) and housefly (*M. domestica*) adults.[10152]

- A multivariate statistical analysis showed that germacrene D and (E,E)-alpha-farnesene are the major contributors to the radical scavenging activity (antioxidant) of ylang ylang essential oil, with eugenol also contributing.[10153]

- Inhalation of ylang ylang essential oil was compared to music therapy for reducing high blood pressure in elderly people with hypertension.[10154] Five drops of ylang ylang essential oil were added to 20 mL of water in a diffuser and diffused four times per week for two weeks. The music therapy group participated in music therapy with sound and MP3 of Java Langgam music four times per week, for two weeks. Blood pressure was taken prior to and immediately following interventions. Both interventions reduced blood pressure during week one, with greater benefits achieved at the end of two weeks. Aromatherapy reduced systolic blood pressure better than music therapy, but music therapy was better for diastolic blood pressure.

- Excessive alcohol consumption can badly damage the liver because the liver is responsible for metabolizing alcohol—over 90% of alcohol is processed by the liver with the rest exiting the body via urine, sweat, and breathing. When more alcohol is consumed than the liver can process, liver cells are destroyed, which results in scarring of the liver (cirrhosis), alcoholic hepatitis, and cellular mutations that can lead to cancer. Oral administration of ylang ylang essential oil reversed serum biomarkers of liver damage caused by alcohol (AST, ALT, TP, TC, TG, and TB), improved antioxidant enzyme activity, and maintained liver health and function in rats with liver damage caused by alcohol consumption.[10155] Further analysis identified sixty-three constituents in ylang ylang that beneficially regulate proteins associated with liver toxicity by altering Toll-like receptor, Adipocytokine, TNF, Sphingolipid, FoxO, AMPK, Relaxin, MAPK, NF-kappa B, HIF-1, Fc epsilon RI, IL-17, VEGF, T cell receptor, NOD-like receptor, mTOR, PI3K- Akt signaling, and more.

- Oral administration of ylang ylang essential oil (30 mg/kg body weight; equivalent to about 4 drops in humans) relieved neuropathic pain in a spared nerve injury model—a preclinical model used to evaluate therapies for neuropathy in a single location—in mice and also alleviated anxiety associated with the pain.[10156]

- The effects of ylang ylang essential oil against acute inflammation was evaluated in several preclinical models (cytotoxicity, neutrophil chemotaxis induced by N-formyl methionyl leucyl phenylalanine, and phagocytic activity tests; zymosan-induced peritonitis, carrageenan-induced leukocyte rolling, and adhesion events in the *in situ* microcirculation model, and in carrageenan-induced paw edema models).[10157] The research showed that ylang ylang was not toxic in the laboratory assay or the acute toxicity test in mice. Laboratory models demonstrated the anti-inflammatory activity of ylang ylang oil in the neutrophil chemotaxis and phagocytic tests. Oral administration of the oil reduced leukocyte recruitment and nitric oxide production in the zymosan-induced peritonitis model, reduced rolling and adherent leukocyte number induced by carrageenan in the *in situ* microcirculation model, and reduced carrageenan-induced edema and mechanical hyperalgesia. Altogether, the results confirm the anti-inflammatory effects of ylang ylang essential oil in acute inflammatory models.

- A randomized controlled clinical trial evaluated the effects of inhaling ylang ylang essential oil among people hospitalized for interventional neuroradiology (INR) procedures.[10158] Ylang ylang (25 mcL) or a placebo (25 mcL of distilled water) were dropped onto two pieces of absorbent mulberry paper and then attached to the person's gown at shoulder level for twelve hours. Trait and state anxiety scores and biological indices—salivary cortisol and alpha-amylase (indicators of stress and anxiety), blood pressure, and heart rate—were measured before and after the intervention. The ylang ylang group experienced significantly less trait and state anxiety and decreased salivary alpha-amylase, showing that inhaling ylang ylang can decrease anxiety related to unfamiliar medical procedures.

- Autism spectrum disorder (ASD) is a brain disorder characterized by a broad range of symptoms that impacts a person's ability to socialize, communicate, learn, think, and problem solve. There are three levels of ASD depending on how severe the disorder is and the requirement for support to function in daily life. Level 1 requires minimal support but expresses difficulty in social interactions, organization, and planning. Level 2 requires substantial support with social interactions limited to narrow special interests and repetitive behaviors. Level 3 has severe verbal and nonverbal social communication skills deficits and expresses great distress and difficulty changing actions or focus that requires very substantial support. One in forty-four children are currently diagnosed with ASD, which has increased from 1 in 150 since 2020. A preclinical model of autism-like behaviors investigated the effects of inhaling ylang ylang essential oil—ten minutes exposure for seven days.[10159] What the researchers found was that lower amounts of ylang ylang oil significantly enhanced social interactions with strangers, while medium exposure to ylang ylang oil improved task performance and anxiety related to the task. Additionally, inhalation of the oil enhanced metabolism of serotonin and dopamine in the prefrontal cortex. The researchers concluded that ylang ylang inhalation alleviates anxiety and improves cognitive and social abilities, suggesting it may improve the quality of life of individuals with ASD.

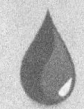

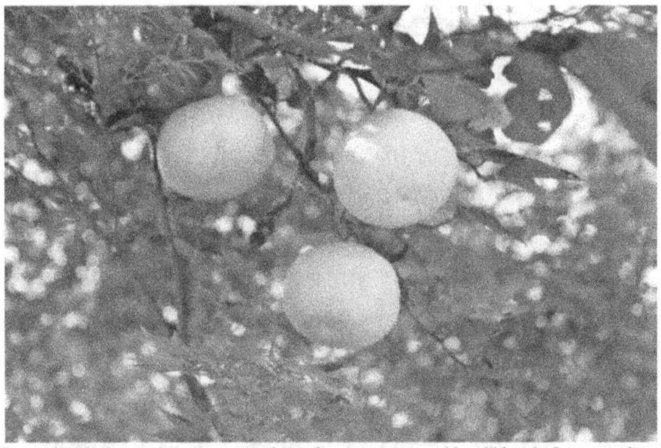

# YUZU
## (Kansu Orange)

*Citrus junos* Sieb. ex Tanaka, *Citrus aurantium* subsp *junos* (Siebold ex Tanaka), *Citrus aurantium* subsp *junos* (Makino); *Citrus ichangensis* × *C. reticulata* var. *austere*

**FAMILY:** Rutaceae
**NOTE:** Top
**AROMA INTENSITY:** Medium
**AROMA:** Citrusy, fresh, sweet, tangy, complex
**COMMON EXTRACTION METHOD:** Cold-pressed/expressed from the rind (peel); may also be steam distilled from the rind (peel)
**POSSIBLE SUBSTITUTE OILS:** Bergamot, grapefruit, tangerine, lime
**BLENDS WELL WITH:** Basil, bay laurel, bergamot, black pepper, blue cypress, cardamom, cedarwood, chamomile (German, Roman), clary sage, clove, copaiba, coriander, cypress, ginger, grapefruit, lavender, lemon, lemon eucalyptus, lime, marjoram, orange, palmarosa, patchouli, petitgrain, pine, rosemary, sandalwood, tangerine, vetiver, ylang ylang
**RECOMMENDED DILUTION RANGE:** 3%–50%; neat for limited conditions

**PRIMARY COMPOUNDS:**[10160,10161,10162]

*Cold-pressed (expressed)*

| | |
|---|---|
| Limonene | 63.1%–79.4% |
| Gamma-Terpinene | 7.6%–12.5% |
| Beta-Phellandrene | 1.6%–5.4% |
| Linalool | 1.4%–4.7% |
| Myrcene | 1.1%–3.2% |
| Alpha-Pinene | 1.1%–2.7% |

**OTHER COMPOUNDS:** Beta-pinene, sabinene, alpha-phellandrene, para-cymene, terpinolene, (E)-beta-farnesene, bicyclogermacrene, germacrene D-4-ol, alpha-terpineol

**PREFERRED COMPOSITION FOR CLINICAL USE:**

| Constituent | |
|---|---|
| **Limonene** | 60%–80% |
| **Gamma-Terpinene** | 3%–13% |
| **Beta-Phellandrene** | 0.1%–6% |
| **Linalool** | 1%–5% |
| **Myrcene** | 1%–5% |
| **Alpha-Pinene** | 1%–4% |
| **Beta-Pinene** | 0.5%–3% |
| **(E)-Beta-Farnesene** | 0.01%–3% |

**REPORTED THERAPEUTIC PROPERTIES:** Analgesic, antiseptic, antibacterial, antifungal, anti-inflammatory, antiseptic, antispasmodic, diuretic, relieves constipation, nervine, relaxing, uplifting, relieves anxiety, **stress management**, antidepressant

**CAUTIONS:**

■ None currently known.

■ Photosensitizing compounds were not identified in analysis of distilled yuzu essential oil and analyses of seven samples of the cold-pressed oil showed no bergapten in three of the samples and only minute levels (0.5–3.8 ppm) in the other four samples.[10163,10164] The distilled oil should not be photosensitizing, but the cold-pressed oil could be mildly photosensitizing (low risk).

**SELECTED EVIDENCE:**

☐ Inhaling yuzu essential oil for ten minutes improved mood state (reduced tension and fatigue) for up to thirty-five minutes in menstruating women.[10165] Another study concluded that inhalation of 10 mcL of yuzu essential oil from a diffuser for ten minutes alleviated negative emotional stress (tension-anxiety, depression-dejection, anger-hostility, and confusion) for up to thirty minutes partly by reducing sympathetic nervous system activity.[10166]

☐ *In vitro* research concluded that limonene from yuzu essential oil may have "potential anti-inflammatory efficacy for the treatment of bronchial asthma" due to its ability to inhibit inflammatory cytokines, ROS (reactive oxygen species) production, and inactivate eosinophil migration (eosinophils migrate to inflammatory sites in tissues, which can trigger an allergic response).[10167]

☐ Inhaling yuzu essential oil for ten minutes significantly reduced heart rate and premenstrual symptoms (tension-anxiety, anger-hostility, and fatigue), with the effects lasting up to thirty-five minutes after inhalation.[10168]

☐ Yuzu, bitter orange, and citron essential oils each exhibited good antioxidant activity in the ABTS and DPPH assays.[10169]

☐ Citrus essential oil such as yuzu and tangerine limited melanin production, suggesting they may be helpful for skin hyperpigmentation.[10170]

# ZDRAVETZ
## (Big-Root Geranium, Wild Geranium)

*Geranium macrorrhizum* L.

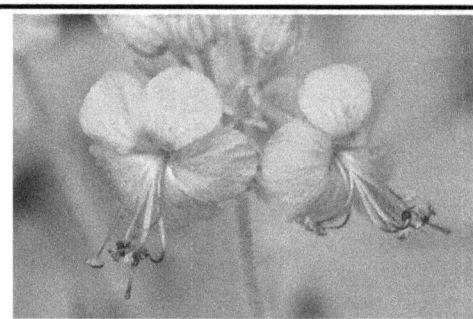

**FAMILY:** Geraniaceae
**NOTE:** Middle-Base
**AROMA INTENSITY:** Medium-Strong
**AROMA:** Green, herbaceous, earthy, sweet-woody, slightly floral
**COMMON EXTRACTION METHOD:** Hydrodistilled from the flowering aerial parts
**POSSIBLE SUBSTITUTE OILS:** Geranium, helichrysum, myrrh, palmarosa, ledum
**BLENDS WELL WITH:** Agarwood, angelica, balsam fir, bergamot, chamomile (German, Roman), cistus, clary sage, coriander, cypress, frankincense, geranium, helichrysum, juniper berry, Phoenician juniper, hyssop, lavender, lemongrass, mastic, Mediterranean mandarin, muhuhu, neroli, petitgrain, pine, rose, rosewood, sandalwood, tangerine, vetiver, white verbena, ylang ylang
**SUBCELLULAR LOCALIZATION | EPIGENETIC INFLUENCE:** Currently unknown | Currently unknown
**RECOMMENDED DILUTION RANGE:** 5%–Neat

**PRIMARY CONSTITUENTS:**[10171,10172,10173]

| | |
|---|---|
| Germacrone | 37.4%–60.1% |
| Germacrene B | 0.0%–11.3% |
| (E)-Beta-Elemenone | 1.6%–5.3% |
| Gamma-Curcumene | 0.0%–4.1% |
| Alpha-Eudesmol | 0.0%–3.9% |
| Piperitone | 0.0%–3.0% |

Note: Zdravetz essential oil is rich in natural plant waxes (similar to rose otto), which makes it crystallize at room temperature.

**OTHER CONSTITUENTS:** Linalool, beta-selinene, amorpha-4,7-dien-11-ol, caryophyllene oxide, eremophila-1(10),11-dien-9beta-ol, selina-3,7(11)-diene, beta-curcumene, geranyl acetate, gamma-elemene, beta-elemene, alpha-terpineol, terpinolene, gamma-terpinene, (Z)-beta-ocimene, 2-phenylethyl isovalerate, alpha-bulnesene, alpha-curcumene, germacrene D

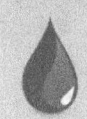

**PREFERRED COMPOSITION FOR CLINICAL USE:**

| Constituent | |
| --- | --- |
| Germacrone | 50%–77% |
| Germacrene B | 0%–10% |
| Gamma-Curcumene | 0%–5% |
| (E)-Beta-Elemenone | 0%–6% |
| Gamma-Terpinene | 0.1%–3% |

**REPORTED THERAPEUTIC PROPERTIES:** Analgesic, relieves headache/migraine, **antispasmodic**, antiseptic, antibacterial, antifungal, antimicrobial, antiallergic, aids female reproductive function, relieves menopausal symptoms, relieves itching, soothes skin irritation and chronic skin conditions, expels excess gas, astringent, wound healing, relieves blisters/boils, relieves hemorrhoids, reduces blood pressure, balances blood sugar, aids circulation, reduces fever, promotes restful sleep, **aphrodisiac**, antidepressant, relieves anxiety, stress management, stimulates creativity, promotes mental clarity

**CAUTIONS:**

■ May interfere with the enzymes responsible for metabolizing medications (NSAIDs, proton-pump inhibitors, acetaminophen, antiepileptics, immune modulators, blood-sugar medications, blood pressure medications, antidepressants, antipsychotics, diabetic medications, antihistamines, antibiotics, and anesthetics) due to germacrone content.[10174]

**SELECTED EVIDENCE:**

☐ *In vitro* research demonstrates that zdravetz essential oil inhibits a number of bacterium (*B. subtilis, S. aureus, E. coli, S. aureus* (clinical isolate), *K. pneumoniae, E. coli* (clinical isolate)).[10175] A very strong inhibition of *B. subtilis* was noted. However, the same researchers noted that its antifungal activity was weak against *P. chrysogenum, A. restrictus, A. fumigatus,* and *C. albicans.*

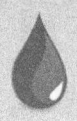

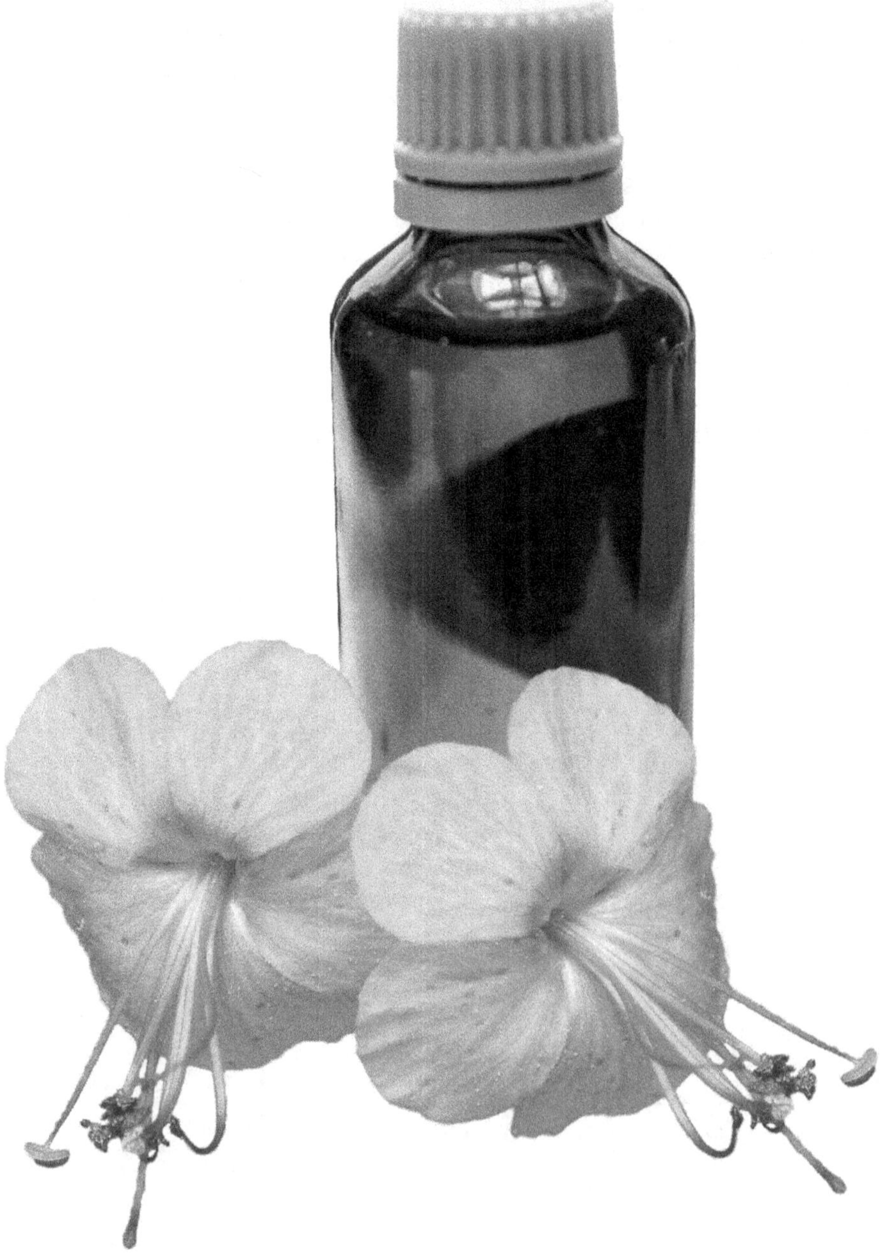

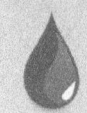

# ESSENTIAL OIL THERAPY FOR HEALTH CONDITIONS

The following protocol suggestions are recommended to preserve life and correct health conditions if modern medicine is not available or with the explicit permission of your healthcare practitioner. They are not meant to be substituted for medical treatment when it is available nor to replace treatment prescribed by your physician or healthcare practitioner. Do not attempt to diagnose or prescribe essential oils for conditions that require professional attention.[10176] Always consult your healthcare professoinal for any health condition, injury, or illness.

If you have more than one condition to address it is usually advised to work on one condition at a time, beginning with the most pressing. The most critical condition may be psychological because of the significant correlation between a person's psychological state and health conditions experienced. In fact, it is estimated that up to 90 percent of all doctor visits are stress-related, and that a number of chronic health conditions are associated with stress.

If the protocols for two or more of your health conditions recommend the same oil or oils, you may be able to address more than one concern with one protocol. In this case, it is recommended to use the protocol with most number of drops recommended. For example, if one health protocol recommends 3 drops of lavender and the other 5, use the protocol that recommends 5 drops for both health conditions, rather than taking 8 drops.

For ease of use, the recommended oils for a specific condition may be mixed together as a blend and used as suggested, rather than mixed together for each application and use.

The number of essential oil drops recommended for topical application should be diluted appropriately before applying unless a neat application is recommended.

The recommendations are based on known protocols, consensus of user testimonials, historical usage, clinical experience, and published scientific research. The protocols are intended to ease symptoms, restore normal function of cells, organs, or systems, reestablish balance or homeostasis, eliminate illness cause, or manage an aspect of the disease or its progression.

***Drops recommended in the protocols of this edition have been adjusted from the first edition to use roughly a 40 to 60 mg drop, rather than the 30 mg drop of the first edition.***

## ABDOMINAL CRAMPS

Topical—Dilute appropriately, and apply one or a combination of peppermint, German chamomile, ginger, or fennel to abdomen every 30 minutes until cramps subside. Recommended dilution: 5%–10%.

Oral—Ingest a combination of 2 drops each of peppermint and ginger and 1 drop of fennel every 2 hours (up to 3 times per day) or until cramps subside.

## ABDOMINAL MIGRAINE

Topical— Dilute appropriately, and apply 1 to 2 drops each of lavender, ginger, peppermint, and German chamomile to the abdomen and cover with a warm wet towel up to 3 times daily. Recommended dilution: 5%–10%.

Oral—Take a capsule filled with 1 drop each of lemon, lemongrass, lavender, and peppermint, and basil up to 3 times daily. Consider taking 1 to 2 drops each of copaiba, lavender, and ginger in a capsule twice daily as a preventive.

Inhalation—Inhale 1 drop each of bergamot, lemon, lavender, and ylang ylang as needed.

## ABSCESS

Topical—Dilute appropriately, and apply one or a combination of frankincense, lavender, and tea tree to the abscess several times daily. Recommended dilution: 5%–10%.

## ACNE

Topical—Dilute appropriately, and apply one or a combination of frankincense, tea tree, German chamomile, geranium, or lavender at least 2 times daily. Recommned diltion: 1%–3% for face, 5% for other areas.

Oral—Purify the blood by taking 2 drops each of geranium, clove, and grapefruit, 2 times daily.

## ACNE, CYSTIC

Topical—Mix together 2 drops each of thyme, lavender, rosemary, and tea tree in three-quarters cup water and one-quarter cup organic apple cider vinegar, and then apply a small amount of this mixture with a cotton ball, 2 to 3 times daily. A trace amount of any of the mentioned oils diluted in 4 drops of jojoba or grapeseed carrier oil may be applied neat to the cysts up to 3 times daily as well.

Oral—Take a capsule filled with 2 drops each of cinnamon, oregano, thyme, and clove, twice daily.

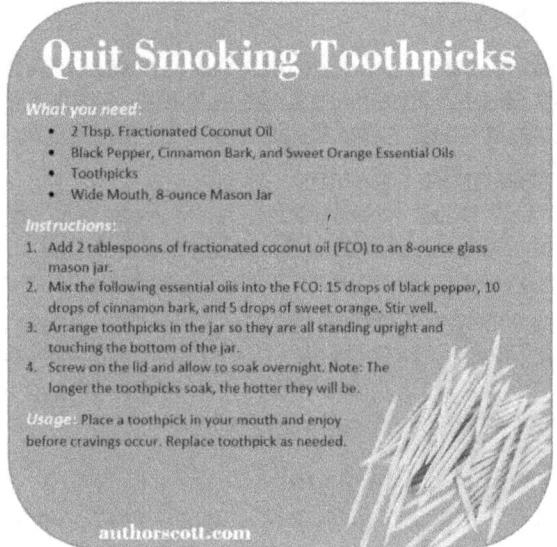

## ADDICTIONS

Inhalation—Add 1 drop of black pepper, clove, and grapefruit to a cotton ball or diffuser jewelry and inhale as needed throughout the day.

Topical—Dilute appropriately, and apply 1 to 3 drops of lavender or German chamomile to the temples, back of the neck, and forehead to relax the mind and body. Recommended dilution: 3%–5%.

Other—Practice deep breathing for 15 minutes as often as needed each day. Use "quit smoking sticks." (see above)

## ADDISON'S DISEASE

Topical—Apply 2 drops each of rosemary and pine and 1 drops each of geranium, blue spruce, balsam fir, and clove one at a time to the adrenal area on the back (about midway). Gently feather each oil up the spine with the back of your fingers, and after applying all of the oils, cover entire back with 20–30 drops of carrier oil and massage into entire back. To improve results, apply a warm washcloth after complete process and leave in place

until cool. Repeat this process up to twice daily. Perform the Waterfall Technique®, once weekly.

Other—Women should also consider the following: apply 2 to 4 drops of clary sage to the forehead or wrists, 1 to 2 times daily. Also, consider a natural bioidentical progesterone or molecular progesterone complex.

## ADENOIDITIS (Inflamed Adenoids)

Topical—Dilute appropriately, and apply frankincense, myrrh, and copaiba to the outside of the jaw just beneath the ears. Recommended dilution: 3%–5%.

Oral—Gargle with a mixture of 1 drop each of copaiba, frankincense, and lemon; 1 teaspoon of honey; and one-quarter teaspoon of salt, 2 to 4 times daily. Take a capsule with 1 drop each of vetiver, lemongrass, clove, and German chamomile, 1 to 3 times daily.

## ADRENAL FATIGUE

Topical—Apply 2 drops each of rosemary and pine and 1 drops each of geranium, blue spruce, balsam fir, and clove 1 at a time to the adrenal area on the back (about midway). Gently feather each oil up the spine with the back of your fingers, and after applying all of the oils, cover entire back with 20–30 drops of carrier oil and massage into entire back. To improve results, apply a warm washcloth after complete process and leave in place until cool. Repeat this process up to 3 times daily. Perform the Waterfall Technique®, once weekly. Women should also consider the following: dilute appropriately, and apply clary sage to the forehead or wrists, 1 to 2 times daily.

Other: Women consider a natural bioidentical progesterone or molecular progesterone complex. Practice deep breathing techniques for 15 minutes, 2 times daily.

## ALLERGIES

Oral—Take 1 capsule filled with 3 drops each of lavender and German chamomile and 1 drop lemon, rosemary, and blue tansy, 1 to 3 times daily. Alternately, take a capsule filled with 3 drops each of peppermint, lemon, and lavender, 1 to 3 times daily.

Topical—Dilute appropriately, and apply 1 drop lavender under the nose and massage 1 to 3 drops into the four small toes of the feet, 3 to 5 times daily. Recommended dilution: 1%-3% under the nose and 5%–10% on the feet.

## ALTITUDE SICKNESS

Oral—Take a capsule filled with 5 drops of lemon, and 1 drops each of frankincense, cedarwood, and peppermint 1 to 3 times daily.

Inhalation—Place 1 drop each of peppermint and eucalyptus on the palm and inhale as needed.

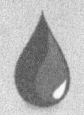

## ALZHEIMER'S DISEASE/DEMENTIA

Topical— Dilute appropriately, and massage 2 to 3 drops of lavender to the shoulders, back, and bottoms of the feet to improve sleep quality. Dilute appropriately, and apply 1 to 2 drops each of frankincense, vetiver, and rosemary to the base of the neck, crown of the head, and behind the ears, 2 to 4 times daily. Apply 3 to 4 drops of orange oil on the bottoms of the feet, 1 to 2 times daily. Recommended dilution: 3%–5%.

Inhalation—Apply 1 drop each of rosemary and peppermint oil on palms, rub together, and cup over nose and mouth to inhale as often as needed. Alternately, diffuse 2 to 3 drops each of rosemary and peppermint oil for at least 30 minutes in the afternoon or evening.

## AMOEBIC DYSENTERY (Amoebiasis)

Oral—Take a capsule filled with 3 drops each of oregano and lemongrass and 1 drop of thyme, 1 to 3 times daily.

Topical—Dilute appropriately, and apply 1 drop each of basil, fennel, copaiba and thyme to the lower abdomen, 2 to 4 times daily. Recommended dilution: 5%–10%.

## AMYOTROPHIC LATERAL SCLEROSIS (ALS)

See LOU GEHRIG'S DISEASE

## ANEMIA

Oral—Take one or a combination of 2 drops each of German chamomile, lemon, frankincense, or helichrysum, 2 times daily.

Topical—Dilute appropriately, and apply 1 drop of German chamomile, frankincense, lemon, and/or helichrysum to the lower back over the kidneys, 2 to 4 times daily. Recommended dilution: 5%–10%.

## ANEURYSM

An aneurysm can be life-threatening and emergency care should be sought as soon as possible.

Topical—Mix 2 drops each of geranium and lavender and 1 drop each of helichrysum and cypress and apply to the head and back of the neck, every 2 hours. Recommended dilution 25%–50%.

## ANGER

Inhalation—Place 1 drop each of ylang ylang, orange, and German chamomile on a tissue and inhale as needed.

Topical—Massage the soles of the feet (focusing on the liver area on the outside of the right foot) with 1 drop each of ylang ylang, orange, German chamomile, and lavender, 1 to 3 times daily. Recommended dilution: 3%–5%.

## ANGINA

Seek medical attention to determine the cause of insufficient blood flow to the heart muscle.

Topical—Dilute appropriately, and apply 1 to 2 drops each of wintergreen, clove, lavender, ylang ylang, and/or helichrysum over heart area, 2 to 4 times daily. Recommended dilution: 5%–10%.

Oral—Take 5 drops of a combination of helichrysum, clove, lemon, or orange, 1 to 3 times daily.

## ANKYLOSING SPONDYLITIS

Oral—Take a capsule filled with 3 drops of frankincense and 1 drop each of balsam fir, copaiba, and ginger, 2 to 4 times daily.

Topical—Dilute appropriately, and apply 2 drops each of basil, balsam fir, cypress, copaiba, and lavender to the back and hips, 1 to 3 times daily. Perform the Waterfall Technique®, once or twice weekly.

Other—Keep the back limber by performing yoga cat-cow poses for 1 to 2 minutes immediately before bedtime.

## ANXIETY

Topical—Dilute appropriately, and apply 1 to 2 drops of lavender and cedarwood to the base of the skull, neck, and head. Recommended dilution: 3%–10%.

Oral—Take 1 capsule filled with 2 drops of lavender, and 1 drop each of Virginia cedarwood and German chamomile, 1 to 3 times daily.

Inhalation—Apply 1 drop each of orange, cedarwood, and lavender to one palm, rub together with the other palm, and cup hands over mouth and nose to inhale as often as needed.

## APNEA, SLEEP

Topical—Dilute appropriately, and massage 1 to 2 drops of eucalyptus and/or black spruce to the bottoms of each big toe and the feet before retiring to bed. Recommended dilution: 5%–10%.

Inhalation—Apply 1 drop each of black spruce and balsam fir on pillowcase before bedtime.

## APPENDICITIS

Appendicitis is considered a medical emergency and professional care should be sought as soon as possible. Severe abdominal pain requires medical attention. The appendix could burst if not treated in a timely manner, which allows its contents to leak out and spreads infection throughout your abdomen.

Oral—Take a capsule filed with 2 drops each of ginger, lemon, and peppermint, and 1 drops each of basil and oregano, 2 to 3 times daily.

Topical—Dilute appropriately, and apply 1 drop each of wintergreen, orange, and lemon to the arch of the right foot and near the heel. Recommended dilution: 5%–10%.

Other—DO NOT massage the abdomen.

## ARACHNOID CYSTS

Topical—Dilute appropriately, and apply 2 drops each of frankincense, vetiver, sandalwood, and blue spruce along the entire spine and to the base of the hairline. Apply 4 to 5 drops of orange oil to the feet, 2 times daily. Recommended dilution: 10%–25%. Perform the Waterfall Technique®, once or twice weekly.

Oral—Take a capsule filled with 3 drops each of frankincense, vetiver, and sandalwood, 2 to 4 times daily.

## ARTHRITIS (RHEUMATOID)

Topical—Dilute appropriately, and apply a blend of peppermint, wintergreen, frankincense, eucalyptus, and copaiba to affected area as needed (cypress and helichrysum may also be added to increase circulation to affected joints). Recommended dilution: 20%–33%.

Oral—Take 1 capsule filled with 3 drops each of frankincense, balsam fir, and copaiba, and 1 drop of nutmeg, 2 times daily.

## ARTHROGRYPOSIS MULTIPLEX CONGENITA (ARTHROGRYPOSIS)

Topical—Mix together 1 drop each of marjoram, cypress, frankincense, lavender, basil, and German chamomile in 4 teaspoons of carrier oil and massage enough of the mixture into the affected areas up to 3 times daily.

## ASPERGER SYNDROME

Topical—Dilute appropriately, and apply 1 drop each of frankincense, cedarwood, vetiver, and ylang ylang to both sides of the neck, 1 to 3 times daily. Applying a mixture of 2 drops each of lavender, ylang ylang, blue tansy, and orange to the bottoms of the feet or by gently stroking the person's head with the oils on your hand may be calming during hyperactive episodes. Recommended dilution: 3%–5%.

Inhalation—Inhaling 1 to 2 drops of lavender may reduce anxious feelings.

Other—Many individuals with Asperger syndrome are opposed to touch and certain odors, so it may be necessary to offer them the recommended oils and allow them to choose which ones to apply.

## ASTHMA

Topical—Dilute appropriately, and apply 1 to 2 drops each of ginger, myrtle, thyme, and pine (or cypress) to the chest as often as needed. Recommended dilution: 3%–5%.

Inhalation—Apply 1 to 2 drops of lavender, ginger, or myrtle to 1 palm, rub together with other palm, cup over mouth and nose and inhale. Place 1 to 2 drops of one or more of myrtle, ginger or lavender in 3 inches of hot water that is not too hot to touch with your hand and cover head with towel to inhale every 4 to 6 hours.

Oral—Take a capsule filled with 1 drop each of copaiba, peppermint, ginger, and lemon, morning and evening.

## ATHEROSCLEROSIS

Oral—Ingest 1 drop each of rosemary, juniper, lemon, lime, and ylang ylang, 2 to 4 times daily.

Topical—Dilute appropriately, and apply ylang ylang, rosemary, and/or juniper on carotid arteries and over heart, 2 to 4 times daily. Recommended dilution: 2%–5%.

Inhale—Add 2 to 3 drops of lavender to a cotton ball, tissue, or cloth and inhale several times daily.

## ATHLETE'S FOOT

Topical—Soak foot in Epsom salts (use coarse sea salt for diabetics) bath with 1 drop each of tea tree, lemongrass, rosemary, and lavender added directly to the salts (not the water), up to 2 times daily. Apply 3 to 5 drops each of oregano, lemongrass, and tea tree to affected areas after soaking. Recommended dilution: 10%–15%.

## ATTENTION DEFICIT DISORDER (ADD) or ATTENTION DEFICIT HYPERACTIVITY DISORDER (ADHD)

Topical—Dilute appropriately, and apply 1 drop each of cedarwood, German chamomile, and lavender and/or frankincense and vetiver to the back of the neck, brain stem, and head up to 4 times daily (frankincense and vetiver increase focus, lavender and German chamomile help calm anxious feelings). Recommended dilution: 3%–5%.

Oral—Take 1 capsule filled with 2 drops each of orange, lavender, and frankincense, 2 times daily.

## AUTISM

Topical—Create a roller bottle with 2 to 3 drops each of melissa, frankincense, ylang ylang, lavender, and vetiver, fill the rest with carrier oil, then apply this blend to the back of the neck/base of the skull, twice daily. Applying a mixture of 2 drops each of lavender, ylang ylang, blue tansy, and orange to the bottoms of the feet or by gently stroking the person's head with the oils on your hand may be calming during hyperactive episodes. Recommended dilution 3%–10%.

Inhalation—Inhaling 1 to 2 drops of lavender may reduce anxious feelings.

Other—Many individuals with autism are opposed to touch and certain odors, so it may be necessary to offer them the recommended oils and allow them to choose which ones to apply.

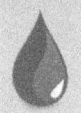

## AUTOIMMUNE DISORDER

(Immune Balancing Protocol) Oral—Take a capsule filled with 2 drops each of frankincense, copaiba, ginger, and spruce, morning and evening.

## BACK PAIN

Topical—Dilute appropriately, and apply a combination of 1 to 2 drops of wintergreen, black spruce, balsam fir, copaiba, peppermint, and frankincense to affected area, 2 to 4 times daily. For muscular back pain, add 1 drop of basil and marjoram as well. Recommended dilution: 15%–50%.

Oral—Take 1 capsule with 2 to 3 drops each of frankincense, copaiba, and balsam fir, 2 times daily.

## BARRETT'S ESOPHAGUS

Oral—Swallow 3 drops each of lemon and 1 drop of ginger mixed in honey and water, 2 to 4 times daily.

Topical—Dilute appropriately, and apply 1 drop each of frankincense, ginger, lavender, and blue tansy externally to the throat and breastbone areas, 2 to 4 times daily. Recommended dilution: 3%–5%.

## BASAL CELL CARCINOMA

*See Chapter 6*

## BED WETTING (NOCTURNAL URINATION)

Topical—Apply 1 to 3 drops of cypress mixed with carrier oil over the stomach and bladder area before going to bed. Recommended dilution: 3%–5%.

## BELL'S PALSY

Topical—Dilute appropriately, and apply 1 drop each of frankincense, helichrysum, geranium, spruce, and copaiba directly behind and underneath both ears and on the affected area of the face, 2 to 3 times daily. Recommended dilution: 1%–5%. Perform the Waterfall Technique®, once or twice weekly.

Oral—Take 1 capsule filled with 1 drop each of clove, oregano, lemon, cinnamon, and melissa, 2 to 3 times daily.

## BENIGN MOTOR NEURON DISORDER

Topical—Perform the Waterfall Technique®, once or twice weekly. Dilute appropriately, and apply 1 drop each of spruce, vetiver, frankincense, and sandalwood behind the ears and at the base of the skull, 2 to 4 times daily. Recommended dilution: 3%–5%. Apply 1 to 1 drop each of marjoram, pine, lavender, and lemongrass to the major muscles, 1 to 3 times daily. Recommended dilution: 5%–10%.

Oral—Take a capsule filled with 5 drops each of frankincense, sandalwood, and myrrh, 1 to 3 times daily.

## BENIGN PROSTATIC HYPERPLASIA (BPH), ENLARGED PROSTATE

Topical—Dilute appropriately, and apply 1 drop of frankincense, myrrh, orange, balsam fir, and copaiba heavily diluted to the area between the anus and scrotum, 2 times daily. Recommended dilution: 1%–3%.

Retention—Mix 2 drops each of frankincense, copaiba, myrrh, and balsam fir in 1 tablespoon of carrier oil and insert rectally; alternately, create a suppository with the same oils. Retain as long as possible.

Oral—Take a capsule filled with 2 drops each of copaiba, lime, vetiver, and rosemary, 1 to 3 times daily.

## BIPOLAR DISORDER

*Only use in conjunction with Western medical options and with approval from a physician.*

Topical—Dilute appropriately, and apply 1 drop each of frankincense, cedarwood, sandalwood, spruce, and lavender to the base of the skull and behind the ears, 2 to 4 times daily. Apply 1 to 2 drops of helichrysum over the liver, 1 to 3 times daily. Recommended dilution: 5%–10%.

Oral—Take a capsule filled with 2 drops each of melissa, orange, and frankincense, 1 to 3 times daily.

## BITES (ANIMAL)

Topical—Dilute appropriately, and apply 1 drop each of thyme, oregano, lavender, German chamomile, and lemongrass every 15 minutes for the first 2 hours, and then 1 time per hour for the next 24 to 48 hours. Apply peppermint to the bite as needed for pain. Recommended dilution: 5%–10%.

Oral—Take a capsule filled with 3 drops of oregano, and 1 drop each of eucalyptus, tea tree, and thyme, 2 to 3 times daily.

## BLADDER INFECTION

*See URINARY TRACT INFECTION (UTI)*

## BLEEDING

*Seek medical attention immediately if the blood spurts from the wound, or if it will not stop bleeding after 10 minutes of direct pressure.*

Topical—After cleansing the wound thoroughly, dilute appropriately, and apply 1 drop of geranium, cypress, helichrysum, or lavender near the wound every 5 minutes until bleeding stops. Recommended dilution; 25%–50%.

Other—Apply direct pressure to the wound.

## BLISTERS

Topical—Dilute appropriately, and apply 1 drop of lavender, German Chamomile, myrrh, copaiaba and/or helichrysum to the blister several times daily. Recommended dilution: 10%–15%.

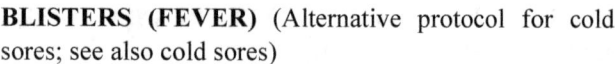

**BLISTERS (FEVER)** (Alternative protocol for cold sores; see also cold sores)

Topical—Dilute appropriately, and apply 1 drop of tea tree, melissa, clove, or rosemary to the blister several times daily. Recommended dilution: 25%–50%.

**BLOATING**

Oral—Take 1 to 2 drops of peppermint, juniper, and/or fennel in a capsule, 2 times daily.

**BLOOD CLOT**

*Abnormal blood clots can be a medical emergency and lead to a stroke, heart attack, or other serious conditions. Only use this protocol in conjunction with Western medical options and with approval from a physician.*

Topical—Dilute appropriately, and massage 4 drops of lavender to the bottoms of the feet up to 3 times daily. Apply 1 drop of geranium, lemon, orange, and helichrysum near the affected area (do not massage the affected area), 3 to 5 times daily. Recommended dilution: 10%–25%.

Oral—Take 2 capsules with 1 drop each of geranium, helichrysum, orange, grapefruit, and lemon, 2 times daily.

**BOILS**

Topical—Dilute appropriately, and apply 1 drop of a combination of one or more of helichrysum, copaiba, lavender, frankincense, myrrh, spruce, peppermint, or tea tree, several times daily. Recommended dilution: 10%–25%.

**BONE SPURS**

Topical—Dilute appropriately, and apply 1 drop each of eucalyptus, myrtle, pine, lavender, balsam fir, oregano, and peppermint to affected area, 2 to 3 times daily. Alternately, apply 2 to 5 drops of wintergreen, balsam fir, or cypress to affected area, 2 to 4 times daily. Recommended dilution: 10%–25%.

**BRAIN INJURY (Traumatic Brain Injury)**

*Only use this protocol in conjunction with Western medical options and with approval from a physician.*

Topical—Dilute appropriately, and apply 1 to 2 drops each of lavender, vetiver, cedarwood, rosemary, and helichrysum to the base of the skull and back of the neck, 3 to 5 times daily. Apply 2 drops each of black spruce, blue tansy, and frankincense to the bottom of the feet, 2 to 3 times daily. Recommended dilution: 5%–10%. When the person recovers enough, perform the Waterfall Technique®, once or twice weekly.

Oral—Take a capsule filled with 3 drops each of frankincense, marjoram, black pepper, cedarwood, and helichrysum, 1 to 3 times daily. Alternately, place 1 drop of each oil on the tongue, 1 to 3 times daily.

**BRITTLE BONES**

Topical—Dilute appropriately, and apply 1 drop each of wintergreen, pine, thyme, frankincense, and balsam fir to affected bones, 2 to 3 times daily. Women apply 1 to 2 drops of clary sage to the forehead or carotid arteries, 3 times daily. Men apply 3 drops of blue spruce or vetiver to the feet, 3 times daily. Recommended dilution: 3%–10%.

**BROKEN BONES**

*Broken bones require more than essential oils. Seek medical attention to have the bone set and casted. This protocol is intended to help relieve pain and encourage normal healing of bones. It should be followed for the duration that the cast is on, applying oils for 3 weeks before resting 1 week, then repeating the application process.*

Topical—Dilute appropriately, and apply 1 drop each of balsam fir, cypress, helichrysum, lemongrass, and wintergreen to the area, 2 to 4 times daily. Recommended dilution: 5%–15%.

Oral—Take a capsule filled with 3 drops each of balsam fir, copaiba, and frankincense, 1 to 3 times daily.

**BRONCHITIS**

Topical—Dilute appropriately, and apply 1 to 2 drops of eucalyptus, ginger, myrtle, and/or copaiba to the chest as needed. Recommended dilution: 5%–10%.

Inhalation—Place 1 to 2 drops each of eucalyptus, myrtle, and copaiba in half cup of hot water in bowl, cover head and bowl with towel and inhale 3 to 6 times daily. To improve outcome, hold your breath for as long as possible during the inhalation then breathe out slowly.

Oral—Take 1 capsule filled with 2 drops each of lemon and peppermint, and 1 drop each of myrtle and rosemary, 1 to 3 times daily.

**BRUCELLOSIS**

Oral—Take a capsule filled with 1 drop each of cinnamon, lemon, peppermint, marjoram, and oregano, 1 to 3 times daily.

Topical—Dilute appropriately, and apply 1 to 2 drops each of lemon and peppermint to the spine as needed for fever. Apply 1 to 2 drops each of basil, marjoram, and ginger to sore muscles as needed. Recommended dilution: 10%–25%.

**BRUISE/BUMPS**

Topical—Dilute appropriately, and apply 1 to 2 drops of helichrysum, blue tansy, lavender, geranium, copaiba, and/or frankincense to the bruise and surrounding area,

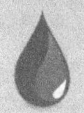

several times daily (it is best to begin application directly after a blow that may cause a bruise). Recommended dilution: 10%–25%.

## BUNIONS
Topical—Dilute appropriately, and apply 1 to 2 drops of lemon, wintergreen, and pine to the bunion, several times daily. Recommended dilution: 10%–25%.

## BURNS
Other—Cool the area in cold water for several minutes. Do not use ice.
Topical—Apply sufficient lavender, tea tree, and German chamomile to the burn every 15 minutes until pain subsides, covering applications with aloe vera, and then apply every two hours or as necessary until healing is complete. Recommended dilution: 25%–50%.

## BURSITIS
Topical—Dilute appropriately, and apply 1 to 2 drops each of wintergreen, balsam fir, lemongrass, and cypress to affected area, 3 to 5 times daily. Recommended dilution: 25%–50%.

## C. DIFF INFECTION
*C. diff infections can be life-threatening. Only use this protocol under the supervision of a healthcare professional. A fecal transplant may be recommended.*
Oral—Take a capsule with 2 drops each of cinnamon, thyme, and oregano, 3 to 4 times daily.
Retention—Create suppositories with 3 drops each of myrrh, patchouli, and melissa in 1 tablespoon of carrier and insert once or twice daily.
Topical—Dilute appropriately, and apply 1 drop each of rosemary, lemon, and ginger to the lower abdomen in a clockwise motion, 2 to 4 times daily for diarrhea. Recommended dilution: 5%–10%.
Other—Take a high-potency, multistrain probiotic 2 to 4 hours after each essential oil capsule.

## CALCIFIC TENDINITIS
Topical—Dilute appropriately, and apply 1 drop each of cypress, balsam fir, eucalyptus, wintergreen, grapefruit, lemongrass, and lemon to and widely around the affected area, 2 to 3 times daily. Recommended dilution: 10%–20%.
Oral—For difficult calcification, take a capsule filled with 4 drops of lemon, 1 drop each of frankincense, balsam fir, and copaiba, 1 to 2 times daily.

## CALLUSES
Topical—Dilute appropriately, and apply 1 drop each of oregano, lavender, or frankincense to the area, 2 to 3 times daily. Recommended dilution 5%–10%.

## CANCER
*See Chapter 6*

## CANDIDA (CANDIDIASIS)
Topical—(cutaneous candidiasis) Dilute appropriately, and apply 1 drop each of lemongrass, clove, eucalyptus, lavender, and tea tree to the affected area, 2 times daily. Recommended dilution: 5%–15%.
Oral—Take 1 to 2 drops each of oregano, lemongrass, lavender, and lemon in a capsule, 3 times daily.

## CANKER SORES
Topical—Apply 1 drop of 1 or more of clove, lemon, copaiba, lavender, tea tree, and/or peppermint directly to the canker sore several times daily. Rotating which oils are used will increase effectiveness. Recommended dilution: 50%–neat.

## CARPAL TUNNEL SYNDROME
Topical—Dilute appropriately, and apply a combination of lemongrass, marjoram, peppermint, cypress, rosemary, and wintergreen to affected area, 3 to 4 times daily. Recommended dilution: 10%–25%.
Oral—For added support, take a capsule filled with 2 drops each of frankincense, copaiba, balsam fir, and 1 drop of lemongrass, 2 to 3 times daily.

## CATARACTS
Topical—Dilute appropriately in castor oil, and apply a blend of lemongrass, frankincense, and lavender widely around the orbit of the eye at night at least 30 minutes before going to bed. Recommended dilution: 1%–3%. Oral—Take a capsule filled with 2 drops each of frankincense, lavender, and lemongrass, 2 times daily.

## CAVITIES
*See your dentist to repair the cavity as soon as possible.*
Topical—Dilute appropriately, and apply 1 drop each of clove and peppermint oil to tooth, 3 times daily. Recommended dilution: 25%–neat.
Other—Consider oil pulling with 1 tablespoon of coconut oil and 1 drop each of spearmint and peppermint essential oil for 5 to 10 minutes daily.

## CELIAC DISEASE
*This protocol is intended to support optimum digestive system function and encourage tighter intestinal junctions. A strict gluten free diet must be adhered to.*
Oral—Take a capsule filled with 2 drops of lemon, and ginger, and 1 drop each of orange, fennel, thyme, and peppermint, 3 times daily, preferably before each meal.

## CELLULITIS

Topical—Dilute appropriately, and apply 1 drop each of helichrysum, lavender, tea tree, eucalyptus, and thyme to the affected area, 2 to 3 times daily. Recommended dilution: 5%–10%.

## CHAPPED SKIN

Topical—Dilute appropriately, and apply 1 to 2 drops of lavender, myrrh, and/or German chamomile to affected area as often as needed. Recommended dilution: 5%–10%.

## CHARCOT FOOT
## (NEUROPATHIC ARTHROPATHY)

Topical—Dilute appropriately, massage 2 drops each of spruce, cypress, balsam fir, and vetiver to the top of the feet and ankles, 2 to 4 times daily. For wounds, apply 1 to 2 drops each of frankincense, copaiba, cedarwood, and lavender to the wound, several times daily. Recommended dilution: 10%–25%.

## CHERRY ANGIOMA

Topical—Dilute appropriately, and apply a 1 to 2 drops of a mixture containing equal portions of frankincense, geranium, lemongrass, German chamomile, lavender, and orange to the affected area, several times daily. Recommended dilution: 3%–5%.

## CHICKEN POX (CHICKENPOX)

Topical—Dilute appropriately, and apply 1 to 2 drops each of tea tree, lavender, lemongrass, and German chamomile to spots, 3 times daily. Recommended dilution: 10%–25%.

Oral—Take a capsule with 2 drops each of lemongrass, oregano, and lemon, 2 to 3 times daily.

## CHILBLAINS (Pernio)

Topical—Dilute appropriately, and apply 1 drop each of German chamomile, lavender, basil, and cypress to the affected area, 1 to 3 times daily. Alternately, add 1 drop of each to each application of lotion. Reccommended dilution: 10%–25%.

## CHOLERA

*Only use in conjunction with Western medical options and with approval from a physician.*

Oral—Take a capsule filled with 2 drops each of oregano and cinnamon, and 1 drop each of eucalyptus, tea tree, and thyme up to 4 times daily.

Other—Drink plenty of water with electrolytes to replenish what has been lost through diarrhea.

## CHRONIC FATIGUE

Topical—Dilute appropriately, and apply 1 drop each of frankincense, sandalwood, and cedarwood to the base of the skull and head, 2 to 4 times daily. Recommended dilution: 5%–10%.

Inhalation—Place 2 drops of peppermint in 1 palm, rub together with other palm, and cup over nose and mouth to inhale as often as necessary.

Oral—Take a capsule filled with 1 drop each of lemongrass, myrrh, clove, and lemon, twice daily.

## CHRONIC OBSTRUCTIVE
## PULMONARY DISEASE (COPD)

Topical—Dilute appropriately, and apply 1 to 2 drops of eucalyptus, myrtle, cedarwood, peppermint, and/or copaiba to the chest as needed. Recommended dilution: 5%–10%.

Inhalation—Place 1 to 2 drops of eucalyptus, rosemary, myrtle, and peppermint in 3 inches of hot water that is not too hot to touch with your hand, and cover head with towel to inhale, 1 or 2 times daily.

Oral—Take 1 capsule filled with 1 drop each of myrtle, rosemary, eucalyptus, thyme, and lemon up to 3 times daily.

## CIRCULATION, POOR

Topical—Dilute appropriately, and apply 1 to 2 drops each of cypress, helichrysum, and cedarwood to the area of poor circulation, 3 to 5 times daily. Recommended dilution: 5%–10%.

Oral—Take a capsule filled with 1 drop each of lemongrass, cypress, bergamot, clove, and fennel, morning and evening.

## COLD (COMMON COLD)

Topical—During early onset of cold, apply 1 to 2 drops each of eucalyptus, tea tree, and lemon to the chest and neck every 15 to 30 minutes for the first 4 hours. Recommended dilution: 5%–10%.

Inhalation—Place 1 drop of eucalyptus or tea tree under the nose, and consider a steam inhalation with 1 to 2 drops of rosemary and eucalyptus.

Oral—At the first signs of cold, drop 1 drop of tea tree under the tongue every 15 minutes for the first hour, swishing it around your mouth and at the back of the throat for 30 to 60 seconds. Take 1 capsule filled with 1 drop each of clove, oregano, lemon, cinnamon, and eucalyptus, 2 to 3 times daily thereafter.

## COLD SORES

Topical—Dilute appropriately, and apply one or more of clove, lemon, tea tree, melissa, and peppermint directly to the cold sore, several times daily. Recommended dilution: 5%–50%.

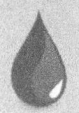

## COLITIS, ULCERATIVE

Oral—Take a capsule filled with 1 drop each of spearmint, rosemary, copaiba, fennel, peppermint, German chamomile, and ginger, 3 times daily.

Topical—Dilute appropriately, and apply peppermint, wintergreen, or fennel on the lower abdomen, 2 to 4 times daily. Recommended dilution: 5%–10%.

## COMPARTMENT SYNDROME

*Permanent damage or disability may occur if pressure is not relieved quickly. Only use this protocol in conjunction with Western medical options and with approval from a physician.*

Topical—Dilute appropriately, and apply 1 drop each of cypress, helichrysum, lemongrass, grapefruit, lemon, wintergreen, geranium, and cypress to affected area, 2 to 4 times daily. Recommended dilution: 10%–20%.

Oral—Take a capsule filled with 1 to 2 drops each of grapefruit, lemon, and lemongrass, 1 to 3 times daily.

## COMPLEX REGIONAL PAIN SYNDROME (REFLEX SYMPATHETIC DYSTROPHY SYNDROME)

Topical—Dilute appropriately, and apply 1 drop each of frankincense, vetiver, helichrysum, and geranium to the spine, 1 to 2 times daily. Apply 1 drop each of lavender, balsam fir, helichrysum, copaiba, and peppermint to areas of discomfort, 2 to 4 times daily. Recommended dilution: 10%–25%.

Oral—Take a capsule filled with 1 to 2 drops each of frankincense, copaiba, balsam fir, vetiver, and helichrysum, 1 to 3 times daily.

## CONCUSSION

*Anyone with a concussion should be assessed by a physician as soon as possible.*

Topical—Dilute appropriately, and apply 2 drops each of frankincense, vetiver, lavender, and rosemary to base of the skull and crown of the head, 1 to 3 times daily. Recommended dilution: 10%–25%.

Oral—Take 2 drops each of frankincense, lavender, bergamot, and rosemary in a capsule, twice daily.

## CONGESTION (SINUS)

Topical—Dilute appropriately, and apply eucalyptus, peppermint, or rosemary to the cheeks, nose, chest, and upper back as often as needed. Recommended dilution: 5%–10%.

Inhalation—Place 1 to 2 drops each of eucalyptus, rosemary, and peppermint in a bowl of hot water, cover head and bowl with towel to inhale.

## CONJUNCTIVITIS (PINK EYE)

Topical—Dilute appropriately, and apply lavender, tea tree, or frankincense in a wide circle around both eyes, up to 3 times daily. Apply 1 drop of lavender to palm and cup over eye for 5 minutes. Recommended dilution: 1%–3%.

Oral—Take 1 capsule filled with 2 drops each of clove and oregano, and 1 drop each of lemon, cinnamon, and eucalyptus, 2 to 3 times daily.

## CONSTIPATION

Oral—Take a capsule with 2 drops each of juniper, ginger, and lemon, 1 to 3 times daily, or until constipation is relieved.

Topical—Dilute appropriately, and apply 1 drop each of lemon, rosemarym and ginger over the abdomen, 1 to 3 times daily, or until constipation is relieved. Recommended dilution: 5%–10%.

Other—Sit on a chair and bring your knees to your chest, 1 leg at a time, 25 to 50 times each leg.

## CONVULSIONS

*A person who experiences a convulsion should have further evaluation by medical professionals to determine the cause.*

Topical—Dilute appropriately, and apply 1 to 2 drops of frankincense, copaiba, lemongrass, and lavender to the base of the skull, across the neck, and the upper part of the spine. Recommended dilution: 5%–10%.

## CORNS

Topical—Dilute appropriately, and apply 1 to 2 drops of clove, oregano, frankincense, or grapefruit to the corn, several times daily. Recommended dilution: 10%–25%.

## COUGH

Topical—Dilute appropriately, and massage 1 to 2 drops each of eucalyptus, myrtle, cedarwood, and peppermint into the chest and upper back, 3 to 4 times daily; cover chest with a warm, wet rag following application. Recommended dilution: 5%–15%.

Oral—Take a capsule with 2 drops each of oregano, cinnamon, rosemary, and lemon, 2 to 3 times daily. Create a cough syrup by adding 5 drops each of lemon and tea tree and 3 drops each of thyme and peppermint to 1 cup of pure maple, yacon, or raw honey (must be 13 months or older for honey) and give 1 teaspoon of this mixture, 4 to 6 times daily.

Inhalation—Place 1 to 2 drops each of eucalyptus, rosemary, and peppermint in a bowl of hot water, cover head and bowl with towel to inhale. For young children, use cedarwood and myrtle instead.

## CRAMPS, MUSCLE

*See MUSCLE CRAMPS*

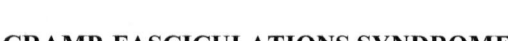

## CRAMP-FASCICULATIONS SYNDROME

Topical—Dilute appropriately, and apply 1 to 2 drops each of geranium, vetiver, basil, lavender, peppermint, and marjoram to the affected area(s), 2 to 4 times daily. Recommended dilution: 5%–10%.

Oral—Take a capsule filled with 1 to 2 drops each of frankincense, vetiver, lavender, and orange, 1 to 3 times daily.

## CROHN'S DISEASE

Oral—Take a capsule filled with 1 to 2 drops each of fennel, copaiba, peppermint, German chamomile, and ginger, 3 times daily.

Topical—Dilute appropriately, and apply 1 drop each of peppermint, ginger, and fennel on the lower abdomen, 2 to 4 times daily. Recommended dilution: 5%–10%.

## CROUP

*See CROUP in Chapter 4*

## CRYPTOSPORIDIOSIS

Oral—Take a capsule filled with 2 drops each of cinnamon and oregano, and drop each of lemongrass, peppermint, and lemon, 1 to 2 times daily.

Retention—For difficult cases, consider creating a suppository with 2 drops each of oregano, lemon, and marjoram in 1 tablespoon of carrier oil and insert into rectum up to twice daily.

## CUTS/SCRAPES

Topical—Dilute appropriately, and apply 1 to 2 drops of a mixture of helichrysum, tea tree, lavender, and frankincense to the area to promote healing every 2 to 4 hours. Recommended dilution: 5%–10%.

## CYST (GANGLION)

Topical—Dilute appropriately, and apply 1 to 2 drops of oregano, thyme, or frankincense to the area, 1 to 3 times daily. Recommended dilution: 3%–5%.

## CYST (SPLENIC)

*A splenic cyst should be evaluated by a physician as rare complications like hemorrhage, rupture, and infection may occur.*

Oral—Take 2 drops of oregano, and 1 drop each of frankincense, lemon, geranium, grapefruit, and sandalwood in a capsule, 1 to 3 times daily.

Topical—Dilute appropriately, and apply 1 to 2 drops each of oregano, thyme, frankincense, and orange under the left breast to the bottom of the rib cage near the edge of the torso, 2 to 3 times daily. Recommended dilution: 3%–5%.

## CYSTITIS

*See URINARY TRACT INFECTION*

## DANDRUFF

Topical—Mix 2 drops each of tea tree, rosemary, lavender, cedarwood, and basil in one tablespoon of carrier oil like jojoba or castor oil and massage into scalp, leaving in for 30 to 60 minutes; wash out with a natural shampoo and/or mild water.

## DARIER DISEASE (KERATOSIS FOLLICULARIS)

Topical—Mix 1 drop each of lavender, tea tree, frankincense, marjoram, lemongrass, and German chamomile in 1 tablespoon of coconut oil and apply to affected area, 1 to 3 times daily.

## DENGUE FEVER

*See YELLOW FEVER*

## DENTAL FILLING, LOST

*This is meant to be performed while waiting to see the dentist to replace the lost filling.*

Topical—Mix together a small amount of beeswax or zinc oxide powder (you can also purchase dental wax or compound) with 2 drops of clove oil and place in tooth where filling fell out.

## DENTAL INFECTION

*See your dentist as soon as possible to identify the extent of the infection.*

Topical—Dilute appropriately, and apply 1 drop of clove, myrrh, thyme, or tea tree diluted to gums and teeth, 2 to 3 times daily. Recommended dilution: 10%–25%.

## DEPRESSION

*Do not quit antidepressant medications without the express consent of your doctor. Use this protocol in conjunction with Western medical options and with approval from a physician.*

Topical—Dilute to 5%–10%, and apply frankincense or ylang ylang to heart center, 3 to 5 times daily. Apply a mixture of up to 10 drops of citrus oils (clinical research used 10 drops of a 2% dilution of orange essential oil, 3 times daily) to a place that won't be exposed to the sun, 1 to 3 times daily.

Inhalation—Apply 2 drops each of lemon and orange to 1 palm, rub together, and cup hands over mouth and nose to inhale as often as needed.

## DERMATITIS

Other—Wash affected skin with a mixture of cool to lukewarm water and 1 tablespoon of sea salt or baking soda (this can sting—like pouring salt in a wound). Some essential oils and carrier oils will exacerbate chronic skin conditions. If this occurs, consider applying homeopathic calendula or cardiospermum instead.

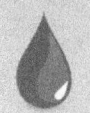

Topical—After washing skin as indicated above, mix together 2 tablespoons of olive oil and 1 drop each of geranium, lavender, frankincense, German chamomile, blue tansy, and tea tree and gently apply to irritated area up to 3 times daily.

## DERMATITIS (SEBORRHEIC)

Other—In a large bowl, mix together several cups of water and up to 1 cup of sea salt, thoroughly wash hair, scalp, and other irritated areas with this mixture, 1 to 2 times daily (this can sting—like pouring salt in a wound). Topical—Apply a mixture of 2 tablespoons of olive oil and 1 to 2 drops each of geranium, lavender, frankincense, German chamomile, blue tansy, and tea tree to the scalp, cover with a shower cap, and leave in place for at least 20 minutes and up to overnight, and then shampoo hair and scalp with a natural shampoo.

## DIABETES

Topical—Dilute appropriately, and massage 1 drop each of cinnamon, lemongrass, fennel, and copaiba to pancreas reflex point on the outer edge of the left foot about midway down, 2 to 4 times daily. Perform the massage for 5 to 10 minutes. Recommended dilution: 5%–10%. Oral—Take 1 capsule with 1 drops each of cinnamon, fennel, lemongrass, and geranium, morning and evening.

## DIARRHEA

Oral—Take a capsule with 2 drops each of peppermint and fennel, 1 to 3 times daily, or until diarrhea is relieved. Topical—Dilute appropriately, and apply 1 to 3 drops of peppermint and fennel over the abdomen every hour or until diarrhea is relieved. Recommended dilution: 5%–10%.
Other—Drink plenty of water to replenish lost fluids.

## DISTAL RENAL TUBULAR ACIDOSIS

Oral—Take a capsule filled with 4 drops of lemon and 1 drop of juniper, 2 to 3 times daily.
Topical—Dilute appropriately, and apply 1 to 2 drops of pine over the kidney area on the back, 3 times daily. Recommended dilution: 5%–10%.

## DIVERTICULITIS

Oral—Take 1 capsule filled with 1 drops each of oregano, peppermint, nutmeg, cypress, copaiba, fennel, and marjoram, 2 to 3 times daily. Topical—Dilute appropriately, and apply copaiba, peppermint, nutmeg, cypress, fennel, and marjoram over the abdomen, 2 to 3 times daily. Recommended dilution: 5%–10%.

## DIZZINESS

Inhalation—Place 1 drop each of peppermint and cypress in 1 palm, rub together with other palm, and cup hands over mouth and nose to inhale as often as necessary.
Topical—Dilute appropriately, and apply peppermint, frankincense, or cypress to the temples, back of the neck and shoulders. Recommended dilution: 3%–5%.

## DOPAMINE DEFICIENCY

Topical—Dilute appropriately, and apply 1 drop each of geranium, eucalyptus, rosemary, and clary sage behind and underneath the ears, 1 to 3 times daily. Recommended dilution: 3%–5%.
Inhalation—Place 1 drop of black pepper and rosemary on a tissue and inhale as needed. Refresh tissue up to 3 times daily.

## DRY SKIN

Topical—Mix 1 to 2 drops of lavender, myrrh, and German chamomile mixed in shea or mango butter to affected area as often as needed. A jojoba and coconut oil mixture can also be used with the mentioned essential oils. Recommended dilution: 1%–3%.

## DUPUYTREN'S CONTRACTURE

Topical—Dilute appropriately, and massage 1 drop each of lemongrass, basil, marjoram, vetiver, helichrysum, and frankincense to the affected area several times daily. Recommended dilution: 25%–50%.

## DYSESTHESIA (CUTANEOUS)

Topical—Dilute appropriately, and apply 1 drop each of vetiver, blue tansy, peppermint, juniper, German chamomile, and helichrysum to the area, 2 to 4 times daily. Recommended dilution: 5%–15%.
Oral—Take a capsule with 2 drops of helichrysum and 1 drop each of vetiver, copaiba, and lavender, 1 to 3 times daily.

## DYSENTERY

*Seek medical attention if symptoms are severe or last longer than a few days.*
Oral—Take 1 capsule with 2 drops each of peppermint, lemongrass, thyme, and oregano, twice daily.
Topical—Dilute appropriately, and apply 1 drop each of peppermint, basil, fennel, and ginger to abdomen, 2 to 3 times daily. Recommended dilution: 5%–10%.

## EAR INFECTION

Topical—Dilute appropriately, and apply 1 drop each of lavender and tea tree around the ear and on the fleshy part of the ear every 30 minutes until pain subsides, and then apply every 2 hours. Recommended dilution: 1%–5%.

Other—Apply 1 drop of tea tree or basil and 10 to 15 drops of carrier oil to a cotton ball and place inside ear, refresh every 30 minutes until pain diminishes, and then refresh every 2 hours; leave a fresh cotton ball in overnight.

## EAR MITES

Topical—Dilute appropriately, and apply 1 to 2 drops each of eucalyptus and tea tree around the ear and on the fleshy part of the ear, 3 to 5 times daily. Recommended dilution: 1%–5%.

Other—Apply 1 drop each of tea tree and eucalyptus and 10 to 15 drops of carrier oil to a cotton ball and place inside ear, and then refresh every hour; leave a fresh cotton ball in overnight. Consider using an ear oil with garlic as instructed on the bottle label.

## EARACHE

Topical—Dilute appropriately, and apply 1 to 2 drops each of peppermint and lavender around the ear and on the fleshy part of the ear every 30 minutes until pain subsides, and then apply every 2 hours. Recommended dilution: 1%–5%.

Other—Apply 1 drop of tea tree or basil and 10 to 15 drops of carrier oil to a cotton ball and place inside ear, refresh every 30 minutes until pain diminishes, and then refresh every 2 hours; leave a fresh cotton ball in overnight. Consider using an ear oil with garlic as instructed on the bottle label.

## EATING DISORDER
### (Anorexia & Bulimia)

*Only use this protocol in conjunction with Western medical options and with approval from a physician.*

Topical—Dilute appropriately, and massage 1 to 2 drops each of orange, German chamomile, and ginger to the ball of both feet and the big toes up to 3 times daily. Place 1 drop of frankincense on the crown of the head and behind the ears 3 times daily. Recommended dilution: 5%–10%.

Inhalation—Put 1 drop each of orange and German chamomile on a tissue or cotton ball and inhale as needed throughout the day.

Oral—Take a capsule with 2 drops each of orange, German chamomile, and ginger, 1 to 3 times daily.

## EBOLA VIRUS DISEASE

*Ebola is life threatening. Only use this protocol if standard medical care or treatment is not available.*

Oral—Take a capsule filled with 2 drops each of cinnamon, clove, and oregano and 1 drop each of eucalyptus and tea tree, 2 to 3 times daily. Take a second capsule with 3 drops each of geranium and helichrysum for hemorrhaging state. If severe nausea or vomiting is occurring, take a capsule filled with 2 drops each of ginger, peppermint, and 1 drop of fennel 1 to 3 times daily.

Topical—Dilute appropriately, and apply 2 drops of peppermint or lemon along the spine, 2 to 4 times daily for fever. Apply 3 drops each of cypress and helichrysum along the spine, 2 to 4 times daily for hemorrhaging.

Inhalation—Apply 1 to 2 drops of peppermint or ginger to your palms, rub together, and cup over your nose and mouth to inhale as needed for nausea.

## ECHINOCOCCOSIS CYSTS, LIVER
### (Hydatid disease)

Oral—Take a capsule filled with 1 drop each of thyme, peppermint, and lemon essential oil, 3 times daily, for 180 days, skipping a day every seven days.

## ECTHYMA

Topical—Dilute appropriately, and apply 1 to 2 drops each of thyme, tea tree, lemongrass, and lavender to the affected area, 2 to 4 times daily. Apply 1 drop each of lavender, geranium, and myrrh, 1 to 3 times daily as the area begins to heal. Recommended dilution: 1%–5%.

Oral—Take 2 drops each of thyme, lemongrass, lavender, and cinnamon, 1 to 3 times daily.

## ECZEMA

Topical—Apply a mixture of 2 to 3 drops each of lavender, frankincense, and tea tree in 2 tablespoons of carrier oil to the affected area as often as needed. Lemon oil may also be beneficial, but you must avoid sun exposure to the area of application for at least 12 hours afterward.

Other—Some essential oils and carrier oils will exacerbate chronic skin conditions. If this occurs, consider applying homeopathic calendula or cardiospermum cream instead.

## EDEMA

*Edema can be a sign of a serious medical condition such as heart failure, kidney disease, or liver issues. Seek medical attention to determine the cause.*

Topical—Dilute appropriately, and massage 1 to 2 drops each of lemongrass, grapefruit, lemon, and cypress in a teaspoon of carrier oil to affected area in strokes toward the heart, 1 to 3 times daily.

Oral—Take a capsule filled with 1 to 2 drops each of grapefruit, lemon, and lemongrass, 1 to 3 times daily.

Other—If swelling is in the ankles or feet, keep feet elevated when sitting.

## EHLERS-DANLOS SYNDROME

Topical—Dilute appropriately, and apply 1 drop each of cypress, helichrysum, frankincense, rosemary, and vetiver

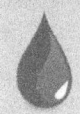

to the long limbs and abdomen, 1 to 2 times daily. For pain, apply 1 to 2 drops each of eucalyptus, balsam fir, peppermint, and wintergreen to areas of discomfort. Recommended dilution: 3%–5%.
Oral—Take a capsule filled with 2 drops each of balsam fir, copaiba, and lavender, 1 to 2 times daily. Take an additional capsule with 1 drop each of fennel, ginger, frankincense, and peppermint daily.

## EMOTIONAL SHOCK
*See SHOCK, EMOTIONAL*

## ENDOMETRIOSIS
Retention—Mix 5 drops each of geranium, frankincense, tea tree, copaiba, and rosemary in 1 ounce of carrier oil, apply to tampon, insert vaginally, and retain overnight. Alternately, create a pessary with the same oils. Topical—Massage the abdomen with 3 drops each of rosemary, copaiba, lavender, and cypress and cover with a hot compress. Perform the Waterfall Technique®, once or twice weekly.
Oral—Take a capsule filled with 4 drops of copaiba and 1 drop each of geranium and clary sage, 1 to 3 times daily. Other: Consider a natural bioidentical progesterone or molecular progesterone complex.

## ENTEROVIRUS
*Only use this protocol in conjunction with Western medical options and with approval from a physician.* Topical—Dilute appropriately, and apply 2 drops each of eucalyptus (preferably *Eucalyptus globulus*), rosemary, basil, and ginger to the chest and upper back and cover with a warm compress, 3 to 5 times daily. Recommended dilution: 5%–10%.
Oral—Take a capsule filled with 2 drops each of oregano and cinnamon, and 1 drop each of ginger, rosemary, eucalyptus and basil, twice daily.
Inhalation—Place 1 to 2 drops each of eucalyptus, rosemary, and basil in 3 inches of hot water that is not too hot to touch with your hand, and cover head with towel to inhale every 2 hours.

## EPIDIDYMITIS
Topical—Mix 2 to 3 drops each of frankincense and copaiba with 1 teaspoon of carrier oil and apply to the scrotum, 1 to 3 times daily. Apply 2 drops each of helichrysum and geranium mixed in 20 drops of carreier oil over the spleen 1 to 3 times daily. For shortness of breath, apply 1 to 2 drops of myrtle mixed in 10 drops of carrier oil to the chest as often as needed.
Oral—Take 1 capsule filled with 2 drops each of clove, oregano, lemon, cinnamon, and 1 drop of eucalyptus, 1 to 2 times daily.

## EOSINOPHILIC ESOPHAGITIS
Oral—Take 2 to 3 drops each of lemon and 1 drop of ginger in water, 2 to 4 times daily.
Topical—Dilute appropriately, and apply 2 drops each of frankincense, ginger, lavender, and blue tansy externally to the throat area, 2 to 4 times daily. Recommended dilution: 3%–5%.

## EPILEPSY
*Always try new essential oils with a companion that can offer help as certain essential oil aromas can trigger an epileptic reaction in those with epilepsy, potenrially even those not listed as triggers.*
Oral—Take 1 capsule with 1 to 2 drops each of frankincense, cedarwood, lemongrass, and lavender, 1 to 3 times daily.
Inhalation—Place 1 to 2 drops of frankincense, cedarwood, or clary sage in 1 palm, rub palms together, and cup over nose and mouth to inhale. Add 1 drop each of clary sage, frankincense, or cedarwood to 3 inches of hot water that is not too hot to touch with your hand, cover your head and the water with a towel over, and breathe deeply.
Other—See the list of oils to avoid in Appendix G.

## EPSTEIN BARR (MONONUCLEOSIS)
Oral—Take a capsule filled with 1 drop each of thyme, oregano, melissa, lemon, and cinnamon, 1 to 3 times daily. For sore throats, gargle with 1 drop each of lemon, peppermint, eucalyptus, and clove every 1 to 3 hours (mix with honey for better results) and swallow mixture.
Topical—Dilute appropriately, and apply 2 drops each of eucalyptus and frankincense on the front of the neck. Recommended dilution: 3%–5%. Perform the Waterfall Technique®, once or twice weekly.

## ERECTILE DYSFUNCTION
Oral—Take 1 drop of geranium or fennel under the tongue nightly. Take a capsule filled with 2 drops each of ginger, marjoram, rosemary, and cypress at least 1 hour before intercourse.
Topical—Dilute appropriately, and apply 4 to 5 drops of spruce on each forearm daily. Recommended dilution: 10%–25%. Dilute heavily and apply 1 drop each of cypress, marjoram, helichrysum, and ginger around the base of the penis approximately 30 minutes before intercourse. Recommended dilution: 1%.

## ESSENTIAL TREMORS
Topical—Dilute appropriately, and apply 1 drop each of lavender, frankincense, lemongrass, vetiver, geranium, and peppermint to the spine, base of the skull, and behind the ears, 1 to 2 times daily. Recommended dilution: 3%–5%.

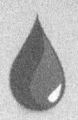

Inhalation—Inhale a blend of 3 drops of frankincense and 1 drop each of lemongrass and vetiver as needed throughout the day.

## EXHAUSTION

Topical—Dilute appropriately, and apply one or a combination of peppermint, rosemary, and/or cypress to the chest and base of the skull, 2 to 4 times daily. Recommended dilution: 3%–5%.

Inhalation—Place 1 to 2 drops of peppermint, rosemary, and/or cypress on palm and rub palms together, cup over nose and mouth, and breathe deeply as needed.

## FAINTING

Inhalation—Place 1 to 2 drops of peppermint and or sandalwood in palms, rub together, and cup over nose and mouth to inhale until symptoms subside.

## FATIGUE (PHYSICAL)

Inhalation—Place 1 to 2 drops of peppermint, rosemary, and/or lemongrass on palm and rub palms together, cup over nose and mouth, and breathe deeply.

Topical—Dilute appropriately, and apply 1 to 2 drops of peppermint, rosemary, and/or lemongrass to the temples, behind the ears, and over the sternum. Recommended dilution: 3%–5%.

## FATIGUE (MENTAL)

Inhalation—Place 1 to 2 drops of balsam fir, peppermint, and/or frankincense, on palms, rub palms together, and cup over nose and mouth to inhale as needed.

Topical—Dilute appropriately, and apply 1 to 2 drops of peppermint, frankincense, and/or balsam fir to the base of the skull, head, and neck. Recommended dilution: 3%–5%.

## FEAR

Topical—Dilute appropriately, and apply 1 to 2 drops of ylang ylang, lavender, and/or melissa to the temples, chest, and forehead as needed. Recommended dilution: 3%–5%.

Inhalation—Place 1 to 2 drops of ylang ylang, lavender, and/or melissa on palms, rub palms together, and cup over nose and mouth to inhale as needed.

## FEVER

Topical—Dilute appropriately, and apply peppermint or eucalyptus to the forehead, temples, back of neck, and tips of the ears as often as needed. Recommended dilution: 10%–25%.

## FIBROMYALGIA

Topical—Dilute appropriately, and apply 1 to 2 drops each of basil, frankincense, rosemary, peppermint, eucalyptus, and copaiba to the most affected areas and along the spine, 2 to 4 times daily. Recommended dilution: 10%–25%. Perform the Waterfall Technique®, once weekly.

Inhalation—Place 2 drops of peppermint in 1 palm, rub together with other palm, and cup over nose and mouth to inhale as often as necessary.

Oral—Take a capsule filled with 2 drops of frankincense and 1 drop each of lemongrass, basil, myrrh, and German chamomile, 2 times daily.

## FLATULENCE

Oral—Take 1 capsule filled with 2 drops of peppermint, and 1 drop each of oregano and lemongrass, 1 to 3 times daily.

Topical—Dilute appropriately, and apply 1 drop each of peppermint, fennel, and ginger to the lower abdomen, 1 to 3 times daily. Recommended dilution: 3%–5%.

## FLU (INFLUENZA)

Oral—Take a capsule filled with 2 drops each of clove, oregano, and cinnamon and 1 drop of eucalyptus, 2 to 3 times daily.

Topical—Dilute appropriately, and apply 1 to 2 drops of eucalyptus, rosemary, or myrtle to the chest several times daily, and cover with a warm, wet towel. Recommended dilution: 5%–10%.

## FOOD INTOLERANCE

Oral—Apply 1 drop of peppermint on the tongue, before each meal. Take 1 capsule with 1 drop each of lavender, lemongrass, ginger, and German chamomile, 1 to 3 times daily.

## FOOD POISONING

Oral—Take 1 capsule filled with 2 drops each of lemongrass, fennel, and peppermint, 1 to 3 times daily, or until symptoms are alleviated.

Topical—Dilute appropriately, and apply 1 to 2 drops of peppermint, lemongrass, and/or juniper to the lower abdomen, 1 to 3 times daily. Recommended dilution: 3%–5%.

## FOX-FORDYCE DISEASE

Topical—Apply a mixture of 1 to 2 drops each of geranium, tea tree, and lavender in equal parts of carrier oil to the affected areas, 2 to 4 times daily. Recommended dilution: 3%–5%. For the groin, dilute the mixture to 1%.

## FRIEDREICH'S ATAXIA

Topical—Dilute appropriately, and massage 1 to 2 drops each of pine, basil, lavender, and balsam fir along spine 2 to 4 times daily. Apply 1 to 2 drops each of marjoram, pine, lavender, and lemongrass to the major muscles, 1 to 3 times daily. Apply 1 drop each of vetiver, geranium, frankincense, and sandalwood behind the ears, 1 to 2 times daily. Recommended dilution: 3%–5%.

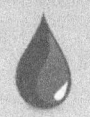

Oral—Take a capsule filled with 2 drops each of orange, frankincense, and vetiver, 1 to 3 times daily.

## FROSTBITE

Topical—Create a warm compress by mixing 2 drops of thyme, cypress, and rosemary in warm water, then dip a cloth in the water, and wrap frostbitten area. Cover with plastic and a hot water bottle for 3 hours. Massage the area with 1 to 2 drops each of thyme, cypress, and rosemary to the area 3 to 5 times daily. Recommended diltuon: 5%–10%. For frostbitten feet soak the feet in warm water with 1 to 2 drops of each oil mixed in half a cup of Epsom salts (use coarse sea salt for diabetics).

## FUNGAL INFECTION

Topical—Dilute appropriately, and apply geranium, lemongrass, tea tree, and/or lavender to area, several times daily. Recommended dilution: 5%–10%.

Oral—Take 1 capsule filled 2 drops each of lemongrass, oregano, and cinnamon, and 1 drop of eucalyptus, 2 to 3 times daily.

## G6PD (GLUCOSE-6-PHOSPHATE DEHYDROGENASE DEFICIENCY)

Topical—Dilute appropriately, and apply 1 drop each of lemon, clove, ginger, helichrysum, cypress, and frankincense to the spine and lower back, 1 to 3 times daily. Recommended dilution: 5%–10%.

Other—Avoid the use of essential oils that contain moderate to significant amounts of camphor and menthol (e.g. rosemary, peppermint, camphor).

## GALLBLADDER INFECTION/INFLAMMATION

Oral—Take 1 capsule filled with 2 drops each of lemon, juniper, and thyme, 2 to 3 times daily.

Topical—Apply 1 to 2 drops each of peppermint, juniper, and German chamomile over the gallbladder area (upper right part of the abdomen), 2 to 3 times daily. Recommended dilution: 3%–5%.

## GALLBLADDER STONES (GALLSTONES)

Oral—Take 1 capsule filled with 4 drops each of lemon and orange, 1 to 3 times daily.

Topical—Dilute appropriately, and apply 2 to 3 drops of peppermint, juniper, and German chamomile over the gallbladder area (upper right part of the abdomen), 2 to 3 times daily. Recommended dilution: 3%–5%.

## GANGRENE

Topical—Dilute appropriately, and apply 1 drop each of lavender, myrrh, sandalwood, geranium, and thyme to affected area, several times daily. Recommended dilution: 10%–25%.

Oral—Take 1 capsule filled with 2 drops each of clove, oregano, lemon, and cinnamon, 3 to 4 times daily.

## GASTRITIS

Oral—Take a capsule filled with 2 drops each of peppermint, fennel, ginger, and lemongrass, 1 to 3 times daily.

Topical—Dilute appropriately, and apply peppermint, lemongrass, and fennel to the stomach area as often as needed. Recommended dilution: 3%–5%.

## GASTROENTERITIS (STOMACH FLU)

Oral—Take a capsule filled with 1 drop each of peppermint, cinnamon, thyme, lemongrass, and oregano, 2 to 4 times daily.

Topical—Dilute appropriately, and apply 1 drop each of peppermint, ginger, and/or juniper to abdomen until symptoms subside. Recommended dilution: 5%–10%.

Inhalation—Apply 1 drop each of ginger and peppermint to 1 palm, rub palms together, and inhale as often as needed.

## GASTROESOPHAGEAL REFLUX DISEASE (GERD, ACID REFLUX)

Oral—Take 1 drops each of lemon, orange, and ginger in water, 2 to 3 times daily. Alternately, take 2 drops of lemon sublingually.

## GENITAL WARTS

Topical—Dilute appropriately, and apply oregano, geranium, or frankincense heavily and apply to warts, 1 to 3 times daily. Recommended dilution: 1%.

## GIARDIASIS (Giardia)

Oral—Take a capsule filled with 1 drop each of basil, eucalyptus, thyme, clove, and oregano, 2 to 3 times daily.

Topical—Dilute appropriately, and apply 1 to 2 drops of lavender and peppermint over the stomach area, several times daily. Recommended dilution: 3%–5%.

## GINGIVITIS

Oral—Gargle with a mixture of 1 drop each of peppermint, myrrh, wintergreen, and clove, several times daily (do not swallow).

Topical—Dilute appropriately, and apply 1 drop of clove on affected area, several times daily. Recommended dilution: 50%.

## GLAUCOMA

Oral—Take 1 to 2 drops each of geranium, frankincense, and cypress in a capsule, 3 times daily.

Topical—Dilute appropriately, and apply cypress or frankincense widely around the eye, 2 to 3 times daily. Recommended dilution: 1%–3%.

## GLIOBLASTOMA

*See Chapter 6*

## GOUT

Oral—Take a capsule filled with 2 drops each of juniper, lemon, lavender, and frankincense 1 to 3 times daily. As an alternative, take a capsule with 1 drop each of peppermint, juniper, pine, and lemon up to 3 times daily.

Topical—Dilute appropriately, and gently apply apply 1 drop each of frankincense, peppermint, and cypress to affected joints, several times daily. Recommended dilution: 25%–50%.

## GRANULOMA ANNULARE

Topical—Dilute appropriately, and apply 1 drop each of tea tree, geranium, German chamomile, and lavender to the area, 1 to 3 times daily. Recommended dilution: 5%–10%.

## GRAVES' DISEASE

Oral—Take a capsule filled with 1 drops each of frankincense, myrtle, myrrh, German chamomile, and clove, 1 to 3 times daily.

Topical—Perform the Waterfall Technique®, once or twice weekly.

## "GREEN NAIL"
## (PSEUDOMONAS AERUGINOSA INFECTION)

Topical—Soak foot or hand in Epsom salts (use coarse sea salt for diabetics) bath by adding 2 drops each of eucalyptus, peppermint, and cypress to a handful of salts and adding to warm water. After soak, apply 1 drop each of lemongrass, oregano, thyme, and eucalyptus to the affected nail 2 to 4 times daily. Recommended ilution: 25%–neat. Once cleared up, apply 1 drop each of grapefruit and lavender, 3 times daily to stimulate repair and growth of nail. Recommended dilution: 5%–10%.

## GROWING PAINS

Topical—Apply 2 drops each of copaiba, balsam fir, lavender, and cypress to the long bones of the body, 1 to 3 times daily. Recommended dilution: 5%–10%.

## GUILLAIN-BARRE SYNDROME

Topical—Dilute appropriately, and apply 1 to 2 drops each of vetiver, sandalwood, cypress, and frankincense behind the ears and at the base of the skull, 2 to 4 times daily. Recommended dilution: 3%–5%. Perform the Waterfall Technique®, twice weekly.

Oral—Take a capsule filled with 2 drops each of German chamomile, lavender, frankincense, morning and evening.

## GUM DISEASE

Oral—Gargle with a mixture of 1 drop each of wintergreen, myrh, tea tree, and clove, several times daily (do not swallow).

Topical—Dilute appropriately, and apply a mixture of clove, rosemary, lemon, and myrrh to the gums, 2 to 4 times daily. Recommended dilution: 10%–15%.

## GYNECOMASTIA

Topical—Apply 1 drop each of lemon, grapefruit, cypress, and frankincense to the breasts up to 3 times daily. Recommended dilution: 3%–5%.

## HAIR LOSS

Topical—Mix 2 drops each of cedarwood, rosemary, cypress, and geranium in ¼ cup each of jojoba and coconut oil and massage mixture into the hair and scalp once daily. Alternately, add 1 drop of each oil with each shampoo or conditioner application (for best results use this daily). Alternately, add 5 drops of each essential oil to an 8-ounce bottle of shampoo or conditioner.

## HAMMER TOE

Topical—Dilute appropriately, and apply 1 drop each of lavender, black spruce, helichrysum, and frankincense to the toe, 1 to 3 times daily. Recommended dilution: 25%–50%.

## HANGOVER

Topical—Dilute appropriately, and apply lavender and peppermint to the temples and back of the neck every 15 to 30 minutes until symptoms subside. Recommended dilution: 3%–5%. Oral—Take a capsule filled with 1 drop each of lemon, grapefruit, lavender, and peppermint, 1 to 2 times.

## HASHIMOTO'S DISEASE

Oral—Take a capsule filled with 1 drop each of frankincense, myrrh, nutmeg, German chamomile, and clove, 1 to 3 times daily.

Topical—Dilute appropriately, and apply 1 drop each of myrtle, sandalwood, frankincense, and peppermint over the thyroid area on the neck, 1 to 3 times daily. Massage 1 drop of myrtle on the tip of the big toe, morning and evening. Recommended dilution: 5%–10%. Perform the Waterfall Technique®, once or twice weekly.

## HAY FEVER

Oral—Take 1 capsule with 2 drops each of lavender and German chamomile, 1 to 3 times daily. Alternately, take 1 capsule filled with 2 drops each of peppermint, lavender and lemon, 1 to 3 times daily.

Inhalation—Apply lavender, eucalyptus, and peppermint to your palms, rub together, and cup over nose and mouth to inhale as often as needed.

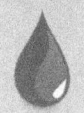

## HEAD LICE

Topical—Mix 3 drops eucalyptus, spearmint, and thyme and 2 drops each of tea tree, geranium, and lavender in 1 teaspoon of carrier oil and massage into scalp; cover with a shower cap and let sit for 30 minutes, and rinse clean with 2 drops each of eucalyptus, lavender, geranium, and rosemary in 16 ounces of warm water. Repeat procedure every other day for at least 7 days.

## HEADACHE

Topical—Dilute appropriately, and apply peppermint, copaiba, and/or lavender to the temples, forehead, and back of the neck as often as needed. Recommended dilution: 10%–25%.

Inhalation—Apply lavender, eucalyptus, and peppermint to your palms, rub together, and cup over nose and mouth to inhale as often as needed.

## HEARING IMPAIRMENT

Topical—Dilute appropriately, and apply a mixture of helichrysum, geranium, and lavender around the ear and on the fleshy part of the ear and then pull ear lobe in a circular motion 10 times to enhance absorption, 3 times daily. Recommended dilution: 3%–5%.

Other—Apply 1 to 2 drops of helichrysum with 10 to 15 drops of ccarrier oil on a cotton ball and leave in overnight.

## HEART ATTACK

*Get professional medical attention as soon as possible.*

Topical—Dilute appropriately, and gently massage 1 drop each of marjoram, helichrysum, rosemary, and ylang ylang over the chest every 10 to 20 minutes until symptoms subside. Recommended dilution: 10%–25%.

Inhalation—Place 1 drop each of lavender, ylang ylang, and German chamomile on a tissue and have the person inhale as necessary.

## HEART FAILURE

*Seek emergency treatment if you experience shortness of breath, chest pain, or irregular heartbeat.*

Topical—Dilute appropriately, and apply 1 drop each of bergamot, rosemary, marjoram, lavender, and ylang ylang diluted in a teaspoon of carrier oil over the heart area of the chest, up to 4 times daily. Recommended dilution: 3%–5%.

Other—For fluid retention see the EDEMA information.

## HEART PALPITATIONS

Topical—Apply 1 to 2 drops of ylang ylang, lavender, and/or rosemary on the chest, morning and night. Recommended dilution: 3%–5%.

Inhalation—Apply lavender to your palms, rub together, and cup over nose and mouth to inhale as often as needed.

## HEARTBURN

Oral—Take a capsule filled with 2 drops each of ginger and lemon, and 1 drop of fennel, 1 to 3 times daily. Take 3 drops of lemon or orange in a 50:50 mixture of apple cider vinegar and water daily (1 teaspoon of each).

## HEAT EXHAUSTION

Topical—Dilute appropriately, and apply 2 to 3 drops of peppermint to the forehead, tips of the ears, shoulders, and back of neck. Recommended dilution: 25%–50%.

Other—Cover forehead with a cool damp cloth after applying peppermint.

## HEEL SPURS

*See PLANTAR FASCIITIS*

## HEMOPHILIA

Oral—Take a capsule with 2 drops each of geranium and helichrysum, 1 to 3 times daily.

## HEMORRHOIDS

Topical—Dilute appropriately, and apply a mixture of 1 drop each of lavender, cypress, geranium, myrrh, and helichrysum to the area at each bowel movement and additionally as needed. Recommended dilution: 3%–5%.

## HEPATITIS

Oral—Take a capsule filled with 2 drops each of orange, helichrysum, and German chamomile, 2 to 4 times daily. Alternately, take 1 drop each of clove, oregano, orange, and black pepper, 2 to 4 times daily.

Topical—Dilute appropriately, and apply 2 drops each of helichrysum and orange over the liver area 2 to 4 times daily; apply a warm, wet towel over the liver after applying these oils, 1 to 2 times daily. Recommended dilution: 10%–15%.

## HERNIA

Topical—Dilute appropriately, and apply 1 drop each of cypress, frankincense, rosemary, basil, lavender, marjoram, and eucalyptus to the area, 2 to 4 times daily. Recommended dilution: 10%–25%.

Oral—Take a capsule filled with 2 drops each of frankincense, lemongrass, and copaiba, 2 to 4 times daily for pain.

## HERPES SIMPLEX VIRUS

Oral—Take a capsule filled with 2 drops of oregano, and 1 drop each of German chamomile, ginger, thyme, eucalyptus, and tea tree, 1 to 2 times daily.

## HICCUPS

Topical—Dilute appropriately, and apply 1 drop each of vetiver, peppermint, and basil to the lower abdomen and on the side of the neck and behind the ears. Recommended dilution: 3%–5%.

Inhalation—Inhale 1 drop each of lavender and ylang ylang for about 10 minutes.

## HIGH BLOOD PRESSURE (HYPERTENSION)

Oral—Take a capsule filled with 2 drops each of ylang ylang, clove, and lavender, 1 to 2 times daily.

Topical—Apply 1 to 3 drops of ylang ylang, marjoram, and lavender to the heart area and over carotid arteries, 1 to 3 times daily. Recommended dilution: 5%–10%.

Inhalation—Apply lavender or ylang ylang to your palms, rub together, and cup over nose and mouth to inhale as often as needed.

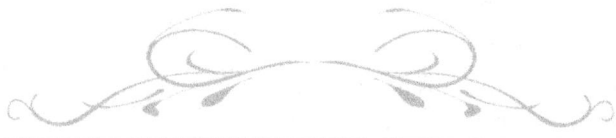

*"My husband had severe reactions to 3 different blood pressure medications . . . using the high blood pressure "recipe," [and] carefully monitoring his BP 3x a day . . . after 2 months of use, he's at a consistent 132/82, which is better than it EVER was on Rx!!!"*

Barb A.

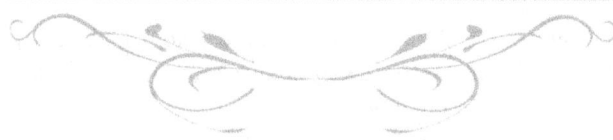

## HIV (HUMAN IMMUNODEFICIENCY VIRUS)

Oral—Take a capsule filled with 1 drop each of ginger, lemon, orange, oregano, and tea tree, and another capsule filled with 2 drops each of frankincense and clove, 2 to 4 times daily.

Topical—Perform the Waterfall Technique®, once or twice weekly.

## HIVES

Oral—Take a capsule filled with 2 drops each of German chamomile, frankincense, and lavender, 1 to 3 times daily.

Topical—Apply a 1 to 2 drops of peppermint, myrrh, German chamomile, or lavender in 2 teaspoons of carrier oil to affected area as often as needed. Lavender with clary sage may work for tough hives. Hives may be aggravated by topical application of essential oils, so apply the oil to a small area first before applying to large areas.

## HORMONAL IMBALANCE (MEN)

Topical—Dilute appropriately, and apply 1 to 2 drops of vetiver and black spruce to the inside of each forearm 2 times daily. Alternately, fennel, myrtle, or a combination of both may be used (3 to 4 drops, 2 to 3 times daily). Recommended dilution: 10%–15%.

Oral—Take 1 drop each of vetiver, basil (linalool CT), tea tree, bergamot, eucalyptus (*E. globulus*), and clove in a capsule, twice daily.

## HORMONAL IMBALANCE (WOMEN)

Topical—Dilute appropriately, and apply 1 to 2 drops of clary sage or fennel to forehead and abdomen, 1 to 2 times daily. Recommended dilution: 10%–15%.

Oral—Take 1 drop each of vetiver, rosemary, lemon, bergamot, and geranium, twice daily.

Other: Consider a natural bioidentical progesterone or molecular progesterone complex.

## HOT FLASHES

Topical—Dilute appropriately, and apply 1 drop of peppermint oil on the tip of each ear, on the outside of the right ankle, and on the back of the neck. Recommended dilution: 25%–50%.

## HUNTINGTON'S DISEASE

*Only use this protocol in conjunction with Western medical options and with approval from a physician.*

Topical—Dilute appropriately, and apply 1 drop each of rosemary, frankincense, lavender, and vetiver behind the ears and at the base of the skull 2 to 4 times daily. Apply 1 drop each of vetiver, geranium, German chamomile, marjoram, pine, frankincense, and helichrysum along the spine and feather lightly up the spine once daily. Recommended dilution: 3%–5%.

Oral—Take a capsule filled with 2 drops each of orange, vetiver, and frankincense, 1 to 3 times daily.

## HYDATID CYSTS, LIVER

*See ECHINOCOCCOSIS CYSTS, LIVER*

## HYDROCEPHALUS

*Only use this protocol in conjunction with Western medical options and with approval from a physician.*

Topical—Dilute appropriately, and massage 1 to 2 drops of rosemary, myrrh, German chamomile, cedarwood, and peppermint layered in that order to both sides of the spine daily. Massage the feet with 2 to 3 drops of lavender, 3 times daily. For headache, apply 1 drop each of peppermint, rosemary, and lavender to the temples, crown of the head, forehead and behind the ears up to 4 times daily. Recommended dilution: 5%–25%.

## HYPERACTIVITY

Topical—Dilute appropriately, and apply 1 to 2 drops each of lavender, cedarwood, and German chamomile to the chest or sole of each foot and toes, 2 to 4 times daily. Recommended dilution: 5%–10%.

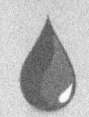

Inhalation—Apply 1 drop of cedarwood and lavender to palms, rub together, and cup over nose and mouth to inhale as often as needed.

## HYPERCHOLESTEROLEMIA (HIGH CHOLESTEROL)

Oral—Take a capsule filled with 2 drops each of lemongrass, lime, clove, and lemon, morning and evening.

Other—Consider a red yeast rice supplement.

## HYPERGLYCEMIA (HIGH BLOOD SUGAR)

Oral—Take a capsule filled with 2 drops each of cinnamon, fennel, geranium, and grapefruit, morning and evening.

Topical—Dilute appropriately, and apply 1 to 2 drops each of cinnamon, fennel, and geranium to the bottoms of the feet, particularly the pancreas reflex point on the outer edge of the left foot about midway down, 1 to 2 times daily. Recommended dilution: 3%–5%.

## HYPERTENSION

*See HIGH BLOOD PRESSURE*

## HYPERTHYROID

Oral—Take a capsule filled with 1 to 2 drops each of frankincense, myrrh, German chamomile, and clove, 1 to 3 times daily.

Topical—Dilute appropriately, and apply 1 drop each of lemongrass, myrtle, and peppermint to over the thyroid area on the chest or the thyroid reflex point on the bottoms of the feet (at the crease of the big toe), 2 to 4 times daily. Recommended dilution: 3%–5%.

## HYPOGLYCEMIA (LOW BLOOD SUGAR)

Oral—Take a capsule filled with 1 drop each of juniper, cypress, and basil, 1 to 3 times daily.

Other—Consume a protein meal or shake at regular intervals (about every 4 hours) to stabilize blood sugar levels. Exercise regularly.

## HYPOTENSION (LOW BLOOD PRESSURE)

Topical—Dilute appropriately, and apply 1 to 2 drops of cypress, geranium, and rosemary to the heart area and over carotid arteries, 1 to 3 times daily. Recommended dilution: 5%–10%.

## HYPOTHERMIA

Topical—Massage the body with 1 to 2 drops of a combination of rosemary, basil, and marjoram in 1 teaspoon of carrier oil. Create a warm compress by adding 2 drops of each oil in 1 cup of warm water and dip a cloth in the mixture. Apply the cloth to hypothermic areas.

Oral—Add 1 drop of each of rosemary, basil, and marjoram to a cup of warm water and drink up to 3 times daily.

## HYPOTHYROID

Oral—Take a capsule filled with 1 drop each of frankincense, myrrh, German chamomile, and clove, 1 to 3 times daily.

Topical—Dilute appropriately, and apply 1 drop each of myrtle, sandalwood, and peppermint over the thyroid area on the chest, 1 to 3 times daily. Apply 3 to 5 drops of orange on the feet, once daily, particularly massaging it into the thyroid reflex area on the feet.

Other—Consider a desiccated natural thyroid supplement.

## HYPOTONIA

Topical—Mix together 1 drop each of frankincense, sandalwood, vetiver, cedarwood, and blue spruce in 2 teaspoons of carrier oil and apply to the base of the skull, behind the ears, and along the spine, 1 to 3 times daily. Mix together 2 drops each of juniper, marjoram, and pine in 1 teaspoon of carrier oil and massage into legs and arms, 1 to 2 times daily. Recommended dilution: 3%–10%.

## IDIOPATHIC THROMBOCYTOPENIA PURPURA (Immune Thrombocytopenia)

Oral—Take a capsule filled with 3 drops of lemon, and 1 drop each of lavender, and helichrysum, 2 to 3 times daily.

Topical—Dilute appropriately, and apply a combination of 1 drop each of helichrysum, blue tansy, lavender, and frankincense to bruises, 3 to 5 times daily. Recommended dilution: 5%–10%.

## IMPETIGO

Topical—Clean the affected area with distilled water (or boiled water that has cooled) and 5 to 10 drops of lavender essential oil. Then, dilute appropriately, and apply 1 to 2 drops each of geranium, tea tree, lavender, and myrtle to affected area, 3 to 5 times daily. Recommended dilution: 3%–15% (depending on location affected).

Oral—Take 1 capsule filled with 1 drops each of clove, oregano, lemon, cinnamon, thyme, and tea tree, 2 to 3 times daily.

## IMPOTENCE

*See ERECTILE DYSFUNCTION*

## INCONTINENCE (URINARY)

Topical—Dilute appropriately, and apply 2 to 3 drops of cypress or balsam fir over the lower abdomen, 2 to 4 times daily; for more support, apply 1 drop each of frankincense and cedarwood diluted to the area between the anus and vagina/scrotum. Recommend dilution: 3%–10% (use 3% for the frankincense and cedarwood).

Other—Perform pelvic floor (Kegel) exercises, 3 to 5 times daily, by squeezing the muscles you would use to stop your urine for 3 seconds then relaxing for 3 seconds; repeat the exercises 15 times.

## INDIGESTION
Oral—Take a capsule filled with 1 drops each of ginger, peppermint, fennel, and nutmeg, 1 to 3 times daily.

Topical—Apply 1 to 2 drops of ginger, peppermint, fennel, or nutmeg to the stomach area as needed. Recommended dilution: 5%–10%.

## INFERTILITY, FEMALE
*This protocol may work best when used from the last day of one period until the next period begins, but success has been reported while performing the protocol through the entire cycle as well.*

Topical—Dilute appropriately, and apply 2 to 4 drops of clary sage to the lower abdomen and mons pubis 2 times daily. Apply 1 drop each of clary sage to the inside and outside of the right ankle. Recommended dilution: 5%–10%.

Oral—Take a capsule filled with 1 drop each of ylang ylang, frankincense, fennel, clary sage, and geranium, 2 times daily.

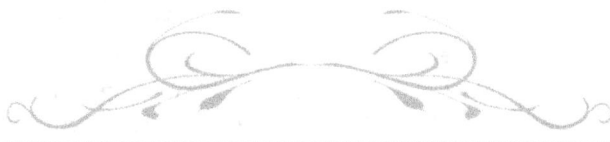

*"My husband and I tried to conceive for almost 2 years, which included the loss of a baby through miscarriage. I started Dr. Johnson's infertility protocol . . . and not two months later I became pregnant. Our daughter is such a joy to our family. I couldn't be more grateful for Dr. Johnson and all of his time, research, and knowledge that he has shared with the world."*

Lauren D.

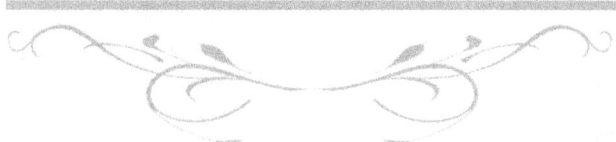

## INFERTILITY, MALE
Topical—Dilute appropriately, and apply 1 drop each of basil, sandalwood, and marjoram to the inside of the ankles and on the wrists. Apply 1 drop each of geranium, basil, and cypress to the lower abdomen above the penis, 2 times daily. Recommended dilution: 5%–10%.

Oral—Take a capsule filled with 1 drop each of vetiver, cinnamon, frankincense, basil, and cypress, 2 times daily.

## INFLAMMATION
Oral—Take a capsule filled with 2 drops each of copaiba and frankincense, and 1 drop each of orange, rosemary, and balsam fir, 1 to 3 times daily.

Topical—Dilute appropriately, and apply 1 to 2 drops each of copaiba, wintergreen, lemongrass, and frankincense to affected area, 1 to 4 times daily. Recommended dilution: 20%–50%.

## INSECT BITE/STING
Topical—Dilute appropriately, and apply repeated doses of 1 drop of lavender, basil, lemongrass, or tea tree to bite or sting until irritation subsides, and then continue applying 1 drop every 2 hours for the next 8 hours. Recommended dilution: 25%–50%, unless applying trace amounts neat.

Other—If the stinger is still present in the skin use a blunt knife, credit card, or other similar object to flick/scrape the stinger out—do not pull it out as this can release more venom from the venom sack.

## INSECT REPELLANT
Topical—Dilute appropriately (witch hazel or sesame oil are good carriers), and apply a mixture of 1 drop each of lemongrass, cedarwood, geranium, peppermint, and thyme to exposed skin and clothes (may stain some clothes) as needed. Citronella and lemon eucalyptus are also excellent choices. Recommended dilution: 3%–5%.

## INSOMNIA
Topical—Dilute appropriately, and apply 1to 2 drops of lavender or German chamomile to the bottoms of feet 15 minutes before retiring to bed. Recommended dilution: 5%–10%

Inhalation—Inhale a mixture of 3 drops lavender, 2 drops orange, and 1 drop vetiver before bed.

Other—Place 2 drops of lavender on your pillow before retiring to bed.

## INTENTION TREMORS
Topical—Dilute appropriately, and apply 1 drop each of lavender, frankincense, lemongrass, vetiver, geranium, and peppermint to the spine, base of the skull, and behind the ears, 1 to 2 times daily. Recommended dilution: 3%–5%. Perform the Waterfall Technique®, once or twice weekly.

Inhalation—Inhale a blend of 3 drops of frankincense and 1 drop each of lemongrass and vetiver as needed throughout the day.

## IRITIS
Topical—Mix 1 drops each of basil, frankincense, lavender, copaiba, and pine in 2 teaspoons of carrier oil (preferable grapeseed) and apply a couple of drops of this

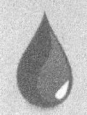

mixture widely around the eye and behind the ears, several times daily.

Oral—Take a capsule filled with 3 drops copaiba, and 1 drop each of frankincense, pine, and cypress, 1 to 3 times daily.

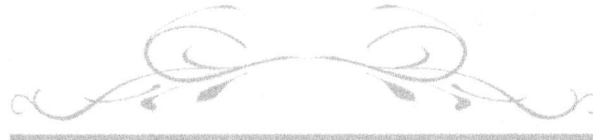

*"With the aid of this book I am now prescription free! I was told I would be on meds the rest of my life but I proved them wrong by following [the] protocols for irritable bowel syndrome."*

Jean W.

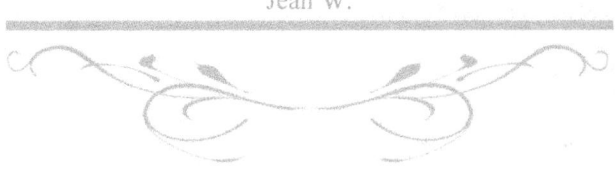

## IRRITABLE BOWEL SYNDROME

Oral—Take 1 capsule filled with 1 to 2 drops each of fennel, peppermint, nutmeg, juniper, and marjoram, 2 to 3 times daily.

Topical—Dilute appropriately, and apply peppermint, fennel, juniper, and marjoram over the abdomen, 2 to 3 times daily. Recommended dilution: 5%–10%.

## ITCHING

Topical—Dilute appropriately, and apply a 1 to 2 drops of peppermint, myrrh, German chamomile, or lavender to affected area as often as needed. Recommended dilution: 3%–5%.

Other—Consider homeopathic calendula or cardiospermum cream.

## JAUNDICE

Topical—Adults: apply 1 to 2 drops of geranium, German chamomile, lemon, and helichrysum over the liver (upper right part of the abdomen), 1 to 3 times daily. Recommended dilution: 10%–20%. For infant jaundice, see the children's section.

## JET LAG

Topical—Dilute appropriately, and apply 1 drop each of eucalyptus, cedarwood, and peppermint to the base of the skull, temples, and head in the morning and early afternoon; dilute and apply 1 drop each of frankincense, geranium, and lavender on temples, head, and neck at night. Recommended dilution: 3%–5%. Perform the Waterfall Technique® on the day of arrival to and/or from the destination.

## JOCK ITCH (Tinea cruris)

Topical—Dilute appropriately, and apply 1 drop each of eucalyptus, vetiver, tea tree, and lavender to the area, 2 to 4 times daily. Recommended dilution: 1%–3%.

Oral—Take a capsule filled with 2 drops each of lemongrass, oregano, and clove, 1 to 3 times daily.

## JOINT PAIN

Topical—Dilute appropriately, and apply a combination of wintergreen, balsam fir, copaiba, and marjoram to the affected area, 2 to 4 times daily. Recommended dilution: 20%–50%.

Oral—Take 1 capsule with 2 drops each of frankincense, copaiba, and balsam fir and 1 drop of rosemary, 2 times daily.

## KELOIDS

Topical—Dilute appropriately, and apply 1 to 2 drops of geranium, lavender, geranium, and helichrysum on and widely around the scar, 2 to 3 times daily until improved; if the scars are painful, apply 1 drop each of copaiba, basil, and balsam fir to the scar, 1 to 3 times daily between scar treatment applications for relief. Reocmmended dilution: 5%–10%.

## KERATOSIS PILARIS

Topical—Mix 1 drop each of lavender, lemongrass, and German chamomile in 1 tablespoon of coconut oil and apply to affected area, 1 to 3 times daily.

## KIDNEY INFECTION

*Kidney infections must be treated quickly to avoid severe complications such as permanent kidney damage and sepsis. Only use this protocol in conjunction with Western medical options and with approval from a physician.*

Topical—Dilute appropriately, and apply 1 to 2 drops of rosemary, vetiver, lemongrass, or marjoram over the kidney areas on the back, 2 to 3 times daily. Recommended dilution: 10%–15%.

Oral—Take a capsule filled with 2 drops each of rosemary, thyme, oregano, lemongrass, and marjoram, 1 to 3 times daily.

## KIDNEY STONES

Oral—Take 1 capsule filled with 4 drops each of lemon and orange, and 1 drop each of juniper, frankincense, and helichrysum 1 to 3 times, daily. To prevent kidney stones, drink a glass of water with 3 to 4 drops of lemon, daily.

Topical—Dilute appropriately, and apply 3 to 5 drops of wintergreen, juniper, and German chamomile over the kidneys, 2 to 3 times daily. Recommended dilution: 25%–50%.

## LARYNGITIS

Oral—Gargle with 1 drop each of lemon, eucalyptus, and vetiver mixed in water and honey 2 to 4 times, daily, and

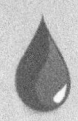

swallow. Add 1 drop of any of the above oils to your water daily for 7 to 14 days after symptoms subside for deeper healing.

Topical—Dilute appropriately, and apply 1 to 3 drops of eucalyptus, copaiba, and frankincense to the neck and chest, 2 to 4 times daily. Recommended dilution: 3%–5%.

## LEG CRAMPS
Topical—Dilute appropriately, and apply 1 to 2 drops of cypress, black spruce, and marjoram to the legs before going to bed or immediately following muscle cramp. Redomended dilution: 10%–15%.

Other—Drink ample fluids with electrolytes (coconut water is a great natural electrolyte) and increase dietary minerals.

## LEISHMANIASIS
Oral—Take a capsule filled with 1 drop each of lemongrass, oregano, clove, frankincense, and German chamomile, 2 to 4 times daily.

Topical—For cutaneous leishmaniasis, dilute appropriately and apply 1 drop each of frankincense, wintergreen, lavender, and German chamomile to the affected area up to 6 times daily. Recommended dilution: 5%–15%.

## LEPROSY
Topical—Dilute appropriately, and apply 2 to 3 drops each of lavender, myrrh, vetiver, and tea tree to the affected area, 2 to 3 times daily. Recommended dilution: 10%–15%.

Oral—Take a capsule with 1 drop each of clove, cinnamon, lemon, oregano, and rosemary, 1 to 3 times daily.

## LEPTOSPIROSIS
Oral—Take a capsule filled with 1 drop each of cinnamon, lemongrass, oregano, peppermint, and lemon, 1 to 2 times daily.

Retention—For difficult cases, consider mixing 2 drops each of oregano, lemon, and eucalyptus in 1 tablespoon of carrier oil and retain in rectum for up to 8 hours; repeat, 2 times daily. Alternately, create a suppository with the above oils.

## LEUKEMIA
See Chapter 6

## LEWY BODY DEMENTIA
Oral—Take a capsule filled with 1 drops each of basil, lavender, rosemary, cedarwood, and frankincense, 1 to 2 times daily.

Topical—Dilute appropriately, and apply 1 to 2 drops of lavender, cedarwood, vetiver, frankincense, and rosemary on the forehead, temples, and behind the ears, 2 to 4 times

daily. For muscle dysfunction, apply 1 to 2 drops each of German chamomile, marjoram, pine, frankincense, and helichrysum to the long bones of the body, 2 to 4 times daily. Recommended dilution: 3%–5%.

## LIBIDO (LOW, FEMALE)
Topical—Dilute appropriately, and apply 2 drops each of ylang ylang, clary sage, geranium, and sandalwood and 1 drop of spruce to the back and shoulders, 1 to 2 times daily. Reccommended dilution: 3%–5%.

## LIBIDO (LOW, MALE)
Topical—Dilute appropriately, and apply 1 to 2 drops of spruce, cedarwood, sandalwood, ylang ylang, and orange to the back and shoulders, 1 to 2 times daily. Recommended dilution: 3%–5%.

## LICE
See HEAD LICE

## LICHEN PLANUS
Oral—Take a capsule filled with 1 drops each of vetiver, frankincense, lavender, and spruce, clove, morning and evening. Take an additional capsule with 1 drop each of clove, oregano, lemon, cinnamon, and tea tree, once midday. For oral lichen planus, add 1 drop each of clove, tea tree, and oregano to half a cup of water and 1 teaspoon of aloe vera, and then swish, gargle, and swallow up to 3 times daily (this would be done in place of the midday capsule recommended above).

Topical—For lichen planus that affects the skin, dilute appropriately and apply 1 to 2 drops each of frankincense, lavender, and tea tree in 1 teaspoon of aloe vera to the affected area as often as needed.

## LICHEN SCLEROSUS
Topical—Dilute appropriately, and apply 2 drops each of lavender, copaiba, German chamomile, and geranium in 1 teaspoon of carrier oil to the affected area up to three times daily.

Oral—Consider the hormone balancing protocol in this chapter.

## LICHEN SIMPLEX CHRONICUS
Topical—Dilute heavily 1 to 2 drops each of frankincense, lavender, and tea tree and apply to affected area as often as needed. Apply 1 drop each of lavender, cedarwood, copaiba, and orange to the wrists, 2 to 4 times daily. Recommended dilution: 1%–3%.

Oral—Take a capsule filled with 3 drops each of lavender and German chamomile, 1 to 3 times daily.

Other—Do not scratch the area as it will make the condition worse.

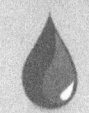

## LIPOMA

Topical—Dilute appropriately, and apply 1 to 2 drops each of frankincense, grapefruit, lemon, and lavender to area, 2 to 4 times daily. Recommended dilution: 5%–10%.

Oral—Take a capsule filled with 1 drop each of frankincense, myrtle, orange, lemongrass, and lemon, 1 to 3 times daily.

## LIVER CIRRHOSIS

Topical—Dilute appropriately, and apply 1 to 2 drops each of helichrysum, nutmeg, and orange over the liver area, 2 times daily. Recommended dilution: 3%–5%.

Oral—Take a capsule filled with 1 drop each of lemon, thyme, ginger, and myrrh, 3 times daily.

## LOU GEHRIG'S DISEASE (ALS)

Topical—Perform the Waterfall Technique®, once or twice weekly. Apply 1 drop each of spruce, vetiver, frankincense, and sandalwood behind the ears and at the base of the skull, 1 to 2 times daily. Apply 1 to 2 drops each of marjoram, pine, lavender, and lemongrass to the major muscles, 1 to 2 times daily. Recommneded dilution: 3%–5%.

Oral—Take a capsule filled with 2 drops each of frankincense, sandalwood, and myrrh, 1 to 3 times daily.

## LOW BLOOD PRESSURE

See HYPOTENSION

## LOW BLOOD SUGAR

See HYPOGLYCEMIA

## LUPUS

Topical—Massage entire body with 3 drops each of lemongrass, copaiba, marjoram, and frankincense mixed with 5 teaspoons of carrier oil, 3 times per week.

Oral—Take a capsule filled with 2 drops each of lemongrass, thyme, helichrysum, and rosemary, morning and evening.

Other—See recommendations for joint pain, rash, and indigestion for support for other common symptoms of lupus.

## LYME DISEASE

Oral—Take a capsule filled with 2 drops each of clove, oregano, and cinnamon and 1 drop each of thyme and thyme, 3 times daily. Alternately, take a capsule with 2 drops each of oregano, lemongrass, lavender, and clove in a capsule 3 times a day for 7 to 10 days, then switch to 2 drops each of ginger, tea tree, rosemary, and thyme in a capsule 3 times a day for 7 to 10 days, then rest 3 to 7 days and repeat.

Topical—Dilute appropriately, and massage 1 to 2 drops of lemongrass, frankincense, and ylang ylang to the bottoms of the feet, 2 to 3 times daily. Recommended dilution: 5%–10%.

## LYMPHEDEMA

Topical—Dilute appropriately, and apply 1 to 3 drops each of lemongrass, juniper, lemon, cypress, and grapefruit to the affected area 1 to 3 times daily. Make sure massage strokes move from the extremities to the center of the body. Recommended dilution: 5%–10%.

Oral—Take a capsule filled with 3 drops each of cypress, grapefruit, and helichrysum, 1 to 3 times daily.

Other—Receive lymphatic drainage massage by a qualified massage therapist if possible.

## LYMPHOMA

See Chapter 6

## MACULAR DEGENERATION

Oral—Take a capsule filled with 3 drops each of lemon and clove, 1 to 2 times daily.

Topical—Dilute appropriately, and apply 1 drop each of frankincense and helichrysum widely around the eye, 2 to 4 times daily. Apply 2 drops of frankincense to the palm and cup over eye (with eye open) for a few minutes, 3 to 5 times daily. Recommended dilution: 1%–3%.

## MALARIA

Life-threatening complications can develop with malaria. Only use this protocol in conjunction with Western medical options and with approval from a physician.

Oral—Take a capsule with 2 drops each of lemon and rosemary and 1 drop each of thyme, marjoram, myrtle, and eucalyptus, 1 to 3 times daily.

Topical—Dilute appropriately, and apply 2 to 3 drops of thyme, rosemary or tea tree, and lemon to the spine before retiring to bed at night. Recommended dilution: 3%–5%.

Other—Take a capsule with 1 drop each of myrtle, rosemary, oregano, lemongrass, and marjoram 1 to 2 times daily, five days per week, as a preventive.

## MASTOCYTOSIS, CUTANEOUS

Topical—Dilute appropriately, and apply 1 to 2 drops each of German chamomile, cedarwood, lavender, frankincense, thyme, and eucalyptus to the affected area, 2 to 4 times daily. Recommended dilution: 3%–5%.

Oral—Take a capsule filled with 2 drops each of lemon, orange, and frankincense, 1 to 3 times daily.

## MEASLES

Only use this protocol in conjunction with Western medical options and with approval from a physician.

Topical—Dilute appropriately, and apply tea tree, lavender, and German chamomile to spots several times daily. Recommended dilution: 5%–10%.

Oral—Take a capsule filled with 2 drops of melissa, and 1 drop each of German chamomile, lavender, and oregano, 2 to 3 times daily.

## MECHANICAL ALLODYNIA

Oral—Take 1 drop each of bergamot, copaiba, German chamomile, lavender, basil (linalool CT), and lemongrass in a capsule morning and evening.

Topical—Dilute appropriately, and massage 2 drops of orange and 1 drop each of lemongrass, geranium, and vetiver into each foot before retiring to bed. Recommended dilution: 5%–10%.

## MEDULLARY SPONGE KIDNEY

Oral—Take a capsule filled with 1 to 2 drops each of lemon, juniper, grapefruit, and geranium, 1 to 3 times daily.

Topical—Dilute appropriately, and apply 2 drops each of marjoram, juniper, and frankincense over the kidney area of the back, 2 to 4 times daily. Recommended dilution: 10%–15%.

## MELANOMA

*See Chapter 6*

## MENIERE'S DISEASE

Topical—Dilute appropriately, and apply 1 to 2 drops of helichrysum and frankincense behind the ears and on the fleshy part of the ear, 2 to 4 times daily. Recommended dilution: 3%–5%.

Other—Apply 1 drop of helichrysum and 10 drops of carrier oil on a cotton ball and place cotton ball in ear overnight; repeat for both ears.

Inhalation—Place 1 drop each of peppermint, ginger, and cypress in 1 palm, rub together with other palm, and cup hands over mouth and nose to inhale as often as necessary.

## MENINGITIS

*Only use this protocol in conjunction with Western medical options and with approval from a physician.*

Topical—Dilute appropriately, and apply 1 to 2 drops each of oregano, eucalyptus, tea tree, lemon, and thyme in along the spine and behind and below the ears up to 3 times daily. Recommended dilution: 5%–10% (spine), 1%–3% (around ears).

Oral—Take a capsule with 2 drops each of oregano, lemon, cinnamon, and clove and 1 drop each of tea tree and thyme 3 times daily.

## MENOPAUSAL SYMPTOMS

Topical—Dilute appropriately, and apply 2 to 3 drops of German chamomile, clary sage, or fennel to the forehead, carotid arteries, lower abdomen, and back, 1 to 3 times daily. Apply 1 drop of peppermint to the tips of the ears, temples and back of the neck for hot flashes. Recommended dilution: 3%–5%.

Inhalation—Apply 1 to 2 drops of frankincense or German chamomile to your palms, rub together, and cup over nose and mouth to inhale as often as needed.

Other—Consider a natural bioidentical progesterone or molecular progesterone complex.

## MENSTRUAL CRAMPS

Topical—Dilute appropriately, and apply 1 drop each of basil, marjoram, clary sage, geranium, and lavender to the lower abdomen, and then cover with warm damp cloth followed by a warm dry towel up to 3 times daily. Recommended dilution: 5%–10%.

## MENSTRUAL PAIN

Topical—Apply 1 to 2 drops of basil, marjoram, clary sage, peppermint, geranium, and lavender to the lower abdomen, lower back, and legs as needed. Recommended dilution: 5%–10%.

## MENSTRUATION, EXCESS

Topical—Dilute appropriately, and massage lower abdomen with 1 to 2 drops each of cinnamon, cypress, helichrysum, and geranium heavily diluted in carrier oil, 1 to 3 times daily. Recommended dilution: 3%–5%.

## MESOTHELIOMA

*See Chapter 6*

## METABOLIC SYNDROME

*See HIGH BLOOD PRESSURE, HYPERGLYCEMIA, HYPERCHOLESTEROLEMIA, and WEIGHT MANAGEMENT*

## METHYLENETETRAHYDROFOLATE REDUCTASE POLYMORPHISM (MTHFR)

Oral—Take a capsule filled with 2 drops each of copaiba, frankincense, and balsam fir and 1 drops each of lemongrass, clove, and cinnamon, morning and evening.

Topical—Dilute appropriately, and massage 4 to 5 drops of orange oil to the bottoms of the feet, daily. Recommended dilution: 10%–15%.

## MIDDLE EAST RESPIRATORY SYNDROME (MERS, CORONAVIRUS)

*Only use this protocol in conjunction with Western medical options and with approval from a physician.*

Oral—Take a capsule filled with 2 drops each of cinnamon and oregano, 1 drop each of thyme, vetiver, eucalyptus, and tea tree, 1 to 3 times daily.

Topical—Dilute appropriately, and apply 1 drop each of myrtle, eucalyptus, and pine to the chest and upper back, 2 to 4 times daily. Recommended dilution: 10%–15%.

Inhalation—Place 1 to 2 drops each of myrtle and eucalyptus in 3 inches of hot water that is not too hot to

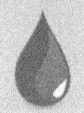

touch with your hand, and cover head with towel to inhale every 2 hours.

Other—Consider taking 600 mg of n-acetyl cysteine morning and evening; 30 mg of zinc, three times daily; 1,000 mg of vitamin C, 5 times daily; 500 mg of quesrcetin daily; and 10,000 IU of vitamin D for 10 to 14 days.

## MIGRAINE

Topical—Dilute appropriately, and apply peppermint, copaiba, basil, and lavender to the temples, forehead, and back of the neck as often as needed. Recommended dilution: 10%–25%. Place 1 drop of peppermint on your thumb and press to the roof of your mouth every 15 to 30 minutes until symptoms subside.

Inhalation—Apply lavender, eucalyptus, and peppermint to your palms, rub together, and cup over nose and mouth to inhale as often as needed.

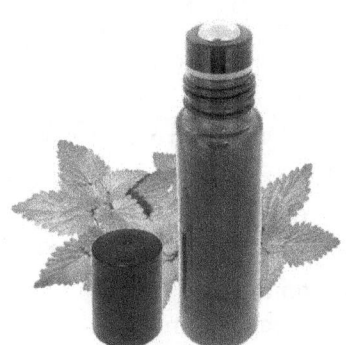

**HEAD TENSION BLEND**

Peppermint – 10 drops
Lavender – 7 drops
Rosemary – 7 drops
Hinoki – 7 drops
Copaiba – 6 drops
German Chamomile – 3 drops
Fill the rest of a 10 mL bottle with carrier oil

*Apply to the temples, back of the neck, forehead, and behind the ears at first signs of visual disturbance or when feeling head tension/pressure.*

## MISOPHONIA (Selective Sound Sensitivity Syndrome)

Topical—Dilute appropriately, and apply 1 drop each of vetiver, cedarwood, cypress and myrrh behind the ears and on the fleshy part of the ear 2 times daily. Apply 1 drop each of lavender, cedarwood, and German chamomile to the wrists, 2 to 4 times daily. Recommended dilution: 3%–5%. Place 1 drop of helichrysum with 10 drops of carrier oil on a cotton ball and place in ear, repeat for other ear and retain overnight.

## MOLES

Topical—Apply 1 drop of frankincense or oregano to the mole, 2 times daily. Recommended dilution 5%–10%.

## MOLLUSCUM CONTAGIOSUM

Topical—Mix 1 drops each of lemongrass, melissa, tea tree, and geranium in carrier oil and apply to affected areas, 3 to 5 times daily. Recommended dilution: 5%–10%.

Oral—Take a capsule filled with 1 drop each of lemongrass, oregano, cinnamon, and lemon, 1 to 2 times daily.

## MONONUCLEOSIS

*See EPSTEIN BARR*

## MONTGOMERY (AREOLAR) GLAND BLOCKAGE/CYST

Topical—Dilute appropriately, and apply 1 to 2 drops each of frankincense, lavender, and helichrysum to the area and cover with a warm compress, 2 to 4 times daily. Recommended dilution: 5%–10%.
Oral—Take a capsule filled with 2 drops each of lemon, frankincense, and lavender, 1 to 2 times daily.

## MOOD DISTURBANCE

Inhalation—Apply frankincense, lavender, or German chamomile to your palms, rub together, and cup over your nose and mouth to inhale as needed.
Topical—Apply frankincense, orange, lavender, or German chamomile to the temples, chest, and neck as often as needed. Recommended dilution: 5%–10%.

## MOTION SICKNESS

Oral—Take a capsule with 1 drop each of fennel, spearmint, lemon, peppermint, and ginger 30 minutes before travel and again every 4 hours while traveling. Inhalation—Apply 1 to 2 drops of peppermint to your palms, rub together, and cup over your nose and mouth to inhale as needed.

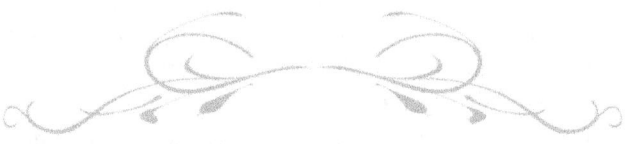

*"[For 13 months] I had a MRSA infection and endured four hospital stays in isolation because of sepsis. Twice I almost died. Then they discovered the infection in my fibula. It ate about 2 inches of my fibula. After months of no progress with antibiotics, a wound care specialist wanted to amputate my foot. I used a protocol designed by Dr. Johnson to close the wound (helichrysum, copaiba, and lavender in aloe and FCO carrier oil) and took cinnamon, tea tree, oregano, lemongrass, lavender, balsam fir, ylang ylang, and ginger orally. Now the wound is almost completely closed."*

Maryann L.

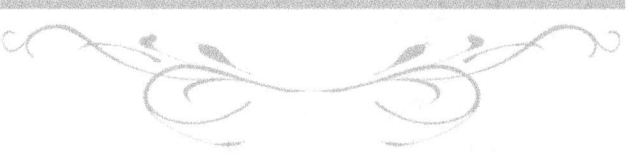

**MRSA (Methicillin-Resistant *Staphylococcus aureus*)**

Topical—Dilute appropriately, and apply 1 to 2 drops each of eucalyptus, lemongrass, thyme, and tea tree to affected area, 2 to 4 times daily. Recommended dilution: 5%–10%.

Oral—Take a capsule filled with 2 drops each of cinnamon and clove, and 1 drop of each lemongrass and eucalyptus, 2 to 3 times daily. Alternately, take 2 drops each of cinnamon and oregano, and 1 drop each of lemongrass, tee tree, balsam fir, ylang ylang, and ginger in a capsule 1 to 2 times daily.

## MULTIPLE SCLEROSIS

*Only use this protocol in conjunction with Western medical options and with approval from a physician.*

Topical—Dilute appropriately, and apply 1 to 2 drops each of frankincense, helichrysum, vetiver, rosemary, marjoram, and wintergreen along the spine, 2 times daily. Apply 1 to 2 drops of vetiver, spruce, cedarwood, and frankincense on temples, forehead, and behind the ears. Recommended dulition: 5%–10%.

Oral—Take a capsule with 1 drops each of rosemary, frankincense, balsam fir, helichrysum, and copaiba morning and night.

## MUMPS

*Only use this protocol in conjunction with Western medical options and with approval from a physician.*

Topical—Dilute appropriately, and apply 1 to 2 drops of tea tree, thyme, or lavender behind the ears, 4 times daily. Recommended dilution: 3%–5%.

Oral—Take a capsule filled with 2 drops each of lemon, lavender, and cypress, 2 times daily.

## MURMUR, HEART

Topical—Mix together 2 drops each of basil, marjoram, frankincense, lavender, and ylang ylang in 10 mL of carrier oil, and apply a small amount of this blend over the heart twice daily.

Oral—Take 1 to 2 drops each of lavender, ylang ylang, and marjoram morning and evening.

## MUSCLE CRAMPS

Topical—Dilute appropriately, and apply 1 drop each of lavender, spearmint, marjoram, myrtle, and basil to the affected area and cover with a warm towel or hot compress. Recommended dilution: 5%–15%.

Other—Stretch the muscle.

## MUSCLE PAIN/SORENESS

Topical—Dilute appropriately, and apply 1 to 2 drops each of pine, peppermint, copaiba, balsam fir, and marjoram to sore muscles, 2 to 3 times daily. Recommended dilution: 10%–20%.

## MUSCLE SPASMS

Topical—Dilute appropriately, and apply 1 to 2 drops each of basil, spearmint, wintergreen, lavender, and marjoram to muscles, 2 to 3 times daily. Recommended dilution: 5%–15%.

## MUSCULAR DYSTROPHY

*Only use this protocol in conjunction with Western medical options and with approval from a physician.* Topical—Dilute appropriately, and massage 1 to 2 drops each of pine, basil, lavender, and balsam fir along spine, 2 to 4 times daily. Apply 1 to 2 drops each of marjoram, pine, lavender, and lemongrass to the major muscles, 1 to 3 times daily. Recommended dilution: 5%–10%.

## MYASTHENIA GRAVIS

Topical—Perform the Waterfall Technique® once or twice weekly.

Oral—Take a capsule filled with 2 drops each of frankincense and copaiba, and 1 drop each of bergamot and vetiver, morning and evening.

## MYELODYSPLASTIC SYNDROME

Oral—Take a capsule filled with 2 drops each of lemon, rosemary, and ginger 2 to 4 times daily.

Topical—Apply 2 to 3 drops each of German chamomile, marjoram, pine, frankincense, and helichrysum to the long bones of the body 2 to 4 times daily. Recommended dilution: 5%–10%.

## MYOCARDITIS (VIRAL)

Oral—Take a capsule filled with 2 drops each of cinnamon and copaiba, and 1 drop each of ginger, frankincense, lavender, and lemongrass every 2 hours until symptoms subside (up to 3 doses); then take the same capsule 1 to 3 times daily for another 5 days.

Topical—Dilute appropriately, and apply 1 drop each of basil, marjoram, lavender, ylang ylang, and frankincense over the heart every 30 minutes until symptoms subside (up to 4 applications). Recommended dilution: 5%–15%.

## MYOSITIS

Oral—Take a capsule filled with 3 drops each of copaiba, frankincense, and orange oil, 1 to 3 times daily.

Topical—Dilute appropriately, and apply 2 drops each of basil, marjoram, balsam fir, and copaiba to area of soreness, 2 to 4 times daily. For skin rashes (dermatomyositis), apply 1 drop each of lavender, German chamomile, and tea tree to affected area, 1 to 3 times daily. Recommended dilution: 5%–15%.

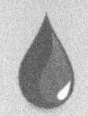

## NAILS, BRITTLE OR WEAK

Topical—Cover nail, particularly the base of the nail(s), with 1 drop each of grapefruit, frankincense, and myrrh mixed in vitamin E oil. Recommended dilution: 50%.

## NARCOLEPSY

Topical—Dilute appropriately, and apply 1 to 2 drops each of peppermint and geranium on the temples up to five times daily during the day. Apply 2 drops each of lavender, orange, blue tansy, and ylang ylang to the bottoms of the feet before going to bed. Recommended dilution: 3%–5%.

Other—Place two drops of lavender on pillow before retiring for bed.

## NAUSEA

Oral—Take a capsule filled with 1 drops each of ginger, peppermint, spearmint, lemon, and fennel, 1 to 3 times daily.

Topical—Dilute appropriately, and apply 1 to 2 drops of ginger, fennel, or peppermint in the navel and behind the ears every 1 to 2 hours. Recommended dilution: 3%–5%.

Inhalation—Apply 1 to 2 drops of peppermint or ginger to your palms, rub together, and cup over your nose and mouth to inhale as needed.

## NERVOUS TICS

Topical—Dilute appropriately, and apply 1 drop each of vetiver, frankincense, cedarwood, and spruce behind the ears and at the base of the skull, 1 to 3 times daily. Recommended dilution: 3%–5%.

Inhalation—Place 2 drops each of lavender and German chamomile on a tissue or cotton ball and inhale as needed.

Oral—Take a capsule filled with 1 drop each of vetiver, frankincense, marjoram, and lavender, 2 to 4 times daily.

## NEURALGIA

Topical—Dilute appropriately, and apply 1 drop each of helichrysum, eucalyptus, spruce, vetiver, peppermint, and copaiba to affected area, 3 to 5 times daily. Recommended diluition: 15%–25%.

Oral—Take a capsule with 2 drops of bergamot, and 1 drop each of frankincense, copaiba, and balsam fir, 2 to 4 times daily.

## NEUROBLASTOMA

*See Chapter 6*

## NEUROMA

Topical—Dilute appropriately, and apply 1 drop each of vetiver, frankincense, orange, helichrysum, and copaiba to the area of discomfort, 3 to 5 times daily. Recommended dilution: 5%–10%.

Oral—Take a capsule filled with 2 drops each of frankincense, orange, and copaiba and 1 drop of vetiver, 2 to 4 times daily.

## NEUROPATHY

Topical—Dilute appropriately, and apply 1 to 2 drops each of frankincense, spruce, peppermint, vetiver, helichrysum, lavender, and eucalyptus to affected area, 3 to 5 times daily. Recommended dilution: 15%–25%.

Oral—Take a capsule filled with 2 drops of bergamot and 1 drop each of coriander, frankincense, copaiba, and nutmeg, 1 to 3 times daily.

## NIGHT TERRORS

Topical—Dilute appropriately, and massage 1 drop each of blue tansy, orange, and ylang ylang to the bottoms of the feet immediately before retiring to bed. Recommended dilution: 5%–10%.

Inhalation—Diffuse 3 drops of frankincense, 2 drops of orange, and 1 drop of vetiver while sleeping.

## NIPPLES, SORE

Topical—Dilute appropriately, and apply 1 to 2 drops of lavender and helichrysum to the sore nipple(s), 1 to 3 times daily. Recommended dilution: 3%–5%.

## NOSEBLEED

Other—Apply direct pressure by gently squeezing the lower soft parts of the nose against the center wall continuously until bleeding stops.

Topical—Apply 1 drop of cypress or helichrysum across the bridge of the nose. Recommended dilution: 50%–neat.

## OBESITY

*See WEIGHT MANAGEMENT*

## OBSESSIVE-COMPULSIVE DISORDER (OCD)

Topical—Dilute appropriately, and apply 1 drop of lavender on each big toe and the bottoms of the feet, 2 to 4 times daily, particularly before going to bed. Apply 1 drop each of frankincense, sandalwood, spruce, and lavender to the base of the skull and behind the ears, 1 to 3 times daily. Recommended dilution: 3%–5%.

## ORTHOSTATIC HYPOTENSION
### (Postural Hypotension)

Topical—Dilute appropriately, and apply 1 drop each of rosemary, sandalwood, and marjoram over the heart area up to three times daily. Recommended dilution: 3%–5%.

Inhalation—Inhale 1 drop each of rosemary, lavender, sandalwood, and lemon as needed. This will work best if the essential oils are applied to a diffuser necklace or bracelet that can be inhaled regularly throughout the day.

## OSTEOARTHRITIS

Topical—Dilute appropriately, and apply 1 to 2 drops each of balsam fir, peppermint, cypress, and wintergreen on affected area, 2 to 3 times daily. Recommended dilution: 5%–10%.

Oral—Take capsule filled with 2 drops of copaiba, and 1 drop each of rosemary, pine, frankincense, and balsam fir, and nutmeg, 2 to 3 times daily.

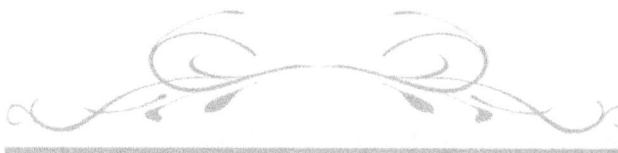

*"[The osteoarthritis] protocol keeps me mobile and away from the doctor's office."*

Jean W.

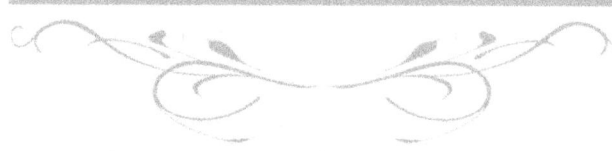

## OSTEOMYELITIS

Topical—Dilute appropriately, and apply 1 to 2 drops each of black spruce, sandalwood, balsam fir, lemongrass, helichrysum, wintergreen, German chamomile, and blue tansy up to 5 times daily. Thyme and eucalyptus can also be considered. Recommended dilution: 5%–10%.

Oral—Take a capsule with 1 to 2 drops each of thyme, oregano, lemongrass, clove, and tea tree, twice daily.

## OSTEOPENIA (Low Bone Mass/Density)

Topical—Create a mixture of 1 to 2 drops each rosemary, eucalyptus, thyme, and pine in 2 tablespoons of carrier oil and apply to the arms and legs, 2 to 4 times daily.

Oral—Take a capsule with 2 drops each of pine, rosemary, thyme, and juniper, 1 to 3 times daily.

## OSTEOPOROSIS

Topical—Apply 1 to 2 drops of clary sage, rosemary, and thyme to affected area (usually the hip, wrist, or spine), 1 to 3 times daily. Men may prefer to use pine in place of clary sage. Recommended dilution: 5%–10%.

Oral—Take a capsule with 1 to 2 drops each of clary sage, rosemary, thyme, and vetiver, 1 to 3 times daily. Men take juniper or pine in place of clary sage.

## OVARIAN CYST

Topical—Dilute appropriately, and apply 1 drop each of orange, frankincense, geranium, and basil over the lower abdomen, 2 to 4 times daily. Mix with grapeseed or evening primrose carrier oil to enhance effects. Recommended dilution: 5%–10%.

Oral—Take a capsule filled with 2 drops each of frankincense, orange, geranium, copaiba, and clove, twice daily.

Retention—Mix 2 to 3 drops each of frankincense, lavender, and cypress with 1 tablespoon of carrier oil, apply mixture to tampon, and retain overnight. Or create vaginal pessaries with the same oils.

## OVERACTIVE BLADDER

Oral—Take a capsule filled with 1 drop each of juniper, cypress, geranium, and German chamomile, morning and evening.

Topical—Dilute appropriately, and apply 1 to 2 drops of ylang ylang and cypress or balsam fir over the bladder area, 3 times daily; for more support, apply 1 drop each of frankincense and cedarwood diluted to the area between the anus and vagina/scrotum at the same time. Recommened dilution: 1%–5%.

Other—Perform pelvic floor (Kegel) exercises 3 to 5 times daily by squeezing the muscles you would use to stop your urine for 3 seconds and then relaxing for 3 seconds; repeat the exercises 15 times. Follow a schedule to go to the bathroom to train your bladder.

## PAGET'S DISEASE

Topical—Dilute appropriately, and apply 1 drop each of rosemary, peppermint, balsam fir, pine, and wintergreen to the affected area, 1 to 2 times daily. Recommended dilution: 3%–5%.

Oral—Take a capsule filled with 1 drops each of vetiver, frankincense, lavender, spruce, nutmeg, and clove, 1 to 3 times daily.

## PAIN

Topical—Dilute appropriately, and apply a combination of wintergreen, balsam fir, copaiba, frankincense, and marjoram to affected area, 2 to 4 times daily. Recommended dilution: 15%–25%.

Oral—Take 1 capsule with 2 drops each of frankincense, copaiba, and balsam fir and 1 drop of rosemary, 1 to 3 times daily.

## PANCREATITIS

*Seek immediate medical attention if your abdominal pain is so severe that you can't find a position that akes you comfortable.*

Topical—Dilute appropriately, and apply 1 to 2 drops each of geranium, peppermint, frankincense, and orange over the pancreas area (upper left abdomen), 2 to 4 times daily. Recommended dilution: 5%–10%.

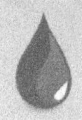

Oral—Take a capsule with 2 drops each of geranium, frankincense, copaiba, peppermint, and orange, 1 to 3 times daily.

Retention—Mix 5 drops each of orange, geranium, and oregano with 1 tablespoon of carrier oil, insert rectally, and retain for 1 hour, 3 times weekly.

## PARANOIA

Topical—Dilute appropriately, and apply 1 drop each of ylang ylang, German chamomile, spruce, and lavender to the temples, forehead, and over the liver area up to 3 times daily. Recommended dilution: 3%–5%.

Inhalation—Place 1 to 2 drops of ylang ylang, lavender, spruce, and German chamomile on palms, rub palms together, and cup over nose and mouth to inhale as needed. Or place the same oils on a tissue or cotton ball and inhale as necessary.

## PARASITES (INTESTINAL)

Oral—Take a capsule filled with 2 drops each of sweet basil, lemongrass, oregano, peppermint, and myrtle, 1 to 2 times daily.

## PARKINSON'S DISEASE

Oral—Take a capsule filled with 2 drops each of clove, lavender, black pepper, and frankincense, 1 to 2 times daily.

Topical—Dilute appropriately, and apply 1 to 2 drops of lavender, cedarwood, peppermint, or myrrh on the forehead, temples, and behind the ears, 2 to 4 times daily. Recommended dilution: 3%–5%.

## PERIPHERAL ARTERIAL DISEASE (PAD)

*PAD can be life-threatening, especially if not treated early. Only use this protocol with the express consent of a healthcare professional.*

Oral—Take a capsule with 2 drops each of lime, juniper, lemon, and ylang ylang, 2 to 4 times daily.

Topical—Dilute appropriately, and gently apply 1 to 2 drops each of cypress, rosemary, ylang ylang, and helichrysum to the lower legs, 2 to 4 times daily. Recommended dilution: 5%–10%.

## PEYRONIE'S DISEASE

Topical—Dilute appropriately, and apply 1 drop of vetiver, frankincense, geranium, and sandalwood to the penis, 1 to 3 times daily. Recommended dilution: 1%–3%.

Oral—Take a capsule filled with 2 drops each of frankincense, vetiver, lemon, and sandalwood, 1 to 2 times daily.

## PHANTOM LIMB PAIN

Topical—Dilute appropriately, and apply 1 drop each of vetiver, spruce, and copaiba to the area above the phantom limb pain. Apply 1 drop each of lavender, German chamomile, and cedarwood to the wrists, rub together, and inhale, 2 to 4 times daily (alternately apply to the feet or spine depending on amputation site). Recommended dilution: 5%–10%.

## PILONIDAL CYST (Pilonidal Abscess)

Topical—Dilute appropriately, and apply 1 drop each of tea tree, lavender, copaiba, and geranium to the affected area 2 to 4 times daily. Consider covering each application with an aloe gel or caster oil. Recommended dilution: 3%–5%.

## PINWORMS

Topical—Dilute appropriately, and apply 1 drop each of tea tree and eucalyptus to the affected area, 3 to 5 times daily. Recommended dilution: 1%–3%.

Oral—Add 1 drop each of lemongrass, basil, clove, and oregano to a capsule and take up to 3 times daily.

Retention—Create suppositories with 3 drops each of myrrh, basil, and melissa in 1 tablespoon of carrier and insert once or twice daily.

## PIRIFORMIS SYNDROME

Topical—Apply 2 to 3 drops each of marjoram, basil, and lavender to the buttocks muscles and hip area, up to 6 times daily. Recommended dilution: 10%–25%.

Oral—Take a capsule filled with 2 drops of bergamot, and 1 drop each of lavender, myrtle, German chamomile, and ginger, 1 to 3 times daily.

Other—Lie on your side and have another person apply pressure to acupressure point GB30, which can be found on the side of the buttocks by locating approximately the middle of the sacrum, and then moving out two-thirds of the way toward the hip. Apply firm pressure to this point (left or right side 1 at a time) with your thumb for about 30 seconds, and then release. Repeat this process until pain is relieved. Then repeat the entire process on the other side.

## PLANTAR FASCIITIS

Topical—Dilute appropriately, and apply 1 drop each of eucalyptus, copaiba, frankincense, spruce, wintergreen, balsam fir, and cypress to the affected area, 2 to 4 times daily. Recommended dilution: 5%–15%.

Other—After applying the essential oils, place a golf ball under the painful area of the foot and roll the golf ball around starting at the front and working to the back of the foot for a total of 3 to 5 minutes. Make sure to use firm pressure. Freeze the golf ball first for better results.

## PLANTAR WARTS

Topical—Apply 1 to 2 drops of oregano, thyme, or frankincense to the wart, up to three times daily. Recommended dilution: 10%–15%.

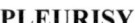
**PLEURISY**

Inhalation—Place 1 to 2 drops each of eucalyptus, myrtle, and cypress in a pot of hot water, and cover head and bowl with towel to inhale.

Topical—Dilute appropriately, and apply 1 to 2 drops each of wintergreen, eucalyptus, and cypress to the neck and chest, 2 to 3 times daily. Recommended dilution: 5%–10%.

Oral—Take a capsule filled with 1 drop each of oregano, thyme, peppermint, ginger, and lemon, 1 to 3 times daily.

**PNEUMONIA**

*Only use this protocol in conjunction with Western medical options and with approval from a physician.*

Topical—Dilute appropriately, and apply 1 to 2 drops of eucalyptus, tea tree, thyme, or oregano to the chest and neck as needed. Recommended dilution: 3%–5%.

Oral—Take 1 capsule filled with 2 drops each of clove, oregano, and cinnamon, eucalyptus, and peppermint, 2 to 3 times daily.

Inhalation—Place 1 to 2 drops each of myrtle and eucalyptus in 3 inches of hot water that is not too hot to touch with your hand, and cover head with towel to inhale every 2 hours.

**PNEUMONIC PLAGUE**

*Only use this protocol in conjunction with Western medical options and with approval from a physician.*

Oral—Take a capsule filled with 2 drops each of cinnamon and oregano, and 1 drop each of thyme, eucalyptus, and tea tree, 2 to 3 times daily.

Topical—Dilute appropriately, and apply 1 to 2 drops of eucalyptus, tea tree, thyme, or oregano to the chest and neck as needed. Recommended dilution: 3%–5%.

Inhalation—Place 1 to 2 drops each of myrtle, rosemary, and eucalyptus in 3 inches of hot water that is not too hot to touch with your hand, and cover head with towel to inhale every 2 hours.

**POLYCYSTIC KIDNEY DISEASE (PKD)**

Topical—Dilute appropriately, and apply 1 to 2 drops each of juniper, geranium, sandalwood, orange, and marjoram over the kidney area on your back, 2 to 4 times daily. Apply 1 to 2 drops each of basil, peppermint, and copaiba over painful areas. Recommended dilution: 5%–15%.

Oral—Take 1 drop each of frankincense, juniper, lemon, geranium, grapefruit, and sandalwood in a capsule, 2 to 4 times daily.

**(PMS) PREMENSTRUAL SYNDROME**

Topical—Dilute appropriately, and apply 1 to 3 drops of clary sage, fennel, marjoram, and geranium to the lower abdomen, 1 to 3 times daily. Recommended dilution: 5%–15%.

Oral—Take a capsule with 1 drop each of fennel, geranium, and copaiba, 1 to 3 times daily.

Inhalation—Apply clary sage and geranium to the palms, cup over nose and mouth, and inhale as needed.

**POISON IVY/OAK**

Topical—Dilute appropriately, and apply 1 to 2 drops each of ginger, lavender, peppermint, and frankincense diluted heavily in a carrier oil (particularly in the weeping stage). Recommended dilution: 0.5%–1%.

**POLIO**

*Only use this protocol in conjunction with Western medical options and with approval from a physician.*

Oral—Take a capsule filled with 2 drops each of frankincense, oregano, lemon, and thyme, 2 times daily.

**POLYCYSTIC OVARY SYNDROME (PCOS)**

Other—Consider using a bioidentical natural progesterone or molecular progesterone complex.

Topical—Dilute appropriately, and apply orange, frankincense, and basil over lower abdomen up to 4 times daily. Mix with grapeseed or castor oil to enhance effects. Recommended dilution: 5%–15%.

Oral—Take a capsule filled with 2 drops each of frankincense, copaiba, orange, and clove, 1 to 3 times daily.

Retention—Mix 2 drops each of frankincense, copaiba, lavender, and cypress with 1 tablespoon of carrier oil, apply mixture to tampon, and retain overnight.

**POLYMYALGIA RHEUMATICA**

Oral—Take a capsule filled with 2 drops each of copaiba and frankincense, and 1 drop each of vetiver, balsam fir, and thyme, 1 to 3 times daily.

Topical—Dilute appropriately, and apply 1 to 2 drops each of peppermint, wintergreen, frankincense, eucalyptus, thyme, and copaiba to affected area as needed (cypress and helichrysum may also be added to increase circulation to affected areas). Recommended dilution: 5%–15%.

**POLYMYOSITIS**

Oral—Take a capsule filled with 2 drops each of copaiba, frankincense, lemon, orange, and sandalwood, 1 to 3 times daily.

Topical—Dilute appropriately, and apply 1 to 2 drops each of marjoram, basil, and lavender to the affected muscles up to 3 times daily. Recommended ilution: 5%–10%.

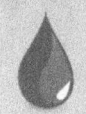

## POSTURAL ORTHOSTATIC TACHYCARDIA SYNDROME

*See ORTHOSTATIC HYPOTENSION*

## PROSTATITIS

Topical—Dilute appropriately, and apply 1 drop each of peppermint, lime, copaiba, and balsam fir to the area between the scrotum and anus, 2 times daily. Recommended dilution: 0.5%–2%.

Retention—Mix 2 drops each of peppermint, thyme, and balsam fir in 1 tablespoon of carrier oil and insert rectally; retain as long as possible.

Oral—Take a capsule filled with 3 drops of lime, and 1 drop each of copaiba, vetiver, and ginger, 1 to 3 times daily.

## PSEUDOMONAS INFECTION

Topical—Dilute appropriately, and apply 1 drop each of geranium, tea tree, lemongrass, pine, basil, and peppermint to the chest/upper back, 2 to 4 times daily. Recommended dilution: 5%–10%.

Oral—Take a capsule filled with 1 drops each of clove, oregano, lemon, cinnamon, and eucalyptus, 2 to 3 times daily.

Inhalation—Place 1 to 2 drops of thyme, cinnamon, and clove in a pot of hot water, and cover head and bowl with towel to inhale, 1 to 2 times daily.

## PSORIASIS

Topical—Apply 1 drop each of lavender, geranium, frankincense, German chamomile, fennel, and sandalwood diluted in 2 tablespoons of carrier oil (preferably a mixture of sweet almond, jojoba, and vitamin E) to the affected area as often as needed. Lemon oil may also be beneficial, but you must avoid sun exposure for at least 12 hours after application.

Oral—Take a capsule with 3 drops of copaiba and 1 drop each of frankincense and lavender, 1 to 2 times daily.

Other—Some essential oils and carrier oils will exacerbate chronic skin conditions. If this occurs, consider applying homeopathic *Berberis aquifolium*, calendula, or cardiospermum cream instead.

## PSORIATIC ARTHRITIS

Topical—Apply 1 to 2 drops each of lavender, geranium, frankincense, and tea tree in a 1 teaspoon of carrier oil (preferably borage seed oil or evening primrose oil) to the affected area as often as needed. Perform the Waterfall Technique®, once or twice per week.

Oral—Take a capsule filled with 3 drops each of copaiba and frankincense, and 1 drop each of nutmeg and vetiver, 2 times daily.

## PTSD (POST-TRAUMATIC STRESS DISORDER)

Topical—Dilute appropriately, and apply 2 drops each of blue tansy, lavender, orange, spruce, and frankincense over the heart area, morning and evening. Dilute and apply 1 drop each of ylang ylang, geranium, and cedarwood over the liver area, 1 to 2 times daily. Dilute and apply 1 drop each of frankincense, vetiver, and German chamomile to the base of the skull and behind the ears, 1 to 2 times daily. Place 1 drop of diluted ylang ylang inside the belly button, morning and evening. Recommended dilution: 3%–5%.

## PULMONARY FIBROSIS

Oral—Take two capsules filled with 10 drops of orange oil and 2 drops of melissa 3 times daily.

Inhalation—Place 2 drops of eucalyptus and 1 drop each of frankincense, peppermint, and lemon in a boiling pot of water, and cover head and bowl with towel to inhale, 1 to 2 times daily.

Topical—Mix 5 drops each of frankincense and eucalyptus and 2 drops wintergreen with 30 mL of carrier oil and apply to the back and chest, 2 times daily.

## PULMONARY HYPERTENSION

*Only use this protocol in conjunction with Western medical options and with approval from a physician.*

Topical—Dilute appropriately, and apply 1 to 3 drops each of eucalyptus, ylang ylang, marjoram, cypress, and lavender to the chest and upper back, 2 to 4 times daily. Recommended dilution: 5%–10%.

Oral—Take a capsule filled with 3 drops of orange, and 1 drop each of clove, lavender, and ylang ylang.

Inhalation—Place 1 drop each of eucalyptus, rosemary, thyme, and lavender in 3 inches of hot water that is not too hot to touch with your hand, and cover head with towel to inhale, 1 or 2 times daily.

## PYTHIOSIS

*Pythiosis is a life-threatening infection that can also require amputation if survived. Emergency medical attention should be sought.*

Oral—Take a capsule filled with 3 drops of oregano, and 1 drop each of marjoram, peppermint, and rosemary, 3 to 4 times daily.

Topical—Dilute appropriately, and apply 1 drop each of oregano, marjoram, peppermint, and rosemary to the affected area up to 3 times a day. Recommended dilution: 5%–7%.

## RABIES

*Only use this protocol in conjunction with Western medical options and with approval from a physician.*

Topical—Dilute appropriately, and apply 1 ro 2 drops each of eucalyptus, thyme, tea tree, and frankincense to the affected area, 2 to 4 times daily. Apply 1 drop each of spruce, vetiver, frankincense, and sandalwood to the base of the skull and behind the ears, 1 to 3 times daily. Recommended dilution: 3%–5%.

Oral—Take a capsule filled with 2 drops each of melissa and oregano and 1 drop each of eucalyptus, tea tree, cinnamon, and thyme, 1 to 3 times daily.

## RADIATION EXPOSURE

Topical—Dilute appropriately, and apply 1 to 2 drops of tea tree, cypress, or sandalwood over the thyroid area, 1 to 3 times daily.

Oral—Take a capsule filled with 2 drops each of frankincense, orange, and clove, and 1 drop of eucalyptus, 2 times daily.

## RASH

Topical—Dilute appropriately, and apply 1 to 4 drops of lavender, German chamomile, or tea tree to affected area as needed. Recommended dilution: 1%–5%.

## RATHKE'S CLEFT CYSTS

Topical—Dilute appropriately, and apply 1 to 2 drops of vetiver, frankincense, cedarwood, helichrysum, and myrrh to the base of the skull and behind the ears, 2 to 4 times daily. Recommended diution: 1%–3%.

Oral—Take a capsule filled with 2 drops each of frankincense, vetiver, and cedarwood, 2 to 3 times daily.

## RAYNAUD'S SYNDROME

Topical—Dilute appropriately, and apply 1 to 2 drops each of cypress, rosemary, and helichrysum to the area of poor circulation, 3 to 5 times daily. Recommended dilution: 3%–10%.

Oral—Take a capsule filled with 1 drop each of spearmint, lemongrass, cypress, clove, ginger, rosemary, marjoram, and cinnamon, morning and evening.

## RESTLESS LEGS SYNDROME

Topical—Massage 1 to 2 drops each of basil, lavender, German chamomile, and/or cedarwood to the lower legs and bottoms of the feet before going to bed. Massage lasting 15 minutes and emphasizing the following reflex points: thyroid, parathyroid, pancreas, adrenal glands, and solar plexus on the feet is particularly helpful. Recommended dilution: 5%–10%.

Other—Check iron and magnesium levels and supplement as necessary.

## RHEUMATIC FEVER

*Only use this protocol in conjunction with Western medical options and with approval from a physician.*

Oral—Take 1 capsule filled with 1 drops each of cinnamon, peppermint, thyme, lemon, eucalyptus, and tea tree oil, 2 to 3 times daily.

Topical—Dilute appropriately, and apply 1 to 2 drops each of marjoram, peppermint, eucalyptus, frankincense, and lavender to painful joints, 1 to 3 times daily. Dilute and apply 1 drop each of bergamot, lavender, and ylang ylang over the heart area, 1 to 2 times daily. Dilute and apply 1 drop each of geranium, vetiver, frankincense, and copaiba to the spine, 1 to 2 times daily. Recommended dilution: 5%–10%.

## RHINITIS (Coryza)

Topical—Dilute appropriately, and apply 1 to 2 drops of lavender, eucalyptus, and peppermint to the forehead and bridge of the nose, 2 to 4 times daily. Recommended dilution: 3%–5%. Add 1 drop each of copaiba and rosemary and 2 drops of carrier oil to a cotton swab and gently rub inside the nose.

Inhalation—Place 1 to 2 drops each of eucalyptus, rosemary, and copaiba in 3 inches of hot water that is not too hot to touch with your hand, and cover head with towel to inhale, 1 or 2 times daily.

## RINGWORM

Topical—Dilute appropriately, and apply 1 to 2 drops each of lemongrass, rosemary, geranium, tea tree, and lavender to the affected area 3 times daily. Recommended dilution: 5%–10%. For ringworm of the scalp, dilute and apply a drop of each oil in 1 teaspoon of carrier oil or shampoo and massage into scalp, once daily.

Oral—Take a capsule with 1 drops each of lemongrass, oregano, cinnamon, and tea tree 2 to 3 times daily.

## ROSACEA

Topical—Create a mixture of 1 drop each of tea tree, lavender, and German chamomile in 1 teaspoon of carrier oil (preferably jojoba) and apply a small amount of this mixture to the affected area up to 3 times daily.

Oral—Take a capsule filled with 1 drop each of German chamomile, lavender, and lemon, morning and evening.

## RSV, ADULT
## (RESPIRATORY SYNCYTIAL VIRUS)

Topical—Dilute appropriately, and apply 1 to 2 drops each of myrtle, rosemary, eucalyptus, and melissa to the chest, 2 to 3 times daily. Recommended dilution: 5%–10%.

Inhalation—Place 1 to 2 drops each of eucalyptus and peppermint in a boiling pot of water, cover head and bowl with towel to inhale, 1 to 3 times daily.

Oral—Take a capsule filled with 1 drops each of clove, oregano, thyme, melissa, cinnamon, eucalyptus, 2 to 3 times daily.

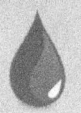

## RUBELLA (GERMAN MEASLES)

*Only use this protocol in conjunction with Western medical options and with approval from a physician.*

Topical—Soak a cloth in 1 drop each of tea tree, eucalyptus, lavender, and German chamomile and 1 cup of cool water and wipe rash with cloth several times daily. For aching joints, dilute appropriately, and apply 1 to 2 drops each of lemongrass, eucalyptus, balsam fir, copaiba, and marjoram to affected area, 2 to 4 times daily. Recommended dilution: 10%–25%.

Oral—Take a capsule filled with 2 drops each of German chamomile, lavender, and oregano and 1 drop each of eucalyptus and tea tree, 2 to 3 times daily.

## SARCOIDOSIS

Oral—Take a capsule filled with 2 drops of ginger, and 1 drop each of copaiba, vetiver, frankincense, and German chamomile, 1 to 2 times daily. Take a second capsule with 2 drops each of orange, peppermint, and lemon, once daily.

Topical—Dilute appropriately, and apply 1 to 2 drops each of ginger, myrtle, and eucalyptus to the chest and upper back, 1 to 2 times daily. Recommended dilution: 5%–10%. Perform the Waterfall Technique®, once or twice weekly.

Inhalation—Place 1 to 2 drops each of eucalyptus, rosemary, and ginger in 3 inches of hot water that is not too hot to touch with your hand, and cover head with towel to inhale, 1 or 2 times daily.

## SCABIES

Topical—Apply 1 to 2 drops each of tea tree, clove, eucalyptus, geranium, and lavender to the area, 2 to 4 times daily. Recommended dilution: 5%–10%.

## SCARLET FEVER (SCARLATINA)

Oral—Take 1 capsule filled with 1 drops each of cinnamon, peppermint, thyme, lemon, eucalyptus, and tea tree oil, 2 to 3 times daily.

Topical—Dilute appropriately, and apply 1 to 2 drops each of marjoram, peppermint, eucalyptus, frankincense, and lavender to painful joints, 1 to 3 times daily. Dilute and apply 1 drop each of bergamot, lavender, and ylang ylang over the heart area, 1 to 2 times daily. Dilute and apply 1 drop each of geranium, vetiver, frankincense, and copaiba to the spine, 1 to 2 times daily. Recommended dilution: 5%–10%.

## SCARRING (SCARS)

Topical—Dilute appropriately, and apply 1 to 2 drops of frankincense, lavender, geranium, and helichrysum on and widely around the scar, 2 to 3 times daily until improved. Recommended dilution: 3%–10%.

## SCHIZOPHRENIA

*Only use this protocol in conjunction with Western medical options and with approval from a physician.*

Topical—Apply 1 to 2 drops each of vetiver, frankincense, and lavender behind the ears and on the crown of the head, and then apply the excess to the top of the big toes, 2 to 4 times daily. Recommended dilution: 3%–5%.

## SCIATICA

Topical—Dilute appropriately, and apply 1 to 3 drops of frankincense, helichrysum, lemongrass, geranium, and balsam fir on sciatic joint and down leg, 2 to 3 times daily. Recommended dilution: 10%–25%.

Oral—Take a capsule filled with 2 drops each of copaiba, balsam fir, lemongrass, and frankincense, 1 to 3 times daily.

## SCLERITIS (EPISCLERITIS)

Topical—Mix 2 drops each of basil, frankincense, German chamomile, lavender, copaiba, and helichrysum in 1.5 to 2 teaspoons of carrier oil (preferable grapeseed) and apply a couple of drops of this mixture widely around the eye and behind the ears, several times daily.

Oral—Take a capsule filled with 3 drops copaiba, and 2 drops each of frankincense and cypress, 1 to 3 times daily.

## SCLERODERMA

Topical—Dilute appropriately, and apply 1 drop each of frankincense, rosemary, lemongrass, myrrh, and German chamomile to affected area, 2 to 4 times daily. Recommended dilution: 3%–5%.

Oral—Take a capsule filled with 2 drops each of copaiba, frankincense, and ginger, 1 to 3 times daily.

## SCOLIOSIS

Topical—Perform the Waterfall Technique®, once or twice weekly.

## SEIZURES

Topical—Dilute appropriately, and apply 1 to 2 drops each of frankincense, vetiver, sandalwood, and copaiba to the scalp, 3 times daily. Recommended dilution: 1%–3%.

Oral—Take a capsule filled with 1 drop each of lavender, copaiba, and myrrh, 1 to 3 times daily.

## SENSORY PROCESSING DISORDER

Topical—Dilute appropriately, and apply 1 to 2 drops each of frankincense, myrtle, vetiver, and sandalwood to the forehead and behind the ears, 1 to 3 times daily. Apply 1 to 3 drops of spruce to both sides of the neck, 1 to 3 times daily. Recommended dilution: 3%–5%.

## SHINGLES

Topical—Dilute appropriately, and apply 1 to 2 drops each of clove, eucalyptus, lemon, peppermint, and tea tree

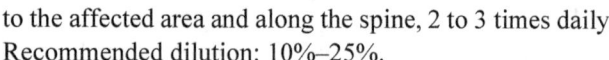

to the affected area and along the spine, 2 to 3 times daily. Recommended dilution: 10%–25%.

Oral—Take a capsule with 4 drops of peppermint, 3 times daily.

## SHIN SPLINTS

Topical—Dilute appropriately, and apply 1 to 2 drops each of balsam fir, copaiba, lemongrass, peppermint, and wintergreen on both shins, 2 to 3 times daily. Recommended dilution: 10%–25%.

Oral—Take a capsule filled with 2 drops each of balsam fir, copaiba, and frankincense, 1 to 3 times daily.

## SHOCK, EMOTIONAL

Inhalation—Apply 1 to 2 drops of lavender or peppermint in palms and place near nose to inhale.

Topical—Place 1 drop of peppermint directly on the sternum. Recommended dilution: 10%–25%.

## SINUS HEADACHE

Topical—Dilute appropriately, and apply 1 to 2 drops rosemary and peppermint over the sinuses and on the temples. Recommended dilution: 5%–10%.

Inhalation—Apply 2 to 3 drops of eucalyptus, rosemary, or peppermint to your hands, rub together, and inhale, several times daily.

## SINUSITIS (SINUS INFECTION)

Topical—Dilute appropriately, and apply 1 to 3 drops of tea tree, eucalyptus, pine, and/or peppermint on forehead, nose, cheeks, chest, and upper back, 3 to 5 times daily. Recommended dilution: 3%–5%.

Oral—Take a capsule filled with 1 to 2 drops each of eucalyptus, pine, myrtle, and lemon 1 to 2 times daily; and take 1 drop of lavender on or under the tongue, 1 to 3 times daily.

Inhalation—Apply 1 to 2 drops of peppermint, eucalyptus, or tea tree in palms and cup over nose and mouth to inhale as often as needed. Add 1 to 2 drops of peppermint, eucalyptus, and tea tree to hot water and breathe deeply through your nose over the mixture. Hold your breath as long as you can and then exhale through your mouth. Repeat this for a few minutes.

## SJOGREN'S SYNDROME

Oral—Take a capsule filled with 2 drops each of frankincense, vetiver, and copaiba and fill the rest of the capsule with evening primrose oil and take this 2 to 4 times daily.

Topical—Dilute appropriately, and apply 1 drop of lavender diluted widely around each eye, 1 to 3 times daily for eye discomfort. Recommended dilution: 1%–3%.

Inhalation—To manage stress, add 1 to 2 drops each of lavender, ylang ylang, and orange to a tissue or cotton ball and inhale as necessary throughout the day.

Other—Chew sugar-free chewing gum to keep the mouth moist.

## SKEETER SYNDROME

Topical—Dilute appropriately, and apply repeated doses of 1 drop each of tea tree, melissa, and basil to affected area until irritation subsides, and then continue applying 1 drop every 2 hours for the next 8 hours. Recommended dilution: 25%–50%.

## SKIN TAG

Topical—Dilute appropriately, and apply 1 drop of oregano, lemon, or frankincense to the skin tag, 2 to 4 times daily until it falls off. Recommended dilution: 3%–5%.

## SKIN ULCER

Topical—Dilute appropriately, and apply 2 to 3 drops of lavender, helichrysum, myrrh, or German chamomile to affected area, 1 to 3 times daily. Recommended dilution: 5%–10%.

## SMALL INTESTINAL BACTERIAL OVERGROWTH (SIBO)

Oral—Take a capsule filled with 2 drops each of peppermint, lemongrass, thyme, and orange, 1 to 3 times daily.

Other—Take a high-potency probiotic, 4 times daily.

## SMELL, LOSS OF SENSE OF (ANOSMIA)

Inhalation—Smell the following oils for at least 15 seconds, twice daily:

Weeks 1-4: Smell geranium, eucalyptus, lemongrass, and clove for 15-20 seconds, twice daily.

Weeks 5-8: Smell fennel, cinnamon, thyme, and lemon for 15-20 seconds, twice daily.

Weeks 9-12: Smell geranium, eucalyptus, lemongrass, and clove for 15-20 seconds, twice daily.

Weeks 13-16: Smell fennel, cinnamon, thyme, and lemon for 15-20 seconds, twice daily.

Weeks 17-20: Smell geranium, eucalyptus, lemongrass, and clove for 15-20 seconds, twice daily.

Weeks 21-24: Smell fennel, cinnamon, thyme, and lemon for 15-20 seconds, twice daily.

Weeks 25-28: Smell geranium, eucalyptus, lemongrass, and clove for 15-20 seconds, twice daily.

Weeks 29-32: Smell fennel, cinnamon, thyme, and lemon for 15-20 seconds, twice daily.

## SMOKING CESSATION

Oral—Lick a trace amount of black pepper off the back of your hand any time you are tempted to smoke.

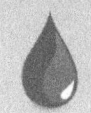

Inhalation—Apply 1 drop of black pepper, lavender, cinnamon, or grapefruit to the palms, cup over nose and mouth, and inhale as needed.

Other—Use quit smoking sticks (see *ADDICTIONS*).

## SNAKE BITE

*If the bite was from a poisonous snake seek medical attention immediately.*

Topical—Dilute appropriately, and apply 1 to 2 drops of clove, eucalyptus, or tea tree to the bite every 15 minutes until medical attention is available.

Oral—Take a capsule filled with 4 drops each of helichrysum, copaiba, and juniper every 2 hours.

## SORE THROAT

Other—Gargle with 1 drop each of lemon, peppermint, tea tree, eucalyptus, and clove every 1 to 3 hours (mix with honey for better results). This can be added to a mouthwash or a water, honey, and lemon juice mixture.

Oral—Take a capsule with 2 drops each of peppermint and lemon, and 1 drop of eucalyptus, thyme, and tea tree, 2 times daily for the next 3 to 4 days.

Topical—Dilute appropriately, and apply 1 to 3 drops of frankincense, tea tree, and/or eucalyptus over the throat area of the neck and cover with a warm wet towel, 2 times daily. Recommended dilution: 3%–5%.

## SPASMODIC DYSPHONIA

Topical—Dilute appropriately, and apply a mixture of 1 drop each of myrrh, copaiba, spruce, vetiver, rosemary, and tea tree to the throat, 3 to 5 times daily. Recommended dilution: 3%–5%.

Oral—Add 1 drop each of lemon and copaiba to a mixture of water, honey, and lemon juice and swallow, twice daily.

## SPRAINS

Topical—Dilute appropriately, and gently apply 1 to 2 drops each of copaiba, basil, wintergreen, lemongrass, and balsam fir into the affected area, up to 5 times daily. Recommended dilution: 10%–25%.

Other—Apply a cold compress, 2 times daily.

## STAPH INFECTION

Topical—Dilute appropriately, and apply 1 to 3 drops each of oregano, thyme, and eucalyptus to affected area, 3 to 5 times daily. Recommended dilution: 3%–5%.

Inhalation—Place 1 to 2 drops each of eucalyptus, tea tree, and juniper in 3 inches of hot water not too hot to touch with your hand, and cover head with towel to inhale every 2 to 4 hours.

Oral—Take 1 capsule filled with 1 drop each of clove, oregano, lemon, cinnamon, eucalyptus, 2 to 3 times daily.

## STOMACH FLU

See *GASTROENTERITIS*

## STOMACHACHE

Topical—Dilute appropriately, and apply 1 drop each of peppermint, ginger, fennel, and juniper to abdomen until stomachache subsides. Recommended dilution: 5%–10%.

Oral—Take a capsule with 1 drop each of juniper, peppermint, fennel, lemon, and ginger every two hours, or until stomachache subsides.

## STREP THROAT

Oral—Take a capsule filled with 1 drops each of clove, oregano, lemon, cinnamon, tea tree, and eucalyptus, 3 to 4 times daily.

Other—Gargle with 1 to 2 drops each of lemon, peppermint, and lavender every 1 to 3 hours (mix with honey and lemon for better results).

## STRESS

Topical—Dilute appropriately, and apply 1 to 2 drops each of cedarwood, lavender, and chamomile to the chest, 1 to 3 times daily. Recommended dilution: 5%–10%.

Inhalation—Apply 1 drop each of lavender, cedarwood, and lime to the palms and cup over nose and mouth to inhale, 2 to 4 times daily.

## STROKE

*Seek medical attention immediately.*

Topical—Dilute appropriately, and apply 1 to 2 drops each of frankincense, cypress, helichrysum, geranium, and lavender to the temples, forehead, back of the neck, and throat, 2 to 4 times daily. Recommended dilution: 5%–10%. Perform the Waterfall Technique®, once or twice weekly, during recovery.

Oral—Take a capsule filled with 1 drop each of frankincense, cypress, helichrysum, and lavender, 1 to 3 times daily, or place 1 drop each of frankincense and lavender on the tongue.

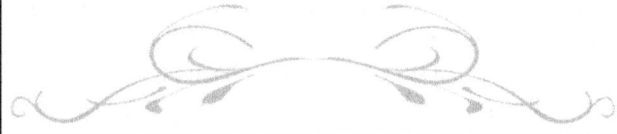

*"I used the protocol for a developing sty in my eye, and in two days the sty was absolutely gone."*

Megan L.

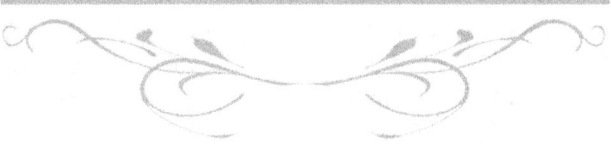

## STY (STYE)

Topical—Apply 1 drop of lavender and frankincense on each palm and rub together, cup palms over eyes with eye open, and allow essential oils to evaporate for 1 minute, 2 to 4 times daily. Apply 1 drop of lavender widely around the eye (following the orbit) diluted to about 1%. Note: Some report good success by placing a drop of lavender on a Q-tip and then swabbing the sty with the Q-tip, though this is not recommended as oils may get in the eye. Other—Apply a warm compress over the eye, several times daily.

## SUN FUNGUS (TINEA VERSICOLOR)

Topical—Dilute appropriately, and apply 1 to 2 drops each of rosemary, tea tree, frankincense, and lavender to the area two to four times daily. Recommended dilution: 5%–10%.

## SUNBURN

Topical—Apply a combination of lavender, tea tree, and peppermint to the affected area and then cover with aloe vera gel or oil as often as needed.

## SUNSCREEN

Topical—Mix together 4 drops each of myrrh, helichrysum, peppermint, and lavender, and 2 drops sandalwood in 2 ounces of zinc oxide cream, sesame seed oil, or coconut oil and apply generously (reapply every 2 to 4 hours). Will not protect as well as a zinc oxide-based sunscreen.

## SWEATING, EXCESS

Topical—Dilute appropriately, and apply 1 to 2 drops of tea tree or rosemary under each arm, 1 to 3 times daily. Recommended dilution: 1%–3%.

## SWIMMER'S EAR (OTITIS EXTERNA)

Topical—Dilute appropriately, and apply 1 drop each of tea tree, basil, and thyme around the ear and on the fleshy part of the ear. Recommended dilution: 3%–5%.
Other—Place 1 drop of tea tree or basil on a cotton ball with 5 drops of carrier oil and place the cotton ball in the ear. Replace every 30 to 60 minutes for the first 4 hours and then every 4 hours thereafter.

## TACHYCARDIA

Topical—Dilute appropriately, and apply 1 to 2 drops of ylang ylang, lavender, and rosemary over the heart, 2 to 4 times daily. Recommended dilution: 3%–5%.
Inhalation—Apply 1 drop each of lavender, cedarwood, and German chamomile to the palms, rub together, and inhale as often as needed.

## TACTILE ALLODYNIA

Oral—Take 1 drop each of bergamot, copaiba, German chamomile, lavender, basil (linalool CT), and lemongrass in a capsule morning and evening.
Topical—Dilute appropriately, and massage 2 drops of orange and 1 drop each of lemongrass, geranium, and vetiver into each foot before retiring to bed. Recommended dilution: 3%–5%.

## TARLOV CYSTS

Topical—Dilute appropriately, and apply 1 drop each of frankincense, basil, sandalwood, vetiver, and lemongrass to the affected area, 1 to 3 times daily. Recommended dilution: 5%–10%.
Oral—Take a capsule filled with 2 drops each of frankincense, orange, and lemongrass, 1 to 3 times daily.

## TEETH, SENSITIVE

Topical—Dilute appropriately, and apply 1 drop of myrrh, clove, or copaiba to the teeth and gums experiencing sensitivity, 1 to 3 times daily. Recommended dilution: 50%–neat.
Other—Consider a sensitive toothpaste with ingredients like L-arginine, hydroxyapatite, and aloe.

## TENDINITIS (TENDONITIS)

Topical—Dilute appropriately, and apply 1 to 2 drops each of lemongrass, marjoram, basil, copaiba, and wintergreen to the affected area, 2 to 3 times daily. Recommended dilution: 10%–25%.

## TETANUS (LOCKJAW)

*Only use this protocol in conjunction with Western medical options and with approval from a physician.*
Topical—To prevent tetanus, thoroughly cleanse all wounds and then apply 1 drop each of tea tree, eucalyptus, and geraniu to the wound before covering with a bandage. Replace bandage and reapply oils, 3 times daily. Recommended dilution: 5%–15%.
Oral—Take 1 capsule filled with 1 drop each of clove, cinnamon, tea tree, oregano, and rosemary, 3 times daily.

## THERMAL ALLODYNIA

Oral—Take 1 drop each of bergamot, copaiba, German chamomile, lavender, basil (linalool CT), and lemongrass in a capsule morning and evening.
Topical—Dilute appropriately, and apply massage 1 drop each of orange, rosemary, lemongrass, geranium, and vetiver into each foot before retiring to bed. Recommended dilution: 3%–5%.

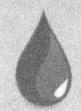

**THRUSH, ORAL (Oral Candidiasis)**
Oral—Gargle with 1 drop each of clove, cinnamon, copaiba, and lemon in 4 ounces of salt water, several times daily. Add half teaspoon of salt to a glass and drop oils on the salt before adding water.

**THRUSH, VAGINAL (Vaginal Candidiasis)** Retention—Mix two tablespoons of carrier oil with 1 drop each of geranium, eucalyptus, and frankincnese, place on tampon, and insert in vagina; replace every 2 to 4 hours. Oral—Take a capsule filled with 2 drops each of clove, cinnamon, lemon, and geranium, 2 to 4 times daily.

**THYROID NODULES**
Topical—Dilute appropriately, and apply 1 drop each of frankincense, balsam fir, myrtle, German chamomile, and nutmeg over the thyroid area of the neck, morning and evening. Recommended dilution: 3%–5%.
Oral—Take a capsule filled with 2 drops of frankincense, and 1 drop each of orange, lemon, grapefruit, and clove, 1 to 3 times daily.

**TICK BITES**
Other—Remove the tick with fine-tipped tweezers by grasping the tick as close to the skin as possible and pulling upward with even, steady pressure. Do not twist or jerk, which may leave the head of the tick in the body. Essential oils should not be used to cause the tick to back out as doing so may cause it to regurgitate its stomach contents (including bacteria) into the person.
Topical—Apply 1 drop of geranium, thyme, lavender, and melissa to tick bite every 15 minutes for the first hour, and then hourly for the next 4 to 8 hours. Recommended dilution: 5%–10%.

**TICK REPELLENT**
Topical—Mix together 12 drops each of geranium, rosemary, marjoram, and lavender with half a cup of distilled water, one-third cup witch hazel extract, and 1 teaspoon of vegetable glycerin. Shake well and apply to exposed skin and clothes before going outdoors.

**TINNITUS**
Topical—Dilute appropriately, and apply a 1 drop each of basil, helichrysum, geranium, and lavender on temples, forehead, back of neck, around the ear, and on the fleshy part of the ear, and then pull earlobe in a circular motion 10 times to enhance absorption, 3 times daily. Recommended dilution: 1%–5%.
Other—Apply 1 to 2 drops of helichrysum with 5 drops of carrier oil on a cotton ball and leave in overnight.

**TMJ (TEMPOROMANDIBULAR JOINT SYNDROME)**
Topical—Dilute appropriately, and massage 1 drop each of wintergreen, peppermint, balsam fir, and spruce to both jaws, 2 to 4 times daily. Recommended dilution: 5%–15%.
Inhalation—Inhale 2-4 drops of lavender for 30 minutes each day.

**TOENAIL FUNGUS**
Topical—Soak foot in Epsom salts (use coarse sea salt for diabetics) bath by adding 1 drop each of geranium, lavender, melissa, and tea tree to a handful of salts and adding to warm water. After soak, apply 1 drop each of oregano, lemongrass, myrrh, and tea tree. Once cleared up, apply 1 drop each of grapefruit and lavender, 3 times daily to stimulate repair and growth of toenail. Recommended dilution: 10%–50%.

**TONSILLITIS**
Oral—Take a capsule filled with 1 drop each of cinnamon, lemongrass, oregano, and eucalyptus, 1 to 3 times daily. Other—Gargle with 1 drop each of lemon, cinnamon, eucalyptus, and clove every 1 to 3 hours (mix with honey for better results).

**TOOTHACHE**
*See a dentist to determine the cause and have the necessary dental work completed.*
Topical—Apply 1 to 2 drops of clove, copaiba, and/or peppermint to the gums and tooth. Recommended dilution: 50%–neat.

**TOURETTE'S SYNDROME**
Topical—Dilute appropriately, and apply 1 to 2 drops of vetiver, frankincense, cedarwood, and spruce behind the ears and at the base of the skull, 1 to 3 times daily. Recommended dilution: 3%–5%.
Oral—Take a capsule filled with 1 drop each of rosemary, basil (linalool CT), black pepper, clove, and frankincense, 2 to 4 times daily.
Inhalation—Add 1 drop each of black pepper, clary sage, and eucalyptus to a tissue or cotton ball and inhale from several times throughought the day (refersh the oils at least once during the day).

**TOXOPLASMOSIS**
Oral—Take a capsule filled with 1 drop each of geranium, lemongrass, oregano, melissa, and marjoram, 1 to 3 times daily.

**TRAUMA RECOVERY**
Topical—Dilute appropriately, and apply 1 drop each of spruce, frankincense, and German chamomile to the

breastbone up to 3 times daily. Recommended dilution: 3%–5%.

Inhalation—Place 1 drop each of spruce, frankincense, and German chamomile on a tissue and inhale as needed.

## TUBERCULOSIS

Inhalation—Place 2 drops each of peppermint, eucalyptus, and myrtle in 3 inches of hot water that is not too hot to touch with your hand and cover head with towel to inhale for 10 minutes, 2 to 3 times daily.

Oral—Take a capsule filled with 1 drop each of myrtle, vetiver, ginger, thyme, geranium, and peppermint, 2 to 3 times daily.

Topical—Dilute appropriately, and apply 1 to 2 drops of eucalyptus, myrtle, and rosemary to chest and upper back, 2 to 3 times daily. Recommended dilution: 5%–10%.

## TYPHOID FEVER

*Only use this protocol in conjunction with Western medical options and with approval from a physician.*

Topical—Dilute appropriately, and apply 1 to 2 drops of basil and/or peppermint to the lower abdomen and along the spine, 2 to 4 times daily. Recommended dilution: 5%–10%.

Oral—Take a capsule filled with 2 drops of thyme, and 1 drop each of oregano, clove, and cinnamon, 1 to 3 times daily.

## ULCERS, DUODENAL/GASTRIC (Peptic Ulcer)

Topical—Dilute appropriately, and apply 1 to 2 drops of frankincense, German chamomile, or lavender to the stomach area, 3 to 5 times daily.

Oral—Take a capsule filled with 2 drops of orange, and 1 drop each of thyme, geranium, spearmint, and lemongrass, 1 to 3 times daily.

Other—Consider taking DGL (deglycyrrhizinated licorice) tablets. Peptic ulcers are frequently caused by *H. pylori* infection. Follow the *H. pylori* protocol after healing the ulcer.

## URINARY RETENTION

Other—Place 3 to 4 drops of peppermint in the toilet or other urine collecting water before sitting over water to urinate.

Oral—Drink 2 drops of juniper oil in a beverage (possibly cranberry juice), 1 to 3 times daily until urine is released.

Topical—Dilute appropriately, and apply 1 to 2 drops of juniper over the pelvic area, 1 to 3 times daily. Recommended dilution: 3%–5%.

## URINARY TRACT INFECTION (UTI)

*Only use this protocol in conjunction with Western medical options and with approval from a physician.*

*Bacteria can travel up the ureters and infect the kidneys, which may cause kidney damage.*

Oral—Take 1 capsule filled with 1 drops each of clove, oregano, marjoram, cinnamon, and rosemary every 20 minutes for 1 hour, and then 3 to 6 times daily thereafter.

Topical—Dilute appropriately, and apply 1 drop each of marjoram, rosemary, and juniper, to the pelvic area, 1 to 3 times daily. Recommended dilution: 3%–5%.

Other—Drink two 8-ounce glasses of unsweetened cranberry or blueberry juice daily for 3 to 5 days.

## UTERINE FIBROIDS

Topical—Dilute appropriately, and apply 1 to 2 drops each of frankincense, lavender, and geranium on the lower abdomen and back, 2 to 4 times daily; place a warm, wet towel over the back after application. Recommended dilution: 5%–10%.

Oral—Take a capsule filled with 2 drops of frankincense and 1 drop each of lavender, copaiba, orange, and geranium, 1 to 3 times daily. Alternately, take a capsule filled with 2 drops each of frankincense, orange, and sandalwood, 1 to 3 times daily.

Retention—Mix 2 drops each of frankincense, sandalwood, copaiba, and cypress with 1 tablespoon of carrier oil, apply mixture to tampon, and retain overnight.

## VARICOCELES

Topical—Mix 2 drops each of copaiba, frankincense, and cypress with 1 drop of German chamomile in 1 tablespoon of carrier oil and apply daily to the scrotum.

## VAGINAL ATROPHY (ATROPHIC VAGINITIS)

Topical—Dilute appropriately, and apply 1 to 2 drops of clary sage on the mons pubis area, 1 to 3 times daily. Recommended dilution: 3%–5%. Apply 1 to 2 drops each of lavender, copaiba, and geranium, diluted in 2 teaspoons of carrier oil, to the labia and around the entrance to the vagina, 1 or 2 times daily.

Other: Consider a natural bioidentical progesterone or molecular progesterone complex.

## VAGINAL YEAST INFECTION

Retention—Mix 2 drops each of rosemary, tea tree, thyme, and marjoram with 1 tablespoon of carrier oil, put on tampon, and insert into vagina, replacing every 4 hours.

Oral—Take a capsule filled with 1 drop each of lemongrass, oregano, and rosemary, and thyme, 1 to 3 times daily.

## VAGINITIS

Retention—Mix 2 drops each of rosemary, tea tree, thyme, and marjoram with 1 tablespoon of carrier oil, put on tampon, and insert into vagina, replacing every 4 hours.

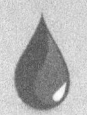

Oral—Take a capsule filled with 1 drop each of cinnamon, oregano, vetiver, and thyme, morning and evening.

## VARICOSE VEINS

Topical—Apply 2 to 3 drops each of lemongrass, geranium, and cypress mixed in some grapeseed carrier oil to the areas around the varicose veins (not directly on them) with massage strokes toward the direction of the heart, 1 to 3 times daily. Recommended dilution: 3%–5%.

## VENOUS REFLUX DISEASE

Topical—Dilute appropriately, and apply 2 drops each of cypress, lemongrass, and helichrysum, and 1 drop of peppermint to both legs, 1 to 3 times daily. Recommended dilution: 3%–5%..

## VERTIGO

Topical—Dilute appropriately, and apply 1 drop each of ginger, frankincense, and cypress behind the ears and to the temples. Recommended dilution: 3%–5%.

Oral—Take a capsule with 2 drops of ginger, and 1 drop each of lemon, cypress, and frankincense up to 3 times daily.

Inhalation—Place 1 drop each of peppermint, ginger, and cypress in 1 palm, rub together with other palm, and cup hands over mouth and nose to inhale as often as necessary.

Other—Apply 1 drop of helichrysum on a cotton ball with 5 to 10 drops of carrier oil and place cotton ball in ear overnight; repeat for both ears.

## VIRAL MENINGITIS

*Only use this protocol in conjunction with Western medical options and with approval from a physician. Viral meinigitis can be fatal if left untreated.*

Topical—Dilute appropriately, and apply a mixture of 1 to 2 drops each of marjoram, lemongrass, tea tree, melissa, and thyme to the spine, 3 to 5 times daily. Apply 1 to 3 drops of lemon or peppermint to the spine, 2 to 4 times daily for fever. Apply 1 to 2 drops each of lavender and marjoram to the neck and forehead for neck pain or headache. Recommended dilution: 5%–10%.

Inhalation—For nausea or vomiting, apply 1 drop each of lemon and ginger to your palms, rub together, and cup over your nose and mouth to inhale as needed.

Oral—Take a capsule filled with 1 drop each of oregano, melissa, lemongrass, and cinnamon, thyme, and tea tree, 2 to 4 times daily.

## VITILIGO

Topical—Create a mixture of 2 drops geranium and 1 drop bergamot in 2 teaspoons of hazelnut oil and apply enough of this mixture to cover the affected area 1 to 3 times daily. Add 5 drops of black cumin to the formula if available.

Oral—Take 2 drops each of lemongrass and copaiba and 1 drop of lavender in a capsule, 1 to 3 times daily.

## VOMITING

Inhalation—Apply 1 drop each of peppermint, lemon, and ginger to a cotton ball and inhale as needed.

Topical—Dilute appropriately, and apply 1 drop each of peppermint, lemon, and ginger to the stomach area as needed. Recommended dilution: 5%–10%.

## WARTS

Topical—Apply 1 drop of oregano, thyme, or frankincense to warts, 3 times daily, being careful to avoid contact with surrounding skin. Recommended dilution: 25%–50%.

## WARTS (SEED)

Other—Apply small squares of duct tape over seed warts and replace each time the duct tape falls off until wart is gone.

Topical—Apply 1 drop of oregano, thyme, or frankincense to seed warts, 3 times daily (do not apply duct tape over oils). Recommended dilution: 3%–5%.

## WEIGHT MANAGEMENT

Oral—Take a capsule filled with 3 drops of grapefruit, and 1 drop each of orange and lemongrass, 2 to 3 times daily.

Other—Decrease caloric intake, increase caloric expenditure, and manage stress.

## WEST NILE VIRUS

*Only use this protocol in conjunction with Western medical options and with approval from a physician.*

Oral—Take a capsule filled with 1 drop each of oregano, lemongrass, frankincense, peppermint, thyme, tea tree, and eucalyptus, 2 to 3 times daily.

Topical—Perform the Waterfall Technique®, once or twice weekly.

## WHOOPING COUGH (PERTUSSIS)

Inhalation—Place 1 to 2 drops each of rosemary or pine, eucalyptus, and/or myrtle in 3 inches of hot water that is not too hot to touch with your hand and cover head with towel to inhale every 2 to 4 hours.

Topical—Dilute appropriately, and apply 1 drop each of thyme, cypress, eucalyptus, and myrtle to the chest and cover with a warm compress, 1 to 3 times daily. Recommended dilution: 3%–5%.

## WOLFF-PARKINSON-WHITE SYNDROME

Topical—Apply 1 to 2 drops of ylang ylang, lavender, and/or rosemary on the chest morning and night. Apply 1 drop each of eucalyptus, myrtle, and peppermint to the upper back if shortness of breath occurs. Recommended dilution: 5%–10%.

Inhalation—Apply 1 drop each of lavender, ginger, and peppermint to your palms, rub together, and cup over nose and mouth to inhale as often as needed during dizzy spells.

## WOUNDS

Topical—Clean area thoroughly with soap and warm water. Dilute and apply 1 to 2 drops each of frankincense, copaiba, cedarwood, and lavender to the wound, several times daily to promote healing. Apply 1 to 2 drops of lemongrass, tea tree, and rosemary to disinfect and protect the wound from germs. Recommended dilution: 3%–5%.

## WRINKLES

Topical—Dilute appropriately, and apply 1 to 2 drops of frankincense, sandalwood, lavender, and/or helichrysum to wrinkles, morning and evening. Mix in avocado or apricot kernel oil to enhance the benefits. Recommended dilution: 1%–3%.

## XANTHOMAS

Topical—For those occurring in the eye, soak a piece of cloth in 1 drop of cypress, a pinch of salt, and 1 cup of tepid water; wring out excess water from cloth and apply over closed eye. For xanthomas in other locations, apply 1 drop each of lemongrass and cypress to the area, several times daily. Recommended dilution: 3%–5%.

## YELLOW FEVER

*Only use this protocol in conjunction with Western medical options and with approval from a physician.*

Oral—Take a capsule with 1 drop each of lemongrass, peppermint, oregano, lemon, basil, and thyme, 3 to 4 times daily. Continue taking capsules for 2 weeks following reversal of symptoms, but no longer than 21 days total.

Topical—Dilute appropriately, and apply 1 drop each of lemongrass, oregano, peppermint, and lemon over the liver area of the abdomen, 2 times daily. Recommended dilution: 1%–5%.

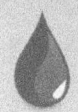

# ESSENTIAL OILS FOR INFANTS AND CHILDREN

Our children are extremely precious, and as parents, we are the first responders when it comes to their health and well-being. Children get sick, and as parents we want to do everything in our power to make them feel better. When our actions don't provide our children relief, it can be a very frustrating experience. Without the proper knowledge and the right tools, caring for children can be an intimidating undertaking. As a parent, it is your right and responsibility to determine what health care your child receives and to determine whether the condition can be safely and effectively managed at home or requires professional care. Even better, an integrative minded pediatrician or family care practitioner trained in the use of natural remedies who properly balances Western and complementary approaches can be an incredible resource for the natural parents.

Essential oils are a valuable tool for the parents who seek to raise their children using what is found in nature. Many parents prefer natural options when it comes to the care of their children, but they may feel ill equipped to employ the healing power natural remedies possess. This hesitancy or uncertainty leads to frequent trips to the pediatrician's office, often to be told that the illness is caused by a virus for which Western medicine provides very limited support. Or the illness has occurred when the doctor's office is closed and you can't get in for several hours. Indeed, many pediatricians and other doctors now outsource their after-hours operations to third-party sources that are less qualified, provide very limited support, and do not know your family and child. These can be long nights for both the parents and the child, unless the parent is prepared to handle the situation at home.

Just as adults realize remarkable results when essential oils are used correctly, essential oils can be of great benefit to infants and children. In fact, children tend to respond to natural remedies more rapidly and completely than adults. However, unintended, adverse consequences can also occur with the use of natural remedies, particularly among children who are more receptive to the profound effects of essential oils. The adage "less is more" is absolutely true with children and essential oils, and very small amounts of essential oils can provide rapid and far-reaching restoration in a child's body.

No parent wants to be responsible for being the cause of a trip to the doctor, and so a few cautions are warranted when using essential oils with children. When it comes to children and infants, it is important to use essential oils responsibly and to err on the side of caution. One need only review the scientific and medical literature—or perhaps talk to their integrative minded physician—to know that unintended reactions to essential oils do occur and are treated in doctor's offices, urgent care facilities, and hospitals.[2384] Because of this, every effort has been made to thoroughly review the available literature and incorporate practical and clinical experience to determine what constitutes the safe use of essential oils for children.

Some believe that parents are incapable of caring for the well-being of their children alone. But the reality is a parent can choose to receive directions for the care of their children from a trained physician (who will intrinsically prescribe what he or she is trained on and comfortable with—synthetic chemical options) or a reliable resource—like a book—that shares detailed instructions about how to use natural remedies effectively and safely.

However, as interest in more natural options grows among parents, so does the interest to learn how to use them safely among savvy physicians. An integrative minded physician trained in the use of essential oils and other natural products can be a huge asset to the natural parent! Ideally, you should work collaboratively and in partnership with an integrative minded physician for the care and treatment of your children.

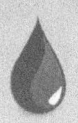 

This section is intended to provide foundational knowledge and a better understanding of the use of essential oils for the care of infants and children. As you discover the ease at which you can use essential oils for many of the common ailments your children face, your confidence will grow. You will also increase your children's acceptance and trust of natural options that they can then pass on to their children and grandchildren. This cycle may lead to healthier generations that have returned to treatment options that past generations used successfully for hundreds of years.

**Safety First!**

As was mentioned earlier in this book, some essential oils should be avoided in young children, particularly those high in 1,8-cineole (eucalyptol), menthol, thujones, camphor, and methyl salicylate (wintergreen). As a review, some common essential oils that contain these constituents include: peppermint, rosemary, eucalyptus, ravintsara, niaouli, camphor, bay laurel, Spanish sage, cardamom, and spike lavender, which should be avoided in children under 3, particularly around the nose and mouth. A very, very small minority of children may respond adversely to the use of these essential oils, including central nervous system problems,[10177,10178,10179] respiratory distress (difficulty or labored breathing), and toxicity,[10180,10181,10182,10183,10184,10185,10186] and this reaction can occur from inhalation only. Very young children, from age birth to 24 months, are more likely to experience adverse reactions because their breathing and airway defensive reflexes are still maturing. Use each of these oils very cautiously, both topically and diffused, for children under age 5, and it is best to avoid them in children under age 3. Wintergreen and birch (both high in methyl salicylate) should not be used topically under age 12, particularly during illness or fever, due to the risk of developing Reye's syndrome.[10187] Reye's syndrome is a rare but serious condition that causes swelling of the liver and brain. It most frequently affects children and teens recovering from a viral illness such as the flu or chickenpox. The use of aspirin has been linked to a higher risk of Reye's syndrome, and since wintergreen and birch are almost entirely methyl salicylate (a compound similar to aspirin) it is best to avoid their use in children under age 12, and even teens experiencing a viral illness.

Oral administration of essential oils is a parent choice—some choose to give their children essential oils orally (in a capsule, mixed with a fatty substance, etc.), while others choose not to. In some cases, oral administration may be unnecessary if topical or aromatic administration is effective.

If you choose to do so, it should generally be reserved to children who are 6 or older, and when the child has the ability to communicate how the essential oils affect the way the child feels internally after taking the oil. This will help identify any gastrointestinal upset or discomfort that they may experience as a result. The smaller the child, the greater the risk for toxicity with oral administration. Please keep in mind that not all essential oils can be taken orally because of their chemical compounds, toxicity degree, or they may be a perfume grade not suitable for oral use. Only take high-quality essential oils intended for therapeutic use orally. Oils not intended for therapeutic use could cause harm if taken internally.

Some essential oils should not be applied on the skin before exposing that skin to the UV rays of the sun. These oils include angelica, bergamot, bitter orange, citron, cumin, garlic, grapefruit, kabosu, khella, kumquat, lemon, lime, Mediterranean mandarin, neroli, petitgrain, Persian lime, rue, tagetes, and tangerine. The relative risk of these essential oils depends on the levels of furocoumarins present in the oil and the distillation method (i.e. cold-pressed/expressed citrus oils versus distilled). These oils should be applied where the skin will not be exposed to sun (where clothes will cover or the soles of the feet), or sun exposure should be avoided for a minimum of 12 hours following their application.

If your child has very sensitive skin or has allergies or a chronic skin condition, it would be best to modify the dilution ratios from teaspoons to tablespoons of carrier oil. For example, if the dilution ratio calls for 2 drops of essential oil per teaspoon, you should mix 2 drops of essential oil per tablespoon of carrier oil.

Keep essential oils away from the eyes, and never apply essential oils directly into the ear canal. Instead, apply essential oils widely around the perimeter of the eyes (usually reserved for older children) or ear, and/or add a drop on a cotton ball and place this in the ear. Essential oils applied around the perimeter of the eyes must be massaged in completely to avoid any migrating into the eye itself. To avoid confusion some herbal oil tonics like garlic and mullein are available and applied directly in the ears. Keep in mind these are herbal extracts not essential oils and that this practice is considered safe.

If your child is currently taking medication, review the essential oils you intend to use for interactions with those medications, and reduce the amount of essential oil recommend by half. It is also wise to use essential oils at least two hours following the administration of

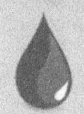

medications when possible. Keep in mind that interactions with drugs are more likely to occur with oral administration.

The preferred and recommended essential oils will vary depending on the age and weight of the child. In general, you will blend the essential oils in the carrier oil before applying them to the skin. Combining the essential oils and carrier oil in a roller bottle is convenient. However, you may also apply the essential oils to the skin first and then cover with the appropriate amount of carrier oil if desired. The following table can be used as a guide for appropriate essential oils and carrier oils as well as reasonable dilution ranges to follow when caring for your child.

| Age/Weight | Essential Oils, Carrier Oils, and Dilution Range* |
|---|---|
| Birth–12 mos. (6–22 lb.) | **Preferred Essential Oils:** Bergamot, chamomile (Roman, German), copaiba, frankincense, geranium, grapefruit, lavender, lemon, lime, tea tree, neroli, orange (sweet), petitgrain, tangerine, thyme (for specific conditions) <br><br> **Preferred Primary Carriers:** Sweet almond, sunflower seed, apricot kernel, coconut, grapeseed <br><br> **Preferred Secondary Carriers (Smaller amounts):** Olive oil (10%), jojoba (10%) <br><br> **Dilution Range:** 0.3% dilution—1 drop of essential oil per 2 teaspoons of carrier oil |
| 1–5 yrs. (23–44 lb.) | **Preferred Essential Oils:** Balsam fir, basil (linalool CT), bergamot, chamomile (Roman, German), cedarwood, cinnamon, cistus, clove, copaiba, cypress, frankincense, geranium, ginger, grapefruit, helichrysum, lavender, lemon, lime, tea tree, myrtle, neroli, orange (sweet), oregano, petitgrain, pine, rose, sandalwood, tangerine, thyme, vetiver, ylang ylang <br><br> **Preferred Primary Carriers:** Sweet almond, sunflower seed, grapeseed, apricot kernel, coconut, aloe vera <br><br> **Preferred Secondary Carriers** Olive oil (10%), jojoba (10%), avocado (10%) |
| | **Dilution Range:** 1.5%–3.0%; neat for some applications—2–4 drops of essential oil per 5 mL of carrier oil; neat applications undiluted |
| 6–11 yrs. (45–77 lb.) | **Preferred Essential Oils:** All essential oils except wintergreen and birch; caution with fennel is advised in prepubertal girls <br><br> **Preferred Primary Carriers:** Sweet almond, grapeseed, apricot kernel, coconut, sesame seed, sunflower, aloe vera <br><br> **Preferred Secondary Carriers** Olive oil (10%), jojoba (10%), avocado (10%) <br><br> **Dilution Range:** 1.5%–5.0%; neat for some applications—2–7 drops of essential oil per 5 mL of carrier oil; neat applications undiluted |
| 12–17 yrs. (78–153 lb.) | **Preferred Essential Oils:** All essential oils <br><br> **Preferred Carrier Oils:** All carrier oils except St. John's wort <br><br> **Dilution Range:** 1.5%–20.0%; neat for some applications —2–30 drops of essential oil per 5 mL of carrier oil; neat applications undiluted |
| 18+ yrs. (154+ lb.) | **Preferred Essential Oils:** All essential oils <br><br> **Preferred Carrier Oils:** All carrier oils <br><br> **Dilution Range:** 1.5%–Neat—2 drops of essential oil per 5 mL of carrier oil to undiluted |

* Unless otherwise recommended in this book or a published clinical study.

Once the appropriate mixture (blend) has been created, a small amount of this blend should be applied to the child. Preferred application sites include the area of discomfort, the soles of the feet, wrists, and abdomen. The face should generally be avoided. The mixture should be applied more regularly for an acute condition (3–6 times or more daily), and less often for a chronic condition (2–3 times daily). In addition, if a range is recommended for the particular condition, the higher number of drops should be used for acute conditions and the lower number for chronic conditions.

### Methods of Application/Use

There are a number of ways in which to administer essential oils to children. Each can provide benefits, improved well-being, restoration of health, and mood enhancement. The method of administration will differ based on what you want to accomplish, but often using more than one method simultaneously can amplify benefits and produce more rapid results.

**Aromatic Baths:**
Birth–12 mos.        1 drop EO/2 tsp. carrier oil
1–2 years 1–2 drops EO/1 tsp. carrier oil
3–4 years 2–3 drops EO/1 tsp. carrier oil
5–6 years 3–4 drops EO/1 tsp. carrier oil
7–12 years        3–5 drops EO/1 tsp. carrier oil
13–17 years        4–7 drops EO/1 tsp. carrier oil

**Aromatic Compress**:
Birth–2 years        Not recommended
2–3 years 1–2 drops EO
4–12 years        2–4 drops EO
13–17 years        2–5 drops EO

**Aromatic Foot Bath**:
Birth–2 years        Not recommended
2–5 years 1–3 drops EO/1 tsp. carrier oil
6–12 years        1–4 drops EO/1 tsp. carrier oil
13–17 years        2–5 drops EO/1 tsp. carrier oil

**Diffusion**:
Birth–12 mos.        1–2 drops EO
1–2 years 1–2 drops EO
3–4 years 2–4 drops EO
5–6 years 2–5 drops EO
7–12 years        2–6 drops EO
13–17 years        3–8 drops EO

**Gargle** (per half-cup warm water):
6–12 years        1 drop
13–17 years        1–3 drops

**Inhalation** (on cotton ball or tissue):
2–5 years 1–2 drops EO
6–12 years        1–3 drops EO
13–17 years        1–4 drops EO

**Oral** (in capsule, or with milk, honey, tea):
Birth–2 years        Not recommended
3–5 years Very limited and only
                mild oils*
6–11 years        1–3 drops/dose
                (8 drops/day max)
12–17 years        1–5 drops/dose
                (15 drops/day max)

**Pillow** (add to underside on corner):
1–5 years 1–2 drops EO
6–17 years        1–3 drops EO

**Spot Treatment** (on a cotton swab or ball):
1–5 years 1 drop EO
6–12 years        1–2 drops EO
13–17 years        1–3 drops EO

**Steam Inhalation** (in 1 pint of hot water):
Birth–12 mos.        1 drop EO
1–2 years 1–2 drops EO
3–5 years 1–3 drops EO
6–12 years        2–4 drops EO
13–17 years        2–6 drops EO

**Sublingual** (under the tongue; mild oils*):
Birth–5 years        Not recommended
6–11 years        1 drop/dose
12–17 years        1–2 drops/dose
*Mild oils may include citrus oils, lavender, copaiba, frankincense, and chamomile.

### Homeopathic Remedies

In addition to essential oils, homeopathic remedies will be recommended when appropriate. It has been my experience that homeopathic remedies work well in conjunction with essential oils, and given their extensive safety record (even in day old infants), they can be used with the smallest of children without fear of side effects or unintended consequences. Oral homeopathic remedies usually come in pellets that dissolve under the tongue or as a liquid. Homeopathics are also available as creams and ointments.

### Homeopathic Remedy Use:

■ Choose oral homeopathic remedies that are 6X, 6C, 30X, or 30C potency for home use.
■ Take homeopathic remedies with a clean mouth—rinsed and free of food. Ideally the teeth should not be brushed for one hour prior to or after taking a homeopathic remedy orally.
■ Allow the remedy to slowly dissolve under the tongue.
■ If pellets are being used for children under 2, crush them between two spoons to create a powder and administer this powder in the mouth.
■ Avoid touching the pellets if possible. Instead, pour the desired number of pellets into the bottle cap, and dump them directly into the mouth.
■ Apply homeopathic creams and ointments directly on and widely around the affected area.
■ For less serious complaints and mild illnesses, take the homeopathic remedy every 4 to 8 hours.
■ The recommended dose should be taken every 30 minutes to 2 hours for more serious acute complaints.
■ Take the remedy 1 to 2 times daily for chronic complaints.

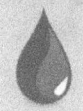

■ Reduce the frequency of the dose as symptoms improve and stop administration when significant improvement of all symptoms is experienced.

■ Be aware that homeopathic remedies may cause a temporary worsening of symptoms before relieving them. This is a good thing and an indication that the remedy is working. If this occurs, you can reduce the dosing frequency.

■ Only take the homeopathic form of the remedies mentioned because some nonhomeopathic forms of the remedies mentioned are highly toxic since they are not diluted infinitesimally.

■ For more information on the homeopathic remedies recommended, see the brief remedy profiles in Appendix B.

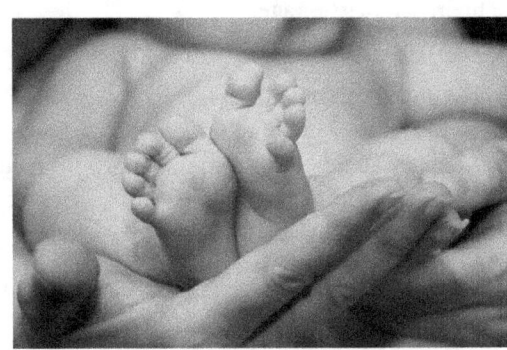

## HEALTH CONDITIONS

### ABDOMINAL MIGRAINE

Topical—Mix together 2 drops each of ginger and lemon, and 1 drop each of lavender and marjoram essential oil in 2 teaspoons of carrier oil and apply a small amount of this mixture to the lower abdomen every 15 to 30 minutes while migraine occurs (3–5 years). Mix together 2 drops each of ginger, lemon, and peppermint, and 1 drop each of lavender, spearmint, and marjoram essential oil in 2 teaspoons of carrier oil and apply a small amount of this mixture to the lower abdomen every 15 to 30 minutes while migraine occurs (6–17 years).
Oral—Take a capsule filled 1 drop each of peppermint, German chamomile, and lavender essential oil, twice daily (6–11 years). Take a capsule filled 1 drop each of peppermint, lemongrass, copaiba, German chamomile, and lavender essential oil, twice daily (12-17 years).
Inhalation—Inhale 1 drop each of bergamot, lemon, lavender, and ylang ylang as needed (all ages).

### ACNE, NEWBORN

Topical—Mix 1 drop each of lavender, orange, and chamomile in 1 pint of water. Dip a cotton ball in this mixture and wring it out, and then rub the cotton ball over the affected area. Shake mixture well before each use. Make sure to avoid areas near the eyes and mouth.

### ACNE, ADOLESCENT/TEENAGE

Topical—Mix together 1 cup of water, 1/2 pint of organic apple cider vinegar, and 2 drops each of basil, orange, and tea tree in a jar. Dip a cotton ball in the mixture and apply to the affected area, morning and evening. Shake the mixture well before each use. Tea tree may also be used neat for tough acne. Keep essential oils away from eyes.

### ANXIETY

Inhalation—Place 1 drop each of lavender, cedarwood, and bergamot on a tissue and allow the child to inhale as desired (1–17 years).
Oral—Take 2 drops of lavender orally up to 3 times daily (6–17 years).
Topical—Mix together 5 drops each of lavender, orange, and cedarwood, and then apply 1 drop of this mixture with equal parts of carrier oil to the wrists; 1 part essential oil to 5 parts carrier may be used for ages 3 to 5 (3–17 years).

### ARTHRITIS (JUVENILE RHEUMATOID)

Topical—Mix together 3 drops each of ginger, frankincense, copaiba, balsam fir, and eucalyptus in 3 teaspoons of sesame seed oil and 1 teaspoon of aloe vera oil and gently apply a small amount of this mixture to the affected joints (age 6+).

Oral—Take 1 drop each of frankincense, ginger, and copaiba orally up to 3 times daily (6–11 years). Take 2 drops each of ginger and copaiba, and 1 drop of frankincense orally up to 3 times daily (12–17 years).
Aromatic Bath—Take a warm bath with 1 drop each of German chamomile, eucalyptus, ginger, and lavender in half a cup of Epsom salts (use coarse sea salt for diabetics) as needed.

### ASTHMA

*These options can be used along with Western treatment options. An acute asthma attack (severe shortness of breath, coughing, wheezing, low peak expiratory flow) requires medical attention if it is more than a minor attack, or may require the use of a rescue inhaler if minor.*
Topical—Mix together 1 drop each of ginger, myrtle, and pine in 1 teaspoon of carrier oil and apply a small amount of this to upper back and chest (1–11 years). Mix together 2 drops each of ginger, myrtle, thyme, and pine in 1 teaspoon of carrier oil and apply a small amount of this to upper back and chest (12–17 years).
Inhalation—Place 1 drop each of frankincense and lavender on a cotton ball or tissue and have child inhale this whenever he/she feels an asthma attack coming on (1–5 years). Place 1 drop each of frankincense, pine, and balsam fir to a cotton ball or tissue and have child inhale this

whenever he/she feels an asthma attack coming on (6–17 years).

## ATHLETE'S FOOT

Aromatic Footbath—Soak foot in a foot bath with 1 drop each of tea tree and lavender in half a cup of Epsom salts (use coarse sea salt for diabetics) and 1 tablespoon of apple cider vinegar, 2 times daily (2–17 years).

Topical—Mix together 1 drop each of tea tree, lemongrass, and oregano in 1 teaspoon of carrier oil and apply a small amount to the affected area after soaking (2–5 years). Mix together 1 drop each of tea tree, lemongrass, and oregano in half a teaspoon of carrier oil and apply a small amount to the affected area after soaking (6–17 years).

## ATTENTION DEFICIT DISORDERS (ADD and ADHD)

Topical—Create a mixture of 1 to 3 (appropriate for age) drops of vetiver and frankincense in 1 teaspoon of carrier oil and apply a small amount of this mixture to the back of the neck, crown of the head, and behind the ears several times daily to increase focus (2–17 years). For a calming effect create a mixture of 1 to 3 (appropriate for age) drops of cedarwood and chamomile in 1 teaspoon of carrier oil and apply a small amount of this mixture to the back of the neck, crown of the head, and behind the ears, several times daily (2–17 years).

Oral—Take a capsule filled with 1 drop each of cedarwood, lavender, and frankincense, 2 times daily (6–11 years). Take a capsule filled with 2 drops each of cedarwood, lavender, and frankincense, 2 times daily (12–17 years).

## AUTISM

Topical—Create a mixture of 1 to 3 (appropriate for age) drops of vetiver, sandalwood, and frankincense in 1 teaspoon of carrier oil and apply a small amount of this mixture to the back of the neck, crown of the head, and behind the ears, several times daily to support healthy nervous system function. Apply 3 drops of orange oil neat to the bottoms of the feet, 3 times daily (6–11 years), dilute in 1 teaspoon of carrier oil (1–5 years) and apply a small amount of the mixture to the feet. For a calming effect create a mixture of 1 to 3 (appropriate for age) drops of cedarwood and chamomile in 1 teaspoon of carrier oil and apply a small amount of this mixture to the back of the neck, crown of the head, and behind the ears, several times daily.

Inhalation—Let the child choose one or more of the following oils and place 1 drop on a cotton ball or tissue to inhale as desired: lavender, ylang ylang, orange, or blue tansy.

## BEDWETTING

Topical—Apply 1 drop of cypress mixed in 5 drops of carrier oil to the lower abdomen prior to retiring for bed.

Homeopathic Remedies—Give the child equisetum 30C if the bedwetting is a habit. Causticum 30C could be considered if the bedwetting is brought on by fear that something bad will happen to him or her.

## BITES (ANIMAL)

*The child should be seen by a physician to rule out rabies.*

Topical—Create a mixture of 1 drop each of thyme, oregano, lavender, lemongrass, and German chamomile and apply this mixture neat to the bite every 15 minutes for the first 2 hours, and then once per hour for the next 24 to 48 hours (2–17 years). Dilute in half a teaspoon of aloe vera oil for children 1 years of age.

## BITES (INSECT)

Topical—Apply repeated doses of a mixture of 1 drop each of lavender, basil, lemongrass, and tea tree in 1 teaspoon of apple cider vinegar to the area until irritation subsides (6–17 years). Use 1 drop each of lavender, German chamomile, and tea tree in 1 teaspoon of apple cider vinegar (1–5 years). Then continue application every 2 hours for the next 8 hours.

Homeopathic Remedies—Give the child apis 6C every 15 minutes until relief is achieved.

## BLEEDING

*Seek medical attention immediately if the blood spurts from the wound or if the wound is in the chest or or abdomen.*

Topical—Apply 1 drop of lavender, cypress, or helichrysum neat near the bleed, and repeat every 5 minutes until bleeding stops (2–17 years). Dilute in 2 teaspoons of carrier oil for children birth to 12 months.

## BLISTERS

Topical—Create a mixture of 1 drop each of lemon, lavender, and tea tree in 5 teaspoons of carrier oil and apply a small amount of this mixture to the blister, several times daily (birth–12 months). Create a mixture of 1 drop each of tea tree, clove, and chamomile in 1 teaspoon of carrier oil and apply to the blister, several times daily (2–17 years).

## BOILS

Topical—Create a mixture of 1 drop each of lavender, tea tree, and frankincense (or chamomile) in 1 teaspoon of carrier oil and apply a small amount of the mixture to the boil, several times daily (1–17 years). Place 1 drop of tea tree on a bandage and apply to the boil for additional relief and healing.

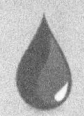

## BONES (BROKEN, FRACTURED)

*Broken bones require more than essential oils. Seek medical attention to have the bone set and casted. This protocol is to help relieve pain and encourage normal healing. It should be followed for the duration that the cast is on, applying oils for 3 weeks before resting 1 week, then repeating the application.*

Topical—Create a mixture of 1 drop each of balsam fir, cypress, ginger, and helichrysum in 1 teaspoon of sesame seed carrier oil and apply a small amount of this mixture to the exposed skin around the cast, several times daily (1–5 years). Create a mixture of 2 drops each of balsam fir, cypress, ginger, lemongrass, and helichrysum in 1 teaspoon of sesame seed carrier oil and apply a small amount of this mixture to the exposed skin around the cast, several times daily (6–17 years).

## BRONCHITIS, BRONCHIOLITIS

*Seek medical attention if your child is experiencing shortness of breath or labored breathing.*

Steam Inhalation—Place a bowl of hot water with 1 drop each of copaiba and frankincense next to, but out of reach of, the infant (birth–12 months) up to 3 times daily. Place a bowl of hot water with 2 drops each of myrtle and copaiba, and 1 drop of frankincense next to, but out of reach of, the child (1–5 years) up to 3 times daily. Place a bowl of hot water with 2 drops each of eucalyptus, myrtle, copaiba, and thyme next to the child up to 3 times daily (6–17 years).

Topical—Create a mixture of 1 drop each of lemon and frankincense in 2 teaspoons of carrier oil and apply a small amount of this mixture to the chest and upper back, 3 to 5 times daily (birth–12 months). Create a mixture of 1 drop each of myrtle, ginger, pine, and thyme in 1 teaspoon of carrier oil and apply a small amount of this mixture to the chest and upper back, 3 to 5 times daily (1–5 years). Create a mixture of 1 to 2 drops each of eucalyptus, myrtle, peppermint, ginger, pine, and thyme in 1 teaspoon of carrier oil and apply a small amount of this mixture to the chest and upper back, 3 to 5 times daily (6–17 years).

Oral—Take 1 drop each of oregano, cinnamon, and lemon orally up to 3 times daily (6–11 years). Take 1 drop each of oregano, tea tree, thyme, lemon, and cinnamon up to 3 times daily (12–17 years).

## BRUISE

Topical—Mix together 1 drop of lavender in 2 teaspoons of carrier oil and apply enough of the mixture to cover the affected area and surrounding area, several times daily (birth–12 months). Mix together 1 drop each of helichrysum, lavender, and frankincense in 1 teaspoon of carrier oil and apply enough of this mixture to the affected area and surrounding area, several times daily (1–5 years). Mix together 1 drop each of helichrysum, lavender, and frankincense in equal parts of carrier oil and apply enough of this mixture to the affected area and surrounding area, several times daily (6–17).

Homeopathic Remedies—Arnica cream can be applied over the essential oils (not to be applied over broken skin).

## BURNS

Other—First cool the area with cold water (not ice) for several minutes. If the burn covers a large area of the body, is on the hands, feet, face, or genitals, seek medical attention as soon as possible.

Topical—Mix together 1 drop of lavender in 2 teaspoons of aloe vera gel and apply to the affected area, several times daily, and keep the area covered with a cool, damp gauze pad (birth–12 months). Apply 1 to 5 drops of lavender and/or German chamomile (enough to cover the area) neat (or with equal parts aloe vera) to the affected area, and then soak a gauze pad in half a pint of cold water with 5 drops of lavender, wring out, and apply to the affected area (1 to 17 years). Change the dressing every hour.

## CANKER SORES

Topical—Mix together 1 drop of lavender, lemon, or tea tree in 1 teaspoon of carrier oil and apply 1 drop of this mixture to the affected area, several times daily (1–5 years). Mix together 1 drop of lavender, lemon, or tea tree in half a teaspoon of carrier oil and apply 1 drop of this mixture to the affected area, several times daily (6–11 years). Apply 1 drop of lavender, lemon, or tea tree neat to the affected area up to four times daily (12–17 years). Rotating the oils used will improve effectiveness.

## CHICKEN POX

Aromatic Bath—Place 1 cup of raw oats in some muslin (or similar cloth) and add 3 drops each of German chamomile, tea tree, and lavender to the oats. Tie the material off or place a rubber band around the top to close securely and run a bath with this mixture under the stream of water. Place the mixture inside the material in the bath and then add 1 drop of each oil in half a cup of baking soda to the bath. Allow the child to soak for several minutes (2–17 years). Use 1 drop of each oil in the oatmeal mixture for infants (birth and up to age 2).

Topical—Mix together 1 drop each of lavender and German chamomile in 3 teaspoons of carrier oil and apply small amounts of this mixture to the spots up to 3 times daily (birth–12 months). Mix together 2 drops each of German chamomile, tea tree, and lavender in 1 teaspoon of carrier oil and apply small amounts of this mixture to the spots, several times daily (1–5 years). Mix together 5 drops each of German chamomile, tea tree, and lavender in equal parts carrier oil and apply small amounts of this mixture to the spots, several times daily (6–17 years).

Oral—Take 1 drop each of lemongrass, oregano, and lemon orally, 3 times daily (6–11 years). Take 2 drops each of oregano and lemon, and 1 drop of lemongrass orally, 3 times daily (12–17 years).

Homeopathic Remedies—Give the child Rhus tox 30C 3 times daily, reducing the frequency of dose as symptoms improve.

## CHILBLAINS

Topical—Mix together 1 drop each of lavender and German chamomile in 3 teaspoons of carrier oil and apply a small amount of this mixture to the affected area up to 3 times daily (birth–12 months). Mix together 1 drop each of lavender, cypress, and German chamomile in 1 teaspoon of carrier oil and apply a small amount of this mixture to the affected area up to 3 times daily (1–5 years). Mix together 1 drop each of lavender and German chamomile in half a teaspoon of carrier oil and apply a small amount of this mixture to the affected area up to 3 times daily (6–17 years).

## CIRCUMCISION

Topical—Mix 1 drop each of lavender and German chamomile in half a pint of water and spray this mixture on the genital area, several times daily.

Homeopathic Remedies—Give the child arnica before and after the procedure.

## COLDS (Common Cold)

Topical—Create a mixture of 10 drops each of tea tree and lemon, and 5 drops of lavender. Add 1 drop of this mixture to 2 teaspoons of carrier oil and massage a small amount of this mixture into the chest and upper back every 30 minutes for the first 4 hours. Then apply every 2 hours until symptoms subside (birth–12 months). Create a mixture of 10 drops each of tea tree and lemon, and 5 drops each of myrtle and thyme. Add 2 to 3 drops of this mixture to 1 teaspoon of carrier oil and massage a small amount of this mixture into the chest and upper back every 30 minutes for the first 4 hours. Then apply every 2 hours until symptoms subside (1–5 years). Create a mixture of 10 drops each of tea tree and lemon, and 3 drops each of myrtle, eucalyptus, and thyme. Add 3 to 5 drops of this mixture to 1 teaspoon of carrier oil and massage a small amount of this mixture into the chest and upper back every 30 minutes for the first 4 hours. Then apply every 2 hours until symptoms subside (6–17 years).

Steam Inhalation—Add 2 to 10 drops of the above-mentioned mixtures (according to age) to 1 pint of hot water and place near the child (but where young children will not be able to touch it).

Aromatic Bath—Add 1 drop of the above mixture (according to age) to 1 teaspoon of carrier oil to a warm bath (birth–12 months). Add 1 to 4 drops of the above mixture in 1 teaspoon of carrier oil to a warm bath (1–5 years). Add 3 to 7 drops of the above mixture in 1 teaspoon of carrier oil to a warm bath (6–17 years).

## COLD SORES (Fever Blisters)

Topical—Mix together 1 drop of lavender, lemon, or tea tree in 1 teaspoon of carrier oil and apply 1 drop of this mixture to the affected area, several times daily (1–5 years). Mix together 1 drop of lavender, lemon, or tea tree in half a teaspoon of carrier oil and apply 1 drop of this mixture to the affected area, several times daily (6–11 years). Apply 1 drop of lavender, lemon, or tea tree neat to the affected area up to four times daily (12–17 years). Rotating the oils used will improve effectiveness.

## COLIC

*There are many underlying reasons a child experiences colic. It is strongly recommended to check for medical causes of irritability such as food sensitivities, acid reflux, etc.*

Topical—Mix together 1 drop of German chamomile and lavender in 3 teaspoons of carrier oil and apply to the infant's abdomen up to 3 times daily (birth–12 months).

Aromatic Bath—Give the infant a bath by adding 1 drop of lavender in 1 teaspoon of carrier oil to the bath water.

Inhalation—Apply 1 drop each of lavender and cedarwood to your body for the infant to inhale.

Homeopathic Remedies—Give the child pulsatilla 30C (if the colic occurs after feeding or in the evening), chamomilla 30C (if accompanying teething or the abdomen is very sensitive to touch), or belladonna (when the baby is very restless and arches backwards).

Other—Consider pediatric chiropractic.

## CONCUSSION

*Seek medical attention as soon as possible if the person lost consciousness, experiences weakness, involuntary movements, or changes in personality as a result of the concussion.*

Topical—Apply 1 drop each of frankincense, vetiver, and sandalwood with 9 drops of carrier oil to the head and back of the neck, 1 to 3 times daily (2–5 years). Apply 1 to 2 drops each of frankincense, vetiver, and sandalwood with equal drops of carrier oil to the head and back of the neck, 1 to 3 times daily (6–17 years).

Oral—Take 1 drop each of frankincense, vetiver, and sandalwood orally, 1 to 3 times daily (6–11 years). Take 1 drop each of frankincense, vetiver (turmeric is also a good option and may be added if available), and sandalwood orally, 2 to 3 times daily (12–17 years).

Homeopathic—Give the child natrum sulphuricum 30C.

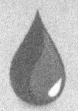

## CONGESTION (SINUS)

*Seek medical attention if your child experiences mucous drainage from the eyes, redness around the eyes, or fever, which may indicate a sinus infection.*

Topical—Mix together 1 drop each of lemon and lavender in 3 teaspoons of carrier oil and massage a small amount of this to the chest and upper back, several times daily (birth–12 months). Mix together 1 drop each of myrtle, pine, and thyme in 1 teaspoon of carrier oil and apply a small amount of this to the chest and upper back, several times daily (1–5 years). Mix together 2 to 3 drops of eucalyptus and 1 to 2 drops each of myrtle, peppermint, and thyme in 1 teaspoon of carrier oil and apply to the chest and upper back, several times daily (6–17 years).

Steam Inhalation—Add 1 drop each of lemon, frankincense, and bergamot to 1 pint of hot water and place near, but out of reach of the infant, up to 3 times daily (birth–12 months). Add 1 to 2 drops each of myrtle, pine, and thyme to 1 pint of hot water and place near, but out of reach of the child, up to 3 times daily (1–5 years). Add 1 to 3 drops each of myrtle, eucalyptus, and peppermint to 1 pint of hot water and place near the child up to 3 times daily (6–17 years).

## CONJUNCTIVITIS (Pink Eye)

*Seek medical attention if fever and pain around the eye occurs, or if pain increases with movement of the eye.*

Topical—Mix together 1/8 teaspoon of raw, organic honey with 2 tablespoons of distilled warm water until dissolved. Place 1 to 3 drops of the mixture in both eyes with a clean eye dropper 2 to 4 times daily until infection clears. Mix together 1 drop each of lavender, frankincense, and tea tree in 1 to 2 teaspoons of carrier oil and apply this mixture widely around both eyes (6–17 years) up to 3 times daily.

## CONSTIPATION

Topical—Mix together 1 drop each of lemon and grapefruit in 3 teaspoons of carrier oil and massage a small amount of this mixture to the abdomen in a clockwise direction up to 3 times daily (birth–12 months). Mix together 1 drop each of lemon, ginger, and grapefruit in 1 teaspoon of carrier oil and massage a small amount of this mixture to the abdomen in a clockwise direction up to 3 times daily (1–5 years). Mix together 1 to 2 drops each of lemon, ginger, and grapefruit in 1 teaspoon of carrier oil and massage a small amount of this mixture to the abdomen in a clockwise direction up to 3 times daily (6–17 years).

Oral—Take 1 drop each of lemon and ginger orally up to 3 times daily (6–11 years). Take 1 to 2 drops each of ginger, lemon, and grapefruit orally up to 3 times daily (12–17 years).

Other—Have the child lie on her back and pump her knees toward the chest (as if riding a bicycle) several times.

## COUGH

*Children under 1 with a cough should be seen by a physician. Seek medical attention for a cough with chest pain, shortness of breath, labored breathing, or fever that lasts more than 3 days.*

Topical—Mix together 1 drop each of tea tree and lavender in 3 teaspoons of carrier oil and apply a small amount of this mixture to the chest and upper back, several times daily (birth–12 months). Mix together 1 drop each of sandalwood, myrtle, pine, and cypress in half a teaspoon of carrier oil and apply a small amount of this mixture to the chest and upper back, several times daily (1–5 years). Apply 1 drop of oregano, thyme, and clove in 10 to 15 drops of carrier oil to the bottoms of the feet up to 3 times daily (1 to 5 years). Mix together 1 to 3 drops each of eucalyptus, myrtle, basil, and peppermint in half a teaspoon of carrier oil and apply a small amount of this mixture to the chest and upper back, several times daily (6–17 years). Apply 1 drop of one of the above oils (within the appropriate age range) to chest area of the child's pajamas before going to bed.

Steam Inhalation—Add 1 drop each of tea tree and lavender to 1 pint of hot water and place near, but out of reach of the infant, up to 3 times daily (birth–12 months). Add 1 to 2 drops each of sandalwood, myrtle, pine, and cypress to 1 pint of hot water and place near, but out of reach of the child, up to 3 times daily (1–5 years). Add 1 to 3 drops each of myrtle, eucalyptus, basil, and peppermint to 1 pint of hot water and place near the child up to 3 times daily (6–17 years).

Oral—Take 1 to 2 drops each of oregano, cinnamon, myrrh, and lemon orally up to 3 times daily (6–17 years). Create a cough syrup by adding 5 drops of lemon, and 3 drops each of German chamomile and tea tree to 1 cup of pure maple syrup and give 1 teaspoon of this mixture up to 3 times daily (6–17 years).

## CRADLE CAP
### (Infantile Seborrheic Dermatitis)

Topical—Massage 1 drop each of lemon, tea tree, lavender, and geranium in 1 tablespoon of carrier oil to the scalp. Leave in place for up to 15 minutes and then rinse with warm water and a mild soap. Do this once daily, being sure to keep mixture away from baby's eyes and face.

## CROUP

Seek medical attention if your child experiences stridor (a harsh, raspy, whooping sound when breathing in) during periods of calm or rest.

Follow the directions for cough, but cover each essential oil application with a warm, damp towel.

Homeopathic Remedies—Give the child aconitum 30C (for croupy coughs that are worse at night and wake the child), spongia 30C (if aconitum is ineffective), or hepar sulphur 30C (for croupy coughs that are worse when exposed to cold).

## CRYPTOSPORIDIOSIS

Topical—Mix together 1 to 2 drops each of German chamomile, lavender, and sandalwood in half a teaspoon of carrier oil, and apply a small amount of the mixture to the lower abdomen up to 6 times daily (1–5 years). Mix together 1 to 2 drops each of lemongrass, clove, oregano, myrtle, and German chamomile in half a teaspoon of carrier oil, and apply to the lower abdomen up to 6 times daily.

Oral—Take 1 drop each of clove, oregano, and lemongrass orally up to 3 times daily (6–11 years). Take 1 drop each of clove, lemongrass, oregano, and German chamomile orally up to 3 times daily (12–17 years).

## CUTS (Minor)

Other—Thoroughly wash/cleanse the area and remove any debris or dirt 2 to 3 times daily.

Topical—Place 1 drop each of lavender and tea tree on a gauze pad and cover the cut (birth–12 months). Place 1 to 2 drops each of lavender and tea tree on a gauze pad and cover the cut (1–5 years). Place 1 to 3 drops of lavender, tea tree, and eucalyptus on a gauze pad and cover the wound with this (6–17 years). Replace all pads, 2 to 4 times daily. Allow the area to breathe for several minutes between each gauze pad change. Alternately, place 1 single drop of chosen oil on a bandage before covering. Apply 1 drop of tea tree in half a teaspoon of carrier oil around the wound up to 3 times daily (birth–5). Apply 1 drop of tea tree and eucalyptus in equal parts of carrier oil around the wound up to 3 times daily (6–17 years).

## DEPRESSION

*Children with depression should be under the care of a licensed professional. Seek medical attention immediately if your child experiences suicidal thoughts.*

Topical—Apply 1 to 4 drops of orange oil to the bottoms of the feet, 3 times daily (2–17 years). Apply 1 drop each of ylang ylang, bergamot, and frankincense in equal parts of carrier oil to the heart area of the chest up to 3 times daily (2–17 years).

Oral—Take 2 drops of lemon and 1 drop of bergamot or neroli orally up to 3 times daily (6–11 years). Take 2 drops of lemon and orange, and 1 drop of bergamot or neroli orally up to 3 times daily (12–17 years).

## DIAPER RASH

Topical—Mix together 1 drop each of lavender, German chamomile, and tea tree in 1 teaspoon of carrier oil and apply at each diaper change.

## DIARRHEA

*A physician can determine if the diarrhea is infectious or non-infectious related.*

Topical—Mix together 1 drop each of German chamomile, lavender, and tea tree in 2 teaspoons of carrier oil and massage a small amount of this mixture over the entire abdomen up to 3 times daily (birth–12 months). Mix together 1 drop each of German chamomile, lavender, and tea tree in 1 teaspoon of carrier oil and massage a small amount of this mixture over the entire abdomen up to 3 times daily (1–5 years). Mix together 1 drop each of peppermint, fennel, and basil in half a teaspoon of carrier oil and massage a small amount of this mixture over the entire abdomen up to 3 times daily (6–17 years).

Oral—Take 1 to 3 drops of peppermint orally up to 3 times daily (6–17 years).

## EAR INFECTION
### (Earache, Otitis Media)

*Seek medical attention if your child experiences drainage from the ear or tenderness of the skull.*

Topical—Mix together 1 drop each of lavender and tea tree in 1 to 2 teaspoons of carrier oil and apply a small amount of this mixture around the ear, then place 1 drop of this mixture on a cotton ball, and place the cotton ball in the ear. Replace the cotton ball every 30 minutes until symptoms are relieved (birth–12 months). Mix together 1 drop each of lavender, basil, thyme, and tea tree in 1 teaspoon of carrier oil and apply a small amount of this mixture around the ear, then place 1 drop of this mixture on a cotton ball, and place the cotton ball in the ear—replace the cotton ball every 30 minutes until symptoms are relieved (1–17 years). In addition, apply 1 drop each of cinnamon, oregano, clove, and lemon in equal parts carrier oil to the bottoms of the feet every 2 to 4 hours (1–17 years).

Oral—Take 1 drop each of oregano, cinnamon, tea tree, and lemon orally up to 3 times daily (6–17 years).

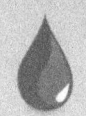

Homeopathic Remedies—Give pulsatilla 30C (if child is more clingy than usual), chamomilla 30C (if the child is very irritable), or hepar sulphur 30C (if severe pain is the major complaint). For chronic ear infections, give the child mercurius.

## ECZEMA

Homeopathic Remedies—Homeopathic cardiospermum should be the first remedy used for eczema. If this does not provide relief, the next option is homeopathic calendula. Essential oils (and some carrier oils) may make the condition worse if not heavily diluted.

Topical—Mix together 1 drop each of lavender, tea tree, German chamomile, and frankincense in 2 tablespoons of sweet almond oil and apply a small amount of this mixture up to 6 times daily.

## EPILEPSY (Seizures)

Other—Please review the list of essential oils and carrier oils that may trigger seizures. Always try new essential oils with a companion that can offer help as certain essential oil aromas can trigger an epileptic reaction in those with epilepsy, even those not listed as triggers.

Topical—Mix together 1 drop each of ylang ylang, Roman chamomile, lavender, and lemongrass in 1 teaspoon of carrier oil and apply a small amount of this mixture to the back of the neck, 2 times daily (6–17 years). Use the same oil in 2 teaspoons of carrier oil for ages 1 to 5.

Oral—Take 3 drops of rose oil orally, 3 times daily (6–11 years). Take 5 to 7 drops of rose oil orally, 3 times daily (6–17 years).

## FEVER

*Fevers can be beneficial by making the body's internal environment less hospitable for harmful organisms. However, it may also be necessary to calm the fever. The American Academy of Pediatrics recommends that you contact your child's doctor when fever temperatures reach the following: under*
*3 months—any fever of 100.4°F or higher, 3 to 6 months— any fever of 101°F or higher, over 6 months—any fever of 103°F or higher.*

Topical—Mix together 1 pint of lukewarm water, 1 tablespoon of apple cider vinegar, 3 drops of lavender, and 1 drop of lemon. Dip a clean cloth in this mixture and gently wring out before applying to the forehead and spine (birth–5 years). Avoid the eyes and ears. Mix together 1 pint of lukewarm water, 1 tablespoon of apple cider vinegar, 3 drops of peppermint, and 1 drop each of eucalyptus and lavender. Dip a clean cloth in this mixture and gently wring out before applying to the forehead and spine (6–17 years).

## FIFTH DISEASE

Aromatic Bath —Place 1 cup of raw oats in some muslin (or similar cloth) and add 3 drops each of German chamomile, tea tree, and lavender to the oats. Tie the material off or place a rubber band around the top to close securely and run a bath with this mixture under the stream of water. Place the mixture inside the material in the bath and then add 1 drop of each oil in half a cup of baking soda to the bath. Allow the child to soak for several minutes (2–17 years). Use 1 drop of each oil in the oatmeal mixture for infants (birth and up to age 2).

Topical—Mix together 1 drop each of thyme, tea tree, lavender, and geranium in 3 teaspoons of carrier oil and apply a small amount of the mixture to the affected area (stay clear of the eyes and mouth) up to 3 times daily (1–17 years).

Oral—Take 1 to 2 drops each of lemon, oregano, cinnamon, and tea tree orally, 1 to 3 times daily (6–17 years).

## FLU (Influenza)

*Seek medical attention if any issues with breathing occur, or if symptoms improve and then return.*

Topical—Create a mixture of 10 drops each of tea tree and lemon, and 5 drops of lavender. Add 1 drop of this mixture to 2 teaspoons of carrier oil and massage a small amount of this mixture into the chest and upper back every 30 minutes for the first 4 hours. Then apply every 2 hours until symptoms subside (birth–12 months). Mix together 1 drop each of myrtle, tea tree, and thyme in 1 teaspoon of carrier oil and apply a small amount of this mixture to the chest and upper back, 3 to 6 times daily (1–5 years). Mix together 1 to 3 drops each of myrtle, eucalyptus, tea tree, lemongrass, and thyme in 1 teaspoon of carrier oil and apply a small amount of this mixture to the chest and upper back, 3 to 6 times daily (6–17 years). Apply 1 drop each of cinnamon, clove, and oregano to the bottoms of the feet in 10 drops of carrier oil every 3 hours (1–17 years).

Oral—Take 1 drop each of tea tree, lemongrass, and cinnamon orally, 3 times daily (6–11 years). Take 1 to 2 drops each of tea tree, cinnamon, oregano, and lemongrass orally, 3 times daily (12–17 years).

Homeopathic Remedies—Take oscillococcinum 200C at the first signs of flu. Gelsemium 30C every 1 to 2 hours until symptoms subside is also a good option.

## FOOD POISONING

*Seek medical attention if your child experiences blood in the stool.*

Topical—Mix together 1 drop each of lemon and German chamomile in half a teaspoon of carrier oil and apply enough of this mixture to cover the abdomen every 2 hours until symptoms subside (1–5 years). Mix together 1 to 2 drops each of peppermint, ginger, and lemongrass in half a teaspoon of carrier oil and apply enough of this mixture to cover the abdomen every 1 to 2 hours until symptoms subside (6–17 years).

Oral—Take 1 drop each of peppermint, lemongrass, and juniper orally up to 3 times daily (6–17 years).

## FROSTBITE

*Seek medical attention especially if your child's skin will not warm, remains numb, blisters, or swells.*

Topical—Mix together 1 pint of warm water and 1 to 3 drops each of thyme, cypress, ginger, and geranium, and dip a clean cloth in the water. Wring out, apply to the frostbitten area, and then cover with plastic wrap and a hot water bottle for up to 3 hours (1–17 years). Massage the area with 1 drop each of thyme, ginger, and cypress in equal parts carrier oil up to five times daily. Seek medical attention as soon as possible.

## G6PD DEFICIENCY
### (Glucose-6-Phosphate Dehydrogenase)

Topical—Mix together 1 drop each of lemon and frankincense in 2 teaspoons of carrier oil and apply this mixture to the spine and lower back up to 3 times daily (birth–12 months). Mix together 1 to 2 drops each of lemon, ginger, clove, helichrysum, and cypress in 1 teaspoon of carrier oil and apply this mixture to the spine and lower back up to 3 times daily (1–17 years).

Other—Avoid the use of essential oils with high menthol and camphor content.

## GASTROESOPHAGEAL REFLUX
## DISEASE (GERD, Acid Reflux)

*It is strongly recommended that a comprehensive analysis be performed including nutrition, allergies, and digestion to determine the root cause of GERD.*

Oral—Take 1 drop each of lemon, orange, and ginger orally up to 3 times daily (6–11 years). Take 2 drops each of lemon, orange, and ginger orally up to 3 times daily (12–17 years).

Topical—Mix together 1 drop each of lemon and chamomile in 1 teaspoon of carrier oil and apply a small amount of this mixture to the abdomen and chest up to 3 times daily (birth–12 months). Mix together 1 drop each of lemon, orange, and ginger in half a teaspoon of carrier oil and apply a small amount of this mixture to the abdomen and chest up to 3 times daily (1–5 years).

Other—Consider hiatal massage for children birth to 5 years.

## GIARDIA

*Seek medical attention if the child experiences malnutrition, weight loss, or dehydration from giardia.*

Topical—Mix together 1 drop each of clove, basil, and thyme in 1 teaspoon of carrier oil and apply a small amount of this mixture to the abdomen up to 6 times daily (1–5 years). Mix together 1 to 2 drops of clove, basil, and thyme in half a teaspoon of carrier oil and apply a small amount of this mixture to the abdomen up to 6 times daily (6–17 years).

Oral—Take 1 drop each of clove, thyme, and basil orally, 1 to 3 times daily (6–11 years). Take 2 drops of clove and thyme, and 1 drop of basil orally, 1 to 3 times daily (12–17 years).

## GROWING PAINS

Topical—Mix together 1 drop each of balsam fir, frankincense, lavender, German chamomile, and ginger in 1 teaspoon of carrier oil and apply some of this mixture to the painful areas up to 6 times daily (1–5 years). Mix together 1 to 2 drops each of balsam fir, lemongrass, marjoram, ginger, and eucalyptus in 1 teaspoon of carrier oil and apply to the painful areas up to 6 times daily (6–17 years).

Aromatic Bath—Mix together 1 drop each of lavender, balsam fir, German chamomile, and ginger to half a cup of Epsom salts (use coarse sea salt for diabetics) and add this to a warm bath (1–5 years). Mix together 1 to 2 drops each of balsam fir, marjoram, lemongrass, basil, and ginger to half a cup of Epsom salts (use coarse sea salt for diabetics) and add this to a warm bath (1–5 years).

Other—Apply heat to the area.

Homeopathic Remedies—Give the child calcarea phos 6X.

## HAND, FOOT, & MOUTH DISEASE

Topical—Mix together 1 drop each of tea tree, lemon, and lavender in 2 teaspoons of carrier oil and apply this mixture to any skin blisters, 2 to 4 times daily (birth–12 months). Mix together 1 drop each of tea tree, lemon, lavender, and thyme in 1 teaspoon of aloe vera oil and apply this mixture to any skin blisters, 2 to 4 times daily (1–6 years). Mix together 2 to 3 drops each of tea tree, lemon, lavender, and thyme in 1 teaspoon of aloe vera oil and apply this mixture to any skin blisters and mouth sores, 2 to 4 times daily (7–17 years). Apply 1 to 2 drops of cinnamon, thyme, and oregano in 12 drops of carrier oil to the feet up to 3 times daily (1–17 years). See fever section for fevers.

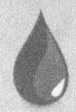

## HAY FEVER

*Experiment with the different formulas to determine which one provides the greatest relief for your child.*

Inhalation—Place 1 drop each of lavender, German chamomile, and lemon on a tissue and have the child inhale as necessary (1–17 years). Children 6 or over can use the above formula or place 1 drop each of eucalyptus, peppermint, and lavender in a tissue and inhale as necessary (6–17 years).

Oral—Take 2 drops each of lavender and German chamomile orally up to 3 times daily (6–11). Take 2 drops each of lavender, lemon, and German chamomile orally up to 3 times daily (12–17 years). Alternately, take 1 to 2 drops each of lavender, lemon, and peppermint orally up to 3 times daily (6–17 years).

Homeopathic Remedies—Give the child sulphur 6C (if most affected in the summer or symptoms are aggravated by heat) or ambrosia 6C (for ragweed allergies).

## HEAD LICE

Topical—Mix together 10 drops each of tea tree and lavender, and 5 drops each of myrtle and thyme, and then add 5 drops of this mixture to 1 tablespoon of carrier oil and massage into scalp. Cover the head with a shower cap and let sit for 30 minutes before rinsing the hair with 16 ounces of warm water and 20 drops of the above mixture (1–5 years). For older children follow the same procedure with the following modifications: use 10 drops of the mixture during the scalp massage, and substitute eucalyptus for myrtle (6–17 years).

## HEADACHE

*Seek medical attention for excruciating headaches accompanied by disorientation or neck stiffness to assess neurological explanations.*

Topical—Mix together 5 drops each of lavender, German chamomile, and basil, and then mix 1 to 2 drops of this mixture with 20 drops of carrier oil and apply to the temples, forehead, and back of the neck up to 3 times daily (1–5 years). Mix together 5 drops each of lavender, peppermint, and basil, and then mix 1 to 2 drops of this mixture with 10 drops of carrier oil and apply to the temples, forehead, and back of the neck up to 3 times daily (6–11 years). Mix together 5 drops each of lavender, peppermint, and basil, and then mix 1 to 2 drops of this mixture with 5 drops of carrier oil and apply to the temples, forehead, and back of the neck up to 3 times daily (12–17 years).

Oral—Place 1 drop of peppermint on your thumb with 2 drops of carrier oil and push this mixture to the roof of your mouth (12–17 years) up to 3 times daily.

Homeopathic Remedies—Give the child kali bichromicum 6C (for headache with nausea or above the eyes), gelsemium 6C (for headache at the back of the head), or bryonia 6C (for headaches that are worse from the slightest motion).

## HEAT EXHAUSTION

*Seek medical attention if your child experiences nausea, vomiting, headache, dizziness, fatigue, rapid heartbeat, hot and dry skin, shortness of breath, or decreased urination.*

Topical—Mix together 1 drop each of lavender and lemon in equal parts carrier oil and apply to the back of the neck, temples, shoulders, and tips of the ears; then soak a cloth in half a cup of cool water and 2 drops each of lavender and lemon and place this over the back of the child's neck (1–5 years). Mix together 2 drops each of lavender and peppermint in equal parts carrier oil and apply to the back of the neck, temples, shoulders, and tips of the ears; then soak a cloth in half a cup of cool water and 3 to 4 drops each of lavender and peppermint and place this over the back of the child's neck (6–17 years).

Homeopathic Remedies—Give the child belladonna 30C.

## HEMORRHOIDS

Topical—Mix together 1 drop each of lavender, cypress, and tea tree in 5 to 10 drops of carrier oil and apply a drop of this mixture to the painful area, several times daily (1–17 years).

## HIVES (Urticaria)

*Seek medical attention if breathing issues, constricted airways, profuse diarrhea, vomiting, fainting, or dizziness occurs with the hives.*

Homeopathic Remedies—Apply calendula to the affected area as indicated on the product label.

Topical—Mix together 2 to 4 drops each of German chamomile and lavender in 1 to 2 teaspoons of carrier oil to the affected area up to 3 times daily (1–17 years). Test on a small area first because essential oils may aggravate hives.

Oral—Take 2 drops of German chamomile and 1 drop of lavender orally, 1 to 3 times daily (6–11 years). Take 2 drops each of German chamomile and lavender, and 1 drop of frankincense orally, 1 to 3 times daily (12–17 years).

Homeopathic Remedies—Give the child apis 30C (for hives that are worse with any heat), pulsatilla 6C (for hives following eating rich or greasy foods, or after emotional trauma), or urtica urens 6C (for hives that burn).

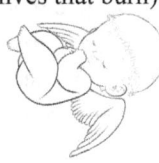

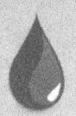 

## IMPETIGO

*Seek medical attention if the area is painful, the redness is spreading, or fever is experienced.*

Topical—Mix together 1 drop each of lavender, German chamomile, and tea tree in 3 teaspoons of carrier oil and apply very small amounts of this mixture to the affected areas up to 3 times daily (birth–12 months). Mix together 1 drop each of lavender, tea tree, thyme, and German chamomile in 1 teaspoon of carrier oil and apply very small amounts of this mixture to the affected areas up to 3 times daily (1–5 years). Mix together 2 drops each of lavender, tea tree, thyme, and lemongrass in 1 teaspoon of carrier oil and apply very small amounts of this mixture to the affected areas up to 3 times daily (6–17 years).

Oral—Take 1 drop each of cinnamon, lemongrass, and peppermint orally up to 3 times daily (6–11 years). Take 1 drop each of cinnamon, lemongrass, tea tree, and peppermint orally up to 3 times daily (12–17 years).

Homeopathic Remedies—Give the child antimonium crudum 6C.

## INDIGESTION

Topical—Mix together 1 drop each of lavender and German chamomile in 2 teaspoons of carrier oil and apply a small amount of this mixture to the abdomen in a clockwise circular motion up to 3 times daily (birth–12 months). Mix together 1 drop each of ginger and basil in 1 teaspoon of carrier oil and apply a small amount of this mixture to the abdomen in a clockwise circular motion up to 3 times daily (1–5 years). Mix together 1 drop each of ginger, peppermint, fennel, and basil in half a teaspoon of carrier oil and apply a small amount of this mixture to the abdomen in a clockwise circular motion up to 3 times daily (6–17 years).

Oral—Take 1 drop each of peppermint and ginger orally up to 3 times daily (6–11 years). Take 2 drops of peppermint, and 1 drop each of ginger and fennel orally up to 3 times daily (12–17 years).

Homeopathic Remedies—Give the child bryonia 30C (if indigestion occurs after eating rich or fatty foods), or nux vomica 30C (if from overindulging or long-term stress).

## INSOMNIA

Inhalation—Place 1 drop of lavender on the crib or bed sheet away from the infant's head before bedtime (birth–12 months). Place 1 drop each of cedarwood and lavender on the pillow away from the child's face, or the upper part of the pajamas before going to bed (1–17 years).

Topical—Massage 1 drop of lavender with 5 drops of carrier oil to the soles of the feet before bedtime (birth–12 months). Massage 1 drop each of cedarwood and lavender in equal parts of carrier oil to the soles of the feet before retiring to bed (1–17 years).

Homeopathic Remedies—Give the child coffea 6C (mentally hyperactive), rhus tox 30C (restless), or kali phosphoricum 6C (if night terrors interrupt sleep).

## JAUNDICE (Infant)

*Only use in conjunction with Western treatment options. Severe jaundice could result in brain damage, breathing problems, and seizures.*

Topical—Mix together 1 drop each of geranium, lemon, and helichrysum in 2 tablespoons of carrier oil and apply a small amount of this mixture on the upper right part of the abdomen (over the liver) and to the bottoms of the feet up to 3 times daily.

## LARYNGITIS

Topical—Mix together 1 drop each of thyme and tea tree in 1 teaspoon of carrier oil and apply to the upper chest and over the throat up to 4 times daily (1–5 years). Mix together 1 drop each of thyme, eucalyptus, and tea tree in 1 teaspoon of carrier oil and apply to the upper chest and over the throat up to 4 times daily (6–17 years).

Oral—Gargle with a mixture of 1 drop each of lemon, German chamomile, and vetiver with 1 teaspoon of honey in 4 ounces of water and spit out up to 3 times daily (2–5 years). Gargle with 1 drop each of lemon, eucalyptus, and vetiver with 1 teaspoon of honey in 4 ounces of water and swallow up to 3 times daily (6–17 years).

## MALARIA

*Life-threatening complications can develop with malaria. Only use this protocol in conjunction with Western medical options and with approval from a physician. Seek medical attention immediately for symptoms such as severe fatigue or shortness of breath.*

Topical—Mix together 1 drop each of lemon, sandalwood, and myrtle in 1 teaspoon of carrier oil and apply a small amount of this mixture to the spine up to 5 times daily (birth–12 months). Mix together 1 drop each of lemongrass, myrtle, sandalwood, tea tree, and lemon in 10 drops of carrier oil and apply this mixture to the spine and bottoms of the feet up to 5 times daily (1–5 years). Mix together 1 drop each of lemongrass, myrtle, sandalwood, rosemary, and oregano in 10 drops of carrier oil and apply to the spine and bottoms of the feet up to 5 times daily (6–17 years).

Oral—Take 1 drop each of rosemary, thyme, tea tree, and oregano orally up to 3 times daily (6–11 years). Take 2 drops each of rosemary and oregano, and 1 drop each of thyme and tea tree up to 3 times daily (12–17 years).

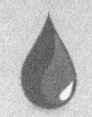

## Symptoms of
# Malaria

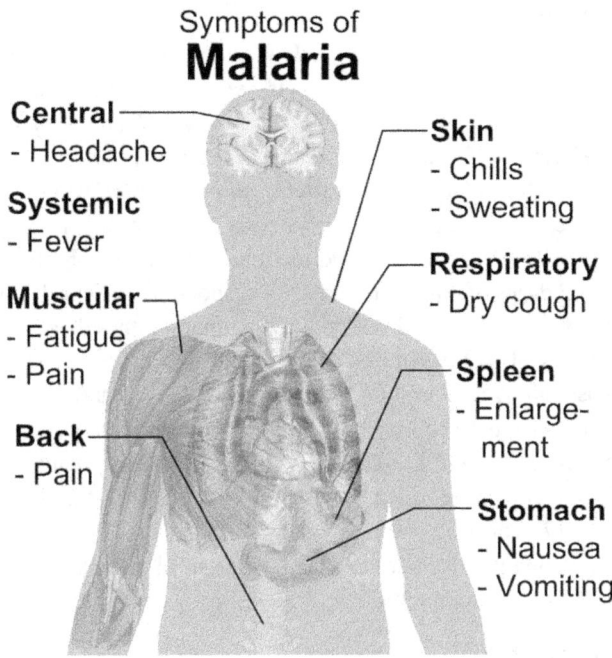

**Central** — Headache

**Systemic** - Fever

**Muscular** - Fatigue - Pain

**Back** - Pain

**Skin** - Chills - Sweating

**Respiratory** - Dry cough

**Spleen** - Enlargement

**Stomach** - Nausea - Vomiting

## MEASLES

*Only use in conjunction with Western medical options and with approval from a physician.*

Aromatic Bath —Place 1 cup of raw oats in some muslin (or similar cloth) and add 3 drops each of German chamomile, tea tree, and lavender to the oats. Tie the material off or place a rubber band around the top to close securely and run a bath with this mixture under the stream of water. Place the mixture inside the material in the bath and then add 1 drop of each oil in half a cup of baking soda to the bath. Allow the child to soak for several minutes (2–17). Use 1 drop of each oil in the oatmeal mixture for infants (birth and up to age 2).

Topical—Mix together 1 drop each of tea tree, lavender, and German chamomile in 4 teaspoons of carrier oil and dab a small amount of this mixture to the affected area with a cotton ball, several times daily (birth–12 months). Mix together 1 drop each of tea tree, lavender, and German chamomile in 1 teaspoon of carrier oil and dab a small amount of this mixture to the affected area with a cotton ball, several times daily (1–5 years). Mix together 1 drop each of tea tree, lavender, and German chamomile in half a teaspoon of carrier oil and dab a small amount of this mixture to the affected area with a cotton ball, several times daily (birth–12 months).

Oral—Take 1 drop each of oregano, lavender, German chamomile, and tea tree orally, 2 to 3 times daily (6–11 years). Take 2 drops of oregano, and 1 drop each of lavender, German chamomile, and tea tree orally, 2 to 3 times daily (12–17 years).

Homeopathic Remedies—Give the child belladonna 30C or aconitum 30C every 2 hours during the beginning stages of the measles. For mild cases, give pulsatilla 30C.

## MENINGITIS, VIRAL

*Only use in conjunction with Western medical options and with approval from a physician.*

Topical—Mix together 1 drop each of tea tree, German chamomile, bergamot, thyme, and lemon in 2 tablespoons of carrier oil and apply a small amount of this mixture to the spine and behind and below the ears up to 3 times daily (birth–12 months). Mix together 1 drop each of thyme, cinnamon, lemongrass, tea tree, and bergamot in 1 teaspoon of carrier oil and apply a small amount of this mixture to the spine and behind and below the ears up to 3 times daily (1–5 years). Mix together 2 drops each of thyme, cinnamon, lemongrass, tea tree, eucalyptus, and bergamot in 1 teaspoon of carrier oil and apply a small amount of this mixture to the spine and behind and below the ears up to 3 times daily (6–17 years).

Oral—Take 1 drop each of oregano, cinnamon, clove, tea tree, and peppermint orally, 3 times daily (6–11 years). Take 1 drop each of oregano, cinnamon, clove, tea tree, eucalyptus, and peppermint orally, 3 times daily (12–17 years).

## MENSTRUAL PAIN,
## PREMENSTRUAL SYNDROME (PMS)

Topical—Massage the lower abdomen with 1 drop each of clary sage, geranium, lavender, and marjoram in 5 drops of carrier oil up to 3 times daily (8–17 years).

Aromatic Bath—Take a warm bath with 2 drops each of bergamot, clary sage, and lavender in half a teaspoon of carrier oil (8–17 years).

Inhalation—Place 1 drop each of lavender, clary sage, and geranium on a tissue and inhale from this as necessary (8–17 years).

## MIGRAINE

Topical—Mix together 1 drop each of peppermint, basil, and lavender in 1 teaspoon of carrier oil and apply a small amount of this mixture to the temples, forehead, back of the neck, and behind the ears every 30 minutes until symptoms subside (1–5 years). Mix together 1 drop each of peppermint, basil, and lavender in half a teaspoon of carrier oil and apply a small amount of this mixture to the temples, forehead, back of the neck, and behind the ears every 30 minutes until symptoms subside (6–17 years).

Oral—Place 1 drop of peppermint on your thumb with 2 drops of carrier oil and push this mixture to the roof of your mouth (12–17 years) up to 3 times daily.

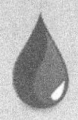

Homeopathic Remedies—Give the child bryonia 6C (for migraine aggravated by slightest motion) or belladonna 6C (for a migraine that makes the head feel like it will burst).

Other—Children 6 and older can consider a feverfew herb supplement (not essential oil) daily as a preventive.

## MOLLUSCUM CONTAGIOSUM

Topical—In a 10 mL roller bottle, mix together 3 drops each of tea tree and lemongrass essential oil and fill the rest of the bottle with an aloe-based carrier oil. Apply enough of this mixture to cover the affected area 3 to 5 times daily (1–5 years). Use the same formula/procedure with 5 to 7 drops of each essential oil for children 6 to 11, and 10 drops each for children 12–17 years.

## MONONUCLEOSIS

*Caution must be exercised with contact sports if the child has an enlarged spleen.*

Topical—Mix together 1 drop each of eucalyptus and frankincense in half a teaspoon of carrier oil and apply to the front of the neck, upper chest, and back (1–5 years). Mix together 2 drops each of eucalyptus and frankincense in half a teaspoon of carrier oil and apply to the front of the neck, upper chest, and back (6–17 years). In addition, mix together 1 drop each of oregano, thyme, basil, cypress, marjoram, and peppermint in 1.5 teaspoons of carrier oil and apply this mixture to the back (1–5 years). In addition, mix together 1 drop each of oregano, thyme, basil, cypress, marjoram, and peppermint in 1 teaspoon of carrier oil and apply this mixture to the back (6–17 years).

Oral—Take 1 drop each of thyme, oregano, lemon, and cinnamon orally, 1 to 3 times daily (6–11 years). Take 1 drop each of thyme, oregano, lemon, and cinnamon orally, 3 times daily (12–17 years).

## MOTION SICKNESS

Topical—Mix together 1 drop each of peppermint, ginger, spearmint, fennel, and lemon in half a teaspoon of carrier oil and apply a small amount of this mixture to the wrists and insides of the ankles (6–17 years). This mixture can also be inhaled from a tissue.

Inhalation—Place 1 drop each of lemon and ginger on a tissue and inhale as necessary (1–5 years).

Oral—Take a capsule with 2 drops of peppermint and 1 drop each of ginger and spearmint orally 30 minutes before travel begins and every 4 hours thereafter (6–17 years).

Homeopathic Remedies—Give the child cocculus 6C.

Other—Make sure the child keeps his/her feet on the ground and eyes open, preferably where they can see the road.

## MUMPS

*Only use in conjunction with Western medical options. Life-threatening complications such as encephalitis (inflammation of the brain), pancreatitis (inflammation of the pancreas), and meningitis may occur with mumps. In addition, swelling of the testicles and ovaries may occur.*

Topical—Mix together 10 drops each of tea tree and thyme, and 5 drops of lavender and German chamomile, and then mix 2 drops of this mixture with 1 teaspoon of carrier oil and apply to the neck and behind the ears up to 4 times daily (1–5 years). Use the same formula with 3 to 5 drops in half a teaspoon of carrier oil for older children (6–17 years).

Oral—Take 1 drop each of lemon, lavender, and cypress orally, 2 times daily (6–11 years). Take 1 drop each of lemon, lavender, eucalyptus, and cypress, 2 times daily (12–17 years).

Homeopathic Remedies—Give the child pilocarpinum 30C or belladonna 30C.

## MUSCLE SORENESS

Topical—Mix together 1 drop each of basil, lavender, ginger, and German chamomile in 1 teaspoon of carrier oil and apply enough of the mixture to cover the sore muscle (1–5 years). Mix together 1 drop each of basil, lavender, marjoram, ginger, and peppermint in half a teaspoon of carrier oil and apply enough of the mixture to cover the sore muscle (6–17 years).

Homeopathic Remedies—Apply arnica cream to the sore muscles. 30C pellets can be taken orally as well.

## NAUSEA

*Seek medical attention if nausea is accompanied by high fever, stiff neck, blurred vision, or a severe headache.*

Topical—Mix together 1 drop each of peppermint, ginger, spearmint, fennel, and lemon in half a teaspoon of carrier oil and apply a small amount of this mixture to the wrists and insides of the ankles (6–17 years). This mixture can also be inhaled from a tissue.

Inhalation—Place 1 drop each of lemon and ginger on a tissue and inhale as necessary (1–5 years).

Oral—Take a capsule with 2 drops of peppermint and 1 drop each of ginger and spearmint orally 30 minutes before travel begins and every 4 hours thereafter (6–17 years).

Homeopathic Remedies—Give the child nux vomica 6C (especially if accompanied by drowsiness and irritability) or antimonium crudum 30C (if associated with overeating or eating rich foods).

## PINWORM (Threadworm)

Topical—Mix together 1 drop each of lavender, oregano, clove, basil, myrtle, and German chamomile in 1 teaspoon

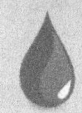

of carrier oil and apply this mixture to the abdomen up to 6 times daily (1–5 years). Mix together 2 drops each of basil, eucalyptus, oregano, clove, and lavender and apply to the abdomen up to 6 times daily (6–17 years).

Oral—Take 1 drop each of clove, oregano, and lavender orally, 2 times daily for 21 days, and then rest 7 days before repeating another 21 days (6–11 years). Take 2 drops of oregano and 1 drop each of clove, basil, and lavender orally, 2 times daily for 21 days, and then rest 7 days before repeating another 21 days (12–17 years).

## PLANTAR WARTS

Topical—Mix together 10 drops each of oregano and thyme, and 5 drops of tea tree, clove, and lemon, and then use a cotton swab to apply 1 drop of this mixture neat to the wart, 1 to 3 times daily (1–17 years).

## PNEUMONIA

*Seek medical attention if the child experiences rapid breathing without fever, painful cough, labored breathing, or has a weakened immune system.*

Topical—Mix together 1 drop each of frankincense, lemon, lavender, and chamomile in 1 teaspoon of carrier oil and use enough of this mixture to cover the upper back and chest up to 3 times daily (birth–12 months). Mix together 1 drop each of myrtle, ginger, lemon, frankincense, thyme, and lavender in half a teaspoon of carrier oil and use enough of this mixture to cover the upper back and chest up to 3 times daily (1–5 years). Mix together 2 drops each of peppermint, eucalyptus, thyme, ginger, and lemongrass in half a teaspoon of carrier oil and use enough of this mixture to cover the upper back and chest up to 3 times daily (6–17 years).

Steam Inhalation—Add 1 drop each of tea tree, frankincense, and lavender to 1 pint of hot water and place near, but out of reach of the infant, up to 3 times daily (birth–12 months). Add 1 to 2 drops each of thyme, myrtle, pine, and cypress to 1 pint of hot water and place near, but out of reach of the child, up to 3 times daily (1–5 years). Add 1 to 2 drops each of cinnamon, eucalyptus, basil, lemongrass, and peppermint to 1 pint of hot water and place near the child up to 3 times daily (6–17 years).

Oral—Take 1 drop each of cinnamon, clove, and oregano orally, 3 times daily (6–11 years). Take 2 drops of cinnamon, and 1 drop each of clove, eucalyptus, and oregano, 3 times daily (12–17 years).

## PSORIASIS

*It is strongly advised that persons who experience psoriasis have further analysis including nutrition, allergies, and autoimmune tests. Some have found a multi-enzyme and probiotic helpful.*

Homeopathic Remedies—Apply berberis aquifolium tincture cream to the affected area as instructed on the product label.

Topical—Mix together 1 drop each of lavender, cistus, frankincense, German chamomile, and tea tree in 2 tablespoons of sesame seed oil and apply a small amount of this mixture up to 6 times daily. Test on a small patch of skin first. Some essential oils and carrier oils will make the condition worse.

## PYLORIC STENOSIS

*Surgery is the frequently required to correct pyloric stenosis, but this can be used for temporary relief with physician approval until surgery can be performed.*

Topical—Mix together 2 drops each of orange and cypress in 2 teaspoons of carrier oil and massage into the abdomen, 1 to 4 times daily (birth–5 years).

## RABIES

*Only use in conjunction with Western medical options and with approval from a physician.*

Topical—Mix together 10 drops each of thyme, tea tree, and frankincense, and then add 2 drops of this to 1 teaspoon of carrier oil and apply to the spine and affected area (birth–5 years). In addition, mix 1 drop of geranium in 10 drops of carrier oil and apply a small amount of this mixture behind the ears, 2 times daily (birth–5 years). Mix together 10 drops each of thyme, eucalyptus, tea tree, and frankincense, and then add 5 drops of this to half a teaspoon of carrier oil and apply to the spine and affected area (6–17 years). In addition, mix 1 drop of vetiver, geranium, and sandalwood in 5 drops of carrier oil and apply a small amount of this mixture behind the ears, 2 times daily (6–17 years).

Oral—Take 1 drop each of cinnamon, oregano, thyme, and tea tree orally, 3 times daily (6–11 years). Take 1 drop each of cinnamon, oregano, eucalyptus, tea tree, and thyme orally, 3 times daily (12–17 years).

## RASH

*Seek medical attention if the rash is accompanied by fever.*

Topical—Mix together 1 drop each of lavender and German chamomile in 3 teaspoons of carrier oil and apply a small amount of this mixture to the affected area up to 3 times daily (birth–5 years).

Mix together 2 drops each of lavender, German chamomile, and tea tree in 1 teaspoon of carrier oil and apply to the affected area up to 3 times daily (6–17 years).

## REACTIVE ATTACHMENT DISORDER

Topical—In a 10 mL roller bottle, add 1 drop each of vetiver, ylang ylang, frankincense, blue tansy, and lavender and fill the rest with carrier oil. Apply this blend to the shoulders and back of the neck, 1 to 3 times daily (1–5). Add 2 drops of each essential oil to the blend for children aged 6 to 17 years.

## RESPIRATORY SYNCYTIAL VIRUS (RSV)

*Only use in conjunction with Western medical options.*

Steam Inhalation—Place a bowl of hot water with 1 to 2 drops of frankincense next to, but out of reach of, the infant (birth–12 months) up to 3 times daily. Place a bowl of hot water with 2 drops each of myrtle and pine, and 1 drop of frankincense next to, but out of reach of, the child (1–5 years) up to 3 times daily. Place a bowl of hot water with 2 drops each of eucalyptus, myrtle, pine, and thyme next to the child up to 3 times daily (6–17 years).

Topical—Create a mixture of 1 drop each of lemon and frankincense in 2 teaspoons of carrier oil and apply a small amount of this mixture to the chest and upper back, 3 to 5 times daily (birth–12 months). Create a mixture of 1 drop each of myrtle, ginger, pine, and thyme in 1 teaspoon of carrier oil and apply a small amount of this mixture to the chest and upper back, 3 to 5 times daily (1–5 years). Create a mixture of 1 to 2 drops each of eucalyptus, myrtle, peppermint, ginger, pine, and thyme in 1 teaspoon of carrier oil and apply a small amount of this mixture to the chest and upper back, 3 to 5 times daily (6–17 years).

Oral—Take 1 drop each of oregano, cinnamon, and lemon orally up to 3 times daily (6–11 years). Take 1 drop each of oregano, tea tree, thyme, lemon, and cinnamon up to 3 times daily (12–17 years).

## RINGWORM

*It is strongly recommended that underlying gastrointestinal causes be investigated.*

Topical—Mix together 1 drop each of lavender, German chamomile, and tea tree in 1 teaspoon of carrier oil and apply a small amount of this mixture to the affected area, 3 times daily (birth–5 years). Mix together 2 drops each of lemongrass, rosemary, tea tree, and lavender in half a teaspoon of carrier oil and apply enough of the mixture to cover the affected area, 3 times daily (6–17 years).

Oral—Take 2 drops of lemongrass, and 1 drop each of German chamomile, cinnamon, and juniper, morning and evening (6–17 years).

## RUBELLA (GERMAN MEASLES)

*Those with rubella should avoid close proximity and contact with women who are pregnant.*

Topical—Soak a clean cloth in 1 cup of cool water with 1 drop each of tea tree, lavender, and German chamomile, wring out, and wipe affected area, several times daily (birth–17 years). For aching joints mix together 1 drop of German chamomile, lavender, and copaiba in 1 teaspoon

of carrier oil and apply a small amount to the affected joints (birth–5 years). For aching joints mix together 1 drop of eucalyptus, ginger, eucalyptus, lavender, German chamomile, and copaiba in half a teaspoon of carrier oil and apply a small amount to the affected joints (6–17 years).

## SHIN SPLINTS

Topical—Mix together 2 drops each of balsam fir, copaiba, lemongrass, and peppermint in half a teaspoon of carrier oil and apply enough of the mixture to cover the shins up to 3 times daily (6–11 years). Mix together 2 drops each of balsam fir, copaiba, lemongrass, wintergreen, and peppermint in half a teaspoon of carrier oil and apply enough of the mixture to cover the shins up to 3 times daily (12–17 years).

## SHOCK, EMOTIONAL

Inhalation—Add 1 to 2 drops each of lavender and lemon to a tissue and place near the child's nose to inhale (1–5 years). Add 1 to 2 drops of lavender and peppermint to a tissue and place near the child's nose to inhale (6–17 years). These oils can also simply be inhaled directly from the bottle.

Homeopathic Remedy—Give the child arnica 30C orally if the shock resulted from an injury or caused by pain.

## SINUSITIS (Sinus Infection)

Topical—Mix together 1 drop each of pine, balsam fir, and tea tree in 1 teaspoon of carrier oil and apply a small amount of this mixture to the forehead, nose, cheekbones, chest, and upper back, 3 to 5 times daily (1–5 years). Make sure to avoid the eyes. Mix together 1 drop each of eucalyptus, peppermint, pine, and tea tree in half a teaspoon of carrier oil and apply a small amount of this mixture to the forehead, nose, cheekbones, chest, and upper back, 3 to 5 times daily (6–17 years).

Oral—Take 1 drop each of pine, myrtle, lemon, and eucalyptus orally up to 3 times daily (6–17 years).

Steam Inhalation—Add 1 to 2 drops each of thyme, myrtle, pine, and cypress to 1 pint of hot water and place near, but out of reach of the child, up to 3 times daily (1–17 years).

## SORE THROAT

Oral—Gargle with a mixture of 1 drop each of lemon, German chamomile, and vetiver with 1 teaspoon of honey in 4 ounces of water and spit out, up to 3 times daily (2–5 years). Gargle with 1 drop each of lemon, bergamot, and peppermint with 1 teaspoon of honey in 4 ounces of water and swallow every 1 to 3 hours until symptoms improve (6–11 years). Gargle with 1 to 2 drops each of lemon,

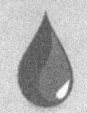

bergamot, and peppermint with 1 teaspoon of honey in 4 ounces of water and swallow every 1 to 3 hours until symptoms improve (12–17 years).

Topical— Mix together 1 drop each of lavender, geranium, and lemon in 1.5 teaspoons of carrier oil and apply to the neck over the throat 2 times daily (birth–12 months). Mix together 10 drops of tea tree, and 5 drops each of thyme and lemon, then dilute 5 drops of the blend in 1 teaspoon of carrier oil, and apply to the front of the throat, 2 times daily (1–5 years). Mix together 10 drops of tea tree, and 5 drops each of thyme eucalyptus, and lemon, then dilute 5 drops of the blend in half a teaspoon of carrier oil, and apply to the front of the throat, 2 times daily (6–17 years).

Homeopathic Remedies—If the tonsils are swollen, give the child belladonna 30C.

## SPRAINS

Topical—Dip a clean cloth in 2 drops each of lavender, German chamomile, and copaiba in 1 pint of cool water, wring out and wrap area of the sprain, 2 times daily the first day of the injury and then 2 times weekly thereafter (1–17 years). Mix together 1 drop each of lavender, copaiba, and German chamomile in half a teaspoon of carrier oil and apply enough of this mixture to cover the sprained area and widely around it up to 3 times daily (1–5 years). Mix together 1 drop each of basil, copaiba, balsam fir, and peppermint in half a teaspoon of carrier oil and apply enough of this mixture to cover the sprained area and widely around it up to 3 times daily (6–11 years). Mix together 1 drop each of basil, copaiba, balsam fir, wintergreen, and peppermint in 10 drops of carrier oil and apply this mixture to the sprained area and widely around it up to 3 times daily (12–17 years).

Homeopathic Remedies—Apply ruta graveolens and arnica cream to the sprain as indicated on the product label. Give the child Rhus tox orally 6C.

## STOMACH FLU (Gastroenteritis)

*Seek medical attention if the child is unable to retain fluids or hydration becomes an issue.*

Topical—Mix together 1 drop each of ginger and basil in 10 teaspoons of carrier oil and massage to the abdomen in a clockwise circular motion up to 3 times daily (1–5 years). Mix together 1 to 2 drops each of peppermint, ginger, and juniper in 10 drops of carrier oil and massage to the abdomen in a clockwise circular motion up to 3 times daily (6–17 years).

Oral—Take a capsule with 1 drop each of lemongrass, peppermint, ginger, and oregano orally up to 3 times daily (6–11 years). Take 1 drop each of peppermint, ginger,

clove, lemongrass, and oregano orally up to 3 times daily (12–17 years).

## STREP THROAT

Oral—Gargle with a mixture of 1 drop each of lemon, thyme, and tea tree with 1 teaspoon of honey in 4 ounces of water and spit out, up to 3 times daily (2–5 years). Gargle with 1 drop each of lemon, bergamot, and peppermint with 1 teaspoon of honey in 4 ounces of water and swallow every 1 to 3 hours until symptoms improve (6–11 years). Gargle with 1 to 2 drops each of lemon, tea tree, thyme, and peppermint with 1 teaspoon of honey in 4 ounces of water and swallow every 1 to 3 hours until symptoms improve (12–17 years). Take a capsule with 1 drop each of cinnamon, peppermint, lemongrass, and thyme, 2 times daily (6–17 years).

Topical—Mix together 1 drop each of lavender, geranium, and lemon in 1.5 teaspoons of carrier oil and apply to the neck over the throat 2 times daily (birth–12 months). Mix together 10 drops of tea tree, and 5 drops each of thyme and lemon, then dilute 5 drops of the blend in 1 teaspoon of carrier oil, and apply to the neck over the throat, 2 times daily (1–5 years). Mix together 10 drops of tea tree, and 5 drops each of thyme, eucalyptus, and lemon, then dilute 5 drops of the blend in half a teaspoon of carrier oil, and apply to the neck over the throat, 2 times daily (6–17 years).

Homeopathic Remedies—If the tonsils are swollen, give the child belladonna 30C.

## STRAWBERRY HEMANGIOMA

Topical—Create a mixture of 1 to 2 drops each of helichrysum, cypress, frankincense, and geranium in 8 teaspoons of carrier oil and apply 1 to 2 drops of this mixture up to 3 times daily.

## STRESS

Inhalation—Place 1 drop each of lavender, ylang ylang, and bergamot on a tissue and allow the child to inhale as desired (1–17 years).

Topical—Mix together 5 drops each of lavender, orange, ylang ylang, chamomile, and cedarwood, and then apply 1 drop of this mixture with equal parts of carrier oil to the wrists, 1 part essential oil to 5 parts carrier may be used for ages 3 to 5 (3–17 years).

## STY (STYE)

*Seek medical attention if redness spreads from the eye, tenderness extends to the skin around the eye, or the child experiences pain when moving the eye.*

Topical—Mix together 1 drop each of lavender and frankincense in 1 teaspoon of carrier oil and apply a very small amount of this mixture widely around the eye—following the orbit—up to 3 times daily (1–17 years).

Other—Cover affected eye with a warm washcloth for several minutes several times daily.

## SUNBURN

Topical—Mix together 5 drops of lavender oil and 1 drop of tea tree in 1 teaspoon of aloe vera and cover the sunburned area up to 3 times daily (1–5 years). Mix together 5 drops of lavender oil and 1 drop each of tea tree and peppermint in 1 teaspoon of aloe vera and cover the sunburned area up to 3 times daily (6–17 years).

## SWIMMER'S EAR (Otitis Externa) *Most of the time swimmer's ear is characterized by pain when you pull the ear lobe. Seek medical attention if no pain occurs when pulling on the ear lobe and it is accompanied by fever.*

Topical—Mix together 1 drop each of lavender and tea tree in 1 to 2 teaspoons of carrier oil and apply a small amount of this mixture around the ear, then place 1 drop of this mixture on a cotton ball, and place the cotton ball in the ear. Replace the cotton ball every 30 minutes until symptoms are relieved (birth–12 months). Mix together 1 drop each of lavender, basil, thyme, and tea tree in 1 teaspoon of carrier oil and apply a small amount of this mixture around the ear and on the fleshy part of the ear, then place 1 drop of this mixture on a cotton ball, and place the cotton ball in the ear—replace the cotton ball every 30 minutes until symptoms for the first 4 hours, then every 4 hours thereafter (2–17 years). In addition, apply 1 drop each of cinnamon, oregano, clove, and lemon in equal parts carrier oil to the bottoms of the feet every 2 to 4 hours (2–17 years).

## SWOLLEN LYMPH GLANDS OR LYMPH NODES

*Seek medical attention if the swollen gland makes breathing or swallowing difficult, or if accompanied by a fever over 104°F, night sweats, or red skin over the swollen lymph node.*

Topical—Mix together 5 drops each of thyme, tea tree, and geranium, and then place 1 drop of this mixture diluted in 3 drops of carrier oil to the swollen lymph node/gland, 2 to 3 times daily (birth–5 years). Mix together 5 drops each of thyme, tea tree, and geranium, and then place 1 drop of this mixture neat on the swollen lymph node/gland up to 3 times daily (6–17 years).

## TEETHING

Homeopathic Remedies—Give the infant chamomilla 30X or 6C orally.

Topical/Oral—Dilute 1 drop of copaiba, frankincense, or German chamomile in 1 tablespoon of carrier oil and rub a very small amount of this mixture on the gums (3 months–5 years) as needed.

## THRUSH (Oral)

Oral—Swish for at least 30 seconds with a mixture of 1 drop each of lemon, geranium, and tea tree in 4 ounces of water, and then spit out, up to 3 times daily (2–5 years). Swish for at least 30 seconds with a mixture of 1 drop each of palmarosa, geranium, and tea tree in 4 ounces of water, and then spit out, up to 3 times daily (6–17 years).

## THRUSH (Vaginal, Anal)

Topical—Mix 5 drops each of tea tree, German chamomile, and orange in 1 to 2 ounces of plain, unsweetened yogurt and apply a small amount to the anus or vagina at each diaper change or after each time using the toilet (birth–11 years). Mix together 5 drops each of tea tree, German chamomile, and orange in 1 tablespoon of carrier oil and apply to the affected area each time after using the toilet, or at least 3 times daily (12–17 years).

## TONSILITIS

Topical—Mix together 10 drops of lavender, and 5 drops each of ginger, thyme, tea tree, and lemon, and then dilute 1 drop of this in half a teaspoon of carrier oil before applying to the outside of the throat and on the back, up to 3 times daily (birth–5 years). Mix together 5 drops each of oregano, thyme, lemongrass, and eucalyptus, and then dilute 2 drops of this in half a teaspoon of carrier oil before applying to the outside of the throat and on the back, up to 6 times daily (6–17 years).

Oral—Gargle with a mixture of 1 drop each of lemon, thyme, and tea tree with 1 teaspoon of honey in 4 ounces of water and spit out up to 3 times daily (2–5 years). Gargle with 1 drop each of lemon, bergamot, and peppermint with 1 teaspoon of honey in 4 ounces of water and swallow every 1 to 3 hours until symptoms improve (6–11 years). Gargle with 1 to 2 drops each of lemon, tea tree, thyme, and peppermint with 1 teaspoon of honey in 4 ounces of water and swallow every 1 to 3 hours until symptoms improve (12–17 years). Take a capsule with 1 drop each of cinnamon, lemongrass, oregano, and eucalyptus, 1 to 3 times daily (6–17 years).

Homeopathic Remedies—Give the child belladonna 30C orally.

Other—Consider taking the probiotic *Streptococcus salivarius* K12 daily as a preventive, possibly with *Streptococcus salivarius* M18.

## TOOTHACHE

Topical/Oral—Dilute 1 drop of copaiba, frankincense, or German chamomile in 1 tablespoon of carrier oil and rub a very small amount of this mixture on the gums (3

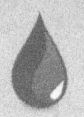

months–5 years). Dilute 1 drop of clove or peppermint in 5 to 10 drops of carrier oil and apply a small amount of this mixture to the sore tooth up to 3 times daily (6–17 years).

## TUBERCULOSIS

*Only use in conjunction with Western medical treatment options.*

Steam Inhalation—Place a bowl of hot water with 1 drop each of myrtle and frankincense next to, but out of reach of, the infant up to 3 times daily (birth–12 months). Place a bowl of hot water with 2 drops each of myrtle, vetiver, and pine next to, but out of reach of, the child up to 3 times daily (1–5 years). Place a bowl of hot water with 2 drops each of eucalyptus, myrtle, peppermint, and myrtle next to the child up to 3 times daily (6–17 years).

Topical—Mix together 10 drops each of lemon and tea tree, and 5 drops each of bergamot and frankincense, and dilute 2 to 5 drops of this mixture in half a teaspoon of carrier oil, and then apply to the chest and upper back, 2 times daily (birth–5 years). Mix together 10 drops of peppermint, and 5 drops each of myrtle, vetiver, ginger, and eucalyptus, and dilute 8 to 15 drops of this mixture in half a teaspoon of carrier oil, and then apply to the chest and upper back, 3 times daily (6–17 years).

Oral—Take 1 drop each of clove, vetiver, peppermint, oregano, and myrtle orally up to 3 times daily (6–17 years).

## UMBILICAL CORD INFECTION

Topical—Place a trace amount of tea tree on your fingertip (less than 1 drop) and apply this trace amount around the umbilical cord. Repeat the process with a trace amount of lavender on your fingertip. Repeat this process 2 times daily.

## URINARY TRACT INFECTION (UTI)

Topical—Mix together 10 drops of thyme, and 5 drops each of tea tree, bergamot, and German chamomile, then dilute 2 to 3 drops of this blend in half a teaspoon of carrier oil, and apply to the pelvic area and lower back (1–5 years). Use the same mixture and apply 3 to 5 drops diluted in half a teaspoon of carrier oil to the pelvic area and lower back (6–17 years).

Oral—Take 1 drop each of oregano, tea tree, lemon, and thyme orally up to 3 times daily (6–17 years).

## VOMITING

*See NAUSEA*

## WARTS (Non-plantar)

Topical— Mix together 10 drops each of oregano, and 5 drops of thyme, tea tree, clove, and lemon, and then use a cotton swab to apply 1 drop of this mixture neat to the wart, 1 to 3 times daily (1–17 years).

## WARTS (Seed)

*Warts that have little black dots in them, leading them to be called "seed warts." These warts don't truly have seeds. The black dots are tiny blood vessels that have grown up into the wart.*

Other—Apply a small piece of duct tape to the seed warts and replace each time it falls off until the seed wart falls off or seed falls out (1–17 years).

Topical—Mix together 10 drops each of oregano, and 5 drops of thyme, tea tree, clove, and lemon, and then use a cotton swab to apply 1 drop of this mixture neat to the wart, 1 to 3 times daily (1–17 years).

Homeopathic Remedies—Apply thuja ointment as directed on the product label.

## WHOOPING COUGH (Pertussis)

*Only use in conjunction with Western treatment options.*

Topical—Mix together 1 drop each of tea tree and lavender in 3 teaspoons of carrier oil and apply a small amount of this mixture to the chest and upper back, several times daily (birth–12 months). Mix together 1 drop each of sandalwood, myrtle, pine, and cypress in half a teaspoon of carrier oil and apply a small amount of this mixture to the chest and upper back, several times daily (1–5 years). Apply 1 drop of oregano, thyme, and clove in 10 to 15 drops of carrier oil to the bottoms of the feet up to 3 times daily (1 to 5 years). Mix together 1 to 3 drops each of eucalyptus, myrtle, basil, and peppermint in half a teaspoon of carrier oil and apply a small amount of this mixture to the chest and upper back, several times daily (6–17 years). Apply 1 drop of one of the above oils (within the appropriate age range) to chest area of the child's pajamas before going to bed.

Steam Inhalation—Add 1 drop each of tea tree and lavender to 1 pint of hot water and place near but out of reach of the infant, up to 3 times daily (birth–12 months). Add 1 to 2 drops each of sandalwood, myrtle, pine, and cypress to 1 pint of hot water and place near, but out of reach of the child, up to 3 times daily (1–5 years). Add 1 to 3 drops each of myrtle, eucalyptus, basil, and peppermint to 1 pint of hot water and place near the child up to 3 times daily (6–17 years).

Oral—Take 1 to 2 drops each of oregano, cinnamon, myrrh, and lemon orally up to 3 times daily (6–17 years). Create a cough syrup by adding 5 drops of lemon, and 3 drops each of German chamomile and tea tree to 1 cup of pure maple syrup and give 1 teaspoon of this mixture up to 3 times daily (6–17 years).

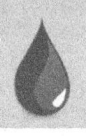 

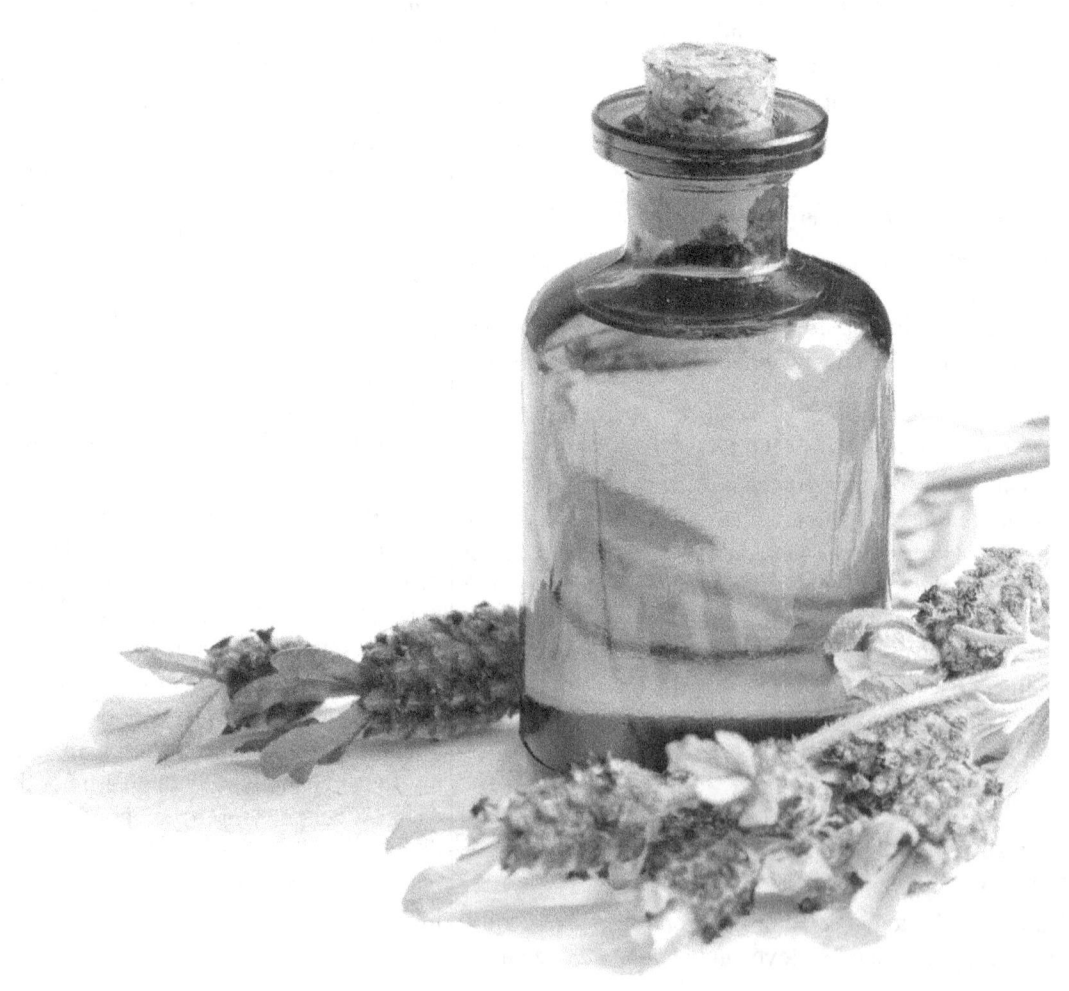

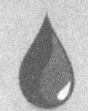

# ESSENTIAL OILS FOR PREGNANCY, LABOR, AND CHILDBIRTH

Pregnancy is an incredible journey filled with joy, delight, and happiness, but along with those pleasant experiences comes emotional challenges, adjustment, and discomfort. Many essential oils can be a vital part of pregnancy and reduce these unpleasant experiences of pregnancy and make the nine months more pleasurable. Empowered with a greater understanding of appropriate essential oils and their use during pregnancy and lactation, mothers can make informed decisions leading to a healthy pregnancy and happy baby.

Most expecting mothers want to take the utmost care for their precious growing baby, and therefore it is always wise to err on the side of caution when it comes to essential oils and pregnancy. The reality is that no mother in their right mind would sign up for an essential oil study that was designed to determine what essential oils, and at what dosage, harm could be caused to their developing baby. Because of this, our knowledge of what may harm fetuses and nursing babies must be inferred from animal studies and case studies of women who attempted to cause an abortion with essential oils. This book has gone to great effort to identify case studies and preclinical research suggesting that certain essential oils have the potential to cause harm to fetuses or nursing babies.

The composition of the essential oil and the method of administration determine the level of risk for an essential oil being used during pregnancy. Oral administration has the greatest potential for toxicity, followed by rectal, vaginal, and topical administration.

According to *The Merck Manual*, most substances with a molecular weight of less than 500 Daltons readily cross the placenta and enter the fetus's bloodstream.[10188] Since most common essential oil constituents are less than 225 Daltons, it is logical to suspect that essential oil molecules diffuse across the placenta similarly to the way they cross other epithelial barriers.

The greatest risk to a fetus from substances that cross the placenta is during the first trimester. Substances that are known to be toxic, cause abortions, or cause birth defects should be strictly avoided during this time.

The use of essential oils during pregnancy is a very controversial, hotly debated, and convoluted subject. There are hundreds of different opinions on which essential oils are safe to use and which are not during pregnancy. Frankly, very little clinical evidence exists that essential oils cause harm to the fetus, except in extreme cases (usually an intentional attempt to induce abortion with extreme amounts of oral ingestion). However, the safety of children and women who are pregnant is not something to take lightly.

The general rule among aromatherapists is that essential oils that are questionable during pregnancy should also be avoided or used cautiously during lactation. This may be conservative, but again, what is more precious than your family and children? The reasoning behind this contraindication is that most of the essential oils contraindicated during pregnancy have moderate toxicity potential, which could be detrimental to a breastfeeding infant. Research also suggests that trace amounts of essential oil constituents do transfer into human breast milk. Metabolites of 1,8-cineole were present in human breast milk at concentrations of traces to 250 mcg/kg after ingestion of 100 mg of this constituent, which can modify the aroma of breast milk.[10189,10190]

Another concern is the potential for essential oils to cause nipple aversion. It is possible that if essential oils are applied directly to the nipples or near the nipples the baby may not enjoy the smell or taste and refuse to latch. Essential oils should be applied away from the nipples to reduce this risk. However, this can be problematic if you are treating cracked nipples, so the best approach is to gently wipe off your nipples before feeding if you are using essential oils to relieve cracked nipples. The bottom line is we want to be cautious when it comes to breastfeeding infants.

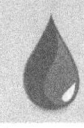 

The following table is meant to be used as a guide in conjunction with your healthcare practitioner's recommendation to determine which oils, if any, should be used during your pregnancy.

### Common Essential Oils to Avoid during Pregnancy and Lactation

Anise, applemint (pulegone CTs), auracaria, basil (methyl chavicol and methyl eugenol CTs), bay (West Indies), bay laurel, betony (bicyclogermacrene CT), birch, blue cypress (wood oil), boldo, buchu, calamus (various CTs), carrot seed, cassia, chaste tree, cinnamon bark, cinnamon leaf, clove, dill (with apiol), elecampane, fennel, Formosan cypress (twig oil), genipi, hairy basil (various CTs), hemp, holy basil (various CTs), hyssop (various CTs), juniper (Chinese), kumquat (linalool CT), ledum (*L. palustre*), lovage, mountain savory, mugwort, myrrh, nutmeg, oregano, parsley, pennyroyal, Ponderosa pine, ravensara (various CTs), rosalina (methyl eugenol CT), rue, sage, savin, savory (wild—carvacrol & thymol CTs), spearmint (pulegone-menthone-isomenthone CT), star anise, summer savory, tamala (various CTs), tansy, tarragon, thuja, western red cedar (leaves), white turmeric, wintergreen, wormseed (American), wormwood, and yarrow

### Common Carrier Oils to Avoid during Pregnancy and Lactation

Borage seed oil (oral), calendula (oral), evening primrose oil (oral)

### Common Essential Oils to Use Cautiously during Pregnancy and Lactation

Allspice, black cumin, black pepper (eugenol CT), blue spruce, camphor, citronella, feverfew, fingerroot ((E)-beta-ocimene and camphor CTs), honey myrtle, hops, hyssop (various CTs), Japanese cedarwood (bark), kanuka (37+ weeks), lemon basil, lemon catnip, lemon myrtle (citral CT), lemon tea tree, lemon verbena, lemongrass, manuka (37+ weeks), may chang, melissa, ocotea, ravintsara (camphor CT), rosemary (1,8-cineole, camphor CTs), Spanish sage, spike lavender, sweet wormwood, wild turmeric, verbena, white sage, white spruce, and white verbena (camphor CT)

### Preferred Essential Oils during the First Trimester

Balsam fir, bergamot, black pepper, cedarwood, chamomile (German, Roman), copaiba, coriander, cypress, frankincense, geranium, ginger, grapefruit, helichrysum, lavender, lemon, tea tree, myrtle, orange, neroli, patchouli, peppermint, petitgrain, pine, sandalwood, tangerine, vetiver, ylang ylang

### Preferred Essential Oils during the Second/Third Trimester and Lactation

Balsam fir, bergamot, black pepper, cedarwood, chamomile (German, Roman), clary sage, copaiba, coriander, cypress, eucalyptus (globulus, radiata), frankincense, geranium, ginger, grapefruit, helichrysum, juniper, lavender, lemon, tea tree, myrtle, orange, neroli, patchouli, peppermint*, petitgrain, pine, sandalwood, tangerine, thyme (linalool CT), vetiver, ylang ylang

### Preferred Carrier Oils during Pregnancy and Lactation

*Primary*: Sweet almond, apricot kernel, coconut, grapeseed, hazelnut, macadamia, peanut, safflower, sunflower, walnut

*Secondary (used in smaller quantities up to 20% of carrier oil total)*: Aloe vera, avocado, jojoba, olive, sesame, wheat germ

\* Some suggest that peppermint essential oil should be avoided during the last trimester and while lactating to reduce the risk of interfering with milk supply. A small number of lactating women have reported that their milk supply decreased when they used peppermint-containing products. However, clinical research using peppermint gel, peppermint water, or menthol essence on the breasts for nipple cracks and soreness during breastfeeding has not reported any adverse effect of this practice, including reduced milk supply.[10191,10192,10193] Based on the available research, it is reasonable to conclude that the topical application of diluted peppermint essential oil poses little risk of drying up milk supply during the third trimester. However, oral use may increase the risk of reducing milk supply in a small percentage of lactating women.

As a cautionary measure, it is suggested that the internal use of essential oils be avoided during the first trimester and that dilutions of no more than 3% be used topically, particularly among women with a prior history of miscarriage. As always, do not use the same oil or oils for more than 21 days without a break (or five to six days per week) to avoid sensitization and the remote possibility of tolerance buildup. Diffusion of the restricted oils during pregnancy and lactation may be safe (as it is the safest route of essential oil administration), but until this is proven definitively it may be wise to avoid diffusion of the questionable oils.

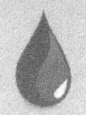

While I personally believe essential oils can be a wonderful part of a healthy pregnancy, the decision of which, if any, essential oils are appropriate for use during pregnancy ultimately remains solely with the mother-to-be and her OBGYN or other healthcare practitioner. ***Always consult your healthcare practitioner before using essential oils during pregnancy and while nursing.***

This resource is meant to provide options for you to discuss with your healthcare practitioner as you determine what is best for you and your treasured baby during this precious time of pregnancy.

| | Topical Dilution | Oral Maximum |
|---|---|---|
| *First Trimester* | 1.0%–3.0% <br><br> *1–4 drops of essential oil per teaspoon of carrier oil* | **Not recommended** |
| *Second & Third Trimester* | 1.0%–5.0% <br><br> *1–7 drops of essential oil per teaspoon of carrier oil* | **1–10 drops total daily,** which should be mild and preferred oils |

Unless otherwise indicated in this book or a published clinical study.

## HEALTH PROTOCOLS FOR GENERAL CONDITIONS OF PREGNANCY, LABOR, AND POST-PREGNANCY

### ALLERGIES (Hay Fever)

Topical—Apply 1 drop of lavender neat under the nose (on the upper lip) up to 3 times daily (all trimesters).

Oral—Take 1 drop each of lavender, peppermint, and German chamomile in a capsule up to 3 times daily (2nd/3rd trimester). Alternately, take a capsule with 1 drop each of peppermint, lemon, and lavender in a capsule up to 3 times daily (2nd/3rd trimester).

### ANXIETY

Topical—Mix together 1 drop each of lavender, orange, and cedarwood in 1 teaspoon of carrier oil and apply a small amount of this mixture to the base of the skull, neck, and wrists (all trimesters).

Oral—Take 1 capsule filled with 2 drops of lavender and 1 drop of orange 1 to 2 times daily (2nd/3rd trimesters).

Inhalation—Apply 1 drop each of cedarwood, orange, and lavender to a tissue or cotton ball and inhale as often as needed (all trimesters).

### BACKACHE

Topical—Mix together 2 drops each of lavender, ginger, copaiba, and German chamomile in 2 teaspoons of carrier oil and massage a small amount of this mixture (enough to cover the back or sore area) in to the back and feet, 2 times daily (all trimesters).

### BLEEDING
### (Reduce During Labor and Delivery)

Topical—Mix together 5 drops each of lavender, cypress, geranium, and helichrysum in 2 teaspoons of carrier oil and apply a small amount of this mixture to the lower back and insides of the ankles daily during the last 1 to 2 weeks of pregnancy (3rd trimester).

### BREASTFEEDING
*See LACTATION PROBLEMS*

### BREAST ABSCESS
*See MASTITIS*

### BREAST ENGORGEMENT

Topical—Mix together 2 drops each of lavender, geranium, cypress, and tangerine in 2 teaspoons of sesame seed carrier oil (or another suitable carrier oil) and apply enough of this mixture to cover the breast, gently massaging the mixture into the breast (all trimesters and post-pregnancy).

### BREAST TENDERNESS

Topical—Mix together 1 drops each of bergamot, geranium, and lavender in 1 teaspoon of carrier oil and apply enough of this mixture to cover the breast up to 3 times daily (1st trimester). Mix together 2 drops each of bergamot and geranium, and 1 drop of clary sage in 1 teaspoon of carrier oil and apply enough of this mixture to cover the breast up to 3 times daily (2nd/3rd trimesters).

### BREECH BABIES

Topical—Under the direction of your healthcare practitioner, apply 3–5 drops of peppermint diluted 25% to 50% to the top of the abdomen in an arcing motion.

### CAESAREAN SECTION SCARS

Topical—Mix together 1 drop each of frankincense, helichrysum, sandalwood, bergamot, and lavender in equal parts of carrier oil and apply a small amount of this mixture to the scars, 3 times daily. Apply the same mixture to the incision before scarring, but after the stitches have been removed.

## CERVICAL SCAR TISSUE, SOFTEN
Topical—Mix together 1 drop each of frankincense, lavender, and helichrysum in half teaspoon of carrier oil and apply a small amount of this mixture to the pubic area up to 3 times daily (all trimesters).

## COLDS/FLU
Oral—Take a capsule with 1 drop each of vetiver, lemon, and thyme up to 3 times daily (2nd/3rd trimester).

Topical—Massage 1 drop each of lemon, thyme, and tea tree in equal parts carrier oil to the feet up to 3 times daily (all trimesters). Mix together 1 drop each of myrtle, pine, and ginger in half a teaspoon of carrier oil and apply a small amount of this mixture to the upper chest and back up to 3 times daily (all trimesters).

Inhalation—Add 1 to 2 drops each of myrtle, eucalyptus, and pine to 1 cup of hot water and inhale up to 3 times daily (all trimesters).

## CONGESTION
Inhalation—Add 1 to 2 drops each of myrtle, eucalyptus, and pine to 1 cup of hot water and inhale up to 3 times daily (all trimesters).

Topical—Mix together 1 drop each of myrtle, pine, and ginger in half a teaspoon of carrier oil and apply a small amount of this mixture to the upper chest, back, and a trace amount across the bridge of the nose up to 3 times daily (all trimesters).

## CONSTIPATION
Oral—Take 2 drops of ginger and 1 drop of lemon orally up to 3 times daily (2nd/3rd trimesters).

Topical—Mix together 1 drop each of lemon and ginger in 1 teaspoon of carrier oil and apply a small amount of this mixture to the lower back and the abdomen in a clockwise direction up to 5 times daily (all trimesters).

## CRACKED NIPPLES
Topical—Mix together 1 400–500 mg capsule of marshmallow root herb, 2 drops each of lavender and chamomile (German or Roman), 1 drop each of helichrysum and peppermint (omit peppermint if you know it decreases your milk supply) in 10 mL of coconut oil and 5 mL of moringa fixed oil (use 15 mL of coconut if moringa is not available) and apply enough of the mixture to cover the nipple and areola up to three times daily. Gently wipe the nipples before nursing.

## CRAMPS, LEG
Topical—Mix together 1 drop each of cypress, grapefruit, bergamot, lavender, and geranium in 1 teaspoon of carrier oil and apply to the legs morning and night (all trimesters).

## CYSTITIS (Urinary Tract Infection)
See **URINARY TRACT INFECTION**

## DEPRESSION (During Pregnancy)
Inhalation—Place 1 drop each of orange, frankincense, and ylang ylang on a tissue or cotton ball and inhale as necessary (all trimesters). A few drops of these oils can also be added to a diffuser.

Topical—Massage 3 drops of orange oil to the feet in equal parts of carrier oil, morning and evening (all trimesters).

## DEPRESSION, POSTPARTUM
Other—Discuss the possibility of a natural bioidentical progesterone or molecular progesterone complex with your healthcare professional and use as directed.

Inhalation—Apply 1 drop of frankincense, ylang ylang, orange, or grapefruit to palms, rub together, and place over nose and mouth to inhale as needed. Alternately, place 1 drop of each on a tissue or cotton ball and inhale as needed throughout the day.

Topical—Apply 1 to 2 drops each of geranium, marjoram, and thyme diluted in half a teaspoon of carrier oil over the liver at night.

## DIABETES, GESTATIONAL
Oral—With your healthcare practitioner's approval, take a capsule with 2 drops of geranium, morning and evening (2nd/3rd trimester).

## DIZZINESS
Inhalation—Place 1 drop each of peppermint and cypress on a tissue or cotton ball and inhale as often as necessary (all trimesters).

Topical—Mix together 1 drop each of peppermint, frankincense, and cypress in 1 teaspoon of carrier oil and apply a small amount of this mixture to the temples, back of the neck, and shoulders up to 3 times daily (all trimesters).

## EDEMA (Swelling)
Oral—Take 1 drop each of grapefruit, lemon, and cypress in a capsule up to 3 times daily (2nd/3rd trimesters).

Topical—Massage 1 drop each of grapefruit, lemon, and cypress in a teaspoon of carrier oil to affected area in strokes toward the heart, 1 to 3 times daily (all trimesters).

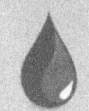

Other—Drink at least half of your body weight of water in ounces daily.

## ENDOMETRIOSIS

Other—Ask your healthcare practitioner about the use of a bioidentical progesterone or molecular progesterone complex product.

Topical—Mix together 2 drops each of lavender, geranium, copaiba, and cypress in 1 to 2 teaspoons of carrier oil and apply a small amount of this mixture to the lower abdomen, followed by a warm towel, up to 3 times daily (all trimesters).

Oral—Take a capsule filled with 2 drops of copaiba and 1 drop of bergamot, 1 to 2 times daily.

## ENERGY BOOST DURING LABOR

Topical—Place 2 to 3 drops of peppermint oil in 1 cup of cool water and dip a clean cloth in this mixture. Apply to the back of the neck, refreshing regularly.

Inhalation—Place 2 drops of peppermint and 1 drop each of lemon and orange on a tissue or cotton ball and inhale as necessary. This mixture can also be diffused.

## FATIGUE

Inhalation—Place 1 drop of peppermint or lemon neat on palm and rub palms together, cup over nose and mouth, and breathe deeply up to 3 times daily (all trimesters). Alternately, 1 drop of each of these oils can be placed on a tissue or cotton ball and inhaled as necessary (all trimesters).

Other—Take an aromatic bath with 2 drops each of bergamot, orange, and tangerine in one teaspoon of carrier oil added to warm water (all trimesters).

## FEAR

Inhalation—Place 1 drop each of ylang ylang, frankincense, and lavender on a tissue or cotton ball and inhale as needed (all trimesters).

## FLATULENCE

Topical—Mix 2 drops each of lemon and lavender in 1 teaspoon of carrier oil and apply to the abdomen in a clockwise direction (all trimesters).

## FLU
See *COLDS/FLU*

## FLUID RETENTION
See *EDEMA (SWELLING)*

## GASTROESOPHAGEAL REFLUX DISEASE (GERD, Acid Reflux)
See *HEARTBURN*

## GROUP B STREP (After positive test to reduce transmission to baby)

Oral—Take a capsule with 2 drops each of lavender and lemon, and 1 drop of thyme, 2 times daily (3rd trimester). Retention—Soak a tampon in 2 drops each of lemon and lavender, and 1 drop of thyme, and 1 tablespoon of carrier oil and insert in the vagina. Leave overnight and remove in the morning, for 7 days (3rd trimester).

## HEADACHE

Topical—Mix together 1 drop each of peppermint, German chamomile, and lavender in half a teaspoon of carrier oil and apply a small amount of this mixture to the temples, forehead, and back of the neck up to 3 times daily (all trimesters).

## HEARTBURN

Oral—Take 1 drop each of lemon, orange, and ginger orally up to 3 times daily (2nd/3rd trimesters).

Topical—Mix together 2 drops each of ginger and lemon in 1 teaspoon of carrier oil and apply a small amount of this mixture on the upper chest (all trimesters).

## HEMORRHOIDS

Topical—Mix together 1 drop each of lavender, cypress, and tea tree in 10 to 20 drops of carrier oil and apply a drop of this mixture to the painful area, several times daily (all trimesters).

## HIGH BLOOD PRESSURE

Inhalation—Place 1 drop each of neroli, ylang ylang, and lavender on a tissue or cotton ball and inhale regularly (all trimesters).

Oral—Take a capsule filled with 1 drop each of lavender, ylang ylang, and bergamot, 2 times daily (2nd/3rd trimester).

## HYPOTHYROIDISM

Topical—Mix together 2 drops of balsam fir and 1 drop of myrtle in half a teaspoon of carrier oil and apply over the throat and breastbone area up to 3 times daily (all trimesters).

## INDUCING LABOR

*Only to be used after the 39th week of pregnancy and with your health care practitioner's approval.*

Oral—Take 60 mL of castor oil in 8 ounces of juice once (may cause diarrhea, nausea, and vomiting).[2399]

Inhalation—Place 5 drops of clary sage on a tissue or cotton ball and inhale regularly (can also be placed under your pillow at night).

## LACTATION PROBLEMS (INCREASING MILK SUPPLY)

Topical—Mix together 1 to 2 drops each of geranium and basil (linalool CT) in half a teaspoon of carrier oil and apply to the breast away from the nipple (between nursing sessions) and on the bottoms of the feet, 1 to 3 times daily. Fennel may also be considered for short periods of time (3 to 5 days), but only if geranium and basil (linalool CT) are ineffective. If fennel is required, mix 2 drops of fennel in one teaspoon of carrier oil and apply a small amount of this mixture after each nursing away from the nipple area. Do not apply these oils where the infant will potential ingest them while nursing, and wipe your breast clean before nursing.

## LACTATION PROBLEMS (DECREASING MILK SUPPLY)

Oral—Take a capsule filled with 2 drops each of peppermint and oregano, 1 to 3 times daily. Alternately, drink one cup of herbal sage tea every 6 hours.

Topical—Cover the breasts with raw cold cabbage leaves by placing them inside your bra. Leave them in place for a couple of hours.

## LABOR PROTOCOLS

*With the exception of the preterm labor protocol, the labor protocols are meant to relax the mother, aid coping ability, ease pain and discomfort, and support normal contractions and transitions through the various stages of labor.*

## LABOR, PRETERM

*Contact your physician, especially labor prior to 37 weeks gestation.*

Topical—Apply 3 to 5 drops of lavender diluted in 10 to 20 drops of carrier oil to the abdomen and pubic area every 8 hours until preterm labor stops (all trimesters).

## LABOR, EARLY STAGES

Topical—Massage the feet and lower back with a mixture of 2 drops each of lavender, tangerine, and copaiba in 1 teaspoon of carrier oil.

Other—Soak a large cloth in 1 cup of warm water and 2 drops each of clary sage, tangerine, and lavender, then wring out, and apply this cloth to the lower back and abdomen. Repeat as needed. Take an aromatic bath with 2 drops each of lavender and cedarwood in half a teaspoon of carrier oil added to the water.

## LABOR, ACTIVE/TRANSITION

Topical—Soak a small towel in cool water and 2 drops each of neroli, lavender, and tangerine, then wring out, and gently wipe forehead, face, neck, arms and any other areas that she desires.

## LABOR, PUSHING

Inhalation—Place 2 drops each of lavender and neroli on a tissue or cotton ball (can be pinned to a bra) and inhale between each contraction. Alternate with another tissue or cotton ball that has 3 drops each of tangerine, orange, and lemon.

## LABOR, PLACENTAL DELIVERY

Topical—Soak a cloth in 2 drops each of lavender and geranium and 1 cup of warm water, then wring out, and apply to the lower abdomen. Cover with a warm towel. Replace each time the cloth cools.

## LEG PAIN (Leg Labor)

Topical—Mix together 1 drop each of lavender, ginger, German chamomile, peppermint, and frankincense in half a teaspoon of carrier oil and apply a small amount of this mixture to the affected area up to 4 times daily (3rd trimester).

## MASTITIS

Topical—Massage a mixture of 2 to 3 drops of tea tree, thyme, and frankincense in 1 teaspoon of carrier oil on the breast and armpits, 1 to 3 times daily; cover with a warm compress after application.

## MENSTRUAL-TYPE CRAMPING

Topical—Mix together 2 drops each of chamomile, lavender, geranium, and frankincense in 2 teaspoons of carrier oil and apply a small amount of this mixture to the lower abdomen up to 3 times daily (all trimesters).

Other—Place 2 drops each of chamomile and frankincense in a capsule (fill the rest of the capsule with olive or coconut oil) and insert the capsule as far back in the vagina as possible nightly until cramping subsides or after 7 days (all trimesters).

## MISCARRIAGE

Topical—If your doctor informs you that you are having a miscarriage, apply 2 to 3 drops of clary sage in equal parts of carrier oil to the lower abdomen to support passing tissue. Apply 1 to 2 drops each of marjoram, basil (linalool CT), and lavender in equal parts carrier oil to the abdomen for pain.

Inhalation—Place 1 to 2 drops each of lavender, bergamot, orange, and ylang ylang on a tissue or cotton ball and inhale as needed.

## MORNING SICKNESS

*See NAUSEA, MORNING SICKNESS*

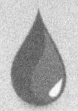

## MUSCLE CRAMPS

Topical—Mix together 1 drop each of lavender, balsam fir, and German chamomile in 1 teaspoon of carrier oil and massage a small amount of this mixture into the muscle up to 3 times daily (all trimesters).

## MUSCLES, SORE

Topical—Mix together 1 to 2 drops each of lavender, ginger, and copaiba in 1 teaspoon of carrier oil and massage a small amount of this mixture into sore muscle(s) up to 3 times daily (all trimesters).

## MUSCLE SPASMS

Topical—Mix together 1 drop each of lavender, petitgrain, and ginger in 1 teaspoon of carrier oil and apply a small amount of this mixture to the affected area up to 3 times daily (1st trimester). Mix together 2 drops each of ginger and lavender, and 1 drop of petitgrain and apply a small amount of this mixture to the affected area up to 3 times daily (2nd/3rd trimesters).

## NASAL CONGESTION

Inhalation—Place 1 to 2 drops each of eucalyptus, lavender, and peppermint in 1 cup of hot water and inhale from the bowl for 10 to 15 minutes up to 3 times daily (all trimesters).

## NAUSEA, MORNING SICKNESS

Inhalation—Place 1 to 2 drops each of peppermint, lemon, and ginger on a tissue or cotton ball and inhale as necessary. Refresh the tissue every 4 hours (all trimesters).
Topical—Mix together 1 drop each of peppermint, lemon, and ginger in 1 teaspoon of carrier oil and apply a small amount of this mixture behind the ears and 1 drop of this mixture in the navel (all trimesters).
Oral—Take 1 drop each of ginger and peppermint in a capsule up to 3 times daily (2nd/3rd trimesters).
Other—Apply firm pressure to a point on your wrist that is three of your finger widths below the wrist and between your two arm bones, several times daily (all trimesters). Make sure to eat a high-protein meal at night.

## NIPPLES (SORE)

Topical—Mix together 2 drops of lavender in 1 teaspoon of carrier oil and apply to the nipples up to 3 times daily. Wipe off before breastfeeding (all trimesters and lactation).

## PALPITATIONS (Heart)

Topical—Mix together 2 drops each of lavender, ylang ylang, and neroli in 1 teaspoon of carrier oil and apply a small amount of this mixture over the heart up to 3 times daily (all trimesters).

## PELVIC PRESSURE

Oral—Take a capsule with 2 drops each of copaiba and tangerine up to 2 times daily (2nd/3rd trimester).
Topical—Mix together 1 drop each of copaiba, tangerine, peppermint, and German chamomile in 1 teaspoon of carrier oil and apply a small amount of this mixture to the pelvic area up to 3 times daily.

## PERINEAL CARE (During Birth)

Topical—Apply a mixture of 1 drop of helichrysum with 10 drops of carrier oil to the perineum while pushing and during crowning.

## PERINEAL CARE (Prior to Delivery)

Topical—To increase the elasticity of the perineum (the area between the anus and vagina that is often cut or torn during delivery) before delivery, mix together 2 drops each of sandalwood, lavender, chamomile, and orange in 1 teaspoon of carrier oil and apply a small amount of this mixture to the perineum and lower part of the vagina daily during the last 6 weeks of your pregnancy (3rd trimester).

## PERINEAL CARE (After Delivery)

Other—Mix together 5 drops each of lavender, neroli, grapefruit, tangerine, orange, and chamomile. Take a sitz bath by filling an ordinary bathtub with enough water to cover the hips and genital area, and then add 3 to 4 drops of the above mixture in equal parts carrier oil to the bath and soak.
Topical—Mix together 5 drops each of lavender, neroli, tangerine, helichrysum, chamomile, and geranium in 1 ounce of organic aloe vera juice and place this mixture in a spray bottle. Spray the vaginal and perineal area after each use of the toilet and as often as desired for soothing comfort.

## POSTPARTUM HEMORRHAGE

*This can be a life-threatening situation. Seek medical care immediately.*
Topical—Apply 1 to 2 drops each of helichrysum, geranium, and cypress over the lower back and lower abdomen on route to medical care.

## PUBIC DIASTASIS

Topical—Mix together 2 drops of balsam fir, and 1 drop each of copaiba and pine in 1 teaspoon of carrier oil and apply a small amount of this to the pubic bones up to 3 times daily (all trimesters).

## REST, PROMOTE DURING LABOR

Inhalation—Place 2 drops each of lavender and cedarwood, and 1 drop of vetiver on a tissue or cotton ball and place near to inhale.

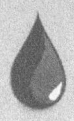

Topical—Massage 1 drop of lavender and 10 drops of carrier oil to the shoulders and upper back every 2 to 4 hours.

## ROUND LIGAMENT PAIN
Topical—Mix together 1 drop each of peppermint, lavender, frankincense, and ginger in 1 teaspoon of carrier oil and apply a small amount of this mixture to the lower abdomen and pelvic area up to 3 times daily (2nd/3rd trimesters).

## SCIATIC PAIN
Other—Lie on your side and have another person apply pressure to acupressure point GB30, which can be found on the side of the buttocks by locating approximately the middle of the sacrum, and then moving out two-thirds of the way toward the hip. Apply firm pressure to this point (left or right side 1 at a time) with your thumb for about 30 seconds, and then release. Repeat this process until pain is relieved. Then repeat the entire process on the other side.

Topical—Mix together 2 drops each of vetiver, German chamomile, geranium, and copaiba in 2 teaspoons of sesame seed oil (or another suitable carrier oil) and apply some of this mixture to the lower back, hip area and down the leg up to 3 times daily.

## SHORTNESS OF BREATH
Topical—Apply 2 drops of frankincense in a teaspoon of carrier oil to the upper chest and back, 2 times daily (all trimesters).

## SKIN BLEMISHES
Topical—Mix together 2 drops each of tea tree, thyme, orange, lavender, and frankincense in 3 teaspoons of carrier oil and apply a very small amount of this mixture to the blemish, morning and evening (all trimesters).

## SLEEP PROBLEMS
Topical—Mix together 5 drops each of lavender, chamomile, and cedarwood and 2 drops of vetiver. Then massage 1 drop of this blend mixed in 5 drops of carrier oil to the bottom of each foot before retiring to bed (all trimesters).

## STRETCH MARKS
Topical—Mix together 3 drops each of frankincense, lemon, sandalwood, and lavender in 2 tablespoons of coconut oil, 2 teaspoons of coconut oil, and 1 teaspoon of avocado oil, and then gently apply a small amount of this mixture to the abdomen and hips daily (2nd/3rd trimesters).

## TOXEMIA
Topical—Mix together 1 to 2 drops each of cypress, lavender, and ylang ylang in a teaspoon of carrier oil and apply to the ankles with massage strokes from the extremities to the middle of the body daily (all trimesters).

Oral—Take a capsule filled with 1 drop each of grapefruit, lemon, and ylang ylang, 1 to 3 times daily (2nd/3rd trimesters).

## URINARY TRACT INFECTION (UTI)
Topical— Mix together 10 drops of thyme, and 5 drops each of tea tree, bergamot, and German chamomile, then dilute 3 to 5 drops of this blend in 1 teaspoon of carrier oil, and apply to the pelvic area and lower back (all trimesters).

Oral—Take 1 drop each of geranium, lemon, and thyme orally, 2 times daily (2nd/3rd trimesters).

Other—Drink at least half your body weight in ounces daily. Take a multistrain probiotic, 4 times daily. Drink two 8-ounce glasses of unsweetened cranberry or blueberry juice daily for 3 to 5 days.

## URINATION (Trouble After Birth)
Other—Place 1 drop of peppermint in the toilet or other urine collecting water before sitting over water to urinate.

Topical—Apply 1 to 2 drops of juniper in 5 drops of carrier oil over the pelvic area.

Inhalation—Place 1 drop each of lavender and orange on a tissue and inhale regularly to calm the body.

## UTERUS, HYPERSTIMULATED
Topical—Apply 3 drops of lavender and 2 drops of orange oil in 10 drops of carrier oil to the lower abdomen and pubic area (all trimesters).

## VAGINA, INFLAMMATION OF
Topical—Mix together 1 drop each of chamomile, lavender, copaiba, and bergamot in 1 teaspoon of carrier oil and apply a small amount of this mixture to the vagina up to 3 times daily (all trimesters).

## VAGINAL YEAST INFECTION
Retention—Soak a tampon in 3 drops each of lavender and tea tree, 1 drop each of thyme and bergamot, and 1 tablespoon of carrier oil and insert in the vagina. Leave in overnight and remove in the morning for 7 days (2nd/3rd trimester).

Other—Take an aromatic bath with 2 drops each of tea tree, bergamot, and lavender in half a teaspoon of carrier oil added to warm bath water (1st trimester).

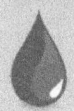

## VARICOSE VEINS

Topical—Mix together 1 to 2 drops each of helichrysum, lemon, geranium, and cypress mixed in 2 teaspoons of grapeseed carrier oil and massage to the areas around the varicose veins (not directly on them) with massage strokes toward the direction of the heart, 1 to 3 times daily.

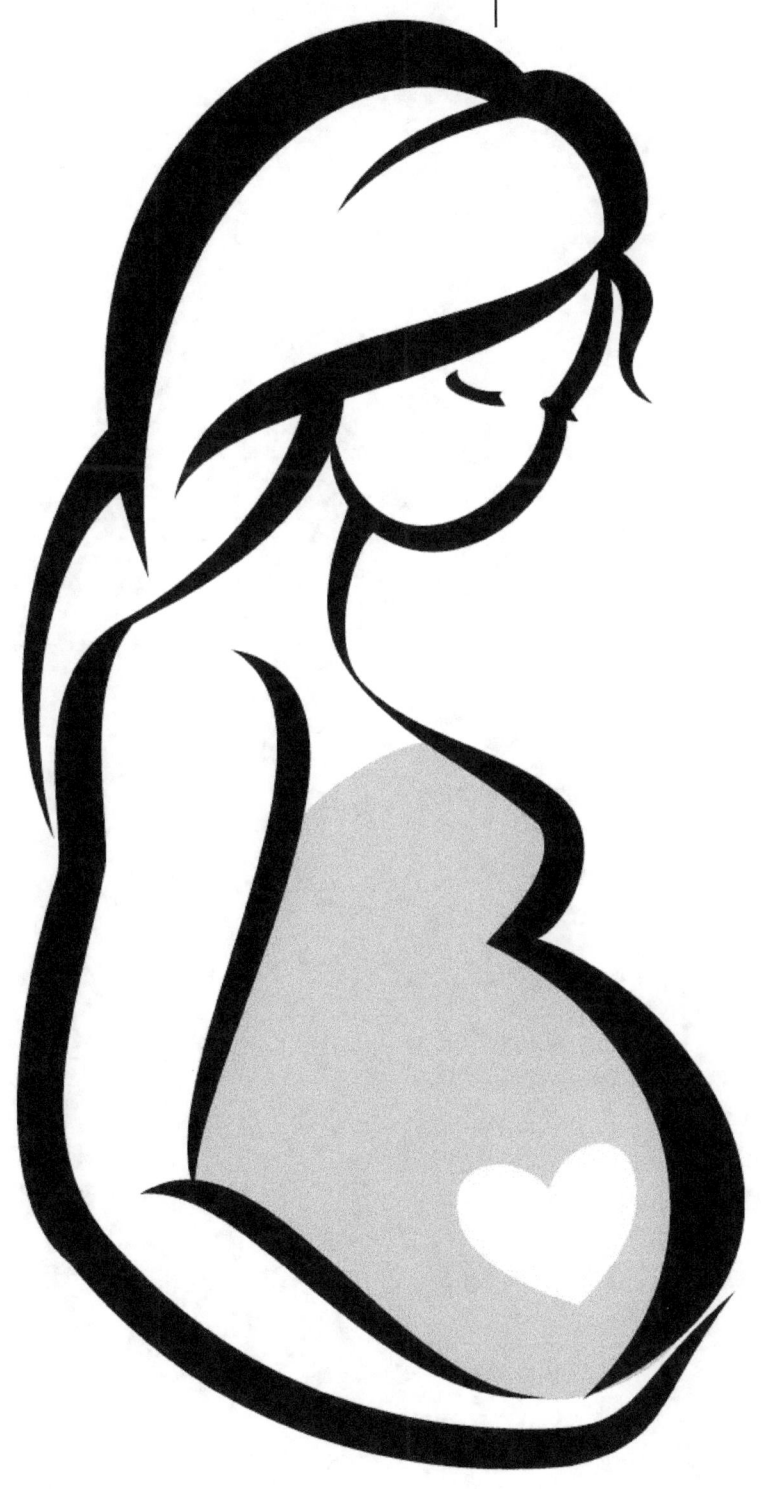

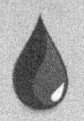

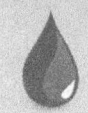

# ESSENTIAL OILS & CANCER

Cancer is a group of over 100 related diseases that takes the lives of an estimated 8.2 million people each year. It affects young and old, men and women, people of all races, and regrettably even children. Most people, especially those in industrialized nations, will be affected by cancer in some way during their lifetime, whether personally or through a friend or loved one. Because of this, cancer is a large focus of today's scientific research, and some of this research is uncovering the remarkable ability of natural products to prevent and treat cancer, including essential oils.

## FOUR STAGES OF CARCINOGENESIS

*Initiation.* A cancer-causing substance (carcinogen) from within or outside the body interacts with DNA to cause an adduct (a segment of DNA binds to the cancer-causing substance, which may cause an incorrect base to be incorporated into the genome of next generation cells) or break (severing of the DNA double helix, which can cause genetic rearrangements). This leads to irreversible changes in the genetic material of a normal target stem cell, and gives this cell immortality.

*Promotion.* Cells acquire genetic features of the cancerous cell, which allows cells that have undergone initiation to become cancerous when exposed to certain microenvironmental factors (i.e. growth factors, cytokines, suppressed immune system, and certain substances—cigarette smoke, alcohol, amines, saccharin, hormones, and mycotoxins).

*Malignant Conversion.* Preneoplastic cells (preceding the formation of abnormal tissue growth—benign or cancerous) transform into cells that are cancerous. Additional genetic changes beyond those that occur during the initial stages is required for malignant conversion to occur. Malignant conversion can be accelerated if preneoplastic cells are exposed to a carcinogenic substance.

*Progression.* The tumor becomes more aggressive and is more likely to spread, rather than remain localized and benign, due to the continuing development of unstable chromosomes.

All types of cancer involve the uncontrolled division and growth of cells. Everyone has cells inside their body that have mutant proteins caused by DNA damage. The immune system usually keeps them from becoming cancerous through checkpoints that determine whether the cell is healthy and should divide, or is damaged and requires repair or destruction. Protective proteins trigger tumor suppression and stop potential cancers by detecting and destroying damaged cells. These damaged cells inside all of us become cancerous when the immune system is overwhelmed or "tricked", or by certain triggers (i.e. toxins, environmental exposures, diet, or activity level). Unhealthy cells start dividing and replicating when this occurs. Therefore, an intact immune system is critical to prevent cancer.

Normally, human cells grow and divide to form new cells only when the body needs them. This process of replacing old or damaged cells with new cells happens in an orderly manner. Cancer occurs when this organized process is disrupted and damaged or abnormal cells survive when they should die, and new cells form unnecessarily. These extra cells then divide uncontrollably, which may lead to the formation of tumors (growths). Leukemias (cancers of the blood) generally do not form solid tumors.

According to the stem cell theory of cancer, small populations of cancerous stem cells allow cancer to survive in the body. A cancer stem cell is defined by the Association for Cancer Research (ACR) as a cell within a tumor that possesses the capacity to self-renew and produce descendants that become the cancer cells that comprise the tumor. The source of these cells is not defined by the ACR, but they could theoretically originate from stem (cells that can develop into and replenish many types of cells and essentially divide

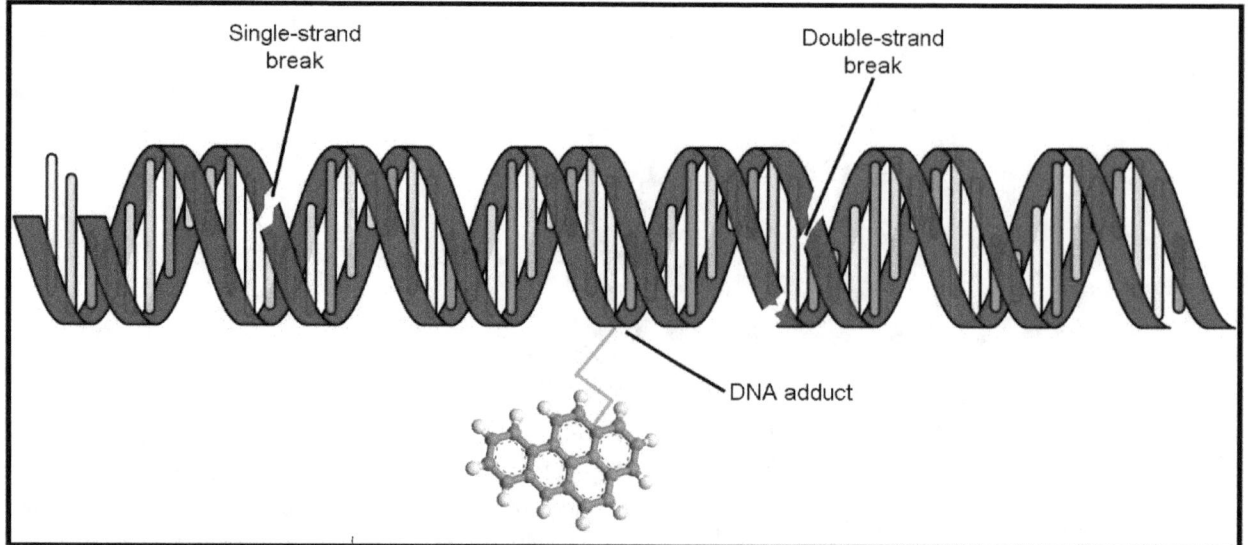

without limit as long as the person remains alive), progenitor (early descendants of stem cells that can develop into many types of cells, but cannot divide and reproduce indefinitely), or differentiated cells (specialized cells that are committed to a specific function and form different tissues and organs).[5009] As such these cells may be called tumor-promoting cells or cancer-initiating cells instead. It has been well-established that these tumor-initiating cells possess sufficiently similar characteristics and properties to stem cells to warrant a comparison.[10194] This theory proposes that of all of the cancerous cells in the body a few act as stem cells that reproduce themselves and sustain the cancer in the body much the same way healthy stem cells renew and sustain healthy organs and tissues. This has significant implications for cancer treatment and the ability of the cancer to spread.

Cancer cells are different from normal healthy cells in many ways. First, they are less specialized than normal cells. Normal cells mature (differentiate) into very specific cells with well-defined functions, whereas cancer cells do not become specialized cells. Second, cancer cells are able to disregard cellular signals that instruct cells to stop dividing or begin the process of programmed cell death (apoptosis). Cancer cells also influence their microenvironment (other nearby cells, molecules, and tissues) differently. For example, they could trigger normal cells to create blood vessels to supply oxygen and nutrients to the cancerous tumor (called angiogenesis). Another way cancer cells are different from normal cells is their ability to evade detection by the immune system. The immune system is a complex network of specialized cells, organs, and tissues designed to protect the body from harmful and invasive organisms. It normally detects and removes damaged or abnormal cells, but some cancer cells are able to "hide" from the immune system and therefore spread rapidly without being detected. Cancer cells also somewhat "hijack" the immune system to stay alive and grow. They may use immune cells that normally prevent abnormal immune responses to keep the immune system from destroying them. It is clear that a number of mechanisms must be considered when attacking cancerous cells.

While cancer is genetic—arising from genes that control the way our cells function—it is largely caused by preventable reasons such as diet, activity level, smoking, and environmental exposures. Cancer cells will generally have more genetic alterations, like DNA mutations, than normal cells. These genetic changes to proto-oncogenes (genes involved in normal cell growth and division), tumor suppressor genes, and DNA repair genes trigger cancer. Alterations (mutations) to proto-oncogenes (HER-2, RAS, MYC, SRC, hTERT) can allow cells to survive that should be destroyed. In this case, they become oncogenes, or genes that produce cancer cells, which do not stop at cell checkpoints that are designed to detect abnormal cells. Tumor suppressor genes (p53, Rb, APC) also participate in regulating cell growth and division. When these genes are altered, uncontrolled growth and division can occur. DNA repair genes (BRCA1, BRCA2) are responsible for repairing damage to DNA. DNA errors are not corrected, allowing subsequent DNA mutations to accumulate when their function is altered.

Cancer can occur virtually anywhere among the body's trillions of cells. Cancerous tumors are malignant, meaning they can spread to nearby tissues and potentially travel to other places in the body through the blood and lymph system to form additional tumors. This is called metastasis. Metastatic cancers retain the same name as the original cancer. For instance, if cancer originated in the breast and forms a metastatic tumor in

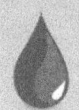

the liver, it is called metastatic breast cancer, not liver cancer.

Cancer may also be described by the type of cell that formed them. Here are some categories of cancers based on the cell that formed them:

- *Astrocytoma.* A brain tumor that begins in the star-shaped brain cells called astrocytes, which are a type of glial cell and the most numerous non-neuronal cells in the central nervous system. They serve to keep neurons healthy and functioning optimally.
- *Carcinoma.* Formed by epithelial (cells that cover the inside and outside surfaces of the body) cells, carcinomas are the most common type of cancer. They can be further divided into: 1) adenocarcinoma—cancer formed in the epithelial cells that produce fluids or mucus; 2) basal cell carcinoma—cancer formed in the lower layer of the epidermis; 3) squamous cell carcinoma—cancer formed in the squamous cells (epithelial cells just beneath the outer layer of the skin); and 4) transitional cell carcinoma—cancer formed in the transitional epithelium (tissue made of multiple layers found in organ linings).
- *Ependymoma.* Cancer that begins in the cells that line the fluid-filled spaces of the central nervous system.
- *Glioblastoma.* A fast-growing and spreading brain tumor that arises from astrocytes. This is a difficult brain tumor to treat because they are highly malignant and supported by a large network of blood vessels.
- *Glioma.* Cancer that begins in glial cells (cells that surround and support nerve cells) and can occur in the brain, brain stem, or spinal column.
- *Leukemia.* Cancers that start in the blood-forming tissue of the bone marrow that produce large quantities of abnormal white blood cells. This increase in abnormal white blood cells overcomes normal cells and can reduce oxygen supply to tissues, reduce clotting, and decrease immune activity.
- *Lymphoma.* Cancer that starts in the lymphocytes (white blood cells—T or B cells—that fight disease) and causes an increase of abnormal cells in the lymph nodes, lymph vessels, and other organs of the body.
- *Medulloblastoma.* A fast-growing brain tumor that forms in the cerebellum (the lower, rear portion of the brain) that occurs most commonly in children.
- *Melanoma.* Cancer that forms in the cells that develop into melanocytes (specialized cells that produce skin pigment called melanin).

- *Multiple myeloma.* Beginning in the plasma cells (white blood cells that secrete antibodies), multiple myeloma causes the accumulation of abnormal cells in the bone marrow and form tumors in bones throughout the body.
- *Neuroblastoma.* A type of cancer that starts in the very early forms of nerve cells that commonly affects children and infants. It frequently occurs in and around the adrenal glands.
- *Oligodendroglialtumor.* Rare brain tumors that begin in the oligodendrocytes (cells that cover and protect nerve cells in the central nervous system) of the brain.
- *Sarcoma.* Cancers that form in bone and soft tissues (muscle, fat, lymph and blood vessels, tendons, and ligaments).

## STAGES OF CANCER

Cancer staging describes the cancer location, whether or where it has spread (metastasized), and if it is affecting other parts of the body. If a cancer returns or spreads the stage doesn't change, it retains the same stage as the first diagnosis and more recent information regarding the size and spread of the cancer is added to the stage.

*Staging*

- **Tumor (T).** The letter "T" plus a number (0–4) describes the location and size of the tumor. A higher number indicates a larger tumor or one that has spread more deeply into nearby tissue.
- **Node (N).** The letter "N" plus a number (0–3) describes whether the cancer has been found in the lymph nodes. The higher the number the more lymph nodes that are involved.
- **Metastasis (M).** Whether the tumor has spread to other parts of the body is indicated by the letter "M." M0 means the cancer hasn't spread. M1 means the cancer has spread.

*Stage Grouping*

- **Stage 0.** Cancer that has not spread from its original location (*in situ*).
- **Stage I.** A small cancer or tumor that hasn't grown deeply into nearby tissues.
- **Stage II and III.** Larger cancers or tumors that have grown deeply into nearby tissue; may have also spread to lymph nodes.
- **Stage IV.** Cancer has spread to other organs or parts of the body; also called metastatic or advanced cancer.

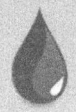

*Recovery Probability/Prognostics*

- **Grade.** The degree to which cancer cells look like healthy cells under a microscope and its likelihood to spread. Well-differentiated (low-grade) tumor cells look more like healthy cells and tend to grow and spread more slowly; whereas poorly differentiated (high-grade, undifferentiated) look less like healthy cells and grow and spread more rapidly.
- **Tumor markers.** Substances found at higher than normal levels in the blood, urine, or body tissues in some people with cancer.
- **Tumor genetics.** Genetic markers that help predict the risk of cancer metastasis and what treatments may work for the cancer.

Conventional Western treatment for cancer often involves chemotherapy, radiation, immunotherapy, or surgery to remove the tumor. While these treatment options are effective for some cancers, they are not completed without serious risks and side effects. When you consider that some researchers estimate that up to ninety percent of all cancers are caused by lifestyle and environmental factors,[5011] a disproportionate amount of time and research is dedicated to profitable drugs rather than promoting preventive measures. Let's address the elephant in the room. Cancer is huge money for drug companies, hospitals, and even physicians. The average annual cost of treating cancer in a single individual with drugs is estimated to exceed $100,000.[10195] The attractive profits even caused a Detroit-area physician, Dr. Farid Fata, to give chemotherapy drugs to patients who didn't need them—including some who didn't even have cancer. For-profit cancer centers aggressively advertise their services to the public seeking their piece of the windfall profits available in the cancer industry. Drug companies' mark up cancer drugs thousands of percent to hospitals, who mark up the drug hundreds of percent to the patient. Highly lucrative revenues from cancer drugs have led to patients being profit centers, not people, and it is costing human lives. The cancer industry has been hijacked and money is driving the industry, not people's health.

Chemotherapy is an invasive and toxic regimen of drugs that is intended to kill cancer cells. Unfortunately, chemotherapy drugs are not able to differentiate between healthy cells/tissues and cancer cells/tissues. This leads to the destruction of healthy cells and tissues by degrees, and those healthy cells that are not killed may be damaged or toxified. It also attacks the immune system, which is vital to fighting cancer. This toxic therapy can produce results because the drugs perform their function of killing cells very well. However, tumor shrinkage is not necessarily killing the cancer itself. Chemotherapy only kills the daughter cells (either of the two cells formed when a cell divides by mitosis) of cancer-initiating cells and not the cancer-initiating cells themselves, and even worse, research suggests both chemotherapy and radiotherapy creates cancer stem cells.[5012,5013] So while the chemotherapy can shrink the tumor, it causes a more aggressive and malignant tumor to form from the cancer stem cells it creates. The bottom line is that chemotherapy is enriching tumor-promoting cells simultaneously as it indiscriminately kills healthy and abnormal cells.

It is also noteworthy that many of the doctors and nurses tasked with prescribing and administering chemotherapy would not take it themselves if they were diagnosed with cancer. A widely-publicized study regarding this is the outdated McGill study of 1986, in which the majority (about 66%) of physicians and oncology nurses stated they would refuse chemotherapy.[10196] This response pertained to the use of cisplatin (a then new chemotherapy drug with considerable side effects) for symptomatic metastatic bone disease for incurable lung cancer. A follow up study in 1997 asked "You are a 60-year-old oncologist with non-small-cell lung cancer, one liver metastasis, and bone metastases. Your performance status is 1. Would you take chemotherapy? Yes or no?" This time the results were reversed with 64.5% of oncologists and hematologists, and 67% of oncology nurses suggesting they would undergo chemotherapy in this situation.[5415] However, only 33% of a mixture of radiation oncologists and other types of physicians also surveyed (listed as "other" on the survey) would accept the chemotherapy. Even with the large increase in oncologists willing to undergo chemotherapy in the second study, it is remarkable that such a high percentage of those who prescribe and administer chemotherapy would be unwilling to take it themselves. This really speaks volumes to their confidence in the safety and efficacy of this form of cancer treatment.

Chemotherapy side effects are also extensive, including reduced immune function, sensory loss, nausea, vomiting, blood disorders, dizziness, diarrhea or constipation, hair loss, loss of appetite/malnutrition, fatigue, pain, mouth/throat sores, organ damage/failure, internal bleeding, cognitive dysfunction, nerve damage, and sexual dysfunction.

Radiation therapy, also called radiotherapy, involves the use of high doses of radiation to kill cancer cells and shrink tumors. The process takes days or weeks of treatment before cancer cells die, and this die off of cancer cells can continue for months after treatment ends. Radiation works by damaging and killing cells that

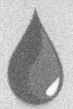

are dividing. Like chemotherapy, it is unable to distinguish healthy cells from cancer cells and so nearby healthy cells that are dividing are also destroyed during treatment. The most common side effect of radiation therapy is fatigue, but other side effects can occur months or years after treatment ends (called late effects). Side effects depend on the site being treated but can include skin problems, development of a second cancer, dry mouth, mouth sores, nausea, vomiting, lymphedema, tooth decay, difficulty swallowing, scarring of the lungs (fibrosis), diarrhea, sexual dysfunction, and infertility.

Sometimes the tumor is removed from the body by surgery. However, cancer can come back after surgery because not all of the cancer cells were removed or they may have broken off from the primary tumor and spread to other parts of the body. This is why surgery may be combined with chemotherapy or radiation treatment. Pain and infection are the two most common risks of surgical removal of cancer. Bleeding, damage to nearby tissues, and adverse reactions to anesthesia are also possible.

Immunotherapy is a biological therapy (a treatment that uses substances from living organisms) designed to help your immune system detect and kill cancer cells. A number of types of immunotherapy are used to treat cancer, such as:

1. **Monoclonal antibodies** (MAs) are drugs that bind to specific cells or proteins and trigger an immune response that destroys cancer cells. Antibodies are proteins that circulate throughout the body until they find and attach to an antigen (foreign substance). MAs are designed to target specific antigens on cancer cells.
2. **Adoptive cell transfer** attempts to boost T cell (white blood cells that are part of the immune system) activity to fight cancer. T cells are removed from the person's tumor and the most active T cells against the cancer are identified, or they are genetically modified to destroy the cancer cells. These T cells are then grown in a lab and injected back into the patient to fight cancer.
3. Two types of **cytokines** (proteins produced by white blood cells that regulate immune responses, inflammation, and blood cell formation) are used to treat cancer: interferons (INFs) and interleukins (ILs). Hematopoietic cytokines are also used to reduce some of the side effects of chemotherapy. INF-α may enhance a person's immune response to cancer by activating white blood cells (natural killer cells and dendritic cells) and inhibiting and killing cancer cells. ILs also enhance immune activity by increasing the proliferation of white blood cells (cytotoxic T cells and natural killer cells) that help destroy cancer cells.
4. **Bacillus Calmette-Guérin (BCG)** therapy involves the insertion of a weakened form of the tuberculosis bacterium directly into the bladder via catheter, which causes an immune response that kills cancer cells. The mechanism behind how BCG triggers an immune response against cancer is poorly understood.

Other cancer treatments may include targeted therapy, hormone therapy, precision medicine, and stem cell transplant. Targeted therapy is a treatment that targets changes in cancer cells that allow them to grow, divide, and spread. Hormone therapy blocks or interferes with hormone functions in the body and is used to treat cancers that use hormones to grow. Precision medicine creates a personalized treatment plan based on an understanding of the genetic causes of a person's cancer. Stem cell transplants serve to restore blood-forming stem cells in people who have had their levels diminished by chemotherapy or radiation.

Aggressive cancer treatments like chemotherapy and radiation should really be a last resort. Reports from medical professionals and individuals battling cancer demonstrate that natural options do work. Varying degrees of success have been reported with non-traditional cancer therapies such as the Hoxsey Therapy, Gerson Therapy, and others. Beginning with these aggressive approaches is akin to burning your house down to get rid of cockroaches. While you may get rid of your cockroach problem, you no longer have a home.

If the best course of action is determined to be chemotherapy or radiation treatment, essential oils may still be a valuable supportive therapy. Indeed, essential oils can be a powerful complementary therapy to support your well-being and to reduce the side effects of conventional cancer treatment. Some research even suggests that essential oils or essential oil constituents can increase the effectiveness of chemotherapy drugs, while simultaneously reducing their toxicity and side effects. The following complementary essential oil therapy options can be helpful and used if the attending physician approves:

- *Nausea and vomiting.* Clinical research suggests that taking two drops each of peppermint and spearmint essential oils orally in a capsule 30 minutes prior to chemotherapy treatment significantly reduces the severity and number of nausea and vomiting episodes.[10197] Simple inhalation of ginger, lemon, peppermint, or spearmint (one drop of each placed on a cotton ball that is inserted in an oxygen mask during

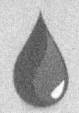

treatment; or diffusion of three to five drops of any combination of lemon, spearmint, or peppermint essential oils in a water diffuser for 30 to 60 minutes immediately following treatment) may also reduce nausea and vomiting.

- *Stress and anxiety.* A 10- to 15-minute shoulder and foot massage with two drops of lavender and one drop of ylang ylang in 5 mL of carrier oil 30 minutes prior to treatment can reduce cortisol levels and encourage a more relaxed state. The same essential oils (possibly with marjoram and bergamot added) may also be diffused or inhaled just prior to treatment.[10198,10199]

- *Depression.* Citrus essential oils are strongly uplifting and can be applied topically or inhaled to encourage a more positive outlook. Combine six drops of orange essential oil with 15 mL of fractionated coconut oil (FCO) and massage ten drops of this blend to the feet and hands (three drops on each foot and two drops on each hand), three times daily.[10200] Alternately, diffuse either of the following combinations of essential oils for 30 minutes, up to three times daily. Combination 1: 3 drops of orange, 3 drops of tangerine, 2 drops of clove. Combination 2: 2 drops each of lemon, tangerine, and orange, and 1 drop each of spearmint, peppermint, and grapefruit.

- *Insomnia.* Vetiver essential oil can increase GABA levels in the brain, which is a calming neurotransmitter and helps promote restful sleep.[10201,10202] Lavender essential oil is commonly used to promote more restful sleep as well.[10203] Massage two drops each of vetiver and lavender essential oil to the feet about 15 minutes prior to retiring for bed, or diffuse the same combination while sleeping (set the diffuser timer for 60 minutes).

- *Fatigue.* Mint oils are energizing and promote greater alertness. Diffuse 2 drops each of peppermint and spearmint and one drop of basil for 30 minutes, up to three times daily to reduce fatigue and tiredness.

- *Pain.* Gargling with equal parts of manuka and kanuka essential oil in water reduced mucositis (painful inflammation of the mucous membranes of the digestive tract after chemotherapy or radiation treatment) and reduced pain in cancer patients.[10204] A combination of ginger and orange essential oil can also be massaged to sore areas of the body as needed. Create a blend of 3 drops ginger and 2 drops orange essential oil in 5 mL of aloe and FCO carrier oil, then massage into sore areas. Inhale marjoram and lavender as needed.[10205,10206]

- *Appetite loss.* Apply one, or a combination of, ginger, spearmint, and peppermint essential oil to a diffuser necklace and wear throughout the day, refresh your chosen essential oil(s) twice daily.[10207,10208]

- *Bowel regularity.* Massage the abdomen in a clockwise motion for five minutes with a blend of one drop each of lemon, peppermint, and rosemary in 5 mL of carrier oil, once or twice daily, to promote bowel regularity.[10209]

- *Memory and concentration problems.* Inhalation of rosemary essential oil has been shown to improve cognition by triggering neurochemical pathways involved in memory.[10210,10211] Diffuse 4 drops of rosemary and two drops of lemon essential oil for two hours each morning.[1998]

- *Immune system suppression.* An aromatic massage with ginger essential oil may restore immune system activity (lymphocyte numbers) following chemotherapy. Patients received a 45-minute massage, three times per week, with 0.05 mL of ginger essential oil diluted in coconut oil, which was massaged to the head, neck, face, back, shoulders, arms, hands, lower legs, and feet.[10212]

- *Reduce radiotherapy side effects and damage.* Some essential oil constituents (alpha-asarone, diallyl disulfide, eugenol, thymol, thymoquinone) have demonstrated protection from radiotherapy-induced damage.[5032] These constituents can protect vital organs, cells, and tissues from the damaging effects of radiation exposure. Other essential oils are potent antioxidants that protect cells from free radical damage (black pepper, marjoram, German chamomile, and nutmeg). With physician approval, and three days following radiotherapy, take two drops each of clove, black pepper, marjoram, and German chamomile, and 1 drop each of nutmeg and thyme in a capsule, morning and evening. If skin side effects occur at the site of radiotherapy, mix together 3 to 5 drops each of clove, marjoram, German chamomile, sandalwood, and patchouli essential oil in 15 mL of carrier oil (sesame is a good choice unless known allergies exist) and apply enough of this mixture to cover the affected area up to three times daily. Continue taking these capsules for 21 days after treatment concludes.

- *Potentiating chemotherapy agents and reducing their side effects.* Multiple essential oil constituents have demonstrated the ability to potentiate chemotherapy agents or reduce the harmful side effects and toxicity they cause.[10213] To reduce the toxic effects of chemotherapy, seek physician approval to take three drops each of cinnamon and lemongrass, and two drops each of marjoram, black pepper, and clove in a capsule three days after chemotherapy concludes, morning and evening. Continue taking these capsules for 21 days after treatment concludes. See *Appendix G* for a list of possible essential oils constituents that could potentially enhance the cytotoxic effects of chemotherapy drugs.

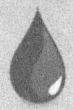

**Essential Oil Therapy for Cancer**

The use of essential oils as a therapy for cancer is controversial and still in its infancy. The majority of cancer research with essential oils has been *in vitro* studies that can't be directly applied to human health without further controlled clinical trials. In reality, the use of essential oils as a cancer therapy may still be a decade or more away from being a truly viable alternative with established therapeutic doses and treatment regimens. Until then, we have to work within the research and clinical experience that is available. The goal is to target multiple mechanisms that prevent cancer promotion and progression and kill existing cancer cells. Experience and limited research tell us that with the right evidence-based approach this can be accomplished within the realm of natural medicine, and perhaps in conjunction with standard treatment options.

This chapter is meant to be a guide and another point of information for individuals to make informed decisions in collaboration with their healthcare professionals regarding the treatment of cancer. It is not meant to be a substitute for reasonable and appropriate care.

Cancer is one of the most common life-threatening illnesses that affects up to half of all people during our lifetime. Decisions regarding cancer treatment should be made with your physician. Together you can determine the best course of action that gives you the most likelihood of successfully healing and overcoming the cancer you are facing. Your physician can also monitor your response to the essential oil regimen (if this is what is selected as an adjunct or primary therapy), including blood markers and any adverse effects experienced. This partnership with your physician provides the greatest possibility of successful treatment and survival. Unfortunately, it is difficult to find a willing licensed physician to support non-standard treatment for cancer. This is because the medical and pharmaceutical associations have such a grip on what physicians can and can't do. If they use standard treatment, like chemotherapy and radiotherapy, and people die it is acceptable; but if they use non-standard treatments and people live they are regarded as "quacks" and heavily persecuted. They also risk losing their license, or in the case of non-licensed professionals risk prison.

Ultimately, treatment decisions should be left to the person diagnosed with cancer, or in the case of a child, in collaboration with his or her parent or legal guardian. The protocols could also become a viable option if standard therapies proved unsuccessful. They are not intended for self-treatment and should only be used under the guidance of a qualified health professional.

Frankincense essential oil has been a leading candidate for use as a cancer therapy largely based on *in vitro* research and unpublished clinical research and case studies. For example, *Boswellia carterii* and *B. sacra* have both been shown to increase capsase 3 activity and cytochrome C in cancer cells to promote apoptosis (programmed cell death).[4972] Some experts believe that an enriched *B. sacra* frankincense—frankincense with the lighter molecules removed through evaporation—is the most viable and potent frankincense essential oil to consider for cancer therapy. These same researchers have seen some success in killing cancer according to their unpublished case studies and clinical experiments. However, a number of other essential oils also have preliminary research for specific types of cancer and are certainly worthy of consideration. In addition, enriched frankincense is not often used in the published studies using frankincense, suggesting that "unenriched" frankincense may also be useful for cancer. Hopefully, courageous and dedicated scientists will notice this preliminary research and continue the pursuit of identifying essential oils that are viable options to treat various types of cancers in humans.

In an ideal world, large clinical trials would establish effective doses. But this is not likely to occur anytime soon given the opposition to using natural medicine that can't be patented and therefore provide huge profits. Since a therapeutic essential oil dose for cancer has not been established in the scientific literature, anecdotal evidence from unpublished experiences must be used to determine a general direction for effective dosing. The doses recommended in this book are adapted from this unpublished data. Large oral doses are frequently suggested and may be difficult and or a shock to the system if introduced too quickly. Therefore, it is prudent to slowly build up to the recommended doses to allow the body to adjust. For instance, you may want to start with twenty-five percent of the therapeutic dose for three to five days; then work up to fifty percent in another three to five days; and finally, the full recommended dose after the first six to ten days. Because the number of drops in an essential oil bottle varies based on the specific gravity of the oil and the size of the orifice in the dropper, it is necessary to adjust the number of drops based on the label of the bottle. More precise dosing can be achieved when a specified amount of essential oil is used based on body weight (mL/kg). This will need to be calculated according to the label of the essential oil you are using. For instance, if you need to take 2.0 mL daily in divided doses, and your bottle says that each drop contains 60 mg of essential oil, you would want to take 30 drops per day in divided doses (see Appendix E for helpful conversion charts and the end

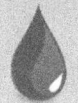

of this chapter for a dosage table). Using a type 2 measuring pipette can improve dosing accuracy.

The following is a list of essential oils that may be useful for the specific types of cancer according to published preliminary research. Please refer to the individual profiles in this book for more information and specific details for each essential oil listed.

### Adenocarcinoma
Basil, wormwood

### Bile Duct
Hemp

### Bladder
Frankincense, mastic, pink pepper, sandalwood, hemlock spruce (tsuga)

### Bone Marrow
Wormwood

### Brain (Astrocytoma)
Lemon

### Brain (Glioblastoma)
Sweet basil, guava leaf, lemongrass, mastic, melissa, oregano (carvacrol), Spanish sage, tagetes, thyme (thymol)

### Brain (Glioma)
Balsam poplar, German chamomile (alpha-bisabolol), juniper (Phoenician), peppermint

### Brain (Neuroblastoma)
Bay laurel, bergamot, cinnamon, citron, hemp, juniper, lavender, lemongrass, may chang, myrtle, rosemary

### Breast
Agarwood, allspice, anise, balsam fir, basil, bay (West Indies), bay laurel, black cumin, cajeput, cardamom, cassia, catnip, chaste tree, cilantro, cinnamon, clary sage (sclareol), clove, coriander, cumin, dwarf pine, fennel (anethole), frankincense, Formosan cypress, geranium, goldenrod, guava leaf, hemp, holy basil, Indian borage (weak), juniper, juniper (Phoenician), katrafay, lavender, leleshwa, lemon verbena, lemongrass, marjoram, mastic, may chang, Mediterranean mandarin, melissa, moringa seed, myrrh, myrtle, orange leaf, oregano, palo santo, palo santo (limonene), patchouli, peppermint, pine, pink pepper, rosemary, sandalwood, spikenard, tagetes, tea tree, thyme, turmeric (turmerones), tuermic leaf, vetiver, wild marjoram, wormwood

### Breast (Drug-resistant)
Black cumin (thymoquinone; enhances chemotherapy)

### Breast (Ductal Cell)
Lemon verbena

### Breast (ER+)
Clove, fennel (anethole), hemp, pine

### Breast (Metastatic)
Formosan cypress, geranium, hemp, mountain savory

### Breast (Triple negative)
Black pepper, fennel, hemp, vetiver

### Cancer (Angiogenesis)
Nutmeg, orange, oregano

### Cancer (Intracellular calcium levels)
Citronella (citronellol, citronellal), garlic (diallyl trisulfide)

### Cancer (Detoxify cancerous molecules)
Orange (d-limonene)

### Cancer (DNA adduct formation)
Black pepper, cardamom, coriander, nutmeg

### Cancer (DNA damage)
Citronella, fennel, ginger, lemongrass, marjoram, parsley, rosemary, summer savory, turmeric (turmerones), white verbena

### Cancer (Genetic Mutation)
German chamomile, ginger, myrtle

### Cancer (Metastasis/proliferation)
Orange (d-limonene), oregano, turmeric (tumerones)

### Cancer (Oncogene activation)
Oregano

### Cancer (Refractor solid tumors)
Orange (d-limonene)

### Cancer (Tumor formation)
Cardamom, coriander (linalool), melissa, oregano

### Cervical
Allspice, bay (West Indies), bergamot mint, black cumin (thymoquinone), chaste tree, clove, coriander, dwarf pine, fennel, feverfew, geranium, ginger, goldenrod, guava leaf, juniper, juniper (Phoenician), kaffir lime, lemon, mastic, Mediterranean mandarin, moringa seed, mountain savory, orange leaf, oregano, patchouli, peppermint, pink pepper, rhododendron, rosemary, sage, tagetes, turmeric, vilayti tulsi, white verbena, wormseed (American)

### Colorectal
Agarwood, ajowan, balsam fir, balsam poplar, caraway, cedarwood (Himalayan), clove, black cumin, dwarf pine, eucalyptus, fennel, frankincense, German chamomile, ginger, grapefruit, hemp, lavender, leleshwa, lemon verbena, lemongrass, lime (distilled), marjoram, mastic, melissa, moringa seed, mugwort,

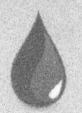

myrrh, myrtle CT linalool, orange, oregano (4-terpineol-rich), orange, oregano, Oriental arborvitae (minor sesquiterpenes), patchouli,peppermint, pink pepper, rhododendron, sage, tagetes, tansy, turmeric (turmerones), vetiver, wormwood

### Endometrial
Turmeric

### Epithelial
Peppermint

### Esophageal
Clove

### Fibroblasts (Cancer-associated)
Black cumin

### Head & Neck
Cinnamon, lovage

### Kidney
Bay laurel, mastic, Oriental arborvitae, sage (1,8-cineole-rich)

### Larynx
Moringa seed

### Leukemia (Acute lymphoblastic)
Feverfew, lavender, thyme

### Leukemia (Acute lymphoblastic, drug-resistant)
Feverfew

### Leukemia (Acute monocytic)
Anise, gobre salla, oregano

### Leukemia (Erythroleukemia)
Cinnamon, may chang, mountain savory

### Leukemia (Lymphoid)
Bay laurel (1,8-cineole), turmeric (tumerones)

### Leukemia (Myeloid)
Basil (sweet), bay laurel, bay laurel (1,8-cineole), cedarwood (Atlas), clove (eugenol), geranium, German chamomile, grapefruit, marjoram, pink pepper, tea tree (terpinen-4-ol), melissa, peppermint, petitgrain, turmeric (turmerones)

### Leukemia (Promyelocytic—acute myeloid)
Black cumin (thymoquinone; enhances chemotherapy), chaste tree, citron (fingered), geranium, hemp, lemongrass, melissa, mugwort, petitgrain, tea tree (terpinen-4-ol)

### Leukemia (T lymphoblast)
Fennel

### Liver
Allspice, anise, bay (West Indies), citronella (citronellal, citronellol), coriander, dill, eucalyptus, fennel, Formosan cypress, geranium, ginger, gobre salla, goldenrod, grapefruit, guava leaf, Indian borage (weak), juniper (Phoenician), lavender, leleshwa, lemon verbena, may chang, Mediterranean mandarin, moringa seed, myrrh, orange, orange leaf, oregano, pink pepper, rosemary, schisandra fruit, sweet wormwood, tagetes, turmeric, turmeric (turmerones)

### Lung
Balsam fir, balsam poplar, cassia, catnip, chaste tree, cistus, cinnamon, clove, cypress, dill, fennel, Formosan cypress, gobre salla, grapefruit, Indian borage (metastatic), juniper, juniper (Phoenician), lavender, leleshwa, lemon, lemongrass, marjoram, mastic (Lewis), may chang (non-small cell), melissa, neroli, oregano, Oriental arborvitae (minor sesquiterpenes), peppermint, sage, tangerine, tansy, thyme, white verbena, wormwood (non-small cell)

### Lymphoma
Copaiba (beta-caryophyllene), turmeric (turmerones)

### Melanoma
Balsam fir, bay laurel, bergamot, cassia (cinnamaldehyde), cinnamon (cinnamaldehyde), citron, clove, cumin, cypress, frankincense, geranium, lemon verbena, mastic, mugwort, myrrh, Oriental arborvitae, pennyroyal, rosemary, tea tree, sage, shell ginger, vetiver, white verbena, wormwood, yarrow

### Mesothelioma (Protective lining of organs)
Tea tree

### Multiple Myeloma
Ginger (beta-sesquiphellandrene)

### Musculoskeletal (Rhabdomyosarcoma)
Blue tansy

### Nasopharangeal
Tagetes

### Oral
Basil (sweet), celery, guava leaf, Japanese cedarwood, may chang, sage, thyme

### Oral (Precancerous submucous fibrosis)
Turmeric

### Ovarian
Cajeput, fennel (anethole), gobre salla, helichrysum, mastic, myrtle, Oriental arborvitae (minor sesquiterpenes), rhododendron, rosemary, turmeric

### Ovarian (ER+)
Rosemary

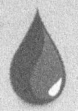

### Pancreatic
Frankincense, mastic, peppermint

### Prostate
Balsam fir, basil, cajeput, cinnamon, clove, gobre salla, kumquat, lavender, lemongrass, marjoram, myrtle, orange, oregano, rosemary, tea tree, thyme, turmeric, vilayti tulsi

### Prostate (Androgen+)
Elemi, frankincense, rosemary

### Prostate (Androgen–)
Frankincense

### Sarcoma
Coriander (linalool)

### Skin
Clove, frankincense, goldenrod, juniper, tea tree, myrrh, rosewood, sandalwood, tea tree

### Skin (Papillomas—HPV)
Sandalwood, shell ginger

### Stomach (Gastric)
Black cumin, fennel, geranium, goldenrod, holy basil, oregano, peppermint, tagetes

### Thyroid
Clove, mastic

### Uterine (ER+, endometrial)
Clary sage (sclareol)

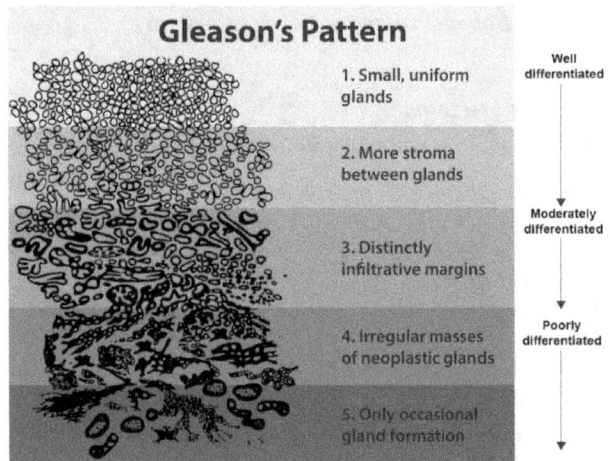

**Gleason's Pattern**

1. Small, uniform glands — Well differentiated

2. More stroma between glands

3. Distinctly infiltrative margins — Moderately differentiated

4. Irregular masses of neoplastic glands — Poorly differentiated

5. Only occasional gland formation

You should always work with your physician or another qualified healthcare professional to determine what is the best course of action if you are diagnosed with cancer. Delaying appropriate action could decrease your survivability odds. Under the supervision of a physician or healthcare professional the following protocols are intended to be used as a guide if the decision has been made to incorporate essential oils and other natural options into your treatment plan. All options that have a significant chance of successful healing and survival, with minimal risk, should be considered.

The protocols listed in this chapter are intended to provide an additional option (outside of simple high-dose frankincense and orange therapy in other works by this author) for you and your healthcare professional to consider. SuperCarrier essential oils (essential oils that are abundant in constituents that enhance bioavailability and efficacy of other constituents found in essential oils) have been included in each protocol to increase the effectiveness of the therapy through enhanced delivery to cells.

In addition, herbal or dietary supplements (listed as DS) are recommended when appropriate based on the available evidence. They may be taken with the essential oils or used only while resting from essential oil administration. Turmeric herb will be recommended frequently largely due to its ability to kill multiple types of cancer without harming normal/healthy cells, its ability to inhibit cancer through multiple pathways, its inhibition of all three stages of cancer (initiation, promotion, and progression), and its wide safety margin.[4481] Up to 8,000 mg of the active compound in turmeric (curcumin) has been administered in clinical trials with good tolerability and no toxicity reported.[4570] Remember, cancer is a complex disease, which requires a multidimensional method of attack for greatest efficacy.

Always check with your physician for any interactions with any current medications you are taking or contraindications based on your current state of health. In addition, it is not completely clear whether certain natural options will interfere with chemotherapy or radiation treatment. As was mentioned in Chapter 1, some essential oil compounds may increase the effectiveness of chemotherapy. You should not use natural remedies in conjunction with chemotherapy or radiation without the express permission of your physician. Always inform your physician of any supplements or essential oils that you are using to avoid potentially harmful interactions.

Most of all, maintain hope. Your cells must "hear" from you that you believe the treatment option you choose will be successful. Miraculous healing can take place when faith is combined with appropriate actions and efficacious treatment options.

## SUPERCARRIER BLEND
This blend contains SuperCarrier essential oils that include constituents that can increase the bioavailability and efficacy of other essential oils used in combination. To create the blend, combine 3 mL each of lemongrass,

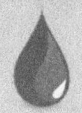

ginger, lavender, ylang ylang, and balsam fir in a 15 mL amber glass bottle. Roll in hands and shake for one to two minutes, then let rest (preferably for twenty-four hours) before using.

## BASAL CELL CARCINOMA

*Never attempt to treat cancer alone. Working with an integrative physician increases your healing potential.*

Oral—Fill a 60-mL amber glass bottle with 10 mL each of frankincense, myrrh, tea tree, and sandalwood, and 5 mL each of clove and tea tree essential oils, and 10 mL of the SuperCarrier blend. Take 0.008 to 0.014 mL/kg of the blend daily in 3 divided doses in capsules (with food and at least eight ounces of water) on days 1 through 5. Take 0.017 to 0.028 mL/kg of the blend daily in 3 divided doses in capsules (with food and at least eight ounces of water) on days 6 through 10. Take 0.035 to 0.056 mL/kg of the blend in capsules daily in 3 to 6 divided doses with food (or fill each capsule with 50% organic olive oil if taking without a meal) and an eight-ounce glass of water on days 11 through 21. Rest from the essential oils days 22 through 28 and then continue another 21-day course of the blend at the maximum dose (0.056 mL/kg). Reevaluate cancer status after the second course and determine whether an additional course at the full dose is necessary or another approach should be considered. Use a type 2 measuring pipette to fill empty capsules for greater accuracy of dosing.

Topical—Create a turmeric and essential oil paste by mixing together 1/2 cup of turmeric powder, 1 cup of distilled water, 1/3 cup of organic coconut oil, and 30 drops each of myrrh, sandalwood, and tea tree essential oil. Apply approximately one teaspoon of the mixture to the affected area up to three times daily.

## CANCER (BLADDER)

*Never attempt to treat cancer alone. Working with an integrative physician increases your healing potential.*

Oral—Fill a 60-mL amber glass bottle with 20 mL of frankincense essential oil, 15 mL each of sandalwood and spruce (black) essential oil, 5 mL of orange essential oil, and 5 mL of the SuperCarrier blend. Take 0.008 to 0.014 mL/kg of the blend daily in 3 divided doses in capsules (with food and at least eight ounces of water) on days 1 through 5. Take 0.017 to 0.028 mL/kg of the blend daily in 3 divided doses in capsules (with food and at least eight ounces of water) on days 6 through 10. Take 0.035 to 0.056 mL/kg of the blend in capsules daily in 3 to 6 divided doses with food (or fill each capsule with 50% organic olive oil if taking without a meal) and an eight-ounce glass of water on days 11 through 21. Rest from the essential oils days 22 through 28 and then continue another 21-day course of the blend at the

maximum dose (0.056 mL/kg). Reevaluate cancer status after the second course and determine whether an additional course at the full dose is necessary or another approach should be considered. Use a type 2 measuring pipette to fill empty capsules for greater accuracy of dosing.

Topical—Apply 5 to 7 drops of the blend diluted (1 part essential oil to 3 parts carrier oil) to the lower abdominal area just above the penis or vagina, once daily.

DS—Take 500 mg of quercetin twice daily for 21 days.[10214,10215]

## CANCER (BONE)

*Never attempt to treat cancer alone. Working with an integrative physician increases your healing potential.*

Oral—Fill a 60-mL amber glass bottle with 15 mL each of frankincense and cedarwood essential oils, 10 mL each of ginger and orange essential oils, and 10 mL of the SuperCarrier blend. Take 0.008 to 0.014 mL/kg of the blend daily in 3 divided doses in capsules (with food and at least eight ounces of water) on days 1 through 5. Take 0.017 to 0.028 mL/kg of the blend daily in 3 divided doses in capsules (with food and at least eight ounces of water) on days 6 through 10. Take 0.035 to 0.056 mL/kg of the blend in capsules daily in 3 to 6 divided doses with food (or fill each capsule with 50% organic olive oil if taking without a meal) and an eight-ounce glass of water on days 11 through 21. Rest from the essential oils days 22 through 28 and then continue another 21-day course of the blend at the maximum dose (0.056 mL/kg). Reevaluate cancer status after the second course and determine whether an additional course at the full dose is necessary or another approach should be considered. Use a type 2 measuring pipette to fill empty capsules for greater accuracy of dosing.

Topical—Apply a mixture of 2 to 3 drops of rosemary essential oil in 10 drops of carrier oil over the affected bone(s) once daily.

DS—Take 750 to 1,000 mg of standardized turmeric (to 95% total curcuminoids) or curcumin extract three times daily with food (preferably with fat).[10216,10217] Take each dose of turmeric/curcumin with 10 mg of piperine (from black pepper) to increase bioavailability and therefore efficacy.[10218]

## CANCER (BRAIN, ASTROCYTOMA)

*Never attempt to treat cancer alone. Working with an integrative physician increases your healing potential.*

Oral—Fill a 60-mL amber glass bottle with 40 mL of lemon essential oil, 10 mL of orange essential oil, and 10 mL of the SuperCarrier blend. Take 0.008 to 0.014

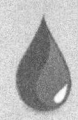

mL/kg of the blend daily in 3 divided doses in capsules (with food and at least eight ounces of water) on days 1 through 5. Take 0.017 to 0.028 mL/kg of the blend daily in 3 divided doses in capsules (with food and at least eight ounces of water) on days 6 through 10. Take 0.035 to 0.056 mL/kg of the blend in capsules daily in 3 to 6 divided doses with food (or fill each capsule with 50% organic olive oil if taking without a meal) and an eight-ounce glass of water on days 11 through 21. Rest from the essential oils days 22 through 28 and then continue another 21-day course of the blend at the maximum dose (0.056 mL/kg). Reevaluate cancer status after the second course and determine whether an additional course at the full dose is necessary or another approach should be considered. Use a type 2 measuring pipette to fill empty capsules for greater accuracy of dosing.

DS—Take 750 to 1,000 mg of standardized turmeric (to 95% total curcuminoids) or curcumin extract three times daily with food (preferably with fat).[10219] Take each dose of turmeric/curcumin with 10 mg of piperine (from black pepper) to increase bioavailability and therefore efficacy.[10220]

DS—Take 1,400 mg of *Boswellia serrata* extract three times daily (primarily to control cerebral edema and reduce inflammation).[10221]

DS—Take 500 mg of berberine three times daily.[10222]

## CANCER (BRAIN, GLIOMA/ GLIOBLASTOMA)

*Never attempt to treat cancer alone. Working with an integrative physician increases your healing potential.*

Oral—Fill a 60-mL amber glass bottle with 10 mL each of myrrh and thyme essential oil, 8 mL each of sweet basil (linalool CT), oregano, juniper berry, and orange essential oils, and 8 mL of the SuperCarrier blend. Take 0.008 to 0.014 mL/kg of the blend daily in 3 divided doses in capsules (with food and at least eight ounces of water) on days 1 through 5. Take 0.017 to 0.028 mL/kg of the blend daily in 3 divided doses in capsules (with food and at least eight ounces of water) on days 6 through 10. Take 0.035 to 0.056 mL/kg of the blend in capsules daily in 3 to 6 divided doses with food (or fill each capsule with 50% organic olive oil if taking without a meal) and an eight-ounce glass of water on days 11 through 21. Rest from the essential oils days 22 through 28 and then continue another 21-day course of the blend at the maximum dose (0.056 mL/kg). Reevaluate cancer status after the second course and determine whether an additional course at the full dose is necessary or another approach should be considered. Use a type 2 measuring pipette to fill empty capsules for greater accuracy of dosing.

Topical—Apply a mixture of 2 to 3 drops of the blend in 10 drops of carrier oil to the base of the skull, crown of the head, forehead, and behind the ears once daily.

DS—Take 750 to 1,000 mg of standardized turmeric (to 95% total curcuminoids) or curcumin extract three times daily with food (preferably with fat).[10223] Take each dose of turmeric/curcumin with 10 mg of piperine (from black pepper) to increase bioavailability and therefore efficacy.[10224]

DS—Take 1,400 mg of *Boswellia serrata* extract three times daily (primarily to control cerebral edema and reduce inflammation).[10225]

DS—Take 500 mg of berberine three times daily.[10226]

## CANCER (BREAST)

*Never attempt to treat cancer alone. Working with an integrative physician increases your healing potential.*

Oral—Fill a 60-mL amber glass bottle with 20 mL of frankincense essential oil, 10 mL each of orange and fennel essential oil, and 5 mL each of clove, thyme, and rosemary essential oils, and 5 mL of the SuperCarrier blend. Take 0.008 to 0.014 mL/kg of the blend daily in 3 divided doses in capsules (with food and at least eight ounces of water) on days 1 through 5. Take 0.017 to 0.028 mL/kg of the blend daily in 3 divided doses in capsules (with food and at least eight ounces of water) on days 6 through 10. Take 0.035 to 0.056 mL/kg of the blend in capsules daily in 3 to 6 divided doses with food (or fill each capsule with 50% organic olive oil if taking without a meal) and an eight-ounce glass of water on days 11 through 21. Rest from the essential oils days 22 through 28 and then continue another 21-day course of the blend at the maximum dose (0.056 mL/kg). Reevaluate cancer status after the second course and determine whether an additional course at the full dose is necessary or another approach should be considered. Use a type 2 measuring pipette to fill empty capsules for greater accuracy of dosing.

Topical—Massage 2 drops of the blend in 15 drops of carrier oil to the breast and armpit area 2 to 3 times daily.

DS—Take 2,000 mg of standardized turmeric (to 95% total curcuminoids) or curcumin extract three times daily with food for 7 days, then rest 7 days before repeating another 7 days, for a total of four cycles (4 weeks taking 6 g of turmeric, with one week rest between each week of turmeric).[10227]

## CANCER (BREAST, ER+)

*Never attempt to treat cancer alone. Working with an integrative physician increases your healing potential.*

Oral—Fill a 60-mL amber glass bottle with 15 mL each of clove and fennel essential oil, and 10 mL each of orange and pine essential oils, and 10 mL of the SuperCarrier blend. Take 0.008 to 0.014 mL/kg of the

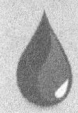

blend daily in 3 divided doses in capsules (with food and at least eight ounces of water) on days 1 through 5. Take 0.017 to 0.028 mL/kg of the blend daily in 3 divided doses in capsules (with food and at least eight ounces of water) on days 6 through 10. Take 0.035 to 0.056 mL/kg of the blend in capsules daily in 3 to 6 divided doses with food (or fill each capsule with 50% organic olive oil if taking without a meal) and an eight-ounce glass of water on days 11 through 21. Rest from the essential oils days 22 through 28 and then continue another 21-day course of the blend at the maximum dose (0.056 mL/kg). Reevaluate cancer status after the second course and determine whether an additional course at the full dose is necessary or another approach should be considered. Use a type 2 measuring pipette to fill empty capsules for greater accuracy of dosing.

Topical—Massage 2 drops of the blend in 15 drops of carrier oil to the breast and armpit area 2 to 3 times daily.

DS—Take 2,000 mg of standardized turmeric (to 95% total curcuminoids) or curcumin extract three times daily with food for 7 days, then rest 7 days before repeating another 7 days, for a total of four cycles (4 weeks taking 6 g of turmeric, with one week rest between each week of turmeric).[10228]

### CANCER (CERVICAL)

*Never attempt to treat cancer alone. Working with an integrative physician increases your healing potential.*

Oral—Fill a 60-mL amber glass bottle with 15 ml each of clove and patchouli essential oil, and 10 mL each of orange and peppermint essential oil, and the SuperCarrier blend. Take 0.008 to 0.014 mL/kg of the blend daily in 3 divided doses in capsules (with food and at least eight ounces of water) on days 1 through 5. Take 0.017 to 0.028 mL/kg of the blend daily in 3 divided doses in capsules (with food and at least eight ounces of water) on days 6 through 10. Take 0.035 to 0.056 mL/kg of the blend in capsules daily in 3 to 6 divided doses with food (or fill each capsule with 50% organic olive oil if taking without a meal) and an eight-ounce glass of water on days 11 through 21. Rest from the essential oils days 22 through 28 and then continue another 21-day course of the blend at the maximum dose (0.056 mL/kg). Reevaluate cancer status after the second course and determine whether an additional course at the full dose is necessary or another approach should be considered. Use a type 2 measuring pipette to fill empty capsules for greater accuracy of dosing.

DS—Take 750 to 1,000 mg of standardized turmeric (to 95% total curcuminoids) or curcumin extract three times daily with food (preferably with fat).[10229,10230] Take each dose of turmeric/curcumin with 10 mg of piperine (from black pepper) to increase bioavailability and therefore efficacy.[10231]

DS—Take 400 mg of green tea extract standardized to deliver 200 mg of EGCG (epigallocatechin gallate) once daily for up to twelve weeks.[10232]

Herbal/Topical—Create an herbal paste by mixing together 1/2 cup of turmeric powder, 1 tablespoon of green tea powder, 1 cup of distilled water, 1/3 cup of organic aloe vera oil, and 25 drops of the essential oil blend.[10233,10234] Apply approximately one teaspoon of the cream inside the vagina at bed time, except when menstruating. Alternately, insert 500 mg of curcumin extract into the vagina at bedtime, excluding the days of menstruation.

DS (Prevention)—Women with a family history of cervical cancer should take a daily multi-strain probiotic with *Bifidobacterium adolescentis* or *Lactobacillus casei* Shirota to aid the clearance of human papilloma virus and reduce lesion formation.[10235,10236]

### CANCER (COLORECTAL)

*Never attempt to treat cancer alone. Working with an integrative physician increases your healing potential.*

Oral—Fill a 60-mL amber glass bottle with 20 mL of orange essential oil, 10 mL each of balsam fir and patchouli, and 5 mL each of clove and oregano essential oil, and 10 mL of the SuperCarrier blend. Take 0.008 to 0.014 mL/kg of the blend daily in 3 divided doses in capsules (with food and at least eight ounces of water) on days 1 through 5. Take 0.017 to 0.028 mL/kg of the blend daily in 3 divided doses in capsules (with food and at least eight ounces of water) on days 6 through 10. Take 0.035 to 0.056 mL/kg of the blend in capsules daily in 3 to 6 divided doses with food (or fill each capsule with 50% organic olive oil if taking without a meal) and an eight-ounce glass of water on days 11 through 21. Rest from the essential oils days 22 through 28 and then continue another 21-day course of the blend at the maximum dose (0.056 mL/kg). Reevaluate cancer status after the second course and determine whether an additional course at the full dose is necessary or another approach should be considered. Use a type 2 measuring pipette to fill empty capsules for greater accuracy of dosing.

DS—Take 2,000 mg of standardized turmeric (to 95% total curcuminoids) or curcumin extract twice daily with food, for 30 days.[10237]

DS—Take 1,000 mg of resveratrol daily for 30 days.[10238]

DS—Take 1,000 mg of ginger herb twice daily for 28 days, then rest for 7 days before taking it for another 28 days.[10239,10240]

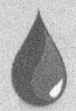

## CANCER (ENDOMETRIAL)
*See* CANCER (UTERINE, ENDOMETRIAL)

## CANCER (ESOPHAGEAL)
*Never attempt to treat cancer alone. Working with an integrative physician increases your healing potential.*

Oral—Fill a 60-mL amber glass bottle with 20 mL each of frankincense and orange essential oil, 10 mL of clove essential oil, and 10 mL of the SuperCarrier blend. Take 0.008 to 0.014 mL/kg of the blend daily in 3 divided doses in capsules (with food and at least eight ounces of water) on days 1 through 5. Take 0.017 to 0.028 mL/kg of the blend daily in 3 divided doses in capsules (with food and at least eight ounces of water) on days 6 through 10. Take 0.035 to 0.056 mL/kg of the blend in capsules daily in 3 to 6 divided doses with food (or fill each capsule with 50% organic olive oil if taking without a meal) and an eight-ounce glass of water on days 11 through 21. Rest from the essential oils days 22 through 28 and then continue another 21-day course of the blend at the maximum dose (0.056 mL/kg). Reevaluate cancer status after the second course and determine whether an additional course at the full dose is necessary or another approach should be considered. Use a type 2 measuring pipette to fill empty capsules for greater accuracy of dosing.

DS—Take one teaspoon of Oregon black raspberry liquid extract (*Rubus occidentalis*) and two teaspoons of raw, organic, unfiltered honey in some water daily for 21 days, then rest for 7 days before repeating for another 21 days.[10241,10242]

DS—Take 750 to 1,000 mg of standardized turmeric (to 95% total curcuminoids) or curcumin extract three times daily with food (preferably with fat).[10243] Take each dose of turmeric/curcumin with 10 mg of piperine (from black pepper) to increase bioavailability and therefore efficacy.[10244]

## CANCER (HEAD & NECK)
*Never attempt to treat cancer alone. Working with an integrative physician increases your healing potential.*

Oral—Fill a 60-mL amber glass bottle with 20 mL each of frankincense and orange essential oil, 10 mL of cinnamon essential oil, and 10 mL of the SuperCarrier blend. Take 0.008 to 0.014 mL/kg of the blend daily in 3 divided doses in capsules (with food and at least eight ounces of water) on days 1 through 5. Take 0.017 to 0.028 mL/kg of the blend daily in 3 divided doses in capsules (with food and at least eight ounces of water) on days 6 through 10. Take 0.035 to 0.056 mL/kg of the blend in capsules daily in 3 to 6 divided doses with food (or fill each capsule with 50% organic olive oil if taking without a meal) and an eight-ounce glass of water on days 11 through 21. Rest from the essential oils days 22 through 28 and then continue another 21-day course of the blend at the maximum dose (0.056 mL/kg). Reevaluate cancer status after the second course and determine whether an additional course at the full dose is necessary or another approach should be considered. Use a type 2 measuring pipette to fill empty capsules for greater accuracy of dosing.

DS—Take 100 mg of grapeseed extract standardized to 95% proanthocyanidins three times daily for 30 days.[10245,10246]

DS—Take 1,000 mg of resveratrol daily for 30 days.[10247]

## CANCER (KIDNEY)
*Never attempt to treat cancer alone. Working with an integrative physician increases your healing potential.*

Oral—Fill a 60-mL amber glass bottle with 20 mL each of frankincense and orange essential oil, 10 mL of the SuperCarrier blend, and 5 mL each of marjoram and rosemary essential oil. Take 0.008 to 0.014 mL/kg of the blend daily in 3 divided doses in capsules (with food and at least eight ounces of water) on days 1 through 5. Take 0.017 to 0.028 mL/kg of the blend daily in 3 divided doses in capsules (with food and at least eight ounces of water) on days 6 through 10. Take 0.035 to 0.056 mL/kg of the blend in capsules daily in 3 to 6 divided doses with food (or fill each capsule with 50% organic olive oil if taking without a meal) and an eight-ounce glass of water on days 11 through 21. Rest from the essential oils days 22 through 28 and then continue another 21-day course of the blend at the maximum dose (0.056 mL/kg). Reevaluate cancer status after the second course and determine whether an additional course at the full dose is necessary or another approach should be considered. Use a type 2 measuring pipette to fill empty capsules for greater accuracy of dosing.

DS—Take 1 mg/kg body weight of Maitake D-fraction twice daily about 20 minutes prior to breakfast and dinner.[10248,10249] In addition, take 2,500 mg of vitamin C four times daily.[10250]

## CANCER (LEUKEMIA, LYMPHOID)
*Never attempt to treat cancer alone. Working with an integrative physician increases your healing potential.*

Oral—Fill a 60-mL amber glass bottle with 20 mL each of frankincense and orange essential oil, 10 mL of the

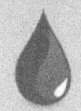

SuperCarrier blend, and 5 mL each of ginger and rosemary essential oil. Take 0.008 to 0.014 mL/kg of the blend daily in 3 divided doses in capsules (with food and at least eight ounces of water) on days 1 through 5. Take 0.017 to 0.028 mL/kg of the blend daily in 3 divided doses in capsules (with food and at least eight ounces of water) on days 6 through 10. Take 0.035 to 0.056 mL/kg of the blend in capsules daily in 3 to 6 divided doses with food (or fill each capsule with 50% organic olive oil if taking without a meal) and an eight-ounce glass of water on days 11 through 21. Rest from the essential oils days 22 through 28 and then continue another 21-day course of the blend at the maximum dose (0.056 mL/kg). Reevaluate cancer status after the second course and determine whether an additional course at the full dose is necessary or another approach should be considered. Use a type 2 measuring pipette to fill empty capsules for greater accuracy of dosing.

DS—Take 750 to 1,000 mg of standardized turmeric (to 95% total curcuminoids) or curcumin extract three times daily with food (preferably with fat).[10251] Take each dose of turmeric/curcumin with 10 mg of piperine (from black pepper) to increase bioavailability and therefore efficacy.[10252]

## CANCER (LEUKEMIA, MYELOID)

*Never attempt to treat cancer alone. Working with an integrative physician increases your healing potential.*

Oral—Fill a 60-mL amber glass bottle with 10 mL each of tangerine, marjoram, geranium, and cedarwood (Atlas) essential oils, 5 mL each of clove, sweet basil, tea tree essential oil, and 5 mL of the SuperCarrier blend. Take 0.008 to 0.014 mL/kg of the blend daily in 3 divided doses in capsules (with food and at least eight ounces of water) on days 1 through 5. Take 0.017 to 0.028 mL/kg of the blend daily in 3 divided doses in capsules (with food and at least eight ounces of water) on days 6 through 10. Take 0.035 to 0.056 mL/kg of the blend in capsules daily in 3 to 6 divided doses with food (or fill each capsule with 50% organic olive oil if taking without a meal) and an eight-ounce glass of water on days 11 through 21. Rest from the essential oils days 22 through 28 and then continue another 21-day course of the blend at the maximum dose (0.056 mL/kg). Reevaluate cancer status after the second course and determine whether an additional course at the full dose is necessary or another approach should be considered. Use a type 2 measuring pipette to fill empty capsules for greater accuracy of dosing.

DS—Take 150 to 200 mg of purified indirubin (from Ganggui Luhui Wan, a traditional Chinese medicine containing plants such as *Indigofera tinctoria* L. and *Isatis tinctoria* L) three times per day for 30 days.[10253,10254] It is common for indirubin to cause gastrointestinal upset.

DS—Take 750 to 1,000 mg of standardized turmeric (to 95% total curcuminoids) or curcumin extract three times daily with food (preferably with fat).[10255] Take each dose of turmeric/curcumin with 10 mg of piperine (from black pepper) to increase bioavailability and therefore efficacy.[10256]

DS—Take 1,200 to 1,500 mg of *Boswellia serrata* extract three times daily for 30 days.[10257]

## CANCER (LEUKEMIA, PROMYELOCYTIC, ACUTE MYELOID)

*Never attempt to treat cancer alone. Working with an integrative physician increases your healing potential.*

Oral—Fill a 60-mL amber glass bottle with 20 mL each of geranium and orange essential oil, 10 mL of tea tree essential oil, and 10 mL of the SuperCarrier blend. Take 0.008 to 0.014 mL/kg of the blend daily in 3 divided doses in capsules (with food and at least eight ounces of water) on days 1 through 5. Take 0.017 to 0.028 mL/kg of the blend daily in 3 divided doses in capsules (with food and at least eight ounces of water) on days 6 through 10. Take 0.035 to 0.056 mL/kg of the blend in capsules daily in 3 to 6 divided doses with food (or fill each capsule with 50% organic olive oil if taking without a meal) and an eight-ounce glass of water on days 11 through 21. Rest from the essential oils days 22 through 28 and then continue another 21-day course of the blend at the maximum dose (0.056 mL/kg). Reevaluate cancer status after the second course and determine whether an additional course at the full dose is necessary or another approach should be considered. Use a type 2 measuring pipette to fill empty capsules for greater accuracy of dosing.

DS—Take 750 to 1,000 mg of standardized turmeric (to 95% total curcuminoids) or curcumin extract three times daily with food (preferably with fat).[10258] Take each dose of turmeric/curcumin with 10 mg of piperine (from black pepper) to increase bioavailability and therefore efficacy.[10259]

DS—Take 1,200 to 1,500 mg of *Boswellia serrata* extract three times daily for 30 days.[10260]

DS—Take 1,000 mg of Korean Red Ginseng (*Panax ginseng*) up to three times per day for 12 weeks.[10261]

## CANCER (LIVER)

*Never attempt to treat cancer alone. Working with an integrative physician increases your healing potential.*

Oral—Fill a 60-mL amber glass bottle with 10 mL each of frankincense, juniper berry, rosemary, marjoram, and

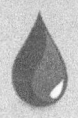

tangerine essential oil, and 10 mL of the SuperCarrier blend. Take 0.008 to 0.014 mL/kg of the blend daily in 3 divided doses in capsules (with food and at least eight ounces of water) on days 1 through 5. Take 0.017 to 0.028 mL/kg of the blend daily in 3 divided doses in capsules (with food and at least eight ounces of water) on days 6 through 10. Take 0.035 to 0.056 mL/kg of the blend in capsules daily in 3 to 6 divided doses with food (or fill each capsule with 50% organic olive oil if taking without a meal) and an eight-ounce glass of water on days 11 through 21. Rest from the essential oils days 22 through 28 and then continue another 21-day course of the blend at the maximum dose (0.056 mL/kg). Reevaluate cancer status after the second course and determine whether an additional course at the full dose is necessary or another approach should be considered. Use a type 2 measuring pipette to fill empty capsules for greater accuracy of dosing.

DS—Take 750 to 1,000 mg of standardized turmeric (to 95% total curcuminoids) or curcumin extract three times daily with food (preferably with fat).[10262,10263] Take each dose of turmeric/curcumin with 10 mg of piperine (from black pepper) to increase bioavailability and therefore efficacy.[10264]

## CANCER (LUNG)

*Never attempt to treat cancer alone. Working with an integrative physician increases your healing potential.*

Oral—Fill a 60-mL amber glass bottle with 10 mL each of peppermint, balsam fir, orange, and frankincense essential oil, 5 mL each of cinnamon, thyme, and clove essential oil, and 5 mL of the SuperCarrier blend. Take 0.008 to 0.014 mL/kg of the blend daily in 3 divided doses in capsules (with food and at least eight ounces of water) on days 1 through 5. Take 0.017 to 0.028 mL/kg of the blend daily in 3 divided doses in capsules (with food and at least eight ounces of water) on days 6 through 10. Take 0.035 to 0.056 mL/kg of the blend in capsules daily in 3 to 6 divided doses with food (or fill each capsule with 50% organic olive oil if taking without a meal) and an eight-ounce glass of water on days 11 through 21. Rest from the essential oils days 22 through 28 and then continue another 21-day course of the blend at the maximum dose (0.056 mL/kg). Reevaluate cancer status after the second course and determine whether an additional course at the full dose is necessary or another approach should be considered. Use a type 2 measuring pipette to fill empty capsules for greater accuracy of dosing.

DS—Take 1,000 mg of ginger herb twice daily for 28 days, then rest for 7 days before taking it for another 28 days.[10265]

## CANCER (LYMPHOMA)

*Never attempt to treat cancer alone. Working with an integrative physician increases your healing potential.*

Oral—Fill a 60-mL amber glass bottle with 20 mL each of copaiba and orange essential oil, 10 mL of frankincense essential oil, and 10 mL of the SuperCarrier blend. Take 0.008 to 0.014 mL/kg of the blend daily in 3 divided doses in capsules (with food and at least eight ounces of water) on days 1 through 5. Take 0.017 to 0.028 mL/kg of the blend daily in 3 divided doses in capsules (with food and at least eight ounces of water) on days 6 through 10. Take 0.035 to 0.056 mL/kg of the blend in capsules daily in 3 to 6 divided doses with food (or fill each capsule with 50% organic olive oil if taking without a meal) and an eight-ounce glass of water on days 11 through 21. Rest from the essential oils days 22 through 28 and then continue another 21-day course of the blend at the maximum dose (0.056 mL/kg). Reevaluate cancer status after the second course and determine whether an additional course at the full dose is necessary or another approach should be considered. Use a type 2 measuring pipette to fill empty capsules for greater accuracy of dosing.

DS—Take 750 to 1,000 mg of standardized turmeric (to 95% total curcuminoids) or curcumin extract three times daily with food (preferably with fat).[10266] Take each dose of turmeric/curcumin with 10 mg of piperine (from black pepper) to increase bioavailability and therefore efficacy.[10267]

## CANCER (MELANOMA)

*Never attempt to treat cancer alone. Working with an integrative physician increases your healing potential.*

Oral—Fill a 60-mL amber glass bottle with 15 mL each of bergamot and cypress essential oil, 5 mL each of cinnamon, rosemary, clove, and tea tree essential oil, and 10 mL of the SuperCarrier blend. Take 0.008 to 0.014 mL/kg of the blend daily in 3 divided doses in capsules (with food and at least eight ounces of water) on days 1 through 5. Take 0.017 to 0.028 mL/kg of the blend daily in 3 divided doses in capsules (with food and at least eight ounces of water) on days 6 through 10. Take 0.035 to 0.056 mL/kg of the blend in capsules daily in 3 to 6 divided doses with food (or fill each capsule with 50% organic olive oil if taking without a meal) and an eight-ounce glass of water on days 11 through 21. Rest from the essential oils days 22 through 28 and then continue another 21-day course of the blend at the maximum dose (0.056 mL/kg). Reevaluate cancer status after the second course and determine whether an additional course at the full dose is necessary or another approach should be

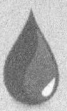

considered. Use a type 2 measuring pipette to fill empty capsules for greater accuracy of dosing.

Topical—Create a turmeric and essential oil paste by mixing together 1/2 cup of turmeric powder, 1 cup of distilled water, 1/3 cup of organic coconut oil, and 30 drops each of sandalwood, vetiver, and tea tree essential oil. Apply approximately one teaspoon of the mixture to the affected area up to three times daily.

DS—Take 600 mg of aged garlic four times daily.[10268,10269] Alternately, eat 1 to 2 segments of a garlic bulb (called a clove) with meals three times daily. Oil of garlic extract may also be applied to the affected area twice daily for two weeks.

DS—Take 750 to 1,000 mg of standardized turmeric (to 95% total curcuminoids) or curcumin extract three times daily with food (preferably with fat).[10270,10271] Take each dose of turmeric/curcumin with 10 mg of piperine (from black pepper) to increase bioavailability and therefore efficacy.[10272]

## CANCER (MESOTHELIOMA)

*Never attempt to treat cancer alone. Working with an integrative physician increases your healing potential.*

Oral—Fill a 60-mL amber glass bottle with 20 mL each of frankincense and orange essential oil, 10 mL of tea tree essential oil, and 10 mL of the SuperCarrier blend. Take 0.008 to 0.014 mL/kg of the blend daily in 3 divided doses in capsules (with food and at least eight ounces of water) on days 1 through 5. Take 0.017 to 0.028 mL/kg of the blend daily in 3 divided doses in capsules (with food and at least eight ounces of water) on days 6 through 10. Take 0.035 to 0.056 mL/kg of the blend in capsules daily in 3 to 6 divided doses with food (or fill each capsule with 50% organic olive oil if taking without a meal) and an eight-ounce glass of water on days 11 through 21. Rest from the essential oils days 22 through 28 and then continue another 21-day course of the blend at the maximum dose (0.056 mL/kg). Reevaluate cancer status after the second course and determine whether an additional course at the full dose is necessary or another approach should be considered. Use a type 2 measuring pipette to fill empty capsules for greater accuracy of dosing.

DS—Take 750 to 1,000 mg of standardized turmeric (to 95% total curcuminoids) or curcumin extract three times daily with food (preferably with fat).[10273,10274] Take each dose of turmeric/curcumin with 10 mg of piperine (from black pepper) to increase bioavailability and therefore efficacy.[10275]

## CANCER (MULTIPLE MYELOMA)

*Never attempt to treat cancer alone. Working with an integrative physician increases your healing potential.*

Oral—Fill a 60-mL amber glass bottle with 15 mL each of frankincense and ginger, 10 mL of orange and 5 mL each of clove, lemongrass, and tea tree essential oils, and 5 mL of the SuperCarrier blend. Take 0.008 to 0.014 mL/kg of the blend daily in 3 divided doses in capsules (with food and at least eight ounces of water) on days 1 through 5. Take 0.017 to 0.028 mL/kg of the blend daily in 3 divided doses in capsules (with food and at least eight ounces of water) on days 6 through 10. Take 0.035 to 0.056 mL/kg of the blend in capsules daily in 3 to 6 divided doses with food (or fill each capsule with 50% organic olive oil if taking without a meal) and an eight-ounce glass of water on days 11 through 21. Rest from the essential oils days 22 through 28 and then continue another 21-day course of the blend at the maximum dose (0.056 mL/kg). Reevaluate cancer status after the second course and determine whether an additional course at the full dose is necessary or another approach should be considered. Use a type 2 measuring pipette to fill empty capsules for greater accuracy of dosing.

DS—Take 1,000 mg of ginger herb twice daily for 28 days, then rest for 7 days before taking it for another 28 days.[10276,10277,10278]

DS—Take 750 to 1,000 mg of standardized turmeric (to 95% total curcuminoids) or curcumin extract three times daily with food (preferably with fat).[10279,10280] Take each dose of turmeric/curcumin with 10 mg of piperine (from black pepper) to increase bioavailability and therefore efficacy.[10281]

DS—Take 1,000 mg of rice bran arabinoxylan three times daily with the turmeric for 28 days, then take 1,000 mg per day as a maintenance dose.[10282]

## CANCER (NEUROBLASTOMA)

*Never attempt to treat cancer alone. Working with an integrative physician increases your healing potential.*

Oral—Fill a 60-mL amber glass bottle with 30 mL of bergamot essential oil, and 10 mL of each of orange and lemongrass essential oil, and 10 mL of the SuperCarrier blend. Take 0.008 to 0.014 mL/kg of the blend daily in 3 divided doses in capsules (with food and at least eight ounces of water) on days 1 through 5. Take 0.017 to 0.028 mL/kg of the blend daily in 3 divided doses in capsules (with food and at least eight ounces of water) on days 6 through 10. Take 0.035 to 0.056 mL/kg of the blend in capsules daily in 3 to 6 divided doses with food (or fill each capsule with 50% organic olive oil if taking without a meal) and an eight-ounce glass of water on

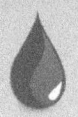 

days 11 through 21. Rest from the essential oils days 22 through 28 and then continue another 21-day course of the blend at the maximum dose (0.056 mL/kg). Reevaluate cancer status after the second course and determine whether an additional course at the full dose is necessary or another approach should be considered. Use a type 2 measuring pipette to fill empty capsules for greater accuracy of dosing.

DS—Take 750 to 1,000 mg of standardized turmeric (to 95% total curcuminoids) or curcumin extract three times daily with food (preferably with fat).[10283] Take each dose of turmeric/curcumin with 10 mg of piperine (from black pepper) to increase bioavailability and therefore efficacy.[10284]

DS—Take 1,400 mg of *Boswellia serrata* extract three times daily (primarily to control cerebral edema and reduce inflammation).[10285]

## CANCER (ORAL)

*Never attempt to treat cancer alone. Working with an integrative physician increases your healing potential.*

Oral—Fill a 60-mL amber glass bottle with 15 mL each of frankincense and orange essential oil, and 10 mL each of thyme and sweet basil (linalool CT) essential oils, and 10 mL of the SuperCarrier blend. Take 0.008 to 0.014 mL/kg of the blend daily in 3 divided doses in capsules (with food and at least eight ounces of water) on days 1 through 5. Take 0.017 to 0.028 mL/kg of the blend daily in 3 divided doses in capsules (with food and at least eight ounces of water) on days 6 through 10. Take 0.035 to 0.056 mL/kg of the blend in capsules daily in 3 to 6 divided doses with food (or fill each capsule with 50% organic olive oil if taking without a meal) and an eight-ounce glass of water on days 11 through 21. Rest from the essential oils days 22 through 28 and then continue another 21-day course of the blend at the maximum dose (0.056 mL/kg). Reevaluate cancer status after the second course and determine whether an additional course at the full dose is necessary or another approach should be considered. Use a type 2 measuring pipette to fill empty capsules for greater accuracy of dosing.

Gargle—Mix together one capsule of ginger root herb (or turmeric herb), one teaspoon of raw, organic, unfiltered honey, 2 drops of sweet basil essential oil and a tablespoon of warm water. Gargle with the mixture and swallow three times daily. Every other day switch the capsule between turmeric herb and ginger herb for greater efficacy.

## CANCER (OSTEOSARCOMA)

*Never attempt to treat cancer alone. Working with an integrative physician increases your healing potential.*

Oral—Fill a 60-mL amber glass bottle with 20 mL each of frankincense and coriander essential oils, 5 mL each of lemongrass and orange essential oils, and 10 mL of the SuperCarrier blend. Take 0.008 to 0.014 mL/kg of the blend daily in 3 divided doses in capsules (with food and at least eight ounces of water) on days 1 through 5. Take 0.017 to 0.028 mL/kg of the blend daily in 3 divided doses in capsules (with food and at least eight ounces of water) on days 6 through 10. Take 0.035 to 0.056 mL/kg of the blend in capsules daily in 3 to 6 divided doses with food (or fill each capsule with 50% organic olive oil if taking without a meal) and an eight-ounce glass of water on days 11 through 21. Rest from the essential oils days 22 through 28 and then continue another 21-day course of the blend at the maximum dose (0.056 mL/kg). Reevaluate cancer status after the second course and determine whether an additional course at the full dose is necessary or another approach should be considered. Use a type 2 measuring pipette to fill empty capsules for greater accuracy of dosing.

Topical—Apply a mixture of 2 to 3 drops of rosemary essential oil in 10 drops of carrier oil over the affected bone(s) once daily.

DS—Take 750 to 1,000 mg of standardized turmeric (to 95% total curcuminoids) or curcumin extract three times daily with food (preferably with fat).[10286,10287] Take each dose of turmeric/curcumin with 10 mg of piperine (from black pepper) to increase bioavailability and therefore efficacy.[10288]

## CANCER (OVARIAN)

*Never attempt to treat cancer alone. Working with an integrative physician increases your healing potential.*

Oral—Fill a 60-mL amber glass bottle with 20 ml of frankincense, 10 mL each of fennel, rosemary, and orange essential oils, and 10 mL of the SuperCarrier blend. Take 0.008 to 0.014 mL/kg of the blend daily in 3 divided doses in capsules (with food and at least eight ounces of water) on days 1 through 5. Take 0.017 to 0.028 mL/kg of the blend daily in 3 divided doses in capsules (with food and at least eight ounces of water) on days 6 through 10. Take 0.035 to 0.056 mL/kg of the blend in capsules daily in 3 to 6 divided doses with food (or fill each capsule with 50% organic olive oil if taking without a meal) and an eight-ounce glass of water on days 11 through 21. Rest from the essential oils days 22 through 28 and then continue another 21-day course of the blend at the maximum dose (0.056 mL/kg). Reevaluate cancer status after the second course and determine whether an additional course at the full dose is necessary or another approach should be considered.

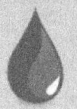

Use a type 2 measuring pipette to fill empty capsules for greater accuracy of dosing.

Retention—Mix 3 drops each of fennel and rosemary essential oil, and 3 drops of the SuperCarrier blend in 1 tablespoon of carrier oil, dip tampon into mixture and insert into vagina, retaining overnight.

DS—Take 750 to 1,000 mg of standardized turmeric (to 95% total curcuminoids) or curcumin extract three times daily with food (preferably with fat).[10289,10290] Take each dose of turmeric/curcumin with 10 mg of piperine (from black pepper) to increase bioavailability and therefore efficacy.[10291]

DS—Take 1,000 mg of ginger herb twice daily for 28 days, then rest for 7 days before taking it for another 28 days.[10292]

## CANCER (OVARIAN, ER+)

*Never attempt to treat cancer alone. Working with an integrative physician increases your healing potential.*

Oral—Fill a 60-mL amber glass bottle with 20 ml of frankincense, 15 mL each of rosemary and orange essential oils, and 10 mL of the SuperCarrier blend. Take 0.008 to 0.014 mL/kg of the blend daily in 3 divided doses in capsules (with food and at least eight ounces of water) on days 1 through 5. Take 0.017 to 0.028 mL/kg of the blend daily in 3 divided doses in capsules (with food and at least eight ounces of water) on days 6 through 10. Take 0.035 to 0.056 mL/kg of the blend in capsules daily in 3 to 6 divided doses with food (or fill each capsule with 50% organic olive oil if taking without a meal) and an eight-ounce glass of water on days 11 through 21. Rest from the essential oils days 22 through 28 and then continue another 21-day course of the blend at the maximum dose (0.056 mL/kg). Reevaluate cancer status after the second course and determine whether an additional course at the full dose is necessary or another approach should be considered. Use a type 2 measuring pipette to fill empty capsules for greater accuracy of dosing.

Retention—Mix 3 drops each of frankincense and rosemary essential oil, and 3 drops of the SuperCarrier blend in 1 tablespoon of carrier oil, dip tampon into mixture and insert into vagina, retaining overnight.

DS—Take 750 to 1,000 mg of standardized turmeric (to 95% total curcuminoids) or curcumin extract three times daily with food (preferably with fat).[10293,10294] Take each dose of turmeric/curcumin with 10 mg of piperine (from black pepper) to increase bioavailability and therefore efficacy.[10295]

DS—Take 1,000 mg of ginger herb twice daily for 28 days, then rest for 7 days before taking it for another 28 days.[10296]

## CANCER (PANCREATIC)

*Never attempt to treat cancer alone. Working with an integrative physician increases your healing potential.*

Oral—Fill a 60-mL amber glass bottle with 25 mL each of frankincense and orange essential oil, and 10 mL of the SuperCarrier blend. Take 0.008 to 0.014 mL/kg of the blend daily in 3 divided doses in capsules (with food and at least eight ounces of water) on days 1 through 5. Take 0.017 to 0.028 mL/kg of the blend daily in 3 divided doses in capsules (with food and at least eight ounces of water) on days 6 through 10. Take 0.035 to 0.056 mL/kg of the blend in capsules daily in 3 to 6 divided doses with food (or fill each capsule with 50% organic olive oil if taking without a meal) and an eight-ounce glass of water on days 11 through 21. Rest from the essential oils days 22 through 28 and then continue another 21-day course of the blend at the maximum dose (0.056 mL/kg). Reevaluate cancer status after the second course and determine whether an additional course at the full dose is necessary or another approach should be considered. Use a type 2 measuring pipette to fill empty capsules for greater accuracy of dosing.

DS—Take 1,200 to 1,500 mg of *Boswellia serrata* extract three times daily for 30 days.[10297,10298]

DS—Take 2,000 mg of standardized turmeric (to 95% total curcuminoids) or curcumin extract four times daily with food.[10299,10300] Take each dose of turmeric/curcumin with 10 mg of piperine (from black pepper) to increase bioavailability and therefore efficacy.[10301]

## CANCER (PROSTATE)

*Never attempt to treat cancer alone. Working with an integrative physician increases your healing potential.*

Oral—Fill a 60-mL amber glass bottle with 10 mL each of frankincense, balsam fir, clove, and orange essential oil, 5 mL each of cinnamon and thyme essential oil, and 10 mL of the SuperCarrier blend. Take 0.008 to 0.014 mL/kg of the blend daily in 3 divided doses in capsules (with food and at least eight ounces of water) on days 1 through 5. Take 0.017 to 0.028 mL/kg of the blend daily in 3 divided doses in capsules (with food and at least eight ounces of water) on days 6 through 10. Take 0.035 to 0.056 mL/kg of the blend in capsules daily in 3 to 6 divided doses with food (or fill each capsule with 50% organic olive oil if taking without a meal) and an eight-ounce glass of water on days 11 through 21. Rest from the essential oils days 22 through 28 and then continue another 21-day course of the blend at the maximum dose

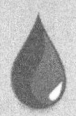

(0.056 mL/kg). Reevaluate cancer status after the second course and determine whether an additional course at the full dose is necessary or another approach should be considered. Use a type 2 measuring pipette to fill empty capsules for greater accuracy of dosing.

DS—Take 100 mg of grapeseed extract standardized to 95% proanthocyanidins three times daily for 30 days.[10302]

DS—Take 750 to 1,000 mg of standardized turmeric (to 95% total curcuminoids) or curcumin extract three times daily with food (preferably with fat).[10303,10304] Take each dose of turmeric/curcumin with 10 mg of piperine (from black pepper) to increase bioavailability and therefore efficacy.[10305]

## CANCER (PROSTATE, ANDROGEN +)

*Never attempt to treat cancer alone. Working with an integrative physician increases your healing potential.*

Oral—Fill a 60-mL amber glass bottle with 10 mL each of rosemary, frankincense, balsam fir, and orange essential oil, 5 mL each of clove, cinnamon, and thyme essential oil, and 5 mL of the SuperCarrier blend. Take 0.008 to 0.014 mL/kg of the blend daily in 3 divided doses in capsules (with food and at least eight ounces of water) on days 1 through 5. Take 0.017 to 0.028 mL/kg of the blend daily in 3 divided doses in capsules (with food and at least eight ounces of water) on days 6 through 10. Take 0.035 to 0.056 mL/kg of the blend in capsules daily in 3 to 6 divided doses with food (or fill each capsule with 50% organic olive oil if taking without a meal) and an eight-ounce glass of water on days 11 through 21. Rest from the essential oils days 22 through 28 and then continue another 21-day course of the blend at the maximum dose (0.056 mL/kg). Reevaluate cancer status after the second course and determine whether an additional course at the full dose is necessary or another approach should be considered. Use a type 2 measuring pipette to fill empty capsules for greater accuracy of dosing.

DS—Take 100 mg of grapeseed extract standardized to 95% proanthocyanidins three times daily for 30 days.[10306,10307]

DS—Take 750 to 1,000 mg of standardized turmeric (to 95% total curcuminoids) or curcumin extract three times daily with food (preferably with fat).[10308] Take each dose of turmeric/curcumin with 10 mg of piperine (from black pepper) to increase bioavailability and therefore efficacy.[10309]

## CANCER (SKIN)

*Never attempt to treat cancer alone. Working with an integrative physician increases your healing potential.*

Oral—Fill a 60-mL amber glass bottle with 10 mL each of frankincense, myrrh, geranium, and sandalwood, and 5 mL each of clove and tea tree essential oils, and 10 mL of the SuperCarrier blend. Take 0.008 to 0.014 mL/kg of the blend daily in 3 divided doses in capsules (with food and at least eight ounces of water) on days 1 through 5. Take 0.017 to 0.028 mL/kg of the blend daily in 3 divided doses in capsules (with food and at least eight ounces of water) on days 6 through 10. Take 0.035 to 0.056 mL/kg of the blend in capsules daily in 3 to 6 divided doses with food (or fill each capsule with 50% organic olive oil if taking without a meal) and an eight-ounce glass of water on days 11 through 21. Rest from the essential oils days 22 through 28 and then continue another 21-day course of the blend at the maximum dose (0.056 mL/kg). Reevaluate cancer status after the second course and determine whether an additional course at the full dose is necessary or another approach should be considered. Use a type 2 measuring pipette to fill empty capsules for greater accuracy of dosing.

Topical—Create a turmeric and essential oil paste by mixing together 1/2 cup of turmeric powder, 1 cup of distilled water, 1/3 cup of organic coconut oil, and 30 drops each of myrrh, sandalwood, and tea tree essential oil. Apply approximately one teaspoon of the mixture to the affected area up to three times daily.

## CANCER (STOMACH, GASTRIC)

*Never attempt to treat cancer alone. Working with an integrative physician increases your healing potential.*

Oral—Fill a 60-mL amber glass bottle with 20 mL of peppermint essential oil, 10 mL each of frankincense, copaiba, and orange essential oil, 5 mL of clove essential oil, and 5 mL of the SuperCarrier blend. Take 0.008 to 0.014 mL/kg of the blend daily in 3 divided doses in capsules (with food and at least eight ounces of water) on days 1 through 5. Take 0.017 to 0.028 mL/kg of the blend daily in 3 divided doses in capsules (with food and at least eight ounces of water) on days 6 through 10. Take 0.035 to 0.056 mL/kg of the blend in capsules daily in 3 to 6 divided doses with food (or fill each capsule with 50% organic olive oil if taking without a meal) and an eight-ounce glass of water on days 11 through 21. Rest from the essential oils days 22 through 28 and then continue another 21-day course of the blend at the maximum dose (0.056 mL/kg). Reevaluate cancer status after the second course and determine whether an additional course at the full dose is necessary or another approach should be considered. Use a type 2 measuring pipette to fill empty capsules for greater accuracy of dosing.

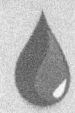

DS—Take 2,000 mg of standardized turmeric (to 95% total curcuminoids) or curcumin extract with 500 mg of quercetin twice daily with food (preferably with fat).[10310,10311,10312] Take turmeric with 20 mg of piperine (from black pepper) to increase bioavailability and therefore efficacy.[10313]

## CANCER (TESTICULAR)

*Never attempt to treat cancer alone. Working with an integrative physician increases your healing potential.*

Oral—Fill a 60-mL amber glass bottle with 15 mL each of frankincense and orange essential oil, and 5 mL each of geranium, cinnamon, ginger, and oregano, and 10 mL of the SuperCarrier blend. Take 0.008 to 0.014 mL/kg of the blend daily in 3 divided doses in capsules (with food and at least eight ounces of water) on days 1 through 5. Take 0.017 to 0.028 mL/kg of the blend daily in 3 divided doses in capsules (with food and at least eight ounces of water) on days 6 through 10. Take 0.035 to 0.056 mL/kg of the blend in capsules daily in 3 to 6 divided doses with food (or fill each capsule with 50% organic olive oil if taking without a meal) and an eight-ounce glass of water on days 11 through 21. Rest from the essential oils days 22 through 28 and then continue another 21-day course of the blend at the maximum dose (0.056 mL/kg). Reevaluate cancer status after the second course and determine whether an additional course at the full dose is necessary or another approach should be considered. Use a type 2 measuring pipette to fill empty capsules for greater accuracy of dosing.

DS—Take 750 to 1,000 mg of standardized turmeric (to 95% total curcuminoids) or curcumin extract three times daily with food (preferably with fat).[10314] Take turmeric with 20 mg of piperine (from black pepper) to increase bioavailability and therefore efficacy.[10315]

## CANCER (THYROID)

*Never attempt to treat cancer alone. Working with an integrative physician increases your healing potential.*

Oral—Fill a 60-mL amber glass bottle with 20 mL each of frankincense and orange essential oil, 10 mL of balsam fir, and 10 mL of the SuperCarrier blend. Take 0.008 to 0.014 mL/kg of the blend daily in 3 divided doses in capsules (with food and at least eight ounces of water) on days 1 through 5. Take 0.017 to 0.028 mL/kg of the blend daily in 3 divided doses in capsules (with food and at least eight ounces of water) on days 6 through 10. Take 0.035 to 0.056 mL/kg of the blend in capsules daily in 3 to 6 divided doses with food (or fill each capsule with 50% organic olive oil if taking without a meal) and an eight-ounce glass of water on days 11 through 21. Rest from the essential oils days 22 through 28 and then continue another 21-day course of the blend

at the maximum dose (0.056 mL/kg). Reevaluate cancer status after the second course and determine whether an additional course at the full dose is necessary or another approach should be considered. Use a type 2 measuring pipette to fill empty capsules for greater accuracy of dosing.

DS—Take 750 to 1,000 mg of standardized turmeric (to 95% total curcuminoids) or curcumin extract three times daily with food (preferably with fat).[10316,10317] Take turmeric with 20 mg of piperine (from black pepper) to increase bioavailability and therefore efficacy.[10318]

## CANCER (UTERINE, ENDOMETRIAL)

*Never attempt to treat cancer alone. Working with an integrative physician increases your healing potential.*

Oral—Fill a 60-mL amber glass bottle with 20 mL each of frankincense and orange essential oil, 10 mL of clary sage, and 10 mL of the SuperCarrier blend. Take 0.008 to 0.014 mL/kg of the blend daily in 3 divided doses in capsules (with food and at least eight ounces of water) on days 1 through 5. Take 0.017 to 0.028 mL/kg of the blend daily in 3 divided doses in capsules (with food and at least eight ounces of water) on days 6 through 10. Take 0.035 to 0.056 mL/kg of the blend in capsules daily in 3 to 6 divided doses with food (or fill each capsule with 50% organic olive oil if taking without a meal) and an eight-ounce glass of water on days 11 through 21. Rest from the essential oils days 22 through 28 and then continue another 21-day course of the blend at the maximum dose (0.056 mL/kg). Reevaluate cancer status after the second course and determine whether an additional course at the full dose is necessary or another approach should be considered. Use a type 2 measuring pipette to fill empty capsules for greater accuracy of dosing.

DS—Take 750 to 1,000 mg of standardized turmeric (to 95% total curcuminoids) or curcumin extract three times daily with food (preferably with fat).[10319,10320] Take turmeric with 20 mg of piperine (from black pepper) to increase bioavailability and therefore efficacy.[10321]

## CANCER (VAGINAL, VULVAR)

*Never attempt to treat cancer alone. Working with an integrative physician increases your healing potential.*

Oral—Fill a 60-mL amber glass bottle with 20 mL each of frankincense and orange essential oil, and 10 mL each of clary sage and the SuperCarrier blend. Take 0.008 to 0.014 mL/kg of the blend daily in 3 divided doses in capsules (with food and at least eight ounces of water) on days 1 through 5. Take 0.017 to 0.028 mL/kg of the blend daily in 3 divided doses in capsules (with food and at least eight ounces of water) on days 6 through 10. Take

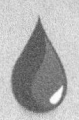

0.035 to 0.056 mL/kg of the blend in capsules daily in 3 to 6 divided doses with food (or fill each capsule with 50% organic olive oil if taking without a meal) and an eight-ounce glass of water on days 11 through 21. Rest from the essential oils days 22 through 28 and then continue another 21-day course of the blend at the maximum dose (0.056 mL/kg). Reevaluate cancer status after the second course and determine whether an additional course at the full dose is necessary or another approach should be considered. Use a type 2 measuring pipette to fill empty capsules for greater accuracy of dosing.

Topical—Create a turmeric and essential oil paste by mixing together 1/2 cup of turmeric powder, 1 cup of distilled water, 1/3 cup of organic coconut oil, and 30 drops each of myrrh, sandalwood, and tea tree essential oil. Apply approximately one teaspoon of the mixture to the affected area up to three times daily.

## BLACK CUMIN PROTOCOLS

Black cumin essential oil contains thymoquinone, which is one of the most potent medicinal molecules ever discovered in nature. This one constituent has been called a panacea drug for good reasons. Thymoquinone has demonstrated anticancer activity against a variety of cancers both as a treatment and as a preventive. It also attacks cancer through multiple mechanisms, making it a valuable natural option for cancer. Most of the research has been preclinical, but the mounting evidence suggests that thymoquinone is worthy of clinical trials for cancer.

Small amounts of thymoquinone are found in the fixed herbal oil, but the essential oil concentrates this powerful constituent, particularly supercritical carbon dioxide extracts from the herbal/fixed oil. Unfortunately, as of this writing, the essential oil is not widely available commercially. Should it become commercially available the following are 60-mL recipes to use for various cancers in place of the 60-mL recipes listed above. These blends would be used the same as listed in the above protocols.

**Breast:** 10 mL each of frankincense, black cumin, orange, and fennel essential oils, and 5 mL each of clove, thyme, and rosemary essential oils, and 5 mL of the SuperCarrier blend.

**Colorectal:** 10 mL each of orange, black cumin, balsam fir, and patchouli essential oils, and 5 mL each of clove and oregano essential oils, and 10 mL of the SuperCarrier blend

**Glioblastoma:** 10 mL each of black cumin and thyme essential oil, 8 mL each of sweet basil (linalool CT), oregano, juniper berry, and orange essential oils, and 8 mL of the SuperCarrier blend.

**Liver:** 10 mL each of frankincense, juniper berry, rosemary, marjoram, and tangerine essential oil, and 10 mL of the SuperCarrier blend

**Lymphoblastic Leukemia:** 15 mL each of frankincense and orange essential oil, 10 mL of black cumin essential oil, 10 mL of the SuperCarrier blend, and 5 mL each of ginger and rosemary essential oil.

**Lymphoma:** 15 mL each of copaiba and orange essential oil, 10 mL each of black cumin and of frankincense essential oil, and 10 mL of the SuperCarrier blend

**Multiple Myeloma:** 10 mL each of black cumin, frankincense, and ginger essential oils, 10 mL of orange and 5 mL each of clove, lemongrass, and tea tree essential oils, and 5 mL of the SuperCarrier blend

**Osteosarcoma:** 15 mL each of frankincense and coriander essential oils, 10 mL of black cumin essential oil, 5 mL each of lemongrass and orange essential oils, and 10 mL of the SuperCarrier blend

**Ovarian:** 10 ml each of frankincense, black cumin, fennel, rosemary, and orange essential oils, and 10 mL of the SuperCarrier blend

**Pancreatic:** 20 mL each of frankincense and orange essential oil, and 10 mL each of black cumin essential oil and the SuperCarrier blend.

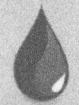

| WEIGHT | | TOTAL DAILY DOSE | | | DIVIDED DOSES, 3 TIMES DAILY (Drops Equivalent 30 mg \| 60 mg droppers) | | |
|---|---|---|---|---|---|---|---|
| | | *(0.008–0.014 mL/kg)* | *(0.017–0.028 mL/kg)* | *(0.035–0.056 mL/kg)* | | | |
| *lb.* | *kg* | *Days 1–5* | *Days 6–10* | *Days 11–21* | *Days 1–5* | *Days 6–10* | *Days 11–21* |
| 100 | 45.5 | 0.36–0.64 mL | 0.77–1.27 mL | 1.59–2.55 mL | 0.12–0.21 mL (4–6 \| 2–3 drops) | 0.26–0.42 mL (8–13 \| 4–6 drops) | 0.53–0.85 mL (16–26 \| 8–13 drops) |
| 105 | 47.7 | 0.38–0.67 mL | 0.81–1.34 mL | 1.67–2.67 mL | 0.13–0.22 mL (4–7 \| 2–3 drops) | 0.27–0.45 mL (8–14 \| 4–7 drops) | 0.56–0.89 mL (17–27 \| 9–14 drops) |
| 110 | 50 | 0.40–0.70 mL | 0.85–1.40 mL | 1.75–2.80 mL | 0.13–0.23 mL (4–7 \| 2–3 drops) | 0.28–0.47 mL (9–14 \| 4–7 drops) | 0.58–0.93 mL (18–28 \| 9–14 drops) |
| 115 | 52.3 | 0.42–0.73 mL | 0.89–1.46 mL | 1.83–2.93 mL | 0.14–0.24 mL (4–7 \| 2–4 drops) | 0.30–0.49 mL (9–14 \| 5–7 drops) | 0.61–0.98 mL (19–30 \| 9–15 drops) |
| 120 | 54.6 | 0.44–0.76 mL | 0.93–1.53 mL | 1.91–3.06 mL | 0.15–0.25 mL (5–8 \| 2–4 drops) | 0.31–0.51 mL (9–15 \| 5–8 drops) | 0.64–1.02 mL (19–31 \| 10–16 drops) |
| 125 | 56.8 | 0.45–0.80 mL | 0.97–1.60 mL | 1.99–3.18 mL | 0.15–0.27 mL (5–8 \| 2–4 drops) | 0.32–0.53 mL (10–16 \| 5–8 drops) | 0.66–1.06 mL (20–32 \| 10–16 drops) |
| 130 | 59.1 | 0.47–0.83 mL | 1.01–1.66 mL | 2.07–3.31 mL | 0.16–0.28 mL (5–9 \| 2–4 drops) | 0.34–0.55 mL (10–17 \| 5–8 drops) | 0.69–1.10 mL (21–33 \| 11–17 drops) |
| 135 | 61.4 | 0.49–0.86 mL | 1.04–1.72 mL | 2.15–3.44 mL | 0.16–0.29 mL (5–9 \| 2–4 drops) | 0.35–0.57 mL (11–17 \| 5–9 drops) | 0.72–1.15 mL (22–35 \| 11–17 drops) |
| 140 | 63.6 | 0.51–0.89 mL | 1.08–1.78 mL | 2.23–3.56 mL | 0.17–0.30 mL (5–9 \| 3–5 drops) | 0.36–0.59 mL (11–18 \| 6–9 drops) | 0.74–1.20 mL (22–36 \| 11–18 drops) |
| 145 | 65.9 | 0.53–0.92 mL | 1.12–1.84 mL | 2.31–3.69 mL | 0.18–0.31 mL (6–9 \| 3–5 drops) | 0.37–0.61 mL (11–19 \| 6–9 drops) | 0.77–1.23 mL (23–37 \| 12–19 drops) |
| 150 | 68.2 | 0.55–0.96 mL | 1.16–1.92 mL | 2.39–3.82 mL | 0.18–0.32 mL (6–10 \| 3–5 drops) | 0.38–0.64 mL (12–19 \| 6–10 drops) | 0.80–1.27 mL (24–39 \| 12–19 drops) |
| ≥ 155 | ≥ 70.5 | 0.56–0.99 mL | 1.20–1.97 mL | 2.50–3.95 mL | 0.19–0.33 mL (6–10 \| 3–5 drops) | 0.40–0.66 mL (12–20 \| 6–10 drops) | 0.83–1.32 mL (25–40 \| 13–20 drops) |

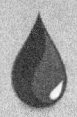

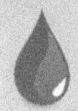

# APPENDIX A:
### ESSENTIAL OIL CONSTITUENTS

**1-Epi-Cubenol**

| | |
|---|---|
| Japanese Cedarwood (Heartwood) | 0.0%–18.9% |
| Japanese Cedarwood (Sapwood) | 0.0%–12.5% |
| Calendula (Alpha-Cadinol/Delta-Cadinene CT) | 0.0%–8.0% |
| Damiana (1,8-Cineole CT) | 0.0%–4.1% |
| Japanese Cedarwood (Twig) | 3.2%–3.3% |
| Muhuhu (Wood) | 0.0%–2.6% |

**1-Terpineol**

| | |
|---|---|
| Saro (1,8-Cineole CT) | 2.1%–4.2% |

**10-Epi-Gamma-Eudesmol**

| | |
|---|---|
| Agarwood (Malaysian) | 7.1%–30.4% |
| Amyris | 6.8%–9.7% |
| Agarwood (*A. malaccensis*) | 0.0%–9.2% |
| Agarwood (*A. crassna*) | 0.0%–9.0% |
| Geranium | 0.0%–5.6% |
| Damiana (1,8-Cineole CT) | 0.0%–4.5% |
| Pink Pepper (*S. molle*, Leaves, Elemol/Beta-Eudesmol CT) | 4.3% |
| Guaiacwood | 0.0%–2.2% |

**10-Isobutyryloxy-8,9-Didehydrothymol Isobutyrate**

| | |
|---|---|
| Arnica (Roots, Thymol Derivatives CT) | 10.3%–12.3% |

**10-Isobutyryloxy-8,9-Didehydrothymol Methyl Ether**

| | |
|---|---|
| Arnica (Roots, Thymol Derivatives CT) | 6.9%–8.6% |

**10-Isocaleroxy-8,9-Dihydrothymol Methyl Ether**

| | |
|---|---|
| Arnica (Roots, Thymol Derivatives CT) | 3.4%–3.6% |

**13-Tridecanolide**

| | |
|---|---|
| Angelica Root | 1.5%–6.1% |

**15-Copaenol**

| | |
|---|---|
| Schisandra Fruit (*S. sphenanthera*, α-Cad. CT) | 3.0% |

**15-Pentadecanolide**

| | |
|---|---|
| Angelica Root | 2.0%–14.9% |

**16-Kaurene (Kaurene, Kaur-16-ene, Ent-Kaurene)**

| | |
|---|---|
| Japanese Cedarwood (16-Kaurene CT) | 11.6%–42.1% |
| Japanese Cedarwood (16-Kaurene/Valencene CT) | 40.6% |

**17-Heptadecanolide**

| | |
|---|---|
| Angelica Root | 0.4%–3.1% |

**1,1,3a-Trimethyl-7-Methyl-ene-Decahydrocyclo-Propa[a]-Naphthalene**

| | |
|---|---|
| Japanese Cedarwood (Sapwood) | 0.0%–7.6% |
| Japanese Cedarwood (Heartwood) | 0.0%–6.8% |

**1,2-Dimethyl-4(2-propenyl)benzene**

| | |
|---|---|
| Moringa (Seeds, Cyclopentane CT) | 8.7% |

**1,2,3-Trimethyl-2-Cyclopentene-1-Carboxylic Acid**

| | |
|---|---|
| Damiana (1,8-Cineole CT) | 0.0%–10.6% |

**1,2,5,5,8a-Pentamethyl-1,2,3,5,6,7,8,8aoctahydronaphthalene-1ol**

| | |
|---|---|
| Agarwood (*A. sinensis*) | 0.0%–5.8% |

**1,3,5-Trimethyl-2-(2,2,2-Trifluoro-Ethoxy-Benzene)**

| | |
|---|---|
| Agarwood (*A. sinensis*) | 0.0%–13.4% |

**1,3,5-Trimethyl-6-Methylidene-Tricyclo [3.2.1.0(2,7)]oct6-3-en-8-exo-ol**

| | |
|---|---|
| Agarwood (*A. crassna*) | 0.0%–10.3% |

**1,3,8-Para-Menthatriene (1,3,8-P-Menthatriene)**

| | |
|---|---|
| Parsley (Leaves, 1,3,8-Para-Menth. CT) | 29.3%–64.7% |
| Parsley (Leaves, Myristicin CT) | 5.4%–24.2% |
| Tagetes (*T. patula*, Aerial Parts) | 3.9% |

**1,3-Cyclopentadiene, 5,5-dimethyl-1-ethyl-**

| | |
|---|---|
| Feverfew | 0.0%–4.8% |

**1,4-Cineole**

| | |
|---|---|
| Western Red Cedar (Wood) | 1.1%–1.3% |

**1,4,7-Cycloundecatrien,1,5,9,9-TetramethylZ,Z,Z-100**

| | |
|---|---|
| Black Pepper (Beta-Caryophyllene CT) | 0.0%–5.1% |

**1,5-Epoxy-Nor-Ketoguaiene**

| | |
|---|---|
| Agarwood (*A. malaccensis*) | 0.0%–4.1% |

**1,6-Germacadien-5-ol**

| | |
|---|---|
| White Verbena (Camphor CT) | 0.0%–8.2% |

**1,7,7-Trimethylbicyclo**

| | |
|---|---|
| Hinoki (needles) | 0.0%–10.2% |

**1,7-Di-Epi-Alpha-Cedrene**

| | |
|---|---|
| Helichrysum (*H. italicum*) | 0.2%–2.9% |

**1,8-Cineole (Eucalyptol)**

| | |
|---|---|
| Blue Mallee (1,8-Cineole CT) | 85.0%–94.2% |
| Gully Gum | 72.2%–86.4% |
| Eucalyptus (*E. globulus*) | 33.6%–83.9% |
| Southern Blue Gum | 44.0%–81.3% |
| Big Badja Gum | 71.7%–81.2% |
| Rosalina (1,8-Cineole CT) | 43.6%–79.5% |
| Hairy Basil (1,8-Cineole CT) | 21.8%–78.3% |
| Niaouli (1,8-Cineole CT) | 19.1%–76.3% |
| Niaouli (1,8-Cineole/Viridiflorol CT) | 0.4%–75.0% |
| Eucalyptus (*E. radiata*) | 22.4%–74.3% |
| Niaouli (*M. viridiflora*, 1,8-cineole CT) | 67.0%–72.9% |
| White Sage | 34.5%–71.7% |
| Saro (1,8-Cineole CT) | 47.3%–71.6% |
| Cajeput (Cajuput) | 44.8%–70.1% |
| Wild Marjoram (1,8-Cineole CT) | 56.8%–69.6% |
| Bay Laurel | 18.8%–68.8% |
| Ravintsara (1,8-Cineole CT) | 53.8%–63.0% |
| Galangal (Greater, 1,8-Cineole CT) | 22.6%–61.9% |
| Ravensara (1,8-Cineole CT) | 31.0%–60.8% |
| Blue Mallee (Cryptone CT) | 41.0%–58.2% |
| Cardamom | 15.9%–55.6% |
| Galangal (Lesser) | 28.1%–55.4% |
| Sweet Inula (1,8-Cineole CT) | 22.4%–54.9% |
| Rosemary (1,8-Cineole CT) | 41.6%–52.4% |
| Sage (1,8-Cineole CT) | 39.5%–50.3% |
| Vilayti Tulsi (1,8-Cineole CT) | 32.0%–47.6% |
| Niaouli (Viridiflorol/ Para-cymene/1,8-cineole CT) | 0.4%–47.0% |
| Guava Leaf (1,8-Cineole) | 42.7% |
| Sweet Nancy (Yomogi Alc.\1,8-Cin. CT) | 20.2%–41.0% |
| Fingerroot (*B. rotunda* 1,8-Cineole CT) | 41.0% |
| Niaouli (Viridiflorol CT) | 0.1%–40.0% |
| Myrtle (1,8-Cineole CT) | 25.7%–40.4% |
| Chaste Tree (Leaves) | 15.6%–35.2% |
| Spike Lavender | 28.0%–34.9% |
| Shell Ginger (1,8-Cineole CT) | 13.8%–37.8% |
| Boldo (*1,8-Cineole\Para-Cymene\Limonene CT*) | 11.8%–36.6% |
| Damiana (1,8-Cineole CT) | 11.4%–35.2% |
| Fragonia (Balanced CT) | 12.4%–34.2% |
| Spanish Sage | 13.0%–33.8% |
| Mugwort (1,8-Cineole CT) | 24.9%–32.2% |
| Rosemary (Camphor CT) | 9.0%–31.6% |
| Myrtle (Alpha-Pinene CT) | 6.5%–30.4% |
| Rosalina (Linalool CT) | 13.3%–29.4% |
| Hairy Basil (1,8-Cineole\Linalool CT) | 17.3%–29.0% |
| Yarrow (1,8-Cineole\Camphor CT) | 8.7%–28.8% |
| Cardamom (Alpha-Terpinyl Acetate CT) | 4.3%–27.2% |
| Rosemary (Alpha-Pinene CT) | 5.3%–26.5% |
| Lavandin (Giant) | 0.0%–26.1% |
| Myrtle (Myrtenyl Acetate CT) | 16.6%–25.7% |
| Holy Basil (aerial parts, beta-bisabolene CT) | 5.1%–24.9% |

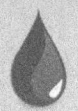
| | |
|---|---|
| Sage (Camphor CT) | 3.6%–24.7% |
| Vilayti Tulsi (Sabinene CT) | 5.2%–24.6% |
| Holy Basil (Aerial Parts, Estragole CT) | 1.1%–23.4% |
| Shell Ginger (Terpinen-4-ol CT) | 10.8%–23.1% |
| White Verbena (Camphor CT) | 0.0%–23.0% |
| Monarda (Carvacrol CT) | 1.0%–22.2% |
| Guava Leaf (Alpha-Pinene CT) | 7.6%–21.4% |
| Thyme (Thuyanol-4 CT) | 0.0%–21.2% |
| Boldo (Ascaridole CT) | 12.0%–21.1% |
| Catnip (1,8-cineole CT) | 21.0% |
| Holy Basil (aerial parts, eugenol CT) | 2.2%–20.8% |
| Rosemary (Borneol CT) | 20.0% |
| Lavender (True English) | 0.0%–19.8% |
| Shell Ginger (Para-Cymene CT) | 18.9% |
| Guava Leaf (Selin-11-en-4-Alpha-ol CT) | 12.8%–18.8% |
| Chaste Tree (Berries) | 8.4%–17.5% |
| Black Pepper (Beta-Pinene CT) | 17.2% |
| Fingerroot ((E)-Beta-Ocimene CT) | 7.5%–17.0% |
| Sage (Wild) | 5.1%–16.8% |
| Leleshwa | 13.1%–16.5% |
| Tea tree | 0.1%–16.5% |
| Kanuka | 3.5%–16.4% |
| Yarrow (Sabinene CT) | 4.7%–16.0% |
| Sage (Alpha-Thujone CT) | 1.9%–15.9% |
| Lavandin (Super) | 0.0%–15.9% |
| White Turmeric (Distilled) | 0.0%–15.9% |
| Guava Leaf ((2E)-Hexenal CT) | 15.9% |
| Sage (Beta-Thujone CT) | 5.0%–15.7% |
| Lavandin (Dutch) | 0.0%–15.6% |
| Yarrow (Beta-Thujone CT) | 0.4%–15.2% |
| Hyssop (Linalool CT) | 12.3%–14.9% |
| Rosemary (Beta-Myrcene CT) | 8.0%–14.5% |
| Kunzea (Alpha-Pinene CT) | 3.6%–14.5% |
| Mugwort (Camphor CT) | 3.9%–14.1% |
| Monarda (Thymol CT) | 0.0%–14.1% |
| Genipi (A. umbelliformis, C-SH\B CT) | 4.1%–14.0% |
| Fingerroot (Camphor CT) | 2.6%–13.9% |
| Sweet Wormwood (Camphor CT) | 1.2%–13.9% |
| Galangal (False, Ethyl-p-Methoxycinnamate CT) | 5.7%–13.6% |
| Catnip (Nepetalactone CT) | 0.0%–13.5% |
| Mugwort (Artemisia Ketone CT) | 3.4%–13.2% |
| Mugwort (Alpha-Thujone CT) | 1.0%–13.2% |
| Thyme (Alpha-Terpineol CT) | 0.1%–13.2% |
| Rosemary (Bornyl Acetate CT) | 5.3%–12.8% |
| Fingerroot (Gamma-Terpinene CT) | 12.8% |
| Guava Leaf (Beta-Caryophyllene CT) | 1.8%–12.4% |
| Camphor (Camphor CT) | 1.0%–12.0% |
| Tansy (Beta-Thujone CT) | 0.5%–11.8% |
| Mugwort (Beta-Thujone CT) | 11.7% |
| Wild Chamomile (C. mixtus, Sant. Alc. CT) | 3.2%–11.6% |
| Vilayti Tulsi (Fenchone CT) | 0.0%–11.5% |
| Ravintsara (Camphor CT) | 1.0%–11.3% |
| Pennyroyal (M. pulegium) | 0.1%–11.1% |
| Ginger | 0.2%–10.9% |
| Blue Mountain Sage (Delta-3-Carene CT) | 0.0%–10.9% |
| Wild Marjoram (Linalool CT) | 1.1%–10.8% |
| Sweer Nancy (Artemisia Ketone CT) | 10.6% |
| Turmeric (Leaves) | 0.0%–10.5% |
| Lavandin (Abrialis) | 6.7%–10.4% |
| Sweet Wormwood (Artemisia Ketone CT) | 0.0%–10.4% |
| Lavandin (Grosso) | 4.0%–10.2% |
| Blue Yarrow (Artemisia Ketone CT) | 10.2% |
| Wild Turmeric (Distilled) | 0.1%–10.1% |
| Yarrow (Chamazulene CT) | 0.1%–9.6% |

| | |
|---|---|
| Genipi (A. umbelliformis, Alpha-Thujone CT) | 0.3%–9.5% |
| Mugwort (Beta-Caryophyllene CT) | 9.5% |
| Fingerroot (B. rotunda Nerol-Camphor CT) | 9.5% |
| White Verbena (Linalool CT) | 4.2%–9.2% |
| Rosemary (Beta-Myrcene CT) | 3.4%–9.0% |
| Myrtle (Limonene CT) | 6.6%–8.7% |
| Helichrysum (H. splendidum, Alpha-Terpinene CT) | 8.6% |
| Applemint (M. suav., Linalool CT) | 8.5% |
| Lavender (Brazilian) | 7.9% |
| Spearmint (Pulegone-Menthone-Isomenthone CT) | 1.6%–7.8% |
| Wild Chamomile (O. multicaulis) | 7.2%–7.4% |
| Hairy Basil (var. pilosum Eugenol CT) | 7.4% |
| Verbena (Linalool CT) | 0.0%–7.0% |
| Hairy Basil ((E)-Methyl Cinnamate CT) | 0.0%–7.0% |
| Spearmint (Carvone CT) | 1.0%–6.8% |
| Peppermint | 4.1%–6.7% |
| Niaouli ((E)-Nerolidol CT) | 0.1%–6.6% |
| Basil (Methyl Eugenol CT) | 0.1%–6.2% |
| Spearmint (Piperitone Oxide CT) | 0.4%–5.8% |
| Ocotea (Leaves) | 5.7% |
| Benzoin (Siam, S-HS Absolute) | 0.5%–5.5% |
| Wormwood (Trans-Sabinyl Acetate CT) | 1.0%–5.2% |
| Petitgrain (Lemon) | 0.0%–5.2% |
| Spearmint (Menthone CT) | 5.2% |
| Basil (Linalool CT) | 0.2%–5.0% |
| Spearmint (Linalool CT) | 4.7%–4.9% |
| Monarda (Linalool CT) | 0.4%–4.8% |
| Cinnamon Bark | 0.0%–4.6% |
| Allspice (Leaves, Eugenol CT) | 0.0%–4.6% |
| Verbena (Myrcene CT) | 0.1%–4.5% |
| Tamala ((E)-Cinnamaldehyde\Cinn. Ac. CT) | 0.1%–4.4% |
| Lavender (Bulgarian) | 0.4%–4.2% |
| Applemint (M. suav., Italian) | 0.0%–4.2% |
| Allspice (Berries, Methyl Eugenol CT) | 1.3%–4.1% |
| Allspice (Leaves, Methyl Eugenol CT) | 4.1% |
| Verbena (Limonene\Piperitenone CT) | 0.0%–4.0% |
| Ravensara (Limonene CT) | 0.1%–3.9% |
| Thyme (Thymol CT) | 0.0%–3.8% |
| Tamala (Linalool\(E)-Cinnamaldehyde CT) | 0.2%–3.7% |
| Holy Basil (Methyl Chavicol CT) | 2.5%–3.5% |
| Spearmint (Piperitenone Oxide CT) | 0.4%–3.5% |
| Lemon Eucalyptus | 1.8%–3.4% |
| Lavender (French) | 0.0%–3.4% |
| Bay (West Indies) | 0.0%–3.2% |
| Thyme (Carvacrol CT) | 0.0%–3.1% |
| Camphor (Linalool CT) | 0.1%–3.0% |
| Damiana (Delta-Cadinene CT) | 1.9%–2.8% |
| Sweet Inula (T-Cadinol CT) | 2.6% |
| Cumin | 0.1%–2.2% |
| Mugwort (Alpha-Phellandrene CT) | 1.8% |
| Mugwort (Germacrene D CT) | 1.8% |
| Honey Myrtle | 0.5%–1.6% |
| Ravensara (Methyl Eugenol CT) | 0.0%–1.4% |
| Rosewood (Wood) | 0.6%–1.2% |
| Spearmint (Cis-Ocimenone CT) | 1.2% |
| Cornmint | 0.0%–0.1% |

**1,8-Cineole + Limonene**

| | |
|---|---|
| Ocotea (Flowers Calices) | 0.0%–8.1% |
| Applemint (M. suav., Pulegone CT) | 5.5% |

**1,10(15)-Furanogermacradien-6-One**

| | |
|---|---|
| Opoponax (C. erythraea) | 4.3%–10.4% |

**1,10 Di-Epi-Cubenol**

| | |
|---|---|
| Holy Basil (aerial parts, eugenol CT) | 0.0%–2.6% |

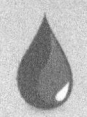

**1-Allyl-2,3,4,5-Tetramethoxybenzene**
| | |
|---|---|
| Parsley Seed | 2.0%–12.8% |
| Parsley (Whole Plant) | 6.5%–10.5% |

**1-Dodecanol**
| | |
|---|---|
| Rue (2-Undecanone CT) | 0.0%–11.0% |

**1-H-Cyclopropa[a]naphthalene Octahydro Compound**
| | |
|---|---|
| Calamus (Beta-Asarone CT) | 0.0%–2.9% |

**1-Methyl-5-(1-Methylethenyl)-Cyclohexene**
| | |
|---|---|
| Chinese Red Pine (Leaves) | 0.0%–6.0% |

**1-Nonene**
| | |
|---|---|
| Rue (2-Undecanone CT) | 0.0%–4.4% |

**1-Octanol**
| | |
|---|---|
| Frankincense (*B. carterii*) | 0.0%–11.9% |

**1-Octan-3-ol**
| | |
|---|---|
| Mugwort (1,8-Cineole CT) | 0.0%–1.8% |

**1-Octene**
| | |
|---|---|
| Mugwort (Chrysanthenyl Acetate CT) | 1.0% |

**1-Octen-3-ol**
| | |
|---|---|
| Monarda (Carvacrol/Para-Cymene CT) | 0.0%–10.3% |
| Mugwort (Alpha-Thujone CT) | 1.4%–1.7% |

**1-Octen-3yl Acetate**
| | |
|---|---|
| Mugwort (Chrysanthenyl Acetate CT) | 1.1% |

**1-Tricosene**
| | |
|---|---|
| Oakmoss Aboslute (Hydro. + Hexane) | 10.1% |

**1[7]2-Mentha-Diene-8-ol**
| | |
|---|---|
| Sweet Inula (Bornyl Acetate CT) | 0.0%–2.1% |

**1(5),3-Aromadendradiene**
| | |
|---|---|
| Indian Borage (Thymol CT) | 0.0%–7.1% |
| Indian Borage (Beta-Caryophyllene CT) | 3.2% |

**1(10)-Aristolen-9beta-ol**
| | |
|---|---|
| Spikenard (Calarene CT, Nepal) | 0.0%–11.6% |

**1(10),4-Furanodien-6-one**
| | |
|---|---|
| Opoponax (*C. erythraea*) | 9.0%–20.6% |

**10(15)-Cadinene-4-ol**
| | |
|---|---|
| Japanese Cedarwood (Alpha-Pinene CT) | 0.0%–7.2% |

**1a,2,3,3a,4,5,6,7b-octahydro-1,1,3a,7-tetramethyl-1H-Cyclopropanaphthelene (Beta-Maaliene)**
| | |
|---|---|
| Spikenard (Calarene CT, Nepal) | 0.0%–5.6% |

**2,5-Dimethylpyrazine**
| | |
|---|---|
| Fenugreek | 6.1% |

**2.6-Dimethylstyrene**
| | |
|---|---|
| Verbena (Myrcene CT) | 1.0%–7.2% |
| Verbena (Linalool CT) | 0.0%–3.8% |

**2,2-Dimethylbutanoic Acid**
| | |
|---|---|
| Khella (Aerial Parts, 2,2-Dimethylbut. CT) | 30.1% |

**2,2,6-Trimethylcyclohexanone**
| | |
|---|---|
| Cistus | 0.9%–11.8% |

**2,5-Dimethoxy-p-Cymene**
| | |
|---|---|
| Arnica (Roots, 2,5-Dimethoxy-p-Cymene CT) | 28.9%–40.6% |

**2,6-Diisopropylanisole**
| | |
|---|---|
| Arnica (Roots, 2,5-Dimethoxy-p-Cymene CT) | 8.9%–14.1% |

**2,6,9,9-Tetramethyl-2,6,10-Cyclodecatrien-1-one**
| | |
|---|---|
| Plai (2,6,9,9-Tetramethyl-2,6,10-Cyclodecatrien-1-one) | 60.8% |

**2-Acetoxy Tetradecanone**
| | |
|---|---|
| Rue (2-Undecanone CT) | 0.0%–14.5% |

**2-Acetyltridecane**
| | |
|---|---|
| Rue (2-Undecanone CT) | 0.0%–12.7% |

**2-Caren-10-al**
| | |
|---|---|
| Cumin | 0.0%–7.9% |

**2-Carene**
| | |
|---|---|
| Turmeric (Rhizome, Distilled) | 5.4%–61.8% |
| Hinoki (needles and twigs) | 17.4% |

**2-Epoxypropane**
| | |
|---|---|
| Rhododendron (Flowers) | 12.5% |

**2-Ethyl-4-Methyl-1,3-Pentadienyl Benzene**
| | |
|---|---|
| Wormwood ((Z)-Epoxy Ocimene CT) | 0.0%–7.4% |

**2-Heptanol Acetate**
| | |
|---|---|
| Rue (2-Undecanone CT) | 0.0%–17.5% |

**2-Hexenal (Tans-2-Hexenal)**
| | |
|---|---|
| Mugwort (Chrysanthenyl Acetate CT) | 5.0% |
| Mugwort (Alpha-Thujone CT) | 0.4%–3.1% |
| Mugwort (Beta-Caryophyllene CT) | 2.3% |
| Mugwort (1,8-Cineole CT) | 0.0%–1.1% |
| Mugwort (Camphor CT) | 0.0%–1.1% |
| Mugwort (Germacrene D CT) | 1.0% |

**2-Hydroxyguaia-1(10),11-Dien-15-oic Acid**
| | |
|---|---|
| Agarwood (*A. malaccensis*) | 0.0%–14.6% |

**2-Methoxycinnamaldehyde (O-Methoxycinnamic Aldehyde, (E)-O-Methoxycinnamaldehyde)**
| | |
|---|---|
| Cassia (Bark) | 0.0%–13.2% |

**2-Methylbutyl Angelate**
| | |
|---|---|
| Chamomile (Roman) | 13.0%–20.3% |

**2-Methylbutyl Butyrate (2-Methylbutyl butanoate, Butanoic acid, 2-methylbutyl ester)**
| | |
|---|---|
| Khella (Aerial Parts, 2-Mehtylbutyl Bu. CT) | 41.8% |

**2-Methylene-5-(1-methylvinyl)-8-methyl-bicyclo[5.3.0]decane**
| | |
|---|---|
| Japanese Cedarwood (Sapwood) | 0.0%–5.6% |

**2-Methylpentan-3-one**
| | |
|---|---|
| Helichrysum (ssp. *italicum*) | 0.0%–8.2% |

**2-Methyl-Cyclohexyl Pentanoate**
| | |
|---|---|
| Helichrysum (*H. italicum*) | 0.0%–11.1% |

**2-methyl-6-methylene-3,7-octadien-2-ol**
| | |
|---|---|
| Ledum (*L. palustre*) | 0.0%–7.9% |

**2-Nonanone**
| | |
|---|---|
| Rue (2-Undecanone CT) | 4.9%–41.7% |

**2-Nonene**
| | |
|---|---|
| Rue (2-Undecanone CT) | 0.0%–3.1% |

**2-Nonyacetate**
| | |
|---|---|
| Rue (2-Undecanone CT) | 0.0%–11.1% |

**2-Phenylethyl Alcohol (2-Phenylethanol)**
| | |
|---|---|
| Rose (Indian) | 0.4%–9.6% |
| Rose (Turkish) | 0.5%–1.2% |
| Rose (Bulgarian) | 0.2%–1.2% |

**2-Pinen-4-ol**
| | |
|---|---|
| Tsauri Grass | 0.0%–8.9% |

**2-Propeonic Acid**
| | |
|---|---|
| Galangal (False, 2-Propeonic Acid CT) | 35.5% |

**2-Undecanone**
| | |
|---|---|
| Rue (2-Undecanone CT) | 30.7%–73.2% |

**2-Vinyl-4H-1,3-Dithiin**
| | |
|---|---|
| Garlic (Vinyldithiins CT) | 17.7%–38.1% |
| Garlic (Sulfides CT) | 0.0%–8.7% |

**(2E)-Hexenal**
| | |
|---|---|
| Guava Leaf ((2E)-Hexenal CT) | 28.4% |

**(2Z,6E)-Farnesol (Cis,Trans-Farnesol, Z,E-Farnesol)**
| | |
|---|---|
| Betony (Bicyclogermacrene CT) | 0.0%–7.4% |
| Guava Leaf ((E)-Nerolidol CT) | 6.7% |

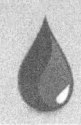

**3-Buthylphthalide**
Celery Seed                                    0.0%–3.5%
Celery Leaf                                    0.0%–3.5%

**3-Methyl-2-Butenyl Acetate**
Ylang Ylang (French I)                         4.2%

**3-Methyl-3-Buten-1-ol Acetate**
Ylang Ylang (French I)                         2.2%

**3-Methyl-5-Phenyl-Isothiazole**
Rhododendron (Flowers)                         6.4%%

**3-Methyl-6-Tert-Butylphenol**
Rhododendron (Flowers)                         10.8%

**3-Methylbutyl Isobutyrate**
Chamomile (Roman)                              5.2%–6.3%

**3-Methylenecyclohexene**
Schisandra Fruit (S. sphenanthera, α-Cad. CT)  4.4%

**3-Octanol**
Applemint (M. suav., Italian)                  0.0%–4.7%

**3-Octanyl Acetate**
Applemint (M. suav., Italian)                  0.0%–4.9%

**3-Undecyne**
Lemongrass (West Indian)                       1.5%–6.1%

**3,4-Decadienal**
Sweet Inula (Borneol CT)                       0.0%–7.5%

**3,4-Epoxy-Para-Menthan-2-One**
Wormseed, American (Ascaridole CT)             0.0%–4.1%

**3,5-Ditert-Butyl Phenol**
Turmeric (Rhizome, Solvent Extracted)          0.0%–5.4%

**3,7,11-Trimethyl-1,6 10-Dodecatrien-3-ol**
Jasmine (Hydrodistilled)                       12.5%

**3,7,11,15-Tetramethyl-Hexadecen-3-ol**
Jasmine (Hydrodistilled)                       12.4%

**3,9-Epoxy-p-Mentha-1,8(10)-Diene**
Tagetes (T. patula, Aerial Parts)              6.2%

**3-(2,3,4-Trithia-5-Heptenyl)-1-Thia-Cyclohex-5-ene**
Garlic (Vinyldithiins CT)                      2.0%–6.7%

**3-Vinyl-4h-1,2-Dithiin**
Garlic (Vinyldithiins CT)                      14.5%–32.7%
Garlic (Sulfides CT)                           0.0%–4.5%

**(3E,6E)-Alpha-Farnesene**
Jasmine Absolute (Benzyl Acetate CT)           0.0%–5.8%

**4-Carene**
Shell Ginger (1,8-Cineole CT)                  0.0%–7.3%

**4-Hydroxy-8,9-Didehydrothymol Dimethyl Ether**
Arnica (Roots, Thymol Derivatives CT)          4.7%–7.4%

**4-Hydroxythymol Dimethyl Ether**
Arnica (Roots, Thymol Derivatives CT)          3.9%–4.8%

**4-Methylhexan-3-one**
Helichrysum (ssp. italicum)                    0.0%–10.5%

**4-Phenyl 2-Butanoate**
Agarwood (A. malaccensis)                      0.4%–32.1%

**4-Vinyl-Guaiacol**
Tagetes (T. patula, Aerial Parts)              8.6%

**4,6,9-Trimethyldec-8-en-3,5-dione**
Helichrysum (ssp. italicum)                    0.3%–19.8%

**4,6-Dimethyloctan-3,5-dione**
Helichrysum (ssp. italicum)                    0.0%–11.3%

**4,7,10-Cycloundecatriene**
Guava Leaf (Limonene CT)                       0.0%–4.4%

**4a,5-Dimethyl-3-(1-ethylidene)-4,4a,5,6,7,8-Hexahydro-2(3H)-Napthalenone**
Agarwood (A. crassna)                          0.0%–9.7%

**4a-Hydroxy-4b-Methyldihydrocostol**
Formosan Cypress (Wood, α-Eudesmol CT) 5.5%

**5-(3-furyl)-2-methyl-1-penten-3-ol=lepalol**
Ledum (L. palustre)                            0.0%–7.9%

**5-(3-furyl)-2-methyl-1-penten-3-one=lepalone**
Ledum (L. palustre)                            0.0%–3.5%

**5-Acetyl Thiazole**
Applemint (M. rotun., Pulegone CT)             0.0%–11.3%

**5-Indanol**
Allspice (Berries, Eugenol CT)                 0.0%–5.9%

**5-Isopropylidene-3,8-Dimethyl-1(5H)-Azulene**
White Turmeric (Solvent Extracted)             4.3%–9.2%

**5-Methyl-2-(2-Hydroxy-2-Propyl)-Cyclohexanol**
Lemon Eucalyptus                               0.0%–4.7%

**5,6-Diethenyl-1-Methyl-Cyclohexene**
Rue (2-Undecanone CT)                          0.0%–3.4%

**5,9-Dimethyl-1-Decanol**
Kaffir Lime Petitgain                          0.0%–5.0%

**6-Camphenone**
Fingerroot (Gamma-Terpinene CT)                18.7%

**6-Methyl-5-Hepten-2-ol**
White Verbena (Citral CT)                      0.0%–6.0%

**6-Methyl-5-Hepten-2-One (6-Methyl Hept-5-ene-2-one)**
Fenugreek                                      4.5%
Petitgrain (Lemon)                             0.7%–3.2%
Petitgrain (Lime)                              1.1%–2.5%
Lemon Myrtle (Citral CT)                       0.1%–2.5%

**7-Epi-Alpha-Eudesmol**
Amyris                                         9.4%–10.7%
Guaiacwood                                     0.0%–3.3%

**7-Isobutyroxy Thymol Isobutyrate**
Arnica (Roots, Thymol Derivatives CT)          2.1%–3.1%

**8-Hydroxy-10(11), Eremophiladien-9-one**
Buddha Wood                                    0.1%–4.1%

**8-Nydroxymenthone**
Buchu (A. crenulata)                           0.0%–4.9%

**8-Mercapto-p-menthan-3-one (cis + trans)**
Buchu (A. betulina, Isomenthone CT)            0.7%–6.6%

**8Beta-Hydroxysandracopimarene**
Japanese Cedarwood (Alpha-Pinene CT)           0.0%–3.6%

**9,1-Eremophiladien-8-One**
Agarwood (A. crassna)                          0.0%–6.3%

**9,12-Octadecadienoic Acid**
Moringa (Flowers)                              12.2%
Moringa (Leaves, (E)-Phytol CT)                7.8%

**9,12,15-Octadecatrienoic Acid**
Jasmine (Hydrodistilled)                       4.8%

**9-Epi-(E)-Caryophyllene**
Pink Pepper (S. terebinthifolius, Leaves, p-Cymen-7-ol CT) 10.1%
Black Sage (Caryophyllene Oxide CT)            0.6%–6.0%

**9-Hydroxy-1,7,9-Eremophilatrien-8-one**
Buddha Wood                                    0.0%–6.7%

**9-Hydroxy-7(11),9-Eremophiladien-8-one**
Buddha Wood                                    18.0%–37.0%

**9-Isobutyryloxy Thymol Isobutyrate**
Arnica (Roots, Thymol Derivatives CT)          5.3%–6.7%

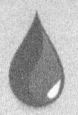

**Abienol**

Chinese Cedarwood — 0.0%–4.5%

**Abietadiene**

Chinese Cedarwood — 0.0%–5.3%

**Abietatriene**

Chaste Tree (Berries) — 0.0%–1.2%

**Acetophenone**

Cassia (Bark) — 0.0%–6.9%

**Acoradiene**

Schisandra Fruit (*S. chinensis*) — 1.8%–3.0%

**Acorenone**

Calamus (Acorenone CT) — 22.4%–27.5%
Calamus (Shyobunones CT) — 9.0%–13.0%

**Acorone + Isoacrone**

Calamus (Shyobunones CT) — 8.0%–10.0%

**AETIB (2-Methyl-propanoic acid-2-[3-[(acetyloxy)methyl]oxiranyl]-5-methylphenyl ester)**

Arnica (Roots, 2,5-Dimethoxy-p-Cymene CT) — 1.0%–4.2%

**Agarospirol**

Agarwood (Malaysian) — 0.0%–24.2%
Agarwood (*A. crassna*) — 3.7%–5.8%
Agarwood (*A. sinensis*) — 0.0%–4.0%

**Alantolactone (Helenine, Helenin)**

Elecampane — 51.3%–55.8%

**Aliphatic Aldehyde**

Monarda (Carvacrol/Para-Cymene CT) — 0.0%–6.3%

**Allo-Ocimene (Neo-Allo-Ocimene)**

Tagetes (*T. patula*, Flowers) — 3.7%
Calendula ((E)-Beta-Ocimene CT) — 3.7%
Black Pepper (Beta-Pinene CT) — 3.4%

**Alloaromadendrene (Allo-Aromadendrene)**

Maritime Pine (Needles, Beta-Cary. CT) — 0.0%–12.5%
Calendula (Alpha-Cadinol/Delta-Cadinene CT) — 0.0%–9.4%
Valerian — 0.0%–6.9%
Gurjun Balsam (*D. turbinatus*) — 4.0%–6.0%
Gurjun Balsam (*D. tuberculatus*) — 4.0%–6.0%
Gurjun Balsam (*D. kerri*) — 5.3%
Ravintsara (Camphor CT) — 0.0%–4.4%
Black Sage (Alpha-Pinene CT) — 0.0%–4.3%
Pink Pepper (*S. molle*, Leaves, Beta-Pinene CT) — 4.0%
Opoponax (*C. erythraea*) — 2.0%–3.6%
Ledum (*L. palustre*) — 0.8%–3.2%
Southern Blue Gum — 0.0%–3.0%
Kunzea (Spathulenol\Globulol CT) — 1.2%–2.9%
Chaste Tree (Leaves) — 0.0%–2.0%
Hyssop (Pinocamphone CT) — 0.0%–1.0%

**Allyl Methyl Disulfide**

Garlic (Sulfides CT) — 0.0%–9.1%

**Allyl Methyl Trisulfide**

Garlic (Sulfides CT) — 7.3%–18.2%

**Alpha-Agarofuran**

Agarwood (Malaysian) — 1.4%–3.5%

**Alpha-Alaskane**

Chinese Cedarwood — 0.0%–4.8%

**Alpha-Amorphene**

Muhuhu (Wood) — 11.9%–16.5%
Hinoki (Taiwan Cypress, wood) — 0.0%–9.4%
Guggul — 0.0%–7.6%
Formosan Cypress (Wood, Myrtenol CT) — 0.0%–6.3%
Rhododendron (Aerial Parts) — 3.2%–5.3%
Indian Borage (Delta-Cadinene CT) — 0.0%–4.8%

Indian Borage (Thymol CT) — 0.0%–4.2%
Indian Borage (Beta-Caryophyllene CT) — 3.0%
Manuka (Selinene/Beta-Elemene CT) — 2.8%

**Alpha-Asarone (Trans-Asarone, Azaron)**

Calamus (Alpha-Asarone CT) — 50.1%
Calamus (Beta-Asarone CT) — 0.1%–17.3%

**Alpha-Bergamotene <Isomer Not Identified>**

Copaiba — 1.0%–11.8%
Basil (Linalool CT) — 2.6%–11.2%
Schisandra Fruit (*S. chinensis*) — 8.6%–10.5%
Basil (Methyl Eugenol CT) — 0.1%–6.8%
Holy Basil (aerial parts, beta-bisabolene CT) — 2.9%–6.6%
Opoponax (*C. guidotti*) — 0.0%–3.0%
Chaste Tree (Berries) — 0.0%–1.9%

**Alpha-Bisabolol & Isomer: Epi-Alpha-Bisabolol**

Blue Mountain Sage (Alpha-Bisabolol CT) — 37.4%–47.6%
German Chamomile — 0.1%–44.2%
Balsam Poplar — 23.5%–25.8%
Blue Mountain Sage (Delta-3-Carene CT) — 8.2%–19.7%
Blue Mountain Sage (Gamma-Terpinene CT) — 17.4%
Katrafay (Alpha-Pinene CT) — 0.0%–16.9%
Lavender (Brazilian) — 13.1%
Sandalwood (*S. spicatum*) — 4.9%–10.7%
Katrafay (Alpha-Eudesmol CT) — 0.0%–7.1%
Katrafay (Ishwarane CT) — 0.0%–5.8%
Yarrow (1,8-Cineole\Camphor CT) — 0.0%–5.5%
Valerian — 0.0%–5.4%
Blue Mountain Sage ((E)-Nerolidol CT) — 1.3%–4.7%
Guava Leaf (β-Cary.\(E)-Nerolidol CT) — 3.2%
Chaste Tree (Leaves) — 0.0%–2.7%

**Alpha-Bulnesene (Delta-Guaiene)**

Patchouli (Brazilian) — 6.9%–55.1%
Patchouli (Indonesian, Malaysian, Vietnamese) — 6.8%–14.7%
Patchouli (Chinese) — 0.9%–11.8%

**Alpha-Cadinene**

Japanese Cedarwood (Heartwood) — 0.0%–18.6%
Schisandra Fruit (*S. sphenanthera*, α-Cad. CT) — 18.3%
Japanese Cedarwood (Heartwood) — 0.0%–17.3%
Helichrysum (*H. splendidum*, Delta-cadinene CT) — 2.3%–7.6%
Damiana (Caryophyllene Oxide CT) — 0.0%–7.3%
Guava Leaf (Beta-Caryophyllene CT) — 0.0%–5.3%

**Alpha-Cadinol**

Calendula (Alpha-Cadinol/Delta-Cadinene CT) — 2.0%–33.6%
Hinoki (wood) — 20.5%
Helichrysum (*H. splendidum*, Delta-cadinene CT) — 5.8%–16.8%
Pink Pepper (*S. terebinthifolius*, Fruits, δ-3-Carene CT) — 0.0%–16.3%
Katrafay ((γ,δ)-Cadinene CT) — 0.0%–15.3%
Guggul — 7.3%–14.5%
Juniper (*J. recurva*, Needles) — 0.8%–13.1%
Hinoki (Taiwan Cypress, wood) — 0.3%–12.9%
Indian Borage (Delta-Cadinene CT) — 5.7%–12.5%
Formosan Cypress (Twig) — 12.4%
Sweet Inula (1,8-Cineole CT) — 0.0%–11.8%
Wild Chamomile (*O. mixta, C. mixtrum*) — 0.1%–8.9%
Cangerana (Leaves) — 0.9%–8.0%
Citronella (*C. winteranius*) — 0.5%–8.0%
Copaiba (Leaves) — 3.2%–7.9%
Pine — 0.0%–7.7%
Pink Pepper (*S. molle*, Fruits, α-Phellandrene CT) — 0.1%–7.2%
Calendula (Alpha-Cadinol/Delta-Cadinene CT) — 0.5%–6.8%
Damiana (Caryophyllene Oxide CT) — 0.0%–6.5%
White Pine — 0.0%–5.7%
Japanese Cedarwood (Heartwood) — 0.0%–5.2%

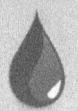

| | |
|---|---|
| Black Pepper (Beta-Caryophyllene CT) | 0.0%–4.9% |
| Juniper (Chinese) | 0.0%–4.8% |
| Gobre Salla | 0.9%–4.3% |
| Formosan Cypress (Wood, Myrtenol CT) | 0.4%–4.1% |
| Hairy Basil (var. *pilosum* Linalool CT) | 0.0%–4.0% |
| Mastic (NT\B, Germacrene D CT) | 3.8% |
| Ghandi Root | 0.0%–3.7% |
| Maritime Pine (Needles, Alpha-Pinene CT) | 0.0%–3.5% |
| Engelmann Spruce | 0.0%–3.3% |
| Allspice (Leaves, Eugenol CT) | 0.0%–3.2% |
| Mastic (Leaves) | 0.0%–3.0% |
| Yarrow (Chamazulene CT) | 0.0%–1.8% |
| Helichrysum (*H. splendidum*, Alpha-Terpinene CT) | 1.6% |
| Ylang Ylang (French IV) | 1.5% |

**Alpha-Calacorene**

| | |
|---|---|
| Muhuhu (Leaves) | 6.0% |
| Muhuhu (Wood) | 4.4%–5.0% |

**Alpha-Camphenal**

| | |
|---|---|
| Juniper, Phoenicia (leaves, isoborneol CT) | 7.9% |

**Alpha-Campholenal (Campholenic Aldehyde)**

| | |
|---|---|
| Hyssop (Alpha-Pinene CT) | 1.1% |

**Alpha-Cedrene**

| | |
|---|---|
| Chinese Cedarwood | 0.7%–44.2% |
| Cedarwood (Virginian, Wood) | 21.1%–35.0% |
| Texas Cedarwood | 1.8%–30.7% |
| Cedarwood (Himalayan, Wood) | 0.0%–15.8% |
| Helichrysum (*H. italicum*) | 0.0%–9.6% |
| Frankincense (*B. carterii*) | 0.0%–6.1% |
| Calamus (Alpha-Asarone CT) | 3.1% |

**Alpha-Chamagrene**

| | |
|---|---|
| Sweet Inula (Bornyl Acetate CT) | 0.0%–2.9% |

**Alpha-Cis-Bergamotene ((Z)-Alpha-Bergamotene)**

| | |
|---|---|
| Holy Basil (aerial parts, eugenol CT) | 1.3%–3.1% |

**Alpha-Copaene (Copaene)**

| | |
|---|---|
| Copaiba | 1.6%–18.2% |
| Katrafay (Ishwarane CT) | 5.9%–15.6% |
| Katrafay ((γ,δ)-Cadinene CT) | 0.1%–13.8% |
| Guggul | 0.0%–10.1% |
| Muhuhu (Leaves) | 9.0% |
| Pink Pepper (*S. terebinthifolius*, Fruits, Myrc/Lim. CT) | 3.5%–8.0% |
| Katrafay (Leaves) | 0.1%–7.7% |
| Betony (MLD-C CT) | 4.8%–7.3% |
| Black Sage (Tricyclene CT) | 7.0% |
| Indian Borage (Beta-Caryophyllene CT) | 6.9% |
| Opoponax (*C. erythraea*) | 4.4%–6.6% |
| Manuka (Leptospermone CT) | 0.6%–6.6% |
| Betony (Bicyclogermacrene CT) | 1.7%–6.5% |
| Cedarwood (Virginian, Wood) | 0.0%–6.3% |
| Black Pepper (Beta-Caryophyllene CT) | 0.2%–5.5% |
| Frankincense (*B. carterii*) | 0.0%–5.5% |
| Myrrh | 0.0%–5.5% |
| Katrafay (Alpha-Pinene CT) | 1.1%–5.1% |
| Maritime Pine (Needles, Beta-Cary. CT) | 0.0%–5.1% |
| Indian Borage (Delta-Cadinene CT) | 2.6%–5.0% |
| Gurjun Balsam (*D. turbinatus*) | 5.0% |
| Black Pepper (Limonene CT) | 0.1%–4.8% |
| Betony (β-Phell.\α-Pinene CT) | 0.0%–4.4% |
| Ocotea (Leaves) | 3.3% |
| Gurjun Balsam (*D. kerri*) | 3.1% |
| Muhuhu (Wood) | 1.2%–3.0% |
| Tarragon (Methyl Chavicol CT) | 0.0%–2.2% |
| Copaiba (Leaves) | 0.1%–1.5% |
| Mugwort (1,8-Cineole CT) | 0.6%–1.3% |

| | |
|---|---|
| Ocotea (Flowers Calices) | 0.0%–1.3% |
| Angelica Root | 0.2%–1.1% |

**Alpha-Copaene-11-ol**

| | |
|---|---|
| Angelica Root | 0.1%–2.5% |

**Alpha-Cubebene**

| | |
|---|---|
| Applemint (*M. suav.*, Italian) | 0.0%–10.1% |
| Japanese Cedarwood (Heartwood) | 0.2%–9.3% |
| Basil (Methyl Eugenol CT) | 0.1%–6.2% |
| Manuka (Leptospermone CT) | 3.0%–4.4% |
| Black Cumin (Thymoquinone CT) | 0.0%–3.0% |
| Rosewood (Wood) | 0.0%–2.8% |
| Ocotea (Flowers Calices) | 0.0%–1.1% |

**Alpha-Curcumene**

| | |
|---|---|
| Guava Leaf (β-Bisabolene\β-Sesqu. CT) | 5.1% |

**Alpha-Eudesmol**

| | |
|---|---|
| Katrafay (Alpha-Eudesmol CT) | 9.9%–37.5% |
| Japanese Cedarwood (Twig) | 10.9%–25.6% |
| Guava Leaf (Limonene CT) | 0.0%–23.3% |
| Formosan Cypress (Wood, α-Eudesmol CT) | 18.1% |
| Agarwood (Malaysian) | 0.0%–17.3% |
| Auracaria | 10.8%–13.3% |
| Japanese Cedarwood (16-Kaurene CT) | 0.0%–12.2% |
| Frankincense (*B. serrata*) | 0.2%–11.5% |
| Katrafay (Alpha-Pinene CT) | 3.9%–11.3% |
| Blue Cypress (Wood) | 7.6%–11.2% |
| Japanese Cedarwood (Heartwood) | 0.0%–10.7% |
| Amyris | 4.8%–9.4% |
| Japanese Cedarwood (Alpha-Pinene CT) | 2.6%–7.1% |
| African Bluegrass (Linalool CT) | 6.5%–6.7% |
| Pink Pepper (*S. molle*, Leaves, α-Phellandrene CT) | 0.0%–6.1% |
| Fragonia (Balanced CT) | 0.0%–5.1% |
| Galangal (Lesser) | 0.0%–4.5% |
| Zdravetz | 0.0%–3.9% |
| Japanese Cedarwood (Sapwood) | 0.0%–3.8% |
| Guaiacwood | 0.0%–3.7% |
| Balsam Poplar | 0.0%–3.7% |
| Japanese Cedarwood (Bark) | 0.0%–3.4% |
| Spikenard (Valeranone CT) | 3.0% |
| Angelica Root | 0.1%–1.1% |

**Alpha-Farnesene ((E,E)-Alpha-Farnesene)**

| | |
|---|---|
| Ylang Ylang (Madagascan III) | > 17.4% |
| Applemint (*M. suav.*, Italian) | 0.0%–16.5% |
| Ylang Ylang Complete | 3.9%–12.9% |
| Ylang Ylang (Madagascan II) | > 12.7% |
| Ylang Ylang (French IV) | 10.1% |
| Ginger | 0.0%–7.0% |
| Ylang Ylang (Solvent Extracted) | 6.2%–6.8% |
| Black Sage (Alpha-Santalene CT) | 6.4% |
| Carrot Seed | 0.2%–5.9% |
| Galangal (Lesser) | 0.0%–5.7% |
| Cananga | 0.1%–3.8% |
| Black Pepper (Beta-Caryophyllene CT) | 0.0%–3.9% |
| Ylang Ylang (French I) | 1.6% |

**Alpha-Fenchene**

| | |
|---|---|
| Valerian | 0.0%–28.3% |
| Mugwort (Camphor CT) | 0.0%–3.9% |

**Alpha-Fenchyl Acetate (Endo-Fenchyl Acetate)**

| | |
|---|---|
| Galangal (Greater, 1,8-Cineole CT) | 0.0%–18.4% |
| Galangal (Lesser) | 0.5%–15.2% |

**Alpha-Guaiene**

| | |
|---|---|
| Patchouli (Chinese) | 1.7%–21.5% |
| Patchouli (Indonesian, Malaysian, Vietnamese) | 4.3%–13.4% Patchouli |
| (Brazilian) | 2.9%–12.0% |

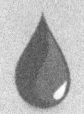

**Alpha-Guiene—continued**

| | |
|---|---|
| Agarwood (*A. crassna*) | 0.0%–8.9% |
| Agarwood (*A. malaccensis*) | 0.0%–5.8% |
| Chinese Red Pine (Leaves) | 0.0%–3.7% |
| Yarrow (Chamazulene CT) | 0.1%–2.0% |
| Chaste Tree (Leaves) | 0.0%–1.2% |
| Hyssop (Alpha-Pinene CT) | 1.0% |

**Alpha-Gurjunene**

| | |
|---|---|
| Gurjun Balsam (*D. tuberculatus*) | 90.0% |
| Gurjun Balsam (*D. kerri*) | 79.2% |
| Gurjun Balsam (*D. turbinatus*) | 20.0%–75.0% |
| Spikenard (Calarene CT) | 0.1%–9.1% |
| Japanese Cedarwood (16-Kaurene/Valencene CT) | 7.9% |
| Black Sage (Beta-Phellandrene CT) | 6.2% |
| Opoponax (*C. erythraea*) | 4.3%–6.0% |
| Guggul | 0.0%–5.5% |
| Tamala (Trans-Sabinene Hydrate CT) | 4.7% |
| Kunzea (Spathulenol\Globulol CT) | 1.1%–4.5% |
| Ferula (Limonene CT) | 3.1% |
| Chaste Tree (Leaves) | 0.0%–1.6% |
| Mugwort (Camphor CT) | 0.0%–1.3% |

**Alpha-Himachalene**

| | |
|---|---|
| Cedarwood (Himalayan, Wood) | 10.4%–30.8% |
| Cedarwood (Atlas) | 4.2%–16.4% |
| Schisandra Fruit (*S. chinensis*) | 8.8%–11.4% |

**Alpha-Humulene (Alpha-Caryophyllene)**

| | |
|---|---|
| Hops | 1.9%–51.2% |
| Plai (2,6,9,9-Tetramethyl-2,6,10-Cyclodecatrien-1-one) | 23.9% |
| Guava Leaf (Beta-Caryophyllene CT) | 1.0%–17.2% |
| Catnip (1,8-cineole CT) | 14.4% |
| Sage (Wild) | 4.0%–13.5% |
| Ledum (*R. groenlandicum*) | 0.0%–12.1% |
| Guava Leaf (Viridiflorol CT) | 0.1%–10.9% |
| Ylang Ylang (Solvent Extracted) | 10.7%–10.8% |
| Aleppo Pine (Aerial Parts) | 0.0%–10.5% |
| Indian Borage (Carvacrol CT) | 0.0%–9.7% |
| Katrafay (Ishwarane CT) | 0.0%–9.5% |
| Japanese Cedarwood (Heartwood) | 0.7%–9.4% |
| Cananga | 4.2%–9.2% |
| Guggul | 0.0%–8.9% |
| Mugwort (Alpha-Phellandrene CT) | 8.8% |
| Formosan Cypress (Neeldes, Germ. D CT) | 4.4%–8.7% |
| Hemp (Myrcene CT) | 0.7%–8.7% |
| Copaiba | 1.1%–8.6% |
| Indian Borage (Delta-Cadinene CT) | 6.3%–8.2% |
| Aleppo Pine (Needles) | 1.4%–8.0% |
| Indian Borage (Beta-Caryophyllene CT) | 8.0% |
| Hemp (Beta-Caryophyllene CT) | 5.4%–7.8% |
| Rhododendron (Leaves) | 7.2% |
| Maritime Pine (Needles, Beta-Cary. CT) | 4.3%–6.9% |
| Juniper (Needles) | 0.8%–6.2% |
| Ylang Ylang (French IV) | 6.2% |
| Tamala (Beta-Caryophyllene CT) | 6.2% |
| Sage (Alpha-Thujone CT) | 0.0%–5.6% |
| Oriental Arborvitae (Needles) | 0.0%–5.6% |
| Holy Basil (Aerial Parts, Estragole CT) | 0.0%–5.5% |
| Mugwort (Germacrene D CT) | 5.0% |
| Black Pepper (Beta-Caryophyllene CT) | 0.0%–4.9% |
| Black Sage (Alpha-Pinene CT) | 1.6%–4.8% |
| Black Sage (Beta-Caryophyllene CT) | 4.8% |
| Juniper Berry | 1.3%–4.6% |
| Silver Fir (*A. alba*) | 0.8%–4.6% |
| Mugwort (Beta-Caryophyllene CT) | 4.4% |
| Wild Chamomile (*O. multicaulis*) | 0.0%–4.1% |
| Formosan Cypress (Wood, α-Eudesmol CT) | 4.1% |
| Applemint (*M. suav.*, Carvone CT) | 0.0%–4.0% |
| Allspice (Leaves, Eugenol CT) | 0.0%–3.9% |
| Applemint (*M. rotun.*, β-Caryophyllene CT) | 3.9% |
| Chinese Red Pine (Leaves) | 1.7%–3.4% |
| Mastic (Leaves) | 0.0%–3.3% |
| Angelica Root | 0.4%–3.2% |
| Mugwort (Alpha-Thujone CT) | 2.6%–3.1% |
| Guava Leaf (β-Cary.\(E)-Nerolidol CT) | 3.1% |
| Calendula (Alpha-Cadinol/Delta-Cadinene CT) | 0.0%–3.0% |
| Chaste Tree (Berries) | 0.0%–2.7% |
| Manuka (Selinene/Beta-Elemene CT) | 2.6% |
| Holy Basil (aerial parts, eugenol CT) | 1.3%–2.3% |
| Sweet Inula (1,8-Cineole CT) | 1.9%–2.0% |
| Mugwort (Camphor CT) | 0.0%–1.9% |
| Ocotea (Flowers Calices) | 0.0%–1.8% |
| Mugwort (1,8-Cineole CT) | 0.5%–1.6% |
| Mugwort (Isobornyl Isobutyrate D CT) | 1.3% |

**Alpha-Humulene Epoxide**

| | |
|---|---|
| Angelica Root | 0.1%–2.0% |

**Alpha-Ionone (Trans-Alpha-Ionone, (E)-Alpha-Ionone)**

| | |
|---|---|
| Arnica (Flowers) | 4.0%–4.3% |

**Alpha-Isocomene**

| | |
|---|---|
| Arnica (Roots, Thymol Derivatives CT) | 6.9%–9.1% |
| Arnica (Roots, 2,5-Dimethoxy-p-Cymene CT) | 1.3%–7.6% |

**Alpha-Longifolene**

| | |
|---|---|
| Pine | 0.0%–9.6% |

**Alpha-Longipinene**

| | |
|---|---|
| Ylang Ylang (Solvent Extracted) | 6.8%–6.9% |
| Vetiver | 0.0%–4.2% |

**Alpha-Muurolene**

| | |
|---|---|
| Siam Wood (Root Bark) | 1.8%–10.4% |
| Kumquat (*F. margarita*, Leaves) | 0.1%–10.3% |
| Japanese Cedarwood (Heartwood) | 1.5%–9.3% |
| Guggul | 0.0%–8.1% |
| Muhuhu (Leaves) | 8.0% |
| Katrafay (Ishwarane CT) | 0.0%–6.7% |
| Rhododendron (Aerial Parts) | 2.7%–5.9% |
| Hinoki (wood) | 5.8% |
| Calendula (Alpha-Cadinol/Delta-Cadinene CT) | 0.0%–5.6% |
| Japanese Cedarwood (Bark) | 1.3%–5.4% |
| Formosan Cypress (Wood, Myrtenol CT) | 1.3%–5.3% |
| Japanese Cedarwood (Sapwood) | 3.4%–4.0% |
| Manuka (Selinene/Beta-Elemene CT) | 3.1% |
| Muhuhu (Wood) | 0.9%–3.0% |
| Angelica Root | 0.2%–1.1% |

**Alpha-Muurolol**

| | |
|---|---|
| Betony (Bicyclogermacrene CT) | 0.0%–7.7% |
| Helichrysum (*H. splendidum*, Delta-cadinene CT) | 3.4%–7.1% |
| Formosan Cypress (Wood, α-Eudesmol CT) | 6.5% |
| Calendula (Alpha-Cadinol/Delta-Cadinene CT) | 0.0%–5.7% |
| Guava Leaf (Beta-Caryophyllene CT) | 0.0%–5.6% |
| Siam Wood (Root Bark) | 0.0%–3.3% |
| Guava Leaf ((E)-Nerolidol CT) | 3.1% |
| Helichrysum (*H. splendidum*, Spathulenol CT) | 0.4%–2.9% |

**Alpha-Myrcene**

| | |
|---|---|
| Tangerine (Distilled) | 0.0%–4.2% |
| Ravintsara (1,8-Cineole CT) | 0.0%–3.2% |

**Alpha-Ocimene**

| | |
|---|---|
| Tagetes (*T. patula*, Aerial Parts) | 3.4% |

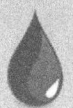

**Alpha-Patchoulene**

| | |
|---|---|
| Patchouli (Chinese) | 0.0%–9.1% |
| Patchouli (Indonesian, Malaysian, Vietnamese) | 1.8%–8.0% |
| Patchouli (Brazilian) | 5.2%–6.7% |
| Calendula (Alpha-Cadinol/Delta-Cadinene CT) | 0.0%–4.3% |

**Alpha-Phellandrene**

| | |
|---|---|
| Dill (Aerial Parts, Alpha-Phellandrene CT) | 31.8%–63.0% |
| Dill Leaves | 62.7% |
| Turmeric (Leaves) | 8.0%–57.8% |
| Pink Pepper (*S. molle*, Fruits, α-Phellandrene CT) | 22.1%–46.5% |
| Pink Pepper (*S. molle*, Leaves, α-Phellandrene CT) | 26.5%–45.7% |
| Pink Pepper (*S. molle*, Fruits/Leaves, α-Phell./Sylv. CT) | 32.8%–45.0% |
| Pink Pepper (*S. molle*, Aerial Parts, α-Phell. CT) | 35.9% |
| Pink Pepper (*S. terebinthifolius*, Fruits, α-Phell. CT) | 34.4% |
| Dill (Flowers) | 30.3% |
| Pink Pepper (*S. terebinthifolius*, Fruits/Leaves, Bicyclogerm. CT) | 11.7%–22.2% |
| Elemi | 8.8%–17.6% |
| Eucalyptus Dives | 0.0%–17.4% |
| Mugwort (Alpha-Phellandrene CT) | 17.3% |
| Wormwood (Beta-Pinene CT) | 9.8%–16.4% |
| Pink Pepper (*S. terebinthifolius*, Fruits, Limonene CT) | 11.9%–15.7% |
| Betony (Alpha-Thujene CT) | 0.1%–14.0% |
| Monarda (Thymol CT) | 0.4%–13.7% |
| Mastic (NT\B, Alpha-Pinene CT) | 1.2%–13.4% |
| Pink Pepper (*S. terebinthifolius*, Fruits, δ-3-Carene CT) | 2.9%–12.9% |
| Fennel (Trans-Anethole CT) | 0.1%–10.5% |
| Wormwood (Sabinene CT) | 5.4%–10.3% |
| Vilayti Tulsi (Sabinene CT) | 0.0%–10.2% |
| Mastic (NT\B, Terpinene-4-ol CT) | 4.3%–10.0% |
| Pink Pepper (*S. terebinthifolius*, Leaves, Sabinene CT) | 9.9% |
| Turmeric (Rhizome, Distilled) | 0.5%–9.4% |
| Blue Tansy (Sabinene CT) | 7.1%–9.2% |
| Angelica Root | 0.8%–9.1% |
| Parsley (Leaves, Myristicin CT) | 0.3%–8.7% |
| Black Pepper (Limonene CT) | 0.5%–8.6% |
| Dill (Aerial Parts, Carvone CT) | 0.1%–8.0% |
| Rosemary (Alpha-Pinene CT) | 0.1%–7.9% |
| Juniper, Phoenicia (leaves, isoborneol CT) | 7.6% |
| Camphor (Camphor CT) | 0.2%–6.3% |
| Mugwort (Beta-Thujone CT) | 6.3% |
| Juniper, Phoenicia (needles) | 0.0%–6.1% |
| Wormwood ((Z)-Epoxy Ocimene CT) | 0.0%–6.0% |
| Nutmeg (East Indian) | 0.0%–5.8% |
| Helichrysum (*H. splendidum*, Alpha-Terpinene CT) | 5.5% |
| Yarrow (1,8-Cineole\Camphor CT) | 0.5%–5.4% |
| Wormwood (Myrcene CT) | 0.0%–5.3% |
| Wormwood (Beta-Thujone CT) | 0.0%–4.9% |
| Wild Marjoram (1,8-Cineole CT) | 0.0%–3.8% |
| Mastic (NT\B, Beta-Myrcene CT) | 1.5%–3.5% |
| Mastic (Leaves) | 0.0%–3.5% |
| Black Pepper (Delta-3-Carene CT) | 2.9%–3.4% |
| Mastic (Twigs, Alpha-Pinene CT) | 3.4% |
| Ravensara (Sabinene CT) | 1.1%–2.8% |
| Cumin | 0.0%–1.9% |
| Ravensara (Alpha-Terpinene CT) | 1.2%–1.3% |

**Alpha-Pinene**

| | |
|---|---|
| Formosan Cypress (Neeldes, α-Pinene CT) | 89.3%–96.9% |
| Turkish Pine (Needles) | 1.4%–90.2% |
| Juniper, Phoenicia (Berries) | 26.9%–86.4% |
| Mastic (Gum Resin) | 21.7%–82.3% |
| Cedarwood (Atlas) | 14.9%–79.4% |
| Frankincense (*B. sacra*) | 5.3%–78.5% |
| Maritime Pine (Gum Resin) | 44.1%–78.0% |

| | |
|---|---|
| Kanuka | 54.5%–72.4% |
| Hyssop (Alpha-Pinene CT) | 70.9% |
| Juniper, Phoenicia (needles) | 20.3%–65.7% |
| Guava Leaf (Alpha-Pinene CT) | 23.9%–65.4% |
| Frankincense (*B. frereana*) | 2.0%–64.7% |
| Cypress | 30.0%–64.2% |
| Myrtle (Alpha-Pinene CT) | 26.4%–64.0% |
| Frankincense (*B. carterii*) | 2.0%–64.0% |
| Kunzea (Alpha-Pinene CT) | 28.3%–62.5% |
| Juniper Berry | 18.3%–62.3% |
| Rosemary (Alpha-Pinene CT) | 14.1%–62.2% |
| White Pine | 17.7%–57.8% |
| Cistus (Alpha-Pinene CT) | 5.3%–56.0% |
| Blue Cypress (Leaves) | 35.9%–55.6% |
| Aleppo Pine (Cones) | 47.1%–53.6% |
| Oriental Arborvitae (Berries) | 23.5%–52.4% |
| Black Sage (Alpha-Pinene CT) | 20.5%–52.3% |
| Pine | 14.8%–51.1% |
| Red Pine | 13.0%–50.1% |
| Aleppo Pine (Aerial Parts) | 0.0%–47.1% |
| Juniper (Leaves) | 1.4%–45.6% |
| Chinese Red Pine (Leaves) | 8.2%–45.5% |
| Turkish Pine (Cones) | 30.9%–40.7% |
| Parsley Seed | 26.0%–40.6% |
| Mastic (NT\B, Alpha-Pinene CT) | 16.5%–40.2% |
| Chinese Red Pine (Twigs) | 28.1%–39.1% |
| Fragonia (Alpha-Pinene CT) | 21.5%–38.5% |
| Betony (β-Phell.\α-Pinene CT) | 8.4%–37.3% |
| Rhododendron (Aerial Parts) | 8.3%–37.4% |
| Ponderosa Pine | 9.1%–37.2% |
| Galbanum | 5.4%–36.6% |
| Rosemary (Borneol Acetate CT) | 7.7%–35.8% |
| Oriental Arborvitae (Needles) | 15.0%–35.7% |
| Angelica Root | 3.8%–35.7% |
| Silver Fir (*A. alba*) | 2.9%–31.7% |
| Hemp (Myrcene CT) | 2.3%–31.0% |
| Pink Pepper (*S. terebinthifolius*, Leaves, Sabinene CT) | 30.3% |
| Katrafay (Alpha-Pinene CT) | 2.1%–30.0% |
| Japanese Cedarwood (Alpha-Pinene CT) | 6.1%–29.5% |
| Guava Leaf (Limonene CT) | 0.0%–29.5% |
| Utah Juniper (Needles/Twigs) | 10.2%–29.2% |
| Goldenrod | 0.0%–29.2% |
| Maritime Pine (Needles, Alpha-Pinene CT) | 10.2%–28.9% |
| Fragonia (Balanced CT) | 11.6%–28.0% |
| Aleppo Pine (Branches) | 27.9% |
| Niaouli (Viridiflorol CT) | 0.2%–27.7% |
| Nutmeg (East Indian) | 10.2%–26.5% |
| Balsam Fir | 6.2%–25.8% |
| Grindelia | 8.3%–25.5% |
| Gobre Salla | 13.8%–25.2% |
| Niaouli (1,8-Cineole CT) | 0.8%–25.0% |
| Wild Chamomile (*O. multicaulis*) | 11.6%–24.9% |
| Siam Wood (Leaves) | 24.9% |
| Rosemary (Camphor CT) | 6.7%–24.7% |
| Engelmann Spruce | 2.3%–24.7% |
| Dwarf Pine (Needles, Needles/Twigs) | 12.9%–24.5% |
| Mastic (Leaves) | 0.0%–24.3% |
| White Spruce (Needles) | 4.1%–24.0% |
| Blue Spruce | 4.1%–23.8% |
| Tsuga | 16.4%–23.7% |
| Pink Pepper (*S. molle*, Leaves, Beta-Pinene CT) | 22.7% |
| Myrtle (1,8-Cineole CT) | 14.7%–22.5% |
| Mastic (NT\B, Terpinene-4-ol CT) | 7.1%–22.4% |
| Aleppo Pine (Needles) | 1.2%–22.2% |

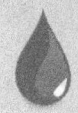

### Alpha-Pinene—continued

| | |
|---|---|
| Helichrysum (*H. italicum*) | 9.3%–21.7% |
| Niaouli (*M. viridiflora*, Terpinen-4-ol CT) | 21.6% |
| Turkish Pine (Resin) | 21.4% |
| Fennel | 0.8%–20.0% |
| Nutmeg (West Indian) | 9.4%–19.9% |
| Mastic (Twigs, Alpha-Pinene CT) | 19.2% |
| Turkish Pine (Needles/Twigs) | 18.1%–19.0% |
| Myrtle (Limonene CT) | 10.7%–18.9% |
| Chaste Tree (Berries) | 1.2%–18.9% |
| Juniper, Phoenicia (leaves, isoborneol CT) | 18.3% |
| Turkish Pine (Twigs) | 14.5%–18.2% |
| Blue Mallee (Cryptone CT) | 5.4%–18.2% |
| Katrafay (Alpha-Eudesmol CT) | 0.0%–18.1% |
| Spanish Sage | 4.9%–17.5% |
| Japanese Cedarwood (Bark) | 0.0%–17.1% |
| Niaouli (Viridiflorol/ Para-cymene/1,8-cineole CT) | 0.0%–17.0% |
| Leleshwa | 6.9%–16.9% |
| Japanese Cedarwood (16-Kaurene CT) | 3.1%–16.8% |
| Black Pepper (Beta-Caryophyllene CT) | 0.3%–16.7% |
| Parsley (Whole Plant) | 15.5%–16.6% |
| Spruce (Black) | 7.4%–16.6% |
| Rosemary (Beta-Myrcene CT) | 8.8%–16.5% |
| Sweet Wormwood (Artemisia Ketone CT) | 0.0%–16.5% |
| Pink Pepper (*S. terebinthifolius*, Fruits, δ-3-Carene CT) | 1.8%–16.3% |
| Wild Chamomile (*O. mixta, C. mixtrum*) | 0.6%–16.0% |
| Rosemary (1,8-Cineole CT) | 5.2%–15.8% |
| Savin (Needles & Branches) | 1.2%–15.8% |
| Myrtle (Myrtenyl Acetate CT) | 14.7%–15.6% |
| Coriander | 1.2%–15.5% |
| Formosan Cypress (Wood, Myrtenol CT) | 1.3%–15.1% |
| Mugwort (Beta-Thujone CT) | 15.1% |
| Turkish Pine (Bark) | 14.9% |
| Valerian | 0.0%–14.8% |
| Rosemary (Verbenone CT) | 2.5%–14.7% |
| Guava Leaf (Beta-Caryophyllene CT) | 0.0%–14.7% |
| Black Sage (Caryophyllene Oxide CT) | 1.1%–14.4% |
| Eucalyptus (*E. globulus*) | 4.5%–14.2% |
| Utah Juniper (Needles/Berries) | 14.2% |
| Chaste Tree (Leaves) | 1.0%–13.9% |
| Black Cumin (Para-Cymene CT) | 0.7%–13.8% |
| Siberian Fir | 6.7%–13.7% |
| White Spruce (Needles & Twigs) | 4.8%–13.7% |
| Black Pepper (Beta-Pinene CT) | 13.6% |
| Formosan Cypress (Neeldes, Germ. D CT) | 8.1%–13.3% |
| Rosalina (Linalool CT) | 6.3%–13.1% |
| Rosalina (1,8-Cineole CT) | 0.0%–13.1% |
| Fennel (Trans-Anethole CT) | 0.0%–12.4% |
| Juniper (*J. wallichiana\J. indica*, Leaves) | 1.8%–12.2% |
| Southern Blue Gum | 1.2%–12.2% |
| White Spruce (Branches) | 12.0%–12.1% |
| Savory (Wild, Linalool CT) | 5.8%–12.0% |
| Eucalyptus (*E. radiata*) | 2.0%–11.9% |
| White Spruce (Oleoresin) | 7.5%–11.8% |
| Tagetes (*T. minuta*, Limonene CT) | 0.5%–11.8% |
| Pink Pepper (*S. molle*, Leaves/Fruits, Sabinene CT) | 0.7%–11.7% |
| Douglas Fir (Needles & Twigs) | 0.1%–11.7% |
| Pink Pepper (*S. molle*, Leaves, Epi-Bicyclosesquiphell. CT) | 11.5% |
| Hinoki (*Needles & Twigs*, α-Terpinene CT) | 11.4% |
| Frankincense (*B. serrata*) | 0.0%–11.2% |
| Hinoki (Taiwan Cypress, wood) | 0.0%–11.1% |
| Manuka (Leptospermone CT) | 1.0%–11.0% |
| Lemon Tea Tree (*L. liversidgei*) | 0.8%–11.0% |
| Galangal (Greater, 1,8-Cineole CT) | 0.5%–10.9% |
| Tamala (Linalool CT) | 10.5% |
| Black Pepper (Limonene CT) | 4.5%–10.4% |
| Black Sage (Beta-Phellandrene CT) | 10.4% |
| Catnip (1,8-cineole CT) | 10.4% |
| Verbena (Linalool CT) | 0.2%–10.3% |
| Hinoki (*Leaves*, Alpha-Terpinolene CT) | 10.1% |
| Dwarf Pine (Twigs) | 5.6%–9.7% |
| Sweet Wormwood (Camphor CT) | 0.0%–9.7% |
| Pink Pepper (*S. terebinthifolius*, Fruits/Leaves, Bicyclogerm. CT) | 5.2%–9.6% |
| Black Sage (Beta-Caryophyllene CT) | 9.5% |
| Mastic (NT\B, Germacrene D CT) | 9.4% |
| Fingerroot (*B. rotunda* 1,8-Cineole CT) | 9.2% |
| White Sage | 5.1%–9.0% |
| Juniper (*J. wallichiana\J. indica*, Berries) | 8.1%–8.8% |
| Helichrysum (ssp. *italicum*) | 0.1%–8.6% |
| Mastic (Aerial parts, Beta-Eudesmol CT) | 8.6% |
| Big Badja Gum | 5.1%–8.4% |
| Betony (MLD-C CT) | 4.9%–8.4% |
| Black Pepper (Delta-3-Carene CT) | 7.4%–8.3% |
| Rosemary (Borneol CT) | 8.3% |
| Juniper (*J. recurva*, Berries) | 8.3% |
| Ferula (Limonene CT) | 8.3% |
| Savin (Berries) | 5.0%–8.1% |
| Ravensara (Sabinene CT) | 4.2%–8.1% |
| Ledum (*R. groenlandicum*) | 0.0%–8.0% |
| Pink Pepper (*S. terebinthifolius*, Fruits, Myrc./Lim. CT) | 6.0%–7.9% |
| White Fir (*A. concolor*) | 4.4%–7.9% |
| Niaouli (1,8-Cineole/Viridiflorol CT) | 1.3%–7.9% |
| Hinoki (needles) | 0.1%–7.8% |
| Bay Laurel | 1.9%–7.7% |
| Hemp (Beta-Caryophyllene CT) | 0.7%–7.7% |
| Douglas Fir (Needles) | 0.0%–7.6% |
| Vilayti Tulsi (Sabinene CT) | 2.0%–7.4% |
| Kumquat (*C. japonica*, Leaves CT Beta-Pinene) | 7.4% |
| Kunzea (Spathulenol\Globulol CT) | 0.6%–7.3% |
| Niaouli (*M. viridiflora*, 1,8-cineole CT) | 5.8%–7.2% |
| Juniper (*J. recurva*, Needles) | 0.5%–6.9% |
| Applemint (*M. suav.*, Carvone CT) | 0.0%–6.6% |
| Benzoin (Siam, SPME Absolute) | 1.8%–6.6% |
| Oakmoss Aboslute (Hydro. + Hexane) | 6.6% |
| Mastic (NT\B, Limonene CT) | 4.9%–6.5% |
| Pink Pepper (*S. molle*, Leaves, α-Phellandrene CT) | 0.2%–6.5% |
| Pink Pepper (*S. terebinthifolius*, Fruits, α-Phell. CT) | 6.5% |
| Ravensara (Limonene CT) | 3.0%–6.4% |
| Juniper (Chinese) | 1.3%–6.4% |
| Aleppo Pine (Aerial Parts) | 0.0%–6.4% |
| Yarrow (Sabinene CT) | 2.8%–6.3% |
| Allspice (Berries, Methyl Eugenol CT) | 0.1%–6.3% |
| Wormwood (Beta-Pinene CT) | 3.2%–5.9% |
| Mugwort (1,8-Cineole CT) | 0.8%–5.9% |
| Sage (Alpha-Thujone CT) | 0.1%–5.9% |
| Mugwort (Alpha-Thujone CT) | 1.8%–5.7% |
| Mastic (NT\B, Beta-Myrcene CT) | 2.5%–5.5% |
| Sage (Beta-Thujone CT) | 0.1%–5.5% |
| African Bluegrass (Myrcene CT) | 2.3%–5.4% |
| Boldo (*1,8-Cineole\Para-Cymene\Limonene CT*) | 4.2%–5.3% |
| Sage (Camphor CT) | 0.1%–5.3% |
| Mediterranean Mandarin (CP\Expressed) | 0.3%–5.2% |
| Caraway | 0.0%–5.2% |
| Pink Pepper (*S. molle*, Aerial Parts, α-Phell. CT) | 5.2% |
| Betony (Bicyclogermacrene CT) | 0.6%–5.1% |
| Kaffir Lime Peel | 0.4%–5.1% |
| Summer Savory (Gamma-Terpinene CT) | 0.0%–5.1% |
| Black Sage (Tricyclene CT) | 5.1% |

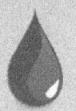

| | |
|---|---|
| Ravintsara (1,8-Cineole CT) | 3.7%–5.0% |
| Opoponax (*C. erythraea*) | 3.4%–5.0% |
| Blue Mountain Sage (Delta-3-Carene CT) | 2.4%–5.0% |
| Ravintsara (Camphor CT) | 2.1%–5.0% |
| Guggul | 2.0%–5.0% |
| Hairy Basil (Camphor CT) | 3.4%–4.9% |
| Blue Tansy (Sabinene CT) | 2.1%–4.9% |
| Wild Chamomile (*C. mixtus*, Sant. Alc. CT) | 2.7%–4.8% |
| Camphor (Camphor CT) | 2.0%–4.7% |
| Gully Gum | 0.4%–4.6% |
| Catnip (Nepetalactone CT) | 0.0%–4.6% |
| Ravensara (Alpha-Terpinene CT) | 3.9%–4.5% |
| Mugwort (Artemisia Ketone CT) | 3.4%–4.5% |
| Cistus (*Viridiflorol-Trans-Pinocarveol CT*) | 0.1%–4.5% |
| Niaouli (E-Nerolidol CT) | 0.0%–4.5% |
| Blue Mountain Sage (Limonene CT) | 4.5% |
| Pink Pepper (*S. molle*, Leaves, Elemol/Beta-Eudesmol CT) | 4.5% |
| Ocotea (Leaves) | 4.4% |
| Pink Pepper (*S. molle*, Fruits, α-Phellandrene CT) | 1.1%–4.3% |
| Wormwood (Trans-Sabinyl Acetate CT) | 0.2%–4.3% |
| Shell Ginger (Terpinene-4-ol CT) | 0.0%–4.1% |
| Tsauri Grass | 0.0%–4.1% |
| Yarrow (Chamazulene CT) | 0.0%–4.1% |
| Mugwort (Isobornyl Isobutyrate D CT) | 4.0% |
| Black Pepper (Eugenol CT) | 0.9%–3.8% |
| Mastic (Twigs, Alpha-Pinene CT) | 3.8% |
| Wild Marjoram (1,8-Cineole CT) | 0.5%–3.6% |
| Fennel (Methyl Chavicol CT) | 0.2%–3.6% |
| Saro (1,8-Cineole CT) | 1.1%–3.5% |
| Applemint (*M. suav.*, Piperitenone CT) | 0.0%–3.4% |
| Sweet Inula (1,8-Cineole CT) | 2.3%–3.2% |
| Kaffir Lime Peel | 2.0%–3.2% |
| Verbena (Myrcene CT) | 0.4%–3.1% |
| Vilayti Tulsi (Fenchone CT) | 0.0%–3.1% |
| Japanese Cedarwood (16-Kaurene/Valencene CT) | 3.1% |
| Tamala (Trans-Sabinene Hydrate CT) | 3.1% |
| Persian Lime (Distilled) | 1.8%–2.8% |
| Petitgrain (Mandarin) | 1.7%–2.8% |
| May Chang (Neral CT) | 2.9% |
| Yuzu | 1.1%–2.7% |
| Hyssop (Linalool CT) | 2.2%–2.5% |
| Yarrow (1,8-Cineole\Camphor CT) | 0.6%–2.5% |
| Orange (Cold-pressed/expressed) | 0.5%–2.4% |
| Persian Lime (Cold Pressed\Expressed) | 1.9%–2.3% |
| Blue Mallee (1,8-Cineole CT) | 0.0%–2.1% |
| Mugwort (Beta-Caryophyllene CT) | 2.1% |
| Mugwort (Camphor CT) | 0.1%–2.0% |
| Hyssop (Pinocamphone CT) | 0.1%–1.8% |
| Mediterranean Mandarin (Hydrodistilled) | 0.6%–1.5% |
| Mugwort (Alpha-Phellandrene CT) | 1.3% |
| Ravensara (Methyl Eugenol CT) | 0.2%–1.2% |
| Cumin | 0.3%–1.0% |

**Alpha-Pinene Isomer**

| | |
|---|---|
| Hinoki (needles) | 0.1%–5.9% |

**Alpha-Pinene Oxide**

| | |
|---|---|
| Cumin | 0.0%–1.6% |

**Alpha-Pulegone ((-)-(E)-Alpha-Pulegone)**

| | |
|---|---|
| Buchu (*A. crenulata*) | 0.0%–4.8% |
| Buchu (*A. betulina*, Isomenthone CT) | 0.4%–4.6% |

**Alpha-Santalene**

| | |
|---|---|
| Black Sage (Alpha-Santalene CT) | 35.6% |
| Opoponax (*C. guidotti*) | 11.1%–21.9% |
| Schisandra Fruit (*S. sphenanthera*, α-Cad. CT) | 13.0% |

| | |
|---|---|
| Black Sage (Alpha-Pinene CT) | 0.0%–10.6% |
| Schisandra Fruit (*S. sphenanthera*, δ-Cad. CT) | 10.1% |
| Turmeric (Rhizome, Distilled) | 0.8%–6.6% |
| Canadian Fleabane | 0.0%–5.8% |

**Alpha-Selinene (Naphthalene, 1,2,3,4,4a,5,6,8a-octahydro-4a,8-dimethyl-2-(1-methylethenyl)-, [2R-(2α,4aα,8aβ)]-)**

| | |
|---|---|
| Guava Leaf (Beta-Caryophyllene CT) | 0.0%–10.0% |
| Ledum (*R. groenlandicum*) | 0.3%–9.9% |
| Guggul | 0.1%–9.3% |
| Spikenard (Nardol CT) | 9.2% |
| Guava Leaf (β-Cary.\(E)-Nerolidol CT) | 8.3% |
| Black Cumin (Para-Cymene CT) | 0.0%–6.5% |
| Manuka (Leptospermone CT) | 2.7%–6.1% |
| Guava Leaf (Selin-11-en-4-Alpha-ol CT) | 3.6%–5.8% |
| Helichrysum (ssp. *microphyllum*) | 3.8%–5.4% |
| Hairy Basil (Camphor CT) | 2.9%–5.3% |
| Helichrysum (*H. italicum*) | 0.0%–4.8% |
| Formosan Cypress (Wood, α-Eudesmol CT) | 4.8% |
| Celery Leaf | 1.2%–4.3% |
| Agarwood (*A. sinensis*) | 0.5%–4.1% |
| Black Pepper (Beta-Caryophyllene CT) | 0.0%–4.1% |
| Hemp (Beta-Caryophyllene CT) | 1.6%–4.0% |
| Opoponax (*C. erythraea*) | 3.2%–3.8% |
| Schisandra Fruit (*S. sphenanthera*, α-Cad. CT) | 3.8% |
| Maritime Pine (Needles, Beta-Cary. CT) | 0.0%–3.5% |
| Cedarwood (Virginian, Wood) | 0.0%–3.0% |
| White Pine | 0.0%–3.0% |
| Celery Seed | 0.0%–2.7% |
| Spearmint (Cis-Ocimenone CT) | 1.7% |
| Rosewood (Wood) | 0.7%–1.3% |
| Rosewood (Leaves) | 1.1% |

**Alpha-Selinene/Viridiflorene**

| | |
|---|---|
| Manuka (Selinene/Beta-Elemene CT) | 13.5% |

**Alpha-Terpinene**

| | |
|---|---|
| Wormseed, American (Alpha-Terpinene CT) | 40.7%–60.4% |
| Hinoki (*Needles & Twigs*, α-Terpinene CT) | 40.6% |
| Ravensara (Alpha-Terpinene CT) | 25.3%–27.7% |
| Wormseed, American (Ascaridole CT) | 0.7%–20.7% |
| Pink Pepper (*S. molle*, Fruits/Leaves, p-Cymene CT) | 2.2%–18.3% |
| Helichrysum (*H. splendidum*, Alpha-Terpinene CT) | 14.9% |
| Ravensara (1,8-Cineole CT) | 0.0%–12.4% |
| Tea tree | 7.9%–10.4% |
| Summer Savory (Gamma-Terpinene CT) | 0.0%–10.2% |
| Marjoram | 2.8%–8.2% |
| Ravensara (Methyl Eugenol CT) | 0.6%–7.8% |
| Petitgrain (Mandarin) | 0.0%–7.4% |
| Ravensara (Limonene CT) | 1.8%–7.1% |
| Plai (Terpinen-4-ol, No Phenylbutanoids CT) | 0.4%–6.4% |
| Plai (Sabinene CT) | 2.0%–6.0% |
| Oregano (Terpinen-4-ol CT) | 2.8%–5.9% |
| Cumin | 0.0%–5.7% |
| Savin (Needles & Branches) | 0.3%–5.4% |
| Nutmeg (East Indian) | 0.1%–5.2% |
| Mastic (NT\B, Terpinene-4-ol CT) | 3.6%–5.0% |
| Indian Borage (Carvacrol CT) | 0.0%–4.8% |
| Shell Ginger (Terpinene-4-ol CT) | 0.7%–4.7% |
| Mugwort (1,8-Cineole CT) | 0.0%–4.6% |
| Juniper (*J. wallichiana\J. indica*, Leaves) | 1.5%–4.5% |
| Ledum (*L. palustre*) | 0.1%–4.5% |
| Douglas Fir (Needles) | 0.9%–4.3% |
| Juniper (*J. wallichiana\J. indica*, Berries) | 0.1%–4.3% |
| Khella (Seeds) | 0.1%–4.0% |
| Mountain Savory (Thymol CT) | 1.7%–3.9% |

### Alpha-Terpinene—continued

| | |
|---|---|
| Maritime Pine (Needles, Alpha-Pinene CT) | 0.0%–3.8% |
| Mastic (Twigs, Alpha-Pinene CT) | 3.6% |
| Black Pepper (Limonene CT) | 0.0%–3.4% |
| Lime (Distilled) | 0.4%–3.0% |
| Spearmint (Linalool CT) | 0.9%–3.0% |
| Ledum (*R. groenlandicum*) | 0.0%–2.3% |
| Angelica Root | 0.1%–2.0% |
| Ravensara (Methyl Chavicol CT) | 0.1%–0.8% |

### Alpha-Terpineol

| | |
|---|---|
| Thyme (Alpha-Terpineol CT) | 40.9%–90.4% |
| Kumquat (*F. margarita*, Fruit CT α-Terpineol) | 55.5% |
| Guava Leaf (1,8-Cineole) | 38.7% |
| Cedarwood (Himalayan, Needles) | 30.2% |
| Lovage (Aerial Parts) | 0.8%–27.9% |
| Bergamot Mint | 1.5%–24.9% |
| Niaouli (Viridiflorol/ Para-cymene/1,8-cineole CT) | 0.5%–24.5% |
| Tagetes (*T. minuta*, Alpha-Terpineol CT) | 20.8% |
| Lavender (Munstead) | 19.2%–20.6% |
| Juniper, Phoenicia (needles) | 0.0%–19.8% |
| Hinoki (Taiwan Cypress, wood) | 2.2%–19.4% |
| Rosewood (Wood) | 0.1%–18.8% |
| Eucalyptus (*E. radiata*) | 0.0%–15.2% |
| Niaouli (1,8-Cineole CT) | 0.0%–15.0% |
| Hairy Basil (var. *pilosum* Eugenol CT) | 15.0% |
| Clary Sage | 1.8%–14.3% |
| Thyme (Linalool CT) | 0.0%–14.2% |
| Neroli (*C. aurantium*) | 4.6%–14.0% |
| Niaouli (1,8-Cineole/Viridiflorol CT) | 0.0%–14.0% |
| Thyme (Thuyanol-4 CT) | 2.0%–13.9% |
| Niaouli (Viridiflorol CT) | 1.5%–13.6% |
| Leleshwa | 0.9%–13.2% |
| Petitgrain (Bergamot/Bitter Orange) | 7.1%–12.9% |
| Galangal (Greater, 1,8-Cineole CT) | 2.1%–12.7% |
| Cajeput | 5.9%–12.5% |
| Monarda (Carvacrol CT) | 0.1%–12.0% |
| Mastic (Leaves) | 0.1%–11.6% |
| Applemint (*M. suav.*, Linalool CT) | 11.1% |
| Palo Santo (Wood) | 5.8%–10.9% |
| Applemint (*M. rotun.*, Piperitenone CT) | 10.9% |
| Juniper, Phoenicia (Berries) | 0.0%–10.8% |
| Fennel | 0.1%–10.5% |
| Ravintsara (1,8-Cineole CT) | 3.8%–10.3% |
| Ponderosa Pine | 0.0%–10.0% |
| Galangal (Lesser) | 6.4%–9.2% |
| Chaste Tree (Leaves) | 1.4%–9.2% |
| Niaouli (*M. viridiflora*, 1,8-cineole CT) | 8.2%–8.4% |
| Kaffir Lime Peel | 0.4%–8.4% |
| Myrtle (1,8-Cineole CT) | 0.0%–8.4% |
| Pink Pepper (*S. molle*, Fruits, α-Phellandrene CT) | 0.0%–8.4% |
| Thyme (Carvacrol CT) | 0.0%–8.2% |
| Niaouli (*M. viridiflora*, Terpinen-4-ol CT) | 8.1% |
| Rosalina (1,8-Cineole CT) | 6.5%–8.0% |
| Frankincense (*B. serrata)* | 1.0%–7.8% |
| Monarda (Thymol CT) | 0.6%–7.8% |
| Oregano (Terpinen-4-ol CT) | 5.0%–7.6% |
| Gully Gum | 0.0%–7.5% |
| Cardamom (Alpha-Terpinyl Acetate CT) | 2.1%–7.4% |
| Lime (Distilled) | 0.0%–7.4% |
| Marjoram | 4.9%–6.9% |
| White Fir (*A. concolor*) | 1.2%–6.9% |
| Turkish Pine (Bark) | 6.7% |
| Persian Lime (Distilled) | 1.4%–6.6% |

| | |
|---|---|
| Fragonia (Balanced CT) | 3.0%–6.3% |
| Japanese Cedarwood (Alpha-Pinene CT) | 0.1%–6.1% |
| Thyme (Thymol CT) | 0.0%–6.1% |
| Wild Marjoram (1,8-Cineole CT) | 1.7 %–6.0% |
| Lavender (True English) | 1.5%–6.0% |
| Yarrow (1,8-Cineole\Camphor CT) | 0.9%–5.9% |
| Kanuka | 0.0%–5.7% |
| Pink Pepper (*S. molle*, Leaves, α-Phellandrene CT) | 0.0%–5.6% |
| Pink Pepper (*S. terebinthifolius*, Fruits, α-Phell. CT) | 5.6% |
| Douglas Fir (Needles & Twigs) | 0.0%–5.4% |
| Boldo (*1,8-Cineole\Para-Cymene\Limonene CT)* | 1.9%–5.2% |
| Mastic (NT\B, Terpinene-4-ol CT) | 3.7%–5.0% |
| Mastic (NT\B, Alpha-Pinene CT) | 2.5%–5.0% |
| Rosemary (Verbenone CT) | 2.4%–4.9% |
| Rosemary (1,8-Cineole CT) | 0.0%–4.9% |
| Verbena (Myrcenone CT) | 0.0%–4.6% |
| Cassia (Leaves) | 0.0%–4.2% |
| Shell Ginger (Terpinene-4-ol CT) | 0.0%–4.2% |
| Kunzea (Alpha-Pinene CT) | 0.0%–4.0% |
| Mastic (NT\B, Germacrene D CT) | 4.0% |
| Lavender (Indian) | 1.2%–3.8% |
| Japanese Cedarwood (Bark) | 0.0%–3.7% |
| Rosalina (Linalool CT) | 0.0%–3.6% |
| Rosewood (Leaves) | 3.6% |
| Chinese Red Pine (Twigs) | 0.1%–3.3% |
| Chinese Red Pine (Leaves) | 0.0%–3.3% |
| Indian Borage (Carvacrol CT) | 0.0%–3.3% |
| Engelmann Spruce | 0.3%–3.2% |
| Sage (1,8-Cineole CT) | 2.6%–3.1% |
| Elemi | 1.1%–2.7% |
| Rose (Indian) | 0.1%–2.7% |
| Chaste Tree (Berries) | 0.2%–2.6% |
| Southern Blue Gum | 0.3%–2.4% |
| Mediterranean Mandarin (Hydrodistilled) | 0.0%–2.2% |
| Sweet Inula (Borneol CT) | 0.0%–2.2% |
| Western Red Cedar (Wood) | 1.8%–1.9% |
| Yarrow (Chamazulene CT) | 0.3%–1.9% |
| Mugwort (1,8-Cineole CT) | 0.0%–1.8% |
| Spike Lavender | 0.8%–1.6% |
| Lemon Eucalyptus | 0.1%–1.0% |

### Alpha-Terpinolene (Terpinolene)

| | |
|---|---|
| Turmeric (Leaves) | 11.5%–26.4% |
| Hemp (Myrcene CT) | 0.1%–23.8% |
| Tagetes (*T. erecta*, Leaves) | 11.2%–22.2% |
| Douglas Fir (Needles) | 15.6%–20.2% |
| Hinoki (*Leaves*, Alpha-Terpinolene CT) | 19.5% |
| Niaouli (Viridiflorol/ Para-cymene/1,8-cineole CT) | 0.1%–19.2% |
| Douglas Fir (Needles & Twigs) | 0.0%–18.8% |
| Parsley (Leaves, 1,3,8-Para-Menth. CT) | 2.1%–13.9% |
| Tagetes (*T. erecta*, Aerial Parts) | 0.1%–13.9% |
| Vilayti Tulsi (Sabinene CT) | 5.6%–13.8% |
| Tagetes (*T. patula*, Limonene CT) | 0.0%–11.2% |
| Tagetes (*T. minuta*, Limonene CT) | 0.0%–11.0% |
| Parsley (Leaves, Myristicin CT) | 0.8%–10.3% |
| Aleppo Pine (Aerial Parts) | 0.0%–10.1% |
| Aleppo Pine (Needles) | 0.0%–9.9% |
| Black Cumin (Para-Cymene CT) | 0.0%–9.1% |
| Niaouli (1,8-Cineole, Viridiflorol CT) | 1.4%–8.3% |
| Tagetes (*T. patula*, Flowers) | 7.8% |
| Cypress | 4.5%–6.6% |
| Tagetes (*T. erecta*, Flowers) | 4.7%–6.3% |
| Hemp (Beta-Caryophyllene CT) | 0.2%–6.0% |
| Oriental Arborvitae (Needles) | 2.1%–5.3% |
| Persian Lime (Distilled) | 0.0%–5.2% |

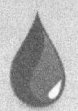

| Petitgrain (Mandarin) | 0.6%–4.6% |
|---|---|
| Kaffir Lime Peel | 0.3%–4.3% |
| Oriental Arborvitae (Berries) | 1.7%–4.0% |
| Sweet Wormwood (Camphor CT) | 0.0%–3.7% |
| Rosalina (Linalool CT) | 0.0%–3.6% |
| Juniper (*J. recurva*, Berries) | 3.6% |
| Plai (Terpinen-4-ol CT) | 0.4%–3.4% |
| Dwarf Pine (Needles, Needles/Twigs) | 0.0%–3.4% |
| Hinoki (*Needles & Twigs*, α-Terpinene CT) | 3.4% |
| Plai (Terpinen-4-ol, No Phenylbutanoids CT) | 2.2%–3.0% |
| Elemi | 2.5%–2.8% |
| Angelica Root | 0.5%–1.9% |
| Mediterranean Mandarin (CP\Expressed) | 0.0%–1.6% |
| Ledum (*R. groenlandicum*) | 0.0%–1.5% |

**Alpha-Terpinyl Acetate (Terpinyl Acetate)**

| Lovage (Leaves) | 26.1%–70.0% |
|---|---|
| Cardamom (Alpha-Terpinyl Acetate CT) | 10.2%–68.2% |
| Lovage (Aerial Parts) | 1.6%–52.4% |
| Lovage (Roots) | 0.0%–46.4% |
| Cardamom (1,8-Cineole CT) | 0.9%–35.3% |
| Wormseed, American (Alpha-Terpinene CT) | 0.0%–31.6% |
| Chaste Tree (Berries) | 2.9%–16.8% |
| Bay Laurel | 0.0%–14.6% |
| Juniper, Phoenicia (needles) | 0.0%–12.9% |
| Hinoki (needles) | 0.0%–12.6% |
| Neroli (*C. aurantium*) | 0.2%–11.7% |
| Niaouli (1,8-Cineole CT) | 0.0%–11.4% |
| Cypress | 0.0%–6.6% |
| Turkish Pine (Needles) | 0.0%–5.3% |
| Niaouli (Viridiflorol/ Para-cymene/1,8-cineole CT) | 0.0%–5.0% |
| Myrtle (Alpha-Pinene CT) | 0.0%–4.9% |
| Oriental Arborvitae (Needles) | 0.0%–4.7% |
| Wild Marjoram (1,8-Cineole CT) | 0.0%–4.5% |
| Genipi (*A. umbelliformis*, C-SH\B CT) | 0.7%–4.2% |
| Juniper, Phoenicia (leaves, isoborneol CT) | 3.5% |
| Tamala (Beta-Caryophyllene CT) | 3.2% |
| Chaste Tree (Leaves) | 0.0%–3.1% |
| Sage (1,8-Cineole CT) | 1.4%–2.9% |
| Ravintsara (Camphor CT) | 0.0%–2.3% |

**Alpha-Thujene**

| Frankincense (*B. serrata*) | 22.5%–69.8% |
|---|---|
| Frankincense (*B. carterii*) | 1.0%–52.4% |
| Frankincense (*B. frereana*) | 0.0%–33.1% |
| Betony (Alpha-Thujene CT) | 13.4%–32.3% |
| Calendula (Alpha-Thujene CT) | 26.9% |
| Pink Pepper (*S. terebinthifolius*, Fruits, Limonene CT) | 3.0%–21.7% |
| Black Cumin (Para-Cymene CT) | 0.0%–15.3% |
| Black Cumin (Thymoquinone CT) | 1.3%–10.5% |
| Frankincense (*B. sacra*) | 0.9%–6.6% |
| Rosalina (1,8-Cineole CT) | 0.0%–5.9% |
| Savin (Berries) | 0.0%–5.4% |
| Black Pepper (Limonene CT) | 0.1%–4.9% |
| Hairy Basil (Camphor CT) | 0.0%–4.9% |
| Savin (Needles & Branches) | 0.6%–4.8% |
| Mastic (NT\B, Alpha-Pinene CT) | 0.8%–4.2% |
| Black Pepper (Delta-3-Carene CT) | 0.0%–4.2% |
| Shell Ginger (1,8-Cineole CT) | 0.0%–4.1% |
| Eucalyptus Dives | 0.0%–3.1% |
| Black Cumin (Trans-Anethole CT) | 2.4%–2.4% |
| Mugwort (Camphor CT) | 0.0%–2.2% |
| Ravensara (Limonene CT) | 0.4%–2.1% |
| Ravensara (Sabinene CT) | 1.2%–1.6% |
| Ravensara (Alpha-Terpinene CT) | 1.2%–1.3% |

| Angelica Root | 0.0%–1.1% |
|---|---|
| Mugwort (1,8-Cineole CT) | 0.0%–1.0% |
| Hyssop (Pinocamphone CT) | 0.0%–1.0% |

**Alpha-Thujone**

| Genipi (*A. genipi*) | 26.0%–79.8% |
|---|---|
| Western Red Cedar (Leaves) | 54.1%–77.5% |
| Thuja | 42.6%–69.8% |
| Genipi (*A. umbelliformis*, Alpha-Thujone CT) | 29.7%–67.5% |
| Sage (Alpha-Thujone CT) | 24.5%–52.9% |
| Mugwort (Alpha-Thujone CT) | 14.4%–48.5% |
| Wormwood (Alpha-Thujone CT) | 17.7%–30.7% |
| Sage (Wild) | 14.1%–29.8% |
| Sage (Camphor CT) | 2.1%–28.6% |
| Sage (Beta-Thujone CT) | 2.2%–18.4% |
| Wormwood (Trans-Sabinyl Acetate CT) | 0.0%–15.9% |
| Boldo (Ascaridole CT) | 0.0%–14.3% |
| Tansy (Beta-Thujone CT) | 0.0%–11.0% |
| Mugwort (Camphor CT) | 10.2%–10.7% |
| Sage (1,8-Cineole CT) | 0.1%–9.9% |
| Wormwood (Trans-Sabinene Hydrate CT) | 0.1%–8.1% |
| Great Mugwort | 0.5%–4.4% |
| Mugwort (Artemisia Ketone CT) | 0.2%–3.1% |
| Mugwort (1,8-Cineole CT) | 0.0%–2.5% |
| Yarrow (Chamazulene CT) | 0.0%–2.1% |
| Mugwort (Camphor CT) | 0.0%–1.3% |

**Alpha-Turmerone**

| Turmeric (Rhizome, Solvent Extracted) | 6.5%–53.4% |
|---|---|
| Turmeric (Rhizome, Distilled) | 0.0%–44.1% |

**Alpha-Vetivone**

| Vetiver | 2.0%–6.3% |
|---|---|

**Alpha-Ylangene (Ylangene)**

| Schisandra Fruit (*S. chinensis*) | 37.7%–50.4% |
|---|---|
| Muhuhu (Leaves) | 5.2% |
| Mastic (Gum Resin) | 0.0%–4.0% |

**Alpha-Zingiberene**

| Ginger | 5.7%–32.2% |
|---|---|
| Mugwort (Germacrene D CT) | 14.9% |
| Betony (Alpha-Zingiberene CT) | 12.2% |
| White Turmeric (Distilled) | 0.0%–12.0% |
| Lemon Verbena (Leaves) | 2.8%–5.7% |
| Hops | 0.0%–5.6% |
| Turmeric (Rhizome, Distilled) | 0.0%–4.4% |
| Lemon Verbena (Stems) | 1.9%–3.7% |
| Black Pepper (Beta-Caryophyllene CT) | 0.0%–3.4% |
| Amyris | 1.2%–2.9% |
| Mugwort (1,8-Cineole CT) | 0.0%–1.0% |

**Amyl Isobutyrate**

| Khella (Seeds) | 13.2%–16.0% |
|---|---|

**Amyl Isovalerate (n-Amyl Isovalerate; Butanoic acid, 3-methyl-, pentyl ester; Pentyl 3-methylbutanoate; Pentyl isovalerate; Pentyl isopentanoate)**

| Khella (Aerial Parts, 2-Mehtylbutyl Bu. CT) | 3.9% |
|---|---|

**Amyl Valerate**

| Khella (Seeds) | 10.0%–13.2% |
|---|---|

**Anethole (isomer not identified)**

| Cedarwood (Himalayan, Needles) | 14.6% |
|---|---|
| Mugwort (1,8-Cineole CT) | 0.0%–2.2% |

**Aristolene**

| Spikenard (Calarene CT) | 6.3%–15.6% |
|---|---|
| Agarwood (*A. sinensis*) | 0.0%–14.8% |
| Damiana (1,8-Cineole CT) | 0.0%–3.5% |

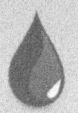

**Aristolenone**

Spikenard (Calarene CT, Nepal)  0.0%–6.5%

**Aristolochene**

Chinese Red Pine (Leaves)  0.0%–3.7%

**Aromadendrene**

Agarwood (Malaysian)  0.0%–25.9%
Southern Blue Gum  2.0%–16.9%
Aleppo Pine (Needles)  0.0%–7.1%
Black Sage (Caryophyllene Oxide CT)  0.0%–6.8%
Guava Leaf (Beta-Caryophyllene CT)  0.2%–6.6%
Rhododendron (Leaves)  6.3%
Opoponax (*C. erythraea*)  3.5%–4.4%
Rosalina (Linalool CT)  2.0%–4.1%
Valerian  0.0%–4.0%
Manuka (Leptospermone CT)  1.6%–2.2%
Ylang Ylang (French IV)  1.5%

**Aromadendrene Oxide**

Mastic (Twigs, Alpha-Pinene CT)  3.8%

**ar-Curcumene**

Wild Turmeric (Distilled)  0.0%–23.2%
Ginger  1.9%–16.7%
White Turmeric (Distilled)  0.0%–12.1%
Katrafay (Leaves)  0.1%–8.6%
Turmeric (Rhizome, Distilled)  0.5%–6.6%
Lemon Verbena (Stems)  1.3%–6.1%
Mugwort (Germacrene D CT)  6.0%
Lemon Verbena (Leaves and stems)  3.0%–5.7%
Helichrysum (ssp. *italicum*)  0.9%–4.6%
Amyris  1.5%–2.7%
Lemon Verbena (Leaves)  0.6%–1.7%

**ar-Turmerone**

Turmeric (Rhizome, Distilled)  5.4%–61.8%
Turmeric (Rhizome, Solvent Extracted)  5.4%–33.2%
Ginger  0.0%–12.8%
Wild Turmeric (Solvent Extracted)  7.0%

**Artemisia Acetate**

Sweet Nancy (Yomogi Alc.\1,8-Cin. CT)  0.0%–7.6%

**Artemisia Alcohol**

Sweet Wormwood (Artemisia Ketone CT)  3.7%–56.0%
Wild Chamomile (*O. mixta, C. mixtrum*)  1.2%–13.2%
Sweet Nancy (Yomogi Alc.\1,8-Cin. CT)  4.1%–8.6%
Mugwort (Beta-Thujone CT)  8.5%
Sweet Nancy (Artemisyl Acetate CT)  3.4%–7.1%
Mugwort (Camphor CT)  0.0%–4.5%
Mugwort (Artemisia Ketone CT)  1.3%–4.1%
Sweer Nancy (Artemisia Ketone CT)  2.7%

**Artemisia Ketone**

Sweet Wormwood (Artemisia Ketone CT)  28.3%–75.5%
Sweer Nancy (Artemisia Ketone CT)  55.7%
African Bluegrass (Artemisia Ketone CT)  37.5%
Mugwort (Artemisia Ketone CT)  18.8%–29.4%
Tansy (Beta-Thujone CT)  0.0%–23.5%
Blue Yarrow (Artemisia Ketone CT)  14.9%
Sweet Wormwood (Camphor CT)  2.7%–6.3%
Calendula ((E)-Beta-Ocimene CT)  3.4%

**Artemisia Triene**

Sweet Nancy (Yomogi Alc.\1,8-Cin. CT)  0.0%–8.3%

**Artemisyl Acetate**

Sweet Nancy (Artemisyl Acetate CT)  62.3%–78.8%

**Ascaridole ((Z)-Ascaridole, Cis-Ascaridole)**

Wormseed, American (Ascaridole CT)  29.7%–61.4%
Boldo (Ascaridole CT)  21.3%–51.2%

Boldo (Ascaridole CT, no 1,8-cineole)  36.5%–46.9%
Wormseed, American (Carvacrol CT)  22.5%
Wormseed, American (Alpha-Terpinene CT)  0.9%–17.9%
Ledum (*L. palustre*)  0.1%–14.2%
Boldo (*1,8-Cineole\Para-Cymene\Limonene CT*)  1.0%–6.3%

**Baimuxinal**

Agarwood (*A. sinensis*)  0.0%–14.8%

**Benzaldehyde**

Benzoin (Siam, S-HS Absolute)  10.2%–46.8%
Benzoin (Siam, HSSE Absolute)  15.0%–30.2%
Benzoin (Siam, SPME Absolute)  17.3%–21.9%
Cinnamon Bark  0.6%–9.9%
Guava Leaf ((2E)-Hexenal CT)  8.2%
Benzoin (Sumatra, S-HS Absolute)  4.7%–6.6%
Benzoin (Sumatra, HSSE Absolute)  3.5%–6.0%
Benzoin (Sumatra, SPME Absolute)  3.1%–4.5%
Tamala ((E)-Cinnamaldehyde\Cinn. Ac. CT)  1.3%–4.1%
Tamala ((E)-Cinnamaldehyde CT)  2.0%–3.2%
Ocotea (Flowers Calices)  0.0%–3.2%

**Benzene Isothiocyanatomethyl**

Moringa (Seeds, Naphthalene CT)  34.9%

**Benzeneacetylaldehyde**

Wormwood ((Z)-Epoxy Ocimene CT)  0.0%–5.5%
Wormwood (Cis-Chrysanthenyl Acetate CT)  1.6%–3.3%

**Benzoic Acid**

Benzoin (Siam, Ethanol Absolute)  31.0%–36.0%
Benzoin (*S. benzoin*, Absolute)  19.2%–28.2%
Benzoin (Siam, Absolute)  18.4%
Benzoin (Siam, SPME Absolute)  8.5%–15.3%
Benzoin (Siam, Hydrodistilled)  12.5%
Peru Balsam  8.1%–8.9%
Benzoin (Sumatra, SPME Absolute)  1.1%–6.8%
Benzoin (Siam, HSSE Absolute)  1.1%–6.8%
Benzoin (Sumatra, Ethanol Absolute)  2.0%–4.0%
Tolu Balsam  2.5%

**Benzyl Acetate**

Jasmine Absolute (Benzyl Acetate CT)  15.0%–31.0%
Ylang Ylang (French I)  27.5%
Ylang Ylang (Madagascan I)  3.3%–8.0%
Jasmine Absolute (Benzyl Benzoate CT)  4.8%–7.7%

**Benzyl Acetone (Benzylacetone)**

Agarwood (*A. sinensis*)  1.4%–19.5%
Shell Ginger (1,8-Cineole CT)  0.1%–4.2%

**Benzyl Alcohol**

Benzoin (Sumatra, Absolute)  43.4%
Tolu Balsam  41.8%
Benzoin (Siam, Absolute)  38.8%
Benzoin (Siam, HSSE Absolute)  1.8%–12.3%
Cananga  0.0%–7.8%
Benzoin (Siam, S-HS Absolute)  0.9%–6.9%
Benzoin (Siam, SPME Absolute)  3.3%–6.7%

**Benzyl Benzoate (Ascabin, Ascabiol)**

Benzoin (Siam, Hydrodistilled)  80.1%
Benzoin (Sumatra, Hydrodistilled)  76.1%
Peru Balsam  56.6%–66.2%
Benzoin (Sumatra, Absolute)  50.7%
Tolu Balsam  46.6%
Peru Balsam (Resinoid Absolute)  25.0%–40.0%
Benzoin (Siam, Absolute)  39.3%
Jasmine Absolute (Benzyl Acetate CT)  2.5%–20.0%
Tamala ((E)-Cinnamaldehyde\Cinn. Ac. CT)  0.0%–15.3%

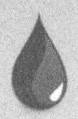

| | |
|---|---|
| Cinnamon Bark | 0.3%–15.1% |
| Ylang Ylang (Madagascan I) | 4.3%–14.9% |
| Ylang Ylang (Madagascan II) | 5.3%–12.3% |
| Ylang Ylang (Madagascan III) | 5.9%–12.8% |
| Cananga | 2.0%–7.6% |
| Ylang Ylang (Complete) | 0.0%–7.6% |
| Ylang Ylang (French I) | 6.1% |
| Jasmine (Hydrodistilled) | 4.9% |
| Benzoin (Siam, HSSE Absolute) | 0.7%–4.8% |
| Cinnamon (leaves) | 3.0%–4.0% |

**Benzyl Benzoate + Phytol**

| | |
|---|---|
| Jasmine Absolute (Benzyl Benzoate CT) | 20.1%–26.6% |

**Benzyl Cinnamate**

| | |
|---|---|
| Peru Balsam (Resinoid Absolute) | 10.0%–25.0% |
| Peru Balsam | 15.9%–22.1% |
| Benzoin (Sumatra, Hydrodistilled) | 3.3% |

**Benzyl Formate**

| | |
|---|---|
| Benzoin (Siam, S-HS Absolute) | 0.5%–3.7% |

**Benzyl Salicylate**

| | |
|---|---|
| Ylang Ylang (French IV) | 4.1% |

**Beta-Acorenol**

| | |
|---|---|
| Calendula (Alpha-Cadinol/Delta-Cadinene CT) | 0.0%–3.6% |

**Beta-Agarofuran**

| | |
|---|---|
| Agarwood (*A. crassna*) | 0.4%–10.3% |
| Agarwood (Malaysian) | 1.0%–5.0% |

**Beta-Asarone ((Z)-Azarone, (Z)-Isoelemicin, Cis-Asarone)**

| | |
|---|---|
| Calamus (Beta-Asarone CT) | 79.4%–95.9% |
| Calamus (Acorenone CT) | 9.3%–10.2% |
| Kumquat (*C. japonica*, Leaves CT Linalool) | 5.0% |
| Calamus (Alpha-Asarone CT) | 3.5% |

**Beta-Bisabolene**

| | |
|---|---|
| Holy Basil (aerial parts, beta-bisabolene CT) | 24.6%–52.0% |
| Holy Basil (aerial parts, eugenol CT) | 0.0%–21.0% |
| Guava Leaf (β-Bisabolene\β-Sesqu. CT) | 19.2% |
| Hairy Basil (1,8-Cineole CT) | 0.0%–15.9% |
| Copaiba | 1.0%–12.7% |
| Ledum (*R. groenlandicum*) | 0.0%–12.6% |
| Blue Mountain Sage (Delta-3-Carene CT) | 0.2%–11.3% |
| Black Pepper (Limonene CT) | 0.2%–8.0% |
| Ginger | 0.0%–7.8% |
| Black Pepper (Beta-Caryophyllene CT) | 0.0%–7.1% |
| Opoponax (*C. guidotti*) | 0.0%–5.1% |
| Lemon (Distilled) | 0.0%–4.9% |
| Guava Leaf (Alpha-Pinene CT) | 0.0%–4.8% |
| Hairy Basil (var. *pilosum* Eugenol CT) | 4.5% |
| Persian Lime (Cold Pressed\Expressed) | 0.8%–2.4% |
| Angelica Root | 0.3%–1.3% |

**Beta-Bisabolenol**

| | |
|---|---|
| Pink Pepper (*S. molle*, Leaves, Elemol/Beta-Eudesmol CT) | 5.1% |

**Beta-Bisabolol**

| | |
|---|---|
| Hops | 0.0%–15.0% |
| Guava Leaf (Alpha-Pinene CT) | 0.0%–9.2% |
| Vetiver | 0.0%–4.7% |
| Guava Leaf (β-Cary.\(E)-Nerolidol CT) | 3.2% |

**Beta-Bourbonene**

| | |
|---|---|
| Juniper, Phoenicia (needles) | 0.0%–12.9% |
| Hyssop (Linalool CT) | 0.1%–5.4% |
| Applemint (*M. suav.*, Carvone CT) | 1.6%–5.2% |

**Beta-Cadinene**

| | |
|---|---|
| Formosan Cypress (Wood, α-Eudesmol CT) | 7.9% |
| Basil (Methyl Eugenol CT) | 0.1%–6.2% |

**Beta-Caryophyllene (Trans-Caryophyllene; *Stereoisomer* Trans-Beta-Caryophyllene, (E)-Beta-Caryophyllene)**

| | |
|---|---|
| Black Pepper (Beta-Caryophyllene CT) | 18.4%–70.4% |
| Copaiba | 36.5%–53.3% |
| Aleppo Pine (Needles) | 0.0%–49.7% |
| Guava Leaf (Beta-Caryophyllene CT) | 12.0%–46.0% |
| Hairy Basil (Trans-Caryophyllene CT) | 43.0% |
| Cananga | 11.0%–38.2% |
| Hemp (Myrcene CT) | 11.0%–37.5% |
| Tagetes (*T. erecta*, Flowers) | 7.1%–35.2% |
| Arnica (Flowers) | 31.6%–34.6% |
| Maritime Pine (Needles, Beta-Cary. CT) | 26.6%–30.9% |
| Vilayti Tulsi (1,8-Cineole CT) | 4.7%–29.0% |
| Cangerana (Wood) | 28.6% |
| Niaouli (1,8-Cineole/Viridiflorol CT) | 0.5%–28.0% |
| Red Pine | 0.7%–27.6% |
| Applemint (*M. rotun.*, β-Caryophyllene CT) | 26.7% |
| Ylang Ylang (Solvent Extracted) | 25.0%–26.1% |
| Hemp (Beta-Caryophyllene CT) | 19.6%–26.1% |
| Holy Basil (aerial parts, eugenol CT) | 0.1%–25.4% |
| Black Sage (Beta-Caryophyllene CT) | 25.4% |
| Tamala (Beta-Caryophyllene CT) | 25.3% |
| Niaouli (Viridiflorol CT) | 1.3%–24.6% |
| Catnip (Nepetalactone CT) | 0.2%–24.6% |
| Yarrow (Chamazulene CT) | 2.5%–22.2% |
| Guava Leaf (β-Cary.\(E)-Nerolidol CT) | 21.6% |
| Ylang Ylang (Madagascan III) | 14.8%–21.5% |
| Guava Leaf (Limonene CT) | 6.2%–21.3% |
| Guggul | 2.7%–20.8% |
| Thyme (Thuyanol-4 CT) | 0.8%–20.3% |
| Sage (Wild) | 5.2%–19.8% |
| Pink Pepper (*S. molle*, Leaves, Bicyclogermacrene CT) | 17.7%–19.7% |
| Ylang Ylang (Madagascan II) | 1.7%–19.6% |
| Muhuhu (Leaves) | 19.1% |
| Ylang Ylang (Complete) | 1.5%–18.8% |
| Chinese Red Pine (Leaves) | 0.7%–18.5% |
| Mugwort (Beta-Caryophyllene CT) | 17.5% |
| Guava Leaf (Alpha-Pinene CT) | 5.2%–17.4% |
| Betony (β-Phell.\α-Pinene CT) | 0.0%–16.9% |
| Mugwort (Alpha-Thujone CT) | 6.3%–16.5% |
| Black Sage (Alpha-Pinene CT) | 11.7%–16.5% |
| Guava Leaf ((E)-Nerolidol CT) | 15.8% |
| Pink Pepper (*S. molle*, Leaves, Limonene CT) | 15.6% |
| Melissa | 0.1%–15.3% |
| Ocotea (Leaves) | 15.1% |
| Black Sage (Caryophyllene Oxide CT) | 7.7%–14.8% |
| Maritime Pine (Needles, Alpha-Pinene CT) | 0.2%–14.8% |
| Fenugreek | 14.6% |
| Hops | 4.1%–14.5% |
| Turkish Pine (Needles) | 0.0%–14.5% |
| Aleppo Pine (Branches) | 14.3% |
| Indian Borage (Carvacrol CT) | 0.0%–14.1% |
| Black Pepper (Limonene CT) | 1.4%–14.0% |
| Holy Basil (aerial parts or seeds, methyl eugenol CT) | 1.3%–13.7% |
| Betony (Bicyclogermacrene CT) | 3.1%–13.4% |
| Clove | 3.1%–13.0% |
| Holy Basil (leaves) | 10.9%–12.9% |
| Mastic (Leaves) | 0.0%–12.8% |
| Indian Borage (Beta-Caryophyllene CT) | 12.6% |
| Thyme (Linalool CT) | 0.5%–12.3% |
| Guava Leaf (Selin-11-en-4-Alpha-ol CT) | 8.2%–12.1% |
| Vilayti Tulsi (Sabinene CT) | 0.0%–11.7% |
| Rhododendron (Leaves) | 11.6% |

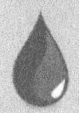

**Beta-Caryophyllene—continued**

| | |
|---|---|
| Aleppo Pine (Cones) | 6.7%–11.2% |
| Ylang Ylang (Madagascan I) | 1.1%–11.2% |
| Aleppo Pine (Aerial Parts) | 0.0%–11.2% |
| Turkish Pine (Bark) | 11.2% |
| Geranium | 0.0%–11.0% |
| Myrrh | 4.4%–10.9% |
| Dwarf Pine (Twigs) | 4.0%–10.9% |
| Carrot Seed | 0.0%–10.7% |
| Black Pepper (Delta-3-Carene CT) | 2.1%–10.6% |
| Katrafay (Ishwarane CT) | 0.8%–10.5% |
| Cinnamon Bark | 0.7%–10.4% |
| Thyme (Carvacrol CT) | 0.0%–10.3% |
| Juniper (Needles) | 0.8%–10.3% |
| Thyme (Thymol CT) | 0.0%–10.3% |
| Hairy Basil (var. *pilosum* Linalool CT) | 1.0%–10.0% |
| Indian Borage (Delta-Cadinene CT) | 5.3%–9.8% |
| Verbena (Linalool CT) | 1.6%–9.8% |
| Turkish Pine (Twigs) | 6.8%–9.7% |
| Clove (Leaves) | 0.5%–9.7% |
| Vilayti Tulsi (Fenchone CT) | 7.0%–9.7% |
| Thyme (Geraniol CT) | 0.3%–9.6% |
| Chaste Tree (Berries) | 0.1%–9.5% |
| Aleppo Pine (Twigs) | 9.5% |
| Savory (Wild, Linalool CT) | 2.8%–9.3% |
| Turkish Pine (Resin) | 9.1% |
| Dwarf Pine (Needles, Needles/Twigs) | 2.4%–9.0% |
| Hairy Basil (var. *pilosum* Terpinen-4-ol CT) | 2.1%–9.0% |
| Copaiba (Leaves) | 1.1%–9.0% |
| Chaste Tree (Leaves) | 2.3%–8.9% |
| Sweet Wormwood (Camphor CT) | 0.3%–8.9% |
| Allspice (Leaves, Eugenol CT) | 1.4%–8.7% |
| Niaouli ((E)-Nerolidol CT) | 0.5%–8.7% |
| Tagetes (*T. erecta*, Aerial Parts) | 1.7%–8.6% |
| Applemint (*M. suav.*, Carvone CT) | 2.5%–8.5% |
| Spanish Sage | 1.2%–8.5% |
| Silver Fir (*A. alba*) | 2.2%–8.4% |
| Ravensara (Limonene CT) | 1.5%–8.4% |
| White Pine | 3.3%–8.2% |
| Black Sage (Tricyclene CT) | 8.2% |
| Tagetes (*T. patula*, Limonene CT) | 0.0%–8.0% |
| Spearmint (Pulegone-Menthone-Isomenthone CT) | 0.0%–8.0% |
| Thyme (Thymol CT) | 0.0%–7.8% |
| Betony (Germacrene D-Spathulenol CT) | 7.8% |
| Allspice (Berries, Eugenol CT) | 3.3%–7.7% |
| Cajeput (Cajuput) | 3.8%–7.6% |
| Oriental Arborvitae (Needles) | 3.0%–7.5% |
| Yarrow (Sabinene CT) | 2.3%–7.5% |
| Blue Mountain Sage (Delta-3-Carene CT) | 0.0%–7.3% |
| Gobre Salla | 1.8%–7.2% |
| Fragonia (Balanced CT) | 0.2%–6.8% |
| Celery Leaf | 3.7%–6.7% |
| Pennyroyal (*M. fruticosa*, Isomenthol CT) | 5.1%–6.6% |
| Allspice (Berries, Methyl Eugenol CT) | 2.7%–6.6% |
| White Verbena (Citral CT) | 0.0%–6.6% |
| Mastic (Aerial parts, Beta-Eudesmol CT) | 6.6% |
| Rhododendron (Aerial Parts) | 2.3%–6.5% |
| Citronella (*C. nardus*) | 0.8%–6.5% |
| Catnip (1,8-cineole CT) | 6.4% |
| Spearmint (Linalool CT) | 4.4%–6.3% |
| Turkish Pine (Needles/Twigs) | 5.6%–6.2% |
| Mastic (Twigs, Alpha-Pinene CT) | 6.2% |
| Lavender (True English) | 2.0%–6.1% |
| Pink Pepper (*S. molle*, Leaves/Fruits, Sabinene CT) | 1.2%–6.1% |

| | |
|---|---|
| Guava Leaf (β-Bisabolene\β-Sesqu. CT) | 6.0% |
| Guava Leaf (Viridiflorol CT) | 5.9%–5.9% |
| Mugwort (Camphor CT) | 0.0%–5.8% |
| Damiana (Caryophyllene Oxide CT) | 0.6%–5.6% |
| Camphor (Camphor CT) | 1.5%–5.5% |
| Sage (1,8-Cineole CT) | 1.4%–5.5% |
| Celery Seed | 0.9%–5.5% |
| Blue Mountain Sage (Limonene CT) | 5.4% |
| Hairy Basil (Linalool CT, Inflorescences) | 2.8%–5.3% |
| Lavender (Bulgarian) | 1.7%–5.2% |
| Mastic (NT\B, Terpinene-4-ol CT) | 1.1%–5.2% |
| Clary Sage | 3.2%–5.1% |
| Turkish Pine (Cones) | 0.0%–5.1% |
| Helichrysum (*H. italicum*) | 2.0%–5.0% |
| Pine | 0.6%–4.9% |
| Neroli (*C. sinensis*) | 0.1%–4.9% |
| Sweet Inula (1,8-Cineole CT) | 1.6%–4.8% |
| Mugwort (Artemisia Ketone CT) | 0.0%–4.8% |
| Galangal (Lesser) | 0.3%–4.7% |
| Sage (Alpha-Thujone CT) | 0.0%–4.7% |
| Pink Pepper (*S. molle*, Leaves, Beta-Pinene CT) | 4.7% |
| Genipi (*A. umbelliformis*, C-SH\B CT) | 1.0%–4.6% |
| Hairy Basil ((E)-Methyl Cinnamate CT) | 0.0%–4.6% |
| Betony (Alpha-Zingiberene CT) | 4.6% |
| Verbena (Limonene\Piperitenone CT) | 1.8%–4.5% |
| Pink Pepper (*S. molle*, Fruits/Leaves, α-Phell./Sylv. CT) | 0.0%–4.5% |
| Black Pepper (Eugenol CT) | 3.5%–4.4% |
| Applemint (*M. rotun.*, Piperitenone CT) | 0.4%–4.4% |
| Sweet Inula (T-Cadinol CT) | 4.4% |
| Hairy Basil (Camphor CT) | 3.1%–4.3% |
| Lemon Verbena (Leaves) | 0.4%–4.3% |
| Kunzea (Spathulenol\Globulol CT) | 2.9%–4.1% |
| Oriental Arborvitae (Berries) | 1.9%–4.1% |
| Cinnamon (leaves) | 1.7%–4.1% |
| Mastic (NT\B, Germacrene D CT) | 4.1% |
| Gurjun Balsam (*D. turbinatus*) | 2.0%–4.0% |
| Lavender (Indian) | 0.9%–4.0% |
| Mountain Savory (Thymol CT) | 1.7%–3.8% |
| Lemon Catnip (Beta-Citronellol CT) | 0.0%–3.7% |
| Tamala (Eugenol CT) | 0.1%–3.6% |
| Lemon Tea Tree (*L. liversidgei*) | 3.0%–3.5% |
| May Chang (Citral CT) | 0.1%–3.5% |
| Maritime Pine (Gum Resin) | 0.1%–3.5% |
| Arnica (Roots, 2,5-Dimethoxy-p-Cymene CT) | 0.0%–3.5% |
| Lemon Basil | 2.1%–3.2% |
| Manuka (Leptospermone CT) | 2.0%–3.2% |
| Applemint (*M. rotun.*, Pulegone CT) | 0.0%–3.2% |
| Manuka (Selinene/Beta-Elemene CT) | 3.2% |
| Yarrow (1,8-Cineole\Camphor CT) | 1.1%–3.1% |
| Ledum (*R. groenlandicum*) | 0.0%–3.1% |
| Magnolia (Leaves) | 0.0%–3.0% |
| Lemon Eucalyptus | 1.8%–2.9% |
| Hyssop (Linalool CT) | 2.4%–2.8% |
| Hyssop (Alpha-Pinene CT) | 2.7% |
| Hyssop (Pinocamphone CT) | 0.3%–2.5% |
| Ravintsara (Linalool CT) | 0.3%–2.5% |
| Allspice (Leaves, Methyl Eugenol CT) | 2.5% |
| Mastic (NT\B, Limonene CT) | 0.7%–2.3% |
| Spike Lavender | 0.5%–1.9 |
| Ravensara (Methyl Chavicol CT) | 0.4%–1.8% |
| Mugwort (Chrysanthenyl Acetate CT) | 1.6% |
| Gurjun Balsam (*D. kerri*) | 1.1% |
| Southern Blue Gum | 0.1%–1.0% |
| Ravensara (Methyl Eugenol CT) | 0.1%–0.9% |

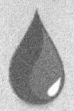

**Beta-Caryophyllene Oxide**

*See Caryophyllene Oxide*

**Beta-Cedrene**

| | |
|---|---|
| Chinese Cedarwood | 0.0%–11.5% |
| Cedarwood (Virginian, Wood) | 0.0%–9.2% |
| Texas Cedarwood | 0.1%–5.5% |

**Beta-Chamigrene**

| | |
|---|---|
| Schisandra Fruit (*S. chinensis*) | 4.9%–6.6% |
| Schisandra Fruit (*S. sphenanthera*, α-Cad. CT) | 3.0% |

**Beta-Copaene**

| | |
|---|---|
| Goldenrod | 0.0%–9.8% |
| Hairy Basil (Camphor CT) | 0.0%–3.7% |

**Beta-Costol**

| | |
|---|---|
| Tamala (Eugenol CT) | 0.0%–3.9% |

**Beta-Cubebene**

| | |
|---|---|
| Goldenrod | 0.0%–26.9% |
| Muhuhu (Leaves) | 15.5% |
| Savory (Wild, Linalool CT) | 1.7%–9.1% |
| Sweet Inula (Borneol CT) | 0.0%–7.1% |
| Calendula (Alpha-Cadinol/Delta-Cadinene CT) | 0.5%–6.5% |
| Galbanum | 0.0%–4.9% |
| Sweet Wormwood (Artemisia Ketone CT) | 0.0%–3.9% |
| Calendula (Alpha-Cadinol/Delta-Cadinene CT) | 0.0%–3.8% |

**Beta-Curcumene**

| | |
|---|---|
| Wild Turmeric (Distilled) | 0.0%–29.9% |
| Balsam Poplar | 0.0%–3.9% |
| Ylang Ylang (French IV) | 2.7% |

**Beta-Curcumene-12-ol**

| | |
|---|---|
| Sandalwood (*S. spicatum*) | 0.0%–7.2% |

**Beta-Davanone-2-ol**

| | |
|---|---|
| Davana | 0.0%–3.1% |

**Beta-Dehydroelsholtzione (Naginata Ketone)**

| | |
|---|---|
| Pink Pepper (*S. terebinthifolius*, Leaves, p-Cymen-7-ol CT) | 4.6% |

**Beta Dihdroagarofuran**

| | |
|---|---|
| African Bluegrass (Linalool CT) | 2.4%–6.4% |

**Beta-Elemene**

| | |
|---|---|
| Holy Basil (aerial parts, eugenol CT) | 0.0%–18.0% |
| Hinoki (Taiwan Cypress, wood) | 0.2%–15.8% |
| Palo Santo (Leaves, Aerial Parts) | 11.3%–14.1% |
| Black Cumin (Para-Cymene CT) | 0.0%–11.0% |
| Manuka (Selinene/Beta-Elemene CT) | 10.8% |
| Myrrh | 4.4%–10.9% |
| Katrafay (Ishwarane CT) | 0.0%–8.9% |
| White Turmeric (Distilled) | 0.0%–8.3% |
| Opoponax (*C. erythraea*) | 5.4%–8.2% |
| Wild Turmeric (Distilled) | 0.4%–7.5% |
| Pink Pepper (*S. terebinthifolius*, Fruits/Leaves, Bicyclogerm. CT) | 0.0%–7.3% |
| Katrafay (Leaves) | 1.1%–7.0% |
| Wild Chamomile (*O. multicaulis*) | 0.0%–6.7% |
| Black Pepper (Beta-Caryophyllene CT) | 0.2%–5.1% |
| Wild Chamomile (*C. mixtus*, Sant. Alc. CT) | 0.0%–5.0% |
| Hairy Basil (Eugenol CT) | 4.3% |
| Magnolia (Flowers) | 1.3%–3.8% |
| Formosan Cypress (Wood, Myrtenol CT) | 1.1%–3.6% |
| Chinese Red Pine (Leaves) | 0.0%–3.4% |
| Damiana (Delta-Cadinene CT) | 2.7%–3.2% |
| Frankincense (*B. frereana*) | 0.0%–2.7% |
| Frankincense (*B. sacra*) | 0.0%–2.6% |
| Ledum (*R. groenlandicum*) | 0.0%–1.6% |
| Mugwort (1,8-Cineole CT) | 0.0%–1.4% |

**Beta-Elemol**

| | |
|---|---|
| Siam Wood (Root Bark) | 3.2%–4.5% |

**Beta-Epi-Eudesmol**

| | |
|---|---|
| Agarwood (*A. crassna*) | 0.0%–4.2% |

**Beta-Eudesmol**

| | |
|---|---|
| Auracaria | 25.9%–31.1% |
| Kumquat (*F. margarita*, Leaves) | 12.4%–28.3% |
| Formosan Cypress (Twig) | 25.1% |
| Mastic (Aerial parts, Beta-Eudesmol CT) | 16.3% |
| Calendula (Alpha-Cadinol/Delta-Cadinene CT) | 0.0%–14.5% |
| Blue Cypress (Wood) | 8.5%–14.0% |
| Balsam Poplar | 3.4%–11.4% |
| Pink Pepper (*S. molle*, Leaves, Elemol/Beta-Eudesmol CT) | 10.3% |
| Japanese Cedarwood (Bark) | 0.0%–9.9% |
| Black Pepper (Eugenol CT) | 0.9%–9.7% |
| Japanese Cedarwood (Sapwood) | 0.0%–9.3% |
| Agarwood (Malaysian) | 0.0%–8.4% |
| Valerian | 0.0%–8.3% |
| Amyris | 7.9%–8.2% |
| Big Badja Gum | 0.0%–7.8% |
| Rabbitbrush (var. *nauseosa*) | 7.7% |
| Blue Tansy (Chamazulene CT) | 3.0%–7.0% |
| Yarrow (1,8-Cineole\Camphor CT) | 0.0%–6.1% |
| Japanese Cedarwood (Heartwood) | 0.0%–6.1% |
| Japanese Cedarwood (16-Kaurene/Valencene CT) | 5.9% |
| Leleshwa | 0.3%–5.8% |
| Japanese Cedarwood (16-Kaurene CT) | 0.0%–5.7% |
| Gully Gum | 0.0%–5.5% |
| Fragonia (Balanced CT) | 0.0%–5.5% |
| Japanese Cedarwood (Alpha-Pinene CT) | 0.0%–4.8% |
| Siam Wood (Root Bark) | 3.2%–4.5% |
| Pink Pepper (*S. molle*, Leaves, α-Phellandrene CT) | 0.0%–4.2% |
| White Spruce (Needles & Twigs) | 0.9%–4.0% |
| Magnolia (Leaves) | 1.7%–3.7% |
| Davana | 0.0%–3.7% |
| Chaste Tree (Berries) | 0.0%–2.4% |
| Angelica Root | 0.4%–1.8% |

**Beta-Farnesene; (E)-Beta-Farnesene**

| | |
|---|---|
| Katrafay (Leaves) | 27.7%–35.6% |
| Wormwood ((E)-Beta-Farnesene CT) | 31.6% |
| Ginger | 0.0%–14.7% |
| German Chamomile | 2.3%–14.0% |
| Chaste Tree (Berries) | 0.1%–11.7% |
| Wild Chamomile (*O. mixta*, *C. mixtrum*) | 1.5%–11.3% |
| Hops | 0.0%–9.5% |
| Chaste Tree (Leaves) | 0.0%–9.4% |
| Hairy Basil (var. *pilosum* Eugenol CT) | 9.2% |
| Wild Chamomile (*O. multicaulis*) | 0.0%–8.6% |
| Hemp (Beta-Caryophyllene CT) | 4.8%–8.5% |
| Lavender (Bulgarian) | 1.0%–4.7% |
| Lavender (True English) | 0.1%–4.2% |
| Carrot Seed | 0.5%–4.0% |
| Guava Leaf (β-Bisabolene\β-Sesqu. CT) | 4.0% |
| Angelica Root | 0.1%–2.7% |
| Applemint (*M. suav.*, Italian) | 0.0%–2.3% |
| Ledum (*R. groenlandicum*) | 0.0%–1.3% |

**Beta-Funebrene**

| | |
|---|---|
| Chinese Cedarwood | 0.0%–3.4% |

**Beta-Guaiene (Trans-Beta-Guaiene)**

| | |
|---|---|
| Formosan Cypress (Wood, α-Eudesmol CT) | 8.0% |
| Guava Leaf (Selin-11-en-4-Alpha-ol CT) | 3.9%–6.7% |
| Agarwood (*A. crassna*) | 0.0%–4.4% |
| Cananga | 0.1%–3.8% |

**Beta-Guajene**

| | |
|---|---|
| Davana | 0.0%–18.4% |

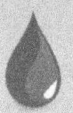

**Beta-Gurjunene (Calarene)**

*See Calarene*

**Beta-Himachalene**

| | |
|---|---|
| Cedarwood (Atlas) | 9.9%–40.4% |
| Cedarwood (Himalayan, Wood) | 12.3%–38.3% |
| Schisandra Fruit (*S. sphenanthera, δ-Cad. CT*) | 19.8% |
| Schisandra Fruit (*S. sphenanthera, α-Cad. CT*) | 11.4% |
| Chinese Cedarwood | 0.0%–6.4% |

**Beta-Himachalene Oxide**

| | |
|---|---|
| Cedarwood (Himalayan, Wood) | 0.0%–14.9% |

**Beta-Humulene**

| | |
|---|---|
| Tamala (Eugenol CT) | 0.0%–4.4% |

**Beta-Ionone (Trans-Beta-Ionone, (E)-Beta-Ionone)**

| | |
|---|---|
| Calendula (Alpha-Cadinol/Delta-Cadinene CT) | 0.0%–3.2% |

**Beta-Longifolene**

| | |
|---|---|
| Schisandra Fruit (*S. sphenanthera, δ-Cad. CT*) | 4.8% |

**Beta-Maaliene**

| | |
|---|---|
| Spikenard (Calarene CT) | 5.6%–10.2% |

**Beta-Oplopenone (Oplopenone)**

| | |
|---|---|
| Damiana (1,8-Cineole CT) | 1.0%–10.3% |
| Damiana (Caryophyllene Oxide CT) | 0.0%–6.0% |
| Muhuhu (Wood) | 0.0%–3.5% |
| Ledum (*L. palustre*) | 0.0%–1.7% |

**Beta-Patchoulene**

| | |
|---|---|
| Patchouli (Chinese) | 0.0%–5.8% |

**Beta-Patchoulol**

| | |
|---|---|
| Calendula (Alpha-Cadinol/Delta-Cadinene CT) | 0.0%–3.4% |

**Beta-Phellandrene**

| | |
|---|---|
| Lovage (Roots) | 0.4%–62.5% |
| Lovage (Leaves) | 9.6%–44.0% |
| Lovage (Aerial Parts) | 12.9%–42.5% |
| Betony (β-Phell.\α-Pinene CT) | 4.6%–37.9% |
| Parsley (Leaves, Myristicin CT) | 6.2%–35.9% |
| Parsley (Leaves, 1,3,8-Para-Menth. CT) | 3.1%–29.8% |
| Pink Pepper (*S. molle*, Aerial Parts, α-Phell. CT) | 29.3% |
| Rabbitbrush (var. *albicaulis*) | 26.0% |
| Black Sage (Beta-Phellandrene CT) | 25.3% |
| Chinese Red Pine (Leaves) | 14.9%–25.2% |
| Juniper (Needles) | 3.7%–25.2% |
| Juniper, Phoenicia (needles) | 0.1%–24.4% |
| Balsam Fir | 4.4%–23.1% |
| Rabbitbrush (var. *nauseosa*) | 22.8% |
| Galbanum | 0.1%–22.7% |
| Pink Pepper (*S. molle*, Fruits, α-Phellandrene CT) | 0.0%–20.8% |
| Pink Pepper (*S. terebinthifolius*, Fruits, δ-3-Carene CT) | 0.0%–18.5% |
| Rabbitbrush (var. *consimilis*) | 18.0% |
| Monarda (Thymol CT) | 0.0%–17.0% |
| Lavender (True English) | 0.0%–16.0% |
| Angelica Root | 0.1%–15.4% |
| Betony (Alpha-Thujene CT) | 1.1%–14.4% |
| Pink Pepper (*S. molle*, Leaves, α-Phellandrene CT) | 9.6%–13.6% |
| Mugwort (Chrysanthenyl Acetate CT) | 11.4% |
| Rabbitbrush (var. *glabratus*) | 10.9% |
| Pink Pepper (*S. terebinthifolius*, Fruits, α-Phell. CT) | 10.6% |
| Bay Laurel | 0.0%–10.5% |
| Siberian Fir | 2.4%–9.3% |
| Spanish Sage | 0.1%–9.3% |
| Parsley Seed | 4.4%–8.8% |
| Boldo (*1,8-Cineole\Para-Cymene\Limonene CT*) | 0.0%–8.4% |
| Juniper, Phoenicia (leaves, isoborneol CT) | 8.1% |
| Blue Mountain Sage (Limonene CT) | 7.8% |
| Dill (Aerial Parts, Alpha-Phellandrene CT) | 7.4%–7.5% |

| | |
|---|---|
| Hyssop (Pinocamphone CT) | 3.4%–7.5% |
| White Fir (*A. concolor*) | 1.1%–6.5% |
| Pink Pepper (*S. terebinthifolius*, Fruits/Leaves, Bicyclogerm. CT) | 0.0%–6.5% |
| Petitgrain (Mandarin) | 0.0%–6.3% |
| Betony (Bicyclogermacrene CT) | 0.0%–5.8% |
| Mastic (NT\B, Alpha-Pinene CT) | 0.0%–5.8% |
| Xanthoxylum | 0.0%–5.7% |
| White Spruce (Needles) | 0.0%–5.5% |
| Oriental Arborvitae (Berries) | 0.0%–5.5% |
| Yuzu | 1.6%–5.4% |
| Boldo (Ascaridole CT) | 0.0%–5.4% |
| White Pine | 1.1%–5.3% |
| Mastic (Leaves) | 0.0%–5.0% |
| Mastic (NT\B, Terpinene-4-ol CT) | 3.7%–4.8% |
| Black Pepper (Delta-3-Carene CT) | 3.2%–4.5% |
| Tsuga | 0.0%–4.4% |
| Ginger | 0.2%–4.3% |
| Parsley (Whole Plant) | 0.0%–4.2% |
| White Spruce (Oleoresin) | 0.1%–4.1% |
| Mugwort (Alpha-Thujone CT) | 2.9%–3.7% |
| Hinoki (*Needles & Twigs*, α-Terpinene CT) | 3.5% |
| Plai (Triquinacene, 1,4-Bis(Methoxy)- CT) | 3.5% |
| Engelmann Spruce | 0.6%–3.3% |
| Spearmint (Pulegone-Menthone-Isomenthone CT) | 0.0%–3.0% |
| Ravensara (Limonene CT) | 1.0%–2.9% |
| Eucalyptus Dives | 0.0%–2.8% |
| Elemi | 1.8%–2.3% |
| Mugwort (1,8-Cineole CT) | 0.0%–2.2% |
| Ledum (*R. groenlandicum*) | 0.0%–1.3% |

**Beta-Pinene**

| | |
|---|---|
| Galbanum | 45.5%–66.3% |
| Ponderosa Pine | 17.0%–66.0% |
| White Fir (*A. Concolor*) | 41.5%–52.2% |
| Turkish Pine (Needles) | 0.0%–47.5% |
| Kumquat (*C. japonica*, Leaves CT Beta-Pinene) | 47.4% |
| Gobre Salla | 18.1%–46.8% |
| Aleppo Pine (Aerial Parts) | 0.2%–46.8% |
| Aleppo Pine (Needles) | 0.2%–46.8% |
| Red Pine | 1.9%–42.4% |
| Black Pepper (Beta-Pinene CT) | 41.2% |
| Turkish Pine (Cones) | 28.3%–39.6% |
| Douglas Fir (Needles) | 21.2%–39.5% |
| Mastic (Gum Resin) | 3.0%–38.7% |
| Balsam Fir | 27.3%–38.0% |
| White Pine | 7.9%–35.5% |
| Wormwood (Beta-Pinene CT) | 12.3%–31.9% |
| Lemon (Distilled) | 0.6%–31.5% |
| Douglas Fir (Needles & Twigs) | 3.7%–31.2% |
| Pink Pepper (*S. molle*, Leaves, Beta-Pinene CT) | 31.1% |
| Kaffir Lime Peel | 13.5%–30.5% |
| Rabbitbrush (var. *glabratus*) | 30.3% |
| Mugwort (Isobornyl Isobutyrate D CT) | 30.1% |
| Engelmann Spruce | 1.2%–29.7% |
| Maritime Pine (Gum Resin) | 17.0%–29.5% |
| Pine | 1.8%–29.4% |
| Parsley Seed | 18.6%–27.2% |
| Turkish Pine (Needles/Twigs) | 20.0%–26.8% |
| Black Pepper (Limonene CT) | 4.7%–25.6% |
| Petitgrain (Lemon) | 10.5%–25.1% |
| Chinese Red Pine (Twigs) | 20.8%–24.3% |
| White Spruce (Oleoresin) | 4.7%–23.8% |
| Maritime Pine (Needles, Alpha-Pinene CT) | 0.9%–21.7% |
| Cedarwood (Atlas) | 2.4%–21.4% |
| White Spruce (Branches) | 20.4%–20.5% |

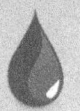

| | | | |
|---|---|---|---|
| Rabbitbrush (var. *nauseosa*) | 19.8% | Kumquat (*F. margarita*, Leaves) | 0.0%–8.3% |
| Yarrow (Chamazulene CT) | 0.1%–19.4% | Saro (1,8-Cineole CT) | 2.1%–8.0% |
| Turkish Pine (Twigs) | 17.5%–19.2% | Pink Pepper (*S. terebinthifolius*, Leaves, Sabinene CT) | 8.0% |
| Lime (Cold-pressed/expressed) | 0.1%–19.2% | Yarrow (Beta-Thujone CT) | 0.0%–7.8% |
| Neroli (*C. aurantium*) | 3.5%–19.1% | Ravensara (Sabinene CT) | 3.9%–7.7% |
| Pink Pepper (*S. molle*, Fruits/Leaves, p-Cymene CT) | 1.8%–19.0% | Sage (Beta-Thujone CT) | 1.0%–7.7% |
| Nutmeg (West Indian) | 7.3%–18.8% | Monarda (Linalool CT) | 0.8%–7.7% |
| Aleppo Pine (Twigs) | 18.7% | Rosemary (1,8-Cineole CT) | 4.8%–7.5% |
| Hyssop (Pinocamphone CT) | 9.9%–18.4% | Sage (1,8-Cineole CT) | 3.3%–7.3% |
| Black Pepper (Delta-3-Carene CT) | 13.2%–18.3% | Niaouli (*M. viridiflora*, Terpinen-4-ol CT) | 7.3% |
| Genipi (*A. genipi*) | 1.3%–17.9% | Hinoki (*Needles & Twigs*, α-Terpinene CT) | 7.2% |
| Nutmeg (East Indian) | 0.0%–17.7% | Sweet Inula (1,8-Cineole CT) | 3.6%–6.9% |
| Spanish Sage | 4.6%–17.3% | Lemon (Distilled) | 0.0%–6.9% |
| Katrafay (Beta-Pinene CT) | 17.1% | Vilayti Tulsi (Sabinene CT) | 0.0%–6.7% |
| Rabbitbrush (var. *albicaulis*) | 16.8% | Vilayti Tulsi (1,8-Cineole CT) | 4.2%–6.6% |
| Cumin | 6.8%–16.3% | Allspice (Berries, Eugenol CT) | 0.0%–6.5% |
| Rhododendron (Aerial Parts) | 6.2%–16.0% | Hinoki (needles) | 0.0%–6.4% |
| Lemon (Cold-pressed/expressed) | 0.1%–15.8% | Camphor (Camphor CT) | 0.0%–6.3% |
| Pink Pepper (*S. molle*, Aerial Parts, α-Phell. CT) | 15.7% | Oakmoss Aboslute (Hydro. + Hexane) | 6.3% |
| Silver Fir (*A. alba*) | 0.5%–15.5% | Sweet Wormwood (Artemisia Ketone CT) | 0.0%–6.0% |
| Chinese Red Pine (Leaves) | 3.0%–15.4% | Hairy Basil (1,8-Cineole CT) | 1.9%–5.8% |
| Dwarf Pine (Twigs) | 2.2%–15.4% | Galangal (Lesser) | 1.0%–5.7% |
| Persian Lime (Cold Pressed\Expressed) | 7.9%–15.3% | Turkish Pine (Bark) | 5.7% |
| White Spruce (Needles & Twigs) | 3.4%–15.1% | Wild Marjoram (1,8-Cineole CT) | 1.7 %–5.6% |
| Fenugreek | 15.1% | Juniper Berry | 1.7%–5.4% |
| Pink Pepper (*S. molle*, Leaves, Epi-Bicyclosesquiphell. CT) | 14.7% | Grindelia | 1.5%–5.2% |
| Sage (Camphor CT) | 1.4%–14.5% | Eucalyptus (*E. globulus*) | 0.3%–5.2% |
| Galangal (Greater, 1,8-Cineole CT) | 0.9%–14.4% | Mastic (NT\B, Terpinene-4-ol CT) | 2.3%–5.1% |
| Pink Pepper (*S. molle*, Leaves, Bicyclogermacrene CT) | 1.1%–14.0% | Niaouli (1,8-Cineole CT) | 0.5%–5.0% |
| Black Pepper (Beta-Caryophyllene CT) | 0.7%–13.6% | Pink Pepper (*S. molle*, Fruits, α-Phellandrene CT) | 0.0%–5.0% |
| Chaste Tree (Berries) | 0.6%–13.2% | Niaouli (Viridiflorol CT) | 0.4%–5.0% |
| Black Sage (Alpha-Pinene CT) | 0.1%–13.1% | Vilayti Tulsi (Fenchone CT) | 3.2%–4.9% |
| Persian Lime (Distilled) | 1.8%–13.0% | Sage (Alpha-Thujone CT) | 0.7%–4.8% |
| Mastic (NT\B, Alpha-Pinene CT) | 2.0%–12.8% | Black Pepper (Eugenol CT) | 1.7%–4.7% |
| Katrafay (Leaves) | 0.2%–12.8% | Bay Laurel | 1.4%–4.7% |
| Pink Pepper (*S. molle*, Leaves/Fruits, Sabinene CT) | 0.6%–12.7% | Turmeric (Leaves) | 0.1%–4.7% |
| Lime (Distilled) | 0.9%–12.6% | Summer Savory (Thymol CT) | 1.2%–4.5% |
| Mastic (Leaves) | 0.0%–12.6% | Bergamot (Distilled) | 0.8%–4.4% |
| Yarrow (Sabinene CT) | 2.3%–12.3% | Spearmint (*M. crispa*, Rotundifolone CT) | 4.4% |
| Bergamot (Cold-pressed/expressed) | 0.1%–12.1% | Mugwort (Artemisia Ketone CT) | 1.8%–4.3% |
| Betony (β-Phell.\α-Pinene CT) | 0.0%–12.1% | Savin (Berries) | 0.6%–4.3% |
| Rosemary (Alpha-Pinene CT) | 1.1%–12.0% | Shell Ginger (Terpinene-4-ol CT) | 0.3%–4.3% |
| Wormwood (Myrcene CT) | 0.1%–11.8% | Damiana (Caryophyllene Oxide CT) | 0.0%–3.9% |
| Parsley (Whole Plant) | 10.4%–11.6% | Plai (Sabinene CT) | 2.3%–3.8% |
| Genipi (*A. umbelliformis*, C-SH\B CT) | 1.8%–11.5% | Blue Mallee (Cryptone CT) | 0.7%–3.8% |
| White Spruce (Needles) | 0.0%–11.3% | Mugwort (Beta-Caryophyllene CT) | 3.8% |
| Monarda (Thymol CT) | 1.6%–10.9% | Black Cumin (Para-Cymene CT) | 0.0%–3.7% |
| Hyssop (Alpha-Pinene CT) | 10.9% | Petitgrain (Bergamot/Bitter Orange) | 1.6%–3.6% |
| Wormwood (Trans-Sabinyl Acetate CT) | 0.2%–10.4% | Pennyroyal (*M. fruticosa*, Pulegone CT) | 1.2%–3.6% |
| Tamala (Linalool CT) | 10.4% | Ajowan (Gamma-Terpinene\P-Cymene CT) | 0.0%–3.6% |
| Helichrysum (*H. splendidum*, Alpha-Terpinene CT) | 10.2% | Ravintsara (1,8-Cineole CT) | 0.0%–3.5% |
| Blue Tansy (Sabinene CT) | 5.3%–10.1% | Rosemary (Camphor CT) | 2.5%–3.4% |
| Tamala (Eugenol CT) | 0.1%–10.1% | Formosan Cypress (Neeldes, α-Pinene CT) | 1.9%–3.4% |
| Turkish Pine (Resin) | 9.7% | Tarragon (Methyl Chavicol CT) | 0.0%–3.4% |
| Hemp (Myrcene CT) | 0.4%–9.3% | Angelica Root | 0.2%–3.1% |
| Goldenrod | 0.0%–9.3% | Hyssop (Linalool CT) | 2.9%–3.0% |
| Peppermint | 0.1%–9.2% | Black Cumin (Thymoquinone CT) | 0.4%–3.0% |
| White Sage | 3.8%–9.1% | Catnip (Nepetalactone CT) | 0.0%–3.0% |
| Wormwood (Alpha-Thujone CT) | 1.3%–9.0% | Ravensara (Alpha-Terpinene CT) | 2.7%–2.9% |
| Ajowan (Gamma-Terpinolene CT) | 8.9% | Ravensara (Limonene CT) | 2.2%–2.9% |
| Blue Spruce | 0.0%–8.8% | Mastic (NT\B, Germacrene D CT) | 2.9% |
| Dwarf Pine (Needles, Needles/Twigs) | 0.0%–8.7% | Spike Lavender | 0.8%–2.6% |
| Ledum (*R. groenlandicum*) | 1.0%–8.4% | Pennyroyal (*M. pulegium*) | 0.4%–2.5% |
| Fragonia (Balanced CT) | 0.9%–8.3% | Celery Leaf | 0.0%–2.5% |

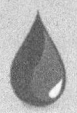

**Beta-Pinene—continued**

| | |
|---|---|
| Chaste Tree (Leaves) | 1.0%–2.4% |
| Mediterranean Mandarin (CP\Expressed) | 0.5%–2.4% |
| Petitgrain (Mandarin) | 0.0%–2.3% |
| Blue Mallee (1,8-Cineole CT) | 0.0%–2.3% |
| Lemon Eucalyptus | 0.9%–2.2% |
| Frankincense (*B. carterii*) | 0.0%–2.1% |
| Mugwort (Camphor CT) | 0.0%–2.1% |
| Spearmint (Piperitenone Oxide CT) | 0.4%–2.0% |
| Spearmint (Piperitone Oxide CT) | 0.4%–2.0% |
| Niaouli (Viridiflorol/ Para-cymene/1,8-cineole CT) | 0.1%–2.0% |
| Mugwort (Alpha-Thujone CT) | 0.7%–1.9% |
| Ocotea (Flowers Calices) | 0.0%–1.7% |

**Beta-Santalene**

| | |
|---|---|
| Sandalwood (*S. album*) | 0.9%–5.9% |

**Beta-Selinene**

| | |
|---|---|
| Celery Leaf | 9.2%–37.4% |
| Ledum (*R. groenlandicum*) | 2.3%–35.4% |
| Celery Seed | 10.1%–27.0% |
| Helichrysum (ssp. *microphyllum*) | 6.6%–17.1% |
| Maritime Pine (Needles, Beta-Cary. CT) | 0.0%–13.5% |
| Guava Leaf (Beta-Caryophyllene CT) | 0.0%–11.0% |
| Ocotea (Flowers Calices) | 2.1%–10.1% |
| Manuka (Selinene/Beta-Elemene CT) | 10.0% |
| Sweet Wormwood (Camphor CT) | 0.0%–9.4% |
| Chaste Tree (Leaves) | 0.0%–9.0% |
| Hairy Basil (var. *pilosum* Terpinen-4-ol CT) | 0.3%–7.7% |
| Hairy Basil (Camphor CT) | 3.3%–7.0% |
| Helichrysum (*H. italicum*) | 2.0%–6.9% |
| Juniper, Phoenicia (Berries) | 0.0%–6.9% |
| Wormwood (Trans-Sabinene Hydrate CT) | 0.0%–6.7% |
| Manuka (Leptospermone CT) | 0.3%–5.8% |
| Hemp (Beta-Caryophyllene CT) | 1.8%–5.4% |
| Wormwood (Chamazulene CT) | 4.5%–5.3% |
| Hinoki (Taiwan Cypress, wood) | 0.4%–5.0% |
| Holy Basil (aerial parts, eugenol CT) | 0.0%–5.0% |
| Mugwort (1,8-Cineole CT) | 2.1%–4.7% |
| Copaiba | 0.5%–4.7% |
| Sweet Wormwood (Artemisia Ketone CT) | 0.0%–4.6% |
| Ocotea (Leaves) | 4.4% |
| Formosan Cypress (Wood, Myrtenol CT) | 0.0%–4.1% |
| Opoponax (*C. erythraea*) | 3.3%–3.6% |
| Camphor (Linalool CT) | 0.5%–2.9% |
| Black Cumin (Para-Cymene CT) | 0.0%–2.7% |
| Mugwort (Germacrene D CT) | 1.2% |
| Mugwort (Chrysanthenyl Acetate CT) | 1.0% |

**Beta-Sesquiphellandrene**

| | |
|---|---|
| Ginger | 1.9%–18.4% |
| Guava Leaf (β-Bisabolene\β-Sesqu. CT) | 14.8% |
| White Turmeric (Distilled) | 0.0%–9.8% |
| Plai (Terpinen-4-ol CT) | 5.9%–7.0% |
| Turmeric (Rhizome, Distilled) | 0.0%–5.6% |
| Galangal (Greater, 1,8-Cineole CT) | 0.0%–5.0% |
| Amyris | 1.5%–4.7% |
| Hemp (Beta-Caryophyllene CT) | 2.0%–4.6% |
| Calamus (Shyobunones CT) | 0.0%–3.0% |

**Beta-Sinensal**

| | |
|---|---|
| Black Sage (Alpha-Santalene CT) | 17.7% |

**Beta-Terpineol**

| | |
|---|---|
| Spearmint (Linalool CT) | 1.0%–3.0% |

**Beta-Thujene**

| | |
|---|---|
| Persian Lime (Distilled) | 0.0%–14.9% |

**Beta-Thujone**

| | |
|---|---|
| Tansy (Beta-Thujone CT) | 28.1%–97.9% |
| Yarrow (Beta-Thujone CT) | 8.3%–96.2% |
| Great Mugwort | 19.6%–71.3% |
| Wormwood (Beta-Thujone CT) | 12.3%–64.6% |
| Sage (Beta-Thujone CT) | 20.4%–49.7% |
| Sage (Camphor CT) | 2.1%–28.6% |
| Wormwood ((Z)-Epoxy Ocimene CT) | 0.0%–27.8% |
| Wormwood (Chamazulene CT) | 17.2%–22.1% |
| Mugwort (Beta-Thujone CT) | 20.8% |
| Genipi (*A. umbelliformis*, Alpha-Thujone CT) | 4.6%–19.5% |
| Sage (Alpha-Thujone CT) | 3.5%–17.9% |
| Mugwort (1,8-Cineole CT) | 0.0%–13.5% |
| Wormwood (Alpha-Thujone CT) | 5.6%–13.4% |
| Genipi (*A. genipi*) | 6.8%–10.4% |
| Thuja | 3.1%–10.0% |
| Mugwort (Alpha-Thujone CT) | 5.2%–8.7% |
| Savin (Needles & Branches) | 0.0%–8.7% |
| Western Red Cedar (Leaves) | 6.8%–8.3% |
| Wormwood (Myrcene CT) | 0.4%–7.3% |
| Boldo (Ascaridole CT) | 0.0%–7.2% |
| Wormwood (Trans-Sabinene Hydrate CT) | 3.7%–6.7% |
| Mugwort (Camphor CT) | 2.8%–5.8% |
| Wormwood (Myrcene-Sabinene CT) | 0.1%–4.5% |
| Sage (1,8-Cineole CT) | 0.1%–3.7% |
| Mugwort (Camphor CT) | 0.0%–1.2% |

**Beta-Turmerone (Curlone)**

| | |
|---|---|
| Turmeric (Rhizomes, Solvent Extracted) | 18.1%–22.7% |
| Turmeric (Rhizomes, Distilled) | 10.6%–18.5% |

**Beta-Vetivenene**

| | |
|---|---|
| Vetiver | 0.0%–9.8% |

**Beyerene**

| | |
|---|---|
| Hinoki (needles and twigs) | 4.7% |

**Bezenaminium**

| | |
|---|---|
| Calamus ((E)-Methylisoeugenol CT) | 4.9% |

**Bicyclo[2.2.1]Hept-2-en-7-ol**

| | |
|---|---|
| Wormwood ((Z)-Epoxy Ocimene CT) | 0.0%–18.9% |
| Wormwood (Cis-Chrysanthenyl Acetate CT) | 3.2%–5.3% |

**Bicyclo[2.2.1]Heptan-2-ol**

| | |
|---|---|
| Hinoki (needles and twigs) | 18.8% |

**Bicyclogermacrene**

| | |
|---|---|
| Pink Pepper (*S. terebinthifolius*, Fruits/Leaves, Bicyclogerm. CT) | 23.6%–35.6% |
| Pink Pepper (*S. molle*, Leaves, Bicyclogermacrene CT) | 20.5%–29.2% |
| Helichrysum (*H. splendidum*, Spathulenol CT) | 7.4%–20.5% |
| Betony (Bicyclogermacrene CT) | 6.8%–18.0% |
| Kunzea (Spathulenol\Globulol CT) | 7.6%–14.0% |
| Black Sage (Alpha-Pinene CT) | 0.0%–13.8% |
| Thuja | 1.1%–13.2% |
| Davana | 0.0%–11.8% |
| Black Sage (Tricyclene CT) | 11.7% |
| Pink Pepper (*S. molle*, Leaves, Limonene CT) | 11.6% |
| Black Sage (Beta-Caryophyllene CT) | 11.3% |
| Betony (Alpha-Thujene CT) | 0.0%–10.7% |
| Helichrysum (*H. splendidum*, Germacrene D-4-ol CT) | 8.8% |
| Chaste Tree (Berries) | 0.0%–8.4% |
| Betony (Germacrene D-Spathulenol CT) | 8.1% |
| Helichrysum (*H. splendidum*, Alpha-Terpinene CT) | 7.9% |
| Vilayti Tulsi (Sabinene CT) | 0.6%–7.5% |
| Fragonia (Balanced CT) | 0.5%–6.7% |
| Helichrysum (*H. splendidum*, Delta-cadinene CT) | 0.8%–6.3% |
| Holy Basil (aerial parts, eugenol CT) | 0.0%–6.3% |
| Pine | 0.0%–6.2% |
| Copaiba (Leaves) | 1.5%–5.7% |

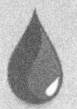

| | |
|---|---|
| Black Pepper (Beta-Caryophyllene CT) | 0.0%–5.1% |
| Ravintsara (Camphor CT) | 0.0%–5.0% |
| Tamala (Eugenol\Eugenyl Acetate CT) | 1.5%–4.9% |
| Betony (MLD-C CT) | 3.1%–4.5% |
| Fragonia (Alpha-Pinene CT) | 2.9%–4.5% |
| Pink Pepper (*S. molle*, Leaves, α-Phellandrene CT) | 0.0%–4.1% |
| Betony (β-Phell.\α-Pinene CT) | 0.0%–4.0% |
| Dwarf Pine (Needles, Needles/Twigs) | 0.0%–3.9% |
| Kunzea (Alpha-Pinene CT) | 0.4%–3.8% |
| Hyssop (Pinocamphone CT) | 0.0%–2.0% |
| Mugwort (Camphor CT) | 0.0%–1.6% |

**Bicyclosesquiphellandrene**

| | |
|---|---|
| White Verbena (Carvone\Limonene CT) | 0.0%–7.7% |
| Applemint (*M. rotun.*, β-Caryophyllene CT) | 4.5% |
| Applemint (*M. rotun.*, Piperitenone CT) | 0.0%–2.5% |
| Applemint (*M. suav.*, Italian) | 0.0%–2.4% |

**Biformen**

| | |
|---|---|
| Japanese Cedarwood (16-Kaurene CT) | 0.0%–3.9% |

**Bisabolatriene-1-ol-4-one**

| | |
|---|---|
| Japanese Cedarwood (Twig) | 5.7%–5.8% |

**Bisabolol Oxide A (Alpha-Bisabolol Oxide A)**

| | |
|---|---|
| German Chamomile | 3.1%–56.0% |

**Bisabolol Oxide B (Alpha-Bisabolol Oxide B)**

| | |
|---|---|
| German Chamomile | 3.9%–27.2% |
| Blue Mountain Sage (Alpha-Bisabolol CT) | 0.0%–5.3% |

**Bisabolone Oxide A (Alpha-Bisabolone Oxide A)**

| | |
|---|---|
| German Chamomile | 0.5%–24.8% |

**Borneol**

| | |
|---|---|
| Sweet Inula (Borneol CT) | 34.5%–43.6% |
| Sweet Inula (Bornyl Acetate CT) | 2.7%–32.2% |
| Lavender (Brazilian) | 22.4% |
| Sweet Inula (1,8-Cineole CT) | 5.4%–20.4% |
| Genipi (*A. umbelliformis*, C-SH\B CT) | 0.1%–19.4% |
| Hinoki (Taiwan Cypress, wood) | 3.0%–16.0% |
| Rosemary (Borneol CT) | 15.6% |
| Rosemary (Alpha-Pinene CT) | 3.4%–13.7% |
| Sweet Inula (T-Cadinol CT) | 12.8% |
| Hinoki (*Needles & Twigs*, α-Terpinene CT) | 12.5% |
| Yarrow (Sabinene CT) | 0.0%–12.4% |
| Rosemary (Camphor CT) | 0.0%–11.6% |
| Mountain Savory (Carvacrol CT) | 0.0%–11.5% |
| Mugwort (Germacrene D CT) | 10.8% |
| Lavandin (Giant) | 7.6%–10.1% |
| Spike Lavender | 0.9%–10.1% |
| African Bluegrass (Myrcene CT) | 1.0%–9.5% |
| Fingerroot (*B. rotunda* 1,8-Cineole CT) | 9.2% |
| Calendula (Alpha-Cadinol/Delta-Cadinene CT) | 0.0%–9.1% |
| Mugwort (1,8-Cineole CT) | 0.0%–9.0% |
| Mugwort (Camphor CT) | 0.8%–8.9% |
| Sage (Beta-Thujone CT) | 1.1%–8.8% |
| Rosemary (Bornyl Acetate CT) | 3.6%–8.4% |
| Galangal (Greater, 1,8-Cineole CT) | 0.0%–8.4% |
| Wild Turmeric (Distilled) | 0.0%–8.2% |
| Spruce (Black) | 0.0%–7.8% |
| Savory (Wild, Linalool CT) | 2.8%–7.6% |
| Rosemary (Verbenone CT) | 0.3%–7.3% |
| Valerian | 0.0%–6.6% |
| Citronella (*C. nardus*) | 0.0%–6.6% |
| Applemint (*M. rotun.*, Piperitenone CT) | 0.0%–6.4% |
| Yarrow (1,8-Cineole\Camphor CT) | 2.9%–6.2% |
| Sage (Camphor CT) | 0.3%–6.2% |
| Siberian Fir | 0.0%–6.1% |
| Lavandin (Dutch) | 3.3%–6.0% |

| | |
|---|---|
| Ginger | 0.0%–5.6% |
| Applemint (*M. suav.*, Pulegone CT) | 5.6% |
| Lavandin (Super) | 1.3%–5.5% |
| Mugwort (Beta-Caryophyllene CT) | 5.4% |
| Blue Yarrow (Artemisia Ketone CT) | 5.4% |
| Galangal (False, Ethyl-p-Methoxycinnamate CT) | 2.6%–5.2% |
| Engelmann Spruce | 0.3%–5.2% |
| Lavender (True English) | 0.4%–5.1% |
| Applemint (*M. rotun.*, Piperitone CT) | 5.1% |
| Rosemary (1,8-Cineole CT) | 2.6%–4.8% |
| Blue Mountain Sage (Delta-3-Carene CT) | 1.3%–4.8% |
| Oregano (*O. onites*) | 0.5%–4.6% |
| Grindelia | 1.5%–4.5% |
| Wild Marjoram (Linalool CT) | 0.1%–4.4% |
| White Spruce (Needles) | 0.0%–4.3% |
| Savory (Wild, Carvacrol CT) | 0.0%–4.2% |
| Mountain Savory (Thymol CT) | 2.4%–4.1% |
| White Spruce (Branches) | 2.7%–3.9% |
| Genipi (*A. umbelliformis*, Alpha-Thujone CT) | 0.1%–3.9% |
| Lavandin (Abrialis) | 2.4%–3.7% |
| Lavandin (Grosso) | 1.6%–3.6% |
| Red Pine | 0.0%–3.5% |
| Applemint (*M. suav.*, PO-PEO CT) | 3.4% |
| Sage (1,8-Cineole CT) | 1.5%–2.4% |
| Oregano (Carvacrol CT) | 0.9%–2.4% |
| Holy Basil (aerial parts or seeds, methyl eugenol CT) | 0.0%–2.4% |
| Mugwort (Beta-Thujone CT) | 2.4% |
| Sage (Alpha-Thujone CT) | 0.8%–2.3% |
| Mugwort (Alpha-Thujone CT) | 0.0%–2.2% |
| Yarrow (Chamazulene CT) | 0.0%–1.8% |
| Tansy (Beta-Thujone CT) | 0.0%–1.0% |

**Bornyl Acetate**

| | |
|---|---|
| Sweet Inula (Bornyl Acetate CT) | 43.1%–72.3% |
| Spruce (Black) | 21.6%–52.0% |
| Tsuga | 26.8%–39.6% |
| Sweet Inula (Borneol CT) | 0.6%–38.3% |
| Siberian Fir | 31.0%–37.6% |
| Valerian | 2.9%–35.5% |
| Douglas Fir (Needles & Twigs) | 0.0%–34.7% |
| White Spruce (Needles) | 0.0%–31.3% |
| Juniper (Chinese) | 12.3%–30.4% |
| Silver Fir (*A. alba*) | 1.0%–30.3% |
| Blue Spruce | 6.7%–29.4% |
| Sweet Inula (T-Cadinol CT) | 25.4% |
| Rosemary (Bornyl Acetate CT) | 14.3%–20.3% |
| White Fir (*A. concolor*) | 0.6%–20.2% |
| White Spruce (Needles & Twigs) | 11.3%–19.6% |
| Utah Juniper (Needles/Twigs) | 9.3%–18.5% |
| Balsam Fir | 4.9%–17.6% |
| Rosemary (Verbenone CT) | 2.0%–17.0% |
| Cistus (*Viridiflorol-Trans-Pinocarveol CT*) | 0.0%–16.7% |
| Yarrow (Chamazulene CT) | 0.1%–15.8% |
| Utah Juniper (Needles/Berries) | 14.9% |
| Rosemary (Alpha-Pinene CT) | 0.0%–14.3% |
| Wild Chamomile (*O. mixta, C. mixtrum*) | 0.1%–12.2% |
| White Spruce (Branches) | 11.7%–11.9% |
| Dwarf Pine (Needles, Needles/Twigs) | 2.3%–11.6% |
| Grindelia | 1.3%–10.8% |
| Mastic (NT\B, Terpinene-4-ol CT) | 0.5%–10.3% |
| Goldenrod | 0.3%–9.2% |
| Chinese Red Pine (Twigs) | 8.4%–8.7% |
| Feverfew | 0.0%–8.7% |
| Calendula (Alpha-Cadinol/Delta-Cadinene CT) | 0.0%–8.7% |
| Ledum (*R. groenlandicum*) | 0.3%–8.4% |

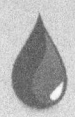
**Bornyl Acetate—continued**

| | |
|---|---|
| Yarrow (Sabinene CT) | 0.0%–8.0% |
| Chinese Red Pine (Leaves) | 0.9%–7.8% |
| Khella (Aerial Parts, 2,2-Dimethylbut. CT) | 7.3% |
| White Spruce (Needles & Twigs) | 0.2%–5.6% |
| Sweet Inula (1,8-Cineole CT) | 0.2%–5.3% |
| Myrtle (1,8-Cineole CT) | 0.0%–5.2% |
| Engelmann Spruce | 1.1%–5.1% |
| Rosemary (Borneol CT) | 5.0% |
| Thuja | 0.8%–4.5% |
| Sage (Alpha-Thujone CT) | 0.0%–4.5% |
| Angelica Root | 0.8%–4.2% |
| Orange (Cold-pressed/expressed) | 0.0%–4.2% |
| May Chang (Citral CT) | 0.0%–4.0% |
| Pine | 0.1%–3.9% |
| Cistus (Alpha-Terpinene CT) | 1.9%–3.7% |
| Mastic (Leaves) | 0.1%–3.3% |
| Ledum (*L. palustre*) | 0.0%–3.3% |
| Applemint (*M. rotun.*, β-Caryophyllene CT) | 3.3% |
| Rosemary (Camphor CT) | 2.9%–3.0% |
| Dwarf Pine (Twigs) | 0.4%–3.0% |
| Frankincense (*B. frereana*) | 0.0%–2.8% |
| Mugwort (Alpha-Thujone CT) | 0.0%–1.0% |
| Mugwort (Germacrene D CT) | 1.0% |

**Brachyl Oxide**

| | |
|---|---|
| Muhuhu (Wood) | 10.0%–10.6% |

**Bulnesol (5-Azulenemethanol 1,2,3,3a,4,5,6,7-octahydro-α,α,3,8-tetramethyl-, [3S-(3α,3aβ,5α)]- Guai-1(10)-en-11-ol)**

| | |
|---|---|
| Guaiacwood | 34.7%–40.5% |
| Palo Santo (Wood) | 13.8%–18.0% |
| Agarwood (*A. malaccensis*) | 0.0%–8.1% |
| Aleppo Pine (Aerial Parts) | 0.0%–7.6% |
| Agarwood (*A. sinensis*) | 0.0%–6.4% |

**Butylated Hydroxutoluene**

| | |
|---|---|
| Valerian | 0.0%–8.0% |
| Moringa (Seeds, Naphthalene CT) | 6.1% |

**Cadalene**

| | |
|---|---|
| Damiana (1,8-Cineole CT) | 0.0%–5.1% |
| Muhuhu (Wood) | 3.0%–3.2% |

**Cadin-1-(10)-en-4,beta-ol**

| | |
|---|---|
| Hinoki (wood) | 6.8% |

**Cadina-1,3,5-Triene**

| | |
|---|---|
| Japanese Cedarwood (Bark) | 0.0%–10.5% |

**Cadina-1.4-Diene**

| | |
|---|---|
| Black Sage (Beta-Caryophyllene CT) | 5.9% |
| Manuka (Leptospermone CT) | 0.0%–5.3% |

**Cadina-3,5-Diene**

| | |
|---|---|
| Manuka (Leptospermone CT) | 0.0%–8.0% |

**Cadinene <γ,δ>**

| | |
|---|---|
| Katrafay ((γ,δ)-Cadinene CT) | 0.5%–35.2% |
| Katrafay (Ishwarane CT) | 0.6%–9.6% |
| Katrafay (Alpha-Pinene CT) | 1.1%–7.4% |

**Calarene (Beta-Gurjunene)**

| | |
|---|---|
| Spikenard (Calarene CT) | 25.9%–35.4% |
| Spikenard (Calarene CT, Nepal) | 9.4%–29.1% |
| Gurjun Balsam (*D. turbinatus*) | 15.0% |
| Kumquat (*F. margarita*, Leaves) | 0.0%–10.0% |
| Vetiver | 0.0%–9.8% |
| Mastic (Leaves) | 0.0%–7.8% |
| Mastic (Twigs, Alpha-Pinene CT) | 6.5% |
| Guggul | 0.0%–4.6% |
| Chaste Tree (Berries) | 0.0%–1.2% |

| | |
|---|---|
| Gurjun Balsam (*D. kerri*) | 0.8% |

**Camphene**

| | |
|---|---|
| Douglas Fir (Needles & Twigs) | 0.1%–29.8% |
| Siberian Fir | 17.5%–28.4% |
| Spruce (Black) | 14.0%–22.0% |
| Silver Fir (*A. alba*) | 5.6%–19.8% |
| White Spruce (Needles) | 6.1%–18.2% |
| Blue Spruce | 7.1%–18.0% |
| Mugwort (Camphor CT) | 3.9%–17.4% |
| Pine | 0.4%–16.8% |
| Tsuga | 11.9%–14.5% |
| Engelmann Spruce | 1.7%–14.3% |
| Canadian Fleabane | 0.0%–14.2% |
| Ginger | 0.6%–12.7% |
| White Spruce (Needles & Twigs) | 8.0%–12.6% |
| Feverfew | 1.6%–12.2% |
| Camphor (Camphor CT) | 0.2%–11.7% |
| Rosemary (Alpha-Pinene CT) | 5.5%–11.5% |
| Rosemary (Camphor CT) | 5.2%–11.2% |
| Rosemary (1,8-Cineole CT) | 3.0%–11.1% |
| Spanish Sage | 5.6%–11.0% |
| Valerian | 0.0%–11.0% |
| Citron (Distilled) | 0.0%–10.9% |
| Wild Turmeric (Distilled) | 0.0%–10.2% |
| Cistus (Alpha-Pinene CT) | 0.9%–10.0% |
| Sage (Beta-Thujone CT) | 1.0%–9.9% |
| Balsam Fir | 3.5%–9.7% |
| Sage (Camphor CT) | 2.1%–9.7% |
| White Fir (*A. concolor*) | 0.5%–9.0% |
| Bay Laurel | 0.2%–8.9% |
| Sage (Alpha-Thujone CT) | 4.8%–8.5% |
| Opoponax (*C. erythraea*) | 0.0%–8.2% |
| Fingerroot ((E)-Beta-Ocimene CT) | 5.4%–8.0% |
| Citronella (*C. nardus*) | 0.0%–8.0% |
| Spanish Sage | 5.2%–7.1% |
| African Bluegrass (Myrcene CT) | 2.6%–7.1% |
| Sweet Inula (Bornyl Acetate CT) | 0.6%–7.1% |
| Rosemary (Bornyl Acetate CT) | 4.2%–7.0% |
| Sweet Wormwood (Camphor CT) | 0.0%–7.0% |
| Black Sage (Tricyclene CT) | 7.0% |
| Leleshwa | 3.8%–6.3% |
| Fingerroot (Camphor CT) | 0.0%–5.8% |
| Sweet Inula (Borneol CT) | 0.0%–5.7% |
| Rosemary (Beta-Myrcene CT) | 1.3%–5.1% |
| Mastic (NT\B, Alpha-Pinene CT) | 1.1%–5.1% |
| Hinoki (needles and twigs) | 5.1% |
| Sweet Wormwood (Artemisia Ketone CT) | 0.0%–5.0% |
| Saro (1,8-Cineole CT) | 1.2%–4.8% |
| White Pine | 1.7%–4.6% |
| Sweet Inula (1,8-Cineole CT) | 0.0%–4.6% |
| Sweet Inula (T-Cadinol CT) | 4.3% |
| Grindelia | 1.9%–4.2% |
| Mugwort (Alpha-Phellandrene CT) | 4.2% |
| Galangal (Greater, 1,8-Cineole CT) | 0.5%–4.1% |
| Mastic (NT\B, Terpinene-4-ol CT) | 2.2%–4.0% |
| Dwarf Pine (Needles, Needles/Twigs) | 1.5%–4.0% |
| Mugwort (Alpha-Thujone CT) | 0.0%–4.0% |
| White Sage | 0.4%–3.9% |
| Sage (1,8-Cineole CT) | 0.2%–3.9% |
| Hairy Basil (Camphor CT) | 0.1%–3.7% |
| Mugwort (Artemisia Ketone CT) | 1.4%–3.6% |
| Kumquat (*C. japonica*, Leaves CT Beta-Pinene) | 3.6% |
| Japanese Cedarwood (16-Kaurene CT) | 0.1%–3.4% |
| Wild Marjoram (Linalool CT) | 0.9%–3.3% |

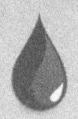 

| | |
|---|---|
| Mugwort (Beta-Caryophyllene CT) | 3.3% |
| May Chang (Neral CT) | 3.1% |
| Ravintsara (Camphor CT) | 0.0%–2.8% |
| Mastic (NT\B, Limonene CT) | 0.9%–2.3% |
| Frankincense (*B. carterii*) | 0.0%–2.1% |
| Hyssop (Linalool CT) | 0.0%–2.0% |
| Angelica Root | 0.2%–1.5% |
| Ledum (*R. groenlandicum*) | 0.0%–1.4% |
| Tansy (Beta-Thujone CT) | 0.0%–1.0% |

**Camphene Hydrate**

| | |
|---|---|
| Engelmann Spruce | 0.3%–5.0% |
| White Fir (*A. concolor*) | 0.1%–4.1% |
| Ravintsara (Linalool CT) | 0.0%–1.5% |

**Camphenilone**

| | |
|---|---|
| Wild Chamomile (*C. mixtus*, Sant. Alc. CT) | 0.0%–4.8% |

**Camphor**

| | |
|---|---|
| Camphor (Camphor CT) | 36.5%–98.0% |
| Feverfew | 42.7%–94.0% |
| Ravintsara (Camphor CT) | 40.5%–72.5% |
| Fingerroot (Camphor CT) | 32.1%–58.0% |
| White Verbena (Camphor CT) | 0.0%–52.0% |
| White Spruce (Needles) | 0.0%–49.6% |
| Japanese Cedarwood (Bark) | 0.0%–48.4% |
| Hairy Basil (Camphor CT) | 38.6%–48.2% |
| Sweet Wormwood (Camphor CT) | 17.7%–48.0% |
| Mugwort (Camphor CT) | 17.3%–47.7% |
| Sage (Camphor CT) | 19.8%–36.5% |
| Fingerroot (*B. rotunda* Nerol-Camphor CT) | 36.0% |
| Rosemary (Camphor CT) | 14.9%–35.8% |
| Camphor (Linalool CT) | 0.7%–33.5% |
| Utah Juniper (Needles/Twigs) | 5.9%–31.3% |
| Spanish Sage | 6.1%–31.0% |
| Sage (Beta-Thujone CT) | 5.2%–29.5% |
| Yarrow (1,8-Cineole\Camphor CT) | 11.0%–28.4% |
| Wild Turmeric (Distilled) | 2.4%–26.9% |
| Blue Spruce | 0.0%–26.4% |
| Sage (Alpha-thujone CT) | 5.5%–26.1% |
| Great Mugwort | 1.1%–25.7% |
| Sage (1,8-Cineole CT) | 8.8%–25.0% |
| White Spruce (Needles & Twigs) | 8.5%–24.5% |
| Fingerroot ((E)-Beta-Ocimene CT) | 16.1%–24.0% |
| Sweet Wormwood (Artemisia Ketone CT) | 0.0%–23.8% |
| Spike Lavender | 10.8%–23.2% |
| Tansy (Beta-Thujone CT) | 0.0%–23.0% |
| Indian Borage (Carvacrol CT) | 0.0%–22.2% |
| White Sage | 2.1%–21.7% |
| White Spruce (Branches) | 20.2%–20.4% |
| Rosemary (1,8-Cineole CT) | 7.9%–18.9% |
| Rosemary (Alpha-Pinene CT) | 2.4%–18.9% |
| Blue Tansy (Chamazulene CT) | 4.0%–18.0% |
| Mugwort (1,8-Cineole CT) | 1.4%–16.3% |
| Fenugreek | 16.3% |
| Rosemary (Borneol CT) | 15.3% |
| Rosemary (Verbenone CT) | 2.9%–14.9% |
| Engelmann Spruce | 1.0%–14.9% |
| Juniper, Phoenicia (Berries) | 0.0%–14.9% |
| Hairy Basil (1,8-Cineole\Linalool CT) | 0.0%–14.1% |
| Galangal (Greater, 1,8-Cineole CT) | 0.0%–14.0% |
| Blue Tansy (Sabinene CT) | 11.7%–13.2% |
| Thuja | 0.7%–13.0% |
| Fingerroot (*B. rotunda* 1,8-Cineole CT) | 13.0% |
| Hairy Basil (Linalool CT, Leaves) | 12.8% |
| Hairy Basil (1,8-Cineole CT) | 0.0%–12.7% |

| | |
|---|---|
| Lavandin (Dutch) | 10.0%–12.5% |
| Lavandin (Abrialis) | 8.2%–12.2% |
| Yarrow (Beta-Thujone CT) | 0.0%–11.7% |
| Blue Yarrow (Artemisia Ketone CT) | 11.5% |
| Lavandin (Super) | 0.0%–11.4% |
| Utah Juniper (Needles/Berries) | 11.4% |
| Mugwort (Alpha-Thujone CT) | 0.0%–10.9% |
| Rosemary (Bornyl Acetate CT) | 6.4%–10.4% |
| White Turmeric (Distilled) | 2.9%–10.3% |
| Hairy Basil (Linalool CT, Inflorescences) | 0.0%–9.5% |
| Rosemary (Beta-Myrcene CT) | 2.1%–9.0% |
| Lavandin (Grosso) | 5.9%–8.8% |
| Mugwort (Beta-Thujone CT) | 8.7% |
| Lavandin (Giant) | 5.3%–8.4% |
| Blue Mountain Sage (Delta-3-Carene CT) | 1.0%–6.0% |
| Wild Marjoram (Linalool CT) | 2.4%–5.3% |
| Verbena (Myrcene CT) | 0.1%–5.0% |
| Blue Mountain Sage (Limonene CT) | 4.7% |
| Yarrow (Chamazulene CT) | 0.1%–4.3% |
| Galangal (False, Ethyl-p-Methoxcinnamate CT) | 0.0%–4.3% |
| Mugwort (Artemisia Ketone CT) | 3.4%–3.5% |
| Lavender (Brazilian) | 3.5% |
| Helichrysum (*H. splendidum*, Alpha-Terpinene CT) | 1.2% |
| Chaste Tree (Berries) | 0.0%–1.1% |

**Carhydranol**

| | |
|---|---|
| Spearmint (Piperitenone Oxide CT) | 1.5%–2.0% |
| Spearmint (Piperitone Oxide CT) | 0.2%–2.0% |

**Carotol**

| | |
|---|---|
| Carrot Seed | 38.9%–66.8% |
| Juniper (Chinese) | 0.0%–11.4% |
| Galangal (Lesser) | 0.0%–8.9% |

**Carvacrol**

| | |
|---|---|
| Indian Borage (Carvacrol CT) | 21.7%–98.0% |
| Thyme (Carvacrol CT) | 21.5%–84.1% |
| Oregano (Carvacrol CT) | 48.5%–83.4% |
| Oregano (*O. onites*) | 65.5%–79.4% |
| Summer Savory (Carvacrol CT) | 44.0%–79.2% |
| Savory (Wild, Carvacrol CT) | 17.7%–71.6% |
| Mountain Savory (Carvacrol CT) | 16.1%–63.4% |
| Wormseed, American (Carvacrol CT) | 62.4% |
| Oregano (*O. syriacum*, Carvacrol CT) | 47.1%–57.7% |
| Summer Savory (Gamma-Terpinene CT) | 12.3%–40.2% |
| Monarda (Carvacrol/Para-Cymene CT) | 23.9%–39.1% |
| Oregano (*O. syriacum*, Thymol CT) | 3.4%–33.8% |
| Monarda (Linalool CT) | 17.8%–33.3% |
| Thyme (Thymol CT) | 0.8%–26.8% |
| Thyme (Thuyanol-4 CT) | 0.0%–21.4% |
| Savory (Wild, Thymol CT) | 2.4%–19.0% |
| Savory (Wild, Linalool CT) | 5.0%–16.3% |
| Summer Savory (Thymol CT) | 11.0%–14.0% |
| Fennel (Trans-Anethole CT) | 0.0%–12.6% |
| Black Cumin (Thymoquinone CT) | 0.0%–10.3% |
| Oregano (Terpinen-4-ol CT) | 4.7%–9.4% |
| Tarragon (Methyl Chavicol CT) | 0.0%–7.7% |
| Mountain Savory (Thymol CT) | 3.8%–6.9% |
| Thyme (Geraniol CT) | 0.0%–6.9% |
| Thyme (Linalool CT) | 0.0%–6.8% |
| Indian Borage (Delta-Cadinene CT) | 0.1%–6.0% |
| Applemint (*M. rotun.*, Piperitenone CT) | 0.0%–6.0% |
| Mountain Savory (Thymol CT) | 4.0%–5.1% |
| Wormseed, American (Ascaridole CT) | 0.0%–4.9% |
| Wormseed, American (Alpha-Terpinene CT) | 0.0%–4.3% |
| Black Cumin (Trans-Anethole CT) | 1.6%–3.7% |

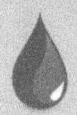

### Carvacrol—continued

| | |
|---|---|
| Black Cumin (Para-Cymene CT) | 0.0%–3.0% |
| Thyme (Alpha-Terpineol CT) | 0.0%–3.0% |
| Rabbitbrush (var. *nauseosa*) | 2.5% |

### Carvacrol Methyl Ether

| | |
|---|---|
| Mountain Savory (Carvacrol CT) | 0.0%–11.0% |
| Monarda (Thymol CT) | 0.0%–9.8% |
| Monarda (Carvacrol/Para-Cymene CT) | 0.2%–5.5% |

### Carvaotanacetone

| | |
|---|---|
| Tsauri Grass | 0.0%–19.9% |

### (E)-Carveol (Trans-Carveol, P-Mentha-6,8-Dien-2-ol)

| | |
|---|---|
| Kumquat (*F. margarita*, Fruit CT α-Terpineol) | 5.7% |
| Tsauri Grass | 0.0%–5.1% |

### Carvone

| | |
|---|---|
| Caraway | 38.0%–80.5% |
| White Verbena (Carvone\Limonene CT) | 25.3%–77.2% |
| Spearmint (Carvone CT) | 48.6%–76.5% |
| Dill Seed | 50.1%–75.9% |
| Spearmint (Scotch, *M. cardiaca*) | 60.9%–74.1% |
| Dill (Aerial Parts, Carvone CT) | 36.1%–73.6% |
| Applemint (*M. suav.*, Carvone CT) | 24.7%–55.7% |
| Applemint (*M. suav.*, Piperitenone CT) | 0.0%–14.0% |
| Galangal (False, Ethyl-p-Methoxycinnamate CT) | 0.0%–11.1% |
| Dill (Flowers) | 10.3% |
| Gingergrass | 1.1%–8.5% |
| Pink Pepper (*S. terebinthifolius*, Leaves, p-Cymen-7-ol CT) | 7.5% |
| Tansy (Beta-Thujone CT) | 0.0%–6.6% |
| Holy Basil (Aerial Parts, Estragole CT) | 0.0%–6.3% |
| Verbena (Myrcenone CT) | 0.0%–5.9% |
| Petitgrain (Bergamot/Bitter Orange) | 0.0%–5.8% |
| Kumquat (*F. margarita*, Fruit CT α-Terpineol) | 5.7% |
| Black Cumin (Trans-Anethole CT) | 2.0%–4.0% |
| Tsauri Grass (var. *madagascariensis*) | 3.1%–3.9% |
| Ledum (*L. palustre*) | 0.0%–2.4% |
| Ledum (*R. groenlandicum*) | 0.0%–1.9% |

### Caryophylla-4(14),8(15)-Dien-5alpha-ol

| | |
|---|---|
| Sweet Inula (Borneol CT) | 0.0%–2.7% |

### Caryophylladienol

| | |
|---|---|
| Wild Chamomile (*O. mixta, C. mixtrum*) | 0.0%–3.1% |

### Caryophyllene

| | |
|---|---|
| Lavender (True English) | 0.0%–24.1% |
| Davana | 0.0%–20.7% |
| Mugwort (Germacrene D CT) | 19.6% |
| Tagetes (*T. patula*, Limonene CT) | 11.9%–17.7% |
| Rosemary (Bornyl Acetate CT) | 0.0%–13.6% |
| Rosemary (Beta-Myrcene CT) | 0.0%–8.3% |
| Patchouli (Chinese) | 0.5%–6.8% |
| Sweet Inula (T-Cadinol CT) | 6.3% |
| Mugwort (1,8-Cineole CT) | 1.2%–5.3% |
| Rosemary (1,8-Cineole CT) | 0.1%–4.2% |
| Spearmint (Menthone CT) | 2.9% |
| Allspice (Leaves, Methyl Eugenol CT) | 2.7% |
| Sweet Inula (Borneol CT) | 0.5%–2.8% |
| Ravintsara (Camphor CT) | 0.0%–2.2% |
| Sweet Inula (Bornyl Acetate CT) | 0.0%–2.1% |

### Caryophyllene Oxide (Caryophyllene Oxide, Caryophyllene Epoxide, Beta-Caryophyllene Epoxide)

| | |
|---|---|
| Aleppo Pine (Aerial Parts) | 0.0%–48.2% |
| Melissa | 1.3%–31.7% |
| Chaste Tree (Berries) | 0.0%–24.9% |
| Black Sage (Caryophyllene Oxide CT) | 15.0%–23.1% |
| White Verbena (Citral CT) | 0.0%–20.5% |

| | |
|---|---|
| Cananga | 0.0%–17.6% |
| Copaiba (Leaves) | 7.4%–16.6% |
| Cangerana (Leaves) | 10.8%–16.5% |
| Catnip (Nepetalactone CT) | 0.0%–14.3% |
| Applemint (*M. suav.*, Italian) | 0.3%–14.2% |
| Hairy Basil (Trans-Caryophyllene CT) | 13.9% |
| Damiana (Caryophyllene Oxide CT) | 9.6%–13.7% |
| Pine | 0.0%–12.6% |
| Hemp (Myrcene CT) | 0.1%–11.3% |
| Hemp (Beta-Caryophyllene CT) | 2.0%–10.7% |
| Shell Ginger (1,8-Cineole CT) | 5.0%–10.4% |
| Tamala (Beta-Caryophyllene CT) | 10.3% |
| Copaiba | 0.3%–10.2% |
| Guava Leaf (Selin-11-en-4-Alpha-ol CT) | 6.9%–9.3% |
| Guava Leaf (Limonene CT) | 1.6%–9.3% |
| Betony (Bicyclogermacrene CT) | 1.2%–8.5% |
| Guava Leaf (β-Cary.\(E)-Nerolidol CT) | 8.2% |
| Aleppo Pine (Cones) | 2.3%–7.5% |
| Black Pepper (Eugenol CT) | 2.6%–7.2% |
| Lemongrass (East Indian) | 1.3%–7.2% |
| Katrafay (Alpha-Pinene CT) | 1.6%–7.1% |
| Hairy Basil (Citral CT) | 0.0%–7.1% |
| Katrafay (Beta-Pinene CT) | 7.0% |
| Turkish Pine (Bark) | 6.9% |
| Mugwort (1,8-Cineole CT) | 3.6%–6.5% |
| Guava Leaf (Beta-Caryophyllene CT) | 3.0%–6.5% |
| Juniper, Phoenicia (Berries) | 0.0%–6.3% |
| Mastic (Leaves) | 0.0%–6.1% |
| Yarrow (Sabinene CT) | 0.0%–6.0% |
| Grindelia | 0.0%–5.9% |
| Indian Borage (Carvacrol CT) | 0.0%–5.9% |
| Wild Turmeric (Solvent Extracted) | 5.9% |
| Sweet Inula (Bornyl Acetate CT) | 1.1%–5.7% |
| Wormseed, American (Carvacrol CT) | 5.6% |
| Verbena (Myrcenone CT) | 0.0%–5.5% |
| Genipi (*A. umbelliformis*, C-SH\B CT) | 2.2%–5.4% |
| Damiana (Delta-Cadinene CT) | 2.9%–5.3% |
| Pink Pepper (*S. molle*, Leaves, Bicyclogermacrene CT) | 0.5%–5.3% |
| Pink Pepper (*S. terebinthifolius*, Leaves, p-Cymen-7-ol CT) | 5.2% |
| Lemon Verbena (Stems) | 1.3%–5.1% |
| Calendula (Alpha-Cadinol/Delta-Cadinene CT) | 0.0%–5.0% |
| Lemon Verbena (Leaves and stems) | 3.1%–4.9% |
| Oregano (Carvacrol CT) | 0.0%–4.9% |
| Black Pepper (Beta-Caryophyllene CT) | 0.0%–4.9% |
| Chaste Tree (Leaves) | 2.2%–4.8% |
| Katrafay ((γ,δ)-Cadinene CT) | 0.6%–4.8% |
| Yarrow (Chamazulene CT) | 0.5%–4.8% |
| Plai (2,6,9,9-Tetramethyl-2,6,10-Cyclodecatrien-1-one) | 4.8% |
| Lavender (Brazilian) | 4.5% |
| Carrot Seed | 0.0%–4.3% |
| Holy Basil (aerial parts, beta-bisabolene CT) | 2.8%–4.2% |
| Sweet Inula (Borneol CT) | 2.5%–4.2% |
| Ocotea (Leaves) | 4.2% |
| Siam Wood (Leaves) | 4.0% |
| Sweet Wormwood (Artemisia Ketone CT) | 0.0%–3.9% |
| Holy Basil (aerial parts, eugenol CT) | 0.0%–3.9% |
| Neroli (*C. sinensis*) | 0.0%–3.9% |
| Sweer Nancy (Artemisia Ketone CT) | 3.8% |
| Mugwort (Artemisia Ketone CT) | 0.6%–3.7% |
| Lemon Basil | 0.0%–3.7% |
| Tagetes (*T. patula*, Aerial Parts) | 3.7% |
| White Verbena (Linalool CT) | 2.9%–3.6% |
| Damiana (1,8-Cineole CT) | 0.9%–3.6% |
| Yarrow (1,8-Cineole\Camphor CT) | 0.2%–3.3% |

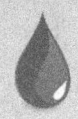

| | |
|---|---|
| Hyssop (Linalool CT) | 0.0%–3.2% |
| Spearmint (Pulegone-Menthone-Isomenthone CT) | 0.0%–3.0% |
| Lemon Verbena (Leaves) | 0.8%–2.5% |
| Mugwort (Camphor CT) | 1.2%–2.3% |
| Hyssop (Alpha-Pinene CT) | 2.1% |
| Spike Lavender | 0.0%–1.6% |
| Mugwort (Germacrene D CT) | 1.1% |

**Cedr-1(15)-en-9-ol**

| | |
|---|---|
| Guava Leaf (β-Cary.\(E)-Nerolidol CT) | 7.9% |

**(-)-Cedreanol (1-Naphthalenol, 1,2,3,4,4a,7,8,8a-octahydro-1,6-dimethyl-4-(1-methylethyl)-, [1R-(1α,4β,4aβ,8aβ)]-)**

| | |
|---|---|
| Mastic (Aerial parts, Beta-Eudesmol CT) | 7.7% |

**Cedrenol**

| | |
|---|---|
| Chinese Cedarwood | 0.0%–6.1% |

**Cedrol (Alpha-Cedrol)**

| | |
|---|---|
| Chinese Cedarwood | 0.0%–54.6% |
| Texas Cedarwood | 12.2%–29.5% |
| Cedarwood (Virginian, Wood) | 4.0%–22.2% |
| Oriental Arborvitae (Needles) | 9.8%–20.3% |
| Savin (Needles & Branches) | 0.0%–15.9% |
| Oriental Arborvitae (Berries) | 6.5%–9.6% |
| Juniper, Phoenicia (leaves, isoborneol CT) | 3.7% |

**Cembrene (Thunbergen)**

| | |
|---|---|
| Aleppo Pine (Needles) | 0.0%–5.4% |
| Guggul | 0.0%–5.3% |

**Cembrene A (3(E)-Cembrene A)**

| | |
|---|---|
| Guggul | 0.0%–8.2% |
| Chaste Tree (Leaves) | 0.0%–1.1% |

**Chamazulene**

| | |
|---|---|
| German Chamomile | 0.7%–61.3% |
| Great Mugwort | 3.6%–49.4% |
| Yarrow (Chamazulene CT) | 15.7%–44.3% |
| Wormwood (Chamazulene CT) | 25.3%–39.9% |
| Blue Tansy (Chamazulene CT) | 17.0%–38.0% |
| Wormwood (Beta-Pinene CT) | 4.2%–13.9% |
| Wormwood (Myrcene CT) | 0.0%–6.8% |
| Blue Cypress | 0.0%–5.6% |
| Yarrow (Sabinene CT) | 0.0%–5.3% |
| Blue Tansy (Sabinene CT) | 2.8%–5.0% |
| Wormwood (Sabinene CT) | 0.0%–4.3% |

**Chavicol**

| | |
|---|---|
| Bay (West Indies) | 7.1%–9.3% |
| Allspice (Leaves, Eugenol CT) | 0.0%–4.8% |

**Chavicol Acetate**

| | |
|---|---|
| Galangal (Greater, 1,8-Cineole CT) | 0.0%–5.9% |

**Chrysanthenol**

| | |
|---|---|
| Feverfew | 0.0%–8.4% |

**Cinerolone**

| | |
|---|---|
| Applemint (M. suav., Italian) | 0.0%–18.8% |

**Cinnamyl Acetate**

| | |
|---|---|
| Tamala ((E)-Cinnamaldehyde\Cinn. Ac. CT) | 18.4%–42.3% |
| Tamala (Linalool\(E)-Cinnamaldehyde CT) | 0.6%–13.7% |
| Ocotea (Leaves) | 11.4% |
| Tamala ((E)-Cinnamaldehyde CT) | 1.3%–11.1% |
| Cassia (Leaves) | 0.0%–9.2% |
| Cinnamon Bark | 0.1%–8.8% |
| Cassia (Bark) | 0.0%–4.2% |
| Ylang Ylang (French IV) | 1.6% |

**Cinnamyl Cinnamate**

| | |
|---|---|
| Benzoin (Sumatra, Ethanol Absolute) | 5.0%–8.0% |
| Benzoin (S. paralleloneurum, Absolute) | 4.6%–6.8% |

**Cis-2-Methoxy Cinnamic Acid**

| | |
|---|---|
| Cassia (Bark) | 0.0%–43.1% |

**Cis-8-Menthene**

| | |
|---|---|
| Applemint (M. suav., Pulegone CT) | 4.2% |
| Applemint (M. suav., PO-PEO CT) | 2.9% |

**Cis-Anethole ((Z)-Anethole)**

| | |
|---|---|
| Fennel (Trans-Anethole CT) | 0.1%–8.6% |

**Cis-Alpha-Atlantone (Turmerone)**

| | |
|---|---|
| Cedarwood (Atlas) | 0.2%–29.5% |

**Cis-Alpha-Bergamotene ((Z)-Alpha-Bergamotene)**

| | |
|---|---|
| Canadian Fleabane | 0.0%–9.9% |

**Cis-Alpha-Bisabolene**

| | |
|---|---|
| Opoponax (C. guidotti) | 2.3%–27.0% |

**Cis-Alpha-Copaene-8-ol ((Z)-Alpha-Copaene-8-ol)**

| | |
|---|---|
| Sweet Nancy (Artemisyl Acetate CT) | 0.0%–7.4% |

**Cis-Beta-Caryophyllene ((Z)-Beta-Caryophyllene)**

| | |
|---|---|
| Aleppo Pine (Needles) | 0.0%–40.3% |
| Aleppo Pine (Aerial Parts) | 0.0%–40.3% |

**Cis-Calamenene ((Z)-Calamenene)**

| | |
|---|---|
| Muhuhu (Leaves) | 10.5% |
| Schisandra Fruit (S. chinensis) | 2.1%–5.3% |

**Cis-Carveol ((Z)-Carveol, (Z)-p-Mentha-6,8-dien-2-ol, Cis-p-Mentha-6,8-dien-2-ol))**

| | |
|---|---|
| Spearmint (Carvone CT) | 14.0%–21.3% |
| Tsauri Grass | 0.0%–6.4% |
| Caraway | 0.0%–5.0% |
| Gingergrass | 1.0%–3.5% |

**Cis-Chrysanthenyl Acetate ((Z)-Chrysanthernyl Acetate)**

| | |
|---|---|
| Wormwood (Cis-Chrysanthenyl Acetate CT) | 3.6%–36.7% |
| Wormwood ((Z)-Epoxy Ocimene CT) | 0.0%–26.4% |
| Wormwood (Myrcene CT) | 7.7%–17.9% |
| Wormwood (Sabinene CT) | 0.0%–11.0% |
| Wormwood (Beta-Thujone CT) | 0.0%–5.2% |

**Cis-Sesquisabinene Hydrate ((Z)-Sesquisabinene Hydrate)**

| | |
|---|---|
| Katrafay (Beta-Pinene CT) | 12.8% |
| Katrafay (Leaves) | 0.0%–9.8% |

**Cis-Davanone ((Z)-Davanone)**

| | |
|---|---|
| Mugwort (Camphor CT) | 0.0%–2.5% |

**Cis-Dihydrotagetone ((Z)-Dihydrotagetone)**

| | |
|---|---|
| Tagetes (T. minuta, Alpha-Terpineol CT) | 5.0% |

**Cis-Enyne-Bicycloether ((Z)-Enyne Biccyloether)**

| | |
|---|---|
| German Chamomile | 8.8%–26.1% |

**Cis-Linalool Oxide ((Z)-Linalool Oxide)**

| | |
|---|---|
| Petitgrain (Bergamot/Bitter Orange) | 0.0%–8.1% |
| Rosewood (Wood) | 1.3%–2.1% |
| Rosewood (Leaves) | 0.8% |

**Cis-M-Mentha-2,8-Diene**

| | |
|---|---|
| Betony (MLD-C CT) | 1.4%–4.3% |

**Cis-Methyl Isoeugenol ((Z)-Methyl Isoeugenol)**

| | |
|---|---|
| Ocotea (Leaves) | 3.5% |

**Cis-Ocimenone ((Z)-Ocimenone, (Z)-Tagetenone)**

| | |
|---|---|
| Spearmint (Cis-Ocimenone CT) | 61.7% |
| Tagetes (T. minuta, Limonene CT) | 0.0%–19.1% |
| Tagetes (T. minuta, (Z)-Beta-Ocimene CT) | 4.0%–15.9% |
| Tagetes (T. patula, Limonene CT) | 10.9%–13.4% |
| Tagetes (T. erecta, Flowers) | 0.0%–7.7% |
| Tagetes (T. minuta, Alpha-Terpineol CT) | 6.1% |
| Tsauri Grass | 0.0%–5.2% |
| Tagetes (T. minuta, Limonene CT) | 2.7%–5.1% |
| Verbena (Myrcenone CT) | 0.0%–4.9% |

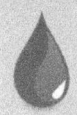

**Cis-P-Mentha-2,3-Dien-1-ol**

| | |
|---|---|
| Ledum (*R. groenlandicum*) | 0.0%–2.9% |

**Cis-P-Mentha-1.7.8 Dien-2-ol (Cis-p-Mentha-1(7),8-Dien-2-ol)**

| | |
|---|---|
| Ledum (*R. groenlandicum*) | 0.0%–6.2% |
| Southern Blue Gum | 0.0%–1.1% |

**Cis-Sabinene Hydrate ((Z)-Sabinene Hydrate)**

*See Thuyanol-4*

**Cis-Sabinol ((Z)-Sabinol)**

| | |
|---|---|
| Mugwort (1,8-Cineole CT) | 0.0%–1.1% |

**Cis-Verbenol ((Z)-Verbenol)**

| | |
|---|---|
| Tsauri Grass | 0.0%–9.6% |
| Boldo (Ascaridole CT) | 0.0%–7.2% |

**Cis-Z-Alpha-Bisabolene Epoxide**

| | |
|---|---|
| Agarwood (*A. sinensis*) | 0.0%–4.7% |

**Citral (Geranial + Neral)**

| | |
|---|---|
| Lemon Myrtle (Citral CT) | < 99% |
| Lemongrass (East Indian) | < 98.8% |
| White Verbena (Citral CT) | < 90.7% |
| Lemon Basil | < 90.7% |
| May Chang (Citral CT) | < 86.3% |
| Hairy Basil (Citral CT) | < 83.9% |
| Lemongrass (West Indian) | < 82.7% |
| Petitgrain (Lime) | < 80.3% |
| Melissa | < 79.0% |
| Lemon Verbena (Stems) | < 67.0% |
| Lemon Verbena (Leaves) | < 65.9% |
| Lemon Tea Tree (*L. petersonii*) | < 64.2% |
| May Chang (Neral CT) | < 63.6% |
| Honey Myrtle | < 62.6% |
| Lemon Tea Tree (*L. liversidgei*) | < 55.6% |
| Petitgrain (Lemon) | < 47.7% |
| Lime (Distilled) | < 47.4% |
| Lemon Verbena (Leaves and Stems) | < 38.0% |
| Lemon Catnip (Beta-Citronellol CT) | < 37.7% |
| Citronella (*C. nardus*) | < 36.9% |
| Tangerine (Distilled) | < 33.5% |
| White Verbena (Carvone\Limonene CT) | < 20.8% |
| Lemon Catnip (Geraniol\Nerol CT) | < 17.0% |
| Citronella (*C. winteranius*) | < 14.1% |
| Citron (Distilled) | < 13.9% |
| Persian Lime (Distilled) | < 11.1% |
| Citron (Cold-pressed/Expressed) | > 10.1% |
| Ocotea (Leaves) | < 10.0% |
| Persian Lime (Cold Pressed\Expressed) | < 6.3% |
| Lemon (Distilled) | < 5.4% |
| Lemon Myrtle (Citronellal CT) | < 5.0% |

**Citronellal (Rhodinal)**

| | |
|---|---|
| Lemon Myrtle (Citronellal CT) | 85.0%–89.2% |
| Lemon Eucalyptus | 40.0%–83.5% |
| Kaffir Lime Petitgain | 65.4%–81.5% |
| May Chang (Citronellal CT) | 44.8%–77.2% |
| Citronella (*C. winteranius*) | 26.5%–42.8% |
| Citronella (*C. nardus*) | 5.2%–41.3% |
| Lemon Tea Tree (*L. petersonii*) | 4.3%–33.9% |
| Melissa | 0.4%–20.3% |
| Kaffir Lime Peel | 0.1%–16.8% |
| May Chang (Citral CT) | 0.0%–6.2% |
| Kumquat (*F. margarita*, Fruit CT α-Terpineol) | 5.0% |
| Honey Myrtle | 0.2%–1.0% |

**Citronellic Acid (3,7-Dimethyl-6-Octenoic Acid)**

| | |
|---|---|
| Chaste Tree (Leaves) | 0.0%–6.6% |
| Lemon Eucalyptus | 0.0%–1.9% |

**Citronellol (Dihydrogeraniol, Beta-Citronellol)**

| | |
|---|---|
| Rose (Iranian) | 12.6%–53.4% |
| Geranium | 2.4%–45.7% |
| Rose (Turkish) | 24.5%–43.0% |
| Lemon Catnip (Beta-Citronellol CT) | 25.2%–39.3% |
| Lemon Tea Tree (*L. petersonii*) | 0.1%–26.8% |
| Lemon Catnip (Geraniol\Nerol CT) | 11.4%–14.1% |
| May Chang (Citronellal CT) | 10.9%–14.0% |
| Lemon Eucalyptus | 12.6%–13.0% |
| Citronella (*C. winteranius*) | 5.2%–11.5% |
| Citronella (*C. nardus*) | 4.6%–9.2% |
| Kaffir Lime Peel | 0.2%–7.8% |
| Melissa | 0.1%–7.7% |
| Kaffir Lime Petitgain | 0.0%–6.6% |
| Savin (Needles & Branches) | 0.0%–6.4% |
| Lemon Myrtle (Citronellal CT) | 2.6%–3.4% |

**Citronellol + Nerol**

| | |
|---|---|
| Rose (Indian) | 2.2%–44.9% |
| Rose (Bulgarian) | 21.6%–31.9% |

**Citronellyl Acetate**

| | |
|---|---|
| Chaste Tree (Leaves) | 0.3%–7.8% |
| Douglas Fir (Needles & Twigs) | 0.2%–5.9% |
| Catnip (Nepetalactone CT) | 0.0%–5.2% |
| Melissa | 0.0%–3.7% |
| Lemon Eucalyptus | 0.0%–2.4% |

**Citronellyl Formate**

| | |
|---|---|
| Geranium | 0.0%–18.1% |
| Rose (Iranian) | 0.0%–14.6% |
| Rhododendron (Leaves) | 5.5% |
| Manuka (Selinene/Beta-Elemene CT) | 2.3% |

**Coniferyl Benzoate**

| | |
|---|---|
| Benzoin (Siam, Ethanol Absolute) | 29.0%–56.0% |
| Benzoin (*S. benzoin*, Absolute) | 15.6%–18.2% |

**Coniferyl Derivatives**

| | |
|---|---|
| Benzoin (Siam, Ethanol Absolute) | 5.0% |

**Copaborneol**

| | |
|---|---|
| Katrafay (Alpha-Pinene CT) | 4.7%–20.0% |
| Katrafay (Alpha-Eudesmol CT) | 0.0%–9.6% |
| Katrafay (Ishwarane CT) | 0.0%–5.2% |

**Copaenal**

| | |
|---|---|
| Muhuhu (Wood) | 7.2%–7.5% |

**Copaenol**

| | |
|---|---|
| Muhuhu (Wood) | 6.3%–7.5% |

**Copalic Acid**

| | |
|---|---|
| Copaiba | 2.1%–7.6% |

**Croweacin**

| | |
|---|---|
| Khella (Aerial Parts, 2,2-Dimethylbut. CT) | 12.2% |

**Cryptomeridiol**

| | |
|---|---|
| Fragonia (Balanced CT) | 0.0%–6.6% |

**Cryptomerione**

| | |
|---|---|
| Japanese Cedarwood (Twig) | 7.5%–7.6% |

**Cryptone**

| | |
|---|---|
| Blue Mallee (Cryptone CT) | 1.3%–4.9% |
| Rabbitbrush (var. *nauseosa*) | 2.6% |

**Cubebol**

| | |
|---|---|
| Japanese Cedarwood (Heartwood) | 0.0%–39.9% |
| Black Sage (Beta-Phellandrene CT) | 23.9% |
| Japanese Cedarwood (Sapwood) | 0.0%–20.5% |
| Cangerana (Leaves) | 0.0%–9.3% |
| Helichrysum (*H. splendidum*, Alpha-Terpinene CT) | 7.3% |
| Japanese Cedarwood (Twig) | 4.3%–4.5% |

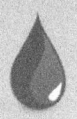

**Cubenol**

| | |
|---|---|
| Japanese Cedarwood (Heartwood) | 0.0%–18.4% |
| Japanese Cedarwood (Bark) | 0.0%–14.0% |
| Japanese Cedarwood (Sapwood) | 0.0%–13.3% |
| Pine | 0.0%–5.1% |
| Juniper, Phoenicia (Berries) | 0.0%–4.9% |
| Guava Leaf (Beta-Caryophyllene CT) | 0.0%–4.4% |
| African Bluegrass (Linalool CT) | 3.5%–4.1% |
| Japanese Cedarwood (Twig) | 0.1%–4.0% |
| Guava Leaf ((E)-Nerolidol CT) | 4.0% |
| Ferula (Limonene CT) | 3.8% |
| Wild Chamomile (*C. mixtus*, Sant. Alc. CT) | 0.0%–3.2% |

**Cuminaldehyde**

| | |
|---|---|
| Cumin | 19.9%–39.5% |

**Cuminyl Alcohol (Cuminol, Para-Cymen-7-ol)**

| | |
|---|---|
| Cumin | 0.2%–30.0% |
| Pink Pepper (*S. terebinthifolius*, Leaves, p-Cymen-7-ol CT) | 22.5% |

**Cuparene**

| | |
|---|---|
| Chinese Cedarwood | 0.0%–10.2% |
| Schisandra Fruit (*S. sphenanthera, α-Cad.* CT) | 8.7% |

**Cupressene**

| | |
|---|---|
| Japanese Cedarwood (Sapwood) | 0.0%–12.6% |

**Curcumol**

| | |
|---|---|
| Wild Turmeric (Solvent Extracted) | 35.8% |

**Curdione**

| | |
|---|---|
| White Turmeric (Distilled) | 0.0%–19.6% |
| White Turmeric (Solvent Extracted) | 7.0%–13.8% |
| Wild Turmeric (Distilled) | 0.0%–4.8% |

**Curzerene**

| | |
|---|---|
| Myrrh | 8.5%–40.1% |
| White Turmeric (Distilled) | 0.0%–29.4% |
| Opoponax (*C. guidotti*) | 0.0%–11.4% |
| White Turmeric (Solvent Extracted) | 0.0%–10.4% |
| Agarwood (*A. malaccensis*) | 0.0%–4.7% |
| Ledum (*R. groenlandicum*) | 0.0%–2.8% |

**Curzerenone**

| | |
|---|---|
| White Turmeric (Distilled) | 0.0%–31.6% |
| Plai (Terpinen-4-ol CT) | 0.1%–3.7% |

**Cyclocolorenone**

| | |
|---|---|
| Ledum (*L. palustre*) | 2.7%–6.5% |
| Ledum (R. groenlandicum) | 0.0%–2.1% |

**Cyclohexanone**

| | |
|---|---|
| Calamus ((E)-Methylisoeugenol CT) | 21.3% |
| Geranium | 0.0%–5.2% |
| Hairy Basil (var. *pilosum* Linalool CT) | 0.0%–4.4% |

**Cycloisolongifolene**

| | |
|---|---|
| Vetiver | 0.0%–5.9% |

**Cyclopentane**

| | |
|---|---|
| Moringa (Seeds, Cyclopentane CT) | 51.5% |

**Daniellic Acid**

| | |
|---|---|
| Copaiba | 2.6%–33.7% |

**Dauc-6(14),11-dien-5-ol**

| | |
|---|---|
| Siam Wood (Root Bark) | 1.8%–3.9% |

**Daucene**

| | |
|---|---|
| Carrot Seed | 0.0%–8.7% |

**Daucol**

| | |
|---|---|
| Carrot Seed | 2.0%–12.6% |
| Guava Leaf (Beta-Caryophyllene CT) | 0.0%–4.8% |

**Davanone**

| | |
|---|---|
| Davana | 32.7%–55.0% |

**Decanal**

| | |
|---|---|
| Arnica (Flowers) | 2.7%–5.3% |

**Decane**

| | |
|---|---|
| Betony (Alpha-Zingiberene CT) | 6.0% |

**Decenal**

| | |
|---|---|
| Cilantro | 6.6%–14.3% |

**Decanoic Acid**

| | |
|---|---|
| German Chamomile | 0.1%–5.1% |

**Dehydro-1,8-Cineole**

| | |
|---|---|
| Lovage (Aerial Parts) | 0.0%–6.8% |

**Dehydro-Aromadendrene**

| | |
|---|---|
| Vetiver | 0.0%–7.3% |

**Dehydroisoferruginol**

| | |
|---|---|
| Japanese Cedarwood (Bark) | 0.0%–5.1% |

**Dehydroisocalamendiol**

| | |
|---|---|
| Calamus (Acorenone CT) | 3.5%–4.5% |

**Dehydronepetalactone**

| | |
|---|---|
| Catnip (Nepetalactone CT) | 0.0%–5.0% |

**Delta-Amorphene**

| | |
|---|---|
| Copaiba | 0.0%–5.4% |
| Manuka (Leptospermone CT) | 0.0%–4.2% |
| Muhuhu (Wood) | 0.0%–2.7% |

**Delta-3-Carene (3-Carene, (+)-3-Carene)**

| | |
|---|---|
| Pink Pepper (*S. terebinthifolius*, Fruits, δ-3-Carene CT) | 5.8%–55.4% |
| Dwarf Pine (Twigs) | 24.0%–51.7% |
| Juniper (*J. recurva*, Berries) | 46.1% |
| Pine | 0.1%–33.7% |
| Black Pepper (Delta-3-Carene CT) | 19.0%–32.6% |
| Dwarf Pine (Needles, Needles/Twigs) | 13.1%–27.9% |
| Balsam Fir | 0.0%–27.7% |
| Turkish Pine (Twigs) | 14.2%–25.1% |
| Blue Mountain Sage (Delta-3-Carene CT) | 18.4%–25.0% |
| Oriental Arborvitae (Berries) | 9.5%–23.8% |
| Cypress | 11.1%–22.7% |
| Juniper (*J. recurva*, Needles) | 13.6%–23.7% |
| Turkish Pine (Needles/Twigs) | 11.3%–21.2% |
| Oriental Arborvitae (Needles) | 6.3%–20.1% |
| Blue Mountain Sage (Alpha-Bisabolol CT) | 7.0%–19.3% |
| Ponderosa Pine | 0.2%–19.3% |
| Japanese Cedarwood (Bark) | 0.0%–18.6% |
| Angelica Root | 3.4%–17.1% |
| Aleppo Pine (Aerial Parts) | 0.0%–16.3% |
| Aleppo Pine (Twigs) | 16.3% |
| Canadian Fleabane | 0.0%–15.9% |
| Hinoki (*Leaves*, Alpha-Terpinolene CT) | 15.2% |
| Indian Borage (Carvacrol CT) | 0.0%–15.0% |
| Silver Fir (*A. alba*) | 0.0%–13.9% |
| Turkish Pine (Cones) | 7.8%–13.4% |
| Red Pine | 0.5%–12.9% |
| Siberian Fir | 6.2%–12.2% |
| Galbanum | 0.6%–12.1% |
| Black Pepper (Limonene CT) | 0.0%–11.3% |
| Juniper, Phoenicia (needles) | 0.4%–10.7% |
| Blue Mountain Sage (Limonene CT) | 10.2% |
| Japanese Cedarwood (16-Kaurene CT) | 0.1%–9.9% |
| Frankincense (*B. serrata*) | 0.5%–9.6% |
| Engelmann Spruce | 0.2%–9.4% |
| Turkish Pine (Bark) | 9.3% |
| Black Pepper (Beta-Caryophyllene CT) | 0.0%–9.2% |
| Galangal (Lesser) | 0.0%–8.9% |
| Galangal (False, Ethyl-p-Methoxycinnamate CT) | 0.0%–7.9% |
| Mastic (Leaves) | 0.0%–7.2% |

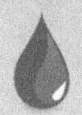

### Delta-3-Carene—continued

| | |
|---|---|
| Black Pepper (Eugenol CT) | 4.2%–6.4% |
| Blue Spruce | 0.0%–6.4% |
| White Sage | 1.3%–6.3% |
| Myrtle (Alpha-Pinene CT) | 0.0%–6.1% |
| White Spruce (Needles) | 0.0%–5.4% |
| Mastic (Twigs, Alpha-Pinene CT) | 5.2% |
| Melissa | 0.0%–5.0% |
| Juniper, Phoenicia (Berries) | 0.0%–4.5% |
| Maritime Pine (Needles, Alpha-Pinene CT) | 0.0%–3.5% |
| Maritime Pine (Gum Resin) | 0.0%–3.3% |
| Opoponax (*C. erythraea*) | 0.4%–3.0% |
| White Pine | 0.0%–3.0% |

### Delta-Cadinene

| | |
|---|---|
| Siam Wood (Root Bark) | 4.2%–32.6% |
| Schisandra Fruit (*S. sphenanthera*, δ-Cad. CT) | 25.6% |
| Calendula (Alpha-Cadinol/Delta-Cadinene CT) | 5.1%–22.5% |
| Goldenrod | 0.0%–20.4% |
| Indian Borage (Delta-Cadinene CT) | 12.5%–18.7% |
| Helichrysum (*H. splendidum*, Delta-cadinene CT) | 9.3%–16.9% |
| Betony (MLD-C CT) | 9.5%–16.0% |
| Japanese Cedarwood (Bark) | 0.0%–15.9% |
| Katrafay (Leaves) | 0.4%–14.5% |
| Calendula (Alpha-Thujene CT) | 13.1% |
| African Bluegrass (Myrcene CT) | 0.0%–12.8% |
| Betony (Bicyclogermacrene CT) | 2.3%–12.2% |
| Formosan Cypress (Wood, Myrtenol CT) | 0.6%–11.9% |
| Betony (Alpha-Thujene CT) | 0.1%–11.6% |
| Pine | 0.0%–11.6% |
| Rhododendron (Aerial Parts) | 9.1%–11.4% |
| Guggul | 0.0%–11.4% |
| Hinoki (wood) | 10.8% |
| Japanese Cedarwood (Twig) | 0.0%–10.4% |
| Formosan Cypress (Neeldes, Germ. D CT) | 6.3%–10.3% |
| Juniper (*J. recurva*, Needles) | 0.8%–10.2% |
| Indian Borage (Beta-Caryophyllene CT) | 9.8% |
| Black Sage (Beta-Caryophyllene CT) | 9.4% |
| Betony (Alpha-Zingiberene CT) | 9.1% |
| Hinoki (Taiwan Cypress, wood) | 2.1%–9.0% |
| Manuka (Leptospermone CT) | 4.8%–8.6% |
| Muhuhu (Leaves) | 8.5% |
| Helichrysum (*H. splendidum*, Germacrene D-4-ol CT) | 8.4% |
| African Bluegrass (Linalool CT) | 0.0%–8.1% |
| Maritime Pine (Needles, Beta-Cary. CT) | 0.0%–7.8% |
| Damiana (Delta-Cadinene CT) | 5.5%–7.7% |
| Ylang Ylang (Solvent Extracted) | 5.4%–7.6% |
| Pink Pepper (*S. molle*, Fruits/Leaves, α-Phell./Sylv. CT) | 1.1%–7.6% |
| White Pine | 0.1%–7.5% |
| Helichrysum (*H. splendidum*, Alpha-Terpinene CT) | 7.4% |
| Cangerana (Wood) | 7.4% |
| Galbanum | 1.5%–7.2% |
| Pink Pepper (*S. terebinthifolius*, Fruits, δ-3-Carene CT) | 0.3%–7.1% |
| Helichrysum (*H. splendidum*, Spathulenol CT) | 1.4%–6.9% |
| Muhuhu (Wood) | 3.3%–6.5% |
| Japanese Cedarwood (Alpha-Pinene CT) | 0.8%–6.5% |
| Betony (Germacrene D-Spathulenol CT) | 6.5% |
| Cananga | 0.5%–6.0% |
| Balsam Poplar | 0.0%–5.7% |
| Juniper (*J. recurva*, Berries) | 5.7% |
| Ghandi Root | 0.1%–5.6% |
| Mastic (Aerial parts, Beta-Eudesmol CT) | 5.6% |
| Savin (Needles & Branches) | 0.1%–5.4% |
| Ylang Ylang (Madagascan II) | 2.1%–5.2% |

| | |
|---|---|
| Mastic (Leaves) | 0.4%–5.2% |
| Maritime Pine (Needles, Alpha-Pinene CT) | 1.4%–5.0% |
| White Spruce (Needles & Twigs) | 1.1%–4.9% |
| Juniper, Phoenicia (Berries) | 0.0%–4.9% |
| Pink Pepper (*S. molle*, Leaves, Epi-Bicyclosesquiphell. CT) | 4.9% |
| Mugwort (Isobornyl Isobutyrate D CT) | 4.8% |
| Gobre Salla | 0.4%–4.6% |
| Ponderosa Pine | 0.0%–4.6% |
| Juniper (*J. wallichiana\J. indica*, Leaves) | 0.6%–4.5% |
| Black Sage (Caryophyllene Oxide CT) | 2.5%–4.1% |
| Pink Pepper (*S. molle*, Fruits, α-Phellandrene CT) | 0.3%–4.0% |
| Vetiver | 0.0%–4.0% |
| Mastic (Twigs, Alpha-Pinene CT) | 4.0% |
| Guava Leaf ((E)-Nerolidol CT) | 4.0% |
| Mugwort (Germacrene D CT) | 3.9% |
| Dwarf Pine (Needles, Needles/Twigs) | 1.0%–3.6% |
| Wild Chamomile (*O. mixta, C. mixtrum*) | 0.1%–3.4% |
| Mastic (NT\B, Germacrene D CT) | 3.4% |
| Japanese Cedarwood (16-Kaurene CT) | 0.5%–3.3% |
| Copaiba (Leaves) | 1.8%–3.1% |
| Ocotea (Flowers Calices) | 1.6%–3.1% |
| Damiana (Caryophyllene Oxide CT) | 1.0%–2.7% |
| Damiana (1,8-Cineole CT) | 1.4%–2.6% |
| Frankincense (*B. carterii*) | 0.0%–2.6% |
| Mugwort (Camphor CT) | 0.0%–2.5% |
| Yarrow (Chamazulene CT) | 0.0%–2.3% |
| Ledum (*R. groenlandicum*) | 0.0%–2.2% |
| Spearmint (Piperitone Oxide CT) | 0.1%–1.9% |
| Ocotea (Leaves) | 1.8% |
| Spearmint (Piperitenone Oxide CT) | 0.1%–1.6% |
| Rosewood (Wood) | 0.1%–1.4% |
| Mugwort (1,8-Cineole CT) | 0.0%–1.3% |

### Delta-Cadinene + Unidentified Sesquiterpene Hydrocarbon

| | |
|---|---|
| Hairy Basil (Eugenol CT) | 9.8% |

### Delta-Cadinol

| | |
|---|---|
| Damiana (Caryophyllene Oxide CT) | 0.0%–2.6% |
| Yarrow (Chamazulene CT) | 0.0%–2.3% |

### Delta-Elemene

| | |
|---|---|
| Goldenrod | 0.0%–7.4% |
| Kumquat (*F. margarita*, Leaves) | 2.3%–5.3% |
| Valerian | 0.0%–4.4% |

### Delta-Fenchol

| | |
|---|---|
| Applemint (*M. suav.*, PO-PEO CT) | 5.9% |

### Delta-Selinene

| | |
|---|---|
| Agarwood (*A. crassna*) | 0.0%–12.4% |
| Ferula (Limonene CT) | 3.5% |

### Delta-Terpineol

| | |
|---|---|
| Spanish Sage | 0.3%–12.0% |
| Wild Marjoram (Linalool CT) | 0.4%–4.4% |

### Demelverine

| | |
|---|---|
| Applemint (*M. suav.*, Italian) | 0.0%–2.2% |

### Diallyl Disulfide

| | |
|---|---|
| Garlic (Sulfides CT) | 17.5%–44.6% |

### Diallyl Sulfide

| | |
|---|---|
| Garlic (Vinyldithiins CT) | 6.0%–17.6% |
| Garlic (Sulfides CT) | 0.0%–7.6% |

### Diallyl Tetrasulfide

| | |
|---|---|
| Garlic (Sulfides CT) | 0.0%–4.1% |

### Diallyl Trisulfide

| | |
|---|---|
| Garlic (Sulfides CT) | 19.9%–45.9% |
| Garlic (Vinyldithiins CT) | 0.2%–14.1% |

**Diepi-Alpha-Cedrene Epoxide**
Agarwood (*A. sinensis*) — 0.4%–6.0%

**Dihydro-Beta-Ionene**
Spikenard (Nardol CT) — 7.9%

**Dihydro-Occidentalol**
Helichrysum (ssp. *microphyllum*) — 7.6%–12.2%

**Dihydrocarvone**
Spearmint (Carvone CT) — 0.0%–21.5%
Applemint (*M. suav.*, Piperitenone CT) — 0.0%–2.8%

**Dihydrocarvylacetate**
Tsauri Grass — 0.0%–4.2%

**Dihydrochamazulene Isomer**
Wormwood (Myrcene CT) — 5.5%–11.6%

**Dihydrocolumellarin**
Blue Cypress (Wood) — 1.3%–14.0%

**Dihydroedulan II**
Applemint (*M. suav.*, Piperitenone CT) — 0.0%–4.1%

**Dihydroeudesmol**
Cangerana (Leaves) — 0.0%–4.0%

**Dihydrojinkoh-Eremol**
Agarwood (*A. crassna*) — 0.0%–7.3%
Agarwood (*A. malaccensis*) — 0.1%–4.8%

**Dihydrolinalool**
Rose (Iranian) — 0.0%–39.2%

**Dihydropyrocurzerenone**
Opoponax (*C. erythraea*) — 1.1%–4.2%

**Dihydrotagetone**
Tagetes (*T. minuta*, Dihydrotagetone CT) — 33.8%–54.2%
Calendula ((E)-Beta-Ocimene CT) — 31.7%
Tagetes (*T. minuta*, (Z)-Beta-Ocimene CT) — 3.0%–16.4%
Tagetes (*T. minuta*, Alpha-Terpineol CT) — 13.7%
Tagetes (*T. patula*, Flowers) — 4.9%
Tagetes (*T. patula*, Limonene CT) — 0.0%–4.5%
Tagetes (*T. patula*, Aerial Parts) — 2.3%

**Diisobutyl Phthalate**
Oakmoss Absolute (Hydro. + Hexane) — 6.5%

**Dill Apiole (Dill Apiol)**
Dill (Aerial Parts, Carvone CT) — 0.0%–16.9%

**Dill Ether**
Dill (Flowers) — 22.0%
Dill (Aerial Parts, Alpha-Phellandrene CT) — 0.9%–20.8%
Dill Leaves — 16.4%
Dill (Aerial Parts, Carvone CT) — 0.0%–13.2%

**Dimethyl Anthranilate (Methyl n-Methyl Anthranilate)**
Petitgrain (Mandarin) — 13.2%–65.3%

**Diphenylamine**
Rhododendron (Flowers) — 4.2%

**Diplophyllin**
Elecampane — 0.0%–5.1%

**Diosphenol**
Buchu (*A. betulina*, Isomenthone CT) — 12.0%–26.3%
Applemint (*M. rotun.*, Pulegone CT) — 0.0%–3.8%

**Disiloxane**
Rose (Iranian) — 0.0%–17.6%

**Docosane**
Moringa (Fruits) — 32.7%
Rose (Iranian) — 0.0%–19.5%
Moringa (Leaves, Pentacosane CT) — 0.3%–6.8%
Tagetes (*T. minuta*, Limonene CT) — 0.0%–5.0%

**Dodecanal (N-Dodecanal)**
Coriander — 0.1%–8.1%
Mediterranean Mandarin (Hydrodistilled) — 0.0%–3.0%
Cilantro — 3.0%–4.4%

**Dodecane**
Chaste Tree (Leaves) — 0.0%–1.0%

**Dodecanoic Acid**
Lemongrass (East Indian) — 0.0%–5.3%

**Drimenol**
Valerian — 0.0%–4.4%

**(E)-1-(3,4-Dimethoxyphenyl)But-1-ene**
Plai (Terpinen-4-ol CT) — 6.0%–7.4%

**(E)-1-(3,4-Dimethoxyphenyl)Butadiene**
Plai (Sabinene CT) — 1.0%–27.5%
Plai (Terpinen-4-ol CT) — 9.8%–19.1%

**(E)-2-Decenal (2-(E)-Decenal)**
Cilantro — 9.1%–15.9%
Moringa (Seeds, Cyclopentane CT) — 4.4%

**(E)-2-Decen-1-ol**
Cilantro — 14.2%–26.0%

**(E)-2-Tetradecenal**
Cilantro — 0.4%–6.8%

**(E)-2-Tridecenal**
Cilantro — 0.0%–7.0%

**(E)-2-Dodecenal**
Cilantro — 5.4%–6.2%

**(E)-2-Dodecenal**
Cilantro — 0.0%–4.6%

**(E)-8-Acetylthio-p-menthan-3-one**
Buchu (*A. crenulata*) — 0.4%–10.4%

**(E)-Alpha-Bisabolene (Trans-Alpha-Bisabolene)**
Hairy Basil (1,8-Cineole CT) — 0.0%–13.7%
Galangal (Lesser) — 0.1%–4.2%
Spike Lavender — 0.2%–2.3%

**(E)-Beta-Elemenone (Trans-Beta-Elemenone)**
Zdravetz — 1.6%–5.3%

**(E)-Beta-Farnesol (Trans-Beta-Farnesol)**
German Chamomile — 0.0%–5.2%

**(E)-Beta-Ocimene (Trans-Beta-Ocimene, Trans-Ocimene)**
Calendula ((E)-Beta-Ocimene CT) — 46.2%
Frankincense (*B. sacra*) — 0.0%–32.3%
Fingerroot ((E)-Beta-Ocimene CT) — 19.0%–27.0%
Palo Santo (Leaves, Aerial Parts) — 13.0%–20.8%
Tagetes (*T. erecta*, Aerial Parts) — 8.7%–14.8%
Hemp (Myrcene CT) — 0.4%–10.2%
Canadian Fleabane — 0.0%–9.1%
Rabbitbrush (var. *glabratus*) — 9.1%
Tarragon (Methyl Chavicol CT) — 1.0%–7.8%
Kumquat (*C. japonica*, Leaves CT Beta-Pinene) — 7.6%
Tagetes (*T. erecta*, Leaves) — 0.6%–7.0%
Mastic (Twigs, Alpha-Pinene CT) — 6.9%
Verbena (Linalool CT) — 1.6%–6.2%
Lavandin (Abrialis) — 4.0%–5.5%
African Bluegrass (Myrcene CT) — 0.1%–5.3%
Catnip (1,8-cineole CT) — 5.0%
Neroli (*C. sinensis*) — 0.1%–4.8%
Lavender (Bulgarian) — 1.0%–4.2%
Petitgrain (Bergamot/Bitter Orange) — 3.1%–4.1%
Hemp (Beta-Caryophyllene CT) — 0.4%–4.1%
Mastic (Leaves) — 0.0%–3.9%

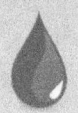

**(E)-Beta-Ocimene—continued**

| | |
|---|---|
| Petitgrain (Lemon) | 1.5%–2.2% |
| Chaste Tree (Leaves) | 0.1%–2.2% |
| Angelica Root | 0.0%–1.8% |
| Mugwort (Chrysanthenyl Acetate CT) | 1.2% |

**(E)-Cadinene (Trans-Cadinene)**

| | |
|---|---|
| Ylang Ylang (Madagascan II) | > 5.8% |
| Ylang Ylang (Madagascan III) | > 5.8% |

**(E)-Cadinene Ether (Trans-Cadinene Ether)**

| | |
|---|---|
| Indian Borage (Thymol CT) | 0.0%–3.9% |

**(E)-Cinnamaldehyde (Trans-Cinnamaldehyde, Cinnamic Aldehyde)**

| | |
|---|---|
| Cassia (Bark) | 24.6%–92.3% |
| Cinnamon Bark | 50.5%–91.0% |
| Tamala ((E)-Cinnamaldehyde CT) | 60.1%–82.0% |
| Cassia (Leaves) | 57.9%–78.4% |
| Tamala (Linalool\(E)-Cinnamaldehyde CT) | 7.7%–61.7% |
| Tamala ((E)-Cinnamaldehyde\Cinn. Ac. CT) | 28.2%–55.0% |
| Ocotea (Flowers Calices) | 27.9%–28.2% |
| Galangal (False, Ethyl-p-Methoxycinnamate CT) | 0.0%–5.3% |
| Ocotea (Leaves) | 5.1% |
| Cinnamon (leaves) | 0.8%–2.7% |

**(E)-Cinnamic Acid (Trans-Cinnamic Acid)**

| | |
|---|---|
| Benzoin (Sumatra, Ethanol Absolute) | 16.0%–26.0% |
| Benzoin (*S. paralleloneurum*, Absolute) | 5.7%–23.2% |
| Benzoin (*S. benzoin*, Absolute) | 1.8%–7.5% |
| Peru Balsam | 3.0%–5.1% |
| Cassia (Bark) | 0.0%–5.0% |
| Benzoin (Sumatra, Hydrodistilled) | 3.5% |
| Tolu Balsam | 2.7% |

**(E)-Citronellyl Tiglate (Citronellyl Tiglate)**

| | |
|---|---|
| Oakmoss Aboslute (Hydro. + Hexane) | 7.8% |

**(E)-Cycloisolongifol-5-ol**

| | |
|---|---|
| Indian Borage (Thymol CT) | 0.0%–8.0% |
| Indian Borage (Delta-Cadinene CT) | 0.0%–5.3% |

**(E)-Dihydrocarvone (Trans-Dyhdrocarvone)**

| | |
|---|---|
| Dill (Aerial Parts, Carvone CT) | 0.0%–14.7% |
| Dill Seed | 0.1%–5.9% |

**(E)-Dehydroterpineol (Trans-Dehydroterpineol)**

| | |
|---|---|
| Chaste Tree (Leaves) | 0.0%–1.8% |

**(E)-Epoxy Ocimene (Trans-Epoxy Ocimene)**

| | |
|---|---|
| Wormwood ((Z)-Epoxy Ocimene CT) | 0.0%–8.4% |

**(E)-Ethyl Cinnamate**

| | |
|---|---|
| Galangal (False, Ethyl-p-Methoxycinnamate CT) | 13.1%–29.5% |

**(E)-Isocitral (Trans-Isocitral)**

| | |
|---|---|
| Honey Myrtle | 0.0%–2.4% |

**(E)-Isopiperitenol (Trans-Isopiperitenol, Trans-p-Mentha-1,8-Dien-3-ol)**

| | |
|---|---|
| Tsauri Grass | 0.0%–7.1% |
| Tsauri Grass (var. *madagascariensis*) | 2.3%–3.9% |

**(E)-Isovalencenol (Trans-Isovalencenol)**

| | |
|---|---|
| Vetiver | 0.0%–15.6% |
| Chaste Tree (Leaves) | 0.0%–1.8% |

**(E)-Muurola-4(14),5-Diene**

| | |
|---|---|
| Juniper (*J. recurva*, Berries) | 4.3% |
| Muhuhu (Wood) | 0.0%–2.9% |

**(E)-Myrtanol (Trans-Myrtanol)**

| | |
|---|---|
| Formosan Cypress (Wood, Myrtenol CT) | 13.1%–19.2% |
| Feverfew | 0.0%–4.7% |

**(E)-p-Mentha-2,8-Dien-1-ol (Trans-para-Mentha-2,8-Dien-1-ol)**

| | |
|---|---|
| Tsauri Grass | 0.0%–26.2% |
| Tsauri Grass (var. *madagascariensis*) | 11.2%–19.0% |
| Gingergrass | 2.4%–9.8% |

**(E)-p-Mentha-1(7),8-Dien-2-ol (Trans-para-Mentha-1(7),8-Dien-2-ol)**

| | |
|---|---|
| Tsauri Grass (var. *madagascariensis*) | 14.7%–22.4% |
| Tsauri Grass | 0.0%–22.3% |
| Gingergrass | 8.6%–20.5% |

**(E)-Pinene Hydrate (Trans-Pinene Hydrate)**

| | |
|---|---|
| Leleshwa | 3.2%–6.5% |

**(E)-Piperitol (Trans-Piperitol)**

| | |
|---|---|
| Tsauri Grass | 0.0%–5.4% |
| Gingergrass | 0.0%–3.6% |

**(E)-Sesquilavandulol**

| | |
|---|---|
| Feverfew | 0.0%–4.8% |

**(E)-Tagetone (Trans-Tagetone)**

| | |
|---|---|
| Tagetes (*T. minuta*, Dihydrotagetone CT) | 6.2%–17.1% |
| Tagetes (*T. erecta*, Aerial Parts) | 0.1%–10.6% |
| Tagetes (*T. minuta*, Limonene CT) | 0.0%–5.7% |
| Tagetes (*T. patula*, Aerial Parts) | 5.3% |

**(E,E)-Farnesol (Farnesol, Trans,Trans-Farnesol)**

| | |
|---|---|
| Sandalwood (*S. spicatum*) | 9.3%–38.7% |
| Niaouli (Viridiflorol/ Para-cymene/1,8-cineole CT) | 0.0%–10.8% |
| Niaouli (Viridiflorol CT) | 0.0%–10.0% |
| Neroli (*C. aurantium*) | 0.0%–8.0% |
| German Chamomile | 0.0%–6.9% |
| Yarrow (Sabinene CT) | 0.0%–6.5% |
| Niaouli (1,8-Cineole CT) | 0.0%–5.0% |
| Cananga | 0.0%–3.9% |

**(E,E)-Farnesyl Acetate ((2E,6E)-Farnesyl Acetate)**

| | |
|---|---|
| Ylang Ylang (French IV) | 2.1% |
| Ylang Ylang (Madagascan I) | 0.5%–7.8% |
| Ylang Ylang (Madagascan II) | 0.7%–6.2% |
| Chaste Tree (Berries) | 0.0%–1.0% |

**Eicosane**

| | |
|---|---|
| Rose (Iranian) | 0.7%–20.5% |
| Moringa (Fruits) | 5.2% |
| Rose (Indian) | 0.1%–5.0% |

**Elemicin**

| | |
|---|---|
| Nutmeg (East Indian) | 0.6%–30.9% |
| Nutmeg (West Indian) | 0.4%–6.1% |
| Elemi | 2.4%–4.7% |
| Parsley (Whole Plant) | 2.7%–4.1% |
| Ravensara (Methyl Eugenol CT) | 0.6%–1.7% |

**Elemol (Alpha-Elemol)**

| | |
|---|---|
| Japanese Cedarwood (16-Kaurene CT) | 8.6%–20.5% |
| Kumquat (*F. margarita*, Leaves) | 0.0%–18.8% |
| Juniper (Chinese) | 0.0%–18.6% |
| Formosan Cypress (Twig) | 15.0% |
| Citronella (*C. winteranius*) | 2.0%–14.5% |
| Japanese Cedarwood (Heartwood) | 0.0%–14.1% |
| Elemi | 6.3%–13.7% |
| Pink Pepper (*S. terebinthifolius*, Fruits, δ-3-Carene CT) | 0.0%–13.6% |
| Pink Pepper (*S. molle*, Leaves, α-Phellandrene CT) | 0.1%–13.3% |
| Japanese Cedarwood (Alpha-Pinene CT) | 0.2%–12.7% |
| Amyris | 8.7%–10.9% |
| Pink Pepper (*S. molle*, Leaves, Elemol/Beta-Eudesmol CT) | 10.3% |
| Savin (Needles & Branches) | 0.0%–8.3% |
| Auracaria | 5.0%–7.6% |
| Wild Marjoram (Linalool CT) | 0.9%–6.6% |

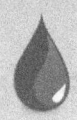
Hyssop (Pinocamphone CT) 0.0%–5.7%
Juniper (*J. recurva*, Needles) 3.9%–5.1%
Citronella (*C. nardus*) 0.0%–4.8%
Pink Pepper (*S. molle*, Fruits/Leaves, α-Phell./Sylv. CT) 0.8%–4.3%
Hinoki (needles) 0.0%–4.2%
Pink Pepper (*S. terebinthifolius*, Fruits/Leaves, Bicyclogerm. CT) 0.0%–4.0%
Yarrow (1,8-Cineole\Camphor CT) 0.0%–3.0%

**Epi-Alpha-Cadinol (T-Cadinol)**
Sweet Inula (T-Cadinol CT) 30.2%
Sweet Inula (Borneol CT) 0.0%–23.8%
Spikenard (Valeranone CT) 22.7%
Sweet Inula (Bornyl Acetate CT) 0.0%–13.4%
Basil (Linalool CT) 3.4%–13.1%
Hinoki (wood) 10.6%
Helichrysum (*H. splendidum*, Delta-cadinene CT) 3.6%–9.0%
Japanese Cedarwood (Twig) 6.8%–8.7%
Guava Leaf (Selin-11-en-4-Alpha-ol CT) 1.2%–8.2%
Pink Pepper (*S. molle*, Leaves, Beta-Pinene CT) 5.6%
Juniper (*J. recurva*, Needles) 0.3%–5.5%
Hairy Basil ((E)-Methyl Cinnamate CT) 0.0%–5.3%
Mastic (Leaves) 0.0%–4.9%
Calendula (Alpha-Cadinol/Delta-Cadinene CT) 0.0%–4.8%
Black Pepper (Eugenol CT) 1.5%–4.7%
Japanese Cedarwood (Alpha-Pinene CT) 0.3%–4.7%
Wild Marjoram (Linalool CT) 1.2%–4.6%
Pink Pepper (*S. terebinthifolius*, Fruits, δ-3-Carene CT) 0.1%–4.6%
Wild Chamomile (*O. mixta, C. mixtrum*) 0.2%–4.4%
White Pine 0.0%–4.0%
Japanese Cedarwood (Heartwood) 0.0%–3.9%
Helichrysum (*H. splendidum*, Spathulenol CT) 0.4%–3.4%
Allspice (Leaves, Eugenol CT) 0.0%–3.1%
Chaste Tree (Berries) 0.6%–3.0%
Chaste Tree (Leaves) 0.0%–2.7%

**Epi-Alpha-Muurolol (T-Muurolol)**
Calendula (Alpha-Thujene CT) 24.9%
Formosan Cypress (Twig) 21.6%
Hinoki (wood) 18.5%
Hinoki (Taiwan Cypress, wood) 0.5%–16.9%
Katrafay (Alpha-Eudesmol CT) 0.0%–13.7%
Lavender (Brazilian) 13.4%
Calendula (Alpha-Cadinol/Delta-Cadinene CT) 0.0%–13.0%
Katrafay ((γ,δ)-Cadinene CT) 0.0%–11.8%
Japanese Cedarwood (Bark) 0.0%–10.7%
Mastic (Leaves) 0.0%–9.1%
Indian Borage (Delta-Cadinene CT) 4.4%–7.3%
Japanese Cedarwood (Heartwood) 0.0%–6.9%
Wild Chamomile (*O. mixta, C. mixtrum*) 0.2%–6.6%
Juniper (*J. recurva*, Needles) 0.5%–5.5%
Ghandi Root 0.0%–5.3%
Juniper (Chinese) 0.0%–5.0%
Ylang Ylang (French IV) 4.4%
Black Pepper (Eugenol CT) 2.6%–3.8%
Sweet Inula (T-Cadinol CT) 3.0%
Yarrow (Chamazulene CT) 0.0%–2.7%

**Epi-Bicyclosesquiphellandrene**
Pink Pepper (*S. molle*, Leaves, Epi-Bicyclosesquiphell. CT) 18.6%
Galbanum 0.0%–4.4%
Valerian 0.0%–4.2%

**Epi-Cedrol (Epicedrol)**
Japanese Cedarwood (16-Kaurene CT) 0.0%–3.8%

**Epi-Cubebol**
Japanese Cedarwood (Heartwood) 0.0%–26.9%
Japanese Cedarwood (Sapwood) 0.0%–3.7%

**Epi-Cubenol**
Frankincense (*B. serrata*) 0.0%–9.1%
Ferula (Limonene CT) 3.2%

**Epi-Curzerenone**
White Turmeric (Solvent Extracted) 24.1%–44.6%
White Turmeric (Distilled) 0.0%–19.0%

**Epi-Zonarene**
Japanese Cedarwood (Bark) 0.0%–5.0%

**Epiglobulol**
Celery Leaf 0.0%–7.7%
Southern Blue Gum 0.0%–1.2%

**Epimanoyl oxide (1H-naphtho (2,1,b) pyran)**
Clary Sage 0.0%–8.6%

**Epixonarene**
Hinoki (needles) 0.0%–4.1%

**Epoxybulnesene**
Agarwood (*A. crassna*) 0.0%–5.3%
Agarwood (*A. malaccensis*) 0.0%–11.0%

**Eremophila-7(11),9-Dien-8-One**
Agarwood (*A. sinensis*) 4.5%–5.4%

**Eremophilene**
Formosan Cypress (Wood, α-Eudesmol CT) 4.3%

**Eremophilone**
Buddha Wood 40.5%–43.0%

**Ethanol**
Rose (Turkish) 0.0%–13.4%
Rose (Bulgarian) 0.0%–0.9%

**Ethyl-2-Methylbutyrate (Ethyl 2-Methylbutanoate)**
Magnolia (Flowers) 1.5%–6.8%

**Ethyl-p-Methoxycinnamate ((E)-Ethyl p-methoxy-cinnamate, Trans-Ethyl p-Methoxycinnamate)**
Galangal (False, Ethyl-p-Methoxycinnamate CT) 18.4%–51.6%
Galangal (False, 2-Propeonic Acid CT) 26.0%

**Ethyl Everninate**
Oakmoss Aboslute 0.0%–3.7%

**Ethyl Hematommate**
Oakmoss Aboslute 1.4%–3.4%

**Ethyl Vinyl Sulfide**
Garlic (Vinyldithiins CT) 0.0%–9.7%
Garlic (Sulfides CT) 0.0%–9.7%

**Eudesma-2,6,8-Triene**
Valerian 0.0%–7.6%

**Eudesma-3,7(11)-Diene (Selina-3,7(11)-Diene)**
Japanese Cedarwood (16-Kaurene/Valencene CT) 8.4%

**Eudesma-3,11-Dien-2-One**
Ledum (*R. groenlandicum*) 0.0%–8.9%

**Eudesma-4(15),7-diene-1-Beta-1-ol**
Indian Borage (Beta-Caryophyllene CT) 9.0%

**Eudesmen-5-en-11-ol**
Helichrysum (ssp. *microphyllum*) 3.7%–23.5%
Helichrysum (ssp. *italicum*) 1.1%–5.8%

**Eudesm-7(11)-en-4alpha-ol**
Agarwood (*A. sinensis*) 0.8%–4.4%

**Eudesmol <α,β>**
Katrafay (Ishwarane CT) 0.0%–8.1%

**Eugenol**
Clove (Leaves) 87.5%–98.8%
Bay (West Indies) 45.2%–92.9%
Tamala (Eugenol CT) 66.1%–91.4%
Clove Bud 69.8%–87.0%
Allspice (Berries, Eugenol CT) 68.8%–86.4%

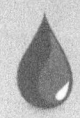

**Eugenol—continued**

| | |
|---|---|
| Allspice (Leaves, Eugenol CT) | 54.3%–85.3% |
| Cinnamon (leaves) | 74.9%–81.7% |
| Tamala (Eugenol\Eugenyl Acetate CT) | 41.8%–77.8% |
| Holy Basil (leaves) | 71.3%–75.1% |
| Hairy Basil (Eugenol CT) | 66.4% |
| Holy Basil (aerial parts, eugenol CT) | 15.7%–51.5% |
| Black Pepper (Eugenol CT) | 12.1%–41.0% |
| Allspice (Berries, Methyl Eugenol CT) | 8.3%–28.8% |
| Hairy Basil (var. *pilosum* Eugenol CT) | 28.5% |
| Hairy Basil (Linalool CT, Leaves) | 17.2% |
| Holy Basil (Aerial Parts, Estragole CT) | 0.0%–17.0% |
| Verbena (Myrcenone CT) | 0.0%–15.3% |
| Kumquat (*C. japonica*, Leaves CT Linalool) | 14.8% |
| Hairy Basil (1,8-Cineole\Linalool CT) | 8.0%–14.7% |
| Indian Borage (Thymol CT) | 0.0%–14.6% |
| Basil (Linalool CT) | 4.7%–11.2% |
| Cinnamon Bark | 1.9%–10.0% |
| Allspice (Leaves, Methyl Eugenol CT) | 8.3% |
| Citronella (*C. nardus*) | 0.0%–8.1% |
| Hairy Basil (Thymol CT) | 8.1% |
| Holy Basil (aerial parts, beta-bisabolene CT) | 2.9%–7.6% |
| Basil (Methyl Eugenol CT) | 0.1%–7.6% |
| Cassia (Leaves) | 0.0%–4.5% |
| Jasmine Absolute (Benzyl Benzoate CT) | 2.0%–4.0% |
| Camphor (Linalool CT) | 0.0%–3.6% |
| Hairy Basil (1,8-Cineole CT) | 0.0%–3.6% |
| Rose (Indian) | 0.0%–3.3% |
| Holy Basil (aerial parts or seeds, methyl eugenol CT) | 0.1%–2.4% |
| Ravensara (Methyl Eugenol CT) | 0.0%–0.6% |

**Eugenyl Acetate**

| | |
|---|---|
| Tamala (Eugenol\Eugenyl Acetate CT) | 12.3%–47.1% |
| Clove Bud | 5.0%–21.3% |
| Tamala (Eugenol CT) | 0.0%–9.8% |
| Clove (Leaves) | 0.1%–2.5% |

**Eugenyl Hexanoate**

| | |
|---|---|
| Valerian | 0.0%–4.9% |

**(E,Z)-Farnesol ((2E,6Z)-Farnesol), Trans-Cis-Farnesol)**

| | |
|---|---|
| Rose (Indian) | 0.3%–5.4% |
| Neroli (*C. sinensis*) | 0.1%–4.6% |
| Palmarosa | 1.6%–3.4% |
| Ylang Ylang (French IV) | 1.4% |

**(E,Z)-Geranyl Linalool**

| | |
|---|---|
| Jasmine Absolute (Benzyl Acetate CT) | 0.0%–5.0% |
| Chaste Tree (Leaves) | 0.0%–2.2 % |

**Farnesal**

| | |
|---|---|
| Valerian | 0.0%–8.0% |

**Farnesol**

| | |
|---|---|
| Magnolia (Leaves) | 0.0%–5.5% |

**Farnesyl Acetate**

| | |
|---|---|
| Valerian | 0.0%–7.1% |

**Fenchol (Fenchyl Alcohol, Alpha-Fenchol)**

| | |
|---|---|
| Leleshwa | 10.9%–29.1% |
| Vilayti Tulsi (Fenchone CT) | 0.7%–8.6% |

**Fenchone (Alpha-Fenchone)**

| | |
|---|---|
| Vilayti Tulsi (Fenchone CT) | 8.1%–42.3% |
| Fennel (Trans Anethole CT) | 1.0%–34.7% |
| Mugwort (Alpha-Thujone CT) | 0.0%–16.6% |
| Western Red Cedar (Leaves) | 0.0%–15.2% |
| Thuja | 0.4%–14.5% |
| Fennel (Methyl Chavicol CT) | 1.0%–10.4% |
| Vilayti Tulsi (Sabinene CT) | 0.0%–8.1% |

| | |
|---|---|
| Applemint (*M. suav.*, Pulegone CT) | 3.6% |
| Engelmann Spruce | 0.0%–3.0% |

**Ferruginol**

| | |
|---|---|
| Japanese Cedarwood (Bark) | 0.0%–11.5% |
| Japanese Cedarwood (Sapwood) | 0.0%–10.8% |
| Japanese Cedarwood (Twig) | 4.3%–4.8% |

**Flavesone**

| | |
|---|---|
| Manuka (Leptospermone CT) | 0.0%–12.3% |

**Fokienol**

| | |
|---|---|
| Siam Wood (Root Bark) | 24.0%–26.4% |

**Formic Acid**

| | |
|---|---|
| Spikenard (Nardol CT) | 9.4% |

**Furanoeudesma-1,3-Diene (Furanoeudsmadiene)**

| | |
|---|---|
| Myrrh | 15.0%–49.1% |
| Opoponax (*C. guidotti*) | 0.0%–18.6% |

**Furanodiene**

| | |
|---|---|
| Myrrh | 0.0%–19.7% |

**Gamma-Atlantone**

| | |
|---|---|
| Cedarwood (Himalayan, Wood) | 6.0%–8.6% |

**Gamma-Bisabolene**

| | |
|---|---|
| Opoponax (*C. guidotti*) | 0.0%–3.9% |

**Gamma-Cadinene**

| | |
|---|---|
| Pink Pepper (*S. terebinthifolius*, Fruits, α-Phell. CT) | 18.0% |
| Siam Wood (Root Bark) | 2.3%–15.6% |
| Hinoki (wood) | 12.5% |
| African Bluegrass (Myrcene CT) | 0.0%–12.3% |
| Hinoki (Taiwan Cypress, wood) | 1.4%–12.1% |
| Calendula (Alpha-Cadinol/Delta-Cadinene CT) | 0.0%–11.9% |
| Formosan Cypress (Wood, Myrtenol CT) | 0.0%–11.4% |
| Pine | 0.0%–11.1% |
| Ylang Ylang (Madagascan III) | < 17.4% |
| Ylang Ylang (Madagascan II) | < 12.7% |
| Juniper, Phoenicia (Berries) | 0.0%–10.2% |
| Galangal (False, Ethyl-p-Methoxycinnamate CT) | 0.0%–9.8% |
| Guggul | 0.0%–8.6% |
| Pink Pepper (*S. molle*, Leaves, Epi-Bicyclosesquiphell. CT) | 6.9% |
| Garlic (Sulfides CT) | 0.0%–6.8% |
| Pink Pepper (*S. molle*, Leaves, Beta-Pinene CT) | 6.0% |
| Formosan Cypress (Neeldes, Germ. D CT) | 2.3%–5.3% |
| Mastic (Aerial parts, Beta-Eudesmol CT) | 5.0% |
| Copaiba | 0.8%–4.6% |
| Hairy Basil (1-8-Cineole\Linalool CT) | 0.0%–4.6% |
| Juniper, Phoenicia (needles) | 0.0%–4.4% |
| Maritime Pine (Needles, Beta-Cary. CT) | 0.0%–3.9% |
| Japanese Cedarwood (Heartwood) | 0.0%–3.7% |
| Muhuhu (Leaves) | 3.5% |
| Sweet Inula (T-Cadinol CT) | 3.3% |
| Ylang Ylang (French IV) | 2.1% |
| Sweet Inula (Bornyl Acetate CT) | 0.0%–2.0% |

**Gamma-Cadinol**

| | |
|---|---|
| Pink Pepper (*S. molle*, Leaves, α-Phellandrene CT) | 0.0%–4.7% |

**Gamma-Costal**

| | |
|---|---|
| Formosan Cypress (Wood, α-Eudesmol CT) | 7.0% |

**Gamma-Curcumene**

| | |
|---|---|
| Helichrysum (*H. italicum*) | 2.3%–22.5% |
| Helichrysum (ssp. *microphyllum*) | 0.8%–18.2% |
| Helichrysum (ssp. *italicum*) | 0.8%–12.9% |
| Balsam Poplar | 4.6%–6.4% |
| Zdravetz | 0.0%–4.1% |

**Gamma-Elemene**

| | |
|---|---|
| Hops | 0.0%–14.0% |
| Holy Basil (aerial parts, eugenol CT) | 7.7%–10.5% |

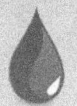 

| | |
|---|---|
| Chaste Tree (Leaves) | 0.0%–9.1% |
| Mugwort (Alpha-Phellandrene CT) | 8.8% |
| Vilayti Tulsi (1,8-Cineole CT) | 0.0%–8.2% |
| Juniper Berry | 0.1%–6.4% |
| Angelica Root | 0.6%–2.2% |

**Gamma-Eudesmol**

| | |
|---|---|
| Auracaria | 19.0%–19.1% |
| Kumquat (*F. margarita*, Leaves) | 8.4%–19.0% |
| Japanese Cedarwood (Twig) | 6.1%–11.8% |
| Katrafay (Alpha-Eudesmol CT) | 0.0%–11.1% |
| Japanese Cedarwood (16-Kaurene CT) | 0.0%–10.6% |
| Blue Cypress (Wood) | 8.0%–9.7% |
| Japanese Cedarwood (Alpha-Pinene CT) | 0.0%–9.1% |
| Amyris | 6.6%–8.5% |
| Japanese Cedarwood (Bark) | 0.0%–7.0% |
| Katrafay (Alpha-Pinene CT) | 0.0%–6.2% |
| African Bluegrass (Linalool CT) | 4.0%–4.5% |
| Siam Wood (Root Bark) | 2.0%–3.0% |
| Guaiacwood | 0.0%–2.6% |
| Angelica Root | 0.1%–1.2% |

**Gamma-Gurjunene**

| | |
|---|---|
| Sweet Wormwood (Camphor CT) | 0.0%–4.3% |
| Mugwort (1,8-Cineole CT) | 0.0%–2.8% |

**Gamma-Gurjunene Epoxide**

| | |
|---|---|
| Indian Borage (Thymol CT) | 0.0%–5.2% |

**Gamma-Himachalene**

| | |
|---|---|
| Cedarwood (Himalayan, Wood) | 7.0%–12.6% |
| Cedarwood (Atlas) | 5.1%–11.0% |
| Anise | 0.0%–8.2% |

**Gamma-Humulene**

| | |
|---|---|
| Mugwort (1,8-Cineole CT) | 0.0%–1.1% |

**Gamma-Muurolene**

| | |
|---|---|
| Japanese Cedarwood (Heartwood) | 0.0%–11.8% |
| Formosan Cypress (Neeldes, Germ. D CT) | 5.8%–9.1% |
| Mugwort (Camphor CT) | 0.0%–9.0% |
| Katrafay (Ishwarane CT) | 0.0%–8.2% |
| Galangal (Lesser) | 0.0%–7.9% |
| Siam Wood (Root Bark) | 0.0%–7.1% |
| Kumquat (*F. margarita*, Leaves) | 0.0%–6.5% |
| Applemint (*M. suav.*, Piperitenone CT) | 0.0%–5.5% |
| Kumquat (*F. margarita*, Fruit CT α-Terpineol) | 5.5% |
| Cangerana (Wood) | 5.0% |
| Yarrow (Chamazulene CT) | 0.1%–4.6% |
| Arnica (Flowers) | 2.7%–3.3% |
| Applemint (*M. rotun.*, β-Caryophyllene CT) | 3.2% |
| Applemint (*M. suav.*, Carvone CT) | 0.0%–3.0% |

**Gamma-Selinene**

| | |
|---|---|
| Agarwood (*A. crassna*) | 0.0%–13.7% |
| Japanese Cedarwood (16-Kaurene CT) | 0.0%–10.6% |
| Vetiver | 0.0%–4.1% |

**Gamma-Terpinene**

| | |
|---|---|
| Summer Savory (Gamma-Terpinene CT) | 27.4%–70.4% |
| Ajowan (Gamma-Terpinene\P-Cymene CT) | 21.3%–48.1% |
| Petitgrain (Mandarin) | 19.8%–47.9% |
| Fingerroot (Gamma-Terpinene CT) | 44.0% |
| Summer Savory (Carvacrol CT) | 9.1%–41.8% |
| Niaouli (Viridiflorol/ Para-cymene/1,8-cineole CT) | 0.0%–32.4% |
| Citron (Fingered, Distilled) | 22.5%–28.4% |
| Tea tree | 10.0%–28.0% |
| Ajowan (Thymol CT) | 11.3%–27.8% |
| Thyme (Carvacrol CT) | 0.0%–26.8% |
| Citron (Cold-pressed/Expressed) | 21.7%–26.2% |
| Citron (Distilled) | 0.3%–24.5% |

| | |
|---|---|
| Thyme (Thymol CT) | 0.0%–23.5% |
| Persian Lime (Cold Pressed\Expressed) | 12.5%–21.5% |
| Mediterranean Mandarin (CP\Expressed) | 13.1%–20.7% |
| Lime (Cold-pressed/expressed) | 0.1%–20.6% |
| Blue Mountain Sage (Gamma-Terpinene CT) | 20.3% |
| Cumin | 0.0%–19.6% |
| Savory (Wild, Thymol CT) | 2.2%–18.7% |
| Summer Savory (Thymol CT) | 16.0%–18.6% |
| Lemon (Cold-pressed/expressed) | 0.1%–18.0% |
| Persian Lime (Distilled) | 11.8%–17.0% |
| Lime (Distilled) | 0.1%–16.5% |
| Shell Ginger (Terpinen-4-ol CT) | 5.7%–16.1% |
| Mediterranean Mandarin (Hydrodistilled) | 0.1%–15.8% |
| Savory (Wild, Carvacrol CT) | 0.8%–14.8% |
| Indian Borage (Carvacrol CT) | 0.0%–14.7% |
| Shell Ginger (1,8-Cineole CT) | 0.0%–14.5% |
| Marjoram | 6.9%–14.3% |
| Lemon (Distilled) | 0.1%–14.1% |
| Coriander | 4.6%–13.6% |
| Mountain Savory (Carvacrol CT) | 0.0%–13.5% |
| Plai (Terpinen-4-ol, No Phenylbutanoids CT) | 5.8%–13.3% |
| Black Cumin (Para-Cymene CT) | 0.2%–12.9% |
| Yuzu | 7.6%–12.5% |
| Ledum (*R. groenlandicum*) | 0.0%–12.2% |
| Bergamot (Cold-pressed/expressed) | 4.3%–11.4% |
| Blue Mountain Sage ((E)-Nerolidol CT) | 0.1%–11.3% |
| Lemon (Distilled) | 9.8%–10.4% |
| Bergamot (Distilled) | 0.1%–10.3% |
| Mountain Savory (Thymol CT) | 5.9%–9.8% |
| Hairy Basil (var. *pilosum* Terpinen-4-ol CT) | 0.1%–9.2% |
| Plai (Sabinene CT) | 5.3%–9.0% |
| Tagetes (*T. patula*, Aerial Parts) | 8.4% |
| Oregano (*O. syriacum*, Thymol CT) | 6.5%–8.0% |
| Mastic (NT\B, Terpinene-4-ol CT) | 4.5%–7.8% |
| Douglas Fir (Needles) | 1.8%–7.4% |
| Vilayti Tulsi (Fenchone CT) | 1.6%–7.0% |
| Petitgrain (Bergamot/Bitter Orange) | 0.0%–7.0% |
| Hinoki (needles) | 0.1%–6.8% |
| Juniper (*J. wallichiana\J. indica*, Berries) | 0.1%–6.6% |
| Juniper (*J. wallichiana\J. indica*, Leaves) | 3.9%–6.4% |
| Oregano (Carvacrol CT) | 0.0%–6.3% |
| Kaffir Lime Peel | 0.9%–6.2% |
| Rhododendron (Leaves) | 6.1% |
| Ravensara (Alpha-Terpinene CT) | 5.7%–5.9% |
| Wild Marjoram (Linalool CT) | 0.2%–5.8% |
| African Bluegrass (Myrcene CT) | 0.0%–5.7% |
| Black Pepper (Beta-Pinene CT) | 5.7% |
| Tangerine (Cold-pressed/expressed) | 0.1%–5.4% |
| Basil (Linalool CT) | 0.0%–5.4% |
| Thyme (Geraniol CT) | 0.0%–5.3% |
| Oregano (*O. onites*) | 1.7%–5.2% |
| Utah Juniper (Needles/Twigs) | 1.0%–5.2% |
| Nutmeg (East Indian) | 0.1%–5.2% |
| Utah Juniper (Needles/Berries) | 5.2% |
| Mugwort (1,8-Cineole CT) | 0.0%–5.1% |
| Oregano (Terpinen-4-ol CT) | 0.0%–5.0% |
| Thyme (Thuyanol-4 CT) | 0.0%–5.0% |
| Lovage (Aerial Parts) | 0.0%–4.9% |
| Oregano (*O. syriacum*, Carvacrol CT) | 3.4%–4.8% |
| Hairy Basil (var. *pilosum* Linalool CT) | 0.0%–4.8% |
| Hinoki (*Leaves*, Alpha-Terpinolene CT) | 4.8% |
| Nutmeg (West Indian) | 1.7%–4.7% |
| Mastic (Leaves) | 0.0%–4.5% |
| Ravensara (Sabinene CT) | 1.9%–4.4% |

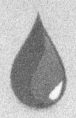
### Gamma-Terpinene—continued

| | |
|---|---|
| Mastic (NT\B, Alpha-Pinene CT) | 2.2%–4.2% |
| Catnip (Nepetalactone CT) | 0.0%–4.2% |
| Ravensara (Limonene CT) | 1.8%–4.1% |
| Savory (Wild, Linalool CT) | 0.0%–4.1% |
| Kanuka | 0.0%–4.1% |
| Shell Ginger (P-Mentha-1,3-Dien-7-al CT) | 4.1% |
| Plai (Triquinacene,1,4-Bis(Methoxy)- CT) | 3.9% |
| Plai (Terpinen-4-ol CT) | 1.8%–3.6% |
| Indian Borage (Thymol CT) | 3.2%–3.5% |
| Japanese Cedarwood (Alpha-Pinene CT) | 0.0%–3.5% |
| Rosalina (Linalool CT) | 0.0%–3.2% |
| Japanese Cedarwood (16-Kaurene CT) | 0.5%–3.1% |
| Angelica Root | 0.4%–3.1% |
| Mastic (NT\B, Germacrene D CT) | 3.1% |
| Thyme (Alpha-Terpineol CT) | 0.0%–3.0% |
| Mugwort (Isobornyl Isobutyrate D CT) | 2.8% |
| Rabbitbrush (var. nauseosa) | 2.6% |
| Mastic (NT\B, Limonene CT) | 1.9%–2.5% |
| Niaouli (1,8-Cineole/Viridiflorol CT) | 0.1%–2.0% |
| Mugwort (Camphor CT) | 0.0%–1.8% |
| Ocotea (Flowers Calices) | 0.0%–1.7% |
| Ravensara (Methyl Eugenol CT) | 0.7%–1.6% |
| Chaste Tree (Leaves) | 0.6%–1.6% |
| Lemon Eucalyptus | 0.3%–1.5% |
| Chaste Tree (Berries) | 0.6%–1.1% |

### Gamma-Terpineol

| | |
|---|---|
| Palo Santo (Wood) | 0.0%–8.7% |

### Gamma-Terpinolene

| | |
|---|---|
| Ajowan (Gamma-Terpinolene CT) | 53.6% |
| Dwarf Pine (Twigs) | 2.5%–4.3% |
| Dwarf Pine (Needles, Needles/Twigs) | 0.0%–4.3% |

### Gamma-Ylangene + Alpha Copaene

| | |
|---|---|
| Manuka (Selinene/Beta-Elemene CT) | 6.0% |

### Geranial (E-Citral, Citral A, Trans-Citral, Alpha-Citral)

| | |
|---|---|
| Lemon Myrtle (Citral CT) | 46.1%–60.7% |
| White Verbena (Citral CT) | 30.5%–54.6% |
| Lemongrass (East Indian) | 25.0%–53.8% |
| Lemon Basil | 31.2%–50.9% |
| May Chang (Citral CT) | 33.2%–50.0% |
| Lemongrass (West Indian) | 27.0%–48.1% |
| Hairy Basil (Citral CT) | 28.6%–47.2% |
| Melissa | 6.6%–45.2% |
| Lemon Tea Tree (L. petersonii) | 29.8%–40.7% |
| Honey Myrtle | 38.0%–40.3% |
| Lemon Verbena (Stems) | 29.5%–39.6% |
| Lemon Verbena (Leaves) | 29.5%–38.5% |
| Lemon Tea Tree (L. liversidgei) | 31.0%–34.6% |
| Petitgrain (Lime) | 11.8%–26.9% |
| Lemon Verbena (Leaves and stems) | 9.9%–26.0% |
| Citronella (C. nardus) | 1.2%–22.7% |
| Petitgrain (Lemon) | 14.3%–22.6% |
| Lemon Catnip (Beta-Citronellol CT) | 4.9%–22.3% |
| Ginger | 1.2%–20.1% |
| Tangerine (Distilled) | 0.1%–19.0% |
| Rose (Iranian) | 0.0%–12.3% |
| White Verbena (Carvone\Limonene CT) | 0.0%–10.4% |
| Lemon Catnip (Geraniol\Nerol CT) | 4.9%–9.9% |
| Citron (Distilled) | 0.1%–8.2% |
| Citronella (C. winteranius) | 1.5%–8.1% |
| Kumquat (C. japonica, Leaves CT Linalool) | 7.9% |
| Persian Lime (Distilled) | 0.0%–6.4% |
| Lime (Cold-pressed/expressed) | 0.0%–6.1% |

| | |
|---|---|
| Ocotea (Leaves) | 5.6% |
| Persian Lime (Cold Pressed\Expressed) | 1.0%–4.0% |
| Palmarosa | 0.0%–2.1% |

### Geraniol

| | |
|---|---|
| Monarda (var. menthaefolia) | 86.8%–93.2% |
| Palmarosa | 63.5%–83.8% |
| Thyme (Geraniol CT) | 23.5%–72.7% |
| Citronella (C. winteranius) | 16.2%–40.1% |
| Geranium | 1.1%–38.4% |
| Citronella (C. nardus) | 2.4%–36.5% |
| Lemon Catnip (Beta-Citronellol CT) | 19.6%–32.9% |
| Lemon Catnip (Geraniol\Nerol CT) | 23.5%–31.0% |
| Thyme (Linalool CT) | 0.0%–30.0% |
| Rose (Indian) | 2.5%–26.5% |
| Fingerroot ((E)-Beta-Ocimene CT) | 11.0%–26.0% |
| Rose (Bulgarian) | 4.8%–25.3% |
| Rose (Iranian) | 0.0%–22.7% |
| Fingerroot (Gamma-Terpinene CT) | 20.6% |
| Rose (Turkish) | 2.1%–18.0% |
| African Bluegrass (Myrcene CT) | 1.7%–17.1% |
| Fingerroot (Camphor CT) | 6.2%–16.2% |
| Ginger | 0.0%–14.5% |
| Kumquat (C. japonica, Leaves CT Linalool) | 12.7% |
| Melissa | 0.1%–11.8% |
| Dill (Aerial Parts, Alpha-Phellandrene CT) | 0.0%–10.6% |
| Thyme (Carvacrol CT) | 0.0%–10.3% |
| Mountain Savory (Carvacrol CT) | 0.0%–10.2% |
| Verbena (Myrcenone CT) | 0.0%–9.5% |
| Thyme (Thymol CT) | 0.0%–8.9% |
| White Verbena (Citral CT) | 0.0%–7.1% |
| Lemongrass (East Indian) | 0.1%–7.0% |
| Citron (Distilled) | 0.3%–6.6% |
| Mountain Savory (Thymol CT) | 0.0%–6.4% |
| Citron (Cold-pressed/Expressed) | 2.9%–6.3% |
| Lemon Verbena (Leaves and stems) | 0.1%–6.0% |
| Honey Myrtle | 2.1%–5.3% |
| Lemon Basil | 0.0%–5.1% |
| Fenugreek | 4.8% |
| May Chang (Citronellal CT) | 1.1%–4.6% |
| Neroli (C. aurantium) | 0.4%–4.3% |
| Lemon Verbena (Leaves) | 0.0%–4.0% |
| Lemon Tea Tree (L. petersonii) | 1.2%–3.9% |
| Petitgrain (Lime) | 1.3%–3.8% |
| Tangerine (Distilled) | 0.0%–3.5% |
| Applemint (M. suav., PO-PEO CT) | 3.4% |
| Calendula (Alpha-Cadinol/Delta-Cadinene CT) | 0.0%–3.0% |
| Applemint (M. suav., Linalool CT) | 2.7% |
| May Chang (Citral CT) | 0.4%–2.6% |
| Petitgrain (Lemon) | 0.8%–2.4% |
| Rosewood (Wood) | 0.7%–1.3% |
| Rosewood (Leaves) | 1.3% |

### Geranyl Acetate

| | |
|---|---|
| Lemongrass (East Indian) | 0.6%–24.0% |
| Ginger | 0.0%–18.8% |
| Palmarosa | 2.3%–14.8% |
| Ylang Ylang Complete | 7.6%–12.6% |
| Clary Sage | 3.8%–12.1% |
| Ylang Ylang (Madagascan I) | 6.2%–11.0% |
| Myrtle (Limonene CT) | 0.9%–10.9% |
| Applemint (M. suav., Linalool CT) | 10.9% |
| Citronella (C. nardus) | 0.0%–9.7% |
| Petitgrain (Bergamot/Bitter Orange) | 0.0%–8.7% |
| Petitgrain (Lime) | 1.7%–8.3% |

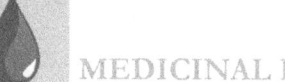

| | |
|---|---|
| Catnip (1,8-cineole CT) | 8.2% |
| Ylang Ylang (Madagascan II) | 2.6%–7.2% |
| Melissa | 0.1%–7.1% |
| Mountain Savory (Carvacrol CT) | 0.0%–6.7% |
| Myrtle (1,8-Cineole CT) | 1.9%–6.3% |
| Neroli (*C. aurantium*) | 2.6%–4.9% |
| Spanish Sage | 0.0%–4.9% |
| Rose (Indian) | 0.1%–4.1% |
| Citronella (*C. winteranius*) | 1.8%–4.0% |
| Lemon Verbena (Leaves) | 0.9%–4.0% |
| Tangerine (Distilled) | 0.0%–3.9% |
| Calendula (Alpha-Cadinol/Delta-Cadinene CT) | 0.0%–3.8% |
| Petitgrain (Lemon) | 0.8%–3.2% |
| Persian Lime (Cold Pressed\Expressed) | 0.2%–2.4% |
| Ledum (*L. palustre*) | 0.2%–1.7% |

### Geranyl Butyrate

| | |
|---|---|
| Sweet Inula (Borneol CT) | 0.0%–2.0% |

### Germacrene

| | |
|---|---|
| Ylang Ylang (Solvent Extracted) | 10.3%–12.0% |
| Vilayti Tulsi (1,8-Cineole CT) | 0.0%–4.9% |

### Germacrene A

| | |
|---|---|
| Tamala (Trans-Sabinene Hydrate CT) | 11.3% |
| Palo Santo (Leaves, Aerial Parts) | 0.0%–3.9% |
| Ledum (*R. groenlandicum*) | 0.0%–1.0% |

### Germacrene B

| | |
|---|---|
| Pink Pepper (*S. terebinthifolius*, Fruits/Leaves, Bicyclogerm. CT) | 0.0%–13.7% |
| Zdravetz | 0.0%–11.3% |
| Ledum (*R. groenlandicum*) | 0.0%–9.4% |
| Juniper, Phoenicia (Berries) | 0.0%–7.3% |
| Citronella (*C. winteranius*) | 0.0%–6.8% |
| Cangerana (Wood) | 6.2% |
| White Turmeric (Distilled) | 0.6%–6.0% |
| Myrrh | 0.9%–4.3% |
| Chaste Tree (Berries) | 0.0%–4.2% |
| Copaiba (Leaves) | 1.4%–1.8% |

### Germacrene D

| | |
|---|---|
| Goldenrod | 28.4%–69.7% |
| Formosan Cypress (Neeldes, Germ. D CT) | 35.1%–41.2% |
| Wild Chamomile (*O. mixta, C. mixtrum*) | 0.5%–28.6% |
| Mugwort (Germacrene D CT) | 25.3% |
| Ylang Ylang (Madagascan II) | 15.1%–25.1% |
| Ylang Ylang Complete | 18.8%–24.4% |
| White Pine | 2.3%–19.6% |
| Ponderosa Pine | 0.1%–19.3% |
| Betony (Germacrene D-Spathulenol CT) | 19.3% |
| Maritime Pine (Needles, Alpha-Pinene CT) | 2.9%–19.2% |
| Copaiba (Leaves) | 4.0%–18.0% |
| Turkish Pine (Needles) | 0.0%–17.9% |
| Guava Leaf (Viridiflorol CT) | 2.7%–16.8% |
| Arnica (Flowers) | 12.5%–16.3% |
| Sweet Wormwood (Camphor CT) | 0.0%–15.6% |
| Mastic (Leaves) | 0.0%–14.3% |
| Betony (MLD-C CT) | 7.5%–13.5% |
| Ylang Ylang (Madagascan I) | 0.1%–13.5% |
| Mastic (NT\B, Germacrene D CT) | 13.5% |
| Clary Sage | 1.3%–13.3% |
| Betony (β-Phell.\α-Pinene CT) | 2.5%–13.2% |
| Betony (Bicyclogermacrene CT) | 4.2%–12.5% |
| Applemint (*M. rotun.*, β-Caryophyllene CT) | 12.3% |
| Pink Pepper (*S. molle*, Leaves, Bicyclogermacrene CT) | 7.4%–12.1% |
| Pink Pepper (*S. terebinthifolius*, Fruits, Myrc./Lim. CT) | 10.9%–11.5% |
| Yarrow (1,8-Cineole\Camphor CT) | 0.7%–11.5% |
| Betony (Alpha-Thujene CT) | 0.4%–11.3% |

| | |
|---|---|
| Canadian Fleabane | 0.0%–11.3% |
| Yarrow (Chamazulene CT) | 0.0%–11.2% |
| Black Pepper (Limonene CT) | 0.0%–11.0% |
| Gobre Salla | 0.0%–10.3% |
| Holy Basil (leaves) | 9.1%–10.2% |
| Helichrysum (*H. splendidum*, Delta-cadinene CT) | 3.4%–10.1% |
| Dwarf Pine (Needles, Needles/Twigs) | 0.7%–9.9% |
| Black Sage (Tricyclene CT) | 9.9% |
| Chinese Red Pine (Leaves) | 0.0%–9.8% |
| Juniper Berry | 1.1%–9.6% |
| Cangerana (Wood) | 9.3% |
| Feverfew | 0.0%–9.2% |
| Helichrysum (*H. splendidum*, Germacrene D-4-ol CT) | 9.0% |
| Kumquat (*F. margarita*, Leaves) | 0.0%–8.9% |
| Pink Pepper (*S. molle*, Leaves, Limonene CT) | 8.9% |
| Aleppo Pine (Needles) | 0.1%–8.8% |
| Aleppo Pine (Aerial Parts) | 0.0%–8.8% |
| Pink Pepper (*S. terebinthifolius*, Fruits, δ-3-Carene CT) | 0.0%–8.7% |
| Applemint (*M. suav.*, Carvone CT) | 0.0%–8.5% |
| Betony (Alpha-Zingiberene CT) | 8.4% |
| Cananga | 1.3%–8.3% |
| Melissa | 0.1%–8.3% |
| Turkish Pine (Needles/Twigs) | 3.3%–8.1% |
| Wormwood (Myrcene CT) | 0.6%–8.0% |
| Juniper (Needles) | 3.0%–7.8% |
| Spearmint (Piperitone Oxide CT) | 2.0%–7.5% |
| Pink Pepper (*S. terebinthifolius*, Fruits/Leaves, Bicyclogerm. CT) | 0.0%–7.4% |
| Spearmint (Piperitenone Oxide CT) | 4.2%–7.2% |
| Pink Pepper (*S. molle*, Leaves/Fruits, Sabinene CT) | 0.0%–7.1% |
| Applemint (*M. suav.*, Piperitenone CT) | 0.0%–7.0% |
| Hairy Basil (1-8-Cineole\Linalool CT) | 0.0%–6.9% |
| Yarrow (Sabinene CT) | 1.0%–6.8% |
| Applemint (*M. rotun.*, Pulegone CT) | 0.0%–6.8% |
| Grindelia | 0.0%–6.8% |
| Black Sage (Alpha-Pinene CT) | 0.0%–6.7% |
| Mugwort (Beta-Caryophyllene CT) | 6.7% |
| Spearmint (*M. crispa*, Rotundifolone CT) | 6.6% |
| Pine | 0.2%–6.5% |
| Wild Chamomile (*O. multicaulis*) | 0.0%–6.3% |
| Hyssop (Pinocamphone CT) | 0.7%–6.2% |
| Dwarf Pine (Twigs) | 0.1%–6.2% |
| Galangal (Greater, 1,8-Cineole CT) | 0.0%–6.1% |
| Kumquat (*F. margarita*, peel SD) | 0.0%–5.9% |
| Turkish Pine (Twigs) | 1.4%–5.5% |
| Spearmint (Pulegone-Menthone-Isomenthone CT) | 0.0%–5.3% |
| Pink Pepper (*S. molle*, Leaves, α-Phellandrene CT) | 0.0%–5.2% |
| Mastic (Twigs, Alpha-Pinene CT) | 5.2% |
| Hairy Basil (var. *pilosum* Terpinen-4-ol CT) | 0.5%–5.0% |
| Tansy (Beta-Thujone CT) | 0.0%–5.0% |
| Red Pine | 0.1%–4.9% |
| Hairy Basil (Linalool CT, Inflorescences) | 0.1%–4.8% |
| Applemint (*M. rotun.*, Piperitenone CT) | 0.6%–4.7% |
| Lavender (True English) | 0.2%–4.7% |
| Spearmint (Carvone CT) | 0.0%–4.7% |
| Copaiba | 1.2%–4.6% |
| Mugwort (Alpha-Thujone CT) | 4.5%–4.5% |
| Black Sage (Beta-Caryophyllene CT) | 4.5% |
| Mugwort (Artemisia Ketone CT) | 0.2%–4.4% |
| Great Mugwort | 0.6%–4.3% |
| Verbena (Myrcenone CT) | 0.0%–4.3% |
| Mastic (NT\B, Terpinene-4-ol CT) | 2.2%–4.1% |
| Tagetes (*T. erecta*, Flowers) | 1.5%–4.1% |
| Mastic (Twigs, Alpha-Pinene CT) | 4.1% |
| Hairy Basil (1,8-Cineole CT) | 0.0%–3.9% |

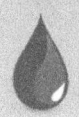

**Germacrene D—continued**

| | |
|---|---|
| Indian Borage (Carvacrol CT) | 0.0%–3.9% |
| Indian Borage (Delta-Cadinene CT) | 0.0%–3.9% |
| Verbena (Linalool CT) | 0.2%–3.8% |
| Maritime Pine (Needles, Beta-Cary. CT) | 0.0%–3.8% |
| Hairy Basil (Linalool CT, Leaves) | 3.5% |
| Wild Chamomile (*C. mixtus,* Sant. Alc. CT) | 1.5%–3.3% |
| Basil (Linalool CT) | 0.8%–3.3% |
| Mugwort (1,8-Cineole CT) | 0.0%–3.2% |
| Mastic (NT\B, Limonene CT) | 1.8%–3.1% |
| Spearmint (Linalool CT) | 1.9%–3.0% |
| Holy Basil (aerial parts, eugenol CT) | 0.1%–2.6% |
| Holy Basil (aerial parts or seeds, methyl eugenol CT) | 0.1%–2.3% |
| Verbena (Limonene\Piperitenone CT) | 0.0%–2.3% |
| Ravensara (Sabinene CT) | 1.5%–2.2% |
| Mastic (NT\B, Beta-Myrcene CT) | 0.8%–2.1% |
| Angelica Root | 0.2%–2.1% |
| Palo Santo (Wood) | 0.0%–2.1% |
| Chaste Tree (Berries) | 0.7%–1.6% |
| Ravensara (Methyl Chavicol CT) | 0.1%–1.6% |
| Ledum (*R. groenlandicum*) | 0.0%–1.5% |
| Ravensara (Alpha-Terpinene CT) | 0.5%–1.1% |

**Germacrene D-4-ol**

| | |
|---|---|
| Helichrysum (*H. splendidum,* Germacrene D-4-ol CT) | 17.1% |
| Galangal (False, Ethyl-p-Methoxycinnamate CT) | 0.0%–8.0% |
| African Bluegrass (Myrcene CT) | 0.8%–9.4% |
| Gobre Salla | 0.0%–6.7% |
| Indian Borage (Thymol CT) | 0.0%–5.7% |
| Pink Pepper (*S. terebinthifolius,* Fruits, δ-3-Carene CT) | 0.0%–5.3% |
| Juniper Berry | 0.0%–4.4% |
| Helichrysum (*H. splendidum,* Alpha-Terpinene CT) | 2.5% |

**Germacrene Isomer**

| | |
|---|---|
| Myrrh | 0.4%–6.5% |
| Ocotea (Leaves) | 1.8% |

**Germacrone ((E,E)-Germacrone)**

| | |
|---|---|
| Zdravetz | 37.4%–60.1% |
| Ledum (*R. groenlandicum*) | 0.0%–29.3% |
| White Turmeric (Distilled) | 0.0%–10.8% |
| Myrrh | 0.0%–5.8% |
| Wild Turmeric (Distilled) | 0.0%–4.9% |

**Geyrene**

| | |
|---|---|
| Rue (2-Undecanone CT) | 0.0%–10.4% |

**Globulol**

| | |
|---|---|
| Kunzea (Spathulenol\Globulol CT) | 15.3%–22.6% |
| Kunzea (Alpha-Pinene CT) | 0.5%–16.6% |
| Guava Leaf ((2E)-Hexenal CT) | 10.3% |
| Cangerana (Leaves) | 0.0%–9.8% |
| Pink Pepper (*S. molle,* Leaves, Bicyclogermacrene CT) | 0.0%–9.5% |
| Southern Blue Gum | 1.8%–5.5% |
| Cistus (*Viridiflorol-Trans-Pinocarveol CT*) | 0.0%–5.0% |
| Guava Leaf (Beta-Caryophyllene CT) | 0.0%–4.0% |
| Hairy Basil (Camphor CT) | 0.0%–3.8% |
| Spikenard (Ledene Oxide CT) | 1.9% |
| Blue Mallee (1,8-Cineole CT) | 0.0%–1.7% |

**Guaia-1(10),11-Dien-15-ol**

| | |
|---|---|
| Agarwood (*A. malaccensis*) | 0.0%–6.5% |

**Guaia-1(10),11-Diene-9-One**

| | |
|---|---|
| Agarwood (*A. sinensis*) | 0.0%–10.9% |

**Guaia-3,9-Dien-11-ol**

| | |
|---|---|
| Agarwood (Malaysian) | 0.0%–4.9% |

**Guaia-3,9-Diene**

| | |
|---|---|
| Agarwood (*A. crassna*) | 0.0%–7.8% |

**Guaiazulene**

| | |
|---|---|
| Blue Cypress | 0.1%–6.2% |

**Guaiadiene (Guaia-6,9-Diene)**

| | |
|---|---|
| Boldo (Ascaridole CT) | 0.0%–8.8% |
| Geranium | 0.0%–5.4% |

**Guaiol**

| | |
|---|---|
| Guaiacwood | 20.3%–26.8% |
| Blue Cypress (Wood) | 13.7%–15.3% |
| Agarwood (*A. sinensis*) | 0.0%–10.7% |
| Damiana (1,8-Cineole CT) | 0.0%–8.9% |
| Auracaria | 6.0%–6.9% |
| Chaste Tree (Leaves) | 0.0%–1.3% |
| Hyssop (Alpha-Pinene CT) | 1.0% |

**(-)-Hanamyol**

| | |
|---|---|
| Guaiacwood | 0.0%–2.5% |

**Hardwickiic Acid**

| | |
|---|---|
| Copaiba | 0.0%–9.0% |

**Hedycariol**

| | |
|---|---|
| Japanese Cedarwood (Bark) | 0.0%–6.2% |
| Japanese Cedarwood (Heartwood) | 0.0%–5.7% |

**Hedycaryol**

| | |
|---|---|
| Black Pepper (Eugenol CT) | 1.3%–9.1% |
| African Bluegrass (Linalool CT) | 5.4%–7.6% |

**Heneicosane**

| | |
|---|---|
| Rose (Indian) | 0.0%–19.7% |
| Rose (Iranian) | 0.0%–18.0% |
| Rose (Turkish) | 2.9%–8.9% |
| Rose (Bulgarian) | 1.1%–8.6% |

**Heptacosane**

| | |
|---|---|
| Moringa (Leaves, Pentacosane CT) | 0.0%–11.4% |

**Heptadecane (N-Heptadecane)**

| | |
|---|---|
| Chaste Tree (Berries) | 0.0%–12.5% |
| Rose (Indian) | 0.5%–6.0% |
| Rose (Bulgarian) | 2.7%–5.1% |
| Rose (Turkish) | 0.2%–0.5% |

**Herniarin**

| | |
|---|---|
| Tarragon (Methyl Chavicol CT) | 0.0%–4.3% |

**Hexacosane**

| | |
|---|---|
| Moringa (Leaves, Pentacosane CT) | 11.2%–13.9% |

**Hexadecane (N-Hexadecane)**

| | |
|---|---|
| Chaste Tree (Berries) | 0.0%–12.4% |

**Hexadecanoic Acid (n-Hexadecanoic Acid)**

| | |
|---|---|
| Moringa (Leaves, (E)-Phytol CT) | 13.8% |
| Moringa (Seeds, Cyclopentane CT) | 11.1% |
| Jasmine (Hydrodistilled) | 9.2% |
| Agarwood (*A. crassna*) | 0.0%–9.0% |
| Arnica (Roots, Thymol Derivatives CT) | 4.1%–7.2% |
| Agarwood (Malaysian) | 0.0%–7.0% |
| Valerian | 0.0%–5.0% |

**Hexadecanol**

| | |
|---|---|
| Rose (Iranian) | 0.0%–7.8% |

**Hexadecyl Acetate**

| | |
|---|---|
| Moringa (Flowers) | 21.0% |

**Hexafarnesyl Acetone**

| | |
|---|---|
| Sweet Inula (Borneol CT) | 0.0%–2.5% |

**Hexahydrofarnesyl Acetone**

| | |
|---|---|
| Moringa (Leaves, (E)-Phytol CT) | 8.5% |
| Arnica (Flowers) | 1.8%–3.1% |

**Himachalene Epoxide**

| | |
|---|---|
| Indian Borage (Beta-Caryophyllene CT) | 8.6% |
| Indian Borage (Thymol CT) | 0.0%–7.9% |

Indian Borage (Delta-Cadinene CT) 1.6%–4.9%

**Himachalol**

Cedarwood (Atlas) 5.3%–66.2%

Cedarwood (Himalayan, Wood) 12.1%–18.2%

**Hinesol**

Agarwood (*A. sinensis*) 0.3%–6.3%

**Hinokitiol (Beta-Thujaplicin)**

Western Red Cedar (Wood) 0.0%–2.0%

**Humulene Epoxide**

Guava Leaf (Beta-Caryophyllene CT) 0.0%–6.9%

Yarrow (Chamazulene CT) 0.1%–1.9%

**Humulene Epoxide II**

Hops 0.0%–7.9%

Black Sage (Caryophyllene Oxide CT) 3.1%–5.0%

Copaiba (Leaves) 1.7%–3.3%

Plai (2,6,9,9-Tetramethyl-2,6,10-Cyclodecatrien-1-one) 3.3%

**Humulene Oxide**

Aleppo Pine (Aerial Parts) 0.0%–6.7%

Wild Turmeric (Solvent Extracted) 6.4%

Mugwort (1,8-Cineole CT) 0.0%–1.2%

**Hydroxy Davanone**

Davana 0.0%–3.0%

**Hydroxy-Copalic Acid**

Copaiba 1.2%–5.1%

**Incensole Acetate**

Frankincense (*B. carterii*) 0.0%–2.3%

**Indole**

Jasmine Absolute (Benzyl Acetate CT) 0.7%–6.5%

**Isocalamendiol**

Calamus (Shyobunones CT) 2.0%–3.0%

**Isocalamendiol Isomer**

Calamus (Acorenone CT) 0.0%–4.7%

**Isoacorone**

Calamus (Acorenone CT) 0.0%–5.0%

**Isoalantolactone**

Elecampane 26.3%–36.9%

**Isoamyl 2-Methylbutyrate (3-Methylbutyl 2-methylbutyrate, 3-Methylbutyl 2-methylbutanoate, Butanoic acid, 2-methyl-, 3-methylbutyl ester)**

Khella (Aerial Parts, Isoamyl 2-Meth. CT) 10.3%–36.0%

Khella (Seeds) 23.4%–27.7%

Khella (Aerial Parts, 2-Mehtylbutyl Bu. CT) 10.0%

Chamomile (Roman) 3.9%–4.5%

**Ishwarane**

Katrafay (Ishwarane CT) 5.8%–22.1%

Katrafay (Alpha-Eudesmol CT) 0.0%–13.1%

**Iso-Alpha-Cedrene**

Chinese Cedarwood 0.0%–32.0%

**Isoamyl Angelate**

Chamomile (Roman) 3.7%–17.9%

**Isoamyl Dodecanoate**

Agarwood (*A. crassna*) 0.0%–13.4%

Agarwood (*A. malaccensis*) 0.0%–55.6%

**Isoamyl Isobutyrate (Isoamyl Isobutanoate, Isoamyl Isoblutyrate, 3-Methylbutyl Isobutyrate, Isoamyl2-Methylpropanoate)**

Chamomile (Roman) 5.3%–23.7%

Khella (Aerial Parts, Isoamyl 2-Meth. CT) 0.0%–6.8%

**Isoamyl Isovalerate (Isopentyl 3-methylbutanoate, 3-Methylbutyl 3-methylbutanoate, Isopentyl Isopentanoate)**

Khella (Aerial Parts, Isoamyl 2-Meth. CT) 0.0%–10.0%

**Isoamyl Tigliate**

Chamomile (Roman) 11.7%–19.9%

**Isoascaridole ((E)-Ascaridole, Trans-Ascaridole)**

Wormseed, American (Ascaridole CT) 0.5%–27.7%

**Isoborneol**

Juniper, Phoenicia (leaves, isoborneol CT) 20.9%

Mugwort (Camphor CT) 0.0%–8.2%

Lemon Catnip (Geraniol\Nerol CT) 0.0%–5.0%

Calendula (Alpha-Cadinol/Delta-Cadinene CT) 0.0%–3.8%

**Isobornyl 2-Methylbutyrate**

Mugwort (Camphor CT) 0.0%–5.3%

**Isobornyl Acetate**

Hinoki (needles) 0.0%–5.7%

**Isobornyl Isobutyrate**

Mugwort (Isobornyl Isobutyrate D CT) 38.1%

**Isobutyl Angelate**

Chamomile (Roman) 24.5%–36.0%

**Isobutyl Isobutyrate**

Chamomile (Roman) 1.4%–5.3%

**Isocaryophyllene**

Schisandra Fruit (*S. sphenanthera*, δ-Cad. CT) 5.6%

**Isocaryophyllene Oxide**

Yarrow (Chamazulene CT) 0.0%–2.6%

**Isofuranodiene**

Opoponax (*C. guidotti*) 0.0%–6.8%

**Isogeraniol**

Khella (Aerial Parts, 2,2-Dimethylbut. CT) 14.0%

Lemon Myrtle (Citral CT) 1.0%–4.2%

**Isogermacrene-D**

Ylang Ylang (French IV) 1.8%

**Isoledene**

Ravensara (Alpha-Terpinene CT) 0.0%–14.2%

Japanese Cedarwood (Heartwood) 0.0%–12.4%

Japanese Cedarwood (Sapwood) 0.0%–5.0%

Katrafay (Ishwarane CT) 0.9%–4.8%

**Isoleptospermone**

Manuka (Leptospermone CT) 1.4%–11.5%

**Isomenthol**

Pennyroyal (*M. fruticosa*, Isomenthol CT) 48.1%–67.1%

**Isomenthone (Cis-Menthone)**

Spearmint (Pulegone-Menthone-Isomenthone CT) 2.6%–31.4%

Buchu (*A. betulina*, Isomenthone CT) 4.6%–29.1%

Buchu (*A. crenulata*) 3.6%–27.6%

Pennyroyal (*M. fruticosa*, Pulegone CT) 15.2%–19.3%

Buchu (*A. betulina*, Menthone CT) 14.2%

Pennyroyal (*M. pulegium*) 0.0%–12.9%

Pennyroyal (*M. pulegioides*) 0.8%–8.6%

Geranium 0.0%–7.9%

Cornmint 2.4%–6.1%

Peppermint 0.0%–5.3%

Pennyroyal (*M. fruticosa*, Isomenthol CT) 0.0%–4.9%

Spearmint (Menthone CT) 2.6%

**Isomyrcenol**

Verbena (Linalool CT) 0.0%–6.2%

**Isoneral**

Lemon Myrtle (Citral CT) 0.6%–2.7%

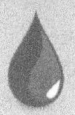

**Isophytol**

| | |
|---|---|
| Jasmine Absolute (Benzyl Acetate CT) | 0.0%–8.0% |
| Yarrow (Chamazulene CT) | 0.0%–2.9% |

**Isopimarol**

| | |
|---|---|
| Japanese Cedarwood (Twig) | 10.9%–25.6% |

**Isopinocamphone (Cis-Pinocamphone)**

| | |
|---|---|
| Hyssop (Pinocamphone CT) | 3.2%–27.5% |
| Hyssop (Linalool CT) | 0.1%–1.5% |

**Isopiperitenol**

| | |
|---|---|
| Gingergrass | 0.0%–13.4% |

**Isopiperitenol A**

| | |
|---|---|
| Ledum (*R. groenlandicum*) | 0.0%–3.1% |

**Isopiperitenol B**

| | |
|---|---|
| Ledum (*R. groenlandicum*) | 0.0%–1.9% |

**Isopropyl Hexadecanoate**

| | |
|---|---|
| German Chamomile | 0.0%–12.7% |

**Isopulegol**

| | |
|---|---|
| Lemon Eucalyptus | 8.2%–14.6% |
| Lemon Tea Tree (*L. petersonii*) | 0.0%–5.2% |

**Isopulegol Isomer (1568)**

| | |
|---|---|
| Lemon Myrtle (Citronellal CT) | 1.6%–2.5% |

**Isopulegol Isomer (1577)**

| | |
|---|---|
| Lemon Myrtle (Citronellal CT) | 0.0%–2.8% |

**Isopulegone**

| | |
|---|---|
| Pennyroyal (*M. pulegium*) | 1.4%–2.5% |

**Isospathulenol**

| | |
|---|---|
| Kunzea (Spathulenol\Globulol CT) | 2.9%–4.1% |
| Indian Borage (Beta-Caryophyllene CT) | 3.0% |

**Isovaleraldehyde**

| | |
|---|---|
| Niaouli (1,8-Cineole/Viridiflorol CT) | 0.0%–32.4% |
| Tea tree | 18.6%–28.0% |
| Thyme (Carvacrol CT) | 0.0%–26.8% |
| Thyme (Thymol CT) | 0.0%–23.5% |
| Lime (Cold-pressed/expressed) | 0.1%–20.6% |
| Lemon (Cold-pressed/expressed) | 1.0%–18.0% |
| Lime (Distilled) | 0.0%–16.5% |
| Marjoram | 6.9%–14.3% |
| Lemon (Distilled) | 0.1%–14.1% |
| Coriander | 4.6%–13.6% |
| Bay Laurel | 0.0%–10.5% |

**Isovaleric Acid**

| | |
|---|---|
| Valerian | 0.0%–13.1% |

**Isovaleric Acid 3-Phenylpropyl Ester**

| | |
|---|---|
| Sweet Inula (Borneol CT) | 0.0%–2.1% |

**Italicene**

| | |
|---|---|
| Helichrysum (*H. italicum*) | 0.0%–7.1% |
| Helichrysum (ssp. *microphyllum*) | 1.4%–5.1% |

**Italidiones**

| | |
|---|---|
| Helichrysum (*H. italicum*) | 0.0%–5.1% |
| Helichrysum (ssp. *italicum*) | 0.0%–4.8% |

**Jasmine Lactone**

| | |
|---|---|
| Jasmine Absolute (Benzyl Benzoate CT) | 3.1%–8.5% |

**Jinkho-Eremol**

| | |
|---|---|
| Agarwood (*A. malaccensis*) | 0.0%–6.5% |
| Agarwood (*A. crassna*) | 2.3%–4.5% |

**Kauran-16-ol**

| | |
|---|---|
| Japanese Cedarwood (Twig) | 0.0%–3.4% |

**Karanone**

| | |
|---|---|
| Agarwood (*A. malaccensis*) | 0.0%–4.9% |

**Kaurenoic Acid**

| | |
|---|---|
| Copaiba | 0.0%–10.1% |

**Kessane**

| | |
|---|---|
| Valerian | 0.0%–8.2% |
| Celery Leaf | 0.0%–3.5% |
| Celery Seed | 0.0%–3.3% |

**Kessyl Acetate**

| | |
|---|---|
| Valerian | 0.0%–4.7% |

**Khusimol (Zizanol)**

| | |
|---|---|
| Vetiver | 3.4%–24.6% |

**Kongol**

| | |
|---|---|
| Yarrow (1,8-Cineole\Camphor CT) | 0.0%–2.3% |

**Lavandulol**

| | |
|---|---|
| Wormwood (Trans-Sabinene Hydrate CT) | 0.0%–5.5% |
| Lavender (French) | 0.0%–4.3% |

**Lavandulyl Acetate (Lavandulol Acetate)**

| | |
|---|---|
| Lavender (True English) | 2.7%–6.4% |
| Lavender (Polish) | 4.5%–5.7% |
| Lavender (Indian) | 0.6%–4.5% |
| Lavender (Bulgarian) | 2.5%–4.4% |
| Lavandin (Grosso) | 1.6%–2.9% |

**Ledene Oxide**

| | |
|---|---|
| Spikenard (Ledene Oxide CT) | 13.0% |

**Ledol**

| | |
|---|---|
| Ledum (*L. palustre*) | 21.0%–32.2% |
| Cistus (Alpha-Pinene CT) | 0.0%–13.8% |
| Valerian | 0.0%–12.1% |
| Spanish Sage | 0.0%–10.8% |
| Cistus (*Viridiflorol-Trans-Pinocarveol CT*) | 0.4%–6.6% |
| Kunzea (Spathulenol\Globulol CT) | 4.8%–6.3% |
| Guava Leaf ((E)-Nerolidol CT) | 5.5% |

**Lendene**

| | |
|---|---|
| Japanese Cedarwood (16-Kaurene CT) | 0.0%–3.8% |

**Leptospermone**

| | |
|---|---|
| Manuka (Leptospermone CT) | 8.7%–29.4% |
| Kunzea (Alpha-Pinene CT) | 0.1%–2.1% |

**Limonene (*d*-Limonene, *l*-limonene)**

| | |
|---|---|
| Orange–Bitter (Cold-pressed/expressed) | 90.3%–98.7% |
| Lemon (Cold-pressed/expressed) | 38.1%–95.8% |
| Orange (Cold-pressed/expressed) | 85.4%–95.4% |
| Grapefruit (Cold-pressed/expressed) | 86.3%–95.3% |
| Kumquat (*F. margarita*, peel CP) | 95.1% |
| Kumquat (*F. margarita*, peel SD) | 41.6%–94.9% |
| Tangerine (Cold-pressed/expressed) | 87.1%–94.7% |
| Kumquat (*F. margarita*, Fruit CT Limonene) | 1.9%–94.6% |
| Lime (Cold-pressed/expressed) | 39.9%–94.4% |
| Orange (Distilled) | 81.5%–93.7% |
| Kumquat (*C. japonica*, Peel CP) | 93.4% |
| Tangerine (Distilled) | 45.7%–92.4% |
| Mediterranean Mandarin (Hydrodistilled) | 70.5%–90.0% |
| Grapefruit (Distilled) | 70.9%–88.6% |
| Canadian Fleabane | 31.2%–81.1% |
| Yuzu | 63.1%–79.4% |
| Mediterranean Mandarin (CP\Expressed) | 65.3%–77.6% |
| Kabosu | 70.5%–75.5% |
| Lemon (Distilled) | 61.8%–73.8% |
| Palo Santo (Wood) | 60.7%–68.7% |
| Citron (Distilled) | 35.4%–67.2% |
| Ledum (*R. groenlandicum*) | 0.3%–67.2% |
| Tagetes (*T. minuta*, Limonene CT) | 13.0%–66.3% |
| Celery Seed | 58.4%–63.5% |
| Celery Leaf | 16.0%–63.1% |
| Persian Lime (Distilled) | 47.5%–62.0% |
| Persian Lime (Cold Pressed\Expressed) | 40.3%–59.8% |

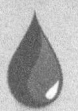

| | |
|---|---|
| Bergamot (Distilled) | 31.7%–59.2% |
| Citron (Fingered, Distilled) | 52.4%–59.0% |
| Citron (Cold-pressed/Expressed) | 44.5%–56.6% |
| Elemi | 54.6%–56.0% |
| Blue Cypress (Leaves) | 35.9%–55.6% |
| Silver Fir (A. alba) | 7.5%–54.7% |
| Juniper (Needles) | 2.8%–53.9% |
| Lime (Distilled) | 49.7%–53.8% |
| Petitgrain (Lime) | 22.1%–53.4% |
| Bergamot (Cold-pressed/expressed) | 10.5%–53.2% |
| Mastic (NT\B, Limonene CT) | 46.2%–51.8% |
| Verbena (Limonene\Piperitenone CT) | 27.5%–51.7% |
| Myrtle (Limonene CT) | 23.4%–44.2% |
| Pink Pepper (S. terebinthifolius, Fruits, Limonene CT) | 31.8%–44.1% |
| Dill Seed | 14.7%–44.1% |
| Guava Leaf (Limonene CT) | 27.1%–42.1% |
| Tsauri Grass | 7.7%–42.0% |
| Pink Pepper (S. molle, Leaves, Limonene CT) | 41.9% |
| Black Pepper (Limonene CT) | 10.3%–38.4% |
| Caraway | 13.1%–35.5% |
| Petitgrain (Lemon) | 17.8%–33.5% |
| Frankincense (B. sacra) | 5.6%–33.5% |
| White Verbena (Carvone\Limonene CT) | 18.5%–33.2% |
| Dill (Flowers) | 33.2% |
| Rabbitbrush (var. consimilis) | 33.2% |
| Palo Santo (Leaves, Aerial Parts) | 26.5%–30.7% |
| Kaffir Lime Peel | 5.3%–30.7% |
| Engelmann Spruce | 1.6%–30.2% |
| Gingergrass | 6.0%–30.1% |
| Galangal (Greater, Piperitenone CT) | 29.6% |
| Applemint (M. suav., Carvone CT) | 22.6%–29.2% |
| Buchu (A. betulina, Isomenthone CT) | 11.6%–28.2% |
| Neroli (C. aurantium) | 9.2%–27.5% |
| White Spruce (Needles) | 8.2%–26.5% |
| Verbena (Linalool CT) | 0.5%–26.2% |
| Ferula (Limonene CT) | 26.0% |
| Spearmint (Carvone CT) | 5.8%–25.2% |
| White Spruce (Needles & Twigs) | 9.8%–25.1% |
| Blue Spruce | 0.0%–24.8% |
| Betony (MLD-C CT) | 15.3%–24.5% |
| Tsauri Grass (var. madagascariensis) | 5.1%–24.0% |
| Myrtle (Alpha-Pinene CT) | 0.3%–23.9% |
| Boldo (Ascaridole CT, no 1,8-cineole) | 18.5%–23.2% |
| White Fir (A. Concolor) | 1.6%–23.0% |
| Chaste Tree (Berries) | 0.8%–23.0% |
| May Chang (Citral CT) | 0.7%–22.9% |
| Ravensara (Limonene CT) | 13.9%–22.5% |
| Fennel (Methyl Chavicol CT) | 0.1%–22.4% |
| Ravensara (Alpha-Terpinene CT) | 14.8%–21.8% |
| Spearmint (Scotch, M. cardiaca) | 6.8%–21.6% |
| Pink Pepper (S. molle, Fruits, α-Phellandrene CT) | 0.0%–20.9% |
| Frankincense (B. carterii) | 1.0%–20.4% |
| Dill (Aerial Parts, Carvone CT) | 6.9%–19.9% |
| Xanthoxylum | 8.2%–19.8% |
| Blue Mountain Sage (Limonene CT) | 19.3% |
| Tagetes (T. patula, Limonene CT) | 13.6%–19.2% |
| Aleppo Pine (Aerial Parts) | 0.0%–18.7% |
| Aleppo Pine (Twigs) | 18.7% |
| Lemon Verbena (Leaves and stems) | 3.7%–18.6% |
| Rabbitbrush (var. albicaulis) | 18.6% |
| Juniper (J. recurva, Needles) | 0.2%–18.4% |
| Mastic (NT\B, Alpha-Pinene CT) | 5.2%–17.8% |
| White Spruce (Oleoresin) | 3.6%–17.8% |
| Black Pepper (Beta-Caryophyllene CT) | 2.0%–17.4% |
| Pink Pepper (S. terebinthifolius, Fruits, δ-3-Carene CT) | 0.0%–17.4% |
| Niaouli (M. viridiflora, Terpinen-4-ol CT) | 17.4% |
| Buchu (A. crenulata) | 2.1%–17.2% |
| Hemp (Myrcene CT) | 0.2%–17.2% |
| Pink Pepper (S. terebinthifolius, Fruits, Myrc./Lim. CT) | 14.2%–17.0% |
| Boldo (1,8-Cineole\Para-Cymene\Limonene CT) | 2.0%–17.0% |
| Cedarwood (Himalayan, Needles) | 17.0% |
| Grindelia | 3.6%–16.8% |
| Fennel (Trans-Anethole CT) | 0.3%–16.5% |
| Rabbitbrush (var. glabratus) | 16.5% |
| Angelica Root | 0.0%–16.4% |
| Boldo (Ascaridole CT) | 0.0%–16.1% |
| Verbena (Myrcenone CT) | 0.0%–16.0% |
| Lemon Verbena (Leaves) | 5.6%–15.9% |
| Hemp (Beta-Caryophyllene CT) | 4.1%–15.8% |
| Balsam Fir | 1.8%–15.6% |
| Black Pepper (Delta-3-Carene CT) | 14.1%–15.2% |
| Niaouli (1,8-Cineole CT) | 0.5%–15.0% |
| Juniper (Chinese) | 3.9%–14.2% |
| Tagetes (T. minuta, Piperitone CT) | 13.7% |
| Vilayti Tulsi (Fenchone CT) | 0.8%–13.5% |
| Tamala ((E)-Cinnamaldehyde\Cinn. Ac. CT) | 0.3%–13.5% |
| Turkish Pine (Twigs) | 1.5%–13.4% |
| Pink Pepper (S. molle, Leaves, α-Phellandrene CT) | 0.0%–13.4% |
| Rhododendron (Aerial Parts) | 7.1%–13.3% |
| Dill Leaves | 13.3% |
| Helichrysum (ssp. italicum) | 0.2%–12.8% |
| Hinoki (Taiwan Cypress, wood) | 0.1%–12.8% |
| Petitgrain (Mandarin) | 0.0%–12.6% |
| Goldenrod | 0.2%–12.5% |
| Tagetes (T. minuta, Dihydrotagetone CT) | 5.4%–12.3% |
| Dill (Aerial Parts, Alpha-Phellandrene CT) | 3.7%–11.8% |
| Savory (Wild, Linalool CT) | 1.8%–11.0% |
| Rhododendron (Leaves) | 11.3% |
| Hinoki (needles) | 2.6%–11.2% |
| Citronella (C. nardus) | 0.0%–11.0% |
| Wild Marjoram (1,8-Cineole CT) | 1.1%–10.8% |
| Peppermint | 0.2%–10.8% |
| Hairy Basil (Camphor CT) | 6.8%–10.6% |
| Rosemary (Beta-Myrcene CT) | 2.9%–10.6% |
| Mastic (Leaves) | 0.0%–10.6% |
| Spearmint (M. crispa, Rotundifolone CT) | 10.6% |
| Tagetes (T. erecta, Leaves) | 1.4%–10.4% |
| Spanish Sage | 0.0%–10.4% |
| White Spruce (Branches) | 8.0%–10.2% |
| Utah Juniper (Needles/Twigs) | 7.5%–10.2% |
| Kumquat (C. japonica, Leaves CT Beta-Pinene) | 10.2% |
| White Verbena (Citral CT) | 0.0%–10.2% |
| Eucalyptus (E. globulus) | 0.4%–10.1% |
| Neroli (C. sinensis) | 4.0%–10.0% |
| Niaouli (Viridiflorol CT) | 1.0%–10.0% |
| Japanese Cedarwood (Bark) | 0.0%–9.7% |
| Mastic (Twigs, Alpha-Pinene CT) | 9.6% |
| Pink Pepper (S. molle, Leaves, Epi-Bicyclosesquiphell. CT) | 9.2% |
| Camphor (Camphor CT) | 0.0%–9.0% |
| Mastic (NT\B, Germacrene D CT) | 9.0% |
| Cajeput (Cajuput) | 4.5%–8.9% |
| Myrtle (Myrtenyl Acetate CT) | 4.1%–8.9% |
| Utah Juniper (Needles/Berries) | 8.9% |
| Tagetes (T. erecta, Aerial Parts) | 7.8%–8.6% |
| Ravensara (Sabinene CT) | 7.2%–8.5% |
| Frankincense (B. serrata) | 0.7%–8.5% |
| Siam Wood (Leaves) | 8.5% |
| Oriental Arborvitae (Needles) | 3.6%–8.2% |

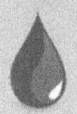

### Limonene—continued

| | |
|---|---|
| Betony (Bicyclogermacrene CT) | 1.9%–8.2% |
| Wild Chamomile (*O. mixta, C. mixtrum*) | 0.1%–8.0% |
| Verbena (Myrcene CT) | 5.3%–7.7% |
| Black Pepper (Eugenol CT) | 4.9%–7.7% |
| Hinoki (needles and twigs) | 7.6% |
| Maritime Pine (Needles, Alpha-Pinene CT) | 0.8%–7.5% |
| Hairy Basil (var. *pilosum* Eugenol CT) | 7.5% |
| May Chang (Neral CT) | 7.4% |
| Blue Yarrow (Artemisia Ketone CT) | 7.4% |
| Rosemary (Verbenone CT) | 0.0%–7.1% |
| Rosalina (1,8-Cineole CT) | 0.0%–7.1% |
| Tagetes (*T. minuta*, (Z)-Beta-Ocimene CT) | 0.0%–7.1% |
| Pink Pepper (*S. molle*, Leaves/Fruits, Sabinene CT) | 3.8%–7.0% |
| Nutmeg (East Indian) | 2.0%–7.0% |
| Tagetes (*T. erecta*, Flowers) | 2.5%–6.9% |
| Japanese Cedarwood (16-Kaurene CT) | 1.1%–6.8% |
| Sage (Beta-Thujone CT) | 1.3%–6.5% |
| Star Anise | 0.4%–6.5% |
| Allspice (Leaves, Eugenol CT) | 0.0%–6.5% |
| Tagetes (*T. patula*, Aerial Parts) | 6.3% |
| Tsuga | 3.4%–6.2% |
| Sage (Camphor CT) | 0.8%–6.2% |
| Applemint (*M. suav.*, Italian) | 0.0%–6.2% |
| Savory (Wild, Carvacrol CT) | 0.0%–6.2% |
| Basil (Methyl Eugenol CT) | 0.1%–6.2% |
| Mugwort (Isobornyl Isobutyrate D CT) | 6.2% |
| Blue Mountain Sage (Delta-3-Carene CT) | 2.8%–6.1% |
| May Chang (Citronellal CT) | 2.2%–6.1% |
| Big Badja Gum | 5.6%–6.0% |
| Hyssop (Linalool CT) | 5.0%–6.0% |
| Niaouli (Viridiflorol/ Para-cymene/1,8-cineole CT) | 1.0%–6.0% |
| Wild Chamomile (*O. multicaulis*) | 0.1%–6.0% |
| Vilayti Tulsi (Sabinene CT) | 0.0%–5.9% |
| Gully Gum | 0.0%–5.9% |
| Juniper (*J. recurva*, Berries) | 5.9% |
| Turkish Pine (Resin) | 5.8% |
| Hyssop (Pinocamphone CT) | 0.0%–5.6% |
| Spruce (Black) | 2.6%–5.5% |
| Siberian Fir | 0.0%–5.5% |
| Lemon Verbena (Stems) | 3.2%–5.4% |
| Tarragon (Methyl Chavicol CT) | 2.8%–5.4% |
| Cypress | 2.0%–5.4% |
| Chinese Red Pine (Twigs) | 1.8%–5.3% |
| Spearmint (Pulegone-Menthone-Isomenthone CT) | 0.7%–5.2% |
| Mastic (NT\B, Terpinene-4-ol CT) | 4.0%–5.2% |
| Juniper Berry | 2.9%–5.1% |
| Juniper, Phoenicia (needles) | 0.0%–5.0% |
| Japanese Cedarwood (Alpha-Pinene CT) | 0.0%–5.0% |
| Mugwort (Artemisia Ketone CT) | 0.9%–4.8% |
| Parsley (Whole Plant) | 0.6%–4.8% |
| Spearmint (Piperitone Oxide CT) | 0.4%–4.8% |
| Chaste Tree (Leaves) | 0.1%–4.8% |
| Cornmint | 0.6%–4.7% |
| Chinese Red Pine (Leaves) | 0.0%–4.7% |
| Oriental Arborvitae (Berries) | 0.0%–4.7% |
| Rabbitbrush (var. *nauseosa*) | 4.7% |
| Turmeric (Leaves) | 0.0%–4.6% |
| Rosemary (Bornyl Acetate CT) | 0.1%–4.6% |
| Blue Mountain Sage (Alpha-Bisabolol CT) | 2.0%–4.5% |
| Ravensara (Methyl Eugenol CT) | 0.7%–4.5% |
| Eucalyptus (*E. radiata*) | 0.5%–4.5% |
| Douglas Fir (Needles & Twigs) | 0.4%–4.5% |
| Ravintsara (Camphor CT) | 0.0%–4.5% |

| | |
|---|---|
| Tagetes (*T. patula*, Flowers) | 4.5 % |
| Nutmeg (West Indian) | 2.9%–4.4% |
| Southern Blue Gum | 0.0%–4.4% |
| Holy Basil (Aerial Parts, Estragole CT) | 0.0%–4.4% |
| Pink Pepper (*S. molle*, Leaves, Elemol/Beta-Eudesmol CT) | 4.4% |
| Black Cumin (Trans-Anethole CT) | 4.3%–4.3% |
| Pennyroyal (*M. pulegium*) | 0.9%–4.3% |
| Savin (Needles & Branches) | 0.6%–4.3% |
| Hairy Basil (var. *pilosum* Terpinen-4-ol CT) | 0.1%–4.3% |
| Rue (2-Undecanone CT) | 0.0%–4.3% |
| Ravensara (Methyl Chavicol CT) | 0.1%–4.2% |
| Catnip (Nepetalactone CT) | 0.0%–4.1% |
| Coriander | 0.1%–4.0% |
| Bay (West Indies) | 0.1%–4.0% |
| Guava Leaf (Beta-Caryophyllene CT) | 0.0%–4.0% |
| Valerian | 0.0%–4.0% |
| Kanuka | 0.0%–3.9% |
| Frankincense (*B. papyrifera*) | 1.4%–3.8% |
| Mastic (Gum Resin) | 0.2%–3.8% |
| Ponderosa Pine | 0.1%–3.7% |
| White Sage | 1.5%–3.5% |
| Mugwort (Chrysanthenyl Acetate CT) | 3.5% |
| Juniper, Phoenicia (leaves, isoborneol CT) | 3.5% |
| Rosalina (Linalool CT) | 0.0%–3.4% |
| Applemint (*M. suav.*, Piperitenone CT) | 0.6%–3.3% |
| Maritime Pine (Gum Resin) | 1.4%–3.2% |
| Tamala (Linalool CT) | 3.2% |
| Rosemary (Camphor CT) | 2.8%–3.1% |
| Pennyroyal (*M. fruticosa*, Pulegone CT) | 1.2%–3.0% |
| White Pine | 1.2%–3.0% |
| Mugwort (Alpha-Thujone CT) | 0.0%–2.7% |
| Hyssop (Alpha-Pinene CT) | 2.7% |
| Black Cumin (Para-Cymene CT) | 0.0%–2.6% |
| Sage (Alpha-Thujone CT) | 1.1%–2.4% |
| Frankincense (*B. frereana*) | 0.0%–2.4% |
| Black Cumin (Thymoquinone CT) | 0.7%–2.3% |
| Spearmint (Piperitenone Oxide CT) | 1.1%–1.8% |
| Spearmint (Cis-Ocimenone CT) | 1.5% |
| Blue Mallee (1,8-Cineole CT) | 0.2%–1.3% |
| Lemon Eucalyptus | 0.5%–1.1% |
| Honey Myrtle | 0.6%–1.0% |
| Ravensara (1,8-Cineole CT) | 0.0%–0.8% |

### Linoleic Acid

| | |
|---|---|
| Arnica (Roots, Thymol Derivatives CT) | 2.9%–3.3% |

### Limonene + Beta-Phellandrene

| | |
|---|---|
| Dwarf Pine (Needles, Needles/Twigs) | 13.1%–27.9% |
| Dwarf Pine (Twigs) | 12.7%–24.3% |

### Linalool (Linalol, Beta-Linalool, Linalyl Alcohol)

| | |
|---|---|
| Rosewood (Wood) | 73.0%–99.0% |
| Saro (1,8-Cineole CT) | 72.5%–95.8% |
| Ravintsara (Linalool CT) | 87.2%–95.3% |
| Thyme (Linalool CT) | 32.2%–93.8% |
| Magnolia (Flowers) | 66.9%–91.7% |
| Hairy Basil (Linalool CT, Inflorescences) | 61.0%–88.1% |
| Camphor (Linalool CT) | 40.3%–87.3% |
| White Verbena (Linalool CT) | 53.4%–84.7% |
| Rosewood (Leaves) | 82.5% |
| Magnolia (Leaves) | 76.6%–80.1% |
| Coriander | 51.0%–79.9% |
| Spearmint (Linalool CT) | 65.2%–75.3% |
| Ghandi Root | 32.4%–71.2% |
| Xanthoxylum | 57.0%–70.6% |
| Basil (Linalool CT) | 45.3%–69.3% |

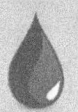

| | |
|---|---|
| Wild Marjoram (Linalool CT) | 59.3%–69.0% |
| Lavender (French) | 9.3%–68.8% |
| Monarda (Linalool CT) | 45.7%–67.0% |
| Petitgrain (Bergamot/Bitter Orange) | 18.6%–66.0% |
| Verbena (Linalool CT) | 27.3%–65.2% |
| Tamala (Linalool\(E)-Cinnamaldehyde CT) | 22.7%–62.0% |
| Bergamot Mint | 4.8%–60.9% |
| Tamala (Linalool CT) | 60.7% |
| Rosalina (Linalool CT) | 36.3%–56.2% |
| Hyssop (Linalool CT) | 48.0%–51.7% |
| Lavender (True English) | 24.5%–50.6% |
| Hairy Basil (var. *pilosum* Linalool CT) | 29.7%–50.1% |
| Lavender (Bulgarian) | 25.4%–47.3% |
| Lavandin (Dutch) | 42.5%–47.0% |
| Lavender (Munstead) | 37.8%–46.1% |
| Lavandin (Giant) | 34.9%–45.7% |
| Lavender (Italian) | 33.3%–45.0% |
| Spike Lavender | 27.2%–43.1% |
| Lavandin (Super) | 23.0%–41.8% |
| Thyme (Geraniol CT) | 0.4%–40.8% |
| Lavandin (Abrialis) | 19.6%–39.6% |
| Clary Sage | 12.8%–38.6% |
| Basil (Methyl Eugenol CT) | 0.1%–37.5% |
| Lavender (Indian) | 26.7%–37.1% |
| Lavandin (Grosso) | 25.7%–35.5% |
| Applemint (*M. suav.*, Linalool CT) | 35.3% |
| Kumquat (*C. japonica*, Leaves CT Linalool) | 35.1% |
| Khella (Seeds) | 22.0%–35.0% |
| Lavender (Polish) | 27.3%–34.7% |
| Neroli (*C. aurantium*) | 26.6%–34.4% |
| Holy Basil (Methyl Chavicol CT) | 23.9%–33.1% |
| Thyme (Thuyanol CT) | 2.4%–32.5% |
| Khella (Aerial Parts, Isoamyl 2-Meth. CT) | 4.9%–32.0% |
| Neroli (*C. sinensis*) | 16.4%–31.8% |
| Bergamot (Distilled) | 9.5%–31.8% |
| Niaouli ((E)-Nerolidol CT) | 0.0%–30.0% |
| Ylang Ylang (I Madagascan) | 11.7%–30.0% |
| Thyme (Carvacrol CT) | 1.1%–29.9% |
| African Bluegrass (Linalool CT) | 28.0%–29.6% |
| Fragonia (Alpha-Pinene CT) | 18.3%–25.3% |
| Mountain Savory (Carvacrol CT) | 0.5%–24.8% |
| Cedarwood (Himalayan, Needles) | 24.5% |
| Khella (Aerial Parts, 2-Mehtylbutyl Bu. CT) | 23.5% |
| Ravintsara (Camphor CT) | 0.5%–22.9% |
| Camphor (Camphor CT) | 0.6%–22.3% |
| Holy Basil (Aerial Parts, Estragole CT) | 0.0%–21.8% |
| Ravensara (Sabinene CT) | 6.5%–21.4% |
| Bergamot (Cold-pressed/expressed) | 1.8%–20.3% |
| Hairy Basil (Linalool CT, Leaves) | 20.2% |
| Hairy Basil (1,8-Cineole\Linalool CT) | 19.1%–19.6% |
| Thyme (Alpha-pinene CT) | 0.4%–19.2% |
| Verbena (Myrcene CT) | 1.7%–19.1% |
| Tamala ((E)-Cinnamaldehyde CT) | 2.9%–18.5% |
| Hairy Basil (var. *pilosum* Terpinen-4-ol CT) | 0.1%–18.5% |
| Myrtle (Alpha-Pinene CT) | 0.7%–18.4% |
| Savory (Wild, Linalool CT) | 17.2%–18.2% |
| Bay Laurel | 0.4%–17.7% |
| Myrtle (1,8-Cineole CT) | 3.2%–17.6% |
| Shell Ginger (1,8-Cineole CT) | 0.0%–17.1% |
| Geranium | 0.3%–16.0% |
| Wild Marjoram (1,8-Cineole CT) | 1.8%–15.7% |
| Myrtle (Limonene CT) | 1.0%–15.4% |
| Oregano (*Terpinen-4-ol CT*) | 2.1%–15.2% |
| Helichrysum (ssp microphyllum) | 0.0%–14.9% |
| Fragonia (Balanced CT) | 1.7%–14.7% |
| Thyme (Thymol CT) | 1.1%–13.4% |
| Tamala (Beta-Caryophyllene CT) | 13.4% |
| Myrtle (Myrtenyl Acetate CT) | 10.1%–13.3% |
| Jasmine Absolute (Benzyl Acetate CT) | 3.0%–12.7% |
| Ylang Ylang (II Madagascan) | 3.9%–12.2% |
| Hairy Basil (Citral CT) | 2.0%–12.2% |
| Khella (Aerial Parts, 2,2-Dimethylbut. CT) | 12.1% |
| Spearmint (Carvone CT) | 0.3%–11.3% |
| Ylang Ylang (Complete) | 1.3%–10.6% |
| Cardamom (Alpha-Terpinyl Acetate CT) | 0.0%–10.2% |
| Black Cumin (Para-Cymene CT) | 0.0%–9.9% |
| Kumquat (*C. japonica*, Leaves CT Beta-Pinene) | 9.8% |
| Petitgrain (Mandarin) | 0.0%–9.6% |
| Ylang Ylang (I French) | 9.0% |
| Basil (Methyl Chavicol CT) | 0.9%–8.6% |
| Cinnamon (leaves) | 2.5%–8.5% |
| Lemon Tea Tree (*L. liversidgei*) | 2.0%–8.5% |
| Verbena (Myrcene CT) | 0.1%–8.4% |
| Kumquat (*F. margarita*, Leaves) | 1.0%–8.2% |
| Petitgrain (Lime) | 0.9%–8.1% |
| Nutmeg (East Indian) | 0.2%–7.4% |
| Wormwood (Beta-Thujone CT) | 0.4%–7.3% |
| Lemon Basil | 4.5%–7.2% |
| Wormwood (Myrcene CT) | 5.3%–7.0% |
| Rosemary (Verbenone CT) | 1.0%–6.6% |
| Savory (Wild, Carvacrol CT) | 0.1%–6.6% |
| Hairy Basil ((E)-Methyl Cinnamate CT) | 0.0%–6.6% |
| Blue Yarrow (Artemisia Ketone CT) | 6.6% |
| Chaste Tree (Berries) | 0.2%–6.5% |
| Engelmann Spruce | 0.0%–6.5% |
| Kaffir Lime Petitgain | 2.9%–6.4% |
| Cardamom (1,8-Cineole CT) | 0.6%–6.4% |
| Wild Turmeric (Solvent Extracted) | 6.4% |
| Cinnamon Bark | 0.0%–6.3% |
| Wormwood ((Z)-Epoxy Ocimene CT) | 0.0%–5.9% |
| Ravensara (Limonene CT) | 3.0%–5.7% |
| Cananga | 1.0%–5.6% |
| Rosalina (1,8-Cineole CT) | 0.0%–5.1% |
| Wormwood (Sabinene CT) | 3.9%–4.9% |
| Wormwood (Trans-Sabinyl Acetate CT) | 0.3%–4.8% |
| Ginger | 0.0%–4.8% |
| Yuzu | 1.4%–4.7% |
| Ravensara (Methyl Eugenol CT) | 0.4%–4.7% |
| Wormwood (Alpha-Thujone CT) | 0.1%–4.7% |
| Ravensara (Alpha-Terpinene CT) | 3.3%–4.5% |
| Kunzea (Spathulenol\Globulol CT) | 0.8%–4.3% |
| White Verbena (Camphor CT) | 0.0%–4.1% |
| Black Pepper (Beta-Caryophyllene CT) | 0.5%–4.0% |
| Wormwood (Trans-Sabinene Hydrate CT) | 0.0%–4.0% |
| Black Pepper (Limonene CT) | 0.6%–3.9% |
| Mountain Savory (Thymol CT) | 0.4%–3.2% |
| Ocotea (Flowers Calices) | 0.0%–3.2% |
| Manuka (Selinene/Beta-Elemene CT) | 3.2% |
| Rosemary (Camphor CT) | 0.0%–3.1% |
| Palmarosa | 0.8%–2.6% |
| Lemon Eucalyptus | 0.1%–2.2% |
| Petitgrain (Lemon) | 1.4%–2.1% |
| Ravensara (Methyl Chavicol CT) | 0.7%–1.9% |
| Orange–Bitter (Cold-pressed/expressed) | 0.0%–1.6% |
| Orange (Distilled) | 0.1%–1.4% |
| Lemon Myrtle (Citral CT) | 0.1%–1.0% |

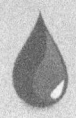

**Linalyl Acetate**

| | |
|---|---|
| Bergamot Mint | 23.8%–67.9% |
| Clary Sage | 16.9%–60.8% |
| Lavender (French) | 1.2%–59.4% |
| Petitgrain (Bergamot/Bitter Orange) | 12.4%–50.0% |
| Lavender (Indian) | 35.4%–47.6% |
| Lavandin (Super) | 20.4%–45.0% |
| Lavender (True English) | 3.7%–45.0% |
| Lavender (Italian) | 31.7%–41.2% |
| Bergamot (Cold-pressed/expressed) | 15.6%–40.5% |
| Lavender (Bulgarian) | 19.9%–37.6% |
| Lavandin (Grosso) | 26.2%–36.7% |
| Lavandin (Abrialis) | 18.6%–28.0% |
| Marjoram | 3.8%–26.1% |
| Lavender (Polish) | 19.7%–22.4% |
| Bergamot (Distilled) | 10.7%–16.8% |
| Basil (Linalool CT) | 0.0%–16.0% |
| Lavender (Munstead) | 6.1%–12.2% |
| Lavandin (Dutch) | 4.5%–11.7% |
| Blue Yarrow (Artemisia Ketone CT) | 11.5% |
| Neroli (*C. aurantium*) | 3.3%–11.3% |
| Myrtle (Limonene CT) | 0.5%–8.2% |
| Basil (Methyl Eugenol CT) | 0.2%–7.2% |
| Wormwood (Myrcene CT) | 0.0%–7.0% |
| Myrtle (1,8-Cineole CT) | 0.0%–5.3% |
| Spanish Sage | 0.0%–4.2% |
| Ghandi Root | 0.0%–3.3% |

**Linalyl Anthanilate**

| | |
|---|---|
| Ponderosa Pine | 0.0%–9.0% |

**Linalyl Formate**

| | |
|---|---|
| Rose (Iranian) | 0.0%–11.9% |

**Linalyl Propionate (1,6-Octadien-3-ol, 3,7-dimethyl-, propanoate; Linalyl n-Propionate)**

| | |
|---|---|
| Kumquat (*F. margarita*, peel SD) | 0.0%–9.6% |

**Lindestrene**

| | |
|---|---|
| Myrrh | 12.0%–12.9% |

**Longifolene (Junipene, 1,4-Methenozaulene)**

| | |
|---|---|
| Black Cumin (Thymoquinone CT) | 1.2%–10.2% |
| Turkish Pine (Resin) | 8.6% |
| Black Cumin (Para-Cymene CT) | 0.0%–6.4% |
| Black Cumin (Trans-Anethole CT) | 0.0%–5.7% |
| Chinese Cedarwood | 0.0%–4.2% |
| Black Cumin (Para-Cymene CT) | 0.0%–2.4% |

**Longipinanol**

| | |
|---|---|
| Hairy Basil (Camphor CT) | 0.0%–6.2% |
| Angelica Root | 1.3%–4.2% |

**Lyratol**

| | |
|---|---|
| Mugwort (Alpha-Phellandrene CT) | 15.1% |

**M-Cresol**

| | |
|---|---|
| Jasmine Absolute (Benzyl Acetate CT) | 0.0%–6.1% |

**M-Cymen-8-ol**

| | |
|---|---|
| Pink Pepper (*S. terebinthifolius*, Leaves, p-Cymen-7-ol CT) | 4.1% |

**Manool**

| | |
|---|---|
| Blue Mountain Sage (Delta-3-Carene CT) | 0.9%–20.9% |
| Blue Mountain Sage ((E)-Nerolidol CT) | 12.1%–12.7% |
| Blue Mountain Sage (Alpha-Bisabolol CT) | 0.0%–8.6% |
| Chinese Cedarwood | 0.0%–7.6% |
| Blue Mountain Sage (Limonene CT) | 6.3% |
| Blue Mountain Sage (Gamma-Terpinene CT) | 5.6% |
| Chaste Tree (Berries) | 0.0%–3.1% |
| Chaste Tree (Leaves) | 0.0%–1.3% |

**Manool Oxide**

| | |
|---|---|
| Chaste Tree (Berries) | 0.0%–1.5% |

**Mentha-1.5-Dien-8-ol**

| | |
|---|---|
| Angelica Root | 0.1%–2.6% |

**Menthatriene**

| | |
|---|---|
| Ledum (*R. groenlandicum*) | 0.0%–4.0% |

**Menthofuran**

| | |
|---|---|
| Palo Santo (Wood) | 0.0%–13.4% |
| Peppermint | 0.1%–11.2% |
| Palo Santo (Leaves, Aerial Parts) | 0.0%–5.1% |

**Menthol**

| | |
|---|---|
| Cornmint | 61.9%–82.2% |
| Peppermint | 25.2%–76.7% |
| Applemint (*M. suav.*, Menthol CT) | 48.3% |
| Pennyroyal (*M. pulegium*) | 0.0%–13.0% |
| Spearmint (Menthone CT) | 5.4% |
| Applemint (*M. rotun.*, Piperitenone CT) | 3.3% |
| Mugwort (1,8-Cineole CT) | 0.0%–1.0% |

**Menthone (Trans-Menthone)**

| | |
|---|---|
| Spearmint (Menthone CT) | 44.5% |
| Spearmint (Pulegone-Menthone-Isomenthone CT) | 15.6%–31.4% |
| Peppermint | 2.5%–30.6% |
| Buchu (*A. betulina*, Menthone CT) | 29.2% |
| Buchu (*A. betulina*, Isomenthone CT) | 2.5%–25.0% |
| Spearmint (Carvone CT) | 0.9%–21.9% |
| Cornmint | 3.4%–19.3% |
| Pennyroyal (*M. pulegium*) | 0.0%–19.2% |
| Buchu (*A. crenulata*) | 1.3%–16.6% |
| Pennyroyal (*M. pulegioides*) | 1.5%–16.0% |
| Geranium | 0.0%–16.0% |
| Applemint (*M. suav.*, Menthol CT) | 8.9% |
| Applemint (*M. suav.*, Piperitenone) | 3.3% |
| Applemint (*M. rotun.*, Piperitenone CT) | 3.1% |
| Applemint (*M. suav.*, Italian) | 0.0%–2.6% |

**Menthyl Acetate**

| | |
|---|---|
| Peppermint | 0.4%–17.4% |
| Cornmint | 0.6%–4.4% |
| Applemint (*M. suav.*, Menthol CT) | 3.4% |

**Methyl-2-Methylbutyrate (Methyl-2-Butanoate, Butanoic acid, 2-methyl-, methyl ester)**

| | |
|---|---|
| Magnolia (Flowers) | 1.3%–7.8% |

**Methyl Allyl Disulfide**

| | |
|---|---|
| Garlic (Vinyldithiins CT) | 0.6%–9.0% |

**Methyl Allyl Trisulfide**

| | |
|---|---|
| Garlic (Vinyldithiins CT) | 0.1%–14.9% |

**Methyl N-Methylanthranilate**

| | |
|---|---|
| Mediterranean Mandarin (Hydrodistilled) | 0.0%–1.5% |

**Methyl Acetate**

| | |
|---|---|
| Basil (Methyl Eugenol CT) | 1.2%–3.6% |

**Methyl Anthranilate**

| | |
|---|---|
| Jasmine Absolute (Benzyl Benzoate CT) | 5.0%–7.8% |

**Methyl Benzoate**

| | |
|---|---|
| Benzoin (Siam, SPME Absolute) | 22.0%–27.7% |
| Benzoin (Siam, HSSE Absolute) | 17.7%–21.9% |
| Benzoin (Siam, S-HS Absolute) | 6.2%–17.5% |
| Jasmine Absolute (Benzyl Acetate CT) | 0.2%–6.9% |
| Ylang Ylang (French I) | 6.1% |
| Ylang Ylang (Madagascan I) | 1.5%–5.6% |

**Methyl Beta-Ocinolcarboxylate**

| | |
|---|---|
| Oakmoss Absolute | 18.6%–30.1% |

**Methyl Caprylate**

| | |
|---|---|
| Ylang Ylang (French IV) | 7.2%. |

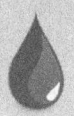

## Methyl Chavicol (Estragole)

| | |
|---|---|
| Fennel (Methyl Chavicol CT) | 61.6%–94.5% |
| Basil (Methyl Chavicol CT) | 78.0%–90.7% |
| Ravensara (Methyl Chavicol CT) | 61.6%–90.0% |
| Tarragon (Methyl Chavicol CT) | 71.3%–84.1% |
| Holy Basil (Aerial Parts, Estragole CT) | 25.1%–75.1% |
| Holy Basil (Methyl Chavicol CT) | 46.4%–56.8% |
| Holy Basil (aerial parts, beta-bisabolene CT) | 3.4%–21.6% |
| Ponderosa Pine | 0.0%–20.4% |
| Hairy Basil (var. *pilosum* Eugenol CT) | 17.3% |
| Hairy Basil (1,8-Cineole CT) | 0.0%–13.4% |
| Ravensara (Limonene CT) | 0.1%–11.9% |
| Holy Basil (aerial parts, eugenol CT) | 10.6%–11.5% |
| Anise | 0.0%–9.1% |
| Fennel (Trans Anethole CT) | 2.6%–8.2% |
| Hairy Basil (var. *pilosum* Terpinen-4-ol CT) | 0.2%–7.2% |
| Ravensara (Sabinene CT) | 1.8%–5.0% |
| Ravensara (Methyl Eugenol CT) | 2.5%–4.5% |
| Moringa (Seeds, Naphthalene CT) | 4.5% |
| Star Anise | 0.0%–2.7% |
| Allspice (Berries, Methyl Eugenol CT) | 0.0%–1.7% |
| Ravensara (Alpha-Terpinene CT) | 0.1%–1.4% |
| Ravensara (1,8-Cineole CT) | 0.0%–0.7% |

## Methyl Cinnamate ((E)-Methyl Cinnamate, Trans-Methyl Cinnamate)

| | |
|---|---|
| Hairy Basil ((E)-Methyl Cinnamate CT) | 45.6%–86.6% |
| Ocotea (Flowers Calices) | 19.5%–21.7% |
| Holy Basil (aerial parts, eugenol CT) | 0.0%–8.7% |
| Hairy Basil (Trans-Caryophyllene CT) | 8.3% |
| Fingerroot (*B. rotunda* Nerol-Camphor CT) | 6.9% |
| Shell Ginger (1,8-Cineole CT) | 4.2%–6.3% |
| Fingerroot (Camphor CT) | 0.0%–5.8% |
| Xanthoxylum | 0.0%–5.7% |
| Galangal (Greater, 1,8-Cineole CT) | 0.0%–5.3% |
| Davana | 0.0%–4.6% |
| Galangal (Lesser) | 0.0%–4.0% |
| Ocotea (Leaves) | 2.1% |

## Methyl Cinnamate (E)/Alpha-Cubebene

| | |
|---|---|
| Manuka (Selinene/Beta-Elemene CT) | 10.6% |

## Methyl Citronellate

| | |
|---|---|
| Lemon Eucalyptus | 0.0%–2.0% |

## Methyl Eugenol (Eugenyl Methyl Ether)

| | |
|---|---|
| Rosalina (Methyl Eugenol CT) | 96.8% |
| Holy Basil (aerial parts or seeds, methyl eugenol CT) | 82.9%–92.4% |
| Ravensara (Methyl Eugenol CT) | 74.0%–81.6% |
| Basil (Methyl Eugenol CT) | 44.6%–78.0% |
| Allspice (Berries, Methyl Eugenol CT) | 43.0%–67.9% |
| Allspice (Leaves, Methyl Eugenol CT) | 62.7% |
| Hairy Basil (Trans-Caryophyllene CT) | 26.0% |
| Bay Laurel | 0.1%–15.8% |
| Allspice (Berries, Eugenol CT) | 0.0%–13.1% |
| Savin (Needles & Branches) | 0.0%–12.1% |
| Calamus (Alpha-Asarone CT) | 8.6% |
| Ravensara (Methyl Eugenol CT) | 0.1%–8.5% |
| Allspice (Leaves, Eugenol CT) | 0.0%–7.1% |
| Tamala (Eugenol CT) | 0.0%–6.4% |
| Ravensara (Limonene CT) | 0.0%–5.2% |
| Myrtle (1,8-Cineole CT) | 0.0%–4.8% |
| Basil (Methyl Chavicol CT) | 0.4%–4.0% |
| Magnolia (Flowers) | 0.0%–3.6% |
| Tarragon (Methyl Chavicol CT) | 0.0%–2.2% |
| Ravensara (Sabinene CT) | 0.3%–1.3% |
| Ravensara (Alpha-Terpinene CT) | 0.1%–1.1% |

## Methyl Heptenone (6-Methyl-5-Hepten-2-one)

| | |
|---|---|
| Lemon Verbena (Leaves and stems) | 1.4%–7.4% |
| Lemon Verbena (Leaves) | 0.3%–4.0% |
| May Chang (Neral CT) | 3.5% |

## Methyl Hexadevenoate

| | |
|---|---|
| Lovage (Roots) | 0.0%–6.1% |

## Methyl Isoeugenol (Trans-Methylisoeugenol, (E)-Methyl Isoeugenol)

| | |
|---|---|
| Calamus (Alpha-Asarone CT) | 50.1% |
| Calamus ((E)-Methylisoeugenol CT) | 41.5% |
| Citronella (*C. nardus*) | 0.0%–11.0% |
| Cinnamon Bark | 0.0%–7.8% |
| Frankincense (*B. serrata*) | 0.0%–3.1% |

## Methyl Myrtenate

| | |
|---|---|
| Western Red Cedar (Wood) | 4.1%–4.5% |

## Methyl Octanoate

| | |
|---|---|
| Pink Pepper (*S. molle*, Fruits, α-Phellandrene CT) | 0.6%–5.2% |

## Methyl Salicylate

| | |
|---|---|
| Wintergreen | 96.9%–99.6% |
| Birch | 97.0%–99.0% |
| Ylang Ylang (Madagascan I) | 1.7%–10.4% |
| Ylang Ylang (Madagascan II) | 0.6%–5.3% |
| Clove (stem) | < 0.6% |
| Clove | < 0.4% |

## Methyl Thujate

| | |
|---|---|
| Western Red Cedar (Wood) | 55.8%–59.1% |

## Myrcene (Beta-Myrcene)

| | |
|---|---|
| Mastic (NT\B, Beta-Myrcene CT) | 75.5%–89.5% |
| Hemp (Myrcene CT) | 12.5%–67.1% |
| Verbena (Myrcene CT) | 33.1%–53.2% |
| Hops | 5.1%–52.4% |
| Wormwood (Myrcene CT) | 8.6%–44.3% |
| Aleppo Pine (Branches) | 42.1% |
| Mastic (Leaves) | 0.2%–39.2% |
| African Bluegrass (Myrcene CT) | 11.6%–35.6% |
| Mastic (Twigs, Alpha-Pinene CT) | 34.1% |
| Bay (West Indies) | 0.3%–30.9% |
| Rosemary (Beta-Myrcene CT) | 17.9%–30.0% |
| Wormwood (Myrcene-Sabinene CT) | 17.7%–29.9% |
| Verbena (Myrcenone CT) | 0.1%–28.8% |
| Aleppo Pine (Aerial Parts) | 0.5%–27.9% |
| Aleppo Pine (Needles) | 0.3%–27.9% |
| White Pine | 1.7%–27.7% |
| Lemongrass (West Indian) | 3.2%–27.0% |
| Juniper Berry | 2.9%–26.5% |
| Hinoki (needles) | 0.0%–26.4% |
| Betony (MLD-C CT) | 4.3%–26.2% |
| Betony (β-Phell.\α-Pinene CT) | 0.7%–23.9% |
| Pink Pepper (*S. terebinthifolius*, Fruits, Myrc./Lim. CT) | 1.6%–20.4% |
| Kabosu | 18.5%–20.2% |
| Allspice (Leaves, Eugenol CT) | 0.0%–19.3% |
| Blue Mountain Sage (Alpha-Bisabolol CT) | 0.0%–18.8% |
| Blue Tansy (Chamazulene CT) | 1.0%–18.4% |
| Blue Tansy (Sabinene CT) | 4.4%–18.4% |
| Pink Pepper (*S. molle*, Fruits, α-Phellandrene CT) | 0.0%–16.8% |
| White Spruce (Needles & Twigs) | 4.8%–16.5% |
| Kumquat (*F. margarita*, peel SD) | 1.8%–16.5% |
| Parsley (Leaves, 1,3,8-Para-Menth. CT) | 2.9%–16.3% |
| Betony (Alpha-Thujene CT) | 0.5%–15.9% |
| Red Pine | 3.5%–14.5% |
| Aleppo Pine (Cones) | 6.3%–13.7% |
| Goldenrod | 0.0%–13.7% |
| Blue Mountain Sage ((E)-Nerolidol CT) | 4.4%–12.3% |

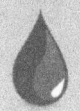

## Myrcene—continued

| | |
|---|---|
| Engelmann Spruce | 5.5%–12.2% |
| Dwarf Pine (Needles, Needles/Twigs) | 1.4%–12.2% |
| Mastic (NT\B, Alpha-Pinene CT) | 1.3%–11.5% |
| Ledum (*L. palustre*) | 0.9%–11.4% |
| Honey Myrtle | 9.8%–11.2% |
| Turkish Pine (Twigs) | 5.5%–11.0% |
| Wormwood (Sabinene CT) | 3.1%–11.0% |
| Savin (Berries) | 5.8%–10.8% |
| White Spruce (Oleoresin) | 3.2%–10.5% |
| Rabbitbrush (var. *glabratus*) | 10.5% |
| Dwarf Pine (Twigs) | 1.6%–10.3% |
| Blue Cypress (Leaves) | 6.0%–10.1% |
| Spanish Sage | 0.1%–10.0% |
| Tamala (Eugenol CT) | 0.0%–9.7% |
| Gobre Salla | 1.2%–9.5% |
| Juniper (Chinese) | 2.8%–9.2% |
| Wormwood (Trans-Sabinyl Acetate CT) | 0.2%–9.2% |
| Verbena (Linalool CT) | 2.6%–9.1% |
| Frankincense (*B. sacra*) | 1.0%–8.9% |
| Frankincense (*B. serrata*) | 0.0%–8.9% |
| Parsley (Leaves, Myristicin CT) | 2.8%–8.7% |
| White Verbena (Citral CT) | 0.0%–8.5% |
| White Spruce (Needles) | 0.0%–8.4% |
| Mastic (Leaves) | 0.0%–8.3% |
| Monarda (Thymol CT) | 2.4%–8.1% |
| Spearmint (*M. crispa*, Rotundifolone CT) | 7.8% |
| Turkish Pine (Needles/Twigs) | 4.9%–7.6% |
| Blue Spruce | 5.1%–7.5% |
| Ponderosa Pine | 0.9%–7.4% |
| Ravensara (Limonene CT) | 5.0%–7.3% |
| Grapefruit (Distilled) | 3.5%–7.3% |
| Juniper (Needles) | 6.5%–6.9% |
| Rabbitbrush (var. *albicaulis*) | 6.9% |
| Great Mugwort | 0.5%–6.8% |
| Pink Pepper (*S. terebinthifolius*, Leaves, Sabinene CT) | 6.6% |
| Grapefruit (Cold-pressed/expressed) | 1.6%–6.3% |
| Lovage (Leaves) | 1.3%–6.2% |
| Maritime Pine (Needles, Alpha-Pinene CT) | 0.4%–6.1% |
| Hinoki (needles and twigs) | 6.1% |
| Hemp (Beta-Caryophyllene CT) | 0.8%–6.0% |
| Spearmint (Linalool CT) | 4.7%–5.9% |
| Angelica Root | 0.3%–5.9% |
| Mugwort (Beta-Caryophyllene CT) | 5.9% |
| Betony (Bicyclogermacrene CT) | 1.7%–5.8% |
| Pink Pepper (*S. terebinthifolius*, Fruits, δ-3-Carene CT) | 1.0%–5.8% |
| Pink Pepper (*S. molle*, Leaves, Bicyclogermacrene CT) | 0.2%–5.5% |
| Rosemary (Verbenone CT) | 0.5%–5.4% |
| Applemint (*M. suav.*, Linalool CT) | 5.3% |
| Mastic (Aerial parts, Beta-Eudesmol CT) | 5.3% |
| Pink Pepper (*S. molle*, Fruits/Leaves, α-Phell./Sylv. CT) | 1.0%–5.1% |
| Wormwood (Alpha-Thujone CT) | 0.1%–5.1% |
| Summer Savory (Gamma-Terpinene CT) | 0.0%–5.1% |
| Mugwort (Alpha-Thujone CT) | 4.9%–5.0% |
| Oriental Arborvitae (Needles) | 1.6%–5.0% |
| Rosemary (Camphor CT) | 2.3%–4.9% |
| Rosemary (Alpha-Pinene CT) | 0.6%–4.9% |
| Juniper (*J. wallichiana\J. indica*, Leaves) | 3.2%–4.7% |
| Oriental Arborvitae (Berries) | 1.6%–4.7% |
| Formosan Cypress (Neeldes, α-Pinene CT) | 0.8%–4.7% |
| Caraway | 0.0%–4.7% |
| Maritime Pine (Gum Resin) | 0.0%–4.7% |
| Tamala (Trans-Sabinene Hydrate CT) | 4.6% |
| Mastic (NT\B, Limonene CT) | 3.0%–4.5% |

| | |
|---|---|
| Pink Pepper (*S. molle*, Leaves, Elemol/Beta-Eudesmol CT) | 4.5% |
| Wormwood (Trans-Sabinene Hydrate CT) | 0.0%–4.4% |
| Black Pepper (Beta-Pinene CT) | 4.4% |
| White Spruce (Branches) | 4.2%–4.3% |
| Savin (Needles & Branches) | 3.0%–4.2% |
| African Bluegrass (Artemisia Ketone CT) | 4.2% |
| Pink Pepper (*S. molle*, Leaves, α-Phellandrene CT) | 0.0%–4.1% |
| Japanese Cedarwood (Alpha-Pinene CT) | 0.0%–3.9% |
| Neroli (*C. sinensis*) | 2.1%–3.7% |
| Wild Chamomile (*O. multicaulis*) | 0.1%–3.7% |
| Juniper (*J. recurva*, Berries) | 3.7% |
| Black Pepper (Limonene CT) | 1.7%–3.6% |
| Mediterranean Mandarin (Hydrodistilled) | 1.5%–3.5% |
| Chaste Tree (Leaves) | 0.0%–3.5% |
| Ravensara (Sabinene CT) | 2.5%–3.4% |
| Pine | 0.2%–3.4% |
| Ravensara (Alpha-Terpinene CT) | 2.8%–3.2% |
| Mastic (Gum Resin) | 1.9%–3.2% |
| Yuzu | 1.1%–3.2% |
| White Sage | 0.5%–3.2% |
| Petitgrain (Mandarin) | 0.0%–3.2% |
| Rabbitbrush (var. *consimilis*) | 3.2% |
| Kumquat (*C. japonica*, Leaves CT Beta-Pinene) | 3.2% |
| Mugwort (Chrysanthenyl Acetate CT) | 2.7% |
| Orange (Cold-pressed/expressed) | 0.7%–2.4% |
| Hyssop (Pinocamphone CT) | 0.0%–2.4% |
| Chaste Tree (Berries) | 1.4%–2.3% |
| Celery Seed | 1.2%–2.3% |
| Tangerine (Cold-pressed/expressed) | 0.7%–2.2% |
| Orange (Distilled) | 0.9%–2.1% |
| Kumquat (*F. margarita*, Fruit CT Limonene) | 1.9%–2.0% |
| Orange–Bitter (Cold-pressed/expressed) | 0.5%–2.0% |
| Kumquat (*F. margarita*, peel CP) | 2.0% |
| Kumquat (*C. japonica*, Peel CP) | 1.9% |
| Mediterranean Mandarin (CP\Expressed) | 0.0%–1.8% |
| Hyssop (Linalool CT) | 0.0%–1.7% |
| Ocotea (Leaves) | 1.4% |
| Mugwort (1,8-Cineole CT) | 0.0%–1.3% |
| Mugwort (Alpha-Phellandrene CT) | 1.3% |
| Cumin | 0.0%–1.2% |

## Myrcenol-8

| | |
|---|---|
| Thyme (Thuyanol-4 CT) | 0.0%–18.7% |
| Thyme (Thuyanol-4 CT) | 0.0%–7.1% |

## Myrcenone

| | |
|---|---|
| Verbena (Myrcenone CT) | 36.2%–71.6% |

## Myristicin

| | |
|---|---|
| Parsley (Leaves, Myristicin CT) | 12.6%–60.5% |
| Nutmeg (East Indian) | 0.3%–45.6% |
| Parsley Seed | 12.4%–42.2% |
| Parsley (Whole Plant) | 32.8%–36.2% |
| Parsley (Leaves, 1,3,8-Para-Menth. CT) | 0.0%–12.2% |

## Myrtenal

| | |
|---|---|
| Verbena (Linalool CT) | 0.0%–6.0% |
| Ledum (*R. groenlandicum*) | 0.3%–4.3% |
| Cumin | 0.0%–3.5% |
| Kunzea (Alpha-Pinene CT) | 0.0%–2.1% |

## Myrtenol

| | |
|---|---|
| Formosan Cypress (Wood, Myrtenol CT) | 20.3%–48.9% |
| Fragonia (Alpha-Pinene CT) | 12.1%–20.0% |
| Fragonia (Balanced CT) | 1.7%–5.5% |
| Tsauri Grass | 0.0%–5.3% |
| Black Cumin (Para-Cymene CT) | 0.0%–3.0% |
| Hyssop (Pinocamphone CT) | 0.7%–2.8% |

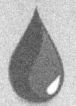

**Myrtenyl Acetate**

| | |
|---|---|
| Myrtle (Myrtenyl Acetate CT) | 20.8%–21.6% |
| Myrtle (1,8-Cineole CT) | 0.0%–7.4% |
| Myrtle (Alpha-Pinene CT) | 0.0%–5.4% |
| Valerian | 0.1%–9.1% |

**Myrtenyl Isovalerate**

| | |
|---|---|
| Valerian | 0.3%–10.5% |

**n-Acetyl-1,2,3,4-Tetrahydro-Isoquinoline**

| | |
|---|---|
| Rhododendron (Flowers) | 29.2% |

**n-Decanol (1-Decanol)**

| | |
|---|---|
| Cilantro | 13.6%–19.6% |

**n-Hex-3-en-2-one**

| | |
|---|---|
| Rue (n-Hex-4-en-3-one CT) | 7.2%–14.1% |

**n-Hex-4-en-3-one**

| | |
|---|---|
| Rue (n-Hex-4-en-3-one CT) | 53.6%–55.1% |

**n-Nonal**

| | |
|---|---|
| Mastic (Gum Resin) | 0.0%–3.5% |

**n-Octabbol**

| | |
|---|---|
| Frankincense (B. papyrifera) | 3.4%–8.8% |

**n-Pent-3-one**

| | |
|---|---|
| Rue (n-Hex-4-en-3-one CT) | 28.2%–37.8% |

**Naphthalene**

| | |
|---|---|
| Moringa (Seeds, Naphthalene CT) | 35.6% |
| African Bluegrass (Artemisia Ketone CT) | 9.6% |
| Red Pine | 0.0%–9.4% |
| Lavender (True English) | 0.0%–4.2% |

**Naphthalenol**

| | |
|---|---|
| White Fir (A. concolor) | 0.0%–6.4% |

**Naphthalenone**

| | |
|---|---|
| Black Cumin (Trans-Anethole CT) | 0.0%–2.6% |

**Nardol (Nardol A)**

| | |
|---|---|
| Spikenard (Nardol CT) | 10.1% |
| Spikenard (Calarene CT, Nepal) | 0.0%–6.0% |

**Neo-Dihydrocaveylacetate**

| | |
|---|---|
| Tsauri Grass | 0.0%–4.2% |

**Neo-Isodihydrocarveol Acetate**

| | |
|---|---|
| Spearmint (Cis-Ocimenone CT) | 1.5% |

**Neoisomenthol**

| | |
|---|---|
| Pennyroyal (M. fruticosa, Isomenthol CT) | 4.5%–10.0% |

**Neoisomenthyl Acetate**

| | |
|---|---|
| Spearmint (Menthone CT) | 8.4% |

**Neomenthol**

| | |
|---|---|
| Applemint (M. suav., Menthol CT) | 3.8% |
| Applemint (M. rotun., Piperitenone CT) | 2.8% |

**Nepetalactone Isomers**

| | |
|---|---|
| Catnip (Nepetalactone CT) | 22.3%–92.2% |
| Lemon Catnip (Beta-Citronellol CT) | 0.0%–25.4% |

**Neral (Z-Citral, Citral B, Cis-Citral, Beta-Citral)**

| | |
|---|---|
| May Chang (Neral CT) | 63.6% |
| Lemongrass (East Indian) | 19.0%–45.0% |
| Rose (Iranian) | 0.0%–44.8% |
| Lemon Myrtle (Citral CT) | 32.0%–40.9% |
| Lemon Basil | 21.8%–39.8% |
| Hairy Basil (Citral CT) | 20.2%–36.6% |
| May Chang (Citral CT) | 26.1%–36.3% |
| White Verbena (Citral CT) | 23.6%–36.1% |
| Lemongrass (West Indian) | 19.3%–34.6% |
| Melissa | 4.6%–33.8% |
| Honey Myrtle | 27.7%–32.3% |
| Lemon Verbena (Leaves) | 25.7%–27.4% |
| Lemon Verbena (Stems) | 23.0%–27.4% |

| | |
|---|---|
| Lemon Tea Tree (L. petersonii) | 17.9%–23.5% |
| Lemon Tea Tree (L. liversidgei) | 19.7%–21.0% |
| Petitgrain (Lime) | 8.3%–20.5% |
| Petitgrain (Lemon) | 10.4%–16.1% |
| Lemon Catnip (Beta-Citronellol CT) | 3.7%–15.4% |
| Tangerine | 0.1%–14.5% |
| Citronella (C. nardus) | 0.0%–14.2% |
| Lemon Verbena (Leaves and stems) | 6.0%–12.0% |
| White Verbena (Carvone\Limonene CT) | 0.0%–10.4% |
| Ginger | 2.6%–9.4% |
| Lemon Catnip (Geraniol\Nerol CT) | 0.4%–7.1% |
| Citronella (C. winteranius) | 0.3%–6.0% |
| Citron (Distilled) | 0.1%–5.7% |
| Ocotea (Leaves) | 4.4% |
| Citron (Cold-pressed/Expressed) | 1.1%–3.8% |
| Persian Lime (Cold Pressed\Expressed) | 1.1%–2.3% |

**Nerol**

| | |
|---|---|
| Fingerroot (B. rotunda Nerol-Camphor CT) | 39.6% |
| Lemon Catnip (Geraniol\Nerol CT) | 24.4%–30.7% |
| Lemon Basil | 0.0%–14.6% |
| Helichrysum (ssp. microphyllum) | 3.7%–14.4% |
| Helichrysum (ssp. italicum) | 1.4%–12.8% |
| Davana | 0.0%–10.0% |
| Melissa | 0.0%–7.9% |
| Rose (Turkish) | 0.8%–7.6% |
| Hairy Basil (Citral CT) | 02.0%–7.2% |
| Cardamom (Alpha-Terpinyl Acetate CT) | 0.0%–6.8% |
| Citron (Distilled) | 0.0%–5.9% |
| Kumquat (C. japonica, Leaves CT Linalool) | 5.3% |
| Lemon Verbena (Leaves) | 0.0%–5.2% |
| Lemongrass (West Indian) | 3.1%–3.7% |
| Honey Myrtle | 0.0%–3.6% |
| Petitgrain (Lemon) | 1.2%–3.4% |
| Petitgrain (Lime) | 1.1%–3.1% |
| Lemongrass (East Indian) | 0.0%–2.9% |
| Rosewood (Wood) | 0.2%–1.7% |

**Nerolidol ((E)-Nerolidol, Trans-Nerolidol)**

| | |
|---|---|
| Niaouli ((E)-Nerolidol CT) | 56.0%–95.0% |
| Blue Mountain Sage ((E)-Nerolidol CT) | 46.7%–53.6% |
| Guava Leaf ((E)-Nerolidol CT) | 35.6% |
| Siam Wood (Root Bark) | 24.0%–35.5% |
| Guava Leaf (β-Cary.\(E)-Nerolidol CT) | 19.2% |
| Neroli (C. aurantium) | 1.8%–17.5% |
| Blue Mountain Sage (Gamma-Terpinene CT) | 15.1% |
| Neroli (C. sinensis) | 2.9%–10.0% |
| Yarrow (Chamazulene CT) | 0.1%–9.6% |
| Yarrow (Sabinene CT) | 0.0%–9.6% |
| Wild Chamomile (C. mixtus, Sant. Alc. CT) | 0.7%–9.0% |
| Cardamom (Alpha-Terpinyl Acetate CT) | 0.3%–8.9% |
| Niaouli (Viridiflorol CT) | 0.1%–8.3% |
| Guava Leaf (Selin-11-en-4-Alpha-ol CT) | 3.3%–8.2% |
| Calendula (Alpha-Cadinol/Delta-Cadinene CT) | 0.0%–8.1% |
| Guava Leaf ((2E)-Hexenal CT) | 6.9% |
| Rhododendron (Leaves) | 5.8% |
| Balsam Poplar | 4.9%–5.4% |
| Peru Balsam (Resinoid Absolute) | 0.0%–5.0% |
| Guava Leaf (Alpha-Pinene CT) | 0.0%–5.0% |
| Boldo (Ascaridole CT) | 0.0%–5.0% |
| Peru Balsam | 3.4%–4.8% |
| Guava Leaf (Beta-Caryophyllene CT) | 0.0%–4.7% |
| Chaste Tree (Leaves) | 0.0%–2.5% |
| Niaouli (1,8-Cineole/Viridiflorol CT) | 0.1%–2.3% |

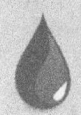

**Neryl-3-Methyl Butanoate**

| | |
|---|---|
| Wormwood (Trans-Sabinyl Acetate CT) | 0.0%–9.1% |
| Wormwood ((Z)-Epoxy Ocimene CT) | 0.0%–5.5% |

**Neryl Acetate**

| | |
|---|---|
| Helichrysum (ssp. *microphyllum*) | 16.9%–56.1% |
| Helichrysum (ssp. *italicum*) | 5.6%–45.9% |
| Fenugreek | 17.3% |
| Coriander | 0.0%–14.2% |
| Helichrysum (*H. italicum*) | 1.4%–11.5% |
| Petitgrain (Lime) | 0.6%–6.1% |
| Applemint (*M. suav.*, Linalool CT) | 6.1% |
| Turkish Pine (Bark) | 5.9% |
| Petitgrain (Lemon) | 0.7%–5.1% |
| Petitgrain (Bergamot/Bitter Orange) | 2.2%–4.5% |
| Lavender (Munstead) | 0.7%–4.4% |
| Lemon Verbena (Leaves) | 0.0%–4.0% |
| Ylang Ylang (French I) | 2.7% |

**Neryl Butanoate**

| | |
|---|---|
| Wormwood (Trans-Sabinyl Acetate CT) | 0.0%–7.9% |
| Wormwood ((Z)-Epoxy Ocimene CT) | 0.0%–4.9% |

**Neryl Isovalerianate**

| | |
|---|---|
| Genipi (*A. umbelliformis*, C-SH\B CT) | 1.4%–10.0% |
| Genipi (*A. umbelliformis*, Alpha-Thujone CT) | 0.0%–6.9% |

**Neryl Propionate**

| | |
|---|---|
| Helichrysum (ssp. *italicum*) | 3.0%–16.4% |
| Helichrysum (ssp. *microphyllum*) | 1.5%–16.4% |

**Nonacosane**

| | |
|---|---|
| Moringa (Leaves, Pentacosane CT) | 0.0%–10.5% |
| Moringa (Flowers) | 10.5% |

**Nonadecane**

| | |
|---|---|
| Rose (Iranian) | 0.0%–51.2% |
| Rose (Indian) | 7.3%–24.7% |
| Rose (Bulgarian) | 8.1%–19.2% |
| Rose (Turkish) | 8.2%–18.9% |
| Moringa (Leaves, (E)-Phytol CT) | 3.7% |

**Nonyl Cyclopropopanecarboxylate**

| | |
|---|---|
| Rue (2-Undecanone CT) | 0.0%–9.2% |

**Nonyl Phenylacetate**

| | |
|---|---|
| Valerian | 0.0%–13.8% |

**Nootkatol**

| | |
|---|---|
| Ledum (*R. groenlandicum*) | 0.0%–2.1% |

**Nootkatone**

| | |
|---|---|
| Grapefruit (Distilled) | 0.0%–8.3% |
| Vetiver | 0.0%–4.1% |

**Norketoagarofuran**

| | |
|---|---|
| Agarwood (*A. malaccensis*) | 0.0%–8.4% |

**Northujane**

| | |
|---|---|
| African Bluegrass (Linalool CT) | 12.3%–16.8% |
| African Bluegrass (Artemisia Ketone CT) | 4.4% |

**O-Cymene (Ortho-Cymene)**

| | |
|---|---|
| White Verbena (Citral CT) | 0.0%–12.4% |
| Cumin | 0.0%–11.8% |
| Pink Pepper (*S. molle*, Fruits/Leaves, α-Phell./Sylv. CT) | 0.0%–8.5% |
| Indian Borage (Carvacrol CT) | 0.0%–7.7% |
| Black Cumin (Para-Cymene CT) | 0.0%–7.3% |
| Blue Yarrow (Artemisia Ketone CT) | 5.3% |

**Occidentalol Acetate**

| | |
|---|---|
| Rose (Iranian) | 0.0%–44.8% |

**Octacosane**

| | |
|---|---|
| Moringa (Fruits) | 19.1% |
| Moringa (Leaves, Pentacosane CT) | 0.0%–10.0% |

**Octadecane (n-Octadecane)**

| | |
|---|---|
| Moringa (Fruits) | 13.1% |
| Rose (Iranian) | 0.0%–6.1% |
| Chaste Tree (Berries) | 0.0%–1.7% |

**Octadecanol**

| | |
|---|---|
| Spearmint (Pulegone-Menthone-Isomenthone CT) | 0.0%–15.0% |

**Octanal**

| | |
|---|---|
| Angelica Root | 0.0%–2.8% |

**Octane-3,3-Dimethyl-2-(1-Buten-3-on-1-yl)**

| | |
|---|---|
| Khella (Aerial Parts, Isoamyl 2-Meth. CT) | 0.0%–6.4% |

**Octanoic Acid**

| | |
|---|---|
| Pink Pepper (*S. molle*, Fruits, α-Phellandrene CT) | 0.0%–4.4% |

**Octanol**

| | |
|---|---|
| Tangerine (Distilled) | 0.0%–6.9% |

**Octyl Acetate**

| | |
|---|---|
| Frankincense (*B. papyrifera*) | 57.1%–65.7% |
| Frankincense (*B. carterii*) | 0.0%–39.3% |

**Osthol**

| | |
|---|---|
| Angelica Root | 1.5%–8.8% |

**P-Allylanisole**

| | |
|---|---|
| Lovage (Roots) | 0.0%–7.0% |

**P-Anisaldehyde (Anisaldehyde, 4-Methoxybenzaldehyde)**

| | |
|---|---|
| Anise | 0.0%–5.4% |
| Star Anise | 0.0%–1.8% |

**P-Diisopropyl-Benzene**

| | |
|---|---|
| Arnica (Roots, 2,5-Dimethoxy-p-Cymene CT) | 1.6%–5.7% |

**P-Mentha-1,3-Dien-7-al (Alpha-Terpinen-7-al)**

| | |
|---|---|
| Shell Ginger (P-Mentha-1,3-Dien-7-al CT) | 40.5% |
| Cumin | 0.0%–17.5% |

**P-Mentha-1,4-Dien-7-al (Gamma-Terpinen-7-al)**

| | |
|---|---|
| Cumin | 0.0%–25.5% |

**P-Menth-1,5-Dien-8-ol**

| | |
|---|---|
| Sweet Inula (Borneol CT) | 0.0%–2.1% |

**P-Mentha-1,5,8-Triene**

| | |
|---|---|
| Ledum (*R. groenlandicum*) | 0.0%–2.2% |

**P-Mentha-2,4,(8)-Diene**

| | |
|---|---|
| Vilayti Tulsi (Fenchone CT) | 0.0%–4.5% |

**P-Mentha-2(7),8-Diene**

| | |
|---|---|
| Vilayti Tulsi (Sabinene CT) | 0.0%–7.9% |

**P-Menth-4,8-Diene**

| | |
|---|---|
| Shell Ginger (P-Mentha-1,3-Dien-7-al CT) | 10.0% |

**P-Menthadienol (Para-Menthadienol)**

| | |
|---|---|
| Gingergrass | 0.0%–5.3% |

**P-Methoxyheptanophenone**

| | |
|---|---|
| Arnica (Roots, 2,5-Dimethoxy-p-Cymene CT) | 6.1%–8.9% |

**Palustrol**

| | |
|---|---|
| Ledum (*L. palustre*) | 26.2%–43.4% |
| Kunzea (Spathulenol\Globulol CT) | 2.5%–2.7% |

**Para-Coumaryl Acetate (P-Coumaryl Acetate)**

| | |
|---|---|
| Benzoin (Sumatra, Ethanol Absolute) | 5.0%–23.0% |

**Para-Coumaryl Cinnamate (P-Coumaryl Cinnamate)**

| | |
|---|---|
| Benzoin (*S. paralleloneurum*, Absolute) | 52.5%–74.1% |

**Para-Coumaryl Benzoate (P-Coumaryl Benzoate)**

| | |
|---|---|
| Benzoin (*S. benzoin*, Absolute) | 30.5%–52.2% |
| Benzoin (*S. paralleloneurum*, Absolute) | 1.3%–3.3% |

**Para-Cresyl Methyl Ether (Methyl-p-Cresol)**

| | |
|---|---|
| Ylang Ylang (French I) | 9.7% |
| Ylang Ylang (French IV) | 1.6% |
| Ylang Ylang (Madagascan I) | 1.1%–10.4% |
| Ylang Ylang (Madagascan II) | 0.6%–5.3% |

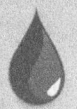

**Para-Cymen-8-ol**

| | |
|---|---|
| Applemint (*M. suav.*, Pulegone CT) | 10.4% |
| Applemint (*M. suav.*, Italian) | 0.0%–9.2% |
| Tagetes (*T. patula*, Limonene CT) | 0.0%–5.4% |
| Eucalyptus Dives | 0.0%–5.1% |
| Applemint (*M. suav.*, PO-PEO CT) | 2.9% |
| Thuja | 0.0%–2.7% |

**Para-Cymene (Paracymene, P-Cymene)**

| | |
|---|---|
| Pink Pepper (*S. molle*, Fruits/Leaves, p-Cymene CT) | 32.8%–69.4% |
| Black Cumin (Para-Cymene CT) | 6.3%–60.2% |
| Ajowan (Gamma-Terpinene\P-Cymene CT) | 33.7%–57.3% |
| Niaouli (Viridiflorol/ Para-cymene/1,8-cineole CT) | 0.4%–40.0% |
| Black Cumin (Thymoquinone CT) | 14.7%–38.0% |
| Monarda (Carvacrol/Para-Cymene CT) | 32.5%–35.4% |
| Thyme (Carvacrol CT) | 0.0%–34.6% |
| Shell Ginger (Para-Cymene CT) | 33.1% |
| Savory (Wild, Carvacrol CT) | 8.1%–31.2% |
| Ajowan (Thymol CT) | 17.9%–30.8% |
| Thyme (Thymol CT) | 0.0%–29.0% |
| Mountain Savory (Carvacrol CT) | 3.0%–28.9% |
| Wormseed, American (Ascaridole CT) | 2.0%–27.2% |
| Wormseed, American (Alpha-Terpinene CT) | 7.3%–26.4% |
| Savory (Wild, Thymol CT) | 7.1%–24.3% |
| Shell Ginger (1,8-Cineole CT) | 0.0%–22.6% |
| Summer Savory (Thymol CT) | 9.0%–19.6% |
| Boldo (Ascaridole CT, no 1,8-cineole) | 12.9%–19.0% |
| Parsley (Leaves, Myristicin CT) | 0.4%–18.9% |
| Blue Mountain Sage (Gamma-Terpinene CT) | 18.4% |
| Mugwort (Chrysanthenyl Acetate CT) | 17.2% |
| Frankincense (*B. carterii*) | 3.0%–17.0% |
| Frankincense (*B. frereana*) | 5.4%–16.9% |
| Petitgrain (Mandarin) | 0.1%–16.3% |
| Sweet Inula (1,8-Cineole CT) | 3.5%–16.2% |
| Monarda (Thymol CT) | 6.0%–14.9% |
| Black Cumin (Trans-Anethole CT) | 9.0%–14.8% |
| Savory (Wild, Linalool CT) | 1.8%–14.8% |
| Ferula (Limonene CT) | 14.3% |
| Mountain Savory (Thymol CT) | 6.4%–13.5% |
| Ajowan (Gamma-Terpinolene CT) | 13.5% |
| Oregano (Carvacrol CT) | 3.0%–12.6% |
| Tea tree | 0.5%–12.0% |
| Indian Borage (Carvacrol CT) | 0.0%–12.0% |
| Aleppo Pine (Aerial Parts) | 0.0%–11.4% |
| Turmeric (Leaves) | 4.8%–11.1% |
| Summer Savory (Gamma-Terpinene CT) | 1.7%–11.1% |
| Mugwort (Alpha-Thujone CT) | 2.7%–10.6% |
| Mastic (NT\B, Terpinene-4-ol CT) | 4.8%–10.2% |
| Niaouli (1,8-Cineole CT) | 0.0%–10.0% |
| Pink Pepper (*S. molle*, Leaves, Elemol/Beta-Eudesmol CT) | 9.4% |
| Blue Tansy (Sabinene CT) | 5.9%–8.9% |
| Eucalyptus Dives | 0.0%–8.5% |
| Mastic (Leaves) | 0.0%–8.5% |
| Oregano (*O. syriacum*, Thymol CT) | 7.0%–8.4% |
| Lavender (Munstead) | 4.8%–8.3% |
| Wormwood (Beta-Pinene CT) | 7.1%–8.2% |
| Pink Pepper (*S. molle*, Fruits/Leaves, α-Phell./Sylv. CT) | 0.0%–8.1% |
| Lemon (Cold-pressed/expressed) | 0.0%–7.8% |
| Mugwort (1,8-Cineole CT) | 0.1%–7.5% |
| Blue Mallee (Cryptone CT) | 3.2%–7.5% |
| Pink Pepper (*S. molle*, Leaves, α-Phellandrene CT) | 0.0%–7.3% |
| Pink Pepper (*S. terebinthifolius*, Fruits, α-Phell. CT) | 7.3% |
| Marjoram | 3.5%–7.0% |
| Mugwort (Beta-Caryophyllene CT) | 6.8% |
| Summer Savory (Carvacrol CT) | 3.1%–6.7% |
| Pink Pepper (*S. molle*, Fruits, α-Phellandrene CT) | 1.8%–6.4% |
| Rosemary (Verbenone CT) | 1.1%–6.3% |
| Wormwood (Sabinene CT) | 4.7%–6.2% |
| Fennel (Trans-Anethole CT) | 0.0%–6.0% |
| Shell Ginger (Terpinen-4-ol CT) | 4.1%–5.9% |
| Citron (Fingered, Distilled) | 0.0%–5.7% |
| Lime (Cold-pressed/expressed) | 0.0%–5.6% |
| Pink Pepper (*S. molle*, Aerial Parts, α-Phell. CT) | 5.4% |
| Dill (Aerial Parts, Alpha-Phellandrene CT) | 0.7%–5.3% |
| Persian Lime (Distilled) | 0.1%–5.3% |
| Oregano (*O. syriacum*, Carvacrol CT) | 3.7%–5.2% |
| Plai (Terpinen-4-ol CT) | 0.0%–5.2% |
| Black Pepper (Limonene CT) | 0.0%–5.2% |
| Eucalyptus (*E. globulus*) | 0.0%–5.1% |
| Myrtle (Limonene CT) | 0.0%–5.1% |
| Thyme (Thuyanol-4 CT) | 0.0%–5.0% |
| Oregano (*O. onites*) | 2.5%–4.9% |
| Arnica (Roots, Thymol Derivatives CT) | 0.1%–4.9% |
| Cistus (Alpha-Pinene CT) | 1.0%–4.8% |
| Ocotea (Flowers Calices) | 0.0%–4.8% |
| Vilayti Tulsi (Fenchone CT) | 2.7%–4.5% |
| Coriander | 0.1%–4.4% |
| Rosalina (Linalool CT) | 0.0%–4.3% |
| Chaste Tree (Berries) | 0.0%–4.2% |
| Blue Mallee (1,8-Cineole CT) | 1.2%–4.1% |
| Angelica Root | 0.6%–3.9% |
| Rosemary (Camphor CT) | 0.0%–3.8% |
| Frankincense (*B. serrata*) | 1.6%–3.5% |
| Black Pepper (Delta-3-Carene CT) | 1.4%–3.5% |
| Mastic (Twigs, Alpha-Pinene CT) | 3.5% |
| Ledum (*R. groenlandicum*) | 0.2%–3.4% |
| Ravensara (Sabinene CT) | 1.4%–3.0% |
| Chaste Tree (Leaves) | 0.0%–3.0% |
| Frankincense (*B. sacra*) | 1.6%–2.7% |
| Mugwort (Camphor CT) | 0.0%–2.4% |
| May Chang (Neral CT) | 2.1% |
| Tansy (Beta-Thujone CT) | 0.0%–1.6% |
| Southern Blue Gum | 0.2%–1.4% |
| Ravensara (Methyl Eugenol CT) | 0.5%–1.2% |
| Lemon Eucalyptus | 0.6%–1.0% |

**Para-Cymene + Limonene**

| | |
|---|---|
| Monarda (Carvacrol CT) | 1.7%–6.0% |

**Para-Cymenene (P-Cymenene)**

| | |
|---|---|
| Boldo (*1,8-Cineole\Para-Cymene\Limonene CT*) | 13.6%–29.8% |
| Juniper, Phoenicia (needles) | 0.0%–25.7% |
| Boldo (Ascaridole CT) | 0.0%–16.3% |
| Cumin | 4.1%–15.6% |
| Mugwort (Artemisia Ketone CT) | 1.7%–7.6% |
| Kanuka | 0.0%–5.1% |
| Ledum (*L. palustre*) | 0.0%–5.0% |
| Angelica Root | 0.0%–4.6% |
| Feverfew | 0.0%–4.2% |
| Japanese Cedarwood (16-Kaurene/Valencene CT) | 3.7% |
| Helichrysum (*H. splendidum*, Alpha-Terpinene CT) | 3.0% |
| Applemint (*M. suav.*, Italian) | 0.0%–2.5% |
| Elemi | 1.1%–1.8% |
| Western Red Cedar (Wood) | 1.1%–1.2% |

**Para-Cymol**

| | |
|---|---|
| Boldo (Ascaridole CT) | 0.0%–7.9% |

**Para-Mentha-1(7),8-Ddiene**

| | |
|---|---|
| Eucalyptus Dives | 0.0%–3.3% |

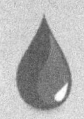

**Para-Menthane-3,8-Diol**

| | |
|---|---|
| Lemon Eucalyptus | 0.0%–2.9% |

**Parsley Apiole (Parsley Apiol)**

| | |
|---|---|
| Parsley (Leaves, 1,3,8-Para-Menth. CT) | 0.0%–22.1% |
| Parsley (Whole Plant) | 17.5%–21.0% |
| Parsley (Leaves, Myristicin CT) | 0.1%–13.5% |
| Parsley Seed | 0.1%–10.2% |

**Patchoulol (Patchouli Alcohol)**

| | |
|---|---|
| Patchouli (Chinese) | 22.9%–78.2% |
| Patchouli (Brazilian) | 36.6%–70.7% |
| Patchouli (Indonesian, Malaysian, Vietnamese) | 37.8%–68.0% |
| Spikenard (Calarene CT) | 0.0%–10.6% |
| Spikenard (Ledene Oxide CT) | 9.6% |

**Pentacosane**

| | |
|---|---|
| Moringa (Leaves, Pentacosane CT) | 13.3%–17.4% |
| Calendula (Alpha-Cadinol/Delta-Cadinene CT) | 0.0%–3.0% |

**Pentadecane (N-Pentadecane)**

| | |
|---|---|
| Galangal (False, 2-Propeonic Acid CT) | 26.1% |
| Galangal (False, Ethyl-p-Methoxycinnamate CT) | 0.0%–9.0% |
| Galangal (Greater, Piperitenone CT) | 5.6% |
| Chaste Tree (Berries) | 0.0%–2.6% |

**Pentadecanol (n-Pentadecanol)**

| | |
|---|---|
| Moringa (Flowers) | 10.5% |

**Pentadecanoic Acid**

| | |
|---|---|
| Yarrow (Chamazulene CT) | 0.0%–2.1% |

**Pentylcyclohexa-1,5-Diene**

| | |
|---|---|
| Lovage (Roots) | 0.0%–12.3% |

**Perhydrofarnesyl Acetone**

| | |
|---|---|
| Jasmine (Hydrodistilled) | 4.9% |

**Perillene**

| | |
|---|---|
| Verbena (Myrcene CT) | 0.1%–4.3% |

**Phellandral**

| | |
|---|---|
| Celery Leaf | 0.0%–17.2% |

**Phenylacetaldehyde**

| | |
|---|---|
| Lovage (Roots) | 0.0%–29.0% |

**Phenylethyl 2-Methylbutanoate (2-Phenylethyl 2-Methylbutanoate)**

| | |
|---|---|
| Aleppo Pine (Needles) | 0.0%–10.3% |

**Phenylethyl 2-Methylbutyrate**

| | |
|---|---|
| Maritime Pine (Needles, Alpha-Pinene CT) | 0.0%–6.1% |

**Phenylethyl 3-Methylbutanoate (2-Phenylethyl 3-Methylbutanoate, 2-Phenylethyl Isovalerate)**

| | |
|---|---|
| Aleppo Pine (Aerial Parts) | 0.0%–8.4% |
| Aleppo Pine (Needles) | 0.0%–6.2% |

**Phenylethyl Acetate**

| | |
|---|---|
| Jasmine Absolute (Benzyl Acetate CT) | 0.0%–6.5% |

**(+)-Phyllocladene**

| | |
|---|---|
| Japanese Cedarwood (Alpha-Pinene CT) | 0.0%–24.1% |

**Phytene-2**

| | |
|---|---|
| Spearmint (Pulegone-Menthone-Isomenthone CT) | 0.0%–3.5% |

**Phytol ((E)-Phytol, Trans-Phytol)**

| | |
|---|---|
| Jasmine (Hydrodistilled) | 25.8% |
| Moringa (Leaves, (E)-Phytol CT) | 21.9% |
| Jasmine Absolute (Benzyl Acetate CT) | 0.0%–12.5% |
| Moringa (Leaves, Pentacosane CT) | 0.0%–7.7% |
| Guava Leaf (Beta-Caryophyllene CT) | 0.0%–4.8% |
| Yarrow (Chamazulene CT) | 0.0%–2.6% |
| Spearmint (Pulegone-Menthone-Isomenthone CT) | 0.0%–2.5% |

**Phytyl Acetate**

| | |
|---|---|
| Jasmine Absolute (Benzyl Acetate CT) | 0.0%–7.0% |

**Pinchotene Acetate**

| | |
|---|---|
| Arnica (Roots, 2,5-Dimethoxy-p-Cymene CT) | 2.5%–4.7% |

**Pinocamphone (Trans-Pinocamphone)**

| | |
|---|---|
| Hyssop (Pinocamphone CT) | 34.0%–53.0% |
| Hyssop (Linalool CT) | 0.1%–1.0% |

**Pinocarvone**

| | |
|---|---|
| Mastic (Gum Resin) | 0.0%–5.3% |
| Wild Chamomile (O. mixta, C. mixtrum) | 0.1%–4.1% |
| Sweet Wormwood (Artemisia Ketone CT) | 0.0%–4.0% |
| Southern Blue Gum | 0.1%–3.9% |
| Hyssop (Pinocamphone CT) | 0.0%–1.4% |
| Ledum (R. groenlandicum) | 0.0%–1.9% |

**Piperidine**

| | |
|---|---|
| Applemint (M. rotun., Pulegone CT) | 0.0%–3.0% |
| Applemint (M. rotun., β-Caryophyllene CT) | 2.7% |

**Piperitenone**

| | |
|---|---|
| Verbena (Limonene\Piperitenone CT) | 32.5%–47.3% |
| Applemint (M. rotun., Piperitenone CT) | 35.6% |
| Galangal (Greater, Piperitenone CT) | 33.3% |
| Applemint (M. suav., Piperitenone) | 33.0% |
| Tagetes (T. patula, Flowers) | 22.9% |
| Pennyroyal (M. pulegium) | 0.0%–16.5% |
| Tagetes (T. minuta, Limonene CT) | 0.0%–12.2% |
| Tagetes (T. erecta, Flowers) | 2.6%–11.0% |
| Pennyroyal (M. fruticosa, Pulegone CT) | 7.1%–10.3% |
| Applemint (M. suav., Piperitenone CT) | 0.0%–10.1% |
| Tagetes (T. erecta, Leaves) | 5.0%–9.7% |
| Tagetes (T. erecta, Aerial Parts) | 0.0%–5.9% |
| Tagetes (T. patula, Limonene CT) | 0.0%–4.9% |
| White Verbena (Carvone\Limonene CT) | 2.2%–4.3% |
| Spearmint (Piperitenone Oxide CT) | 1.0%–2.8% |
| Pennyroyal (M. pulegioides) | 0.5%–2.5% |
| Spearmint (Piperitone Oxide CT) | 0.1%–1.3% |

**Piperitenone Oxide**

| | |
|---|---|
| Applemint (M. suav., Italian) | 35.6%–87.3% |
| Applemint (M. suav., Piperitenone CT) | 55.5%–81.7% |
| Applemint (M. rotun., Piperitenone CT) | 23.5%–80.8% |
| Spearmint (Piperitenone Oxide CT) | 63.5%–70.3% |
| Applemint (M. suav., PO-PEO CT) | 26.0% |
| Applemint (M. rotun., Piperitone CT) | 17.6% |
| Applemint (M. rotun., Pulegone CT) | 0.0%–17.3% |
| Tagetes (T. erecta, Flowers) | 0.0%–7.2% |
| Spearmint (Piperitone Oxide CT) | 0.1%–4.8% |
| Applemint (M. rotun., Piperitenone CT) | 4.0% |
| Applemint (M. rotun., β-Caryophyllene CT) | 3.4% |

**Piperitone**

| | |
|---|---|
| Eucalyptus Dives | 29.2%–88.4% |
| Tagetes (T. minuta, Piperitone CT) | 86.3% |
| Applemint (M. rotun., Piperitone CT) | 54.9% |
| Tagetes (T. erecta, Leaves) | 8.9%–52.4% |
| Tagetes (T. erecta, Aerial Parts) | 3.4%–45.7% |
| Tagetes (T. erecta, Flowers) | 0.6%–28.5% |
| Tagetes (T. patula, Flowers) | 24.7% |
| Applemint (M. rotun., Piperitenone CT) | 21.2% |
| Applemint (M. suav., Piperitenone) | 9.2% |
| Pennyroyal (M. pulegium) | 0.0%–6.4% |
| Tagetes (T. patula, Limonene CT) | 0.0%–6.1% |
| Tagetes (T. minuta, Limonene CT) | 0.0%–6.0% |
| Yarrow (Chamazulene CT) | 0.0%–5.1% |
| Wormseed, American (Ascaridole CT) | 0.0%–5.0% |
| Engelmann Spruce | 0.0%–4.6% |
| White Verbena (Carvone\Limonene CT) | 0.0%–4.4% |
| Cinnamon (leaves) | 0.0%–3.3% |

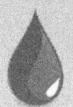

| | |
|---|---|
| Zdravetz | 0.0%–3.0% |
| Applemint (*M. suav.*, Menthol CT) | 3.0% |
| Applemint (*M. rotun.*, Piperitenone CT) | 0.0%–2.6% |
| Spearmint (Piperitone Oxide CT) | 0.1%–1.8% |

**Piperitone Oxide**

| | |
|---|---|
| Spearmint (Piperitone Oxide CT) | 54.2%–72.3% |
| Applemint (*M. rotun.*, Piperitenone CT) | 0.0%–31.4% |
| Applemint (*M. suav.*, PO-PEO CT) | 25.0% |

**Pogostol**

| | |
|---|---|
| Patchouli (Indonesian, Malaysian, Vietnamese) | 3.7%–5.5% |

**Pogostone**

| | |
|---|---|
| Patchouli (Chinese) | 6.0%–32.7% |

**Precocene I**

| | |
|---|---|
| Lavender (Brazilian) | 13.0% |

**Preisocalamendiol**

| | |
|---|---|
| Calamus (Shyobunones CT) | 7.0%–12.0% |
| Calamus (Acorenone CT) | 8.1%–8.1% |

**Propyl Allyl Disulfide**

| | |
|---|---|
| Garlic (Sulfides CT) | 0.0%–7.2% |

**Propyl Tigliate**

| | |
|---|---|
| Chamomile (Roman) | 10.8%–13.1% |

**psi-Diosphenol (ψ-Diosphenol)**

| | |
|---|---|
| Buchu (*A. betulina*, Isomenthone CT) | 10.3%–23.3% |
| Buchu (*A. betulina*, Menthone CT) | 2.9% |

**Pulegol**

| | |
|---|---|
| Pennyroyal (*M. fruticosa*, Isomenthol CT) | 11.1%–15.3% |

**Pulegone ((1R)-(+)-Beta-Pulegone)**

| | |
|---|---|
| Pennyroyal (*M. pulegioides*) | 67.6%–86.7% |
| Applemint (*M. rotun.*, Pulegone CT) | 32.1%–85.5% |
| Pennyroyal (*M. pulegium*) | 38.8%–73.4% |
| Buchu (*A. crenulata*) | 31.6%–73.2% |
| Spearmint (Pulegone-Menthone-Isomenthone CT) | 26.7%–72.1% |
| Pennyroyal (*M. fruticosa*, Pulegone CT) | 56.6%–62.9% |
| Applemint (*M. suav.*, Pulegone CT) | 50.0% |
| Pennyroyal (*M. fruticosa*, Isomenthol CT) | 0.0%–22.5% |
| Applemint (*M. suav.*, Menthol CT) | 20.3% |
| Applemint (*M. suav.*, Piperitenone) | 17.6% |
| Betony (Bicyclogermacrene CT) | 0.0%–15.1% |
| Buchu (*A. betulina*, Menthone CT) | 8.4% |
| Applemint (*M. rotun.*, Piperitenone CT) | 6.5% |
| Buchu (*A. betulina*, Isomenthone CT) | 0.6%–4.5% |
| Peppermint | 0.3%–4.4% |
| Applemint (*M. suav.*, Piperitenone CT) | 0.0%–2.4% |
| Applemint (*M. rotun.*, β-Caryophyllene CT) | 2.4% |
| Cornmint | 0.0%–0.8% |

**rel-2R-Methoxy-4R-Furanogermacdra-1(10)E-en-6-One**

| | |
|---|---|
| Opoponax (*C. erythraea*) | 0.9%–3.1% |

**rel-3R-Methoxy-4S-Furanogermacdra-1E,10(15)-Dien-6-One**

| | |
|---|---|
| Opoponax (*C. erythraea*) | 0.9%–3.9% |

**Rimuene**

| | |
|---|---|
| Thuja | 0.3%–5.0% |
| Siam Wood (Leaves) | 3.3% |

**Rosifoliol**

| | |
|---|---|
| Helichrysum (ssp. *microphyllum*) | 0.0%–20.2% |
| Ledum (*R. groenlandicum*) | 0.0%–4.3% |
| Kunzea (Spathulenol\Globulol CT) | 0.0%–2.0% |

**Rotundifolene**

| | |
|---|---|
| Tagetes (*T. patula*, Aerial Parts) | 4.6% |

**Rotundifolone (Cis-Piperitenone epoxide)**

| | |
|---|---|
| Spearmint (*M. crispa*, Rotundifolone CT) | 58.1% |

**Sabinene**

| | |
|---|---|
| Savin (Berries) | 46.8%–82.9% |

| | |
|---|---|
| Nutmeg (West Indian) | 33.0%–57.0% |
| Savin (Needles & Branches) | 18.3%–56.7% |
| Plai (Sabinene CT) | 34.0%–53.5% |
| Pink Pepper (*S. molle*, Leaves/Fruits, Sabinene CT) | 34.7%–51.7% |
| Juniper (*J. wallichiana\J. indica*, Leaves) | 27.8%–51.0% |
| Juniper (*J. wallichiana\J. indica*, Berries) | 23.2%–50.2% |
| Kaffir Lime Peel | 1.7%–45.6% |
| Nutmeg (East Indian) | 6.3%–44.8% |
| Chaste Tree (Berries) | 3.5%–44.1% |
| Neroli (*C. sinensis*) | 31.4%–41.4% |
| Yarrow (Sabinene CT) | 6.7%–41.3% |
| Pink Pepper (*S. terebinthifolius*, Leaves, Sabinene CT) | 40.7% |
| Ledum (*R. groenlandicum*) | 0.1%–35.0% |
| Ravensara (Sabinene CT) | 25.0%–34.4% |
| Juniper (Needles) | 0.2%–33.6% |
| Vilayti Tulsi (Sabinene CT) | 7.3%–31.3% |
| Wormwood (Myrcene-Sabinene CT) | 18.0%–30.1% |
| Douglas Fir (Needles & Twigs) | 0.0%–29.7% |
| Wormwood (Sabinene CT) | 17.6%–24.5% |
| Juniper, Phoenicia (Berries) | 0.0%–24.3% |
| Blue Tansy (Sabinene CT) | 13.3%–22.3% |
| Wormwood (Myrcene CT) | 0.0%–21.1% |
| Douglas Fir (Needles) | 11.2%–21.0% |
| Japanese Cedarwood (Alpha-Pinene CT) | 0.5%–19.9% |
| Juniper (Chinese) | 15.6%–19.8% |
| Lime (Cold-pressed/expressed) | 0.1%–19.6% |
| Ravensara (Alpha-Terpinene CT) | 16.8%–19.4% |
| Black Pepper (Limonene CT) | 0.8%–18.1% |
| Vilayti Tulsi (Fenchone CT) | 10.3%–18.0% |
| Plai (Terpinen-4-ol, No Phenylbutanoids CT) | 0.0%–17.4% |
| Ravensara (1,8-Cineole CT) | 11.0%–17.2% |
| Chaste Tree (Leaves) | 2.3%–17.1% |
| Lavandin (Giant) | 0.0%–16.9% |
| Ravintsara (1,8-Cineole CT) | 14.1%–16.8% |
| Lavandin (Dutch) | 0.0%–16.7% |
| Ravensara (Limonene CT) | 3.9%–16.4% |
| Pink Pepper (*S. terebinthifolius*, Fruits, Limonene CT) | 0.0%–15.8% |
| Yarrow (Chamazulene CT) | 0.0%–15.2% |
| Melissa (Greek, subsp. Altissima) | 0.9%–14.7% |
| Mugwort (1,8-Cineole CT) | 0.0%–13.7% |
| Juniper (*J. recurva*, Needles) | 0.4%–13.4% |
| Pink Pepper (*S. molle*, Leaves, Bicyclogermacrene CT) | 0.0%–12.9% |
| Hinoki (needles and twigs) | 12.8% |
| Shell Ginger (1,8-Cineole CT) | 0.0%–12.5% |
| Black Pepper (Eugenol CT) | 0.0%–12.1% |
| Marjoram | 4.9%–12.0% |
| Juniper Berry | 2.8%–11.8% |
| Oriental Arborvitae (Berries) | 2.1%–11.1% |
| Japanese Cedarwood (16-Kaurene CT) | 1.2%–11.1% |
| Lavender (True English) | 0.1%–11.0% |
| Mastic (NT\B, Terpinene-4-ol CT) | 4.2%–10.5% |
| Bay Laurel | 0.1%–10.2% |
| Plai (Terpinen-4-ol CT) | 3.7%–10.1% |
| Shell Ginger (Terpinen-4-ol CT) | 1.4%–10.1% |
| Oriental Arborvitae (Needles) | 0.5%–10.0% |
| Black Pepper (Beta-Caryophyllene CT) | 0.0%–10.0% |
| Aleppo Pine (Needles) | 0.1%–9.4% |
| Aleppo Pine (Aerial Parts) | 0.0%–9.4% |
| Wormwood ((Z)-Epoxy Ocimene CT) | 0.0%–9.3% |
| Yarrow (Beta-Thujone CT) | 0.0%–8.9% |
| Wormwood (Beta-Pinene CT) | 0.0%–8.8% |
| Blue Tansy (Chamazulene CT) | 4.0%–8.6% |
| Ghandi Root | 0.0%–8.3% |
| Thuja | 1.4%–7.6% |

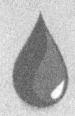

**Sabinene—continued**

| | |
|---|---|
| Ocotea (Leaves) | 7.6% |
| Angelica Root | 0.4%–7.0% |
| Mastic (Leaves) | 0.0%–7.0% |
| Wormwood (Trans-Sabinyl Acetate CT) | 1.0%–6.9% |
| Mastic (NT\B, Alpha-Pinene CT) | 1.0%–6.8% |
| Mastic (NT\B, Germacrene D CT) | 6.7% |
| Lavandin (Super) | 0.0%–6.5% |
| Western Red Cedar (Leaves) | 4.2%–6.4% |
| Boldo (*1,8-Cineole\Para-Cymene\Limonene CT*) | 5.1%–6.3% |
| Hinoki (*Leaves*, Alpha-Terpinolene CT) | 6.3% |
| Pink Pepper (*S. molle*, Leaves, Limonene CT) | 5.9% |
| Elemi | 3.4%–5.7% |
| Rabbitbrush (var. *nauseosa*) | 5.7% |
| Frankincense (*B. sacra*) | 1.1%–5.2% |
| Petitgrain (Lemon) | 1.9%–5.1% |
| Frankincense (*B. carterii*) | 0.0%–4.9% |
| Lemon (Cold-pressed/expressed) | 0.1%–6.3% |
| Wormwood (Beta-Thujone CT) | 0.0%–6.3% |
| Frankincense (*B. serrata*) | 0.4%–5.9% |
| Lemon (Distilled) | 0.0%–5.8% |
| Mastic (Aerial parts, Beta-Eudesmol CT) | 5.5% |
| Pink Pepper (*S. molle*, Fruits/Leaves, α-Phell./Sylv. CT) | 0.9%–5.1% |
| Rosemary (Camphor CT) | 0.0%–5.1% |
| Black Sage (Alpha-Pinene CT) | 0.0%–5.0% |
| Betony (Alpha-Thujene CT) | 0.0%–4.7% |
| Rosemary (Alpha-Pinene CT) | 0.0%–4.6% |
| Cardamom (Alpha-Terpinyl Acetate CT) | 2.6%–4.3% |
| Summer Savory (Thymol CT) | 1.3%–4.3% |
| Silver Fir (*A. alba*) | 0.0%–4.3% |
| Black Pepper (Delta-3-Carene CT) | 0.0%–4.1% |
| Applemint (*M. suav.*, Carvone CT) | 0.0%–4.0% |
| Wormwood (Trans-Sabinene Hydrate CT) | 0.0%–4.0% |
| Vilayti Tulsi (1,8-Cineole CT) | 2.5%–3.9% |
| Wild Chamomile (*C. mixtus*, Sant. Alc. CT) | 0.3%–3.9% |
| Ravensara (Methyl Chavicol CT) | 0.1%–3.4% |
| Wild Chamomile (*O. multicaulis*) | 0.1%–3.4% |
| Rabbitbrush (var. *albicaulis*) | 3.4% |
| Japanese Cedarwood (Bark) | 0.0%–3.3% |
| Mastic (NT\B, Limonene CT) | 2.2%–3.2% |
| Saro (1,8-Cineole CT) | 1.8%–3.2% |
| Great Mugwort | 0.1%–3.0 % |
| Frankincense (*B. frereana*) | 0.0%–2.6% |
| May Chang (Citronellal CT) | 0.8%–2.4% |
| Helichrysum (*H. splendidum*, Alpha-Terpinene CT) | 2.4% |
| Tansy (Beta-Thujone CT) | 0.0%–2.1% |
| Yarrow (1,8-Cineole\Camphor CT) | 0.1%–2.0% |
| Hyssop (Pinocamphone CT) | 1.3%–1.9% |
| Mediterranean Mandarin (Hydrodistilled) | 0.2%–1.4% |
| Hyssop (Linalool CT) | 0.8%–1.0% |
| Ravensara (Methyl Eugenol CT) | 0.4%–0.5% |

**Sabinene Hydrate**

| | |
|---|---|
| Galangal (Greater, 1,8-Cineole CT) | 0.0%–8.8% |
| Hairy Basil (var. *pilosum* Linalool CT) | 0.0%–6.1% |
| Lavandin (Super) | 0.0%–4.6% |
| Spearmint (Pulegone-Menthone-Isomenthone CT) | 0.0%–2.8% |

**Sabinol**

| | |
|---|---|
| Genipi (*A. umbelliformis*, Alpha-Thujone CT) | 0.0%–4.1% |

**Sabinyl Acetate**

| | |
|---|---|
| Wormwood (Chamazulene CT) | 0.1%–5.0% |

**Sabinyl Isovalerinate**

| | |
|---|---|
| Genipi (*A. umbelliformis*, Alpha-Thujone CT) | 0.0%–7.1% |

**Sabinyl Valerianate**

| | |
|---|---|
| Genipi (*A. umbelliformis*, Alpha-Thujone CT) | 0.0%–7.3% |

**Safranal**

| | |
|---|---|
| Cumin | 0.0%–26.8% |

**Safrole**

| | |
|---|---|
| Nutmeg (East Indian) | 0.0%–22.1% |
| Savin (Needles & Branches) | 0.0%–6.6% |
| Ravintsara (Camphor CT) | 0.1%–5.0% |
| Nutmeg (West Indian) | 0.1%–1.4% |

**Sandaracopimarinal**

| | |
|---|---|
| Japanese Cedarwood (Sapwood) | 0.0%–3.7% |
| Japanese Cedarwood (Twig) | 3.2%–3.4% |

**Santal-10-en-2-ol**

| | |
|---|---|
| Petitgrain (Lime) | 0.0%–8.5% |

**Santalcamphor (Santal Camphor)**

| | |
|---|---|
| Buddha Wood | 0.0%–17.5% |

**Santalene** <isomer not identified, likely alpha>

| | |
|---|---|
| Lavender (True English) | 0.4%–4.5% |

**Santene**

| | |
|---|---|
| Douglas Fir (Needles & Twigs) | 0.0%–5.5% |
| Silver Fir (*A. alba*) | 0.0%–5.0% |

**Santolina Alcohol**

| | |
|---|---|
| Wild Chamomile (*O. mixta, C. mixtrum*) | 12.5%–55.1% |
| Wild Chamomile (*C. mixtus*, Sant. Alc. CT) | 17.4%–37.7% |
| Wild Chamomile (*O. multicaulis*) | 10.2%–15.2% |
| Sweet Nancy (Artemisyl Acetate CT) | 4.9%–11.8% |
| Sweet Nancy (Yomogi Alc.\1,8-Cin. CT) | 0.0%–10.0% |

**Santolinatriene (Santolina Triene)**

| | |
|---|---|
| Mugwort (Beta-Caryophyllene CT) | 10.0% |
| Wormwood ((E)-Beta-Farnesene CT) | 4.9% |
| Formosan Cypress (Wood, α-Eudesmol CT) | 4.6% |
| Mugwort (Artemisia Ketone CT) | 4.0%–4.0% |
| Mugwort (1,8-Cineole CT) | 2.2%–4.0% |
| Mugwort (Chrysanthenyl Acetate CT) | 3.6% |

**Sativene (1,4-Methano-1 H-Indene)**

| | |
|---|---|
| Betony (Alpha-Thujene CT) | 0.0%–10.1% |

**Sclarene**

| | |
|---|---|
| Japanese Cedarwood (Sapwood) | 0.0%–27.6% |
| Chaste Tree (Leaves) | 0.0%–3.3% |
| Chaste Tree (Berries) | 0.0%–2.0% |

**Sclareol (13-Epi-Sclareol)**

| | |
|---|---|
| Clary Sage | 1.3%–11.5% |

**Sedanenolide**

| | |
|---|---|
| Celery Seed | 0.0%–2.8% |
| Celery Leaf | 0.0%–2.8% |

**Selin-11-en-4-Alpha-ol**

| | |
|---|---|
| Guava Leaf (Selin-11-en-4-Alpha-ol CT) | 21.0%–22.2% |
| Guava Leaf (β-Cary.\(E)-Nerolidol CT) | 13.4% |
| Guava Leaf (Beta-Caryophyllene CT) | 0.0%–8.3% |

**Selina-3,11-Dien-14-al**

| | |
|---|---|
| Agarwood (*A. sinensis*) | 0.4%–5.5% |
| Agarwood (*A. malaccensis*) | 0.0%–4.9% |
| Agarwood (*A. crassna*) | 0.0%–4.0% |

**Selina-3,11-Dien-14-ol**

| | |
|---|---|
| Agarwood (Malaysian) | 0.0%–7.1% |

**Selina-3,11-Dien-9-One**

| | |
|---|---|
| Agarwood (*A. crassna*) | 1.1%–17.2% |
| Agarwood (*A. malaccensis*) | 0.0%–6.2% |

**Selina-4,11-Dien-14-oic Acid**

| | |
|---|---|
| Agarwood (*A. malaccensis*) | 0.0%–5.2% |

**Selina-6-en-4-ol <isomer>**

| | |
|---|---|
| Damiana (1,8-Cineole CT) | 0.0%–12.0% |

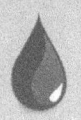

**Selinene <α,β,δ>**

| | |
|---|---|
| Katrafay (Alpha-Eudesmol CT) | 3.4%–17.2% |
| Katrafay (Ishwarane CT) | 0.7%–13.0% |
| Katrafay ((γ,δ)-Cadinene CT) | 0.0%–5.6% |
| Katrafay (Alpha-Pinene CT) | 1.1%–4.5% |

**Sesquiterpene (MW 204)**

| | |
|---|---|
| Ylang Ylang (French IV) | 7.5% |

**Seychellene**

| | |
|---|---|
| Patchouli (Chinese) | 0.0%–9.6% |
| Patchouli (Indonesian, Malaysian, Vietnamese) | 3.7%–7.5% |

**Shyobunones**

| | |
|---|---|
| Calamus (Shyobunones CT) | 13.0%–54.0% |
| Calamus (Acorenone CT) | 13.1%–19.1% |
| Calamus (Beta-Asarone CT) | 0.0%–3.3% |

**Silvestrene**

| | |
|---|---|
| Shell Ginger (1,8-Cineole CT) | 0.0%–4.6% |

**Spathulenol**

| | |
|---|---|
| Copaiba (Leaves) | 12.6%–35.7% |
| Kunzea (Spathulenol\Globulol CT) | 12.2%–34.8% |
| Helichrysum (H. splendidum, Spathulenol CT) | 12.2%–30.7% |
| Pink Pepper (S. molle, Leaves, Bicyclogermacrene CT) | 0.0%–19.2% |
| Tamala (Eugenol CT) | 0.6%–12.7% |
| Betony (Bicyclogermacrene CT) | 3.3%–12.0% |
| Betony (Germacrene D-Spathulenol CT) | 11.1% |
| Agarwood (A. crassna) | 0.0%–9.9% |
| Cangerana (Leaves) | 2.2%–9.8% |
| Applemint (M. suav., Italian) | 0.8%–9.0% |
| Pink Pepper (S. terebinthifolius, Fruits/Leaves, Bicyclogerm. CT) | 0.6%–8.3% |
| Valerian | 0.0%–7.3% |
| Betony (β-Phell.\α-Pinene CT) | 0.0%–7.2% |
| Helichrysum (H. splendidum, Delta-cadinene CT) | 1.6%–6.1% |
| Indian Borage (Delta-Cadinene CT) | 4.9%–5.7% |
| Black Sage (Beta-Caryophyllene CT) | 5.7% |
| Grindelia | 0.0%–5.4% |
| Lemon Verbena (Leaves) | 2.5%–5.2% |
| Yarrow (Chamazulene CT) | 0.0%–5.1% |
| Sweet Wormwood (Camphor CT) | 0.0%–4.9% |
| German Chamomile | 1.7%–4.8% |
| Chaste Tree (Berries) | 0.1%–4.7% |
| Betony (MLD-C CT) | 1.6%–4.3% |
| Spikenard (Calarene CT) | 0.0%–4.3% |
| Betony (Alpha-Zingiberene CT) | 4.1% |
| Blue Mallee (Cryptone CT) | 2.0%–3.8% |
| Tamala (Beta-Caryophyllene CT) | 2.8% |
| Spikenard (Ledene Oxide CT) | 2.7% |
| Chaste Tree (Leaves) | 0.0%–1.8% |
| Mugwort (Isobornyl Isobutyrate D CT) | 1.5% |
| Mugwort (Camphor CT) | 0.0%–1.1% |

**Squalene**

| | |
|---|---|
| Jasmine Absolute (Benzyl Acetate CT) | 0.0%–6.0% |

**Squalene 2,3-Oxide**

| | |
|---|---|
| Jasmine Absolute (Benzyl Acetate CT) | 0.0%–12.0% |

**Styrene**

| | |
|---|---|
| Benzoin (Sumatra, S-HS Absolute) | 90.0%–93.2% |
| Benzoin (Sumatra, HSSE Absolute) | 83.4%–93.1% |
| Benzoin (Sumatra, SPME Absolute) | 72.0%–89.0% |

**Sylvestrene**

| | |
|---|---|
| Pink Pepper (S. molle, Fruits/Leaves, α-Phell./Sylv. CT) | 22.3%–38.5% |
| Pink Pepper (S. terebinthifolius, Fruits, δ-3-Carene CT) | 0.0%–10.7% |

**Terpinen-4-ol (4-Terpineol, Terpineol-4-ol, Terpinene-4-ol)**

| | |
|---|---|
| Plai (Terpinen-4-ol, No Phenylbutanoids CT) | 40.5%–67.1% |
| Shell Ginger (Terpinen-4-ol CT) | 17.3%–55.7% |
| Hairy Basil (var. pilosum Terpinen-4-ol CT) | 25.0%–52.8% |
| Plai (Terpinen-4-ol CT) | 10.2%–50.5% |
| Oregano (Terpinen-4-ol CT) | 41.2%–48.0% |
| Tea tree | 37.0%–46.9% |
| Mastic (NT\B, Terpinene-4-ol CT) | 25.1%–43.8% |
| Marjoram | 28.9%–38.4% |
| Plai (Sabinene CT) | 11.5%–30.0% |
| Mastic (Leaves) | 1.6%–29.9% |
| Thyme (Thuyanol-4 CT) | 2.2%–29.6% |
| Niaouli (M. viridiflora, Terpinen-4-ol CT) | 29.1% |
| Hairy Basil (var. pilosum Linalool CT) | 0.5%–26.8% |
| Juniper (J. wallichiana\J. indica, Berries) | 2.2%–23.6% |
| Lavender (Munstead) | 0.3%–19.5% |
| Shell Ginger (Para-Cymene CT) | 18.8% |
| Plai (Triquinacene,1,4-Bis(Methoxy)- CT) | 18.5% |
| Nutmeg (West Indian) | 5.8%–17.8% |
| Kaffir Lime Peel | 0.0%–17.4% |
| Shell Ginger (1,8-Cineole CT) | 0.0%–17.4% |
| Ghandi Root | 4.6%–16.7% |
| Juniper (J. wallichiana\J. indica, Leaves) | 4.5%–16.1% |
| Mastic (NT\B, Limonene CT) | 10.2%–15.3% |
| Mastic (NT\B, Alpha-Pinene CT) | 6.4%–14.8% |
| Savin (Needles & Branches) | 1.1%–14.4% |
| Lavender (French) | 0.1%–13.5% |
| Genipi (A. genipi) | 1.0%–12.2% |
| Douglas Fir (Needles) | 0.0%–12.2% |
| Ravensara (Methyl Eugenol CT) | 6.0%–12.0% |
| Vilayti Tulsi (Sabinene CT) | 2.9%–11.4% |
| Pink Pepper (S. molle, Leaves, Bicyclogermacrene CT) | 1.2%–10.6% |
| Mastic (NT\B, Germacrene D CT) | 10.0% |
| Japanese Cedarwood (Alpha-Pinene CT) | 0.1%–9.8% |
| Lavender (True English) | 7.8%–9.6% |
| Japanese Cedarwood (16-Kaurene CT) | 0.0%–9.1% |
| Black Pepper (Eugenol CT) | 0.0%–8.8% |
| Thyme (Linalool CT) | 0.0%–8.5% |
| Genipi (A. umbelliformis, C-SH\B CT) | 3.3%–8.2% |
| Eucalyptus Dives | 0.1%–7.9% |
| Chaste Tree (Leaves) | 1.4%–7.8% |
| Great Mugwort | 1.0%–7.7% |
| Mugwort (1,8-Cineole CT) | 2.2%–7.6% |
| Hairy Basil (1-8-Cineole\Linalool CT) | 0.7%–7.5% |
| Lavender (Bulgarian) | 0.1%–7.4% |
| Ravensara (1,8-Cineole CT) | 7.0%–7.2% |
| Petitgrain (Mandarin) | 0.1%–7.1% |
| Thyme (Carvacrol CT) | 0.1%–7.1% |
| Lavandin (Super) | 1.0%–6.7% |
| Savory (Wild, Linalool CT) | 2.8%–6.4% |
| Cistus (Viridiflorol-Trans-Pinocarveol CT) | 0.7%–6.4% |
| Juniper Berry | 0.1%–6.3% |
| Mastic (Twigs, Alpha-Pinene CT) | 6.3% |
| Yarrow (Sabinene CT) | 0.4%–6.2% |
| Thyme (Alpha-Terpineol CT) | 0.0%–6.2% |
| Yarrow (Beta-Thujone CT) | 0.0%–5.8% |
| Ferula (Limonene CT) | 5.8% |
| Neroli (C. sinensis) | 2.3%–5.6% |
| Pink Pepper (S. molle, Leaves/Fruits, Sabinene CT) | 0.8%–5.5% |
| Boldo (1,8-Cineole\Para-Cymene\Limonene CT) | 4.4%–5.3% |
| Hinoki (needles) | 2.1%–5.3% |
| Utah Juniper (Needles/Twigs) | 1.7%–5.2% |
| Angelica Root | 0.9%–5.1% |
| Ledum (R. groenlandicum) | 0.1%–5.1% |
| Niaouli (Viridiflorol/ Para-cymene/1,8-cineole CT) | 0.5%–5.0% |
| Thyme (Thymol CT) | 0.0%–5.0% |
| Ravensara (Limonene CT) | 1.7%–4.8% |

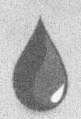

## Terpinen-4-ol—continued

| | |
|---|---|
| Utah Juniper (Needles/Berries) | 4.8% |
| Leleshwa | 2.0%–4.7% |
| Western Red Cedar (Leaves) | 1.6%–4.7% |
| Wormwood (Sabinene CT) | 1.4%–4.5% |
| Savin (Berries) | 1.1%–4.3% |
| Black Cumin (Para-Cymene CT) | 0.0%–4.3% |
| Galbanum | 0.0%–4.1% |
| Mastic (Aerial parts, Beta-Eudesmol CT) | 4.1% |
| Applemint (*M. rotun.*, Piperitenone CT) | 0.3%–4.0% |
| Lavandin (Dutch) | 1.5%–3.9% |
| Guava Leaf (1,8-Cineole) | 3.9% |
| Lavender (Italian) | 1.1%–3.6% |
| Rosalina (Linalool CT) | 0.0%–3.6% |
| Honey Myrtle | 0.0%–3.4% |
| Chaste Tree (Berries) | 0.3%–3.3% |
| Yarrow (1,8-Cineole\Camphor CT) | 1.9%–3.1% |
| Yarrow (Chamazulene CT) | 0.2%–3.1% |
| Thuja | 2.0%–3.0% |
| Niaouli (1,8-cineole CT) | 0.0%–3.0% |
| Applemint (*M. rotun.*, Piperitone CT) | 3.0% |
| Rabbitbrush (var. *consimilis*) | 3.0% |
| Tamala (Linalool CT) | 2.8% |
| Mediterranean Mandarin (Hydrodistilled) | 0.0%–2.4% |
| Rabbitbrush (var. *nauseosa*) | 2.4% |
| Rabbitbrush (var. *glabratus*) | 2.3% |
| Ravensara (Methyl Chavicol CT) | 0.0%–2.2% |
| Lavender (Polish) | 1.1%–2.0% |
| Mastic (NT\B, Beta-Myrcene CT) | 0.5%–2.0% |
| Western Red Cedar (Wood) | 1.4%–1.7% |
| Blue Mallee (1,8-Cineole CT) | 0.6%–1.5% |
| Lemon Eucalyptus | 0.0%–1.0% |

## Terpinen-4-yl Acetate (4-Terpineol Acetate, 4-Terpinenyl Acetate)

| | |
|---|---|
| Ferula (Limonene CT) | 3.4% |

## Tetracosane

| | |
|---|---|
| Moringa (Flowers) | 27.4% |
| Moringa (Fruits) | 24.0% |
| Moringa (Leaves, Pentacosane CT) | 1.5%–9.7% |

## Tetradecane (N-Tetradecane)

| | |
|---|---|
| Chaste Tree (Berries) | 0.0%–3.3% |

## Tetradecenal

| | |
|---|---|
| Agarwood (*A. crassna*) | 0.0%–8.6% |
| Agarwood (*A. malaccensis*) | 0.0%–6.1% |

## Tetra-Dihydrolinalool

| | |
|---|---|
| Frankincense (*B. serrata*) | 0.0%–10.6% |

## Thunbergol (Isocembrol)

| | |
|---|---|
| Guggul | 0.0%–8.7% |
| Aleppo Pine (Aerial Parts) | 0.0%–8.3% |

## Thujic Acid

| | |
|---|---|
| Western Red Cedar (Wood) | 1.8%–25.0% |

## Thujic Acid Isomer

| | |
|---|---|
| Western Red Cedar (Wood) | 0.0%–1.9% |

## Thujol

| | |
|---|---|
| Black Cumin (Para-Cymene CT) | 0.0%–11.2% |

## Thujopsene (Cis-Thujopsene, Widdrene)

| | |
|---|---|
| Texas Cedarwood | 25.0%–60.4% |
| Chinese Cedarwood | 0.0%–37.4% |
| Cedarwood (Virginian, Wood) | 21.3%–30.0% |
| Oriental Arborvitae (Needles) | 0.0%–5.0% |

## Thujyl Alcohol

| | |
|---|---|
| Tansy (Beta-Thujone CT) | 0.0%–8.7% |

## Thuyanol-4 (Cis-Sabinene Hydrate)

| | |
|---|---|
| Thyme (Thuyanol-4 CT) | 1.6%–52.2% |
| Marjoram | 3.0%–30.2% |
| Thyme (Linalool CT) | 0.0%–20.6% |
| Genipi (*A. umbelliformis*, C-SH\B CT) | 2.7%–20.1% |
| Thyme (Alpha-Terpineol CT) | 0.0%–13.9% |
| Thyme (Carvacrol CT) | 0.0%–12.2% |
| Thyme (Thymol CT) | 0.0%–3.3% |
| Plai (Triquinacene,1,4-Bis(Methoxy)- CT) | 3.0% |

## Thymol

| | |
|---|---|
| Thyme (Thymol CT) | 21.4%–72.9% |
| Ajowan (Thymol CT) | 39.1%–67.4% |
| Oregano (*O. syriacum*, Thymol CT) | 36.3%–65.6% |
| Indian Borage (Thymol CT) | 8.8%–58.9% |
| Savory (Wild, Thymol CT) | 22.0%–57.9% |
| Mountain Savory (Thymol CT) | 30.9%–46.0% |
| Black Cumin (Para-Cymene CT) | 0.1%–45.0% |
| Monarda (Thymol CT) | 20.8%–43.6% |
| Hairy Basil (Thymol CT) | 43.5% |
| Summer Savory (Thymol CT) | 28.2%–40.5% |
| Thyme (Alpha-Terpineol CT) | 0.0%–27.4% |
| Thyme (Carvacrol CT) | 0.0%–27.2% |
| Thyme (Linalool CT) | 0.0%–23.6% |
| Oregano (Terpinen-4-ol CT) | 8.4%–22.0% |
| Indian Borage (Carvacrol CT) | 0.0%–21.7% |
| Oregano (*O. syriacum*, Carvacrol CT) | 19.2%–21.0% |
| Mountain Savory (Carvacrol CT) | 0.0%–20.6% |
| Ajowan (Gamma-Terpinene\P-Cymene CT) | 1.5%–17.4% |
| Ajowan (Gamma-Terpinolene CT) | 16.8% |
| Savory (Wild, Carvacrol CT) | 0.1%–15.7% |
| Monarda (Carvacrol/Para-Cymene CT) | 0.2%–12.6% |
| Moringa (Leaves, (E)-Phytol CT) | 9.7% |
| Thyme (Thuyanol-4 CT) | 0.0%–9.3% |
| Thyme (Geraniol CT) | 0.0%–7.9% |
| Wormseed, American (Alpha-Terpinene CT) | 0.0%–7.9% |
| Geranium | 0.0%–7.8% |
| Camphor (Camphor CT) | 0.0%–6.3% |
| Indian Borage (Delta-Cadinene CT) | 2.9%–6.0% |
| Khella (Aerial Parts, 2,2-Dimethylbut. CT) | 6.0% |
| Oregano (Carvacrol CT) | 0.9%–5.9% |
| Helichrysum (*H. italicum*) | 0.0%–5.4% |
| Indian Borage (Beta-Caryophyllene CT) | 3.0% |
| Oregano (*O. onites*) | 0.2%–2.8% |
| Chaste Tree (Leaves) | 0.0%–1.0% |

## Thymol Methyl Ether

| | |
|---|---|
| Arnica (Roots, 2,5-Dimethoxy-p-Cymene CT) | 9.6%–27.2% |
| Mountain Savory (Carvacrol CT) | 0.0%–12.8% |
| Mountain Savory (Thymol CT) | 3.9%–5.1% |

## Thymoquinone (Para-Cymene-2,5-Dione, P-Mentha-3,6-Diene-2,5-Dione)

| | |
|---|---|
| Black Cumin (Thymoquinone CT) | 26.8%–54.8% |
| Black Cumin (Para-Cymene CT) | 0.1%–13.7% |
| Black Cumin (Trans-Anethole CT) | 0.6%–11.8% |
| Savory (Wild, Thymol CT) | 0.0%–4.5% |

## Toluene

| | |
|---|---|
| Benzoin (Siam, S-HS Absolute) | 5.2%–79.6% |
| Benzoin (Siam, SPME Absolute) | 1.7%–28.5% |

## Totarol

| | |
|---|---|
| Formosan Cypress (Twig) | 14.9% |

## Trans-4-Methoxythujane ((E)-4-Methoxythujane)

| | |
|---|---|
| Black Cumin (Para-Cymene CT) | 0.0%–4.0% |

## Trans-Alpha-Bergamotene ((E)-Alpha-Bergamotene)

| | |
|---|---|
| Hairy Basil (var. *pilosum* Terpinen-4-ol CT) | 2.7%–11.4% |

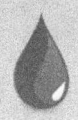
| | |
|---|---|
| Opoponax (*C. guidotti*) | 0.0%–9.3% |
| Canadian Fleabane | 0.0%–8.9% |
| Hairy Basil (Linalool CT, Inflorescences) | 0.0%–8.2% |
| Indian Borage (Carvacrol CT) | 0.0%–8.2% |
| Hairy Basil (var. *pilosum* Linalool CT) | 0.0%–7.6% |
| Hairy Basil ((E)-Methyl Cinnamate CT) | 0.0%–6.8% |
| Hemp (Beta-Caryophyllene CT) | 2.1%–3.9% |
| Hairy Basil (1-8-Cineole\Linalool CT) | 2.0%–3.5% |

**Trans-Beta-Bergamotene ((E)-Beta-Bergamotene)**

| | |
|---|---|
| Opoponax (*C. guidotti*) | 0.0%–9.0% |

**Trans-Anethole ((E)-Anethole)**

| | |
|---|---|
| Anise | 76.9%–95.6% |
| Fennel (Trans-Anethole CT) | 31.0%–94.6% |
| Star Anise | 87.4%–94.1% |
| Black Cumin (Trans-Anethole CT) | 27.1%–38.3% |
| Ravensara (Methyl Chavicol CT) | 0.0%–20.1% |
| Fennel (Methyl Chavicol CT) | 1.4%–19.0% |

**Trans-Ascaridole Glycol**

| | |
|---|---|
| Wormseed, American (Ascaridole CT) | 0.0%–4.5% |

**Trans-Beta-Guaiene ((E)-Beta-Guaiene)**

| | |
|---|---|
| Holy Basil (aerial parts, eugenol CT) | 0.0–19.2% |

**Trans-Cadina-1(6),4-Diene**

| | |
|---|---|
| Japanese Cedarwood (Sapwood) | 0.0%–4.1% |

**Trans-Calamenene (Calamenene, (E)-Calamenene)**

| | |
|---|---|
| Manuka (Leptospermone CT) | 3.1%–22.7% |
| Japanese Cedarwood (Heartwood) | 0.0%–5.3% |
| Kunzea (Alpha-Pinene CT) | 0.6%–4.6% |
| Japanese Cedarwood (Sapwood) | 0.0%–4.6% |
| Chinese Cedarwood | 0.0%–3.9% |
| Manuka (Selinene/Beta-Elemene CT) | 3.3% |
| Kanuka | 0.0%–3.0% |
| Applemint (*M. suav.*, Piperitenone CT) | 0.0%–2.7% |
| Applemint (*M. suav.*, Italian) | 0.4%–2.5% |

**Trans-Carveol ((E)-Carveol, (E)-p-Mentha-6,8-dien-2-ol, Trans-p-Mentha-6,8-dien-2-ol)**

| | |
|---|---|
| Spearmint (Carvone CT) | 0.2%–14.0% |
| Petitgrain (Bergamot/Bitter Orange) | 0.0%–11.9% |
| Applemint (*M. rotun.*, β-Caryophyllene CT) | 7.3% |
| Spearmint (Cis-Ocimenone CT) | 5.0% |
| Gingergrass | 2.1%–4.8% |
| Cumin | 0.0%–4.5% |
| Tagetes (*T. patula*, Aerial Parts) | 3.7% |

**Trans-Caryophyllene (Trans-Beta-Caryophyllene)**

*See Beta-Caryophyllene*

**Trans-Caryophyllene Oxide**

*See Beta-Carophyllene Oxide*

**Trans-Gamma-Bisabolene ((E)-Gamma-Bisabolene)**

| | |
|---|---|
| Guava Leaf (β-Bisabolene\β-Sesqu. CT) | 5.3% |

**Trans-Isoelemicin ((E)-Isoelemicin)**

| | |
|---|---|
| Mugwort (Alpha-Phellandrene CT) | 15.1% |

**Trans-Isodavanaone ((E)-Isodavanaone)**

| | |
|---|---|
| Davana | 0.0%–3.7% |

**Trans-Isolimonene ((E)-Isolimonene)**

| | |
|---|---|
| Petitgrain (Mandarin) | 0.0%–5.9% |

**Trans-Linalool Oxide ((E)-Linalool Oxide)**

| | |
|---|---|
| Wormwood (Chamazulene CT) | 0.1%–6.0% |
| Rosewood (Wood) | 1.2%–2.1% |
| Rosewood (Leaves) | 0.8% |

**(E)-Limonene Oxide (Trans-Limonene Oxide)**

| | |
|---|---|
| Gingergrass | 0.6%–3.8% |

**Trans-Methyl Jasmonates ((E)-Methyl Jasmonates)**

| | |
|---|---|
| Jasmine Absolute (Benzyl Benzoate CT) | 5.0%–7.8% |

**Trans-Ocimenone ((E)-Ocimenone)**

| | |
|---|---|
| Opoponax (*C. guidotti*) | 6.7%–52.6% |
| Tagetes (*T. minuta*, (Z)-Beta-Ocimene CT) | 5.8%–34.8% |
| Tagetes (*T. patula*, Limonene CT) | 10.8%–13.4% |
| Tagetes (*T. minuta*, Alpha-Terpineol CT) | 13.3% |
| Verbena (Myrcenone CT) | 0.0%–11.2% |
| Tagetes (*T. erecta*, Flowers) | 0.0%–9.8% |

**Trans-P-Mentha-1(7),8-Dien-2-ol**

| | |
|---|---|
| Ledum (*R. groenlandicum*) | 0.0%–7.0% |
| Sweet Inula (Borneol CT) | 2.2%–2.2% |
| Southern Blue Gum | 0.0%–1.1% |

**Trans-P-Mentha-2.8-Diene**

| | |
|---|---|
| Angelica Root | 0.0%–1.5% |

**Trans-P-Mentha-2,3-Dien-1-ol**

| | |
|---|---|
| Ledum (*R. groenlandicum*) | 0.0%–1.5% |

**Trans-Pinocarveol ((E)-Pinocarveol)**

| | |
|---|---|
| Cistus (*Viridiflorol-Trans-Pinocarveol CT*) | 1.2%–20.0% |
| Sweet Wormwood (Camphor CT) | 0.0%–10.96% |
| Eucalyptus (*E. radiata*) | 0.0%–4.8% |
| Sweet Wormwood (Artemisia Ketone CT) | 0.0%–4.8% |
| Southern Blue Gum | 0.2%–4.6% |
| Chamomile (Roman) | 0.1%–4.5% |
| Wild Chamomile (*O. mixta, C. mixtrum*) | 0.1%–3.7% |
| Ledum (*R. groenlandicum*) | 0.0%–2.3% |

**Trans-Pinocarveol Acetate ((E)-Pinocarveol Acetate)**

| | |
|---|---|
| Valerian | 0.0%–6.2% |

**Trans-Pseudoisoeugenyl 2-Methylbutyrate**

| | |
|---|---|
| Anise | 0.0%–6.4% |

**Trans-Rose-Oxide ((E)-Rose Oxide)**

| | |
|---|---|
| Mugwort (Isobornyl Isobutyrate D CT) | 2.0% |

**Trans-Sabinene Hydrate ((E)-Sabinene Hydrate)**

| | |
|---|---|
| Tamala (Trans-Sabinene Hydrate CT) | 29.8% |
| Wormwood (Trans-Sabinene Hydrate CT) | 11.0%–21.8% |
| Shell Ginger (P-Mentha-1,3-Dien-7-al CT) | 15.4% |
| Wormwood (Chamazulene CT) | 5.3%–12.6% |
| Marjoram | 3.5%–4.4% |
| Angelica Root | 0.0%–1.2% |

**Trans-Sabinol ((E)-Sabinol)**

| | |
|---|---|
| Wormwood (Alpha-Thujone CT) | 0.1%–6.4% |
| Ledum (*R. groenlandicum*) | 0.0%–1.9% |

**Trans-Sabinenehydrate Acetate ((E)-Sabinenehydrate Acetate)**

| | |
|---|---|
| Mugwort (1,8-Cineole CT) | 0.0%–2.5% |

**Trans-Sabinyl Acetate ((E)-Sabinyl Acetate)**

| | |
|---|---|
| Wormwood (Trans-Sabinyl Acetate CT) | 13.7%–84.5% |
| Savin (Needles & Branches) | 0.0%–54.4% |
| Wormwood ((Z)-Epoxy Ocimene CT) | 0.0%–23.6% |
| Wormwood (Alpha-Thujone CT) | 9.8%–22.1% |
| Wormwood (Beta-Thujone CT) | 0.9%–18.2% |
| Wormwood (Sabinene CT) | 7.8%–13.6% |
| Lovage (Roots) | 0.0%–12.1% |
| Juniper (Chinese) | 0.0%–11.0% |
| Wormwood (Trans-Sabinene Hydrate CT) | 0.0%–8.8% |
| Yarrow (Chamazulene CT) | 0.0%–2.1% |

**Trans-Chrysanthenyl Acetate (Chrysanthenyl Acetate, (E)-Chrysanthenyl Acetate)**

| | |
|---|---|
| Mugwort (Chrysanthenyl Acetate CT) | 39.6% |
| Feverfew | 0.0%–25.1% |
| Tansy (Beta-Thujone CT) | 0.0%–20.0% |
| Great Mugwort | 0.0%–3.2% |
| Angelica Root | 0.3%–1.1% |

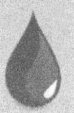

**Trans-Verbenol (Verbenol, (E)-Verbenol)**

| | |
|---|---|
| Frankincense (*B. frereana*) | 0.0%–8.1% |
| Mugwort (Camphor CT) | 0.0%–7.0% |
| Pine | 0.1%–3.5% |
| Mastic (Leaves) | 0.0%–3.1% |
| Angelica Root | 0.1%–1.3% |

**Tremetone**

| | |
|---|---|
| Japanese Cedarwood (Sapwood) | 0.0%–3.1% |

**Tricosane**

| | |
|---|---|
| Rose (Indian) | 0.0%–11.3% |
| Moringa (Leaves, Pentacosane CT) | 0.0%–8.1% |
| Tagetes (*T. minuta*, Limonene CT) | 0.0%–4.2% |
| Oakmoss Aboslute (Hydro. + Hexane) | 4.3% |

**Tricyclene**

| | |
|---|---|
| Black Sage (Tricyclene CT) | 23.9% |
| Silver Fir (*A. alba*) | 0.8%–12.9% |
| Parsley (Leaves, Myristicin CT) | 0.0%–8.8% |
| Mastic (Twigs, Alpha-Pinene CT) | 8.2% |
| Mastic (Leaves) | 0.0%–7.7% |
| Tsuga | 0.0%–6.2% |
| Spruce (Black) | 0.0%–4.6% |
| Pine | 0.1%–4.3% |
| Siberian Fir | 2.3%–3.1% |

**Tridecanol**

| | |
|---|---|
| Rue (2-Undecanone CT) | 0.0%–4.2% |

**Triquinacene,1,4-Bis(Methoxy)-**

| | |
|---|---|
| Plai (Triquinacene,1,4-Bis(Methoxy)- CT) | 26.5% |

**Undecanal**

| | |
|---|---|
| Indian Borage (Carvacrol CT) | 0.0%–8.3% |

**Undecane**

| | |
|---|---|
| Rue (2-Undecanone CT) | 0.0%–3.5% |

**Undecanol**

| | |
|---|---|
| Rose (Iranian) | 0.0%–5.5% |

**Undetermined Non-Volatiles**

| | |
|---|---|
| Benzoin (Sumatra, Ethanol Absolute) | 19.0%–40.0% |
| Benzoin (Sumatra, Ethanol Absolute) | 1.0%–10.0% |

**Undetermined Volatiles**

| | |
|---|---|
| Benzoin (Sumatra, Ethanol Absolute) | 6.0%–20.0% |
| Benzoin (Sumatra, Ethanol Absolute) | 0.0%–20.0% |

**Valencene**

| | |
|---|---|
| Japanese Cedarwood (16-Kaurene/Valencene CT) | 19.9% |
| Japanese Cedarwood (Sapwood) | 0.0%–9.9% |
| Japanese Cedarwood (Bark) | 0.0%–3.9% |

**Valerenal**

| | |
|---|---|
| Valerian | 0.1%–15.6% |
| Spikenard (Calarene CT, Nepal) | 0.0%–5.6% |

**Valerenol**

| | |
|---|---|
| Guava Leaf (Viridiflorol CT) | 0.1%–10.6% |
| Vetiver | 0.0%–3.9% |

**Valeranone (Jatamansone)**

| | |
|---|---|
| Spikenard (Valeranone CT) | 36.7% |
| Valerian | 0.5%–10.9% |
| Spikenard (Calarene CT, Nepal) | 7.9%–9.7% |
| Spikenard (Calarene CT) | 3.7%–9.7% |

**Valerena-4,7-Diene**

| | |
|---|---|
| Spikenard (Calarene CT) | 0.0%–6.6% |

**Valerena-4,7(11)-Diene**

| | |
|---|---|
| Spikenard (Calarene CT, Nepal) | 7.9%–9.7% |

**Valerenic Acid**

| | |
|---|---|
| Valerian | 0.0%–9.8% |

**Valerianol (Kusunol)**

| | |
|---|---|
| Valerian | 0.2%–33.9% |
| Amyris | 21.5%–26.0% |
| Agarwood (Malaysian) | 0.0%–19.4% |
| Agarwood (*A. crassna*) | 0.0%–8.2% |
| Agarwood (*A. malaccensis*) | 0.0%–4.3% |

**Vanillin**

| | |
|---|---|
| Benzoin (Siam, SPME Absolute) | 4.3%–8.0% |
| Benzoin (Siam, HSSE Absolute) | 2.0%–6.1% |

**Veramoss**

| | |
|---|---|
| Oakmoss Aboslute (Hydro. + Hexane) | 11.5% |

**Verbenone**

| | |
|---|---|
| Rosemary (Verbenone CT) | 7.6%–24.9% |
| Rosemary (Alpha-Pinene CT) | 2.3%–15.3% |
| African Bluegrass (Artemisia Ketone CT) | 13.5% |
| Rosemary (Borneol CT) | 8.4% |
| Pink Pepper (*S. terebinthifolius*, Leaves, p-Cymen-7-ol CT) | 7.4% |
| Rosemary (Bornyl Acetate CT) | 0.0%–5.7% |

**Verticiol**

| | |
|---|---|
| Khella (Aerial Parts, Isoamyl 2-Meth. CT) | 0.0%–9.9% |
| Japanese Cedarwood (Sapwood) | 0.0%–3.5% |

**Vetiselinenol**

| | |
|---|---|
| Vetiver | 0.0%–5.6% |

**Viridiflorene (Ledene)**

| | |
|---|---|
| Guava Leaf (β-Cary.\(E)-Nerolidol CT) | 8.8% |
| Kunzea (Spathulenol\Globulol CT) | 3.0%–5.1% |
| Manuka (Leptospermone CT) | 0.7%–4.4% |
| Kunzea (Alpha-Pinene CT) | 0.3%–4.0% |

**Viridiflorol**

| | |
|---|---|
| Niaouli (Viridiflorol CT) | 10.0%–67.4% |
| Niaouli (1,8-Cineole/Viridiflorol CT) | 8.4%–66.0% |
| Niaouli (Viridiflorol/ Para-cymene/1,8-cineole CT) | 4.0%–50.0% |
| Niaouli (1,8-Cineole CT) | 0.0%–47.9% |
| Kunzea (Alpha-Pinene CT) | 0.3%–38.0% |
| Guava Leaf (Viridiflorol CT) | 36.4%–36.4% |
| Sage (Wild) | 9.9%–16.4% |
| Cistus | 0.0%–11.8% |
| Spanish Sage | 0.0%–12.0% |
| Guava Leaf (Limonene CT) | 0.0%–11.3% |
| Kanuka | 0.0%–7.2% |
| Kunzea (Spathulenol\Globulol CT) | 3.9%–6.4% |
| Blue Mountain Sage (Limonene CT) | 5.7% |
| Applemint (*M. rotun.*, β-Caryophyllene CT) | 3.8% |
| Ghandi Root | 0.0%–3.7% |
| Sage (1,8-Cineole CT) | 0.5%–2.9% |
| Muhuhu (Wood) | 0.0%–2.9% |
| Applemint (*M. suav.*, Italian) | 0.0%–2.5% |
| Southern Blue Gum | 0.2%–1.4% |
| Hyssop (Alpha-Pinene CT) | 1.1% |

**Widdrol**

| | |
|---|---|
| Cedarwood (Virginian, Wood) | 1.0%–2.3% |

**Xanthorrhizol**

| | |
|---|---|
| Wild Turmeric (Distilled) | 4.8%–25.7% |

**Xanthotoxine**

| | |
|---|---|
| Rue (2-Undecanone CT) | 0.0%–7.2% |

**Ylangenol**

| | |
|---|---|
| Muhuhu (Wood) | 0.5%–4.0% |

**Yomogi Alcohol**

| | |
|---|---|
| Sweet Nancy (Yomogi Alc.\1,8-Cin. CT) | 22.3%–44.1% |
| Wild Chamomile (*O. mixta, C. mixtrum*) | 0.7%–16.2% |
| Sweet Nancy (Artemisyl Acetate CT) | 4.9%–12.4% |
| Blue Yarrow (Artemisia Ketone CT) | 6.4% |

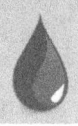

| | |
|---|---|
| Sweet Wormwood (Artemisia Ketone CT) | 0.0%–6.1% |
| Mugwort (Artemisia Ketone CT) | 4.4%–5.5% |
| Wild Chamomile (*C. mixtus,* Sant. Alc. CT) | 0.4%–4.5% |

**(Z)-1-(3,4-Dimethoxyphenyl)Butadiene**

| | |
|---|---|
| Plai (Terpinen-4-ol CT) | 0.0%–3.7% |

**(Z)-3-Butyldene Phthalide ((Z)-3-butylidenephthalide, Trans-3-Butyldenephthalide)**

| | |
|---|---|
| Lovage (Roots) | 0.0%–28.6% |

**(Z)-3-Hex-1Enyl Benzoate**

| | |
|---|---|
| Mastic (Leaves) | 0.0%–6.7% |

**(Z)-3-Hexanol (Cis-3-Hexanol)**

| | |
|---|---|
| Holy Basil (aerial parts, eugenol CT) | 0.0%–8.1% |

**(Z)-3-Hexenyl Butyrate (Cis-3-Hexenyl Butyrate)**

| | |
|---|---|
| Wormwood (Cis-Chrysanthenyl Acetate CT) | 1.5%–4.8% |

**(Z)-Alpha-Santalol (Cis-Alpha-Santalol)**

| | |
|---|---|
| Sandalwood (*S. album*) | 40.4%–57.1% |
| Sandalwood (*S. austrocaledonicum*) | 28.9%–48.4% |
| Sandalwood (*S. paniculatum*) | 39.8%–42.6% |
| Sandalwood (*S. spicatum*) | 5.5%–27.3% |
| Opoponax (*C. guidotti*) | 0.0%–4.0% |

**(Z)-Alpha-Trans-Bergamotol**

| | |
|---|---|
| Sandalwood (*S. album*) | 2.2%–17.2% |
| Black Sage (Alpha-Santalene CT) | 12.9% |
| Sandalwood (*S. austrocaledonicum*) | 0.2%–9.0% |
| Sandalwood (*S. paniculatum*) | 4.2%–5.1% |

**(Z)-Beta-Farnesene (Cis-Beta-Farnesene)**

| | |
|---|---|
| German Chamomile | 0.0%–15.9% |
| Canadian Fleabane | 0.0%–11.1% |
| Black Sage (Alpha-Santalene CT) | 8.8% |
| Mugwort (Alpha-Thujone CT) | 0.0%–8.1% |
| Mugwort (Beta-Caryophyllene CT) | 7.1% |
| Black Sage (Beta-Caryophyllene CT) | 4.2% |
| Holy Basil (aerial parts, eugenol CT) | 0.0%–4.1% |
| Catnip (Nepetalactone CT) | 0.0%–3.6% |

**(Z)-Beta-Ocimene (Cis-Beta-Ocimene, (Z)-Ocimene, Cis-Ocimene)**

| | |
|---|---|
| Tagetes (*T. minuta,* (Z)-Beta-Ocimene CT) | 8.3%–51.7% |
| Wormwood ((E)-Beta-Farnesene CT) | 27.8% |
| Monarda (Carvacrol CT) | 6.2%–27.1% |
| Plai (Triquinacene,1,4-Bis(Methoxy)- CT) | 22.0% |
| Tagetes (*T. erecta,* Aerial Parts) | 5.0%–18.5% |
| Lavender (French) | 0.2%–18.1% |
| Tamala (Trans-Sabinene Hydrate CT) | 17.9% |
| Tagetes (*T. minuta,* Alpha-Terpineol CT) | 17.7% |
| Rabbitbrush (var. *consimilis*) | 14.6% |
| Tagetes (*T. erecta,* Flowers) | 2.8%–13.7% |
| Verbena (Linalool CT) | 0.0%–13.0% |
| African Bluegrass (Myrcene CT) | 0.0%–12.2% |
| Hairy Basil (1,8-Cineole CT) | 0.0%–11.4% |
| Tarragon (Methyl Chavicol CT) | 1.3%–8.3% |
| Tagetes (*T. patula,* Limonene CT) | 0.0%–8.3% |
| Tagetes (*T. minuta,* Dihydrotagetone CT) | 0.0%–7.9% |
| Lavender (True English) | 0.0%–7.8% |
| Lavender (Bulgarian) | 1.7%–7.7% |
| Lovage (Aerial Parts) | 0.0%–7.5% |
| Douglas Fir (Needles) | 0.0%–7.1% |
| Tagetes (*T. erecta,* Leaves) | 0.3%–7.0% |
| Monarda (Linalool CT) | 2.3%–6.9% |
| Vilayti Tulsi (Sabinene CT) | 0.0%–6.9% |
| Neroli (*C. aurantium*) | 0.0%–6.6% |
| Galangal (Greater, 1,8-Cineole CT) | 0.0%–6.4% |
| Lovage (Leaves) | 0.0%–6.2% |

| | |
|---|---|
| Monarda (Thymol CT) | 0.0%–5.9% |
| Betony (β-Phell.\α-Pinene CT) | 0.2%–5.8% |
| Douglas Fir (Needles & Twigs) | 0.0%–5.6% |
| Rhododendron (Aerial Parts) | 3.7%–5.3% |
| Angelica Root | 0.0%–4.8% |
| Tamala (Eugenol CT) | 0.0%–4.5% |
| Savory (Wild, Linalool CT) | 0.0%–4.2% |
| Verbena (Myrcene CT) | 1.9%–3.8% |
| Vilayti Tulsi (1,8-Cineole CT) | 0.0%–3.6% |
| Black Pepper (Beta-Pinene CT) | 3.6% |
| Rabbitbrush (var. *albicaulis*) | 3.3% |
| Black Pepper (Limonene CT) | 0.0%–3.2% |
| Catnip (Nepetalactone CT) | 0.0%–3.1% |
| Lavender (Polish) | 1.9%–2.9% |
| Catnip (1,8-cineole CT) | 2.7% |
| Tagetes (*T. patula,* Aerial Parts) | 2.3% |

**(Z)-Beta-Santalol (Cis-Beta-Santalol)**

| | |
|---|---|
| Sandalwood (*S. album*) | 20.3%–30.5% |
| Sandalwood (*S. austrocaledonicum*) | 13.5%–22.0% |
| Sandalwood (*S. paniculatum*) | 13.7%–16.2% |
| Sandalwood (*S. spicatum*) | 2.1%–10.5% |

**(Z)-Cadina-1(6),4-Diene (Cis-Cadina-1(6),4-Diene)**

| | |
|---|---|
| Juniper (*J. recurva,* Berries) | 8.3% |

**(Z)-Cinnamaldehyde (Cis-Cinnamaldehyde, Cinnamic Aldehyde)**

| | |
|---|---|
| Cassia (Bark) | 4.4%–10.5% |

**(Z)-Cinnamic Acid Methyl Ester**

| | |
|---|---|
| Hairy Basil (var. *pilosum* Linalool CT) | 0.0%–21.5% |

**(Z)-Dihydrocarvone (Cis-Dyhdrocarvone)**

| | |
|---|---|
| Tsauri Grass | 0.0%–17.2% |
| Dill Seed | 0.1%–5.9% |

**(Z)-En-yn-Dicycloether (Cis-Spiroether, (Z)-Spiroether)**

| | |
|---|---|
| Wormwood ((E)-Beta-Farnesene CT) | 11.1% |

**(Z)-Epi-Beta-Santalol**

| | |
|---|---|
| Sandalwood (*S. album*) | 4.9%–11.2% |
| Sandalwood (*S. austrocaledonicum*) | 1.9%–5.4% |
| Sandalwood (*S. paniculatum*) | 3.1%–4.2% |

**(Z)-Epoxy Ocimene (Cis-Epoxy-Ocimene)**

| | |
|---|---|
| Wormwood ((Z)-Epoxy Ocimene CT) | 20.6%–59.7% |
| Wormwood (Cis-Chrysanthenyl Acetate CT) | 24.2%–25.6% |
| Wormwood (Beta-Thujone CT) | 0.2%–23.1% |
| Tagetes (*T. patula,* Aerial Parts) | 2.7% |

**(Z)-Heptadeca-9,16-Dien-7-One**

| | |
|---|---|
| Wild Chamomile (*O. mixta, C. mixtrum*) | 0.0%–12.7% |

**(Z)-Hex-3Enyl Tiglate**

| | |
|---|---|
| Betony (Bicyclogermacrene CT) | 0.0%–8.4% |

**(Z)-Isocitral (Cis-Isocitral)**

| | |
|---|---|
| Honey Myrtle | 0.0%–1.6% |

**(Z)-Isopiperitenol (Cis-Isopiperitenol, Cis-p-Mentha-1,8-Dien-3-ol)**

| | |
|---|---|
| Tsauri Grass | 0.0%–4.2% |

**(Z)-Jasmone (Cis-Jasmone)**

| | |
|---|---|
| Jasmine Absolute (Benzyl Benzoate CT) | 1.8%–7.1% |
| Spearmint (Cis-Ocimenone CT) | 1.3% |

**(Z)-Lanceol (Cis-Lanceol)**

| | |
|---|---|
| Sandalwood (*S. austrocaledonicum*) | 0.0%–9.1% |
| Blue Mountain Sage (Alpha-Bisabolol CT) | 0.2%–8.7% |

**(Z)-Ligustilide (Cis-Ligustilide, Ligustilide A)**

| | |
|---|---|
| Lovage (Roots) | 9.4%–79.7% |
| Lovage (Leaves) | 3.9%–32.1% |
| Lovage (Aerial Parts) | 0.0%–29.7% |

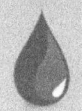

**(Z)-Limonene Oxide (Cis-Limonene Oxide)**

| | |
|---|---|
| Tsauri Grass | 0.0%–19.2% |

**(Z)-Methyl Cinnamate (Cis-Methyl Cinnamate)**

| | |
|---|---|
| Hairy Basil ((E)-Methyl Cinnamate CT) | 5.8%–11.0% |
| Xanthoxylum | 0.0%–4.9% |

**(Z)-Myroxide (Cis-Myroixide)**

| | |
|---|---|
| Tagetes (*T. erecta*, Flowers) | 0.0%–7.9% |
| Wormwood (Sabinene CT) | 0.0%–5.8% |
| Tagetes (*T. erecta*, Leaves) | 0.0%–4.2% |

**(Z)-Myrtanol (Cis-Myrtanol)**

| | |
|---|---|
| Formosan Cypress (Wood, α-Eudesmol CT) | 4.1% |

**(Z)-Nerolidol (Cis-Nerolidol)**

| | |
|---|---|
| Peru Balsam (Resinoid Absolute) | 0.0%–5.0% |
| Tagetes (*T. patula*, Aerial Parts) | 3.2% |

**(Z)-Nuciferol (Cis-Nuciferol)**

| | |
|---|---|
| Sandalwood (*S. austrocaledonicum*) | 1.6%–8.7% |
| Sandalwood (*S. spicatum*) | 5.6%–6.5% |
| Sandalwood (*S. paniculatum*) | 3.2%–4.8% |
| Sandalwood (*S. album*) | 1.8%–5.2% |

**(Z)-*p*-Mentha-2,8-Dien-1-ol**
**(Cis-para-Mentha-2,8-Dien-1-ol)**

| | |
|---|---|
| Gingergrass | 9.1%–27.0% |
| Tsauri Grass | 0.0%–16.3% |
| Tsauri Grass (var. *madagascariensis*) | 8.3%–9.8% |

**(Z)-*p*-Mentha-1(7),8-Dien-2-ol**
**(Cis-para-Mentha-1(7),8-Dien-2-ol)**

| | |
|---|---|
| Gingergrass | 13.0%–31.1% |
| Tsauri Grass | 0.0%–27.7% |
| Tsauri Grass (var. *madagascariensis*) | 12.3%–19.0% |

**(Z)-Piperitol (Cis-Piperitol)**

| | |
|---|---|
| Gingergrass | 0.0%–11.3% |
| Tsauri Grass | 0.0%–3.9% |

**(Z)-Tagetone (Cis-Tagetone)**

| | |
|---|---|
| Tagetes (*T. minuta*, Dihydrotagetone CT) | 0.2%–23.0% |
| Tagetes (*T. minuta*, (Z)-Beta-Ocimene CT) | 1.8%–17.7% |
| Tagetes (*T. minuta*, Alpha-Terpineol CT) | 8.4% |
| Tagetes (*T. patula*, Limonene CT) | 4.3%–7.0% |
| Calendula ((E)-Beta-Ocimene CT) | 4.6% |
| Tagetes (*T. patula*, Flowers) | 4.6% |

**(Z)-Valerinic Acid (Cis-Valerinic Acid)**

| | |
|---|---|
| Spikenard (Calarene CT, Nepal) | 0.0%–5.7% |

**(Z,Z)-Alpha-Farnesene (Cis-Alpha-Farnesene, Cis, Cis-Alpha-Farnesene)**

| | |
|---|---|
| Cananga | 0.4%–4.4% |

**Zingiberene (Alpha-Zingiberene)**

*See Alpha-Zingiberene*

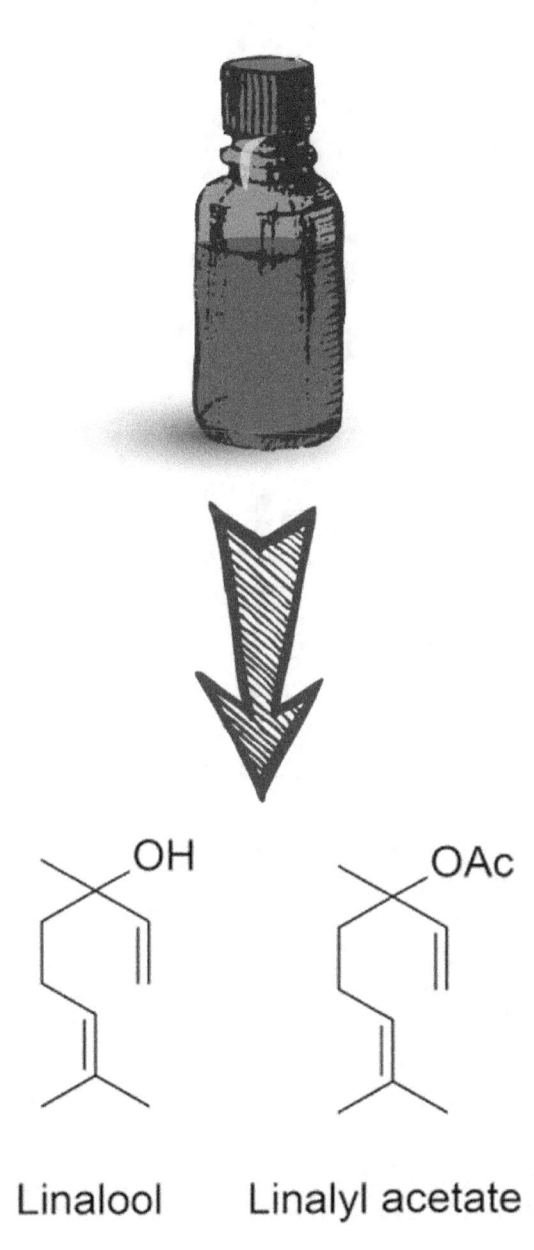

Linalool    Linalyl acetate

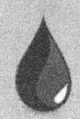

*Aconitum*: Generally used during the initial stages of illness or injury. Symptoms are sudden, often worse from exposure to cold, and sometimes intense. Anxiety, fear, restlessness, and grief are often present.

*Apis Mellifica*: Commonly used for insect stings or bites and burning or stinging pains. Symptoms are characterized by swelling, aggravation by warmth, and relief by cold.

*Ambrosia*: This is a common remedy for hay fever with intensely itchy eyelids and profuse watery nasal discharge. It is also used for whooping cough. In addition, the throat may be irritated and breathing labored in people who need this remedy.

*Antimonium Crudum*: This remedy acts very powerfully on the mucous membranes and skin. A thick, white coating is almost always present on the tongue when this remedy is needed. Symptoms include severe irritability, especially in children, who don't even want to be looked at. Digestive problems are usually present.

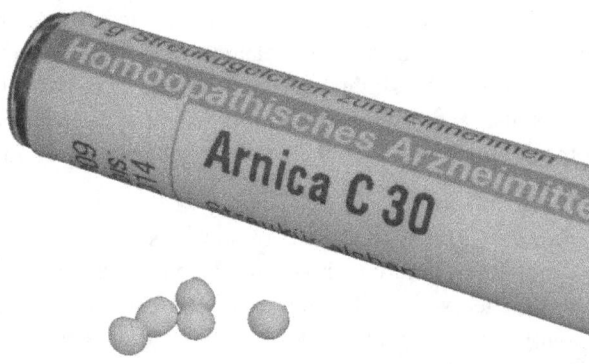

*Arnica (Arnica Montana)*: This is an excellent remedy for common injuries, trauma, bruising, swelling, and muscle soreness. Arnica may relieve old injuries that still cause discomfort. It is frequently used before and after surgery.

*Belladonna*: This remedy is commonly given to those with a flushed, red face and glassy eyes. It is useful when symptoms appear and vanish suddenly. Throbbing pains, hypersensitivity to touch, fever, and hot, red mucous membranes are also key symptoms.

*Bryonia (Bryonia Alba)*: This remedy is usually given when symptoms are made worse by motion. Key symptoms include sharp pain, dry mouth and/or rectum, thirst for cold drinks, and relief from pressure to painful area. The person who needs this remedy is frequently irritable and wants to be left alone.

*Calcarea Phos (Calcarea Phosphorica, Calc Phos)*: People who need this remedy are usually friendly but insecure. They become fatigued and bored easily. Nutritional deficiencies and weak or brittle bones may also be a problem.

*Calendula*: This remedy prevents wound infections and aids tissue regeneration to speed the healing of wounds and burns. It should not be used for a deep wound because it may cause the outer layers of the skin to heal more quickly than the deeper layers.

*Cardiospermum*: Extracted from the flowering tropical balloon vine, this gel or cream helps relieve itching and inflammation of the skin. It is considered a natural alternative to cortisone creams and is widely used for the relief of eczema and rashes.

*Causticum Hahnemanni*: This remedy is useful for individuals who are very serious and introspective. They may experience mental exhaustion and sadness after a specific event. It is particularly useful for injuries that involve decreased muscle power, tendon injuries, and rheumatic conditions. It is predominantly used for chronic conditions, as opposed to acute conditions.

*Chamomilla*: People who need this remedy are usually hypersensitive (physically and psychologically) and hard to please. Infants may only be comforted if they are held and carried. Key symptoms include sour discharges from the body (stool, vomit, and sweat) and pain that is not proportional to the condition experienced.

*Coffea*: This remedy helps relieve hyperactivity, restlessness, over-sensitivity, and exaggerated senses. It may be useful for people who become overanxious prior to an event, or who are unable to sleep because of overactivity. Other tell-tale symptoms of this remedy include unusual activity of mind/body and hypersensitivity to the symptoms of the condition being experienced.

*Cocculus*: In general, this remedy is used for travel sickness experienced in a car, boat, or airplane. It may also be useful for nausea during pregnancy.

*Equisetum*: This remedy may be useful for bedwetting and other symptoms involving the urinary system. The person may feel a constant desire to urinate. Symptoms are usually worse with pressure, movement, or touch.

*Gelsemium*: This remedy is for those with general fatigue (physical and mental). The eyelids and extremities may feel heavy and the person may be drowsy and lethargic.

*Hepar Sulphur*: People who need this remedy are usually hyper and excitable (physically and psychologically). They are also very irritable, impulsive, anger easily, and argumentative. Key symptoms include highly sensitive skin, dislike of cold weather, a low pain threshold, and offensive discharges and perspiration.

*Kali Bichromicum (Kali Bic)*: This remedy is best suited for detail-oriented individuals that tend to see things only in black and white. Key symptoms include thick, yellowish or greenish discharges, pain that migrates from place to place, and symptoms that get worse in the cold.

*Mercurius*: This remedy is well suited to handle advanced stages of acute conditions. Symptoms are usually worst at night, during wet weather, or with extreme temperature changes. The person often experiences excess perspiration and salivation, as well as copious and unpleasant discharges.

*Natrum Sulphuricum*: This remedy is considered a preferred remedy for liver and gallbladder problems, like gallstones. It is also valuable for head injuries—particularly headaches and mental troubles caused by them. People who need this remedy tend to experience worsening of their symptoms in dry weather, from pressure, or when changing positions.

*Nux Vomica*: This remedy should be the first thought when symptoms occur after overindulgence in rich foods or beverages. Symptoms may also occur after long-term stress. The person is very irritable and may experience constipation.

*Oscillococcinum (Anas Barbariae)*: A very popular flu remedy in France used during the first 48 hours of flu-like symptoms. Sometimes used for the common cold also.

*Pilocarpinum*: This remedy potently stimulates glandular function. It effectively relieves excessive perspiration and salivation. Many homeopaths consider this the best remedy for mumps and its associated symptoms, particularly if excess perspiration or salivation is present.

*Pulsatilla*: This is the most often used remedy for acute conditions in children. Symptoms are usually worse in warm rooms or hot weather and may begin after eating rich or fatty foods. Children who need this remedy may be generally easygoing but may crave attention and be moody and sensitive.

*Rhus Tox (Rhus Toxicodendron)*: A key symptom that this remedy relieves is stiffness after rest that is worse after initial movement but improves with more motion. Symptoms may be aggravated by cold, wet weather and at night. The person who needs this remedy is usually restless and has achy joints and ligaments (like those caused by rheumatoid arthritis or other joint disorders).

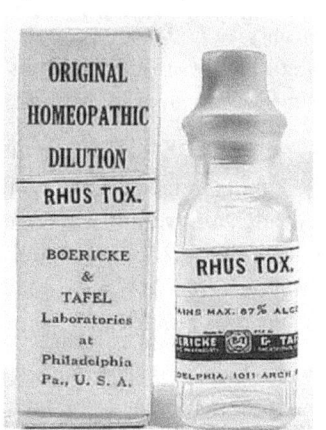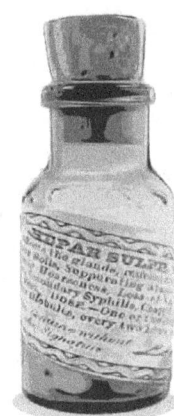

*Ruta Graveolens (Ruta or Rue)*: This remedy is effective for injuries to bones, tendons, and ligaments (fractures, sprains). It may be helpful after joint surgery (knee, elbow) and for bruises that leave a hard spot.

*Spongia (Spongia Tosta)*: Typical characteristics of people who need this remedy include fear of death (especially dying of heart-related causes), late risers, exhaustion after slight exertion, and waking up fearful, anxious, and grumpy. Spongia is very useful for respiratory conditions and is commonly prescribed for children with a croupy cough.

*Sulphur*: This remedy is commonly used for chronic conditions. Children who need this remedy are usually very messy, intelligent, and self-centered. Key symptoms include feeling warm, symptoms aggravated by heat, red mucous membranes, face, and lips, and dry skin.

*Thuja occidentalis*: This cream or gel is primarily used to treat a variety of skin conditions including warts, fungal infections, and skin cancer. It has also been used topically to soothe the pains of arthritis and rheumatism.

**Urtica Urens**: Key symptoms of this remedy include burning, stinging, red, irritated skin rashes. People who need this remedy may be impatient, irritable, and restless. It is useful for hives, particularly hive-like eruptions associated with rheumatic conditions.

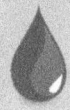

# APPENDIX C:

*Underlined essential oils are considered a primary remedy for the condition or a primary property of the essential oil.*

**Abscesses, Heals**: Tea tree, moringa, mountain savory, niaouli, savory (wild), verbena

**Acne, Combats**: *See Blemishes, Scars, Wrinkles, Acne—Reduces Appearance of*

**Acceptance, Encourages**: Sandalwood, spruce (black), wintergreen

**Adaptogenic**: Lavender, lemon

**Adrenal Function, Supports**: Basil, nutmeg, red pine, rhododendron, Siam wood, spruce (black)

**Addiction (Food, Sugar), Combats**: Dill seed

**Addictions (General), Reduces**: Jasmine absolute

**Agitation, Eases**: Melissa

**Aggression, Combats**: Bergamot, sandalwood

**Alertness, Promotes**: Genipi, peppermint, rabbitbrush, wild marjoram, wintergreen

**Analgesic (Pain Relief)**: African bluegrass, ajowan, agarwood, Aleppo pine, allspice, amyris, anise, applemint, arnica, auracaria, balsam fir, basil, bay (West Indies), bay laurel, benzoin absolute, bergamot, bergamot mint, betony, big badja gum, birch, black cumin, black pepper, black sage, blue cypress, blue mallee, blue spruce, blue tansy, boldo, buchu, Buddha wood, cajeput, calamus, calendula, camphor, Canadian fleabane, cangerana, Cape chamomile, cassia, catnip, celery, chaste tree, Chinese red pine, cilantro, cinnamon, citron, citronella, clove, copaiba, coriander, damiana, davana, dill seed, Douglas fir, dwarf pine, elemi, Engelmann spruce, eucalyptus, eucalyptus dives, fennel, ferula, feverfew, fingerroot, Formosan cypress, Fragonia, frankincense, galbanum, galangal, garlic, geranium, German chamomile, Ghandi root, ginger, gingergrass, guava leaf, guggul, gully gum, gurjun balsam, helichrysum, hemp, hinoki, holy basil, honey myrtle, hops, Indian borage, Japanese cedarwood, jasmine absolute, juniper berry, juniper (Chinese), juniper (Himalayan), juniper (Phoenician), kabosu, kaffir lime, kanuka, katrafay, kunzea, lavandin, lavender, leleshwa, lemon, lemon verbena, ledum, lemon catnip, lemon eucalyptus,

lemon tea tree, lemongrass, lovage, manuka, maritime pine, marjoram, mastic, may chang, tea tree, monarda, moringa, muhuhu, neroli, niaouli, nutmeg, oakmoss absolute, opoponax, oregano, palo santo, parsley seed, peppermint, peta, pine, pink pepper, plai, ponderosa pine, rabbitbrush, ravensara, ravintsara, red pine, rhododendron, Roman chamomile, rosalina, rosemary, rosewood, rue, sandalwood, saro, savin, savory (wild), shell ginger, Siam wood, Siberian fir, silver fir, Southern blue gum, Spanish sage, spearmint, spike lavender, spruce (black), star anise, summer savory, sweet inula, sweet nancy, sweet wormwood, tagetes, tamala, tansy, tarragon, Texas cedarwood, thyme, tolu balsam, tsauri grass, tsuga, Turkish pine, turmeric, verbena, vetiver, vilayti tulsi, Virginian cedarwood, white fir, white pine, white spruce, white verbena, wild chamomile, wild marjoram, wintergreen, wormseed (American), xanthoxylum, yarrow, yuzu, zdravetz

**Anesthetic**: Allspice, bay laurel, clove, eucalyptus, peppermint, Southern blue gum, thyme

**Anger\Rage, Reduces**: Ajowan, Aleppo pine, allspice, blue tansy, davana, garlic, German chamomile, kabosu, kanuka, ledum, Mediterranean mandarin, melissa, peppermint, peta, petitgrain, Peru balsam, pine, plai, Roman chamomile, rose, sweet nancy, sweet wormwood, tagetes, tolu balsam, Turkish pine, vetiver, ylang ylang

**Antiaging**: African bluegrass, allspice, amyris, applemint, calendula, Canadian fleabane, clove, frankincense, galbanum, kumquat, moringa, rosalina, schisandra fruit, shell ginger, Siam wood, yarrow

**Antiallergic**: Auracaria, black cumin, black sage, blue cypress, blue tansy, calamus, caraway, dill seed, fingerroot, Formosan cypress, Fragonia, German chamomile, gingergrass, goldenrod, grindelia, gurjun balsam, helichrysum, hemp, hinoki, hops, juniper (Chinese), kanuka, khella, ledum, lemon may chang, myrtle, lemongrass, manuka, moringa, oregano, palo santo, parsley seed, plai, ravensara, rosalina, schisandra fruit, shell ginger, spikenard, sweet inula, tansy, vilayti tulsi, white pine, white verbena, wild chamomile, yarrow, zdravetz

**Antiarthritic**: Allspice, arnica, balsam poplar, big badja gum, black sage, blue mallee, buchu, calamus, cangerana, caraway, cassia, catnip, celery, Chinese cedarwood, Chinese red pine, cilantro, citron, dwarf pine, feverfew, fingerroot, frankincense, galangal, galbanum, German chamomile, gingergrass, gobre salla, guggul, gully gum, Japanese cedarwood, jasmine absolute, juniper berry, juniper (Chinese),

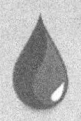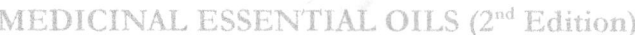

juniper (Himalayan), juniper (Phoenician), kaffir lime, katrafay, kunzea, marjoram, mountain savory, parsley seed, pennyroyal, Peru balsam, peta, pink pepper, plai, ponderosa pine, rabbitbrush, ravintsara, red pine, rosemary, rue, savory (wild), silver fir, summer savory, tamala, tarragon, Texas cedarwood, thyme, tolu balsam, tsauri grass, turmeric, verbena, vetiver, vilayti tulsi, Virginian cedarwood, white fir, white pine, wild chamomile, wild marjoram, wintergreen, xanthoxylum

**Antibacterial**: African bluegrass, agarwood, ajowan, Aleppo pine, allspice, amyris, anise, applemint, arnica, auracaria, balsam fir, balsam poplar, basil, bay (West Indies), bay laurel, benzoin absolute, bergamot, bergamot mint, betony, big badja gum, black cumin, black pepper, black sage, blue cypress, blue mallee, blue mountain sage, blue spruce, blue tansy, boldo, Buddha wood, cajeput, calamus, calendula, camphor, Canadian fleabane, cangerana, caraway, cassia, celery, chaste tree, cilantro, cinnamon, cistus, citron, citronella, clary sage, copaiba, coriander, cumin, cypress, davana, dill seed, Douglas fir, dwarf pine, elecampane, elemi, Engelmann spruce, eucalyptus dives, eucalyptus, ferula, feverfew, fingerroot, Formosan cypress, Fragonia, galangal, garlic, geranium, genipi, German chamomile, Ghandi root, ginger, gingergrass, gobre salla, grapefruit, grindelia, guava leaf, guggul, gully gum, gurjun balsam, hairy basil, helichrysum, hemp, hinoki, holy basil, honey myrtle, Indian borage, Japanese cedarwood, jasmine absolute, juniper (Phoenician), kaffir lime, kabosu, kanuka, katrafay, khella, kumquat, kunzea, lavandin, lavender, lemon, lemon basil, lemon verbena, ledum, leleshwa, lemon catnip, lemon eucalyptus, lemon myrtle, lemon tea tree, lemongrass, lime, lovage, manuka, maritime pine, magnolia, marjoram, mastic, Mediterranean mandarin, tea tree, melissa, monarda, moringa, mountain savory, muhuhu, myrtle, neroli, niaouli, oakmoss absolute, ocotea, opoponax, orange, oregano, Oriental arborvitae, palmarosa, palo santo, parsley seed, patchouli, pennyroyal, peppermint, Persian lime, Peru balsam, peta, petitgrain, pine, pink pepper, plai, ponderosa pine, rabbitbrush, ravensara, ravintsara, red pine, rhododendron, Roman chamomile, rosalina, rose, rosemary, rosewood, rue, sage, sandalwood, saro, savory (wild), schisandra fruit, shell ginger, Siberian fir, Southern blue gum, spearmint, spikenard, star anise, summer savory, sweet inula, sweet nancy, sweet wormwood, tagetes, tamala, tansy, tarragon, Texas cedarwood, thuja, thyme, tolu balsam, tsauri grass, Turkish pine, turmeric, valerian, verbena, vetiver, vilayti tulsi, Virginian cedarwood, Western red cedar, white pine, white sage, white

spruce, white verbena, wild chamomile, wild marjoram, wormseed (American), wormwood, xanthoxylum, ylang ylang, yuzu, zdravetz

**Anticancer**: African bluegrass, agarwood, allspice, balsam fir, basil, bay laurel, bergamot, betony, black cumin, Buddha wood, camphor, cardamom, citron, clove, fenugreek, fingerroot, frankincense, galangal, garlic, Ghandi root, ginger, gobre salla, guava leaf, guggul, hemp, Japanese cedarwood, juniper (Phoenician), kabosu, kumquat, lavender, lemongrass, may chang, Mediterranean mandarin, tea tree, moringa, orange, orange (bitter), oregano, Oriental arborvitae, palo santo, parsley seed, peppermint, pink pepper, rosemary, savin, silver fir, tagetes, tamala, thuja, tsauri grass, turmeric, white verbena, wormwood

**Anticonvulsive (Anti-epileptic)**: Anise, applemint, black cumin, caraway, citronella, guava leaf, honey myrtle, lemongrass, neroli, rose, rue, spearmint, star anise, white verbena

**Antidepressant**: African bluegrass, ajowan, allspice, amyris, anise, bay (West Indies), benzoin absolute, bergamot, bergamot mint, birch, black cumin, blue mountain sage, Buddha wood, calamus, caraway, carrot seed, cassia, chaste tree, citron, clary sage, coriander, damiana, davana, Douglas fir, frankincense, galangal, galbanum, geranium, German chamomile, Ghandi root, gingergrass, gobre salla, grapefruit, grindelia, hairy basil, helichrysum, hemp, honey myrtle, hops, Japanese cedarwood, jasmine absolute, kabosu, kaffir lime, kanuka, kumquat, lavandin, lavender, lemon, lemon basil, lemon tea tree, lemon verbena, lemongrass, lime, may chang, Mediterranean mandarin, melissa, monarda, moringa, muhuhu, neroli, ocotea, orange, orange (bitter), oregano, palmarosa, patchouli, Persian lime, petitgrain, pink pepper, ravensara, ravintsara, rhododendron, Roman chamomile, rosalina, rose, rosemary, rosewood, rue, saro, schisandra fruit, shell ginger, Spanish sage, spearmint, spike lavender, star anise, sweet inula, sweet wormwood, tagetes, tangerine, tansy, tarragon, thyme, tolu balsam, valerian, verbena, vetiver, white spruce, white verbena, wormwood, xanthoxylum, yuzu, zdravetz

**Antifungal**: African bluegrass, agarwood, ajowan, Aleppo pine, allspice, amyris, anise, applemint, arnica, auracaria, balsam fir, balsam poplar, bay (West Indies), bay laurel, benzoin absolute, bergamot mint, betony, big badja gum, black cumin, black sage, blue cypress, blue mallee, blue tansy, cajeput, calamus, calendula, Canadian fleabane, catnip, cedarwood, celery, cilantro, citron, citronella, clove, copaiba, coriander, cumin,

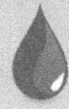

davana, dill seed, Douglas fir, elecampane, elemi, eucalyptus, eucalyptus dives, fennel, ferula, feverfew, fingerroot, Formosan cypress, Fragonia, galangal, garlic, genipi, German chamomile, Ghandi root, gingergrass, gobre salla, grindelia, guaiacwood, guava leaf, gully gum, gurjun balsam, helichrysum, hemp, hinoki, holy basil, honey myrtle, Indian borage, Japanese cedarwood, jasmine absolute, kaffir lime, kanuka, khella, kumquat, kunzea, lavandin, lavender, leleshwa, lemon, lemon basil, lemon catnip, lemon eucalyptus, lemon tea tree, lemongrass, lovage, manuka, maritime pine, marjoram, mastic, may chang, Mediterranean mandarin, tea tree, melissa, monarda, moringa, mountain savory, myrrh, neroli, oakmoss absolute, ocotea, opoponax, orange, orange (bitter), oregano, Oriental arborvitae, parsley seed, patchouli, pennyroyal, peppermint, Persian lime, Peru balsam, peta, petitgrain, pine, pink pepper, plai, ponderosa pine, rabbitbrush, ravensara, ravintsara, red pine, rhododendron, rosalina, rosemary, rue, sage, sandalwood, saro, savory (wild), schisandra fruit, shell ginger, Siam wood, Siberian fir, Southern blue gum, spearmint, spike lavender, spikenard, star anise, sweet inula, sweet nancy, sweet wormwood, summer savory, tagetes, tamala, Texas cedarwood, thuja, thyme, tolu balsam, tsauri grass, tsuga, Turkish pine, turmeric, vetiver, vilayti tulsi, Virginian cedarwood, Western red cedar, white pine, white sage, white spruce, white verbena, wild chamomile, wild marjoram, wormseed (American), wormwood, ylang ylang, yuzu, zdravetz

**Anti-Infectious**: Ajowan, applemint, big badja gum, blue cypress, blue mallee, buchu, Cape chamomile, cinnamon, davana, Fragonia, genipi, Ghandi root, goldenrod, gully gum, holy basil, honey myrtle, Indian borage, Japanese cedarwood, kunzea, lemon tea tree, may chang, tea tree, monarda, mountain savory, mugwort, neroli, oregano, pine, ponderosa pine, ravensara, ravintsara, red pine, rosalina, Siberian fir, spikenard, tagetes, tamala, tansy, tsuga, Virginian cedarwood, white pine, white sage

**Anti-Inflammatory**: African bluegrass, agarwood, ajowan, Aleppo pine, allspice, amyris, anise, applemint, arnica, auracaria, balsam fir, basil, bay laurel, benzoin absolute, bergamot, bergamot mint, betony, big badja gum, birch, black cumin, black pepper, black sage, blue cypress, blue mallee, blue mountain sage, blue spruce, blue tansy, boldo, buchu, Buddha wood, calamus, calendula, camphor, Canadian fleabane, cangerana, Cape chamomile, catnip, cedarwood, celery, Chinese cedarwood, Chinese red pine, cistus, citron, citronella, clove, copaiba, cumin, cypress, davana, dill seed, dwarf pine, Engelmann

spruce, fenugreek, ferula, feverfew, fingerroot, Formosan cypress, Fragonia, frankincense, galangal, galbanum, geranium, German chamomile, Ghandi root, ginger, gingergrass, gobre salla, goldenrod, grindelia, guaiacwood, guava leaf, guggul, gully gum, gurjun balsam, hairy basil, helichrysum, hemp, hinoki, honey myrtle, hops, hyssop, Indian borage, Japanese cedarwood, juniper (Chinese), juniper (Himalayan), kabosu, kaffir lime, kanuka, katrafay, kumquat, kunzea, lavender, ledum, lemon, lemon catnip, lemon eucalyptus, lemon tea tree, lemon verbena, lemongrass, lime, lovage, manuka, maritime pine, marjoram, mastic, may chang, tea tree, monarda, moringa, muhuhu, myrrh, neroli, oakmoss absolute, ocotea, opoponax, orange, orange (bitter), oregano, palo santo, parsley seed, patchouli, pennyroyal, Persian lime, Peru balsam, peta, petitgrain, pine, pink pepper, plai, ponderosa pine, rabbitbrush, ravintsara, red pine, rhododendron, Roman chamomile, rosalina, rose, sage, sandalwood, saro, savory (wild), schisandra fruit, shell ginger, Siam wood, Siberian fir, silver fir, Spanish sage, spearmint, spike lavender, spikenard, spruce (black), star anise, summer savory, sweet inula, sweet nancy, sweet wormwood, tagetes, tangerine, tamala, tansy, Texas cedarwood, thyme, tolu balsam, tsauri grass, tsuga, Turkish pine, turmeric, valerian, verbena, vetiver, vilayti tulsi, Virginian cedarwood, white fir, white pine, white spruce, white verbena, wintergreen, wild chamomile, wild marjoram, wormseed (American), xanthoxylum, yarrow, ylang ylang, yuzu

**Antimicrobial**: Agarwood, Aleppo pine, allspice, arnica, balsam fir, bay (West Indies), bay laurel, benzoin absolute, bergamot mint, betony, birch, black cumin, boldo, buchu, Buddha wood, cajeput, camphor, caraway, cardamom, cassia, catnip, cinnamon, cistus, clove, davana, Douglas fir, elecampane, Engelmann spruce, eucalyptus dives, fenugreek, feverfew, Fragonia, galbanum, galangal, garlic, genipi, grindelia, guava leaf, hairy basil, helichrysum, holy basil, honey myrtle, hyssop, Indian borage, jasmine absolute, juniper berry, juniper (Chinese), juniper (Himalayan), juniper (Phoenician), khella, kunzea, lavender, lemon, lemon basil, lemon catnip, lemon myrtle, lemon tea tree, lemongrass, manuka, maritime pine, pink pepper, mastic, may chang, tea tree, monarda, moringa, mountain savory, muhuhu, myrrh, myrtle, oakmoss absolute, oregano, parsley seed, pennyroyal, peppermint, pine, plai, ravensara, Roman chamomile, rosalina, saro, savin, savory (wild), shell ginger, silver fir, Spanish sage, spike lavender, spruce (black), summer savory, sweet wormwood, tagetes, tangerine,

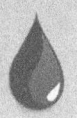

tamala, tansy, thuja, thyme, tsuga, Turkish pine, turmeric, valerian, vetiver, white fir, white sage, white spruce, white verbena, wild chamomile, wormwood, xanthoxylum, zdravetz

**Antineuralgic:** Ajowan, Aleppo pine, bay (West Indies), bay laurel, betony, blue spruce, cajeput, Chinese red pine, cistus, coriander, eucalyptus, geranium, German chamomile, ginger, hairy basil, hemp, hops, katrafay, lemon, lemongrass, maritime pine, marjoram, peppermint, pine, pink pepper, Roman chamomile, rosemary, sandalwood, Southern blue gum, spearmint, Turkish pine, valerian, white verbena

**Antioxidant:** African bluegrass, ajowan, allspice, anise, applemint, balsam fir, balsam poplar, basil, bay (West Indies), benzoin absolute, bergamot mint, betony, black cumin, black pepper, blue spruce, blue tansy, calamus, calendula, Canadian fleabane, carrot seed, celery, Chinese red pine, cilantro, citronella, clove, davana, dill seed, Douglas fir, dwarf pine, Engelmann spruce, fenugreek, ferula, fingerroot, Formosan cypress, Fragonia, frankincense, garlic, geranium, German chamomile, ginger, gobre salla, grapefruit, guaiacwood, guava leaf, guggul, helichrysum, hinoki, holy basil, honey myrtle, Japanese cedarwood, juniper berry, juniper (Phoenician), kaffir lime, kumquat, kunzea, lemon tea tree, lemongrass, maritime pine, may chang, monarda, moringa, mountain savory, nutmeg, oakmoss absolute, oregano, palo santo, parsley seed, Persian lime, Peru balsam, peta, pine, pink pepper, ponderosa pine, rosemary, savory (wild), schisandra fruit, shell ginger, Siam wood, silver fir, star anise, summer savory, sweet inula, sweet nancy, sweet wormwood, tamala, tarragon, thyme, tolu balsam, tsuga, Turkish pine, turmeric, vetiver, white fir, white pine, white spruce, white verbena, wild marjoram, wormwood, xanthoxylum

**Antioxidant Production\Activity, Increases:** Black cumin, black pepper, clove, lemon myrtle, orange, Siberian fir

**Antiparasitic:** African bluegrass, ajowan, anise, bergamot, bergamot mint, big badja gum, black cumin, black sage, blue mallee, boldo, cajeput, calamus, calendula, camphor, Cape chamomile, carrot seed, cassia, cinnamon, citronella, clove, davana, dwarf pine, elecampane, fennel, ferula, galbanum, garlic, gingergrass, gully gum, holy basil, juniper (Chinese), juniper (Himalayan), lemon, lemon verbena, lemongrass, lovage, maritime pine, mastic, monarda, mugwort, niaouli, ocotea, opoponax, pennyroyal, Peru balsam, pine, ponderosa pine,

rabbitbrush, Roman chamomile, saro, savin, star anise, summer savory, tagetes, tansy, tarragon, thuja, thyme, tolu balsam, tsauri grass, turmeric, verbena, vetiver, Western red cedar, wormseed (American), wormwood

**Antirheumatic:** Agarwood, Aleppo pine, allspice, anise, applemint, arnica, balsam fir, balsam poplar, bay laurel, benzoin absolute, betony, big badja gum, birch, black cumin, black sage, blue mallee, boldo, buchu, calamus, camphor, Canadian fleabane, cangerana, cassia, cedarwood, celery, Chinese cedarwood, Chinese red pine, cilantro, citron, citronella, coriander, Douglas fir, elemi, eucalyptus, feverfew, fingerroot, frankincense, galbanum, galangal, garlic, German chamomile, Ghandi root, gingergrass, gobre salla, guaiacwood, guggul, gully gum, gurjun balsam, hyssop, juniper berry, juniper (Chinese), juniper (Himalayan), juniper (Phoenician), katrafay, kunzea, ledum, lemon, lovage, maritime pine, marjoram, may chang, niaouli, nutmeg, parsley seed, pennyroyal, Peru balsam, peta, pine, pink pepper, plai, rabbitbrush, ravintsara, Roman chamomile, rosemary, rue, savin, Siam wood, Siberian fir, silver fir, Southern blue gum, Spanish sage, star anise, sweet nancy, sweet wormwood, tamala, tansy, tarragon, Texas cedarwood, thuja, thyme, tolu balsam, tsauri grass, Turkish pine, turmeric, verbena, vetiver, vilayti tulsi, Virginian cedarwood, Western red cedar, white fir, white pine, white spruce, wild chamomile, wild marjoram, wintergreen, wormseed (American), xanthoxylum, yarrow

**Anti-Seizure:** *See Anticonvulsive (Anti-epileptic)*

**Antiseptic:** African bluegrass, ajowan, Aleppo pine, allspice, amyris, anise, applemint, balsam poplar, bay (West Indies), bay laurel, benzoin absolute, bergamot, big badja gum, black cumin, blue mallee, blue mountain sage, blue spruce, boldo, buchu, cajeput, calendula, camphor, Cape chamomile, caraway, cardamom, carrot seed, catnip, cedarwood, Chinese cedarwood, Chinese red pine, cinnamon, cistus, citronella, clary sage, clove, copaiba, cumin, cypress, damiana, davana, Douglas fir, dwarf pine, elemi, eucalyptus, eucalyptus dives, fennel, fingerroot, frankincense, galangal, galbanum, geranium, German chamomile, ginger, gingergrass, gobre salla, goldenrod, grapefruit, guaiacwood, guava leaf, guggul, gully gum, gurjun balsam, hyssop, Indian borage, jasmine absolute, juniper berry, juniper (Chinese), juniper (Himalayan), juniper (Phoenician), kaffir lime, kabosu, lavandin, lavender, leleshwa, lemon, lemon catnip, lemon eucalyptus, lemon myrtle, lemon tea tree, lemon verbena, lemongrass, lime, lovage, maritime pine, marjoram, mastic, may

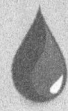

chang, Mediterranean mandarin, tea tree, melissa, moringa, muhuhu, myrrh, myrtle, neroli, niaouli, nutmeg, oakmoss absolute, opoponax, orange, orange (bitter), Oriental arborvitae, palmarosa, palo santo, parsley seed, patchouli, pennyroyal, peppermint, Persian lime, Peru balsam, peta, petitgrain, pine, pink pepper, plai, ponderosa pine, rabbitbrush, ravensara, ravintsara, Roman chamomile, rose, rosemary, rosewood, sage, sandalwood, saro, shell ginger, Siberian fir, silver fir, Southern blue gum, spearmint, spike lavender, spikenard, spruce (black), star anise, summer savory, sweet nancy, sweet wormwood, tagetes, tangerine, thyme, tolu balsam, tsauri grass, tsuga, Turkish pine, turmeric, vetiver, vilayti tulsi, Western red cedar, white fir, white sage, white spruce, white verbena, wild marjoram, wintergreen, yarrow, ylang ylang, yuzu, zdravetz

**Antispasmodic:** African bluegrass, ajowan, angelica, anise, applemint, arnica, balsam fir, basil, bay (West Indies), bay laurel, bergamot, bergamot mint, birch, black cumin, blue mountain sage, blue tansy, buchu, cajeput, calamus, calendula, camphor, Canadian fleabane, Cape chamomile, caraway, cardamom, cassia, catnip, cedarwood, celery, chaste tree, cilantro, citronella, clove, coriander, cumin, cypress, damiana, davana, dill seed, Douglas fir, Engelmann spruce, eucalyptus, fenugreek, ferula, feverfew, fingerroot, Fragonia, galangal, galbanum, genipi, German chamomile, Ghandi root, ginger, grindelia, guava leaf, gurjun balsam, hairy basil, helichrysum, hemp, honey myrtle, hops, hyssop, jasmine absolute, juniper berry, juniper (Chinese), juniper (Himalayan), juniper (Phoenician), kabosu, khella, kunzea, lavandin, lavender, lemon catnip, lemon myrtle, lemon verbena, lime, lovage, manuka, marjoram, mastic, may chang, Mediterranean mandarin, melissa, monarda, moringa, mugwort, myrrh, neroli, niaouli, nutmeg, opoponax, orange, orange (bitter), oregano, palo santo, pennyroyal, peppermint, Persian lime, peta, petitgrain, plai, ponderosa pine, rabbitbrush, ravensara, red pine, rhododendron, Roman chamomile, rose, rosemary, rue, sage, sandalwood, shell ginger, Siberian fir, silver fir, Southern blue gum, Spanish sage, spearmint, spike lavender, spikenard, spruce (black), star anise, summer savory, sweet nancy, sweet wormwood, tagetes, tamala, tangerine, thyme, turmeric, valerian, verbena, vetiver, Western red cedar, white fir, white pine, white spruce, white verbena, wild chamomile, wintergreen, xanthoxylum, yarrow, ylang ylang, yuzu, zdravetz

**Antitumor:** Fennel, frankincense, ledum, melissa, myrrh, sandalwood, thyme, turmeric

**Antiviral:** African bluegrass, ajowan, allspice, applemint, balsam poplar, basil, big badja gum, black cumin, black pepper, blue cypress, blue mallee, blue mountain sage, blue tansy, Buddha wood, cajeput, camphor, cassia, cinnamon, cistus, clary sage, clove, davana, Douglas fir, elemi, Engelmann spruce, eucalyptus, fenugreek, Fragonia, gingergrass, gully gum, holy basil, honey myrtle, Indian borage, kaffir lime, kanuka, katrafay, kumquat, kunzea, lavandin, leleshwa, lemon verbena, lemon eucalyptus, lemon myrtle, lemon tea tree, lemongrass, lime, manuka, maritime pine, marjoram, mastic, Mediterranean mandarin, tea tree, melissa, monarda, mountain savory, myrrh, oregano, Oriental arborvitae, palmarosa, patchouli, Persian lime, peta, pine, pink pepper, plai, ravensara, ravintsara, rosalina, rose, rue, sage, saro, savory (wild), shell ginger, Southern blue gum, star anise, summer savory, sweet inula, sweet wormwood, tansy, thuja, thyme, tsauri grass, turmeric, white pine, white sage, white spruce, white verbena, xanthoxylum

**Anxiolytic (Reduces Anxiety):** African bluegrass, agarwood, Aleppo pine, amyris, angelica, anise, applemint, balsam fir, basil, bergamot, bergamot mint, betony, black cumin, black sage, blue mountain sage, blue tansy, Buddha wood, calendula, Cape chamomile, caraway, carrot seed, catnip, cedarwood, cilantro, cistus, citron, clary sage, copaiba, coriander, damiana, davana, dill seed, Douglas fir, dwarf pine, elemi, eucalyptus dives, fennel, feverfew, Formosan cypress, Fragonia, frankincense, galangal, German chamomile, Ghandi root, gingergrass, guava leaf, gurjun balsam, hairy basil, hemp, hinoki, holy basil, honey myrtle, hops, hyssop, Japanese cedarwood, jasmine absolute, kabosu, kaffir lime, kanuka, khella, kumquat, kunzea, lavandin, lavender, lemon basil, lemon catnip, lemon tea tree, lemon verbena, lime, magnolia, maritime pine, marjoram, mastic, may chang, Mediterranean mandarin, melissa, monarda, moringa, mugwort, muhuhu, neroli, nutmeg, opoponax, orange, orange (bitter), palmarosa, palo santo, Persian lime, Peru balsam, petitgrain, pine, pink pepper, plai, rabbitbrush, ravensara, ravintsara, red pine, Roman chamomile, rosalina, rue, saro, schisandra fruit, shell ginger, Siberian fir, Spanish sage, spearmint, spike lavender, spikenard, spruce (black), star anise, sweet inula, tamala, tangerine, tansy, Texas cedarwood, tolu balsam, tsauri grass, Turkish pine, turmeric, valerian, vetiver, Virginian cedarwood, white pine, white spruce, white verbena, wormseed (American), wormwood, xanthoxylum, ylang ylang, yuzu, zdravetz

**Aphrodisiac:** Agarwood, amyris, cardamom, cedarwood, celery, clary sage, clove, coriander,

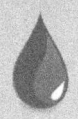 

cumin, damiana, fingerroot, galangal, Ghandi root, ginger, gingergrass, jasmine absolute, juniper (Chinese), juniper (Himalayan), lovage, moringa, muhuhu, myrtle, neroli, nutmeg, orange, patchouli, ravensara, rose, rosemary, rosewood, sandalwood, Siam wood, vetiver, ylang ylang, zdravetz

**Appetite, Stimulates**: Ajowan, bay laurel, caraway, cardamom, cilantro, coriander, fingerroot, genipi, hemp, lime, Persian lime, tamala, tarragon, vilayti tulsi

**Appetite, Balances**: Celery, grapefruit, ocotea

**Asthma, Relieves**: Khella

**Astringent**: African bluegrass, benzoin absolute, birch, black sage, cajeput, Canadian fleabane, cassia, catnip, cedarwood, Chinese cedarwood, cistus, citronella, clary sage, cypress, damiana, davana, elecampane, geranium, ginger, grapefruit, grindelia, guava leaf, guggul, helichrysum, hyssop, juniper berry, juniper (Chinese), juniper (Himalayan), juniper (Phoenician), leleshwa, lemon, lemon catnip, lemongrass, lime, maritime pine, mastic, may chang, myrrh, myrtle, orange (bitter), Oriental arborvitae, palmarosa, parsley seed, pennyroyal, peppermint, Persian lime, Peru balsam, pink pepper, plai, rose, rosemary, sage, sandalwood, spruce (black), sweet nancy, sweet wormwood, thuja, tolu balsam, tsauri grass, tsuga, Virginian cedarwood, Western red cedar, white sage, wintergreen, yarrow, zdravetz

**Awareness, Increases**: Engelmann spruce, garlic

**Bile, Stimulates Release\Flow of**: Applemint, bay laurel, catnip, Mediterranean mandarin, melissa, peppermint, rosemary, spike lavender, yarrow

**Bites (Snake), Relieves\Antidotes**: Rue, turmeric, wormseed (American)

**Bleeding, Stops Excess**: Black sage, Canadian fleabane, Chinese cedarwood, cistus, cypress, geranium, lime, maritime pine, Oriental arborvitae, Persian lime, pink pepper, rosemary, sweet nancy, sweet wormwood, yarrow

**Blemishes, Scars, Wrinkles, Acne—Reduces Appearance of**: Amyris, applemint, balsam poplar, bergamot, big badja gum, black cumin, blue mallee, cajeput, calendula, camphor, caraway, carrot seed, cedarwood, Chinese cedarwood, cistus, clove, elecampane, elemi, fennel, fenugreek, frankincense, galbanum, garlic, geranium, German chamomile, gingergrass, grapefruit, gully gum, helichrysum, holy basil, hyssop, Japanese cedarwood, jasmine absolute, juniper berry, juniper (Phoenician), kabosu, kaffir

lime, kanuka, kumquat, lavandin, lavender, leleshwa, lemon, lemon verbena, lime, manuka, may chang, Mediterranean mandarin, tea tree, melissa, moringa, mountain savory, muhuhu, myrtle, neroli, niaouli, opoponax, orange (bitter), palmarosa, patchouli, Persian lime, petitgrain, ravintsara, rhododendron, Roman chamomile, rosalina, rose, rosemary, rosewood, sandalwood, savory (wild), sweet inula, tangerine, Texas cedarwood, thyme, tsauri grass, vetiver, Virginian cedarwood, white spruce, wild chamomile, yarrow

**Blisters, Heals**: Big badja gum, blue mallee, dwarf pine, elecampane, fenugreek, German chamomile, gully gum, gurjun balsam, lavender, lemon tea tree, tea tree, parsley seed, pennyroyal, rabbitbrush, rosalina, Roman chamomile, savin, white verbena, zdravetz

**Blood Clots, Helps Clear**: Fennel, helichrysum, ocotea

**Blood Pressure (High), Normalizes\ Balances**: Amyris, applemint, bergamot mint, black cumin, Canadian fleabane, caraway, catnip, celery, cumin, fenugreek, galangal, garlic, hairy basil, honey myrtle, khella, lavender, lemon, lemon basil, lemon catnip, marjoram, may chang, melissa, moringa, mugwort, neroli, ocotea, parsley seed, pink pepper, rabbitbrush, sandalwood, shell ginger, sweet inula, sweet nancy, tagetes, tsauri grass, valerian, white verbena, yarrow, ylang ylang, zdravetz

**Blood, Purifies**: Angelica, birch, cinnamon, clove, spike lavender, coriander, rose, tangerine

**Blood Sugar, Supports Normal Levels**: Anise, black cumin, Canadian fleabane, cassia, cilantro, cinnamon, citron, clove, coriander, eucalyptus, dill seed, fennel, fenugreek, geranium, guava leaf, guggul, kumquat, lemon basil, lemon tea tree, moringa, ocotea, parsley seed, Southern blue gum, star anise, tamala, tarragon, white verbena, zdravetz

**Boils, Supports Healing of**: Cape chamomile, dwarf pine, fenugreek, Gurjun balsam, lavender, lemon, mastic, tea tree, moringa, niaouli, pennyroyal, rabbitbrush, rosalina, Roman chamomile, rue, zdravetz

**Bone Growth (Abnormal), Reduces**: Eucalyptus, Southern blue gum

**Bone Pain, Relieves**: Balsam fir, wintergreen

**Bone Turnover, Promotes Healthy**: Pine, rosemary, sage, thyme

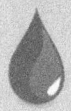

**Brain Function\Cognition, Aids\Protects**: *See Memory\Cognition, Aids\Protects*

**Brain Neurons, Regenerates**: Turmeric

**Breasts (Swollen), Relieves**: Parsley seed

**Bronchodilator (Increases Airflow to the Lungs)**: Ginger, khella, myrtle, oregano, peppermint

**Bruises, Relieves**: Arnica, balsam poplar, calendula, cinnamon, genipi, geranium, gurjun balsam, helichrysum, kunzea, lavender, lemon tea tree, lemongrass, mastic, mountain savory, plai, savory (wild), white verbena, wild marjoram

**Burnout, Reduces**: Basil, rosemary

**Burns\Sunburns, Soothes**: Calendula, lavender, tea tree, niaouli, peta, Roman chamomile, tagetes, wild chamomile, yarrow

**Burns (Radiation), Heals**: Tea tree, niaouli

**Cardiovascular\Endothelial Function Supports\Protects**: Amyris, bergamot, black cumin, black sage, Buddha wood, calamus, caraway, citron, Formosan cypress, dwarf pine, garlic, goldenrod, hemp, hairy basil, holy basil, honey myrtle, lavender, marjoram, may chang, melissa, nutmeg, orange (bitter), parsley seed, pink pepper, rhododendron, rose, rosemary, sandalwood, shell ginger, spikenard, sweet inula, thyme, valerian, Virginian cedarwood, white verbena, wormwood, ylang ylang

**Cell Cycle (Healthy), Supports**: Frankincense, helichrysum, tangerine, thyme, vetiver, ylang ylang

**Cellular Regeneration, Supports**: Carrot seed, cistus, frankincense, geranium, kanuka, myrrh, neroli, palmarosa, rosalina, spikenard, turmeric, wintergreen

**Cellulitis, Reduces**: Parsley seed

**Change, Encourages Acceptance of and Adaptation to**: Muhuhu, wild chamomile

**Cholesterol (High), Balances**: Basil, orange (bitter), black cumin, calamus, cinnamon, dill seed, garlic, guggul, holy basil, lavender, lemon basil, lemongrass, moringa, orange, shell ginger, tamala, turmeric, yarrow

**Circulation, Aids\Stimulates**: Ajowan, anise, arnica, basil, benzoin absolute, birch, black pepper, cajeput, calamus, calendula, carrot seed, cassia, cedarwood, cinnamon, clove, coriander, cumin, cypress, damiana, dwarf pine, elemi, fenugreek, galbanum, garlic, ginger, gingergrass, goldenrod, helichrysum, jasmine absolute, lemongrass, lime, lovage, magnolia, maritime pine, marjoram, mastic, mountain savory, myrrh, opoponax, niaouli, palmarosa, pennyroyal, Persian lime, Peru balsam, pink pepper, rhododendron, savory (wild), Siberian fir, silver fir, Spanish sage, star anise, summer savory, tamala, tarragon, tolu balsam, tsauri grass, verbena, vilayti tulsi, white fir, white pine, white spruce, wild marjoram, yarrow, zdravetz

**Circulation\Redness, Increases Localized**: Allspice, camphor, dwarf pine, juniper (Chinese), juniper (Himalayan), nutmeg, patchouli, ponderosa pine, red pine, rosemary, Siberian fir, silver fir, spike lavender, spruce (black), thuja, thyme, tsuga, vetiver, white fir, wintergreen

**Colic, Soothes**: Cumin, fennel, German chamomile, lavender, Roman chamomile

**Communication, Encourages Open**: Fennel

**Compassion\Empathy, Encourages**: Calendula

**Concentration\Focus\Attention, Aids**: Balsam fir, bay laurel, big badja gum, blue mallee, cardamom, copaiba, Douglas fir, eucalyptus, fenugreek, frankincense, galbanum, genipi, gully gum, honey myrtle, hyssop, ledum, lemon, mugwort, myrrh, niaouli, palo santo, peppermint, sandalwood, Southern blue gum, Spanish sage, tsauri grass, vetiver, wild marjoram

**Confidence, Enhances**: *See Self-confidence, Encourages*

**Confusion, Reduces**: Basil, bay laurel, cajeput, clary sage, rosemary, Siam wood

**Constipation, Relieves**: African bluegrass, cardamom, fennel, fingerroot, ginger, kabosu, lemon, marjoram, Mediterranean mandarin, nutmeg, Oriental arborvitae, parsley seed, patchouli, plai, rose, spikenard, tangerine, yuzu

**Corns, Removes**: Garlic, kanuka

**Cough, Eases\Soothes**: Ajowan, Aleppo pine, allspice, amyris, anise, applemint, balsam fir, basil, benzoin absolute, big badja gum, black cumin, black sage, blue mallee, blue mountain sage, buchu, cajeput, calamus, camphor, cassia, cedarwood, Chinese red pine, cistus, cypress, damiana, davana, Douglas fir, elecampane, Engelmann spruce, eucalyptus, fennel, feverfew, fingerroot, Formosan cypress, frankincense, galangal, gingergrass, gobre salla, goldenrod, grindelia, gully gum, hemp, hops (spasmodic), Indian borage, kanuka, khella, lavender, ledum, leleshwa, lovage, magnolia, manuka, maritime pine, tea tree,

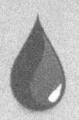 
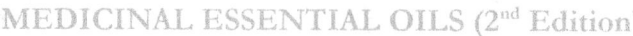

mountain savory, muhuhu, <u>myrtle</u>, nutmeg, oakmoss absolute, opoponax, Oriental arborvitae, palo santo, parsley seed, pennyroyal, Peru balsam, pine, ponderosa <u>pine</u>, <u>rabbitbrush</u>, ravensara, ravintsara, red pine, rhododendron, rose, saro, savory (wild), shell ginger, Siberian fir, silver fir, <u>Southern blue gum</u>, Spanish sage, spruce (black), star anise, summer savory, tarragon, Texas cedarwood, thuja, <u>thyme</u>, tolu balsam, tsauri grass, <u>tsuga</u>, Turkish pine, turmeric, <u>verbena</u>, vilayti tulsi, Virginian cedarwood, Western red cedar, white fir, <u>white pine</u>, white sage, <u>white sage</u>, wild marjoram, wintergreen

**Courage\Valor Increases:** Black pepper, cilantro, cinnamon, clove, ginger, mugwort

**Cramps\Spasms (Intestinal), Relieves:** Mountain savory, savory (wild), summer savory, white verbena

**Creativity, Stimulates:** Gurjun balsam, helichrysum, hemp, myrrh, neroli, opoponax, palo santo, peppermint, petitgrain, ravensara, white sage, zdravetz

**Cystitis, Reduces:** Amyris

**Dandruff, Relieves:** Tolu balsam, Virginian cedarwood

gobre salla, **gestant:** Amyris, anise, balsam fir, basil, bay laurel, bergamot, big badja gum, black pepper, <u>blue mallee</u>, cajeput, caraway, chaste tree, clove, copaiba, <u>eucalyptus</u>, eucalyptus dives, galbanum, genipi, <u>gobre salla</u>, hinoki, <u>hyssop</u>, khella, manuka, marjoram, myrtle, niaouli, <u>palo santo</u>, patchouli, pennyroyal, peppermint, <u>pine</u>, ponderosa pine, rosalina, rosemary, sage, sandalwood, Southern blue gum, Spanish sage, <u>spearmint</u>, star anise, sweet inula, verbena, white fir, white pine, <u>white sage</u>, white spruce, wild marjoram

**Denial, Reduces:** Douglas fir

**Deodorant:** <u>Citronella</u>, cypress, honey myrtle, kanuka, lemongrass, magnolia, may chang, neroli, nutmeg, orange (bitter), petitgrain, rosewood, wintergreen

**Despondency, Combats:** Bergamot, clary sage, sandalwood, thyme, ylang ylang

**Detoxification, Aids:** Birch, black cumin, buchu, carrot seed, <u>cilantro</u>, <u>cumin</u>, fingerroot, galbanum, <u>grapefruit</u>, helichrysum, Japanese cedarwood, guggul, kaffir lime, <u>ledum</u>, lemon, lemongrass, lovage, tea tree, nutmeg, parsley seed, Peru balsam, pine, rhododendron, Roman chamomile, tarragon, thuja, tolu balsam, vetiver

**Diarrhea, Relieves:** Ajowan, amyris, calamus, <u>Canadian fleabane</u>, cassia, cilantro, <u>cinnamon</u>, fennel, galangal, garlic, <u>ginger</u>, <u>guava leaf</u>, Indian borage, juniper (Chinese), lemongrass, <u>tea tree</u>, moringa, mountain savory, ocotea, orange (bitter), peppermint, Peru balsam, plai, rabbitbrush, savory (wild), shell ginger, summer savory, tamala, tolu balsam, <u>verbena</u>, white verbena

**Digestive Aid:** African bluegrass, agarwood, Aleppo pine, allspice, angelica, <u>anise</u>, applemint, <u>basil</u>, bay (West Indies), <u>bergamot</u>, betony, birch, <u>black pepper</u>, black sage, blue mountain sage, boldo, cajeput, calamus, cangerana, <u>cardamom</u>, <u>caraway</u>, cassia, catnip, celery, <u>cinnamon</u>, <u>cilantro</u>, citron, citronella, clary sage, <u>clove</u>, copaiba, <u>coriander</u>, <u>cumin</u>, dill seed, elecampane, <u>fennel</u>, <u>fingerroot</u>, frankincense, galangal, genipi, <u>German chamomile</u>, ginger, gobre salla, grapefruit, grindelia, guava leaf, guggul, hemp, holy basil, hops, hyssop, juniper berry, juniper (Chinese), juniper (Himalayan), juniper (Phoenician), kabosu, kaffir lime, kumquat, lavender, lemon, lemon catnip, lemon tea tree, lemon verbena, lemongrass, magnolia, maritime pine, mastic, may chang, <u>Mediterranean mandarin</u>, melissa, monarda, mountain savory, mugwort, neroli, <u>nutmeg</u>, ocotea, opoponax, <u>orange</u>, orange (bitter), Oriental arborvitae, palmarosa, patchouli, pennyroyal, <u>peppermint</u>, petitgrain, pink pepper, rabbitbrush, rhododendron, Roman chamomile, <u>rosemary</u>, rue, savory (wild), schisandra fruit, shell ginger, <u>spearmint</u>, star anise, summer savory, sweet nancy, sweet wormwood, tangerine, tamala, tarragon, Turkish pine, <u>turmeric</u>, valerian, vilayti tulsi, white verbena, wild chamomile, wild marjoram, wormwood, yarrow

**Digestive Juices, Stimulates:** <u>Allspice</u>, catnip, yarrow

**Disappointment, Combats:** Manuka

**Disinfectant:** Applemint, benzoin absolute, bergamot, caraway, catnip, davana, dill seed, Douglas fir, galangal, leleshwa, lemon, lemon catnip, lime, orange, Persian lime, pine, Roman chamomile, rosalina, sandalwood, silver fir, tagetes, white fir, ylang ylang

**Distractions (Mental), Reduces:** Myrrh

**Diuretic:** Agarwood, Aleppo pine, angelica, basil, bay laurel, benzoin absolute, <u>birch</u>, buchu, camphor, Canadian fleabane, caraway, cardamom, carrot seed, catnip, celery, cedarwood, chaste tree, citron, citronella, cumin, <u>cypress</u>, damiana, Douglas fir, dwarf pine, elecampane, eucalyptus, fennel, ferula,

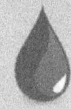

frankincense, galangal, genipi, geranium, ginger, goldenrod, grapefruit, guaiacwood, helichrysum, hyssop, Indian borage, juniper berry, juniper (Phoenician), kabosu, lavender, ledum, lemon, lemon catnip, lemongrass, lovage, maritime pine, Mediterranean mandarin, moringa, mugwort, orange, oregano, Oriental arborvitae, parsley seed, Peru balsam, pine, pink pepper, ravensara, Roman chamomile, rosemary, sage, sandalwood, savin, shell ginger, Southern blue gum, spearmint, spike lavender, spruce (black), sweet inula, tagetes, tangerine, thuja, thyme, tolu balsam, tolu balsam, tsuga, Turkish pine, turmeric, wintergreen, wormseed (American), yuzu

**Dizziness, Reduces**: Black cumin, shell ginger

**Drug Withdrawal, Reduces**: Anise, black pepper, rose

**Earache, Relieves**: Basil, cajeput, lavender, tea tree

**Edema, Reduces**: *See Fluid Retention, Reduces Excess*

**Ego, Reduces Excess**: Indian borage, mountain savory, savory (wild)

**Emotionally Stabilizing\Balancing**: Balsam fir, calendula, fennel, geranium, helichrysum, khella, Texas cedarwood, Virginian cedarwood

**Empowerment, Encourages Feelings of**: Silver fir, white fir

**Endocrine System, Supports**: Balsam fir, chaste tree, elemi, Engelmann spruce, red pine, Siam wood, tansy, tsuga, white spruce, wormwood

**Energizing**: Cassia, fennel, grapefruit, katrafay, lemongrass, ocotea, plai, ravensara, rosemary, saro, silver fir, spearmint, white fir, white sage

**Erectile Dysfunction, Reduces**: *See Impotence (Male), Reduces*

**Euphoria, Promotes**: Clary sage, gingergrass, ylang ylang

**Exhaustion\Fatigue (Mental), Relieves**: Ajowan, bay (West Indies), Aleppo pine, black cumin, black pepper, cajeput, caraway, damiana, eucalyptus, ferula, galangal, genipi, ginger, holy basil, hyssop, katrafay, lemon basil, lemongrass, maritime pine, nutmeg, peppermint, pine, rosemary, schisandra fruit, shell ginger, Southern blue gum, spearmint, spruce (black), tagetes, tamala, thyme, Turkish pine

**Expectorant**: Angelica, anise, black pepper, camphor, cedarwood, cistus, clove, copaiba, cypress, eucalyptus, fennel, frankincense, genipi, ginger,

goldenrod, helichrysum, holy basil, lavandin, marjoram, tea tree, myrtle, niaouli, orange, oregano, palo santo, peppermint, pine, ravensara, rosemary, sage, silver fir, Southern blue gum, spearmint, spike lavender, star anise, thyme, tsuga, white fir, ylang ylang

**Eye Health, Protects\Improves**: Frankincense, hemp, lemongrass, pine, white verbena

**Fats, Breaks Down\Metabolizes**: Coriander, genipi, sage

**Fear, Combats**: Amyris, black pepper, Cape chamomile, cedarwood, frankincense, grapefruit, lavender, maritime pine, mountain savory, niaouli, parsley seed, ravintsara, savory (wild), Spanish sage, summer savory, tarragon, Texas cedarwood, vetiver, Virginian cedarwood, ylang ylang

**Fever, Reduces**: Agarwood, ajowan, angelica, bay (West Indies), bay laurel, bergamot, birch, black cumin, black sage, buchu, cajeput, Canadian fleabane, cangerana, chaste tree, cumin, eucalyptus, eucalyptus dives, German chamomile, gully gum, hairy basil, helichrysum, hemp, holy basil, hyssop, katrafay, lavender, lemon, lemon basil, lemon eucalyptus, lemon verbena, lemon myrtle, lemon tea tree, lemongrass, lime, lovage, may chang, melissa, monarda, niaouli, palmarosa, parsley seed, patchouli, peppermint, Persian lime, Roman chamomile, rose, rosewood, sandalwood, shell ginger, Siberian fir, silver fir, Southern blue gum, Spanish sage, spearmint, valerian, verbena, vilayti tulsi, Western red cedar, white fir, white verbena, wormwood, yarrow, zdravetz

**Fluid Retention, Reduces Excess**: Cypress, grapefruit, juniper berry, juniper (Phoenician), mastic, tangerine

**Forgiveness, Fosters**: Engelmann spruce, helichrysum, spruce (black), wintergreen

**Frustration, Removes\Reduces**: Amyris, German chamomile, ginger, lemon, ylang ylang

**Gallbladder Supportive**: Bay (West Indies), boldo, German chamomile, juniper berry, juniper (Chinese), juniper (Himalayan), juniper (Phoenician), lemon verbena, Mediterranean mandarin, monarda, pennyroyal, peppermint, rosemary, wild chamomile, wintergreen

**Gallbladder, Reduces Inflammation**: Pine

**Gallstones, Eliminates\Dissolves**: Boldo, celery, maritime pine, pine

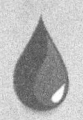 

**Gas, Expels Excess**: Agarwood, ajowan, allspice, angelica, anise, applemint, basil, bay laurel, bergamot mint, birch, black cumin, blue mountain sage, buchu, cajeput, calamus, caraway, cardamom, carrot seed, cassia, catnip, celery, cilantro, clary sage, clove, coriander, cumin, davana, dill seed, fennel, fingerroot, frankincense, galangal, German chamomile, ginger, guava leaf, hairy basil, ledum, lemon, lemon catnip, lemongrass, lovage, marjoram, may chang, mountain savory, myrrh, neroli, nutmeg, orange, orange (bitter), oregano, parsley seed, patchouli, pennyroyal, peppermint, petitgrain, plai, rabbitbrush, ravensara, Roman chamomile, rosemary, sandalwood, savory (wild), shell ginger, spearmint, spike lavender, star anise, sweet nancy, sweet wormwood, tangerine, tarragon, thyme, turmeric, valerian, vilayti tulsi, wintergreen, zdravetz

**Gastrointestinal Tract, Heals\Protects**: Black pepper, cardamom, cedarwood, clove, copaiba, German chamomile, ginger, lemon myrtle, lemongrass, marjoram, myrtle, neroli, orange (bitter), oregano, turmeric

**Glands, Reduces Inflammation of**: Bay laurel, lemon, lemongrass

**Gout, Relieves** (*See also Uric Acid, Clears Body of*): Guaiacwood, lovage, maritime pine, peppermint, pink pepper

**Gratitude, Encourages Feelings of**: Arnica

**Grief\Despair, Combats**: Cypress, frankincense, lemon basil, marjoram, melissa, rhododendron, rose, rue, Siam wood, Spanish sage, vetiver

**Grounding**: Aleppo pine, balsam fir, balsam poplar, blue cypress, blue spruce, cedarwood, Chinese red pine, cinnamon, Engelmann spruce, guaiacwood, gurjun balsam, khella, maritime pine, mastic, muhuhu, oakmoss absolute, palo santo, pine, red pine, savin, spruce (black), tsuga, Turkish pine, vetiver, Virginian cedarwood, Western red cedar, white pine, white verbena

**Guilt, Diminishes**: Cardamom, cypress, juniper, juniper (Chinese), juniper (Himalayan), juniper (Phoenician), sandalwood, thyme

**Gum (Inflammation), Reduces**: Tea tree

**Hair, Nourishes\Strengthens**: Auracaria, carrot seed, lemon, lemon verbena, Peru balsam, rosemary, Texas cedarwood, Virginian cedarwood, yarrow, ylang ylang

**Hair Loss, Slows\Reverses**: Black cumin, cedarwood, chaste tree, garlic, hinoki, kaffir lime, tea tree, rosemary, thyme, ylang ylang

**Headache\Migraine Relief**: African bluegrass, allspice, basil, betony, big badja gum, black cumin, blue mallee, catnip, chaste tree, cilantro, coriander, damiana, davana, feverfew, gully gum, hairy basil, hemp, holy basil, hops, Indian borage, kaffir lime, kanuka, katrafay, kunzea, lavender, leleshwa, lemon basil, lemon catnip, lemon myrtle, lemon tea tree, lemongrass, manuka, may chang, monarda, pennyroyal, peppermint, rabbitbrush, Roman chamomile, rosemary, savin, shell ginger, spearmint, spikenard, thyme, tolu balsam, valerian, vilayti tulsi, white verbena, wild chamomile, wild marjoram, yarrow, zdravetz

**Heart, Stimulates**: Camphor

**Hemorrhoids\Anal Fissures, Relieves**: Amyris, cistus, cypress, Ghandi root, tea tree, neroli, parsley seed, Texas cedarwood, Virginian cedarwood, wormseed (American), yarrow, zdravetz

**Hives, Relieves**: Grindelia

**Hormones, Stimulates Release\Balances**: Benzoin absolute, bergamot, betony, blue spruce (male, testosterone), Canadian fleabane, cardamom, catnip, chaste tree (female, progesterone; thyroid), clary sage (female, estrogen), elecampane, Fragonia, geranium, hemp, holy basil, jasmine absolute, lemon catnip, tea tree, melissa, mugwort, myrtle (thyroid), pennyroyal, rose (female), rosewood, sage, Spanish sage, spikenard, tansy, vetiver (male, testosterone), vilayti tulsi, wormwood

**Hysteria, Combats\Reduces**: Buchu, gurjun balsam, jasmine absolute, melissa, mugwort, pennyroyal, wormseed (American)

**Imagination, Stimulates**: Geranium

**Immune Supportive**: African bluegrass, ajowan, angelica, applemint, balsam fir, benzoin absolute, bergamot mint, black cumin, blue tansy, buchu, Buddha wood, Chinese cedarwood, Chinese red pine, citron, copaiba, damiana, Douglas fir, dwarf pine, elecampane, elemi, Engelmann spruce, fenugreek, Formosan cypress, Fragonia, galbanum, garlic, genipi, Ghandi root, gingergrass, grapefruit, grindelia, guava leaf, guggul, gurjun balsam, hyssop, kaffir lime, kunzea, lavender, ledum, lemon, lemon myrtle, lime, manuka, maritime pine, plai, tea tree, moringa, mountain savory, oregano, palo santo, parsley seed, peppermint, Persian lime, ponderosa pine, red pine,

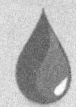

rosalina, rosemary, sage, saro, savory (wild), summer savory, sweet inula, tansy, tsauri grass, white fir, white pine, white spruce, wormwood

**Immune Modulator:** Cistus, Fragonia, frankincense

**Impotence (Male), Reduces:** Amyris, damiana, garlic, goldenrod, lemon catnip

**Injury (Sports), Recovery from:** Arnica, camphor, ginger, kunzea, lemongrass, tea tree, ocotea, plai, thyme, white verbena, wintergreen

**Insect Bites\Stings, Relieves:** Allspice, basil, blue mountain sage, calendula, cardamom, Indian borage, kanuka, manuka, tea tree, mountain savory, niaouli, rue, savory (wild), spike lavender, sweet inula, turmeric, verbena

**Insect Repellent:** African bluegrass, Aleppo pine, amyris, big badja gum, blue mallee, blue mountain sage, Buddha wood, calamus, Canadian fleabane, catnip, Chinese cedarwood, citronella, clove, davana, eucalyptus, feverfew, fingerroot, Formosan cypress, garlic, genipi, Ghandi root, gingergrass, guaiacwood, guava leaf, gully gum, hemp, hinoki, honey myrtle, Japanese cedarwood, kaffir lime, lavandin, leleshwa, lemon catnip, lemon eucalyptus, lemon tea tree, lemongrass, maritime pine, mountain savory, pennyroyal, pink pepper, plai, rosemary, savory (wild), Siam wood, Southern blue gum, star anise, sweet nancy, sweet wormwood, tagetes, tansy, Texas cedarwood, tsauri grass, vetiver, vilayti tulsi, Virginian cedarwood, Western red cedar. White verbena, wormseed (American), wormwood

**Insecticide:** African bluegrass, ajowan, Aleppo pine, amyris, anise, applemint, auracaria, basil, bay (West Indies), bay laurel, big badja gum, black cumin, black sage, blue mallee, boldo, buchu, Buddha wood, calamus, camphor, cardamom, Canadian fleabane, cassia, catnip, celery, Chinese cedarwood, cilantro, cinnamon, eucalyptus, eucalyptus dives, dill seed, fingerroot, Formosan cypress, galangal, garlic, geranium, Ghandi root, goldenrod, Japanese cedarwood, juniper (Chinese), juniper (Phoenician), kaffir lime, leleshwa, lemon catnip, lemon tea tree, Oriental arborvitae, parsley seed, patchouli, pennyroyal, peppermint, Peru balsam, pink pepper, plai, ledum, may chang, niaouli, ravintsara, rue, Siam wood, spikenard, star anise, sweet nancy, sweet wormwood, tagetes, tangerine, tolu balsam, Turkish pine, vilayti tulsi, Western red cedar, white verbena, wild marjoram, wormseed (American), wormwood, yarrow

**Inspiration, Promotes:** Clary sage, Formosan cypress

**Introspection, Promotes:** Copaiba

**Intuition, Increases:** Opoponax

**Invigorating:** Cumin, eucalyptus, myrtle, orange (bitter), peppermint, Southern blue gum

**Irritability (Emotional), Reduces:** Cape chamomile, coriander, lavender, kabosu, Mediterranean mandarin, myrrh, sandalwood, sweet nancy, sweet wormwood, wild chamomile

**Jealousy, Reduces:** Buchu, pennyroyal

**Jet Lag, Relieves:** Fragonia

**Joy\Pleasure, Increases:** Ylang ylang

**Kidney Stones, Prevents\Eliminates:** Celery, Goldenrod, holy basil, juniper berry, juniper (Phoenician), khella, lemon

**Kidneys, Supports or Protects:** Aleppo pine, black cumin, Canadian fleabane, damiana, fenugreek, juniper, ledum, lovage, maritime pine, rhododendron, white pine

**Lactation, Stimulates:** Caraway, dill seed, fennel, fenugreek

**Libido, Enhances:** Cassia, clary sage, nutmeg, parsley seed, rose, ylang ylang

**Libido, Decreases:** Chaste tree, marjoram

**Lice, Kills:** Eucalyptus, tea tree, Peru balsam

**Liver Supportive or Protective:** Agarwood, Aleppo pine, angelica, applemint, bay (West Indies), black cumin, boldo, cajeput, Canadian fleabane, caraway, carrot seed, celery, copaiba, cypress, fenugreek, fingerroot, geranium, German chamomile, goldenrod, guava leaf, gurjun balsam, helichrysum, Japanese cedarwood, juniper berry, juniper (Chinese), juniper (Himalayan), juniper (Phoenician), ledum, lemon verbena, lovage, monarda, moringa, nutmeg, ocotea, pennyroyal, peppermint, petitgrain, Roman chamomile, rose, rosemary, schisandra fruit, shell ginger, spearmint, tamala, turmeric, wild chamomile, wintergreen, wormwood, yarrow

**Loneliness, Reduces:** Bergamot, frankincense, Roman chamomile, rose

**Love, Encourages Feelings of:** Juniper, juniper (Himalayan), juniper (Phoenician), lavender, rhododendron, rose, ylang ylang

**Lymph System Supportive:** Angelica, bay laurel, celery, cistus, galbanum, geranium, goldenrod, grapefruit, guaiacwood, hinoki, katrafay, ledum,

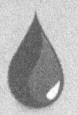 

mastic, Mediterranean mandarin, orange, ravensara, rhododendron, sandalwood, spikenard

**Meditation, Aids**: Agarwood, balsam fir, blue mountain sage, Buddha wood, frankincense, guaiacwood, guggul, muhuhu, myrrh, palo santo, rhododendron, sweet inula, vilayti tulsi, Western red cedar

**Memory\Cognition, Aids\Protects**: Aleppo pine, black cumin, black pepper, calamus, cinnamon, citron, clove, coriander, fenugreek, hairy basil, marjoram, mastic, mugwort, nutmeg, rosemary, rosemary, sage, Siberian fir, Spanish sage, sandalwood, savory (wild), thyme, Turkish pine, turmeric, valerian

**Menopausal Symptoms, Relieves**: Bergamot mint, chaste tree, zdravetz

**Menstrual Pain\PMS\Cramps, Alleviates**: African bluegrass, anise, bergamot mint, betony, blue mountain sage, chaste tree, celery, cinnamon, clary sage, coriander, cypress, damiana, davana, fenugreek, German chamomile, guava leaf, hairy basil, hemp, hops, Indian borage, jasmine absolute, juniper berry, juniper (Chinese), juniper (Himalayan), juniper (Phoenician), lavender, lovage, marjoram, nutmeg, oregano, palo santo, pennyroyal, Peru balsam, pink pepper, Roman chamomile, rose, rosemary, star anise, tarragon, tolu balsam, valerian, verbena, wild chamomile, wild marjoram, wormwood, xanthoxylum

**Menstruation, Balances\Regulates**: Ajowan, angelica, bay (West Indies), cajeput, calendula, caraway, catnip, chaste tree, Chinese cedarwood, cumin, damiana, davana, fennel, feverfew, galangal, galbanum, geranium, guaiacwood, guggul, hyssop, khella, lavandin, lemon basil, lemon catnip, lovage, melissa, mugwort, Oriental arborvitae, rose, Spanish sage, summer savory, tamala, Western red cedar, wild chamomile, wintergreen, wormwood

**Menstruation, Stimulates**: Parsley seed, pennyroyal, savin, thuja, wormseed (American)

**Mental Clarity, Promotes**: Amyris, basil, bergamot mint, calamus, citronella, gingergrass, grindelia, honey myrtle, maritime pine, myrtle, patchouli, peta, rabbitbrush, rhododendron, tsauri grass, turmeric, Virginian cedarwood, white sage, white spruce, zdravetz

**Mentally Refreshing**: Applemint

**Mentally Stimulating**: Anise, basil, big badja gum, blue mallee, eucalyptus dives, garlic, gully gum,

kaffir lime, kumquat, leleshwa, peppermint, rosemary, sage, tarragon, white sage, wild marjoram

**Metabolism, Enhances**: Cardamom, cinnamon, elecampane, fennel, pine

**Mind, Calming to**: Myrrh, palmarosa

**Mindfulness, Increases**: Vilayti tulsi

**Mood Swings, Reduces**: Bergamot, carrot seed, marjoram, ocotea, spruce (black), ylang ylang

**Morale, Enhances**: Cinnamon

**Motion Sickness, Relieves**: Cardamom, chamomile (Roman), citron, coriander, fennel, galangal, ginger, grapefruit, lemon, patchouli, peppermint, spearmint

**Motivation, Encourages**: Agarwood, basil, ginger, Indian borage, manuka, mountain savory, savory (wild)

**Mouth Sores, Reduces\Heals**: Lavender, lemon, tea tree, peppermint

**Mucus, Removes\Expels Excess**: Ajowan, Aleppo pine, amyris, balsam fir, bay laurel, benzoin absolute, big badja gum, blue mallee, blue tansy, cajeput, Chinese cedarwood, Chinese red pine, citron, davana, dill seed, Douglas fir, dwarf pine, elecampane, elemi, Engelmann spruce, eucalyptus dives, fenugreek, ferula, feverfew, fingerroot, Fragonia, garlic, gingergrass, gobre salla, grindelia, gully gum, gurjun balsam, jasmine absolute, kunzea, lemon eucalyptus, lovage, magnolia, manuka, maritime pine, mastic, monarda, mountain savory, niaouli, oakmoss absolute, opoponax, Peru balsam, pine, ponderosa pine, rabbitbrush, red pine, rhododendron, rosalina, sage, saro, savory (wild), shell ginger, Siberian fir, silver fir, summer savory, sweet inula, sweet nancy, sweet wormwood, tagetes, Texas cedarwood, thuja, tolu balsam, tsauri grass, tsuga, Turkish pine, Virginian cedarwood, Western red cedar, white fir, white pine, white sage, white spruce, wild marjoram, wormseed (American), yarrow

**Muscles, Relaxes\Soothes**: African bluegrass, balsam fir, basil, birch, German chamomile, elemi, katrafay, lavender, marjoram, mountain savory, palmarosa, peppermint, sage, saro, tarragon, verbena, white fir, wintergreen, yarrow

**Muscle Tone, Improves**: Cumin, basil, marjoram

**Nails, Strengthens**: Carrot seed, grapefruit, lemon, myrrh, ravensara

**Nausea\Vomiting, Relieves**: Agarwood, ajowan, basil, cassia, davana, feverfew, fingerroot, galangal,

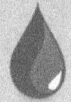

German chamomile, ginger, hemp, ledum, lemon, patchouli, peppermint, petitgrain, white verbena

**Negative Emotions, Past Trauma, Corrects\ Releases\Heals:** Balsam fir, balsam poplar, bergamot, blue spruce, cangerana, copaiba, cumin, elecampane, eucalyptus, Fragonia, frankincense, garlic, helichrysum, kunzea, leleshwa, lemon myrtle, lovage, marjoram, oakmoss absolute, Peru balsam, rose, Southern blue gum, sweet nancy, sweet wormwood, tolu balsam, tsuga

**Nervine (Soothes and\or Supports Nerves):** Aleppo pine, allspice, angelica, basil, bergamot, betony, blue spruce, boldo, calamus, cardamom, catnip, celery, chaste tree, Chinese red pine, cilantro, cistus, citronella, clary sage, cumin, damiana, davana, Douglas fir, eucalyptus, ferula, geranium, German chamomile, guaiacwood, gurjun balsam, hairy basil, helichrysum, hemp, hinoki, holy basil, hops, hyssop, juniper (Chinese), juniper (Himalayan), katrafay, lavender, lemon catnip, lemon tea tree, lemongrass, lovage, maritime pine, marjoram, may chang, melissa, monarda, mugwort, myrtle, patchouli, peppermint, petitgrain, pine, pink pepper, rhododendron, Roman chamomile, rose, rosemary, rue, sage, Southern blue gum, spearmint, spike lavender, spruce (black), tsuga, Turkish pine, turmeric, valerian, vetiver, white verbena, xanthoxylum, ylang ylang, yuzu

**Nightmares, Combats:** Betony, lemon, lemon basil, melissa

**Nutrient Absorption, Improves:** Black pepper, galbanum, tea tree, niaouli

**Oppressive Feelings, Reduces:** Tea tree

**Oral Cleanliness\Health, Promotes:** Black sage, calendula, cumin, elecampane, eucalyptus, frankincense, holy basil, Japanese cedarwood, kaffir lime, mastic, tea tree, peppermint, Peru balsam, rosemary, Siberian fir, Southern blue gum, summer savory, tolu balsam, vilayti tulsi, white verbena

**Overactive Mind, Calms:** Patchouli

**Oversensitivity (Emotional), Reduces:** Roman chamomile

**Overwhelming Feelings, Reduces:** Cardamom, cypress, juniper berry, juniper (Chinese), juniper (Himalayan), juniper (Phoenician), nutmeg

**Panic Attacks, Relieves:** Lavender

**Pancreas Function, Supports:** Canadian fleabane, copaiba, dill seed, juniper berry, juniper (Phoenician), lemon verbena, peppermint, wild chamomile

**Paranoia, Combats:** Parsley seed

**Peaceful Feelings, Fosters:** Chinese cedarwood, cistus, myrrh, spikenard

**Penetration Through Skin (Other Essential Oils or Substances), Enhances:** Balsam fir, camphor, ginger, kanuka, lavender, lemongrass, ylang ylang

**Perfectionism, Reduces:** Cypress, orange

**Perspective, Encourages:** Angelica, catnip, peppermint, petitgrain

**Perspiration (Excess), Reduces:** Citronella, cypress, hyssop, petitgrain, sage, Spanish sage, yarrow

**Perspiration, Promotes:** Bay (West Indies), birch, camphor, juniper (Himalayan), lemon catnip, rosemary, spike lavender

**Pessimism, Removes:** Auracaria, Blue cypress, galangal, orange

**Pituitary, Supports:** Bergamot, chast tree, Siam wood

**Poisoning, Counters:** Rue

**Possessive\Jealous Feelings, Combats:** Ledum, palmarosa

**Prostate Health\Function, Supports:** Mastic

**Purification\Purifies:** Angelica, anise, betony, big badja gum, blue mallee, cumin, Douglas fir, gully gum, hyssop, leleshwa, lemon tea tree, opoponax, pennyroyal, star anise, Western red cedar, white sage

**Radiation Damage, Protects Against:** Cajeput, tea tree, patchouli

**Red Blood Cells, Encourages Production of:** Helichrysum, lemon

**Refreshing:** Eucalyptus, lemon, pine, peppermint, Southern blue gum

**Regenerative\Restorative:** Cedarwood, geranium, grapefruit, lime, neroli, patchouli, Persian lime, rosemary, rosewood, tangerine

**Regret, Combats:** Rue

**Relaxing\Calming:** Agarwood, amyris, angelica, applemint, auracaria, balsam fir, basil, benzoin absolute, bergamot, betony, blue cypress, blue spruce, blue tansy, buchu, Buddha wood, calamus, cangerana, catnip, celery, chaste tree, citronella, davana, dill seed, elemi, Formosan cypress, Fragonia, galbanum, German chamomile, gingergrass, goldenrod, hairy basil, hemp, hinoki, honey myrtle, kanuka, lavandin,

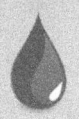

lemon catnip, lemon eucalyptus, lemon myrtle, lemon tea tree, magnolia, manuka, may chang, melissa, monarda, palo santo, pennyroyal, petitgrain, pink pepper, ponderosa pine, Roman chamomile, rosalina, rosewood, rue, savin, spikenard, sweet nancy, sweet wormwood, tagetes, Texas cedarwood, tsauri grass, tsuga, valerian, verbena, Virginian cedarwood, Western red cedar, white spruce, white verbena, wild chamomile, wintergreen

**Reproductive Health, Supports**: Frankincense, leleshwa, mugwort, zdravetz

**Reproductive System (Male), Protects**: Celery, cinnamon

**Respiratory Supportive**: Agarwood, ajowan, Aleppo pine, amyris, anise, applemint, balsam fir, balsam poplar, basil, benzoin absolute, betony, big badja gum, black cumin, black pepper, black sage, blue cypress, blue mallee, blue mountain sage, blue spruce, cajeput, camphor, catnip, celery, Chinese cedarwood, Chinese red pine, cistus, cypress, damiana, davana, dill seed, Douglas fir, dwarf pine, elecampane, Engelmann spruce, eucalyptus, eucalyptus dives, fenugreek, ferula, feverfew, fingerroot, Formosan cypress, Fragonia, frankincense, galangal, garlic, ginger, gingergrass, genipi, gobre salla, grindelia, guaiacwood, gully gum, gurjun balsam, hemp, hinoki, holy basil, honey myrtle, hops, Indian borage, Japanese cedarwood, jasmine absolute, juniper (Chinese), juniper (Himalayan), kaffir lime, kanuka, katrafay, khella, kunzea, lavandin, leleshwa, lemon basil, lemon catnip, lemon eucalyptus, lovage, magnolia, manuka, maritime pine, mastic, may chang, melissa, monarda, moringa, muhuhu, myrtle, niaouli, oakmoss absolute, opoponax, Oriental arborvitae, palo santo, Peru balsam, peta, pine, pink pepper, plai, ponderosa pine, rabbitbrush, ravensara, ravintsara, red pine, rhododendron, rosalina, saro, schisandra fruit, Siberian fir, silver fir, Southern blue gum, star anise, summer savory, sweet inula, sweet nancy, sweet wormwood, tagetes, tolu balsam, tsauri grass, tsuga, Turkish pine, verbena, vilayti tulsi, Western red cedar, white fir, white pine, white sage, white spruce, wild marjoram, wormseed (American), xanthoxylum, ylang ylang

**Restlessness, Reduces**: Kabosu, Mediterranean mandarin

**Revitalizing**: Cilantro, Spanish sage

**Rigidity (Emotional), Combats**: Galbanum

**Security, Promotes Sense of**: Bergamot, cedarwood, cypress, geranium, Indian borage, oregano, Roman chamomile, spruce (black)

**Sedating**: Anise, bay laurel, benzoin absolute, bergamot, bergamot mint, blue tansy, Buddha wood, cedarwood, chaste tree, clary sage, cypress, frankincense, geranium, German chamomile, hairy basil, hinoki, hops, jasmine absolute, juniper berry, juniper (Chinese), juniper (Himalayan), juniper (Phoenician), lavender, lemon, lemongrass, marjoram, myrrh, myrtle, neroli, Oriental arborvitae, sandalwood, Siam wood, spikenard, tagetes, valerian, ylang ylang

**Self-Acceptance, Encourages**: Engelmann spruce

**Self-Confidence, Encourages**: Ajowan, anise, basil, bay laurel, blue cypress, clove, cypress, fennel, Formosan cypress, hemp, tea tree, niaouli, peppermint, ravintsara, rosalina, rosemary, Siam wood, spruce (black), star anise, thyme, vilayti tulsi, wintergreen

**Self-Destructive Behavior, Reduces**: Myrtle

**Self-Esteem\Self-Love, Encourages**: Fragonia, parsley seed, red pine, rosalina, ylang ylang

**Shame, Lessens**: Cardamom

**Shock, Relieves**: Calaway, cistus, galbanum, lavandin, lavender, tea tree, neroli, spike lavender, summer savory

**Sinusitis, Relieves**: Big badja gum, blue mallee, eucalyptus dives, gully gum, hinoki, ravintsara, sweet inula

**Skin, Brightens**: Cajeput, white verbena

**Skin, Encourages Pigment Production**: Black pepper

**Skin, Heals/Regenerates**: Cape chamomile, cistus, guggul, lavender, myrrh, rose

**Skin, Improves Luster**: Basil, lemon

**Skin, Nourishes**: Auracaria, balsam poplar, blue tansy, carrot seed, Formosan cypress, gingergrass, guggul, jasmine absolute, lemon, lemon verbena, may chang, moringa, patchouli, Peru balsam, rose, sandalwood, tsauri grass, turmeric, Western red cedar, wild chamomile, yarrow

**Skin, Protects from UV Damage**: Black pepper, calendula, patchouli, tolu balsam

**Skin, Relieves Itching\Irritation\Rashes**: Applemint, auracaria, blue cypress, calendula, caraway, cilantro, fenugreek, kanuka, oakmoss absolute, peppermint, white sage, zdravetz

**Skin, Softens\Moisturizes**: Amyris, blue mountain sage, galbanum, guaiacwood, helichrysum, kanuka,

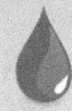

katrafay, moringa, Oriental arborvitae, palmarosa, patchouli, rose, sandalwood, yarrow

**Skin Conditions, Helps Relieve Chronic:** African bluegrass, Aleppo pine, amyris, applemint, auracaria, balsam poplar, black cumin, black sage, blue mountain sage, calendula, cangerana, Cape chamomile, Chinese cedarwood, cistus, elemi, Engelmann spruce, feverfew, galangal, garlic, Ghandi root, gingergrass, grindelia, guaiacwood, guggul, gurjun balsam, hairy basil, helichrysum, hemp, hops, Japanese cedarwood, juniper berry, juniper (Phoenician), khella, kumquat, kunzea, ledum, leleshwa, lovage, magnolia, manuka, may chang, melissa, mugwort, monarda, moringa, muhuhu, myrrh, Oriental arborvitae, patchouli, peta, pine, ponderosa pine, rabbitbrush, ravintsara, Roman chamomile, rosalina, rosemary, sandalwood, Siam wood, Spanish sage, spike lavender, sweet inula, sweet nancy, sweet wormwood, tagetes, Texas cedarwood, tsauri grass, Turkish pine, valerian, Virginian cedarwood, white verbena, wild chamomile, zdravetz

**Skin (Oily), Reduces:** Citronella, cypress, ylang ylang

**Skin Tone, Evens:** Bergamot, Mediterranean mandarin, patchouli

**Sleep, Encourages Restful:** Ajowan, amyris, angelica, anise, auracaria, benzoin absolute, bergamot, black sage, calamus, Cape chamomile, catnip, cedarwood, Chinese cedarwood, clary sage, celery, fingerroot, fragonia, Ghandi root, guava leaf, hairy basil, hemp, holy basil, hops, Indian borage, jasmine absolute, kabosu, lavender, leleshwa, lemon, lemon catnip, lemon myrtle, lemon tea tree, lime, magnolia, marjoram, may chang, Mediterranean mandarin, melissa, monarda, moringa, myrtle, neroli, orange (bitter), Persian lime, petitgrain, rhododendron, rosalina, rose, rue, star anise, tangerine, Texas cedarwood, valerian, vetiver, Virginian cedarwood, white verbena, wild chamomile, wormwood, xanthoxylum, yarrow, zdravetz

**Smoking Cessation, Addictions:** Black pepper, ledum

**Sore Throat, Relieves:** Bergamot, big badja gum, blue mountain sage, Chinese red pine, cinnamon, gingergrass, gully gum, hyssop, Indian borage, lemon myrtle, lovage, mountain savory, orange (bitter), opoponax, red pine, savory (wild), summer savory, tsauri grass, verbena, white sage, xanthoxylum

**Spleen Function, Supports:** Helichrysum

**Sprains\Strains, Relieves:** African bluegrass, arnica, balsam poplar, buchu, kunzea, lemongrass, pink pepper, plai, tamala, tolu balsam, wild chamomile, wild marjoram, wintergreen

**Stability\Balance, Encourages Feelings of:** Ginger, silver fir, turmeric, silver fir, white fir

**Stimulating:** Ajowan, Aleppo pine, angelica, bay (West Indies), birch, boldo, cajeput, camphor, cardamom, carrot seed, cassia, cilantro, clove, copaiba, coriander, elemi, eucalyptus, ginger, grapefruit, helichrysum, hyssop, lavender, mugwort, niaouli, nutmeg, ocotea, orange, orange (bitter), patchouli, peppermint, pine, ravensara, rosewood, Siam wood, silver fir, Southern blue gum, spearmint, spike lavender, tangerine, tansy, thyme, Turkish pine, white fir, wintergreen

**Stomachache\Stomach Upset, Relieves:** Ajowan, allspice, bergamot mint, Cape chamomile, ferula, galangal, guaiacwood, gurjun balsam, hairy basil, lovage, moringa, pennyroyal, plai, rabbitbrush, valerian, xanthoxylum

**Stomach Acid, Stimulates Production:** Black pepper

**Stomach/Intestines, Protects/Supports Function:** Black sage, caraway, celery, copaiba, fenugreek, katrafay, moringa, orange (bitter), Japanese cedarwood, juniper (Himalayan), juniper (Phoenician), Siam wood

**Stress Management:** African bluegrass, agarwood, Aleppo pine, amyris, angelica, applemint, balsam poplar, basil, benzoin absolute, bergamot mint, betony, blue mountain sage, black sage, blue tansy, calendula, Canadian fleabane, cangerana, Cape chamomile, caraway, cardamom, catnip, cedarwood, Chinese cedarwood, Chinese red pine, cilantro, citron, clary sage, clove, copaiba, davana, dill seed, Douglas fir, dwarf pine, elemi, Engelmann spruce, fenugreek, ferula, feverfew, fingerroot, Formosan cypress, frankincense, German chamomile, Ghandi root, gobre salla, grapefruit, guaiacwood, guava leaf, guggul, gurjun balsam, hairy basil, helichrysum, hemp, hinoki, holy basil, honey myrtle, hops, hyssop, Japanese cedarwood, jasmine absolute, juniper (Chinese), kabosu, kaffir lime, kanuka, khella, kunzea, lavandin, lavender, lemon, lemon verbena, lemon catnip, lemon tea tree, lemongrass, lime, magnolia, manuka, maritime pine, marjoram, mastic, may chang, mugwort, muhuhu, neroli, nutmeg, orange, opoponax, Oriental arborvitae, palmarosa, palo santo, patchouli, Persian lime, Peru balsam, peta, pine, ponderosa pine, rabbitbrush, ravensara, ravintsara,

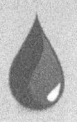 

red pine, rhododendron, Roman chamomile, rosalina, rose, rosemary, rosewood, rue, sandalwood, schisandra fruit, shell ginger, Siberian fir, Spanish sage, spearmint, spike lavender, spikenard, spruce (black), summer savory, sweet nancy, sweet wormwood, tamala, tangerine, tansy, tarragon, Texas cedarwood, thuja, tolu balsam, Turkish pine, turmeric, valerian, verbena, vetiver, Virginian cedarwood, Western red cedar, white pine, white sage, white spruce, white verbena, wild chamomile, wormwood, xanthoxylum, yarrow, ylang ylang, yuzu, zdravetz

**Sweating, Promotes\Encourages:** *See Perspiration, Encourages*

**Sweating, Decreases:** *See Perspiration, Decreases*

**Sweating, Relieves Excess:** Citronella, may chang, petitgrain, sage, Spanish sage

**Tantrums, Calms:** German chamomile, Roman chamomile

**Tendonitis, Relieves:** Balsam fir, balsam poplar, lemongrass, wintergreen

**Thinking (Obsessive), Reduces:** Marjoram

**Thyroid Function, Supports:** Balsam fir, chaste tree, ledum, lemon verbena, myrtle, spruce (black)

**Tissue, Supports Regeneration:** Blue tansy, cistus, lavender

**Toothache, Tooth Pain, Relieves:** Allspice, bay (West Indies), clove, pink pepper, tsauri grass, xanthoxylum

**Traumatic Events, Helps Manage Better:** Cistus, cypress

**Transitions Difficult (Emotionally), Aids:** Cypress, lemongrass, palmarosa, tamala

**Uplifting:** Balsam fir, bergamot, cinnamon, Canadian fleabane, catnip, celery, cumin, Engelmann spruce, fingerroot, Formosan cypress, kanuka, lemon, lemon catnip, lemon eucalyptus, lemon myrtle, lime, may chang, melissa, niaouli, orange, palmarosa, Persian lime, petitgrain, tamala, tarragon, tsuga, vilayti tulsi, white spruce, yuzu

**Urinary Tract Health, Supports or Cleanses:** Agarwood, ajowan, allspice, buchu, dill seed, dwarf pine, goldenrod, juniper berry, juniper (Phoenician), leleshwa, maritime pine, mastic, myrtle, parsley seed

**Uric Acid, Clears Body of:** Celery, juniper berry, juniper (Phoenician), peppermint, pine

**Uterus Function, Supports:** Parsley seed

**Vaginal Health, Supports:** Amyris, applemint

**Varicose Veins, Reduces\Relieves:** Grapefruit, mastic, yarrow

**Vasodilator:** Arnica, Canadian fleabane, davana, goldenrod, kunzea, lemon catnip, marjoram

**Vertigo, Relieves:** Frankincense, ginger, lavender, melissa, valerian, ylang ylang

**Warming:** Balsam fir, basil, bay laurel, cajeput, cardamom, coriander, cypress, marjoram, melissa, mugwort, oregano, spruce (black), turmeric, wintergreen

**Warts, Removes:** Cinnamon, clove, frankincense, garlic, kanuka, tea tree, oregano, pink pepper, rosalina, rue, savin, thuja, Western red cedar

**Weight Management:** Black cumin, black pepper, catnip, coriander, garlic, grapefruit, guggul, hairy basil, ledum, lemon, lemon catnip, kumquat, lemon tea tree, lime, orange (bitter), Persian lime, turmeric, valerian, white verbena

**Well-being (General Feeling), Encourages:** Bergamot, oregano

**Worrisome\Negative Thoughts, Combats:** Arnica, Chinese cedarwood, juniper berry, juniper (Chinese), juniper (Himalayan), juniper (Phoenician), nutmeg, Roman chamomile, tagetes, thuja, white sage

**Wound Healing:** Aleppo pine, amyris, auracaria, bergamot, blue cypress, balsam poplar, benzoin absolute, bergamot mint, betony, big badja gum, black cumin, black sage, blue mallee, blue mountain sage, blue tansy, cajeput, calendula, cangerana, Cape chamomile, Chinese cedarwood, cistus, clary sage, copaiba, davana, dill seed, Douglas fir, dwarf pine, elecampane, elemi, eucalyptus, Formosan cypress, frankincense, galbanum, garlic, genipi, geranium, German chamomile, goldenrod, guaiacwood, guggul, gully gum, gurjun balsam, helichrysum, hyssop, Indian borage, jasmine absolute, kanuka, kunzea, lavandin, lemon eucalyptus, lemon tea tree, marjoram, mastic, monarda, moringa, myrrh, niaouli, oakmoss absolute, opoponax, palmarosa, parsley seed, patchouli, peta, pink pepper, ponderosa pine, rabbitbrush, ravensara, Roman chamomile, rosemary, rosewood, sage, savin, Southern blue gum, Spanish sage, spike lavender, spikenard, sweet inula, sweet nancy, sweet wormwood, tagetes, thyme, tolu balsam, verbena, vetiver, wormseed (American), yarrow, ylang ylang, zdravetz

**Wrinkles, Reduces Appearance of:** *See Blemishes, Scars, Wrinkles, Acne—Reduces Appearance of*

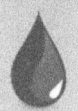

# APPENDIX D:
## USAGE QUICK REFERENCE GUIDE

| ESSENTIAL OIL | Oral Administration | Children | Pregnancy & Lactation | Drug Interaction | Health Contraindication | Photosensitizing | Epilepsy, Convulsions | Compromised Liver or Kidneys |
|---|---|---|---|---|---|---|---|---|
| AFRICAN BLUEGRASS CT ARTEMISIA KETONE | ● | ● | ● | ● | ● | ● | ● | ● |
| AFRICAN BLUEGRASS CT LINALOOL | ● | ● | ● | ● | ● | ● | ● | ● |
| AFRICAN BLUEGRASS CT MYRCENE | ● | ● | ● | ● | ● | ● | ● | ● |
| AGARWOOD | ● | ● | ● | ● | ● | ● | ● | ● |
| AJOWAN | ▪ | ● | ● | ● | ▪ | ● | ● | ● |
| ALEPPO PINE | ● | ● | ● | ▪ | ● | ● | ● | ● |
| ALLSPICE CT EUGENOL | ● | ● | ● | ● | ▪ | ● | ● | ● |
| ALLSPICE CT METHYL EUGENOL | ▲ | ▲ | ▪ | ▪ | ▪ | ● | ● | ● |
| AMYRIS | ● | ● | ● | ● | ● | ▪ | ● | ● |
| ANGELICA ROOT | ● | ● | ● | ● | ● | ▪ | ● | ● |
| ANISE | ● | ▪ | ▲ | ▪ | ● | ● | ● | ● |
| APPLEMINT | ● | ● | ● | ● | ● | ● | ● | ● |
| APPLEMINT CT CARVONE | ● | ● | ● | ● | ● | ● | ● | ● |
| APPLEMINT CT MENTHOL | ● | ▲ | ● | ▪ | ▪ | ● | ● | ● |
| APPLEMINT CTs WITH PULEGONE | ▲ | ▲ | ▲ | ▲ | ▲ | ● | ▲ | ▲ |
| ARNICA (FLOWERS) | ● | ● | ● | ● | ● | ● | ● | ● |
| AURACARIA | ● | ● | ▪ | ▪ | ● | ● | ● | ● |
| BALSAM FIR | ● | ● | ● | ▪ | ● | ● | ● | ● |
| BALSAM POPLAR | ● | ● | ● | ▪ | ● | ● | ● | ● |
| BASIL (SWEET) CT LINALOOL | ● | ● | ● | ▪ | ▪ | ● | ● | ● |
| BASIL CT METHYL CHAVICOL/METHYLEUGENOL | ▲ | ▲ | ▲ | ▪ | ▪ | ● | ● | ● |
| BAY (WEST INDIES) | ● | ● | ▪ | ▪ | ▪ | ● | ● | ● |
| BAY LAUREL | ▲ | ▲ | ▲ | ▪ | ▪ | ● | ● | ● |
| BAY LAUREL ABSOLUTE | ▲ | ▲ | ▲ | ● | ● | ▪ | ● | ● |
| BENZOIN ABSOLUTE | ▲ | ● | ● | ▪ | ● | ▪ | ● | ● |
| BERGAMOT | ● | ● | ● | ▪ | ● | ▪ | ● | ● |
| BERGAMOT MINT | ● | ● | ● | ● | ● | ● | ● | ● |
| BETONY (ALL OTHER CTs) | ● | ● | ● | ● | ● | ● | ● | ● |
| BETONY CT ALPHA-ZINGIBERENE | ● | ● | ● | ● | ● | ● | ● | ● |
| BETONY CT BETA-PHELLANDRENE | ● | ● | ● | ▪ | ● | ● | ● | ● |
| BETONY CT BICYCLOGERMACRENE | ▲ | ▪ | ▲ | ▲ | ▲ | ● | ▲ | ▲ |
| BIG BADJA GUM | ▪ | ▲ | ● | ▪ | ▲ | ● | ▲ | ● |
| BIRCH | ▪ | ▲ | ▲ | ▲ | ▲ | ● | ▲ | ● |
| BITTER ORANGE | ● | ● | ● | ● | ● | ▪ | ● | ● |
| BLACK CUMIN SEED CT PARA-CYMENE | ▪ | ● | ▪ | ▪ | ▪ | ● | ● | ● |
| BLACK CUMIN SEED CT THYMOQUINONE | ● | ● | ▪ | ▪ | ▪ | ● | ● | ● |
| BLACK CUMIN SEED CT TRANS-ANETHOLE | ● | ▪ | ▪ | ▪ | ▪ | ● | ● | ● |
| BLACK PEPPER CT BETA-CARYOPHYLLENE | ● | ● | ● | ● | ● | ● | ● | ● |
| BLACK PEPPER CT BETA-PINENE | ● | ● | ▪ | ▪ | ● | ● | ● | ● |
| BLACK PEPPER CT EUGENOL | ● | ● | ● | ▪ | ▲ | ● | ▲ | ● |
| BLACK SAGE | ● | ● | ● | ▪ | ● | ● | ● | ● |

*Please review the individual essential oil monographs for more detail.*

● Recommended, no known risk warranted        ▪ Caution warranted        ▲ Avoid or great caution

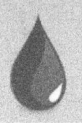

| ESSENTIAL OIL | Oral Administration | Children | Pregnancy & Lactation | Drug Interaction | Health Contraindication | Photosensitizing | Epilepsy, Convulsions | Compromised Liver or Kidneys |
|---|---|---|---|---|---|---|---|---|
| BLUE CYPRESS (LEAVES) | ● | ● | ● | ● | ● | ● | ● | ● |
| BLUE CYPRESS (WOOD) | ● | ● | ▲ | ▲ | ▲ | ● | ● | ● |
| BLUE MALLEE | ■ | ▲ | ● | ● | ▲ | ● | ▲ | ● |
| BLUE MOUNTAIN SAGE CT ALPHA-BISABOLOL | ● | ● | ● | ■ | ● | ● | ● | ● |
| BLUE MOUNTAIN SAGE CT (E)-NEROLIDOL | ● | ● | ● | ■ | ● | ● | ● | ● |
| BLUE MOUNTAIN SAGE (ALL OTHER CTS) | ● | ● | ● | ● | ● | ● | ● | ● |
| BLUE SPRUCE | ■ | ■ | ● | ● | ▲ | ● | ▲ | ● |
| BLUE TANSY CT CHAMZULENE | ● | ● | ● | ■ | ● | ● | ▲ | ● |
| BLUE TANSY CT SABINENE | ● | ● | ● | ● | ▲ | ● | ▲ | ● |
| BOLDO | ▲ | ▲ | ▲ | ▲ | ▲ | ● | ▲ | ▲ |
| BUCHU | ▲ | ▲ | ▲ | ▲ | ▲ | ● | ▲ | ▲ |
| BUDDHA WOOD | ● | ● | ● | ● | ● | ● | ● | ● |
| CALAMUS CT ALPHA- OR BETA-ASARONE | ▲ | ▲ | ▲ | ■ | ▲ | ● | ● | ▲ |
| CALAMUS CT ACORENONE | ▲ | ▲ | ▲ | ■ | ▲ | ● | ● | ▲ |
| CALAMUS CT (E)-METHYLISOEUGENOL | ● | ● | ● | ● | ● | ● | ● | ● |
| CALAMUS CT SHYOBUNONES | ● | ● | ● | ● | ● | ● | ● | ● |
| CALENDULA | ● | ● | ● | ● | ● | ● | ● | ● |
| CAPE CHAMOMILE | ● | ● | ● | ● | ● | ● | ● | ● |
| CAJEPUT | ■ | ▲ | ● | ■ | ▲ | ● | ▲ | ● |
| CAMPHOR | ■ | ▲ | ■ | ▲ | ▲ | ● | ▲ | ▲ |
| CANADIAN FLEABANE | ● | ● | ● | ● | ● | ● | ● | ● |
| CANGERANA | ● | ● | ● | ● | ● | ● | ● | ● |
| CARAWAY | ● | ● | ● | ● | ● | ● | ● | ● |
| CARDAMOM | ■ | ▲ | ● | ■ | ▲ | ● | ▲ | ● |
| CARROT SEED | ● | ● | ▲ | ● | ● | ● | ● | ● |
| CASSIA BARK | ● | ● | ▲ | ■ | ■ | ● | ● | ● |
| CASSIA LEAVES | ● | ● | ▲ | ■ | ■ | ● | ● | ● |
| CATNIP | ● | ● | ● | ■ | ● | ● | ● | ● |
| CEDARWOOD | ● | ● | ● | ● | ● | ● | ● | ● |
| CELERY | ● | ● | ● | ● | ● | ■ | ● | ● |
| CHASTE TREE | ● | ● | ▲ | ■ | ▲ | ● | ▲ | ● |
| CHINESE CEDARWOOD | ● | ● | ● | ■ | ● | ● | ● | ● |
| CHINESE RED PINE | ● | ● | ● | ■ | ● | ● | ● | ● |
| CILANTRO | ● | ● | ● | ● | ● | ● | ● | ● |
| CINNAMON BARK | ● | ● | ▲ | ■ | ■ | ● | ● | ● |
| CINNAMON LEAVES | ● | ● | ▲ | ■ | ■ | ● | ● | ● |
| CISTUS | ● | ● | ● | ● | ● | ● | ● | ● |
| CITRON (INCLUDES FINGERED CITRON) | ● | ● | ● | ■ | ● | ■ | ● | ● |
| CITRONELLA | ● | ● | ■ | ■ | ● | ● | ● | ● |
| CLARY SAGE | ● | ● | ▲ | ● | ● | ● | ● | ● |
| CLOVE BUD | ● | ● | ● | ■ | ■ | ● | ● | ● |
| COPAIBA BALSAM | ● | ● | ● | ● | ● | ● | ● | ● |
| COPAIBA (LEAVES) | ● | ● | ● | ● | ● | ● | ● | ● |
| CORIANDER SEED | ● | ● | ● | ■ | ● | ● | ● | ● |
| CUMIN | ● | ● | ● | ■ | ● | ■ | ● | ● |

*Please review the individual essential oil monographs for more detail.*

● Recommended, no known risk warranted    ■ Caution warranted    ▲ Avoid or great caution

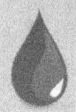

| ESSENTIAL OIL | Oral Administration | Children | Pregnancy & Lactation | Drug Interaction | Health Contraindication | Photosensitizing | Epilepsy, Convulsions | Compromised Liver or Kidneys |
|---|---|---|---|---|---|---|---|---|
| CYPRESS | ● | ● | ● | ▪ | ▪ | ● | ● | ● |
| DAMIANA CT 1,8-CINEOLE | ● | ● | ● | ▪ | ▲ | ● | ● | ● |
| DAMIANA CT CARYOPHYLLENE OXIDE | ● | ● | ● | ● | ● | ● | ● | ● |
| DAMIANA CT DELTA-CADINENE | ● | ● | ● | ● | ● | ● | ● | ● |
| DAVANA | ● | ● | ● | ● | ● | ● | ● | ● |
| DILL (AERIAL PARTS) CT CARVONE | ▲ | ▲ | ▲ | ▪ | ▲ | ● | ● | ▲ |
| DILL SEED | ● | ● | ● | ● | ● | ● | ● | ● |
| DOUGLAS FIR | ● | ● | ● | ● | ● | ● | ● | ● |
| DWARF PINE | ● | ● | ● | ● | ● | ● | ● | ● |
| ELECAMPANE | ● | ▲ | ● | ● | ● | ● | ● | ● |
| ELEMI | ● | ● | ● | ▪ | ● | ● | ● | ● |
| ENGELMANN SPRUCE | ● | ● | ● | ● | ▲ | ● | ● | ▲ |
| EUCALYPTUS | ▪ | ▲ | ● | ▪ | ▲ | ● | ▲ | ● |
| EUCALYPTUS DIVES | ● | ● | ● | ▪ | ● | ● | ● | ● |
| FENNEL (SWEET) CT METHYL CHAVICOL | ▪ | ▪ | ▲ | ▪ | ▲ | ▪ | ▲ | ● |
| FENNEL (SWEET) CT TRANS-ANETHOLE | ● | ▪ | ▲ | ▪ | ▲ | ▪ | ▲ | ● |
| FENUGREEK | ● | ● | ● | ▪ | ▲ | ● | ● | ● |
| FEVERFEW | ▪ | ▲ | ▪ | ● | ▲ | ● | ▲ | ▲ |
| FERULA | ● | ● | ● | ● | ● | ● | ● | ● |
| FINGERROOT CT 1,8-CINEOLE | ● | ● | ● | ▪ | ▲ | ● | ▲ | ▲ |
| FINGERROOT CT CAMPHOR | ▪ | ▪ | ▪ | ▪ | ▲ | ● | ▲ | ▲ |
| FINGERROOT CT (E)-BETA-OCIMENE | ▪ | ▪ | ▪ | ▪ | ▲ | ● | ▲ | ▲ |
| FINGERROOT CT GAMMA-TERPINENE | ● | ● | ● | ▪ | ▲ | ● | ▲ | ▲ |
| FINGERROOT CT NEROL | ▪ | ▪ | ▪ | ● | ▲ | ● | ▲ | ▲ |
| FORMOSAN CYPRESS (TWIG) | ● | ● | ▲ | ● | ● | ● | ● | ● |
| FORMOSAN CYPRESS (WOOD) CT ALPHA-EUDESMOL | ● | ● | ● | ● | ● | ● | ● | ● |
| FORMOSAN CYPRESS (WOOD) CT GERMACRENE D | ● | ● | ● | ● | ● | ● | ● | ● |
| FORMOSAN CYPRESS (WOOD) CT MYRTENOL | ● | ● | ● | ▪ | ● | ● | ● | ● |
| FRAGONIA CT ALPHA-PINENE | ● | ● | ● | ● | ● | ● | ● | ● |
| FRAGONIA CT BALANCED | ● | ● | ● | ▪ | ▲ | ● | ▲ | ● |
| FRANKINCENSE | ● | ● | ● | ▪ | ● | ● | ● | ● |
| GALANGAL CT 1,8-CINEOLE (GREATER/LESSER) | ▪ | ▲ | ● | ▪ | ▲ | ● | ▲ | ● |
| GALANGAL CT PIPERITENONE OXIDE (GREATER) | ● | ● | ● | ● | ● | ● | ● | ● |
| GALANGAL (FALSE) | ● | ● | ● | ▪ | ● | ● | ● | ● |
| GALBANUM | ● | ● | ● | ● | ● | ● | ● | ● |
| GARLIC CT SULFIDES | ● | ● | ▪ | ▪ | ▪ | ▪ | ● | ● |
| GARLIC CT VINYLDITHIINS | ● | ● | ▪ | ▪ | ● | ▪ | ● | ● |
| GENIPI | ▲ | ▲ | ▲ | ▲ | ▲ | ● | ▲ | ▲ |
| GERANIUM | ● | ● | ● | ● | ● | ● | ● | ● |
| GERMAN CHAMOMILE | ● | ● | ● | ▪ | ● | ● | ● | ● |
| GHANDI ROOT | ● | ● | ● | ● | ● | ● | ● | ● |
| GINGER | ● | ● | ● | ▪ | ● | ▪ | ● | ● |
| GOBRE SALLA | ● | ● | ● | ▪ | ● | ● | ● | ● |
| GOLDENROD | ● | ● | ● | ● | ● | ● | ● | ● |
| GRAPEFRUIT | ● | ● | ● | ▪ | ● | ● | ▪ | ● |

*Please review the individual essential oil monographs for more detail.*

● Recommended, no known risk warranted    ▪ Caution warranted    ▲ Avoid or great caution

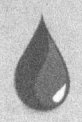

| ESSENTIAL OIL | Oral Administration | Children | Pregnancy & Lactation | Drug Interaction | Health Contraindication | Photosensitizing | Epilepsy, Convulsions | Compromised Liver or Kidneys |
|---|---|---|---|---|---|---|---|---|
| GRINDELIA | • | • | • | • | • | • | • | • |
| GUAIACWOOD | • | • | • | • | • | • | • | • |
| GUAVA LEAF ALL OTHER CTs | • | • | • | • | • | • | • | • |
| GUAVA LEAF CT 1,8-CINEOLE | • | • | • | ◦ | ▲ | • | ▲ | • |
| GUAVA LEAF CT ALPHA-PINENE | • | • | • | ◦ | ▲ | • | ▲ | • |
| GUAVA LEAF CT (E)-NEROLIDOL | • | • | • | ◦ | • | • | • | • |
| GUGGUL | • | • | • | • | • | • | • | • |
| GULLY GUM | ◦ | ▲ | • | ◦ | ▲ | • | ▲ | • |
| GURJUN BALSAM | • | • | • | • | • | • | • | • |
| HAIRY BASIL CT 1,8-CINEOLE | ◦ | ▲ | ▲ | ◦ | ▲ | • | ▲ | • |
| HAIRY BASIL CT 1,8-CINEOLE\LINALOOL | ◦ | ▲ | ▲ | ◦ | ▲ | • | ▲ | • |
| HAIRY BASIL CT CAMPHOR | ◦ | ◦ | ◦ | • | ▲ | • | ▲ | ▲ |
| HAIRY BASIL CT CITRAL | • | ◦ | • | ◦ | • | • | • | • |
| HAIRY BASIL CT (E)-METHYL CINNAMATE | • | • | • | ◦ | ◦ | ◦ | • | • |
| HAIRY BASIL CT EUGENOL | ▲ | ◦ | ▲ | ◦ | ◦ | • | • | • |
| HAIRY BASIL (INFLORESCENCES) CT LINALOOL | • | • | • | • | • | • | • | • |
| HAIRY BASIL (LEAVES) CT LINALOOL | • | • | ▲ | ◦ | • | • | • | • |
| HAIRY BASIL (VAR. PILOSUM) CT LINALOOL | • | • | • | • | • | • | • | • |
| HAIRY BASIL CT METHYL CHAVICOL | ▲ | ◦ | ▲ | ◦ | ◦ | • | • | • |
| HAIRY BASIL CT TERPINEN-4-OL | ▲ | ◦ | ▲ | ◦ | • | • | • | • |
| HAIRY BASIL CT THYMOL | ◦ | • | • | ◦ | ◦ | • | • | • |
| HAIRY BASIL CT TRANS-CARYOPHYLLENE | ▲ | ▲ | ▲ | ◦ | • | • | • | • |
| HELICHRYSUM (ITALICUM) | • | • | • | • | • | • | • | • |
| HELICHRYSUM (SPLENDIDUM) CT SPATHULENOL | • | • | • | • | • | • | • | • |
| HEMP | • | • | • | ◦ | ◦ | • | • | • |
| HINOKI | • | • | • | ◦ | • | • | • | • |
| HOLY BASIL CT BETA-BISABOLENE | ▲ | ▲ | ▲ | ◦ | • | • | • | • |
| HOLY BASIL CT EUGENOL | • | • | ◦ | ◦ | • | • | • | • |
| HOLY BASIL CT METHYL EUGENOL | ▲ | ◦ | ▲ | ◦ | ▲ | • | ▲ | • |
| HOLY BASIL CT METHYL CHAVICOL | ▲ | ▲ | ▲ | ◦ | • | • | • | • |
| HONEY MYRTLE | • | • | ◦ | ◦ | • | • | • | • |
| HOPS | • | • | • | • | • | • | • | • |
| HYSSOP CT ALPHA-PINENE | • | • | • | • | • | • | • | • |
| HYSSOP CT LINALOOL | • | • | • | • | • | • | • | • |
| HYSSOP CT MYRTENYL ACETATE | • | • | • | • | ◦ | • | • | • |
| HYSSOP CT PINOCAMPHONE & ALL OTHERS | ▲ | ▲ | ▲ | ◦ | ▲ | • | ▲ | • |
| INDIAN BORAGE CT BETA-CARYOPHYLLENE | • | • | • | • | • | • | • | • |
| INDIAN BORAGE CT CARVACROL | ◦ | ◦ | ▲ | ◦ | ◦ | • | ▲ | • |
| INDIAN BORAGE CT DELTA-CADINENE | • | • | • | • | • | • | • | • |
| INDIAN BORAGE CT THYMOL | ◦ | • | ▲ | ◦ | ◦ | • | • | • |
| JAPANESE CEDARWOOD | ◦ | ▲ | ◦ | • | ▲ | • | ▲ | ▲ |
| JAPANESE CEDARWOOD (BARK) | • | • | • | ◦ | • | • | • | • |
| JASMINE ABSOLUTE | ▲ | ◦ | • | • | ◦ | • | • | • |

*Please review the individual essential oil monographs for more detail.*

• Recommended, no known risk warranted    ◦ Caution warranted    ▲ Avoid or great caution

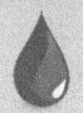

| ESSENTIAL OIL | Oral Administration | Children | Pregnancy & Lactation | Drug Interaction | Health Contraindication | Photosensitizing | Epilepsy, Convulsions | Compromised Liver or Kidneys |
|---|---|---|---|---|---|---|---|---|
| JUNIPER BERRY | ● | ● | ● | ▪ | ● | ● | ● | ● |
| JUNIPER LEAVES (NEEDLES) | ● | ● | ● | ▪ | ● | ● | ● | ● |
| JUNIPER (CHINESE) LEAVES | ▲ | ▲ | ▲ | ● | ▲ | ● | ▲ | ▲ |
| JUNIPER (HIMALAYAN) BERRIES | ● | ● | ● | ▪ | ● | ● | ● | ● |
| JUNIPER (HIMALAYAN) LEAVES | ● | ● | ● | ▪ | ● | ● | ● | ● |
| JUNIPER (PHOENICIAN) BERRIES OR LEAVES | ● | ● | ● | ● | ▲ | ● | ▲ | ● |
| JUNIPER (UTAH) | ▲ | ▲ | ▲ | ● | ▲ | ● | ▲ | ● |
| KABOSU | ● | ● | ● | ● | ● | ▪ | ● | ● |
| KAFFIR LIME (PEEL) DISTILLED | ● | ● | ● | ● | ● | ▪ | ● | ● |
| KAFFIR LIME PETITGRAIN | ● | ● | ● | ● | ● | ▪ | ● | ● |
| KANUKA | ● | ● | ▪ | ● | ● | ● | ● | ● |
| KATRAFAY | ● | ● | ● | ● | ● | ● | ● | ● |
| KHELLA | ● | ● | ● | ● | ● | ▪ | ● | ● |
| KUMQUAT (LEAVES) | ● | ● | ● | ● | ● | ▪ | ● | ● |
| KUMQUAT (PEEL) | ● | ● | ● | ● | ● | ▪ | ● | ● |
| KUMQUAT (LEAVES) *C. JAPONICA* CT LINALOOL | ▲ | ▲ | ▲ | ▪ | ▲ | ▪ | ● | ▲ |
| KUNZEA | ● | ● | ▪ | ● | ● | ● | ● | ● |
| LAVANDIN | ● | ● | ● | ▪ | ▲ | ● | ▲ | ● |
| LAVENDER | ● | ● | ● | ▪ | ● | ● | ● | ● |
| LEDUM (*LEDUM PALUSTRE*) | ▲ | ▲ | ▲ | ● | ● | ● | ● | ● |
| LEDUM (*RHODODENDRON GROENLANDICUM*) | ● | ● | ● | ● | ● | ● | ● | ● |
| LELESHWA | ● | ● | ● | ● | ● | ● | ● | ● |
| LEMON (COLD-PRESSED/EXPRESSED) | ● | ● | ● | ● | ● | ▪ | ● | ● |
| LEMON (DISTILLED) | ● | ● | ● | ● | ● | ● | ● | ● |
| LEMON BASIL | ● | ● | ▪ | ▪ | ● | ● | ● | ● |
| LEMON CATNIP CT BETA-CITRONELLOL | ● | ● | ▪ | ▪ | ● | ● | ● | ● |
| LEMON CATNIP CT GERANIOL/NEROL | ● | ● | ▪ | ● | ● | ● | ● | ● |
| LEMON EUCALYPTUS | ● | ● | ● | ● | ● | ● | ● | ● |
| LEMON MYRTLE CT CITRAL | ● | ● | ▪ | ● | ● | ● | ● | ● |
| LEMON MYRTLE CT CITRONELLAL | ● | ● | ● | ▪ | ● | ● | ● | ● |
| LEMON TEA TREE CT CITRAL | ● | ● | ▪ | ▪ | ● | ● | ● | ● |
| LEMON VERBENA | ● | ● | ▪ | ▪ | ● | ● | ● | ● |
| LEMONGRASS | ● | ● | ▪ | ▪ | ● | ● | ● | ● |
| LIME (COLD-PRESSED/EXPRESSED) | ● | ● | ● | ● | ● | ▪ | ● | ● |
| LIME (DISTILLED) | ● | ● | ● | ▪ | ● | ● | ● | ● |
| LOVAGE | ● | ● | ▲ | ▪ | ● | ● | ● | ● |
| LOVAGE (ROOT) | ▲ | ● | ▲ | ▪ | ▲ | ● | ▲ | ● |
| MAGNOLIA (FLOWERS OR LEAVES) | ● | ● | ● | ▪ | ● | ● | ● | ● |
| MANUKA CT LEPTOSPERMONE | ● | ● | ▪ | ● | ● | ● | ● | ● |
| MANUKA CT SELINENE/BETA-ELEMENE | ● | ● | ▪ | ● | ● | ● | ● | ● |
| MARITIME PINE | ● | ● | ● | ● | ● | ● | ● | ● |
| MARJORAM (SWEET) | ● | ● | ● | ● | ● | ● | ● | ● |
| MASTIC (BETA-EUDESMOL CT) | ● | ● | ● | ● | ● | ● | ● | ● |

*Please review the individual essential oil monographs for more detail.*

● Recommended, no known risk warranted  ▪ Caution warranted  ▲ Avoid or great caution

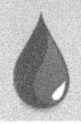

| ESSENTIAL OIL | Oral Administration | Children | Pregnancy & Lactation | Drug Interaction | Health Contraindication | Photosensitizing | Epilepsy, Convulsions | Compromised Liver or Kidneys |
|---|---|---|---|---|---|---|---|---|
| MASTIC (BETA-MYRCENE CT) | ● | ● | ● | ■ | ● | ● | ● | ● |
| MASTIC (ALL OTHER CTs) | ● | ● | ● | ● | ● | ● | ● | ● |
| MAY CHANG | ● | ● | ● | ■ | ● | ● | ● | ● |
| MEDITERRANEAN MANDARIN (COLD-PRESSED/EXPRESSED) | ● | ● | ● | ● | ● | ■ | ● | ● |
| MEDITERRANEAN MANDARIN (DISTILLED) | ● | ● | ● | ● | ● | ● | ● | ● |
| TEA TREE | ■ | ● | ● | ■ | ● | ● | ● | ● |
| MELISSA | ● | ● | ■ | ● | ● | ● | ● | ● |
| MONARDA CT CARVACROL & CARVACROL/P-CYMENE | ● | ● | ● | ● | ● | ● | ● | ● |
| MONARDA CT GERANIOL & LINALOOL | ● | ● | ● | ● | ● | ● | ● | ● |
| MONARDA CT THYMOL | ● | ● | ● | ● | ● | ● | ● | ● |
| MORINGA | ● | ● | ● | ● | ● | ● | ● | ● |
| MORINGA ((E)-PHYTOL CT) | ● | ● | ● | ● | ■ | ● | ● | ● |
| MOUNTAIN SAVORY CT CARVACROL | ● | ● | ▲ | ● | ● | ● | ● | ● |
| MOUNTAIN SAVORY CT THYMOL | ■ | ● | ▲ | ● | ■ | ● | ● | ● |
| MUGWORT CT 1,8-CINEOLE | ▲ | ▲ | ▲ | ● | ▲ | ● | ▲ | ▲ |
| MUGWORT CT ALPHA-PHELLANDRENE | ● | ● | ● | ● | ● | ● | ● | ● |
| MUGWORT CT ALPHA-THUJONE | ▲ | ▲ | ▲ | ● | ▲ | ● | ▲ | ▲ |
| MUGWORT CT ARTEMISIA KETONE | ● | ● | ● | ● | ● | ● | ● | ● |
| MUGWORT CT BETA-CARYOPHYLLENE | ● | ● | ● | ● | ● | ● | ● | ● |
| MUGWORT CT BETA-THUJONE | ▲ | ▲ | ▲ | ● | ▲ | ● | ▲ | ▲ |
| MUGWORT CT CAMPHOR | ▲ | ▲ | ▲ | ● | ▲ | ● | ▲ | ▲ |
| MUGWORT CT CHRYSANTHENYL ACETATE | ● | ● | ● | ● | ● | ● | ● | ● |
| MUGWORT CT GERMACRENE D | ● | ● | ● | ● | ● | ● | ● | ● |
| MUGWORT CT ISOBORNYL ISOBUTYRATE | ● | ● | ● | ● | ● | ● | ● | ● |
| MUGWORT (GREAT) | ▲ | ▲ | ▲ | ● | ▲ | ● | ▲ | ▲ |
| MUHUHU | ● | ● | ● | ● | ● | ● | ● | ● |
| MYRRH | ● | ● | ▲ | ● | ● | ● | ● | ● |
| MYRTLE CT 1,8-CINEOLE | ● | ● | ● | ■ | ▲ | ● | ▲ | ● |
| MYRTLE CT ALPHA-PINENE | ● | ● | ● | ■ | ▲ | ● | ▲ | ● |
| MYRTLE CT LIMONENE | ● | ● | ● | ■ | ▲ | ● | ● | ● |
| MYRTLE CT MYRTENYL ACETATE | ● | ● | ● | ■ | ▲ | ● | ▲ | ● |
| NEROLI | ● | ● | ● | ● | ● | ■ | ● | ● |
| NIAOULI CT 1,8-CINEOLE \| 1,8-CINEOLE/VIRIDIFLOROL | ■ | ▲ | ● | ■ | ▲ | ● | ▲ | ● |
| NIAOULI CT (E)-NEROLIDOL | ● | ● | ● | ● | ● | ● | ● | ● |
| NIAOULI CT TERPINENE-4-OL | ● | ● | ● | ● | ● | ● | ● | ● |
| NIAOULI CT VIRIDIFLOROL | ● | ● | ● | ■ | ▲ | ● | ▲ | ● |
| NIAOULI CT VIRIDIFLOROL/P-CYMENE/1,8-CINEOLE | ■ | ■ | ● | ● | ▲ | ● | ▲ | ● |
| NUTMEG (EAST INDIAN) | ■ | ▲ | ▲ | ■ | ● | ● | ● | ● |
| NUTMEG (WEST INDIAN) | ■ | ▲ | ▲ | ● | ● | ● | ● | ● |
| OAKMOSS ABSOLUTE | ▲ | ● | ● | ● | ● | ● | ● | ● |
| OCOTEA | ● | ● | ■ | ■ | ● | ● | ● | ● |

*Please review the individual essential oil monographs for more detail.*

● Recommended, no known risk warranted    ■ Caution warranted    ▲ Avoid or great caution

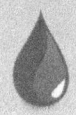

## ESSENTIAL OIL

| ESSENTIAL OIL | Oral Administration | Children | Pregnancy & Lactation | Drug Interaction | Health Contraindication | Photosensitizing | Epilepsy, Convulsions | Compromised Liver or Kidneys |
|---|---|---|---|---|---|---|---|---|
| OPOPONAX | ● | ● | ● | ● | ● | ● | ● | ● |
| ORANGE (SWEET, COLD-PRESSED/EXPRESSED) | ● | ● | ● | ● | ● | ■ | ● | ● |
| ORANGE (SWEET, DISTILLED) | ● | ● | ● | ● | ● | ● | ● | ● |
| OREGANO CT CARVACROL | ● | ● | ▲ | ● | ■ | ● | ● | ● |
| OREGANO CT TERPINENE-4-OL | ● | ● | ▲ | ■ | ■ | ● | ● | ● |
| OREGANO CT THYMOL | ■ | ● | ▲ | ● | ● | ● | ● | ● |
| ORIENTAL ARBORVITAE | ● | ● | ● | ● | ● | ● | ● | ● |
| PALMAROSA | ● | ● | ● | ● | ■ | ● | ● | ● |
| PALO SANTO (LEAVES, AERIAL PARTS) | ● | ● | ● | ● | ● | ● | ● | ● |
| PALO SANTO (WOOD) | ■ | ● | ● | ● | ● | ● | ● | ● |
| PARSLEY (LEAVES, AERIAL PARTS) | ▲ | ▲ | ▲ | ■ | ▲ | ● | ● | ▲ |
| PARSLEY (SEED) | ▲ | ▲ | ▲ | ■ | ▲ | ■ | ● | ▲ |
| PATCHOULI | ● | ● | ● | ■ | ● | ● | ● | ● |
| PENNYROYAL | ▲ | ▲ | ▲ | ■ | ▲ | ● | ▲ | ▲ |
| PEPPERMINT | ● | ▲ | ● | ■ | ■ | ● | ● | ● |
| PERSIAN LIME (COLD-PRESSED/EXPRESSED) | ● | ● | ● | ■ | ● | ■ | ● | ● |
| PERSIAN LIME (DISTILLED) | ● | ● | ● | ● | ● | ● | ● | ● |
| PERU BALSAM | ■ | ● | ● | ● | ● | ● | ● | ● |
| PETITGRAIN OF BERGAMOT | ● | ● | ● | ● | ● | ● | ● | ● |
| PETTGRAIN OF MANDARIN | ● | ● | ● | ● | ● | ■ | ● | ● |
| PINE | ● | ● | ● | ● | ● | ● | ● | ● |
| PINK PEPPER (*S. MOLLE*, α-PHELL. CT, AERIAL PARTS) | ● | ● | ● | ■ | ● | ● | ● | ● |
| PINK PEPPER (*S. TEREB.*, FRUITS, CT Δ-3-CARENE) | ● | ● | ● | ■ | ● | ● | ● | ● |
| PINK PEPPER (ALL OTHER CTS) | ● | ● | ● | ● | ● | ● | ● | ● |
| PLAI CT SABINENE | ● | ● | ● | ■ | ● | ● | ● | ● |
| PLAI CT TERPINEN-4-OL (BOTH TYPES) | ● | ● | ● | ■ | ● | ● | ● | ● |
| PLAI CT 2,6,9,9-TETRAMETHYL-2,6,10-CYCLOUNDECATRIEN-1-ONE | ● | ● | ● | ● | ● | ● | ● | ● |
| PLAI CT TRIQUINACENE,1,4-BIS(METHOXY)- | ● | ● | ● | ● | ● | ● | ● | ● |
| PONDEROSA PINE | ▲ | ■ | ▲ | ● | ● | ● | ● | ● |
| RABBITBRUSH (ALL OTHER VARITIES) | ● | ● | ● | ● | ● | ● | ● | ● |
| RABBITBRUSJ (VAR. ALBICAULIS) | ● | ● | ● | ■ | ● | ● | ● | ● |
| RAVENSARA CT 1,8-CINEOLE | ■ | ▲ | ● | ■ | ▲ | ● | ▲ | ● |
| RAVENSARA CT ALPHA-TERPINENE | ● | ● | ● | ● | ● | ● | ● | ● |
| RAVENSARA CT LIMONENE | ▲ | ● | ▲ | ■ | ● | ● | ● | ● |
| RAVENSARA CT METHYL CHAVICOL | ▲ | ● | ▲ | ● | ● | ● | ● | ● |
| RAVENSARA CT METHYL EUGENOL | ▲ | ▲ | ▲ | ● | ● | ● | ● | ● |
| RAVENSARA CT SABINENE | ● | ● | ● | ● | ● | ● | ● | ● |
| RAVINTSARA CT 1,8-CINEOLE | ■ | ▲ | ● | ■ | ▲ | ● | ▲ | ● |
| RAVINTSARA CT CAMPHOR | ■ | ▲ | ■ | ● | ▲ | ● | ▲ | ▲ |
| RAVINTSARA CT LINALOOL | ● | ● | ● | ■ | ● | ● | ● | ● |
| RED PINE | ● | ● | ● | ● | ● | ● | ● | ● |

*Please review the individual essential oil monographs for more detail.*

● Recommended, no known risk warranted     ■ Caution warranted     ▲ Avoid or great caution

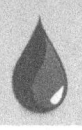

| ESSENTIAL OIL | Oral Administration | Children | Pregnancy & Lactation | Drug Interaction | Health Contraindication | Photosensitizing | Epilepsy, Convulsions | Compromised Liver or Kidneys |
|---|---|---|---|---|---|---|---|---|
| RHODODENDRON | ● | ● | ● | ● | ● | ● | ● | ● |
| ROMAN CHAMOMILE | ● | ● | ● | ● | ● | ● | ● | ● |
| ROSALINA CT 1,8-CINEOLE | ■ | ▲ | ● | ● | ▲ | ● | ▲ | ● |
| ROSALINA CT LINALOOL | ● | ● | ● | ■ | ▲ | ● | ▲ | ● |
| ROSALINA CT METHYL EUGENOL | ▲ | ▲ | ▲ | ● | ● | ● | ● | ● |
| ROSE OTTO | ● | ● | ● | ■ | ● | ● | ● | ● |
| ROSE ABSOLUTE | ▲ | ● | ● | ■ | ● | ● | ● | ● |
| ROSEMARY CT 1,8-CINEOLE | ■ | ▲ | ▲ | ■ | ▲ | ● | ▲ | ● |
| ROSEMARY CT ALPHA-PINENE | ■ | ▲ | ▲ | ● | ▲ | ● | ▲ | ● |
| ROSEMARY CT BETA-MYRCENE | ■ | ● | ● | ● | ▲ | ● | ▲ | ● |
| ROSEMARY CT BORNEOL | ■ | ● | ● | ● | ▲ | ● | ▲ | ● |
| ROSEMARY CT BORNYL ACETATE | ■ | ● | ● | ● | ▲ | ● | ▲ | ● |
| ROSEMARY CT CAMPHOR | ▲ | ▲ | ▲ | ● | ▲ | ● | ▲ | ▲ |
| ROSEMARY CT VERBENONE | ■ | ● | ● | ● | ▲ | ● | ▲ | ● |
| ROSEWOOD | ● | ● | ● | ■ | ● | ● | ● | ● |
| RUE | ▲ | ● | ▲ | ● | ● | ■ | ● | ● |
| SAGE | ▲ | ▲ | ▲ | ■ | ▲ | ● | ▲ | ▲ |
| SANDALWOOD (EAST INDIAN, HAWAIIAN) | ● | ● | ● | ● | ● | ● | ● | ● |
| SANDALWOOD (NEW CALEDONIAN, PACIFIC ISLAND) | ● | ● | ● | ● | ● | ● | ● | ● |
| SANDALWOOD (WEST AUSTRALIAN) | ● | ● | ● | ■ | ● | ● | ● | ● |
| SARO CT 1,8-CINEOLE | ■ | ● | ● | ■ | ▲ | ● | ▲ | ● |
| SARO CT LINALOOL | ● | ● | ● | ● | ● | ● | ● | ● |
| SAVIN (BERRIES) | ● | ● | ● | ● | ● | ● | ● | ● |
| SAVIN (NEEDLES & BRANCHES) | ▲ | ● | ▲ | ● | ● | ● | ▲ | ▲ |
| SAVORY (WILD) CT CARVACROL | ● | ● | ▲ | ■ | ● | ● | ● | ● |
| SAVORY (WILD) CT LINALOOL | ● | ● | ● | ● | ● | ● | ● | ● |
| SAVORY (WILD) CT THYMOL | ■ | ● | ▲ | ■ | ● | ● | ● | ● |
| SCHISANDRA FRUIT | ● | ● | ● | ● | ● | ● | ● | ● |
| SHELL GINGER CT 1,8-CINEOLE | ● | ● | ● | ● | ▲ | ● | ▲ | ▲ |
| SHELL GINGER CT P-MENTHA-1,3-DIEN-7-AL | ● | ● | ● | ● | ● | ● | ● | ● |
| SHELL GINGER CT PARA-CYMENE | ● | ● | ● | ■ | ● | ● | ● | ● |
| SHELL GINGER CT TERPINEN-4-OL | ● | ● | ● | ■ | ▲ | ● | ▲ | ● |
| SIAM WOOD (LEAVES) | ● | ● | ● | ● | ● | ● | ● | ● |
| SIAM WOOD (ROOT BARK) | ● | ● | ● | ● | ● | ● | ● | ● |
| SIBERIAN FIR | ● | ● | ● | ● | ● | ● | ● | ● |
| SILVER FIR | ● | ● | ● | ● | ● | ● | ● | ● |
| SOUTHERN BLUE GUM | ■ | ▲ | ● | ● | ▲ | ● | ▲ | ● |

*Please review the individual essential oil monographs for more detail.*

● Recommended, no known risk warranted     ■ Caution warranted     ▲ Avoid or great caution

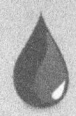

| ESSENTIAL OIL | Oral Administration | Children | Pregnancy & Lactation | Drug Interaction | Health Contraindication | Photosensitizing | Epilepsy, Convulsions | Compromised Liver or Kidneys |
|---|---|---|---|---|---|---|---|---|
| SPANISH SAGE | ◼ | ◼ | ◼ | ◼ | ▲ | ● | ▲ | ● |
| SPEARMINT CT CARVONE | ● | ● | ● | ◼ | ◼ | ● | ● | ● |
| SPEARMINT CT CIS-OCIMENONE | ● | ● | ● | ● | ◼ | ● | ● | ● |
| SPEARMINT CT LINALOOL | ● | ● | ● | ◼ | ◼ | ● | ● | ● |
| SPEARMINT CT MENTHONE | ● | ● | ● | ● | ◼ | ● | ● | ● |
| SPEARMINT CT PIPERITENONE OXIDE | ● | ● | ● | ● | ◼ | ● | ● | ● |
| SPEARMINT CT PIPERITONE | ● | ● | ● | ● | | ● | ● | ● |
| SPEARMINT CT PULEGONE/MENTHONE/ISOMENTHONE | ▲ | ▲ | ▲ | ● | ▲ | ● | ▲ | ▲ |
| SPEARMINT CT ROTUNDIFOLONE | ● | ● | ● | ● | ◼ | ● | ● | ● |
| SPIKE LAVENDER | ◼ | ▲ | ◼ | ◼ | ▲ | ● | ▲ | ▲ |
| SPIKENARD | ● | ● | ● | ● | ● | ● | ● | ● |
| SPRUCE (BLACK) | ● | ● | ● | ● | ● | ● | ● | ● |
| STAR ANISE | ● | ◼ | ▲ | ◼ | ◼ | ● | ● | ● |
| SUMMER SAVORY CT CARVACROL | ● | ● | ▲ | ◼ | ◼ | ● | ● | ● |
| SUMMER SAVORY CT GAMMA-TERPINENE | ● | ● | ▲ | ● | ● | ● | ● | ● |
| SUMMER SAVORY CT THYMOL | ◼ | ● | ▲ | ◼ | ◼ | ● | ● | ● |
| SWEET INULA CT 1,8-CINEOLE | ● | ▲ | ● | ◼ | ▲ | ● | ▲ | ● |
| SWEET INULA CT BORNEOL | ● | ● | ● | ◼ | ● | ● | ● | ● |
| SWEET INULA CT BORNYL ACETATE | ● | ● | ● | ◼ | ● | ● | ● | ● |
| SWEET INULA CT T-CADINOL | ● | ● | ● | ● | ● | ● | ● | ● |
| SWEET NANCY CT YOMOGI ALCOHOL/1,8-CINEOLE | ● | ● | ● | ◼ | ▲ | ● | ▲ | ● |
| SWEET NANCY CT ARTEMISYL ACETATE | ● | ● | ● | ◼ | ◼ | ● | ● | ● |
| SWEET NANCY CT ARTEMISIA KETONE | ● | ● | ● | ◼ | ◼ | ● | ● | ● |
| SWEET WORMWOOD CT ARTEMISIA KETONE | ◼ | ▲ | ◼ | ◼ | ◼ | ● | ● | ▲ |
| SWEET WORMWOOD CT CAMPHOR | ◼ | ▲ | ◼ | ● | ◼ | ● | ● | ▲ |
| TAGETES | ● | ● | ● | ◼ | ● | ◼ | ● | ● |
| TAMALA CT BETA-CARYOPHYLLENE | ● | ● | ● | ● | ● | ● | ● | ● |
| TAMALA CT (E)-CINNAMALDEHYDE | ● | ● | ▲ | ◼ | ◼ | ● | ● | ● |
| TAMALA CT (E)-CINNAMALDEHYDE/CINNAMYL ACETATE | ● | ● | ▲ | ◼ | ◼ | ● | ● | ● |
| TAMALA CT EUGENOL | ● | ● | ▲ | ◼ | ◼ | ● | ● | ● |
| TAMALA CT EUGENOL/EUGENYL ACETATE | ● | ● | ▲ | ◼ | ◼ | ● | ● | ● |
| TAMALA CT LINALOOL/(E)-CINNAMALDEHYDE | ● | ● | ▲ | ◼ | ◼ | ● | ● | ● |
| TAMALA CT LINALOOL | ● | ● | ● | ● | ● | ● | ● | ● |
| TAMALA CT TRANS-SABINENE HYDRATE | ● | ● | ● | ● | ● | ● | ● | ● |
| TANGERINE (COLD-PRESSED/EXPRESSED) | ● | ● | ● | ◼ | ● | ◼ | ● | ● |
| TANGERINE (DISTILLED) | ● | ● | ● | ◼ | ● | ● | ● | ● |
| TANSY CT BETA-THUJONE | ▲ | ▲ | ▲ | ● | ▲ | ● | ▲ | ▲ |

*Please review the individual essential oil monographs for more detail.*

● Recommended, no known risk warranted     ◼ Caution warranted     ▲ Avoid or great caution

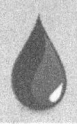

| ESSENTIAL OIL | Oral Administration | Children | Pregnancy & Lactation | Drug Interaction | Health Contraindication | Photosensitizing | Epilepsy, Convulsions | Compromised Liver or Kidneys |
|---|---|---|---|---|---|---|---|---|
| TARRAGON CT METHYL CHAVICOL | ▲ | ▪ | ▲ | ● | ● | ● | ● | ● |
| TEXAS CEDARWOOD | ● | ● | ● | ▪ | ● | ● | ● | ● |
| THUJA | ▲ | ▲ | ▲ | ● | ▲ | ● | ▲ | ▲ |
| THYME CT ALPHA-TERPINEOL | ● | ● | ● | ▪ | ▲ | ● | ▲ | ● |
| THYME CT CARVACROL | ● | ● | ● | ▪ | ▪ | ● | ● | ● |
| THYME CT GERANIOL | ● | ● | ● | ▪ | ▪ | ● | ● | ● |
| THYME CT LINALOOL | ● | ● | ● | ▪ | ▲ | ● | ▲ | ● |
| THYME CT THUYANOL-4 | ● | ● | ● | ▪ | ▲ | ● | ▲ | ● |
| THYME CT THYMOL | ▪ | ● | ● | ▪ | ▪ | ● | ● | ● |
| TOLU BALSAM | ▪ | ● | ● | ● | ● | ● | ● | ● |
| TOLU BALSAM ABSOLUTE | ▲ | ● | ● | ● | ● | ● | ● | ● |
| TSAURI GRASS | ● | ● | ● | ● | ● | ● | ● | ● |
| TSAURI GRASS (VAR. MADAGASCARIENSIS) | ● | ● | ● | ● | ● | ● | ● | ● |
| TSUGA | ● | ● | ● | ● | ● | ● | ● | ● |
| TURKISH PINE | ● | ● | ● | ● | ● | ● | ● | ● |
| TURMERIC (ABSOLUTE) | ▲ | ● | ● | ▪ | ▪ | ● | ● | ● |
| TURMERIC (LEAVES) | ● | ● | ● | ● | ● | ● | ● | ● |
| TURMERIC (RHIZOME) | ▪ | ● | ● | ▪ | ▪ | ● | ● | ● |
| TURMERIC (WHITE) | ● | ● | ▲ | ● | ● | ● | ● | ● |
| TURMERIC (WILD) | ● | ▲ | ▪ | ● | ▲ | ● | ● | ● |
| VALERIAN | ● | ● | ● | ▪ | ● | ● | ● | ● |
| VERBENA CT LIMONENE | ● | ● | ● | ● | ● | ● | ● | ● |
| VERBENA CT LINALOOL | ● | ● | ● | ● | ● | ● | ● | ● |
| VERBENA CT MYRCENE | ● | ● | ▪ | ▪ | ● | ● | ● | ● |
| VERBENA CT MYRCENONE | ● | ● | ● | ● | ● | ● | ● | ● |
| VETIVER | ● | ● | ● | ● | ● | ● | ● | ● |
| VILAYTI TULSI CT 1,8-CINEOLE | ● | ● | ● | ● | ▲ | ● | ▲ | ● |
| VILAYTI TULSI CT FENCHONE | ● | ● | ● | ▪ | ▲ | ● | ▲ | ● |
| VILAYTI TULSI CT SABINENE | ● | ● | ● | ● | ▲ | ● | ▲ | ● |
| VIRGINIAN CEDARWOOD | ● | ● | ● | ▪ | ● | ● | ● | ● |
| WESTERN RED CEDAR (NEEDLES) | ▲ | ▲ | ▲ | ● | ▲ | ● | ▲ | ▲ |
| WESTERN RED CEDAR (WOOD) | ● | ● | ● | ● | ● | ● | ● | ● |
| WHITE FIR | ● | ● | ● | ● | ● | ● | ● | ● |
| WHITE PINE | ● | ● | ● | ● | ● | ● | ● | ● |
| WHITE SAGE | ▪ | ▲ | ● | ▪ | ▲ | ● | ▲ | ● |

*Please review the individual essential oil monographs for more detail.*

● Recommended, no known risk warranted      ▪ Caution warranted      ▲ Avoid or great caution

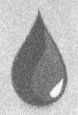

| ESSENTIAL OIL | Oral Administration | Children | Pregnancy & Lactation | Drug Interaction | Health Contraindication | Photosensitizing | Epilepsy, Convulsions | Compromised Liver or Kidneys |
|---|---|---|---|---|---|---|---|---|
| WHITE SPRUCE (BRANCHES) | ● | ▲ | ■ | ● | ▲ | ● | ▲ | ▲ |
| WHITE SPRUCE (NEEDLES) | ■ | ▲ | ■ | ● | ▲ | ● | ▲ | ▲ |
| WHITE SPRUCE (NEEDLES & TWIGS) | ■ | ▲ | ■ | ● | ▲ | ● | ▲ | ▲ |
| WHITE SPRUCE (OLEORESIN) | ● | ● | ● | ● | ● | ● | ● | ● |
| WHITE VERBENA CT CAMPHOR | ▲ | ■ | ■ | ● | ▲ | ● | ▲ | ▲ |
| WHITE VERBENA CT CARVONE/LIMONENE | ● | ● | ● | ■ | ■ | ● | ● | ● |
| WHITE VERBENA CT CITRAL | ● | ● | ■ | ■ | ● | ● | ● | ● |
| WHITE VERBENA CT LINALOOL | ● | ● | ● | ■ | ● | ● | ● | ● |
| WILD CHAMOMILE | ● | ● | ● | ● | ● | ● | ● | ● |
| WILD MARJORAM CT 1,8-CINEOLE | ■ | ▲ | ● | ■ | ▲ | ● | ▲ | ● |
| WILD MARJORAM CT LINALOOL | ● | ● | ● | ● | ● | ● | ● | ● |
| WINTERGREEN | ■ | ▲ | ▲ | ▲ | ▲ | ● | ▲ | ● |
| WORMSEED (AMERICAN) CT ALPHA-TERPINENE | ▲ | ▲ | ▲ | ● | ▲ | ● | ▲ | ▲ |
| WORMSEED (AMERICAN) CT ASCARIDOLE | ▲ | ▲ | ▲ | ■ | ▲ | ● | ▲ | ▲ |
| WORMSEED (AMERICAN) CT CARVACROL | ▲ | ▲ | ▲ | ● | ▲ | ● | ▲ | ▲ |
| WORMWOOD CT ALPHA-THUJONE | ▲ | ▲ | ▲ | ● | ▲ | ● | ▲ | ▲ |
| WORMWOOD CT BETA-PINENE | ● | ● | ● | ● | ● | ● | ● | ● |
| WORMWOOD CT BETA-THUJONE | ▲ | ▲ | ▲ | ● | ▲ | ● | ▲ | ▲ |
| WORMWOOD CT CHAMAZULENE | ▲ | ▲ | ▲ | ● | ▲ | ● | ▲ | ▲ |
| WORMWOOD CT CIS-CHRYSANTHENYL ACETATE | ● | ● | ● | ● | ● | ● | ● | ● |
| WORMWOOD CT (E)-BETA-FARNESENE | ● | ● | ● | ● | ● | ● | ● | ● |
| WORMWOOD CT MYRCENE | ● | ● | ▲ | ■ | ▲ | ● | ▲ | ▲ |
| WORMWOOD CT MYRCENE/SABINENE | ● | ● | ▲ | ● | ▲ | ● | ▲ | ▲ |
| WORMWOOD CT SABINENE | ▲ | ▲ | ▲ | ● | ▲ | ● | ▲ | ▲ |
| WORMWOOD CT TRANS-SABINENE HYDRATE | ▲ | ▲ | ▲ | ● | ▲ | ● | ▲ | ▲ |
| WORMWOOD CT TRANS-SABINYL ACETATE | ▲ | ▲ | ▲ | ● | ▲ | ● | ▲ | ▲ |
| WORMWOOD CT (Z)-EPOXY OCIMENE | ▲ | ▲ | ▲ | ● | ▲ | ● | ▲ | ▲ |
| XANTHOXYLUM | ● | ● | ● | ■ | ● | ● | ● | ● |
| YARROW CT 1,8-CINEOLE/CAMPHOR | ▲ | ■ | ■ | ■ | ▲ | ● | ▲ | ▲ |
| YARROW CT ARTEMESIA KETONE | ● | ● | ■ | ● | ▲ | ● | ▲ | ● |
| YARROW CT BETA THUJONE | ▲ | ▲ | ▲ | ● | ▲ | ● | ▲ | ▲ |
| YARROW CT CHAMAZULENE | ■ | ■ | ■ | ■ | ▲ | ● | ▲ | ● |
| YARROW CT SABINENE | ● | ● | ● | ● | ▲ | ● | ▲ | ● |
| YLANG YLANG | ● | ● | ● | ● | ● | ● | ● | ● |
| YLANG YLANG (I FRACTIONS) | ■ | ● | ● | ● | ● | ● | ● | ● |
| YUZU | ● | ● | ● | ● | ● | ■ | ● | ● |
| ZDRAVETZ | ● | ● | ● | ■ | ● | ● | ● | ● |

*Please review the individual essential oil monographs for more detail.*

● Recommended, no known risk warranted      ■ Caution warranted      ▲ Avoid or great caution

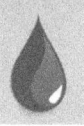 

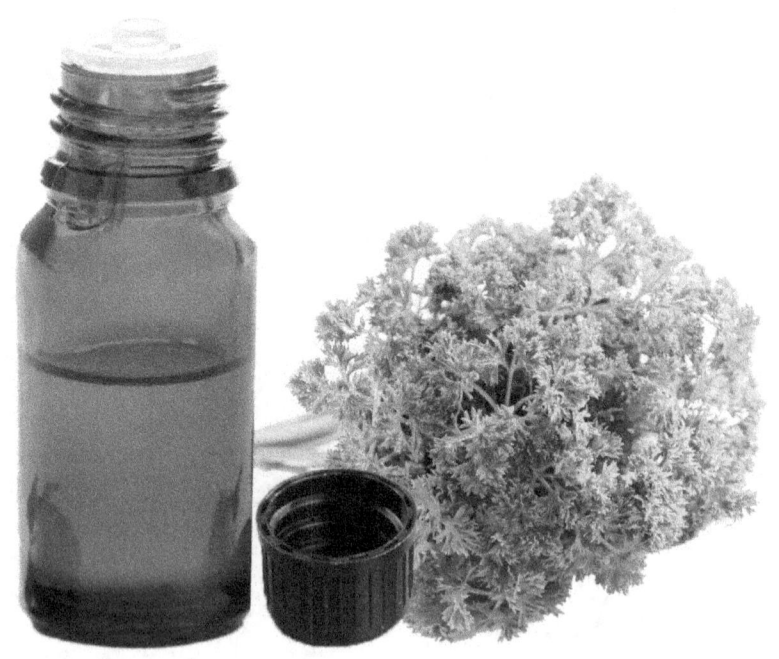

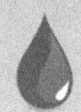

# APPENDIX E:
## CONVERSION CHART, ABBREVIATIONS, AND DEFINITIONS

Depending on the specific gravity of the essential oil and the orificer reducer, the number of drops per milliliter (mL) ranges from 15 to 40. This chart uses an average of 30 drops per mL and 30 milligrams (mg) per drop.

| DROPS | ML | MG |
|---|---|---|
| 1 | 0.033 | 30 |
| 2 | 0.066 | 60 |
| 3 | 0.10 | 90 |
| 4 | 0.13 | 120 |
| 5 | 0.17 | 150 |
| 6 | 0.20 | 180 |
| 7 | 0.23 | 210 |
| 8 | 0.26 | 240 |
| 9 | 0.30 | 270 |
| 10 | 0.33 | 300 |
| 15 | 0.50 | 450 |
| 20 | 0.66 | 600 |
| 25 | 0.83 | 750 |
| 30 | 1.0 | 900 |
| 35 | 1.16 | 1,050 |
| 40 | 1.32 | 1,200 |
| 45 | 1.49 | 1,350 |
| 50 | 1.65 | 1,500 |
| 100 | 3.30 | 3,000 |
| 150 | 4.95 | 4,500 |
| 200 | 6.60 | 6,000 |
| 250 | 8.25 | 7,500 |
| 300 | 9.90 | 9,000 |
| 350 | 11.55 | 10,500 |
| 400 | 13.20 | 12,000 |
| 450 | 14.95 | 13,500 |
| 500 | 16.50 | 15,000 |

Some modern essential oil orifice reducers dispense roughly 60 mg per drop. This chart uses about 17 drops per mL and 60 mg per drop.

| DROPS | ML | MG |
|---|---|---|
| 1 | 0.066 | 60 |
| 2 | 0.132 | 120 |
| 3 | 0.198 | 180 |
| 4 | 0.264 | 240 |
| 5 | 0.330 | 300 |
| 6 | 0.396 | 360 |
| 7 | 0.462 | 420 |
| 8 | 0.528 | 480 |

| DROPS | ML | MG |
|---|---|---|
| 9 | 0.594 | 540 |
| 10 | 0.660 | 600 |
| 15 | 0.990 | 900 |
| 16 | 1.056 | 960 |
| 20 | 1.32 | 1,200 |
| 25 | 1.65 | 1.500 |
| 30 | 1.98 | 1,800 |
| 35 | 2.31 | 2,100 |
| 40 | 2.64 | 2,400 |
| 45 | 2.97 | 2,700 |
| 50 | 3.3 | 3,000 |
| 76 | 5.02 | 4,560 |
| 100 | 6.6 | 6,000 |
| 150 | 9.9 | 9,000 |
| 200 | 13.2 | 12,000 |
| 228 | 15.05 | 13,680 |
| 250 | 16.5 | 15,000 |
| 300 | 19.8 | 18,500 |
| 350 | 23.1 | 21,000 |

## Symbols and Abbreviations

| | |
|---|---|
| α, A | Alpha |
| ar- | Aromatic |
| β, B | Beta |
| (Z) | Cis, Beta |
| (+) | Clockwise rotation (polarized light) |
| d- | Clockwise rotation (polarized light) |
| (R)- | Clockwise rotation (chirality center) |
| (−) | Counterclockwise rotation (polarized light) |
| l- | Clockwise rotation (polarized light) |
| (S)- | Counterclockwise rotation (chirality center) |
| δ, Δ | Delta |
| ε, E | Epsilon |
| γ, Γ | Gamma |
| n- | "Normal"—an unbranched chain with the functional group (if present) on the 1-position |
| o- | Ortho |
| p- | Para |
| π, Π | Pi |
| ψ, Ψ | psi |
| s- | "Secondary" |
| σ, Σ | Sigma |
| τ, T | Tau |
| t- | "Tert" |
| (E) | Trans, Alpha |
| mono | 1 |

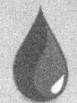
| | |
|---|---|
| meth- | (carbons: 1; alkyl group: methyl) |
| di | 2 |
| eth- | (carbons: 2; alkyl group: ethyl) |
| tri | 3 |
| prop- | (carbons: 3; alkyl group: propyl) |
| tetra | 4 |
| but- | (carbons: 4; alkyl group: butyl) |
| penta | 5 |
| pent- | (carbons: 5; alkyl group: pentyl) |
| hexa | 6 |
| hex- | (carbons: 6; alkyl group: hexyl) |
| hepta | 7 |
| hept- | (carbons: 7; alkyl group: heptyl) |
| octa | 8 |
| oct- | (carbons: 8; alkyl group: octyl) |
| ennea | 9 |
| nona | 9 |
| non- | (carbons: 9; alkyl group: nonyl) |
| deca | 10 |
| dec- | (carbons: 10; alkyl group: decyl) |
| hendeca | 11 |
| undeca | 11 |
| dodeca | 12 |
| henicosa | 21 |
| > | More/Greater than |
| < | Less than |
| a, a. | Before |
| a.c. | Before meals |
| ad lib | As desired |
| bid | Twice daily |
| CT | Chemotype |
| Dx | Diagnosis |
| g | Grams |
| g/kg | Grams of administered substance per kilogram (2.2 pounds) of body weight. |
| gtt | Drop |
| im | Intramuscular (administered directly into a muscle) |
| inj. | Injection (administration of a substance into the body either under or through the skin) |
| ip | Intraperitoneal (administered into the abdominal cavity) |
| iv | Intravenous (administered into a vein or veins) |
| lb. | Pound |
| $LC_{50}$ | Median lethal concentration. The concentration of a substance that is lethal to 50 percent of the tested population during a toxicity test. |
| $LD_{50}$ | Median Lethal Dose. A measurement of acute toxicity that represents the individual dose that is lethal to 50 percent of the tested population. |
| $LD_{LO}$ | The lowest dose of a substance at which the death of the exposed organism occurs. |
| μg, mcg | Micrograms (millionths of a gram) |

| | |
|---|---|
| mg | Milligrams (thousandths of a gram) |
| μl | Microliters (millionths of a liter) |
| mL | Milliliters (thousandths of a liter) |
| mL/Kg | Milliliters of administered substance per kilogram (2.2 pounds) of body weight. |
| MRSA | Methicillin-resistant *Staphylococcus aureus*. A strain of staph bacteria that is resistant to common antibiotics. |
| p or p. | After, per |
| po | By mouth |
| prn | As needed |
| pr, r. | Rectally, per rectum |
| qid | Four times per day |
| Qqds | Four times per day |
| q1h | Every hour |
| q2h | Every 2 hours |
| q3h | Every 3 hours |
| q4h | Every 4 hours |
| q6h | Every 6 hours |
| q8h | Every 8 hours |
| q12h | Every 12 hours |
| qs | As much as needed |
| $RD_{50}$ | The exposure concentration of a substance that reduces the respiratory rate of a population by 50 percent. |
| Rx | Prescription |
| sc, sq | Subcutaneous. Applied under the skin. |
| tid, tds | Three times per day |

## Studies Definitions

*Case Report or Series*: Collections of reports regarding the treatment of patients (or a single patient) that do not involve a control group.

*Case Control:* Studies that use existing data to compare people with a specific condition to those who do not have the condition to identify contributing factors or exposures associated with the condition.

*Cohort:* An observational study that evaluates a group of people over a period of time to determine the effects of particular variables (such as sun exposure) among one group versus another group that has not been exposed to the same variable.

*Cross Sectional Surveys*: Data collection at a single point in time over a short period to estimate the prevalence of a condition for a specific population. Data can also be used to evaluate the cause of disease or the results of intervention.

*Double-blinding*: Group assignment (treatment or control) is hidden from the study participants and the researchers.

*Hierarchy of Research Evidence*: An approach used to determine the best available evidence and the use of this

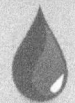

evidence to establish a recommended approach for the care of individual patients.

*in silico*: By computer modeling.

*in suto:* In its original place (especially of a malignant tumor); undisturbed.

*in toto:* As a whole; in all; overall.

*in vitro:* Studies performed with cells of biological molecules outside a living organism, such as a test tube or culture dish.

*in vivo:* Studies performed within a living organism or natural setting.

*Meta-analysis*: A thorough examination of published and valid studies that mathematically combines the results of the individual studies to produce results as if it were one large study.

*Randomized Controlled Trial*: Studies that evaluate treatments or exposure outcomes in real patients using methodologies that reduce bias and compare treatment versus a control group that is not exposed to the treatment being evaluated in the study.

*Single-blinding*: The study participants do not know if they are in the treatment or control group.

*Systematic Review*: The extensive evaluation of published literature to answer a specific clinical question. The literature is critically evaluated for quality according to specific criteria.

*Triple-blinding*: Group (treatment or control) assignments are hidden from the study participants, researchers, and tasked with analyzing the data.

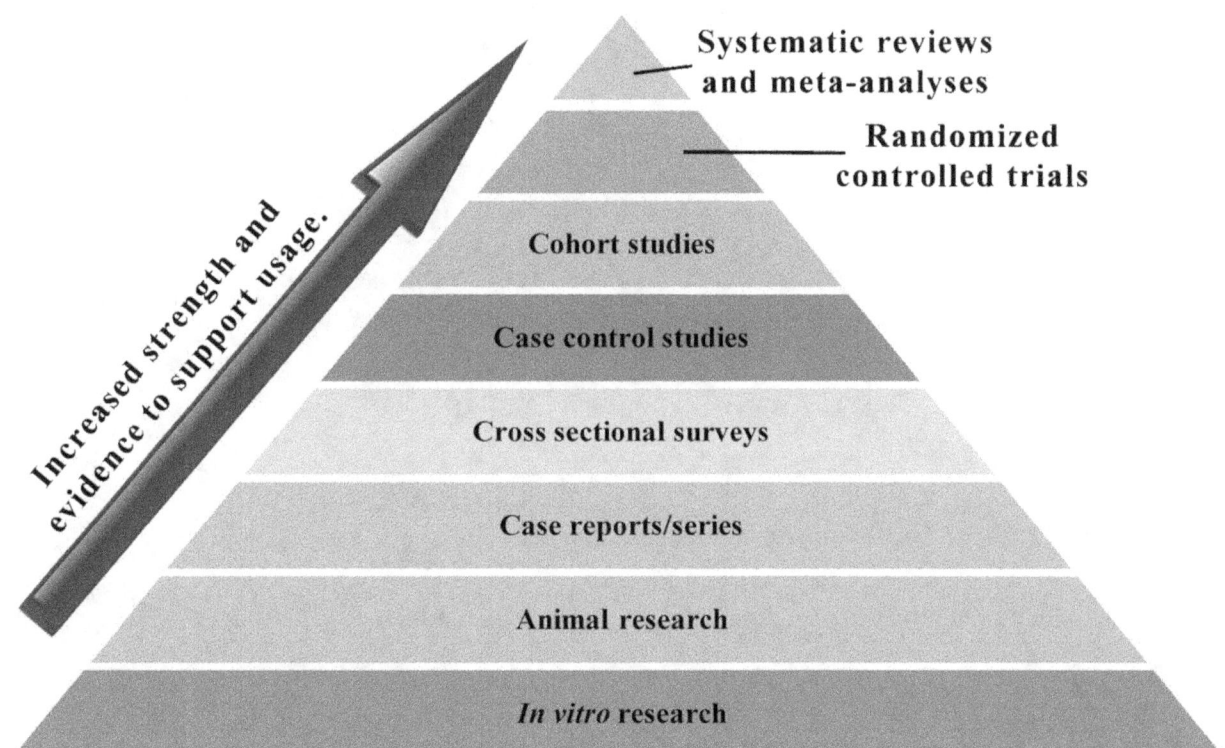

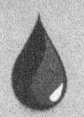

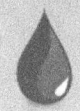

# APPENDIX F:
## ESSENTIAL OIL NOTES

Base notes are the least volatile and contain larger molecules, which take the longest to evaporate—up to days. They are relaxing, sedating, and soothing. Base notes are effective for chronic health conditions. In addition, they affect the spirit and are often used as aphrodisiacs. Base notes are typically about 10 to 30 percent of the blend (though this a guideline and not a firm rule for evidence-based essential oil therapy).

Middle notes are more volatile and contain medium-sized molecules that are estimated to evaporate in 2 to 48 hours. Middle notes are highly valuable because they aid the function of body systems, help regulate metabolism, and balance the production of hormones by the endocrine system. They are also helpful for regulating the reproductive system. Middle notes typically about 30 to 50 percent of the blend (though this a guideline and not a firm rule for evidence-based essential oil therapy).

Top notes are highly volatile with very small molecules that are estimated to evaporate in 1 to 24 hours. They strongly influence the mind and emotions, and encourage relaxation, a positive outlook on life, calm anxiety, and help reduce the negative effects of stress. They also affect the body by stimulating circulation and digestion. Top notes are often very effective for acute health conditions. Top notes typically about 15 to 30 percent of the blend (though this a guideline and not a firm rule for evidence-based essential oil therapy).

## ESSENTIAL OIL NOTES

**Top Notes:**

Ajowan, bergamot, big badja gum, birch, bitter orange, blue mallee, blue mountain, camphor, Chinese red pine, cilantro, citron, coriander, dwarf pine, eucalyptus, eucalyptus dives, garlic, genipi, gobre salla, grapefruit, gully gum, kabosu, kanuka, kumquat, lemon, lemon basil, lemon myrtle, lemon verbena, lime, Mediterranean mandarin, orange (sweet), Oriental arborvitae, peppermint, Persian lime, pine, Ponderosa pine, red pine, rue, sage, saro, Southern blue gum, spearmint, tangerine, thuja, Western red cedar (needles), white pine, yuzu

**Top/Middle Notes:**

Aleppo pine, anise, applemint, basil (sweet), bay (West Indies), bay laurel, bergamot mint, black pepper, blue cypress, citronella, Douglas fir, Engelmann spruce, feverfew, Formosan cypress, galbanum, guava leaf, hairy basil, hemp, hinoki, holy basil, honey myrtle, kaffir lime petitgrain, lavandin, lavender, leleshwa, lemon catnip, lemon tea tree, lemongrass, magnolia, maritime pine, may chang, myrtle, petitgrain (bergamot, mandarin), ravensara, rosemary, Siberian fir, silver fir, spruce (black), sweet nancy, sweet wormwood, tagetes, thyme, tsuga, Turjish pine, vilayti tulsi, white fir, white spruce, wild chamomile, wintergreen

**Middle Notes:**

African bluegrass, allspice, arnica, balsam fir, betony, black sage, blue spruce, blue tansy, boldo, buchu, calendula, cajeput, Canadian fleabane, cangerana, Cape chamomile, caraway, cardamom, carrot seed, cassia, catnip, celery, chaste tree, cinnamon, clary sage, clove, cypress, daminana, dill, elecampane, elemi, fennel (sweet), fenugreek, ferula, Fragonia, geranium, German chamomile, goldenrod, grindelia, hops, hyssop, Indian borage, juniper berry, juniper (Chinese), juniper (Himalayan), juniper (Phoenician), katrafay, khella, kunzea, ledum, lemon eucalyptus, manuka, marjoram, tea tree, melissa, monarda, moringa, mountain savory, mugwort, neroli, niaouli, nutmeg, ocotea, oregano, palmarosa, palo santo, parsley, patchouli, pennyroyal, peta, pink pepper, plai, rabbitbrush, ravintsara, rhododendron, Roman chamomile, rose, rosewood, savin, savory (wild), schisandra fruit, shell ginger, Spanish sage, spike lavender, star anise, summer savory, sweet inula, tamala, tarragon, verbena, white sage, white verbena, wild marjoram, wormseed (American), xanthoxylum, yarrow

**Middle/Base Notes:**

Agarwood, angelica root, auracaria, calamus, cedarwood, cistus, cumin, fingerroot, ginger, helichrysum, jasmine absolute, mastic, opoponax, rosalina, tansy, ylang ylang, zdravetz

**Base Notes:**

Amyris, balsam poplar, benzoin absolute, black cumin seed, Buddha wood, Chinese cedarwood, copaiba, davana, frankincense, Ghandi root, guaiacwood, guggul, gurjun balsam, muhuhu, myrrh, oakmoss absolute, Peru balsam, sandalwood, Siam wood, spikenard, Texas cedarwood, tolu balsam, turmeric, valerian, vetiver, Virginian cedarwood, Western red cedar (wood), white turmeric, wild turmeric, wormwood

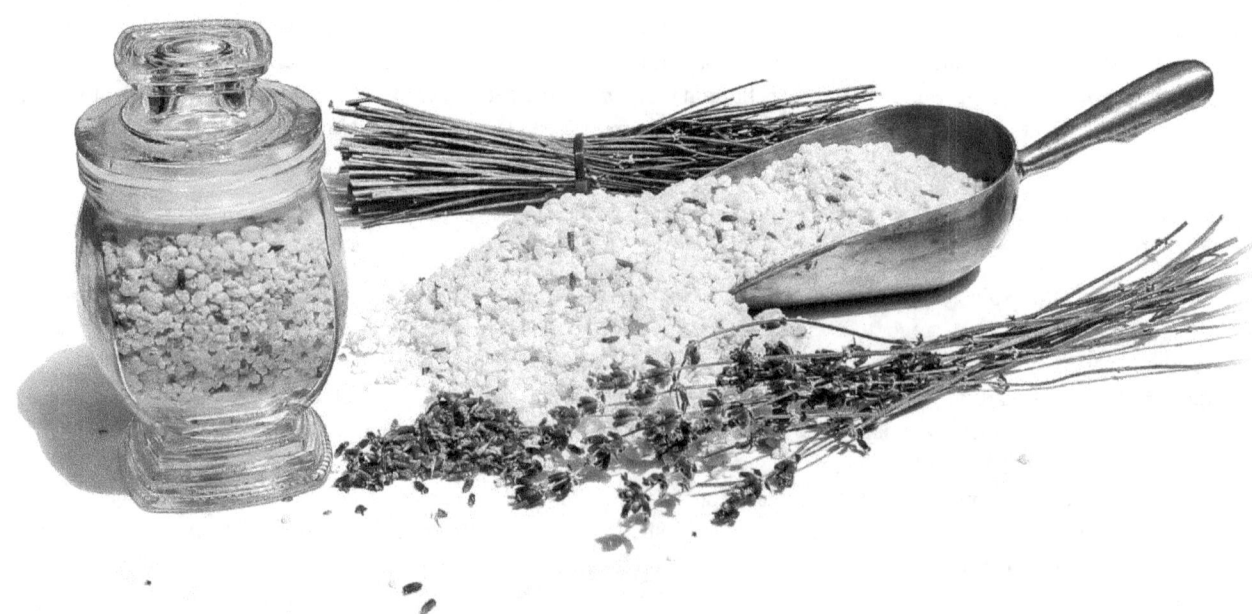

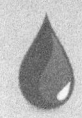

# APPENDIX G:
## CAUTIONS QUICK REFERENCE GUIDE

This guide is meant to help quickly identify an essential oil or essential oils that may interfere with medications or possibly be contraindicated with certain health conditions. While every effort has been made to identify these interactions and contraindications, it may not list all possible cautions. Always consult your physician or pharmacist before using essential oils with medications or if you have a known health condition, or believe you may have a health condition.

Interaction risk will vary based on method of administration with risk from greatest to least being: oral > retention > topical > diffusion. Some interactions may only occur when used orally, but interactions are possible with other methods of administration as well (i.e. topical application of wintergreen).

| CAUTION | ESSENTIAL OILS |
|---|---|
| ACETAMINOPHEN: | Anise, star anise |
| ALCOHOL: | Tansy, valerian |
| ANEMIA, IRON-DEFICIENCY: | Applemint (menthol CTs), peppermint, spearmint |
| ANTIBIOTICS, ANTIFUNGALS, ANTIVIRALS: | Ajowan, allspice, applemint (various CTs), basil (various CTs), bay (West Indies), bay laurel, benzoin absolute, black cumin, black pepper (eugenol CT), black sage, blue mountain sage ((E)-nerolidol CT), camphor (linalool CT), cassia, cinnamon bark, cinnamon leaf, citronella, clove, coriander, cumin, eucalyptus, *Eucalyptus dives*, fennel, fingerroot ((E)-beta-ocimene CT), garlic, geranium, ghandi root, guava ((E)-nerolidol CT), hairy basil (various CTs), holy basil (various CTs), honey myrtle, Indian borage (carvacrol & thymol CTs), lavender (terpinene-4-ol rich), lemon catnip, lemon myrtle (citral CT), lemon tea tree, lemon verbena, lemongrass, lime (distilled), magnolia, mastic (beta-eudesmol CT), may chang, melaleuca, monarda (various CTs), mountain savory, myrtle, niaouli ((E)-nerolidol CT), ocotea, oregano, palmarosa, pennyroyal, peppermint, plai (various CTs), ravintsara, (linalool CT), ravensara (various CTs), rose, rosemary, rosewood, rosalina (methyl eugenol CT), sandalwood (Australian), saro, savin, savory (wild, carvacrol, & thymol CTs), shell ginger, saim wood (root bark), spearmint (various CTs), summer savory (carvacrol & thymol CTs), sweet inula, tagetes (various CTs), tamala (various CTs), tangerine (distilled), tarragon (methyl chavicol CT), thyme, white verbena (linalool CT), wild marjoram (linalool CT), wormseed (American), xanthoxylum |
| ANTICHOLINERGIC MEDS: *Antihistamines, antipsychotics, antispasmodics, antiarrythmics, antiemetics, muscle relaxers, tricyclic antidepressants* | Ajowan, Aleppo pine, allspice, applemint, balsam poplar, basil (methyl eugenol CT), bay (West Indies), bergamot, bitter orange, black cumin, blue mountain sage (alpha-bisabolol CT), calamus, cinnamon (leaves), citron, clove, dill, dwarf pine (twigs), German chamomile, hairy basil (various CTs), hinoki, holy basil (various CTs), Indian borage (carvacrol & thymol CTs), juniper (Himalayan), kaffir lime petitgrain, lemon, lime, lovage, marjoram, melissa, monarda (various CTs), mountain savory, oregano, pink pepper (various CTs), plai (various CTs), ravensara (methyl eugenol CT), rosalina (methyl eugenol CT), savory (wild), Spanish sage, summer savory, sweet inula, sweet wormwood, tamala (various CTs), tarragon, thyme, wild marjoram, wormseed (American) |

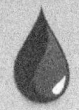

| | |
|---|---|
| *ANTICOAGULANT/ ANTIPLATELET*<br>*MEDS*<br>*(Blood Thinners):*<br>*Heparin, warfarin (Coumadin),*<br>*NSAIDs, heparin, aspirin, apixaban,*<br>*dabigatran, rivaroxaban, clopidogrel*<br>*(Plavix), prausugrel, dipyramole,*<br>*glycoprotein IIb/IIIa antagonists* | Ajowan, allspice, anise, applemint (carvone CT), auracaria, basil, bay (West Indies), bay laurel (low risk), benzoin absolute, big badja gum, birch, black cumin, black pepper (eugenol CT), blue cypress (wood oil)—low risk, blue mallee, boldo, cajeput, calamus (beta-sarone CT), caraway (carvone CT), cassia, chaste tree, cinnamon bark, cinnamon leaf, clove, cypress, dill (carvone CT), eucalyptus, fennel, Formosan cypress (twig oil), garlic, German chamomile, ginger, gully gum, hairy basil (various CTs), holy basil (various CTs), Indian borage (carvacrol & thymol CTs), lavandin, lovage, melissa, monarda (various CTs), mountain savory, niaouli (various CTs), nutmeg (East Indian), ocotea, oregano, patchouli, ravensara (various CTs), rosalina (1,8-cineole CT), saro (1,8-cineole CT), savory (wild, carvacrol & thymol CTs), spearmint (carvone CT), Southern blue gum, star anise, summer savory (carvacrol & thymol CTs), sweet inula (bornyl acetate, borneol CTs) tamala (various CTs), tarragon, thyme, turmeric, vilayti tulsi, white sage, white verbena (carvone-limonene CT), wintergreen, wormseed (American), yarrow; aloe vera (oral),[10322] avocado oil (oral),[10323] borage seed oil,[10324] DMSO,[10325] evening primrose oil,[10326] grapeseed oil,[10327,10328] olive oil (oral)[10329] |
| *ANTIDEPRESSANTS:*<br>*Fluoxetine (Prozac), paroxetine*<br>*(Paxil), sertraline (Zoloft), citalopram*<br>*(Celexa), escitalopram (Lexapro);*<br>*duloxetine (Cymbalta), venlafaxine*<br>*(Effexor XR), desvenlafaxine,*<br>*levomilnacipran (Fetzima); bupropiom*<br>*(Wellbutrin); trazadone, mirtazapine,*<br>*voritioxetine; imipramine,*<br>*nortriptyline, doxepin, amitriptyline,*<br>*trimipramine, desipramine,*<br>*protriptyline; MAOIs* | Anise, basil (methyl chavicol CT), clove, nutmeg, star anise |
| *ANTIFUNGALS:* | See ANTIBIOTICS, ANTIFUNGALS, ANTIVIRALS |
| *ANTIPARASITICS (Pentamidine):* | Wormseed (American) |
| *ANTIPSYCHOTICS:*<br>*Olanzapine, paliperidone, asenapine,*<br>*clozapine, ariprazole, ziprasidone,*<br>*rispasidone, iloperidone,*<br>*thioxanthenes, phenothiazines, lithium,*<br>*haloperidol, loxapine, molindone, etc.* | Chaste tree, nutmeg, parsley |
| *ANTISEIZURE DRUGS (Valproate):* | Black Cumin (Thymoquinone CT) |
| *ANTIVIRALS:* | See ANTIBIOTICS, ANTIFUNGALS, ANTIVIRALS |
| *ASPIRIN (Acetylsalicylic Acid):* | Ajowan, allspice, anise, applemint (carvone CT), auracaria, basil, bay (West Indies), bay laurel (low risk), benzoin absolute, big badja gum, birch, black cumin, black pepper (eugenol CT), blue cypress (wood oil)—low risk, blue mallee, boldo, cajeput, calamus (beta-sarone CT), caraway (carvone CT), cassia, chaste |

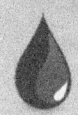

| | |
|---|---|
| | tree, cinnamon bark, cinnamon leaf, clove, cypress, dill (carvone CT), eucalyptus, fennel, Formosan cypress (twig oil), garlic, German chamomile, ginger, gully gum, hairy basil (various CTs), holy basil (various CTs), Indian borage (carvacrol & thymol CTs), lavandin, lovage, melissa, monarda (various CTs), mountain savory, niaouli (various CTs), nutmeg (East Indian), ocotea, oregano, patchouli, ravensara (various CTs), rosalina (1,8-cineole CT), saro (1,8-cineole CT), savory (wild, carvacrol & thymol CTs), spearmint (carvone CT), Southern blue gum, star anise, summer savory (carvacrol & thymol CTs), sweet inula (bornyl acetate, borneol CTs) tamala (various CTs), tarragon, thyme, turmeric, vilayti tulsi, white sage, white verbena (carvone-limonene CT), wintergreen, wormseed (American), yarrow; aloe vera (oral),[10330] avocado oil (oral),[10331] borage seed oil,[10332] DMSO,[10333] evening primrose oil,[10334] grapeseed oil,[10335,10336] olive oil (oral)[10337] |
| *ASPIRIN, SALICYLATE, & NSAID ALLERGIES:* | Birch, wintergreen; may also want to be cautious with ylang ylang (up to 10.4%); other essential oils with very low contents and risk include: clove (<0.6%), jasmine absolute (<3.4%) |
| *BARBITURATES:* *Pentobarbital, secobarbital, mephobarbital, phenobarbital, butabarbital, amobarbital, hexobarbital, etc.* | Aleppo pine, anise, applemint (carvone CT), bay laurel, bay (West Indies), big badja gum, blue mallee, boldo (1,8-cineole and 1,8-Cineole\Para-Cymene\Limonene CTs), cajeput, calamus (various CTs), caraway, cardamom, catnip, chaste tree, clary sage, damiana (1,8-cineole CT), dill (carvone CT), eucalyptus, fingerroot (1,8-cineole CT), Formosan cypress (Myrtenol CT), Fragonia (balanced CT), galangal (1,8-cineole CTs), guava leaf (1,8-Cineole CT), gully gum, hairy basil (various CTs), hemp, holy basil (eugenol CTs), kumquat (linalool CT), lavandin, lemon basil, lemon catnip (beta-citronellol CT), lemon myrtle, lemon tea tree, lemon verbena, lemongrass, lovage, mastic, may chang, myrtle, mugwort (1,8-cineole CT), niaouli (various CTs), nutmeg, peppermint, ravensara (1,8-cineole CT), ravintsara, rosalina (various CTs), rosemary, rosewood (large doses), sage (various CTs), saro (1,8-cineole CT), shell ginger (various CTs), Southern blue gum, Spanish sage, spearmint (carvone CT), spike lavender, star anise, sweet inula, sweet nancy (yomogi alcohol/1,8-cineole CT), tarragon, valerian, verbena, vilayti tulsi, white sage, white verbena (various CTs), wild marjoram (1,8-cineole CT), wormwood, yarrow |
| *BENZODIAZEPINES:* *Diazepam, clonazepam, alprazolam, lorazepam, flurazepam, etc.* | Anise, applemint (carvone CT), caraway, catnip, dill (carvone CT), lemon catnip (beta-citronellol CT), nutmeg, peppermint, star anise, tagetes, valerian |
| *BLEEDING DISORDERS* *(von Willbrand Disease (VWD), Hemophilia A, Hemophilia B):* | Ajowan, allspice, anise, applemint (carvone CT), auracaria, basil, bay (West Indies), bay laurel (low risk), benzoin absolute, big badja gum, birch, black cumin, black pepper (eugenol CT), blue cypress (wood oil)—low risk, blue mallee, boldo, cajeput, calamus (beta-sarone CT), caraway (carvone CT), cassia, chaste tree, cinnamon bark, cinnamon leaf, clove, cypress, dill (carvone CT), eucalyptus, fennel, Formosan cypress (twig oil), garlic, German chamomile, ginger, gully gum, hairy basil (various CTs), holy basil (various CTs), Indian borage (carvacrol & thymol |

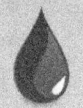

CTs), lavandin, lovage, melissa, monarda (various CTs), mountain savory, niaouli (various CTs), nutmeg (East Indian), ocotea, oregano, patchouli, ravensara (various CTs), rosalina (1,8-cineole CT), saro (1,8-cineole CT), savory (wild, carvacrol & thymol CTs), spearmint (carvone CT), Southern blue gum, star anise, summer savory (carvacrol & thymol CTs), sweet inula (bornyl acetate, borneol CTs) tamala (various CTs), tarragon, thyme, turmeric, vilayti tulsi, white sage, white verbena (carvone-limonene CT), wintergreen, wormseed (American), yarrow; aloe vera (oral),[10338] avocado oil (oral),[10339] borage seed oil,[10340] DMSO,[10341] evening primrose oil,[10342] grapeseed oil,[10343,10344] olive oil (oral)[10345]

| | |
|---|---|
| *BLOOD PRESSURE MEDS:*<br>*Diuretics, alpha-blockers, alpha-2 receptor agonist, beta-blockers, ACE inhibitors, angiotensin II receptor blockers, calcium channel blockers, central agonists, combined alpha/beta blockers, peripheral adrenergic inhibitors, vasodilators* | Ajowan, allspice, anise, applemint (carvone CT), auracaria, basil, bay (West Indies), bay laurel (low risk), benzoin absolute, big badja gum, birch, black cumin, black pepper (eugenol CT), blue cypress (wood oil)—low risk, blue mallee, boldo, cajeput, calamus (beta-sarone CT), caraway (carvone CT), cassia, chaste tree, cinnamon bark, cinnamon leaf, citronella, clove, cypress, dill (carvone CT), eucalyptus, fennel, Formosan cypress (twig oil), garlic, German chamomile, ginger, gully gum, hairy basil (various CTs), holy basil (various CTs), Indian borage (carvacrol & thymol CTs), lavandin, lovage, melissa, monarda (various CTs), mountain savory, niaouli (various CTs), nutmeg (East Indian), ocotea, oregano, patchouli, ravensara (various CTs), rosalina (1,8-cineole CT), saro (1,8-cineole CT), savory (wild, carvacrol & thymol CTs), spearmint (carvone CT), Southern blue gum, star anise, summer savory (carvacrol & thymol CTs), sweet inula (bornyl acetate, borneol CTs) tamala (various CTs), tarragon, thyme, turmeric, vilayti tulsi, white sage, white verbena (carvone-limonene CT), wintergreen, wormseed (American), yarrow; aloe vera (oral),[10346] avocado oil (oral),[10347] borage seed oil,[10348] DMSO,[10349] evening primrose oil,[10350] grapeseed oil,[10351,10352] olive oil (oral)[10353,10354,10355] |
| *BROKEN SKIN:* | Camphor, feverfew, fingerroot (camphor CT), hairy basil (various CTs), Japanese cedarwood (bark), ravintsara (camphor CT), sweet wormwood, white spruce, white verbena (camphor CT) |
| *CAFFEINE:* | Anise, applemint, peppermint, star anise |
| *CARDIAC DRUGS:* | Aloe vera (oral)[10356] |
| *CHEMOTHERAPY/ RADIOTHERAPY DRUGS, POTENTIATES (Essential oil constituent: Cancer/Drug):* | Alpha-pinene (lung/paclitaxel); aromadendrene (leukemia, colorectal/doxorubicin, digitonin/breast, leukemia); beta-caryophyllene (multiple cancers/multidrug); beta-elemene (multiple cancers/multidrug); beta-pinene (lung/paclitaxel); borneol (brain/facilitates delivery across BBB); bornyl acetate (gastric/5-fluouracil); camphor (breast/radiotherapy); citral (lymphoma/doxorubicin, multiple cancers/5-fluorouracil); diallyl disulfide (colorectal/oncogene expression, cervical/radiotherapy); diallyl trisulfide (osteosarcoma/multidrug, colorectal/multiple drugs, leukemia/multidrug, multiple cancers/modifies p-glycoprotein, gastric/docetaxel); cinnamaldehyde (colorectal/5-fluorouracil, |

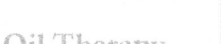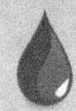

oxaliplatin); farnesol (refractory tumors/multiple drugs, prostate/docetaxel); eugenol (cervical/gemcitabine); geraniol (pancreatic/gemcitabine, colon/5-fluorouracil); germacrone (breast/Adriamycin); limonene (breast/multidrug, prostate/docetaxel); linalool (breast/doxorubicin); menthol (colorectal/methotrexate); nerolidol (colon/doxorubicin); sclareol (breast/multidrug); terpinene-4-ol (multiple cancers/multidrug); thymoquinone (gastric/5-fluorouracil, osteosarcoma/5-fluorouracil, oxaliplatin, leukemia/topotecan, doxorubicin, breast/tamoxifen, paclitaxel, doxorubicin, radiotherapy, ovarian/oxaliplatin, cisplatin, glioblastoma/temozolomide, colon/cisplatin, topotecan, pancreas/gemcitabine, nasopharyngeal/5-fluouracil, prostate/zoledronic acid, docetaxel, multiple myeloma/bortezomib, thalidomide); trans-anethole (ovarian/cisplatin, oxaliplatin); tricosane (colon/doxorubicin)

| | |
|---|---|
| *CHILDREN:* | Allspice (methyl eugenol CT), anise, applemint (pulegone and menthol CTs), basil (methyl chavicol and methyl eugenol CTs), bay laurel, betony (bicyclogermacrene CT), big badja gum, birch, black cumin, blue mallee, blue spruce, boldo, buchu, cajeput, calamus (various CTs), camphor, cardamom (1,8-Cineole CT), dill (with apiol), elecampane, eucalyptus, fennel, feverfew, fingerroot ((E)-beta-ocimene and camphor CTs), galangal (1,8-cineole CTs), genipi, gully gum, hairy basil (various CTs), holy basil (various CTs), hyssop (various CTs), Indian borage (carvacrol CT), Japanese cedarwood (bark), juniper (Utah), kumquat (linalool CT), ledum (*L. palustre*), mugwort, niaouli (various CTs), nutmeg, parsley, pennyroyal, peppermint, Ponderosa pine, ravensara (various CTs), ravintsara, rosalina (various CTs), rosemary (1,8-cineole, camphor CTs), sage, savin, Southern blue gum, Spanish sage, spearmint (pulegone-menthone-isomenthone CT), spike lavender, star anise, sweet inula, sweet wormwood, tansy, tarragon, thuja, western red cedar (leaves), white sage, white spruce, white verbena (camphor CT), wild marjoram (1,8-cineole CT), wild turmeric, wintergreen, wormseed (American), wormwood, yarrow; borage seed oil, evening primrose oil |
| *CHOLINERGIC MEDS:* <br> *Chloride, edrophonium chloride,* <br> *neostigmine, piridogstimina* | Ajowan, Aleppo pine, allspice, applemint, balsam poplar, basil (methyl eugenol CT), bay (West Indies), bergamot, bitter orange, black cumin, blue mountain sage (alpha-bisabolol CT), calamus, cinnamon (leaves), citron, clove, dill, dwarf pine (twigs), German chamomile, hairy basil (various CTs), hinoki, holy basil (various CTs), Indian borage (carvacrol & thymol CTs), juniper (Himalayan), kaffir lime petitgrain, lemon, lime, lovage, marjoram, melissa, monarda (various CTs), mountain savory, oregano, pink pepper (various CTs), plai (various CTs), ravensara (methyl eugenol CT), rosalina (methyl eugenol CT), savory (wild), Spanish sage, summer savory, sweet inula, sweet wormwood, tamala (various CTs), tarragon, thyme, wild marjoram, wormseed (American) |
| *CODEINE:* | Anise, peppermint (very large doses), rosemary, star anise |

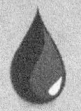

*CYTOCHROME P450 (CYP450) ENZYMES INTERFERENCE:*
*NSAIDs, proton-pump inhibitors, acetaminophen, anti-epileptics, immune modulators, blood sugar medications, blood pressure medications, antidepressants, antipsychotics, diabetic medications, antihistamines, antibiotics, anesthetics*

*Interaction risk is greatest with oral administration, although some essential oils contain constituents (methyl salicylate, safrole, citral, geraniol, chamazulene, and alpha-bisabolol) that could potentially interact when used topically as well.*

Aleppo pine, allspice, anise, applemint (various CTs), arnica, balsam fir (low risk), balsam poplar, basil, bay (West Indies), bergamot, betony (alpha-zingiberene CT), big badja gum, black cumin, black pepper (eugenol CT, beta-caryophyllene CT), black sage, blue mallee, blue mountain sage (alpha-bisabolol CT), blue tansy (chamazulene CT)—low risk, boldo (1,8-cineole and 1,8-Cineole\Para-Cymene\Limonene CTs), cajeput, calendula (low risk), cananga, cangerana, cardamom, cassia, chaste tree, Chinese cedarwood, cinnamon bark, cinnamon leaf, citronella (low risk), clove, copaiba, damiana (1,8-cineole CT), elecampane, eucalyptus (low risk), fennel, fingerroot (1,8-cineole CT and (E)-beta-ocimene CT), fragonia (balanced CT), frankincense, geranium, galangal (1,8-cineole CTs), garlic, genepi, German chamomile, ginger, grapefruit (low risk), guava leaf (1,8-Cineole CT, beta-caryophyllene CT), gully gum, hairy basil (various CTs), hemp, hinoki (low risk), holy basil, honey myrtle, hops, Japanese cedarwood (low risk), lavandin (Giant), ledum (*L. groenlandicum*), lemon basil, lemon catnip, lemon myrtle (citral CT), lemon tea tree, lemon verbena, lemongrass, lime, Maritime pine, mastic (various CTs), may chang, melissa, monarda (geraniol CT), mugwort (1,8-cineole CT and Great Mugwort), myrtle, niaouli (various CTs), nutmeg, ocotea, palmarosa, parsley, peppermint, Persian lime, ravensara (various CTs), red pine, ravintsara, rosalina (various CTs), rosemary, sage (various CTs), sandalwood (Australian), saro (1,8-cineole CT), shell ginger (various CTs), Southern blue gum, Spanish sage, spike lavender, star anise, sweet inula, sweet nancy (yomogi alcohol/1,8-cineole CT), tagetes (*T. erecta, flowers*), tangerine, tarragon, Texas cedarwood, thuja, thyme, turmeric, verbena, vilayti tulsi, Virginian cedarwood, western red cedar, white sage, white verbena (citral CT), wild marjoram (1,8-cineole CT), wormwood (alpha-thujone CT), yarrow, ylang ylang, zdravetz; aloe vera (oral),[10357] DMSO[10358,10359]

*DIABETIC MEDS (Antidiabetics):*
*Metformin, sulfonylureas, meglitinides, thiazidinediones, DPP-4 inhibitors, GLP-1 receptor agonists, SGLT2 inhibitors, insulin*

African bluegrass (myrcene CT), anise, applemint (carvone CT), basil, bay laurel, big badja gum, black cumin, black pepper (eugenol CT), blue mallee, caraway, cassia, cinnamon bark, citron, citronella, coriander, dill (carvone CT), eucalyptus, fennel, fenugreek, fingerroot ((E)-beta-ocimene CT), galangal (1,8-cineole CTs), geranium, gully gum, hairy basil (various CTs), honey myrtle, Indian borage (carvacrol & thymol CTs), juniper berry, juniper (Phoenician), lemon basil, lemon catnip, lemon myrtle (citral CT), lemon verbena, lemongrass, lime (distilled), lovage, may chang, melissa, monarda (various CTs), mountain savory, myrtle, niaouli (various CTs), ocotea, oregano, palmarosa, rosalina (1,8-cineole CT), rose, rosemary, sage, saro (1,8-cineole CT), savory (wild, carvacrol CT), Southern blue gum, spearmint (carvone CT), star anise, summer savory (carvacrol CT), sweet inula, tamala (various CTs), tangerine (distilled), thyme (geraniol and linalool CTs), turmeric, white sage, white verbena (various CTs), wild marjoram (1,8-cineole CT), wormseed (American, carvacrol CT); Epsom salts, olive oil (oral),[10360] sunflower oil (oral),[10361] sweet almond oil (oral)[10362]

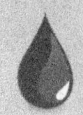

| | |
|---|---|
| *DIURETIC MEDS:*<br>**Amiloride, eplerenone, chlorothiazide, hydrochlorothiazide, bumetanide, fursemide, torsemide, etc.** | Indian borage (beta-caryophyllene CT), juniper berry, juniper (Phoenician), parsley, star anise; aloe vera (oral)[10363,10364] |
| *DRIVING/OPERATING MACHINERY:* | Bay laurel |
| *DRUGS THAT MAY CAUSE LIVER DAMAGE:*<br>*Acetaminophen, statins, NSAIDs, methotrexate, imipramine, steroids, oral contraceptives, sulfa drugs, etc.* | Applemint (with >14.9% Pulegone), betony (bicyclogermacrene CT), boldo (1,8-cineole and 1,8-Cineole\Para-Cymene\Limonene CTs), buchu, camphor, dill (aerial parts, carvone CT), feverfew, fingerroot, genipi, Japanese cedarwood (bark), juniper (Chinese), kumquat (linalool CT), mugwort, parsley, pennyroyal, ravintsara (camphor CT), rosemary (camphor CT), sage, savin, spearmint (pulegone-menthone-isomenthone CT), spike lavender, sweet wormwood, tansy, thuja, western red cedar (leaves), white spruce, white spruce, white verbena (camphor CT), wormwood, yarrow |
| *EPILEPSY (CONVULSIONS, SEIZURES):* | Ajowan, applemint (pulegone CTs), artemesia, bay laurel, betony (bicyclogermacrene CT), big badja gum, birch, blue spruce, blue mallee, blue tansy, boldo, buchu, cajeput, calamint, camphor, cardamom, chaste tree, damiana (1,8-cineole CT), eucalyptus, Engelmann spruce, fennel, fenugreek, feverfew, fingerroot, Fragonia (balanced CT), galangal (1,8-cineole CTs), guava leaf (1,8-Cineole and Alpha-Pinene CTs), gully gum, hairy basil (various CTs), holy basil (various CTs), hyssop (various CTs), Indian borage (carvacrol CT), genipi, Japanese cedarwood (bark), juniper (Chinese), juniper (Phoenician), juniper (Utah), lavandin, lovage, mugwort, myrtle, niaouli (various CTs), pennyroyal, ravensara (various CTs), ravintsara, rosalina (various CTs), rosemary, sage, saro (1,8-cineole CT), savin, shell ginger (various CTs), Southern blue gum, Spanish sage, spearmint (pulegone-menthone-isomenthone CT), spike lavender, sweet inula, sweet nancy (yomogi alcohol/1,8-cineole CT), sweet wormwood, tansy, thuja, thyme, vilayti tulsi, western red cedar (leaves), white sage, white spruce, white verbena (camphor CT), wild marjoram (1,8-cineole CT), wild turmeric, wintergreen, wormseed (American), wormwood, yarrow; borage seed oil,[10365,10366] evening primrose oil[10367] |
| *ESTROGEN RECEPTORS, INTERACT WITH:*<br><br>*Attach to estrogen receptors and mimic or block the action of estrogen (trans-anethole, sclareol, methyl chavicol (estragole)); or attach to estrogen receptors and displace estrogen (citral— geranial + neral, geraniol, nerol) or have an anti-estrogenic effect (eugenol)*<br><br>*Strong: Trans-anethole, sclareol, methyl chavicol (estragole)*<br><br>*High concentrations only: Citral (geranial + neral), geraniol, nerol, eugenol* | Strong: Anise (trans-anethole, methyl chavicol), allspice—berries methyl eugenol CT (methyl chavicol), basil—methyl chavicol CT (methyl chavicol), clary sage (sclareol), fennel (trans-anethole, methyl chavicol), Himalayan cedarwood—needles (trans-anethole), holy basil (methyl chavicol), Japanese cedarwood (16-Kaurene/Valencene CT; scalreol), moringa—seeds Naphthalene CT (methyl chavicol), mugwort (trans-anethole), ravensara (methyl chavicol), star anise (trans-anethole), tarragon (methyl chavicol); Only in high concentrations: African bluegrass—myrcene CT (geraniol), allspice (eugenol), applemint (geraniol), basil—sweet (eugenol), black pepper (eugenol), calendula (geraniol), camphor (eugenol), cardamom—alpha-terpinyl acetate CT (nerol), cassia (eugenol), cinnamon bark (eugenol), citronella (citral, geraniol), clove (eugenol), davana (nerol), dill (geraniol), fenugreek (geraniol), fingerroot (geraniol, nerol), geranium (geraniol), ginger (geraniol), hairy basil (nerol, eugenol), |

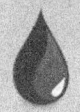 

helichrysum (nerol), holy basil (eugenol), honey myrtle (geraniol, nerol), jasmine absolute—benzyl benzoate CT (eugenol), lemon—distilled (citral), lemon catnip (citral, geraniol, nerol), lemon myrtle (citral), lemon tea tree (citral, geraniol), lemon verbena (citral, geraniol, nerol), lemongrass (citral, nerol), lime (distilled; citral), may chang—citronellal CT (geraniol), melissa (citral, geraniol, nerol), mountain savory (geraniol), neroli (geraniol), ocotea—leaves (citral), palmarosa (geraniol), Persian lime (citral), ravensara (eugenol), rose (geraniol, nerol, eugenol), rosewood (geraniol, nerol), tamala (eugenol), tangerine (citral, geraniol), thyme—carvacrol, geraniol, linalool, and thymol CTs (geraniol), verbena (geraniol, eugenol), white verbena (citral, geraniol)

| | |
|---|---|
| *FLUOROURACIL:* | Eucalyptus, peppermint |
| *GASTROESOPHAGEAL REFLUX DISEASE (GERD):* | Birch, peppermint (low risk), wintergreen |
| *GLUTEN INTOLERANCE:* | Wheat germ oil[10368,10369] |
| *G6PD (GLUCOSE-6-PHOSPHATE DEHYDROGENASE DEFICIENCY:* | Applemint (menthol CTs), blue spruce, blue tansy, camphor, cinnamon bark, Engelmann spruce, fenugreek, feverfew, fingerroot ((E)-beta-ocimene and camphor CTs), galangal (1,8-cineole CTs), hairy basil (various CTs), Indian borage (carvacrol CTs), Japanese cedarwood (bark), juniper (Utah), lavandin, mugwort, peppermint, ravintsara (camphor CT), rosemary (various CTs), sage (various CTs), Spanish sage, spearmint (menthone CT—low risk), spike lavender, sweet wormwood, tansy, thuja, white sage, white spruce, white verbena (camphor CT), wild turmeric, yarrow |
| *HORMONE REPLACEMENT THERAPY:* | Anise (low risk), chaste tree, clary sage |
| *IBUPROFEN* | Anise, fennel (trans-anethole CTs), star anise |
| *IMMUNOSUPPRESSANTS:* *Azathioprine, mycophenolate mofetil, cyclosporine, methotrexate, leflunomide, cyclophosphamide, chlorambucil, nitrogen mustards* | Peppermint; any essential oil that may stimulate the immune system should be used cautiously |
| *IRON DEFICIENCY:* | Peppermint, spearmint (all CTs) |
| *KIDNEY DISORDERS/ COMPROMISED KIDNEY FUNCTION:* | Applemint (with >14.9% Pulegone), betony (bicyclogermacrene CT), boldo, buchu, calamus, dill (aerial parts, carvone CT), genipi, kumquat (linalool CT), juniper (Chinese), mugwort, parsley, pennyroyal, sage, savin, spearmint (pulegone-menthone-isomenthone CT), sweet wormwood, tansy, thuja, western red cedar (leaves), wormseed (American), wormwood, yarrow |

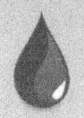

| | |
|---|---|
| *LEVODOPA (L-DOPA):* | Lovage |
| *LIVER DISORDERS/ COMPROMISED LIVER FUNCTION:* | Applemint (with >14.9% Pulegone), betony (bicyclogermacrene CT), boldo (1,8-cineole and 1,8-Cineole\Para-Cymene\Limonene CTs), buchu, camphor, dill (aerial parts, carvone CT), feverfew, fingerroot, genipi, Japanese cedarwood (bark), juniper (Chinese), kumquat (linalool CT), mugwort, parsley, pennyroyal, ravintsara (camphor CT), rosemary (camphor CT), sage, savin, spearmint (pulegone-menthone-isomenthone CT), spike lavender, sweet wormwood, tansy, thuja, western red cedar (leaves), white spruce, white spruce, white verbena (camphor CT), wormseed (American), wormwood, yarrow |
| *LONG-TERM USE (TOXICITY):* | Birch, hyssop (various CTs), tansy, wintergreen; borage seed oil,[10370] DMSO[10371] |
| *MAOI ANTIDEPRESSANTS:* *Tranylcypromine (**Parnate**), phenelzine (Nardil), isocarboxazid (Marplan)* | Allspice, bay (West Indies), black pepper (eugenol CT), cinnamon leaf, clove, hairy basil (various CTs), holy basil (eugenol CT), nutmeg, parsley, tamala (various CTs) |
| *MUCOUS MEMBRANE IRRITATION:* | Ajowan, allspice, bay (West Indies), black pepper (eugenol CT), cassia, cinnamon bark, cinnamon leaf, clove, hairy basil (various CTs), holy basil (various CTs), Indian borage (carvacrol & thymol CTs), lemon tea tree, may chang, melissa, monarda (various CTs), mountain savory, ocotea, oregano, peppermint, savory (wild, carvacrol & thymol CTs), summer savory, tamala (various CTs), thyme, wormseed (American, carvacrol CT) |
| *NCAA BANNED SUBSTANCE:* | Bitter orange extracts (not essential oils; seek legal counsel) |
| *ORAL CAUTIONS:* | Allspice (methyl eugenol CT), applemint (pulegone CTs), basil (methyl chavicol and methyl eugenol CTs), bay laurel, benzoin absolute, betony (bicyclogermacrene CT), big badja gum, birch, black cumin, blue mallee, blue spruce, boldo, buchu, cajeput, calamus (various CTs), camphor, cardamom, dill (carvone CT), eucalyptus, fennel (methyl chavicol CT), feverfew, fingerroot (camphor CT), galangal (1,8-cineole CTs), genipi, gully gum, hairy basil (various CTs), holy basil (various CTs), hyssop (various CTs), Indian borage (carvacrol & thymol CTs), Japanese cedarwood (bark), jasmine absolute, juniper (Chinese), juniper (Utah), kumquat (linalool CT), ledum (*L. palustre*), lovage (root), monarda (thymol CT), mountain savory, mugwort, niaouli (various CTs), nutmeg, oakmoss absolute, oregano (thymol CT), palo santo, parsley, pennyroyal, Peru balsam, Ponderosa pine, ravensara (various CTs), ravintsara, rosalina (various CTs), rosemary (various CTs), rue, sage, saro (1,8-cineole CT), savin, savory (wild, thymol CT), Southern blue gum, Spanish sage, |

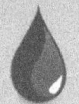

spearmint (pulegone-menthone-isomenthone CT), spike lavender, summer savory (thymol CT), sweet inula, sweet wormwood, tansy, tarragon, thuja, thyme, tolu balsam, vilayti tulsi, western red cedar (leaves), white sage, white spruce, white verbena (camphor CT), wild marjoram (1,8-cineole CT), wild turmeric, wintergreen, wormseed (American), wormwood, yarrow, ylang ylang (I fractions); kukui nut[10372,10373]

| | |
|---|---|
| *PARACETAMOL:* | Rosemary |

*PARKINSON'S DISEASE:* Ajowan, applemint (pulegone CTs), artemesia, bay laurel, betony (bicyclogermacrene CT), big badja gum, birch, blue spruce, blue mallee, blue tansy, boldo, buchu, cajeput, calamint, camphor, cardamom, chaste tree, damiana (1,8-cineole CT), eucalyptus, Engelmann spruce, fennel, fenugreek, feverfew, fingerroot, Fragonia (balanced CT), galangal (1,8-cineole CTs), guava leaf (1,8-Cineole and Alpha-Pinene CTs), gully gum, hairy basil (various CTs), holy basil (various CTs), hyssop (various CTs), genipi, Japanese cedarwood (bark), juniper (Chinese), juniper (Phoenician), juniper (Utah), lavandin, lovage, mugwort, myrtle, niaouli (various CTs), pennyroyal, ravensara (various CTs), ravintsara, rosalina (various CTs), rosemary, sage, saro (1,8-cineole CT), savin, shell ginger (various CTs), Southern blue gum, Spanish sage, spearmint (pulegone-menthone-isomenthone CT), spike lavender, sweet inula, sweet nancy (yomogi alcohol/1,8-cineole CT), sweet wormwood, tansy, thuja, thyme, vilayti tulsi, western red cedar (leaves), white sage, white spruce, white verbena (camphor CT), wild marjoram (1,8-cineole CT), wild turmeric, wintergreen, wormseed (American), wormwood, yarrow; borage seed oil,[10374,10375] evening primrose oil[10376]

*PHOTOSENSITIZING:* Amyris, angelica, bay laurel (absolute), bergamot, bitter orange, celery seed, citron, cumin, fennel, garlic, ginger (very, very low risk), grapefruit (mild), kabosu, kaffir lime petitgrain, khella, kumquat, lemon, lime (cold-pressed\expressed), Mediterranean mandarin, neroli (very low risk), orange (sweet), Persian lime, petitgrain (low risk), rue (moderate risk), tagetes, tangerine (very low risk), yuzu (cold-pressed; low risk)

*PHYTOESTROGENS:*

*Interact with estrogen receptors to mimic or block the action of estrogen.*

**1)** *Trans-anethole, sclareol, methyl chavicol (estragole), (Z)-ligustilide*
**2)** *Xanthorrhizol (enhances estrogenic gene expression)*
3) *High concentrations only (displace estrogen from receptors)—citral (geranial + neral), geraniol, nerol, eugenol*

1) Anise (trans-anethole, methyl chavicol), allspice—berries methyl eugenol CT (methyl chavicol), basil—methyl chavicol CT (methyl chavicol), clary sage (sclareol), fennel (trans-anethole, methyl chavicol), Japanese cedarwood (16-Kaurene/Valencene CT; scalreol), hairy basil (methyl chavicol), Himalayan cedarwood—needles (trans-anethole), holy basil (methyl chavicol), lovage (ligustilide), moringa—seeds Naphthalene CT (methyl chavicol), mugwort (trans-anethole), ponderosa pine (methyl chavicol), ravensara (methyl chavicol), star anise (trans-anethole), tarragon (methyl chavicol);
2) Wild turmeric (distilled);
3) African bluegrass—myrcene CT (geraniol), allspice (eugenol), applemint (geraniol), basil—sweet (eugenol), bay—West Indies (eugenol), black pepper (eugenol), calendula (geraniol), camphor (eugenol), cardamom—

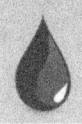

alpha-terpinyl acetate CT (nerol), cassia (eugenol), cinnamon bark (eugenol), citronella (citral, geraniol), clove (eugenol), davana (nerol), dill (geraniol), fenugreek (geraniol), fingerroot (geraniol, nerol), geranium (geraniol), ginger (geraniol), hairy basil (nerol, eugenol), helichrysum (nerol), holy basil (eugenol), honey myrtle (geraniol, nerol), jasmine absolute—benzyl benzoate CT (eugenol), lemon—distilled (citral), lemon basil (citral, geraniol, nerol), lemon catnip (citral, geraniol, nerol), lemon myrtle (citral), lemon tea tree (citral, geraniol), lemon verbena (citral, geraniol, nerol), lemongrass (citral, nerol), lime (distilled; citral), may chang—citronellal CT (geraniol), melissa (citral, geraniol, nerol), mountain savory (geraniol), neroli (geraniol), ocotea—leaves (citral), palmarosa (geraniol), Persian lime (citral), ravensara (eugenol), rose (geraniol, nerol, eugenol), rosewood (geraniol, nerol), tamala (eugenol), tangerine (citral, geraniol), thyme—carvacrol, geraniol, linalool, and thymol CTs (geraniol), verbena (geraniol, eugenol), white verbena (citral, geraniol)

| | |
|---|---|
| *PREGNANCY & LACTATION:* | Allspice, anise, applemint (pulegone CTs), auracaria, bay laurel, basil (methyl chavicol and methyl eugenol CTs), bay (West Indies), betony (bicyclogermacrene CT), birch, black cumin, black pepper (eugenol CT), blue cypress (wood oil)—low risk, blue spruce, boldo, buchu, calamus (various CTs), camphor, carrot seed, cassia, chaste tree, cinnamon bark, cinnamon leaf, citronella (low risk), clove, dill (with apiol), elecampane, fennel, feverfew, fingerroot ((E)-beta-ocimene and camphor CTs), Formosan cypress (twig oil), garlic, genipi, hairy basil (various CTs), hemp, holy basil (various CTs), honey myrtle, hops, hyssop (various CTs), Indian borage (carvacrol & thymol CTs), Japanese cedarwood (bark), juniper (Chinese), juniper (Utah), kanuka (37+ weeks), kumquat (linalool CT), ledum (*L. palustre*), lemon basil, lemon catnip, lemon myrtle (citral CT), lemon tea tree, lemon verbena, lemongrass, manuka (37+ weeks), lovage, may chang, melissa, mountain savory, mugwort, myrrh, nutmeg, ocotea, oregano, parsley, pennyroyal, Ponderosa pine, ravensara (various CTs), ravintsara (camphor CT), rosalina (methyl eugenol CT), rosemary (1,8-cineole, camphor CTs), rue, sage, savin, savory (wild, carvacrol & thymol CTs), Spanish sage, spearmint (pulegone-menthone-isomenthone CT), spike lavender, star anise, summer savory, sweet wormwood, tamala (various CTs), tansy, tarragon, thuja, verbena, western red cedar (leaves), white sage, white spruce, white turmeric, white verbena (camphor CT), wild turmeric, wintergreen, wormseed (American), wormwood, yarrow; calendula (oral),[10377] borage seed oil (oral),[10378,10379] evening primrose oil (oral)[10380,10381] |
| *PREMATURE BREAST DEVELOPMENT (Premature Thelarche):* | Anise, black cumin, fennel, star anise |
| *PSYCHOTROPIC DRUGS:* | See ANTIPSYCHOTICS |

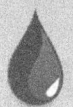
| | |
|---|---|
| *REFSUM DISEASE, AMACR DEFICIENCY:* | Jasmine absolute, moringa ((E)-phytol CT) |
| *SALICYLATE SENSITIVITIES:* | *Avoid (15%+):* Birch, wintergreen<br><br>*Caution (amounts of 0.5%–14.9%):* Clove bud (< 0.6%), clove stem (< 0.4%), jasmine absolute (< 3.4%), ylang ylang I Madagascan (< 10.5%), ylang ylang II Madagascan (< 5.4%) |
| *TAMOXIFEN:* | Wild turmeric (distilled) |
| *TOPICAL APPLICATION (SENSITIZATION):* | African bluegrass (myrcene CT), benzoin absolute, cassia, cinnamon bark, citronella, elecampane, fingerroot (CTs with geraniol), garlic, geranium, hairy basil (citral CT), honey myrtle, jasmine absolute, lemon basil, lemon tea tree, lemon verbena, lemon catnip, lemon myrtle (citral CT), lemon tea tree, lemongrass, lime (distilled), may chang, melissa, monarda (geraniol CT), oakmoss absolute, palmarosa, Peru balsam, rose, tamala, tangerine (distilled), thyme (various CTs), tolu balsam, white verbena (citral CT), wormseed (American, carvacrol CT), ylang ylang |
| *VENTRICULAR FIBRILLATION:* | Applemint (menthol CT), peppermint |

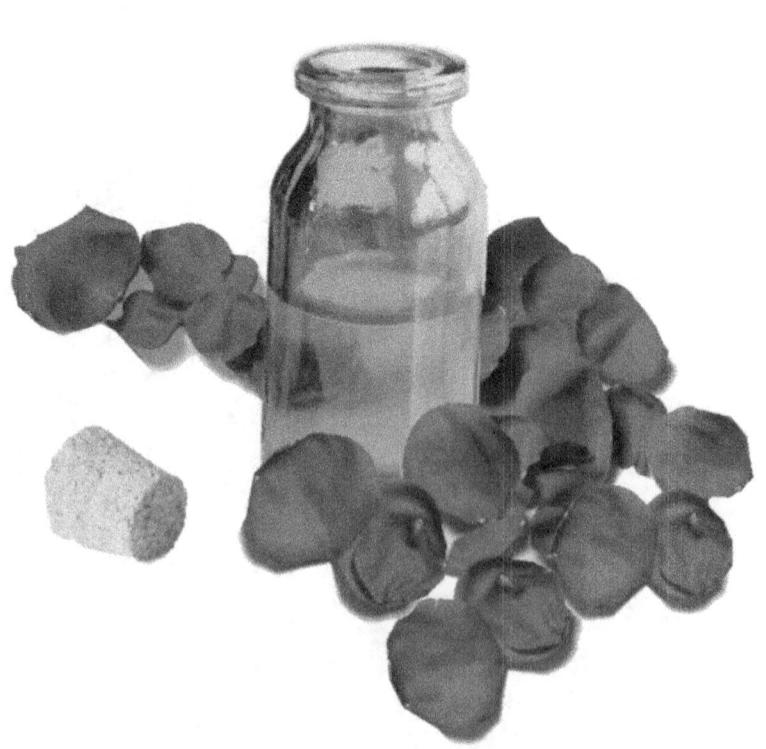

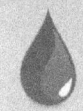

# APPENDIX H:

10382,10383,10384,10385,10386,10387,10388,10389,10390,10391,10392,10393, 10394

## POSSIBLE ESSENTIAL OIL ADULTERATIONS

The adulteration of essential oils is all about profits. Adulteration reduces the costs of the end product, which allows the unscrupulous vendor to provide more "essential oil" and therefore acquire more profits. The costlier the raw materials from which an essential oil is obtained (or the difficulty obtaining good yields from these materials), the more likely it is to be adulterated. Rose and melissa are two great examples of essential oils that are very costly to produce and therefore often adulterated. Adulterated essential oils will be more likely to cause skin irritation, undesirable effects, and toxicity, especially if used long-term. There are several ways to adulterate an essential oil including:

1) The addition of undetectable materials such as vegetable or mineral oil. These materials are generally not detectable by GC-MS analysis except by observing a reduced "total area" of detectable components, alcohol solubility tests, or derivatization (the transformation of compounds into a product with a similar structure).

2) The addition of detectable materials such as solvents and perfumery materials (Abitol, benzyl alcohol, benzyl benzoate, carbitol, diacetone alcohol, dipropylene glycol, dipropylene glycol methyl ether, ethanol, isopropyl myristate, kerosene fractions, methylene chloride, methyl ethyl ketone, nitrobenzene, phenyl ethyl alcohol, phthalate esters, propylene glycol, rosin hydrogenated methyl ester, toluene, tracetin, and tripropylene clycol methyl ether). These adulterants are generally detectable by GC-MS analysis.

3) The addition of cheaper, but chemically identical (called nature identical), synthetic compounds such as technical grade anethole to anise oil, limonene or carvone to caraway.

4) The addition of isolated or natural compounds to essential oils (i.e. isolated menthol to peppermint, isolated 1,8-cineole to eucalyptus).

5) The addition of cheaper essential oils or fractions of essential oils (i.e. lemon oil to bergamot oil, lavandin oil to lavender oil, turpentine fractions to fir needles oils).

6) The addition of unnatural synthetic fragrance compounds that do not exist in nature during manufacturing (hydroxycitronellal, synthetic white musk).

7) The addition of bases (jamine absolute base, bergamit base) or reconstituted essential oils (basically chemical copies of genuine essential oils created from various chemicals) to genuine essential oils. This is particularly a problem with floral absolutes like jasmine and rose.

8) Passing off one essential oil as another. For example, cornmint may be de-mentholized and then passed off as peppermint, or star anise for anise.

The following are known or common adulterations of the essential oils in this work.

**African Bluegrass:** Unknown or not commonly adulterated.

**Agarwood:** Added patchouli, white oil, vetiver, sandalwood, synthetic white musk, soa-soa, or buaya oil. White oil adulteration may be detected by swiping the oil across the neck. If a warm sensation is produced it is likely adulterated. A greasy feel or a strong alcohol smell are also signs of adulteration.

**Ajowan:** Addition of ajowan chaff oil, which can be detected by thymol content below 35% in the thymol CT.

**Aleppo Pine:** Unknown or not commonly adulterated.

**Allspice:** Cheaper pimento leaf may be added to berry (allspice) oil, which increases the specific gravity and the phenol content; clove stem or leaf, or fractions from the isolation of eugenol, may also be added to berry oil. Pimenta leaf may be adulterated with clove stem or leaf, or combination and fractions.

**Amyris:** Fractions of the oils sold as the whole oil or addition of cedarwood or copaiba balsam. Amyris may be used to adulterate sandalwood oil.

**Angelica Root:** Added angelica leaf or seed oil, phellandrene, added lovage root (*Levisticumn officinale*)—would increase specific gravity and refractive index.

**Anise:** Added cheaper star anise oil or technical grade (USP) anethole.

**Applemint:** Unknown or not commonly adulterated.

**Arnica:** Unknown or not commonly adulterated.

**Auracaria:** Unknown or not commonly adulterated.

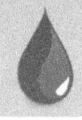 

**Balsam Fir:** Added turpentine oil fractions, camphene, or bornyl acetate.

**Balsam Poplar:** Unknown or not commonly adulterated.

**Basil (sweet, tropical):** Added Reunion basil (methyl chavicol CT of sweet basil)—would increase specific gravity and refractive index; added α-linalool; added linalool or methyl chavicol.

**Bay (West Indies):** Addition of clove leaf essential oil, rose terpenes, lime oil terpenes, synthetic myrcene or other terpenes.

**Bay Laurel:** Added kerosene or alcohol.

**Benzoin Absolute:** Addition of vanillin, benzyl benzoate, ethyl cinnamate, benzyl cinnamate, or benzoic acid.

**Bergamot:** Added linalool or linalyl acetate.

**Bergamot Mint:** Added linalool or linalyl acetate.

**Betony:** Unknown or not commonly adulterated.

**Big Badja Gum:** Essential oils high in 1,8-cineole are not typically adulterated, but alpha-terpineol may be added to convert another eucalyptus species to *E. radiata.*

**Birch:** Added methyl salicylate or wintergreen.

**Bitter Orange:** Added sweet orange oil; added citrus terpenes or traces of other typical compounds; added fatty aldehydes, monoterpene alcohols, and esters to terpeneless and folded citrus oils.

**Black Cumin Seed:** Added black cumin chaff oil.

**Black Pepper:** Added phellandrene, pinene, limonene, dipentene, clove sesquiterpenes, or caryophyllene; or added *Schinus molle* oil, atractyulis concrete oil, elemi, *Eucalyptus dives*, or copaiba balsam.

**Black Sage:** Unknown or not commonly adulterated.

**Blue Cypress:** Unknown or not commonly adulterated.

**Blue Mallee:** Essential oils high in 1,8-cineole are not typically adulterated, but alpha-terpineol may be added to convert another eucalyptus species to *E. radiata.*

**Blue Mountain Sage:** Unknown or not commonly adulterated.

**Blue Spruce:** Unknown or not commonly adulterated.

**Blue Tansy:** Unknown or not commonly adulterated.

**Boldo:** Unknown or not commonly adulterated.

**Buchu:** May be adulterated with monoterpene sulfides, like *p*-mentha-8-thiol-3-one.

**Buddha Wood:** Unknown or not commonly adulterated.

**Cajeput:** Added eucalyptus (or substituted completely), niaouli, or *Melaleuca symphyocarpa.*

**Calamus:** Added amyris, copaiba balsam, cedarwood fractions, sesquiterpenes fractions from various sources, or limonene.

**Calendula:** Substituting another *Tagetes* spp.

**Camphor:** Added camphor fractions.

**Canadian Fleabane:** Added synthetic compounds (terpinyl acetate, d-limonene, etc.) or cajeput or eucalyptus oil, which can be detected by a decrease in the characteristic fresh-herbaceous odor of Canadian fleabane.

**Cangerana:** Unknown or not commonly adulterated.

**Cape Chamomile:** Unknown or not commonly adulterated.

**Caraway:** Added synthetic carvone or limonene, or caraway chaff oil (distilled from the waste material from the threshing of caraway fruits). The chaff oil will be higher in terpenes and lower in carvone.

**Cardamom:** Added linalyl acetate, 1,8-cineole, or alpha-terpinyl acetate.

**Carrot Seed:** Added d-limonene or oil from siftings (a process used to separate the seeds from the chaff.

**Cassia:** Added kerosene or rosin; added cinnamaldehyde, methyl cinnamic aldehyde, or coumarin.

**Catnip:** Unknown or not commonly adulterated.

**Cedarwood:** Added Chinese cedarwood (*Cupressus funebris*). May also be confused with Himalayan cedarwood oil.

**Celery:** Addition of synthetic limonene and traces of alkyl phthalides. Maraniol and cyclotene may also be added to fortify or enrich poorer oils.

**Chaste Tree:** Added Asiatic species such as *V. negundo, V. rotundifolia,* or *V. trifolia.*

**Chinese Cedarwood:** Substituted with Texas or Virginian cedarwood, or either of these essential oils added to Chinese cedarwood.

**Chinese Red Pine:** Unknown or not commonly adulterated.

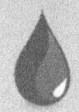

**Cilantro:** Unknown or not commonly adulterated.

**Cinnamon:** Mixing cinnamon leaves in with cinnamon bark—would increase specific gravity and eugenol content; added cassia oil—would increase the specific gravity and cinnamic aldehyde content; added benzaldehyde, eugenol, or cinnamaldehyde.

**Cistus:** Adulteration of the flowering plant oil is not common; however, the resinoid may be adulterated with added Abitol with small amounts of ambroxan and para-methyl acetophenone.

**Citron:** Unknown or not commonly adulterated.

**Citronella:** Added dipentene or citronella terpenes.

**Clary sage:** Added linalool or linalyl acetate, or addition of *Mentha citrata*.

**Clove Bud:** Added clove leaf oil; added eugenol or eugenyl acetate; added terpineol, dibenzyl, dibenzyl ether, or acetins.

**Copaiba:** Added Gurjun balsam (*Dipterocarpus alantus*).

**Coriander:** Added combinations of linalool, certain pyrazines, decyl aldehyde, decyl alcohol, linalyl acetate, phellandrene, and limonene.

**Cumin:** Added cuminaldehyde, para-cymene and other compounds typically present in cumin—would affect optical rotation.

**Cypress:** Added alpha-pinene, camphene, delta-3-carene, or myrcene; or added juniper berry, juniper wood, pine needle oils, and cypress oil from different species.

**Damiana:** Added rose fragrance chemicals or aroma chemcials (phenylethyl alcohol, ionones, phenylethyl formate, damascenone, damascene).

**Davana:** Unknown or not commonly adulterated.

**Dill:** Added alpha-phellandrene and limonene.

**Douglas Fir:** Fir needles oils may be adulterated with added turpentine oil fractions, camphene, or bornyl acetate.

**Dwarf Pine:** Unknown or not commonly adulterated.

**Elecampane:** Unknown or not commonly adulterated.

**Elemi:** Added limonene or alpha-phellandrene.

**Engelmann Spruce:** Unknown or not commonly adulterated.

**Eucalyptus:** Essential oils high in 1,8-cineole are not typically adulterated, but alpha-terpineol may be added to convert another eucalyptus species to *E. radiata*.

**Eucalyptus Dives:** Unknown or not commonly adulterated.

**Fennel:** Added anethole, limonene, estragole, fenchone, phellandrene, or other monoterpenes; Added bitter fennel oil.

**Fenugreek:** Unknown or not commonly adulterated.

**Ferula:** Unknown or not commonly adulterated.

**Feverfew:** Unknown or not commonly adulterated.

**Fingerroot:** Unknown or not commonly adulterated.

**Formosan Cypress:** Unknown or not commonly adulterated.

**Fragonia:** Unknown or not commonly adulterated.

**Frankincense:** Unknown or not commonly adulterated.

**Galangal:** Unknown or not commonly adulterated.

**Galbanum:** Added beta-pinene, undecatrienes, camphene, and others; Added foreruns of galbanol.

**Garlic:** Added aliphatic sulphide mixtures containing 2-propenyl disulphide, 1-propenyl disulphide, etc.

**Genipi:** Unknown or not commonly adulterated.

**Geranium:** Added citronellol or geraniol.

**German Chamomile:** Added azulenes or bisabolol; less expensive chamomiles.

**Ghandi Root:** Unknown or not commonly adulterated.

**Ginger:** Added galangal oil.

**Gingergrass:** Added geraniol.

**Gobre Salla:** Unknown or not commonly adulterated.

**Goldenrod:** Unknown or not commonly adulterated.

**Grapefruit:** Added citrus terpenes, nootkatone, or traces of other typical compounds; added fatty aldehydes, monoterpene alcohols, and esters to terpeneless and folded citrus oils.

**Grindelia:** Unknown or not commonly adulterated.

**Guaiacwood:** Unknown or not commonly adulterated.

**Guava Leaf:** Unknown or not commonly adulterated.

**Guggul:** Unknown or not commonly adulterated.

**Gully Gum:** Essential oils high in 1,8-cineole are not typically adulterated, but alpha-terpineol may be added to convert another eucalyptus species to E. radiata.

**Gurjun Balsam:** Unknown or not commonly adulterated.

**Hairy Basil:** Unknown or not commonly adulterated.

**Helichrysum:** Added species or subspecies of *Helichrysum* oils.

**Hemp:** Unknown or not commonly adulterated.

**Hinoki:** Unknown or not commonly adulterated.

**Holy Basil:** Added methyl chavicol and linalool.

**Honey Myrtle:** Unknown or not commonly adulterated.

**Hops:** Unknown or not commonly adulterated.

**Hyssop:** Added cedar leaf, camphor, camphor fractions, lavandin, myrtle, or sage oils.

**Indian Borage:** Unknown or not commonly adulterated.

**Japanese Cedarwood:** Unknown or not commonly adulterated.

**Jasmine Absolute:** Added indole, alpha-amyl cinnamaldehyde, ylang ylang fractions, jasmones, or jasmine bases.

**Juniper Berry:** Added terpene hydrocarbon mixtures containing alpha-pinene, camphene, and delta-3-carene; Added juniper leaf/branch oil or spoiled juniper berries; Poor oil from the fermentation process; or added turpentine oil fractions.

**Juniper (Chinese):** Unknown or not commonly adulterated.

**Juniper (Himalayan):** Unknown or not commonly adulterated.

**Juniper (Phoenician):** Unknown or not commonly adulterated.

**Kabosu:** Unknown or not commonly adulterated.

**Kaffir Lime Petitgrain:** Unknown or not commonly adulterated.

**Kanuka:** Unknown or not commonly adulterated.

**Katrafay:** Unknown or not commonly adulterated.

**Khella:** Unknown or not commonly adulterated.

**Kumquat:** The adulteration of kumquat is not reported, but it is possible it is adulterated similarly to other citrus fruits with the addition of citrus terpenes.

**Kunzea:** Unknown or not commonly adulterated.

**Lavandin:** Unknown or not commonly adulterated.

**Lavender:** Added lavandin, spike lavender, or rectified *Cinnamomum* spp. with acetylated *Cinnamomum* spp. or acetylated lavandin oils, rosemary fractions; added linalool (dihydolinalool marker), linalyl acetate (dihydrolinalyl acetate marker), lavandulol, lavandulyl acetate, terpinyl propionate, isobornyl acetate, and terpineol.

**Ledum:** Unknown or not commonly adulterated.

**Leleshwa:** Unknown or not commonly adulterated.

**Lemon:** Added citrus terpenes, citral, or traces of other typical compounds; added fatty aldehydes, monoterpene alcohols, and esters to terpeneless and folded citrus oils.

**Lemon Basil:** Unknown or not commonly adulterated.

**Lemon Catnip:** Unknown or not commonly adulterated.

**Lemon Eucalyptus:** Unknown or not commonly adulterated.

**Lemon Myrtle:** Added synthetic citral.

**Lemon Tea Tree:** Unknown or not commonly adulterated.

**Lemon Verbena:** Lemon verbena oil distilled over lemon oil.

**Lemongrass:** Added citral.

**Lime:** Added citrus terpenes or traces of other typical compounds; added fatty aldehydes, monoterpene alcohols, and esters to terpeneless and folded citrus oils.

**Lovage:** Added lovage seed or herb oil, or added cyclotene, maraniol, n-butyl phthalide, nbutylidene phthalide, or synthetic compounds of compounds naturally present in lovage oil.

**Magnolia:** Codistilled with ylang ylang flowers.

**Manuka:** Unknown or not commonly adulterated.

**Maritime Pine:** Unknown or not commonly adulterated.

**Marjoram:** Added terpineol, turpentine-terpineol fractions, carvacrol, or para-cymene; added *Melaleuca alternifolia*.

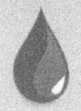

**Mastic:** Added alpha-pienne, myrcene, or limonene.

**May Chang:** Unknown or not commonly adulterated.

**Mediterranean Mandarin:** The adulteration of Mediterranean Mandarin is not reported, but it is possible it is adulterated similarly to other citrus fruits with the addition of citrus terpenes.

**Tea tree:** Added terpinen-4-ol, alpha-terpinene, or gamma-terpinene.

**Melissa:** Reconstructed from mixtures of citronella, lemon, and May chang (*Litsea cubeba*) oils with other compounds; added lemon eucalyptus or citronella oil.

**Monarda:** Unknown or not commonly adulterated.

**Moringa:** Unknown or not commonly adulterated.

**Mountain Savory:** Added oregano or thyme oils.

**Mugwort:** Unknown or not commonly adulterated.

**Muhuhu:** Unknown or not commonly adulterated.

**Myrrh:** Refined myrrh with both essential oil and extracted matter.

**Myrtle:** Essential oils high in 1,8-cineole are not typically adulterated, but alpha-terpineol may be added to convert another eucalyptus species to *E. radiata*.

**Neroli:** Complete reconstruction with synthetic compounds.

**Niaouli:** Substituted with eucalyptus, to which trace amounts of terpinyl esters, aldehydes, terpineol, terpinolene, benzaldehyde, borneol, etc. are added.

**Nutmeg:** Added limonene, alpha-pinene, myrcene, camphene, terpinolene, dipentene, or turpentine fractions; added *Melaleuca alternifolia*.

**Oakmoss Absolute:** Unknown or not commonly adulterated.

**Ocotea:** Unknown or not commonly adulterated.

**Opoponax:** Added myrrh, copaiba balsam, traces of lovage, and Siberian pine fractions.

**Orange (sweet):** Added citrus terpenes or traces of other typical compounds; added fatty aldehydes, monoterpene alcohols, and esters to terpeneless and folded citrus oils.

**Oregano:** added carvacrol, para-cymene, or dimethyl sulfide—may be detected by "by-note" of oil evaporating on test paper; or added thyme oil.

**Oriental Arborvitae:** Unknown or not commonly adulterated.

**Palmarosa:** Added geraniol, mixtures of geraniol, citronellol, and nerol, or gingergrass oil.

**Palo Santo:** Unknown or not commonly adulterated.

**Parsley:** Unknown or not commonly adulterated.

**Patchouli:** Added cedarwood, Chinese patchouli, or clove oils; Added terpenes, methyl abietate, hydroabietic alcohols, camphor oil residues, or vetiver fractions/residues; added castor oil.

**Pennyroyal:** Unknown or not commonly adulterated.

**Peppermint:** Added menthol, menthyl acetate, or phellandrene; added cottonseed, spearmint, or corn mint (*Mentha arvensis)* oil; or cruder adulterations with benzyl alcohol, triacetin, nopol, 2-cyclohexyl-cyclohexanone, and trimethyl cyclohexanol.

**Persian Lime:** Added citrus terpenes or traces of other typical compounds; added fatty aldehydes, monoterpene alcohols, and esters to terpeneless and folded citrus oils.

**Peru Balsam:** Added benzyl benzoate, benzyl salicylate, benzyl alcohol, high-boiling, low cost solvents, vanillin, dibenzyl, ethyl benzoate, ethyl cinnamate, and cinnamic alcohol.

**Petitgrain:** Added mixtures of linalool, linalyl acetate, alpha-terpineol, geranyl acetate, neral acetate, nerone, and pyrazines.

**Pine:** Added bornyl acetate, isobornyl acetate, limonene, alpha-pinene, or camphene.

**Pink Pepper:** Unknown or not commonly adulterated.

**Plai:** Unknown or not commonly adulterated.

**Ponderosa Pine:** Unknown or not commonly adulterated.

**Rabbitbrush:** Unknown or not commonly adulterated.

**Ravensara:** May be confused and substituted with ravintsara.

**Ravintsara:** May be confused and substituted with ravensara.

**Red Pine:** Unknown or not commonly adulterated.

**Rhododendron:** Unknown or not commonly adulterated.

**Roman Chamomile:** Added isobutyl angelate and bisabolols.

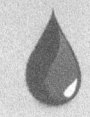 

**Rosalina:** Unknown or not commonly adulterated.

**Rose Otto:** Reconstructions using damascones, beta-ionone plus citronellol, other rose alcohols, and rose steroetenes; addition of a few percent of phenylethyl alcohol, ethyl alcohol, rhodinol fractions; Added cheaper Moroccan or Crimea rose oils; formerly adulterated with palmarosa and guaiacwood essential oil, and spermaceti.

**Rosemary:** Added camphor, turpentine, or isobornyl acetate with eucalyptus and turpentine oil fractions; added fractions of camphor, cedarwood, or pine oil; added Spanish sage oil.

**Rosewood:** Added linalool, plus trace amounts of methyl heptenone, methyl heptenol, 3-octanol, or para-methyl acetophenone.

**Rue:** Unknown or not commonly adulterated.

**Sage:** Added cedar leaf, thuja oil fractions, Spanish sage fractions, rosemary oil, and various Artemisia oils.

**Sandalwood:** East Indian sandalwood is frequently adulterated with Australian sandalwood, araucaria oil, copaiba oil, amyris oil, bleached copaiba balsam with odorless solvents (benzyl benzoate, benzyl alcohol, diethyl phthalate, isopropyl myristate, and liquid paraffin), or added sandalwood terpenes or fragrance chemicals. Australian sandalwood is not commonly adulterated, but in the past it was cut with *Eucaria spicata* and *Eremophila mitchell*. New Caledonian and Hawaiian sandalwood essential oils may be subject to similar adulterations as above.

**Saro:** Unknown or not commonly adulterated.

**Savin:** Unknown or not commonly adulterated.

**Savory (wild):** Added oregano or thyme oils.

**Schisandra Fruit:** Unknown or not commonly adulterated.

**Shell Ginger:** Unknown or not commonly adulterated.

**Saim Wood:** Unknown or not commonly adulterated.

**Siberian Fir:** Fir needles oils may be adulterated with added turpentine oil fractions, camphene, or bornyl acetate.

**Silver Fir:** Added turpentine oil fractions, camphene, or bornyl acetate.

**Southern Blue Gum:** Essential oils high in 1,8-cineole are not typically adulterated, but alpha-terpineol may be added to convert another eucalyptus species to *E. radiata*.

**Spanish Sage:** Unknown or not commonly adulterated.

**Spearmint:** Added carvone or Chinese spearmint.

**Spike Lavender:** Added whole oils or fractions of eucalyptus, camphor, rosemary, lavandin or Spanish sage oils.

**Spikenard:** Added *Valeriana wallichii* oil, patchouli oil, cajeput oil, borneol, isobornyl valerianate, terpinyl valerianate, terpineol, or eugenol.

**Spruce (black):** Added bornyl acetate, isobornyl acetate, limonene, alpha-pinene, or camphene.

**Star Anise:** Unknown or not commonly adulterated.

**Summer Savory:** Added oregano or thyme oils.

**Sweet Inula:** Unknown or not commonly adulterated.

**Sweet Nancy:** Unknown or not commonly adulterated.

**Sweet Wormwood:** Unknown or not commonly adulterated.

**Tagetes:** Unknown or not commonly adulterated.

**Tamala:** Unknown or not commonly adulterated.

**Tangerine:** Added citrus terpenes, dimethyl anthranilate, alpha-sinesal, perilla aldehyde, or traces of other typical compounds; added fatty aldehydes, monoterpene alcohols, and esters to terpeneless and folded citrus oils.

**Tansy:** Added cedar leaf or sage oil.

**Tarragon:** Added estragole (sometimes 50% or more) along with small amounts of phellandrene and other terpenes, which will decrease the time it will show on a perfume blotter.

**Texas Cedarwood:** Added Virginian cedarwood.

**Thuja:** Unknown or not commonly adulterated.

**Thyme:** Adding wild thyme (*Thymus mastichina*) to thyme (*Thymus vulgaris*); added thymol, carvacrol, para-cymene, or a commercial product called thymene.

**Tolu Balsam:** Added rosin or resinous residues from other balsams (copaiba balsam, Peru balsam, acaroid, colophonium).

**Tsuga:** Added bornyl acetate, isobornyl acetate, limonene, alpha-pinene, or camphene.

**Turkish Pine:** Unknown or not commonly adulterated.

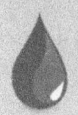

**Turmeric:** Unknown or not commonly adulterated.

**Valerian:** Added bornyl isovalerate or kesso root oil.

**Verbena:** Unknown or not commonly adulterated.

**Vetiver:** Added cedarwood derivatives, amyris oil, caryophyllene, vetiverol, cyperus oil, other grasses, or diluted with non-aromatic substances.

**Vilayti Tulsi:** Unknown or not commonly adulterated.

**Virginian Cedarwood:** Unknown or not commonly adulterated. Although, it may be used to adulterate other cedarwood oils.

**Western Red Cedar:** Unknown or not commonly adulterated.

**White Fir:** Added turpentine oil fractions, camphene, or bornyl acetate.

**White Pine:** Unknown or not commonly adulterated.

**White Sage:** Unknown or not commonly adulterated.

**White Spruce:** Unknown or not commonly adulterated.

**White Turmeric:** Unknown or not commonly adulterated.

**White Verbena:** Unknown or not commonly adulterated.

**Wild Chamomile:** Unknown or not commonly adulterated.

**Wild Marjoram:** Unknown or not commonly adulterated.

**Wild Turmeric:** Unknown or not commonly adulterated.

**Wintergreen:** Added methyl salicylate.

**Wormseed (American):** Unknown or not commonly adulterated.

**Wormwood:** Unknown or not commonly adulterated.

**Yarrow:** Unknown or not commonly adulterated.

**Yuzu:** Mixtures of grapefruit and tangerine essential oil; added citrus terpenes.

**Ylang ylang:** Added benzyl acetate, methyl benzoate, para-cresyl methyl ether, geranyl acetate, benzyl benzoate, or benzyl cinnamate; Complete reconstruction with synthetic compounds; Added cedarwood, lower ylang ylang grades, or Gurjun balsam oil; added *Artabotrys unicinatus* flowers.

**Zdravetz:** Unknown or not commonly adulterated.

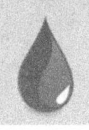

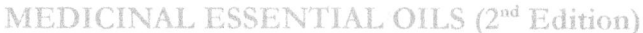

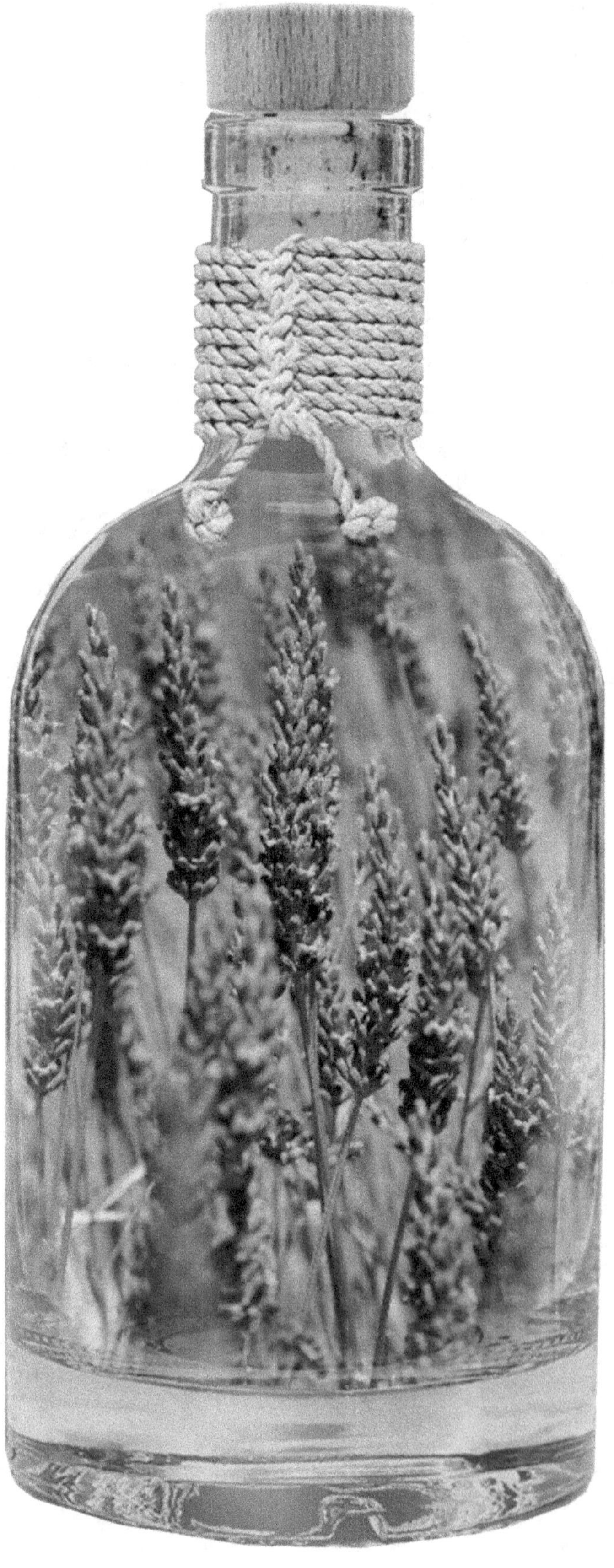

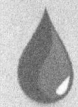

Use this chart to apply oils to the feet to support specific organs, body parts, or systems.

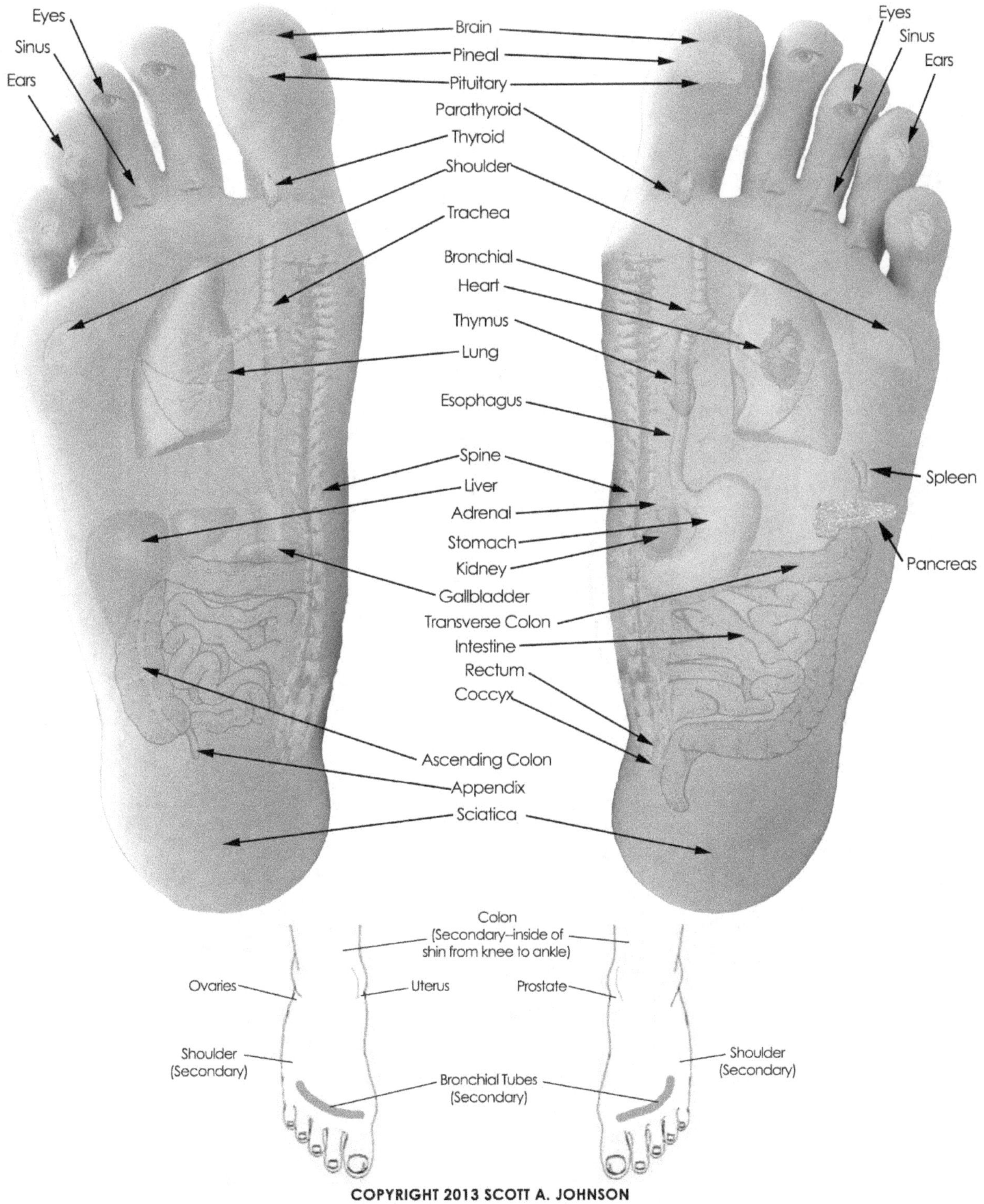

Eyes
Sinus
Ears

Brain
Pineal
Pituitary
Parathyroid
Thyroid
Shoulder
Trachea
Bronchial
Heart
Thymus
Lung
Esophagus
Spine
Liver
Adrenal
Stomach
Kidney
Gallbladder
Transverse Colon
Intestine
Rectum
Coccyx
Ascending Colon
Appendix
Sciatica

Eyes
Sinus
Ears

Spleen

Pancreas

Colon
(Secondary–inside of
shin from knee to ankle)

Ovaries

Uterus

Prostate

Shoulder
(Secondary)

Bronchial Tubes
(Secondary)

Shoulder
(Secondary)

**COPYRIGHT 2013 SCOTT A. JOHNSON**

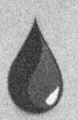

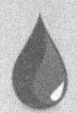

About the Author:

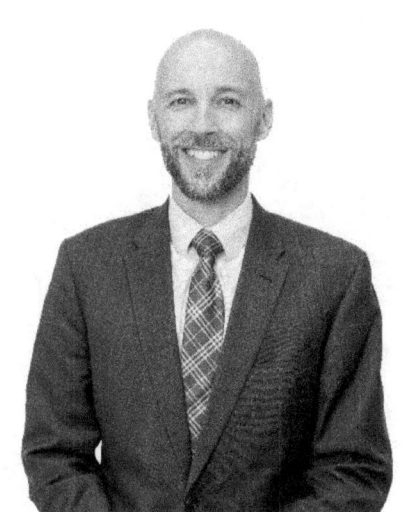

As one of the most prolific natural medicine writers of the 21st century, Dr. Scott A. Johnson has empowered tens of thousands of individuals to realize greater wellness naturally through more than a twenty evidence-based books. His research emphasis is medicinal essential oils and their clinical application for the leading ailments afflicting modern man. He is one of the world's leading experts on essential oils and supercritical essential oils. Dr. Johnson pioneered evidence-based essential oil therapy, which combines the art of ancient healing with modern science to maximize their therapeutic benefits. One of his research focuses is the safety of essential oils, and he has published internationally on the subject.

His diverse educational background—doctor of naturopathy, board-certified alternative medical practitioner, Certified Elite Essential Oil Specialist (CEEOS), Certified Clinical Master Aromatherapist (CCMA), and Certified Professional Coach (CPC) and critical mind allow him to take complex health topics to any audience. He is an acclaimed international speaker and has delivered keynote presentations across North America, Europe, Australia, and Asia. He travels the globe carrying his passion for people and natural medicine and sharing the secrets of natural healing.

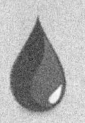

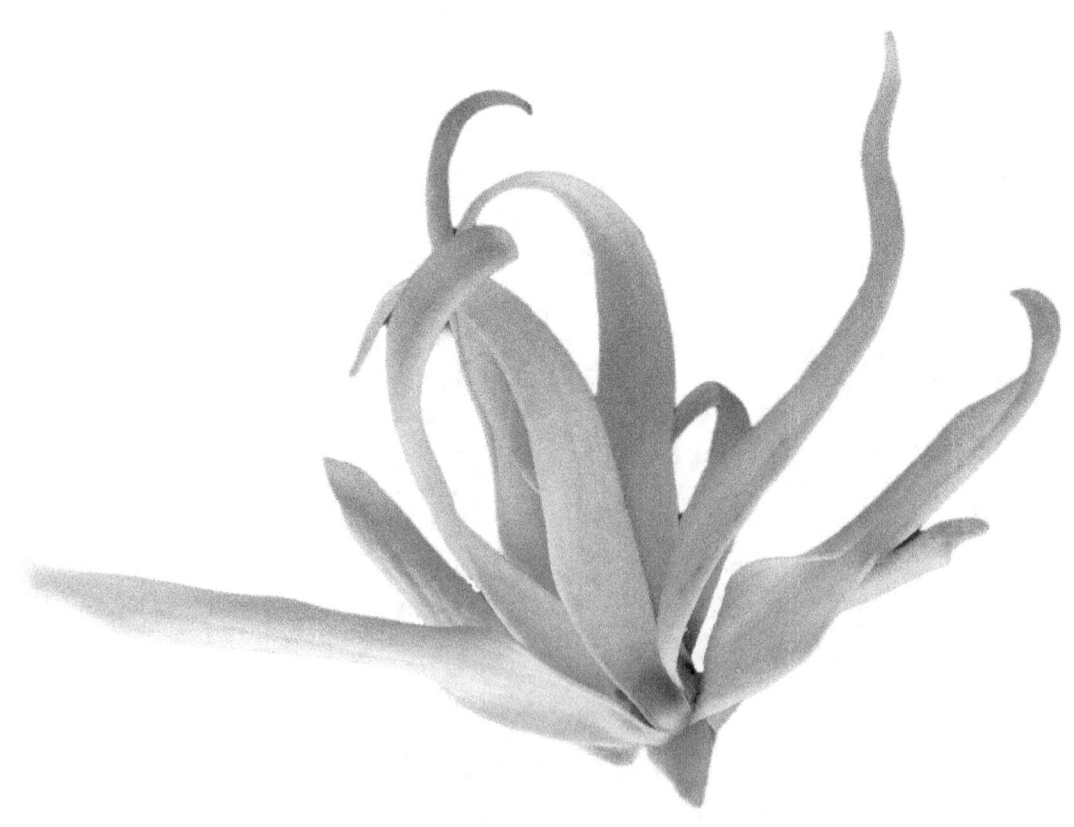

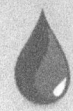

# REFERENCES

[1] Gochev V, Stoyanova A, Girova T, et al. Chemical composition and antimicrobial activity of Bulgarian peppermint oils. *Sci Papers*. 2008;36(5):83-89. Available at: https://blogs.uni-plovdiv.net/argon/files/2008/03/010_NT36_2008.pdf

[2] Satyal P, Pappas RS. Antique lavender essential oil from 1945, its chemical composition and enantiomeric distribution. *Nat Volatiles Essent Oils*. 2016;3(2):20-25.

[3] Kubeczka KH. Possibilities of quality determination of essential oils which are used as medicine. In: Kubeczka KH, editor. Vorkommen und Analytik atherischer Ole. Stuttgart, Germany: Thieme. p 60–71.

[4] Crowell PL. Prevention and therapy of cancer by dietary monoterpenes. *J Nutr*. 1999 Mar;129(3):775S-779S.

[5] Chidambara Murthy KN, Jayaprakasha GK, Patill BS. D-limonene rich volatile oil from blood oranges inhibits angiogenesis, metastasis and cell death in human colon cancer cells. *Life Sci*. 2012 Oct 5;91(11-12).

[6] Lahlou M. Essential oils and fragrance constituents: bioactivity and mechanism of action. *Flav Frag J*. 2004 Mar/Apr;19(2):159-165.

[7] Buchbauer G, Jirovetz L. Aromatherapy - use of fragrances and essential oils as medicaments. 1994 Sep/Oct; 9(5):217- 22.

[8] Abdel-Maksoud G, El-min AR. A review on the materials used during mummification process in ancient Egypt. *Med Archaeology Archaeometry*. 2011;11(2):129-50.

[9] Charrié-Duhaut A, Connan J, Rouquette N, et al. The canopic jars of Rameses II: real use revealed by molecular study of organic residues. *J Archaeological Sci*. 2007;34:957-67.

[10] Colombini MP, Modugno Fr, Silvano Fl, et al. Characterization of the Balm of an Egyptian Mummy from the Seventh Century B.C. *Studies in Conservation*. 2000;45(1):19-29.

[11] David, A. R. (2007). 'Imhotep: founder of medical science in ancient Egypt,' in W F Bynum and H Bynum (eds.), Biographical Dictionary of the History of Medicine. Westport, CT: Greenwood Publishing Group.

[12] Indiana University. Medicine In Ancient Egypt. Available at: http://www.indiana. edu/~ancmed/egypt.HTM.

[13] Curran J. The Yellow Emperor's Classic of Internal Medicine. *BMJ*. 2008 Apr 5;336(7647):777.

[14] Grammaticos PC, Diamantis A. Useful known and unknown views of the father of medicine, Hippocrates and his teacher Democritus. *Hell J Nucl Med*. 2008 Jan-Apr;11(1):2-4.

[15] Bassolé IHN, Juliani HR. Essential Oils in Combination and Their Antimicrobial Properties. *Molecules*. 2012;17:3989-4006.

[16] Chamberlain M. Les essences au point de vue de leurs propriétes antiseptiques. *Ann Inst Pasteur 1*. 1887;153-64.

[17] Danon A, Ben-Shimon, Z. Ben-Zvi. Effect of exercise and heat exposure on percutaneous absorption of methyl salicylate. *Eur J Clin Pharm*. 1986;31(1):49-52.

[18] Millar RJ, Bowman J. Oil of wintergreen (methyl salicylate) poisoning treated by exchange transfusion. *Can Med Assoc J*. 1961 Apr 29;84(17):956-7.

[19] Caseley RT. Salicylate poisoning: a case in infancy treated by exchange transfusion. *N Z Med J*. 1962 Mar;61:149-53.

[20] Chyka PA. et al. Salicylate poisoning: an evidence-based consensus guideline for out-of-hospital management. *Clin Toxicol (Phila)*. 2007;45(2):95-13.

[21] Chan TY. Potential dangers from topical preparations containing methyl salicylate. *Hum Exp Toxicol*. 1996 Sep;15(9):747-5.

[22] Davis JE. Are one or two dangerous? Methyl salicylate exposure in toddlers. *J Emerg Med*. 2007 Jan;32(1):63-9.

[23] Stevenson CS. Oil of wintergreen (methyl salicylate) poisoning. Report of three cases, one with autopsy, and a review of the literature. *Am J Med Sci*. 1937;193:772-799.

[24] Eimas A. Methyl salicylate poisoning in an infant. Report of patient with partial necropsy. *J Pediatr*. 1938;13:500-54.

[25] Darben T, Cominos B, Lee CT. Topical eucalyptus oil poisoning. *Australas J Dermatol*. 1998 Nov;39(4):265-7.

[26] Myott E. Case of eucalyptus poisoning. *Brit M J*. 1906;1:558.

[27] Eikholt TH, Box RH. Toxicities of peppermint and Pycnanthemun albescens oils, Fam. Labiateae. *J Pharm Sci*. 1965;54:1071-72.

[28] O'Mullane NM, Joyce P, Kamath SV, et al. Adverse CNS effects of menthol-containing olbas oil [letter]. *Lancet*. 1982;1(8281):1121.

[29] Halicioglu O, Astarcioglu G, Yaprak I, et al. Epileptic seizures caused by accidental ingestion of sage (Salvia officinalis L.) oil in children: A rare, exceptional case of a threat to public health. *Ped Neurol*. 2011 Oct;45(1):259-60. [13] Craig JO. Poisoning by the volatile oils in childhood. *Arch Dis Child*. 1953;28:259-67.

[30] Craig JO. Poisoning by the volatile oils in childhood. *Arch Dis Child*. 1953;28:259-67.

[31] Hindle RC. Eucalyptus oil ingestion. *N Z Med J*. 1994 May 11;107(977)185-6.

[32] Tibballs J. Clinical effects and management of eucalyptus oil ingestion in infants and small children. *Med J Aust*. 1995 Aug;163(4):177-80.

[33] Melis K. Bochner A, Janssens G. Accidental nasal eucalyptol and menthol instillation. *Eur J Pediatr*. 1989 Aug;148(8):786-7.

[34] Reynolds JEF. Martindale: The Extra Pharmacopoeia. *The Pharmaceutical Press, London*. 1993.

[35] No author listed. Monographs on the medicinal uses of plants. *Exeter: European Scientific Cooperative on Phytotherapy*. 1997.

[36] Javorka K, Tomori Z, Zavarska L. Protective and defensive airway reflexes in premature infants. *Physiol Bohemoslov*. 1980;29(1):29-35.

[37] Pereira EJ, Sim L, Driver HS, et al. The effect of inhaled menthol on upper airway resistance in humans: A randomized controlled crossover study. *Can Respir*. 2013 Jan-Feb;20(1):e1-e4.

[38] Henley DV, Lipson N, Korach KS, et al. Prepubertal gynecomastia linked to lavender and tea tree oils. *N Engl J Med*. 2007 Feb;356(5):479-85.

[39] Politano VT, McGinty D, Lewis EM, et al. Uterotrophic assay of percutaneous lavender oil in immature female rats. *Int J Toxicol*. 2013 Mar-Apr;32(2):123-29.

[40] Albini A, Rosano C, Angelini G, et al. Exogenous hormonal regulation in breast cancer cells by phytoestrogens and endocrine disruptors. *Curr Med Chem*. 2014 Feb;21:1129-45.

[41] Sashidhara KV, Rosaiah JN, Kumar A, et al. Cell growth inhibitory action of an unusual labdane diterpene, 13-epi- sclareol in breast and uterine cancers in vitro. *Phytother Res*. 2007 Nov;21(11):1105-07.

[42] Chen C, De Gasperi M, Salcedo R, et al. Evaluation of the phytochemical anethole as an anti-tumor agent in MCF-7 cells. *Cancer Res*. 2009 Dec;69:3100.

[43] Trock BJ, Hilakivi-Clarke L, Clarke R. Metaanalysis of soy intake and breast cancer risk. *J Natl Cancer Inst*. 2006;98:459–471.

[44] This P, De La Rochefordiere A, Clough K, et al. Phytoestrogens after breast cancer. *Endocr Relat Cancer*. 2001;8:129–134.

[45] Lazennec G, Bresson D, Lucas A, et al. ER beta inhibits proliferation and invasion of breast cancer cells. *Endocrinology*. 2011 Sep;142(9):4120-30.

[46] Dip R, Lenz S, Antignac JP, et al. Global gene expression profiles induced by phytoestrogens in human breast cancer cells. *Endocr Relat Cancer*. 2008 Mar;15(1):161-73.

[47] Wang C, Kurzer Ms. Phytoestrogen concentration determines effects on DNA synthesis in human breast cancer cells. *Nutr Cancer*. 1997;28(3):236-47.

[48] Mahaira LG, Tsimplouli C, Sakellaridis N, et al. The labdane diterpene sclareol (labd-14-ene-8. 13-diol) induces apoptosis in human tumor cell lines and suppression of tumor growth in vivo via a p53-independent mechanism of action. *Eur J Pharmacol*. 2011 Sep;666(1-3):173-82.

[49] Dimas K, Hatziantoniou S, Tseleni S, et al. Sclareol induces apoptosis in human HCT116 colon cancer cells in vitro and suppression of HCT116 tumor growth in immunodeficient mice. *Apoptosis*. 2007 Apr;12(4):685-94.

[50] Noori S, Hassan ZM, Salehian O. Sclareol reduces CD4+ CD25+ FoxP3+ treg cells in breast cancer model in vivo. *Iran J Immunol*. 2013 Mar;10(1):10-21.

[51] Sashidhara KV, Rosaiah JN, Kumar A, et al. Cell growth inhibitory action of an unusual labdane diterpene, 13-epi-sclareol in breast and uterine cancers in vitro. *Phytother Res*. 2007 Nov;21(11):1105-8.

[52] Chen FP, Chien MH, Chern IY. Impact of lower concentrations of phytoestrogens on the effects of estradiol in breast cancer cells. *Taiwan J Obstet Gynecol*. 2016 Dec;55(6):826-834.

[53] Satih S, Chalabi N, Rabiau N, et al. Transcriptional profiling of breast cancer cells exposed to soy phytoestrogens after BRCA1 knockdown with a whole human genome microarray approach. *Nutr Cancer*. 2010;62(5):659-67.

[54] Cotterchio M, Boucher BA, Manno M, et al. Dietary phytoestrogen intake is associated with reduced colorectal cancer risk. *J Nutr*. 2006 Dec;136(12):346-53.

[55] Fritz H, Seely D, Flower G, et al. Soy, red clover, and isoflavones and breast cancer: a systematic review. *PLoS One*. 2013 Nov;8(11):e81968.

[56] Melzig MF, Moller I, Jarry H. New investigations of the in vitro pharmacological activity of essential oils from Apiaceae. *Zeitschrift fur Phytotherapie*. 2003;24:112-16.

[57] Howees MJ, Houghton PJ, Barlow DJ, et al. Assessment of estrogenic activity in some common essential oil constituents. *J Pharm Pharmacol*. 2002 Nov;54(11):1521-28.

[58] Dixon RA, Ferreira D. Genistein. *Phytochemistry*. 2002 Jun;60(3):205-11.

[59] Ko KP. Isoflavones: chemistry, analysis, functions and effects on health and cancer. *Asian Pac J Cancer Prev*. 2014;15(17):7001-10.

[60] Martini MC, Dancisak BB, Haggans CJ, et al. Effects of soy intake on sex hormone metabolism in premenopausal women. *Nutr Cancer*. 1999;34(2):133-39.

[61] Forschmidt P. Teratogenic activity of flavor additives. *Teratology*. 1979;19:26A.

[62] Domaracky M, Rehak P, Juhas S, et al. Effects of selected plant essential oils on the growth and development of mouse preimplantation embryos in vivo. *Physiol Res*. 2007;56(1):97-104.

[63] Vesselinovitch SD, Rao KVN, Mihailovich N. Transplacental and lactational carcinogenesis by safrole. *Cancer Res*. 1979 Nov;39(11):4378-80.

[64] Zhou L, Zhang K, Li J, et al. Inhibition of vascular endothelial growth factor-mediated angiogenesis involved in reproductive toxicity induced by sesquiterpenoids of Curcuma zedoaria in rats. *Reprod Toxicol*. 2013 Jun;37:62-9.

[65] Wilson JG. Present status of drugs as teratogens in man. *Teratology*. 1973 Feb;7(1):3-15.

[66] Chu YH, Chen HW, Li Q, et al. Antifertility effect of volatile oil of Daucus carota seeds. *Reproductive & Contraception*. 1985;5:37-40.

[67] Dong JY, Xue LQ, Zhu XW, et al. Antifertility agents form seeds of Daucus carota. *Zhongcaoyao*. 1981;12:61.

[68] Sharma MM, Lal G, Jacob D. Estrogenic and pregnancy interceptor effects of carrot seed daucus carota seeds. *Indian J Exp Biol*. 1976 Jul;14(4):506-8.

[69] Keenan DL, Dharmarajan AM, Zacur HA. Dietary carrot seed results in diminished ovarian progesterone secretion, whereas a metabolite, retinoic acid, stimulates progesterone secretion in the in vitro perfused rabbit ovary. *Fertil Steril*. 1997 Aug;68(2):358-63.

[70] Ostad SN, Khakinegard B, Sabzevari O. Evaluation of the teratogenicity of fennel essential oil (FEO) on the rat embryo limb buds culture. *Toxicol*. 2004 Oct;18(5):623-7.

[71] Karabulut AK, Ulger H, Pratten MK. Protection by free oxygen radical scavenging enzymes against salicylate- induced embryonic malformation in vitro. *Toxicol In Vitro*. 2000 Aug;14(4):297-307.

[72] Overman DO, White JA. Comparative teratogenic effects of methyl salicylate applied orally or topically to hamsters. *Teratology*. 1983 Dec;28(3):421-6.

[73] European Medicines Agency. Public statement on the use of herbal medicinal products containing estragole. Available at: http://www.ema.europa.eu/docs/en_GB/document_library/Scientific_guideline/2010/04/WC500089960.pdf.

[74] Forschmidt P. Teratogenic activity of flavor additives. *Teratology*. 1979;19:26A.

[75] Toaff ME, Hunt TP, Andersen ME. Selective oocyte degeneration and impaired fertility in rats with aliphatic monoterpene, citral. *J Reprod Fertil.* 1979;55:347-52.
[76] Randerath K, Putman KL, Randerath E. Flavor constituents in cola drinks induce hepatic DNA adducts in adult and fetal mice. *Biochem Biophys Res Commun.* 1993 Apr 15;192(1):61-8.
[77] Tisserand R, Young R. *Essential Oil Safety* (Second Edition). 2014 Churchill Livingstone Elsevier.
[78] Burkhard PR, Burkhardt K, Haenggeli CA, et al. Plant-induced seizures: reappearance of an old problem. *J Neurol.* 1999 Aug;246(8):667-70.
[79] Skalli S, Bencheikh RS. Epileptic seizures induced by fennel essential oil. *Epileptic Discord.* 2011;13:345-347.
[80] Early DF. Pennyroyal: a rare case of epilepsy. *Lancet.* 1961;281:580-81.
[81] Koutroumanidou E, Kimbaris A, Kortsaris A, et al. Increased seizure latency and decreased severity of pentylenetetrazol-induced seizures in mice after essential oil administration. *Epilepsy Res Treat.* 2013;2013:532657.
[82] Waldman N. Seizure caused by dermal application of over-the-counter eucalyptus oil head lice preparation. *Clin Toxicol (Phila).* 2011 Oct;49(8):750-1.
[83] Darben T, Cominos B, Lee CT. Topical eucalyptus poisoning. *Australas J Dermatol.* 1998 Nov;39(4):265-7.
[84] Miller LG. Herbal medicinals: selected clinical considerations focusing on known or potential drug-herb interactions. *Arch Intern Med.* 1998;158(20):2200-2211.
[85] Adams MKM, Sparrow JM, Tole DM. Inadvertent administration of Olbas oil into the eye: a surprisingly frequent presentation. *Eye.* 2009;23(1):244.
[86] Naganuma M, Hirose S, Nakayama Y, et al. A study of the phototoxicity of lemon oil. *Arch Dermatol Res.* 1985;278(1):31-6.
[87] Placzek M, Froemel W, Eberlein B, et al. Evaluation of phototoxic properties of fragrances. *Acta Derm Venereol.* 2007;87(4):312-6.
[88] Kejlova K, Jirova D, Bendova H, et al. Phototoxicity of essential oils intended for cosmetic use. *Toxicol In Vitro.* 2010 Dec;24(8):2084-9.
[89] Opdyke DIJ. Monographs on fragrance raw materials. *Food Cosmet Toxicol.* 1974;12(Suppl.):509.
[90] Dugrand-Judek A, Olry A, Hehn A, et al. The distribution of coumarins and furanocoumarins in Citrus species closely matches citrus phylogeny and reflects the organization of biosynthetic pathways. *PLoS One.* 2015 Nov;10(11):e0142757.
[91] Kohlert C, Schindler G, Marz RW, et al. Systemic availability and pharmacokinetics of thymol in humans. *J Clin Pharmacol.* 2002 Jul;42(7):731-7.
[92] Jager W, Nasel B, Nasel C, et al. Pharmacokinetic studies of the fragrance constituent 1,8-cineole in humans during inhalation. *Chem Senses.* 1996 Aug;21(4):191-97.
[93] Fillipson AF. Short-term inhalation exposure to turpentine: toxicokinetics and acute effects in men. *Occup Environ Med.* 1996 Feb;53(2):100-5.
[94] Fillipson AF. Short-term inhalation exposure to turpentine: toxicokinetics and acute effects in men. *Occup Environ Med.* 1996 Feb;53(2):100-5.
[95] Falk-Filipsson A, Lof A, Hagberg M, et al. d-limonene exposure to humans by inhalation: uptake, distribution, elimination, and effects on the pulmonary function. *J Toxicol Environ Health.* 1993 Jan;38(1):77-88.
[96] Jager W, Buchbauer G, Jirovetz L, et al. Percutaneous absorption of lavender oil from massage oil. *J Soc Cosmetic Chemists.* 1992;43(1):49-54.
[97] Gelal A, Jacob P 3rd, Yu L, et al. Disposition kinetics and effects of menthol. *Clin Pharmacol Ther.* 1999 Aug;66(2):128-35.
[98] Pratzel HG, Schubert E, Muhanna N. Pharmacokinetic study of percutaneous absorption of salicylic acid from baths with salicylate methyl ether and salicylic acid. *Z Rheumatol.* 1990 Jul-Aug;49(4):185-91.
[99] Kohlert C, Schindler G, Marz RW, et al. Systemic availability and pharmacokinetics of thymol in humans. *J Clin Pharmacol.* 2002 Jul;42(7):731-7.
[100] Davis L, Kuttan G. Effect of Withania somnifera on cyclophosphamide-induced urotoxicity. *Cancer Lett.* 2000 Jan 1;148(1):9-17.
[101] Davis L, Kuttan G. Suppressive effect of cyclophosphamide-induced toxicity by Withania somnifera extract in mice. *J Ethnopharmacol.* 1998;62:209-14.
[102] Mrozikiewicz PM, Bogacz A, Karaiewicz M, et al. The effect of standardized Echinacea pupurea extract on rat cytochrome P450 expression level. *Phytomedicine.* 2010 Aug;17(10):830-3.
[103] Nowack R, Andrassy J, Fischereder M, et al. Effects of dietary factors on drug transport and metabolism: the impact on dosage guidelines in transplant. *Clin Pharmacol Ther.* 2009 Apr;85(4):439-43.
[104] Xiaochun W, Qing L, Huawen X, et al. Effects of berberine on the blood concentration of cyclosporine A in renal transplanted recipients: clinical and pharmacokinetic study. *Eur J Clin Pharmacol.* 2005 Sep;61(8):567-72.
[105] Miyashita M, Sadzuka Y. Effect of linalool as a component of Humulus lupulus on doxorubicin-induced antitumor activity. *Food Chem Toxicol.* 2013 Mar;53:174-9.
[106] Wu M, Li T, Chen L, et al. Essential oils from Inula japonica and Angelicae dahuricae enhance sensitivity of MCF-7/ADR breast cancer cells to doxorubicin via multiple mechanisms. *J Ethnopharmacol.* 2016 Mar 2;180:18-27.
[107] Effenberger-Neidnicht K, Schobert R. Combinatorial effects of thymoquinone on the anticancer activity of doxorubicin. *Cancer Chemother Pharmacol.* 2011 Apr;67(4):867-74.
[108] Carnesecchi S, Bras-Gonçalves R, Bradaia A, et al. Geraniol, a component of plant essential oils, modulates DNA synthesis and potentiates 5-fluorouracil efficacy on human colon tumor xenografts. *Cancer Lett.* 2004 Nov 8;215(1):53-9.
[109] Abdullah D, Ping QN, Liu GJ. Enhancing effect of essential oils on the penetration of 5-fluorouracil through rat skin. *Yao Xue Xue Bao.* 1996;31(3):214-21.
[110] Simone CB 2nd, Simone NL, Simone V, et al. Antioxidants and other nutrients do not interfere with chemotherapy or radiation therapy and can increase kill and increase survival, part 1. *Altern Ther Health Med.* 2007 Jan-Feb;13(1):22-8.
[111] Lawenda BD, Kelly KM, Ladas EJ, et al. Should supplemental antioxidant administration be avoided during chemotherapy and radiation therapy? *JNCI J Natl Cancer Inst.* 2008;100(11):773-83.
[112] Tayarani-Najaran Z, Talasaz-Firoozi E, Jalali N, et al. Antiemetic activity of volatile oil from Mentha spicata and Mentha X piperita in chemotherapy-induced nausea and vomiting. *Ecancermedicalscience.* 2013;7:290.
[113] Lua PL, Salihah N, Mazlan N. Effects of inhaled ginger aromatherapy on chemotherapy-induced nausea and vomiting and health-related quality of life in women with breast cancer. *Complement Ther Med.* 2015 Jun;23(3):396-404.
[114] Klauke AL, Racz I, Pradier B, et al. The cannabinoid CB2 receptor-selective phytocannabinoid beta-caryophyllene exerts analgesic effects in mouse models of inflammatory and neuropathic pain. *Euro Neuropsychopharmacol.* 2014 Apr;24(4):608-20.
[115] Russo EB. Taming THC: potential cannabis synergy and phytocannabinoid-terpenoid entourage effects. *Br J Pharmacol.* 2011 Aug;163(7):1344-64.
[116] Passosa GF, Fernandesa ES, da Cunha FM, et al. Anti-inflammatory and anti-allergic properties of the essential oil and active constituents from Cordia verbenacea. *J Ethnopharmacology.* 2007 Mar;110(2):323–33.
[117] Leson G, Pless P, Grotenhermen F, et al. Evaluating the impact of hemp food consumption on workplace drug tests. *J Anal Toxicol.* 2001 Nov-Dec;25(8):691-8.
[118] Leson G, Pless P, Grotenhermen F, et al. Evaluating the impact of hemp food consumption on workplace drug tests. *J Anal Toxicol.* 2001 Nov-Dec;25(8):691-8.
[119] Fortner N, Fogerson R, Lindman D, et al. Marijuana-positive urine test results from consumption of hemp seeds in food products. *J Anal Toxicol.* 1997 Oct;21(6):476-81.
[120] NCAA. 2014–2015 Banned Drugs. Available at: http://www.ncaa.org/health-and-safety/policy/2014-15-ncaa- banned-drugs.
[121] Burt SA, Reinders RD. Antibacterial activity of selected plant essential oils against Escherichia coli O157:H7. *Lett Appl Microbiol.* 2003;36(3):162-7.
[122] Williams LR, Stockley JK, Yan W, et al. Essential oils with high antimicrobial activity for therapeutic use. *Int J of Aromatherapy.* 1998;8(4):30-40.
[123] Thomsen NA, Hammer KA, Riley TV, et al. Effect of habituation to tea tree (Melaleuca alternifolia) oil on the subsequent susceptibility of Staphylococcus spp. to antimicrobials, triclosan, tea tree oil, terpinen-4-ol and carvacrol. *Int H Antimicrob Agents.* 2013 Apr;41(4):343-51.
[124] Becerril R, Nerin C, Gomez-Lus R. Evaluation of bacterial resistance to essential oils after exposure to oregano and cinnamon essential oils. *Foodborne Pathogens Disease.* 2012 Aug;9(8):699-705.
[125] Singh BR, Singh V, Ebibeni N, et al. Antimicrobial and herbal drug resistance in enteric bacteria isolated from faecal droppings of common house lizard/Gecko (Hemidactylus frenatus). *Int J Microbiol.* 2013;2013:340848.
[126] Becerril R, Nerin C, Gomez-Lus R. Evaluation of bacterial resistance to essential oils after exposure to oregano and cinnamon essential oils. *Foodborne Pathogens Disease.* 2012 Aug;9(8):699-705.
[127] Royal College of Psychiatrists. Coming off antidepressants. Available at: http://www.rcpsych.ac.uk/expertadvice/treatments/antidepressants/comingoffantidepressants.aspx.
[128] Wiesenthal A, Hunter L, Wang S, et al. Nanoparticles: small and mighty. *Int J Dermatol.* 2011 Mar;50(3):247-54.
[129] Francomme P, Penoel D. *L'Aromatherapie Exactment.* 1990, pg. 197. Roger Jolois, Editeur Limoges.
[130] Jager W, Buchbauer G, Jirovetz L, et al. Percutaneous absorption of lavender oil from massage oil. *Journal of the Society of Cosmetic Chemists.* 1992;43(1):49-54.
[131] Becker KL, Bilezikian JP, Bremmer WJ, et al. Principles and Practice of Endocrinology and Metabolism (Prin & Practice of Endocrinolo) Third Edition. 2001 Apr. Wolters Kluwer Health: Riverwoods, IL.
[132] Thompson TM, Toerne T, Erickson TB. Salicylate Toxicity from Genital Exposure to a Methylsalicylate-Containing Rubefacient. *West J Emerg Med.* 2016 Mar;17(2):181-3.
[133] Oriba HA, Bucks DA, Maibach HI. Percutaneous absorption of hydrocortisone and testosterone on the vulva and forearm: effect of the menopause and site. *Bristish J Dermatology.* 1996;134:229-33.
[134] Prausnitz MR, Elias PM, Franz TJ, et al. Medical Therapy. Skin Barrier and Transdermal Drug Delivery. Available at: http://drugdelivery.chbe.gatech.edu/Papers/2012/Prausnitz%20Derm%20Book%20Chapter%202012.pdf
[135] Baynes, RE and Hodgson E. Absorption and Distribution of Toxicants. in Chapter 6 of A Textbook of modern toxicology. 3rd edition. 2004, John Wiley & Sons, Inc.
[136] Sharma N, Agarwal G, Rana AC, et al. A Review: Transdermal Drug Delivery System: A Tool For Novel Drug Delivery System. *Int J Drug Devel Res.* 2011 Jul-Sep;3(3):70-84.
[137] Yamamoto R, Takasuga S, Kominami K, et al. Iontophoretic transdermal delivery of glycyrrhizin: effects of pH, drug concentration, co-ions, current intensity, and chemical enhancers. *Chem Pharm Bull (Tokyo).* 2013;61(12):1275-81.
[138] Man MQ, Lin TK, Santiago JL, et al. Basis for enhanced barrier function of pigmented skin. *J Invest Dermatol.* 2014 Sep;134(9):2399-2407.
[139] Colquhoun A. Gamma-linolenic acid inhibits both tumor cell cycle progression and angiogenesis in the orthotopic C6 glioma model through changes in VEGF, ERK1/2, MMP2, cyclin, D1, pRb and p27 protein expression. *Lipids Health Dis.* 2009 Mar 17;8:8.
[140] Challoner KR, McCarron MM. Castor bean intoxication. *Ann Emerg Med.* 1990;19:1177-83.
[141] Korac RR, Khambholja KM. Potential of herbs in skin protection from ultraviolet radiation. *Pharmacogn Rev.* 2001 Jul;5(10):164-73.
[142] Pearson TW, Dawson HJ, Lackey HB. Naturally occurring levels of dimethyl sulfoxide in selected fruits, vegetables, grains and beverages. *J Agric Food Chem.* 1981;29(5):1089-91.
[143] Ahn H, Kim J, Jeung EB, et al. Dimethyl sulfoxide inhibits NLRP3 inflammasome activation. *Immunobiology.* 2014 Apr;219(4):315-22.
[144] American Cancer Society. Available at: http://www.cancer.org/treatment/treatmentsandsideeffects/complementaryandalternativemedicine/pharmacologicalandbiologicaltreatment/dmso.

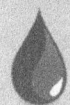

[145] Lucas L, Russell A, Keast R. Molecular mechanisms of inflammation. Anti-inflammatory benefits of virgin olive oil and the phenolic constituent oleocanthal. *Curr Pharm Des.* 2011;17(8):754-68.
[146] Korac RR, Khambholja KM. Potential of herbs in skin protection from ultraviolet radiation. *Pharmacogn Rev.* 2001 Jul;5(10):164-73.
[147] Prasad NR, Menon VP, Vasudev V, et al. Radioprotective effect of sesamol on gamma-radiation induced DNA damage, lipid peroxidation and antioxidants levels in cultured human lymphocytes. *Toxicology.* 2005 May 5;209(3):225-35.
[148] Mishra K, Srivastava PS, Chaudhury NK. Sesamol as a potential radioprotective agent: in vitro studies. *Radiat Res.* 2011 Nov;176(5):613-23.
[149] Bleasel N, Tate B, Rademaker M. Allergic contact dermatitis following exposure to essential oils. *Australas J Dermatol.* 2002 Aug;43(3):211-3.
[150] Rutherford T, Nixon R, Tam M, et al. Allergy to tea tree oil: retrospective review of 41 cases with positive patch test over 4.5 years. *Australas J Dermatol.* 2007 May;48(2):83-7.
[151] Ahlin M, Dingizian V, Svenssson A. High frequency of contact allergy caused by alternative medicine substances. Tea tree oil tops the list. *Lakartidingen.* 2011 Aug 10-23;108(32-33):1487-90.
[152] Uter W, Schmidt E, Geier J, et al. Contact allergy to essential oils: current patch test results (2000-2008) from the Information Network of Departments of Dermatology (IVDK). *Contact Dermatitis.* 2010 Nov;63(5):277-83.
[153] Garcia-Abujeta JL, de Larramendi CH, Berna JP, et al. Mud bath dermatitis due to cinnamon oil. *Contact Dermatitis.* 2005 Apr;52(4):234.
[154] Karlberg AT, Borje A, Duus Johansen J, et al. Activation of non-sensitizing or low-sensitizing fragrance substances into potent sensitizers - prehaptens and prohaptens. *Contact Dermatitis.* 2013 Dec;69(6):323-34.
[155] Trattner A, David M, Lazarov A. Occupational contact dermatitis due to essential oils. *Contact Dermatitis.* 2008 May;58(5):282-4.
[156] Jung P, Sesztak-Greinecker G, Wantke F, et al. Mechanical irritation triggering allergic contact dermatitis from essential oils in a masseur. *Contact Dermatitis.* 2006 May;54(5):397-9.
[157] Keane FM, Smith HR, White IR, et al. Occupational allergic contact dermatitis in two aromatherapists. *Contact Dermatitis.* 2000 Jul;43(1):49-51.
[158] Rutherford T, Nixon R, Tam M, et al. Allergy to tea tree oil: retrospective review of 41 cases with positive patch test over 4.5 years. *Australas J Dermatol.* 2007 May;48(2):83-7.
[159] Uter W, Johansen JD, Borje A, et al. Categorization of fragrance contact allergens for prioritization of preventive measures: clinical and experimental data and consideration of structure-activity relationships. *Contact Dermatitis.* 2013 Oct;69(4):196-230.
[160] Ahlin M, Dingizian V, Svenssson A. High frequency of contact allergy caused by alternative medicine substances. Tea tree oil tops the list. *Lakartidingen.* 2011 Aug 10-23;108(32-33):1487-90.
[161] Karlberg AT, Bergsterom MA, Borje A, et al. Allergic contact dermatitis—formation, structural requirements, and reactivity of skin sensitizers. *Chem Res Toxicol.* 2008 Jan;21(1):53-69.
[162] Smith Pease CK, Basketter DA, Patlewicz GY. Contact allergy: the role of skin chemistry and metabolism. *Clin Exp Dematol.* 2003 Mar;28(2):177-83.
[163] Basketter D, Dooms-Goossens A, Karlberg AT, et al. The chemistry of contact allergy: why is a molecule allergenic? *Contact Dermatitis.* 1995 Feb;32(2):65-73.
[164] Dikovic M, Pease CK, Gerberick GF, et al. Hapten-protein binding: from theory to practical application in the in vitro prediction of skin sensitization. *Contact Dermatitis.* 2005;53(4):189.
[165] Larsen W, Nakayama H, Fischer T, et al. Fragrance contact dermatitis - a worldwide multicenter investigation (Part I). *Contact Dermatitis. Am J Contact Dermat.* 1996 Jun;7(2):77-83.
[166] Larsen W, Nakayama H, Fischer T, et al. Fragrance contact dermatitis - a worldwide multicenter investigation (Part II). *Contact Dermatitis.* 2001 Jun;44(6):344-6.
[167] Larsen W, Nakayama H, Fischer T, et al. Fragrance contact dermatitis - a worldwide multicenter investigation (Part III). *Contact Dermatitis.* 2002 Mar;46(3):141-4.
[168] Rudback J, Bergstrom MA, Borje A, et al. a-Terpinene, an antioxidant in tea tree oil autoxidizes rapidly to skin allergens on air exposure. *Chem Res Toxicol.* 2012 Mar 19;25(3):713-21.
[169] Skold M, Haqvall L, Karlberg AT. Autoxidation of linalyl acetate, the main component of lavender oil, creates potent contact allergens. *Contact Dermatitis.* 2008 Jan;58(1):9-14.
[170] Haqvall L, Backtorp C, Svensson S, et al. Fragrance constituent geraniol forms contact allergens on air exposure. Identification and quantification of oxidation produces and effect on skin sensitization. *Chem Res Toxicol.* 2007 May;20(5):807-14.
[171] Matura M, Skold M, Borje A, et al. Selected oxidized fragrance terpenes are common contact allergens. *Contact Dermatitis.* 2005 Jun;52(6):320-8.
[172] Rudback J, Ramzy A, Karlberg AT, et al. Determination of allergic hydroperoxides in essential oils using gas chromatography with electron ionization mass spectrometry. *J Sep Science.* 2014 Apr;37(8):982-9.
[173] Sciarrone D, Ragonese C, Carnovale C, et al. Evaluation of tea tree oil quality and ascaridole: a deep study by means of chiral and multi heart-cuts multidimensional gas chromatography system coupled to mass spectrometry detection. *J Chromatogr A.* 2010 Oct 8;1217(41):6422-7. Epub 2010 Aug 13.
[174] Krutz NL, Hennen J1, Korb C, et al. Activation of the Endoperoxide Ascaridole Modulates Its Sensitizing Capacity. *Toxicol Sci.* 2015 Oct;147(2):515-23.
[175] Uter W, Johansen JD, Borje A, et al. Categorization of fragrance contact allergens for prioritization of preventive measures: clinical and experimental data and consideration of structure-activity relationships. *Contact Dermatitis.* 2013 Oct;69(4):196-230.
[176] Bleasel N, Tate B, Rademaker N. Allergic contact dermatitis following exposure to essential oils. *Australas J Dermatol.* 2002 Aug;43(3):211-13.
[177] Keane FM, Smith HR, White IR, et al. Occupational allergic contact dermatitis in two aromatherapists. *Contact Dermatitis.* 2000 Jul;43(1):49-51.
[178] Cockayne SE, Gawkrodger DJ. Occupational contact dermatitis in an aromatherapist. *Contact Dermatitis.* 1997 Dec;37(6):306-07.
[179] Selvag E, Holm, JO, Thune P. Allergic contact dermatitis in an aroma therapist with multiple sensitizations to essential oils. *Contact Dermatitis.* 1995 Nov;33(5):354-55.
[180] Mozelsio NBm Harris KE, McGrath KG, et al. Immediate systemic hypersensitivity reaction associated with topical application of Australian tea tree oil. *Allergy Asthma Proc.* 2003 Jan-Feb;24(1):73-75.
[181] Kim HM, Cho SH. Lavender oil inhibits immediate-type allergic reactions in mice and rats. *J Pharm Pharmacol.* 1999 Feb;51(2):221-26.
[182] Cariddi L, Excobar F, Moser M, et al. Monoterpenes isolated from Minthostachys verticillata (Griseb.) Epiling essential oil modulates immediate-type hypersensitivity responses in vitro and in vivo. *Planta Med.* 2011 Oct;77(15):1687-94.
[183] Hosokawa H, Ogwana T. Study of skin irritations caused by perfumery materials. *Perfumer and Flavorist.* 1979;4(4):7-8.
[184] Bhalla AK, Amento EP, Clemens TL, et al. Specific high-affinity receptors for 1,25-dihydroxyvitamin D3 in human peripheral blood mononuclear cells: presence in monocytes and induction in T lymphocytes following activation. *J Clin Endocrinol Metab.* 1983 Dec;57(6):1308-10.
[185] Boonstra A, Barrat FJ, Crain C, et al. 1alpha,25-Dihydroxyvitamin d3 has a direct effect on naive CD4(+) T cells to enhance the development of Th2 cells. J Immunol. 2001 Nov 1;167(9):4974-80.
[186] Searing DA, Leung DYM. Vitamin D in Atopic Dermatitis, Asthma and Allergic Diseases. *Immunol Allergy Clin North Am.* 2010 Aug;30(3):397–409.
[187] Hennino A, Vocanson M, Toussaint Y, et al. Skin-infiltrating CD8+ T cells initiate atopic dermatitis lesions. *J Immunol.* 2007 May 1;178(9):5571-7.
[188] Schwenck J, Griessinger CM, Fuchs K, et al. In vivo optical imaging of matrix metalloproteinase activity detects acute and chronic contact hypersensitivity reactions and enables monitoring of the antiinflammatory effects of N- acetylcysteine. *Mol Imaging.* 214 Nov;13(0):1-12.
[189] Lee YH, Su SB, Huang CC, et al. N-acetylcysteine attenuates hexavalent chromium-induced hypersensitivity through inhibition of cell death, ROS-related signaling and cytokine expression. *PLoS One.* 2014 Sep;9(9):e108317.
[190] Norback D, Bjornsson E, Janson C, et al. Asthmatic symptoms and volatile organic constituents, formaldehyde, and carbon dioxide in dwellings. *Occup Environ Med.* 1995;52:388-95.
[191] Mangprayool T, Kupittayanant S, Chudapongse N. Participation of citral in the bronchodilatory effect of ginger oil and possible mechanism of action. *Fitoterapia.* 2013 Sep;89:68-73.
[192] Janbaz KH, Nisa M, Saqib F, et al. Bronchodilator, vasodilator and spasmolytic activities of methanolic extract of Myrtus communis L. *J Physiol Pharmacol.* 2013 Aug;64(4):479-84.
[193] Ueno-lio T, Shibakura M, Yokota K, et al. Lavender essential oil inhalation suppresses allergic airway inflammation and mucous cell hyperplasia in a murine model of asthma. *Life Sci.* 2014 Jul 17;108(2):19-15.
[194] Ueno-lio T, Shibakura M, Yokota K, et al. Lavender essential oil inhalation suppresses allergic airway inflammation and mucous cell hyperplasia in a murine model of asthma. *Life Sci.* 2014 Jul 17;18(2):19-15.
[195] Shusterman D, Murphy MA, Blames J. Differences in nasal irritant sensitivity by age, gender, and allergic rhinitis status. *Int Arch Occup Environ Health.* 2003 Oct;76(8):577-83.
[196] Shusterman D. Individual factors in nasal chemesthesis. *Chem Senses.* 2002 Jul;27(6):551-64.
[197] Shusterman D. Trigeminally-mediated health effects of air pollutants: sources of inter-individual variability. *Hum Exp Toxicol.* 2007 Mar;26(3):149-57.
[198] Otto D, Molhave L, Rose G, et al. Neurobehavioral and sensory irritant effects of controlled exposure to a complex mixture of volatile organic constituents. *Neurotoxicol Teratol.* 1990 Nov-Dec;12(6):649-52.
[199] Cornetto-Muniz JE, Cain WS, Abraham MH, et al. Sensory properties of selected terpenes. Thresholds for odor, nasal pungency, nasal localization, and eye irritation. *Ann N Y Acad Sci.* 1998 Nov;855:648-51.
[200] Molhave L, Kjaergaard SK, Hempel-Jorgensen A, et al. The eye irritation and odor potencies of four terpenes which are major constituents of the emissions of VOCs from Nordic soft woods. *Indoor Air.* 2000 Dec;10(4):315-18.
[201] Nielsen GD, Larsen ST, Hougaard KS, et al. Mechanisms of acute inhalation effects of (+) and (-)-alpha-pinene in BALB/c mice. *Basic Clin Pharmacol Toxicol.* 2005 Jun;96(6):420-28.
[202] California Air Resources Board and the California Environmental Protection Agency: California Air Resources Board Research Division Indoor Air Chemistry: Cleaning Agents, Ozone and Toxic Air Contaminants. 2006 Apr.
[203] Rohr AC, Wilkins CK, Clausen PA, et al. Upper airway and pulmonary effects of oxidation products of (+)-alpha- pinene, d-limonene, and isoprene in BALB/c mice. *Inhal Toxicol.* 2002 Jul;14(7):663-84.
[204] Geiss O, Giannopoulos G, Tirendi S, et al. The AIRMEX study VOC measurements in public buildings and schools/kindergartens in eleven European cities; Statistical analysis of the data. *Atmos Environ.* 2011;45:3676-84.
[205] Chioca LR, Antunes VD, Ferro MM, et al. Anosmia does not impair the anxiolytic-like effect of lavender essential oil inhalation in mice. *Life Sci.* 2013 May 30;92(20-21):971-5.
[206] Hummel T, Rissom K, Reden J, et al. Effects of olfactory training in patients with olfactory loss. *Laryngoscope.* 2009 Mar;119(3):496-9.
[207] Konstantinidis I, Tsakiropoulou E, Bekiaridou P, et al. Use of olfactory training in post-traumatic and postinfectious olfactory dysfunction. *Laryngoscope.* 2013 Dec;123(12):E85-90.
[208] Morton CA, Garioch J, Todd P, et al. Contact sensitivity to menthol and peppermint in patients with intra-oral symptoms. *Contact Dermatitis.* 1995 May;32(5):281-4.
[209] Tremblay S, Avon SL. Contact allergy to cinnamon: a case report. *J Can Den Assoc.* 2008 Jun;74(5):445-61.
[210] Biron JF, Lovion JP, Bailey JR, et al. Cinnamon-induced oral contact stomatitis. *Dent Today.* 2013 Feb;32(2):82.
[211] Cappello G, Spezzaferro M, Grossi L, et al. Peppermint oil (Mintoil) in the treatment of irritable bowel syndrome: a prospective double blind placebo-controlled randomized trial. *Dig Liver Dis.* 2007 Jun;39(6):530-6.

[212] Kehrl W, Sonnemann U, Dethlefsen U. Therapy for acute nonpurulent rhinosinusitis with cineole: results of a double-blind, randomized, placebo-controlled trial. *Laryngoscope.* 2004 Apr;114(4):738-42.
[213] Fandohan P, Gronlonfin B, Laleye A, et al. Toxicity and gastric tolerance of essential oils from Cymbopogon citratus, Ocimum gratissimum and Ocimum basilicum in Wistar rats. *Food Chem Toxicol.* 2008 Jul;46(7):2493-7.
[214] Jamal A, Javed K, Aslam M, et al. Gastroprotective effect of cardamom, Elettaria cardamomum Maton. fruits in rats. *J Ethnopharmacol.* 2006 Jan 16;103(2):149-53.
[215] Khushtar M, Kumar V, Javed K, et al. Protective effect of ginger oil on aspirin and pylorus ligation-induced gastric ulcer model in rats. *Indian J Pharm Sci.* 2009 Sep;71(5):554-8.
[216] Bonamin F, Moraes TM, Dos Santos RC, et al. The effect of a minor constituent of essential oil from Citrus aurantium: the role of B-myrcene in preventing peptic ulcer disease. *Chem Biol Interact.* 2014 Apr 5;212:11-9.
[217] Rozza AL, Pellizzon CH. Essential oils from medicinal and aromatic plants: a review of the gastroprotective and ulcer-healing activities. *Fundam Clin Pharmacol.* 2013 Feb;27(1):51-63.
[218] Liju VB, Jeena K, Kuttan R. Gastroprotective activity of essential oils from turmeric and ginger. *J Basic Clin Physiol Pharmacol.* 2015 Jan;26(1):95-103.
[219] Oliveira IS, da Silva FV, Viana AF, et al. Gastroprotective activity of carvacrol ion experimentally induced gastric lesions in rodents. *Naunyn-Schmiedeberg's Arch Pharmacol.* 2012 Sep;385(9):899-908.
[220] Santin JR, Lemos M, Klein-Junior LC, et al. Gastroprotective activity of essential oil of the Syzygium aromaticum and its major component eugenol in different animal models. *Naunyn-Schmiedeberg's Arch Pharmacol.* 2011 Feb;383(2):149-58.
[221] Silva FV, Guimaraes AG, Silva ER, et al. Anti-inflammatory and anti-ulcer activities of carvacrol, a monoterpene present in the essential oil of oregano. *J Med Food.* 2012 Nov;15(11):984-91.
[222] Al-Howiriny T, Alsheikh A, Alqasoumi S, et al. Protective effect of Origanum marjorana L. 'Marjoram' in various models of gastric mucosal injury in rats. *Am J Chin Med.* 2009;37(3):531-45.
[223] Thompson Coon J, Ernst E. Systematic review: herbal medicinal plants for non-ulcer dyspepsia. *Aliment Pharmacol Ther.* 2002 Oct;16(10):1689-99.
[224] Joshi J, Ghaisas S, Vaidya A, et al. Early human safety study of turmeric oil (Curcuma longa) administered orally in healthy volunteers. *JAPI.* 2003 Nov;51:1055-60.
[225] Nozaki Y. [Clinical studies of essential oil of Pelargonium Graveolens]. *Aroma Res.* 2011;2(1):61-65.
[226] Uehleke H, Brinkschultze-Freitas M. Oral toxicity of an essential oil from myrtle and adaptive liver stimulation. *Toxicology.* 1979 Mar-Apr;12(3):335-42.
[227] Gavura S. Gold mine or dumpster dive? A closer look at adverse event reports. Available at: https://www.sciencebasedmedicine.org/gold-mine-or-dumpster-dive-a-closer-look-at-adverse-event-reports/.
[228] Mitsikostas DD, Chalarakis NG, Mantonakis LI, et al. Nocebo In Fibromyalgia: Meta-Analysis Of Placebo-Controlled Clinical Trials And Implications For Practice. *Arthritis and Rheumatism.* 2011 Nov;63(Suppl 10):739.
[229] Liccardi G1, Senna G, Russo M, et al. Evaluation of the nocebo effect during oral challenge in patients with adverse drug reactions. *J Investig Allergol Clin Immunol.* 2004;14(2):104-7.
[230] Baldinger P, Hoflich AS, Mitterhauser M, et al. Effects of Silexan on the serotonin-1a receptor and microstructure of the human brain: a randomized, placebo-controlled, double-blind, cross-over study with molecular and structural imaging. *Int J Neuropsychopharmacol.* 2014 Oct 31;18(4):pyu063.
[231] Kasper S, Gastpar M, Muller WE, et al. Lavender oil preparation Silexan is effective in generalized anxiety- disorder--a randomized, double-blind comparison to placebo and paroxetine. *Int J Neuropsychopharmacol.* 2014 Jun;17(6):859-69.
[232] Kasper S. An orally administered Lavandula oil preparation (Silexan) for anxiety disorder and related conditions: an evidence based review. *Int J Psychiatry Clin Pract.* 2013 Nov;17 Suppl 1:15-22.
[233] Schuwald AM, Noldner M, Wilmes T, et al. Lavender oil-potent anxiolytic properties via modulating dependent calcium channels. *PloS One.* 2013 Apr 29;8(4):e59998.
[234] Uehleke B, Schaper S, Dienel A, et al. Phase II trial on the effects of Silexan in patients with neurasthenia, post- traumatic stress disorder or somatization disorder. *Phytomedicine.* 2012 Jun;19(8):665-71.
[235] Kasper S, Gastpar M, Muller WE, et al. Silexan, an orally administered Lavandula oil preparation, is effective in the treatment of 'subsyndromal' anxiety disorder: a randomized, double-blind, placebo controlled trial. *Int Clin Psychopharmacol.* 201 Sep;25(5):277-87.
[236] Woelk H, Schlafke S. A multi-center, double-blind, randomised study of the Lavender oil preparation Silexan in comparison to Lorazepam for generalized anxiety disorder). *Phytomedicine.* 2010 Feb;17(2):94-99.
[237] Amato A, Liotta R, Mule F. Effects of menthol on circular smooth muscle of human colon: analysis of the mechanism of action. *Eur J Pharmacol.* 2014 Oct 5;740:295-301.
[238] Grundmann O, Yoon SL. Complementary and alternative medicines in irritable bowel syndrome: an integrative view. *World J Gastroenterol.* 2014 Jan;20(2):346-62.
[239] Khanna R, MacDonald JK, Levensque BG. Peppermint oil for the treatment of irritable bowel syndrome: a systematic review and meta-analysis. *J Clin Gasteroenterol.* 2014 Jul;48(6):505-12.
[240] Kline RM, Kline JJ, Di Palma J, et al. Enteric-coated, pH-dependent peppermint oil capsules for the treatment of irritable bowel syndrome in children. *J Pediatr.* 2001;138:125-28.
[241] Dew MJ, Evans BK, Rhodes J. Peppermint oil for the irritable bowel syndrome: a multicentre trial. *Br J Clin Pract.* 1984;38:394-98.
[242] Merat S, Khalili S, Mostajabi P, et al. The effect of enteric-coated, delayed-release peppermint oil on irritable bowel syndrome. *Dig Dis Sci.* 201 May;55(5):1385-90.
[243] Si W, Gong J, Tsao R, et al. Antimicrobial activity of essential oils and structurally related synthetic food additives towards selected pathogenic and beneficial gut bacteria. *J Appl Microbiol.* 2006 Feb;100(2):296-305.
[244] Moritz CM, Rall VL, Saeki MJ, et al. Inhibitory effect of essential oils against Lactobacillus rhamnosus and starter culture in fermented milk during its shelf-life period. *Braz J Microbiol.* 2012 Jul;43(3):1147-56.
[245] Feniman CM, Rall VL, Doyama JT, et al. Cell enumeration and visualisation by transmission electron microscopy of Lactobacillus rhamnosus treated with cinnamon (Cinnamomum zeylanicum B.) essential oil. *Nat Prod Res.* 2012;26(18):1721-23.
[246] Lee HS, Ahn YJ. Growth-inhibiting effects of Cinnamomum cassia bark-derived materials on human intestinal bacteria. *J Agric Food Chem.* 1998;46(1):8-12.
[247] Thaweboon S, Thaweboon B. In vitro antimicrobial activity of Ocimum americanum L. essential oil against oral microorganisms. *Southeast Asian J trop Med Public Health.* 2009 Sep;40(5):1025-33.
[248] Hammer KA, Dry L, Johnson M, et al. Susceptibility of oral bacteria to Melaleuca alternifolia (tea tree) oil in vitro. *Oral Microbiol Immunol.* 2003 Dec;18(6):389-92.
[249] Hammer KA, Carson CF. In vitro susceptibilities of Lactobacilli and organisms associated with bacterial vaginosis to Melaleuca alternifolia (Tea Tree) oil. *Antimicrob Agents Chemother.* 1999 Jan;43(1):196.
[250] Li AL, Ni WW, Zhang QM, et al. Effect of cinnamon essential oil on gut microbiota in the mouse model of dextran sodium sulfate-induced colitis. *Microbiol Immunol.* 2020 Jan;64(1):23-32.
[251] Wang L, Zhang Y, Fan G, et al. Effects of orange essential oil on intestinal microflora in mice. *J Sci Food Agric.* 2019 Jun;99(8):4019-4028.
[252] Leong W, Huang G, Liao W, et al. Traditional Patchouli essential oil modulates the host's immune responses and gut microbiota and exhibits potent anti-cancer effects in ApcMin /+ mice. *Pharmacol Res.* 2022 Jan 13;176:106082.
[253] Thapa S, Luna RA, Chumpitazi BP, et al. Peppermint oil effects on the gut microbiome in children with functional abdominal pain. *Clin Transl Sci.* 2022 Apr;15(4):1036-1049.
[254] Johnson JD, Ryan MJ, Toft JD II, et al. Two-year toxicity and carcinogenicity study of methyl eugenol in F344/N rats and B6C3F(1) mice. *J Agric Food Chem.* 2000 Aug;48(8):3620-32.
[255] Williams GM, Latropoulos MJ, Jeffrey AM, et al. Methyl eugenol hepatocellular cancer initiating effects in rat liver. *Food Chem Toxicol.* 2013 Mar;53:187-96.
[256] Evans JG, Gaunt IF, Lake BG. Two-year toxicity study on coumarin in the baboon. *Food Cosmet Toxicol.* 1979 Jun;17(3):187-93.
[257] Janes SE, Price CS, Thomas D. Essential oil poisoning: N-acetylcysteine for eugenol-induced hepatic failure and analysis of national database. *Fur J Pediatr.* 2005 Aug;164(8):520-2.
[258] Brown SA, Biggerstaff J, Savidge GF. Disseminated intravascular coagulation and hepatocellular necrosis due to clove oil. *Blood Coagul Fibrinolysis.* 1992 Oct;3(5):665-8.
[259] Alam K, Nagi MN, Badary OA, et al. The protective action of thymol against carbon tetrachloride hepatotoxicity in mice. *Pharmacol Res.* 1999 Aug;40(2):159-63.
[260] Aristatile B, Al-Numair KS, Veeramani C, et al. Effect of carvacrol on hepatic marker enzymes and antioxidant status in D-galactosamine-induced hepatotoxicity in rats. *Fundam Clin Pharmacol.* 2009 Dec;23(6):757-65.
[261] Marshall AD, Caldwell. Influence of epoxide metabolism on the cytotoxicity of trans-anethole in freshly isolated rat hepatocytes. *Food Chem Toxicol.* 1992 Jun;30(6):467-73.
[262] Birdane FM, Cemek M, Birdane YO, et al. Beneficial effects of Foeniculum vulgare on ethanol-induced acute gastric mucosal injury in rats. *World J Gastroenterol.* 2007 Jan 28;13(4):607-11.
[263] Ozbek H, Ugras S, Dulger H, et al. Hepatoprotective effect of Foeniculum vulgare essential oil. *Fitoterapia.* 2003 Apr;74(3):317-9.
[264] Friedman M, Preti G, Deems R, et al. Limonene in expired lung air of patients with liver disease. *Dig Dis Sci.* 1994 Aug;39(8):1672-6.
[265] Janes SE, Price CS, Thomas D. Essential oil poisoning: N-acetylcysteine for eugenol-induced hepatic failure and analysis of national database. *Eur J Pediatr.* 2005 Aug;164(8):520-2.
[266] Bicchi C, Liberto E, Matteodo M, et al. Quantitative analysis of essential oils: a complex task. *Flavour Fragr J.* 2008;23:382–91.
[267] Adams RP, Weyerstahl P. cis- and trans-Sabinene Hydrate: Comparisons of quadrupole and ion trap mas spectra. *J Essent Oil Res.* 1992 Mar/Apr;4:197–200.
[268] Chagonda LS, Makanda C, Chalchat JC. The essential oils of wild and cultivated Cymbopogon validus (Stapf) Stapf ex Burtt Davy and Elionurus muticus (Spreng.) Kunth from Zimbabwe. *Flavour Frag J.* 2000 Mar;15(2):100-04.
[269] Rungqu P, Oyedeji O, Nkeh-Chungag B, et al. Anti-inflammatory activity of the essential oils of Cymbopogon validus (Stapf) Stapf ex Burtt Davy from Eastern Cape, South Africa. *Asian Pac J Tropical Med.* 2016 May;9(5):426-31.
[270] Boukhris M, Bouaziz M, Feki I, et al. Hypoglycemic and antioxidant effects of leaf and essential oil of Pelargonium graveolens L'Her. in alloxan induced diabetic rats. *Lipids Health Dis.* 2012 Jun 26;11:81.
[271] Adeneye AA, Agbaje EO. Hypoglycemic and hypolipidemic effects of fresh leaf aqueous extract of Cymbopogon citratus Stapf. in rats. *J Ethnopharmacol.* 2007 Jul 25; 112(3):440-4.
[272] Bharti SK, Kumar A, Prakash O, et al. Essential Oil of Cymbopogon Citratus Against Diabetes: Validation by In vivo Experiments and Computational Studies. *J Bioanal Biomed.* 2013;5:194-203.
[273] Hagvall L. Cytochrome P450-mediated activation of the fragrance constituent geraniol forms potent contact allergens. *Tox Appl Pharm.* 2008 Dec;233(2):308-13.
[274] Rungqu P, Oyedeji O, Nkeh-Chungag B, et al. Anti-inflammatory activity of the essential oils of Cymbopogon validus (Stapf) Stapf ex Burtt Davy from Eastern Cape, South Africa. *Asian Pac J Tropical Med.* 2016 May;9(5):426-31.
[275] Naidoo N. The essential oil from Cymbopogon validus. Masters Dissertation. Available at: http://ir.dut.ac.za/bitstream/handle/10321/308/Naidoo_2007.pdf?sequence=1.
[276] Naidoo N. The essential oil from Cymbopogon validus. Masters Dissertation. Available at: http://ir.dut.ac.za/bitstream/handle/10321/308/Naidoo_2007.pdf?sequence=1
[277] Naidoo N. The essential oil from Cymbopogon validus. Masters Dissertation. Available at: http://ir.dut.ac.za/bitstream/handle/10321/308/Naidoo_2007.pdf?sequence=1.

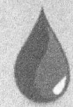
[278] Wetwitayaklung P, Thavanapong N, and Charoenteeraboon J. Chemical Constituents and Antimicrobial Activity of Essential Oil and Extracts of Heartwood of Aquilaria crassna Obtained from Water Distillation and Supercritical Fluid Carbon Dioxide Extraction. *Silpakorn U Science & Tech J.* 2009;3(1):25-33.

[279] No author listed. King of Scents—Agarwood. *Perfume & Flavorist.* 2019 Mar;44(3):42-56.

[280] Dharmadasa RM, Siriwardana A, Samarasinghe K, et al. Standardization of Gyrinops Walla Gaertn. (Thymalaeaceae): Newly Discovered, Fragrant Industrial Potential, Endemic Plant from Sri Lanka. *World J Agric Res.* 2013;1(6):101-3.

[281] Ma S, Fu Y, Li Y, et al. The formation and quality evaluation of agarwood induced by the fungi in Aquilaria sinensis. *Ind Crops Prod.* 2021;173:114129.

[282] Pripdeevech P, Khummueng W, Park SK. Identification of Odor-active Components of Agarwood Essential Oils from Thailand by Solid Phase Microextraction-GC/MS and GC-O. *J Esent Oil Res.* 2011 July/Aug;23:46-53.

[283] Wang S, Wang C, Peng D, et al. Agarwood Essential Oil Displays Sedative-Hypnotic Effects through the GABAergic System. *Molecules.* 2017;22:2190.

[284] Takemoto H, Ito M, Shiraki T, et al. Sedative effects of vapor inhalation of agarwood oil and spikenard extract and identification of their active components. *J Nat Med.* 2008;62:41–46.

[285] Ngan TTK, Thuy DTT, Tuyen TT, et al. Chemical Components of Agarwood (Aquilaria crassna) Essential Oils Grown in Various Regions of Asia. *Asian J Chem.* 2020;32(1):36-40.

[286] Yoswathana N. Extraction of agarwood (Aquilaria crassna) oil by using supercritical carbon dioxide extraction and enzyme pretreatment on hydrodistillation. *J Food Agric Environ.* 2013;11(2):1055-59.

[287] Nor Azah MA, Ismail N, Mailina J, et al. Chemometric study of selected agarwood oils by gas chromatography-mass spectrometry. *J Tropical Forest Sci.* 2014;26(3):382-88.

[288] Pripdeevech P, Khummueng W, Park SK. Identification of Odor-active Components of Agarwood Essential Oils from Thailand by Solid Phase Microextraction-GC/MS and GC-O. *J Essent Oil Res.* 2011 Jul-Aug;(23):46-53.

[289] Tajuddin SN, Yusoff MM. Chemical composition of volatile oils of Aquilaria malaccensis (Thymelaeaceae) from Malaysia. *Nat Prod Commun.* 2010 Dec;5(12):1965-8.

[290] NA Mat Yusof, Tajuddin SN, Hisyam A, et al. Production of Agarwood Essential Oil: Study on Effectiveness Pre-Treatment Technique of Hydrodistillation Extraction. *Borneo J Resource Sci Tech.* 2015;5(2):62-69.

[291] Ismail N, Mohd Ali NA, Jamil M, et al. A review study of agarwood oil and its quality analysis. *J Teknologi.* 2014;68(1):37-42.

[292] Jok VA, Radzi NC, Ku Hamid KH. Agarwood Oil Yield As A Result of Changes in Cell Morphology Due To Soaking Process. *Procedia Social Behav Sci.* 2015 Jul;195:2443-50.

[293] Chen H, Yang Y, Xue J, et al. Comparison of Compositions and Antimicrobial Activities of Essential Oils from Chemically Stimulated Agarwood, Wild Agarwood and Healthy Aquilaria sinensis (Lour.) Gilg Trees. *Molecules.* 2011;16(6):4884-4896.

[294] Zhang Z, Han XM, Wei JH. Compositions and antifungal activities of essential oils from agarwood of Aquilaria sinensis (Lour.) Gilg induced by Lasiodiplodia theobromae (Pat.) Griffon. & Maubl. *J Braz Chem Soc.* 2014 Jan;25(1):0103-5053.

[295] Ngan TTK, Thuy DTT, Tuyen TT, et al. Chemical Components of Agarwood (Aquilaria crassna) Essential Oils Grown in Various Regions of Asia. *Asian J Chem.* 2020;32(1):36-40.

[296] Sen S, Dehingia M, Talukdar NC, et al. Chemometric analysis reveals links in the formation of fragrant bio-molecules during agarwood (Aquilaria malaccensis) and fungal interactions. *Sci Rep.* 2017 Mar 14;7:44406.

[297] Ma S, Fu Y, Li Y, et al. The formation and quality evaluation of agarwood induced by the fungi in Aquilaria sinensis. *Ind Crops Prod.* 2021;173:114129.

[298] Ismail N, Mohd Ali NA, Jamil M, et al. A review study of agarwood oil and its quality analysis. *J Teknologi.* 2014;68(1):37-42.

[299] Hashim YZ, Phirdaous A, Azura A, et al. Screening of anticancer activity from agarwood essential oil. *Pharmacognosy Res.* 2014 Jul;6(3):191-4.

[300] Dahham SS, Hassan LE, Ahamed MB, et al. In vivo toxicity and antitumor activity of essential oils extract from agarwood (Aquilaria crassna). *BMC Complement Altern Med.* 2016 Jul 22;16(1):236.

[301] Wang S, Wang C, Peng D, et al. Agarwood Essential Oil Displays Sedative-Hypnotic Effects through the GABAergic System. *Molecules.* 2017;22:2190.

[302] Takemoto H, Ito M, Shiraki T, et al. Sedative effects of vapor inhalation of agarwood oil and spikenard extract and identification of their active components. *J Nat Med.* 2008;62:41–46.

[303] Chen H, Yang Y, Xue J, et al. Comparison of Compositions and Antimicrobial Activities of Essential Oils from Chemically Stimulated Agarwood, Wild Agarwood and Healthy Aquilaria sinensis (Lour.) Gilg Trees. *Molecules.* 2011;16(6):4884-4896.

[304] Wetwitayaklung P, Thavanapong N, and Charoenteeraboon J. Chemical Constituents and Antimicrobial Activity of Essential Oil and Extracts of Heartwood of Aquilaria crassna Obtained from Water Distillation and Supercritical Fluid Carbon Dioxide Extraction. *Silpakorn U Science & Tech J.* 2009;3(1):25-33.

[305] Zhang Z, Han XM, Wei JH. Compositions and antifungal activities of essential oils from agarwood of Aquilaria sinensis (Lour.) Gilg induced by Lasiodiplodia theobromae (Pat.) Griffon. & Maubl. *J Braz Chem Soc.* 2014 Jan;25(1):0103-5053.

[306] Takemoto H, Ito M, Shiraki T, et al. Sedative effects of vapor inhalation of agarwood oil and spikenard extract and identification of their active components. *J Nat Med.* 2008 Jan;62(1):41-46.

[307] Ga'al H, Fouad H, Mao G, et al. Larvicidal and pupicidal evaluation of silver nanoparticles synthesized using Aquilaria sinensis and Pogostemon cablin essential oils against dengue and zika viruses vector Aedes albopictus mosquito and its histopathological analysis. *Artif Cells Nanomed Biotechnol.* 2018 Sep;46(6):1171-1179.

[308] De Rubis G, Paudel KR, Manandhar B, et al. Agarwood Oil Nanoemulsion Attenuates Cigarette Smoke-Induced Inflammation and Oxidative Stress Markers in BCi-NS1.1 Airway Epithelial Cells. *Nutrients.* 2023 Feb;15(4):1019.

[309] Seo SM. Park HM, Park IK. Larvicidal Activity of Ajowan (Trachyspermum ammi) and Peru Balsam (Myroxylon pereira) Oils and Blends of Their Constituents against Mosquito, Aedes aegypti, Acute Toxicity on Water Flea, Daphnia magna, and Aqueous Residue. *J Agric Food Chem.* 2012;60(23):5909–5914.

[310] Abbasxabeh S, Gandomi H, Ashkan J, et al. Chemical Constituents, Antimicrobial and Antioxidative Effects of Trachyspermum ammi Essential Oil. *J Food Processing and Preservation.* 2014 Aug;38(4):1690-95.

[311] Vitali LA, Beghelli D, Biapa Nya PC, et al. Diverse biological effects of the essential oil from Iranian Trachyspermum ammi. *Arabian J Chem.* 2015 Jun;1-12.

[312] Singh G, Maurya S, Catalan C, et al. Chemical Constituents, Antifungal and Antioxidative Effects of Ajwain Essential Oil and Its Acetone Extract. *J Agric Food Chem.* 2004;52(11):3292-96.

[313] Zarshenas MM, Samani SM Petramfar P, et al. Analysis of the essential oil components from different Carum copticum L. samples from Iran. *Pharmacognosy Res.* 2014 Mar;6(1):62-66.

[314] Kohlert C, Schindler G, Marz RW, et al. Systemic availability and pharmacokinetics of thymol in humans. *J Clin Pharmacol.* 2002 Jul;42(7):731-7.

[315] US Centers for Disease Control and Prevention. ATSDR, Agency for Toxic Substances and Disease Registry. Medical Management Guidelines for Phenol. Available at: https://www.atsdr.cdc.gov/MHMI/mmg115.pdf.

[316] Jukic M, Politeo O, Maksimmovic M, et al. In vitro acetylcholinesterase inhibitory properties of thymol, carvacrol and their derivatives thymoquinone and thymohydroquinone. *Phytother Res.* 2007;21(3):259-61.

[317] Tognolini M, Barocelli E, Ballabeni V, et al. Comparative screening of plant essential oils; phenylpropanoid moiety as basic core for antiplatelet activity. *Life Sci.* 2006 Feb 23;78(13):1419-32.

[318] Okazaki K, Kawazoe K, Takaishi Y. Human platelet aggregation inhibitors from thyme (Thymus vulgaris L.). *Phytother Res.* 2002 Jun;16(4):398-9.

[319] Jukic M, Politeo O, Maksimmovic M, et al. In vitro acetylcholinesterase inhibitory properties of thymol, carvacrol and their derivatives thymoquinone and thymohydroquinone. *Phytother Res.* 2007;21(3):259-61.

[320] Boskabady MH, Rakhshandah H, Moetamedshariati V. Bronchodilatory and anticholinergic effects of Carum copticum on isolated guinea pig tracheal chains. *Medical Journal of the Islamic Republic of Iran.* 1998;11:329–334.

[321] Boskabady MH, Shaikhi J. Inhibitory effect of Carum copticum on histamine (H1) receptors of isolated guinea-pig tracheal chains. *J Ethnopharmacol.* 2000 Mar;69(3):217-27.

[322] Langeveld WT, Veldhuizen EJ, Burt SA. Synergy between essential oil constituents and antibiotics. *Crit Rev Microbiol.* 2014 Feb;40(1);76-94.

[323] Palaniappan K, Holley Ra. Use of natural antimicrobials to increase antibiotic susceptibility of drug resistant bacteria. *In J Food Microbiol.* 2010 Jun 15;140(2-3):164-8.

[324] Ilic BS, Kocic BD, Ciric VM, et al. An in vitro synergistic interaction of combinations of Thymus glabrescens essential oil and its main constituents with chloramphenicol. *ScientificWorldJournal.* 2014 Jan 28;2014:826219.

[325] Miladinovic DL, Ilic BS, Kocic BD, et al. Antibacterial investigation of thyme essential oil and its main constituents on combination with tetracycline. *J Med Food.* 2015 Aug;18(8):935-7.

[326] Petramfar P, Moein M, Samani SM, et al. Trachyspermum ammi 10% topical cream versus placebo on neuropathic pain, a randomized, double-blind, placebo-controlled trial. *Neurol Sci.* 2016 Sep;37(9):1449-55.

[327] Roy S, Chaurvedi P, Chowdhary A, et al. Evaluation of antiviral activity of essential oil of Trachyspermum Ammi against Japanese encephalitis virus. *Pharmacognosy Res.* 2015 Jul-Sep;7(3):263-7.

[328] Hosseinkhani F, Jabalameli F, Banar M, et al. Monoterpene isolated from the essential oil of Trachyspermum ammi is cytotoxic to multidrug-resistant Pseudomonas aeruginosa and Staphylococcus aureus strains. *Rev Soc Bras Med Trop.* 2016 Apr;49(2):172-6.

[329] Soni R, Sharma G, Jasuja ND. Essential Oil Yield Pattern and Antibacterial and Insecticidal Activities of Trachyspermum ammi and Myristica fragrans. *Scientifica (Cairo).* 2016;2016:1428194.

[330] Soni R, Sharma G, Jasuja ND. Essential Oil Yield Pattern and Antibacterial and Insecticidal Activities of Trachyspermum ammi and Myristica fragrans. *Scientifica (Cairo).* 2016;2016:1428194.

[331] Moein MR, Zomorodian K, Pakshir K, et al. Trachyspermum ammi (L.) sprague: chemical composition of essential oil and antimicrobial activities of respective fractions. *J Evid Based Complementary Altern Med.* 2015 Jan;20(1):50-6.

[332] Kavoosi G, Tafsiry A, Ebdam AA, et al. Evaluation of antioxidant and antimicrobial activities of essential oils from Carum copticum seed and Ferula assafoetida latex. *J Food Sci.* 2013 Feb;78(2):T356-61.

[333] Zomorodian K, Ghadiri P, Saharkhiz MJ, et al. Antimicrobial activity of seven essential oils from Iranian aromatic plants against common causes of oral infections. *Jundishapur J Microbiol.* 2015 Feb 19;8(2):e17766.

[334] Kahkha MR, Amanloo S, Kaykhaii M. Antiaflatoxigenic activity of Carum copticum essential oil. *Environ Chem Lett.* 2014;12:231-234.

[335] Boskabady MH, Shaikhi J. Inhibitory effect of Carum copticum on histamine (H1) receptors of isolated guinea-pig tracheal chains. *J Ethnopharmacol.* 2000 Mar;69(3):217-27.

[336] Sharifzadeh A, Khosravi AR, Shokri H, et al. Antifungal effect of Trachyspermum ammi against susceptible and fluconazole-resistant strains of Candida albicans. *J Mycol Med.* 2015 Jun;25(2):143-50.

[337] Moein MR, Zomorodian K, Pakshir K, et al. Trachyspermum ammi (L.) sprague: chemical composition of essential oil and antimicrobial activities of respective fractions. *J Evid Based Complementary Altern Med.* 2015 Jan;20(1):50-6.

338 Gemeda N, Woldeamanuel Y, Asrat D, et al. Effect of essential oils on Aspergillus spore germination, growth and mycotoxin production: a potential source of botanical food preservative. *Asian Pac J Trop Biomed.* 2014 May;4(Suppl 1):S373-81.

339 Kazemi M. Effect of Carum copticum essential oil on growth and aflatoxin formation by Aspergillus strains. *Nat Prod Res.* 2015;29(11):1065-8.

340 Khan MS, Ahmad I, Cameotra SS. Carum copticum and Thymus vulgaris oils inhibit virulence in Trichophyton rubrum and Aspergillus spp. *Braz J Microbiol.* 2014 Aug 29;45(2):523-31.

341 Kahkha MR, Amanloo S, Kaykhaii M. Antiaflatoxigenic activity of Carum copticum essential oil. *Environ Chem Lett.* 2014;12:231-234.

342 Uniyal V, Saxena S, Bhatt RP. Screening of some essential oils against Trichosporon species. *J Environ Biol.* 2013 Jan;34(1):17-22.

343 Singh Sp, Dubey P, Tripathi SC. Fungitoxic properties of the essential oil of Trachyspermum ammi Sprague. *Mykosen.* 1986 Jan;29(1):37-40.

344 Moazeni M, Saharkhiz MJ, Hosseini AA. In vitro lethal effect of ajowan (Trachyspermum ammi L.) essential oil on hydatid cyst protoscoleces. *Vet Parasitol.* 2012 Jun 8;187(1-2):203-8.

345 Soni R, Sharma G, Jasuja ND. Essential Oil Yield Pattern and Antibacterial and Insecticidal Activities of Trachyspermum ammi and Myristica fragrans. *Scientifica (Cairo).* 2016;2016:1428194.

346 Seo SM, Jung CS2, Kang J, et al. Larvicidal and acetylcholinesterase inhibitory activities of apiaceae plant essential oils and their constituents against aedes albopictus and formulation development. *J Agric Food Chem.* 2015 Nov 18;63(45):9977-86.

347 Yeom HJ, Kang JS, Kim GH, et al. Insecticidal and acetylcholine esterase inhibition activity of Apiaceae plant essential oils and their constituents against adults of German cockroach (Blattella germanica). *J Agric Food Chem.* 2012 Jul 25;60(29):7194-203.

348 Seo SM, Park HM, Park IK. Larvicidal activity of ajowan (Trachyspermum ammi) and Peru balsam (Myroxylon pereira) oils and blends of their constituents against mosquito, Aedes aegypti, acute toxicity on water flea, Daphnia magna, and aqueous residue. *J Agric Food Chem.* 2012 Jun 13;60(23):5909-14.

349 Seo SM, Kim J, Lee SG, et al. Fumigant antitermitic activity of plant essential oils and components from Ajowan (Trachyspermum ammi), Allspice (Pimenta dioica), caraway (Carum carvi), dill (Anethum graveolens), Geranium (Pelargonium graveolens), and Litsea (Litsea cubeba) oils against Japanese termite (Reticulitermes speratus Kolbe). *J Agric Food Chem.* 2009 Aug 12;57(15):6596-602.

350 Pandey SK, Upadhyay S, Tripathi AK. Insecticidal and repellent activities of thymol from the essential oil of Trachyspermum ammi (Linn) Sprague seeds against Anopheles stephensi. *Parasitol Res.* 2009 Aug;105(2):507-12.

351 Chaubey MK. Fumigant toxicity of essential oils from some common spices against pulse beetle, Callosobruchus chinensis (Coleoptera: Bruchidae). *J Oleo Sci.* 2008;57(3):171-9.

352 Paul S, Kang SC. Studies on the viability and membrane integrity of human spermatozoa treated with essential oil of Trachyspermum ammi (L.) Sprague ex Turrill fruit. *Andrologia.* 2012 May;44 Suppl 1:117-25.

353 Paul S, Kang SC. In vitro determination of the contraceptive spermicidal activity of essential oil of Trachyspermum ammi (L.) Sprague ex Turrill fruits. *N Biotechnol.* 2011 Oct;28(6):684-90.

354 Sargazi Zadeh G, Panahi N. Endothelium-independent vasorelaxant activity of Trachyspermum ammi essential oil on rat aorta. *Clin Exp Hypertens.* 2017;39(2):133-138.

355 Shakeri G, Jamshidi A, Khanzadi S, et al. Modeling of Salmonella typhimurium growth under the effects of Carum copticum essential oil, temperature, pH and inoculum size. *Vet Res Forum.* 2017 Winter;8(1):59-65.

356 Lee HR, Kim GH, Choi WS, et al. Repellent Activity of Apiaceae Plant Essential Oils and their Constituents Against Adult German Cockroaches. *J Econ Entomol.* 2017 Apr 1;110(2):552-557.

357 Talei GR, Mohammadi M, Bahmani M, et al. Synergistic effect of Carum copticum and Mentha piperita essential oils with ciprofloxacin, vancomycin, and gentamicin on Gram-negative and Gram-positive bacteria. *Int J Pharm Investig.* 2017 Apr-Jun;7(2):82-87.

358 Singh A, Ahmad A, et al. Antioxidant Activity of Essential Oil Extracted by SC-CO₂ from Seeds of Trachyspermum ammi. *Medicines (Basel).* 2017 Jul 11;4(3).

359 Snoussi M, Noumi E, Punchappady-Devasya R, et al. Antioxidant properties and anti-quorum sensing potential of Carum copticum essential oil and phenolics against Chromobacterium violaceum. *J Food Sci Technol.* 2018 Aug;55(8):2824-2832.

360 Grǎdinaru AC, Trifan A, Şpac A, et al. Antibacterial activity of traditional spices against lower respiratory tract pathogens: combinatorial effects of Trachyspermum ammi essential oil with conventional antibiotics. *Lett Appl Microbiol.* 2018 Nov;67(5):449-457.

361 Eftekhari M, Hoseinsalari A, Mansourian M, et al. Trachyspermum ammi (L.) Sprague, superb essential oil and its major components on peptic ulcers: in vivo combined in silico studies. *Daru.* 2019 Jun;27(1):317-327.

362 Javan AJ, Salimiraad S, Khorshidpour B, et al. Combined Effect of Trachyspermum ammi Essential Oil and Propolis Ethanolic Extract on Some Foodborne Pathogenic Bacteria. *Vet Res Forum.* 2019 Summer;10(3):235-40.

363 Kardan-Yamchi J, Mahboubi M, Kazemian H, et al. The Chemical composition and anti-mycobacterial activities of Trachyspermum copticum and Pelargonium graveolens essential oils. *Recent Pat Antiinfect Drug Discov.* 2019 Oct 28. [Epub ahead of print]

364 Lee SC, Seo SM, Huh MJ, et al. Behavioral and Electrophysiological Effects of Ajowan (Trachyspermum ammi Sprague) (Apiales: Apiaceae) Essential Oil and Its Constituents on Nymphal and Adult Bean Bugs, Riptortus clavatus (Thunberg) (Hemiptera: Alydidae). *Insects.* 2020 Feb 4;11(2):104.

365 Omidpanah S, Aliakbari F, Nabavi SM, et al. Effects of Monoterpenes of Trachyspermum ammi on the Viability of Spermatogonia Stem Cells In Vitro. *Plants (Basel).* 2020 Mar 9;9(3).

366 Mahmoudzadeh M, Hosseini H, Mahmoudzadeh L, et al. Comparative Effects of Carum copticum Essential Oil on Bacterial Growth and Shiga-Toxin Gene Expression of Escherichia coli O157:H7 at Abused Refrigerated Temperatures. *Curr Microbiol.* 2020 Apr 13. [Epub ahead of print]

367 Piri A, Sahebzadeh N, Zibaee A, et al. Toxicity and Physiological Effects of Ajwain (Carum Copticum, Apiaceae) Essential Oil and Its Major Constituents Against Tuta Absoluta (Meyrick) (Lepidoptera: Gelechiidae). *Chemosphere.* 2020 May 17;256:127103.

368 Almnhawy M, Jebur M, Alhajamee M, et al. PLGA-Based Nano-Encapsulation of Trachyspermum Ammi Seed Essential Oil (TSEO-PNP) as a Safe, Natural, Efficient, Anticancer Compound in Human HT-29 Colon Cancer Cell Line. *Nutr Cancer.* 2020 Dec 15;1-13.

369 Zare MR, Khorram M, Barzeger S, et al. Antimicrobial core-shell electrospun nanofibers containing Ajwain essential oil for accelerating infected wound healing. *Int J Pharm.* 2021 May 12;603:120698.

370 Khorsandi K, Kianmehr Z, Ghelichkhani E. Combination effect of red light irradiation and Traychspermum ammi essential oil on colorectal cancer cells (SW480). *Lasers Med Sci.* Online ahead of print.

371 Hejazi M, Zareshahrabadi Z, Ashayeri S, et al. Characterization and Physical and Biological Properties of Tissue Conditioner Incorporated with Carum copticum L. *Biomed Res Int.* 2021 Aug 12;2021:5577760.

372 Trifan A, Luca SV, Bostǎnaru AC, et al. Apiaceae Essential Oils: Boosters of Terbinafine Activity against Dermatophytes and Potent Anti-Inflammatory Effectors. *Plants (Basel).* 2021 Nov 4;10(11):2378.

373 Aouadhi C, Jouini A, Mechichi D, et al. Characterization of Primary Action Mode of Eight Essential Oils and Evaluation of Their Antibacterial Effect against Extended-Spectrum β-Lactamase (ESBL)-Producing Escherichia coli Inoculated in Turkey Meat. *Molecules.* 2022 Apr 18;27(8):2588.

374 Dabowl AE, Mohsenzadeh M. Physicochemical, antioxidant, antibacterial and antibiofilm activity of Carum copticum essential oil nanoemulsion on Escherichia coli O157:H7 and Listeria monocytogenes. *Vet Res Forum.* 2021 Dec;12(4):437-444.

375 Subaharan K, Senthamarai Selvan P, et al. Ultrasound-assisted nanoemulsion of Trachyspermum ammi essential oil and its constituent thymol on toxicity and biochemical aspect of Aedes aegypti. *Environ Sci Pollut Res Int.* 2022 May 21. Online ahead of print.

376 Sachan N, Saraswat N, Chandra P, et al. Isolation of Thymol from Trachyspermum ammi Fruits for Treatment of Diabetes and Diabetic Neuropathy in STZ-Induced Rats. *Biomed Res Int.* 2022 Apr 28;2022:8263999.

377 Modareskia M, Fattahi M, Mirjalili MH. Thymol screening, phenolic contents, antioxidant and antibacterial activities of Iranian populations of Trachyspermum ammi (L.) Sprague (Apiaceae). *Sci Rep.* 2022 Sep 19;12(1):15645.

378 Mirniyam G, Rahimmalek M, Arzani A, et al. Changes in Essential Oil Composition, Polyphenolic Compounds and Antioxidant Capacity of Ajowan (Trachyspermum ammi L.) Populations in Response to Water Deficit. *Foods.* 2022 Oct 5;11(19):3084.

379 Tumen I, Hafizoglu H, Kilic A, et al. Yields and Constituents of Essential Oil from Cones of Pinaceae spp. Natively Grown in Turkey. *Molecules.* 2010;15:5797-806.

380 Ustun O, Senol FS, Kurkcuoglu M, et al. Investigation on chemical composition, anticholinesterase and antioxidant activities of extracts and essential oils of Turkish Pinus species and pycnogenol [J]. *Ind Crop Prod.* 2012;38:115-23.

381 Koutsaviti K, Giatropoulos A, Pitarokili D, et al. Greek Pinus essential oils: larvicidal activity and repellency against Aedes albopictus (Diptera: Culicidae). *Parasitol Res.* 2015 Feb;114(2):583-92.

382 Macchioni F, Cioni P, Flamini G, et al. Chemical composition of essential oils from needles, branches and cones of Pinus pinea, P. halepensis, P. pinaster and P. nigra from central Italy. *Flavour Frag J.* 2003;18(2):139-43.

383 Badjah-Hadj-Ahmed Y, Tazerouti F, Meklati BY. Analysis of pine needles essential oils by GC-MS and GC-FTIR. Availble at: https://www.google.com/url?sa=t&rct=j&q=&esrc=s&source=web&cd=1&cad=rja&uact=8&ved=0ahUKEwjJwI3T1pzQAhUG9GMKHXPOB3AQFggoMAA&url=http%3A%2F%2Ffaculty.ksu.edu.sa%2Fbadjah%2FDocuments%2520Badjah%2FPinus%2520essential%2520oil%2520analysis.pdf&usg=AFQjCNESmZtTmoXbVTChR4__mUMbIHCc8Q&sig2=ioP1sLVZKNFGiFhsLObfBA

384 Fekih N, Allali H, Merghache S, et al. Chemical composition and antibacterial activity of Pinus halepensis Miller growing in West Northern of Algeria. *Asian Pac J Trop Dis.* 2014 Apr;4(2):97-103.

385 Dob T, Berramdane T, Chelgoum C. Chemical composition of essential oil of Pinus halepensis Miller growing in Algeria. *C.R. Chimie.* 2005;8:1939-45.

386 Nam A, Tomi F, Gibernau M, et al. Composition and Chemical Variability of the Needle Oil from Pinus halepensis growing in Corsica. *Chem Biodiversity.* 2016;13(4):380-86.

387 Tundis R, Loizzo MR, Bonesi M, et al. Comparative study on the antioxidant capacity and cholinesterase inhibitory activity of Citrus aurantifolia Swingle, C. aurantium L., and C. bergamia Risso and Poit. Peel oils. *J Food Sci.* 2012 Jan;77(1):H40-46.

388 Nguyen LT, Mysliveckova Z, Szotakova B, et al. The inhibitory effects of β-caryophyllene, β-caryophyllene oxide and α-humulene on the activities of the main drug-metabolizing enzymes in rat and human liver in vitro. *Chem-Biol Interactoins.* 2017 Dec 25;278:123-8.

389 De Olivera AC, Ribeiro-Pinto LF, Paumgartten JR. In vitro inhibition of CYP2B1 monoxygenase by beta-myrcene and other monoterpenoid constituents. *Br J Nutr.* 1999;81:289-95.

390 De-Oliveira AC1, Ribeiro-Pinto LF, Otto SS, et al. Induction of liver monooxygenases by beta-myrcene. *Toxicology.* 1997 Dec 26;124(2):135-40.

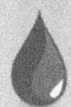

391 Nguyen LT, Mysliveckova Z, Szotakova B, et al. The inhibitory effects of β-caryophyllene, β-caryophyllene oxide and α-humulene on the activities of the main drug-metabolizing enzymes in rat and human liver in vitro. *Chem-Biol Interactoins.* 2017 Dec 25;278:123-8.
392 Freitas JC1, Presgrave OA, Fingola FF, et al. Effect of beta-myrcene on pentobarbital sleeping time. *Braz J Med Biol Res.* 1993 May;26(5):519-23.
393 Süntar I, Tumen I, Ustün O, et al. Appraisal on the wound healing and anti-inflammatory activities of the essential oils obtained from the cones and needles of Pinus species by in vivo and in vitro experimental models. *J Ethnopharmacol.* 2012 Jan 31;139(2):533-40.
394 Fekih N, Allali H, Merghache S, et al. Chemical composition and antibacterial activity of Pinus halepensis Miller growing in West Northern of Algeria. *Asian Pac J Trop Dis.* 2014 Apr;4(2):97-103.
395 Ustun O, Senol FS, Kurkcuoglu M, et al. Investigation on chemical composition, anticholinesterase and antioxidant activities of extracts and essential oils of Turkish Pinus species and pycnogenol [J]. *Ind Crop Prod.* 2012;38:115-23.
396 Darvesh S, Hopkins DA, Geula C, Neurobiology of butyrylcholinesterase. *Nat Rev Neurosci.* 2003 Feb;4:131–38. 2494 Carvalho-Freitas MIR, Costa M. Anxiolytic and sedative effects of extracts and essential oil from Citrus aurantium L. Biolog Pharm Bull. 2002;25(12):1629–33.
397 Bouzenna H, Samout N, Amani E, et al. Protective Effects of Pinus halepensis L. Essential Oil on Aspirin-induced Acute Liver and Kidney Damage in Female Wistar Albino Rats. *J Oleo Sci.* 2016 Aug 1;65(8):701-12.
398 Ustun O, Senol FS, Kurkcuoglu M, et al. Investigation on chemical composition, anticholinesterase and antioxidant activities of extracts and essential oils of Turkish Pinus species and pycnogenol [J]. *Ind Crop Prod.* 2012;38:115-23.
399 Ahmed SBH, Sghaier RM, Guesmi F, et al. Evaluation of anti-leishmanial, cytotoxic and antioxidant activities of essential oils extracted from plants issued from the leishmaniasis-endemic region of Sned (Tunisia). *Nat Prod Res.* 2011 Jul;25(12):1195-201.
400 Koutsaviti K, Giatropoulos A, Pitarokili D, et al. Greek Pinus essential oils: larvicidal activity and repellency against Aedes albopictus (Diptera: Culicidae). *Parasitol Res.* 2015 Feb;114(2):583-92.
401 Macchioni F, Cioni PL, Flamini G, et al. Acaricidal activity of pine essential oils and their main components against Tyrophagus putrescentiae, a stored food mite. *J Agric Food Chem.* 2002 Jul 31;50(16):4586-8.
402 Padmakumari KP, Sasidharan I, Sreekumar MM. Composition and antioxidant activity of essential oil of pimento (Pimenta dioica (L) Merr.) from Jamaica. *Nat Prod Res.* 2011 Jan;25(2):152-60.
403 Jirovetz L, Buchbauer G, Stoilova I, et al. Spice plants: Chemical composition and antioxidant properties of Pimenta Lindl. essential oils, part 1: Pimenta dioica (L.) Merr. leaf oil from Jamaica. *ERNÄHRUNG/NUTRITION.* 2007;31:55-63.
404 Dharmadasa RM, Abeysinghe DC, Dissanayake DMN, et al. Leaf Essential Oil Composition, Antioxidant Activity, Total Phenolic Content and Total Flavonoid Content of Pimenta Dioica (L.) Merr (Myrtaceae): A Superior Quality Spice Grown in Sri Lanka. *Universal J Agric Res.* 2015;3(2):49-52.
405 Monteiro O, Souza A, Soledade L, et al. Chemical evaluation and thermal analysis of the essential oil from the fruits of the vegetable species Pimenta dioica Lindl. *J Thermal Analysis Calorimetry.* 2011 Nov;106(2):595-600.
406 Martinez-Velazquez M, Castillo-Herrera G, Rosario-Cruz R, et al. Acaricidal effect and chemical composition of essential oils extracted from Cuminum cyminum, Pimenta dioica and Ocimum basilicum against the cattle tick Rhipicephalus (Boophilus) microplus (Acari). *Parasitol Res.* 2011 Feb;108(2):481-87.
407 Pino JA, Rosado A. Chemical Composition of the Leaf Oil of Pimenta dioica L. from Cuba. *J Essent Oil Res.* 1996;8(3):331-32.
408 Faria LR, Machado RD, Pimenta PH, et al. Structural organization and phytochemical analysis of Pimenta dioica (L.) Merrill (Myrtaceae) leaves collected from Goias State, Brazil. *J Med Plant Res.* 2014 Oct;8(38):1134-47.
409 Jiang ZT, Feng X, Li R, et al. Composition Comparison of Essential Oils Extracted by Classical Hydro distillation and Microwave-assisted Hydrodistillation from Pimenta dioica. *J Essential Oil Bearing Plants.* 2013;16(1):45-50.
410 Minott DA, Brown HA. Differentiation of fruiting and non-fruiting Pimenta dioica(L.) merr trees based on composition of leaf volatiles. *J Essent Oil Res.* 2007;19:354-57.
411 García-Fajardoa J, Martínez-Sosaa M, Estarrón-Espinosa M. Comparative Study of the Oil and Supercritical CO2 Extract of Mexican Pimento (Pimenta dioica Merrill). *J Essent Oil Res* 1997;9(2):181-85.
412 Park IK, Kim J, Lee SG, et al. Nematicidal Activity of Plant Essential Oils and Components From Ajowan (Trachyspermum ammi), Allspice (Pimenta dioica) and Litsea (Litsea cubeba) Essential Oils Against Pine Wood Nematode (Bursaphelenchus Xylophilus). *J Nematol.* 2007 Sep;39(3):275–79.
413 Seo MI, Kim J, Chin SH, et al. Fumigant antitermitic activity of plant essential oils and components from Ajowan (Trachyspermum ammi), Allspice (Pimenta dioica), caraway (Carum carvi), dill (Anethum graveolens), Geranium (Pelargonium graveolens), and Litsea (Litsea cubeba ) oils against Japanese termite (Reticulitermes speratus Kolbe). *J Agric Food Chem.* 2009;57:6596-6602.
414 Johnson JD, Ryan MJ, Toft JD II, et al. Two-year toxicity and carcinogenicity study of methyl eugenol in F344/N rats and B6C3F(1) mice. *J Agric Food Chem.* 2000 Aug;48(8):3620-32.
415 European Commission. Opinion of the Scientific Committee on Food on methyl eugenol (4-Allyl-1,2- dimethoxybenzene). Available at: http://ec.europa.eu/food/fs/sc/scf/out102_en.pdf.
416 National Toxicology Program. NTP Toxicology and Carcinogenesis Studies of Methyleugenol (CAS NO. 93-15-2) in F344/N Rats and B6C3F1 Mice (Gavage Studies). *Natl Toxicol Program Tech Rep Ser.* 2000 Jul;491:1-412.
417 National Toxicology Program. Carcinogenesis Studies of Eugenol (CAS No. 97-53-0) in F344/N Rats and B6C3F1 Mice (Feed Studies). Technical Report Series No. 223. NIH Publication No. 84-1779. 1983. U.S. DHHS, PHS, NIH, NTP, Research Triangle Park, NC.
418 Domaracky M, Rehak P, Juhas S, et al. Effects of selected plant essential oils on the growth and development of mouse preimplantation embryos in vivo. *Physiol Res.* 2007;56(1):97-104.
419 Vrskova D, Modra H. Evaluation of the developmental toxicity of 2-phenoxyethanol and clove oil anesthetics using the Frog Embryo Teratogenesis Assay: Xenopus (FETAX). *Veterinarami Medicina.* 2012;57(5):245-50.
420 Amini A, Cheraghi E, Safaee MR, et al. The role of eugenol in the reduction of teratogenic effects of retinoic acid on skeletal morphology of mice embryo. *Yakhteh Medical Journal.* 2003;4:195-200.
421 Chen R, Chen J, Cheng S, et al. Assessment of embryotoxicity of constituents in cosmetics by the embryonic stem cell tes. *Toxicol Mech Methods.* 2010 Mar;20(3):112-18.
422 Price CJ, George JD, Marr MC, et al. Developmental toxicity evaluation of methyleugenol (MEUG) administered to Sprague-Dawley rats on gestational days (gd) 6 through 19. *Birth Defects Res A Clin Mol Teratol.* 2006 Jun;76:395.
423 Johnson JD, Ryan MJ, Toft JD II, et al. Two-year toxicity and carcinogenicity study of methyl eugenol in F344/N rats and B6C3F(1) mice. *J Agric Food Chem.* 2000 Aug;48(8):3620-32.
424 National Toxicology Program. NTP Toxicology and Carcinogenesis Studies of Methyleugenol (CAS NO. 93-15-2) in F344/N Rats and B6C3F1 Mice (Gavage Studies). *Natl Toxicol Program Tech Rep Ser.* 2000 Jul;491:1-412.
425 Kerckaert GA, Brauninger R, LeBoeuf RA, et al. Use of the Syrian hamster embryo cell transformation assay for carcinogenicity prediction of chemicals currently being tested by the National Toxicology Program in rodent bioassays. *Environ Health Perspect.* 1996;104:1075-84.
426 National Toxicology Program. Carcinogenesis Studies of Eugenol (CAS No. 97-53-0) in F344/N Rats and B6C3F1 Mice (Feed Studies). Technical Report Series No. 223. NIH Publication No. 84-1779. 1983. U.S. DHHS, PHS, NIH, NTP, Research Triangle Park, NC.
427 Delgado IF, Carvalho RR, Nogueira, et al. Study on embryofetotoxicity of b-myrcene in the rat. *Food and Chemical Toxicology.* 1993;31(1):31-5.
428 Paumgartten FJ, De-Carvalho RR, Souza CA, et al. Study of the effects of beta-myrcene on rat fertility and general reproductive performance. *Braz J Med Biol Res.* 1998 Jul;31(7):955-65.
429 Johnson JD, Ryan MJ, Toft JD II, et al. Two-year toxicity and carcinogenicity study of methyl eugenol in F344/N rats and B6C3F(1) mice. *J Agric Food Chem.* 2000 Aug;48(8):3620-32.
430 European Commission. Opinion of the Scientific Committee on Food on methyl eugenol (4-Allyl-1,2- dimethoxybenzene). Available at: http://ec.europa.eu/food/fs/sc/scf/out102_en.pdf.
431 National Toxicology Program. NTP Toxicology and Carcinogenesis Studies of Methyleugenol (CAS NO. 93-15-2) in F344/N Rats and B6C3F1 Mice (Gavage Studies). *Natl Toxicol Program Tech Rep Ser.* 2000 Jul;491:1-412.
432 National Toxicology Program. Carcinogenesis Studies of Eugenol (CAS No. 97-53-0) in F344/N Rats and B6C3F1 Mice (Feed Studies). Technical Report Series No. 223. NIH Publication No. 84-1779. 1983. U.S. DHHS, PHS, NIH, NTP, Research Triangle Park, NC.
433 Chen SJ, Wang MH, Chen IJ. Antiplatelet and calcium inhibitory properties of eugenol and sodium eugenol acetate. *Gen Pharmacol.* 1996 Jun;27(4):629-33.
434 Tognolini M, Barocelli E, Ballabeni V, et al. Comparative screening of plant essential oils; phenylpropanoid moiety as basic core for antiplatelet activity. *Life Sci.* 2006 Feb 23;78(13):1419-32.
435 Heck AM, DeWitt BA, Lukes AL. Potential interactions between alternative therapies and warfarin. *Am J Health Syst Pharm.* 2000;57(13):1221-1227.
436 Saaeed SA, Gilani AH. Antithrombotic activity of clove oil. *J Pak Med Assoc.* 1994;44(5):112-15.
437 Kamatou GP, Vermaak I, Viljoen AM. Eugenol—from the remote Maluku Islands to the international market place: A review of a remarkable and versatile molecule. *Molecules.* 2012;17:6953-81.
438 Cochrane ML. Inhibition of Cytochrome P450 2C9 by essential oils. Available at: https://libres.uncg.edu/ir/uncg/listing.aspx?id=18102.
439 Dohi S, Terasaki M, Makino M. Acetylcholinesterase inhibitory activity and chemical composition of commercial essential oils. *J Agric Food Chem.* 2009 May 27;57(10):4313-8.
440 Lee SE, Lee BH, Choi WS, et al. Fumigant toxicity of volatile natural products from Korean spices and medicinal plants towards the rice weevil, Sitophilus oryzae (L). *Pest Manag Sci.* 2001;57:548-53.
441 Langeveld WT, Veldhuizen EJ, Burt SA. Synergy between essential oil constituents and antibiotics. *Crit Rev Microbiol.* 2014 Feb;40(1);76-94.
442 Hemaiswarya S, Doble M. Synergistic interaction of eugenol with antibiotics against Gram negative bacteria. *Phytomedicine.* 2009 Nov;16(11):997-1005.
443 Ahmad A, Khan A, Ahmad Khan L, et al. In vitro synergy of eugenol and methyleugenol with fluconazole against clinical Candida isolates. *J Med Microbiol.* 2010;59:1178-84.
444 Sarrami N, Pemberton MN, Thornhill MH, et al. Adverse reactions associated with the use of eugenol in dentistry. *British Dental J.* 2002;193:253-55.
445 Tammannavar P, Pushpalatha C, Jain S, et al. An unexpected positive hypersensitive reaction to eugenol. *BMJ Case Rep.* 2013; 2013: bcr2013009464.
446 Padmakumari KP, Sasidharan I, Sreekumar MM. Composition and antioxidant activity of essential oil of pimento (Pimenta dioica (L) Merr.) from Jamaica. *Nat Prod Res.* 2011 Jan;25(2):152-60.
447 Jirovetz L, Buchbauer G, Stoilova I, et al. Spice plants: Chemical composition and antioxidant properties of Pimenta Lindl. essential oils, part 1: Pimenta dioica (L.) Merr. leaf oil from Jamaica. *ERNÄHRUNG/NUTRITION.* 2007;31:55-63.

[448] Dharmadasa RM, Abeysinghe DC, Dissanayake DMN, et al. Leaf Essential Oil Composition, Antioxidant Activity, Total Phenolic Content and Total Flavonoid Content of Pimenta Dioica (L.) Merr (Myrtaceae): A Superior Quality Spice Grown in Sri Lanka. *Universal J Agric Res*. 2015;3(2):49-52.
[449] Misharina TA, Alinkina ES, Medvedeva IB. [Antiradical properties of essential oils and extracts from clove bud and pimento]. *Prikl Biokhim Mikrobiol*. 2015 Jan-Feb;51(1):99-104.
[450] Padmakumari Amma KP, Rani MP, Sasidharan I, et al. Comparative chemical composition and in vitro antioxidant activities of essential oil isolated from the leaves of Cinnamomum tamala and Pimenta dioica. *Nat Prod Res*. 2013;27(3):290-4.
[451] Ramos A, Visozo A, Piloto J, et al. Screening of antimutagenicity via antioxidant activity in Cuban medicinal plants. *J Ethnopharmacol*. 2003 Aug;87(2-3):241-6.
[452] Martinez-Velazquez M, Castillo-Herrera G, Rosario-Cruz R, et al. Acaricidal effect and chemical composition of essential oils extracted from Cuminum cyminum, Pimenta dioica and Ocimum basilicum against the cattle tick Rhipicephalus (Boophilus) microplus (Acari). *Parasitol Res*. 2011 Feb;108(2):481-87.
[453] Park IK, Kim J, Lee SG, et al. Nematicidal Activity of Plant Essential Oils and Components From Ajowan (Trachyspermum ammi), Allspice (Pimenta dioica) and Litsea (Litsea cubeba) Essential Oils Against Pine Wood Nematode (Bursaphelenchus Xylophilus). *J Nematol*. 2007 Sep;39(3):275–79.
[454] Kim JR, Haribalan P, Son BK, et al. Fumigant toxicity of plant essential oils against Camptomyia corticalis (Diptera: Cecidomyiidae). *J Econ Entomol*. 2012 Aug;105(4):1329-34.
[455] Oussalah M, Caillet S, Saucier L, et al. Antimicrobial effects of selected plant essential oils on the growth of a Pseudomonas putida strain isolated from meat. *Meat Sci*. 2006 Jun;73(2):236-44.
[456] Oussalah M, Caillet S, Saucier L, et al. Inhibitory effects of selected plant essential oils on the growth of four pathogenic bacteria: E. coli O157:H7, Salmonella Typhimurium, Staphylococcus aureus and Listeria monocytogenes. *Food Control*. 2007 May;18(5):414-20.
[457] Zabka M, Pavela R, Slezakova L. Antifungal effect of Pimenta dioica essential oil against dangerous pathogenic and toxinogenic fungi. *Industrial Crops Products*. 2009 Sep;30(2):250-53.
[458] Feng J, Shi W, Miklossy J, et al. Identification of Essential Oils with Strong Activity against Stationary Phase Borrelia burgdorferi. *Antibiotics (Basel)*. 2018 Oct 16;7(4).
[459] Chaudhari AK, Singh VK, Dwivedy AK, et al. Chemically characterised Pimenta dioica (L.) Merr. essential oil as a novel plant based antimicrobial against fungal and aflatoxin B1 contamination of stored maize and its possible mode of action. *Nat Prod Res*. 2018 Nov 13:1-5.
[460] Lorenzo-Leal AC, Palou E, López-Malo A. Evaluation of the efficiency of allspice, thyme and rosemary essential oils on two foodborne pathogens in in-vitro and on alfalfa seeds, and their effect on sensory characteristics of the sprouts. *Int J Food Microbiol*. 2019 Feb 12;295:19-24.
[461] Gomes da Rocha Voris D, Dos Santos Dias L, Alencar Lima J, et al. Evaluation of larvicidal, adulticidal, and anticholinesterase activities of essential oils of Illicium verum Hook. f., Pimenta dioica (L.) Merr., and Myristica fragrans Houtt. against Zika virus vectors. *Environ Sci Pollut Res Int*. 2018 Aug;25(23):22541-22551.
[462] Lorenzo-Leal AC, Palou E, López-Malo A, et al. Antimicrobial, Cytotoxic, and Anti-Inflammatory Activities of Pimenta dioica and Rosmarinus officinalis Essential Oils. *Biomed Res Int*. 2019 May 7;2019:1639726.
[463] Mahomoodally F, Aumeeruddy-Elafi Z, Venugopala KN, et al. Antiglycation, Comparative Antioxidant Potential, Phenolic Content and Yield Variation of Essential Oils From 19 Exotic and Endemic Medicinal Plants. *Saudi J Biol Sci*. 2019 Nov;26(7):1779-88.
[464] Xao S, Cui P, Shi W, et al. Identification of Essential Oils With Strong Activity Against Stationary Phase Uropathogenic Escherichia Coli. Discov Med. 2019 Oct;28(154):179-188.
[465] Xiao S, Cui P, Shi W, et al. Identification of essential oils with activity against stationary phase Staphylococcus aureus. *BMC Complement Med Ther*. 2020 Mar 24;20(1):99.
[466] Merida-Reyes MS, Munoz-Wug MA, Oliva-Hernandez BE, et al. Composition and Antibacterial Activity of the Essential Oil from Pimenta dioica (L.) Merr. from Guatemala. *Medicines (Basel)*. 2020 Sep 23;7(10):E59.
[467] Marques CS, Carvalho SG, Bertoli LD, et al. β-Cyclodextrin inclusion complexes with essential oils: Obtention, characterization, antimicrobial activity and potential application for food preservative sachets. *Food Res Int*. 2019 May;119:499-509.
[468] Ismail MM, Samir R, Saber FR, et al. Pimenta Oil as A Potential Treatment for Acinetobacter Baumannii Wound Infection: In Vitro and In Vivo Bioassays in Relation to Its Chemical Composition. *Antibiotics (Basel)*. 2020 Oct 7;9(10):679.
[469] Youssef FS, Labib RM, Gad HA, et al. Pimenta dioica and Pimenta racemosa: GC-based metabolomics for the assessment of seasonal and organ variation in their volatile components, in silico and in vitro cytotoxic activity estimation. *Food Funct*. 2021 May 14. Online ahead of print.
[470] Sarathambal C, Rajagopal S, Viswanathan R. Mechanism of antioxidant and antifungal properties of Pimenta dioica (L.) leaf essential oil on Aspergillus flavus. *J Food Sci Technol*. 2021 Jul;58(7):2497-2506.
[471] Sarathambal C, Rajagopal S, Viswanathan R. Mechanism of antioxidant and antifungal properties of Pimenta dioica(L.) leaf essential oil on Aspergillus flavus. *J Food Sci Technol*. 2021 Jul;58(7):2497-2506.
[472] Chaudhari AK, Sing VK, Das S, et al. Fabrication, characterization, and bioactivity assessment of chitosan nanoemulsion containing allspice essential oil to mitigate Aspergillus flavus contamination and aflatoxin B 1 production in maize. *Food Chem*. 2021 Sep 25;372:131221.
[473] Narayanankutty A, Kuttithodi AM, Alfarhan A, et al. Chemical Composition, Insecticidal and Mosquito Larvicidal Activities of Allspice (Pimenta dioica) Essential Oil. *Molecules*. 2021 Nov 5;26(21):6698.
[474] Peter R, Josende ME, da Silva Barreto J, et al. Effect of Illicium verum (Hook) essential oil on cholinesterase and locomotor activity of Alphitobius diaperinus (Panzer). *Pestic Biochem Physiol*. 2022 Feb;181:105027.
[475] Alrashidi AA, Noumi E, Snoussi M, et al. Chemical Composition, Antibacterial and Anti-Quorum Sensing Activities of Pimenta dioica L. Essential Oil and Its Major Compound (Eugenol) against Foodborne Pathogenic Bacteria. *Plants (Basel)*. 2022 Feb 17;11(4):540.
[476] Soonwera M, Moungthipmalai T, Takawirapat W, et al. Ovicidal and repellent activities of several plant essential oils against Periplaneta americana L. and enhanced activities from their combined formulation. *Sci Rep*. 2022 Jul 15;12(1):12070.
[477] Van Beek TA, Kleis R, Posthumus MA, et al. Essential oil of Amyris balsamifera. *Phytochemistry*. 1989;28(7):1909-11.
[478] Howes MJR, Simmonds MSJ, Kite GC. Evaluation of the quality of sandalwood essential oils by gas chromatography–mass spectrometry. *J Chromatography A*. 2004;1028:307-12.
[479] Edens Garden. Chromatogram Amyris. Available at: https://cdn.shopify.com/s/files/1/0380/8537/files/Amyris_8_15.pdf?8518045739611058027.
[480] Stillpoint Aromatics. Amyris Essential Oil. Available at: http://www.stillpointaromatics.com/amyris-Amyris-balsamiferaessential-oil-aromatherapy.
[481] Mauerman B, Ahmed N, Tambhar N, et al. Trends in Furanocoumarin Profiles Among Commerical-Scale Essential Oils. International Conference on the Science of Botanicals, Poster. Mar 2022.
[482] Jirovetz L, Buchbauer G, Denkova Z, et al. Comparative study on the antimicrobial activities of different sandalwood essential oils of various origin. *Flavour Frag J*. 2006 May-Jun;21(3):465-68.
[483] Baylac S, Racine P. Inhibition of 5-lipoxygenase by essential oils and other natural fragrant extracts. *Int J Aromatherapy*. 2003;13(2-3):138-42.
[484] Carroll JF, Paluch G, Coats J, et al. Elemol and amyris oil repel the ticks Ixodes scapularis and Amblyomma americanum (Acari: Ixodidae) in laboratory bioassays. *Exp Appl Acarol*. 2010 Aug;51(4):383-92.
[485] Amer A, Mehlhorn H. Larvicidal effects of various essential oils against Aedes, Anopheles, and Culex larvae (Diptera, Culicidae). *Parasitology Res*. 2006 Apr;99(4):466-72.
[486] Zhu J, Zeng X, Yanma, et al. Adult repellency and larvicidal activity of five plant essential oils against mosquitoes. *J Am Mosq Control Assoc*. 2006 Sep;22(3):515-22.
[487] Feng J, Shi W, Miklossy J, et al. Identification of Essential Oils with Strong Activity against Stationary Phase Borrelia burgdorferi. *Antibiotics (Basel)*. 2018 Oct 16;7(4).
[488] Xiao S, Cui P, Shi W, et al. Identification of essential oils with activity against stationary phase Staphylococcus aureus. *BMC Complement Med Ther*. 2020 Mar 24;20(1):99.
[489] Rapper SL, Tankeu S, Kamatou G, et al. The use of chemometric modelling to determine chemical composition-antimicrobial activity relationships of essential oils used in respiratory tract infections. *Fitoterapia*. 2021 Aug 26;105024.
[490] Fraternale D, Flamini G, Ricci D. Essential oil composition and antimicrobial activity of Angelica adchangelica L. (Apiaceae) roots. *J Med Food*. 2014 Sep;17(9):1043–47.
[491] Nivinskiene O, Butkiene R, Mockute D. Changes in the chemical composition of essential oil of Angelica archangelica L. roots during storage. *Chemija* (Vilnius). 2003;14(1):52–56.
[492] Pasqua G, Monacelli B. Silvestrini A. Accumulation of essential oils in relation to root differentiation in Angelica archangelica L. *Eur J Histochemistry*. 2003Jan-Mar;47(1):87–90.
[493] Wu MJ, Sun XJ, Dai YH, et al. Determination of constituents of essential oil from Angelica sinensis by gas chromatography — mass spectrometry. *J Central South Univeristy Tech*. 2005 Aug;12(4):430-36.
[494] Tabanaca N, Wedge DE, Wang X, et al. Chemical Composition and Antifungal Activity of Angelica sinensis Essential Oil against three Colletotrichum species. *Nat Prod Commun*. 2008;7(3):1073-78.
[495] Raquet N, Schrenk D. Application of the equivalency factor concept to the phototoxicity and genotoxicity of furocoumarin mixtures. *Food Chem Toxicol*. 2014 Jun;68:257–66.
[496] Scientific Committee on Consumer Products. Opinion on furocoumarins in cosmetic products. 2005 Dec. Available at:
http://ec.europa.eu/health/ph_risk/committees/04_sccp/docs/sccp_o_036.pdf.
[497] Qang K, Cao P, Shui W, et al. Angelica sinensis polysaccharide regulates glucose and lipid metabolism disorder in prediabetic and streptozotocin-induced diabetic mice through the elevation of glycogen levels and reduction of inflammatory factors. *Food Funct*. 2015 Mar;6(3):902–09.
[498] Tang Y, Zhu M, Yu S, et al. Identification and comparative quantification of bio-active phthalides in essential oils from Si-Wu-Tang, Fo-Shou-San, Radix Angelica and Rhizoma Chuanziong. *Molecules*. 2010;15:341–51.
[499] Lao SC, Li SP, Kan KKW, et al. Identification and quantification of 13 components in Angelica sinensis (Danggui) by gas chromatography-mass spectrometry coupled with pressurized liquid extraction. *Analytica Chimica Acta*. 2004;526:131–37.
[500] Circosta C, Pasquale RD, Palumbo DR, et al. Estrogenic activity of standardized extract of Angelica sinensis. *Phytother Res*. 2006 Aug;20(8):665–69.
[501] Zhu DPQ. Dong quai. *Am J Chinese Med*. 1987;15:117-125.
[502] Fraternale D, Flamini G, Ricci D. Essential oil composition and antimicrobial activity of Angelica adchangelica L. (Apiaceae) roots. *J Med Food*. 2014 Sep;17(9):1043–47.
[503] Fraternale D, Teodori L, Rudov A, et al. The In Vitro Activity of Angelica archangelica L. Essential Oil on Inflammation. *J Med Food*. 2018 Aug 29;21(12):1238-43.
[504] Korpinen RI, Valimaa AL, Liimatainen J, et al. Essential Oils and Supercritical CO 2 Extracts of Arctic Angelica ( Angelica archangelica L.), Marsh Labrador Tea ( Rhododendron tomentosum) and Common Tansy ( Tanacetum vulgare)-Chemical Compositions and Antimicrobial Activities. *Molecules*. 2021 Nov 25;26(23):7121.
[505] Pathak S, Wanjari MM, Jain SK, et al. Evaluation of antiseizure activity of essential oil from roots of Angelica archangelica Linn. in mice. *Indian J Pharm Sci*. 2010 May;72(3):371–75.
[506] Orav A1, Raal A, Arak E. Essential oil composition of Pimpinella anisum L. fruits from various European countries. *Nat Prod Res*. 2008 Feb 15;22(3):227-32.
[507] Ozcan MM, Chalchat JC. Chemical composition and antifungal effect of anise (Pimpinella anisum L.) fruit oil at ripening stage. *Physiology Metab Orig Art*. 2006 Dec;56(4):353-58.

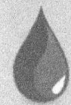

[508] Ullah H, Mahmood A, Honermeier B. Essential oil and composition of anise (Pimpinella anisum L.) with varying seed rates and row spacing. *Pak J Bot.* 2014;46(5):1859-64.

[509] Kimbaris AC, Koliopoulos G, Michaelakis, et al. Bioactivity of Dianthus caryophyllus, Lepidium sativum, Pimpinella anisum, and Illicium verum essential oils and their major components against the West Nile vector Culex pipiens. *Parasitol Res.* 2012;111:2403-10.

[510] Acimovic M, Tesevic V, Todosijevic M, et al. Compositional characteristics of the essential oil of Pimpinella anisum and Foeniculum vulgare grown in Serbia. *Botanica Serbica.* 2015;39(1):9-14.

[511] Radaelli M, da Silva BP, Weidlich L, et al. Antimicrobial activities of six essential oils commonly used as condiments in Brazil against Clostridium perfringens. *Braz J Microbiol.* 2016 Apr-Jun;47(2):424-30.

[512] Akdemir Evrendilek G. Empirical prediction and validation of antibacterial inhibitory effects of various plant essential oils on common pathogenic bacteria. *Int J Food Microbiol.* 2015 Jun 2;202:35-41.

[513] European Medicines Agency. Public statement on the use of herbal medicinal products containing estragole. Available at: http://www.ema.europa.eu/docs/en_GB/document_library/Scientific_guideline/2010/04/WC500089960.pdf.

[514] Tabanca N, Khan SI, Bedir E, et al. Estrogenic activity of isolated constituents and essential oils of Pimpinella species from Turkey, evaluated using a recombinant yeast screen. *Planta Med.* 2004 Aug;70(8):728-35.

[515] Albert-Puleo M. Fennel and anise as estrogenic agents. *J Ethnopharmacol.* 1980 Dec;2(4):337-44.

[516] Malini T, Vanithakumari G, Megala N, et al. Effect of Foeniculum vulgare Mill. seed extract on the genital organs of male and female rats. *Indian J Physiol Pharmacol.* 1985 Jan-Mar;29(1):21-6.

[517] Howes MJ, Houghton PJ, Barlow DJ, et al. Assessment of estrogenic activity in some common essential oil constituents. *J Pharm Pharmacol.* 2002 Nov;54(11):1521-28.

[518] Ostad SN, Soodi M, Shariffzadeh M, et al. The effect of fennel essential oil on uterine contraction as a model for dysmenorrhea, pharmacology and toxicology study. *J Ethnopharmacol.* 2001 Aug;76(3):299-304.

[519] Rosti L, Nardini A, Bettini ME, et al. Toxic effects of a herbal tea mixture in two newborns. *Acta Paediatrica.* 1994;83:683.

[520] Turkyilmaz Z, Karabulut R, Sonmez K, et al. A striking and frequent cause of premature thelarche in children: Foeniculum vulgare. *J Pediatr Surg.* 2008 Nov;43(11):2109-11.

[521] Tognolini M, Barocelli E, Ballabeni V, et al. Comparative screening of plant essential oils; phenylpropanoid moiety as basic core for antiplatelet activity. *Life Sci.* 2006 Feb 23;78(13):1419-32.

[522] Yoshioka M, Tamada TT. Aromatic factors of anti-platelet aggregation in fennel oil. *Biogenic Amines.* 2005 Apr;19(2):89-96.

[523] Tognolini M, Ballabeni V, Bertoni S, et al. Protective effect of Foeniculum vulgare essential oil and anethole in an experimental model of thrombosis. *Pharm Res.* 2007;56:254-60.

[524] Dhar SK. Anti-fertility activity and hormonal profile of trans-anethole in rats. *Indian J Physiol Pharmacol.* 1995;39(1):63-67.

[525] Kreydiyyeh SI, Usta J, Knio K, et al. Aniseed oil increases glucose absorption and reduces urine output in the rat. *Life Sci.* 2003 Dec 19;74(5):663-73.

[526] Sheikh BA, Pari L, Rathinham A, et al. Trans-anethole, a terpenoid ameliorates hyperglycemia by regulating key enzymes of carbohydrate metabolism in streptozotocin induced diabetic rats. *Biochimie.* 2015 May;112:57-65.

[527] Pari L, Sheikh BA. Antihyperglycemic effect of trans-anethole in streptozotocin induced diabetic rats with special reference to glycoprotein components. *Int J Adv Res Biol Sci.* 2015;2(5):28-34.

[528] Kreydiyyeh SI, Usta J, Knio K, et al. Aniseed oil increases glucose absorption and reduces urine output in the rat. *Life Sci.* 2003 Dec 19;74(5):663-73.

[529] Samojlik I, Petković S, Stilinović N, et al. Pharmacokinetic Herb-Drug Interaction between Essential Oil of Aniseed (Pimpinella anisum L., Apiaceae) and Acetaminophen and Caffeine: A Potential Risk for Clinical Practice. *Phytother Res.* 2016 Feb;30(2):253-9.

[530] Wisniewski-Rebecca ES, Rocha BA, Wiirzler LA, et al. Synergistic effects of anethole and ibuprofen in acute inflammatory response. *Chem Biol Interact.* 2015 Dec 5;242:247-53.

[531] Samojlik I, Mijatović V, Petković S, et al. The influence of essential oil of aniseed (Pimpinella anisum, L.) on drug effects on the central nervous system. *Fitoterapia.* 2012 Dec;83(8):1466-73.

[532] Samojlik I, Mijatović V, Petković S, et al. The influence of essential oil of aniseed (Pimpinella anisum, L.) on drug effects on the central nervous system. *Fitoterapia.* 2012 Dec;83(8):1466-73.

[533] Samojlik I, Mijatović V, Petković S, et al. The influence of essential oil of aniseed (Pimpinella anisum, L.) on drug effects on the central nervous system. *Fitoterapia.* 2012 Dec;83(8):1466-73.

[534] Samojlik I, Mijatović V, Petković S, et al. The influence of essential oil of aniseed (Pimpinella anisum, L.) on drug effects on the central nervous system. *Fitoterapia.* 2012 Dec;83(8):1466-73.

[535] Howes MJ, Houghton PJ, Barlow DJ, et al. Assessment of estrogenic activity in some common essential oil constituents. *J Pharm Pharmacol.* 2002 Nov;54(11):1521-28.

[536] Chen CH, deGraffenreid LA. Anethole suppressed cell survival and induced apoptosis in human breast cancer cells independent of estrogen receptor status. *Phytomedicine.* 2012 Jun 15;19(8-9):763-7.

[537] Nessa MU, Beale P, Chan C, et al. Studies on combination of platinum drugs cisplatin and oxaliplatin with phytochemicals anethole and curcumin in ovarian tumor models. *Anticancer Res.* 2012 Nov;32(11):4843-50.

[538] Ostad SN, Soodi M, Shariffzadeh M, et al. The effect of fennel essential oil on uterine contraction as a model for dysmenorrhea, pharmacology and toxicology study. *J Ethnopharmacol.* 2001 Aug;76(3):299-304.

[539] Khorshidi N, Ostad SN, Mosaddegh M, et al. Clinical effects of fennel essential oil on primary dysmenorrhea. *Iran J Pharm Res.* 2003 Spring;2(2):89-93.

[540] Nahidi F1, Kariman N, Simbar M, et al. The Study on the Effects of Pimpinella anisum on Relief and Recurrence of Menopausal Hot Flashes. *Iran J Pharm Res.* 2012 Fall;11(4):1079-85.

[541] Subehan UT, Iwata H, Kadota S, et al. Mechanism-based inhibition of CYP3A4 and CYP2D6 by Indonesian medicinal plants. *J Ethnopharmacol.* 2006 May;105(3):449-55.

[542] Subehan Z, Kadota SF, Tezuka Y. Inhibition on human liver cytochrome P450 3A4 by constituents of fennel (Foeniculum vulgare): Identification and characterization of a mechanism-based inactivator. *J Agric Food Chem.* 2007 Dec;55(25):10162-67.

[543] Yarnell E, Abascal K. Interaction of Herbal Constituents with Cytochrome P450 Enzymes. *Alt Complement Ther.* 2007 Nov;13(5):239-47.

[544] Sinitskaia ZF, Lashneva NV, Chichilanova GV, et al. [Effect of trans-anethole on liver monooxygenase system and its induction of polychlorinated diphenyls]. *Vopr Pitan.* 1994;(5):24-7.

[545] Rompelberg CJ, Verhagen H, van Bladeren PJ. Effects of the naturally occurring alkenylbenzenes eugenol and trans-anethole on drug-metabolizing enzymes in the rat liver. *Food Chem Toxicol.* 1993 Sep;31(9):637-45.

[546] Rompelberg CJ, Verhagen H, van Bladeren PJ. Effects of the naturally occurring alkenylbenzenes eugenol and trans-anethole on drug-metabolizing enzymes in the rat liver. *Food Chem Toxicol.* 1993 Sep;31(9):637-45.

[547] Fitsiou E, Mitropoulou G, Spyridopoulou K, et al. Phytochemical Profile and Evaluation of the Biological Activities of Essential Oils Derived from the Greek Aromatic Plant Species Ocimum basilicum, Mentha spicata, Pimpinella anisum and Fortunella margarita. *Molecules.* 2016 Aug 16;21(8).

[548] Koriem KM, Arbid MS, El-Gendy NF, et al. The Protective Role of Anise Oil in Oxidative Stress and Genotoxicity Produced in Favism. *J Diet Suppl.* 2016;13(5):505-21.

[549] Radaelli M, da Silva BP, Weidlich L, et al. Antimicrobial activities of six essential oils commonly used as condiments in Brazil against Clostridium perfringens. *Braz J Microbiol.* 2016 Apr-Jun;47(2):424-30.

[550] Akdemir Evrendilek G. Empirical prediction and validation of antibacterial inhibitory effects of various plant essential oils on common pathogenic bacteria. *Int J Food Microbiol.* 2015 Jun 2;202:35-41.

[551] Shukla HS, Tripathi SC. Antifungal substance in the essential oil of anise (Pimpinella anisum L.). *Ultural and Biological Chemistry.* 1987;51(7):1991–1993.

[552] Felšöciová S, Kačániová M, Horská E, et al. Antifungal activity of essential oils against selected terverticillate penicillia. *Ann Agric Environ Med.* 2015;22(1):38-42.

[553] Kosalec I, Pepeljnjak S, Kuatrak D. Antifungal activity of fluid extract and essential oil from anise fruits (Pimpinella anisum L., Apiaceae). *Acta Pharmaceutica.* 2005;55(4):377–385.

[554] Özcan MM, Chalchat JC. Chemical composition and antifungal effect of anise (Pimpinella anisum L.) fruit oil at ripening stage. *Annals of Microbiology.* 2006;56(4):353–358.

[555] Fitsiou E, Mitropoulou G, Spyridopoulou K, et al. Phytochemical Profile and Evaluation of the Biological Activities of Essential Oils Derived from the Greek Aromatic Plant Species Ocimum basilicum, Mentha spicata, Pimpinella anisum and Fortunella margarita. *Molecules.* 2016 Aug 16;21(8).

[556] Gradinaru AC, Miron A, Trifan A, et al. Screening of antibacterial effects of anise essential oil alone and in combination with conventional antibiotics against Streptococcus pneumoniae clinical isolates. *Rev Med Chir Soc Med Nat Iasi.* 2014 Apr-Jun;118(2):537-43.

[557] Pourgholami MH, Majzoob S, Javadi M, et al. The fruit essential oil of Pimpinella anisum exerts anticonvulsant effects in mice. *J Ethnopharmacol.* 1999 Aug;66(2):211-5.

[558] Koch C, Reichling J, Kehm R, et al. Efficacy of anise oil, dwarf-pine oil and chamomile oil against thymidine- kinase-positive and thymidine-kinase-negative herpesviruses. *J Pharm Pharmacol.* 2008 Nov;60(11):1545-50.

[559] Ferreira A, Proenca C, Serralheiro ML, et al. The in vitro screening for acetylcholinesterase inhibition and antioxidant activity of medicinal plants from Portugal. *J Ethnopharmacol.* 2006 Nov 3;108(1):31-37.

[560] Tas A. Analgesic effect of Pimpinella anisum L. essential oil extract in mice. *Indian Veterinary Journal.* 2009;86(2):145–147.

[561] Tas A, Özbek H, Atasoy N, Altug ME, Ceylan E. Evaluation of analgesic and antiinflammatory activity of Pimpinella anisum fixed oil extract. *Indian Veterinary Journal.* 2006;83(8):840–843.

[562] Karimzadeh F, Hosseini M, Mangeng D, et al. Anticonvulsant and neuroprotective effects of Pimpinella anisum in rat brain. *BMC Complement Altern Med.* 2012 Jun 18;12:76.

[563] Mosaffa-Jahromi M, Tamaddon AM, Afsharypuor S, et al. Effectiveness of Anise Oil for Treatment of Mild to Moderate Depression in Patients With Irritable Bowel Syndrome: A Randomized Active and Placebo-Controlled Clinical Trial. *J Evid Based Complementary Altern Med.* 2017 Jan;22(1):41-46.

[564] Koch C, Reichling J, Kehm R, et al. Efficacy of anise oil, dwarf-pine oil and chamomile oil against thymidine- kinase-positive and thymidine-kinase-negative herpesviruses. *J Pharm Pharmacol.* 2008 Nov;60(11):1545-50.

[565] Koch C, Reichling J, Schneele J, et al. Inhibitory effect of essential oils against herpes simplex virus type 2. *Phytomedicine.* 2008 Jan;15(1-2):71-8.

[566] Veal L. The potential effectiveness of essential oils as a treatment for headlice, Pediculus humanus capitis. *Complement Ther Nurs Midwifery.* 1996 Aug;2(4):97-101.

[567] Yones DA, Bakir HY, Bayoumi SA, et al. Chemical composition and efficacy of some selected plant oils against Pediculus humanus capitis in vitro. *Parasitol Res.* 2016 Aug;115(8):3209-18.

[568] Tavallali V, Rahmati S, Bahmanzadegan A, et al. Antioxidant activity, polyphenolic contents and essential oil composition of Pimpinella anisum L. as affected by zinc fertilizer. *J Sci Food Agric*. 2017 Nov;97(14):4883-4889.

[569] Asadollahpoor A, Abdollahi M, Rahimi R, et al. Pimpinella anisum L. fruit: Chemical composition and effect on rat model of nonalcoholic fatty liver disease. *J Res Med Sci*. 2017 Mar 15;22:37.

[570] Mosvat SH, Jaberi AR, Sobhani Z, et al. Efficacy of Anise (Pimpinella anisum L.) oil for migraine headache: A pilot randomized placebo-controlled clinical trial. *J Ethnopharmacol*. 2019 May 23;236:155-160.

[571] Mosaffa-Jahromi M, Lankarani KB, Pasalar M, et al. Efficacy and safety of enteric coated capsules of anise oil to treat irritable bowel syndrome. *J Ethnopharmacol*. 2016 Dec 24;194:937-946.

[572] Mosaffa-Jahromi M, Tamaddon AM, Afsharypuor S, et al. Effectiveness of Anise Oil for Treatment of Mild to Moderate Depression in Patients With Irritable Bowel Syndrome: A Randomized Active and Placebo-Controlled Clinical Trial. *J Evid Based Complementary Altern Med*. 2016 Feb 11;22(1):41-6.

[573] Bartoňková I, Dvořák Z. Essential oils of culinary herbs and spices display agonist and antagonist activities at human aryl hydrocarbon receptor AhR. *Food Chem Toxicol*. 2018 Jan;111:374-384.

[574] Hashem AS, Awadalla SS, Zayed GM, et al. Pimpinella anisum essential oil nanoemulsions against Tribolium castaneum-insecticidal activity and mode of action. *Environ Sci Pollut Res Int*. 2018 Jul;25(19):18802-18812.

[575] Vieira JN, Gonçalves CL, Villarreal JPV, et al. Chemical composition of essential oils from the apiaceae family, cytotoxicity, and their antifungal activity in vitro against candida species from oral cavity. *Braz J Biol*. 2019 Jul-Sep;79(3):432-437.

[576] Skuhrovec J, Douda O, Zouhar M, et al. Insecticidal and Behavioral Effect of Microparticles of Pimpinella Anisum Essential Oil on Larvae of Leptinotarsa Decemlineata (Coleoptera: Chrysomelidae). *J Econ Entomol*. 2020 Feb 8;113(1):255-262.

[577] Hashem AS, Ramadan MM, Abdel-Hady AAA, et al. Pimpinella anisum Essential Oil Nanoemulsion Toxicity against Tribolium castaneum? Shedding Light on Its Interactions with Aspartate Aminotransferase and Alanine Aminotransferase by Molecular Docking. *Molecules*. 2020 Oct 20;25(20):4841.

[578] Das S, Singh VK, Dwivedy AK, et al. Nanostructured Pimpinella anisum essential oil as novel green food preservative against fungal infestation, aflatoxin B 1 contamination and deterioration of nutritional qualities. *Food Chem*. 2020 Nov 8;128574.

[579] Trifan A, Luca SV, Bostǎnaru AC, et al. Apiaceae Essential Oils: Boosters of Terbinafine Activity against Dermatophytes and Potent Anti-Inflammatory Effectors. *Plants (Basel)*. 2021 Nov 4;10(11):2378.

[580] Alomar HA, Fathallah N, Abdel-Aziz MM, et al. GC-MS Profiling, Anti-Helicobacter pylori, and Anti-Inflammatory Activities of Three Apiaceous Fruits' Essential Oils. *Plants (Basel)*. 2022 Oct 5;11(19):2617.

[581] Denett GO, Comelli NC, Rodriguez MR, et al. Chemical composition and insecticidal activity of essential oils from cultivated and native aromatic plants of Argentina against Carpophilus dimidiatus (Fabricius) (Nitidulidae) and Oryzaephilus mercator (L.) (Silvanidae). *Nat Prod Res*. 2023 Jan 9:1-5.

[582] Azam F, Alqarni MH, Alnasser SM, et al. Formulation, In Vitro and In Silico Evaluations of Anise (Pimpinella anisum L.) Essential Oil Emulgel with Improved Antimicrobial Effects. *Gels*. 2023 Jan 28;9(2):111.

[583] Bakhshi M, Kamalinejad M, Shokri M, et al. In vitro antibacterial effect of Pimpinella anisum essential oil on Enterococcus faecalis, Lactobacillus casei, Actinomyces naeslundii, and Aggregatibacter actinomycetemcomitans. *Folia Med (Plovdiv)*. 2022 Oct 31;64(5):799-806.

[584] Božović M, Pirolli A, Ragno R. Mentha suaveolens Ehrh. (Lamiaceae) Essential Oil and Its Main Constituent Piperitenone Oxide: Biological Activities and Chemistry. *Molecules*. 2015;20:9605-33.

[585] El-Kashoury EA, El-Askary HI, Kandil ZA, et al. Chemical Composition and Biological Activities of the Essential Oil of Mentha suaveolens Ehrh. *Z Naturforsch*. 2012;67c:571–79.

[586] Benyad N, Ebrahim W, Hakiki A, et al. Chemical characterization and insecticidal evaluation of the essential oil of Mentha suaveolens L. and Mentha puelgium L. growing in Morocco. *Studii şi Cercetări Ştiinţifice, Chimie şi Inginerie Chimică, Biotehnologii, Industrie Alimentară*. 2012;13(1):27-32.

[587] Pavela R, Kaffkova K, Kumsta. Chemical Composition and Larvicidal Activity of Essential Oils from Different Mentha L. and Pulegium Species against Culex quinquefasciatus Say (Diptera: Culicidae). *Plant Protect Sci*. 2014;50(1):36-42.

[588] Koliopoulos G, Pitarokili D, Kioulos E, et al. Chemical composition and larvicidal evaluation of Mentha, Salvia, and Melissa essential oils against the West Nile virus misquito Culex pipiens. *Parasitol Res*. 2010;107:327-35.

[589] Zekri N, Sabri H, Khannouchi S, et al. Phytochemical study and fumigant toxicity of Mentha suaveolens Ehrh essential oil from Morocco against adults of S. oryzae. *Australian J Basic Appl Sci*. 2013 Dec;7(14):499-606.

[590] Brada M, Bezzina M, Marlier M, et al. Variabilité de la composition chimique des huiles essentielles de Mentha rotundifolia du nord de l'Algérie. *Biotechnol Agron Soc Environ*. 2007;11(1):3-7.

[591] Sutour S, Bradesi P, Casanova J, et al. Composition and chemical variability of Mentha suaveolens ssp. suaveolens and M. suaveolens ssp. insularis from Corsica. *Chem Biodivers*. 2010 Apr;7(4):1002-8.

[592] Aziz EE, Craker LE. Essential oil constituents of peppermint, pennyroyal and applemint grown in a desert agrosystem. *J Herbs Spices Med Plants*. 2009;15:361-67.

[593] Velasco-Negueruela A, Perez-Alonso MJ. Essential oils of Calamintha nepeta (L.) Savi and Mentha aff suaveolens Ehrh. grown in Córdoba, Argentina. *J Essent Oil Res*. 1996;8:81–84.

[594] El Arch M, Satrani B, Farah A, et al. Composition chimique et activités antimicrobienne et insecticide de l'huile essentielle de Mentha rotundifolia du Maroc. *Acta Bot Gallica*. 2003;150:267-74.

[595] Derwich E, Benziane Z, Taouil R, et al. Comparative Essential Oil Composition of Leaves of Mentha rotundifolia and Mentha pulegium a Traditional Herbal Medicine in Morocco. *American-Eurasian J Sustainable Agric*. 2012;4(1):47-54.

[596] Petretto GL, Fancello F, Zara S, et al. Antimicrobial activity against beneficial microorganisms and chemical composition of essential oil of Mentha suaveolens ssp. insularis grown in Sardinia. *J Food Sci*. 2014 Mar;79(3):M369-77.

[597] Lorenzo D, Paz D, Dellacassa E, et al. Essential oil of Mentha pulegium and Mentha rotundifolia from Uruguay. *Braz Archives Biology Tech*. 2002 Dec;45(4):519-24.

[598] Brada M, Bezzina M, Marlier M, et al. Chemical composition of the leaf oil of Mentha rotundifolia (L.) from Algeria. *J Essent Oil Res*. 2006 Nov-Dec;18:663-65.

[599] Oumzil H, Ghoulami S, Rhajaoui M, et al. Antibacterial and antifungal activity of essential oils of Mentha suaveolens. *Phytother Res*. 2002;16:727–31.

[600] Garzoli S, Pirolli A, Vavala E, et al. Multidisciplinary Approach to Determine the Optimal Time and Period for Extracting the Essential Oil from Mentha suaveolens Ehrh. *Molecules*. 2015 May 26;20(6):9640-55.

[601] Bakerink JA, Gospe SM Jr, Dimand RJ, et al. Multiple organ failure after ingestion of pennyroyal oil from herbal tea in two infants. *Pediatrics*. 1996;98(5):944-47.

[602] Sudekum M, Poppenga RH, Raju N, et al. Pennyroyal oil toxicosis in a dog. *J Am Vet Med Assoc*. 1992;200:817-8.

[603] Anderson IB, Mullen WH, Meeker JE, et al. Pennyroyal toxicity: measurement of toxic metabolite levels in two cases and review of the literature. *Ann Intern Med*. 1996;124:726-34.

[604] Seeff L, Stickel F, Navarro VJ. Hepatotoxicity of herbals and dietary supplements. In, Kaplowitz N, DeLeve LD, eds. Drug-induced liver disease. 3rd ed. Amsterdam: Elsevier, 2013, pp. 631-58.

[605] Moolla A. A phytochemical and pharmacological investigation of indigenous Agathosma species. MSc Dissertation, University of the Witwatersrand. 2006.

[606] Mullen W, Anderson I, Oishii S, et al. Accidental pennyroyal oil ingestion in a toddler with the first human serum metabolite detection. *Vet Hum Toxicol*. 1994;36:342.

[607] Melis K. Bochner A, Janssens G. Accidental nasal eucalyptol and menthol instillation. *Eur J Pediatr*. 1989 Aug;148(8)786-7.

[608] Reynolds JEF. Martindale: The Extra Pharmacopoeia. The Pharmaceutical Press, London. 1993.

[609] No author listed. Monographs on the medicinal uses of plants. *Exeter: European Scientific Cooperative on Phytotherapy*. 1997.

[610] Javorka K, Tomori Z, Zavarska L. Protective and defensive airway reflexes in premature infants. *Physiol Bohemoslov*. 1980;29(1):29-35.

[611] Barnes J, Anderson LA, Philpson JD. Herbal Medicine: A Guide for Healthcare Professionals. London, UK: The Pharmaceutical Press, 1996.

[612] Zimmerman HJ. Unconventional drugs. Miscellaneous drugs and diagnostic chemicals. In, Zimmerman, HJ. Hepatotoxicity: the adverse effects of drugs and other chemicals on the liver. 2nd ed. Philadelphia: Lippincott,1999; pp. 731-34.

[613] Bakerink JA, Gospe SM Jr, Dimand RJ, et al. Multiple organ failure after ingestion of pennyroyal oil from herbal tea in two infants. *Pediatrics*. 1996;98(5):944-47.

[614] Anderson IB, Mullen WH, Meeker JE, et al. Pennyroyal toxicity: measurement of toxic metabolite levels in two cases and review of the literature. *Ann Intern Med*. 1996;124:726-34.

[615] Seeff L, Stickel F, Navarro VJ. Hepatotoxicity of herbals and dietary supplements. In, Kaplowitz N, DeLeve LD, eds. Drug-induced liver disease. 3rd ed. Amsterdam: Elsevier, 2013, pp. 631-58.

[616] Lassila T, Mattila S, Turpeinen M, et al. Tandem mass spectrometric analysis of S- and N-linked glutathione conjugates of pulegone and menthofuran and identification of P450 enzymes mediating their formation. *Rapid Commun Mass Spectrom*. 2016 Apr 15;30(7):917-26.

[617] Nelson SD, McClanahan RH, Thomassen D, et al. Investigations of mechanisms of reactive metabolite formation from (R)-(+)-pulegone. *Xenobiotica*. 1992 Sep-Oct;22(9-10):1157-64.

[618] Moorthy B, Madyastha P, Madyastha KM. Metabolism of a monoterpene ketone, R-(+)-pulegone--a hepatotoxin in rat. *Xenobiotica*. 1989 Feb;19(2):217-24.

[619] Madyastha KM, Raj CP. Effects of menthofuran, a monoterpene furan on rat liver microsomal enzymes, in vivo. *Toxicology*. 1994 Apr 18;89(2):119-25.

[620] Nelson SD. Mechanisms of the formation and disposition of reactive metabolites that can cause acute liver injury. *Drug Metab Rev*. 1995;27(1-2):147-77.

[621] Moorthy B, Madyastha P, Madyastha KM. Hepatotoxicity of pulegone in rats: its effects on microsomal enzymes, in vivo. *Toxicology*. 1989 May 15;55(3):327-37.

[622] Madyastha KM, Raj CP. Effects of menthofuran, a monoterpene furan on rat liver microsomal enzymes, in vivo. *Toxicology*. 1994 Apr 18;89(2):119-25.

[623] Burkhard PR, Burkhardt K, Haenggeli CA, et al. Plant-induced seizures: reappearance of an old problem. *J Neurol*. 1999 Aug;246(8):667-70.

[624] Olowe SA, Ransome-Kuti O. The risk of jaundice in glucose-6-phosphate dehydrogenase deficient babies exposed to menthol. *Acta Paediatr Scand*. 1980 May;69(3):341-5.

[625] Dillon Remy M, Manning Alleyne P, Bratt DE, et al. Neonatal jaundice at Port-of-Spain General Hospital abstract. *West Indian Med J*. 1987;36(Suppl):28.

[626] Akdogan M, Gultekin F, Yontem M. Effect of Mentha piperita (Labiatae) and Mentha spicata (Labiatae) on iron absorption in rats. *Toxicol Ind Health*. 2004 Sep;20(6-10):119-22.

[627] Murayama M, Kumaroo KK. Inhibitors of ex vivo aggregation of human platelets induced by decompression, during reduced barometric pressure. *Thromb Res*. 1986 May 15;42(4):511-6.

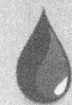

[628] Unger M, Frank A. Simultaneous determination of the inhibitory potency of herbal extracts on the activity of six major cytochrome P450 enzymes using liquid chromatography/mass spectrometry and automated online extraction. *Rapid Commun Mass Spectrom.* 2004;18(19):2273-81.

[629] Hoshino M, Ikarashi N, Tsukui M, et al. Menthol reduces the anticoagulant effect of warfarin by inducing cytochrome P450 2C expression. *Eur J Pharm Sci.* 2014 Jun 2;56:92-101.

[630] Gelal A, Guven H, Balkan D, et al. Influence of menthol on caffeine disposition and pharmacodynamics in healthy female volunteers. *Eur J Clin Pharmacol.* 2003 Sep;59(5-6):417-22.

[631] Gelal A, Jacob P 3rd, Yu L, et al. Disposition kinetics and effects of menthol. *Clin Phramacol Ther.* 1999 Aug;66(2):128-35.

[632] Sullivan JB Jr, Rumack BH, Thomas H Jr, et al. Pennyroyal oil poisoning and hepatotoxicity. *JAMA.* 1979;242:2873-4.

[633] Bakerink JA, Gospe SM Jr, Dimand RJ, et al. Multiple organ failure after ingestion of pennyroyal oil from herbal tea in two infants. *Pediatrics.* 1996;98(5):944-47.

[634] Anderson IB, Mullen WH, Meeker JE, et al. Pennyroyal toxicity: measurement of toxic metabolite levels in two cases and review of the literature. *Ann Intern Med.* 1996;124:726-34.

[635] Zimmerman HJ. Unconventional drugs. Miscellaneous drugs and diagnostic chemicals. In, Zimmerman, HJ. Hepatotoxicity: the adverse effects of drugs and other chemicals on the liver. 2nd ed. Philadelphia: Lippincott,1999: pp. 731-34.

[636] Seeff L, Stickel F, Navarro VJ. Hepatotoxicity of herbals and dietary supplements. In, Kaplowitz N, DeLeve LD, eds. Drug-induced liver disease. 3rd ed. Amsterdam: Elsevier, 2013, pp. 631-58.

[637] Muruganathan U, Srinivasan S, Indumathi D. Antihyperglycemic effect of carvone: Effect on the levels of glycoprotein components in streptozotocin-induced diabetic rats. *J Acute Disease.* 2013;2(4):310-15.

[638] Souza FV, da Rocha MB, de Souza DP, et al. (-)-Carvone: antispasmodic effect and mode of action. *Fitoterapia.* 2013 Mar;85:20-24.

[639] Lee HS. Anticoagulant properties of constituents derived from fennel (Foeniculum vulgare Gaertner) fruits. *Food Sci Biotech.* 2006 Oct;15(5):763-67.

[640] de Sousa DP, Farias Nobrega FF, de Almeida RN. Influence of the chirality of (R)-(-)- and (S)-(+)-carvone in the central nervous system: a comparative study. *Chirality.* 2007 May;19(4):264-268.

[641] Langeveld WT, Veldhuizen EJ, Burt SA. Synergy between essential oil constituents and antibiotics. *Crit Rev Microbiol.* 2014 Feb;40(1);76-94.

[642] Sessa R, Di Pietro M, De Santis F, et al. Effects of Mentha suaveolens essential oil on Chlamydia trachomatis. *Biomed Res Int.* 2015;2015:508071.

[643] Stringaro A, Vavala E, Colone M, et al. Effects of Mentha suaveolens Essential Oil Alone or in Combination with Other Drugs in Candida albicans. *Evid Based Complement Alternat Med.* 2014;2014:125904.

[644] Civitelli L, Panella S, Marcocci ME, et al. In vitro inhibition of herpes simplex virus type 1 replication by Mentha suaveolens essential oil and its main component piperitenone oxide. *Phytomedicine.* 2014 May 15;21(6):857-65.

[645] Shahverdi AR, Mirzaie S, Rafii F, et al. Monoterpenes as nitrofurantoin resistance modulating agents: minimal structural requirements, molecular dynamics simulations, and the effect of piperitone on the emergence of nitrofurantoin resistance in Enterobacteriaceae. *J Mol Model.* 2015 Aug;21(8):198.

[646] Shahverdi AR, Rafii F, Tavassoli F, et al. Piperitone from Mentha longifolia var. chorodictya Rech F. reduces the nitrofurantoin resistance of strains of enterobacteriaceae. *Phytother Res.* 2004 Nov;18(11):911-4.

[647] Scazzocchio F, Garzoli S, Conti C, et al. Properties and limits of some essential oils: chemical characterisation, antimicrobial activity, interaction with antibiotics and cytotoxicity. *Nat Prod Res.* 2016 Sep;30(17):1909-18.

[648] Ferreira A, Proença C, Serralheiro ML, et al. The in vitro screening for acetylcholinesterase inhibition and antioxidant activity of medicinal plants from Portugal. *J Ethnopharmacol.* 2006 Nov 3;108(1):31-7.

[649] Nguyen LT, Mysliveckova Z, Szotakova B, et al. The inhibitory effects of β-caryophyllene, β-caryophyllene oxide and α-humulene on the activities of the main drug-metabolizing enzymes in rat and human liver in vitro. *Chem-Biol Interactoins.* 2017 Dec 25;278:123-8.

[650] Oumzil H, Ghoulami S, Rhajaoui M, et al. Antibacterial and antifungal activity of essential oils of Mentha suaveolens. *Phytother Res.* 2002;16:727–31.

[651] El Arch M, Satrani B, Farah A, et al. Composition chimique et activités antimicrobienne et insecticide de l'huile essentielle de Mentha rotundifolia du Maroc. *Acta Bot Gallica.* 2003;150:267-74.

[652] Riahi L, Elferchichi M, Ghazghazi H, et al. Phytochemistry, antioxidant and antimicrobial activities of the essential oils of Mentha rotundifolia L. in Tunisia. *Ind Crops Prod.* 2013 Aug;49:883-89.

[653] Sessa R, Di Pietro M, De Santis F, et al. Effects of Mentha suaveolens essential oil on Chlamydia trachomatis. *Biomed Res Int.* 2015;2015:508071.

[654] Garzoli S, Pirolli A, Vavala E, et al. Multidisciplinary Approach to Determine the Optimal Time and Period for Extracting the Essential Oil from Mentha suaveolens Ehrh. *Molecules.* 2015 May 26;20(6):9640-55.

[655] Pietrella D, Angiolella L, Vavala E, et al. Beneficial effect of Mentha suaveolens essential oil in the treatment of vaginal candidiasis assessed by real-time monitoring of infection. *BMC Complement Altern Med.* 2011;11:18.

[656] Pietrella D, Angiolella L, Vavala E, et al. Beneficial effect of Mentha suaveolens essential oil in the treatment of vaginal candidiasis assessed by real-time monitoring of infection. *BMC Complement Altern Med.* 2011 Feb 28;11:18.

[657] Stringaro A, Vavala E, Colone M, et al. Effects of Mentha suaveolens Essential Oil Alone or in Combination with Other Drugs in Candida albicans. *Evid Based Complement Alternat Med.* 2014;2014:125904.

[658] Civitelli L, Panella S, Marcocci ME, et al. In vitro inhibition of herpes simplex virus type 1 replication by Mentha suaveolens essential oil and its main component piperitenone oxide. *Phytomedicine.* 2014 May 15;21(6):857-65.

[659] Ferreira A, Proença C, Serralheiro ML, et al. The in vitro screening for acetylcholinesterase inhibition and antioxidant activity of medicinal plants from Portugal. *J Ethnopharmacol.* 2006 Nov 3;108(1):31-7.

[660] Kasrati A, Alaoui Jamali C, Bekkouche K, et al. Comparative evaluation of antioxidant and insecticidal properties of essential oils from five Moroccan aromatic herbs. *J Food Sci Technol.* 2015 Apr;52(4):2312-9.

[661] Sitzmann J, Habegger R, Schnitzler WH, et al. Comparative analysis of antioxidant activities of fourteen mentha essential oils and their components. *Chem Biodivers.* 2014 Dec;11(12):1978-89.

[662] Riahi L, Elferchichi M, Ghazghazi H, et al. Phytochemistry, antioxidant and antimicrobial activities of the essential oils of Mentha rotundifolia L. in Tunisia. *Ind Crops Prod.* 2013 Aug;49:883-89.

[663] Benyad N, Ebrahim W, Hakiki A, et al. Chemical characterization and insecticidal evaluation of the essential oil of Mentha suaveolens L. and Mentha puelgium L. growing in Morocco. *Studii şi Cercetări Ştiinţifice, Chimie şi Inginerie Chimică, Biotehnologii, Industrie Alimentară.* 2012;13(1):27-32.

[664] Pavela R, Kaffkova K, Kumsta. Chemical Composition and Larvicidal Activity of Essential Oils from Different Mentha L. and Pulegium Species against Culex quinquefasciatus Say (Diptera: Culicidae). *Plant Protect Sci.* 2014;50(1):36-42.

[665] Koliopoulos G, Pitarokili D, Kioulos E, et al. Chemical composition and larvicidal evaluation of Mentha, Salvia, and Melissa essential oils against the West Nile virus misquito Culex pipiens. *Parasitol Res.* 2010;107:327-35.

[666] Zekri N, Sabri H, Khannouchi S, et al. Phytochemical study and fumigant toxicity of Mentha suaveolens Ehrh essential oil from Morocco against adults of S. oryzae. *Australian J Basic Appl Sci.* 2013 Dec;7(14):499-606.

[667] El Arch M, Satrani B, Farah A, et al. Composition chimique et activités antimicrobienne et insecticide de l'huile essentielle de Mentha rotundifolia du Maroc. *Acta Bot Gallica.* 2003;150:267-74.

[668] Kasrati A, Alaoui Jamali C, Bekkouche K, et al. Chemical characterization and insecticidal properties of essential oils from different wild populations of Mentha suaveolens subsp. timija (Briq.) Harley from Morocco. *Chem Biodivers.* 2015 May;12(5):823-31.

[669] Kasrati A, Alaoui Jamali C, Bekkouche K, et al. Comparative evaluation of antioxidant and insecticidal properties of essential oils from five Moroccan aromatic herbs. *J Food Sci Technol.* 2015 Apr;52(4):2312-9.

[670] Kasrati A, Alaoui Jamali C, Spooner-Hart R, et al. Chemical Characterization and Biological Activities of Essential Oil Obtained from Mint Timija Cultivated under Mineral and Biological Fertilizers. *J Anal Methods Chem.* 2017;2017:6354532.

[671] Poli JP, Guinoiseau E, de Rocca Serra D, et al. Anti-Quorum Sensing Activity of 12 Essential Oils on chromobacterium violaceum and Specific Action of cis-cis-p-Menthenolide from Corsican Mentha suaveolens ssp. Insularis. *Molecules.* 2018 Aug 23;23(9).

[672] El-Mustapha L, Abderrafea E, Ayoub K, et al. Toxicity of essential oils obtained from Juniperus thurifera var. africana and Mentha suaveolens subsp. timija chemotypes against pre-adult stages of Hyalomma aegyptium tick (Acari: Ixodidae). *Nat Prod Res.* 2019 Oct 17:1-6.

[673] Ed-Dra A, Filali FR, Lo Presti V, et al. Chemical composition, antioxidant capacity and antibacterial action of five Moroccan essential oils against Listeria monocytogenes and different serotypes of Salmonella enterica. *Microb Pathog.* 2020 Dec;149:104510.

[674] Aldogman B, Bilel H, Moustafa SMN, et al. Investigation of Chemical Compositions and Biological Activities of Mentha suaveolens L. from Saudi Arabia. *Molecules.* 2022 May 5;27(9):2949.

[675] Fazal H, Akram M, Ahmad N, et al. Nutritionally rich biochemical profile in essential oil of various Mentha species and their antimicrobial activities. *Protoplasma.* 2022 Aug 9. Online ahead of print.

[676] Zerkani H, Kharchoufa L, Tagnaout I, et al. Chemical Composition and Bioinsecticidal Effects of Thymus zygis L., Salvia officinalis L. and Mentha suaveolens Ehrh. Essential Oils on Medfly Ceratitis capitata and Tomato Leaf Miner Tuta absoluta. *Plants (Basel).* 2022 Nov 14;11(22):3084.

[677] Zerkani H, Kharchoufa L, Tagnaout I, et al. Chemical Composition and Bioinsecticidal Effects of Thymus zygis L., Salvia officinalis L. and Mentha suaveolens Ehrh. Essential Oils on Medfly Ceratitis capitata and Tomato Leaf Miner Tuta absoluta. *Plants (Basel).* 2022 Nov 14;11(22):3084.

[678] Ristić M, Krivokuća-Đokić D, Radanović D, et al. Essential oil of Arnica montana and Arnica chamissonis. *Hemijska Industija.* 2007 Jan;61(5):272-77.

[679] Pljevljakusica D, Rancic D, Ristic M, et al. Rhizome and root yield of the cultivated Arnica montana L., chemical composition and histochemical localization of essential oil. *Ind Crops Prod.* 2012;39:177-89.

[680] Weremczuk-Jezyna I, Wysokinska H, Kalemba D. Constituents of the Essential Oil from Hairy Roots and Plant Roots of Arnica montana L. *J Essent Oils Res.* 2011;23:91-97.

[681] Nguyen LT, Mysliveckova Z, Szotakova B, et al. The inhibitory effects of β-caryophyllene, β-caryophyllene oxide and α-humulene on the activities of the main drug-metabolizing enzymes in rat and human liver in vitro. *Chem-Biol Interactoins.* 2017 Dec 25;278:123-8.
[682] Foster S, Tyler VE. Tyler's Honest Herbal: A Sensible Guide to the Use of Herbs and Related Remedies. 3rd ed., Binghamton, NY: Haworth Herbal Press, 1993.
[683] No authors listed. Final report on the safety assessment of Arnica montana extract and Arnica montana. *Int J Toxicol.* 2001;20:1-11.
[684] Ciganda C, Laborde A. Herbal infusions used for induced abortion. *J Toxicol Clin Toxicol.* 2003;41:235-239.
[685] Yones DA, Bakir HY, Bayoumi SA, et al. Chemical composition and efficacy of some selected plant oils against Pediculus humanus capitis in vitro. *Parasitol Res.* 2016 Aug;115(8):3209-18.
[686] Lebouvier N, Hue T, Hnawia E, et al. Acaricidal activity of essential oils from five endemic conifers of New Caledonia on the cattle tick Rhipicephalus (Boophilus) microplus. *Parasitol Res.* 2013 Apr;112(4):1379-84.
[687] Raharivelomanana P, Cambron A, Azzaro M, et al. Volatile Constituents of Neocallitropsis pancheri (Carrière) de Laubenfels Heartwood Extracts (Cupressaceae). *J Essent Oil Res.* 1993;5(6):587-95.
[688] Tsuneki H, Ma EL, Kobayashi S, et al. Antiangiogenic activity of beta-eudesmol in vitro and in vivo. *Eur J Pharmacol.* 2005 Apr 11;512(2-3):105-15.
[689] Arora CK, Arora RB, Mesta CK, et al. Hypotensive activity of beta-eudesmol and some related sesquiterpenes. *Ind J Med Res.* 1967 May;55(5):463-72.
[690] Wang BG, Hong X, Li L, Zhou J, et al. Chemical constituents of two Chinese Magnoliaceae plants, Tsoongiodendron odorum and Manglietiastrum sinicum, and their inhibition of platelet aggregation. *Planta Med.* 2000 Aug;66(6):511-5.
[691] Lebouvier N, Hue T, Hnawia E, et al. Acaricidal activity of essential oils from five endemic conifers of New Caledonia on the cattle tick Rhipicephalus (Boophilus) microplus. *Parasitol Res.* 2013 Apr;112(4):1379-84.
[692] Pichette A, Larouche PL, Lebrun M, et al. Composition and antibacterial activity of Abies balsamea essential oil. *Phytother Res.* 2006 May;20(5):371-73.
[693] Regimbal JM, Collin G. Essential oil analysis of Balsam Fir Abies balsamea (L.) Mill. *J Essential Oil Res.* 1994;6(3):229-38.
[694] Ross J, Gagnon H, Girard D, et al. Chemical composition of the bark oil of Balsam Fir Abies balsamea (L.) Mill. *J Essential Oil Res.* 1996 May;8(4):343-46.
[695] Guenther E. The essential oils. 6 vols. 1948-1952. D. van Nostrand Co., Inc. Toronto, New York, London.
[696] Garneau FX, Collin G, Gagnon H, et al. Chemical composition of the hydrosol and the essential oil of three different species of the Pinaceae family: Picea glauca (Moench) Voss., Picea mariana (Mill.) B.S.P., and Abies balsamea (L.) Mill. *J Essential Oil Bearing Plants.* 2012;15(2):227-36.
[697] Pichette A, Larouche PL, Lebrun M, et al. Composition and antibacterial activity of Abies balsamea essential oil. *Phytother Res.* 2006 May;20(5):371-73.
[698] Legault J, Dahl W, Debiton E, et al. Antitumor activity of balsam fir oil: Production of reactive oxygen species possible mechanism of action. *Planta Med.* 2003;69(5):402-07.
[699] Legault J, Dahl W, Debiton E, et al. Antitumor activity of balsam fir oil: Production of reactive oxygen species possible mechanism of action. *Planta Med.* 2003;69(5):402-07.
[700] Pichette A, Larouche PL, Lebrun M, et al. Composition and antibacterial activity of Abies balsamea essential oil. *Phytother Res.* 2006 May;20(5):371-73.
[701] Adamo SA, El Nabbout A, Ferguson LV, et al. Balsam fir (Abies balsamea) needles and their essential oil kill overwintering ticks (Ixodes scapularis) at cold temperatures. *Sci Rep.* 2022 Jul 29;12(1):12999.
[702] Aromatics International. Balsam Poplar. Available at: https://www.aromatics.com/products/essential-oils/balsam-poplar.
[703] Stillpoint Aromatics. Balsam Poplar Essential Oil. Available at: http://www.stillpointaromatics.com/balsam-poplar-Populus-balsamifera-essential-oil.
[704] Piochon-Gauthier M, Legault J, Sylvestre M, et al. The essential oil of Populus balsamifera buds: its chemical composition and cytotoxic activity. *Nat Prod Commun.* 2014 Feb;9(2):257-60.
[705] Piochon-Gauthier M, Legault J, Sylvestre M, et al. The essential oil of Populus balsamifera buds: its chemical composition and cytotoxic activity. *Nat Prod Commun.* 2014 Feb;9(2):257-60.
[706] Hussain AI, Anwar F, Sherrazi STH, et al. Chemical composition, antioxidant and antimicrobial activities of basil (Ocimum basilicum) essential oil depends on seasonal variations. *Food Chem.* 2008 Jun 1;108(3):986-95.
[707] Carvalho Filho JLS, Blank AF, Alves PB, et al. Influence of harvesting time, temperature and drying period on basil (Ocimum basilicum L.) essential oil. *Rev Bras Farmacogn.* 2006 Jan-Mar;16(1):24-30.
[708] Giachino RRA, Sonmez C, Tonk FA, et al. RAPD and essential oil characterization of Turkish basil (Ocimum basilicum L.). *Plant Systemics Evolution.* 2014 Oct;300(8):1779-91.
[709] Koba K, Poutouli PW, Raynaud C, et al. Chemical composition and antimicrobial properties of different basil essential oils chemotypes from Togo. *J Bangledesh Pharm Soc.* 2009;4:1-8.
[710] Ozcan M, Chalchat JC. Essential oil composition of Ocimum basilicum L. and Ocimum minimum L. in Turkey. *Czech J Food Sci.* 2002 Nov;20(6):223-28.
[711] Liber Z, Carovic-Stanko K, Politeo O, et al. Chemical composition and genetic relationship among Ocimum basilicum L cultivars. *Chem & Biodivers.* 2011 Nov;8(11):1978-89.
[712] European Medicines Agency. Public statement on the use of herbal medicinal products containing estragole. Available at: http://www.ema.europa.eu/docs/en_GB/document_library/Scientific_guideline/2010/04/WC500089960.pdf.
[713] Johnson JD, Ryan MJ, Toft JD II, et al. Two-year toxicity and carcinogenicity study of methyl eugenol in F344/N rats and B6C3F(1) mice. *J Agric Food Chem.* 2000 Aug;48(8):3620-32.
[714] European Commission. Opinion of the Scientific Committee on Food on methyl eugenol (4-Allyl-1,2- dimethoxybenzene). Availableat: http://ec.europa.eu/food/fs/sc/scf/out102_en.pdf.
[715] National Toxicology Program. NTP Toxicology and Carcinogenesis Studies of Methyleugenol (CAS NO. 93-15-2) in F344/N Rats and B6C3F1 Mice (Gavage Studies). *Natl Toxicol Program Tech Rep Ser.* 2000 Jul;491:1-412.
[716] National Toxicology Program. Carcinogenesis Studies of Eugenol (CAS No. 97-53-0) in F344/N Rats and B6C3F1 Mice (Feed Studies). Technical Report Series No. 223. NIH Publication No. 84-1779. 1983. U.S. DHHS, PHS, NIH, NTP, Research Triangle Park, NC.
[717] European Medicines Agency. Public statement on the use of herbal medicinal products containing estragole. Available at: http://www.ema.europa.eu/docs/en_GB/document_library/Scientific_guideline/2010/04/WC500089960.pdf.
[718] Ding W, Levy DD, Bishop ME, et al. In vivo genotoxicity of estragole in male F344 rats. *Environ Mol Mutagen.* 2015 May;56(4):356-65.
[719] Eisenmann SW, Poulev A, Struwe L, et al. Qualitative variation of anti-diabetic constituents in different tarragon (Artemisia dracunculus L.) cytotypes. *Fitoterapia.* 2011 Oct;82(7):1062–74.
[720] European Medicines Agency. Public statement on the use of herbal medicinal products containing estragole. Available at: http://www.ema.europa.eu/docs/en_GB/document_library/Scientific_guideline/2010/04/WC500089960.pdf.
[721] Johnson JD, Ryan MJ, Toft JD II, et al. Two-year toxicity and carcinogenicity study of methyl eugenol in F344/N rats and B6C3F(1) mice. *J Agric Food Chem.* 2000 Aug;48(8):3620-32.
[722] National Toxicology Program. NTP Toxicology and Carcinogenesis Studies of Methyleugenol (CAS NO. 93-15-2) in F344/N Rats and B6C3F1 Mice (Gavage Studies). *Natl Toxicol Program Tech Rep Ser.* 2000 Jul;491:1-412.
[723] Kerckaert GA, Brauninger R, LeBoeuf RA, et al. Use of the Syrian hamster embryo cell transformation assay for carcinogenicity prediction of chemicals currently being tested by the National Toxicology Program in rodent bioassays. *Environ Health Perspect.* 1996;104:1075-84.
[724] National Toxicology Program. Carcinogenesis Studies of Eugenol (CAS No. 97-53-0) in F344/N Rats and B6C3F1 Mice (Feed Studies). Technical Report Series No. 223. NIH Publication No. 84-1779. 1983. U.S. DHHS, PHS, NIH, NTP, Research Triangle Park, NC.
[725] European Commission. Opinion of the Scientific Committee on Food on methyl eugenol (4-Allyl-1,2- dimethoxybenzene). Availableat: http://ec.europa.eu/food/fs/sc/scf/out102_en.pdf.
[726] European Commission. Opinion of the Scientific Committee on Food on estragole (1-Allyl-4-methoxybenzene). Available at: http://ec.europa.eu/food/fs/sc/scf/out104_en.pdf.
[727] California Environmental Protection Agency. Evidence of the carcinogenicity of estragole. Available at: http:// oehha.ca.gov/prop65/pdf/estragf.pdf.
[728] Drinkwater NR, Miller EC, Miller JA, et al. Hepatocarcinogenicity of estragole (1-allyl-4-methoxybenzene) and 1'-hydroxyestragole in the mouse and mutagenicity of 1'-acetoxyestragole in bacteria. *J Natl Cancer Inst.* 1976 Dec;57(6):1323-31.
[729] Zeller A, Horst K, Rychlik M. Study of the metabolism of estragole in humans consuming fennel tea. *Chem Res Toxicol.* 2009 Dec;22(12):1929-37.
[730] Johnson JD, Ryan MJ, Toft JD II, et al. Two-year toxicity and carcinogenicity study of methyl eugenol in F344/N rats and B6C3F(1) mice. *J Agric Food Chem.* 2000 Aug;48(8):3620-32.
[731] European Commission. Opinion of the Scientific Committee on Food on methyl eugenol (4-Allyl-1,2- dimethoxybenzene). Availableat: http://ec.europa.eu/food/fs/sc/scf/out102_en.pdf.
[732] National Toxicology Program. NTP Toxicology and Carcinogenesis Studies of Methyleugenol (CAS NO. 93-15-2) in F344/N Rats and B6C3F1 Mice (Gavage Studies). *Natl Toxicol Program Tech Rep Ser.* 2000 Jul;491:1-412.
[733] National Toxicology Program. Carcinogenesis Studies of Eugenol (CAS No. 97-53-0) in F344/N Rats and B6C3F1 Mice (Feed Studies). Technical Report Series No. 223. NIH Publication No. 84-1779. 1983. U.S. DHHS, PHS, NIH, NTP, Research Triangle Park, NC.
[734] Maltzman TH, Christou M, Gould MN, et al. Effects of monoterpenoids on in vivo DMBA-DNA adduct formation and on phase I hepatic metabolizing enzymes. *Carcinogenesis.* 1989;12:2081-87.
[735] Kim NH, Hyun SH, Jin CH, et al. Pretreatment with 1,8-cineole potentiates thioacetamide-induced hepatotoxicity and immunosuppression. *Arch Pharm Res.* 2004 Jul;27(7):781-9.
[736] Khan MM. Masters Thesis: Inhibition of Cytochrome P450 2E1 and Cytochrome P450 2A6 by Essential Oils: Tarragon (Artemisia dracunculus) and Basil (Ocimum basilicum). 2014. Available at: https://libres.uncg.edu/ir/uncg/f/Khan_uncg_0154M_11587.pdf
[737] Tognolini M, Barocelli E, Ballabeni V, et al. Comparative screening of plant essential oils; phenylpropanoid moiety as basic core for antiplatelet activity. *Life Sci.* 2006 Feb 23;78(13):1419-32.
[738] Lee HS. Anticoagulant properties of constituents derived from fennel (Foeniculum vulgare Gaertner) fruits. *Food Sci Biotech.* 2006 Oct;15(5):763-67.
[739] Drinkwater NR, Miller EC, Miller JA, et al. Hepatocarcinogenicity of estragole (1-allyl-4-methoxybenzene) and 1'-hydroxyestragole in the mouse and mutagenicity of 1'-acetoxyestragole in bacteria. *J Natl Cancer Inst.* 1976 Dec;57(6):1323-31.
[740] Zeggwagh NA, Eddouks M. Anti-hyperglycaemic and hypolipidemic effects of Ocimum basilicum aqueous extract in diabetic rats. 2007;2(3):123-29.
[741] Lee SE, Lee BH, Choi WS, et al. Fumigant toxicity of volatile natural products from Korean spices and medicinal plants towards the rice weevil, Sitophilus oryzae (L). *Pest Manag Sci.* 2001;57:548-53.
[742] Hemaiswarya S, Doble M. Synergistic interaction of eugenol with antibiotics against Gram negative bacteria. *Phytomedicine.* 2009 Nov;16(11):997-1005.
[743] Ahmad A, Khan A, Ahmad Khan L, et al. In vitro synergy of eugenol and methyleugenol with fluconazole against clinical Candida isolates. *J Med Microbiol.* 2010;59:1178-84.
[744] Cardoso NN, Alviano CS, Blank AF, et al. Synergism Effect of the Essential Oil from Ocimum basilicum var. Maria Bonita and Its Major Components with Fluconazole and Its Influence on Ergosterol Biosynthesis. *Evid Based Complement Alternat Med.* 2016;2016:5647182.
[745] Shin S, Pyun MS. Anti-Candida effects of estragole in combination with ketoconazole or amphotericin B. *Phytother Res.* 2004 Oct;18(10):827-30.
[746] Shin S. Essential oil compounds from Agastache rugosa as antifungal agents against Trichophyton species. *Arch Pharm Res.* 2004 Mar;27(3):295-9.

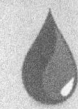
[747] Shin S, Kang CA. Antifungal activity of the essential oil of Agastache rugosa Kuntze and its synergism with ketoconazole. *Lett Appl Microbiol.* 2003;36(2):111-5.

[748] Bayla B, Bassole IH, Gnoula C, et al. Chemical composition, antioxidant, anti-inflammatory and anti-proliferative activity of essential oils of plants for Burkina Faso. *PLoS One.* 2014 Mar 24;9(3):e92122.

[749] Manosroi J, Dhumtanom P, Manosroi A. Anti-proliferative activity of essential oil extracted from Thai medicinal plants on KB and P388 cell lines. *Cancer Lett.* 2006 Apr 8;235(11):114-20.

[750] Okamoto A, Kuriyama H, Watanabe S, et al. The effect of aromatherapy massage on mild depression: A pilot study. *Psych Clin Neurosci.* 2005 Jun;59(3):363.

[751] Matiz G, Osorio MR, Camacho F, et al. Effectiveness of antimicrobial formulations for acne based on orange (Citrus sinensis) and sweet basil (Ocimum basilicum L) essential oils. *Biomedica.* 2012 Jan-Mar;32(1):125-33.

[752] Nascimento SS, Araujo AA, Brito RG, et al. Cyclodextrin-complexed Ocimum basilicum leaves essential oil increases Fos protein expression in the central nervous system and produce an antihyperalgesic effect in animal models for fibromyalgia. *Int J Mol Sci.* 2014 Dec 29;16(1):547-63.

[753] Nascimento SS, Camargo EA, DeSantana JM, et al. Linalool and linalool complexed in β-cyclodextrin produce anti-hyperalgesic activity and increase Fos protein expression in animal model for fibromyalgia. *Naunyn-Schmiedeberg's Arch Pharmacol.* 2014 Oct;387(10):935-42.

[754] Ahmad AH, Ismail Z. cFos and its consequences in pain. *Malays J Med Sci.* 2002 Jan;9(1):3-8.

[755] Venancio AM, Onfre AS, Lira AF, et al. Chemical composition, acute toxicity, and antinociceptive activity of the essential oil of plant breeding cultivar of basil (Ocimum basilicum L.). *Planta Med.* 2011 May;77(8):825-29.

[756] Varney E, Buckle J. Effect of inhaled essential oils on mental exhaustion and moderate burnout: a small pilot study. *J Altern Complement Med.* 2013;19(1):69-71.

[757] Beric T, Nikolic B, Stanojevic J, Vukovic-Gacic B, et al. Protective effect of basil (Ocimum basilicum L.) against oxidative damage and mutagenesis. *Food Chem Toxicol.* 2008 Feb;46(2):724-32.

[758] Fathiazad F, Matlobi A, Khorrami A, et al. Phytochemical screening and evaluation of cardioprotective activity of ethanolic extract of Ocimum basilicum L. (basil) against isoproterenol induced myocardial infarction in rats. *DARU J Pharm Sci.* 2012;20:87.

[759] Kristinsson KG, Magnusdottir AB, Petersen H, et al. Effective treatment of experimental acute otitis media by application of volatile fluids into the ear canal. *J Infect Dis.* 2005 Jun 1;191(11):1876-80.

[760] Joshri RK. Chemical composition and antimicrobial activity of the essential oil of Ocimum basilicum L. (sweet basil) from Western Ghats of North West Karnataka, India. *Anc Sci Life.* 2014 Jan;33(3):151-56.

[761] Sienkiewicz M, Lysakowska M, Pastuszka M, et al. The potential use of basil and rosemary essential oils as effective antibacterial agents. *Molecules.* 2013 Aug 5;18(8):9334-51.

[762] Opalchenova G, Obreshkova D. Comparative studies on the activity of basil—an essential oil from Ocimum basilicum L.—against multidrug resistant clinical isolates of the genera Staphylococcus, Enterococcus and Pseudomonas by using different test methods. *J Microbiol Methods.* 2003 Jul;54(1):105-10.

[763] De Almeida I, Alviano DS, Vieira DP, et al. Antigiardial activity of Ocimum basilicum essential oil. *Parasitol Res.* 2007 Jul;101(2):443-52.

[764] Sanchez-Suarez J, Riveros I, Delgado G. Evaluation of the leishmanicidal and cytotoxic potential of essential oils derived from ten Columbian plants. *Iran J Parasitol.* 2013 Jan;8(1):129-36.

[765] Císarová M, Tančinová D, Medo J, et al. The in vitro effect of selected essential oils on the growth and mycotoxin production of Aspergillus species. *J Environ Sci Health B.* 2016 Oct 2;51(10):668-674.

[766] Sakkas H, Gousia P, Economou V, et al. In vitro antimicrobial activity of five essential oils on multidrug resistant Gram-negative clinical isolates. *J Intercult Ethnopharmacol.* 2016 Jun-Aug;5(3):212–18.

[767] Nikolaevskii VV, Kononova NS, Pertsovskii AI, et al. Effect of essential oils on the course of experimental atherosclerosis. *Patol Fiziol Eksp Ter.* 1990 Sep-Oct;(5):52-53.

[768] Perumalasamy H, Kim JY, Kim JR, et al. Toxicity of basil oil constituents and related constituents and the efficacy of spray formulations to Dermatophagoides farine (Acari: Pyroglyphidae). *J Med Entomol.* 2014 May;51(3):650-57.

[769] Akono Ntonga P, Baldovini N, Mouray E, et al. Activity of Ocimum basilicum, Ocimum canum, and Cymbopogon citratus essential oils against Plasmodium falciparum and mature-stage larvae of Anopheles funestus s.s. *Parasite.* 2014;21:33.

[770] Satoh T, Sugawara Y. Effects on humans elicited by inhaling the fragrance of essential oils: sensory test, multi- channel thermometric study and forehead surface potential wave measurement on basil and peppermint. *Anal Sci.* 2003 Jan;19(1):139-46.

[771] Ezz Eldin HM, Badawy AF. In vitro anti-Trichomonas vaginalis activity of Pistacia lentiscus mastic and Ocimum basilicum essential oil. *J Parasitol Dis.* 2015 Sep;39(3):465-73.

[772] Plant J. Effects of essential oils on telomere length in human cells. *Med Aromat Plants.* 2016;5(2):1-6.

[773] Ozdikmenli S, Demirel Zorba NN. Evaluation of usage of essential oils instead of spices in meat ball formulation for controlling Salmonella spp. *Food Sci Technol Int.* 2016 Mar;22(2):93-101.

[774] Ergüden C, Özkoç S, Öztürk B, et al. [Investigation of the in vitro effects of Melissa officinalis L., Mentha x piperita L. and Ocimum basilicum L. (Lamiaceae) essential oils on the cysts and trophozoites of Acanthamoeba castellani]. *Mikrobiyol Bul.* 2016 Oct;50(4):569-579.

[775] Hovijitra RS, Choonharuangdej S, Srithavaj T. Effect of essential oils prepared from Thai culinary herbs on sessile Candida albicans cultures. *J Oral Sci.* 2016;58(3):365-71.

[776] Yarou BB, Bawin T, Boullis A, et al. Oviposition deterrent activity of basil plants and their essentials oils against Tuta absoluta (Lepidoptera: Gelechiidae). *Environ Sci Pollut Res Int.* 2018 Oct;25(30):29880-29888.

[777] Wiwattanaratanabut K, choonharuangdej S, Srithava T. In Vitro Anti-Cariogenic Plaque Effects of Essential Oils Extracted from Culinary Herbs. *J Clin Diagnostic Res.* 2017 Sep;11(9):DC30-5.

[778] Gucwa K, Milewski S, Dymerski T, et al. Investigation of the Antifungal Activity and Mode of Action of Thymus vulgaris, Citrus limonum, Pelargonium graveolens, Cinnamomum cassia, Ocimum basilicum, and Eugenia caryophyllus Essential Oils. *Molecules.* 2018 May 8;23(5).

[779] Giatropoulos A, Kimbaris A, Michaelakis A, et al. Chemical composition and assessment of larvicidal and repellent capacity of 14 Lamiaceae essential oils against Aedes albopictus. *Parasitol Res.* 2018 Jun;117(6):1953-1964.

[780] Pierattini EC, Bedini S, Venturi F, et al. Sensory Quality of Essential Oils and Their Synergistic Effect with Diatomaceous Earth, for the Control of Stored Grain Insects. *Insects.* 2019 Apr 20;10(4).

[781] Rezzoug M, Bakhiche B, Gherib A, et al. Chemical composition and bioactivity of essential oils and Ethanolic extracts of Ocimum basilicum L. and Thymus algeriensis Boiss. & Reut. from the Algerian Saharan Atlas. *BMC Complement Altern Med.* 2019 Jun 21;19(1):146.

[782] Pejcic M, Stojanovic-Radic Z, Gencic M, et al. Anti-virulence Potential of Basil and Sage Essential Oils: Inhibition of Biofilm Formation, Motility and Pyocyanin Production of Pseudomonas Aeruginosa Isolates. *Food Chem Toxicol.* 2020 May 14;141:111431.

[783] Liu M, Luo F, Qing Z, et al. Chemical Composition and Bioactivity of Essential Oil of Ten Labiatae Species. *Molecules.* 2020 Oct 21;25(20):4862.

[784] Jaber H, Oubiji A, Ouryemchi I, et al. Chemical Composition and Antibacterial Activities of Eight Plant Essential Oils from Morocco against Escherichia coli Strains Isolated from Different Turkey Organs. *Biochem Res Int.* 2021 Mar 15;2021:6685800.

[785] Sentari M, Harahap U, Wahmurti T, et al. Blood Cortisol Level and Blood Serotonin Level in Depression Mice with Basil Leaf Essential Oil Treatment. *Open Access Macedonian J Med Sci.* 2019 Aug 30;7(16):2652-5.

[786] Brozyna M, Paleczny J, Kozlowska W, et al. The Antimicrobial and Antibiofilm In Vitro Activity of Liquid and Vapour Phases of Selected Essential Oils against Staphylococcus aureus. *Pathogens.* 2021 Sep 17;10(9):1207.

[787] Harčárová M, Čonková E, Proškovcová M, et al. Comparison of antifungal activity of selected essential oils against Fusarium graminearum in vitro. *Ann Agric Environ Med.* 2021 Sep 16;28(3):414-418.

[788] Lisboa FP, Silvestre WP, Castro JO, et al. In Vitro Antimicrobial Activity of Selected Essential Oils Against Endometritis-Causing Microorganisms in Mares. *J Equine Vet Sci.* 2022 Mar;110:103840.

[789] Kim DS, Hong SJ, Yoon S, et al. Olfactory Stimulation with Volatile Aroma Compounds of Basil (Ocimum basilicum L.) Essential Oil and Linalool Ameliorates White Fat Accumulation and Dyslipidemia in Chronically Stressed Rats. *Nutrients.* 2022 Apr;14(9):1822.

[790] Mahran HA. Using nanoemulsions of the essential oils of a selection of medicinal plants from Jazan, Saudi Arabia, as a green larvicidal against Culex pipiens. *PLoS One.* 2022 May 23;17(5):e0267150.

[791] Man A, Mare AD, Mares M, et al. Antifungal and anti-virulence activity of six essential oils against important Candida species - a preliminary study. *Future Microbiol.* 2022 Jul;17:737-753.

[792] Galgano M, Capozza P, Pellegrini F, et al. Antimicrobial Activity of Essential Oils Evaluated In Vitro against Escherichia coli and Staphylococcus aureus. *Antibiotics (Basel).* 2022 Jul 20;11(7):979.

[793] Km DS, Hong SJ, Yoon S, et al. Olfactory Stimulation with Volatile Aroma Compounds of Basil (Ocimum basilicum L.) Essential Oil and Linalool Ameliorates White Fat Accumulation and Dyslipidemia in Chronically Stressed Rats. *Nutrients.* 2022;14:1822.

[794] Luca SV, Zengin G, Sinan KI, et al. Post-Distillation By-Products of Aromatic Plants from Lamiaceae Family as Rich Sources of Antioxidants and Enzyme Inhibitors. *Antioxidants (Basel).* 2023 Jan 16;12(1):210.

[795] Prasannakumar NR, Jyothi N, Saroja S, et al. Insecticidal properties of Ocimum basilicum and Mentha piperita essential oils against South American Tomato moth, Phthorimaea absoluta (Meyrick) (Lepidoptera: Gelichiidae). *Pestic Biochem Physiol.* 2023 Feb;190:105329.

[796] Prasannakumar NR, Jyothi N, Saroja S, et al. Insecticidal properties of Ocimum basilicum and Mentha piperita essential oils against South American Tomato moth, Phthorimaea absoluta (Meyrick) (Lepidoptera: Gelichiidae). *Pestic Biochem Physiol.* 2023 Feb;190:105329.

[797] Jirovetz L, Buchbauer G, Stoilova I, et al. Spice plants: Chemical composition and antioxidant properties of Pimenta Lindl. essential oils, part 2: Pimenta racemosa (Mill.) J.W. Moore leaf oil from Jamaica. *ERNÄHRUNG/NUTRITION.* 2007;37:293-300.

[798] Alitonou GA, Noudogbessi JP, Sessou P, et al. Chemical composition and biological activities of essential oils of Pimenta racemosa (Mill.) J. W. Moore. from Benin. *Int J Biosci.* 2012;2(9):1-12.

[799] Pradadheesh VS, Yadav A, Singh SC, et al. Leaf Essential Oil of Cultivated Pimenta Racemosa (Mill.) J.W. Moore from North India: Distribution of Phenylpropanoids and Chiral Terpenoids. *Med Aromat Plants.* 2013;2(1):1-4.

[800] Domaracky M, Rehak P, Juhas S, et al. Effects of selected plant essential oils on the growth and development of mouse preimplantation embryos in vivo. *Physiol Res.* 2007;56(1):97-104.

801 Vrskova D, Modra H. Evaluation of the developmental toxicity of 2-phenoxyethanol and clove oil anesthetics using the Frog Embryo Teratogenesis Assay: Xenopus (FETAX). *Veterinarami Medicina*. 2012;57(5):245-50.

802 Amini A, Cheraghi E, Safaee MR, et al. The role of eugenol in the reduction of teratogenic effects of retinoic acid on skeletal morphology of mice embryo. *Yakhteh Medical Journal*. 2003;4:195-200.

803 Chen R, Chen J, Cheng S, et al. Assessment of embryotoxicity of constituents in cosmetics by the embryonic stem cell tes. *Toxicol Mech Methods*. 2010 Mar;20(3):112-18.

804 Price CJ, George JD, Marr MC, et al. Developmental toxicity evaluation of methyleugenol (MEUG) administered to Sprague-Dawley rats on gestational days (gd) 6 through 19. *Birth Defects Res A Clin Mol Teratol*. 2006 Jun;76:395.

805 Chen SJ, Wang MH, Chen IJ. Antiplatelet and calcium inhibitory properties of eugenol and sodium eugenol acetate. *Gen Pharmacol*. 1996 Jun;27(4):629-33.

806 Tognolini M, Barocelli E, Ballabeni V, et al. Comparative screening of plant essential oils; phenylpropanoid moiety as basic core for antiplatelet activity. *Life Sci*. 2006 Feb 23;78(13):1419-32.

807 Heck AM, DeWitt BA, Lukes AL. Potential interactions between alternative therapies and warfarin. *Am J Health Syst Pharm*. 2000;57(13):1221-1227.

808 Saaeed SA, Gilani AH. Antithrombotic activity of clove oil. *J Pak Med Assoc*. 1994;44(5):112-15.

809 Kamatou GP, Vermaak I, Viljoen AM. Eugenol—from the remote Maluku Islands to the international market place: A review of a remarkable and versatile molecule. *Molecules*. 2012;17:6953-81.

810 de Olivera AC, Ribeiro-Pinto LF, Paumgartten JR. In vitro inhibition of CYP2B1 monoxygenase by beta-myrcene and other monoterpenoid constituents. *Br J Nutr*. 1999;81:289-95.

811 Cochrane ML. Inhibition of Cytochrome P450 2C9 by essential oils. Available at: https://libres.uncg.edu/ir/uncg/listing.aspx?id=18102.

812 de-Oliveira AC1, Ribeiro-Pinto LF, Otto SS, et al. Induction of liver monooxygenases by beta-myrcene. *Toxicology*. 1997 Dec 26;124(2):135-40.

813 Freitas JC1, Presgrave OA, Fingola FF, et al. Effect of beta-myrcene on pentobarbital sleeping time. *Braz J Med Biol Res*. 1993 May;26(5):519-23.

814 Dohi S, Terasaki M, Makino M. Acetylcholinesterase inhibitory activity and chemical composition of commercial essential oils. *J Agric Food Chem*. 2009 May 27;57(10):4313-8.

815 Lee SE, Lee BH, Choi WS, et al. Fumigant toxicity of volatile natural products from Korean spices and medicinal plants towards the rice weevil, Sitophilus oryzae (L). *Pest Manag Sci*. 2001;57:548-53.

816 Langeveld WT, Veldhuizen EJ, Burt SA. Synergy between essential oil constituents and antibiotics. *Crit Rev Microbiol*. 2014 Feb;40(1);76-94.

817 Hemaiswarya S, Doble M. Synergistic interaction of eugenol with antibiotics against Gram negative bacteria. *Phytomedicine*. 2009 Nov;16(11):997-1005.

818 Ahmad A, Khan A, Ahmad Khan L, et al. In vitro synergy of eugenol and methyleugenol with fluconazole against clinical Candida isolates. *J Med Microbiol*. 2010;59:1178-84.

819 Sarrami N, Pemberton MN, Thornhill MH, et al. Adverse reactions associated with the use of eugenol in dentistry. *British Dental J*. 2002;193:253-55.

820 Tammannavar P, Pushpalatha C, Jain S, et al. An unexpected positive hypersensitive reaction to eugenol. *BMJ Case Rep*. 2013; 2013: bcr2013009464.

821 Alitonou GA, Noudogbessi JP, Sessou P, et al. Chemical composition and biological activities of essential oils of Pimenta racemosa (Mill.) J. W. Moore. from Benin. *Int J Biosci*. 2012;2(9):1-12.

822 Burt SA, Reinders RD. Antibacterial activity of selected plant essential oils against Escherichia coli O157:H7. *Lett Appl Microbiol*. 2003;36(3):162-7.

823 Noel TS, Kifouli A, Boniface Y, et al. Antimicrobial and physico-chemical effects of essential oils on fermented milk during preservation. *J Appl Biosci*. 2016 Mar;99:9467-75.

824 Sessou P, Farougou S, Ahounou S, et al. Comparative study of antifungal activities of six selected essential oils against fungal isolates from cheese wagashi in Benin. *Pak J Biol Sci*. 2013 Dec 1;16(23):1751-7.

825 Jirovetz L, Buchbauer G, Stoilova I, et al. Spice plants: Chemical composition and antioxidant properties of Pimenta Lindl. essential oils, part 2: Pimenta racemosa (Mill.) J.W. Moore leaf oil from Jamaica. *ERNÄHRUNG/NUTRITION*. 2007;37:293-300.

826 Alitonou GA, Noudogbessi JP, Sessou P, et al. Chemical composition and biological activities of essential oils of Pimenta racemosa (Mill.) J. W. Moore. from Benin. *Int J Biosci*. 2012;2(9):1-12.

827 Alitonou GA, Noudogbessi JP, Sessou P, et al. Chemical composition and biological activities of essential oils of Pimenta racemosa (Mill.) J. W. Moore. from Benin. *Int J Biosci*. 2012;2(9):1-12.

828 Kim JR, Haribalan P, Son BK, et al. Fumigant toxicity of plant essential oils against Camptomyia corticalis (Diptera: Cecidomyiidae). *J Econ Entomol*. 2012 Aug;105(4):1329-34.

829 Leyva M, Tacoronte JE, Marquetti Mdel C. [Chemical composition and lethal effect of essential oil from Pimenta racemosa (Myrtales: Myrtaceae) on Blatella germanica (Dictyoptera: Blattellidae)]. *Rev Cubana Med Trop*. 2007 May-Aug;59(2):154-8.

830 Lee HS. Mosquito larvicidal activity of aromatic medicinal plant oils against Aedes aegypti and Culex pipiens pallens. *J Am Mosq Control Assoc*. 2006 Jun;22(2):292-5.

831 Alitonou GA, Noudogbessi JP, Sessou P, et al. Chemical composition and biological activities of essential oils of Pimenta racemosa (Mill.) J. W. Moore. from Benin. *Int J Biosci*. 2012;2(9):1-12.

832 Ismail MM, Samir R, Saber FR, et al. Pimenta Oil as A Potential Treatment for Acinetobacter Baumannii Wound Infection: In Vitro and In Vivo Bioassays in Relation to Its Chemical Composition. *Antibiotics (Basel)*. 2020 Oct 7;9(10):679.

833 Ayoub IM, Abdel-Aziz MM, Elhady SS, et al. Valorization of Pimenta racemosa Essential Oils and Extracts: GC-MS and LC-MS Phytochemical Profiling and Evaluation of Helicobacter pylori Inhibitory Activity. *Molecules*. 2022 Nov 17;27(22):7965.

834 Yalcin H, Anik M, Sanda MA, et al. Gas chromatography/mass spectrometry analysis of Laurus nobilis essential oil composition of northern Cyprus. *J Med Food*. 2008;10(4):715-19.

835 Basak SS, Candan F. Effect of Laurus nobilis L. essential oil and its main components on alpha-glucosidase and reactive oxygen species scavenging activity. *Iran J Pharm Res*. 2013 Spring;12(2):367-79.

836 Marzouki H, Elaissi A, Khaldi A, et al. Seasonal and geographical variation of Laurus nobilis L. essential oil from Tunisia. *Open Nat Prod J*. 20009;2:86-91.

837 Ben Jamaa JM, Tersim N, Toudert KT, et al. Insecticidal activities of essential oils from leaves of Laurus nobilis L. from Tunisia, Algeria and Morocco, and comparative chemical composition. *J Stored Prod Res*. 2012 Jan;48:97-104.

838 Kovacevic NN, Simic MD, Ristic MS. Essential oil of Laurus nobilis from Montenegro. *Chem Nat Constituents*. 2007;43(4):408-11.

839 Ben Jemaa JM, Tersim N. Composition and repellent efficacy of essential oil from Laurus nobilis against adults of the cigarette beetle Lasioderma serricorne (Coleoptera: Anobiidae). *Tunisian J Plant Prot*. 2011;6(1):29-42.

840 Johnson JD, Ryan MJ, Toft JD II, et al. Two-year toxicity and carcinogenicity study of methyl eugenol in F344/N rats and B6C3F(1) mice. *J Agric Food Chem*. 2000 Aug;48(8):3620-32.

841 European Commission. Opinion of the Scientific Committee on Food on methyl eugenol (4-Allyl-1,2- dimethoxybenzene). Available at: http://ec.europa.eu/food/fs/sc/scf/out102_en.pdf.

842 National Toxicology Program. NTP Toxicology and Carcinogenesis Studies of Methyleugenol (CAS NO. 93-15-2) in F344/N Rats and B6C3F1 Mice (Gavage Studies). *Natl Toxicol Program Tech Rep Ser*. 2000 Jul;491:1-412.

843 National Toxicology Program. Carcinogenesis Studies of Eugenol (CAS No. 97-53-0) in F344/N Rats and B6C3F1 Mice (Feed Studies). Technical Report Series No. 223. NIH Publication No. 84-1779. 1983. U.S. DHHS, PHS, NIH, NTP, Research Triangle Park, NC.

844 Craig JO. Poisoning by the volatile oils in childhood. *Arch Dis Child*. 1953;28:259-67.

845 Melis K. Bochner A, Janssens G. Accidental nasal eucalyptol and menthol instillation. *Eur J Pediatr*. 1989 Aug;148(8)786-7.

846 Day LM, Ozanne-Smith J, Parsons BJ, et al. Eucalyptus oil poisoning among young children: mechanisms of access and the potential prevention. *Aust N Z J Public Health*. 1997 Jun;21(3):297-302.

847 Chandar SD, Prashanti M, Kumar CL, et al. Eucalyptus Oil-Induced Seizures in Children: A Single-Center Prospective Study. *Cureus*. 2021 Mar 25;13(3):e14109.

848 Johnson JD, Ryan MJ, Toft JD II, et al. Two-year toxicity and carcinogenicity study of methyl eugenol in F344/N rats and B6C3F(1) mice. *J Agric Food Chem*. 2000 Aug;48(8):3620-32.

849 National Toxicology Program. NTP Toxicology and Carcinogenesis Studies of Methyleugenol (CAS NO. 93-15-2) in F344/N Rats and B6C3F1 Mice (Gavage Studies). *Natl Toxicol Program Tech Rep Ser*. 2000 Jul;491:1-412.

850 Kerckaert GA, Brauninger R, LeBoeuf RA, et al. Use of the Syrian hamster embryo cell transformation assay for carcinogenicity prediction of chemicals currently being tested by the National Toxicology Program in rodent bioassays. *Environ Health Perspect*. 1996;104:1075-84.

851 National Toxicology Program. Carcinogenesis Studies of Eugenol (CAS No. 97-53-0) in F344/N Rats and B6C3F1 Mice (Feed Studies). Technical Report Series No. 223. NIH Publication No. 84-1779. 1983. U.S. DHHS, PHS, NIH, NTP, Research Triangle Park, NC.

852 Price CJ, George JD, Marr MC, et al. Developmental toxicity evaluation of methyleugenol (MEUG) administered to Sprague-Dawley rats on gestational days (gd) 6 through 19. *Birth Defects Res A Clin Mol Teratol*. 2006 Jun;76:395.

853 Johnson JD, Ryan MJ, Toft JD II, et al. Two-year toxicity and carcinogenicity study of methyl eugenol in F344/N rats and B6C3F(1) mice. *J Agric Food Chem*. 2000 Aug;48(8):3620-32.

854 European Commission. Opinion of the Scientific Committee on Food on methyl eugenol (4-Allyl-1,2- dimethoxybenzene). Available at: http://ec.europa.eu/food/fs/sc/scf/out102_en.pdf.

855 National Toxicology Program. NTP Toxicology and Carcinogenesis Studies of Methyleugenol (CAS NO. 93-15-2) in F344/N Rats and B6C3F1 Mice (Gavage Studies). *Natl Toxicol Program Tech Rep Ser*. 2000 Jul;491:1-412.

856 National Toxicology Program. Carcinogenesis Studies of Eugenol (CAS No. 97-53-0) in F344/N Rats and B6C3F1 Mice (Feed Studies). Technical Report Series No. 223. NIH Publication No. 84-1779. 1983. U.S. DHHS, PHS, NIH, NTP, Research Triangle Park, NC.

857 Tsai HH, Lin HW, Chen YL, et al. A review of potential harmful interactions between anticoagulant/antiplatelet agents and Chinese herbal medicines. *PLoS One*. 2013 May 9;8(5):e64255.

858 Moharam BA, Jantan I, bin Ahmad F, et al. Antiplatelet Aggregation and Platelet Activating Factor (PAF) Receptor Antagonistic Activities of the Essential Oils of Five Goniothalamus Species. *Molecules*. 2010;15:5124-38.

859 Gray AM, Flatt PR. Antihyperglycemic actions of Eucalyptus globulus (Eucalyptus) are associated with pancreatic and extra pancreatic effects in mice. *J Nutr*. 1998 Dec;128(12):2319–23.

860 Basak SS, Candan F. Effect of Laurus nobilis L. Essential Oil and its Main Components on α-glucosidase and Reactive Oxygen Species Scavenging Activity. *Iran J Pharm Res*. 2013 Spring;12(2):367-79.

861 Dey B. Chemo-profiling of eucalyptus and study of its hypoglycemic potential. *World J Diabetes*. 2013 Oct 15;4(5):170–76.

862 Sayyah M, Valizadeh J, Kamalinejad M. Anticonvulsant activity of the leaf oil of Laurus nobilis against pentylentetrazole- and maximal electroshock-induced seizure. *Phytomedicine*. 2002 Apr;9(3):212-16.

863 Culic M, Kekovic G, Grbic G, et al. Wavelet and fractal analysis of rat brain activity in seizures evoked by camphor oil and 1,8-cineole. *Gen Physiol Biophys*. 2009;28 Sec No:33-40.

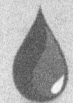

[864] Burkhard PR, Burkhardt K, Haenggeli CA, et al. Plant-induced seizures: reappearance of an old problem. *J Neurol.* 1999 Aug;246(8):667-70.

[865] Waldman N. Seizure caused by dermal application of over-the-counter eucalyptus oil head lice preparation. *Clin Toxicol (Phila).* 2011 Oct;49(8):750-1.

[866] Craig JO. Poisoning by the volatile oils in childhood. *Arch Dis Child.* 1953;28:259-67.

[867] Mathew T, Kamath V, Kumar RS, et al. Eucalyptus oil inhalation-induced seizure: A novel, underrecognized, preventable cause of acute symptomatic seizure. *Epilepsia Open.* 2017 Jul 4;2(3):350-354.

[868] Sayyah M, Valizadeh J, Kamalinejad M. Anticonvulsant activity of the leaf oil of Laurus nobilis against pentylentetrazole- and maximal electroshock-induced seizure. *Phytomedicine.* 2002 Apr;9(3):212-16.

[869] Sayyah M, Valizadeh J, Kamalinejad M. Anticonvulsant activity of the leaf oil of Laurus nobilis against pentylentetrazole- and maximal electroshock-induced seizure. *Phytomedicine.* 2002 Apr;9(3):212-16.

[870] Jori A, Bianchetti A, Prestini PE, et al. Effect of eucalyptol (1,8-cineole) on the metabolism of other drugs in rats and in man. *Eur J Pharmacol.* 1970;9(3):362-66.

[871] de Sousa DP, Raphael E, Brocksom U, et al. Sedative effect of monoterpene alcohols in mice: A preliminary screening. *Verlag der Zeitschrift fur Naturforschung.* 2007;62c:563-66.

[872] Ahmad A, Khan A, Ahmad Khan L, et al. In vitro synergy of eugenol and methyleugenol with fluconazole against clinical Candida isolates. *J Med Microbiol.* 2010;59:1178-84.

[873] Placzek M, Froemel W, Eberlein B, et al. Evaluation of phototoxic properties of fragrances. *Acta Derm Venereol.* 2007;87(4):312-6.

[874] Saab AM, Tundis R, Loizzo MR, et al. Antioxidant and antiproliferative activity of Laurus nobilis L. (Lauraceae) leaves and seeds essential oils against K562 human chronic myelogenous leukaemia cells. *Nat Prod Res.* 2012;26(18):1741-45.

[875] Al-Kalaldeh JZ, Abu-Dahab R, Afifi FU. Volatile oil composition and antiproliferative activity of Laurus nobilis, Origanum syriacum, Origanum vulgare, and Salvia triloba against human breast adenocarcinoma cells. *Nutr Res.* 2010 Apr;30(4):271-78.

[876] Loizzo MR, Tundis R, Menichini F, et al. Cytotoxic activity of essential oils from Labiatae and Lauraceae families against in vitro human tumor models. *Anticancer Res.* 2007 Sep-Oct;27(5A):3293-99.

[877] Moteki H, Hibasami H, Yamada Y, et al. Specific induction of apoptosis by 1,8-cineole in two human leukemia cell lines, but not in human stomach cancer cell line. *Oncol Rep.* 2002 Jul-Aug;9(4):757-60.

[878] Sayyah M, Saroukhani G, Peirovi A, et al. Analgesic and anti-inflammatory activity of the leaf essential oil of Laurus nobilis Linn. *Phytother Res.* 2003 Aug;17(7):733-36.

[879] Matsubara E, Fukagawa M, Okmoto T, et al. Volatiles emitted from the leaves of Laurus nobilis L. improve vigilance performance in visual discrimination task. *Biomed Res.* 2011 Feb;32(1):19-28.

[880] Ferreira A, Proenca C, Serralheiro ML, et al. The in vitro screening for acetylcholinesterase inhibition and antioxidant activity of medicinal plants from Portugal. *J Ethnopharmacol.* 2006 Nov 3;108(1):31-37.

[881] Chmit M, Kanaan H, Habib J, et al. Antibacterial and antibiofilm activities of polysaccharides, essential oil, and fatty oil extracted from Laurus nobilis growing in Lebanon. *Asian Pac J Trop Med.* 2014 Sep;7S1:S546-52.

[882] Dadalioglu I, Evrendilek GA. Chemical compositions and antibacterial effects of essential oils of Turkish oregano (Origanum minutiflorum), bay laurel (Laurus nobilis), Spanish Lavender (Lavandula stoechas L.) and fennel (Foeniculum vulgare) on common foodborne pathogens. *J Agric Food Chem.* 2004 Dec 29;52(26):8255-60.

[883] Loizzo MR, Saab AM, Tundis R, et al. Phytochemical analysis and in vitro antiviral activities of the essential oils of seven Lebanon species. *Chem Biodivers.* 2008 Mar;5(3):461-70.

[884] Loizzo MR, Saab AM, Tundis R, et al. Phytochemical analysis and in vitro antiviral activities of the essential oils of seven Lebanon species. *Chem Biodivers.* 2008 Mar;5(3):461-70.

[885] Peixoto LR, Rosalen PL, Ferreira GL, et al. Antifungal activity, mode of action and anti-biofilm effects of Laurus nobilis Linnaeus essential oil against Candida spp. *Arch Oral Biol.* 2016 Oct 18;73:179-185.

[886] Houicher A, Hechachna H, Teldji H, et al. In vitro study of the antifungal activity of essential oils obtained from Mentha spicata, Thymus vulgaris and Laurus nobilis. *Recent Pat Food Nutr Agric.* 2016;8(2):99-106.

[887] Caputo L, Nazzaro F, Souza LF, et al. Laurus nobilis: Composition of Essential Oil and Its Biological Activities. *Molecules.* 2017 Jun 3;22(6). PLoS One. 2022 May 23;17(5):e0267150.

[888] Caputo L, Nazzaro F, Souza LF, et al. Laurus nobilis: Composition of Essential Oil and Its Biological Activities. *Molecules.* 2017 Jun 3;22(6).

[889] Bartoňková I, Dvořák Z. Essential oils of culinary herbs and spices display agonist and antagonist activities at human aryl hydrocarbon receptor AhR. *Food Chem Toxicol.* 2018 Jan;111:374-384.

[890] Fernandez CMM, da Rosa MF, Fernandez ACAM, et al. Essential oil and fractions isolated of Laurel to control adults and larvae of cattle ticks. *Nat Prod Res.* 2020 Mar;34(5):731-735.

[891] Fidan H, Stefanova G, Kostova I, et al. Chemical Composition and Antimicrobial Activity of Laurus nobilis L. Essential Oils from Bulgaria. *Molecules.* 2019 Feb 22;24(4).

[892] Mahomoodally F, Aumeeruddy-Elafi Z, Venugopala KN, et al. Antiglycation, Comparative Antioxidant Potential, Phenolic Content and Yield Variation of Essential Oils From 19 Exotic and Endemic Medicinal Plants. *Saudi J Biol Sci.* 2019 Nov;26(7):1779-88.

[893] Mahomoodally F, Aumeeruddy-Elafi Z, Venugopala KN, et al. Antiglycation, Comparative Antioxidant Potential, Phenolic Content and Yield Variation of Essential Oils From 19 Exotic and Endemic Medicinal Plants. *Saudi J Biol Sci.* 2019 Nov;26(7):1779-88.

[894] Córdoba S, Vivot W, Szusz W, et al. Antifungal Activity of Essential Oils Against Candida Species Isolated from Clinical Samples. *Mycopathologia.* 2019 Oct;184(5):615-623.

[895] Nafis A, Kasrati A, Jamali CAA, et al. Comparative Study of the in Vitro Antimicrobial and Synergistic Effect of Essential Oils from Laurus nobilis L. and Prunus armeniaca L. from Morocco with Antimicrobial Drugs: New Approach for Health Promoting Products. *Antibiotics (Basel).* 2020 Mar 25;9(4).

[896] Rebickova K, Bajer T, Silha D, et al. Comparison of Chemical Composition and Biological Properties of Essential Oils Obtained by Hydrodistillation and Steam Distillation of Laurus nobilis L. *Plant Foods Hum Nutr.* 2020 Jul 24. Online ahead of print.

[897] Capetti F, Cagliero C, Marengo A, et al. Bio-Guided Fractionation Driven by In Vitro α-Amylase Inhibition Assays of Essential Oils Bearing Specialized Metabolites with Potential Hypoglycemic Activity. *Plants (Basel).* 2020 Sep 21;9(9):E1242.

[898] Al-Mijalli SH, Mrabti HN, Ouassou H, et al. Chemical Composition, Antioxidant, Anti-Diabetic, Anti-Acetylcholinesterase, Anti-Inflammatory, and Antimicrobial Properties of Arbutus unedo L. and Laurus nobilis L. Essential Oils. *Life (Basel).* 2022 Nov 14;12(11):1876.

[899] Nabila B, Piras A, Fouzia B, et al. Chemical composition and antibacterial activity of the essential oil of Laurus nobilis leaves. *Nat Prod Res.* 2020 Oct 28;1-5.

[900] Belasli A, Miri YB, Aboudaou M, et al. Antifungal, antitoxigenic, and antioxidant activities of the essential oil from laurel ( Laurus nobilis L.): Potential use as wheat preservative. *Food Sci Nutr.* 2020 Jul 23;8(9):4717-4729.

[901] Stefanova G, Girova T, Gochev V, et al. Comparative study on the chemical composition of laurel (Laurus nobilis L.) leaves from Greece and Georgia and the antibacterial activity of their essential oil. *Heliyon.* 2020 Dec 21;6(12):e05491.

[902] Vinturelle R, Mattos C, Meloni J, et al. Evaluation of essential oils as an ecological alternative in the search for control Rhipicephalus microplus (Acari: Ixodidae). *Vet Parasitol Reg Stud Reports.* 2021 Jan;23:100523.

[903] Ozogul Y, El Abed N, Ozogul F. Antimicrobial effect of laurel essential oil nanoemulsion on food-borne pathogens and fish spoilage bacteria. *Food Chem.* 2021 Aug 11;368:130831.

[904] Alimi D, Hajri A, Jallouli S, et al. In vitro acaricidal activity of essential oil and crude extracts of Laurus nobilis, (Lauraceae) grown in Tunisia, against arthropod ectoparasites of livestock and poultry: Hyalomma scupense and Dermanyssus gallinae. *Vet Parasitol.* 2021 Jun 24;298:109507.

[905] Ercin E, Kecel-Gunduz S, Gok B, et al. Laurus nobilis L. Essential Oil-Loaded PLGA as a Nanoformulation Candidate for Cancer Treatment. *Molecules.* 2022 Mar 15;27(6):1899.

[906] Odeh D, Oršolić N, Berendika M, et al. Antioxidant and Anti-Atherogenic Activities of Essential Oils from Myrtus communis L. and Laurus nobilis L. in Rat. *Nutrients.* 2022 Mar 31;14(7):1465.

[907] Haouel-Hamdi S, Soltani A, Ben Hamedou M, et al. Laurel essential oil: biological activities and application for semolina preservation against the red flour beetle Tribolium castaneum (Tenebrionidae). *Int J Environ Health Res.* 2022 Jun 29:1-11.

[908] Razzouk S, Mazri MA, Jeldi L, et al. Chemical Composition and Antimicrobial Activity of Essential Oils from Three Mediterranean Plants against Eighteen Pathogenic Bacteria and Fungi. *Pharmaceutics.* 2022 Aug 1;14(8):1608.

[909] Jiang C, Hong J, Meng J, et al. Antibacterial activity of essential oils extracted from the unique Chinese spices cassia bark, bay fruits and cloves. *Arch Microbiol.* 2022 Oct 18;204(11):674.

[910] Moyler DA. The flavour gum resins: their chemistry and uses. *Riv Ital EPPOS.* 1998;(Special Number):351–360.

[911] Fernandez X, Lizzani-Cuvelier L, Loiseau AM, et al. Volatile constituents of benzoin gums: Siam and Sumatra. Part 1. *Flavour Frag J.* 2003;18:328-3.

[912] Pastorova I, de Koster CG, Boon JJ. Analytical study of free ad ester bound benzoic and cinnamic acids of gum benzoin resins by GC-MS and HPLC-frit FAB-MS. *Phytochem Anal.* 1997 Mar;8(2):63-73.

[913] Castel C, Fernandez X, Lizzani-Cuveiler L, et al. Volatile constituents of benzoin gums: Siam and Sumatra, part 2. Study of headspace sampling methods. *Flavour Frag J.* 2006 Jan-Feb;21(1):59-67.

[914] Burger P, Casale A, Kerdudo A, et al. New insights in the chemical composition of benzoin balsams. *Food Chem.* 2016 Nov 1;210:613-22.

[915] Paterson JR, Baxter G, Dreyer JS, et al. Salicylic acid sans aspirin in animals and man: persistence in fasting and biosynthesis from benzoic acid. *J Agric Food Chem.* 2008;56:11648–52.

[916] Tsai HH, Lin HW, Chen YL, et al. A review of potential harmful interactions between anticoagulant/antiplatelet agents and Chinese herbal medicines. *PLoS One.* 2013 May 9;8(5):e64255.

[917] Lin WY, Kuo YH, Chang YL, et al. Anti-platelet aggregation and chemical constituents from the rhizome of Gynura japonica. *Planta Med.* 2003 Aug;69(8):757-64.

[918] Basu S, Jana S, Patel VB, et al. Effects of piperine, cinnamic acid and gallic acid on rosuvastatin pharmacokinetics in rats. *Phytother Res.* 2013 Oct;27(10):1548-56. doi: 10.1002/ptr.4894. Epub 2012 Dec 3.

[919] Langeveld WT, Veldhuizen EJ, Burt SA. Synergy between essential oil constituents and antibiotics. *Crit Rev Microbiol.* 2014 Feb;40(1);76-94.

[920] Rastogi N, Goh KS, Horgen L, et al. Synergistic activities of antituberculous drugs with cerulenin and trans-cinnamic acid against Mycobacterium tuberculosis. *FEMS Immunol Med Microbiol.* 1998 Jun;21(2):149-57.

[921] Arya SH, Doble M. Synergisitic interaction of cinnamic acid with amikacin against Escherichia coli under in vitro conditions. *Adv Biomed Res.* Available at: http://www.wseas.us/e-library/conferences/2010/Cambridge/MABIPH/MABIPH-06.pdf.

[922] Sasseville D, Saber M, Lessard L. Allergic contact dermatitis from tincture of benzoin with multiple concomitant reactions. *Contact Dermatitis.* 2009 Dec;61(6):358-60.

[923] Fettig J, Taylor J, Sood A. Post-surgical allergic contact dermatitis to constituent tincture of benzoin and association with reactions to fragrances and essential oils. *Dermatitis.* 2014 Jul-Aug;25(4):211-2.

[924] Lakshmi C, Srinivas CR. Contact dermatitis to constituent tincture of benzoin applied under occlusion. *Indian J Dermatol Venereol Leprol.* 2006 Jan-Feb;72(1):62-3.

[925] Scardamaglia L, Nixon R, Fewings J. Constituent tincture of benzoin: a common contact allergen? *Australas J Dermatol.* 2003 Aug;44(3):180-4.

[926] James WD, White SW, Yanklowitz B. Allergic contact dermatitis to constituent tincture of benzoin. *J Am Acad Dermatol.* 1984 Nov;11(5 Pt 1):847-50.

[927] Shin S. Anti-Aspergillus activities of plant essential oils and their combination effects with ketoconazole or amphotericin B. *Arch Pharm Res.* 2003 May;26(5):389-93.

[928] Jantapan K, Poapolathep A, Imsilp K, et al. Inhibitory Effects of Thai Essential Oils on Potentially Aflatoxigenic Aspergillus parasiticus and Aspergillus flavus. *Biocontrol Sci.* 2017;22(1):31-40.

[929] Dugo G, Cotroneo A, Verzera A, et al. Genuineness characters of Calabrian bergamot essential oil. *Flavour Frag J.* 1991 Mar;6(1):39-56.

[930] Eleni M, Antonios M, Koliopoulos G, Alexios-Leandros S, et al. High quality bergamot oil from Greece: Chemical analysis using gas chromatography and larvicidal activity against the West Nile Virus vector. *Molecule.* 2009;14:839-49.

[931] Nabiha B, Adelfatteh EO, Faten K, et al. Chemical composition of bergamot (Citrus Bergamia Risso) essential oil obtained by hydrodistillation. *J Chem Chemical Eng.* 2010 Apr;4(4):60-62.

[932] Verzera A, Trozzi A, Stagno d' Alcontes I, et al. The composition of the volatile fraction of Calabrian bergamot essential oil. *Rivista Italiana EPPOS.* 1998;25:17-38.

[933] Eleni M, Antonios M, Koliopoulos G, Alexios-Leandros S, et al. High quality bergamot oil from Greece: Chemical analysis using gas chromatography and larvicidal activity against the West Nile Virus vector. *Molecule.* 2009;14:839-49.

[934] Knott E, Hofmann H. Purely natural: phototoxic dermatitis. *MMW Fortschr Med.* 2007 Feb 8;149(6):36.

[935] Dubertret L, Serraf-Ticazes D, Jeammougin M, et al. Phototoxic properties of perfumes containing bergamot oil on human skin: photoprotective effect of UVA and UVB sunscreen. *J Photochem Photobiol B.* 1990 Nov;7(2-4):251-59.

[936] Williamson EA. Inhibition of cytochrome P450 2E1, cytochrome P450 3A6 and cytochrome P450 2A6 by citrus essential oils. University of North Carolina Thesis. Available at: http://libres.uncg.edu/ir/uncg/f/Williamson_uncg_0154M_10494.pdf.

[937] Tundis R, Loizzo MR, Bonesi M, et al. Comparative study on the antioxidant capacity and cholinesterase inhibitory activity of Citrus aurantifolia Swingle, C. aurantium L., and C. bergamia Risso and Poit. Peel oils. *J Food Sci.* 2012 Jan;77(1):H40-46.

[938] Russo R, Cassiano MG, Ciociaro A, et al. Role of D-limonene in autophagy induced by bergamot essential oil in SH- SY5Y neuroblastomas cells. *PLoS One.* 2014 Nov;9(11):e113682.

[939] Russo R, Ciociaro A, Berliocchi L, et al. Implication of limonene and linalyl acetate in cytotoxicity induced by bergamot essential oil in human neuroblastoma cells. *Fitoterapia.* 2013 Sep;89:48-57.

[940] Berliocchi L, Ciociaro A, Russo R, et al. Toxic profile of bergamot essential oil on survival and proliferation of SH- SY5Y neuroblastoma cells. *Food Chem Toxicol.* 2011 Nov;49(11):2780-92.

[941] Celia C, Trapasso E, Locatelli M, et al. Anticancer activity of liposomal bergamot essential oil (BEO) on human neuroblastoma cells. *Colloids Surf B Biointerfaces.* 2013 Dec;112:548-53.

[942] Navarra M, Ferlazzo N, Cimi S, et al. Effects of bergamot essential oil and its extractive fractions on SH-SY5Y human neuroblastoma cell growth. *J Pharm Pharmacol.* 2015 Aug;67(8):1042-53.

[943] Kang P, Han SH, Moon HK, et al. Citrus bergamia Risso elevates intracellular CA (2+) in human vascular endothelial cells due to release of Ca (2+) from primary intracellular stores. *Evid Based Complement Altern Med.* 2013;2013:759615.

[944] Kang P, Suh SH, Min SS, et al. The essential oil of Citrus bergamia Risso induces vasorelaxation of the mouse aorta by activating K(+) channels and inhibiting Ca(2+) influx. *J Pharm Pharmacol.* 2013 May;65(5):745-49.

[945] You JH, Kang P, Min SS, et al. Bergamot essential oil differentially modulates intracellular Ca2+ levels in vascular endothelial and smooth muscle cells: a new finding seen with fura-2. *J Cardiovasc Pharmacol.* 2013 Apr;61(4):324-28.

[946] Trombetta D, Cimino F, Cristani M, et al. In vitro protective effects of two extracts from bergamot peels on human endothelial cells exposed to tumor necrosis factor-alpha (TNF-alpha). *J Agric Food Chem.* 2010 Jul 28;58(14):8430-36.

[947] Hwang JH. The effects of the inhalation method using essential oils on blood pressure and stress responses of clients with essential hypertension. *Taehan Kanho Hakhoe Chi.* 2006 Dec;36(7):1123-34.

[948] Graziano AC, Cardile V, Crasci L, et al. Protective effects of an extract from Citrus bergamia against inflammation injury in interferon-y and histamine exposed human keratinocytes. *Life Sci.* 2012 Jun 27;90(25-26):968-74.

[949] Menichini F, Tundis R, Loizzo MR, et al. In vitro photo-induced cytotoxic activity of Citrus bergamia and C. medica L. cv. Diamante peel essential oils and identified active coumarins. *Pharm Biol.* 2010 Sep;48(9):1059-65.

[950] Furneri PM, Mondello L, Mandalari G, et al. In vitro antimycoplasmal activity of citrus bergamia essential oil and its major components. *Eur J Med Chme.* 2012 Jun;52:66-69.

[951] Bagetta G, Morrone LA, Rombola L, et al. Neuropharmacology of the essential oil of bergamot. *Fitoterapia.* 2010 Sep;81(6):453-61.

[952] Rombola L, Corasanti MT, Rotiroti D, et al. Effects of systemic administration of the essential oil of bergamot (BEO) on gross behavior and EEG power spectra recorded from the rat hippocampus and cerebral cortex. *Funct Neurol.* 2009 Apr-Jun;24(2):107-12.

[953] Amantea D, Fratto V, Maida S, Rotiroti D, et al. Prevention of glutamate accumulation and upregulation of phospho- Akt may account for neuroprotection afforded by bergamot essential oil against brain injury induced by focal cerebral ischemia in rat. *Int Rev Neurobiol.* 2009;85:389-405.

[954] Sakurada T, Kuwahata H, Katsuyama S, et al. Intraplantar injection of bergamot essential oil into mouse hindpaw: effects on capsaicin-induced nociceptive behaviors. *Int Rev Neurobiol.* 2009;85:237-48.

[955] Corasaniti MT, Maiuolo J, Maida S, et al. Cell signaling pathways in the mechanisms of neuroprotection afforded by bergamot essential oil against NMDA-induced cell death in vitro. *Br J Pharmacol.* 2007 Jun;151(4):518-29.

[956] Kuwahata H, Komatsu T, Katsuyama S, et al. Peripherally injected linalool and bergamot essential oil attenuate mechanical allodynia via inhibiting spinal ERK phosphorylation. *Pharmacol Biochem Behav.* 2013 Fen;103(4):735-41.

[957] Watanabe E, Kuchta K, Rauwald HW, et al. Mood enhancement by bergamot (Citrus bergamia (Risso) Wright & Arn.) volatile vapor with regards to personality and lifestyle related changes in salivary cortisol levels: A randomized cross-over trial. *Planta Med.* 2013;79:PN116.

[958] Lemon K. An assessment of treating depression and anxiety with aromatherapy. *Int J Aromatherapy.* 2004 Jul;14(2):63-69.

[959] Liu SH, Lin TH, Chang KM. The physical effects of aromatherapy in alleviating work-related stress on elementary school teachers in Taiwan. *Evid Based Complement Altern Med.* 2013;2013:853809.

[960] Watanabe E, Kuchta K, Kimura M, et al. Effects of bergamot (citrus bergamia (Risso) Wright & Arn.) essential oil aromatherapy on mood states, parasympathetic nervous system activity, and salivary cortisol levels in 41 healthy females. *Forsch Komplementmed.* 2015;22(1)43-49.

[961] Saiyudthong S, Marsden CA. Acute effects of bergamot oil on anxiety-related behaviour and corticosterone level in rats. *Phytother Res.* 2011 Jun;25(6):858-62.

[962] Chang SY. Effects of aroma hand massage on pain, state anxiety and depression in hospice patients with terminal cancer. *Taehan Kanho Hakhoe Chi.* 2008 Aug;38(4):493-502.

[963] Tundis R, Loizzo MR, Bonesi M, et al. Comparative study on the antioxidant capacity and cholinesterase inhibitory activity of Citrus aurantifolia Swingle, C. aurantium L., and C. bergamia Risso and Poit. Peel oils. *J Food Sci.* 2012 Jan;77(1):H40-46.

[964] Darvesh S, Hopkins DA, Geula C, Neurobiology of butyrylcholinesterase. *Nat Rev Neurosci.* 2003 Feb;4:131-38.

[965] Fisher K, Phillips C. In vitro inhibition of vancomycin-susceptible and vancomycin-resistant Enterococcus faecium and E. faecalis in the presence of citrus essential oils. *Br J Biomed Sci.* 2009;66(4):180-85.

[966] Fisher K, Phillips C. The mechanism of action of a citrus oil blend against Enterococcus faecium and Enterococcus faecalis. *J Appl Microbiol.* 2009 Apr;106(4):1343-49.

[967] Dyer J, Cleary L, McNeill S, et al. The use of aromasticks to help with sleep problems: A patient experience survey. Complement Ther Clin Pract. 2016 Feb;22:51-8.

[968] Campolo O, Romeo FV, Algeri GM, et al. Larvicidal Effects of Four Citrus Peel Essential Oils Against the Arbovirus Vector Aedes albopictus (Diptera: Culicidae). *J Econ Entomol.* 2016 Feb;109(1):360-5.

[969] Pazinato R, Volpato A, Baldissera MD, et al. In vitro effect of seven essential oils on the reproduction of the cattle tick Rhipicephalus microplus. *J Adv Res.* 2016 Nov;7(6):1029-1034.

[970] Han X, Beaumont C, Stevens N. Chemical composition analysis and in vitro biological activities of ten essential oils in human skin cells. *Biochim Open.* 2017 Apr 26;5:1-7.

[971] Restuccia C, Oliveri Conti G, Zuccarello P, et al. Efficacy of different citrus essential oils to inhibit the growth and B1 aflatoxin biosynthesis of Aspergillus flavus. *Environ Sci Pollut Res Int.* 2019 Oct;26(30):31263-31272.

[972] Rombolà L, Scuteri D, Adornetto A, et al. Anxiolytic-Like Effects of Bergamot Essential Oil Are Insensitive to Flumazenil in Rats. *Evid Based Complement Alternat Med.* 2019 Aug 14;2019:2156873.

[973] Scuteri D, Rombolia L, Tridico L, et al. Neuropharmacological Properties of the Essential Oil of Bergamot for the Clinical Management of Pain-Related BPSDs. *Curr Med Chem.* 2018;25:1-10.

[974] Caputo L, Cornara L, Bazzicalupo M, et al. Chemical Composition and Biological Activities of Essential Oils from Peels of Three Citrus Species. *Molecules.* 2020 Apr 19;25(8).

[975] Lombardo GE, Crimi S, Muscumeci L, et al. Mechanisms Underlying the Anti-Inflammatory Activity of Bergamot Essential Oil and Its Antinociceptive Effects. *Plants (Basel).* 2020 Jun 1;9(6):E704.

[976] Filipovic G, Stevanovic MD, Stojanovic-Radic Z, et al. Choosing the right essential oil for a mouthwash: chemical, antimicrobial and cytotoxicity study. *Chem Biodivers.* Online ahead of print.

[977] Garbin VP, Munguia B, Saldana JC, et al. Chemical characterization and in vitro anthelmintic activity of Citrus bergamia Risso and Citrus X paradisii Macfad essential oil against Haemonchus contortus Kirby isolate. *Acta Trop.* 2021 Feb 22;105869.

[978] Maugeri A, Lombardo GE, Musumeci L, et al. Bergamottin and 5-Geranyloxy-7-methoxycoumarin Cooperate in the Cytotoxic Effect of Citrus bergamia (Bergamot) Essential Oil in Human Neuroblastoma SH-SY5Y Cell Line. *Toxins (Basel).* 2021 Apr 10;13(4):275.

[979] Chen SJ, Chen CH, Chang HY. [Effects of Inhaling Essential Oil on Headache-Related Quality of Life Among Nurses Working in Emergency and Critical Care Units]. *Hu Li Za Zhi.* 2021 Oct;68(5):51-64.

[980] Hongratanaworakit T. Aroma-therapeutic Effects of Massage Blended Essential Oils on Humans. *Nat Prod Commun.* 2011;6(8):1199-1204.

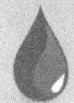

[981] Zhang N, Kong F, Zhao L, et al. Essential oil, juice, and ethanol extract from bergamot confer improving effects against primary dysmenorrhea in rats. *J Food Biochem*. 2021 Feb;45(2):e13614.
[982] Chen ML, Chen YE, Lee HF. The Effect of Bergamot Essential Oil Aromatherapy on Improving Depressive Mood and Sleep Quality in Postpartum Women: A Randomized Controlled Trial. *J Nursing Res*. 2021. Online ahead of print.
[983] Ridha AF, Komalasari, Sina CI, et al. PENGARUH AROMATERAPI BERGAMOT (CITRUS BERGAMIA) TERHADAP TINGKAT DEPRESI POST PARTUMDI RS BLUD KOTA TANJUNGPINANG. *MALAHAYATI NURSING JOURNAL*. 2023;5(3):756-73.
[984] Alexa VT, Galuscan A, Soica CM, et al. In Vitro Assessment of the Cytotoxic and Antiproliferative Profile of Natural Preparations Containing Bergamot, Orange and Clove Essential Oils. *Molecules*. 2022 Feb 1;27(3):990.
[985] Catalano R, Procopio F, Chavarria D, et al. Molecular Modeling and Experimental Evaluation of Non-Chiral Components of Bergamot Essential Oil with Inhibitory Activity against Human Monoamine Oxidases. *Molecules*. 2022;27:2467.
[986] Rombola L, Straface M, Scuteri D, et al. Antispasmodic Effect of Bergamot Essential Oil on Rat Isolated Gut Tissues. *Pharmaceuticals*. 2022 Apr;14(4):775.
[987] Tian L, Hu T, Zhang S, Zhang H, et al. A Comparative Study on Relieving Exercise-Induced Fatigue by Inhalation of Different Citrus Essential Oils. *Molecules*. 2022 May 18;27(10):3239.
[988] Lin L, Yang Q, Li TT, et al. Effect of aromatherapy in patients with Alzheimer's disease: a randomised controlled clinical trial. 2022 Apr. Online ahead of print.
[989] Madia VN, Toscanelli W, De Vita D, et al. Ultrastructural Damages to H1N1 Influenza Virus Caused by Vapor Essential Oils. *Molecules*. 2022 Jun 9;27(12):3718.
[990] Mojtehedi M, Salehi-Pourmehr H, Ostadrahimi A, et al. Effect of Aromatherapy with Essential oil of Lavandula Angustifolia Mill- Citrus Bergamia and Mindfulness-Based Intervention on Sexual Function, Anxiety, and Depression in Postmenopausal Women: A Randomized Controlled Trial with Factorial Design. *Iran J Nurs Midwifery Res*. 2022;27:392-405.
[991] Hung CL, Lin YL, Chou CM, et al. Efficacy of Aromatherapy at Relieving the Work-Related Stress of Nursing Staff from Various Hospital Departments during COVID-19. *Healthcare*. 2023;11:157.
[992] Cebi N, Erarslan A. Determination of the Antifungal, Antibacterial Activity and Volatile Compound Composition of Citrus bergamia Peel Essential Oil. *Foods*. 2023 Jan 3;12(1):203.
[993] Padilia RC, Verma RS, Chauhan A, et al. Essential oil composition of sixteen elite cultivars of Mentha from western Himalayan region, India. *Majeo Int Sci Technol*. 2013;7(10):83-93.
[994] Verma SK. Goswami P, Verma RS, et al. Chemical composition and antimicrobial activity of bergamot-mint (Mentha citrata Ehrh.) essential oils isolated from the herbage and aqueous distillate using different methods. *Ind Crops Prod*. 2016;91:152-60.
[995] Malizia RA, Molli JS, Cardell DA, et al. Essential Oil of Mentha citrata Grown in Argentina. Variation in the Composition and Yield at Full- and Post-Flowering. *J Essent Oil Res*. 1996;8(4):347-49.
[996] Verma SK. Goswami P, Verma RS, et al. Chemical composition and antimicrobial activity of bergamot-mint (Mentha citrata Ehrh.) essential oils isolated from the herbage and aqueous distillate using different methods. *Ind Crops Prod*. 2016;91:152-60.
[997] Pavela R. Insecticidal activity of some essential oils against larvae of Spodoptera littoralis. *Fitoterapia*. 2005 Dec;76(7-8):691-6.
[998] Ouakouak H, Benchikha N, hassani A, et al. Chemical Composition and Biological Activity of Mentha citrata Ehrh., Essential Oils Growing in Southern Algeria. *J Food Sci Technol*. 2019 Dec;56(12):5346-53.
[999] Fazal H, Akram M, Ahmad N, et al. Nutritionally rich biochemical profile in essential oil of various Mentha species and their antimicrobial activities. *Protoplasma*. 2022 Aug 9. Online ahead of print.
[1000] Pirbalouti AG, Mohammadi M. Phytochemical composition of the essential oil of different populations of Stachys lavandulifolia Vahl. *Asian Pac J Trop Biomed*. 2013 Feb;3(2):123–28.
[1001] Aghaei Y, Hossein Mirjalili M, Nazeri V. Chemical diversity among the essential oils of wild populations of Stachys lavandulifolia Vahl. (Lamiaceae) from Iran. *Chem Biodivers*. 2013;10(2):262-73.
[1002] Yavari A, Shahgolzari SM. Chemical Composition of Essential Oil of Stachys lavandulifolia Vahl. From Iran. *Int J Pharmacognosy Phytochem Res*. 2015;7(4):673-76.
[1003] Javidnia K, Mojab F, Mojahedi SA. Chemical Constituents of the Essential Oil of Stachys lavandulifolia Vahl from Iran. *J Essent Oil Res*. 2004 Winter;3(1):61-63.
[1004] Mahzooni-kachapi, Mahdavi M, Roozbeh-nasira'ei L, et al. Antimicrobial activity and chemical composition of essential oils of Stachys lavandulifolia Vahl. from Mazandaran, Iran. *J Med Plant Res*. 2012 Jun;6(24):4149-58.
[1005] Feizbaksh a, Saber Tehrani M, Rustaiyan A. Composition of the Essential Oil of Stachys lavandulifolia Vahl. from Iran. *J Essent Oil Res*. 2003 Mar-Apr;15(2):72-73.
[1006] Meshkatalsadat MH, Sajjadi E, and Amiri H. Chemical Constituents of the Essential Oils of Different Stages of the Growth of Stachys lavandulifolia Vahl. From Iran. *Pak J Biol Sci*. 2007;10:2784-86.
[1007] Bakerink JA, Gospe SM Jr, Dimand RJ, et al. Multiple organ failure after ingestion of pennyroyal oil from herbal tea in two infants. *Pediatrics*. 1996;98(5):944-47.
[1008] Sudekum M, Poppenga RH, Raju N, et al. Pennyroyal oil toxicosis in a dog. *J Am Vet Med Assoc*. 1992;200:817-8.
[1009] Anderson IB, Mullen WH, Meeker JE, et al. Pennyroyal toxicity: measurement of toxic metabolite levels in two cases and review of the literature. *Ann Intern Med*. 1996;124:726-34.
[1010] Seeff L, Stickel F, Navarro VJ. Hepatotoxicity of herbals and dietary supplements. In, Kaplowitz N, DeLeve LD, eds. Drug-induced liver disease. 3rd ed. Amsterdam: Elsevier, 2013, pp. 631-58.
[1011] Moolla A. A phytochemical and pharmacological investigation of indigenous Agathosma species. MSc Dissertation, University of the Witwatersrand. 2006.
[1012] Mullen W, Anderson I, Oishii S, et al. Accidental pennyroyal oil ingestion in a toddler with the first human serum metabolite detection. *Vet Hum Toxicol*. 1994;36:342.
[1013] Barnes J, Anderson LA, Philpson JD. Herbal Medicine: A Guide for Healthcare Professionals. London, UK: The Pharmaceutical Press, 1996.
[1014] Anderson IB, Mullen WH, Meeker JE, et al. Pennyroyal toxicity: measurement of toxic metabolite levels in two cases and review of the literature. *Ann Intern Med*. 1996;124:726-34.
[1015] Zimmerman HJ. Unconventional drugs. Miscellaneous drugs and diagnostic chemicals. In, Zimmerman, HJ. Hepatotoxicity: the adverse effects of drugs and other chemicals on the liver. 2nd ed. Philadelphia: Lippincott,1999: pp. 731-34.
[1016] Centers for Disease Control. Fatality and illness associated with consumption of pennyroyal oil - Colorado. *MMWR*. 1978;27:511-13.
[1017] Delgado IF, Carvalho RR, Nogueira, et al. Study on embryofetotoxicity of b-myrcene in the rat. *Food and Chemical Toxicology*. 1993;31(1):31-5.
[1018] Paumgartten FJ, De-Carvalho RR, Souza CA, et al. Study of the effects of beta-myrcene on rat fertility and general reproductive performance. *Braz J Med Biol Res*. 1998 Jul;31(7):955-65.
[1019] Barnes J, Anderson LA, Philpson JD. Herbal Medicine: A Guide for Healthcare Professionals. London, UK: The Pharmaceutical Press, 1996.
[1020] Zimmerman HJ. Unconventional drugs. Miscellaneous drugs and diagnostic chemicals. In, Zimmerman, HJ. Hepatotoxicity: the adverse effects of drugs and other chemicals on the liver. 2nd ed. Philadelphia: Lippincott,1999: pp. 731-34.
[1021] Gordon WP, Huitric AC, Seth CL, et al. The metabolism of the abortifacient terpene, (R)-(+)-pulegone, to a proximate toxin, menthofuran. *Drug Metab Dispos*. 1987;15:589–94.
[1022] Khojasteh-Bakht SC, Chen W, Koenigs LL, et al. Metabolism of (R)-(+)-pulegone and (R)-(+)-menthofuran by human liver cytochrome P-450s: evidence for formation of a furan epoxide. *Drug Metab Dispos*. 1999 May;27(5):574-80.
[1023] Gordon P, Khojasteh SC. A decades-long investigation of acute metabolism-based hepatotoxicity by herbal constituents: a case study of pennyroyal oil. *Drug Metab Rev*. 2015 Feb;47(1):12-20.
[1024] National Toxicology Program. Toxicology and carcinogenesis studies of pulegone (CAS No. 89-82-7) in F344/N rats and B6C3F1 mice (gavage studies). *Natl Toxicol Program Tech Rep Ser*. 2011 Aug;(563):1-201.
[1025] National Toxicology Program. Toxicology and carcinogenesis studies of pulegone (CAS No. 89-82-7) in F344/N rats and B6C3F1 mice (gavage studies). *Natl Toxicol Program Tech Rep Ser*. 2011 Aug;(563):1-201.
[1026] National Toxicology Program. Toxicology and carcinogenesis studies of pulegone (CAS No. 89-82-7) in F344/N rats and B6C3F1 mice (gavage studies). *Natl Toxicol Program Tech Rep Ser*. 2011 Aug;(563):1-201.
[1027] Sullivan JB Jr, Rumack BH, Thomas H Jr, et al. Pennyroyal oil poisoning and hepatotoxicity. *JAMA*. 1979;242:2873-4.
[1028] Moorthy B, Madyastha P, Madyastha KM. Hepatotoxicity of pulegone in rats: its effects on microsomal enzymes, in vivo. *Toxicology*. 1989 May 15;55(3):327-37.
[1029] Madyastha KM, Raj CP. Effects of menthofuran, a monoterpene furan on rat liver microsomal enzymes, in vivo. *Toxicology*. 1994 Apr 18;89(2):119-25.
[1030] Burkhard PR, Burkhardt K, Haenggeli CA, et al. Plant-induced seizures: reappearance of an old problem. *J Neurol*. 1999 Aug;246(8):667-70.
[1031] Bonesi M, Menichini F, Tundis R, et al. Acetylcholinesterase and butyrylcholinesterase inhibitory activity of Pinus species essential oils and their constituents. *J Enzyme Inhib Med Chem*. 2010 Oct;25(5):622-8.
[1032] Sullivan JB Jr, Rumack BH, Thomas H Jr, et al. Pennyroyal oil poisoning and hepatotoxicity. *JAMA*. 1979;242:2873-4.
[1033] Sudekum M, Poppenga RH, Raju N, et al. Pennyroyal oil toxicosis in a dog. *J Am Vet Med Assoc*. 1992;200:817-8.
[1034] Anderson IB, Mullen WH, Meeker JE, et al. Pennyroyal toxicity: measurement of toxic metabolite levels in two cases and review of the literature. *Ann Intern Med*. 1996;124:726-34.
[1035] Zimmerman HJ. Unconventional drugs. Miscellaneous drugs and diagnostic chemicals. In, Zimmerman, HJ. Hepatotoxicity: the adverse effects of drugs and other chemicals on the liver. 2nd ed. Philadelphia: Lippincott,1999: pp. 731-34.
[1036] Seeff L, Stickel F, Navarro VJ. Hepatotoxicity of herbals and dietary supplements. In, Kaplowitz N, DeLeve LD, eds. Drug-induced liver disease. 3rd ed. Amsterdam: Elsevier, 2013, pp. 631-58.
[1037] Jeena K, Liju VB, Viswanathan R, et al. Antimutagenic potential and modulation of carcinogen-metabolizing enzymes by ginger essential oil. *Phytother Res*. 2014 Jun;28(6):849-55.
[1038] Qiu JX1, Zhou ZW2, He ZX, et al. Estimation of the binding modes with important human cytochrome P450 enzymes, drug interaction potential, pharmacokinetics, and hepatotoxicity of ginger components using molecular docking, computational, and pharmacokinetic modeling studies. *Drug Des Devel Ther*. 2015 Feb 16;9:841-66.
[1039] Mahzooni-kachapi, Mahdavi M, Roozbeh-nasira'ei L, et al. Antimicrobial activity and chemical composition of essential oils of Stachys lavandulifolia Vahl. from Mazandaran, Iran. *J Med Plant Res*. 2012 Jun;6(24):4149-58.
[1040] Barreto RSS, Quintana JSS, Amarante RKL, et al. Evidence for the involvement of TNF-α and IL-1β in the antinociceptive and anti-inflammatory activity of Stachys lavandulifolia Vahl. (Lamiaceae) essential oil and (-)-α-bisabolol, its main compound, in mice. *J Ethnopharmacol*. 2016 Sep 15;191:9-18.
[1041] Hazarti S, Lotfi K, Govahi M, et al. A comparative study: Influence of various drying methods on essential oil components and biological properties of Stachys lavandulifolia. *Food Sci Nutr*. 2021 Mar 8;9(5):2612-2619.
[1042] Iqbal Z, Akhtar M, Mahmood T, et al. Variation in Composition and Yield of Foliage Oil of Eucalyptus Polybractea. *J Chem Soc Pakistan*. 2011 Mar;33(2):183-187.

[1043] Juan LW, Lucia A, Zerba EN, et al. Chemical composition and fumigant toxicity of the essential oils from 16 species of Eucalyptus against Haematobia irritans (Diptera: Muscidae) adults. *J Econ Entomol.* 2011 Jun;104(3):1087-92.
[1044] Antonio RD. [Federal University of Prana, Rodrigo Damian Antony phytochemical characterization, morphology, anatomy and organic activities-GICAS of Eucalyptus badjensis Beuzev. & M.B. Welch, Myrtaceae. 2011. http://acervodigital.ufpr.br/bitstream/handle/1884/26303/DissertacaoFinalRDAntonio.pdf?sequence=1.
[1045] Craig JO. Poisoning by the volatile oils in childhood. *Arch Dis Child.* 1953;28:259-67.
[1046] Melis K. Bochner A, Janssens G. Accidental nasal eucalyptol and menthol instillation. *Eur J Pediatr.* 1989 Aug;148(8)786-7.
[1047] Day LM, Ozanne-Smith J, Parsons BJ, et al. Eucalyptus oil poisoning among young children: mechanisms of access and the potential prevention. *Aust N Z J Public Health.* 1997 Jun;21(3):297-302.
[1048] Chandar SD, Prashanti M, Kumar CL, et al. Eucalyptus Oil-Induced Seizures in Children: A Single-Center Prospective Study. *Cureus.* 2021 Mar 25;13(3):e14109.
[1049] Burkhard PR, Burkhardt K, Haenggeli CA, et al. Plant-induced seizures: reappearance of an old problem. *J Neurol.* 1999 Aug;246(8):667-70.
[1050] Waldman N. Seizure caused by dermal application of over-the-counter eucalyptus oil head lice preparation. *Clin Toxicol (Phila).* 2011 Oct;49(8):750-1.
[1051] Craig JO. Poisoning by the volatile oils in childhood. *Arch Dis Child.* 1953;28:259-67.
[1052] Newall CA, Anderson LA, Phillipson JD. "Herbal Medicines: A Guide for Health-care Professionals." London: The Pharmaceutical Press, 1996, 108.
[1053] European Medicines Agency. Community herbal monograph on Eucalyptus globulus Labill., Eucalyptus polybractea R.T. Baker and/or
Eucalyptus smithii R.T. Baker, aetheroleum. 2013 Jun. Available at: http://www.ema.europa.eu/docs/en_GB/document_library/Herbal_-_Community_herbal_monograph/2013/07/WC500147008.pdf
[1054] Fischer JH, Dethlefsen U. Efficacy of cineole in patients suffering from acute bronchitis: a placebo-controlled double-blind trial. *Cough.* 2013; 9: 25.
[1055] Worth W, Dethlefsen U. Patients with asthma benefit from concomitant therapy with cineole: a placebo-controlled, double-blind trial. *J Asthma.* 2012 Oct;49(8):849-53.
[1056] Day LM, Ozanne-Smith J, Parsons BJ, et al. Eucalyptus oil poisoning among young children: mechanisms of access and the potential prevention. *Aust N Z J Public Health.* 1997 Jun;21(3):297-302.
[1057] Myott E. Case of eucalyptus poisoning. *Brit M J.* 1906;1:558.
[1058] Hindle RC. Eucalyptus oil ingestion. *N Z Med J.* 1994 May 11;107(977)185-6.
[1059] Tibballs J. Clinical effects and management of eucalyptus oil ingestion in infants and small children. *Med J Aust.* 1995 Aug;163(4):177-80.
[1060] Waldman W, Barwina M, Sein Anand J. Accidental ontoxication with eucalyptus oil—a case report. *Przeql Lek.* 2011;68(8):555-6.
[1061] Day LM, Ozanne-Smith J, Parsons BJ, et al. Eucalyptus oil poisoning among young children: mechanisms of access and the potential prevention. *Aust N Z J Public Health.* 1997 Jun;21(3):297-302.
[1062] De Vincenzi M, Silano M, De Vincenzi A, et al. Constituents of aromatic plants: eucalyptol. *Fitoterapia.* 2002 Jun;73(3):269-75.
[1063] Unger M, Frank A. Simultaneous determination of the inhibitory potency of herbal extracts on the activity of six major cytochrome P450 enzymes using liquid chromatography/mass spectrometry and automated online extraction. *Rapid Commun Mass Spectrom.* 2004;18(19):2273-81.
[1064] Jori A, Bianchetti A, Prestini PE, et al. Effect of eucalyptol (1,8-cineole) on the metabolism of other drugs in rats and in man. *Eur J Pharmacol.* 1970;9(3):362-66.
[1065] Kim NH, Hyun SH, Jin CH, et al. Pretreatment with 1,8-cineole potentiates thioacetamide-induced hepatotoxicity and immunosuppression. *Arch Pharm Res.* 2004 Jul;27(7):781-9.
[1066] Gray AM, Flatt PR. Antihyperglycemic actions of Eucalyptus globulus (Eucalyptus) are associated with pancreatic and extra pancreatic effects in mice. *J Nutr.* 1998 Dec;128(12):2319–23.
[1067] Basak SS, Candan F. Effect of Laurus nobilis L. Essential Oil and its Main Components on α-glucosidase and Reactive Oxygen Species Scavenging Activity. *Iran J Pharm Res.* 2013 Spring;12(2):367-79.
[1068] Dey B. Chemo-profiling of eucalyptus and study of its hypoglycemic potential. *World J Diabetes.* 2013 Oct 15;4(5):170–76.
[1069] Tsai HH, Lin HW, Chen YL, et al. A review of potential harmful interactions between anticoagulant/antiplatelet agents and Chinese herbal medicines. *PLoS One.* 2013 May 9;8(5):e64255.
[1070] Moharam BA, Jantan I, bin Ahmad F, et al. Antiplatelet Aggregation and Platelet Activating Factor (PAF) Receptor Antagonistic Activities of the Essential Oils of Five Goniothalamus Species. *Molecules.* 2010;15:5124-38.
[1071] Jori A, Bianchetti A, Prestini PE, et al. Effect of eucalyptol (1,8-cineole) on the metabolism of other drugs in rats and in man. *Eur J Pharmacol.* 1970;9(3):362-66.
[1072] de Sousa DP, Raphael E, Brocksom U, et al. Sedative effect of monoterpene alcohols in mice: A preliminary screening. *Verlag der Zeitschrift fur Naturforschung.* 2007;62c:563-66.
[1073] Juan LW, Lucia A, Zerba EN, et al. Chemical composition and fumigant toxicity of the essential oils from 16 species of Eucalyptus against Haematobia irritans (Diptera: Muscidae) adults. *J Econ Entomol.* 2011 Jun;104(3):1087-92.
[1074] Lucia A1, Juan LW, Zerba EN, et al. Validation of models to estimate the fumigant and larvicidal activity of Eucalyptus essential oils against Aedes aegypti (Diptera: Culicidae). *Parasitol Res.* 2012 May;110(5):1675-86.
[1075] Morton JF, Thomas CC. Major medicinal plants: Botany, culture and uses. *J Pharm Sci.* 1978 Nov;67(11):1649.
[1076] Green Valley Aromatherapy. Material safety data sheet. Birch. Available at: https://www.57aromas.com/media/pdf-sheets/birch.pdf.
[1077] National Institutes of Health, Medline Plus. Reye Syndrome. Available at: http://www.nlm.nih.gov/medlineplus/ency/article/001565.htm.
[1078] Karabulut AK, Ulger H, Pratten MK. Protection by free oxygen radical scavenging enzymes against salicylate- induced embryonic malformation in vitro. *Toxicol In Vitro.* 2000 Aug;14(4):297-307.
[1079] Overman DO, White JA. Comparative teratogenic effects of methyl salicylate applied orally or topically to hamsters. *Teratology.* 1983 Dec;28(3):421-6.
[1080] Chan TY. Potential dangers from topical preparations containing methyl salicylate. *Hum Exp Toxicol.* 1996 Sep;15(9):747-5.
[1081] Botma M, Colquhoun-Flannery W, Leighton S. Laryngeal oedema caused by accidental ingestion of Oil of Wintergreen. *Int J Pediatr Otorhinolaryngol.* 2001 May 11;58(3):229-32.
[1082] Chyka PA. et al. Salicylate poisoning: an evidence-based consensus guideline for out-of-hospital management. *Clin Toxicol (Phila).* 2007;45(2):95-13.
[1083] Johnson PN. Methyl salicylate/aspirin (salicylate) equivalence: who do you trust? *Vet Hum Toxicol.* 1984 Aug; 26(4):317-318.
[1084] Howrie DL, Moriarty R, Breit R. Candy flavoring as a source of salicylate poisoning. *Pediatrics.* 1985 May 1;75(5):869-71.
[1085] Tisserand R, Young R. *Essential Oil Safety* (Second Edition). 2014 Churchill Livingstone Elsevier.
[1086] Burkhard PR, Burkhardt K, Haenggeli CA, et al. Plant-induced seizures: reappearance of an old problem. *J Neurol.* 1999 Aug;246(8):667-70.
[1087] Tanen DA, Danish DC, Reardon JM, et al. Comparison of oral aspirin versus topical applied methyl salicylate for platelet inhibition. *Ann Pharmacother.* 2008 Oct;42(10):1396-401.
[1088] Le Bourhis B, Soenen AM. Recherches sur l'action psychotrope de quelques substances aromatiques utilisees en alimentation. *Food Cosmet Toxicol.* 1973;11:1-9.
[1089] Joss JD, LeBlond RF. Potentiation of warfarin anticoagulation associated with topical methyl salicylate. *Ann Pharmacother.* 2000 Jun;34(6):729-33.
[1090] Chan TY. Potential dangers from topical preparations containing methyl salicylate. *Hum Exp Toxicol.* 1996;15:747- 50.
[1091] Orra P, Bartle WR, Walker SE, et al. Serum concentrations of salicylic acid following topically applied salicylate derivatives. *Ann Pharmacother.* 1996 Sep;30(9):935-40.
[1092] Botma M, Colquhoun-Flannery W, Leighton S. Laryngeeal oedema caused by accidental ingestion of oil of wintergreen. *Int J Ped Otorhinolaryngology.* 2001 May;58(3):229-32.
[1093] Parker D, Martinez C, Stanley C, et al. The analysis of methyl salicylate and salicylic acid from Chinese herbal medicine ingestion. *J Analytical Tox.* 2004 Apr;28:214-16.
[1094] Demirci F, Demirci B, Baser KHC, et al. The composition and antifungal bioassay of the essential oils of different Betula species growing in Turkey. *Chem Nat Comp.* 2000 Mar-Apr; 36(2):159-65.
[1095] Goc A, Niedzwiecki A, Rath M. Anti-borreliae efficacy of selected organic oils and fatty acids. *BMC Complement Altern Med.* 2019 Fen;19(1):40.
[1096] Tanabe H, Doi T, Akai M, et al. Effect and usability of anti-inflammatory drug plasters for knee osteoarthritis: A crossover double-blind, repeated measures, randomized controlled trial. *J Orthop Sci.* 2021 May;26(3):421-429.
[1097] Sarrou E, Chatzopoulou P, Dimassi-Theriou K, et al. Volatile constituents and antioxidant activity of peel, flowers and leaf oils of Citrus aurantium L. growing in Greece. *Molecules.* 2013;18:10639–10647.
[1098] Costa CA, Cury TC, Cassettari BO, et al. Citrus aurantium L. essential oil exhibits anxiolytic-like activity mediated by 5-HT(1A)-receptors and reduces cholesterol after repeated oral treatment. *BMC Complement Altern Med.* 2013 Feb 23;13:42.
[1099] Jabiri Karoui I, Marzouk B. Characterization of bioactive constituents in Tunisian bitter orange (Citrus aurantium L.) peel and juice and determination of their antioxidant activities. *BioMed Res Int.* 2013;2013:345415.
[1100] Opdyke DIJ. Monographs on fragrance raw materials. *Food Cosmet Toxicol.* 1974;12(Suppl.):901–02.
[1101] IFRA. Citrus oils and other furocoumarins containing essential oils. Available at: https://ifrafragrance.org/standards/IFRA_STD_089.pdf.
[1102] Tundis R, Loizzo MR, Bonesi M, et al. Comparative study on the antioxidant capacity and cholinesterase inhibitory activity of Citrus aurantifolia Swingle, C. aurantium L., and C. bergamia Risso and Poit. Peel oils. *J Food Sci.* 2012 Jan;77(1):H40–46.
[1103] NCAA. 2014–2015 Banned Drugs. Available at: http://www.ncaa.org/health-and-safety/policy/2014-15-ncaa- banned-drugs.
[1104] Costa CA, Cury TC, Cassettari BO, et al. Citrus aurantium L. essential oil exhibits anxiolytic-like activity mediated by 5-HT(1A)-receptors and reduces cholesterol after repeated oral treatment. *BMC Complement Altern Med.* 2013 Feb 23;13:42.
[1105] Hawrelak JA, Cattley T, Myers SP. Essential oils in the treatment of intestinal dysbiosis: A preliminary in vitro study. *Altern Med Rev.* 2009 Dec;14(4)380-84.
[1106] Polo CM, Moraes TM, Pellizzon CH, et al. Gastric ulcers in Middle-aged rats: The healing effect of essential oil from Citrus aurantium L. (Rutaceae). *Evid Based Complement Altern Med.* 2012;2012:509451.
[1107] Moraes TM, Kushima H, Moleiro FC, et al. Effects of limonene and essential oil from Citrus aurantium on gastric mucosa: role of prostaglandins and gastric mucus secretion. *Chem Biol Interact.* 2009 Aug 14;180(3):499–505.
[1108] Tundis R, Loizzo MR, Bonesi M, et al. Comparative study on the antioxidant capacity and cholinesterase inhibitory activity of Citrus aurantifolia Swingle, C. aurantium L., and C. bergamia Risso and Poit. Peel oils. *J Food Sci.* 2012 Jan;77(1):H40–46.
[1109] Darvesh S, Hopkins DA, Geula C, Neurobiology of butyrylcholinesterase. *Nat Rev Neurosci.* 2003 Feb;4:131–38.
[1110] Yip YB, Tam AC. An experimental study on the effectiveness of massage with aromatic ginger and orange essential oil for moderate-to-severe knee pain among the elderly in Hong Kong. *Complement Ther Med.* 2008 Jun;16(3):131-38.

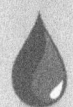

[1111] Sanei-Dehkordi A, Sedaghat MM, Vatandoost H, et al. Chemical Compositions of the Peel Essential Oil of Citrus aurantium and Its Natural Larvicidal Activity against the Malaria Vector Anopheles stephensi (Diptera: Culicidae) in Comparison with Citrus paradisi. *J Arthropod Borne Dis.* 2016 Oct 4;10(4):577-585.
[1112] Martins MH, Fracarolli L, Vieira TM, et al. Schistosomicidal Effects of the Essential Oils of Citrus limonia and Citrus reticulata Against Schistosoma mansoni. *Chem Biodivers.* 2017 Jan;14(1).
[1113] Ben Hsouna A, Gargouri M, Dhifi W, et al. Potential anti-inflammatory and antioxidant effects of Citrus aurantium essential oil against carbon tetrachloride-mediated hepatotoxicity: A biochemical, molecular and histopathological changes in adult rats. *Environ Toxicol.* 2019 Apr;34(4):388-400.
[1114] Teneva D, Denkova-Kostova R, Goranov B, et al. Chemical composition, antioxidant activity and antimicrobial activity of essential oil from Citrus aurantium L zest against some pathogenic microorganisms. *Z Naturforsch C.* 2019 May 27;74(5-6):105-111.
[1115] Restuccia C, Oliveri Conti G, Zuccarello P, et al. Efficacy of different citrus essential oils to inhibit the growth and B1 aflatoxin biosynthesis of Aspergillus flavus. *Environ Sci Pollut Res Int.* 2019 Oct;26(30):31263-31272.
[1116] Di Vito M, Bellardi MG, Sanguinetti M, et al. Potent In Vitro Activity of Citrus aurantium Essential Oil and Vitis vinifera Hydrolate Against Gut Yeast Isolates From Irritable Bowel Syndrome Patients-The Right Mix for Potential Therapeutic Use. *Nutrients.* 2020 May 7;12(5):E1329.
[1117] Karimzadeh Z, Forouzi MA, Rahiminexhad E, et al. The Effects of Lavender and Citrus aurantium on Anxiety and Agitation of the Conscious Patients in Intensive Care Units: A Parallel Randomized Placebo-Controlled Trial. *Biomed Res Int.* 2021 Jun 15;2021:5565956.
[1118] Benayad O, Bouhrim M, Tiji S, et al. Phytochemical Profile, α-Glucosidase, and α-Amylase Inhibition Potential and Toxicity Evaluation of Extracts from Citrus aurantium (L) Peel, a Valuable By-Product from Northeastern Morocco. *Biomolecules.* 2021 Oct 20;11(11):1555.
[1119] Vitalini S, Iriti M, Vinciguerra V, Garzoli S. A Comparative Study of the Chemical Composition by SPME-GC/MS and Antiradical Activity of Less Common Citrus Species. *Molecules.* 2021 Sep 4;26(17):5378.
[1120] Badalamenti N, Bruno M, Schicchi R, et al. Chemical Compositions and Antioxidant Activities of Essential Oils, and Their Combinations, Obtained from Flavedo By-Product of Seven Cultivars of Sicilian Citrus aurantium L. *Molecules.* 2022 Feb 27;27(5):1580.
[1121] Ebrahimi A, Eslami J, Darvishi I, et al. An overview of the comparison of inhalation aromatherapy on emotional distress of female and male patients in preoperative period. *J Complement Integr Med.* 2021 May 12;19(1):111-119.
[1122] Hajlaoui H, Arrouadi S, Aouadi K, et al. GC-MS Profile, α-glucosidase Inhibition Potential, Antibacterial and Antioxidant Evaluation of Peels Citrus aurantium (L), Essential Oil. *J Pharm Res Int.* 2021;33(60N):1580-91.
[1123] Changbunjong T, Boonmasawai S, Sungpradit S, et al. Contact and Fumigant Activities of Citrus aurantium Essential Oil against the Stable Fly Stomoxys calcitrans (Diptera: Muscidae). *Plants (Basel).* 2022 Apr 21;11(9):1122.
[1124] Chen L, Xie T. Effect of Citrus aurantium on Pain Intensity and Blood Pressure in Gastrectomy. *Indian J Pharm Sci.* 2022;84(2) Spl Issue:174-9.
[1125] Jian R, Lin Y, Li Y, et al. Larvicidal Activity of Two Rutaceae Plant Essential Oils and Their Constituents Against Aedes albopictus (Diptera: Culicidae) in Multiple Formulations. *J Med Entomol.* 2022 Jul 4:tjac083.
[1126] Jugreet BS, Lall N, Anina Lambrechts I, et al. In Vitro and In Silico Pharmacological and Cosmeceutical Potential of Ten Essential Oils from Aromatic Medicinal Plants from the Mascarene Islands. *Molecules.* 2022 Dec 8;27(24):8705.
[1127] Toma CC, Sima GM, Hanganu D, et al. Chemical composition of the Tunisian Nigella sativa. Note I. Profile on essential oil. *Farmacia.* 2010;58(4):458-64.
[1128] D'Antuono LF, Moretti A, Lovato AFS. Seed yield, yield components, oil content and essential oil content and composition of Nigella satia L. and Nigella damascena L. *Industrial Crops Prod.* 2002;15:59-69.
[1129] Gerige SJ, Yadav Gerige MK, Rao M, et al. GC-MS Analysis of Nigella sativa Seeds and Antimicrobial Activity of its Volatile oil. *Brazilian Arch Biol Tech.* 2009 Sep-Oct;52(50:1189-92.
[1130] Nickavar B, Mojab F, Javidnia K, et al. Chemical Composition of the Fixed and Volatile Oils of Nigella sativa L. from Iran. *Verlag der Zeitschrift für Naturforschung, Tübinge.* 2003;629-31. Mozaffari FS, GhorbaniM, Babai A, et al. The Effect of Water Stress on the Seed Oil of Nigella sativa L. *J Essent Oil Res.* 2000;12(1):36-38.
[1131] Wajs A, Bonikowski R, Kalemna D. Composition of essential oil from seeds of Nigella sativa L. cultivated in Poland. *Flavour Frag J.* 2008;23:126-32.
[1132] Singh RK, Jhunjhunwalla KN. Chemical composition of volatile oils of Nigella sativa seeds. *World J Pharmacy Pharmaceutical Sci.* 2014;3(10):1588-94.
[1133] Hajhashemi V, Ghannadi A, Jafarabadi H. Black cumin seed essential oil, as a potent analgesic and antiinflammatory drug. *Phytother Res.* 2004;18:195–99.
[1134] Shokri H, Sharifzadeh A, Ashrafi Tamai I. Anti-Candida zeylanoides activity of some Iranian plants used in traditional medicine. *J Mycol Méd.* 2012;22:211–16.
[1135] Mahmoudvand H, Dezaki ES, Kheirandish F, et al. Scolicidal effects of black cumin seed (Nigella sativa) essential oil on hydatid cysts. *Korean J Parasitol.* 2014 Dec;52(6):653-9.
[1136] Kokoska L, Havlik J, Valterova I, et al. Comparison of chemical composition and antibacterial activity of Nigella sativa seed essential oils obtained by different extraction methods. *J Food Prot.* 2008 Dec;71(12):2475-80.
[1137] Ostad SN, Khakinegard B, Sabzevari O. Evaluation of the teratogenicity of fennel essential oil (FEO) on the rat embryo limb buds culture. *Toxicol.* 2004 Oct;18(5):623-7.
[1138] Tabanca N, Khan SI, Bedir E, et al. Estrogenic activity of isolated constituents and essential oils of Pimpinella species from Turkey, evaluated using a recombinant yeast screen. *Planta Med.* 2004 Aug;70(8):728-35.
[1139] Albert-Puleo M. Fennel and anise as estrogenic agents. *J Ethnopharmacol.* 1980 Dec;2(4):337-44.
[1140] Malini T, Vanithakumari G, Megala N, et al. Effect of Foeniculum vulgare Mill. seed extract on the genital organs of male and female rats. *Indian J Physiol Pharmacol.* 1985 Jan-Mar;29(1):21-6.
[1141] Dhar SK. Anti-fertility activity and hormonal profile of trans-anethole in rats. *Indian J Physiol Pharmacol.* 1995;39(1):63-67.
[1142] Paramasivam A, Kalaimangai M, Sambantham S, et al. Anti-angiogenic activity of thymoquinone by the down-regulation of VEGF using zebrafish (Danio rerio) model. *Biomed Prevent Nutr.* 2012 Jul-Sep;2(3):169-73.
[1143] Yi T, Cho SG, Yi A, et al. Thymoquinone inhibits tumor angiogenesis and tumor growth through suppressing AKT and ERK signaling pathways. *Mol Cancer Ther.* 2008 Jul;7(7):1789-96.
[1144] Peng L, Liu A, Shen Y, et al. Antitumor and anti-angiogenesis effects of thymoquinone on osteosarcoma through the NF-κB pathway. *Oncol Rep.* 2013 Feb;29(2):571-8.
[1145] AbuKhader MM, Khater SH, Al-Matubsi HY. Acute effects of thymoquinone on the pregnant rat and embryo-fetal development. *Drug Chem Toxicol.* 2013 Jan;36(1):27-34.
[1146] European Medicines Agency. Public statement on the use of herbal medicinal products containing estragole. Available at: http://www.ema.europa.eu/docs/en_GB/document_library/Scientific_guideline/2010/04/WC500089960.pdf.
[1147] Turkyilmaz Z, Karabulut R, Sonmez K, et al. A striking and frequent cause of premature thelarche in children: Foeniculum vulgare. *J Pediatr Surg.* 2008 Nov;43(11):2109-11.
[1148] Kohlert C, Schindler G, Marz RW, et al. Systemic availability and pharmacokinetics of thymol in humans. *J Clin Pharmacol.* 2002 Jul;42(7):731-7.
[1149] Toxicology Data Network, National Library of Medicine. Thymol. Available at: http://toxnet.nlm.nih.gov/cgi-bin/sis/search/a?dbs+hsdb:@term+@DOCNO+866.
[1150] Bamosa AO. A review on the hypoglycemic effect of nigella sativa and thymoquinone. *Rev Articles.* 2015;3(1):2-7.
[1151] Ali Sangi SM, Sulaiman MI, Abd El-wahab MF, et al. Antihyperglycemic effect of thymoquinone and oleuropein, on streptozotocin-induced diabetes mellitus in experimental animals. *Pharmacogn Mad.* 2015 Oct;11(Suppl 2):S251-57.
[1152] El-Dakhakhny M, Mady N, Lembert N, et al. The hypoglycemic effect of Nigella sativa oil is mediated by extrapancreatic actions. *Planta Med.* 2002 May;68(5):465-6.
[1153] Fararh KM, Shimizu Y, Shiina T, et al. Thymoquinone reduces hepatic glucose production in diabetic hamsters. *Res Vet Sci.* 2005 Dec;79(3):219-23.
[1154] Razavi BM, Hosseinzadeh H. A review of the effects of Nigella sativa L. and its constituent, thymoquinone, in metabolic syndrome. *J Endocrinol Invest.* 2014 Nov;37(11):1031-40.
[1155] Sheikh BA, Pari L, Rathinham A, et al. Trans-anethole, a terpenoid ameliorates hyperglycemia by regulating key enzymes of carbohydrate metabolism in streptozotocin induced diabetic rats. *Biochimie.* 2015 May;112:57-65.
[1156] Pari L, Sheikh BA. Antihyperglycemic effect of trans-anethole in streptozotocin induced diabetic rats with special reference to glycoprotein components. *Int J Adv Res Biol Sci.* 2015;2(5):28-34.
[1157] AbuKhader MM. Thymoquinone: a promising antidiabetic agent. *Int J Diabetes Dev Countries.* 2012 Jun;32(2):65-68.
[1158] Jukic M, Politeo O, Maksimmovic M, et al. In vitro acetylcholinesterase inhibitory properties of thymol, carvacrol and their derivatives thymoquinone and thymohydroquinone. *Phytother Res.* 2007;21(3):259-61.
[1159] Tognolini M, Barocelli E, Ballabeni V, et al. Comparative screening of plant essential oils; phenylpropanoid moiety as basic core for antiplatelet activity. *Life Sci.* 2006 Feb 23;78(13):1419-32.
[1160] Okazaki K, Kawazoe K, Takaishi Y. Human platelet aggregation inhibitors from thyme (Thymus vulgaris L.). *Phytother Res.* 2002 Jun;16(4):398-9.
[1161] Lee HS. Anticoagulant properties of constituents derived from fennel (Foeniculum vulgare Gaertner) fruits. *Food Sci Biotech.* 2006 Oct;15(5):763-67.
[1162] Thushara RM, Hemshekhar M, Santhosh MS, et al. Differential action of phytochemicals on platelet apoptosis: a biological overview. *Curr Med Chem.* 2013;20(8):1018-27.
[1163] Towhid ST, Schmidt EM, Schmid E, et al. Thymoquinone-induced platelet apoptosis. *J Cell Biochem.* 2011 Nov;112(11):3112-21.
[1164] Jukic M, Politeo O, Maksimmovic M, et al. In vitro acetylcholinesterase inhibitory properties of thymol, carvacrol and their derivatives thymoquinone and thymohydroquinone. *Phytother Res.* 2007;21(3):259-61.
[1165] Subehan UT, Iwata H, Kadota S, et al. Mechanism-based inhibition of CYP3A4 and CYP2D6 by Indonesian medicinal plants. *J Ethnopharmacol.* 2006 May;105(3):449-55.
[1166] Subehan Z, Kadota SF, Tezuka Y. Inhibition on human liver cytochrome P450 3A4 by constituents of fennel (Foeniculum vulgare): Identification and characterization of a mechanism-based inactivator. *J Agric Food Chem.* 2007 Dec;55(25):10162-67.
[1167] Yarnell E, Abascal K. Interaction of Herbal Constituents with Cytochrome P450 Enzymes. *Alt Complement Ther.* 2007 Nov;13(5):239-47.
[1168] Sinitskaia ZF, Lashneva NV, Chichilanova GV, et al. [Effect of trans-anethole on liver monooxygenase system and its induction of polychlorinated diphenyls]. *Vopr Pitan.* 1994;(5):24-7.
[1169] Rompelberg CJ, Verhagen H, van Bladeren PJ. Effects of the naturally occurring alkenylbenzenes eugenol and trans-anethole on drug-metabolizing enzymes in the rat liver. *Food Chem Toxicol.* 1993 Sep;31(9):637-45.
[1170] Elbarbry F, Ragheb A, Marfleet T, et al. Modulation of hepatic drug metabolizing enzymes by dietary doses of thymoquinone in female New Zealand White rabbits. *Phytother Res.* 2012 Nov;26(11):1726-30.
[1171] Al-Jenoobi FI, Al-Thukair AA, Abbas FA, et al. Effect of black seed on dextromethorphan o- and n-demethylation in human liver microsomes and healthy human subjects. *Drug Metabolism Letters.* 2010;4(1):51–55.

[1172] Liu X, Park JH, Abd El-Aty AM, et al. Isolation of volatiles from Nigella sativa seeds using microwave-assisted extraction: effect of whole extracts on canine and murine CYP1A. *Biomed Chromatogr*. 2013 Jul;27(7):938-45.

[1173] Ahmad A, Khan RM, Alkharfy KM, et al. Effects of Thymoquinone on the Pharmacokinetics and Pharmacodynamics of Glibenclamide in a Rat Model. *Nat Prod Commun*. 2015 Aug;10(8):1395-8.

[1174] Rompelberg CJ, Verhagen H, van Bladeren PJ. Effects of the naturally occurring alkenylbenzenes eugenol and trans-anethole on drug-metabolizing enzymes in the rat liver. *Food Chem Toxicol*. 1993 Sep;31(9):637-45.

[1175] Langeveld WT, Veldhuizen EJ, Burt SA. Synergy between essential oil constituents and antibiotics. *Crit Rev Microbiol*. 2014 Feb;40(1);76-94.

[1176] Kouidhi B, Zmantar T, Jrah H, et al. Antibacterial and resistance-modifying activities of thymoquinone against oral pathogens. *Ann Clin Microbiol Antimicrob*. 2011 Jun 27;10:29.

[1177] Raza M, Alghasham AA, Alorainy MS, et al. Potentiation of Valproate-induced Anticonvulsant Response by Nigella sativa Seed Constituents: The Role of GABA Receptors. *Int J Health Sci (Qassim)*. 2008 Jan;2(1):15-25.

[1178] Periasamy VS, Athinarayanan J, Alshatwi AA. Anticancer activity of an ultrasonic nanoemulsion formulation of Nigella sativa L. essential oil on human breast cancer cells. *Ultrason Sonochem*. 2016 Jul;31:449-55.

[1179] Islam SN, Begum P, Ahsan T, et al. Immunosuppressive and cytotoxic properties of Nigella sativa. *Phytother Res*. 2004 May;18(5):395-8.

[1180] Salim EI, Fukushima S. Chemopreventive potential of volatile oil from black cumin (Nigella sativa L.) seeds against rat colon carcinogenesis. *Nutr Cancer*. 2003;45(2):195-202.

[1181] Ichwan SJ, Al-Ani IM, Bilal HG, et al. Apoptotic activities of thymoquinone, an active ingredient of black seed (Nigella sativa), in cervical cancer cell lines. *Chin J Physiol*. 2014 Oct 31;57(5):249-55.

[1182] Sakalar C, Yuruk M, Kaya T, et al. Pronounced transcriptional regulation of apoptotic and TNF-NF-kappa-B signaling genes during the course of thymoquinone mediated apoptosis in HeLa cells. *Mol Cell Biochem*. 2013 Nov;383(1-2):243-51.

[1183] Lang M, Borgmann M, Oberhuber G, et al. Thymoquinone attenuates tumor growth in ApcMin mice by interference with Wnt-signaling. *Mol Cancer*. 2013 May 13;12(1):41.

[1184] Effenberger-Neidnicht K, Schobert R. Combinatorial effects of thymoquinone on the anticancer activity of doxorubicin. *Cancer Chemother Pharmacol*. 2011 Apr;67(4):867-74.

[1185] Ait Mbarek L, Ait Mouse H, Elabbadi N, et al. Anti-tumor properties of blackseed (Nigella sativa L.) extracts. *Braz J Med Biol Res*. 2007 Jun;40(6):839-47.

[1186] Boskabady MH, Javan H, Sajady M, et al. The possible prophylactic effect of Nigella sativa seed extract in asthmatic patients. *Fundam Clin Pharmacol*. 2007 Oct;21(5):559-66.

[1187] Dehkordi FR, Kamkhah AF. Antihypertensive effect of Nigella sativa seed extract in patients with mild hypertension. *Fundam Clin Pharmacol*. 2008 Aug;22(4):447-52.

[1188] el Tahir KE, Ashour MM, al-Harbi MM. The cardiovascular actions of the volatile oil of the black seed (Nigella sativa) in rats: elucidation of the mechanism of action. *Gen Pharmacol*. 1993 Sep;24(5):1123-31.

[1189] Hajhashemi V, Ghannadi A, Jafarabadi H. Black cumin seed essential oil, as a potent analgesic and antiinflammatory drug. *Phytother Res*. 2004;18:195–99.

[1190] Amin B, Hosseinzadeh H. Black Cumin (Nigella sativa) and Its Active Constituent, Thymoquinone: An Overview on the Analgesic and Anti-inflammatory Effects. *Planta Med*. 2016 Jan;82(1-2):8-16.

[1191] Hajhashemi V, Ghannadi A, Jafarabadi H. Black cumin seed essential oil, as a potent analgesic and antiinflammatory drug. *Phytother Res*. 2004;18:195–99.

[1192] Asdadi A, Harhar H, Gharby S, et al. Chemical composition and antifungal activity of Nigella Sativa L. oil seed cultivated in Morocco. *Int J Pharma Sci Invent*. 2014;3:9–15.

[1193] Khosravi AR, Minooeianhaghighi MH, Shokri H, et al. The potential inhibitory effect of Cuminum cyminum, Ziziphora clinopodioides and Nigella sativa essential oils on the growth of Aspergillus fumigatus and Aspergillus flavus. *Braz J Microbiol*. 2011;42:216–24.

[1194] Naeini A, Khosravi AR, Chitsaz M, et al. Anti-Candida albicans activity of some Iranian plants used in traditional medicine. *J Mycol Méd*. 2009;19:168–72.

[1195] Shokri H, Sharifzadeh A, Ashrafi Tamai I. Anti-Candida zeylanoides activity of some Iranian plants used in traditional medicine. *J Mycol Méd*. 2012;22:211–16.

[1196] Singh G, Marimuthu P, de Heluani CS, et al. Chemical constituents and antimicrobial and antioxidant potentials of essential oil and acetone extract of Nigella sativa seeds. *J Sci Food Agric*. 2005;85:2297–2306.

[1197] Singh SS, Singh DG, Schuff C, et al. Composition, in vitro antioxidant and antimicrobial activities of essential oil and oleoresins obtained from black cumin seeds (Nigella sativa L.) *BioMed Res Int*. 2015 In Press.

[1198] Sitara U, Niaz I, Naseem J, et al. Antifungal effect of essential oils on in vitro growth of pathogenic fungi. *Pak J Bot*. 2008;40:409–14.

[1199] Rath CC, Mohapatra S. Susceptibility characterisation of Candida spp. to four essential oils. *Indian J Med Microbiol*. 2015 Feb;33 Suppl:93-6.

[1200] Ichwan SJ, Al-Ani IM, Bilal HG, et al. Apoptotic activities of thymoquinone, an active ingredient of black seed (Nigella sativa), in cervical cancer cell lines. *Chin J Physiol*. 2014 Oct 31;57(5):249-55.

[1201] Islam SK, Ahsan M, Hassan CM, et al. Antifungal activities of the oils of Nigella sativa seeds. *Pak J Pharm Sci*. 1989 Jan;2(1):25-8.

[1202] Toama MA, El-Alfy TS, El-Fatatry HM. Antimicrobial activity of the volatile oil of Nigella sativa Linneaus seeds. *Antimicrob Agents Chemother*. 1974 Aug;6(2):225-6.

[1203] Toppozada HH, Mazloum HA, el-Dakhakhny M. The antibacterial properties of the Nigella sativa l. seeds. Active principle with some clinical applications. *J Egypt Med Assoc*. 1965;48:Suppl:187-202.

[1204] Shokri H. A review on the inhibitory potential of Nigella sativa against pathogenic and toxigenic fungi. *Avicenna J Phytomed*. 2016 Jan-Feb;6(1):21–33.

[1205] Khan MA, Dhaded S, Joshi S, et al. Commercial and Plant Extract Denture Cleansers in Prevention of Candida albicans Growth on Soft Denture Reliner: In Vitro Study. *J Clin Diagn Res*. 2016 Feb;10(2):ZC42-5.

[1206] Hassanien MF, Assiri AM, Alzohairy AM, et al. Health-promoting value and food applications of black cumin essential oil: an overview. *J Food Sci Technol*. 2015 Oct;52(10):6136-42.

[1207] Shaaban HA, Sadek Z, Edris AE, et al. Analysis and antibacterial activity of Nigella sativa essential oil formulated in microemulsion system. *J Oleo Sci*. 2015;64(2):223-32.

[1208] Kokoska L, Havlik J, Valterova I, et al. Comparison of chemical composition and antibacterial activity of Nigella sativa seed essential oils obtained by different extraction methods. *J Food Prot*. 2008 Dec;71(12):2475-80.

[1209] Toama MA, El-Alfy TS, El-Fatatry HM. Antimicrobial activity of the volatile oil of Nigella sativa Linneaus seeds. *Antimicrob Agents Chemother*. 1974 Aug;6(2):225-6.

[1210] Toppozada HH, Mazloum HA, el-Dakhakhny M. The antibacterial properties of the Nigella sativa l. seeds. Active principle with some clinical applications. *J Egypt Med Assoc*. 1965;48:Suppl:187-202.

[1211] Cherkaoui-Tangi K, Israili ZH, Lyoussi B, et al. Vasorelaxant effect of essential oil isolated from Nigella sativa L. seeds in rat aorta: Proposed mechanism. *Pak J Pharm Sci*. 2016 Jan;29(1):1-8.

[1212] Singh SS, Singh DG, Schuff C, et al. Composition, in vitro antioxidant and antimicrobial activities of essential oil and oleoresins obtained from black cumin seeds (Nigella sativa L.) *BioMed Res Int*. 2015 In Press.

[1213] Hassanien MF, Assiri AM, Alzohairy AM, et al. Health-promoting value and food applications of black cumin essential oil: an overview. *J Food Sci Technol*. 2015 Oct;52(10):6136-42.

[1214] Abdel-Wahhab MA, Aly SE. Antioxidant property of Nigella sativa (black cumin) and Syzygium aromaticum (clove) in rats during aflatoxicosis. *J Appl Toxicol*. 2005 May-Jun;25(3):218-23.

[1215] Burits M, Bucar F. Burits M, Bucar F. Antioxidant activity of Nigella sativa essential oil. *Phytother Res*. 2000 Aug;14(5):323-8.

[1216] Sultan MT, Butt MS, Karim R, et al. Nigella sativa fixed and essential oil improves antioxidant status through modulation of antioxidant enzymes and immunity. *Pak J Pharm Sci*. 2015 Mar;28(2):589-95.

[1217] Sultan MT, Butt MS, Karim R, et al. Effect of Nigella sativa fixed and essential oils on antioxidant status, hepatic enzymes, and immunity in streptozotocin induced diabetes mellitus. *BMC Complement Altern Med*. 2014 Jun 17;14:193.

[1218] Sultan MT, Butt MS, Karim R, et al. Nigella sativa Fixed and Essential Oil Supplementation Modulates Hyperglycemia and Allied Complications in Streptozotocin-Induced Diabetes Mellitus. *Evid Based Complement Alternat Med*. 2014;2014:826380.

[1219] Kanter M, Akpolat M, Aktas C. Protective effects of the volatile oil of Nigella sativa seeds on beta-cell damage in streptozotocin-induced diabetic rats: a light and electron microscopic study. *J Mol Histol*. 2009 Oct;40(5-6):379-85.

[1220] Sultan MT, Butt MS, Ahmad RS, et al. Supplementation of Nigella sativa fixed and essential oil mediates potassium bromate induced oxidative stress and multiple organ toxicity. *Pak J Pharm Sci*. 2012 Jan;25(1):175-81.

[1221] Boskabady MH, Vahedi N, Amery S, et al. The effect of Nigella sativa alone, and in combination with dexamethasone, on tracheal muscle responsiveness and lung inflammation in sulfur mustard exposed guinea pigs. *J Ethnopharmacol*. 2011 Sep 2;137(2):1028-34.

[1222] Mahmoudvand H, Dezaki ES, Kheirandish F, et al. Scolicidal effects of black cumin seed (Nigella sativa) essential oil on hydatid cysts. *Korean J Parasitol*. 2014 Dec;52(6):653-9.

[1223] Mahmoudvand H, Tavakoli R, Sharififar F, et al. Leishmanicidal and cytotoxic activities of Nigella sativa and its active principle, thymoquinone. *Pharm Biol*. 2015 Jul;53(7):1052-7.

[1224] Agarwal R, Kharya MD, Shrivastava R. Antimicrobial & anthelmintic activities of the essential oil of Nigella sativa Linn. *Indian J Exp Biol*. 1979 Nov;17(11):1264-5.

[1225] Kacem R, Meraihi Z. The effect of essential oil extracted from Nigella sativa (L.) seeds on human neutrophil functions. *Nat Prod Res*. 2009;23(13):1168-75.

[1226] Islam SN, Begum P, Ahsan T, et al. Immunosuppressive and cytotoxic properties of Nigella sativa. *Phytother Res*. 2004 May;18(5):395-8.

[1227] Kacem RI, Meraihi Z. Effects of essential oil extracted from Nigella sativa (L.) seeds and its main components on human neutrophil elastase activity. *Yakugaku Zasshi*. 2006 Apr;126(4):301-5.

[1228] Hoenderdos K, Condliffe A. The neutrophil in chronic obstructive pulmonary disease. *Am J Respir Cell Mol Biol*. 2013 May;48(5):531-9.

[1229] Chua F, Laurent GJ. Neutrophil Elastase. *Proc Am Thoracic Soc*. 2006;3(5):424-27.

[1230] el Tahir KE, Ashour MM, al-Harbi MM. The respiratory effects of the volatile oil of the black seed (Nigella sativa) in guinea-pigs: elucidation of the mechanism(s) of action. *Gen Pharmacol*. 1993 Sep;24(5):1115-22.

[1231] Aqel M, Shaheen R. Effects of the volatile oil of Nigella sativa seeds on the uterine smooth muscle of rat and guinea pig. *J Ethnopharmacol*. 1996 May;52(1):23-6.

[1232] Alhebshi AH, Odawara A1, Gotoh M, et al. Thymoquinone protects cultured hippocampal and human induced pluripotent stem cells-derived neurons against α-synuclein-induced synapse damage. *Neurosci Lett*. 2014 Jun 6;570:126-31.

[1233] Erboga M, Kanter M, Aktas C, et al. Thymoquinone Ameliorates Cadmium-Induced Nephrotoxicity, Apoptosis, and Oxidative Stress in Rats is Based on its Anti-Apoptotic and Anti-Oxidant Properties. *Biol Trace Elem Res*. 2016 Mar;170(1):165-72.

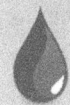

[1234] Nagi MN, Almakki HA. Thymoquinone supplementation induces quinone reductase and glutathione transferase in mice liver: possible role in protection against chemical carcinogenesis and toxicity. *Phytother Res.* 2009 Sep;23(9):1295-8.

[1235] Khattab MM, Nagi MN. Thymoquinone supplementation attenuates hypertension and renal damage in nitric oxide deficient hypertensive rats. *Phytother Res.* 2007 May;21(5):410-4.

[1236] Mansour MA, Ginawi OT, El-Hadiyah T, et al. Effects of volatile oil constituents of Nigella sativa on carbon tetrachloride-induced hepatotoxicity in mice: evidence for antioxidant effects of thymoquinone. *Res Commun Mol Pathol Pharmacol.* 2001;110(3-4):239-51.

[1237] Tekeoglu I, Dogan A, Ediz L, et al. Effects of thymoquinone (volatile oil of black cumin) on rheumatoid arthritis in rat models. *Phytother Res.* 2007 Sep;21(9):895-7.

[1238] Raj GA, Chandrasekaran M, Krishnamoorthy S, et al. Phytochemical profile and larvicidal properties of seed essential oil from Nigella sativa L. (Ranunculaceae), against Aedes aegypti, Anopheles stephensi, and Culex quinquefasciatus (Diptera: Culicidae). *Parasitol Res.* 2015 Sep;114(9):3385-91.

[1239] Abedi AS, Rismanchi M, Shahdoostkhany M, et al. Microwave-assisted extraction of Nigella sativa L. essential oil and evaluation of its antioxidant activity. *J Food Sci Technol.* 2017 Nov;54(12):3779-3790.

[1240] Ashraf SA, Al-Shammari E, Hussain T, et al. In-vitro antimicrobial activity and identification of bioactive components using GC-MS of commercially available essential oils in Saudi Arabia. *J Food Sci Technol.* 2017 Nov;54(12):3948-3958.

[1241] Shanmugam MK, Arfuso F, Kumar AP, et al. Modulation of diverse oncogenic transcription factors by thymoquinone, an essential oil compound isolated from the seeds of Nigella sativa Linn. *Pharmacol Res.* 2018 Mar;129:357-364.

[1242] Ashraf S, Anjum AA, Ahmad A, et al. In vitro activity of Nigella sativa against antibiotic resistant Salmonella enterica. *Environ Toxicol Pharmacol.* 2017 Dec 17;58:54-58.

[1243] Al-Okbi SY, Mohamed DA, Hamed TE, et al. Hepatic Regeneration and Reno-Protection by Fish oil, Nigella sativa Oil and Combined Fish Oil/Nigella sativa Volatiles in CCl4 Treated Rats. *J Oleo Sci.* 2018 Mar 1;67(3):345-353.

[1244] Mouwakeh A, Telbisz Á, Spengler G, et al. Antibacterial and Resistance Modifying Activities of Nigella sativa Essential Oil and its Active Compounds Against Listeria monocytogenes. *In Vivo.* 2018 Jul-Aug;32(4):737-743.

[1245] Kiari FZ, Meddah B, Tir Touil Meddah A. In vitro study on the activity of essential oil and methanolic extract from Algerian Nigella sativa L. Seeds on the growth kinetics of micro-organisms isolated from the buccal cavities of periodontal patients. *Saudi Dent J.* 2018 Oct;30(4):312-323.

[1246] Mouwakeh A, Kincses A, Nové M, et al. Nigella sativa essential oil and its bioactive compounds as resistance modifiers against Staphylococcus aureus. *Phytother Res.* 2019 Apr;33(4):1010-1018.

[1247] Hetta HF, Meshaal AK, Algammal AM, et al. In-vitro Antimicrobial Activity of Essential Oils and Spices Powder of some Medicinal Plants Against Bacillus Species Isolated from Raw and Processed Meat. *Infect Drug Resist.* 2020 Dec 4;13:4367-4378.

[1248] Landucci E, Mazzantini C, Buonvicino D, et al. Neuroprotective Effects of Thymoquinone by the Modulation of ER Stress and Apoptotic Pathway in In Vitro Model of Excitotoxicity. *Molecules.* 2021 Mar 13;26(6):1592.

[1249] Dalli M, Azizi SE, Benouda H, et al. Molecular Composition and Antibacterial Effect of Five Essential Oils Extracted from Nigella sativa L. Seeds against Multidrug-Resistant Bacteria: A Comparative Study.

[1250] Avci G, Ulutas E, Ozdemir V, et al. The positive effect of black seed (Nigella sativa L.) essential oil on thyroid hormones in rats with hypothyroidism and hyperthyroidism. *J Food Biochem.* 2021 Jun 3;e13801.

[1251] Alfaiz FA. Molecular studies of immunological enzyme clumping factor B for the inhibition of Staphylococcus aureus with essential oils of Nigella sativa. *J Mol Recognit.* 2021 Oct 8;e2941.

[1252] Ciesielska-Figlon K, Daca A, Kokotkiewicz A, et al. The influence of Nigella sativa essential oil on proliferation, activation, and apoptosis of human T lymphocytes in vitro. *Biomed Pharmacother.* 2022 Jun 29;153:113349.

[1253] Zouirech O, Alyousef AA, El Barnossi A, et al. Phytochemical Analysis and Antioxidant, Antibacterial, and Antifungal Effects of Essential Oil of Black Caraway (Nigella sativa L.) Seeds against Drug-Resistant Clinically Pathogenic Microorganisms. *Biomed Res Int.* 2022 Jul 26;2022:5218950.

[1254] Dalli M, Daoudi NE, Abrigach F, et al. In vitro α-amylase and hemoglobin glycation inhibitory potential of Nigella sativa essential oil, and molecular docking studies of its principal components. *Front Pharmacol.* 2022 Oct 20;13:1036129.

[1255] Orac A, Stulova I, Lailas T, et al. Effect of storage on the essential oil composition of Piper nigrum L. fruits of different ripening states. *J Agric Food Chem.* 2004 May 5;52(9):2582-86.

[1256] Aziz S, Naher S, Abukawasar MD, et al. Comparative studies on physicochemical properties and GC-MS analysis of essential oil of the two varieties of the black pepper (Piper nigrum Linn.). *Int J Pharm Phytopharm Res.* 2012;2(2):67- 70.

[1257] Sruthi D, Zachariah J, Leela NK, et al. Correlation between chemical profiles of black pepper (Piper nigrum L.) var. Panniur-1 collected from different locations. *J Med Plants Res.* 2013 Aug;7(31):2349-57.

[1258] Jirovetz L, Buchbauer G, Benoit Ngassoum M, et al. Aroma constituent analysis of Piper nigrum and Piper guineense essential oils from Cameroon using solid-phase microextraction—gas chromatography, solid-phase microextraction—gas chromatography—mass spectrometry and olfactometry. *J Chrom A.* 2002;976:265-75.

[1259] Oboh G, Ademosun AO, Odubanjo OV, et al. Antioxidative properties and inhibition of key enzymes relevant to type-2 diabetes and hypertension by essential oils from black pepper. *Adv Pharmacol Sci.* 2013;2013:926047.

[1260] Nguyen LT, Mysliveckova Z, Szotakova B, et al. The inhibitory effects of β-caryophyllene, β-caryophyllene oxide and α-humulene on the activities of the main drug-metabolizing enzymes in rat and human liver in vitro. *Chem-Biol Interactoins.* 2017 Dec 25;278:123-8.

[1261] Domaracky M, Rehak P, Juhas S, et al. Effects of selected plant essential oils on the growth and development of mouse preimplantation embryos in vivo. *Physiol Res.* 2007;56(1):97-104.

[1262] Vrskova D, Modra H. Evaluation of the developmental toxicity of 2-phenoxyethanol and clove oil anesthetics using the Frog Embryo Teratogenesis Assay: Xenopus (FETAX). *Veterinarami Medicina.* 2012;57(5):245-50.

[1263] Amini A, Cheraghi E, Safaee MR, et al. The role of eugenol in the reduction of teratogenic effects of retinoic acid on skeletal morphology of mice embryo. *Yakhteh Medical Journal.* 2003;4:195-200.

[1264] Chen R, Chen J, Cheng S, et al. Assessment of embryotoxicity of constituents in cosmetics by the embryonic stem cell tes. *Toxicol Mech Methods.* 2010 Mar;20(3):112-18.

[1265] Chen SJ, Wang MH, Chen IJ. Antiplatelet and calcium inhibitory properties of eugenol and sodium eugenol acetate. *Gen Pharmacol.* 1996 Jun;27(4):629-33.

[1266] Tognolini M, Barocelli E, Ballabeni V, et al. Comparative screening of plant essential oils; phenylpropanoid moiety as basic core for antiplatelet activity. *Life Sci.* 2006 Feb 23;78(13):1419-32.

[1267] Heck AM, DeWitt BA, Lukes AL. Potential interactions between alternative therapies and warfarin. *Am J Health Syst Pharm.* 2000;57(13):1221-1227.

[1268] Saaeed SA, Gilani AH. Antithrombotic activity of clove oil. *J Pak Med Assoc.* 1994;44(5):112-15.

[1269] Kamatou GP, Vermaak I, Viljoen AM. Eugenol—from the remote Maluku Islands to the international market place: A review of a remarkable and versatile molecule. *Molecules.* 2012;17:6953-81.

[1270] Cochrane ML. Inhibition of Cytochrome P450 2C9 by essential oils. Available at: https://libres.uncg.edu/ir/uncg/listing.aspx?id=18102.

[1271] Nguyen LT, Mysliveckova Z, Szotakova B, et al. The inhibitory effects of β-caryophyllene, β-caryophyllene oxide and α-humulene on the activities of the main drug-metabolizing enzymes in rat and human liver in vitro. *Chem-Biol Interactoins.* 2017 Dec 25;278:123-8.

[1272] Langeveld WT, Veldhuizen EJ, Burt SA. Synergy between essential oil constituents and antibiotics. *Crit Rev Microbiol.* 2014 Feb;40(1):76-94.

[1273] Oboh G, Ademosun AO, Odubanjo OV, et al. Antioxidative properties and inhibition of key enzymes relevant to type-2 diabetes and hypertension by essential oils from black pepper. *Adv Pharmacol Sci.* 2013;2013:926047.

[1274] Sarrami N, Pemberton MN, Thornhill MH, et al. Adverse reactions associated with the use of eugenol in dentistry. *British Dental J.* 2002;193:253-55.

[1275] Tammannavar P, Pushpalatha C, Jain S, et al. An unexpected positive hypersensitive reaction to eugenol. *BMJ Case Rep.* 2013; 2013: bcr2013009464.

[1276] Burkhard PR, Burkhardt K, Haenggeli CA, et al. Plant-induced seizures: reappearance of an old problem. *J Neurol.* 1999 Aug;246(8):667-70.

[1277] Waldman N. Seizure caused by dermal application of over-the-counter eucalyptus oil head lice preparation. *Clin Toxicol (Phila).* 2011 Oct;49(8):750-1.

[1278] Craig JO. Poisoning by the volatile oils in childhood. *Arch Dis Child.* 1953;28:259-67.

[1279] Oboh G, Ademosun AO, Odubanjo OV, et al. Antioxidative properties and inhibition of key enzymes relevant to type-2 diabetes and hypertension by essential oils from black pepper. *Adv Pharmacol Sci.* 2013;2013:926047.

[1280] Gray AM, Flatt PR. Antihyperglycemic actions of Eucalyptus globulus (Eucalyptus) are associated with pancreatic and extra pancreatic effects in mice. *J Nutr.* 1998 Dec;128(12):2319–23.

[1281] Basak SS, Candan F. Effect of Laurus nobilis L. Essential Oil and its Main Components on α-glucosidase and Reactive Oxygen Species Scavenging Activity. *Iran J Pharm Res.* 2013 Spring;12(2):367-79.

[1282] Fathiazad F, Mazandarani M, Hamedeyazdan. Phytochemical analysis and antioxidant activity of Hyssopus officinalis L. from Iran. *Adv Pharm Bull.* 2011 Dec;1(2):63–67.

[1283] Haze S, Sakai K, Gozu Y. Effects of fragrance inhalation on sympathetic activity in normal adults. *Jpn J Pharmacol.* 2002 Nov;90(3):247-53.

[1284] Kitikannakorn N, Chaiyakunapruk N, Nimpitakpong P, et al. An overview of the evidences of herbals for smoking cessation. *Complement Ther Med.* 2013 Oct;21(5):557-64.

[1285] Cordell B, Buckle J. The effects of aromatherapy on nicotine craving on a U.S. campus: a small comparison study. *J Altern Complement Med.* 2013 Aug;19(8):709-13.

[1286] Rose JE, Behm FM. Inhalation of vapor from black pepper extract reduces smoking withdrawal symptoms. *Drug Alcohol Depend.* 1994 Feb;34(3):225-29.

[1287] Kristiniak S, Harpel J, Breckenridge DM, et al. Black pepper essential oil to enhance intravenous catheter insertion in patients with poor vein visibility: a controlled study. *J Altern Complement Med.* 2012 Nov;18(11):1003-07.

[1288] Ou MC, Lee YF, Li CC, et al. The effectiveness of essential oils for patients with neck pain: a randomized controlled study. *J Altern Complement Med.* 2014 Oct;20(10):771-79.

[1289] Ebihara T, Ebihara S, Maruyama M, et al. A randomized trial of olfactory stimulation using black pepper oil in older people with swallowing dysfunction. *J Am Geriatr Soc.* 2006 Sep;54(9):1401-06.

[1290] Hashim S, Aboobaker VS, Madhubala R, et al. Modulatory effects of essential oils from spices on the formation of DNA adduct by aflatoxin B1 in vitro. *Nutr Cancer.* 1994;21(2):169-75.

[1291] Jeen K, Liju VB, Umadevi NP, et al. Antioxidant, anti-inflammatory and antinociceptive properties of black pepper essential oil (Piper nigrum Linn). *JEOP.* 2014 Mar;17(1):1-12.

[1292] Dorman HJ, Deans SG. Antimicrobial agents from plants: antibacterial activity of plant volatile oils. *J Appl Microbiol.* 2000 Feb;88(2):308-16.

[1293] Plant J. Effects of essential oils on telomere length in human cells. *Med Aromat Plants.* 2016;5(2):1-6.

[1294] Zhang J, Wang Y, Pan DD, et al. Effect of black pepper essential oil on the quality of fresh pork during storage. *Meat Sci.* 2016 Jul;117:130-6.

[1295] Costa R, Abreu C, Machado J. Effectiveness of Piper nigrum essential oil in the treatment of back pain. *Exp Pathol Health Sci*. 2016;8(2):81-84.

[1296] Costa R, Machado J, Abreu C. Evaluation of Analgesic Properties of Piper Nigrum Essential Oil: a Randomized, Double-blind, Placebo-controlled Study. *World J Tradit Chin Med*. 2016;2(2):60-4.

[1297] Nikolić MM, Jovanović KK, Marković TL, et al. Antimicrobial synergism and cytotoxic properties of Citrus limon L., Piper nigrum L. and Melaleuca alternifolia (Maiden and Betche) Cheel essential oils. *J Pharm Pharmacol*. 2017 Nov;69(11):1606-1614.

[1298] Vinturelle R, Mattos C, Meloni J, et al. In Vitro Evaluation of Essential Oils Derived from Piper nigrum (Piperaceae) and Citrus limonum (Rutaceae) against the Tick Rhipicephalus (Boophilus) microplus (Acari: Ixodidae). *Biochem Res Int*. 2017;2017:5342947.

[1299] Wiwattanaratanabut K, choonharuangdej S, Srithava T. In Vitro Anti-Cariogenic Plaque Effects of Essential Oils Extracted from Culinary Herbs. *J Clin Diagnostic Res*. 2017 Sep;11(9):DC30-5.

[1300] Han X, Beaumont C, Rodriguez D, et al. Black pepper (Piper nigrum) essential oil demonstrates tissue remodeling and metabolism modulating potential in human cells. *Phytother Res*. 2018 Sep;32(9):1848-1852.

[1301] Castellanos LM, Olivas NA, Ayala-Soto J, et al. In Vitro and In Vivo Antifungal Activity of Clove ( Eugenia caryophyllata) and Pepper ( Piper nigrum L.) Essential Oils and Functional Extracts Against Fusarium oxysporum and Aspergillus niger in Tomato ( Solanum lycopersicum L.). *Int J Microbiol*. 2020 Apr 30;2020:1702037.

[1302] Zhang C, Zhao J, Famous E, et al. Antioxidant, hepatoprotective and antifungal activities of black pepper (Piper nigrum L.) essential oil. *Food Chem*. 2020 Dec 16;346:128845.

[1303] Ghosh S, Kumar A, Sachan N, et al. Anxiolytic and antidepressant-like effects of essential oil from the fruits of Piper nigrum Linn. (Black pepper) in mice: involvement of serotonergic but not GABAergic transmission system. *Heliyon*. 2021 Apr 25;7(4):e06884.

[1304] Wang Y, Wang L, Tan J, et al. Comparative Analysis of Intracellular and in vitro Antioxidant Activities of Essential Oil From White and Black Pepper (Piper nigrum L.). *Front Pharmacol*. 2021 Jun 25;12:680754.

[1305] Eren H, Turkmen AS, Aslan A. Effect of topical application of black pepper essential oil on peripheral intravenous catheter insertion: A randomized controlled study. *Explore*. 2021 Jun 8;

[1306] Chen SX, Xiang JY, Han JX, et al. Essential Oils from Spices Inhibit Cholinesterase Activity and Improve Behavioral Disorder in AlCl3 Induced Dementia. *Chem Biodivers*. 2022 Jan;19(1):e202100443.

[1307] Tomaš N, Myszka K, Wolko Ł. Black pepper and tarragon essential oils suppress the lipolytic potential and the type II secretion system of P. psychrophila KM02. *Sci Rep*. 2022 Mar 31;12(1):5487.

[1308] Aleksic A, Stojanovic-Radic Z, Harmanus C, et al. In vitro anti-clostridial action and potential of the spice herbs essential oils to prevent biofilm formation of hypervirulent Clostridioides difficile strains isolated from hospitalized patients with CDI. *Anaerobe*. 2022 Auf;76:102604.

[1309] Mahmoud MF, Elmaghraby AM, Ali N, et al. Black pepper oil (Piper nigrum L.) mitigates dexamethasone induced pancreatic damage via modulation of oxidative and nitrosative stress. *Biomed Phramcother*. 2022 Sep;153:113456.

[1310] Zhang M, Qiu B, Sun M, et al. Preparation of Black pepper (Piper nigrum L.) essential oil nanoparticles and its antitumor activity on triple negative breast cancer in vitro. *J Food Biochem*. 2022 Sep 19:e14406.

[1311] Marcião Vieira AC, Azevedo SG, Linhares RA, et al. Biodefensive Based on Piper nigrum Essential Oil for Controlling of Anopheles aquasalis Larvae: Influence of Temperature (35 °C) and Preservatives. *Biomolecules*. 2022 Nov 18;12(11):1711.

[1312] Weluwanarak T, Changbunjong T, Leesombun A, et al. Effects of Piper nigrum L. Fruit Essential Oil Toxicity against Stable Fly (Diptera: Muscidae). *Plants (Basel)*. 2023 Feb 24;12(5):1043.

[1313] Santos RP, Nunes EP, Nascimento RF, et al. Chemical composition and larvicidal activity of the essential oils of Cordia leucomalloides and Cordia curassavica from the Northeast of Brazil. *J Braz Chem Soc*. 2006 Sep-Oct;17(5):ISSN 1678-4790.

[1314] Ferreira LLC, Coelho-Mattos JL, Vieira CRM, et al. Chemical Composition of the Essential Oil of Varronia curassavica Jacq. (Boraginaceae) from Instituto Vital Brazil Farm. *Rev Virtual de Quim*. 2009 Apr;8(1):ISSN 1984-6835.

[1315] da S. Feijo EVR, de Oliveira RA, do B. Costa LC. Light affects Varronia curassavica essential oil yield by increasing trichomes frequency. *Rev Bras Farmacogn*. 2014 Sep-Oct;24(5):ISSN 0102-695X.

[1316] Rodriguez FFG, Oliveira LGS, Rodrigues FFG, et al. Chemical composition, antibacterial and antifungal activities of essential oil from Cordia verbenacea DC leaves. *Pharmacognosy Res*. 2012 Jul-Sep;4(3):161-65.

[1317] Meccia G, Rojas LB, Velasco J, et al. Chemical composition and antibacterial activity of the essential oil of Cordia verbenacea from the Venezuelan Andes. *Nat Prod Commun*. 2009 Aug;4(8):1119-22.

[1318] Vila R, Queiroz EF, Canigueral S. Composition of the essential oil of the leaves of Cordia verbenacea. *Planta Med*. 2009;75:PG17.

[1319] Alves MS, Santos DP, Silva LCP, et al. Essential Oils Composition and Toxicity Tested by Fumigation Against Callosobruchus maculatus Coleoptera: Bruchidae) Pest of Stored Cowpea. *Rev Virtual Quim*. 2015 Nov-Dec;7(6):ISSN 1984-6835.

[1320] Nizio DAC, Brito FA, Sampaio TS, et al. Chemical Characterization of Essential Oils from Varronia curassavica Jacq. Germplasm. *Rev Virtual de Quim*. 2009 Apr;8(1):ISSN 1984-6835.

[1321] Matias EFF, Alves EF, Silva MKN, et al. Seasonal variation, chemical composition and biological activity of the essential oil of Cordia verbenacea DC (Boraginaceae) and the sabinene. *Industrial Crops Prod*. 2016 Sep;87:45-53.

[1322] de Castro Nizio DA, Blank AF, Sampaio TS, et al. Distillation methods affect the chemical composition of Varronia curassavica Jacq. Essential oil. *Biosci J*. 2018 May/June;34(3):629-39.

[1323] Da S. Feijo EVR, de Oliveira RA, do B. Costa LC. Light affects Varronia curassavica essential oil yield by increasing trichomes frequency. *Rev Bras Farmacogn*. 2014;24:516-523.

[1324] Queiroz TB, Mendes ADR, Silva JCRL, et al. Content and chemical composition of the essential oil of 'erva-baleeira' (Varronia curassavica Jaqc.) as a function of harvesting times. *Rev Bras Plantas Med*. 2016; 18(Supl. 1):356-62.

[1325] Brandao DS, Costa KP, Vieira JTR, et al. Growing of tropical black sage and chemical composition of the essential oil. *Revista de Ciencias Agrarias*. 2017;40(4):823-9.

[1326] Hernandez T, Canales M, Teran B, et al. Antimicrobial activity of the essential oil and extracts of Cordia curassavica (Boraginaceae). *J Ethnopharmacology*. 2007;111:137-41.

[1327] Santos AV, Antunes e Defaveri AC, Bizzo HR, et al. In vitro propagation, histochemistry, and analysis of essential oil from conventionally propagated and in vitro-propagated plants of Varronia curassavica Jacq. *In Vitro Cell Dev Biol—Plant*. 2013;49:405–413.

[1328] de Castro Nizio DA, de Andrade Brito F, Sampaio TS, et al. Chemical diversity of native populations of Varronia curassavica Jacq. and antifungal activity against Lasiodoplodia theobromae. *Ind Crops Prod*. 2015 Dec 15;76:437-48.

[1329] de Castro Nizio DA, Fujimoto RY, Maria AN, et al. Essential oils of Varronia curassavica accessions have different activity against white spot disease in freshwater fish. *Parasitol Res*. 2018 Jan;117(1):97-105.

[1330] Rodriguez FFG, Oliveira LGS, Rodrigues FFG, et al. Chemical composition, antibacterial and antifungal activities of essential oil from Cordia verbenacea DC leaves. *Pharmacognosy Res*. 2012 Jul-Sep;4(3):161-65.

[1331] Bonesi M, Menichini F, Tundis R, et al. Acetylcholinesterase and butyrylcholinesterase inhibitory activity of Pinus species essential oils and their constituents. *J Enzyme Inhib Med Chem*. 2010 Oct;25(5):622-8

[1332] Nguyen LT, Mysliveckova Z, Szotakova B, et al. The inhibitory effects of β-caryophyllene, β-caryophyllene oxide and α-humulene on the activities of the main drug-metabolizing enzymes in rat and human liver in vitro. *Chem-Biol Interactoins*. 2017 Dec 25;278:123-8.

[1333] Passos GF, Fernandes ES, da Cunha FM, et al. Anti-inflammatory and anti-allergic properties of the essential oil and active constituents from Cordia verbenacea. *J Ethnopharmacol*. 2007 Mar 1;110(2):323-33.

[1334] Pulli B, Ali M, Forghani R, et al. Measuring Myeloperoxidase Activity in Biological Samples. *PLoS One*. 2013;8(7):e67976.

[1335] Pimentel SP, Barrella GE, Casarin RC, et al. Protective effect of topical Cordia verbenacea in a rat periodontitis model: immune-inflammatory, antibacterial and morphometric assays. *BMC Complement Altern Med*. 2012 Nov 21;12:224.

[1336] Rodriguez FFG, Oliveira LGS, Rodrigues FFG, et al. Chemical composition, antibacterial and antifungal activities of essential oil from Cordia verbenacea DC leaves. *Pharmacognosy Res*. 2012 Jul-Sep;4(3):161-65.

[1337] Meccia G, Rojas LB, Velasco J, et al. Chemical composition and antibacterial activity of the essential oil of Cordia verbenacea from the Venezuelan Andes. *Nat Prod Commun*. 2009 Aug;4(8):1119-22.

[1338] Hernandez T, Canales M, Teran B, et al. Antimicrobial activity of the essential oil and extracts of Cordia curassavica (Boraginaceae). *J Ethnopharmacology*. 2007;111:137-41.

[1339] Rosales HFA, Mejia JJ, Cordoba Y, et al. Antioxidant Activity and Chemical Composition of Cordia curassavica Essential Oil Collected in Santander, Colombia. *Rev Virtual de Quim*. 2009 Apr;8(1):ISSN 1984-6835.

[1340] Santos RP, Nunes EP, Nascimento RF, et al. Chemical composition and larvicidal activity of the essential oils of Cordia leucomalloides and Cordia curassavica from the Northeast of Brazil. *J Braz Chem Soc*. 2006 Sep-Oct;17(5):ISSN 1678-4790.

[1341] Ogunwande IA, Olawore NO, Kasali AA, et al. Chemical composition of the leaf oils of Callitris intratropica R.T. Baker & H.G. Smith from Nigeria. *Flav Frag J*. 2003 Sep-Oct;18(5):387-89.

[1342] Doimo L. Azulenes, costols and y-lactones from cypress-pines (Callitris columellaris, C. glaucophylla and C. intratropica) distilled and methanol extracts. *J Essent Oil Res*. 2001;13(1):25-29.

[1343] Aromatics International. Blue Cypress - Callitris intratropica. Available at: http://www.aromaticsinternational.com/products/essential-oils/blue-cypress.

[1344] Tsuneki H, Ma EL, Kobayashi S, et al. Antiangiogenic activity of beta-eudesmol in vitro and in vivo. *Eur J Pharmacol*. 2005 Apr 11;512(2-3):105-15.

[1345] Arora CK, Arora RB, Mesta CK, et al. Hypotensive activity of beta-eudesmol and some related sesquiterpenes. *Ind J Med Res*. 1967 May;55(5):463-72.

[1346] Wang BG, Hong X, Li L, Zhou J, et al. Chemical constituents of two Chinese Magnoliaceae plants, Tsoongiodendron odorum and Manglietiastrum sinicum, and their inhibition of platelet aggregation. *Planta Med*. 2000 Aug;66(6):511-5.

[1347] Baylac S, Racine P. Inhibition of 5-lipoxygenase by essential oils and other natural fragrant extracts. *Int J Aromatherapy*. 2003;13(2-3):138-42.

[1348] Destryana RA, Young DG, Woolley CL, et al. Antioxidant and anti-inflammation activities of ocotea, copaiba and blue cypress essential oils in vitro and in vivo. *J Am Oil Chem Soc*. 2014 Sep;91(9):1531-42.

[1349] Chao S, Young G, Oberg C, et al. Inhibition of methicillin-resistant Staphylococcus aureus (MRSA) by essential oils. *Flav Frag J*. 2008;23:444-49.

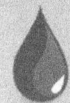

1350 Iqbal Z, Akhtar M, Mahmood T, et al. Variation in Composition and Yield of Foliage Oil of Eucalyptus Polybractea. *J Chem Soc Pakistan.* 2011 Mar;33(2):183-187.
1351 King DJ, Gleadow RM, Woodrwo IE. Regulation of oil accumulation in single glands of Eucalyptus polybractea. *New Phytologist.* 2006;172:440-51.
1352 Juan LW, Lucia A, Zerba EN, et al. Chemical composition and fumigant toxicity of the essential oils from 16 species of Eucalyptus against Haematobia irritans (Diptera: Muscidae) adults. *J Econ Entomol.* 2011 Jun;104(3):1087-92.
1353 Craig JO. Poisoning by the volatile oils in childhood. *Arch Dis Child.* 1953;28:259-67.
1354 Melis K. Bochner A, Janssens G. Accidental nasal eucalyptol and menthol instillation. *Eur J Pediatr.* 1989 Aug;148(8)786-7.
1355 Day LM, Ozanne-Smith J, Parsons BJ, et al. Eucalyptus oil poisoning among young children: mechanisms of access and the potential prevention. *Aust N Z J Public Health.* 1997 Jun;21(3):297-302.
1356 Chandar SD, Prashanti M, Kumar CL, et al. Eucalyptus Oil-Induced Seizures in Children: A Single-Center Prospective Study. *Cureus.* 2021 Mar 25;13(3):e14109.
1357 Burkhard PR, Burkhardt K, Haenggeli CA, et al. Plant-induced seizures: reappearance of an old problem. *J Neurol.* 1999 Aug;246(8):667-70.
1358 Waldman N. Seizure caused by dermal application of over-the-counter eucalyptus oil head lice preparation. *Clin Toxicol (Phila).* 2011 Oct;49(8):750-1.
1359 Craig JO. Poisoning by the volatile oils in childhood. *Arch Dis Child.* 1953;28:259-67.
1360 Newall CA, Anderson LA, Phillipson JD. "Herbal Medicines: A Guide for Health-care Professionals." London: The Pharmaceutical Press, 1996, 108.
1361 Day LM, Ozanne-Smith J, Parsons BJ, et al. Eucalyptus oil poisoning among young children: mechanisms of access and the potential prevention. *Aust N Z J Public Health.* 1997 Jun;21(3):297-302.
1362 Myott E. Case of eucalyptus poisoning. *Brit M J.* 1906;1:558.
1363 Hindle RC. Eucalyptus oil ingestion. *N Z Med J.* 1994 May 11;107(977)185-6.
1364 Tibballs J. Clinical effects and management of eucalyptus oil ingestion in infants and small children. *Med J Aust.* 1995 Aug;163(4):177-80.
1365 Waldman W, Barwina M, Sein Anand J. Accidental ontoxication with eucalyptus oil—a case report. *Przeql Lek.* 2011;68(8):555-6.
1366 Day LM, Ozanne-Smith J, Parsons BJ, et al. Eucalyptus oil poisoning among young children: mechanisms of access and the potential prevention. *Aust N Z J Public Health.* 1997 Jun;21(3):297-302.
1367 De Vincenzi M, Silano M, De Vincenzi A, et al. Constituents of aromatic plants: eucalyptol. *Fitoterapia.* 2002 Jun;73(3):269-75.
1368 Unger M, Frank A. Simultaneous determination of the inhibitory potency of herbal extracts on the activity of six major cytochrome P450 enzymes using liquid chromatography/mass spectrometry and automated online extraction. *Rapid Commun Mass Spectrom.* 2004;18(19):2273-81.
1369 Jori A, Bianchetti A, Prestini PE, et al. Effect of eucalyptol (1,8-cineole) on the metabolism of other drugs in rats and in man. *Eur J Pharmacol.* 1970;9(3):362-66.
1370 Kim NH, Hyun SH, Jin CH, et al. Pretreatment with 1,8-cineole potentiates thioacetamide-induced hepatotoxicity and immunosuppression. *Arch Pharm Res.* 2004 Jul;27(7):781-9.
1371 Gray AM, Flatt PR. Antihyperglycemic actions of Eucalyptus globulus (Eucalyptus) are associated with pancreatic and extra pancreatic effects in mice. *J Nutr.* 1998 Dec;128(12):2319–23.
1372 Basak SS, Candan F. Effect of Laurus nobilis L. Essential Oil and its Main Components on α-glucosidase and Reactive Oxygen Species Scavenging Activity. *Iran J Pharm Res.* 2013 Spring;12(2):367-79.
1373 Dey B. Chemo-profiling of eucalyptus and study of its hypoglycemic potential. *World J Diabetes.* 2013 Oct 15;4(5):170–76.
1374 Gray AM, Flatt PR. Antihyperglycemic actions of Eucalyptus globulus (Eucalyptus) are associated with pancreatic and extra pancreatic effects in mice. *J Nutr.* 1998 Dec;128(12):2319-23.
1375 Dey B. Chemo-profiling of eucalyptus and study of its hypoglycemic potential. *World J Diabetes.* 2013 Oct 15;4(5):170–76.
1376 Tsai HH, Lin HW, Chen YL, et al. A review of potential harmful interactions between anticoagulant/antiplatelet agents and Chinese herbal medicines. *PLoS One.* 2013 May 9;8(5):e64255.
1377 Moharam BA, Jantan I, bin Ahmad F, et al. Antiplatelet Aggregation and Platelet Activating Factor (PAF) Receptor Antagonistic Activities of the Essential Oils of Five Goniothalamus Species. *Molecules.* 2010;15:5124-38.
1378 Jori A, Bianchetti A, Prestini PE, et al. Effect of eucalyptol (1,8-cineole) on the metabolism of other drugs in rats and in man. *Eur J Pharmacol.* 1970;9(3):362-66.
1379 de Sousa DP, Raphael E, Brocksom U, et al. Sedative effect of monoterpene alcohols in mice: A preliminary screening. *Verlag der Zeitschrift fur Naturforschung.* 2007;62c:563-66.
1380 Juan LW, Lucia A, Zerba EN, et al. Chemical composition and fumigant toxicity of the essential oils from 16 species of Eucalyptus against Haematobia irritans (Diptera: Muscidae) adults. *J Econ Entomol.* 2011 Jun;104(3):1087-92.
1381 Lucia A1, Juan LW, Zerba EN, et al. Validation of models to estimate the fumigant and larvicidal activity of Eucalyptus essential oils against Aedes aegypti (Diptera: Culicidae). *Parasitol Res.* 2012 May;110(5):1675-86.
1382 Hammer KA, Carson CF, Riley TV. Antimicrobial activity of essential oils and other plant extracts. *J Appl Microbiology.* 1999 Jun;86(6):985-90.
1383 Aldoghaim FS, Flematti GR, Hammer KA, et al. Antimicrobial Activity of Several Cineole-Rich Western Australian Eucalyptus Essential Oils. *Microorganisms.* 2018 Dec 3;6(4).
1384 Fisher VL. Indigenous Salvia species - an investigation of the antimicrobial activity, antioxidant activity and chemical composition of leaf extracts. Masters Thesis, University of Witwatersrand. Available at: http://wiredspace.wits.ac.za/bitstream/handle/10539/1619/Fisher%20research%20report%20FINAL.pdf?sequence=2.
1385 Viljoen AM, Gono-Bwalya A, Kamatou GPP, et al. The Essential Oil Composition and Chemotaxonomy of Salvia stenophylla and its Allies S. repens and S. runcinata. *J Essent Oil Res.* 2006;18:37-45.
1386 Ganzera M, Schneider P, Stuppner H. Inhibitory effects of the essential oil of chamomile (Matricaria recutita L.) and its major constituents on human cytochrome P450 enzymes. *Life Sci.* 2006 Jan 18;78(8):856-61.
1387 Shanmuganathan B, Sheeja Malar D, Sathya S, et al. Antiaggregation Potential of Padina gymnospora against the Toxic Alzheimer's Beta-Amyloid Peptide 25-35 and Cholinesterase Inhibitory Property of Its Bioactive Compounds. *PLoS One.* 2015 Nov 4;10(11):e0141708.
1388 Brehm-Stecher BF, Johnson EA. Sensitization of Staphylococcus aureus and Escherichia coli to antibiotics by the sesquiterpenoids nerolidol, farnesol, bisabolol, and apritone. *Antimicrob Agents Chemother.* 2003 Oct;47(10):3357-60.
1389 Kamatou GP, Viljoen AM, Gono-Bwalya AB, et al. The in vitro pharmacological activities and a chemical investigation of three South African Salvia species. *J Ethnopharmacol.* 2005 Dec 1;102(3):382-90.
1390 Kamatou GP, Viljoen AM, Gono-Bwalya AB, et al. The in vitro pharmacological activities and a chemical investigation of three South African Salvia species. *J Ethnopharmacol.* 2005 Dec 1;102(3):382-90.
1391 Fisher VL. Indigenous Salvia species - an investigation of the antimicrobial activity, antioxidant activity and chemical composition of leaf extracts. Masters Thesis, University of Witwatersrand. Available at: http://wiredspace.wits.ac.za/bitstream/handle/10539/1619/Fisher%20research%20report%20FINAL.pdf?sequence=2.
1392 Kamatou GP, Viljoen AM, Gono-Bwalya AB, et al. The in vitro pharmacological activities and a chemical investigation of three South African Salvia species. *J Ethnopharmacol.* 2005 Dec 1;102(3):382-90.
1393 Kocak A, Kilic O. Identification of essential oil composition of four Picea Mill. (Pinaceae) species from Canada. *J Agric Sci Tech.* 2014:209-14.
1394 Baath MH, Burzo I. Quantitative and qualitative seasonal variation of volatile oil from 16 Conifer species. *Analele stiintifice ale Universitatii.* 2009;2:103-10.
1395 Young Living Essential Oils. Patent: Composition containing an essential oil product and method for using such to maintain normal levels of testosterone. Available at: http://www.google.com/patents/WO2014078590A1?cl=en.
1396 Khine H, Weiss D, Graber N, et al. A cluster of children with seizures caused by camphor poisoning. *Pediatrics.* 2009 May;123(5):1269-72.
1397 Michiels EA, Mazor SS. Toddler with seizures due to ingesting camphor at an Indian celebration. *Pediatr Emerg Care.* 2010 Aug;26(8):574-75.
1398 Koren G. Medications which can kill a toddler with one tablet or teaspoonful. *J toxicol Clin Toxicol.* 1993;31(3):407- 13.
1399 Bar-Oz B, Levicheck Z, Koren G. Medications that can kill a toddler with one tablet or teaspoonfull – A 2004 update. *Paediatr Drugs.* 2004;6(2):123-6.
1400 Rabl W, Katzgraber F, Steinlechner M. Camphor ingestion for abortion (case report). *Forensic Sci Int.* 1997 Sep 19;89(1-2):137-40.
1401 Flaman Z, Pellechia-Clarke S, Bailey B, et al. Unintentional exposure of young children to camphor and eucalyptus oils. *Paediatr Child Health.* 2001 Feb;6(2):80-83.
1402 Burkhard PR, Burkhardt K, Haenggeli CA, et al. Plant-induced seizures: reappearance of an old problem. *J Neurol.* 1999 Aug;246(8):667-70.
1403 Narayan S, Singh N. Camphor poisoning-An unusual cause of seizure. *Med J Armed Forces India.* 2012 Jul;68(3):252-53.
1404 Chanaranaj KJ, G MV, S M. Camphor poisoning in a child. *Natl Med J India.* 2013 Jan-Feb;26(1):60.
1405 Manoguerra AS, Erdman AR, Wax PM, et al. Camphor poisoning: an evidence-based practice guideline for out-of- hospital management. *Clin Toxicol (Phila).*2006;44(4):357-70.
1406 Gibson DE, Moore GP, Pfaff JA. Camphor ingestion. *Am J Emerg Med.* 1989 Jan;7(1):41-43.
1407 Koppel C, Martends F, Schirop T, et al. Hemoperfusion in acute camphor poisoning. *Intensive Care Med.* 1988;14(4):431-33.
1408 Olowe SA, Ransome-Kuti O. The risk of jaundice in glucose-6-phosphate dehydrogenase deficient babies exposed to menthol. *Acta Paediatr Scand.* 1980 May;69(3):341-5.
1409 Dillon Remy M, Manning Alleyne P, Bratt DE, et al. Neonatal jaundice at Port-of-Spain General Hospital abstract. *West Indian Med J.* 1987;36(Suppl):28.
1410 Young Living Essential Oils. Patent: Composition containing an essential oil product and method for using such to maintain normal levels of testosterone. Available at: http://www.google.com/patents/WO2014078590A1?cl=en.
1411 Chen N, Sun G, Yuan X, et al. Inhibition of lung inflammatory responses by bornyl acetate is correlated with regulation of myeloperoxidase activity. *J Surg Res.* 2014 Jan;186(1):436-45.
1412 Wu X, Li X, Xiao F, et al. Studies on the analgesic anti-inflammatory effect of bornyl acetate in volatile oil from Amomum villosum. *Zhong Yao Cai.* 2004 Jun;27(6):438-39.
1413 Wajs-Bonikowska A, Szoka L, Karna E, et al. Composition and Biological Activity of Picea pungens and Picea orientalis Seed and Cone Essential Oils. *Chem Biodivers.* 2017 Mar;14(3).
1414 Greche H, Hajjaji N, Ismaili-Alaoui M, et al. Chemical composition and antifungal properties of the essential oil of Tanacetum annuum. *J Essential Oil Res.* 2000;12(1):122-24.
1415 Greche H, Ismaili-Alaouri, Zrirs S, et al. Composition of Tanacetum annuum L. oil from Morocco. *J Essential Oil Res.* 1999;11(3):343-48.
1416 Haddar S, Greche H, Bakri H, et al. Chemical composition and anti-proliferative properties of the essential oil of Tanacetum annuum L. *Moroccan J Biol.* 2008;4(5):17-23.
1417 Aromatics International. Blue Tansy - Tanacetum annuum. Available at: http://www.aromaticsinternational.com/products/essential-oils/blue-tansy.
1418 Ganzera M, Schneider P, Stuppner H. Inhibitory effects of the essential oil of chamomile (Matricaria recutita L.) and its major constituents on human cytochrome P450 enzymes. *Life Sci.* 2006 Jan 18;78(8):856-61.
1419 Olowe SA, Ransome-Kuti O. The risk of jaundice in glucose-6-phosphate dehydrogenase deficient babies exposed to menthol. *Acta Paediatr Scand.* 1980 May;69(3):341-5.
1420 Dillon Remy M, Manning Alleyne P, Bratt DE, et al. Neonatal jaundice at Port-of-Spain General Hospital abstract. *West Indian Med J.* 1987;36(Suppl):28.
1421 Khine H, Weiss D, Graber N, et al. A cluster of children with seizures caused by camphor poisoning. *Pediatrics.* 2009 May;123(5):1269-72.

1422 Agarwal A, Mallhotra HS. Camphor ingestion: an unusual cause of seizure. *J Assoc Physicians India.* 2008 Feb;56:123-24.
1423 Haddar S, Greche H, Bakri H, et al. Chemical composition and anti-proliferative properties of the essential oil of Tanacetum annuum L. *Moroccan J Biol.* 2008;4(5):17-23.
1424 Baylac S, Racine P. Inhibition of 5-lipoxygenase by essential oils and other natural fragrant extracts. *Int J Aromatherapy.* 2003;13(2-3):138-42.
1425 Greche H, Hajjaji N, Ismaili-Alaoui M, et al. Chemical composition and antifungal properties of the essential oil of Tanacetum annuum. *J Essent Oil Res.* 2000;12(1):122-24.
1426 Miraldi E, Ferri S, Franchi GG, et al. Peumus boldus essential oil: New constituents and comparison of oils from leaves of different origin. *Fitoterapia.* 1996;67:227-30.
1427 Verdeguer M, Garcia-Rellan D, Boira H, et al. Herbicidal Activity of Peumus boldus and Drimys winterii Essential Oils from Chile. *Molecules.* 2011;16:403-11.
1428 Bittner M, Aguilera MA, Hernandez V, et al. Fungistatic Activity Of Essential Oils Extracted from Peumus boldus Mol., Laureliopsis philippiana (Looser) Schodde and Laurelia sempervirens (Ruiz & Pav.) Tul. (Chilean Monimiaceae). *Chilean J Agric Res.* 2009;69(1):ISSN 0718-5839.
1429 Vila R, Valenzuela L, Bello H, et al. Composition and Antimicrobial Activity of the Essential Oil of Peumus boldus Leaves. *Planta Med.* 1999;65:178-79.
1430 Urzua A, Santander R, Echeverria J, et al. Insecticidal Properties of Peumus boldus Mol. Essential Oil on the House Fly, Musca domestica L. *Boletín Latinoamericano y del Caribe de Plantas Medicinales y Aromáticas.* 2010;9(6):465-469.
1431 Petigny L, Périno S, Minuti M, et al. Simultaneous microwave extraction and separation of volatile and non-volatile organic constituents of boldo leaves. From lab to industrial scale. *Int J Mol Sci.* 2014 Apr 25;15(5):7183-98.
1432 European Medicines Agency. Assessment report on Peumus boldus Molina, folium. Available at: http://www.ema.europa.eu/docs/en_GB/document_library/Herbal_-_HMPC_assessment_report/2009/12/WC500018102.pdf.
1433 Haliciglu O, Astarcioglu G, Yaprak I, et al. Toxicity of Salvia officinalis in a newborn and a child: an alarming report. *Pediatr Neurol.* 2011 Oct;45(4):259-60.
1434 Lachenmeier DW, Walch SG. Epileptic seizure caused by accidental ingestion of sage (Salvia officinalis L.) oil in children: a rare, exceptional case or a threat to public health. *Pediatr Neurol.* 2012 Mar;46(3):201.
1435 European Medicines Agency. Assessment report on Peumus boldus Molina, folium. Available at: http://www.ema.europa.eu/docs/en_GB/document_library/Herbal_-_HMPC_assessment_report/2009/12/WC500018102.pdf.
1436 Almeida ER, Melo AM, Xavier H. Toxicological evaluation of the hydro-alcohol extract of the dry leaves of Peumus boldus and boldine in rats. *Phytother Res.* 2000 Mar;14(2):99-102.
1437 Mitchell EMH, Heumann S, Araujo A, et al. Brazilian adolescents' knowledge and beliefs about abortion methods: a school-based internet inquiry. *BMC Womens Health.* 2014;14:27.
1438 da Silva Costa KC, Bexerra SB, Norte CM, et al. Medicinal plants with teratogenic potential: current considerations. *Braz J Pharm Sci.* 2012;48(3):427-33.
1439 Brinker F. Herb Contraindications and Drug Interactions. 2nd ed. Sandy, OR. Eclectic Medical Publications. 1998.
1440 Osol A, ed. The Dispensatory of the United States of America. 25th ed. Philadelphia, PA: Lippincott, 1955.
1441 Piscaglia F, Leoni S, Venturi A, et al. Caution in the use of boldo in herbal laxatives: a case of hepatotoxicity. *Scand J Gastroenterol.* 2005;40:236-39.
1442 Monzon S, Lezaun A, Saenz D, et al. Anaphylaxis to boldo infusion, a herbal remedy. *Allergy.* 2004;59:1019-20.
1443 European Medicines Agency. Assessment report on Peumus boldus Molina, folium. Available at: http://www.ema.europa.eu/docs/en_GB/document_library/Herbal_-_HMPC_assessment_report/2009/12/WC500018102.pdf.
1444 European Medicines Agency. Public statement on the use of herbal medicinal products containing thujone. Available at: http://www.ema.europa.eu/docs/en_GB/document_library/Public_statement/2011/02/WC500102294.pdf.
1445 Millet Y, Jouglard J, Steinmetz MD, et al. Toxicity of some essential plant oils. Clinical and experimental study. *Clin Toxicol.* 1981 Dec;18(12):1485-98.
1446 Cristovao L, Carvalho F, Bastos MDL, et al. Hepatotoxicity of an essential oil of Salvia officinalis L.: an in vitro study using freshly isolated rat hepatocytes. *Congress Biomarkers.* 2001 Sep:165.
1447 Opdyke DLJ, Letizia C. Monographs on fragrance raw materials. *Food Cosmet Toxicol.* 1982:643-644.
1448 Lambert J, Cormier J. Potential interaction between warfarin and boldo-fenugreek. *Pharmacotherapy.* 2001;21:509-12.
1449 Al-Jaber HI, Hammad HM, Al-Qudah MA, et al. Volatile Oil Composition and Antiplatelet Activity of Jordanian Achillea biebersteinii Collected at Different Growth Stages. *J Essential Oil Bearing Plants.* 2014 Sep;17(4):584-98.
1450 Uc A, Bishop WP, Sanders KD. Camphor hepatotoxicity. *South Med J.* 2000;93:596-98.
1451 Frohne D. Giftpflanzen: Cupressaceae. Stuttgart: Wissenschaftliche Verlagsgesellschaft mbH; 1997. pp. 153–6.
1452 Dolan LC, Matulka RA, Burdock GA. Naturally Occurring Food Toxins. *Toxins (Basel).* 2010 Sep;2(9):2289–2332.
1453 Piscaglia F, Leoni S, Venturi A, et al. Caution in the use of boldo in herbal laxatives: a case of hepatotoxicity. *Scand J Gastroenterol.* 2005;40:236-39.
1454 United States National Toxicology Program (NTP). Alpha-Thujone. Dec 10, 1997. Available at: http://ntp.niehs.nih.gov/index.cfm?objectid=03DB8C36-E7A1-9889-3BDF8436F2A8C51F.
1455 Chittiboyina AG, Avonto C, Khan IA. What Happens after Activation of Ascaridole? Reactive Constituents and Their Implications for Skin Sensitization. *Chem Res Toxicol.* 2016 Sep 19;29(9):1488-92.
1456 Sciarrone D, Ragonese C, Carnovale C, et al. Evaluation of tea tree oil quality and ascaridole: a deep study by means of chiral and multi heart-cuts multidimensional gas chromatography system coupled to mass spectrometry detection. *J Chromatogr A.* 2010 Oct 8;1217(41):6422-7.
1457 Krutz NL, Hennen J1, Korb C, et al. Activation of the Endoperoxide Ascaridole Modulates Its Sensitizing Capacity. *Toxicol Sci.* 2015 Oct;147(2):515-23.
1458 Jori A, Bianchetti A, Prestini PE, et al. Effect of eucalyptol (1,8-cineole) on the metabolism of other drugs in rats and in man. *Eur J Pharmacol.* 1970;9(3):362-66.
1459 de Sousa DP, Raphael E, Brocksom U, et al. Sedative effect of monoterpene alcohols in mice: A preliminary screening. *Verlag der Zeitschrift fur Naturforschung.* 2007;62c:563-66.
1460 Lamborn LL. Modern soaps, candles and glycerin: A practical manual of modern methods of utilization of fats and oils in the manufacture of soaps and candles, and of the recovery of glycerin. Library of the University of Wisconsin.
1461 Oyen LP, Dung NX. Plant resources of South-East Asia. 1999. Backhyus, Leiden.
1462 Kim NH, Hyun SH, Jin CH, et al. Pretreatment with 1,8-cineole potentiates thioacetamide-induced hepatotoxicity and immunosuppression. *Arch Pharm Res.* 2004 Jul;27(7):781-9.
1463 Passone MA, Girardi NS, Etcheverry M. Evaluation of the control ability of five essential oils against Aspergillus section Nigri growth and ochratoxin A accumulation in peanut meal extract agar conditioned at different water activities levels. *Int J Food Microbiol.* 2012 Oct 15;159(3):198-206.
1464 Bluma R, Amaiden MR, Daghero J, et al. Control of Aspergillus section Flavi growth and aflatoxin accumulation by plant essential oils. *J Appl Microbiol.* 2008 Jul;105(1):203-14.
1465 Bluma RV, Etcheverry MG. Application of essential oils in maize grain: impact on Aspergillus section Flavi growth parameters and aflatoxin accumulation. *Food Microbiol.* 2008 Apr;25(2):324-34.
1466 Bittner M, Aguilera MA, Hernandez V, et al. Fungistatic Activity Of Essential Oils Extracted from Peumus boldus Mol., Laureliopsis philippiana (Looser) Schodde and Laurelia sempervirens (Ruiz & Pav.) Tul. (Chilean Monimiaceae). *Chilean J Agric Res.* 2009;69(1):ISSN 0718-5839.
1467 Vila R, Valenzuela L, Bello H, et al. Composition and Antimicrobial Activity of the Essential Oil of Peumus boldus Leaves. *Planta Med.* 1999;65:178-79.
1468 Urzua A, Santander R, Echeverria J, et al. Insecticidal Properties of Peumus boldus Mol. Essential Oil on the House Fly, Musca domestica L. *Boletín Latinoamericano y del Caribe de Plantas Medicinales y Aromáticas.* 2010;9(6):465-469.
1469 Posthumus MA, van Beek TA, Collins NF, et al. Chemical Composition of the Essential Oils of Agathosma betulina, A. crenulata and an A. betulina x crenulata Hybrid (Buchu). *J Essent Oil Res.* 1996 Apr;8:223-228.
1470 Collins NF, Graven EH, van Beek TA. Chemotaxonomy of Commercial Buchu Species (Agathosma betulina and A. crenulata). *J Essent Oil Res.* 1996;8(3):229-35.
1471 Viljoen AM, Moolla A, van Vuuren SF, et al. The biological activity and essential oil composition of 17 Agathosma (Rutaceae) species. *J Essent Oil Res.* 2006;18:2–16.
1472 Bakerink JA, Gospe SM Jr, Dimand RJ, et al. Multiple organ failure after ingestion of pennyroyal oil from herbal tea in two infants. *Pediatrics.* 1996;98(5):944-47.
1473 Sudekum M, Poppenga RH, Raju N, et al. Pennyroyal oil toxicosis in a dog. *J Am Vet Med Assoc.* 1992;200:817-8.
1474 Anderson IB, Mullen WH, Meeker JE, et al. Pennyroyal toxicity: measurement of toxic metabolite levels in two cases and review of the literature. *Ann Intern Med.* 1996;124:726-34.
1475 Seeff L, Stickel F, Navarro VJ. Hepatotoxicity of herbals and dietary supplements. In, Kaplowitz N, DeLeve LD, eds. Drug-induced liver disease. 3rd ed. Amsterdam: Elsevier, 2013, pp. 631-58.
1476 Moolla A. A phytochemical and pharmacological investigation of indigenous Agathosma species. MSc Dissertation, University of the Witwatersrand. 2006.
1477 Mullen W, Anderson I, Oishii S, et al. Accidental pennyroyal oil ingestion in a toddler with the first human serum metabolite detection. *Vet Hum Toxicol.* 1994;36:342.
1478 Barnes J, Anderson LA, Philpson JD. Herbal Medicine: A Guide for Healthcare Professionals. London, UK: The Pharmaceutical Press, 1996.
1479 Zimmerman HJ. Unconventional drugs. Miscellaneous drugs and diagnostic chemicals. In, Zimmerman, HJ. Hepatotoxicity: the adverse effects of drugs and other chemicals on the liver. 2nd ed. Philadelphia: Lippincott,1999: pp. 731-34.
1480 Anderson IB, Mullen WH, Meeker JE, et al. Pennyroyal toxicity: measurement of toxic metabolite levels in two cases and review of the literature. *Ann Intern Med.* 1996;124:726-34.
1481 Centers for Disease Control. Fatality and illness associated with consumption of pennyroyal oil - Colorado. *MMWR.* 1978;27:511-13.
1482 Ciganda C, Laborde A. Herbal infusions used for induced abortion. *J Toxicol Clin Toxicol.* 2003;41(3):235-9.
1483 Valance WB. Pennyroyal poisoning: a fatal case. *Lancet.* 1955;266 (6895):850-51.
1484 Gold J, Cates W Jr. Herbal abortifacients. *JAMA.* 1980;243:1365-66.
1485 Khojasteh-Bakht SC, Chen W, Koenigs LL, et al. Metabolism of (R)-(+)-pulegone and (R)-(+)-menthofuran by human liver cytochrome P-450s: evidence for formation of a furan epoxide. *Drug Metab Dispos.* 1999 May;27(5):574-80
1486 Gordon P, Khojasteh SC. A decades-long investigation of acute metabolism-based hepatotoxicity by herbal constituents: a case study of pennyroyal oil. *Drug Metab Rev.* 2015 Feb;47(1):12-20.
1487 National Toxicology Program. Toxicology and carcinogenesis studies of pulegone (CAS No. 89-82-7) in F344/N rats and B6C3F1 mice (gavage studies). *Natl Toxicol Program Tech Rep Ser.* 2011 Aug;(563):1-201.
1488 National Toxicology Program. Toxicology and carcinogenesis studies of pulegone (CAS No. 89-82-7) in F344/N rats and B6C3F1 mice (gavage studies). *Natl Toxicol Program Tech Rep Ser.* 2011 Aug;(563):1-201.
1489 National Toxicology Program. Toxicology and carcinogenesis studies of pulegone (CAS No. 89-82-7) in F344/N rats and B6C3F1 mice (gavage studies). *Natl Toxicol Program Tech Rep Ser.* 2011 Aug;(563):1-201.

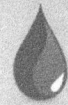

[1490] Sullivan JB Jr, Rumack BH, Thomas H Jr, et al. Pennyroyal oil poisoning and hepatotoxicity. *JAMA*. 1979;242:2873-4.
[1491] The Review of Natural Products by Facts and Comparisons. St. Louis, MO: Wolters Kluwer Co., 1999.
[1492] Foster S, Tyler VE. Tyler's Honest Herbal: A Sensible Guide to the Use of Herbs and Related Remedies. 3rd ed., Binghamton, NY: Haworth Herbal Press, 1993.
[1493] Martindale W. Martindale the Extra Pharmacopoeia. Pharmaceutical Press, 1999.
[1494] McGuffin M, Hobbs C, Upton R, Goldberg A, eds. American Herbal Products Association's Botanical Safety Handbook. Boca Raton, FL: CRC Press, LLC 1997.
[1495] Sullivan JB Jr, Rumack BH, Thomas H Jr, et al. Pennyroyal oil poisoning and hepatotoxicity. *JAMA*. 1979;242:2873-4.
[1496] Anderson IB, Mullen WH, Meeker JE, et al. Pennyroyal toxicity: measurement of toxic metabolite levels in two cases and review of the literature. *Ann Intern Med*. 1996;124:726-34.
[1497] Allen WT. Note on a case of supposed poisoning by pennyroyal. *Lancet*. 1897;1(3841):1022-23.
[1498] Braithwaite PF. A case of poisoning by pennyroyal: recovery. *Br Med J*. 1906;2:865.
[1499] Girling J. Poisoning by pennyroyal. *Br Med J*. 1887;1:1214.
[1500] Buechel DW, Haverlah VC, Gardner ME. Pennyroyal oil ingestion: report of a case. *J Am Osteopath Assoc*. 1983;82:793-4.
[1501] Flynn EF. Poisoning by essence of pennyroyal. *Br Med J*. 1893;2:1270.
[1502] Sayyah M, Valizadeh J, Kamalinejad M. Anticonvulsant activity of the leaf oil of Laurus nobilis against pentylentetrazole- and maximal electroshock-induced seizure. *Phytomedicine*. 2002 Apr;9(3):212-16.
[1503] Culic M, Kekovic G, Grbic G, et al. Wavelet and fractal analysis of rat brain activity in seizures evoked by camphor oil and 1,8-cineole. *Gen Physiol Biophys*. 2009;28 Sec No:33-40.
[1504] Burkhard PR, Burkhardt K, Haenggeli CA, et al. Plant-induced seizures: reappearance of an old problem. *J Neurol*. 1999 Aug;246(8):667-70.
[1505] Waldman N. Seizure caused by dermal application of over-the-counter eucalyptus oil head lice preparation. *Clin Toxicol (Phila)*. 2011 Oct;49(8):750-1.
[1506] Craig JO. Poisoning by the volatile oils in childhood. *Arch Dis Child*. 1953;28:259-67.
[1507] Mathew T, Kamath V, Kumar RS, et al. Eucalyptus oil inhalation-induced seizure: A novel, underrecognized, preventable cause of acute symptomatic seizure. *Epilepsia Open*. 2017 Jul 4;2(3):350-354.
[1508] Sullivan JB Jr, Rumack BH, Thomas H Jr, et al. Pennyroyal oil poisoning and hepatotoxicity. *JAMA*. 1979;242:2873-4.
[1509] Sudekum M, Poppenga RH, Raju N, et al. Pennyroyal oil toxicosis in a dog. *J Am Vet Med Assoc*. 1992;200:817-8.
[1510] Anderson IB, Mullen WH, Meeker JE, et al. Pennyroyal toxicity: measurement of toxic metabolite levels in two cases and review of the literature. *Ann Intern Med*. 1996;124:726-34.
[1511] Zimmerman HJ. Unconventional drugs. Miscellaneous drugs and diagnostic chemicals. In, Zimmerman, HJ. Hepatotoxicity: the adverse effects of drugs and other chemicals on the liver. 2nd ed. Philadelphia: Lippincott,1999: pp. 731-34.
[1512] Seeff L, Stickel F, Navarro VJ. Hepatotoxicity of herbals and dietary supplements. In, Kaplowitz N, DeLeve LD, eds. Drug-induced liver disease. 3rd ed. Amsterdam: Elsevier, 2013, pp. 631-58.
[1513] Moolla A. A phytochemical and pharmacological investigation of indigenous Agathosma species. MSc Dissertation, University of the Witwatersrand. 2006.
[1514] Lambert MI, Burgess T, Noakes TO. BuchuLife Research. The efficacy of Buchu (Agathosma Betulina) in treating symptoms of pain and
swelling from exercise-induced muscle damage. Available at: http://www.buchulife.com/researchdoc/efficacy-buchu-treating-symptoms-pain-and-swelling.
[1515] Lis-Balchin M, Hart S, Simspon E. Buchu (Agathosma betulina and A. crenulata, Rutaceae) essential oils: their pharmacological action on guinea-pig ileum and antimicrobial activity on microorganisms. *J Pharmacy Pharmacol*. 2001 Apr;53(4):579-82.
[1516] Viljoen AM, Moolla A, van Vuuren SF, et al. The biological activity and essential oil composition of 17 Agathosma (Rutaceae) species. *J Essent Oil Res*. 2006;18:2–16.
[1517] Lis-Balchin M, Hart S, Simspon E. Buchu (Agathosma betulina and A. crenulata, Rutaceae) essential oils: their pharmacological action on guinea-pig ileum and antimicrobial activity on microorganisms. *J Pharmacy Pharmacol*. 2001 Apr;53(4):579-82.
[1518] Lee JH, Lee JS. Chemical Composition and Antifungal Activity of Plant Essential Oils against Malassezia furfur. *Kor J Microbiol Biotechnol*. 2010;38(3):315-21.
[1519] Viljoen AM, Moolla A, van Vuuren SF, et al. The biological activity and essential oil composition of 17 Agathosma (Rutaceae) species. *J Essent Oil Res*. 2006;18:2–16.
[1520] Moolla A. A phytochemical and pharmacological investigation of indigenous Agathosma species. MSc Dissertation, University of the Witwatersrand. 2006.
[1521] Moolla A, van Vuuren SF, van Zyl RL, et al. Biological activity and toxicity profile of 17 Agathosma (Ruataceae) species. *South African J Botany*. 2007;73:588–92.
[1522] Beattie KD, Waterman PG, Forster PI, et al. Chemical composition and cytotoxicity of oils and eremophilanes derived from various parts of Eremophila mitchellii Benth. (Myoporaceae). *Phytochemistry*. 2011 Apr;72(4-5):400-8.
[1523] Stillpoint Aromatics. Buddha Wood Essential Oil. Avialbale at: http://www.stillpointaromatics.com/essential-oils/buddha-wood-Eremophilla-mitchelli-essential-oil-aromatherapy.
[1524] Beattie KD, Waterman PG, Forster PI, et al. Chemical composition and cytotoxicity of oils and eremophilanes derived from various parts of Eremophila mitchellii Benth. (Myoporaceae). *Phytochemistry*. 2011 Apr;72(4-5):400-8.
[1525] Saleh MA, Clark S, Woodaard B, et al. Antioxidant and free radical scavenging activities of essential oils. *Ehtnicity & Disease*. 2010 Spring;20(S1):78-82.
[1526] Kumar A, Tandon S, Yadav A. Chemical composition of the essential oil from fresh leaves of Melaleuca leucadendron L. from North India. *J Essent Oil Bearing Plants*. 2005;8(1):19-22.
[1527] Pujiarti R, Ohtani Y, Ichiura H. Physicochemical properties and chemical compositions of Melaleuca leucadendron leaf oils taken from the plantations of Java, Indonesia. *J Wood Sci*. 2011 oct;57(5):446-51.
[1528] Pujiarti R, Ohtani Y, Ichiura H. Chemical compositions, antioxidant and antifungal activities of Melaleuca leucadendron Linn. leaf oils from Indonesia. *Wood Res J*. 2012;3(1):23-29.
[1529] Pujiarti R, Ohtani Y, Widowati TB, et al. Utilization of Melaleuca leucadendron essential oil. *Wood Res J*. 2012 2(2):94-99.
[1530] Falci SP, Teixeira MA, Chagas PF, et al. Antimicrobial activity of Melaleuca sp. oil against clinical isolates of antibiotics resistant Staphylococcus aureus. *Acta Cir Bras*. 2015 Jul;30(7):491-6.
[1531] Craig JO. Poisoning by the volatile oils in childhood. *Arch Dis Child*. 1953;28:259-67.
[1532] Melis K. Bochner A, Janssens G. Accidental nasal eucalyptol and menthol instillation. *Eur J Pediatr*. 1989 Aug;148(8)786-7.
[1533] Day LM, Ozanne-Smith J, Parsons BJ, et al. Eucalyptus oil poisoning among young children: mechanisms of access and the potential prevention. *Aust N Z J Public Health*. 1997 Jun;21(3):297-302.
[1534] Chandar SD, Prashanti M, Kumar CL, et al. Eucalyptus Oil-Induced Seizures in Children: A Single-Center Prospective Study. *Cureus*. 2021 Mar 25;13(3):e14109.
[1535] Burkhard PR, Burkhardt K, Haenggeli CA, et al. Plant-induced seizures: reappearance of an old problem. *J Neurol*. 1999 Aug;246(8):667-70.
[1536] Waldman N. Seizure caused by dermal application of over-the-counter eucalyptus oil head lice preparation. *Clin Toxicol (Phila)*. 2011 Oct;49(8):750-1.
[1537] Craig JO. Poisoning by the volatile oils in childhood. *Arch Dis Child*. 1953;28:259-67.
[1538] Day LM, Ozanne-Smith J, Parsons BJ, et al. Eucalyptus oil poisoning among young children: mechanisms of access and the potential prevention. *Aust N Z J Public Health*. 1997 Jun;21(3):297-302.
[1539] Myott E. Case of eucalyptus poisoning. *Brit M J*. 1906;1:558.
[1540] Hindle RC. Eucalyptus oil ingestion. *N Z Med J*. 1994 May 11;107(977)185-6.
[1541] Tibballs J. Clinical effects and management of eucalyptus oil ingestion in infants and small children. *Med J Aust*. 1995 Aug;163(4):177-80.
[1542] Waldman W, Barwina M, Sein Anand J. Accidental ontoxication with eucalyptus oil—a case report. *Przeql Lek*. 2011;68(8):555-6.
[1543] Day LM, Ozanne-Smith J, Parsons BJ, et al. Eucalyptus oil poisoning among young children: mechanisms of access and the potential prevention. *Aust N Z J Public Health*. 1997 Jun;21(3):297-302.
[1544] De Vincenzi M, Silano M, De Vincenzi A, et al. Constituents of aromatic plants: eucalyptol. *Fitoterapia*. 2002 Jun;73(3):269-75.
[1545] Jori A, Bianchetti A, Prestini PE, et al. Effect of eucalyptol (1,8-cineole) on the metabolism of other drugs in rats and in man. *Eur J Pharmacol*. 1970;9(3):362-66.
[1546] Kim NH, Hyun SH, Jin CH, et al. Pretreatment with 1,8-cineole potentiates thioacetamide-induced hepatotoxicity and immunosuppression. *Arch Pharm Res*. 2004 Jul;27(7):781-9.
[1547] Tsai HH, Lin HW, Chen YL, et al. A review of potential harmful interactions between anticoagulant/antiplatelet agents and Chinese herbal medicines. *PLoS One*. 2013 May 9;8(5):e64255.
[1548] Moharam BA, Jantan I, bin Ahmad F, et al. Antiplatelet Aggregation and Platelet Activating Factor (PAF) Receptor Antagonistic Activities of the Essential Oils of Five Goniothalamus Species. *Molecules*. 2010;15:5124-38.
[1549] Jori A, Bianchetti A, Prestini PE, et al. Effect of eucalyptol (1,8-cineole) on the metabolism of other drugs in rats and in man. *Eur J Pharmacol*. 1970;9(3):362-66.
[1550] de Sousa DP, Raphael E, Brocksom U, et al. Sedative effect of monoterpene alcohols in mice: A preliminary screening. *Verlag der Zeitschrift fur Naturforschung*. 2007;62c:563-66.
[1551] Farag RS, Shalaby AS, El-Baroty GA, et al. Chemical and biological evaluation of the essential oils of different Melaleuca species. *Phytother Res*. 2004 Jan;18(1):30-35.b
[1552] Hammer KA, Carson CF, Riley TV. Antimicrobial activity of essential oils and other plant extracts. *J Appl Microbiol*. 1999 Jun;86(6):985-90.
[1553] Falci SP, Teixeira MA, Chagas PF, et al. Antimicrobial activity of Melaleuca sp. oil against clinical isolates of antibiotics resistant Staphylococcus aureus. *Acta Cir Bras*. 2015 Jul;30(7):491-6.
[1554] Pino JA, Regalado EL, Rodriguez JL, et al. Phytochemical analysis and in vitro free radical-scavenging activities of the essential oils from leaf and fruit of Melaleuca leucadendra L. *Chem Biodivers*. 2010 Sep;7(9):2281-88.
[1555] Amer A, Mehlhorn H, et al. Repellency of forty-one essential oils against Aedes, Anopheles, and Culex mosquitoes. *Parasitol Res*. 2006 Sep;99(4):478-90.
[1556] Noosidum A, Prabaripal A, Chareonviriyaphap, et al. Excito-repellancy properties of essential oils from Melaleuca leucadendron L., Listea cubeba (Lour.) Persoon, and Listea salicifolia (Nees) on Aedes aegypti (L.) mosquitoes. *J Vector Ecol*. 2008;33(2):305-12.
[1557] Bua A, Molicotti P, Donadu MG, et al. "In vitro" activity of Melaleuca cajuputi against mycobacterial species. *Nat Prod Res*. 2018 Dec 5:1-4.
[1558] Krzyśko-Łupicka T, Sokół S, Piekarska-Stachowiak A. Evaluation of Fungistatic Activity of Eight Selected Essential Oils on Four Heterogeneous Fusarium Isolates Obtained From Cereal Grains in Southern Poland. *Molecules*. 2020 Jan 10;25(2):292.
[1559] An NTG, Huong LT, Satyal P, et al. Mosquito Larvicidal Activity, Antimicrobial Activity, and Chemical Compositions of Essential Oils from Four Species of Myrtaceae from Central Vietnam. *Plants (Basel)*. 2020 Apr 22;9(4).
[1560] Septiana S, Bachtiar BM, Yuliana ND, et al. Cajuputs candy impairs Candida albicans and Streptococcus mutans mixed biofilm formation in vitro. Version 2. *F1000Res*. 2019;8:1923.
[1561] Monzote L, Scherbakov AM, Scull R, et al. Essential Oil from Melaleuca leucadendra: Antimicrobial, Antikinetoplastid, Antiproliferative and Cytotoxic Assessment. *Molecules*. 2020 Nov 25;25(23):5514.

1562 Gretšušnikova T, Koel M, Orav A. Comparison of the essential oil composition of Acorus calamus obtained by supercritical carbon dioxide extraction and hydrodistillation methods. Available at: http://www.isasf.net/fileadmin/files/Docs/Arcachon/posters/p153-P12%20full%20text.pdf.
1563 Raina VK, Srivastava SK, Syamasunder KV. Essential oil composition of Acorus calamus L. from the lower region of the Himalayas. *Flavour Frag J.* 2003 Jan-Feb;18(1):18-20.
1564 Kumari R, Agrawal SB, Singh S, et al. Supplemental ultraviolet-B induced changes in essential oil composition and total phenolics of Acorus calamus L. (sweet flag). *Ecotoxicol Environ Saf.* 2009 Oct;72(7):2013-9.
1565 Radusiene J, Judžentienė A, Pečiulytė D, et al. Essential oil composition and antimicrobial assay of Acorus calamus leaves from different wild populations. *Plant Genetic Res.* 2007 Apr;5(01):37-44.
1566 Raal A, Orav A, Gretchushnikova T. β-Asarone content and essential oil composition of Acorus calamus L. rhizomes from Estonia. *J Essent Oil Res.* 2006;28(4):299-304.
1567 Lohani H, Chandra Andola H, Chauhan N, et al. Variations of Essential oil composition of Acorus calamus: from Uttarakhand Himalaya. *J Pharm Res.* 2012;5(2):1246-47.
1568 Lawrence BM. Essential oils 1981-1987. Allured Publishing, Wheaton. 1981. p. 77-78.
1569 Rana TS, Mahar KS, Pandey MM, et al. Molecular and chemical profiling of 'sweet flag' (Acorus calamus L.) germplasm from India. *Physiol Mol Biol Plants.* 2013 Apr;19(2):231–37.
1570 Liu XC, Zhou LG, Liu ZL, et al. Identification of insecticidal constituents of the essential oil of Acorus calamus rhizomes against Liposcelis bostrychophila Badonnel. *Molecules.* 2013 May 15;18(5):5684-96.
1571 Kim WJ, Hwang KH, Park DG, et al. Major constituents and antimicrobial activity of Korean herb Acorus calamus. *Nat Prod Res.* 2011 Aug;25(13):1278-81.
1572 Lawrence BM. Essential oils 1979-1980. Allured Publishing, Wheaton. 1981. p. 47-48.
1573 Mazza G. Determination of β-asarone in essential oil of A. calamus L. and in alcoholic beverages by high performance liquid chromatography. *Sci Ailment.* 1984;4:233-45.
1574 Mazza G. Gas chromatographic and mass spectrometric studies of the constituents of the rhizome of calamus: II. The volatile constituents of alcoholic extracts. *J Chromatography A.* 1985;328:195-206.
1575 Rost LCM, Bos R. Biosystematic invesgations with Acorus calamus L.3. Communication. Constituents of essential oils. *Planta Med.* 1979;27:350-361.
1576 Marongiu B, Piras A, Porcedda S, et al. Chemical Composition of the Essential Oil and Supercritical CO2 Extract of Commiphora myrrha (Nees) Engl. and of Acorus calamus L. J Agric Food Chem. 2005;53(20):7939–43.
1577 Lawrence BM. Essential oils 1979-1980. Allured Publishing, Wheaton. 1981. p. 47-48.
1578 Lawrence BM. Essential oils 1981-1987. Allured Publishing, Wheaton. 1981. p. 77-78.
1579 Ogra RK, Mohanpuria P, Sharma UK, et al. Indian calamus (Acorus calamus L.): Not a tetraploid. *Curr Sci.* 2009 Dec;97(11):1644-47.
1580 Rana TS, Mahar KS, Pandey MM, et al. Molecular and chemical profiling of 'sweet flag' (Acorus calamus L.) germplasm from India. *Physiol Mol Biol Plants.* 2013 Apr;19(2):231–37.
1581 Johnson JD, Ryan MJ, Toft JD II, et al. Two-year toxicity and carcinogenicity study of methyl eugenol in F344/N rats and B6C3F(1) mice. *J Agric Food Chem.* 2000 Aug;48(8):3620-32.
1582 European Medicines Agency. Public statement on the use of herbal medicinal products containing estragole. Available at: http://www.ema.europa.eu/docs/en_GB/document_library/Scientific_guideline/2010/04/WC500089960.pdf.
1583 European Commission. Opinion of the Scientific Committee on Food on methyl eugenol (4-Allyl-1,2- dimethoxybenzene). Available at: http://ec.europa.eu/food/fs/sc/scf/out102_en.pdf.
1584 Kerckaert GA, Brauninger R, LeBoeuf RA, et al. Use of the Syrian hamster embryo cell transformation assay for carcinogenicity prediction of chemicals currently being tested by the National Toxicology Program in rodent bioassays. *Environ Health Perspect.* 1996;104:1075-84.
1585 National Toxicology Program. Carcinogenesis Studies of Eugenol (CAS No. 97-53-0) in F344/N Rats and B6C3F1 Mice (Feed Studies). Technical Report Series No. 223. NIH Publication No. 84-1779. 1983. U.S. DHHS, PHS, NIH, NTP, Research Triangle Park, NC.
1586 López ML, Hernández A, Chamorro G, et al. alpha-Asarone toxicity in long-term cultures of adult rat hepatocytes. *Planta Med.* 1993 Apr;59(2):115-20.
1587 Chamorro G, Salazar M, Salazar S, et al. [Pharmacology and toxicology of Guatteria gaumeri and alpha-asarone.] *Rev Invest Clin.* 1993;45(6):597-604.
1588 European Medicines Agency. Public statement on the use of herbal medicinal products containing asarone. Available at: http://www.ema.europa.eu/docs/en_GB/document_library/Scientific_guideline/2010/04/WC500089956.pdf.
1589 Yabiku HK. Calamus oil - Toxicological aspects and their control in alcoholic beverages. M. S. Thesis, Sao Paulo, Brazil, Submitted to FAO/WHO. 1980.
1590 Price CJ, George JD, Marr MC, et al. Developmental toxicity evaluation of methyleugenol (MEUG) administered to Sprague-Dawley rats on gestational days (gd) 6 through 19. *Birth Defects Res A Clin Mol Teratol.* 2006 Jun;76:395.
1591 Johnson JD, Ryan MJ, Toft JD II, et al. Two-year toxicity and carcinogenicity study of methyl eugenol in F344/N rats and B6C3F(1) mice. *J Agric Food Chem.* 2000 Aug;48(8):3620-32.
1592 National Toxicology Program. NTP Toxicology and Carcinogenesis Studies of Methyleugenol (CAS NO. 93-15-2) in F344/N Rats and B6C3F1 Mice (Gavage Studies). *Natl Toxicol Program Tech Rep Ser.* 2000 Jul;491:1-412.
1593 Kerckaert GA, Brauninger R, LeBoeuf RA, et al. Use of the Syrian hamster embryo cell transformation assay for carcinogenicity prediction of chemicals currently being tested by the National Toxicology Program in rodent bioassays. *Environ Health Perspect.* 1996;104:1075-84.
1594 National Toxicology Program. Carcinogenesis Studies of Eugenol (CAS No. 97-53-0) in F344/N Rats and B6C3F1 Mice (Feed Studies). Technical Report Series No. 223. NIH Publication No. 84-1779. 1983. U.S. DHHS, PHS, NIH, NTP, Research Triangle Park, NC.
1595 Unger P, Melzig MF. Comparative Study of the Cytotoxicity and Genotoxicity of Alpha- and Beta-Asarone. *Sci Pharm.* 2012 Jul-Sep; 80(3): 663–668.
1596 Hagan EC, Hansen WH, Fitzhugh OG, et al. Food flavourings and constituents of related structure. II. Subacute and chronic toxicity. *Food Cosmet Toxicol.* 1967 Apr;5(2):141-57.
1597 Taylor JM. (Food and Drug Administration) Personal communication to the World Health Organization concerning unpublished studies on beta-asarone and calamus oils. 1981. Found at: http://www.inchem.org/documents/jecfa/jecmono/v16je04.htm.
1598 Taylor JM, et al. Toxicity of oil of calamus (Jammus variety). *Toxicol Exptl Pharmacol.* 1967;10:405.
1599 Weinberg M. Studies conducted with Calamus. Unpublished report from Foster D. Snell, Inc. submitted to the World Health Organization by Comitato Per Lo Studio Delle Bevande Alcooliche Aromatizzate. 1969. Found at: http://www.inchem.org/documents/jecfa/jecmono/v16je04.htm.
1600 Zuba D, Bogumila B. Alpha- and beta-asarone in herbal medicinal products. A case study. *Forensic Sci Int.* 2012 Nov 30;223(1-3):e5-9.
1601 Meyer F, Meyer E. Percutaneous absorption of essential oils and their constituents. *Arzneimittel-Forsch.* 1965;9:516.
1602 National Institutes of Health. Report on carcinogens. Available at: http://ntp.niehs.nih.gov/ntp/roc/content/profiles/methyleugenol.pdf.
1603 Rubio-Póo C, Lemini C, García-Mondragón J, et al. The anticoagulant effect of beta-asarone in the mouse and the rat. *Proc West Pharmacol Soc.* 1991;34:107-12.
1604 Dandiya PC, Cullumbine H. Studies on Acorus calamus. III. Some pharmacological actions of the volatile oil. *J Pharmacol Exptl Therap.* 1959;125:353-59.
1605 Menon MK, Dandiya PC. The mechanism of the tranquillizing action of asarone from Acorus calamus Linn. *J Pharm Pharmacol.* 1967 Mar;19(3):170-5.
1606 Baxter RM, Dandiya PC, Kandel SI, et al. Separation of the hypnotic-potentiating principles from the essential oil of Acorus calamus L. of Indian origin by liquid-gas chromatograph. *Nature.* 1960 Feb;185:466-67.
1607 Dandiya PC, Baxter RM, Walker GC, et al. Studies on Acorns calamus. II. Investigation of volatile oil. *J Pharm Pharmacol.* 1959;11:163-68.
1608 Unger P, Melzig MF. Comparative Study of the Cytotoxicity and Genotoxicity of Alpha- and Beta-Asarone. *Sci Pharm.* 2012 Jul-Sep; 80(3): 663–668.
1609 Hagan EC, Hansen WH, Fitzhugh OG, et al. Food flavourings and constituents of related structure. II. Subacute and chronic toxicity. *Food Cosmet Toxicol.* 1967 Apr;5(2):141-57.
1610 Taylor JM. (Food and Drug Administration) Personal communication to the World Health Organization concerning unpublished studies on beta-asarone and calamus oils. 1981. Found at: http://www.inchem.org/documents/jecfa/jecmono/v16je04.htm.
1611 Taylor JM, et al. Toxicity of oil of calamus (Jammus variety). *Toxicol Exptl Pharmacol.* 1967;10:405.
1612 Weinberg M. Studies conducted with Calamus. Unpublished report from Foster D. Snell, Inc. submitted to the World Health Organization by Comitato Per Lo Studio Delle Bevande Alcooliche Aromatizzate. 1969. Found at: http://www.inchem.org/documents/jecfa/jecmono/v16je04.htm.
1613 Zuba D, Bogumila B. Alpha- and beta-asarone in herbal medicinal products. A case study. *Forensic Sci Int.* 2012 Nov 30;223(1-3):e5-9.
1614 Mukherjee PK, Kumar V, Mal M, et al. In vitro acetylcholinesterase inhibitory activity of the essential oil from Acorus calamus and its main constituents. *Planta Med.* 2007 Mar;73(3):283-5. Epub 2007 Feb 7.
1615 Meyer F, Meyer E. Percutaneous absorption of essential oils and their constituents. *Arzneimittel-Forsch.* 1965;9:516.
1616 Bisht D, Pal A, Chanotiya CS, et al. Terpenoid composition and antifungal activity of three commercially important essential oils against Aspergillus flavus and Aspergillus niger. *Nat Prod Res.* 2011 Dec;25(20):1993-8.
1617 Mahboubi M, Kazempour N, Mahboubi A. The efficacy of essential oils as natural preservatives in vegetable oil. *J Diet Suppl.* 2014 Dec;11(4):334-46.
1618 Satyal P, Paudel P, Poudel A, et al. Chemical compositions, phytotoxicity, and biological activities of Acorus calamus essential oils from Nepal. *Nat Prod Commun.* 2013 Aug;8(8):1179-81.
1619 Kim WJ, Hwang KH, Park DG, et al. Major constituents and antimicrobial activity of Korean herb Acorus calamus. *Nat Prod Res.* 2011 Aug;25(13):1278-81.
1620 Thobunluepop P. Implementation of bio-fungicides and seed treatment in organic rice cv. KDML 105 farming. *Pak J Biol Sci.* 2009 Aug 15;12(16):1119-26.
1621 Mukherjee PK, Kumar V, Mal M, et al. In vitro acetylcholinesterase inhibitory activity of the essential oil from Acorus calamus and its main constituents. *Planta Med.* 2007 Mar;73(3):283-5.
1622 Kumar R, Prakash O, Pan AK, et al. Compositional variations and anthelmentic activity of essential oils from rhizomes of different wild populations of Acorus calamus L. and its major component, beta-Asarone. *Nat Prod Commun.* 2009 Feb;4(2):275-8.
1623 Chaudhari GN, Kokate CK, Nimbkar AY. Search for anthelmintics of plant origin: Activities of volatile principles of Acorus calamus against Ascaris lumbricoides. *Anc Sci Life.* 1981 Oct;1(2):103-5.
1624 Chen HP, Yang K, Zheng LS, et al. Repellent and insecticidal activities of shyobunone and isoshyobunone derived from the essential oil of Acorus calamus rhizomes. *Pharmacogn Mag.* 2015 Oct-Dec;11(44):675-81.
1625 Liu XC, Zhou LG, Liu ZL, et al. Identification of insecticidal constituents of the essential oil of Acorus calamus rhizomes against Liposcelis bostrychophila Badonnel. *Molecules.* 2013 May 15;18(5):5684-96.
1626 Sharma PR, Sharma OP, Saxena BP. Effect of sweet flag rhizome oil (Acorus calamus) on hemogram and ultrastructure of hemocytes of the tobacco armyworm, Spodoptera litura (Lepidoptera: Noctuidae). *Micron.* 2008 Jul;39(5):544-51.
1627 Gupta H, Deeksha, Urvashi, et al. Insecticidal and Detoxification Enzyme Inhibition Activities of Essential Oils for the Control of Pulse Beetle, Callosobruchus maculatus (F.) and Callosobruchus chinensis (L.) (Coleoptera: Bruchidae). *Molecules.* 2023 Jan 4;28(2):492.

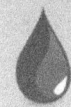

[1628] Gazim ZC, Rezende CM, Fraga SR, et al. Analysis of the essential oils from Calendula officinalis growing in Brazil using three different extraction procedures. *Rev Bras de Ciências Farm.* 2008 Jul-Sep;44(3):391-95.

[1629] Chalchat JC, Garry RP, Michet A. Chemical composition of essential oil of Calendula officinalis L. (Pot Marigold). *Flavour Frag J.* 1991;6:189-92.

[1630] Okoh OO, Sadimenko AP, Asekun OT, et al. The effects of drying on the chemical components of essential oils of Calendula officinalis L. *African J Biotech.* 2008 May;7(10):1500-02.

[1631] Salome-Abarca LF, Soto-Hernandez RM, Cruz-Huerta N, et al. Chemical composition of scented extracts obtained from Calendual officinalis by three extraction methods. *Botanical Sci.* 2015;93(3):633-38.

[1632] Khalid KA. Effect of potassium uptake on the composition of essential oil content in Calendula officinalis L. flowers. *Emir J Food Agric.* 2013;25(3):189-95.

[1633] Mishra A, Mishra A, Chattopadhyay P. Assessment of In vitro Sun Protection Factor of Calendula Officinalis L. (Asteraceae) Essential Oil Formulation. *J Young Pharm.* 2012 Jan;4(1):17-21.

[1634] Tavassoli M, Shayeghi M, Abai M, et al. Repellency Effects of Essential Oils of Myrtle (Myrtus communis), Marigold (Calendula officinalis) Compared with DEET against Anopheles stephensi on Human Volunteers. *Iran J Arthropod Borne Dis.* 2011;5(2):10-22.

[1635] Hiroi T, Miyazaki Y, Kobayashi Y, et al. Induction of hepatic P450s in rat by essential oil wood leaf oils. *Xenobiotica.* 1995 May;25(5):457-67.

[1636] Mishra AK, Mishra A, Verma A, et al. Effects of Calendula Essential Oil-Based Cream on Biochemical Parameters of Skin of Albino Rats against Ultraviolet B Radiation. *Sci Pharm.* 2012 Sep;80(3):669-83.

[1637] Mishra A, Mishra A, Chattopadhyay P. Assessment of In vitro Sun Protection Factor of Calendula Officinalis L. (Asteraceae) Essential Oil Formulation. *J Young Pharm.* 2012 Jan;4(1):17-21.

[1638] Tavassoli M, Shayeghi M, Abai M, et al. Repellency Effects of Essential Oils of Myrtle (Myrtus communis), Marigold (Calendula officinalis) Compared with DEET against Anopheles stephensi on Human Volunteers. *Iran J Arthropod Borne Dis.* 2011;5(2):10-22.

[1639] Gazim ZC, Rezende CM, Fraga SR, et al. Antifungal activity of the essential oil from Calendula officinalis L. (asteraceae) growing in Brazil. *Braz J Microbiol.* 2008 Jan;39(1):61-3.

[1640] Lohani A, Mishra AK, Verma A, et al. Cosmeceutical potential of geranium and calendula essential oil: Determination of antioxidant activity and in vitro sun protection factor. *J Cosmet Dermatol.* 2019 Apr;18(2):550-557.

[1641] Satyal P, Paudel P, Poudel A, et al. Bioactivities and compositional analyses of Cinnamomum essential oils from Nepal: C. camphora, C. tamala, and C. glaucescens. *Nat Prod Comm.* 2013 Sep;8(12):1777-84.

[1642] Chen HP, Yang K, You CX, et al. Chemical constituents and insecticidal activities of the essential oil of Cinnamomum camphora leaves against lasioderma serricorne. *J Chem.* 2014;2014(2014):963729.

[1643] Frizzo C, Santos A, Paroul N, et al. Essential oils of camphor tree (Cinnamomum camphora Nees & Eberm) cultivated in Southern Brazil. *Brazilian Arch Biol Tech.* 2000 Jan;43(3):1590.

[1644] Pino JA, Fuentes V. Leaf oil of Cinnamomum camphora (L.) J Presl. From Cuba. *J Essential Oil Res.* 1998;10(5):531-32.

[1645] Pandey AK, Bora HR, Deka SC, et al. Composition of the essential oil of the bark of Cinnamomum camphora. *J Med Aromatic Plant Sci.* 1997;19(2):408-09.

[1646] Pelissier Y, Marion C, Prunac S, et al. Volatile components of leaves, stems and bark of Cinnamomum camphora Nees et Ebermaier. *J Essential Oil Res.* 1995;7(3):313-15.

[1647] Ho CL, Wang EIC, Su YC. Essential oil composition and bioactivities of the various parts of Cinnamomum camphora Sieb var linaloolifera Fujuta. *Research Paper.* 2009;31(2):77-96.

[1648] Khine H, Weiss D, Graber N, et al. A cluster of children with seizures caused by camphor poisoning. *Pediatrics.* 2009 May;123(5):1269-72.

[1649] Michiels EA, Mazor SS. Toddler with seizures due to ingesting camphor at an Indian celebration. *Pediatr Emerg Care.* 2010 Aug;26(8):574-75.

[1650] Koren G. Medications which can kill a toddler with one tablet or teaspoonful. *J toxicol Clin Toxicol.* 1993;31(3):407-13.

[1651] Bar-Oz B, Levicheck Z, Koren G. Medications that can kill a toddler with one tablet or teaspoonfull – A 2004 update. *Paediatr Drugs.* 2004;6(2):123-6.

[1652] Craig JO. Poisoning by the volatile oils in childhood. *Arch Dis Child.* 1953;28:259-67.

[1653] Melis K. Bochner A, Janssens G. Accidental nasal eucalyptol and menthol instillation. *Eur J Pediatr.* 1989 Aug;148(8)786-7.

[1654] Day LM, Ozanne-Smith J, Parsons BJ, et al. Eucalyptus oil poisoning among young children: mechanisms of access and the potential prevention. *Aust N Z J Public Health.* 1997 Jun;21(3):297-302.

[1655] Chandar SD, Prashanti M, Kumar CL, et al. Eucalyptus Oil-Induced Seizures in Children: A Single-Center Prospective Study. *Cureus.* 2021 Mar 25;13(3):e14109.

[1656] Rabl W, Katzgraber F, Steinlechner M. Camphor ingestion for abortion (case report). *Forensic Sci Int.* 1997 Sep 19;89(1-2):137-40.

[1657] Flaman Z, Pellechia-Clarke S, Bailey B, et al. Unintentional exposure of young children to camphor and eucalyptus oils. *Paediatr Child Health.* 2001 Feb;6(2):80-83.

[1658] Burkhard PR, Burkhardt K, Haenggeli CA, et al. Plant-induced seizures: reappearance of an old problem. *J Neurol.* 1999 Aug;246(8):667-70.

[1659] Narayan S, Singh N. Camphor poisoning-An unusual cause of seizure. *Med J Armed Forces India.* 2012 Jul;68(3):252-53.

[1660] Chanaranaj KJ, G MV, S M. Camphor poisoning in a child. *Natl Med J India.* 2013 Jan-Feb;26(1):60.

[1661] Manoguerra AS, Erdman AR, Wax PM, et al. Camphor poisoning: an evidence-based practice guideline for out-of- hospital management. *Clin Toxicol (Phila).*2006;44(4):357-70.

[1662] Gibson DE, Moore GP, Pfaff JA. Camphor ingestion. *Am J Emerg Med.* 1989 Jan;7(1):41-43.

[1663] Koppel C, Martends F, Schirop T, et al. Hemoperfusion in acute camphor poisoning. *Intensive Care Med.* 1988;14(4):431-33.

[1664] Olowe SA, Ransome-Kuti O. The risk of jaundice in glucose-6-phosphate dehydrogenase deficient babies exposed to menthol. *Acta Paediatr Scand.* 1980 May;69(3):341-5.

[1665] Dillon Remy M, Manning Alleyne P, Bratt DE, et al. Neonatal jaundice at Port-of-Spain General Hospital abstract. *West Indian Med J.* 1987;36(Suppl):28.

[1666] Uc A, Bishop WP, Sanders KD. Camphor hepatotoxicity. *South Med J.* 2000;93:596-98.

[1667] Cardoso NN, Alviano CS, Blank AF, et al. Synergism Effect of the Essential Oil from Ocimum basilicum var. Maria Bonita and Its Major Components with Fluconazole and Its Influence on Ergosterol Biosynthesis. *Evid Based Complement Alternat Med.* 2016;2016:5647182.

[1668] Covington TR, et al. Handbook of Nonprescription Drugs. 11<sup>th</sup> ed. Washington, D.C.: American Pharmaceutical Association. 1996.

[1669] Lee HJ, Hyun EA, Yoon WJ, et al. In vitro anti-inflammatory and anti-oxidative effects of Cinnamomum camphora extracts. *J Ethnopharmacology.* 2006 Jan;103(2):208-16.

[1670] Chen W, Vermaak I, Viljoen A. Camphor--a fumigant during the black death and a coveted fragrant wood in ancient Egypt and Babylon--a review. *Molecules.* 2013 May;18(5):5434-54.

[1671] Jiang H, Wang J, Song L, et al. GC×GC-TOFMS Analysis of Essential Oils Composition from Leaves, Twigs and Seeds of Cinnamomum camphora L. Presl and Their Insecticidal and Repellent Activities. *Molecules.* 2016;21(4):423.

[1672] Guo S, Geng Z, Zhang W, et al. The Chemical Composition of Essential Oils from Cinnamomum camphora and Their Insecticidal Activity against the Stored Product Pests. *Int J Mol Sci.* 2016 Nov 4;17(11).

[1673] Abu El Ezz NMT, Hassan NMF, El Namaky AH, et al. Efficacy of some essential oils on Cephalopina titillator with special concern to nasal myiasis prevalence among camels and its consequent histopathological changes. *J Parasit Dis.* 2018 Jun;42(2):196-203.

[1674] Moayedi Y, Greenberg SA, Jenkins BA, et al. Camphor white oil induces tumor regression through cytotoxic T cell-dependent mechanisms. *Mol Carcinog.* 2019 May;58(5):722-734.

[1675] Wu K, Lin Y, Chai X, et al. Mechanisms of vapor-phase antibacterial action of essential oil from Cinnamomum camphora var. linaloofera Fujita against Escherichia coli. *Food Sci Nutr.* 2019 Jul 4;7(8):2546-2555.

[1676] Wang L, Zhang K, Zhang K, et al, et al. Antibacterial Activity of Cinnamomum camphora Essential Oil on Escherichia coli During Planktonic Growth and Biofilm Formation. *Front Microbiol.* 2020 Nov 12;11:561002.

[1677] Poudel DK, Rokaya A, Ojha PK, et al. The Chemical Profiling of Essential Oils from Different Tissues of Cinnamomum camphora L. and Their Antimicrobial Activities. *Molecules.* 2021 Aug 24;26(17):5132.

[1678] Xiao S, Liu S, Yu H, et al. A Study on the Mechanism of the Sedative-hypnotic Effect of Cinnamomum camphora chvar. Borneol Essential Oil Based on Network Pharmacology. *J Oleo Sci.* 2022 Jul 1;71(7):1063-1073.

[1679] Veres K, Csupor-Loffler B, Lazar A, et al. Antifungal Activity and Composition of Essential Oils of Conyza canadensis Herbs and Roots. *Sci World J.* 2012;2012(2012):489646.

[1680] Lis A, Piggott JR, Gora J. Chemical composition variability of the essential oil of Conyza canadensis Cronq. *Flavour Frag J.* 2003 Sep-Oct;118(5):364-67.

[1681] Curini M, Bianchi A, Epifano F, et al. Composition and in vitro Antifungal Activity of Essential Oils of Erigeron canadensis and Myrtus communis from France. *Chem Nat Constituents.* 2003 Mar;39(2):191-94.

[1682] Gora J, Lis A, Kula J, et al. Chemical composition variability of the essential oils in the ontogenesis of some plants. *Flavour Frag J.* 2002;17:445-51.

[1683] Miyazawa M, Yamamoto K, Kameoka H. The essential oil of Erigeron Canadensis L. *J Essent Oil Res.* 1992 May-Jun;4:227-230.

[1684] Unnithan CR, Muuz M, Woldu A, et al. Chemical analysis of the essential oil of Erigeron Canadensis L. *UJPBS.* 2014;2(2):8-10.

[1685] Choi HJ, Wang HY, Kim YN, et al. Composition and Cytotoxicity of Essential Oil Extracted by Steam Distillation from Horseweed (Erigeron canadensis L.) in Korea. *J Korean Soc Appl Biological Chem.* 2008 Mar;51(1):55-59.

[1686] Veres K, Csupor-Loffler B, Lazar A, et al. Antifungal Activity and Composition of Essential Oils of Conyza canadensis Herbs and Roots. *Sci World J.* 2012;2012(2012):489646.

[1687] de las Heras B, Slowing K, Benedi J, et al. Antiinflammatory and antioxidant activity of plants used in traditional medicine in Ecuador. *J Ethnopharmacology.* 1998 Jun;61(2):161-66.

[1688] Mohammad SA, Venkateshwarlu K, Noor Ahmed VH, et al. Investigation of neuroprotective effects of Conyza Canadensis ethanolic extract on scopolamine induced cognitive impairment and oxidative stress in Swiss mice. *Int J Exp Pharmacology.* 2013;3(1)L1-10.

[1689] Hoi TM, Huong LT, Chinh HV, et al. Essential Oil Compositions of Three Invasive Conyza Species Collected in Vietnam and Their Larvicidal Activities against Aedes aegypti, Aedes albopictus, and Culex quinquefasciatus. *Molecules.* 2020 Oct 7;25(19):4576.

[1690] Weyerstahl P, Schneider S, Marschall H. Constituents of the Brazilian Cangerana oil. *Flavour Frag J.* 1996;11:81-84.

[1691] Piva AD, Ferronato R, Flach A, et al. Seasonal variation of the essential oil of Cabralea canjerana. *Chem Nat Comp.* 2014 Mar;50(1):151-52.

[1692] Nguyen LT, Mysliveckova Z, Szotakova B, et al. The inhibitory effects of β-caryophyllene, β-caryophyllene oxide and α-humulene on the activities of the main drug-metabolizing enzymes in rat and human liver in vitro. *Chem-Biol Interactoins.* 2017 Dec 25;278:123-8.

[1693] Piva AD, Ferronato R, Flach A, et al. Seasonal variation of the essential oil of Cabralea canjerana. *Chem Nat Comp.* 2014 Mar;50(1):151-52.

[1694] Mierendorff HG, Stahl-Biskup E, Posthumus MA, et al. Composition of commercial Cape chamomile oil (Eriocephalus punctulatus / Eriocephalus tenuifolius). *Flavour Frag J.* 2003 Nov;18(6):510-14.

[1695] Seo SM, Kim J, Kang J, et al. Fumigant toxicity and acetylcholinesterase inhibitory activity of 4 Asteraceae plant essential oils and their constituents against Japanese termite (Reticulitermes speratus Kolbe). *Pestic Biochem Physiol.* 2014 Jul;113:55-61.

[1696] Seo SM, Kim J, Kang J, et al. Fumigant toxicity and acetylcholinesterase inhibitory activity of 4 Asteraceae plant essential oils and their constituents against Japanese termite (Reticulitermes speratus Kolbe). *Pestic Biochem Physiol.* 2014 Jul;113:55-61.

[1697] Meshkatalsadat MH, Aalahvarzi S, Aminiradpoor R, et al. Identification of essential oil constituents of caraway (Carum carvi) using ultrasonic assist with headspace solid phase microextraction (UA-HS-SPME). *Digest J Nanonmaterials Biostructures.* 2012 Jun;7(2):637-40.

[1698] Laribi B, Kouki K, Mougou A, et al. Fatty acid and essential oil composition of three Tunisian caraway (Carum carvi L.) seed ecotypes. *J Sci Food Agric.* 2010 Feb;90(3):391-96.

[1699] Fang R, Jiang CH, Wang XY, et al. Insecticidal Activity of Essential Oil of Carum Carvi Fruits from China and Its Main Components against Two Grain Storage Insects. *Molecules.* 2010;15:9391-9402.

[1700] Raal A, Arak E, Orav A. The content and composition of the essential oil Found in Carum carvi L. commercial fruits obtained from different countries. *J Essent Oil Res.* 2012;24(1):53-59.

[1701] Fang R, Jiang CH, Wang XY, et al. Insecticidal Activity of Essential Oil of Carum Carvi Fruits from China and Its Main Components against Two Grain Storage Insects. *Molecules.* 2010;15:9391-9402.

[1702] Ene AC, Nwankwo EA, Samdi LM. Alloxan-induced diabetes in rats and the effects of black caraway (Carum carvi L.) oil on their body weight. *Res J Med Med Sci.* 2007;2:48–52.

[1703] Eddouks M, Lemhadri A, Michel JB. Caraway and caper: potential anti-hyperglycaemic plants in diabetic rats. *J Ethnopharmacol.* 2004;94:143–8.

[1704] Souza FV, da Rocha MB, de Souza DP, et al. (-)-Carvone: antispasmodic effect and mode of action. *Fitoterapia.* 2013 Mar;85:20-24.

[1705] Rajeshwari T, Raja B. Antihypertensive, antihyperlipidemicand antioxidantinfluence of D-carvone in L-NAME induced hypertensive rats. *Int J Pharmaceutical Biol Arch.* 2014;5(4):82-88.

[1706] de Sousa DP, Farias Nobrega FF, de Almeida RN. Influence of the chirality of (R)-(-)- and (S)-(+)-carvone in the central nervous system: a comparative study. *Chirality.* 2007 May;19(4):264-268.

[1707] Hawrelak JA, Cattley T, Myers SP. Essential oils in the treatment of intestinal dysbiosis: A preliminary in vitro study. *Altern Med Rev.* 2009 Dec;14(4):380-4.

[1708] Baananou S, Bagdonaite E, Marongiu B, et al. Extraction of the volatile oil from Carum carvi of Tunisia and Lithuania by supercritical carbon dioxide: chemical composition and antiulcerogenic activity. *Nat Prod Res.* 2013;27(22):2132-6.

[1709] Seo SM, Jung CS, Kang J, et al. Larvicidal and acetylcholinesterase inhibitory activities of Apiaceae plant essential oils and their constituents against Aedes albopictus and formulation development. *J Agric Food Chem.* 2015 Nov 18;63(45):9977-86.

[1710] Yeom HJ, Kang JS, Kim GH, et al. Insecticidal and acetylcholine esterase inhibition activity of Apiaceae plant essential oils and their constituents against adults of German cockroach (Blattella germanica). *J Agric Food Chem.* 2012 Jul 25;60(29):7194-203.

[1711] Pitasawat B, Champakaew D, Choochote W, et al. Aromatic plant-derived essential oil: an alternative larvicide for mosquito control. *Fitoterapia.* 2007 Apr;78(3):205-10.

[1712] Chaiyasit D, Choochote W, Rattanachanpichai E, et al. Essential oils as potential adulticides against two populations of Aedes aegypti, the laboratory and natural field strains, in Chiang Mai province, northern Thailand. *Parasitol Res.* 2006 Nov;99(6):715-21.

[1713] Dadkhah A, Fatemi F. Heart and kidney oxidative stress status in septic rats treated with caraway extracts. *Pharm Biol.* 2011 Jul;49(7):679-86.

[1714] Samojlik I, Lakić N, Mimica-Dukić N, et al. Antioxidant and hepatoprotective potential of essential oils of coriander (Coriandrum sativum L.) and caraway (Carum carvi L.) (Apiaceae). *J Agric Food Chem.* 2010 Aug 11;58(15):8848-53.

[1715] Fazlara A, Najafzadeh H, Lak E. The potential application of plant essential oils as natural preservatives against Escherichia coli O157:H7. *Pak J Biol Sci.* 2008 Sep 1;11(17):2054-61.

[1716] Mohsenzadeh M. Evaluation of antibacterial activity of selected Iranian essential oils against Staphylococcus aureus and Escherichia coli in nutrient broth medium. *Pak J Biol Sci.* 2007 Oct 15;10(20):3693-7.

[1717] Freise J, Köhler S. [Peppermint oil-caraway oil fixed combination in non-ulcer dyspepsia--comparison of the effects of enteric preparations]. *Pharmazie.* 1999 Mar;54(3):210-5.

[1718] May B, Kuntz HD, Kieser M, et al. Efficacy of a fixed peppermint oil/caraway oil combination in non-ulcer dyspepsia. *Arzneimittelforschung.* 1996 Dec;46(12):1149-53.

[1719] Madisch A, Heydenreich CJ, Wieland V, et al. Treatment of functional dyspepsia with a fixed peppermint oil and caraway oil combination preparation as compared to cisapride. A multicenter, reference-controlled double-blind equivalence study. *Arzneimittelforschung.* 1999 Nov;49(11):925-32.

[1720] May B, Köhler S, Schneider B. Efficacy and tolerability of a fixed combination of peppermint oil and caraway oil in patients suffering from functional dyspepsia. *Aliment Pharmacol Ther.* 2000 Dec;14(12):1671-7.

[1721] Holtmann G, Haag S, Adam B, et al. Effects of a fixed combination of peppermint oil and caraway oil on symptoms and quality of life in patients suffering from functional dyspepsia. *Phytomedicine.* 2003;10 Suppl 4:56-7.

[1722] Showraki A, Emamghoreishi M, Oftadegan S. Anticonvulsant Effect of the Aqueous Extract and Essential Oil of Carum Carvi L. Seeds in a Pentylenetetrazol Model of Seizure in Mice. *Iran J Med Sci.* 2016 May;41(3):200-208.

[1723] Bartoňková I, Dvořák Z. Essential oils of culinary herbs and spices display agonist and antagonist activities at human aryl hydrocarbon receptor AhR. *Food Chem Toxicol.* 2018 Jan;111:374-384.

[1724] Khatamian N, Homayouni Tabrizi M, Ardalan P, et al. Synthesis of Carum Carvi essential oil nanoemulsion, the cytotoxic effect, and expression of caspase 3 gene. *J Food Biochem.* 2019 Aug;43(8):e12956.

[1725] Khatamian N, Homayouni Tabrizi M, Ardalan P, et al. Synthesis of Carum Carvi essential oil nanoemulsion, the cytotoxic effect, and expression of caspase 3 gene. *J Food Biochem.* 2019 Aug;43(8):e12956.

[1726] Ben Salha G, Herrera Díaz R, Lengliz O, et al. Effect of the Chemical Composition of Free-Terpene Hydrocarbons Essential Oils on Antifungal Activity. *Molecules.* 2019 Sep 29;24(19).

[1727] Klys M, Izdebska A, Malejky-Klusek N. Repellent Effect of the Caraway Carum carvi L. on the Rice Weevil Sitophilus oryzae L. (Coleoptera, Dryophthoridae). *Insects.* 2020 Nov 26;11(12):E836.

[1728] Nasiri S, Ghahfarokhi MS, Abyaneh MR. Effect of Carum carvi essential oil on ERG6 gene expression and virulence factors in Candida albicans. *Curr Med Mycol.* 2020 Jun;6(2):30-36.

[1729] Maurya A, Kumar S, Singh BK, et al. Mechanistic investigations on antifungal and antiaflatoxigenic activities of chemically characterised Carum carvi L. essential oil against fungal infestation and aflatoxin contamination of herbal raw materials. *Nat Prod Res.* 2021 Oct 21;1-6.

[1730] Trifan A, Luca SV, Bostănaru AC, et al. Apiaceae Essential Oils: Boosters of Terbinafine Activity against Dermatophytes and Potent Anti-Inflammatory Effectors. *Plants (Basel).* 2021 Nov 4;10(11):2378.

[1731] Ghannay S, Aouadi K, Kadri A, et al. GC-MS Profiling, Vibriocidal, Antioxidant, Antibiofilm, and Anti-Quorum Sensing Properties of Carum carvi L. Essential Oil: In Vitro and In Silico Approaches. *Plants (Basel).* 2022 Apr 14;11(8):1072.

[1732] Dabowl AE, Mohsenzadeh M. Physicochemical, antioxidant, antibacterial and antibiofilm activity of Carum copticum essential oil nanoemulsion on Escherichia coli O157:H7 and Listeria monocytogenes. *Vet Res Forum.* 2021 Dec;12(4):437-444.

[1733] Alomar HA, Fathallah N, Abdel-Aziz MM, et al. GC-MS Profiling, Anti-Helicobacter pylori, and Anti-Inflammatory Activities of Three Apiaceous Fruits' Essential Oils. *Plants (Basel).* 2022 Oct 5;11(19):2617.

[1734] Aouini J, Bachrouch O, Msaada K, et al. Screening of antimicrobial and insecticidal properties of essential oils extracted from three Tunisian aromatic and medicinal plants. *Int J Environ Health Res.* 2023 Mar 9:1-11.

[1735] Liu C, Cheng F, Aisa HA, et al. Comprehensive Study of Components and Antimicrobial Properties of Essential Oil Extracted from Carum carvi L. Seeds. *Antibiotics (Basel).* 2023 Mar 16;12(3):591.

[1736] Alqarni MH, Foudah AI, Aodah AH, et al. Caraway Nanoemulsion Gel: A Potential Antibacterial Treatment against Escherichia coli and Staphylococcus aureus. *Gels.* 2023 Mar 3;9(3):193.

[1737] Abbasipour H, Mahmoudvand M, Rastegar F, et al. Fumigant toxicity and oviposition deterrency of the essential oil from cardamom, Elettaria cardamomum, against three stored—product insects. *J Insect Sci.* 2011;11:165.

[1738] Leela NK, Prasath D, Venugopal MN. Essential oil composition of selected cardamom genotypes at different maturity levels. *Indian J Hort.* 2008;65(3):366-69.

[1739] Padmakumari Amma KPA, Priya Rani M, Sasidharan I, et al. Chemical composition, flavonoid-phenolic contents and radical scavenging activity of four major varieties of cardamom. *Int J Biol Med Res.* 2010;1(3):20-24.

[1740] Asadollahi-Baboli M, Mani-Varnosfaderani A. Chemometrics-assisted GC-MS analysis of volatile and semi-volatile constituents of Elettaria cardamomum. *Food Anal Methods.* 2014 Oct;7(9):1745-54.

[1741] Leela NK, Prasath D, Venugopal MN. Essential oil composition of selected cardamom genotypes at different maturity levels. *Ind J Hort.* 2008 Aug;65(3):366-69.

[1742] Craig JO. Poisoning by the volatile oils in childhood. *Arch Dis Child.* 1953;28:259-67.

[1743] Melis K. Bochner A, Janssens G. Accidental nasal eucalyptol and menthol instillation. *Eur J Pediatr.* 1989 Aug;148(8)786-7.

[1744] Day LM, Ozanne-Smith J, Parsons BJ, et al. Eucalyptus oil poisoning among young children: mechanisms of access and the potential prevention. *Aust N Z J Public Health.* 1997 Jun;21(3):297-302.

[1745] Chandar SD, Prashanti M, Kumar CL, et al. Eucalyptus Oil-Induced Seizures in Children: A Single-Center Prospective Study. *Cureus.* 2021 Mar 25;13(3):e14109.

[1746] Burkhard PR, Burkhardt K, Haenggeli CA, et al. Plant-induced seizures: reappearance of an old problem. *J Neurol.* 1999 Aug;246(8):667-70.

[1747] Waldman N. Seizure caused by dermal application of over-the-counter eucalyptus oil head lice preparation. *Clin Toxicol (Phila).* 2011 Oct;49(7):750-1.

[1748] Craig JO. Poisoning by the volatile oils in childhood. *Arch Dis Child.* 1953;28:259-67.

[1749] Day LM, Ozanne-Smith J, Parsons BJ, et al. Eucalyptus oil poisoning among young children: mechanisms of access and the potential prevention. *Aust N Z J Public Health.* 1997 Jun;21(3):297-302.

[1750] Myott E. Case of eucalyptus poisoning. *Brit M J.* 1906;1:558.

[1751] Hindle RC. Eucalyptus oil ingestion. *N Z Med J.* 1994 May 11;107(977)185-6.

[1752] Tibballs J. Clinical effects and management of eucalyptus oil ingestion in infants and small children. *Med J Aust.* 1995 Aug;163(4):177-80.

[1753] Waldman W, Barwina M, Sein Anand J. Accidental ontoxication with eucalyptus oil—a case report. *Przeql Lek.* 2011;68(8):555-6.

[1754] Day LM, Ozanne-Smith J, Parsons BJ, et al. Eucalyptus oil poisoning among young children: mechanisms of access and the potential prevention. *Aust N Z J Public Health.* 1997 Jun;21(3):297-302.

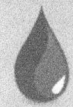

[1755] De Vincenzi M, Silano M, De Vincenzi A, et al. Constituents of aromatic plants: eucalyptol. *Fitoterapia.* 2002 Jun;73(3):269-75.
[1756] Banjeree S, Sharma R, Kale RK, et al. Influence of certain essential oils on carcinogen-metabolizing enzyme soluble sulfhydryls in mouse liver. *Nutr Cancer.* 1994;21(3):263-69.
[1757] Kim NH, Hyun SH, Jin CH, et al. Pretreatment with 1,8-cineole potentiates thioacetamide-induced hepatotoxicity and immunosuppression. *Arch Pharm Res.* 2004 Jul;27(7):781-9.
[1758] Jori A, Bianchetti A, Prestini PE, et al. Effect of eucalyptol (1,8-cineole) on the metabolism of other drugs in rats and in man. *Eur J Pharmacol.* 1970;9(3):362-66.
[1759] de Sousa DP, Raphael E, Brocksom U, et al. Sedative effect of monoterpene alcohols in mice: A preliminary screening. *Verlag der Zeitschrift fur Naturforschung.* 2007;62c:563-66.
[1760] Bhattacharjee B, Chatterjee J. Identification of proapoptopic, anti-inflammatory, anti-proliferative anti-invasive and anti-angiogenic targets of essential oils in cardamom by dual reverse virtual screening and binding pose analysis. *Asian Pac J Cancer Prev.* 2013;14(6):3735-42.
[1761] Acharya A, Das I, Singh S, et al. Chemopreventive properties of indole-3-carbinol, diindolylmethane and other constituents of cardamom against carcinogenesis. *Recent Pat Food Nutr Agric.* 2010 Jun;2(20:166-77.
[1762] Jamal A, Farah, Siddiqui A, et al. Antiulcerogenic activity of Elettaria cardamomum Maton. and Amomum subulatum Roxb. Seeds. *Ind J Trad Knowledge.* 2005 July;4(3):0972-5938.
[1763] Hashim S, Aboobaker VS, Madhubala R, et al. Modulatory effects of essential oils from spices on the formation of DNA adduct by aflatoxin B1 in vitro. *Nutr Cancer.* 1994;21(2):169-75.
[1764] Al-Zuhair H, el-Sayeh B, Ameen HA, et al. Pharmacological studies of cardamom oil in animals. *Pharmacol Res.* 1996 Jul-Aug;34(1-2):79-82.
[1765] Singh G, Kiran S, Marimuthu P, et al. Antioxidant and antimicrobial activities of the essential oil and various oleoresins of Elettaria cardamomum (seeds and pods). *J Sci Food Agric.* 2008 Jan;88(2):280-89.
[1766] Aneja KR, Joshi R. Antimicrobial Activity of Amomum subulatum and Elettaria cardamomum against dental caries causing microorganisms. *EBL.* 2009;2009(7):840-49.
[1767] Mutlu-Ingok A, Karbancioglu-Guler F. Cardamom, Cumin, and Dill Weed Essential Oils: Chemical Compositions, Antimicrobial Activities, and Mechanisms of Action against Campylobacter spp. *Molecules.* 2017 Jul 15;22(7).
[1768] Heimesaat MM, Mousavi S, Weschka D, et al. Anti-Pathogenic and Immune-Modulatory Effects of Peroral Treatment with Cardamom Essential Oil in Acute Murine Campylobacteriosis. *Microorganisms.* 2021;9(1):169.
[1769] Alam A, Rehman NU, Ansari MN, et al. Effects of Essential Oils of Elettaria cardamomum Grown in India and Guatemala on Gram-Negative Bacteria and Gastrointestinal Disorders. *Molecules.* 2021 Apr 27;26(9):2546.
[1770] Pourkhosravani E, Nayeri FD, Bazargani MM. Decoding antibacterial and antibiofilm properties of cinnamon and cardamom essential oils: a combined molecular docking and experimental study. *AMB Express.* 2021 Oct 26;11(1):143.
[1771] Khatiban M, Mirzaie M, Fazeli A, et al. Effect of Cardamom Inhalation Therapy on Intra-and Postoperative Nausea and Vomiting of Mothers Undergoing Spinal Anesthesia for Elective Cesarean Section. *J PeriAnesthesia Nursing.* 2022 May 14;000:1-6.
[1772] Alanazi AD, Ben Said M, Shater AF, et al. Acaricidal, Larvacidal, and Repellent Activity of Elettaria cardamomum Essential Oil against Hyalomma anatolicum Ticks Infesting Saudi Arabian Cattle. *Plants (Basel).* 2022 Apr 30;11(9):1221.
[1773] Almohammed HI, Alkhaibari AM, Alanazi AD. Antiparasitic effects of Elettaria cardamomum L. essential oil and its main compounds, 1-8 Cineole alone and in combination with albendazole against Echinococcus granulosus protoscoleces. *Saudi J Biol Sci.* 2022 Apr;29(4):2811-2818.
[1774] Tarfaoui K, Brhadda N, Ziri R, et al. Chemical Profile, Antibacterial and Antioxidant Potential of Zingiber officinale Roscoe and Elettaria cardamomum (L.) Maton Essential Oils and Extracts. *Plants (Basel).* 2022 May 31;11(11):1487.
[1775] Noumi E, Alshammari GS, Zmantar T, et al. Antibiofilm Potential and Exoenzyme Inhibition by Elattaria cardamomum Essential Oil in Candida spp. Strains. *Life (Basel).* 2022 Nov 1;12(11):1756.
[1776] Vukovic NL, Vukic MD, Obradovic AD, et al. GC, GC/MS Analysis, and Biological Effects of Essential Oils from Thymus mastchina and Elettaria cardamomum. *Plants (Basel).* 2022 Nov 23;11(23):3213.
[1777] Castillo NET, Teresa-Martínez GD, Alonzo-Macías M, et al. Antioxidant Activity and GC-MS Profile of Cardamom (Elettaria cardamomum) Essential Oil Obtained by a Combined Extraction Method-Instant Controlled Pressure Drop Technology Coupled with Sonication. *Molecules.* 2023 Jan 21;28(3):1093.
[1778] Ozcan MM, Chalchat JC. Chemical composition of carrot seed seeds (Daucus carota L.) cultivated in Turkey: characterization of the seed oil and essential oil. *Grasas y Aceites.* 20007;58(4):359-65.
[1779] Misiak IJ, Lipok J, Nowakowska EM, et al. Antifungal activity of the carrot seed oil and its major sesquiterpene constituents. *Verlag der Zeitschrift fur Naturforschung, Tubingen.* 2004;59c:791-96.
[1780] Sharma MM, Lal G, Jacob D. Estrogenic and pregnancy interceptor effects of carrot seed daucus carota seeds. *Indian J Exp Biol.* 1976 Jul;14(4):506-8.
[1781] Keenan DL, Dharmarajan AM, Zacur HA. Dietary carrot seed results in diminished ovarian progesterone secretion, whereas a metabolite, retinoic acid, stimulates progesterone secretion in the in vitro perfused rabbit ovary. *Fertil Steril.* 1997 Aug;68(2):358-63.
[1782] Dong JY, Xue LQ, Zhu XW, et al. Antifertility agents from seeds of Daucus carota. *Zhongcaoyao.* 1981;12:61.
[1783] Abad MJ, Ansuategui M, Bermejo P. Active antifungal substances from natural sources. *ARKIVOC.* 2007;7:116-45.
[1784] Muturi EJ, Doll K, Ramirez JL, et al. Bioactivity of Wild Carrot (Daucus carota, Apiaceae) Essential Oil Against Mosquito Larvae. *J Med Entomol.* 2019 Apr 16;56(3):784-789.
[1785] Chiboub W, Sassi AB, Amina CM, et al. Valorization of the Green Waste from Two Varieties of Fennel and Carrot Cultivated in Tunisia by Identification of the Phytochemical Profile and Evaluation of the Antimicrobial Activities of Their Essentials Oils. *Chem Biodivers.* 2019 Jan;16(1):e1800546.
[1786] Ali A, Radwan MM, Wanas AS, et al. Repellent Activity of Carrot Seed Essential Oil and Its Pure Compound, Carotol, Against Mosquitoes. *J Am Mosq Control Assoc.* 2018 Dec;34(4):272-280.
[1787] Luc D, Michel BJ, Vanina L, et al. Antibacterial Mode of Action of the Daucus carota Essential Oil Active Compounds against Campylobacter jejuni and Efflux-Mediated Drug Resistance in Gram-Negative Bacteria. *Molecules.* 2020 Nov 20;25(22):5448.
[1788] Badalamenti N, Modica A, Ilardi V, et al. Daucus carota subsp. maximus (Desf.) Ball from Pantelleria, Sicily (Italy): isolation of essential oils and evaluation of their bioactivity. *Nat Prod Res.* 2021 Dec 19:1-6.
[1789] Koroch A, Ranarivelo L, Behr O, et al. Quality attributes of ginger and cinnamon essential oils from Madagascar. *Bot Med.* 2007:338-41.
[1790] Liu XC, Cheng J, Zhao NN, et al. Insecticidal activity of essential oil of Cinnamomum cassia and its main constituent, trans-cinnamaldehyde, against the Booklice, Liposcelis bostrychophila. *Trop J Pharm Res.* 2014 Oct;13(10):1697-1702.
[1791] Kong JO, Lee SM, Moon YS, et al. Nematicidal activity of cassia and cinnamon oil constituents and related constituents toward Bursaphelenchus xylophilus (Nematoda: Parasitaphelenchidae). *J Nematol.* 2007 Mar;39(1):31-36.
[1792] Chang CT, Chang WL, Hsu JC, et al. Chemical composition and tyrosine inhibitory activity of Cinnamomum cassia essential oil. *Botanical Studies.* 2012;54(10):1-7.
[1793] Kocevski D, Du M, Kan J, et al. Antifungal effect of Allium tuberosum, Cinnamomum cassia, and Pogostemon cablin essential oils and their components against population of Aspergillus species. *Food Microbiol Safety.* 2013 May;78(5):M731-37.
[1794] Pannee C, Chandhanee I, Wacharee L. Anti-inflammatory effects of essential oil from the leaves of Cinnamomum cassia and cinnamaldehyde on lipopolysaccharide-stimulated J774A.1 cells. *J Adv Pharm Technol Res.* 2014;5(4):164- 70.
[1795] Mith H, Dure R, Delcenserie V, et al. Antimicrobial activities of commercial essential oils and their components against food-borne pathogens and food spoilage bacteria. *Food Sci Nutr.* 2014 Jul;2(4):403-16.
[1796] Li YQ, Kong DX, Huang RS, et al. Variations in essential oil yields and compositions of Cinnamomum cassia leaves at different developmental stages. *Ind Crops Prod.* 2013 May;47:91-101.
[1797] Domaracky M, Rehak P, Juhas S, et al. Effects of selected plant essential oils on the growth and development of mouse preimplantation embryos in vivo. *Physiol Res.* 2007;56(1):97-104.
[1798] Forschmidt P. Teratogenic activity of flavor additives. *Teratology.* 1979;19:26A.
[1799] Mantovani A, Stazi AV, Macri C, et al. Pre-natal (segment II) toxicity study of cinnamic aldehyde in the Sprague- Dawley rat. *Food Chem Toxicol.* 1989;27:781-86.
[1800] Huang J, Wang S, Luo X, et al. Cinnamaldehyde reduction of platelet aggregation and thrombosis in rodents. *Thromb Res.* 2007;119(3):337-42.
[1801] Kim SY, Koo YK, Koo JY, et al. Platelet anti-aggregation activities of constituents from Cinnamomum cassia. *J Med Food.* 2010 Oct;13(5):1069-74.
[1802] Takenaga M, Hirai A, Terano T, et al. In vitro effect of cinnamic aldehyde, a main component of Cinnamomi Cortex, on human platelet aggregation and arachidonic acid metabolism. *J Pharmacobiodyn.* 1987 May;10(5):201-208.
[1803] Mack TS, Raner GM. Regulation of cytochrome P450 2A6 and phase II enzymes by unsaturated aldehydes. University of North Carolina at Greensboro. Available at: http://libres.uncg.edu/ir/uncg/listing.aspx?id=2343.
[1804] Wickramasinghe RH, Muller G, Norpoth K. Spectral evidence of interaction of spice constituents with hepatic microsomal cytochrome P-450. *Cytobios.* 1980;29(113):25-27.
[1805] Singh G, Maurya S, deLampasona MP, et al. A comparison of chemical antioxidant and antimicrobial studies of cinnamon leaf and bark volatile oils, oleoresins and their constituents. *Food Chem Toxicol.* 2007;45:1650–61.
[1806] Verspohl EJ, Bauer K, Neddermann E. Antidiabetic effect of Cinnamomum cassia and Cinnamomum zeylanicum in vivo and in vitro. *Phytother. Res.* 2005 Mar;19(3):203-06.
[1807] Hua P, Guijun Z, Guixing R. Antidiabetic effects of cinnamon oil in diabetic KK-A mice. *Food Chem Toxicol.* 2010 Aug-Sep;48(8-9):2344-9.
[1808] Sung HK, Sun HH, Choung SY. Anti-diabetic effect of cinnamon extract on blood glucose in db/db mice. *J Ethnopharmacol.* 2006 Mar 8;104(1-2):119-23.
[1809] Langeveld WT, Veldhuizen EJ, Burt SA. Synergy between essential oil constituents and antibiotics. *Crit Rev Microbiol.* 2014 Feb;40(1);76-94.
[1810] Palaniappan K, Holley RA. Use of natural antimicrobials to increase antibiotic susceptibility of drug resistant bacteria. *In J Food Microbiol.* 2010 Jun 15;140(2-3):164-8.
[1811] National Toxicology Program. Cinnamaldehyde. 1989 Dec. Available at: https://ntp.niehs.nih.gov/ntp/htdocs/chem_background/exsumpdf/cinnamaldehyde_508.pdf.
[1812] National Toxicology Program. Cinnamaldehyde. 1989 Dec. Available at: https://ntp.niehs.nih.gov/ntp/htdocs/chem_background/exsumpdf/cinnamaldehyde_508.pdf.
[1813] Pannee C, Chandhanee I, Wacharee L. Anti-inflammatory effects of essential oils from the leaves of Cinnamomum cassia and cinnamaldehyde on lipopolysaccharide-stimulated J774A.1 cells. *J Adv Pharm Technol Res.* 2014 Oct;5(4):164-70.
[1814] Sun L, Zong SB, Li JC, et al. The essential oil from the twigs of Cinnamomum cassia Presl alleviates pain and inflammation in mice. *J Ethnopharmacol.* 2016 Dec 24;194:904-912.
[1815] Naveed R, Hussain I, Tawab A, et al. Antimicrobial activity of the bioactive components of essential oils from Pakistani species against Salmonella and other multi-drug resistant bacteria. *BMC Complement Altern Med.* 2013 Oct;13:265.
[1816] Ooi LSM, Li Y, Kam SL, et al. Antimicrobial activities of cinnamon oil and cinnamaldehyde from the Chinese medicinal herb Cinnamomum cassia Blume. *Am J Chin Med.* 2006;34(3):511.

1817 Raffaella C, Casettari L, Fagioli L, et al. Activity of essential oil-based microemulsions against Staphylococcus aureus biofilms developed on stainless steel surface in different culture media and growth conditions. *Int J Food Microbiol*. 2016 Oct 17;241:132-140.

1818 Oussalah M, Caillet S, Lacroix M. Mechanism of action of Spanish oregano, Chinese cinnamon, and savory essential oils against cell membranes and walls of Escherichia coli O157:H7 and Listeria monocytogenes. *J Food Prot*. 2006 May;69(5):1046-55.

1819 Verspohl EJ, Bauer K, Neddermann E. Antidiabetic effect of Cinnamomum cassia and Cinnamomum zeylanicum in vivo and in vitro. *Phytother Res*. 2005 Mar;19(3):203-06.

1820 Dugoua JJ, Seely D, Perri D, et al. From type 2 diabetes to antioxidant activity: a systematic review of the safety and efficacy of common and cassia cinnamon bark. *Can J Phys Pharm*. 2007;85(9):837-47.

1821 Hayashi K, Imanishi N, Kashiwayama Y, et al. Inhibitory effect of cinnamaldehyde, derived from Cinnamoni cortex, on the growth of influenza A/PR/8 virus in vitro and in vivo. *Antiviral Res*. 2007 Apr;74(1):1-8.

1822 Chou ST, Chang WL, Chang CT, et al. Cinnamomum cassia essential oil inhibits α-MSH-induced melanin production and oxidative stress in murine B16 melanoma cells. *Int J Mol Sci*. 2013 Sep 18;14(9):19186-201.

1823 García P, Ramallo IA, Furlan RL. Reverse Phase Compatible TLC-Bioautography for Detection of Tyrosinase Inhibitors. *Phytochem Anal*. 2017 Mar;28(2):101-105.

1824 Hayashi K, Imanishi N, Kashiwayama Y, et al. Inhibitory effect of cinnamaldehyde, derived from Cinnamomi cortex, on the growth of influenza A/PR/8 virus in vitro and in vivo. *Antiviral Res*. 2007 Apr;74(1):1-8.

1825 Yones DA, Bakir HY, Bayoumi SA, et al. Chemical composition and efficacy of some selected plant oils against Pediculus humanus capitis in vitro. *Parasitol Res*. 2016 Aug;115(8):3209-18.

1826 Almeida Lde F, Paula JF, Almeida RV, et al. Efficacy of citronella and cinnamon essential oils on Candida albicans biofilms. *Acta Odontol Scand*. 2016 Jul;74(5):393-8.

1827 Kim J, Jang M, Shin E, et al. Fumigant and contact toxicity of 22 wooden essential oils and their major components against Drosophila suzukii (Diptera: Drosophilidae). *Pestic Biochem Physiol*. 2016 Oct;133:35-43.

1828 Jeon YJ, Lee SG, Yang YC, et al. Insecticidal activities of their components derived from the essential oils of Cinnamomum sp. barks and against Ricania sp. (Homoptera: Ricaniidae), a newly recorded pest. *Pest Manag Sci*. 2017 Oct;73(10):2000-2004.

1829 Le TB, Beaufay C, Nghiem DT, et al. In Vitro Anti-Leishmanial Activity of Essential Oils Extracted from Vietnamese Plants. *Molecules*. 2017 Jun 27;22(7).

1830 Gucwa K, Milewski S, Dymerski T, et al. Investigation of the Antifungal Activity and Mode of Action of Thymus vulgaris, Citrus limonum, Pelargonium graveolens, Cinnamomum cassia, Ocimum basilicum, and Eugenia caryophyllus Essential Oils. *Molecules*. 2018 May 8;23(5).

1831 Firmino DF, Cavalcante TTA, Gomes GA, et al. Antibacterial and Antibiofilm Activities of Cinnamomum Sp. Essential Oil and Cinnamaldehyde: Antimicrobial Activities. *ScientificWorldJournal*. 2018 Jun 6;2018:7405736.

1832 Ács K, Balázs VL, Kocsis B, et al. Antibacterial activity evaluation of selected essential oils in liquid and vapor phase on respiratory tract pathogens. *BMC Complement Altern Med*. 2018 Jul 27;18(1):227.

1833 Powers CN, Osier JL, McFeeters RL, et al. Antifungal and Cytotoxic Activities of Sixty Commercially-Available Essential Oils. *Molecules*. 2018 Jun 27;23(7).

1834 El Atki Y, Aouam I, El Kamari F, et al. Antibacterial activity of cinnamon essential oils and their synergistic potential with antibiotics. *J Adv Pharm Technol Res*. 2019 Apr-Jun;10(2):63-67.

1835 Onder A, Yilmaz-Oral D, Jarkovic I, et al. Evaluation of relaxant responses properties of cinnamon essential oil and its major component, cinnamaldehyde on human and rat corpus cavernosum. *Int Braz J Urol*. 2019 Jun 20;45.

1836 Kozics K, Buckova M, Puskarova A, et al. The Effect of Ten Essential Oils on Several Cutaneous Drug-Resistant Microorganisms and Their Cyto/Genotoxic and Antioxidant Properties. Molecules. 2019 Dec 13;24(24):24244570.

1837 Cheng WX, Zhong S, Meng XB, et al. Cinnamaldehyde Inhibits Inflammation of Human Synoviocyte Cells Through Regulation of Jak/Stat Pathway and Ameliorates Collagen-Induced Arthritis in Rats. *J Pharmacol Exp Ther*. 2020 May;373(2):302-310.

1838 Ramazani E, YazdFazeli M, Emami SA, et al. Protective effects of Cinnamomum verum, Cinnamomum cassia and cinnamaldehyde against 6-OHDA-induced apoptosis in PC12 cells. *Mol Biol Rep*. 2020 Mar 12. [Epub ahead of print]

1839 Netopilova M, Houdkova M, Urbanova K, et al. In vitro antimicrobial combinatory effect of Cinnamomum cassia essential oil with 8-hydroxyquinoline against Staphylococcus aureus in liquid and vapour phase. *J Appl Microbiol*. 2020 Apr 29. [Epub ahead of print]

1840 Kozics K, Buckova M, Puskarova A, et al. The Effect of Ten Essential Oils on Several Cutaneous Drug-Resistant Microorganisms and Their Cyto/Genotoxic and Antioxidant Properties. *Molecules*. 2019 Dec 13;24(24):4570.

1841 Vasconcelos NG, de Sa Queiroz JHF, da Silva KE, et al. Synergistic effects of Cinnamomum cassia L. essential oil in combination with polymyxin B against carbapenemase-producing Klebsiella pneumoniae and Serratia marcescens. *PLoS One*. 2020 Jul 23;15(7):e0236505.

1842 Vasconcelos NG, Silva KE, Croda J, et al. Antibacterial activity of Cinnamomum cassia L. essential oil in a carbapenem- and polymyxin-resistant Klebsiella aerogenes strain. *Rev Soc Bras Med Trop*. 2020 Oct 5;53:e20200032.

1843 Dumas E, Degraeve P, Trinh NTT, et al. Inter-strains comparison of the antimicrobial effect and mode of action of a Vietnamese Cinnamomum cassia essential oil from leaves and its principal component against Listeria monocytogenes. *Lett Appl Microbiol*. 2021 Feb 17. Online ahead of print.

1844 Huang Y, Liu H, Liu S, et al. Cinnamon Cassia Oil Emulsions Stabilized by Chitin Nanofibrils: Physicochemical Properties and Antibacterial Activities. *J Agric Food Chem*. 2020 Dec 9;68(49):14620-14631.

1845 Nwanade CF, Wang M, Wang T, et al. Acaricidal activity of Cinnamomum cassia (Chinese cinnamon) against the tick Haemaphysalis longicornis is linked to its content of (E)-cinnamaldehyde. *Parasit Vectors*. 2021 Jun 22;14(1):330.

1846 Li C, Luo Y, Zhang W, et al. A comparative study on chemical compositions and biological activities of four essential oils: Cymbopogon citratus (DC.) Stapf, Cinnamomum cassia (L.) Presl, Salvia japonica Thunb. and Rosa rugosa Thumb. *J Ethnopharmacol*. 2021 Jul 28;114472.

1847 Bordin C, Alves DS, Alves LFA, et al. Fumigant activity of essential oils from Cinnamomum and Citrus spp. and pure compounds against Dermanyssus gallinae (De Geer) (Acari: Dermanyssidae) and toxicity toward the nontarget organism Beauveria bassiana (Vuill.). *Vet Parasitol*. 2021 Feb;290:109341.

1848 Ginting EV, Retnaningrum E, Widiasih DA. Antibacterial activity of clove (Syzygium aromaticum) and cinnamon (Cinnamomum burmannii) essential oil against extended-spectrum β-lactamase-producing bacteria. *Vet World*. 2021 Aug;14(8):2206-2211.

1849 Lang M, Montjarret A, Duteil E, et al. Cinnamomum cassia and Syzygium aromaticum Essential Oils Reduce the Colonization of Salmonella Typhimurium in an In Vivo Infection Model Using Caenorhabditis elegans. *Molecules*. 2021 Sep 15;26(18):5598.

1850 Rodriguez Diaz C, Mith H, Bernard T, et al. In vitro study of antimicrobial activity of essential oils and their components against the main Clostridioides difficile PCR-ribotypes isolated in Belgium. *IAFP Eur Congress*. 2021.

1851 Dos Santos LR, Alía A, Martin I, et al. Antimicrobial activity of essential oils and natural plant extracts against Listeria monocytogenes in a dry-cured ham-based model. *J Sci Food Agric*. 2021 Aug 11. Online ahead of print.

1852 Liang D, Feng B, Li N, et al. Preparation, characterization, and biological activity of Cinnamomum cassia essential oil nano-emulsion. *Ultrason Sonochem*. 2022 Apr 20;86:106009.

1853 Xu X, Li Q, Dong W, et al. Cinnamon cassia oil chitosan nanoparticles: Physicochemical properties and anti-breast cancer activity. *Int J Biol Macromol*. 2022 Nov 7:S0141-8130(22)02433-3.

1854 Rosato R, Napoli E, Granata G, et al. Study of the Chemical Profile and Anti-Fungal Activity against Candida auris of Cinnamomum cassia Essential Oil and of Its Nano-Formulations Based on Polycaprolactone. *Plants (Basel)*. 2023 Jan 12;12(2):358.

1855 Alam A, Ansari MJ, Alqarni MH, et al. Antioxidant, Antibacterial, and Anticancer Activity of Ultrasonic Nanoemulsion of Cinnamomum Cassia L. Essential Oil. *Plants (Basel)*. 2023 Feb 13;12(4):834.

1856 Zomorodian K, Jamal Saharkhiz M, Javad Rahimi M, et al. Chemical Composition and Antimicrobial Activities of Essential Oil of Nepeta Cataria L. Against Common Causes of Oral Infections. *J Dent (Tehran)*. 2013 Jul;10(4):329–37.

1857 De Pooter HL, Nicolai B, De Laet J, et al. The essential oils of five Nepeta Species. A preliminary evaluation of their use in chemotaxonomy by cluster analysis. *Flavour Frag J*. 1988 Dec;3(4):155-59.

1858 Srifi A, Rahmoudi B, Bouisisa El, et al. Étude phytochimique et activité antifongique in vitro des huiles essentielles de quatre espèces du genre Nepeta du Maroc. *Phytothérapie*. 2013 Jun;11(3):161-71.

1859 Mortexa-Semnani K, Saeeedi M. Essential oils composition of Nepeta cataria L. and Nepeta crassifolia Boiss. and Buhse from Iran. *J Essent Oil Res*. 2007;7(2):120-24.

1860 Bourrel C, Perineau F, Michel G, et al. Catnip (Nepeta cataria L.) Essential Oil: Analysis of Chemical Constituents, Bacteriostatic and Fungistatic Properties. *J Essent Oil Res*. 1993;5(2):159-67.

1861 Mohammadi S, Jamal Saharkhiz M. Changes in Essential Oil Content and Composition of Catnip (Nepeta cataria L.) During Different Developmental Stages. *J Essent Oil-Bearing Plants*. 2013 Mar;14(2):396-400.

1862 Filani A, Shah AJ, Zubair A, et al. Chemical composition and mechanisms underlying the spasmolytic and bronchodilatory properties of the essential oil of Nepeta cataria L. *J Ethnopharmacology*. 2009;121(3):405-11.

1863 Adiguzel A, Ozer H, Sokmen M, et al. Antimicrobial and antioxidant activity of the essential oil and methanol extract of Nepeta cataria. *Polish J Microbiol*. 2009;58(1):69-76.

1864 Sharma A, Singh Cannoo D. Phytochemical composition of essential oils isolated from different species of genus Nepeta of Labiatae family: A review. *Pharmacophore*. 2013;4(6):181-211.

1865 Harney JW, Barofsky IM, Leary JD. Behavioral and toxicological studies of cyclopentanoid monoterpenes from Nepeta cataria. *Lloydia*. 1978 Jul-Aug;41(4):367-74.

1866 McElvain SM, Bright RD, Johnson PR. The Constituents of the Volatile Oil of Catnip. I. Nepetalic Acid, Nepetalactone and Related Constituents. *J American Chemical Society*. 1941;63(6):1558-63.

1867 Sharma A, Singh Cannoo D. Phytochemical composition of essential oils isolated from different species of genus Nepeta of Labiatae family: A review. *Pharmacophore*. 2013;4(6):181-211.

1868 Saeidnia S, Gohari AR, Haddadi A, et al. Presence of monoterpene synthase in four Labiatae species and Solid-Phase Microextraction- Gas chromatography-Mass Spectroscopy analysis of their aroma profiles. *Pharmacognosy Res*. 2014 Apr;6(2):138-42.

1869 Saeidnia S, Gohari AR, Hadjiakhoondi A. Trypanocidal Activity of Oil of the Young Leaves of Nepeta cataria L. Obtained by Solvent Extraction. *J Med Plants*. 2007 Dec;7(Suppl 4):54-57.

1870 Sherry CJ, Hunter PS. The effect of an ethanol extract of catnip (Nepeta cataria) on the behavior of the young chick. *Experientia*. 1979 Feb 15;35(2):237-8.

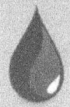

[1871] Harney JW, Barofsky IM, Leary JD. Behavioral and toxicological studies of cyclopentanoid monoterpenes from Nepeta cataria. *Lloydia*. 1978 Jul-Aug;41(4):367-74.

[1872] Massoco CO, Silva MR, Gorniak SL, et al. Behavioral effects of acute and long-term administration of catnip (Nepeta cataria) in mice. *Vet Hum Toxicol*. 1995 Dec;37(6):530-3.

[1873] Osterhoudt KC, Lee SK, Callahan JM, et al. Catnip and the alteration of human consciousness. *Vet Hum Toxicol*. 1997 Dec;39(6):373-5.

[1874] Jackson B, Reed A. Catnip and the alteration of consciousness. *JAMA*. 1969 Feb 17;207(7):1349-50.

[1875] Zomorodian K, Jamal Saharkhiz M, Javad Rahimi M, et al. Chemical Composition and Antimicrobial Activities of Essential Oil of Nepeta Cataria L. Against Common Causes of Oral Infections. *J Dent (Tehran)*. 2013 Jul;10(4):329–37.

[1876] Srifi A, Rahmoudi B, Bouisisa El, et al. Étude phytochimique et activité antifongique in vitro des huiles essentielles de quatre espèces du genre Nepeta du Maroc. *Phytothérapie*. 2013 Jun;11(3):161-71.

[1877] Bourrel C, Perineau F, Michel G, et al. Catnip (Nepeta cataria L.) Essential Oil: Analysis of Chemical Constituents, Bacteriostatic and Fungistatic Properties. *J Essent Oil Res*. 1993;5(2):159-67.

[1878] Adiguzel A, Ozer H, Sokmen M, et al. Antimicrobial and antioxidant activity of the essential oil and methanol extract of Nepeta cataria. *Polish J Microbiol*. 2009;58(1):69-76.

[1879] Filani A, Shah AJ, Zubair A, et al. Chemical composition and mechanisms underlying the spasmolytic and bronchodilatory properties of the essential oil of Nepeta cataria L. *J Ethnopharmacology*. 2009;121(3):405-11.

[1880] Ricci EL, Toyama DO, Guilardi Lago JH, et al. Anti-nociceptive and anti-inflammatory actions of Nepeta cataria L. var. citriodora (Becker) Balb. essential oil in mice. *J Health Sci Inst*. 2010;28(3):289-93. (*Note, the title misidentifies the essential oil as *N. cataria* L. var. *citriodora* Balbis. when the composition and the rest of the study identifies it as *N. cataria* nepetalactone CT).

[1881] Obermayr U, Ruther J, Bernier UR, et al. Evaluation of a Push-Pull Approach for Aedes aegypti (L.) Using a Novel Dispensing System for Spatial Repellents in the Laboratory and in a Semi-Field Environment. *PLoS One*. 2015 Jun 26;10(6):e0129878.

[1882] Khan MA, Jones I, Loza-Reyes E, et al. Interference in foraging behaviour of European and American house dust mites Dermatophagoides pteronyssinus and Dermatophagoides farinae (Acari: Pyroglyphidae) by catmint, Nepeta cataria (Lamiaceae). *Exp Appl Acarol*. 2012 May;57(1):65-74.

[1883] Zhu JJ, Berkebile DR, Dunlap CA, et al. Nepetalactones from essential oil of Nepeta cataria represent a stable fly feeding and oviposition repellent. *Med Vet Entomol*. 2012 Jun;26(2):131-8.

[1884] Birkett MA, Hassanali A, Hoglund S, et al. Repellent activity of catmint, Nepeta cataria, and iridoid nepetalactone isomers against Afro-tropical mosquitoes, ixodid ticks and red poultry mites. *Phytochemistry*. 2011 Jan;72(1):109-14.

[1885] Zhu JJ, Zeng XP, Berkebile D, et al. Efficacy and safety of catnip (Nepeta cataria) as a novel filth fly repellent. *Med Vet Entomol*. 2009 Sep;23(3):209-16.

[1886] Spero NC, Gonzalez YI, Scialdone MA, et al. Repellency of hydrogenated catmint oil formulations to black flies and mosquitoes in the field. *J Med Entomol*. 2008 Nov;45(6):1080-6.

[1887] Amer A, Mehlhorn H. Repellency effect of forty-one essential oils against Aedes, Anopheles, and Culex mosquitoes. *Parasitol Res*. 2006 Sep;99(4):478-90.

[1888] Peterson CJ, Ems-Wilson J. Catnip essential oil as a barrier to subterranean termites (Isoptera: Rhinotermitidae) in the laboratory. *J Econ Entomol*. 2003 Aug;96(4):1275-82.

[1889] Spero NC, Gonzalez YI, Scialdone MA, et al. Repellency of hydrogenated catmint oil formulations to black flies and mosquitoes in the field. *J Med Entomol*. 2008 Nov;45(6):1080-6.

[1890] Amer A, Mehlhorn H. Repellency effect of forty-one essential oils against Aedes, Anopheles, and Culex mosquitoes. *Parasitol Res*. 2006 Sep;99(4):478-90.

[1891] Peterson CJ, Nemetz LT, Jones LM, et al. Behavioral activity of catnip (Lamiaceae) essential oil components to the German cockroach (Blattodea: Blattellidae). *J Econ Entomol*. 2002 Apr;95(2):377-80.

[1892] Sparks JT, Bohbot JD, Ristic M, et al. Chemosensory Responses to the Repellent Nepeta Essential Oil and Its Major Component Nepetalactone by Aedes aegypti (Diptera: Culicidae), a Vector of Zika Virus. *J Med Entomol*. 2017 Jul 1;54(4):957-963.

[1893] Patience GS, Karirekinyana G, Galli F, et al. Sustainable manufacture of insect repellents derived from Nepeta cataria. *Sci Rep*. 2018 Feb 2;8(1):2235.

[1894] Reichert W, Ejercito J, Guda T, et al. Repellency Assessment of Nepeta cataria Essential Oils and Isolated Nepetalactones on Aedes aegypti. *Sci Rep*. 2019 Feb 6;9(1):1524.

[1895] Tan J, Qiao F. Hepatoprotective Effect of Essential Oils of Nepeta cataria L. on Acetaminophen-induced Liver Dysfunction. *Biosci Rep*. 2019 Aug 7;39(8).

[1896] Stepanycheva E, Petrova M, Chermensjaya T, et al. Fumigant Effect of Essential Oils on Mortality and Fertility of Thrips Frankliniella Occidentalis Perg. *Environ Sci Pollut Res Int*. 2019 Oct;26(30):30885-30892.

[1897] Arantes SM. Picarra A, Guerreiro M, et al. Toxicological and Pharmacological Properties of Essential Oils of Calamintha Nepeta, Origanum Virens and Thymus Mastichina of Alentejo (Portugal). *Food Chem Toxicol*. 2019 Nov;133:110747.

[1898] Zahirnia A, Boroomand M, Nasirian H, et al. Comparing Cytotoxicity of Propoxur and Nepeta crispa (Lamiales: Lamiaceae) Essential Oil Against Invertebrate (Sf9) and Vertebrate (L929) Cell Lines. *Vet World*. 2019 Nov;12(11):1698-1706.

[1899] Yang S, Bai M, Yang J, et al. Chemical Composition and Larvicidal Activity of Essential Oils From Peganum harmala, Nepeta cataria and Phellodendron amurense Against Aedes aegypti (Diptera: Culicidae). *Saudi Pharm J*. 2020 May;28(5):560-564.

[1900] Shi X, Wang C, Simon JE, et al. Repellency of Novel Catnip Oils Against the Bed Bug (Hemiptera: Cimicidae). *J Med Entomol*. 2021 Mar 12;58(2):528-534.

[1901] Hogenbom J, Istanbouli M, Faraone N. Novel β-Cyclodextrin and Catnip Essential Oil Inclusion Complex and Its Tick Repellent Properties. *Molecules*. 2021 Dec 6;26(23):7391.

[1902] Ghasemzadeh S, Messelink GJ, Avila GA, et al. Sublethal impacts of essential plant oils on biochemical and ecological parameters of the predatory mite Amblyseius swirskii. *Front Plant Sci*. 2022 Sep 16;13:923802.

[1903] Kilinc BI, Godelek D, Sufer O, et al. Essential Oils from Some Lamiaceae Plants: Antioxidant and Anticancer Potentials besides Thermal Properties. *Chem Biodiversity*. 2022;19:e202200418.

[1904] Patel HK, Gomes EN, Wu Q, et al. Volatile metabolites from new cultivars of catnip and oregano as potential antibacterial and insect repellent agents. *Front Plant Sci*. 2023 Feb 23;14:1124305.

[1905] Paoli M, Nam AM, Castola V, et al. Chemical variability of the wood essential oil of Cedrus atlantica Manetti from Corsica. *Chem Biodivers*. 2011 Feb;8(2):344-51.

[1906] Derwich E, Benziane Z, Boukir A. Chemical composition and in vitro antibacterial activity of the essential oil of Cedrus atlantica. *Int J Agric Biol*. 2010;12:381-85.

[1907] Aberchane M, Fechtal M, Abdelaziz C. Analysis of Moroccan Atlas cedarwood oil (Cedrus atlantica Manetti). *J Essent Oil Res*. 2004;16(6):542-47.

[1908] Zeng WC, Zhang Z, Gao H, et al. Chemical composition, antioxidant, and antimicrobial activities of essential oil from pine needle (Cedrus deodara). *J Food Sci*. 2012 Jul;77(7):C824-29.

[1909] Chaudry A, Kaur P, Singh B, et al. Chemical composition of hydrodistilled and solvent volatiles extracted from woodchips of Himalayan Cedrus: Cedrus deodara (Roxb.) Loud. *Nat Prod Comm*. 2009 Sep;4(9):1257-60.

[1910] Nigam MC, Ateeque A, Misra LN. Composition of the essential oil of Cedrus deodara. *Indian Perf*. 1990;34(4):278- 81.

[1911] Aromatics International. Cedarwood (Indian) Cedrus deodora. Available at: http://www.aromaticsinternational.com/products/essential-oils/cedarwood-indian.

[1912] Menin L, Sepulveda F, Tsybin YO. Analyse d'une huile essentielle de Cèdre. *Service De Spectrometrie De Masse De L'Isic (SSMI)*. 2012 Dec. Available at: http://www.gedane.com/files/documents/Cedre_CED501F090228_121213.pdf.

[1913] Lawrence BM. Progress in essential oils. *Perf Flavorist*. 1998;23(5):67-68.

[1914] Adams RP. Cedar wood oil – analyses and properties. *Essent Oils Waxes*. 1991;12:159-73.

[1915] Zhu K. Extraction of fir wood oil from fir wood waste and synthesis of Cedar series perfumes. *Division of Fine Chemicals, College of Chemical Engineering, Nanjing Forestry University, Nanjing, Jiangsu, China*. Available at: http://www3.aiche.org/proceedings/content/Annual-2013/extended-abstracts/P346313.pdf.

[1916] Saab AM, Lampronti I, Borgatti M, et al. In vitro evaluation of the anti-proliferative activities of the wood essential oils of three Cedrus species against K562 human chronic myelogenous leukaemia cells. *Nat Prod Res*. 2012;26(23):2227-31.

[1917] Baylac S, Racine P. Inhibition of 5-lipoxygenase by essential oils and other natural fragrant extracts. *Int J Aromatherapy*. 2003;13(2-3):138-42.

[1918] Kumar A, Singh C, Chaudhary AK. Gastric antisecretory and antiulcer activities of Cedrus deodara (Roxb.) Loud. In Wistar rats. *J Ethnopharmacol*. 2011 Mar;134(2):294-97.

[1919] Shinde UA, Kulkarni KR, Phadke AS, et al. Mast cell stabilizing and lipoxygenase inhibitory activity of Cedrus deodara (Roxb.) Loud. Wood oil. *Indian J Exp Biol*. 1999 Mar;37(30:258-61.

[1920] Shinde UA, Phadke AS, Nair AM, et al. Studies on the anti-inflammatory and analgesic activity of Cedrus deodara (Roxb.) Loud. Wood oil. *J Ethnopharmacol*. 1999 Apr;65(1):21-27.

[1921] Shinde UA, Phadke AS, Nair AM, et al. Stabilizing activity - a possible mechanism of action for the anti- inflammatory activity of Cedrus deodara wood oil. *Fitoterapia*.1999 Jun;70(3):251-57.

[1922] Baylac S, Racine P. Inhibition of 5-lipoxygenase by essential oils and other natural fragrant extracts. *Int J Aromatherapy*. 2003;13(2-3):138-42.

[1923] Shinde UA, Phadke AS, Nair AM, et al. Preliminary studies on the immunomodulatory activity of Cedrus deodara wood oil. *Fitoterapia*. 1999 Aug;70(4):333-39.

[1924] Hay IC, Jamieson M, Ormerod AD. Randomized trial of aromatherapy. Successful treatment for alopecia areata. *Arch Dermatol*. 1998 Nov;134(11):1349-52.

[1925] Martins DF, Emer AA, Paula Batisti A, et al. Inhalation of Cedrus atlantica essential oil alleviates pain behavior through activation of descending pain modulation pathways in a mouse model of postoperative pain. *J Ethnopharmacol*. 2015 Dec 4;175:30-8.

[1926] Pazinato R, Volpato A, Baldissera MD, et al. In vitro effect of seven essential oils on the reproduction of the cattle tick Rhipicephalus microplus. *J Adv Res*. 2016 Nov;7(6):1029-1034.

[1927] Emer AA, Donatello NN, Batisti AP, et al. The role of the endocannabinoid system in the antihyperalgesic effect of Cedrus atlantica essential oil inhalation in a mouse model of postoperative pain. *J Ethnopharmacol*. 2017 Sep 14;210:477-484.

[1928] Bhagat M, Kumar A, Suravajhala R. Cedrus deodara (bark) essential oil induces apoptosis in human colon cancer cells by inhibiting Nuclear Factor kappa B. *Curr Top Med Chem*. 2020 Jul 22. Online ahead of print.

[1929] Al Kamaly O, Saleh A, Sfouk AA, et al. Cedrus atlantica (Endl.) Manetti ex Carrière Essential Oil Alleviates Pain and Inflammation with No Toxicity in Rodent. *Process*. 2022;10:581.

[1930] Hassanen NHM, Eisa AMF, Hafez SAM, et al. Antioxidant and antimicrobial activity of celery (Apium graveolens) and coriander (Coriandrum sativum) herb and seed essential oils. *Int J Current Micribiol Appl Sci*. 2015;4(3):284-96.

[1931] Al-Din Helaly A, Pill Bael J, Mady E, et al. Phytochemical Analysis of Some Celery Accessions. *J Medicinally Active Plants*. 2015 Jun;4(1-2):1-7.

[1932] Alves-Silva JM, Dias dos Santos SM, Pintado ME, et al. Chemical composition and in vitro antimicrobial, antifungal and antioxidant properties of essential oils obtained from some herbs widely used in Portugal. *Food Control*. 2013 Aug;32(2):371-78.

[1933] Donovan A, Isaac S, Collin HA. Inhibitory effects of essential oil components extracted from celery (Apium graveolens) on the growth of Septoria apiicola, causal agent of leaf spot disease. *Plant Pathology*. 1993 Oct;42(5):691-700.

[1934] Mauerman B, Ahmed N, Tambhar N, et al. Trends in Furanocoumarin Profiles Among Commerical-Scale Essential Oils. International Conference on the Science of Botanicals, Poster. Mar 2022.

[1935] Hassanen NHM, Eisa AMF, Hafez SAM, et al. Antioxidant and antimicrobial activity of celery (Apium graveolens) and coriander (Coriandrum sativum) herb and seed essential oils. *Int J Current Micribiol Appl Sci.* 2015;4(3):284-96.

[1936] Alves-Silva JM, Dias dos Santos SM, Pintado ME, et al. Chemical composition and in vitro antimicrobial, antifungal and antioxidant properties of essential oils obtained from some herbs widely used in Portugal. *Food Control.* 2013 Aug;32(2):371-78.

[1937] Nagella P, Ahmad A, Kim SJ, et al. Chemical composition, antioxidant activity and larvicidal effects of essential oil from leaves of Apium graveolens. *Immunopharmacol Immunotoxicol.* 2012;34(2):205-09.

[1938] Hassanen NHM, Eisa AMF, Hafez SAM, et al. Antioxidant and antimicrobial activity of celery (Apium graveolens) and coriander (Coriandrum sativum) herb and seed essential oils. *Int J Current Micribiol Appl Sci.* 2015;4(3):284-96.

[1939] Alves-Silva JM, Dias dos Santos SM, Pintado ME, et al. Chemical composition and in vitro antimicrobial, antifungal and antioxidant properties of essential oils obtained from some herbs widely used in Portugal. *Food Control.* 2013 Aug;32(2):371-78.

[1940] Baananou S, Bouftira I, Mahmoud A, et al. Antiulcerogenic and antibacterial activities of Apium graveolens essential oil and extract. *Nat Prod Res.* 2013;27(12):1075-83.

[1941] Helal MA. Celery oil modulates DEHP-induced reproductive toxicity in male rats. *Reprod Biol.* 2014 Sep;14(3):182-9.

[1942] Friedman M, Henika PR, Mandrell RE. Bactericidal activities of plant essential oils and some of their isolated constituents against Campylobacter jejuni, Escherichia coli, Listeria monocytogenes, and Salmonella enterica. *J Food Prot.* 2002 Oct;65(10):1545-60.

[1943] Baananou S, Bouftira I, Mahmoud A, et al. Antiulcerogenic and antibacterial activities of Apium graveolens essential oil and extract. *Nat Prod Res.* 2013;27(12):1075-83.

[1944] Al-Howiriny T, Alsheikh A, Alqasoumi S, et al. Gastric antiulcer, antisecretory and cytoprotective properties of celery (Apium graveolens) in rats. *Pharm Biol.* 2010 Jul;48(7):786-93.

[1945] Baananou S, Piras A, Marongiu B, et al. Antiulcerogenic activity of Apium graveolens seeds oils isolated by supercritical CO2. *African J Pharmacy Pharamcol.* 2012 Mar 15;6(10):756-62.

[1946] Nagella P, Ahmad A, Kim SJ, et al. Chemical composition, antioxidant activity and larvicidal effects of essential oil from leaves of Apium graveolens. *Immunopharmacol Immunotoxicol.* 2012;34(2):205-09.

[1947] Kumar S, Mishra M1, Wahab N, et al. Larvicidal, Repellent, and Irritant Potential of the Seed-Derived Essential oil of Apium graveolens Against Dengue Vector, Aedes aegypti L. (Diptera: Culicidae). *Front Public Health.* 2014 Sep 18;2:147.

[1948] Nirmala MJ, Durai L, Gopakumar V, et al. Preparation of Celery Essential Oil-Based Nanoemulsion by Ultrasonication and Evaluation of Its Potential Anticancer and Antibacterial Activity. *Int J Nanomedicine.* 2020 Oct 8;15:7651-7666.

[1949] Zorga J, Kunicka-Styczynska A, Gruska R, et al. Ultrasound-Assisted Hydrodistillation of Essential Oil from Celery Seeds ( Apium graveolens L.) and Its Biological and Aroma Profiles. *Molecules.* 2020 Nov 14;25(22):5322.

[1950] Foudah AI, Alqarni MH, Alam A, et al. Determination of Chemical Composition, In Vitro and In Silico Evaluation of Essential Oil from Leaves of Apium graveolens Grown in Saudi Arabia. *Molecules.* 2021 Dec 4;26(23):7372.

[1951] Ghannadi A, Bagherinejad M, Abedi D, et al. Antibacterial activity and composition of essential oils from Pelargonium graveolens L'Her and Vitex agnus-castus L. *Iran J Microbiol.* 2012 Dec;4(4):171–76.

[1952] Sorensen JM, Katsiotis ST. Parameters influencing the yield and composition of the essential oil from Cretan Vitex agnus-castus fruits. *Planta Med.* 2000 Apr;66(3):245–50.

[1953] Stojkovic D, Marina S, Glamoclija J, et al. Chemical composition and antimicrobial activity of Vitex agnus-castus L. fruits and leaves essential oils. *Food Chem.* 2011 Oct;128(4):1017–22.

[1954] Taziki S, Hamedeyazdan S, Pasandi AN. Variations in essential oils of Vitex agnus castus fruits growing in Qum, Khorasan and Tehran in Iran. *Annals Biol Res.* 2013;4(2):308–12.

[1955] Habbab A, Sekkoum K, Belboukhari N. Chemical constituents and biological evaluation of leaves essential oils of Vitex agnus-castus L. growing in the southern-west Algeria. *Int Sci Index.* 1999 Jan:26113.

[1956] Senatore F, Della Porta G, Reverchon E. Constituents of Vitex agnus-castus L essential oil. *Flavour Frag J.* 1996 May/June;11(3):179–82.

[1957] Brinker F. The toxicology of botanical medicines. 3rd ed. 2000, Sandy, Oregon: Eclectic Medical Publications. p. 296.

[1958] Jellin JM, Batz F, Hitchens K. Natural medicines comprehensive database 3rd Edition. 2002, Stockton, CA: Therapeutic Research Faculty. p. 1530.

[1959] Dugoua JJ, Seely D, Perri D, et al. Safety and efficacy of chaste tree (Vitex agnus-castus) during pregnancy and lactation. *Can J Clin Pharmacol.* 2008 Winter;15(1):e74–79.

[1960] Wuttke W, Jarry H, Christoffel V, et al. Chaste tree (Vitex agnus-castus)--pharmacology and clinical indications. *Phytomedicine.* 2003 May;10(4):348–57.

[1961] Luecha P, Umehara K, Miyase T, et al. Antiestrogenic constituents of the Thai medicinal plants Capparis flavicans and Vitex glabrata. *J Nat Prod.* 2009 Nov;72(11):1954–59.

[1962] Lucks BC. Vitex agnus castus essential oil and menopausal balance: a self-care survey. *Complement Ther Nurs Midwifery.* 2002;8:148–54.

[1963] Lucks BC. Vitex agnus castus essential oil and menopausal balance: a research update. *Complement Ther Nurs Midwifery.* 2003;9:157–60.

[1964] Wuttke W. Dopaminergic action of extracts of Agnus Castus. *Forschende Komplementarmedizen.* 1996;3:329–30.

[1965] Sayyah M, Valizadeh J, Kamalinejad M. Anticonvulsant activity of the leaf oil of Laurus nobilis against pentylentetrazole- and maximal electroshock-induced seizure. *Phytomedicine.* 2002 Apr;9(3):212-16.

[1966] Culic M, Kekovic G, Grbic G, et al. Wavelet and fractal analysis of rat brain activity in seizures evoked by camphor oil and 1,8-cineole. *Gen Physiol Biophys.* 2009;28 Sec No:33-40.

[1967] Burkhard PR, Burkhardt K, Haenggeli CA, et al. Plant-induced seizures: reappearance of an old problem. *J Neurol.* 1999 Aug;246(8):667-70.

[1968] Waldman N. Seizure caused by dermal application of over-the-counter eucalyptus oil head lice preparation. *Clin Toxicol (Phila).* 2011 Oct;49(8):750-1.

[1969] Craig JO. Poisoning by the volatile oils in childhood. *Arch Dis Child.* 1953;28:259-67.

[1970] Mathew T, Kamath V, Kumar RS, et al. Eucalyptus oil inhalation-induced seizure: A novel, underrecognized, preventable cause of acute symptomatic seizure. *Epilepsia Open.* 2017 Jul 4;2(3):350-354.

[1971] Jori A, Bianchetti A, Prestini PE, et al. Effect of eucalyptol (1,8-cineole) on the metabolism of other drugs in rats and in man. *Eur J Pharmacol.* 1970;9(3):362–66.

[1972] de Sousa DP, Raphael E, Brocksom U, et al. Sedative effect of monoterpene alcohols in mice: A preliminary screening. *Verlag der Zeitschrift fur Naturforschung.* 2007;62c:563–66.

[1973] Lin WY, Kuo YH, Chang YL, et al. Anti-platelet aggregation and chemical constituents from the rhizome of Gynura japonica. *Planta Med.* 2003 Aug;69(8):757-64.

[1974] Wuttke W, Jarry H, Christoffel V, et al. Chaste tree (Vitex agnus-castus)--pharmacology and clinical indications. *Phytomedicine.* 2003 May;10(4):348–57.

[1975] Wuttke W. Dopaminergic action of extracts of Agnus Castus. *Forschende Komplementarmedizen.* 1996;3:329–30.

[1976] Ganzera M, Schneider P, Stuppner H. Inhibitory effects of the essential oil of chamomile (Matricaria recutita L.) and its major constituents on human cytochrome P450 enzymes. *Life Sci.* 2006 Jan 18;78(8):856–61.

[1977] Nguyen LT, Mysliveckova Z, Szotakova B, et al. The inhibitory effects of β-caryophyllene, β-caryophyllene oxide and α-humulene on the activities of the main drug-metabolizing enzymes in rat and human liver in vitro. *Chem-Biol Interactoins.* 2017 Dec 25;278:123-8.

[1978] Šošić-Jurjević B, Ajdžanović V, Filipović B, et al. Functional morphology of pituitary-thyroid and -adrenocortical axes in middle-aged male rats treated with Vitex agnus castus essential oil. *Acta Histochem.* 2016 Jul 28;118(7):736-45.

[1979] Jasmina P, Filipović B, Šošić-Jurjević B, et al. Vitex agnus-castus essential oil affects thyroid C cells and bone metabolism in middle-aged male rats. *Acta Vet.* 2013;63(1):23-35.

[1980] Ghannadi A, Bagherinejad M, Abedi D, et al. Antibacterial activity and composition of essential oils from Pelargonium graveolens L'Her and Vitex agnus-castus L. *Iran J Microbiol.* 2012 Dec;4(4):171–76.

[1981] Blumenthal M., ed. The Complete German Commission E Monographs: Therapeutic Guide to Herbal Medicines. Austin: American Botanical Council, 1998.

[1982] Khalilzadeh E, Vafaei Saiah G, Hasannejad H, et al. Antinociceptive effects, acute toxicity and chemical composition of Vitex agnus-castus essential oil. *Avicenna J Phytomed.* 2015 May-Jun;5(3):218–30.

[1983] Wuttke W, Jarry H, Christoffel V, et al. Chaste tree (Vitex agnus-castus)--pharmacology and clinical indications. *Phytomedicine.* 2003 May;10(4):348–57.

[1984] Lucks BC. Vitex agnus castus essential oil and menopausal balance: a research update. *Complement Ther Nurs Midwifery.* 2003;9:157–60.

[1985] Asdadi A, Hamdouch A, Oukacha A, et al. Study on chemical analysis, antioxidant and in vitro antifungal activities of essential oil from wild Vitex agnus-castus L. seeds growing in area of Argan Tree of Morocco against clinical strains of Candida responsible for nosocomial infections. J Mycol Med. 2015 Dec;25(4):e118-27.

[1986] Neves RC, Camara CA. Chemical composition and acaricidal activity of the essential oils from Vitex agnus-castus L. (Verbenaceae) and selected monoterpenes. *An Acad Bras Cienc.* 2016 Aug 4;0:0.

[1987] Gonçalves R, Ayres VFS, Carvalho CE, et al. Chemical Composition and Antibacterial Activity of the Essential Oil of Vitex agnus-castus L. (Lamiaceae). *An Acad Bras Cienc.* 2017 Oct-Dec;89(4):2825-2832.

[1988] Ilhan S. Essential Oils from Vitex agnus castus L. Leaves Induces Caspase-Dependent Apoptosis of Human Multidrug-Resistant Lung Carcinoma Cells through Intrinsic and Extrinsic Pathways. *Nutr Cancer.* 2020 Sep 25;1-9.

[1989] Ayres VFS, Oliveira MR, Baldin ELL, et al. Chemical composition and insecticidal activity of the essential oils of Piper marginatum , Piper callosum and Vitex agnus-castus. *An Acad Bras Cienc.* 2021 Jul 19;93(3):e20200616.

[1990] Zhelev I, Petkova Z, Kostova I, et al. Chemical Composition and Antimicrobial Activity of Essential Oil of Fruits from Vitex agnus-castus L., Growing in Two Regions in Bulgaria. *Plants (Basel).* 2022 Mar 28;11(7):896.

[1991] Zhu L, Li Y, Li B, et al. Aromatic plants and essential constituents. South China Institute of Botany, Hong Kong. 1993.

[1992] Carroll JF, Tabanaca N, Kramer M, et al. Essential oils of Cupressus funebris, Juniperus communis, and J. chinensis (Cupressaceae) as repellents against ticks (Acari: Ixodidae) and mosquitoes (Diptera: Culicidae) and as toxicants against mosquitoes. *J Vector Ecol.* 2011 Dec;36(2):258-68.

[1993] Adams RP, Li S. The botanical source of Chinese Cedarwood oil: Cupressus funebris or Cupressaceae Species? *J Essent Oil Res.* May-Jun 2008;20:235-42.

[1994] Tabanaca N, Wedge DE, Carroll JF, et al. Activity of Cupressus funebris, Juniperus communis, and J. chinensis (Cupressaceae) Essential Oils as Repellents against Ticks (Acari: Ixodidae) and as Repellents and Toxicants against Mosquitoes (Diptera: Culicidae). *Planta Med.* 2011;77:42.

[1995] Jeong HU, Kwon SS, Kong TY, et al. Inhibitory effects of cedrol, β-cedrene, and thujopsene on cytochrome P450 enzyme activities in human liver microsomes. *J Toxicol Environ Health A.* 2014;77(22-24):1522-32.

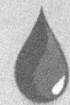

[1996] Carroll JF, Tabanaca N, Kramer M, et al. Essential oils of Cupressus funebris, Juniperus communis, and J. chinensis (Cupressaceae) as repellents against ticks (Acari: Ixodidae) and mosquitoes (Diptera: Culicidae) and as toxicants against mosquitoes. *J Vector Ecol.* 2011 Dec;36(2):258-68.

[1997] Tabanaca N, Wedge DE, Carroll JF, et al. Activity of Cupressus funebris, Juniperus communis, and J. chinensis (Cupressaceae) Essential Oils as Repellents against Ticks (Acari: Ixodidae) and as Repellents and Toxicants against Mosquitoes (Diptera: Culicidae). *Planta Med.* 2011;77:42.

[1998] Manivannan R, Kumar MS, Jawahar N, et al. A comparative antimicrobial study on the essential oil of the leaves of various species of cupressus. *Anc Sci Life.* 2005 Jan;24(3):131-3.

[1999] Xie Q, Liu Z, Li Z. Chemical Composition and Antioxidant Activity of Essential Oil of Six Pinus Taxa Native to China. *Molecules.* 2015;20:9380-92.

[2000] Yatagai M, Hong Y. Chemical composition of the essential oil of Pinus massoniana Lamb. *J Essent Oil Res.* 1997 Jul-Aug;9:485-87.

[2001] Changmao S, Wengui D, Cen B, et al. Comparison of chemical components of essential oils in needles of Pinus massoniana Lambb and Pinus elliottottii Engelm from Guangxi. *Chinese J Chromatography.* 2006 Nov;24(6):619-24.

[2002] Bonesi M, Menichini F, Tundis R, et al. Acetylcholinesterase and butyrylcholinesterase inhibitory activity of Pinus species essential oils and their constituents. *J Enzyme Inhib Med Chem.* 2010 Oct;25(5):622-8.

[2003] Xie Q, Liu Z, Li Z. Chemical Composition and Antioxidant Activity of Essential Oil of Six Pinus Taxa Native to China. *Molecules.* 2015;20:9380-92.

[2004] Eyres G, Dufour JP, Hallifax G, et al. Identification of character-impact odorants in coriander and wild coriander leaves using gas-chromatography-olfactory (GCO) and comprehensive two-dimensional gas chromatography-time—of- flight mass spectrometry (GCxGC-TOFMS). *J Separation Sci.* 2005 Jun;28(9-10):1061-74.

[2005] Matasyoh JC, Maiyo ZC, Ngure RM, et al. Chemical composition and antimicrobial activity of the essential oil of Coriandrum sativum. *Food Chem.* 2009 Mar;113(2):526-29.

[2006] Freires Ide A, Murata RM, Furletti VF, et al. Coriandrum sativum L. (Coriander) essential oil: antifungal activity and mode of action on Candida spp., and molecular targets affected in human whole-genome expression. *PLoS One.* 2014 Jun;9(6):e99086.

[2007] Chung IM, Ahmad A, Kim SJ, et al. Composition of the essential oil constituents from leaves and stems of Korean Coriandrum sativum and their immunotoxicity activity on the Aedes aegypti L. *Immunopharmacol Immunotoxicol.* 2012 Feb;34(1):152-6.

[2008] Freires IA, Denny C, Benso B, et al. Antibacterial Activity of Essential Oils and Their Isolated Constituents against Cariogenic Bacteria: A Systematic Review. *Molecules.* 2015 Apr 22;20(4):7329-58.

[2009] Han X, Beaumont C, Stevens N. Chemical composition analysis and in vitro biological activities of ten essential oils in human skin cells. *Biochim Open.* 2017 Apr 26;5:1-7.

[2010] Powers CN, Osier JL, McFeeters RL, et al. Antifungal and Cytotoxic Activities of Sixty Commercially-Available Essential Oils. *Molecules.* 2018 Jun 27;23(7).

[2011] Foudah AI, Alqarni MH, Alam A, et al. Evaluation of the composition and in vitro antimicrobial, antioxidant, and anti-inflammatory activities of Cilantro ( Coriandrum sativum L. leaves) cultivated in Saudi Arabia (Al-Kharj). *Saudi J Biol Sci.* 2021 Jun;28(6):3461-3468.

[2012] Raveau R, Fontaine J, Verdin A, et al. Chemical Composition, Antioxidant and Anti-Inflammatory Activities of Clary Sage and Coriander Essential Oils Produced on Polluted and Amended Soils-Phytomanagement Approach. *Molecules.* 2021;26(17):5321.

[2013] Unlu M, Ergene E, Unlu GV, et al. Composition, antimicrobial activity and in vitro cytotoxicity of essential oil from Cinnamomum zeylanicum Blume (Lauraceae). *Food Chem Toxicol.* 2012 Nov;48(11):3274-80.

[2014] Zouheyr H, Rachida A, Perry MG. Effect of essential oil of Cinnamomum zeylanicum on some pathogenic bacteria. *African J Microbio Res.* 2014 Mar 5;8(110):1026-31.

[2015] Jham G, Dhingra O, Jardin C, et al. Identification of the major fungitoxic component of cinnamon bark oil. *Fitopatologia Brasileira.* 2005 Jul-Aug;30(4):4158.

[2016] Paranagama PA, Wimalasena S, Jayatilake GS, et al. A comparison of essential oil constituents of bark, leaf, root and fruit of cinnamon (cinnamomum zeylanicum Blum) grown in Sri Lanka. *J Natn Sci Foundation Sri Lanka.* 201;29(3&4):147-53.

[2017] Petrovic GM, Stojanovic GS, Radulovic NS. Encapsulation of cinnamon oil in β-cyclodextrin. *J Med Plants Res.* 2010 Jul;4(14):1382-90.

[2018] Baruah A, Nath SC, Hazarika AK. Investigation of the essential oils of Cinnamomum verum Presl. Grown at lower Brahmaputra valley of Assam. *Indian Perfumer.* 2010;54(3):21-23.

[2019] Domaracky M, Rehak P, Juhas S, et al. Effects of selected plant essential oils on the growth and development of mouse preimplantation embryos in vivo. *Physiol Res.* 2007;56(1):97-104.

[2020] Forschmidt P. Teratogenic activity of flavor additives. *Teratology.* 1979;19:26A.

[2021] Mantovani A, Stazi AV, Macri C, et al. Pre-natal (segment II) toxicity study of cinnamic aldehyde in the Sprague- Dawley rat. *Food Chem Toxicol.* 1989;27:781-86.

[2022] Huang J, Wang S, Luo X, et al. Cinnamaldehyde reduction of platelet aggregation and thrombosis in rodents. *Thromb Res.* 2007;119(3):337-42.

[2023] Kim SY, Koo YK, Koo JY, et al. Platelet anti-aggregation activities of constituents from Cinnamomum cassia. *J Med Food.* 2010 Oct;13(5):1069-74.

[2024] Takenaga M, Hirai A, Terano T, et al. In vitro effect of cinnamic aldehyde, a main component of Cinnamomi Cortex, on human platelet aggregation and arachidonic acid metabolism. *J Pharmacobiodyn.* 1987 May;10(5):201-208.

[2025] Mack TS, Raner GM. Regulation of cytochrome P450 2A6 and phase II enzymes by unsaturated aldehydes. University of North Carolina at Greensboro. Available at: http://libres.uncg.edu/ir/uncg/listing.aspx?id=2343.

[2026] Wickramasinghe RH, Muller G, Norpoth K. Spectral evidence of interaction of spice constituents with hepatic microsomal cytochrome P-450. *Cytobios.* 1980;29(113):25-27.

[2027] Singh G, Maurya S, deLampasona MP, et al. A comparison of chemical antioxidant and antimicrobial studies of cinnamon leaf and bark volatile oils, oleoresins and their constituents. *Food Chem Toxicol.* 2007;45:1650–61.

[2028] Verspohl EJ, Bauer K, Neddermann E. Antidiabetic effect of Cinnamomum cassia and Cinnamomum zeylanicum in vivo and in vitro. *Phytother. Res.* 2005 Mar;19(3):203-06.

[2029] Hua P, Guijun Z, Guixing R. Antidiabetic effects of cinnamon oil in diabetic KK-A mice. *Food Chem Toxicol.* 2010 Aug-Sep;48(8-9):2344-9.

[2030] Sung HK, Sun HH, Choung SY. Anti-diabetic effect of cinnamon extract on blood glucose in db/db mice. *J Ethnopharmacol.* 2006 Mar 8;104(1-2):119-23.

[2031] Langeveld WT, Veldhuizen EJ, Burt SA. Synergy between essential oil constituents and antibiotics. *Crit Rev Microbiol.* 2014 Feb;40(1):76-94.

[2032] Palaniappan K, Holley RA. Use of natural antimicrobials to increase antibiotic susceptibility of drug resistant bacteria. *In J Food Microbiol.* 2010 Jun 15;140(2-3):164-8.

[2033] National Toxicology Program. Cinnamaldehyde. 1989 Dec. Available at: https://ntp.niehs.nih.gov/ntp/htdocs/chem_background/exsumpdf/cinnamaldehyde_508.pdf.

[2034] National Toxicology Program. Cinnamaldehyde. 1989 Dec. Available at: https://ntp.niehs.nih.gov/ntp/htdocs/chem_background/exsumpdf/cinnamaldehyde_508.pdf.

[2035] Domaracky M, Rehak P, Juhas S, et al. Effects of selected plant essential oils on the growth and development of mouse preimplantation embryos in vivo. *Physiol Res.* 2007;56(1):97-104.

[2036] Vrskova D, Modra H. Evaluation of the developmental toxicity of 2-phenoxyethanol and clove oil anesthetics using the Frog Embryo Teratogenesis Assay: Xenopus (FETAX). *Veterinarami Medicina.* 2012;57(5):245-50.

[2037] Amini A, Cheraghi E, Safaee MR, et al. The role of eugenol in the reduction of teratogenic effects of retinoic acid on skeletal morphology of mice embryo. *Yakhteh Medical Journal.* 2003;4:195-200.

[2038] Chen R, Chen J, Cheng S, et al. Assessment of embryotoxicity of constituents in cosmetics by the embryonic stem cell tes. *Toxicol Mech Methods.* 2010 Mar;20(3):112-18.

[2039] Chen SJ, Wang MH, Chen IJ. Antiplatelet and calcium inhibitory properties of eugenol and sodium eugenol acetate. *Gen Pharmacol.* 1996 Jun;27(4):629-33.

[2040] Tognolini M, Barocelli E, Ballabeni V, et al. Comparative screening of plant essential oils; phenylpropanoid moiety as basic core for antiplatelet activity. *Life Sci.* 2006 Feb 23;78(13):1419-32.

[2041] Heck AM, DeWitt BA, Lukes AL. Potential interactions between alternative therapies and warfarin. *Am J Health Syst Pharm.* 2000;57(13):1221-1227.

[2042] Saaeed SA, Gilani AH. Antithrombotic activity of clove oil. *J Pak Med Assoc.* 1994;44(5):112-15.

[2043] Kamatou GP, Vermaak I, Viljoen AM. Eugenol—from the remote Maluku Islands to the international market place: A review of a remarkable and versatile molecule. *Molecules.* 2012;17:6953-81.

[2044] Cochrane ML. Inhibition of Cytochrome P450 2C9 by essential oils. Available at: https://libres.uncg.edu/ir/uncg/listing.aspx?id=18102

[2045] Dohi S, Terasaki M, Makino M. Acetylcholinesterase inhibitory activity and chemical composition of commercial essential oils. *J Agric Food Chem.* 2009 May 27;57(10):4313-8.

[2046] Langeveld WT, Veldhuizen EJ, Burt SA. Synergy between essential oil constituents and antibiotics. *Crit Rev Microbiol.* 2014 Feb;40(1):76-94.

[2047] Sarrami N, Pemberton MN, Thornhill MH, et al. Adverse reactions associated with the use of eugenol in dentistry. *British Dental J.* 2002;193:253-55.

[2048] Tammannavar P, Pushpalatha C, Jain S, et al. An unexpected positive hypersensitive reaction to eugenol. *BMJ Case Rep.* 2013; 2013: bcr2013009464.

[2049] Naveed R, Hussain I, Tawab A, et al. Antimicrobial activity of the bioactive components of essential oils from Pakistani species against Salmonella and other multi-drug resistant bacteria. *BMC Complement Altern Med.* 2013 Oct;13:265.

[2050] Ooi LSM, Li Y, Kam SL, et al. Antimicrobial activities of cinnamon oil and cinnamaldehyde from the Chinese medicinal herb Cinnamomum cassia Blume. *Am J Chin Med.* 2006;34(3):511.

[2051] Urbaniak A, Glowacka A, Kowalczyk E, et al. The antibacterial activity of cinnamon oil on the selected gram- positive and gram-negative bacteria. *Med Dosw Mikrobiol.* 2014;66(2):131-41.

[2052] Miller AB, Cates RG, Lawrence M, et al. The antibacterial and antifungal activity of essential oils extracted from Guatemalan medicinal plants. *Pharm Biol.* 2014 Oct 21:1-7.

[2053] Tampieri MP, Galuppi R, Macchioni F, et al. The inhibition of Candida albicans by selected essential oils and their major components. *Mycopathologia.* 2005 Apr;159(3):339-45.

[2054] Cisarová M, Tančinová D, Medo J, et al. The in vitro effect of selected essential oils on the growth and mycotoxin production of Aspergillus species. *J Environ Sci Health B.* 2016 Oct 2;51(10):668-674.

[2055] Abbaszadegan A, Dadolahi S, Gholami A, et al. Antimicrobial and Cytotoxic Activity of Cinnamomum zeylanicum, Calcium Hydroxide, and Triple Antibiotic Paste as Root Canal Dressing Materials. *J Contemp Dent Pract.* 2016 Feb 1;17(2):105-13.

[2056] Seo HS, Beuchat LR, Kim H, et al. Development of an experimental apparatus and protocol for determining antimicrobial activities of gaseous plant essential oils. *Int J Food Microbiol.* 2015 Dec 23;215:95-100.

[2057] Hili P, Evans CS, Veness RG. Antimicrobial action of essential oils: the effect of dimethylsulfoxide on the activity of cinnamon essential oil. *Lett Appl Microbiol.* 1997 Apr;24(4):269-75.

[2058] Warnke PH, Becker ST, Podschun R, et al. The battle against multi-resistant strains: Renaissance of antimicrobial essential oils as a promising force to fight hospital-acquired infections. *J Craniomaxillofac Surg.* 2009 Oct;37(7):392- 97.

[2059] Verspohl EJ, Bauer K, Neddermann E. Antidiabetic effect of Cinnamomum cassia and Cinnamomum zeylanicum in vivo and in vitro. *Phytother. Res.* 2005 Mar;19(3):203-06.

[2060] Ping H, Zhang G, Ren G. Antidiabetic effects of cinnamon oil in diabetic KK-A$^Y$ mice. *Food Chem Toxicol.* 2010 Aug-Sep;48(8-9):2344-49.

[2061] Kim SH, Hyun SH, Choung SY. Anti-diabetic effect of cinnamon extract on blood glucose in db/db mice. *J Ethnopharmacol.* 2006 Mar;104(1-2):119-123.

[2062] Zu Y, Yu H, Liang L, et al. Activities of ten essential oils towards Propionibacterium acnes and PC-3, A-549 and MCF-7 cancer cells. *Molecules.* 2010;15:3200-10.

[2063] Yang XQ, Zheng H, Ye Q, et al. Essential oil of Cinnamon exerts anti-cancer activity against head and neck squamous cell carcinoma via attenuating epidermal growth factor receptor - tyrosine kinase. *J BUON.* 2015 Nov-Dec;20(6):1518-25.

[2064] Hayashi K, Imanishi N, Kashiwayama Y, et al. Inhibitory effect of cinnamaldehyde, derived from Cinnamoni cortex, on the growth of influenza A/PR/8 virus in vitro and in vivo. *Antiviral Res.* 2007 Apr;74(1):1-8.

[2065] Chou ST, Chang WL, Chang CT, et al. Cinnamomum cassia essential oil inhibits α-MSH-induced melanin production and oxidative stress in murine B16 melanoma cells. *Int J Mol Sci.* 2013 Sep 18;14(9):19186-201.

[2066] Yuce A, Turk G, Ceribasi S, et al. Effects of cinnamon (Cinnamon zeylanicum) bark oil on testicular antioxidant values, apoptotic germ cell and sperm quality. *Andrologia.* 2013 Aug;45(4):248-55.

[2067] Sariözkan S, Türk G, Güvenç M, et al. Effects of Cinnamon (C. zeylanicum) Bark Oil Against Taxanes-Induced Damages in Sperm Quality, Testicular and Epididymal Oxidant/Antioxidant Balance, Testicular Apoptosis, and Sperm DNA Integrity. *Nutr Cancer.* 2016;68(3):481-94.

[2068] Inouye S, Uchida K, Nishiyama Y, et al. Combined effect of heat, essential oils and salt on fungicidal activity against Trichophyton mentagrophytes in a foot bath. *Nihon Ishinjin Gakkai Zasshi.*2007;48(1):27-36.

[2069] Guerra FQ, Mendes JM, Sousa JP, et al. Increasing antibiotic activity against multidrug-resistant Acinetobacter spp by essential oils of Citrus limon and Cinnamomum zeylanicum. *Nat Prod Res.* 2012;26(23):2235-38.

[2070] Mishra A, Bhatti R, Singh A, et al. Ameliorative effect of the cinnamon oil from Cinnamomum zeylanicum upon early stage diabetic nephropathy. *Planta Med.* 2010 Mar;76(5):412-17.

[2071] Shaverdi AR, Monsef-Esfahani HR, Tavasoli F, et al. Trans-cinnamaldehyde from Cinnamomum zeylanicum bark essential oil reduces clindamycin resistance of Clostridium difficile in vitro. *J Food Sci.* 2007 Jan;72(10:S055-58.

[2072] Al-Mariri A, Saour G, Hamou R. In vitro antibacterial effects of five volatile oil extracts against intramacrophage Brucella abortus 544. *Iran J Med Sci.* 2012 Jun;37(2):119-25.

[2073] Inouye S, Takizawa T, Yamaguchi H. Antibacterial activity of essential oils and their major constituents against respiratory tract pathogens by gaseous contact. *J Antimicrobi Chemother.* 2001 May;47(5):565-73.

[2074] Prabuseenivasan S, Jayakumar M, Ignacimuthu S. In vitro antibacterial activity of some plant essential oils. *BMC Complement Altern Med.* 2006 Nov;6:39.

[2075] Yap PS, Krishnan T, Chan KG, et al. Antibacterial Mode of Action of Cinnamomum verum Bark Essential Oil, Alone and in Combination with Piperacillin, Against a Multi-Drug-Resistant Escherichia coli Strain. *J Microbiol Biotechnol.* 2015 Aug;25(8):1299-306.

[2076] Cui H, Li W, Li C, et al. Liposome containing cinnamon oil with antibacterial activity against methicillin-resistant Staphylococcus aureus biofilm. *Biofouling.* 2016;32(2):215-25.

[2077] Inouye S, Yamaguchi H, Takizawa. Screening of the antibacterial effects of a variety of essential oils on respiratory tract pathogens, using a modified dilution assay method. *J Infect Chemother.* 201 Dec;7(4):251-54.

[2078] Herman A. Comparison of antimicrobial activity of essential oils, plant extracts and methylparaben in cosmetic emulsions: 2 months study. *Indian J Microbiol.* 2014 Sep;54(3):361-64.

[2079] Wu S, Patel KB, Booth LJ, et al. Protective essential oil attenuates influenza virus infection: an in vitro study in MDCK cells. *BMC Complement Altern Med.* 2010 Nov;10:69.

[2080] Hayashi K, Imanishi N, Kashiwayama Y, et al. Inhibitory effect of cinnamaldehyde, derived from Cinnamomi cortex, on the growth of influenza A/PR/8 virus in vitro and in vivo. *Antiviral Res.* 2007 Apr;74(1):1-8.

[2081] Hili P, Evans CS, Veness RG. Antimicrobial action of essential oils: the effect of dimethylsulfoxide on the activity of cinnamon essential oil. *Lett Appl Microbiol.* 1997 Apr;24(4):269-75.

[2082] Zoldaz PR, Raudenbush B. Cognitive Enhancement Through Stimulation of the Chemical Senses. *North AM J Psychology.* 2005;7(1):125.

[2083] Budri PE, Silva NC, Bonsaglia EC, et al. Effect of essential oils of Syzygium aromaticum and Cinnamomum zeylanicum and their major components on biofilm production in Staphylococcus aureus strains isolated from milk of cows with mastitis. *J Dairy Sci.* 2015 Sep;98(9):5899-904.

[2084] Monteiro IN, Monteiro OD, Costa-Junior LM, et al. Chemical composition and acaricide activity of an essential oil from a rare chemotype of Cinnamomum verum Presl on Rhipicephalus microplus (Acari: Ixodidae). *Vet Parasitol.* 2017 Apr 30;238:54-57.

[2085] Han X, Parker TL. Antiinflammatory Activity of Cinnamon (Cinnamomum zeylanicum) Bark Essential Oil in a Human Skin Disease Model. *Phytother Res.* 2017 Jul;31(7):1034–1038.

[2086] Hovijitra RS, Choonharuangdej S, Srithavaj T. Effect of essential oils prepared from Thai culinary herbs on sessile Candida albicans cultures. *J Oral Sci.* 2016;58(3):365-71.

[2087] Intorasoot A, Chornchoem P, Sookkhee S, et al. Bactericidal activity of herbal volatile oil extracts against multidrug-resistant Acinetobacter baumannii. *J Intercult Ethnopharmacol.* 2017 Apr 21;6(2):218-222.

[2088] Jeon YJ, Lee SG, Yang YC, et al. Insecticidal activities of their components derived from the essential oils of Cinnamomum sp. barks and against Ricania sp. (Homoptera: Ricaniidae), a newly recorded pest. *Pest Manag Sci.* 2017 Oct;73(10):2000-2004.

[2089] LeBel G, Haas B, Adam AA, et al. Effect of cinnamon (Cinnamomum verum) bark essential oil on the halitosis-associated bacterium Solobacterium moorei and in vitro cytotoxicity. *Arch Oral Biol.* 2017 Jul 12;83:97-104.

[2090] Mateo EM, Gómez JV, Dominguez I, et al. Impact of bioactive packaging systems based on EVOH films and essential oils in the control of aflatoxigenic fungi and aflatoxin production in maize. *Int J Food Microbiol.* 2017 Aug 2;254:36-46.

[2091] Mahmoudvand H, Mahmoudvand H, Oliaee RT, et al. In vitro Protoscolicidal Effects of Cinnamomum zeylanicum Essential Oil and Its Toxicity in Mice. *Pharmacogn Mag.* 2017 Oct; 13(Suppl 3): S652–S657.

[2092] Monteiro IN, Monteiro ODS, Costa-Junior LM, et al. Chemical composition and acaricide activity of an essential oil from a rare chemotype of Cinnamomum verum Presl on Rhipicephalus microplus (Acari: Ixodidae). *Vet Parasitol.* 2017 Apr 30;238:54-57.

[2093] Sheng L, Rasco B, Zhu MJ, et al. Cinnamon Oil Inhibits Shiga Toxin Type 2 Phage Induction and Shiga Toxin Type 2 Production in Escherichia coli O157:H7. *Appl Environ Microbiol.* 2016 Oct 27;82(22):6531-6540.

[2094] Wiwattanaratanabut K, choonharuangdej S, Srithava T. In Vitro Anti-Cariogenic Plaque Effects of Essential Oils Extracted from Culinary Herbs. *J Clin Diagnostic Res.* 2017 Sep;11(9):DC30-5.

[2095] Wang Y, Zhang Y, Shi YQ, et al. Antibacterial effects of cinnamon (Cinnamomum zeylanicum) bark essential oil on Porphyromonas gingivalis. *Microb Pathog.* 2018 Mar;116:26-32.

[2096] Khater HF, Ali AM, Abouelella GA, et al. Toxicity and growth inhibition potential of vetiver, cinnamon, and lavender essential oils and their blends against larvae of the sheep blowfly, Lucilia sericata. *Int J Dermatol.* 2018 Apr;57(4):449-457.

[2097] Shahina Z, El-Ganiny AM, Minion J, et al. Cinnamomum zeylanicum bark essential oil induces cell wall remodelling and spindle defects in Candida albicans. *Fungal Biol Biotechnol.* 2018 Feb 9;5:3.

[2098] Essid R, Hammami M, Gharbi D, et al. Antifungal mechanism of the combination of Cinnamomum verum and Pelargonium graveolens essential oils with fluconazole against pathogenic Candida strains. *Appl Microbiol Biotechnol.* 2017 Sep;101(18):6993-7006.

[2099] Solarte AL, Astorga RJ, Aguiar F, et al. Combination of Antimicrobials and Essential Oils as an Alternative for the Control of Salmonella enterica Multiresistant Strains Related to Foodborne Disease. *Foodborne Pathog Dis.* 2017 Oct;14(10):558-563.

[2100] Brnawi WI, Hettiarachchy NS, Horax R, et al. Comparison of Cinnamon Essential Oils from Leaf and Bark with Respect to Antimicrobial Activity and Sensory Acceptability in Strawberry Shake. *J Food Sci.* 2018 Feb;83(2):475-480.

[2101] Firmino DF, Cavalcante TTA, Gomes GA, et al. Antibacterial and Antibiofilm Activities of Cinnamomum Sp. Essential Oil and Cinnamaldehyde: Antimicrobial Activities. *ScientificWorldJournal.* 2018 Jun 6;2018:7405736.

[2102] Plata-Rueda A, Campos JM, da Silva Rolim G, et al. Terpenoid constituents of cinnamon and clove essential oils cause toxic effects and behavior repellency response on granary weevil, Sitophilus granarius. *Ecotoxicol Environ Saf.* 2018 Jul 30;156:263-270.

[2103] Gómez JV, Tarazona A, Mateo-Castro R, et al. Selected plant essential oils and their main active components, a promising approach to inhibit aflatoxigenic fungi and aflatoxin production in food. *Food Addit Contam Part A Chem Anal Control Expo Risk Assess.* 2018 Aug;35(8):1581-1595.

[2104] Condò C, Anacarso I, Sabia C, et al. Antimicrobial activity of spices essential oils and its effectiveness on mature biofilms of human pathogens. *Nat Prod Res.* 2018 Oct 13:1-8.

[2105] Powers CN, Osier JL, McFeeters RL, et al. Antifungal and Cytotoxic Activities of Sixty Commercially-Available Essential Oils. *Molecules.* 2018 Jun 27;23(7).

[2106] Viteri Jumbo LO, Haddi K, Faroni LRD, et al. Toxicity to, oviposition and population growth impairments of Callosobruchus maculatus exposed to clove and cinnamon essential oils. *PLoS One.* 2018 Nov 16;13(11):e0207618.

[2107] Rangel ML, de Aquino SG, de Lima JM, et al. In Vitro Effect of Cinnamomum zeylanicum Blume Essential Oil on Candida spp. Involved in Oral Infections. *Evid Based Complement Alternat Med.* 2018 Oct 17;2018:4045013.

[2108] Khater HF, Geden CJ. Potential of essential oils to prevent fly strike and their effects on the longevity of adult Lucilia sericata. *J Vector Ecol.* 2018 Dec;43(2):261-270.

[2109] Chansang A, Champakaew D, Junkum A, et al. Synergy in the adulticidal efficacy of essential oils for the improvement of permethrin toxicity against Aedes aegypti L. (Diptera: Culicidae). *Parasit Vectors.* 2018 Jul 13;11(1):417.

[2110] Teles AM, Rosa TDDS, Mouchrek AN, et al. Cinnamomum zeylanicum, Origanum vulgare, and Curcuma longa Essential Oils: Chemical Composition, Antimicrobial and Antileishmanial Activity. *Evid Based Complement Alternat Med.* 2019 Jan 15;2019:2421695.

[2111] Gabriel KT, Kartforosh L, Crow SA Jr, et al. Antimicrobial Activity of Essential Oils Against the Fungal Pathogens Ascosphaera apis and Pseudogymnoascus destructans. *Mycopathologia.* 2018 Dec;183(6):921-934.

[2112] Bellassoued K, Ghrab F, Hamed H, et al. Protective effect of essential oil of Cinnamomum verum bark on hepatic and renal toxicity induced by carbon tetrachloride in rats. *Appl Physiol Nutr Metab.* 2019 Apr 17:1-13.

[2113] Yang SK, Yusoff K, Ajat M, et al. Disruption of KPC-producing Klebsiella pneumoniae membrane via induction of oxidative stress by cinnamon bark (Cinnamomum verum J. Presl) essential oil. *PLoS One.* 2019 Apr 2;14(4):e0214326.

[2114] Li Y, Yao JH, Shu YT, et al. [Comparative study of penetration-enhancing effect in vitro of cinnamon oil and cinnamaldehyde on ibuprofen]. *Zhongguo Zhong Yao Za Zhi.* 2018 Sep;43(17):3493-3497.

[2115] Uzair B, Niaz N, Bano A, et al. Essential oils showing in vitro anti MRSA and synergistic activity with penicillin group of antibiotics. *Pak J Pharm Sci.* 2017 Sep;30(5(Supplementary)):1997-2002.

[2116] Kerekes EB, Vidács A, Takó M, et al. Antibiofilm Effect of Selected Essential Oils and Main Components on Mono- and Polymicrobic Bacterial Cultures. *Microorganisms.* 2019 Sep 12;7(9).

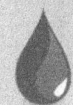

[2117] Ebani VV, Nardoni S, Bertelloni F, et al. In Vitro Antimicrobial Activity of Essential Oils Against Salmonella enterica Serotypes Enteritidis and Typhimurium Strains Isolated from Poultry. *Molecules*. 2019 Mar 4;24(5).
[2118] Niknezhad F, Sayad-Fathi S, Karimzadeh A, et al. Improvement in histology, enzymatic activity, and redox state of the liver following administration of Cinnamomum zeylanicum bark oil in rats with established hepatotoxicity. *Anat Cell Biol*. 2019 Sep;52(3):302-311.
[2119] Onder A, Yilmaz-Oral D, Jerkovic I, et al. Evaluation of relaxant responses properties of cinnamon essential oil and its major component, cinnamaldehyde on human and rat corpus cavernosum. *Int Braz J Urol*. 2019 Sep-Oct;45(5):1033-1042.
[2120] Khater HF, Geden GJ. Efficacy and Repellency of Some Essential Oils and Their Blends Against Larval and Adult House Flies, Musca Domestica L. (Diptera: Muscidae). *J Vector Ecol*. 2019 Dec;44(2):256-63.
[2121] Najar B, Pistelli L, Shortrede JE, et al. Chemical Composition and in Vitro Cytotoxic Screening of Sixteen Commercial Essential Oils on Five Cancer Cell Lines. *Chem Biodivers*. 2020 Jan;17(1):e1900478.
[2122] Mahomoodally F, Aumeeruddy-Elafi Z, Venugopala KN, et al. Antiglycation, Comparative Antioxidant Potential, Phenolic Content and Yield Variation of Essential Oils From 19 Exotic and Endemic Medicinal Plants. *Saudi J Biol Sci*. 2019 Nov;26(7):1779-88.
[2123] Elcocks ER, Spencer-Phillips PTN, Adukwu EC. Rapid Bactericidal Effect Of Cinnamon Bark Essential Oil Against Pseudomonas Aeruginosa. *J Appl Microbiol*. 2020 Apr;128(4):1025-37.
[2124] Yang SK, Yusoff K, Ajat M, et al. Disruption of KPC-producing Klebsiella Pneumoniae Membrane via Induction of Oxidative Stress by Cinnamon Bark (Cinnamomum Verum J. Presl) Essential Oil. PLoS One. 2019;14(4):e0214326.
[2125] Kallel I, Hadrich B, Gargouri B, et al. Optimization of Cinnamon (Cinnamomum zeylanicum Blume) Essential Oil Extraction: Evaluation of Antioxidant and Antiproliferative Effects. *Evid Based Complement Alternat Med*. 2019;2019:6498347.
[2126] Lang M, Ferron PJ, Bursztyka J, et al. Evaluation of Immunomodulatory Activities of Essential Oils by High Content Analysis. J Biotechnol. 2019 Sep 10;303:65-71.
[2127] Xao S, Cui P, Shi W, et al. Identification of Essential Oils With Strong Activity Against Stationary Phase Uropathogenic Escherichia Coli. Discov Med. 2019 Oct;28(154):179-188.
[2128] Al-Nabusi AA, Osali TM, Olaimat AN, et al. Inactivation of Salmonella Spp. In Tahini Using Plant Essential Oil Extracts. *Food Microbiol*. 2020 Apr;86:103338.
[2129] Tepe AS, Ozaslan M. Anti-Alzheimer, anti-diabetic, skin-whitening, and antioxidant activities of the essential oil of Cinnamomum zeylanicum. *Ind Crops Prod*. 2020 Mar;145:112069.
[2130] Xiao S, Cui P, Shi W, et al. Identification of essential oils with activity against stationary phase Staphylococcus aureus. *BMC Complement Med Ther*. 2020 Mar 24;20(1):99.
[2131] Alibi S, Ben Selma W, Ramos-Vivas J, et al. Anti-oxidant, antibacterial, antibiofilm, and anti-quorum sensing activities of four essential oils against multidrug-resistant bacterial clinical isolates. *Curr Res Transl Med*. 2020 Mar 16. [Epub ahead of print]
[2132] Li AL, Ni WW, Zhang QM, et al. Effect of cinnamon essential oil on gut microbiota in the mouse model of dextran sodium sulfate-induced colitis. *Microbiol Immunol*. 2020 Jan;64(1):23-32.
[2133] Seyed Ahmadi SG, Farahpour MR, Hamishehkar H, et al. Topical application of Cinnamon verum essential oil accelerates infected wound healing process by increasing tissue antioxidant capacity and keratin biosynthesis. *Kaohsiung J Med Sci*. 2019 Nov;35(11):686-694.
[2134] Peach DAH, Almond M, Gries R, et al. Lemongrass and Cinnamon Bark: Plant Essential Oil Blend as a Spatial Repellent for Mosquitoes in a Field Setting. *J Med Entomol*. 2019 Sep 3;56(5):1346-1352.
[2135] Somrani M, Ingles MC, Debbabi H, et al. Garlic, Onion, and Cinnamon Essential Oil Antibiofilms' Effect Against Listeria monocytogenes. *Foods*. 2020 May 4;9(5):E567.
[2136] Behbahani BA, Falah F, Arab FL, et al. Chemical Composition and Antioxidant, Antimicrobial, and Antiproliferative Activities of Cinnamomum zeylanicum Bark Essential Oil. *Evid Based Complement Alternat Med*. 2020 Apr 29;2020:5190603.
[2137] Fabbri J, Maggiore MA, Pensel PE, et al. In Vitro Efficacy Study of Cinnamomum Zeylanicum Essential Oil and Cinnamaldehyde Against the Larval Stage of Echinococcus Granulosus. *Exp Parasitol*. 2020 Jul;214:107904.
[2138] Mohammed KAA, Ahmed HMS, Sharaf HA, et al. Encapsulation of Cinnamon Oil in Whey Protein Counteracts the Disturbances in Biochemical Parameters, Gene Expression, and Histological Picture of the Liver and Pancreas of Diabetic Rats. *Environ Sci Pollut Res Int*. 2020 Jan;27(3):2829-2843.
[2139] Yang Y, Islam MB, Tak JH. Insecticidal Activity of 28 Essential Oils and a Commercial Product Containing Cinnamomum cassia Bark Essential Oil against Sitophilus zeamais Motschulsky. *Insects*. 2020 Jul 27;11(8):E474.
[2140] Csikos E, Cseko K, Ashraf AR, et al. Effects of Thymus vulgaris L., Cinnamomum verum J.Presl and Cymbopogon nardus (L.) Rendle Essential Oils in the Endotoxin-induced Acute Airway Inflammation Mouse Model. *Molecules*. 2020 Aug 4;25(15):3553.
[2141] Wijesinghe GK, Maia FC, de Oliveira TR. Effect of Cinnamomum verum leaf essential oil on virulence factors of Candida species and determination of the in-vivo toxicity with Galleria mellonella model. *Mem Inst Oswaldo Cruz*. 2020 Sep 25;115:e200349.
[2142] Tran HNH, Graham L, Adukwu EC. In vitro antifungal activity of Cinnamomum zeylanicum bark and leaf essential oils against Candida albicans and Candida auris. *Appl Microbiol Biotechnol*. 2020 Oct;104(20):8911-8924.
[2143] Hetta HF, Meshaal AK, Algammal AM, et al. In-vitro Antimicrobial Activity of Essential Oils and Spices Powder of some Medicinal Plants Against Bacillus Species Isolated from Raw and Processed Meat. *Infect Drug Resist*. 2020 Dec 4;13:4367-4378.
[2144] De Arujo MRC, Maciel PP, Castellano LRC, et al. Efficacy of essential oil of cinnamon for the treatment of oral candidiasis: A randomized trial. *Spec Care Dentist*. 2021 Jan 21. Online ahead of print.
[2145] Hurtado R, Peltroche N, Mauricio F, et al. Antifungal Efficacy of Four Different Concentrations of the Essential Oil of Cinnamomum zeylanicum (Canela) against Candida albicans: An In Vitro Study. *J Int Soc Prev Community Dent*. 2020 Nov 24;10(6):724-730.
[2146] Ahmed WMS, Abdel-Azeem NM, Ibrahim MA, et al. Neuromodulatory effect of cinnamon oil on behavioural disturbance, CYP1A1, iNOStranscripts and neurochemical alterations induced by deltamethrin in rat brain. *Ecotoxicol Environ Saf*. 2021 Feb;209:111820.
[2147] Osanloo M, Ghaznavi G, Abdollahi A. Surveying the chemical composition and antibacterial activity of essential oils from selected medicinal plants against human pathogens. *Iran J Microbiol*. 2020 Dec;12(6):577-583.
[2148] Akrami S, Amin M, Saki M. In vitro evaluation of the antibacterial effects of Cinnamomum zeylanicum essential oil against clinical multidrug-resistant Shigella isolates. *Mol Biol Rep*. 2021 Apr 1. doi: 10.1007/s11033-021-06309-w.
[2149] Wijesinghe GK, Feirira SB, Maia FC, et al. In-vitro Antibacterial and Antibiofilm Activity of Cinnamomum verum Leaf Oil against Pseudomonas aeruginosa, Staphylococcus aureus and Klebsiella pneumoniae. *An Acad Bras Cienc*. 2021 Feb 24;93(1):e20201507.
[2150] Denkova-Kostova R, Teneva D, Tomova T, et al. Chemical composition, antioxidant and antimicrobial activity of essential oils from tangerine ( Citrus reticulata L.), grapefruit ( Citrus paradisi L.), lemon ( Citrus lemon L.) and cinnamon ( Cinnamomum zeylanicum Blume). *Z Naturforsch C J Biosci*. 2020 Nov 23;76(5-6):175-185.
[2151] Firooziyan S, Amani A, Osanloo M, et al. Preparation of nanoemulsion of Cinnamomum zeylanicum oil and evaluation of its larvicidal activity against a main malaria vector Anopheles stephensi. *J Environ Health Sci Eng*. 2021 Apr 29;19(1):1025-1034.
[2152] Castro JC, Pante GC, Centenaro BM, et al. Antifungal and antimycotoxigenic effects of Zingiber officinale, Cinnamomum zeylanicum and Cymbopogon martinii essential oils against Fusarium verticillioides. *Food Addit Contam Part A Chem Anal Control Expo Risk Assess*. 2020 Sep;37(9):1531-1541.
[2153] Unalan I, Fuggerer T, Slavik B, et al. Antibacterial and antioxidant activity of cinnamon essential oil-laden 45S5 bioactive glass/soy protein composite scaffolds for the treatment of bone infections and oxidative stress. *Mater Sci Eng C Mater Biol Appl*. 2021 Sep;128:112320.
[2154] Abd El-Aziz NK, Ammar AM, El-Naenaeey EYM, et al. Antimicrobial and antibiofilm potentials of cinnamon oil and silver nanoparticles against Streptococcus agalactiae isolated from bovine mastitis: new avenues for countering resistance. *BMC Vet Res*. 2021 Mar 31;17(1):136.
[2155] Marchesini P, de Oliveira DR, Gomes GA, et al. Acaricidal activity of essential oils of Cinnamomum zeylanicum and Eremanthus erythropappus, major compounds and cinnamyl acetate in Rhipicephalus microplus. *Rev Bras Parasitol Vet*. 2021 Sep 6;30(3):e009221.
[2156] Pourkhosravani E, Nayeri FD, Bazargani MM. Decoding antibacterial and antibiofilm properties of cinnamon and cardamom essential oils: a combined molecular docking and experimental study. *AMB Express*. 2021 Oct 26;11(1):143.
[2157] Narayanankutty A, Kunnath K, Alfarhan A, et al. Chemical Composition of Cinnamomum verum Leaf and Flower Essential Oils and Analysis of Their Antibacterial, Insecticidal, and Larvicidal Properties. *Molecules*. 2021 Oct 19;26(20):6303.
[2158] Wijesinghe GK, de Oliveira TR, Maia FC, et al. Efficacy of true cinnamon (Cinnamomum verum) leaf essential oil as a therapeutic alternative for Candida biofilm infections. *Iran J Basic Med Sci*. 2021 Jun;24(6):787-795.
[2159] Michalczky A, Ostrowska P. Essential oils and their components in combating fungal pathogens of animal and human skin. *J Mycol Med*. 2021 Jun;31(2):101118.
[2160] Guo Y, Pizzol R, Gabbanini S, et al. Absolute Antioxidant Activity of Five Phenol-Rich Essential Oils. *Molecules*. 2021 Aug 29;26(17):5237.
[2161] de Aguiar FC, Solarte AL, Gómez-Gascón L, et al. Antimicrobial susceptibility of cinnamon and red and common thyme essential oils and their main constituent compounds against Streptococcus suis. *Lett Appl Microbiol*. 2022 Jan;74(1):63-72.
[2162] Anandhi P, Tharani M, Rajeshkumar S, et al. Antibacterial activity of cinnamon and clove oil against wound pathogens. *J Popul Ther Clin Pharmacol*. 2022 Jan 6;28(2):e41-e46.
[2163] Wen MM, Abdelwahab IA, Aly RG, et al. Nanophyto-gel against multi-drug resistant Pseudomonas aeruginosa burn wound infection. *Drug Deliv*. 2021 Dec;28(1):463-477.
[2164] Rodriguez Diaz C, Mith H, Bernard T, et al. In vitro study of antimicrobial activity of essential oils and their components against the main Clostridioides difficile PCR-ribotypes isolated in Belgium. *IAFP Eur Congress*. 2021.
[2165] Ali SS, Abd Elnabi MK, Alkherkhisy MM, et al. Exploring the potential of Cinnamomum zeylanicum oil against drug resistant Helicobacter pylori-producing cytotoxic genes. *J Appl Biomed*. 2022 Feb 16. Online ahead of print.
[2166] Stevens N, Allred K. Antidiabetic Potential of Volatile Cinnamon Oil: A Review and Exploration of Mechanisms Using In Silico Molecular Docking Simulations. *Molecules*. 2022 Jan 27;27(3):853.
[2167] Ali T. Anjum AA, Sattar MMK, et al. Antibacterial activity of plant essential oils against indigenously characterized methicillin-resistant Staphylococcus aureus (MRSA). *Trop Biomed*. 2022 Mar 1;39(1):17-25.
[2168] Nakamura A, Kawahara A, Takahashi H, et al. Comparison between the Antimicrobial Activity of Essential Oils and Their Components in the Vapor Phase against Food-related Bacteria. *J Oleo Sci*. 2022;71(3):411-417.

2169 Altun M, Yapici BM. Determination of chemical compositions and antibacterial effects of selected essential oils against human pathogenic strains. *An Acad Bras Cienc.* 2022 Mar 11;94(1):e20210074.

2170 Hussein MAM, Gunduz O, Sahin A, et al. Dual Spinneret Electrospun Polyurethane/PVA-Gelatin Nanofibrous Scaffolds Containing Cinnamon Essential Oil and Nanoceria for Chronic Diabetic Wound Healing: Preparation, Physicochemical Characterization and In-Vitro Evaluation. *Molecules.* 2022 Mar 26;27(7):2146.

2171 El-Zehery HRA, Zaghloul RA, Abdel-Rahman HM, et al. Novel strategies of essential oils, chitosan, and nano- chitosan for inhibition of multi-drug resistant: E. coli O157:H7 and Listeria monocytogenes. *Saudi J Biol Sci.* 2022 Apr;29(4):2582-2590.

2172 Esmaeili F, Zahmatkeshan M, Yousefpoor Y, et al. Anti-inflammatory and anti-nociceptive effects of Cinnamon and Clove essential oils nanogels: an in vivo study. *BMC Complement Med Ther.* 2022 May 20;22(1):143.

2173 Andriantsoanirina V, Guillot J, Ratsimbason M, et al. In vitro efficacy of essential oils against Sarcoptes scabiei. *Sci Rep.* 2022 May 3;12(1):7176.

2174 Man A, Mare AD, Mares M, et al. Antifungal and anti-virulence activity of six essential oils against important Candida species - a preliminary study. *Future Microbiol.* 2022 Jul;17:737-753.

2175 Xin R, Wang G, Qiu Z, et al. Screening of essential oils with acaricidal activity against Haemaphysalis longicornis (Acari: Ixodidae) and analysis of active components. *Vet Parasitol.* 2022 Jul;307-308:109712.

2176 Soonwera M, Moungthipmalai T, Takawirapat W, et al. Ovicidal and repellent activities of several plant essential oils against Periplaneta americana L. and enhanced activities from their combined formulation. *Sci Rep.* 2022 Jul 15;12(1):12070.

2177 Foda AM, Kalaba MH, El-Sherbiny GM, et al. Antibacterial activity of essential oils for combating colistin-resistant bacteria. *Expert Rev Anti Infect Ther.* 2022 Jul 22:1-14.

2178 Morsi DS, El-Nabi SH, Elmaghraby MA, et al. Anti-proliferative and immunomodulatory potencies of cinnamon oil on Ehrlich ascites carcinoma bearing mice. *Sci Rep.* 2022 Jul 12;12(1):11839.

2179 Osanloo M, Firoozian S, Zarenezhad E, et al. A Nanoliposomal Gel Containing Cinnamomum zeylanicum Essential Oil with Effective Repellent against the Main Malaria Vector Anopheles stephensi. *Interdiscip Perspect Infect Dis.* 2022 Jun 22;2022:1645485.

2180 Alibi S, Selma WB, Mansour HB, et al. Activity of Essential Oils Against Multidrug-Resistant Salmonella enteritidis. *Curr Microbiol.* 2022 Jul 30;79(9):273.

2181 Bukhari S, Siddique MH, Naeem A, et al. Combined efficacy of Cinnamomum zeylanicum and doxorubicin against leukemia through regulation of TRAIL and NF-kappa B pathways in rat model. *Mol Biol Rep.* 2022 Jul;49(7):6495-6507.

2182 Jiang C, Hong J, Meng J, et al. Antibacterial activity of essential oils extracted from the unique Chinese spices cassia bark, bay fruits and cloves. *Arch Microbiol.* 2022 Oct 18;204(11):674.

2183 Sarwar W, Ali Q, Ahmed S. Microscopic visualization of the antibiofilm potential of essential oils against Staphylococcus aureus and Klebsiella pneumoniae. *Microsc Res Tech.* 2022 Oct 17. Online ahead of print.

2184 Devecioglu D, Turker M, Karbancioglu-Guler F. Antifungal Activities of Different Essential Oils and Their Electrospun Nanofibers against Aspergillus and Penicillium Species Isolated from Bread. *ACS Omega.* 2022 Oct 14;7(42):37943-37953.

2185 Saeedi M, Iraji A, Vahedi-Mazdabadi Y, Alizadeh A, et al. Cinnamomum verum J. Presl. Bark essential oil: in vitro investigation of anti-cholinesterase, anti-BACE1, and neuroprotective activity. *BMC Complement Med Ther.* 2022 Nov 18;22(1):303.

2186 Nguyen LTH, Nguyen NPK, Tran KN, et al. Anxiolytic-like Effect of Inhaled Cinnamon Essential Oil and Its Main Component Cinnamaldehyde in Animal Models. *Molecules.* 2022 Nov 18;27(22):7997.

2187 Barbarossa A, Sblano S, Rosato A, et al. Synergistic Action of Cinnamomum verum Essential Oil with Sertraline. *Antibiotics (Basel).* 2022 Nov 13;11(11):1617.

2188 Paiano RB, de Sousa RLM, Bonilla J, et al. In vitro effects of cinnamon, oregano, and thyme essential oils against Escherichia coli and Trueperella pyogenes isolated from dairy cows with clinical endometritis. *Theriogenology.* 2022 Nov 7;196:106-111.

2189 Nemattalab M, Rohani M, Evazalipour M, et al. Formulation of Cinnamon (Cinnamomum verum) oil loaded solid lipid nanoparticles and evaluation of its antibacterial activity against Multi-drug Resistant Escherichia coli. *BMC Complement Med Ther.* 2022 Nov 9;22(1):289.

2190 de la Rosa-Garcia JM, Cordero-Perez P, Jimenez-Torres CA, et al. Evaluation of the hypolipidemic effect of cinnamon essential oil in a model of acute damage induced by triton WR-1339. *Annals Hepatology.* 2022 Dec;27(Sup 3):100862

2191 Moungthipmalai T, Puwanard C, Aungtikun J, et al. Ovicidal toxicity of plant essential oils and their major constituents against two mosquito vectors and their nontarget aquatic predators. *Sci Rep.* 2023 Feb 6;13(1):2119.

2192 Choonharuangdej S, Srithavaj T, Thummawanit S. Fungicidal and inhibitory efficacy of cinnamon and lemongrass essential oils on Candida albicans biofilm established on acrylic resin: An in vitro study. *J Prosthet Dent.* 2021 Apr;125(4):707.e1-707.e6.

2193 Wang Y, Yuan C, Liu Y, et al. Fabrication of kappa-carrageenan hydrogels with cinnamon essential oil/hydroxypropyl-β-cyclodextrin composite: Evaluation of physicochemical properties, release kinetics and antimicrobial activity. *Int J Biol Macromol.* 2021 Feb 15;170:593-601.

2194 Moungthipmalai T, Puwanard C, Aungtikun J, et al. Ovicidal toxicity of plant essential oils and their major constituents against two mosquito vectors and their nontarget aquatic predators. *Sci Rep.* 2023 Feb 6;13(1):2119.

2195 Cappelli G, Giovannini D, Vilardo L, et al. Cinnamomum zeylanicum Blume Essential Oil Inhibits Metastatic Melanoma Cell Proliferation by Triggering an Incomplete Tumour Cell Stress Response. *Int J Mol Sci.* 2023 Mar 16;24(6):5698.

2196 Di Vito M, Garzoli S, Rosato R, et al. A New Potential Resource in the Fight against Candida auris: the Cinnamomum zeylanicum Essential Oil in Synergy with Antifungal Drug. *Microbiol Spectr.* 2023 Mar 28:e0438522.

2197 Refaey MS, A A Fayed M, Kutkat O, et al. Bio-guided chemical characterization and nano-formulation studies of selected edible volatile oils with potentials antibacterial and anti-SARS-CoV-2 activities. *Arab J Chem.* 2023 Jul;16(7):104813.

2198 Osanloo M, Noori F, Tavassoli A, et al. Effect of PCL nanofiber mats coated with chitosan microcapsules containing cinnamon essential oil for wound healing. *BMC Complement Med Ther.* 2023 Mar 18;23(1):84.

2199 Attia RG, Khalil MMH, Hussein MA, et al. Cinnamon Oil Encapsulated with Silica Nanoparticles: Chemical Characterization and Evaluation of Insecticidal Activity Against the Rice Moth, Corcyra cephalonica. *Neotrop Entomol.* 2023 Mar 13. Online ahead of print.

2200 Verdeguer M, Blazquez MA, Boira H. Chemical composition and herbicidal activity of the essential oil from Cistus ladanifer L. population from Spain. *Nat Prod Res.* 2012;26(17):1602-09.

2201 Gomes PB, Mata VG, Rodriguez AE. Characterization of the Portuguese-Grown Cistus ladanifer essential oil. *J Essential Oil Res.* 2005;17(2):160-65.

2202 Viuda-Martos M, Sendra E, Perez-Alvarez JA, et al. Identification of flavonoid content and chemical composition on the essential oils of Moroccan herbs: Myrtle (Myrtus communis L.), Rockrose (Cistus ladanifer L.) and Montpellier cistus (Cistus monospeliensis L.). *J Essential Oil Res.* 2011;23(2):1-9.

2203 Greche H, Mrabet N, Zrira S, et al. The volatiles of the leaf of Cistus ladanifer L. var. albiflorus and Labdanum Extracts of Moroccan origin and their antimicrobial activities. *J Essential Oil Res.* 2009;21(2):166-73.

2204 Simon-Fuentes A, Sendra JM, Cunat P. Neutral volatiles of Cistus ladaniferus L. essential oil. *An Quim, Ser. C.* 1987;83:201-204.

2205 Lawrence BM. Progress in Essential Oils. *Perfum Flavor.* 1999;24(4):31-50.

2206 Regino JMB, Frazao S, Carmo MM, et al. Study of the volatile concrete (Cistus ladanifer L.) compared with the essential oil. *J Natl Aromatic Plants and Oils.* 1987.

2207 Guinoiseau E, Lorenzi V, Luciani A, et al. Susceptibility of the multi-drug resistant strain of Enterobacter aerogenes EA289 to the terpene alcohols from Cistus ladaniferus essential oil. *Nat Prod Commun.*2011 Aug;6(8):1159-62.

2208 Mediavilla I, Guillamon E, Ruiz A, et al. Essential Oils from Residual Foliage of Forest Tree and Shrub Species: Yield and Antioxidant Capacity. *Molecules.* 2021 May 28;26(11):3257.

2209 Karkouri JE, Bouhrim M, Al Kamaly OM, et al. Chemical Composition, Antibacterial and Antifungal Activity of the Essential Oil from Cistus ladanifer L. *Plants (Basel).* 2021 Sep 30;10(10):2068.

2210 Xavier V, Finimundy TC, Heleno SA, et al. Chemical and Bioactive Characterization of the Essential Oils Obtained from Three Mediterranean Plants. *Molecules.* 2021 Dec 10;26(24):7472.

2211 Oliveira AS, Rolo J, Gaspar C, et al. Thymus mastichina (L.) L. and Cistus ladanifer L. for skin application: chemical characterization and in vitro bioactivity assessment. *J Ethnopharmacol.* 2023 Feb 10;302(Pt A):115830.

2212 Boy FR, Benito MJ, Córdoba MG, et al. Antimicrobial Properties of Essential Oils Obtained from Autochthonous Aromatic Plants. *Int J Environ Res Public Health.* 2023 Jan 17;20(3):1657.

2213 Aliberti L, Caputo L, De Feo V, et al. Chemical Composition and in Vitro Antimicrobial, Cytotoxic, and Central Nervous System Activities of the Essential Oils of Citrus medica L. cv. 'Liscia' and C. medica cv. 'Rugosa' Cultivated in Southern Italy. *Molecules.* 2016 Sep 18;21(9).

2214 Menichini F, Tundis R, Bonesi M, et al. Chemical composition and bioactivity of Citrus medica L. cv. Diamante essential oil obtained by hydrodistillation, cold-pressing and supercritical carbon dioxide extraction. *Nat Prod Res.* 2011 Apr;25(8):789-99.

2215 Gabriele B, Fazio A, Dugo P, et al. Essential oil composition of Citrus medica L. Cv. Diamante (Diamante citron) determined after using different extraction methods. *J Separation Science.* 2009;32(1):99-108.

2216 Venturini N, Barboni T, Curk F, et al. Volatile and Flavonoid Composition of the Peel of Citrus medica L. var. Corsican Fruit for Quality Assessment of Its Liqueur. *Food Techno Biotechnol.* 2014;52(4):403-10.

2217 Kim KN, Ko YJ, Yang HM, et al. Anti-inflammatory effect of essential oil and its constituents from fingered citron (Citrus medica L. var. sarcodactylis) through blocking JNK, ERK and NF-κB signaling pathways in LPS-activated RAW 264.7 cells. *Food Chem Toxicol.* 2013 Jul;57:126-31.

2218 Menchini F, Tundis R, Loizzo MR, et al. Chemical composition and in vitro anticholinesterase inhibitory activity of Citrus medica L. cv. Diamante essential oil. *Planta Med.* 2009;74:PJ3.

2219 Kim KN, Ko YJ, Yang HM, et al. Anti-inflammatory effect of essential oil and its constituents from 4 fingered citron (Citrus medica L. var. sarcodactylis) through blocking JNK, 5 ERK and NF-jB signaling pathways in LPS-activated RAW 264.7 cells. *Food Chem Toxicol.* 2013 Jul;57:126-31.

2220 Dung NX, Pha NM, Lo VN, et al. Chemical investigation of the fruit peel of Citrus medica L. var. sarcadactylis (Noot.) Swingle from Vietnam. *J Essent Oil Res.* 1996 Jan-Feb;8:15-18.

2221 Dugrand-Judek A, Olry A, Hehn A, et al. The distribution of coumarins and furanocoumarins in citrus cpecies closely matches phylogeny and reflects the organization of biosynthetic pathways. *PLoS One.* 2015;10(11):e0142757.

2222 Menichini F, Tundis R, Loizzo MR, et al. In vitro photo-induced cytotoxic activity of Citrus bergamia and C. medica L. cv. Diamante peel essential oils and identified active coumarins. *Pharm Biol.* 2010 Sep;48(9):1059-65.

2223 Menchini F, Tundis R, Loizzo MR, et al. Chemical composition and in vitro anticholinesterase inhibitory activity of Citrus medica L. cv. Diamante essential oil. *Planta Med.* 2009;74:PJ3.

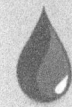

[2224] Peng CH1, Ker YB, Weng CF, et al. Insulin secretagogue bioactivity of finger citron fruit (Citrus medica L. var. Sarcodactylis Hort, Rutaceae). *J Agric Food Chem.* 2009 Oct 14;57(19):8812-9.
[2225] Dang NH, Nhung PH, Mai Anh, et al. Chemical Composition and α-Glucosidase Inhibitory Activity of Vietnamese Citrus Peels Essential Oils. *J Chem.* 2016;2016:6787952.
[2226] Aliberti L, Caputo L, De Feo V, et al. Chemical Composition and in Vitro Antimicrobial, Cytotoxic, and Central Nervous System Activities of the Essential Oils of Citrus medica L. cv. 'Liscia' and C. medica cv. 'Rugosa' Cultivated in Southern Italy. *Molecules.* 2016 Sep 18;21(9).
[2227] Menichini F, Tundis R, Loizzo MR, et al. In vitro photo-induced cytotoxic activity of Citrus bergamia and C. medica L. cv. Diamante peel essential oils and identified active coumarins. *Pharm Biol.* 2010 Sep;48(9):1059-65.
[2228] Aliberti L, Caputo L, De Feo V, et al. Chemical Composition and in Vitro Antimicrobial, Cytotoxic, and Central Nervous System Activities of the Essential Oils of Citrus medica L. cv. 'Liscia' and C. medica cv. 'Rugosa' Cultivated in Southern Italy. *Molecules.* 2016 Sep 18;21(9):1244.
[2229] Peng CH1, Ker YB, Weng CF, et al. Insulin secretagogue bioactivity of finger citron fruit (Citrus medica L. var. Sarcodactylis Hort, Rutaceae). *J Agric Food Chem.* 2009 Oct 14;57(19):8812-9.
[2230] Dang NH, Nhung PH, Mai Anh, et al. Chemical Composition and α-Glucosidase Inhibitory Activity of Vietnamese Citrus Peels Essential Oils. *J Chem.* 2016;2016:6787952.
[2231] Aliberti L, Caputo L, De Feo V, et al. Chemical Composition and in Vitro Antimicrobial, Cytotoxic, and Central Nervous System Activities of the Essential Oils of Citrus medica L. cv. 'Liscia' and C. medica cv. 'Rugosa' Cultivated in Southern Italy. *Molecules.* 2016 Sep 18;21(9).
[2232] Al-Kalifawi EJ. The Antimicrobial Activity of Essential Oils of Al-Abbas's (AS) Hand Fruit Peel (Citrus Medica) var. Sarcodactylis Swingle. *J Nat Sci Res.* 2015;5(12):19-27.
[2233] Menchini F, Tundis R, Loizzo MR, et al. Chemical composition and in vitro anticholinesterase inhibitory activity of Citrus medica L. cv. Diamante essential oil. *Planta Med.* 2009;74:PJ3.
[2234] Darvesh S, Hopkins DA, Geula C, Neurobiology of butyrylcholinesterase. *Nat Rev Neurosci.* 2003 Feb;4:131–38. [2494] Carvalho-Freitas MIR, Costa M. Anxiolytic and sedative effects of extracts and essential oil from Citrus aurantium L. Biolog Pharm Bull. 2002;25(12):1629–33.
[2235] Menchini F, Tundis R, Loizzo MR, et al. Chemical composition and in vitro anticholinesterase inhibitory activity of Citrus medica L. cv. Diamante essential oil. *Planta Med.* 2009;74:PJ3.
[2236] Sharma JN, AL-Omran A, Parvathy SS. Role of nitric oxide in inflammatory diseases. *Inflammopharmacology.* 2007 Dec;15(6):252-59.
[2237] Kim KN, Ko YJ, Yang HM, et al. Anti-inflammatory effect of essential oil and its constituents from 4 fingered citron (Citrus medica L. var. sarcodactylis) through blocking JNK, 5 ERK and NF-jB signaling pathways in LPS-activated RAW 264.7 cells. *Food Chem Toxicol.* 2013 Jul;57:126-31.
[2238] Deng G, Craft JD, Steinberg KM, et al. Influence of Different Isolation Methods on Chemical Composition and Bioactivities of the Fruit Peel Oil of Citrus medica L. var. sarcodactylis (Noot.) Swingle. *Medicines (Basel).* 2017 Jan 4;4(1).
[2239] Li ZH, Cai M, Liu YS, et al. Antibacterial Activity and Mechanisms of Essential Oil from Citrus medica L. var. sarcodactylis. *Molecules.* 2019 Apr 22;24(8).
[2240] Guo J, Hu X, Gao Z, et al. Global transcriptomic response of Listeria monocytogenes exposed to Fingered Citron (Citrus medica L. var. sarcodactylis Swingle) essential oil. *Food Res Int.* 2021 May;143:110274.
[2241] Vitalini S, Iriti M, Vinciguerra V, Garzoli S. A Comparative Study of the Chemical Composition by SPME-GC/MS and Antiradical Activity of Less Common Citrus Species. *Molecules.* 2021 Sep 4;26(17):5378.
[2242] Vitalini S, Iriti M, Ovidi E, et al. Detection of Volatiles by HS-SPME-GC/MS and Biological Effect Evaluation of Buddha's Hand Fruit. *Molecules.* 2022 Mar 3;27(5):1666.
[2243] Ghani A, Taghvaeefard N, Hosseinifarahi M, et al. Essential oil composition and antioxidant activity of citron fruit (Citrus medica var. macrocarpa Risso.) peel as relation to ripening stages. *Int J Environ Health Res.* 2022 Jun 18:1-11.
[2244] Aquilano C, Baccari L, Caprari C, et al. Effects of EOs vs. Antibiotics on E. coli Strains Isolated from Drinking Waters of Grazing Animals in the Upper Molise Region, Italy. *Molecules.* 2022 Nov 24;27(23):8177.
[2245] Rodrigues KA, Dias CN, do Amaral FM, et al. Molluscicidal and larvicidal activities and essential oil composition of Cymbopogon winterianus. *Pharm Biol.* 2013 Oct;51(10):1293-97.
[2246] Cassel E, Varbgas EMF. Experiments and modeling of the Cymbopogon winterianus essential oil extraction by steam distillation. *J Mex Chem Soc.* 206;50(3):126-29.
[2247] Quintanas-Junior LJ, Souza TT, Leite BS, et al. Phytochemical screening and anticonvulsant activity of Cymbopogon winterianus Jowitt (Poaceae) leaf essential oil in rodents. *Phytomedicine.* 208 Aug 1;15(8):619-24.
[2248] Carlin JT, Kramer S, Ho CT. Comparison of commercial citronella oils from various origins. *Flavor and Fragrance: A World Perspective.* 1988. pp. 495-504.
[2249] Rao BR, Kaul PN, Bhattacharya AK. Java citronella (Cymbopogon winterianus Jowitt) cultivation in a tribal area of Andhra Pradesh. *J Essential Oil Bearing Plants.* 1998;1:114-18.
[2250] Nakahara K, Alzoreky NS, Yoshihashi T, et al. Chemical Composition and Antifungal Activity of Essential Oil from Cymbopogon nardus (Citronella Grass). *Japan Agric Res Quarterly.* 2012 Dec;37(4):249-252.
[2251] Khanuja SPS, Shasany AK, Pawar A, et al. Essential oil constituents and RAPD markers to establish species relationship in Cymbopogon Spreng. (Poaceae). *Biochem Syst Ecol.* 2005;33:171-86.
[2252] Wany A, Jha S, Nigram VK, et al. Chemical analysis and therapeutic uses of citronella oil from Cymbopogon winteranius: A short review. *Int J Adv Res.* 2013;1(6):504-21.
[2253] Abena AA, Gbenou JD, Yayi E, et al. Comparative chemical and analgesic properties of essential oils of Cymbopogon nardus (L.) Rendle of Benin and Congo. *Afr J Trad CAM.* 2007;4(2):267-72.
[2254] Nogueira AC, Carvalho RR, Souza CA, et al. Study on the embryofeto-toxicity of citral in the rat. *Toxicology.* 1995;96(2):105-13.
[2255] Boukhris M, Bouaziz M, Feki I, et al. Hypoglycemic and antioxidant effects of leaf and essential oil of Pelargonium graveolens L'Her. in alloxan induced diabetic rats. *Lipids Health Dis.* 2012 Jun 26;11:81.
[2256] Adeneye AA, Agbaje EO. Hypoglycemic and hypolipidemic effects of fresh leaf aqueous extract of Cymbopogon citratus Stapf. in rats. *J Ethnopharmacol.* 2007 Jul 25; 112(3):440-4.
[2257] Bharti SK, Kumar A, Prakash O, et al. Essential Oil of Cymbopogon Citratus Against Diabetes: Validation by In vivo Experiments and Computational Studies. *J Bioanal Biomed.* 2013;5:194-203.
[2258] Kshirsagan R, Reddy GB, Bakshi V, et al. Geraniol a major component of essential oil ameliorates endothelial dysfunction induced by high-fat diet fed rats. *Atherosclerosis.* 2015 Jun;241(1):e154-e155.
[2259] Ibrahim SM, El-Denshary ES, Abdallah DM. Geraniol, Alone and in Combination with Pioglitazone, Ameliorates Fructose-Induced Metabolic Syndrome in Rats via the Modulation of Both Inflammatory and Oxidative Stress Status. *PLoS One.* 2015 Feb 13;10(2):e0117516.
[2260] Srinivasan S, Muruganathan U. Antidiabetic efficacy of citronellol, a citrus monoterpene by ameliorating the hepatic key enzymes of carbohydrate metabolism in streptozotocin-induced diabetic rats. *Chem Biol Interact.* 2016 Apr 25;250:38-46.
[2261] Seo KA, Kim H, Ku HY, et al. The monoterpenoids citral and geraniol are moderate inhibitors of the CYP2B6 hydroxylase activity. *Chem Biol Interact.* 2008;174:141-46.
[2262] Sheweita SA, Newairy AA, Mansour HA, et al. Effect of some hypoglycemic herbs on the activity of phase I and II drug-metabolizing enzymes in alloxan-induced diabetic rats. *Toxicology.* 2002 May 24;17(2):131-39.
[2263] Seo KA, Kim H, Ku HY, et al. The monoterpenoids citral and geraniol are moderate inhibitors of the CYP2B6 hydroxylase activity. *Chem Biol Interact.* 2008;174:141-46.
[2264] Sheweita SA, Newairy AA, Mansour HA, et al. Effect of some hypoglycemic herbs on the activity of phase I and II drug-metabolizing enzymes in alloxan-induced diabetic rats. *Toxicology.* 2002 May 24;17(2):131-39.
[2265] Raner GM, Vaz AD, Coon MJ. Metabolism of all-trans, 9-cis, and 13-cis isomers of retinal by purified isozymes of microsomal cytochrome P450 and mechanism-based inhibition of retinoid oxidation by citral. *Mol Pharmacol.* 1996;49(3):515-22.
[2266] De Olivera AC, Ribeiro-Pinto LF, Paumgartten JR. In vitro inhibition of CYP2B1 monoxygenase by beta-myrcene and other monoterpenoid constituents. *Br J Nutr.* 1999;81:289-95.
[2267] De Menezes IA, Moreira IJ, de Paula JW, et al. Cardiovascular effects induced by Cymbopogon winterianus essential oil in rats: involvement of calcium channels and vagal pathway. *J Pharm Pharmacol.* 2010 Feb;62(2):215-21.
[2268] Choi JY, Damte D, Seung-Jin L, et al. Antimicrobial activity of lemongrass and oregano essential oil against standard antibiotic resistant Staphylococcus aureus and field isolates from chronic mastitis cow. *International Journal of Phytomedicine.* 2012;4(1):134-39.
[2269] Hagvall L. Cytochrome P450-mediated activation of the fragrance constituent geraniol forms potent contact allergens. *Tox Appl Pharm.* 2008 Dec;233(2):308-13.
[2270] Kuhn GO, McCampbell P, Singmaster G, et al. Application of microencapsulation technology to improve the stability of citral in rodent diets. *Fundam Appl Toxicol.* 1991 Oct;17(3):635-40.
[2271] De Mozzi P, Johnston GA. An outbreak of allergic contact dermatitis caused by citral in beauticians working in a health spa. *Contact Dermatitis.* 2014 Jun;70(6):377-9.
[2272] MaBberg D, Simon A, Haussinger D, et al. Monoterpene (-)-citronellal affects hepatocarcinoma cell signaling via an olfactory receptor. *Arch Biochem Biophys.* 2015 Jan 15;566:10-9.
[2273] Schwarz EC, Qu B, Hoth M. Calcium, cancer and killing: The role of calcium in killing cancer cells by cytotoxic T lymphocytes and natural killer cells. *Biochimica et Biophysica Acta (BBA) - Mol Cell Res.* 2013 Jul;1883(7):1603-11.
[2274] De Santana MT, de Oliveira MG, Santana MF, et al. Citronellal, a monoterpene present in Java citronella oil, attenuates mechanical nociception response in mice. *Pharm Biol.* 2013 Sep;51(9):1144-49.
[2275] Leite BL, Bonfim RR, Antoniolli AR, et al. Assessment of antinociceptive, anti-inflammatory and antioxidant properties of Cymbopogon winterianus leaf. *Pharm Biol.* 2010 Oct;48(10):1164-69.
[2276] Quintans-Junior L, da Rocha RF, Caregnato FF, et al. Antinociceptive and redox properties of citronellal, an essential oil present in lemongrass. *J Med Food.* 2011 Jun;14(6):630-39.
[2277] de Menezes IA, Moreira IJ, de Paula JW, et al. Cardiovascular effects induced by Cymbopogon winterianus essential oil in rats: involvement of calcium channels and vagal pathway. *J Pharm Pharmacol.* 2010 Feb;62(2):215-21.
[2278] de Oliveira WA, de Oliveira Preira F, de Luna GC, et al. Antifungal activity of Cymbopogon winterianus jowitt ex bor against Candida albicans. *Braz J Microbiol.* 2011 Apr;42(2):433-41.
[2279] Duarte MC, Figueira GM, Sartoratto A, et al. Anti-candida activity of Brazilian medicinal plants. *J Ethnopharmacol.* 2005 Feb 28;97(2):305-11.
[2280] Almeida Lde F, Paula JF, Almeida RV, et al. Efficacy of citronella and cinnamon essential oils on Candida albicans biofilms. *Acta Odontol Scand.* 2016 Jul;74(5):393-8.
[2281] Silva MR, Ximenes RM, da Costa JG, et al. Comparative anticonvulsant activities of the essential oil (Eos) from Cymbopogon winterianus Jowitt and Cymbopogon citratus (DC) Stapf. in mice. *Naunyn Schmiedebergs Arch Pharmacol.* 2010 May;381(5):415-26.
[2282] Tawatsin A, Wratten SD, Scott RR, et al. Repellency of volatile oils from pants against three mosquito vectors. *J Vector Ecol.* 2001 Jun;26(1):76-82.
[2283] Sinha S, Biswas D, Mukherjee A. Antigenotoxic and antioxidant activities of palmarosa and citronella essential oils. *J Ethnopharmacol.* 2011 Oct;137(3):1521-27.

[2284] Brito RG, Santos PL, Prado DS, et al. Citronellol reduces orofacial nociceptive behaviors in mice - evidence of involvement of retrosplenial cortex and periaqueductal grey areas. *Basic Clin Pharmacol Toxicol*. 2013 Apr;112(4):215- 21.

[2285] Bastos JF, Noreira IJ, Ribeiro TP, et al. Hypotensive and vasorelaxant effects of citronellol, a monoterpene alcohol, in rats. *Basic Clin Pharamacol Toxicol*. 2010 Apr;106(4):331-37.

[2286] Nararak J, Sathantriphop S, Chauhan K, et al. Avoidance Behavior to Essential Oils by Anopheles minimus, a Malaria Vector in Thailand. *J Am Mosq Control Assoc*. 2016 Mar;32(1):34-43.

[2287] Adams TF, Wongchai C, Chaidee A, et al. "Singing in the Tube"--audiovisual assay of plant oil repellent activity against mosquitoes (Culex pipiens). *Parasitol Res*. 2016 Jan;115(1):225-39.

[2288] Boonyuan W, Grieco JP, Bangs MJ, et al. Excito-repellency of essential oils against an Aedes aegypti (L.) field population in Thailand. *J Vector Ecol*. 2014 Jun;39(1):112-22.

[2289] Warikoo R, Wahab N, Kumar S. Oviposition-altering and ovicidal potentials of five essential oils against female adults of the dengue vector, Aedes aegypti L. *Parasitol Res*. 2011 Oct;109(4):1125-31.

[2290] Phasomkusolsil S, Soonwera M. Potential larvicidal and pupacidal activities of herbal essential oils against Culex quinquefasciatus say and Anopheles minimus (Theobald). *Southeast Asian J Trop Med Public Health*. 2010 Nov;41(6):1342-51.

[2291] Phasomkusolsil S, Soonwera M. Insect repellent activity of medicinal plant oils against Aedes aegypti (Linn.), Anopheles minimus (Theobald) and Culex quinquefasciatus Say based on protection time and biting rate. *Southeast Asian J Trop Med Public Health*. 2010 Jul;41(4):831-40.

[2292] Trongtokit Y, Rongsriyam Y, Komalamisra N, et al. Comparative repellency of 38 essential oils against mosquito bites. *Phytother Res*. 2005 Apr;19(4):303-9.

[2293] Hsu WS, Yen JH, Wang YS. Formulas of components of citronella oil against mosquitoes (Aedes aegypti). *J Environ Sci Health B*. 2013;48(11):1014-9.

[2294] Batubara I, Suparto IH, Sa'diah S, et al. Effects of inhaled citronella oil and related constituents on rat body weight and brown adipose tissue sympathetic nerve. *Nutrients*. 2015 Mar 12;7(3):1859-70.

[2295] Lopatina IuV, Eremina OIu. [Peculicidal activity of plant essential oils and their based preparations]. *Med Parazitol (Mosk)*. 2014 Apr-Jun;(2):37-42.

[2296] Ocheng F, Bwanga F, Joloba M, et al. Essential Oils from Ugandan Aromatic Medicinal Plants: Chemical Composition and Growth Inhibitory Effects on Oral Pathogens. *Evid Based Complement Alternat Med*. 2015;2015:230832.

[2297] Trindade LA, de Araújo Oliveira J, de Castro RD, et al. Inhibition of adherence of C. albicans to dental implants and cover screws by Cymbopogon nardus essential oil and citronellal. *Clin Oral Investig*. 2015 Dec;19(9):2223-31.

[2298] de Billerbeck VG, Roques CG, Bessière JM, et al. Effects of Cymbopogon nardus (L.) W. Watson essential oil on the growth and morphogenesis of Aspergillus niger. *Can J Microbiol*. 2001 Jan;47(1):9-17.

[2299] Kpoviessi S, Bero J, Agbani P, et al. Chemical composition, cytotoxicity and in vitro antitrypanosomal and antiplasmodial activity of the essential oils of four Cymbopogon species from Benin. *J Ethnopharmacol*. 2014;151(1):652-9.

[2300] Clemente MA, de Oliveira Monteiro CM, Scoralik MG, et al. Acaricidal activity of the essential oils from Eucalyptus citriodora and Cymbopogon nardus on larvae of Amblyomma cajennense (Acari: Ixodidae) and Anocentor nitens (Acari: Ixodidae). *Parasitol Res*. 2010 Sep;107(4):987-92.

[2301] Abena AA, Gbenou JD, Yayi E, et al. Comparative chemical and analgesic properties of essential oils of Cymbopogon nardus (L) Rendle of Benin and Congo. *Afr J Tradit Complement Altern Med*. 2007 Feb 16;4(3):267-72.

[2302] Oussalah M, Caillet S, Saucier L, et al. Antimicrobial effects of selected plant essential oils on the growth of a Pseudomonas putida strain isolated from meat. *Meat Sci*. 2006 Jun;73(2):236-44.

[2303] Gaire S, O'Connell M, Holguin FO, et al. Insecticidal Properties of Essential Oils and Some of Their Constituents on the Turkestan Cockroach (Blattodea: Blattidae). *J Econ Entomol*. 2017 Apr 1;110(2):584-592.

[2304] Gabriel KT, Kartforosh L, Crow SA Jr, et al. Antimicrobial Activity of Essential Oils Against the Fungal Pathogens Ascosphaera apis and Pseudogymnoascus destructans. *Mycopathologia*. 2018 Dec;183(6):921-934.

[2305] da Silva LC, de Souza Perinoot WM, Sa FA, et al. In vitro acaricidal activity of Cymbopogon citratus, Cymbopogon nardus and Mentha arvensis against Rhipicephalus microplus (Acari: Ixodidae). *Exp Parasitol*. 2020 Sep;216:107937.

[2306] Elazab ST, Soliman AF, Nishikawa Y. Effect of some plant extracts from Egyptian herbal plants against Toxoplasma gondii tachyzoites in vitro. *J Vet Med Sci*. 2020 Dec 1. Online ahead of print.

[2307] Kundu A, Dutta A, Mandal A, et al. A Comprehensive in vitro and in silico Analysis of Nematicidal Action of Essential Oils. *Front Plant Sci*. 2021 Jan 8;11:614143.

[2308] Tavares LA, Rezende AA, Santos JL, et al. Cymbopogon winterianus Essential Oil Attenuates Bleomycin-Induced Pulmonary Fibrosis in a Murine Model. *Pharmaceutics*. 2021 May 9;13(5):679.

[2309] Piasecki B, Biernasiuk A, Skiba A, et al. Composition, Anti-MRSA Activity and Toxicity of Essential Oils from Cymbopogon Species. *Molecules*. 2021 Dec 13;26(24):7542.

[2310] Mota TF, Silva CMA, Conceição MDS, et al. Screening organic repellent compounds against Lutzomyia longipalpis (Diptera: Psychodidae) present in plant essential oils: Bioassay plus an in silico approach. *Acta Trop*. 2022 Feb 12;229:106367.

[2311] Chelaghema A, Durand N, Servent A, et al. Antifungal and antimycotoxic activities of 3 essential oils against 3 mycotoxinogenic fungi. *Arch Microbiol*. 2022 Jul 19;204(8):504.

[2312] Wang T, Ren Y, Zhao J, et al. Research on the Bioactivity of Plant Essential Oils on Armyworm [Mythimna separata (Walker)] Larvae. *Front Chem*. 2022 Jun 29;10:936873.

[2313] Dangol S, Poudel DK, Ojha PK, et al. Essential Oil Composition Analysis of Cymbopogon Species from Eastern Nepal by GC-MS and Chiral GC-MS, and Antimicrobial Activity of Some Major Compounds. *Molecules*. 2023 Jan 5;28(2):543.

[2314] Yuce E, Yildirim N, Yildirim NC, et al. Essential oil composition, antioxidant and antifungal activities of Salvia sclarea L. from Munzur Valley in Tunceli Turkey. *Cell Mol Biol )Noisy-le-grand)*. 2014 Jun 15;60(2):1-5.

[2315] Pitarokili D, Couladis M, Petsikos-Panayotarou N, et al. Composition and antifungal activity on soil-borne pathogens of the essential oil of Salvia sclarea from Greece. *J Agric Food Chem*. 2002 Nov 6;50(23):6688-91.

[2316] Dzumayev KK, Tsibulskaya IA, Zenkevich IG, et al. Essential oils of Salvia sclarea L. produced from plants grown in Southern Uzbekistan. *J Essential Oil res*. 1995;7(6):597-604.

[2317] Torres ME, Velasco-Negueruela A, Perez-Alonso MJ, Et al. Volatile constituents of two Salvia species grown wild in Spain. *J Essential Oil Res*. 1997;9(1):27-33.

[2318] Nasermoadeli S, Rowshan V. Comparison of Salvia sclarea L. essential oil components in wild and field population. *Int J Agric Crop Sci*. 2013;5(8):828-31.

[2319] Hristova Y, Gochev V, Juerfen W, et al. Chemical composition and antifungal activity of essential oil of Salvia sclarea L. from Bulgaria against clinical isolates of Candida species. *J BioSci Biotech*. 2013;2(1):39.

[2320] Yadav A, Chanotiya CS, Singh AK. Terpenoid compositions and enantio-differentiation of linalool and sclareol in Salvia sclarea L. from three different climatic regions of India. *J Essent Oil Res*. 2010;22(6):589-92.

[2321] Wang C, Kurzer Ms. Phytoestrogen concentration determines effects on DNA synthesis in human breast cancer cells. *Nutr Cancer*. 1997;28(3):236-47.

[2322] Mahaira LG, Tsimplouli C, Sakellaridis N, et al. The labdane diterpene sclareol (labd-14-ene-8. 13-diol) induces apoptosis in human tumor cell lines and suppression of tumor growth in vivo via a p53-independent mechanism of action. *Eur J Pharmacol*. 2011 Sep;666(1-3):173-82.

[2323] Dimas K, Hatziantoniou S, Tseleni S, et al. Sclareol induces apoptosis in human HCT116 colon cancer cells in vitro and suppression of HCT116 tumor growth in immunodeficient mice. *Apoptosis*. 2007 Apr;12(4):685-94.

[2324] Noori S, Hassan ZM, Salehian O. Sclareol reduces CD4+ CD25+ FoxP3+ treg cells in breast cancer model in vivo. *Iran J Immunol*. 2013 Mar;10(1):10-21.

[2325] Sashidhara KV, Rosaiah JN, Kumar A, et al. Cell growth inhibitory action of an unusual labdane diterpene, 13-epi- sclareol in breast and uterine cancers in vitro. *Phytother Res*. 2007 Nov;21(11):1105-8.

[2326] Chen FP, Chien MH, Chern IY. Impact of lower concentrations of phytoestrogens on the effects of estradiol in breast cancer cells. *Climacteric*.

[2327] Saith S, Chalabi N, Rabiau N, et al. Transcriptional profiling of breast cancer cells exposed to soy phytoestrogens after BRCA1 knockdown with a whole human genome microarray approach. *Nutr Cancer*. 2010;62(5):659-67.

[2328] Imanshahidi M, Hosseinzadeh H. The pharmacological effects of Salvia species on the central nervous system. *Phytother Res*. 2006 Jun;20(6):427-37.

[2329] Ou MC, Hsu TF, Lai AC, et al. Pain relief assessment by aromatic essential oil massage on outpatients with primary dysmenorrhea: a randomized, double blind clinical trial. *J Obstet Gynaecol Res*. 2012 May;38(5):817-22.

[2330] Han SH, Hur MH, Buckle J, et al. Effect of aromatherapy on symptoms of dysmenorrhea in college students: A randomized placebo-controlled clinical trial. *J Alt Complement Med*. 2006 Jul-Aug;12(6):535-41.

[2331] Hur MH, Lee MS, Seong KY, et al. Aromatherapy massage on the abdomen for alleviating menstrual pain in high school girls: a preliminary controlled clinical study. *Evid Based Complement Alternat Med*. 2012;2012:187163.

[2332] Pemberton E, Turpin PG. The effect of essential oils on work-related stress in intensive care unit nurses. *Holist Nurs Pract*. 2008 Mar-Apr;22(2):97-102.

[2333] Seol GH, Shim HS, Kim PJ, et al. Antidepressant-like activity effect of Salvia sclarea is explained by modulation of dopamine activities in rats. *J Ethnopharmacol*. 2010 Jul 6;130(1):187-90.

[2334] Burns E, Blamey C, Ersser SJ, et al. The use of aromatherapy in intrapartum midwifery practice an observational study. *Complement Ther Nurs Midwifery*. 2000 Feb;6(1):33-4.

[2335] Moretti MDL, Peana AT, Satta M. A study on anti-inflammatory and peripheral analgesic action of Salvia sclarea oil and its main components. *J Essent Oil Res*. 1997;9(2):199-204.

[2336] Chovanova R, Mezovska J, Vaverkova S, et al. The inhibition of the Tet(K) efflux pump of tetracycline resistant staphylococcus epidermidis by essential oils from three Salvia species. *Lett Appl Microbiol*. 2015 Jul;61(1):58-62.

[2337] Andrade MA, Azevedo CD, Motta FN, et al. Essential oils: in vitro activity against Leishmania amazonensis, cytotoxicity and chemical composition. *BMC Complement Altern Med*. 2016 Nov 8;16(1):444.

[2338] Raafat K, Habib J. Phytochemical Compositions and Antidiabetic Potentials of Salvia sclarea L. Essential Oils. *J Oleo Sci*. 2018 Aug 1;67(8):1015-1025.

[2339] Sienkiewicz M, Głowacka A, Poznańska-Kurowska K, et al. The effect of clary sage oil on staphylococci responsible for wound infections. *Postepy Dermatol Alergol*. 2015 Feb;32(1):21–26.

[2340] Lee KB, Cho E, Kang YS. Changes in 5-hydroxytryptamine and Cortisol Plasma Levels in Menopausal Women After Inhalation of Clary Sage Oil. *Phytother Res*. 2014 Nov;28(11):1599-605.

[2341] Mitc M, Zrnic A, Wanner J, et al. Clary Sage Essential Oil and Its Effect on Human Mood and Pulse Rate: An in vivo Pilot Study. *Planta Med*. 2020 Jul 20. Online ahead of print.

[2342] Najar B, Pistelli L, Venturi F, et al. Salvia Spp. Essential Oils against the Arboviruses Vector Aedes albopictus (Diptera: Culicidae): Bioactivity, Composition, and Sensorial Profile-Stage 1. *Biology (Basel)*. 2020 Aug 4;9(8):E206.

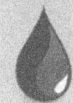

[2343] Wong J, Chiang YF, Shih YH, et al. Salvia sclarea L. Essential Oil Extract and Its Antioxidative Phytochemical Sclareol Inhibit Oxytocin-Induced Uterine Hypercontraction Dysmenorrhea Model by Inhibiting the Ca 2+-MLCK-MLC20 Signaling Cascade: An Ex Vivo and In Vivo Study. *Antioxidants (Basel).* 2020 Oct 14;9(10):991.
[2344] Shanaida M, Hudz N, Białoń M, et al. Chromatographic profiles and antimicrobial activity of the essential oils obtained from some species and cultivars of the Mentheae tribe (Lamiaceae). *Saudi J Biol Sci.* 2021 Nov;28(11):6145-6152.
[2345] Gad HA, Mamadalieva RZ, Khalil N, et al. GC-MS Chemical Profiling, Biological Investigation of Three Salvia Species Growing in Uzbekistan. *Molecules.* 2022 Aug 23;27(17):5365.
[2346] Kačániová M, Vukovic NL, Čmiková N, et al. Salvia sclarea Essential Oil Chemical Composition and Biological Activities. *Int J Mol Sci.* 2023 Mar 8;24(6):5179.
[2347] Fayemiwo KA, Adeleke MA, Okoro OP, et al. Larvicidal efficacies and chemical composition of essential oils of Pinus sylvestris and Syzygium aromaticum against mosquitoes. *Asian Pac J Trop Biomed.* 2014 Jan;4(1):30-34.
[2348] Alma MH, Ertas M, Nitz S, et al. Chemical composition and content of essential oil from the bud of cultivated Turkish clove (Syzygium aromaticum L.). *BioResources.* 2007;2(2):265-69.
[2349] Gaylor R, Michel J, Thierry D, et al. Bud, leaf and stem essential oil composition of clove (Syzygium aromaticum L.) from Indonesia, Madagascar and Zanzibar. *Int J Bas Appl Sci.* 2014;3(3):2473.
[2350] Pino JA, Marbot R, Aguero J, et al. Essential oil from buds and leaves of clove (Syzygium aromaticum (L.) Merr. Et Perry) grown in in Cuba. *J Essential Oil Res.* 2001;13(4):278-79.
[2351] Razafimamonjison G, Jahiel M, Duclos T, et al. Bud, leaf and stem essential oil composition of clove (Syzygium aromaticum L.) from Indonesia, Madagascar and Zanzibar. *Int J Basic Appl Sci.* 2014;3(3):1-22.
[2352] Sohilait HJ. Chemical Composition of the Essential Oils in Eugenia caryophyllata, Thunb from Amboina Island. *Sci J Chem.* 2015;3(6):95-99.
[2353] Domaracky M, Rehak P, Juhas S, et al. Effects of selected plant essential oils on the growth and development of mouse preimplantation embryos in vivo. *Physiol Res.* 2007;56(1):97-104.
[2354] Vrskova D, Modra H. Evaluation of the developmental toxicity of 2-phenoxyethanol and clove oil anesthetics using the Frog Embryo Teratogenesis Assay: Xenopus (FETAX). *Veterinarami Medicina.* 2012;57(5):245-50.
[2355] Amini A, Cheraghi E, Safaee MR, et al. The role of eugenol in the reduction of teratogenic effects of retinoic acid on skeletal morphology of mice embryo. *Yakhteh Medical Journal.* 2003;4:195-200.
[2356] Chen R, Chen J, Cheng S, et al. Assessment of embryotoxicity of constituents in cosmetics by the embryonic stem cell tes. *Toxicol Mech Methods.* 2010 Mar;20(3):112-18.
[2357] Chen SJ, Wang MH, Chen IJ. Antiplatelet and calcium inhibitory properties of eugenol and sodium eugenol acetate. *Gen Pharmacol.* 1996 Jun;27(4):629-33.
[2358] Tognolini M, Barocelli E, Ballabeni V, et al. Comparative screening of plant essential oils; phenylpropanoid moiety as basic core for antiplatelet activity. *Life Sci.* 2006 Feb 23;78(13):1419-32.
[2359] Heck AM, DeWitt BA, Lukes AL. Potential interactions between alternative therapies and warfarin. *Am J Health Syst Pharm.* 2000;57(13):1221-1227.
[2360] Saaeed SA, Gilani AH. Antithrombotic activity of clove oil. *J Pak Med Assoc.* 1994;44(5):112-15.
[2361] Kamatou GP, Vermaak I, Viljoen AM. Eugenol—from the remote Maluku Islands to the international market place: A review of a remarkable and versatile molecule. *Molecules.* 2012;17:6953-81.
[2362] Langeveld WT, Veldhuizen EJ, Burt SA. Synergy between essential oil constituents and antibiotics. *Crit Rev Microbiol.* 2014 Feb;40(1);76-94.
[2363] Cochrane ML. Inhibition of Cytochrome P450 2C9 by essential oils. Available at: https://libres.uncg.edu/ir/uncg/listing.aspx?id=18102
[2364] Dohi S, Terasaki M, Makino M. Acetylcholinesterase inhibitory activity and chemical composition of commercial essential oils. *J Agric Food Chem.* 2009 May 27;57(10):4313-8.
[2365] Sarrami N, Pemberton MN, Thornhill MH, et al. Adverse reactions associated with the use of eugenol in dentistry. *British Dental J.* 2002;193:253-55.
[2366] Tammannavar P, Pushpalatha C, Jain S, et al. An unexpected positive hypersensitive reaction to eugenol. *BMJ Case Rep.* 2013; 2013: bcr2013009464.
[2367] Janes SE, Price CS, Thomas D. Essential oil poisoning: N-acetylcysteine for eugenol-induced hepatic failure and analysis of national database. *Fur J Pediatr.* 2005 Aug;164(8):520-2.
[2368] Eisen JS, Koren G, Juurlink DN, N-acetylcysteine for the treatment of clove oil-induced fulminant hepatic failure. *J Toxicol Clin Toxicol.* 2004;42(1):89-92.
[2369] Brown SA, Biggerstaff J, Savidge GF. Disseminated intravascular coagulation and hepatocellular necrosis due to clove oil. *Blood Coagul Fibrinolysis.* 1992 Oct;3(5):665-68.
[2370] Hartnoll G, Moore D, Douek D. Near fatal ingestion of oil of cloves. *Arch Dis. Child.* 1993;69(3):392-93.
[2371] Kumar PS, Febriyant RM, Sofyan FF, et al. Anticancer potential of Syzygium aromaticum L. in MCF-7 human breast cancer cell lines. *Pharmacognosy Res.* 2014 Oct;6(4):350-54.
[2372] Yoo CB, Han KT, Cho Ks, et al. Eugenol isolated from the essential oil of Eugenia caryophyllata induces a reactive oxygen species-mediated apoptosis in HL-60 human promyeolocytic leukemia cells. *Cancer Lett.* 2005 Jul;225(1):41-52.
[2373] Kouidhi B, Zmantar T, Bakhrouf A. Anticariogenic and cytotoxic activity of clove essential oil (Eugenia caryophyllata) against a large number of oral pathogens. *Ann Microbiol.* 2010 Dec;60(4):599-604.
[2374] Dwivedi V, Shrivastava R, Hussain S, et al. Comparative anticancer potential of clove (Syzygium aromaticum)--an Indian spice--against cancer cell lines of various anatomical origin. *Asian Pac J Cancer Prev.* 2011;12(8):1989-93.
[2375] Pal D, Banerjee S, Mukherjee S, et al. Eugenol restricts DMBA croton oil induced skin carcinogenesis in mice: down regulation of c-Myc and H-ras, and activation of p53 dependent apoptotic pathway. *J Dermatol Sci.* 2010 Jul;59(1):31-39.
[2376] Dalai MK, Bhadra S, Chaudhary SK, et al. Anti-cholinesterase activity of the standardized extract of Syzygium aromaticum L. *Pharmacogn Mag.* 2014 Apr;10(Suppl 2):S276-82.
[2377] Islamuddin M, Sahal D, Afrin F. Apoptosis-like death in Leishmania donovani promastigotes induced by eugenol- rich oil of Syzygium aromaticum. *J Med Microbiol.* 2014 Jan;63(Pt 1):74-85.
[2378] Machado M, Sousa Mdo C, Salgueiro L, et al. Effects of essential oils on the growth of Giardia lamblia trophozoites. *Nat Prod Commun.* 2010 Jan;5(1):137-41.
[2379] Fu YJ, Chen LY, Zu YG, et al. Against propionibacterium acnes and its mechanism of action. *i.* 2009;145(1):86-88.
[2380] Grespan R, Paludo M, Lemos Hde P, et al. Anti-arthritic effect of eugenol on collagen-induced arthritis experimental model. *Biol Pharm Bull.* 2012;35(10):1818-20.
[2381] Abdurrahman O, Hanefi O. The anti-inflammatory activity of Eugenia caryophyllata essential oil: AN animal model of anti-inflammatory action. *Eur J Gen Med.* 2005 Dec;2(4):1304-3897.
[2382] Bachiega TF, de Sousa JP, Bastos JK, et al. Clove and eugenol in noncytotoxic concentrations exert immunomodulatory/anti-inflammatory action on cytokine production by murine macrophages. *J Pharm Pharmacol.* 2012 Apr;64(4):610-16.
[2383] Carrasco FR, Schmidt G, Romero AL, et al. Immunomodulatory activity of Zingiber officinale Roscoe, Salvia officinalis L. and Syzygium aromaticum L. essential oils: evidence for humor- and cell-mediated responses. *J Pharm Pharmacol.* 2009 Jul;61(7):961-67.
[2384] Halder S, Mehta AK, Mediratta PK, et al. Essential oil of clove (Eugenia caryophyllata) augments the humoral immune response but decreases cell mediated immunity. *Phytother Res.* 2011 Aug;25(8):1254-56.
[2385] Santin JR, Lemos M, Kelin-Junior LC, et al. Gastroprotective activity of essential oils of the Syzygium aromaticum and its major component eugenol in different animal models. *Naunyn-Schmiedeberg's Arch Pharmacol.* 2011 Feb;383(2):149-58.
[2386] Khan MS, Ahmad I. Biofilm inhibition by Cymbopogon citratus and Syzygium aromaticum essential oils in the strains of Candida albicans. *J Ethnopharmacol.* 2012 Mar 27;140(2):416-23.
[2387] Pinto E, Vale-Silva L, Cavaleiro C, et al. Antifungal activity of the clove essential oil from Syzygium aromaticum on Candida, Aspergillus and dermatophyte species. *J Med Microbiol.* 2009 Nov;58(Pt 11):1454-62.
[2388] Císarová M, Tančinová D, Medo J, et al. The in vitro effect of selected essential oils on the growth and mycotoxin production of Aspergillus species. *J Environ Sci Health B.* 2016 Oct 2;51(10):668-674.
[2389] Sharma A, Rajendran S, Srivastava A, et al. Antifungal activities of selected essential oils against Fusarium oxysporum f. sp. lycopersici 1322, with emphasis on Syzygium aromaticum essential oil. *J Biosci Bioeng.* 2017 Mar;123(3):308-313.
[2390] Elizaquivel P, Azizkhani M, Aznar R, et al. The effect of essential oils on norovirus surrogates. *Food Control.* 2013 Jul;32(1):275-278.
[2391] Misharina TA, Fatkullina LD, Alinkina ES, et al. Effects of low doses of essential oil on the antioxidant state of the erythrocytes, liver, and the brains of mice. *Prikl Biokhim Mikrobiol.*2014 Jan-Feb;50(1):101-07.
[2392] Halder S, Mehta AK, Mediratta PK, et al. Acute effect of essential oil of Eugenia caryophyllata on cognition and pain in mice. *Naunyn-Schmiedeberg's Arch Pharmacol.* 2012 Jun;385(6):587-93.
[2393] Sherry E, Boeck H, Warnke PH. Percutaneous treatment of chronic MRSA osteomyelitis with a novel plant-derived antiseptic. *BMC Surgery.* 2001;1:1.
[2394] Machado M, Dinis AM, Salgueiro L, et al. Anti-giardia activity of Syzygium aromaticum essential oil and eugenol: effects on growth, viability, adherence and ultrastructure. *Exp Parasitol.* 2011 Apr;127(4):732-39.
[2395] Liu BB, Luo L, Liu XL, et al. Essential oil of Syzygium aromaticum reverses the deficits of stress-induced behaviors and hippocampal p-ERK/p-CREB/brain-derived neurotrophic factor expression. *Planta Med.* 2015 Feb;81(3):185-92.
[2396] Inouye S, Uchida K, Nishiyama Y, et al. Combined effect of heat, essential oils and salt on fungicidal activity against Trichpphyton mentagrophytes in a foot bath. *Nihon Ishinjin Gakkai Zasshi.*2007;48(1):27-36.
[2397] Baylac S, Racine P. Inhibition of 5-lipoxygenase by essential oils and other natural fragrant extracts. *Int J Aromatherapy.* 2003;13(2-3):138-42.
[2398] Prabuseenivasan S, Jayakumar M, Ignacimuthu S. In vitro antibacterial activity of some plant essential oils. *BMC Complement Altern Med.* 2006 Nov;6:39.
[2399] Hili P, Evans CS, Veness RG. Antimicrobial action of essential oils: the effect of dimethylsulfoxide on the activity of cinnamon essential oil. *Lett Appl Microbiol.* 1997 Apr;24(4):269-75.
[2400] Rajkowska K, Kunicka-Styczyńska A, Maroszyńska M, et al. Selected Essential Oils as Antifungal Agents Against Antibiotic-Resistant Candida spp.: In Vitro Study on Clinical and Food-Borne Isolates. *Microb Drug Resist.* 2017 Jan;23(1):18-24.
[2401] Kovács JK, Felső P, Makszin L, et al. Antimicrobial and virulence modulating effect of clove essential oil on the food-borne pathogen Campylobacter jejuni. *Appl Environ Microbiol.* 2016 Sep 30;82(20):6158-6166.
[2402] Arung ET, Matsubara E, Kusuma IW, et al. Inhibitory components from the buds of clove (Syzygium aromaticum) on melanin formation in B16 melanoma cells. *Fitoterapia.* 2011 Mar;82(20:198-202.
[2403] Noonan FP, Zaidi MR, Wolnicka-Glubisz A, et al, Melanoma induction by ultraviolet A but not ultraviolet B radiation requires melanin pigment. *Nat Prod Commun.* 2012 Jun;3:884.
[2404] Wei A, Shibamoto T. Antioxidant activities of essential oil mixtures toward skin lipid squalene oxidized by UV irradiation. *Cutan Ocul Toxicol.* 2007;26(3):227-33.
[2405] Zheng GQ, Kenney PM, Lam LKT. Sesquiterpenes from clove (Eugenia caryophyllata) as potential anticariogenic agents. *J Nat Prod.* 1992;55(7):999-1003

[2406] Kouidhi B, Zmantar T, Bakhrouf A. Anticariogenic and cytotoxic activity of clove essential oil (Eugenia caryophyllata) against a large number of oral pathogens. *Ann Microbiol.* 2010 Dec;60(4):599-604.

[2407] Sarikaya M, Filik L, Ergul B, et al. Favourable effect of Eugenol on liver histology in acute cholestasis in rats after bile duct ligation. *Bratisl Lek Listy.* 2014;115(10):622-24.

[2408] Pasay C, Mounsey K, Stevenson G, et al. Acaricidal activity of eugenol-based constituents against scabies mites. *PLoS One.* 2010 Aug 11;5(8):e12079.

[2409] Hili P, Evans CS, Veness RG. Antimicrobial action of essential oils: the effect of dimethylsulfoxide on the activity of cinnamon essential oil. *Lett Appl Microbiol.* 1997 Apr;24(4):269-75.

[2410] Khalilzadeh E, Hazrati R, Saiah GV. Effects of topical and systemic administration of Eugenia caryophyllata buds essential oil on corneal anesthesia and analgesia. *Res Pharm Sci.* 2016 Jul;11(4):293-302.

[2411] Plant J. Effects of essential oils on telomere length in human cells. *Med Aromat Plants.* 2016;5(2):1-6.

[2412] Yones DA, Bakir HY, Bayoumi SA, et al. Chemical composition and efficacy of some selected plant oils against Pediculus humanus capitis in vitro. *Parasitol Res.* 2016 Aug;115(8):3209-18.

[2413] Labib GS, Aldawsari H. Innovation of natural essential oil-loaded Orabase for local treatment of oral candidiasis. *Drug Des Devel Ther.* 2015 Jun 29;9:3349-59.

[2414] Oboh G, Akinbola IA, Ademosun AO, et al. Essential Oil from Clove Bud (Eugenia aromatica Kuntze) Inhibit Key Enzymes Relevant to the Management of Type-2 Diabetes and Some Pro-oxidant Induced Lipid Peroxidation in Rats Pancreas in vitro. *J Oleo Sci.* 2015;64(7):775-82.

[2415] Pérez-Rosés R, Risco E, Vila R, et al. Biological and Nonbiological Antioxidant Activity of Some Essential Oils. *J Agric Food Chem.* 2016 Jun 15;64(23):4716-24.

[2416] Choi MS, Choi BS, Kim SH, et al. Essential Oils from the Medicinal Herbs Upregulate Dopamine Transporter in Rat Pheochromocytoma Cells. *J Med Food.* 2015 Oct;18(10):1112-20.

[2417] Cwikla C, Schmidt K, Matthias A, et al. Investigation into the antibacterial activities of phytotherapeutics against Helicobacter pylori and Campylobacter jejuni. *Phytother Res.* 2010 May;24(5):649-56.

[2418] Fang F, Candy K, Melloul E, et al. In vitro activity of ten essential oils against Sarcoptes scabiei. *Parasit Vectors.* 2016 Nov 22;9(1):594.

[2419] D'Amato S, Mazzarrino G, Rossi C, et al. Thymus Vulgaris (Red Thyme) and Caryophyllus Aromaticus (Clove) Essential Oils to Control Spoilage Microorganisms in Pork Under Modified Atmosphere. *Ital J Food Saf.* 2016 Aug 3;5(3):5785.

[2420] Soonwera M, Phasomkusolsil S. Effect of Cymbopogon citratus (lemongrass) and Syzygium aromaticum (clove) oils on the morphology and mortality of Aedes aegypti and Anopheles dirus larvae. *Parasitol Res.* 2016 Apr;115(4):1691-703.

[2421] Iwamatsu T, Miyamoto D, Mitsuno H, et al. Identification of repellent odorants to the body louse, Pediculus humanus corporis, in clove essential oil. *Parasitol Res.* 2016 Apr;115(4):1659-66.

[2422] Xu JG, Liu T, Hu QP, et al. Chemical Composition, Antibacterial Properties and Mechanism of Action of Essential Oil from Clove Buds against Staphylococcus aureus. *Molecules.* 2016 Sep 8;21(9).

[2423] Rajkowska K, Kunicka-Styczyńska A, Maroszyńska M, et al. Selected Essential Oils as Antifungal Agents Against Antibiotic-Resistant Candida spp.: In Vitro Study on Clinical and Food-Borne Isolates. *Microb Drug Resist.* 2017 Jan;23(1):18-24.

[2424] Intorasoot A, Chornchoem P, Sookkhee S, et al. Bactericidal activity of herbal volatile oil extracts against multidrug-resistant Acinetobacter baumannii. *J Intercult Ethnopharmacol.* 2017 Apr 21;6(2):218-222.

[2425] Basholli-Salihu M, Schuster R, Hajdari A, et al. Phytochemical composition, anti-inflammatory activity and cytotoxic effects of essential oils from three Pinus spp. *Pharm Biol.* 2017 Dec;55(1):1553-1560.

[2426] Yones DA, Bakir HY, Bayoumi SA, et al. Chemical composition and efficacy of some selected plant oils against Pediculus humanus capitis in vitro. *Parasitol Res.* 2016 Aug;115(8):3209-18.

[2427] Ferreira FM, Delmonte CC, Novato TLP, et al. Acaricidal activity of essential oil of Syzygium aromaticum, hydrolate and eugenol formulated or free on larvae and engorged females of Rhipicephalus microplus. *Med Vet Entomol.* 2018 Mar;32(1):41-47.

[2428] Beltrán-Villalobos KL, Déciga-Campos M, Aguilar-Mariscal H, et al. Synergistic antinociceptive interaction of Syzygium aromaticum or Rosmarinus officinalis coadministered with ketorolac in rats. *Biomed Pharmacother.* 2017 Aug 9;94:858-864.

[2429] Kumar P, Mishra S, Kumar A, et al. In vivo and in vitro control activity of plant essential oils against three strains of Aspergillus niger. *Environ Sci Pollut Res Int.* 2017 Sep;24(27):21948-21959.

[2430] Gaire S, O'Connell M, Holguin FO, et al. Insecticidal Properties of Essential Oils and Some of Their Constituents on the Turkestan Cockroach (Blattodea: Blattidae). *J Econ Entomol.* 2017 Apr 1;110(2):584-592.

[2431] Zhang Y, Wang Y, Zhu X, et al. Antibacterial and antibiofilm activities of eugenol from essential oil of Syzygium aromaticum (L.) Merr. & L. M. Perry (clove) leaf against periodontal pathogen Porphyromonas gingivalis. *Microb Pathog.* 2017 Dec;113:396-402.

[2432] Yan X, Zhang G, Bie F, et al. Eugenol inhibits oxidative phosphorylation and fatty acid oxidation via downregulation of c-Myc/PGC-1β/ERRα signaling pathway in MCF10A-ras cells. *Sci Rep.* 2017 Oct 10;7(1):12920.

[2433] Han X, Parker TL. Anti-inflammatory activity of clove (Eugenia caryophyllata) essential oil in human dermal fibroblasts. *Pharm Biol.* 2017 Dec;55(1):1619-1622.

[2434] Whiley H, Gaskin S, Schroder T, et al. Antifungal properties of essential oils for improvement of indoor air quality: a review. *Rev Environ Health.* 2017 Dec;113:396-402.

[2435] Zanusso Junior G, Massago M, Kian D, et al. Efficacy of essential oil of Syzygium aromaticum alone and in combination with benznidazole on murine oral infection with Trypanosoma cruzi IV. *Exp Parasitol.* 2018 Feb;185:92-97.

[2436] Bakour M, Soulo N, Hammas N, et al. The Antioxidant Content and Protective Effect of Argan Oil and Syzygium aromaticum Essential Oil in Hydrogen Peroxide-Induced Biochemical and Histological Changes. *Int J Mol Sci.* 2018 Jun 18;19(2).

[2437] Fang F, Candy K, Melloul E, et al. In vitro activity of ten essential oils against Sarcoptes scabiei. *Parasites & Vectors.* 216;9:954.

[2438] Bartoňková I, Dvořák Z. Essential oils of culinary herbs and spices display agonist and antagonist activities at human aryl hydrocarbon receptor AhR. *Food Chem Toxicol.* 2018 Jan;111:374-384.

[2439] Mohamed MSM, Abdallah AA, Mahran MH, et al. Potential Alternative Treatment of Ocular Bacterial Infections by Oil Derived from Syzygium aromaticum Flower (Clove). *Curr Eye Res.* 2018 Jul;43(7):873-881.

[2440] Gucwa K, Milewski S, Dymerski T, et al. Investigation of the Antifungal Activity and Mode of Action of Thymus vulgaris, Citrus limonum, Pelargonium graveolens, Cinnamomum cassia, Ocimum basilicum, and Eugenia caryophyllus Essential Oils. *Molecules.* 2018 May 8;23(5).

[2441] Solarte AL, Astorga RJ, Aguiar F, et al. Combination of Antimicrobials and Essential Oils as an Alternative for the Control of Salmonella enterica Multiresistant Strains Related to Foodborne Disease. *Foodborne Pathog Dis.* 2017 Oct;14(10):558-563.

[2442] Besra M, Kumar V. In vitro investigation of antimicrobial activities of ethnomedicinal plants against dental caries pathogens. *3 Biotech.* 2018 May;8(5):257.

[2443] Ács K, Balázs VL, Kocsis B, et al. Antibacterial activity evaluation of selected essential oils in liquid and vapor phase on respiratory tract pathogens. *BMC Complement Altern Med.* 2018 Jul 27;18(1):227.

[2444] Fazly Bazzaz BS, Khameneh B, Namazi N, et al. Solid lipid nanoparticles carrying Eugenia caryophyllata essential oil: the novel nanoparticulate systems with broad-spectrum antimicrobial activity. *Lett Appl Microbiol.* 2018 Jun;66(6):506-513.

[2445] Plata-Rueda A, Campos JM, da Silva Rolim G, et al. Terpenoid constituents of cinnamon and clove essential oils cause toxic effects and behavior repellency response on granary weevil, Sitophilus granarius. *Ecotoxicol Environ Saf.* 2018 Jul 30;156:263-270.

[2446] Elezzayat E, Elleboudy N, Moustafa A, et al. Insecticidal, Oxidative, and Genotoxic Activities of Syzygium aromaticum and Eucalyptus globulus on Culex pipiens Adults and Larvae. *Turkiye Parazitol Derg.* 2018 Sep;42(3):213-222.

[2447] Wan J, Zhong S, Schwarz P, et al. Influence of oil phase composition on the antifungal and mycotoxin inhibitory activity of clove oil nanoemulsions. *Food Funct.* 2018 May 23;9(5):2872-2882.

[2448] Rajkowska K, Nowicka-Krawczyk P, Kunicka-Styczynska. Effect of Clove and Thyme Essential Oils on Candida Biofilm Formation and the Oil Distribution in Yeast Cells. *Molecules.* 2019 May 21;24(10):24101954.

[2449] Condò C, Anacarso I, Sabia C, et al. Antimicrobial activity of spices essential oils and its effectiveness on mature biofilms of human pathogens. *Nat Prod Res.* 2018 Oct 13:1-8.

[2450] Viteri Jumbo LO, Haddi K, Faroni LRD, et al. Toxicity to, oviposition and population growth impairments of Callosobruchus maculatus exposed to clove and cinnamon essential oils. *PLoS One.* 2018 Nov 16;13(11):e0207618.

[2451] Radünz M, da Trindade MLM, Camargo TM, et al. Antimicrobial and antioxidant activity of unencapsulated and encapsulated clove (Syzygium aromaticum, L.) essential oil. *Food Chem.* 2019 Mar 15;276:180-186.

[2452] Leal Pinto SM, Herrera Sandoval LV, Vargas LY. In vitro susceptibility of Microsporum spp. and mammalian cells to Eugenia caryophyllus essential oil, eugenol and semisynthetic derivatives. *Mycoses.* 2019 Jan;62(1):41-51.

[2453] Maness LR, Zubov T. The Inhibitory Effect of Essential Oils on Rhizopus stolonifer, Trichophyton mentagrophytes, and Microsporum gypseum. *Lab Med.* 2019 Apr;50(2):e18-e22.

[2454] Muchembled J, Deweer C, Sahmer K, et al. Gene expression responses of Listeria monocytogenes Scott A exposed to sub-lethal concentrations of natural antimicrobials. *Environ Sci Pollut Res Int.* 2018 Oct;25(30):29921-29928.

[2455] Castillo-Morales RM, Carreño Otero AL, Mendez-Sanchez SC, et al. Mitochondrial affectation, DNA damage and AChE inhibition induced by Salvia officinalis essential oil on Aedes aegypti larvae. *Comp Biochem Physiol C Toxicol Pharmacol.* 2019 Jul;221:29-37.

[2456] Khosravi AR, Sharifzadeh A, Nikaein D, et al. Chemical composition, antioxidant activity and antifungal effects of five Iranian essential oils against Candida strains isolated from urine samples. *J Mycol Med.* 2018 Jun;28(2):355-360.

[2457] Rodrigues AM, Sampaio CG, Souza JSN, et al. Different susceptibilities of Aedes aegypti and Aedes albopictus larvae to plant-derived products. *Rev Soc Bras Med Trop.* 2019 Apr 11;52:e20180197.

[2458] Ribes S, Fuentes A, Barat JM, et al. Effect of oregano (Origanum vulgare L. ssp. hirtum) and clove (Eugenia spp.) nanoemulsions on Zygosaccharomyces bailii survival in salad dressings. *Food Chem.* 2019 Oct 15;295:630-636.

[2459] Anacarso I, Sabia C, de Niederhäusern S, et al. In vitro evaluation of the amoebicidal activity of rosemary (Rosmarinus officinalis L.) and cloves (Syzygium aromaticum L. Merr. & Perry) essential oils against Acanthamoeba polyphaga trophozoites. *Nat Prod Res.* 2019 Feb;33(4):606-611.

[2460] Mandava K, Batchu UR, Kakulavaram S, et al. Design and study of anticaries effect of different medicinal plants against S.mutans glucosyltransferase. *BMC Complement Altern Med.* 2019 Aug 2;19(1):197.

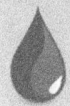

[2461] El-Garawani IM, Hassab El-Nabi S, Dawoud GT, et al. Triggering of apoptosis and cell cycle arrest by fennel and clove oils in Caco-2 cells: The role of combination. *Toxicol Mech Methods*. 2019 Jul 31:1-32.
[2462] Pereira Dos Santos E, Nicácio PHM, Coêlho Barbosa F, et al. Chitosan/Essential Oils Formulations for Potential Use as Wound Dressing: Physical and Antimicrobial Properties. *Materials (Basel)*. 2019 Jul 10;12(14).
[2463] Nirmala MJ, Durai L, Gopakumar V, et al. Anticancer and antibacterial effects of a clove bud essential oil-based nanoscale emulsion system. *Int J Nanomedicine*. 2019 Aug 12;14:6439-6450.
[2464] Ebani VV, Nardoni S, Bertelloni F, et al. In Vitro Antimicrobial Activity of Essential Oils Against Salmonella enterica Serotypes Enteritidis and Typhimurium Strains Isolated from Poultry. *Molecules*. 2019 Mar 4;24(5).
[2465] Wongsawan K, Chaisri W, Tangtrongsup S, et al. Bactericidal Effect of Clove Oil Against Multidrug-Resistant Streptococcus suis Isolated From Human Patients and Slaughtered Pigs. Pathogens. 2019 Dec 21;9(1):9010014.
[2466] Yan G, Zhu BR, Tian FL, et al. Inhibitory Activity of Plant Essential Oils Against E. coli 1-Deoxy-d-xylulose-5-phosphate Reductoisomerase. *Molecules*. 2019 Jul;24(14):24142518.
[2467] Lang M, Ferron PJ, Bursztyka J, et al. Evaluation of Immunomodulatory Activities of Essential Oils by High Content Analysis. J Biotechnol. 2019 Sep 10;303:65-71.
[2468] Xao S, Cui P, Shi W, et al. Identification of Essential Oils With Strong Activity Against Stationary Phase Uropathogenic Escherichia Coli. Discov Med. 2019 Oct;28(154):179-188.
[2469] Ngo-Mback MNL, Babii C, Jazet Dongmo PM, et al. Anticandidal and synergistic effect of essential oil fractions from three aromatic plants used in Cameroon. *J Mycol Med*. 2020 Mar 3:100940.
[2470] Guz L, Ziętek J, Puk K, et al. Inhibitory activities of essential oils against Babesia canis. *Pol J Vet Sci*. 2020 Mar;23(1):161-163.
[2471] Alibi S, Ben Selma W, Ramos-Vivas J, et al. Anti-oxidant, antibacterial, antibiofilm, and anti-quorum sensing activities of four essential oils against multidrug-resistant bacterial clinical isolates. *Curr Res Transl Med*. 2020 Mar 16. [Epub ahead of print]
[2472] Yilmaz-Oral D, Onder A, Gur S, et al. The beneficial effect of clove essential oil and its major component, eugenol, on erectile function in diabetic rats. *Andrologia*. 2020 Apr 30:e13606.
[2473] Lambert MM, Campos DR, Borges DA, et al. Activity of Syzygium Aromaticum Essential Oil and Its Main Constituent Eugenol in the Inhibition of the Development of Ctenocephalides Felis Felis and the Control of Adults. *Vet Parasitol*. 2020 May 12;282:109126.
[2474] Castellanos LM, Olivas NA, Ayala-Soto J, et al. In Vitro and In Vivo Antifungal Activity of Clove ( Eugenia caryophyllata) and Pepper ( Piper nigrum L.) Essential Oils and Functional Extracts Against Fusarium oxysporum and Aspergillus niger in Tomato ( Solanum lycopersicum L.). *Int J Microbiol*. 2020 Apr 30;2020:1702037.
[2475] Toledo PFS, Viteri Jumbo LO, Rezende SM, et al. Disentangling the ecotoxicological selectivity of clove essential oil against aphids and nontarget ladybeetles. *Sci Total Environ*. 2020 May 20;718:137328.
[2476] Alfikri FN, Pujiarti R, Wibisono MG, et al. Yield, Quality, and Antioxidant Activity of Clove ( Syzygium aromaticum L.) Bud Oil at the Different Phenological Stages in Young and Mature Trees. *Scientifica (Cairo)*. 2020 Jun 2;2020:9701701.
[2477] Aman RM, Hashim IIA, Meshali MM. Novel Clove Essential Oil Nanoemulgel Tailored by Taguchi's Model and Scaffold-Based Nanofibers: Phytopharmaceuticals With Promising Potential as Cyclooxygenase-2 Inhibitors in External Inflammation. *Int J Nanomedicine*. 2020 Mar 30;15:2171-2195.
[2478] Mizan MFR, Ashrafudoulla M, Hossain MI, et al. Effect of Essential Oils on Pathogenic and Biofilm-Forming Vibrio parahaemolyticus Strains. *Biofouling*. 2020 Apr;36(4):467-478.
[2479] Rinaldi F, Oliva A, Sabatino M, et al. Antimicrobial Essential Oil Formulation: Chitosan Coated Nanoemulsions for Nose to Brain Delivery. *Pharmaceutics*. 2020 Jul 17;12(7):E678.
[2480] Zhang L, Gu B, Wang Y, et al. Clove essential oil confers antioxidant activity and lifespan extension in C. elegans via the DAF-16/FOXO transcription factor. *Comp Biochem Physiol C Toxicol Pharmacol*. 2020 Nov 7;242:108938.
[2481] Hetta HF, Meshaal AK, Algammal AM, et al. In-vitro Antimicrobial Activity of Essential Oils and Spices Powder of some Medicinal Plants Against Bacillus Species Isolated from Raw and Processed Meat. *Infect Drug Resist*. 2020 Dec 4;13:4367-4378.
[2482] Kujur A, Kumar A, Prakash B. Elucidation of antifungal and aflatoxin B 1 inhibitory mode of action of Eugenia caryophyllata L. essential oil loaded chitosan nanomatrix against Aspergillus flavus. *Pestic Biochem Physiol*. 2021 Feb;172:104755.
[2483] Teles AM, Silva-Silva JV, Fernandes JMP, et al. GC-MS Characterization of Antibacterial, Antioxidant, and Antitrypanosomal Activity of Syzygium aromaticum Essential Oil and Eugenol. *Evid Based Complement Alternat Med*. 2021 Feb 20;2021:6663255.
[2484] Vazquez-Ucha JC, Martinez-Guitian M, Lasarte-Monterrubio C, et al. Syzygium aromaticum (clove) and Thymus zygis (thyme) essential oils increase susceptibility to colistin in the nosocomial pathogens Acinetobacter baumannii and Klebsiella pneumoniae. *Biomed Pharmacother*. 2020 Oct;130:110606.
[2485] Jaber H, Oubiji A, Ouryemchi I, et al. Chemical Composition and Antibacterial Activities of Eight Plant Essential Oils from Morocco against Escherichia coli Strains Isolated from Different Turkey Organs. *Biochem Res Int*. 2021 Mar 15;2021:6685800.
[2486] Dudek-Wicher R, Paleczny J, Kowalska-Krochmal B, et al. Activity of Liquid and Volatile Fractions of Essential Oils against Biofilm Formed by Selected Reference Strains on Polystyrene and Hydroxyapatite Surfaces. *Pathogens*. 2021 Apr 23;10(5):515.
[2487] Booq RY, Alshehri AA, Almughem FA, et al. Formulation and Evaluation of Alcohol-Free Hand Sanitizer Gels to Prevent the Spread of Infections during Pandemics. *Int J Environ Res Public Health*. 2021 Jun 9;18(12):6252.
[2488] Ikawati S, Himawan T, Abadi AL, et al. Toxicity nanoinsecticide based on clove essential oil against Tribolium castaneum (Herbst). *J Pestic Sci*. 2021 May 20;46(2):222-228.
[2489] Hassine DBm El Euch SK, Rahmani R, et al. Clove Buds Essential Oil: The Impact of Grinding on the Chemical Composition and Its Biological Activities Involved in Consumer's Health Security. *Biomed Res Int*. 2021 Aug 2;2021:9940591.
[2490] Sarto MPM, Lucas da Silva HF, de Souza Fernandes N, et al. Essential oils from Syzygium aromaticum and Zingiber officinale, administered alone or in combination with benznidazole, reduce the parasite load in mice orally inoculated with Trypanosoma cruzi II. *BMC Complement Med Ther*. 2021 Feb 25;21(1):77.
[2491] Harčárová M, Čonková E, Proškovcová M, et al. Comparison of antifungal activity of selected essential oils against Fusarium graminearum in vitro. *Ann Agric Environ Med*. 2021 Sep 16;28(3):414-418.
[2492] Michalczky A, Ostrowska P. Essential oils and their components in combating fungal pathogens of animal and human skin. *J Mycol Med*. 2021 Jun;31(2):101118.
[2493] Kačániová M, Galovičová L, Borotová P, et al. Chemical Composition, In Vitro and In Situ Antimicrobial and Antibiofilm Activities of Syzygium aromaticum (Clove) Essential Oil. *Plants (Basel)*. 2021 Oct 15;10(10):2185.
[2494] Vasconcelos PGS, de Almeida Maia CM, Vascolcelos VMD, et al. In vitro inhibition of a multispecies oral cavity biofilm by Syzygium aromaticum essential oil. *Gerodontology*. 2021 Oct 11. Online ahead of print.
[2495] Lang M, Montjarret A, Duteil E, et al. Cinnamomum cassia and Syzygium aromaticum Essential Oils Reduce the Colonization of Salmonella Typhimurium in an In Vivo Infection Model Using Caenorhabditis elegans. *Molecules*. 2021 Sep 15;26(18):5598.
[2496] Guo Y, Pizzol R, Gabbanini S, et al. Absolute Antioxidant Activity of Five Phenol-Rich Essential Oils. *Molecules*. 2021 Aug 29;26(17):5237.
[2497] Selka MA, Chenafa A, Achouri MY. [Developement and biological activity evaluation of clove essential oil based emulsion]. *Ann Pharm Fr*. 2021 Dec 9:S0003-4509(21)00177-2.
[2498] Shakeel F, Alam P, Ali A, et al. Investigating Antiarthritic Potential of Nanostructured Clove Oil (Syzygium aromaticum) in FCA-Induced Arthritic Rats: Pharmaceutical Action and Delivery Strategies. *Molecules*. 2021 Dec 2;26(23):7327.
[2499] Tabari MA, Rostami A, Khodashenas A, et al. Acaricidal activity, mode of action, and persistent efficacy of selected essential oils on the poultry red mite (Dermanyssus gallinae). *Food Chem Toxicol*. 2020 Apr;138:111207.
[2500] Elnabawy EM, Hassan S, Taha EA. Repellent and Toxicant Effects of Eight Essential Oils against the Red Flour Beetle, Tribolium castaneum Herbst (Coleoptera: Tenebrionidae). *Biology (Basel)*. 2021 Dec 21;11(1):3.
[2501] Anandhi P, Tharani M, Rajeshkumar S, et al. Antibacterial activity of cinnamon and clove oil against wound pathogens. *J Popul Ther Clin Pharmacol*. 2022 Jan 6;28(2):e41-e46.
[2502] Lauteri C, Maggio F, Serio A, et al. Overcoming Multidrug Resistance in Salmonella spp. Isolates Obtained From the Swine Food Chain by Using Essential Oils: An in vitro Study. *Front Microbiol*. 2022 Feb 9;12:808286.
[2503] Maocha IG, Carvalho J, Lopes-Nunes J, et al. Drug formulations for localized treatment of Human Papillomavirus-induced lesions. *J Pharm Sci*. 2022 Feb 16:S0022-3549(22)00068-5.
[2504] Irahal IN, Guenaou I, Lahlou FA, et al. Syzygium aromaticum bud (clove) essential oil is a novel and safe aldose reductase inhibitor: in silico, in vitro, and in vivo evidence. *Hormones (Athens)*. 2022 Feb 25. Online ahead of print.
[2505] Abadi AVM, Karimi E, Oskoueian E, et al. Chemical investigation and screening of anti-cancer potential of Syzygium aromaticum L. bud (clove) essential oil nanoemulsion. *3 Biotech*. 2022 Feb;12(2):49.
[2506] Ali T. Anjum AA, Sattar MMK, et al. Antibacterial activity of plant essential oils against indigenously characterized methicillin-resistant Staphylococcus aureus (MRSA). *Trop Biomed*. 2022 Mar 1;39(1):17-25.
[2507] Dos Santos LR, Alía A, Martin I, et al. Antimicrobial activity of essential oils and natural plant extracts against Listeria monocytogenes in a dry-cured ham-based model. *J Sci Food Agric*. 2021 Aug 11. Online ahead of print.
[2508] Al-Zereini WA, Al-Trawneh IN, Al-Qudah MA, et al. Antibacterial, antioxidant, and cytotoxic activities of Syzygium aromaticum (L.) Merr. & Perry essential oil with identification of its chemical constituents. *Z Naturforsch C J Biosci*. 2022 May 23. Online ahead of print.
[2509] Esmaeili F, Zahmatkeshan M, Yousefpoor Y, et al. Anti-inflammatory and anti-nociceptive effects of Cinnamon and Clove essential oils nanogels: an in vivo study. *BMC Complement Med Ther*. 2022 May 20;22(1):143.
[2510] El-Zehery HRA, Zaghloul RA, Abdel-Rahman HM, et al. Novel strategies of essential oils, chitosan, and nano- chitosan for inhibition of multi-drug resistant: E. coli O157:H7 and Listeria monocytogenes. *Saudi J Biol Sci*. 2022 Apr;29(4):2582-2590.
[2511] Esmaeili F, Zahmatkeshan M, Yousefpoor Y, et al. Anti-inflammatory and anti-nociceptive effects of Cinnamon and Clove essential oils nanogels: an in vivo study. *BMC Complement Med Ther*. 2022 May 20;22(1):143.
[2512] Man A, Mare AD, Mares M, et al. Antifungal and anti-virulence activity of six essential oils against important Candida species - a preliminary study. *Future Microbiol*. 2022 Jul;17:737-753.
[2513] Csikós E, Csekő K, Kemény Á, et al. Pinus sylvestris L. and Syzygium aromaticum (L.) Merr. & L. M. Perry Essential Oils Inhibit Endotoxin-Induced Airway Hyperreactivity despite Aggravated Inflammatory Mechanisms in Mice. *Molecules*. 2022 Jun 16;27(12):3868.
[2514] Uchewa OO, Egwuagu CB, Egwu OA, et al. Neuromodulatory Potency of Essential Oil in Cadmium Induced Cognitive Impairment on the Prefrontal Cortex of Wistar Rats. JTEMB-D-22-00398, Available at SSRN: https://ssrn.com/abstract=4173960 or http://dx.doi.org/10.2139/ssrn.4173960.

[2515] Alibi S, Selma WB, Mansour HB, et al. Activity of Essential Oils Against Multidrug-Resistant Salmonella enteritidis. *Curr Microbiol.* 2022 Jul 30;79(9):273.
[2516] Razzouk S, Mazri MA, Jeldi L, et al. Chemical Composition and Antimicrobial Activity of Essential Oils from Three Mediterranean Plants against Eighteen Pathogenic Bacteria and Fungi. *Pharmaceutics.* 2022 Aug 1;14(8):1608.
[2517] Uto T, Ohta T, Nakayama E, et al. Bioassay-guided Fractionation of Clove Buds Extract Identifies Eugenol as Potent Melanogenic Inducer in Melanoma Cells. *J Oleo Sci.* 2022;71(9):1403-1412.
[2518] von Thadden C, Altun E, Aydogdu M, et al. Antimicrobial Fibrous Bandage-like Scaffolds Using Clove Bud Oil. J *Funct Biomater.* 2022 Aug 30;13(3):136.
[2519] Glorίková N, Skuhrovec J, Nový P, et al. Attraction or Repelling Effects of Commercial Plant Essential Oils on the Synanthropic Cheiracanthium mildei (Araneae: Cheiracanthiidae). *J Econ Entomol.* 2022 Oct 12;115(5):1472-1479.
[2520] Jiang C, Hong J, Meng J, et al. Antibacterial activity of essential oils extracted from the unique Chinese spices cassia bark, bay fruits and cloves. *Arch Microbiol.* 2022 Oct 18;204(11):674.
[2521] Farooq M, Bangonan L, Xue RD, et al. Evaluation of essential oils as spatial repellents against Aedes aegypto in an olfactometer. *J Am Mosq Control Assoc.* 2022 Nov 9. Online ahead of print.
[2522] Costa LV, Moreira JMAR, Menezes IG, et al. Antibiotic resistance profiles and activity of clove essential oil (Syzygium aromaticum) against Pseudomonas aeruginosa isolated of canine otitis. *Vet World.* 2022 Oct;15(10):2499-2505.
[2523] Hekmatpanah A, Sharifzadeh A, Shokri H, et al. Efficacy of Syzygium aromaticum essential oil on the growth and enzymatic activity of pathogenic Candida albicans strains. *Curr Med Mycol.* 2022 Mar;8(1):12-19.
[2524] Alanazi AK, Alqasmi MH, Alrouji M, et al. Antibacterial Activity of Syzygium aromaticum (Clove) Bud Oil and Its Interaction with Imipenem in Controlling Wound Infections in Rats Caused by Methicillin-Resistant Staphylococcus aureus. *Molecules.* 2022 Dec 5;27(23):8551.
[2525] Susurluk H. Potential use of essential oils from Origanum vulgare and Syzygium aromaticum to control Tetranychus urticae Koch (Acari: Tetranychidae) on two host plant species. *PeerJ.* 2023 Jan 20;11:e14475.
[2526] Biernasiuk A, Baj T, Malm A. Clove Essential Oil and Its Main Constituent, Eugenol, as Potential Natural Antifungals against Candida spp. Alone or in Combination with Other Antimycotics Due to Synergistic Interactions. *Molecules.* 2022 Dec 26;28(1):215.
[2527] Refaey MS, A A Fayed M, Kutkat O, et al. Bio-guided chemical characterization and nano-formulation studies of selected edible volatile oils with potentials antibacterial and anti-SARS-CoV-2 activities. *Arab J Chem.* 2023 Jul;16(7):104813.
[2528] Elbestawy MKM, El-Sherbiny GM, Moghannem SA. Antibacterial, Antibiofilm and Anti-Inflammatory Activities of Eugenol Clove Essential Oil against Resistant Helicobacter pylori. *Molecules.* 2023 Mar 7;28(6):2448.
[2529] Kiki MJ. In Vitro Antiviral Potential, Antioxidant, and Chemical Composition of Clove (Syzygium aromaticum) Essential Oil. *Molecules.* 2023 Mar 7;28(6):2421.
[2530] Soares DC, Portella NA, Ramos MF, et al. Trans-B-Caryophyllene: An effective antileishmanial constituent found in commercial copaiba oil (Copaifera spp.). *Evid Based Compl Altern Med.* 2013;2013(2013):761323.
[2531] Silveira ER. Volatile constituents of Copaifera langsdorffii from the Brazilian northeast. *J Essential Oil Res.* 2005 Mar-Apr;17(2):130-32.
[2532] Almeida MR, Darin JDC, Hernandes LC, et al. Genotoxicity assessment of Copaiba oil and its fractions in Swiss mice. *Genr Mol Biol.* 2012 Aug 2;35(3):1415-17.
[2533] Rolim de Almeida LF, de Oliveira Portella R, Bufalo J, et al. Non-oxygenated sesquiterpenes in the essential oil of Copaifera langsdofrrii Desf. increase during the day in the dry season. *PLoS One.* 2016;11(2):e0149332.
[2534] Veiga Jr VF, Rosas EC, Carvalho MV, et al. Chemical composition and anti-inflammatory activity of copaiba oils from Copaifera cearensis Huber ex Ducke, Copaifera reticulata Ducke and Copaifera multijuga Hayne—A comparative study. *J Ethnopharm.* 2007;112:248-54.
[2535] Zoghbi MDGB, Andrade EHA, Martins-da-Silva RCV, et al. Chemical Variation in the Volatiles of Copaifera reticulata Ducke (Leguminosae) Growing Wild in the States of Pará and Amapá, Brazil. *J Essent Oil Res.* 2009 Nov/Dec;21:501-3.

[2536] Lameira OA, Martins-da-Silva RCV. Seasonal Variation in the Volatiles of Copaifera duckei Dwyer Growing Wild in the State of Para Brazil. *J Essent Oil Res.* 2009 Mar/Apr;21:105-7.
[2537] Zoghbi MDGB, Martins-da-Silva RCV, Trigo JR. Volatiles of Oleoresins of Copaifera paupera (Herzog) Dwyer, C. piresii Dwyer and C. pubiflora Benth. (Leguminosae). *J Essent Oil Res.* 2009 Sep/Oct;21:403-4.
[2538] Santos AO, Ueda-Nakamura T, Dias Filho BP, et al. Effect of Brazilian copaiba oils on Leishmania amazonensis. *J Ethnopharmacol.* 2008;120:204-8.
[2539] Sant'Anna BMP, Fontes SP, Pinto AC, et al. Characterization of woody odorant contributors in copaiba oil (Copaifera multijuga Hayne). *J Braz Chem Soc.* 2007;18(5):984-9.
[2540] Barbosa PCS, Medeiros RS, Sampaio PTB, et al. Influence of abiotic factors on the chemical composition of copaiba oil (Copaifera multijuga Hayne): Soil composition, seasonality and diameter at breast height. *J Braz Chem Soc.* 2012;23(10:1823-33.
[2541] Cascon V, Gilbert B. Characterization of the chemical composition of oleoresins of Copaifera guianensis Desf., Copaifera duckei Dwyer and Copaifera multijuga Hayne. *Phytochem.* 2000;55:773-8.
[2542] Herrero-Jauregui C, Casado MA, Zoghbi MDGB, et al. Chemical Variability of Copaifera reticulata Ducke Oleoresin. *Chem Biodivers.* 2011;8:674-85.
[2543] Guimaraes-Santos A, Santos DS, Santos IR, et al. Copaiba oil-resin treatment is neuroprotective and reduces neutrophil recruitment and microglia activation after motor cortex excitotoxic injury. *Evidence-Based Complement Altern Med.* 2012;2012:918174.
[2544] Bardaji DKR, da Silva JJM, Bianchi TC, et al. Copaifera reticulata oleoresin: Chemical characterization and antibacterial properties against oral pathogens. *Anaerobe.* 2016;40:18-27.
[2545] Souza Barbosa P, Moreira Wiedemann L, da Silva Medeiros R, et al. Phytochemical Fingerprints of Copaiba Oils (Copaifera multijuga Hayne) Determined by Multivariate Analysis. *Chem Biodiversity.* 2013;10(7):1350-60.
[2546] Zoghbi MDGB, Lameira OA, Oliveira ECP. Seasonal Variation of Oleoresin and Volatiles from Copaifera martii Hayne Growing Wild in the State of Pará, Brazil. *J Essent Oil Res.* 2007;19(6):504-6.
[2547] Silva MT, Borges LL, de Sousa Fiuza T, et al. Viscosity of the Oil-resins and Chemical Composition of the Essential Oils from Oils-resins of Copaifera multijuga Hayne Growing in the National Forest Saracá-Taquera Brazil. 2017;20(5):1226-34.
[2548] Nguyen LT, Mysliveckova Z, Szotakova B, et al. The inhibitory effects of β-caryophyllene, β-caryophyllene oxide and α-humulene on the activities of the main drug-metabolizing enzymes in rat and human liver in vitro. *Chem-Biol Interactoins.* 2017 Dec 25;278:123-8.
[2549] Lin WY, Kuo YH, Chang YL, et al. Anti-platelet aggregation and chemical constituents from the rhizome of Gynura japonica. *Planta Med.* 2003 Aug;69(8):757-64.
[2550] Nascimento AM, Brandão MG, Oliveira GB, et al. Synergistic bactericidal activity of Eremanthus erythropappus oil or beta-bisabolene with ampicillin against Staphylococcus aureus. *Antonie Van Leeuwenhoek.* 2007 Jul;92(1):95-100.
[2551] Basile AC, Sertie JAA, Freitas PCD, et al. Anti-inflammatory activity of oleoresin from Brazilian copaifera. *J Ethnopharmacol.* 1988;22(1):101-09.
[2552] Veiga VF, Zunino L, Calixto JB, et al. Phytochemical and antioedematogenic studies of commercial copaiba oils available in Brazil. *Phytother Res.* 2001;15:476-80.
[2553] Gomes NM, Rezende CM, Fontes SP, et al. Antinociceptive activity of Amazonian copaiba oils. *J Ethnopharmacol.* 2007 Feb;19(3):486-92.
[2554] Nogueira Neto J, Lindoso MJ, Coelho LF, et al. Changes in the volume and histology of endometriosis foci in rats treated with copaiba oil (Copaiferalangsdorffii). *Acta Cir Bras.* 2011;26 Suppl 2:20-24.
[2555] Gelmini F, Beretta G, Anselmi C, et al. GC-MS profiling of the phytochemical constituents of the oleoresin from Copaifera langsdorffii Desf. and preliminary in vivo evaluation of its antipsoriatic effect. *Int J Pharm.* 2013 Jan 20;440(2):170-78.
[2556] Souza AB, Martins CH, Souza MG, et al. Antimicrobial activity of terpenoids from Copaifera lansdorffii Desf. against cariogenic bacteria. *Phytother Res.* 2011 Feb;25(2):215-20.
[2557] Pieri FA, Mussi MCM, Fiorini JA, et al. Bacteriostatic effect of copaiba oil (Copaifera officinalis) against Streptococcus mutans. *Braz Dent J.* 2012;23(1):0103-6440.
[2558] Da Silva AG, Puziol Pde F, Leitao RN, et al. Application of the essential oil from copaiba (Copaifera langsdorffi Desf.) for acne vulgaris: a double blind, placebo-controlled clinical trial. *Altern Med Rev.* 2012 Mar;17(1):69-75.
[2559] Paiva LA, de Alencar Cunha KM, Santos FA, et al. Investigation on the wound healing activity of ole-resin from Copaifera langsdorffi in rats. *Phytother Res.* 2002Dec;16(8):737-39.
[2560] Estevao LR, Medeiros JP, Bartella-Evencio L, et al. Effects of the topical administration of copaiba oil ointment (Copaifera langsdorfii) in skin flaps viability of rats. *Acta Cir Bras.* 2013 Dec;28(12):863-69.
[2561] de Lima Silva JJ, Guimaraes SB, da Silveira ER, et al. Effects of Copaifera langsdorfii Desf. on ischemia-reperfusion of randomized skin flaps in rats. *Aesthetic Plast Surg.* 2009 Jan;33(1):104-09.
[2562] Paiva LA, Gurgel LA, Campos AR, et al. Attenuation of ischemia/reperfusion-induced intestinal injury by oleo-resin from Copaifera langsdorffii in rats. *Life Sci.* 2004 sep;75(16):1979-87.
[2563] Paiva LA, Rao VS, Garmosa NV, et al. Gastroprotective effect of Copaifera langsdorffii ole-resin on experimental gastric ulcer models in rats. *J Ethnopharmacol.* 1998 Aug;62(1):73-78.
[2564] Paiva LA, Gurgel LA, De Sousa ET, et al. Protective effect of Copaifera lansdorffii ole-resin against acetic acid-induced colitis in rats. *J Ethnopharmacol.* 2004 Jul;93(1):51-56.
[2565] Baylac S, Racine P. Inhibition of 5-lipoxygenase by essential oils and other natural fragrant extracts. *Int J Aromatherapy.* 2003;13(2-3):138-42.
[2566] Amiel E, Ofir R, Dudai N, et al. β-caryophyllene, a constituent isolated from the Biblical balm of Gilead (Commiphora gileadensis), is a selective apoptosis inducer for tumor cell lines. *Evid Based Complement Altern Med.* 2012;2012:872394.
[2567] Veiga Jr VF, Rosas EC, Carvalho MV, et al. Chemical composition and anti-inflammatory activity of copaiba oils from Copaifera cearensis Huber ex Ducke, Copaifera reticulata Ducke and Copaifera multijuga Hayne—A comparative study. *J Ethnopharm.* 2007;112:248-54.
[2568] Lima SRM, Veiga Jr. VF, Christo HB, et al. In vivo and in vitro studies on the anticancer activity of Copaifera multijuga Hayne and its fractions. *Phytother Res.* 2003;17:1048–53.
[2569] Kobayashi C, Fontanive TO, Enzweiler BG, et al. Pharmacological evaluation of Copaifera multijuga oil in rats. *Pharm Biol.* 2011;49(3):306-13.
[2570] Guimaraes-Santos A, Santos DS, Santos IR, et al. Copaiba oil-resin treatment is neuroprotective and reduces neutrophil recruitment and microglia activation after motor cortex excitotoxic injury. *Evidence-Based Complement Altern Med.* 2012;2012:918174.
[2571] Gonçalves Dias FG, Jorge AT, de Freitas Pereira L, et al. Use of Copaifera multijuga for acute corneal repair after chemical injury: A clinical, histopathological and toxicogenetic study. *Biomed Pharmacother.* 2017 Dec;96:1193-1198.
[2572] Liu H, Song Z, Liao D, et al. Neuroprotective effects of trans-caryophyllene against kainic acid induced seizure activity and oxidative stress in mice. *Neurochem Res.* 2015 Jan;40(1):118-23.

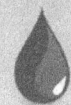

[2573] Bardaji DKR, da Silva JJM, Bianchi TC, et al. Copaifera reticulata oleoresin: Chemical characterization and antibacterial properties against oral pathogens. *Anaerobe*. 2016;40:18-27.
[2574] Santos AO, Ueda-Nakamura T, Dias Filho BP, et al. Effect of Brazilian copaiba oils on Leishmania amazonensis. *J Ethnopharmacol*. 2008;120:204-8.
[2575] Rondon FC, Bevilaqua CM, Accioly MP, et al. In vitro efficacy of Coriandrum sativum, Lippia sidoides and Copaifera reticulata against Leishmania chagasi. *Rev Bras Parasitol Vet*. 2012 Jul-Sep;21(3):185-91.
[2576] Kobayashi C, Fontanive TO, Enzweiler BG, et al. Pharmacological evaluation of Copaifera multijuga oil in rats. *Pharm Biol*. 2011;49(3):306-13.
[2577] Diefenbach AL, Muniz FWMG, Oballe HJR, et al. Antimicrobial activity of copaiba oil (Copaifera ssp.) on oral pathogens: Systematic review. *Phytother Res*. 2018 Apr;32(4):586-596.
[2578] Ribeiro VP, Arruda C, da Silva JJM, et al. Use of spinning band distillation equipment for fractionation of volatile compounds of Copaifera oleoresins for developing a validated Gas Chromatographic method and evaluating antimicrobial activity. *Biomed Chromatogr*. 2018 Oct 26:e4412.
[2579] Campos-Carraro C, Turck P, de Lima-Seolin BG, et al. Copaiba Oil Attenuates Right Ventricular Remodeling by Decreasing Myocardial Apoptotic Signaling in Monocrotaline-Induced Rats. *J Cardiovasc Pharmacol*. 2018 Nov;72(5):214-221.
[2580] Campos C, de Castro AL, Tavares AMV, et al. Effect of Free and Nanoencapsulated Copaiba Oil on Monocrotaline-induced Pulmonary Arterial Hypertension. *J Cardiovasc Pharmacol*. 2017 feb;69(2):79-85.
[2581] Quiñones OG, Hossy BH, Padua TA, et al. Copaiba oil enhances in vitro/in vivo cutaneous permeability and in vivo anti-inflammatory effect of celecoxib. *J Pharm Pharmacol*. 2018 Jul;70(7):964-975.
[2582] Quinones OG, Abranches RP, Nakamura MJ, et al. Copaiba Oil: Chemical Composition and Influence on In-vitro Cutaneous Permeability of Celecoxib. *Curr Drug Deliv*. 2018;15(3):357-366.
[2583] Barbosa MMC, Vicentini FA, Castro-Ghizoni CV, et al. Copaiba Oil Decreases Oxidative Stress and Inflammation But not Colon Damage in Rats with TNBS-Induced Colitis. *Endocr Metab Immune Disord Drug Targets*. 2018;18(3):268-280.
[2584] Feitosa DJS Junior, de Carvalho LTF, Rocha IRO, et al. Effects of Copaiba oil in the healing process of urinary bladder in rats. *Int Braz J Urol*. 2018 Mar-Apr;44(2):384-389.
[2585] de Oliveira RVM, Ohara MT, Carvahalo Vila MMD, et al. In vitro evaluation of copaiba oil as a kojic acid skin enhancer. *Brazilian J Pharm Sci*. 2010 Apr/Jun;46(2):363-70.
[2586] Biondo-Simoes MDLP, Jenning Jr. L, Boel BEDO, et al. Comparative Analysis of the Effects of Honey, Copaiba Oil-Resin and a Commercial Product (Fibrinolysin, Deoxyribonuclease and Chloramphenicol) on Second Intention Healing, in Rats. *Rev Col Bras Cir*. 2019 Nov 25;46(5):e20192245.
[2587] Dalenogare DP, Ferro AR, De Pra SDT, et al. Antinociceptive Activity of Copaifera Officinalis Jacq. L Oil and Kaurenoic Acid in Mice. *Inflammopharmacology*. 2019 Auf;27(4):829-844.
[2588] Urasaki Y, Beaumont C, Workman M, et al. Fast-Acting and Receptor-Mediated Regulation of Neuronal Signaling Pathways by Copaiba Essential Oil. *Int J Mol Sci*. 2020 Mar 25;21(7).
[2589] Urasaki Y, Beaumont C, Talnot JN, et al. Akt3 Regulates the Tissue-Specific Response to Copaiba Essential Oil. *Int J Mol Sci*. 2020;21(8):2851.
[2590] Caputo LS, Campos MIC, Dias HJ, et al. Copaiba oil suppresses inflammation in asthmatic lungs of BALB/c mice induced with ovalbumin. *Int Immunopharmacol*. 2020 Mar;80:106177.
[2591] Lima LR, Andrade FK, Alves DR, et al. Anti-acetylcholinesterase and toxicity against Artemia salina of chitosan microparticles loaded with essential oils of Cymbopogon flexuosus, Pelargonium x ssp and Copaifera officinalis. *Int J Biol Macromol*. 2020 Nov 17;S0141-8130(20)35015-7.
[2592] Vinturelle R, Mattos C, Meloni J, et al. Evaluation of essential oils as an ecological alternative in the search for control Rhipicephalus microplus (Acari: Ixodidae). *Vet Parasitol Reg Stud Reports*. 2021 Jan;23:100523.
[2593] Lima LR, Andtrade FK, Alves DR, et al. Anti-acetylcholinesterase and toxicity against Artemia salina of chitosan microparticles loaded with essential oils of Cymbopogon flexuosus, Pelargonium x ssp and Copaifera officinalis. *Int J Biol Macromolecules*. 2021 Jan 15;167:1361-70.
[2594] De Araujo Silva E, Prada AL, Boechat AL, et al. Anti-inflammatory effects and acute oral toxicity of Copaifera spp. essential oil-loaded nanoemulsion. *Bol Latinoam Caribe Plant Med Aromat*. 2022;21(3):323-42.
[2595] Zhang N, Chen J, Dong W, et al. The Effect of Copaiba Oil Odor on Anxiety Relief in Adults under Mental Workload: A Randomized Controlled Trial. *Evidence-Based Complement Alternat Med*. 2022;2022:3874745.
[2596] Pinto EP, Menezes RP, de S Tavares W, et al. Copaiba essential oil loaded-nanocapsules film as a potential candidate for treating skin disorders: preparation, characterization, and antibacterial properties. *Int J Pharm*. 2023 Jan 12;633:122608.
[2597] Zhelijazkov VD, Astatkie T, Schlegel V. Hydrodistillation extraction time effect on essential oil yield, composition, and bioactivity of coriander oil. *J Oleo Sci*. 2014;63(9):857-865.
[2598] Ebrahimi SN, Hadian J, Ranjbar H. Essential oil compositions of different accessions of Coriandrum sativum L. *Nat Prod Res*. 2010 Sep;24(14):1287-94.
[2599] de Figueiredo RO, Nakagawa J, Ming LC. Composition of coriander essential oil from Brazil. *Acta Hort*. 2004;629:135-37.
[2600] Gray AM, Flatt PR. Insulin-releasing and insulin-like activity of the traditional anti-diabetic plant Coriandrum sativum (coriander). *Br J Nutr*. 1999;81(3):203-09.
[2601] Srivastava N, Tiwari G, Tiwari R. Polyherbal preparation for anti-diabetic activity: a screening study. *Indian J Med Sci*. 2010 Apr;64(4):163-76.
[2602] Eidi M, Eidi A, Saeidi A, et al. Effect of coriander seed (Coriandrum sativum L.) ethanol extract on insulin release from pancreatic beta cells in streptozotocin-induced diabetic rats. *Phytother Res*. 2009 Mar;23(3):404-06.
[2603] Duarte A, Ferreira S, Silva F, et al. Synergistic activity of coriander oil and conventional antibiotics against Acinetobacter baumannii. *Phytomedicine*. 2012 Feb;19(3-4):236-38.
[2604] Cardoso NN, Alviano CS, Blank AF, et al. Synergism Effect of the Essential Oil from Ocimum basilicum var. Maria Bonita and Its Major Components with Fluconazole and Its Influence on Ergosterol Biosynthesis. *Evid Based Complement Alternat Med*. 2016;2016:5647182.
[2605] Scazzocchio F, Garzoli S, Conti C, et al. Properties and limits of some essential oils: chemical characterisation, antimicrobial activity, interaction with antibiotics and cytotoxicity. *Nat Prod Res*. 2016 Sep;30(17):1909-18.
[2606] Jana S, Patra K, Sarkar S, et al. Antitumorigenic potential of linalool is accompanied by modulation of oxidative stress: an in vivo study in sarcoma-180 solid tumor model. *Nutr Cancer*. 2014;66(5):835-48.
[2607] Thompson A, Meah D, Ahmed N, et al. Comparison of the antibacterial activity of essential oils and extracts of medicinal and culinary herbs to investigate potential new treatments for irritable bowel syndrome. *BMC Complement Altern Med*. 2013 Nov;13:338.
[2608] Cioanca O, Hritcu L, Mihasan M, et al. Cognitive-enhancing and antioxidant activities of inhaled coriander volatile oil in amyloid β(1-42) rat model of Alzheimer's disease. *Physiol Behav*. 2013 Aug;120:193-202.
[2609] Freires Ide A, Murata RM, Furletti VF, et al. Coriandum sativum L. (Coriander) essential oil: antifungal activity and mode of action on Candida spp., and molecular targets affected in human whole-genome expression. *PloS One*. 2014 Jun;9(6):e99086.
[2610] Jana S, Patra K, Sarkar S, et al. Antitumorigenic potential oil linalool is accompanied by modulation of oxidative stress: an in vivo study in sarcoma-180 solid tumor. *Nutr Cancer*. 2014;66(5):835-48.
[2611] Hashim S, Aboobaker VS, Madhubala R, et al. Modulatory effects of essential oils from spices on the formation of DNA adduct by aflatoxin B1 in vitro. *Nutr Cancer*. 1994;21(2):169-75.
[2612] Duarte A, Ferreira S, Silva F, et al. Synergistic activity of coriander oil and conventional antibiotics against Acinetobacter baumannii. *Phytomedicine*. 2012 Feb;19(3-4):236-38.
[2613] Casetti F, Bartelke S, Biehler K, et al. Antimicrobial activity against bacteria with dermatological relevance and skin tolerance of the essential oil from Coriandrum sativum L. fruits. *Phytother Res*. 201 2Mar;26(3):420-24.
[2614] Bag A, Chattopadhyay RR. Evaluation of Synergistic Antibacterial and Antioxidant Efficacy of Essential Oils of Spices and Herbs in Combination. *PLoS One*. 2015 Jul 1;10(7):e0131321.
[2615] Silva F, Ferreira S, Duarte A, et al. Antifungal activity of Coriandrum sativum essential oil, its mode of action against Candida species and potential synergism with amphotericin B. *Phytomedicine*. 2011 Dec;19(1):42-47.
[2616] Furletti VF, Teixeira IP, Obando-Pereda G, et al. Action of Coriandrum sativum L. essential oil upon oral Candida albicans biofilm formation. *Evid Based Complement Altern Med*. 2011;2011:9858232.
[2617] Reuter J, Juyke C, Casetti F, et al. Anti-inflammatory potential of lipolotion containing coriander oil in the ultraviolet erythema test. *J Dtsch Dermat Ges*. 2008 Oct;6(10):847-51.
[2618] Aissoi A, Zizi S, Israili ZH, et al. Hypoglycemic and hypolipidemic effects of Coriandrum sativum L. in Meriones shawi rats. *J Ethnopharmacology*. 2011 Sep;137(1):652-61.
[2619] Brindis F, Gonzalez-Andrade M, Gonzalez-Tujano ME, et al. Postprandial glycaemia and inhibition of α-glucosidase activity by aqueous extract from Coriandrum sativum. *Nat Prod Res*. 2014;28(22):2021-25.
[2620] Heidari B, Sajjadi SE, Minaiyan M. Effect of Coriandrum sativum hydroalcoholic extract and its essential oil on acetic acid- induced acute colitis in rats. *Avicenna J Phytomed*. 2016 Mar-Apr;6(2):205-14.
[2621] Mansouri N, Aoun L, Dalichaouche N, et al. Yields, chemical composition, and antimicrobial activity of two Algerian essential oils against 40 avian multidrug-resistant Escherichia coli strains. *Vet World*. 2018 Nov;11(11):1539-1550.
[2622] Altınok-Yipel F, Ozan Tekeli İ, Özsoy ŞY, et al. Hepatoprotective Activity of Linalool in Rats Against Liver Injury Induced by Carbon Tetrachloride. *Int J Vitam Nutr Res*. 2019 Apr 1:1-7.
[2623] Ben Miri Y, Djenane D. Evaluation of Protective Impact of Algerian Cuminum cyminum L. and Coriandrum sativum L. Essential Oils on Aspergillus flavus Growth and Aflatoxin B1 Production. *Pak J Biol Sci*. 2018;21(2):67-77.
[2624] Monzote L, Herrera I, Satyal P, et al. In-Vitro Evaluation of 52 Commercially-Available Essential Oils Against Leishmania amazonensis. Molecules. 2019 Mar 20;24(7):24071248.
[2625] Kačániová M, Galovičová L, Ivanišová E, et al. Antioxidant, Antimicrobial and Antibiofilm Activity of Coriander (Coriandrum sativum L.) Essential Oil for Its Application in Foods. *Foods*. 2020 Mar 4;9(3).
[2626] Can E, Kızak V, Can ŞS, et al. Anesthetic Efficiency of Three Medicinal Plant Oils for Aquatic Species: Coriander Coriandrum sativum, Linaloe Tree Bursera delpechiana, and Lavender Lavandula hybrida. *J Aquat Anim Health*. 2019 Sep;31(3):266-273.
[2627] Caputo L, Piccialli I, Ciccone R, et al. Lavender and coriander essential oils and their main component linalool exert a protective effect against amyloid-β neurotoxicity. *Phytother Res*. 2021 Jan;35(1):486-493.
[2628] Hajlaoui H, Arraouadi S, Noumi E, et al. Antimicrobial, Antioxidant, Anti-Acetylcholinesterase, Antidiabetic, and Pharmacokinetic Properties of Carum carvi L. and Coriandrum sativum L. Essential Oils Alone and in Combination. *Molecules*. 2021 Jun 13;26(12):3625.
[2629] Rapper SL, Tankeu S, Kamatou G, et al. The use of chemometric modelling to determine chemical composition-antimicrobial activity relationships of essential oils used in respiratory tract infections. *Fitoterapia*. 2021 Aug 26;105024.
[2630] Trifan A, Luca SV, Bostănaru AC, et al. Apiaceae Essential Oils: Boosters of Terbinafine Activity against Dermatophytes and Potent Anti-Inflammatory Effectors. *Plants (Basel)*. 2021 Nov 4;10(11):2378.

[2631] Eid AM, Issa L, Al-Kharouf O, et al. Development of Coriandrum sativum Oil Nanoemulgel and Evaluation of Its Antimicrobial and Anticancer Activity. *Biomed Res Int.* 2021 Oct 11;2021:5247816.

[2632] Salem MA, Manaa EG, Osama N, et al. Coriander (Coriandrum sativum L.) essential oil and oil-loaded nano-formulations as an anti-aging potentiality via TGFβ/SMAD pathway. *Sci Rep.* 2022 Apr 21;12(1):6578.

[2633] Abbas A, Anwar F, Ahmad N, et al. Characterization of Bioactives and Nutra-Pharmaceutical Potential of Supercritical Fluid and Hydro-Distilled Extracted Coriander Leaves Essential Oil. *Dose Response.* 2022 Nov 8;20(4):15593258221130749.

[2634] Das S, Pradhan C, Pillai D. Dietary coriander (Coriandrum sativum L) oil improves antioxidant and anti-inflammatory activity, innate immune responses and resistance to Aeromonas hydrophila in Nile tilapia (Oreochromis niloticus). *Fish Shellfish Immunol.* 2022 Dec 10;132:108486.

[2635] Barbosa DHX, Gondim CR, Silva-Henriques MQ, et al. Coriandrum sativum L. essential oil obtained from organic culture shows antifungal activity against planktonic and multi-biofilm Candida. *Braz J Biol.* 2023 Jan 16;83:e264875.

[2636] Albuquerque KRS, Purgato GA, Piccolo MS, et al. Formulations of essential oils obtained from plants traditionally used as condiments or traditional medicine active against Staphylococcus aureus isolated from dairy cows with mastitis. *Lett Appl Microbiol.* 2023 Mar 1;76(3):ovad034.

[2637] Aouini J, Bachrouch O, Msaada K, et al. Screening of antimicrobial and insecticidal properties of essential oils extracted from three Tunisian aromatic and medicinal plants. *Int J Environ Health Res.* 2023 Mar 9:1-11.

[2638] Chaudhry AH, Tanveer A, Shar A, et al. Physico-chemical investigation and antimicrobial activity of essential oil of Cuminum cyminum L. *World App Sci J.* 2012;19(3):330–33.

[2639] Hajlaoui H, Mighri, Noumi E, et al. Chemical composition and biological activities of Tunisian Cuminum cyminum L. essential oil: a high effectiveness against Vibrio spp. strains. *Food Chem toxicol.* 2010 Aug-Sep;48(8–9):2186–92.

[2640] Hashemian N, Ghasemi Pirbalouti A, Hashemi M, et al. Diversity in chemical composition and antibacterial activity of essential oils of cumin (Cuminum cyminum L.) diverse from northeast of Iran. *Aust J Crop Sci.* 2013;7(11):1752–1760.

[2641] Kan Y, Kartal M, Ozek T, et al. Composition of essential oil of Cumin cyminum L. according to harvesting times. *Turkish J Pharm Sci.* 2007;4(1):25–29.

[2642] Opdyke DIJ. Monographs on fragrance raw materials. *Food Cosmet Toxicol.* 1974;12(Suppl.):869–70.

[2643] Toroglu S. In-vitro antimicrobial activity and synergistic/antagonistic effect of interactions between antibiotics and some spice essential oils. *J Environ Biol.* 2011 Jan;32(1):23-9.

[2644] Chaudhry AH, Tanveer A, Shar A, et al. Physico-chemical investigation and antimicrobial activity of essential oil of Cuminum cyminum L. *World App Sci J.* 2012;19(3):330–33.

[2645] Singh G, Kapoor IP, Pandey SK, et al. Studies on essential oils: part 10; antibacterial activity of volatile oils of some spices. *Phytother Res.* 2002 Nov;16(7):16(7):680–82.

[2646] Bag A, Chattopadhyay RR. Evaluation of Synergistic Antibacterial and Antioxidant Efficacy of Essential Oils of Spices and Herbs in Combination. *PLoS One.* 2015 Jul 1;10(7):e0131321.

[2647] Hajlaoui H, Mighri, Noumi E, et al. Chemical composition and biological activities of Tunisian Cuminum cyminum L. essential oil: a high effectiveness against Vibrio spp. strains. *Food Chem toxicol.* 2010 Aug-Sep;48(8–9):2186–92.

[2648] Naeini A, Naderi NJ, Shokri H. Analysis and in vitro anti-Candida antifungal activity of Cumimum cyminum and Salvadora persica herbs extracts against pathogenic Candida strains. *J Mycol Med.* 2014 Mar;24(1):13–18.

[2649] Minooeianhaghighi MH, Sepehrian L, Shokri H, et al. Antifungal effects of Lavandula binaludensis and Cuminum cyminum essential oils against Candida albicans strains isolated from patients with recurrent vulvovaginal candidiasis. *J Mycol Med.* 2017 Mar;27(1):65-71.

[2650] Pajohi MR, Tajik H, Farshid AA, et al. Synergistic antibacterial activity of the essential oil of Cuminum cyminum L. seed and nisin in a food model. *J Appl Microbiol.* 2011 Apr;110(4):943–51.

[2651] Irkin R, Korukuoglu M. Growth inhibition of pathogenic bacteria and some yeasts by selected essential oils and survival of L. monocytogenes and C. albicans in apple-carrot juice. *Foodborne Pathog Dis.* 2009 Apr;6(3):387–94.

[2652] Shayegh S, Rasooli I, Taghizadeh M, et al. Phytotherapeutic inhibition of supragingival dental plaque. *Nat Prod Res.* 2008 Mar;22(5)428–39.

[2653] Janahmadi M, Niazi F, Danyali S, et al. Effects of the fruit essential oil of Curcuminum cyminum Linn. (Apiaceae) on pentylenetetrazol-induced epileptiform activity in F1 neurones of Helix aspersa. *J Ethnopharmacol.* 2006 Mar;104(1–2):278–82.

[2654] Wei J, Zhang X, Bi Y, et al. Anti-inflammatory effects of cumin essential oil by blocking JNK, ERK, and NF-KB signaling pathways in LPS-stimulated RAW 264.7 cells. *Evid Based Complement Alt Med.* 2015;(2015):474509.

[2655] Gómez-Mateos Pérez M, Navarro Moll C1, Merino Espinosa G, et al. Evaluation of different Mediterranean essential oils as prophylactic agents in anisakidosis. *Pharm Biol.* 2017 Dec;55(1):456-461.

[2656] Jafari S, Sattari R, Ghavamzadeh S, et al. Evaluation the effect of 50 and 100 mg doses of Cuminum cyminum essential oil on glycemic indices, insulin resistance and serum inflammatory factors on patients with diabetes type II: A double-blind randomized placebo-controlled clinical trial. *J Tradit Complement Med.* 2016 Dec 21;7(3):332-338.

[2657] Villarreal JPV, Santos PRD, Silva MAMPD, et al. Evaluation of phytotherapy alternatives for controlling Rhipicephalus (Boophilus) microplus in vitro. *Rev Bras Parasitol Vet.* 2017 Jul-Sep;26(3):299-306.

[2658] Ebade ME. Essential oils of green cumin and chamomile partially protect against acute acetaminophen hepatotoxicity in rats. *An Acad Bras Cienc.* 2018 Jun 25:0.

[2659] Feng J, Shi W, Miklossy J, et al. Identification of Essential Oils with Strong Activity against Stationary Phase Borrelia burgdorferi. *Antibiotics (Basel).* 2018 Oct 16;7(4).

[2660] Vieira JN, Gonçalves CL, Villarreal JPV, et al. Chemical composition of essential oils from the apiaceae family, cytotoxicity, and their antifungal activity in vitro against candida species from oral cavity. *Braz J Biol.* 2019 Jul-Sep;79(3):432-437.

[2661] Bartoňková I, Dvořák Z. Essential oils of culinary herbs and spices display agonist and antagonist activities at human aryl hydrocarbon receptor AhR. *Food Chem Toxicol.* 2018 Jan;111:374-384.

[2662] Ghasemi G, Fattahi M, Alirezalu A, et al. A new source of oxygenated monoterpenes with phytotoxic activity: essential oil of Cuminum Cyminum L. from Iran. *Nat Prod Res.* 2018 Nov 6:1-4.

[2663] Morovati A, Pourghassem Gargari B, Sarbakhsh P, et al. The effect of cumin supplementation on metabolic profiles in patients with metabolic syndrome: A randomized, triple blind, placebo-controlled clinical trial. *Phytother Res.* 2019 Apr;33(4):1182-1190.

[2664] Morovati A, Pourghassem Gargari B, et al. Effects of cumin (Cuminum cyminum L.) essential oil supplementation on metabolic syndrome components: A randomized, triple-blind, placebo-controlled clinical trial. *Phytother Res.* 2019 Dec;33(12):3261-3269.

[2665] Khorram Z, Hakimaneh SM, Naeini A, et al. The Antifungal Effects of Two Herbal Essences in Comparison with Nystatin on the Candida Strains Isolated from the Edentulous Patients. *J Contemp Dent Pract.* 2019 Jun 1;20(6):716-719.

[2666] Ben Miri Y, Djenane D. Evaluation of Protective Impact of Algerian Cuminum cyminum L. and Coriandrum sativum L. Essential Oils on Aspergillus flavus Growth and Aflatoxin B1 Production. *Pak J Biol Sci.* 2018;21(2):67-77.

[2667] Mutlu-Ingok A, Karbancioglu-Guler F. Cardamom, Cumin, and Dill Weed Essential Oils: Chemical Compositions, Antimicrobial Activities, and Mechanisms of Action against Campylobacter spp. *Molecules.* 2017 Jul 15;22(7).

[2668] Alizadeh Behbahani B, Noshad M, Falah F, et al. Cumin essential oil: Phytochemical analysis, antimicrobial activity and investigation of its mechanism of action through scanning electron microscopy. *Microb Pathog.* 2019 Sep 5;136:103716.

[2669] Elisa B, Aldo A, Ludovica G, et al. Chemical Composition and Antimycotic Activity of Six Essential Oils (Cumin, Fennel, Manuka, Sweet Orange, Cedar and Juniper) Against Different Candida Spp. *Nat Prod res.* 2019 Nov 29:1-6.

[2670] Nirmala NJ, Duria L, Rao KA, et al. Ultrasonic Nanoemulsification of Cuminum cyminum Essential Oil and Its Applications in Medicine. *Int J Nanomedicine.* 2020 Feb 5;17:759-807.

[2671] Babashahi M, Mirlohi M, Ghiasvand R, et al. Effects of Probiotic Soy Milk Fermented by Lactobacillus plantarum A7 (KC 355240) Added With Cuminum Cyminum Essential Oil on Fasting Blood Glucose Levels, Serum Lipid Profile and Body Weight in Diabetic Wistar Rats. *Int J Prev Med.* 2020 Jan 24;11:8.

[2672] Amiri A, Mousakhani-Ganjeh A, Amiri Z, et al. Fabrication of Cumin Loaded-Chitosan Particles: Characterized by Molecular, Morphological, Thermal, Antioxidant and Anticancer Properties as Well as Its Utilization in Food System. *Food Chem.* 2020 Apr 25;310:125821.

[2673] Tanhaieian A, Pourgonabadi S, Akbari M, et al. The effective and safe method for preventing and treating bacteria-induced dental diseases by herbal plants and a recombinant peptide. *J Clin Exp Dent.* 2020 Jun 1;12(6):e523-e532.

[2674] Rosa JS, Oliveira L, Sousa RMOF, et al. Bioactivity of some Apiaceae essential oils and their constituents against Sitophilus zeamais (Coleoptera: Curculionidae). *Bull Entomol Res.* 2020 Jun;110(3):406-416.

[2675] da Silva MAMP, Zehetmeyr FK, Pereira KM, et al. Ovicidal in vitro activity of the fixed oil of Helianthus annus L. and the essential oil of Cuminum cyminum L. against Fasciola hepatica (Linnaeus, 1758). *Exp Parasitol.* 2020 Aug 29;218:107984.

[2676] Tanapichatsakul C, Khruengsai S, Pripdeevech P, et al. In vitro and in vivo antifungal activity of Cuminum cyminum essential oil against Aspergillus aculeatus causing bunch rot of postharvest grapes. *PLoS One.* 2020 Nov 24;15(11):e0242862.

[2677] Morteza-Semnani K, Saeedi M, Akbari J, et al. Development of a novel nanoemulgel formulation containing cumin essential oil as skin permeation enhancer. *Drug Deliv Transl Res.* 2021 Jul 17. Online ahead of print.

[2678] Sharifi A, Mohammadzadeh A, Salehi TZ, et al. Cuminum cyminum L. Essential Oil: A Promising Antibacterial and Antivirulence Agent Against Multidrug-Resistant Staphylococcus aureus. *Front Microbiol.* 2021 Aug 4;12:667833.

[2679] Qiao Y, Yu Z, Bai L, et al. Chemical composition of essential oils from Thymus mongolicus, Cinnamomum verum, and Origanum vulgare and their acaricidal effects on Haemaphysalis longicornis (Acari: Ixodidae). *Ecotoxicol Environ Saf.* 2021 Aug 17;224:112672.

[2680] Korinek M, Handoussa H, Tsai YH, et al. Anti-Inflammatory and Antimicrobial Volatile Oils: Fennel and Cumin Inhibit Neutrophilic Inflammation via Regulating Calcium and MAPKs. *Front Pharmacol.* 2021 Oct 11;12:674095.

[2681] Pajohi Alamoti M, Bazargani-Gilani B, Mahmoudi R, et al. Essential Oils from Indigenous Iranian Plants: A Natural Weapon vs. Multidrug-Resistant Escherichia coli. *Microorganisms.* 2022 Jan 5;10(1):109.

[2682] Ghannay S, Aouadi K, Kadri A, et al. In Vitro and In Silico Screening of Anti-Vibrio spp., Antibiofilm, Antioxidant and Anti-Quorum Sensing Activities of Cuminum cyminum L. Volatile Oil. *Plants (Basel).* 2022 Aug 29;11(17):2236.

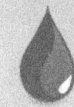

2683 Alomar HA, Fathallah N, Abdel-Aziz MM, et al. GC-MS Profiling, Anti-Helicobacter pylori, and Anti-Inflammatory Activities of Three Apiaceous Fruits' Essential Oils. *Plants (Basel)*. 2022 Oct 5;11(19):2617.

2684 Denett GO, Comelli NC, Rodriguez MR, et al. Chemical composition and insecticidal activity of essential oils from cultivated and native aromatic plants of Argentina against Carpophilus dimidiatus (Fabricius) (Nitidulidae) and Oryzaephilus mercator (L.) (Silvanidae). *Nat Prod Res*. 2023 Jan 9:1-5.

2685 Ranjbar R, Zarenezhad E, Abdollahi A, et al. Nanoemulsion and Nanogel Containing Cuminum cyminum L Essential Oil: Antioxidant, Anticancer, Antibacterial, and Antilarval Properties. *J Trop Med*. 2023 Feb 6;2023:5075581.

2686 Selim SA, Adam ME, Hassan SM, et al. Chemical composition, antimicrobial and antibiofilm activity of the essential oil and methanol extract of the Mediterranean cypress (Cupressus sempervirens L.). *BMC Complement Altern Med*. 2014 Jun 2;14:179.

2687 El Hamrouni-Aschi K, Khouja ML, Boussaid M, et al. Essential-oil composition of the Tunisian endemic cypress (Cupressus sempervirens L. var. numidica TRAB.). *Chem Biodivers*. 2013 Jun;10(6):989-1003.

2688 Asgary S, Naderi GA, Shams Ardekani MR, et al. Chemical analysis and biological activities of Cupressus sempervirens var. horizontalis essential oils. *Pharm Biol*. 2013 Feb;51(2):137-44.

2689 Boukhris M, Regane G, Yangui T, et al. Chemical composition and biological potential of essential oil from Tunisian Cupressus sempervirens L. *J Arid Land Studies*. 2012;22(1):329-32.

2690 Khayyat MH, Enami SA, Rahimizadeh M, et al. Chemical constituents of Cupressus sempervirens L. cv. Cereiformis Rehd. Essential oils. *Iranian J Pharm Sci*. 2005;6(1):39-42.

2691 Tognolini M, Barocelli E, Ballabeni V, et al. Comparative screening of plant essential oils; phenylpropanoid moiety as basic core for antiplatelet activity. *Life Sci*. 2006 Feb 23;78(13):1419-32.

2692 Loizzo MR, Tundis R, Menichini F, et al. Antiproliferative effects of essential oils and their major constituents in human renal adenocarcinoma and amelanotic melanoma cells. *Cell Prolif*. 2008 Dec;41(6):1002-12.

2693 Aazza S, Lyoussi B, Megias C, et al. Anti-oxidant anti-inflammatory and anti-proliferative activities of Moroccan commercial essential oils. *Nat Prod Commun*. 2014 Apr;9(4):587-94.

2694 Asgary S, Naderi GA, Shams Ardekani MR, et al. Chemical analysis and biological activities of Cupressus sempervirens var. horizontalis essential oils. *Pharm Biol*. 2013 Feb;51(2):137-44.

2695 Mazari K, Bendimerad N, Bekhechi C, et al. Chemical composition and antimicrobial activity of essential oils isolated from Algerian Juniperus phoenicea L. and Cupressus sempervirens L. *J Med Plants Res*. 2010 May;4(10):959- 64.

2696 Ibrahim TA, El-Hela AA, El-Hefnawy HM, et al. Chemical Composition and Antimicrobial Activities of Essential Oils of Some Coniferous Plants Cultivated in Egypt. *Iran J Pharm Res*. 2017 Winter;16(1):328-337.

2697 Pedroso RDS, Balbino BL, Andrade G, et al. In Vitro and In Vivo Anti- Candida Spp. Activity of Plant-Derived Products. *Plants (Basel)*. 2019 Nov;8(11):494.

2698 Almadiy AA, Nenaah GE. Bioactivity and safety evaluations of Cupressus sempervirens essential oil, its nanoemulsion and main terpenes against Culex quinquefasciatus Say. *Environ Sci Pollut Res Int*. 2021 Sep 30. Online ahead of print.

2699 Alimi D, Hajri A, Jallouli S, et al. Phytochemistry, anti-tick, repellency and anti-cholinesterase activities of Cupressus sempervirens L. and Mentha pulegium L. combinations against Hyalomma scupense (Acari: Ixodidae). *Vet Parasitol*. 2022 Jan 31;303:109665.

2700 Xavier V, Finimundy TC, Heleno SA, et al. Chemical and Bioactive Characterization of the Essential Oils Obtained from Three Mediterranean Plants. *Molecules*. 2021 Dec 10;26(24):7472.

2701 Galovicova L, Cmikova N, Schwarzova M, et al. Biological Activity of Cupressus sempervirens Essential Oil. *Plants*. 2023;12:1097.

2702 Alcaraz-Meléndez, Delgado-Rodríguez J, Real-Cosío S. Analysis of essential oils from wild and micropropagated plants of damiana (Turnera diffusa). *Fitoterapia*. 2004 Dec;75(7-8):696-701.

2703 Alcaraz-Meléndez, Delgado-Rodríguez J, Real-Cosío S. Differences in Essential Oil Production and Leaf Structure in Phenotypes of Damiana (Turnera diffusa Willd.). *J Plant Biol*. 2007 Jun;50(3):378-82.

2704 Papas R. Chromatogram Damiana. 2014 Jun. Available at: https://www.facebook.com/EssentialOilUniversity/photos/pcb.10152557097573083/10152557043498083/?type=3&theater.

2705 Bicchi C, Ribiolo P, Saranz Camargo EE, et al. Components of Turnera diffusa Willd. var. afrodisiaca (Ward) Urb. Essential Oil. *Flavour Frag J*. 2003 Jan;18(1):59-61.

2706 Burkhard PR, Burkhardt K, Haenggeli CA, et al. Plant-induced seizures: reappearance of an old problem. *J Neurol*. 1999 Aug;246(8):667-70.

2707 Culic M, Kekovic G, Grbic G, et al. Wavelet and fractal analysis of rat brain activity in seizures evoked by camphor essential oil and 1,8-cineole. *Gen Physiol Biophys*. 2009;Special Issue(28):33–40.

2708 Mathew T, Kamath V, Kumar RS, et al. Eucalyptus oil inhalation–induced seizure: A novel, underrecognized, preventable cause of acute symptomatic seizure. *Epilepsia Open*. 2017 Sep;2(3):350–354.

2709 Jori A, Bianchetti A, Prestini PE, et al. Effect of eucalyptol (1,8-cineole) on the metabolism of other drugs in rats and in man. *Eur J Pharmacol*. 1970;9(3):362-66.

2710 de Sousa DP, Raphael E, Brocksom U, et al. Sedative effect of monoterpene alcohols in mice: A preliminary screening. *Verlag der Zeitschrift fur Naturforschung*. 2007;62c:563-66.

2711 Birhanie MW, Walle B, Rebba K, et al. Hypnotic effect of the essential oil from the leaves of Myrtus communis on mice. *Nat Sci Sleep*. 2016 Aug 16;8:267-75.

2712 Lamborn LL. Modern soaps, candles and glycerin: A practical manual of modern methods of utilization of fats and oils in the manufacture of soaps and candles, and of the recovery of glycerin. Library of the University of Wisconsin.

2713 Oyen LP, Dung NX. Plant resources of South-East Asia. 1999. Backhyus, Leiden.

2714 Kim NH, Hyun SH, Jin CH, et al. Pretreatment with 1,8-cineole potentiates thioacetamide-induced hepatotoxicity and immunosuppression. *Arch Pharm Res*. 2004 Jul;27(7):781-9.

2715 Bueno J, Escobar P, Martínez JR, et al. Composition of three essential oils, and their mammalian cell toxicity and antimycobacterial activity against drug resistant-tuberculosis and nontuberculous mycobacteria strains. *Nat Prod Commun*. 2011 Nov;6(11):1743-8.

2716 Silva-Trujillo L, Quintero-Rueda E, Stashenko EE, et al. Essential Oils from Colombian Plants: Antiviral Potential against Dengue Virus Based on Chemical Composition, In Vitro and In Silico Analyses. *Molecules*. 2022 Oct 12;27(20):6844.

2717 Duque JE, Urbina DL, Vesga LC, et al. Insecticidal activity of essential oils from American native plants against Aedes aegypti (Diptera: Culicidae): an introduction to their possible mechanism of action. *Sci Rep*. 2023 Feb 20;13(1):2989.

2718 Carreño H, Stashenko EE, Escobar P. Essential Oils Distilled from Colombian Aromatic Plants and Their Constituents as Penetration Enhancers for Transdermal Drug Delivery. *Molecules*. 2023 Mar 22;28(6):2872.

2719 Isidorov1 VA, Zenkevich IG, Krajewska U. Gas chromatography of essential oils with preliminary partition of components. *Phytochemical Analysis*. 2001 March-Apr;12(2):87-90.

2720 Roman Wanner JK, Bail S, Buchbauer G, et al. GC-MS-analysis, antimicrobial activities and olfactory evaluation of essential Davana (Artemisia pallens Wall. ex DC) oil from India. *Nat Prod Communications*. 2007 Dec;3(7):1057-62.

2721 Krishna District. Davana Oil. Available at: http://krishna.nic.in/PDFfiles/MSME/Chemical/davana[1].pdf.

2722 Mallavarapu GR, Kulkarni RN, Baskaran K, et al. Influence of plant growth stage on the essential oil content and composition in Davana (Artemisia pallens wall.). *J Agric Food Chem*. 1999 Jan;47(1):254-8.

2723 Kamath A, Asha MR, Ravi R, et al. Comparative study of odour and GC-olfactometric profiles of selected essential oils. *Flavour Frag J*. 2001 Nov;16(6):401-407.

2724 Aromatics International. Davana oil. Available at: https://www.aromatics.com/products/essential-oils/davana.

2725 Mallavarapu GR, Kulkarni RN, Baskaran K, et al. Influence of plant growth stage on the essential oil content and composition in Davana (Artemisia pallens wall.). *J Agric Food Chem*. 1999 Jan;47(1):254-8.

2726 Roman Wanner JK, Bail S, Buchbauer G, et al. GC-MS-analysis, antimicrobial activities and olfactory evaluation of essential Davana (Artemisia pallens Wall. ex DC) oil from India. *Nat Prod Communications*. 2007 Dec;3(7):1057-62.

2727 Nakhare S, Garg SC. Anthelmintic activity of the essential oil of Artemisia pallens Wall. *Ancient Sci Life*. 1991 Jan;X(3):185-186.

2728 Singh S, Bhatt D, Singh MK, et al. New Insights into the Chemical Composition, Proinflammatory Cytokine Inhibition Profile of Davana (Artemisia pallens Wall. ex DC.) Essential Oil and cis-Davanone in Primary Macrophage Cells. *Chem Biodivers*. 2021 Oct 20:e2100531.

2729 Sharopov FS, Wink M, Gulmurodov IS, et al. Composition and bioactivity of the essential oil of Anethum graveolens L. from Tajikstan. *Int J Med Arom Plants*. 2013 Jun;3(2):125-30.

2730 Radulescu V, Popescu ML, Ilies DC. Chemical composition of the volatile oil from different plant parts of Anethum graveolens L. (Umbelliferae) cultivated in Romania. *Farmacia*. 2012;58(5):594-600.

2731 Jirovetz L, Buchbauer G, Stoyanova AS, et al. Composition, quality control, and antimicrobial activity of the essential oil of long-time stored dill (Anethum graveolens L.) seeds from Bulgaria. *J Agric Food Chem*. 2003 Jun 18;51(13):3854-7.

2732 Rana VS, Blazquez MA. Chemical Composition of the Essential Oil of Anethum graveolens Aerial Parts. *J Essent Oil-Bearing Plants*. 2014 Nov;17(6):1219-23.

2733 Yili A, Aisa HA, Maksimov VV, et al. Chemical composition and antimicrobial activity of essential oil from seeds of Anethum graveolens growing in Uzbekistan. Chem Nat Constituents. 2009;45(2):280-81.

2734 Lowenstein L, Ballew DH. Fatal acute hemolytic anemia, thrombocytopenic purpura, nephrosis and hepatitis resulting from ingestion of a constituent containing apiol. *Can Med Assoc J*. 1958 Feb 1;78(3):195-8.

2735 Basso U. [Study of death caused by apiol and experimental study of its toxic action]. *Arch Patol Clin Med*. 1957;34(4):308-22.

2736 Barni B, Barni I. [The apiol poisoning]. Rassegna casistica. 1967;3(2):197-221.

2737 Newall CA, Anderson LA, Philpson JD. Herbal Medicine: A Guide for Healthcare Professionals. London, UK: The Pharmaceutical Press, 1996.

2738 Colalillo R. Apiol poisoning in 7 women and 2 children. *Rivista di Tossicologia Sperimentale e Clinica*. 1988;18(2):125-130.

2739 Hermann K, Le Roux A, Fiddes FS. Death from apiol used as abortifacient. *Lancet*. 1956 Jun 16;270(6929):937-9.

2740 Lowenstein L, Ballew DH. Fatal acute hemolytic anemia, thrombocytopenic purpura, nephrosis and hepatitis resulting from ingestion of a constituent containing apiol. *Can Med Assoc J*. 1958 Feb 1;78(3):195-8.

2741 Basso U. [Study of death caused by apiol and experimental study of its toxic action]. *Arch Patol Clin Med*. 1957;34(4):308-22.

2742 Mumolo M. [On a case of acute and fatal poisoning caused by apiol]. *Recenti Prog Med*. 1964 Feb;36:139-51.

2743 Barni B, Barni I. [The apiol poisoning]. Rassegna casistica. 1967;3(2):197-221.

2744 D'Aprile F. [Clinical study-Experimental apiol poisoning]. *Annali di Ostetricia Ginecologia*. 1928;50:1204-27.

2745 Ciganda C, Laborde A. Herbal infusions used for induced abortion. *J Toxicol Clin Toxicol*. 2003;41:235-239.

2746 Hermann K, Le Roux A, Fiddes FS. Death from apiol used as abortifacient. *Lancet*. 1956 Jun 16;270(6929):937-9.

2747 Lowenstein L, Ballew DH. Fatal acute hemolytic anemia, thrombocytopenic purpura, nephrosis and hepatitis resulting from ingestion of a constituent containing apiol. *Can Med Assoc J*. 1958 Feb 1;78(3):195-8.

2748 Basso U. [Study of death caused by apiol and experimental study of its toxic action]. *Arch Patol Clin Med*. 1957;34(4):308-22.

2749 Mumolo M. [On a case of acute and fatal poisoning caused by apiol]. *Recenti Prog Med*. 1964 Feb;36:139-51.

2750 Barni B, Barni I. [The apiol poisoning]. Rassegna casistica. 1967;3(2):197-221.

2751 D'Aprile F. [Clinical study-Experimental apiol poisoning]. *Annali di Ostetricia Ginecologia*. 1928;50:1204-27.

2752 Souza FV, da Rocha MB, de Souza DP, et al. (-)-Carvone: antispasmodic effect and mode of action. *Fitoterapia*. 2013 Mar;85:20-24.

2753 Rajeshwari T, Raja B. Antihypertensive, antihyperlipidemicand antioxidantinfluence of D-carvone in L-NAME induced hypertensive rats. *Int J Pharmaceutical Biol Arch*. 2014;5(4):82-88.

2754 Lowenstein L, Ballew DH. Fatal acute hemolytic ahemia, thrombocytopenic purpura, nephrosis and hepatitis resulting from ingestion of a constituent containing apiol. *Can Med Assoc J*. 1958 Feb 1;78(3):195-8.

2755 Basso U. [Study of death caused by apiol and experimental study of its toxic action]. *Arch Patol Clin Med*. 1957;34(4):308-22.

2756 Barni B, Barni I. [The apiol poisoning]. Rassegna casistica. 1967;3(2):197-221.

2757 Newall CA, Anderson LA, Philpson JD. Herbal Medicine: A Guide for Healthcare Professionals. London, UK: The Pharmaceutical Press, 1996.

2758 Colalillo R. Apiol poisoning in 7 women and 2 children. *Rivista di Tossicologia Sperimentale e Clinica*. 1988;18(2):125-130.

2759 Ene AC, Nwankwo EA, Samdi LM. Alloxan-induced diabetes in rats and the effects of black caraway (Carum carvi L.) oil on their body weight. *Res J Med Med Sci*. 2007;2:48–52.

2760 Eddouks M, Lemhadri A, Michel JB. Caraway and caper: potential anti-hyperglycaemic plants in diabetic rats. *J Ethnopharmacol*. 2004;94:143–8.

2761 Essway GS, Sobbhy HM, El-Banna HA. The hypoglycaemic effect of volatile oils of some Egyptian plants. Veterinary Medical Journal. 1995;43(2):167-72.

2762 Muruganathan U, Srinivasan S, Indumathi D. Antihyperglycemic effect of carvone: Effect on the levels of glycoprotein components in streptozotocin-induced diabetic rats. *J Acute Disease*. 2013;2(4):310-15.

2763 de Sousa DP, Farias Nobrega FF, de Almeida RN. Influence of the chirality of (R)-(-)- and (S)-(+)-carvone in the central nervous system: a comparative study. *Chirality*. 2007 May;19(4):264-268.

2764 Orhan I, Kartal M, Kan Y, et al. Activity of essential oils and individual components against acetyl- and butyrylcholinesterase. *Z Naturforsch C*. 2008 Jul-Aug;63(7-8):547-53.

2765 Kazemi M. Phenolic profile, antioxidant capacity and anti-inflammatory activity of Anethum graveolens L. essential oil. *Nat Prod Res*. 2015;29(6):551-3.

2766 Sousa RM, Rosa JS, Oliveira L, et al. Activities of Apiaceae essential oils against armyworm, Pseudaletia unipuncta (Lepidoptera: Noctuidae). *J Agric Food Chem*. 2013 Aug 14;61(32):7661-72.

2767 Song JE, Kim JM, Lee NH, et al. Acaricidal and Insecticidal Activities of Essential Oils against a Stored-Food Mite and Stored-Grain Insects. *J Food Prot*. 2016 Jan;79(1):174-8.

2768 Seo SM, Jung CS, Kang J, et al. Larvicidal and acetylcholinesterase inhibitory activities of apiaceae plant essential oils and their constituents against aedes albopictus and formulation development. *J Agric Food Chem*. 2015 Nov 18;63(45):9977-86.

2769 Yeom HJ, Kang JS, Kim GH, et al. Insecticidal and acetylcholine esterase inhibition activity of Apiaceae plant essential oils and their constituents against adults of German cockroach (Blattella germanica). *J Agric Food Chem*. 2012 Jul 25;60(29):7194-203.

2770 Chaubey MK. Fumigant toxicity of essential oils from some common spices against pulse beetle, Callosobruchus chinensis (Coleoptera: Bruchidae). *J Oleo Sci*. 2008;57(3):171-9.

2771 Mazyad SA, El-Serougi AO, Morsy TA. The efficacy of the volatile oils of three plants for controlling Lucilia sericata. *J Egypt Soc Parasitol*. 1999;29(1):91-100.

2772 Choochote W, Chaithong U, Kamsuk K, et al. Repellent activity of selected essential oils against Aedes aegypti. *Fitoterapia*. 2007 Jul;78(5):359-64.

2773 Chen Y, Zeng H, Tian J, et al. Dill (Anethum graveolens L.) seed essential oil induces Candida albicans apoptosis in a metacaspase-dependent manner. *Fungal Biol*. 2014 Apr;118(4):394-401.

2774 Anghel I, Holban AM, Andronescu E, et al. Efficient surface functionalization of wound dressings by a phytoactive nanocoating refractory to Candida albicans biofilm development. *Biointerphases*. 2013 Dec;8(1):12.

2775 Chen Y, Zeng H, Tian J, et al. Antifungal mechanism of essential oil from Anethum graveolens seeds against Candida albicans. *J Med Microbiol*. 2013 Aug;62(Pt 8):1175-83.

2776 Tian J, Ban X, Zeng H, et al. The mechanism of antifungal action of essential oil from dill (Anethum graveolens L.) on Aspergillus flavus. *PLoS One*. 2012;7(1):e30147.

2777 Jirovetz L, Buchbauer G, Stoyanova AS, et al. Composition, quality control, and antimicrobial activity of the essential oil of long-time stored dill (Anethum graveolens L.) seeds from Bulgaria. *J Agric Food Chem*. 2003 Jun 18;51(13):3854-7.

2778 Kumar P, Mishra S, Kumar A, et al. Antifungal efficacy of plant essential oils against stored grain fungi of Fusarium spp. *J Food Sci Technol*. 2016 Oct;53(10):3725-3734.

2779 Zeng H, Tian J, Zheng Y, et al. In Vitro and In Vivo Activities of Essential Oil from the Seed of Anethum graveolens L. against Candida spp. *Evid Based Complement Alternat Med*. 2011;2011:659704.

2780 Takahashi N, Yao L, Kim M, et al. Dill seed extract improves abnormalities in lipid metabolism through peroxisome proliferator-activated receptor-α (PPAR-α) activation in diabetic obese mice. *Mol Nutr Food Res*. 2013 Jul;57(7):1295-9.

2781 Hajhashemi V, Abbasi N. Hypolipidemic activity of Anethum graveolens in rats. *Phytother Res*. 2008 Mar;22(3):372-5.

2782 Jana S, Shekhawat. Anethum graveolens: An Indian traditional medicinal herb and spice. *Pharmacogn Rev*. 2010 Jul;4(8):179-84.

2783 Orhan I, Kartal M, Kan Y, et al. Activity of essential oils and individual components against acetyl- and butyrylcholinesterase. *Z Naturforsch C*. 2008 Jul-Aug;63(7-8):547-53.

2784 Darvesh S, Hopkins DA, Geula C. Neurobiology of butyrylcholinesterase. *Nat Rev Neurosci*. 2003 Feb;4:131-38.

2785 Lee HR, Kim GH, Choi WS, et al. Repellent Activity of Apiaceae Plant Essential Oils and their Constituents Against Adult German Cockroaches. *J Econ Entomol*. 2017 Apr 1;110(2):552-557.

2786 Osanloo M, Sereshti H, Sedaghat MM, et al. Nanoemulsion of Dill essential oil as a green and potent larvicide against Anopheles stephensi. *Environ Sci Pollut Res Int*. 2018 Mar;25(7):6466-6473.

2787 Mutlu-Ingok A, Karbancioglu-Guler F. Cardamom, Cumin, and Dill Weed Essential Oils: Chemical Compositions, Antimicrobial Activities, and Mechanisms of Action against Campylobacter spp. *Molecules*. 2017 Jul 15;22(7).

2788 Bartoňková I, Dvořák Z. Essential oils of culinary herbs and spices display agonist and antagonist activities at human aryl hydrocarbon receptor AhR. *Food Chem Toxicol*. 2018 Jan;111:374-384.

2789 Vieira JN, Gonçalves CL, Villarreal JPV, et al. Chemical composition of essential oils from the apiaceae family, cytotoxicity, and their antifungal activity in vitro against candida species from oral cavity. *Braz J Biol*. 2019 Jul-Sep;79(3):432-437.

2790 Manzuoerh R, Farahpour MR, Oryan A, et al. Effectiveness of topical administration of Anethum graveolens essential oil on MRSA-infected wounds. *Biomed Pharmacother*. 2019 Jan;109:1650-1658.

2791 Kaur N, Chahal KK, Kumar A, et al. Antioxidant activity of Anethum graveolens L. essential oil constituents and their chemical analogues. *J Food Biochem*. 2019 Apr;43(4):e12782.

2792 Fazel N, Pejhan A, Taghizadeh M, et al. Effects of Anethum graveolens L. (Dill) essential oil on the intensity of retained intestinal gas, flatulence and pain after cesarean section: A randomized, double-blind placebo-controlled trial. *J Herbal Med*. 2017 Jun;8:8-13.

2793 Al-Sheddi ES, Al-Zaid NA, Al-Oqail MM, et al. Evaluation of Cytotoxicity, Cell Cycle Arrest and Apoptosis Induced by Anethum graveolens L . Essential Oil in Human Hepatocellular Carcinoma Cell Line. *Saudi Pharm J*. 2019 Nov;27(7):1053-1060.

2794 Rosa JS, Oliveira L, Sousa RMOF, et al. Bioactivity of some Apiaceae essential oils and their constituents against Sitophilus zeamais (Coleoptera: Curculionidae). *Bull Entomol Res*. 2020 Jun;110(3):406-416.

2795 Tavakkol Afshari HS, Homayouni Tabrizi M, Ardalan T, et al. Anethum Graveolens Essential Oil Nanoemulsions (AGEO-NE) as an Exclusive Apoptotic Inducer in Human Lung Adenocarcinoma (A549) Cells. *Nutr Cancer*. 2021 Jul 20:1-9. Online ahead of print.

2796 Ellah NHA, Shaltout AS, El Aziz SMMA, et al. Vaginal suppositories of cumin seeds essential oil for treatment of vaginal candidiasis: Formulation, in vitro, in vivo, and clinical evaluation. *Eur J Pharm Sci*. 2021 Feb 1;157:105602.

2797 Aati HY, Perveen S, Aati S, et al. Headspace solid-phase microextraction method for extracting volatile constituents from the different parts of Saudi Anethum graveolens L. and their antimicrobial activity. *Heliyon*. 2022 Mar 5;8(3):e09051.

2798 Ghasemzadeh S, Messelink GJ, Avila GA, et al. Sublethal impacts of essential plant oils on biochemical and ecological parameters of the predatory mite Amblyseius swirskii. *Front Plant Sci*. 2022 Sep 16;13:923802.

2799 Tesevic V, Milosavljevic S, Vajs V, et al. Chemical composition and antifungal activity of the essential oil of Douglas fir (Pseudosuga menziesii Mirb. Franco) from Serbia. *J Serb Chem Soc*. 2009;74(10):1035-40.

2800 Adams RP. Chemosystematics of Douglas Fir (Pseudotsuga menziesii): Effects of leaf drying on essential oil composition. *Phytologia*. 2012 Apr;94(1):133-38.

2801 Jirovetz L, Puschmann C, Stojanova A, et al. Analysis of the essential oil volatiles of Douglas fir (Pseudotsuga menziesii) from Bulgaria. *Flavour Frag J*. 2000;15(6):434-37.

2802 Tesevic V, Milosavljevic S, Vajs V, et al. Chemical composition and antifungal activity of the essential oil of Douglas fir (Pseudosuga menziesii Mirb. Franco) from Serbia. *J Serb Chem Soc*. 2009;74(10):1035-40.

2803 Mitic ZS, Stojanovic-Radic Z, Cvetkovic VJ, et al. Pseudotsuga menziesii (Pinaceae): Volatile Profiles, Antimicrobial Activity and Toxicological Evaluation of Its Essential Oil. *Chem Biodivers*. 2021 Jul 3. Online ahead of print.

2804 Visan DC, Oprea E, Radulescu V, et al. Original Contributions to the Chemical Composition, Microbicidal, Virulence-Arresting and Antibiotic-Enhancing Activity of Essential Oils from Four Coniferous Species. *Pharmaceuticals (Basel)*. 2021 Nov 13;14(11):1159.

2805 Chung YH, Chen SJ, Lee CL, et al. Relaxing Effects of Breathing Pseudotsuga menziesii and Lavandula angustifolia Essential Oils on Psychophysiological Status in Older Adults. *Int J Environ Res Public Health*. 2022 Nov 18;19(22):15251.

2806 Hajdari A, Mustafa B, Ahmeti G, et al. Essential oil composition variability among natural populations of Pinus mugo Turra in Kosovo. *Springerplus*. 2015;4:828.

2807 Stevanovic T, Garneau FX, Jean FI, et al. The essential oil composition of Pinus mugo Turra from Serbia. *Flavour Frag J*. 2005 Jan-Feb;20(1):96-97.

2808 Bojović S, Jurc M, Ristić M, et al. Essential-Oil Variability in Natural Populations of Pinus mugo Turra from the Julian Alps. *Chem Biodivers*. 2016 Feb;13(2):181-7.

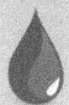

2809 Celiński K, Bonikowski R, Wojnicka-Półtorak A, et al. Volatiles as Chemosystematic Markers for Distinguishing Closely Related Species within the Pinus mugo Complex. *Chem Biodivers.* 2015 Aug;12(8):1208-13.

2810 Aazza S, Lyoussi B, Miguel MG. Antioxidant and antiacetylcholinesterase activities of some commercial essential oils and their major compounds. *Molecules.* 2011 Sep 7;16(9):7672-90.

2811 Miyazawa M, Yamafuji C. Inhibition of acetylcholinesterase activity by bicyclic monoterpenoids. *J Agric Food Chem.* 2005 Mar 9;53(5):1765-8.

2812 Grassmann J, Hippeli S, Vollmann R, et al. Antioxidative properties of the essential oil from Pinus mugo. *J Agric Food Chem.* 2003 Dec 17;51(26):7576-82.

2813 Grassmann J, Hippeli S, Spitzenberger R, et al. The monoterpene terpinolene from the oil of Pinus mugo L. in concert with alpha-tocopherol and beta-carotene effectively prevents oxidation of LDL. *Phytomedicine.* 2005 Jun;12(6-7):416-23.

2814 Kačániová M, Vukovič N, Horská E, et al. Antibacterial activity against Clostridium genus and antiradical activity of the essential oils from different origin. *J Environ Sci Health B.* 2014;49(7):505-12.

2815 Kačániová M, Vukovič N, Horská E, et al. Antibacterial activity against Clostridium genus and antiradical activity of the essential oils from different origin. *J Environ Sci Health B.* 2014;49(7):505-12.

2816 Basholli-Salihu M, Schuster R, Hajdari A, et al. Phytochemical composition, anti-inflammatory activity and cytotoxic effects of essential oils from three Pinus spp. *Pharm Biol.* 2017 Dec;55(1):1553-1560.

2817 Thalappil MA, Butturini E, Carcereri de Prati A, et al. Pinus mugo Essential Oil Impairs STAT3 Activation through Oxidative Stress and Induces Apoptosis in Prostate Cancer Cells. *Molecules.* 2022 Jul 28;27(15):4834.

2818 Basholli-Salihu M, Schuster R, Hajdari A, et al. Phytochemical composition, anti-inflammatory activity and cytotoxic effects of essential oils from three Pinus spp. *Pharm Biol.* 2017 Dec;55(1):1553-1560.

2819 Garzoli S, Lasci VL, Caradonna V, et al. Liquid and Vapor Phase of Four Conifer-Derived Essential Oils: Comparison of Chemical Compositions and Antimicrobial and Antioxidant Properties. *Pharmaceuticals (Basel).* 2021 Feb 8;14(2):134.

2820 Stojanović-Radić Z, Čomić LJ, Radulović N, et al. Antistaphylococcal activity of Inula helenium L. root essential oil: eudesmane sesquiterpene lactones induce cell membrane damage. *Eur J Clin Microbiol Infect Dis.* 2012;31:1015-25.

2821 Bourrel C, Vilarem G, Perineau F. Chemical Analysis, Bacteriostatic and Fungistatic Properties of the Essential Oil of Elecampane (Inula helenium L.). *J Essent Oil Res.* 1993 Jul-Aug;5:411-17.

2822 Deriu A, Zanetti S, Sechi LA, et al. Antimicrobial activity of Inula helenium L. essential oil against Gram-positive and Gram-negative bacteria and Candida spp. *Int J Antimicrob Agents.* 2008 Jun;31(6):588-90.

2823 Opdyke DIJ. Monographs on fragrance raw materials. *Food Cosmet Toxicol.* 1976;14(Suppl):307-08. *Int J Antimicrob Agents.* 2008 Jun;31(6):588-90.

2824 Qin CZ, Lv QL, Wu NY, et al. Mechanism-based inhibition of Alantolactone on human cytochrome P450 3A4 in vitro and activity of hepatic cytochrome P450 in mice. *J Ethnopharmacol.* 2015 Jun 20;168:146-9.

2825 Chapman DE, Holbrook DJ, Chaney SG, et al. In vitro inhibition of mouse hepatic mixed-function oxidase enzymes by helenalin and alantolactone. *Biochem Pharmacol.* 1989 Nov 15;38(22):3913-23.

2826 Stojanović-Radić Z, Čomić LJ, Radulović N, et al. Antistaphylococcal activity of Inula helenium L. root essential oil: eudesmane sesquiterpene lactones induce cell membrane damage. *Eur J Clin Microbiol Infect Dis.* 2012;31:1015-25.

2827 Bourrel C, Vilarem G, Perineau F. Chemical Analysis, Bacteriostatic and Fungistatic Properties of the Essential Oil of Elecampane (Inula helenium L.). *J Essent Oil Res.* 1993 Jul-Aug;5:411-17.

2828 Deriu A, Zanetti S, Sechi LA, et al. Antimicrobial activity of Inula helenium L. essential oil against Gram-positive and Gram-negative bacteria and Candida spp. *Int J Antimicrob Agents.* 2008 Jun;31(6):588-90.

2829 Bourrel C, Vilarem G, Perineau F. Chemical Analysis, Bacteriostatic and Fungistatic Properties of the Essential Oil of Elecampane (Inula helenium L.). *J Essent Oil Res.* 1993 Jul-Aug;5:411-17.

2830 Deriu A, Zanetti S, Sechi LA, et al. Antimicrobial activity of Inula helenium L. essential oil against Gram-positive and Gram-negative bacteria and Candida spp. *Int J Antimicrob Agents.* 2008 Jun;31(6):588-90.

2831 Rasul A, Khan M, Ali M, et al. Targeting Apoptosis Pathways in Cancer with Alantolactone and Isoalantolactone. *Sci World J.* 2013;(2013):248532.

2832 Villanueva MA, Torres RC. The composition of Manila elemi oil. *Flavour Frag J.* 1993;8:35–37.

2833 Yang H, Jung EM, Ahn C, et al. Elemol from Chamaecyparis obtusa ameliorates 2,4-dinitrochlorobenzene-induced atopic dermatitis. *Int J Mol Med.* 2015 Aug;36(2):463-72.

2834 Servi H, Demir U, Servi EY, et al. Antiproliferative and Antibacterial Activities of Four Commercial Essential Oil Samples from Boswellia carteri, B. serrata, and two chemotypes of Canarium luzonicum. *J Essent Oil Bearing Plants.* 2023. Online ahead of print.

2835 Mardarowicz M, Wianowska D, Dawidowicz AL, et al. Comparison of terpene composition in Engelmann spruce (Picea engelmannii) using hydrodistillation, SPME and PLE. *Z Naturforsch C.* 2004 Sep-Oct;59(9-10):641-8.

2836 Wagner MR, Clancy KM, Tinus RW. Maturational variation in needle essential oils from Pseudotsuga menziesii, Abies concolor and Picea englemannii. *Phytochemistry.* 1989;28(3):765-70.

2837 Stillpoint Aromatics. Engelmann Spruce Essential Oil. Available at: www.stillpointaromatics.com/engelmann-spruce-Picea-engelmannii-essential-oil-aromatherapy.

2838 Aromatics International. Engelmann Spruce. Available at: https://www.aromatics.com/products/essential-oils/engelman-spruce.

2839 Burkhard PR, Burkhardt K, Haenggeli CA, et al. Plant-induced seizures: reappearance of an old problem. *J Neurol.* 1999 Aug;246(8):667-70.

2840 Narayan S, Singh N. Camphor poisoning-An unusual cause of seizure. *Med J Armed Forces India.* 2012 Jul;68(3):252-53.

2841 Chanaranaj KJ, G MV, S M. Camphor poisoning in a child. *Natl Med J India.* 2013 Jan-Feb;26(1):60.

2842 Olowe SA, Ransome-Kuti O. The risk of jaundice in glucose-6-phosphate dehydrogenase deficient babies exposed to menthol. *Acta Paediatr Scand.* 1980 May;69(3):341-5.

2843 Dillon Remy M, Manning Alleyne P, Bratt DE, et al. Neonatal jaundice at Port-of-Spain General Hospital abstract. *West Indian Med J.* 1987;36(Suppl):28.

2844 Kumar P, Mishra S, Malik A, et al. Compositional analysis and insecticidal activity of Eucalyptus globulus (family: Myrtaceae) essential oil against housefly (Musca domestica). *Acta Trop.* 2012 May;122(2):212-18.

2845 Ait-Ouazzou A, Loran S, Bakkali M, et al. Chemical composition and antimicrobial activity of essential oils for Thymus algeriensis, Eucalyptus globulus and Rosmarinus officinalis from Morocco. *J Sci Food Agric.* 2011 Nov;91(14):2643-51.

2846 Song A, Wang Y, Liu Y. Study on the chemical constituents of the essential oil of the leaves of Eucalyptus globulus Labill from China. *Traditional Med.* 2009;4(4):134-40.

2847 Maciel MV, Morais SM, Bevilaqua CML, et al. Chemical composition of Eucalyptus spp. essential oils and their insecticidal effects of Lutzomyia longipalpis. *Vet Parasitol.* 2010;167:1-10.

2848 Singh AK. Chemical composition of the leaf oil of Eucalyptus radiata Sieb, ex DC subsp. Robertsonii (Blakely) L. Johnson et D. Blaxell: A rich source of Eucalyptus oil of Pharmacopoeia grade. *J Essential Oil Res.* 1994;6(6):657-59.

2849 Bendaoud H, Bouajila J, Rhouma A, et al. GC/MS analysis and antimicrobial and antioxidant activities of essential oil of Eucalyptus radiata. *J Sci Food Agric.* 2009 Jun;89(8):1292-97.

2850 Bignell AM, Dunlop PJ, Brophy JJ, et al. Volatile leaf oils of some South-western and Southern Australian species of the Genus Eucalyptus (Series 1). Part XIII. (a) Series Subulatae, (b) Series Curviptera, (c) Series Contorae, (d) Series Incognitae, (e) Series Terminaliptera, (f) Series Inclusae, (g) Series Microcorythae and (h) Series Cornutae. *Flav Frag J.* 1996 Nov-Dec;11(6):339-47.

2851 Derwich E, Benziane Z, Boukir A. GC/MS analysis of volatile constituents and antimicrobial activity of the essential oil of the leaves of Eucalyptus radiata in Atlas Median from Morocco. *Adv Nat Appl Sci.* 2009;3(3):305-13.

2852 Craig JO. Poisoning by the volatile oils in childhood. *Arch Dis Child.* 1953;28:259-67.

2853 Melis K. Bochner A, Janssens G. Accidental nasal eucalyptol and menthol instillation. *Eur J Pediatr.* 1989 Aug;148(8)786-7.

2854 Day LM, Ozanne-Smith J, Parsons BJ, et al. Eucalyptus oil poisoning among young children: mechanisms of access and the potential prevention. *Aust N Z J Public Health.* 1997 Jun;21(3):297-302.

2855 Chandar SD, Prashanti M, Kumar CL, et al. Eucalyptus Oil-Induced Seizures in Children: A Single-Center Prospective Study. *Cureus.* 2021 Mar 25;13(3):e14109.

2856 Burkhard PR, Burkhardt K, Haenggeli CA, et al. Plant-induced seizures: reappearance of an old problem. *J Neurol.* 1999 Aug;246(8):667-70.

2857 Waldman N. Seizure caused by dermal application of over-the-counter eucalyptus oil head lice preparation. *Clin Toxicol (Phila).* 2011 Oct;49(8):750-1.

2858 Craig JO. Poisoning by the volatile oils in childhood. *Arch Dis Child.* 1953;28:259-67.

2859 Mathew T, Kamath V, Kumar RS, et al. Eucalyptus oil inhalation–induced seizure: A novel, underrecognized, preventable cause of acute symptomatic seizure. *Epilepsia Open.* 2017 Jul;2(3):350-4.

2860 Newall CA, Anderson LA, Phillipson JD. "Herbal Medicines: A Guide for Health-care Professionals." London: The Pharmaceutical Press, 1996, 108.

2861 European Medicines Agency. Community herbal monograph on Eucalyptus globulus Labill., Eucalyptus polybractea R.T. Baker and/or Eucalyptus smithii R.T. Baker, aetheroleum. 2013 Jun. Available at: http://www.ema.europa.eu/docs/en_GB/document_library/Herbal_-_Community_herbal_monograph/2013/07/WC500147008.pdf

2862 Fischer JH, Dethlefsen U. Efficacy of cineole in patients suffering from acute bronchitis: a placebo-controlled double-blind trial. *Cough.* 2013; 9: 25.

2863 Worth W, Dethlefsen U. Patients with asthma benefit from concomitant therapy with cineole: a placebo-controlled, double-blind trial. *J Asthma.* 2012 Oct;49(8):849-53.

2864 Day LM, Ozanne-Smith J, Parsons BJ, et al. Eucalyptus oil poisoning among young children: mechanisms of access and the potential prevention. *Aust N Z J Public Health.* 1997 Jun;21(3):297-302.

2865 Myott E. Case of eucalyptus poisoning. *Brit M J.* 1906;1:558.

2866 Hindle RC. Eucalyptus oil ingestion. *N Z Med J.* 1994 May 11;107(977)185-6.

2867 Tibballs J. Clinical effects and management of eucalyptus oil ingestion in infants and small children. *Med J Aust.* 1995 Aug;163(4):177-80.

2868 Waldman W, Barwina M, Sein Anand J. Accidental ontoxication with eucalyptus oil—a case report. *Przegl Lek.* 2011;68(8):555-6.

2869 Day LM, Ozanne-Smith J, Parsons BJ, et al. Eucalyptus oil poisoning among young children: mechanisms of access and the potential prevention. *Aust N Z J Public Health.* 1997 Jun;21(3):297-302.

[2870] De Vincenzi M, Silano M, De Vincenzi A, et al. Constituents of aromatic plants: eucalyptol. *Fitoterapia.* 2002 Jun;73(3):269-75.
[2871] Unger M, Frank A. Simultaneous determination of the inhibitory potency of herbal extracts on the activity of six major cytochrome P450 enzymes using liquid chromatography/mass spectrometry and automated online extraction. *Rapid Commun Mass Spectrom.* 2004;18(19):2273-81.
[2872] Jori A, Bianchetti A, Prestini PE, et al. Effect of eucalyptol (1,8-cineole) on the metabolism of other drugs in rats and in man. *Eur J Pharmacol.* 1970;9(3):362-66.
[2873] Kim NH, Hyun SH, Jin CH, et al. Pretreatment with 1,8-cineole potentiates thioacetamide-induced hepatotoxicity and immunosuppression. *Arch Pharm Res.* 2004 Jul;27(7):781-9.
[2874] Gray AM, Flatt PR. Antihyperglycemic actions of Eucalyptus globulus (Eucalyptus) are associated with pancreatic and extra pancreatic effects in mice. *J Nutr.* 1998 Dec;128(12):2319–23.
[2875] Basak SS, Candan F. Effect of Laurus nobilis L. Essential Oil and its Main Components on α-glucosidase and Reactive Oxygen Species Scavenging Activity. *Iran J Pharm Res.* 2013 Spring;12(2):367-79.
[2876] Fathiazad F, Mazandarani M, Hamedeyazdan. Phytochemical analysis and antioxidant activity of Hyssopus officinalis L. from Iran. *Adv Pharm Bull.* 2011 Dec;1(2):63–67.
[2877] Gray AM, Flatt PR. Antihyperglycemic actions of Eucalyptus globulus (Eucalyptus) are associated with pancreatic and extra pancreatic effects in mice. *J Nutr.* 1998 Dec;128(12):2319-23.
[2878] Tsai HH, Lin HW, Chen YL, et al. A review of potential harmful interactions between anticoagulant/antiplatelet agents and Chinese herbal medicines. *PLoS One.* 2013 May 9;8(5):e64255.
[2879] Moharam BA, Jantan I, bin Ahmad F, et al. Antiplatelet Aggregation and Platelet Activating Factor (PAF) Receptor Antagonistic Activities of the Essential Oils of Five Goniothalamus Species. *Molecules.* 2010;15:5124-38.
[2880] Hendry ER, Worthington T, Conway BR, et al. Antimicrobial efficacy of eucalyptus oil and 1,8-cineole alone and in combination with chlorhexidine digluconate against microorganisms grown in planktonic and biofilm cultures. *J Antimicrob Chemother.* 2009;64(6):1219-25.
[2881] Kifer D, Muzinic V, Segvic Klaric S. Antimicrobial potency of single and combined mupirocin and monoterpenes, thymol, menthol and 1,8-cineole against Staphylococcus aureus planktonic and biofilm growth. *J Antibiotics (Tokyo).* 2016 Sep;69(9):689-96.
[2882] Pereira V, Dias C, Vasconcelos MC, et al. Antibacterial activity and synergistic effects between Eucalyptus globulus leaf residues (essential oils and extracts) and antibiotics against several isolates of respiratory tract infections (Pseudomonas aeruginosa). *Industrial Crops Prod.* 2014 Jan;52:1-7.
[2883] Hendry ER, Worthinton T, Conway BR, et al. Antimicrobial efficacy of eucalyptus oil and 1,8-cineole alone and in combination with chlorhexidine digluconate against microorganisms grown in planktonic and biofilm cultures. *J Antimicrob Chemother.* 2009;64(6):1219-25.
[2884] Jori A, Bianchetti A, Prestini PE, et al. Effect of eucalyptol (1,8-cineole) on the metabolism of other drugs in rats and in man. *Eur J Pharmacol.* 1970;9(3):362-66.
[2885] de Sousa DP, Raphael E, Brocksom U, et al. Sedative effect of monoterpene alcohols in mice: A preliminary screening. *Verlag der Zeitschrift fur Naturforschung.* 2007;62c:563-66.
[2886] Carnesecchi S, Bras-Gonçalves R, Bradaia A, et al. Geraniol, a component of plant essential oils, modulates DNA synthesis and potentiates 5-fluorouracil efficacy on human colon tumor xenografts. *Cancer Lett.* 2004 Nov 8;215(1):53-9.
[2887] Juergens JR. Anti-inflammatory properties of the monoterpene 1,8-cineole: Current evidence for co-medication in inflammatory airway diseases. *Drug Res (Stuttg).*2014 Dec;64(12):638-46.
[2888] Bachir RG, Benali M. Antibacterial activity of the essential oils from the leaves of Eucalyptus radiata against Escherichia coli and Staphylococcus aureus. *Asian Pac J Trop Biomed.* 2012 Sep;2(9):739-42.
[2889] Tohidpour A, Sattari M, Omidbaigi R, et al. Antibacterial effect of essential oils from two medicinal plants against Methicillin-resistant Staphylococcus aureus (MRSA). *Phytomedicine.* 2010 Feb;17(2):142-45.
[2890] Mayaud L, Carricajo A, Zhiri A, et al. Comparison of bacteriostatic and bactericidal activity of 13 essential oils against strains with varying sensitivity to antibiotics. *Lett Appl Microbiol.* 2008 Sep;47(3):167-73.
[2891] Toloza AC, Lucia A, Zerba E, et al. Eucalyptus essential oil toxicity against permethrin-resistant Pediculus humanus capitis (Phthiraptera: Pediculidae). *Parisatol Res.* 2010 Jan;106(2):409-14.
[2892] Yones DA, Bakir HY, Bayoumi SA, et al. Chemical composition and efficacy of some selected plant oils against Pediculus humanus capitis in vitro. *Parasitol Res.* 2016 Aug;115(8):3209-18.
[2893] Avello M, Fernández P, Fernández M, et al. [Pediculicide effect of a Eucaliptus globulus L formulation]. *Rev Chilena Infectol.* 2016 Aug;33(4):433-437.
[2894] Sherry E, Boeck H, Warnke PH. Percutaneous treatment of chronic MRSA osteomyelitis with a novel plant-derived antiseptic. *BMC Surgery.* 2001;1:1.
[2895] Ben-Arye E, Dudai N, Eini A, et al. Treatment of upper respiratory tract infections in primary care: A randomized study using aromatic herbs. *Evid-Based Complement Altern Med.* 2011;2011:690346.
[2896] Kako H, Fukumoto S, Kobayashi Y, et al. Effects of direct exposure of green odour components on dopamine release from rat brain striatal slices and PC12 cells. *Brain Res Bull.* 2008 Mar;75(5):706-12.
[2897] Cermelli C, Fabio A, Fabio G, et al. Effect of eucalyptus essential oil on respiratory bacteria and viruses. *Curr Microbiol.* 2008 Jan;56(1):89-92.
[2898] Salari MH, Amine G, Shirazi MH, et al. Antibacterial effects of Eucalyptus globulus leaf extract on pathogenic bacteria isolated from specimens of patients with respiratory tract disorders. *Clin Microbiol Infect.* 2006 Feb;12(2):194- 96.
[2899] Ghaffar A, Yameen M, Kiran S, et al. Chemical Composition and in-Vitro Evaluation of the Antimicrobial and Antioxidant Activities of Essential Oils Extracted from Seven Eucalyptus Species. *Molecules.* 2015 Nov 18;20(11):20487-98.
[2900] Hammad H, Chieppa M, Perros F, et al. House dust mite allergen induces asthmas via Toll-like receptor 4 triggering of airway structural cells. *Nat Med.*2009 Apr;15(4):410-16.
[2901] Lu XQ, Tang FD, Wang Y, et al. Effect of Eucalyptus globulus oil on lipopolysaccharide-induced chronic bronchitis and mucin hypersecretion in rats. *Zhonggou Zhong Yao ZA Zhi.* 2004 Feb;29(2):168-71.
[2902] Kim MJ, Nam ES, Paik SI. The effects of aromatherapy in pain, depression, and life satisfaction of arthritis patients. *Taehan Kanho Hakhoe Chi.* 2005 Feb;35(1):186-94.
[2903] Silva J, Abebe W, Sousa SM, et al. Analgesic and anti-inflammatory effects of essential oils of eucalyptus. *J Ethnopharmacol.* 2003 Dec;89(2-3):277-83.
[2904] Ait-Ouazzou A, Loran S, Bakkali M, et al. Chemical composition and antimicrobial activity of essential oils of Thymus algeriensis, Eucalyptus globulus and Rosmarinus officinalis from Morocco. *J Sci Food Agric.* 2011 Nov;91(14):2643-51.
[2905] Bansod S, Rai M. Antifungal activity of essential oils from Indian medicinal plants against human pathogenic Aspergillus fumigatus and A. niger. *World J Med Sci.* 2008;3(2):81-88.
[2906] Perczak A, Juś K, Marchwińska K, et al. Degradation of Zearalenone by Essential Oils under In vitro Conditions. *Front Microbiol.* 2016 Aug 11;7:1224.
[2907] Turcotte JC, Hunt PJB, Blaustein JD. Estrogenic effects of zearalenone on the expression of progestin receptors and sexual behavior in female rats. *Hormones and Behavior.* 2005;47:178-84.
[2908] Takemura H, Shim JY, Sayama K, et al. Characterization of the estrogenic activities of zearalenone and zeranol in vivo and in vitro. *J Steroid Biochem Mol Biol.* 2007 Feb;103(2):170-7.
[2909] Frizzell C, Ndossi D, Verhaegen S, et al. Endocrine disrupting effects of zearalenone, alpha- and beta-zearalenol at the level of nuclear receptor binding and steroidogenesis. *Toxicol Lett.* 2011 Oct 10;206(2):210-7.
[2910] Vigo E, Cepeda A, Gualillo O, et al. In-vitro anti-inflammatory effect of Eucalyptus globulus and Thymus vulgaris: nitric oxide inhibition in J774A.1 murine macrophages. *J Pharm Pharmacol.* 2004 Feb;56(2):257-63.
[2911] Sharma JN, AL-Omran A, Parvathy SS. Role of nitric oxide in inflammatory diseases. *Inflammopharmacology.* 2007 Dec;15(6):252-59.
[2912] Gobel H, Schmidt G, Dworschak M, et al. Essential plant oils and headache mechanism. *Phytomedicine.* 1995 Oct;2(2):93-12.
[2913] Kaur CD, Saraf S. In vitro sun protection factor determination of herbal oils used in cosmetics. *Pharmacognosy Res.* 2010 Jan;2(1):22-25.
[2914] Plant J. Effects of essential oils on telomere length in human cells. *Med Aromat Plants.* 2016;5(2):1-6.
[2915] Fang F, Candy K, Melloul E, et al. In vitro activity of ten essential oils against Sarcoptes scabiei. *Parasit Vectors.* 2016 Nov 22;9(1):594.
[2916] Sharififard M, Safdari F, Siahpoush A, et al. Evaluation of Some Plant Essential Oils against the Brown-Banded Cockroach, Supella longipalpa (Blattaria: Ectobiidae): A Mechanical Vector of Human Pathogens. *J Arthropod Borne Dis.* 2016 Oct 4;10(4):528-537.
[2917] Lalthazuali, Mathew N. Mosquito repellent activity of volatile oils from selected aromatic plants. *Parasitol Res.* 2017 Feb;116(2):821-825.
[2918] Vieira M, Bessa LJ, Martins MR, et al. Chemical Composition, Antibacterial, Antibiofilm and Synergistic Properties of Essential Oils from Eucalyptus globulus Labill. and Seven Mediterranean Aromatic Plants. *Chem Biodivers.* 2017 Jun;14(6).
[2919] Saporito F, Sandri G, Bonferoni MC, et al. Essential oil-loaded lipid nanoparticles for wound healing. *Int J Nanomedicine.* 2017 Dec 27;13:175-186.
[2920] Yadav M, Jindal DK, Parle M, et al. Targeting oxidative stress, acetylcholinesterase, proinflammatory cytokine, dopamine and GABA by eucalyptus oil (Eucalyptus globulus) to alleviate ketamine-induced psychosis in rats. *Inflammopharmacology.* 2019 Apr;27(2):301-311.
[2921] Sharafati Chaleshtori F, Saholi M, Sharafati Chaleshtori R. Chemical Composition, Antioxidant and Antibacterial Activity of Bunium persicum, Eucalyptus globulus, and Rose Water on Multidrug-Resistant Listeria Species. *J Evid Based Integr Med.* 2018 Jan-Dec;23:2515690X17751314.
[2922] Ambrosio CMS, De Alencar SM, Moreno AM, et al. Evaluation of the selective antibacterial activity of Eucalyptus globulus and Pimenta pseudocaryophyllus essential oils individually and in combination on Enterococcus faecalis and Lactobacillus rhamnosus. *Can J Microbiol.* 2018 Nov;64(11):844-855.
[2923] Alam P, Shakeel F, Anwer MK, et al. Wound Healing Study of Eucalyptus Essential Oil Containing Nanoemulsion in Rat Model. *J Oleo Sci.* 2018 Aug 1;67(8):957-968.
[2924] Quatrin PM, Verdi CM, de Souza ME, et al. Antimicrobial and antibiofilm activities of nanoemulsions containing Eucalyptus globulus oil against Pseudomonas aeruginosa and Candida spp. *Microb Pathog.* 2017 Nov;112:230-242.
[2925] Clavijo-Romero A, Quintanilla-Carvajal MX, Ruiz Y, et al. Stability and antimicrobial activity of eucalyptus essential oil emulsions. *Food Sci Technol Int.* 2019 Jan;25(1):24-37.
[2926] Galli GM, Roza LF, Santos RCV, et al. Low Dose of Nanocapsules Containing Eucalyptus Oil Has Beneficial Repellent Effect Against Horn Fly (Diptera: Muscidae). *J Econ Entomol.* 2018 Sep 20.
[2927] Elzayyat E, Elleboudy N, Moustafa A, et al. Insecticidal, Oxidative, and Genotoxic Activities of Syzygium aromaticum and Eucalyptus globulus on Culex pipiens Adults and Larvae. *Turkiye Parazitol Derg.* 2018 Sep;42(3):213-222.
[2928] Lin TC, Wang SH, Huang CC, et al. Anti-Fatigue, Antioxidation, and Anti-Inflammatory Effects of Eucalyptus Oil Aromatherapy in Swimming-Exercised Rats. *Chin J Physiol.* 2018 Oct 31;61(5):257-265.
[2929] Aldoghaim FS, Flematti GR, Hammer KA, et al. Antimicrobial Activity of Several Cineole-Rich Western Australian Eucalyptus Essential Oils. *Microorganisms.* 2018 Dec 3;6(4).
[2930] Vivekanandhan P, Usha-Raja-Nanthini A, Valli G, et al. Comparative efficacy of Eucalyptus globulus (Labill) hydrodistilled essential oil and temephos as mosquito larvicide. *Nat Prod Res.* 2019 Jan 9:1-4.
[2931] Muchembled J, Deweer C, Sahmer K, et al. Gene expression responses of Listeria monocytogenes Scott A exposed to sub-lethal concentrations of natural antimicrobials. *Environ Sci Pollut Res Int.* 2018 Oct;25(30):29921-29928.

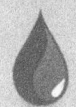

[2932] Madreseh-Ghahfarokhi S, Pirali Y, Dehghani-Samani A, et al. The insecticidal and repellent activity of ginger (Zingiber officinale) and eucalyptus (Eucalyptus globulus) essential oils against Culex theileri Theobald, 1903 (Diptera: Culicidae). *Ann Parasitol.* 2018;64(4):351-360.
[2933] Moazeni M, Hosseini SV, Al-Qanbar MH, et al. In vitro evaluation of the protoscolicidal effect of Eucalyptus globulus essential oil on protoscolices of hydatid cyst compared with hypertonic saline, povidone iodine and silver nitrate. *J Visc Surg.* 2019 Sep;156(4):291-295.
[2934] Lee G, Park J, Kim MS, et al. Analgesic effects of eucalyptus essential oil in mice. *Korean J Pain.* 2019 Apr 1;32(2):79-86.
[2935] Kaura T, Mewara A, Zaman K, et al. Utilizing larvicidal and pupicidal efficacy of Eucalyptus and neem oil against Aedes mosquito: An approach for mosquito control. *Trop Parasitol.* 2019 Jan-Jun;9(1):12-17.
[2936] Djebir S, Ksouri S, Trigui M, et al. Chemical Composition and Acaricidal Activity of the Essential Oils of Some Plant Species of Lamiaceae and Myrtaceae against the Vector of Tropical Bovine Theileriosis: Hyalomma scupense (syn. Hyalomma detritum). *Biomed Res Int.* 2019 Feb 7;2019:7805467.
[2937] Dehghani-Samani A, Madreseh-Ghahfarokhi S, Dehghani-Samani A, et al. In-vitro antigiardial activity and GC-MS analysis of Eucalyptus globulus and Zingiber officinalis essential oils against Giardia lamblia cysts in simulated condition to human's body. *Ann Parasitol.* 2019;65.
[2938] Bonde JP, Giwercman A, Ernst E. Review Identifying environmental risk to male reproductive function by occupational sperm studies: logistics and design options. *Occup Environ Med.* 1996 Aug; 53(8):511-9.
[2939] Mbaye MM, Khalifi BE, Addoum B, et al. The Effect of Supplementation with Some Essential Oils on the Mobility and the Vitality of Human Sperm. *ScientificWorldJournal.* 2019;2019:4878912.
[2940] Madreseh-Ghahfarokhi D, Dehghani-Samani A, Pirali Y, et al. Zingiber officinalis and Eucalyptus globulus, Potent Lethal/Repellent Agents Against Rhipicephalus bursa, Probable Carrier for Zoonosis. *J Arthropod Borne Dis.* 2019 Jun;13(2):214-223.
[2941] Omari KE, Hamze M, Alwan S, et al. In-vitro Evaluation of the Antibacterial Activity of the Essential Oils of Micromeria Barbata, Eucalyptus Globulus and Juniperus Excelsa Against Strains of Mycobacterium Tuberculosis (Including MDR), Mycobacterium Kansasii and Mycobacterium Gordonae. *J Infect Public Health.* 2016 Sep-Oct;12(5):615-618.
[2942] Soonwera M, Sittichok S. Adulticidal activities of Cymbopogon citratus (Stapf.) and Eucalyptus globulus (Labill.) essential oils and of their synergistic combinations against Aedes aegypti (L.), Aedes albopictus (Skuse), and Musca domestica (L.). *Environ Sci Pollut Res Int.* 2020 Apr 1. [Epub ahead of print]
[2943] Lou CW, Hsieh MC, Lu CT, et al. Evaluation of Repellent Effectiveness of Polyvinyl Alcohol/Eucalyptus globules Nanofibrous Membranes against Forcipomyia taiwana. *Polymers (Basel).* 2020 Apr 10;12(4).
[2944] Capetti F, Cagliero C, Marengo A, et al. Bio-Guided Fractionation Driven by In Vitro α-Amylase Inhibition Assays of Essential Oils Bearing Specialized Metabolites with Potential Hypoglycemic Activity. *Plants (Basel).* 2020 Sep 21;9(9):E1242.
[2945] Schneider R. Essential oil inhaler (AromaStick®) improves heat tolerance in the Hot Immersion Test (HIT). Results from two randomized, controlled experiments. *J Therm Biol.* 2020 Jan;87:102478.
[2946] Adenubi OT, Abolaji AO, Salihu T, et al. Chemical composition and acaricidal activity of Eucalyptus globulus essential oil against the vector of tropical bovine piroplasmosis, Rhipicephalus (Boophilus) annulatus. *Exp Appl Acarol.* 2021 Jan 3. Online ahead of print.
[2947] Khazraei H, Shamsdin SA, Zamani M. In Vitro Cytotoxicity and Apoptotic Assay of Eucalyptus globulus Essential Oil in Colon and Liver Cancer Cell Lines. *J Gastrointest Cancer.* 2021 Mar 3. Online ahead of print.
[2948] Mediavilla I, Guillamon E, Ruiz A, et al. Essential Oils from Residual Foliage of Forest Tree and Shrub Species: Yield and Antioxidant Capacity. *Molecules.* 2021 May 28;26(11):3257.
[2949] Brozyna M, Paleczny J, Kozlowska W, et al. The Antimicrobial and Antibiofilm In Vitro Activity of Liquid and Vapour Phases of Selected Essential Oils against Staphylococcus aureus. *Pathogens.* 2021 Sep 17;10(9):1207.
[2950] Boumendjel M, Boucheker A, Feknous S, et al. Adaptogenic activity of Cinnamomum camphora, Eucalyptus globulus, Lavandula stœchas and Rosmarinus officinalis essential oil used in North-African folk medicine. *Cell Mol Biol (Noisy-le-grand).* 2021 Aug 31;67(2):83-88.
[2951] Sheikh Z, Amani A, Basseri HR, et al. Repellent Efficacy of Eucalyptus globulus and Syzygium aromaticum Essential Oils against Malaria Vector, Anopheles stephensi (Diptera: Culicidae). *Iran J Public Health.* 2021 Aug;50(8):1668-1677.
[2952] Zhao C, Cao Y, Zhang Z, et al. Cinnamon and Eucalyptus Oils Suppress the Inflammation Induced by Lipopolysaccharide In Vivo. *Molecules.* 2021 Dec 6;26(23):7410.
[2953] Infante V, Campos PM, Gaspar LR, et al. Safety and efficacy of combined essential oils for the skin barrier properties: in vitro, ex vivo and clinical studies. *Int J Cosmet Sci.* 2022 Jan 5. Online ahead of print.
[2954] Kobenan KC, Ochou GEC, Kouadio IS, et al. Chemical Composition, Antioxidant Activity, Cholinesterase Inhibitor and in Vitro Insecticidal Potentiality of Essential Oils of Lippia multiflora Moldenke and Eucalyptus globulus Labill. on the Main Carpophagous Pests of Cotton Plant in Ivory Coast. *Chem Biodivers.* 2022 Feb 2:e202100993.
[2955] Ali T. Anjum AA, Sattar MMK, et al. Antibacterial activity of plant essential oils against indigenously characterized methicillin-resistant Staphylococcus aureus (MRSA). *Trop Biomed.* 2022 Mar 1;39(1):17-25.
[2956] Moreira P, Sousa FJ, Matos P, et al. Chemical Composition and Effect against Skin Alterations of Bioactive Extracts Obtained by the Hydrodistillation of Eucalyptus globulus Leaves. *Pharmaceutics.* 2022 Mar 3;14(3):561.
[2957] Rizg WY, Hosny KM, Mahmoud SS, et al. Repurposing Lovastatin Cytotoxicity against the Tongue Carcinoma HSC3 Cell Line Using a Eucalyptus Oil-Based Nanoemulgel Carrier. *Gels.* 2022 Mar 12;8(3):176.
[2958] Horváth A, Pandur E, Sipos K, et al. Anti-inflammatory effects of lavender and eucalyptus essential oils on the in vitro cell culture model of bladder pain syndrome using T24 cells. *BMC Complement Med Ther.* 2022 Apr 30;22(1):119.
[2959] Belkhodja H, Meddah B, Sidelarbi K, et al. In vitro and in vivo anti-inflammatory profile of Eucalyptus globulus essential oil. *J Appl Biol Sci.* 2022;16(1):80-8.
[2960] Madia VN, Toscanelli W, De Vita D, et al. Ultrastructural Damages to H1N1 Influenza Virus Caused by Vapor Essential Oils. *Molecules.* 2022 Jun 9;27(12):3718.
[2961] Ruas A, Graça A, Marto J, et al. Chemical Characterization and Bioactivity of Commercial Essential Oils and Hydrolates Obtained from Portuguese Forest Logging and Thinning. *Molecules.* 2022 Jun 2;27(11):3572.
[2962] Roczeń-Karczmarz M, Demkowska-Kutrzepa M, Zdybel J, et al. Comparison of the effectiveness of selected essential oils with mineral oil and spinosad on Dermanyssus gallinae. *Pol J Vet Sci.* 2022 Jun;25(2):261-268.
[2963] Brinsi C, Abidi A, Hosni K, et al. Protective Effect of Eucalyptus globulus Extracts Against Bleomycin-Induced Pulmonary Fibrosis in Rats. *J Med Food.* 2022 Jul;25(7):741-750.
[2964] Ziyadi S, Iddar A, Errafiy N, et al. Protective Effect of Some Essential Oils Against Gamma-Radiation Damages in Tetrahymena pyriformis Exposed to Cobalt-60 Source. *Curr Microbiol.* 2022 Aug 3;79(9):279.
[2965] Rekioua N, Boumendjel M, Taibi F, et al. Insecticidal effect of Eucalyptus globulus and Rosmarinus officinalis essential oils on a stored food pest Ephestia kuehniella (Lepidoptera, Pyralidea). *Cell Mol Biol (Noisy-le-grand).* 2022 Apr 30;68(4):144-157.
[2966] Assaggaf HM, Naceiri Mrabti H, Rajab BS, et al. Singular and Combined Effects of Essential Oil and Honey of Eucalyptus Globulus on Anti-Inflammatory, Antioxidant, Dermatoprotective, and Antimicrobial Properties: In Vitro and In Vivo Findings. *Molecules.* 2022 Aug 11;27(16):5121.
[2967] Alemu S, Bayu Y, Wasihun P, et al. Prevalence, Phytochemical Investigation, and In Vitro Acaricidal Efficacy Evaluation of Dodonaea angustifolia, Eucalyptus globulus, Millettia ferruginea, and Euphorbia abyssinica against Sarcoptic Mange of Camel, Babile District, Ethiopia. *J Parasitol Res.* 2022 Aug 11;2022:8639370.
[2968] Alipanah H, Abdollahi A, Firooziyan S, et al. Nanoemulsion and Nanogel Containing Eucalyptus globulus Essential Oil; Larvicidal Activity and Antibacterial Properties. *Interdiscip Perspect Infect Dis.* 2022 Aug 31;2022:1616149.
[2969] Öztürk Yaşa G, Safçi Berik S. Effects of Eucalyptus Essential Oil in Post-COVID Syndrome: A Pilot Study. *J Immunol Clin Microbiol.* 2022;7(4):82-87
[2970] Landeo-Villanueva GE, Salazar-Salvatierra ME, Ruiz-Quiroz JR, et al. Inhibitory Activity of Essential Oils of Mentha spicata and Eucalyptus globulus on Biofilms of Streptococcus mutans in an In Vitro Model. *Antibiotics (Basel).* 2023 Feb 10;12(2):369.
[2971] Iseppi R, Mariani M, Benvenuti S, et al. Effects of Melaleuca alternifolia Chell (Tea Tree) and Eucalyptus globulus Labill. Essential Oils on Antibiotic-Resistant Bacterial Biofilms. *Molecules.* 2023 Feb 9;28(4):1671.
[2972] Cai K, Liu Y, Yue Y, et al. Essential Oil Nanoemulsion Hydrogel with Antibiofilm Activity for the Treatment of Infected Wounds. *Molecules.* 2023 Mar 14;28(6):2638.
[2973] Čmiková N, Galovičová L, Schwarzová M, et al. Chemical Composition and Biological Activities of Eucalyptus globulus Essential Oil. *Plants (Basel).* 2023 Feb 28;12(5):1076.
[2974] Gilles M, Zhao J, Agboola S. Chemical composition and antimicrobial properties of essential oils of three Australian Eucalyptus species. *Food Chem.* 2010 May;119(2):731-37.
[2975] Lim E, Lee BH, Park CG. Fumigant activity of essential oils and their components from Eucalyptus codonocarpa and E. dives against Tetranychus urticae (Acari: Tetranychidae) at three temperatures. *J Appl Entomology.* 2012 Nov;136(9):698-703.
[2976] Weber B, Hartmann B, Stockigt D, et al. Extensive Study on the Minor Constituents of the Essential Oil of Eucalyptus dives Schau. Type. *J Essent Oil Res.* 2006 Nov-Dec;18(6):607-10.
[2977] Bignell CM, Dunlop PJ, Brophy JJ. Volatile leaf oils of some south-western and southern Australian species of the genus Eucalyptus (series I). Part XVI: Subgenus Symphyomyrtus, Section Bisectaria, Series Cneorifoliae, Series Porantherae and Series Falcatae. *Flavour Frag J.* 1997 Jul;12(4):261-67.
[2978] Delaquis PJ, Stanich K, Girard B, et al. Antimicrobial activity of individual and mixed fractions of dill, cilantro, coriander and eucalyptus essential oils. *Int J Food Microbiol.* 2002 Mar 25;74(1-2):101-9.
[2979] Shahverdi AR, Mirzaie S, Rafii F, et al. Monoterpenes as nitrofurantoin resistance modulating agents: minimal structural requirements, molecular dynamics simulations, and the effect of piperitone on the emergence of nitrofurantoin resistance in Enterobacteriaceae. *J Mol Model.* 2015 Aug;21(8):198.
[2980] Shahverdi AR, Rafii F, Tavassoli F, et al. Piperitone from Mentha longifolia var. chorodictya Rech F. reduces the nitrofurantoin resistance of strains of enterobacteriaceae. *Phytother Res.* 2004 Nov;18(11):911-4.
[2981] Gilles M, Zhao J, Agboola S. Chemical composition and antimicrobial properties of essential oils of three Australian Eucalyptus species. *Food Chem.* 2010 May;119(2):731-37.
[2982] Delaquis PJ, Stanich K, Girard B, et al. Antimicrobial activity of individual and mixed fractions of dill, cilantro, coriander and eucalyptus essential oils. *Int J Food Microbiol.* 2002 Mar 25;74(1-2):101-9.
[2983] Lim E, Lee BH, Park CG. Fumigant activity of essential oils and their components from Eucalyptus codonocarpa and E. dives against Tetranychus urticae (Acari: Tetranychidae) at three temperatures. *J Appl Entomology.* 2012 Nov;136(9):698-703.

[2984] Song JE, Kim JM, Lee NH, et al. Acaricidal and Insecticidal Activities of Essential Oils against a Stored-Food Mite and Stored-Grain Insects. *J Food Prot.* 2016 Jan;79(1):174-8.
[2985] Park IK, Shin SC. Fumigant activity of plant essential oils and components from garlic (Allium sativum) and clove bud (Eugenia caryophyllata) oils against the Japanese termite (Reticulitermes speratus Kolbe). *J Agric Food Chem.* 2005 Jun 1;53(11):4388-92.
[2986] Zhelijazkov VD, Horgan T, Astakie T, et al. Distillation time modifies essential oil yield, composition, and antioxidant capacity of fennel (Foeniculum vulgare Mill). *J Oleo Sci.* 2013;62(9):665-72.
[2987] Raal A, Orav A, Arak E. Essential oil composition of Foeniculum vulgare Mill. Fruits from pharmacies in different countries. *Nat Prod Res.* 2012;26(13):1173-78.
[2988] Miguel MG, Cruz X, Faleiro L, et al. Foeniculum vulgare essential oils: chemical composition, antioxidant and antimicrobial activities. *Nat Prod Commun.* 2012 Feb;5(2):319-28.
[2989] Tognolimi M, Ballabeni V, Bertoni S, et al. Protective effect of Foeniculum vulgare essential oil and anethole in an experimental model of thrombosis. *Pharm Res.* 2007;56:254-60.
[2990] Shahat AA, Ibrahim AY, Hendawy SF, et al. Chemical composition, antimicrobial and antioxidant activities of essential oils from Organically cultivated fennel cultivars. *Molecules.* 2011;16:1366-77.
[2991] Bajan M, Aprotosoaie AC, Spac A, et al. Chemical composition of essential oil obtained from Romanian fennel fruits. *Rev Med Chir Soc Med Nat Iasi.* 2011 Apr-Jun;115(2):590-94.
[2992] Aprotosoaie AC, Spac A, Hancianu M, et al. The chemical profile of essential oils obtained from fennel fruits (Foeniculum Vulgare Mill.). *Farmacia.* 2010;58(1):46-53.
[2993] Miraldi E. Comparison of the essential oils from ten Foeniculum vulgare Miller samples of fruits of different origin. *Flav Frag J.* 1999;14:379-82.
[2994] Acimovic M, Tesevic V, Todosijevic M, et al. Compositional characteristics of the essential oil of Pimpinella anisum and Foeniculum vulgare grown in Serbia. *Botanica Serbica.* 2015;39(1):9-14.
[2995] Singh G, Maurya S, de Lampasona MP, et al. Chemical constituents, antifungal and antioxidative potential of Foeniculum vulgare volatile oil and its acetone extract. *Food Cont.* 2006;17:745-52.
[2996] Lopes VR, Barata AM, Farias R. Morphological and Essential Oil Variability from Nine Portuguese Fennel (Foeniculum vulgare Mill.) Accessions. *Acta Hort.* 2010 Feb;860:33-50.
[2997] European Medicines Agency. Public statement on the use of herbal medicinal products containing estragole. Available at: http://www.ema.europa.eu/docs/en_GB/document_library/Scientific_guideline/2010/04/WC500089960.pdf.
[2998] Turkyilmaz Z, Karabulut R, Sonmez K, et al. A striking and frequent cause of premature thelarche in children: Foeniculum vulgare. *J Pediatr Surg.* 2008 Nov;43(11):2109-11.
[2999] Ostad SN, Khakinegard B, Sabzevari O. Evaluation of the teratogenicity of fennel essential oil (FEO) on the rat embryo limb buds culture. *Toxicol.* 2004 Oct;18(5):623-7.
[3000] European Medicines Agency. Public statement on the use of herbal medicinal products containing estragole. Available at: http://www.ema.europa.eu/docs/en_GB/document_library/Scientific_guideline/2010/04/WC500089960.pdf.
[3001] Rosti L, Nardini A, Bettini ME, et al. Toxic effects of a herbal tea mixture in two newborns. *Acta Paediatrica.* 1994;83:683.
[3002] Dhar SK. Anti-fertility activity and hormonal profile of trans-anethole in rats. *Indian J Physiol Pharmacol.* 1995;39(1):63-67.
[3003] European Commission. Opinion of the Scientific Committee on Food on estragole (1-Allyl-4-methoxybenzene). Available at: http://ec.europa.eu/food/fs/sc/scf/out104_en.pdf.
[3004] California Environmental Protection Agency. Evidence of the carcinogenicity of estragole. Available at: http://oehha.ca.gov/prop65/pdf/estragf.pdf.
[3005] Gori L, Gallo E, Mascherini V, et al. Can estragole in fennel seed decoctions really be considered a danger for human health? A fennel safety update. *Evid Based Complement Altern Med.* 2012;2012:860542.
[3006] Mauerman B, Ahmed N, Tambhar N, et al. Trends in Furanocoumarin Profiles Among Commerical-Scale Essential Oils. International Conference on the Science of Botanicals, Poster. Mar 2022.
[3007] Burkhard PR, Burkhardt K, Haenggeli CA, et al. Plant-induced seizures: reappearance of an old problem. *J Neurol.* 1999 Aug;246(8):667-70.
[3008] Skalli S, Bencheikh RS. Epileptic seizure induced by fennel essential oil. *Epileptic Discord.* 2011;13:345-347.
[3009] Tognolini M, Barocelli E, Ballabeni V, et al. Comparative screening of plant essential oils; phenylpropanoid moiety as basic core for antiplatelet activity. *Life Sci.* 2006 Feb 23;78(13):1419-32.
[3010] Yoshioka M, Tamada TT. Aromatic factors of anti-platelet aggregation in fennel oil. *Biogenic Amines.* 2005 Apr;19(2):89-96.
[3011] Rather MA, Dar BA, Sofi SN, et al. Foeniculum vulgare: A comprehensive review of its traditional use, phytochemistry, pharmacology, and safety. *Arabian J Chem.* 2012 Apr;XX:1-10.
[3012] Tognolini M, Ballabeni V, Bertoni S, et al. Protective effect of Foeniculum vulgare essential oil and anethole in an experimental model of theombosis. *Pharm Res.* 2007;56:254-60.
[3013] Kilic O, Kocak A. Volatile constituents of Juniperus communis L., Taxus Canadensis Marshall. and Tsuga Canadensis (L.) Carr. From Canada. *J Agric Sci Tech.* 2014;B4:135-40.
[3014] El-Soud N, El-Laithy N, El-Saeed G, et al. Antidiabetic activities of Foeniculum vulgare Mill. Essential oil in streptozotocin-induced diabetic rats. *Macedonian J Med.* 2011;173:1857-5773.
[3015] Wisniewski-Rebecca ES, Rocha BA, Wiirzler LA, et al. Synergistic effects of anethole and ibuprofen in acute inflammatory response. *Chem Biol Interact.* 2015 Dec 5;242:247-53.
[3016] Howes MJ, Houghton PJ, Barlow DJ, et al. Assessment of estrogenic activity in some common essential oil constituents. *J Pharm Pharmacol.* 2002 Nov;54(11):1521-28.
[3017] Chen CH, deGraffenreid LA. Anethole suppressed cell survival and induced apoptosis in human breast cancer cells independent of estrogen receptor status. *Phytomedicine.* 2012 Jun 15;19(8-9):763-7.
[3018] Nessa MU, Beale P, Chan C, et al. Studies on combination of platinum drugs cisplatin and oxaliplatin with phytochemicals anethole and curcumin in ovarian tumor models. *Anticancer Res.* 2012 Nov;32(11):4843-50.
[3019] Ostad SN, Soodi M, Shariffzadeh M, et al. The effect of fennel essential oil on uterine contraction as a model for dysmenorrhea, pharmacology and toxicology study. *J Ethnopharmacol.* 2001 Aug;76(3):299-304.
[3020] Khorshidi N, Ostad SN, Mosaddegh M, et al. Clinical effects of fennel essential oil on primary dysmenorrhea. *Iran J Pharm Res.* 2003 Spring;2(2):89-93.
[3021] Cao LX. Endometriosis as treated by traditional Chinese medicine. *J Am Coll Trad Chin Med.* 1983;1:54-57.
[3022] Zhu M, Wong PY, Li RC. Effect of oral administration of fennel (Foeniculum vulgare) on ciprofloxacin absorption and disposition in the rat. *J Pharm Pharmacol.* 1999;51:1391-96.
[3023] Shin S, Pyun MS. Anti-Candida effects of estragole in combination with ketoconazole or amphotericin B. *Phytother Res.* 2004 Oct;18(10):827-30.
[3024] Shin S. Essential oil compounds from Agastache rugosa as antifungal agents against Trichophyton species. *Arch Pharm Res.* 2004 Mar;27(3):295-9.
[3025] Shin S, Kang CA. Antifungal activity of the essential oil of Agastache rugosa Kuntze and its synergism with ketoconazole. *Lett Appl Microbiol.* 2003;36(2):111-5.
[3026] Kubo I, Fujita K. Naturally occurring anti-Salmonella agents. *J Agric Food Chem.* 2001 Dec;49(12):5750-4.
[3027] Subehan UT, Iwata H, Kadota S, et al. Mechanism-based inhibition of CYP3A4 and CYP2D6 by Indonesian medicinal plants. *J Ethnopharmacol.* 2006 May;105(3):449-55.
[3028] Subehan Z, Kadota SF, Tezuka Y. Inhibition on human liver cytochrome P450 3A4 by constituents of fennel (Foeniculum vulgare): Identification and characterization of a mechanism-based inactivator. *J Agric Food Chem.* 2007 Dec;55(25):10162-67.
[3029] Khan MM. Masters Thesis: Inhibition of Cytochrome P450 2E1 and Cytochrome P450 2A6 by Essential Oils: Tarragon (Artemisia dracunculus) and Basil (Ocimum basilicum). 2014. Available at: https://libres.uncg.edu/ir/uncg/f/Khan_uncg_0154M_11587.pdf
[3030] Rompelberg CJ, Verhagen H, van Bladeren PJ. Effects of the naturally occurring alkenylbenzenes eugenol and trans-anethole on drug-metabolizing enzymes in the rat liver. *Food Chem Toxicol.* 1993 Sep;31(9):637-45.
[3031] Zeng H, Chen X, Liang J. In Vitro antifungal activity and mechanism of essential oil from fennel (Foeniculum vulgare L.) on dermatophyte species. *J Med Microbiol.* 2015 Jan;64(Pt 1):93-103.
[3032] Mesfin M, Asres K, Shibeshi W. Evaluation of anxiolytic activity of the essential oil of the aerial part of Foeniculum vulgare Miller in mice. *BMC Complement Altern Med.* 2014 Aug 23;14:310.
[3033] Orhan IE, Ozcelik B, Kan Y, et al. Inhibitory effects of various essential oils and individual components against extended-spectrum beta-lactamase (ESBL) produced by Klebsiella pneumoniae and their chemical compositions. *J Food Sci.* 2011 Oct;76(8):M538-46.
[3034] Tripathi P, Tripathi R, Patel RK, et al. Investigation of antimutagenic potential of Foeniculum vulgare essential oil on cyclophosphamide induced genotoxicity and oxidative stress in mice. *Drug Chem Toxicol.* 2013 Jan;36(1):35-41.
[3035] Khaldun AO. Antibacterial action of ether oils of some plants. *Zh Mikrobiol Epidemiol Immunobiol.* 2006;3:92-93.
[3036] Patra M, Shahi SMidgely G, et al. Utilization of essential oil as natural antifungal against nail-infective fungi. *Flavour Frag J.* 2002 Mar/Apr;17(2):91-94.
[3037] Tognolini M, Ballabeni V, Bertoni S, et al. Protective effect of Foeniculum vulgare essential oil and anethole in an experimental model of thrombosis. *Pharm Res.* 2007;56:254-60.
[3038] Haze S, Sakai K, Gozu Y. Effects of fragrance inhalation on sympathetic activity in normal adults. *Jpn J Pharmacol.* 2002 Nov;90(3):247-53.
[3039] Chen CH, deGraffenreid LA. Anethole suppressed cell survival and induced apoptosis in human breast cancer cells independent of estrogen receptor status. *Phytomedicine.* 2012 Jun 15;19(8-9):763-7.
[3040] Nessa MU, Beale P, Chan C, et al. Studies on combination of platinum drugs cisplatin and oxaliplatin with phytochemicals anethole and curcumin in ovarian tumor models. *Anticancer Res.* 2012 Nov;32(11):4843-50.
[3041] Ostad SN, Soodi M, Shariffzadeh M, et al. The effect of fennel essential oil on uterine contraction as a model for dysmenorrhea, pharmacology and toxicology study. *J Ethnopharmacol.* 2001 Aug;76(3):299-304.
[3042] Khorshidi N, Ostad SN, Mosaddegh M, et al. Clinical effects of fennel essential oil on primary dysmenorrhea. *Iran J Pharm Res.* 2003 Spring;2(2):89-93.
[3043] Omidvar S, Esmalizabdeh S, Baradaran M, et al. Effect of fennel on pain intensity in dysmenorrhoea: A placebo-controlled trial. *Ayu.* 2012 Apr-Jun; 33(2): 311–313.
[3044] Mohebbi-kian E, Mohammad-Alizadeh S, Bekhradi R. Efficacy of fennel and combined oral contraceptive on depot medroxy-progesterone acetate induced amenorrhea: A randomized placebo-controlled trial. *Contraception.* 2014;90:440-46.
[3045] Mohebbi-kian E, Mohammad-Alizadeh S, Bekhradi R. Efficacy of fennel and combined oral contraceptive on depot medroxy-progesterone acetate induced amenorrhea: A randomized placebo-controlled trial. *Contraception.* 2014;90:440-46.
[3046] Jazani NH, Zartoshti M, Babazadeh H, et al. Antibacterial effects of Iranian fennel essential oil isolates of Acinetobacter baumannii. *Pak J Biol Sci.* 2009 May 1;12(9):738-41.
[3047] Aprotosoaie AC, Hancianu M, Poiata A, et al. In vitro antimicrobial activity and chemical composition of the essential oil of Foeniculum vulgare Mill. *Rev Med Chir Soc Med Nat Iasi.* 2008 Jul-Sep;112(3):832-36.
[3048] Dadalioglu I, Evrendilek GA. Chemical compositions and antibacterial effects of essential oils of Turkish oregano (Origanum minutiflorum), bay laurel (Laurus nobilis), Spanish Lavender (Lavendula stoechas L.) and fennel (Foeniculum vulgare) on common foodborne pathogens. *J Agric Food Chem.* 2004 Dec 29;52(26):8255-60.
[3049] Boskabady MH, KhatamiA, Nazari A. Possible mechanism(s) for relaxant effects of Foeniculum vulgare on guinea pig tracheal chains. *Pharmazie.* 2004 Jul;59(7):561-64.

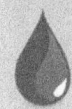

[3050] Ozbek H, Ugras S, Dulger H, et al. Hepatoprotective effect of Foeniculum vulgare essential oil. *Fitoterapia*. 2003 Apr;74(3)317-19.

[3051] Han AY, Lee HS, Seol GH, et al. Foeniculum vulgare Mill. increases cytosolic Ca2+ concentration and inhibits store-operated Ca2+ entry in vascular endothelial cells. *Biomed Pharmacother*. 2016 Oct 6;84:800-805.

[3052] Caleja C, Barros L, Antonio AL, et al. Fortification of yogurts with different antioxidant preservatives: A comparative study between natural and synthetic additives. *Food Chem*. 2016 Nov 1;210:262-8.

[3053] Portincasa P, Bonfrate L, Scribano ML, et al. Curcumin and Fennel Essential Oil Improve Symptoms and Quality of Life in Patients with Irritable Bowel Syndrome. *J Gastrointest Liver Dis*. 2016 Jun;25(2):151-7.

[3054] Garzoli S, Božović M, Baldisserotto A, et al. Essential oil extraction, chemical analysis and anti-Candida activity of Foeniculum vulgare Miller - new approaches. *Nat Prod Res*. 2017 Jun 15:1-6.

[3055] Sharopov F, Valiev A, Satyal P, et al. Cytotoxicity of the Essential Oil of Fennel (Foeniculum vulgare) from Tajikistan. *Foods*. 2017 Aug 28;6(9).

[3056] Rezayat SM, Dehpour AR, Motamed SM, et al. Foeniculum vulgare essential oil ameliorates acetic acid-induced colitis in rats through the inhibition of NF-kB pathway. *Inflammopharmacology*. 2018 Jun;26(3):851-859.

[3057] Wiwattanaratanabut K, choonharuangdej S, Srithava T. In Vitro Anti-Cariogenic Plaque Effects of Essential Oils Extracted from Culinary Herbs. *J Clin Diagnostic Res*. 2017 Sep;11(9):DC30-5.

[3058] Pavela R. Essential oils from Foeniculum vulgare Miller as a safe environmental insecticide against the aphid Myzus persicae Sulzer. *Environ Sci Pollut Res Int*. 2018 Apr;25(11):10904-10910.

[3059] Levorato S, Dominici L, Fatigoni C, et al. In vitro toxicity evaluation of estragole-containing preparations derived from Foeniculum vulgare Mill. (fennel) on HepG2 cells. *Food Chem Toxicol*. 2017 Dec 9;111:616-622.

[3060] Akhbari M, Kord R, Jafari Nodooshan S, et al. Analysis and evaluation of the antimicrobial and anticancer activities of the essential oil isolated from Foeniculum vulgare from Hamedan, Iran. *Nat Prod Res*. 2018 Jan 7:1-4.

[3061] Bartoňková I, Dvořák Z. Essential oils of culinary herbs and spices display agonist and antagonist activities at human aryl hydrocarbon receptor AhR. *Food Chem Toxicol*. 2018 Jan;111:374-384.

[3062] Kwiatkowski P, Mnichowska-Polanowska M, Pruss A, et al. The effect of fennel essential oil in combination with antibiotics on Staphylococcus aureus strains isolated from carriers. *Burns*. 2017 Nov;43(7):1544-1551.

[3063] Rahimikian F, Rahimi R, Golzareh P, et al. Effect of Foeniculum vulgare Mill. (fennel) on menopausal symptoms in postmenopausal women: a randomized, triple-blind, placebo-controlled trial. *Menopause*. 2017 Sep;24(9):1017-1021.

[3064] Vieira JN, Gonçalves CL, Villarreal JPV, et al. Chemical composition of essential oils from the apiaceae family, cytotoxicity, and their antifungal activity in vitro against candida species from oral cavity. *Braz J Biol*. 2019 Jul-Sep;79(3):432-437.

[3065] Mafakheri H, Mirghazanfari SM. Antifungal activity of the essential oils of some medicinal plants against human and plant fungal pathogens. *Cell Mol Biol (Noisy-le-grand)*. 2018 Dec 31;64(15):13-19.

[3066] Mostafa DM, Abd El-Alim SH, Asfour MH, et al. Transdermal fennel essential oil nanoemulsions with promising hepatic dysfunction healing effect: In vitro and in vivo study. *Pharm Dev Technol*. 2019 Feb 18:1-33.

[3067] Chiboub W, Sassi AB, Amina CM, et al. Valorization of the Green Waste from Two Varieties of Fennel and Carrot Cultivated in Tunisia by Identification of the Phytochemical Profile and Evaluation of the Antimicrobial Activities of Their Essentials Oils. *Chem Biodivers*. 2019 Jan;16(1):e1800546.

[3068] Ghasemian A, Al-Marzoqi AH, Mostafavi SKS, et al. Chemical Composition and Antimicrobial and Cytotoxic Activities of Foeniculum vulgare Mill Essential Oils. *J Gastrointest Cancer*. 2020 Mar;51(1):260-266.

[3069] El-Garawani IM, Hassab El-Nabi S, Dawoud GT, et al. Triggering of apoptosis and cell cycle arrest by fennel and clove oils in Caco-2 cells: The role of combination. *Toxicol Mech Methods*. 2019 Jul 31:1-32.

[3070] Khorram Z, Hakimaneh SM, Naeini A, et al. The Antifungal Effects of Two Herbal Essences in Comparison with Nystatin on the Candida Strains Isolated from the Edentulous Patients. *J Contemp Dent Pract*. 2019 Jun 1;20(6):716-719.

[3071] Kalleli F, Bettaieb Rebey I, Wannes WA, et al. Chemical composition and antioxidant potential of essential oil and methanol extract from Tunisian and French fennel (Foeniculum vulgare Mill.) seeds. *J Food Biochem*. 2019 Aug;43(8):e12935.

[3072] Al-Okbi SY, Hussein AMS, Elbakry HFH, et al. Health Benefits of Fennel, Rosemary Volatile Oils and their Nano-Forms in Dyslipidemic Rat Model. *Pak J Biol Sci*. 2018 Jan;21(7):348-358.

[3073] Karami F, Dastan D, Fallah M, et al. In Vitro Activity of Foeniculum vulgare and Its Main Essential Oil Component Trans-Anethole on Trichomonas vaginalis. *Iran J Parasitol*. 2019 Oct-Dec;14(4):631-638.

[3074] Chen F, Guo Y, Yang X, et al. Insight into the essential oil isolation from Foeniculum vulgare Mill. fruits using double-condensed microwave-assisted hydrodistillation and evaluation of its antioxidant, antifungal and cytotoxic activity. *Ind Crops Prod*. 2020 Feb;144:112052.

[3075] Sabzi Nojadeh M, Pouresmaeil M, Younessi-Hamzekhanlu M, et al. Phytochemical profile of fennel essential oils and possible applications for natural antioxidant and controlling Convolvulus arvensis L. *Nat Prod Res*. 2020 Mar 16:1-5.

[3076] Timoumi R, Salem IB, Amara I, et al. Protective effects of fennel essential oil against oxidative stress and genotoxicity induced by the insecticide triflumuron in human colon carcinoma cells. *Environ Sci Pollut Res Int*. 2020 Mar;27(8):7957-7966.

[3077] Pala A, Serdar O, Yonar SM, et al. Ameliorative effect of Fennel (Foeniculum vulgare) essential oil on chlorpyrifos toxicity in Cyprinus carpio. *Environ Sci Pollut Res Int*. 2020 Aug 21. Online ahead of print.

[3078] Abbasi-Maleki S, Maleki SG. Antidepressant-like effects of Foeniculum vulgare essential oil and potential involvement of dopaminergic and serotonergic systems on mice in the forced swim test. *PharmaNutrition*. 2021;15:100241.

[3079] Korinek M, Handoussa H, Tsai YH, et al. Anti-Inflammatory and Antimicrobial Volatile Oils: Fennel and Cumin Inhibit Neutrophilic Inflammation via Regulating Calcium and MAPKs. *Front Pharmacol*. 2021 Oct 11;12:674095.

[3080] Oviedo-Sarmiento JS, Cortes JJB, Avila WAD, et al. Fumigant toxicity and biochemical effects of selected essential oils toward the red flour beetle, Tribolium castaneum (Coleoptera: Tenebrionidae). *Pestic Biochem Physiol*. 2021 Nov;179:104941.

[3081] Aboelhadid SM, Arafa WM, Abdel-Baki AS, et al. Acaricidal activity of Foeniculum vulgare against Rhipicephalus annulatus is mainly dependent on its constituent from trans-anethone. *PLoS One*. 2021 Dec 2;16(12):e0260172.

[3082] D'Aquila P, Paparazzo E, Crudo M, et al. Antibacterial Activity and Epigenetic Remodeling of Essential Oils from Calabrian Aromatic Plants. *Nutrients*. 2022 Jan 17;14(2):391.

[3083] Štrbac F, Bosco A, Maurelli MP, et al. Anthelmintic Properties of Essential Oils to Control Gastrointestinal Nematodes in Sheep-In Vitro and In Vivo Studies. *Vet Sci*. 2022 Feb 19;9(2):93.

[3084] Hong SJ, Yoon S, Jo SM, et al. Olfactory Stimulation by Fennel (Foeniculum vulgare Mill.) Essential Oil Improves Lipid Metabolism and Metabolic Disorders in High Fat-Induced Obese Rats. *Nutrients*. 2022 Feb 10;14(4):741.

[3085] Karadağ AE, Çaşkurlu A, Demirci B, et al. Binary Synergistic Combinations of Lavender and Fennel Essential Oils with Amoxicillin. *Planta Med*. 2022 Jul 4. Online ahead of print.

[3086] Lauricella M, Maggio A, Badalamenti N, et al. Essential oil of Foeniculum vulgare subsp. piperitum fruits exerts an anti-tumor effect in triple-negative breast cancer cells. *Mol Med Rep*. 2022 Jul;26(1):243.

[3087] Karadağ AE, Çaşkurlu A, Demirci B, et al. Binary Synergistic Combinations of Lavender and Fennel Essential Oils with Amoxicillin. *Planta Med*. 2022 Jul 4. Online ahead of print.

[3088] Li C, Cai Q, Wu X, et al. Anti-inflammatory Study on the Constituents of Angelica sinensis (Oliv.) Diels, Angelica dahurica (Hoffm.) Benth. & Hook.f. ex Franch. & Sav., Angelica pubescence Maxim and Foeniculum vulgare Mill. Essential Oils. *J Oleo Sci*. 2022 Jul 6. Online ahead of print.

[3089] Di Napoli M, Castagliuolo G, Badalamenti N, et al. Antimicrobial, Antibiofilm, and Antioxidant Properties of Essential Oil of Foeniculum vulgare Mill. Leaves. *Plants (Basel)*. 2022 Dec 17;11(24):3573.

[3090] Coimbra A, Miguel S, Ribeiro M, et al. Chemical composition, antioxidant, and antimicrobial activities of six commercial essential oils. *Lett Appl Microbiol*. 2023 Jan 23;76(1):ovac042.

[3091] Jahanifard E, Ghofleh-Maramazi H, Sharififard M, et al. Pediculicidal Activity of Foeniculum vulgare Essential Oil in Treatment of Pediculus capitis as a Public Health Problem. *J Arthropod Borne Dis*. 2022 Mar 31;16(1):61-71.

[3092] Hamden K, Keskes H, Belhaj S, et al. Inhibitory potential of omega-3 fatty and fenugreek essential oil on key enzymes of carbohydrate-digestion and hypertension in diabetes rats. *Lipids Health Dis*. 2011 Dec 5;10:226.

[3093] Hamden K, Keskes H, Belhaj S, et al. Inhibitory potential of omega-3 fatty and fenugreek essential oil on key enzymes of carbohydrate-digestion and hypertension in diabetes rats. *Lipids Health Dis*. 2011 Dec 5;10:226.

[3094] Burkhard PR, Burkhardt K, Haenggeli CA, et al. Plant-induced seizures: reappearance of an old problem. *J Neurol*. 1999 Aug;246(8):667-70.

[3095] Narayan S, Singh N. Camphor poisoning-An unusual cause of seizure. *Med J Armed Forces India*. 2012 Jul;68(3):252-53.

[3096] Chanaranaj KJ, G MV, S M. Camphor poisoning in a child. *Natl Med J India*. 2013 Jan-Feb;26(1):60.

[3097] Olowe SA, Ransome-Kuti O. The risk of jaundice in glucose-6-phosphate dehydrogenase deficient babies exposed to menthol. *Acta Paediatr Scand*. 1980 May;69(3):341-5.

[3098] Dillon Remy M, Manning Alleyne P, Bratt DE, et al. Neonatal jaundice at Port-of-Spain General Hospital abstract. *West Indian Med J*. 1987;36(Suppl):28.

[3099] Hamden K, Keskes H, Belhaj S, et al. Inhibitory potential of omega-3 fatty and fenugreek essential oil on key enzymes of carbohydrate-digestion and hypertension in diabetes rats. *Lipids Health Dis*. 2011 Dec 5;10:226.

[3100] Garg SN, Misra LM, Agarwal SK. Essential oil from rhizomes of Ferula jaeschkeana. *Phytochemistry*. 1989;28(2):634-36.

[3101] Lawrence BM. Progress in essential oils. *Perf Flavorist*. 2012;37:42-43.

[3102] Hendricks H, Bos R, Woerdenbag HJ. The essential oil of Tanacetum parthenium (L). Schultz-Bip. *Flavour Frag J*. 1996 Nov;11(6):367-71.

[3103] Izadi Z, Esna-Ashari M, Piri K, et al. Chemical Composition and Antimicrobial Activity of Feverfew (Tanacetum parthenium) Essential Oil. *Int J Agric Biology*. 2010 Sep;12:759-63.

3104 Sharopov FS, Setzer WN, Salomiddin JI, et al. Composition and bioactivity of the essential oil of Tanacetum parthenium from a wild population growing in Tajikistan. *Am J Essential Oils Nat Prod.* 2012;2(4):32-34.

3105 Haziri A, Govori-Odai S, Ismaili M, et al. Essential Oil of Tanacetum parthenium (L.) from East Part of Kosova. *Am J Biochem Biotech.* 2009;5(4):226-28.

3106 Dajić Stevanović ZP, Nastovski TLj., Ristić MS, et al. Variability of Essential Oil Composition of Cultivated Feverfew (Tanacetum parthenium (L.) Schultz Bip.) Populations. *J Essent Oil Res.* 2009;21(4):292-94.

3107 Stanković N, Mihajilov-Krstev T, Zlatković B, et al. Comparative Study of Composition, Antioxidant, and Antimicrobial Activities of Essential Oils of Selected Aromatic Plants from Balkan Peninsula. *Planta Med.* 2016 May;82(7):650-61.

3108 Polatoglu K, Demirci F, Demirci B, et al. Antibacterial activity and the variation of Tanacetum parthenium (L.) Schultz Bip. essential oils from Turkey. *J Oleo Sci.* 2010;59(4):177-84.

3109 Khine H, Weiss D, Graber N, et al. A cluster of children with seizures caused by camphor poisoning. *Pediatrics.* 2009 May;123(5):1269-72.

3110 Michiels EA, Mazor SS. Toddler with seizures due to ingesting camphor at an Indian celebration. *Pediatr Emerg Care.* 2010 Aug;26(8):574-75.

3111 Koren G. Medications which can kill a toddler with one tablet or teaspoonful. *J toxicol Clin toxicol.* 1993;31(3):407- 13.

3112 Flaman Z, Pellechia-Clarke S, Bailey B, et al. Unintentional exposure of young children to camphor and eucalyptus oils. *Paediatr Child Health.* 2001 Feb;6(2):80-83.

3113 Rabl W, Katzgraber F, Steinlechner M. Camphor ingestion for abortion (case report). *Forensic Sci Int.* 1997 Sep 19;89(1-2):137-40.

3114 Flaman Z, Pellechia-Clarke S, Bailey B, et al. Unintentional exposure of young children to camphor and eucalyptus oils. *Paediatr Child Health.* 2001 Feb;6(2):80-83.

3115 Burkhard PR, Burkhardt K, Haenggeli CA, et al. Plant-induced seizures: reappearance of an old problem. *J Neurol.* 1999 Aug;246(8):667-70.

3116 Narayan S, Singh N. Camphor poisoning-An unusual cause of seizure. *Med J Armed Forces India.* 2012 Jul;68(3):252-53.

3117 Chanaranaj KJ, G MV, S M. Camphor poisoning in a child. *Natl Med J India.* 2013 Jan-Feb;26(1):60.

3118 Uc A, Bishop WP, Sanders KD. Camphor hepatotoxicity. *South Med J.* 2000;93:596-98.

3119 Olowe SA, Ransome-Kuti O. The risk of jaundice in glucose-6-phosphate dehydrogenase deficient babies exposed to menthol. *Acta Paediatr Scand.* 1980 May;69(3):341-5.

3120 Dillon Remy M, Manning Alleyne P, Bratt DE, et al. Neonatal jaundice at Port-of-Spain General Hospital abstract. *West Indian Med J.* 1987;36(Suppl):28.

3121 Manoguerra AS, Erdman AR, Wax PM, et al. Camphor poisoning: an evidence-based practice guideline for out-of- hospital management. *Clin Toxicol (Phila).*2006;44(4):357-70.

3122 Gibson DE, Moore GP, Pfaff JA. Camphor ingestion. *Am J Emerg Med.* 1989 Jan;7(1):41-43.

3123 Koppel C, Martends F, Schirop T, et al. Hemoperfusion in acute camphor poisoning. *Intensive Care Med.* 1988;14(4):431-33.

3124 Covington TR, et al. Handbook of Nonprescription Drugs. 11th ed. Washington, D.C.: American Pharmaceutical Association. 1996.

3125 Sharopov FS, Setzer WN, Salomiddin JI, et al. Composition and bioactivity of the essential oil of Tanacetum parthenium from a wild population growing in Tajikistan. *Am J Essential Oils Nat Prod.* 2012;2(4):32-34.

3126 Stanković N, Mihajilov-Krstev T, Zlatković B, et al. Comparative Study of Composition, Antioxidant, and Antimicrobial Activities of Essential Oils of Selected Aromatic Plants from Balkan Peninsula. *Planta Med.* 2016 May;82(7):650-61.

3127 Izadi Z, Esna-Ashari M, Piri K, et al. Chemical Composition and Antimicrobial Activity of Feverfew (Tanacetum parthenium) Essential Oil. *Int J Agric Biology.* 2010 Sep;12:759-63.

3128 Polatoglu K, Demirci F, Demirci B, et al. Antibacterial activity and the variation of Tanacetum parthenium (L.) Schultz Bip. essential oils from Turkey. *J Oleo Sci.* 2010;59(4):177-84.

3129 Shafaghat A, Sadeghi H, Oji K. Composition and antibacterial activity of essential oils from leaf, stem and root of Chrysanthemum parthenium (L.) Bernh. from Iran. *Nat Prod Commun.* 2009 Jun;4(6):859-60.

3130 Izadi Z, Aghaalikhani M, Esna-Ahari M, et al. Determining Chemical Composition and Antimicrobial Activity of Feverfew (Tanacetum parthenium L.) Essential Oil on Some Microbial Strains. *Zahedan J Res Med Sci.* 2013;15(6):8-13.

3131 Sharopov FS, Setzer WN, Salomiddin JI, et al. Composition and bioactivity of the essential oil of Tanacetum parthenium from a wild population growing in Tajikistan. *Am J Essential Oils Nat Prod.* 2012;2(4):32-34.

3132 Stanković N, Mihajilov-Krstev T, Zlatković B, et al. Comparative Study of Composition, Antioxidant, and Antimicrobial Activities of Essential Oils of Selected Aromatic Plants from Balkan Peninsula. *Planta Med.* 2016 May;82(7):650-61.

3133 Polatoglu K, Demirci F, Demirci B, et al. Antibacterial activity and the variation of Tanacetum parthenium (L.) Schultz Bip. essential oils from Turkey. *J Oleo Sci.* 2010;59(4):177-84.

3134 Sukari MA, Moahd Sharif NW, Yap ALC, et al. Chemical constituents variations of essential oils from rhizomes of four Zingiberacea species. *Malaysian J Analytic Sci.* 2008;12(3):638-44.

3135 Phanthonga P, Lomarat P, Traidej Chomnawang M, et al. Antibacterial activity of essential oils and their active components from Thai spices against foodborne pathogens. *ScienceAsia.* 2013;39:472-76.

3136 Natta L, Orapin K, Krittika N, et al. Essential oil from five Zingiberaceae for anti food-borne bacteria. *Int Food Res J.* 2008;15(3):337-46.

3137 Jantan BJ, Basni I, Said Ahmad A, et al. Constituents of the rhizome oils of Boesenbergia pandurata (Roxb.) Schlecht from Malaysia, Indonesia and Thailand. *Flavour Frag J.* 2001 Mar-Apr;16(2):110-12.

3138 Baharudin MKA, Hamid SA, Susanti D. Chemical Composition and Antibacterial Activity of Essential Oils from Three Aromatic Plants of the Zingiberaceae Family in Malaysia. *J Phys Sci.* 2015;26(1):71-81.

3139 Khine H, Weiss D, Graber N, et al. A cluster of children with seizures caused by camphor poisoning. *Pediatrics.* 2009 May;123(5):1269-72.

3140 Michiels EA, Mazor SS. Toddler with seizures due to ingesting camphor at an Indian celebration. *Pediatr Emerg Care.* 2010 Aug;26(8):574-75.

3141 Koren G. Medications which can kill a toddler with one tablet or teaspoonful. *J toxicol Clin toxicol.* 1993;31(3):407- 13.

3142 Craig JO. Poisoning by the volatile oils in childhood. *Arch Dis Child.* 1953;28:259-67.

3143 Melis K. Bochner A, Janssens G. Accidental nasal eucalyptol and menthol instillation. *Eur J Pediatr.* 1989 Aug;148(8)786-7.

3144 Day LM, Ozanne-Smith J, Parsons BJ, et al. Eucalyptus oil poisoning among young children: mechanisms of access and the potential prevention. *Aust N Z J Public Health.* 1997 Jun;21(3):297-302.

3145 Chandar SD, Prashanti M, Kumar CL, et al. Eucalyptus Oil-Induced Seizures in Children: A Single-Center Prospective Study. *Cureus.* 2021 Mar 25;13(3):e14109.

3146 Flaman Z, Pellechia-Clarke S, Bailey B, et al. Unintentional exposure of young children to camphor and eucalyptus oils. *Paediatr Child Health.* 2001 Feb;6(2):80-83.

3147 Rabl W, Katzgraber F, Steinlechner M. Camphor ingestion for abortion (case report). *Forensic Sci Int.* 1997 Sep 19;89(1-2):137-40.

3148 Burkhard PR, Burkhardt K, Haenggeli CA, et al. Plant-induced seizures: reappearance of an old problem. *J Neurol.* 1999 Aug;246(8):667-70.

3149 Uc A, Bishop WP, Sanders KD. Camphor hepatotoxicity. *South Med J.* 2000;93:596-98.

3150 Olowe SA, Ransome-Kuti O. The risk of jaundice in glucose-6-phosphate dehydrogenase deficient babies exposed to menthol. *Acta Paediatr Scand.* 1980 May;69(3):341-5.

3151 Dillon Remy M, Manning Alleyne P, Bratt DE, et al. Neonatal jaundice at Port-of-Spain General Hospital abstract. *West Indian Med J.* 1987;36(Suppl):28.

3152 Manoguerra AS, Erdman AR, Wax PM, et al. Camphor poisoning: an evidence-based practice guideline for out-of- hospital management. *Clin Toxicol (Phila).*2006;44(4):357-70.

3153 Gibson DE, Moore GP, Pfaff JA. Camphor ingestion. *Am J Emerg Med.* 1989 Jan;7(1):41-43.

3154 Koppel C, Martends F, Schirop T, et al. Hemoperfusion in acute camphor poisoning. *Intensive Care Med.* 1988;14(4):431-33.

3155 Jori A, Bianchetti A, Prestini PE, et al. Effect of eucalyptol (1,8-cineole) on the metabolism of other drugs in rats and in man. *Eur J Pharmacol.* 1970;9(3):362-66.

3156 de Sousa DP, Raphael E, Brocksom U, et al. Sedative effect of monoterpene alcohols in mice: A preliminary screening. *Verlag der Zeitschrift fur Naturforschung.* 2007;62c:563-66.

3157 Lamborn LL. Modern soaps, candles and glycerin: A practical manual of modern methods of utilization of fats and oils in the manufacture of soaps and candles, and of the recovery of glycerin. Library of the University of Wisconsin.

3158 Oyen LP, Dung NX. Plant resources of South-East Asia. 1999. Backhyus, Leiden.

3159 Seo KA, Kim H, Ku HY, et al. The monoterpenoids citral and geraniol are moderate inhibitors of the CYP2B6 hydroxylase activity. *Chem Biol Interact.* 2008;174:141-46.

3160 Kim NH, Hyun SH, Jin CH, et al. Pretreatment with 1,8-cineole potentiates thioacetamide-induced hepatotoxicity and immunosuppression. *Arch Pharm Res.* 2004 Jul;27(7):781-9.

3161 Ibrahim SM, El-Denshary ES, Abdallah DM. Geraniol, Alone and in Combination with Pioglitazone, Ameliorates Fructose-Induced Metabolic Syndrome in Rats via the Modulation of Both Inflammatory and Oxidative Stress Status. *PLoS One.* 2015 Feb 13;10(2):e0117516.

3162 Srinivasan S, Muruganathan U. Antidiabetic efficacy of citronellol, a citrus monoterpene by ameliorating the hepatic key enzymes of carbohydrate metabolism in streptozotocin-induced diabetic rats. *Chem Biol Interact.* 2016 Apr 25;250:38-46.

3163 Shin S, Lim S. Antifungal effects of herbal essential oils alone and in combination with ketoconazole against Trichophyton spp. *J Appl Micribiol.* 2004;97:1289-96.

3164 Boukhris M, Bouaziz M, Feki I, et al. Hypoglycemic and antioxidant effects of leaf and essential oil of Pelargonium graveolens L'Her. in alloxan induced diabetic rats. *Lipids Health Dis.* 2012 Jun 26;11:81.

3165 Adeneye AA, Agbaje EO. Hypoglycemic and hypolipidemic effects of fresh leaf aqueous extract of Cymbopogon citratus Stapf. in rats. *J Ethnopharmacol.* 2007 Jul 25; 112(3):440-4.

3166 Bharti SK, Kumar A, Prakash O, et al. Essential Oil of Cymbopogon Citratus Against Diabetes: Validation by In vivo Experiments and Computational Studies. *J Bioanal Biomed.* 2013;5:194-203.

3167 Hagvall L. Cytochrome P450-mediated activation of the fragrance constituent geraniol forms potent contact allergens. *Tox Appl Pharm.* 2008 Dec;233(2):308-13.

3168 Covington TR, et al. Handbook of Nonprescription Drugs. 11th ed. Washington, D.C.: American Pharmaceutical Association. 1996.

3169 Phanthonga P, Lomarat P, Traidej Chomnawang M, et al. Antibacterial activity of essential oils and their active components from Thai spices against foodborne pathogens. *ScienceAsia.* 2013;39:472-76.

3170 Natta L, Orapin K, Krittika N, et al. Essential oil from five Zingiberaceae for anti food-borne bacteria. *Int Food Res J.* 2008;15(3):337-46.

3171 Baharudin MKA, Hamid SA, Susanti D. Chemical Composition and Antibacterial Activity of Essential Oils from Three Aromatic Plants of the Zingiberaceae Family in Malaysia. *J Phys Sci.* 2015;26(1):71-81.

3172 Wannissorn B, Maneesin P, Tubtimted S, et al. Antimicrobial activity of essential oils extracted from Thai herbs and spices. *As J Food Ag-Ind.* 2009;2(4):677-89.

3173 Jantapan K, Poapolathep A, Imsilp K, et al. Inhibitory Effects of Thai Essential Oils on Potentially Aflatoxigenic Aspergillus parasiticus and Aspergillus flavus. *Biocontrol Sci.* 2017;22(1):31-40.

3174 Phukerd U, Soonwera M. Repellency of essential oils extracted from Thai native plants against Aedes aegypti (Linn.) and Culex quinquefasciatus (Say). *Parasitol Res.* 2014 Sep;113(9):3333-40.

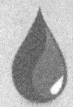

[3175] Phukerd U, Soonwera M. Larvicidal and pupicidal activities of essential oils from Zingiberaceae plants against Aedes aegypti (Linn.) and Culex quinquefasciatus say mosquitoes. *Southeast Asian J Trop Med Public Health*. 2013 Sep;44(5):761-71.
[3176] Wang SY, Wu CL, Chu FH, et al. Chemical composition and antifungal activity of essential oil isolated from Chamaecyparis formosensis Matsum. wood. *Holzforschung*. 2005;59:295–99.
[3177] Kuo PM, Chu FH, Chang ST, et al. Insecticidal activity of essential oil from Chamaecyparis formosensis Matsum. *Holzforschung*. 2007;61:595–99.
[3178] Hsu CY, Lin CY, Chang ST. Antitermitic activities of wood essential oil and its constituents from Chamaecyparis formosensis. *Wood Sci Tech*. 2016 Mar;50(4):663-76.
[3179] Wang SY, Wang YS, Tseng YH, et al. Analysis of fragrance compositions of precious coniferous woods grown in Taiwan. *Holzforschung*. 2006;60:528-32.
[3180] Satyal, P. Private communication, 2016.
[3181] Bernart, M. Private communication, 2016.
[3182] Lin CY, Chen YJ, Cheng SS, et al. Rapid Differentiation of Three Chamaecyparis Species (Cupressaceae) Grown in Taiwan Using Solid-Phase Microextraction—Gas Chromatography/Mass Spectrometry, Cluster Analysis, and Principal Component Analysis. *J Agric Food Chem*. 2011;59:10854-59.
[3183] Chen YJ, Lin CY, Cheng SS, et al. Rapid Discrimination and Feature Extraction of Three Chamaecyparis Species by Static-HS/GC−MS. *J Agric Food Chem*. 2015;63:810-20.
[3184] Ho CL, Hua KF, Hsu KP, et al. Composition and antipathogenic activities of the twig essential oil of Chamaecyparis formosensis from Taiwan. *Nat Prod Commun*. 2012 Jul;7(7):933-6.
[3185] Tsuneki H, Ma EL, Kobayashi S, et al. Antiangiogenic activity of beta-eudesmol in vitro and in vivo. *Eur J Pharmacol*. 2005 Apr 11;512(2-3):105-15.
[3186] Arora CK, Arora RB, Mesta CK, et al. Hypotensive activity of beta-eudesmol and some related sesquiterpenes. *Ind J Med Res*. 1967 May;55(5):463-72.
[3187] Wang BG, Hong X, Li L, Zhou J, et al. Chemical constituents of two Chinese Magnoliaceae plants, Tsoongiodendron odorum and Manglietiastrum sinicum, and their inhibition of platelet aggregation. *Planta Med*. 2000 Aug;66(6):511-5.
[3188] de Sousa DP, Raphael E, Brocksom U, et al. Sedative effect of monoterpene alcohols in mice: A preliminary screening. *Verlag der Zeitschrift fur Naturforschung*. 2007;62c:563-66.
[3189] Yen HF, Wang SY, Wu CC, et al. Cytotoxicity, Anti-Platelet Aggregation Assay and Chemical Components Analysis of Thirty-Eight Kinds of Essential Oils. *J Food Drug Analysis*. 2012;20(2):478-83.
[3190] Chen CJ, Kumar KJ, Chen YT, et al. Effect of Hinoki and Meniki Essential Oils on Human Autonomic Nervous System Activity and Mood States. *Nat Prod Commun*. 2015 Jul;10(7):1305-8.
[3191] Hsu CY, Lin CY, Chang ST. Antitermitic activities of wood essential oil and its constituents from Chamaecyparis formosensis. *Wood Sci Tech*. 2016 Mar;50(4):663-76.
[3192] Lowe RF, Russell MF, Southwell IA. Composition of an Essential Oil from Agonis fragrans J.R.Wheeler et N.G.Marchant. *J Essent Oil Res*. 2007 Jul-Aug;19:342-44.
[3193] Robinson CJ. A New Essential oil – Agonis fragrans. Chemotype Selection and Evaluation. 2006 Aug. Available at:
https://www.google.com/url?sa=t&rct=j&q=&esrc=s&source=web&cd=1&cad=rja&uact=8&ved=0ahUKEwjT3f6U-PbPAhXhyVQKHePHAEsQFggtMAA&url=https%3A%2F%2Frirdc.infoservices.com.au%2Fdownloads%2F06-090&usg=AFQjCNGYgbDCQBlU7G8UxfFXww6BJ6E9qg&sig2=qizd35u_CrONdETw1UuWmg.
[3194] Burkhard PR, Burkhardt K, Haenggeli CA, et al. Plant-induced seizures: reappearance of an old problem. *J Neurol*. 1999 Aug;246(8):667-70.
[3195] Culic M, Kekovic G, Grbic G, et al. Wavelet and fractal analysis of rat brain activity in seizures evoked by
camphor essential oil and 1,8-cineole. *Gen Physiol Biophys*. 2009;Special Issue(28):33–40.
[3196] Mathew T, Kamath V, Kumar RS, et al. Eucalyptus oil inhalation–induced seizure: A novel, underrecognized, preventable cause of acute symptomatic seizure. *Epilepsia Open*. 2017 Sep;2(3):350–354.
[3197] Jori A, Bianchetti A, Prestini PE, et al. Effect of eucalyptol (1,8-cineole) on the metabolism of other drugs in rats and in man. *Eur J Pharmacol*. 1970;9(3):362-66.
[3198] de Sousa DP, Raphael E, Brocksom U, et al. Sedative effect of monoterpene alcohols in mice: A preliminary screening. *Verlag der Zeitschrift fur Naturforschung*. 2007;62c:563-66.
[3199] Birhanie MW, Walle B, Rebba K, et al. Hypnotic effect of the essential oil from the leaves of Myrtus communis on mice. *Nat Sci Sleep*. 2016 Aug 16;8:267-75.
[3200] Lamborn LL. Modern soaps, candles and glycerin: A practical manual of modern methods of utilization of fats and oils in the manufacture of soaps and candles, and of the recovery of glycerin. Library of the University of Wisconsin.
[3201] Oyen LP, Dung NX. Plant resources of South-East Asia. 1999. Backhyus, Leiden.
[3202] Kim NH, Hyun SH, Jin CH, et al. Pretreatment with 1,8-cineole potentiates thioacetamide-induced hepatotoxicity and immunosuppression. *Arch Pharm Res*. 2004 Jul;27(7):781-9.
[3203] Carson CF, Hammer KA, Riley TV. Antimicrobial activity of Agonis fragrans oil. In: Robinson CJ. A New Essential oil – Agonis fragrans. Chemotype Selection and Evaluation.
[3204] Dunstan J, Hale J, Lehman H, et al. Effects of Agonis fragrans oil on mononuclear cell immune responses. In: Robinson CJ. A New Essential oil – Agonis fragrans. Chemotype Selection and Evaluation.
[3205] Suhail MM, Wu W, Cao A, et al. Boswellia sacra essential oil induces tumor cell-specific apoptosis and suppresses tumor aggressiveness in cultured human breast cancer cells. *BMC Complement Altern Med*. 2011;11:129.
[3206] Ni X, Suhail MM, Yang Q, et al. Frankincense essential oil prepared from hydrodistillation of Boswellia sacra gum resin induces human pancreatic cancer cell death in cultures and in xenograft murine model. *BMC Complement Altern Med*. 2012;12:253.
[3207] Al-Harrasi A, Al-Saidi S. Phytochemical analysis of the essential oil from botanically certified oleogum resin of Boswellia sacra (Omani Luban). *Molecules*. 2008;13(9):2181-89.
[3208] Woolley CL, Suhail MM, Smith BL, et al. Chemical differentiation of Boswellia sacra and Boswellia carterii oils by gas chromatography and chiral gas chromatography-mass spectrometry. *J Chromatogr A*. 212 Oct 26;1261:158-63.
[3209] Kamatou GP, Viljoen A, van Vuuren S. Variation in essential oil composition of Boswellia carterii Birdw. and its antimicrobial activity. *African J Trad Complement Altern Med*. 2008.
[3210] Van Vuuren SF, Kamatou GPP, Viljoen AM. Volatile composition and antimicrobial activity of twenty commercial frankincense essential oils samples. *S African J Botany*. 2012;76:686-91.
[3211] Basar S. Phytochemical investigations on Boswellia species. Available at: http://www.chemie.uni-hamburg.de/bibliothek/2005/DissertationBasar.pdf.
[3212] Al-Saidi S, Rameshkumar KB, Hisham A, et al. Composition and antibacterial activity of the essential oils of four commercial grades of Omani luban, the ole-gum resin of Boswellia sacra Flueck. *Chem Biodiv*. 2012 Mar;9(3):615-24.
[3213] Hall L. Chemotaxinomical investigation of frankincense producing Boswellia spp. from Somalia and a quest for quality standards. Thesis. University of Strathclyde.
[3214] Camarda L, Talya D, Stefano VD, et al. Chemical composition and antimicrobial activity of some oleogum resin essential oils from Boswellia Spp. (Burseraceae). *Annali Di Chimica*. 2007;97:837.
[3215] Bekana D, Kenede Tesfahun, Assefa M, et al. Comparative Phytochemical Analyses of Resins of Boswellia Species (B. papyrifera (Del.) Hochst., B. neglecta S. Moore, and B. rivae Engl.) from Northwestern, Southern, and Southeastern Ethiopia. *Analytic Chem*. 2014;2014:374678.
[3216] Gupta M, Rout PK, Misra LN, et al. Chemical composition and bioactivity of Boswellia serrata Roxb. essential oil in relation to geographical variation. *Plant Biosys*. 2016 Jun;21:1-7.
[3217] Singh B, Kumar R, Bhandari S, et al. Volatile constituents of natural Boswellia serrata oleo-gum-resin and commercial samples. *Flavour Frag J*. 2007 Mar;22(2):145-47.
[3218] Niebler J, Buettner A. Frankincense Revisited, Part I: Comparative Analysis of Volatiles in Commercially Relevant Boswellia Species. *Chemistry & Biodiversity*. 2016;13(5):613-29.
[3219] Frank A, Unger M. Analysis of frankincense from various Boswellia species with inhibitory activity on human drug metabolizing cytochrome P450 enzymes using liquid chromatography mass spectrometry after automated on-line extraction. *J Chromatogra A*. 2006 Apr 21;1112(1-2):255-62.
[3220] Dozmorov MG, Yang Q, Wu W, et al. Differential effects of selective frankincense (Ru Ziang) essential oil versus non-selective sandalwood (Tan Xiang) essential oil on cultured bladder cancer cells: a microarray and bioinformatics study. *Chin Med*. 2014 Jul;9:18.
[3221] Frank MB, Yang Q, Osban J, et al. Frankincense oil derived from Boswellia carteri induces tumor cell specific cytotoxicity. *BMC Complement Altern Med*. 2009;9:6.
[3222] Ni X, Suhail MM, Yang Q, et al. Frankincense essential oil prepared from hydrodistillation of Boswellia sacra gum resins induces human pancreatic cancer cell death in cultures and in a xenograft murine model. *BMC Complement Altern Med*. 2012 Dec;12:253.
[3223] Suhail MM, Wu W, Cao A, et al. Boswellia sacra essential oil induces tumor cell-specific apoptosis and suppresses tumor aggressiveness in cultured human breast cancer cells. *BMC Complement Alt Med*. 2011;11:29.
[3224] Al-Harrasi A, Ali L, Hussain J, et al. Analgesic effects of crude extracts and fractions of Omani frankincense obtained from traditional medicinal plant Boswellia sacra on animal models. *Asian Pac J Trop Med*. 2014 Sep;7S1:S485-90.
[3225] Chang SY. Effects of aroma hand massage on pain, state anxiety and depression in hospice patients with terminal cancer. *Taehan Kanho Hakhoe Chi*. 2008 Aug;38(4):493-502.
[3226] Dyer J, Cleary L, McNeill S, et al. The use of aromasticks to help with sleep problems: A patient experience survey. *Complement Ther Clin Pract*. 2016 Feb;22:51-8.
[3227] Blain EJ, Ali AY, Duance VC. Boswellia frereana (frankincense) suppresses cytokine-induced matrix metalloproteinase expression and production of proinflammatory molecules in articular cartilage. *Phytother Res*.2010 jun;24(6):905-12.
[3228] Al-Saidi S, Rameshkumar KB, Hisham A, et al. Composition and antibacterial activity of the essential oils of four commercial grades of Omani luban, the ole-gum resin of Boswellia sacra Flueck. *Chem Biodiv*. 2012 Mar;9(3):615-24.
[3229] Gupta M, Rout PK, Misra LN, et al. Chemical composition and bioactivity of Boswellia serrata Roxb. essential oil in relation to geographical variation. *Plant Biosys*. 2016 Jun;21:1-7.
[3230] Choi WS, Kwon MH, Kim YC. Inhibition effects of frankincense oil on skin aging (I): Focused on gross examination. *J Environ Toxicol*. 2008;23(20:119-27.
[3231] Mikhaeil BR, Maatooq GT, Badira FA, et al. Chemistry and immunomodulatory activity of frankincense oil. *Z Naturforsch C*. 2003 Mar-Apr;58(3-4):230-38.
[3232] Hou Q, He WJ, Hao HJ, et al. The four-herb Chinese medicine ANBP enhances wound healing and inhibits scar formation via bidirectional regulation of transformation growth factor pathway. *PloS One*.2014 Dec 9;9(12):e112274.
[3233] Lee DH, Kim SS, Seong S, et al. A case of metastatic bladder cancer in both lungs treated with Korean medicine therapy alone. *Case Rep Oncol*. 2014 Jul;7(2):534-40.
[3234] Rufino AT, Ribeiro M, Judas F, et al. Anti-inflammatory and chondroprotective activity of (+)-α-pinene: structural and enantiomeric selectivity. *J Nat Prod*. 2014 Feb;77(2):264-69.
[3235] Neves A, Rosa S, Goncalves J, et al. Screening of five essential oils for identification of potential inhibitors of IL-1- induced Nf-kappaB activation and NO production in human chondrocytes: characterization of the inhibitory activity of alpha-pinene. *Planta Med*. 2010 Feb;76(3):303-08.
[3236] Zaki AA, Hashish NE, Amer MA, et al. Cardioprotective and antioxidant effects of oleogum resin "Olibanum" from Bos Boswellia carteri Birdw. (Bursearceae). *Chin J Nat Med*.2014 May;12(5):345-50.
[3237] de Rapper S, Van Vuuren SF, Kamatou GP, et al. The additive and synergistic antimicrobial effects of select frankincense and myrrh oils—a combination from the pharaonic pharmacopoeia. *Lett Appl Microbiol*. 2012 Apr;54(4):352-58.
[3238] Schillaci D, Arizza V, Dayton T, et al. In vitro anti-biofilm activity of Boswellia spp. oleogum resin essential oils. *Lett Appl Microbiol*. 2008 Nov;47(5):433-8.

3239 Yagi S, Babiker R, Tzanova T, et al. Chemical composition, antiproliferative, antioxidant and antibacterial activities of essential oils from aromatic plants growing in Sudan. *Asian Pac J Trop Med.* 2016 Aug;9(8):763-70.

3240 Sadhasivam S, Palanivel S, Ghosh S. Synergistic antimicrobial activity of Boswellia serrata Roxb. ex Colebr. (Burseraceae) essential oil with various azoles against pathogens associated with skin, scalp & nail infections. *Lett Appl Microbiol.* 2016 Dec;63(6):495-501.

3241 Nikolic M, Smiljkovic M, Markovic T, et al. Sensitivity of clinical isolates of Candida to essential oils from Burseraceae family. *EXCLI J.* 2016 Apr 19;15:280-9.

3242 S K, Kujur A, Patel L, et al. Assessment of toxicity and biochemical mechanisms underlying the insecticidal activity of chemically characterized Boswellia carterii essential oil against insect pest of legume seeds. *Pestic Biochem Physiol.* 2017 Jun;139:17-23.

3243 Ren P, Ren X, Cheng L, et al. Frankincense, pine needle and geranium essential oils suppress tumor progression through the regulation of the AMPK/mTOR pathway in breast cancer. *Oncol Rep.* 2018 Jan;39(1):129-137.

3244 Reis D, Jones TT. Frankincense Essential Oil as a Supportive Therapy for Cancer-Related Fatigue: A Case Study. *Holist Nurs Pract.* 2018 May/Jun;32(3):140-142.

3245 Al-Otaibi WA, Alkhatib MH, Wali AN, et al. Cytotoxicity and apoptosis enhancement in breast and cervical cancer cells upon coadministration of mitomycin C and essential oils in nanoemulsion formulations. *Biomed Pharmacother.* 2018 Oct;106:946-955.

3246 Hakkim FL, Bakshi HA, Khan S, et al. Frankincense essential oil suppresses melanoma cancer through down regulation of Bcl-2/Bax cascade signaling and ameliorates heptotoxicity via phase I and II drug metabolizing enzymes. *Oncotarget.* 2019 May 28;10(37):3472-3490.

3247 Okano S, Honda Y, Kodama T, et al. The Effects of Frankincense Essential Oil on Stress in Rats. *J Oleo Sci.* 2019;68(10):1003-1009.

3248 Monzote L, Herrera I, Satyal P, et al. In-Vitro Evaluation of 52 Commercially-Available Essential Oils Against Leishmania amazonensis. Molecules. 2019 Mar 20;24(7):24071248.

3249 Di Stefano V, Schillaci D, Cusimano MG, et al. In Vitro Antimicrobial Activity of Frankincense Oils from Boswellia sacra Grown in Different Locations of the Dhofar Region (Oman). *Antibiotics (Basel).* 2020 Apr 20;9(4).

3250 Hosny EN, Elhadidy ME, Sawie HG, et al. Effect of frankincense oil on the neurochemical changes induced in rat model of status epilepticus. *Clin Phytosci.* 2020;6(3):1189.

3251 Aldahlawi AM, Alzahrani AT, Elshal MF. Evaluation of immunomodulatory effects of Boswellia sacra essential oil on T-cells and dendritic cells. *BMC Complement Med Ther.* 2020 Nov 19;20(1):352.

3252 TC Erciyes University. Massage With Frankincense and Myrrh Oil in Treating Chronic Low Back Pain. The Effects of Massage With Frankincense and Myrrh Oil in Treating Chronic Low Back Pain: A Randomized Controlled Trial. Available at: https://ichgcp.net/clinical-trials-registry/NCT04494165. Accessed April 7, 2021.

3253 Dudek-Wicher R, Paleczny J, Kowalska-Krochmal B, et al. Activity of Liquid and Volatile Fractions of Essential Oils against Biofilm Formed by Selected Reference Strains on Polystyrene and Hydroxyapatite Surfaces. *Pathogens.* 2021 Apr 23;10(5):515.

3254 Becer E, Kabadayi H, Baser KHC, et al. Boswellia sacra essential oil manages colon cancer stem cells proliferation and apoptosis: a new perspective for cure. *J Essent Oil Res.* 2021;1(33):53-62.

3255 Ayub MA, Hanif MA, Blanchfield J, et al. Chemical composition and antimicrobial activity of Boswellia serrata oleo-gum-resin essential oil extracted by superheated steam. *Nat Prod Res.* 2022 Feb 24:1-6.

3256 Xia D, Lou W, Fung KM, et al. Cancer Chemopreventive Effects of Boswellia sacra Gum Resin Hydrodistillates on Invasive Urothelial Cell Carcinoma: Report of a Case. *Integr Cancer Ther.* 2017 Dec;16(4):605–611.

3257 Fung KM, Suhail MM, McClendon B, et al. Management of basal cell carcinoma of the skin using frankincense (Boswellia sacra) essential oil: A case study. Available at: https://essentialoilscienceeducation.org/management-of-basal-cell-carcinoma-of-the-skin-using-frankincense-boswellia-sacra-essential-oil-a-case-study/.

3258 Almutairi MBF, Alrouji M, Almuhanna Y, et al. In-Vitro and In-Vivo Antibacterial Effects of Frankincense Oil and Its Interaction with Some Antibiotics against Multidrug-Resistant Pathogens. *Antibiotics (Basel).* 2022 Nov 10;11(11):1591.

3259 Bogavac MA, Perić TM, Mišković J, et al. Antimicrobial and Toxic Effects of Boswellia serrata Roxb. and Mentha piperita Linn. Essential Oils on Vaginal Inhabitants. *Medicines (Basel).* 2022 Dec 9;9(12):62.

3260 Azzazy HME, Abdelnaser A, Al Mulla H, et al. Essential Oils Extracted from Boswellia sacra Oleo Gum Resin Loaded into PLGA-PCL Nanoparticles: Enhanced Cytotoxic and Apoptotic Effects against Breast Cancer Cells. *ACS Omega.* 2022 Dec 19;8(1):1017-1025.

3261 Borotova P, Cmikova N, Galovicova L, et al. Antioxidant, Antimicrobial, and Anti-Insect Properties of Boswellia carterii Essential Oil for Food Preservation Improvement. *Horticulturae.* 2023 Mar;9(3):333.

3262 Servi H, Demir U, Servi EY, et al. Antiproliferative and Antibacterial Activities of Four Commercial Essential Oil Samples from Boswellia carteri, B. serrata, and two chemotypes of Canarium luzonicum. *J Essent Oil Bearing Plants.* 2023. Online ahead of print.

3263 Wu Y, Wang Y, Li ZH, et al. Composition of the essential oil from Alpinia galanga rhizomes and its bioactivity on Lasioderma serricorne. *Bull Insectol.* 2014;67(2):247-54.

3264 Mallavarapu GR, Rao L, Ramesh S, et al. Composition of the Volatile Oils of Alpinia galanga Rhizomes and Leaves from India. *J Essent Oil Res.* 2002 Nov;14(6):397-99.

3265 Nampoothiri SV, Menon AN, Esakkidurai T, et al. Essential Oil Composition of Alpinia calcarata and Alpinia galanga Rhizomes-A Comparative Study. 2016 Jan;19(1):82-87.

3266 Padalia RC, Verma RS, Sundaresan V, et al. Chemical diversity in the Genus Alpinia (Zingiberaceae): Comparative composition of four Alpinia species grown in Northern India. *Chem Biodiv.* 2010 Apr;7(8):2076-87.

3267 Rana VS, Verdeguer M, Blazquez A. GC and GC/MS Analysis of the Volatile Constituents of the Oils of Alpinia galanga (L.) Willd and A. officinarum Hance Rhizomes. *J Essent Oil Res.* 2010 Nov-Dec;22:521-24.

3268 Raina AP, Walia S, Abraham Z, et al. Essential oil constituents of rhizome oil of Alpinia species from South India. *Planta Med.* 2009;75:PI40.

3269 Zhang J, Dou J, Zhang J, et al. Chemical composition and antioxidant properties of the essential oil and methanol extracts of rhizoma Alpinia officinarum from China in vitro. *African J Biotech.* 2010 Jul;9(27):4264-71.

3270 Indrayan AK, Garg SN, Rathi AK, et al. Chemical composition and antimicrobial activity of the essential oil of Alpinia officinarum rhizome. *Indian J Chem Section B.* 2007 Dec;46(12):2060-63.

3271 Indrayan AK, Kurian A, Tyagi PK, et al. Comparative chemical study of two varities of attractive medicinal plant Kaempferia galanga Linn. *Nat Product Radiance.* 2007;6(4):327-33.

3272 Kumar A. Chemical composition of essential oil isolated from the rhizomes of Kaempferia galanga L. *Int J Pharma Bio Sci.* 2014 Jan;5(1):(P)225-31.

3273 Tewtrakul S, Yuenyongsawad S, Kummee S, et al. Chemical components and biological activities of volatile oil of Kaempferia galanga Linn. *Songklanakarin J Sci Technol.* 2005;27(Suppl. 2):503-07.

3274 Wong KC, Ong KS, Lim CL. Composition of the essential oil of rhizomes of Kaempferia galanga L. *Flavour Frag J.* 1992;7:263-66.

3275 Liu ZC, Liang Y, Shi Wp, et al. Repellent and Insecticidal Effects of the Essential Oil of Kaempferia galanga Rhizomes to Liposcelis bostrychophila (Psocoptera: Liposcelidae) *J Economic Entomol.* 2014 Aug;107(4):1706-12.

3276 Abdullah F, Subramanian P2, Ibrahim H, et al. Chemical composition, antifeedant, repellent, and toxicity activities of the rhizomes of galangal, Alpinia galanga against Asian subterranean termites, Coptotermes gestroi and Coptotermes curvignathus (Isoptera: Rhinotermitidae). *J Insect Sci.* 2015 Feb 16;15:175.

3277 Jirovetz L, Buchbauer G, Shafi MP, et al. Analysis of the essential oils of the leaves, stems, rhizomes and roots of the medicinal plant Alpinia galanga from southern India. *Acta Pharm.* 2003 Jun;53(2):73-81.

3278 Craig JO. Poisoning by the volatile oils in childhood. *Arch Dis Child.* 1953;28:259-67.

3279 Melis K. Bochner A, Janssens G. Accidental nasal eucalyptol and menthol instillation. *Eur J Pediatr.* 1989 Aug;148(8)786-7.

3280 Day LM, Ozanne-Smith J, Parsons BJ, et al. Eucalyptus oil poisoning among young children: mechanisms of access and the potential prevention. *Aust N Z J Public Health.* 1997 Jun;21(3):297-302.

3281 Chandar SD, Prashanti M, Kumar CL, et al. Eucalyptus Oil-Induced Seizures in Children: A Single-Center Prospective Study. *Cureus.* 2021 Mar 25;13(3):e14109.

3282 Khine H, Weiss D, Graber N, et al. A cluster of children with seizures caused by camphor poisoning. *Pediatrics.* 2009 May;123(5):1269-72.

3283 Michiels EA, Mazor SS. Toddler with seizures due to ingesting camphor at an Indian celebration. *Pediatr Emerg Care.* 2010 Aug;26(8):574-75.

3284 Koren G. Medications which can kill a toddler with one tablet or teaspoonful. *J toxicol Clin toxicol.* 1993;31(3):407- 13.

3285 Flaman Z, Pellechia-Clarke S, Bailey B, et al. Unintentional exposure of young children to camphor and eucalyptus oils. *Paediatr Child Health.* 2001 Feb;6(2):80-83.

3286 Burkhard PR, Burkhardt K, Haenggeli CA, et al. Plant-induced seizures: reappearance of an old problem. *J Neurol.* 1999 Aug;246(8):667-70.

3287 Waldman N. Seizure caused by dermal application of over-the-counter eucalyptus oil head lice preparation. *Clin Toxicol (Phila).* 2011 Oct;49(8):750-1.

3288 Craig JO. Poisoning by the volatile oils in childhood. *Arch Dis Child.* 1953;28:259-67.

3289 Newall CA, Anderson LA, Phillipson JD. "Herbal Medicines: A Guide for Health-care Professionals." London: The Pharmaceutical Press, 1996, 108.

3290 European Medicines Agency. Community herbal monograph on Eucalyptus globulus Labill., Eucalyptus polybractea R.T. Baker and/or Eucalyptus smithii R.T. Baker, aetheroleum. 2013 Jun. Available at: http://www.ema.europa.eu/docs/en_GB/document_library/Herbal_-_Community_herbal_monograph/2013/07/WC500147008.pdf

3291 Fischer JH, Dethlefsen U. Efficacy of cineole in patients suffering from acute bronchitis: a placebo-controlled double-blind trial. *Cough.* 2013; 9: 25.

3292 Worth W, Dethlefsen U. Patients with asthma benefit from concomitant therapy with cineole: a placebo-controlled, double-blind trial. *J Asthma.* 2012 Oct;49(8):849-53.

3293 Day LM, Ozanne-Smith J, Parsons BJ, et al. Eucalyptus oil poisoning among young children: mechanisms of access and the potential prevention. *Aust N Z J Public Health.* 1997 Jun;21(3):297-302.

3294 Myott E. Case of eucalyptus poisoning. *Brit M J.* 1906;1:558.

3295 Hindle RC. Eucalyptus oil ingestion. *N Z Med J.* 1994 May 11;107(977)185-6.

3296 Tibballs J. Clinical effects and management of eucalyptus oil ingestion in infants and small children. *Med J Aust.* 1995 Aug;163(4):177-80.

3297 Waldman W, Barwina M, Sein Anand J. Accidental ontoxication with eucalyptus oil—a case report. *Przegl Lek.* 2011;68(8):555-6.

3298 Day LM, Ozanne-Smith J, Parsons BJ, et al. Eucalyptus oil poisoning among young children: mechanisms of access and the potential prevention. *Aust N Z J Public Health.* 1997 Jun;21(3):297-302.

3299 De Vincenzi M, Silano M, De Vincenzi A, et al. Constituents of aromatic plants: eucalyptol. *Fitoterapia.* 2002 Jun;73(3):269-75.

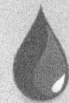

[3300] Manoguerra AS, Erdman AR, Wax PM, et al. Camphor poisoning: an evidence-based practice guideline for out-of- hospital management. *Clin Toxicol (Phila)*.2006;44(4):357-70.

[3301] Gibson DE, Moore GP, Pfaff JA. Camphor ingestion. *Am J Emerg Med*. 1989 Jan;7(1):41-43.

[3302] Koppel C, Martends F, Schirop T, et al. Hemoperfusion in acute camphor poisoning. *Intensive Care Med*. 1988;14(4):431-33.

[3303] Olowe SA, Ransome-Kuti O. The risk of jaundice in glucose-6-phosphate dehydrogenase deficient babies exposed to menthol. *Acta Paediatr Scand*. 1980 May;69(3):341-5.

[3304] Dillon Remy M, Manning Alleyne P, Bratt DE, et al. Neonatal jaundice at Port-of-Spain General Hospital abstract. *West Indian Med J*. 1987;36(Suppl):28.

[3305] Lamborn LL. Modern soaps, candles and glycerin: A practical manual of modern methods of utilization of fats and oils in the manufacture of soaps and candles, and of the recovery of glycerin. Library of the University of Wisconsin.

[3306] Oyen LP, Dung NX. Plant resources of South-East Asia. 1999. Backhyus, Leiden.

[3307] Kim NH, Hyun SH, Jin CH, et al. Pretreatment with 1,8-cineole potentiates thioacetamide-induced hepatotoxicity and immunosuppression. *Arch Pharm Res*. 2004 Jul;27(7):781-9.

[3308] Gray AM, Flatt PR. Antihyperglycemic actions of Eucalyptus globulus (Eucalyptus) are associated with pancreatic and extra pancreatic effects in mice. *J Nutr*. 1998 Dec;128(12):2319–23.

[3309] Basak SS, Candan F. Effect of Laurus nobilis L. Essential Oil and its Main Components on α-glucosidase and Reactive Oxygen Species Scavenging Activity. *Iran J Pharm Res*. 2013 Spring;12(2):367-79.

[3310] Fathiazad F, Mazandarani M, Hamedeyazdan. Phytochemical analysis and antioxidant activity of Hyssopus officinalis L. from Iran. *Adv Pharm Bull*. 2011 Dec;1(2):63–67.

[3311] Jori A, Bianchetti A, Prestini PE, et al. Effect of eucalyptol (1,8-cineole) on the metabolism of other drugs in rats and in man. *Eur J Pharmacol*. 1970;9(3):362-66.

[3312] de Sousa DP, Raphael E, Brocksom U, et al. Sedative effect of monoterpene alcohols in mice: A preliminary screening. *Verlag der Zeitschrift fur Naturforschung*. 2007;62c:563-66.

[3313] Huang J, Wang S, Luo X, et al. Cinnamaldehyde reduction of platelet aggregation and thrombosis in rodents. *Thromb Res*. 2007;119(3):337–42.

[3314] Ballabeni V, Tognolini M, Bertoni S, et al. Antiplatelet and antithrombotic activities of essential oil from wild Ocotea quixos (Lam.) Kostern. (Lauraceae) calices from Amazonian Ecuador. *Pharmacol Res*. 2007 Jan;55(1):23–30.

[3315] Noro T, Miyase T, Kuroyanagi M, et al. Monoamine Oxidase Inhibitor from the Rhizomes of Kaempferia galanga L. *Chem Pharm Bull*. 1983;31(8):2708-11.

[3316] Noro T, Miyase T, Kuroyanagi M, et al. Monoamine Oxidase Inhibitor from the Rhizomes of Kaempferia galanga L. *Chem Pharm Bull*. 1983;31(8):2708-11.

[3317] Indrayan AK, Garg SN, Rathi AK, et al. Chemical composition and antimicrobial activity of the essential oil of Alpinia officinarum rhizome. *Indian J Chem Section B*. 2007 Dec;46(12):2060-63.

[3318] Tadtong S, Watthanachaiyingcharoen R, Kamkaen N. Antimicrobial constituents and synergism effect of the essential oils from Cymbopogon citratus and Alpinia galanga. *Nat Prod Commun*. 2014 Feb;9(2):277-80.

[3319] Tadtong S, Watthanachaiyingcharoen R, Kamkaen N. Antimicrobial constituents and synergism effect of the essential oils from Cymbopogon citratus and Alpinia galanga. *Nat Prod Commun*. 2014 Feb;9(2):277-80.

[3320] Tadtong S, Watthanachaiyingcharoen R, Kamkaen N. Antimicrobial constituents and synergism effect of the essential oils from Cymbopogon citratus and Alpinia galanga. *Nat Prod Commun*. 2014 Feb;9(2):277-80.

[3321] Tewtrakul S, Yuenyongsawad S, Kummee S, et al. Chemical components and biological activities of volatile oil of Kaempferia galanga Linn. *Songklanakarin J Sci Technol*. 2005;27(Suppl. 2):503-07.

[3322] Tewtrakul S, Yuenyongsawad S, Kummee S, et al. Chemical components and biological activities of volatile oil of Kaempferia galanga Linn. *Songklanakarin J Sci Technol*. 2005;27(Suppl. 2):503-07.

[3323] Zhang J, Dou J, Zhang J, et al. Chemical composition and antioxidant properties of the essential oil and methanol extracts of rhizoma Alpinia officinarum from China in vitro. *African J Biotech*. 2010 Jul;9(27):4264-71.

[3324] Tewtrakul S, Yuenyongsawad S, Kummee S, et al. Chemical components and biological activities of volatile oil of Kaempferia galanga Linn. *Songklanakarin J Sci Technol*. 2005;27(Suppl. 2):503-07.

[3325] Wu Y, Wang Y, Li ZH, et al. Composition of the essential oil from Alpinia galanga rhizomes and its bioactivity on Lasioderma serricorne. *Bull Insectol*. 2014;67(2):247-54.

[3326] Abdullah F, Subramanian P2, Ibrahim H, et al. Chemical composition, antifeedant, repellent, and toxicity activities of the rhizomes of galangal, Alpinia galanga against Asian subterranean termites, Coptotermes gestroi and Coptotermes curvignathus (Isoptera: Rhinotermitidae). *J Insect Sci*. 2015 Feb 16;15:175.

[3327] Liu ZC, Liang Y, Shi Wp, et al. Repellent and Insecticidal Effects of the Essential Oil of Kaempferia galanga Rhizomes to Liposcelis bostrychophila (Psocoptera: Liposcelidae). *J Economic Entomol*. 2014 Aug;107(4):1706-12.

[3328] Sutthanont N, Choochote W, Tuetun B, et al. Chemical composition and larvicidal activity of edible plant-derived essential oils against the pyrethroid-susceptible and -resistant strains of Aedes aegypti (Diptera: Culicidae). *J Vector Ecol*. 2010 Jun;35(1):106-15.

[3329] Misni N, Nor ZM, Ahmad R. New Candidates for Plant-Based Repellents Against Aedes aegypti. *J Am Mosq Control Assoc*. 2016 Jun;32(2):117-23.

[3330] Chansang A, Champakaew D, Junkum A, et al. Synergy in the adulticidal efficacy of essential oils for the improvement of permethrin toxicity against Aedes aegypti L. (Diptera: Culicidae). *Parasit Vectors*. 2018 Jul 13;11(1):417.

[3331] Kanani MR, Rahiminejad MR, Sonboli A, et al. Chemotaxonomic significance of the essential oils of 18 Ferula species (Apiaceae) from Iran. *Chem Biod*. 2011 Mar;8(3):503-17.

[3332] Aromatics International. Galbanum - Ferula galbaniflua. Available at: http://www.aromaticsinternational.com/products/essential-oils/galbanum.

[3333] Mahboubi M, Kazempour N, Mahboubi M. Antimicrobial activity of Rosemary, Fennel and Galbanum essential oil against clinical isolates of Staphylococcus aureus. *Biharean Biologist*. 2011;5(1):4-7.

[3334] Sadraei H, Asghari GR, Hajhashemi V, et al. Spasmolytic activity of essential oil and various extracts of Ferula gummosa Boiss. On ileum contractions. *Phytomedicine*. 2001 Sep;8(5):370-76.

[3335] Eftekhar F, Yousefzadi M, Borhani K. Antibacterial activity of the essential oil from Ferula gummosa seed. *Fitoterapia*. 2004 Dec;75(7-8):758-59.

[3336] Ghasemi Y, Faridi P, Mehregan I, et al. Ferula gummosa fruits: An aromatic antimicrobial agent. *Chem Nat Constituents*. 2005 May;41(13):311-14.

[3337] Abedi D, Jalali M, Sadeghi N. Compositional and antimicrobial activity of oleogumresin of Ferula gumosa Bioss. Essential oil using Alamar Blue™. *Res Pharm Sci*. 2008 Apr;3(1):41-45.

[3338] Afshar FF, Saffarian P, Hosseini HM, et al. Antimicrobial effects of Ferula gummosa Boiss gum against extended-spectrum β-lactamase producing Acinetobacter clinical isolates. *Iran J Microbiol*. 2016 Aug;8(4):263-273.

[3339] Andrade MA, Azevedo CD, Motta FN, et al. Essential oils: in vitro activity against Leishmania amazonensis, cytotoxicity and chemical composition. *BMC Complement Altern Med*. 2016 Nov 8;16(1):444.

[3340] Satarian F, Hosseini HM, Ghadaksaz A, et al. Multi-Drug Resistant Clinical Pseudomonas aeruginosas Inhibited by Ferula gummosa Boiss. *Recent Pat Antiinfect Drug Discov*. 2018;13(1):89-99.

[3341] Tabari MA, Youssefi MR, Nasiri M, et al. Towards green drugs against cestodes: Effectiveness of Pelargonium roseum and Ferula gummosa essential oils and their main component on Echinococcus granulosus protoscoleces. *Vet Parasitol*. 2019 Feb;266:84-87.

[3342] Najafi MN, Arianmehr A, Sani AM. Preparation of Barije (Ferula Gummosa) Essential Oil-Loaded Liposomes and Evaluation of Physical and Antibacterial Effect on Escherichia Coli O157:H7. *J Food Prot*. 2020 Mar 1;83(3):511-517.

[3343] Pavela R, Morshedloo MR, Lupidi G, et al. The volatile oils from the oleo-gum-resins of Ferula assa-foetida and Ferula gummosa: A comprehensive investigation of their insecticidal activity and eco-toxicological effects. *Food Chem Toxicol*. 2020 Apr 2;140:111312.

[3344] Bashiri-Nahnjeh M, Sarihi A, Ebadi A, et al. In silico molecular modeling, neuro-behavioral profile, and toxicity assessment of the essential oil of Ferula gummosa Boiss. as an anti-seizure agent. *J Ethnopharmacol*. 2023 Jun 12;309:116347.

[3345] Chekki RZ, Snoussi A, Hamrouni I, et al. Chemical composition, antibacterial and antioxidant activities of Tunisian garlic (Allium sativum) essential oil and ethanol extract. *Mediterranean J Chem*. 2014;3(4):947-56.

[3346] Dziri S, Casabianca H, Hanchi B, et al. Composition of garlic essential oil (Allium sativum L.) as influenced by drying method. *J Essent Oil Res*. 2014;26(2):91-96.

[3347] Mnayer D, Fabiano-Tixier AS, Petitcolas E, et al. Chemical Composition, Antibacterial and Antioxidant Activities of Six Essentials Oils from the Alliaceae Family. *Molecules*. 2014;19:20034-53.

[3348] Rao PGP, Rao LJ, Raghavan B. Chemical composition of essential oils fog ariel (Allium sativum L.). *J Spices Aromatic Crops*. 1999;8(1):41-47.

[3349] ZKimbaris AC, Siatis NG, Pappas CS, et al. Quantitative analysis of garlic (Allium sativum) oil unsaturated acyclic components using FT-Raman spectroscopy. 2006;94:287-95.

[3350] Farnsworth NR, Bingel AS, Cordell GA, et al. Potential value of plants as sources of new antifertility agents I. *J Pharm Sci*. 1975 Apr;64(4):535-98.

[3351] Mennella JA, Johnson A, Beauchamp GK. Garlic ingestion by pregnant women alters the odor of amniotic fluid. *Chem Senses*. 1995;20:207-9.

[3352] Ziaei S, Hantoshzadeh S, Rezasoltani P, et al. The effect of garlic tablet on plasma lipids and platelet aggregation in nulliparous pregnants at high risk of preeclampsia. *Eur J Obstet Gynecol Reprod Biol*. 2001;99:201-6.

[3353] Soltani PR. Preeclampisia is an important complication of pregnancy which can result in morbidity and mortality in mother, fetus and the neonate. *J Med Counc Islamic Repub Iran*. 2005;23(3):319.

[3354] Kim SH, Lee IC, Baek HS, et al. Induction of cytochrome P450 3A1 expression by diallyl disulfide: protective effects against cyclophosphamide-induced embryo-fetal developmental toxicity. *Food Chem Toxicol*. 2014 Jul;69:312-9.

[3355] El Sayyad HI, Abou_El-Naga AM, Gadallah AA, et al. Protective effects of Allium sativum against defects of hypercholesterolemia on pregnant rats and their offspring. *Int J Clin Exp Med*. 2010; 3(2): 152–163.

[3356] Mennella JA, Beauchamp GK. The effects of repeated exposure to garlic-flavored milk on the nursling's behavior. *Pediatr Res*. 1993;34:805-8.

[3357] Mennella JA, Beauchamp GK. Maternal diet alters the sensory qualities of human milk and the nursling's behavior. *Pediatrics*. 1991;88:737-44.

[3358] [No authors listed]. The effect of essential oil of garlic on hyperlipemia and platelet aggregation--an analysis of 308 cases. Cooperative Group for Essential Oil of Garlic. *J Tradit Chin Med*. 1986 Jun;6(2):117-20.

[3359] Barrie SA, Wright JV, Pizzorno JE. Effects of Garlic Oil on Platelet Aggregation, Serum Lipids and Blood Pressure in Humans. *J Orthomolecular Med*. 1987;2(1):15-21.

[3360] Makheja AN, Vanderhoek JY, Bailey JM. Inhibition of platelet aggregation and thromboxane synthesis by onion and garlic. *Lancet*. 979 Apr 7;1(8119):781.

[3361] Boullin DJ. Garlic as a platelet inhibitor. *Lancet*. 1981 Apr 4;1(8223):776-7.

3362 Fenwick GR, Hanley AB. The genus Allium--Part 3. *Crit Rev Food Sci Nutr*. 1985;23(1):1-73.

3363 Lawson LD, Hughes BG. Characterization of the formation of allicin and other thiosulfinates from garlic. *Planta Med*. 1992 Aug;58(4):345-50.

3364 Bordia A, Verma SK, Srivastava KC. Effect of garlic (Allium sativum) on blood lipids, blood sugar, fibrinogen and fibrinolytic activity in patients with coronary artery disease. *Prostaglandins Leukot Essent Fatty Acids*. 1998 Apr;58(4):257-63.

3365 Bordia A. Effect of garlic on human platelet aggregation in vitro. *Atherosclerosis*. 1978 Aug;30(4):355-60.

3366 Qi R, Liao F, Inoue K, et al. Inhibition by diallyl trisulfide, a garlic component, of intracellular Ca(2+) mobilization without affecting inositol-1,4, 5-trisphosphate (IP(3)) formation in activated platelets. *Biochem Pharmacol*. 2000 Nov 15;60(10):1475-83.

3367 Ariga T, Takeda A, Teramoto S, et al. Inhibition Site of Methylallyl Trisulfide: A Volatile Oil Component of Garlic, in the Platelet Arachidonic Acid Cascade. *Food Factors for Cancer Prevention*. 1997:231-34.

3368 Lawson LD, Ransom DK, Hughes BG. Inhibition of whole blood platelet-aggregation by compounds in garlic clove extracts and commercial garlic products. *Thromb Res*. 1992 Jan 15;65(2):141-56.

3369 Lai YS, Chen WC, Ho CT, et al. Garlic essential oil protects against obesity-triggered nonalcoholic fatty liver disease through modulation of lipid metabolism and oxidative stress. *J Agric Food Chem*. 2014 Jun 25;62(25):5897-906.

3370 Taubert D, Glöckner R, Müller D, et al. The garlic ingredient diallyl sulfide inhibits cytochrome P450 2E1 dependent bioactivation of acrylamide to glycidamide. *Toxicol Lett*. 2006 Jun 20;164(1):1-5.

3371 Davenport DM, Wargovich MJ. Modulation of cytochrome P450 enzymes by organosulfur constituents from garlic. *Food Chem Toxicol*. 2005 Dec;43(12):1753-62.

3372 Fisher CD, Augustine LM, Maher JM, et al. Induction of drug-metabolizing enzymes by garlic and allyl sulfide compounds via activation of constitutive androstane receptor and nuclear factor E2-related factor 2. *Drug Metab Dispos*. 2007 Jun;35(6):995-1000.

3373 Lii CK, Tsai CW, Wu CC. Garlic allyl sulfides display differential modulation of rat cytochrome P450 2B1 and the placental form glutathione S-transferase in various organs. *J Agric Food Chem*. 2006 Jul 12;54(14):5191-6.

3374 Johnson S. Supercritical Essential Oils. 2017. Scott A Johnson Professional Writing Services, LLC: Orem, Utah.

3375 Pyun MS, Shin S. Antifungal effects of the volatile oils from Allium plants against Trichophyton species and synergism of the oils with ketoconazole. *Phytomedicine*. 2006 Jun;13(6):394-400.

3376 Scheman A, Gupta S. Photoallergic contact dermatitis from diallyl disulfide. *Contact Dermatitis*. 2001 Sep;45(3):179.

3377 Alvarez MS, Jacobs S, Jiang SB, Brancaccio RR, et al. Photocontact allergy to diallyl disulfide. *Am J Contact Dermat*. 2003 Sep;14(3):161-5.

3378 Lee TY, Lam TH. Contact dermatitis due to topical treatment with garlic in Hong Kong. *Contact Dermatitis*. 1991 Mar;24(3):193-6.

3379 Cabanillas M, Fernandez-Redondo V, Toribio J. Allergic contact dermatitis to plants in a Spanish dermatology department: a 7-year review. *Contact Dermatitis*. 2006 Aug;55(2):84-91.

3380 Lai YS, Chen WC, Ho CT, et al. Garlic essential oil protects against obesity-triggered nonalcoholic fatty liver disease through modulation of lipid metabolism and oxidative stress. *J Agric Food Chem*. 2014 Jun 25;62(25):5897-906.

3381 Jan CR, Lo HR, Chen CY, et al. Effect of allyl sulfides from garlic essential oil on intracellular ca2+ levels in renal tubular cells. *J Nat Prod*. 2012 Dec 28;75(12):2101-7.

3382 Tsai HH, Lin HW, Chen YL, et al. A review of potential harmful interactions between anticoagulant/antiplatelet agents and Chinese herbal medicines. *PLoS One*. 2013 May 9;8(5):e64255.

3383 Chekki RZ, Snoussi A, Hamrouni I, et al. Chemical composition, antibacterial and antioxidant activities of Tunisian garlic (Allium sativum) essential oil and ethanol extract. *Mediterranean J Chem*. 2014;3(4):947-56.

3384 Mnayer D, Fabiano-Tixier AS, Petitcolas E, et al. Chemical Composition, Antibacterial and Antioxidant Activities of Six Essentials Oils from the Alliaceae Family. *Molecules*. 2014;19:20034-53.

3385 Casella S, Leonardi M, Melai B, et al. The role of diallyl sulfides and dipropyl sulfides in the in vitro antimicrobial activity of the essential oil of garlic, Allium sativum L., and leek, Allium porrum L. *Phytother Res*. 2013 Mar;27(3):380-3.

3386 El-Sayed HS, Chizzola R, Ramadan AA, et al. Chemical composition and antimicrobial activity of garlic essential oils evaluated in organic solvent, emulsifying, and self-microemulsifying water based delivery systems. *Food Chem*. 2017 Apr 15;221:196-204.

3387 Kocić-Tanackov S, Dimić G, Lević J, et al. Effects of onion (Allium cepa L.) and garlic (Allium sativum L.) essential oils on the Aspergillus versicolor growth and sterigmatocystin production. *J Food Sci*. 2012 May;77(5):M278-84.

3388 Kloucek P, Smid J, Flesar J, et al. In vitro inhibitory activity of essential oil vapors against Ascosphaera apis. *Nat Prod Commun*. 2012 Feb;7(2):253-6.

3389 Pyun MS, Shin S. Antifungal effects of the volatile oils from Allium plants against Trichophyton species and synergism of the oils with ketoconazole. *Phytomedicine*. 2006 Jun;13(6):394-400.

3390 Ndoye Foe FM, Tchinang TF, Nyegue AM, et al. Chemical composition, in vitro antioxidant and anti-inflammatory properties of essential oils of four dietary and medicinal plants from Cameroon. *BMC Complement Altern Med*. 2016 Apr 7;16:117.

3391 Barrie SA, Wright JV, Pizzorno JE. Effects of Garlic Oil on Platelet Aggregation, Serum Lipids and Blood Pressure in Humans. *J Orthomolecular Med*. 1987;2(1):15-21.

3392 [No authors listed]. The effect of essential oil of garlic on hyperlipemia and platelet aggregation--an analysis of 308 cases. Cooperative Group for Essential Oil of Garlic. *J Tradit Chin Med*. 1986 Jun;6(2):117-20.

3393 Bordia A. Effect of garlic on blood lipids in patients with coronary heart disease. *Am J Clin Nutr*. 1981 Oct;34(10):2100-3.

3394 Bordia A, Verma SK, Srivastava KC. Effect of garlic (Allium sativum) on blood lipids, blood sugar, fibrinogen and fibrinolytic activity in patients with coronary artery disease. *Prostaglandins Leukot Essent Fatty Acids*. 1998 Apr;58(4):257-63.

3395 Saxena KK, Gupta B, Kulshrestha VK, et al. Effect of garlic pretreatment on isoprenaline-induced myocardial necrosis in albino rats. *Indian J Physiol Pharmacol*. 1980 Jul-Sep;24(3):233-6.

3396 Bordia A, Verma SK. Effect of garlic feeding on regression of experimental atherosclerosis in rabbits. *Artery*. 1980;7(5):428-37.

3397 Singh TU, Kumar D, Tandan SK, et al. Inhibitory effect of essential oils of Allium sativum and Piper longum on spontaneous muscular activity of liver fluke, Fasciola gigantica. *Exp Parasitol*. 2009 Dec;123(4):302-8.

3398 Lai YS, Chen WC, Ho CT, et al. Garlic essential oil protects against obesity-triggered nonalcoholic fatty liver disease through modulation of lipid metabolism and oxidative stress. *J Agric Food Chem*. 2014 Jun 25;62(25):5897-906.

3399 Jung HY, Lee KY, Yoo DY, et al. Essential oils from two Allium species exert effects on cell proliferation and neuroblast differentiation in the mouse dentate gyrus by modulating brain-derived neurotrophic factor and acetylcholinesterase. *BMC Complement Altern Med*. 2016 Nov 3;16(1):431.

3400 Chekki RZ, Snoussi A, Hamrouni I, et al. Chemical composition, antibacterial and antioxidant activities of Tunisian garlic (Allium sativum) essential oil and ethanol extract. *Mediterranean J Chem*. 2014;3(4):947-56.

3401 Mnayer D, Fabiano-Tixier AS, Petitcolas E, et al. Chemical Composition, Antibacterial and Antioxidant Activities of Six Essentials Oils from the Alliaceae Family. *Molecules*. 2014;19:20034-53.

3402 Ndoye Foe FM, Tchinang TF, Nyegue AM, et al. Chemical composition, in vitro antioxidant and anti-inflammatory properties of essential oils of four dietary and medicinal plants from Cameroon. *BMC Complement Altern Med*. 2016 Apr 7;16:117.

3403 Misharina TA, Terenina MB, Krikunova NI. [Antioxidant properties of essential oils]. *Prikl Biokhim Mikrobiol*. 2009 Nov-Dec;45(6):710-6.

3404 Kiralan M, Bayrak A, Abdulaziz OF, et al. Essential oil composition and antiradical activity of the oil of Iraq plants. *Nat Prod Res*. 2012;26(2):132-9.

3405 Park IK, Shin SC. Fumigant activity of plant essential oils and components from garlic (Allium sativum) and clove bud (Eugenia caryophyllata) oils against the Japanese termite (Reticulitermes speratus Kolbe). *J Agric Food Chem*. 2005 Jun 1;53(11):4388-92.

3406 Zhao NN, Zhang H, Zhang XC, et al. Evaluation of acute toxicity of essential oil of garlic (Allium sativum) and its selected major constituent constituents against overwintering Cacopsylla chinensis (Hemiptera: Psyllidae). *J Econ Entomol*. 2013 Jun;106(3):1349-54.

3407 Martinez-Velazquez M, Rosario-Cruz R, Castillo-Herrera G, et al. Acaricidal effect of essential oils from Lippia graveolens (Lamiales: Verbenaceae), Rosmarinus officinalis (Lamiales: Lamiaceae), and Allium sativum (Liliales: Liliaceae) against Rhipicephalus (Boophilus) microplus (Acari: Ixodidae). *J Med Entomol*. 2011 Jul;48(4):822-7.

3408 Machial CM, Shikano I, Smirle M, et al. Evaluation of the toxicity of 17 essential oils against Choristoneura rosaceana (Lepidoptera: Tortricidae) and Trichoplusia ni (Lepidoptera: Noctuidae). *Pest Manag Sci*. 2010 Oct;66(10):1116-21.

3409 Park IK, Choi KS, Kim DH, et al. Fumigant activity of plant essential oils and components from horseradish (Armoracia rusticana), anise (Pimpinella anisum) and garlic (Allium sativum) oils against Lycoriella ingenua (Diptera: Sciaridae). *Pest Manag Sci*. 2006 Aug;62(8):723-8.

3410 Ranger CM, Reding ME, Oliver JB, et al. Acute toxicity of plant essential oils to scarab larvae (Coleoptera: Scarabaeidae) and their analysis by gas chromatography-mass spectrometry. *J Econ Entomol*. 2013 Feb;106(1):159-67.

3411 Kimbaris AC, Kioulos E, Koliopoulos G, et al. Coactivity of sulfide ingredients: a new perspective of the larvicidal activity of garlic essential oil against mosquitoes. *Pest Manag Sci*. 2009 Mar;65(3):249-54.

3412 Plata-Rueda A, Martinez LC, Santos MHD, et al. Insecticidal activity of garlic essential oil and their constituents against the mealworm beetle, Tenebrio molitor Linnaeus (Coleoptera: Tenebrionidae). *Sci Rep*. 2017 Apr 20;7:46406.

3413 Mendoza-Juache A, Aranda-Romo S, Bermeo-Escalona JR, et al. The essential oil of Allium sativum as an alternative agent against Candida isolated from dental prostheses. *Rev Iberoam Micol*. 2017 Jul-Sep;34(3):158-164.

3414 Mossa AH, Afia SI, Mohafrash SMM, et al. Formulation and characterization of garlic (Allium sativum L.) essential oil nanoemulsion and its acaricidal activity on eriophyid olive mites (Acari: Eriophyidae). *Environ Sci Pollut Res Int*. 2018 Apr;25(11):10526-10537.

3415 Muturi EJ, Ramirez JL, Zilkowski B, et al. Ovicidal and Larvicidal Effects of Garlic and Asafoetida Essential Oils Against West Nile Virus Vectors. *J Insect Sci*. 2018 Mar 1;18(2).

3416 Li WR, Ma YK, Shi QS, et al. Diallyl disulfide from garlic oil inhibits Pseudomonas aeruginosa virulence factors by inactivating key quorum sensing genes. *Appl Microbiol Biotechnol*. 2018 Sep;102(17):7555-7564.

3417 Yang C, Li L, Yang L1, Lü H, et al. Anti-obesity and Hypolipidemic effects of garlic oil and onion oil in rats fed a high-fat diet. *Nutr Metab (Lond)*. 2018 Jun 20;15:43.

3418 Feng J, Shi W, Miklossy J, et al. Identification of Essential Oils with Strong Activity against Stationary Phase Borrelia burgdorferi. *Antibiotics (Basel)*. 2018 Oct 16;7(4).

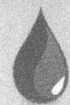

[3419] Alkhatib MH, Al-Otaibi WA, Wali AN. Antineoplastic activity of mitomycin C formulated in nanoemulsions-based essential oils on HeLa cervical cancer cells. *Chem Biol Interact.* 2018 Aug 1;291:72-80.
[3420] Huang YJ, Lu KH, Lin YE, et al. Garlic Essential Oil Mediates Acute and Chronic Mild Stress-Induced Depression in Rats via Modulation of Monoaminergic Neurotransmission and Brain-Derived Neurotrophic Factor Levels. *Food Funct.* 2019 Dec 11;10(12):8094-8105.
[3421] Krzyśko-Łupicka T, Sokół S, Piekarska-Stachowiak A. Evaluation of Fungistatic Activity of Eight Selected Essential Oils on Four Heterogeneous Fusarium Isolates Obtained From Cereal Grains in Southern Poland. *Molecules.* 2020 Jan 10;25(2):292.
[3422] Bedini S, Guarino S, Echeverria MC, et al. Allium sativum, Rosmarinus officinalis, and Salvia officinalis Essential Oils: A Spiced Shield Against Blowflies. *Insects.* 2020 Feb 25;11(3):143.
[3423] Paraskevis D, Kostaki EG, Magiorkinis G, et al. Full-genome evolutionary analysis of the novel coronavirus (2019-nCoV) rejects the hypothesis of emergence as a result of a recent recombination event. Infect Genet Evol. 2020;79: 104212.
[3424] Wang X, Xu W, Hu G, et al. SARS-CoV-2 infects T lymphocytes through its spike protein-mediated membrane fusion. *Cell Mol Immunol.* 2020 Apr 7. [Epub ahead of print]
[3425] National Center for Biotechnology Information. 6LU7: The crystal structure of COVID-19 main protease in complex with an inhibitor N3. Available at: https://www.ncbi.nlm.nih.gov/Structure/pdb/6LU7. Accessed April 9, 2020.
[3426] Thuy BTP, My TTA, Hai NTT, et al. Investigation into SARS-CoV-2 Resistance of Compounds in Garlic Essential Oil. *ACS Omega.* 2020 Mar 31. [Epub ahead of print]
[3427] Shaghadi N. Molecular Docking study of novel COVID-19 Protease with low risk Terpenoides Compounds of Plants. *ChemRxiv.* 2020 Apr 3;14:28.
[3428] Sharma AD, Kaur I. Eucalyptol (1,8 cineole) from Eucalyptus Essential Oil a Potential Inhibitor of COVID 19 Corona Virus Infection by Molecular Docking Studies. *Preprints.* 2020:2020030455.
[3429] My TTA, Loan HTP,Hai NTT, et al. Evaluation of the Inhibitory Activities of COVID-19 of Melaleuca cajuputi Oil Using Docking Simulation. *ChemistrySelect.* 2020 Jun 8;5(21):6312-6320.
[3430] Kumar, KJS, Vani MG, Wang CS, et al. Geranium and Lemon Essential Oils and Their Active Compounds Downregulate Angiotensin-Converting Enzyme 2 (ACE2), a SARS-CoV-2 Spike Receptor-Binding Domain, in Epithelial Cells. *Plants.* 2020;9(6):770.
[3431] Panikar S, Shoba G, Arum M, et al. Essential oils as an effective alternative for the treatment of COVID-19: Molecular interaction analysis of protease (M pro) with pharmacokinetics and toxicological properties. *J Infect Public Health.* 2021 Feb 10;14(5):601-610.
[3432] Demirci F, Karadag AE, Biltekin SN, et al. In vitro ACE2 and 5-LOX Inhibition of Rosmarinus officinalis L. Essential Oil and its Major Component 1,8-Cineole. *Rec Nat Prod.* 2021. Online ahead of print.
[3433] Zareie A, Soleimani D, Askari G, et al. Cinnamon: A Promising Natural Product Against COVID-19. *Adv Exp Med Biol.* 2021;1327:191-195.
[3434] Torres Neto L, Monteiro MLG, Galvan D, et al. An Evaluation of the Potential of Essential Oils against SARS-CoV-2 from In Silico Studies through the Systematic Review Using a Chemometric Approach. *Pharmaceuticals (Basel).* 2021 Nov 10;14(11):1138.
[3435] Taysi S, Algburi FS, Mohammed Z, et al. Thymoquinone: A Review of Pharmacological Importance, Oxidative Stress, COVID-19, and Radiotherapy. *Mini Rev Med Chem.* 2022 Jan 4. Online ahead of print.
[3436] Costa RBGM, Martins RMG, de Lima GS, et al. Molecular Docking in silico Analysis of Brazilian Essential Oils Against Host Targets and SARS-CoV-2 Proteins. *J Braz Chem Soc.* 2022;00(00):1-17.
[3437] Teymoori S. Evaluation of the effects of peppermint on improving the function of the respiratory system in COVID-19 infection. *5th Int Conf Agric Sci Med Plants Tradit Med.* 2022 Mar. Available at: https://www.sid.ir/FileServer/SE/693E20220502.
[3438] Torres Neto L, Monteiro MLG, Fernández-Romero J, et al. Essential oils block cellular entry of SARS-CoV-2 delta variant. *Sci Rep.* 2022 Nov 30;12(1):20639.
[3439] Wang Y, Wu Y, Fu P, et al. Effect of garlic essential oil in 97 patients hospitalized with covid-19: A multi-center experience. *Pak J Pharm Sci.* 2022 Jul;35(4):1077-1082.
[3440] Somrani M, Ingles MC, Debbabi H, et al. Garlic, Onion, and Cinnamon Essential Oil Antibiofilms' Effect Against Listeria monocytogenes. *Foods.* 2020 May 4;9(5):E567.
[3441] Mizan MFR, Ashrafudoulla M, Hossain MI, et al. Effect of Essential Oils on Pathogenic and Biofilm-Forming Vibrio parahaemolyticus Strains. *Biofouling.* 2020 Apr;36(4):467-478.
[3442] Agassi SFT, Yeh TM, Chang CD, et al. Potentiation of Differentiation and Apoptosis in a Human Promyelocytic Leukemia Cell Line by Garlic Essential Oil and Its Organosulfur Compounds. *Anticancer Res.* 2020 Nov;40(11):6345-6354.
[3443] Demeter S, Lebbe O, Hecq F, et al. Insecticidal Activity of 25 Essential Oils on the Stored Product Pest, Sitophilus granaries. *Foods.* 2021 Jan 20;10(2):E200.
[3444] Heimesaat MM, Mousavi S, Weschja D, et al. Garlic Essential Oil as Promising Option for the Treatment of Acute Campylobacteriosis-Results from a Preclinical Placebo-Controlled Intervention Study. *Microorganisms.* 2021 May 25;9(6):1140.
[3445] Yoshioka Y, Matsumura S, Morimoto M, et al. Inhibitory Activities of Sulfur Compounds in Garlic Essential Oil against Alzheimer's Disease-Related Enzymes and Their Distribution in the Mouse Brain. *J Agric Food Chem.* 2021 Aug 30. Online ahead of print.
[3446] Herrera-Calderon O, Chacaltana-Ramos LJ, Huayanca-Gutierrez IC, et al. Chemical Constituents, In Vitro Antioxidant Activity and In Silico Study on NADPH Oxidase of Allium sativum L. (Garlic) Essential Oil. *Antioxidants (Basel).* 2021 Nov 20;10(11):1844.
[3447] Mondéjar-López M, Rubio-Moraga A, López-Jimenez AJ, et al. Chitosan nanoparticles loaded with garlic essential oil: A new alternative to tebuconazole as seed dressing agent. *Carbohydr Polym.* 2022 Feb 1;277:118815.
[3448] Gong X, Su X, Liu H. Diallyl Trisulfide, the Antifungal Component of Garlic Essential Oil and the Bioactivity of Its Nanoemulsions Formed by Spontaneous Emulsification. *Molecules.* 2021 Nov 26;26(23):7186.
[3449] Hsu CN, Hou CY, Chang-Chien GP, et al. Maternal Garlic Oil Supplementation Prevents High-Fat Diet-Induced Hypertension in Adult Rat Offspring: Implications of H2S-Generating Pathway in the Gut and Kidneys. *Mol Nutr Food Res.* 2021 Jun;65(11):e2001116.
[3450] Elnabawy EM, Hassan S, Taha EA. Repellent and Toxicant Effects of Eight Essential Oils against the Red Flour Beetle, Tribolium castaneum Herbst (Coleoptera: Tenebrionidae). *Biology (Basel).* 2021 Dec 21;11(1):3.
[3451] Morshdy AEMA, El-Tahlawy AS, Qari SH, et al. Antibiofilms' Activity of Garlic and Thyme Essential Oils against Salmonella typhimurium. *Molecules.* 2022 Mar 28;27(7):2182.
[3452] Polito F, Amato G, Caputo L, et al. Chemical Composition and Agronomic Traits of Allium sativum and Allium ampeloprasum Leaves and Bulbs and Their Action against Listeria monocytogenes and Other Food Pathogens. *Foods.* 2022 Mar 29;11(7):995.
[3453] El-Zehery HRA, Zaghloul RA, Abdel-Rahman HM, et al. Novel strategies of essential oils, chitosan, and nano- chitosan for inhibition of multi-drug resistant: E. coli O157:H7 and Listeria monocytogenes. *Saudi J Biol Sci.* 2022 Apr;29(4):2582-2590.
[3454] Galisteo A, González-Coloma A, Castillo P, et al. In vitro anti-clostridial action and potential of the spice herbs essential oils to prevent biofilm formation of hypervirulent Clostridioides difficile strains isolated from hospitalized patients with CDI. *Anaerobe.* 2022 Jun 14;76:102604.
[3455] Aleksic A, Stojanovic-Radic Z, Harmanus C, et al. In vitro anti-clostridial action and potential of the spice herbs essential oils to prevent biofilm formation of hypervirulent Clostridioides difficile strains isolated from hospitalized patients with CDI. *Anaerobe.* 2022 Auf;76:102604.
[3456] Ibrar M, Ayub Y, Nazir R, et al. Garlic and ginger essential oil-based neomycin nano-emulsions as effective and accelerated treatment for skin wounds' healing and inflammation: In-vivo and in-vitro studies. *Saudi Pharm J.* 2022 Dec;30(12):1700-1709.
[3457] Rubiolo P, Matteodo M, Bicchi C, et al. Chemical and biomolecular characterization of Artemisia umbelliformis Lam., an important ingredient of the Alpine liqueur "Genepi." *J Agric Food Chem.* 2009 May 13;57(9):3436-43.
[3458] Bicchi C, Mario Nano G, Frattini C. On the composition of essential oils of Artemisia genipi Weber and Artemisia umbelliformis Lam. *Zeitschrift für Lebensmittel-Untersuchung und Forschung.* 1982 May;175(3):182-85.
[3459] Mucciarelli M, Caramiello R, Maffei ME, et al. Essential Oils from some Artemisia species growing spontaneously in North-West Italy. *Flavour Frag J.* 1995;10:25-32.
[3460] Haliciglu O, Astarcioglu G, Yaprak I, et al. Toxicity of Salvia officinalis in a newborn and a child: an alarming report. *Pediatr Neurol.* 2011 Oct;45(4):259-60.
[3461] Lachenmeier DW, Walch SG. Epileptic seizure caused by accidental ingestion of sage (Salvia officinalis L.) oil in children: a rare, exceptional case or a threat to public health. *Pediatr Neurol.* 2012 Mar;46(3):201.
[3462] Stafstrom CE. Seizures in a 7-month-old child after exposure to the essential plant oil thuja. *Pediatr Neurol.* 2007 Dec;37(6):446-8.
[3463] da Silva Costa KC, Bexerra SB, Norte CM, et al. Medicinal plants with teratogenic potential: current considerations. *Braz J Pharm Sci.* 2012;48(3):427-33.
[3464] Brinker F. Herb Contraindications and Drug Interactions. 2nd ed. Sandy, OR. Eclectic Medical Publications. 1998.
[3465] European Medicines Agency. Public statement on the use of herbal medicinal products containing thujone. Available at: http://www.ema.europa.eu/docs/en_GB/document_library/Public_statement/2011/02/WC500102294.pdf.
[3466] Millet Y, Jouglard J, Steinmetz MD, et al. Toxicity of some essential plant oils. Clinical and experimental study. *Clin Toxicol.* 1981 Dec;18(12):1485-98.
[3467] Cristovao L, Carvalho F, Bastos MDL, et al. Hepatotoxicity of an essential oil of Salvia officinalis L.: an in vitro study using freshly isolated rat hepatocytes. *Congress Biomarkers.* 2001 Sep:165.
[3468] Millet Y, Jouglard J, Steinmetz MD, et al. Toxicity of some essential plant oils. Clinical and experimental study. *Clin Toxicol.* 1981 Dec;18(12):1485–98.
[3469] Burkhard PR, Burkhardt K, Haenggeli CA, et al. Plant-induced seizures: reappearance of an old problem. *J Neurol.* 1999 Aug;246(8):667–70.
[3470] Weisbord SD, Soule JB, Kimmel PL. Poison on line-acute renal failure caused by oil of wormwood purchased through the internet. *N Engl J Med.* 1997;337:825-7.
[3471] Arditti J, Faizende JJ, Bernard J, et al. Trois observations d'intoxication par des essences végétales convulsivantes. *Ann Med.* 1978;17:371-74.
[3472] Burkhard PR, Burkhardt K, Haenggeli CA, et al. Plant-induced seizures: reappearance of an old problem. *J Neurol.* 1999 Aug;246(8):667-70.
[3473] Waldman N. Seizure caused by dermal application of over-the-counter eucalyptus oil head lice preparation. *Clin Toxicol (Phila).* 2011 Oct;49(8):750-1.
[3474] Craig JO. Poisoning by the volatile oils in childhood. *Arch Dis Child.* 1953;28:259-67.
[3475] Narayan S, Singh N. Camphor poisoning-An unusual cause of seizure. *Med J Armed Forces India.* 2012 Jul;68(3):252-53.
[3476] Chanaranaj KJ, G MV, S M. Camphor poisoning in a child. *Natl Med J India.* 2013 Jan-Feb;26(1):60.
[3477] Perry NB, Anderson RE, Brennan NJ, et al. Essential oils from dalmatian sage (Salvia officinalis L.) variations among individuals, plant parts, seasons, and sites. *J Agric Food Chem.* 1999;47:2048-54.
[3478] Millet Y, Jouglard J, Steinmetz MD, et al. Toxicity of some essential plant oils. Clinical and experimental study. *Clin Toxicol.* 1981 Dec;18(12):1485-98.

3479 Abass K, Reponen P, Mattila S, et al. Metabolism of α-thujone in human hepatic preparations in vitro. *Xenobiotica*. 2011 Feb;41(2):101-11.

3480 Frohne D. Giftpflanzen: Cupressaceae. Stuttgart: Wissenschaftliche Verlagsgesellschaft mbH; 1997. pp. 153–6.

3481 Dolan LC, Matulka RA, Burdock GA. Naturally Occurring Food Toxins. *Toxins (Basel)*. 2010 Sep;2(9):2289–2332.

3482 United States National Toxicology Program (NTP). Alpha-Thujone. Dec 10, 1997. Available at: http://ntp.niehs.nih.gov/index.cfm?objectid=03DB8C36-E7A1-9889-3BDF8436F2A8C51F.

3483 Boukhris M, Simmonds, Sayadi S, et al. Chemical composition and biological activities of polar extracts and essential oil of rose-scented geranium, Pelargonium graveolens. *Phytother Res.* 2013 Aug;27(8):1206-13.

3484 Bouzenna H, Krichen L. Pelargonium graveolens L'Her. and Artemesia arborescens L. essential oils: chemical composition, antifungal activity against Rhizoctonia solani and insecticidal activity against Rhyzopertha dominica. *Nat Prod Res.* 213;27(9):841-46.

3485 Boukhatem MN, Kameli A, Saidi F. Essential oil of Algerian rose-scented geranium (Pelargonium graveolens): Chemical composition and antimicrobial activity against food spoilage pathogens. *Food Control.* 2013 Nov;34(1):208- 13.

3486 Verma RS, Verma RK, Yadav AK, et al. Changes in the essential oil composition of rose-scented geranium (Pelargonium graveolens L'Herit. ex Ait) due to date of transplanting under hill conditions of Uttarakhand. *Indian J Nat Prod Res.* 2010 Sep;1(3):367-70.

3487 Dyubeni L, Mayekiso B, Magwa ML. A comparative study on essential oil yield and composition of rose-scented geranium (P.c.v. Rose) commercially grown on three different sites of the Amathole region in the Eastern Cape, South Africa. *African J Agric Res.* 2012 Nov;7(43):5842-48.

3488 Ben Slima A, Ali MB, Barkallah M, et al. Antioxidant properties of Pelargonium graveolens L'Her essential oil on the reproductive damage induce by deltamethrin in mice as compared to alpha-tocopherol. *Lipids Health Dis.* 2013 Mar;12:30.

3489 Sea KA, Kim H, Ku HY, et al. The monoterpenoids citral and geraniol are moderate inhibitors of CYP2B6 hydroxylase activity. *Chem Biol Interact.* 2008 Aug 11;174(3):141-6.

3490 Boukhris M, Bouaziz M, Feki I, et al. Hypoglycemic and antioxidant effects of leaf and essential oil of Pelargonium graveolens L'Her. in alloxan induced diabetic rats. *Lipids Health Dis.* 2012 Jun 26;11:81.

3491 Rosato A, Piarulli M, Corbo F, et al. In vitro synergistic antibacterial action of certain combinations of gentamicin and essential oils. *Curr Med Chem.* 2010;17(28):3289-95.

3492 Malik T, Singh P, Pant S, et al. Potentiation of antimicrobial activity of ciproloxacin by Pelargonium graveolens essential oil against selected uropathogens. *Phytother Res.* 2011 Aug;25(8):1225-28.

3493 Rosato A, Vitali C, Gallo D, et al. The inhibition of Candida species by selected essential oils and their synergism with Aamphotericin B. *Phytomedicine.* 2008 Aug;15(8):635-38.

3494 Rosato A, Vitali C, De Laurentis N, et al. Antibacterial effect of some essential oils administered alone or in combination with Norfloxacin. *Phytomedicine.* 2007 Nov;14(11):727-32.

3495 Shin S, Lim S. Antifungal effects of herbal essential oils alone or in combination with ketoconazole against Trichophyton spp. *J Appl Microbiol.* 2004;97(6):1289-96.

3496 Shin S. Anti-aspergillus activities of plant essential oils and their combination effects with ketoconazole or amphotericin B. *Arch Pharm Res.* 2003 May;26(5):389-93.

3497 Hagvall L. Cytochrome P450-mediated activation of the fragrance constituent geraniol forms potent contact allergens. *Tox Appl Pharm.* 2008 Dec;233(2):308-13.

3498 Fayed SA. Antioxidant and anticancer activities of Citrus reticulata (Petitgrain Mandarin) and Pelargonium graveolens (Geranium) essential oils. *Res J Agric Biol Sci.* 2009;5(5):740-47.

3499 Ben Slima A, Ali MB, Barkallah M, et al. Antioxidant properties of Pelargonium graveolens L'Her essential oil on the reproductive damage induce by deltamethrin in mice as compared to alpha-tocopherol. *Lipids Health Dis.* 2013 Mar;12:30.

3500 Ghannadi A, Bagherinejad M. Abedi D, et al. Antibacterial activity and composition of essential oils from Pelargonium graveolens L'Her and Vitex agnus-castus L. *Iran J Microbiol.* 2012 Dec;4(4):171-76.

3501 Rafiq R, Hayek SA, Anyanwu U, et al. Antibacterial and Antioxidant Activities of Essential Oils from Artemisia herba-alba Asso., Pelargonium capitatum × radens and Laurus nobilis L. *Foods.* 2016 Apr 11;5(2).

3502 Malik T, Singh P, Pant S, et al. Potentiation of antimicrobial activity of ciproloxacin by Pelargonium graveolens essential oil against selected uropathogens. *Phytother Res.* 2011 Aug;25(8):1225-28.

3503 Rosato A, Vitali C, De Laurentis N, et al. Antibacterial effect of some essential oils administered alone or in combination with Norfloxacin. *Phytomedicine.* 2007 Nov;14(11):727-32.

3504 Shin S, Lim S. Antifungal effects of herbal essential oils alone or in combination with keoconazole against Trichophyton spp. *J Appl Microbiol.* 2004;97(6):1289-96.

3505 Rosato A, Vitali C, Gallo D, et al. The inhibition of Candida species by selected essential oils and their synergism with Aamphotericin B. *Phytomedicine.* 2008 Aug;15(8):635-38.

3506 Rosaro A, Piarulli M, Corbo F, et al. In vitro synergistic antibacterial action of certain combination of gentamicin and essential oils. *Curr Med Chem.* 2010;17(28):3289-95.

3507 Shin S. Anti-aspergillus activities of plant essential oils and their combination effects with ketoconazole or amphotericin B. *Arch Pharm Res.* 2003 May;26(5):389-93.

3508 Boukhris M, Bouaziz M, Feki I, et al. Hypoglycemic and antioxidant effects of leaf essential oil of Pelargonium graveolens L'Her, in alloxan induced diabetic rats. *Lipids Health Dis.* 2012 Jun 26;11:81.

3509 Suijun W, Zhen Y, Ying G, et al. A role for trans-caryophyllene in the moderation of insulin secretion. *Biochem Biophys Res Commun.* 2014 Feb;444(4):451-54.

3510 Sabzghabaee AM, Shirdare Z, Ebadian B, et al. Clinical evaluation of the essential oil of Pelargonium graveolens for the treatment of denture stomatitis. *Dent Res J (Isfahan).* 2011 Dec;8(Suppl 1):S105-08.

3511 Kang HY, Na SS, Kim YK. Effects of oral care with essential oil on improvement in oral health status of hospice patients. *J Korean Acad Nurs.* 2010 Aug;40(4):473-81.

3512 Maruyamma N, Takizawa T, Ishibashi H, et al. Protective activity of geranium oil and its component, geraniol, in combination with vaginal washing against vaginal candidiasis in mice. *Biol Pharm Bull.* 2008 Aug;31(8):1501-06.

3513 Inouye S, Uchida K, Nishiyama Y, et al. Combined effect of heat, essential oils and salt on fungicidal activity against Trichiphyton mentagrophytes in a foot bath. *Nihon Ishinjin Gakkai Zasshi.* 2007;48(1):27-36.

3514 Maruyama N, Sekimoto Y, Ishibashi H, et al. Suppression of neutrophil accumulation in mice by cutaneous application of geranium essential oil. *J Inflamm (Lond).* 2005 Feb 10;2(1):1.

3515 Abe S, Maruyama N, Hayama K, et al. Suppression of neutrophil recruitment in mice by geranium essential oil. *Mediators Inflamm.* 2004 Feb;13(1):21-24.

3516 Boukhris M, Simmonds MS, Sayadi S, et al. Chemical composition and biological activities of polar extracts and essential oil of rose-scented geranium, Pelargonium graveolens. *Phytother Res.* 2013 Aug;27(8):1206-13.

3517 Sun W, Xu Z, Wang C, et al. Study on antioxidant activity of essential oils and its monomer from Pelargonium graveolens. *Zhong Yao Cai.* 2005 Feb;28(2):87-89.

3518 Brito RG, Santos PL, Prado DS, et al. Citronellol reduces orofacial nociceptive behaviors in mice - evidence of involvement of retrosplenial cortex and periaqueductal grey areas. *Basic Clin Pharmacol Toxicol.* 2013 Apr;112(4):215- 21.

3519 Bastos JF, Noreira IJ, Ribeiro TP, et al. Hypotensive and vasorelaxant effects of citronellol, a monoterpene alcohol, in rats. *Basic Clin Pharamacol Toxicol.* 2010 Apr;106(4):331-37.

3520 Nozaki Y. [Clinical studies of essential oil of Pelargonium Graveolens]. *Aroma Res.* 2011;2(1):61-65.

3521 Mizuno D, Konoha-Mizuno K, Mori M, et al. An in vitro system comprising immortalized hypothalamic neuronal cells (GT1-7 Cells) for evaluation of the neuroendocrine effects of essential oils. *Evid Based Complement Alternat Med.* 2015;2015:343942.

3522 Tabanca N, Wang M, Avonto C, et al. Bioactivity-guided investigation of geranium essential oils as natural tick repellents. *J Agric Food Chem.* 2013 May;61(17):4101-07.

3523 Domingos Tda S, Braga EM. Massage with aromatherapy: effectiveness on anxiety of users with personality disorders in psychiatric hospitalization. *Rev Esc Enferm USP.* 2015 May-Jun;49(3):450-6.

3524 Pazinato R, Volpato A, Baldissera MD, et al. In vitro effect of seven essential oils on the reproduction of the cattle tick Rhipicephalus microplus. *J Adv Res.* 2016 Nov;7(6):1029-1034.

3525 Fang F, Candy K, Melloul E, et al. In vitro activity of ten essential oils against Sarcoptes scabiei. *Parasit Vectors.* 2016 Nov 22;9(1):594.

3526 Boukhatem MN, Kameli A, Ferhat MA, et al. Rose geranium essential oil as a source of new and safe anti-inflammatory drugs. *Libyan J Med.* 2013 Oct 7;8:22520.

3527 Shinohara K, Doi H, Kumagai C, et al. Effects of essential oil exposure on salivary estrogen concentration in perimenopausal women. *Neuro Endocrinol Lett.* 2017 Jan;37(8):567-572.

3528 Shakeri G, Jamshidi A, Khanzadi S, et al. Modeling of Salmonella typhimurium growth under the effects of Carum copticum essential oil, temperature, pH and inoculum size. *Vet Res Forum.* 2017 Winter;8(1):59-65.

3529 Ouedrhiri W, Balouiri M, Bouhdid S, et al. Antioxidant and antibacterial activities of Pelargonium asperum and Ormenis mixta essential oils and their synergistic antibacterial effect. *Environ Sci Pollut Res Int.* 2018 Oct;25(30):29860-29867.

3530 Abd-Rabou A, Edris AE. Evaluation of the Antiproliferative Activity of Some Nanoparticulate Essential Oils Formulated in Microemulsion on Selected Human Carcinoma Cell Lines. *Curr Clin Pharmacol.* 2017;12(4):231-244.

3531 Essid R, Hammami M, Gharbi D, et al. Antifungal mechanism of the combination of Cinnamomum verum and Pelargonium graveolens essential oils with fluconazole against pathogenic Candida strains. *Appl Microbiol Biotechnol.* 2017 Sep;101(18):6993-7006.

3532 Mahboubi M, Taghizadeh M, Khamechian T, et al. The Wound Healing Effects of Herbal Cream Containing Oliveria Decumbens and Pelargonium Graveolens Essential Oils in Diabetic Foot Ulcer Model. *World J Plast Surg.* 2018 Jan;7(1):45–50.

3533 Simoes BM, Kohler B, Clarke RB, et al. Estrogenicity of essential oils is not required to relieve symptoms of urogenital atrophy in breast cancer survivors. *Ther Adv Med Oncol.* 2018;10:1758835918766189.

3534 Gucwa K, Milewski S, Dymerski T, et al. Investigation of the Antifungal Activity and Mode of Action of Thymus vulgaris, Citrus limonum, Pelargonium graveolens, Cinnamomum cassia, Ocimum basilicum, and Eugenia caryophyllus Essential Oils. *Molecules.* 2018 May 8;23(5).

3535 Ralambondrainy M, Belarbi E, Viranaicken W, et al. In vitro comparison of three common essential oils mosquito repellents as inhibitors of the Ross River virus. *PLoS One.* 2018 May 17;13(5):e0196757.

3536 Lohani A, Mishra AK, Verma A, et al. Cosmeceutical potential of geranium and calendula essential oil: Determination of antioxidant activity and in vitro sun protection factor. *J Cosmet Dermatol.* 2019 Apr;18(2):550-557.

3537 Montibeler J, Domingos TDS, Braga EM, et al. Effectiveness of aromatherapy massage on the stress of the surgical center nursing team: a pilot study. *Rev Esc Enferm USP.* 2018 Aug 23;52:03348.

3538 Kardan-Yamchi J, Mahboubi M, Kazemian H, et al. The Chemical composition and anti-mycobacterial activities of Trachyspermum copticum and Pelargonium graveolens essential oils. *Recent Pat Antiinfect Drug Discov.* 2019 Oct 28. [Epub ahead of print]

3539 Angilella L. Synergistic activity of Pelargonium capitatum and Cymbopogon martini essential oils against C. albicans. *Nat Prod Res.* 2020 Aug 25;1-5.

[3540] Amine KM, Kahina C, Nawel H, et al. Protective Effects of Pelargonium graveolens Essential Oil on Methomyl-Induced Oxidative Stress and Spatial Working Memory Impairment in Association with Histopathological Changes in the Hippocampus of Male Wistar Rats. *Basic Clin Neurosci.* Jul-Aug 2020;11(4):433-446.

[3541] Huang SY, Yao N, He JK, et al. In vitro Anti-parasitic Activity of Pelargonium X. asperum Essential Oil Against Toxoplasma gondii. *Front Cell Dev Biol.* 2021 Feb 18;9:616340.

[3542] Dudek-Wicher R, Paleczny J, Kowalska-Krochmal B, et al. Activity of Liquid and Volatile Fractions of Essential Oils against Biofilm Formed by Selected Reference Strains on Polystyrene and Hydroxyapatite Surfaces. *Pathogens.* 2021 Apr 23;10(5):515.

[3543] Kafa AHT, Aslan R, Celik C, et al. Antimicrobial synergism and antibiofilm activities of Pelargonium graveolens, Rosemary officinalis, and Mentha piperita essential oils against extreme drug-resistant Acinetobacter baumannii clinical isolates. *Z Naturforsch C J Biosci.* 2021 Jun 17. Online ahead of print.

[3544] Boukhatem MN, Sufha T, Darwish NH, et al. [Rose-scented geranium essential oil from Algeria (Pelargonium graveolens L'Hérit.): Assessment of antioxidant, anti-inflammatory and anticancer properties against different metastatic cancer cell lines]. *Ann Pharm Fr.* 2021 Jul 23;S0003-4509(21)00096-1.

[3545] Ibrahim MA, Sallem OW, Abdelhassib MR, et al. Potentiation of anti-Helicobacter pylori activity of clarithromycin by Pelargonium graveolens oil. *Arab J Gastroenterol.* 2021 Sep;22(3):224-228.

[3546] Michalczky A, Ostrowska P. Essential oils and their components in combating fungal pathogens of animal and human skin. *J Mycol Med.* 2021 Jun;31(2):101118.

[3547] Lima LR, Andtrade FK, Alves DR, et al. Anti-acetylcholinesterase and toxicity against Artemia salina of chitosan microparticles loaded with essential oils of Cymbopogon flexuosus, Pelargonium x ssp and Copaifera officinalis. *Int J Biol Macromolecules.* 2021 Jan 15;167:1361-70.

[3548] Okla MK, Rubnawaz S, Dawoud TM, et al. Laser Light Treatment Improves the Mineral Composition, Essential Oil Production and Antimicrobial Activity of Mycorrhizal Treated Pelargoniumgraveolens. *Molecules.* 2022 Mar 8;27(6):1752.

[3549] Said AA, Nasr Y, Galal AAA, et al. Concerns with Male Infertility Induced by Exposure to Titanium Nanoparticles and the Supporting Impact of Pelargonium graveolens Essential Oil: Morphometric Records in Male-Wistar Rats. *Life.* 2022;12(5):639.

[3550] Mobarakeh MA, Ziaeirad M. Comparing the Effect of Aromatherapy With Geranium and Lemon Essential Oil on Situational Anxiety and Physiological Indices of Patients After Coronary Angioplasty. *Complement Med J Arak University Med Sci.* 2022 Jan;11(4):316-28.

[3551] Satou T, Kawata A, Hasegawa A, et al. Effects of Inhalation of Essential Oil From Pelargonium graveolens on the Autonomic Nervous System of Awake Mice. *Nat Prod Commun.* 2022;17(6):1-5.

[3552] Ibrahium SM, Aboelhadid SM, Wahba AA, et al. Preparation of geranium oil formulations effective for control of phenotypic resistant cattle tick Rhipicephalus annulatus. *Sci Rep.* 2022 Jul 8;12(1):11693.

[3553] Jaradat N, Hawash M, Qadi M, et al. Chemical Markers and Pharmacological Characters of Pelargonium graveolens Essential Oil from Palestine. Molecules. 2022 Sep 5;27(17):5721.

[3554] Al-Mijalli SH, Mrabti HN, Assaggaf H, et al. Chemical Profiling and Biological Activities of Pelargonium graveolens Essential Oils at Three Different Phenological Stages. *Plants (Basel).* 2022 Aug 27;11(17):2226.

[3555] Jamalian A, Shams-Ghahfarokhi M, Jaimand K, et al. Chemical composition and antifungal activity of Matricaria recutita flower essential oil against medically important dermatophytes and soil-borne pathogens. *J Mycol Med.* 2012 Dec;22(4):308-15.

[3556] Orav A, Raal A, Arak E. Content and composition of the essential oil of Chamomilla recutita (L.) Rauschert from some European countries. *Nat Prod Res.* 210;24(1):48-55.

[3557] Sashidhara KV, Verma RS, Ram P. Essential oil composition of Matricaria recutita L. from the lower region of the Himalayas. *Flav Frag J.* 2006 Mar-Apr;21(2):274-76.

[3558] Can OD, Demir Ozkay U, Kiyan HT, et al. Psychopharmacological profile of Chamomile (Matricaria recutita L.) essential oil in mice. *Phytomedicine.* 2012 Feb 15;19(3-4):306-10.

[3559] Orav A, Kailas T, Ivask K. Volatile constituents of Matricaria recutita L. from Estonia. *Proc Estonian Acad Sci Chem.* 2001;50(1):39-45.

[3560] Ganzera M, Schneider P, Stuppner H. Inhibitory effects of the essential oil of chamomile (Matricaria recutita L.) and its major constituents on human cytochrome P450 enzymes. *Life Sci.* 2006 Jan 18;78(8):856-61.

[3561] Heck AM, DeWitt BA, Lukes AL. Potential interactions between alternative therapies and warfarin. *Am J Health Syst Pharm.* 2000;57(13):1221-1227.

[3562] Tsai HH, Lin HW, Chen YL, et al. A review of potential harmful interactions between anticoagulant/antiplatelet agents and Chinese herbal medicines. *PLoS One.* 2013 May 9;8(5):e64255.

[3563] Segal R, Pilote L. Warfarin interaction with Matricaria chamomilla. *CMAJ.* 2006;174:1281-82.

[3564] Shanmuganathan B, Sheeja Malar D, Sathya S, et al. Antiaggregation Potential of Padina gymnospora against the Toxic Alzheimer's Beta-Amyloid Peptide 25-35 and Cholinesterase Inhibitory Property of Its Bioactive Compounds. *PLoS One.* 2015 Nov 4;10(11):e0141708.

[3565] Mitoshi M, Kuryama I, Nakayama H, et al. Effects of essential oils from herbal plants and citrus fruits on DNA polymerase, cancer cell growth inhibitory, anti-allergenic, and antioxidant activities. *J Agric Food Chem.* 2012 nov;60(145):11343-50.

[3566] Romeilah RM. Anticancer and antioxidant activities of Matricaria chamomilla L. and Majorana hortensis essential oils. *Res J Medicine Med Sci.* 2009;4(2):332-39.

[3567] Zargaran A, Borhani-Haghighi A, Faridi P, et al. Potential effect and mechanism of action of topical chamomile (Matricaria chamomilla L.) oil on migraine headache: A medical hypothesis. *Med Hypotheses.* 2014 Nov;83(5):566-69.

[3568] Niederhofer H. Observational study: Matricaria chamomilla may improve some symptoms of attention-deficit hyperactivity disorder. *Phytomedicine.* 2009 Apr;16(4):284-86.

[3569] Mitoshi M, Kuryama I, Nakayama H, et al. Effects of essential oils from herbal plants and citrus fruits on DNA polymerase, cancer cell growth inhibitory, anti-allergenic, and antioxidant activities. *J Agric Food Chem.* 2012 nov;60(145):11343-50.

[3570] Romero Mdel C, Valero A, Martin-Sanchez J, et al. Activity of Matricaria chamomilla essential oil against anisakiasis. *Phytomedicine.* 2012 Apr;19(6):520-23.

[3571] Capuzzo A, Occhipinti A, Maffei ME. Antioxidant and radical scavenging activities of chamazulene. *Nat Prod Res.* 2014;28(24):2321-23.

[3572] Caleja C, Barros L, Antonio AL, et al. Fortification of yogurts with different antioxidant preservatives: A comparative study between natural and synthetic additives. *Food Chem.* 2016 Nov 1;210:262-8.

[3573] Tomic M, Popovic V, Petrovic S, et al. Antihyperalgesic and antiedematous activities of bisabolol-oxides-rich matricaria oil in a rat model of inflammation. *Phytother Res.* 2014 May;28(5):759-66.

[3574] Rocha NF, Rios ER, Carvalho AM, et al. Anti-nociceptive and anti-inflammatory activities of (-)-α-bisabolol in rodents. *Naunyn-Schmiedeberg's Arch Pharmacol.* 2011 Dec;384(6):525-33.

[3575] Baylac S, Racine P. Inhibition of 5-lipoxygenase by essential oils and other natural fragrant extracts. *Int J Aromatherapy.* 2003;13(2-3):138-42.

[3576] Hernandez-Ceruelos A, Madrigal-Santillan E, Morales-Gonzalez JA, et al. Antigenotoxic effect of Chamomilla recutita (L.) Rauschert essential oil in mouse spermatogonial cells, and determination of its antioxidant capacity in vitro. *Int J Mol Sci.* 2010 Sep;11(10):3793-802.

[3577] Moura Rocha NF, Venancio ET, Noura BA, et al. Gastroprotection of (-)-alpha-bisabolol on acute gastric mucosal lesions in mice: the possible involved pharmacological mechanisms. *Fundam Clin Pharmacol.* 2010 Feb;24(11):63-71.

[3578] Hernandez-Ceruelos A, Madrigal-Bujaidar E, de la Cruz C. Inhibitory effect of chamomile essential oil on the sister chromatid exchanges induced by daunorubicin and methyl methanesulfonate in mouse bone marrow. *Toxicol Lett.* 2002 Sep;135(1-2):103-10.

[3579] Morales-Yuste M, Morillas-Marquez F, Martin-Sanchez J, et al. Activity of (-)-alpha-bisabolol against Leishmania infantum promastigotes. *Phytomedicine.* 2010 Mar;17(3-4):279-81.

[3580] Koch C, Reichling J, Kehm R, et al. Efficacy of anise oil, dwarf-pine oil and chamomile oil against thymidine- kinase-positive and thymidine-kinase-negative herpesviruses. *J Pharm Pharmacol.* 2008 Nov;60(11):1545-50.

[3581] Koch C, Reichling J, Schneele J, et al. Inhibitory effect of essential oils against herpes simplex virus type 2. *Phytomedicine.* 2008 Jan;15(1-2):71-78.

[3582] Kobayashi Y, Takahashi R, Ogino F. Antipruritic effect of the single oral administration of German chamomile flower extract and its combined effect with anti-allergenic agents in ddY mice. *J Ethnopharmacol.* 2005 Oct;101(1-3):308-12.

[3583] Owlia P, Rasooli I, Saderi H, et al. Antistreptococcal and antioxidant activity of essential oil from Matricaria chamomilla L. *Res J Biol Sci.* 2007;2(2):155-60.

[3584] Hans VM, Grover HS, Deswal H, et al. Antimicrobial Efficacy of Various Essential Oils at Varying Concentrations against Periopathogen Porphyromonas gingivalis. *J Clin Diagn Res.* 2016 Sep;10(9):ZC16-ZC19.

[3585] Weseler A, Geiss HK, Saller R, et al. A novel colorimetric broth microdilution method to determine the minimum inhibitory concentration (MIC) of antibiotics and essential oils absent Helicobacter pylori. *Pharmazie.* 2005 Jul;60(7):498-502.

[3586] Presibella MM, Villas-Boas LDB, de Silva Belletti KM, et al. Comparison of chemical constituents of Chamomilla recutita (L.) rauschert essential oil and its anti-chemotactic activity. *Braz Arch Biol Technol.* 2006 Sep;49(5):1516-8913.

[3587] Domingues Martins M, Martins Marques M, Kalil Bussadori S, et al. Comparative analysis between Chamomilla recutita and corticosteroids on wound healing. AN in vitro and in vivo study. *Phytother Res.* 2009;23:274-78.

[3588] Cavalieri E, Mariotto S, Fabrizi C, et al. alpha-Bisabolol, a non-toxic natural constituent, strongly induces apoptosis in glioma cells. *Biochem Biophys Res Commun.* 2004 Mar;315(3):589-94.

[3589] Andrade MA, Azevedo CD, Motta FN, et al. Essential oils: in vitro activity against Leishmania amazonensis, cytotoxicity and chemical composition. *BMC Complement Altern Med.* 2016 Nov 8;16(1):444.

[3590] Hashempur MH, Ghasemi MS, Daneshfard B, et al. Efficacy of topical chamomile oil for mild and moderate carpal tunnel syndrome: A randomized double-blind placebo-controlled clinical trial. *Complement Ther Clin Pract.* 2017;26:61-7.

[3591] A Al-Tamimi M, Rastall B, M Abu-Reidah I, et al. Chemical Composition, Cytotoxic, Apoptotic and Antioxidant Activities of Main Commercial Essential Oils in Palestine: A Comparative Study. *Medicines (Basel).* 2016 Oct 25;3(4).

[3592] Awaad AA, El-Meligy RM, Zain GM, et al. Experimental and clinical antihypertensive activity of Matricaria chamomilla extracts and their angiotensin-converting enzyme inhibitory activity. *Phytother Res.* 2018 Aug;32(8):1564-1573.

[3593] Zargaran A, Borhani-Haghighi A, Salehi-Marzijarani M, et al. Evaluation of the effect of topical chamomile (Matricaria chamomilla L.) oleogel as pain relief in migraine without aura: a randomized, double-blind, placebo-controlled, crossover study. *Neurol Sci.* 2018 Aug;39(8):1345-1353.

[3594] Shakya VK, Luqman S, Tikku AP, et al. A relative assessment of essential oil of Chrysopogon zizanioides and Matricaria chamomilla along with calcium hydroxide and chlorhexidine gel against Enterococcus faecalis in ex vivo root canal models. *J Conserv Dent.* 2019 Jan-Feb;22(1):34-39.

[3595] Piri E, Mahmoodi Sourestani M, Khaleghi E, et al. Chemo-Diversity and Antiradical Potential of Twelve Matricaria chamomilla L. Populations from Iran: Proof of Ecological Effects. *Molecules.* 2019 Apr 3;24(7).

[3596] Karam TK, Ortega S, Nakamura TU, et al. Development of Chitosan Nanocapsules Containing Essential Oil of Matricaria Chamomilla L. For the Treatment of Cutaneous Leishmaniasis. *Int J Biol Macromol.* 2020 Jun 18;162:199-208.
[3597] Yuan R, Zhang D, Yang J, et al. Review of aromatherapy essential oils and their mechanism of action against migraines. *J Ethnopharmacol.* 2021 Jan 30;265:113326.
[3598] Ebrahimi H, Mardani A, Basirinezhad MH, et al. The effects of Lavender and Chamomile essential oil inhalation aromatherapy on depression, anxiety and stress in older community-dwelling people: A randomized controlled trial. *Explore (NY).* 2021 Jan 9;S1550-8307(21)00001-X.
[3599] Karam TK, Ortega S, Nakamura TU, et al. Development of chitosan nanocapsules containing essential oil of Matricaria chamomilla L. for the treatment of cutaneous leishmaniasis. *Int J Biol Macromol.* 2020 Nov 1;162:199-208.
[3600] Frydeysiak E, Kunicka-Styczyńska A, Śmigielski K, et al. The Impact of Selected Essential Oils Applied to Non-Woven Viscose on Bacteria That Cause Lower Urinary Tract Infections-Preliminary Studies. *Molecules.* 2021 Nov 13;26(22):6854.
[3601] Elnabawy EM, Hassan S, Taha EA. Repellent and Toxicant Effects of Eight Essential Oils against the Red Flour Beetle, Tribolium castaneum Herbst (Coleoptera: Tenebrionidae). *Biology (Basel).* 2021 Dec 21;11(1):3.
[3602] Qasem A, Assaggaf H, Montesano D, et al. Determination of Chemical Compounds and Investigation of Biological Properties of Matricaria chamomilla Essential Oils, Honey, and Their Mixture. *Molecules.* 2022 Sep 9;27(18):5850.
[3603] Zardosht R, Basiri A, Sahebkar A, et al. Effect of Chamomile Oil on Cesarean Section Pain in Primiparous Women: A Randomized Clinical Trial. *Curr Rev Clin Exp Pharmacol.* 2021;16(4):369-374.
[3604] Gladikostić N, Ikonić B, Teslić N, et al. Essential Oils from Apiaceae, Asteraceae, Cupressaceae and Lamiaceae Families Grown in Serbia: Comparative Chemical Profiling with In Vitro Antioxidant Activity. *Plants (Basel).* 2023 Feb 7;12(4):745.
[3605] De Cicco P, Ercolano G, Sirignano C, et al. Chamomile essential oils exert anti-inflammatory effects involving human and murine macrophages: Evidence to support a therapeutic action. *J Ethnopharmacol.* 2023 Mar 20:116391.
[3606] Mahmujianah, Furiani ES, Murtiani F, et al. Lavender and Chamomile Aromatherapy Effectivity on Sleep Quality in the Third Trimester Pregnant Women. Jurnal Ilmiah Kedokteran *Wijaya Kusuma (JIKW).* 2023 Mar;12(1):51-58.
[3607] Singh G, Kapoor IPS, Singh OP, et al. Studies on essential oils, part 28: Chemical composition, antifungal and insecticidal activities of rhizome volatile oil of Homalomena aromatica Schott. *Flavour Frag J.* 200 Jul-Aug;15(4):278-80.
[3608] Todorova M, Thi Tho PT, Ognyanov I, et al. The composition of Homalomena aromatica Schott. Oil of Vietnamese origin. *Flavour Frag J.* 1988;3:179-81.
[3609] Jarikasem S, Drophy JJ, Thubthimthed S, et al. Chemical Composition of the Essential Oil from Homalomena aromatica Schott Rhizome. 28th Congress on Science and Technology of Thailand. Available at: http://www.thaiscience.info/Article%20for%20ThaiScience/Article/5/10007403.pdf.
[3610] Rana VS, Pukhrambam M, Singh HB, et al. Essential oil composition of Homalomena aromatica roots. *Indian Perfumer.* 2009 Oct-Dec;53:43-45.
[3611] Policegoudra RS, Goswami S, Aradhya SM, et al. Bioactive constituents of Homalomena aromatica essential oil and its antifungal activity against dermatophytes and yeasts. *J Mycol Med.* 2012 Mar;22(1):83-7.
[3612] Cardoso NN, Alviano CS, Blank AF, et al. Synergism Effect of the Essential Oil from Ocimum basilicum var. Maria Bonita and Its Major Components with Fluconazole and Its Influence on Ergosterol Biosynthesis. *Evid Based Complement Alternat Med.* 2016;2016:5647182.
[3613] Policegoudra RS, Goswami S, Aradhya SM, et al. Bioactive constituents of Homalomena aromatica essential oil and its antifungal activity against dermatophytes and yeasts. *J Mycol Med.* 2012 Mar;22(1):83-7.
[3614] Singh G, Kapoor IPS, Singh OP, et al. Studies on essential oils, part 28: Chemical composition, antifungal and insecticidal activities of rhizome volatile oil of Homalomena aromatica Schott. *Flavour Frag J.* 200 Jul-Aug;15(4):278-80.
[3615] Singh G, Kapoor IPS, Singh OP, et al. Studies on essential oils, part 28: Chemical composition, antifungal and insecticidal activities of rhizome volatile oil of Homalomena aromatica Schott. *Flavour Frag J.* 200 Jul-Aug;15(4):278-80.
[3616] Hazarika S, Dhiman S, Rabha B, et al. Repellent activity of some essential oils against Simulium species in India. *J Insect Sci.* 2012;12:5.
[3617] Tiwari S, Upadhyay N, Singh BK, et al. Chemically characterized nanoencapsulatedHomalomena aromatica Schott. essential oil as green preservative against fungal and aflatoxin B 1 contamination of stored spices based on in vitro and in situ efficacy and favorable safety profile on mice. *Environ Sci Pollut Res Int.* 2021 Aug 12. Online ahead of print.
[3618] Sasidharan I, Venugopal VV, Menon AN. Essential oil composition of two unique ginger (Zingiber officinale Roscoe) cultivars from Sikkim. *Nat Prod Res.* 2012;26(19):1759-64.
[3619] Gupta S, Pandotra P, Ram G, et al. Composition of a monoterpenoid-rich essential oil from the rhizome of Zingiber officinale from north Western Himalayas. *Nat Prod Commun.* 2011 Jan;6(1):93-96.
[3620] Bayala B, Bassole IFN, Gnoula C, et al. Chemical composition, antioxidant, anti-inflammatory and anti-proliferative activities of essential oils of plants from Burkina Faso. *PLoS One.* 2014;9(3):e92122.
[3621] Martins AP, Salqueira L, Goncalves MJ, et al. Essential oil composition and antimicrobial activity of three Zingiberaceae from S. Tome e Principe. *Planta Med.* 2001 Aug;67(6):580-84.
[3622] Onyenekwe PC, Hasimoto S. The composition of the essential oil of dried Nigerian ginger (Zingiber officinale Roscoe). *Eur Food Res Tech.* 1999 Oct;209(6):407-10.
[3623] Nampoothiri SV, Venugopalan VV, Joy B, et al. Comparison of essential oil composition of three ginger cultivars from sub Himalayan region. *Asian Pac J Trop Biomed.* 2012:S1347-50.
[3624] Kizhakkayil J, Sasikumar B. Characterization of ginger (Zingiber officinale Rosc.) germplasm based on volatile and non-volatile components. *African J Biotech.* 2012 Jan 12;11(4):777-86.
[3625] Wohlmuth H, Smith MK, Brooks LO, et al. Essential oil composition of diploid and tetraploid clones of ginger (Zingiber officinale Roscoe) grown in Australia. *J Agric Food Chem.* 2006;54:1414-9.
[3626] Tognolini M, Barocelli E, Ballabeni V, et al. Comparative screening of plant essential oils; phenylpropanoid moiety as basic core for antiplatelet activity. *Life Sci.* 2006 Feb 23;78(13):1419-32.
[3627] Heck AM, DeWitt BA, Lukes AL. Potential interactions between alternative therapies and warfarin. *Am J Health Syst Pharm.* 2000;57(13):1221-1227.
[3628] Jeena K, Liju VB, Viswanathan R, et al. Antimutagenic potential and modulation of carcinogen-metabolizing enzymes by ginger essential oil. *Phytother Res.* 2014 Jun;28(6):849-55.
[3629] Sritoomma N, Moyle W, Cooke M, et al. The effectiveness of Swedish massage with aromatic ginger oil in treating chronic low back pain in older adults: a randomized controlled trial. *Complement Ther Med.* 2014 Feb;22(1):26-33.
[3630] Yip YB, Tam AC. An experimental study on the effectiveness of massage with aromatic ginger and orange essential oil for moderate-to-severe knee pain among the elderly in Hong Kong. *Complement Ther Med.* 2008 Jun;16(3):131-38.
[3631] Jeena K, Liju VB, Viswanathan R, et al. Antimutagenic potential and modulation of carcinogen-metabolizing enzymes by ginger essential oil. *Phytother Res.* 2014 Jun;28(6):849-55.
[3632] Mangprayool T, Kupittayanant S, Chudapongse N. Participation of citral in the bronchodilatory effect of ginger oil and possible mechanism of action. *Fitoterapia.* 2013 Sep;89:68-73.
[3633] Podlogar JA, Verspohl EJ. Antiinflammatory effects of ginger and some of its components in human bronchial epithelial (BEAS-2B) cells. *Phytother Res.* 2012 Mar;26(3):333-36.
[3634] Bayala B, Bassole IH, Gnoula C, et al. Chemical composition, antioxidant, anti-inflammatory and anti-proliferative activities of essential oils of plants from Burkina Faso. *PLoS One.* 2014 Mar 24;9(3):e92122.
[3635] Pidgeon GP, Kandouz M, Meram A, et al. Mechanisms controlling cell cycle arrest and induction of apoptosis after 12-lipoxygenase inhibition in prostate cancer cells. *Cancer Res.* 2002 May 1; 62(9):2721-7.
[3636] Nogueira de Melo GA, Grespan R, Fonseca JP, et al. Inhibitory effects of ginger (Zingiber officinale Roscoe) essential oil on leukocyte migration in vivo and in vitro. *J Nat Med.* 2011 Jan;65(10):241-46.
[3637] Funk JL, Frye JB, Oyarzo JN, et al. Anti-Inflammatory Effects of the Essential Oils of Ginger (Zingiber officinale Roscoe) in Experimental Rheumatoid Arthritis. *PharmaNutrition.* 2016 Jul;4(3):123-131.
[3638] Bachiega TF, de Sousa JP, Bastos JK, et al. Clove and eugenol in noncytotoxic concentrations exert immunomodulatory/anti-inflammatory action on cytokine production by murine macrophages. *J Pharm Pharmacol.* 2012 Apr;64(4):610-16.
[3639] Zhou HL, Deng YM, Xie QM. The modulatory effects of the volatile oil of ginger on the cellular immune response in vitro and in vivo in mice. *J Ethnopharmacol.* 2006 Apr 21;105(1-2):301-05.
[3640] Carrasco FR, Schmidt G, Romero AL, et al. Immunomodulatory activity of Zingiber officinale Roscoe, Salvia officinalis L. and Syzygium aromaticum L. *J Pharm Pharmacol.* 209 Jul;61(7):961-67.
[3641] Khiewkhern S, Promthet S, Sukprasert A, et al. Effectiveness of aromatherapy with light Thai massage for cellular immunity improvement in colorectal cancer patients receiving chemotherapy. *Asian Pac J Cancer Prev.* 2013;14(6):3903-07.
[3642] Calvert I. Ginger: an essential oil for shortening labour? *Pract Midwife.* 2005 Jan;8(1):30-34.
[3643] Hashim S, Aboobaker VS, Madhubala R, et al. Modulatory effects of essential oils from spices on the formation of DNA adduct by aflatoxin B1 in vitro. *Nutr Cancer.* 1994;21(2):169-75.
[3644] Lua PL, Zakaria NS. A brief review of current scientific evidence involving aromatherapy use for nausea and vomiting. *J Altern Complement Med.* 2012 Jun;18(6):534-40.
[3645] Hunt R, Dienemann J, Norton HJ, et al. Aromatherapy as treatment for postoperative nausea: a randomized trial. *Anesth Analg.* 2013 Sep;117(3):597-604.
[3646] Misharina TA, Fatkullina LD, Alinkina ES, et al. Effects of low doses of essential oil on the antioxidant state of the erythrocytes, liver, and the brains of mice. *Prikl Biokhim Mikrobiol.*2014 Jan-Feb;50(1):101-07.
[3647] Pérez-Rosés R, Risco E, Vila R, et al. Biological and Nonbiological Antioxidant Activity of Some Essential Oils. *J Agric Food Chem.* 2016 Jun;64:4716-24.
[3648] Koch C, Reichling J, Schneele J, et al. Inhibitory effect of essential oils against herpes simplex virus type 2. *Phytomedicine.* 2008 Jan;15(1-2):71-78.
[3649] Schnitzler P, Koch C, Reichling J. Susceptibility of drug-resistant clinical herpes simplex virus type 1 strain to essential oils of ginger, thyme, hyssop, and sandalwood. *Antimicrob Agents Chemother.* 2007 May;51(5):1859-62.
[3650] Liju VB, Jeena K, Kuttan R. Gastroprotective activity of essential oils from turmeric and ginger. *J Basic Clin Physiol Pharmacol.* 2015 Jan;26(1):95-103.
[3651] Liu CT, Raghu R, Lin SH, et al. Metabolomics of ginger essential oil against alcoholic fatty liver in mice. *J Agric Food Chem.* 2013 Nov;61(46):11231-40.
[3652] Buddhakala N, Talubmook C, Sriyotha P, et al. Inhibitory effects of ginger oil on spontaneous and PGF2alpha- induced contraction of rat myometrium. *Planta Med.* 2008 Mar;74(4):385-91.
[3653] Weseler A, Geiss HK, Saller R, et al. A novel colorimetric broth microdilution method to determine the minimum inhibitory concentration (MIC) of antibiotics and essential oils absent Helicobacter pylori. *Pharmazie.* 2005 Jul;60(7):498-502.

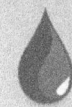

[3654] Riyazi A, Hensel A, Bauer K, et al. The effect of the volatile oil from ginger rhizomes (Zingiber officinale), its fractions and isolated constituents on the 5-HT3 receptor complex and the serotoninergic system of the rat ileum. *Planta Med.* 2007 Apr;73(4):355-62.
[3655] Qiang LQ, Wang CP, Wang FM, et al. Combined administration of the mixture of honokiol and magnolol and ginger evokes antidepressant-like synergism in rats. *Arch Pharm Res.* 2009 Sep;32(9):1281-92.
[3656] Yi LT, Xu Q, Li YC, et al. Antidepressant-like synergism of extracts from magnolia bark and ginger rhizome alone and in combination in mice. *Prog Neuropsychopharmacol Biol Psychiatry.* 2009 Jun;33(4):616-24.
[3657] Plant J. Effects of essential oils on telomere length in human cells. *Med Aromat Plants.* 2016;5(2):1-6.
[3658] Císarová M, Tančinová D, Medo J, et al. The in vitro effect of selected essential oils on the growth and mycotoxin production of Aspergillus species. *J Environ Sci Health B.* 2016 Oct 2;51(10):668-674.
[3659] Johnson JR, Rivard RL, Griffin KH, et al. The effectiveness of nurse-delivered aromatherapy in an acute care setting. *Complement Ther Med.* 2016 Apr;25:164-9.
[3660] Lee YR, Shin HS. Effectiveness of Ginger Essential Oil on Postoperative Nausea and Vomiting in Abdominal Surgery Patients. *J Altern Complement Med.* 2017 Mar;23(3):196-200.
[3661] Geiger JL. The essential oil of ginger, Zingiber officinale, and anesthesia. *Int J Aromatherapy.* 2005;15:7-14.
[3662] Pazinato R, Volpato A, Baldissera MD, et al. In vitro effect of seven essential oils on the reproduction of the cattle tick Rhipicephalus microplus. *J Adv Res.* 2016 Nov;7(6):1029-1034.
[3663] Nakayama M, Okizaki A, Takahashi K, et al. A Randomized Controlled Trial for the Effectiveness of Aromatherapy in Decreasing Salivary Gland Damage following Radioactive Iodine Therapy for Differentiated Thyroid Cancer. *Biomed Res Int.* 2016;2016:9509810.
[3664] Eissa FA, Choudhry H, Abdulaal WH, et al. Possible hypocholesterolemic effect of ginger and rosemary oils in rats. *Afr J Tradit Complement Altern Med.* 2017 Jun 5;14(4):188-200.
[3665] Avcioglu NH, Sahal G, Bilkay IS, et al. Antibiofilm effects of Citrus limonum and Zingiber officinale Oils on biofilm formation of Klebsiella ornithinolytica, Klebsiella oxytoca and Klebsiella terrigena species. *Afr J Tradit Complement Altern Med.* 2016 Sep 29;13(6):61-67.
[3666] A Al-Tamimi M, Rastall B, M Abu-Reidah I, et al. Chemical Composition, Cytotoxic, Apoptotic and Antioxidant Activities of Main Commercial Essential Oils in Palestine: A Comparative Study. *Medicines (Basel).* 2016 Oct 25;3(4).
[3667] Ashraf SA, Al-Shammari E, Hussain T, et al. In-vitro antimicrobial activity and identification of bioactive components using GC-MS of commercially available essential oils in Saudi Arabia. *J Food Sci Technol.* 2017 Nov;54(12):3948-3958.
[3668] Santos PASR, Avanco GB, Nerilo SB, et al. Assessment of Cytotoxic Activity of Rosemary (Rosmarinus officinalis L.), Turmeric (Curcuma longa L.), and Ginger (Zingiber officinale R.) Essential Oils in Cervical Cancer Cells (HeLa). *ScientificWorldJournal.* 2016; 2016: 9273078.
[3669] El-Shouny WA, Ali SS, Sun J, et al. Drug resistance profile and molecular characterization of extended spectrum beta-lactamase (ESβL)-producing Pseudomonas aeruginosa isolated from burn wound infections. Essential oils and their potential for utilization. *Microb Pathog.* 2018 Feb 3;116:301-312.
[3670] Herve T, Raphaël KJ, Ferdinand N, et al. Growth Performance, Serum Biochemical Profile, Oxidative Status, and Fertility Traits in Male Japanese Quail Fed on Ginger (Zingiber officinale, Roscoe) Essential Oil. *Vet Med Int.* 2018 Jun 28;2018:7682060.
[3671] Wang LX, Qian J, Zhao LN, et al. Effects of volatile oil from ginger on the murine B16 melanoma cells and its mechanism. *Food Funct.* 2018 Feb 21;9(2):1058-1069.
[3672] Al-Otaibi WA, Alkhatib MH, Wali AN, et al. Cytotoxicity and apoptosis enhancement in breast and cervical cancer cells upon coadministration of mitomycin C and essential oils in nanoemulsion formulations. *Biomed Pharmacother.* 2018 Oct;106:946-955.
[3673] Akinyemi AJ, Faboya OL, Paul AA, et al. Nephroprotective Effect of Essential Oils from Ginger (Zingiber officinale) and Turmeric (Curcuma longa) Rhizomes against Cadmium-induced Nephrotoxicity in Rats. *J Oleo Sci.* 2018;67(10):1339-1345.
[3674] Ferreira FMD, Hirooka EY, Ferreira FD, et al. Effect of Zingiber officinale Roscoe essential oil in fungus control and deoxynivalenol production of Fusarium graminearum Schwabe in vitro. *Food Addit Contam Part A Chem Anal Control Expo Risk Assess.* 2018 Oct 3:1-7.
[3675] Degan D, Ornello R, Tiseo C, et al. The Role of Inflammation in Neurological Disorders. *Curr Pharm Des.* 2018;24(14):1485-1501.
[3676] Miller AH, Raison CL. The role of inflammation in depression: from evolutionary imperative to modern treatment target. *Nat Rev Immunol.* 2016 Jan;16(1):22-34.
[3677] Akinyemi AJ, Adeniyi PA. Effect of Essential Oils from Ginger (Zingiber officinale) and Turmeric (Curcuma longa) Rhizomes on Some Inflammatory Biomarkers in Cadmium Induced Neurotoxicity in Rats. *J Toxicol.* 2018 Oct 8;2018:4109491.
[3678] Karaman S, Karaman T, Tapar H, et al. A randomized placebo-controlled study of aromatherapy for the treatment of postoperative nausea and vomiting. *Complement Ther Med.* 2019 Feb;42:417-421.
[3679] Madreseh-Ghahfarokhi S, Pirali Y, Dehghani-Samani A, et al. The insecticidal and repellent activity of ginger (Zingiber officinale) and eucalyptus (Eucalyptus globulus) essential oils against Culex theileri Theobald, 1903 (Diptera: Culicidae). *Ann Parasitol.* 2018;64(4):351-360.
[3680] Camero M, Lanave G, Catella C, et al. Virucidal activity of ginger essential oil against caprine alphaherpesvirus-1. *Vet Microbiol.* 2019 Mar;230:150-155.
[3681] Fahmi A, Hassanen N, Abdur-Rahman M, et al. Phytochemicals, antioxidant activity and hepatoprotective effect of ginger (Zingiber officinale) on diethylnitrosamine toxicity in rats. *Biomarkers.* 2019 Jul;24(5):436-447.
[3682] Pehlivan S, Karadakovan A. Effects of aromatherapy massage on pain, functional state, and quality of life in an elderly individual with knee osteoarthritis. *Jpn J Nurs Sci.* 2019 Oct;16(4):450-458.
[3683] Baldin VP, Bertin de Lima Scodro R, Mariano Fernandez CM, et al. Ginger essential oil and fractions against Mycobacterium spp. *J Ethnopharmacol.* 2019 Jul 17:112095.
[3684] De Lima DAN, Pelegrini BB, Uechi FAA, et al. Evaluation of Antineoplasic Activity of Zingiber Officinale Essential Oil in the Colorectal Region of Wistar Rats. *Asian Pac J Cancer Prev.* 2020 Jul 1;21(7):2141-2147.
[3685] Wang X, Shen Y, Thankur K, et al. Antibacterial Activity and Mechanism of Ginger Essential Oil against Escherichia coli and Staphylococcus aureus. *Molecules.* 2020 Aug 30;25(17):3955.
[3686] Faria TRB, Furletti-Goes VF, Franzini CM, et al. Anti-inflammatory and antimicrobial effects of Zingiber officinale mouthwash on patients with fixed orthodontic appliances. *Am J Orthod Dentofacial Orthop.* 2020 Oct 20;S0889-5406(20)30527-8.
[3687] Sing PP, Jaiswal AK, Kumar A, et al. Untangling the multi-regime molecular mechanism of verbenol-chemotype Zingiber officinale essential oil against Aspergillus flavus and aflatoxin B1. *Sci Rep.* 2021 Mar 25;11(1):6832.
[3688] De Lima DAN, Pelegrini BB, Uechi FAA, et al. Evaluation of Antineoplasic Activity of Zingiber Officinale Essential Oil in the Colorectal Region of Wistar Rats. *Asian Pac J Cancer Prev.* 2020 Jul 1;21(7):2141-2147.
[3689] Castro JC, Pante GC, Centenaro BM, et al. Antifungal and antimycotoxigenic effects of Zingiber officinale, Cinnamomum zeylanicum and Cymbopogon martinii essential oils against Fusarium verticillioides. *Food Addit Contam Part A Chem Anal Control Expo Risk Assess.* 2020 Sep;37(9):1531-1541.
[3690] Sarto MPM, Lucas da Silva HF, de Souza Fernandes N, et al. Essential oils from Syzygium aromaticum and Zingiber officinale, administered alone or in combination with benznidazole, reduce the parasite load in mice orally inoculated with Trypanosoma cruzi II. *BMC Complement Med Ther.* 2021 Feb 25;21(1):77.
[3691] Shirooye P, Hashem-Dabaghian F, Hamzeloo-Moghdam M, et al. A clinical comparative study of oral and topical ginger on severity and duration of primary dysmenorrhea. *Res J Pharmacognosy.* 2017;4(1):23-32.
[3692] Zaid A, Haw XR, Alkatib HH, et al. Phytochemical Constituents and Antiproliferative Activities of Essential Oils from Four Varieties of Malaysian Zingiber officinale Roscoe against Human Cervical Cancer Cell Line. *Plants (Basel).* 2022 May 10;11(10):1280.
[3693] Sulistyarini WD, Handayani FN, Astobudi TE. Management of chemotherapy-induced nausea and vomiting using ginger aromatherapy in cancer patients. *Husaga Mahakal Jurnal Kesehatan.* 2022;12(1):53-64.
[3694] Tarfaoui K, Brhadda N, Ziri R, et al. Chemical Profile, Antibacterial and Antioxidant Potential of Zingiber officinale Roscoe and Elettaria cardamomum (L.) Maton Essential Oils and Extracts. *Plants (Basel).* 2022 May 31;11(11):1487.
[3695] Williams AS, Dove J, Krock JE, et al. Efficacy of Inhaled Essential Oil Use on Selected Symptoms Affecting Quality of Life in Patients With Cancer Receiving Infusion Therapies. *ONF.* 2022;49(4):349-58.
[3696] Aydinli A, Karadag S. Effects of abdominal massage applied with ginger and lavender oil for elderly with constipation: A randomized controlled trial. *Explore.* 2023 Jan-Feb;19(1):115-120.
[3697] You Z, Li Y, Zhang K, Zheng X, et al. Inhibitory effect of plant essential oils on α-glucosidase. *Food Sci Biotechnol.* 2022 Aug 9;31(12):1593-1602.
[3698] Zhang S, Zhang L, Yu M, et al. Essential oils of Zingiber officinale: Chemical composition, in vivo alleviation effects on TPA induced ear swelling in mice and in vitro bioactivities. *Front Nutr.* 2022 Oct 24;9:1043175.
[3699] Mabrouk DM, El Makawy AI, Ahmed KA, et al. Topiramate potential neurotoxicity and mitigating role of ginger oil in mice brain. *Environ Sci Pollut Res Int.* 2022 Dec;29(58):87184-87199.
[3700] Mathela CS, Lohani H, Pande C, et al. Chemosystematics of terpenoids in Cymbopogon martinii. *Biochem System Ecol.* 1988;16(2):167-69.
[3701] Nigam MC, Nigam IC, Levi L. Essential oils and their constituents XXVII. Composition of oil of gingergrass. *Can J Chem.* 1965;43:521-25.
[3702] Boelens MH. Sensory and chemical evaluation of tropical grass oils. *Perfum Flavor.* 1994;19:29–45.
[3703] Das MK, Ansari MA. Evaluation of repellent action of Cymbopogan martinii martinii Stapf var sofia oil against Anopheles sundaicus in tribal villages of Car Nicobar Island, Andaman & Nicobar Islands, India. *J Vector Borne Dis.* 2003 Sep-Dec;40(3-4):100-4.
[3704] Ansari MA, Razdan RK. Repellent action of Cymbopogan martinii martini Stapf var sofia oil against mosquitoes. *Indian J Malariol.* 1994;31(3):95–102.
[3705] Vitalini S, Nalbone L, Bernardi C, et al. Ginger and parsley essential oils: chemical composition, antimicrobial activity, and evaluation of their application in cheese preservation. *Nat Prod Res.* 2022 Sep 22:1-6.
[3706] Guerrini A, Tacchini M, Chiocchio I, et al. A Comparative Study on Chemical Compositions and Biological Activities of Four Amazonian Ecuador Essential Oils: Curcuma longa L. (Zingiberaceae), Cymbopogon citratus (DC.) Stapf, (Poaceae), Ocimum campechianum Mill. (Lamiaceae), and Zingiber officinale Roscoe (Zingiberaceae). *Antibiotics (Basel).* 2023 Jan 15;12(1):177.
[3707] Ibrar M, Ayub Y, Nazir R, et al. Garlic and ginger essential oil-based neomycin nano-emulsions as effective and accelerated treatment for skin wounds' healing and inflammation: In-vivo and in-vitro studies. *Saudi Pharm J.* 2022 Dec;30(12):1700-1709.
[3708] Yousuf Dar M, Shah WA, Mubashir S, et al. Chromatographic analysis, anti-proliferative and radical scavenging activity of Pinus wallichiana essential oil growing in high altitude areas of Kashmir, India. *Phytomedicine.* 2012 Oct 15;19(13):1228-33.

3709 Ioannou E, Koutsaviti A, Tzakou O, et al. The genus Pinus: a comparative study on the needle essential oil composition of 46 pine species. *Phytochem Rev.* 2014 Dec;13(4):741-68.

3710 Yousuf Dar M, Shah WA, Mubashir S, et al. Chromatographic analysis, anti-proliferative and radical scavenging activity of Pinus wallichiana essential oil growing in high altitude areas of Kashmir, India. *Phytomedicine.* 2012 Oct 15;19(13):1228-33.

3711 Yousuf Dar M, Shah WA, Mubashir S, et al. Chromatographic analysis, anti-proliferative and radical scavenging activity of Pinus wallichiana essential oil growing in high altitude areas of Kashmir, India. *Phytomedicine.* 2012 Oct 15;19(13):1228-33.

3712 De Qiang L, Pan SH, Zhu XW, et al. Anticancer activity and chemical composition of leaf oil from Solidago Canadensis L. in China. *Adv Mat Res.* 2011 Oct;1584:347-53.

3713 Mishra D, Shivani J, Sah P, et al. Chemical composition, analgesic and antimicrobial activity of Solidago canadensis essential oil from India. *J Pharm Res.* 2011 Jan;4(1):63.

3714 Huang B, Lei Y, Qin L, et al. Chemical composition and cytotoxic activities of the essential oil from the inflorescences of Solidago Canadensis L., an invasive weed in Southeastern China. *J Essential Oil Bearing Plants.* 2012;15(4):667-71.

3715 Kasali AA, Ekundayo O, Paul C, et al. epi-Cubebanes from Solidago Canadensis. *Phytochemistry.* 2002 Apr;59(8):805-10.

3716 Chanotiya CS, Yadav A. Natural variability in enantiomeric composition of bioactive chiral terpenoids in the essential oil of Solidago Canadensis L. from Uttarakhand, India. *Nat Prod Comm.* 2008;3(2):263-66.

3717 YeCheng D, RuiYu L, LinLin Y, et al. Insecticidal activities and chemical constituents of essential oils from alien invasive plants Solidago Canadensis and Wedelia triolobata. *J Guangxi Normal Univ.* 2014;32(2):122-29.

3718 Ibrahim NA, Mohamed SM, Faraif MA, et al. Chemical composition, antiviral and antimicrobial activities of the essential oils of Aster Novi-Belgii, Solidago Canadensis, and Myoporum Laetum growing in Egypt. *Bull Faculty Pharm (Cairo University).* 2006;44(1):103-110.

3719 El-Sherei M, Khaleel A, Motaal AA, et al. Effect of Seasonal Variation on the Composition of the Essential Oil of Solidago canadensis Cultivated in Egypt. *J Essential Oil Bear Plants.* 2014;17(5):891-98.

3720 Ibrahim NA, Mohamed SM, Faraif MA, et al. Chemical composition, antiviral and antimicrobial activities of the essential oils of Aster Novi-Belgii, Solidago Canadensis, and Myoporum Laetum growing in Egypt. *Bull Faculty Pharm (Cairo University).* 2006;44(1):103-110.

3721 De Qiang L, Pan SH, Zhu XW, et al. Anticancer activity and chemical composition of leaf oil from Solidago Canadensis L. in China. *Adv Mat Res.* 2011 Oct;1584:347-53.

3722 Huang B, Lei Y, Qin L, et al. Chemical composition and cytotoxic activities of the essential oil from the inflorescences of Solidago Canadensis L., an invasive weed in Southeastern China. *J Essential Oil Bearing Plants.* 2012;15(4):667-71.

3723 Mishra D, Joshi S, Bisht G, et al. Chemical composition and antimicrobial activity of Solidago canadensis linn. Root essential oil. *J Basic Clin Pharm.* 2010 Jun;1(3):187-90.

3724 Duarte MC, Figueira GM, Sartoratto A, et al. Anti-Candida activity of Brazilian medicinal plants. *J Ethnopharmacol.* 2005 Feb 28;97(2):305-11.

3725 Liu S, Shao X, Wei Y, et al. Solidago canadensis L. Essential Oil Vapor Effectively Inhibits Botrytis cinerea Growth and Preserves Postharvest Quality of Strawberry as a Food Model System. *Front Microbiol.* 2016 Aug 2;7:1179.

3726 Regnault-Roger C, Hamraoui A, Holeman M, et al. Insecticidal effect of essential oils from Mediterranean plants upon Acanthoscelides Obtectus Say (Coleoptera, Bruchidae), a pest of kidney bean (Phaseolus vulgaris L.). *J Chem Ecol.* 1993;19(6):1233-44.

3727 Kalemba D, Gora J, Kurowska A, et al. Study of essential oils with regard to their effects on insects. Part III. Essential oil of goldenrod (Solidago canadensis L.). *Tecnologia I Chemia Spozywcza.* 1990;47:91-97.

3728 Regnault-Roger C. The potential of botanical essential oil for insect pest control. *Integrated Pest Manag Rev.* 1997;2:25-34.

3729 Elshafie HS, Gruľová D, Baranová B, et al. Antimicrobial Activity and Chemical Composition of Essential Oil Extracted from Solidago canadensis L. Growing Wild in Slovakia. *Molecules.* 2019 Mar 27;24(7). pii: E1206. doi: 10.3390/molecules24071206.

3730 Uysal B, Sozmen F, Aktas O, et al. Essential oil composition and antibacterial activity of the grapefruit (Citrus Paradisi. L) peel essential oils obtained by solvent-free microwave extraction: comparison with hydrodistillation. *Int J Food Sci Tech.* 2011 Jul;46(7):1455-61.

3731 Okunowo WO, Oyedeji O, Agloabi L, et al. Essential oil of grape fruit (Citrus paradise) peels and its antimicrobial activities. *Sci Res.* 2013 Jul;4(7B):1-9.

3732 Pino JA, Acevedo A, Rabelo J, et al. Chemical composition of distilled grapefruit oil. *J Essential Oil Res.* 1999;11(1):75-76.

3733 Njoroge SM, Koaze H, Karanja PN, et al. Volatile constituents of redblush grapefruit (Citrus paradisi) and pummelo (Citrus grandis) peel essential oils from Kenya. *J Agric Food Chem.* 2005 Dec;53(25):9790-94.

3734 Ahmad MM, Rehman SU, Iqbal Z, et al. Genetic variability to essential oil composition in four citrus fruit species. *Pak J Bot.* 2006;38(2):319-24.

3735 Darroudi A, Fadaee J. Gas chromatography/mass spectrometry for separation and identification of cold- pressed/expressed constituents in grapefruit essential oil from Iran. *Asian J Chemistry.* 2012;24(6):2817-18.

3736 Kamal GM, Anwar F, Hussain AI, et al. Yield and chemical composition of Citrus essential oils as affected by drying pretreatment of peels. *Int Food Res J.* 2011;18(4):1275-82.

3737 Kejlova K, Jirova D, Bendova H, et al. Phototoxicity of essential oils intended for cosmetic use. *Toxicol In Vitro.* 2010 Dec;24(8):2084-9.

3738 Placzek M, Froemel W, Eberlein B, et al. Evaluation of phototoxic properties of fragrances. *Acta Derm Venereol.* 2007;87(4):312-6.

3739 Stanley WL, Leonard J. Citrus coumarins. *J Agr Food Chem.* 1971;19:1106-1110.

3740 Ho PC, Saville DJ, Wanwimolruk S. Inhibition of hyman CUP3A4 activity by grapefruit flavonoids, furanocoumarins and related constituents. *J Pharm Pharm Sci.* 2001 Sep-Dec;4(3):217-27.

3741 Crivello J, Bulut U. Curcumin: A naturally occurring long-wavelength photosensitizer for diaryliodanium salts. *J of Polymer Scie Part A: Polymer Chem.* 2005 Sep;43(21):5217-31.

3742 Araki N, Tsuroka S, Hasegawa G, et al. Inhibition of CYP3A4 by 6',7'-dihydroxybergamottin in human CYP3A4 over-expressed hepG2 cells. *J Pharm Pharmacol.* 2012 Dec;64(12):1715-21.

3743 Messer A, Raquet N, Lohr C, et al. Major furanocoumarins in grapefruit juice II: phototoxicity, photogenotoxicity, and inhibitory potency vs. cytochrome P450 3A4 activity. *Food Chem Toxciol.* 2012 Mar;50(3-4):756-60.

3744 Dugo P, Russo M, Saro M, et al. Multidimensional liquid chromatography for the determination of chiral coumarins and furocoumarins in citrus essential oils. *J Sep Sci.* 2012 Jul;34(14):1828-36.

3745 Sea KA, Kim H, Ku HY, et al. The monoterpenoids citral and geraniol are moderate inhibitors of CYP2B6 hydroxylase activity. *Chem Biol Interact.* 2008 Aug 11;174(3):141-6.

3746 Wangensteen H, Molden E, Christensen H, et al. Identification of epoxybergamottin as a CYP3A4 inhibitor in grapefruit peel. *Eur J Clin Pharamacol.* 2003 Feb;58(10):663-68.

3747 Ho PC, Saville DJ, Wanwimolruk S. Inhibition of human CYP3A4 activity by grapefruit flavonoids, furanocoumarins and related constituents. *J Pharm Pharm Sci.* 2001 Sep-Dec;4(3):217-27.

3748 Hata T, Sakaguchi I, Mori M, et al. Induction of apoptosis by Citrus paradisi essential oil in human leukemic (HL-60) cells. *In Vitro.* 2003 Nov-Dec;17(6):553-59.

3749 Hur MH, Han SH. Clinical trial of aromatherapy on postpartum mother's perineal healing. *Taehan Kanho Hakhoe Chi.* 2004 Feb;34(1):53-62.

3750 Haze S, Sakai K, Gozu Y, et al. Grapefruit oil attenuates adipogenesis in cultured subcutaneous adipocytes. *Planta Med.* 2010 Jul;76(10:950-55.

3751 Shen J, Niijima A, Tanida M, et al. Mechanism of changes induced in plasma glycerol by scent stimulation with grapefruit and lavender essential oils. *Neurosci Lett.* 2007 Apr;416(3):241-46.

3752 Shen J, Niijima A, Tanida M, et al. Olfactory stimulation with scent of grapefruit oil affects autonomic nerves, lipolysis and appetite in rats. *Neurosci Lett.* 2005 Jun;380(3):289-94.

3753 Mori M, Ikeda N, Kato Y, et al. Inhibition of elastase activity by essential oils in vitro. *J Cosmetic Dermatol.* 2002;1(4):183-87.

3754 Uysal B, Sozmen F, Aktas O, et al. Essential oil composition and antibacterial activity of the grapefruit (Citrus Paradisi. L) peel essential oils obtained by solvent-free microwave extraction: comparison with hydrodistillation. *Int J Food Sci Tech.* 2011;46:1455-61.

3755 Tanida M, Niijima A, Shen J, et al. Olfactory stimulation with scent of essential oil of grapefruit affects autonomic neurotransmission and blood pressure. *Brain Res.* 2005 Oct;1058(1-2):44-55.

3756 Perczak A, Juś K, Marchwińska K, et al. Degradation of Zearalenone by Essential Oils under In vitro Conditions. *Front Microbiol.* 2016 Aug 11;7:1224.

3757 Turcotte JC, Hunt PJB, Blaustein JD. Estrogenic effects of zearalenone on the expression of progestin receptors and sexual behavior in female rats. *Hormones and Behavior.* 2005;47:178-84.

3758 Takemura H, Shim JY, Sayama K, et al. Characterization of the estrogenic activities of zearalenone and zeranol in vivo and in vitro. *J Steroid Biochem Mol Biol.* 2007 Feb;103(2):170-7.

3759 Frizzell C, Ndossi D, Verhaegen S, et al. Endocrine disrupting effects of zearalenone, alpha- and beta-zearalenol at the level of nuclear receptor binding and steroidogenesis. *Toxicol Lett.* 2011 Oct 10;206(2):210-7.

3760 Hozumi H, Hasegawa S, Tsunenari T, et al. Aromatherapies using Osmanthus fragrans oil and grapefruit oil are effective complementary treatments for anxious patients undergoing colonoscopy: A randomized controlled study. *Complement Ther Med.* 2017 Oct;34:165-169.

3761 Maness LR, Zubov T. The Inhibitory Effect of Essential Oils on Rhizopus stolonifer, Trichophyton mentagrophytes, and Microsporum gypseum. *Lab Med.* 2019 Apr 8;50(2):e18-e22.

3762 Battistini R, Rossini I, Ercolini C, et al. Antiviral Activity of Essential Oils Against Hepatitis A Virus in Soft Fruits. *Food Environ Virol.* 2019 Mar;11(1):90-95.

3763 Luciardi M, Blazquez MA, Alberto MR, et al. Grapefruit Essential Oils Inhibit Quorum Sensing of Pseudomonas Aeruginosa. *Food Sci Technol Int.* 2020 Apr;26(3):231-241.

3764 Deng W, Liu K, Cao S, et al. Chemical Composition, Antimicrobial, Antioxidant, and Antiproliferative Properties of Grapefruit Essential Oil Prepared by Molecular Distillation. *Molecules.* 2020 Jan 5;25(1):217.

3765 Garbin VP, Munguia B, Saldana JC, et al. Chemical characterization and in vitro anthelmintic activity of Citrus bergamia Risso and Citrus X paradisii Macfad essential oil against Haemonchus contortus Kirby isolate. *Acta Trop.* 2021 Feb 22;105869.

3766 Denkova-Kostova R, Teneva D, Tomova T, et al. Chemical composition, antioxidant and antimicrobial activity of essential oils from tangerine ( Citrus reticulata L.), grapefruit ( Citrus paradisi L.), lemon ( Citrus lemon L.) and cinnamon ( Cinnamomum zeylanicum Blume). *Z Naturforsch C J Biosci.* 2020 Nov 23;76(5-6):175-185.

3767 Miya G, Nyalambisa M, Oyedeji O, et al. Chemical Profiling, Toxicity and Anti-Inflammatory Activities of Essential Oils from Three Grapefruit Cultivars from KwaZulu-Natal in South Africa. *Molecules.* 2021 Jun 3;26(11):3387.

3768 Zhang N, Liao Y, Xie L, et al. Using essential oils from Citrus paradisi as a fumigant for Solenopsis invicta workers and evaluating the oils' effect on worker behavior. *Environ Sci Pollut Res Int.* 2021 Jun 18. Online ahead of print.

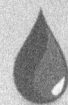

[3769] Li C, Cai Q, Wu X, et al. Variation in compositions and biological activities of essential oils from four Citrus species: Citrus limon, Citrus sinensis, Citrus paradisi, and Citrus reticulata. *Chem Biodivers.* 2022 Feb 10. Online ahead of print.
[3770] Zhang X, Xu H, Hua J, et al. Protective Effects of Grapefruit Essential Oil against Staphylococcus Aureus-Induced Inflammation and Cell Damage in Human Epidermal Keratinocytes. *Chme Biodiversity.* 2022 May:e202200205.
[3771] Jian R, Lin Y, Li Y, et al. Larvicidal Activity of Two Rutaceae Plant Essential Oils and Their Constituents Against Aedes albopictus (Diptera: Culicidae) in Multiple Formulations. *J Med Entomol.* 2022 Jul 4:tjac083.
[3772] Li C, Zhu H, Zhao K, et al. Chemical constituents, biological activities and anti-rheumatoid arthritic properties of four citrus essential oils. *Phytother Res.* 2022 Jul;36(7):2908-2920.
[3773] Kaltenbach G, Schafer M, Schimmer O. Volatile Constituents of the Essential Oil of Grindelia robusta Nutt. and Grindelia squarrosa Dun. *J Essent Oil Res.* 1993;5(1):107-08.
[3774] El-Shamy AM, Rl-Hawary SS, El-Shabrawy AO, et al. Essential oil composition of three Grindelia species. *J Essent Oil Res.* 2000;12(5):631-34.
[3775] Veres K, Roza O, Laczkó-Zöld E, et al. Chemical composition of essential oils of Grindelia squarrosa and G. hirsutula. *Nat Prod Commun.* 2014 Apr;9(4):573-4.
[3776] Veres K, Roza O, Laczko-Zold E, et al. Chemical composition of essential oils of Grindelia squarrosa (Pursh) Dunal and Grindelia oregana A. Gray. *Planta Med.* 2013;79(13):1191.
[3777] Rodilla JM, Silva LA, Martinez N, et al. Advances in the identification and agrochemical importance of sesquiterpenoids from Bulnesia sarmientoi essential oil. *Ind Crops Prod.* 2011;3:497-503.
[3778] Prudent D, Perineaeu F, Bravo R, et al. Preparation er caracterisation d'extraits volatils de bois de Gaiac (Bulnesia samienti Lor.) *Rivist Ital.* 1991;5:35-43.
[3779] Prudent D, Perineaeu F, Bravo R, et al. Preparation er caracterisation d'extraits volatils de bois de Gaiac (Bulnesia samienti Lor.) *Rivist Ital.* 1991;5:35-43.
[3780] Prudent D, Perineaeu F, Bravo R, et al. Preparation er caracterisation d'extraits volatils de bois de Gaiac (Bulnesia samienti Lor.) *Rivist Ital.* 1991;5:35-43.
[3781] Hiebert MR, Flores-Guibi ME, Baru JE, et al. Antimycobacterial activity of the ethanolic extract of the wood of Bulnesia sarmientoi Lorentz ex. Griseb. *Revista Latinoamericanca de Quimica.* 2011 Dec;40(1):7-12.
[3782] Andrade MA, Azevedo CD, Motta FN, et al. Essential oils: in vitro activity against Leishmania amazonensis, cytotoxicity and chemical composition. *BMC Complement Altern Med.* 2016 Nov 8;16(1):444.
[3783] Luns DAR, Martins R, Pombal S, et al. Effect of essential oils against acaricide-susceptible and acaricide-resistant Rhipicephalus ticks. *Exp Appl Acarol.* 2021 Feb 24. Online ahead of print.
[3784] El-Ahmady SH, Ashour ML, Wink M. Chemical composition and anti-inflammatory activity of the essential oils of Psidium guajava fruits and leaves. *J Essent Oil Res.* 2013;25(6):475-81.
[3785] de Lima RK, das Gracas Cardoso M, Andrade MA, et al. Composition of the essential oil from the leaves of tree domestic varieties and one wild variety of the guava plant (Psidium guajava L., Myrtaceae). *Rev Bras Farmacogn.* 2010 Jan-Mar;20(1):0102-695X.
[3786] Satyal P, Paudel P, Lamichhane B, et al. Leaf essential oil composition and bioactivity of Psidium guajava from Kathmandu, Nepal. *Am J Essential Oils Nat Prod.* 2015;3(2):11-14.
[3787] Bhalke RD, Patel SJ, Girme AS, et al. Major volatile constituent of bark and leaves of Psidium guajava Linn. (Myrtacae). *Pharmacologyonlin.* 2008;3:187-90.
[3788] Cole RA, Setzer WN. Chemical Composition of the Leaf Essential Oil of Psidium guajava from Monteverde, Costa Rica. *J Essent Oil Res.* 2007;10(5):365-73.
[3789] Tucker AO, Maciarello MJ, Landrum LR. Volatile leaf oils of American Myrtaceae. III. Psidium cattleianum Sabine, P. friedrichsthalianum (Berg) Niedenzu, P. guajava L., P. guineense Sw., and P. sartorianum (Berg) Niedenzu. *J Essent Oil Research.* 1995;7:187-90.
[3790] Santos FA, Rao VSN, Silveira ER. Investigations on the antinociceptive effect of Psidium guajava leaf essential oil and its major constituents. *Phytother Res.* 1998;12:24-27.
[3791] da Silva JD, Luz AIR, da Silva MHL, et al. Essential oil of the leaves and stems of four Psidium spp. *Flavour Frag J.* 2003;18:240-43.
[3792] Siani AC, Souza MC, Henriques MGMO, et al. Anti-inflammatory activity of essential oils from Syzygium cumini and Psidium guajava. *Pharmaceutical Biol.* 2013;51:881-87.
[3793] Ji X, Pu Q, Garraffo HM, et al. The essential oil of the leaves of Psidium guajava L. *J Essent Oil Res.* 1991;3:187-89.
[3794] Ogunwande IA, Olawore NO, Adeleke KA, et al. Chemical composition of the leaf volatile oil of Psidium guajava L. growing in Nigeria. *Flavour Fragr J.* 2003;18:136-38.
[3795] Khadhri A, El Mokni RE, Almeida C, et al. Chemical composition of essential oil of Psidium guajava L. growing in Tunisia. *Industrial Crops Prod.* 2014;52:29-31.
[3796] Sacchetti G, Maietti S, Muzzoli M, et al. Comparative evaluation of 11 essential oils of different origin as functional antioxidants, antiradicals and antimicrobials in foods. *Food Chem.* 2005;91:621-32.
[3797] Smith RM, Oliveros-Belardo L. The composition of leaf essential oils of Psidium guajava L. from Manila, Philippines. *As J Pharm.* 1977;3:5-9.
[3798] Pino JA, Aguero J, Marbot R, et al. Leaf oil of Psidium guajava L. from Cuba. *J Essent Oil Res.* 2001 Jan-Feb;13:61-62.
[3799] Torres AM, Ricciari GAL, Agrela de Nassiff AE, et al. Estudio comparativo de aceites esenciales de species de Psidium (Myrtaceae) del Nordeste. *Reunión de Comunicaciones Científicas y Tecnológicas.* 1999;8:8111-14.
[3800] Chen HC, Sheu MJ, Lin LY, et al. Chemical composition of the leaf essential oil of Psidium guajava L. from Taiwan. *J Essent Oil Res.* 2007;19:345-47.
[3801] Adam F, Vahirua-Lechat I, Deslandes E, et al. Aromatic plants of French Polynesia. V. Chemical composition of essential oils of leaves of Psidium guajava L. and Psidium cattleyanum Sabine. *J Essent Oil Research.* 2011;23:98-101.
[3802] Khadhri A, El Mokni R, Almeida C, et al. Chemical composition of essential oil of Psidium guajava L. growing in Tunisia. *Industrial Crops Prod.* 2014;52:29-31.
[3803] Nguyen LT, Mysliveckova Z, Szotakova B, et al. The inhibitory effects of β-caryophyllene, β-caryophyllene oxide and α-humulene on the activities of the main drug-metabolizing enzymes in rat and human liver in vitro. *Chem-Biol Interactoins.* 2017 Dec 25;278:123-8.
[3804] Burkhard PR, Burkhardt K, Haenggeli CA, et al. Plant-induced seizures: reappearance of an old problem. *J Neurol.* 1999 Aug;246(8):667-70.
[3805] Culic M, Kekovic G, Grbic G, et al. Wavelet and fractal analysis of rat brain activity in seizures evoked by
camphor essential oil and 1,8-cineole. *Gen Physiol Biophys.* 2009;Special Issue(28):33–40.
[3806] Mathew T, Kamath V, Kumar RS, et al. Eucalyptus oil inhalation–induced seizure: A novel, underrecognized, preventable cause of acute symptomatic seizure. *Epilepsia Open.* 2017 Sep;2(3):350–354.
[3807] Sayyah M, Valizadeh J, Kamalinejad M. Anticonvulsant activity of the leaf oil of Laurus nobilis against pentylentetrazole- and maximal electroshock-induced seizure. *Phytomedicine.* 2002 Apr;9(3):212-16.
[3808] Culic M, Kekovic G, Grbic G, et al. Wavelet and fractal analysis of rat brain activity in seizures evoked by camphor oil and 1,8-cineole. *Gen Physiol Biophys.* 2009;28 Sec No:33-40.https://pubmed.ncbi.nlm.nih.gov/25599399/
[3809] Burkhard PR, Burkhardt K, Haenggeli CA, et al. Plant-induced seizures: reappearance of an old problem. *J Neurol.* 1999 Aug;246(8):667-70.
[3810] Waldman N. Seizure caused by dermal application of over-the-counter eucalyptus oil head lice preparation. *Clin Toxicol (Phila).* 2011 Oct;49(8):750-1.
[3811] Craig JO. Poisoning by the volatile oils in childhood. *Arch Dis Child.* 1953;28:259-67.
[3812] Mathew T, Kamath V, Kumar RS, et al. Eucalyptus oil inhalation-induced seizure: A novel, underrecognized, preventable cause of acute symptomatic seizure. *Epilepsia Open.* 2017 Jul 4;2(3):350-354.
[3813] Jori A, Bianchetti A, Prestini PE, et al. Effect of eucalyptol (1,8-cineole) on the metabolism of other drugs in rats and in man. *Eur J Pharmacol.* 1970;9(3):362-66.
[3814] de Sousa DP, Raphael E, Brocksom U, et al. Sedative effect of monoterpene alcohols in mice: A preliminary screening. *Verlag der Zeitschrift fur Naturforschung.* 2007;62c:563-66.
[3815] Lamborn LL. Modern soaps, candles and glycerin: A practical manual of modern methods of utilization of fats and oils in the manufacture of soaps and candles, and of the recovery of glycerin. Library of the University of Wisconsin.
[3816] Oyen LP, Dung NX. Plant resources of South-East Asia. 1999. Backhyus, Leiden.
[3817] Kim NH, Hyun SH, Jin CH, et al. Pretreatment with 1,8-cineole potentiates thioacetamide-induced hepatotoxicity and immunosuppression. *Arch Pharm Res.* 2004 Jul;27(7):781-9.
[3818] Brehm-Stecher BF, Johnson EA. Sensitization of Staphylococcus aureus and Escherichia coli to antibiotics by the sesquiterpenoids nerolidol, farnesol, bisabolol, and apritone. *Antimicrob Agents Chemother.* 2003 Oct;47(10):3357-60.
[3819] El-Ahmady SH, Ashour ML, Wink M. Chemical composition and anti-inflammatory activity of the essential oils of Psidium guajava fruits and leaves. *J Essent Oil Res.* 2013;25(6):475-81.
[3820] Manosroi J, Dhumtanom P, Manosroi A. Anti-proliferative activity of essential oil extracted from Thai medicinal plants on KB and P388 cell lines. *Cancer Lett.* 2006;235:114–20.
[3821] El-Ahmady SH, Ashour ML, Wink M. Chemical composition and anti-inflammatory activity of the essential oils of Psidium guajava fruits and leaves. *J Essent Oil Res.* 2013;25(6):475-81.
[3822] Siani AC, Souza MC, Henriques MGMO, et al. Anti-inflammatory activity of essential oils from Syzygium cumini and Psidium guajava. *Pharmaceutical Biol.* 2013;51:881-87.
[3823] Ngoula F, Guemdjo Tekam M, Kenfack A, et al. Effects of heat stress on some reproductive parameters of male cavie (Cavia porcellus) and mitigation strategies using guava (Psidium guajava) leaves essential oil. *J Therm Biol.* 2017 Feb;64:67-72.
[3824] El-Ahmady SH, Ashour ML, Wink M. Chemical composition and anti-inflammatory activity of the essential oils of Psidium guajava fruits and leaves. *J Essent Oil Res.* 2013;25(6):475-81.
[3825] Santos FA, Rao VSN, Silveira ER. Investigations on the antinociceptive effect of Psidium guajava leaf essential oil and its major constituents. *Phytother Res.* 1998;12:24-27.
[3826] Little JW, Ford A, Symons-Liguori AM, et al. Endogenous adenosine A3 receptor activation selectively alleviates persistent pain states. *Brain.* 2015 Jan;138(Pt 1):28-35.
[3827] Gonçalves FA, Andrade Neto M, Bezerra JN, et al. Antibacterial activity of GUAVA, Psidium guajava Linnaeus, leaf extracts on diarrhea-causing enteric bacteria isolated from Seabob shrimp, Xiphopenaeus kroyeri (Heller). *Rev Inst Med Trop Sao Paulo.* 2008 Jan-Feb;50(1):11-5.
[3828] Joseph B, Priya RM, Helen PAM, et al. Bio-active constituents in essential oil and its effects of antimicrobial, cytotoxic activity from the Psidium guajava (L.) Leaf. *J Adv Biotechnol.* 2010;9:10-14.
[3829] Santos FA, Rao VS, Silveira ER. The leaf essential oil of Psidium guyanensis offers protection against pentylenetetrazole-induced seizures. *Planta Med.* 1997 Apr;63(2):133-5.
[3830] Satyal P, Paudel P, Lamichhane B, et al. Leaf essential oil composition and bioactivity of Psidium guajava from Kathmandu, Nepal. *Am J Essential Oils Nat Prod.* 2015;3(2):11-14.
[3831] Rajkumar S, Jebanesan A. Repellent activity of selected plant essential oils against the malarial fever mosquito Anopheles stephensi. *Trop Biomed.* 2007 Dec;24(2):71-5.
[3832] Wang L, Wu Y1, Huang T, et al. Chemical compositions, antioxidant and antimicrobial activities of essential oil of Psidium guajava L. leaves from different geographic regions in China. *Chem Biodivers.* 2017 Sep;14(9).
[3833] Silva EAJ, Estevam EBB, Silva TS, et al. Antibacterial and antiproliferative activities of the fresh leaf essential oil of Psidium guajava L. (Myrtaceae). *Braz J Biol.* 2019 Oct-Dec;79(4):697-702.
[3834] Silva EAJ, Estevam EBB, Silva TS, et al. Antibacterial and antiproliferative activities of the fresh leaf essential oil of Psidium guajava L. (Myrtaceae). *Braz J Biol.* 2019 Oct-Dec;79(4):697-702.
[3835] Chaturvedi T, Singh S, Nishad I, et al. Chemical composition and antimicrobial activity of the essential oil of senescent leaves of guava (Psidium guajava L.). *Nat Prod Res.* 2019 Aug 12:1-5.

3836 Mandal AK, Paudel S, Pandey A, et al. Guava Leaf Essential Oil as a Potent Antioxidant and Anticancer Agent: Validated through Experimental and Computational Study. *Antioxidants (Basel)*. 2022 Nov 7;11(11):2204.

3837 Mahomoodally F, Aumeeruddy-Elafi Z, Venugopala KN, et al. Antiglycation, Comparative Antioxidant Potential, Phenolic Content and Yield Variation of Essential Oils From 19 Exotic and Endemic Medicinal Plants. *Saudi J Biol Sci*. 2019 Nov;26(7):1779-88.

3838 Fernandes CC, Rezende JL, Silva EAJ, et al. Chemical composition and biological activities of essential oil from flowers of Psidium guajava (Myrtaceae). *Braz J Biol*. 2020 Aug 14;S1519-69842020005022213.

3839 de Souza WFC, de Lucena FA, de Castro RJS, et al. Exploiting the chemical composition of essential oils from Psidium cattleianum and Psidium guajava and its antimicrobial and antioxidant properties. *J Food Sci*. 2021 Sep 5. Online ahead of print.

3840 Jhaiaun P, Panthawong A, Sukkanon C, et al. Avoidance Behavior to Guava Leaf Volatile Oil by Three Medically Important Mosquito Vectors. *J Econ Entomol*. 2021 Dec 6;114(6):2534-2542.

3841 Zhang X, Wang J, Zhu H, et al. Chemical composition, antibacterial, antioxidant and enzyme inhibitory activities of the essential oil from leaves of Psidium guajava L. *Chem Biodivers*. 2022 Mar 28. Online ahead of print.

3842 Lahlou Y, El Amraoui B, El-Wahidi M, et al. Chemical composition, antioxidant and antimicrobial activities of Moroccan species of Psidium guajava extracts. *Rocz Panstw Zakl Hig*. 2022;73(1):65-77.

3843 Silva Maiolini TC, Rosa W, de Oliveira Miranda D, et al. Essential Oils from Different Myrtaceae Species from Brazilian Atlantic Forest Biome - Chemical Dereplication and Evaluation of Antitrypanosomal Activity. *Chem Biodivers*. 2022 Jun;19(6):e202200198.

3844 Aly SH, Eldahshan OA, Al-Rashood ST, et al. Chemical Constituents, Antioxidant, and Enzyme Inhibitory Activities Supported by In-Silico Study of n-Hexane Extract and Essential Oil of Guava Leaves. *Molecules*. 2022 Dec 16;27(24):8979.

3845 Varamini S, Sakhteman A, Yousefi G, et al. Volatile composition analysis of five different Commiphora mukul (Hook. ex Stocks) Engl. gum samples. *Trends Pharm Sci*. 2016;2(3):219-22.

3846 Bhati A. Essential oil from the resin of Commiphora mukul. *J Indian Chem Soc*. 1950;27:436–40.

3847 Sarbhoy AK, Varshney JL, Maheshwari ML, et al. Efficacy of some essential oils and their constituents on few ubiquitous molds. *Zentralbl Bakteriol Naturwiss*. 1978;133(7-8):723-5.

3848 Saeed MA, Sabir AW. Antibacterial activities of some constituents from oleo-gum-resin of Commiphora mukul. *Fitoterapia*. 2004 Mar;75(2):204-8.

3849 Siddiqui MZ, Thomas M, Prasad N. Physicochemical Characterization and Antioxidant Activity of Essential Oils of Guggul (Commiphora wightii) Collected from Madhya Pradesh. *Indian J Pharm Sci*. 2013 May;75(3):368-72.

3850 Juan LW, Lucia A, Zerba EN, et al. Chemical composition and fumigant toxicity of the essential oils from 16 species of Eucalyptus against Haematobia irritans (Diptera: Muscidae) adults. *J Econ Entomol*. 2011 Jun;104(3):1087-92.

3851 Baptista EB, Zimmermann-Franco D, Barros Ltaliza AA, et al. Chemical composition and antifungal activity of essential oil from Eucalyptus smithii against dermatophytes. *Rev Soc Bras Med Trop*. 2015 Nov-Dec;48(6):ISSN 1678-9849.

3852 Chisowa EH. Chemical Composition of Essential Oils of Three Eucalyptus Species Grown in Zambia. *J Essent Oil Res*. 1997 Nov-Dec;9:653-55.

3853 Bignell CM, Dunlop PJ, Brophy JJ. Volatile leaf oils of some south-western and southern Australian species of the genus Eucalyptus (series 1). Part XIX. *Flavour Frag J*. 1998 Mar;13(2):131-39.

3854 Craig JO. Poisoning by the volatile oils in childhood. *Arch Dis Child*. 1953;28:259-67.

3855 Melis K. Bochner A, Janssens G. Accidental nasal eucalyptol and menthol instillation. *Eur J Pediatr*. 1989 Aug;148(8)786-7.

3856 Day LM, Ozanne-Smith J, Parsons BJ, et al. Eucalyptus oil poisoning among young children: mechanisms of access and the potential prevention. *Aust N Z J Public Health*. 1997 Jun;21(3):297-302.

3857 Chandar SD, Prashanti M, Kumar CL, et al. Eucalyptus Oil-Induced Seizures in Children: A Single-Center Prospective Study. *Cureus*. 2021 Mar 25;13(3):e14109.

3858 Sayyah M, Valizadeh J, Kamalinejad M. Anticonvulsant activity of the leaf oil of Laurus nobilis against pentylentetrazole- and maximal electroshock-induced seizure. *Phytomedicine*. 2002 Apr;9(3):212-16.

3859 Culic M, Kekovic G, Grbic G, et al. Wavelet and fractal analysis of rat brain activity in seizures evoked by camphor oil and 1,8-cineole. *Gen Physiol Biophys*. 2009;28 Sec No:33-40.

3860 Burkhard PR, Burkhardt K, Haenggeli CA, et al. Plant-induced seizures: reappearance of an old problem. *J Neurol*. 1999 Aug;246(8):667-70.

3861 Waldman N. Seizure caused by dermal application of over-the-counter eucalyptus oil head lice preparation. *Clin Toxicol (Phila)*. 2011 Oct;49(8):750-1.

3862 Craig JO. Poisoning by the volatile oils in childhood. *Arch Dis Child*. 1953;28:259-67.

3863 Mathew T, Kamath V, Kumar RS, et al. Eucalyptus oil inhalation-induced seizure: A novel, underrecognized, preventable cause of acute symptomatic seizure. *Epilepsia Open*. 2017 Jul 4;2(3):350-354.

3864 Newall CA, Anderson LA, Phillipson JD. "Herbal Medicines: A Guide for Health-care Professionals." London: The Pharmaceutical Press, 1996, 108.

3865 European Medicines Agency. Community herbal monograph on Eucalyptus globulus Labill., Eucalyptus polybractea R.T. Baker and/or Eucalyptus smithii R.T. Baker, aetheroleum. 2013 Jun. Available at: http://www.ema.europa.eu/docs/en_GB/document_library/Herbal_-_Community_herbal_monograph/2013/07/WC500147008.pdf

3866 Fischer JH, Dethlefsen U. Efficacy of cineole in patients suffering from acute bronchitis: a placebo-controlled double-blind trial. *Cough*. 2013; 9: 25.

3867 Worth W, Dethlefsen U. Patients with asthma benefit from concomitant therapy with cineole: a placebo-controlled, double-blind trial. *J Asthma*. 2012 Oct;49(8):849-53.

3868 Fischer JH, Dethlefsen U. Efficacy of cineole in patients suffering from acute bronchitis: a placebo-controlled double-blind trial. *Cough*. 2013; 9: 25.

3869 Worth W, Dethlefsen U. Patients with asthma benefit from concomitant therapy with cineole: a placebo-controlled, double-blind trial. *J Asthma*. 2012 Oct;49(8):849-53.

3870 Day LM, Ozanne-Smith J, Parsons BJ, et al. Eucalyptus oil poisoning among young children: mechanisms of access and the potential prevention. *Aust N Z J Public Health*. 1997 Jun;21(3):297-302.

3871 Myott E. Case of eucalyptus poisoning. *Brit M J*. 1906;1:558.

3872 Hindle RC. Eucalyptus oil ingestion. *N Z Med J*. 1994 May 11;107(977)185-6.

3873 Tibballs J. Clinical effects and management of eucalyptus oil ingestion in infants and small children. *Med J Aust*. 1995 Aug;163(4):177-80.

3874 Waldman W, Barwina M, Sein Anand J. Accidental ontoxication with eucalyptus oil—a case report. *Przeql Lek*. 2011;68(8):555-6.

3875 Day LM, Ozanne-Smith J, Parsons BJ, et al. Eucalyptus oil poisoning among young children: mechanisms of access and the potential prevention. *Aust N Z J Public Health*. 1997 Jun;21(3):297-302.

3876 De Vincenzi M, Silano M, De Vincenzi A, et al. Constituents of aromatic plants: eucalyptol. *Fitoterapia*. 2002 Jun;73(3):269-75.

3877 Unger M, Frank A. Simultaneous determination of the inhibitory potency of herbal extracts on the activity of six major cytochrome P450 enzymes using liquid chromatography/mass spectrometry and automated online extraction. *Rapid Commun Mass Spectrom*. 2004;18(19):2273-81.

3878 Kim NH, Hyun SH, Jin CH, et al. Pretreatment with 1,8-cineole potentiates thioacetamide-induced hepatotoxicity and immunosuppression. *Arch Pharm Res*. 2004 Jul;27(7):781-9.

3879 Gray AM, Flatt PR. Antihyperglycemic actions of Eucalyptus globulus (Eucalyptus) are associated with pancreatic and extra pancreatic effects in mice. *J Nutr*. 1998 Dec;128(12):2319–23.

3880 Basak SS, Candan F. Effect of Laurus nobilis L. Essential Oil and its Main Components on α-glucosidase and Reactive Oxygen Species Scavenging Activity. *Iran J Pharm Res*. 2013 Spring;12(2):367-79.

3881 Dey B. Chemo-profiling of eucalyptus and study of its hypoglycemic potential. *World J Diabetes*. 2013 Oct 15;4(5):170–76.

3882 Tsai HH, Lin HW, Chen YL, et al. A review of potential harmful interactions between anticoagulant/antiplatelet agents and Chinese herbal medicines. *PLoS One*. 2013 May 9;8(5):e64255.

3883 Moharam BA, Jantan I, bin Ahmad F, et al. Antiplatelet Aggregation and Platelet Activating Factor (PAF) Receptor Antagonistic Activities of the Essential Oils of Five Goniothalamus Species. *Molecules*. 2010;15:5124-38.

3884 Jori A, Bianchetti A, Prestini PE, et al. Effect of eucalyptol (1,8-cineole) on the metabolism of other drugs in rats and in man. *Eur J Pharmacol*. 1970;9(3):362-66.

3885 de Sousa DP, Raphael E, Brocksom U, et al. Sedative effect of monoterpene alcohols in mice: A preliminary screening. *Verlag der Zeitschrift fur Naturforschung*. 2007;62c:563-66.

3886 Baptista EB, Zimmermann-Franco D, Barros Ltaliza AA, et al. Chemical composition and antifungal activity of essential oil from Eucalyptus smithii against dermatophytes. *Rev Soc Bras Med Trop*. 2015 Nov-Dec;48(6):ISSN 1678-9849.

3887 Camporese A. [In vitro activity of Eucalyptus smithii and Juniperus communis essential oils against bacterial biofilms and efficacy perspectives of complementary inhalation therapy in chronic and recurrent upper respiratory tract infections]. *Infez Med*. 2013 Jun;21(2):117-24.

3888 Juan LW, Lucia A, Zerba EN, et al. Chemical composition and fumigant toxicity of the essential oils from 16 species of Eucalyptus against Haematobia irritans (Diptera: Muscidae) adults. *J Econ Entomol*. 2011 Jun;104(3):1087-92.

3889 Lucia A1, Juan LW, Zerba EN, et al. Validation of models to estimate the fumigant and larvicidal activity of Eucalyptus essential oils against Aedes aegypti (Diptera: Culicidae). *Parasitol Res*. 2012 May;110(5):1675-86.

3890 Lawrence BM. Essential oils 1979-1980. Allured Publishing. p. 34-35.

3891 Ehret C, Ourisson G. Le y-gurjunene structure et configuration isomerisation de L'α-gurjunene. *Terahedron*. 1969;25:1785-99.

3892 Jantan IB. The essential oil of Dipterocarpus kerrii. *J Trop Forest Sci*. 1988;1(1):1-11.

3893 Stillpoint Aromatics. Balsam Gurjun Essential Oil. Available at: http://www.stillpointaromatics.com/balsam-gurjun-Dipterocarpus-turbinatus-essential-oil-aromatherapy.

3894 Carovic-Stanko K, Orlic S, Politeo O, et al. Composition and antibacterial activities of essential oils of seven Ocimum taxa. *Food Chem*. 2010 Mar;119(1):196-201.

3895 Vina A, Murillo E. Essential oil composition from twelve varieties of basil (Ocimum spp) grown in Colombia. *J Braz Chem Soc*. 2003 Sep/Oct;14(5):ISSN 1678-4790.

3896 de Vasconcelos MG, Dos Santos RD, Abreu Matos FJ, et al. Volatile constituents from leaf, inflorescence and root oils of Ocimum americanum L. grown in north-eastern Brazil. *Flavour Frag J*. 2003 Jul/Aug;18(4):303-04.

3897 Mondello L, Zappia G, Cotroneo A, et al. Studies on the essential oil-bearing plants of Bangladesh. Part VIII. Composition of some Ocimum oils O. basilicum L. var. purpurascens; O. sanctum L. green; O. sanctum L. purple; O. americanum L., citral type; O. americanum L., camphor type. *Flavour Frag J*. 2002 Sep/Oct;17(5):335-340.

3898 Padalia RC, Verma RS, Chauhan A, et al. Changes in aroma profiles of 11 Indian Ocimum taxa during plant ontogeny. Acta Physil Plant. 2013 Aug;35(8):2567-87.

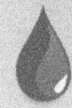

[3899] Abd El-Aziz SE, Omer E. Chemical Composition of Ocimum americanum Essential Oil and Its Biological Effects Against, Agrotis ipsilon, (Lepidoptera: Noctuidae). *Res J Agric Biol Sci.* 2007;3(6):740-47.
[3900] Parida R, Sandeep S, Sethy BK, et al. Chemical composition, antioxidant and antimicrobial activities of essential oil from lime basil (Ocimum Americanum): A potent source for natural antioxidant. *Int J Pharmacy Pharmaceutical Sci.* 2014 Jan;6(7):487-90.
[3901] Zhang JW, Li SK, Wu WJ. The Main Chemical Composition and in vitro Antifungal Activity of the Essential Oils of Ocimum basilicum Linn. var. pilosum (Willd.) Benth. *Molecules.* 2009;14:273-78.
[3902] Yayi E, Moudachirou M, Chlchat JC. Chemotyping of Three Ocimum Species from Benin: O. basilicum, O. canum and O. gratissimum. *J Essent Oil Res.* 2001 Jan;13(1):13-17.
[3903] Sishu R, Tadese S, Bucar F, et al. Chemical composition and antioxidant activity of the essential oils of Ocimum americanum and Ocimum basillicum var. thyrsiflorum. *Int J Essent Oil Ther.* 2010;4:64-68.
[3904] Zollo PH, Biyiti L, Tchoumbougnang F, et al. Aromatic plants of tropical Africa. Part XXXII. Chemical composition and antifungal activity of thirteen essential oils from aromatic plants of Cameroon. *Flavour Frag J.* 1998;13:107-14.
[3905] Fun CE, Baerheim Svendsen A. Composition of the essential oils of Ocimum basilicum var. canum Sims and O. gratissimum L. Grown on Aruba. *Flavour Frag J.* 1990 sep;5(3):173-77.
[3906] Ekundayo O, Laakso I, Hiltunen R. Constituents of the volatile oil from leaves of Ocimum canum sims. *Flavour Frag J.* 1989 Mar;4(1):17-18.
[3907] Akono Ntonga P, Baldovini N, Mouray E, et al. Activity of Ocimum basilicum, Ocimum canum, and Cymbopogon citratus essential oils against Plasmodium falciparum and mature-stage larvae of Anopheles funestus s.s. *Parasite.* 2014;21:33.
[3908] Nascimento JC, Barbosa LC, Paula VF, et al. Chemical composition and antimicrobial activity of essential oils of Ocimum canum Sims. and Ocimum selloi Benth. *An Acad Bras Cienc.* 2011 Sep;83(3):787-99
[3909] Martins AP, Salgueiro LR, Vila R, et al. Composition of the essential oils of Ocimum canum, O. gratissimum and O. minimum. *Planta Med.* 1999 Mar;65(2):187-9.
[3910] Ntezurubanza L, Scheffer JJ, Looman A. Composition of the essential oil of Ocimum canum grown in Rwanda. *Pharm Weekbl Sci.* 1985 Dec 13;7(6):273-6.
[3911] Yamada AN, Grespan R, Yamada ÁT, et al. Anti-inflammatory activity of Ocimum americanum L. essential oil in experimental model of zymosan-induced arthritis. *Am J Chin Med.* 2013;41(4):913-26.
[3912] Bayala B, Bassole IH, Gnoula C, et al. Chemical composition, antioxidant, anti-inflammatory and anti-proliferative activities of essential oils of plants from Burkina Faso. *PLoS One.* 2014 Mar 24;9(3):e92122.
[3913] Cavalcanti ES, Morais SM, Lima MA, et al. Larvicidal activity of essential oils from Brazilian plants against Aedes aegypti L. *Mem Inst Oswaldo Cruz.* 2004 Aug;99(5):541-4.
[3914] Cimanga K, Kambu K, Tona L, et al. Correlation between chemical composition and antibacterial activity of essential oils of some aromatic medicinal plants growing in the Democratic Republic of Congo. *J Ethnopharmacol.* 2002 Feb;79(2):213-20.
[3915] de Lima Silva L, Garlet QI, Koakoski G, et al. Anesthetic activity of the essential oil of Ocimum americanum in Rhamdia quelen (Quoy & Gaimard, 1824) and its effects on stress parameters. *Neotropical Ichthyology.* 2015;13(4):715-22.
[3916] Cardoso NN, Alviano CS, Blank AF, et al. Synergism Effect of the Essential Oil from Ocimum basilicum var. Maria Bonita and Its Major Components with Fluconazole and Its Influence on Ergosterol Biosynthesis. *Evid Based Complement Alternat Med.* 2016;2016:5647182.
[3917] Domaracky M, Rehak P, Juhas S, et al. Effects of selected plant essential oils on the growth and development of mouse preimplantation embryos in vivo. *Physiol Res.* 2007;56(1):97-104.
[3918] Vrskova D, Modra H. Evaluation of the developmental toxicity of 2-phenoxyethanol and clove oil anesthetics using the Frog Embryo Teratogenesis Assay: Xenopus (FETAX). *Veterinarami Medicina.* 2012;57(5):245-50.
[3919] Amini A, Cheraghi E, Safaee MR, et al. The role of eugenol in the reduction of teratogenic effects of retinoic acid on skeletal morphology of mice embryo. *Yakhteh Medical Journal.* 2003;4:195-200.
[3920] Chen SJ, Wang MH, Chen IJ. Antiplatelet and calcium inhibitory properties of eugenol and sodium eugenol acetate. *Gen Pharmacol.* 1996 Jun;27(4):629-33.
[3921] Tognolini M, Barocelli E, Ballabeni V, et al. Comparative screening of plant essential oils; phenylpropanoid moiety as basic core for antiplatelet activity. *Life Sci.* 2006 Feb 23;78(13):1419-32.
[3922] Heck AM, DeWitt BA, Lukes AL. Potential interactions between alternative therapies and warfarin. *Am J Health Syst Pharm.* 2000;57(13):1221-1227.
[3923] Saaeed SA, Gilani AH. Antithrombotic activity of clove oil. *J Pak Med Assoc.* 1994;44(5):112-15.
[3924] Kamatou GP, Vermaak I, Viljoen AM. Eugenol—from the remote Maluku Islands to the international market place: A review of a remarkable and versatile molecule. *Molecules.* 2012;17:6953-81.
[3925] Tao G, Irie Y, Li DJ, et al. Eugenol and its structural analogs inhibit monoamine oxidase A and exhibit antidepressant-like activity. *Bioorg Med Chem.* 2005 Aug 1;13(15):4777-88.
[3926] Olowe SA, Ransome-Kuti O. The risk of jaundice in glucose-6-phosphate dehydrogenase deficient babies exposed to menthol. *Acta Paediatr Scand.* 1980 May;69(3):341-5.
[3927] Dillon Remy M, Manning Alleyne P, Bratt DE, et al. Neonatal jaundice at Port-of-Spain General Hospital abstract. *West Indian Med J.* 1987;36(Suppl):28.
[3928] Langeveld WT, Veldhuizen EJ, Burt SA. Synergy between essential oil constituents and antibiotics. *Crit Rev Microbiol.* 2014 Feb;40(1);76-94.
[3929] Nogueira AC, Carvalho RR, Souza CA, et al. Study on the embryofeto-toxicity of citral in the rat. *Toxicology.* 1995;96(2):105-13.
[3930] Seo KA, Kim H, Ku HY, et al. The monoterpenoids citral and geraniol are moderate inhibitors of the CYP2B6 hydroxylase activity. *Chem Biol Interact.* 2008;174:141-46.
[3931] Hagvall L, Baron JM, Börje A, et al. Cytochrome P450-mediated activation of the fragrance constituent geraniol forms potent contact allergens. *Toxicol Appl Pharmacol.* 2008 Dec 1;233(2):308-13.
[3932] Chen CJ, Tseng YH, Chu FH, et al. Neuropharmacological activities of fruit essential oil from Litsea cubeba Persoon. *J Wood Sci.* 2012;58:538-43.
[3933] Modak T, Mukhopadhaya A. Effects of citral, a naturally occurring antiadipogenic molecule, on an energy-intense diet model of obesity. *Indian J Pharmacol.* 2011 May-Jun;43(3):300-05.
[3934] Najafian M, Ebrahim-Habibi A, Yaghmaei P, et al. Citral as a potential antihyperlipidemic medicine in diabetes: a study on streptozotocin-induced diabetic rats. *J Diabetes Metabolic Disorders.* 2011;10(1):3.
[3935] Choi JY, Damte D, Seung-Jin L, et al. Antimicrobial activity of lemongrass and oregano essential oil against standard antibiotic resistant Staphylococcus aureus and field isolates from chronic mastitis cow. *International Journal of Phytomedicine.* 2012;4(1):134-39.
[3936] Shin S, Lim S. Antifungal effects of herbal essential oils alone and in combination with ketoconazole against Trichophyton spp. *J Appl Micribiol.* 2004;97:1289-96.
[3937] Lalko J, Api AM. Investigation of the dermal sensitization potential of various essential oils in the local lymph node assay. *Food Chem Toxicol.* 2006 May;44(5):739-46.
[3938] Huang J, Wang S, Luo X, et al. Cinnamaldehyde reduction of platelet aggregation and thrombosis in rodents. *Thromb Res.* 2007;119(3):337–42.
[3939] Ballabeni V, Tognolini M, Bertoni S, et al. Antiplatelet and antithrombotic activities of essential oil from wild Ocotea quixos (Lam.) Kostern. (Lauraceae) calices from Amazonian Ecuador. *Pharmacol Res.* 2007 Jan;55(1):23–30.
[3940] European Medicines Agency. Public statement on the use of herbal medicinal products containing estragole. Available at: http://www.ema.europa.eu/docs/en_GB/document_library/Scientific_guideline/2010/04/WC500089960.pdf.
[3941] European Medicines Agency. Public statement on the use of herbal medicinal products containing estragole. Available at: http://www.ema.europa.eu/docs/en_GB/document_library/Scientific_guideline/2010/04/WC500089960.pdf.
[3942] Ding W, Levy DD, Bishop ME, et al. In vivo genotoxicity of estragole in male F344 rats. *Environ Mol Mutagen.* 2015 May;56(4):356-65.
[3943] European Commission. Opinion of the Scientific Committee on Food on estragole (1-Allyl-4-methoxybenzene). Available at: http://ec.europa.eu/food/fs/sc/scf/out104_en.pdf.
[3944] California Environmental Protection Agency. Evidence of the carcinogenicity of estragole. Available at: http:// oehha.ca.gov/prop65/pdf/estragf.pdf.
[3945] Mertas A, Garbusińska A, Szliszka E, et al. The influence of tea tree oil (Melaleuca alternifolia) on fluconazole activity against fluconazole-resistant Candida albicans strains. *Biomed Res Int.* 2015;2015:590470.
[3946] Khine H, Weiss D, Graber N, et al. A cluster of children with seizures caused by camphor poisoning. *Pediatrics.* 2009 May;123(5):1269-72.
[3947] Michiels EA, Mazor SS. Toddler with seizures due to ingesting camphor at an Indian celebration. *Pediatr Emerg Care.* 2010 Aug;26(8):574-75.
[3948] Koren G. Medications which can kill a toddler with one tablet or teaspoonful. *J toxicol Clin toxicol.* 1993;31(3):407- 13.
[3949] Flaman Z, Pellechia-Clarke S, Bailey B, et al. Unintentional exposure of young children to camphor and eucalyptus oils. *Paediatr Child Health.* 2001 Feb;6(2):80-83.
[3950] Rabl W, Katzgraber F, Steinlechner M. Camphor ingestion for abortion (case report). *Forensic Sci Int.* 1997 Sep 19;89(1-2):137-40.
[3951] Narayan S, Singh N. Camphor poisoning-An unusual cause of seizure. *Med J Armed Forces India.* 2012 Jul;68(3):252-53.
[3952] Chanaranaj KJ, G MV, S M. Camphor poisoning in a child. *Natl Med J India.* 2013 Jan-Feb;26(1):60.
[3953] Uc A, Bishop WP, Sanders KD. Camphor hepatotoxicity. *South Med J.* 2000;93:596-98.
[3954] Olowe SA, Ransome-Kuti O. The risk of jaundice in glucose-6-phosphate dehydrogenase deficient babies exposed to menthol. *Acta Paediatr Scand.* 1980 May;69(3):341-5.
[3955] Dillon Remy M, Manning Alleyne P, Bratt DE, et al. Neonatal jaundice at Port-of-Spain General Hospital abstract. *West Indian Med J.* 1987;36(Suppl):28.
[3956] Manoguerra AS, Erdman AR, Wax PM, et al. Camphor poisoning: an evidence-based practice guideline for out-of- hospital management. *Clin Toxicol (Phila).*2006;44(4):357-70.
[3957] Gibson DE, Moore GP, Pfaff JA. Camphor ingestion. *Am J Emerg Med.* 1989 Jan;7(1):41-43.
[3958] Koppel C, Martends F, Schirop T, et al. Hemoperfusion in acute camphor poisoning. *Intensive Care Med.* 1988;14(4):431-33.
[3959] Covington TR, et al. Handbook of Nonprescription Drugs. 11$^{th}$ ed. Washington, D.C.: American Pharmaceutical Association. 1996.
[3960] Johnson JD, Ryan MJ, Toft JD II, et al. Two-year toxicity and carcinogenicity study of methyl eugenol in F344/N rats and B6C3F(1) mice. *J Agric Food Chem.* 2000 Aug;48(8):3620-32.
[3961] European Commission. Opinion of the Scientific Committee on Food on methyl eugenol (4-Allyl-1,2- dimethoxybenzene).Availableat:http://ec.europa.eu/food/fs/sc/scf/out102_en.pdf.
[3962] National Toxicology Program. NTP Toxicology and Carcinogenesis Studies of Methyleugenol (CAS NO. 93-15-2) in F344/N Rats and B6C3F1 Mice (Gavage Studies). *Natl Toxicol Program Tech Rep Ser.* 2000 Jul;491:1-412.
[3963] National Toxicology Program. Carcinogenesis Studies of Eugenol (CAS No. 97-53-0) in F344/N Rats and B6C3F1 Mice (Feed Studies). Technical Report Series No. 223. NIH Publication No. 84-1779. 1983. U.S. DHHS, PHS, NIH, NTP, Research Triangle Park, NC.
[3964] Johnson JD, Ryan MJ, Toft JD II, et al. Two-year toxicity and carcinogenicity study of methyl eugenol in F344/N rats and B6C3F(1) mice. *J Agric Food Chem.* 2000 Aug;48(8):3620-32.

[3965] National Toxicology Program. NTP Toxicology and Carcinogenesis Studies of Methyleugenol (CAS NO. 93-15-2) in F344/N Rats and B6C3F1 Mice (Gavage Studies). *Natl Toxicol Program Tech Rep Ser*. 2000 Jul;491:1-412.

[3966] Kerckaert GA, Brauninger R, LeBoeuf RA, et al. Use of the Syrian hamster embryo cell transformation assay for carcinogenicity prediction of chemicals currently being tested by the National Toxicology Program in rodent bioassays. *Environ Health Perspect*. 1996;104:1075-84.

[3967] National Toxicology Program. Carcinogenesis Studies of Eugenol (CAS No. 97-53-0) in F344/N Rats and B6C3F1 Mice (Feed Studies). Technical Report Series No. 223. NIH Publication No. 84-1779. 1983. U.S. DHHS, PHS, NIH, NTP, Research Triangle Park, NC.

[3968] Johnson JD, Ryan MJ, Toft JD II, et al. Two-year toxicity and carcinogenicity study of methyl eugenol in F344/N rats and B6C3F(1) mice. *J Agric Food Chem*. 2000 Aug;48(8):3620-32.

[3969] European Commission. Opinion of the Scientific Committee on Food on methyl eugenol (4-Allyl-1,2- dimethoxybenzene). Available at: http://ec.europa.eu/food/fs/sc/scf/out102_en.pdf.

[3970] National Toxicology Program. NTP Toxicology and Carcinogenesis Studies of Methyleugenol (CAS NO. 93-15-2) in F344/N Rats and B6C3F1 Mice (Gavage Studies). *Natl Toxicol Program Tech Rep Ser*. 2000 Jul;491:1-412.

[3971] National Toxicology Program. Carcinogenesis Studies of Eugenol (CAS No. 97-53-0) in F344/N Rats and B6C3F1 Mice (Feed Studies). Technical Report Series No. 223. NIH Publication No. 84-1779. 1983. U.S. DHHS, PHS, NIH, NTP, Research Triangle Park, NC.

[3972] Ahmad A, Khan A, Ahmad Khan L, et al. In vitro synergy of eugenol and methyleugenol with fluconazole against clinical Candida isolates. *J Med Microbiol*. 2010;59:1178-84.

[3973] Nguyen LT, Mysliveckova Z, Szotakova B, et al. The inhibitory effects of β-caryophyllene, β-caryophyllene oxide and α-humulene on the activities of the main drug-metabolizing enzymes in rat and human liver in vitro. *Chem-Biol Interactoins.* 2017 Dec 25;278:123-8.

[3974] Craig JO. Poisoning by the volatile oils in childhood. *Arch Dis Child*. 1953;28:259-67.

[3975] Melis K. Bochner A, Janssens G. Accidental nasal eucalyptol and menthol instillation. *Eur J Pediatr*. 1989 Aug;148(8)786-7.

[3976] Day LM, Ozanne-Smith J, Parsons BJ, et al. Eucalyptus oil poisoning among young children: mechanisms of access and the potential prevention. *Aust N Z J Public Health*. 1997 Jun;21(3):297-302.

[3977] Chandar SD, Prashanti M, Kumar CL, et al. Eucalyptus Oil-Induced Seizures in Children: A Single-Center Prospective Study. *Cureus*. 2021 Mar 25;13(3):e14109.

[3978] European Medicines Agency. Public statement on the use of herbal medicinal products containing estragole. Available at: http://www.ema.europa.eu/docs/en_GB/document_library/Scientific_guideline/2010/04/WC500089960.pdf.

[3979] European Medicines Agency. Public statement on the use of herbal medicinal products containing estragole. Available at: http://www.ema.europa.eu/docs/en_GB/document_library/Scientific_guideline/2010/04/WC500089960.pdf.

[3980] Ding W, Levy DD, Bishop ME, et al. In vivo genotoxicity of estragole in male F344 rats. *Environ Mol Mutagen*. 2015 May;56(4):356-65.

[3981] Sayyah M, Valizadeh J, Kamalinejad M. Anticonvulsant activity of the leaf oil of Laurus nobilis against pentylentetrazole- and maximal electroshock-induced seizure. *Phytomedicine*. 2002 Apr;9(3):212-16.

[3982] Culic M, Kekovic G, Grbic G, et al. Wavelet and fractal analysis of rat brain activity in seizures evoked by camphor oil and 1,8-cineole. *Gen Physiol Biophys*. 2009;28 Sec No:33-40.

[3983] Burkhard PR, Burkhardt K, Haenggeli CA, et al. Plant-induced seizures: reappearance of an old problem. *J Neurol*. 1999 Aug;246(8):667-70.

[3984] Waldman N. Seizure caused by dermal application of over-the-counter eucalyptus oil head lice preparation. *Clin Toxicol (Phila)*. 2011 Oct;49(8):750-1.

[3985] Craig JO. Poisoning by the volatile oils in childhood. *Arch Dis Child*. 1953;28:259-67.

[3986] Mathew T, Kamath V, Kumar RS, et al. Eucalyptus oil inhalation-induced seizure: A novel, underrecognized, preventable cause of acute symptomatic seizure. *Epilepsia Open*. 2017 Jul 4;2(3):350-354.

[3987] Newall CA, Anderson LA, Phillipson JD. "Herbal Medicines: A Guide for Health-care Professionals." London: The Pharmaceutical Press, 1996, 108.

[3988] European Medicines Agency. Community herbal monograph on Eucalyptus globulus Labill., Eucalyptus polybractea R.T. Baker and/or Eucalyptus smithii R.T. Baker, aetheroleum. 2013 Jun. Available at: http://www.ema.europa.eu/docs/en_GB/document_library/Herbal_-_Community_herbal_monograph/2013/07/WC500147008.pdf

[3989] Fischer JH, Dethlefsen U. Efficacy of cineole in patients suffering from acute bronchitis: a placebo-controlled double-blind trial. *Cough*. 2013; 9: 25.

[3990] Worth W, Dethlefsen U. Patients with asthma benefit from concomitant therapy with cineole: a placebo-controlled, double-blind trial. *J Asthma*. 2012 Oct;49(8):849-53.

[3991] Day LM, Ozanne-Smith J, Parsons BJ, et al. Eucalyptus oil poisoning among young children: mechanisms of access and the potential prevention. *Aust N Z J Public Health*. 1997 Jun;21(3):297-302.

[3992] Myott E. Case of eucalyptus poisoning. *Brit M J*. 1906;1:558.

[3993] Hindle RC. Eucalyptus oil ingestion. *N Z Med J*. 1994 May 11;107(977)185-6.

[3994] Tibballs J. Clinical effects and management of eucalyptus oil ingestion in infants and small children. *Med J Aust*. 1995 Aug;163(4):177-80.

[3995] Waldman W, Barwina M, Sein Anand J. Accidental ontoxication with eucalyptus oil—a case report. *Przeql Lek*. 2011;68(8):555-6.

[3996] Day LM, Ozanne-Smith J, Parsons BJ, et al. Eucalyptus oil poisoning among young children: mechanisms of access and the potential prevention. *Aust N Z J Public Health*. 1997 Jun;21(3):297-302.

[3997] De Vincenzi M, Silano M, De Vincenzi A, et al. Constituents of aromatic plants: eucalyptol. *Fitoterapia*. 2002 Jun;73(3):269-75.

[3998] European Commission. Opinion of the Scientific Committee on Food on estragole (1-Allyl-4-methoxybenzene). Available at: http://ec.europa.eu/food/fs/sc/scf/out104_en.pdf.

[3999] California Environmental Protection Agency. Evidence of the carcinogenicity of estragole. Available at: http://oehha.ca.gov/prop65/pdf/estragf.pdf.

[4000] Gray AM, Flatt PR. Antihyperglycemic actions of Eucalyptus globulus (Eucalyptus) are associated with pancreatic and extra pancreatic effects in mice. *J Nutr*. 1998 Dec;128(12):2319–23.

[4001] Basak SS, Candan F. Effect of Laurus nobilis L. Essential Oil and its Main Components on α-glucosidase and Reactive Oxygen Species Scavenging Activity. *Iran J Pharm Res*. 2013 Spring;12(2):367-79.

[4002] Fathiazad F, Mazandarani M, Hamedeyazdan. Phytochemical analysis and antioxidant activity of Hyssopus officinalis L. from Iran. *Adv Pharm Bull*. 2011 Dec;1(2):63–67.

[4003] Jori A, Bianchetti A, Prestini PE, et al. Effect of eucalyptol (1,8-cineole) on the metabolism of other drugs in rats and in man. *Eur J Pharmacol*. 1970;9(3):362-66.

[4004] de Sousa DP, Raphael E, Brocksom U, et al. Sedative effect of monoterpene alcohols in mice: A preliminary screening. *Verlag der Zeitschrift fur Naturforschung*. 2007;62c:563-66.

[4005] Tsai HH, Lin HW, Chen YL, et al. A review of potential harmful interactions between anticoagulant/antiplatelet agents and Chinese herbal medicines. *PLoS One*. 2013 May 9;8(5):e64255.

[4006] Moharam BA, Jantan I, bin Ahmad F, et al. Antiplatelet Aggregation and Platelet Activating Factor (PAF) Receptor Antagonistic Activities of the Essential Oils of Five Goniothalamus Species. *Molecules*. 2010;15:5124-38.

[4007] Olowe SA, Ransome-Kuti O. The risk of jaundice in glucose-6-phosphate dehydrogenase deficient babies exposed to menthol. *Acta Paediatr Scand*. 1980 May;69(3):341-5.

[4008] Dillon Remy M, Manning Alleyne P, Bratt DE, et al. Neonatal jaundice at Port-of-Spain General Hospital abstract. *West Indian Med J*. 1987;36(Suppl):28.

[4009] Jori A, Bianchetti A, Prestini PE, et al. Effect of eucalyptol (1,8-cineole) on the metabolism of other drugs in rats and in man. *Eur J Pharmacol*. 1970;9(3):362-66.

[4010] Kim NH, Hyun SH, Jin CH, et al. Pretreatment with 1,8-cineole potentiates thioacetamide-induced hepatotoxicity and immunosuppression. *Arch Pharm Res*. 2004 Jul;27(7):781-9.

[4011] European Medicines Agency. Public statement on the use of herbal medicinal products containing estragole. Available at: http://www.ema.europa.eu/docs/en_GB/document_library/Scientific_guideline/2010/04/WC500089960.pdf.

[4012] European Medicines Agency. Public statement on the use of herbal medicinal products containing estragole. Available at: http://www.ema.europa.eu/docs/en_GB/document_library/Scientific_guideline/2010/04/WC500089960.pdf.

[4013] Ding W, Levy DD, Bishop ME, et al. In vivo genotoxicity of estragole in male F344 rats. *Environ Mol Mutagen*. 2015 May;56(4):356-65.

[4014] Domaracky M, Rehak P, Juhas S, et al. Effects of selected plant essential oils on the growth and development of mouse preimplantation embryos in vivo. *Physiol Res*. 2007;56(1):97-104.

[4015] Vrskova D, Modra H. Evaluation of the developmental toxicity of 2-phenoxyethanol and clove oil anesthetics using the Frog Embryo Teratogenesis Assay: Xenopus (FETAX). *Veterinarami Medicina*. 2012;57(5):245-50.

[4016] Amini A, Cheraghi E, Safaee MR, et al. The role of eugenol in the reduction of teratogenic effects of retinoic acid on skeletal morphology of mice embryo. *Yakhteh Medical Journal*. 2003;4:195-200.

[4017] European Medicines Agency. Public statement on the use of herbal medicinal products containing estragole. Available at: http://www.ema.europa.eu/docs/en_GB/document_library/Scientific_guideline/2010/04/WC500089960.pdf.

[4018] Ding W, Levy DD, Bishop ME, et al. In vivo genotoxicity of estragole in male F344 rats. *Environ Mol Mutagen*. 2015 May;56(4):356-65.

[4019] Eisenmann SW, Poulev A, Struwe L, et al. Qualitative variation of anti-diabetic constituents in different tarragon (Artemisia dracunculus L.) cytotypes. *Fitoterapia*. 2011 Oct;82(7):1062–74.

[4020] European Medicines Agency. Public statement on the use of herbal medicinal products containing estragole. Available at: http://www.ema.europa.eu/docs/en_GB/document_library/Scientific_guideline/2010/04/WC500089960.pdf.

[4021] European Commission. Opinion of the Scientific Committee on Food on estragole (1-Allyl-4-methoxybenzene). Available at: http://ec.europa.eu/food/fs/sc/scf/out104_en.pdf.

[4022] California Environmental Protection Agency. Evidence of the carcinogenicity of estragole. Available at: http://oehha.ca.gov/prop65/pdf/estragf.pdf.

[4023] Drinkwater NR, Miller EC, Miller JA, et al. Hepatocarcinogenicity of estragole (1-allyl-4-methoxybenzene) and 1'-hydroxyestragole in the mouse and mutagenicity of 1'-acetoxyestragole in bacteria. *J Natl Cancer Inst*. 1976 Dec;57(6):1323-31.

[4024] Zeller A, Horst K, Rychlik M. Study of the metabolism of estragole in humans consuming fennel tea. *Chem Res Toxicol*. 2009 Dec;22(12):1929-37.

[4025] Chen SJ, Wang MH, Chen IJ. Antiplatelet and calcium inhibitory properties of eugenol and sodium eugenol acetate. *Gen Pharmacol*. 1996 Jun;27(4):629-33.

[4026] Tognolini M, Barocelli E, Ballabeni V, et al. Comparative screening of plant essential oils; phenylpropanoid moiety as basic core for antiplatelet activity. *Life Sci*. 2006 Feb 23;78(13):1419-32.

[4027] Heck AM, DeWitt BA, Lukes AL. Potential interactions between alternative therapies and warfarin. *Am J Health Syst Pharm*. 2000;57(13):1221-1227.

[4028] Saaeed SA, Gilani AH. Antithrombotic activity of clove oil. *J Pak Med Assoc*. 1994;44(5):112-15.

[4029] Lee HS. Anticoagulant properties of constituents derived from fennel (Foeniculum vulgare Gaertner) fruits. *Food Sci Biotech*. 2006 Oct;15(5):763-67.

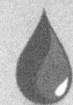

4030 Kamatou GP, Vermaak I, Viljoen AM. Eugenol—from the remote Maluku Islands to the international market place: A review of a remarkable and versatile molecule. *Molecules.* 2012;17:6953-81.

4031 Tao G, Irie Y, Li DJ, et al. Eugenol and its structural analogs inhibit monoamine oxidase A and exhibit antidepressant-like activity. *Bioorg Med Chem.* 2005 Aug 1;13(15):4777-88.

4032 Cochrane ML. Inhibition of Cytochrome P450 2C9 by essential oils. Available at: https://libres.uncg.edu/ir/uncg/listing.aspx?id=18102

4033 Dohi S, Terasaki M, Makino M. Acetylcholinesterase inhibitory activity and chemical composition of commercial essential oils. *J Agric Food Chem.* 2009 May 27;57(10):4313-8.

4034 Langeveld WT, Veldhuizen EJ, Burt SA. Synergy between essential oil constituents and antibiotics. *Crit Rev Microbiol.* 2014 Feb;40(1):76-94.

4035 Sarrami N, Pemberton MN, Thornhill MH, et al. Adverse reactions associated with the use of eugenol in dentistry. *British Dental J.* 2002;193:253-55.

4036 Tammannavar P, Pushpalatha C, Jain S, et al. An unexpected positive hypersensitive reaction to eugenol. *BMJ Case Rep.* 2013; 2013: bcr2013009464.

4037 European Medicines Agency. Public statement on the use of herbal medicinal products containing estragole. Available at: http://www.ema.europa.eu/docs/en_GB/document_library/Scientific_guideline/2010/04/WC500089960.pdf.

4038 European Medicines Agency. Public statement on the use of herbal medicinal products containing estragole. Available at: http://www.ema.europa.eu/docs/en_GB/document_library/Scientific_guideline/2010/04/WC500089960.pdf.

4039 Ding W, Levy DD, Bishop ME, et al. In vivo genotoxicity of estragole in male F344 rats. *Environ Mol Mutagen.* 2015 May;56(4):356-65.

4040 Eisenmann SW, Poulev A, Struwe L, et al. Qualitative variation of anti-diabetic constituents in different tarragon (Artemisia dracunculus L.) cytotypes. *Fitoterapia.* 2011 Oct;82(7):1062–74.

4041 European Medicines Agency. Public statement on the use of herbal medicinal products containing estragole. Available at: http://www.ema.europa.eu/docs/en_GB/document_library/Scientific_guideline/2010/04/WC500089960.pdf.

4042 European Commission. Opinion of the Scientific Committee on Food on estragole (1-Allyl-4-methoxybenzene). Available at: http://ec.europa.eu/food/fs/sc/scf/out104_en.pdf.

4043 California Environmental Protection Agency. Evidence of the carcinogenicity of estragole. Available at: http://oehha.ca.gov/prop65/pdf/estragf.pdf.

4044 Drinkwater NR, Miller EC, Miller JA, et al. Hepatocarcinogenicity of estragole (1-allyl-4-methoxybenzene) and 1'-hydroxyestragole in the mouse and mutagenicity of 1'-acetoxyestragole in bacteria. *J Natl Cancer Inst.* 1976 Dec;57(6):1323-31.

4045 Zeller A, Horst K, Rychlik M. Study of the metabolism of estragole in humans consuming fennel tea. *Chem Res Toxicol.* 2009 Dec;22(12):1929-37.

4046 Lee HS. Anticoagulant properties of constituents derived from fennel (Foeniculum vulgare Gaertner) fruits. *Food Sci Biotech.* 2006 Oct;15(5):763-67.

4047 Kohlert C, Schindler G, Marz RW, et al. Systemic availability and pharmacokinetics of thymol in humans. *J Clin Pharmacol.* 2002 Jul;42(7):731-7.

4048 US Centers for Disease Control and Prevention. ATSDR, Agency for Toxic Substances and Disease Registry. Medical Management Guidelines for Phenol. Available at: https://www.atsdr.cdc.gov/MHMI/mmg115.pdf.

4049 Jukic M, Politeo O, Maksimmovic M, et al. In vitro acetylcholinesterase inhibitory properties of thymol, carvacrol and their derivatives thymoquinone and thymohydroquinone. *Phytother Res.* 2007;21(3):259-61.

4050 Tognolini M, Barocelli E, Ballabeni V, et al. Comparative screening of plant essential oils; phenylpropanoid moiety as basic core for antiplatelet activity. *Life Sci.* 2006 Feb 23;78(13):1419-32.

4051 Okazaki K, Kawazoe K, Takaishi Y. Human platelet aggregation inhibitors from thyme (Thymus vulgaris L.). *Phytother Res.* 2002 Jun;16(4):398-9.

4052 Jukic M, Politeo O, Maksimmovic M, et al. In vitro acetylcholinesterase inhibitory properties of thymol, carvacrol and their derivatives thymoquinone and thymohydroquinone. *Phytother Res.* 2007;21(3):259-61.

4053 Boskabady MH, Rakhshandah H, Moetamedshariati V. Bronchodilatory and anticholinergic effects of Carum copticum on isolated guinea pig tracheal chains. *Medical Journal of the Islamic Republic of Iran.* 1998;11:329–334.

4054 Boskabady MH, Shaikhi J. Inhibitory effect of Carum copticum on histamine (H1) receptors of isolated guinea-pig tracheal chains. *J Ethnopharmacol.* 2000 Mar;69(3):217-27.

4055 Langeveld WT, Veldhuizen EJ, Burt SA. Synergy between essential oil constituents and antibiotics. *Crit Rev Microbiol.* 2014;40(1):76-94.

4056 Palaniappan K, Holley Ra. Use of natural antimicrobials to increase antibiotic susceptibility of drug resistant bacteria. *In J Food Microbiol.* 2010 Jun 15;140(2-3):164-8.

4057 Ilic BS, Kocic BD, Ciric VM, et al. An in vitro synergistic interaction of combinations of Thymus glabrescens essential oil and its main constituents with chloramphenicol. *ScientificWorldJournal.* 2014 Jan 28;2014:826219.

4058 Miladinovic DL, Ilic BS, Kocic BD, et al. Antibacterial investigation of thyme essential oil and its main constituents on combination with tetracycline. *J Med Food.* 2015 Aug;18(8):935-7.

4059 Yamada AN, Grespan R, Yamada ÁT, et al. Anti-inflammatory activity of Ocimum americanum L. essential oil in experimental model of zymosan-induced arthritis. *Am J Chin Med.* 2013;41(4):913-26.

4060 Bayala B, Bassole IH, Gnoula C, et al. Chemical composition, antioxidant, anti-inflammatory and anti-proliferative activities of essential oils of plants from Burkina Faso. *PLoS One.* 2014 Mar 24;9(3):e92122.

4061 Pidgeon GP, Kandouz M, Meram A, et al. Mechanisms controlling cell cycle arrest and induction of apoptosis after 12-lipoxygenase inhibition in prostate cancer cells. *Cancer Res.* 2002 May 1; 62(9):2721-7.

4062 Parida R, Sandeep S, Sethy BK, et al. Chemical composition, antioxidant and antimicrobial activities of essential oil from lime basil (Ocimum Americanum): A potent source for natural antioxidant. *Int J Pharmacy Pharmaceutical Sci.* 2014 Jan;6(7):487-90.

4063 Sishu R, Tadese S, Bucar F, et al. Chemical composition and antioxidant activity of the essential oils of Ocimum americanum and Ocimum basillicum var. thyrsiflorum. *Int J Essent Oil Ther.* 2010;4:64-68.

4064 Bayala B, Bassole IH, Gnoula C, et al. Chemical composition, antioxidant, anti-inflammatory and anti-proliferative activities of essential oils of plants from Burkina Faso. *PLoS One.* 2014 Mar 24;9(3):e92122.

4065 Carovic-Stanko K, Orlic S, Politeo O, et al. Composition and antibacterial activities of essential oils of seven Ocimum taxa. *Food Chem.* 2010 Mar;119(1):196-201.

4066 Parida R, Sandeep S, Sethy BK, et al. Chemical composition, antioxidant and antimicrobial activities of essential oil from lime basil (Ocimum Americanum): A potent source for natural antioxidant. *Int J Pharmacy Pharmaceutical Sci.* 2014 Jan;6(7):487-90.

4067 Zhang JW, Li SK, Wu WJ. The Main Chemical Composition and in vitro Antifungal Activity of the Essential Oils of Ocimum basilicum Linn. var. pilosum (Willd.) Benth. *Molecules.* 2009;14:273-78.

4068 Zollo PH, Biyiti L, Tchoumbougnang F, et al. Aromatic plants of tropical Africa. Part XXXII. Chemical composition and antifungal activity of thirteen essential oils from aromatic plants of Cameroon. *Flavour Frag J.* 1998;13:107-14.

4069 Vyry Wouatsa NA, Misra L, Venkatesh Kumar R. Antibacterial activity of essential oils of edible spices, Ocimum canum and Xylopia aethiopica. *J Food Sci.* 2014 May;79(5):M972-7.

4070 Nascimento JC, Barbosa LC, Paula VF, et al. Chemical composition and antimicrobial activity of essential oils of Ocimum canum Sims. and Ocimum selloi Benth. *An Acad Bras Cienc.* 2011 Sep;83(3):787-99.

4071 Thaweboon S, Thaweboon B. In vitro antimicrobial activity of Ocimum americanum L. essential oil against oral microorganisms. *Southeast Asian J Trop Med Public Health.* 2009 Sep;40(5):1025-33.

4072 Freires IA, Denny C, Benso B, et al. Antibacterial Activity of Essential Oils and Their Isolated Constituents against Cariogenic Bacteria: A Systematic Review. *Molecules.* 2015 Apr 22;20(4):7329-58.

4073 Cimanga K, Kambu K, Tona L, et al. Correlation between chemical composition and antibacterial activity of essential oils of some aromatic medicinal plants growing in the Democratic Republic of Congo. *J Ethnopharmacol.* 2002 Feb;79(2):213-20.

4074 de Lima Silva L, Garlet QI, Koakoski G, et al. Anesthetic activity of the essential oil of Ocimum americanum in Rhamdia quelen (Quoy & Gaimard, 1824) and its effects on stress parameters. *Neotropical Ichthyology.* 2015;13(4):715-22.

4075 Abd El-Aziz SE, Omer E. Chemical Composition of Ocimum americanum Essential Oil and Its Biological Effects Against, Agrotis ipsilon, (Lepidoptera: Noctuidae). *Res J Agric Biol Sci.* 2007;3(6):740-47.

4076 Akono Ntonga P, Baldovini N, Mouray E, et al. Activity of Ocimum basilicum, Ocimum canum, and Cymbopogon citratus essential oils against Plasmodium falciparum and mature-stage larvae of Anopheles funestus s.s. *Parasite.* 2014;21:33.

4077 Nararak J, Sathantriphop S, Chauhan K, et al. Avoidance Behavior to Essential Oils by Anopheles minimus, a Malaria Vector in Thailand. *J Am Mosq Control Assoc.* 2016 Mar;32(1):34-43.

4078 Sathantriphop S, Kongmee M, Tainchum K, et al. Comparison of Field and Laboratory-Based Tests for Behavioral Response of Aedes aegypti (Diptera: Culicidae) to Repellents. *J Econ Entomol.* 2015 Dec;108(6):2770-8.

4079 Boonyuan W, Grieco JP, Bangs MJ, et al. Excito-repellency of essential oils against an Aedes aegypti (L.) field population in Thailand. J *Vector Ecol.* 2014 Jun;39(1):112-22.

4080 Cavalcanti ES, Morais SM, Lima MA, et al. Larvicidal activity of essential oils from Brazilian plants against Aedes aegypti L. *Mem Inst Oswaldo Cruz.* 2004 Aug;99(5):541-4.

4081 Cimanga K, Kambu K, Tona L, et al. Correlation between chemical composition and antibacterial activity of essential oils of some aromatic medicinal plants growing in the Democratic Republic of Congo. *J Ethnopharmacol.* 2002 Feb;79(2):213-20.

4082 Chokechaijaroenporn O, Bunyapraphatsara N, Kongchuensin S. Mosquito repellent activities of ocimum volatile oils. *Phytomedicine.* 1994 Sep;1(2):135-9.

4083 Tawatsin A, Wratten SD, Scott RR, et al. Repellency of volatile oils from pants against three mosquito vectors. *J Vector Ecol.* 2001 Jun;26(1):76-82.

4084 Bianchini A, Tomi P, Costa J, et al. Composition of Helichrysum italicum (Roth) G. Don fil. subsp. italicum essential oil from Corsica (France). *Flav Frag J.* 2001 Jan-Feb;16(1):30-34.

4085 Leonardi M, Ambryszewska KE, Melai B, et al. Essential-oil composition of Helichrysum italicum (ROTH) G.DON ssp. Italicum from Elba Island (Tuscany, Italy). *Chem Biodviers.* 2013 Mar;10(3):343-55.

4086 Cristofari G, Znini M, Majidi L, et al. Helichrysum italicum subsp. italicum essential oil as environmentally friendly inhibitor on the corrosion of mil steel in hydrochloric acid. *Int J Electrochem Sci.* 2012;7:9024-41.

4087 Satta M, Tuberoso CIG, Angioni A, et al. Analysis of the essential oil of Helichrysum italicum G. Don ssp. microphyllum (Willd) Nym. *J Essential Oil Res.* 1999;11(6):711-15.

4088 Guinoiseau E, Lorenzi V, Luciani A, et al. Biological properties and resistance reversal effect of Helichrysum italicum (Roth) G. Don. *Micro Pathogens and Strat Combat: Sci Tech.* 2013:1073-80.

4089 Mastelic J, Politeo O, Jerkovic I. Contribution to the analysis of the essential oil of Helichrysum italicum (Roth) G. Don. - determination of ester bonded acids and phenols. *Molecules.* 208;13:795-803.

4090 Antunes Castela Viega DM. Formulacoes topicas de Helichrysum italicum e sua aplicabilidade. *Covilha.* 2011 Jun:ii-63.

4091 Mastelic J, Politeo O, Jerkovic I, et al. Composition and antimicrobial activity of Helichrysum italicum essential oil and its terpene fractions. *Chem Nat Constituents.* 2005 Jan;41(10:35-40.

4092 Weyerstahl P. Isolation and synthesis of constituents from the essential oil of Helichrysum italicum. In: Brunke EJ. Progress in essential oil research. De Gruyter, Berlin:177-95.

4093 Mashigo MF, Combrinck S, Regnier T, et al. Chemical variations, trichome structure and antifungal activities of essential oils of Helichrysum splendidum from South Africa. *South African J Botany.* 2015 Jan;96:78-84.

4094 Marongui B, Piras A, Porcedda S. Comparative analysis of the oil and supercritical CO(2) extract of Artemisia arborescens L. and Helichrysum splendidum (Thunb.) Less. *Nat Prod Res.* 2006 May;20(5):421-28.

4095 Chagonda LS, Makanda C, Chalchat JC. Essential Oils of Four Wild and Semi-Wild Plants from Zimbabwe: Colospermum mopane (Kirk ex Benth.) Kirk ex Leonard, Helichrysum splendidum (Thunb.) Less, Myrothamnus flabellifolia (Welw.) and Tagetes minuta L. *J Essent Oil Res.* 1999;11(5):573-78.

4096 Mastelic J, Politeo O, Jerkovic I. Contribution to the Analysis of the Essential Oil of Helichrysum italicum (Roth) G. Don. – Determination of Ester Bonded Acids and Phenols. *Molecules.* 2008;13:795-803.

4097 Lozina V. Private Communication. 2016.

4098 Lorenzi V, Muselli A, Bernardini AF, et al. Geraniol restores antibiotic activities against multidrug-resistant isolates from gram-negative species. *Antimicrobial Agents Chemother.* 2009 May;53(5):2209-11.

4099 Appendino G, Ottino M, Marquez N, et al. Arzanol, an anti-inflammatory and anti-HIV-1 phloroglucinol alpha- Pyrone from helichrysum italicum ssp. Microphyllum. *J Nat Prod.* 2007;70(4):608-12.

4100 Sala A, Recio M, Giner RM, et al. Anti-inflammatory and antioxidant properties of Helichrysum italicum. *J Pharm Pharmacol.* 2002;54(3):365-71.

4101 Baylac S, Racine P. Inhibition of 5-lipoxygenase by essential oils and other natural fragrant extracts. *Int J Aromatherapy.* 2003;13(2-3):138-42.

4102 Varney E, Buckle J. Effect of inhaled essential oils on mental exhaustion and moderate burnout: a small pilot study. *J Altern Complement Med.* 2013;19(1):69-71.

4103 Matsumoto T, Kimura T, Hayashi T, et al. Does Japanese Citrus Fruit Yuzu (Citrus junos Sieb. ex Tanaka) Fragrance Have Lavender-Like Therapeutic Effects That Alleviate Premenstrual Emotional Symptoms? A Single-Blind Randomized Crossover Study. *J Altern Complement Med.* 2017 Jun;23(6):461-470.

4104 Han X, Beaumont C, Stevens N. Chemical composition analysis and in vitro biological activities of ten essential oils in human skin cells. *Biochim Open.* 2017 Apr 26;5:1-7.

4105 Oliva A, Garzoli S, Sabatino, et al. Chemical composition and antimicrobial activity of essential oil of Helichrysum italicum (Roth) G. Don fil. (Asteraceae) from Montenegro. *Nat Prod Res.* 2019 Jan 3:1-4.

4106 Fraternale D, Flamini G, Ascrizzi R, et al. In Vitro Anticollagenase and Antielastase Activities of Essential Oil of Helichrysum italicum subsp. italicum (Roth) G. Don. *J Med Food.* 2019 Oct;22(10):1041-1046.

4107 Peruc D, Ticac B, Broznic D, et al. Juniper and immortelle essential oils synergistically inhibit adhesion of nontuberculous mycobacteria to Acanthamoeba castellanii. *Arh Hig Rada Toksikol.* 2020 Oct 6;71(3):223-230.

4108 Contini A, Di Bello D, Azzara A, et al. Assessing the cytotoxic/genotoxic activity and estrogenic/antiestrogenic potential of essential oils from seven aromatic plants. *Food Chem Toxicol.* 2020 Apr;138:111205.

4109 Genčić MS, Aksić JM, Živković Stošić MZ, et al. Linking the antimicrobial and anti-inflammatory effects of immortelle essential oil with its chemical composition - The interplay between the major and minor constituents. *Food Chem Toxicol.* 2021 Nov 9;158:112666.

4110 Judzentiene A, Budiene J, Nedveckyte I, et al. Antioxidant and Toxic Activity of Helichrysum arenarium (L.) Moench and Helichrysum italicum (Roth) G. Don Essential Oils and Extracts. *Molecules.* 2022 Feb 15;27(4):1311.

4111 Andjić M, Draginić N, Kočović A, et al. Immortelle essential oil-based ointment improves wound healing in a diabetic rat model. *Biomed Pharmacother.* 2022 Apr 13;150:112941.

4112 Zheljazkov VD, Semerdjieva I, Yankova-Tsvetkova E, et al. Chemical Profile and Antimicrobial Activity of the Essential Oils of Helichrysum arenarium (L.) Moench. and Helichrysum italicum (Roth). G. Don. *Plants (Basel).* 2022 Mar 31;11(7):951.

4113 Węglarz Z, Kosakowska O, Pióro-Jabrucka E, et al. Antioxidant and Antibacterial Activity of Helichrysum italicum (Roth) G. Don. from Central Europe. *Pharmaceuticals (Basel).* 2022 Jun 10;15(6):735.

4114 Balázs VL, Filep R, Répás F, et al. Immortelle (Helichrysum italicum (Roth) G. Don) Essential Oil Showed Antibacterial and Biofilm Inhibitory Activity against Respiratory Tract Pathogens. *Molecules.* 2022 Aug 27;27(17):5518.

4115 Lemaire G, Olivero M, Rouquet V, et al. Neryl acetate, the major component of Corsican Helichrysum italicum essential oil, mediates its biological activities on skin barrier. *PLoS One.* 2023 Mar 3;18(3):e0268384.

4116 Mediavilla V, Steinemann S. Essential oil of Cannabis sativa L. strains. J Int Hemp Assoc. 1997;4(2):80-82.

4117 Nissen L, Zatta A, Stefanini I, et al. Characterization and antimicrobial activity of essential oils of industrial hemp varieties (Cannabis sativa L.). *Fitoterapia.* 2010 Jul;81(5):413-9.

4118 Novak J, Zitterl-Eglseer K, Deans SG, et al. Essential oils of different cultivars of Cannabis sativa L. and their antimicrobial activity. *Flavour Frag J.* 2001 Jul-Aug;16(4):259-62.

4119 Verma RS, Padalia RC, Verma SK, et al. The essential oil of 'bhang' (Cannabis sativa L.) for non-narcotic applications. *Curr Sci.* 2014 Aug;4(25):645-50.

4120 Ross SA, El Sohly MA. The volatile oil composition of fresh and air-dried buds of Cannabis sativa. *J Nat Prod.* 1996;59:49–51.

4121 Delgado IF, Carvalho RR, Nogueira, et al. Study on embryofetotoxicity of b-myrcene in the rat. *Food and Chemical Toxicology.* 1993;31(1):31-5.

4122 Paumgartten FJ, De-Carvalho RR, Souza CA, et al. Study of the effects of beta-myrcene on rat fertility and general reproductive performance. *Braz J Med Biol Res.* 1998 Jul;31(7):955-65.

4123 do Vale TG, Furtado EC, Santos JG Jr, et al. Central effects of citral, myrcene and limonene, constituents of essential oil chemotypes from Lippia alba (Mill.) n.e. Brown. *Phytomedicine.* 2002 Dec;9(8):709-14.

4124 Segelman AB, Sofia RD, Segelman FP, et al. Cannabis sativa L. (marijuana). V. Pharmacological evaluation of marijuana aqueous extract and volatile oil. *J Pharm Sci.* 1974 Jun;63(6):962-4.

4125 Freitas JC1, Presgrave OA, Fingola FF, et al. Effect of beta-myrcene on pentobarbital sleeping time. *Braz J Med Biol Res.* 1993 May;26(5):519-23.

4126 De Olivera AC, Ribeiro-Pinto LF, Paumgartten JR. In vitro inhibition of CYP2B1 monoxygenase by beta-myrcene and other monoterpenoid constituents. *Br J Nutr.* 1999;81:289-95.

4127 De-Oliveira AC1, Ribeiro-Pinto LF, Otto SS, et al. Induction of liver monooxygenases by beta-myrcene. *Toxicology.* 1997 Dec 26;124(2):135-40.

4128 Nguyen LT, Mysliveckova Z, Szotakova B, et al. The inhibitory effects of β-caryophyllene, β-caryophyllene oxide and α-humulene on the activities of the main drug-metabolizing enzymes in rat and human liver in vitro. *Chem-Biol Interactoins.* 2017 Dec 25;278:123-8.

4129 Nissen L, Zatta A, Stefanini I, et al. Characterization and antimicrobial activity of essential oils of industrial hemp varieties (Cannabis sativa L.). *Fitoterapia.* 2010 Jul;81(5):413-9.

4130 Verma RS, Padalia RC, Verma SK, et al. The essential oil of 'bhang' (Cannabis sativa L.) for non-narcotic applications. *Curr Sci.* 2014 Aug;4(25):645-50.

4131 Paula-Freire LI, Andersen ML, Gama VS, et al. The oral administration of trans-caryophyllene attenuates acute and chronic pain in mice. *Phytomedicine.* 2014 Feb 15;21(3):356-62.

4132 Gertsch J, Leonti M, Raduner S, et al. Beta-caryophyllene is a dietary cannabinoid. *Proc Natl Acad Sci USA.* 2008 Jul 1;105(26):9099-104.

4133 Marini E, Magi G, Ferretti G, et al. Attenuation of Listeria monocytogenes Virulence by Cannabis sativa L. Essential Oil. *Front Cell Infect Microbiol.* 2018 Aug 22;8:293.

4134 Zengin G, Menghini L, Di Sotto A, et al. Chromatographic Analyses, In Vitro Biological Activities, and Cytotoxicity of Cannabis sativa L. Essential Oil: A Multidisciplinary Study. *Molecules.* 2018 Dec 10;23(12).

4135 Iseppi R, Brighenti V, Licata M, et al. Chemical Characterization and Evaluation of the Antibacterial Activity of Essential Oils from Fibre-Type Cannabis sativa L. (Hemp). *Molecules.* 2019 Jun 21;24(12).

4136 Smeriglio A, Trombetta D, Alloisio S, et al. Promising in vitro antioxidant, anti-acetylcholinesterase and neuroactive effects of essential oil from two non-psychotropic Cannabis sativa L. biotypes. *Phytother Res.* 2020 Apr 20. [Epub ahead of print]

4137 Pellegrini M, Palmieri S, Ricci A, et al. In vitro antioxidant and antimicrobial activity of Cannabis sativa L. cv 'Futura 75' essential oil. *Nat Prod Res.* 2020 Aug 31;1-5.

4138 Rossi P, Cappelli A, Marinelli O, et al. Mosquitocidal and Anti-Inflammatory Properties of The Essential Oils Obtained from Monoecious, Male, and Female Inflorescences of Hemp (Cannabis sativa L.) and Their Encapsulation in Nanoemulsions. *Molecules.* 2020 Jul 29;25(15):3451.

4139 Zheliazkov VD, Sikora V, Dincheva I, et al. Industrial, CBD, and Wild Hemp: How Different Are Their Essential Oil Profile and Antimicrobial Activity? *Molecules.* 2020 Oct 12;25(20):4631.

4140 Menghini L, Ferrante C, Carradori S, et al. Chemical and Bioinformatics Analyses of the Anti-Leishmanial and Anti-Oxidant Activities of Hemp Essential Oil. *Biomolecules.* 2021 Feb 12;11(2):272.

4141 Mazzara E, Torresi J, Fico G, et al. A Comprehensive Phytochemical Analysis of Terpenes, Polyphenols and Cannabinoids, and Micromorphological Characterization of 9 Commercial Varieties of Cannabis sativa L. *Plants (Basel).* 2022 Mar 27;11(7):891.

4142 Ovidi E, Laghezza Masci V, et al. Hemp (Cannabis sativa L., Kompolti cv.) and Hop (Humulus lupulus L., Chinook cv.) Essential Oil and Hydrolate: HS-GC-MS Chemical Investigation and Apoptotic Activity Evaluation. *Pharmaceuticals (Basel).* 2022 Aug 8;15(8):976.

4143 Soares EFMS, Carlos DFLP, Epifanio NMM, et al. Insecticidal activity of essential oil of Cannabis sativa against the immature and adult stages of Ctenocephalides felis felis. *Rev Bras Parasitol Vet.* 2023 Jan 13;32(1):e015122.

4144 Chien TC, Lo SF, Ho CL. Chemical composition and anti-inflammatory activity of Chamaecyparis obtusa f. formosana wood essential oil from Taiwan. *Nat Prod Commun.* 2014 May;9(5):723-26.

4145 Lee JH, Lee BK, Kim JH, et al. Comparison of chemical compositions and antimicrobial activities of essential oils from three conifer trees; Pinus densiflora, Crytpomeria japonica, and Chamaecyparis obtusa. *J Microbiol Biotechnol.* 2009;19(4):391-96.

4146 Suh HR, Chung HJ, Park EH, et al. The effects of Chamaecyparis obtusa essential oil on pain-related behavior and expression of pro-inflammatory cytokines in carrageenan-induced arthritis in rats. *Biosci Biotechnol Biochem.* 2015 Jan;80(1):203-09.

4147 Kang YM, Min JY, Choi MS. Essential oil yields and chemical composition of Chamaecyparis obtusa obtained from various populations and environmental factors. *J Forest Environ Sci.* 2014 Aug;30(3):285-92.

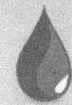

4148 Wang SY, Wang YS, Tseng YH, et al. Analysis of fragrance composition of precious coniferous woods grown in Taiwan. *Holzforschung*. 2006;60:528-32.

4149 Shieh B, Lizuka Y, Matsubara Y. Monoterpenoid and Sesquiterpenoid Constituents of the Essential Oil of Hinoki (Chamaecyparis obtusa (Sieb. et Zucc.) Endl.). *J Agric Biol Chem*. 1981;45(6):1497-99.

4150 Kim EH, Kang SY, Park BI, et al. Chamaecyparis obtusa Suppresses Virulence Genes in Streptococcus mutans. *Evid Based Complement Alternat Med*. 2016;2016:2396404.

4151 Kasuya H, Iida S, Ono K, et al. Intracerebral distribution of alpha-pinene and the anxiolytic-like effect in mice following inhaled administration of essential oil from Chamaecyparis obtusa. *Nat Prod Commun*. 2015 Aug;10(8):1479- 82.

4152 Eltayeb LMH, Yagi S, Mohamed HMM, et al. Essential Oils Composition and Biological Activity of Chamaecyparis obtusa, Chrysopogon nigritanus and Lavandula coronopifolia Grown Wild in Sudan. *Molecules*. 2023 Feb;28(3):1005.

4153 Hiroi T, Miyazaki Y, Kobayashi Y, et al. Induction of hepatic P450s in rat by essential oil wood leaf oils. *Xenobiotica*. 1995 May;25(5):457-67.

4154 Bae D, Seol H, Yoon HG, et al. Inhaled essential oil from Chamaecyparis obtusa ameliorates the impairments of cognitive function induced by injection of β-amyloid in rats. *Pharm Biol*. 2012 Jul;50(7):900-10.

4155 Park Y, Jung SM, Yoo SA, et al. Antinociceptive and anti-inflammatory effects of essential oil extracted from Chamaecyparis obtusa in mice. *Int Immunopharmacol*. 2015 Dec;29(2):320-325.

4156 Suh HR, Chung HJ, Park EH, et al. The effects of Chamaecyparis obtusa essential oil on pain-related behavior and expression of pro-inflammatory cytokines in carrageenan-induced arthritis in rats. *Biosci Biotechnol Biochem*. 2015 Jan;80(1):203-09.

4157 Chien TC, Lo SF, Ho CL. Chemical composition and anti-inflammatory activity of Chamaecyparis obtusa f. formosana wood essential oil from Taiwan. *Nat Prod Commun*. 2014 May;9(5):723-26.

4158 Park Y, Yoo SA, Kim WU, et al. Anti-inflammatory effects of essential oils extracted from Chamaecyparis obtusa on murine models of inflammation and RAW 264.7 cells. *Mol Med Rep*. 2016 Apr;13(4):3335-41.

4159 An BS, Kang JH, Yang H, et al. Anti-inflammatory effects of essential oils from Chamaecyparis obtusa via the cyclooxygenase-2 pathway in rats. *Mol Med Rep*. 2013 Jul;8(1):255-9.

4160 Lee GS, Hong EJ, Gwak KS, et al. The essential oils of Chamaecyparis obtusa promotes hair growth through the induction of vascular endothelial growth factor gene. *Fitoterapia*. 2012 Jan;81(1):17-24.

4161 Kasuya H, Iida S, Ono K, et al. Intracerebral distribution of alpha-pinene and the anxiolytic-like effect in mice following inhaled administration of essential oil from Chamaecyparis obtusa. *Nat Prod Commun*. 2015 Aug;10(8):1479- 82.

4162 Chen CJ, Kumar KJ, Chen YT, et al. Effect of hinoki and meniki essential oils on human autonomic nervous system activity and mood states. *Nat Prod Commun*. 2015 Jul;10(7):1305-08.

4163 Kim ES, Kang SY, Kim YH, et al. Chamaecyparis obtusa essential oil inhibits methicillin-resistant staphylococcus aureus biofilm formation and expression of virulence factors. *J Med Food*. 2015 Jul;18(7):810-17.

4164 Bae MS, Park DH, Choi CY, et al. Essential Oils and Non-volatile Constituents Derived from Chamaecyparis obtusa: Broad Spectrum Antimicrobial Activity against Infectious Bacteria and MDR (multidrug resistant) Strains. *Nat Prod Commun*. 2016 May;11(5):693-4.

4165 Kim EH, Kang SY, Park BI, et al. Chamaecyparis obtusa Suppresses Virulence Genes in Streptococcus mutans. *Evid Based Complement Alternat Med*. 2016;2016:2396404.

4166 Kwon HH, Yoon JY, Park SY, et al. Comparison of clinical and histological effects between lactobacillus-fermented Chamaecyparis obtusa and tea tree essential oil for the treatment of acne: an eight-week double-blind randomized controlled split-face study. *Dermatology*. 2014;229(2):102-09.

4167 Park HJ, Kim SK, Kang WS, et al. Effects of essential oil from Chamaecyparis obtusa on cytokine genes in the hippocampus of maternal separation rats. *Can J Physiol Pharmacol*. 2014 Feb;92(2):95-101.

4168 Kasuya H, Hata E, Satou T, et al. Effect on emotional behavior and stress by inhalation of the essential oil from Chamaecyparis obtusa. *Nat Prod Commun*. 2013 Apr;8(4):515-18.

4169 Bae D, Seol H, Yoon HG, et al. Inhaled essential oil from Chamaecyparis obtusa ameliorates the impairments of cognitive function induced by injection of β-amyloid in rats. *Pharm Biol*. 2012 Jul;50(7):900-10.

4170 Hong EJ, Na KJ, Choi IG, et al. Antibacterial and antifungal effects of essential oils from coniferous trees. *Biol Pharm Bull*. 2004 Jun;27(6):863-66.

4171 Lee SH, Do HS1, Min KJ, et al. Effects of Essential Oil from Hinoki Cypress, Chamaecyparis obtusa, on Physiology and Behavior of Flies. *PLoS One*. 2015 Dec 1;10(12):e0143450.

4172 Shin SH, Ye MK, Lee DW, et al. Effect of microencapsulated essential oil form Chamaecyparis obtusa on monocyte-derived dendritic cell activation and CD4+ T cell polarization. *PLoS One*. 2018 Jul 27;13(7):e0201233.

4173 Raha S, Kim SM, Lee HJ, et al. Essential oil from Korean Chamaecyparis obtusa leaf ameliorates respiratory activity in Sprague-Dawley rats and exhibits protection from NF-κB-induced inflammation in WI38 fibroblast cells. *Int J Mol Med*. 2019 Jan;43(1):393–403.

4174 Yoo KH, Kwon TR, Kim YU, et al. The Effects of Fabric Containing Chamaecyparis Obtusa Essential Oil on Atopic Dermatitis-Like Lesions: A Functional Clothing Possibility. *Skin Pharmacol Physiol*. 2020 Jun 12;1-11.

4175 Shin SH, Ye MK, Lee DW, et al. Immunomodulative Effects of Chamaecyparis obtusa Essential Oil in Mouse Model of Allergic Rhinitis. *Molecules*. 2020 Oct 2;25(19):4517.

4176 Shin SH< Ye MK, Chae MH, et al. Chamaecyparis obtusa Essential Oil Inhibits House Dust Mite Induced Nasal Epithelial Cell Activation and Immune Responses. *J Oleo Sci*. 2021;70(3):431-438.

4177 Eltayeb LMH, Yagi S, Mohamed HMM, et al. Essential Oils Composition and Biological Activity of Chamaecyparis obtusa, Chrysopogon nigritanus and Lavandula coronopifolia Grown Wild in Sudan. *Molecules*. 2023 Jan 19;28(3):1005.

4178 Saharkhiz MJ, Kamyab AA, Kazerani NK, et al. Chemical compositions and antimicrobial activities of Ocimum sanctum L. essential oils at different harvest stages. *Jundishapur J Microbiol*. 2015 Jan; 8(1): e13720.

4179 Kumari R, Agrawal S. Comparative analysis of essential oil composition and oil containing glands in Ocimum sanctum L. (Holy basil) under ambient and supplemental level of UV-B through gas chromatography–mass spectrometry and scanning electron microscopy. *Acta Physiologiae Plantarum*. 2011 Jul;33(4):1093-1101.

4180 Joshi RK, Hoti SL. Chemical composition of the essential oil of Ocimum tenuiflorum L. (Krishna Tulsi) from North West Karnataka, India. *Plant Science Today*. 2014;1(3):99-102.

4181 Sims C, Juliana HR, Mentreddy SR, et al. Essential Oils in Holy Basil (Ocimum tenuiflorum L.) as Influenced by Planting Dates and Harvest Times in North Alabama. *J Med Active Plants*. 2014 Oct;3(2):33-41.

4182 Archana R, Ashok K, Dutta M. Chemical characterization of aroma constituents in essential oil isolated from "Holy Basil" (Ocimum tenuiflorum L.) grown in India. *Genetic Res Crop Evol*. 2013 Jun;60(5):1727-35.

4183 Klaudija CS, Zlatko L, Olivera P, et al. Molecular and chemical characterization of the most widespread Ocimum species. 2011 Jul;294(3):253-62.

4184 Joshi RK. Chemical Composition, In Vitro Antimicrobial and Antioxidant Activities of the Essential Oils of Ocimum Gratissimum, O. Sanctum and their Major Constituents. *Indian J Pharm Sci*. 2013 Jul;75(4):457-62.

4185 Domaracky M, Rehak P, Juhas S, et al. Effects of selected plant essential oils on the growth and development of mouse preimplantation embryos in vivo. *Physiol Res*. 2007;56(1):97-104.

4186 Vrskova D, Modra H. Evaluation of the developmental toxicity of 2-phenoxyethanol and clove oil anesthetics using the Frog Embryo Teratogenesis Assay: Xenopus (FETAX). *Veterinarami Medicina*. 2012;57(5):245-50.

4187 Amini A, Cheraghi E, Safaee MR, et al. The role of eugenol in the reduction of teratogenic effects of retinoic acid on skeletal morphology of mice embryo. *Yakhteh Medical Journal*. 2003;4:195-200.

4188 Chen R, Chen J, Cheng S, et al. Assessment of embryotoxicity of constituents in cosmetics by the embryonic stem cell tes. *Toxicol Mech Methods*. 2010 Mar;20(3):112-18.

4189 Kamatou GP, Vermaak I, Viljoen AM. Eugenol—from the remote Maluku Islands to the international market place: A review of a remarkable and versatile molecule. *Molecules*. 2012;17:6953-81.

4190 Chen SJ, Wang MH, Chen IJ. Antiplatelet and calcium inhibitory properties of eugenol and sodium eugenol acetate. *Gen Pharmacol*. 1996 Jun;27(4):629-33.

4191 Tognolini M, Barocelli E, Ballabeni V, et al. Comparative screening of plant essential oils; phenylpropanoid moiety as basic core for antiplatelet activity. *Life Sci*. 2006 Feb 23;78(13):1419-32.

4192 Heck AM, DeWitt BA, Lukes AL. Potential interactions between alternative therapies and warfarin. *Am J Health Syst Pharm*. 2000;57(13):1221-1227.

4193 Saaeed SA, Gilani AH. Antithrombotic activity of clove oil. *J Pak Med Assoc*. 1994;44(5):112-15.

4194 Langeveld WT, Veldhuizen EJ, Burt SA. Synergy between essential oil constituents and antibiotics. *Crit Rev Microbiol*. 2014 Feb;40(1);76-94.

4195 Amber K, Aijaz A, Immaculata X, et al. Anticandidal effect of Ocimum sanctum essential oil and its synergy with fluconazole and ketoconazole. *Phytomedicine*. 2010 Oct;17(12):921-5.

4196 Ahmad A, Khan A, Ahmad Khan L, et al. In vitro synergy of eugenol and methyleugenol with fluconazole against clinical Candida isolates. *J Med Microbiol*. 2010;59:1178-84.

4197 Singh S, Rehan HM, Majumdar DK. Effect of Ocimum sanctum fixed oil on blood pressure, blood clotting time and pentobarbitone-induced sleeping time. *J Ethnopharmacol*. 2001;78:139-43.

4198 Sakina MR, Dandiya PC, Hamdard ME, Hameed A. Preliminary psychopharmacological evaluation of Ocimum sanctum leaf extract. *J Ethnopharmacol*. 1990;28:143-50.

4199 Jori A, Bianchetti A, Prestini PE, et al. Effect of eucalyptol (1,8-cineole) on the metabolism of other drugs in rats and in man. *Eur J Pharmacol*. 1970;9(3):362-66.

4200 de Sousa DP, Raphael E, Brocksom U, et al. Sedative effect of monoterpene alcohols in mice: A preliminary screening. *Verlag der Zeitschrift fur Naturforschung*. 2007;62c:563-66.

4201 Dohi S, Terasaki M, Makino M. Acetylcholinesterase inhibitory activity and chemical composition of commercial essential oils. *J Agric Food Chem*. 2009 May 27;57(10):4313-8.

4202 Nguyen LT, Mysliveckova Z, Szotakova B, et al. The inhibitory effects of β-caryophyllene, β-caryophyllene oxide and α-humulene on the activities of the main drug-metabolizing enzymes in rat and human liver in vitro. *Chem-Biol Interactoins*. 2017 Dec 25;278:123-8.

4203 European Medicines Agency. Public statement on the use of herbal medicinal products containing estragole. Available at: http://www.ema.europa.eu/docs/en_GB/document_library/Scientific_guideline/2010/04/WC500089960.pdf.

4204 European Commission. Opinion of the Scientific Committee on Food on methyl eugenol (4-Allyl-1,2- dimethoxybenzene). Available at: http://ec.europa.eu/food/fs/sc/scf/out102_en.pdf.

4205 European Medicines Agency. Public statement on the use of herbal medicinal products containing estragole. Available at: http://www.ema.europa.eu/docs/en_GB/document_library/Scientific_guideline/2010/04/WC500089960.pdf.

4206 European Medicines Agency. Public statement on the use of herbal medicinal products containing estragole. Available at: http://www.ema.europa.eu/docs/en_GB/document_library/Scientific_guideline/2010/04/WC500089960.pdf.

4207 Ding W, Levy DD, Bishop ME, et al. In vivo genotoxicity of estragole in male F344 rats. *Environ Mol Mutagen.* 2015 May;56(4):356-65.

4208 Eisenmann SW, Poulev A, Struwe L, et al. Qualitative variation of anti-diabetic constituents in different tarragon (Artemisia dracunculus L.) cytotypes. *Fitoterapia.* 2011 Oct;82(7):1062–74.

4209 Buck DS, Nidorf DM, Addino JG. Comparison of two topical preparations for the treatment of onchomycosis: Melaleuca alternifolia (tea tree) oil and clotrimazole. *J Fam Pract.* 1994 Jun;38(6):601-05.

4210 European Commission. Opinion of the Scientific Committee on Food on estragole (1-Allyl-4-methoxybenzene). Available at: http://ec.europa.eu/food/fs/sc/scf/out104_en.pdf.

4211 California Environmental Protection Agency. Evidence of the carcinogenicity of estragole. Available at: http://oehha.ca.gov/prop65/pdf/estragf.pdf.

4212 Drinkwater NR, Miller EC, Miller JA, et al. Hepatocarcinogenicity of estragole (1-allyl-4-methoxybenzene) and 1'-hydroxyestragole in the mouse and mutagenicity of 1'-acetoxyestragole in bacteria. *J Natl Cancer Inst.* 1976 Dec;57(6):1323-31.

4213 Zeller A, Horst K, Rychlik M. Study of the metabolism of estragole in humans consuming fennel tea. *Chem Res Toxicol.* 2009 Dec;22(12):1929-37.

4214 Heck AM, DeWitt BA, Lukes AL. Potential interactions between alternative therapies and warfarin. *Am J Health Syst Pharm.* 2000;57(13):1221-1227.

4215 Chen SJ, Wang MH, Chen IJ. Antiplatelet and calcium inhibitory properties of eugenol and sodium eugenol acetate. *Gen Pharmacol.* 1996 Jun;27(4):629-33.

4216 Tognolini M, Barocelli E, Ballabeni V, et al. Comparative screening of plant essential oils; phenylpropanoid moiety as basic core for antiplatelet activity. *Life Sci.* 2006 Feb 23;78(13):1419-32.

4217 Lee HS. Anticoagulant properties of constituents derived from fennel (Foeniculum vulgare Gaertner) fruits. *Food Sci Biotech.* 2006 Oct;15(5):763-67.

4218 Sayyah M, Valizadeh J, Kamalinejad M. Anticonvulsant activity of the leaf oil of Laurus nobilis against pentylentetrazole- and maximal electroshock-induced seizure. *Phytomedicine.* 2002 Apr;9(3):212-16.

4219 Culic M, Kekovic G, Grbic G, et al. Wavelet and fractal analysis of rat brain activity in seizures evoked by camphor oil and 1,8-cineole. *Gen Physiol Biophys.* 2009;28 Sec No:33-40.

4220 Burkhard PR, Burkhardt K, Haenggeli CA, et al. Plant-induced seizures: reappearance of an old problem. *J Neurol.* 1999 Aug;246(8):667-70.

4221 Waldman N. Seizure caused by dermal application of over-the-counter eucalyptus oil head lice preparation. *Clin Toxicol (Phila).* 2011 Oct;49(8):750-1.

4222 Craig JO. Poisoning by the volatile oils in childhood. *Arch Dis Child.* 1953;28:259-67.

4223 Mathew T, Kamath V, Kumar RS, et al. Eucalyptus oil inhalation-induced seizure: A novel, underrecognized, preventable cause of acute symptomatic seizure. *Epilepsia Open.* 2017 Jul 4;2(3):350-354.

4224 Lamborn LL. Modern soaps, candles and glycerin: A practical manual of modern methods of utilization of fats and oils in the manufacture of soaps and candles, and of the recovery of glycerin. Library of the University of Wisconsin.

4225 Oyen LP, Dung NX. Plant resources of South-East Asia. 1999. Backhyus, Leiden.

4226 Khan MM. Masters Thesis: Inhibition of Cytochrome P450 2E1 and Cytochrome P450 2A6 by Essential Oils: Tarragon (Artemisia dracunculus) and Basil (Ocimum basilicum). 2014. Available at: https://libres.uncg.edu/ir/uncg/f/Khan_uncg_0154M_11587.pdf

4227 Sarrami N, Pemberton MN, Thornhill MH, et al. Adverse reactions associated with the use of eugenol in dentistry. *British Dental J.* 2002;193:253-55.

4228 Tammannavar P, Pushpalatha C, Jain S, et al. An unexpected positive hypersensitive reaction to eugenol. *BMJ Case Rep.* 2013; 2013: bcr2013009464.

4229 Nascimento AM, Brandão MG, Oliveira GB, et al. Synergistic bactericidal activity of Eremanthus erythropappus oil or beta-bisabolene with ampicillin against Staphylococcus aureus. *Antonie Van Leeuwenhoek.* 2007 Jul;92(1):95-100.

4230 Shin S, Pyun MS. Anti-Candida effects of estragole in combination with ketoconazole or amphotericin B. *Phytother Res.* 2004 Oct;18(10):827-30.

4231 Shin S. Essential oil compounds from Agastache rugosa as antifungal agents against Trichophyton species. *Arch Pharm Res.* 2004 Mar;27(3):295-9.

4232 Shin S, Kang CA. Antifungal activity of the essential oil of Agastache rugosa Kuntze and its synergism with ketoconazole. *Lett Appl Microbiol.* 2003;36(2):111-5.

4233 Johnson JD, Ryan MJ, Toft JD II, et al. Two-year toxicity and carcinogenicity study of methyl eugenol in F344/N rats and B6C3F(1) mice. *J Agric Food Chem.* 2000 Aug;48(8):3620-32.

4234 European Commission. Opinion of the Scientific Committee on Food on methyl eugenol (4-Allyl-1,2- dimethoxybenzene). Available at: http://ec.europa.eu/food/fs/sc/scf/out102_en.pdf.

4235 National Toxicology Program. NTP Toxicology and Carcinogenesis Studies of Methyleugenol (CAS NO. 93-15-2) in F344/N Rats and B6C3F1 Mice (Gavage Studies). *Natl Toxicol Program Tech Rep Ser.* 2000 Jul;491:1-412.

4236 National Toxicology Program. Carcinogenesis Studies of Eugenol (CAS No. 97-53-0) in F344/N Rats and B6C3F1 Mice (Feed Studies). Technical Report Series No. 223. NIH Publication No. 84-1779. 1983. U.S. DHHS, PHS, NIH, NTP, Research Triangle Park, NC.

4237 Johnson JD, Ryan MJ, Toft JD II, et al. Two-year toxicity and carcinogenicity study of methyl eugenol in F344/N rats and B6C3F(1) mice. *J Agric Food Chem.* 2000 Aug;48(8):3620-32.

4238 National Toxicology Program. NTP Toxicology and Carcinogenesis Studies of Methyleugenol (CAS NO. 93-15-2) in F344/N Rats and B6C3F1 Mice (Gavage Studies). *Natl Toxicol Program Tech Rep Ser.* 2000 Jul;491:1-412.

4239 Kerckaert GA, Brauninger R, LeBoeuf RA, et al. Use of the Syrian hamster embryo cell transformation assay for carcinogenicity prediction of chemicals currently being tested by the National Toxicology Program in rodent bioassays. *Environ Health Perspect.* 1996;104:1075-84.

4240 National Toxicology Program. Carcinogenesis Studies of Eugenol (CAS No. 97-53-0) in F344/N Rats and B6C3F1 Mice (Feed Studies). Technical Report Series No. 223. NIH Publication No. 84-1779. 1983. U.S. DHHS, PHS, NIH, NTP, Research Triangle Park, NC.

4241 Johnson JD, Ryan MJ, Toft JD II, et al. Two-year toxicity and carcinogenicity study of methyl eugenol in F344/N rats and B6C3F(1) mice. *J Agric Food Chem.* 2000 Aug;48(8):3620-32.

4242 European Commission. Opinion of the Scientific Committee on Food on methyl eugenol (4-Allyl-1,2- dimethoxybenzene). Available at: http://ec.europa.eu/food/fs/sc/scf/out102_en.pdf.

4243 National Toxicology Program. NTP Toxicology and Carcinogenesis Studies of Methyleugenol (CAS NO. 93-15-2) in F344/N Rats and B6C3F1 Mice (Gavage Studies). *Natl Toxicol Program Tech Rep Ser.* 2000 Jul;491:1-412.

4244 National Toxicology Program. Carcinogenesis Studies of Eugenol (CAS No. 97-53-0) in F344/N Rats and B6C3F1 Mice (Feed Studies). Technical Report Series No. 223. NIH Publication No. 84-1779. 1983. U.S. DHHS, PHS, NIH, NTP, Research Triangle Park, NC.

4245 Ahmad A, Khan A, Ahmad Khan L, et al. In vitro synergy of eugenol and methyleugenol with fluconazole against clinical Candida isolates. *J Med Microbiol.* 2010;59:1178-84.

4246 Lee SE, Lee BH, Choi WS, et al. Fumigant toxicity of volatile natural products from Korean spices and medicinal plants towards the rice weevil, Sitophilus oryzae (L). *Pest Manag Sci.* 2001;57:548-53.

4247 Manaharan T, Thirugnanasampandan R, Jayakumar R, et al. Purified Essential Oil from Ocimum sanctum Linn. Triggers the Apoptotic Mechanism in Human Breast Cancer Cells. *Pharmacogn Mag.* 2016 May;12(Suppl 3):S327-31.

4248 Zomorodian K, Ghadiri P, Saharkhiz MJ, et al. Antimicrobial activity of seven essential oils from Iranian aromatic plants against common causes of oral infections. *Jundishapur J Microbiol.* 2015 Feb 19;8(2):e17766.

4249 Rao BR, Kotharia SK, Rajput DK, et al. Chemical and biological diversity in fourteen selections of four Ocimum species. *Nat Prod Commun.* 2011 Nov;6(11):1705-10.

4250 Saharkhiz MJ, Kamyab AA, Kazerani NK, et al. Chemical Compositions and Antimicrobial Activities of Ocimum sanctum L. Essential Oils at Different Harvest Stages. *Jundishapur J Microbiol.* 2015 Jan;8(1):e13720.

4251 Yamani HA, Pang EC, Mantri N, et al. Antimicrobial activity of Tulsi (Ocimum tenuiflorum) essential oil and their major constituents against three species of bacteria. *Front Microbiol.* 2016;7:681.

4252 Saharkhiz MJ, Kamyab AA, Kazerani NK, et al. Chemical compositions and antimicrobial activities of Ocimum sanctum L. essential oils at different harvest stages. *Jundishapur J Microbiol.* 2015 Jan; 8(1): e13720.

4253 Kumar A, Shukla R, Singh P, et al. Chemical composition, antifungal and antiaflatoxigenic activities of Ocimum sanctum L. essential oil and its safety assessment as plant based antimicrobial. *Food Chem Toxicol.* 2010 Feb;48(2):539-43.

4254 Khan A, Ahmad A, Khan LA, et al. Ocimum sanctum (L.) essential oil and its lead molecules induce apoptosis in Candida albicans. *Res Microbiol.* 2014 Jul-Aug;165(6):411-9.

4255 Khan A, Ahmad A, Akhtar F, et al. Ocimum sanctum essential oil and its active principles exert their antifungal activity by disrupting ergosterol biosynthesis and membrane integrity. *Res Micribiol.* 2010 Dec;161(10):816-23.

4256 Khan A, Ahmad A, Xess I, et al. Ocimum sanctum essential oil inhibits virulence attributes in Candida albicans. *Phytomedicine.* 2014 Mar 15;21(4):448-52.

4257 Amber K, Aijaz A, Immaculata X, et al. Anticandidal effect of Ocimum sanctum essential oil and its synergy with fluconazole and ketoconazole. *Phytomedicine.* 2010 Oct;17(12):921-5.

4258 Navin MI, Ajay L, Naseem S, et al. Preliminary ex-vivo and an animal model evaluation of Ocimum sanctum's essential oil extract for its antibacterial and anti- inflammatory properties. *Oral Health Dent Manag.* 2013 Sep;12(3):174-9.

4259 Joshi RK. Chemical Composition, In Vitro Antimicrobial and Antioxidant Activities of the Essential Oils of Ocimum Gratissimum, O. Sanctum and their Major Constituents. *Indian J Pharm Sci.* 2013 Jul;75(4):457-62.

4260 Saeio K, Chaiyana W, Okonogi S. Antityrosinase and antioxidant activities of essential oils of edible Thai plants. *Drug Discov Ther.* 2011 Jun;5(3):144-9.

4261 Trevisan MT, Vasconcelos Silva MG, Pfundstein B, et al. Characterization of the volatile pattern and antioxidant capacity of essential oils from different species of the genus Ocimum. *J Agric Food Chem.* 2006 Jun 14;54(12):4378-82.

4262 Suanarunsawat T1, Devakul Na Ayutthaya W, Songsak T, et al. Antioxidant Activity and Lipid-Lowering Effect of Essential Oils Extracted from Ocimum sanctum L. Leaves in Rats Fed with a High Cholesterol Diet. *J Clin Biochem Nutr.* 2010 Jan;46(1):52-9.

4263 Dohi S, Terasaki M, Makino M. Acetylcholinesterase inhibitory activity and chemical composition of commercial essential oils. *J Agric Food Chem.* 2009 May 27;57(10):4313-8.

4264 Charoo NA, Shamsher AA, Kohli K, et al. Improvement in bioavailability of transdermally applied flurbiprofen using tulsi (Ocimum sanctum) and turpentine oil. *Colloids Surf B Biointerfaces.* 2008 Sep 1;65(2):300-7.

4265 Viyoch J, Pisutthanan N, Faikreua A, et al. Evaluation of in vitro antimicrobial activity of Thai basil oils and their micro-emulsion formulas against Propionibacterium acnes. *Int J Cosmet Sci.* 2006 Apr;28(2):125-33.

4266 Zheljazkov VD, Cantrell CL, Tekwani B, et al. Content, composition, and bioactivity of the essential oils of three basil genotypes as a function of harvesting. *J Agric Food Chem.* 2008 Jan 23;56(2):380-5.

4267 Asha MK, Prashanth D, Murali B, et al. Anthelmintic activity of essential oil of Ocimum sanctum and eugenol. *Fitoterapia.* 2001 Aug;72(6):669-70.

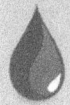

[4268] Singh S, Rehan HM, Majumdar DK. Effect of Ocimum sanctum fixed oil on blood pressure, blood clotting time and pentobarbitone-induced sleeping time. *J Ethnopharmacol.* 2001;78:139-43.
[4269] Lalthazuali, Mathew N. Mosquito repellent activity of volatile oils from selected aromatic plants. *Parasitol Res.* 2017 Feb;116(2):821-825.
[4270] Ahirwar P, Shashikiran ND, Sundarraj RK, et al. A clinical trial comparing antimicrobial efficacy of "essential oil of Ocimum sanctum" with triple antibiotic paste as an intracanal medicament in primary molars. *J Indian Soc Pedod Prev Dent.* 2018 Apr-Jun;36(2):191-197.
[4271] Bhavya ML, Obulkaxmi S, Devi SS. Efficacy of Ocimum tenuiflorum essential oil as grain protectant against coleopteran beetle, infesting stored pulses. *J Food Sci Technol.* 2021 Apr;58(4):1611-1616.
[4272] Boonyanugomol W, Rukseree K, Prapatpong P, et al. An In Vitro Anti-Cancer Activity of Ocimum tenuiflorum Essential Oil by Inducing Apoptosis in Human Gastric Cancer Cell Line. *Medicina (Kaunas).* 2021 Jul 30;57(8):784.
[4273] Zabka M, Pavela R, Kovarikova K, et al. Antifungal and Insecticidal Potential of the Essential Oil from Ocimum sanctum L. against Dangerous Fungal and Insect Species and Its Safety for Nontarget Useful Soil Species Eisenia fetida (Savigny, 1826). *Plants (Basel).* 2021 Oct 14;10(10):2180.
[4274] Jayapal V, Vidya Raj CK, Muthaiah M, et al. In-vitro anti-Mycobacterium tuberculosis effect of essential oil of Ocimum sanctum L. (Tulsi/Basil) leaves. *Indian J Tuberc.* 2021 Oct;68(4):470-473.
[4275] Andriantsoanirina V, Guillot J, Ratsimbason M, et al. In vitro efficacy of essential oils against Sarcoptes scabiei. *Sci Rep.* 2022 May 3;12(1):7176.
[4276] Southwell IA, Russell M, Smith RL, et al. Melaleuca teretifolia, a Novel Aromatic and Medicinal Plant from Australia. *Acta Hort.* 2004 Dec:677.10.
[4277] Southwell IA, Russell M, Smith RL, et al. Melaleuca teretifolia Chemovars: New Australian Sources of Citral and 1,8-Cineole. *J Essent Oil Res.* 2003;15(3):339-41.
[4278] Aromatics International. Honey Myrtle. Available at: https://www.aromatics.com/products/essential-oils/honey-myrtle.
[4279] Nogueira AC, Carvalho RR, Souza CA, et al. Study on the embryofeto-toxicity of citral in the rat. *Toxicology.* 1995;96(2):105-13.
[4280] Seo KA, Kim H, Ku HY, et al. The monoterpenoids citral and geraniol are moderate inhibitors of the CYP2B6 hydroxylase activity. *Chem Biol Interact.* 2008;174:141-46.
[4281] Sheweita SA, Newairy AA, Mansour HA, et al. Effect of some hypoglycemic herbs on the activity of phase I and II drug-metabolizing enzymes in alloxan-induced diabetic rats. *Toxicology.* 2002 May 24;17(2):131-39.
[4282] Raner GM, Vaz AD, Coon MJ. Metabolism of all-trans, 9-cis, and 13-cis isomers of retinal by purified isozymes of microsomal cytochrome P450 and mechanism-based inhibition of retinoid oxidation by citral. *Mol Pharmacol.* 1996;49(3):515-22.
[4283] De Olivera AC, Ribeiro-Pinto LF, Paumgartten JR. In vitro inhibition of CYP2B1 monoxygenase by beta-myrcene and other monoterpenoid constituents. *Br J Nutr.* 1999;81:289-95.
[4284] Modak T, Mukhopadhaya A. Effects of citral, a naturally occurring antiadipogenic molecule, on an energy-intense diet model of obesity. *Indian J Pharmacol.* 2011 May-Jun;43(3):300-05.
[4285] Najafian M, Ebrahim-Habibi A, Yaghmaei P, et al. Citral as a potential antihyperlipidemic medicine in diabetes: a study on streptozotocin-induced diabetic rats. *J Diabetes Metabolic Disorders.* 2011;10(1):3.
[4286] Choi JY, Damte D, Seung-Jin L, et al. Antimicrobial activity of lemongrass and oregano essential oil against standard antibiotic resistant Staphylococcus aureus and field isolates from chronic mastitis cow. *International Journal of Phytomedicine.* 2012;4(1):134-39.
[4287] do Vale TG, Furtado EC, Santos JG Jr, et al. Central effects of citral, myrcene and limonene, constituents of essential oil chemotypes from Lippia alba (Mill.) n.e. Brown. *Phytomedicine.* 2002 Dec;9(8):709-14.
[4288] Kuhn GO, McCampbell P, Singmaster G, et al. Application of microencapsulation technology to improve the stability of citral in rodent diets. *Fundam Appl Toxicol.* 1991 Oct;17(3):635-40.
[4289] De Mozzi P, Johnston GA. An outbreak of allergic contact dermatitis caused by citral in beauticians working in a health spa. *Contact Dermatitis.* 2014 Jun;70(6):377-9.
[4290] Hidayat Y, Neil H, Hassan E. Repellency and oviposition deterrence effects of plant essential and vegetable oils against female Queensland fruit fly Bactrocera tryoni (Froggatt) (Diptera: Tephritidae). *Aust J Entomology.* 2013 Nov;52(4):379-86.
[4291] Jang M, Kim J, Yoon KA, et al. Biological activity of Myrtaceae plant essential oils and their major components against Drosophila suzukii (Diptera: Drosophilidae). *Pest Manag Sci.* 2017 Feb;73(2):404-409.
[4292] Nance MR, Setzer WN. Volatile components of aroma hops (Humulus lupulus L.) commonly used in beer brewing. *J Brewing Distilling.* 2011 Apr;2(2):16-22.
[4293] Bernatiene G, Nivinskiene O, Butjiene R, et al. Chemical composition of essential oils of hops (Humulus lupus L.) growing wild in Aukstaitija. *Chemija.* 2004;15(2):31-36.
[4294] Katsiotis ST, Langezaal CR, Scheffer JJC, et al. Comparative study of the essential oils from hops of various Humulus lupulus L. cultivars. *Flacour Frag J.* 1989;4:187-91.
[4295] Delgado IF, Carvalho RR, Nogueira, et al. Study on embryofetotoxicity of b-myrcene in the rat. *Food and Chemical Toxicology.* 1993;31(1):31-5.
[4296] Paumgartten FJ, De-Carvalho RR, Souza CA, et al. Study of the effects of beta-myrcene on rat fertility and general reproductive performance. *Braz J Med Biol Res.* 1998 Jul;31(7):955-65.
[4297] do Vale TG, Furtado EC, Santos JG Jr, et al. Central effects of citral, myrcene and limonene, constituents of essential oil chemotypes from Lippia alba (Mill.) n.e. Brown. *Phytomedicine.* 2002 Dec;9(8):709-14.
[4298] Segelman AB, Sofia RD, Segelman FP, et al. Cannabis sativa L. (marijuana). V. Pharmacological evaluation of marijuana aqueous extract and volatile oil. *J Pharm Sci.* 1974 Jun;63(6):962-4.
[4299] Freitas JC1, Presgrave OA, Fingola FF, et al. Effect of beta-myrcene on pentobarbital sleeping time. *Braz J Med Biol Res.* 1993 May;26(5):519-23.
[4300] De Olivera AC, Ribeiro-Pinto LF, Paumgartten JR. In vitro inhibition of CYP2B1 monoxygenase by beta-myrcene and other monoterpenoid constituents. *Br J Nutr.* 1999;81:289-95.
[4301] De-Oliveira AC1, Ribeiro-Pinto LF, Otto SS, et al. Induction of liver monooxygenases by beta-myrcene. *Toxicology.* 1997 Dec 26;124(2):135-40.
[4302] Nguyen LT, Mysliveckova Z, Szotakova B, et al. The inhibitory effects of β-caryophyllene, β-caryophyllene oxide and α-humulene on the activities of the main drug-metabolizing enzymes in rat and human liver in vitro. *Chem-Biol Interactoins.* 2017 Dec 25;278:123-8.
[4303] Akdemir Evrendilek G. Empirical prediction and validation of antibacterial inhibitory effects of various plant essential oils on common pathogenic bacteria. *Int J Food Microbiol.* 2015 Jun 2;202:35-41.
[4304] Langezaal CR, Chandra A, Scheffer JJ. Antimicrobial screening of essential oils and extracts of some Humulus lupulus L. cultivars. *Pharm Weekbl Sci.* 1992 Dec 11;14(6):353-56.
[4305] Akdemir Evrendilek G. Empirical prediction and validation of antibacterial inhibitory effects of various plant essential oils on common pathogenic bacteria. *Int J Food Microbiol.* 2015 Jun 2;202:35-41.
[4306] Mitic V, Dordevic S. Essential oil composition of Hyssopus officinalis L. cultivated in Serbia. *Facta Universitatis.* 2000;2(2):105–08.
[4307] Fatemeh F, Hamedeyazdan S. A review on Hyssopus officinalis L.: Composition and biological activities. *African J Pharm Pharmacol.* 2011 Nov;5(8):1959–66.
[4308] Zawislak G. The chemical composition of essential hyssop oil depending on plant growth stage. *Acta Sci Pol, Hortorum Cultus.* 2013;12(3):161–70.
[4309] Garg SN, Naqvi AA, Singh A, et al. Composition of essential oil from an annual crop of Hyssopus officinals grown in Indian plains. *Flavour Frag J.* 1999 May;14(3):170–72.
[4310] Mazzanti G, Battinelli L, Salvatore G. Antimicrobial properties of the linalol-rich essential oil of Hyssopus officinalis L. var decumbens (Lamiaceae). *Flavour Frag J.* 1998 Sep;13(5):289–94.
[4311] Ogunwande IA, Flamini G, Alese OO, et al. A new chemical form of essential oil of Hyssopus officinalis L. (Lamiaceae) from Nigeria. *Int J Biol Chem Sci.* 2011 Feb;5(1):46-55.
[4312] Millet Y, Jouglard J, Steinmetz MD, et al. Toxicity of some essential plant oils. Clinical and experimental study. *Clin Toxicol.* 1981 Dec;18(12):1485–98.
[4313] O'Mullane NM, Joyce P, Kamath SV, et al. Adverse CNS effects of menthol-containing Olbas Oil. *Lancet.* 1982 May;1(8281):1121.
[4314] Millet Y, Tognetti P, Lavaire-Perlovisi M, et al. Experimental study of the toxic convulsant properties of commercial preparations of essences of sage and hyssop (author's transl). *Rev Electroencephalogr Neurophysiol Clin.* 1979 Jan-Mar;9(1):12–18.
[4315] McGuffin M, Hobbs C, Upton R, Goldberg A, eds. American Herbal Products Association's Botanical Safety Handbook. Boca Raton, FL: CRC Press, LLC 1997.
[4316] Blumenthal M, ed. The Complete German Commission E Monographs: Therapeutic Guide to Herbal Medicines. Trans. S. Klein. Boston, MA: American Botanical Council, 1998.
[4317] Gruenwald J, Brendler T, Jaenicke C. PDR for Herbal Medicines. 1st ed. Montvale, NJ: Medical Economics Company, Inc., 1998.
[4318] Salvator G, D'Andrea A, Nicoletti M. A pinocamphone poor oil of Hyssopus officinalis L. var. decumbens from France (Barton). *J Essential Oil Res.* 1998 Sep;10(5):563–67.
[4319] Kizil S, Hasimi N, Tolam V, et al. Chemical Composition, Antimicrobial and Antioxidant Activities of Hyssop (Hyssopus officinalis L.) Essential Oil. *Not Bot Hort Agrobot Cluj.* 2010;38:99-103.
[4320] Marino M, Bersani C, Comi G. Impedance measurements to study the antimicrobial activity of essential oils from Lamiaceae and Compositae. *Int J Food Microbiol.* 2001;67:187–95.
[4321] Motiejunaite O, Kalediene L. Antimicrobial activity of Lamiaceae plant essential oils on Aspergillus niger growth. *Biol Sci.* 2003;51:237-42.
[4322] Mazzanti G, Lu M, Salvatore G. Spasmolytic action of the essential oil from Hyssopus officinalis L. var. decumbens and its major components. *Phytother Res.* 1998 Sep;12(S1):S92–S94.
[4323] Lu M, Battinelli L, Daniele C, et al. Muscle relaxing activity of Hyssopus officinalis essential oil on isolated intestinal preparations. *Planta Med.* 2002 Mar;68(3):213-16.
[4324] Kim SW, Lee HR2, Jang MJ, et al. Fumigant Toxicity of Lamiaceae Plant Essential Oils and Blends of Their Constituents against Adult Rice Weevil Sitophilus oryzae. *Molecules.* 2016 Mar 16;21(3):361.
[4325] de Elguea-Culebras GO, Sánchez-Vioque R, Berruga MI, et al. Biocidal potential and chemical composition of industrial essential oils from Hyssopus officinalis, Lavandula x intermedia var. super and Santolina chamaecyparissus. *Chem Biodivers.* 2018 Jan;15(1).
[4326] Ahmadi H, Babalar M, Sarcheshmeh MAA, et al. Effects of exogenous application of citrulline on prolonged water stress damages in hyssop (Hyssopus officinalis L.): Antioxidant activity, biochemical indices, and essential oils profile. *Food Chem.* 2020 Dec 15;333:127433.
[4327] Harčárová M, Čonková E, Proškovcová M, et al. Comparison of antifungal activity of selected essential oils against Fusarium graminearum in vitro. *Ann Agric Environ Med.* 2021 Sep 16;28(3):414-418.
[4328] Mićović T, Katanić Stanković JS, Bauer R, et al.
In vitro, in vivo and in silico evaluation of the anti-inflammatory potential of Hyssopus officinalis L. subsp. aristatus (Godr.) Nyman (Lamiaceae). *J Ethnopharmacol.* 2022 Mar 28;293:115201.
[4329] Gharakhani-Beni A, Ghasemi Pirbalouti A, Javanmard H, et al. Chemical compositions, yield and antioxidant activity of the essential oil of hyssop (Hyssopus officinalis L.) under intercropping with fenugreek (Trigonella foenum-graecum L.). *Nat Prod Res.* 2022 May 26:1-6.
[4330] Proškovcová M, Čonková E, Váczi P, et al. Efficacy of Lamiaceae essential oils with selected azoles against Candida albicans clinical isolates. *Pol J Vet Sci.* 2022 Jun;25(2):279-285.
[4331] Gharakhani-Beni A, Ghasemi Pirbalouti A, Javanmard H, et al. Chemical compositions, yield and antioxidant activity of the essential oil of hyssop (Hyssopus officinalis L.) under intercropping with fenugreek (Trigonella foenum-graecum L.). *Nat Prod Res.* 2023 Feb;37(4):675-680.
[4332] Arumugam G, Swamy MK, Sinniah UR. Plectranthus amboinicus (Lour.) Spreng: Botanical,Phytochemical, Pharmacological and Nutritional Significance. *Molecules.* 2016;21:369.

[4333] dos Santos NO, Mariane B, Lago JHG, et al. Assessing the Chemical Composition and Antimicrobial Activity of Essential Oils from Brazilian Plants—Eremanthus erythropappus (Asteraceae), Plectrantuns barbatus, and P. amboinicus (Lamiaceae). *Molecules.* 2015;20:8440-452.
[4334] Hassani MS, Zainati I, Zrira S, et al. Chemical Composition and Antimicrobial Activity of Plectranthus amboinicus (Lour) Spring. Essential Oil from Archipelago of Comoros. 2012;15(4):637-44.
[4335] Senthilkumar A, Venkatesalu V. Chemical composition and larvicidal activity of the essential oil of Plectranthus amboinicus (Lour.) Spreng against Anopheles stephensi: a malarial vector mosquito. *Parasitol Res.* 2012;107:1275-78.
[4336] Goncalves TB, Braga MA, de Oliveira FFM, et al. Effect of subinihibitory and inhibitory concentrations of Plectranthus amboinicus (Lour.) Spreng essential oil on Klebsiella pneumoniae. *Phytomedicine.* 2012;19:962-68.
[4337] El-hawary SS, El-sofany RH, Abdel-Monem AR, et al. Seasonal variation in the composition of Plectranthus amboinicus (Lour.) Spreng essential oil and its biological activities. *Am J Essential Oils Nat Prod.* 2013;1(2):11-18.
[4338] Erny Sabrina MN, Razali M, Mirfat AHS, et al. Antimicrobial activity and bioactive evaluation of Plectranthus amboinicus essential oil. *Am J Res Commun.* 2014;2(12):121-27.
[4339] Velasco J, Rojas LB, Diaz T, et al. Chemical composition and antibacterial activity of essential oil of Coleus amboinicus Lour., against enteric pathogens. *J Essential Oil Bear Plants.* 2009;12(4):453-61.
[4340] Su LC, Huang CG, Chang ST, et al. An improved bioassay facilitates the screening of repellents against cat flea, Ctenocephalides felis (Siphonaptera: Pulicidae). *Pest Manag Sci.* 2014 Feb;70(2):264-70.
[4341] El-hawary SS, El-sofany RH, Abdel-Monem AR, et al. Seasonal variation in the composition of Plectranthus amboinicus (Lour.) Spreng essential oil and its biological activities. *Am J Essential Oils Nat Prod.* 2013;1(2):11-18.
[4342] Khine H, Weiss D, Graber N, et al. A cluster of children with seizures caused by camphor poisoning. *Pediatrics.* 2009 May;123(5):1269-72.
[4343] Michiels EA, Mazor SS. Toddler with seizures due to ingesting camphor at an Indian celebration. *Pediatr Emerg Care.* 2010 Aug;26(8):574-75.
[4344] Koren G. Medications which can kill a toddler with one tablet or teaspoonful. *J toxicol Clin Toxicol.* 1993;31(3):407- 13.
[4345] Bar-Oz B, Levicheck Z, Koren G. Medications that can kill a toddler with one tablet or teaspoonfull – A 2004 update. *Paediatr Drugs.* 2004;6(2):123-6.
[4346] Domaracky M, Rehak P, Juhas S, et al. Effects of selected plant essential oils on the growth and development of mouse preimplantation embryos in vivo. *Physiol Res.* 2007;56(1):97-104.
[4347] Rabl W, Katzgraber F, Steinlechner M. Camphor ingestion for abortion (case report). *Forensic Sci Int.* 1997 Sep 19;89(1-2):137-40.
[4348] Flaman Z, Pellechia-Clarke S, Bailey B, et al. Unintentional exposure of young children to camphor and eucalyptus oils. *Paediatr Child Health.* 2001 Feb;6(2):80-83.
[4349] Chen R, Chen J, Cheng S, et al. Assessment of embryotoxicity of constituents in cosmetics by the embryonic stem cell tes. *Toxicol Mech Methods.* 2010 Mar;20(3):112-18.
[4350] Kohlert C, Schindler G, Marz RW, et al. Systemic availability and pharmacokinetics of thymol in humans. *J Clin Pharmacol.* 2002 Jul;42(7):731-7.
[4351] Toxicology Data Network, National Library of Medicine. Thymol. Available at: http://toxnet.nlm.nih.gov/cgi-bin/sis/search/a?dbs+hsdb:@term+@DOCNO+866.
[4352] Manoguerra AS, Erdman AR, Wax PM, et al. Camphor poisoning: an evidence-based practice guideline for out-of- hospital management. *Clin Toxicol (Phila).*2006;44(4):357-70.
[4353] Gibson DE, Moore GP, Pfaff JA. Camphor ingestion. *Am J Emerg Med.* 1989 Jan;7(1):41-43.
[4354] Koppel C, Martends F, Schirop T, et al. Hemoperfusion in acute camphor poisoning. *Intensive Care Med.* 1988;14(4):431-33.
[4355] Lemhadri A, Zeggwagh NA, Maghrani M, et al. Anti-hypoglycaemic activity of the aqueous extract of Origanum vulgare growing wild in Tafilalet region. *J Ethnopharmacol.* 2004 Jun;92(2-3):251-6.
[4356] Mirazi N, Rezaei M, Mirhoseini M. Hypoglycemic effect of Satureja montanum L. hydroethanolic extract on diabetic rats. *J HerbMed Pharm.* 2016;5(1):17-22.
[4357] Ezhumalai M, Radhiga T, Pugalendi KV. Antihyperglycemic effect of carvacrol in combination with rosiglitazone in high-fat diet-induced type 2 diabetic C57BL/6J mice. *Mol Cell Biochem.* 2014 Jan;385(1-2):23-31.
[4358] Chen SJ, Wang MH, Chen IJ. Antiplatelet and calcium inhibitory properties of eugenol and sodium eugenol acetate. *Gen Pharmacol.* 1996 Jun;27(4):629-33.
[4359] Tognolini M, Barocelli E, Ballabeni V, et al. Comparative screening of plant essential oils; phenylpropanoid moiety as basic core for antiplatelet activity. *Life Sci.* 2006 Feb 23;78(13):1419-32.
[4360] Heck AM, DeWitt BA, Lukes AL. Potential interactions between alternative therapies and warfarin. *Am J Health Syst Pharm.* 2000;57(13):1221-1227.
[4361] Saaeed SA, Gilani AH. Antithrombotic activity of clove oil. *J Pak Med Assoc.* 1994;44(5):112-15.
[4362] Gutierrez J, Rodriguez G, Barry-Ryan C, et al. Efficacy of plant essential oils against foodborne pathogens and spoilage bacteria associated with ready-to-eat vegetables: antimicrobial and sensory screening. *J Food Prot.* 2008 Sep;71(9):1846-54.
[4363] Karkabounas S, Kostoula OK, Daskalou T, et al. Anticarcinogenic and antiplatelet effects of carvacrol. *Exp Oncol.* 2006 Jun;28(2):121-5.
[4364] Burkhard PR, Burkhardt K, Haenggeli CA, et al. Plant-induced seizures: reappearance of an old problem. *J Neurol.* 1999 Aug;246(8):667-70.
[4365] Narayan S, Singh N. Camphor poisoning-An unusual cause of seizure. *Med J Armed Forces India.* 2012 Jul;68(3):252-53.
[4366] Chanaranaj KJ, G MV, S M. Camphor poisoning in a child. *Natl Med J India.* 2013 Jan-Feb;26(1):60.
[4367] Olowe SA, Ransome-Kuti O. The risk of jaundice in glucose-6-phosphate dehydrogenase deficient babies exposed to menthol. *Acta Paediatr Scand.* 1980 May;69(3):341-5.
[4368] Dillon Remy M, Manning Alleyne P, Bratt DE, et al. Neonatal jaundice at Port-of-Spain General Hospital abstract. *West Indian Med J.* 1987;36(Suppl):28.
[4369] Langeveld WT, Veldhuizen EJ, Burt SA. Synergy between essential oil constituents and antibiotics. *Crit Rev Microbiol.* 2014 Feb;40(1);76-94.
[4370] Langeveld WT, Veldhuizen EJ, Burt SA. Synergy between essential oil constituents and antibiotics. *Crit Rev Microbiol.* 2014 Feb;40(1);76-94.
[4371] Jukic M, Politeo O, Maksimmovic M, et al. In vitro acetylcholinesterase inhibitory properties of thymol, carvacrol and their derivatives thymoquinone and thymohydroquinone. *Phytother Res.* 2007;21(3):259-61.
[4372] Dohi S, Terasaki M, Makino M. Acetylcholinesterase inhibitory activity and chemical composition of commercial essential oils. *J Agric Food Chem.* 2009 May 27;57(10):4313-8.
[4373] El-hawary SS, El-sofany RH, Abdel-Monem AR, et al. Seasonal variation in the composition of Plectranthus amboinicus (Lour.) Spreng essential oil and its biological activities. *Am J Essential Oils Nat Prod.* 2013;1(2):11-18.
[4374] Manjamalai A, Grace VM. The chemotherapeutic effect of essential oil of Plectranthus amboinicus (Lour) on lung metastasis developed by B16F-10 cell line in C57BL/6 mice. *Cancer Invest.* 2013 Jan;31(1):74-82.
[4375] dos Santos NO, Mariane B, Lago JHG, et al. Assessing the Chemical Composition and Antimicrobial Activity of Essential Oils from Brazilian Plants—Eremanthus erythropappus (Asteraceae), Plectrantuns barbatus, and P. amboinicus (Lamiaceae). *Molecules.* 2015;20:8440-452.
[4376] El-hawary SS, El-sofany RH, Abdel-Monem AR, et al. Seasonal variation in the composition of Plectranthus amboinicus (Lour.) Spreng essential oil and its biological activities. *Am J Essential Oils Nat Prod.* 2013;1(2):11-18.
[4377] Erny Sabrina MN, Razali M, Mirfat AHS, et al. Antimicrobial activity and bioactive evaluation of Plectranthus amboinicus essential oil. *Am J Res Commun.* 2014;2(12):121-27.
[4378] Hassani MS, Zainati I, Zrira S, et al. Chemical Composition and Antimicrobial Activity of Plectranthus amboinicus (Lour) Spring. Essential Oil from Archipelago of Comoros. 2012;15(4):637-44.
[4379] Velasco J, Rojas LB, Diaz T, et al. Chemical composition and antibacterial activity of essential oil of Coleus amboinicus Lour., against enteric pathogens. *J Essential Oil Bear Plants.* 2009;12(4):453-61.
[4380] Goncalves TB, Braga MA, de Oliveira FFM, et al. Effect of subinihibitory and inhibitory concentrations of Plectranthus amboinicus (Lour.) Spreng essential oil on Klebsiella pneumoniae. *Phytomedicine.* 2012;19:962-68.
[4381] El-hawary SS, El-sofany RH, Abdel-Monem AR, et al. Seasonal variation in the composition of Plectranthus amboinicus (Lour.) Spreng essential oil and its biological activities. *Am J Essential Oils Nat Prod.* 2013;1(2):11-18.
[4382] Erny Sabrina MN, Razali M, Mirfat AHS, et al. Antimicrobial activity and bioactive evaluation of Plectranthus amboinicus essential oil. *Am J Res Commun.* 2014;2(12):121-27.
[4383] Nogueira JC1, Dniz Mde F, Lima EO. In vitro antimicrobial activity of plants in Acute Otitis Externa. *Braz J Otorhinolaryngol.* 2008 Jan-Feb;74(1):118-24.
[4384] El-hawary SS, El-sofany RH, Abdel-Monem AR, et al. Seasonal variation in the composition of Plectranthus amboinicus (Lour.) Spreng essential oil and its biological activities. *Am J Essential Oils Nat Prod.* 2013;1(2):11-18.
[4385] El-hawary SS, El-sofany RH, Abdel-Monem AR, et al. Seasonal variation in the composition of Plectranthus amboinicus (Lour.) Spreng essential oil and its biological activities. *Am J Essential Oils Nat Prod.* 2013;1(2):11-18.
[4386] El-hawary SS, El-sofany RH, Abdel-Monem AR, et al. Seasonal variation in the composition of Plectranthus amboinicus (Lour.) Spreng essential oil and its biological activities. *Am J Essential Oils Nat Prod.* 2013;1(2):11-18.
[4387] Senthilkumar A, Venkatesalu V. Chemical composition and larvicidal activity of the essential oil of Plectranthus amboinicus (Lour.) Spreng against Anopheles stephensi: a malarial vector mosquito. *Parasitol Res.* 2012;107:1275-78.
[4388] Kweka EJ, Senthilkumar A, Venkatesalu V. Toxicity of essential oil from Indian borage on the larvae of the African malaria vector mosquito, Anopheles gambiae. *Parasit Vectors.* 2012 Dec 3;5:277.
[4389] Su LC, Huang CG, Chang ST, et al. An improved bioassay facilitates the screening of repellents against cat flea, Ctenocephalides felis (Siphonaptera: Pulicidae). *Pest Manag Sci.* 2014 Feb;70(2):264-70.
[4390] Velasco J, Rojas LB, Diaz T, et al. Chemical composition and antibacterial activity of essential oil of Coleus amboinicus Lour., against enteric pathogens. *J Essential Oil Bear Plants.* 2009;12(4):453-61.
[4391] Huang HT, Lin CC, Kuo TC, et al. Phytochemical composition and larvicidal activity of essential oils from herbal plants. *Planta.* 2019 Jul;250(1):59-68.
[4392] Antonio-Gutiérrez O, Alvízar-Martínez JA, Solano R, et al. Microwave-Assisted Hydrodistillation of Essential Oil from Plectranthus amboinicus: Evaluation of Its Antifungal Effect and Chemical Composition. *Life (Basel).* 2023 Feb 15;13(2):528.
[4393] Cha JD, Kim JY. Essential Oil from Cryptomeria japonica Induces Apoptosis in Human Oral Epidermoid Carcinoma Cells via Mitochondrial Stress and Activation of Caspases. *Molecules.* 2012;17:3890-901.
[4394] Cha JD, Jeong MR, Jeong SI, et al. Chemical composition and antimicrobial activity of the essential oil of Cryptomeria japonica. *Phytother Res.* 2007 Mar;21(3):295-99.
[4395] Yoon WJ, Kim SS, Oh TH, et al. Cryptomeria japonica essential oil inhibits the growth of drug-resistant skin pathogens and LPS-induced nitric oxide and pro-inflammatory cytokine production. *Polish J Microbiol.* 2009;58(1):61-68.
[4396] Wang SY, Lai WC, Chu FH, et al. Essential oil from the leaves of Cryptomeria japonica acts as a silverfish (Lepisma saccharina) repellent and insecticide. *J Wood Sci.* 2006;52:522-26.
[4397] Ho CL, Wang EIC, Yu HT, et al. Compositions and antioxidant activities of essential oils of different tissues from Cryptomeria japonica D. Don. *Forestry Res Quarterly.* 2010;32(1):63-76.
[4398] Satyal P, Setzer WN. Chemical composition of Cryptomeria japonica leaf oil from Nepal. *Am J Essent Oils Nat Prod.* 2015;3(2):7-10.
[4399] Cheng SS, Lin HY, Chang ST. Chemical Composition and Antifungal Activity of Essential Oils from Different Tissues of Japanese Cedar (Cryptomeria japonica). *J Agric Food Chem.* 2005;53:614-19.
[4400] Lee JH, Lee BK, Kim JH, et al. Comparison of Chemical Compositions and Antimicrobial Activities of Essential Oils from Three Conifer Trees; Pinus densiflora, Cryptomeria japonica, and Chamaecyparis obtusa. *J Microbiol Biotechnol.* 2009;19(4):391-96.

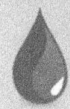

[4401] Kim SH, Lee SY, Hong CY, et al. Antifungal Effect of Elemol and Eudesmol from Cryptomeria japonica Essential Oil against Trichophyton rubrum. *Academia J Agric Res.* 2016 Aug;4(8):511-17.
[4402] Mdoe FP, Cheng SS, Lyaruu L, et al. Larvicidal efficacy of Cryptomeria japonica leaf essential oils against Anopheles gambiae. *Parasit Vectors.* 2014 Sep 4;7:426.
[4403] Moiteiro C, Esteves T, Ramalho L, et al. Essential oil characterization of two Azorean Cryptomeria japonica populations and their biological evaluations. *Nat Prod Commun.* 2013 Dec;8(12):1785-90.
[4404] Cheng SS, Lin CY, Chung MJ, et al. Chemical composition and antitermitic activity against Coptotermes formosanus Shiraki of Cryptomeria japonica leaf essential oil. *Chem Biodivers.* 2012 Feb;9(2):352-8.
[4405] Cheng SS, Chua MT, Chang EH, et al. Variations in insecticidal activity and chemical compositions of leaf essential oils from Cryptomeria japonica at different ages. *Bioresour Technol.* 2009 Jan;100(1):465-70.
[4406] Cheng SS, Chang HT, Wu CL, et al. Anti-termitic activities of essential oils from coniferous trees against Coptotermes formosanus. *Bioresour Technol.* 2007 Jan;98(2):456-9.
[4407] Hiroi T, Miyazaki Y, Kobayashi Y, et al. Induction of hepatic P450s in rat by essential oil wood leaf oils. *Xenobiotica.* 1995 May;25(5):457-67.
[4408] Khine H, Weiss D, Graber N, et al. A cluster of children with seizures caused by camphor poisoning. *Pediatrics.* 2009 May;123(5):1269-72.
[4409] Michiels EA, Mazor SS. Toddler with seizures due to ingesting camphor at an Indian celebration. *Pediatr Emerg Care.* 2010 Aug;26(8):574-75.
[4410] Koren G. Medications which can kill a toddler with one tablet or teaspoonful. *J toxicol Clin toxicol.* 1993;31(3):407- 13.
[4411] Flaman Z, Pellechia-Clarke S, Bailey B, et al. Unintentional exposure of young children to camphor and eucalyptus oils. *Paediatr Child Health.* 2001 Feb;6(2):80-83.
[4412] Rabl W, Katzgraber F, Steinlechner M. Camphor ingestion for abortion (case report). *Forensic Sci Int.* 1997 Sep 19;89(1-2):137-40.
[4413] Flaman Z, Pellechia-Clarke S, Bailey B, et al. Unintentional exposure of young children to camphor and eucalyptus oils. *Paediatr Child Health.* 2001 Feb;6(2):80-83.
[4414] Narayan S, Singh N. Camphor poisoning-An unusual cause of seizure. *Med J Armed Forces India.* 2012 Jul;68(3):252-53.
[4415] Chanaranaj KJ, G MV, S M. Camphor poisoning in a child. *Natl Med J India.* 2013 Jan-Feb;26(1):60.
[4416] Uc A, Bishop WP, Sanders KD. Camphor hepatotoxicity. *South Med J.* 2000;93:596-98.
[4417] Olowe SA, Ransome-Kuti O. The risk of jaundice in glucose-6-phosphate dehydrogenase deficient babies exposed to menthol. *Acta Paediatr Scand.* 1980 May;69(3):341-5.
[4418] Dillon Remy M, Manning Alleyne P, Bratt DE, et al. Neonatal jaundice at Port-of-Spain General Hospital abstract. *West Indian Med J.* 1987;36(Suppl):28.
[4419] Manoguerra AS, Erdman AR, Wax PM, et al. Camphor poisoning: an evidence-based practice guideline for out-of- hospital management. *Clin Toxicol (Phila).*2006;44(4):357-70.
[4420] Gibson DE, Moore GP, Pfaff JA. Camphor ingestion. *Am J Emerg Med.* 1989 Jan;7(1):41-43.
[4421] Koppel C, Martends F, Schirop T, et al. Hemoperfusion in acute camphor poisoning. *Intensive Care Med.* 1988;14(4):431-33.
[4422] Covington TR, et al. Handbook of Nonprescription Drugs. 11th ed. Washington, D.C.: American Pharmaceutical Association. 1996.
[4423] Cha JD, Kim JY. Essential Oil from Cryptomeria japonica Induces Apoptosis in Human Oral Epidermoid Carcinoma Cells via Mitochondrial Stress and Activation of Caspases. *Molecules.* 2012;17:3890-901.
[4424] Yoon WJ, Kim SS, Oh TH, et al. Cryptomeria japonica essential oil inhibits the growth of drug-resistant skin pathogens and LPS-induced nitric oxide and pro-inflammatory cytokine production. *Polish J Microbiol.* 2009;58(1):61-68.
[4425] Cha JD, Jeong MR, Jeong SI, et al. Chemical composition and antimicrobial activity of the essential oil of Cryptomeria japonica. *Phytother Res.* 2007 Mar;21(3):295-99.
[4426] Lee JH, Lee BK, Kim JH, et al. Comparison of Chemical Compositions and Antimicrobial Activities of Essential Oils from Three Conifer Trees; Pinus densiflora, Cryptomeria japonica, and Chamaecyparis obtusa. *J Microbiol Biotechnol.* 2009;19(4):391-96.
[4427] Moiteiro C, Esteves T, Ramalho L, et al. Essential oil characterization of two Azorean Cryptomeria japonica populations and their biological evaluations. *Nat Prod Commun.* 2013 Dec;8(12):1785-90.
[4428] Cheng SS, Lin HY, Chang ST. Chemical Composition and Antifungal Activity of Essential Oils from Different Tissues of Japanese Cedar (Cryptomeria japonica). *J Agric Food Chem.* 2005;53:614-19.
[4429] Lee JH, Lee BK, Kim JH, et al. Comparison of Chemical Compositions and Antimicrobial Activities of Essential Oils from Three Conifer Trees; Pinus densiflora, Cryptomeria japonica, and Chamaecyparis obtusa. *J Microbiol Biotechnol.* 2009;19(4):391-96.
[4430] Kim SH, Lee SY, Hong CY, et al. Antifungal Effect of Elemol and Eudesmol from Cryptomeria japonica Essential Oil against Trichophyton rubrum. *Academia J Agric Res.* 2016 Aug;4(8):511-17.
[4431] Moiteiro C, Esteves T, Ramalho L, et al. Essential oil characterization of two Azorean Cryptomeria japonica populations and their biological evaluations. *Nat Prod Commun.* 2013 Dec;8(12):1785-90.
[4432] Takao Y, Kuriyama I, Yamada T, et al. Antifungal properties of Japanese cedar essential oil from waste wood chips made from used sake barrels. *Mol Med Rep.* 2012 May;5(5):1163-8.
[4433] Ho CL, Wang EIC, Yu HT, et al. Compositions and antioxidant activities of essential oils of different tissues from Cryptomeria japonica D. Don. *Forestry Res Quarterly.* 2010;32(1):63-76.
[4434] Kim SH, Lee SY, Hong CY, et al. Whitening and antioxidant activities of bornyl acetate and nezukol fractionated from Cryptomeria japonica essential oil. *Int J Cosmet Sci.* 2013 Oct;35(5):484-90.
[4435] Wang SY, Lai WC, Chu FH, et al. Essential oil from the leaves of Cryptomeria japonica acts as a silverfish (Lepisma saccharina) repellent and insecticide. *J Wood Sci.* 2006;52:522-26.
[4436] Barbosa P, Lima AS, Vieira P, et al. Nematicidal activity of essential oils and volatiles derived from Portuguese aromatic flora against the pinewood nematode, Bursaphelenchus xylophilus. *J Nematol.* 2010 Mar;42(1):8-16.
[4437] Mdoe FP, Cheng SS, Lyaruu L, et al. Larvicidal efficacy of Cryptomeria japonica leaf essential oils against Anopheles gambiae. *Parasit Vectors.* 2014 Sep 4;7:426.
[4438] Cheng SS, Lin CY, Chung MJ, et al. Chemical composition and antitermitic activity against Coptotermes formosanus Shiraki of Cryptomeria japonica leaf essential oil. *Chem Biodivers.* 2012 Feb;9(2):352-8.
[4439] Cheng SS, Chang HT, Wu CL, et al. Anti-termitic activities of essential oils from coniferous trees against Coptotermes formosanus. *Bioresour Technol.* 2007 Jan;98(2):456-9.
[4440] Cheng SS, Chang HT, Chang ST, et al. Bioactivity of selected plant essential oils against the yellow fever mosquito Aedes aegypti larvae. *Bioresour Technol.* 2003 Aug;89(1):99-102.
[4441] Cheng SS, Lin CY, Chung MJ, et al. Chemical composition and antitermitic activity against Coptotermes formosanus Shiraki of Cryptomeria japonica leaf essential oil. *Chem Biodivers.* 2012 Feb;9(2):352-8.
[4442] Gu HJ, Cheng SS, Lin CY, et al. Repellency of essential oils of Cryptomeria japonica (Pinaceae) against adults of the mosquitoes Aedes aegypti and Aedes albopictus (Diptera:Culicidae). *J Agric Food Chem.* 2009 Dec 9;57(23):11127-33.
[4443] Cheng SS, Chua MT, Chang EH, et al. Variations in insecticidal activity and chemical compositions of leaf essential oils from Cryptomeria japonica at different ages. *Bioresour Technol.* 2009 Jan;100(1):465-70.
[4444] Kim SH, Lee SY, Hong CY, et al. Whitening and antioxidant activities of bornyl acetate and nezukol fractionated from Cryptomeria japonica essential oil. *Int J Cosmet Sci.* 2013 Oct;35(5):484-90.
[4445] Matsunaga T, Hasegawa C, Kawasuji T, et al. Isolation of the antiulcer constituent in essential oil from the leaves of Cryptomeria japonica. *Biol Pharm Bull.* 2000 May;23(5):595-8.
[4446] Fang F, Candy K, Melloul E, et al. In vitro activity of ten essential oils against Sarcoptes scabiei. *Parasit Vectors.* 2016 Nov 22;9(1):594.
[4447] Matsubara E, Ohira T. Inhalation of Japanese cedar (Cryptomeria japonica) wood odor causes psychological relaxation after monotonous work among female participants. *Biomed Res (Tokyo).* 2018;39(5):241-9.
[4448] Ruas A, Graça A, Marto J, et al. Chemical Characterization and Bioactivity of Commercial Essential Oils and Hydrolates Obtained from Portuguese Forest Logging and Thinning. *Molecules.* 2022 Jun 2;27(11):3572.
[4449] Wei FH, Chen FL, Tan XM. Gas Chromatographic-Mass Spectrometric Analysis of Essential Oil of Jasminum officinale L var Grandiflorum Flower. *Tropical J Pharm Res.* 2015 Jan;14(1):149-52.
[4450] Eid RA, Taha LS, Soad MM. Physiological properties studies on essential oil of Jasminum grandiflorum L. as affected by some vitamins. *Ozean J Appl Sci.* 2010;3(1):87-96.
[4451] Basset F. Journées de Digne, Le jasmin, la fleur le roi. *Parfums Cosmétiques Arômes.* 1994;119:58-64.
[4452] Bera P, Reddy Kotamreddy JN, Samanta T, et al. Inter-specific variation in headspace scent volatiles composition of four commercially cultivated jasmine flowers. *Nat Prod Res.* 2015;29(14):1328-35.
[4453] Rout PK, Naik SN, Rao YR. Composition of Absolutes of Jasminum sambac L. Flowers Fractionated with Liquid CO2 and Methanol and Comparison with Liquid CO2 Extract. *J Essent Oil Res.* 2010 Sep/Oct ;22 :398-406
[4454] Edris AE, Chizzola R, Franz C. Isolation and characterization of the volatile aroma compounds from the concrete headspace and the absolute of Jasminum sambac (L.) Ait. (Oleaceae) flowers grown in Egypt. *Eur Food Res Technol.* 2008 ;226 :621-6.
[4455] National Library of Medicine. TOXNET. Benzyl acetate. Available at: https://toxnet.nlm.nih.gov/cgi-bin/sis/search/a?dbs+hsdb:@term+@DOCNO+2851.
[4456] van den Brink DM, van Miert JNI, Dacremont G, et al. Characterization of the Final Step in the Conversion of Phytol into Phytanic Acid. *J Biol Chem.* 2005 Jul 22;280(29):26838-44.
[4457] Selkälä EM, Nair RR, Schmitz W, et al. Phytol is lethal for Amacr-deficient mice. *Biochim Biophys Acta.* 2015 Oct;1851(10):1394-405.
[4458] McGinty D, Letizia CS, Api AM. Fragrance material review on phytol. *Food Chem Toxicol.* 2010;48:S59–S63.
[4459] National Institutes of Health. U.S. National Library of Medicine. Alpha-methylacyl-CoA racemase deficiency. Available at: https://ghr.nlm.nih.gov/condition/alpha-methylacyl-coa-racemase-deficiency.
[4460] Kagoura M, Matsui C, Morohashi M. Phytol is a novel tumor promoter on ICR mouse skin. *Jpn J Cancer Res.* 1999 Apr;90(4):377-84.
[4461] Larsen W, Nakayama H, Fischer T, et al. Fragrance contact dermatitis: A worldwide multicentre investigation (part II). *Contact Dermatitis.* 2002;46:141-44.
[4462] Larsen WG. Perfume dermatitis: a study of 20 patients. *Arch Dermat.* 1977;113:623-26.
[4463] Bouhlal K, Meynadier J, Peyron JL, et al. The cutaneous effects of the common concretes and absolutes used in the perfume industry. 1988. In: Lawrence BM. The antimicrobial/biological activity of essential oils Allured Pub. Corp: Carol Stream, Illinois, pp. 10-23.
[4464] Uter W, Schmidt E, Heier J, et al. Contact allergy to essential oils: current patch test results (2000-2008) from the Information Network of Departments of Dermatology (IVDK). *Contact Dermatitis.* 2010;63:277-83.
[4465] González-de-Olano D, Córdoba-Guijarro S, Marín-Manzano E, et al. Allergy to jasmine is not always delayed contact allergy. *Dermatitis.* 2012 Mar-Apr;23(2):94-5.

4466 de Groot AC1, Schmidt E. Essential Oils, Part I: Introduction. *Dermatitis.* 2016 Mar-Apr;27(2):39-42.
4467 Kieć-Swierczyńska M1, Krecisz B, Swierczyńska-Machura D. [Contact allergy to fragrances]. *Med Pr.* 2006;57(5):431-7.
4468 Belsito DV, Fowler JF Jr, Sasseville D, et al. Delayed-type hypersensitivity to fragrance materials in a select North American population. *Dermatitis.* 2006 Mar;17(1):23-8.
4469 Frosch PJ, Johansen JD, Menné T, et al. Further important sensitizers in patients sensitive to fragrances. *Contact Dermatitis.* 2002 Nov;47(5):279-87.
4470 Lis-Balchin M, Hart S, Wan Hang Lo B. Jasmine absolute (Jasminum grandiflora L.) and its mode of action on guinea-pig ileum in vitro. *Phytother Res.* 2002 Aug;16(5):437-9.
4471 Lis-Balchin M, Hart S, Deans SG, et al. Comparison of the Pharmacological and Antimicrobial Action of Commercial Plant Essential Oils. *J Herbs Spices Med Plants.* 1996;4(2):69-86.
4472 Lis-Balchin M, Hart S. A preliminary study of the effect of essential oils on skeletal and smooth muscle in vitro. *J Ethnopharmacol.* 1997 Nov;58(3):183-7.
4473 Lis-Balchin M, Hart S. The effect of essential oils on the uterus compared to that of other muscles. Proc 27th Int Symp Ess Oils. Vienna, Austria, 8-11 Sep. Franz Ch, Mathe A, Buchbauer G. Allured Pub. Corp: Carol Stream, Illinois, pp. 29-32.
4474 Weber ST, Heuberger E. The impact of natural odors on affective states in humans. *Chem Senses.* 2008 Mar;33(5):441-47.
4475 Shekhar S, Prasad MP. Evaluation of antimicrobial activity of Jasminum species using solvent extracts against clinical pathogens. *World J Pharmacy Pharmaceutical Sci.* 2015;4(05):1247-56.
4476 Císarová M, Tančinová D, Medo J, et al. The in vitro effect of selected essential oils on the growth and mycotoxin production of Aspergillus species. *J Environ Sci Health B.* 2016 Oct 2;51(10):668-674.
4477 Bartoňková I, Dvořák Z. Essential oils of culinary herbs and spices display agonist and antagonist activities at human aryl hydrocarbon receptor AhR. *Food Chem Toxicol.* 2018 Jan;111:374-384.
4478 Farouk S, Almutairi AB, Alharbi YO, et al. Acaricidal Efficacy of Jasmine and Lavender Essential Oil or Mustard Fixed Oil against Two-Spotted Spider Mite and Their Impact on Growth and Yield of Eggplants. *Biology (Basel).* 2021 May 6;10(5):410.
4479 Mansour KA, El-Neketi M, Lahloub MF, et al. Nanoemulsions of Jasminum humile L. and Jasminum grandiflorum L. Essential Oils: An Approach to Enhance Their Cytotoxic and Antiviral Effects. *Molecules.* 2022 Jun 6;27(11):3639.
4480 Pthran R, Zhang MWB, Tam WW, et al. Prevalence of depression amongst medical students: a meta-analysis. *Med Educ.* 2016 Apr;50(4):456-68.
4481 Sukarman TL, Gani IP, Jasputra DK. The Comparisons of Lavender and Jasmine Aromatherapy Effectiveness on Depression Level for Medical Students. *Berkala Ilmiah Kedokteran Duta Wacana.* 2022 Aug;7(1):19-22.
4482 Ariani A, Yusita I, Nurlaelasari D. Kombinasi Aromaterapy Jasmine Sambac dan Loving Yoga terhadap
Disfungsi Seksual pada Akseptor KB Suntik DMPA. *Jurnal Ilmiah Universitas Batanghari Jambi.* 2022 Oct;22(3):1923-7.
4483 Cabral C, Francisco V, Cavaleiro C, et al. Essential oil of Juniperus communis subsp. Alpina (Suter) Celak needles: chemical composition, antifungal activity and cytotoxicity. *Phytother Res.* 2012 Sep;26(9):1352-57.
4484 Ottavioli J, Gonny M, Casanova J, et al. Chemical variability of the needles oil of Juniperus communis ssp. alpine from Corsica. *Chem Biodivers.* 2009 Dec;6(12):2192-99.
4485 Orav A, Kailas T, Muurisepp M. Chemical investigation of the essential oil from berries and needles of common juniper (Juniperus communis L.) growing wild in Estonia. *Nat Prod Res.* 2010 Nov;24(19):1789-99.
4486 Hoferl M, Stoilova I, Schmidt E, et al. Chemical composition and antioxidant properties of Juniper Berry (Juniperus communis L.) essential oil. Action of the essential oil on the antioxidant protection of Saccharomyces cerevisiae model organism. *Antioxidants.* 2014;3(1):81-98.
4487 Sela F, Karapandzova M, Stefkov G, et al. Chemical composition of berry essential oils from Juniperus communis L. (Cupressaceae) growing wild in Republic of Macedonia and assessment of the chemical composition in accordance to European Pharmacopoeia. *Macedonian Pharm Bull.* 2011;57(1,2):43-51.
4488 Stillpoint Aromatics. Juniper, Utah Essential Oil. Available at: http://www.stillpointaromatics.com/utah-juniper-Juniperus-osteosperma-essential-oils-aroamtherapy?keyword=juniper.
4489 Aromatics International. Utah Juniper. Available at: https://www.aromatics.com/products/essential-oils/utah-juniper.
4490 Schilcher H, Leuschner F. The potential nephrotoxic effects of essential juniper oil. *Arzneimittelforschung.* 1997 Jul;47(7):855-8.
4491 Ali SA, Rizk MZ, Ibrahim NA, et al. Protective role of Juniperus phoenicea and Cupressus sempervirens against CCl(4). *World J Gastrointest Pharmacol Ther.* 2012 Dec 6;1(6):123-31.
4492 Butani L, Afshinnik A, Johnson J, et al. Amelioration of tacrolimus-induced nephrotoxicity in rats using juniper oil. *Transplantation.* 2003 Jul 27;76(2):306-11.
4493 Dearing DM, Mangione AM, Karasov WH. Ingestion of plant secondary constituents causes diuresis in desert herbivores. *Oecologia.* 2002 Feb;130(4):576-584.
4494 Ju JB, Kim JS, Choi CW, et al. Comparison between ethanolic and aqueous extracts from Chinese juniper berries for hypoglycaemic and hypolipidemic effects in alloxan-induced diabetic rats. *J Ethnopharmacol.* 2008 Jan 4;115(1):110- 15.
4495 Bonesi M, Menichini F, Tundis R, et al. Acetylcholinesterase and butyrylcholinesterase inhibitory activity of Pinus species essential oils and their constituents. *J Enzyme Inhib Med Chem.* 2010 Oct;25(5):622-8.
4496 Khine H, Weiss D, Graber N, et al. A cluster of children with seizures caused by camphor poisoning. *Pediatrics.* 2009 May;123(5):1269-72.
4497 Michiels EA, Mazor SS. Toddler with seizures due to ingesting camphor at an Indian celebration. *Pediatr Emerg Care.* 2010 Aug;26(8):574-75.
4498 Koren G. Medications which can kill a toddler with one tablet or teaspoonful. *J toxicol Clin toxicol.* 1993;31(3):407- 13.
4499 Flaman Z, Pellechia-Clarke S, Bailey B, et al. Unintentional exposure of young children to camphor and eucalyptus oils. *Paediatr Child Health.* 2001 Feb;6(2):80-83.
4500 Rabl W, Katzgraber F, Steinlechner M. Camphor ingestion for abortion (case report). *Forensic Sci Int.* 1997 Sep 19;89(1-2):137-40.
4501 Flaman Z, Pellechia-Clarke S, Bailey B, et al. Unintentional exposure of young children to camphor and eucalyptus oils. *Paediatr Child Health.* 2001 Feb;6(2):80-83.
4502 Burkhard PR, Burkhardt K, Haenggeli CA, et al. Plant-induced seizures: reappearance of an old problem. *J Neurol.* 1999 Aug;246(8):667-70.
4503 Narayan S, Singh N. Camphor poisoning-An unusual cause of seizure. *Med J Armed Forces India.* 2012 Jul;68(3):252-53.
4504 Chanaranaj KJ, G MV, S M. Camphor poisoning in a child. *Natl Med J India.* 2013 Jan-Feb;26(1):60.
4505 Olowe SA, Ransome-Kuti O. The risk of jaundice in glucose-6-phosphate dehydrogenase deficient babies exposed to menthol. *Acta Paediatr Scand.* 1980 May;69(3):341-5.
4506 Dillon Remy M, Manning Alleyne P, Bratt DE, et al. Neonatal jaundice at Port-of-Spain General Hospital abstract. *West Indian Med J.* 1987;36(Suppl):28.
4507 Manoguerra AS, Erdman AR, Wax PM, et al. Camphor poisoning: an evidence-based practice guideline for out-of- hospital management. *Clin Toxicol (Phila).*2006;44(4):357-70.
4508 Gibson DE, Moore GP, Pfaff JA. Camphor ingestion. *Am J Emerg Med.* 1989 Jan;7(1):41-43.
4509 Koppel C, Martends F, Schirop T, et al. Hemoperfusion in acute camphor poisoning. *Intensive Care Med.* 1988;14(4):431-33.
4510 Mori M, Ikeda N, Kato Y, et al. Inhibition of elastase activity by essential oils in vitro. *J Cosmetic Dermatol.* 2002;1(4):183-87.
4511 Asgary S, Naderi GA, Shams Ardekani MR, et al. Inhibition of protein glycation by essential oils of branchlets and fruits of Juniperus communis subsp. Hemisphaerica. *Res Pharm Sci.* 2014;9(3):179-85.
4512 Camporese A. In vitro activity of Eucalyptus smithii and Juniperus communis oils against bacterial biofilms and efficacy perspectives of complementary inhalation therapy in chronic and recurrent upper respiratory tract infections. *Infez Med.* 2013 Jun;21(2):117-24.
4513 Ozogul Y, Kuley E, Ucar Y, et al. Antimicrobial Impacts of Essential Oils on Food Borne-Pathogens. Recent Pat Food Nutr Agric. 2015;7(1):53-61.
4514 Cavaleiro C, Pinto E, Goncalves MJ, et al. Antifungal activity of Juniperus essential oils against dermatophyte, Aspergillus and Candida strains. *J Appl Microbiol.* 2006 Jun;100(6):1333-38.
4515 Pepeljnak S, Kosalec I, Kalodera Z, et al. Antimicrobial activity of juniper berry essential oil (Juniperus communis L., Cupressaceae). *Acta Pharm.* 2005 Dec;55(4):417-22.
4516 Baylac S, Racine P. Inhibition of 5-lipoxygenase by essential oils and other natural fragrant extracts. *Int J Aromatherapy.* 2003;13(2-3):138-42.
4517 Elmastas M, Gulcin I, Beydemir S, et al. A study on the in vitro antioxidant activity of juniper (Juniperus communis L.) fruit extracts. *Analytical Lett.* 2006;39(1):47-65.
4518 Pazinato R, Volpato A, Baldissera MD, et al. In vitro effect of seven essential oils on the reproduction of the cattle tick Rhipicephalus microplus. *J Adv Res.* 2016 Nov;7(6):1029-1034.
4519 Luís Â, Duarte AP, Pereira L, et al. Chemical Profiling and Evaluation of Antioxidant and Anti-Microbial Properties of Selected Commercial Essential Oils: A Comparative Study. *Medicines (Basel).* 2017 Jun 5;4(2).
4520 Vasilijević B, Knežević-Vukčević J, Mitić-Ćulafić D, et al. Chemical characterization, antioxidant, genotoxic and in vitro cytotoxic activity assessment of Juniperus communis var. saxatilis. *Food Chem Toxicol.* 2018 Feb;112:118-125.
4521 Klančnik A, Zorko Š, Toplak N, et al. Antiadhesion activity of juniper (Juniperus communis L.) preparations against Campylobacter jejuni evaluated with PCR-based methods. *Phytother Res.* 2018 Mar;32(3):542-550.
4522 Moreno ÉM, Leal SM, Stashenko EE, et al. Induction of programmed cell death in Trypanosoma cruzi by Lippia alba essential oils and their major and synergistic terpenes (citral, limonene and caryophyllene oxide). *BMC Complement Altern Med.* 2018 Jul 27;18(1):225.
4523 Peruč D, Tićac B, Broznić D, et al. Juniperus communis essential oil limit the biofilm formation of Mycobacterium avium and Mycobacterium intracellulare on polystyrene in a temperature-dependent manner. *Int J Environ Health Res.* 2020 Mar 20:1-14.
4524 Elshafie HS, Caputo L, Martino LD, et al. Biological Investigations of Essential Oils Extracted From Three Juniperus Species and Evaluation of Their Antimicrobial, Antioxidant and Cytotoxic Activities. *J Appl Microbiol.* 2020 May 23. Online ahead of print.
4525 Darwish RS, Hammoda HM, Ghareeb DA, et al. Efficacy-directed discrimination of the essential oils of three Juniperus species based on their in-vitro antimicrobial and anti-inflammatory activities. *J Ethnopharmacol.* 2020 Sep 15;259:112971.
4526 Peruc D, Ticac B, Broznic D, et al. Juniper and immortelle essential oils synergistically inhibit adhesion of nontuberculous mycobacteria to Acanthamoeba castellanii. *Arh Hig Rada Toksikol.* 2020 Oct 6;71(3):223-230.
4527 Najar B, Nardi V, Stincarelli MA, et al. Screening of the essential oil effects on human H1N1 influenza virus infection: an in vitro study in MDCK cells. *Nat Prod Res.* 2021 Jun 26;1-4.
4528 Semerdjieva I, Zheljazkov VD, Radoukova T, et al. Biological Activity of Essential Oils of Four Juniper Species and Their Potential as Biopesticides. *Molecules.* 2021 Oct 21;26(21):6358.
4529 Xavier V, Finimundy TC, Heleno SA, et al. Chemical and Bioactive Characterization of the Essential Oils Obtained from Three Mediterranean Plants. *Molecules.* 2021 Dec 10;26(24):7472.
4530 Maurya AK, Devi K, Agnihotri VK. Chemical profiling and α-glucosidase inhibitory activity of essential oils extracted with two methods from some North Western Himalayan aromatic crops. *Nat Prod Res.* 2022 Apr 28:1-4.
4531 Peruc D, Gobin I, Abram M, et al. Antimycobacterial potential of the juniper berry essential oil in tap water. *Arh Hig Rada Toksikol.* 2018 Mar 1;69(1):46-54.
4532 Raina VK, Srivastava S, Kv S. Essential oil composition of Juniperus chinensis from the plains of northern India. *Flavour Frag J.* 2005 Jan;20(1):57-59.
4533 Kim MG, Lee NH, Kim JM, et al. Chemical Composition of Essential Oils Extracted from Five Juniperus chinensis Varieties in Korea. *J Essential Oil Bear Plants.* 2015;18(4):852-56.

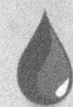

[4534] Afsharypuor S, Rahiminexhad M, Ghaemmaghami L, et al. Essential oil constituents of leaves of the male and female shrubs of Juniperus chinensis L. from Isfahan. *Iranian J Pharmaceutical Sci.* 2007;3(3):177-80.

[4535] Casares R. Juniperus sabina. *Food Cosmet Toxicol.* 1964;2:680-81. Found in U.S. Food and Drug Administration. FDA Poisonous Plant Database. Available at: http://www.accessdata.fda.gov/scripts/plantox/detail.cfm?id=5133.

[4536] Radulović NS, Mladenović MZ, Randjelovic PJ, et al. Toxic essential oils. Part IV: The essential oil of Achillea falcata L. as a source of biologically/pharmacologically active trans-sabinyl esters. *Food Chem Toxicol.* 2015 Jun;80:114-29.

[4537] Judzentiene A, Budiene J, Gircyte R, et al. Toxic activity and chemical composition of Lithuanian wormwood (Artemisia absinthium L.) essential oils. *Rec Nat Prod.* 2012;6(2):180-83.

[4538] Pages N, Fournier G, Chamorro G, et al. Teratological evaluation of Juniperus sabina essential oil in mice. *Planta Med.* 1989 Apr;55(2):144-46.

[4539] Pages N, Fournier G, Baudel C, et al. Sabinyl Acetate, the Main Component of Juniperus sabina L'Hérit. Essential Oil, is Responsible for Antiimplantation Effect. *Phytother Res.* 1996 Aug;10(5):438-440.

[4540] Pages N, Fournier G, Velut V, et al. Potential teratogenicity in mice of the essential oil of Salvia lavandulifolia Vahl. Study of a fraction rich in sabinyl acetate. *Phytother Res.* 1992 Mar;6(2):80-83.

[4541] Casares R. Juniperus sabina. *Food Cosmet Toxicol.* 1964;2:680-81. Found in U.S. Food and Drug Administration. FDA Poisonous Plant Database. Available at: http://www.accessdata.fda.gov/scripts/plantox/detail.cfm?id=5133.

[4542] Burkhard PR, Burkhardt K, Haenggeli CA, et al. Plant-induced seizures: reappearance of an old problem. *J Neurol.* 1999 Aug;246(8):667-70.

[4543] Patoir A, Patoir G, Bedrine H. Note sur l'action de l'essence de rue sur l'organisme animal. *Computes Rendues Société Bologique.* 1938;127:1324-25.

[4544] Pages N, Fournier G, Chamorro G, et al. Teratological evaluation of Juniperus sabina essential oil in mice. *Planta Med.* 1989 Apr;55(2):144-46.

[4545] Casares R. Juniperus sabina. *Food Cosmet Toxicol.* 1964;2:680-81. Found in U.S. Food and Drug Administration. FDA Poisonous Plant Database. Available at: http://www.accessdata.fda.gov/scripts/plantox/detail.cfm?id=5133.

[4546] Lee CH, Park JM, Song HY, et al. Acaricidal activities of major constituents of essential oil of Juniperus chinensis leaves against house dust and stored food mites. *J Food Prot.* 2009 Aug;72(8):1686-91.

[4547] Adams RP, Thappa RK, Agarwal SG, et al. The Leaf Essential Oil of Juniperus recurva Buch.-Ham. ex D. Don from India and Nepal Compared with J. recurva var. squamata (D. Don) Parl. *J Essent Oil Res.* 1998 Jan;10(1):21-24.

[4548] Oda J, Ando N, Nakajima Y, et al. Studies on Insecticidal Constituents of Juniperus recurva Buch. *Agric Biol Chme.* 1977;41(1):201-04.

[4549] Lohani H, Haider SZ, Chauhan NK, et al. Aroma profile of two Juniperus species from Alpine region in Uttarakhand. *J Nat Prod.* 2013;6:38-43.

[4550] Lohani H, Haider SZ, Nirpendra K, et al. Essential oil composition of leaves and berries of Juniperus communis and Juniperus indica from Uttarakhand Himalaya. *J Med Aromatic Plant Sci.* 2010;32(3):199-201.

[4551] Chanotiya CS, Mathela CS. Essential oil composition of Juniperus wallichiana from north western region of Kumaon Himalaya. *J Essent Oil Res.* 2007;19:422.

[4552] Buffa G, Caramiello R, Canoca D, et al. Chemotaxonomy of Juniperus indica Bertol. and J. recurva Buch. - Ham. ex D. Don from Nepal. *Giornale botanico italiano.* 1996;130(1):56.

[4553] Plant J. Private communication. 2016.

[4554] Aazza S, Lyoussi B, Miguel MG. Antioxidant and antiacetylcholinesterase activities of some commercial essential oils and their major compounds. *Molecules.* 2011 Sep 7;16(9):7672-90.

[4555] Miyazawa M, Yamafuji C. Inhibition of acetylcholinesterase activity by bicyclic monoterpenoids. *J Agric Food Chem.* 2005 Mar 9;53(5):1765-8.

[4556] Ennajar M, Bouajila J, Lebrihi A, et al. The influence of organ, season and drying method on chemical composition and antioxidant and antimicrobial activities of Juniperus phoenicea L. essential oils. *J Sci Food Agric.* 2010 Feb 1;90(3):462-70.

[4557] Ait-Ouazzou A, Loran S, Arakrak A, et al. Evaluation of the chemical composition and antimicrobial activity of Mentha pulegium, Juniperus Phoenicia, and Cyperus longus essential oils from Morocco. *Food Res Int.* 2012 Jan;45(1):313-19.

[4558] Medini H, Elaissi A, Farhat F, et al. Seasonal and geographical influences on the chemical composition of Juniperus phoeniciea l. essential oil leaves from Northern Tunisia. *Chem Biodiversity.* 2009 Seo;6(9):1378-1387.

[4559] Ennajar M, Bouajila J, Lebrihi A, et al. Chemical composition and antimicrobial and antioxidant activities of essential oils and various extracts of Juniperus phoenicea L. (Cupressaceae). *Food Microbiol Safety.* 2009 Sep;74(7):M364-71.

[4560] Chaftar N, Girardot M, Quellard N, et al. Activity of Six Essential Oils Extracted from Tunisian Plants against Legionella pneumophila. *Chem Biodivers.* 2015 Oct;12(10):1565-74.

[4561] el-Sawi SA, Motawae HM, Ali AM. Chemical composition, cytotoxic activity and antimicrobial activity of essential oils of leaves and berries of Juniperus phoenicea L. grown in Egypt. *Afr J Tradit Complement Altern Med.* 2007 Jun 10;4(4):417-26.

[4562] Schilcher H, Leuschner F. The potential nephrotoxic effects of essential juniper oil. *Arzneimittelforschung.* 1997 Jul;47(7):855-8.

[4563] Ali SA, Rizk MZ, Ibrahim NA, et al. Protective role of Juniperus phoenicea and Cupressus sempervirens against CCl(4). *World J Gastrointest Pharmacol Ther.* 2012 Dec 6;1(6):123-31.

[4564] Butani L, Afshinnik A, Johnson J, et al. Amelioration of tacrolimus-induced nephrotoxicity in rats using juniper oil. *Transplantation.* 2003 Jul 27;76(2):306-11.

[4565] Olowe SA, Ransome-Kuti O. The risk of jaundice in glucose-6-phosphate dehydrogenase deficient babies exposed to menthol. *Acta Paediatr Scand.* 1980 May;69(3):341-5.

[4566] Dillon Remy M, Manning Alleyne P, Bratt DE, et al. Neonatal jaundice at Port-of-Spain General Hospital abstract. *West Indian Med J.* 1987;36(Suppl):28.

[4567] Dearing DM, Mangione AM, Karasov WH. Ingestion of plant secondary constituents causes diuresis in desert herbivores. *Oecologia.* 2002 Feb;130(4):576-584.

[4568] Burkhard PR, Burkhardt K, Haenggeli CA, et al. Plant-induced seizures: reappearance of an old problem. *J Neurol.* 1999 Aug;246(8):667-70.

[4569] Narayan S, Singh N. Camphor poisoning-An unusual cause of seizure. *Med J Armed Forces India.* 2012 Jul;68(3):252-53.

[4570] Chanaranaj KJ, G MV, S M. Camphor poisoning in a child. *Natl Med J India.* 2013 Jan-Feb;26(1):60.

[4571] Ju JB, Kim JS, Choi CW, et al. Comparison between ethanolic and aqueous extracts from Chinese juniper berries for hypoglycaemic and hypolipidemic effects in alloxan-induced diabetic rats. *J Ethnopharmacol.* 2008 Jan 4;115(1):110- 15.

[4572] el-Sawi SA, Motawae HM, Ali AM. Chemical composition, cytotoxic activity and antimicrobial activity of essential oils of leaves and berries of Juniperus phoenicea L. grown in Egypt. *Afr J Tradit Complement Altern Med.* 2007 Jun 10;4(4):417-26.

[4573] Mazari K, Bendimerad N, Bekhechi C, et al. Chemical composition and antimicrobial activity of essential oils isolated from Algerian Juniperus phoenicea L. and Cupressus sempervirens L. *J Med Plants Res.* 2010 May;4(10):959- 64.

[4574] Ennajar M, Bouajila J, Lebrihi A, et al. The influence of organ, season and drying method on chemical composition and antioxidant and antimicrobial activities of Juniperus phoenicea L. essential oils. *J Sci Food Agric.* 2010 Feb 1;90(3):462-70.

[4575] Ait-Ouazzou A, Loran S, Arakrak A, et al. Evaluation of the chemical composition and antimicrobial activity of Mentha pulegium, Juniperus Phoenicia, and Cyperus longus essential oils from Morocco. *Food Res Int.* 2012 Jan;45(1):313-19.

[4576] Ennajar M, Bouajila J, Lebrihi A, et al. Chemical composition and antimicrobial and antioxidant activities of essential oils and various extracts of Juniperus phoenicea L. (Cupressaceae). *Food Microbiol Safety.* 2009 Sep;74(7):M364-71.

[4577] Fouad B, Abderrahmane R, Youssef A, et al. Chemical composition and antibacterial activity of the essential oil of Moroccan Juniperus phoenicea. *Nat Prod Commun.* 2011 Oct;6(10):1515-8.

[4578] Bouyahyaoui A, Bahri F, Romane A, et al. Antimicrobial Activity and Chemical Analysis of the Essential Oil of Algerian Juniperus phoenicea. *Nat Prod Commun.* 2016 Apr;11(4):519-22.

[4579] el-Sawi SA, Motawae HM, Ali AM. Chemical composition, cytotoxic activity and antimicrobial activity of essential oils of leaves and berries of Juniperus phoenicea L. grown in Egypt. *Afr J Tradit Complement Altern Med.* 2007 Jun 10;4(4):417-26.

[4580] Chaftar N, Girardot M, Quellard N, et al. Activity of Six Essential Oils Extracted from Tunisian Plants against Legionella pneumophila. *Chem Biodivers.* 2015 Oct;12(10):1565-74.

[4581] Ennajar M, Bouajila J, Lebrihi A, et al. The influence of organ, season and drying method on chemical composition and antioxidant and antimicrobial activities of Juniperus phoenicea L. essential oils. *J Sci Food Agric.* 2010 Feb 1;90(3):462-70.

[4582] Ennajar M, Bouajila J, Lebrihi A, et al. Chemical composition and antimicrobial and antioxidant activities of essential oils and various extracts of Juniperus phoenicea L. (Cupressaceae). *Food Microbiol Safety.* 2009 Sep;74(7):M364-71.

[4583] Yvon Y, Raoelison EG, Razafindrazaka R, et al. Relation between chemical composition or antioxidant activity and antihypertensive activity for six essential oils. *J Food Sci.* 2012 Aug;77(8):H184-91.

[4584] Medini H, Elaissi A, Larbi Khouja M, et al. Chemical composition and antioxidant activity of the essential oil of Juniperus phoenicea L. berries. *Nat Prod Res.* 2011 Oct;25(18):1695-706.

[4585] Bouyahyaoui A, Bahri F, Romane A, et al. Antimicrobial Activity and Chemical Analysis of the Essential Oil of Algerian Juniperus phoenicea. *Nat Prod Commun.* 2016 Apr;11(4):519-22.

[4586] Giatropoulos A, Pitarokili D, Papaioannou F, et al. Essential oil composition, adult repellency and larvicidal activity of eight Cupressaceae species from Greece against Aedes albopictus (Diptera: Culicidae). *Parasitol Res.* 2013 Mar;112(3):1113-23.

[4587] Garboui SS, Borg-Karlson AK, Pålsson K. Tick repellent properties of three Libyan plants. *J Med Entomol.* 2009 Nov;46(6):1415-9.

[4588] Njoroge SM, Ukeda H, Kusunose H, et al. Volatile components of the essential oils from Kabosu, Daidai, and Yuko, Japanese sour citrus fruits. *Flavour Frag J.* 1994;9(6):289-97.

[4589] Minh Tu NT, Onishi Y, Choi HS, et al. Characteristic odor components of Citrus sphaerocarpa Tanaka (Kabosu) cold-pressed peel oil. *J Agric Food Chem.* 2002 May 8;50(10):2908-13.

[4590] Dugrand-Judek A, Olry A, Hehn A, et al. The distribution of coumarins and furanocoumarins in Citrus species closely matches citrus phylogeny and reflects the organization of biosynthetic pathways. *PLoS One.* 2015 Nov;10(11):e0142757.

[4591] Sato A, Asano K, Sato T. The chemical composition of Citrus hystrix DC (Swangi). *J Essent Oil Res.* 1990 Jul-Aug;2:179-83.

[4592] Loh FS, Awang RM, Omar D, et al. Insecticidal properties of Citrus hystrix DC leaves essential oil against Spodoptera litura fabricius. *J Med Plant Res.* 2011 Aug;5(16):3739-44.

[4593] Lawrence B, Hogg JW, Terhune SJ, et al. Constituents of the leaf and peel oil of Citrus Hystrix, D.C. *Phytochemistry.* 1971 Jun;10(6):1404-05.

[4594] Hongratanaworakit T, Buchbauer G. Chemical composition and stimulating effect of Citrus hystrix oil on humans. *Flavour Frag J.* 2007 Sep;22(5):443-49.

[4595] Kasuan N, Muhammad Z, Yusoff Z, et al. Extraction of Citrus hystrix D.C. (Kaffir Lime) essential oil using automated steam distillation process: Analysis of volatile constituents. *Malaysian J Aanalytical Sci.* 2013;17(3):359-69.

[4596] Sutthanont N, Choochote W, Tuetun, et al. Chemical composition and larvicidal activity of edible plant-derived essential oils against the pyrethroid-susceptible and -resistant strains of Aedes aegypti (Diptera: Culicidae). *J Vector Ecol.* 2010 Jun;35(1):106-15.

4597 Orhan I, Kartal M, Kan Y, et al. Activity of essential oils and individual components against acetyl- and butyrylcholinesterase. *Z Naturforsch C.* 2008 Jul-Aug;63(7-8):547-53.

4598 Chaiyana W, Saeio K, Hennink WE, et al. Characterization of potent anticholinesterase plant oil based microemulsion. *Int J Pharm.* 2010 Nov 30;401(1-2):32-40.

4599 Bonesi M, Menichini F, Tundis R, et al. Acetylcholinesterase and butyrylcholinesterase inhibitory activity of Pinus species essential oils and their constituents. *J Enzyme Inhib Med Chem.* 2010 Oct;25(5):622-8.

4600 Mauerman B, Ahmed N, Tambhar N, et al. Trends in Furanocoumarin Profiles Among Commerical-Scale Essential Oils. International Conference on the Science of Botanicals, Poster. Mar 2022.

4601 Hongratanaworakit T, Buchbauer G. Chemical composition and stimulating effect of Citrus hystrix oil on humans. *Flavour Frag J.* 2007 Sep;22(5):443-49.

4602 Wongsariya K, Phanthong P, Bunyapraphatsara N, et al. Synergistic interaction and mode of action of Citrus hystrix essential oil against bacteria causing periodontal diseases. *Pharm Biol.* 2014 Mar;52(3):273-80.

4603 Srisukh V, tribuddharat C, Nukoolkarn V, et al. Antibacterial activity of essential oils from Citrus hystrix (makrut lime) against respiratory tract pathogens. *Science Asia.* 2012;38:212-17.

4604 Chaiyana W, Saeio K, Hennink WE, et al. Characterization of potent anticholinesterase plant oil based microemulsion. *Int J Pharm.* 2010 Nov 30;401(1-2):32-40.

4605 Darvesh S, Hopkins DA, Geula C. Neurobiology of butyrylcholinesterase. *Nat Rev Neurosci.* 2003 Feb;4:131-38.

4606 Sutthanont N, Choochote W, Tuetun, et al. Chemical composition and larvicidal activity of edible plant-derived essential oils against the pyrethroid-susceptible and -resistant strains of Aedes aegypti (Diptera: Culicidae). *J Vector Ecol.* 2010 Jun;35(1):106-15.

4607 Loh FS, Awang RM, Omar D, et al. Insecticidal properties of Citrus hystrix DC leaves essential oil against Spodoptera litura fabricius. *J Med Plant Res.* 2011 Aug;5(16):3739-44.

4608 Thavara U, Tawatsin A, Bhakdeenuan P, et al. Repellent activity of essential oils against cockroaches (Dictyoptera: Blattidae, Blattellidae, and Blaberidae) in Thailand. *Southeast Asian J Trop Med Public Health.* 2007 Jul;38(4):663-73.

4609 Nararak J, Sathantriphop S, Kongmee M, et al. Excito-Repellency of Citrus hystrix DC Leaf and Peel Essential Oils Against Aedes aegypti and Anopheles minimus (Diptera: Culicidae), Vectors of Human Pathogens. *J Med Entomol.* 2017 Jan;54(1):178-186.

4610 Nararak J, Sathantriphop S, Chauhan K, et al. Avoidance Behavior to Essential Oils by Anopheles minimus, a Malaria Vector in Thailand. *J Am Mosq Control Assoc.* 2016 Mar;32(1):34-43.

4611 Tawatsin A, Wratten SD, Scott RR, et al. Repellency of volatile oils from pants against three mosquito vectors. *J Vector Ecol.* 2001 Jun;26(1):76-82.

4612 Wiwattanaratanabut K, choonharuangdej S, Srithava T. In Vitro Anti-Cariogenic Plaque Effects of Essential Oils Extracted from Culinary Herbs. *J Clin Diagnostic Res.* 2017 Sep;11(9):DC30-5.

4613 Aumeeruddy-Elalfi Z, Lall N, et al. Selected essential oils inhibit key physiological enzymes and possess intracellular and extracellular antimelanogenic properties in vitro. *J Food Drug Anal.* 2018 Jan;26(1):232-243.

4614 Mahomoodally F, Aumeeruddy-Elafi Z, Venugopala KN, et al. Antiglycation, Comparative Antioxidant Potential, Phenolic Content and Yield Variation of Essential Oils From 19 Exotic and Endemic Medicinal Plants. *Saudi J Biol Sci.* 2019 Nov;26(7):1779-88.

4615 Kulig M, Galanty A, Grabowska K, et al. Assessment of safety and health-benefits of Citrus hystrix DC. peel essential oil, with regard to its bioactive constituents in an in vitro model of physiological and pathological skin conditions. *Biomed Pharmacother.* 2022 May 20;151:113151.

4616 Othman HIA, Alkatib HH, Zaid A, et al. Phytochemical Composition, Antioxidant and Antiproliferative Activities of Citrus hystrix, Citrus limon, Citrus pyriformis, and Citrus microcarpa Leaf Essential Oils against Human Cervical Cancer Cell Line. *Plants (Basel).* 2022 Dec 27;12(1):134.

4617 Maddocks-Jennings W, Wilkinson JM, Shillinton D, et al. A fresh look at manuka and kanuka essential oils from New Zealand. *Int J Aromatherapy.* 2005;15:141-46.

4618 Silva CJ, Barbosa LCA, Demuner AJ, et al. Chemical composition and antibacterial activities from the essential oils of myrtaceae species planted in Brazil. *Quimica Nova.* 2010;33(1):ISSN 1678-7064.

4619 Porter NG, Wilkins AL. Chemical, physical and antimicrobial properties of essential oils of Leptospermum scoparium and Kunzea ericoides. *Phytochemistry.* 1998;50:407-15.

4620 Schnitzler P, Wiesenhofer K, Reichling J. Comparative study on the cytotoxicity of different Myrtaceae essential oils on cultured Vero and RC-37 cells. *Pharmazie.* 2008;63:830-85.

4621 Lis-Balchin M, Hart SL, Deans SG. Pharmacological and antimicrobial studies on different tea-tree oils (Melaleuca alternifolia, Leptospermum scoparium or Manuka and Kunzea ericoides or Kanuka), originating in Australia and New Zealand. *Phytother Res.* 2000 Dec;14(8):623-9.

4622 Maddocks-Jennings W, Wilkinson JM, Cavanagh HM, et al. Evaluating the effects of the essential oils Leptospermum scoparium (manuka) and Kunzea ericoides (kanuka) on radiotherapy induced mucositis: a randomized, placebo controlled feasibility study. *Eur J Oncol Nurs.* 2009 Apr;13(2):87-93.

4623 Lis-Balchin M, Hart SL, Deans SG. Pharmacological and antimicrobial studies on different tea-tree oils (Melaleuca alternifolia, Leptospermum scoparium or Manuka and Kunzea ericoides or Kanuka), originating in Australia and New Zealand. *Phytother Res.* 2000 Dec;14(8):623-9.

4624 Chen CC, Yan SH, Yen MY, et al. Investigations of kanuka and manuka essential oils for in vitro treatment of disease and cellular inflammation caused by infectious microorganisms. *J Microbiol Immunol Infect.* 2016 Feb;49(1):104-11.

4625 Lis-Balchin M, Hart SL. An investigation of the actions of the essential oils of Manuka (Leptospermum scoparium) and Kanuka (Kunzea ericoides), Myrtaceae on guinea-pig smooth muscle. *J Pharm Pharmacol.* 1998 Jul;50(7):809-11.

4626 Lis-Balchin M, Hart SL, Deans SG. Pharmacological and antimicrobial studies on different tea-tree oils (Melaleuca alternifolia, Leptospermum scoparium or Manuka and Kunzea ericoides or Kanuka), originating in Australia and New Zealand. *Phytother Res.* 2000 Dec;14(8):623-9.

4627 Chen CC, Yan SH, Yen MY, et al. Investigations of kanuka and manuka essential oils for in vitro treatment of disease and cellular inflammation caused by infectious microorganisms. *J Microbiol Immunol Infect.* 2016 Feb;49(1):104-11.

4628 Afoulous S, Ferhout H, Guy Raoelison E, et al. Chemical composition and anticancer, antiinflammatory, antioxidant and antimalarial activities of leaves essential oil of Cedrelopsis grevei. *Food Chem Toxicol.* 2013;56:352-62.

4629 Rakotobe M, Menut C, Sahondra H, et al. The Bark Essential Oil Composition and Chemotaxonomical Appraisal of Cedrelopsis grevei H. Baillon from Madagascar. *Nat Prod Commun.* 2008;3(0):1-6.

4630 Gauvin A, Ravaomanarivo H, Smadja J. Comparative analysis by gas chromatography-mass spectrometry of the essential oils from bark and leaves of Cedrelopsis grevei Baill, an aromatic and medicinal plant from Madagascar. *J Chromatogr A.* 2004 Mar 12;1029(1-2):279-82.

4631 Rakotobe M, Menut C, Andrianoelisoa H, et al. Bark Essential Oil of Cedrelopsis grevei from Madagascar: Investigation of Steam-Distillation Conditions. *Chem Biodiversity.* 2014;11(2):323-31.

4632 Afoulous S, Ferhout H, Guy Raoelison E, et al. Chemical composition and anticancer, antiinflammatory, antioxidant and antimalarial activities of leaves essential oil of Cedrelopsis grevei. *Food Chem Toxicol.* 2013;56:352-62.

4633 Afoulous S, Ferhout H, Guy Raoelison E, et al. Chemical composition and anticancer, antiinflammatory, antioxidant and antimalarial activities of leaves essential oil of Cedrelopsis grevei. *Food Chem Toxicol.* 2013;56:352-62.

4634 Afoulous S, Ferhout H, Guy Raoelison E, et al. Chemical composition and anticancer, antiinflammatory, antioxidant and antimalarial activities of leaves essential oil of Cedrelopsis grevei. *Food Chem Toxicol.* 2013;56:352-62.

4635 Afoulous S, Ferhout H, Guy Raoelison E, et al. Chemical composition and anticancer, antiinflammatory, antioxidant and antimalarial activities of leaves essential oil of Cedrelopsis grevei. *Food Chem Toxicol.* 2013;56:352-62.

4636 Sellami HK, Flamini G, Cioni PL, et al. Composition of the essential oils in vrious organs at different developmental staghes of Ammi visnaga (L.) La,. From Tunisia. *Chem Biodivers.* 2011 Nov;8(11):1990-2004.

4637 Khadhri A, El Mokni R, Mguis K, et al. Variability of two essential oils of Ammi visnaga (L.) Lam. a traditional Tunisian medicinal plant. *J Med Plants Res.* 2011 Sept;5(20):5079-82.

4638 Khalfallah A, Labed A, Semra Z, et al. Antibacterial activity and chemical composition of the essential oil of Ammi visnaga. (Apiaceae) from Constantine, Algeria. *Int J Med Arom Plants.* 2011 Dec;1(3):302-05.

4639 Fairouz B, Salima KG. Antibacterial Activity and Chemical Composition of Ammi visnaga L. Essential Oil Collected from Boumerdes (Algeria) During Three Periods of the Plant Growth. *J Essent Oil Bearing Plants.* 2014;17(6):1317-28.

4640 Al-Snafi AE. Chemical constituents and pharmacological activities of Ammi majus and Ammi visnaga. A review. *Int J Pharm Ind Res.* 2013;3(3):257-65.

4641 Satrani B, Farah A, Fechtal M, et al. Chemical Composition, Antimicrobial and antifungal Activities of the Essential oil of Ammi visnaga (L.) Lam from Morocco. *Acta Bot Gal.* 2004;15(1):65-71.

4642 Ibrahim SM, Kadry HA, El Olemy MM. Use of acid-dye technique in the analysis of natural products. Part 3. Spectrophotometric microdetermination of khellin and bergapten. *Lloydia.* 1979;42:366-373.

4643 Penoel D, Franchomme P. L'Aromatherapie Exactement. 1990. Rogers Jollois.

4644 Penoel D, Franchomme P. L'Aromatherapie Exactement. 1990. Rogers Jollois.

4645 Aromatic Apothecary. Ammi visnaga. Available at: https://www.wingedseed.com/11001/AMMI+VISNAGA+ESSENTIAL+OIL.html.

4646 Ossenkoppele PM, van der Sluis WG, van Vloten WA. [Phototoxic dermatitis following the use of Ammi majus fruit for vitiligo]. *Ned Tijdschr Geneeskd.* 1991 Mar 16;135(11):478-80.

4647 Khalfallah A, Labed A, Semra Z, et al. Antibacterial activity and chemical composition of the essential oil of Ammi visnaga L. (Apiaceae) from Constantine, Algeria. *Int J Med Arom Plants.* 2011 Dec;1(3):302-05.

4648 Fairouz B, Salima KG. Antibacterial Activity and Chemical Composition of Ammi visnaga L. Essential Oil Collected from Boumerdes (Algeria) During Three Periods of the Plant Growth. *J Essent Oil Bearing Plants.* 2014;17(6):1317-28.

4649 Satrani B, Farah A, Fechtal M, et al. Chemical Composition, Antimicrobial and antifungal Activities of the Essential oil of Ammi visnaga (L.) Lam from Morocco. *Acta Bot Gal.* 2004;15(1):65-71.

4650 Soro KN, Sbri L, Amalich S, et al. Chemical composition of Moroccan Ammi visnaga L. (Lam.) and antibacterial activity of its essential oil against extended-spectrum beta-lactamase-producing and not producing bacteria. *Phytothérapie.* 2015 Jun;13(3):168-75.

4651 Satrani B, Farah A, Fechtal M, et al. Chemical Composition, Antimicrobial and antifungal Activities of the Essential oil of Ammi visnaga (L.) Lam from Morocco. *Acta Bot Gal.* 2004;15(1):65-71.

4652 Kamal FZ, Stanciu GD, Lefter R, et al. Chemical Composition and Antioxidant Activity of Ammi visnaga L. Essential Oil. *Antioxidants (Basel).* 2022 Feb 10;11(2):347.

[4653] Ibrahim NA, El-Hawary SS, Mohammed MMD, et al. Chemical Composition, Antiviral against avian Influenza (H5N1) Virus and Antimicrobial activities of the Essential Oils of the Leaves and Fruits of Fortunella margarita, Lour. Swingle, Growing in Egypt. *J Appl Pharm Sci.* 2015 Jan;5(01):006-012.
[4654] Quijano CE, Pino JA. Volatile Constituents of Kumquat (Fortunella margarita (Lour.) Swingle) Leaf Oil. *J Essent Oil Res.* 2009 May-Jun;21(3):194-96.
[4655] Peng LW, Sheu MJ, Lin LY, et al. Effect of heat treatments on the essential oils of kumquat (Fortunella margarita Single). *Food Chem.* 2013 Jan 15;136:532-37.
[4656] Wang YW, Zeng WC, Xu PY, et al. Chemical Composition and Antimicrobial Activity of the Essential Oil of Kumquat (Fortunella crassifolia Swingle) Peel. *Int J Mol Sci.* 2012;13(3):3382-93.
[4657] Satyal P, Paudel P, Limbu K, et al. Leaf Essential Oil Composition of Citrus japonica from Nepal. *J Essent Oil Bear Plants.* 2012;15(3):357-59.
[4658] Bunrathep S, Soodvilai S, Settharaksa S, et al. Chemical constituents and biological activities of Fortunella japonica essential oils. *BHST.* 2013;13(1):43-49.
[4659] Choi HS. Characteristic Odor Components of Kumquat (Fortunella japonica Swingle) Peel Oil. *J Agric Food Chem.* 2005;53(5):1642-47.
[4660] Jayaprakasha GK, Murthy KN, Demarais R, et al. Inhibition of prostate cancer (LNCaP) cell proliferation by volatile components from Nagami kumquats. *Planta Med.* 2012 Jun;78(10):974-80.
[4661] Nouri A, Shafaghatlonbar A. Chemical constituents and antioxidant activity of essential oil and organic extract from the peel and kernel parts of Citrus japonica Thunb. (kumquat) from Iran. *Nat Prod Res.* 2016;30(9):1093-7.
[4662] Abu-Gabal NS, Abd-Alla HI, Mohamed NZ, et al. Phytophenolics composition, hypolipidemic, hypoglycemic and antioxidative effects of the leaves of Fortunella japonica (Thunb.) Swingle. *Int J Pharmacy Pharmaceutical Sci.* 2015;7(12):ISSN-0975-1491.
[4663] Unger P, Melzig MF. Comparative Study of the Cytotoxicity and Genotoxicity of Alpha- and Beta-Asarone. *Sci Pharm.* 2012 Jul-Sep; 80(3): 663–668.
[4664] Taylor JM. (Food and Drug Administration) Personal communication to the World Health Organization concerning unpublished studies on beta-asarone and calamus oils. 1981. Found at: http://www.inchem.org/documents/jecfa/jecmono/v16je04.htm.
[4665] Zuba D, Bogumila B. Alpha- and beta-asarone in herbal medicinal products. A case study. *Forensic Sci Int.* 2012 Nov 30;223(1-3):e5-9.
[4666] European Commission. Scientific Committee on Food. Opinion of the Scientific Committee on Food on the presence of beta-asarone in flavourings and other food ingredients with flavouring properties. 2002 Jan. Available at: http://ec.europa.eu/food/fs/sc/scf/out111_en.pdf.
[4667] European Medicines Agency. Public statement on the use of herbal medicinal products containing asarone. Available at: http://www.ema.europa.eu/docs/en_GB/document_library/Scientific_guideline/2010/04/WC500089956.pdf.
[4668] Salazar M1, Salazar S, Ulloa V, et al. [Teratogenic action of alpha-asarone in the mouse]. *J Toxicol Clin Exp.* 1992 Aug;12(3):149-54.
[4669] Yabiku HK. Calamus oil - Toxicological aspects and their control in alcoholic beverages. M. S. Thesis, Sao Paulo, Brazil, Submitted to FAO/WHO. 1980.
[4670] Unger P, Melzig MF. Comparative Study of the Cytotoxicity and Genotoxicity of Alpha- and Beta-Asarone. *Sci Pharm.* 2012 Jul-Sep; 80(3): 663–668.
[4671] Hagan EC, Hansen WH, Fitzhugh OG, et al. Food flavourings and constituents of related structure. II. Subacute and chronic toxicity. *Food Cosmet Toxicol.* 1967 Apr;5(2):141-57.
[4672] Taylor JM. (Food and Drug Administration) Personal communication to the World Health Organization concerning unpublished studies on beta-asarone and calamus oils. 1981. Found at: http://www.inchem.org/documents/jecfa/jecmono/v16je04.htm.
[4673] Taylor JM, et al. Toxicity of oil of calamus (Jammus variety). *Toxicol Exptl Pharmacol.* 1967;10:405.
[4674] Weinberg M. Studies conducted with Calamus. Unpublished report from Foster D. Snell, Inc. submitted to the World Health Organization by Comitato Per Lo Studio Delle Bevande Alcooliche Aromatizzate. 1969. Found at: http://www.inchem.org/documents/jecfa/jecmono/v16je04.htm.
[4675] Zuba D, Bogumila B. Alpha- and beta-asarone in herbal medicinal products. A case study. *Forensic Sci Int.* 2012 Nov 30;223(1-3):e5-9.
[4676] Meyer F, Meyer E. Percutaneous absorption of essential oils and their constituents. *Arzneimittel-Forsch.* 1965;9:516.
[4677] Unger P, Melzig MF. Comparative Study of the Cytotoxicity and Genotoxicity of Alpha- and Beta-Asarone. *Sci Pharm.* 2012 Jul-Sep; 80(3): 663–668.
[4678] Taylor JM. (Food and Drug Administration) Personal communication to the World Health Organization concerning unpublished studies on beta-asarone and calamus oils. 1981. Found at: http://www.inchem.org/documents/jecfa/jecmono/v16je04.htm.
[4679] Zuba D, Bogumila B. Alpha- and beta-asarone in herbal medicinal products. A case study. *Forensic Sci Int.* 2012 Nov 30;223(1-3):e5-9.
[4680] European Commission. Scientific Committee on Food. Opinion of the Scientific Committee on Food on the presence of beta-asarone in flavourings and other food ingredients with flavouring properties. 2002 Jan. Available at: http://ec.europa.eu/food/fs/sc/scf/out111_en.pdf.
[4681] European Medicines Agency. Public statement on the use of herbal medicinal products containing asarone. Available at: http://www.ema.europa.eu/docs/en_GB/document_library/Scientific_guideline/2010/04/WC500089956.pdf.
[4682] Dandiya PC, Cullumbine H. Studies on Acorus calamus. III. Some pharmacological actions of the volatile oil. *J Pharmacol Exptl Therap.* 1959;125:353-59.
[4683] Menon MK, Dandiya PC. The mechanism of the tranquillizing action of asarone from Acorus calamus Linn. *J Pharm Pharmacol.* 1967 Mar;19(3):170-5.
[4684] Baxter RM, Dandiya PC, Kandel SI, et al. Separation of the hypnotic-potentiating principles from the essential oil of Acorus calamus L. of Indian origin by liquid-gas chromatograph. *Nature.* 1960 Feb;185:466-67.
[4685] Dandiya PC, Baxter RM, Walker GC, et al. Studies on Acorns calamus. II. Investigation of volatile oil. *J Pharm Pharmacol.* 1959;11:163-68.
[4686] Jayaprakasha GK, Murthy KN, Demarais R, et al. Inhibition of prostate cancer (LNCaP) cell proliferation by volatile components from Nagami kumquats. *Planta Med.* 2012 Jun;78(10):974-80.
[4687] Jayaprakasha GK, Murthy KN, Demarais R, et al. Inhibition of prostate cancer (LNCaP) cell proliferation by volatile components from Nagami kumquats. *Planta Med.* 2012 Jun;78(10):974-80.
[4688] Yang EJ, Kim SS, Moon JY, et al. Inhibitory effects of Fortunella japonica var. margarita and Citrus sunki essential oils on nitric oxide production and skin pathogens. *Acta Microbiol Immunol Hung.* 2010 Mar;57(1):15-27.
[4689] Yang EJ, Kim SS, Moon JY, et al. Inhibitory effects of Fortunella japonica var. margarita and Citrus sunki essential oils on nitric oxide production and skin pathogens. *Acta Microbiol Immunol Hung.* 2010 Mar;57(1):15-27.
[4690] Ibrahim NA, El-Hawary SS, Mohammed MMD, et al. Chemical Composition, Antiviral against avian Influenza (H5N1) Virus and Antimicrobial activities of the Essential Oils of the Leaves and Fruits of Fortunella margarita, Lour. Swingle, Growing in Egypt. *J Appl Pharm Sci.* 2015 Jan;5(01):006-012.
[4691] Wang YW, Zeng WC, Xu PY, et al. Chemical Composition and Antimicrobial Activity of the Essential Oil of Kumquat (Fortunella crassifolia Swingle) Peel. *Int J Mol Sci.* 2012;13(3):3382-93.
[4692] Bunrathep S, Soodvilai S, Settharaksa S, et al. Chemical constituents and biological activities of Fortunella japonica essential oils. *BHST.* 2013;13(1):43-49.
[4693] Ibrahim NA, El-Hawary SS, Mohammed MMD, et al. Chemical Composition, Antiviral against avian Influenza (H5N1) Virus and Antimicrobial activities of the Essential Oils of the Leaves and Fruits of Fortunella margarita, Lour. Swingle, Growing in Egypt. *J Appl Pharm Sci.* 2015 Jan;5(01):006-012.
[4694] Bunrathep S, Soodvilai S, Settharaksa S, et al. Chemical constituents and biological activities of Fortunella japonica essential oils. *BHST.* 2013;13(1):43-49.
[4695] Jayaprakasha GK, Murthy KN, Demarais R, et al. Inhibition of prostate cancer (LNCaP) cell proliferation by volatile components from Nagami kumquats. *Planta Med.* 2012 Jun;78(10):974-80.
[4696] Nouri A, Shafaghatlonbar A. Chemical constituents and antioxidant activity of essential oil and organic extract from the peel and kernel parts of Citrus japonica Thunb. (kumquat) from Iran. *Nat Prod Res.* 2016;30(9):1093-7.
[4697] Thomas J, Webb CE, Narkowicz C, et al. Evaluation of repellent properties of volatile extracts from the Australian native plant Kunzea ambigua against Aedes aegypti (Diptera: Culcidae). *J Med Entomol.* 2009 Nov;46(6):1387-91.
[4698] Thomas J, Narkowicz CK, Jacobson GA. An Examination of the Essential Oils of Tasmanian Kunzea ambigua, Other Kunzea spp. and Commercial Kunzea Oil. *J Essent Oil Res.* 2010;22(5):381-85.
[4699] Thomas J, Webb CE, Narkowicz C, et al. Evaluation of repellent properties of volatile extracts from the Australian native plant Kunzea ambigua against Aedes aegypti (Diptera: Culcidae). *J Med Entomol.* 2009 Nov;46(6):1387-91.
[4700] Kara N, Baydar H. Determination of lavender and lavandin cultivars (Lavandula sp.) containing high quality essential oil in Isparta, Turkey. *Turkish J Field Crops.* 2013;18(1):58-65.
[4701] Jianu C, Pop G, Gruia AT, et al. Chemical composition and antimicrobial activity of essential oils of lavender (Lavandula angustifolia) and lavandin (Lavandula x intermedia) grown in Western Romania. *Int J Agric Biol.* 2013;15:772-76.
[4702] Chatzopoulou PS, Goliaris AH. Contribution to the analysis of the volatile constituents from some lavender and lavandin cultivars grown in Greece. *Scientia Pharmaceutica (Sci. Pharm).* 2003;71:229-34.
[4703] Bombarda I, Dupuy N, Da JPLV, et al. Comparative chemometric analyses of geographic origins and compositions of lavandin var. Grosso essential oils by mid infrared spectroscopy and gas chromatography. *Analytica Chimica Acta.* 2008 Apr;613(1):31-39.
[4704] Piccaglia R, Marotti M. Characterization of several aromatic plants grown in northern Italy. *Flav Frag J.* 1993 Mar;8(2):115-22.
[4705] Gitsopoulis TK, Chatzopoulou P, Georgoulas I. Effects of essential oils of Lavandula x hybrida Rev, Foeniculum vulgare Mill and thymus capitatus L. on aestivum L., Hordeum vulgare L., Lolium rigidum L. and Phalaris brachystachys L. *J Essent Oil Res.* 2013;16(6):817-25.
[4706] Burkhard PR, Burkhardt K, Haenggeli CA, et al. Plant-induced seizures: reappearance of an old problem. *J Neurol.* 1999 Aug;246(8):667-70.
[4707] Narayan S, Singh N. Camphor poisoning-An unusual cause of seizure. *Med J Armed Forces India.* 2012 Jul;68(3):252-53.
[4708] Chanaranaj KJ, G MV, S M. Camphor poisoning in a child. *Natl Med J India.* 2013 Jan-Feb;26(1):60.
[4709] Olowe SA, Ransome-Kuti O. The risk of jaundice in glucose-6-phosphate dehydrogenase deficient babies exposed to menthol. *Acta Paediatr Scand.* 1980 May;69(3):341-5.
[4710] Dillon Remy M, Manning Alleyne P, Bratt DE, et al. Neonatal jaundice at Port-of-Spain General Hospital abstract. *West Indian Med J.* 1987;36(Suppl):28.
[4711] Ballabeni V, Tognolini M, Chiavarini M, et al. Novel antiplatelet and antithrombotic activities of essential oil from Lavandula hybrida Reverchon "grosso". *Phytomedicine.*2004 Nov;11(7-8):596-601.
[4712] Jori A, Bianchetti A, Prestini PE, et al. Effect of eucalyptol (1,8-cineole) on the metabolism of other drugs in rats and in man. *Eur J Pharmacol.* 1970;9(3):362-66.
[4713] de Sousa DP, Raphael E, Brocksom U, et al. Sedative effect of monoterpene alcohols in mice: A preliminary screening. *Verlag der Zeitschrift fur Naturforschung.* 2007;62c:563-66.
[4714] Jori A, Bianchetti A, Prestini PE, et al. Effect of eucalyptol (1,8-cineole) on the metabolism of other drugs in rats and in man. *Eur J Pharmacol.* 1970;9(3):362-66.

[4715] Kim NH, Hyun SH, Jin CH, et al. Pretreatment with 1,8-cineole potentiates thioacetamide-induced hepatotoxicity and immunosuppression. *Arch Pharm Res.* 2004 Jul;27(7):781-9.
[4716] Hancianu M, Cioanca O, Mihasan M, et al. Neuroprotective effects of inhaled lavender oil on scopolamine-induced dementia via anti-oxidative activities in rats. *Phytomedicine.* 2013 Mar;20(5):446-52.
[4717] Hritcu L, Cianca O, Hancianu M. Effects of lavender oil inhalation on improving scopolamine-induced spatial memory impairment in laboratory rats. *Phytomedicine.* 2012 Apr 15;19(6):529-34.
[4718] Barocelli E, Calcina F, Chivarini M, et al. Antinociceptive and gastroprotective effects of inhaled and orally administered Lavandula hybrida Reverchon "Grosso" essential oil. *Life Sci.* 2004 Nov;76(2):213-23.
[4719] Aridogan BC, Baydar H, Kaya S, et al. Antimicrobial activity and chemical composition of some essential oils. *Arch Pharm Res.* 2002 Dec;25(6):860-64.
[4720] Vegh A, Bencsik T, Molnar P, et al. Composition and antipseudomonal effect of essential oils isolated from different lavender species. *Nat Prod Commun.* 2012 Oct;7(10:1393-96.
[4721] Moon T, Wilkinson JM, Cavanagh HM. Antiparasitic activity of two Lavandula essential oils against Giardia duodenalis, Trichomonas vaginalis and Hexamita inflata. *Parasitol Res.* 2006 Nov;99(6):722-28.
[4722] McCaffrey R, Thomas D, Kinzelman A. The effects of lavender and rosemary essential oils on test-taking anxiety among graduate nursing students. *Holistic Nurs Prac.* 2009 Mar-Apr;23(2):88-93.
[4723] Braden R, Reichow S, Halm MA. The use of the essential oil Lavandin to reduce preoperative anxiety in surgical patients. *J PeriAnesthesia Nurs.* 2009 Dec;24(6):348-55.
[4724] Carrasco A, Martinez-Gutierrez R, Thomas V, et al. Lavandin (Lanandula x intermedia Emeric ex Loiseleur) essential oil from Spain: determination of aromatic profile by gas chromatography-mass-spectrometry, antioxidant and lipoxygenase inhibitory bioactivities. *Nat Prod Res.* 2016;30(10):1123-30.
[4725] Bajalan I, Rouzbahani R, Ghasemi Pirbalouti A, et al. Chemical composition and antibacterial activity of Iranian Lavandula x hybrid. *Chem Biodivers.* 2017 Jul;14(7).
[4726] de Elguea-Culebras GO, Sánchez-Vioque R, Berruga MI, et al. Biocidal potential and chemical composition of industrial essential oils from Hyssopus officinalis, Lavandula x intermedia var. super and Santolina chamaecyparissus. *Chem Biodivers.* 2018 Jan;15(1).
[4727] Tardugno R, Serio A, Pellati F, et al. Lavandula x intermedia and Lavandula angustifolia essential oils: phytochemical composition and antimicrobial activity against foodborne pathogens. *Nat Prod Res.* 2018 May 21:1-6.
[4728] Ayik C, Özden D. The effects of preoperative aromatherapy massage on anxiety and sleep quality of colorectal surgery patients: A randomized controlled study. *Complement Ther Med.* 2018 Feb;36:93-99.
[4729] Garzoli S, Turchetti G, Giacomello P, et al. Liquid and Vapour Phase of Lavandin (Lavandula × intermedia) Essential Oil: Chemical Composition and Antimicrobial Activity. *Molecules.* 2019 Jul 25;24(15).
[4730] Can E, Kızak V, Can ŞS, et al. Anesthetic Efficiency of Three Medicinal Plant Oils for Aquatic Species: Coriander Coriandrum sativum, Linaloe Tree Bursera delpechiana, and Lavender Lavandula hybrida. *J Aquat Anim Health.* 2019 Sep;31(3):266-273.
[4731] Iseppi R, Tardugno R, Brighenti V, et al. Phytochemical Composition and In Vitro Antimicrobial Activity of Essential Oils from the Lamiaceae Family against Streptococcus agalactiae and Candida albicans Biofilms. *Antibiotics (Basel).* 2020 Sep 10;9(9):E592.
[4732] Masci VL, Ovidi E, Taddei AR, et al. Apoptotic Effects on HL60 Human Leukaemia Cells Induced by Lavandin Essential Oil Treatment. *Molecules.* 2020 Jan 26;25(3):538.
[4733] D'Addanno T, Laquale S, Argentieri MP, et al. Nematicidal Activity of Essential Oil from Lavandin ( Lavandula × intermedia Emeric ex Loisel.) as Related to Chemical Profile. *Molecules.* 2021 Oct 26;26(21):6448.
[4734] Wainer J, Thomas A, Chimhau T, et al. Extraction of Essential Oils from Lavandula × intermedia 'Margaret Roberts' Using Steam Distillation, Hydrodistillation, and Cellulase-Assisted Hydrodistillation: Experimentation and Cost Analysis. *Plants (Basel).* 2022 Dec 12;11(24):3479.
[4735] Kara N, Baydar H. Determination of lavender and lavandin cultivars (Lavandula sp.) containing high quality essential oil in Isparta, Turkey. *Turkish J Field Crops.* 2013;18(1):58-65.
[4736] Aromatics International. Lavender (Indian) - Lavandula angustifolia. Available at: http://www.aromaticsinternational.com/products/floral/lavender-india.
[4737] Schmidt E, GmbH KK. The Characteristics of Lavender Oils from Eastern Europe. *Perfum Flavor.* 2003 Jul-Aug;28:48-60.
[4738] Cardoso NN, Alviano CS, Blank AF, et al. Synergism Effect of the Essential Oil from Ocimum basilicum var. Maria Bonita and Its Major Components with Fluconazole and Its Influence on Ergosterol Biosynthesis. *Evid Based Complement Alternat Med.* 2016;2016:5647182.
[4739] de Rapper S, Viljoen A, van Vuuren S, et al. The In Vitro Antimicrobial Effects of Lavandula angustifolia Essential Oil in Combination with Conventional Antimicrobial Agents. *Evid Based Complement Alternat Med.* 2016;2016:2752739.
[4740] Tayarani-Najaran Z, Amiri A, et al. Comparative studies of cytotoxic and apoptotic properties of different extracts and thee essential oil of Lavandula angustifolia on malignant and normal cells. *Nutr Cancer.* 2014;66(3):424-34.
[4741] Zhao Y, Chen R, Wang Y, et al. In Vitro and In Vivo Efficacy Studies of Lavender angustifolia Essential Oil and Its Active Constituents on the Proliferation of Human Prostate Cancer. *Integr Cancer Ther.* 2017 Jun;16(2):215-226.
[4742] Niksic H, Kovac-Besovic E, Sober M, et al. Phytochemical and pharmacological (antiproliferative) effects of essential oil of Lavandula angustifolia Mill. Lamiaceae. *Planta Med.* 2016 Dec;81(S 01):S1-S381.
[4743] Donadu MG, Usai D1, Mazzarello V, et al. Change in Caco-2 cells following treatment with various lavender essential oils. *Nat Prod Res.* 2017 Jan 23:1-4.
[4744] Ou MC, Hsu TF, Lai AC, et al. Pain relief assessment by aromatic essential oil massage on outpatients with primary dysmenorrhea: a randomized, double blind clinical trial. *J Obstet Gynaecol Res.* 2012 May;38(5):817-22.
[4745] Hur MH, Han SH. Clinical trial of aromatherapy on postpartum mother's perineal healing. *Taehan Kanho Hakhoe Chi.* 2004 Feb;34(1):53-62.
[4746] Vakilian K, Atarha M, Bekradi R, et al. Healing advantages of lavender essential oil during episiotomy recovery: A clinical trial. *Complement Ther Clin Pract.* 2011;17:50-53.
[4747] Sheikhan F, Jahdi F, Khoei EM, et al. Episiotomy pain relief: Use of lavender essence in primiparous Iranian women. *Complement Ther Clin Pract.* 2012 Feb;18(1):66-70.
[4748] Vakilian K, Atarha M, Bekhradi R, et al. Healing advantages of lavender essential oil during episiotomy recovery: a clinical trial. *Complement Ther Clin Pract.* 2011 Feb;17(1):50-53.
[4749] Marzouk TM, El-Nemer AM, Baraka HN. The effect of aromatherapy abdominal massage on alleviating menstrual pain in nursing students: a prospective randomized cross-over study. *Evid Based Complement Altern Med.* 2013;2013:742421.
[4750] Han SH, Hur MH, Buckle J, et al. Effect of aromatherapy on symptoms of dysmenorrhea in college students: A randomized placebo-controlled clinical trial. *J Altern Complement Med.* 2006 Jul-Aug;12(6):535-41.
[4751] Hancianu M, Cioanca O, Mihasan M, et al. Neuroprotective effects of inhaled lavender oil on scopolamine-induced dementia via anti-oxidative activities in rats. *Phytomedicine.* 2013 Mar;20(5):446-52.
[4752] Smallwood J, Brown R, Coulter F, et al. Aromatherapy and behavior disturbances in dementia: a randomized controlled trial. *Int J Geriatr Psychiatry.* 2001;16:1010-13.
[4753] Hritcu L, Cianca O, Hancianu M. Effects of lavender oil inhalation on improving scopolamine-induced spatial memory impairment in laboratory rats. *Phytomedicine.* 2012 Apr 15;19(6):529-34.
[4754] Hawrelak JA, Cattley T, Myers SP. Essential oils in the treatment of intestinal dysbiosis: A preliminary in vitro study. *Altern Med Rev.* 2009 Dec;14(4)380-84.
[4755] Baker J, Brown K, Rajendiran E, et al. Medicinal lavender modulates the enteric microbiota to protect against Citrobacter rodentium-induced colitis. *AM J Physiol Gastrointest Liver Physiol.* 2012 Oct;303(7):G825-36.
[4756] Baldinger P, Hoflich AS, Mitterhauser M, et al. Effects of Silexan on the serotonin-1a receptor and microstructure of the human brain: a randomized, placebo-controlled, double-blind, cross-over study with molecular and structural imaging. *Int J Neuropsychopharmacol.* 2014 Oct 31;18(4):pyu063.
[4757] Kasper S, Gastpar M, Muller WE, et al. Lavender oil preparation Silexan is effective in generalized anxiety- disorder--a randomized, double-blind comparison to placebo and paroxetine. *Int J Neuropsychopharmacol.* 2014 Jun;17(6):859-69.
[4758] Kasper S. AN orally administered Lavandula oil preparation (Silexan) for anxiety disorder and related conditions: an evidence based review. *Int J Psychiatry Clin Pract.* 2013 Nov;17 Suppl 1:15-22.
[4759] Schuwald AM, Noldner M, Wilmes T, et al. Lavender oil-potent anxiolytic properties via modulating dependent calcium channels. *PloS One.* 2013 Apr 29;8(4):e59998.
[4760] Uehleke B, Schaper S, Dienel A, et al. Phase II trial on the effects of Silexan in patients with neurasthenia, post- traumatic stress disorder or somatization disorder. *Phytomedicine.* 2012 Jun;19(8):665-71.
[4761] Kasper S, Gastpar M, Muller WE, et al. Silexan, an orally administered Lavandula oil preparation, is effective in the treatment of 'subsyndromal' anxiety disorder: a randomized, double-blind, placebo controlled trial. *Int Clin Psychopharmacol.* 201 Sep;25(5):277-87.
[4762] Woelk H, Schlafke S. A multi-center, double-blind, randomised study of the Lavender oil preparation Silexan in comparison to Lorazepam for generalized anxiety disorder). *Phytomedicine.* 2010 Feb;17(2):94-99.
[4763] Donelli D, Antonelli M, Bellinazzi C, et al. Effects of lavender on anxiety: A systematic review and meta-analysis.
[4764] Kasper S, Muller WE, Volz HP, et al. Silexan in anxiety disorders: Clinical data and pharmacological background. *World J Biol Psychiatry.* 2018 Sep;19(6):412-420.
[4765] Bartova L, Dold M, Volz HP, et al. Beneficial effects of Silexan on co-occurring depressive symptoms in patients with subthreshold anxiety and anxiety disorders: randomized, placebo-controlled trials revisited. *Eur Arch Psychiatry Clin Neurosci.* 2022 Mar 9. Online ahead of print.
[4766] Chang SY. Effects of aroma hand massage on pain, state anxiety and depression in hospice patients with terminal cancer. *Taehan Kanho Hakhoe Chi.* 2008 Aug;38(4):493-502.
[4767] Morris N, The effects of lavender (Lavandula angustifolium) baths on psychological well-being: two exploratory randomized control trials. *Complement Ther Med.* 2002 Dec;10(4):223-28.
[4768] Lee SY. The effect of lavender aromatherapy on cognitive function, emotion, aggressive behavior of elderly with dementia. *Taehan Kanho Hakhoe Chi.* 2005 Apr;35(2):303-12.
[4769] Inouye S, Uchida K, Nishiyama Y, et al. Combined effect of heat, essential oils and salt on fungicidal activity against Trichohyton mentagrophytes in a foot bath. *Nihon Ishinjin Gakkai Zasshi.*2007;48(1):27-36.
[4770] Imura M, Misao H, Ushijima H. The psychological effects of aromatherapy-massage in healthy postpartum mothers. *J Midwifery Womens Health.* 2006 Mar-Apr;51(2):e21-27.
[4771] Ziaee M, Khorrami A, Nourafcan H, et al. Cardioprotective effects of essential oil of Lavandula angustifolia on isoproterenol-induced acute myocardial infarction in rat. *Iran J Pharm Res.* 2015 Jan;14(1):279-89.
[4772] Nikolaevskii VV, Kononova NS, Pertsovskii AI, et al. Effect of essential oils on the course of experimental atherosclerosis. *Patol Fiziol Eksp Ter.* 1990 Sep-Oct;(5):52-53.
[4773] Umezu T. Behavioral effects of plant-derived essential oils in the Geller type conflict test in mice. *Jpn J Pharmacol.* 2000 Jun;83(2):150-53.

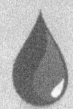

4774 Umezu T, Nagano K, Ito H, et al. Anticonflict effects of lavender oil and identification of its active constituents. *Pharmacol Biochem Behav.*2006 Dec;85(4):713-21.
4775 Chioca LR, Ferro MM, Baretta IP, et al. Anxiolytic-like effect of lavender essential oil inhalation in mice: participation of serotonergic but not GABBAA/benzodiazepine neurotransmission. *J Ethnopharmacol.* 2013 May;147(2):412-18.
4776 Yap PS, Krishnan T, Yiap BC, et al. Membrane disruption and anti-quorum sensing effects of synergistic interaction between Lavandula angustifolia (lavender oil) in combination with antibiotic against plasmid-conferred multi-drug- resistant Escherichia coli. *J Appl Microbiol.* 2014 May;116(50):1119-28.
4777 Moon T, Wilkinson JM, Cavanagh HM. Antiparasitic activity of two Lavandula essential oils against Giardia duodenalis, Trichomonas vaginalis and Hexamita inflata. *Parasitol Res.* 2006 Nov;99(6):722-28.
4778 S'Auria FD, Tecca M, Strippoli V, et al. Antifungal activity of Lavandula angustifolia essential oil against Candida albicans yeast and mycelial form. *Med Mycol.* 2005 Aug;43(5):391-96.
4779 Bona E, Cantamessa S, Pavan M, et al. Sensitivity of Candida albicans to essential oils: are they an alternative to antifungal agents? *J Appl Microbiol.* 2016 Dec;121(6):1530-1545.
4780 Tirabassi G, Giovannini L, Paggi F, et al. Possible efficacy of lavender and tea tree oils in the treatment of young women affected by mild idiopathic hirsutism. *J Endocrinol Invest.* 2013 Jan;36(1):50-54.
4781 Conrad P, Adams C. The effects of clinical aromatherapy for anxiety and depression in the high risk postpartum woman - a pilot study. *Complement Ther Clin Pract.* 2012 Aug;18(3):164-68.
4782 Matsumoto T, Asakura H, Hyashi T. Does lavender aromatherapy alleviate premenstrual emotional symptoms?: a randomized crossover trial. *Biopsychosoc Med.* 2013 May;7:12.
4783 Bradley BF, Brown SL, Chu S, et al. Effects of orally administered lavender essential oil on responses to anxiety- provoking film clips. *Hum Psychopharm Clin Exper.* 2009 Jun;24(4):319-30.
4784 Wang D, Yuan X, Liu T, et al. Neuroprotective activity of lavender oil on transient focal cerebral ischemia in mice. *Molecules.* 2012 Aug;17(8):9803-17.
4785 Vakili A, Sharifat S, Akhavan MM, et al. Effect of lavender oil (Lavandula angustifolia) on cerebral edema and its possible mechanisms in an experimental model of stroke. *Brain Res.* 2014 Feb;1548:56-62.
4786 Kaur CD, Saraf S. In vitro sun protection factor determination of herbal oils used in cosmetics. *Pharmacognosy Res.* 2010 Jan;2(1):22-25.
4787 Apay SE, Arslan S, Akpinar RB, et al. Effect of aromatherapy massage on dysmenorrhea in Turkish students. *Pain Manag Nurs.* 2012 Dec;13(4):236-40.
4788 Soltani R, Soheilipour S, Hajhashemi V, et al. Evaluation of the effect of aromatherapy with lavender essential oil on post-tonsillectomy pain in pediatric patients: a randomized controlled trial. *Int J Pediatr Otorhinolaryngol.* 2013 Sep;77(9):1579-81.
4789 Dyer J, Cleary L, McNeill S, et al. The use of aromasticks to help with sleep problems: A patient experience survey. Complement Ther Clin Pract. 2016 Feb;22:51-8.
4790 Cha JH, Lee SH, Too YS. Effects of aromatherapy on changes in the autonomic nervous system, aortic pulse wave velocity and aortic augmentation index in patients with essential hypertension. *J Korean Acad Nurs.* 2010 Oct;40(5):705-13.
4791 Hwang JH. The effects of the inhalation method using essential oils on blood pressure and stress responses of clients with essential hypertension. *Taehan Kanho Hakhoe Chi.* 2006 Dec;36(7):1123-34.
4792 Kim IH, Kim C, Seong K, et al. Essential oil inhalation on blood pressure and salivary cortisol levels in prehypertensive and hypertensive subjects. *Evid Based Complement Alternat Med.* 2012;2012:984203.
4793 Toda M, Morimoto K. Effect of lavender aroma on salivary endocrinological stress markers. *Arch Oral Biol.* 2008 Oct;53(10):964-68.
4794 Sayorwan W, Siripornpanich V, Piriyapunyaporn T, et al. The effects of lavender oil inhalation on emotional states, autonomic nervous system, and brain electrical activity. *J Med Assoc Thai.* 2012 Apr;95(4):598-606.
4795 Huang L, Abuhamdah S, Howes MJ, et al. Pharmacological profile of essential oils derived from Lavandula angustifolia and Melissa officinalis with anti-agitation properties: focus on ligand-gated channels. *J Pharm Pharmacol.* 2008 Nov;60(11):1515-22.
4796 Olapour A, Behaeen K, Akhondzadeh R, et al. The effect of inhalation of aromatherapy blend containing lavender essential oil on cesarean postoperative pain. *Anesth Pain Med.* 2013 Summer;3(1):203-07.
4797 Altaei DT. Topical lavender oil for the treatment of recurrent aphthous ulceration. *Am J Dent.* 2012 Feb;25(1):39-43.
4798 Pemberton E, Turpin PG. The effect of essential oils on work-related stress in intensive care unit nurses. *Holist Nurs Pract.* 2008 Mar-Apr;22(2):97-102.
4799 Chen MC, Fang SH, Fang L. The effects of aromatherapy in relieving symptoms related to job stress among nurses. *Int J Nurs Pract.* 2015 Feb;21(1):87-93.
4800 Sasannejad P, Saeedi M, Shoeibi A, et al. Lavender essential oil in the treatment of migraine headache: a placebo- controlled clinical trial. *Eur Neurol.* 2012;67(5):288-91.
4801 Yamaguchi M, Tahara Y, Kosaka S. Influence of concentration of fragrances on salivary alpha-amylase. *Int J Cosmetic Sci.* 2009 Oct;31(5):391-95.
4802 Bradley BF, Starkey NJ, Brown SL, et al. Anxiolytic effects of Lavandula angustifolia odour on the Mongolian gerbil elevated plus maze. *J Ethnopharmacol.* 2007 May 22;111(3):517-25.
4803 Shubina LP, Siurin SA, Savchenko VM. Inhalation of essential oils in the combined treatment of patients with chronic bronchitis. *Crach Delo.* 1990 May;(5):66-67.
4804 Evandri MG, Battinelli L, Daniele C, et al. The antimutagenic activity of Lavandula angustifolia (lavender) essential oil in the bacterial reverse mutation assay. *Food Chem Toxicol.* 2005 Sep;43(9):1381-87.
4805 Ueno-lio T, Shibakura M, Yokota K, et al. Lavender essential oil inhalation suppresses allergic airway inflammation and mucous cell hyperplasia in a murine model of asthma. *Life Sci.* 2014 Jul 17;18(2):19-15.
4806 Huang MY, Liao MH, Wang YK, et al. Effect of lavender essential oil on LPS-stimulated inflammation. *Am J Chin Med.* 2012;40(4):845-59.
4807 Hajhashemi V, Ghannadi A, Sharif B. Anti-inflammatory and analgesic properties of the leaf extracts and essential oil of Lavandula angustifolia Mill. *J Ethnopharmacol.* 2003 Nov;89:67-71.
4808 Carrasco A, Martinez-Gutierrez R, Tomas V, et al. Lavandula angustifolia and Lavandula latifolia Essential Oils from Spain: Aromatic Profile and Bioactivities. *Planta Med.* 2016 Jan;82(1-2):163-70.
4809 Johannessen B. Nurses experience of aromatherapy use with dementia patients experiencing disturbed sleep patterns. AN action research project. *Complement Ther Clin Pract.* 2013 Nov;19(4):209-13.
4810 Lis-Balchin M. Studies on the mode of action of the essential oil of lavender (Lavandula angustifolia P. Miller). *Phytother Res.* 1999 Sep;13(6):540-42.
4811 Buchbauer G, Jirovetz L, Jager W, et al. Aromatherapy: evidence for sedative effects of the essential oil of lavender after inhalation. *Z Naturforsch C.*1991 Nov-Dec;46(11-12):1067-72.
4812 Ghelardini C, Galeotti N, Salvatore G, et al. Local anesthetic activity of essential oil of Lavandula angustifolia. *Planta Med.* 1999 Dec;65(8):700-03.
4813 Guillemain J, Rousseau A, Delaveau P. Neurodepressive effects of the essential oil of Lavandula angustifolia Mill. *Ann Pharm Fr.* 1989;47(6):337-43.
4814 Takhashi M, Yoshino A, Yamanaka A, et al. Effects of inhaled lavender essential oil on stress-loaded animals: changes in anxiety-related behavior and expression levels of selected mRNAs and proteins. *Nat Prod Commun.* 2012 Nov;7(11):1539-44.
4815 Kim S, Kim HJ, Yeo JS, et al. The effect of lavender oil on stress, bispectral index values, and needle insertion pain in volunteers. *J Altern Complement Med.* 2011 Sep;17(9):823-26.
4816 Shimada K, Fukada S, Maeda K, et al. Aromatherapy alleviates endothelial dysfunction of medical staff night-shift work: preliminary observations. *Hypertens Res.* 2011 Feb;34(2):264-67.
4817 Kang HY, Na SS, Kim YK. Effects of oral care with essential oil on improvement in oral health status of hospice patients. *J Korean Acad Nurs.*2010 Aug;40(4):473-81.
4818 Louis M, Kowalski SD. Use of aromatherapy with hospice patients to decrease pain, anxiety, and depression and to promote an increased sense of well-being. *Am J Hosp Palliat Care.* 2002 Nov-Dec;19(6):381-86.
4819 Barker SC, Altman PM. A randomised, assessor blind, parallel group comparative efficacy trial of three products for the treatment of head lice in children—melaleuca oil and lavender oil, pyretrins and piperonyl butoxide, and a "suffocation" product. *BMC Dermatol.* 2010 Aug;10:6.
4820 Barker SC, Altman PM. An ex vivo, assessor blind, randomised, parallel group, comparative efficacy trial of the ovicidal activity of three pediculicides after a single application--melaleuca oil and lavender oil, eucalyptus oil and lemon tea tree oil, and a "suffocation" pediculicide. *BMC Dermatol.* 2011 Aug 24;11:14.
4821 Kritsidima M, Newton T, Asimakopoulou K. The effects of lavender scent on dental patient anxiety levels: a cluster randomised-controlled trial. *Community Dent Oral Epidemiol.* 2010 Feb;38(1):83-87.
4822 Lehrner J, Marwinski G, Lehr S, et al. Ambient odors of orange and lavender reduce anxiety and improve mood in a dental office. *Physiol Behav.* 2005 Sep 15;86(1-2):92-95.
4823 Arzi A, Sela L, Green A, et al. The influence of odorants on respiratory patterns in sleep. *Chem Senses.* 2010 Jan;35(1):31-40.
4824 Field T, Field T, Cullen C, et al. Lavender bath oil reduces stress and crying and enhances sleep in very young infants. *Early Hum Dev.*2008 Jun;84(6):399-401.
4825 Kim JT, Ren CJ, Fielding GA, et al. Treatment with lavender aromatherapy in the post-anesthesia care unit reduces opioid requirements of morbidly obese patients undergoing laparoscopic adjustable gastric banding. *Obes Surg.* 2007 Jul;17(7):920-25.
4826 Shiina Y, Funabashi N, Lee K, et al. Relaxation effects of lavender aromatherapy improve coronary flow velocity reserve in healthy men evaluated by transthoracic Doppler echocardiography. *Int J Cardiol.* 2008 Sep;129(2):193-97.
4827 Goel N, Kim H, Lao RP. An olfactory stimulus modifies sleep in young men and women. *ChronobiolInt.* 2005;22(5):889-904.
4828 Lewith GT, Godfrey AD, Prescott P. A single-blinded, randomized pilot study evaluating the aroma of Lavandula angustifolia as a treatment for mild insomnia. *J Altern Complement Med.* 2005 Aug;11(4):631-17.
4829 Kim MJ, Nam ES, Paik SI. The effects of aromatherapy in pain, depression, and life satisfaction of arthritis patients. *Taehan Kanho Hakhoe Chi.* 2005 Feb;35(1):186-94.
4830 Holmes C, Hopkins V, Hensford C, et al. Lavender oil as a treatment for agitated behaviour in severe dementia: a placebo controlled study. *Int J Geriatr Psychiatry.* 2002 Apr;17(4):305-08.
4831 Kim HM, Cho Sh. Lavender oil inhibits immediate-type allergic reaction in mice and rats. *J Pharm Pharmacol.* 1999 Feb;51(2):221-26.
4832 Hay IC, Jamieson M, Ormerod AD. Randomized trial of aromatherapy. Successful treatment for alopecia areata. *Arch Dermatol.* 1998 Nov;134(11):1349-52.
4833 Mkolo MN, Magano SR. Repellent effects of the essential oil if Lavandula angustifolia against adults of Hyalomma marginatum rufipes. *J S Afr Vet Assoc.* 2007 Sep;78(3):149-52.
4834 Giovannini D, Gismondi A, Basso A, et al. Lavandula angustifolia Mill. Essential Oil Exerts Antibacterial and Anti-Inflammatory Effect in Macrophage Mediated Immune Response to Staphylococcus aureus. Immunol Invest. 2016 Jan;45(1):11-28.
4835 Domingos Tda S, Braga EM. Massage with aromatherapy: effectiveness on anxiety of users with personality disorders in psychiatric hospitalization. *Rev Esc Enferm USP.* 2015 May-Jun;49(3):450-6.
4836 Xu P, Wang K, Lu C, et al. Protective effect of lavender oil on scopolamine induced cognitive deficits in mice and H2O2 induced cytotoxicity in PC12 cells. *J Ethnopharmacol.* 2016 Dec 4;193:408-415.
4837 Carrasco A, Martinez-Gutierrez R, Tomas V, et al. Lavandula angustifolia and Lavandula latifolia Essential Oils from Spain: Aromatic Profile and Bioactivities. *Planta Med.* 2016 Jan;82(1-2):163-70.

[4838] Marin I, Sayas-Barberá E, Viuda-Martos M, et al. Chemical Composition, Antioxidant and Antimicrobial Activity of Essential Oils from Organic Fennel, Parsley, and Lavender from Spain. *Foods*. 2016 Mar 4;5(1).

[4839] Nikolova G, Karamalakova Y, Kovacheva N, et al. Protective effect of two essential oils isolated from Rosa damascena Mill. and Lavandula angustifolia Mill, and two classic antioxidants against L-dopa oxidative toxicity induced in healthy mice. *Regul Toxicol Pharmacol*. 2016 Jul 2;81:1-7.

[4840] Cisarová M, Tančinová D, Medo J, et al. The in vitro effect of selected essential oils on the growth and mycotoxin production of Aspergillus species. *J Environ Sci Health B*. 2016 Oct 2;51(10):668-674.

[4841] Domingos Tda S, Braga EM. Massage with aromatherapy: effectiveness on anxiety of users with personality disorders in psychiatric hospitalization. *Rev Esc Enferm USP*. 2015 May-Jun;49(3):450-6.

[4842] Hasanzadeh F, Kashouk NM, Amini S, et al. The effect of cold application and lavender oil inhalation in cardiac surgery patients undergoing chest tube removal. *EXCLI J*. 2016 Jan 22;15:64-74.

[4843] Johnson JR, Rivard RL, Griffin KH, et al. The effectiveness of nurse-delivered aromatherapy in an acute care setting. *Complement Ther Med*. 2016 Apr;25:164-9.

[4844] Seo YM, Jeong SH. [Effects of Blending Oil of Lavender and Thyme on Oxidative Stress, Immunity, and Skin Condition in Atopic Dermatitis Induced Mice]. *J Korean Acad Nurs*. 2015 Jun;45(3):367-77.

[4845] Nasiri A, Mahmodi MA, Nobakht Z, et al. Effect of aromatherapy massage with lavender essential oil on pain in patients with osteoarthritis of the knee: A randomized controlled clinical trial. *Complement Ther Clin Pract*. 2016 Nov;25:75-80.

[4846] Mori HM, Kawanami H, Kawahata H, et al. Wound healing potential of lavender oil by acceleration of granulation and wound contraction through induction of TGF-β in a rat model. *BMC Complement Altern Med*. 2016 May 26;16:144.

[4847] Fang F, Candy K, Melloul E, et al. In vitro activity of ten essential oils against Sarcoptes scabiei. *Parasit Vectors*. 2016 Nov 22;9(1):594.

[4848] de Rapper S, Viljoen A, van Vuuren S, et al. The In Vitro Antimicrobial Effects of Lavandula angustifolia Essential Oil in Combination with Conventional Antimicrobial Agents. *Evid Based Complement Alternat Med*. 2016;2016:2752739.

[4849] Marin I, Sayas-Barberá E, Viuda-Martos M, et al. Chemical Composition, Antioxidant and Antimicrobial Activity of Essential Oils from Organic Fennel, Parsley, and Lavender from Spain. *Foods*. 2016 Mar 4;5(1).

[4850] Kim W, Hur MH. [Inhalation Effects of Aroma Essential Oil on Quality of Sleep for Shift Nurses after Night Work]. *J Korean Acad Nurs*. 2016 Dec;46(6):769-779

[4851] Xu P, Wang K, Lu C, et al. The Protective Effect of Lavender Essential Oil and Its Main Component Linalool against the Cognitive Deficits Induced by D-Galactose and Aluminum Trichloride in Mice. *Evid Based Complement Alternat Med*. 2017;2017:7426538.

[4852] Kozics K, Srancikova A, Sedlackova E, et al. Antioxidant potential of essential oil from Lavandula angustifolia in in vitro and ex vivo cultured liver cells. *Neoplasma*. 2017 May 9;64.

[4853] Yazdkhasti M, Pirak A. The Effect of Aromatherapy With Lavender Essence on Severity of Labor Pain and Duration of Labor in Primiparous Women. *Complement Ther Clin Pract*. 2016 Nov;25:81-86.

[4854] Nasiri A, Mahmodi MA, Nobakht Z. Effect of aromatherapy massage with lavender essential oil on pain in patients with osteoarthritis of the knee: A randomized controlled clinical trial. *Complement Ther Clin Pract*. 2016 Nov;25:75-80.

[4855] Andrys D, Adaszynska-Skwirzyńska M, Kulpa D. Essential oil obtained from micropropagated lavender, its effect on HSF cells and application in cosmetic emulsion as a natural protective substance. *Nat Prod Res*. 2018;32(7):849-53.

[4856] Luís Â, Duarte AP, Pereira L, et al. Chemical Profiling and Evaluation of Antioxidant and Anti-Microbial Properties of Selected Commercial Essential Oils: A Comparative Study. *Medicines (Basel)*. 2017 Jun 5;4(2).

[4857] Donadu MG, Usai D, Mazzarello V, et al. Change in Caco-2 cells following treatment with various lavender essential oils. *Nat Prod Res*. 2017 Sep;31(18):2203-2206.

[4858] Yayla EM, Ozdemir L. Effect of Inhalation Aromatherapy on Procedural Pain and Anxiety After Needle Insertion Into an Implantable Central Venous Port Catheter: A Quasi-Randomized Controlled Pilot Study. *Cancer Nurs*. 2019 Jan/Feb;42(1):35-41.

[4859] Khater HF, Geden CJ. Potential of essential oils to prevent fly strike and their effects on the longevity of adult Lucilia sericata. *J Vector Ecol*. 2018 Dec;43(2):261-270.

[4860] El Alaoui C, Chemin J, Fechtali T, et al. Modulation of T-type Ca2+ channels by Lavender and Rosemary extracts. *PLoS One*. 2017 Oct 26;12(10):e0186864.

[4861] Coelho LS, Correa-Netto NF, Masukawa MY, et al. Inhaled Lavandula angustifolia essential oil inhibits consolidation of contextual- but not tone-fear conditioning in rats. *J Ethnopharmacol*. 2018 Apr 6;215:34-41.

[4862] Shokri A, Saeedi M, Fakhar M, et al. Antileishmanial Activity of Lavandula angustifolia and Rosmarinus Officinalis Essential Oils and Nano-emulsions on Leishmania major (MRHO/IR/75/ER). *Iran J Parasitol*. 2017 Oct-Dec;12(4):622-631.

[4863] Simoes BM, Kohler B, Clarke RB, et al. Estrogenicity of essential oils is not required to relieve symptoms of urogenital atrophy in breast cancer survivors. *Ther Adv Med Oncol*. 2018;10:1758835918766189.

[4864] Adaszyńska-Skwirzyńska M, Szczerbińska D. The antimicrobial activity of lavender essential oil (Lavandula angustifolia) and its influence on the production performance of broiler chickens. *J Anim Physiol Anim Nutr (Berl)*. 2018 Aug;102(4):1020-1025.

[4865] Ferreira LE, Benincasa BI, Fachin AL, et al. Essential oils of Citrus aurantifolia, Anthemis nobile and Lavandula officinalis: in vitro anthelmintic activities against Haemonchus contortus. *Parasit Vectors*. 2018; 11: 269.

[4866] Cardia GFE, Silva-Filho SE, Silva EL, et al. Effect of Lavender (Lavandula angustifolia) Essential Oil on Acute Inflammatory Response. *Evid Based Complement Alternat Med*. 2018 Mar 18;2018:1413940.

[4867] Nasiri A, Mahmodi MA. Aromatherapy massage with lavender essential oil and the prevention of disability in ADL in patients with osteoarthritis of the knee: A randomized controlled clinical trial. *Complement Ther Clin Pract*. 2018 Feb;30:116-121.

[4868] Vasireddy L, Bingle LEH, Davies MS. Antimicrobial activity of essential oils against multidrug-resistant clinical isolates of the Burkholderia cepacia complex. *PLoS One*. 2018 Aug 2;13(8):e0201835.

[4869] Hassanzadeh M, Kiani F, Bouya S, et al. Comparing the effects of relaxation technique and inhalation aromatherapy on fatigue in patients undergoing hemodialysis. *Complement Ther Clin Pract*. 2018 May;31:210-214.

[4870] Caputo L, Reguilon MD, Miñarro J, et al. Lavandula angustifolia Essential Oil and Linalool Counteract Social Aversion Induced by Social Defeat. *Molecules*. 2018 Oct 19;23(10).

[4871] Duan X, Tashiro M, Wu D, et al. Autonomic nervous function and localization of cerebral activity during lavender aromatic immersion. *Technol Health Care*. 2007;15(2):69-78.

[4872] Bikmoradi A, Khaleghverdi M, Seddighi I, et al. Effect of inhalation aromatherapy with lavender essence on pain associated with intravenous catheter insertion in preschool children: A quasi-experimental study. *Complement Ther Clin Pract*. 2017 Aug;28:85-91.

[4873] Tugut N, Demirel G, Baser M, et al. Effects of lavender scent on patients' anxiety and pain levels during gynecological examination. *Complement Ther Clin Pract*. 2017 Aug;28:65-69.

[4874] Karaman S, Karaman T, Tapar H, et al. A randomized placebo-controlled study of aromatherapy for the treatment of postoperative nausea and vomiting. *Complement Ther Med*. 2019 Feb;42:417-421.

[4875] Sánchez-Vidaña DI, Po KK, Fung TK, et al. Lavender essential oil ameliorates depression-like behavior and increases neurogenesis and dendritic complexity in rats. *Neurosci Lett*. 2019 May 14;701:180-192.

[4876] Bedini S, Flamini G, Cosci F, et al. Toxicity and oviposition deterrence of essential oils of Clinopodium nubigenum and Lavandula angustifolia against the myiasis-inducing blowfly Lucilia sericata. *PLoS One*. 2019 Feb 20;14(2):e0212576.

[4877] Bakhtiari S, Paki S, Khalili A, et al. Effect of lavender aromatherapy through inhalation on quality of life among postmenopausal women covered by a governmental health center in Isfahan, Iran: A single-blind clinical trial. *Complement Ther Clin Pract*. 2019 Feb;34:46-50.

[4878] Aboutaleb N, Jamali H, Abolhasani M, et al. Lavender oil (Lavandula angustifolia) attenuates renal ischemia/reperfusion injury in rats through suppression of inflammation, oxidative stress and apoptosis. *Biomed Pharmacother*. 2019 Feb;110:9-19.

[4879] Sanna MD, Les F, Lopez V, et al. Lavender (Lavandula angustifolia Mill.) Essential Oil Alleviates Neuropathic Pain in Mice With Spared Nerve Injury. *Front Pharmacol*. 2019 May 9;10:472.

[4880] Petrosino S, Di Marzo V. FAAH and MAGL inhibitors: therapeutic opportunities from regulating endocannabinoid levels. *Curr Opin Investig Drugs*. 2010 Jan;11(1):51-62.

[4881] Donatello NN, Emer AA, Salm DC, et al. Lavandula Angustifolia Essential Oil Inhalation Reduces Mechanical Hyperalgesia in a Model of Inflammatory and Neuropathic Pain: The Involvement of Opioid and Cannabinoid Receptors. *J Neuroimmunol*. 2020 Jan 10;340:577145.

[4882] Zhu LY, Gao YS, Song LZ, et al. [Research on improving memory impairment of blue lavender volatile oil]. *Zhongguo Zhong Yao Za Zhi*. 2017 Dec;42(24):4819-4826.

[4883] Sánchez-Vidaña DI, Po KK, Fung TK, et al. Lavender essential oil ameliorates depression-like behavior and increases neurogenesis and dendritic complexity in rats. *Neurosci Lett*. 2019 May 14;701:180-192.

[4884] Qadeer S, Emad S, Perveen T, et al. Role of ibuprofen and lavender oil to alter the stress induced psychological disorders: A comparative study. *Pak J Pharm Sci*. 2018 Jul;31(4(Supplementary)):1603-1608.

[4885] Karan NB. Influence of lavender oil inhalation on vital signs and anxiety: A randomized clinical trial. *Physiol Behavior*. 2019;211:112676.

[4886] Montibeler J, Domingos TDS, Braga EM, et al. Effectiveness of aromatherapy massage on the stress of the surgical center nursing team: a pilot study. *Rev Esc Enferm USP*. 2018 Aug 23;52:03348.

[4887] Kazemzadeh R, Nikjou R, Rostamnegad M, et al. Effect of lavender aromatherapy on menopause hot flushing: A crossover randomized clinical trial. *J Chinese Med Assoc*. 2016 Sep;79(9):489-92.

[4888] Chien LW, Cheng SL, Liu CF. The Effect of Lavender Aromatherapy on Autonomic Nervous System in Midlife Women with Insomnia. *Evidence-Based Complement Altern Med*. 2012;2012:740813.

[4889] Khater HF, Geden GJ. Efficacy and Repellency of Some Essential Oils and Their Blends Against Larval and Adult House Flies, Musca Domestica L. (Diptera: Muscidae). *J Vector Ecol*. 2019 Dec;44(2):256-63.

[4890] Velasco-Rodriquez, R, Perez-Hernandez MGP, Maturano-Melgoza JA, et al. The Effect of Aromatherapy With Lavender (Lavandula Angustifolia) on Serum Melatonin Levels. *Complement Ther Med*. 2019 Dec;47:102208.

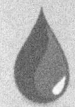

4891 Lari ZN, Hajimonfarednejad M, Riasatian M, et al. Efficacy of Inhaled Lavandula Angustifolia Mill. Essential Oil on Sleep Quality, Quality of Life and Metabolic Control in Patients With Diabetes Mellitus Type II and Insomnia. *J Ethnopharmacol*. 2020 Jan;251:112560.

4892 Bialori M, Krzysko-Lupicka T, et al. Chemical Composition of Two Different Lavender Essential Oils and Their Effect on Facial Skin Microbiota. *Molecules*. 2019 Sep;24(18):3270.

4893 Duluklu B, Celik SS. Effects of Lavender Essential Oil for Colorectal Cancer Patients With Permanent Colostomy on Elimination of Odor, Quality of Life, and Ostomy Adjustment: A Randomized Controlled Trial. *Eur J Oncol Nurs*. 2019 Oct;42:90-96.

4894 Souri F, Rakhshan K, Erfani S, et al. Natural Lavender Oil (Lavandula Angustifolia) Exerts Cardioprotective Effects Against Myocardial Infarction by Targeting Inflammation and Oxidative Stress. *Inflammopharmacology*. 2019 Aug;27(4):799-807.

4895 Cathey K, Gunyon N, Chung N, et al. A Feasibility Study of Lavender Aromatherapy in an Awake Craniotomy Environment. *J Patient Cent Res Rev*. 2020 Winter;7(1):19–30.

4896 Arslan I, Aydinoglu S, Karan NB. Can Lavender Oil Inhalation Help to Overcome Dental Anxiety and Pain in Children? A Randomized Clinical Trial. *Eur J Pediatr*. 2020 Feb 6 [Online ahead of print].

4897 Toda M, Matsuse R. Endocrinological effect of lavender aromatherapy on stressful visual stimuli. *Contemp Clin Trials Commun*. 2020 Mar;17:100547.

4898 Abbaszadeh R, Tabari F, Asadpour A. The Effect of Lavender Aroma on Anxiety of Patients Having Bone Marrow Biopsy. *Asian Pac J Cancer Prev*. 2020 Mar 1;21(3):771-775.

4899 Carbone C, Caddeo C, Grimaudo MA, et al. Ferulic Acid-NLC With Lavandula Essential Oil: A Possible Strategy for Wound-Healing? *Nanomaterials (Basel)*. 2020 May 8;10(5):E898.

4900 Kwiatkowski P, Lopusiewixz L, Kostek M, et al. The Antibacterial Activity of Lavender Essential Oil Alone and In Combination With Octenidine Dihydrochloride Against MRSA Strains. *Molecules*. 2019 Dec 26;25(1):95.

4901 Rai VK, Sinha P, Yadav KS, et al. Anti-psoriatic Effect of Lavandula Angustifolia Essential Oil and Its Major Components Linalool and Linalyl Acetate. *J Ethnopharmacol*. 2020 Jul 2;113127.

4902 Lai PJ, Ng EV, Yang SK, et al. Transcriptomic Analysis of Multi-Drug Resistant Escherichia coli K-12 Strain in Response to Lavandula angustifolia Essential Oil. *3 Biotech*. 2020 Jul;10(7):313.

4903 Manganiello-Terra FA, Correa-Netto NF, Masukawa MY, et al. Inhaled Lavandula Angustifolia Essential Oil Enhances Extinction Learning and Inhibits Memory Updating in Mice Submitted to the Contextual Fear Conditioning. *J Ethnopharmacol*. 2020 Jun 7;260:113048.

4904 Gullickson M, Hodge CF, Hegeman A, et al. Deterrent Effects of Essential Oils on Spotted-Wing Drosophila ( Drosophila suzukii): Implications for Organic Management in Berry Crops. *Insects*. 2020 Aug 15;11(8):E536.

4905 Gurler M, Kizilirmak A, Baser M. The Effect of Aromatherapy on Sleep and Quality of Life in Menopausal Women with Sleeping Problems: A Non-Randomized, Placebo-Controlled Trial. *Complement Med Res*. 2020 Jun 9;1-10.

4906 Arbianingsih A, Amal AA, Hidayah N, et al. Massage with lavender aromatherapy reduced sleep disturbances on infant. *Enferm Clin*. 2020 Mar;30 Suppl 3:62-65.

4907 Mohammadpourhodki R, Sadeghnezhad H, Ebrahimi H, et al. The Effect of Aromatherapy Massage with Lavender and Citrus Aurantium Essential Oil on Quality of Life of Patients on Chronic Hemodialysis: A Parallel Randomized Clinical Trial Study. *J Pain Symptom Manage*. 2020 Sep 1:S0885-3924(20)30718-1.

4908 Döner A, Taşcı S. Effect of massage therapy with lavender oil on severity of restless legs syndrome and quality of life in hemodialysis patients. *J Nurs Scholarsh*. 2022 May;54(3):304-314.

4909 Sara A, Dhibi S, Bouzenna H, et al. Leaves of Lavender Protect Adult Mice from Hydrogen Peroxide-induced Injury: Evidence fromin vitro and in vivo Tests. *J Oleo Sci*. 2020;69(9):1107-1115.

4910 Benli M, Olson J, Huck O, et al. A novel treatment modality for myogenous temporomandibular disorders using aromatherapy massage with lavender oil: A randomized controlled clinical trial. *Cranio*. 2020 Sep 5;1-11.

4911 Nasiri M, Asayesh H, Khosroabadi ZY, et al. Effects of Aromatherapy with Lavender (Lavandula angustifolia MILL) on Post-Dural Puncture Headache: A Randomized Placebo-Controlled Trial. *Altern Ther Health Med*. 2020 Nov 27;AT6279.

4912 Usta C, Tanyeri-Bayraktar B, Bayraktar S. Pain Control with Lavender Oil in Premature Infants: A Double-Blind Randomized Controlled Study. *J Altern Complement Med*. 2020 Dec 1. Online ahead of print.

4913 Ghaderi F, Solhjou N. The effects of lavender aromatherapy on stress and pain perception in children during dental treatment: A randomized clinical trial. *Complement Ther Clin Pract*. 2020 Aug;40:101182.

4914 Cheraif K, Bakchiche B, Gherib A, et al. Chemical Composition, Antioxidant, Anti-Tyrosinase, Anti-Cholinesterase and Cytotoxic Activities of Essential Oils of Six Algerian Plants. *Molecules*. 2020 Apr 8;25(7):1710.

4915 Welden LMS, Leatherland P, Schitter MB, et al. Abdominal Surgical Patients Randomized to Aromatherapy for Pain Management. *J Perianesth Nurs*. 2021 Jan 24;S1089-9472(20)30251-3.

4916 Karimzadeh Z, Forouzi MA, Tajadini H, et al. Effects of lavender and Citrus aurantium on pain of conscious intensive care unit patients: A parallel randomized placebo-controlled trial. *J Integr Med*. 2021 Jan 14;S2095-4964(21)00006-6.

4917 Ozkaraman A, Dugum O, Yilmaz HO, et al. Aromatherapy: The Effect of Lavender on Anxiety and Sleep Quality in Patients Treated With Chemotherapy. *Clin J Oncology Nursing*. 2018 Apr;22(2):203-10.

4918 Miastkowska M, Kantyka T, Bielexka E, et al. Enhanced Biological Activity of a Novel Preparation of Lavandula angustifolia Essential Oil. *Molecules*. 2021 Apr 23;26(9):2458.

4919 Miastkowska M, Sikora E, Kulawik-Pioro A, et al. Bioactive Lavandula angustifolia essential oil-loaded nanoemulsion dressing for burn wound healing. In vitro and in vivo studies. *Biomaterials Adv*. 2023 Mar;213362.

4920 Dos Reis Lucena L, Dos Santos-Junior JG, Tufik S, et al. Lavender essential oil on postmenopausal women with insomnia: Double-blind randomized trial. *Complement Ther Med*. 2021 Apr 24;59:102726.

4921 Manor R, Kumarnsit E, Samerphob N, et al. Characterization of pharmaco-EEG fingerprint and sleep-wake profiles of Lavandula angustifolia Mill. essential oil inhalation and diazepam administration in rats. *J Ethnopharmacol*. 2021 May 8;276:114193.

4922 Nafis A, Puedrhiri W, Iriti I, et al. Chemical composition and synergistic effect of three Moroccan lavender EOs with ciprofloxacin against foodborne bacteria: a promising approach to modulate antimicrobial resistance. *Lett Appl Microbiol*. 2021 Jun;72(6):698-705.

4923 Sayed AM, Morsy S, Tawfik GM, et al. The best route of administration of lavender for anxiety: a systematic review and network meta-analysis. *Gen Hosp Psychiatry*. May-Jun 2020;64:33-40.

4924 Rivaz M, Rahpeima M, Khademian Z, et al. The effects of aromatherapy massage with lavender essential oil on neuropathic pain and quality of life in diabetic patients: a randomized clinical trial. *Complement Ther Clin Pract*. 2021 Jun. Online ahead of print.

4925 Puvaca N, Milenkovic J, Coghill TG, et al. Antimicrobial Activity of Selected Essential Oils against Selected Pathogenic Bacteria: In Vitro Study. *Antibiotics (Basel)*. 2021 May 8;10(5):546.

4926 Akgul EA, Karakul A, Altin A, et al. Effectiveness of lavender inhalation aromatherapy on pain level and vital signs in children with burns: a randomized controlled trial. *Complement Ther Med*. 2021;60:102758.

4927 Ramić D, Bucar F, Kunej U, et al. Antibiofilm potential of Lavandula preparations against Campylobacter jejuni. *Appl Environ Microbiol*. 2021 Jul 28:AEM0109921. Online ahead of print.

4928 Bonaccorso A, Cimino C, Manno DE, et al. Essential Oil-Loaded NLC for Potential Intranasal Administration. *Pharmaceutics*. 2021 Jul 28;13(8):1166.

4929 Garzoli S, Laghezza Masci V, Franceschi S, et al. Headspace/GC-MS Analysis and Investigation of Antibacterial, Antioxidant and Cytotoxic Activity of Essential Oils and Hydrolates from Rosmarinus officinalis L. and Lavandula angustifolia Miller. *Foods*. 2021 Jul 30;10(8):1768.

4930 Ciocaraln A, Lupascu L, Aricu A, et al. Chemical Composition and Assessment of Antimicrobial Activity of Lavender Essential Oil and Some By-Products. *Plants (Basel)*. 2021 Sep 3;10(9):1829.

4931 Chen SJ, Chen CH, Chang HY. [Effects of Inhaling Essential Oil on Headache-Related Quality of Life Among Nurses Working in Emergency and Critical Care Units]. *Hu Li Za Zhi*. 2021 Oct;68(5):51-64.

4932 Capari C, Fantasma F, Divino F, et al. Chemical Profile, In Vitro Biological Activity and Comparison of Essential Oils from Fresh and Dried Flowers of Lavandula angustifolia L. *Molecules*. 2021 Sep 1;26(17):5317.

4933 Mahdavikian S, Fallahi M, Khatony A. Comparing the Effect of Aromatherapy with Peppermint and Lavender Essential Oils on Fatigue of Cardiac Patients: A Randomized Controlled Trial. *Evidence-Based Compl Alt Med*. 2021;2021:9925945.

4934 Yogi W, Tsukada M, Sato Y, et al. Influences of Lavender Essential Oil Inhalation on Stress Responses during Short-Duration Sleep Cycles: A Pilot Study. *Healthcare*. 2021;9(7):909.

4935 Pasias IN, Ntakoulas DD, Raptopoulou K, et al. Chemical Composition of Essential Oils of Aromatic and Medicinal Herbs Cultivated in Greece-Benefits and Drawbacks. *Foods*. 2021 Oct 3;10(10):2354.

4936 Yao N, He JK, Pan M, et al. In Vitro Evaluation of Lavandula angustifolia Essential Oil on Anti- Toxoplasma Activity. *Front Cell Infect Microbiol*. 2021 Sep 29;11:755715.

4937 Karimzadeh Z, Forouzi MA, Rahiminexhad E, et al. The Effects of Lavender and Citrus aurantium on Anxiety and Agitation of the Conscious Patients in Intensive Care Units: A Parallel Randomized Placebo-Controlled Trial. *Biomed Res Int*. 2021 Jun 15;2021:5565956.

4938 Creezer MF, Nedel SS, Christmann M, et al. Lavender essential oil for spinal pain in obese women: A clinical trial. *Columna*. 2021;20(3):192-6.

4939 Jones T, Purdy M, Stewart EA, et al. Lavender Aromatherapy to Reduce Anxiety During Intrauterine Insemination: A Randomized Controlled Trial. *Glob Adv Health Med*. 2021 Nov 17;10:21649561211059074.

4940 Pandur E, Balatinacz A, Micalizzi G, et al. Anti-inflammatory effect of lavender (Lavandula angustifolia Mill.) essential oil prepared during different plant phenophases on THP-1 macrophages. *BMC Complement Med Ther*. 2021 Nov 24;21(1):287.

4941 Şahin S, Tokgöz B, Demir G. Effect of Lavender Aromatherapy On Arteriovenous Fistula Puncture Pain and the Level of State and Trait Anxiety in Hemodialysis Patients: A Randomized Controlled Trial. *Pain Manag Nurs*. 2021 Aug;22(4):509-515.

4942 Ghasemi M, Rejeh N, Bahrami T, et al. Aromatherapy Massage vs. Foot Reflexology on the Severity of Restless Legs Syndrome in Female Patients Undergoing Hemodialysis. *Geriatrics*. 2021;6(4):99.

4943 Abo Eleneen AABI, Abd-Allah IM, Ibrahim AK. Aromatic Abdominal Massage for Alleviating Menstrual Pain in Nursing Students at Suez Canal University. *Egyptian J Health Care*. 2018;9(3):429-39.

4944 Seo E, Shin YK, Hsieh YS, et al. Linalyl acetate as a potential preventive agent against muscle wasting in rheumatoid arthritis rats chronically exposed to nicotine. *J Pharmacol Sci*. 2021 Sep;147(1):27-32.

[4945] Resmiati, Handayani ND, Violita, et al. Application of foot massage therapy procedures using lavender essential oil on clients with hypertension. *Indonesian Nurs Sci J.* 2021;3(11):159-64.

[4946] de Alteriis E, Maione A, Falanga A, et al. Activity of Free and Liposome-Encapsulated Essential Oil from Lavandula angustifolia against Persister-Derived Biofilm of Candida auris. *Antibiotics (Basel).* 2021 Dec 27;11(1):26.

[4947] Moghadam ZE, Delmoradi F, Aemmi SZ, et al. Effectiveness of aromatherapy with inhaled lavender essential oil and breathing exercises on ECT-related anxiety in depressed patients. *Explore (NY).* 2021 Dec 30:S1550-8307(21)00273-1.

[4948] Rahmadhani DY. The Effectiveness of Lavender Aromatherapy on Blood Pressure among Elderly with Essential Hypertension. *J Palembang Nurs Stud.* 2022;1(1):1-8.

[4949] Infante V, Campos PM, Gaspar LR, et al. Safety and efficacy of combined essential oils for the skin barrier properties: in vitro, ex vivo and clinical studies. *Int J Cosmet Sci.* 2022 Jan 5. Online ahead of print.

[4950] Rezaie SM, Shahabinejad M, Loripoor M, et al. The effect of aromatherapy with lavender essential oil on the working memory of women with multiple sclerosis. *J Med Life.* 2021 Nov-Dec;14(6):776–781.

[4951] Burgess A, Harris A, Wheeling J. A Pilot Randomized Control Trial to Assess the Impact of Lavender on Anxiety and Comfort After Cesarean Birth and the Barriers Encountered. *MCN Am J Matern Child Nurs.* 2022 Mar-Apr 01;47(2):85-91.

[4952] Varaei S, Jalalian Z, Nejad MSY, et al. Comparison the effects of inhalation and massage aromatherapy with lavender and sweet orange on fatigue in hemodialysis patients: a randomized clinical trial. *J Complement Integr Med.* 2020 May 28;18(1):193-200.

[4953] Rahimi E, Sedighi Chafjiri A, et al. Evaluation of the Effect of Lavender Aroma on Fatigue Among Hemodialysis Patients. *Holist Nurs Pract.* 2022 Mar-Apr 01;36(2):76-84.

[4954] Özel BZ, Quevedo A, Jung C, et al. Lavender Aromatherapy for Anxiety and Pain During Multichannel Urodynamics: A Randomized Controlled Pilot Trial. *Female Pelvic Med Reconstr Surg.* 2021 Nov 1;27(11):654-658.

[4955] Swathi G, Kanagaraj P. Effectiveness of aromatherapy on post-operative pain and discomfort among orthopaedic patients: Experimental study. *Int J Applied Res.* 2022;8(2):19-26.

[4956] Fahmy MA, Farghaly AA, Hassan EE, et al. Evaluation of the Anti-Cancer/Anti-Mutagenic Efficiency of Lavandula officinalis Essential Oil. *Asian Pac J Cancer Prev.* 2022 Apr 1;23(4):1215-1222.

[4957] Irlinia RR, Susilawati, Sari NE. Pemberian Inhalasi Aromatherapy Lavender Mempengaruhi Nyeri Menstruasi Pada Remaja Putri. *Midwifery J.* 2022;2(1):37-40.

[4958] Choi NY, Wu YT, Park SA. Effects of Olfactory Stimulation with Aroma Oils on Psychophysiological Responses of Female Adults. *Int J Environ Res Public Health.* 2022;18(9):5196.

[4959] Najar B, Pistelli L, Fratini F. Exploitation of Marginal Hilly Land in Tuscany through the Cultivation of Lavandula angustifolia Mill.: Characterization of Its Essential Oil and Antibacterial Activity. *Molecules.* 2022 May 17;27(10):3216.

[4960] Xie Q, Wang Y, Zou GL. Protective effects of lavender oil on sepsis-induced acute lung injury via regulation of the NF-κB pathway. *Pharm Biol.* 2022 Dec;60(1):968-978.

[4961] Deng X, Lu Z, Chen J, Chen W. Essential Oil Compositions, Antioxidant Activities, and Procollagen Synthesis Abilities of Four Lavandula angustifolia Varieties. *Curr Pharm Biotechnol.* 2022 May 17. Online ahead of print.

[4962] El-Kasem Bosly HA. Larvicidal and adulticidal activity of essential oils from plants of the Lamiaceae family against the West Nile virus vector, Culex pipiens (Diptera: Culicidae). *Saudi J Biol Sci.* 2022 Aug;29(8):103350.

[4963] Said NE, Shehata NS, El Haleem SA. Effect of Aromatic Massage on Somatic Problems among a Cohort of Menopausal Women. *Evidence-Based Nurs Res.* 2022 Jul-Sep;4(3):22-33.

[4964] Fella C, Amina D, Latifa A, et al. The effects of lavender essential oil and gallic acid pre-treatment on the neurocognitive assessment of post-stroke Wistar rats. *Uttar Pradesh J Zoology.* 2022;43(12):37-47.

[4965] Aponso M, Patti A, Hearn MTW, et al. Anxiolytic effects of essential oils may involve anti-oxidant regulation of the pro-oxidant effects of ascorbate in the brain. *Neurochem Int.* 2021 Nov;150:105153.

[4966] Lestari KP, Oktaviana AW, Sulistyowati DID, et al. Effleurage Massage With Lavender (Lavandula Lamiaceae) Essential Oil Aromatherapy Reduces Pregnant Women's Lower Back Pain. *Int Virtual Conference Nurs.* 2022;2022:270-84.

[4967] Citlik Saritas S, Buyukbayram Z, Kaplan Serin E, et al. Effects of lavender oil intervention before endoscopic retrograde cholangiopancreatography on patients' vital signs, pain and anxiety: A randomized controlled study. *Explore (NY).* 2021 Sep-Oct;17(5):446-450.

[4968] Maya-Enero S, Fabregas-Mithans M, Llufriu-Marques RM, et al. Analgesic effect of inhaled lavender essential oil for frenotomy in healthy neonates: a randomized clinical trial. *World J Pediatrics.* 2022. Online ahead of print.

[4969] Horváth A, Pandur E, Sipos K, et al. Anti-inflammatory effects of lavender and eucalyptus essential oils on the in vitro cell culture model of bladder pain syndrome using T24 cells. *BMC Complement Med Ther.* 2022 Apr 30;22(1):119.

[4970] El-Sayed SM, Hassan KM, Abdelhamid AN, et al. Exogenous Paclobutrazol Reinforces the Antioxidant and Antimicrobial Properties of Lavender (Lavandula officinalis L.) Oil through Modulating Its Composition of Oxygenated Terpenes. *Plants (Basel).* 2022 Jun 19;11(12):1607.

[4971] van der Heijden MJE, O'Flaherty LA, van Rosmalen J, et al. Aromatherapy massage seems effective in critically ill children: an observational before-after study. *Paediatr Neonatal Pain.* 2022 Feb 7;4(2):61-68.

[4972] Can Çiçek S, Demir Ş, Yılmaz D, et al. The Effect of Aromatherapy on Blood Pressure and Stress Responses by Inhalation and Foot Massage in Patients With Essential Hypertension: Randomized Clinical Trial. *Holist Nurs Pract.* 2022 Jul-Aug 01;36(4):209-222.

[4973] Dimitriou T, Papatriantafyllou J, Konsta A, et al. Assess of Combinations of Non-Pharmacological Interventions for the Reduction of Irritability in Patients with Dementia and their Caregivers: A Cross-Over RCT. *Brain Sci.* 2022;12(6):691.

[4974] Jadagheeshwari, Vaitheswari. Outcome of aromatherapy to reduce afterpain and fatigue among postnatal mothers. *IJ Social Rehab.* 2022;7(1):21-28

[4975] Gismondi A, Marco GD, Redi EL, et al. The antimicrobial activity of Lavandula angustifolia Mill. essential oil against Staphylococcus species in a hospital environment. *J Herb Med.* 2021 Apr;26:100426.

[4976] Bogdan MA, Bungau S, Tit DM, et al. Chemical Profile, Antioxidant Capacity, and Antimicrobial Activity of Essential Oils Extracted from Three Different Varieties (Moldoveanca 4, Vis Magic 10, and Alba 7) of Lavandula angustifolia. *Molecules.* 2021 Jul 20;26(14):4381.

[4977] Kavurmaci M, Sarıaslan A, Yıldız İ. Determination the effects of lavender oil quality of sleep and fatigue of students. *Perspect Psychiatr Care.* 2022 Jul;58(3):1013-1020.

[4978] Seddighi-Khavidak M, Tahan N, Akbarzadeh-Baghban A. Comparing the effects of vestibular rehabilitation with and without lavender oil scents as an olfactory stimulus on balance, fear of falling down and activities of daily living of people with multiple sclerosis: a randomized clinical trial. *Disabil Rehabil.* 2022 Jun;44(13):3132-3138.

[4979] Pthran R, Zhang MWB, Tam WW, et al. Prevalence of depression amongst medical students: a meta-analysis. *Med Educ.* 2016 Apr;50(4):456-68.

[4980] Sukarman TL, Gani IP, Jasputra DK. The Comparisons of Lavender and Jasmine Aromatherapy Effectiveness on Depression Level for Medical Students. *Berkala Ilmiah Kedokteran Duta Wacana.* 2022 Aug;7(1):19-22.

[4981] Nategh M, Heidari MR, Ebadi A, et al. Lavender aromatherapy on anxiety and depression in patients with Acute Coronary Syndrome: a single-blind randomized clinical trial. *Front Nurs.* 2022;9(2):233-239.

[4982] Hudhariana RN, Yunnani, Ristani A. The effect of massage effleurage with lavender aromatherapy on the intensity of dymenorore pain in adolescent women in the Pabelan Health Center. *Jurnal Ilmu dan Teknologi Kesehatan STIKES Widya Husada.* 2022 Jun;13(2):75-79.

[4983] Aydinli A, Karadag S. Effects of abdominal massage applied with ginger and lavender oil for elderly with constipation: A randomized controlled trial. *Explore.* 2023 Jan-Feb;19(1):115-120.

[4984] Sun J, Sun P, Kang C, et al. Chemical composition and biological activities of essential oils from six lamiaceae folk medicinal plants. *Front Plant Sci.* 2022 Aug 1;13:919294.

[4985] Li J, Wang X, Xun S, et al. Study of the Mechanism of Antiemetic Effect of Lavandula angustifolia Mill. Essential Oil Based on Ca2+/CaMKII/ERK1/2 Pathway. *Drug Des Devel Ther.* 2022 Jul 26;16:2407-2422.

[4986] Ziyadi S, Iddar A, Errafiy N, et al. Protective Effect of Some Essential Oils Against Gamma-Radiation Damages in Tetrahymena pyriformis Exposed to Cobalt-60 Source. *Curr Microbiol.* 2022 Aug 3;79(9):279.

[4987] Biltekin SN, Karadağ AE, Demirci B, et al. ACE2 and LOX Enzyme Inhibitions of Different Lavender Essential Oils and Major Components Linalool and Camphor. *ACS Omega.* 2022 Oct 5;7(41):36561-36566.

[4988] Chung YH, Chen SJ, Lee CL, et al. Relaxing Effects of Breathing Pseudotsuga menziesii and Lavandula angustifolia Essential Oils on Psychophysiological Status in Older Adults. *Int J Environ Res Public Health.* 2022 Nov 18;19(22):15251.

[4989] Elmali Şi Mşek H, Ecevi T Alpar Ş. The effect of aromatherapy and Su Jok interventions on post-cesarean pain. *Complement Ther Clin Pract.* 2022 Nov;49:101642.

[4990] Rostamkalaei SS, Iman M, Ataee R, et al. The effects of Lavandula angustifolia essential oil on analgesic effects and percutaneous absorption of naproxen sodium gel; an in vivo and in vitro study. *Clin Exp Pharmacol Physiol.* 2022 Dec 27. Online ahead of print.

[4991] Wei M, Liu F, Raka RN, et al. In vitro and in silico analysis of 'Taikong blue' lavender essential oil in LPS-induced HaCaT cells and RAW264.7 murine macrophages. *BMC Complement Med Ther.* 2022 Dec 6;22(1):324.

[4992] Ebrahimi S, Paryad E, Ghanbari Khanghah A, et al. The effects of lavandula aromatherapy on pain relief after coronary artery bypass graft surgery: A randomized clinical trial. *Appl Nurs Res.* 2022 Dec;68:151638.

[4993] Lak F, Zandi-Sohani N, Ghodoum Parizipour MH, et al. Synergic effects of some plant-derived essential oils and Iranian isolates of entomopathogenic fungus Metarhizium anisopliae Sorokin to control Acanthoscelides obtectus (Say) (Coleoptera: Chrysomelidae). *Front Plant Sci.* 2022 Dec 9;13:1075761.

[4994] Alkana SAM, Alhaweri HS, Khalifa GA, et al. Dental Pain Perception and Emotional Changes: On The Relationship Between Dental Anxiety And Olfaction. 2022 Dec. Available at: https://assets.researchsquare.com/files/rs-2317977/v1/db96c3aa-ea07-4933-8231-d8c092669129.pdf?c=1672240431.

[4995] Xu Y, Ma L, Liu F, et al. Lavender essential oil fractions alleviate sleep disorders induced by the combination of anxiety and caffeine in mice. *J Ethnopharmacol.* 2022 Oct 26:115868.

[4996] Mijatovic S, Stankovic JA, Calovski IC, et al. Antifungal Activity of Lavandula angustifolia Essential Oil against Candida albicans: Time-Kill Study on Pediatric Sputum Isolates. *Molecules.* 2022 Sep 24;27(19):6300.

[4997] Martella N, Colardo M, Sergio W, et al. Lavender Essential Oil Modulates Hepatic Cholesterol Metabolism in HepG2 Cells. *Curr Issues Mol Biol.* 2023;45(1):364-378.

[4998] Lejeune VBP, Lopes RV, Baggio DF, et al. Antinociceptive and anxiolytic-like effects of Lavandula angustifolia essential oil on rat models of orofacial pain. *J Appl Oral Sci.* 2023 Jan 6;30:e20220304.

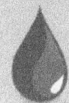

4999 Caprari C, Fantasma F, Monaco P, et al. Chemical Profiles, In Vitro Antioxidant and Antifungal Activity of Four Different Lavandula angustifolia L. EOs. *Molecules.* 2023 Jan 2;28(1):392.
5000 Farida DF. The effect of combination of perineum massage with lavender aromatherapy on the degree of perineum rain and anxiety in pregnant mothers 24 weeks in Mandir Dyah's self-practice, Kalasan Sleman. *J Appl Health Manag Tech.* 2023;5(1):23-9.
5001 Adaszyńska-Skwirzyńska M, Dzięcioł M, Szczerbińska D. Lavandula angustifolia Essential Oils as Effective Enhancers of Fluconazole Antifungal Activity against Candida albicans. *Molecules.* 2023 Jan 25;28(3):1176.
5002 Demirağ H, Hintistan S, Bulut E. The effect of topically administered lavender aromatherapy on the pain of insulin injection in diabetic patients: a double-blind randomized controlled clinical trial. *Turk J Med Sci.* 2022 Dec;52(6):1845-1853.
5003 Mahmujianah, Furiani ES, Murtiani F, et al. Lavender and Chamomile Aromatherapy Effectivity on Sleep Quality in the Third Trimester Pregnant Women. Jurnal Ilmiah Kedokteran *Wijaya Kusuma (JIKW).* 2023 Mar;12(1):51-58.
5004 Meutia RTM, Marlindawani J, Ritarwan K, et al. INTERVENSI MASSAGE AROMATERAPI (LAVENDER) TERHADAP PENURUNAN INTENSITAS NYERI PENDERITA NEUROPATHY DIABETIC. *J Telenursing.* 2023 Jan-Jun;5:279-289.
5005 Collin G. Aromas from Quebec. IV. Chemical composition of the essential oil of Ledum groenlandicum: A review. *Am J Essential Oils Nat Prod.* 2015;2(3):6–11.
5006 Baananou S, Bagdonaite E, Marongiu B, et al. Supercritical CO2 extract and essential oil or aerial part of Ledum palustre L.—chemical composition and anti-inflammatory activity. *Nat Prod res.* 2015;29(11):999–1005.
5007 Butkiene R, Mockute D. The Variability of the Essential Oil Composition of Wild Ledum palustre L. Shoots During Vegetation Period. *J Essent Oil Res.* 2011;23(1):9-13.
5008 European Medicines Agency. Assessment report on Peumus boldus Molina, folium. Available at: http://www.ema.europa.eu/docs/en_GB/document_library/Herbal_-_HMPC_assessment_report/2009/12/WC500018102.pdf.
5009 European Medicines Agency. Assessment report on Peumus boldus Molina, folium. Available at: http://www.ema.europa.eu/docs/en_GB/document_library/Herbal_-_HMPC_assessment_report/2009/12/WC500018102.pdf.
5010 Almeida ER, Melo AM, Xavier H. Toxicological evaluation of the hydro-alcohol extract of the dry leaves of Peumus boldus and boldine in rats. *Phytother Res.* 2000 Mar;14(2):99-102.
5011 Mitchell EMH, Heumann S, Araujo A, et al. Brazilian adolescents' knowledge and beliefs about abortion methods: a school-based internet inquiry. *BMC Womens Health.* 2014;14:27.
5012 Osol A, ed. The Dispensatory of the United States of America. 25th ed. Philadelphia, PA: Lippincott, 1955.
5013 Piscaglia F, Leoni S, Venturi A, et al. Caution in the use of boldo in herbal laxatives: a case of hepatotoxicity. *Scand J Gastroenterol.* 2005;40:236-39.
5014 Monzon S, Lezaun A, Saenz D, et al. Anaphylaxis to boldo infusion, a herbal remedy. *Allergy.* 2004;59:1019-20.
5015 European Medicines Agency. Assessment report on Peumus boldus Molina, folium. Available at: http://www.ema.europa.eu/docs/en_GB/document_library/Herbal_-_HMPC_assessment_report/2009/12/WC500018102.pdf.
5016 Chittiboyina AG, Avonto C, Khan IA. What Happens after Activation of Ascaridole? Reactive Constituents and Their Implications for Skin Sensitization. *Chem Res Toxicol.* 2016 Sep 19;29(9):1488-92.
5017 Sciarrone D, Ragonese C, Carnovale C, et al. Evaluation of tea tree oil quality and ascaridole: a deep study by means of chiral and multi heart-cuts multidimensional gas chromatography system coupled to mass spectrometry detection. *J Chromatogr A.* 2010 Oct 8;1217(41):6422-7.
5018 Krutz NL, Hennen J1, Korb C, et al. Activation of the Endoperoxide Ascaridole Modulates Its Sensitizing Capacity. *Toxicol Sci.* 2015 Oct;147(2):515-23.
5019 Pimkaew P1, Küblbeck J, Petsalo A, et al. Interactions of sesquiterpenes zederone and germacrone with the human cytochrome P450 system. *Toxicol In Vitro.* 2013 Sep;27(6):2005-12.
5020 Baananou S, Bagdonaite E, Marongiu B, et al. Supercritical CO2 extract and essential oil or aerial part of Ledum palustre L.—chemical composition and anti-inflammatory activity. *Nat Prod res.* 2015;29(11):999–1005.
5021 Baananou S, Bagdonaite E, Marongiu B, et al. Supercritical CO2 extract and essential oil or aerial part of Ledum palustre L.—chemical composition and anti-inflammatory activity. *Nat Prod res.* 2015;29(11):999–1005.
2662 Jaenson TGT, Palsson K, Borg-Karlson AK. Evaluation of extracts and oils of tick-repellent plants from Sweden. *Med Vet Entomology.* 2005 Dec;19(4):345–52.
5022 Chao S, Young G, Oberg C, et al. Inhibition of methicillin-resistant Staphylococcus aureus (MRSA) by essential oils. *Flav Frag J.* 2008 Nov-Dec;23(6):444-49.
5023 Dampc A1, Luczkiewicz M. Rhododendron tomentosum (Ledum palustre). A review of traditional use based on current research. *Fitoterapia.* 2013 Mar;85:130-43.
5024 Jesionek A, Kokotkiewicz A, Mikosik-Roczynska A, et al. Chemical variability of Rhododendron tomentosum (Ledum palustre) essential oils and their pro-apoptotic effect on lymphocytes and rheumatoid arthritis synoviocytes. *Fitoterapia.* 2019 Oct 28:104402.
5025 Benelli G, Pavela R, Cianfaglione K, et al. Ascaridole-rich Essential Oil From Marsh Rosemary (Ledum Palustre) Growing in Poland Exerts Insecticidal Activity on Mosquitoes, Moths and Flies Without Serious Effects on Nontarget Organisms and Human Cells. *Food Chem Toxicol.* 2020 Feb 13;138:111184. [Online ahead of print].
5026 Lagha AB, Vaillancourt K, Huacho PM, et al. Effects of Labrador Tea, Peppermint, and Winter Savory Essential Oils on Fusobacterium nucleatum. *Antibiotics (Basel).* 2020 Nov 10;9(11):794.
5027 Korpinen RI, Valimaa AL, Liimatainen J, et al. Essential Oils and Supercritical CO 2 Extracts of Arctic Angelica ( Angelica archangelica L.), Marsh Labrador Tea ( Rhododendron tomentosum) and Common Tansy ( Tanacetum vulgare)-Chemical Compositions and Antimicrobial Activities. *Molecules.* 2021 Nov 25;26(23):7121.
5028 Jepkorir KJ. Chemical composition and anti-microbial activity of essential oils of the plants: Tarchonanthus camphoratus, Leonotis nepetifolia and Satureja biflora. Masters Thesis, Egerton University. 2007. Available at: http://ir-library.egerton.ac.ke/jspui/bitstream/123456789/254/1/Chemical%20composition%20%20anti-microbial%20activity%20of%20essential%20oils%20of%20the%20plantTARCHONANTHUS%20CAMPHORATUS,.pdf.
5029 Kiwanuka NS. Chemical composition and biological potential of the volatile constituents of Tarchanthus camphoratus and Tarchanthus trilobus var galpinni of Kwazulu – Natal Province. Doctoral Thesis, University of Zululand. 2009. Avialable at: http://uzspace.uzulu.ac.za/bitstream/handle/10530/1355/CHEMICAL+COMPOSITION+AND+BIOLOGICAL+POTENTIAL.pdf;jsessionid=58B8B3F3190ADEA9DFCF050410D12E1F?sequence=1.
5030 Costa R, d'Acampora Zellner B, Crupi ML, et al. GC-MS, GC-O and enantio-GC investigation of the essential oil of Tarchananthus canphoratus L. *Flavour Frag J.* 2008;23:40-48.
5031 Matasyoh JC, Kiplimo JJ, Karubiu NM, et al. Chemical composition and antimicrobial activity of essential oil of Tarchanthus camphoratus. *Food Chem.* 2007;101:1183-1187.
5032 van Vuren S. The Antimicrobial Activity and Essential Oil Composition of Medicinal Aromatic Plants Used in African Traditional Healing. Doctoral Thesis, University of the Witwatersrand. Available at: http://wiredspace.wits.ac.za/bitstream/handle/10539/4505/PhDthesisSvanVuuren1.pdf?sequence=3&isAllowed=y
5033 Nanyonga SK, Opoku A, Lewu FB, et al. Chemical composition, antioxidant activity and cytotoxicity of the essential oils of the leaves and stem of Tarchonanthus camphoratus. *African J Pharm Pharmacol.* 2013 Feb;7(7):360-67.
5034 Nanyonga SK, Opoku A, Lewu FB, et al. Variation in chemical composition and antibacterial activity of the essential oil of fresh and dry leaves and dry stem of Tarchonanthus camphoratus. *J Med Plants Res.* 2013 Feb;7(8):442-47.
5035 Awadh Ali NA, Al-Fatimi MA, Crouch RA, et al. Antimicrobial, Antioxidant, and Cytotoxic Activities of the Essential Oil of Tarchonanthus camphoratus. *Nat Prod Commun.* 2013;8(5):683-86.
5036 Mwangi JW, Achola KJ, Lwande W, et al. Volatile constituents of essential oil of Tarchonanthus camphoratus L. *J Essent Oil Res.* 1994;6:183-85.
5037 Omolo MO, Okinyo D, Ndiege IO, et al. Repellency of essential oils of some Kenyan plants against Anopheles gambiae. *Phytochemistry.* 2004 Oct;65(20):2797-802.
5038 Awadh Ali NA, Al-Fatimi MA, Crouch RA, et al. Antimicrobial, Antioxidant, and Cytotoxic Activities of the Essential Oil of Tarchonanthus camphoratus. *Nat Prod Commun.* 2013;8(5):683-86.
5039 Jepkorir KJ. Chemical composition and anti-microbial activity of essential oils of the plants: Tarchonanthus camphoratus, Leonotis nepetifolia and Satureja biflora. Masters Thesis, Egerton University. 2007. Available at: http://ir-library.egerton.ac.ke/jspui/bitstream/123456789/254/1/Chemical%20composition%20%20anti-microbial%20activity%20of%20essential%20oils%20of%20the%20plantTARCHONANTHUS%20CAMPHORATUS,.pdf.
5040 Matasyoh JC, Kiplimo JJ, Karubiu NM, et al. Chemical composition and antimicrobial activity of essential oil of Tarchanthus camphoratus. *Food Chem.* 2007;101:1183-1187.
5041 Nanyonga SK, Opoku A, Lewu FB, et al. Variation in chemical composition and antibacterial activity of the essential oil of fresh and dry leaves and dry stem of Tarchonanthus camphoratus. *J Med Plants Res.* 2013 Feb;7(8):442-47.
5042 Awadh Ali NA, Al-Fatimi MA, Crouch RA, et al. Antimicrobial, Antioxidant, and Cytotoxic Activities of the Essential Oil of Tarchonanthus camphoratus. *Nat Prod Commun.* 2013;8(5):683-86.
5043 van Vuuren SF1, Naidoo D. An antimicrobial investigation of plants used traditionally in southern Africa to treat sexually transmitted infections. *J Ethnopharmacol.* 2010 Aug 9;130(3):552-8.
5044 Nanyonga SK, Opoku A, Lewu FB, et al. Chemical composition, antioxidant activity and cytotoxicity of the essential oils of the leaves and stem of Tarchonanthus camphoratus. *African J Pharm Pharmacol.* 2013 Feb;7(7):360-67.
5045 Awadh Ali NA, Al-Fatimi MA, Crouch RA, et al. Antimicrobial, Antioxidant, and Cytotoxic Activities of the Essential Oil of Tarchonanthus camphoratus. *Nat Prod Commun.* 2013;8(5):683-86.
5046 van Vuuren SF1, Naidoo D. An antimicrobial investigation of plants used traditionally in southern Africa to treat sexually transmitted infections. *J Ethnopharmacol.* 2010 Aug 9;130(3):552-8.
5047 Nasr FA, Noman OM, Alqahtani AS, et al. Phytochemical constituents and anticancer activities of Tarchonanthus camphoratus essential oils grown in Saudi Arabia. *Saudi Pharm J.* 2020 Nov;28(11):1474-1480.
5048 Bourgou S, Rahali FZ, Ourghemmi I, et al. Changes of peel essential oil composition of four Tunisian citrus during fruit maturation. *Sci World J.* 2012;2012:528593.
5049 Jomaa S, Rahmo A, Alnori AS, et al. The cytotoxic effect of essential oil of Syrian Citrus limon peel on human colorectal carcinoma cell line. *Middle E J Cancer.* 2012;3(1):15-21.
5050 Lota ML, Serra DDR, Tomi F, et al. Volatile components of peel and leaf oils of lemon and lime. *J Agric Food Chem.* 2002;50:796-805.
5051 Kejlova K, Jirova D, Bendova H, et al. Phototoxicity of essential oil intended for cosmetic use. *Toxicol In Vitro.* 2010 Dec;24(8):2084-9.
5052 Naganuma M, Hirose S, Nakayama Y, et al. A study of the phototoxicity of lemon oil. *Arch Dermatol Res.* 1985;278(1):31-6.
5053 Placzek M, Fromel W, Eberlein B, et al. Evaluation of phototoxic properties of fragrances. *Acta Derm Venereol.* 2007;87(4):312-6.

[5054] Oboh G, Olasehinde TA, Ademosun AO. Essential oil from lemon peels inhibit key enzymes linked to neurodegenerative conditions and pro-oxidant induced lipid peroxidation. *J Oleo Sci.* 2014;63(4):373-81.
[5055] Koo HN, Hong SH, Kim CY, et al. Inhibitory effect of apoptosis in human astrocytes CCF-STTG1 by lemon oil. *Pharmacol Res.* 2002 Jun;45(6):469-73.
[5056] Mori M, Ikeda N, Kato Y, et al. Inhibition of elastase activity by essential oils in vitro. *J Cosmetic Dermatol.* 2002;1(4):183-87.
[5057] Cha JH, Lee SH, Too YS. Effects of aromatherapy on changes in the autonomic nervous system, aortic pulse wave velocity and aortic augmentation index in patients with essential hypertension. *J Korean Acad Nurs.* 2010 Oct;40(5):705-13.
[5058] Komiya M, Takeuchi T, Harada E. Lemon oil vapor causes an antistress effect via modulating the 5-HT and DA activities in mice. *Behav Brain Res.* 2006 Sep;172(2):240-49.
[5059] Yavari Kia P, Safajou M, Shahnazi M, et al. The effect of lemon inhalation aromatherapy on nausea and vomiting of pregnancy: a double-blinded, randomized, controlled clinical trial. *Iran Red Crescent Med J.* 2014 Mar;16(3):e14360.
[5060] Forbes MA, Schmid MM. Use of OTC essential oils to clear plantar warts. *Nurse Pract.* 2006 Mar;31(3):53-55.
[5061] Zhou W, Fukumoto S, Yokogoshi H. Components of lemon essential oil attenuate dementia induced by scopolamine. *Nutr Neurosci.* 2009 Apr;12(2):57-64.
[5062] Ferrara L, Navigilio D, Armone Caruso A. Cytological aspects on the effects of a nasal spray consisting of standardized extract of citrus lemon and essential oils in allergic rhinopathy. *ISRN Pharm.* 2012;2012:404606.
[5063] Valgimigli L, Gabbanini S, Berlini E, et al. Lemon (Citrus limon, Burm.f.) essential oil enhances the trans-epidermal release of lipid-(A, E) and water-(B6, C) soluble vitamins from topical emulsions in reconstructed human epidermis. *Int J Cosmet Sci.* 2012 Aug;34(4):347-56.
[5064] Kim MA, Sakong JK, Kim EJ, et al. Effect of aromatherapy massage for the relief of constipation in the elderly. *Taehan Kanho Hakhoe Chi.* 2005 Feb;35(1):56-64.
[5065] Hur MH, Park J, Maddock-Jennings W, et al. Reduction of mouth malodour and volatile sulphur constituents in intensive care patients using an essential oil mouthwash. *Phytother Res.* 2007 Jul;21(7):641-43.
[5066] Forrer M, Kulik EM, Filippi A, et al. The antimicrobial activity of alpha-bisabolol and tea tree oil against Solobacterium moorei, a gram-positive bacterium associated with halitosis. *Arch Oral Biol.* 2013 Jan;58(1):10-16.
[5067] Oboh G, Olasehinde TA, Ademosun AO. Essential oil from lemon peels inhibit key enzymes linked to neurodegenerative conditions and pro-oxidant induced lipid peroxidation. *J Oleo Sci.* 2014;63(4):373-81.
[5068] Darvesh S, Hopkins DA, Geula C. Neurobiology of butyrylcholinesterase. *Nat Rev Neurosci.* 2003 Feb;4:131-38.
[5069] Igimi G, Watanabe D, Yanamoto F, et al. A useful cholesterol solvent for medical dissolution of gallstones. *Am J Dig Dis.* 1976;27:536-45.
[5070] Igma H, Tamura R, Toraishi K, et al. Medical dissolution of gallstones. Clinical experience of d-limonene as a simple, safe, and effective solvent. *Dig Dis Sci.* 1991;36:200-08.
[5071] Wilkins J Jr. Method for treating gastrointestinal disorder.US patent (642045). 2002.
[5072] Willette RC, Barrow L, Doster R, et al. Purified d-limonene: an effective agent for the relief of occasional symptoms of heartburn. Proprietary study. WRC Laboratories, Inc. Galveston, TX.
[5073] Guerra FQ, Mendes JM, Sousa JP, et al. Increasing antibiotic activity against multidrug-resistant Acinetobacter spp by essential oils of Citrus limon and Cinnamomum zeylanicum. *Nat Prod Res.* 2012;26(23):2235-38.
[5074] Hamdan D, Ashour ML, Mulyaningsih S, et al. Chemical composition of the essential oils of variegated pink-fleshed lemon (Citrus x limon L. Burm. F.) and their antiinflammatory and antimicrobial activities. *Z Naturforsch C.* 2013 Jul- Aug;68(7-8):275-84.
[5075] Campelo LM, Goncalves FC, Feitosa CM, et al. Antioxidant activity of Citrus limon essential oil in mouse hippocampus. *Pharm Biol.* 2011 Jul;49(7):709-15.
[5076] Baylac S, Racine P. Inhibition of 5-lipoxygenase by essential oils and other natural fragrant extracts. *Int J Aromatherapy.* 2003;13(2-3):138-42.
[5077] Amorim JL, Simas DL, Pinheiro MM, et al. Anti-Inflammatory Properties and Chemical Characterization of the Essential Oils of Four Citrus Species. *PLoS One.* 2016 Apr 18;11(4):e0153643.
[5078] Campelo LM, de Almeida AA, de Freitas RL, et al. Antioxidant and antinociceptive effects of Citrus limon essential oil in mice. *J Biomed Biotechnol.* 2011;2011:678673.
[5079] Bouzenna H, Hfaiedh N, Giroux-Metges MA, et al. Protective effects of essential oil of Citrus limon against aspirin-induced toxicity in IEC-6 cells. *Appl Physiol Nutr Metab.* 2017 May;42(5):479-486.
[5080] L M Lopes C, Goncalves e Sa C, de Almeida AA, et al. Sedative anxiolytic and antidepressant activities of Citrus limon (Burn) essential oil in mice. *Pharmazie.* 2011 Aug;66(8):623-27.
[5081] Kiecolt-Glaser JK, Graham JE, Malarkey WB, et al. Olfactory influences on mood and autonomic, endocrine, and immune function. *Psychoneuroendocinology.* 2008 Apr;33(3):328-39.
[5082] Komori T. Effects of lemon and valerian inhalation on autonomic nerve activity in depressed and healthy subjects. *Int J Essent Oil Ther.* 2009;3(1):3-8.
[5083] Kaur CD, Saraf S. In vitro sun protection factor determination of herbal oils used in cosmetics. *Pharmacognosy Res.* 2010 Jan;2(1):22-25.
[5084] Dutta BK, Karmakar S, Naglot A, et al. Anticandidal activity of some essential oils of a mega biodiversity hotspot in India. *Mycoses.* 2007 Mar;50(2):121-24.
[5085] Jing L, Zhang Y, Fan S, et al. Preventive and ameliorating effects of citrus D-limonene on dyslipidemia and hyperglycemia in mice with high-fat diet-induced obesity. *Eur J Pharmacol.* 2013 Sep 5;715(1-3):46-55.
[5086] Shi YF, Zhang XY, Han H, et al. Effect of lemon essential oil on caries factors of Streptococcus sobrinus. *Ahonqhua Kou Qiang Yi Xue Za Zhi.* 2012 Dec;47(12):739-42.
[5087] Ogeturk M, Kose E, Sarsilmaz M, et al. Effects of lemon essential oil aroma on the learning behavior of rats. *Neurosciences (Riyadh).* 2010 Oct;15(4):292-93.
[5088] Warnke PH, Becker ST, Podschun R, et al. The battle against multi-resistant strains: Renaissance of antimicrobial essential oils as a promising force to fight hospital-acquired infections. *J Craniomaxillofac Surg.* 2009 Oct;37(7):392- 97.
[5089] Ceccarelli I, Lariviere WR, Fiorenzani P, et al. Effects of long-term exposure of lemon essential oil odor on behavioral, hormonal and neuronal parameters in male and female rats. *Brain Res.* 2004 Mar 19;1001(1-2):78-86.
[5090] Aloisa AM, Ceccarelli I, Masi F, et al. Effects of the essential oil from citrus lemon in male and female rats exposed to a persistent painful stimulation. *Behav Brain Res.* 2002;136;127-35.
[5091] Ceccarelli I, Masi F, Fiorenzani P, Sex differences in the citrus lemon essential oil-induced increase of hippocampal acetylcholine release in rats exposed to a persistent painful stimulation. *Neurosci Lett.* 2002 Sep 13;330(1):25-28.
[5092] Bouzenna H, Dhibi S, Samout N, et al. The protective effect of Citrus limon essential oil on hepatotoxicity and nephrotoxicity induced by aspirin in rats. *Biomed Pharmacother.* 2016 Oct;83:1327-1334.
[5093] Plant J. Effects of essential oils on telomere length in human cells. *Med Aromat Plants.* 2016;5(2):1-6.
[5094] Císarová M, Tančinová D, Medo J, et al. The in vitro effect of selected essential oils on the growth and mycotoxin production of Aspergillus species. *J Environ Sci Health B.* 2016 Oct 2;51(10):668-674.
[5095] Perczak A, Juś K, Marchwińska K, et al. Degradation of Zearalenone by Essential Oils under In vitro Conditions. *Front Microbiol.* 2016 Aug 11;7:1224.
[5096] Turcotte JC, Hunt PJB, Blaustein JD. Estrogenic effects of zearalenone on the expression of progestin receptors and sexual behavior in female rats. *Hormones and Behavior.* 2005;47:178-84.
[5097] Takemura H, Shim JY, Sayama K, et al. Characterization of the estrogenic activities of zearalenone and zeranol in vivo and in vitro. *J Steroid Biochem Mol Biol.* 2007 Feb;103(2):170-7.
[5098] Frizzell C, Ndossi D, Verhaegen S, et al. Endocrine disrupting effects of zearalenone, alpha- and beta-zearalenol at the level of nuclear receptor binding and steroidogenesis. *Toxicol Lett.* 2011 Oct 10;206(2):210-7.
[5099] Loizzo MR, Tundis R1, Bonesi M, et al. Chemical Profile and Antioxidant Properties of Extracts and Essential Oils from Citrus x limon (L.) Burm. cv Femminello Comune. *Chem Biodivers.* 2016 May;13(5):571-81.
[5100] Campolo O, Romeo FV, Algeri GM, et al. Larvicidal Effects of Four Citrus Peel Essential Oils Against the Arbovirus Vector Aedes albopictus (Diptera: Culicidae). *J Econ Entomol.* 2016 Feb;109(1):360-5.
[5101] Nakayama M, Okizaki A, Takahashi K, et al. A Randomized Controlled Trial for the Effectiveness of Aromatherapy in Decreasing Salivary Gland Damage following Radioactive Iodine Therapy for Differentiated Thyroid Cancer. *Biomed Res Int.* 2016;2016:9509810.
[5102] Nikolić MM, Jovanović KK, Marković TL, et al. Antimicrobial synergism and cytotoxic properties of Citrus limon L., Piper nigrum L. and Melaleuca alternifolia (Maiden and Betche) Cheel essential oils. *J Pharm Pharmacol.* 2017 Nov;69(11):1606-1614.
[5103] Avcioglu NH, Sahal G, Bilkay IS, et al. Antibiofilm effects of Citrus limonum and Zingiber officinale Oils on biofilm formation of Klebsiella ornithinolytica, Klebsiella oxytoca and Klebsiella terrigena species. *Afr J Tradit Complement Altern Med.* 2016 Sep 29;13(6):61-67.
[5104] Vinturelle R, Mattos C, Meloni J, et al. In Vitro Evaluation of Essential Oils Derived from Piper nigrum (Piperaceae) and Citrus limonum (Rutaceae) against the Tick Rhipicephalus (Boophilus) microplus (Acari: Ixodidae). *Biochem Res Int.* 2017;2017:5342947.
[5105] Mojtahedin A, Seifdavati J, Seyedsharifi R. Effects of different levels of dietary Citrus Limon essential oil on some blood parameters and antioxidant status in Afshari Ewes. *Cell Mol Biol (Noisy-le-grand).* 2018 Jan 31;64(1):47-51.
[5106] Gucwa K, Milewski S, Dymerski T, et al. Investigation of the Antifungal Activity and Mode of Action of Thymus vulgaris, Citrus limonum, Pelargonium graveolens, Cinnamomum cassia, Ocimum basilicum, and Eugenia caryophyllus Essential Oils. *Molecules.* 2018 May 8;23(5).
[5107] Bouzenna H, Samout N, Dhibi S, et al. Protective effect of essential oil from Citrus limon against aspirin-induced toxicity in rats. *Hum Exp Toxicol.* 2018 Dec 19:960327118819044.
[5108] Lanzerstorfer A, Hackl M, Schlömer M, et al. The influence of air-dispersed essential oils from lemon (Citrus limon) and silver fir (Abies alba) on airborne bacteria and fungi in hospital rooms. *J Environ Sci Health A Tox Hazard Subst Environ Eng.* 2019;54(3):256-260.
[5109] Restuccia C, Oliveri Conti G, Zuccarello P, et al. Efficacy of different citrus essential oils to inhibit the growth and B1 aflatoxin biosynthesis of Aspergillus flavus. *Environ Sci Pollut Res Int.* 2019 Oct;26(30):31263-31272.
[5110] Pedroso RDS, Balbino BL, Andrade G, et al. In Vitro and In Vivo Anti- Candida Spp. Activity of Plant-Derived Products. *Plants (Basel).* 2019 Nov;8(11):494.
[5111] Liu B, Kou J, Li F, et al. Lemon essential oil ameliorates age-associated cognitive dysfunction via modulating hippocampal synaptic density and inhibiting acetylcholinesterase. *Aging (Albany NY).* 2020 May 11;12.
[5112] Rambod M, Rakhshan M, Tohidinik S, et al. The effect of lemon inhalation aromatherapy on blood pressure, electrocardiogram changes, and anxiety in acute myocardial infarction patients: A clinical, multi-centered, assessor-blinded trial design. *Complement Ther Clin Pract.* 2020 May;39:101155.
[5113] Safajou F, Soltani N, Taghizadeh M, et al. The Effect of Combined Inhalation Aromatherapy with Lemon and Peppermint on Nausea and Vomiting of Pregnancy: A Double-Blind, Randomized Clinical Trial. *Iranian J Nursing Midwifery Res.* 2020;25(5):401-6.

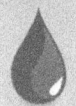

5114 Putri RD, Astrina Natalia DA, et al. Giving aromatherapy combination of lemon and peppermint affects the intensity of nausea and vomiting in pregnant women in trimester 1. *JKM*. 2022 Apr;8(2):2476-8944.
5115 Maaroufi Z, Cokean S, Loiseau PM, et al. In vitro antileishmanial potentialities of essential oils from Citrus limon and Pistacia lentiscus harvested in Tunisia. *Parasitol Res*. 2021 Jan 10. Online ahead of print.
5116 Denkova-Kostova R, Teneva D, Tomova T, et al. Chemical composition, antioxidant and antimicrobial activity of essential oils from tangerine ( Citrus reticulata L.), grapefruit ( Citrus paradisi L.), lemon ( Citrus lemon L.) and cinnamon ( Cinnamomum zeylanicum Blume). *Z Naturforsch C J Biosci*. 2020 Nov 23;76(5-6):175-185.
5117 Soroh A, Owen LL, Rahim N, et al. Microemulsification of essential oils for the development of antimicrobial and mosquito repellent functional coatings for textiles. *J Appl Microbiol*. 2021 May 22. Online ahead of print.
5118 Wu P, Tang X, Jian R, et al. Insecticidal Activities of Essential Oils of Discarded Perfume Lemon and Leaves ( Citrus Limon (L.) Burm. F.) as Possible Sources of Functional Botanical Agents. *Front Chem*. 2021 May 24;9:679116.
5119 Luciardi MC, Blazquez MA, Alberto MR, et al. Lemon Oils Attenuate the Pathogenicity of Pseudomonas aeruginosa by Quorum Sensing Inhibition. *Molecules*. 2021 May 12;26(10):2863.
5120 Zarenezhad E, Agholi M, Ghanbariasad A, et al. A nanoemulsion-based nanogel of Citrus limon essential oil with leishmanicidal activity against Leishmania tropica and Leishmania major. *J Parasit Dis*. 2021 Jun;45(2):441-448.
5121 Oyeleye SI, Ogunsuyi OB, Adedeji V, et al. Citrus spp. essential oils improve behavioral pattern, repressed cholinesterases and monoamine oxidase activities, and production of reactive species in fruit fly (Drosophila melanogaster) model of Alzheimer's Disease. *J Food Biochem*. 2021 Mar;45(3):e13558.
5122 Brozyna M, Paleczny J, Kozlowska W, et al. The Antimicrobial and Antibiofilm In Vitro Activity of Liquid and Vapour Phases of Selected Essential Oils against Staphylococcus aureus. *Pathogens*. 2021 Sep 17;10(9):1207.
5123 Pasias IN, Ntakoulas DD, Raptopoulou K, et al. Chemical Composition of Essential Oils of Aromatic and Medicinal Herbs Cultivated in Greece-Benefits and Drawbacks. *Foods*. 2021 Oct 3;10(10):2354.
5124 Elnabawy EM, Hassan S, Taha EA. Repellent and Toxicant Effects of Eight Essential Oils against the Red Flour Beetle, Tribolium castaneum Herbst (Coleoptera: Tenebrionidae). *Biology (Basel)*. 2021 Dec 21;11(1):3.
5125 Li C, Cai Q, Wu X, et al. Variation in compositions and biological activities of essential oils from four Citrus species: Citrus limon, Citrus sinensis, Citrus paradisi, and Citrus reticulata. *Chem Biodivers*. 2022 Feb 10. Online ahead of print.
5126 Goncalves S. Effects of plaster therapy on thigh fat. *Our Dermatol Online*. 2022;13(1):32-5.
5127 Ozer Z, Teke N, Bahcecioglu G, et al. Effectiveness of lemon essential oil in reducing test anxiety in nursing Students. *Explore*. 2022;000:1-7.
5128 Galgano M, Capozza P, Pellegrini F, et al. Antimicrobial Activity of Essential Oils Evaluated In Vitro against Escherichia coli and Staphylococcus aureus. *Antibiotics (Basel)*. 2022 Jul 20;11(7):979.
5129 Li C, Zhu H, Zhao K, et al. Chemical constituents, biological activities and anti-rheumatoid arthritic properties of four citrus essential oils. *Phytother Res*. 2022 Jul;36(7):2908-2920.
5130 Kusumawati DA, Prasetyorini H. Giving lemon aromatherapy to reduce nausea for pregnant women in the first trimester at the Limbangan Health Center. *Jurnal Ilmu dan Teknologi Kesehatan STIKES Widya Husada*. 2022 Apr;13(2):40-45.
5131 Bouabdallah S, Cianfaglione K, Azzouz M, et al. Sustainable Extraction, Chemical Profile, Cytotoxic and Antileishmanial Activities In-Vitro of Some Citrus Species Leaves Essential Oils. *Pharmaceuticals (Basel)*. 2022 Sep 19;15(9):1163.
5132 Riaz M, Qadir R, Akhtar MT, et al. Chemical Characterization, Antioxidant, Antimicrobial, Cytotoxicity and In-silico Studies of n-hexane Extract and Essential Oils from Citrus limon Leaves. *Chem Biodivers*. 2022 Nov 15. Online ahead of print.
5133 Ibrahium SM, Wahba AA, Farghali AA, et al. Acaricidal Activity of Tea Tree and Lemon Oil Nanoemulsions against Rhipicephalus annulatus. *Pathogens*. 2022 Dec 9;11(12):1506.
5134 Ueda K, Horita T, Suzuki T. Effects of inhaling essential oils of Citrus limonum L., Santalum album, and Cinnamomum camphora on human brain activity. *Brain Behav*. 2023 Jan 9:e2889.
5135 Othman HIA, Alkatib HH, Zaid A, et al. Phytochemical Composition, Antioxidant and Antiproliferative Activities of Citrus hystrix, Citrus limon, Citrus pyriformis, and Citrus microcarpa Leaf Essential Oils against Human Cervical Cancer Cell Line. *Plants (Basel)*. 2022 Dec 27;12(1):134.
5136 Cozzi L, Vicenza T, Battistini R, et al. Effects of Essential Oils and Hydrolates on the Infectivity of Murine Norovirus. *Viruses*. 2023 Mar 4;15(3):682.
5137 Grayer RJ, Kite GC, Goldstone FJ, et al. Intraspecific taxonomy and essential oil chemotypes in Sweet Basil, Ocimum basilicum. *Phytochem*. 1996;43(5):1033-39.
5138 Carovic-Stanko K, Orlic S, Politeo O, et al. Composition and antibacterial activities of essential oils of seven Ocimum taxa. *Food Chem*. 2010;19:196-201.
5139 Nogueira AC, Carvalho RR, Souza CA, et al. Study on the embryofeto-toxicity of citral in the rat. *Toxicology*. 1995;96(2):105-13.
5140 De Olivera AC, Ribeiro-Pinto LF, Paumgartten JR. In vitro inhibition of CYP2B1 monoxygenase by beta-myrcene and other monoterpenoid constituents. *Br J Nutr*. 1999;81:289-95.
5141 Seo KA, Kim H, Ku HY, et al. The monoterpenoids citral and geraniol are moderate inhibitors of the CYP2B6 hydroxylase activity. *Chem Biol Interact*. 2008;174:141-46.
5142 Raner GM, Vaz AD, Coon MJ. Metabolism of all-trans, 9-cis, and 13-cis isomers of retinal by purified isozymes of microsomal cytochrome P450 and mechanism-based inhibition of retinoid oxidation by citral. *Mol Pharmacol*. 1996;49(3):515-22.
5143 Modak T, Mukhopadhaya A. Effects of citral, a naturally occurring antiadipogenic molecule, on an energy-intense diet model of obesity. *Indian J Pharmacol*. 2011 May-Jun;43(3):300-05.
5144 Najafian M, Ebrahim-Habibi A, Yaghmaei P, et al. Citral as a potential antihyperlipidemic medicine in diabetes: a study on streptozotocin-induced diabetic rats. *J Diabetes Metabolic Disorders*. 2011;10(1):3.
5145 Choi JY, Damte D, Seung-Jin L, et al. Antimicrobial activity of lemongrass and oregano essential oil against standard antibiotic resistant Staphylococcus aureus and field isolates from chronic mastitis cow. *International Journal of Phytomedicine*. 2012;4(1):134-39.
5146 Shin S, Lim S. Antifungal effects of herbal essential oils alone and in combination with ketoconazole against Trichophyton spp. *J Appl Micribiol*. 2004;97:1289-96.
5147 do Vale TG, Furtado EC, Santos JG Jr, et al. Central effects of citral, myrcene and limonene, constituents of essential oil chemotypes from Lippia alba (Mill.) n.e. Brown. *Phytomedicine*. 2002 Dec;9(8):709-14.
5148 Kuhn GO, McCampbell P, Singmaster G, et al. Application of microencapsulation technology to improve the stability of citral in rodent diets. *Fundam Appl Toxicol*. 1991 Oct;17(3):635-40.
5149 De Mozzi P, Johnston GA. An outbreak of allergic contact dermatitis caused by citral in beauticians working in a health spa. *Contact Dermatitis*. 2014 Jun;70(6):377-9.
5150 Carovic-Stanko K, Orlic S, Politeo O, et al. Composition and antibacterial activities of essential oils of seven Ocimum taxa. *Food Chem*. 2010;19:196-201.
5151 Wesolowska A, Jadczak D, Grzeszczuk M. GC–MS Analysis of Lemon Catnip (Nepeta cataria L. var. citriodora Balbis) Essential Oil. *Acta Chromatographica*. 2011 Feb;23(1):169-80.
5152 Suschke U, Sporer F, Schneele J, et al. Antibacterial and cytotoxic activity of Nepeta cataria L., N. cataria var. citriodora (Beck.) Balb. and Melissa officinalis L. essential oils. *Nat Prod Commun*. 2006 Dec;2(12):1277-86.
5153 Chalchat J C, Lamy J. Chemical composition of the essential oil isolated from wild catnip Nepeta cataria L. cv. Citriodora from Dro^me region of France. *J Essent Oil Res*. 1997;9:527-32.
5154 Klimek B, Modnicki D. Terpenoids and sterols from Nepeta cataria L. var. citriodora (Lamiaceae). *Acta Pol Pharm*. 2005 May-Jun;62(3):231-5.
5155 Nogueira AC, Carvalho RR, Souza CA, et al. Study on the embryofeto-toxicity of citral in the rat. *Toxicology*. 1995;96(2):105-13.
5156 Boukhris M, Bouaziz M, Feki I, et al. Hypoglycemic and antioxidant effects of leaf and essential oil of Pelargonium graveolens L'Her. in alloxan induced diabetic rats. *Lipids Health Dis*. 2012 Jun 26;11:81.
5157 Adeneye AA, Agbaje EO. Hypoglycemic and hypolipidemic effects of fresh leaf aqueous extract of Cymbopogon citratus Stapf. in rats. *J Ethnopharmacol*. 2007 Jul 25; 112(3):440-4.
5158 Bharti SK, Kumar A, Prakash O, et al. Essential Oil of Cymbopogon Citratus Against Diabetes: Validation by In vivo Experiments and Computational Studies. *J Bioanal Biomed*. 2013;5:194-203.
5159 Kshirsagan R, Reddy GB, Bakshi V, et al. Geraniol a major component of essential oil ameliorates endothelial dysfunction induced by high-fat diet fed rats. *Atherosclerosis*. 2015 Jun;241(1):e154-e155.
5160 Ibrahim SM, El-Denshary ES, Abdallah DM. Geraniol, Alone and in Combination with Pioglitazone, Ameliorates Fructose-Induced Metabolic Syndrome in Rats via the Modulation of Both Inflammatory and Oxidative Stress Status. *PLoS One*. 2015 Feb 13;10(2):e0117516.
5161 Srinivasan S, Muruganathan U. Antidiabetic efficacy of citronellol, a citrus monoterpene by ameliorating the hepatic key enzymes of carbohydrate metabolism in streptozotocin-induced diabetic rats. *Chem Biol Interact*. 2016 Apr 25;250:38-46.
5162 Sea KA, Kim H, Ku HY, et al. The monoterpenoids citral and geraniol are moderate inhibitors of CYP2B6 hydroxylase activity. *Chem Biol Interact*. 2008 Aug 11;174(3):141-6.
5163 Seo KA, Kim H, Ku HY, et al. The monoterpenoids citral and geraniol are moderate inhibitors of the CYP2B6 hydroxylase activity. *Chem Biol Interact*. 2008;174:141-46.
5164 Sheweita SA, Newairy AA, Mansour HA, et al. Effect of some hypoglycemic herbs on the activity of phase I and II drug-metabolizing enzymes in alloxan-induced diabetic rats. *Toxicology*. 2002 May 24;17(2):131-39.
5165 Raner GM, Vaz AD, Coon MJ. Metabolism of all-trans, 9-cis, and 13-cis isomers of retinal by purified isozymes of microsomal cytochrome P450 and mechanism-based inhibition of retinoid oxidation by citral. *Mol Pharmacol*. 1996;49(3):515-22.
5166 De Olivera AC, Ribeiro-Pinto LF, Paumgartten JR. In vitro inhibition of CYP2B1 monoxygenase by beta-myrcene and other monoterpenoid constituents. *Br J Nutr*. 1999;81:289-95.
5167 Seo KA, Kim H, Ku HY, et al. The monoterpenoids citral and geraniol are moderate inhibitors of the CYP2B6 hydroxylase activity. *Chem Biol Interact*. 2008;174:141-46.
5168 do Vale TG, Furtado EC, Santos JG Jr, et al. Central effects of citral, myrcene and limonene, constituents of essential oil chemotypes from Lippia alba (Mill.) n.e. Brown. *Phytomedicine*. 2002 Dec;9(8):709-14.
5169 Sherry CJ, Hunter PS. The effect of an ethanol extract of catnip (Nepeta cataria) on the behavior of the young chick. *Experientia*. 1979 Feb 15;35(2):237-8.
5170 Harney JW, Barofsky IM, Leary JD. Behavioral and toxicological studies of cyclopentanoid monoterpenes from Nepeta cataria. *Lloydia*. 1978 Jul-Aug;41(4):367-74.
5171 Massoco CO, Silva MR, Gorniak SL, et al. Behavioral effects of acute and long-term administration of catnip (Nepeta cataria) in mice. *Vet Hum Toxicol*. 1995 Dec;37(6):530-3.
5172 Osterhoudt KC, Lee SK, Callahan JM, et al. Catnip and the alteration of human consciousness. *Vet Hum Toxicol*. 1997 Dec;39(6):373-5.
5173 Jackson B, Reed A. Catnip and the alteration of consciousness. *JAMA*. 1969 Feb 17;207(7):1349-50.
5174 Choi JY, Damte D, Seung-Jin L, et al. Antimicrobial activity of lemongrass and oregano essential oil against standard antibiotic resistant Staphylococcus aureus and field isolates from chronic mastitis cow. *International Journal of Phytomedicine*. 2012;4(1):134-39.
5175 Shin S, Lim S. Antifungal effects of herbal essential oils alone and in combination with ketoconazole against Trichophyton spp. *J Appl Micribiol*. 2004;97:1289-96.

5176 Hagvall L. Cytochrome P450-mediated activation of the fragrance constituent geraniol forms potent contact allergens. *Tox Appl Pharm*. 2008 Dec;233(2):308-13.

5177 Kuhn GO, McCampbell P, Singmaster G, et al. Application of microencapsulation technology to improve the stability of citral in rodent diets. *Fundam Appl Toxicol*. 1991 Oct;17(3):635-40.

5178 De Mozzi P, Johnston GA. An outbreak of allergic contact dermatitis caused by citral in beauticians working in a health spa. *Contact Dermatitis*. 2014 Jun;70(6):377-9.

5179 Suschke U, Sporer F, Schneele J, et al. Antibacterial and cytotoxic activity of Nepeta cataria L., N. cataria var. citriodora (Beck.) Balb. and Melissa officinalis L. essential oils. *Nat Prod Commun*. 2006 Dec;2(12):1277-86.

5180 Ali A, Khan MM, Uddin M, et al. Radiolytically depolymerized sodium alginate improves physiological activities, yield attributes and composition of essential oil of Eucalyptus citriodora Hook. *Carbohydr Polym*. 2014 Nov;112:134– 44.

5181 Gbenou JD, Ahounou JF, Akakpo HB, et al. Phytochemical composition of Cymbopogon citratus and Eucalyptus citriodora essential oils and their anti-inflammatory and analgesic properties on Wistar rats. *Mol Biol Rep*. 2013 Feb;40(2):1127–34.

5182 Olivero-Verbel J, Nerio LS, Stashenko EE. Bioactivity against Tribolium castaneum Herbst (Coleoptera: Tenebrionidae) of Cymbopogon citratus and Eucalyptus citriodora essential oils grown in Colombia. *Pest Manag Sci*. 2010 Jun;66(6):664–68.

5183 Gbenou JD, Ahounou JF, Akakpo HB, et al. Phytochemical composition of Cymbopogon citratus and Eucalyptus citriodora essential oils and their anti-inflammatory and analgesic properties on Wistar rats. *Mol Biol Rep*. 2013 Feb;40(2):1127–34.

5184 Ramos Alvarenga RF, Wan B, Inui T, et al. Airborne antituberculosis activity of Eucalyptus citriodora essential oil. *J Nat Prod*. 2014 Mar;77(3):603–10.

5185 Adesina AB, Josephine OO. Inhibitory effects of the volatile oils of Callistemon citrinus (Curtis) Skeels and Eucalyptus citriodora Hook (Myrtaceae) on the acetylcholine induced contraction of isolated rat ileum. *Pak J Phark Sci*. 2012 Apr;25(2):435–39.

5186 Silva J, Abebe W, Sousa SM, et al. Analgesic and anti-inflammatory effects of essential oils of eucalyptus. *J Ethnopharmacol*. 2003 Dec;89(2–3):277–83.

5187 Lu XQ, Tang FD, Wang Y, et al. Effect of Eucalyptus globulus oil on lipopolysaccharide-induced chronic bronchitis and mucin hypersecretion in rats. *Zhongguo Zhong Yao ZA Zhi*. 2004 Feb;29(2):168–71.

5188 Dutta BK, Karmakar S, Naglot A, et al. Anticandidal activity of some essential oils of a mega biodiversity hotspot in India. *Mycoses*. 2007 Mar;50(2):121–24.

5189 Ramezani H, Singh HP, Batish DR, et al. Antifungal activity of the volatile oil of Eucalyptus citriodora. *Fitoterapia*. 2002 Jun;73(3):261–62.

5190 Luqman S, RAJ Dwivedi G, Darokar M, et al. Antimicrobial activity of Eucalyptus citriodora essential oil. *Int J Essential Oil Ther*. 2008 Jan;2(2):69-75.

5191 Ghaffar A, Yameen M, Kiran S, et al. Chemical Composition and in-Vitro Evaluation of the Antimicrobial and Antioxidant Activities of Essential Oils Extracted from Seven Eucalyptus Species. *Molecules*. 2015 Nov 18;20(11):20487-98.

5192 Olivero-Verbel J, Nerio LS, Stashenko EE. Bioactivity against Tribolium castaneum Herbst (Coleoptera: Tenebrionidae) of Cymbopogon citratus and Eucalyptus citriodora essential oils grown in Colombia. *Pest Manag Sci*. 2010 Jun;66(6):664–68.

5193 Vera SS, Zambrano DF, Méndez-Sanchez SC, et al. Essential oils with insecticidal activity against larvae of Aedes aegypti (Diptera: Culicidae). *Parasitol Res*. 2014 Jul;113(7):2647-54.

5194 Bossou AD, Mangelinckx S, Yedomonhan H, et al. Chemical composition and insecticidal activity of plant essential oils from Benin against Anopheles gambiae (Giles). *Parasit Vectors*. 2013 Dec 3;6:337.

5195 Singh RK, Dhiman RC, Mittal PK. Studies on mosquito larvicidal properties of Eucalyptus citriodora Hook (family-Myrtaceae). *J Commun Dis*. 2007 Dec;39(4):233-6.

5196 Rudin W. [Protection against insects]. *Ther Umsch*. 2005 Nov;62(11):713-8.

5197 Hans VM, Grover HS, Deswal H, et al. Antimicrobial Efficacy of Various Essential Oils at Varying Concentrations against Periopathogen Porphyromonas gingivalis. *J Clin Diagn Res*. 2016 Sep;10(9):ZC16-ZC19.

5198 Luís Â, Duarte AP, Pereira L, et al. Chemical Profiling and Evaluation of Antioxidant and Anti-Microbial Properties of Selected Commercial Essential Oils: A Comparative Study. *Medicines (Basel)*. 2017 Jun 5;4(2).

5199 Castillo RM, Stashenko E, Duque JE. Insecticidal and Repellent Activity of Several Plant-Derived Essential Oils Against Aedes aegypti. *J Am Mosq Control Assoc*. 2017 Mar;33(1):25-35.

5200 Benchaa S, Hazzit M, Abdelkrim H. Allelopathic Effect of Eucalyptus citriodora Essential Oil and its Potential Use as Bioherbicide. *Chem Biodivers*. 2018 Aug;15(8):e1800202.

5201 Feng J, Shi W, Miklossy J, et al. Identification of Essential Oils with Strong Activity against Stationary Phase Borrelia burgdorferi. *Antibiotics (Basel)*. 2018 Oct 16;7(4).

5202 Jang M, Kim J, Yoon KA, et al. Biological activity of Myrtaceae plant essential oils and their major components against Drosophila suzukii (Diptera: Drosophilidae). *Pest Manag Sci*. 2017 Feb;73(2):404-409.

5203 Salem MZM, Elansary HO, Ali HM, et al. Bioactivity of essential oils extracted from Cupressus macrocarpa branchlets and Corymbia citriodora leaves grown in Egypt. *BMC Complement Altern Med*. 2018 Jan 22;18(1):23.

5204 Araujo-Filho JVD, Ribeiro WLC, Andre WPP, et al. Anthelmintic Activity of Eucalyptus Citriodora Essential Oil and Its Major Component, Citronellal, on Sheep Gastrointestinal Nematodes. *Rev Bras Parasitol Vet*. 2019 Oct-Dec;28(4):644-651.

5205 Pinheiro REE, Chaves TP, Melo ES, et al. Modulatory-antibiotic Activity of the Essential Oil From Eucalyptus Citriodora Against MDR Bacterial Strains. *Cell Mol Biol (Noisy-le-grand)*. 2020 Jun 25;66(4):60-64.

5206 Ho CL, Li LH, Weng YC, et al. Eucalyptus essential oils inhibit the lipopolysaccharide-induced inflammatory response in RAW264.7 macrophages through reducing MAPK and NF-κB pathways. *BMC Complement Med Ther*. 2020 Jun 29;20(1):200.

5207 Amri I, Khammassi M, Ben Ayed R, et al. Essential Oils and Biological Activities of Eucalyptus falcata, E. sideroxylon and E. citriodora Growing in Tunisia. *Plants (Basel)*. 2023 Feb 11;12(4):816.

5208 Southwell IA, Russell M, Smith RL, et al. Backhousia citriodora F. Muell. (Myrtaceae), A superior source of citral. *J Essent Oil Res*. 2000;12(5):735–41.

5209 Doran JC, Brophy JJ, Lassak EV, et al. Backhousia citriodora F. Muell.—Rediscovery and chemical characterization of the L-citronellal form and aspects of its breeding system. *Flavour Frag J*. 2001;16:325–328.

5210 Nogueira AC, Carvalho RR, Souza CA, et al. Study on the embryofeto-toxicity of citral in the rat. *Toxicology*. 1995;96(2):105-13.

5211 Modak T, Mukhopadhaya A. Effects of citral, a naturally occurring antiadipogenic molecule, on an energy-intense diet model of obesity. *Indian J Pharmacol*. 2011 May-Jun;43(3):300-05.

5212 Najafian M, Ebrahim-Habibi A, Yaghmaei P, et al. Citral as a potential antihyperlipidemic medicine in diabetes: a study on streptozotocin-induced diabetic rats. *J Diabetes Metabolic Disorders*. 2011;10(1):3.

5213 Seo KA, Kim H, Ku HY, et al. The monoterpenoids citral and geraniol are moderate inhibitors of the CYP2B6 hydroxylase activity. *Chem Biol Interact*. 2008;174:141-46.

5214 Sheweita SA, Newairy AA, Mansour HA, et al. Effect of some hypoglycemic herbs on the activity of phase I and II drug-metabolizing enzymes in alloxan-induced diabetic rats. *Toxicology*. 2002 May 24;17(2):131-39.

5215 Raner GM, Vaz AD, Coon MJ. Metabolism of all-trans, 9-cis, and 13-cis isomers of retinal by purified isozymes of microsomal cytochrome P450 and mechanism-based inhibition of retinoid oxidation by citral. *Mol Pharmacol*. 1996;49(3):515-22.

5216 De Olivera AC, Ribeiro-Pinto LF, Paumgartten JR. In vitro inhibition of CYP2B1 monoxygenase by beta-myrcene and other monoterpenoid constituents. *Br J Nutr*. 1999;81:289-95.

5217 Choi JY, Damte D, Seung-Jin L, et al. Antimicrobial activity of lemongrass and oregano essential oil against standard antibiotic resistant Staphylococcus aureus and field isolates from chronic mastitis cow. *International Journal of Phytomedicine*. 2012;4(1):134-39.

5218 Shin S, Lim S. Antifungal effects of herbal essential oils alone and in combination with ketoconazole against Trichophyton spp. *J Appl Micribiol*. 2004;97:1289-96.

5219 do Vale TG, Furtado EC, Santos JG Jr, et al. Central effects of citral, myrcene and limonene, constituents of essential oil chemotypes from Lippia alba (Mill.) n.e. Brown. *Phytomedicine*. 2002 Dec;9(8):709-14.

5220 Kuhn GO, McCampbell P, Singmaster G, et al. Application of microencapsulation technology to improve the stability of citral in rodent diets. *Fundam Appl Toxicol*. 1991 Oct;17(3):635-40.

5221 De Mozzi P, Johnston GA. An outbreak of allergic contact dermatitis caused by citral in beauticians working in a health spa. *Contact Dermatitis*. 2014 Jun;70(6):377-9.

5222 Burke BE, Baillie JE, Olson RD. Essential oil of Australian lemon myrtle (Backhousia citriodora) in the treatment of molluscum contagiosum in children. *Biomed Pharmacother*. 2004 May;58(4):245–47.

5223 Wilkinson JM, Hipwell M, Ryan T, et al. Bioactivity of Backhousia citriodora: antibacterial and antifungal activity. *J Agric Food Chem*. 2003 Jan;51(1):76–81.

5224 Hayes AJ, Markovic B. Toxicity of Australian essential oil Backhousia citriodora (Lemon myrtle). Part 1. Antimicrobial activity and in vitro toxicity. *Food Chem Toxicol*. 2002 Apr;40(4):535–43.

5225 Zouhir A, Jridi T, Nefzi A, et al. Inhibition of methicillin-resistant Staphylococcus aureus (MRSA) by antimicrobial peptides (AMPs) and plant essential oils. *Pharm Biol*. 2016 Dec;54(12):3136-3150.

5226 Lunguinho ADS, Cardoso MDG, Ferreira CRF, et al. Acaricidal and repellent activity of the essential oils of Backhousia citriodora, Callistemon viminalis and Cinnamodendron dinisii against Rhipicephalus spp. *Vet Parasitol*. 2021 Oct 13;300:109594.

5227 Lim AC, Tang SGH, Zin NM, et al. Chemical Composition, Antioxidant, Antibacterial, and Antibiofilm Activities of Backhousia citriodora Essential Oil. *Molecules*. 2022 Jul 31;27(15):4895.

5228 Kim E, Park IK. Fumigant Antifungal Activity of Myrtaceae Essential Oils and Constituents from Leptospermum petersonii against Three Aspergillus Species. *Molecules*. 2012;17:10459-69.

5229 Demuner AJ, Almeida Barbosa LC, Magalhaes CG, et al. Seasonal Variation in the Chemical Composition and Antimicrobial Activity of Volatile Oils of Three Species of Leptospermum (Myrtaceae) Grown in Brazil. *Molecules*. 2011;16:1181-91.

5230 Van Vuuren SF, Docrat Y, Kamatou GPP, et al. Essential oil composition and antimicrobial interactions of understudiedtea tree species. *South African J Botany*. 2014;92:7-14.

5231 Windsor SAM, Brooks P. Essential oils from Leptospermums of the Sunshine Coast and Northern Rivers Regions. *Chem Central J*. 2012;6:38.

5232 Nogueira AC, Carvalho RR, Souza CA, et al. Study on the embryofeto-toxicity of citral in the rat. *Toxicology*. 1995;96(2):105-13.

5233 Seo KA, Kim H, Ku HY, et al. The monoterpenoids citral and geraniol are moderate inhibitors of the CYP2B6 hydroxylase activity. *Chem Biol Interact*. 2008;174:141-46.

5234 Sheweita SA, Newairy AA, Mansour HA, et al. Effect of some hypoglycemic herbs on the activity of phase I and II drug-metabolizing enzymes in alloxan-induced diabetic rats. *Toxicology*. 2002 May 24;17(2):131-39.

5235 Raner GM, Vaz AD, Coon MJ. Metabolism of all-trans, 9-cis, and 13-cis isomers of retinal by purified isozymes of microsomal cytochrome P450 and mechanism-based inhibition of retinoid oxidation by citral. *Mol Pharmacol*. 1996;49(3):515-22.

5236 De Olivera AC, Ribeiro-Pinto LF, Paumgartten JR. In vitro inhibition of CYP2B1 monoxygenase by beta-myrcene and other monoterpenoid constituents. *Br J Nutr*. 1999;81:289-95.

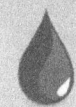

[5237] Modak T, Mukhopadhaya A. Effects of citral, a naturally occurring antiadipogenic molecule, on an energy-intense diet model of obesity. *Indian J Pharmacol.* 2011 May-Jun;43(3):300-05.
[5238] Najafian M, Ebrahim-Habibi A, Yaghmaei P, et al. Citral as a potential antihyperlipidemic medicine in diabetes: a study on streptozotocin-induced diabetic rats. *J Diabetes Metabolic Disorders.* 2011;10(1):3.
[5239] do Vale TG, Furtado EC, Santos JG Jr, et al. Central effects of citral, myrcene and limonene, constituents of essential oil chemotypes from Lippia alba (Mill.) n.e. Brown. *Phytomedicine.* 2002 Dec;9(8):709-14.
[5240] Zanini SF, Silva-Angulo AB, Rosenthal A, et al. Effect of citral and carvacrol on the susceptibility of Listeria monocytogenes and Listeria innocua to antibiotics. *Lett Appl Microbiol.* 2014 May;58(5):486-92.
[5241] Veras HN, Campos AR, Rodrigues FF, et al. Enhancement of the antibiotic activity of erythromycin by volatile constituents of Lippia alba (Mill.) N.E. Brown against Staphylococcus aureus. *Pharmacogn Mag.* 2011 Oct;7(28):334-7.
[5242] Kuhn GO, McCampbell P, Singmaster G, et al. Application of microencapsulation technology to improve the stability of citral in rodent diets. *Fundam Appl Toxicol.* 1991 Oct;17(3):635-40.
[5243] De Mozzi P, Johnston GA. An outbreak of allergic contact dermatitis caused by citral in beauticians working in a health spa. *Contact Dermatitis.* 2014 Jun;70(6):377-9.
[5244] Kim E1, Park IK. Fumigant antifungal activity of Myrtaceae essential oils and constituents from Leptospermum petersonii against three Aspergillus species. *Molecules.* 2012 Sep 3;17(9):10459-69.
[5245] Hood JR, Burton DM, Wilkinson JM, et al. The effect of Leptospermum petersonii essential oil on Candida albicans and Aspergillus fumigatus. *Med Mycol.* 2010 Nov;48(7):922-31.
[5246] Hood JR, Burton D, Wilkinson JM, et al. Antifungal activity of Leptospermum petersonii oil volatiles against Aspergillus spp. in vitro and in vivo. *J Antimicrob Chemother.* 2010 Feb;65(2):285-8.
[5247] Park MJ, Gwak KS, Yang I, et al. Antifungal activities of the essential oils in Syzygium aromaticum (L.) Merr. Et Perry and Leptospermum petersonii Bailey and their constituents against various dermatophytes. *J Microbiol.* 2007 Oct;45(5):460-5.
[5248] Atkinson N, Brice HE. Antibacterial substances produced by flowering plants. II. The antibacterial action of essential oils from some Australian plants. *Aust J Exp Biol Med Sci.* 1955 Oct;33(5):547-54.
[5249] Purwatiningsih, Heather N, Hassan E. Efficacy of Leptospermum petersonii oil, on Plutella xylostella, and its parasitoid, Trichogramma pretiosum. *J Econ Entomol.* 2012 Aug;105(4):1379-84.
[5250] Maguranyi SK, Webb CE, Mansfield S, et al. Are commercially available essential oils from Australian native plants repellent to mosquitoes? *J Am Mosq Control Assoc.* 2009 Sep;25(3):292-300.
[5251] Caputo L, Smeriglio A, Trombetta D, et al. Chemical Composition and Biological Activities of the Essential Oils of Leptospermum petersonii and Eucalyptus gunnii. *Front Microbiol.* 2020 Apr 15;11:409.
[5252] de Figueiredo RO, Stefanini MB, Ming LC, et al. Essential oil composition of Aloysia triphylla (L'Herit) Britton leaves cultivated in Botucatu, Sao Paulo Brazil. *ISHS Acta Horticulturae.* 2004;629:131-34.
[5253] Ozek T, Kirimer N, Baser KHC, et al. Composition of the essential oil of Aloysia triphylla (L'Herit) Britton grown in Turkey. *J Essent Oil Res.* 1996;8(5):581-85.
[5254] Gomes PCS, Oliveira HRC, Vicente AMS, et al. Production, transformation and essential oils composition of leaves and stems of lemon verbena [Aloysia triphylla (L'Herit.) Britton] grown in Portugal. *Rev Bras Pl Med.* 2006;8:130-35.
[5255] Nogueira AC, Carvalho RR, Souza CA, et al. Study on the embryofeto-toxicity of citral in the rat. *Toxicology.* 1995;96(2):105-13.
[5256] De Olivera AC, Ribeiro-Pinto LF, Paumgartten JR. In vitro inhibition of CYP2B1 monoxygenase by beta-myrcene and other monoterpenoid constituents. *Br J Nutr.* 1999;81:289-95.
[5257] Seo KA, Kim H, Ku HY, et al. The monoterpenoids citral and geraniol are moderate inhibitors of the CYP2B6 hydroxylase activity. *Chem Biol Interact.* 2008;174:141-46.
[5258] Raner GM, Vaz AD, Coon MJ. Metabolism of all-trans, 9-cis, and 13-cis isomers of retinal by purified isozymes of microsomal cytochrome P450 and mechanism-based inhibition of retinoid oxidation by citral. *Mol Pharmacol.* 1996;49(3):515-22.
[5259] Modak T, Mukhopadhaya A. Effects of citral, a naturally occurring antiadipogenic molecule, on an energy-intense diet model of obesity. *Indian J Pharmacol.* 2011 May-Jun;43(3):300-05.
[5260] Najafian M, Ebrahim-Habibi A, Yaghmaei P, et al. Citral as a potential antihyperlipidemic medicine in diabetes: a study on streptozotocin-induced diabetic rats. *J Diabetes Metabolic Disorders.* 2011;10(1):3.
[5261] Choi JY, Damte D, Seung-Jin L, et al. Antimicrobial activity of lemongrass and oregano essential oil against standard antibiotic resistant Staphylococcus aureus and field isolates from chronic mastitis cow. *International Journal of Phytomedicine.* 2012;4(1):134-39.
[5262] Shin S, Lim S. Antifungal effects of herbal essential oils alone and in combination with ketoconazole against Trichophyton spp. *J Appl Micribiol.* 2004;97:1289-96.
[5263] do Vale TG, Furtado EC, Santos JG Jr, et al. Central effects of citral, myrcene and limonene, constituents of essential oil chemotypes from Lippia alba (Mill.) n.e. Brown. *Phytomedicine.* 2002 Dec;9(8):709-14.
[5264] Kuhn GO, McCampbell P, Singmaster G, et al. Application of microencapsulation technology to improve the stability of citral in rodent diets. *Fundam Appl Toxicol.* 1991 Oct;17(3):635-40.
[5265] De Mozzi P, Johnston GA. An outbreak of allergic contact dermatitis caused by citral in beauticians working in a health spa. *Contact Dermatitis.* 2014 Jun;70(6):377-9.
[5266] Oukerrou MA, Tilaoui M, Ait Mouse H, et al. Differential in vitro antitumor activity of essential oil of Lippia citriodora from different regions in Morocco. *Chem Biodivers.* 2017 Jul;14(7).
[5267] Rojas J, Palacios O, Ronceros S. The effect of the essential oil from Aloysia triphylla britton (lemon verbena) on Trypanosoma cruzi in mice. *Rev Peru Med Exp Salud Publica.* 2012 Mar;29(1):61-68.
[5268] Escobar P, Leal SM, Herrera LV, et al. Chemical composition and antiprotozoal activities of Colombian Lippia spp essential oils and their major constituents. *Mem Inst Oswaldo Cruz.* 2010 Mar;105(2):0074-0276.
[5269] Ohno T, Kita M, Yaaoka Y, et al. Antimicrobial activity of essential oils against Helicobacter pylori. *Helicobacter.* 2003 Jun;8(3):207-15.
[5270] Gomez LA, Stashenko E, Ocazionez RE. Comparative study on in vitro activities of citral, limonene and essential oils from Lippia citriodora and L. alba on yellow fever virus. *Nat Prod Commun.* 2013 Feb;8(2):249-52.
[5271] Ocazionez RE, Meneses R, Torres FA, et al. Virucidal activity of Colombian Lippia essential oils on dengue virus replication in vitro. *Mem Inst Oswaldo Cruz.* 2010 Mar;105(3):304-09.
[5272] Oliva Mde L, Carezzano ME, Gallucci MN, et al. Antimycotic effect of the essential oil of Aloysia triphylla against Candida species obtained from human pathologies. *Nat Prod Commun.* 2011 Jul;6(7):1039-43.
[5273] Duarte MC, Figueira GM, Sartoratto A, et al. Anti-Candida activity of Brazilian medicinal plants. *J Ethnopharmacol.* 2005 Feb 28;97(2):305-11.
[5274] Demo M, de las Olivia M, Lopez ML, et al. Antimicrobial activity of essential oils obtained from aromatic plants of Argentina. *Pharm Biol.* 2005;43(2):129-34.
[5275] Ragone MI, Sella M, Conforti P, et al. The spasmolytic effect of Aloysia citridora, Palau (South American cedron) is partially due to its vitexin but not isovitexin on rat duodenums. *J Ethnopharmacol.* 2007 Sep;113(2):258-66.
[5276] Benelli G, Pavela R, Canale A, et al. Acute larvicidal toxicity of five essential oils (Pinus nigra, Hyssopus officinalis, Satureja montana, Aloysia citrodora and Pelargonium graveolens) against the filariasis vector Culex quinquefasciatus: Synergistic and antagonistic effects. *Parasitol Int.* 2017 Apr;66(2):166-171.
[5277] Castro KNC, Canuto KM, Brito ES, et al. In vitro efficacy of essential oils with different concentrations of 1,8-cineole against Rhipicephalus (Boophilus) microplus. *Rev Bras Parasitol Vet.* 2018 Apr-Jun;27(2):203-210.
[5278] Farahmandfar R, Asnaashari M, Pourshayegan M, et al. Evaluation of antioxidant properties of lemon verbena (Lippia citriodora) essential oil and its capacity in sunflower oil stabilization during storage time. *Food Sci Nutr.* 2018 Apr 2;6(4):983-990.
[5279] de Souza RC, da Costa MM, Baldisserotto B, et al. Antimicrobial and synergistic activity of essential oils of Aloysia triphylla and Lippia alba against Aeromonas spp. *Microb Pathog.* 2017 Dec;113:29-33.
[5280] Afrasiabian F, Mirabzadeh Ardakani M, Rahmani K, et al. Aloysia citriodora Palau (lemon verbena) for insomnia patients: A randomized, double-blind, placebo-controlled clinical trial of efficacy and safety. *Phytother Res.* 2019 Feb;33(2):350-359.
[5281] Quintero Ruiz N, Córdoba Campo Y, Stashenko EE, et al. Antigenotoxic Effect Against Ultraviolet Radiation-induced DNA Damage of the Essential Oils from Lippia Species. *Photochem Photobiol.* 2017 Jul;93(4):1063-1072.
[5282] Oukerrou MA, Tilaoui M, Mouse HA, et al. Chemical Composition and Cytotoxic and Antibacterial Activities of the Essential Oil of Aloysia citriodora Palau Grown in Morocco. *Adv Pharmacol Sci.* 2017;2017:7801924.
[5283] Oukerrou MA, Tilaoui M, Mouse HA, et al. Chemical Composition and Cytotoxic and Antibacterial Activities of the Essential Oil of Aloysia citriodora Palau Grown in Morocco. *Adv Pharmacol Sci.* 2017;2017:7801924.
[5284] Tanhaeian A, Nazifi N, Ahmadi FS, et al. Comparative study of antimicrobial activity between some medicine plants and recombinant Lactoferrin peptide against some pathogens of cultivated button mushroom. *Arch Microbiol.* 2020 Nov;202(9):2525-2532.
[5285] Jardat N, Hawash M, Abdulhasan MN, et al. Spectral characterization, antioxidant, antimicrobial, cytotoxic, and cyclooxygenase inhibitory activities of Aloysia citriodora essential oils collected from two Palestinian regions. *BMC Complement Med Ther.* 2021 May 17;21(1):143.
[5286] Spyridopoulou K, Aravidou T, Lampri E, et al. Antitumor Potential of Lippia citriodora Essential Oil in Breast Tumor-Bearing Mice. *Antioxidants (Basel).* 2021 May 30;10(6):875.
[5287] de Brito GA, de Oliveira PFR, de Andrade Silva CM, et al. Identification of Bioactive Compounds against Aedes aegypti (Diptera: Culicidae) by Bioassays and in Silico Assays. *Chem Biodivers.* Online ahead of print.
[5288] Quintero WL, Moreno EM, Pinto SML, et al. Immunomodulatory, trypanocide, and antioxidant properties of essential oil fractions of Lippia alba (Verbenaceae). *BMC Complement Med Ther.* 2021 Jul 2;21(1):187.
[5289] Pagotti MC, Candido ACBB, Marçal MG, et al. Trypanocidal Activity of Dysphania ambrosioides, Lippia alba, and Tetradenia riparia Essential Oils against Trypanosoma cruzi. *Chem Biodivers.* 2021 Dec;18(12):e2100678.
[5290] Gbneou JD, Ahounou JF, Akakpo HB, et al. Phytochemical composition of Cymbopogon citratus and Eucalyptus citriodora essential oils and their anti-inflammatory and analgesic properties on Wistar rats. *Mol Biol Rep.* 2013 Feb;40(2):1127-34.
[5291] Bassole IH, Lamien-Meda A, Bayala B, et al. Chemical composition and antimicrobial activity of Cymbopogon citratus and Cymbopogon giganteus essential oils alone and in combination. *Phytomedicine.* 211 Sep 15;18(12):107-74.
[5292] Zheljazkov VD, Cantrell CL, Astatkie T, et al. Lemongrass productivity, oil content, and composition as a function of nitrogen, sulfur, and harvest time. *Agronomy J.* 2010;103(3):805-12.

[5293] Tajidin NE, Ahmad Sh, Rsenani AB, et al. Chemical composition and citral content in lemongrass (Cymbopogon citratus) essential oil at three maturity stages. *African J Biotech*. 2012 Feb;11(11):2685-93.

[5294] Gupta AK, Ganjewala. A study on developmental changes in essential oil content and composition in Cymbopogon flexuosus cultivar Suvarna. *Acta Biologica Szegediensis*. 2015;59(2):119-125.

[5295] Bossou AD, Mangelinckx S, Yedomonhan H, et al. Chemical composition and insecticidal activity of plant essential oils from Benin against Anopheles gambiae (Giles). *Parasit Vectors*. 2013 Dec 3;6:337.

[5296] Nogueira AC, Carvalho RR, Souza CA, et al. Study on the embryofeto-toxicity of citral in the rat. *Toxicology*. 1995;96(2):105-13.

[5297] Delgado IF, Carvalho RR, Nogueira, et al. Study on embryofetotoxicity of b-myrcene in the rat. *Food and Chemical Toxicology*. 1993;31(1):31-5.

[5298] Seo KA, Kim H, Ku HY, et al. The monoterpenoids citral and geraniol are moderate inhibitors of the CYP2B6 hydroxylase activity. *Chem Biol Interact*. 2008;174:141-46.

[5299] Sheweita SA, Newairy AA, Mansour HA, et al. Effect of some hypoglycemic herbs on the activity of phase I and II drug-metabolizing enzymes in alloxan-induced diabetic rats. *Toxicology*. 2002 May 24;17(2):131-39.

[5300] Raner GM, Vaz AD, Coon MJ. Metabolism of all-trans, 9-cis, and 13-cis isomers of retinal by purified isozymes of microsomal cytochrome P450 and mechanism-based inhibition of retinoid oxidation by citral. *Mol Pharmacol*. 1996;49(3):515-22.

[5301] De Olivera AC, Ribeiro-Pinto LF, Paumgartten JR. In vitro inhibition of CYP2B1 monoxygenase by beta-myrcene and other monoterpenoid constituents. *Br J Nutr*. 1999;81:289-95.

[5302] Modak T, Mukhopadhaya A. Effects of citral, a naturally occurring antiadipogenic molecule, on an energy-intense diet model of obesity. *Indian J Pharmacol*. 2011 May-Jun;43(3):300-05.

[5303] Najafian M, Ebrahim-Habibi A, Yaghmaei P, et al. Citral as a potential antihyperlipidemic medicine in diabetes: a study on streptozotocin-induced diabetic rats. *J Diabetes Metabolic Disorders*. 2011;10(1):3.

[5304] Choi JY, Damte D, Seung-Jin L, et al. Antimicrobial activity of lemongrass and oregano essential oil against standard antibiotic resistant Staphylococcus aureus and field isolates from chronic mastitis cow. *International Journal of Phytomedicine*. 2012;4(1):134-39.

[5305] do Vale TG, Furtado EC, Santos JG Jr, et al. Central effects of citral, myrcene and limonene, constituents of essential oil chemotypes from Lippia alba (Mill.) n.e. Brown. *Phytomedicine*. 2002 Dec;9(8):709-14.

[5306] Kuhn GO, McCampbell P, Singmaster G, et al. Application of microencapsulation technology to improve the stability of citral in rodent diets. *Fundam Appl Toxicol*. 1991 Oct;17(3):635-40.

[5307] De Mozzi P, Johnston GA. An outbreak of allergic contact dermatitis caused by citral in beauticians working in a health spa. *Contact Dermatitis*. 2014 Jun;70(6):377-9.

[5308] Sharma PR, Mondhe DM, Muthiah S, et al. Anticancer activity of an essential oil from Cymbopogon flexuosus. *Chem Biol Interact*. 2009 May 15;179(2-3):160-68.

[5309] Bidinotto LT, Costa CA, Salvadori DM, et al. Protective effects of lemongrass (Cymbopogon citratus STAPF) essential oil on DNA damage and carcinogenesis in female Balb/C mice. *J Appl Toxicol*. 2011 Aug;31(6):536-44.

[5310] Kumar A, Malik F, Bhushan S, et al. An essential oil and its major constituent isointermedeol induce apoptosis by increased expression of mitochondrial cytochrome c and apical death receptors in human leukaemia HL-60 cells. *Chem Biol Interact*. 2008 Feb;171(3):332-47.

[5311] Sherry E, Boeck H, Warnke PH. Percutaneous treatment of chronic MRSA osteomyelitis with a novel plant-derived antiseptic. *BMC Surgery*. 2001;1:1.

[5312] Ohno T, Kita M, Yamaoka Y, et al. Antimicrobial activity of essential oils against Helicobacter pylori. *Helicobacter*. 2003 Jun;8(3):207-15.

[5313] Silva MR, Ximenes RM, da Costa JG, et al. Comparative anticonvulsant activities of the essential oil (Eos) from Cymbopogon winterianus Jowitt and Cymbopogon citratus (DC) Stapf. in mice. *Naunyn-Schmiedeberg's Arch Pharmacol*. 2010 May;381(5):415-26.

[5314] Mitoshi M, Kuriyama I, Nakayama H, et al. Suppression of allergic and inflammatory responses by essential oils derived from herbal plants and citrus fruits. *Int J Mol Med*. 2014 Jun;33(6):1643-51.

[5315] Khan MS, Ahmad I. Biofilm inhibition by Cymbopogon citratus and Syzygium aromaticum essential oils in the strains of Candida albicans. *J Ethnopharmacol*. 2012 Mar 27;140(2):416-23.

[5316] Tampieri MP, Galuppi R, Macchioni F, et al. The inhibition of Candida albicans by selected essential oils and their major components. *Mycopathologia*. 2005 Apr;159(3):339-45.

[5317] Tyagi AK, Malik A. Liquid and vapour-phase antifungal activities of selected essential oils against Candida albicans: microscopic observations and chemical characterizations of Cymbopogon citratus. *BMB Complement Altern Med*. 2010 Nov;10:65.

[5318] Amornvit P, Choonharuangdej S, Srithavaj T. Lemongrass-incorporated tissue conditioner against Candida albicans culture. *J Clin Diagn Res*. 2014 Jul;8(7):ZC50-52.

[5319] Choonharuangdej S, Amornvit P, Srithavaj T, et al. Lemongrass-Incorporated Tissue Conditioner Against Candida albicans Culture. *J Clin Diag Res*. 2015 Jul;8(7):50-52.

[5320] Iqbal Z, Zafar MS. Role of antifungal medicaments added to tissue conditioners: A systematic review. J Prosthodont Res. 2016 Oct;60(4):231-239.

[5321] Abe S, Sato Y, Inoue S, et al. Anti-Candida albicans activity of essential oils including lemongrass (Cymbopogon citratus) oil and its component, citral. *Nihon Ishinkin Gakkai Zasshi*. 2003;44(4):285-91.

[5322] Bonferoni MC, Sandri G, Rossi S, et al. A novel ionic amphiphilic chitosan derivative as a stabilizer of nanoemulsions: Improvement of antimicrobial activity of Cymbopogon citratus essential oil. *Colloids Surf B Biointerfaces*. 2017 Jan 24;152:385-392.

[5323] Tayebook GS, Tavakoli F, Hassani S, et al. Effects of Cymbopogon citratus and Ferula assa-foetida extracts on glutamate-induced neurotoxicity. *In Vitro Cell Dev Biol Anim*. 2013 Oct;49(9):706-15.

[5324] Dutta BK, Karmakar S, Naglot A, et al. Anticandidal activity of some essential oils of a mega biodiversity hotspot in India. *Mycoses*. 2007 Mar;50(2):121-24.

[5325] Warnke PH, Becker ST, Podschun R, et al. The battle against multi-resistant strains: Renaissance of antimicrobial essential oils as a promising force to fight hospital-acquired infections. *J Craniomaxillofac Surg*. 2009 Oct;37(7):392-97.

[5326] Inouye S, Takizawa T, Yamaguchi H. Antibacterial activity of essential oils and their major constituents against respiratory tract pathogens by gaseous contact. *J Antimicrobi Chemother*. 2001 May;47(5):565-73.

[5327] Tadtong S, Watthanachaiyingcharoen R, Kamkaen N. Antimicrobial constituents and synergism effect of the essential oils from Cymbopogon citratus and Alpinia galanga. *Nat Prod Commun*. 2014 Feb;9(2):277-80.

[5328] Adukwu EC, Bowles M, Edwards-Jones V, et al. Antimicrobial activity, cytotoxicity and chemical analysis of lemongrass essential oil (Cymbopogon flexuosus) and pure citral. *Appl Microbiol Biotechnol*. 2016 Nov;100(22):9619-9627.

[5329] Irkin R, Korukluoglu M. Effectiveness of Cymbopogon citratus L. essential oil to inhibit the growth of some filamentous fungi and yeasts. *J Med Food*. 2009 Feb;12(1):193-97.

[5330] Dias N, Dias MC, Cavaleiro C, et al. Oxygenated monoterpenes-rich volatile oils as potential antifungal agents for dermatophytes. *Nat Prod Res*. 2016 Jun 16:1-5.

[5331] Sivamani P, Singaravelu G, Thiagarajan V, et al. Comparative molecular docking analysis of essential oil constituents as elastase inhibitors. *Bioinformation*. 2012;8(10):457-60.

[5332] Soonwera M, Phasomkusolsil S. Efficacy of Thai herbal essential oils as green repellent against mosquito vectors. *Acta Trop*. 2015 Feb;142:127-30.

[5333] Carmo ES, Pereira Fde O, Cavalcante NM, et al. Treatment of pityriasis versicolor with topical application of essential oil of Cymbopogon citratus (DC) Stapf - therapeutic pilot study. *An Bras Dermatol*. 2013 May-Jun;88(3):381-85.

[5334] Warad SB, Kolar SS, Kalburgi V, et al. Lemongrass essential oil gel as a local drug delivery agent for the treatment of periodontitis. *Anc Scie Life*. 2013 Apr;32(4):205-11.

[5335] Fernandes C, De Souza H, De Oliveria G, et al. Investigation of the mechanisms underlying the gastroprotective effect of Cymbopogon citratus essential oil. *J Young Pharm*. 2012 Jan;4(1):28-32.

[5336] Kaur CD, Saraf S. In vitro sun protection factor determination of herbal oils used in cosmetics. *Pharmacognosy Res*. 2010 Jan;2(1):22-25.

[5337] Gbenou JD, Ahounou JF, Akakpo HB, et al. Phytochemical composition of Cymbopogon citratus and Eucalyptus citriodora essential oils and their anti-inflammatory and analgesic properties on Wistar rats. *Mol Biol Rep*. 2013 Feb;40(2):1127-34.

[5338] Viana GS, Vale TG, Pinho RS, et al. Antinociceptive effect of the essential oil from Cymbopogon citratus in mice. *J Ethnopharmacol*. 2000 Jun;70(3):323-27.

[5339] Machado M, Pires P, Dinis AM, Monoterpenic aldehydes as potential anti-Leishmania agents: activity of Cymbopogon citratus and citral on L. infantum, L. tropica and L. major. *Exp Parasitol*. 2012 Mar;130(3):223-31.

[5340] Santin MR, dos Santos AO, Nakamura CV, et al. In vitro activity of the essential oil of Cymbopogon citratus and its major component (citral) on Leishmania amazonensis. *Parasitol Res*. 2009 Nov;105(6):1489-96.

[5341] Oliveira VC, Moura DM, Lopes JA, et al. Effects of essential oils from Cymbopogon citratus (DC) Stapf., Lippia sidoides Cham., and Ocimum gratissimum L. on growth and ultrastructure of Leishmania chagasi Promastigotes. *Parasitol Res*. 2009 Apr;104(5):153-59.

[5342] Blasi DV, Debrot S, Menound PA, Gendre L, Schowing J. Amoebicidal effect of essential oils *in vitro*. J Toxicol Clin Exp. 1990;10:361-73.

[5343] Bidnotto LT, Costa CA, Costa M, et al. Modifying effects of lemongrass essential oil on specific tissue response to the carcinogen N-methyl-N-nitrosurea in female BALB/c mice. *J Med Food*. 2012 Feb;15(2):161-68.

[5344] Costa CA, Kohn DO, de Lima VM, et al. The GABAergic system contributes to the anxiolytic-like effect of essential oil from Cymbopogon citratus (lemongrass). *J Ethnopharmacol*. 211 Sep;137(1):828-36.

[5345] Wuthi-Udomlert M, Chotipatoomwam P, Panyadee S, et al. Inhibitory effect of formulated lemongrass shampoo on Malassezia furfur: a yeast associated with dandruff. *Southeast Asian J Trop Med Public Health*. 2011 Mar;42(2):363-69.

[5346] Costa CA, Bidnotto LT, Takahira RK, et al. Cholesterol reduction and lack of genotoxic or toxic effects in mice after repeated 21-day oral intake of lemongrass (Cymbopogon citratus) essential oil. *Food Chem Toxicol*. 2011 Sep;49(9):2268-72.

[5347] Sforcin JM, Amaral JT, Fernandes A Jr, et al. Lemongrass effects on IL-1beta and IL-6 production by macrophages. *Nat Prod Res*. 2009;23(12):1151-59.

[5348] Katsukawa M, Nakata R, Takizawa Y, et al. Citral, a component of lemongrass oil, activates PPARa and y and suppressed COX-2 expression. *Biochem Biophys Acta*. 2010 Nov;1801(110:1214-20.

[5349] Santoro GF, Cardoso MG, Guimaraes LG, et al. Anti-proliferative effect of the essential oil of Cymbopogon citratus (DC) Stapf (lemongrass) on intracellular amastigotes, bloodstream trypomastigotes and culture epimastigotes of Trypanosoma cruzi (Protozoa: Kinetoplastida). *Parasitology*. 2007 Oct;134(Pt 11):1649-56.

[5350] Blanco MM, Costa CA, Freire AO, et al. Neurobehavioral effect of essential oil of Cymbopogon citratus in mice. *Phytomedicine*. 2009 Mar;16(2-3):265-70.

[5351] Bharti SK, Kumar A, Prakash O, et al. Essential Oil of Cymbopogon Citratus Against Diabetes: Validation by In vivo Experiments and Computational Studies. *J Bioanal Biomed*. 2013;5:194-203.

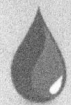

[5352] Bharti SK, Kumar A, Prakash O, et al. Essential Oil of Cymbopogon Citratus Against Diabetes: Validation by In vivo Experiments and Computational Studies. *J Bioanal Biomed.* 2013;5:194-203.

[5353] Inouye S, Yamaguchi H, Takizawa. Screening of the antibacterial effects of a variety of essential oils on respiratory tract pathogens, using a modified dilution assay method. *J Infect Chemother.* 201 Dec;7(4):251-54.

[5354] Tchoumbougnang F, Zollo PH, Dagne E, et al. In vivo antimalarial activity of essential oil from Cymbopogon citratus and Ocimum gratissium on mice infected with Plasmodium berghei. *Planta Med.* 2005 Jan;71(1):20-23.

[5355] Pereira RS, Sumita TC, Furlan MR, et al. Antibacterial activity of essential oils on microorganisms isolated from urinary tract infection. *Rev Saude Publica.* 2004 Apr;38(2):326-28.

[5356] Karbach J, Ebenezer S, Warnke PH, et al. Antimicrobial effect of Australian antibacterial essential oils as alternative to common antiseptic solutions against clinically relevant oral pathogens. *Clin Lab.* 2015;61(1-2):61-68.

[5357] De Oliveira TL, Soares Rde A, Piccoli RH. A Weibull model to describe antimicrobial kinetics of oregano and lemongrass oils against Salmonella Enteritidis in ground beef during refrigerated storage. *Meat Sci.* 2013 Mar;93(3):645-51.

[5358] Onawunmi GO. In vitro studies on the antibacterial activity of phenoxyethanol in combination with lemongrass oil. *Pharmazie.*1988 Jan;43(1):42-44.

[5359] Chaisripipat W, Lourith N, Kanlayavattanakul M. Anti-dandruff hair tonic containing lemongrass (Cymbopogon flexuosus) oil. *Forsch Komplementmed.* 2015;22(4):226-29.

[5360] Dany SS, Mohanty P, Tangade P, et al. Efficacy of 0.25% lemongrass oil mouthwash: A three arm prospective parallel clinical study. *J Clin Diagn Res.* 2015 Oct;9(10):ZC13-17.

[5361] Azad MF, Schwiertz A, Jentsch HF. Adjunctive use of essential oils following scaling and root planing -a randomized clinical trial. *BMC Complement Altern Med.* 2016 Jun 7;16(1):171.

[5362] Goes TC, Ursulino FR, Almeida-Souza TH, et al. Effect of lemongrass aroma on experimental anxiety in humans. *J Altern Complement Med.* 2015 Dec;21(12):766-73.

[5363] Adukwu EC, Bowles M, Edwards-Jones V, et al. Antimicrobial activity, cytotoxicity and chemical analysis of lemongrass essential oil (Cymbopogon flexuosus) and pure citral. *Appl Microbiol Biotechnol.* 2016 Nov;100(22):9619-9627.

[5364] Soonwera M, Phasomkusolsil S. Effect of Cymbopogon citratus (lemongrass) and Syzygium aromaticum (clove) oils on the morphology and mortality of Aedes aegypti and Anopheles dirus larvae. *Parasitol Res.* 2016 Apr;115(4):1691-703.

[5365] Bossou AD, Mangelinckx S, Yedomonhan H, et al. Chemical composition and insecticidal activity of plant essential oils from Benin against Anopheles gambiae (Giles). *Parasit Vectors.* 2013 Dec 3;6:337.

[5366] Tofiño-Rivera A, Ortega-Cuadros M, Galvis-Pareja D, et al. Effect of Lippia alba and Cymbopogon citratus essential oils on biofilms of Streptococcus mutans and cytotoxicity in CHO cells. *J Ethnopharmacol.* 2016 Dec 24;194:749-754.

[5367] Mishra S, Kumar P, Malik A, et al. Microscopic investigation to determine the effect of Beauveria bassiana (Bals.) Vuill. and Cymbopogon citratus (DC.) Stapf. treatment on different life stages of Musca domestica (L.). *J Parasit Dis.* 2017 Jun;41(2):543-550.

[5368] De Silva BCJ, Jung WGl, Hossain S, et al. Antimicrobial property of lemongrass (Cymbopogon citratus) oil against pathogenic bacteria isolated from pet turtles. *Lab Anim Res.* 2017 Jun;33(2):84-91.

[5369] Luis Â, Duarte AP, Pereira L, et al. Chemical Profiling and Evaluation of Antioxidant and Anti-Microbial Properties of Selected Commercial Essential Oils: A Comparative Study. *Medicines (Basel).* 2017 Jun 5;4(2).

[5370] Rossi GG, Guterres KB, Bonez PC, et al. Antibiofilm activity of nanoemulsions of Cymbopogon flexuosus against rapidly growing mycobacteria. *Microb Pathog.* 2017 Nov 6;113:335-341.

[5371] Costa S, Cavadas C, Cavaleiro C, et al. In vitro susceptibility of Trypanosoma brucei brucei to selected essential oils and their major components. *Exp Parasitol.* 2018 Jul;190:34-40.

[5372] Oliveira MAC, Borges AC, Brighenti FL, et al. Cymbopogon citratus essential oil: effect on polymicrobial caries-related biofilm with low cytotoxicity. *Braz Oral Res.* 2017 Nov 6;31:e89.

[5373] Giordana F, Nicola M, Valentina C, et al. Chemical composition of essential oils from Thymus vulgaris, Cymbopogon citratus and Rosmarinus officinalis and their effects on the HIV-1 Tat protein function. *Chem Biodivers.* 2018 Feb;15(2).

[5374] Venzon L, Mariano LNB, Somensi LB, et al. Essential oil of Cymbopogon citratus (lemongrass) and geraniol, but not citral, promote gastric healing activity in mice. *Biomed Pharmacother.* 2017 Dec 14;98:118-124.

[5375] Li CC, Yu HF, Chang CH, et al. Effects of lemongrass oil and citral on hepatic drug-metabolizing enzymes, oxidative stress, and acetaminophen toxicity in rats. *J Food Drug Anal.* 2018 Jan;26(1):432-438.

[5376] Bayala B, Bassole IHN, Maqdasy S, et al. Cymbopogon citratus and Cymbopogon giganteus essential oils have cytotoxic effects on tumor cell cultures. Identification of citral as a new putative anti-proliferative molecule. *Biochimie.* 2018 Oct;153:162-170.

[5377] Mani López E, Valle Vargas GP, Palou E, et al. Penicillium expansum Inhibition on Bread by Lemongrass Essential Oil in Vapor Phase. *J Food Prot.* 2018 Feb 23:467-471.

[5378] Ralambondrainy M, Belarbi E, Viranaicken W, et al. In vitro comparison of three common essential oils mosquito repellents as inhibitors of the Ross River virus. *PLoS One.* 2018 May 17;13(5):e0196757.

[5379] Koseki Y, Tanaka R, Murata H. Development of antibacterial denture cleaner for brushing containing tea tree and lemongrass essential oils. *Dent Mater J.* 2018 Jul 29;37(4):659-666.

[5380] Gaonkar R, Shiralgi Y, Lakkappa DB, et al. Essential oil from Cymbopogon flexuosus as the potential inhibitor for HSP90. *Toxicol Rep.* 2018 Apr 5;5:489-496.

[5381] Damos PT. An in vitro ULV olfactory bioassay method for testing the repellent activity of essential oils against moths. *MethodsX.* 2018 Apr 20;5:375-394.

[5382] Vasireddy L, Bingle LEH, Davies MS. Antimicrobial activity of essential oils against multidrug-resistant clinical isolates of the Burkholderia cepacia complex. *PLoS One.* 2018 Aug 2;13(8):e0201835.

[5383] Quendera AP, Barreto AS, Semedo-Lemsaddek T. Antimicrobial activity of essential oils against foodborne multidrug-resistant enterococci and aeromonads in planktonic and biofilm state. *Food Sci Technol Int.* 2018 Sep 7:1082013218799027.

[5384] Powers CN, Osier JL, McFeeters RL, et al. Antifungal and Cytotoxic Activities of Sixty Commercially-Available Essential Oils. *Molecules.* 2018 Jun 27;23(7).

[5385] Gabriel KT, Kartforosh L, Crow SA Jr, et al. Antimicrobial Activity of Essential Oils Against the Fungal Pathogens Ascosphaera apis and Pseudogymnoascus destructans. *Mycopathologia.* 2018 Dec;183(6):921-934.

[5386] Zouhir A, Jridi T, Nefzi A, et al. Inhibition of methicillin-resistant Staphylococcus aureus (MRSA) by antimicrobial peptides (AMPs) and plant essential oils. *Pharm Biol.* 2016 Dec;54(12):3136-3150.

[5387] Brügger BP, Martínez LC, Plata-Rueda A, et al. Bioactivity of the Cymbopogon citratus (Poaceae) essential oil and its terpenoid constituents on the predatory bug, Podisus nigrispinus (Heteroptera: Pentatomidae). *Sci Rep.* 2019 Jun 7;9(1):8358.

[5388] Oliveira JB, Teixeira MA, Paiva LF, et al. In Vitro and In Vivo Antimicrobial Activity of Cymbopogon citratus (DC.) Stapf. Against Staphylococcus spp. Isolated from Newborn Babies in an Intensive Care Unit. *Microb Drug Resist.* 2019 Dec;25(10):1490-1496.

[5389] Macedo ITF, Oliveira LMB, André WPP, et al. Anthelmintic effect of Cymbopogon citratus essential oil and its nanoemulsion on sheep gastrointestinal nematodes. *Rev Bras Parasitol Vet.* 2019 Aug 29;28(3):522-527.

[5390] Kozics K, Buckova M, Puskarova A, et al. The Effect of Ten Essential Oils on Several Cutaneous Drug-Resistant Microorganisms and Their Cyto/Genotoxic and Antioxidant Properties. *Molecules.* 2019 Dec 13;24(24):24244570.

[5391] Krzyško-Łupicka T, Sokół S, Piekarska-Stachowiak A. Evaluation of Fungistatic Activity of Eight Selected Essential Oils on Four Heterogeneous Fusarium Isolates Obtained From Cereal Grains in Southern Poland. *Molecules.* 2020 Jan 10;25(2):292.

[5392] Korona-Glowniak I, Glowniak-Lipa A, Ludwiczuk A, et al. The In Vitro Activity of Essential Oils Against Helicobacter Pylori Growth and Urease Activity. *Molecules.* 2020 Jan 29;25(3):586.

[5393] Ortega-Ramirez LA, Gutierrez-Pacheco MM, Vargas-Arispuro I, et al. Inhibition of Glucosyltransferase Activity and Glucan Production as an Antibiofilm Mechanism of Lemongrass Essential Oil Against Escherichia coli O157:H7. *Antibiotics (Basel).* 2020 Feb 29;9(3).

[5394] Xiao S, Cui P, Shi W, et al. Identification of essential oils with activity against stationary phase Staphylococcus aureus. *BMC Complement Med Ther.* 2020 Mar 24;20(1):99.

[5395] Soonwera M, Sittichok S. Adulticidal activities of Cymbopogon citratus (Stapf.) and Eucalyptus globulus (Labill.) essential oils and of their synergistic combinations against Aedes aegypti (L.), Aedes albopictus (Skuse), and Musca domestica (L.). *Environ Sci Pollut Res Int.* 2020 Apr 1. [Epub ahead of print]

[5396] Li M, Liu B, Bernigaud C, et al. Lemongrass (Cymbopogon citratus) oil: A promising miticidal and ovicidal agent against Sarcoptes scabiei. *PLoS Negl Trop Dis.* 2020 Apr 6;14(4):e0008225.

[5397] Agwunobi DO, Pei T, Wang K1, et al. Effects of the essential oil from Cymbopogon citratus on mortality and morphology of the tick Haemaphysalis longicornis (Acari: Ixodidae). *Exp Appl Acarol.* 2020 Apr 3. [Epub ahead of print]

[5398] Kozics K, Buckova M, Puskarova A, et al. The Effect of Ten Essential Oils on Several Cutaneous Drug-Resistant Microorganisms and Their Cyto/Genotoxic and Antioxidant Properties. *Molecules.* 2019 Dec 13;24(24):4570.

[5399] Plata-Rueda A, Rolim GDS, Wilcken CF, et al. Acute Toxicity and Sublethal Effects of Lemongrass Essential Oil and Their Components Against the Granary Weevil, Sitophilus granaries. *Insects.* 2020 Jun 18;11(6):E379.

[5400] Ngo-Mback MNL, Babii C, Jazet Dongmo PM, et al. Anticandidal and synergistic effect of essential oil fractions from three aromatic plants used in Cameroon. *J Mycol Med.* 2020 Mar 3:100940.

[5401] Sahal G, Woerdenbag HJ, Hinrichs WLJ, et al. Antifungal and biofilm inhibitory effect of Cymbopogon citratus (lemongrass) essential oil on biofilm forming by Candida tropicalis isolates; an in vitro study. *J Ethnopharmacol.* 2019 Aug 27:112188.

[5402] Hacke ACM, Miyoshi E, Marques JA, et al. Anxiolytic Properties of Cymbopogon Citratus (DC.) Stapf Extract, Essential Oil and Its Constituents in Zebrafish (Danio Rerio). *J Ethnopharmacol.* 2020 May 27;113036.

[5403] Trang DT, Hoang TKV, Nguyen TTM, et al. Essential Oils of Lemongrass ( Cymbopogon citratus Stapf) Induces Apoptosis and Cell Cycle Arrest in A549 Lung Cancer Cells. *Biomed Res Int.* 2020 Jan 11;2020:5924856.

[5404] Rojas-Armas JP, Arroyo-Acevedo JL, Palomino-Pacheco M, et al. The Essential Oil of Cymbopogon citratus Stapt and Carvacrol: An Approach of the Antitumor Effect on 7,12-Dimethylbenz-[α]-anthracene (DMBA)-Induced Breast Cancer in Female Rats. *Molecules.* 2020 Jul 20;25(14):E3284.

[5405] Temitayo GI, Olawande B, Emmanuel YO, et al. Inhibitory potentials of Cymbopogon citratus oil against aluminium-induced behavioral deficits and neuropathology in rats. *Anat Cell Biol.* 2020 Aug 25. Online ahead of print.

[5406] Pereira EC, Oliveira EC, Sousa EMO, et al. Lethal concentration of Cymbopogon citratus (Poaceae) essential oil for Dolops discoidalis and Argulus sp. (Crustacea: Argulidae). *J Fish Dis.* 2020 Sep 13. Online ahead of print.

[5407] da Silva LC, de Souza Perinoot WM, Sa FA, et al. In vitro acaricidal activity of Cymbopogon citratus, Cymbopogon nardus and Mentha arvensis against Rhipicephalus microplus (Acari: Ixodidae). *Exp Parasitol.* 2020 Sep;216:107937.

[5408] Elazab ST, Soliman AF, Nishikawa Y. Effect of some plant extracts from Egyptian herbal plants against Toxoplasma gondii tachyzoites in vitro. *J Vet Med Sci.* 2020 Dec 1. Online ahead of print.

[5409] Gao S, Liu G, Li J, et al. Antimicrobial Activity of Lemongrass Essential Oil (Cymbopogon flexuosus) and Its Active Component Citral Against Dual-Species Biofilms of Staphylococcus aureus and Candida Species. *Front Cell Infect Microbiol.* 2020 Dec 22;10:603858.

[5410] Martins WDS, de Arajuo JSF, Feitosa BF, et al. Lemongrass (Cymbopogon citratus DC. Stapf) essential oil microparticles: Development, characterization, and antioxidant potential. *Food Chem.* 2021 Mar 22;355:129644.

[5411] Choonharuangdej S, Srithavaj T, Thummawanit S. Fungicidal and inhibitory efficacy of cinnamon and lemongrass essential oils on Candida albicans biofilm established on acrylic resin: An in vitro study. *J Prosthet Dent.* 2021 Apr;125(4):707.e1-707.e6.

[5412] Hacke ACM, Miyoshi E, Marques JA, et al. Cymbopogon citratus (DC.) Stapf, citral and geraniol exhibit anticonvulsant and neuroprotective effects in pentylenetetrazole-induced seizures in zebrafish. *J Ethnopharmacol.* 2021 Apr 25;275:114142.

[5413] Pereira EC, Oliveira EC, Sousa EMO, et al. Lethal concentration of Cymbopogon citratus (Poaceae) essential oil for Dolops discoidalis and Argulus sp. (Crustacea: Argulidae). *J Fish Dis.* 2020 Dec;43(12):1497-1504.

[5414] Ngamdokmai N, Paracha TU, Waranuch N, et al. Effects of Essential Oils and Some Constituents from Ingredients of Anti-Cellulite Herbal Compress on 3T3-L1 Adipocytes and Rat Aortae. *Pharmaceuticals (Basel).* 2021 Mar 11;14(3):253.

[5415] Meenapriya M, Priya J. Effect of Lemongrass Oil on Rheumatoid Arthritis. *Pharm Sci Res.* 2017;9(2):237-9.

[5416] Marinkovic J, Nikolic B, Markovic T, et al. Cymbopogon citratus essential oil: an active principle of nanoemulsion against Enterococcus faecalis root canal biofilm. *Future Microbiol.* 2021 Aug;16:907-918.

[5417] Kobenan KC, Bini KKN, Kouakou M, et al. Chemical composition and spectrum of insecticidal activity of the essential oils of Ocimumgratissimum L. and Cymbopogoncitratus Stapf on the main insects of the cotton entomofauna in Côte d'Ivoire. *Chem Biodivers.* 2021 Aug 27. Online ahead of print.

[5418] Moustafa MAM, Awad M, Amer A, et al. Insecticidal Activity of Lemongrass Essential Oil as an Eco-Friendly Agent against the Black Cutworm Agrotis ipsilon (Lepidoptera: Noctuidae). *Insects.* 2021 Aug 17;12(8):737.

[5419] Silva FDOE, Soares JCM, Valdez A, et al. Cymbopogon citratus protects erythrocytes from lipid peroxidation in vitro. *Cardiovasc Hematol Agents Med Chem.* 2021 Sep 6. Online ahead of print.

[5420] Selvati Rezende DADC, Cardoso MDG, Alves E, et al. Effect of the essential oils of Satureja montana L., Myristica fragrans H. and Cymbopogon flexuosus S. on mycotoxin-producing Aspergillus flavus and Aspergillus ochraceus Antifungal properties of essential oils. *FEMS Microbiol Lett.* 2021 Oct 30;fnab137.

[5421] Yan J, Wu H, Chen K, et al. Antifungal Activities and Mode of Action of Cymbopogon citratus, Thymus vulgraris, and Origanum heracleoticum Essential Oil Vapors against Botrytis cinerea and Their Potential Application to Control Postharvest Strawberry Gray Mold. *Foods.* 2021 Oct 15;10(10):2451.

[5422] Shzryna S, Anisah N, Saleh I, et al. Acaricidal activity of the essential oils from Citrus hystrix (Rutaceae) and Cymbopogon citratus (Poaceae) on the cattle tick Rhipicephalus (Boophilus) microplus larvae (Acari: Ixodidae). *Trop Biomed.* 2020 Jun 1;37(2):433-442.

[5423] Agwunobi DO, Zhang M, Zhang X, et al. Transcriptome profile of Haemaphysalis longicornis (Acari: Ixodidae) exposed to Cymbopogon citratus essential oil and citronellal suggest a cytotoxic mode of action involving mitochondrial Ca 2+ overload and depolarization. *Pestic Biochem Physiol.* 2021 Nov;179:104971.

[5424] Salaria D, Rolta R, Sharma N, et al. In vitro and in silico antioxidant and anti-inflammatory potential of essential oil of Cymbopogon citratus (DC.) Stapf. of North-Western Himalaya. *J Biomol Struct Dyn.* 2022;40(24):14131-14145.

[5425] Wang MX, Wei A, Yuan J, et al. Expression and regulation of peroxiredoxin 5 in human osteoarthritis. *FEBS Lett.* 2002;531:359-362.

[5426] Wang MX, Wei A, Yuan J, et al. Antioxidant enzyme peroxiredoxin 5 is upregulated in degenerative human tendon. *Biochem Biophys Res Commun.* 2001;284:667-673.

[5427] Uzawa A, Kawaguchi N, Kanai T, et al. Increased serum peroxiredoxin 5 levels in myasthenia gravis. *J Neuroimmun.* 2015 Oct 15;287:16-18.

[5428] Abruzzo PM, Matte A, Bolotta A, et al. Plasma peroxiredoxin changes and inflammatory cytokines support the involvement of neuro-inflammation and oxidative stress in Autism Spectrum Disorder. *J Transl Med.* 2019 Oct 2;17(1):332.

[5429] Mat-Rani S, Chotprasert N, Srimaneekarn N, et al. Fungicidal Effect of Lemongrass Essential Oil on Candida albicans Biofilm Pre-established on Maxillofacial Silicone Specimens. *J Int Soc Prev Community Dent.* 2021 Aug 13;11(5):525-530.

[5430] Sprenger S, Woldemariam T, Kotchoni S, et al. Lemongrass essential oil and its major constituent citral isomers modulate adipogenic gene expression in 3T3-L1 cells. *J Food Biochem.* 2022 Jan 3:e14037.

[5431] Piasecki B, Biernasiuk A, Skiba A, et al. Composition, Anti-MRSA Activity and Toxicity of Essential Oils from Cymbopogon Species. *Molecules.* 2021 Dec 13;26(24):7542.

[5432] Castillo-Morales RM, Serrano SO, Villamizar ALR, et al. Impact of Cymbopogon flexuosus (Poaceae) essential oil and primary components on the eclosion and larval development of Aedes aegypti. *Sci Rep.* 2021 Dec 21;11(1):24291.

[5433] Kumar A, Singh PP, Prakash B. Assessing the efficacy of chitosan nanomatrix incorporated with Cymbopogon citratus (DC.) Stapf essential oil against the food-borne molds and aflatoxin B1 production in food system. *Pestic Biochem Physiol.* 2022 Jan;180:105001.

[5434] Ishijima SA, Ezawa K, Abe S. Lemongrass and Perilla Essential Oils Synergistically Increased Antimicrobial Activity. *Med Mycol J.* 2021;62(4):79-87.

[5435] Paiva LF, Teixeira-Loyola ABA, Schnaider TB, et al. Association of the essential oil of Cymbopogon citratus (DC) Stapf with nystatin against oral cavity yeasts. *An Acad Bras Cienc.* 2022 Feb 18;94(1):e20200681.

[5436] Sharma AD, Kaur I. Essential oil from Cymbopogon citratus exhibits "anti-aspergillosis" potential: in-silico molecular docking and in vitro studies. *Bull Natl Res Cent.* 2022;46(1):23.

[5437] Brandão RM, Cardoso MDG, de Oliveira JE, et al. Antifungal and antiocratoxigenic potential of Alpinia speciosa and Cymbopogon flexuosus essential oils encapsulated in poly(lactic acid) nanofibers against Aspergillus fungi. *Lett Appl Microbiol.* 2022 Mar 21. Online ahead of print.

[5438] de Oliveira Alencar DD, de Souza EL, da Cruz Almeida ET, et al. Microencapsulation of Cymbopogon citratus D.C. Stapf Essential Oil with Spray Drying: Development, Characterization, and Antioxidant and Antibacterial Activities. *Foods.* 2022 Apr 13;11(8):1111.

[5439] Radünz AL, Radünz M, Bizollo AR, et al. Insecticidal and repellent activity of native and exotic lemongrass on Maize weevil. *Braz J Biol.* 2022 Apr 8;84:e252990.

[5440] Yasir M, Nawaz A, Ghazanfar S, et al. Anti-bacterial activity of essential oils against multidrug-resistant foodborne pathogens isolated from raw milk. *Braz J Biol.* 2022 May 9;84:e259449.

[5441] da Silva AMS, Chagas EC, Chaves FCM, et al. Prospecting of essential oils in combination with florfenicol against motile Aeromonas isolated from tambaqui (Colossoma macropomum). *Arch Microbiol.* 2022 Jun 15;204(7):392.

[5442] Kabotso DEK, Neglo D, Kwashie P, et al. GC/MS Composition and Resistance Modulatory Inhibitory Activities of Three Extracts of Lemongrass: Citral Modulates the Activities of Five Antibiotics at Sub-Inhibitory Concentrations on Methicillin-Resistant Staphylococcus aureus. *Chem Biodivers.* 2022 Aug 26:e202200296.

[5443] Jin C, Han H, Xie Y, et al. Toxicity, Behavioral Effects, and Chitin Structural Chemistry of Reticulitermes flaviceps Exposed to Cymbopogon citratus EO and Its Major Constituent Citral. *Insects.* 2022 Sep 6;13(9):812.

[5444] Mouta LFGL, Marques RS, Koga-Ito CY, et al. Cymbopogon citratus Essential Oil Increases the Effect of Digluconate Chlorhexidine on Microcosm Biofilms. *Pathogens.* 2022 Sep 20;11(10):1067.

[5445] de Melo AM, Barbi RCT, Chaves Almeida FL, et al. Effect of Microencapsulation on Chemical Composition and Antimicrobial, Antioxidant and Cytotoxic Properties of Lemongrass (Cymbopogon flexuosus) Essential Oil. *Food Technol Biotechnol.* 2022 Sep;60(3):386-395.

[5446] Tanveer M, Ejaz S, Zaka SM, et al. Toxicology of diatomaceous earth, phyto oils and their admixed emulsions against adults of Tribolium castaneum (Herbst). *Toxicol Rep.* 2022 May 16;9:1172-1179.

[5447] Lak F, Zandi-Sohani N, Ghodoum Parizipour MH, et al. Synergic effects of some plant-derived essential oils and Iranian isolates of entomopathogenic fungus Metarhizium anisopliae Sorokin to control Acanthoscelides obtectus (Say) (Coleoptera: Chrysomelidae). *Front Plant Sci.* 2022 Dec 9;13: 1075761.

[5448] Guerrini A, Tacchini M, Chiocchio I, et al. A Comparative Study on Chemical Compositions and Biological Activities of Four Amazonian Ecuador Essential Oils: Curcuma longa L. (Zingiberaceae), Cymbopogon citratus (DC.) Stapf, (Poaceae), Ocimum campechianum Mill. (Lamiaceae), and Zingiber officinale Roscoe (Zingiberaceae). *Antibiotics (Basel).* 2023 Jan 15;12(1):177.

[5449] Chowdhury H, Bera AK, Raut SS, et al. In vitro antibacterial efficacy of Cymbopogon flexuosus essential oil against Aeromonas hydrophila of fish origin and in silico molecular docking of the essential oil components against DNA gyrase-B and their drug-likeness. *Chem Biodivers.* 2023 Feb 17:e202200668.

[5450] Spadaro F, Costa R, Circosta C, et al. Volatile composition and biological activity of new Lime Citrus aurantifolia essential oil. *Nat Prod Commun.* 2012 Nov;7(11):1523-26.

[5451] Gamarra FMC, Sakanaka LS, Tambourgi EG, et al. Influence of the quality of essential oil lemon (Citrus aurantifolia) oil by distillation process. *Braz J Chem Eng.* 2006 Jan-Mar;23(1):014-6632.

[5452] Costa R, Bisignano C, Filocamo A, et al. Antimicrobial activity and chemical composition of Citrus aurantifolia (Christm.) Swingle essential oil from Italian organic crops. *J Essent Oil Res.* 2014;26(6):400-08.

[5453] Lota ML, Serra DDR, Tomi F, et al. Volatile components of peel and leaf oils of lemon and lime. *J Agric Food Chem.* 2002;50:796-805.

[5454] Lee JH, Lee JS. Chemical composition and antifungal activity of plant essential oils against Malassezia furfur. *Kor J Microbiol Biotechnol.* 2010;38(3):315-21.

[5455] Dugrand-Judek A, Olry A, Hehn A, et al. The distribution of coumarins and furanocoumarins in citrus cpecies closely matches phylogeny and reflects the organization of biosynthetic pathways. *PLoS One.* 2015;10(11):e0142757.

[5456] Williamson EA. Inhibition of cytochrome P450 2E1, cytochrome P450 3A6 and cytochrome P450 2A6 by citrus essential oils. University of North Carolina Thesis. Available at: http://libres.uncg.edu/ir/uncg/f/Williamson_uncg_0154M_10494.pdf.

[5457] Chaiyana W, Okonogi S. Inhibition of cholinesterase by essential oil from food plant. *Phytomedicine.* 2012 Jun;19(8-9):836-39.

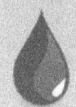

5458 Tundis R, Loizzo MR, Bonesi M, et al. Comparative study on the antioxidant capacity and cholinesterase inhibitory activity of Citrus aurantifolia Swingle, C. aurantium L., and C. bergamia Risso and Poit. Peel oils. *J Food Sci.* 2012 Jan;77(1):H40-46.

5459 Asnaashari S, Delazar A, Habibi B, et al. Essential oil from Citrus aurantifolia prevents ketotifen-induced weight- gain in mice. *Phytother Res.* 2010 Dec;24(12):1893-97.

5460 Van Hung P, Chi PT, Phi NT. Comparison of antifungal activities of Vietnamese citrus essential oils. *Nat Prod Res.* 2013 Mar;27(4-5):506-08.

5461 Patil JR, Jayaprakasha GK, Chidambara M, et al. Apoptosis-mediated proliferation inhibition of human colon cancer cells by volatile principles of Citrus aurantifolia. *Food Chem.* 2009 Jun;114(4):1351-58.

5462 Chaiyana W, Okonogi S. Inhibition of cholinesterase by essential oil from food plant. *Phytomedicine.* 2012 Jun;19(8-9):836-39.

5463 Tundis R, Loizzo MR, Bonesi M, et al. Comparative study on the antioxidant capacity and cholinesterase inhibitory activity of Citrus aurantifolia Swingle, C. aurantium L., and C. bergamia Risso and Poit. Peel oils. *J Food Sci.* 2012 Jan;77(1):H40-46.

5464 Darvesh S, Hopkins DA, Geula C, Neurobiology of butyrylcholinesterase. *Nat Rev Neurosci.* 2003 Feb;4:131-38.

5465 Prabuseenivasan S, Jayakumar M, Ignacimuthu S. In vitro antibacterial activity of some plant essential oils. *BMC Complement Altern Med.* 2006 Nov;6:39.

5466 Amorim JL, Simas DL, Pinheiro MM, et al. Anti-Inflammatory Properties and Chemical Characterization of the Essential Oils of Four Citrus Species. *PLoS One.* 2016 Apr 18;11(4):e0153643.

5467 Mirzaei-Najafgholi H, Tarighi S, Golmohammadi M, et al. The Effect of Citrus Essential Oils and Their Constituents on Growth of Xanthomonas citri subsp. citri. *Molecules.* 2017 Apr 14;22(4).

5468 Ferreira LE, Benincasa BI, Fachin AL, et al. Essential oils of Citrus aurantifolia, Anthemis nobile and Lavandula officinalis: in vitro anthelmintic activities against Haemonchus contortus. *Parasit Vectors.* 2018; 11: 269.

5469 Lemes RS, Alves CCF, Estevam EBB, et al. Chemical composition and antibacterial activity of essential oils from Citrus aurantifolia leaves and fruit peel against oral pathogenic bacteria. *An Acad Bras Cienc.* 2018 Apr-Jun;90(2):1285-1292.

5470 Ibrahim FA, Usman LA, Akolade JO, et al. Antidiabetic Potentials of Citrus aurantifolia Leaf Essential Oil. *Drug Res (Stuttg).* 2019 Apr;69(4):201-206.

5471 Lin LY, Chuang CH, Chen HC, et al. Lime (Citrus aurantifolia (Christm.) Swingle) Essential Oils: Volatile Compounds, Antioxidant Capacity, and Hypolipidemic Effect. *Foods.* 2019 Sep 7;8(9).

5472 Acheampong DO, Barffour IK, Boye A, et al. Histoprotective Effect of Essential Oil from Citrus aurantifolia in Testosterone-Induced Benign Prostatic Hyperplasia Rat. *Adv Urol.* 2019 Sep 25;2019:3031609.

5473 Sarma R, Adhikari K, Mahanta S, et al. Insecticidal Activities of Citrus aurantifolia Essential Oil Against Aedes aegypti (Diptera: Culicidae). *Toxicol Rep.* 2019 Oct 14;6:1091-96.

5474 Dos SDantos EGG, Bezerra WADS, Temeyer KB, et al. Effects of essential oils on native and recombinant acetylcholinesterases of Rhipicephalus microplus. *Rev Bras Parasitol Vet.* 2021 May 28;30(2):e002221.

5475 Song BW, Lee CY, Park JH, et al. Cold-pressed oil from Citrus aurantifolia inhibits the proliferation of vascular smooth muscle cells via regulation of PI3K/MAPK signaling pathways. *Exp Ther Med.* 2022 Jan;23(1):21.

5476 Toulemonde B, Noleau I. Volatile constituents of lovage (Levisticum officinale Koch.). *Dev Food Sci.* 1988;18:641-57. In: Lawrence BM, Mookherjee BD, Willis BJ. Flavors and Fragrances; a World Perspective. Elsevier, Amsterdam, p. 641-56.

5477 Bylaite E, Roozen JP, Legger A, et al. Dynamic Headspace-Gas Chromatography-Olfactometry Analysis of Different Anatomical Parts of Lovage (Levisticum officinale Koch.) at Eight Growing Stages. *J Agric Food Chem.* 2000;448:6183-90.

5478 Roslon W, Osinska E, Wajs-Bonikowska A. Effect of plantation establishment and raw material stabilization on the useful traits of lovage leaves (Levisticum officinale Koch.). *Acta Sci Pol Hortorum Cultus.* 2013;12(1):141-55.

5479 Sertel S, Eichhorn T, Plinkert PK, et al. Chemical Composition and Antiproliferative Activity of Essential Oil from the Leaves of a Medicinal Herb, Levisticum officinale, against UMSCC1 Head and Neck Squamous Carcinoma Cells. *Anticancer Res.* 2011;31:185-92.

5480 Mohammad Reza VR, Abbas H. The Essential Oil Composition of Levisticum officinalis from Iran. *Asian J Biochem.* 2007;2(2);161-63.

5481 Raal A, Arak E. Composition of the Essential Oil of Levisticum Officinale W.D.J. Koch from Some European Countries. *J Essent Oil Res.* 2008 Jul-Aug;20:318-22.

5482 Heidarpour O, Souri MK, Omidbagi R, et al. Changes in Content and Constituents of Essential Oil in Different Plant Parts of Lovage (Levisticum officinale Koch. Cv. Budakalaszi) Cultivated in Iran. *J Essent Oil Bear Plants.* 2013 Sep;16(3):318-22.

5483 Circosta C, Pasquale RD, Palumbo DR, et al. Estrogenic activity of standardized extract of Angelica sinensis. *Phytother Res.* 2006 Aug;20(8):665–69.

5484 Circosta C, Pasquale RD, Palumbo DR, et al. Estrogenic activity of standardized extract of Angelica sinensis. *Phytother Res.* 2006 Aug;20(8):665–69.

5485 Shi M, Chang L, He G. [Stimulating action of Carthamus tinctorius L., Angelica sinensis (Oliv.) Diels and Leonurus sibiricus L. on the uterus]. *Zhongguo Zhong Yao Za Zhi.* 1995 Mar;20(3):173-5, 192.

5486 Pages N, Fournier G, Chamorro G, et al. Teratological evaluation of Juniperus sabina essential oil in mice. *Planta Med.* 1989 Apr;55(2):144-46.

5487 Pages N, Fournier G, Baudel C, et al. Sabinyl Acetate, the Main Component of Juniperus sabina L'Hérit. Essential Oil, is Responsible for Antiimplantation Effect. *Phytother Res.* 1996 Aug;10(5):438-440.

5488 Pages N, Fournier G, Velut V, et al. Potential teratogenicity in mice of the essential oil of Salvia lavandulifolia Vahl. Study of a fraction rich in sabinyl acetate. *Phytother Res.* 1992 Mar;6(2):80-83.

5489 Casares R. Juniperus sabina. *Food Cosmet Toxicol.* 1964;2:680-81. Found in U.S. Food and Drug Administration. FDA Poisonous Plant Database. Available at: http://www.accessdata.fda.gov/scripts/plantox/detail.cfm?id=5133.

5490 Brindis F, Rodríguez R, Bye R, et al. (Z)-3-butylidenephthalide from Ligusticum porteri, an α-glucosidase inhibitor. *J Nat Prod.* 2011 Mar 25;74(3):314-20.

5491 Zhang L, Du JR, Wang J, et al. Z-ligustilide extracted from Radix Angelica Sinensis decreased platelet aggregation induced by ADP ex vivo and arterio-venous shunt thrombosis in vivo in rats. *Yakugaku Zasshi.* 2009 Jul;129(7):855-9.

5492 Qi H, Zhao J, Han Y, et al. Z-ligustilide potentiates the cytotoxicity of dopamine in rat dopaminergic PC12 cells. *Neurotox Res.* 2012 Nov;22(4):345-54.

5493 Matsumoto K, Kohno S, Ojima K, et al. Effects of methylenechloride-soluble fraction of Japanese angelica root extract, ligustilide and butylidenephthalide, on pentobarbital sleep in group-housed and socially isolated mice. *Life Sci.* 1998;62(23):2073-82.

5494 Kuang X, Du JR, Liu YX, et al. Postischemic administration of Z-Ligustilide ameliorates cognitive dysfunction and brain damage induced by permanent forebrain ischemia in rats. *Pharmacol Biochem Behav.* 2008 Jan;88(3):213-21.

5495 Bonesi M, Menichini F, Tundis R, et al. Acetylcholinesterase and butyrylcholinesterase inhibitory activity of Pinus species essential oils and their constituents. *J Enzyme Inhib Med Chem.* 2010 Oct;25(5):622-8.

5496 Yarnell E. Botanical medicines for the urinary tract. *World J Urol.* 2002 Nov;20(5):285-93.

5497 Burkhard PR, Burkhardt K, Haenggeli CA, et al. Plant-induced seizures: reappearance of an old problem. *J Neurol.* 1999 Aug;246(8):667-70.

5498 Sertel S, Eichhorn T, Plinkert PK, et al. Chemical Composition and Antiproliferative Activity of Essential Oil from the Leaves of a Medicinal Herb, Levisticum officinale, against UMSCC1 Head and Neck Squamous Carcinoma Cells. *Anticancer Res.* 2011;31:185-92.

5499 Kuang X, Du JR, Liu YX, et al. Postischemic administration of Z-Ligustilide ameliorates cognitive dysfunction and brain damage induced by permanent forebrain ischemia in rats. *Pharmacol Biochem Behav.* 2008 Jan;88(3):213-21.

5500 Bartoňková I, Dvořák Z. Essential oils of culinary herbs and spices display agonist and antagonist activities at human aryl hydrocarbon receptor AhR. *Food Chem Toxicol.* 2018 Jan;111:374-384.

5501 Punjee P, Dilokkunanant U, Sukkatta U, et al. Scented Extracts and Essential Oil Extraction from Michelia alba D.C. *Kasetsart J (Nat Sci).* 2009;43:197-203.

5502 Pensuk W, Padumanonda T, Pichaensoonthon C. Comparison of the Chemical Constituents in Michelia alba Flower Oil Extracted by Steam Distillation, Hexane Extraction and Enfleurage Method. *J Thai Traditional Alternative Med.* 2007 Jan-Apr;5(1).

5503 Ueyama Y, Hashimoto S, Nii H, et al. The Chemical Composition of the Flower Oil and the Leaf Oil of Michelia alba D.C. *J Essent Oil Res.* 1992;4(1):15-23.

5504 Shau NA. Chemical constituents and biological activities of essential oil from Champaka (Michelia alba de canolle). Doctoral thesis, University Purtra Malaysia. Available at: http://psasir.upm.edu.my/38912/1/FBSB%202013%208R.pdf.

5505 Cardoso NN, Alviano CS, Blank AF, et al. Synergism Effect of the Essential Oil from Ocimum basilicum var. Maria Bonita and Its Major Components with Fluconazole and Its Influence on Ergosterol Biosynthesis. *Evid Based Complement Alternat Med.* 2016;2016:5647182.

5506 Koomhin P, Sattayakhom A, Chandharakool S, et al. Michelia Essential Oil Inhalation Increases Fast Alpha Wave Activity. *Sci Pharm.* 2020;88:23.

5507 Songsamoe S, Koomhin P, Matan N. The effects of Michelia alba oil against mould on brown rice and assessing the brain response using electroencephalogram (EEG). *J Food Sci Technol.* 2021 May;58(5):1776-1787.

5508 Porter NG, Wilkins AL. Chemical, physical and antimicrobial properties of essential oils of Leptospermum scoparium and Kunzea ericoides. *Phytochemistry.* 1998;50:407-15.

5509 Schnitzler P, Wiesenhofer K, Reichling J. Comparative study on the cytotoxicity of different Myrtaceae essential oils on cultured Vero and RC-37 cells. *Pharmazie.* 2008;63:830-85.

5510 Douglas MH, van Klink JW, Smallfield BM, et al. Essential oils from New Zealand manuka: triketone and other chemotypes of Leptospermum scoparium. *Phytochemistry.* 2004 May;65(9):1255-64.

5511 Christoph F, Kubeczka KH, Stahl-Biskup E. The Composition of Commercial Manuka Oils from New Zealand. *J Essent Oil Res.* 1999 Nov-Dec;11:705-10.

5512 Lis-Balchin M, Hart SL, Deans SG. Pharmacological and antimicrobial studies on different tea-tree oils (Melaleuca alternifolia, Leptospermum scoparium or Manuka and Kunzea ericoides or Kanuka), originating in Australia and New Zealand. *Phytother Res.* 2000 Dec;14(8):623-9.

5513 Maddocks-Jennings W, Wilkinson JM, Cavanagh HM, et al. Evaluating the effects of the essential oils Leptospermum scoparium (manuka) and Kunzea ericoides (kanuka) on radiotherapy induced mucositis: a randomized, placebo controlled feasibility study. *Eur J Oncol Nurs.* 2009 Apr;13(2):87-93.

5514 Takarada K, Kimizuka R, Takahashi N, et al. A comparison of the antibacterial efficacies of essential oils against oral pathogens. *Oral Microbiol Immunol.* 2004 Feb;19(1):61-4.

5515 Filoche SK, Soma K, Sissons CH. Antimicrobial effects of essential oils in combination with chlorhexidine digluconate. Oral Microbiol Immunol. 2005 Aug;20(4):221-5.

5516 Vervelle A, Mouhyi J, Del Corso M, et al. [Mouthwash solutions with microencapsuled natural extracts: Efficiency for dental plaque and gingivitis]. *Rev Stomatol Chir Maxillofac.* 2010 Jun;111(3):148-51.

5517 Mouhyi J, Del Corso M, Hippolyte MP, et al. [Mouthwash solutions containing microencapsulated natural extracts: Clinical results on dental plaque and gingivitis]. *Rev Stomatol Chir Maxillofac.* 2010 Jun;111(3):144-7.

5518 Schnitzler P, Wiesenhofer K, Reichling J. Comparative study on the cytotoxicity of different Myrtaceae essential oils on cultured Vero and RC-37 cells. *Pharmazie.* 2008;63:830-85.

5519 Reichling J, Koch C, Stahl-Biskup E, et al. Virucidal activity of a beta-triketone-rich essential oil of Leptospermum scoparium (manuka oil) against HSV-1 and HSV-2 in cell culture. *Planta Med.* 2005 Dec;71(12):1123-7.

5520 Kwon OS1, Jung SH, Yang BS. Topical Administration of Manuka Oil Prevents UV-B Irradiation-Induced Cutaneous Photoaging in Mice. *Evid Based Complement Alternat Med.* 2013;2013:930857.

5521 Song CY, Nam EH, Park SH, et al. In vitro efficacy of the essential oil from Leptospermum scoparium (manuka) on antimicrobial susceptibility and biofilm formation in Staphylococcus pseudintermedius isolates from dogs. *Vet Dermatol.* 2013 Aug;24(4):404-8, e87.

5522 Chen CC, Yan SH, Yen MY, et al. Investigations of kanuka and manuka essential oils for in vitro treatment of disease and cellular inflammation caused by infectious microorganisms. *J Microbiol Immunol Infect.* 2016 Feb;49(1):104-11.

5523 Fang F, Candy K, Melloul E, et al. In vitro activity of ten essential oils against Sarcoptes scabiei. *Parasit Vectors.* 2016 Nov 22;9(1):594.

5524 Turchi B, Mancini S, Pistelli L, et al. Sub-inhibitory stress with essential oil affects enterotoxins production and essential oil susceptibility in Staphylococcus aureus. *Nat Prod Res.* 2017 Jun 8:1-7.

5525 Muturi EJ, Selling GW, Doll KM, et al. Leptospermum Scoparium Essential Oil Is a Promising Source of Mosquito Larvicide and Its Toxicity Is Enhanced by a Biobased Emulsifier. *PLoS One.* 2020 Feb 20;15(2):e0229076.

5526 Porter GC, Safii SH, Medlicott NJ, et al. Formulation of a Semisolid Emulsion Containing Leptospermum scoparium Essential Oil and Evaluation of In Vitro Antimicrobial and Antibiofilm Efficacy. *Planta Med.* 2021 Jan 12. Online ahead of print.

5527 Michalczky A, Ostrowska P. Essential oils and their components in combating fungal pathogens of animal and human skin. *J Mycol Med.* 2021 Jun;31(2):101118.

5528 Duque LS, Marchesini P, Monteiro C, et al. Acaricidal activity of the essential oils from Leptospermum scoparium, Origanum vulgare and Litsea cubeba on Rhipicephalus microplus: Influence of the solvents and search for fractions with higher bioactivity. *Vet Parasitol.* 2021 Dec;300:109606.

5529 Pedonese F, Longo E, Torracca B, et al. Antimicrobial and antibiofilm activity of manuka essential oil against Listeria monocytogenes and Staphylococcus aureus of food origin. *Ital J Food Saf.* 2022 Feb 22;11(1):10039.

5530 Gray BH, Green KJ, Haines RR, et al. Antibacterial interactions between two monofloral honeys and several topical antiseptics, including essential oils. *BMC Complement Med Ther.* 2022 Aug 26;22(1):228.

5531 Noites A, Araújo B, Machado J, et al. Antifungal Potential of Some Herb Decoctions and Essential Oils on Candida Species. *Healthcare (Basel).* 2022 Sep 21;10(10):1820.

5532 Kubeczka KH, Schultze W. Biology and chemistry of conifer oils. *Flav Frag J.* 1987;2:137-48.

5533 Leseche B, Levisalles J, Rudler H. L'essence de térébenthine du pin maritime (Pinus pinaster de Portugal). *Parfumes Cosmetiques et Aromes.* 1984;58:53-58.

5534 Dob T, Berramdane T, Chelghoum C. Analysis of Essential Oil from the Needles of Pinus pinaster Growing in Algeria. *Chem Nat Constituents.* 2005 Sep;41(5):545-48.

5535 Mimoune NA, Mimoune DA, Yataghene A. Chemical composition and antimicrobial activity of the essential oils of Pinus pinaster. *J Coastal Life Med.* 2013;1(1):55-59.

5536 Hmamouchi M, Hamamouchi J, Zouhdi M. Chemical and Antimicrobial Properties of Essential Oils of Five Moroccan Pinaceae. *J Essent Oil Res.* 2011 Ju-Aug;13:298-302.

5537 Macchioni F, Flamini G, Maccioni S, et al. Chemical composition of essential oils from needles, branches and cones of Pinus pinea, Phalepensis, P-pinaster and P. nigra from central Italy. *Flavour Frag J.* 2003 Mar;18:139-43.

5538 Petrakis PV, Tsitsimpikou C, Tzakou O, et la. Needle volatiles from five Pinus species growing in Greece. *Flavour Frag J.* 2001 Jul;16(4):249-52.

5539 Pauly G, Gleizes M, Bernard-Dagan C. Identification des constituants de l'essence des aiguilles de Pinus pinaster. *Phytochemistry.* 1973;12(6):1395-98.

5540 Nguyen LT, Mysliveckova Z, Szotakova B, et al. The inhibitory effects of β-caryophyllene, β-caryophyllene oxide and α-humulene on the activities of the main drug-metabolizing enzymes in rat and human liver in vitro. *Chem-Biol Interactoins.* 2017 Dec 25;278:123-8.

5541 Mimoune NA, Mimoune DA, Yataghene A. Chemical composition and antimicrobial activity of the essential oils of Pinus pinaster. *J Coastal Life Med.* 2013;1(1):55-59.

5542 Jantapan K, Poapolathep A, Imsilp K, et al. Inhibitory Effects of Thai Essential Oils on Potentially Aflatoxigenic Aspergillus parasiticus and Aspergillus flavus. *Biocontrol Sci.* 2017;22(1):31-40.

5543 Tümen İ, Akkol EK, Taştan H, et al. Research on the Antioxidant, Wound Healing, and Anti-inflammatory Activities and the Phytochemical Composition of Maritime Pine (Pinus pinaster Ait). *J Ethnopharmacol.* 2018 Jan 30;211:235-246.

5544 Ruas A, Graça A, Marto J, et al. Chemical Characterization and Bioactivity of Commercial Essential Oils and Hydrolates Obtained from Portuguese Forest Logging and Thinning. *Molecules.* 2022 Jun 2;27(11):3572.

5545 Coimbra A, Miguel S, Ribeiro M, et al. Chemical composition, antioxidant, and antimicrobial activities of six commercial essential oils. *Lett Appl Microbiol.* 2023 Jan 23;76(1):ovac042.

5546 Soliman FM, Yousif MF, Zagloul SS, et al. Seasonal variation in the essential oil composition of Origanum majorana L. cultivated in Egypt. *Z Naturforsch C.* 2009 Sep-Oct;64(9-10):611-14.

5547 Vera RR, Chane-Ming J. Chemical composition of the essential oil of marjoram (Origanum majorana L.) from Reunion Island. *Food Chem.* 1999 Aug;66(2):143-45.

5548 Freire JM, Cardoso MG, Batista LR, et al. Essential oil of Origanum majorana L., Illicium verum Hook. F. and Cinnamomum zeylanicum Blume: chemical and antimicrobial characterization. *Revista Brasileira de Plantas Medicinais.* 2011;13(2):1516-0572.

5549 Ramos S, Rojas LB, Lucena ME, et al. Chemical composition and antibacterial activity of Origanum majorana L. essential oil from the Venezuelan Andes. *J Essential Oil Res.* 2011;23(5):45-49.

5550 Barazandeh MM. Essential oil composition of Origanum majorana L. from Iran. *J Essential Oil Res.* 2001;13(2):76- 77.

5551 Baser KHC, Krimer N. Composition of the essential oil of Origanum majorana L. from Turkey. *J Essent Oil Res.* 1993 Sep/Oct;5:577-9.

5552 Bagci Y, Kan Y, Dogu S, et al. The essential oil compositions of Origanum majroana L. cultivated in Konya and collected from Mersin-Turkey. *Indian J Pharm Education Res.* 2017 Jul/Sep;51(3):S463-9.

5553 Mossa AT, Nawwar GA. Free radical scavenging and antiacetylcholinesterase activities of Origanum majorana L. essential oil. *Hum Exp Toxicol.* 2011 Oct;30(10):1501-13.

5554 Mertas A, Garbusińska A, Szliszka E, et al. The influence of tea tree oil (Melaleuca alternifolia) on fluconazole activity against fluconazole-resistant Candida albicans strains. *Biomed Res Int.* 2015;2015:590470.

5555 Romeilah RM. Anticancer and antioxidant activities of Matricaria chamomilla L. and Mafjopana hortensis essential oils. *Res J Medicine Med Sci.* 2009;4(2):332-39.

5556 Hussain AI, Anwar F, Rasheed Sh, et al. Composition, antioxidant and chemotherapeutic properties of the essential oils from two Origanum species growing in Pakistan. *Rev Bras Farmacogn.* 2011;21(6).

5557 Kim IH, Kim C, Seong K, et al. Essential oil inhalation on blood pressure and salivary cortisol levels in prehypertensive and hypertensive subjects. *Evid Based Complement Alternat Med.* 2012;2012:984203.

5558 Ou MC, Hsu TF, Lai AC, et al. Pain relief assessment by aromatic essential oil massage on outpatients with primary dysmenorrhea: a randomized, double blind clinical trial. *J Obstet Gynaecol Res.* 2012 May;38(5):817-22.

5559 Kim MJ, Nam ES, Paik SI. The effects of aromatherapy in pain, depression, and life satisfaction of arthritis patients. *Taehan Kanho Hakhoe Chi.* 2005 Feb;35(1):186-94.

5560 Fonseca AO, Pereira DI, Jacob RG, et al. In vitro susceptibility of Brazilian Pythium insidiosum isolates to essential oils of some Lamiaceae family. *Mycopathologia.* 2016 Aug;181(7-8):617-22.

5561 Refaie AA, Ramadan A, Mossa AT. Oxidative damage and nephrotoxicity induced by prallethrin in rat and the protective effect of Origanum majorana essential oil. *Asian Pac J Trop Med.* 2014 Sep;7S1:S506-13.

5562 Mossa AT, Refaie AA, Ramadan A, Bouajila J. Amelioration of prallethrin-induced oxidative stress and hepatotoxicity in rat by the administration of Origanum majorana essential oil. *Biomed Res Int.* 2013;2013:859085

5563 Mossa AT, Refaie AA, Ramadan A, et al. Antimutagenic effect of Origanum majorana L. essential oil against prallethirn-induced genotoxic damage in rat bone marrow cells. *J Med Food.* 2013 Dec;16(12):1101-07.

5564 El-Ashmawy IM, Saleh A, Salama OM. Effects of marjoram volatile oil and grape seed extract on ethanol toxicity in male rats. *Basic Clin Pharmacol Toxicol.* 2007 Nov;101(5):320-27.

5565 Mossa AT, Nawwar GA. Free radical scavenging and antiacetylcholinesterase activities of Origanum majorana L. essential oil. *Hum Exp Toxicol.* 2011 Oct;30(10):1501-13.

5566 Hussain AI, Anwar F, Rasheed Sh, et al. Composition, antioxidant and chemotherapeutic properties of the essential oils from two Origanum species growing in Pakistan. *Rev Bras Farmacogn.* 2011;21(6).

5567 Guerra-Boone L, Alvarez-Roman R, Salazar-Aranda R, et al. Antimicrobial and antioxidant activities and chemical characterization of essential oils of Thymus vulgaris, Rosmarinus officinalis, and Origanum majorana from northeastern Mexico. *Pak J Pharm Sci.* 2015;28:363S-369S.

5568 Al-Howiriny T, Alsheikh A, Alqasoumi S, et al. Protective effect of Origanum majorana L. 'Marjoram' on various models of gastric mucosal injury in rats. *Am J Chin Med.* 2009;37(3):531-45.

5569 El-Ashmawy IM, el-Nahas AF, Salama OM. Protective effect of volatile oil, alcoholic and aqueous extracts of Origanum majorana on lead acetate toxicity in mice. *Basic Clin Pharmacol Toxicol.* 2005 Oct;97(4):238-43.

5570 Deans SG, Svoboda KP. The antimicrobial properties of marjoram (Origanum majorana L.) volatile oil. *Flav Frag J.* 1990 Sep;5(3):187-90.

5571 Kim SW, Lee HR2, Jang MJ, et al. Fumigant Toxicity of Lamiaceae Plant Essential Oils and Blends of Their Constituents against Adult Rice Weevil Sitophilus oryzae. *Molecules.* 2016 Mar 16;21(3):361.

5572 Olfa B, Mariem A, Salah AM, et al. Chemical content, antibacterial and antioxidant properties of essential oil extract from Tunisian Origanum majorana L. cultivated under saline condition. *Pak J Pharm Sci.* 2016 Nov;29(6):1951-1958.

5573 Grzesiak B, Kołodziej B, Głowacka A, et al. The Effect of Some Natural Essential Oils Against Bovine Mastitis Caused by Prototheca zopfii Isolates In Vitro. *Mycopathologia.* 2018 Jun;183(3):541-550.

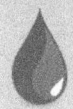

[5574] Vasireddy L, Bingle LEH, Davies MS. Antimicrobial activity of essential oils against multidrug-resistant clinical isolates of the Burkholderia cepacia complex. *PLoS One*. 2018 Aug 2;13(8):e0201835.

[5575] Giatropoulos A, Kimbaris A, Michaelakis A, et al. Chemical composition and assessment of larvicidal and repellent capacity of 14 Lamiaceae essential oils against Aedes albopictus. *Parasitol Res*. 2018 Jun;117(6):1953-1964.

[5576] Makrane H, Aziz M, Berrabah M, et al. Myorelaxant Activity of essential oil from Origanum majorana L. on rat and rabbit. *J Ethnopharmacol*. 2018 Sep 8;228:40-49.

[5577] Merino JJ, Parmigiani-Izquierdo JM, López-Oliva ME, et al. Origanum majorana Essential Oil Inhalation during Neurofeedback Training Reduces Saliva Myeloperoxidase Activity at Session-1 in Bruxistic Patients. *J Clin Med*. 2019 Jan 31;8(2).

[5578] Lagha R, Ben Abdallah F, Al-Sarhan BO, et al. Antibacterial and Biofilm Inhibitory Activity of Medicinal Plant Essential Oils Against Escherichia coli Isolated from UTI Patients. *Molecules*. 2019 Mar 23;24(6).

[5579] Kerekes EB, Vidács A, Takó M, et al. Antibiofilm Effect of Selected Essential Oils and Main Components on Mono- and Polymicrobic Bacterial Cultures. *Microorganisms*. 2019 Sep 12;7(9).

[5580] Waller SB, Cleff MB, de Mattos CB, et al. In vivo protection of the marjoram (Origanum majorana Linn.) essential oil in the cutaneous sporotrichosis by Sporothrix brasiliensis. *Nat Prod Res*. 2019 Oct 17:1-5.

[5581] Ben Salha G, Herrera Díaz R, Lengliz O, et al. Effect of the Chemical Composition of Free-Terpene Hydrocarbons Essential Oils on Antifungal Activity. *Molecules*. 2019 Sep 29;24(19).

[5582] Son HK, So WY, Kim M. Effects of Aromatherapy Combined with Music Therapy on Anxiety, Stress, and Fundamental Nursing Skills in Nursing Students: A Randomized Controlled Trial. *Int J Environ Res Public Health*. 2019 Oct 29;16(21).

[5583] Moumni S, Elaissi A, Trabelsi A, et al. Correlation between chemical composition and antibacterial activity of some Lamiaceae species essential oils from Tunisia. *BMC Complement Med Ther*. 2020 Apr 3;20(1):103.

[5584] Athamneh K, Alneyadi A, Alsamri H, et al. Origanum majorana Essential Oil Triggers p38 MAPK-Mediated Protective Autophagy, Apoptosis, and Caspase-Dependent Cleavage of P70S6K in Colorectal Cancer Cells. *Biomolecules*. 2020 Mar 6;10(3).

[5585] Amor G, Caputo L, La Storia A, et al. Chemical Composition and Antimicrobial Activity of Artemisia herba-alba and Origanum majorana Essential Oils from Morocco. *Molecules*. 2019 Nov 6;24(22).

[5586] Chaves RDSB, Martins RL, Rodrigues ABL, et al. Evaluation of larvicidal potential against larvae of Aedes aegypti (Linnaeus, 1762) and of the antimicrobial activity of essential oil obtained from the leaves of Origanum majorana L. *PLoS One*. 2020 Jul 17;15(7):e0235740.

[5587] Chaudhari AK, Singh VK, Deeplika SD, et al. Improvement of in vitro and in situ antifungal, AFB 1 inhibitory and antioxidant activity of Origanum majorana L. essential oil through nanoemulsion and recommending as novel food preservative. *Food Chem Toxicol*. 2020 Jul 5;111536.

[5588] Guler E, Ozbilgin A, Becer E, et al. [An Endemic Plant of Cyprus, Origanum majorana: Is It A New Alternative Natural Product for Malaria Treatment?] *Mikrobiyol Bul*. 2020 Jul;54(3):463-478.

[5589] Postu PA, Gorgon DL, Cioanca O, et al. Memory-Enhancing Effects of Origanum majorana Essential Oil in an Alzheimer's Amyloid beta1-42 Rat Model: A Molecular and Behavioral Study. *Antioxidants (Basel)*. 2020 Sep 26;9(10):E919.

[5590] Elazab ST, Soliman AF, Nishikawa Y. Effect of some plant extracts from Egyptian herbal plants against Toxoplasma gondii tachyzoites in vitro. *J Vet Med Sci*. 2020 Dec 1. Online ahead of print.

[5591] Hetta HF, Meshaal AK, Algammal AM, et al. In-vitro Antimicrobial Activity of Essential Oils and Spices Powder of some Medicinal Plants Against Bacillus Species Isolated from Raw and Processed Meat. *Infect Drug Resist*. 2020 Dec 4;13:4367-4378.

[5592] Lei D, Hong T, Li L, et al. Isobaric tags for relative and absolute quantitation-based proteomics analysis of the effect of ginger oil on bisphenol A-induced breast cancer cell proliferation. *Oncol Lett*. 2021 Feb;21(2):101.

[5593] Mohamend AA, El-Hefny M, El-Shanhorey N, et al. Foliar Application of Bio-Stimulants Enhancing the Production and the Toxicity of Origanum majorana Essential Oils Against Four Rice Seed-Borne Fungi. *Molecules*. 2020 May 19;25(10):2363.

[5594] Elmhalli F, Garboui SS, Karlson AKB, et al. Acaricidal activity against Ixodes ricinus nymphs of essential oils from the Libyan plants Artemisia herba alba, Origanum majorana and Juniperus phoenicea. *Vet Parasitol Reg Stud Reports*. 2021 Apr;24:100575.

[5595] Ed-Dra A, Filali FR, Lo Presti V, et al. Chemical composition, antioxidant capacity and antibacterial action of five Moroccan essential oils against Listeria monocytogenes and different serotypes of Salmonella enterica. *Microb Pathog*. 2020 Dec;149:104510.

[5596] Guler E, Ozbilgin A, Cavus I, et al. In vitro Anti-Leishmanial Activity of Essential Oils Extracted from Plants Growing in Northern Cyprus Against Leishmania tropica. *Turkiye Parazitol Derg*. 2021 Jun 7;45(2):101-107.

[5597] Farouk A, Mohsen M, Ali H, et al. Antioxidant Activity and Molecular Docking Study of Volatile Constituents from Different Aromatic Lamiaceous Plants Cultivated in Madinah Monawara, Saudi Arabia. *Molecules*. 2021 Jul 7;26(14):4145.

[5598] Kaskatepe B, Aslan Erdem S, Ozturk S, et al. Antifungal and Anti-Virulent Activity of Origanum majorana L. Essential Oil on Candida albicans and In Vivo Toxicity in the Galleria mellonella Larval Model. *Molecules*. 2022 Jan 20;27(3):663.

[5599] Ghazal TSA, Schelz Z, Vidács L, et al. Antimicrobial, Multidrug Resistance Reversal and Biofilm Formation Inhibitory Effect of Origanum majorana Extracts, Essential Oil and Monoterpenes. *Plants (Basel)*. 2022 May 27;11(11):1432.

[5600] Arafat K, Sulaiman S, Al-Azawi AM, et al. Origanum majorana essential oil decreases lung tumor growth and metastasis in vitro and in vivo.

[5601] Paudel PN, Satyal P, Satyal R, et al. Chemical Composition, Enantiomeric Distribution, Antimicrobial and Antioxidant Activities of Origanum majorana L. Essential Oil from Nepal. *Molecules*. 2022 Sep 19;27(18):6136.

[5602] Mehanna S, Issa MY, Hassan NH, et al. Origanum majorana essential oil improves the rat's sexual behavior and testicular oxidative damage induced by imidacloprid via modulating the steroidogenesis pathways. *Saudi Pharm J*. 2022 Sep;30(9):1315-1326.

[5603] Aboelhadid SM, Abdel-Baki AS, Hassan KM, et al. Role of antioxidant activity of essential oils in their acaricidal activities against Rhipicephalus annulatus. *Exp Appl Acarol*. 2022 Oct;88(2):209-224.

[5604] Hussein Z, Yasir SM. Origanum majorana attenuates ciprofloxacin-induced nephropathy in rats. *Wiad Lek*. 2022;75(12):3046-3049.

[5605] Rathore S, Mukhia S, Kumar R, et al. Essential oil composition and antimicrobial potential of aromatic plants grown in the mid-hill conditions of the Western Himalayas. *Sci Rep*. 2023 Mar 25;13(1):4878.

[5606] Boelens MH, Jimenez R, et al. Chemical composition of the essential oils from the gum and from various parts of Pistacia lentiscus l. (mastic gum tree). *Flavour Frag J*. 1991 Dec;6(4):271-75.

[5607] Kivcak B, Akay S, Demirci B, et al. Chemical Composition of Essential Oils from Leaves and Twigs of Pistacia lentiscus, Pistacia lentiscus var. chia, and Pistacia terebinthus from Turkey. *Pharmac Biol*. 2008 Sep;42(4-5):360-66.

[5608] Gardeli C, Vassiliki P, Athanasios M, et al. Essential oil composition of Pistacia lentiscus L. and Myrtus communis L.: Evaluation of antioxidant capacity of methanolic extracts. *Food Chem*. 2008 Apr;107(3):1120-30.

[5609] Amhamdi H, Aouinti F, Wathelet JP, et al. Chemical Composition of the Essential Oil of Pistacia lentiscus L. from Eastern Morocco. *Rec Nat Prod*. 2009;3(2):90-95.

[5610] Llorens-Molina JA, Gonzalez SV, Martinez JS. Essential oil composition of leaves of Pistacia lentiscus L. growing wild in Valencia (Spain). *Nat Volatiles Essent Oils*. 2015;2(40:17-26.

[5611] Nahida SHA, Siddiqui AN. Pistacia lentiscus: A review on phytochemistry and pharmacological properties. *Int J Pharm Pharmaceutical Sci*. 2012;2(Suppl 4):16-20.

[5612] Haloui T, Farrah A, Balouiri M, et al. Bacteriostatic and Bactericidal Profile of Leaves and Twigs Essential oils of Moroccan Pistacia lentiscus L. *J Appl Pharm Sci*. 2015 Jun;5(06):50-53.

[5613] Duru ME, Cakir A, Kordali S, et al. Chemical composition and antifungal properties of essential oils of three Pistacia species grown in Turkey. *Fitoterapia*. 2003 Mar;74:170-76.

[5614] Castola V, Bighelli A, Casanova J. Intraspecific chemical variability of the essential oil of Pistacia lentiscus L. from Corsica. *Biochem Systematics Ecol*. 2000 Jan;28(1):79-88.

[5615] Miyamoto T, Okimoto T, Kuwano M. Chemical Composition of the Essential Oil of Mastic Gum and their Antibacterial Activity Against Drug-Resistant Helicobacter pylori. *Nat Prod Bioprospect*. 2014 Aug 4(4):227-31.

[5616] Vidrich V, Fusi P, Graziano A, et al. Chemical Composition of the Essential Oil of Pistacia lentiscus L. *J Essential Oil Res*. 2004;16(3):223-26.

[5617] Zrira S, Elamrani A, Benjilali B. Chemical composition of the essential oil of Pistacia lentiscus L. from Morocco—a seasonal variation. *Flavour Frag J*. 2003;18(6):475-80.

[5618] Hafsé M, Benbrahim KF, Saidi A, et al. Volatile Components and Antibacterial Profile of Essential Oils Extracted from Leaves and Twigs of Lentiscus L. *British Microbiol Res J*. 2013;3(4):602-11.

[5619] Chryssavgi G, Vassiliki P, Athanasios M, et al. Essential oil composition of Pistacia lentiscus L. and Myrtus communic L.: Evaluation of antioxidant capacity of methanolic extracts. *Food Chem*. 2008;107:1120-30.

[5620] Lahmar A, Bedoui A, Mokdad-Bzeouich I, et al. Reversal of resistance in bacteria underlies synergistic effect of essential oils with conventional antibiotics. *Microb Pathog*. 2017 May;106:50-59.

[5621] De Olivera AC, Ribeiro-Pinto LF, Paumgartten JR. In vitro inhibition of CYP2B1 monoxygenase by beta-myrcene and other monoterpenoid constituents. *Br J Nutr*. 1999;81:289-95.

[5622] De-Oliveira AC1, Ribeiro-Pinto LF, Otto SS, et al. Induction of liver monooxygenases by beta-myrcene. *Toxicology*. 1997 Dec 26;124(2):135-40.

[5623] Nguyen LT, Mysliveckova Z, Szotakova B, et al. The inhibitory effects of β-caryophyllene, β-caryophyllene oxide and α-humulene on the activities of the main drug-metabolizing enzymes in rat and human liver in vitro. *Chem-Biol Interactoins*. 2017 Dec 25;278:123-8.

[5624] Freitas JC1, Presgrave OA, Fingola FF, et al. Effect of beta-myrcene on pentobarbital sleeping time. *Braz J Med Biol Res*. 1993 May;26(5):519-23.

[5625] Zaraa I, Ben Taazayet S, Trojjet S, et al. Acute generalized exanthematous pustulosis induced by the essential oil of Pistacia lentiscus. *Clin Exp Dermatol*. 2012 Jun;37(4):361-3.

[5626] Magkouta S, Stathopoulos GT, Psallidas I, et al. Protective effects of mastic oil from Pistacia lentiscus variation chia against experimental growth of lewis lung carcinoma. *Nutr Cancer*. 2009;61(5):640-8.

[5627] Catalani S, Palma F, Battistelli S, et al. Oxidative stress and apoptosis induction in human thyroid carcinoma cells exposed to the essential oil from Pistacia lentiscus aerial parts. *PLoS One*. 2017 Feb 14;12(2):e0172138.

[5628] Haloui T, Farrah A, Balouiri M, et al. Bacteriostatic and Bactericidal Profile of Leaves and Twigs Essential oils of Moroccan Pistacia lentiscus L. *J Appl Pharm Sci*. 2015 Jun;5(06):50-53.

5629 Hafsé M, Benbrahim KF, Saidi A, et al. Volatile Components and Antibacterial Profile of Essential Oils Extracted from Leaves and Twigs of Lentiscus L. *British Microbiol Res J.* 2013;3(4):602-11.

5630 Mharti FZ, Lyoussi B, Abdellaoui A. Antibacterial activity of the essential oils of Pistacia lentiscus used in Moroccan folkloric medicine. *Nat Prod Commun.* 2011 Oct;6(10):1505-6.

5631 Lahmar A, Bedoui A, Mokdad-Bzeouich I, et al. Reversal of resistance in bacteria underlies synergistic effect of essential oils with conventional antibiotics. *Microb Pathog.* 2017 May;106:50-59.

5632 Duru ME, Cakir A, Kordali S, et al. Chemical composition and antifungal properties of essential oils of three Pistacia species grown in Turkey. *Fitoterapia.* 2003 Mar;74:170-76.

5633 Barra A, Coroneo V, Dessi S, et al. Characterization of the volatile constituents in the essential oil of Pistacia lentiscus L. from different origins and its antifungal and antioxidant activity. *J Agric Food Chem.* 2007 Aug 22;55(17):7093-8.

5634 Ezz Eldin HM, Badawy AF. In vitro anti-Trichomonas vaginalis activity of Pistacia lentiscus mastic and Ocimum basilicum essential oil. *J Parasit Dis.* 2015 Sep;39(3):465-73.

5635 Klibet F, Boumendjel A, Khiari M, et al. Oxidative stress-related liver dysfunction by sodium arsenite: Alleviation by Pistacia lentiscus oil. *Pharm Biol.* 2016;54(2):354-63.

5636 Saidi SA, Ncir M, Chaaben R, et al. Liver injury following small intestinal ischemia reperfusion in rats is attenuated by Pistacia lentiscus oil: antioxidant and anti-inflammatory effects. *Arch Physiol Biochem.* 2017 Mar 24:1-7.

5637 Zaraa I, Ben Taazayet S, Trojjet S, et al. Acute generalized exanthematous pustulosis induced by the essential oil of Pistacia lentiscus. *Clin Exp Dermatol.* 2012 Jun;37(4):361-3.

5638 Maxia A, Sanna C, Frau MA, et al. Anti-inflammatory activity of Pistacia lentiscus essential oil: involvement of IL-6 and TNF-alpha. *Nat Prod Commun.* 2011 Oct;6(10):1543-4.

5639 Barra A, Coroneo V, Dessi S, et al. Characterization of the volatile constituents in the essential oil of Pistacia lentiscus L. from different origins and its antifungal and antioxidant activity. *J Agric Food Chem.* 2007 Aug 22;55(17):7093-8.

5640 Traboulsi AF, Taoubi K, el-Haj S, et al. Insecticidal properties of essential plant oils against the mosquito Culex pipiens molestus (Diptera: Culicidae). *Pest Manag Sci.* 2002 May;58(5):491-5.

5641 Miyamoto T, Okimoto T, Kuwano M. Chemical Composition of the Essential Oil of Mastic Gum and their Antibacterial Activity Against Drug-Resistant Helicobacter pylori. *Nat Prod Bioprospect.* 2014 Aug 4(4):227–31.

5642 Buriani A, Fortinguerra S, Sorrenti V, et al. Human Adenocarcinoma Cell Line Sensitivity to Essential Oil Phytocomplexes from Pistacia Species: a Multivariate Approach. *Molecules.* 2017 Aug 11;22(8).

5643 Marengo A, Piras A, Falconieri D, et al. Chemical and biomolecular analyses to discriminate three taxa of Pistacia genus from Sardinia Island (Italy) and their antifungal activity. *Nat Prod Res.* 2017 Sep 20:1-9.

5644 Spyridopoulou K, Tiptiri-Kourpeti A, Lampri E, et al. Dietary mastic oil extracted from Pistacia lentiscus var. chia suppresses tumor growth in experimental colon cancer models. *Sci Rep.* 2017 Jun 19;7(1):3782.

5645 Mohamed K, Zine K, Fahima K, et al. NiO nanoparticles induce cytotoxicity mediated through ROS generation and impairing the antioxidant defense in the human lung epithelial cells (A549): Preventive effect of Pistacia lentiscus essential oil. *Toxicol Rep.* 2018 Mar 21;5:480-488.

5646 Fathollahi M, Aminzare M, Mohseni M, et al. Antioxidant capacity, antimicrobial activities and chemical composition of Pistacia atlantica subsp. kurdica essential oil. *Vet Res Forum.* 2019 Fall;10(4):299-305.

5647 Milia E, Usai M, Szotakova B, et al. The Pharmaceutical Ability of Pistacia lentiscus L. Leaves Essential Oil Against Periodontal Bacteria and Candida Sp. And Its Anti-Inflammatory Potential. *Antibiotics (Basel).* 2020 May 26;9(6):E281.

5648 Contini A, Di Bello D, Azzara A, et al. Assessing the cytotoxic/genotoxic activity and estrogenic/antiestrogenic potential of essential oils from seven aromatic plants. *Food Chem Toxicol.* 2020 Apr;138:111205.

5649 Xanthis V, Fitsiou E, Voulgaridou GP, et al. Antioxidant and Cytoprotective Potential of the Essential Oil Pistacia lentiscus var. chia and Its Major Components Myrcene and α-Pinene. *Antioxidants (Basel).* 2021 Jan 18;10(1):127.

5650 Pasias IN, Ntakoulas DD, Raptopoulou K, et al. Chemical Composition of Essential Oils of Aromatic and Medicinal Herbs Cultivated in Greece-Benefits and Drawbacks. *Foods.* 2021 Oct 3;10(10):2354.

5651 Souilah N, Amina B, Hamdi B, et al. Ethnobotanical investigation of Pistacia lentiscus L. grown in El Kala (Algeria), and phytochemical study and antioxidant activity of its essential oil and extracts. *Nat Prod Res.* 2022 Jan 11:1-6.

5652 Si L, Chen Y, Han X, et al. Chemical Composition of Essential Oils of Litsea cubeba Harvested from Its Distribution Areas in China. *Molecules.* 2012;17:7057-7066.

5653 Hu L, Du M, Zhang J, et al. Chemistry of the Main Component of Essential Oil of Litsea cubeba and Its Derivatives. *Open J Forestry.* 2014;4:457-66.

5654 Chen CJ, Tseng YH, Chu FH, et al. Neuropharmacological activities of fruit essential oil from Litsea cubeba Persoon. *J Wood Sci.* 2012;58:538-43.

5655 Leclercq PA. Composition of the Stem, Flower and Fruit Oils of Litsea cubeba Pers. from Two Locations of Assam, India. *J Essent Oil Res.* 1998;10(4):381-86.

5656 Nhu-Trang TT, Casabianca H, Grenier-Loustalot MF. Authenticity control of essential oils containing citronellal and citral by chiral and stable-isotope gas-chromatographic analysis. *Anal Bioanal Chem.* 2006 Dec;386(7-8):2141-52.

5657 Wang H, Liu Y. Chemical composition and antibacterial activity of essential oils from different parts of Litsea cubeba. *Chem Biodivers.* 2010 Jan;7(1):229-35.

5658 Nogueira AC, Carvalho RR, Souza CA, et al. Study on the embryofeto-toxicity of citral in the rat. *Toxicology.* 1995;96(2):105-13.

5659 Seo KA, Kim H, Ku HY, et al. The monoterpenoids citral and geraniol are moderate inhibitors of the CYP2B6 hydroxylase activity. *Chem Biol Interact.* 2008;174:141-46.

5660 Hagvall L, Baron JM, Börje A, et al. Cytochrome P450-mediated activation of the fragrance constituent geraniol forms potent contact allergens. *Toxicol Appl Pharmacol.* 2008 Dec 1;233(2):308-13.

5661 Chen CJ, Tseng YH, Chu FH, et al. Neuropharmacological activities of fruit essential oil from Litsea cubeba Persoon. *J Wood Sci.* 2012;58:538-43.

5662 Modak T, Mukhopadhaya A. Effects of citral, a naturally occurring antiadipogenic molecule, on an energy-intense diet model of obesity. *Indian J Pharmacol.* 2011 May-Jun;43(3):300-05.

5663 Najafian M, Ebrahim-Habibi A, Yaghmaei P, et al. Citral as a potential antihyperlipidemic medicine in diabetes: a study on streptozotocin-induced diabetic rats. *J Diabetes Metabolic Disorders.* 2011;10(1):3.

5664 Choi JY, Damte D, Seung-Jin L, et al. Antimicrobial activity of lemongrass and oregano essential oil against standard antibiotic resistant Staphylococcus aureus and field isolates from chronic mastitis cow. *International Journal of Phytomedicine.* 2012;4(1):134-39.

5665 Shin S, Lim S. Antifungal effects of herbal essential oils alone and in combination with ketoconazole against Trichophyton spp. *J Appl Micribiol.* 2004;97:1289-96.

5666 Lalko J, Api AM. Investigation of the dermal sensitization potential of various essential oils in the local lymph node assay. *Food Chem Toxicol.* 2006 May;44(5):739-46.

5667 Kuhn GO, McCampbell P, Singmaster G, et al. Application of microencapsulation technology to improve the stability of citral in rodent diets. *Fundam Appl Toxicol.* 1991 Oct;17(3):635-40.

5668 De Mozzi P, Johnston GA. An outbreak of allergic contact dermatitis caused by citral in beauticians working in a health spa. *Contact Dermatitis.* 2014 Jun;70(6):377-9.

5669 Seal S, Chatterjee P, Bhattacharya S, et al. Vapor of volatile oils from Litsea cubeba seed induces apoptosis and causes cell cycle arrest in lung cancer cells. *PLoS One.* 2012;7(10):e47014.

5670 Ho CL, Jie-Pinge O, Liu YC, et al. Compositions and in vitro anticancer activities of the leaf and fruit oils of Litsea cubeba from Taiwan. *Nat Prod Commun.* 2010 Apr;5(4):617-20.

5671 Nardoni S, Giovanelli S, Pistelli L, et al. In Vitro Activity of Twenty Commercially Available, Plant-Derived Essential Oils against Selected Dermatophyte Species. *Nat Prod Commun.* 2015 Aug;10(8):1473-8.

5672 Chen CJ, Tseng YH, Chu FH, et al. Neuropharmacological activities of fruit essential oil from Litsea cubeba Persoon. *J Wood Sci.* 2012;58:538-43.

5673 Abdul Hammid S, Ahmad F. Chemotype of Litsea cubeba Essential Oil and Its Bioactivity. *Nat Prod Commun.* 2015 Jul;10(7):1301-4.

5674 Li WR, Shi QS, Liang Q, et al. Antibacterial activity and kinetics of Litsea cubeba oil on Escherichia coli. *PLoS One.* 2014 Nov 5;9(11):e110983.

5675 Wang H, Liu Y. Chemical composition and antibacterial activity of essential oils from different parts of Litsea cubeba. *Chem Biodivers.* 2010 Jan;7(1):229-35.

5676 Van Nguyen H, Caruso D, Lebrun M, et al. Antibacterial activity of Litsea cubeba (Lauraceae, May Chang) and its effects on the biological response of common carp Cyprinus carpio challenged with Aeromonas hydrophila. *J Appl Microbiol.* 2016 Aug;121(2):341-51.

5677 Nardoni S, Tortorano A, Mugnaini L, et al. Susceptibility of Microsporum canis arthrospores to a mixture of chemically defined essential oils: a perspective for environmental decontamination. *Z Naturforsch C.* 2015;70(1-2):15- 24.

5678 Zhang SY, Guo Q, Gao XL, et al. [A phytochemical and pharmacological advance on medicinal plant Litsea cubeba (Lauraceae)]. *Zhongguo Zhong Yao Za Zhi.* 2014 Mar;39(5):769-76.

5679 Qian BC, Gong WG, Chen J, et al. [Pharmacological studies on anti-asthmatic and anti-anaphylactic activities of the essential oil of Litsea cubeba (Lour.) Pers. (author's transl)]. *Yao Xue Xue Bao.* 1980 Oct;15(10):584-9.

5680 Wang CY. [The active principles of Litsea cubeba in the treatment of coronary heart disease]. *Zhong Yao Tong Bao.* 1985 Sep;10(9):30-2.

5681 Zhou J. [Progress of Litsea cubeba emulsion in the pharmacological and therapeutic research]. *Zhong Xi Yi Jie He Za Zhi.* 1991 Aug;11(8):509-12.

5682 Noosidum A, Chareonviriyaphap T, Chandrapatya A. Synergistic repellent and irritant effect of combined essential oils on Aedes aegypti (L.) mosquitoes. *J Vector Ecol.* 2014 Dec;39(2):298-305.

5683 Wang X, Li Q, Shen L, et al. Fumigant, contact, and repellent activities of essential oils against the darkling beetle, Alphitobius diaperinus. *J Insect Sci.* 2014 May 30;14:75.

5684 Seo SM, Kim J, Lee SG, et al. Fumigant antitermitic activity of plant essential oils and components from Ajowan (Trachyspermum ammi), Allspice (Pimenta dioica), caraway (Carum carvi), dill (Anethum graveolen), Geranium (Pelargonium graveolens), and Litsea (Litsea cubeba) oils against Japanese termite (Reticulitermes speratus Kolbe). *J Agric Food Chem.* 2009 Aug 12;57(15):6596-602.

5685 Jiang Z, Akhtar Y, Bradbury R, et al. Comparative toxicity of essential oils of Litsea pungens and Litsea cubeba and blends of their major constituents against the cabbage looper, Trichoplusia ni. *J Agric Food Chem.* 2009 Jun 10;57(11):4833-7.

5686 Wang X, Hao Q, Chen Y, et al. The Effect of Chemical Composition and Bioactivity of Several Essential Oils on Tenebrio molitor (Coleoptera: Tenebrionidae). *J Insect Sci.* 2015 Aug 7;15.

5687 Hennino A, Vocanson M, Toussaint Y, et al. Skin-infiltrating CD8+ T cells initiate atopic dermatitis lesions. *J Immunol.* 2007 May 1;178(9):5571-7.

5688 Ka SM, Lin JC, Lin TJ, et al. Citral alleviates an accelerated and severe lupus nephritis model by inhibiting the activation signal of NLRP3 inflammasome and enhancing Nrf2 activation. *Arthritis Res Ther.* 2015 Nov 19;17:331.

5689 Lewis KN, Mele J, Hayes JD, et al. Nrf2, a guardian of healthspan and gatekeeper of species longevity. *Integr Comp Biol.* 2010 Nov;50(5):829-43.

5690 Van Nguyen H, Meile JC, Lebrun M, et al. Litsea cubeba leaf essential oil from Vietnam: chemical diversity and its impacts on antibacterial activity. *Lett Appl Microbiol.* 2018 Mar;66(3):207-214.

5691 Candy K, Nicolas P, Andriantsoanirina V, et al. In vitro efficacy of five essential oils against Pediculus humanus capitis. *Parasitol Res.* 2018 Feb;117(2):603-609.

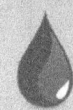

5692 Feng J, Shi W, Miklossy J, et al. Identification of Essential Oils with Strong Activity against Stationary Phase Borrelia burgdorferi. *Antibiotics (Basel)*. 2018 Oct 16;7(4).
5693 She QH, Li WS, Jiang YY, et al. Chemical composition, antimicrobial activity and antioxidant activity of Litsea cubeba essential oils in different months. *Nat Prod Res*. 2019 Mar 31:1-4.
5694 Nguyen QH, Nguyen HV, Vu TH, et al. Characterization of Endophytic Streptomyces griseorubens MPT42 and Assessment of Antimicrobial Synergistic Interactions of its Extract and Essential Oil from Host Plant Litsea cubeba. *Antibiotics (Basel)*. 2019 Oct 28;8(4).
5695 Pedroso RDS, Balbino BL, Andrade G, et al. In Vitro and In Vivo Anti- Candida Spp. Activity of Plant-Derived Products. *Plants (Basel)*. 2019 Nov;8(11):494.
5696 Najar B, Pistelli L, Shortrede JE, et al. Chemical Composition and in Vitro Cytotoxic Screening of Sixteen Commercial Essential Oils on Five Cancer Cell Lines. *Chem Biodivers*. 2020 Jan;17(1):e1900478.
5697 Krzyśko-Łupicka T, Sokół S, Piekarska-Stachowiak A. Evaluation of Fungistatic Activity of Eight Selected Essential Oils on Four Heterogeneous Fusarium Isolates Obtained From Cereal Grains in Southern Poland. *Molecules*. 2020 Jan 10;25(2):292.
5698 Chaiyasut C, Sivamaruthi BS, Wongwan J, et al. Effects of Litsea cubeba (Lour.) Persoon Essential Oil Aromatherapy on Mood States and Salivary Cortisol Levels in Healthy Volunteers. *Evid Based Complement Alternat Med*. 2020 Jul 26;2020:4389239.
5699 Yang Y, Chen Y, Zhang G, et al. Transcriptomic Analysis of Staphylococcus aureus Under the Stress Condition Caused by Litsea cubeba L. Essential Oil via RNA Sequencing. *Front Microbiol*. 2020 Sep 8;11:1693.
5700 Mothana R, Alsaid M, Khlad JM, et al. Assessment of antinociceptive, antipyretic and antimicrobial activity of Piper cubeba L. essential oil in animal models. *Pak J Pharm Sci*. 2016 Mat;29(2, Suppl):671-7.
5701 Dai J, Li, C, Cui H, et al. Unraveling the anti-bacterial mechanism of Litsea cubeba essential oil against E. coli O157:H7 and its application in vegetable juices. *Int J Food Microbiol*. 2021 Jan 2;338:108989.
5702 Thielmann J, Theobald M, Wutz A, et al. Litsea cubeba fruit essential oil and its major constituent citral as volatile agents in an antimicrobial packaging material. *Food Microbiol*. 2021 Jun;96:103725.
5703 Pante GC, Castro JC, Lini RS, et al. Litsea cubeba essential oil: chemical profile, antioxidant activity, cytotoxicity, effect against Fusarium verticillioides and fumonisins production. *J Environ Sci Health B*. 2021 Feb 27;1-9.
5704 Santos AA, Wanderley-Teixeira V, Dos Santos Cruz G, et al. Essential oil toxicity on biological and reproductive parameters of Alabama argillacea (Hübner) (Lepidoptera: Erebidae). *Acta Histochem*. 2021 Apr 12;123(4):151714.
5705 Guo Y, Li Y, Li Z, et al. Deep eutectic solvent-homogenate based microwave-assisted hydrodistillation of essential oil from Litsea cubeba (Lour.) Pers. fruits and its chemical composition and biological activity. *J Chromatogr A*. 2021 Mar 22;1646:462089.
5706 Soroh A, Owen LL, Rahim N, et al. Microemulsification of essential oils for the development of antimicrobial and mosquito repellent functional coatings for textiles. *J Appl Microbiol*. 2021 May 22. Online ahead of print.
5707 Sattayakhom A, Songsamoe S, Yusakul G, et al. Effects of Thai Local Ingredient Odorants, Litsea cubeba and Garlic Essential Oils, on Brainwaves and Moods. *Molecules*. 2021 May 15;26(10):2939.
5708 Duque LS, Marchesini P, Monteiro C, et al. Acaricidal activity of the essential oils from Leptospermum scoparium, Origanum vulgare and Litsea cubeba on Rhipicephalus microplus: Influence of the solvents and search for fractions with higher bioactivity. *Vet Parasitol*. 2021 Dec;300:109606.
5709 Chen J, Zhang J, Zhu L, et al. Antibacterial Activity of the Essential Oil From Litsea cubeba Against Cutibacterium acnes and the Investigations of Its Potential Mechanism by Gas Chromatography-Mass Spectrometry Metabolomics. *Front Microbiol*. 2022 Mar 2;13:823845.
5710 Li A, Shi C, Qian S, Wang Z, et al. Evaluation of antibiotic combination of Litsea cubeba essential oil on Vibrio parahaemolyticus inhibition mechanism and antibiofilm ability. *Microb Pathog*. 2022 May 11;168:105574.
5711 Li H, Kong Y, Hu W, et al. Litsea cubeba Essential Oil: Component Analysis, Anti-Candida albicans Activity and Mechanism Based on Molecular Docking. *J Oleo Sci*. 2022 Jul 6. Online ahead of print.
5712 Songsang N, Anunmana C, Pudla M, et al. Effects of Litsea cubeba Essential Oil Incorporated into Denture Soft Lining Materials. *Polymers (Basel)*. 2022 Aug 10;14(16):3261.
5713 Silva-Trujillo L, Quintero-Rueda E, Stashenko EE, et al. Essential Oils from Colombian Plants: Antiviral Potential against Dengue Virus Based on Chemical Composition, In Vitro and In Silico Analyses. *Molecules*. 2022 Oct 12;27(20):6844.
5714 Nuiden N, Siripornpanich V, Sayorwan W, et al. The effects of Litsea cubeba essential oil inhalation on brain wave activity. *Indian J Trad Knowledge*. 2022 Oct;21(4):797-801.
5715 Qiu Y, Wang Y, Li Y. Solvent-Free Microwave Extraction of Essential Oils from Litsea cubeba (Lour.) Pers. at Different Harvesting Times and Their Skin-Whitening Cosmetic Potential. *Antioxidants (Basel)*. 2022 Dec 1;11(12):2389.
5716 Bai X, Chen T, Liu X, Liu Z, et al. Antibacterial Activity and Possible Mechanism of Litsea cubeba Essential Oil Against Shigella sonnei and Its Application in Lettuce. *Foodborne Pathog Dis*. 2023 Apr 3. Online ahead of print.
5717 El-Hawary SS, Taha KF, Abdel-Monem AR, et al. Chemical composition and biological activities of peels and leaves essential oils of four cultivars of Citrus deliciosa var. tangarina. *Am J Essent Oils Nat Prod*. 2013;1(2):1-6.
5718 El-Hawary SS, Taha KF, Abdel-Monem AR, et al. Chemical composition and biological activities of peels and leaves essential oils of four cultivars of Citrus deliciosa var. tangarina. *Am J Essent Oils Nat Prod*. 2013;1(2):1-6.
5719 Dugo P, Bonaccorsi I, Ragonese C, et al. Analytical characterization of mandarin (Citrus deliciosa Ten.) essential oil. *Flavour Frag J*. 2011 Jan;26(1):34-46.
5720 Steuer B, Schulz H, Lager E. Classification and analysis of citrus oils by NIR spectroscopy. *Food Chem*. 2001;72(1):113-17.
5721 Bonaccorsi I, Sciarrone D, Cotroneo A, et al. Enantiomeric distribution of key volatile components in Citrus essential oils. *Rev Bras Farmacogn*. 2011 Sept-Oct;21(5):ISSN 0102-695X.
5722 Frizzo CD, Lorenzo D, Dellacassa E. Composition and Seasonal Variation of the Essential Oils fromTwo Mandarin Cultivars of Southern Brazil. *J Agric Food Chem*. 2004 ;52:3036-41.
5723 Dugrand-Judek A, Olry A, Hehn A, et al. The distribution of coumarins and furanocoumarins in Citrus species closely matches citrus phylogeny and reflects the organization of biosynthetic pathways. *PLoS One*. 2015 Nov;10(11):e0142757.
5724 El-Hawary SS, Taha KF, Abdel-Monem AR, et al. Chemical composition and biological activities of peels and leaves essential oils of four cultivars of Citrus deliciosa var. tangarina. *Am J Essent Oils Nat Prod*. 2013;1(2):1-6.
5725 El-Hawary SS, Taha KF, Abdel-Monem AR, et al. Chemical composition and biological activities of peels and leaves essential oils of four cultivars of Citrus deliciosa var. tangarina. *Am J Essent Oils Nat Prod*. 2013;1(2):1-6.
5726 El-Hawary SS, Taha KF, Abdel-Monem AR, et al. Chemical composition and biological activities of peels and leaves essential oils of four cultivars of Citrus deliciosa var. tangarina. *Am J Essent Oils Nat Prod*. 2013;1(2):1-6.
5727 El-Hawary SS, Taha KF, Abdel-Monem AR, et al. Chemical composition and biological activities of peels and leaves essential oils of four cultivars of Citrus deliciosa var. tangarina. *Am J Essent Oils Nat Prod*. 2013;1(2):1-6.
5728 Nurzynska-Wierdak R, Bogucka-Kocka A, Symczak G. Volatile constituents of Melissa officinalis leaves determined by plant age. *Nat Prod Commun*. 2014 May;9(5):703-06.
5729 Taherpour AA, Maroofi H, Rafie Z, et al. Chemical composition analysis of the essential oil of Melissa officinalis L. from Kurdistan, Iran by HS/SPME method and calculation of the biophysicochemical coefficients of the components. *Nat Prod Res*. 2012;62(2):152-60.
5730 Patora J, Majda T, Gora J, et al. Variability in the content and composition of essential oil from lemon balm (Melissa officinalis L.) cultivated in Poland. *Acta Poloniae Pharmaccutica - Drug Research*. 2003;60(5):395-400.
5731 Abdellatif F, Boudjella H, Zitouni A, et al. Chemical composition and antimicrobial activity of the essential oil from leaves of Algerian Melissa officinalis L. *EXCLI J*.2014;13:772-81.
5732 Rehman SU, Latief R, Bhat K, et al. Comparative analysis of the aroma chemicals of Melissa officinalis using hydrodistillation and HS-SPME techniques. *Arabian J Chem*. 2013 Sep;917(S2).
5733 Nogueira AC, Carvalho RR, Souza CA, et al. Study on the embryofeto-toxicity of citral in the rat. *Toxicology*. 1995;96(2):105-13.
5734 De Olivera AC, Ribeiro-Pinto LF, Paumgartten JR. In vitro inhibition of CYP2B1 monoxygenase by beta-myrcene and other monoterpenoid constituents. *Br J Nutr*. 1999;81:289-95.
5735 Seo KA, Kim H, Ku HY, et al. The monoterpenoids citral and geraniol are moderate inhibitors of the CYP2B6 hydroxylase activity. *Chem Biol Interact*. 2008;174:141-46.
5736 Raner GM, Vaz AD, Coon MJ. Metabolism of all-trans, 9-cis, and 13-cis isomers of retinal by purified isozymes of microsomal cytochrome P450 and mechanism-based inhibition of retinoid oxidation by citral. *Mol Pharmacol*. 1996;49(3):515-22.
5737 Nguyen LT, Mysliveckova Z, Szotakova B, et al. The inhibitory effects of β-caryophyllene, β-caryophyllene oxide and α-humulene on the activities of the main drug-metabolizing enzymes in rat and human liver in vitro. *Chem-Biol Interactoins*. 2017 Dec 25;278:123-8.
5738 Modak T, Mukhopadhaya A. Effects of citral, a naturally occurring antiadipogenic molecule, on an energy-intense diet model of obesity. *Indian J Pharmacol*. 2011 May-Jun;43(3):300-05.
5739 Najafian M, Ebrahim-Habibi A, Yaghmaei P, et al. Citral as a potential antihyperlipidemic medicine in diabetes: a study on streptozotocin-induced diabetic rats. *J Diabetes Metabolic Disorders*. 2011;10(1):3.
5740 Chung MJ, Cho SY, Bhuiyan MJ, et al. Anti-diabetic effects of lemon balm (Melissa officinalis) essential oil on glucose- and lipid-regulating enzymes in type 2 diabetic mice. *Br J Nutr*. 2010 Jul;104(2):180-88.
5741 Lin WY, Kuo YH, Chang YL, et al. Anti-platelet aggregation and chemical constituents from the rhizome of Gynura japonica. *Planta Med*. 2003 Aug;69(8):757-64.
5742 Ferrieira A, Proenca C, Serralheiro ML, et al. The in vitro screening for acetylcholinesterase inhibition and antioxidant activity of medicinal plants from Portugal. *J Ethnopharmacol*. 2006 Nov 3;108(1):31-37.
5743 Chaiyana W, Okonogi S. Inhibition of cholinesterase by essential oil from food plant. *Phytomedicine*. 2012 Jun;19(8-9):836-39.
5744 Choi JY, Damte D, Seung-Jin L, et al. Antimicrobial activity of lemongrass and oregano essential oil against standard antibiotic resistant Staphylococcus aureus and field isolates from chronic mastitis cow. *International Journal of Phytomedicine*. 2012;4(1):134-39.
5745 Shin S, Lim S. Antifungal effects of herbal essential oils alone and in combination with ketoconazole against Trichophyton spp. *J Appl Micribiol*. 2004;97:1289-96.
5746 do Vale TG, Furtado EC, Santos JG Jr, et al. Central effects of citral, myrcene and limonene, constituents of essential oil chemotypes from Lippia alba (Mill.) n.e. Brown. *Phytomedicine*. 2002 Dec;9(8):709-14.
5747 Kuhn GO, McCampbell P, Singmaster G, et al. Application of microencapsulation technology to improve the stability of citral in rodent diets. *Fundam Appl Toxicol*. 1991 Oct;17(3):635-40.

5748 De Mozzi P, Johnston GA. An outbreak of allergic contact dermatitis caused by citral in beauticians working in a health spa. *Contact Dermatitis*. 2014 Jun;70(6):377-9.
5749 de Sousa AC, Alviano DS, Blank AF, et al. Melissa officinalis L. essential oil: antitumoral and antioxidant activities. *J Pharm Pharmacol*. 2004 May;56(5):677-81.
5750 Queiroz RM, Takiya CM, Guimaraes LP, et al. Apoptosis-inducing effects of Melissa officinalis L. essential oil in glioblastoma multiforme cells. *Cancer Invest*. 2014 Jul;32(6):226-35.
5751 Ballard CG, O'Brien JT, Reichelt K, et al. Aromatherapy as a safe and effective treatment for the management of agitation in sever dementia: the results of a double-blind, placebo-controlled trial with Melissa. *J Clin Psychiatry*. 2002 Jul;63(7):553-58.
5752 Abuhamdah S, Huang L, Elliott MS, et al. Pharmacological profile of essential oil derived from Melissa officinalis with anti-agitation properties: focus on ligand-gated channels. *J Pharm Pharmacol*. 2008 Mar;60(3):377-84.
5753 Huang L, Abuhamdah S, Howes MJ, et al. Pharmacological profile of essential oils derived from Lavandula angustifolia and Melissa officinalis with anti-agitation properties: focus on lignand-gated channels. *J Pharm Pharmacol*. 28 Nov;60(11):1515-22.
5754 Kennedy DO, Scholey AB. The psychopharmacology of European herbs with cognition-enhancing properties. *Curr Pharm Des*. 206;12(35):4613-23.
5755 Hasanein P, Riahi H. Antinociceptive and antihyperglycemic effects of Melissa officinalis essential oil in an experimental model of diabetes. *Med Princ Pract*. 2015;24(1):47-52.
5756 Ferrieira A, Proenca C, Serralheiro ML, et al. The in vitro screening for acetylcholinesterase inhibition and antioxidant activity of medicinal plants from Portugal. *J Ethnopharmacol*. 2006 Nov 3;108(1):31-37.
5757 Chaiyana W, Okonogi S. Inhibition of cholinesterase by essential oil from food plant. *Phytomedicine*. 2012 Jun;19(8-9):836-39.
5758 Darvesh S, Hopkins DA, Geula C, Neurobiology of butyrylcholinesterase. *Nat Rev Neurosci*. 2003 Feb;4:131-38.
5759 Chung MJ, Cho Sy, Bhuiyan MJ, et al. Anti-diabetic effects of lemon balm (Melissa officinalis) essential oil on glucose- and lipid-regulating enzymes in type 2 diabetic mice. *Br J Nutr*. 2010 Jul;10492):180-88.
5760 Schnitzler P, Schumacher A, Astani A, et al. Melissa officinalis oil affects infectivity of enveloped herpesviruses. *Phytomedicine*. 2008 Sep;15(9):734-40.
5761 Astani A, Reichling J, Schnitzler P. Melissa officinalis extract inhibits attachment of herpes simplex virus in vitro. *Chemotherapy*. 2012;58(1):70-77.
5762 Schnitzler P, Schumacher A, Astani A, et al. Melissa officinalis oil affects infectivity of enveloped herpesviruses. *Phytomedicine*. 2008 Sep;15(9):734-40.
5763 Allahverdiyev A, Duran N, Ozguven M, et al. Antiviral activity of the volatile oils of Melissa officinalis L. against Herpes simplex virus type-2. *Phytomedicine*. 2004 Nov;11(7-8):657-61.
5764 Baylac S, Racine P. Inhibition of 5-lipoxygenase by essential oils and other natural fragrant extracts. *Int J Aromatherapy*. 2003;13(2-3):138-42.
5765 Ballard CG, O'Brien JT, Reichelt K, et al. Aromatherapy as a safe and effective treatment for the management of agitation in severe dementia: the results of a double-blind, placebo-controlled trial with Melissa. *J Clin Psychiatry*. 2002 Jul;63(7):553-58.
5766 Bounihi A, Hajjaj G, Alnamer R, et al. In vivo potential anti-inflammatory activity of Melissa officinalis L. essential oil. *Adv Pharmacol Sci*. 2013;2013:101759.
5767 Pourghanbari G, Nili H, Moattari A, et al. Antiviral activity of the oseltamivir and Melissa officinalis L. essential oil against avian influenza A virus (H9N2). *Virusdisease*. 2016 Jun;27(2):170-8.
5768 Jun HJ, Lee JH, Jia Y, et al. Melissa officinalis essential oil reduces plasma triglycerides in human apolipoprotein E2 transgenic mice by inhibiting sterol regulatory element-binding protein-1c-dependent fatty acid synthesis. *J Nutr*. 2012 Mar;142(3):432-40.
5769 Hancianu M, Aprotosoaie AC, Gille E, et al. Chemical composition and in vitro antimicrobial activity of essential oil of Melissa officinalis L. from Romania. *Rev Med Chir Soc Med Nat Iasi*. 2008 Jul-Sep;112(3):843-47.
5770 Mikus J, Harkenthal M, Steverding D, et al. In vitro effect of essential oils and isolated mono- and sesquiterpenes on Leishmania major and Trypanosoma brucei. *Planta Med*. 2000 May;66(4):366-68.
5771 Mimica-Dukic N, Bozin B, Sokovic M, et al. Antimicrobial and antioxidant activities of Melissa officinalis L. (Lamiaceae) essential oil. *J Food Agric Chem*. 2004 May 5;52(9):2485-89.
5772 Sadraei H, Ghannadi A, Malekshahi K. Relaxant effects of essential oil of Melissa officinalis and citral on rat ileum contractions. *Fitoterapia*. 2003 Jul;774(5):445-52.
5773 Schnitzler P, Reichling J. Efficacy of plant products against herpetic infections. *HNO*. 2011 Dec;59(12):1176-84.
5774 Andrade MA, Azevedo CD, Motta FN, et al. Essential oils: in vitro activity against Leishmania amazonensis, cytotoxicity and chemical composition. *BMC Complement Altern Med*. 2016 Nov 8;16(1):444.
5775 Ergüden C, Özkoç S, Öztürk B, et al. [Investigation of the in vitro effects of Melissa officinalis L., Mentha x piperita L. and Ocimum basilicum L. (Lamiaceae) essential oils on the cysts and trophozoites of Acanthamoeba castellani]. *Mikrobiyol Bul*. 2016 Oct;50(4):569-579.
5776 Giatropoulos A, Kimbaris A, Michaelakis A, et al. Chemical composition and assessment of larvicidal and repellent capacity of 14 Lamiaceae essential oils against Aedes albopictus. *Parasitol Res*. 2018 Jun;117(6):1953-1964.
5777 Powers CN, Osier JL, McFeeters RL, et al. Antifungal and Cytotoxic Activities of Sixty Commercially-Available Essential Oils. *Molecules*. 2018 Jun 27;23(7).
5778 Watson K, Hatcher D, Good A. A randomised controlled trial of Lavender (Lavandula Angustifolia) and Lemon Balm (Melissa Officinalis) essential oils for the treatment of agitated behaviour in older people with and without dementia. *Complement Therapies Med*. 2019 Feb;42:366-373.
5779 Serra E, Saubade F, Ligorio C, et al. Methylcellulose Hydrogel With Melissa officinalis Essential Oil as a Potential Treatment for Oral Candidiasis. Microorganisms. 2020 Feb 6;8(2):215.
5780 Korona-Glowniak I, Glowniak-Lipa A, Ludwiczuk A, et al. The In Vitro Activity of Essential Oils Against Helicobacter Pylori Growth and Urease Activity. *Molecules*. 2020 Jan 29;25(3):586.
5781 Vanti G, Ntallis SG, Panagiotidis CA, et al. Glycerosome of Melissa officinalis L. Essential Oil for Effective Anti-HSV Type 1. *Molecules*. 2020 Jul 8;25(14):E3111.
5782 Veiskaramin A, Gholami M, Yarahmadi S, et al. Effect of aromatherapy with Melissa essential oil on stress and hemodynamic parameters in acute coronary syndrome patients: A clinical trial in the emergency department. *Complement Ther Clin Pract*. 2021 Aug;44:101436.
5783 Radulexcu M, Jianu C, Lukinich-Gruia AT, et al. Chemical Composition, In Vitro and In Silico Antioxidant Potential of Melissa officinalis subsp. officinalis Essential Oil. *Antioxidants (Basel)*. 2021 Jul 5;10(7):1081.
5784 Chindo BA, Howes MJR, Abuhamdah S, et al. New Insights Into the Anticonvulsant Effects of Essential Oil From Melissa officinalis L. (Lemon Balm). *Front Pharmacol*. 2021 Oct 14;12:760674.
5785 Stojanovic NM, Mladenovic MZ, Maslovaric A, et al. Lemon balm (Melissa officinalis L.) essential oil and citronellal modulate anxiety-related symptoms - In vitro and in vivo studies. *J Ethnopharmacol*. 2021 Oct 27;114788.
5786 Yu H, Pei J, Qiu W, et al. The Antimicrobial Effect of Melissa officinalis L. Essential Oil on Vibrio parahaemolyticus: Insights Based on the Cell Membrane and External Structure. *Front Microbiol*. 2022 Mar 10;13:812792.
5787 Galgano M, Capozza P, Pellegrini F, et al. Antimicrobial Activity of Essential Oils Evaluated In Vitro against Escherichia coli and Staphylococcus aureus. *Antibiotics (Basel)*. 2022 Jul 20;11(7):979.
5788 Arbab S, Ullah H, Bano I, et al. Evaluation of in vitro antibacterial effect of essential oil and some herbal plant extract used against mastitis pathogens. *Vet Med Sci*. 2022 Oct 17. Online ahead of print.
5789 Karpiński TM, Ożarowski M, Seremak-Mrozikiewicz A, et al. Anti-Candida and Antibiofilm Activity of Selected Lamiaceae Essential Oils. *Front Biosci (Landmark Ed)*. 2023 Feb 16;28(2):28.
5790 Mazza G, Kiehn FA, Marshall HH. 1993. Monarda: A source of geraniol, linalool, thymol and carvacrol-rich essential oils. p. 628-631. In: J. Janick and J.E. Simon (eds.), New crops. Wiley, New York.
5791 Zamureenko VA, Klyuev NA, Bocharov BV, et al. An investigation of the component composition of the essential oil of Monarda fistulosa. *Chem Nat Compd*. 1989:549-51.
5792 Tabanca N, Bernier UR, Ali A, et al. Bioassay-guided investigation of two Monarda essential oils as repellents of yellow fever mosquito Aedes aegypti. *J Agric Food Chem*. 2013 Sep 11;61(36):8573-80.
5793 Contaldo N, Bellardi MG, Cavicchi L, et al. Phytochemical effects of phytoplasma infections on essential oil of Monarda fistulosa L. *Bull Insectology*. 2011;64(Supplement):S177-78.
5794 Mazza G, Chubey BB, Kiehn F. Essential oil of Monardafistulosa L. var. Menthaefolia, a potential source of geraniol. *Flavour Frag J*. 1987 Sep;2(3):129-362.
5795 Lawrence BM. Essential oils 1981-1987. Allured Publishing, Wheaton. 1981. p. 68-76.
5796 Seo KA, Kim H, Ku HY, et al. The monoterpenoids citral and geraniol are moderate inhibitors of the CYP2B6 hydroxylase activity. *Chem Biol Interact*. 2008;174:141-46.
5797 Tognolini M, Barocelli E, Ballabeni V, et al. Comparative screening of plant essential oils; phenylpropanoid moiety as basic core for antiplatelet activity. *Life Sci*. 2006 Feb 23;78(13):1419-32.
5798 Ibrahim SM, El-Denshary ES, Abdallah DM. Geraniol, Alone and in Combination with Pioglitazone, Ameliorates Fructose-Induced Metabolic Syndrome in Rats via the Modulation of Both Inflammatory and Oxidative Stress Status. *PLoS One*. 2015 Feb 13;10(2):e0117516.
5799 Srinivasan S, Muruganathan U. Antidiabetic efficacy of citronellol, a citrus monoterpene by ameliorating the hepatic key enzymes of carbohydrate metabolism in streptozotocin-induced diabetic rats. *Chem Biol Interact*. 2016 Apr 25;250:38-46.
5800 Shin S, Lim S. Antifungal effects of herbal essential oils alone and in combination with ketoconazole against Trichophyton spp. *J Appl Micribiol*. 2004;97:1289-96.
5801 Hagvall L. Cytochrome P450-mediated activation of the fragrance constituent geraniol forms potent contact allergens. *Tox Appl Pharm*. 2008 Dec;233(2):308-13.
5802 Lemhadri A, Zeggwagh NA, Maghrani M, et al. Anti-hypoglycaemic activity of the aqueous extract of Origanum vulgare growing wild in Tafilalet region. *J Ethnopharmacol*. 2004 Jun;92(2-3):251-6.
5803 Mirazi N, Rezaei M, Mirhoseini M. Hypoglycemic effect of Satureja montanum L. hydroethanolic extract on diabetic rats. *J HerbMed Pharm*. 2016;5(1):17-22.
5804 Ezhumalai M, Radhiga T, Pugalendi KV. Antihyperglycemic effect of carvacrol in combination with rosiglitazone in high-fat diet-induced type 2 diabetic C57BL/6J mice. *Mol Cell Biochem*. 2014 Jan;385(1-2):23-31.
5805 Tognolini M, Barocelli E, Ballabeni V, et al. Comparative screening of plant essential oils; phenylpropanoid moiety as basic core for antiplatelet activity. *Life Sci*. 2006 Feb 23;78(13):1419-32.
5806 Tsai HH, Lin HW, Chen YL, et al. A review of potential harmful interactions between anticoagulant/antiplatelet agents and Chinese herbal medicines. *PLoS One*. 2013 May 9;8(5):e64255.
5807 Karkabounas S, Kostoula OK, Daskalou T, et al. Anticarcinogenic and antiplatelet effects of carvacrol. *Exp Oncol*. 2006 Jun;28(2):121-5.
5808 Langeveld WT, Veldhuizen EJ, Burt SA. Synergy between essential oil constituents and antibiotics. *Crit Rev Microbiol*. 2014 Feb;40(1);76-94.

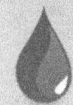

[5809] Jukic M, Politeo O, Maksimmovic M, et al. In vitro acetylcholinesterase inhibitory properties of thymol, carvacrol and their derivatives thymoquinone and thymohydroquinone. *Phytother Res.* 2007;21(3):259-61.

[5810] Kohlert C, Schindler G, Marz RW, et al. Systemic availability and pharmacokinetics of thymol in humans. *J Clin Pharmacol.* 2002 Jul;42(7):731-7.

[5811] US Centers for Disease Control and Prevention. ATSDR, Agency for Toxic Substances and Disease Registry. Medical Management Guidelines for Phenol. Available at: https://www.atsdr.cdc.gov/MHMI/mmg115.pdf.

[5812] Jukic M, Politeo O, Maksimmovic M, et al. In vitro acetylcholinesterase inhibitory properties of thymol, carvacrol and their derivatives thymoquinone and thymohydroquinone. *Phytother Res.* 2007;21(3):259-61.

[5813] Tognolini M, Barocelli E, Ballabeni V, et al. Comparative screening of plant essential oils; phenylpropanoid moiety as basic core for antiplatelet activity. *Life Sci.* 2006 Feb 23;78(13):1419-32.

[5814] Okazaki K, Kawazoe K, Takaishi Y. Human platelet aggregation inhibitors from thyme (Thymus vulgaris L.). *Phytother Res.* 2002 Jun;16(4):398-9.

[5815] Jukic M, Politeo O, Maksimmovic M, et al. In vitro acetylcholinesterase inhibitory properties of thymol, carvacrol and their derivatives thymoquinone and thymohydroquinone. *Phytother Res.* 2007;21(3):259-61.

[5816] Boskabady MH, Rakhshandah H, Moetamedshariati V. Bronchodilatory and anticholinergic effects of Carum copticum on isolated guinea pig tracheal chains. *Medical Journal of the Islamic Republic of Iran.* 1998;11:329–334.

[5817] Boskabady MH, Shaikhi J. Inhibitory effect of Carum copticum on histamine (H1) receptors of isolated guinea-pig tracheal chains. *J Ethnopharmacol.* 2000 Mar;69(3):217-27.

[5818] Langeveld WT, Veldhuizen EJ, Burt SA. Synergy between essential oil constituents and antibiotics. *Crit Rev Microbiol.* 2014 Feb;40(1);76-94.

[5819] Palaniappan K, Holley Ra. Use of natural antimicrobials to increase antibiotic susceptibility of drug resistant bacteria. *In J Food Microbiol.* 2010 Jun 15;140(2-3):164-8.

[5820] Ilic BS, Kocic BD, Ciric VM, et al. An in vitro synergistic interaction of combinations of Thymus glabrescens essential oil and its main constituents with chloramphenicol. *ScientificWorldJournal.* 2014 Jan 28;2014:826219.

[5821] Miladinovic DL, Ilic BS, Kocic BD, et al. Antibacterial investigation of thyme essential oil and its main constituents on combination with tetracycline. *J Med Food.* 2015 Aug;18(8):935-7.

[5822] Zhilyakova ET, Novikov OO, Naumenko EN, et al. Study of Monarda fistulosa essential oil as a prospective antiseborrheic agent. *Bull Exp Biol Med.* 2009 Oct;148(4):612-4.

[5823] Shubina LP, Siurin SA, Savchenko VM. Inhalation of essential oils in the combined treatment of patients with chronic bronchitis. *Crach Delo.* 1990 May;(5):66-67.

[5824] Nikolaevskii VV, Kononova NS, Pertsovskii AI, et al. Effect of essential oils on the course of experimental atherosclerosis. *Patol Fiziol Eksp Ter.* 1990 Sep-Oct;(5):52-53.

[5825] Baylac S, Racine P. Inhibition of 5-lipoxygenase by essential oils and other natural fragrant extracts. *Int J Aromatherapy.* 2003;13(2-3):138-42.

[5826] Zhilyakova ET, Novikov OO, Naumenko EN, et al. Study of Monarda fistulosa essential oil as a prospective antiseborrheic agent. *Bull Exp Biol Med.* 2009 Oct;148(4):612-4.

[5827] Tabanca N, Bernier UR, Ali A, et al. Bioassay-guided investigation of two Monarda essential oils as repellents of yellow fever mosquito Aedes aegypti. *J Agric Food Chem.* 2013 Sep 11;61(36):8573-80.

[5828] Ghosh M, Schepetkin IA, Ozek G, et al. Essential Oils from Monarda fistulosa: Chemical Composition and Activation of Transient Receptor Potential A1 (TRPA1) Channels. *Molecules.* 2020 Oct 22;25(21):E4873.

[5829] Cote H, Pichette A, St-Gelais A, et al. The Biological Activity of Monarda didyma L. Essential Oil and Its Effect as a Diet Supplement in Mice and Broiler Chicken. *Molecules.* 2021 Jun 2;26(11):3368.

[5830] Shanaida M, Hudz N, Białoń M, et al. Chromatographic profiles and antimicrobial activity of the essential oils obtained from some species and cultivars of the Mentheae tribe (Lamiaceae). *Saudi J Biol Sci.* 2021 Nov;28(11):6145-6152.

[5831] Fraternale D, Dufat H, Albertini MC, et al. Chemical composition, antioxidant and anti-inflammatory properties of Monarda didyma L. essential oil. *PeerJ.* 2022 Nov 21;10:e14433.

[5832] Marrufo T, Nazzaro F, Mancini E, et al. Chemical composition and biological activity of the essential oil from leaves of Moringa oleifera Lam. cultivated in Mozambique. *Molecules.* 2013 Sep 9;18(9):10989-1000.

[5833] Chuang PH1, Lee CW, Chou JY, et al. Anti-fungal activity of crude extracts and essential oil of Moringa oleifera Lam. *Bioresour Technol.* 2007 Jan;98(1):232-6.

[5834] Baker MB, de Freitas JV, Silveira ER, et al. Volatile and non-volatile chemical constituents of Moringa oleifera Lam., Moringaceae. *Rev Bras Farmacogn.* 2009 Oct/Dec;19(4):ISSN 0102-695X.

[5835] Pino JA. Floral Scent Composition of Moringa oleifera Lam. *J Essent Oil Res.* 2013;16(3):315-17.

[5836] Kayode RMO, Afolayan AJ. Cytotoxicity and effect of extraction methods on the chemical composition of essential oils of Moringa oleifera seeds. *J Zhejiang Univ-Sci B (Biomed & Biotechnol).* 2015;16(8):680-89.

[5837] van den Brink DM, van Miert JNI, Dacremont G, et al. Characterization of the Final Step in the Conversion of Phytol into Phytanic Acid. *J Biol Chem.* 2005 Jul 22;280(29):26838-44.

[5838] Selkälä EM, Nair RR, Schmitz W, et al. Phytol is lethal for Amacr-deficient mice. *Biochim Biophys Acta.* 2015 Oct;1851(10):1394-405.

[5839] McGinty D, Letizia CS, Api AM. Fragrance material review on phytol. *Food Chem Toxicol.* 2010;48:S59–S63.

[5840] National Institutes of Health. U.S. National Library of Medicine. Alpha-methylacyl-CoA racemase deficiency. Available at: https://ghr.nlm.nih.gov/condition/alpha-methylacyl-coa-racemase-deficiency.

[5841] Kagoura M, Matsui C, Morohashi M. Phytol is a novel tumor promoter on ICR mouse skin. *Jpn J Cancer Res.* 1999 Apr;90(4):377-84.

[5842] Hussein MA, Gobba NA, El Bishbishy MH. Composition, in vitro antioxidant and antitumor properties of essential oil from the seeds of Moringa oleifera. *Int J Pharma Sci.* 2014;4(3):532-40.

[5843] Chuang PH1, Lee CW, Chou JY, et al. Anti-fungal activity of crude extracts and essential oil of Moringa oleifera Lam. *Bioresour Technol.* 2007 Jan;98(1):232-6.

[5844] Marrufo T, Nazzaro F, Mancini E, et al. Chemical composition and biological activity of the essential oil from leaves of Moringa oleifera Lam. cultivated in Mozambique. *Molecules.* 2013 Sep 9;18(9):10989-1000.

[5845] Marrufo T, Nazzaro F, Mancini E, et al. Chemical composition and biological activity of the essential oil from leaves of Moringa oleifera Lam. cultivated in Mozambique. *Molecules.* 2013 Sep 9;18(9):10989-1000.

[5846] Milos M, Radonic A, Bezic N, et al. Localities and seasonal variations in the chemical composition of essential oils from Satureha montana L. and S. cuneifolia Ten. *Flav Frag J.* 2001 May;16(3):157-60.

[5847] Miladi H, Ben Slama R, Mili D, et al. Chemical Composition and Cytotoxic and Antioxidant Activities of Satureja montana L. Essential Oil and Its Antibacterial Potential against Salmonella Spp. Strains. *J Chem.* 2013;(2013):275698.

[5848] Trifan A, Aprotosoaie AC, Brebu M, et al. Chemical composition and antioxidant activity of essential oil from Romanian Saturjea montana L. *Farmacia.* 2015;63(3):413-16.

[5849] Bezic N, Skocibusic M, Dunkic V. Phytochemical composition and antimicrobial activity of Satureja montana L. and Satureja cuneifolia Ten. essential oils. *Acta Bot Croat.* 2005;64(2):313-22.

[5850] Mastelic J, Jerkovic I. Gas chromatography-mass spectrometry analysis of free and glycoconjugated aroma constituents of seasonally collected Satureja montana L. *Food Chem.* 2003 Jan;80(1):135-40.

[5851] Radonic A, Milos M. Chemical composition and in vitro evaluation of antioxidant effect of free volatile constituents from Satureja montana L. *Free Radic Res.* 2003 Jun;37(6):673-9.

[5852] Domaracky M, Rehak P, Juhas S, et al. Effects of selected plant essential oils on the growth and development of mouse preimplantation embryos in vivo. *Physiol Res.* 2007;56(1):97-104.

[5853] Kohlert C, Schindler G, Marz RW, et al. Systemic availability and pharmacokinetics of thymol in humans. *J Clin Pharmacol.* 2002 Jul;42(7):731-7.

[5854] Toxicology Data Network, National Library of Medicine. Thymol. Available at: http://toxnet.nlm.nih.gov/cgi-bin/sis/search/a?dbs+hsdb:@term+@DOCNO+866.

[5855] Lemhadri A, Zeggwagh NA, Maghrani M, et al. Anti-hypoglycaemic activity of the aqueous extract of Origanum vulgare growing wild in Tafilalet region. *J Ethnopharmacol.* 2004 Jun;92(2-3):251-6.

[5856] Mirazi N, Rezaei M, Mirhoseini M. Hypoglycemic effect of Satureja montanum L. hydroethanolic extract on diabetic rats. *J HerbMed Pharm.* 2016;5(1):17-22.

[5857] Ezhumalai M, Radhiga T, Pugalendi KV. Antihyperglycemic effect of carvacrol in combination with rosiglitazone in high-fat diet-induced type 2 diabetic C57BL/6J mice. *Mol Cell Biochem.* 2014 Jan;385(1-2):23-31.

[5858] Tognolini M, Barocelli E, Ballabeni V, et al. Comparative screening of plant essential oils; phenylpropanoid moiety as basic core for antiplatelet activity. *Life Sci.* 2006 Feb 23;78(13):1419-32.

[5859] Tsai HH, Lin HW, Chen YL, et al. A review of potential harmful interactions between anticoagulant/antiplatelet agents and Chinese herbal medicines. *PLoS One.* 2013 May 9;8(5):e64255.

[5860] Karkabounas S, Kostoula OK, Daskalou T, et al. Anticarcinogenic and antiplatelet effects of carvacrol. *Exp Oncol.* 2006 Jun;28(2):121-5.

[5861] Langeveld WT, Veldhuizen EJ, Burt SA. Synergy between essential oil constituents and antibiotics. *Crit Rev Microbiol.* 2014 Feb;40(1);76-94.

[5862] Jukic M, Politeo O, Maksimmovic M, et al. In vitro acetylcholinesterase inhibitory properties of thymol, carvacrol and their derivatives thymoquinone and thymohydroquinone. *Phytother Res.* 2007;21(3):259-61.

[5863] Kundaković T, Stanojković T, Kolundzija B, et al. Cytotoxicity and antimicrobial activity of the essential oil from Satureja montana subsp. pisidica (Lamiceae). *Nat Prod Commun.* 2014 Apr;9(4):569-72.

[5864] Lampronti I, Saab AM, Gambari R. Antiproliferative activity of essential oils derived from plants belonging to the Magnoliophyta division. *Int J Oncol.* 2006 Oct;29(4):989-95.

[5865] Fratini F, Casella S, Leonardi M, et al. Antibacterial activity of essential oils, their blends and mixtures of their main constituents against some strains supporting livestock mastitis. *Fitoterapia.* 2014 Jul;96:1-7.

[5866] Serrano C, Matos O, Teixeira B, et al. Antioxidant and antimicrobial activity of Satureja montana L. extracts. *J Sci Food Agric.* 2011 Jul;91(9):1554-60.

[5867] Carramiñana JJ, Rota C, Burillo J, et al. Antibacterial efficiency of Spanish Satureja montana essential oil against Listeria monocytogenes among natural flora in minced pork. *J Food Prot.* 2008 Mar;71(3):502-8.

[5868] Oussalah M, Caillet S, Salmiéri S, et al. Antimicrobial effects of alginate-based films containing essential oils on Listeria monocytogenes and Salmonella typhimurium present in bologna and ham. *J Food Prot.* 2007 Apr;70(4):901-8.

[5869] Oussalah M, Caillet S, Saucier L, et al. Antimicrobial effects of selected plant essential oils on the growth of a Pseudomonas putida strain isolated from meat. *Meat Sci.* 2006 Jun;73(2):236-44.

[5870] Oussalah M1, Caillet S, Lacroix M. Mechanism of action of Spanish oregano, Chinese cinnamon, and savory essential oils against cell membranes and walls of Escherichia coli O157:H7 and Listeria monocytogenes. *J Food Prot.* 2006 May;69(5):1046-55.

[5871] Oussalah M1, Caillet S, Lacroix M. Mechanism of action of Spanish oregano, Chinese cinnamon, and savory essential oils against cell membranes and walls of Escherichia coli O157:H7 and Listeria monocytogenes. *J Food Prot.* 2006 May;69(5):1046-55.

[5872] Skocibusić M, Bezić N. Phytochemical analysis and in vitro antimicrobial activity of two Satureja species essential oils. *Phytother Res.* 2004 Dec;18(12):967-70.

[5873] D'Amato S, Mazzarrino G, Rossi C, et al. Thymus Vulgaris (Red Thyme) and Caryophyllus Aromaticus (Clove) Essential Oils to Control Spoilage Microorganisms in Pork Under Modified Atmosphere. *Ital J Food Saf.* 2016 Aug 3;5(3):5785.

[5874] Miladi H, Mili D, Ben Slama R, et al. Antibiofilm formation and anti-adhesive property of three mediterranean essential oils against a foodborne pathogen Salmonella strain. *Microb Pathog.* 2016 Apr;93:22-31.

[5875] Michaelakis A, Theotokatos SA, Koliopoulos G, et al. Essential oils of Satureja species: insecticidal effect on Culex pipiens larvae (Diptera: Culicidae). *Molecules.* 2007 Dec 10;12(12):2567-78.

[5876] Tampieri MP, Galuppi R, Macchioni F, et al. The inhibition of Candida albicans by selected essential oils and their major components. *Mycopathologia.* 2005 Apr;159(3):339-45.

[5877] Skocibusić M, Bezić N. Phytochemical analysis and in vitro antimicrobial activity of two Satureja species essential oils. *Phytother Res.* 2004 Dec;18(12):967-70.

[5878] Bona E, Cantamessa S, Pavan M, et al. Sensitivity of Candida albicans to essential oils: are they an alternative to antifungal agents? *J Appl Microbiol.* 2016 Dec;121(6):1530-1545.

[5879] Radonic A, Milos M. Chemical composition and in vitro evaluation of antioxidant effect of free volatile constituents from Satureja montana L. *Free Radic Res.* 2003 Jun;37(6):673-9.

[5880] Benelli G, Pavela R, Canale A, et al. Acute larvicidal toxicity of five essential oils (Pinus nigra, Hyssopus officinalis, Satureja montana, Aloysia citrodora and Pelargonium graveolens) against the filariasis vector Culex quinquefasciatus: Synergistic and antagonistic effects. *Parasitol Int.* 2017 Apr;66(2):166-171.

[5881] Pellegrini M, Ricci A, Serio A, et al. Characterization of Essential Oils Obtained from Abruzzo Autochthonous Plants: Antioxidant and Antimicrobial Activities Assessment for Food Application. *Foods.* 2018 Feb 2;7(2).

[5882] Lagha AB, Vaillancourt K, Huacho PM, et al. Effects of Labrador Tea, Peppermint, and Winter Savory Essential Oils on Fusobacterium nucleatum. *Antibiotics (Basel).* 2020 Nov 10;9(11):794.

[5883] Caprioli G, Lupidi G, Maggi F, et al. Comparison of chemical composition and antioxidant activities of two Winter savory subspecies (Satureja montana subsp. variegata and Satureja montana subsp. montana) cultivated in Northern Italy. *Nat Prod Res.* 2018 Nov 23:1-5.

[5884] Vitanza L, Maccelli A, Marazzato M, et al. Satureja montana L. essential oil and its antimicrobial activity alone or in combination with gentamicin. *Microb Pathog.* 2018 Nov 17;126:323-331.

[5885] Maccellu A, Vitanza L, Imbriano A, et al. Satureja montana L. Essential Oils: Chemical Profiles/Phytochemical Screening, Antimicrobial Activity and O/W NanoEmulsion Formulations. *Pharmaceutics.* 2019 Dec 19;12(1):12010007.

[5886] Šimunović K, Bucar F, Klančnik A, et al. In Vitro Effect of the Common Culinary Herb Winter Savory (Satureja montana) against the Infamous Food Pathogen Campylobacter jejuni. *Foods.* 2020 Apr 24;9(4).

[5887] Rinaldi F, Maurizi L, Conte AL, et al. Nanoemulsions of Satureja montana Essential Oil: Antimicrobial and Antibiofilm Activity against Avian Escherichia coli Strains. *Pharmaceutics.* 2021 Jan 21;13(2):134.

[5888] Reis AC, Konig IFM, Elvati Rezende DADC, et al. Cytotoxic effects of Satureja montana L. essential oil on oocytes of engorged Rhipicephalus microplus female ticks (Acari: Ixodidae). *Microsc Res Tech.* 2021 Jan 6. Online ahead of print.

[5889] Garcia-Diaz M, Gil-Serna J, Patino B, et al. Assessment of the Effect of Satureja montana and Origanum virens Essential Oils on Aspergillus flavus Growth and Aflatoxin Production at Different Water Activities. *Toxins (Basel).* 2020 Feb 25;12(3):142.

[5890] Selvati Rezende DADC, Cardoso MDG, Alves E, et al. Effect of the essential oils of Satureja montana L., Myristica fragrans H. and Cymbopogon flexuosus S. on mycotoxin-producing Aspergillus flavus and Aspergillus ochraceus Antifungal properties of essential oils. *FEMS Microbiol Lett.* 2021 Oct 30;fnab137.

[5891] Kovačević Z, Kladar N, Čabarkapa I, et al. New Perspective of Origanum vulgare L. and Satureja montana L. Essential Oils as Bovine Mastitis Treatment Alternatives. *Antibiotics (Basel).* 2021 Nov 27;10(12):1460.

[5892] Capatina L, Napoli EM, Ruberto G, et al. Origanum vulgare ssp. hirtum (Lamiaceae) Essential Oil Prevents Behavioral and Oxidative Stress Changes in the Scopolamine Zebrafish Model. *Molecules.* 2021 Nov 23;26(23):7085.

[5893] Yao N, Xu Q, Hw JK, et al. Evaluation of Origanum vulgare Essential Oil and Its Active Ingredients as Potential Drugs for the Treatment of Toxoplasmosis. *Front Cell Infect Microbiol.* 2021 Nov 29;11:793089.

[5894] Duque LS, Marchesini P, Monteiro C, et al. Acaricidal activity of the essential oils from Leptospermum scoparium, Origanum vulgare and Litsea cubeba on Rhipicephalus microplus: Influence of the solvents and search for fractions with higher bioactivity. *Vet Parasitol.* 2021 Dec;300:109606.

[5895] Guo Y, Pizzol R, Gabbanini S, et al. Absolute Antioxidant Activity of Five Phenol-Rich Essential Oils. *Molecules.* 2021 Aug 29;26(17):5237.

[5896] Štrbac F, Bosco A, Maurelli MP, et al. Anthelmintic Properties of Essential Oils to Control Gastrointestinal Nematodes in Sheep-In Vitro and In Vivo Studies. *Vet Sci.* 2022 Feb 19;9(2):93.

[5897] Rezende DADCS, Oliveira CD, Batista LR, et al. Bactericidal and antioxidant effects of essential oils from Satureja montana L., Myristica fragrans H. and Cymbopogon flexuosus. *Lett Appl Microbiol.* 2022 May;74(5):741-751.

[5898] Aćimović M, Šovljanski O, Pezo L, et al. Variability in Biological Activities of Satureja montana Subsp. montana and Subsp. variegata Based on Different Extraction Methods. *Antibiotics (Basel).* 2022 Sep 11;11(9):1235.

[5899] Ebani VV, Pieracci Y, Cagnoli G, et al. In Vitro Antimicrobial Activity of Thymus vulgaris, Origanum vulgare, Satureja montana and Their Mixture against Clinical Isolates Responsible for Canine Otitis Externa. *Vet Sci.* 2023 Jan 1;10(1):30.

[5900] Williams JD, Campbell MA, Jaskolka MC, et al. Artemisia vulgaris L. chemotypes. *Am J Plant Sci.* 2013;4:1265– 69.

[5901] Tajadod G, Mazooji A, Salimpour F, et al. The essential oil composition of Artemisia vulgaris L. in Iran. *Annals Biol Res.* 2012;3(1):385–89.

[5902] Govindaraj S, RanjithaKumari BD. Composition and larvicidal activity of Artemisia vulgaris L. stem essential oil against Aedes aegypti. *Jordan J Biol Sci.* 2013 Mar;6(1):11–16.

[5903] Williams JD, Saled AM, Acharya DN. Composition of the essential oil of wild growing Artemisia vulgaris from Erie, Pennsylvnia. *Nat Prod Commun.* 2012 May;7(5):637–40.

[5904] Judzentiene A, Buzelyte J. Chemical composition of essential oils of Artemisia vulgaris L. (mugwort) from North Lithuania. *Chemija.* 200617(1):12–15.

[5905] Said ME, Militello M, Saia S, et al. Artemisia arborescens essential oil composition, enantiomeric distribution and antimicrobial activity from different wild populations from the Mediterranean Area. *Chem Biodivers.* 2016 Aug;13(8):1095-1102.

[5906] Mitello M, Carrubba A, Amparo Blazquez M. Artemisia arborescens L.: essential oil composition and effects of plant growth stage in some genotypes from Sicily. *J Essent Oil Res.* 2012 Jun;24(3):229-235.

[5907] Lohani H, Gwari G, Bhandari U, et al. Variability in the Essential Oils from Aerial Parts of Artemisia vulgaris L. Grown in Uttarakhand (India). *J Essent Oil Bearing Plants.* 2016;19(1):103-07.

[5908] Plant J. Private communication. 2016.

[5909] Sharopov FS, Sulaimonova VA, Setzer WN. Composition of the essential oil of Artemisia absinthium from Tajikstan. *Rec Nat Prod.* 2012;6(2):127–34.

[5910] Millet Y, Jouglard J, Steinmetz MD, et al. Toxicity of some essential plant oils. Clinical and experimental study. *Clin Toxicol.* 1981 Dec;18(12):1485–98.

[5911] Halicioglu O, Astarlioglu G, Yaprak I, et al. Toxicity of Salvia officinalis in a newborn and a child: an alarming report. *Pediatr Neurol.* 2011 Oct;45(4):259–60.

[5912] Lachenmeier DW, Walch SG. Epileptic seizure caused by accidental ingestion of sage (Salvia officinalis L.) oil in children: a rare, exceptional case or a threat to public health. *Pediatr Neurol.* 2012 Mar;46(3):201.

[5913] Khine H, Weiss D, Graber N, et al. A cluster of children with seizures caused by camphor poisoning. *Pediatrics.* 2009 May;123(5):1269–72.

[5914] Michiels EA, Mazor SS. Toddler with seizures due to ingesting camphor and in camphor celebration. *Pediatr Emerg Care.* 2010 Aug;26(8):574–75.

[5915] Craig JO. Poisoning by the volatile oils in childhood. *Arch Dis Child.* 1953;28:259–67.

[5916] Melis K. Bochner A, Janssens G. Accidental nasal eucalyptol and menthol instillation. *Eur J Pediatr.* 1989 Aug;148(8)786–7.

[5917] Day LM, Ozanne-Smith J, Parsons BJ, et al. Eucalyptus oil poisoning among young children: mechanisms of access and the potential prevention. *Aust N Z J Public Health.* 1997 Jun;21(3):297–302.

[5918] Burkhard PR, Burkhardt K, Haenggeli CA, et al. Plant-induced seizures: reappearance of an old problem. *J Neurol.* 1999 Aug;246(8):667–70.

[5919] Waidyanatha S, Johnson JD, Hong SP, et al. Toxicokinetics of α-thujone following intravenous and gavage administration of α-thujone or α- and β-thujone mixture in male and female F344/N rats and B6C3F1 mice. *Toxicol Appl Pharmacol.* 2013 Sep;271(2):216–28.

[5920] Albert-Puleo M. Van Gogh's vision: thujone intoxication. *JAMA.* 1981;246:42.

[5921] Koren G. Medications which can kill a toddler with one tablet or teaspoonful. *J toxicol Clin Toxicol.* 1993;31(3):407- 13.

[5922] Bar-Oz B, Levicheck Z, Koren G. Medications that can kill a toddler with one tablet or teaspoonfull – A 2004 update. *Paediatr Drugs.* 2004;6(2):123-6.

[5923] Arnold W. Vincent van Gogh and thujone connection. *JAMA.* 1988;260:3042–3044.

[5924] Flaman Z, Pellechia-Clarke S, Bailey B, et al. Unintentional exposure of young children to camphor and eucalyptus oils. *Paediatr Child Health.* 2001 Feb;6(2):80-83.

[5925] Rabl W, Katzgraber F, Steinlechner M. Camphor ingestion for abortion (case report). *Forensic Sci Int.* 1997 Sep 19;89(1-2):137-40.

[5926] Blumenthal M, ed. The Complete German Commission E Monographs: Therapeutic Guide to Herbal Medicines. Trans. S. Klein. Boston, MA: American Botanical Council, 1998.

[5927] da Silva Costa KC, Bezerra SB, Norte CM, et al. Medicinal plants with teratogenic potential: current considerations. *Braz J Pharm Sci.* 2012;48(3):427–33.

[5928] Brinker F. Herb Contraindications and Drug Interactions. 2nd ed. Sandy, OR: Eclectic Medical Publications. 1998.

[5929] European Medicines Agency. Public statement on the use of herbal medicinal products containing thujone. Available at: http://www.ema.europa.eu/docs/en_GB/document_library/Public_statement/2011/02/WC500102294.pdf.

[5930] Cristovao L, Carvalho F, Bastos MDL, et al. Hepatotoxicity of an essential oil of Salvia officinalis L.: an in vitro study using freshly isolated rat hepatocytes. *Congress Biomarkers.* 2001 Sep:165.

[5931] Millet Y, Jouglard J, Steinmetz MD, et al. Toxicity of some essential plant oils. Clinical and experimental study. *Clin Toxicol.* 1981 Dec;18(12):1485–98.

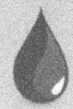

[5932] Manoguerra AS, Erdman AR, Wax PM, et al. Camphor poisoning: an evidence-based practice guideline for out-of- hospital management. *Clin Toxicol (Phila).*2006;44(4):357-70.
[5933] Gibson DE, Moore GP, Pfaff JA. Camphor ingestion. *Am J Emerg Med.* 1989 Jan;7(1):41-43.
[5934] Koppel C, Martends F, Schirop T, et al. Hemoperfusion in acute camphor poisoning. *Intensive Care Med.* 1988;14(4):431-33.
[5935] Millet Y, Jouglard J, Steinmetz MD, et al. Toxicity of some essential plant oils. Clinical and experimental study. *Clin Toxicol.* 1981 Dec;18(12):1485–98.
[5936] Burkhard PR, Burkhardt K, Haenggeli CA, et al. Plant-induced seizures: reappearance of an old problem. *J Neurol.* 1999 Aug;246(8):667–70.
[5937] Charanraj KJ, G MV, S M. Camphor poisoning in a child. *Natl Med J India.* 2013 Jan-Feb;26(1):60.
[5938] Narayan S, Singh N. Camphor poisoning-An unusual cause of seizure. *Med J Armed Forces India.* 2012 Jul;68(3):252–53.
[5939] Perry NB, Anderson RE, Brennan NJ, et al. Essential oils from Dalmatian sage (Salvia officinalis L.) variations among individuals, plant parts, seasons, and sites. *J Agric Food Chem.* 1999;47:2048–54.
[5940] Olowe SA, Ransome-Kuti O. The risk of jaundice in glucose-6-phosphate dehydrogenase deficient babies exposed to menthol. *Acta Paediatr Scand.* 1980 May;69(3):341-5.
[5941] Dillon Remy M, Manning Alleyne P, Bratt DE, et al. Neonatal jaundice at Port-of-Spain General Hospital abstract. *West Indian Med J.* 1987;36(Suppl):28.
[5942] Uc A, Bishop WP, Sanders KD. Camphor hepatotoxicity. *South Med J.* 2000;93:596-98.
[5943] Frohne D. Giftpflanzen: Cupressaceae. Stuttgart: Wissenschaftliche Verlagsgesellschaft mbH; 1997. pp. 153–6.
[5944] Dolan LC, Matulka RA, Burdock GA. Naturally Occurring Food Toxins. *Toxins (Basel).* 2010 Sep;2(9):2289–2332.
[5945] United States National Toxicology Program (NTP). Alpha-Thujone. Dec 10, 1997. Available at: http://ntp.niehs.nih.gov/index.cfm?objectid=03DB8C36-E7A1-9889-3BDF8436F2A8C51F.
[5946] Jori A, Bianchetti A, Prestini PE, et al. Effect of eucalyptol (1,8-cineole) on the metabolism of other drugs in rats and in man. *Eur J Pharmacol.* 1970;9(3):362-66.
[5947] de Sousa DP, Raphael E, Brocksom U, et al. Sedative effect of monoterpene alcohols in mice: A preliminary screening. *Verlag der Zeitschrift fur Naturforschung.* 2007;62c:563-66.
[5948] Jori A, Bianchetti A, Prestini PE, et al. Effect of eucalyptol (1,8-cineole) on the metabolism of other drugs in rats and in man. *Eur J Pharmacol.* 1970;9(3):362-66.
[5949] Ganzera M, Schneider P, Stuppner H. Inhibitory effects of the essential oil of chamomile (Matricaria recutita L.) and its major constituents on human cytochrome P450 enzymes. *Life Sci.* 2006 Jan 18;78(8):856-61.
[5950] Kim NH, Hyun SH, Jin CH, et al. Pretreatment with 1,8-cineole potentiates thioacetamide-induced hepatotoxicity and immunosuppression. *Arch Pharm Res.* 2004 Jul;27(7):781-9.
[5951] Saleh AM, Aljada A, Rizvi SA, et al. In vitro cytotoxicity of Artemisia vulgaris L. essential oil is mediated by a mitochondria-dependent apoptosis in HL-60 leukemic cell line. *BMC Complement Altern Med.* 2014 Jul;14:226.
[5952] Bhatt LR, Lim JA, Chai KY, et al. Antioxidative, and antimicrobial activities of essential oils from Artemisia vulgaris. *Nat Prod Sci.* 2006;12(4):226–31.
[5953] Said ME, Militello M, Saia S, et al. Artemisia arborescens essential oil composition, enantiomeric distribution and antimicrobial activity from different wild populations from the Mediterranean Area. *Chem Biodivers.* 2016 Aug;13(8):1095-102.
[5954] Militello M, Settanni L, Aleo A, et al. Chemical composition and antibacterial potential of Artemisia arborescens L. essential oil. *Curr Microbiol.* 2011 Apr;62(4):1274-81.
[5955] Dhibi S, Ettaya A, Elfeki A, et al. Protective effects of Artemisia arborescens essential oil on oestroprogestative treatment induced hepatotoxicity. *Nutr Res Pract.* 2015 Oct;9(5):466-71.
[5956] Ornano L, Venditti A, Ballero M, et al. Chemopreventive and antioxidant activity of the chamazulene-rich essential oil obtained from Artemisia arborescens L. growing on the Isle of La Maddalena, Sardinia, Italy. *Chem Biodivers.* 2013 Aug;10(8):1464-74.
[5957] Yeom HJ, Jung CS, Kang J, et al. Insecticidal and acetylcholine esterase inhibition activity of Asteraceae plant essential oils and their constituents against adults of the German cockroach (Blattella germanica). *J Agric Food Chem.* 2015 Mar 4;63(8):2241-8.
[5958] Bouzenna H, Krichen L. Pelargonium graveolens L'Her. and Artemisia arborescens L. essential oils: chemical composition, antifungal activity against Rhizoctonia solani and insecticidal activity against Rhysopertha dominica. *Nat Prod Res.* 2013;27(9):841-6.
[5959] Bouzenna H, Krichen L. Pelargonium graveolens L'Her. and Artemisia arborescens L. essential oils: chemical composition, antifungal activity against Rhizoctonia solani and insecticidal activity against Rhysopertha dominica. *Nat Prod Res.* 2013;27(9):841-6.
[5960] Lai F, Sinico C, De Logu A, et al. SLN as a topical delivery system for Artemisia arborescens essential oil: in vitro antiviral activity and skin permeation study. *Int J Nanomedicine.* 2007;2(3):419-25.
[5961] Saddi M, Sanna A, Cottiglia F, et al. Antiherpevirus activity of Artemisia arborescens essential oil and inhibition of lateral diffusion in Vero cells. *Ann Clin Microbiol Antimicrob.* 2007 Sep 26;6:10.
[5962] Sinico C, De Logu A, Lai F, et al. Liposomal incorporation of Artemisia arborescens L. essential oil and in vitro antiviral activity. *Eur J Pharm Biopharm.* 2005 Jan;59(1):161-8.
[5963] Dessí MA, Deiana M, Rosa A, et al. Antioxidant activity of extracts from plants growing in Sardinia. *Phytother Res.* 2001 Sep;15(6):511-8.
[5964] Pandey BP, Thapa R, Upreti A. Chemical composition, antioxidant and antibacterial activities of essential oil and methanol extract of Artemisia vulgaris and Gaultheria fragrantissima collected from Nepal. *Asian Pac J Tropical Med.* 2017 Oct;10(10):952-9.
[5965] Balasubramani S, Sabapathi G, Moola AK, et al. Evaluation of the Leaf Essential Oil from Artemisia vulgaris and Its Larvicidal and Repellent Activity against Dengue Fever Vector Aedes aegypti-An Experimental and Molecular Docking Investigation. *ACS Omega.* 2018 Nov 30;3(11):15657-15665.
[5966] Malik S, de Mesquita LSS, Silva CR, et al. Chemical Profile and Biological Activities of Essential Oil from Artemisia vulgaris L. Cultivated in Brazil. *Pharmaceuticals (Basel).* 2019 Apr 1;12(2).
[5967] Jiang Z, Guo X, Zhang K, et al. The Essential Oils and Eucalyptol From Artemisia vulgaris L. Prevent Acetaminophen-Induced Liver Injury by Activating Nrf2-Keap1 and Enhancing APAP Clearance Through Non-Toxic Metabolic Pathway. *Front Pharmacol.* 2019 Jul 25;10:782.
[5968] Gao S, Zhang K, Wei L, et al. Insecticidal Activity of Artemisia vulgaris Essential Oil and Transcriptome Analysis of Tribolium castaneum in Response to Oil Exposure. *Front Genet.* 2020 Jun 25;11:589.
[5969] Singh NB, Devi ML, Biona T, et al. Phytochemical Composition and Antimicrobial Activity of Essential Oil from the Leaves of Artemisia vulgaris L. *Molecules.* 2023 Feb 28;28(5):2279.
[5970] Lawrence BM. Essential oils 1979-1980. Allured Publishing, Wheaton. 1981. p. 30.
[5971] Edens Garden. Chromatogram Muhuhu. Available at: https://cdn.shopify.com/s/files/1/0380/8537/files/Muhuhu_8_15.pdf?8518045739611058027.
[5972] Oliva MM, Demo MS, Malele RS, et al. Essential oil of Brachylaena hutchinsii Hutch from Tansania: Antimicrobial activity and composition. *East Central African J Pharm Sci.* 2003;6:61-63.
[5973] Oliva MM, Demo MS, Malele RS, et al. Essential oil of Brachylaena hutchinsii Hutch from Tansania: Antimicrobial activity and composition. *East Central African J Pharm Sci.* 2003;6:61-63.
[5974] Marongiu B, Piras A, Porcedda S, et al. Chemical composition of the essential oil and supercitricidal extract of Commiphora myrrha (Nees) Ebgl. and of Acorus calamus L. *J Agric Food Chem.* 205 Oct 5;53(20):7939-43.
[5975] Hanus LO, Rezanka T, Dembitsky VM, et al. Myrrh - Commiphora chemistry. *Biomed Papers.* 2005;149(1):3-28. [1447] Morteza-Semnani K, Saeedi M. Constituents of the essential oil of Commiphora myrrha (Nees( Engl. Var molmol. *J Essent Oil Res.* 2003;15(1):50-51.
[5976] Morteza-Semnani K, Saeedi M. Constituents of the essential oil of Commiphora myrrha (Nees( Engl. Var molmol. *J Essent Oil Res.* 2003;15(1):50-51.
[5977] Aromatics International. Myrrh - Commiphora myrrha. Available at: http://www.aromaticsinternational.com/products/essential-oils/myrrh.
[5978] Zhou L, Zhang K, Li J, et al. Inhibition of vascular endothelial growth factor-mediated angiogenesis involved in reproductive toxicity induced by sesquiterpenoids of Curcuma zedoaria in rats. *Reprod Toxicol.* 2013 Jun;37:62-9.
[5979] Chaiworapongsa T, Romero R, Kusanovic JP, et al. Unexplained fetal death is associated with increased concentrations of anti-angiogenic factors in amniotic fluid. *J Matern Fetal Neonatal Med.* 2010 Aug;23(8):794-805.
[5980] Chen W, Lu Y, Gao J, et al. Beta-elemene inhibits melanoma growth and metastasis via suppressing vascular endothelial growth factor-mediated angiogenesis. *Cancer Chemo Pharmacol.* 2011 Apr;67(4):799-808.
[5981] Chen Y, Zhou C, Ge A, et al. Composition and potential anticancer activities of essential oils obtained from myrrh and frankincense. *Oncol Lett.* 2013;6:1140-46.
[5982] Hur MH, Han SH. Clinical trial of aromatherapy on postpartum mother's perineal healing. *Taehan Kanho Hakhoe Chi.* 2004 Feb;34(1):53-62.
[5983] de Rapper S, Van Vuuren SF, Kamatou GP, et al. The additive and synergistic antimicrobial effects of select frankincense and myrrh oils—a combination from the pharaonic pharmacopoeia. *Lett Appl Microbiol.* 2012 Apr;54(4):352-58.
[5984] Auffray B. Protection against singlet oxygen, the main actor of sebum squalene peroxidation during sun exposure, using Commiphora myrrha essential oil. *Int J Cosmet Sci.* 2007 Feb;29(1):23-29.
[5985] Racine P, Auffray B. Quenching of singlet molecular oxygen by Commiphora myrrha extracts and menthofuran. *Fitoterapia.* 2005 Jun;76(3-4):316-23.
[5986] Massoud A, El Sisi S, Salama O, et al. Preliminary study of therapeutic efficacy of a new fasciolicidal drug derived from Commiphora molmol (myrrh). *Am J Trop Med Hyg.* 2001 Aug;65(2):96-99.
[5987] Tripton DA, Lyle B, Babich H, et al. In vitro cytotoxic and anti-inflammatory effects of myrrh oil on human gingival fibroblasts and epithelial cells. *Tox In Vitro.* 2003 Jun;17(3):301-10.
[5988] Baylac S, Racine P. Inhibition of 5-lipoxygenase by essential oils and other natural fragrant extracts. *Int J Aromatherapy.* 2003;13(2-3):138-42.
[5989] El-Sherbiny GM, El-Sherbiny GM. The effect of Commiphora molmol (Myrrh) in treatment of Trichomoniasis vaginalis infection. *Iranian Red Cresc Med J.* 2011 Jul;13(7):480-86.
[5990] Mahboubi M, Mohammad Taghizadeh L. The anti-dermatophyte activity of Commiphora molmol. *Pharm Biol.* 2016;54(4):720-5.
[5991] Feng J, Shi W, Miklossy J, et al. Identification of Essential Oils with Strong Activity against Stationary Phase Borrelia burgdorferi. *Antibiotics (Basel).* 2018 Oct 16;7(4).
[5992] Orchard A, Viljoen A, van Vuuren S. Wound Pathogens: Investigating Antimicrobial Activity of Commercial Essential Oil Combinations against Reference Strains. *Chem Biodivers.* 2018 Dec;15(12):e1800405.
[5993] Khali N, Fikry S, Salama O. Bactericidal Activity of Myrrh Extracts and Two Dosage Forms Against Standard Bacterial Strains and Multidrug-Resistant Clinical Isolates With GC/MS Profiling. *AMB Express.* 2020 Jan 28;10(1):21.
[5994] Younis NS, Mohamed ME. Protective effects of myrrh essential oil on isoproterenol-induced myocardial infarction in rats through antioxidant, anti-inflammatory, Nrf2/HO-1 and apoptotic pathways. *J Ethnopharmacol.* 2021 Jan 7;270:113793.
[5995] Lenka B, Mohanty R, Satpathy A. Myrrh Oil Reduces Gingival Inflammation and Inhibits Gram Negative Dental Plaque Bacteria at Early Stages – A Randomized Control Trial. *Indian J Forensic Med Toxicol.* 2021;15(2):3795-3804.

5996 Mostafa RE, Taha NM, Lebda MA, et al. Effect of Commiphora Myrrh oil and Extract on Experimentally Induced Gastritis in Rats. *Alexandria J Vet Sci.* 2021 Jul;70(2):1-6.
5997 Abdelsalam AH, Ila HB. In vitro cytogenotoxic and mutagenic effects of Commiphora myrrha essential oil. *Drug Chem Toxicol.* 2021 Oct 4;1-9.
5998 Hamed AM, Awad AA, Abdel-Mobdy AE, et al. Buffalo Yogurt Fortified with Eucalyptus ( Eucalyptus camaldulensis) and Myrrh ( Commiphora Myrrha) Essential Oils: New Insights into the Functional Properties and Extended Shelf Life. *Molecules.* 2021 Nov 13;26(22):6853.
5999 Ulrich J, Stiltz S, St-Gelais A, et al. Phytochemical Composition of Commiphora Oleogum Resins and Their Cytotoxicity against Skin Cancer Cells. *Molecules.* 2022 Jun 17;27(12):3903.
6000 Younis NS. Myrrh Essential Oil Mitigates Renal Ischemia/Reperfusion-Induced Injury. *Curr Issues Mol Biol.* 2023 Feb 1;45(2):1183-1196.
6001 Viuda-Martos M, Sendra E, Perez-Alvarez JA, et al. Identification of flavonoid content and chemical composition on the essential oils of Moroccan herbs: Myrtle (Myrtus communis L.), Rockrose (Cistus ladanifer L.) and Montpellier cistus (Cistus monspeliensis L.). *J Essential Oil Res.* 2011;23(2):1-9.
6002 Nabavizadeh M, Abbaszadegan A, Gholami A, et al. Chemical composition and antimicrobial effect of essential oil from Myrtus communis leaves on microorganisms involved in persistent endodontic infection compared to two common endodontic irrigants: An in vitro study. *J Conserv Dent.* 2014 Sep;17(5):449-53.
6003 Ben Hsouna A, Hamdi N, Miladi R, et al. Myrtus communis essential oil: chemical composition and antimicrobial activities against food spoilage. *Chem Biodivers.* 2014 Apr;11(4):571-80.
6004 Bouzabata A, Castola V, Bighelli A, et al. Chemical variability of Algerian Myrtus communis L. *Chem Biodivers.* 2013 Jan;10(1):129-37.
6005 Bouzabata A, Boussaha F, Casanova J, et al. Composition and chemical variability of leaf oil Myrtus communis from north-eastern Algeria. *Nat Prod Commun.* 2010 Oct;5(10):1659-62.
6006 Tuberoso CI, Barra A, Angioni A, et al. Chemical composition of volatiles in Sardinian myrtle (Myrtus communis L.) alcoholic extracts and essential oils. *J Agric Food Chem.* 2006 Feb 22;54(4):1420-26.
6007 Mimica-Dukic N, Bugarin D, Grbovic S, et al. Essential oil of Myrtus communis L. as a potential antioxidant and antimutagenic agents. *Molecules.* 2010;15:2759-79.
6008 Mahboubi M, Ghazian Bidgoli F. In vitro synergistic efficacy of combination of amphotericin B with Myrtus communis essential oil against clinical isolates of Candida albicans. *Phytomedicine.* 2010 Aug;17(10):771-74.
6009 Zomorodian K, Moein M, Lori ZG, et al. Chemical Composition and Antimicrobial Activities of the Essential Oil from Myrtus communis Leaves. *J Essent Oil Bearing Plants.* 2013;16(1):76-84.
6010 Hennia A, Brada M, Nemmiche S, et al. Chemical Composition and Antimicrobial Activities of the Essential Oil from Myrtus communis Leaves. *J Essent Oil Res.* 2013;16(1):1-6.
6011 Martins C, Cacao R, Cole KJ, et al. Estragole: a weak direct-acting food-borne genotoxin and potential carcinogen. *Mutat Res.* 2012 Aug 30;747(1):86-92.
6012 Jin M, Kijima A, Hibi D, et al. In vivo genotoxicity of methyl eugenol in gpt delta transgenic rats following medium-term exposure. *Toxicol Sci.* 2013 Feb;131(2):387-94.
6013 Uehleke H, Brinkschultze-Freitas M. Oral toxicity of an essential oil from myrtle and adaptive liver stimulation. *Toxicology.* 1979 Mar-Apr;12(3):335-42.
6014 Burkhard PR, Burkhardt K, Haenggeli CA, et al. Plant-induced seizures: reappearance of an old problem. *J Neurol.* 1999 Aug;246(8):667-70.
6015 Culic M, Kekovic G, Grbic G, et al. Wavelet and fractal analysis of rat brain activity in seizures evoked by camphor essential oil and 1,8-cineole. *Gen Physiol Biophys.* 2009;Special Issue(28):33–40.
6016 Mathew T, Kamath V, Kumar RS, et al. Eucalyptus oil inhalation–induced seizure: A novel, underrecognized, preventable cause of acute symptomatic seizure. *Epilepsia Open.* 2017 Sep;2(3):350–354.
6017 Jori A, Bianchetti A, Prestini PE, et al. Effect of eucalyptol (1,8-cineole) on the metabolism of other drugs in rats and in man. *Eur J Pharmacol.* 1970;9(3):362-66.
6018 de Sousa DP, Raphael E, Brocksom U, et al. Sedative effect of monoterpene alcohols in mice: A preliminary screening. *Verlag der Zeitschrift fur Naturforschung.* 2007;62c:563-66.
6019 Birhanie MW, Walle B, Rebba K, et al. Hypnotic effect of the essential oil from the leaves of Myrtus communis on mice. *Nat Sci Sleep.* 2016 Aug 16;8:267-75.
6020 Sepici A, Gurbuz I, Cevik C, et al. Hypoglycemic effects of myrtle oil in normal and alloxan-diabetic rats. *J Ethnopharmacol.* 2004 Aug;9(2-3):311-8.
6021 Gray AM, Flatt PR. Antihyperglycemic actions of Eucalyptus globulus (Eucalyptus) are associated with pancreatic and extra pancreatic effects in mice. *J Nutr.* 1998 Dec;128(12):2319–23.
6022 Basak SS, Candan F. Effect of Laurus nobilis L. Essential Oil and its Main Components on α-glucosidase and Reactive Oxygen Species Scavenging Activity. *Iran J Pharm Res.* 2013 Spring;12(2):367-79.
6023 Fathiazad F, Mazandarani M, Hamedeyazdan. Phytochemical analysis and antioxidant activity of Hyssopus officinalis L. from Iran. *Adv Pharm Bull.* 2011 Dec;1(2):63–67.
6024 Lamborn LL. Modern soaps, candles and glycerin: A practical manual of modern methods of utilization of fats and oils in the manufacture of soaps and candles, and of the recovery of glycerin. Library of the University of Wisconsin.
6025 Oyen LP, Dung NX. Plant resources of South-East Asia. 1999. Backhyus, Leiden.
6026 Kim NH, Hyun SH, Jin CH, et al. Pretreatment with 1,8-cineole potentiates thioacetamide-induced hepatotoxicity and immunosuppression. *Arch Pharm Res.* 2004 Jul;27(7):781-9.
6027 Aleksic V, Mimica-Dukic N, Simin N, et al. Synergistic effect of Myrtus communis L. essential oils and conventional antibiotics against multi-drug resistant Acinetobacter baumannii wound isolates. *Phytomed.* 2014 Oct 15;21;(21):1666-74.
6028 Nakayama M, Okizaki A, Takahashi K, et al. A Randomized Controlled Trial for the Effectiveness of Aromatherapy in Decreasing Salivary Gland Damage following Radioactive Iodine Therapy for Differentiated Thyroid Cancer. *Biomed Res Int.* 2016;2016:9509810.
6029 Nejad BS, Nejad ME, Maanaie SY, et al. Antifungal efficacy og Myrtus communis Linn. *Jentashapir J Health Res.* 2014 August;5(4):e21879.
6030 Mahboubi M, Ghazian Bidgoli F. In vitro synergistic efficacy of combination of amphotericin B with Myrtus communis essential oil against clinical isolates of Candida albicans. *Phytomedicine.* 2010 Aug;17(10):771-74.
6031 Zanetti S, Cannas S, Molicotti P, et al. Evaluation of the antimicrobial properties of the essential oil of Myrtus communis L. against clinical strains of Mycobacterium spp. *Interdiscip Perspect Infect Dis.* 2010;2010.
6032 Maxia A, Frau MA, Falconieri D, et al. Essential oil of Myrtus communis inhibits inflammation in rats by reducing serum IL-6 and TNF-alpha. *Nat Prod Commun.* 2011 Oct;6(10):1545-48.
6033 Bouzabata A, Cabral C, Goncalves MJ, et al. Myrtus communis L. as source of a bioactive and safe essential oil. *Food Chem Toxicol.* 2015 Jan;75:166-72.
6034 Pribalouti AG, Mirbagheri H, Hamedi B, et al. Antibacterial activity of the essential oils of myrtle leaves against Erysipelothrix rhusiopathiae. *Asian Pac J Trop Biomed.* 2014 May;4(Suppl 1):S505-09.
6035 Hedayati A, Khosropanah H, Bazargani A, et al. Assessing the antimicrobial effect of the essential oil of Myrtus communis on the clinical isolates of Porphyromonas gingivalis: An in vitro study. *Jundishapur J Nat Pharm Prod.* 2013 Nov;8(4):165-68.
6036 Cannas S, Molicotti P, Usai D, et al. Antifungal, anti-biofilm and adhesion activity of the essential oil of Myrtus communis L. against Candida species. *Nat Prod Res.* 2014;28(23):2173-77.
6037 Cannas S, Molicotti P, Ruggeri M, et al. Antimycotic activity of Myrtus communis L. towards Candida spp. from isolates. *J Infect Dev Ctries.* 2013 Mar 14;7(3):295-98.
6038 Nassar MI, Aboutabl el-SA, Ahmed RF, et al. Secondary metabolites and bioactives of Myrtus communis. *Pharmacognosy Res.* 2010 Nov;2(6):325-29.
6039 Sepici A, Gurbuz, Cevik C, et al. Hypoglycaemic effects of myrtle oil in normal and alloxan-diabetic rabbits. *J Ethnopharmacol.* 2004 Aug;93(2-3):311-18.
6040 Mimica-Dukic N, Burgarin D, Grbovic S, et al. Essential oil of Myrtus communis L. as a potential antioxidant and antimutagenic agent. *Molecules.* 2010 Apr;15(4):2759-70.
6041 Hayder N, Abdelwahed A, Kilani S, et al. Anti-genotoxic and free-radical scavenging activities of extracts from (Tunisian) Myrtus communis. *Mutat Res.* 2004 Nov 14;564(1):89-95.
6042 Hayder N, Kilani S, Abdelwahed A, et al. Antimutagenic activity of aqueous extracts and essential oil isolated from Myrtus communis. *Pharmazie.* 2003 Jul;58(7):523-24.
6043 Deriu A, Branca G, Molicotti P, et al. In vitro activity of essential oil of Myrtus communis L. against Helicobacter pylori. *Int J Antimicrob Agents.* 2007 Dec;30(6):562-63.
6044 Milhau G, Valentin A, Benoit, et al. In vitro antimalarial activity of eight essential oils. *J Essent Oil Res.* 1997;9(3):329-33.
6045 Anwar S, Crouch RA, Awadh Ali NA, et al. Hierarchical cluster analysis and chemical characterisation of Myrtus communis L. essential oil from Yemen region and its antimicrobial, antioxidant and anti-colorectal adenocarcinoma properties. *Nat Prod Res.* 2017 Jan 9:1-6.
6046 Azadbakht M, Ziai H, Shaban Khani B. Effect of essential oils of Artemisia aucheri Boiss. Zataria multiflora Boiss. And Myrtus communis L. on Trichomonas vaginalis. *J Med Plants.*2003 Dec;2(8):35-40.
6047 Lai Y, Dilidaer D, Chen B, et al. In vitro studies of a distillate of rectified essential oils on sinonasal components of mucociliary clearance. *Am J Rhino Allergy.* 2014 May-Jun;28(3):244-48.
6048 Janbaz KH, Nisa M, Saqib F, et al. Bronchodilator, vasodilator and spasmolytic activities of methanolic extract of Myrtus communis L. *J Physiol Pharmacol.* 2013 Aug;64(4):479-84.
6049 Mahboubi M. Myrtus communis L. and its application in treatment of Recurrent Aphthous Stomatitis. *J Ethnopharmacol.* 2016 Dec 4;193:481-489.
6050 Azimihosaini S, Badiie B. Assessment of the effect of Myrtle drug in the treatment of aphthous stomatitis. *J Ghazvin Univ Med Sci.* 1999;2:4-9. In: Mahboubi M. Myrtus communis L. and its application in treatment of Recurrent Aphthous Stomatitis. *J Ethnopharmacol.* 2016 Dec 4;193:481-489.
6051 Khazaeli P, Chamani G, Mehrabani M, et al. Formulation and clinical evaluation of Myrtus Mucoadhesive paste in the treatment of recurrent aphthous stomatitis. *J Dental School Shahid Beheshti Univ Med Sci.* 2005;23:429-37.
6052 Rad F. Yaghmaee R, Mehdi Abadi P, et al. A comparative clinical trial of topical Triamcinolone (Adcortyle) and a herbal solution for the treatment of minor Aphthous Stomatitis. *Armagan Daneash.* 2010;15:191-95.
6053 Taheri JB, Tavakoli MA. The effect of herbal medicine and Adcortyle in the treatment of aphthous ulcers in oral cavity. *J Dental School Shahid Beheshti Univ Med Sci.* 2002;20:608-16.
6054 Anwar S, Crouch RA, Awadh Ali NA, et al. Hierarchical cluster analysis and chemical characterisation of Myrtus communis L. essential oil from Yemen region and its antimicrobial, antioxidant and anti-colorectal adenocarcinoma properties. *Nat Prod Res.* 2017 Jan 9:1-6.
6055 Yangui I, Zouaoui Boutiti M, Boussaid M, et al. Essential oils of Myrtaceae species growing wild in Tunisia: Chemical variability and antifungal activity against Biscogniauxia Mediterranea, the causative agent of charcoal canker. *Chem Biodivers.* 2017 Jul;14(7).
6056 Mahboubi M. Effectiveness of Myrtus communis in the treatment of hemorrhoids. *J Integr Med.* 2017 Sep;15(5):351-358.
6057 Ebrahimi H. Therapeutic effects of MG topical lotion in patients in hospitals related to Islamic Azad University of Mashhad during the years 1381 to 1382. Khorasan Razavi: Islamic Azad University of Mashhad. 2003.
6058 Farahvash MJ, Sharif H, Kashanian M, Akbari H. Determine the effect of anti-hemorrhoid ointment to treat the symptoms of and compare them with the ointment. In: Hejazi H. Research and Development Center of Barij Report. Kashan: Barij Essence Pharmaceutical Company. 2001:70–89.
6059 Panahi Y, Mousavi-nayeeni SM, Sahebkar A, et al. Myrtus communis essential oil for the treatment of hemorrhoids: a randomized double-blind double-dummy parallel-group comparative study. *Turkish J Pharm Sci.* 2014;11(1):1–8.
6060 Barac A, Donadu M, Usai D, et al. Antifungal activity of Myrtus communis against Malassezia sp. isolated from the skin of patients with pityriasis versicolor. *Infection.* 2018 Apr;46(2):253-257.

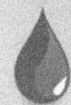
6061 Raeiszadeh M, Pardakhty A, Sharififar F, et al. Development, physicochemical characterization, and antimicrobial evaluation of niosomal myrtle essential oil. *Res Pharm Sci.* 2018 Jun;13(3):250-261.

6062 Harassi Y, Tilaoui M, Idir A, et al. Phytochemical analysis, cytotoxic and antioxidant activities of Myrtus communis essential oil from Morocco. *J Complement Integr Med.* 2019 Jan 19;16(3).

6063 Kutlu Z, Gulaboglu M, Halici Z, et al. Biochemical Research of the Effects of Essential Oil Obtained from the Fruit of Myrtus communis L. on Cell Damage Associated with Lipopolysaccharide-Induced Endotoxemia in a Human Umbilical Cord Vein Endothelial Cells. *Biochem Genet.* 2020 Oct 12. Online ahead of print.

6064 Contini A, Di Bello D, Azzara A, et al. Assessing the cytotoxic/genotoxic activity and estrogenic/antiestrogenic potential of essential oils from seven aromatic plants. *Food Chem Toxicol.* 2020 Apr;138:111205.

6065 Atik H, Bulbul T, Ozdemir V, et al. Effect of myrtle (Myrtus communis L.) essential oil on oxidant–antioxidant balance in rats with propylthiouracil-induced hypothyroidism. *J Food Biochem.* 2020 Oct 4. Online ahead of print.

6066 Mansour RB, Beji RS, Wasli H, et al. Gastroprotective Effect of Microencapsulated Myrtus communis Essential Oil against Ethanol/HCl-Induced Acute Gastric Lesions. *Molecules.* 2022 Feb 26;27(5):1566.

6067 Nikakhtar Z, Hasanzadeh M, Hamedi SS, et al. The efficacy of vaginal suppository based on myrtle in patients with cervicovaginal human papillomavirus infection: A randomized, double-blind, placebo trial. *Phytother Res.* 2018:1-7.

6068 Odeh D, Oršolić N, Berendika M, et al. Antioxidant and Anti-Atherogenic Activities of Essential Oils from Myrtus communis L. and Laurus nobilis L. in Rat. *Nutrients.* 2022 Mar 31;14(7):1465.

6069 Shaapan RM, Al-Abodi HR, Alanazi AD, et al. Myrtus communis Essential Oil; Anti-Parasitic Effects and Induction of the Innate Immune System in Mice with Toxoplasma gondii Infection. *Molecules.* 2021;26:819.

6070 Sebai E, Abidi A, Serairi R, et al. Assessment of anthelmintic potentials of Myrtus communis against Haemonchus contortus and Heligmosomoides polygyrus. *Exp Parasitol.* 2022 Jun 29:108320.

6071 Giuliani C, Moretti RM, Bottoni M, et al. The Leaf Essential Oil of Myrtus communis subsp. tarentina (L.) Nyman: From Phytochemical Characterization to Cytotoxic and Antimigratory Activity in Human Prostate Cancer Cells. *Plants (Basel).* 2023 Mar 13;12(6):1293.

6072 Ammar AH, Bouajila J, Lebrihi A, et al. Chemical composition and in vitro antimicrobial and antioxidant activities of Citrus aurantium l. flowers essential oil (Neroli oil). *Pak J Biol Sci.* 2012 Nov 1;15(21):1034-40.

6073 Sarrou E, Chatzopoulou P, Dimassi-Theriou K, et al. Volatile constituents and antioxidant activity of peel, flowers and leaf oils of Citrus aurantium L. growing in Greece. *Molecules.* 2013;18:10639-10647.

6074 Boussaada O, Chemli R. Chemical composition of essential oils from flowers, leaves and peel of Citrus aurantium L. var. amara from Tunisia. *J Essential Oil Bearing Plants.* 2006;9(2):133-39.

6075 Kai W, Zhu RZ, Qu RF, et al. Comprehensive two-dimensional gas chromatography-time-of-flight mass spectrometry for the analysis of volatile components in neroli essential oil. *Mendeleev Comm.* 2012 Jan;22(1):45-4.

6076 Miguel MG, Dandlen S, Figueiredo AC, et al. Essential Oils of Flowers of Citrus sinensis and Citrus clementina Cultivated in Algarve, Portugal. *Acta Hort.* 2008 Sep;773:89-94.

6077 Mauerman B, Ahmed N, Tambhar N, et al. Trends in Furanocoumarin Profiles Among Commerical-Scale Essential Oils. International Conference on the Science of Botanicals, Poster. Mar 2022.

6078 Bouhlal K, Meynadier JM, Peyron JL, et al. The cutaneous effects of the common concretes and absolutes used in the perfume industry. *J Essent Oil Res.* 1989;1(4):169-95.

6079 Hur MH, Han SH. Clinical trial of aromatherapy on postpartum mother's perineal healing. *Taehan Kanho Hakhoe Chi.* 2004 Feb;34(1):53-62.

6080 Namazi M, Amir Ali Akbari S, Mojab F, et al. Aromatherapy with citrus aurantium oil and anxiety during the first stage of labor. *Iran Red Crescent Med J.* 2014 Jun;16(6):e18371.

6081 Choi SY, Kang P, Lee HS, et al. Effects of inhalation of essential oil of Citrus aurantium L. var amara on menopausal symptoms, stress, and estrogen in postmenopausal women: A randomized controlled trial. *Evid Based Complement Alternat Med.*2014;2014:796518.

6082 Azanchi T, Shafaroodi H, Asgarpanah J. Anticonvulsant activity of Citrus aurantium blossom essential oil (neroli): involvement of the GABAergic system. *Nat Prod Commun.* 2014 Nov;9(11):1615-18.

6083 Kim IH, Kim C, Seong K, et al. Essential oil inhalation on blood pressure and salivary cortisol levels in prehypertensive and hypertensive subjects. *Evid Based Complement Alternat Med.* 2012;2012:984203.

6084 Weseler A, Geiss HK, Saller R, et al. A novel colorimetric broth microdilution method to determine the minimum inhibitory concentration (MIC) of antibiotics and essential oils against Helicobacter pylori. *Pharmazie.* 2005 Jul;60(7):498-502.

6085 Imura M, Misao H, Ushijima H. The psychological effects of aromatherapy-massage in healthy postpartum mothers. *J Midwifery Womens Health.* 2006 Mar-Apr;51(2):e21-27.

6086 Cho MY, Min ES, Hur MH, et al. Effects of aromatherapy on the anxiety, vital signs, and sleep quality of percutaneous coronary intervention patients in intensive care units. *Evid Based Complement Altern Med.* 2013(2013):1- 6.

6087 Baylac S, Racine P. Inhibition of 5-lipoxygenase by essential oils and other natural fragrant extracts. *Int J Aromatherapy.* 2003;13(2-3):138-42.

6088 Sarrou E, Chatzopoulou P, Dimassi-Theriou K, et al. Volatile constituents and antioxidant activity of peel, flowers and leaf oils of Citrus aurantium L. growing in Greece. *Molecules.* 2013;18:1639-47.

6089 Ben Hsouna A, Hamdi N, Ben Halima N, et al. Characterization of essential oil from Citrus aurantium L. flowers: antimicrobial and antioxidant activities. *J Oleo Sci.* 2013;62(10):763-72.

6090 Stevenson C. The psychophysiological effects of aromatherapy massage following cardiac surgery. *Complement Ther Med.* 1994 Jan;2(1):27-35.

6091 Buchbauer G, Jirovetz L, Jager W, et al. Fragrance constituents and essential oils with sedative effects upon inhalation. *J Pharm Sci.* 1993 Jun;82(6):660-64.

6092 Jager W, Buchbauer G, Jirovetz L, et al. Evidence of the sedative effect of neroli oil, citronellal and phenylethyl acetate on mice. *J Essent Oil Res.* 1992;4(4):387-94.

6093 Jaradat NA, Al Zabadi H, Rahhal B, et al. The effect of inhalation of Citrus sinensis flowers and Mentha spicata leave essential oils on lung function and exercise performance: a quasi-experimental uncontrolled before-and-after study. *J Int Soc Sports Nutr.* 2016 Sep 22;13:36.

6094 Kang P, Ryu KH1, Lee JM, et al. Endothelium- and smooth muscle-dependent vasodilator effects of Citrus aurantium L. var. amara: Focus on Ca(2+) modulation. *Biomed Pharmacother.* 2016 Aug;82:467-71.

6095 Khodabakhsh P, Shafaroodi H, Asgarpanah J. Analgesic and anti-inflammatory activities of Citrus aurantium L. blossoms essential oil (neroli): involvement of the nitric oxide/cyclic-guanosine monophosphate pathway. *J Nat Med.* 2015 Jul;69(3):324-31.

6096 Shen CY, Jiang JG, Zhu W, et al. Anti-inflammatory Effect of Essential Oil from Citrus aurantium L. var. amara Engl. *J Agric Food Chem.* 2017 Oct 4;65(39):8586-8594.

6097 Heydari N, Abootalebi M, Jamalimoghadam N, et al. Investigation of the effect of aromatherapy with Citrus aurantium blossom essential oil on premenstrual syndrome in university students: A clinical trial study. *Complement Ther Clin Pract.* 2018 Aug;32:1-5.

6098 Heydari N, Abootalebi M, Tayebi N, et al. The effect of aromatherapy on mental, physical symptoms, and social functions of females with premenstrual syndrome: A randomized clinical trial. *J Family Med Prim Care.* 2019 Sep 30;8(9):2990-2996.

6099 Moslemi F, Alijaniha F, Naseri M, et al. Citrus aurantium Aroma for Anxiety in Patients with Acute Coronary Syndrome: A Double-Blind Placebo-Controlled Trial. *J Altern Complement Med.* 2019 Aug;25(8):833-839.

6100 Huffman JC, Celano CM, Januzzi JL. The relationship between depression, anxiety, and cardiovascular outcomes in patients with acute coronary syndromes. *Neuropsychiatr Dis Treat.* 2010;6:123–136.

6101 Değirmenci H, Erkurt H. Relationship between volatile components, antimicrobial and antioxidant properties of the essential oil, hydrosol and extracts of Citrus aurantium L. flowers. *J Infect Public Health.* 2020 Jan;13(1):58-67.

6102 Navaei Shoorvarzi S, Shahraki F, Shafaei N, et al. Citrus aurantium L. bloom essential oil nanoemulsion: Synthesis, characterization, cytotoxicity, and its potential health impacts on mice. *J Food Biochem.* 2020 Mar 15:e13181.

6103 Moreadi K, Ashtarian H, Danzima NY, et al. Essential Oil from Citrus aurantium Alleviates Anxiety of Patients Undergoing Coronary Angiography: A Single-Blind, Randomized Controlled Trial. *Chin J Integr Med.* 2020 Jun 22. Online ahead of print.

6104 Nidhi P, Rolta R, Kumar V, et al. Synergistic potential of Citrus aurantium L. essential oil with antibiotics against Candida albicans. *J Ethnopharmacol.* 2020 Jul 18;113135.

6105 Abbaspoor Z, Siahposh A, Javadifar N, et al. The Effect of Citrus Aurantium Aroma on the Sleep Quality in Postmenopausal Women: A Randomized Controlled Trial. *Int J Community Based Nurs Midwifery.* 2022 Apr;10(2):86-95.

6106 Mohammadi F, Moradi M, Niazi A, et al. The Impact of Aromatherapy with Citrus Aurantium Essential Oil on Sleep Quality in Pregnant Women with Sleep Disorders: A Randomized Controlled Clinical Trial. *IJCBNM.* 2022 May:1-13.

6107 Abbaspoor Zm Sharifipour F, Siahposh A, et al. Effects of Aromatherapy With Citrus Aurantium Lavender on Sexual Function of Postmenopausal Women: A Randomized Controlled Trial. *J Family Reprod Health.* 2022 Jun;16(2):147-54.

6108 Sharifipour F, Heydarpour S, Salari N. Comparison of Aromatherapy with Citrus aurantium and Lavender on Sexual Satisfaction in Breastfeeding Women: A Randomized Controlled Trial. *Breastfeed Med.* 2023 Jan;18(1):23-29.

6109 Ramanoelina PAR, Viano J, Bianchini JP, et al. Occurrence of various chemotypes in niaouli (Melaleuca quinquenervia) essential oil from Madagascar using multivariate statistical analysis. *J Agric Food Chem.* 1994;42(5):1177-82.

6110 Trilles BL, Bombarda I, Bouraima-Madjebi S, et al. Occurrence of various chemotypes in niaouli [Melaleuca quinquenervia (Cav.) S.T. Blake] essential oil from New Caledonia. *Flav Frag J.* 2006 Jul-Aug;21(4):677-82.

6111 Gaydo EM. Main industrial niaouli (Melaleuca quinquenervia) oil chemotype productions from Madagascar. *J Essent Oil Res.* 2008 Jan;20:261-66.

6112 Gbenou JD, Moudachirou M, Chalchat JC. Chemotypes in Melaleuca quinquenervia (Cav.) S.T. Blake (Niaouli) from Benin using multivariate statistical analysis of their essential oils. *J Essent Oil Res.* 2007;19(2):101-04.

6113 Ireland BF, Hibbert DB, Goldsack RJ, et al. Chemical variation in the leaf essential oil of Melaleuca quinquenervia (Cav.) S.T. Blake. *Biochem Syst Ecol.* 2002;30(5):457-70.

6114 Wheeler GS. Chemotype variation of the weed Melaleuca quinquenervia influences the biomass and fecundity of the biological control agent Oxyops vitiosa. *Biol Control.* 2006;36:121-28.

[6115] Fuselli SR, Garcia de la Rosa SB, Eguaras MJ, et al. In vitro antibacterial effect of exotic plants essential oils on the honeybee pathogen Paenibacillus larvae, causal agent of American foulbrood. *Spanish J Agric Res.* 2010;8(3):651-57.

[6116] De Medici D, Pieretti S, Salvatore G, et al. Chemical analysis of essential oils of malagasy medicinal plants by gas chromatography and NMR spectroscopy. *Flavour Frag J.* 1992 Oct;7(5):275-81.

[6117] Carson CF, Hammer KA, Riley TV. Melaleuca alternifolia (Tea Tree) Oil: a Review of Antimicrobial and Other Medicinal Properties. *Clin Microbiol Rev.* 2006 Jan;19(1):50–62.

[6118] Craig JO. Poisoning by the volatile oils in childhood. *Arch Dis Child.* 1953;28:259-67.

[6119] Melis K. Bochner A, Janssens G. Accidental nasal eucalyptol and menthol instillation. *Eur J Pediatr.* 1989 Aug;148(8)786-7.

[6120] Day LM, Ozanne-Smith J, Parsons BJ, et al. Eucalyptus oil poisoning among young children: mechanisms of access and the potential prevention. *Aust N Z J Public Health.* 1997 Jun;21(3):297-302.

[6121] Chandar SD, Prashanti M, Kumar CL, et al. Eucalyptus Oil-Induced Seizures in Children: A Single-Center Prospective Study. *Cureus.* 2021 Mar 25;13(3):e14109.

[6122] Sayyah M, Valizadeh J, Kamalinejad M. Anticonvulsant activity of the leaf oil of Laurus nobilis against pentylentetrazole- and maximal electroshock-induced seizure. *Phytomedicine.* 2002 Apr;9(3):212-16.

[6123] Culic M, Kekovic G, Grbic G, et al. Wavelet and fractal analysis of rat brain activity in seizures evoked by camphor oil and 1,8-cineole. *Gen Physiol Biophys.* 2009;28 Sec No:33-40.

[6124] Burkhard PR, Burkhardt K, Haenggeli CA, et al. Plant-induced seizures: reappearance of an old problem. *J Neurol.* 1999 Aug;246(8):667-70.

[6125] Waldman N. Seizure caused by dermal application of over-the-counter eucalyptus oil head lice preparation. *Clin Toxicol (Phila).* 2011 Oct;49(8):750-1.

[6126] Craig JO. Poisoning by the volatile oils in childhood. *Arch Dis Child.* 1953;28:259-67.

[6127] Mathew T, Kamath V, Kumar RS, et al. Eucalyptus oil inhalation-induced seizure: A novel, underrecognized, preventable cause of acute symptomatic seizure. *Epilepsia Open.* 2017 Jul 4;2(3):350-354.

[6128] Day LM, Ozanne-Smith J, Parsons BJ, et al. Eucalyptus oil poisoning among young children: mechanisms of access and the potential prevention. *Aust N Z J Public Health.* 1997 Jun;21(3):297-302.

[6129] Myott E. Case of eucalyptus poisoning. *Brit M J.* 1906;1:558.

[6130] Hindle RC. Eucalyptus oil ingestion. *N Z Med J.* 1994 May 11;107(977)185-6.

[6131] Tibballs J. Clinical effects and management of eucalyptus oil ingestion in infants and small children. *Med J Aust.* 1995 Aug;163(4):177-80.

[6132] Waldman W, Barwina M, Sein Anand J. Accidental ontoxication with eucalyptus oil—a case report. *Przeql Lek.* 2011;68(8):555-6.

[6133] Day LM, Ozanne-Smith J, Parsons BJ, et al. Eucalyptus oil poisoning among young children: mechanisms of access and the potential prevention. *Aust N Z J Public Health.* 1997 Jun;21(3):297-302.

[6134] De Vincenzi M, Silano M, De Vincenzi A, et al. Constituents of aromatic plants: eucalyptol. *Fitoterapia.* 2002 Jun;73(3):269-75.

[6135] Gray AM, Flatt PR. Antihyperglycemic actions of Eucalyptus globulus (Eucalyptus) are associated with pancreatic and extra pancreatic effects in mice. *J Nutr.* 1998 Dec;128(12):2319–23.

[6136] Basak SS, Candan F. Effect of Laurus nobilis L. Essential Oil and its Main Components on α-glucosidase and Reactive Oxygen Species Scavenging Activity. *Iran J Pharm Res.* 2013 Spring;12(2):367-79.

[6137] Fathiazad F, Mazandarani M, Hamedeyazdan. Phytochemical analysis and antioxidant activity of Hyssopus officinalis L. from Iran. *Adv Pharm Bull.* 2011 Dec;1(2):63–67.

[6138] Tsai HH, Lin HW, Chen YL, et al. A review of potential harmful interactions between anticoagulant/antiplatelet agents and Chinese herbal medicines. *PLoS One.* 2013 May 9;8(5):e64255.

[6139] Moharam BA, Jantan I, bin Ahmad F, et al. Antiplatelet Aggregation and Platelet Activating Factor (PAF) Receptor Antagonistic Activities of the Essential Oils of Five Goniothalamus Species. *Molecules.* 2010;15:5124-38.

[6140] Jori A, Bianchetti A, Prestini PE, et al. Effect of eucalyptol (1,8-cineole) on the metabolism of other drugs in rats and in man. *Eur J Pharmacol.* 1970;9(3):362-66.

[6141] Kim NH, Hyun SH, Jin CH, et al. Pretreatment with 1,8-cineole potentiates thioacetamide-induced hepatotoxicity and immunosuppression. *Arch Pharm Res.* 2004 Jul;27(7):781-9.

[6142] Nguyen LT, Mysliveckova Z, Szotakova B, et al. The inhibitory effects of β-caryophyllene, β-caryophyllene oxide and α-humulene on the activities of the main drug-metabolizing enzymes in rat and human liver in vitro. *Chem-Biol Interactoins.* 2017 Dec 25;278:123-8.

[6143] Jori A, Bianchetti A, Prestini PE, et al. Effect of eucalyptol (1,8-cineole) on the metabolism of other drugs in rats and in man. *Eur J Pharmacol.* 1970;9(3):362-66.

[6144] de Sousa DP, Raphael E, Brocksom U, et al. Sedative effect of monoterpene alcohols in mice: A preliminary screening. *Verlag der Zeitschrift fur Naturforschung.* 2007;62c:563-66.

[6145] Brehm-Stecher BF, Johnson EA. Sensitization of Staphylococcus aureus and Escherichia coli to antibiotics by the sesquiterpenoids nerolidol, farnesol, bisabolol, and apritone. *Antimicrob Agents Chemother.* 2003 Oct;47(10):3357-60.

[6146] Ferrara L, Navigilio D, Armone Caruso A. Cytological aspects on the effects of a nasal spray consisting of standardized extract of citrus lemon and essential oils in allergic rhinopathy. *ISRN Pharm.* 2012;2012:404606.

[6147] Nam SY, Chang MH, Do JS, et al. Essential oil of niaouli preferentially potentiates antigen-specific cellular immunity and cytokine production by macrophages. *Immunopharmacol Immunotoxicol.* 2008;30(3):459-74.

[6148] Park HM, Kim J, Chang KS, et al. Larvicidal activity of Myrtaceae essential oils and their component against Aedes aegypti, acute toxicity on Daphnia magna, and aqueous residue. *J Med Entomol.* 2011 Mar;48(2):405-10.

[6149] Monti D, Tampucci S, Chetoni P, et al. Niaouli oils from different sources: analysis and influence on cutaneous permeation of estradiol in vitro. *Drug Deliv.*2009 Jul;16(5):237-42.

[6150] Nokhodchi A, Sharabiani K, Rashidi MR, et al. The effect of terpene concentrations on the skin penetration of diclofenac sodium. *Int J Pharm.* 207 Apr 20;335(1-2):97-105.

[6151] Monti D, Chetoni P, Burgalassi S, et al. Effect of different terpene-containing essential oils on permeation of estradiol through hairless mouse skin. *Int J Pharm.* 2002 Apr 26;237(1-2):209-14.

[6152] Leyva M, French-Pacheco L, Quintana F, et al. Melaleuca quinquenervia (Cav.) S.T. Blake (Myrtales: Myrtaceae): Natural alternative for mosquito control. *Asian Pac J Trop Med.* 2016 Oct;9(10):979-984.

[6153] Chao WW, Su CC, Peng HY, et al. Melaleuca quinquenervia essential oil inhibits α-melanocyte-stimulating hormone-induced melanin production and oxidative stress in B16 melanoma cells. *Phytomedicine.* 2017 Oct 15;34:191-201.

[6154] Cilingir-Kaya OT, Gurler EB. Therapeutic potential of essential oil of Melaleuca quinquenervia (Myrtaceae) in a rat model of ethanolinduced peptic ulcer. *Trop J Pharm Res.* 2021 May;20(5):981-6.

[6155] Shakeel F, Salem-Bekhit MM, Haq N, et al. Nanoemulsification Improves the Pharmaceutical Properties and Bioactivities of Niaouli Essential Oil ( Melaleuca quinquenervia L.). *Molecules.* 2021 Aug 5;26(16):4750.

[6156] Valková V, Ďuranová H, Vukovic NL, et al. Assessment of Chemical Composition and Anti-Penicillium Activity of Vapours of Essential Oils from Abies Alba and Two Melaleuca Species in Food Model Systems. *Molecules.* 2022 May 12;27(10):3101.

[6157] Ogunwande IA, Olawore NO, Adeleke KA, et al. Chemical composition of essential oil of Myristica Fragrans Houtt (Nutmeg) from Nigeria. *J Essential Oil Bearing Plants.* 2003;6(1):21-26.

[6158] Kapoor IPS, Singh B, Singh G, et al. Chemical composition and antioxidant activity of essential oil and oleoresins of nutmeg (Myristica fragrans Houtt.) fruits. *Int J Food Prop.* 2013;16(5):1059-70.

[6159] Muchtaridi, Subarnas A, Apriyantono A, et al. Identification of constituents in the essential oil of nutmeg seeds (Myristica fragrans Houtt.) that inhibit locomotor activity in mice. *Int J Mol Sci.* 2010;11(11):4771-81.

[6160] Simpson GIC, Jackson YA. Comparison of the chemical composition of East Indian, Jamaican and other West Indian essential oil of Myristica fragrans Houtt. *J Essential Oil Res.* 2002;14(1):6-9.

[6161] Maya KM, Zachariah TJ, Krishnamoorthy B. Chemical composition of essential oil of nutmeg (Myristica fragrans Houtt.) accessions. *J Spices Aromatic Crops.* 2004;13(2):135-39.

[6162] Pal M, Srivastava M, Soni DK, et al. Composition and antimicrobial activity of essential oil of Myristica fragrans from Andaman Nicobar Island. *Int J Pharm Life Sci.* 2011 Oct;2(10):1115-17.

[6163] Ehlers D, Kirchhoff J, Gerard D, et al. High-performance liquid chromatography analysis of nutmeg and mace oils produced by supercritical CO2 extraction - comparison with steam-distilled oils - comparison of East Indian, West Indian and Papuan oils. *Int J Food Sci Tech.* 1998 Jun;33(3):215-23.

[6164] Ehrenpreis JE, DesLauriers, Lank P, et al. Nutmeg poisonings: A retrospective review of 10 years experience from the Illinois Poison Control center, 2001-2011. *J Med Toxicol.* 2014 Jun;10(2):148-51.

[6165] Sivathanu S, Sampath S, Suresh David H, et al. Myristicin and phenytoin toxicity in an infant. *BMJ Case Rep.* 2014 Jun;2014.

[6166] Carstairs SD, Cantrell FL. The spice of life: an analysis of nutmeg exposures in California. *Clin Toxicol (Phila).* 2011 Mar;49(3):177-80.

[6167] Randerath K, Putman KL, Randerath E. Flavor constituents in cola drinks induce hepatic DNA adducts in adult and fetal mice. *Biochem Biophys Res Commun.* 1993 Apr 15;192(1):61-8.

[6168] Vesselinovitch SD, Rao KVN, Mihailovich N. Transplacental and lactational carcinogenesis by safrole. *Cancer Res.* 1979 Nov;39(11):4378-80.

[6169] Murray M. Toxicological actions of plant-derived and anthropogenic methylenedioxyphenyl-substituted chemicals in mammals and insects. *J Toxicol Environ Health B Crit Rev.* 2012;15(6):365-95.

[6170] Jin M, Kijima A, Hibi D, et al. In vivo genotoxicity of methyl eugenol in gpt delta transgenic rats following medium-term exposure. *Toxicol Sci.* 2013 Feb;131(2):387-94.

[6171] Jin M, Kijima A, Suzuki Y, et al. Comprehensive toxicity study of safrole using medium-term animal model with gpt delta rats. *Toxicology.* 2011 Dec 18;290(2-3):312-21.

[6172] Hallstrom H, Thuvander A. Toxicological evaluation of myristicin. *Natural Toxins* 1997;5:186-92.

[6173] Brenner N, Frank OS, Knight E. Chronic nutmeg psychosis, *J R Soc Med.* 1993;86:179-80.

[6174] Sangalli BC, Sangalli B, Chiang W. Toxicology of nutmeg abuse. *Clin Toxicol.* 2000;38(6):671-78.

[6175] Tsai HH, Lin HW, Chen YL, et al. A review of potential harmful interactions between anticoagulant/antiplatelet agents and Chinese herbal medicines. *PLoS One.* 2013 May 9;8(5):e64255.

[6176] Forrest JE, Heacock RA. Nutmeg and mace, the psychotropic spices from Myristica fragrans. *Lloydia.* 1972 Dec;35(4):440-9.

[6177] Leiter E1, Hitchcock G, Godwin S, et al. Evaluation of the anxiolytic properties of myristicin, a component of nutmeg, in the male Sprague-Dawley rat.*AANA J.* 2011 Apr;79(2):109-14.

[6178] Truitt EB Jr, Duritz G, Ebersberger EM. Evidence of monoamine oxidase inhibition by myristicin and nutmeg. *Proc Soc Exp Biol Med.* 1963 Mar;112:647-50.

[6179] Banjeree S, Sharma R, Kale RK, et al. Influence of certain essential oils on carcinogen-metabolizing enzyme soluble sulfhydryls in mouse liver. *Nutr Cancer.* 1994;21(3):263-69.

[6180] Kimura Y, Ito H, Hatano T. Effects of mace and nutmeg on human cytochrome P450 3A4 and 2C9 activity. *Biol Pharm Bull.* 2012;33(12):1977-87.

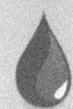

6181 Jeong HG, Yun CH. Induction of rat hepatic cytochrome P450 enzymes by myristicin. *Biochem Biophys Res Commun.* 1995 Dec26;217(3):966-71.
6182 Zhao R, Wang W, Zhao L, et al. Effect of volatile oil from nutmeg on liver licrosomal cytochrome P450 in mice. *Zhonqquo Zhonq Yao Za Zhi.* 2009Feb;34(4):447-49.
6183 Zhao R. [Effect of volatile oil from nutmeg on liver microsomal cytochrome P450 in mice.] *Zhongguo Zhong Yao Za Zhi.* 2009 Feb;34(4):447-9.
6184 Yang AH, He X, Chen JX, et al. Identification and characterization of reactive metabolites in myristicin-mediated mechanism-based inhibition of CYP1A2. *Chem Biol Interact.* 2015 Jul 25;237:133-40.
6185 Ioannides C, Delaforge M, Parke DV. Interactions of safrole and isosafrole and their metabolites with cytochromes P-450. *Chem Biol Interact.* 1985 May;53(3):303-11.
6186 Hashim S, Aboobaker VS, Madhubala R, et al. Modulatory effects of essential oils from spices on the formation of DNA adduct by aflatoxin B1 in vitro. *Nutr Cancer.* 1994;21(2):169-75.
6187 Piaru SP, Mahmud R, Abdul Majid AM, et al. Antioxidant and antiangiogenic activities of the essential oils of Myristica fragrans and Morinda citifolia. *Asian Pac J Trop Med.* 2012 Apr;5(4):294-98.
6188 Firouzi R, Shekarforoush SS, Nazer AH, et al. Effects of essential oils of oregano and nutmeg on growth and survival of Yersinia enterocolitica and Listeria monocytogenes in barbecued chicken. *J Food Prot.* 2007 Nov;70(11):2626-30.
6189 Soni R, Sharma G, Jasuja ND. Essential Oil Yield Pattern and Antibacterial and Insecticidal Activities of Trachyspermum ammi and Myristica fragrans. *Scientifica (Cairo).* 2016;2016:1428194.
6190 Wahab A, Ul Haq R, Ahmed A, et al. Anticonvulsant activities of nutmeg oil of Myristica fragrans. *Phytother Res.* 2009 Feb;23(2):153-58.
6191 Dorman HJD, Deans SG. Antimicrobial agents from plants: antibacterial activity of plant volatiles oils. *J Appl Microbiol.* 2000 Feb;88(2):308-16.
6192 Morita T, Jinno K, Kawagishi H, et al. Hepatoprotective effect of myristicin from nutmeg (Myristica fragrans) on lipopolysaccharide/d-galactosamine-induced liver injury. *J Agric Food Chem.* 2003 Mar;51(6):1560-65.
6193 Pérez-Rosés R, Risco E, Vila R, et al. Biological and Nonbiological Antioxidant Activity of Some Essential Oils. *J Agric Food Chem.* 2016 Jun 15;64(23):4716-24.
6194 Bartoňková I, Dvořák Z. Essential oils of culinary herbs and spices display agonist and antagonist activities at human aryl hydrocarbon receptor AhR. *Food Chem Toxicol.* 2018 Jan;111:374-384.
6195 Das S, Kumar Singh V, Kumar Dwivedy A, et al. Assessment of chemically characterised Myristica fragrans essential oil against fungi contaminating stored scented rice and its mode of action as novel aflatoxin inhibitor. *Nat Prod Res.* 2020 Jan;13(1):58-67.
6196 Gomes da Rocha Voris D, Dos Santos Dias L, Alencar Lima J, et al. Evaluation of larvicidal, adulticidal, and anticholinesterase activities of essential oils of Illicium verum Hook. f., Pimenta dioica (L.) Merr., and Myristica fragrans Houtt. against Zika virus vectors. *Environ Sci Pollut Res Int.* 2018 Aug;25(23):22541-22551.
6197 Ogawa K, Ito M. Appetite-enhancing effects of nutmeg oil and structure-activity relationship of habituation to phenylpropanoids. *J Nat Med.* 2019 Jun;73(3):513-522.
6198 Wang J, Zhang HH, Liu F, et al. Preparation, Characterization and Antimicrobial Activity of Inclusion Complexes of Myristica fragrans Hott. Essential Oil in β-Cyclodextrins. *Pharmzie.* 2019 Oct 1;74(10):590-4.
6199 Matulyte I, Jekabsone A, Jankauskaite L, et al. The Essential Oil and Hydrolats From Myristica fragrans Seeds With Magnesium Aluminometasilicate as Excipient: Antioxidant, Antibacterial, and Anti-inflammatory Activity. *Foods.* 2020 Jan 2;9(1):37.
6200 Ibrahim MA, Cantrell CL, Jeliazokova EA, et al. Utilization of Nutmeg ( Myristica fragrans Houtt.) Seed Hydrodistillation Time to Produce Essential Oil Fractions With Varied Compositions and Pharmacological Effects. *Molecules.* 2020 Jan 28;25(3):565.
6201 Setty JV, Srinivasan I, Sathiesh RT, et al. In vitro evaluation of antimicrobial effect of Myristica fragrans on common endodontic pathogens. *J Indian Soc Pedod Prev Dent.* 2020;38:145-51.
6202 Capetti F, Cagliero C, Marengo A, et al. Bio-Guided Fractionation Driven by In Vitro α-Amylase Inhibition Assays of Essential Oils Bearing Specialized Metabolites with Potential Hypoglycemic Activity. *Plants (Basel).* 2020 Sep 21;9(9):E1242.
6203 Wong C, Crystal K, Coats J. Three molecules found in rosemary or nutmeg essential oils repel ticks (Dermacentor variabilis) more effectively than DEET in a no-human assay. *Pest Manag Sci.* 2021 Mar;77(3):1348-1354.
6204 Cossetin LF, Santi EM, Garlet QI, et al. Comparing the Efficacy of Nutmeg Essential Oil and a Chemical Pesticide against Musca domestica and Chrysomya albiceps for Selecting a New Insecticide Agent against Synantropic Vectors. *Exp Parasitol.* 2021 Apr 1;108104.
6205 Oo T, Saiboonjan B, Srijampa S, et al. Inhibition of Bacterial Efflux Pumps by Crude Extracts and Essential Oil from Myristica fragrans Houtt. (Nutmeg) Seeds against Methicillin-Resistant Staphylococcus aureus. *Molecules.* 2021 Jul 31;26(15):4662.
6206 Harčárová M, Čonková E, Proškovcová M, et al. Comparison of antifungal activity of selected essential oils against Fusarium graminearum in vitro. *Ann Agric Environ Med.* 2021 Sep 16;28(3):414-418.
6207 Selvati Rezende DADC, Cardoso MDG, Alves E, et al. Effect of the essential oils of Satureja montana L., Myristica fragrans H. and Cymbopogon flexuosus S. on mycotoxin-producing Aspergillus flavus and Aspergillus ochraceus Antifungal properties of essential oils. *FEMS Microbiol Lett.* 2021 Oct 30;fnab137.
6208 Seo SM, Lee JW, Shin J, et al. Development of cellulose nanocrystal-stabilized Pickering emulsions of massoia and nutmeg essential oils for the control of Aedes albopictus. *Sci Rep.* 2021 Jun 8;11(1):12038.
6209 Rezende DADCS, Oliveira CD, Batista LR, et al. Bactericidal and antioxidant effects of essential oils from Satureja montana L., Myristica fragrans H. and Cymbopogon flexuosus. *Lett Appl Microbiol.* 2022 May;74(5):741-751.
6210 Terajima Y, Ichikawa H, Tokua K, et al. Quantitative analysis of oakmoss. 1988. In: Lawrence BM, Mookherjee BD, Wilis BJ, Flavors & Fragranaces: A world perspective. Elsevier: Amsterdam. Pp 685-95.
6211 Joulain D, Tabacchi R. Lichen extracts as raw materials in perfumery. Part 1: oakmoss. *Flavour Frag J,* 2009;24:49-61.
6212 Kahriman N, Yazici K, Arslan T, et al. Chemical Composition and Antimicrobial Activity of the Essential Oils from Evernia prunastri (L.) Ach. and Evernia divaricata (L.) Ach. *Asian J Chem.* 2011;23(5):1937-39.
6213 Gavin J, Tabacchi R. Isolement et identification de composés phénoliques et monoterpéniques de la mousse de chêne (Evernia prunastri (L.) Arch.). *Helvetica Chimica Acta.* 1975;58(1):190-94.
6214 Gavin J, Nicollier G, Tabacchi R. Composants volatils de la «mousse de chêne» (Evernia Prunastri (L.) ACH.) 3e communication. Helvetica Chimica Acta. 1978;61:352-57.
6215 Stojanovic IZ, Radulovic NS, Mitrovic TLJ, et al. Volatile constituents of selected Parmeliaceae lichens. *J Serb Chem Soc.* 2011;76(7):987-94.
6216 Hiserodt RD, Swijter DF, Mussinan CJ. Identification of atranorin and related potential allergens in oakmoss absolute by high-performance liquid chromatography-tandem mass spectrometry using negative ion atmospheric pressure chemical ionization. *J Chromatogr A.* 2000 Aug 4;888(1-2):103-11.
6217 Bernard G, Giménez-Arnau E, Rastogi SC, et al. Contact allergy to oak moss: search for sensitizing molecules using combined bioassay-guided chemical fractionation, GC-MS, and structure-activity relationship analysis. *Arch Dermatol Res.* 2003 Nov;295(6):229-35.
6218 Hiserodt RD, Swijter DF, Mussinan CJ. Identification of atranorin and related potential allergens in oakmoss absolute by high-performance liquid chromatography-tandem mass spectrometry using negative ion atmospheric pressure chemical ionization. *J Chromatogr A.* 2000 Aug 4;888(1-2):103-11.
6219 Bernard G, Giménez-Arnau E, Rastogi SC, et al. Contact allergy to oak moss: search for sensitizing molecules using combined bioassay-guided chemical fractionation, GC-MS, and structure-activity relationship analysis. *Arch Dermatol Res.* 2003 Nov;295(6):229-35.
6220 Mowitz M, Zimerson E, Svedman C, et al. Patch testing with serial dilutions and thin-layer chromatograms of oak moss absolutes containing high and low levels of atranol and chloroatranol. *Contact Dermatitis.* 2013 Dec;69(6):342-9.
6221 Gonçalo S, Cabral F, Gonçalo M. Contact sensitivity to oak moss. *Contact Dermatitis.* 1988 Nov;19(5):355-7.
6222 Heisterberg MV, Menné T, Johansen JD. Contact allergy to the 26 specific fragrance ingredients to be declared on cosmetic products in accordance with the EU cosmetics directive. *Contact Dermatitis.* 2011 Nov;65(5):266-75.
6223 Nardelli A, Giménez-Arnau E, Bernard G, et al. Is a low content in atranol/chloroatranol safe in oak moss-sensitized individuals? *Contact Dermatitis.* 2009 Feb;60(2):91-5.
6224 Bonefeld CM, Nielsen MM, Gimenéz-Arnau E, et al. An immune response study of oakmoss absolute and its constituents atranol and chloroatranol. *Contact Dermatitis.* 2014 May;70(5):282-90.
6225 Rastogi SC, Bossi R, Johansen JD, et al. Content of oak moss allergens atranol and chloroatranol in perfumes and similar products. *Contact Dermatitis.* 2004 Jun;50(6):367-70.
6226 Andersen F, Andersen KH, Bernois A, et al. Reduced content of chloroatranol and atranol in oak moss absolute significantly reduces the elicitation potential of this fragrance material. *Contact Dermatitis.* 2015 Feb;72(2):75-83.
6227 Kahriman N, Yazici K, Arslan T, et al. Chemical Composition and Antimicrobial Activity of the Essential Oils from Evernia prunastri (L.) Ach. and Evernia divaricata (L.) Ach. *Asian J Chem.* 2011;23(5):1937-39.
6228 Gianni S, Guerrini A, Noriega P, et al. Essential oil of wild Ocotea quixos (Lam.) Kosterm. (Lauraceae) leaves from Amazonian Ecuador. *Flavour Frag J.* 2006 Jul;21(4):674–76.
6229 Renato B, Alessandro M, Andreotti E, et al. Chemical composition and biological activities of Ishpingo essential oil, a traditional Ecuadorian spice from Ocotea Quixos (Lam.) Kosterm. (Lauraceae) flower calices. *Food Chem.* 2004 May;85(3):415–21.
6230 Bruni R, Medici A, Andreotti E, et al. Chemical composition and biological activities of Ishpingo essential oil, a traditional Ecuadorian spice from Ocotea quixos (Lam.) Kosterm. (Lauraceae) flower calices. *Food Chem.* 2004 May;85(3):415-21.
6231 Domaracky M, Rehak P, Juhas S, et al. Effects of selected plant essential oils on the growth and development of mouse preimplantation embryos in vivo. *Physiol Res.* 2007;56(1):97-104.
6232 Forschmidt P. Teratogenic activity of flavor additives. *Teratology.* 1979;19:26A.
6233 Mantovani A, Stazi AV, Macri C, et al. Pre-natal (segment II) toxicity study of cinnamic aldehyde in the Sprague- Dawley rat. *Food Chem toxicol.* 1989;27:781-86.
6234 Huang J, Wang S, Luo X, et al. Cinnamaldehyde reduction of platelet aggregation and thrombosis in rodents. *Thromb Res.* 2007;119(3):337–42.
6235 Ballabeni V, Tognolini M, Bertoni S, et al. Antiplatelet and antithrombotic activities of essential oil from wild Ocotea quixos (Lam.) Kostern. (Lauraceae) calices from Amazonian Ecuador. *Pharmacol Res.* 2007 Jan;55(1):23–30.
6236 Singh G, Maurya S, deLampasona MP, et al. A comparison of chemical antioxidant and antimicrobial studies of cinnamon leaf and bark volatile oils, oleoresins and their constituents. *Food Chem Toxicol.* 2007;45:1650–61.
6237 Ballabeni V, Tognolini M, Bertoni S, et al. Antiplatelet and antithrombotic activities of essential oil from wild Ocotea quixos (Lam.) Kostern. (Lauraceae) calices from Amazonian Ecuador. *Pharmacol Res.* 2007 Jan;55(1):23–30.

6238 Tognolini M, Barocelli E, Ballaberi E, et al. Comparative screening of plant essential oils: phenylpropanoid moiety as basic core for antiplatelet activity. *Life Sci.* 2006 Feb;78(13):1419–32.
6239 Babu PS, Prabuseenivasan S, Lgnacimuthu S. Cinnamaldehyde-A potential antidiabetic agent. *Phytomedicine.* 2007;14(1):15–22.
6240 Plaisier C, Cok A, Scott J, et al. Effects of cinnamaldehyde on the glucose transport activity of GLUT1. *Biochimie.* 2010 Oct;93(2):339–44.
6241 Langeveld WT, Veldhuizen EJ, Burt SA. Synergy between essential oil components and antibiotics. *Crit Rev Microbiol.* 2014 Feb;40(1);76–94.
6242 National Toxicology Program. Cinnamaldehyde. 1989 Dec. Available at: https://ntp.niehs.nih.gov/ntp/htdocs/chem_background/exsumpdf/cinnamaldehyde_508.pdf
6243 Ballabeni V, Tognolini M, Giorgio C, et al. Ocotea quixos Lam. Essential oil: in vitro and in vivo investigation on its anti-inflammatory properties. *Fitoterapia.* 2010 Jun;81(4):289–95.
6244 Ballabeni V, Tognolini M, Bertoni S, et al. Antiplatelet and antithrombotic activities of essential oil from wild Ocotea quixos (Lam.) Kostern. (Lauraceae) calices from Amazonian Ecuador. *Pharmacol Res.* 2007 Jan;55(1):23–30.
6245 Bruni R, Medici A, Andreotti E, et al. Chemical composition and biological activities of Ishpingo essential oil, a traditional Ecuadorian spice from Ocotea quixos (Lam.) Kosterm. (Lauraceae) flower calices. *Food Chem.* 2004 May;85(3):415-21.
6246 Scalvenzi L, Radice M, Toma L, et al. Larvicidal activity of Ocimum campechianum, Ocotea quixos and Piper aduncum essential oils against Aedes aegypti. *Parasite.* 2019;26:23.
6247 Hanus LO, Rezanaka T, Dembitsky VM, et al. Myrrh-Commiphora chemistry. *Biomed Papers.* 2005;149(1):3-28.
6248 de Rapper S, Van Vuuren SF, Kamatou GP, et al. The additive and synergistic antimicrobial effects of select frankincense and myrrh oils--a combination from the pharaonic pharmacopoeia. *Lett Appl Microbiol.* 2012 Apr;54(4):352-8.
6249 Başer KHC, Demirci B, Dekebo A, et al. Essential oils of some Boswellia spp., myrrh and opopanax. *Flavour Frag J.* 2003;18(2):153–156.
6250 Yeo SK, Ahmed AY, Hayward OA, et al. β-Bisabolene, a Sesquiterpene from the Essential Oil Extract of Opoponax (Commiphora guidottii), Exhibits Cytotoxicity in Breast Cancer Cell Lines. *Phytotherapy Res.* 2016 Mar;30(3):418-25.
6251 Marcotullio MC, Santi C, Mwankie GNOM, et al. Chemical composition of the essential oil of Commiphora erythraea. *Nat Prod Commun.* 2009;4(12):1751-54.
6252 ANLAP Database. Via Cropwatch.org. Available at: http://cropwatch.org.uk/Myrrh%20oil%20biblio%20v1.01.pdf.
6253 Faternale D, Sosa S, Ricci D, et al. Anti-inflammatory, antioxidant and antifungal furanosesquiterpenoids isolated from Commiphora erythraea (Ehrenb.) Engl. Resin. *Fitoterapia.* 2011 Jan;82(4):654-61.
6254 Dekebo A, Dagne E, Sterner O. Furanosesquiterpenes from Commiphora sphaerocarpa and related adulterants of true myrrh. *Fitoterapia.* 2002;73:48-55.
6255 Appendino G, Bianchi F, Bader A, et al. Coumarins from Opopanax chironium. New Dihydrofuranocoumarins and Differential Induction of Apoptosis by Imperatorin and Heraclenin. *J Nat Prod.* 2004;67:532-36.
6256 de Rapper S, Van Vuuren SF, Kamatou GP, et al. The additive and synergistic antimicrobial effects of select frankincense and myrrh oils--a combination from the pharaonic pharmacopoeia. *Lett Appl Microbiol.* 2012 Apr;54(4):352-8.
6257 Gebrehiwot M, Asres K2, Bisrat D, et al. Evaluation of the wound healing property of Commiphora guidottii Chiov. ex. Guid. *BMC Complement Altern Med.* 2015 Aug 18;15:282.
6258 Dekebo A, Dagne E, Sterner O. Furanosesquiterpenes from Commiphora sphaerocarpa and related adulterants of true myrrh. *Fitoterapia.* 2002;73:48-55.
6259 Gebrehiwot M, Asres K2, Bisrat D, et al. Evaluation of the wound healing property of Commiphora guidottii Chiov. ex. Guid. *BMC Complement Altern Med.* 2015 Aug 18;15:282.
6260 Dekebo A, Dagne E, Sterner O. Furanosesquiterpenes from Commiphora sphaerocarpa and related adulterants of true myrrh. *Fitoterapia.* 2002;73:48-55.
6261 Baylac S, Racine P. Inhibition of 5-lipoxygenase by essential oils and other natural fragrant extracts. *Int J Aromatherapy.* 2003;13(2-3):138-42.
6262 Muturi EJ, Hay WT, Doll KM, et al. Insecticidal Activity of Commiphora Erythraea Essential Oil and Its Emulsions Against Larvae of Three Mosquito Species. *J Med Entomol.* 2020 May 30. Online ahead of print.
6263 Bourgou S, Rahail FZ, Ourghemmi I, et al. Changes of peel essential oil composition of four Tunisian citrus during fruit maturation. *ScientificWorldJournal.* 2012;2012:528593.
6264 Tan QLP, Ai MV, Minh NTT. Volatile constituents of essential oil from Citrus sinensis grown in Tien Giang Province, Vietnam. *As J Food Ag-Ind.* 2011;4(03):183-86.
6265 Njoroge SM, Phi NTL, Sawamura M. Chemical composition of peel essential oils of sweet oranges (Citrus sinensis) from Uganda and Rwanda. *J Essential Oil Bearing Plants.*209;12(1):26-33.
6266 Haypek E, Silva LHM, Batista E, et al. Recovery of aroma constituents from orange essential oil. *Braz J Chem Eng.* 2000 Dec;1.17(4-7):0104-6632.
6267 Palacios SM, Bertoni A, Rossi Y, et al. Efficacy of essential oils from edible plants as insecticides against the house fly, Musca Domestica L. *Molecules.* 2009;14:1938-47.
6268 Opdyke DIJ. Monographs on fragrance raw materials. *Food Cosmet Toxicol.* 1974;12(Suppl.):733-34.
6269 Sawamura M, Hasegawa K, Kashiwagi T, et al. Determination of bergapten in Japanese citrus essential oils. *Jap J Aromatherapy.* 2009;9:3-37.
6270 Mauerman B, Ahmed N, Tambhar N, et al. Trends in Furanocoumarin Profiles Among Commerical-Scale Essential Oils. International Conference on the Science of Botanicals, Poster. Mar 2022.
6271 Crowell PL. Prevention and therapy of cancer by dietary monoterpenes. *J Nutr.* 1999 Mar;129(3):775S-778S.
6272 Bodake HB, Panicker KN, Kailaje VV, et al. Chemopreventive effect of orange oil on the development of hepatic preneoplastic lesions induced by N-nitrosodiethylamine in rats: an ultrastructural study. *Indian J Exp Biol.* 2002 Mar;40(3):245-51.
6273 Maltzman TH, Hurt LM, Elson CE, et al. The prevention of nitrosomethylurea-induced mammary tumors by d-limonene and orange oil. *Carcinogenesis.* 1989 Apr;10(4):781-3.
6274 Chidambara Murthy KN, Jayaprakasha GK, Patil BS. D-limonene rich volatile oil from blood oranges inhibits angiogenesis, metastasis and cell death in human colon cancer cells. *Life Sci.* 2010 Oct 5;91(11-12):429-39.
6275 Sargolzaee MR, Faayyazi Bordbar MR, Shakiba M, et al. The comparison of the efficacy of Citrus Fragrance and Fluoxetine in the treatment of major depressive disorder. *J of Gonabad University of Med Sci and Health Sci.* 2004;10(3):43-48.
6276 Matiz G, Osorio MR, Camacho F, et al. Effectiveness of antimicrobial formulations for acne based on orange (Citrus sinensis) and sweet basil (Ocimum basilicum L) essential oils. *Biomedica.* 2012 Jan-Mar;32(1):125-33.
6277 Yip YB, Tam AC. An experimental study on the effectiveness of massage with aromatic ginger and orange essential oil for moderate-to-severe knee pain among the elderly in Hong Kong. *Complement Ther Med.* 2008 Jun;16(3):131-38.
6278 Hur MH, Han SH. Clinical trial of aromatherapy on postpartum mother's perineal healing. *Taehan Kanho Hakhoe Chi.* 2004 Feb;34(1):53-62.
6279 Kaur CD, Saraf S. In vitro sun protection factor determination of herbal oils used in cosmetics. *Pharmacognosy Res.* 2010 Jan;2(1):22-25.
6280 Muthaiyan a, Biswas D, Crandall PG, et al. Application of orange essential oil as an antistaphylococcal agent in a dressing model. *BMC Complement Altern Med.* 2012 Aug;12:125.
6281 Lehrner J, Marwinski G, Lehr S, et al. Ambient odors of orange and lavender reduce anxiety and improve mood in a dental office. *Physiol Behav.* 2005 Sep 15;86(1-2):92-95.
6282 Jafarzadeh M, Arman S, Pour FF, et al. Effect of aromatherapy with orange essential oil on salivary cortisol and pulse rate in children during dental treatment: A randomized controlled clinical trial. *Physiol Behav.* 2005 Mar;2:10.
6283 Lehrner J, Eckersberger C, Walla P, et al. Ambient odor of orange in a dental office reduces anxiety and improves mood in female patients. *Physiol Behav.* 2000 Oct 1-15;1(1-2):83-86.
6284 Faturi CB, Leite JR, Alves PB, et al. Anxiolytic-like effect of sweet orange aroma in Wistar rats. *Prog Neuropsychopharmacol Biol Psychaitry.*2010 May 30;34(4):605-09.
6285 Goes TC, Antunes FD, Alves PB, et al. Effect of sweet orange aroma on experimental anxiety in humans. *J Altern Complement Med.* 2012 Aug;18(8):798-804.
6286 Fisher K, Phillips C. In vitro inhibition of vancomycin-susceptible and vancomycin-resistant Enterococcus faecium and E. faecalis in the presence of citrus essential oils. *Br J Biomed Sci.* 2009;66(4):180-85.
6287 Fisher K, Phillips C. The mechanism of action of a citrus oil blend against Enterococcus faecium and Enterococcus faecalis. *J Appl Microbiol.* 2009 Apr;106(4):1343-49.
6288 O'Bryan CA, Crandall PG, Chalova VI, et al. Orange essential oils antimicrobial activities against Salmonella spp. *J Food Sci.* 2008 Aug;73(6):M264-67.
6289 Sharma N, Tripathi A. Effects of Citrus sinensis (L.) Osbeck epicarp essential oil on growth and morphogenesis of Aspergillus niger (L.) Van Tieghem. *Microbiol Res.* 2008;163(3):337-44.
6290 Cisarová M, Tančinová D, Medo J, et al. The in vitro effect of selected essential oils on the growth and mycotoxin production of Aspergillus species. *J Environ Sci Health B.* 2016 Oct 2;51(10):668-674.
6291 Baylac S, Racine P. Inhibition of 5-lipoxygenase by essential oils and other natural fragrant extracts. *Int J Aromatherapy.* 2003;13(2-3):138-42.
6292 Lv YX, Zhao SP, Zhang JY, et al. Effect of orange peel essential oil on oxidative stress in AOM animals. *Int J Biol Macromol.*2012 May;50(4):1144-50.
6293 Singh P, Shukla R, Prakash B, et al. Chemical profile, antifungal, antiaflatoxigenic and antioxidant activity of Citrus maxima Burm. And Citrus sinensis (L.) Osbeck essential oils and their cyclic monoterpene, DL-limonene. *Food Chem Toxicol.* 2010 Jun;48(6):1734-40.
6294 Murali R, Karthikeyan A, Saravanan R. Protective effects of D-limonene on lipid peroxidation and antioxidant enzymes in streptozotoxin-induced diabetic rats. *Basic Clin Pharmacol Toxicol.* 2013 Mar;112(3):175-81.
6295 Chaudhary SC, Siddiqui MS, Athar M, et al. D-limonene modulates inflammation, oxidative stress and Ras-ERK pathway to inhibit murine skin tumorigenesis. *Hum Exp Toxicol.* 2012 Aug;31(8):799-811.
6296 Cisarová M, Tančinová D, Medo J, et al. The in vitro effect of selected essential oils on the growth and mycotoxin production of Aspergillus species. *J Environ Sci Health B.* 2016 Oct 2;51(10):668-674.
6297 Campolo O, Romeo FV, Algeri GM, et al. Larvicidal Effects of Four Citrus Peel Essential Oils Against the Arbovirus Vector Aedes albopictus (Diptera: Culicidae). *J Econ Entomol.* 2016 Feb;109(1):360-5.
6298 Geraci A, Di Stefano V, Di Martino E, et al. Essential oil components of orange peels and antimicrobial activity. *Nat Prod Res.* 2016 Aug 18:1-7.
6299 Moshfegh C, Swiercz A, Hopkins L, et al. Effects of Essential Oil on Fear Memory and the Immune Response: A Potential Alternative Therapy for Post Traumatic Stress Disorder (PSTD). *Experimental Biol.* 2017. Available at: https://app.core-apps.com/eb2017/abstract/887f0321f580739f713710619ba85f6c.
6300 Badawy MEI, Taktak NEM, El-Aswad AF, et al. Chemical composition of the essential oils isolated from peel of three citrus species and their mosquitocidal activity against Culex pipiens. *Nat Prod Res.* 2018 Dec;32(23):2829-2834.
6301 Abrahamyan HT, Minasyan SM. [Corrective effect of aromatherapy on indices of heart rate variability in students under exam stress conditions]. *Gig Sanit.* 2016;95(6):563-8.
6302 Wolffenbüttel AN, Zamboni A, Becker G, et al. Citrus essential oils inhalation by mice: Behavioral testing, GCMS plasma analysis, corticosterone, and melatonin levels evaluation. *Phytother Res.* 2018 Jan;32(1):160-169.
6303 Shi Y, Huang SA, He Y, et al. Navel Orange Peel Essential Oil To Control Food Spoilage Molds in Potato Slices. *J Food Prot.* 2018 Sep;81(9):1496-1502.

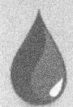

6304 Guo Q, Liu K, Deng W, et al. Chemical composition and antimicrobial activity of Gannan navel orange (Citrus sinensis Osbeck cv. Newhall) peel essential oils. *Food Sci Nutr*. 2018 Jun 14;6(6):1431-1437.

6305 Yang C, Chen H, Chen H, et al. Antioxidant and Anticancer Activities of Essential Oil from Gannan Navel Orange Peel. *Molecules*. 2017 Aug 22;22(8).

6306 Hocayen PAS, Wendler E, Vecchia DD, et al. The nitrergic neurotransmission contributes to the anxiolytic-like effect of Citrus sinensis essential oil in animal models. *Phytother Res*. 2019 Apr;33(4):901-909.

6307 Wang L, Zhang Y, Fan G, et al. Effects of orange essential oil on intestinal microflora in mice. *J Sci Food Agric*. 2019 Jun;99(8):4019-4028.

6308 Zhang L, Yang Z, Fan G, et al. Antidepressant-like effect of Citrus sinensis (L.) Osbeck essential oil and its main component limonene on mice. *J Agric Food Chem*. 2019 Dec 18;67(50):13817-13828.

6309 Liu K, Deng W, Hu W, et al. Extraction of 'Gannanzao' Orange Peel Essential Oil by Response Surface Methodology and its Effect on Cancer Cell Proliferation and Migration. *Molecules*. 2019 Jan 30;24(3).

6310 Toscano-Garibay JD, Arriaga-Alba M, Sánchez-Navarrete J, et al. Antimutagenic and antioxidant activity of the essential oils of Citrus sinensis and Citrus latifolia. *Sci Rep*. 2017 Sep 13;7(1):11479.

6311 Li D, Wu H, Dou H. Weight loss effect of sweet orange essential oil microcapsules on obese SD rats induced by high-fat diet. *Biosci Biotechnol Biochem*. 2019 May;83(5):923-932.

6312 Son HK, So WY, Kim M. Effects of Aromatherapy Combined with Music Therapy on Anxiety, Stress, and Fundamental Nursing Skills in Nursing Students: A Randomized Controlled Trial. *Int J Environ Res Public Health*. 2019 Oct 29;16(21).

6313 Oyedeji AO, Okunowo WO, Osuntiki AA, et al. Insecticidal and biochemical activity of essential oil from Citrus sinensis peel and constituents on Callosobrunchus maculatus and Sitophilus zeamais. *Pestic Biochem Physiol*. 2020 Sep;168:104643.

6314 Bento R, Pagan E, Berdjo D, et al. Chitosan nanoemulsions of cold-pressed orange essential oil to preserve fruit juices. *Int J Food Microbiol*. 2020 Jul 6;331:108786.

6315 Kundu A, Dutta A, Mandal A, et al. A Comprehensive in vitro and in silico Analysis of Nematicidal Action of Essential Oils. *Front Plant Sci*. 2021 Jan 8;11:614143.

6316 Osanloo M, Ghaznavi G, Abdollahi A. Surveying the chemical composition and antibacterial activity of essential oils from selected medicinal plants against human pathogens. *Iran J Microbiol*. 2020 Dec;12(6):577-583.

6317 Gomes B, Ogelil H, Brant F, et al. High larvicidal efficacy of yeast-encapsulated orange oil against Aedes aegypti strains from Brazil. *Parasit Vectors*. 2021 May 22;14(1):272.

6318 Lin X, Cao S, Sun J, et al. The Chemical Compositions, and Antibacterial and Antioxidant Activities of Four Types of Citrus Essential Oils. *Molecules*. 2021 Jun 4;26(11):3412.

6319 Kammoun AK, Altyar AE, Gad HA. Comparative metabolic study of Citrus sinensis leaves cultivars based on GC-MS and their cytotoxic activity. *J Pharm Biomed Anal*. 2021 May 10;198:113991.

6320 Youcef-Ettoumi K, Zouambia Y, Moulai-Mostefa N. Chemical composition, antimicrobial and antioxidant activities of Algerian Citrus sinensis essential oil extracted by hydrodistillation assisted by electromagnetic induction heating. *J Food Sci Technol*. 2021 Aug;58(8):3049-3055.

6321 Noruzi Zamenjani M, Farmahini Farahani M, Amirmohseni L, et al. The Effects of Inhalation Aromatherapy on Postoperative Abdominal Pain: A Three-Arm Randomized Controlled Clinical Trial. *J Perianesth Nurs*. 2021 Apr;36(2):147-152.

6322 Varaei S, Jalalian Z, Nejad MSY, et al. Comparison the effects of inhalation and massage aromatherapy with lavender and sweet orange on fatigue in hemodialysis patients: a randomized clinical trial. *J Complement Integr Med*. 2020 May 28;18(1):193-200.

6323 Bhandari DP, Poudel DK, Satyal P, et al. Volatile Compounds and Antioxidant and Antimicrobial Activities of Selected Citrus Essential Oils Originated from Nepal. *Molecules*. 2021 Nov 4;26(21):6683.

6324 Arrout A, El Ghallab Y, Lefriyekh MR, et al. Citrus essential oils and main terpenes: chemical composition and good litholytic activity on gallstones. *Vegetos*. 2021;34:600-5.

6325 Ma Y. The influence of ambient aroma on the middle school students' academic emotions. *Int J Psych*. 2022 Jan 21:1-6.

6326 Wang QS, Li M, Li X, et al. Protective effect of orange essential oil on the formation of non-alcoholic fatty liver disease caused by high-fat diet. *Food Function*. 2022;2. Online ahead of print.

6327 Li C, Cai Q, Wu X, et al. Variation in compositions and biological activities of essential oils from four Citrus species: Citrus limon, Citrus sinensis, Citrus paradisi, and Citrus reticulata. *Chem Biodivers*. 2022 Feb 10. Online ahead of print.

6328 Kozlova AD. Effect of aromatherapy (orange and pine oils) on human visual-motor response. *Youth Inn Bull*. 2022;11:537-9.

6329 Qu SS, Zhang Y, Ren JN, et al. Effect of different ways of ingesting orange essential oil on blood immune index and intestinal microflora in mice. *J Sci Food Agric*. 2022 Jul 27. Online ahead of print.

6330 Li C, Zhu H, Zhao K, et al. Chemical constituents, biological activities and anti-rheumatoid arthritic properties of four citrus essential oils. *Phytother Res*. 2022 Jul;36(7):2908-2920.

6331 Yousafi Q, Bibi S, Saleem S, et al. Identification of Novel and Safe Fungicidal Molecules against Fusarium oxysporum from Plant Essential Oils: In Vitro and Computational Approaches. *Biomed Res Int*. 2022 Jul 26;2022:5347224.

6332 Laudani F, Campolo O, Caridi R, et al. Aphicidal Activity and Phytotoxicity of Citrus sinensis Essential-Oil-Based Nano-Insecticide. *Insects*. 2022 Dec 13;13(12):1150.

6333 Manzur M, Luciardi MC, Blázquez MA, et al. Citrus sinensis Essential Oils an Innovative Antioxidant and Antipathogenic Dual Strategy in Food Preservation against Spoliage Bacteria. *Antioxidants (Basel)*. 2023 Jan 21;12(2):246.

6334 Salarfad M, Zarei B, Younsesi Z, et al. The Effect of Orange Essential Oil Aromatherapy on Sleep Quality in Hospitalized Children. *Preventive Care Nurs Midwifery J*. 2023;13(1):83-90.

6335 Bejaoui A, Chaabane H, Jemli M, et al. Essential oil composition and antibacterial activity of Origanum vulgare subsp. Glandulosum Desf. at different phenological stages. *J Med Food*. 2013 Dec;16(12):1115-20.

6336 Elezi F, Plaku F, Ibraliu A, et al. Genetic variation of oregano (Origanum vulgare L.) for etheric oil in Albania. *Sci Res*. 2013 Sep;4(9):449-54.

6337 Ekren S, Yerlikaya O, Tokul HE, et al. Chemical composition, antimicrobial activity and antioxidant capacity of some medicinal and aromatic plant extracts. *African J Microbiol Res*. 2013 Jan 29;7(5):383-88.

6338 Lukas B, Schmiderer C, Novak J. Conservation and characterization of oregano (Origanum vulgare L.) wild populations in Europe genetic structure and variability of the essential oil. Available at: http://www.ecpgr.cgiar.org/fileadmin/templates/ecpgr.org/upload/PROJECT_REPORTS/Origanum_vulgare_Final_report.pdf.

6339 Lagouri V, Blekas G, Tsimidou M, et al. Composition and antioxidant activity of essential oils from oregano plants grown in Greece. *A Lebensm Unters Forsch*. 1993;197:20-23.

6340 Begnini KR, Nedel F, Lund RG, et al. Composition and antiproliferative effect of essential oil of Origanum vulgare against tumor cell lines. *J Med Food*. 2014 Oct;17(10):1129-33.

6341 Cleff MB, Meinerz AR, Xavier M, et al. In vitro activity of Origanum vulgare essential oil against Candida species. *Braz J Microbiol*. 2010 Jan-Mar;41(1):1517-8382.

6342 Al-Kalaldeh JZ, Abu-Dahab R, Afifi FU. Volatile oil composition and antiproliferative activity of Laurus nobilis, Origanum syriacum, Origanum vulgare, and Salvia triloba against human breast adenocarcinoma cells. *Nutr Res*. 2010 Apr;30(4):271-78.

6343 Figueredo G, Cabassu P, Chalchat JC, et al. Studies of Mediterranean oregano populations—V. Chemical composition of essential oils of oregano: Origanum syriacum L. var bevanii (Holmes) letswaart, O. syriacum L. var. sinaicum (Boiss.) letswaart, and O. syriacum L. var syriacum from Lebanon and Israel. *Flav Frag J*. 2005 Mar;20(2):164-68.

6344 Baser KH, Kurkcuoglu M, Demirci D, et al. The essential oil of Origanum syriacum L. var. sinaicum (Boiss.) letswaart. *Flav Frag J*. 2003 Mar;18(2):98-99.

6345 Russo M, Suraci F, Postorino S, et al. Essential oil chemical composition and antifungal effects on Sclerotium cepivorum of Thymus capitatus wild populations from Calabria, southern Italy. *Revista Brasileira de Farmacognosia*. 2013 Mar-Apr;23:2:0102-695X.

6346 Lassaad H, Mehrez R, Abderrabba A, et al. Variability in essential oil composition of Tunisian Thymus capitatus (L.) Hoffmans. et Link. *Flavour Frag J*. 2002 Jan;17(1):26-28.

6347 Maissa BJ, Walid H. Antifungal activity of chemically different essential oils from wild Tunisian Thymus spp. *Nat Prod Res*. 2015;29(9):869-73.

6348 Ali IB, Guetat A, Boussaid M. Variation of volatiles in Tunisian populations of Thymbra capitata (L.) Cav. (Lamiaceae). *Chem Biodivers*. 2012 Jul;9(7):1272-85.

6349 Sezik E, Tumen G, , Kirimer N, et al. Essential Oil Composition of Four Origanum vulgare Subspecies of Antolian Origin. *J Essent Oil Res*. 1993 Jul/Aug;5:425-31.

6350 Capatina L, Napoli EM, Ruberto G, et al. Origanum vulgare ssp. hirtum (Lamiaceae) Essential Oil Prevents Behavioral and Oxidative Stress Changes in the Scopolamine Zebrafish Model. *Molecules*. 2021;26:7085.

6351 Novak I, Sipos L, Kokai Z, et al. Effect of the drying method on the composition of Origanum L. subsp. hirtum essential oil analysed by GC-mS and sensory profile method. *Acta Alimentaria*. 2011;40(Suppl.):130-8.

6352 Sarikurkcu C, Zengin G, Oskay M, et al. Composition, antioxidant, antimicrobial and enzyme inhibition activities of two Origanum vulgare subspecies (subsp. vulgare and subsp. hirtum) essential oils. *Ind Crop Prod*. 2015;70:178-84.

6353 Ozcan MM, Pedro LG, Al-Juhaimi F, et al. Constituents of the Essential oil of Origanum vulgare subsp. hirtum Growing Wild in Turkey. *J Essent Oil Bear Plants*. 2012;15(4):572-6.

6354 Soliman FM, Yousif SS, Zaghloul SS, et al. Seasonal variation in the essential oil composition of Origanum syriacum L. subsp. Sinaicum Greuter and Burdet; evaluation of its tocolytic activity. *Egypt J Biomed Sci*. 2007 Mar;23:121-34.

6355 Miguel MG, Gago C, Antunes MD, et al. Antioxidant and Antiproliferative Activities of the Essential Oils from Thymbra capitata and Thymus Species Grown in Portugal. *Evid Based Complement Alternat Med*. 2015;2015:851721.

6356 Domaracky M, Rehak P, Juhas S, et al. Effects of selected plant essential oils on the growth and development of mouse preimplantation embryos in vivo. *Physiol Res*. 2007;56(1):97-104.

6357 Lemhadri A, Zeggwagh NA, Maghrani M, et al. Anti-hypoglycaemic activity of the aqueous extract of Origanum vulgare growing wild in Tafilalet region. *J Ethnopharmacol*. 2004 Jun;92(2-3):251-6.

6358 Tognolini M, Barocelli E, Ballabeni V, et al. Comparative screening of plant essential oils; phenylpropanoid moiety as basic core for antiplatelet activity. *Life Sci*. 2006 Feb 23;78(13):1419-32.

6359 Tsai HH, Lin HW, Chen YL, et al. A review of potential harmful interactions between anticoagulant/antiplatelet agents and Chinese herbal medicines. *PLoS One*. 2013 May 9;8(5):e64255.

6360 Langeveld WT, Veldhuizen EJ, Burt SA. Synergy between essential oil constituents and antibiotics. *Crit Rev Microbiol*. 2014 Feb;40(1);76-94.

6361 Langeveld WT, Veldhuizen EJ, Burt SA. Synergy between essential oil constituents and antibiotics. *Crit Rev Microbiol*. 2014 Feb;40(1);76-94.

6362 Palaniappan K, Holley Ra. Use of natural antimicrobials to increase antibiotic susceptibility of drug resistant bacteria. *In J Food Microbiol*. 2010 Jun 15;140(2-3):164-8.

6363 Kissels W, Wu X, Santos RR, et al. Short communication: Interaction of the isomers carvacrol and thymol with the antibiotics doxycycline and tilmicosin: In vitro effects against pathogenic bacteria commonly found in the respiratory tract of calves. *J Dairy Sci*. 2017 Feb;100(2):970-974.

[6364] Valente JS, Fonseca AO1, Denardi LB, et al. In vitro activity of antifungals in combination with essential oils against the oomycete Pythium insidiosum. *J Appl Microbiol.* 2016 Oct;121(4):998-1003.

[6365] Mertas A, Garbusińska A, Szliszka E, et al. The influence of tea tree oil (Melaleuca alternifolia) on fluconazole activity against fluconazole-resistant Candida albicans strains. *Biomed Res Int.* 2015;2015:590470.

[6366] Kohlert C, Schindler G, Marz RW, et al. Systemic availability and pharmacokinetics of thymol in humans. *J Clin Pharmacol.* 2002 Jul;42(7):731-7.

[6367] Toxicology Data Network, National Library of Medicine. Thymol. Available at: http://toxnet.nlm.nih.gov/cgi-bin/sis/search/a?dbs+hsdb:@term+@DOCNO+866.

[6368] Jukic M, Politeo O, Maksimmovic M, et al. In vitro acetylcholinesterase inhibitory properties of thymol, carvacrol and their derivatives thymoquinone and thymohydroquinone. *Phytother Res.* 2007;21(3):259-61.

[6369] Bostancioglu RB, Kurkcuoglu M, Baser KH, et al. Assessment of anti-angiogenic and anti-tumoral potentials of Origanum onites L. essential oil. *Food Chem Toxicol.* 2012 Jun;50(6):2002-08.

[6370] Zeytinoglu H, Incesu Z, Baser KH. Inhibition of DNA synthesis by carvacrol in mouse myoblast cells bearing a human N-RAS oncogene. *Phytomedicine.* 2003 May;10(4):292-99.

[6371] Liang WZ, Lu CH. Carvacrol-induced [Ca2+]I rise and apoptosis in human glioblastoma cells. *Life Sci.* 2012 May 15;90(17-18):703-11.

[6372] Boskabady MH, Jandaghi P. Relaxant effects of carvacrol on guinea pig tracheal chains and its possible mechanisms. *Pharmazie.* 2003;58(9):661–63.

[6373] Begnini KR, Nedel F, Lund RG, et al Composition and antiproliferative effect of essential oil of Origanum vulgare against tumor cell lines. *J Med Food.* 2014 Oct;17(10):1129-33.

[6374] Misharina TA, Burlakova EB, Fatkullina LD, et al. Effect of oregano essential oil on the engraftment and development of Lewis carcinoma in F1 DBA c57 black hybrid mice. *Prikl Biokhim Mikrobiol.* 2013 Jul-Aug;49(4):423- 28.

[6375] Meneses R, Ocazionez RE, Martinez JR, et al. Inhibitory effect of essential oils obtained from plants grown in Colombian on yellow fever virus replication in intro. *Ann Clin Microbiol Antimicrob.* 2009 Mar 6;8:8.

[6376] Force M, Sparks WS, Ronzio RA. Inhibition of enteric parasites by emulsified oil of oregano in vivo. *Phytother Res.* 2000 May;14(3):213-14.

[6377] Gómez-Mateos Pérez M, Navarro Moll C1, Merino Espinosa G, et al. Evaluation of different Mediterranean essential oils as prophylactic agents in anisakidosis. *Pharm Biol.* 2017 Dec;55(1):456-461.

[6378] Dundar E, Olgun EG, Isiksoy S, et al. The effect of intra-rectal and intra-peritoneal application of Origanum onites L. essential oil on 2,4,6-trinitrobenzenesulfonic acid-induced colitis in the rat. *Exp Toxicol Pathol.* 2008 Apr;59(6):399- 408.

[6379] Elizaquivel P, Azizkhani M, Aznar R, et al. The effect of essential oils on norovirus surrogates. *Food Control.* 2013 Jul;32(1):275-278.

[6380] Gilling DH, Kitajima M, Torrey JR, et al. Antiviral efficacy and mechanisms of action of oregano essential oil and its primary component carvacrol against murine norovirus. *J Appl Microbiol.* 2014 May;116(5):1149-63.

[6381] Tampieri MP, Galuppi R, Macchioni F, et al. The inhibition of Candida albicans by selected essential oils and their major components. *Mycopathologia.*2005 Apr;159(3):339-45.

[6382] Miller AB, Cates RG, Lawrence M, et al. The antimicrobial and antifungal activity of essential oils extracted from Guatemalan medicinal plants. *Pharm Biol.* 2015 Apr;53(4):548-54.

[6383] Alexopoulos A, Kimbaris AC, Plessas S, et al. Antíbacterial activities of essential oils from eight Greek aromatic plants against clinical isolates of Staphylococcus aureus. *Anaerobe.* 2011 Dec;17(6):399-402.

[6384] Karakaya S, El SN, Karagozlu N, et al. Antioxidant and antimicrobial activities of essential oils obtained from oregano (Origanum vulgare ssp. Hirtum) by using different extraction methods. *J Med Food.* 2011 Jun;14(6):645-52.

[6385] Saeed S, Tariq P. Antibacterial activity of oregano (Origanum vulgare Linn.) against gram positive bacteria. *Pak J Pharm Sci.* 2009 Oct;22(4):421-24.

[6386] Cleff MB, Meinerz AR, Xavier M, et al. In vitro activity of Origanum vulgare essential oil against Candida species. *Braz J Microbiol.* 2010 Jan;41(10:116-23.

[6387] Císarová M, Tančinová D, Medo J, et al. The in vitro effect of selected essential oils on the growth and mycotoxin production of Aspergillus species. *J Environ Sci Health B.* 2016 Oct 2;51(10):668-674.

[6388] Seo HS, Beuchat LR, Kim H, et al. Development of an experimental apparatus and protocol for determining antimicrobial activities of gaseous plant essential oils. *Int J Food Microbiol.* 2015 Dec 23;215:95-100.

[6389] Scandorieiro S, de Camargo LC, Lancheros CA, et al. Synergistic and Additive Effect of Oregano Essential Oil and Biological Silver Nanoparticles against Multidrug-Resistant Bacterial Strains. *Front Microbiol.* 2016 May 23;7:760.

[6390] Sakkas H, Gousia P, Economou V, et al. In vitro antimicrobial activity of five essential oils on multidrug resistant Gram-negative clinical isolates. *J Intercult Ethnopharmacol.* 2016 Jun-Aug;5(3):212–18.

[6391] Pesavento G, Maggini V, Maida I, et al. Essential Oil from Origanum vulgare Completely Inhibits the Growth of Multidrug-Resistant Cystic Fibrosis Pathogens. *Nat Prod Commun.* 2016 Jun;11(6):861-4.

[6392] Fratini F, Mancini S, Turchi B, et al. A novel interpretation of the Fractional Inhibitory Concentration Index: The case Origanum vulgare L. and Leptospermum scoparium J. R. et G. Forst essential oils against Staphylococcus aureus strains. *Microbiol Res.* 2017 Jan;195:11-17.

[6393] Iqbal Z, Zafar MS. Role of antifungal medicaments added to tissue conditioners: A systematic review. J Prosthodont Res. 2016 Oct;60(4):231-239.

[6394] Srivatstava A1, Ginjupalli K, Perampalli NU, et al. Evaluation of the properties of a tissue conditioner containing origanum oil as an antifungal additive. *J Prosthet Dent.* 2013 Oct;110(4):313-9.

[6395] Santoro GF, das Gracas Cardoso M, Guimaraes LG, et al. Effect of oregano (Origanum vulgure L.) and thyme (Thymus vulgaris L.) essential oil on Trypanosoma cruzi (Protozoa: Kinetoplastida) growth and ultrastructure. *Parasitol.* 2007 Mar;100(4):783-90.

[6396] de Souza EL, de Barros JC, de Oliveira CE, et al. Influence of Origanum vulgare essential oil on enterotoxin production, membrane permeability and surface characteristics of Staphylococcus aureus. *Int J Food Microbiol.* 2010 Feb 28;137(2-3):308-11.

[6397] Fonseca AO, Pereira DI, Jacob RG, et al. In vitro susceptibility of Brazilian Pythium insidiosum isolates to essential oils of some Lamiaceae family. *Mycopathologia.* 2014 Nov;179(3-4):253-8.

[6398] Firouzi R, Shekarforoush SS, Nazer AH, et al. Effects of essential oils of oregano and nutmeg on growth and survival of Yersinia enterocolitica and Listeria monocytogenes in barbecued chicken. *J Food Prot.* 2007 Nov;70(11):2626-30.

[6399] Ozogul Y, Kuley E, Ucar Y, et al. Antimicrobial Impacts of Essential Oils on Food Borne-Pathogens. Recent Pat Food Nutr Agric. 2015;7(1):53-61.

[6400] Esper RH, Goncalez E, Marques MO, et al. Potential of essential oils for protection of grains contaminated by aflatoxin produced by Aspergillus flavus. *Front Microbiol.* 2014 Jun 4;5:269.

[6401] de Sousa LL, de Andrade SC, Athayde AJ, et al. Efficacy of Origanum vulgare and Rosmarinus officinalis L. essential oils in combination to control postharvest pathogenic Aspergilli and autochthonous mycoflora in Vitis labrusca L. (table grapes). *Int J Food Microbiol.* 2013 Aug 1;165(3):312-18.

[6402] Alinkina ES, Misharina TA, Fatkullina LD. Antiradical properties of oregano, thyme, and savory essential oils. *Prikl Biokhim Mikrobiol.* 2013 Jan-Feb;49(1):82-87.

[6403] Albano SM, Lima AS, Miguel MG, et al. Antioxidant, anti-5-lipoxygenase and antiacetylcholinesterase activities of essential oils and decoction waters of some aromatic plants. Rec Nat Prod. 2012;6(1):35-48.

[6404] Han F, Ma GQ, Yang M, et al. Chemical composition and antioxidant activities of essential oils from different parts of the oregano. *J Zhejiang Univ Sci B.* 2017 Jan.;18(1):79-84.

[6405] Kulisic T, Krisko A, Dragovic-Uzelac V, et al. The effects of essential oils and aqueous tea infusions of oregano (Origanum vulgare L. spp hirtum), thyme (Thymus vulgaris L.) and wild thyme (Thymus serpyllum L.) on the copper- induced oxidation of human low-density lipoprotein. *Int J Food Sci Nutr.* 2007 Mar;58(2):87-93.

[6406] Meisinger C, Baumert J, Khuseyinova N, et al. Plasma oxidized low-density lipoprotein, a strong predictor for acute coronary heart disease events in apparently healthy, middle-aged med from the general population. *Circulation.* 2005 Aug 2;112(5):651-57.

[6407] Pérez-Rosés R, Risco E, Vila R, et al. Biological and Nonbiological Antioxidant Activity of Some Essential Oils. *J Agric Food Chem.* 2016 Jun 15;64(23):4716-24.

[6408] Teixeira B, Marques A, Ramos C, et al. Chemical composition and bioactivity of different oregano (Origanum vulgare) extracts and essential oil. *J Sci Food Agric.* 2013 Aug;93(11):2707-14.

[6409] De Oliveira TL, Soares Rde A, Piccoli RH. A Weibull model to describe antimicrobial kinetics of oregano and lemongrass oils against Salmonella Enteritidis in ground beef during refrigerated storage. *Meat Sci.* 2013 Mar;93(3):645-51.

[6410] Asensio CM, Nepote V, Grosso NR. Chemical stability of extra virgin olive oil added with oregano essential oil. *J Food Sci.* 2011 Sep;76(7):S445-50.

[6411] Krkic N, Sojic B, Lazic V, et al. Lipid oxidative changes in chitosan-oregano coated traditional dry fermented sausage Petrovska klobasa. *Meat Sci.* 2013 Mar;93(3):767-70.

[6412] Chaves-Lopez C, Martin-Sanchez AM, Fuentes-Zaragoza E, et al. Role of oregano (Origanum vulgare) essential oil as a surface fungus inhibitor on fermented sausages: evaluation of its effect on microbial and physicochemical characteristics. *J Food Prot.* 2012 Jan;75(1):104-11.

[6413] Carmo ES, de Oliveira Lima E, de Souza EL. The potential of Origanum vulgare L. (Lamiaceae) essential oil in inhibiting the growth of some food-related Aspergillus species. *Braz J Microbiol.* 2008 Apr;39(2):362-67.

[6414] Nostro A, Blanco AR, Cannatelli MA, et al. Susceptibility of methicillin-resistant staphylococci to oregano essential oil, carvacrol and thymol. *FEMS Microbiol Mett.* 2004 Jan 30;230(2):191-95.

[6415] Inouye S, Uchida K, Nishiyama Y, et al. Combined effect of heat, essential oils and salt on fungicidal activity against Trichophyton mentagrophytes in a foot bath. *Nihon Ishinjin Gakkai Zasshi.*2007;48(1):27-36.

[6416] Lermioglu F, Bagci S, Onderoglu S, et al. Evaluation of the long-term effects of oleum origani on the toxicity induced by administration of streptozotocin in rats. *J Pharm Pharmacol.* 1997 Nov;49(11):1157-61.

[6417] Alma MH, Mavi A, Yildirim A, et al. Screening chemical composition and in vitro antioxidant and antimicrobial activities of the essential oils from Origanum syriacum L. growing in Turkey. *Biol Pharm Bull.* 2003;26(12):1725-29.

[6418] Soylu S, Yigitbas H, Soylu EM, et al. Antifungal effects of essential oils from oregano and fennel on Sclerotinia sclerotiorum. *J Appl Microbiol.* 2007 Oct;103(4):1021-30.

[6419] Miguel MG, Gago C, Antunes MD, et al. Antioxidant and Antiproliferative Activities of the Essential Oils from Thymbra capitata and Thymus Species Grown in Portugal. *Evid Based Complement Alternat Med.* 2015;2015:851721.

[6420] Džamić AM, Nikolić BJ, Giweli AA, et al. Libyan Thymus capitatus essential oil: antioxidant, antimicrobial, cytotoxic and colon pathogen adhesion-inhibition properties. *J Appl Microbiol.* 2015 Aug;119(2):389-99.

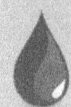

[6421] Usai M, Foddai M, Sechi B, et al. Comparison of antibacterial activity of natural and hydroformylated essential oil of Thymus capitatus growing wild in north Sardinia with commercial Thymus essential oils. *Nat Prod Commun.* 2010 Dec;5(12):1985-9.

[6422] Qaralleh HN, Abboud MM, Khleifat KM, et al. Antibacterial activity in vitro of Thymus capitatus from Jordan. *Pak J Pharm Sci.* 2009 Jul;22(3):247-51.

[6423] Figueiredo AC, Barroso JG, Pedro LG, et al. Portuguese Thymbra and Thymus species volatiles: chemical composition and biological activities. *Curr Pharm Des.* 2008;14(29):3120-40.

[6424] Faleiro L, Miguel G, Gomes S, et al. Antibacterial and antioxidant activities of essential oils isolated from Thymbra capitata L. (Cav.) andOriganum vulgare L. *J Agric Food Chem.* 2005 Oct 19;53(21):8162-8.

[6425] Benbelaïd F, Khadir A, Abdoune MA, et al. Antimicrobial activity of some essential oils against oral multidrug-resistant Enterococcus faecalis in both planktonic and biofilm state. *Asian Pac J Trop Biomed.* 2014 Jun;4(6):463-72.

[6426] Maissa BJ, Walid H. Antifungal activity of chemically different essential oils from wild Tunisian Thymus spp. *Nat Prod Res.* 2015;29(9):869-73.

[6427] Palmeira-de-Oliveira A, Gaspar C, Palmeira-de-Oliveira R, et al. The anti-Candida activity of Thymbra capitata essential oil: effect upon pre-formed biofilm. *J Ethnopharmacol.* 2012 Mar 27;140(2):379-83.

[6428] Bona E, Cantamessa S, Pavan M, et al. Sensitivity of Candida albicans to essential oils: are they an alternative to antifungal agents? *J Appl Microbiol.* 2016 Dec;121(6):1530-1545.

[6429] Figueiredo AC, Barroso JG, Pedro LG, et al. Portuguese Thymbra and Thymus species volatiles: chemical composition and biological activities. *Curr Pharm Des.* 2008;14(29):3120-40.

[6430] Salgueiro LR, Pinto E, Gonçalves MJ, et al. Chemical composition and antifungal activity of the essential oil of Thymbra capitata. *Planta Med.* 2004 Jun;70(6):572-5.

[6431] Machado M, Dinis AM, Salgueiro L, et al. Anti-Giardia activity of phenolic-rich essential oils: effects of Thymbra capitata, Origanum virens, Thymus zygis subsp. sylvestris, and Lippia graveolens on trophozoites growth, viability, adherence, and ultrastructure. *Parasitol Res.* 2010 Apr;106(5):1205-15.

[6432] Machado M, Sousa Mdo C, Salgueiro L, et al. Effects of essential oils on the growth of Giardia lamblia trophozoites. *Nat Prod Commun.* 2010 Jan;5(1):137-41.

[6433] Džamić AM, Nikolić BJ, Giweli AA, et al. Libyan Thymus capitatus essential oil: antioxidant, antimicrobial, cytotoxic and colon pathogen adhesion-inhibition properties. *J Appl Microbiol.* 2015 Aug;119(2):389-99.

[6434] Miguel MG, Gago C, Antunes MD, et al. Antioxidant and Antiproliferative Activities of the Essential Oils from Thymbra capitata and Thymus Species Grown in Portugal. *Evid Based Complement Alternat Med.* 2015;2015:851721.

[6435] Hortigón-Vinagre MP, Blanco J, Ruiz T, et al. Thymbra capitata essential oil prevents cell death induced by 4-hydroxy-2-nonenal in neonatal rat cardiac myocytes. *Planta Med.* 2014 Oct;80(15):1284-90.

[6436] Salama MM, Taher EE, El-Bahy MM. Molluscicidal and Mosquitocidal activities of the essential oils of Thymus capitatus Hoff. et Link. and Marrubium vulgare L. *Rev Inst Med Trop Sao Paulo.* 2012 Sep-Oct;54(5):281-6.

[6437] Salama MM, Taher EE, El-Bahy MM. Molluscicidal and Mosquitocidal activities of the essential oils of Thymus capitatus Hoff. et Link. and Marrubium vulgare L. *Rev Inst Med Trop Sao Paulo.* 2012 Sep-Oct;54(5):281-6.

[6438] Barbosa P, Lima AS, Vieira P, et al. Nematicidal activity of essential oils and volatiles derived from Portuguese aromatic flora against the pinewood nematode, Bursaphelenchus xylophilus. *J Nematol.* 2010 Mar;42(1):8-16.

[6439] Hortigón-Vinagre MP, Blanco J, Ruiz T, et al. Thymbra capitata essential oil prevents cell death induced by 4-hydroxy-2-nonenal in neonatal rat cardiac myocytes. *Planta Med.* 2014 Oct;80(15):1284-90.

[6440] Harmati M, Gyukity-Sebestyen E, Dobra G, et al. Binary mixture of Satureja hortensis and Origanum vulgare subsp. hirtum essential oils: in vivo therapeutic efficiency against Helicobacter pylori infection. *Helicobacter.* 2017 Apr;22(2).

[6441] Cwikla C, Schmidt K, Matthias A, et al. Investigation into the antibacterial activities of phytotherapeutics against Helicobacter pylori and Campylobacter jejuni. *Phytother Res.* 2010 May;24(5):649-56.

[6442] Carrasco A, Perez E, Cutillas AB, et al. Origanum vulgare and Thymbra capitata Essential Oils from Spain: Determination of Aromatic Profile and Bioactivities. *Nat Prod Commun.* 2016 Jan;11(1):113-20.

[6443] Barreto TA, Andrade SC, Maciel JF, et al. A Chitosan Coating Containing Essential Oil from Origanum vulgare L. to Control Postharvest Mold Infections and Keep the Quality of Cherry Tomato Fruit. *Front Microbiol.* 2016 Nov 8;7:1724.

[6444] Kraśniewska K, Gniewosz M, Kosakowska O, et al. Preservation of Brussels Sprouts by Pullulan Coating Containing Oregano Essential Oil. *J Food Prot.* 2016 Mar;79(3):493-500.

[6445] Ozdikmenli S, Demirel Zorba NN. Evaluation of usage of essential oils instead of spices in meat ball formulation for controlling Salmonella spp. *Food Sci Technol Int.* 2016 Mar;22(2):93-101.

[6446] Karaman M, Bogavac M, Radovanović B, et al. Origanum vulgare essential oil affects pathogens causing vaginal infections. *J Appl Microbiol.* 2017 May;122(5):1177-1185.

[6447] Sharififard M, Safdari F, Siahpoush A, et al. Evaluation of Some Plant Essential Oils against the Brown-Banded Cockroach, Supella longipalpa (Blattaria: Ectobiidae): A Mechanical Vector of Human Pathogens. *J Arthropod Borne Dis.* 2016 Oct 4;10(4):528-537.

[6448] Gonçalves JC, de Meneses DA, de Vasconcelos AP, et al. Essential oil composition and antinociceptive activity of Thymus capitatus. *Pharm Biol.* 2017 Dec;55(1):782-786.

[6449] de Souza Silveira Valente J, de Oliveira da Silva Fonseca A, Denardi LB, et al. In Vitro Susceptibility of Pythium insidiosum to Melaleuca alternifolia, Mentha piperita and Origanum vulgare Essential Oils Combinations. *Mycopathologia.* 2016 Aug;181(7-8):617-22.

[6450] Sarikurkcu C, Zengin G, Oskay M, et al. Composition, antioxidant, antimicrobial and enzyme inhibition activities of two Origanum vulgare subspecies (subsp. vulgare and subsp. hirtum) essential oils. *Ind Crop Prod.* 2015;70:178-84.

[6451] Capatina L, Napoli EM, Ruberto G, et al. Origanum vulgare ssp. hirtum (Lamiaceae) Essential Oil Prevents Behavioral and Oxidative Stress Changes in the Scopolamine Zebrafish Model. *Molecules.* 2021;26:7085.

[6452] Turchi B, Mancini S, Pistelli L, et al. Sub-inhibitory stress with essential oil affects enterotoxins production and essential oil susceptibility in Staphylococcus aureus. *Nat Prod Res.* 2017 Jun 8:1-7.

[6453] Szczepanik M, Walczak M, Zawitowska B, et al. Chemical composition, antimicrobial and insecticidal activity against the lesser mealworm Alphitobius diaperinus (Panzer) (Coleoptera: Tenebrionidae) of Origanum vulgare L. ssp. hirtum (Link) and Artemisia dracunculus L. essential oils. *J Sci Food Agric.* 2018 Jan;98(2):767-774.

[6454] Ballester-Costa C, Sendra E, Fernández-López J, et al. Assessment of Antioxidant and Antibacterial Properties on Meat Homogenates of Essential Oils Obtained from Four Thymus Species Achieved from Organic Growth. *Foods.* 2017 Jul 28;6(8).

[6455] Ashraf SA, Al-Shammari E, Hussain T, et al. In-vitro antimicrobial activity and identification of bioactive components using GC-MS of commercially available essential oils in Saudi Arabia. *J Food Sci Technol.* 2017 Nov;54(12):3948-3958.

[6456] Saoudi S, Sifaoui I, Chammem N, et al. Anti-Acanthamoeba activity of Tunisian Thymus capitatus essential oil and organic extracts. *Exp Parasitol.* 2017 Dec;183:231-235.

[6457] Kaskatepe B, Yildiz SS, Kiymaci ME, et al. Chemical composition and antimicrobial activity of the commercial Origanum onites L. oil against nosocomial carbapenem resistant extended spectrum beta lactamase producer Escherichia coli isolates. *Acta Biol Hung.* 2017 Dec;68(4):466-476.

[6458] Grzesiak B, Kołodziej B, Głowacka A, et al. The Effect of Some Natural Essential Oils Against Bovine Mastitis Caused by Prototheca zopfii Isolates In Vitro. *Mycopathologia.* 2018 Jun;183(3):541-550.

[6459] Pellegrini M, Ricci A, Serio A, et al. Characterization of Essential Oils Obtained from Abruzzo Autochthonous Plants: Antioxidant and Antimicrobial Activities Assessment for Food Application. *Foods.* 2018 Feb 2;7(2).

[6460] Han X, Parker TL. Anti-inflammatory, tissue remodeling, immunomodulatory, and anticancer activities of oregano (Origanum vulgare) essential oil in a human skin disease model. *Biochim Open.* 2017 Mar 3;4:73-77.

[6461] Pradebon Brondani L, Alves da Silva Neto T, Antonio Freitag R, et al. Evaluation of anti-enzyme properties of Origanum vulgare essential oil against oral Candida albicans. *J Mycol Med.* 2018 Mar;28(1):94-100.

[6462] Tardugno R, Pellati F1, Iseppi R, et al. Phytochemical composition and in vitro screening of the antimicrobial activity of essential oils on oral pathogenic bacteria. *Nat Prod Res.* 2018 Mar;32(5):544-551.

[6463] Scalas D, Mandras N, Roana J, et al. Use of Pinus sylvestris L. (Pinaceae), Origanum vulgare L. (Lamiaceae), and Thymus vulgaris L. (Lamiaceae) essential oils and their main components to enhance itraconazole activity against azole susceptible/not-susceptible Cryptococcus neoformans strains. *BMC Complement Altern Med.* 2018; 18: 143.

[6464] Bartoňková I, Dvořák Z. Essential oils of culinary herbs and spices display agonist and antagonist activities at human aryl hydrocarbon receptor AhR. *Food Chem Toxicol.* 2018 Jan;111:374-384.

[6465] Vinciguerra V, Rojas F, Tedesco V, et al. Chemical characterization and antifungal activity of Origanum vulgare, Thymus vulgaris essential oils and carvacrol against Malassezia furfur. *Nat Prod Res.* 2018 May 4:1-5.

[6466] Solarte AL, Astorga RJ, Aguiar F, et al. Combination of Antimicrobials and Essential Oils as an Alternative for the Control of Salmonella enterica Multiresistant Strains Related to Foodborne Disease. *Foodborne Pathog Dis.* 2017 Oct;14(10):558-563.

[6467] Schlösser I, Prange A. Antifungal activity of selected natural preservatives against the foodborne molds Penicillium verrucosum and Aspergillus westerdijkiae. *FEMS Microbiol Lett.* 2018 Jul 1;365(13).

[6468] Imtara H, Elamine Y, Lyoussi B, et al. Honey Antibacterial Effect Boosting Using Origanum vulgare L. Essential Oil. *Evid Based Complement Alternat Med.* 2018 Mar 15;2018:7842583.

[6469] Elshafie HS, Armentano MF, Carmosino M, et al. Cytotoxic Activity of Origanum Vulgare L. on Hepatocellular Carcinoma cell Line HepG2 and Evaluation of its Biological Activity. *Molecules.* 2017 Aug 30;22(9).

[6470] Ebani VV, Nardoni S, Bertelloni F, et al. Antimicrobial Activity of Five Essential Oils against Bacteria and Fungi Responsible for Urinary Tract Infections. *Molecules.* 2018 Jul 9;23(7).

[6471] Elansary HO, Abdelgaleil SAM, Mahmoud EA, et al. Effective antioxidant, antimicrobial and anticancer activities of essential oils of horticultural aromatic crops in northern Egypt. *BMC Complement Altern Med.* 2018 Jul 13;18(1):214.

[6472] Taleb MH, Abdeltawab NF, Shamma RN, et al. Origanum vulgare L. Essential Oil as a Potential Anti-Acne Topical Nanoemulsion-In Vitro and In Vivo Study. *Molecules.* 2018 Aug 28;23(9).

[6473] Giatropoulos A, Kimbaris A, Michaelakis A, et al. Chemical composition and assessment of larvicidal and repellent capacity of 14 Lamiaceae essential oils against Aedes albopictus. *Parasitol Res.* 2018 Jun;117(6):1953-1964.

[6474] Wijesundara NM, Rupasinghe HPV. Essential oils from Origanum vulgare and Salvia officinalis exhibit antibacterial and antibiofilm activities against Streptococcus pyogenes. *Microb Pathog*. 2018 Apr;117:118-127.

[6475] Gómez JV, Tarazona A, Mateo-Castro R, et al. Selected plant essential oils and their main active components, a promising approach to inhibit aflatoxigenic fungi and aflatoxin production in food. *Food Addit Contam Part A Chem Anal Control Expo Risk Assess*. 2018 Aug;35(8):1581-1595.

[6476] El Khoury R, Michael Jubeli R, El Beyrouthy M, et al. Phytochemical screening and antityrosinase activity of carvacrol, thymoquinone, and four essential oils of Lebanese plants. *J Cosmet Dermatol*. 2019 Jun;18(3):944-952.

[6477] Balusamy SR, Perumalsamy H, Huq MA, et al. Anti-proliferative activity of Origanum vulgare inhibited lipogenesis and induced mitochondrial mediated apoptosis in human stomach cancer cell lines. *Biomed Pharmacother*. 2018 Oct 18;108:1835-1844.

[6478] Toujani MM, Rittà M, Civra A, et al. Inhibition of HSV-2 infection by pure compounds from Thymus capitatus extract in vitro. *Phytother Res*. 2018 Aug;32(8):1555-1563.

[6479] Massa N, Cantamessa S, Novello G, et al. Antifungal activity of essential oils against azole-resistant and azole-susceptible vaginal Candida glabrata strains. *Can J Microbiol*. 2018 Oct;64(10):647-663.

[6480] Sharifi A, Ahmadi A, Mohammadzadeh A, et al. Streptococcus pneumoniae quorum sensing and biofilm formation are affected by Thymus daenensis, Satureja hortensis, and Origanum vulgare essential oils. *Acta Microbiol Immunol Hung*. 2018 Aug 1;65(3):345-359.

[6481] Solarte AL, Astorga RJ, de Aguiar FC, et al. Susceptibility Distribution to Essential Oils of Salmonella enterica Strains Involved in Animal and Public Health and Comparison of the Typhimurium and Enteritidis Serotypes. *J Med Food*. 2018 Sep;21(9):946-950.

[6482] Muchembled J, Deweer C, Sahmer K, et al. Gene expression responses of Listeria monocytogenes Scott A exposed to sub-lethal concentrations of natural antimicrobials. *Environ Sci Pollut Res Int*. 2018 Oct;25(30):29921-29928.

[6483] Teles AM, Rosa TDDS, Mouchrek AN, et al. Cinnamomum zeylanicum, Origanum vulgare, and Curcuma longa Essential Oils: Chemical Composition, Antimicrobial and Antileishmanial Activity. *Evid Based Complement Alternat Med*. 2019 Jan 15;2019:2421695.

[6484] Sharififard M, Alizadeh I, Jahanifard E, et al. Chemical Composition and Repellency of Origanum vulgare Essential Oil against Cimex lectularius under Laboratory Conditions. *J Arthropod Borne Dis*. 2018 Dec 25;12(4):387-397.

[6485] Fikry S, Khalil N, Salama O. Chemical profiling, biostatic and biocidal dynamics of Origanum vulgare L. essential oil. *AMB Express*. 2019 Mar 26;9(1):41.

[6486] Hizem A, Lundström-Stadelmann B, M'rad S, et al. Activity of Thymus capitatus essential oil components against in vitro cultured Echinococcus multilocularis metacestodes and germinal layer cells. *Parasitology*. 2019 Jun;146(7):956-967.

[6487] Čabarkapa I, Čolović R, Đuragić O, et al. Antibiofilm activities of essential oils rich in carvacrol and thymol against Salmonella Enteritidis. *Biofouling*. 2019 Mar;35(3):361-375.

[6488] Helal IM, El-Bessoumy A, Al-Bataineh E, et al. Antimicrobial Efficiency of Essential Oils from Traditional Medicinal Plants of Asir Region, Saudi Arabia, over Drug Resistant Isolates. *Biomed Res Int*. 2019 Jan 17;2019:8928306.

[6489] Ribes S, Fuentes A, Barat JM, et al. Effect of oregano (Origanum vulgare L. ssp. hirtum) and clove (Eugenia spp.) nanoemulsions on Zygosaccharomyces bailii survival in salad dressings. *Food Chem*. 2019 Oct 15;295:630-636.

[6490] Xie Y, Huang Q, Rao Y, et al. Efficacy of Origanum vulgare essential oil and carvacrol against the housefly, Musca domestica L. (Diptera: Muscidae). *Environ Sci Pollut Res Int*. 2019 Aug;26(23):23824-23831.

[6491] Qneibi M, Jaradat N, Hawash M, et al. The Neuroprotective Role of Origanum syriacum L. and Lavandula dentata L. Essential Oils through Their Effects on AMPA Receptors. *Biomed Res Int*. 2019 Mar 11;2019:5640173.

[6492] Spyridopoulou K, Fitsiou E, Bouloukosta E, et al. Extraction, Chemical Composition, and Anticancer Potential of Origanum onites L. Essential Oil. *Molecules*. 2019 Jul 18;24(14).

[6493] López V, Pavela R, Gómez-Rincón C, et al. Efficacy of Origanum syriacum Essential Oil against the Mosquito Vector Culex quinquefasciatus and the Gastrointestinal Parasite Anisakis simplex, with Insights on Acetylcholinesterase Inhibition. *Molecules*. 2019 Jul 15;24(14).

[6494] Lofa A, Velasco V, Gerding M, et al. Antibiotic-resistant Staphylococcus aureus strains of swine origin: molecular typing and susceptibility to oregano (Origanum vulgare L.) essential oil and maqui (Aristotelia chilensis (Molina) Stuntz) extract. *J Appl Microbiol*. 2019 Oct;127(4):1048-1056

[6495] Vasconcelos NG, Croda J, Silva KE, et al. Origanum vulgare L. essential oil inhibits the growth of carbapenem-resistant gram-negative bacteria. *Rev Soc Bras Med Trop*. 2019 Jun 27;52:e20180502.

[6496] Boskovic M, Glisic M, Djordjevic J, et al. Antioxidative Activity of Thyme (Thymus vulgaris) and Oregano (Origanum vulgare) Essential Oils and Their Effect on Oxidative Stability of Minced Pork Packaged Under Vacuum and Modified Atmosphere. *J Food Sci*. 2019 Sep;84(9):2467-2474.

[6497] Uzair B, Niaz N, Bano A, et al. Essential oils showing in vitro anti MRSA and synergistic activity with penicillin group of antibiotics. *Pak J Pharm Sci*. 2017 Sep;30(5(Supplementary)):1997-2002.

[6498] Khan M, Khan ST, Khan M, et al. Chemical diversity in leaf and stem essential oils of Origanum vulgare L. and their effects on microbicidal activities. *AMB Express*. 2019 Oct 31;9(1):176.

[6499] Bonde JP, Giwercman A, Ernst E. Review Identifying environmental risk to male reproductive function by occupational sperm studies: logistics and design options. *Occup Environ Med*. 1996 Aug; 53(8):511-9.

[6500] Mbaye MM, Khalifi BE, Addoum B, et al. The Effect of Supplementation with Some Essential Oils on the Mobility and the Vitality of Human Sperm. *ScientificWorldJournal*. 2019;2019:4878912.

[6501] Kozics K, Buckova M, Puskarova A, et al. The Effect of Ten Essential Oils on Several Cutaneous Drug-Resistant Microorganisms and Their Cyto/Genotoxic and Antioxidant Properties. Molecules. 2019 Dec 13;24(24):24244570.

[6502] Ma X, Shi W, Zhang Y. Essential Oils with High Activity against Stationary Phase Bartonella henselae. Antibiotics (Basel). 2019 Nov 30;8(4):8040246.

[6503] El Khoury R, Michael-Jubeli R, Bakar J, et al. Origanum Essential Oils Reduce the Level of Melanin in B16-F1 Melanocytes. Eur J Dermatol. 2019 Dec;29(6):596-602.

[6504] Tasdemir D, Kaiser M, Demirci B, et al. Antiprotozoal Activity of Turkish Origanum onites Essential Oil and Its Components. Molecules. 2019 Dec;24(23):24234421.

[6505] Zairi A, Nouir S, Zarrouk A, et al. Chemical Composition, Fatty Acids Profile and Biological Properties of Thymus Capitatus (L.) Hoffmanns, Essential Oil. Sci Rep. 2019 Dec 27;9(1):20134.

[6506] Yan G, Zhu BR, Tian FL, et al. Inhibitory Activity of Plant Essential Oils Against E. coli 1-Deoxy-d-xylulose-5-phosphate Reductoisomerase. *Molecules*. 2019 Jul;24(14):24142518.

[6507] Arantes SM. Picarra A, Guerreiro M, et al. Toxicological and Pharmacological Properties of Essential Oils of Calamintha Nepeta, Origanum Virens and Thymus Mastichina of Alentejo (Portugal). *Food Chem Toxicol*. 2019 Nov;133:110747.

[6508] Xao S, Cui P, Shi W, et al. Identification of Essential Oils With Strong Activity Against Stationary Phase Uropathogenic Escherichia Coli. Discov Med. 2019 Oct;28(154):179-188.

[6509] Cho Y, Kim H, Beuchart LR, et al. Synergistic Activities of Gaseous Oregano and Thyme Thymol Essential Oils Against Listeria Monocytogenes on Surfaces of a Laboratory Medium and Radish Sprouts. *Food Microbiol*. 2020 Apr;86:103357.

[6510] Korona-Glowniak I, Glowniak-Lipa A, Ludwiczuk A, et al. The In Vitro Activity of Essential Oils Against Helicobacter Pylori Growth and Urease Activity. *Molecules*. 2020 Jan 29;25(3):586.

[6511] Laothaweerungsawat N, Sirithunyalug J, Chaiyana W, et al. Chemical Compositions and Anti-Skin-Ageing Activities of Origanum vulgare L. Essential Oil From Tropical and Mediterranean Region. *Molecules*. 2020 Mar 1;25(5).

[6512] Xiao S, Cui P, Shi W, et al. Identification of essential oils with activity against stationary phase Staphylococcus aureus. *BMC Complement Med Ther*. 2020 Mar 24;20(1):99.

[6513] Akkaoui S, Johansson A, Yagoubi M, et al. Chemical Composition, Antimicrobial activity, in Vitro Cytotoxicity and Leukotoxin Neutralization of Essential Oil from Origanum vulgare against Aggregatibacter actinomycetemcomitans. *Pathogens*. 2020 Mar 5;9(3).

[6514] Gong X, Ren Y. Larvicidal and ovicidal activity of carvacrol, p-cymene, and γ-terpinene from Origanum vulgare essential oil against the cotton bollworm, Helicoverpa armigera (Hübner). *Environ Sci Pollut Res Int*. 2020 Mar 23. [Epub ahead of print]

[6515] Moumni S, Elaissi A, Trabelsi A, et al. Correlation between chemical composition and antibacterial activity of some Lamiaceae species essential oils from Tunisia. *BMC Complement Med Ther*. 2020 Apr 3;20(1):103.

[6516] Jan S, Rashid M, Abd Allah EF, et al. Biological Efficacy of Essential Oils and Plant Extracts of Cultivated and Wild Ecotypes of Origanum vulgare L. *Biomed Res Int*. 2020 Apr 6;2020:8751718.

[6517] Kozics K, Buckova M, Puskarova A, et al. The Effect of Ten Essential Oils on Several Cutaneous Drug-Resistant Microorganisms and Their Cyto/Genotoxic and Antioxidant Properties. *Molecules*. 2019 Dec 13;24(24):4570.

[6518] Mbaye MM, Khalfi BE, Ouzamode S, et al. Effect of Origanum vulgare Essential Oil Supplementation on the Advanced Parameters of Mobility and on the Integrity of Human Sperm DNA. *Int J Reprod Med*. 2020 May 13;2020:1230274.

[6519] Anastasiou TI, Mandalakis M, Krigas N, et al. Comparative Evaluation of Essential Oils from Medicinal-Aromatic Plants of Greece: Chemical Composition, Antioxidant Capacity and Antimicrobial Activity against Bacterial Fish Pathogens. *Molecules*. 2020 Jan;25(1):148.

[6520] Avola R, Granata G, Geraci C, et al. Oregano (Origanum vulgare L.) essential oil provides anti-inflammatory activity and facilitates wound healing in a human keratinocytes cell model. *Food Chem Toxicol*. 2020 Jul 14;111586.

[6521] Khoury RE, Michael-Jubelo R, Bakar J, et al. Origanum essential oils reduce the level of melanin in B16-F1 melanocytes. *Eur J Dermatol*. 2019 Dec 1;29(6):596-602.

[6522] Shamseddine L, Chidian JJ. Composition's effect of Origanum Syriacum essential oils in the antimicrobial activities for the treatment of denture stomatitis. *Odontology*. 2020 Aug 17;1-9.

[6523] Liu M, Luo F, Qing Z, et al. Chemical Composition and Bioactivity of Essential Oil of Ten Labiatae Species. *Molecules*. 2020 Oct 21;25(20):4862.

[6524] Simirgiotis MJ, Burton D, Parra F, et al. Antioxidant and Antibacterial Capacities of Origanum vulgare L. Essential Oil from the Arid Andean Region of Chile and its Chemical Characterization by GC-MS. *Metabolites*. 2020 Oct 16;10(10):414.

[6525] Acimovic M, Zoric M, Zheljazkov VD, et al. Chemical Characterization and Antibacterial Activity of Essential Oil of Medicinal Plants from Eastern Serbia. *Molecules*. 2020 Nov 23;25(22):5482.

[6526] Amaral SC, Pruski BB, de Freitas SB, et al. Origanum vulgare essential oil: antibacterial activities and synergistic effect with polymyxin B against multidrug-resistant Acinetobacter baumannii. *Mol Biol Rep*. Online ahead of print.

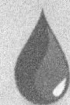

6527 Asensio CM, Quiroga PR, Al-Gburi A, et al. Rheological Behavior, Antimicrobial and Quorum Sensig Inhibition Study of an Argentinean Oregano Essential Oil Nanoemulsion. *Front Nutr.* 2020 Oct 9;7:569913.
6528 Grul'ova D, Pl'uchtova M, Fejer J, et al. Influence of six essential oils on invasive Solidago canadensis L. seed germination. *Nat Prod Res.* 2020 Nov;34(22):3231-3233.
6529 Bedini S, Farina P, Napoli E, et al. Bioactivity of Different Chemotypes of Oregano Essential Oil against the Blowfly Calliphora vomitoria Vector of Foodborne Pathogens. *Insects.* 2021 Jan 11;12(1):52.
6530 Ghitea TC, El-Kharoubi A, Ganea M, et al. The Antimicrobial Activity of Origanum vulgare L. Correlated with the Gastrointestinal Perturbation in Patients with Metabolic Syndrome. *Molecules.* 2021 Jan 8;26(2):283.
6531 Imtara H, Al-Waili N, Aboulghazi A, et al. Chemical composition and antioxidant content of Thymus vulgaris honey and Origanum vulgare essential oil; their effect on carbon tetrachloride-induced toxicity. *Vet World.* 2021 Jan;14(1):292-301.
6532 Kakhki MT, Sedaghat N, Mohsenzadeh M. Chemical composition, antioxidative, antibacterial, and time-kill activities of some selected plant essential oils against foodborne pathogenic and spoilage organisms. *Vet Res Forum.* Fall 2020;11(4):339-346.
6533 Netopilova M, Houdkova M, Urbanova K, et al. Validation of Qualitative Broth Volatilization Checkerboard Method for Testing of Essential Oils: Dual-Column GC-FID/MS Analysis and In Vitro Combinatory Antimicrobial Effect of Origanum vulgare and Thymus vulgaris against Staphylococcus aureus in Liquid and Vapor Phases. *Plants (Basel).* 2021 Feb 18;10(2):393.
6534 Kosakowska O, Wglarz Z, Pioro-Jabrucka E, et al. Antioxidant and Antibacterial Activity of Essential Oils and Hydroethanolic Extracts of Greek Oregano ( O. vulgare L. subsp. hirtum (Link) Ietswaart) and Common Oregano ( O. vulgare L. subsp. vulgare). *Molecules.* 2021 Feb 13;26(4):988.
6535 Vanti G, Tomou EM, Stojovic D, et al. Nanovesicles Loaded with Origanum onites and Satureja thymbra Essential Oils and Their Activity against Food-Borne Pathogens and Spoilage Microorganisms. *Molecules.* 2021 Apr 7;26(8):2124.
6536 Hacioglu M, Oyardi O, Kirinti A. Oregano essential oil inhibits Candida spp. biofilms. *Z Naturforsch C J Biosci.* 2021 Apr 29.
6537 Pusceddu M, Floris I, Mangia NP, et al. In Vitro Activity of Several Essential Oils Extracted from Aromatic Plants against Ascosphaera apis. *Vet Sci.* 2021 May 10;8(5):80.
6538 Benameur Q, Gervasi T, Pellizzeri V, et al. Comparison of sensitivity to a commercial Origanum vulgare essential oil between extended-spectrum β-lactamases (ESBL-) and non-ESBL-producing Enterobacteriaceae isolates. *Nat Prod Res.* 2021 Jun 14;1-6.
6539 Zhao Y, Yang YH, Ye M, et al. Chemical composition and antifungal activity of essential oil from Origanum vulgare against Botrytis cinerea. *Food Chem.* 2021 Jul 1;365:130506.
6540 Proškovcová M, Čonková E, Váczi P, et al. Antibiofilm activity of selected plant essential oils from the Lamiaceae family against Candida albicans clinical isolates. *Ann Agric Environ Med.* 2021 Jun 14;28(2):260-266.
6541 Qiao Y, Yu Z, Bai L, et al. Chemical composition of essential oils from Thymus mongolicus, Cinnamomum verum, and Origanum vulgare and their acaricidal effects on Haemaphysalis longicornis (Acari: Ixodidae). *Ecotoxicol Environ Saf.* 2021 Aug 17;224:112672.
6542 Maral H, Ulupinar S, Baydir AT, et al. Effect of Origanum dubium, Origanum vulgare subsp. hirtum, and Lavandula angustifolia essential oils on lipid profiles and liver biomarkers in athletes. *Z Naturforsch C J Biosci.* 2021 Sep 9. Online ahead of print.
6543 Harčárová M, Čonková E, Proškovcová M, et al. Comparison of antifungal activity of selected essential oils against Fusarium graminearum in vitro. *Ann Agric Environ Med.* 2021 Sep 16;28(3):414-418.
6544 Pasias IN, Ntakoulas DD, Raptopoulou K, et al. Chemical Composition of Essential Oils of Aromatic and Medicinal Herbs Cultivated in Greece-Benefits and Drawbacks. *Foods.* 2021 Oct 3;10(10):2354.
6545 Plata-Rueda A, Zanuncio JC, Serrao JE, et al. Origanum vulgare Essential Oil against Tenebrio molitor (Coleoptera: Tenebrionidae): Composition, Insecticidal Activity, and Behavioral Response. *Plants (Basel).* 2021 Nov 19;10(11):2513.
6546 Hao Y, Li J, Shi L. A Carvacrol-Rich Essential Oil Extracted From Oregano (Origanum vulgare "Hot & Spicy") Exerts Potent Antibacterial Effects Against Staphylococcus aureus. *Front Microbiol.* 2021 Nov 5;12:741861.
6547 Silva ECAD, Leuthier LL, Almeida Júnior A, et al. Physicochemical characteristics and antimicrobial activity of Origanum vulgare L. essential oil and carvacrol on cariogenic bacteria: an in vitro and in silico study. *Nat Prod Res.* 2022 Jan 30;1-4.
6548 D'Aquila P, Paparazzo E, Crudo M, et al. Antibacterial Activity and Epigenetic Remodeling of Essential Oils from Calabrian Aromatic Plants. *Nutrients.* 2022 Jan 17;14(2):391.
6549 Mekkaoui M, Assaggaf H, Qasem A, et al. Ethnopharmacological Survey and Comparative Study of the Healing Activity of Moroccan Thyme Honey and Its Mixture with Selected Essential Oils on Two Types of Wounds on Albino Rabbits. *Foods.* 2021 Dec 23;11(1):28.
6550 Rodriguez Diaz C, Mith H, Bernard T, et al. In vitro study of antimicrobial activity of essential oils and their components against the main Clostridioides difficile PCR-ribotypes isolated in Belgium. *IAFP Eur Congress.* 2021.
6551 Štrbac F, Bosco A, Maurelli MP, et al. Anthelmintic Properties of Essential Oils to Control Gastrointestinal Nematodes in Sheep-In Vitro and In Vivo Studies. *Vet Sci.* 2022 Feb 19;9(2):93.
6552 Cid-Chevecich C, Müller-Sepúlveda A, Jara JA, et al. Origanum vulgare L. essential oil inhibits virulence patterns of Candida spp. and potentiates the effects of fluconazole and nystatin in vitro. *BMC Complement Med Ther.* 2022 Feb 9;22(1):39.
6553 Aykac A, Teralı K, Özbeyli D, et al. A multi-parameter evaluation of the neuroprotective and cognitive-enhancing effects of Origanum onites L. (Turkish Oregano) essential oil on scopolamine-induced amnestic rats. *Metab Brain Dis.* 2022 Feb 24. Online ahead of print.
6554 Nakamura A, Kawahara A, Takahashi H, et al. Comparison between the Antimicrobial Activity of Essential Oils and Their Components in the Vapor Phase against Food-related Bacteria. *J Oleo Sci.* 2022;71(3):411-417.
6555 Altun M, Yapici BM. Determination of chemical compositions and antibacterial effects of selected essential oils against human pathogenic strains. *An Acad Bras Cienc.* 2022 Mar 11;94(1):e20210074.
6556 Moghrovyan A, Parseghyan L, Sevoyan G, et al. Antinociceptive, anti-inflammatory, and cytotoxic properties of Origanum vulgare essential oil, rich with β-caryophyllene and β-caryophyllene oxide. *Korean J Pain.* 2022 Apr 1;35(2):140-151.
6557 Dos Santos LR, Alía A, Martin I, et al. Antimicrobial activity of essential oils and natural plant extracts against Listeria monocytogenes in a dry-cured ham-based model. *J Sci Food Agric.* 2021 Aug 11. Online ahead of print.
6558 Aouadhi C, Jouini A, Mechichi D, et al. Characterization of Primary Action Mode of Eight Essential Oils and Evaluation of Their Antibacterial Effect against Extended-Spectrum β-Lactamase (ESBL)-Producing Escherichia coli Inoculated in Turkey Meat. *Molecules.* 2022 Apr 18;27(8):2588.
6559 Benoutman A, Erbiai EH, Edderdaki FZ, et al. Phytochemical Composition, Antioxidant and Antifungal Activity of Thymus capitatus, a Medicinal Plant Collected from Northern Morocco. *Antibiotics (Basel).* 2022 May 18;11(5):681.
6560 Man A, Mare AD, Mares M, et al. Antifungal and anti-virulence activity of six essential oils against important Candida species - a preliminary study. *Future Microbiol.* 2022 Jul;17:737-753.
6561 Perumalsamy H, Shanmugam R, Kim JR, et al. Nanoemulsion and Encapsulation Strategy of Hydrophobic Oregano Essential Oil Increased Human Prostate Cancer Cell Death via Apoptosis by Attenuating Lipid Metabolism. *Bioinorg Chem Appl.* 2022 May 26;2022:9569226.
6562 Chen WN, Chin KW, Tang KS, et al. Neuroprotective, Neurite Enhancing and Cholinesterase Inhibitory Effects of Lamiaceae Family Essential Oils in Alzheimer's Disease Model. HERMED-D-22-00403. Available at: https://ssrn.com/abstract=4112137 or http://dx.doi.org/10.2139/ssrn.4112137.
6563 Kryeziu TL, Haloci E, Loshaj-Shala A, et al. Nanoencapsulation of Origanum vulgare essential oil into liposomes with anticancer potential. *Pharmazie.* 2022 Jun 1;77(6):172-178.
6564 Aboelhadid SM, Abdel-Tawab H, Mahran HA, et al. Synergistic larvicidal and repellent effects of essential oils of three Origanum species on Rhipicephalus annulatus tick. *Exp Appl Acarol.* 2022 Jul;87(2-3):273-287.
6565 Ziyadi S, Iddar A, Errafiy N, et al. Protective Effect of Some Essential Oils Against Gamma-Radiation Damages in Tetrahymena pyriformis Exposed to Cobalt-60 Source. *Curr Microbiol.* 2022 Aug 3;79(9):279.
6566 Assouguem A, Kara M, Ramzi A, et al. Evaluation of the Effect of Four Bioactive Compounds in Combination with Chemical Product against Two Spider Mites Tetranychus urticae and Eutetranychus orientalis(Acari: Tetranychidae). *Evid Based Complement Alternat Med.* 2022 Aug 22;2022:2004623.
6567 Merghni A, Haddaji N, Bouali N, et al. Comparative Study of Antibacterial, Antibiofilm, Antiswarming and Antiquorum Sensing Activities of Origanum vulgare Essential Oil and Terpinene-4-ol against Pathogenic Bacteria. *Life (Basel).* 2022 Oct 17;12(10):1616.
6568 Iqbal S, Khan FA, Haris A, et al. Essential oils of four wild plants inhibit the blood seeking behaviour of female Aedes aegytpi. *Exp Parasitol.* 2022 Nov 12;244:108424.
6569 Sidiropoulou E, Marugán-Hernández V, Skoufos I, et al. In Vitro Antioxidant, Antimicrobial, Anticoccidial, and Anti-Inflammatory Study of Essential Oils of Oregano, Thyme, and Sage from Epirus, Greece. *Life (Basel).* 2022 Nov 4;12(11):1783.
6570 Bora L, Burkard T, Juan MHS, et al. Phytochemical Characterization and Biological Evaluation of Origanum vulgare L. Essential Oil Formulated as Polymeric Micelles Drug Delivery Systems. *Pharmaceutics.* 2022 Nov 8;14(11):2413.
6571 Mollea C, Bosco F, Fissore D. Agar Plate Methods for Assessing the Antibacterial Activity of Thyme and Oregano Essential Oils against S. epidermidis and E. coli. *Antibiotics (Basel).* 2022 Dec 13;11(12):1809.
6572 Susurluk H. Potential use of essential oils from Origanum vulgare and Syzygium aromaticum to control Tetranychus urticae Koch (Acari: Tetranychidae) on two host plant species. *PeerJ.* 2023 Jan 20;11:e14475.
6573 Ebani VV, Pieracci Y, Cagnoli G, et al. In Vitro Antimicrobial Activity of Thymus vulgaris, Origanum vulgare, Satureja montana and Their Mixture against Clinical Isolates Responsible for Canine Otitis Externa. *Vet Sci.* 2023 Jan 1;10(1):30.
6574 Luca SV, Zengin G, Sinan KI, et al. Post-Distillation By-Products of Aromatic Plants from Lamiaceae Family as Rich Sources of Antioxidants and Enzyme Inhibitors. *Antioxidants (Basel).* 2023 Jan 16;12(1):210.
6575 Silva SL, Araújo FSM, Silva POA, et al. Evaluation of the antimicrobial effect of the Origanum vulgare L essential oil on strains of Klebsiella pneumoniae. *Braz J Biol.* 2023 Jan 30;83:e269317.
6576 Hassan MA, Abo-Elmaaty AMA, Zaglool AW, et al. Origanum vulgare Essential Oil Modulates the AFB1-Induced Oxidative Damages, Nephropathy, and Altered Inflammatory Responses in Growing Rabbits. *Toxins (Basel).* 2023 Jan 12;15(1):69.
6577 Karpiński TM, Ożarowski M, Seremak-Mrozikiewicz A, et al. Anti-Candida and Antibiofilm Activity of Selected Lamiaceae Essential Oils. *Front Biosci (Landmark Ed).* 2023 Feb 16;28(2):28.

[6578] Ersanli C, Tzora A, Skoufos I, et al. The Assessment of Antimicrobial and Antibiofilm Activity of Essential Oils against Staphylococcus aureus Strains. *Antibiotics (Basel)*. 2023 Feb 13;12(2):384.
[6579] Yuan Y, Sun J, Song Y, et al. Antibacterial activity of oregano essential oils against Streptococcus mutans in vitro and analysis of active components. *BMC Complement Med Ther*. 2023 Feb 21;23(1):61.
[6580] Maniki E, Kostoglou D, Paterakis N, et al. Chemical Composition, Antioxidant, and Antibiofilm Properties of Essential Oil from Thymus capitatus Plants Organically Cultured on the Greek Island of Lemnos. *Molecules*. 2023 Jan 24;28(3):1154.
[6581] Rathore S, Mukhia S, Kumar R, et al. Essential oil composition and antimicrobial potential of aromatic plants grown in the mid-hill conditions of the Western Himalayas. *Sci Rep*. 2023 Mar 25;13(1):4878.
[6582] Zinno P, Guantario B, Lombardi G, et al. Chemical Composition and Biological Activities of Essential Oils from Origanum vulgare Genotypes Belonging to the Carvacrol and Thymol Chemotypes. *Plants (Basel)*. 2023 Mar 16;12(6):1344.
[6583] Angiolella L, Rojas F, Mussin J, et al. Modulatory effect of Origanum vulgare essential oil and carvacrol on Malassezia spp. virulence factors. *Med Mycol*. 2023 Mar 2;61(3):myad026.
[6584] Patel HK, Gomes EN, Wu Q, et al. Volatile metabolites from new cultivars of catnip and oregano as potential antibacterial and insect repellent agents. *Front Plant Sci*. 2023 Feb 23;14:1124305.
[6585] Hashemi SM, Safavi SA. Fumigant toxicity of essential oils of leaves and fruits of Platycladus orientalis to Lasioderma serricorne (F.). *Biharean Biologist*. 2012;6(1):65-69.
[6586] Hassanzadeh MK, Rahimizadeh M, Bazzaz BSF, et al. Chemical and Antimicrobial Studies of Platycladus orientalis Essential Oils. *Pharmaceutical Biol*. 2001;39(5):388-90.
[6587] Hashemi SM, Safari SA. Chemical constituents and toxicity of essential oils of oriental Aborvitae, Platycladus orientalis (L.) Franco, against three stored-product beetles. *Chilean J Agric Res*. 2012 Apr-Jun;72(2):188-94.
[6588] Guleria S, Kumar A, Tiku AK. Chemical Composition and Fungitoxic Activity of Essential Oil of Thuja orientalis L. Grown in the North-Western Himalaya. *Z Naturforsch*. 2008;63c:211-14.
[6589] Loizzo M, Tundis R, Menichini F, et al. Antiproliferative effects of essential oils and their major constituents in human renal adenocarcinoma and amelanotic melanoma cells. *Cell Proliferation*. 2008;41(6):1002-12.
[6590] Loizzo MR, Saab AM, Tundis R, et al. Phytochemical analysis and in vitro antiviral activities of the essential oils of seven Lebanon species. *Chem Biodivers*. 2008 Mar;5(3):461-70.
[6591] Nickavar B, Amin G, Parhami S. Volatile constituents of the fruit and leaf oils of Thuja orientalis L. grown in Iran. *Z Naturforsch C*. 2003 Mar-Apr;58(3-4):171-2.
[6592] Worldforestry.org. Platycladus orientalis. Available at: http://www.worldagroforestry.org/treedb/AFTPDFS/Platycladus_orientalis.PDF.
[6593] Loizzo M, Tundis R, Menichini F, et al. Antiproliferative effects of essential oils and their major constituents in human renal adenocarcinoma and amelanotic melanoma cells. *Cell Proliferation*. 2008;41(6):1002-12.
[6594] Kim KH, Moon E, Kim SY, et al. Bioactive sesquiterpenes from the essential oil of Thuja orientalis. *Planta Med*. 2013 Nov;79(17):1680-4.
[6595] Guleria S, Kumar A, Tiku AK. Chemical Composition and Fungitoxic Activity of Essential Oil of Thuja orientalis L. Grown in the North-Western Himalaya. *Z Naturforsch*. 2008;63c:211-14.
[6596] Jain RK, Garg SC. Antimicrobial activity of the essential oil of thuja orientalis L. *Anc Sci Life*. 1997 Jan;16(3):186-9.
[6597] Jain RK, Garg SC. Antimicrobial activity of the essential oil of thuja orientalis L. *Anc Sci Life*. 1997 Jan;16(3):186-9.
[6598] Loizzo MR, Saab AM, Tundis R, et al. Phytochemical analysis and in vitro antiviral activities of the essential oils of seven Lebanon species. *Chem Biodivers*. 2008 Mar;5(3):461-70.
[6599] Emami SA, Asili J, Malekian M, et al. Antioxidant Effects of the Essential Oils of Different Parts of Platycladus orientalis L. (Franco) and Their Components. *J Essential Oil Bearing Plants*. 2011;14:334-44.
[6600] Hashemi SM, Safavi SA. Fumigant toxicity of essential oils of leaves and fruits of Platycladus orientalis to Lasioderma serricorne (F.). *Biharean Biologist*. 2012;6(1):65-69.
[6601] Hashemi SM, Safari SA. Chemical constituents and toxicity of essential oils of oriental Aborvitae, Platycladus orientalis (L.) Franco, against three stored-product beetles. *Chilean J Agric Res*. 2012 Apr-Jun;72(2):188-94.
[6602] Sanei-Dehkordi A, Gholami S, Abai MR, et al. Essential Oil Composition and Larvicidal Evaluation of Platycladus orientalis against Two Mosquito Vectors, Anopheles stephensi and Culex pipiens. *J Arthropod Borne Dis*. 2018 Jun 13;12(2):101-107.
[6603] Zhang Y, Chen S, Qu F, et al. In vivo and in vitro evaluation of hair growth potential of Cacumen Platycladi, and GC-MS analysis of the active constituents of volatile oil. *J Ethnopharmacol*. 2019 Mar 24:111835.
[6604]Gan DL, Yao Y, Su HW, et al. Volatile Oil of Platycladus Orientalis (L.) Franco Leaves Exerts Strong Anti-inflammatory Effects via Inhibiting the IκB/NF-κB Pathway. *Curr Med Sci*. 2021 Feb;41(1):180-186.
[6605] Yasir M, Nawaz A, Ghazanfar S, et al. Anti-bacterial activity of essential oils against multidrug-resistant foodborne pathogens isolated from raw milk. *Braz J Biol*. 2022 May 9;84:e259449.
[6606] Guo X, Hao Y, Zhang W, et al. Comparison of Origanum Essential Oil Chemical Compounds and Their Antibacterial Activity against Cronobacter sakazakii. *Molecules*. 2022 Oct 8;27(19):6702.
[6607] Raina VK, Srivastava SK, Aggarwal KK, et al. Essential oil composition of Cymbopogon martini from different places in India. *Flav Frag J*. 2003 Jul-Aug;18(4):312-15.
[6608] Rajeswara Rao BR, Rajput DK, Patel RP. Essential oil profiles of different parts of palmarosa (Cymbopogon martinii (Roxb.) Wats. Var motia Burk.). *J Essent Oil Res*. 2009;21(6):519-21.
[6609] Rajeswara Rao BR, Kaul PN, Syamasundar KV, et al. Chemical profiles of primary and secondary essential oils of palmarosa (Cymbopogon martini (Roxb.) Wats var, motia Burk.). *Ind Crops Prod*. 2005 Jan;21(1):121-27.
[6610] Cannon JB, Cantrell CL, Astatkie T, et al. Modification of yield and composition of essential oils by distillation time. *Ind Crops Prod*. 2013;41:214-20.
[6611] Katiki LM, Chagas ACS, Bizzo HR, et al. Antihelmintic activity of Cymbopogon martinii, Cymbopogon schoenathus and Mentha piperita essential oils evaluated in four different in vitro tests. *Vet Parasitol*. 2011:1-6.
[6612] Seo KA, Kim H, Ku HY, et al. The monoterpenoids citral and geraniol are moderate inhibitors of the CYP2B6 hydroxylase activity. *Chem Biol Interact*. 2008;174:141-46.
[6613] Ibrahim SM, El-Denshary ES, Abdallah DM. Geraniol, Alone and in Combination with Pioglitazone, Ameliorates Fructose-Induced Metabolic Syndrome in Rats via the Modulation of Both Inflammatory and Oxidative Stress Status. *PLoS One*. 2015 Feb 13;10(2):e0117516.
[6614] Srinivasan S, Muruganathan U. Antidiabetic efficacy of citronellol, a citrus monoterpene by ameliorating the hepatic key enzymes of carbohydrate metabolism in streptozotocin-induced diabetic rats. *Chem Biol Interact*. 2016 Apr 25;250:38-46.
[6615] Shin S, Lim S. Antifungal effects of herbal essential oils alone and in combination with ketoconazole against Trichophyton spp. *J Appl Micribiol*. 2004;97:1289-96.
[6616] Hagvall L. Cytochrome P450-mediated activation of the fragrance constituent geraniol forms potent contact allergens. *Tox Appl Pharm*. 2008 Dec;233(2):308-13.
[6617] Andrade BF, Braga CP, Dos Santos KC, et al. Effect of inhaling Cymbopogon martinii essential oil and geraniol on serum biochemistry parameters and oxidative stress in rats. *Biochem Res Int*. 2014;2014:493183.
[6618] Murbach Teles Andrade BF, Conti BJ, Santiago KB, et al. Cymbopogon martinii essential oil and geraniol at noncytotoxic concentrations exerted immunomodulatory/anti-inflammatory effects in human monocytes. *J Pharm Phamracol*. 2014 Oct;66(10):1491-96.
[6619] Ohkawara S, Tanaka-Kagawa T, Furukawa Y, et al. Activation of the human transient receptor potential vanilloid subtype 1 by essential oils. *Biol Pharm Bull*. 2010;33(8):1434-37.
[6620] Tsai ML, Lin CC, Lin WC, et al. Antimicrobial, antioxidant, and antiinflammatory activities of essential oils from five selected herbs. *Biosci Biotechnol Biochem*.2011;75(10):1977-83.
[6621] Sinha S, Biswas D, Mukherjee A. Antigenotixic and antioxidant activities of palmarosa and citronella essential oils. *J Ethnopharmacol*. 2011 Oct;137(3):1521-27.
[6622] Sivamani P, Singaravelu G, Thiagarajan V, et al. Comparative molecular docking analysis of essential oil constituents as elastase inhibitors. *Bioinformation*. 2012;8(10):457-60.
[6623] Buch P, Patel V, Ranpariya V, et al. Neuroprotective activity of Cymbopogon martinii against cerebral ischemia/reperfusion-induced oxidative stress in rats. *J Ethnopharmacol*. 2012 Jun 26;142(1):35-40.
[6624] Prasad CS, Shukla R, Kumar A, et al. In vitro and in vivo antifungal activity of essential oils of Cymbopogon martini and Chenopodium ambrosioides and their synergism against dermatophytes. *Mycoses*. 2010 Mar 1;53(2):123- 29.
[6625] Prasad SN, Muralidhara. Protective effects of geraniol (a monoterpene) in diabetic nephropathy rat model: attenuation of behavioral impairments and biochemical perturbations. *J Neurosci Res*. 2014 Sep;92(9):1205-16.
[6626] Inouye S, Uchida K, Nishiyama Y, et al. Combined effect of heat, essential oils and salt on fungicidal activity against Trichophyton mentagrophytes in a foot bath. *Nihon Ishinjin Gakkai Zasshi*.2007;48(1):27-36.
[6627] Duarte MC, Leme EE, Delarmelina C, et al. Activity of essential oils from Brazilian medicinal plants. *J Ethnopharmacol*. 2007 May;111(2):197-201.
[6628] Duarte MC, Figueira GM, Sartoratto A, et al. Anti-Candida activity of Brazilian medicinal plants. *J Ethnopharmacol*. 2005 Feb 28;97(2):305-11.
[6629] Tsai ML, Lin CC, Lin WC, et al. Antimicrobial, antioxidant, and antiinflammatory activities of essential oils from five selected herbs. *Biosci Biotechnol Biochem*. 2011;75(10):1977-83.
[6630] Oussalah M, Caillet S, Saucier L, et al. Antioxidant effects of selected plant essential oils on the growth of Pseudomonas putida strain isolated from meat. *Meat Sci*. 206 Jun;73(2):236-44.
[6631] Lodhia MH, Bhatt KR, Thaker VS. Antibacterial activity of essential oils from palmarosa, evening primrose, lavender and tuberose. *Indian J Pharm Sco*. 2009 Mar;71(2):134-36.
[6632] Khan MS, Malik A, Ahmad I. Anti-candidal activity of essential oils alone and in combination with amphotericin or fluconazole against multi-drug resistant isolates of Candida albicans. *Med Mycol*. 2012 Jan;50(1):33-42.
[6633] Gemeda N, Woldeamanuel Y, Asrat D, et al. Effect of essential oils on Aspergillus spore germination, growth and mycotoxin production: a potential source of botanical food preservative. *Asian Pac J Biomed*. 2014 May;4(Suppl 1):S373-81.
[6634] Perczak A, Juś K, Marchwińska K, et al. Degradation of Zearalenone by Essential Oils under In vitro Conditions. *Front Microbiol*. 2016 Aug 11;7:1224.
[6635] Turcotte JC, Hunt PJB, Blaustein JD. Estrogenic effects of zearalenone on the expression of progestin receptors and sexual behavior in female rats. *Hormones and Behavior*. 2005;47:178-84.
[6636] Takemura H, Shim JY, Sayama K, et al. Characterization of the estrogenic activities of zearalenone and zeranol in vivo and in vitro. *J Steroid Biochem Mol Biol*. 2007 Feb;103(2):170-7.
[6637] Frizzell C, Ndossi D, Verhaegen S, et al. Endocrine disrupting effects of zearalenone, alpha- and beta-zearalenol at the level of nuclear receptor binding and steroidogenesis. *Toxicol Lett*. 2011 Oct 10;206(2):210-7.
[6638] de Menezes-Filho JE, Gondim AN, Cruz JS, et al. Geraniol blocks calcium and potassium channels in the Mammalian myocardium: useful effects to treat arrhythmias. *Basic Clin Pharmacol Toxicol*. 2014 Dec;115(6):554-44.
[6639] Pérez-Rosés R, Risco E, Vila R, et al. Biological and Nonbiological Antioxidant Activity of Some Essential Oils. *J Agric Food Chem*. 2016;64(23):4716-24.

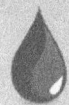

6640 Pazinato R, Volpato A, Baldissera MD, et al. In vitro effect of seven essential oils on the reproduction of the cattle tick Rhipicephalus microplus. *J Adv Res.* 2016 Nov;7(6):1029-1034.
6641 Fang F, Candy K, Melloul E, et al. In vitro activity of ten essential oils against Sarcoptes scabiei. *Parasit Vectors.* 2016 Nov 22;9(1):594.
6642 Simoes BM, Kohler B, Clarke RB, et al. Estrogenicity of essential oils is not required to relieve symptoms of urogenital atrophy in breast cancer survivors. Ther Adv Med Oncol. 2018;10:1758835918766189.
6643 Feng J, Shi W, Miklossy J, et al. Identification of Essential Oils with Strong Activity against Stationary Phase Borrelia burgdorferi. *Antibiotics (Basel).* 2018 Oct 16;7(4).
6644 Murbach Teles Andrade BF, Nunes Barbosa L, Bérgamo Alves FC, et al. The impact of Cymbopogon martinii essential oil on Cutibacterium (formerly Propionibacterium) acnes strains and its interaction with keratinocytes. *J Pharm Pharmacol.* 2018 Dec;70(12):1688-1699.
6645 Gemeda N, Tadele A, Lemma H, et al. Development, Characterization, and Evaluation of Novel Broad-Spectrum Antimicrobial Topical Formulations from Cymbopogon martini (Roxb.) W. Watson Essential Oil. *Evid Based Complement Alternat Med.* 2018 Sep 10;2018:9812093.
6646 Xiao S, Cui P, Shi W, et al. Identification of essential oils with activity against stationary phase Staphylococcus aureus. *BMC Complement Med Ther.* 2020 Mar 24;20(1):99.
6647 Marinkovic J, Culafic DM, Nikolic B, et al. Antimicrobial potential of irrigants based on essential oils of Cymbopogon martinii and Thymus zygis towards in vitro multispecies biofilm cultured in ex vivo root canals. *Arch Oral Biol.* 2020 Jul 16;117:104842.
6648 Angilella L. Synergistic activity of Pelargonium capitatum and Cymbopogon martini essential oils against C. albicans. *Nat Prod Res.* 2020 Aug 25;1-5.
6649 Castro JC, Pante GC, Centenaro BM, et al. Antifungal and antimycotoxigenic effects of Zingiber officinale, Cinnamomum zeylanicum and Cymbopogon martinii essential oils against Fusarium verticillioides. *Food Addit Contam Part A Chem Anal Control Expo Risk Assess.* 2020 Sep;37(9):1531-1541.
6650 Piasecki B, Biernasiuk A, Skiba A, et al. Composition, Anti-MRSA Activity and Toxicity of Essential Oils from Cymbopogon Species. *Molecules.* 2021 Dec 13;26(24):7542.
6651 Monzote L, Hill GM, Cuellar A, et al. Chemical composition and anti-proliferative properties of Bursera graveolens essential oil. *Nat Prod Commun.* 2012 Nov;7(11):1531-34.
6652 Carmona R, Quijano-Celis CE, Pino JA. Leaf oil composition of Bursera graveolens (Kunth) Triana et Planch. *J Essent Oil Res.* 2009;21(5):387-89.
6653 Young DG, Chao S, Casabianca H, et al. Essential oil of Bursera graveolens (Kunth) Triana et Planch from Ecuador. *J Essent Oil Res.* 2007;19(6):525-26.
6654 Aromatics International. Palo Santo (Holy Wood) - Bursera graveolens. Available at: http://www.aromaticsinternational.com/products/essential-oils/palo-santo-holy-wood.
6655 Thomassed D, Slattery JT, Nelson SD. Contribution of menthofuran to the hepatotoxicity of pulegone: assessment based on matched area under the curve and on matched time course. *J Pharmacol Exp Ther.* 1988 Mar;244(3):825-29.
6656 Gordon WP, Forte AJ, McMurtry RJ, et al. Hepatotoxicity and pulmonary toxicity of pennyroyal oil and its constituent terpenes in the mouse. *Toxicol Appl Pharmacol.* 1982;65:413-24.
6657 Carratu B, Federici E, Gallo FR, et al. Plants and parts of plants used in food supplements: an approach to their safety assessment. *Ann Ist Super Sanita.* 2010 Oct-Dec;46(4):0021-2571.
6658 Khojasteh AC, Oishi S, Nelson SD. The metabolism and toxicity of menthofuran in rat liver slices and in rats. *Chem Res Toxicol.* 2010 Nov;23(11):1824-32.
6659 Sun J. D-limonene: safety and clinical applications. *Altern Med Rev.* 2007 Sep;12(3):259-64.
6660 Monzote L, Hill GM, Cuellar A, et al. Chemical composition and anti-proliferative properties of Bursera graveolens essential oil. *Nat Prod Commun.* 2012 Nov;7(11):1531-34.
6661 Monzote L, Hill GM, Cuellar A, et al. Chemical composition and anti-proliferative properties of Bursera graveolens essential oil. *Nat Prod Commun.* 2012 Nov;7(11):1531-34.
6662 Espinoza LC, Sosa L, Granda PC, et al. Development of a Topical Amphotericin B and Bursera graveolens Essential Oil-Loaded Gel for the Treatment of Dermal Candidiasis. *Pharmaceuticals (Basel).* 2021 Oct 12;14(10):1033.
6663 Zhang H, Chen F, Wang X, et al. Evaluation of antioxidant activity of parsley (Petroselinum crispum) essential oil and identification of its antioxidant constituents. *Food Res Int.* 2006;39:833-39.
6664 Voll R, Lougas T, Mets K, et al. Dill (Anethum graveolens L.) and Parsley (Petroselinum crispum (Mill.) Fuss) from Estonia: Seasonal Differences in Essential Oil Composition. *Agronomy Res.* 2011;9(Special Issue II):515-20.
6665 Kurowska A, Galazka I. Essential oil composition of the parsley seed of cultivars marketed in Poland. *Flavour Frag J.* 2006 Jan-Feb;21(1):143-47.
6666 Snoussi M, Dehmani A, Noumi E, et al. Chemical composition and antibiofilm activity of Petroselinum crispum and Ocimum basilicum essential oils against Vibrio spp. strains. *Microbial Pathogenesis.* 2016 Jan;90:13-21.
6667 Marin I, Sayas-Barbera E, Viuda-Martos M, et al. Chemical Composition, Antioxidant and Antimicrobial Activity of Essential Oils from Organic Fennel, Parsley, and Lavender from Spain. *Foods.* 2016;5(18):1-10.
6668 Mulugeta T, Unnithan CR, Tesfay D. Phytochemical screening, characterization and biological activities of Petroselinum crispum (Parsley) leaf oil. *World J Pharmacy Pharmaceutical Sci.* 2015;4(09):142-51.
6669 Simon JE, Quinn J. Characterization of essential oil of parsley. *J Agric Food Chem.* 1988;36:467-72.
6670 Freeman GG, Whenham RJ, Self R, et al. Volatile flavour components of parsley leaves (Petroselinum crispum (mill.) nyman). *J Sci Food Agric.* 1975 Apr;26(4):465-70.
6671 Lowenstein L, Ballew DH. Fatal acute hemolytic anemia, thrombocytopenic purpura, nephrosis and hepatitis resulting from ingestion of a constituent containing apiol. *Can Med Assoc J.* 1958 Feb 1;78(3):195-8.
6672 Basso U. [Study of death caused by apiol and experimental study of its toxic action]. *Arch Patol Clin Med.* 1957;34(4):308-22.
6673 Barni B, Barni I. [The apiol poisoning]. Rassegna casistica. 1967;3(2):197-221.
6674 Newall CA, Anderson LA, Philpson JD. Herbal Medicine: A Guide for Healthcare Professionals. London, UK: The Pharmaceutical Press, 1996.
6675 Colalillo R. Apiol poisoning in 7 women and 2 children. *Rivista di Tossicologia Sperimentale e Clinica.* 1988;18(2):125-130.
6676 Hermann K, Le Roux A, Fiddes FS. Death from apiol used as abortifacient. *Lancet.* 1956 Jun 16;270(6929):937-9.
6677 Lowenstein L, Ballew DH. Fatal acute hemolytic anemia, thrombocytopenic purpura, nephrosis and hepatitis resulting from ingestion of a constituent containing apiol. *Can Med Assoc J.* 1958 Feb 1;78(3):195-8.
6678 Basso U. [Study of death caused by apiol and experimental study of its toxic action]. *Arch Patol Clin Med.* 1957;34(4):308-22.
6679 Mumolo M. [On a case of acute and fatal poisoning caused by apiol]. *Recenti Prog Med.* 1964 Feb;36:139-51.
6680 Barni B, Barni I. [The apiol poisoning]. Rassegna casistica. 1967;3(2):197-221.
6681 D'Aprile F. [Clinical study-Experimental apiol poisoning]. *Annali di Ostetricia Ginecologia.* 1928;50:1204-27.
6682 Ciganda C, Laborde A. Herbal infusions used for induced abortion. *J Toxicol Clin Toxicol.* 2003;41:235-239.
6683 Pecevski J, Savković D, Radivojević D, et al. Effect of oil of nutmeg on the fertility and induction of meiotic chromosome rearrangements in mice and their first generation. *Toxicol Lett.* 1981 Jan;7(3):239-43.
6684 Randerath K, Putman KL, Randerath E. Flavor constituents in cola drinks induce hepatic DNA adducts in adult and fetal mice. *Biochem Biophys Res Commun.* 1993 Apr 15;192(1):61-8.
6685 Hermann K, Le Roux A, Fiddes FS. Death from apiol used as abortifacient. *Lancet.* 1956 Jun 16;270(6929):937-9.
6686 Lowenstein L, Ballew DH. Fatal acute hemolytic anemia, thrombocytopenic purpura, nephrosis and hepatitis resulting from ingestion of a constituent containing apiol. *Can Med Assoc J.* 1958 Feb 1;78(3):195-8.
6687 Basso U. [Study of death caused by apiol and experimental study of its toxic action]. *Arch Patol Clin Med.* 1957;34(4):308-22.
6688 Mumolo M. [On a case of acute and fatal poisoning caused by apiol]. *Recenti Prog Med.* 1964 Feb;36:139-51.
6689 Barni B, Barni I. [The apiol poisoning]. Rassegna casistica. 1967;3(2):197-221.
6690 D'Aprile F. [Clinical study-Experimental apiol poisoning]. *Annali di Ostetricia Ginecologia.* 1928;50:1204-27.
6691 Hallstrom H, Thuvander A. Toxicological evaluation of myristicin. *Natural Toxins* 1997;5:186-92.
6692 Brenner N, Frank OS, Knight E. Chronic nutmeg psychosis, *J R Soc Med.* 1993;86:179-80.
6693 Sangalli BC, Sangalli B, Chiang W. Toxicology of nutmeg abuse. *Clin Toxicol.* 2000;38(6):671-78.
6694 Forrest JE, Heacock RA. Nutmeg and mace, the psychotropic spices from Myristica fragrans. *Lloydia.* 1972 Dec;35(4):440-9.
6695 Leiter E1, Hitchcock G, Godwin S, et al. Evaluation of the anxiolytic properties of myristicin, a component of nutmeg, in the male Sprague-Dawley rat.*AANA J.* 2011 Apr;79(2):109-14.
6696 Truitt EB Jr, Duritz G, Ebersberger EM. Evidence of monoamine oxidase inhibition by myristicin and nutmeg. *Proc Soc Exp Biol Med.* 1963 Mar;112:647-50.
6697 Ozsoy-Sacan O, Yanardag R, Orak H, et al. Effects of parsley (Petroselinum crispum) extract versus glibornuride on the liver of streptozotocin-induced diabetic rats. *J Ethnopharmacol.* 2006 Mar 8;104(1-2):175-81.
6698 Bolkent S, Yanardag R, Ozsoy-Sacan O, et al. Effects of parsley (Petroselinum crispum) on the liver of diabetic rats: a morphological and biochemical study. *Phytother Res.* 2004 Dec;18(12):996-9.
6699 Yanardag R, Bolkent S, Tabakoglu-Oguz A, et al. Effects of Petroselinum crispum extract on pancreatic B cells and blood glucose of streptozotocin-induced diabetic rats. *Biol Pharm Bull.* 2003;26(8):1206-1210.
6700 Bonesi M, Menichini F, Tundis R, et al. Acetylcholinesterase and butyrylcholinesterase inhibitory activity of Pinus species essential oils and their constituents. *J Enzyme Inhib Med Chem.* 2010 Oct;25(5):622-8.
6701 Kreydiyyeh SI, Usta J. Diuretic effect and mechanism of action of parsley. *J Ethnopharmacol.* 2002 Mar;79(3):353-7.
6702 Seo SM, Jung CS2, Kang J, et al. Larvicidal and acetylcholinesterase inhibitory activities of apiaceae plant essential oils and their constituents against aedes albopictus and formulation development. *J Agric Food Chem.* 2015 Nov 18;63(45):9977-86.
6703 Banjeree S, Sharma R, Kale RK, et al. Influence of certain essential oils on carcinogen-metabolizing enzyme soluble sulfhydryls in mouse liver. *Nutr Cancer.* 1994;21(3):263-69.
6704 Kimura Y, Ito H, Hatano T. Effects of mace and nutmeg on human cytochrome P450 3A4 and 2C9 activity. *Biol Pharm Bull.* 2012;33(12):1977-87.
6705 Jeong HG, Yun CH. Induction of rat hepatic cytochrome P450 enzymes by myristicin. *Biochem Biophys Res Commun.* 1995 Dec26;217(3):966-71.
6706 Zhao R, Wang W, Zhao L, et al. Effect of volatile oil from nutmeg on liver licrosomal cytochrome P450 in mice.
*Zhonqquo Zhonq Yao Za Zhi.* 2009Feb;34(4):447-49.
6707 Zhao R. [Effect of volatile oil from nutmeg on liver microsomal cytochrome P450 in mice.] *Zhongguo Zhong Yao Za Zhi.* 2009 Feb;34(4):447-9.
6708 Yang AH, He X, Chen JX, et al. Identification and characterization of reactive metabolites in myristicin-mediated mechanism-based inhibition of CYP1A2. *Chem Biol Interact.* 2015 Jul 25;237:133-40.
6709 Ioannides C, Delaforge M, Parke DV. Interactions of safrole and isosafrole and their metabolites with cytochromes P-450. *Chem Biol Interact.* 1985 May;53(3):303-11.

6710 Lowenstein L, Ballew DH. Fatal acute hemolytic anemia, thrombocytopenic purpura, nephrosis and hepatitis resulting from ingestion of a constituent containing apiol. *Can Med Assoc J.* 1958 Feb 1;78(3):195-8.

6711 Basso U. [Study of death caused by apiol and experimental study of its toxic action]. *Arch Patol Clin Med.* 1957;34(4):308-22.

6712 Barni B, Barni I. [The apiol poisoning]. Rassegna casistica. 1967;3(2):197-221.

6713 Newall CA, Anderson LA, Philpson JD. Herbal Medicine: A Guide for Healthcare Professionals. London, UK: The Pharmaceutical Press, 1996.

6714 Colalillo R. Apiol poisoning in 7 women and 2 children. *Rivista di Tossicologia Sperimentale e Clinica.* 1988;18(2):125-130.

6715 Mauerman B, Ahmed N, Tambhar N, et al. Trends in Furanocoumarin Profiles Among Commerical-Scale Essential Oils. International Conference on the Science of Botanicals, Poster. Mar 2022.

6716 Opdyke DLJ. Monographs on fragrance raw materials. p. 615.

6717 Wei A, Shibamoto T. Antioxidant activities and volatile constituents of various essential oils. *J Agric Food Chem.* 2007 Mar 7;55(5):1737-42.

6718 Ayala A, Munoz MF, Arguelles S. Lipid Peroxidation: Production, Metabolism, and Signaling Mechanisms of Malondialdehyde and 4-Hydroxy-2-Nonenal. *Oxidative Med Cell Longevity.* 2014;2014:360438.

6719 Snoussi M, Dehmani A, Noumi E, et al. Chemical composition and antibiofilm activity of Petroselinum crispum and Ocimum basilicum essential oils against Vibrio spp. strains. *Microbial Pathogenesis.* 2016 Jan;90:13-21.

6720 Marin I, Sayas-Barbera E, Viuda-Martos M, et al. Chemical Composition, Antioxidant and Antimicrobial Activity of Essential Oils from Organic Fennel, Parsley, and Lavender from Spain. *Foods.* 2016;5(18):1-10.

6721 Mulugeta T, Unnithan CR, Tesfay D. Phytochemical screening, characterization and biological activities of Petroselinum crispum (Parsley) leaf oil. *World J Pharmacy Pharmaceutical Sci.* 2015;4(09):142-51.

6722 Sharafati Chaleshtori R, Rafieian Kopaei M, Salehi E, et al. Bioactivity of Apium petroselinum and Portulaca oleracea Essential Oils as Natural Preservatives. *Jundishapur J Microbiol.* 2015 Jan 14;8(3):e20128.

6723 Gutierrez J, Rodriguez G, Barry-Ryan C, et al. Efficacy of plant essential oils against foodborne pathogens and spoilage bacteria associated with ready-to-eat vegetables: antimicrobial and sensory screening. *J Food Prot.* 2008 Sep;71(9):1846-54.

6724 Linde GA, Gazim ZC, Cardoso BK, et al. Antifungal and antibacterial activities of Petroselinum crispum essential oil. *Genet Mol Res.* 2016 Jul 29;15(3).

6725 Marin I, Sayas-Barberá E, Viuda-Martos M, et al. Chemical Composition, Antioxidant and Antimicrobial Activity of Essential Oils from Organic Fennel, Parsley, and Lavender from Spain. *Foods.* 2016 Mar 4;5(1).

6726 Zhang H, Chen F, Wang X, et al. Evaluation of antioxidant activity of parsley (Petroselinum crispum) essential oil and identification of its antioxidant constituents. *Food Res Int.* 2006;39:833-39.

6727 Marin I, Sayas-Barbera E, Viuda-Martos M, et al. Chemical Composition, Antioxidant and Antimicrobial Activity of Essential Oils from Organic Fennel, Parsley, and Lavender from Spain. *Foods.* 2016;5(18):1-10.

6728 Marin I, Sayas-Barberá E, Viuda-Martos M, et al. Chemical Composition, Antioxidant and Antimicrobial Activity of Essential Oils from Organic Fennel, Parsley, and Lavender from Spain. *Foods.* 2016 Mar 4;5(1).

6729 Fejes S, Kéry A, Blázovics A, et al. [Investigation of the in vitro antioxidant effect of Petroselinum crispum (Mill.) Nym. ex A. W. Hill]. *Acta Pharm Hung.* 1998 May;68(3):150-6.

6730 Yousofi A, Daneshmandi S, Soleimani N, et al. Immunomodulatory effect of Parsley (Petroselinum crispum) essential oil on immune cells: mitogen-activated splenocytes and peritoneal macrophages. *Immunopharmacol Immunotoxicol.* 2012;34(2):303-08.

6731 Karimi MH, Ebadi P, Amirghofran Z. Parsley and immunomodulation. *Expert Rev Clin Immunol.* 2012 May;8(4):295-7.

6732 Baylac S, Racine P. Inhibition of 5-lipoxygenase by essential oils and other natural fragrant extracts. *Int J Aromatherapy.* 2003;13(2-3):138-42.

6733 Seo SM, Jung CS2, Kang J, et al. Larvicidal and acetylcholinesterase inhibitory activities of apiaceae plant essential oils and their constituents against aedes albopictus and formulation development. *J Agric Food Chem.* 2015 Nov 18;63(45):9977-86.

6734 Intirach J, Junkum A, Lumjuan N, et al. Antimosquito property of Petroselinum crispum (Umbelliferae) against the pyrethroid resistant and susceptible strains of Aedes aegypti (Diptera: Culicidae). *Environ Sci Pollut Res Int.* 2016 Dec;23(23):23994-24008.

6735 Leal Pinto SM, Herrera Sandoval LV, Vargas LY. In vitro susceptibility of Microsporum spp. and mammalian cells to Eugenia caryophyllus essential oil, eugenol and semisynthetic derivatives. *Mycoses.* 2019 Jan;62(1):41-50.

6736 Piras A, Porcedda S, Falconieri D, et al. Supercritical extraction of volatile and fixed oils from Petroselinum crispum L. seeds: chemical composition and biological activity. *Nat Prod Res.* 2020 Aug 21;1-6.

6737 Rosa JS, Oliveira L, Sousa RMOF, et al. Bioactivity of some Apiaceae essential oils and their constituents against Sitophilus zeamais (Coleoptera: Curculionidae). *Bull Entomol Res.* 2020 Jun;110(3):406-416.

6738 Junkum A, Intirach J, Chansang A, et al. Enhancement of Temephos and Deltamethrin Toxicity by Petroselinum crispum Oil and its Main Constituents Against Aedes aegypti (Diptera: Culicidae). *J Med Entomol.* 2021 Feb 11;tjab008.

6739 Jugreet BS, Ibrahime SK, Zengin G, et al. GC/MS Profiling, In Vitro and In Silico Pharmacological Screening and Principal Component Analysis of Essential Oils from Three Exotic and Two Endemic Plants from Mauritius. *Chem Biodivers.* 2021 Mar;18(3):e2000921.

6740 Jugreet BS, Ibrahime SK, Zengin G, et al. GC/MS Profiling, In Vitro and In Silico Pharmacological Screening and Principal Component Analysis of Essential Oils from Three Exotic and Two Endemic Plants from Mauritius. *Chem Biodivers.* 2021 Mar;18(3):e2000921.

6741 Badr GM, Algefare AI, Alfwuaires MA. Antioxidant Potential of Parsley Leaf ( Petroselinum crispum) Essential Oil on Hypothyroidism and Testicular Injury in Mice Intoxicated by Carbon Tetrachloride. *Biomed Res Int.* 2021 Aug 30;2021:9989174.

6742 Foudah AI, Alqarni MH, Alam A, et al. Phytochemical Screening, In Vitro and In Silico Studies of Volatile Compounds from Petroselinum crispum (Mill) Leaves Grown in Saudi Arabia. *Molecules.* 2022 Jan 29;27(3):934.

6743 Vitalini S, Nalbone L, Bernardi C, et al. Ginger and parsley essential oils: chemical composition, antimicrobial activity, and evaluation of their application in cheese preservation. *Nat Prod Res.* 2022 Sep 22:1-6.

6744 Sánchez-Quintero MJ, Delgado J, et al. Beneficial Effects of Essential Oils from the Mediterranean Diet on Gut Microbiota and Their Metabolites in Ischemic Heart Disease and Type-2 Diabetes Mellitus. *Nutrients.* 2022 Nov 3;14(21):4650.

6745 Albuquerque EL, Lima JK, Souza FH, et al. Insecticidal activity of the essential oil of Pogostemon cablin against urban ants species. *Acta Trop.* 2013 Ser;127(3):181-86.

6746 Dung NX, Leclercq PA, Thai TH, et al. Chemical composition of patchouli oil from Vietnam. *J Essent Oil Res.* Mar- Apr 1989:1.

6747 Silva MAS, EHLERT PAD Ming LC. Composition and chemical variation during daytime of constituents of the essential oil of Pogostemon patchouli Pellet leaves. *Acta Hort.* 2006;629:145-47.

6748 Karimi A. Characterization and antimicrobial activity of patchouli essential oil extracted from Pogostemon cablin [Blanco] Benth. [Lamiaceae]. *Adv Environ Biol.* 2014 May;8(7):231-09.

6749 Rakotonirainy O, Gaydou EM, Faure R, et al. Sesquiterpenes from patchouli (Pogostemon cablin) essential oil. Assignment of the proton and carbon-13 NMR spectra. *J Essent Oil Res.* 1997 May-Jun;9:321-27.

6750 Hussin N, Mondello L, Costa R, et al. Quantitative and physical evaluation of patchouli essential oils obtained from different sources of Pogostemon cablin. *Nat Prod Commun.* 2012;7(7):927-30.

6751 Milchard MJ, Clery R, Esdale R, et al. Application of gas-liquid chromatography to the analysis of essential oil oils. *Perfumer Flav.* 2004;29:28-36.

6752 Hu LF, Li SP, Cao H, et al. GC-MS fingerprint of Pogostemon cablin in China. *J Pharm Biomed Analysis.* 2006;42:200-06.

6753 Tsai HH, Lin HW, Chen YL, et al. A review of potential harmful interactions between anticoagulant/antiplatelet agents and Chinese herbal medicines. *PLoS One.* 2013 May 9;8(5):e64255.

6754 Hsu HC, Yang WC, Tsai WJ, et al. α-Bulnesene, a novel PAF receptor antagonist isolated from Pogostemon cablin. *Biochem Biophys Res Comm.* 2006;345:1033-38.

6755 Jeong JB, Choi J, Lou Z, et al. Patchouli alcohol, an essential oil of Pogostemon cablin, exhibits anti-tumorigenic activity in human colorectal cancer cells. *Int Immunopharmacol.* 2013 Jun;16(2):184-90.

6756 YuJ, Qi Y, Luo G, et al. Extraction and analysis of the essential oil in Pogostemon cablin by enzymatic hydrolysis and inhibitory activity against Hela cell proliferation. *Zhong Yao Cai.* 2012 May;35(5):796-99.

6757 Baylac S, Racine P. Inhibition of 5-lipoxygenase by essential oils and other natural fragrant extracts. *Int J Aromatherapy.* 2003;13(2-3):138-42.

6758 Silva-Filho SE, Wiirzler LA, Cavalcante HA, et al. Effect of patchouli (Pogostemon cablin) essential oil on in vitro and in vivo leukocytes behavior in acute inflammatory response. *Biomed Pharmacother.* 2016 Dec;84:1697-1704.

6759 Lin RF, Feng XX, Li CW, et al. Prevention of UV-radiation-induced cutaneous photoaging in mice by topical administration of patchouli oil. *J Ethnopharmacol.* 2014 Jun 11;154(2):408-18.

6760 Fujiwara Y, Ito M. Synergistic effect of fragrant herbs in Japanese scent sachets. *Planta Med.* 2015 Feb;81(3):193-99.

6761 Swamy MK, Sinniah UR. A comprehensive review on the phytochemical constituents and pharmacological activities of Pogostemon cablin Benth.: An aromatic medicinal plant of industrial importance. *Molecules.* 2015 May 12;20(5):8521-47.

6762 Li YC, Liang HC, Chen HM, et al. Anti-Candida albicans activity and pharmacokinetics of pogostone isolated from Pogostemonis Herba. *Phytomedicine.* 2012 Dec 15;20(1):77-83.

6763 Yi YY, He JJ, Su JQ, et al. Synthesis and antimicrobial evaluation of pogostone and its analogues. *Fitoterapia.* 2013 Jan;84:135-39.

6764 Vázquez-Sánchez D, Cabo ML, Rodríguez-Herrera JJ, et al. Antimicrobial activity of essential oils against Staphylococcus aureus biofilms. *Food Sci Technol Int.* 2015 Dec;21(8):559-70.

6765 Shan-shan QI, Li-ping HU, Wen-na C, et al. Immunological regulation effects of essential oil in leaves of Cablin Patchouli Herb on mice. *Chinese Arch Trad Chinese Med.* 2009 Apr.

6766 Liao JB, Wu DW, Peng SZ, et al. Immunomodulatory potential of patchouli alcohol isolated from Pogostemon cablin (Blanco) Benth (Lamiaceae) in mice. *Trop J Pharm Res.* 2013 Aug;12(4):559-65.

6767 Depo Y, Chaumont J-P, Millet J. Antibacterial activity on skin and chemical composition of the volatile oils from Agastache rugosa and Pogostemon cablin. *J Microbiol.* 1998 Jan 1;18(4):1-4,16.

6768 Albuquerque EL, Lima JK, Souza FH, et al. Insecticidal and repellence activity of the essential oil of Pogostemon cablin against urban ants species. *Acta Trop.* 2013 Sep;127(3):181-86.

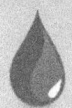

[6769] Machial CM, Shikano I, Smirle M, et al. Evaluation of the toxicity of 17 essential oils against Choristoneura rosaceana (Lepidoptera: Toticidae) and Trichoplusia in (Lepidoptera: Noctuidae). *Pest Manag Sci.* 2010 Oct;66(10):1116-21.

[6770] Wu HQ, Li J, He ZD, et al. Acaricidal activities of traditional Chinese medicine against the house dust mite, Dematophagoides farinae. *Parasitology.* 2010 May;137(6):975-83.

[6771] Ga'al H, Fouad H, Mao G, et al. Larvicidal and pupicidal evaluation of silver nanoparticles synthesized using Aquilaria sinensis and Pogostemon cablin essential oils against dengue and zika viruses vector Aedes albopictus mosquito and its histopathological analysis. *Artif Cells Nanomed Biotechnol.* 2018 Sep;46(6):1171-1179.

[6772] Yu X, Yang G, Jiang H, et al. Patchouli oil ameliorates acute colitis: A targeted metabolite analysis of 2,4,6-trinitrobenzenesulfonic acid-induced rats. *Exp Ther Med.* 2017 Aug;14(2):1184-1192.

[5258] Mahboubi M. Effectiveness of Myrtus communis in the treatment of hemorrhoids. *J Integr Med.* 2017 Sep;15(5):351-358.

[6773] Su J, He J, Su Z, et al. T cell inhibition by pogostone from Pogostemon cablin (Blanco) Benth: In vitro and in vivo immunosuppressive analysis. *Mol Med Rep.* 2017 Oct;16(4):4511-4520.

[6774] Rocha AG, Oliveira BMS1, Melo CR, et al. Lethal Effect and Behavioral Responses of Leaf-Cutting Ants to Essential Oil of Pogostemon cablin (Lamiaceae) and Its Nanoformulation. *Neotrop Entomol.* 2018 Dec;47(6):769-779.

[6775] Powers CN, Osier JL, McFeeters RL, et al. Antifungal and Cytotoxic Activities of Sixty Commercially-Available Essential Oils. *Molecules.* 2018 Jun 27;23(7).

[6776] Yang HM, Zhuo JY, Sun CY, et al. Pogostone attenuates TNF-α-induced injury in A549 cells via inhibiting NF-κB and activating Nrf2 pathways. *Int Immunopharmacol.* 2018 Sep;62:15-22.

[6777] Lima Santos L, Barreto Brandão L, Lopes Martins R, et al. Evaluation of the Larvicidal Potential of the Essential Oil Pogostemon cablin (Blanco) Benth in the Control of Aedes aegypti. *Pharmaceuticals (Basel).* 2019 Apr 8;12(2).

[6778] Leong W, Huang G, Khan I, et al. Patchouli Essential Oil and Its Derived Compounds Revealed Prebiotic-Like Effects in C57BL/6J Mice. *Front Pharmacol.* 2019 Oct 17;10:1229.

[6779] Hong SJ, Cho J, Boo CG, et al. Inhalation of Patchouli ( Pogostemon Cablin Benth.) Essential Oil Improved Metabolic Parameters in Obesity-Induced Sprague Dawley Rats. *Nutrients.* 2020 Jul 13;12(7):E2077.

[6780] Mansuri A, Lokhande K, Kore S, et al. Antioxidant, anti-quorum sensing, biofilm inhibitory activities and chemical composition of Patchouli essential oil: in vitro and in silico approach. *J Biomol Struct Dyn.* 2020 Aug 24:1-12.

[6781] Luchesi L, Paulus D, Busso C, et al. Chemical composition, antifungal and antioxidant activity of essential oils from Baccharis dracunculifolia and Pogostemon cablin against Fusarium graminearum. *Nat Prod Res.* 2020 Aug 6;1-4.

[6782] Gan Y, Ai G, Wu J, et al. Patchouli oil ameliorates 5-fluorouracil-induced intestinal mucositis in rats via protecting intestinal barrier and regulating water transport. *J Ethnopharmacol.* 2020 Mar 25;250:112519.

[6783] Hong SJ, Cho J, Boo CG, et al. Inhalation of Patchouli ( Pogostemon Cablin Benth.) Essential Oil Improved Metabolic Parameters in Obesity-Induced Sprague Dawley Rats. *Nutrients.* 2020 Jul 13;12(7):2077.

[6784] Keerthiraj M, Mandal A, Dutta TK, et al. Nematicidal and Molecular Docking Investigation of Essential Oils from Pogostemon cablin Ecotypes against Meloidogyne incognita. *Chem Biodivers.* 2021 Jul 10. Online ahead of print.

[6785] Leong W, Huang G, Liao W, et al. Traditional Patchouli essential oil modulates the host's immune responses and gut microbiota and exhibits potent anti-cancer effects in ApcMin /+ mice. *Pharmacol Res.* 2022 Jan 13;176:106082.

[6786] Santos AA, Farder-Gomes CF, Ribeiro AV, et al. Lethal and sublethal effects of an emulsion based on Pogostemon cablin (Lamiaceae) essential oil on the coffee berry borer, Hypothenemus hampei. *Environ Sci Pollut Res Int.* 2022 Feb 12. Online ahead of print.

[6787] Astuti P, Khairan K, Marthoenis M, Hasballah K. Antidepressant-like Activity of Patchouli Oil var. Tapak Tuan (Pogostemon cablin Benth) via Elevated Dopamine Level: A Study Using Rat Model. *Pharmaceuticals (Basel).* 2022 May 15;15(5):608.

[6788] Sun J, Sun P, Kang C, et al. Chemical composition and biological activities of essential oils from six lamiaceae folk medicinal plants. *Front Plant Sci.* 2022 Aug 1;13:919294.

[6789] da Silva Temperini MB, Fortunato ABR, Campos DR, et al. Insecticidal activity in vitro of the essential oil of Pogostemon cablin against Ctenocephalides felis felis. *Braz J Vet Med.* 2022 Sep 30;44:e003422.

[6790] Lorenzo D, Paz D, Dellacassa E, et al. Essential oils of Mentha pulegium and Mentha rotundifolia from Uruguay. *Braz Archives Biol Tech.* 2002 Dec;45(4):519-24.

[6791] Boukhebti H, Chaker AN, Belhadj H, et al. Chemical composition and antibacterial activity of Mentha pulegium L. and Mentha spicata L. essential oils. *Der Pharmacia Lettre.* 2011;3(4):267-75.

[6792] Lawrence BM. Essential oils 1976-78, p. 21. Allured Publishing, Wheaton. 1979.

[6793] Telci I, Ceylan M. Essential oil composition of Micromeria fruticosa Druce from Turkey. *Chem Nat Constituents.* 2007 Sep;43(5):629-31.

[6794] Baser KHC, Kirimer N, Ozek T, et al. Essential Oil Composition of Three Labiatae Endemic to Turkey (Micromeria fruticosa (L.) Druce subsp. giresunica P. H. Davis, Sideritis lycia Boiss. et Heldr. and S. arguta Boiss. et Heldr.) *J Essent Oil Res.* 1996 Oct;8(6):699-701.

[6795] Arslan M. Effects of intra-row spacing on herbage yield, essential oil content, and composition of Micromeria fruticosa. *Farmacia.* 2012;60(6):925-31.

[6796] Dudai N, Larkov O, Ravid U, et al. Developmental Control of Monoterpene Content and Composition in Micromeria fruticosa(L.) Druce. *Annals of Botany.* 2001;88:349-54.

[6797] Koutrouanidou E, Kimbaris A, Kortsaris A, et al. Increased Seizure Latency and Decreased Severity of Pentylenetetrazol-Induced Seizures in Mice after Essential Oil Administration. *Epilepsy Res Treat.* 2013;2013:532657.

[6798] Boukhebti H, Chaker AN, Belhadj H, et al. Chemical composition and antibacterial activity of Mentha pulegium L. and Mentha spicata L. essential oils. *Der Pharmacia Lettre.* 2011;3(4):267-75.

[6799] Bakerink JA, Gospe SM Jr, Dimand RJ, et al. Multiple organ failure after ingestion of pennyroyal oil from herbal tea in two infants. *Pediatrics.* 1996;98(5):944-47.

[6800] Sudekum M, Poppenga RH, Raju N, et al. Pennyroyal oil toxicosis in a dog. *J Am Vet Med Assoc.* 1992;200:817-8.

[6801] Anderson IB, Mullen WH, Meeker JE, et al. Pennyroyal toxicity: measurement of toxic metabolite levels in two cases and review of the literature. *Ann Intern Med.* 1996;124:726-34.

[6802] Seeff L, Stickel F, Navarro VJ. Hepatotoxicity of herbals and dietary supplements. In, Kaplowitz N, DeLeve LD, eds. Drug-induced liver disease. 3rd ed. Amsterdam: Elsevier, 2013, pp. 631-58.

[6803] Moolla A. A phytochemical and pharmacological investigation of indigenous Agathosma species. MSc Dissertation, University of the Witwatersrand. 2006.

[6804] Mullen W, Anderson I, Oishii S, et al. Accidental pennyroyal oil ingestion in a toddler with the first human serum metabolite detection. *Vet Hum Toxicol.* 1994;36:342.

[6805] Barnes J, Anderson LA, Philpson JD. Herbal Medicine: A Guide for Healthcare Professionals. London, UK: The Pharmaceutical Press, 1996.

[6806] Zimmerman HJ. Unconventional drugs. Miscellaneous drugs and diagnostic chemicals. In, Zimmerman, HJ. Hepatotoxicity: the adverse effects of drugs and other chemicals on the liver. 2nd ed. Philadelphia: Lippincott,1999; pp. 731-34.

[6807] Anderson IB, Mullen WH, Meeker JE, et al. Pennyroyal toxicity: measurement of toxic metabolite levels in two cases and review of the literature. *Ann Intern Med.* 1996;124:726-34.

[6808] Centers for Disease Control. Fatality and illness associated with consumption of pennyroyal oil - Colorado. *MMWR.* 1978;27:511-13.

[6809] Soares PM, Assreuy AM, Souza EP, et al. Inhibitory effects of the essential oil of Mentha pulegium on the isolated rat myometrium. *Planta Med.* 2005 Mar;71(3):214-8.

[6810] Ciganda C, Laborde A. Herbal infusions used for induced abortion. *J Toxicol Clin Toxicol.* 2003;41(3):235-9.

[6811] Valance WB. Pennyroyal poisoning: a fatal case. *Lancet.* 1955;266 (6895):850-51.

[6812] Gold J, Cates W Jr. Herbal abortifacients. *JAMA.* 1980;243:1365-66.

[6813] Gordon WP, Huitric AC, Seth CL, et al. The metabolism of the abortifacient terpene, (R)-(+)-pulegone, to a proximate toxin, menthofuran. *Drug Metab Dispos.* 1987;15:589–94.

[6814] Khojasteh-Bakht SC, Chen W, Koenigs LL, et al. Metabolism of (R)-(+)-pulegone and (R)-(+)-menthofuran by human liver cytochrome P-450s: evidence for formation of a furan epoxide. *Drug Metab Dispos.* 1999 May;27(5):574-80

[6815] Gordon P, Khojasteh SC. A decades-long investigation of acute metabolism-based hepatotoxicity by herbal constituents: a case study of pennyroyal oil. *Drug Metab Rev.* 2015 Feb;47(1):12-20.

[6816] National Toxicology Program. Toxicology and carcinogenesis studies of pulegone (CAS No. 89-82-7) in F344/N rats and B6C3F1 mice (gavage studies). *Natl Toxicol Program Tech Rep Ser.* 2011 Aug;(563):1-201.

[6817] National Toxicology Program. Toxicology and carcinogenesis studies of pulegone (CAS No. 89-82-7) in F344/N rats and B6C3F1 mice (gavage studies). *Natl Toxicol Program Tech Rep Ser.* 2011 Aug;(563):1-201.

[6818] National Toxicology Program. Toxicology and carcinogenesis studies of pulegone (CAS No. 89-82-7) in F344/N rats and B6C3F1 mice (gavage studies). *Natl Toxicol Program Tech Rep Ser.* 2011 Aug;(563):1-201.

[6819] Sullivan JB Jr, Rumack BH, Thomas H Jr, et al. Pennyroyal oil poisoning and hepatotoxicity. *JAMA.* 1979;242:2873-4.

[6820] The Review of Natural Products by Facts and Comparisons. St. Louis, MO: Wolters Kluwer Co., 1999.

[6821] Foster S, Tyler VE. Tyler's Honest Herbal: A Sensible Guide to the Use of Herbs and Related Remedies. 3rd ed., Binghamton, NY: Haworth Herbal Press, 1993.

[6822] Martindale W. Martindale the Extra Pharmacopoeia. Pharmaceutical Press, 1999.

[6823] McGuffin M, Hobbs C, Upton R, Goldberg A, eds. American Herbal Products Association's Botanical Safety Handbook. Boca Raton, FL: CRC Press, LLC 1997.

[6824] Sullivan JB Jr, Rumack BH, Thomas H Jr, et al. Pennyroyal oil poisoning and hepatotoxicity. *JAMA.* 1979;242:2873-4.

[6825] Anderson IB, Mullen WH, Meeker JE, et al. Pennyroyal toxicity: measurement of toxic metabolite levels in two cases and review of the literature. *Ann Intern Med.* 1996;124:726-34.

[6826] Allen WT. Note on a case of supposed poisoning by pennyroyal. *Lancet.* 1897;1(3841):1022-23.

[6827] Braithwaite PF. A case of poisoning by pennyroyal: recovery. *Br Med J.* 1906;2:865.

[6828] Girling J. Poisoning by pennyroyal. *Br Med J.* 1887;1:1214.

[6829] Buechel DW, Haverlah VC, Gardner ME. Pennyroyal oil ingestion: report of a case. *J Am Osteopath Assoc.* 1983;82:793-4.

[6830] Flynn EF. Poisoning by essence of pennyroyal. *Br Med J.* 1893;2:1270.

[6831] Sayyah M, Valizadeh J, Kamalinejad M. Anticonvulsant activity of the leaf oil of Laurus nobilis against pentylentetrazole- and maximal electroshock-induced seizure. *Phytomedicine.* 2002 Apr;9(3):212-16.

[6832] Culic M, Kekovic G, Grbic G, et al. Wavelet and fractal analysis of rat brain activity in seizures evoked by camphor oil and 1,8-cineole. *Gen Physiol Biophys.* 2009;28 Sec No:33-40.

[6833] Burkhard PR, Burkhardt K, Haenggeli CA, et al. Plant-induced seizures: reappearance of an old problem. *J Neurol.* 1999 Aug;246(8):667-70.

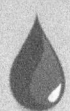

6834 Waldman N. Seizure caused by dermal application of over-the-counter eucalyptus oil head lice preparation. *Clin Toxicol (Phila)*. 2011 Oct;49(8):750-1.

6835 Craig JO. Poisoning by the volatile oils in childhood. *Arch Dis Child*. 1953;28:259-67.

6836 Mathew T, Kamath V, Kumar RS, et al. Eucalyptus oil inhalation-induced seizure: A novel, underrecognized, preventable cause of acute symptomatic seizure. *Epilepsia Open*. 2017 Jul 4;2(3):350-354.

6837 Sullivan JB Jr, Rumack BH, Thomas H Jr, et al. Pennyroyal oil poisoning and hepatotoxicity. *JAMA*. 1979;242:2873-4.

6838 Sudekum M, Poppenga RH, Raju N, et al. Pennyroyal oil toxicosis in a dog. *J Am Vet Med Assoc*. 1992;200:817-8.

6839 Anderson IB, Mullen WH, Meeker JE, et al. Pennyroyal toxicity: measurement of toxic metabolite levels in two cases and review of the literature. *Ann Intern Med*. 1996;124:726-34.

6840 Zimmerman HJ. Unconventional drugs. Miscellaneous drugs and diagnostic chemicals. In, Zimmerman, HJ. Hepatotoxicity: the adverse effects of drugs and other chemicals on the liver. 2nd ed. Philadelphia: Lippincott,1999: pp. 731-34.

6841 Seeff L, Stickel F, Navarro VJ. Hepatotoxicity of herbals and dietary supplements. In, Kaplowitz N, DeLeve LD, eds. Drug-induced liver disease. 3rd ed. Amsterdam: Elsevier, 2013, pp. 631-58.

6842 Moolla A. A phytochemical and pharmacological investigation of indigenous Agathosma species. MSc Dissertation, University of the Witwatersrand. 2006.

6843 Toroglu S. In-vitro antimicrobial activity and synergistic/antagonistic effect of interactions between antibiotics and some spice essential oils. *J Environ Biol*. 2011 Jan;32(1):23-9.

6844 Boukhebti H, Chaker AN, Belhadj H, et al. Chemical composition and antibacterial activity of Mentha pulegium L. and Mentha spicata L. essential oils. *Der Pharmacia Lettre*. 2011;3(4):267-75.

6845 Jazani NH, Ghasemnejad-Berenji H, Sadegpoor S. Antibacterial effects of Iranian Mentha pulegium essential oil on isolates of Klebsiella sp. *Pak J Biol Sci*. 2009 Jan 15;12(2):183-5.

6846 Mahboubi M, Haghi G. Antimicrobial activity and chemical composition of Mentha pulegium L. essential oil. *J Ethnopharmacol*. 2008 Sep 26;119(2):325-7.

6847 Ait-Ouazzou A, Loran S, Arakrak S, et al. Evaluation of the chemical composition and antimicrobial activity of Mentha pulegium, Juniperus phoenicea, and Cyperus longus essential oils from Morocco. *Food Res Int*. 2012 Jan;45(1):313-19.

6848 Toroglu S. In-vitro antimicrobial activity and synergistic/antagonistic effect of interactions between antibiotics and some spice essential oils. *J Environ Biol*. 2011 Jan;32(1):23-9.

6849 Silva N, Alves S, Gonçalves A, et al. Antimicrobial activity of essential oils from Mediterranean aromatic plants against several foodborne and spoilage bacteria. *Food Sci Technol Int*. 2013 Dec;19(6):503-10.

6850 Sarac N, Ugur A. The in vitro antimicrobial activities of the essential oils of some Lamiaceae species from Turkey. *J Med Food*. 2009 Aug;12(4):902-7.

6851 Bouchra C, Achouri M, Idrissi Hassani LM, et al. Chemical composition and antifungal activity of essential oils of seven Moroccan Labiatae against Botrytis cinerea Pers: Fr. *J Ethnopharmacol*. 2003 Nov;89(1):165-9.

6852 Koutrouanidou E, Kimbaris A, Kortsaris A, et al. Increased Seizure Latency and Decreased Severity of Pentylenetetrazol-Induced Seizures in Mice after Essential Oil Administration. *Epilepsy Res Treat*. 2013;2013:532657.

6853 Soares PM, de Freitas Pires A, de Souza EP, et al. Relaxant effects of the essential oil of Mentha pulegium L. in rat isolated trachea and urinary bladder. *J Pharm Pharmacol*. 2012 Dec;64(12):1777-84.

6854 Soares PM, Assreuy AM, Souza EP, et al. Inhibitory effects of the essential oil of Mentha pulegium on the isolated rat myometrium. *Planta Med*. 2005 Mar;71(3):214-8.

6855 Toloza AC, Zygadlo J, Cueto GM, et al. Fumigant and repellent properties of essential oils and component constituents against permethrin-resistant Pediculus humanus capitis (Anoplura: Pediculidae) from Argentina. *J Med Entomol*. 2006 Sep;43(5):889-95.

6856 Yang YC1, Lee HS, Clark JM, et al. Insecticidal activity of plant essential oils against Pediculus humanus capitis (Anoplura: Pediculidae). *J Med Entomol*. 2004 Jul;41(4):699-704.

6857 Maggiore MA, Albanese AA, Gende LB, et al. Anthelmintic effect of Mentha spp. essential oils on Echinococcus granulosus protoscoleces and metacestodes. *Parasitol Res*. 2012 Mar;110(3):1103-12.

6858 Kim JR, Haribalan P, Son BK, et al. Fumigant toxicity of plant essential oils against Camptomyia corticalis (Diptera: Cecidomyiidae). *J Econ Entomol*. 2012 Aug;105(4):1329-34.

6859 Zhang QH, Schneidmiller RG, Hoover DR. Essential oils and their compositions as spatial repellents for pestiferous social wasps. *Pest Manag Sci*. 2013 Apr;69(4):542-52.

6860 Han J, Choi BR, Lee SG, et al. Toxicity of plant essential oils to acaricide-susceptible and -resistant Tetranychus urticae (Acari: Tetranychidae) and Neoseiulus californicus (Acari: Phytoseiidae). *J Econ Entomol*. 2010 Aug;103(4):1293-8.

6861 Yi CG, Choi BR, Park HM, et al. Fumigant toxicity of plant essential oils to Thrips palmi (Thysanoptera: Thripidae) and Orius strigicollis (Heteroptera: Anthocoridae). *J Econ Entomol*. 2006 Oct;99(5):1733-8.

6862 Choi WI, Lee SG, Park HM, et al. Toxicity of plant essential oils to Tetranychus urticae (Acari: Tetranychidae) and Phytoseiulus persimilis (Acari: Phytoseiidae). *J Econ Entomol*. 2004 Apr;97(2):553-8.

6863 Rutledge LC, Lawson MA, Young LL. Tests of repellents against Diamanus montanus (Siphonaptera: Ceratophyllidae). *J Med Entomol*. 1982 Jul 28;19(4):361-5.

6864 Choi WI, Lee EH, Choi BR, et al. Toxicity of plant essential oils to Trialeurodes vaporariorum (Homoptera: Aleyrodidae). *J Econ Entomol*. 2003 Oct;96(5):1479-84.

6865 Rim IS, Jee CH. Acaricidal effects of herb essential oils against Dermatophagoides farinae and D. pteronyssinus (Acari: Pyroglyphidae) and qualitative analysis of a herb Mentha pulegium(pennyroyal). *Korean J Parasitol*. 2006 Jun;44(2):133-8.

6866 Santana-Méridas O, González-Coloma A, Fe Andrés M, et al. Biocidal compounds from Mentha sp essential oils and their structure-activity relationships. *Chem Biodivers*. 2017 Mar;14(3).

6867 Vieira M, Bessa LJ, Martins MR, et al. Chemical Composition, Antibacterial, Antibiofilm and Synergistic Properties of Essential Oils from Eucalyptus globulus Labill. and Seven Mediterranean Aromatic Plants. *Chem Biodivers*. 2017 Jun;14(6).

6868 Bouyahya A, Et-Touys A, Bakri Y, et al. Chemical composition of Mentha pulegium and Rosmarinus officinalis essential oils and their antileishmanial, antibacterial and antioxidant activities. *Microb Pathog*. 2017 Aug 15;111:41-49.

6869 Ebadollahi A, Davari M, Razmjou J, et al. Separate and Combined Effects of Mentha piperata and Mentha pulegium Essential Oils and a Pathogenic Fungus Lecanicillium muscarium Against Aphis gossypii (Hemiptera: Aphididae). *J Econ Entomol*. 2017 Jun 1;110(3):1025-1030.

6870 Kavetsou E, Koutsoukos S, Daferera D, et al. Encapsulation of Mentha pulegium Essential Oil in Yeast Cell Microcarriers: An Approach to Environmentally Friendly Pesticides. *J Agric Food Chem*. 2019 May 1;67(17):4746-4753.

6871 Piras A, Porcedda S, Falconieri D, et al. Antifungal activity of essential oil from Mentha spicata L. and Mentha pulegium L. growing wild in Sardinia island (Italy). *Nat Prod Res*. 2019 Jul 19:1-7.

6872 Uzair B, Niaz N, Bano A, et al. Essential oils showing in vitro anti MRSA and synergistic activity with penicillin group of antibiotics. *Pak J Pharm Sci*. 2017 Sep;30(5(Supplementary)):1997-2002.

6873 Stepanycheva E, Petrova M, Chermensjaya T, et al. Fumigant Effect of Essential Oils on Mortality and Fertility of Thrips Frankliniella Occidentalis Perg. *Environ Sci Pollut Res Int*. 2019 Oct;26(30):30885-30892.

6874 Cheraif K, Bakchiche B, Gherib A, et al. Chemical Composition, Antioxidant, Anti-Tyrosinase, Anti-Cholinesterase and Cytotoxic Activities of Essential Oils of Six Algerian Plants. *Molecules*. 2020 Apr 8;25(7):1710.

6875 Sebai SE, Abidi A, Serairi R, et al. Essential oil of Mentha pulegium induces anthelmintic effects and reduces parasite-associated oxidative stress in rodent model. *Exp Parasitol*. 2021 Apr 1;225:108105.

6876 Ed-Dra A, Filali FR, Lo Presti V, et al. Chemical composition, antioxidant capacity and antibacterial action of five Moroccan essential oils against Listeria monocytogenes and different serotypes of Salmonella enterica. *Microb Pathog*. 2020 Dec;149:104510.

6877 De Albuqyerque Lima T, de Queiroz Baptista NM, de Oliveira APS, et al. Insecticidal activity of a chemotype VI essential oil from Lippia alba leaves collected at Caatinga and the major compound (1,8-cineole) against Nasutitermes corniger and Sitophilus zeamais. *Pestic Biochem Physiol*. 2021 Aug;177:104901.

6878 Messaoudi M, Rebiai A, Sawicka B, et al. Effect of Extraction Methods on Polyphenols, Flavonoids, Mineral Elements, and Biological Activities of Essential Oil and Extracts of Mentha pulegium L. *Molecules*. 2021 Dec 21;27(1):11.

6879 Alimi D, Hajri A, Jallouli S, et al. Phytochemistry, anti-tick, repellency and anti-cholinesterase activities of Cupressus sempervirens L. and Mentha pulegium L. combinations against Hyalomma scupense (Acari: Ixodidae). *Vet Parasitol*. 2022 Jan 31;303:109665.

6880 Aouadhi C, Jouini A, Mechichi D, et al. Characterization of Primary Action Mode of Eight Essential Oils and Evaluation of Their Antibacterial Effect against Extended-Spectrum β-Lactamase (ESBL)-Producing Escherichia coli Inoculated in Turkey Meat. *Molecules*. 2022 Apr 18;27(8):2588.

6881 Ramzi A, El Ouali Lalami A, Ez Zoubi Y, et al. Insecticidal Effect of Wild-Grown Mentha pulegium and Rosmarinus officinalis Essential Oils and Their Main Monoterpenes against Culex pipiens (Diptera: Culicidae). *Plants (Basel)*. 2022 Apr 28;11(9):1193.

6882 Fazal H, Akram M, Ahmad N, et al. Nutritionally rich biochemical profile in essential oil of various Mentha species and their antimicrobial activities. *Protoplasma*. 2022 Aug 9. Online ahead of print.

6883 Assouguem A, Kara M, Ramzi A, et al. Evaluation of the Effect of Four Bioactive Compounds in Combination with Chemical Product against Two Spider Mites Tetranychus urticae and Eutetranychus orientalis(Acari: Tetranychidae). *Evid Based Complement Alternat Med*. 2022 Aug 22;2022:2004623.

6884 Coimbra A, Miguel S, Ribeiro M, et al. Chemical composition, antioxidant, and antimicrobial activities of six commercial essential oils. *Lett Appl Microbiol*. 2023 Jan 23;76(1):ovac042.

6885 Azadi S, Osanloo M, Zarenezhad E, et al. Nano-scaled emulsion and nanogel containing Mentha pulegium essential oil: cytotoxicity on human melanoma cells and effects on apoptosis regulator genes. *BMC Complement Med Ther*. 2023 Jan 9;23(1):6.

6886 Saharkhiz MJ, Motamedi M, Zomorodian K, et al. Chemical composition, antifungal and antibiofilm activities of the essential oil of Mentha piperita L. *ISRN Pharm*. 2012;2012:718645.

6887 Bassole IHN, Lamien-Meda A, Bayala B, et al. Composition and antimicrobial activities of Lippia multiflora Moldenke, Mentha x piperita L. and Ocimum basilicum L. essential oils and their major monoterpene alcohols alone and in combination. *Molecules*. 2010;15:7825-39.

6888 Sokovic MD, Vukojevic J, Marin PD, et al. Chemical composition of essential oils of Thymus and Mentha species and tier antifungal activities. *Molecules*. 209;14:238-49.

6889 Moghaddam M, Pourbaige M, Tabar HK, et al. Composition and antifungal activity of peppermint (Mentha piperita) essential oil from Iran. *J Essent Oil Bearing Plants*. 2013;16(4):506-12.

6890 Grulova D, De Martino L, Mancini E, et al. Seasonal variability of the main components in essential oil of Mentha x piperita L. *J Sc Food Agric*. 2015 Feb;95(3):621-27.

6891 Verma RS, Rahman L, Verma RK, et al. Essential Oil Composition of Menthol Mint (Mentha arvensis) and Peppermint (Mentha piperita) Cultivars at Different Stages of Plant Growth from Kumaon Region of Western Himalaya. *J Medicinal Aromatic Plants*. 2010;1(1):13-18.

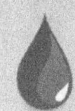

6892 Boren KE, Young DG, Woolley CL, et al. Detecting essential oil adulteration. *J Environ Anal Chem.* 2015;2(2):1-3.
6893 Melis K. Bochner A, Janssens G. Accidental nasal eucalyptol and menthol instillation. *Eur J Pediatr.* 1989 Aug;148(8)786-7.
6894 Reynolds JEF. Martindale: The Extra Pharmacopoeia. *The Pharmaceutical Press, London.* 1993.
6895 No author listed. Monographs on the medicinal uses of plants. *Exeter: European Scientific Cooperative on Phytotherapy.* 1997.
6896 Javorka K, Tomori Z, Zavarska L. Protective and defensive airway reflexes in premature infants. *Physiol Bohemoslov.* 1980;29(1):29-35.
6897 Olowe SA, Ransome-Kuti O. The risk of jaundice in glucose-6-phosphate dehydrogenase deficient babies exposed to menthol. *Acta Paediatr Scand.* 1980 May;69(3):341-5.
6898 Dillon Remy M, Manning Alleyne P, Bratt DE, et al. Neonatal jaundice at Port-of-Spain General Hospital abstract. *West Indian Med J.* 1987;36(Suppl):28.
6899 Gelal A, Jacob P III, Yu L, et al. Disposition kinetics and effects of menthol. *Clin Phramacol Ther.* 1999 Aug;66(2):128-35.
6900 Akdogan M, Gultekin F, Yontem M. Effect of Mentha piperita (Labiatae) and Mentha spicata (Labiatae) on iron absorption in rats. *Toxicol Ind Health.* 2004 Sep;20(6-10):119-22.
6901 Wacher VJ, Wong S, Wong HT. Peppermint oil enhances cyclosporine oral bioavailability in rats: comparison with D-alpha-tocopheryl poly(ethylene glycol 1000) succinate (TPGS) and ketoconazole. *J Pharm Sci.* 2002 Jan;91(1):77-90.
6902 Wacher VJ, Wong S, Wong HT. Peppermint oil enhances cyclosporine oral bioavailability in rats: comparison with D-alpha-tocopheryl poly(ethylene glycol 1000) succinate (TPGS) and ketoconazole. *J Pharm Sci.* 2002 Jan;91(1):77-90.
6903 Samojlik I, Petkovic S, Mimica-Dukic N, et al. Acute and chronic pretreatment with essential oil of peppermint (Mentha X piperita L., Lamiaceae) influences drug effects. *Phytother Res.* 2012 Jun;26(6):820-5.
6904 Samojlik I, Petkovic S, Mimica-Dukic N, et al. Acute and chronic pretreatment with essential oil of peppermint (Mentha X piperita L., Lamiaceae) influences drug effects. *Phytother Res.* 2012 Jun;26(6):820-5.
6905 Abdullah D, Ping QN, Liu GJ. Enhancing effect of essential oils on the penetration of 5-fluorouracil through rat skin. *Yao Xue Xue Bao [Acta Pharm Sinica].* 1996;31(3):214-221.
6906 Schelz Z, Molnar, Hohmann J. Antimicrobial and antiplasmid activates of essential oils. *Fitoterapia.* 2006 Jun;77(4):279-85.
6907 Toroglu S. In-vitro antimicrobial activity and synergistic/antagonistic effect of interactions between antibiotics and some spice essential oils. *J Environ Biol.* 2011 Jan;32(1):23-9.
6908 Valente JS, Fonseca AO1, Denardi LB, et al. In vitro activity of antifungals in combination with essential oils against the oomycete Pythium insidiosum. *J Appl Microbiol.* 2016 Oct;121(4):998-1003.
6909 Dresser GK, Wacher V, Wong S, et al. Evaluation of peppermint oil and ascorbyl palmitate as inhibitors of cytochrome P4503A4 activity in vitro and in vivo. *Clin Pharmacol Ther.* 2002 Sep;72(3):247-55.
6910 Murayama M, Kumaroo KK. Inhibitors of ex vivo aggregation of human platelets induced by decompression, during reduced barometric pressure. *Thromb Res.* 1986 May 15;42(4):511-6.
6911 Unger M, Frank A. Simultaneous determination of the inhibitory potency of herbal extracts on the activity of six major cytochrome P450 enzymes using liquid chromatography/mass spectrometry and automated online extraction. *Rapid Commun Mass Spectrom.* 2004;18(19):2273-81.
6912 Hoshino M, Ikarashi N, Hirobe R, et al. Effects of menthol on the pharmacokinetics of triazolam and phenytoin. *Biol Pharm Bull.* 2015;38(3):454-60.
6913 Hoshino M, Ikarashi N, Tsukui M, et al. Menthol reduces the anticoagulant effect of warfarin by inducing cytochrome P450 2C expression. *Eur J Pharm Sci.* 2014 Jun 2;56:92-101.
6914 Gelal A, Guven H, Balkan D, et al. Influence of menthol on caffeine disposition and pharmacodynamics in healthy female volunteers. *Eur J Clin Pharmacol.* 2003 Sep;59(5-6):417-22.
6915 Inamori M, Akiyama T, Akimoto K, et al. Early effects of peppermint oil on gastric emptying: a crossover study using a continuous real0time 13C breath test (BreathID system). *J Gastroenterol.* 2007 Jul;42(7):539-42.
6916 Kligler B, Chaudhary S. Peppermint oil. *Am Fam Physician.* 2007 Apr 1;75(7):1027-30.
6917 Thomassed D, Slattery JT, Nelson SD. Contribution of menthofuran to the hepatotoxicity of pulegone: assessment based on matched area under the curve and on matched time course. *J Pharmacol Exp Ther.* 1988 Mar;244(3):825-29.
6918 Gordon WP, Forte AJ, McMurtry RJ, et al. Hepatotoxicity and pulmonary toxicity of pennyroyal oil and its constituent terpenes in the mouse. *Toxicol Appl Pharmacol.* 1982;65:413-24.
6919 Carratu B, Federici E, Gallo FR, et al. Plants and parts of plants used in food supplements: an approach to their safety assessment. *Ann Ist Super Sanita.* 2010 Oct-Dec;46(4):0021-2571.
6920 Thorup I, Wurtzen G, Carstensen J, et al. Short term toxicity study in rats dosed with pulegone and menthol. *Toxicol Lett.* 1983 Dec;19(3):207-10.
6921 Madsen C, Wurtzen G, Carstensen J. Short-term toxicity study in rats dosed with menthone. *Toxicol Lett.* 1986 Jul- Aug;32(1-2):147-52.
6922 Eickolt TH, Box RH. Toxicities of peppermint and Pycnanthemun albescens oils, fam Labiateae. *J Pharm Sci.* 1965;54:1071-72.
6923 Nair B, Final report on the safety assessment of Mentha piperita (Peppermint) oil, Mentha piperita (Peppermint) leaf extract, Mentha piperita (Peppermint) leaf, and Mentha piperita (Peppermint) leaf water. *Int J Toxicol.*2001;20 Suppl 3:61-73.
6924 Liu JH, Chen GH, Yeh HZ, et al. Enteric-coated peppermint-oil capsules in the treatment of irritable bowel syndrome: a prospective, randomized trial. *J Gastroenterol.* 1997;32:765-68.
6925 Asao T, Mochiki E, Suzuki H, et al. An easy method for the intraluminal administration of peppermint oil before colonoscopy and its effectiveness in reducing colon spasms. *Gastrointest Endosc.* 2001 Feb;53(2):172-77.
6926 Sun Z, Wang H, Wang J, et al. Chemical composition and anti-inflammatory, cytotoxic and antioxidant activities of essential oil from leaves of Mentha piperita grown in China. *PloS One.* 2014 Dec 10;9(12):e114767.
6927 Thompson A, Meah D, Ahmed N, et al. Comparison of the antibacterial activity of essential oils and extracts of medicinal and culinary herbs to investigate potential new treatments for irritable bowel syndrome. *BMC Complement Altern Med.* 2013 Nov;13:338.
6928 Sharafi SM, Rasooli I, Owlia P, et al. Protective effects of bioactive phytochemicals from Mentha piperita with multiple health potentials. *Pharmacogn Mag.* 2010 Jul;6(23):147-53.
6929 Seo HS, Beuchat LR, Kim H, et al. Development of an experimental apparatus and protocol for determining antimicrobial activities of gaseous plant essential oils. *Int J Food Microbiol.* 2015 Dec 23;215:95-100.
6930 Amato A, Liotta R, Mule F. Effects of menthol on circular smooth muscle of human colon: analysis of the mechanism of action. *Eur J Pharmacol.* 2014 Oct 5;740:295-301.
6931 Grundmann O, Yoon SL. Complementary and alternative medicines in irritable bowel syndrome: an integrative view. *World J Gastroenterol.* 2014 Jan;20(2):346-62.
6932 Khanna R, MacDonald JK, Levensque BG. Peppermint oil for the treatment of irritable bowel syndrome: a systematic review and meta-analysis. *J Clin Gasteroenterol.* 2014 Jul;48(6):505-12.
6933 Kline RM, Kline JJ, Di Palma J, et al. Enteric-coated, pH-dependent peppermint oil capsules for the treatment of irritable bowel syndrome in children. *J Pediatr.* 2001;138:125-28.
6934 Dew MJ, Evans BK, Rhodes J. Peppermint oil for the irritable bowel syndrome: a multicentre trial. *Br J Clin Pract.* 1984;38:394-98.
6935 Merat S, Khalili S, Mostajabi P, et al. The effect of enteric-coated, delayed-release peppermint oil on irritable bowel syndrome. *Dig Dis Sci.* 201 May;55(5):1385-90.
6936 Lua PL, Zakaria NS. A brief review of current scientific evidence involving aromatherapy use for nausea and vomiting. *J Altern Complement Med.* 2012 Jun;18(6):534-40.
6937 Stea S, Beraudi A, De Pasquale D. Essential oils for complementary treatment of surgical patients: state of the art. *Evid Based Complement Altern Med.* 2014;2014:726341.
6938 Hunt R, Dienemann J, Norton HJ, et al. Aromatherapy as treatment for postoperative nausea: a randomized trial. *Anesth Analg.* 2013 Sep;117(3):597-604.
6939 Wright CE, Laude EA, Grattan TJ, et al. Capsaicin and neurokinin A-induced bronchoconstriction in the anaesthetized guinea-pig: evidence for a direct action of menthol on isolated bronchial smooth muscle. *Br J Pharmacol.* 1997 Aug;121(8):1645-50.
6940 Meamarbashi A, Rajabi A. The effects of peppermint on exercise performance. *J Int Sci Sports Nutr.* 2013 Mar 21;10(1):15.
6941 Schumacher A, Reichling J, Schnitzler P. Virucidal effect of peppermint oil on the enveloped viruses herpes simplex virus type 1 and type 2 in vitro. *Phytomedicine.* 2003;10:504-10.
6942 Schnitzler P, Reichling J. Efficacy of plant products against herpetic infections. *HNO.* 2011 Dec;59(12):1176-84.
6943 Romero MC, Navarro MC, Martin-Sanchez J, et al. Peppermint (Mentha piperita) and albendazole anisakiasis in an animal model. *Trop Med Int Health.* 2014 Dec;19(12):1430-36.
6944 Varney E, Buckle J. Effect of inhaled essential oils on mental exhaustion and moderate burnout: a small pilot study. *J Altern Complement Med.* 2013;19(1):69-71.
6945 Kang HY, Na SS, Kim YK. Effects of oral care with essential oil on improvement in oral health status of hospice patients. *J Korean Acad Nurs.*2010 Aug;40(4):473-81.
6946 Barker S, Grayhem P, Koon J, et al. Improved performance on clerical tasks associated with administration of peppermint odor. *Percept Mot Skills.* 2003 Dec;97(3 Pt 1):1007-10.
6947 Kim MJ, Nam ES, Paik SI. The effects of aromatherapy in pain, depression, and life satisfaction of arthritis patients. *Taehan Kanho Hakhoe Chi.* 2005 Feb;35(1):186-94.
6948 Kim MA, Sakong JK, Kim EJ, et al. Effect of aromatherapy massage for the relief of constipation in the elderly. *Taehan Kanho Hakhoe Chi.* 2005 Feb;35(1):56-64.
6949 Duarte MC, Figueira GM, Sartoratto A, et al. Anti-Candida activity of Brazilian medicinal plants. *J Ethnopharmacol.* 2005 Feb 28;97(2):305-11.
6950 Tampieri MP, Galuppi R, Macchioni F, et al. The inhibition of Candida albicans by selected essential oils and their major components. *Mycopathologia.*2005 Apr;159(3):339-45.
6951 Rachitha P, Krupashree K, Jayashree GV, et al. Growth Inhibition and Morphological Alteration of Fusarium sporotrichioides by Mentha piperita Essential Oil. *Pharmacognosy Res.* 2017 Jan-Mar;9(1):74-79.
6952 Uniyal V, Saxena S, Bhatt RP. Screening of some essential oils against Trichosporon species. *J Environ Biol.*2015 Jan;34(1):17-22.
6953 Fonseca AO, Pereira DI, Jacob RG, et al. In vitro susceptibility of Brazilian Pythium insidiosum isolates to essential oils of some Lamiaceae family. *Mycopathologia.* 2015 Jan;179:253-8.
6954 Sivamani P, Singaravelu G, Thiagarajan V, et al. Comparative molecular docking analysis of essential oil constituents as elastase inhibitors. *Bioinformation.* 2012;8(10):457-60.
6955 Koutroumanidou E, Kimbaris A, Kortsaris A, et al. Increased seizure latency and decreased severity of pentylenetetrazol-induced seizures in mice after essential oil administration. *Epilepsy Res Treat.* 2013;2013:532657.
6956 Kumar S, Wahab N, Warikoo R. Bioefficacy of Mentha piperita essential oil against dengue fever mosquito Aedes aegypti L. *Asian Pac J Trop Biomed.* 2011 Apr;1(2):85-88.
6957 Warikoo R, Wahab N, Kumar S. Oviposition-altering and ovicidal potentials of five essential oils against female adults of the dengue vector, Aedes aegypti L. *Parasitol Res.* 2011 Oct;109(4):1125-31.
6958 Tayarani-Najaran Z, Talasaz-Firoozi E, Nasiri R, et al. Antiemetic activity of volatile oil from Mentha spicata and Mentha x piperita in chemotherapy-induced nausea and vomiting. *Ecancermedicalscience.* 2013;7:290.
6959 Herro E, Jacob SE. Mentha piperita (peppermint). *Dematitis.* 2010 Nov-Dec;21(6):327-29.
6960 Sharafi SM, Rasooli I, Owlia P, et al. Protective effects of bioactive phytochemicals from Mentha piperita with multiple health potentials. *Pharmacogn Mag.* 2010 Jul;6(23):147-53.
6961 Schmidt E, Bail S, Buchbauer G, et al. Chemical composition, olfactory evaluation and antioxidant effects of essential oil from Mentha x piperita. *Nat Prod Commun.* 2009 Aug;4(8):1107-12.
6962 Mimica-Dukic N, Bozin B, Sokovic M, et al. Antimicrobial and antioxidant activities of three Mentha species essential oils. *Planta Med.* 2003 May;69(5):413-19.
6963 De Sousa AA, Soares PM, de Almeida AN, et al. Antispasmodic effect of Mentha piperita essential oil on tracheal smooth muscle of rats. *J Ethnopharmacol.* 2010 Jul 20;130(2):433-36.

[6964] Rakover Y, Ben-Arye E, Goldstein LH. The treatment of respiratory ailments with essential oils of some aromatic medicinal plants. *Harefuah*. 2008 Oct;147(10):783-88.

[6965] Inouye S, Yamaguchi H, Takizawa. Screening of the antibacterial effects of a variety of essential oils on respiratory tract pathogens, using a modified dilution assay method. *J Infect Chemother*. 201 Dec;7(4):251-54.

[6966] Rasooli I, Shayegh S, Taghizadeh M, et al. Phytotherapeutic prevention of dental biofilm formation. *Phytother Res*. 2008 Sep;22(9):1162-67.

[6967] Shayegh S, Rasooli I, Taghizadeh M, et al. Phytotherapeutic inhibition of supragingival dental plaque. *Nat Prod Res*. 2008 Mar 20;22(5):428-39.

[6968] Inouye S, Yamaguchi H, Takizawa. Screening of the antibacterial effects of a variety of essential oils on respiratory tract pathogens, using a modified dilution assay method. *J Infect Chemother*. 201 Dec;7(4):251-54.

[6969] Moss M, Hewitt S, Moss L, et al. Modulation of cognitive performance and mood by aromas of peppermint and ylang ylang. *Int J Neurosci*. 2008 Jan;118(1):59-77

[6970] Shavakhi A, Ardenstani SK, Taki M, et al. Premedication with peppermint oil capsules in colonoscopy: a double blind placebo controlled randomized trial study. *Acta Gastroenterol Belq*. 2012 Sep;75(3):349-53.

[6971] Hiki N, Kaminishi M, Yasuda K, et al. Multicenter phase II randomized study evaluating dose-response of antiperistaltic effect of L-menthol sprayed onto gastric mucosa for upper gastrointestinal endoscopy. *Giq Endosc*.2012 Mar;24(2):79-86.

[6972] Sparks MJ, O'Sullivan P, Herrington AA, et al. Does peppermint oil relieve spasm during barium enema? *Br J Radiol*.1995 Aug;68(812):841-43.

[6973] Hur MH, Park J, Maddock-Jennings W, et al. Reduction of mouth malodour and volatile sulphur constituents in intensive care patients using an essential oil mouthwash. *Phytother Res*. 2007 Jul;21(7):641-43.

[6974] Shkurupii VA, Odintsova OA, Kazarinova NV, et al. Use of essential oil of peppermint (Mentha piperita) in complex treatment of patients with infiltrative pulmonary tuberculosis. *Probl Tuberk Bolezn Leqk*.2006;(9):43-45.

[6975] Shkurupii VA, Kazarinova NV, Ogirenko AP, et al. Efficiency of the use of peppermint (Mentha piperita L) essential oil inhalation in the combined multi-drug therapy for pulmonary tuberculosis. *Probl Tuberk*. 2002;(4):36-39.

[6976] Kaur CD, Saraf S. In vitro sun protection factor determination of herbal oils used in cosmetics. *Pharmacognosy Res*. 2010 Jan;2(1):22-25.

[6977] Goerg KJ, Spilker T. Effect of peppermint oil and caraway oil on gastrointestinal motility in healthy volunteers: a pharmacodynamic study using simultaneous determination of gastric and gall-bladder emptying and orocaecal transit time. *Ailment Pharmacol Ther*. 2003 Feb;17(3):445-51.

[6978] Wang LH, Wang CC, Kuo SC. Vehicle and enhancer effects of human skin penetration of aminophylline from cream formulations: evaluation in vivo. *J Cosmet Sci*. 2007 May-Jun;58(3):245-54.

[6979] Nielsen JB. Natural oils affect the human skin integrity and the percutaneous penetration of benzoic acid dose dependently. *Basic Clin Pharmacol Toxicol*. 2006 Jun;98(6):575-81.

[6980] Inouye S, Uchida K, Nishiyama Y, et al. Combined effect of heat, essential oils and salt on fungicidal activity against Trichophyton mentagrophytes in a foot bath. *Nihon Ishinjin Gakkai Zasshi*.2007;48(1):27-36.

[6981] Schelz Z, Molnar, Hohmann J. Antimicrobial and antiplasmid activates of essential oils. *Fitoterapia*. 2006 Jun;77(4):279-85.

[6982] Adam B, Liebregts T, Best J, et al. A combination of peppermint oil and caraway oil attenuates the post-inflammatory visceral hyperalgesia in a rat model. *Scand J Gastroenterol*. 2006 Feb;41(2):155-60.

[6983] Norrish MI, Dwyer KL. Preliminary investigation of the effect of peppermint oil on an objective measure of daytime sleepiness. *Int J Psychophysiol*. 2005 Mar;55(3):291-98.

[6984] Gobel H, Schmidt G, Dworschak M, et al. Essential plant oils and headache mechanism. *Phytomedicine*. 1995 Oct;2(2):93-12.

[6985] Oh JY, Park MA, Kim YC. Peppermint Oil Promotes Hair Growth without Toxic Signs. *Toxicol Res*. 2014 Dec;30(4):297-304.

[6986] Ergüden C, Özkoç S, Öztürk B, et al. [Investigation of the in vitro effects of Melissa officinalis L., Mentha x piperita L. and Ocimum basilicum L. (Lamiaceae) essential oils on the cysts and trophozoites of Acanthamoeba castellani]. *Mikrobiyol Bul*. 2016 Oct;50(4):569-579.

[6987] de Sousa Guedes JP, da Costa Medeiros JA, de Souza E Silva RS, et al. The efficacy of Mentha arvensis L. and M. piperita L. essential oils in reducing pathogenic bacteria and maintaining quality characteristics in cashew, guava, mango, and pineapple juices. *Int J Food Microbiol*. 2016 Dec 5;238:183-192.

[6988] Cwikla C, Schmidt K, Matthias A, et al. Investigation into the antibacterial activities of phytotherapeutics against Helicobacter pylori and Campylobacter jejuni. *Phytother Res*. 2010 May;24(5):649-56.

[6989] Sharififard M, Safdari F, Siahpoush A, et al. Evaluation of Some Plant Essential Oils against the Brown-Banded Cockroach, Supella longipalpa (Blattaria: Ectobiidae): A Mechanical Vector of Human Pathogens. *J Arthropod Borne Dis*. 2016 Oct 4;10(4):528-537.

[6990] Lalthazuali, Mathew N. Mosquito repellent activity of volatile oils from selected aromatic plants. *Parasitol Res*. 2017 Feb;116(2):821-825.

[6991] Masoumi SZ, Asl HR, Poorolajal J, et al. Evaluation of mint efficacy regarding dysmenorrhea in comparison with mefenamic acid: A double blinded randomized crossover study. *Iran J Nurs Midwifery Res*. 2016 Jul-Aug;21(4):363-7.

[6992] de Souza Silveira Valente J, de Oliveira da Silva Fonseca A, Denardi LB, et al. In Vitro Susceptibility of Pythium insidiosum to Melaleuca alternifolia, Mentha piperita and Origanum vulgare Essential Oils Combinations. *Mycopathologia*. 2016 Aug;181(7-8):617-22.

[6993] Marwa C, Fikri-Benbrahim K, Ou-Yahia D, et al. African peppermint (Mentha piperita) from Morocco: Chemical composition and antimicrobial properties of essential oil. *J Adv Pharm Technol Res*. 2017 Jul-Sep;8(3):86-90.

[6994] Talei GR, Mohammadi M, Bahmani M, et al. Synergistic effect of Carum copticum and Mentha piperita essential oils with ciprofloxacin, vancomycin, and gentamicin on Gram-negative and Gram-positive bacteria. *Int J Pharm Investig*. 2017 Apr-Jun;7(2):82-87.

[6995] Ebadollahi A, Davari M, Razmjou J, et al. Separate and Combined Effects of Mentha piperata and Mentha pulegium Essential Oils and a Pathogenic Fungus Lecanicillium muscarium Against Aphis gossypii (Hemiptera: Aphididae). *J Econ Entomol*. 2017 Jun 1;110(3):1025-1030.

[6996] Vendan SE, Manivannan S, Sunny AM, et al. Phytochemical residue profiles in rice grains fumigated with essential oils for the control of rice weevil. *PLoS One*. 2017 Oct 12;12(10):e0186020.

[6997] Chauhan N, Malik A, Sharma S, et al. Repellency potential of essential oils against housefly, Musca domestica L. *Environ Sci Pollut Res Int*. 2018 Feb;25(5):4707-4714.

[6998] Wiwattanaratanabut K, choonharuangdej S, Srithava T. In Vitro Anti-Cariogenic Plaque Effects of Essential Oils Extracted from Culinary Herbs. *J Clin Diagnostic Res*. 2017 Sep;11(9):DC30-5.

[6999] Bellassoued K, Ben Hsouna A, Athmouni K, et al. Protective effects of Mentha piperita L. leaf essential oil against CCl4 induced hepatic oxidative damage and renal failure in rats. *Lipids Health Dis*. 2018 Jan 9;17(1):9.

[7000] Ogaly HA, Eltablawy NA, Abd-Elsalam RM. Antifibrogenic Influence of Mentha piperita L. Essential Oil against CCl4-Induced Liver Fibrosis in Rats. *Oxid Med Cell Longev*. 2018 Apr 19;2018:4039753.

[7001] Rosato A, Carocci A, Catalano A, et al. Elucidation of the synergistic action of Mentha Piperita essential oil with common antimicrobials. *PLoS One*. 2018 Aug 1;13(8):e0200902.

[7002] Modarresi M, Farahpour MR, Baradaran B, et al. Topical application of Mentha piperita essential oil accelerates wound healing in infected mice model. *Inflammopharmacology*. 2019 Jun;27(3):531-537.

[7003] Vasireddy L, Bingle LEH, Davies MS. Antimicrobial activity of essential oils against multidrug-resistant clinical isolates of the Burkholderia cepacia complex. *PLoS One*. 2018 Aug 2;13(8):e0201835.

[7004] Kennedy D, Okello E, Chazot P, et al. Volatile Terpenes and Brain Function: Investigation of the Cognitive and Mood Effects of Mentha × Piperita L. Essential Oil with In Vitro Properties Relevant to Central Nervous System Function. *Nutrients*. 2018 Aug 7;10(8).

[7005] de Sousa Guedes JP, de Souza EL. Investigation of damage to Escherichia coli, Listeria monocytogenes and Salmonella Enteritidis exposed to Mentha arvensis L. and M. piperita L. essential oils in pineapple and mango juice by flow cytometry. *Food Microbiol*. 2018 Dec;76:564-571.

[7006] Abdolshahi A, Naybandi-Atashi S, Heydari-Majd M, et al. Antibacterial activity of some Lamiaceae species against Staphylococcus aureus in yoghurt-based drink (Doogh). *Cell Mol Biol (Noisy-le-grand)*. 2018 Jun 25;64(8):71-77.

[7007] Štefanidesová K, Špitalská E, Csicsay F, et al. Evaluation of the possible use of genus Mentha derived essential oils in the prevention of SENLAT syndrome caused by Rickettsia slovaca. *J Ethnopharmacol*. 2018 Dec 6;232:55-61.

[7008] Mafakheri H, Mirghazanfari SM. Antifungal activity of the essential oils of some medicinal plants against human and plant fungal pathogens. *Cell Mol Biol (Noisy-le-grand)*. 2018 Dec 31;64(15):13-19.

[7009] Benzaid C, Belmadani A, Djeribi R, et al. The Effects of Mentha × piperita Essential Oil on C. albicans Growth, Transition, Biofilm Formation, and the Expression of Secreted Aspartyl Proteinases Genes. *Antibiotics (Basel)*. 2019 Jan 30;8(1).

[7010] Rajkumar V, Gunasekaran C, Christy IK, et al. Toxicity, antifeedant and biochemical efficacy of Mentha piperita L. essential oil and their major constituents against stored grain pest. *Pestic Biochem Physiol*. 2019 May;156:138-144.

[7011] Kovács JK, Felsö P, Horváth G, et al. Stress Response and Virulence Potential Modulating Effect of Peppermint Essential Oil in Campylobacter jejuni. *Biomed Res Int*. 2019 Jan 3;2019:2971741.

[7012] Ashrafi B, Rashidipour M, Marzban A, et al. Mentha piperita essential oils loaded in a chitosan nanogel with inhibitory effect on biofilm formation against S. mutans on the dental surface. *Carbohydr Polym*. 2019 May 15;212:142-149.

[7013] Mandava K, Batchu UR, Kakulavaram S, et al. Design and study of anticaries effect of different medicinal plants against S.mutans glucosyltransferase. *BMC Complement Altern Med*. 2019 Aug 2;19(1):197.

[7014] Tullio V, Roana J, Scalas D, et al. Evaluation of the Antifungal Activity of Mentha x piperita (Lamiaceae) of Pancalieri (Turin, Italy) Essential Oil and Its Synergistic Interaction with Azoles. *Molecules*. 2019 Aug 29;24(17).

[7015] Rafieian-Kopaei M, Hasanpour AH, Lorigooini Z, et al. Comparing the Effect of Intranasal Lidocaine 4% With Peppermint Essential Oil Drop 1.5% on Migraine Attacks: A Double-Blind Clinical Trial. *Int J Prev Med*. 2019 Jul 5;10:121.

[7016] Pang X, Feng YX, Qi XJ, et al. Toxicity and Repellent Activity of Essential Oil From Mentha Piperita Linn. Leaves and Its Major Monoterpenoids Against Three Stored Product Insects. *Environ Sci Pollut Res Int*. 2020 Mar;27(7):7618-7627.

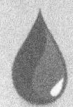

7017 Heydari M, Amirjani A, Bagheri M, et al. Eco-friendly Pesticide Based on Peppermint Oil Nanoemulsion: Preparation, Physicochemical Properties, and Its Aphicidal Activity Against Cotton Aphid. *Environ Sci Pollut Res Int*. 2020 Feb;27(6):6667-6679.

7018 Ahmadi Y, Rezaei J, Rezaei M, et al. Comparison of the Effect of Inhalation Aromatherapy with 10% and 30% Peppermint Essential Oils on the Severity of Nausea in Abdominal Surgery Patients. *Evid Based Complement Alternat Med*. 2020 Apr 20;2020:5897465.

7019 Pavlic B, Teslic N, Zengin G, et al. Antioxidant and enzyme-inhibitory activity of peppermint extracts and essential oils obtained by conventional and emerging extraction techniques. *Food Chem*. 2020 Aug 2;338:127724.

7020 Rajkumar V, Gunasekaran C, Paul CA, et al. Development of encapsulated peppermint essential oil in chitosan nanoparticles: characterization and biological efficacy against stored-grain pest control. *Pestic Biochem Physiol*. 2020 Nov;170:104679.

7021 Lagha AB, Vaillancourt K, Huacho PM, et al. Effects of Labrador Tea, Peppermint, and Winter Savory Essential Oils on Fusobacterium nucleatum. *Antibiotics (Basel)*. 2020 Nov 10;9(11):794.

7022 Kim MH, Park SJ, Yang WM. Inhalation of Essential Oil from Mentha piperita Ameliorates PM10-Exposed Asthma by Targeting IL-6/JAK2/STAT3 Pathway Based on a Network Pharmacological Analysis. *Pharmaceuticals (Basel)*. 2020 Dec 22;14(1):E2.

7023 Abedinpour N, Ghanbariasad A, Taghinexhad A, et al. Preparation of Nanoemulsions of Mentha piperita Essential Oil and Investigation of Their Cytotoxic Effect on Human Breast Cancer Lines. *BioNanoScience*. 2021 Jan. Online ahead of print.

7024 Habibi Q, Maghvan MA. The effect of peppermint essential oil on shigella dysenteriae in wistar rats with regard to the health of working people. *Work Health*. 2020;2020:1-6.

7025 Borzoui E, Khaghani R, Nouri-Ganbalani G. Lethal and Sublethal Effects of Eucalyptus camaldulensis and Mentha piperita Essential Oils on the Khapra Beetle (Coleoptera: Dermestidae) in Terms of Feeding Inhibition, Oviposition, and Seed Damage. *Environ Entomol*. 2021 Mar 25;nvab023.

7026 Kafa AHT, Aslan R, Celik C, et al. Antimicrobial synergism and antibiofilm activities of Pelargonium graveolens, Rosemary officinalis, and Mentha piperita essential oils against extreme drug-resistant Acinetobacter baumannii clinical isolates. *Z Naturforsch C J Biosci*. 2021 Jun 17. Online ahead of print.

7027 Hoult L, Longstaff L, Moss M. Prolonged Low-Level Exposure to the Aroma of Peppermint Essential Oil Enhances Aspects of Cognition and Mood in Healthy Adults. *Am J Pant Sci*. 2019;10:1002-12.

7028 Camele I, Gruľová D, Elshafie HS. Chemical Composition and Antimicrobial Properties of Mentha × piperita cv. 'Kristinka' Essential Oil. *Plants (Basel)*. 2021 Jul 30;10(8):1567.

7029 Mahdavikian S, Fallahi M, Khatony A. Comparing the Effect of Aromatherapy with Peppermint and Lavender Essential Oils on Fatigue of Cardiac Patients: A Randomized Controlled Trial. *Evidence-Based Compl Alt Med*. 2021;2021:9925945.

7030 Jamshed A, Jabeen Q. Prophylactic and curative potential of peppermint oil against calcium oxalate kidney stones. *Pak J Pharm Sci*. 2021 Sep;34(5(Supplementary)):1867-1872.

7031 Silva WMF, Bona NP, Pedra NS, et al. Risk assessment of in vitro cytotoxicity, antioxidant and antimicrobial activities of Mentha piperita L. essential oil. *J Toxicol Environ Health A*. 2021 Nov 15;1-13.

7032 Soleimani M, Kashfi LS, Mirmohamadkhani M, et al. The effect of aromatherapy with peppermint essential oil on anxiety of cardiac patients in emergency department: A placebo-controlled study. *Complement Ther Clin Pract*. 2022 Jan 5;46:101533.

7033 Thapa S, Luna RA, Chumpitazi BP, et al. Peppermint oil effects on the gut microbiome in children with functional abdominal pain. *Clin Transl Sci*. 2022 Jan 20. Online ahead of print.

7034 Altun M, Yapici BM. Determination of chemical compositions and antibacterial effects of selected essential oils against human pathogenic strains. *An Acad Bras Cienc*. 2022 Mar 11;94(1):e20210074.

7035 Lv X, Feng Y, Ma R, et al. Effects of Peppermint Essential Oil on Learning and Memory Ability in APP/PS1 Transgenic Mice. *Molecules*. 2022;27(7):2051.

7036 Han A, Kim J, Hur MH, et al. Effects of Foot Bath and Spray Application of Peppermint and Grapefruit Essential Oils on Lower Extremity Edema, Pain, and Fatigue. *J Korea Convergence Soc*. 2022;13(1):375-86.

7037 Balyan V, Mahantesha S, Talwar V, et al. Clinical Evaluation of an Essential Oil Intraoral Spray for Treatment of Dry Mouth. *World J Dentistry*. 2022;13(2):10015-1916.

7038 Chen WN, Chin KW, Tang KS, et al. Neuroprotective, Neurite Enhancing and Cholinesterase Inhibitory Effects of Lamiaceae Family Essential Oils in Alzheimer's Disease Model. HERMED-D-22-00403. Available at: https://ssrn.com/abstract=4112137 or http://dx.doi.org/10.2139/ssrn.4112137.

7039 Grandi G, Ferrari S, Xholli A, et al. Prevalence of menstrual pain in young women: what is dysmenorrhea? *J Pain Res*. 2012;5:169–174.

7040 Kartikasari R, Suryajaya IW, Sintoro HP. Effect Of Peppermint Aromatherapy On Menstruation Scale Of Pain In Fakultas Kedokteran Hang Tuah Surabaya Students(Msg). *Agri-TEK*. 2020;21(1):10-3.

7041 El-Kasem Bosly HA. Larvicidal and adulticidal activity of essential oils from plants of the Lamiaceae family against the West Nile virus vector, Culex pipiens (Diptera: Culicidae). *Saudi J Biol Sci*. 2022 Aug;29(8):103350.

7042 Hamad Al-Mijalli S, ELsharkawy ER, Abdallah EM, et al. Determination of Volatile Compounds of Mentha piperita and Lavandula multifida and Investigation of Their Antibacterial, Antioxidant, and Antidiabetic Properties. *Evid Based Complement Alternat Med*. 2022 Jun 14;2022:9306251.

7043 Lin S, Wang Y, Wu K, et al. Study on the Effect of Mentha × piperita L. Essential Oil on Electroencephalography upon Stimulation with Different Visual Effects. *Molecules*. 2022 Jun 24;27(13):4059.

7044 Fazal H, Akram M, Ahmad N, et al. Nutritionally rich biochemical profile in essential oil of various Mentha species and their antimicrobial activities. *Protoplasma*. 2022 Aug 9. Online ahead of print.

7045 Dolghi A, Coricovac D, Dinu S, et al. Chemical and Antimicrobial Characterization of Mentha piperita L. and Rosmarinus officinalis L. Essential Oils and In Vitro Potential Cytotoxic Effect in Human Colorectal Carcinoma Cells. *Molecules*. 2022 Sep 19;27(18):6106.

7046 Sanei-Dehkordi A, Abdollahi A, et al. Nanogels Containing Foeniculum vulgare Mill. and Mentha piperita L. Essential Oils: Mosquitoes' Repellent Activity and Antibacterial Effect. *Interdiscip Perspect Infect Dis*. 2022 Aug 31;2022:4510182.

7047 Abdulsahib WK, Kathem SH, Al-Radeef MY, et al. Mentha piperita Oil Exerts an Antiepileptic Effect in Pilocarpine and Pentylenetetrazol-Induced Seizures in Mice. *Vet Med Int*. 2022 Sep 22;2022:4431317.

7048 Bogavac MA, Perić TM, Mišković J, et al. Antimicrobial and Toxic Effects of Boswellia serrata Roxb. and Mentha piperita Linn. Essential Oils on Vaginal Inhabitants. *Medicines (Basel)*. 2022 Dec 9;9(12):62.

7049 Souza LP, Zuim V, Stinguel P, et al. Toxicity of Essential Oil of Mentha piperita (Lamiaceae) and its Monoterpenoid Menthol Against Tetranychus urticae Kogan 1836 (Acari: Tetranychidae). *An Acad Bras Cienc*. 2022 Dec 2;94(suppl 4):e20200427.

7050 Prasannakumar NR, Jyothi N, Saroja S, et al. Insecticidal properties of Ocimum basilicum and Mentha piperita essential oils against South American Tomato moth, Phthorimaea absoluta (Meyrick) (Lepidoptera: Gelichiidae). *Pestic Biochem Physiol*. 2023 Feb;190:105329.

7051 Srief M, Bani M, Mokrani EH, et al. Evaluation of In Vitro and In Silico Anti-Alzheimer Potential of Nonpolar Extracts and Essential Oil from Mentha piperita. *Foods*. 2023 Jan 1;12(1):190.

7052 Moss M, Ho J, Swinburne S, Turner A. Aroma of the essential oil of peppermint reduces aggressive driving behaviour in healthy adults. *Hum Psychopharmacol*. 2023 Mar;38(2):e2865.

7053 Prasannakumar NR, Jyothi N, Saroja S, et al. Insecticidal properties of Ocimum basilicum and Mentha piperita essential oils against South American Tomato moth, Phthorimaea absoluta (Meyrick) (Lepidoptera: Gelichiidae). *Pestic Biochem Physiol*. 2023 Feb;190:105329.

7054 Al-Tawarah NM, Al-Dmour RH, Abu Hajleh MN, et al. Rosmarinus officinalis and Mentha piperita Oils Supplementation Enhances Memory in a Rat Model of Scopolamine-Induced Alzheimer's Disease-like Condition. *Nutrients*. 2023 Mar 22;15(6):1547.

7055 Floare AD, Dumitrescu R, Alexa VT, et al. Enhancing the Antimicrobial Effect of Ozone with Mentha piperita Essential Oil. *Molecules*. 2023 Feb 21;28(5):2032.

7056 Atti-Santos AC, Rossato M, Serafini LA, et al. Extraction of Essential Oils from Lime (Citrus latifolia Tanaka) by Hydrodistillation and Supercritical Carbon Dioxide. *Brazilian Arch Biol Tech*. 2005 Jan;48(1):155-60.

7057 Kummer R, Fachini-Queiroz FC, Estevao-Silva CF, et al. Evaluation of Anti-Inflammatory Activity of Citrus latifolia Tanaka Essential Oil and Limonene in Experimental Mouse Models. *Evid Based Complement Alternat Med*. 2013;2013:859083.

7058 Gargano AC, Almeida Costa CAR, Costa M. Essential oils from Citrus latifolia and Citrus reticulata reduce anxiety and prolong ether sleeping time in mice. *Tree For Sci Biotechnol*. 2008;2(Special Issue 1):121-24.

7059 Pino JA, Rosado A. Comparative investigation of the distilled lime oils (Citrus aurantifolia Swingle and Citrus latifolia Tanaka) from Cuba. *J Essent Oil Res*. 2001 May-Jun;13:179-80.

7060 Njoroge SM, Ukeda H, Kusunose H, et al. Japanese Sour Citrus Fruits. Part IV. Volatile Constituents of Naoshichi and Tahiti Lime Essential Oils. *Flavour Frag J*. 1996 Jan-Feb;11(1):25-29.

7061 Dugo G, Mondello L, Lamonica G, et al. Characterization of Cold-Pressed Key and Persian Lime Oils by Gas Chromatography, Gas Chromatography/Mass Spectroscopy, High-Performance Liquid Chromatography, and Physicochemical Indices. *J Agric Food Chem*. 1997;45(9):3608-16.

7062 Lota ML, de Rocca Serra D, Tomi F, et al. Volatile components of peel and leaf oils of lemon and lime species. *J Agric Food Chem*. 2002 Feb 13;50(4):796-805.

7063 Ruiz-Pérez NJ, González-Ávila M, Sánchez-Navarrete J, et al. Antimycotic Activity and Genotoxic Evaluation of Citrus sinensis and Citrus latifolia Essential Oils. *Sci Rep*. 2016 May 3;6:25371.

7064 Dugrand-Judek A, Olry A, Hehn A, et al. The distribution of coumarins and furanocoumarins in citrus cpecies closely matches phylogeny and reflects the organization of biosynthetic pathways. *PLoS One*. 2015;10(11):e0142757.

7065 Williamson EA. Inhibition of cytochrome P450 2E1, cytochrome P450 3A6 and cytochrome P450 2A6 by citrus essential oils. University of North Carolina Thesis. Available at: http://libres.uncg.edu/ir/uncg/f/Williamson_uncg_0154M_10494.pdf.

7066 Kummer R, Fachini-Queiroz FC, Estevao-Silva CF, et al. Evaluation of Anti-Inflammatory Activity of Citrus latifolia Tanaka Essential Oil and Limonene in Experimental Mouse Models. *Evid Based Complement Alternat Med*. 2013;2013:859083.

7067 Gargano AC, Almeida Costa CAR, Costa M. Essential oils from Citrus latifolia and Citrus reticulata reduce anxiety and prolong ether sleeping time in mice. *Tree For Sci Biotechnol*. 2008;2(Special Issue 1):121-24.

7068 Ruiz-Pérez NJ, González-Ávila M, Sánchez-Navarrete J, et al. Antimycotic Activity and Genotoxic Evaluation of Citrus sinensis and Citrus latifolia Essential Oils. *Sci Rep*. 2016 May 3;6:25371.

[7069] Choi HS, Song HS, Ukeda H, et al. Radical-scavenging activities of citrus essential oils and their components: detection using 1,1-diphenyl-2-picrylhydrazyl. *J Agric Food Chem.* 2000 Sep;48(9):4156-61.

[7070] Toscano-Garibay JD, Arriaga-Alba M, Sánchez-Navarrete J, et al. Antimutagenic and antioxidant activity of the essential oils of Citrus sinensis and Citrus latifolia. *Sci Rep.* 2017 Sep 13;7(1):11479.

[7071] Seo SM. Park HM, Park IK. Larvicidal Activity of Ajowan (Trachyspermum ammi) and Peru Balsam (Myroxylon pereira) Oils and Blends of Their Constituents against Mosquito, Aedes aegypti, Acute Toxicity on Water Flea, Daphnia magna, and Aqueous Residue. *J Agric Food Chem.* 2012;60(23):5909–5914.

[7072] Mammerler V. Contribution to the analysis and quality control of Peru Balsam. Doctoral Thesis. Available at: http://othes.univie.ac.at/4056/1/2009-03-23_0201578.pdf

[7073] Stillpoint Aromatics. Peru Balsam. Available at: https://cdn.shopify.com/s/files/1/0380/8537/files/Peru_Balsam_9_15.pdf?10162884826279448017.

[7074] National Library of Medicine. TOXNET. Benzyl acetate. Available at: https://toxnet.nlm.nih.gov/cgi-bin/sis/search/a?dbs+hsdb:@term+@DOCNO+2851.

[7075] JECFA. Summary of evaluations performed by the Joint FAO/WHO Expert Committee on Food Additives. 2001. Available at: https://toxnet.nlm.nih.gov/cgi-bin/sis/search/a?dbs+hsdb:@term+@DOCNO+2851.

[7076] Thyssen JP, Carlsen BC, Menne T, et al. Trends of contact allergy to fragrance mix I and Myroxylon pereirae among Danish eczema patients tested between 1985 and 2007. *Contact Dermatitis.* 2008 Oct;59(4):238-44.

[7077] Sabroe RA, Holden CR, Gawkrodger DJ. Contact allergy to essential oils cannot always be predicted from allergy to fragrance markers in the baseline series. *Contact Dermatitis.* 2016 Apr;74(4):236-41.

[7078] Boonchai W, Iamtharachai P, Sunthonpalin P. Prevalence of allergic contact dermatitis in Thailand. Dermatitis. 2008;19:142-45.

[7079] Seo SM. Park HM, Park IK. Larvicidal Activity of Ajowan (Trachyspermum ammi) and Peru Balsam (Myroxylon pereira) Oils and Blends of Their Constituents against Mosquito, Aedes aegypti, Acute Toxicity on Water Flea, Daphnia magna, and Aqueous Residue. *J Agric Food Chem.* 2012;60(23):5909–5914.

[7080] Saleh MA, Clark S, Woodard B, et al. Antioxidant and free radical scavenging activities of essential oils. *Ethnicity & Disease.* 2010 Spring;20:S78-S82.

[7081] Bianchini A, Tomi P, Costa J, et al. Composition of Helichrysum italicum (Roth) G. Don fil. subsp. italicum essential oil from Corsica (France). *Flav Frag J.* 2001 Jan-Feb;16(1):30-34.

[7082] Leonardi M, Ambryszewska KE, Melai B, et al. Essential-oil composition of Helichrysum italicum (ROTH) G.DON ssp. Italicum from Elba Island (Tuscany, Italy). *Chem Biodviers.* 2013 Mar;10(3):343-55.

[7083] Cristofari G, Znini M, Majidi L, et al. Helichrysum italicum subsp. italicum essential oil as environmentally friendly inhibitor on the corrosion of mil steel in hydrochloric acid. *Int J Electrochem Sci.* 2012;7:9024-41.

[7084] Satta M, Tuberoso CIG, Angioni A, et al. Analysis of the essential oil of Helichrysum italicum G. Don ssp. microphyllum (Willd) Nym. *J Essential Oil Res.* 1999;11(6):711-15.

[7085] Guinoiseau E, Lorenzi V, Luciani A, et al. Biological properties and resistance reversal effect of Helichrysum italicum (Roth) G. Don. *Micro Pathogens and Strat Combat: Sci Tech.* 2013:1073-80.

[7086] Mastelic J, Politeo O, Jerkovic I. Contribution to the analysis of the essential oil of Helichrysum italicum (Roth) G. Don. - determination of ester bonded acids and phenols. *Molecules.* 208;13:795-803.

[7087] Antunes Castela Viega DM. Formulacoes topicas de Helichrysum italicum e sua aplicabilidade. *Covilha.* 2011 Jun:ii-63.

[7088] Mastelic J, Politeo O, Jerkovic I, et al. Composition and antimicrobial activity of Helichrysum italicum essential oil and its terpene fractions. *Chem Nat Constituents.* 2005 Jan;41(10:35-40.

[7089] Weyerstahl P. Isolation and synthesis of constituents from the essential oil of Helichrysum italicum. In: Brunke EJ. Progress in essential oil research. De Gruyter, Berlin:177-95.

[7090] Mashigo MF, Combrinck S, Regnier T, et al. Chemical variations, trichome structure and antifungal activities of essential oils of Helichrysum splendidum from South Africa. *South African J Botany.* 2015 Jan;96:78-84.

[7091] Marongui B, Piras A, Porcedda S. Comparative analysis of the oil and supercritical CO(2) extract of Artemisia arborescens L. and Helichrysum splendidum (Thunb.) Less. *Nat Prod Res.* 2006 May;20(5):421-28.

[7092] Chagonda LS, Makanda C, Chalchat JC. Essential Oils of Four Wild and Semi-Wild Plants from Zimbabwe: Colospermum mopane (Kirk ex Benth.) Kirk ex Leonard, Helichrysum splendidum (Thunb.) Less, Myrothamnus flabellifolia (Welw.) and Tagetes minuta L. *J Essent Oil Res.* 1999;11(5):573-78.

[7093] Mastelic J, Politeo O, Jerkovic I. Contribution to the Analysis of the Essential Oil of Helichrysum italicum (Roth) G. Don. – Determination of Ester Bonded Acids and Phenols. *Molecules.* 2008;13:795-803.

[7094] Lozina V. Private Communication. 2016.

[7095] Ellouze I, Abderrabba M, Sabaou N, et al. Season's variation impact on Citrus aurantium leaves essential oil: chemical composition and biological activities. *J Food Sci.* 2012 Sep;77(9):T173-80.

[7096] Sarrou E, Chatzopoulou P, Dimassi-Theriou K, et al. Volatile constituents and antioxidant activity of peel, flowers and leaf oils of Citrus aurantium L. growing in Greece. *Molecules.* 2013;18:10639-10647.

[7097] Mondello L, Dugo G, Dugo P, et al. Italian Citrus Petitgrain oils. Part 1. Composition bitter orange petitgrain oil. *J Essent Oil Res.* 1996;8(6):597-609.

[7098] Abderrezak MK, Abaza I, Aburjai T, et al. Comparative compositions of essential oils of Citrus aurantium growing in different soils. *J Mater Environ Sci.* 2014;6:1913-18.

[7099] Fayed SA. Antioxidant and anticancer activities of Citrus reticulata (Petitgrain Mandarin) and Pelargonium graveolens (Geranium) essential oils. *Res J Agric Biol Sci.* 2009;5(5):740-47.

[7100] Dugo G, Mondello L, Cotroneo A, et al. Characterization of Italian citrus petitgrain oils. *Perf Flav.* 1996;21:17-28.

[7101] Ekundayo O, Bakare O, Adesomoju A, et al. Leaf volatile oil composition of Mandarin (Citrus reticulata) from Nigeria. *J Essent Oil Res.* 1990;2(6):329-330.

[7102] Eldahshan OA. Comparison of chemical and antimicrobial studies of Egyptian Mandarin leaves and green branches volatile oil. *Eur J Med Plants.* 2015;5(3):248-54.

[7103] Scientific Committee on Consumer Safety. Opinion on methyl-N-methylanthranilate (phototoxicity only). Available at: http://ec.europa.eu/health/scientific_committees/consumer_safety/docs/sccs_o_075.pdf.

[7104] Mauerman B, Ahmed N, Tambhar N, et al. Trends in Furanocoumarin Profiles Among Commerical-Scale Essential Oils. International Conference on the Science of Botanicals, Poster. Mar 2022.

[7105] Fayed SA. Antioxidant and anticancer activities of Citrus reticulata (Petitgrain Mandarin) and Pelargonium graveolens (Geranium) essential oils. *Res J Agric Biol Sci.* 2009;5(5):740-47.

[7106] Carvalho-Freitas MI, Costa M. Anxiolytic and sedative effects of extracts and essential oil from Citrus aurantium L. *Biol Pharm Bull.* 2002 Dec;25(12):1629-33.

[7107] Huang L, Capdevila L. Aromatherapy Improves Work Performance Through Balancing the Autonomic Nervous System. *J Altern Complement Med.* 2017 Mar;23(3):214-221.

[7108] Sarrou E, Chatzopoulou P, Dimassi-Theriou K, et al. Volatile constituents and antioxidant activity of peel, flowers and leaf oils of Citrus aurantium L. growing in Greece. *Molecules.* 2013 Sep 2;18(9):10639-47.

[7109] A Ellouze I, Abderrabba M, Sabaou N, et al. Season's variation impact on Citrus aurantium leaves essential oil: chemical composition and biological activities. *J Food Sci.* 2012 Sep;77(9):T173-80.

[7110] Misni N, Nor ZM, Ahmad R. New Candidates for Plant-Based Repellents Against Aedes aegypti. *J Am Mosq Control Assoc.* 2016 Jun;32(2):117-23.

[7111] Fang F, Candy K, Melloul E, et al. In vitro activity of ten essential oils against Sarcoptes scabiei. *Parasit Vectors.* 2016 Nov 22;9(1):594.

[7112] Kačániová M, Terentjeva M, Galovičová L, et al. Biological Activity and Antibiofilm Molecular Profile of Citrus aurantium Essential Oil and Its Application in a Food Model. *Molecules.* 2020 Aug 30;25(17):3956.

[7113] Jugreet BS, Lall N, Anina Lambrechts I, et al. In Vitro and In Silico Pharmacological and Cosmeceutical Potential of Ten Essential Oils from Aromatic Medicinal Plants from the Mascarene Islands. *Molecules.* 2022 Dec 8;27(24):8705.

[7114] Fahmy NM, Elhady SS, Bannan DF, et al. Citrus reticulata Leaves Essential Oil as an Antiaging Agent: A Comparative Study between Different Cultivars and Correlation with Their Chemical Compositions. *Plants (Basel).* 2022 Dec 1;11(23):3335.

[7115] Abd Elghani EM, El Sayed AM, Abdel-Aziz Emam MM, et al. Seasonal metabolic profiling of Valencia orange leaf essential oil using GC coupled with chemometrics, nano-formulation, and insecticidal evaluation: in vivo and in silico. *RSC Adv.* 2023 Jan 9;13(3):1659-1671.

[7116] Fayemiwo KA, Adeleke MA, Okoro OP, et al. Larvicidal efficacies and chemical composition of essential oils of Pinus sylvestris and Syzygium aromaticum against mosquitoes. *Asian Pac J Trop Biomed.* 2014 Jan;4(1):30-34.

[7117] Ustun O, Sezik E, Kurkcuoglu M, et al. Study of the essential oil composition Pinus sylvestris from Turkey. *Chem Nat Constituents.* 2006;42(1):26-31.

[7118] Venskutonis PR, Vyskupaityte K, Plausinaitis R. Composition of essential oils of Pinus sylvestris L. from different locations of Lithuania. *J Essent Oil Res.* 2000;12(5):559-65.

[7119] Judzentiene A, Slizyte J, Stikliene A, et al. Characteristics of essential oil composition in the needles of young stand of Scots pine (Pinus sylvestris L.) growing along aerial ammonia gradient. *Chemija.* 2006;17(4):67-73

[7120] Tumen I, Hafizoglu H, Kilic A, et al. Yields and constituents of essential oil from cones of Pinaceae spp. natively grown in Turkey. *Molecules.* 2010;15:5797-5806.

[7121] Tumen I, Reunnanen M. A comparative study on turpentine oils of oleoresins of Pinus sylvestris L. from three districts of Denizli. *Rec Nat Prod.* 2010;4(4):224-29.

[7122] Hoai NT, Duc HV, Thao do T, et al. Selectivity of Pinus sylvestris extract and essential oil to estrogen-insensitive breast cancer cells Pinus sylvestris against cancer cells. *Pharmacogn Mag.* 2015 Oct;11(Suppl 2):S290-5.

[7123] Muhlbauer RC, Lozano A, Palacio S, et al. Common herbs, essential oils, and monoterpenes potently modulate bone metabolism. *Bone.* 2003 Apr;32(4):372-80.

[7124] Kacaniova M, Vukovic N, Horska E, et al. Antibacterial activity against Clostridium genus and antiradical activity of the essential oils from different origin. *J Environ Sci Health B.* 2014;49(7):505-12.

[7125] Boschi F, Nicolato E, Benati D, et al. Drug targeting of airway surface liquid: a pharmacological MRI approach. *Biomed Pharmacother.* 2008 Jul-Aug;62(6):410-19.

[7126] Motiejunaite O, Peciulyte D. Fungicidal properties of Pinus sylvestris L. for improvement of air quality. *Medicina (Kaunas).* 204;40(8):787-94.

[7127] Mandras N, Nostro A, Roana J, et al. Liquid and vapour-phase antifungal activities of essential oils against Candida albicans and non-albicans Candida. *BMC Complement Altern Med.* 2016 Aug 30;16(1):330.

[7128] Scalas D, Mandras N, Roana J, et al. Use of Pinus sylvestris L. (Pinaceae), Origanum vulgare L. (Lamiaceae), and Thymus vulgaris L. (Lamiaceae) essential oils and their main components to enhance itraconazole activity against azole susceptible/not-susceptible Cryptococcus neoformans strains. *BMC Complement Altern Med.* 2018; 18: 143.

[7129] Korona-Glowniak I, Glowniak-Lipa A, Ludwiczuk A, et al. The In Vitro Activity of Essential Oils Against Helicobacter Pylori Growth and Urease Activity. *Molecules.* 2020 Jan 29;25(3):586.

[7130] Mediavilla I, Guillamon E, Ruiz A, et al. Essential Oils from Residual Foliage of Forest Tree and Shrub Species: Yield and Antioxidant Capacity. *Molecules.* 2021 May 28;26(11):3257.

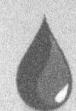

7131 Csikós E, Csekő K, Kemény Á, et al. Pinus sylvestris L. and Syzygium aromaticum (L.) Merr. & L. M. Perry Essential Oils Inhibit Endotoxin-Induced Airway Hyperreactivity despite Aggravated Inflammatory Mechanisms in Mice. *Molecules*. 2022 Jun 16;27(12):3868.
7132 Kozlova AD. Effect of aromatherapy (orange and pine oils) on human visual-motor response. *Youth Inn Bull.* 2022;11:537-9.
7133 Galgano M, Capozza P, Pellegrini F, et al. Antimicrobial Activity of Essential Oils Evaluated In Vitro against Escherichia coli and Staphylococcus aureus. *Antibiotics (Basel)*. 2022 Jul 20;11(7):979.
7134 Nesrine Z, Hosni K, Brahim NB, et al. Essential oil composition of Schinus molle L. fruits: An ornamental species used as condiment. *J Food Biochem.* 2011 Apr;35(2):400-09.
7135 Hamdan SI, Al-Gendy AA, El-Shazly AM. Chemical Composition and Cytotoxic Activity of the Essential Oils of Schinus molle Growing in Egypt. *J Pharm Sci & Res.* 2016 Aug;8(8):779-93.
7136 Baser KHC, Kurkcuoglu M, Demircakmak B. Composition of the essential oil of Schinum molle L. grown in Turkey. *J Essent Oil Res.* 1997 Nov-Dec;9:693-96.
7137 Diaz C, Quesada S, Brenes O, et al. Chemical composition of Schinus molle essential oil and its cytotoxic activity on tumour cell lines. *Nat Prod Res.* 2008 Nov;22(17):1521-34.
7138 Doleski Muhd PS, Ferreira Cuelho CH, Calil Bronadani J, et al. Chemical composition of the Schinus molle L. essential oil and their biological activities. *Revista Cubana de Farmacia.* 2015 Dec;49(1):1-10.
7139 Chamorro ER, Zambon SN, Morales WG, et al. Gas Chromatography in Plant Science Wine Technology, Toxicology and Some Specific Actions. InTech, Rijeka, Coratia. 2012. p. 307-24.
7140 Bendaoud H, Romdhane M, Souchard JP, et al. Chemical composition and anticancer and antioxidant activities of Schinus molle L. and Schinus terebinthifolius Raddi berries essential oils. *J Food Sci.* 2010 Aug 1;75(6):C466-72.
7141 Abdel-Sattar E, Zaitoun AA, Farag MA, et al. Chemical composition, insecticidal and insect repellent activity of Schinus molle L. leaf and fruit essential oils against Trogoderma granarium and Tribolium castaneum. *Nat Prod Res.* 2010 Feb;24(3):226-35.
7142 Hayouni el A, Chraief I, Abedrabba M, et al. Tunisian Salvia officinalis L. and Schinus molle L. essential oils: their chemical compositions and their preservative effects against Salmonella inoculated in minced beef meat. *Int J Food Microbiol.* 2008 Jul 31;125(3):242-51.
7143 Guerra-Boone L, Alvarez-Román R, Salazar-Aranda R, et al. Chemical compositions and antimicrobial and antioxidant activities of the essential oils from Magnolia grandiflora, Chrysactinia mexicana, and Schinus molle found in northeast Mexico. *Nat Prod Commun.* 2013 Jan;8(1):135-8.
7144 Silva AB, Silva T, Franco ES, et al. Antibacterial activity, chemical composition, and cytotoxicity of leaf's essential oil from Brazilian pepper tree (Schinus terebinthifolius, Raddi). *Brazilian J Microbiol.* 2010 Jan-Mar;41(1):ISSN 1517-8832.
7145 Gundidza M, Gweru N, Magwa ML, et al. The chemical composition and biological activities of essential oil from the fresh leaves of Schinus terebinthifolius from Zimbabwe. *African J Biotechnol.* 2009 Dec;8924):7164-69.
7146 Ennigrou A, Hosni K, Casabianca H, et al. Leaf volatile oil constituents of Schinus tereninthifolius and Schninus mollee from Tunisia. *Foodbalt.* 2011:90-92.
7147 Jeribi C, Karoui IJ, Hassine DB, et al. Comparative Study of Bioactive Compounds and Antioxidant Activity of Schinus terebinthifolius RADDI Fruits and Leaves Essential Oils. *Int J Sci Res.* 2014 Dec;3(12):453-58.
7148 Fonesca do Nascimento A, Gomes da Camara CA, Martins de Moraes M, et al. Essential Oil Composition and Acaricidal Activity of Schinus terebinthifolius from Atlantic Forest of Pernambuco, Brazil against Tetranychus urticae. *Nat Prod Commun.* 2012;7(1):129-32.
7149 Almeida Barbosa LC, Demuner AJ, Clemente AD, et al. Seasonal variation in the composition of volatile oils from Schinus terebinthifolius raddi. *Quimica Nova.* 2007;30(8):ISSN 1678-7064.
7150 Atti dos Santos AC, Rossato M, Agostini F, et al. Chemical Composition of the Essential Oils from Leaves and Fruits of Schinus molle L. and Schinus terebinthifolius Raddi from Southern Brazil. *J Essent Oil Bearing Plants.* 2009 Jan:ISSN 0972-060X.
7151 Cole ER, dos Santos RB, Lacerda Junior V, et al. Chemical composition of essential oil from ripe fruit of Schinus terebinthifolius Raddi and evaluation of its activity against wild strains of hospital origin. *Braz J Microbiol.* 2014; 45(3): 821–828.
7152 de Mendonça Rocha PM, Rodilla JM, Díez D, et al. Synergistic antibacterial activity of the essential oil of aguaribay (Schinus molle L.). *Molecules.* 2012 Oct 12;17(10):12023-36.
7153 Bonesi M, Menichini F, Tundis R, et al. Acetylcholinesterase and butyrylcholinesterase inhibitory activity of Pinus species essential oils and their constituents. *J Enzyme Inhib Med Chem.* 2010 Oct;25(5):622-8.
7154 Aazza S, Lyoussi B, Miguel MG. Antioxidant and antiacetylcholinesterase activities of some commercial essential oils and their major compounds. *Molecules.* 2011 Sep 7;16(9):7672-90.
7155 Miyazawa M, Yamafuji C. Inhibition of acetylcholinesterase activity by bicyclic monoterpenoids. *J Agric Food Chem.* 2005 Mar 9;53(5):1765-8.
7156 Hamdan SI, Al-Gendy AA, El-Shazly AM. Chemical Composition and Cytotoxic Activity of the Essential Oils of Schinus molle Growing in Egypt. *J Pharm Sci & Res.* 2016 Aug;8(8):779-93.
7157 Diaz C, Quesada S, Brenes O, et al. Chemical composition of Schinus molle essential oil and its cytotoxic activity on tumour cell lines. *Nat Prod Res.* 2008 Nov;22(17):1521-34.
7158 Bendaoud H, Romdhane M, Souchard JP, et al. Chemical composition and anticancer and antioxidant activities of Schinus molle L. and Schinus terebinthifolius Raddi berries essential oils. *J Food Sci.* 2010 Aug 1;75(6):C466-72.
7159 Santana JS, Sartorelli P, Guadagnin RC, et al. Essential oils from Schinus terebinthifolius leaves - chemical composition and in vitro cytotoxicity evaluation. *Pharm Biol.* 2012 Oct;50(10):1248-53.
7160 Belhamel K, Abderrahim A, Ludwig R. Chemical composition and antibacterial activity of the essential oil of Schinus molle L. grown in Algeria. *Int J Essent Oil Ther.* 2008;2:175-77.
7161 Hayouni el A, Chraief I, Abedrabba M, et al. Tunisian Salvia officinalis L. and Schinus molle L. essential oils: their chemical compositions and their preservative effects against Salmonella inoculated in minced beef meat. *Int J Food Microbiol.* 2008 Jul 31;125(3):242-51.
7162 Guerra-Boone L, Alvarez-Román R, Salazar-Aranda R, et al. Chemical compositions and antimicrobial and antioxidant activities of the essential oils from Magnolia grandiflora, Chrysactinia mexicana, and Schinus molle found in northeast Mexico. *Nat Prod Commun.* 2013 Jan;8(1):135-8.
7163 Silva AB, Silva T, Franco ES, et al. Antibacterial activity, chemical composition, and cytotoxicity of leaf's essential oil from Brazilian pepper tree (Schinus terebinthifolius, Raddi). *Brazilian J Microbiol.* 2010 Jan-Mar;41(1):ISSN 1517-8832.
7164 Gundidza M, Gweru N, Magwa ML, et al. The chemical composition and biological activities of essential oil from the fresh leaves of Schinus terebinthifolius from Zimbabwe. *African J Biotechnol.* 2009 Dec;8924):7164-69.
7165 Cole ER, dos Santos RB, Lacerda Junior V, et al. Chemical composition of essential oil from ripe fruit of Schinus terebinthifolius Raddi and evaluation of its activity against wild strains of hospital origin. *Braz J Microbiol.* 2014; 45(3): 821–828.
7166 Martins Mdo R, Arantes S, Candeias F, et al. Antioxidant, antimicrobial and toxicological properties of Schinus molle L. essential oils. *J Ethnopharmacol.* 2014;151(1):485-92.
7167 de Mendonça Rocha PM, Rodilla JM, Díez D, et al. Synergistic antibacterial activity of the essential oil of aguaribay (Schinus molle L.). Molecules. 2012 Oct 12;17(10):12023-36.
7168 Lopez-Meneses AK, Plascencia-Jatomea M, Lizardi-Mendoza J, et al. Antifungal and antimycotoxigenic activity of essential oils from Eucalyptus globulus, Thymus capitatus and Schinus molle. *Food Sci Technol.* 2015 Oct-Dec;35(4):664-71.
7169 Montanari RM, Barbosa LC, Demuner AJ, et al. Exposure to Anacardiaceae volatile oils and their constituents induces lipid peroxidation within food-borne bacteria cells. *Molecules.* 2012 Aug 14;17(8):9728-40.
7170 Elshafie HS, Ghanney N, Mang SM, et al. An In Vitro Attempt for Controlling Severe Phytopathogens and Human Pathogens Using Essential Oils from Mediterranean Plants of Genus Schinus. *J Med Food.* 2016 Mar;19(3):266-73.
7171 Bendaoud H, Romdhane M, Souchard JP, et al. Chemical composition and anticancer and antioxidant activities of Schinus molle L. and Schinus terebinthifolius Raddi berries essential oils. *J Food Sci.* 2010 Aug 1;75(6):C466-72.
7172 Guerra-Boone L, Alvarez-Román R, Salazar-Aranda R, et al. Chemical compositions and antimicrobial and antioxidant activities of the essential oils from Magnolia grandiflora, Chrysactinia mexicana, and Schinus molle found in northeast Mexico. *Nat Prod Commun.* 2013 Jan;8(1):135-8.
7173 Gundidza M, Gweru N, Magwa ML, et al. The chemical composition and biological activities of essential oil from the fresh leaves of Schinus terebinthifolius from Zimbabwe. *African J Biotechnol.* 2009 Dec;8924):7164-69.
7174 Jeribi C, Karoui IJ, Hassine DB, et al. Comparative Study of Bioactive Compounds and Antioxidant Activity of Schinus terebinthifolius RADDI Fruits and Leaves Essential Oils. *Int J Sci Res.* 2014 Dec;3(12):453-58.
7175 Martins Mdo R, Arantes S, Candeias F, et al. Antioxidant, antimicrobial and toxicological properties of Schinus molle L. essential oils. *J Ethnopharmacol.* 2014;151(1):485-92.
7176 Baldissera MD, Da Silva AS, Oliveira CB, et al. Trypanocidal activity of the essential oils in their conventional and nanoemulsion forms: in vitro tests. *Exp Parasitol.* 2013 Jul;134(3):356-61.
7177 Estevão LR, Medeiros JP, Simões RS, et al. Mast cell concentration and skin wound contraction in rats treated with Brazilian pepper essential oil (Schinus terebinthifolius Raddi). *Acta Cir Bras.* 2015 Apr;30(4):289-95.
7178 Piccinelli AC, Santos JA, Konkiewitz EC, et al. Antihyperalgesic and antidepressive actions of (R)-(+)-limonene, α-phellandrene, and essential oil from Schinus terebinthifolius fruits in a neuropathic pain model. *Nutr Neurosci.* 2015 Jul;18(5):217-24.
7179 Abdel-Sattar E, Zaitoun AA, Farag MA, et al. Chemical composition, insecticidal and insect repellent activity of Schinus molle L. leaf and fruit essential oils against Trogoderma granarium and Tribolium castaneum. *Nat Prod Res.* 2010 Feb;24(3):226-35.
7180 Fonesca do Nascimento A, Gomes da Camara CA, Martins de Moraes M, et al. Essential Oil Composition and Acaricidal Activity of Schinus terebinthifolius from Atlantic Forest of Pernambuco, Brazil against Tetranychus urticae. *Nat Prod Commun.* 2012;7(1):129-32.
7181 Batista LC, Cid YP1, De Almeida AP, et al. In vitro efficacy of essential oils and extracts of Schinus molle L. against Ctenocephalides felis felis. *Parasitology.* 2016 Apr;143(5):627-38.
7182 Pellegrini MC, Alonso-Salces RM, Umpierrez ML, et al. Chemical Composition, Antimicrobial Activity, and Mode of Action of Essential Oils against Paenibacillus larvae, Etiological Agent of American Foulbrood on Apis mellifera. *Chem Biodivers.* 2017 Apr;14(4).
7183 Salem MZM, El-Hefny M, Ali HM, et al. Antibacterial activity of extracted bioactive molecules of Schinus terebinthifolius ripened fruits against some pathogenic bacteria. *Microb Pathog.* 2018 Apr 27;120:119-127.
7184 Rey-Valeirón C, Pérez K, Guzmán L, et al. Acaricidal effect of Schinus molle (Anacardiaceae) essential oil on unengorged larvae and engorged adult females of Rhipicephalus sanguineus (Acari: Ixodidae). *Exp Appl Acarol.* 2018 Nov;76(3):399-411.

7185 do Prado AC, Garces HG, Bagagli E, et al. Schinus molle essential oil as a potential source of bioactive compounds: antifungal and antibacterial properties. *J Appl Microbiol*. 2019 Feb;126(2):516-522.
7186 Duarte JA, Zambrano LAB, Quintana LD, et al. Immunotoxicological Evaluation of Schinus molle L. (Anacardiaceae) Essential Oil in Lymphocytes and Macrophages. *Evid Based Complement Alternat Med*. 2018 Oct 16;2018:6541583.
7187 Andriana Y, Xuan TD, Quy TN, et al. Biological Activities and Chemical Constituents of Essential Oils from Piper cubeba Bojer and Piper nigrum L. *Molecules*. 2019 May 15;24(10).
7188 Afifi F, Aboalhaija NH, Awwad O, et al. Chemodiversity and Antiproliferative Activity of the Essential Oil of Schinus molle L. Growing in Jordan. *Chem Biodivers*. 2019 Nov;16(11):e1900388.
7189 Todirascu-Ciornea E, El-Nashar HAS, Mostada NM, et al. Schinus terebinthifolius Essential Oil Attenuates Scopolamine-Induced Memory Deficits via Cholinergic Modulation and Antioxidant Properties in a Zebrafish Model. *Evid Based Complement Alternat Med*. 2019 Dec:5256781.
7190 Lima MDCL, Ismael JFD, Mota CG, et al. Antinociceptive Effect of the Essential Oil of Schinus terebinthifolius (Female) Leaves on Adult Zebrafish (Danio rerio). *Zebrafish*. 2020 Apr;17(2):112-119.
7191 Nennaah GE, Almadiy AA, Al-Assiuty BA, et al. The essential oil of Schinus terebinthifolius and its nanoemulsion and isolated monoterpenes: investigation of their activity against Culex pipiens with insights into the adverse effects on nontarget organisms. *Pest Manag Sci*. 2021 Nov 13. Online ahead of print.
7192 de Castro Oliveira JA, Ferreira LS, et al. Eugenia uniflora, Melaleuca armillaris, and Schinus molle essential oils to manage larvae of the filarial vector Culex quinquefasciatus (Diptera: Culicidae). *Environ Sci Pollut Res Int*. 2022 Jan 18. Online ahead of print.
7193 Belhoussaine O, El Kourchi C, Harhar H, et al. Chemical Composition, Antioxidant, Insecticidal Activity, and Comparative Analysis of Essential Oils of Leaves and Fruits of Schinus molle and Schinus terebinthifolius. *Evid Based Complement Alternat Med*. 2022 May 30;2022:4288890.
7194 Chaaban SB, Haouel-Hamdi S, Bachrouch O, et al. Fumigant toxicity of four essential oils against the carob moth Ectomyelois ceratoniae Zeller and the Mediterranean flour moth Ephestia kuehniella. *Int J Environ Health Res*. 2022 Dec 4:1-13.
7195 Sukatta U, Rugthaworn P, Punjee P, et al. Chemical Composition and Physical Properties of Oil from Plai (Zingiber cassumunar Roxb.) Obtained by Hydro Distillation and Hexane Extraction. *Kasetsart J (Nat. Sci.)*. 2009;43:212-17.
7196 Bua-in S, Paisooksantivatana. Essential Oil and Antioxidant Activity of Cassumunar Ginger (Zingiberaceae: Zingiber montanum (Koenig) Link ex Dietr.) Collected from Various Parts of Thailand. *Kasetsart J (Nat. Sci.)*. 2009;43:467-75.
7197 Taroeno, Brophy J, Zwaving J. Analysis of the essential oil of Zingiber cassumunar Roxb. from Indonesia. *Flavour Frag J*. 1991;6(2):161-63.
7198 Bordoloi AL, Sperkova J, Leclercq PA. Essential oils of Zingiber cassumunar Roxb. from Northeast India. *J Essent Oil Res*. 1999 Jul-Aug;11:441-45.
7199 Singh CB, Manglembi N, Swapana N, et al. Ethnobotany, Phytochemistry and Pharmacology of Zingiber cassumunar Roxb. (Zingiberaceae). *J Pharmacog Phytochem*. 2015;4(1):1-6.
7200 Islam Bhuiyan MN, Chowdhury JU, Begum J. Volatile constituents of essential oils isolated from leaf and rhizome of Zingiber cassumunar Roxb. *Bangladesh J Pharmacol Soc*. 2008;3:69-73.
7201 Kamazeri TS, Samah O, Taher M, et al. Antimicrobial activity and essential oils of Curcuma aeruginosa, Curcuma mangga, and Zingiber cassumunar from Malaysia. *Asian Pac J Tropical Med*. 2012;(2012):202-09.
7202 Pongprayoon U, Soontornsaratune P, Jarikasem S, et al. Topical antiinflammatory activity of the major lipophilic constituents of the rhizome of Zingiber cassumunar. Part I: The essential oil. *Phytomedicine*. 1997 Feb;3(4):319-22.
7203 Okonogi S, Chaiyana W. Enhancement of anti-cholinesterase activity of Zingiber cassumunar essential oil using a microemulsion technique. *Drug Discov Ther*. 2012 Oct;6(5):249-55.
7204 Chaiyana W, Anuchapreeda S, Leelapornpisid P, et al. Development of Microemulsion Delivery System of Essential Oil from Zingiber cassumunar Roxb. Rhizome for Improvement of Stability and Anti-Inflammatory Activity. *AAPS PharmSciTech*. 2017 May;18(4):1332-1342.
7205 Chaiyana W, Saeio K, Hennink WE, et al. Characterization of potent anticholinesterase plant oil based microemulsion. *Int J Pharm*. 2010 Nov 30;401(1-2):32-40.
7206 Bonesi M, Menichini F, Tundis R, et al. Acetylcholinesterase and butyrylcholinesterase inhibitory activity of Pinus species essential oils and their constituents. *J Enzyme Inhib Med Chem*. 2010 Oct;25(5):622-8.
7207 Menichini F, Tundis R, Loizzo MR, et al. Acetylcholinesterase and butyrylcholinesterase inhibition of ethanolic extract and monoterpenes from Pimpinella anisoides V Brig. (Apiaceae). *Fitoterapia*. 2009 Jul;80(5):297-300.
7208 Perry NS, Houghton PJ, Theobald A, et al. In-vitro inhibition of human erythrocyte acetylcholinesterase by salvia lavandulaefolia essential oil and constituent terpenes. *J Pharm Pharmacol*. 2000 Jul;52(7):895-902.
7209 Mertas A, Garbusińska A, Szliszka E, et al. The influence of tea tree oil (Melaleuca alternifolia) on fluconazole activity against fluconazole-resistant Candida albicans strains. *Biomed Res Int*. 2015;2015:590470.
7210 Boonyanugomol W, Kraisriwattana K, Rukseree K, et al. In vitro synergistic antibacterial activity of the essential oil from Zingiber cassumunar Roxb against extensively drug-resistant Acinetobacter baumannii strains. *J Infect Public Health*. 2017 Feb 2;S1876-0341(17):30008-4.
7211 Pithayanukul P, Tubprasert J, Wuthi-Udomlert M. In vitro antimicrobial activity of Zingiber cassumunar (Plai) oil and a 5% Plai oil gel. *Phytother Res*. 2007 Feb;21(2):164-9.
7212 Wasuwat S, Wanisorn P, Mahintorntep B, et al. Studies on antimicrobial and antifungal activities of terpinen-4-ol extracted from Zingiber cassumunar Roxb. Thailand Institute of Scientific and Technological Research. Research Project. 1989. p.30-32. In: Singh CB, Manglembi N, Swapana N, et al. Ethnobotany, Phytochemistry and Pharmacology of Zingiber cassumunar Roxb. (Zingiberaceae). *J Pharmacog Phytochem*. 2015;4(1):1-6.
7213 Giwanon R, Thubthimthed S, Rerk-am U, et al. Antimicrobial activity of terpinen-4-ol and sabinene. *Thai J Pharm Sci*. 2000;24:27. In: Singh CB, Manglembi N, Swapana N, et al. Ethnobotany, Phytochemistry and Pharmacology of Zingiber cassumunar Roxb. (Zingiberaceae). *J Pharmacog Phytochem*. 2015;4(1):1-6.
7214 Boonyanugomol W, Kraisriwattana K, Rukseree K, et al. In vitro synergistic antibacterial activity of the essential oil from Zingiber cassumunar Roxb against extensively drug-resistant Acinetobacter baumannii strains. *J Infect Public Health*. 2017 Feb 2;S1876-0341(17):30008-4.
7215 Kamazeri TS, Samah O, Taher M, et al. Antimicrobial activity and essential oils of Curcuma aeruginosa, Curcuma mangga, and Zingiber cassumunar from Malaysia. *Asian Pac J Tropical Med*. 2012;(2012):202-09.
7216 Pongprayoon U, Soontornsaratune P, Jarikasem S, et al. Topical antiinflammatory activity of the major lipophilic constituents of the rhizome of Zingiber cassumunar. Part I: The essential oil. *Phytomedicine*. 1997 Feb;3(4):319-22.
7217 Ozaki Y, Kawahara N, Harada M. Anti-inflammatory effect of Zingiber cassumunar Roxb. and its active principles. *Chem Pharm Bull (Tokyo)*. 1991 Sep;39(9):2353-6.
7218 Kaewchoothong A, Tewtrakul S, Panichayupakaranant P. Inhibitory effect of phenylbutanoid-rich Zingiber cassumunar extracts on nitric oxide production by murine macrophage-like RAW264.7 cells. *Phytother Res*. 2012 Dec;26(12):1789-92.
7219 Chaiyana W, Anuchapreeda S, Leelapornpisid P, et al. Development of Microemulsion Delivery System of Essential Oil from Zingiber cassumunar Roxb. Rhizome for Improvement of Stability and Anti-Inflammatory Activity. *AAPS PharmSciTech*. 2017 May;18(4):1332-1342.
7220 Okonogi S, Chaiyana W. Enhancement of anti-cholinesterase activity of Zingiber cassumunar essential oil using a microemulsion technique. *Drug Discov Ther*. 2012 Oct;6(5):249-55.
7221 Chaiyana W, Rades T, Okonogi S. Characterization and in vitro permeation study of microemulsions and liquid crystalline systems containing the anticholinesterase alkaloidal extract from Tabernaemontana divaricata. *Int J Pharm*. 2013 Aug 16;452(1-2):201-10.
7222 Darvesh S, Hopkins DA, Geula C, Neurobiology of butyrylcholinesterase. *Nat Rev Neurosci*. 2003 Feb;4:131-38.
7223 Bua-in S, Paisooksantivatana. Essential Oil and Antioxidant Activity of Cassumunar Ginger (Zingiberaceae: Zingiber montanum (Koenig) Link ex Dietr.) Collected from Various Parts of Thailand. *Kasetsart J (Nat. Sci.)*. 2009;43:467-75.
7224 Phonsena P, Banchong Y, Rawanghet C. Efficacy of essential oils from Phlai (Zingiber montanum), Turmeric (Curcuma longa) and Wan nang Kham (C. aromatic) against Brown Dog. In Proceedings of 44th Kasetsart University Annual Conference. Animal, Veterinary Medicine Bangkok, Thailand. 2006. p. 539-543.
7225 Phasomkusolsil S, Soonwera M. Insect repellent activity of medicinal plant oils against Aedes aegypti (Linn.), Anopheles minimus (Theobald) and Culex quinquefasciatus Say based on protection time and biting rate. *Southeast Asian J Trop Med Public Health*. 2010 Jul;41(4):831-40.
7226 Boonyuan W, Grieco JP, Bangs MJ, et al. Excito-repellency of essential oils against an Aedes aegypti (L.) field population in Thailand. *J Vector Ecol*. 2014 Jun;39(1):112-22.
7227 Eamsobhana P, Yoolek A, Kongkaew W, et al. Laboratory evaluation of aromatic essential oils from thirteen plant species as candidate repellents against Leptotrombidium chiggers (Acari: Trombiculidae), the vector of scrub typhus. *Exp Appl Acarol*. 2009 Mar;47(3):257-62.
7228 Verma RS, Joshi N, Padalia RC, et al. Chemical composition and antibacterial, antifungal, allelopathic and acetylcholinesterase inhibitory activities of cassumunar-ginger. *J Sci Food Agric*. 2018 Jan;98(1):321-327.
7229 Li MX, Ma YP, Zhang HX, et al. Repellent, larvicidal and adulticidal activities of essential oil from Dai medicinal plant Zingiber cassumunar against Aedes albopictus. *Plant Divers*. 2020 Dec 3;43(4):317-323.
7230 Zheljazkov VD. Effects of Distillation Time on the Pinus ponderosa essential Oil Yield, Composition, and Antioxidant Activity. *Hort Sci*. 2012;47(6):785-89.
7231 Kurose K, Okamura D, Yatagi M. Composition of the essential oils from the leaves of nine Pinus species and the cones of three of Pinus species. *Flavour Frag J*. 2007 Jan;22(1):10-20.
7232 Krauze-Baranowska M, Mardarowicz M, Wiwart M. Antifungal activity of the essential oils from some species of the genus Pinus. *Zeitschrift fur Naturforschung C*. 2002 May;57(5-6):478-82.
7233 Kelkar VM, Geils BW, Becker DR, et al. How to recover more value from small pine trees: Essential oils and resins. *Biomass & Bioenergy*. 2006;30:316-20.
7234 Adams RP, Edmunds Jr GF. A re-examination of the volatile leaf oils of Pinus ponderosa Dougl. Ex P. Lawson using ion trap mass spectrometry. *Flavour Frag J*. 1989;4:19-23.
7235 European Medicines Agency. Public statement on the use of herbal medicinal products containing estragole. Available at: http://www.ema.europa.eu/docs/en_GB/document_library/Scientific_guideline/2010/04/WC500089960.pdf.
7236 European Medicines Agency. Public statement on the use of herbal medicinal products containing estragole. Available at: http://www.ema.europa.eu/docs/en_GB/document_library/Scientific_guideline/2010/04/WC500089960.pdf.
7237 Ding W, Levy DD, Bishop ME, et al. In vivo genotoxicity of estragole in male F344 rats. *Environ Mol Mutagen*. 2015 May;56(4):356-65.
7238 Eisenmann SW, Poulev A, Struwe L, et al. Qualitative variation of anti-diabetic constituents in different tarragon (Artemisia dracunculus L.) cytotypes. *Fitoterapia*. 2011 Oct;82(7):1062–74.

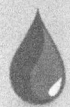

[7239] European Medicines Agency. Public statement on the use of herbal medicinal products containing estragole. Available at: http://www.ema.europa.eu/docs/en_GB/document_library/Scientific_guideline/2010/04/WC500089960.pdf.

[7240] Stegelmeier BL, Gardner DR, James LF, et al. The toxic and abortifacient effects of ponderosa pine. Vet Pathol. 1996 Jan;33(1):22-8.

[7241] California Cattleman. Pine Needle Abortion. UCD Vet News. 1996 Apr. Available at: http://ucanr.edu/sites/UCCE_LR/files/151746.pdf

[7242] European Commission. Opinion of the Scientific Committee on Food on estragole (1-Allyl-4-methoxybenzene). Available at: http://ec.europa.eu/food/fs/sc/scf/out104_en.pdf.

[7243] California Environmental Protection Agency. Evidence of the carcinogenicity of estragole. Available at: http:// oehha.ca.gov/prop65/pdf/estragf.pdf.

[7244] Drinkwater NR, Miller EC, Miller JA, et al. Hepatocarcinogenicity of estragole (1-allyl-4-methoxybenzene) and 1'-hydroxyestragole in the mouse and mutagenicity of 1'-acetoxyestragole in bacteria. J Natl Cancer Inst. 1976 Dec;57(6):1323-31.

[7245] Zeller A, Horst K, Rychlik M. Study of the metabolism of estragole in humans consuming fennel tea. Chem Res Toxicol. 2009 Dec;22(12):1929-37.

[7246] Krauze-Baranowska M, Mardarowicz M, Wiwart M. Antifungal activity of the essential oils from some species of the genus Pinus. Zeitschrift fur Naturforschung C. 2002 May;57(5-6):478-82.

[7247] Tabanca N, Demirci B, Crockett SL, et al. Chemical Composition and Antifungal Activity of Arnica longifolia, Aster hesperius, and Chrysothamnus nauseosus Essential Oils. J Agric Food Chem. 2007 Oct;55(21):8430-35.

[7248] Chao S, Young DG, Casabianca H, et al. Composition of the Oils of Three Chrysothamnus nauseousus Varieties. J Essent Oil Res. 2003 Nov-Dec;15:425-27.

[7249] Bonesi M, Menichini F, Tundis R, et al. Acetylcholinesterase and butyrylcholinesterase inhibitory activity of Pinus species essential oils and their constituents. J Enzyme Inhib Med Chem. 2010 Oct;25(5):622-8.

[7250] Tabanca N, Demirci B, Crockett SL, et al. Chemical Composition and Antifungal Activity of Arnica longifolia, Aster hesperius, and Chrysothamnus nauseosus Essential Oils. J Agric Food Chem. 2007 Oct;55(21):8430-35.

[7251] Gaydou EM. Chemical composition of Ravensara aromatica Sonn Leaf essential oils from Madagascar. J Essent Oil Res. 2006;18:215-17.

[7252] Andrianoelisoa HS, Menut C, de Chatelperron PC, et al. Intraspecific chemical variability and highlighting of chemotypes of leaf essential oils from Ravensara aromatica Sonnerat, a tree endemic to Madagascar. Flav Frag J. 2006 Sep-Oct;21(5):833-38.

[7253] De Medici D, Pieretti S, Salvatore G, et al. Chemical analysis of essential oil of Malagasy medicinal plants by gas chromatography and NMR spectrometry. Flav Frag J. 1992;7:275-281.

[7254] Rosoanaivo P. Ravensara aromatica: a Threatened Aromatic Species of Madagascar. Med Plant Conservation. 1997;4:9.

[7255] Tucker AO, Maciarello MJ. Two commercial oils of Ravensara from Madagascar: R. anisata and R. aromatica. J Essent Oil Res. 1995;7(3): 327-329.

[7256] Behra O, Rakotoarison C, Harris R. Ravintsara vs ravensara, a taxonomic classification. Int J Aromatherapy. 2001;11:4-7.

[7257] Craig JO. Poisoning by the volatile oils in childhood. Arch Dis Child. 1953;28:259-67.

[7258] Melis K. Bochner A, Janssens G. Accidental nasal eucalyptol and menthol instillation. Eur J Pediatr. 1989 Aug;148(8)786-7.

[7259] Day LM, Ozanne-Smith J, Parsons BJ, et al. Eucalyptus oil poisoning among young children: mechanisms of access and the potential prevention. Aust N Z J Public Health. 1997 Jun;21(3):297-302.

[7260] Chandar SD, Prashanti M, Kumar CL, et al. Eucalyptus Oil-Induced Seizures in Children: A Single-Center Prospective Study. Cureus. 2021 Mar 25;13(3):e14109.

[7261] European Medicines Agency. Public statement on the use of herbal medicinal products containing estragole. Available at: http://www.ema.europa.eu/docs/en_GB/document_library/Scientific_guideline/2010/04/WC500089960.pdf.

[7262] Johnson JD, Ryan MJ, Toft JD II, et al. Two-year toxicity and carcinogenicity study of methyl eugenol in F344/N rats and B6C3F(1) mice. J Agric Food Chem. 2000 Aug;48(8):3620-32.

[7263] European Commission. Opinion of the Scientific Committee on Food on methyl eugenol (4-Allyl-1,2- dimethoxybenzene).Availableat:http://ec.europa.eu/food/fs/sc/scf/out102_en.pdf.

[7264] National Toxicology Program. NTP Toxicology and Carcinogenesis Studies of Methyleugenol (CAS NO. 93-15-2) in F344/N Rats and B6C3F1 Mice (Gavage Studies). Natl Toxicol Program Tech Rep Ser. 2000 Jul;491:1-412.

[7265] National Toxicology Program. Carcinogenesis Studies of Eugenol (CAS No. 97-53-0) in F344/N Rats and B6C3F1 Mice (Feed Studies). Technical Report Series No. 223. NIH Publication No. 84-1779. 1983. U.S. DHHS, PHS, NIH, NTP, Research Triangle Park, NC.

[7266] European Medicines Agency. Public statement on the use of herbal medicinal products containing estragole. Available at: http://www.ema.europa.eu/docs/en_GB/document_library/Scientific_guideline/2010/04/WC500089960.pdf.

[7267] Ding W, Levy DD, Bishop ME, et al. In vivo genotoxicity of estragole in male F344 rats. Environ Mol Mutagen. 2015 May;56(4):356-65.

[7268] European Medicines Agency. Public statement on the use of herbal medicinal products containing estragole. Available at: http://www.ema.europa.eu/docs/en_GB/document_library/Scientific_guideline/2010/04/WC500089960.pdf.

[7269] Johnson JD, Ryan MJ, Toft JD II, et al. Two-year toxicity and carcinogenicity study of methyl eugenol in F344/N rats and B6C3F(1) mice. J Agric Food Chem. 2000 Aug;48(8):3620-32.

[7270] National Toxicology Program. NTP Toxicology and Carcinogenesis Studies of Methyleugenol (CAS NO. 93-15-2) in F344/N Rats and B6C3F1 Mice (Gavage Studies). Natl Toxicol Program Tech Rep Ser. 2000 Jul;491:1-412.

[7271] Kerckaert GA, Brauninger R, LeBoeuf RA, et al. Use of the Syrian hamster embryo cell transformation assay for carcinogenicity prediction of chemicals currently being tested by the National Toxicology Program in rodent bioassays. Environ Health Perspect. 1996;104:1075-84.

[7272] National Toxicology Program. Carcinogenesis Studies of Eugenol (CAS No. 97-53-0) in F344/N Rats and B6C3F1 Mice (Feed Studies). Technical Report Series No. 223. NIH Publication No. 84-1779. 1983. U.S. DHHS, PHS, NIH, NTP, Research Triangle Park, NC.

[7273] European Commission. Opinion of the Scientific Committee on Food on methyl eugenol (4-Allyl-1,2- dimethoxybenzene).Availableat:http://ec.europa.eu/food/fs/sc/scf/out102_en.pdf.

[7274] European Commission. Opinion of the Scientific Committee on Food on estragole (1-Allyl-4-methoxybenzene). Available at: http://ec.europa.eu/food/fs/sc/scf/out104_en.pdf.

[7275] California Environmental Protection Agency. Evidence of the carcinogenicity of estragole. Available at: http:// oehha.ca.gov/prop65/pdf/estragf.pdf.

[7276] Drinkwater NR, Miller EC, Miller JA, et al. Hepatocarcinogenicity of estragole (1-allyl-4-methoxybenzene) and 1'-hydroxyestragole in the mouse and mutagenicity of 1'-acetoxyestragole in bacteria. J Natl Cancer Inst. 1976 Dec;57(6):1323-31.

[7277] Zeller A, Horst K, Rychlik M. Study of the metabolism of estragole in humans consuming fennel tea. Chem Res Toxicol. 2009 Dec;22(12):1929-37.

[7278] Day LM, Ozanne-Smith J, Parsons BJ, et al. Eucalyptus oil poisoning among young children: mechanisms of access and the potential prevention. Aust N Z J Public Health. 1997 Jun;21(3):297-302.

[7279] Myott E. Case of eucalyptus poisoning. Brit M J. 1906;1:558.

[7280] Hindle RC. Eucalyptus oil ingestion. N Z Med J. 1994 May 11;107(977)185-6.

[7281] Tibballs J. Clinical effects and management of eucalyptus oil ingestion in infants and small children. Med J Aust. 1995 Aug;163(4):177-80.

[7282] Waldman W, Barwina M, Sein Anand J. Accidental ontoxication with eucalyptus oil—a case report. Przeql Lek. 2011;68(8):555-6.

[7283] Day LM, Ozanne-Smith J, Parsons BJ, et al. Eucalyptus oil poisoning among young children: mechanisms of access and the potential prevention. Aust N Z J Public Health. 1997 Jun;21(3):297-302.

[7284] De Vincenzi M, Silano M, De Vincenzi A, et al. Constituents of aromatic plants: eucalyptol. Fitoterapia. 2002 Jun;73(3):269-75.

[7285] Johnson JD, Ryan MJ, Toft JD II, et al. Two-year toxicity and carcinogenicity study of methyl eugenol in F344/N rats and B6C3F(1) mice. J Agric Food Chem. 2000 Aug;48(8):3620-32.

[7286] European Commission. Opinion of the Scientific Committee on Food on methyl eugenol (4-Allyl-1,2- dimethoxybenzene).Availableat:http://ec.europa.eu/food/fs/sc/scf/out102_en.pdf.

[7287] National Toxicology Program. NTP Toxicology and Carcinogenesis Studies of Methyleugenol (CAS NO. 93-15-2) in F344/N Rats and B6C3F1 Mice (Gavage Studies). Natl Toxicol Program Tech Rep Ser. 2000 Jul;491:1-412.

[7288] National Toxicology Program. Carcinogenesis Studies of Eugenol (CAS No. 97-53-0) in F344/N Rats and B6C3F1 Mice (Feed Studies). Technical Report Series No. 223. NIH Publication No. 84-1779. 1983. U.S. DHHS, PHS, NIH, NTP, Research Triangle Park, NC.

[7289] Sayyah M, Valizadeh J, Kamalinejad M. Anticonvulsant activity of the leaf oil of Laurus nobilis against pentylentetrazole- and maximal electroshock-induced seizure. Phytomedicine. 2002 Apr;9(3):212-16.

[7290] Culic M, Kekovic G, Grbic G, et al. Wavelet and fractal analysis of rat brain activity in seizures evoked by camphor oil and 1,8-cineole. Gen Physiol Biophys. 2009;28 Sec No:33-40.

[7291] Burkhard PR, Burkhardt K, Haenggeli CA, et al. Plant-induced seizures: reappearance of an old problem. J Neurol. 1999 Aug;246(8):667-70.

[7292] Waldman N. Seizure caused by dermal application of over-the-counter eucalyptus oil head lice preparation. Clin Toxicol (Phila). 2011 Oct;49(8):750-1.

[7293] Craig JO. Poisoning by the volatile oils in childhood. Arch Dis Child. 1953;28:259-67.

[7294] Mathew T, Kamath V, Kumar RS, et al. Eucalyptus oil inhalation-induced seizure: A novel, underrecognized, preventable cause of acute symptomatic seizure. Epilepsia Open. 2017 Jul 4;2(3):350-354.

[7295] Ahmad A, Khan A, Ahmad Khan L, et al. In vitro synergy of eugenol and methyleugenol with fluconazole against clinical Candida isolates. J Med Microbiol. 2010;59:1178-84.

[7296] Shin S, Pyun MS. Anti-Candida effects of estragole in combination with ketoconazole or amphotericin B. Phytother Res. 2004 Oct;18(10):827-30.

[7297] Shin S. Essential oil compounds from Agastache rugosa as antifungal agents against Trichophyton species. Arch Pharm Res. 2004 Mar;27(3):295-9.

[7298] Shin S, Kang CA. Antifungal activity of the essential oil of Agastache rugosa Kuntze and its synergism with ketoconazole. Lett Appl Microbiol. 2003;36(2):111-5.

[7299] Tognolini M, Barocelli E, Ballabeni V, et al. Comparative screening of plant essential oils; phenylpropanoid moiety as basic core for antiplatelet activity. Life Sci. 2006 Feb 23;78(13):1419-32.

[7300] Shahriyary L, Yazdanparast R. Tarragon (Artemisia d. has anti-platelet, anticoagulant activity. J Ethnopharmacol. 2007 Nov 1;114(2):194-8.

[7301] Duric K, Kovac Besovic EE, Niksic H, et al. Anticoagulant activity of some Artemisia dracunculus leaf extracts. Bosnian J Basic Med Sci. 2015;15(2):9-14.

[7302] Yazdanparast R, Shahriyary L. Comparative effects of Artemisia dracunculus, Satureja hortensis and Origanum majorana on inhibition of blood platelet adhesion, aggregation and secretion. Vascul Pharmacol. 2008 Jan;48(1):32-37.

[7303] Lee HS. Anticoagulant properties of constituents derived from fennel (Foeniculum vulgare Gaertner) fruits. Food Sci Biotech. 2006 Oct;15(5):763-67.

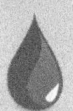
[7304] Lee SE, Lee BH, Choi WS, et al. Fumigant toxicity of volatile natural products from Korean spices and medicinal plants towards the rice weevil, Sitophilus oryzae (L). *Pest Manag Sci.* 2001;57:548-53.

[7305] Khan MM. Masters Thesis: Inhibition of Cytochrome P450 2E1 and Cytochrome P450 2A6 by Essential Oils: Tarragon (Artemisia dracunculus) and Basil (Ocimum basilicum). 2014. Available at: https://libres.uncg.edu/ir/uncg/f/Khan_uncg_0154M_11587.pdf

[7306] Lamborn LL. Modern soaps, candles and glycerin: A practical manual of modern methods of utilization of fats and oils in the manufacture of soaps and candles, and of the recovery of glycerin. Library of the University of Wisconsin.

[7307] Oyen LP, Dung NX. Plant resources of South-East Asia. 1999. Backhyus, Leiden.

[7308] Kim NH, Hyun SH, Jin CH, et al. Pretreatment with 1,8-cineole potentiates thioacetamide-induced hepatotoxicity and immunosuppression. *Arch Pharm Res.* 2004 Jul;27(7):781-9.

[7309] Jori A, Bianchetti A, Prestini PE, et al. Effect of eucalyptol (1,8-cineole) on the metabolism of other drugs in rats and in man. *Eur J Pharmacol.* 1970;9(3):362-66.

[7310] de Sousa DP, Raphael E, Brocksom U, et al. Sedative effect of monoterpene alcohols in mice: A preliminary screening. *Verlag der Zeitschrift fur Naturforschung.* 2007;62c:563-66.

[7311] Ferrara L, Naviglio D, Armone Caruso A. Cytological aspects on the effects of a nasal spray consisting of standardized extract of citrus lemon and essential oils in allergic rhinopathy. *ISRN Pharm.* 2012;2012:404606.

[7312] Sfeir J, Lefrancois C, Baudoux D, et al. In vitro antibacterial activity of essential oils against Streptococcus pyogenes. *Evid Based Complement Alternat Med.* 2013;2013:269161.

[7313] Chalchat JC, Valade I. Chemical composition of leaf oils of Cinnamomum from Madagascar: C. zeylanicum Blume, C. camphora L., C fragrans Baillon and C. angustifolia. *J Essent Oil Res.* 2000;12:537-40.

[7314] Zhu L, Li Y, Li B, et al. Aromatic plants and essential constituents. South China Institute of Botany, Hong Kong. 1993.

[7315] Chen HP, Yang K, You CX, et al. Chemical constituents and insecticidal activities of the essential oil of Cinnamomum camphora leaves against Lasioderma serricorne. *J Chem.* 2014 Jun;2014:1-6.

[7316] Stubbs BJ, Specht A. The essential oil of Cinnamomum camphora (L.) Nees and Eberm.-Variation in oil composition throughout the tree in two chemotypes from Eastern Australia. *J Essent Oil Res.* 2004 May-Jun;16:200-05.

[7317] Pelissier Y, Marion C, Prunac S, et al. Volatile components of leaves, stems and bark of Cinnamomum camphora Ness et Ebermaier. *J Essent Oil Res.* 1995;7:313-15.

[7318] Frizzo CD, Santos AC, Paroul N, et al. Essential oils of Camphor tree (Cinnamomum camphora Nees & Eberm) cultivated in southern Brazil. *Braz Arch Biol Tech.* 2000;43(3).

[7319] Ho CL, Wang EIC, Su YC. Essential oil compositions and bioactives of the various parts of Cinnamomum camphora Sieb. Var linaloolifera Frujuta. *Forest Res Quarterly.* 2009;31(2):77-96.

[7320] Andrianoelisoa H, Menut C, Danthu P. Ravensara aromatica or Ravintsara: a continuing confusion among distributors of essential oils in Europe and North America. *Phytotherapie.* 2012 Jun;10(3):161-69.

[7321] Xiao S, Yu H, Xie Y, et al. Evaluation of the analgesic potential and safety of Cinnamomum camphora chvar. Borneol essential oil. *Bioengineered.* 2021;12(2):9860-71.

[7322] Shi S, Wu Q, Su J, et al. Composition analysis of volatile oils from flowers, leaves and branches of Cinnamomum camphora chvar. Borneol in China. *J Essent Oil Res.* 2013;25(5):394-400.

[7323] Su J, Chen J, Liao S, et al. Composition and biological activities of the essential oil extracted from a novel plant of Cinnamomum camphora Chvar. Borneol. *J Med Plants Res.* 2012 May 16;6(18):3487-94.

[7324] Yu H, Ren X, Liu Y, et al. Extraction of Cinnamomum camphora chvar. Borneol essential oil using neutral cellulase assisted-steam distillation: optimization of extraction, and analysis of chemical constituents. *Ind Crop Prod.* 2019;141:111794.

[7325] Craig JO. Poisoning by the volatile oils in childhood. *Arch Dis Child.* 1953;28:259-67.

[7326] Melis K. Bochner A, Janssens G. Accidental nasal eucalyptol and menthol instillation. *Eur J Pediatr.* 1989 Aug;148(8)786-7.

[7327] Day LM, Ozanne-Smith J, Parsons BJ, et al. Eucalyptus oil poisoning among young children: mechanisms of access and the potential prevention. *Aust N Z J Public Health.* 1997 Jun;21(3):297-302.

[7328] Chandar SD, Prashanti M, Kumar CL, et al. Eucalyptus Oil-Induced Seizures in Children: A Single-Center Prospective Study. *Cureus.* 2021 Mar 25;13(3):e14109.

[7329] Koren G. Medications which can kill a toddler with one tablet or teaspoonful. *J toxicol Clin Toxicol.* 1993;31(3):407- 13.

[7330] Bar-Oz B, Levicheck Z, Koren G. Medications that can kill a toddler with one tablet or teaspoonful – A 2004 update. *Paediatr Drugs.* 2004;6(2):123-6.

[7331] Rabl W, Katzgraber F, Steinlechner M. Camphor ingestion for abortion (case report). *Forensic Sci Int.* 1997 Sep 19;89(1-2):137-40.

[7332] Flaman Z, Pellechia-Clarke S, Bailey B, et al. Unintentional exposure of young children to camphor and eucalyptus oils. *Paediatr Child Health.* 2001 Feb;6(2):80-83.

[7333] Burkhard PR, Burkhardt K, Haenggeli CA, et al. Plant-induced seizures: reappearance of an old problem. *J Neurol.* 1999 Aug;246(8):667-70.

[7334] Narayan S, Singh N. Camphor poisoning-An unusual cause of seizure. *Med J Armed Forces India.* 2012 Jul;68(3):252-53.

[7335] Chanaranaj KJ, G MV, S M. Camphor poisoning in a child. *Natl Med J India.* 2013 Jan-Feb;26(1):60.

[7336] Day LM, Ozanne-Smith J, Parsons BJ, et al. Eucalyptus oil poisoning among young children: mechanisms of access and the potential prevention. *Aust N Z J Public Health.* 1997 Jun;21(3):297-302.

[7337] Myott E. Case of eucalyptus poisoning. *Brit M J.* 1906;1:558.

[7338] Hindle RC. Eucalyptus oil ingestion. *N Z Med J.* 1994 May 11;107(977)185-6.

[7339] Tibballs J. Clinical effects and management of eucalyptus oil ingestion in infants and small children. *Med J Aust.* 1995 Aug;163(4):177-80.

[7340] Waldman W, Barwina M, Sein Anand J. Accidental ontoxication with eucalyptus oil—a case report. *Przeql Lek.* 2011;68(8):555-6.

[7341] Day LM, Ozanne-Smith J, Parsons BJ, et al. Eucalyptus oil poisoning among young children: mechanisms of access and the potential prevention. *Aust N Z J Public Health.* 1997 Jun;21(3):297-302.

[7342] De Vincenzi M, Silano M, De Vincenzi A, et al. Constituents of aromatic plants: eucalyptol. *Fitoterapia.* 2002 Jun;73(3):269-75.

[7343] Manoguerra AS, Erdman AR, Wax PM, et al. Camphor poisoning: an evidence-based practice guideline for out-of- hospital management. *Clin Toxicol (Phila).* 2006;44(4):357-70.

[7344] Gibson DE, Moore GP, Pfaff JA. Camphor ingestion. *Am J Emerg Med.* 1989 Jan;7(1):41-43.

[7345] Koppel C, Martends F, Schirop T, et al. Hemoperfusion in acute camphor poisoning. *Intensive Care Med.* 1988;14(4):431-33.

[7346] Olowe SA, Ransome-Kuti O. The risk of jaundice in glucose-6-phosphate dehydrogenase deficient babies exposed to menthol. *Acta Paediatr Scand.* 1980 May;69(3):341-5.

[7347] Dillon Remy M, Manning Alleyne P, Bratt DE, et al. Neonatal jaundice at Port-of-Spain General Hospital abstract. *West Indian Med J.* 1987;36(Suppl):28.

[7348] Lamborn LL. Modern soaps, candles and glycerin: A practical manual of modern methods of utilization of fats and oils in the manufacture of soaps and candles, and of the recovery of glycerin. Library of the University of Wisconsin.

[7349] Oyen LP, Dung NX. Plant resources of South-East Asia. 1999. Backhyus, Leiden.

[7350] Kim NH, Hyun SH, Jin CH, et al. Pretreatment with 1,8-cineole potentiates thioacetamide-induced hepatotoxicity and immunosuppression. *Arch Pharm Res.* 2004 Jul;27(7):781-9.

[7351] Cardoso NN, Alviano CS, Blank AF, et al. Synergism Effect of the Essential Oil from Ocimum basilicum var. Maria Bonita and Its Major Components with Fluconazole and Its Influence on Ergosterol Biosynthesis. *Evid Based Complement Alternat Med.* 2016;2016:5647182.

[7352] Jori A, Bianchetti A, Prestini PE, et al. Effect of eucalyptol (1,8-cineole) on the metabolism of other drugs in rats and in man. *Eur J Pharmacol.* 1970;9(3):362-66.

[7353] de Sousa DP, Raphael E, Brocksom U, et al. Sedative effect of monoterpene alcohols in mice: A preliminary screening. *Verlag der Zeitschrift fur Naturforschung.* 2007;62c:563-66.

[7354] Uc A, Bishop WP, Sanders KD. Camphor hepatotoxicity. *South Med J.* 2000;93:596-98.

[7355] Covington TR, et al. Handbook of Nonprescription Drugs. 11th ed. Washington, D.C.: American Pharmaceutical Association. 1996.

[7356] Tang Y, Lv X, Liu Y, et al. Metabonomics Study in Mice With Learning and Memory Impairment on the Intervention of Essential Oil Extracted From Cinnamomum camphora Chvar. Borneol. *Front Pharmacol.* 2022 Mar 10;13:770411.

[7357] Xiao S, Yu H, Xie Y, et al. Evaluation of the analgesic potential and safety of Cinnamomum camphora chvar. Borneol essential oil. *Bioengineered.* 2021;12(2):9860-71.

[7358] Satyal P, Paudel P, Poudel A, et al. Bioactives and compositional analyses of Cinnamomum essential oils from Nepal: C. camphora, C. tamala, and C. glaucescens. *Nat Prod Commun.* 2013 Dec;8(12):1777-84.

[7359] Srivastava B, Singh P, Shukla R, et al. A novel combination of the essential oils of Cinnamomum camphora and Alpinia galanga in checking aflatoxin B1 production by a toxigenic strain of Aspergillus flavus. *World J Microbiol Biotech.* 2008;24(5):693-97.

[7360] Su J, Chen J, Liao S, et al. Composition and biological activities of the essential oil extracted from a novel plant of Cinnamomum camphora Chvar. Borneol. *J Med Plants Res.* 2012 May 16;6(18):3487-94.

[7361] Yu H, Ren X, Yang F, et al. Antimicrobial and anti-dust mite efficacy of Cinnamomum camphora chvar. Borneol essential oil using pilot-plant neutral cellulase-assisted steam distillation. *Lett Appl Microbiol.* 2022 Feb;74(2):258-267.

[7362] Su J, Chen J, Liao S, et al. Composition and biological activities of the essential oil extracted from a novel plant of Cinnamomum camphora Chvar. Borneol. *J Med Plants Res.* 2012 May 16;6(18):3487-94.

[7363] Satyal P, Paudel P, Poudel A, et al. Bioactives and compositional analyses of Cinnamomum essential oils from Nepal: C. camphora, C. tamala, and C. glaucescens. *Nat Prod Commun.* 2013 Dec;8(12):1777-84.

[7364] Jiang H, Wang J, Song L, et al. GC×GC-TOFMS Analysis of Essential Oils Composition from Leaves, Twigs and Seeds of Cinnamomum camphora L. Presl and Their Insecticidal and Repellent Activities. *Molecules.* 2016;21(4):423.

[7365] Yu H, Ren X, Yang F, et al. Antimicrobial and anti-dust mite efficacy of Cinnamomum camphora chvar. Borneol essential oil using pilot-plant neutral cellulase-assisted steam distillation. *Lett Appl Microbiol.* 2022 Feb;74(2):258-267.

[7366] Dutta BK, Karmakar S, Naglot A, et al. Anticandidal activity of some essential oils of mega biodiversity hotspot in India. *Mycoses.* 2007 Mar;50(2):121-24.

[7367] Sfeir J, Lefrancois C, Baudoux D, et al. In vitro antibacterial activity of essential oils against Streptococcus pyogenes. *Evid Based Complement Alternat Med.* 2013;2013:269161.

[7368] Guo S, Geng Z, Zhang W, et al. The Chemical Composition of Essential Oils from Cinnamomum camphora and Their Insecticidal Activity against the Stored Product Pests. *Int J Mol Sci.* 2016 Nov 4;17(11).

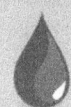

[7369] Wang W, Li D, Huang X, et al. Study on Antibacterial and Quorum-Sensing Inhibition Activities of Cinnamomum camphora Leaf Essential Oil. *Molecules.* 2019 Oct 21;24(20).
[7370] Xu Y, Qin J, Wang P, et al. Chemical Composition and Larvicidal Activities of Essential Oil of Cinnamomum Camphora (L.) Leaf Against Anopheles Stephensi. *Rev Soc Bras Med Trop.* 2020 Jan 27;53:e20190211.
[7371] Chen J, Tang C, Zhang R, et al. Metabolomics Analysis to Evaluate the Antibacterial Activity of the Essential Oil From the Leaves of Cinnamomum Camphora (Linn.) Presl. *J Ethnopharmacol.* 2020 Feb 6;253:112652.
[7372] Xiao S, Yu H, Xie Y, et al. The anti-inflammatory potential of Cinnamomum camphora (L.) J.Presl essential oil in vitro and in vivo. *J Ethnopharmacol.* 2020 Oct 23;113516.
[7373] Chen J, Tang C, Zhou Y, et al. Anti-Inflammatory Property of the Essential Oil from Cinnamomum camphora (Linn.) Presl Leaves and the Evaluation of Its Underlying Mechanism by Using Metabolomics Analysis. *Molecules.* 2020 Oct 19;25(20):4796.
[7374] Bottoni M, Milani F, Mozzo M, et al. Sub-Tissue Localization of Phytochemicals in Cinnamomum camphora (L.) J. Presl. Growing in Northern Italy. *Plants (Basel).* 2021 May 19;10(5):1008.
[7375] Poudel DK, Rokaya A, Ojha PK, et al. The Chemical Profiling of Essential Oils from Different Tissues of Cinnamomum camphora L. and Their Antimicrobial Activities. *Molecules.* 2021 Aug 24;26(17):5132.
[7376] Boumendjel M, Boucheker A, Feknous S, et al. Adaptogenic activity of Cinnamomum camphora, Eucalyptus globulus, Lavandula stœchas and Rosmarinus officinalis essential oil used in North-African folk medicine. *Cell Mol Biol (Noisy-le-grand).* 2021 Aug 31;67(2):83-88.
[7377] Tang Y, Lv X, Liu Y, et al. Metabonomics Study in Mice With Learning and Memory Impairment on the Intervention of Essential Oil Extracted From Cinnamomum camphora Chvar. Borneol. *Front Pharmacol.* 2022 Mar 10;13:770411.
[7378] Mujawah AAH, Abdallah EM, Alshoumar SA, et al. GC-MS and in vitro antibacterial potential of Cinnamomum camphora essential oil against some clinical antibiotic-resistant bacterial isolates. *Eur Rev Med Pharmacol Sci.* 2022 Aug;26(15):5372-5379.
[7379] Ling Q, Zhang B, Wang Y, et al. Chemical Composition and Antioxidant Activity of the Essential Oils of Citral-Rich Chemotype Cinnamomum camphora and Cinnamomum bodinieri. *Molecules.* 2022 Oct 29;27(21):7356.
[7380] Jugreet BS, Ibrahime SK, Zengin G, et al. GC/MS Profiling, In Vitro and In Silico Pharmacological Screening and Principal Component Analysis of Essential Oils from Three Exotic and Two Endemic Plants from Mauritius. *Chem Biodivers.* 2021 Mar;18(3):e2000921.
[7381] Xiao S, Yu H, Xie Y, et al. Evaluation of the analgesic potential and safety of Cinnamomum camphora chvar. Borneol essential oil. *Bioengineered.* 2021 Oct 26. Online ahead of print.
[7382] Jugreet BS, Lall N, Anina Lambrechts I, et al. In Vitro and In Silico Pharmacological and Cosmeceutical Potential of Ten Essential Oils from Aromatic Medicinal Plants from the Mascarene Islands. *Molecules.* 2022 Dec 8;27(24):8705.
[7383] Kilic O, Kocak A. Essential Oil Composition of Six Pinus L. Taxa (Pinaceae) from Canada and Their Chemotaxonomy. *J Aric Sci Tech B.* 2014;4:67-73.
[7384] Krauze-Baranowska M, Mardarowicz M, Wiwart M. Antifungal activity of the essential oils from some species of the genus Pinus. *Zeitschrift fur Naturforschung C.* 2002 May;57(5-6):478-82.
[7385] Aromatics International. Norway Pine (Red Pine). Available at: https://www.aromatics.com/products/balsamic/norway-pine-red-pine.
[7386] Stillpoint Aromatics. Red Pine (Norway Pine) Essential Oil. Available at: http://www.stillpointaromatics.com/red-pine-essential-oil-aromatherapy
[7387] Nguyen LT, Myslivečkova Z, Szotakova B, et al. The inhibitory effects of β-caryophyllene, β-caryophyllene oxide and α-humulene on the activities of the main drug-metabolizing enzymes in rat and human liver in vitro. *Chem-Biol Interactoins.* 2017 Dec 25;278:123-8.
[7388] Krauze-Baranowska M, Mardarowicz M, Wiwart M. Antifungal activity of the essential oils from some species of the genus Pinus. *Zeitschrift fur Naturforschung C.* 2002 May;57(5-6):478-82.
[7389] Innocenti G, Dall'Acqua S, Scialino G, et al. Chemical Composition and Biological Properties of Rhododendron anthopogon Essential Oil. *Molecules.* 2010;15:2326-38.
[7390] Guleria S, Jaitak V, Saini R, et al. Comparative studies of volatileoil composition of Rhododendron anthopogon by hydrodistillation, supercritical carbon dioxide extractionand head space analysis. *Nat Prod Res.* 2011 Aug;25(13):1271-77.
[7391] Gurung K, Innocenti G, Dall'Acqua, et al. GC-MS of Essential Oil of Rhododendron anthopogon D. Don and Its Biological Properties. Available at: https://www.scribd.com/document/5656017/GC-MS-of-Essential-Oil-of-Rhododendron-anthopogon-D-Don-and-Its-Biological-Properties.
[7392] Yonzon M, Lee DJ, Yokochi T, et al. Antimicrobial Activities of Essential Oils of Nepal. *J Essent Oil Res.* 2005 Jan-Feb;17(1):107-11.
[7393] Zhou XL, Lai YX, Ping A, et al. [Study on the chemical constituents in the volatile oils of the flowers of Tibetan medicine Rhododendron anthopogon]. *Zhong Yao Cai.* 2010 Jan;33(1):50-3.
[7394] Gurung K, Innocenti G, Dall'Acqua, et al. GC-MS of Essential Oil of Rhododendron anthopogon D. Don and Its Biological Properties. Available at: https://www.scribd.com/document/5656017/GC-MS-of-Essential-Oil-of-Rhododendron-anthopogon-D-Don-and-Its-Biological-Properties.
[7395] Gurung K, Innocenti G, Dall'Acqua, et al. GC-MS of Essential Oil of Rhododendron anthopogon D. Don and Its Biological Properties. Available at: https://www.scribd.com/document/5656017/GC-MS-of-Essential-Oil-of-Rhododendron-anthopogon-D-Don-and-Its-Biological-Properties.
[7396] Yonzon M, Lee DJ, Yokochi T, et al. Antimicrobial Activities of Essential Oils of Nepal. *J Essent Oil Res.* 2005 Jan-Feb;17(1):107-11.
[7397] Sharafzadeh S, Alizadeh O. German and Roman chamomile. *J Appl Pharm Sci.* 2011;10:01-05.
[7398] European Medicines Agency. Assessment report on Chamaemelum nobile (L.) All., flos. 2011. Available from:
from http://www.ema.europa.eu/docs/en_GB/document_library/Herbal_-_HMPC_assessment_report/2011/03/WC500102591.pdf.
[7399] Bail S, Buchbauer G, Jirovetz L, et al. Antimicrobial activities of Roman chamomile oil from France and its main constituents. *J Essent Oil Res.* 2009;21(3):283-86.
[7400] Omnidbaigi R, Sefidkon F, Kazemi F. Influence of drying methods on the essential oil content and composition of Roman chamomile. *Flav Frag J.* 2004 May;19(3):196-98.
[7401] Baylac S, Racine P. Inhibition of 5-lipoxygenase by essential oils and other natural fragrant extracts. *Int J Aromatherapy.* 2003;13(2-3):138-42.
[7402] Cho MY, Min ES, Hur MH, et al. Effects of aromatherapy on the anxiety, vital signs, and sleep quality of percutaneous coronary intervention patients in intensive care units. *Evid Based Complement Altern Med.* 2013(2013):1-6.
[7403] Hur MH, Han SH. Clinical trial of aromatherapy on postpartum mother's perineal healing. *Taehan Kanho Hakhoe Chi.* 2004 Feb;34(1):53-62.
[7404] Rossi T, Melegari M, Bianchi A, et al. Sedative, anti-inflammatory and anti-diuretic effects induced in rats by essential oils of varieties of Anthemis nobilis: a comparative study. *Pharmacol Res Commun.* 1988 Dec;20 Suppl 5:71-74.
[7405] Della Loggia R. Chamomile extracts exerted anti-inflammatory effects when applied topically in animal models of inflammation. *Plant Med.* 1990;56:657-58.
[7406] Gilligan NP. The palliation of nausea in hospice and palliative care patients with essential oils of Pimpinella anisum (aniseed), Foeniculum vulgare var. dulce (sweet fennel), Anthemis nobilis (Roman chamomile) and Mentha x piperita (peppermint). *Int J Aromather.* 2005;15(4):163-67.
[7407] Merfort I, Heilmann J, Hagedorn-Leweke U, et al. In vitro skin penetration studies of camomile flavones. *Pharmazie.* 1994 Jul;49(7):509-11.
[7408] Srivastava JK, Pandey M, Gupta S. Chamomile, a novel and selective CoX-2 inhibitor with anti-inflammatory activity. *Life Sci.* 2009 Nov;85(19-20):663-69.
[7409] Wilkinson S, Aldridge J, Salmon I, et al. An evaluation of aromatherapy massage in palliative care. *Palliative Med.* 1999;13:409-17.
[7410] Simoes BM, Kohler B, Clarke RB, et al. Estrogenicity of essential oils is not required to relieve symptoms of urogenital atrophy in breast cancer survivors. Ther Adv Med Oncol. 2018;10:1758835918766189.
[7411] Ferreira LE, Benincasa BI, Fachin AL, et al. Essential oils of Citrus aurantifolia, Anthemis nobile and Lavandula officinalis: in vitro anthelmintic activities against Haemonchus contortus. *Parasit Vectors.* 2018; 11: 269.
[7412] Hashikawa-Hobara N, Otsuka A, Ishikawa R, et al. Roman Chamomile Inhalation Combined With Clomipramine Treatment Improves Treatment-Resistant Depression-Like Behavior in Mice. *Biomed Pharmacother.* 2019 Oct;118:109263.
[7413] Silveira V, Rubio KTS, Martucci MEP. Anxiolytic effect of Anthemis nobilis L. (roman chamomile) and Citrus reticulata Blanco (tangerine) essential oils using the light-dark test in zebrafish (Danio rerio). *J Ethnopharmacol.* 2022 Nov;298(15):115580.
[7414] Silva CJ, Barbosa LCA, Maltha CRA, et al. Comparative study of the essential oils of seven Melaleuca (Myrtaceae) species grown in Brazil. *Flavour Frag J.* 2007;22:474-78.
[7415] Sayyah M, Valizadeh J, Kamalinejad M. Anticonvulsant activity of the leaf oil of Laurus nobilis against pentylentetrazole- and maximal electroshock-induced seizure. *Phytomedicine.* 2002 Apr;9(3):212-16.
[7416] Culic M, Kekovic G, Grbic G, et al. Wavelet and fractal analysis of rat brain activity in seizures evoked by camphor oil and 1,8-cineole. *Gen Physiol Biophys.* 2009;28 Sec No:33-40.
[7417] Burkhard PR, Burkhardt K, Haenggeli CA, et al. Plant-induced seizures: reappearance of an old problem. *J Neurol.* 1999 Aug;246(8):667-70.
[7418] Waldman N. Seizure caused by dermal application of over-the-counter eucalyptus oil head lice preparation. *Clin Toxicol (Phila).* 2011 Oct;49(8):750-1.
[7419] Craig JO. Poisoning by the volatile oils in childhood. *Arch Dis Child.* 1953;28:259-67.
[7420] Mathew T, Kamath V, Kumar RS, et al. Eucalyptus oil inhalation-induced seizure: A novel, underrecognized, preventable cause of acute symptomatic seizure. *Epilepsia Open.* 2017 Jul 4;2(3):350-354.
[7421] Jori A, Bianchetti A, Prestini PE, et al. Effect of eucalyptol (1,8-cineole) on the metabolism of other drugs in rats and in man. *Eur J Pharmacol.* 1970;9(3):362-66.
[7422] Kim NH, Hyun SH, Jin CH, et al. Pretreatment with 1,8-cineole potentiates thioacetamide-induced hepatotoxicity and immunosuppression. *Arch Pharm Res.* 2004 Jul;27(7):781-9.
[7423] Jori A, Bianchetti A, Prestini PE, et al. Effect of eucalyptol (1,8-cineole) on the metabolism of other drugs in rats and in man. *Eur J Pharmacol.* 1970;9(3):362-66.
[7424] de Sousa DP, Raphael E, Brocksom U, et al. Sedative effect of monoterpene alcohols in mice: A preliminary screening. *Verlag der Zeitschrift fur Naturforschung.* 2007;62c:563-66.
[7425] Craig JO. Poisoning by the volatile oils in childhood. *Arch Dis Child.* 1953;28:259-67.
[7426] Melis K. Bochner A, Janssens G. Accidental nasal eucalyptol and menthol instillation. *Eur J Pediatr.* 1989 Aug;148(8)786-7.
[7427] Day LM, Ozanne-Smith J, Parsons BJ, et al. Eucalyptus oil poisoning among young children: mechanisms of access and the potential prevention. *Aust N Z J Public Health.* 1997 Jun;21(3):297-302.
[7428] Chandar SD, Prashanti M, Kumar CL, et al. Eucalyptus Oil-Induced Seizures in Children: A Single-Center Prospective Study. *Cureus.* 2021 Mar 25;13(3):e14109.
[7429] Burkhard PR, Burkhardt K, Haenggeli CA, et al. Plant-induced seizures: reappearance of an old problem. *J Neurol.* 1999 Aug;246(8):667-70.
[7430] Waldman N. Seizure caused by dermal application of over-the-counter eucalyptus oil head lice preparation. *Clin Toxicol (Phila).* 2011 Oct;49(8):750-1.
[7431] Craig JO. Poisoning by the volatile oils in childhood. *Arch Dis Child.* 1953;28:259-67.
[7432] Newall CA, Anderson LA, Phillipson JD. "Herbal Medicines: A Guide for Health-care Professionals." London: The Pharmaceutical Press, 1996, 108.
[7433] European Medicines Agency. Community herbal monograph on Eucalyptus globulus Labill., Eucalyptus polybractea R.T. Baker and/or

Eucalyptus smithii R.T. Baker, aetheroleum. 2013 Jun. Available at: http://www.ema.europa.eu/docs/en_GB/document_library/Herbal_-_Community_herbal_monograph/2013/07/WC500147008.pdf

[7434] Fischer JH, Dethlefsen U. Efficacy of cineole in patients suffering from acute bronchitis: a placebo-controlled double-blind trial. *Cough*. 2013; 9: 25.

[7435] Worth W, Dethlefsen U. Patients with asthma benefit from concomitant therapy with cineole: a placebo-controlled, double-blind trial. *J Asthma*. 2012 Oct;49(8):849-53.

[7436] Day LM, Ozanne-Smith J, Parsons BJ, et al. Eucalyptus oil poisoning among young children: mechanisms of access and the potential prevention. *Aust N Z J Public Health*. 1997 Jun;21(3):297-302.

[7437] Myott E. Case of eucalyptus poisoning. *Brit M J*. 1906;1:558.

[7438] Hindle RC. Eucalyptus oil ingestion. *N Z Med J*. 1994 May 11;107(977)185-6.

[7439] Tibballs J. Clinical effects and management of eucalyptus oil ingestion in infants and small children. *Med J Aust*. 1995 Aug;163(4):177-80.

[7440] Waldman W, Barwina M, Sein Anand J. Accidental ontoxication with eucalyptus oil—a case report. *Przeql Lek*. 2011;68(8):555-6.

[7441] Day LM, Ozanne-Smith J, Parsons BJ, et al. Eucalyptus oil poisoning among young children: mechanisms of access and the potential prevention. *Aust N Z J Public Health*. 1997 Jun;21(3):297-302.

[7442] De Vincenzi M, Silano M, De Vincenzi A, et al. Constituents of aromatic plants: eucalyptol. *Fitoterapia*. 2002 Jun;73(3):269-75.

[7443] Gray AM, Flatt PR. Antihyperglycemic actions of Eucalyptus globulus (Eucalyptus) are associated with pancreatic and extra pancreatic effects in mice. *J Nutr*. 1998 Dec;128(12):2319–23.

[7444] Basak SS, Candan F. Effect of Laurus nobilis L. Essential Oil and its Main Components on α-glucosidase and Reactive Oxygen Species Scavenging Activity. *Iran J Pharm Res*. 2013 Spring;12(2):367-79.

[7445] Fathiazad F, Mazandarani M, Hamedeyazdan. Phytochemical analysis and antioxidant activity of Hyssopus officinalis L. from Iran. *Adv Pharm Bull*. 2011 Dec;1(2):63–67.

[7446] Jori A, Bianchetti A, Prestini PE, et al. Effect of eucalyptol (1,8-cineole) on the metabolism of other drugs in rats and in man. *Eur J Pharmacol*. 1970;9(3):362-66.

[7447] Kim NH, Hyun SH, Jin CH, et al. Pretreatment with 1,8-cineole potentiates thioacetamide-induced hepatotoxicity and immunosuppression. *Arch Pharm Res*. 2004 Jul;27(7):781-9.

[7448] Tsai HH, Lin HW, Chen YL, et al. A review of potential harmful interactions between anticoagulant/antiplatelet agents and Chinese herbal medicines. *PLoS One*. 2013 May 9;8(5):e64255.

[7449] Moharam BA, Jantan I, bin Ahmad F, et al. Antiplatelet Aggregation and Platelet Activating Factor (PAF) Receptor Antagonistic Activities of the Essential Oils of Five Goniothalamus Species. *Molecules*. 2010;15:5124-38.

[7450] Jori A, Bianchetti A, Prestini PE, et al. Effect of eucalyptol (1,8-cineole) on the metabolism of other drugs in rats and in man. *Eur J Pharmacol*. 1970;9(3):362-66.

[7451] de Sousa DP, Raphael E, Brocksom U, et al. Sedative effect of monoterpene alcohols in mice: A preliminary screening. *Verlag der Zeitschrift fur Naturforschung*. 2007;62c:563-66.

[7452] Johnson JD, Ryan MJ, Toft JD II, et al. Two-year toxicity and carcinogenicity study of methyl eugenol in F344/N rats and B6C3F(1) mice. *J Agric Food Chem*. 2000 Aug;48(8):3620-32.

[7453] European Commission. Opinion of the Scientific Committee on Food on methyl eugenol (4-Allyl-1,2- dimethoxybenzene). Available at:http://ec.europa.eu/food/fs/sc/scf/out102_en.pdf.

[7454] National Toxicology Program. NTP Toxicology and Carcinogenesis Studies of Methyleugenol (CAS NO. 93-15-2) in F344/N Rats and B6C3F1 Mice (Gavage Studies). *Natl Toxicol Program Tech Rep Ser*. 2000 Jul;491:1-412.

[7455] National Toxicology Program. Carcinogenesis Studies of Eugenol (CAS No. 97-53-0) in F344/N Rats and B6C3F1 Mice (Feed Studies). Technical Report Series No. 223. NIH Publication No. 84-1779. 1983. U.S. DHHS, PHS, NIH, NTP, Research Triangle Park, NC.

[7456] Johnson JD, Ryan MJ, Toft JD II, et al. Two-year toxicity and carcinogenicity study of methyl eugenol in F344/N rats and B6C3F(1) mice. *J Agric Food Chem*. 2000 Aug;48(8):3620-32.

[7457] National Toxicology Program. NTP Toxicology and Carcinogenesis Studies of Methyleugenol (CAS NO. 93-15-2) in F344/N Rats and B6C3F1 Mice (Gavage Studies). *Natl Toxicol Program Tech Rep Ser*. 2000 Jul;491:1-412.

[7458] Kerckaert GA, Brauninger R, LeBoeuf RA, et al. Use of the Syrian hamster embryo cell transformation assay for carcinogenicity prediction of chemicals currently being tested by the National Toxicology Program in rodent bioassays. *Environ Health Perspect*. 1996;104:1075-84.

[7459] National Toxicology Program. Carcinogenesis Studies of Eugenol (CAS No. 97-53-0) in F344/N Rats and B6C3F1 Mice (Feed Studies). Technical Report Series No. 223. NIH Publication No. 84-1779. 1983. U.S. DHHS, PHS, NIH, NTP, Research Triangle Park, NC.

[7460] Johnson JD, Ryan MJ, Toft JD II, et al. Two-year toxicity and carcinogenicity study of methyl eugenol in F344/N rats and B6C3F(1) mice. *J Agric Food Chem*. 2000 Aug;48(8):3620-32.

[7461] European Commission. Opinion of the Scientific Committee on Food on methyl eugenol (4-Allyl-1,2- dimethoxybenzene). Available at:http://ec.europa.eu/food/fs/sc/scf/out102_en.pdf.

[7462] National Toxicology Program. NTP Toxicology and Carcinogenesis Studies of Methyleugenol (CAS NO. 93-15-2) in F344/N Rats and B6C3F1 Mice (Gavage Studies). *Natl Toxicol Program Tech Rep Ser*. 2000 Jul;491:1-412.

[7463] National Toxicology Program. Carcinogenesis Studies of Eugenol (CAS No. 97-53-0) in F344/N Rats and B6C3F1 Mice (Feed Studies). Technical Report Series No. 223. NIH Publication No. 84-1779. 1983. U.S. DHHS, PHS, NIH, NTP, Research Triangle Park, NC.

[7464] Ahmad A, Khan A, Ahmad Khan L, et al. In vitro synergy of eugenol and methyleugenol with fluconazole against clinical Candida isolates. *J Med Microbiol*. 2010;59:1178-84.

[7465] Lee SE, Lee BH, Choi WS, et al. Fumigant toxicity of volatile natural products from Korean spices and medicinal plants towards the rice weevil, Sitophilus oryzae (L). *Pest Manag Sci*. 2001;57:548-53.

[7466] Farag RS, Shalaby AS, El-Baroty GA, et al. Chemical and biological evaluation of the essential oils of different Melaleuca species. *Phytother Res*. 2004 Jan;18(1):30-5.

[7467] Pellati F, Orlandini G, van Leeuwen KA, et al. Gas chromatography combined with mass spectrometry, flame ionization detection and elemental analyzer/isotope ratio mass spectrometry for characterizing and detecting the authenticity of commercial essential oils of Rosa damascena Mill. *Rapid Commun Mass Spectrom*. 2013 Mar 15;27(5):591-602.

[7468] Boskabady MH, Shafei MN, Saberi Z, et al. Pharmacological effects of Rosa damascena. *Iran J Basic Med Sci*. 2011 Jul-Aug;14(4):295-307.

[7469] Kovatcheva N, Zhelijazkov VD, Astatkie T. Productivity, oil content composition, and bioactivity of oil-bearing rose accessions. *Hort Science*. 2011;46(5):710-14.

[7470] Mostafavi A, Afzali D. Chemical composition of the essential oils of Rosa damascena from two different locations in Iran. *Chem Nat Constituents*. 2009 Jan;45(1):110-13.

[7471] Loughmani-Khouzani H, Fini OS, Safari J. Essential oil composition of Rosa damascena Mill cultivated in Central Iran. *Scientia Iranica*. 2007;14(4):316-19.

[7472] Verma RS, Padalia RC, Chauhan A. Chemical investigation of the volatile components of shade-dried petals of damask rose (Rosa damascena Mill.). *Arch Biol Sci*. 2011;63(4):1111-15.

[7473] Babu KGD, Singh B, Joshi VP, et al. Essential oil composition of Damask Rose (Rosa damascena Mill.) distilled under different pressures and temperatures. *Flav Frag J*. 2002;17:136-40.

[7474] Bayrak A, Akgul A. Volatile oil composition of Turkish rose (Rosa damascena). *J Sc Food Agric*. 1994 Apr;64(4):441-48.

[7475] Karami A, Zandi P, Khosh Kui M, et al. Analysis of essential oil from nine distinct genotypes of Iranian Damask rose (Rosa damascena Mill). *J Medicinal Plants Res*.2012 Nov;6(42):5495-98.

[7476] Ibrahim SM, El-Denshary ES, Abdallah DM. Geraniol, Alone and in Combination with Pioglitazone, Ameliorates Fructose-Induced Metabolic Syndrome in Rats via the Modulation of Both Inflammatory and Oxidative Stress Status. *PLoS One*. 2015 Feb 13;10(2):e0117516.

[7477] Srinivasan S, Muruganathan U. Antidiabetic efficacy of citronellol, a citrus monoterpene by ameliorating the hepatic key enzymes of carbohydrate metabolism in streptozotocin-induced diabetic rats. *Chem Biol Interact*. 2016 Apr 25;250:38-46.

[7478] Lim S, Shin S. Effects of citronellol and thymol on cell membrane composition of Candida albicans. *Korean J Pharmacognosy*. 2009 Dec;40(4):357-64.

[7479] Shin S, Lim S. Antifungal effects of herbal essential oils alone and in combination with ketoconazole against Trichophyton spp. *J Appl Micribiol*. 2004;97:1289-96.

[7480] Hagvall L. Cytochrome P450-mediated activation of the fragrance constituent geraniol forms potent contact allergens. *Tox Appl Pharm*. 2008 Dec;233(2):308-13.

[7481] Hur MH, Han SH. Clinical trial of aromatherapy on postpartum mother's perineal healing. *Taehan Kanho Hakhoe Chi*. 2004 Feb;34(1):53-62.

[7482] Marzouk TM, El-Nemer AM, Baraka HN. The effect of aromatherapy abdominal massage on alleviating menstrual pain in nursing students: a prospective randomized cross-over study. *Evid Based Complement Altern Med*. 2013;2013:742421.

[7483] Han SH, Hur MH, Buckle J, et al. Effect of aromatherapy on symptoms of dysmenorrhea in college students: A randomized placebo-controlled clinical trial. *J Altern Complement Med*. 2006 Jul-Aug;12(6):535-41.

[7484] Conrad P, Adams C. The effects of clinical aromatherapy for anxiety and depression in the high risk postpartum woman - a pilot study. *Complement Ther Clin Pract*. 2012 Aug;18(3):164-68.

[7485] Brito RG, Santos PL, Prado DS, et al. Citronellol reduces orofacial nociceptive behaviors in mice - evidence of involvement of retrosplenial cortex and periaqueductal grey areas. *Basic Clin Pharmacol Toxicol*. 2013 Apr;112(4):215- 21.

[7486] Bastos JF, Noreira IJ, Ribeiro TP, et al. Hypotensive and vasorelaxant effects of citronellol, a monoterpene alcohol, in rats. *Basic Clin Pharamacol Toxicol*. 2010 Apr;106(4):331-37.

[7487] Baylac S, Racine P. Inhibition of 5-lipoxygenase by essential oils and other natural fragrances. *Int J Aromatherapy*. 2003;13(2-3):138-42.

[7488] Sadraei H, Asghari G, Emami S. Inhibitory effect of Rosa damascena Mill flower essential oil, geraniol and citronellol on rat ileum contraction. *Res Pharm Sci*. 2013 Jan;8(1):17-23.

[7489] Ohkawara S, Tanaka-Kagawa T, Furukawa Y, et al. Activation of the human transient receptor potential vanilloid subtype 1 by essential oils. *Biol Pharm Bull*. 2010;33(8):1434-37.

[7490] Abbasi Maleki N, Abbasi Maleki S, Bekhradi R. Suppressive effects of Rosa damascena essential oil on naloxone-precipitated morphine withdrawal signs in male mice. *Iran J Pharm Res*. 2013 Summer;12(3):357-61.

[7491] Masoumeh K, Ali M, Hassan R, et al. Evaluation of the anticonvulsant activities of Rosa damascena on the PTZ induced seizures in Wistar rats. *J Biol Sci*. 2008 Feb;8:426-430.

[7492] Ramexani R, Moghimi A, Rakhshandeh H, et al. The effect of Rosa damascena essential oil on the amygdala electrical kindling seizures in rat. *Pak J Biol Sci*. 2008 Mar 1;11(5):746-51.

[7493] Ashrafzadeh F, Rakhshandah H, Mahmoudi E. Rosa damascena oil: an adjunctive therapy for pediatric refractory seizure. *Iranian J Child Neurology*. 2007;1:13-17.

[7494] Boskabady MH, Kiani S, Rakhshandah H. Relaxant effects of Rosa damascena on guinea pig tracheal chains and its possible mechanism(s). *J Ethnopharmacol*. 2006;106:377-382.

[7495] Ulusoy S, Bosgelmex-Tinaz G, Secilmis-Canbay H. Tocopherol, carotene, phenolic contents and antibacterial properties of rose essential oil, hydrosol and absolute. *Curr Microbiol*.2009 Nov;59(5):554-58.

[7496] Ayan M, Tas U, Sogut E, et al. Investigating the effect of aromatherapy in patients with renal colic. *J Altern Complement Med*. 2013 Apr;19(4):329-33.

[7497] Fukada M, Kano E, Miyoshi M, et al. Effect of "rose essential oil" inhalation on stress-induced skin barrier disruption in rats and humans. *Chem Senses*. 2012 May;37(4):347-56.

[7498] Umezu T, Ito H, Nagano K, et al. Anticonflict effects of rose oil and identification of its active constituents. *Life Sci*. 2002 Nov 22;72(1):91-102.

[7499] Norbrega de Almeida R, Cristina Motta S, de Brito Faturi C, et al. Anxiolytic-like effects of rose oil inhalation on the elevated plus-maze test in rats. *Pharmacol Biochem Behav*. 2004 Feb;77(2):361-64.

[7500] Umezu T. Behavioral effects of plant-derived essential oils in the geller type conflict test in mice. *Jpn J Pharmacol*. 2000 Jun;83(2):150-53.

[7501] Mizuno D, Konoha-Mizuno K, Mori M, et al. An in vitro system comprising immortalized hypothalamic neuronal cells (GT1-7 Cells) for evaluation of the neuroendocrine effects of essential oils. *Evid Based Complement Alternat Med*. 2015;2015:343942.

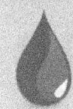
7502 Nikolova G, Karamalakova Y, Kovacheva N, et al. Protective effect of two essential oils isolated from Rosa damascena Mill. and Lavandula angustifolia Mill, and two classic antioxidants against L-dopa oxidative toxicity induced in healthy mice. *Regul Toxicol Pharmacol*. 2016 Jul 2;81:1-7.

7503 Kim J, Jang M, Shin E, et al. Fumigant and contact toxicity of 22 wooden essential oils and their major components against Drosophila suzukii (Diptera: Drosophilidae). *Pestic Biochem Physiol*. 2016 Oct;133:35-43.

7504 Uysal M, Doğru HY, Sapmaz E, et al. Investigating the effect of rose essential oil in patients with primary dysmenorrhea. *Complement Ther Clin Pract*. 2016 Aug;24:45-9.

7505 Shinohara K, Doi H, Kumagai C, et al. Effects of essential oil exposure on salivary estrogen concentration in perimenopausal women. *Neuro Endocrinol Lett*. 2017 Jan;37(8):567-572.

7506 Shakeri G, Jamshidi A, Khanzadi S, et al. Modeling of Salmonella typhimurium growth under the effects of Carum copticum essential oil, temperature, pH and inoculum size. *Vet Res Forum*. 2017 Winter;8(1):59-65.

7507 Shirazi M, Mohebitabar S, Bioos S, et al. The Effect of Topical Rosa damascena (Rose) Oil on Pregnancy-Related Low Back Pain: A Randomized Controlled Clinical Trial. *J Evid Based Complementary Altern Med*. 2017 Jan;22(1):120-126.

7508 Hamedi S, Shomali T, Haghighat A. Rosa damascena Mill. Essential Oil Has Protective Effect Against Testicular Damage in Diabetic Rats. *J Diet Suppl*. 2017 Aug 9:1-7.

7509 Heydari N, Abootalebi M, Jamalimoghadam N, et al. Evaluation of aromatherapy with essential oils of Rosa damascena for the management of premenstrual syndrome. *Int J Gynaecol Obstet*. 2018 Aug;142(2):156-161.

7510 Keyhanmehr AS, Movahhed M, Sahranavard S, et al. The effect of aromatherapy with Rosa damascena essential oil on sleep quality in children. *Res J Pharmacognosy*. 2018;5(1):41-6.

7511 Niazi M, Hashempur MH, Taghizadeh M, et al. Efficacy of topical Rose (Rosa damascena Mill.) oil for migraine headache: A randomized double-blinded placebo-controlled cross-over trial. *Complement Ther Med*. 2017 Oct;34:35-41.

7512 Hamdamian S, Nazarpour S, Simbar M, et al. Effects of aromatherapy with Rosa damascena on nulliparous women's pain and anxiety of labor during first stage of labor. *J Integr Med*. 2018 Mar;16(2):120-125.

7513 Nikolova G, Karamalakova Y, Gadjeva V. Reducing oxidative toxicity of L-dopa in combination with two different antioxidants: an essential oil isolated from Rosa Damascena Mill., and vitamin C. *Toxicol Rep*. 2019 Mar 22;6:267-271.

7514 Farnia V, Tatari F, Alikhani M, et al. Rosa Damascena oil improved sexual function and testosterone in male patients with opium use disorder under methadone maintenance therapy–results from a double-blind, randomized, placebo-controlled clinical trial. *Drug Alcohol Depend*. 2017 Jul 1;176:117-25.

7515 Bahmani DS, Farnia V, Hojatitabar S, et al. Adjuvant Rosa damascena has a small effect on SSRI-induced sexual dysfunction in female patients suffering from MDD. *Pharmacopsychiatry*. 2015;48(4-5):156-63.

7516 Fatemi F, Golbodagh A, Hojihosseini R, Dadkhah A, et al. Anti-inflammatory Effects of Deuterium-Depleted Water Plus Rosa Damascena Mill. Essential Oil Via Cyclooxygenase-2 Pathway in Rats. *Turk J Pharm Sci*. 2020 Feb;17(1):99–107.

7517 Dadkhah A, Fatemi F, Malayeri MRM, et al. Considering the Effect of Rosa damascena Mill. Essential Oil on Oxidative Stress and COX-2 Gene Expression in the Liver of Septic Rats. *Turk J Pharm Sci*. 2019 Dec;16(4):416-424.

7518 Jodaki K, Abdi K, Mousavi MS, et al. Effect of rosa damascene aromatherapy on anxiety and sleep quality in cardiac patients: A randomized controlled trial. *Complement Ther Clin Pract*. 2020 Dec 29;42:101299.

7519 Ghavam M. Relationships of irrigation water and soil physical and chemical characteristics with yield, chemical composition and antimicrobial activity of Damask rose essential oil. *PLoS One*. 2021 Apr 16;16(4):e0249363.

7520 Ghavam M, Afzali A, Manca ML. Chemotype of damask rose with oleic acid (9 octadecenoic acid) and its antimicrobial effectiveness. *Sci Rep*. 2021 Apr 13;11(1):8027.

7521 Vilhelmova-Ilieva N, Dobreva A, Doynovska R, et al. Antiviral Activity of Rosa damascena Mill. and Rosa alba L. Essential Oils against the Multiplication of Herpes Simplex Virus Type 1 Strains Sensitive and Resistant to Acyclovir. *Biology (Basel)*. 2021 Aug 4;10(8):746.

7522 Hashemi F, Nikfarid L, HeydariRad G, et al. The effect of aromatherapy on anxiety in mothers with premature hospitalized infants: a clinical trial study. *Evidence Based Care J*. 2022. Available at: https://ebcj.mums.ac.ir/article_20136.html.

7523 Bahadori H, Amiri MH, Sharafi H, et al. The Effect of Aromatherapy with Damask Rose on Anxiety, Accuracy and Job Stress in Operating Room Nurses. *Evidence Based Care J*. 2022;12(1):56-62.

7524 Mahdood B, Imani B, Khazaei S. Effects of Inhalation Aromatherapy With Rosa damascena (Damask Rose) on the State Anxiety and Sleep Quality of Operating Room Personnel During the COVID-19 Pandemic: A Randomized Controlled Trial. *J Perianesth Nurs*. 2022 Aug;37(4):493-500.

7525 Demirel S. Rosa damascena Miller essential oil relaxes rat thoracic aorta through the NO-cGMP-dependent pathway. *Prostaglandins Other Lipid Mediat*. 2022 Jun 21;162:106661.

7526 Demirel S. Geraniol and β-citronellol participate in the vasorelaxant effects of Rosa damascena Miller essential oil on the rat thoracic aorta. *Fitoterapia*. 2022 Jun 18;161:105243.

7527 Inagaki T, Oguchi E, Murayama M, et al. Stress-relieving and anxiolytic effects of neck and shoulder aromatherapy treatment with rose essential oil. *Showa Univ J Med Sci*. 2022 Jun;34(2):95-101.

7528 Demirel S. Rosa damascena Miller essential oil relaxes rat trachea via KV channels, KATP channels, and BKCa channels. *Prostaglandins Other Lipid Mediat*. 2022 Sep 14;163:106673.

7529 Bikmoradi A, Roshanaei G, Moradkhani S, et al. Impact of inhalation aromatherapy with Damask Rose (Rosa damascena) on stress, anxiety and hemodynamic parameters of patients undergoing coronary angiography: a single blind randomized clinical trial. *J Complement Integr Med*. 2021 May 20;19(3):753-761.

7530 Ardela MP, Puspita NLM, Sustamy RP, et al. Rose Aromatherapy Affects Blood Pressurein Menopausal Women. *J Global Red Public Health*. 2022 dec;7(2):145-8.

7531 Dagli SS, Dagli R. Pain relief effects of aromatherapy with rose oil (Rosa damascena Mill.) inhalation in patients with primary dysmenorrhea: A randomized controlled clinical trial. *J Herbal Med*. 2023;38:100637.

7532 Da Silva Bomfim N, Nakassugi LP, Faggion Pinheiro Oliveira J, et al. Antifungal activity and inhibition of fumonisin production by Rosmarinus officinalis L. essential oil in Fusarium verticillioides (Sacc.) Nirenberg. *Food Chem*. 2015 Jan 1;166:330-36.

7533 Raskovic A, Milanovic I, Pavlovic N, et al. Antioxidant activity of rosemary (Rosemary officinalis L.) essential oil and its hepatoprotective potential. *BMC Complement Altern Med*. 2014 Jul 7;14:225.

7534 Mathlouthi N, Bouzaienne T, Oueslati I, et al. Use of rosemary, oregano, and a commercial blend of essential oils in broiler chickens: In vitro antimicrobial activities and effects on growth performance. *J Anim Sci*. 2012 Mar;90(3):813- 23.

7535 Martinez-Velazquez M, Rosario-Cruz R, Castillo-Herrera G, et al. Acaricidal effect of essential oils from Lippia graveolens (Lamiales: Verbenaceae), Rosmarinus officinalis (Lamiales: Lamiaceae), and Allium sativum (Liliales: Liliaceae) against Rhipicephalus (Boophilus) microplus (Acari: Ixodidae). *J Med Entomol*. 2011 Jul;48(4):822-27.

7536 Jiang Y, Wu N, Fu YJ, et al. Chemical composition and antimicrobial activity of the essential oil of Rosemary. *Environ Toxicol Pharmacol*. 211 Jul;32(1):63-68.

7537 Tschiggerl C, Bucar F. Investigation of the volatile fraction of rosemary infusion extracts. *Sci Pharm*. 2010;78(3):483-92.

7538 Angelini LG, Carpanese G, Cioni PL, et al. Essential oils from Mediterranean Lamiaceae as weed germination inhibitors. *J Agric Food Chem*. 2003 Oct 8;51(21):6158-64.

7539 Jamshidi R, Afzali Z, Afzali D. Chemical composition of hydrodistillation essential oil of rosemary in different origins in Iran and comparison with other countries. *American-Eurasian J Agric & Environ Sci*. 2009;5(1):78-81.

7540 Miladi H, Ben Slama R, Mili D, et al. Essential oil of Thymus vulgaris L. and Rosmarinus officinalis L.: Gas chromatography-mass spectrometry analysis, cytotoxicity and antioxidant properties and antibacterial activities against foodborne pathogens. *Nat Sci*. 2013;5(6):729-39.

7541 Alnamer R, Alaoui K, Bouidida EH, et al. Psychostimulant activity of Rosmarinus officinalis essential oils. *J Nat Prod*. 2012;5:83-92.

7542 Elhassan IA, Osman NM. New chemotype Rosmarinus officinalis L. (Rosemary) "R. officinalis ct. bornyl acetate." *Am J Res Commun*. 2014;2(4):232-40.

7543 Reverchon E, Senatore F. Isolation of rosemary oil, comparison between hydrodistilled and supercritical fluid CO2 extraction. *Flav Frag J*. 1992;7:227-30.

7544 Soliman FM, El-Cashoury EA, Fathy MM. Analysis and biological activity of the essential oil of Rosmarinus officinalis L. from Egypt. *Flav Frag J*. 1994;9:29-33.

7545 Martinez AL, Gonzalez-Trujano ME, Pellicer F, et al. Antinociceptive effect and GC/MS analysis of Rosmarinus officinalis L. essential oil from its aerial parts. *Planta Med*. 2009 Apr;75(5):508-11.

7546 Craig JO. Poisoning by the volatile oils in childhood. *Arch Dis Child*. 1953;28:259-67.

7547 Melis K. Bochner A, Janssens G. Accidental nasal eucalyptol and menthol instillation. *Eur J Pediatr*. 1989 Aug;148(8)786-7.

7548 Day LM, Ozanne-Smith J, Parsons BJ, et al. Eucalyptus oil poisoning among young children: mechanisms of access and the potential prevention. *Aust N Z J Public Health*. 1997 Jun;21(3):297-302.

7549 Chandar SD, Prashanti M, Kumar CL, et al. Eucalyptus Oil-Induced Seizures in Children: A Single-Center Prospective Study. *Cureus*. 2021 Mar 25;13(3):e14109.

7550 Khine H, Weiss D, Graber N, et al. A cluster of children with seizures caused by camphor poisoning. *Pediatrics*. 2009 May;123(5):1269-72.

7551 Michiels EA, Mazor SS. Toddler with seizures due to ingesting camphor at an Indian celebration. *Pediatr Emerg Care*. 2010 Aug;26(8):574-75.

7552 Koren G. Medications which can kill a toddler with one tablet or teaspoonful. *J toxicol Clin Toxicol*. 1993;31(3):407- 13.

7553 Bar-Oz B, Levicheck Z, Koren G. Medications that can kill a toddler with one tablet or teaspoonfull – A 2004 update. *Paediatr Drugs*. 2004;6(2):123-6.

7554 Rabl W, Katzgraber F, Steinlechner M. Camphor ingestion for abortion (case report). *Forensic Sci Int*. 1997 Sep 19;89(1-2):137-40.

7555 Flaman Z, Pellechia-Clarke S, Bailey B, et al. Unintentional exposure of young children to camphor and eucalyptus oils. *Paediatr Child Health*. 2001 Feb;6(2):80-83.

7556 Day LM, Ozanne-Smith J, Parsons BJ, et al. Eucalyptus oil poisoning among young children: mechanisms of access and the potential prevention. *Aust N Z J Public Health*. 1997 Jun;21(3):297-302.

7557 Myott E. Case of eucalyptus poisoning. *Brit M J*. 1906;1:558.

7558 Hindle RC. Eucalyptus oil ingestion. *N Z Med J*. 1994 May 11;107(977)185-6.

7559 Tibballs J. Clinical effects and management of eucalyptus oil ingestion in infants and small children. *Med J Aust*. 1995 Aug;163(4):177-80.

7560 Waldman W, Barwina M, Sein Anand J. Accidental ontoxication with eucalyptus oil—a case report. *Przeql Lek*. 2011;68(8):555-6.

7561 Day LM, Ozanne-Smith J, Parsons BJ, et al. Eucalyptus oil poisoning among young children: mechanisms of access and the potential prevention. *Aust N Z J Public Health*. 1997 Jun;21(3):297-302.

7562 De Vincenzi M, Silano M, De Vincenzi A, et al. Constituents of aromatic plants: eucalyptol. *Fitoterapia*. 2002 Jun;73(3):269-75.

7563 Manoguerra AS, Erdman AR, Wax PM, et al. Camphor poisoning: an evidence-based practice guideline for out-of- hospital management. *Clin Toxicol (Phila)*.2006;44(4):357-70.

7564 Gibson DE, Moore GP, Pfaff JA. Camphor ingestion. *Am J Emerg Med.* 1989 Jan;7(1):41-43.
7565 Koppel C, Martends F, Schirop T, et al. Hemoperfusion in acute camphor poisoning. *Intensive Care Med.* 1988;14(4):431-33.
7566 Sayyah M, Valizadeh J, Kamalinejad M. Anticonvulsant activity of the leaf oil of Laurus nobilis against pentylentetrazole- and maximal electroshock-induced seizure. *Phytomedicine.* 2002 Apr;9(3):212-16.
7567 Culic M, Kekovic G, Grbic G, et al. Wavelet and fractal analysis of rat brain activity in seizures evoked by camphor oil and 1,8-cineole. *Gen Physiol Biophys.* 2009;28 Sec No:33-40.
7568 Burkhard PR, Burkhardt K, Haenggeli CA, et al. Plant-induced seizures: reappearance of an old problem. *J Neurol.* 1999 Aug;246(8):667-70.
7569 Waldman N. Seizure caused by dermal application of over-the-counter eucalyptus oil head lice preparation. *Clin Toxicol (Phila).* 2011 Oct;49(8):750-1.
7570 Craig JO. Poisoning by the volatile oils in childhood. *Arch Dis Child.* 1953;28:259-67.
7571 Mathew T, Kamath V, Kumar RS, et al. Eucalyptus oil inhalation-induced seizure: A novel, underrecognized, preventable cause of acute symptomatic seizure. *Epilepsia Open.* 2017 Jul 4;2(3):350-354.
7572 Olowe SA, Ransome-Kuti O. The risk of jaundice in glucose-6-phosphate dehydrogenase deficient babies exposed to menthol. *Acta Paediatr Scand.* 1980 May;69(3):341-5.
7573 Dillon Remy M, Manning Alleyne P, Bratt DE, et al. Neonatal jaundice at Port-of-Spain General Hospital abstract. *West Indian Med J.* 1987;36(Suppl):28.
7574 de Olivera AC, Ribeiro-Pinto LF, Paumgartten JR. In vitro inhibition of CYP2B1 monoxygenase by beta-myrcene and other monoterpenoid constituents. *Br J Nutr.* 1999;81:289-95.
7575 Subehan, Usia T, Iwata H, et al. Mechanism-based inhibition of CYP3A4 and CYP2D6 by Indonesian medicinal plants. *J Ethnopharmacol.* 2006 May;15(3):449-55.
7576 Unger M, Frank A. Simultaneous determination of the inhibitory potency of herbal extracts on the activity of six major cytochrome P450 enzymes using liquid chromatography/mass spectrometry and automated online extraction. *Rapid Commun Mass Spectrom.* 2004;18(19):2273-81.
7577 de-Oliveira AC, Ribeiro-Pinto LF, Otto SS, et al. Induction of liver monooxygenases by beta-myrcene. *Toxicology.* 1997 Dec 26;124(2):135-40.
7578 Jori A, Bianchetti A, Prestini PE, et al. Effect of eucalyptol (1,8-cineole) on the metabolism of other drugs in rats and in man. *Eur J Pharmacol.* 1970;9(3):362-66.
7579 de Sousa DP, Raphael E, Brocksom U, et al. Sedative effect of monoterpene alcohols in mice: A preliminary screening. *Verlag der Zeitschrift fur Naturforschung.* 2007;62c:563-66.
7580 Freitas JC1, Presgrave OA, Fingola FF, et al. Effect of beta-myrcene on pentobarbital sleeping time. *Braz J Med Biol Res.* 1993 May;26(5):519-23.
7581 Gray AM, Flatt PR. Antihyperglycemic actions of Eucalyptus globulus (Eucalyptus) are associated with pancreatic and extra pancreatic effects in mice. *J Nutr.* 1998 Dec;128(12):2319–23.
7582 Basak SS, Candan F. Effect of Laurus nobilis L. Essential Oil and its Main Components on α-glucosidase and Reactive Oxygen Species Scavenging Activity. *Iran J Pharm Res.* 2013 Spring;12(2):367-79.
7583 Dey B. Chemo-profiling of eucalyptus and study of its hypoglycemic potential. *World J Diabetes.* 2013 Oct 15;4(5):170–76.
7584 Toroglu S. In-vitro antimicrobial activity and synergistic/antagonistic effect of interactions between antibiotics and some spice essential oils. *J Environ Biol.* 2011 Jan;32(1):23-9.
7585 Raskovic A, Milanovic I, Pavlovic N, et al. Analgesic effects of rosemary essential oil and its interactions with codeine and paracetamol in mice. *Eur Rev Med Pharmacol Sci.* 2015 Jan;19(1):165-72.
7586 Uc A, Bishop WP, Sanders KD. Camphor hepatotoxicity. *South Med J.* 2000;93:596-98.
7587 Wang W, Li N, Luo M, et al. Antibacterial activity and anticancer of Rosmarinus officinalis L. essential oil compared to that of its main components. *Molecules.* 2012 Mar 5;17(3):2704-13.
7588 Ngo SN, Williams DB, Head RJ. Rosemary and cancer prevention: preclinical perspectives. *Crit Rev Food Sci Nutr.* 2011 Dec;51(10):946-54.
7589 Hussain AI, Anwar F, Chatha SA, et al. Rosmarinus officinalis essential oil: antiproliferative, antioxidant and antibacterial activities. *Braz J Microbiol.* 2010 Oct;41(4):1070-78.
7590 Melusova M, Slamenova D, Kozics K, Carvacrol and rosemary essential oil manifest cytotoxic, DNA-protective and pro-apoptotic effect having no effect on DNA repair. *Neopasma.* 2014;61(6):690-99.
7591 Wei FX, Liu JX, Wang L, et al. Expression of bcl-2 and bax genes in the liver cancer cell line HepG2 after apoptosis induced by essential oils from Rosmarinus officinalis. *Zhong Yao Cai.* 2008 Jun;31(6):877-79.
7592 Kim MJ, Nam ES, Paik SI. The effects of aromatherapy in pain, depression, and life satisfaction of arthritis patients. *Taehan Kanho Hakhoe Chi.* 2005 Feb;35(1):186-94.
7593 Fernandez LF, Palomino OM, Frutos G. Effectiveness of Rosmarinus officinalis essential oil as antihypotensive agent in primary hypotensive patients and its influence on health-related quality of life. *J Ethnopharmacol.* 2014;151(1):509-16.
7594 Hay IC, Jamieson M, Ormerod AD. Randomized trial of aromatherapy. Successful treatment for alopecia areata. *Arch Dermatol.* 1998 Nov;134(11):1349-52.
7595 Kim MA, Sakong JK, Kim EJ, et al. Effect of aromatherapy massage for the relief of constipation in the elderly. *Taehan Kanho Hakhoe Chi.* 2005 Feb;35(1):56-64.
7596 Fonseca AO, Pereira DI, Jacob RG, et al. In vitro susceptibility of Brazilian Pythium insidiosum isolates to essential oils of some Lamiaceae family. *Mycopathologia.* 2015 Apr;179(3-4):253-8.
7597 Martinez AL, Gonzalez-Trujano ME, Pellicer F, et al. Antinociceptive effect and GC/MS analysis of Rosmarinus officinalis L. essential oil from its aerial parts. *Planta Med.* 2009 Apr;75(5):508-11.
7598 Sivamani P, Singaravelu G, Thiagarajan V, et al. Comparative molecular docking analysis of essential oil constituents as elastase inhibitors. *Bioinformation.* 2012;8(10):457-60.
7599 Baylac S, Racine P. Inhibition of 5-lipoxygenase by essential oils and other natural fragrant extracts. *Int J Aromatherapy.* 2003;13(2-3):138-42.
7600 Sagorchev P, Lukanov J, Beer AM. Investigations into the specific effects of rosemary oil at the receptor level. *Phytomedicine.* 2010 Jul;17(8-9):693-97.
7601 Milhau G, Valentin A, Benoit, et al. In vitro antimalarial activity of eight essential oils. *J Essent Oil Res.* 1997;9(3):329-33.
7602 Sebai H, Selmi S, Rtibi K, et al. Protective effect of Lavandula stoechas and Rosmarinus officinalis oils against reproductive damage and oxidative stress in alloxan-induced diabetic rats. *J Med Food.* 2015 Feb;18(2):241-9.
7603 Gauch LM, Silveira-Gomes F, Esteves RA, et al. Effects of Rosmarinus officinalis essential oil on germ tube formation by Candida albicans isolated from denture wearers. *Rev Soc Bras Med Trop.* 2014 May-Jun;47(3):389-91.
7604 Sayorwan W, Ruangrungsi N, Piriyapunyporn T, et al. Effects of inhaled rosemary oil on subjective feelings and activities of the nervous system. *Sci Pharm.* 2013 Jun;81(2):531-42.
7605 Minaiyan M, Ghannadi AR, Afsharipour M, et al. Effects of extráct and essential oil of Rosmarinus officinalis L. on TNBS-induced colitis. *Res Pharm Sci.* 2011 Jan;6(1):13-21.
7606 Muhlbauer RC, Lozano A, Palacio S, et al. Common herbs, essential oils, and monoterpenes potently modulate bone metabolism. *Bone.* 2003 Apr;32(4):372-80.
7607 Nogueira de Melo GA, Grespan R, Fonseca JP, et al. Rosmarinus officinalis L. essential oil inhibits in vivo and in vitro leukocyte migration. *J med Food.* 2011 Sep;14(9):944-46.
7608 Takaki I, Bersani-Amado LE, Vendruscolo A, et al. Anti-inflammatory and antinociceptive effects of Rosmarinus officinalis L. essential oil in experimental animal models. *J Med Food.* 2008 Dec;11(4):741-46.
7609 Chen CC, Chen HL, Hsieh CW, et al. Upregulation of NF-E2-related factor-2-dependent glutathione by carnosol provokes a cytoprotective response and enhances cell survival. *Acta Pharmacol Sin.* 2011 Jan;32(1):62-69.
7610 Lewis KN, Mele J, Hayes JD, et al. Nrf2, a guardian of healthspan and gatekeeper of species longevity. *Integr Comp Biol.* 2010 Nov;50(5):829-43.
7611 Abu-Al-Basal MA. Healing potential of Rosmarinus officinalis L. in full thickness excision cutaneous wounds in alloxan-induced-diabetic BALB/c mice. *J Ethnopharmcol.* 2010 Sep 15;131(2):443-50.
7612 Jimbo D, Kimura Y, Taniguchi M, et al. Effect of aromatherapy on patients with Alzheimer's disease. *Psychogeriatrics.* 209 Dec;9(4):173-79.
7613 McCaffrey R, Thomas DJ, Kinzelman AO. The effects of lavender and rosemary essential oils on test-taking anxiety among graduate nursing students. *Holist Nurs Pract.* 2009 Mar-Apr;23(2):88-93.
7614 Lugman S, Dwivedi GR, Darokar MP, et al. Potential of rosemary oil to be used in drug-resistant infections. *Altern Ther Health Med.* 2007 Sep-Oct;13(5):54-59.
7615 Bozin B, Mimica-Dukic N, Samojlik I, et al. Antimicrobial and antioxidant properties of rosemary and sage (Rosmarinus officinalis L. and Salvia officinalis L., Lamiaceae) essential oils. *J Agric Food Chem.* 2007 Sep;55(19):7879-85.
7616 Mangena T, Muyima NY. Comparative evaluation of the antimicrobial activities of essential oils of Artemisian afra, Pteronia icana and Rosmarinus officinalis on selected bacterial and yeast strains. *Lett Appl Microbiol.* 1999 Apr;28(4):291-96.
7617 Císarová M, Tančinová D, Medo J, et al. The in vitro effect of selected essential oils on the growth and mycotoxin production of Aspergillus species. *J Environ Sci Health B.* 2016 Oct 2;51(10):668-674.
7618 Satyal P, Jones TH, Lopez EM, et al. Chemotypic Characterization and Biological Activity of Rosmarinus officinalis. *Foods.* 2017 Mar 5;6(3).
7619 Fu Y, Zu Y, Chen L, et al. Investigation of antibacterial activity of rosemary essential oil against Propionbacterium acnes with the atomic force microscopy. *Planta Med.* 207 Oct;73(12):1275-80.
7620 Atsumi T, Tonosaki K. Smelling lavender and rosemary increases free-radical-scavenging activity and decreases cortisol level in saliva. *Psychiatry Res.* 2007 Feb 28;150(1):89-96.
7621 Vijayan P, Raghu C, Ashok G, et al. Antiviral activity of medicinal plants of Nilgiris. *Indian J Med Res.* 2004 Jul;120(1):24-29.
7622 Moss M, Cook J, Wesnes K, et al. Aromas of rosemary and lavender essential oils differentially affect cognition and mood in healthy adults. *Int J Neurosci.* 2003 Jan;113(1):15-38.
7623 Moss M, Oliver L. Plasma 1,8-cineole correlates with cognitive performance following exposure to rosemary essential oil aroma. *Ther Adv Psychopharmacol.* 2012 Jun;2(3):103-13.
7624 Fahim FA, Esmat AY, Fadel HM, et al. Allied studies on the effect of Rosmarinus officinalis L. on experimental hepatotoxicity and mutagenesis. *Int J Food Sci Nutr.* 1999 Nov;50(6):413-27.
7625 Agel MB. Relaxant effect of the volatile oil of Rosmarinus officinalis on tracheal smooth muscle. *J Ethnopharmacol.* 1991 May-Jun;33(1-2):57-62.
7626 El-Seed HR, Khalil NS, Azeem M, et al. Chemical composition and repellency of essential oils from four medicinal plants against Ixodes nymphs (Acari: Ixodidae). *J Med Entomol.* 2012 Sep;49(5):1067-75.
7627 Mizuno D, Konoha-Mizuno K, Mori M, et al. An in vitro system comprising immortalized hypothalamic neuronal cells (GT1-7 Cells) for evaluation of the neuroendocrine effects of essential oils. *Evid Based Complement Alternat Med.* 2015;2015:343942.
7628 Plant J. Effects of essential oils on telomere length in human cells. *Med Aromat Plants.* 2016;5(2):1-6.
7629 Azad MF, Schwiertz A, Jentsch HF. Adjunctive use of essential oils following scaling and root planing -a randomized clinical trial. *BMC Complement Altern Med.* 2016 Jun 7;16(1):171.
7630 Sharififard M, Safdari F, Siahpoush A, et al. Evaluation of Some Plant Essential Oils against the Brown-Banded Cockroach, Supella longipalpa (Blattaria: Ectobiidae): A Mechanical Vector of Human Pathogens. *J Arthropod Borne Dis.* 2016 Oct 4;10(4):528-537.
7631 Sirocchi V, Devlieghere F, Peelman N, et al. Effect of Rosmarinus officinalis L. essential oil combined with different packaging conditions to extend the shelf life of refrigerated beef meat. *Food Chem.* 2017 Apr 15;221:1069-1076.

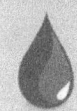

[7632] Satyal P, Jones TH, Lopez EM, et al. Chemotypic Characterization and Biological Activity of Rosmarinus officinalis. *Foods.* 2017 Mar 5;6(3).
[7633] Ksouri S, Djebir S, Bentorki AA, et al. Antifungal activity of essential oils extract from Origanum floribundum Munby, Rosmarinus officinalis L. and Thymus ciliatus Desf. against Candida albicans isolated from bovine clinical mastitis. *J Mycol Med.* 2017 Apr 25. pii: S1156-5233(17)30017-3.
[7634] Filiptsova OV, Gazzavi-Rogozina LV, Timoshyna IA, et al. The essential oil of rosemary and its effect on the human image and numerical short-term memory. *Egyptia J Basic Appl Sci.* 2017 Jun;4(2):107-11.
[7635] Borges RS, Lima ES, Keita H, et al. Anti-inflammatory and antialgic actions of a nanoemulsion of Rosmarinus officinalis L. essential oil and a molecular docking study of its major chemical constituents. Inflammopharmacology. 2018 Feb;26(1):183-195.
[7636] Eissa FA, Choudhry H, Abdulaal WH, et al. Possible hypocholesterolemic effect of ginger and rosemary oils in rats. *Afr J Tradit Complement Altern Med.* 2017 Jun 5;14(4):188-200.
[7637] Bouyahya A, Et-Touys A, Bakri Y, et al. Chemical composition of Mentha pulegium and Rosmarinus officinalis essential oils and their antileishmanial, antibacterial and antioxidant activities. *Microb Pathog.* 2017 Aug 15;111:41-49.
[7638] Luís Â, Duarte AP, Pereira L, et al. Chemical Profiling and Evaluation of Antioxidant and Anti-Microbial Properties of Selected Commercial Essential Oils: A Comparative Study. *Medicines (Basel).* 2017 Jun 5;4(2).
[7639] Selmi S, Rtibi K, Grami D, et al. Rosemary (Rosmarinus officinalis) essential oil components exhibit anti-hyperglycemic, anti-hyperlipidemic and antioxidant effects in experimental diabetes. *Pathophysiology.* 2017 Dec;24(4):297-303.
[7640] Jardak M, Elloumi-Mseddi J, Aifa S, et al. Chemical composition, antibiofilm activity and potential cytotoxic effect on cancer cells of Rosmarinus officinalis L. essential oil from Tunisia. *Lipids Health Dis.* 2017 Oct 2;16(1):190.
[7641] Giordana F, Nicola M, Valentina C, et al. Chemical composition of essential oils from Thymus vulgaris, Cymbopogon citratus and Rosmarinus officinalis and their effects on the HIV-1 Tat protein function. *Chem Biodivers.* 2018 Feb;15(2).
[7642] Villareal MO, Ikeya A, Sasaki K, et al. Anti-stress and neuronal cell differentiation induction effects of Rosmarinus officinalis L. essential oil. *BMC Complement Altern Med.* 2017 Dec 22;17(1):549.
[7643] Limoncu ME, Balcıoğlu C, Oyur T, et al. In vitro Investigation of the Pediculicidal Activities of the Volatile Oil Components of Some Medical Plants Raised in Turkey. *Turkiye Parazitol Derg.* 2017 Dec;41(4):208-213.
[7644] Shokri A, Saeedi M, Fakhar M, et al. Antileishmanial Activity of Lavandula angustifolia and Rosmarinus Officinalis Essential Oils and Nano-emulsions on Leishmania major (MRHO/IR/75/ER). *Iran J Parasitol.* 2017 Oct-Dec;12(4):622-631.
[7645] Pellegrini M, Ricci A, Serio A, et al. Characterization of Essential Oils Obtained from Abruzzo Autochthonous Plants: Antioxidant and Antimicrobial Activities Assessment for Food Application. *Foods.* 2018 Feb 2;7(2).
[7646] Borges RS, Keita H, Ortiz BLS, et al. Anti-inflammatory activity of nanoemulsions of essential oil from Rosmarinus officinalis L.: in vitro and in zebrafish studies. *Inflammopharmacology.* 2018 Aug;26(4):1057-1080.
[7647] Tardugno R, Pellati F1, Iseppi R, et al. Phytochemical composition and in vitro screening of the antimicrobial activity of essential oils on oral pathogenic bacteria. *Nat Prod Res.* 2018 Mar;32(5):544-551.
[7648] Damos PT. An in vitro ULV olfactory bioassay method for testing the repellent activity of essential oils against moths. *MethodsX.* 2018 Apr 20;5:375-394.
[7649] Elansary HO, Abdelgaleil SAM, Mahmoud EA, et al. Effective antioxidant, antimicrobial and anticancer activities of essential oils of horticultural aromatic crops in northern Egypt. *BMC Complement Altern Med.* 2018 Jul 13;18(1):214.
[7650] von Schoen-Angerer T, Deckers B, Henes J, et al. Effect of topical rosemary essential oil on Raynaud phenomenon in systemic sclerosis. *Complement Ther Med.* 2018 Oct;40:191-194.
[7651] Maness LR, Zubov T. The Inhibitory Effect of Essential Oils on Rhizopus stolonifer, Trichophyton mentagrophytes, and Microsporum gypseum. *Lab Med.* 2019 Apr 8;50(2):e18-e22.
[7652] Lorenzo-Leal AC, Palou E, López-Malo A. Evaluation of the efficiency of allspice, thyme and rosemary essential oils on two foodborne pathogens in in-vitro and on alfalfa seeds, and their effect on sensory characteristics of the sprouts. *Int J Food Microbiol.* 2019 Feb 12;295:19-24.
[7653] Lagha R, Ben Abdallah F, Al-Sarhan BO, et al. Antibacterial and Biofilm Inhibitory Activity of Medicinal Plant Essential Oils Against Escherichia coli Isolated from UTI Patients. *Molecules.* 2019 Mar 23;24(6).
[7654] Elmhalli F, Garboui SS, Borg-Karlson AK, et al. The repellency and toxicity effects of essential oils from the Libyan plants Salvadora persica and Rosmarinus officinalis against nymphs of Ixodes ricinus. *Exp Appl Acarol.* 2019 Apr;77(4):585-599.
[7655] Pehlivan S, Karadakovan A. Effects of aromatherapy massage on pain, functional state, and quality of life in an elderly individual with knee osteoarthritis. *Jpn J Nurs Sci.* 2019 Oct;16(4):450-458.
[7656] Lorenzo-Leal AC, Palou E, López-Malo A, et al. Antimicrobial, Cytotoxic, and Anti-Inflammatory Activities of Pimenta dioica and Rosmarinus officinalis Essential Oils. *Biomed Res Int.* 2019 May 7;2019:1639726.
[7657] Battistini R, Rossini I, Ercolini C, et al. Antiviral Activity of Essential Oils Against Hepatitis A Virus in Soft Fruits. *Food Environ Virol.* 2019 Mar;11(1):90-95.
[7658] Benberkane A, Khellouf A, Benhenia K, et al. Rosmarinus officinalis Essential Oil Preloaded in β-Cyclodextrin: Effect on Ram Spermatozoa Motility, Membrane Integrity and Oxidative Status During 4°C Storage. *Cryo Letters.* 2019 Jul/Aug;40(4):219-225.
[7659] Al-Okbi SY, Hussein AMS, Elbakry HFH, et al. Health Benefits of Fennel, Rosemary Volatile Oils and their Nano-Forms in Dyslipidemic Rat Model. *Pak J Biol Sci.* 2018 Jan;21(7):348-358.
[7660] Labib RM, Ayoub IM, Michel HE, et al. Appraisal on the wound healing potential of Melaleuca alternifolia and Rosmarinus officinalis L. essential oil-loaded chitosan topical preparations. *PLoS One.* 2019 Sep 16;14(9):e0219561.
[7661] Pinto NB, Castro LM, Azambuja RHM, et al. Ovicidal and larvicidal potential of Rosmarinus officinalis to control gastrointestinal nematodes of sheep. *Rev Bras Parasitol Vet.* 2019 Oct-Dec;28(4):807-811.
[7662] da Silva Bomfim N, Kohiyama CY, Nakasugi LP, et al. Antifungal and antiaflatoxigenic activity of rosemary essential oil (Rosmarinus officinalis L.) against Aspergillus flavus. *Food Addit Contam Part A Chem Anal Control Expo Risk Assess.* 2019 Oct 23:1-9.
[7663] Iseppi R, Sabia C, de Neiderhausern S, et al. Antibacterial Activity of Rosmarinus officinalis L. And Thymus vulgaris L. Essential Oils and Their Combination Against Food-Borne Pathogens and Spoilage Bacteria in Ready-To-Eat Vegetables. Nat Prod Res. 2019 Dec;33(24):3568-3572.
[7664] Esmael A, Hassan MG, Amer MM, et al. Antimicrobial activity of certain natural-based plant oils against the antibiotic-resistant acne bacteria. *Saudi J Biol Sci.* 2020 Jan;27(1):448–455.
[7665] Capatina L, Boiangiu RS, Dumitru G, et al. Rosmarinus officinalis Essential Oil Improves Scopolamine-Induced Neurobehavioral Changes via Restoration of Cholinergic Function and Brain Antioxidant Status in Zebrafish ( Danio rerio). *Antioxidants (Basel).* 2020 Jan 10;9(1):62.
[7666] Bedini S, Guarino S, Echeverria MC, et al. Allium sativum, Rosmarinus officinalis, and Salvia officinalis Essential Oils: A Spiced Shield Against Blowflies. *Insects.* 2020 Feb 25;11(3):143.
[7667] Hassanen NH, Fahmi A, Shams-Eldin E, et al. Protective Effect of Rosemary ( Rosmarinus officinalis) Against Diethylnitrosamine-Induced Renal Injury in Rats. *Biomarkers.* 2020 Mar 2:1-9. [Online ahead of print].
[7668] Moumni S, Elaissi A, Trabelsi A, et al. Correlation between chemical composition and antibacterial activity of some Lamiaceae species essential oils from Tunisia. *BMC Complement Med Ther.* 2020 Apr 3;20(1):103.
[7669] Chraibi M, Farah A, Elamin O, et al. Characterization, antioxidant, antimycobacterial, antimicrobial effcts of Moroccan rosemary essential oil, and its synergistic antimicrobial potential with carvacrol. *J Adv Pharm Technol Res.* 2020 Jan-Mar;11(1):25-29.
[7670] Silva S, Alves N, Silva P, et al. Antibacterial Activity of Rosmarinus Officinalis, Zingiber Officinale, Citrus Aurantium bergamia, and Copaifera officinalis Alone and in Combination With Calcium Hydroxide Against Enterococcus faecalis. *Biomed Res Int.* 2019 Dec 12;2019:8129439.
[7671] Leporini M, Bonesi M, Loizzo MR, et al. The Essential Oil of Salvia rosmarinus Spenn. From Italy as a Source of Health-Promoting Compounds: Chemical Profile and Antioxidant and Cholinesterase Inhibitory Activity. *Plants (Basel).* 2020 Jun 26;9(6):E798.
[7672] Kryzowski M, Baran B, Lozowski B, et al. The Effect of Rosmarinus officinalis Essential Oil Fumigation on Biochemical, Behavioral, and Physiological Parameters of Callosobruchus maculatus. *Insects.* 2020 Jun 3;11(6):E344.
[7673] Liu T, Wang J, Gong X, et al. Rosemary and Tea Tree Essential Oils Exert Antibiofilm Activities In Vitro Against Staphylococcus Aureus and Escherichia Coli. *J Food Prot.* 2020 Jul 1;83(7):1261-1267.
[7674] Leporini M, Bonesi M, Loizzo MR, et al. The Essential Oil of Salvia rosmarinus Spenn. from Italy as a Source of Health-Promoting Compounds: Chemical Profile and Antioxidant and Cholinesterase Inhibitory Activity. *Plants (Basel).* 2020 Jun 26;9(6):798.
[7675] El-Demerdash FM, El-Sayed RA, Abdel-Daim MM. Hepatoprotective potential of Rosmarinus officinalis essential oil against hexavalent chromium-induced hematotoxicity, biochemical, histological, and immunohistochemical changes in male rats. *Environ Sci Pollut Res Int.* 2021 Jan 4. Online ahead of print.
[7676] Mohammadifar M, Arabi MH, Aghighi F, et al. Anti-osteoarthritis potential of peppermint and rosemary essential oils in a nanoemulsion form: behavioral, biochemical, and histopathological evidence. *BMC Complement Med Ther.* 2021 Feb 9;21(1):57.
[7677] Nasiri A, Boroomand MM. The effect of rosemary essential oil inhalation on sleepiness and alertness of shift-working nurses: A randomized, controlled field trial. *Complement Ther Clin Pract.* 2021;43:101326.
[7678] El-Demerdash FM, El-Sayed RA, Abdel-Daim MM. Rosmarinus officinalis essential oil modulates renal toxicity and oxidative stress induced by potassium dichromate in rats. *J Trace Elem Med Biol.* 2021 May 15;67:126791.
[7679] Ed-Dra A, Filali FR, Lo Presti V, et al. Chemical composition, antioxidant capacity and antibacterial action of five Moroccan essential oils against Listeria monocytogenes and different serotypes of Salmonella enterica. *Microb Pathog.* 2020 Dec;149:104510.
[7680] Puvaca N, Milenkovic J, Coghill TG, et al. Antimicrobial Activity of Selected Essential Oils against Selected Pathogenic Bacteria: In Vitro Study. *Antibiotics (Basel).* 2021 May 8;10(5):546.
[7681] Kafa AHT, Aslan R, Celik C, et al. Antimicrobial synergism and antibiofilm activities of Pelargonium graveolens, Rosemary officinalis, and Mentha piperita essential oils against extreme drug-resistant Acinetobacter baumannii clinical isolates. *Z Naturforsch C J Biosci.* 2021 Jun 17. Online ahead of print.
[7682] Mediavilla I, Guillamon E, Ruiz A, et al. Essential Oils from Residual Foliage of Forest Tree and Shrub Species: Yield and Antioxidant Capacity. *Molecules.* 2021 May 28;26(11):3257.
[7683] Bonaccorso A, Cimino C, Manno DE, et al. Essential Oil-Loaded NLC for Potential Intranasal Administration. *Pharmaceutics.* 2021 Jul 28;13(8):1166.

[7684] Garzoli S, Laghezza Masci V, Franceschi S, et al. Headspace/GC-MS Analysis and Investigation of Antibacterial, Antioxidant and Cytotoxic Activity of Essential Oils and Hydrolates from Rosmarinus officinalis L. and Lavandula angustifolia Miller. *Foods*. 2021 Jul 30;10(8):1768.
[7685] Waller SB, Cleff MB, Dalla Lana DF, et al. Can the essential oil of rosemary (Rosmarinus officinalis Linn.) protect rats infected with itraconazole-resistant Sporothrix brasiliensis from fungal spread? *J Mycol Med*. 2021 Aug 16;31(4):101199.
[7686] Brozyna M, Paleczny J, Kozlowska W, et al. The Antimicrobial and Antibiofilm In Vitro Activity of Liquid and Vapour Phases of Selected Essential Oils against Staphylococcus aureus. *Pathogens*. 2021 Sep 17;10(9):1207.
[7687] Boumendjel M, Boucheker A, Feknous S, et al. Adaptogenic activity of Cinnamomum camphora, Eucalyptus globulus, Lavandula stœchas and Rosmarinus officinalis essential oil used in North-African folk medicine. *Cell Mol Biol (Noisy-le-grand)*. 2021 Aug 31;67(2):83-88.
[7688] Christopoulou SD, Androutsopoulou C, Hahalis P, et al. Rosemary Extract and Essential Oil as Drink Ingredients: An Evaluation of Their Chemical Composition, Genotoxicity, Antimicrobial, Antiviral, and Antioxidant Properties. *Foods*. 2021 Dec 18;10(12):3143.
[7689] Santos Rodrigues AP, Faria E Souza BS, et al. The effects of Rosmarinus officinalis L. essential oil and its nanoemulsion on dyslipidemic Wistar rats. *J Appl Biomed*. 2020 Dec;18(4):126-135.
[7690] Farsi Z, Rajai N, Teymouri F, et al. Effect of Aromatherapy with Rosa Damascena Essential Oil on Nurses' Occupational Stress in the Emergency Department: A Randomized Controlled Trial. *Prev Care Nurs Midwifery J*. 2021;11(3):46-54.
[7691] Mekkaoui M, Assaggaf H, Qasem A, et al. Ethnopharmacological Survey and Comparative Study of the Healing Activity of Moroccan Thyme Honey and Its Mixture with Selected Essential Oils on Two Types of Wounds on Albino Rabbits. *Foods*. 2021 Dec 23;11(1):28.
[7692] Vagedes J, Henes J, Deckers B, et al. Topical Rosmarinus officinalis L. in Systemic Sclerosis-Related Raynaud's Phenomenon: An Open-Label Pilot Study. *Complement Med Res*. 2022 Feb 9. Online ahead of print.
[7693] Aponso M, Patti A, Hearn MTW, et al. Anxiolytic effects of essential oils may involve anti-oxidant regulation of the pro-oxidant effects of ascorbate in the brain. *Neurochem Int*. 2021 Nov;150:105153.
[7694] Rezk S, Lashen S, El-Adl M, et al. Effects of Rosemary Oil (Rosmarinus officinalis) supplementation on the fate of the transplanted human olfactory bulb neural stem cells against ibotenic acid-induced neurotoxicity (Alzheimer model) in rat. *Metab Brain Dis*. 2022 Apr;37(4):973-988.
[7695] Annemer S, Farah A, Stambouli H, et al. Chemometric Investigation and Antimicrobial Activity of Salvia rosmarinus Spenn Essential Oils. *Molecules*. 2022 May 3;27(9):2914.
[7696] Yasir M, Nawaz A, Ghazanfar S, et al. Anti-bacterial activity of essential oils against multidrug-resistant foodborne pathogens isolated from raw milk. *Braz J Biol*. 2022 May 9;84:e259449.
[7697] Chen WN, Chin KW, Tang KS, et al. Neuroprotective, Neurite Enhancing and Cholinesterase Inhibitory Effects of Lamiaceae Family Essential Oils in Alzheimer's Disease Model. HERMED-D-22-00403. Available at: https://ssrn.com/abstract=4112137 or http://dx.doi.org/10.2139/ssrn.4112137.
[7698] El-Kasem Bosly HA. Larvicidal and adulticidal activity of essential oils from plants of the Lamiaceae family against the West Nile virus vector, Culex pipiens (Diptera: Culicidae). *Saudi J Biol Sci*. 2022 Aug;29(8):103350.
[7699] Zhaeintan P, Nickfarjam A, Shams A, et al. Radioprotective Effect of Rosmarinus officinalis L (Rosemary) Essential Oil on Apoptosis, Necrosis and Mitotic Death of Human Peripheral Lymphocytes (PBMCs). *J Biomed Phys Eng*. 2022 Jun 1;12(3):245-256.
[7700] Brożyna M, Paleczny J, Kozłowska W, et al. Chemical Composition and Antibacterial Activity of Liquid and Volatile Phase of Essential Oils against Planktonic and Biofilm-Forming Cells of Pseudomonas aeruginosa. *Molecules*. 2022 Jun 25;27(13):4096.
[7701] Shawer R, El-Shazly MM, Khider AM, et al. Botanical Oils Isolated from Simmondsia chinensis and Rosmarinus officinalis Cultivated in Northern Egypt: Chemical Composition and Insecticidal Activity against Sitophilus oryzae (L.) and Tribolium castaneum (Herbst). *Molecules*. 2022 Jul 8;27(14):4383.
[7702] Sun J, Sun P, Kang C, et al. Chemical composition and biological activities of essential oils from six lamiaceae folk medicinal plants. *Front Plant Sci*. 2022 Aug 1;13:919294.
[7703] Ziyadi S, Iddar A, Errafiy N, et al. Protective Effect of Some Essential Oils Against Gamma-Radiation Damages in Tetrahymena pyriformis Exposed to Cobalt-60 Source. *Curr Microbiol*. 2022 Aug 3;79(9):279.
[7704] Rekioua N, Boumendjel M, Taibi F, et al. Insecticidal effect of Eucalyptus globulus and Rosmarinus officinalis essential oils on a stored food pest Ephestia kuehniella (Lepidoptera, Pyralidea). *Cell Mol Biol (Noisy-le-grand)*. 2022 Apr 30;68(4):144-157.
[7705] Oualdi I, Diass K, Azizi SE, et al. Rosmarinus officinalis essential oils from Morocco: new advances on extraction, GC/MS analysis, and antioxidant activity. *Nat Prod Res*. 2022 Aug 12:1-6.
[7706] Dolghi A, Coricovac D, Dinu S, et al. Chemical and Antimicrobial Characterization of Mentha piperita L. and Rosmarinus officinalis L. Essential Oils and In Vitro Potential Cytotoxic Effect in Human Colorectal Carcinoma Cells. *Molecules*. 2022 Sep 19;27(18):6106.
[7707] Assouguem A, Kara M, Ramzi A, et al. Evaluation of the Effect of Four Bioactive Compounds in Combination with Chemical Product against Two Spider Mites Tetranychus urticae and Eutetranychus orientalis(Acari: Tetranychidae). *Evid Based Complement Alternat Med*. 2022 Aug 22;2022:2004623.
[7708] Lopes RP, Parreira LA, Venancio AN, et al. Chemical characterization and evaluation of acaricidal potential of rosemary essential oil and its main compound α-pinene on the two-spotted spider mite, Tetranychus urticae. *Nat Prod Res*. 2022 Oct 26:1-5.
[7709] Sánchez-Quintero MJ, Delgado J, et al. Beneficial Effects of Essential Oils from the Mediterranean Diet on Gut Microbiota and Their Metabolites in Ischemic Heart Disease and Type-2 Diabetes Mellitus. *Nutrients*. 2022 Nov 3;14(21):4650.
[7710] Shahina Z, Al Homsi R, Price JDW, et al. Rosemary essential oil and its components 1,8-cineole and α-pinene induce ROS-dependent lethality and ROS-independent virulence inhibition in Candida albicans. *PLoS One*. 2022 Nov 16;17(11):e0277097.
[7711] Mohamed ME, Younis NS, El-Beltagi HS, et al. The Synergistic Hepatoprotective Activity of Rosemary Essential Oil and Curcumin: The Role of the MEK/ERK Pathway. *Molecules*. 2022 Dec 15;27(24):8910.
[7712] Saied M, Ali K, Mosayeb A. Rosemary (Rosmarinus officinalis L.) essential oil alleviates testis failure induced by Etoposide in male rats. *Tissue Cell*. 2023 Apr;81:102016.
[7713] Hajhashemi V, Salimian M, Hajihashemi O. Involvement of the NO/cGMP/KATP pathway in the antinociceptive effect of rosemary (Rosmarinus officinalis) essential oil in mice. *Behav Pharmacol*. 2022 Nov 3. Online ahead of print.
[7714] Huang Y, Xu H, Ding M, et al. Screening of Rosemary Essential Oils with Different Phytochemicals for Antioxidant Capacity, Keratinocyte Cytotoxicity, and Anti-Proliferative Activity. *Molecules*. 2023 Jan 6;28(2):586.
[7715] Dhouibi I, Flamini G, Bouaziz M. Comparative Study on the Essential Oils Extracted from Tunisian Rosemary and Myrtle: Chemical Profiles, Quality, and Antimicrobial Activities. *ACS Omega*. 2023 Feb 10;8(7):6431-6438.
[7716] Bowbe KH, Salah KBH, Moumni S, et al. Anti-Staphylococcal Activities of Rosmarinus officinalis and Myrtus communis Essential Oils through ROS-Mediated Oxidative Stress. *Antibiotics (Basel)*. 2023 Jan 28;12(2):266.
[7717] Fareed SA, Yousef EM, El-Moneam SM, et al. Assessment of Effects of Rosemary Essential Oil on the Kidney Pathology of Diabetic Adult Male Albino Rats. *Cureus*. 2023;15(3):e35736.
[7718] Al-Tawarah NM, Al-Dmour RH, Abu Hajleh MN, et al. Rosmarinus officinalis and Mentha piperita Oils Supplementation Enhances Memory in a Rat Model of Scopolamine-Induced Alzheimer's Disease-like Condition. *Nutrients*. 2023 Mar 22;15(6):1547.
[7719] Yang X, Jin C, Wu Z, Han H, et al. Toxicity and Physiological Effects of Nine Lamiaceae Essential Oils and Their Major Compounds on Reticulitermes dabieshanensis. *Molecules*. 2023 Feb 21;28(5):2007.
[7720] Fidelis C, Augusto F, de Tarso Barbosa Sampaio P, et al. Chemical characterization of rosewood (aniba rosaeodora Ducke) leaf essential oil by comprehensive two-dimensional gas chromatography coupled with quadrupole mass spectrometry. *J Essent Oil Res*. 2012 Jun;24(3):245–51.
[7721] Chantraine JM, Dhenin JM, Moretti C. Chemical variability of rosewood (Aniba rosaeodora Ducke) essential oil in French Guiana. *J Essent Oil res*. 2009 Dec;21(6):486–95.
[7722] Essential Oil University. *Aniba rosaedora var amazonica Ducke (A. duckei Kostemans), fam. Lauraceae*. Available at: http://essentialoil.university/eoudb/view/oil/2958.
[7723] Rosato A, Piarulli M, Corbo F, et al. In vitro synergistic antibacterial action of certain combination of gentamicin and essential oils. *Curr Med Chem*. 2010;17(28):3289–95.
[7724] Cardoso NN, Alviano CS, Blank AF, et al. Synergism Effect of the Essential Oil from Ocimum basilicum var. Maria Bonita and Its Major Components with Fluconazole and Its Influence on Ergosterol Biosynthesis. *Evid Based Complement Alternat Med*. 2016;2016:5647182.
[7725] de Almeida RN, Araujo DA, Goncalves JC, et al. Rosewood oil induces sedation and inhibits constituent action potential in rodents. *J Ethnopharmacol*. 2009 Jul;124(3):440–43.
[7726] Soeur J, Marrot L, Perex P, et al. Selective cytotoxicity of Aniba rosaeodora essential oil towards epidermoid cancer cells through induction of apoptosis. *Mutat Res*. 2011 Jan;718(1–2):24–32.
[7727] Sampaio Lde F, Maia JG, de Parijos AM, et al. Linalool from rosewood (Aniba rosaeodora Ducke) oil inhibits adebylate cyclase in the retina, contributing to understanding tis biological activity. *Phytother Res*. 2012 Jan;26(1):73–77.
[7728] Rosato A, Piarulli M, Corbo F, et al. In vitro synergistic antibacterial action of certain combination of gentamicin and essential oils. *Curr Med Chem*. 2010;17(28):3289–95.
[7729] de Almeida RN, Araujo DA, Goncalves JC, et al. Rosewood oil induces sedation and inhibits constituent action potential in rodents. *J Ethnopharmacol*. 2009 Jul;124(3):440–43.
[7730] de Siqueira RJ1, Rodrigues KM, da Silva MT, et al. Linalool-rich rosewood oil induces vago-vagal bradycardic and depressor reflex in rats. *Phytother Res*. 2014 Jan;28(1):42-8.
[7731] Jantapan K, Poapolathep A, Imsilp K, et al. Inhibitory Effects of Thai Essential Oils on Potentially Aflatoxigenic Aspergillus parasiticus and Aspergillus flavus. *Biocontrol Sci*. 2017;22(1):31-40.
[7732] dos Santos ÉRQ, Maia CSF, Fontes Junior EA, et al. Linalool-rich essential oils from the Amazon display antidepressant-type effect in rodents. *J Ethnopharmacol*. 2018 Feb 15;212:43-49.
[7733] Vasireddy L, Bingle LEH, Davies MS. Antimicrobial activity of essential oils against multidrug-resistant clinical isolates of the Burkholderia cepacia complex. *PLoS One*. 2018 Aug 2;13(8):e0201835.
[7734] Okuda M, Fujita Y, Takada-Takatori Y, et al. Aromatherapy improves cognitive dysfunction in senescence-accelerated mouse prone 8 by reducing the level of amyloid beta and tau phosphorylation. *PLoS One*. 2020 Oct 14;15(10):e0240378.
[7735] Teles AM, Silva-Silva JV, Fernandes JMP, Calabrese KDS, et al. Aniba rosaeodora (Var. amazonica Ducke) Essential Oil: Chemical Composition, Antibacterial, Antioxidant and Antitrypanosomal Activity. *Antibiotics (Basel)*. 2020 Dec 30;10(1):24.
[7736] Singh BK, Chaudhari AK, Das S, et al. Chitosan encompassed Aniba rosaeodora essential oil as innovative green candidate for antifungal and antiaflatoxigenic activity in millets with emphasis on cellular and its mode of action. *Front Microbiol*. 2022 Aug 9;13:970670.

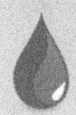
[7737] Malik AA, Mir SR, Ahmad J. Ruta graveolens L. Essential Oil Composition under Different Nutritional Treatments. *American-Eurasian J Agric Environ Sci.* 2013;13(10):1390-95.

[7738] Dzhurmanski A, Zhekova G, Angelova D. Accumulation dynamic of Ruta graveolens L. essential oil. *Agric Sci Tech.* 2011;3(4):343-45.

[7739] Haddouchi F, Chaouche TM, Zaouali Y, et al. Chemical composition and antimicrobial activity of the essential oils from four Ruta species growing in Algeria. *Food Chem.* 2013;14:253-58.

[7740] Ferhat M, Kabouche A, Kabouche Z. Comparative compositions of essential oils of three Ruta species growing in different soils. *J Mater Environ Sci.* 2014;5(3):735-38.

[7741] Hilawie M, Unnithan CR, Muuz M, et al. Extraction, isolation and chemical composition of the essential oil of Ruta graveolens L of Mekelle, Norther Ethiopia. *Int J Pharmacol.* 2015;5(1):5-7.

[7742] Fredj MBH, Marzouk B, Chraief I, et al. Analysis of Tunisian Ruta graveolens L. oils from Jemmel. *J Food Agric Environ.* 2007;5(1):52-55.

[7743] Tampe J, Parra L, Huaiquil K, et al. Potential repellent activity of the essential oil of ruta chalepensis (linnaeus) from chile against aegorhinus superciliosus (guérin) (Coleoptera: Curculionidae). *J Soil Sci Plant Nutr.* 2016;16(1):ISSN 0718-9516.

[7744] Chaftar N, Girardot M, Quellard N, et al. Activity of Six Essential Oils Extracted from Tunisian Plants against Legionella pneumophila. *Chem Biodivers.* 2015 Oct;12(10):1565-74.

[7745] Dzhurmanski A, Zhekova G, Angelova D. Accumulation dynamic of Ruta graveolens L. essential oil. *Agric Sci Tech.* 2011;3(4):343-45.

[7746] Blumenthal M. The Complete German Commission E Monographs: Therapeutic Guide to Herbal Medicines. Trans. S. Klein. Boston, MA: American Botanical Council, 1998.

[7747] Rabaev E, Zeller L, Biton A, et al. [Toxic hepatitis due to the use of Ruta herbal medicine]. *Harefuah.* 2011 Mar;150(3):235-6, 305.

[7748] Ciganda C, Laborde A. Herbal Infusions Used for Induced Abortion. *J Toxicol Clin Toxicol.* 2003 Jan;41(3):235-39.

[7749] Conway GA, Slocumb JC. Plants used as abortifacients and emmenagogues by Spanish New Mexicans. *J Ethnopharmacol.* 1979 Oct;1(3):241-61.

[7750] Maurya R, Srivastava S, Kulshreshta DK, et al. Traditional Remedies for Fertility Regulation. Curr Med Chem. 2004;11:1431-50.

[7751] Ciganda C, Laborde A. Herbal Infusions Used for Induced Abortion. *J Toxicol Clin Toxicol.* 2003 Jan;41(3):235-39.

[7752] Farnsworth NP, bingel AS, Cordell Ga, et al. Potential value of plants as source of new antifertility agents I. *J Pharm Sci.* 1975 Apr;64(4):535-98.

[7753] Gandhi M, Lal R, Sankaranarayanan A, et al. Post-coital antifertility action of Ruta graveolens in female rats and hamsters. *J Ethnopharmacol.* 1991 Aug;34(1):49-59.

[7754] Kong YC, Lau CP, Wat KH, et al. Antifertility principle of Ruta graveolens. *Planta Med.* 1989 Apr;55(2):176-78.

[7755] Kong YC, Lau CP, Wat KH, et al. Antifertility principle of Ruta graveolens. *Planta Med.* 1989 Apr;55(2):176-78.

[7756] Farnsworth NP, bingel AS, Cordell Ga, et al. Potential value of plants as source of new antifertility agents I. *J Pharm Sci.* 1975 Apr;64(4):535-98.

[7757] Gandhi M, Lal R, Sankaranarayanan A, et al. Post-coital antifertility action of Ruta graveolens in female rats and hamsters. *J Ethnopharmacol.* 1991 Aug;34(1):49-59.

[7758] Patoir A, Patoir G, Bedrine H. Note sur l'action de l'essence de rue sur l'organisme animal. *Computes Rendues Société Bologique.* 1938;127:1324-25.

[7759] No author listed. Oil of rue: proposed affirmation of GRAS status with specific limitations as direct human food ingredient. *Fed Regist.* 1974;39:34215.

[7760] The European Agency for the Evaluation of Medicinal Products. Committee for Veterinary Medicinal Products. Ruta graveolens Summary Report. Available at: http://www.ema.europa.eu/docs/en_GB/document_library/Maximum_Residue_Limits_-_Report/2009/11/WC500015840.pdf.

[7761] The European Agency for the Evaluation of Medicinal Products. Committee for Veterinary Medicinal Products. Ruta graveolens Summary Report. Available at: http://www.ema.europa.eu/docs/en_GB/document_library/Maximum_Residue_Limits_-_Report/2009/11/WC500015840.pdf.

[7762] Maurya R, Srivastava S, Kulshreshta DK, et al. Traditional Remedies for Fertility Regulation. Curr Med Chem. 2004;11:1431-50.

[7763] Opdyke DIJ. Monographs on fragrance raw materials. *Food Cosmet Toxicol.* 1974;12(Suppl.):455-56.

[7764] Leung AY, Foster S. Encyclopedia of common natural ingredients used in food, drugs and cosmetics. Second edition. New Jersey: Jon Wiley. 2003.

[7765] The European Agency for the Evaluation of Medicinal Products. Committee for Veterinary Medicinal Products. Ruta graveolens Summary Report. Available at: http://www.ema.europa.eu/docs/en_GB/document_library/Maximum_Residue_Limits_-_Report/2009/11/WC500015840.pdf.

[7766] Seak CJ, Lin CC. Ruta graveolens intoxication. *Clin Toxicol.* 2007;45:173-75.

[7767] DerMarderosian A, Beutler JA. The Review of Natural Products. The Most Complete Source of Natural Product Information. 7th Edition. p. 1405. Wolters Kluwer Health: St. Louis, Missouri. 2012.

[7768] Morais P, Mota A, Cunha AP, et al. Phytophotodermatitis due to homemade ointment for pediculosis capitis. *Contact Dermatitis.* 2008 Dec;59(6):373-74.

[7769] Scientific Committee on Consumer Products. Opinion on furocoumarins in cosmetic products. Available at: http://ec.europa.eu/health/ph_risk/committees/04_sccp/docs/sccp_o_036.pdf.

[7770] Eickhorst K, DeLeo V, Csaposs J. Rue the herb: Ruta graveolens--associated phytophototoxicity. Dermatitis. 2007 Mar;18(1):52-5.

[7771] Schempp CM, Schöpf E, Simon JC. [Bullous phototoxic contact dermatitis caused by Ruta graveolens L. (garden rue), Rutaceae. Case report and review of literature]. *Hautarzt.* 1999 Jun;50(6):432-4.

[7772] Chaftar N, Girardot M, Quellard N, et al. Activity of Six Essential Oils Extracted from Tunisian Plants against Legionella pneumophila. *Chem Biodivers.* 2015 Oct;12(10):1565-74.

[7773] Al-Shuneigat JM, Al-Tarawneh IN, Al-Qudah MA, et al. The Chemical Composition and the Antibacterial Properties of Ruta graveolens L. Essential Oil Grown in Northern Jordan. *Jordan J Biol Sci.* 2015 Jun;8(2):139-43.

[7774] Haddouchi F, Chaouche TM, Zaouali Y, et al. Chemical composition and antimicrobial activity of the essential oils from four Ruta species growing in Algeria. *Food Chem.* 2013;14:253-58.

[7775] Tampe J, Parra L, Huaiquil K, et al. Potential repellent activity of the essential oil of ruta chalepensis (linnaeus) from chile against aegorhinus superciliosus (guérin) (Coleoptera: Curculionidae). *J Soil Sci Plant Nutr.* 2016;16(1):ISSN 0718-9516.

[7776] Faria JM, Barbosa P, Bennett RN, et al. Bioactivity against Bursaphelenchus xylophilus: Nematotoxics from essential oils, essential oils fractions and decoction waters. *Phytochemistry.* 2013 Oct;94:220-8.

[7777] Tabanaca N, Demirci B, Kiyan HT, et al. Repellent and Larvicidal Activity of Ruta graveolens Essential Oil and its Major Individual Constituents Against Aedes aegypti. *Planta Med.* 2012;78-90.

[7778] Donadu MG, Peralta-Ruiz Y, Usai D, Maggio F, et al. Colombian Essential Oil of Ruta graveolens against Nosocomial Antifungal Resistant Candida Strains. *J Fungi (Basel).* 2021 May 14;7(5):383.

[7779] Wang S, Li SC, Cheng FS, et al. Antifungal, Repellency, and Insecticidal Activities of Cymbopogon distans and Ruta graveolens Essential Oils and Their Main Chemical Constituents. *Chem Biodivers.* 2022 Sep 2:e202200351.

[7780] Coimbra A, Miguel S, Ribeiro M, et al. Chemical composition, antioxidant, and antimicrobial activities of six commercial essential oils. *Lett Appl Microbiol.* 2023 Jan 23;76(1):ovac042.

[7781] Bouabida H, Dris D. Biological toxicity of Ruta graveolens essential oil against three species of diptera Drosophila melanogaster, Culex pipiens and Culiseta longiareolata. *J Vector Borne Dis.* 2022 Oct-Dec;59(4):320-326.

[7782] Stesevic D, Ristic M, Nikolic V, et al. Chemotype diversity of indigenous Dalmatian sage (Salvia officinalis L.) populations in Montenegro. *Chem Biodivers.* 2014 Jan;11(1):101-14.

[7783] Bouajaj S, Benyamma A, Bouamama H, et al. Antibacterial, allelopathic and antioxidant activities of essential oil of Salvia officinalis L. growing wild in the Atlas Mountains of Morocco. *Nat Prod Res.* 2013;27(18):1673-76.

[7784] Oniga I, Oprean R, Toiu A, et al. Chemical composition of the essential oil of Salvia officinalis L. from Romania. *Rev Med Chir Soc Med Nat Lasi.* 2010 Apr-Jun;114(2):593-95.

[7785] Porte A, Godoy RLO, Maia-Porte LH. Chemical composition of sage (Salvia officinalis L.) essential oil from the Rio de Janeiro State (Brazil). *Rev Bras Pl Med.* 2013;15(3):438-41.

[7786] Abu-Darwish MS, Cabral C, Ferreira IV, et al. Essential oil of Common Sage (Salvia officinalis L.) from Jordan Assessment of safety in mammalian cells and its antifungal and anti-inflammatory potential. *BioMed Res Int.* 2013;2013:538940.

[7787] Lakhal H, Ghorab H, Chibani S, et al. Chemical composition and biological activities of the essential oils of Salvia officinalis from Batna (Algeria). *Der Pharmacia Lettre.* 2013;5(3):310-14.

[7788] Viuda-Martos M, Ruiz-Navajas Y, Fernandez-Lopez J, et al. Chemical composition of the essential oils obtained from some spices widely used in Mediterranean region. *Acta Chim Slov.* 2007;54:921-26.

[7789] Santos-Gomez PC, Fernandez-Ferreira. Essential oils produced by in vitro shoots of sage (Salvia officinalis L.). *J Agric Food Chem.* 2003 Apr 9;51(8):2260-66.

[7790] Raina AP, Negi KS, Dutta M. Variability in essential oil composition of sage (Salvia officinalis L.) grown under North Western Himalayan region of India. *J Med Pl Res.* 2013 Mar;7(11):683-88.

[7791] Jug-Dujakovic M, Ristic M, Pljevljakusic D, et al. High diversity of indigenous populations of Dalmatian Sage (Salvia officinalis L.) in essential-oil composition. *Chem Biodiv.* 2012;9:2309-23.

[7792] Haliciglu O, Astarcioglu G, Yaprak I, et al. Toxicity of Salvia officinalis in a newborn and a child: an alarming report. *Pediatr Neurol.* 2011 Oct;45(4):259-60.

[7793] Lachenmeier DW, Walch SG. Epileptic seizure caused by accidental ingestion of sage (Salvia officinalis L.) oil in children: a rare, exceptional case or a threat to public health. *Pediatr Neurol.* 2012 Mar;46(3):201.

[7794] Stafstrom CE. Seizures in a 7-month-old child after exposure to the essential plant oil thuja. *Pediatr Neurol.* 2007 Dec;37(6):446-8.

[7795] Khine H, Weiss D, Graber N, et al. A cluster of children with seizures caused by camphor poisoning. *Pediatrics.* 2009 May;123(5):1269-72.

[7796] Michiels EA, Mazor SS. Toddler with seizures due to ingesting camphor at an Indian celebration. *Pediatr Emerg Care.* 2010 Aug;26(8):574-75.

[7797] Koren G. Medications which can kill a toddler with one tablet or teaspoonful. *J toxicol Clin Toxicol.* 1993;31(3):407- 13.

[7798] Bar-Oz B, Levicheck Z, Koren G. Medications that can kill a toddler with one tablet or teaspoonfull – A 2004 update. *Paediatr Drugs.* 2004;6(2):123-6.

[7799] Craig JO. Poisoning by the volatile oils in childhood. *Arch Dis Child.* 1953;28:259-67.

[7800] Melis K. Bochner A, Janssens G. Accidental nasal eucalyptol and menthol instillation. *Eur J Pediatr.* 1989 Aug;148(8)786-7.

[7801] Day LM, Ozanne-Smith J, Parsons BJ, et al. Eucalyptus oil poisoning among young children: mechanisms of access and the potential prevention. *Aust N Z J Public Health.* 1997 Jun;21(3):297-302.

[7802] Chandar SD, Prashanti M, Kumar CL, et al. Eucalyptus Oil-Induced Seizures in Children: A Single-Center Prospective Study. *Cureus.* 2021 Mar 25;13(3):e14109.

[7803] Rabl W, Katzgraber F, Steinlechner M. Camphor ingestion for abortion (case report). *Forensic Sci Int.* 1997 Sep 19;89(1-2):137-40.

[7804] Blumenthal M, ed. The Complete German Commission E Monographs: Therapeutic Guide to Herbal Medicines. Trans. S. Klein. Boston, MA: American Botanical Council, 1998.

[7805] da Silva Costa KC, Bezerra SB, Norte CM, et al. Medicinal plants with teratogenic potential: current considerations. *Braz J Pharm Sci.* 2012;48(3):427–33.

[7806] Brinker F. Herb Contraindications and Drug Interactions. 2nd ed. Sandy, OR. Eclectic Medical Publications. 1998.

[7807] Flaman Z, Pellechia-Clarke S, Bailey B, et al. Unintentional exposure of young children to camphor and eucalyptus oils. *Paediatr Child Health.* 2001 Feb;6(2):80-83.

7808 European Medicines Agency. Public statement on the use of herbal medicinal products containing thujone. Available at: http://www.ema.europa.eu/docs/en_GB/document_library/Public_statement/2011/02/WC500102294.pdf.
7809 Millet Y, Jouglard J, Steinmetz MD, et al. Toxicity of some essential plant oils. Clinical and experimental study. *Clin Toxicol.* 1981 Dec;18(12):1485-98.
7810 Cristovao L, Carvalho F, Bastos MDL, et al. Hepatotoxicity of an essential oil of Salvia officinalis L.: an in vitro study using freshly isolated rat hepatocytes. *Congress Biomarkers.* 2001 Sep:165.
7811 Burkhard PR, Burkhardt K, Haenggeli CA, et al. Plant-induced seizures: reappearance of an old problem. *J Neurol.* 1999 Aug;246(8):667-70.
7812 Manoguerra AS, Erdman AR, Wax PM, et al. Camphor poisoning: an evidence-based practice guideline for out-of- hospital management. *Clin Toxicol (Phila).*2006;44(4):357-70.
7813 Gibson DE, Moore GP, Pfaff JA. Camphor ingestion. *Am J Emerg Med.* 1989 Jan;7(1):41-43.
7814 Koppel C, Martends F, Schirop T, et al. Hemoperfusion in acute camphor poisoning. *Intensive Care Med.* 1988;14(4):431-33.
7815 Burkhard PR, Burkhardt K, Haenggeli CA, et al. Plant-induced seizures: reappearance of an old problem. *J Neurol.* 1999 Aug;246(8):667-70.
7816 Narayan S, Singh N. Camphor poisoning-An unusual cause of seizure. *Med J Armed Forces India.* 2012 Jul;68(3):252-53.
7817 Chanaranaj KJ, G MV, S M. Camphor poisoning in a child. *Natl Med J India.* 2013 Jan-Feb;26(1):60.
7818 Perry NB, Anderson RE, Brennan NJ, et al. Essential oils from dalmatian sage (Salvia officinalis L.) variations among individuals, plant parts, seasons, and sites. *J Agric Food Chem.* 1999;47:2048-54.
7819 Millet Y, Jouglard J, Steinmetz MD, et al. Toxicity of some essential plant oils. Clinical and experimental study. *Clin Toxicol.* 1981 Dec;18(12):1485-98.
7820 Olowe SA, Ransome-Kuti O. The risk of jaundice in glucose-6-phosphate dehydrogenase deficient babies exposed to menthol. *Acta Paediatr Scand.* 1980 May;69(3):341-5.
7821 Dillon Remy M, Manning Alleyne P, Bratt DE, et al. Neonatal jaundice at Port-of-Spain General Hospital abstract. *West Indian Med J.* 1987;36(Suppl):28.
7822 Uc A, Bishop WP, Sanders KD. Camphor hepatotoxicity. *South Med J.* 2000;93:596-98.
7823 Frohne D. Giftpflanzen: Cupressaceae. Stuttgart: Wissenschaftliche Verlagsgesellschaft mbH; 1997. pp. 153–6.
7824 Dolan LC, Matulka RA, Burdock GA. Naturally Occurring Food Toxins. *Toxins (Basel).* 2010 Sep;2(9):2289–2332.
7825 United States National Toxicology Program (NTP). Alpha-Thujone. Dec 10, 1997. Available at: http://ntp.niehs.nih.gov/index.cfm?objectid=03DB8C36-E7A1-9889-3BDF8436F2A8C51F.
7826 Jori A, Bianchetti A, Prestini PE, et al. Effect of eucalyptol (1,8-cineole) on the metabolism of other drugs in rats and in man. *Eur J Pharmacol.* 1970;9(3):362-66.
7827 de Sousa DP, Raphael E, Brocksom U, et al. Sedative effect of monoterpene alcohols in mice: A preliminary screening. *Verlag der Zeitschrift fur Naturforschung.* 2007;62c:563-66.
7828 Lamborn LL. Modern soaps, candles and glycerin: A practical manual of modern methods of utilization of fats and oils in the manufacture of soaps and candles, and of the recovery of glycerin. Library of the University of Wisconsin.
7829 Oyen LP, Dung NX. Plant resources of South-East Asia. 1999. Backhyus, Leiden.
7830 Kim NH, Hyun SH, Jin CH, et al. Pretreatment with 1,8-cineole potentiates thioacetamide-induced hepatotoxicity and immunosuppression. *Arch Pharm Res.* 2004 Jul;27(7):781-9.
7831 Abass K, Reponen P, Mattila S, et al. Metabolism of α-thujone in human hepatic preparations in vitro. *Xenobiotica.* 2011 Feb;41(2):101-11.
7832 Miroddi M, Navarra M, Quattropani MC, et al. Systematic review of clinical trials assessing pharmacological properties of Salvia species on memory, cognitive impairment and Alzheimer's disease. *CNS Neurosci Ther.* 2014 Jun;20(6):485-95.
7833 Kennedy DO, Scholey AB. The psychopharmacology of European herbs with cognition-enhancing properties. *Curr Pharm Des.* 2006;12(35):4613-23.
7834 Russo A, Formisano C, Rigano D, et al. Chemical composition and anticancer activity of essential oils of Mediterranean sage (Salvia officinalis L.) grown in different environmental conditions. *Food Chem Toxicol.* 2013 May;55:45-47.
7835 Loizzo MR, Tundis R, Menichini F, et al. Cytotoxic activity of essential oils from Labiatae and Lauraceae families against in vitro human tumor models. *Anticancer Res.* 2007 Sep-Oct;27(5A):3293-99.
7836 Sertel S, Eichorn T, Plinkert PK, et al. Anticancer activity of Salvia officinalis essential oil against HNSCC cell line (UMSCC1). *HNO.* 2011 Dec;59(12):1203-08.
7837 Pereira RS, Sumita TC, Furlan MR, et al. Antibacterial activity of essential oils on microorganisms isolated from urinary tract infection. *Rev Saude Publica.* 2004 Apr;38(2):326-28.
7838 Suntar I, Akkol EK, Keles J, et al. A novel wound healing ointment: a formulation of Hypericum perforatum oil and sage and oregano essential oils based on traditional Turkish knowledge. *J Ethnopharmacol.* 2011 Mar 8;134(1):89-96.
7839 Stojanović-Radić Z, Pejčić M, Stojanović N, et al. Potential of Ocimum basilicum L. and Salvia officinalis L. essential oils against biofilms of P. aeruginosa clinical isolates. *Cell Mol Biol (Noisy-le-grand).* 2016 Aug 29;62(9):27-33.
7840 Abu-Darwish MS, Cabral C, Ferreira IV, et al. Essential oil of Common Sage (Salvia officinalis L.) from Jordan Assessment of safety in mammalian cells and its antifungal and anti-inflammatory potential. *BioMed Res Int.* 2013;2013:538940.
7841 Muhlbauer RC, Lozano A, Palacio S, et al. Common herbs, essential oils, and monoterpenes potently modulate bone metabolism. *Bone.* 2003 Apr;32(4):372-80.
7842 Abu-Darwish MS, Cabral C, Ferreira IV, et al. Essential oil of Common Sage (Salvia officinalis L.) from Jordan Assessment of safety in mammalian cells and its antifungal and anti-inflammatory potential. *BioMed Res Int.* 2013;2013:538940.
7843 Chovanova R, Mikulasova M, Vaverkova S. In vitro antibacterial and antibiotic resistance modifying effect of bioactive plant extracts on methicillin-resistant staphylococcus epidermidis. *Int J Microbiol.* 2013;2013:760969.
7844 Raffaella C, Casettari L, Fagioli L, et al. Activity of essential oil-based microemulsions against Staphylococcus aureus biofilms developed on stainless steel surface in different culture media and growth conditions. *Int J Food Microbiol.* 2016 Oct 17;241:132-140.
7845 Sookto T, Srithavaj T, Thaweboon S, et al. In vitro effects of Salvia officinalis L. essential oil on Candida albicans. *Asian Pac J Trop Biomed.* 2013 May;3(5):376-80.
7846 Bouaziz M, Yangui T, Sayadi S, et al. Disinfectant properties of essential oils from Salvia officinalis L. cultivated in Tunisia. *Food Chem Toxicol.* 2009 Nov;47(11):2755-60.
7847 Lima CF, Azevedo MF, Araujo R, et al. Metformin-like effect of Salvia officinalis (common sage): is it useful in diabetes prevention? *Br J Nutr.* 2006 Aug;96(2):326-33.
7848 Shubina LP, Siurin SA, Savchenko VM. Inhalation of essential oils in the combined treatment of patients with chronic bronchitis. *Crach Delo.*1990 May;(5):66-67.
7849 Badiee P, Nasirzadeh AR, Motaffaf. Comparison of Salvia officinalis L. essential oil and antifungal agents against candida species. *Pharm Tech Drug Res.* 2012:1-7.
7850 El-Hosseiny LS, Alqurashy NN, Sheweita SA. Oxidative Stress Alleviation by Sage Essential Oil in Co-amoxiclav induced Hepatotoxicity in Rats. *Int J Biomed Sci.* 2016 Jun;12(2):71-8.
7851 Ghorbanpour M, Hatami M, Kariman K, et al. Phytochemical Variations and Enhanced Efficiency of Antioxidant and Antimicrobial Ingredients in Salvia officinalis as Inoculated with Different Rhizobacteria. *Chem Biodivers.* 2016 Mar;13(3):319-30.
7852 Khedher MRB, Khedher SB, Chaieb I, et al. Chemical composition and biological activities of Salvia officinalis essential oil from Tunisia. *EXCLI J.* 2017 Mar 6;16:160-173.
7853 Khedher MRB, Khedher SB, Chaieb I, et al. Chemical composition and biological activities of Salvia officinalis essential oil from Tunisia. *EXCLI J.* 2017 Mar 6;16:160-173.
7854 Cutillas AB, Carrasco A, Martinez-Gutierrez R, et al. Salvia officinalis L. Essential Oil from Spain: Determination of Composition, Antioxidant Capacity, Antienzymatic and Antimicrobial Bioactivities. *Chem Biodivers.* 2017 Aug;14(8)
7855 Koubaa FG, Abdennabi R, Soussi Ben Salah A, et al. Microwave extraction of Salvia officinalis essential oil and assessment of its GC-MS identification and protective effects versus vanadium-induced nephrotoxicity in Wistar rats models. *Arch Physiol Biochem.* 2019 Dec;125(5):404-413.
7856 Bendifallah L, Belguendouz R, Hamoudi L, et al. Biological Activity of the Salvia officinalis L. (Lamiaceae) Essential Oil on Varroa destructor Infested Honeybees. *Plants (Basel).* 2018 Jun 6;7(2).
7857 Khedher MRB, Khedher SB, Chaieb I, et al. Chemical composition and biological activities of Salvia officinalis essential oil from Tunisia. *EXCLI J.* 2017 Mar 6;16:160-173.
7858 Cutillas AB, Carrasco A, Martinez-Gutierrez R, et al. Salvia officinalis L. Essential Oil from Spain: Determination of Composition, Antioxidant Capacity, Antienzymatic and Antimicrobial Bioactivities. *Chem Biodivers.* 2017 Aug;14(8).
7859 Cutillas AB, Carrasco A, Martinez-Gutierrez R, et al. Salvia officinalis L. Essential Oil from Spain: Determination of Composition, Antioxidant Capacity, Antienzymatic and Antimicrobial Bioactivities. *Chem Biodivers.* 2017 Aug;14(8).
7860 Cutillas AB, Carrasco A, Martinez-Gutierrez R, et al. Salvia officinalis L. Essential Oils from Spain: Determination of Composition, Antioxidant Capacity, Antienzymatic, and Antimicrobial Bioactivities. *Chem Biodivers.* 2017 Aug;14(8).
7861 Diab KA, Fahmy MA, Hassan ZM, et al. Genotoxicity of carbon tetrachloride and the protective role of essential oil of Salvia officinalis L. in mice using chromosomal aberration, micronuclei formation, and comet assay. *Environ Sci Pollut Res Int.* 2018 Jan;25(2):1621-1636.
7862 Vetas D, Dimitropoulou E, Mitropoulou G, et al. Disinfection efficiencies of sage and spearmint essential oils against planktonic and biofilm Staphylococcus aureus cells in comparison with sodium hypochlorite. *Int J Food Microbiol.* 2017 Sep 18;257:19-25.
7863 Živković J, Ristić M, Kschonsek J, et al. Comparison of Chemical Profile and Antioxidant Capacity of Seeds and Oils from Salvia sclarea and Salvia officinalis. *Chem Biodivers.* 2017 Dec;14(12).
7864 Alexa E, Sumalan RM, Danciu C, et al. Synergistic Antifungal, Allelopatic and Anti-Proliferative Potential of Salvia officinalis L., and Thymus vulgaris L. Essential Oils. *Molecules.* 2018 Jan 16;23(1).
7865 Fahmy MA, Diab KA, Abdel-Samie NS, et al. Carbon tetrachloride induced hepato/renal toxicity in experimental mice: antioxidant potential of Egyptian Salvia officinalis L essential oil. *Environ Sci Pollut Res Int.* 2018 Jan;25(2):1621-1636.
7866 Wijesundara NM, Rupasinghe HPV. Essential oils from Origanum vulgare and Salvia officinalis exhibit antibacterial and antibiofilm activities against Streptococcus pyogenes. *Microb Pathog.* 2018 Apr;117:118-127.
7867 Castillo-Morales RM, Carreño Otero AL, Mendez-Sanchez SC, et al. Mitochondrial affectation, DNA damage and AChE inhibition induced by Salvia officinalis essential oil on Aedes aegypti larvae. *Comp Biochem Physiol C Toxicol Pharmacol.* 2019 Jul;221:29-37.
7868 Belhadj S, Hentati O, Hammami M, et al. Metabolic impairments and tissue disorders in alloxan-induced diabetic rats are alleviated by Salvia officinalis L. essential oil. *Biomed Pharmacother.* 2018 Sep 27;108:985-995.
7869 Bonde JP, Giwercman A, Ernst E. Review Identifying environmental risk to male reproductive function by occupational sperm studies: logistics and design options. *Occup Environ Med.* 1996 Aug; 53(8):511-9.
7870 Mbaye MM, Khalifi BE, Addoum B, et al. The Effect of Supplementation with Some Essential Oils on the Mobility and the Vitality of Human Sperm. *ScientificWorldJournal.* 2019;2019:4878912.

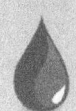

[7871] Bedini S, Guarino S, Echeverria MC, et al. Allium sativum, Rosmarinus officinalis, and Salvia officinalis Essential Oils: A Spiced Shield Against Blowflies. *Insects*. 2020 Feb 25;11(3):143.
[7872] Koubaa-Ghorbel F, Chaabane M, Turki M, et al. The Protective Effects of Salvia Officinalis Essential Oil Compared to Simvastatin Against Hyperlipidemia, Liver, and Kidney Injuries in Mice Submitted to a High-Fat Diet. *J Food Biochem*. 2020 Feb 3;e13160.
[7873] Moumni S, Elaissi A, Trabelsi A, et al. Correlation between chemical composition and antibacterial activity of some Lamiaceae species essential oils from Tunisia. *BMC Complement Med Ther*. 2020 Apr 3;20(1):103.
[7874] Farahpour MR, Pirkhezr E, Ashrafian A, et al. Accelerated Healing by Topical Administration of Salvia Officinalis Essential Oil on Pseudomonas Aeruginosa and Staphylococcus Aureus Infected Wound Model. *Biomed Pharmacother*. 2020 May 24;128:110120.
[7875] Pejcic M, Stojanovic-Radic Z, Gencic M, et al. Anti-virulence Potential of Basil and Sage Essential Oils: Inhibition of Biofilm Formation, Motility and Pyocyanin Production of Pseudomonas Aeruginosa Isolates. *Food Chem Toxicol*. 2020 May 14;141:111431.
[7876] Luca T, Napoli E, Privitera G, et al. Antiproliferative effect and cell cycle alterations induced by Salvia officinalis essential oil and its three main components in human colon cancer cell lines. Chem Biodivers. 2020 Jun 12. [Epub ahead of print]
[7877] Koubaa FG, Chaabane M, Turki M, et al. Anti-oxidant and hepatoprotective effects of Salvia officinalis essential oil against vanadium-induced oxidative stress and histological changes in the rat liver. *Environ Sci Pollut Res Int*. 2020 Oct 27. Online ahead of print.
[7878] Tundis R, Leporini M, Bonesi M, et al. Salvia officinalis L. from Italy: A Comparative Chemical and Biological Study of Its Essential Oil in the Mediterranean Context. *Molecules*. 2020 Dec 10;25(24):5826.
[7879] Madeddu S, Marongiu A, Sanna G, et al. Bovine Viral Diarrhea Virus (BVDV): A Preliminary Study on Antiviral Properties of Some Aromatic and Medicinal Plants. *Pathogens*. 2021 Mar 29;10(4):403.
[7880] Tundis R, Leporini M, Bonesi M, et al. Salvia officinalis L. from Italy: A Comparative Chemical and Biological Study of Its Essential Oil in the Mediterranean Context. *Molecules*. 2020 Dec 10;25(24):5826.
[7881] Ed-Dra A, Filali FR, Lo Presti V, et al. Chemical composition, antioxidant capacity and antibacterial action of five Moroccan essential oils against Listeria monocytogenes and different serotypes of Salmonella enterica. *Microb Pathog*. 2020 Dec;149:104510.
[7882] Mohammed HA, Eldeeb HM, Khan RA, et al. Sage, Salvia officinalis L., Constituents, Hepatoprotective Activity, and Cytotoxicity Evaluations of the Essential Oils Obtained from Fresh and Differently Timed Dried Herbs: A Comparative Analysis. *Molecules*. 2021 Sep 23;26(19):5757.
[7883] de Souza MT, de Souza MT, Bernardi D, et al. Essential Oil of Rosmarinus officinalis Ecotypes and Their Major Compounds: Insecticidal and Histological Assessment Against Drosophila suzukii and Their Impact on a Nontarget Parasitoid. *J Econ Entomol*. 2021 Dec 1;toab230.
[7884] Micić D, Đurović S, Riabov P, et al. Rosemary Essential Oils as a Promising Source of Bioactive Compounds: Chemical Composition, Thermal Properties, Biological Activity, and Gastronomical Perspectives. *Foods*. 2021 Nov 9;10(11):2734.
[7885] Tambur Z, Miljković-Selimović B, Opačić D, et al. Inhibitory effects of propolis and essential oils on oral bacteria. *J Infect Dev Ctries*. 2021 Jul 31;15(7):1027-1031.
[7886] Đurović S, Micić D, Pezo L, et al. The effect of various extraction techniques on the quality of sage (Salvia officinalis L.) essential oil, expressed by chemical composition, thermal properties and biological activity. *Food Chem X*. 2022 Jan 19;13:100213.
[7887] Selim S, Almuhayawi MS, Alqhtani H, et al. Anti-Salmonella and Antibiofilm Potency of Salvia officinalis L. Essential Oil against Antibiotic-Resistant Salmonella enterica. *Antibiotics (Basel)*. 2022 Apr 6;11(4):489.
[7888] Baz MM, Selim A, Radwan IT, et al. Larvicidal and adulticidal effects of some Egyptian oils against Culex pipiens. *Sci Rep*. 2022 Mar 15;12(1):4406.
[7889] Mot MD, Gavrilaş S, Lupitu AI, et al. Salvia officinalis L. Essential Oil: Characterization, Antioxidant Properties, and the Effects of Aromatherapy in Adult Patients. *Antioxidants (Basel)*. 2022 Apr 21;11(5):808.
[7890] Chen WN, Chin KW, Tang KS, et al. Neuroprotective, Neurite Enhancing and Cholinesterase Inhibitory Effects of Lamiaceae Family Essential Oils in Alzheimer's Disease Model. HERMED-D-22-00403. Available at: https://ssrn.com/abstract=4112137 or http://dx.doi.org/10.2139/ssrn.4112137.
[7891] Ghorbel Koubaa F, Chaâbane M, Chiab N, et al. Beneficial effects of Salvia officinalis essential oil on vanadium-induced testicular injury, DNA damage and histological alterations in Wistar rats. *Biometals*. 2022 Jun 28. doi: Online ahead of print.
[7892] Assaggaf HM, Naceiri Mrabti H, Rajab BS, et al. Chemical Analysis and Investigation of Biological Effects of Salvia officinalis Essential Oils at Three Phenological Stages. *Molecules*. 2022 Aug 12;27(16):5157.
[7893] Gad HA, Mamadalieva RZ, Khalil N, et al. GC-MS Chemical Profiling, Biological Investigation of Three Salvia Species Growing in Uzbekistan. *Molecules*. 2022 Aug 23;27(17):5365.
[7894] Zerkani H, Kharchoufa L, Tagnaout I, et al. Chemical Composition and Bioinsecticidal Effects of Thymus zygis L., Salvia officinalis L. and Mentha suaveolens Ehrh. Essential Oils on Medfly Ceratitis capitata and Tomato Leaf Miner Tuta absoluta. *Plants (Basel)*. 2022 Nov 14;11(22):3084.
[7895] Misra BB, Dey S. Quantitative and qualitative evaluation of sesquiterpenoids from essential oil and in vitro somatic embryos of east Indian Sandalwood (Santalum album) tree by HPTLC and GC. *J Med Aroma Plants*. 2013;4(1):1-9.
[7896] Brand JE, Fox JED, Pronk G, et al. Comparison of oil concentration and oil quality from Santalum spicatum and S. album plantations, 8-25 years old, with those from mature S. spicatum natural stands. *Aust Forest*. 2007;70(4):235-41.
[7897] Valder C, Neugebauer M, Meier M, et al. Western Australian sandalwood oil - new constituents of Santalum spicatum (R. Br.) A. DC. (Santalaceae). *J Essent Oil Res*. 2003;15(3):178-86.
[7898] Misra B, Dey S. Biological activities of East Indian sandalwood tree, Santalum album. *Peer J PrePrints*. 2013 Nov 12;1;1-30.
[7899] Bhat KV, Balasundaran M, Balagopalan M. Identification of Santalum album and Osyris Lanceolata through morphological and biochemical characteristics and molecular markers to check adulteration. *KFRI Research Report No. 307*. Available at: http://docs.kfri.res.in/KFRI-RR/KFRI-RR307.pdf.
[7900] Aromatics International. Sandalwood (Hawaiian) - Santalum paniculatum. Available at: http://www.aromaticsinternational.com/products/essential-oils/sandalwood-hawaiian.
[7901] AromatheraChi. Gas chromatography/mass spectrometry report. Available at: http://www.aromatherachi.com/GCMS/SandalwoodGCMSreport.pdf.
[7902] Brophy JJ, Fookes CJR, Lassak EV. Constituents of Santalum spicatum (R.Br.) A. DC. wood oil. *J Essent Oil Res*. 1991;3(6):381-85.
[7903] Roh HS, Kim J, Shin ES, et al. Bioactivity of sandalwood oil (Santalum austrocaledonicum) and its main components against the cotton aphid, Aphis gossypii. *J Pest Sci*. 2014 Nov;88:621-27.
[7904] Baldovini N, Delasalle C, Joulain D. Phytochemistry of the heartwood from fragrant Santalum species: a review. *Flav Frag J*. 2011 Jan;26(1):7-26.
[7905] Braun NA, Meier M, Hammerschmidt FJ, et al. New Caledonian sandalwood oil-a substitute for East Indian sandalwood oil? *J Essent Oil Res*. 2011 Nov;17(5):477-80.
[7906] Proceedings of the regional workshop on sandalwood research, development and extensions in the Pacific Islands. Available at: http://www.spc.int/lrd/publications/doc_download/1423-sandalwood2005-report.
[7907] Yang SP, Raner Gm. Cytochrome P450 expression and activities in human tongue cells and their modulation by green tea Extract. *Toxicol Appl Pharmacol*. 2005;202:140-150.
[7908] Johnson S. Supercritical Essential Oils. 2017. Scott A Johnson Professional Writing Services, LLC: Orem, Utah.
[7909] Dozmorov MG, Yang Q, Wu W, et al. Differential effects of selective frankincense (Ru Ziang) essential oil versus non-selective sandalwood (Tan Xiang) essential oil on cultured bladder cancer cells: a microarray and bioinformatics study. *Chin Med*. 2014 Jul;9:18.
[7910] Dickinson SE, Olson ER, Levenson C, et al. A novel chemopreventive mechanism for a traditional medicine: East Indian sandalwood oil induces autophagy and cell death in proliferating keratinocytes. *Arch Biochem Biophys*. 2014 Sep 15;558:143-52.
[7911] Benencia F, Courreges MC. Antiviral activity of sandalwood oil against Herpes simplex viruses-1 and -2. *Phytomedicine*. 1999;6(2):119-23.
[7912] Koch C, Reichling J, Schneele J, et al. Inhibitory effect of essential oils against herpes simplex virus type 2. *Phytomedicine*. 2008 Jan 25;15(1-2):71-78.
[7913] Schnitzler P, Koch C, Reichling J. Susceptibility of drug-resistant clinical herpes simplex virus type 1 strain to essential oils of ginger, thyme, hyssop, and sandalwood. *Antimicrob Agents Chemother*. 2007 May;51(5):1859-62.
[7914] Baylac S, Racine P. Inhibition of 5-lipoxygenase by essential oils and other natural fragrant extracts. *Int J Aromatherapy*. 2003;13(2-3):138-42.
[7915] Dwivedi C, Abu-Ghazaleh A. Chemopreventive effects of sandalwood oil on skin papillomas in mice. *Eur J Cancer Prev*. 1997 Aug;6(4):399-401.
[7916] Dwivedi C, Zhang Y. Sandalwood oil prevents skin tumor development in CD1 mice. *Eur J Cancer Prev*. 1999 Oct;8(5):449-55.
[7917] Sharma M, Levenson C, Bell RH, et al. Suppression of liposaccharide-stimulated cytokine/chemokine production in skin cells by sandalwood oils. *Phyther Res*. 2014 Jun;28(6):925-32.
[7918] Fujisaki R, Kamei K, Yamamra M, et al. In vitro and in vivo anti-plasmodial activity of essential oils, including hinokitiol. *Southeast Asian J Trop Med public Health*. 2012 Mar;43(2):270-79.
[7919] Heuberger E, Hongratanaworakit T, Buchbauer G. East Indian sandalwood and alpha-santalol odor increase physiological and self-rated arousal in humans. *Planta Med*. 2006 Jul;72(9):792-800.
[7920] Hongratanaworakit T, Heuberger E, Buchbauer G. Evaluation of the effects of East Indian sandalwood oil and α- santalol on humans after transdermal absorption. *Planta Med*. 2004;70:3-7.
[7921] Dyer J, Cleary L, McNeill S, et al. The use of aromasticks to help with sleep problems: A patient experience survey. Complement Ther Clin Pract. 2016 Feb;22:51-8.
[7922] Kim J, Jang M, Shin E, et al. Fumigant and contact toxicity of 22 wooden essential oils and their major components against Drosophila suzukii (Diptera: Drosophilidae). *Pestic Biochem Physiol*. 2016 Oct;133:35-43.
[7923] Moy RL, Levenson C. Sandalwood Album Oil as a Botanical Therapeutic in Dermatology. *J Clin Aesthet Dermatol*. 2017 Oct;10(10):34-39.
[7924] Powers CN, Osier JL, McFeeters RL, et al. Antifungal and Cytotoxic Activities of Sixty Commercially-Available Essential Oils. *Molecules*. 2018 Jun 27;23(7).
[7925] Orchard A, Viljoen A, van Vuuren S. Wound Pathogens: Investigating Antimicrobial Activity of Commercial Essential Oil Combinations against Reference Strains. *Chem Biodivers*. 2018 Dec;15(12):e1800405.
[7926] Younis NS. Doxorubicin-Induced Cardiac Abnormalities in Rats: Attenuation via Sandalwood Oil. *Pharmacol*. 2019 Nov 20:1-9.
[7927] Khan RA, van Vuuren SF. Essential oil combinations against Clostridium perfringens and Clostridium septicum - the causative agents of gas gangrene. *J Appl Microbiol*. 2021 Feb 8. Online ahead of print.
[7928] Rapper SL, Tankeu S, Kamatou G, et al. The use of chemometric modelling to determine chemical composition-antimicrobial activity relationships of essential oils used in respiratory tract infections. *Fitoterapia*. 2021 Aug 26;105024.
[7929] Ueda K, Horita T, Suzuki T. Effects of inhaling essential oils of Citrus limonum L., Santalum album, and Cinnamomum camphora on human brain activity. *Brain Behav*. 2023 Jan 9:e2889.

[7930] Randrianarivelo R, Sarter S, Odoux E, et al. Composition and antimicrobial activity of essential oils of Cinnamosma fragrans. *Food Chemistry*. 2009;114(2):680-84.
[7931] Cardoso NN, Alviano CS, Blank AF, et al. Synergism Effect of the Essential Oil from Ocimum basilicum var. Maria Bonita and Its Major Components with Fluconazole and Its Influence on Ergosterol Biosynthesis. *Evid Based Complement Alternat Med*. 2016;2016:5647182.
[7932] Burkhard PR, Burkhardt K, Haenggeli CA, et al. Plant-induced seizures: reappearance of an old problem. *J Neurol*. 1999 Aug;246(8):667-70.
[7933] Culic M, Kekovic G, Grbic G, et al. Wavelet and fractal analysis of rat brain activity in seizures evoked by camphor essential oil and 1,8-cineole. *Gen Physiol Biophys*. 2009;Special Issue(28):33–40.
[7934] Mathew T, Kamath V, Kumar RS, et al. Eucalyptus oil inhalation–induced seizure: A novel, underrecognized, preventable cause of acute symptomatic seizure. *Epilepsia Open*. 2017 Sep;2(3):350–354.
[7935] Newall CA, Anderson LA, Phillipson JD. "Herbal Medicines: A Guide for Health-care Professionals." London: The Pharmaceutical Press, 1996, 108.
[7936] European Medicines Agency. Community herbal monograph on Eucalyptus globulus Labill., Eucalyptus polybractea R.T. Baker and/or Eucalyptus smithii R.T. Baker, aetheroleum. 2013 Jun. Available at: http://www.ema.europa.eu/docs/en_GB/document_library/Herbal_-_Community_herbal_monograph/2013/07/WC500147008.pdf
[7937] Fischer JH, Dethlefsen U. Efficacy of cineole in patients suffering from acute bronchitis: a placebo-controlled double-blind trial. *Cough*. 2013; 9: 25.
[7938] Worth W, Dethlefsen U. Patients with asthma benefit from concomitant therapy with cineole: a placebo-controlled, double-blind trial. *J Asthma*. 2012 Oct;49(8):849-53.
[7939] Day LM, Ozanne-Smith J, Parsons BJ, et al. Eucalyptus oil poisoning among young children: mechanisms of access and the potential prevention. *Aust N Z J Public Health*. 1997 Jun;21(3):297-302.
[7940] Myott E. Case of eucalyptus poisoning. *Brit M J*. 1906;1:558.
[7941] Hindle RC. Eucalyptus oil ingestion. *N Z Med J*. 1994 May 11;107(977)185-6.
[7942] Tibballs J. Clinical effects and management of eucalyptus oil ingestion in infants and small children. *Med J Aust*. 1995 Aug;163(4):177-80.
[7943] Waldman W, Barwina M, Sein Anand J. Accidental ontoxication with eucalyptus oil—a case report. *Przeql Lek*. 2011;68(8):555-6.
[7944] Day LM, Ozanne-Smith J, Parsons BJ, et al. Eucalyptus oil poisoning among young children: mechanisms of access and the potential prevention. *Aust N Z J Public Health*. 1997 Jun;21(3):297-302.
[7945] De Vincenzi M, Silano M, De Vincenzi A, et al. Constituents of aromatic plants: eucalyptol. *Fitoterapia*. 2002 Jun;73(3):269-75.
[7946] Jori A, Bianchetti A, Prestini PE, et al. Effect of eucalyptol (1,8-cineole) on the metabolism of other drugs in rats and in man. *Eur J Pharmacol*. 1970;9(3):362-66.
[7947] de Sousa DP, Raphael E, Brocksom U, et al. Sedative effect of monoterpene alcohols in mice: A preliminary screening. *Verlag der Zeitschrift fur Naturforschung*. 2007;62c:563-66.
[7948] Sepici A, Gurbuz I, Cevik C, et al. Hypoglycemic effects of myrtle oil in normal and alloxan-diabetic rats. *J Ethnopharmacol*. 2004 Aug;9(2-3):311-8.
[7949] Gray AM, Flatt PR. Antihyperglycemic actions of Eucalyptus globulus (Eucalyptus) are associated with pancreatic and extra pancreatic effects in mice. *J Nutr*. 1998 Dec;128(12):2319–23.
[7950] Basak SS, Candan F. Effect of Laurus nobilis L. Essential Oil and its Main Components on α-glucosidase and Reactive Oxygen Species Scavenging Activity. *Iran J Pharm Res*. 2013 Spring;12(2):367-79.
[7951] Fathiazad F, Mazandarani M, Hamedeyazdan. Phytochemical analysis and antioxidant activity of Hyssopus officinalis L. from Iran. *Adv Pharm Bull*. 2011 Dec;1(2):63–67.
[7952] Lamborn LL. Modern soaps, candles and glycerin: A practical manual of modern methods of utilization of fats and oils in the manufacture of soaps and candles, and of the recovery of glycerin. Library of the University of Wisconsin.
[7953] Oyen LP, Dung NX. Plant resources of South-East Asia. 1999. Backhyus, Leiden.
[7954] Kim NH, Hyun SH, Jin CH, et al. Pretreatment with 1,8-cineole potentiates thioacetamide-induced hepatotoxicity and immunosuppression. *Arch Pharm Res*. 2004 Jul;27(7):781-9.
[7955] Tsai HH, Lin HW, Chen YL, et al. A review of potential harmful interactions between anticoagulant/antiplatelet agents and Chinese herbal medicines. *PLoS One*. 2013 May 9;8(5):e64255.
[7956] Moharam BA, Jantan I, bin Ahmad F, et al. Antiplatelet Aggregation and Platelet Activating Factor (PAF) Receptor Antagonistic Activities of the Essential Oils of Five Goniothalamus Species. *Molecules*. 2010;15:5124-38.
[7957] Randrianarivelo R, Sarter S, Odoux E, et al. Composition and antimicrobial activity of essential oils of Cinnamosma fragrans. *Food Chemistry*. 2009;114(2):680-84.
[7958] Adams RP, Nguyen S, Liu J. Geographical variation in the leaf essential oils of Juniperus Sabina L. and J. Sabina var. arenaria (E.H. Wilson) Farjon. *J Essent Oil Res*. 2006 Sep-Oct;18:497-502.
[7959] Asili J, Emami SA, Rahimizadeh M, et al. Chemical and Antimicrobial Studies of Juniperus sabina L. and Juniperus foetidissima Willd. Essential Oils. *J Essent Oil Bearing Plants*. 2012;13(1):25-36.
[7960] Zeraib A, Ramdani M, Boudjedjou L, et al. Chemical composition and antibacterial activity of Juniperus thurifera L. essential oils. *J BioSci Biotech*. 2014;3(2):147-54.
[7961] Fournier G, Pages N, Fournier C, et al. Contribution to the Study of the Essential Oil of Various Cultivars of Juniperus sabina. *Planta Med*. 1991 Aug;57(4):392-3.
[7962] Hernandez EG, Lopez Martinez MDC, Villanova RG. Determination by gas chromatography of terpenes in the berries of the species Juniperus oxycedrus L., J. thurifera L. and J. sabina L. *J Chromatography A*. 1987;396:416-20.
[7963] Johnson JD, Ryan MJ, Toft JD II, et al. Two-year toxicity and carcinogenicity study of methyl eugenol in F344/N rats and B6C3F(1) mice. *J Agric Food Chem*. 2000 Aug;48(8):3620-32.
[7964] European Medicines Agency. Public statement on the use of herbal medicinal products containing estragole. Available at: http://www.ema.europa.eu/docs/en_GB/document_library/Scientific_guideline/2010/04/WC500089960.pdf.
[7965] European Commission. Opinion of the Scientific Committee on Food on methyl eugenol (4-Allyl-1,2- dimethoxybenzene). Availableat:http://ec.europa.eu/food/fs/sc/scf/out102_en.pdf.
[7966] Casares R. Juniperus sabina. *Food Cosmet Toxicol*. 1964;2:680-81. Found in U.S. Food and Drug Administration. FDA Poisonous Plant Database. Available at: http://www.accessdata.fda.gov/scripts/plantox/detail.cfm?id=5133.
[7967] National Toxicology Program. NTP Toxicology and Carcinogenesis Studies of Methyleugenol (CAS NO. 93-15-2) in F344/N Rats and B6C3F1 Mice (Gavage Studies). *Natl Toxicol Program Tech Rep Ser*. 2000 Jul;491:1-412.
[7968] National Toxicology Program. Carcinogenesis Studies of Eugenol (CAS No. 97-53-0) in F344/N Rats and B6C3F1 Mice (Feed Studies). Technical Report Series No. 223. NIH Publication No. 84-1779. 1983. U.S. DHHS, PHS, NIH, NTP, Research Triangle Park, NC.
[7969] Haliciglu O, Astarcioglu G, Yaprak I, et al. Toxicity of Salvia officinalis in a newborn and a child: an alarming report. *Pediatr Neurol*. 2011 Oct;45(4):259-60.
[7970] Lachenmeier DW, Walch SG. Epileptic seizure caused by accidental ingestion of sage (Salvia officinalis L.) oil in children: a rare, exceptional case or a threat to public health. *Pediatr Neurol*. 2012 Mar;46(3):201.
[7971] Stafstrom CE. Seizures in a 7-month-old child after exposure to the essential plant oil thuja. *Pediatr Neurol*. 2007 Dec;37(6):446-8.
[7972] Pages N, Fournier G, Chamorro G, et al. Teratological evaluation of Juniperus sabina essential oil in mice. *Planta Med*. 1989 Apr;55(2):144-46.
[7973] Pages N, Fournier G, Baudel C, et al. Sabinyl Acetate, the Main Component of Juniperus sabina L'Hérit. Essential Oil, is Responsible for Antiimplantation Effect. *Phytother Res*. 1996 Aug;10(5):438-440.
[7974] Pages N, Fournier G, Velut V, et al. Potential teratogenicity in mice of the essential oil of Salvia lavandulifolia Vahl. Study of a fraction rich in sabinyl acetate. *Phytother Res*. 1992 Mar;6(2):80-83.
[7975] Price CJ, George JD, Marr MC, et al. Developmental toxicity evaluation of methyleugenol (MEUG) administered to Sprague-Dawley rats on gestational days (gd) 6 through 19. *Birth Defects Res A Clin Mol Teratol*. 2006 Jun;76:395.
[7976] Johnson JD, Ryan MJ, Toft JD II, et al. Two-year toxicity and carcinogenicity study of methyl eugenol in F344/N rats and B6C3F(1) mice. *J Agric Food Chem*. 2000 Aug;48(8):3620-32.
[7977] National Toxicology Program. NTP Toxicology and Carcinogenesis Studies of Methyleugenol (CAS NO. 93-15-2) in F344/N Rats and B6C3F1 Mice (Gavage Studies). *Natl Toxicol Program Tech Rep Ser*. 2000 Jul;491:1-412.
[7978] Kerckaert GA, Brauninger R, LeBoeuf RA, et al. Use of the Syrian hamster embryo cell transformation assay for carcinogenicity prediction of chemicals currently being tested by the National Toxicology Program in rodent bioassays. *Environ Health Perspect*. 1996;104:1075-84.
[7979] National Toxicology Program. Carcinogenesis Studies of Eugenol (CAS No. 97-53-0) in F344/N Rats and B6C3F1 Mice (Feed Studies). Technical Report Series No. 223. NIH Publication No. 84-1779. 1983. U.S. DHHS, PHS, NIH, NTP, Research Triangle Park, NC.
[7980] Blumenthal M, ed. The Complete German Commission E Monographs: Therapeutic Guide to Herbal Medicines. Trans. S. Klein. Boston, MA: American Botanical Council, 1998.
[7981] da Silva Costa KC, Bezerra SB, Norte CM, et al. Medicinal plants with teratogenic potential: current considerations. *Braz J Pharm Sci*. 2012;48(3):427–33.
[7982] Brinker F. Herb Contraindications and Drug Interactions. 2nd ed. Sandy, OR. Eclectic Medical Publications. 1998.
[7983] Randerath K, Putman KL, Randerath E. Flavor constituents in cola drinks induce hepatic DNA adducts in adult and fetal mice. *Biochem Biophys Res Commun*. 1993 Apr 15;192(1):61-8.
[7984] Vesselinovitch SD, Rao KVN, Mihailovich N. Transplacental and lactational carcinogenesis by safrole. *Cancer Res*. 1979 Nov;39(11):4378-80.
[7985] Casares R. Juniperus sabina. *Food Cosmet Toxicol*. 1964;2:680-81. Found in U.S. Food and Drug Administration. FDA Poisonous Plant Database. Available at: http://www.accessdata.fda.gov/scripts/plantox/detail.cfm?id=5133.
[7986] Frohne D. Giftpflanzen: Cupressaceae. Stuttgart: Wissenschaftliche Verlagsgesellschaft mbH; 1997. pp. 153–6.
[7987] European Medicines Agency. Public statement on the use of herbal medicinal products containing thujone. Available at: http://www.ema.europa.eu/docs/en_GB/document_library/Public_statement/2011/02/WC500102294.pdf.
[7988] Millet Y, Jouglard J, Steinmetz MD, et al. Toxicity of some essential plant oils. Clinical and experimental study. *Clin Toxicol*. 1981 Dec;18(12):1485-98.
[7989] Cristovao L, Carvalho F, Bastos MDL, et al. Hepatotoxicity of an essential oil of Salvia officinalis L.: an in vitro study using freshly isolated rat hepatocytes. *Congress Biomarkers*. 2001 Sep:165.
[7990] Millet Y, Jouglard J, Steinmetz MD, et al. Toxicity of some essential plant oils. Clinical and experimental study. *Clin Toxicol*. 1981 Dec;18(12):1485–98.
[7991] Burkhard PR, Burkhardt K, Haenggeli CA, et al. Plant-induced seizures: reappearance of an old problem. *J Neurol*. 1999 Aug;246(8):667–70.
[7992] Weisbord SD, Soule JB, Kimmel PL. Poison on line-acute renal failure caused by oil of wormwood purchased through the internet. *N Engl J Med*. 1997;337:825-7.
[7993] Arditti J, Faizende JJ, Bernard J, et al. Trois observations d'intoxication par des essences végétales convulsivantes. *Ann Med*. 1978;17:371-74.
[7994] Murray M. Toxicological actions of plant-derived and anthropogenic methylenedioxyphenyl-substituted chemicals in mammals and insects. *J Toxicol Environ Health B Crit Rev*. 2012;15(6):365-95.

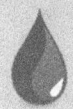

[7995] Jin M, Kijima A, Hibi D, et al. In vivo genotoxicity of methyl eugenol in gpt delta transgenic rats following medium-term exposure. *Toxicol Sci.* 2013 Feb;131(2):387-94.
[7996] Jin M, Kijima A, Suzuki Y, et al. Comprehensive toxicity study of safrole using medium-term animal model with gpt delta rats. *Toxicology.* 2011 Dec 18;290(2-3):312-21.
[7997] Johnson JD, Ryan MJ, Toft JD II, et al. Two-year toxicity and carcinogenicity study of methyl eugenol in F344/N rats and B6C3F(1) mice. *J Agric Food Chem.* 2000 Aug;48(8):3620-32.
[7998] European Commission. Opinion of the Scientific Committee on Food on methyl eugenol (4-Allyl-1,2- dimethoxybenzene). Available at: http://ec.europa.eu/food/fs/sc/scf/out102_en.pdf.
[7999] National Toxicology Program. NTP Toxicology and Carcinogenesis Studies of Methyleugenol (CAS NO. 93-15-2) in F344/N Rats and B6C3F1 Mice (Gavage Studies). *Natl Toxicol Program Tech Rep Ser.* 2000 Jul;491:1-412.
[8000] National Toxicology Program. Carcinogenesis Studies of Eugenol (CAS No. 97-53-0) in F344/N Rats and B6C3F1 Mice (Feed Studies). Technical Report Series No. 223. NIH Publication No. 84-1779. 1983. U.S. DHHS, PHS, NIH, NTP, Research Triangle Park, NC.
[8001] Burkhard PR, Burkhardt K, Haenggeli CA, et al. Plant-induced seizures: reappearance of an old problem. *J Neurol.* 1999 Aug;246(8):667-70.
[8002] Perry NB, Anderson RE, Brennan NJ, et al. Essential oils from dalmatian sage (Salvia officinalis L.) variations among individuals, plant parts, seasons, and sites. *J Agric Food Chem.* 1999;47:2048-54.
[8003] Patoir A, Patoir G, Bedrine H. Note sur l'action de l'essence de rue sur l'organisme animal. *Computes Rendues Société Bologique*. 1938;127:1324-25.
[8004] Pages N, Fournier G, Chamorro G, et al. Teratological evaluation of Juniperus sabina essential oil in mice. *Planta Med.* 1989 Apr;55(2):144-46.
[8005] Dolan LC, Matulka RA, Burdock GA. Naturally Occurring Food Toxins. *Toxins (Basel).* 2010 Sep;2(9):2289–2332.
[8006] Ahmad A, Khan A, Ahmad Khan L, et al. In vitro synergy of eugenol and methyleugenol with fluconazole against clinical Candida isolates. *J Med Microbiol.* 2010;59:1178-84.
[8007] Asili J, Emami SA, Rahimizadeh M, et al. Chemical and Antimicrobial Studies of Juniperus sabina L. and Juniperus foetidissima Willd. Essential Oils. *J Essent Oil Bearing Plants.* 2012;13(1):25-36.
[8008] Zeraib A, Ramdani M, Boudjedjou L, et al. Chemical composition and antibacterial activity of Juniperus thurifera L. essential oils. *J BioSci Biotech.* 2014;3(2):147-54.
[8009] Sampietro DA, Gomez AL, Jimenez CM, et al. Chemical composition and antifungal activity of essential oils from medicinal plants of Kazakhstan. *Nat Prod Res.* 2017 Jun;31(12):1464-1467.
[8010] Abdel-Kader MS, Soliman GA, Alquarni MH, et al. Juniperus sabina L. Essential Oil Against CCl 4 Induced Hepatotoxicity. *Saudi Pharm J.* 2019 Nov;27(7):945–951.
[8011] Zhelijazkov V, Cantrell CL, Semerdjieva I, et al. Essential Oil Composition and Bioactivity of Two Juniper Species from Bulgaria and Slovakia. *Molecules.* 2021 Jun 15;26(12):3659.
[8012] Skočibušić M, Bezić N, Dunkić V. Variability of Satureja cuneifolia Ten. essential oils and their antimicrobial activity depending on the stage of development. *Eur Food Res Tech.* 2004 Mar;218(4):367-71.
[8013] Kan Y, Ucan US, Kartal M, et al. GC-MS Analysis and Antibacterial Activity of Cultivated Satureja cuneifolia Ten. Essential Oil. *Turk J Chem.* 2006;30:253-59.
[8014] Bezić N, Šamanić I, Dunkić V, et al. Essential Oil Composition and Internal Transcribed Spacer (ITS) Sequence Variability of Four South-Croatian Satureja Species (Lamiaceae). *Molecules.* 2009;14:925-38
[8015] Oke F, Aslim B, Ozturk S, et al. Essential oil composition, antimicrobial and antioxidant activities of Satureja cuneifolia Ten. *Food Chem.* 2009 Feb;112:874-79.
[8016] Altun M, Goren AC. Essential Oil Composition of Satureja cuneifolia by Simultaneous Distillation-Extraction and Thermal Desorption GC-MS Techniques. *J Essent Oils Bear Plants.* 2013 Mar;10(2):139-44.
[8017] Kosar M, Demirci B, Demirci F, et al. Effect of Maturation on the Composition and Biological Activity of the Essential Oil of a Commercially Important Satureja Species from Turkey: Satureja cuneifolia Ten. (Lamiaceae). *J Agric Food Chem.* 2008;56:2260-65.
[8018] Tümen G, Kirimer N, Ermin N, et al. The essential oil of Satureja cuneifolia. *Planta Med.* 1998 Feb;64(1):81-3.
[8019] Domaracky M, Rehak P, Juhas S, et al. Effects of selected plant essential oils on the growth and development of mouse preimplantation embryos in vivo. *Physiol Res.* 2007;56(1):97-104.
[8020] Kohlert C, Schindler G, Marz RW, et al. Systemic availability and pharmacokinetics of thymol in humans. *J Clin Pharmacol.* 2002 Jul;42(7):731-7.
[8021] Toxicology Data Network, National Library of Medicine. Thymol. Available at: http://toxnet.nlm.nih.gov/cgi-bin/sis/search/a?dbs+hsdb:@term+@DOCNO+866.
[8022] Lemhadri A, Zeggwagh NA, Maghrani M, et al. Anti-hypoglycaemic activity of the aqueous extract of Origanum vulgare growing wild in Tafilalet region. *J Ethnopharmacol.* 2004 Jun;92(2-3):251-6.
[8023] Mirazi N, Rezaei M, Mirhoseini M. Hypoglycemic effect of Satureja montanum L. hydroethanolic extract on diabetic rats. *J HerbMed Pharm.* 2016;5(1):17-22.
[8024] Ezhumalai M, Radhiga T, Pugalendi KV. Antihyperglycemic effect of carvacrol in combination with rosiglitazone in high-fat diet-induced type 2 diabetic C57BL/6J mice. *Mol Cell Biochem.* 2014 Jan;385(1-2):23-31.
[8025] Tognolini M, Barocelli E, Ballabeni V, et al. Comparative screening of plant essential oils; phenylpropanoid moiety as basic core for antiplatelet activity. *Life Sci.* 2006 Feb 23;78(13):1419-32.
[8026] Tsai HH, Lin HW, Chen YL, et al. A review of potential harmful interactions between anticoagulant/antiplatelet agents and Chinese herbal medicines. *PLoS One.* 2013 May 9;8(5):e64255.
[8027] Karkabounas S, Kostoula OK, Daskalou T, et al. Anticarcinogenic and antiplatelet effects of carvacrol. *Exp Oncol.* 2006 Jun;28(2):121-5.
[8028] Langeveld WT, Veldhuizen EJ, Burt SA. Synergy between essential oil constituents and antibiotics. *Crit Rev Microbiol.* 2014 Feb;40(1);76-94.
[8029] Jukic M, Politeo O, Maksimmovic M, et al. In vitro acetylcholinesterase inhibitory properties of thymol, carvacrol and their derivatives thymoquinone and thymohydroquinone. *Phytother Res.* 2007;21(3):259-61.
[8030] Orhan I, Kartal M, Kan Y, et al. Activity of essential oils and individual components against acetyl- and butyrylcholinesterase. *Z Naturforsch C.* 2008 Jul-Aug;63(7-8):547-53.
[8031] Skočibušić M, Bezić N, Dunkić V. Variability of Satureja cuneifolia Ten. essential oils and their antimicrobial activity depending on the stage of development. *Eur Food Res Tech.* 2004 Mar;218(4):367-71.
[8032] Kan Y, Ucan US, Kartal M, et al. GC-MS Analysis and Antibacterial Activity of Cultivated Satureja cuneifolia Ten. Essential Oil. *Turk J Chem.* 2006;30:253-59.
[8033] Oke F, Aslim B, Ozturk S, et al. Essential oil composition, antimicrobial and antioxidant activities of Satureja cuneifolia Ten. *Food Chem.* 2009 Feb;112:874-79.
[8034] Kosar M, Demirci B, Demirci F, et al. Effect of Maturation on the Composition and Biological Activity of the Essential Oil of a Commercially Important Satureja Species from Turkey: Satureja cuneifolia Ten. (Lamiaceae). *J Agric Food Chem.* 2008;56:2260-65.
[8035] Orhan IE, Ozcelik B, Kan Y, et al. Inhibitory effects of various essential oils and individual components against extended-spectrum beta-lactamase (ESBL) produced by Klebsiella pneumoniae and their chemical compositions. *J Food Sci.* 2011 Oct;76(8):M538-46.
[8036] Skocibusić M, Bezić N. Phytochemical analysis and in vitro antimicrobial activity of two Satureja species essential oils. *Phytother Res.* 2004 Dec;18(12):967-70.
[8037] Oke F, Aslim B, Ozturk S, et al. Essential oil composition, antimicrobial and antioxidant activities of Satureja cuneifolia Ten. *Food Chem.* 2009 Feb;112:874-79.
[8038] Kosar M, Demirci B, Demirci F, et al. Effect of Maturation on the Composition and Biological Activity of the Essential Oil of a Commercially Important Satureja Species from Turkey: Satureja cuneifolia Ten. (Lamiaceae). *J Agric Food Chem.* 2008;56:2260-65.
[8039] Dunkić V, Mikrut A, Bezić N. Anti-Legionella activity of essential oil of Satureja cuneifolia. *Nat Prod Commun.* 2014 May;9(5):713-14.
[8040] Orhan I, Kartal M, Kan Y, et al. Activity of essential oils and individual components against acetyl- and butyrylcholinesterase. *Z Naturforsch C.* 2008 Jul-Aug;63(7-8):547-53.
[8041] Darvesh S, Hopkins DA, Geula C, Neurobiology of butyrylcholinesterase. *Nat Rev Neurosci.* 2003 Feb;4:131-38.
[8042] Wang Z, Chen H, Zhang W, et al. Comparative studies on the chemical composition and antioxidant activities of Schisandra chinensis and Schisandra sphenanthera fruits. *J Med Plants Res.* 2011 Apr;5(7):107-16.
[8043] Chen X, Zhang Y, Zu Y, et al. Composition and biological activities of the essential oil from Schisandra chinensis obtained by solvent-free microwave extraction. *Food Sci Tech.* 2011;44(10):2047-52.
[8044] Chen X, Zhang Y, Zu Y, et al. Chemical composition and antioxidant activity of the essential oil of Schisandra chinensis fruits. *Nat Prod Res.* 2011 May;26(9):842-49.
[8045] Song L, Ding JY, Tang C, et al. Compositions and biological activities of essential oils of Kadsura longepedunculata and Schisandra sphenanthera. *Am J Chin Med.* 2007;35(2):353-64.
[8046] Liu CJ, Zhang SQ, Zhang JS, et al. Chemical composition and antioxidant activity of essential oil from berries of Schisandra chinensis (Turcz.) Baill. *Nat Prod Res.* 2012;26(23):2199-203.
[8047] Song L, Ding JY, Tang C, et al. Compositions and biological activities of essential oils of Kadsura longepedunculata and Schisandra sphenanthera. *Am J Chin Med.* 2007;35(2):353-64.
[8048] Chen X, Zhang Y, Zu Y, et al. Composition and biological activities of the essential oil from Schisandra chinensis obtained by solvent-free microwave extraction. *Food Sci Tech.* 2011;44(10):2047-52.
[8049] Song L, Ding JY, Tang C, et al. Compositions and biological activities of essential oils of Kadsura longepedunculata and Schisandra sphenanthera. *Am J Chin Med.* 2007;35(2):353-64.
[8050] Chen X, Zhang Y, Zu Y, et al. Composition and biological activities of the essential oil from Schisandra chinensis obtained by solvent-free microwave extraction. *Food Sci Tech.* 2011;44(10):2047-52.
[8051] Chen X, Zhang Y, Zu Y, et al. Chemical composition and antioxidant activity of the essential oil of Schisandra chinensis fruits. *Nat Prod Res.* 2011 May;26(9):842-49.
[8052] Liu CJ, Zhang SQ, Zhang JS, et al. Chemical composition and antioxidant activity of essential oil from berries of Schisandra chinensis (Turcz.) Baill. *Nat Prod Res.* 2012;26(23):2199-203.
[8053] Wang Z, Chen H, Zhang W, et al. Comparative studies on the chemical composition and antioxidant activities of Schisandra chinensis and Schisandra sphenanthera fruits. *J Med Plants Res.* 2011 Apr;5(7):107-16.
[8054] Song L, Ding JY, Tang C, et al. Compositions and biological activities of essential oils of Kadsura longepedunculata and Schisandra sphenanthera. *Am J Chin Med.* 2007;35(2):353-64.
[8055] Wang X, Liu Y, Niu Y, et al. The Chemical Composition and Functional Properties of Essential Oils from Four Species of Schisandra Growing Wild in the Qinling Mountains, China. *Molecules.* 2018 Jul 5;23(7).
[8056] Tan L, Yang Y, Peng J, et al. Spectrum-effect relationship between GC-MS fingerprints and antidepressant-like effect of Schisandra chinensis (Turcz.) Baill. essential oil. *Metab Brain Dis.* 2022 Apr. Online ahead of print.
[8057] Victorio CP, Leitao SG, Lage CLS. Chemical Composition of the Leaf Oils of Alpinia zerumbet (Pers.) Burtt et Smith and A. purpurata (Vieill) K. Schum. From Rio de Janeiro, Brazil. *J Essent Oil Res.* 2010 Jan;22(1):52-54.
[8058] Jezler CN, Batista RS, Alves PB, et al. Histochemistry, content and chemical composition of essential oil in different organs of Alpinia zerumbet. *Cienc Rural.* 2013 Oct;43(10):0103-8478.
[8059] Mendes FRS, Silva FGE, Sousa EO, et al. Essential oil of Alpinia zerumbet (Pers.) B.L. Burtt. & R.M. Sm. (Zingiberaceae): chemical composition and modulation of the activity of aminoglycoside antibiotics. *J Essent Oil Res.* 2015;27(3):259-63.
[8060] de Pooter HL, Aboutabl EA, El-Shabrawy AO. Chemical composition and antimicrobial activity of essential oil of leaf, stem and rhizome of Alpinia speciosa. *Flavour Frag J.* 1995 Mar-Apr;10(2):63-67.

8061 Tu PT, Tawata S. Anti-Oxidant, Anti-Aging, and Anti-Melanogenic Properties of the Essential Oils from Two Varieties of Alpinia zerumbet. *Molecules*. 2015 Sep 14;20(9):16723-40.

8062 Bezerra MA, Leal-Cardoso JH, Coelho-De-Souza AN, et al. Myorelaxant and antispasmodic effects of the essential oil of Alpinia speciosa on rat ileum. *Phytother Res*. 2000 Nov;14(7):549-51.

8063 Sayyah M, Valizadeh J, Kamalinejad M. Anticonvulsant activity of the leaf oil of Laurus nobilis against pentylentetrazole- and maximal electroshock-induced seizure. *Phytomedicine*. 2002 Apr;9(3):212-16.

8064 Culic M, Kekovic G, Grbic G, et al. Wavelet and fractal analysis of rat brain activity in seizures evoked by camphor oil and 1,8-cineole. *Gen Physiol Biophys*. 2009;28 Sec No:33-40.

8065 Burkhard PR, Burkhardt K, Haenggeli CA, et al. Plant-induced seizures: reappearance of an old problem. *J Neurol*. 1999 Aug;246(8):667-70.

8066 Waldman N. Seizure caused by dermal application of over-the-counter eucalyptus oil head lice preparation. *Clin Toxicol (Phila)*. 2011 Oct;49(8):750-1.

8067 Craig JO. Poisoning by the volatile oils in childhood. *Arch Dis Child*. 1953;28:259-67.

8068 Mathew T, Kamath V, Kumar RS, et al. Eucalyptus oil inhalation-induced seizure: A novel, underrecognized, preventable cause of acute symptomatic seizure. *Epilepsia Open*. 2017 Jul 4;2(3):350-354.

8069 Jori A, Bianchetti A, Prestini PE, et al. Effect of eucalyptol (1,8-cineole) on the metabolism of other drugs in rats and in man. *Eur J Pharmacol*. 1970;9(3):362-66.

8070 Kim NH, Hyun SH, Jin CH, et al. Pretreatment with 1,8-cineole potentiates thioacetamide-induced hepatotoxicity and immunosuppression. *Arch Pharm Res*. 2004 Jul;27(7):781-9.

8071 Mendes FRS, Silva FGE, Sousa EO, et al. Essential oil of Alpinia zerumbet (Pers.) B.L. Burtt. & R.M. Sm. (Zingiberaceae): chemical composition and modulation of the activity of aminoglycoside antibiotics. *J Essent Oil Res*. 2015;27(3):259-63.

8072 Mertas A, Garbusińska A, Szliszka E, et al. The influence of tea tree oil (Melaleuca alternifolia) on fluconazole activity against fluconazole-resistant Candida albicans strains. *Biomed Res Int*. 2015;2015:590470.

8073 Jori A, Bianchetti A, Prestini PE, et al. Effect of eucalyptol (1,8-cineole) on the metabolism of other drugs in rats and in man. *Eur J Pharmacol*. 1970;9(3):362-66.

8074 de Sousa DP, Raphael E, Brocksom U, et al. Sedative effect of monoterpene alcohols in mice: A preliminary screening. *Verlag der Zeitschrift fur Naturforschung*. 2007;62c:563-66.

8075 Mendes FRS, Silva FGE, Sousa EO, et al. Essential oil of Alpinia zerumbet (Pers.) B.L. Burtt. & R.M. Sm. (Zingiberaceae): chemical composition and modulation of the activity of aminoglycoside antibiotics. *J Essent Oil Res*. 2015;27(3):259-63.

8076 de Pooter HL, Aboutabl EA, El-Shabrawy AO. Chemical composition and antimicrobial activity of essential oil of leaf, stem and rhizome of Alpinia speciosa. *Flavour Frag J*. 1995 Mar-Apr;10(2):63-67.

8077 Lima EO, Gompertz OF, Giesbrecht AM, et al. In vitro antifungal activity of essential oils obtained from officinal plants against dermatophytes. *Mycoses*. 1993 Sep-Oct;36(9-10):333-6.

8078 Kerdudo A, Ellong EN, Burger P, et al. Chemical composition, antimicrobial and insecticidal activities of flowers essential oils of Alpinia zerumbet (Pers.) from Martinique Island. *Chem Biodivers*. 2017 Apr;14(4).

8079 de Sousa DP, de Almeida Soares Hocayen P, Andrade LN, et al. A Systematic Review of the Anxiolytic-Like Effects of Essential Oils in Animal Models. *Molecules*. 2015 Oct 14;20(10):18620-60.

8080 Satou T, Murakami S, Matsuura M, et al. Anxiolytic effect and tissue distribution of inhaled Alpinia zerumbet essential oil in mice. *Nat Prod Commun*. 2010 Jan;5(1):143-6.

8081 Pinto NV, Assreuy AM, Coelho-de-Souza AN, et al. Endothelium-dependent vasorelaxant effects of the essential oil from aerial parts of Alpinia zerumbet and its main constituent 1,8-cineole in rats. *Phytomedicine*. 2009 Dec;16(12):1151-5.

8082 Tu PT, Tawata S. Anti-Oxidant, Anti-Aging, and Anti-Melanogenic Properties of the Essential Oils from Two Varieties of Alpinia zerumbet. *Molecules*. 2015 Sep 14;20(9):16723-40.

8083 Cavalcanti BC, Ferreira JR, Cabral IO, et al. Genetic toxicology evaluation of essential oil of Alpinia zerumbet and its chemoprotective effects against H(2)O(2)-induced DNA damage in cultured human leukocytes. *Food Chem Toxicol*. 2012 Nov;50(11):4051-61.

8084 de Araújo FY, de Oliveira GV, Gomes PX, et al. Inhibition of ketamine-induced hyperlocomotion in mice by the essential oil of Alpinia zerumbet: possible involvement of an antioxidant effect. *J Pharm Pharmacol*. 2011 Aug;63(8):1103-10.

8085 Tu PT, Tawata S. Anti-Oxidant, Anti-Aging, and Anti-Melanogenic Properties of the Essential Oils from Two Varieties of Alpinia zerumbet. *Molecules*. 2015 Sep 14;20(9):16723-40.

8086 Noonan FP, Zaidi MR, Wolnicka-Glubisz A, et al, Melanoma induction by ultraviolet A but not ultraviolet B radiation requires melanin pigment. *Nat Prod Commun*. 2012 Jun;3:884.

8087 Tu PT, Tawata S. Anti-Oxidant, Anti-Aging, and Anti-Melanogenic Properties of the Essential Oils from Two Varieties of Alpinia zerumbet. *Molecules*. 2015 Sep 14;20(9):16723-40.

8088 Maia MO, Dantas CG, Xavier Filho L, et al. The Effect of Alpinia zerumbet Essential Oil on Post-Stroke Muscle Spasticity. *Basic Clin Pharmacol Toxicol*. 2016 Jan;118(1):58-62.

8089 Bezerra MA, Leal-Cardoso JH, Coelho-De-Souza AN, et al. Myorelaxant and antispasmodic effects of the essential oil of Alpinia speciosa on rat ileum. *Phytother Res*. 2000 Nov;14(7):549-51.

8090 Xiao T, Zeng Y, Xu Y, et al. The endothelial protective properties of essential oil from Fructus Alpiniae zerumbet via the Akt/NOS-NO signaling pathway in vitro. *Planta Med*. 2014 Nov;80(17):1628-34.

8091 Shen XC, Tao L, Li WK, et al. Evidence-based antioxidant activity of the essential oil from Fructus A. zerumbet on cultured human umbilical vein endothelial cells' injury induced by ox-LDL. *BMC Complement Altern Med*. 2012 Oct 7;12:174.

8092 Santos BA, Roman-Campos D, Carvalho MS, et al. Cardiodepressive effect elicited by the essential oil of Alpinia speciosa is related to L-type Ca²+ current blockade. *Phytomedicine*. 2011 May 15;18(7):539-43.

8093 Pinto NV, Assreuy AM, Coelho-de-Souza AN, et al. Endothelium-dependent vasorelaxant effects of the essential oil from aerial parts of Alpinia zerumbet and its main constituent 1,8-cineole in rats. *Phytomedicine*. 2009 Dec;16(12):1151-5.

8094 Lahlou S, Interaminense LF, Leal-Cardoso JH, et al. Antihypertensive effects of the essential oil of Alpinia zerumbet and its main constituent, terpinen-4-ol, in DOCA-salt hypertensive conscious rats. *Fundam Clin Pharmacol*. 2003 Jun;17(3):323-30.

8095 Lahlou S, Galindo CA, Leal-Cardoso JH, et al. Cardiovascular effects of the essential oil of Alpinia zerumbet leaves and its main constituent, Terpinen-4-ol, in rats: role of the autonomic nervous system. *Planta Med*. 2002 Dec;68(12):1097-102.

8096 Macedo IT, de Oliveira LM, Camurça-Vasconcelos AL, et al. In vitro effects of Coriandrum sativum, Tagetes minuta, Alpinia zerumbet and Lantana camara essential oils on Haemonchus contortus. *Rev Bras Parasitol Vet*. 2013 Oct-Dec;22(4):463-9.

8097 Kerdudo A, Ellong EN, Burger P, et al. Chemical composition, antimicrobial and insecticidal activities of flowers essential oils of Alpinia zerumbet (Pers.) from Martinique Island. *Chem Biodivers*. 2017 Apr;14(4).

8098 de Araújo FY, de Oliveira GV, Gomes PX, et al. Inhibition of ketamine-induced hyperlocomotion in mice by the essential oil of Alpinia zerumbet: possible involvement of an antioxidant effect. *J Pharm Pharmacol*. 2011 Aug;63(8):1103-10.

8099 de Araújo FY, Silva MI, Moura BA, et al. Central nervous system effects of the essential oil of the leaves of Alpinia zerumbet in mice. *J Pharm Pharmacol*. 2009 Nov;61(11):1521-7.

8100 de Araújo PF, Coelho-de-Souza AN, Morais SM, et al. Antinociceptive effects of the essential oil of Alpinia zerumbet on mice. *Phytomedicine*. 2005 Jun;12(6-7):482-6.

8101 Leal-Cardoso JH, Moreira MR, da Cruz GM, et al. Effects of essential oil of Alpinia zerumbet on the constituent action potential of the rat sciatic nerve. *Phytomedicine*. 2004 Sep;11(6):549-53.

8102 Santos-Júnior L, Oliveira TVC, Cândido JF, et al. Effects of the essential oil of Alpinia zerumbet (Pers.) B.L. Burtt & R.M. Sm. on healing and tissue repair after partial Achilles tenotomy in rats. *Acta Cir Bras*. 2017 Jun;32(6):449-458.

8103 Xiao RY, Wu LJ, Hong XX, et al. Screening of analgesic and anti-inflammatory active component in Fructus Alpiniae zerumbet based on spectrum-effect relationship and GC-MS. *Biomed Chromatogr*. 2018 Mar;32(3).

8104 de Souza TA, Lopes MBP, Ramos AS, et al. Alpinia Essential Oils and Their Major Components against Rhodnius nasutus, a Vector of Chagas Disease. *ScientificWorldJournal*. 2018 Feb 15;2018:2393858.

8105 Huang N, Xu Y, Zhou H, et al. Essential Oil from Fructus Alpiniae Zerumbet Protects Human Umbilical Vein Endothelial Cells In Vitro from Injury Induced by High Glucose Levels by Suppressing Nuclear Transcription Factor-Kappa B Signaling. *Med Sci Monit*. 2017 Oct 4;23:4760-4767.

8106 Ji YP, Shi TY, Zhang YY, et al. Essential oil from Fructus Alpinia zerumbet (fruit of Alpinia zerumbet (Pers.) Burtt.et Smith) protected against aortic endothelial cell injury and inflammation in vitro and in vivo. *J Ethnopharmacol*. 2019 Mar 14;237:149-158.

8107 Zhang Y, Li C, Huang Y, et al. EOFAZ inhibits endothelial-to-mesenchymal transition through downregulation of KLF4. *Int J Mol Med*. 2020 Apr 9. [Epub ahead of print]

8108 de Araújo FYR, Chaves Filho AJM, Nunes AM, et al. Involvement of anti-inflammatory, antioxidant, and BDNF up-regulating properties in the antipsychotic-like effect of the essential oil of Alpinia zerumbet in mice: a comparative study with olanzapine. *Metab Brain Dis*. 2021 Sep 7. Online ahead of print.

8109 Batista TSC, Barros GS, Damasceno FC, et al. Chemical characterization and effects of volatile oil of Alpinia zerumbet on the quality of collagen deposition and caveolin-1 expression in a muscular fibrosis murine model. *Braz J Biol*. 2021 Dec 20;84:e253616.

8110 Batista TSC, Oliveira AFR, Santana LB, et al. Gait analysis with muscular fibrosis and treatment with Alpinia zerumbet essential oil in immobilized rats. *An Acad Bras Cienc*. 2022 Jun 13;94(2):e20211164.

8111 Zhang Y, Zhao S, Tu M, et al. Inhibitory Effect of Essential Oil From Fructus of Alpinia zerumbet on Endothelial-to-Mesenchymal Transformation Induced by TGF-β1 and Downregulation of KLF4. *J Cardiovasc Pharmacol*. 2022 Jul 1;80(1):82-94.

8112 Leseur D, Ban NK, Bighelli A, et al. Analysis of the root oil of Fokienia hodginsii (Dunn) Henry et Thomas (Cupressaceae) by GC, GC–MS and 13C-NMR. *Flavour Frag J*. 2006;21:171-74.

8113 Weyerstahl P, Marschall H, Phan T, et al. Constituents of Vietnamese pemou oil—a reinvestigation. *Flavour Frag J*. 1999;14(6):409-10.

8114 Jiong-guang P, Zhi-ling X, Zhong-wu M, et al. Studies on the Essential Oil Composition in Leaves of Fokienia Hodginsii (Dunn) Henry et Thomas. *Chineses Bull Botany*. 1991;8(4):48-49.

8115 Brehm-Stecher BF, Johnson EA. Sensitization of Staphylococcus aureus and Escherichia coli to antibiotics by the sesquiterpenoids nerolidol, farnesol, bisabolol, and apritone. *Antimicrob Agents Chemother*. 2003 Oct;47(10):3357-60.

8116 Paluch GE, Zhu J, Bartholomay L, et al. Amyris and Siam-wood essential oils: Insect activity of sesquiterpenes. *Entomology*. 2010;Chapter 2:5-18.

8117 Orav A, Kuningas K, Kailas T. Computerized capillary gas chromatographic identification and determination of Siberian fir oil constituents. *J Chromatopgraphy A*. 1995 Apr;697(1-2):495-99.

8118 Pokrovsky LM, Tkachev AV. Study of Composition of Volatile Constituents of Siberian and Far East Conifers by Gas Chromatography - Mass-Spectrometry. Novosibirsk Institute of Organic Chemistry. 1998. Available at: http://www.nioch.nsc.ru/icnpas98/pdf/posters1/136.pdf.

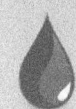

[8119] Polyakov NA, Dubinskaya VA, Efremov AA, et al. Biological Activity of Abies Sibirica Essential Oil and its Major Constituents for Several Enzymes In Vitro. *Pharm Chem J.* 2014;48(7):456-60.
[8120] Petrichenko VM, Molokhova EI, Sukhinina TV. Chemical composition of volatile components and fatty acids in a CO2 extract and the essential oil of the siberian fir. *Medicinal Plants.* 2011 Oct;45(7):412-14.
[8121] Matsubara E, Fukagawa E, Okamoto T, et al. The essential oil of Abies sibirica (Pinaceae) reduces arousal levels after visual display terminal work. *Flavour Frag J.* 2011 May;26(3):204-10.
[8122] Polyakov NA, Dubinskaya VA, Efremov AA, et al. Biological Activity of Abies Sibirica Essential Oil and its Major Constituents for Several Enzymes In Vitro. *Pharm Chem J.* 2014;48(7):456-60.
[8123] Noreikaitė A, Ayupova R, Satbayeva E, et al. General Toxicity and Antifungal Activity of a New Dental Gel with Essential Oil from Abies Sibirica L. *Med Sci Monit.* 2017 Jan 29;23:521-527.
[8124] Yang SA, Jeon SK, Lee EJ, et al. Radical scavenging activity of the essential oil of silver fir (Abies alba). *J Clin Biochem Nutr.* 2009 May;44(3):253-59.
[8125] Alexandru M, Romeo I, Cornelia M, et al. Composition of the volatile oil extracted from Abies alba Miller leaves parasitized by Melampsorella caryophyllacearum (DC.) J. Schrot. *J Plant Develop.* 2011;18:81-86.
[8126] Kubeczka KH, Schultze W. Biology and chemistry of conifer oils. *Flav Frag J.* 1987;2:137-48.
[8127] USDA Natural Resource Conservation Service. Available at: http://plants.usda.gov/core/profile?symbol=ABCO and http://plants.usda.gov/core/profile?symbol=abal3.
[8128] Warren R, Johnson EW. A guide to firs (Abies spp.) of the Arnold Arboretum. Firs of the Arnold Arboretum. Available at: http://arnoldia.arboretum.harvard.edu/pdf/articles/730.pdf.
[8129] Wajs-Bonikowska A1, Sienkiewicz M, Stobiecka A, et al. Chemical composition and biological activity of Abies alba and A. koreana seed and cone essential oils and characterization of their seed hydrolates. *Chem Biodivers.* 2015 Mar;12(3):407-18.
[8130] Kacaniova M, Vukovic N, Horska E, et al. Antibacterial activity against Clostridium genus and antiradical activity of the essential oils from different origin. *J Environ Sci Health B.* 2014;49(7):505-12.
[8131] Yang SA, Jeon SK, Lee SJ, et al. Radical scavenging activity of the essential oil of Silver Fir (Abies alba). *J Clin Biochem Nutr.* 2009 May;44(3):253-59.
[8132] Wajs-Bonikowska A1, Sienkiewicz M, Stobiecka A, et al. Chemical composition and biological activity of Abies alba and A. koreana seed and cone essential oils and characterization of their seed hydrolates. *Chem Biodivers.* 2015 Mar;12(3):407-18.
[8133] Yang SA, Jeon SK, Lee SJ, et al. Radical scavenging activity of the essential oil of Silver Fir (Abies alba). *J Clin Biochem Nutr.* 2009 May;44(3):253-59.
[8134] Wajs-Bonikowska A1, Sienkiewicz M, Stobiecka A, et al. Chemical composition and biological activity of Abies alba and A. koreana seed and cone essential oils and characterization of their seed hydrolates. *Chem Biodivers.* 2015 Mar;12(3):407-18.
[8135] Lanzerstorfer A, Hackl M, Schlömer M, et al. The influence of air-dispersed essential oils from lemon (Citrus limon) and silver fir (Abies alba) on airborne bacteria and fungi in hospital rooms. *J Environ Sci Health A Tox Hazard Subst Environ Eng.* 2019;54(3):256-260.
[8136] Korona-Glowniak I, Glowniak-Lipa A, Ludwiczuk A, et al. The In Vitro Activity of Essential Oils Against Helicobacter Pylori Growth and Urease Activity. *Molecules.* 2020 Jan 29;25(3):586.
[8137] Garzoli S, Lasci VL, Caradonna V, et al. Liquid and Vapor Phase of Four Conifer-Derived Essential Oils: Comparison of Chemical Compositions and Antimicrobial and Antioxidant Properties. *Pharmaceuticals (Basel).* 2021 Feb 8;14(2):134.
[8138] Valková V, Ďúranová H, Vukovic NL, et al. Assessment of Chemical Composition and Anti-Penicillium Activity of Vapours of Essential Oils from Abies Alba and Two Melaleuca Species in Food Model Systems. *Molecules.* 2022 May 12;27(10):3101.
[8139] Dunlop PJ, Bignell CM, Hibbert DB, et al. Use of gas chromatograms of the essential leaf oils of the genus Eucalyptus for taxonomic purposes: E. subser. Euglobulares (Blakely). *Flavour Frag J.* 2003;18:162–69.
[8140] Sebei K, Sakouhi F, Herchi W, et al. Chemical composition and antibacterial activities of seven Eucalyptus species essential oils leaves. *Biol Res.* 2015;48(1):7.
[8141] Elaissi A, Rouis A, Ben Salem NA, et al. Chemical composition of 8 eucalyptus species' essential oils and the evaluation of their antibacterial, antifungal and antiviral activities. *BMC Complement Altern Med.* 2012;21:81.
[8142] Craig JO. Poisoning by the volatile oils in childhood. *Arch Dis Child.* 1953;28:259-67.
[8143] Melis K. Bochner A, Janssens G. Accidental nasal eucalyptol and menthol instillation. *Eur J Pediatr.* 1989 Aug;148(8)786-7.
[8144] Day LM, Ozanne-Smith J, Parsons BJ, et al. Eucalyptus oil poisoning among young children: mechanisms of access and the potential prevention. *Aust N Z J Public Health.* 1997 Jun;21(3):297-302.
[8145] Chandar SD, Prashanti M, Kumar CL, et al. Eucalyptus Oil-Induced Seizures in Children: A Single-Center Prospective Study. *Cureus.* 2021 Mar 25;13(3):e14109.
[8146] Burkhard PR, Burkhardt K, Haenggeli CA, et al. Plant-induced seizures: reappearance of an old problem. *J Neurol.* 1999 Aug;246(8):667–70.
[8147] Waldman N. Seizure caused by dermal application of over-the-counter eucalyptus oil head lice preparation. *Clin Toxicol (Phila).* 2011 Oct;49(8):750–1.
[8148] Craig JO. Poisoning by the volatile oils in childhood. *Arch Dis Child.* 1953;28:259–67.
[8149] Newall CA, Anderson LA, Phillipson JD. "Herbal Medicines: A Guide for Health-care Professionals." London: The Pharmaceutical Press, 1996, 108.
[8150] European Medicines Agency. Community herbal monograph on Eucalyptus globulus Labill., Eucalyptus polybractea R.T. Baker and/or Eucalyptus smithii R.T. Baker, aetheroleum. 2013 Jun. Available at: http://www.ema.europa.eu/docs/en_GB/document_library/Herbal_-_Community_herbal_monograph/2013/07/WC500147008.pdf
[8151] Fischer JH, Dethlefsen U. Efficacy of cineole in patients suffering from acute bronchitis: a placebo-controlled double-blind trial. *Cough.* 2013; 9: 25.
[8152] Worth W, Dethlefsen U. Patients with asthma benefit from concomitant therapy with cineole: a placebo-controlled, double-blind trial. *J Asthma.* 2012 Oct;49(8):849-53.
[8153] Day LM, Ozanne-Smith J, Parsons BJ, et al. Eucalyptus oil poisoning among young children: mechanisms of access and the potential prevention. *Aust N Z J Public Health.* 1997 Jun;21(3):297-302.
[8154] Myott E. Case of eucalyptus poisoning. *Brit M J.* 1906;1:558.
[8155] Hindle RC. Eucalyptus oil ingestion. *N Z Med J.* 1994 May 11;107(977)185-6.
[8156] Tibballs J. Clinical effects and management of eucalyptus oil ingestion in infants and small children. *Med J Aust.* 1995 Aug;163(4):177-80.
[8157] Waldman W, Barwina M, Sein Anand J. Accidental ontoxication with eucalyptus oil—a case report. *Przeql Lek.* 2011;68(8):555-6.
[8158] Day LM, Ozanne-Smith J, Parsons BJ, et al. Eucalyptus oil poisoning among young children: mechanisms of access and the potential prevention. *Aust N Z J Public Health.* 1997 Jun;21(3):297-302.
[8159] De Vincenzi M, Silano M, De Vincenzi A, et al. Constituents of aromatic plants: eucalyptol. *Fitoterapia.* 2002 Jun;73(3):269-75.
[8160] Jori A, Bianchetti A, Prestini PE, et al. Effect of eucalyptol (1,8-cineole) on the metabolism of other drugs in rats and in man. *Eur J Pharmacol.* 1970;9(3):362-66.
[8161] Kim NH, Hyun SH, Jin CH, et al. Pretreatment with 1,8-cineole potentiates thioacetamide-induced hepatotoxicity and immunosuppression. *Arch Pharm Res.* 2004 Jul;27(7):781-9.
[8162] Gray AM, Flatt PR. Antihyperglycemic actions of Eucalyptus globulus (Eucalyptus) are associated with pancreatic and extra pancreatic effects in mice. *J Nutr.* 1998 Dec;128(12):2319–23.
[8163] Basak SS, Candan F. Effect of Laurus nobilis L. Essential Oil and its Main Components on α-glucosidase and Reactive Oxygen Species Scavenging Activity. *Iran J Pharm Res.* 2013 Spring;12(2):367-79.
[8164] Dey B. Chemo-profiling of eucalyptus and study of its hypoglycemic potential. *World J Diabetes.* 2013 Oct 15;4(5):170–76.
[8165] Tsai HH, Lin HW, Chen YL, et al. A review of potential harmful interactions between anticoagulant/antiplatelet agents and Chinese herbal medicines. *PLoS One.* 2013 May 9;8(5):e64255.
[8166] Moharam BA, Jantan I, bin Ahmad F, et al. Antiplatelet Aggregation and Platelet Activating Factor (PAF) Receptor Antagonistic Activities of the Essential Oils of Five Goniothalamus Species. *Molecules.* 2010;15:5124-38.
[8167] Jori A, Bianchetti A, Prestini PE, et al. Effect of eucalyptol (1,8-cineole) on the metabolism of other drugs in rats and in man. *Eur J Pharmacol.* 1970;9(3):362-66.
[8168] de Sousa DP, Raphael E, Brocksom U, et al. Sedative effect of monoterpene alcohols in mice: A preliminary screening. *Verlag der Zeitschrift fur Naturforschung.* 2007;62c:563-66.
[8169] Sebei K, Sakouhi F, Herchi W, et al. Chemical composition and antibacterial activities of seven Eucalyptus species essential oils leaves. *Biol Res.* 2015;48(1):7.
[8170] Usano-Alemany J, Herraiz-Penalver D, Cuadrado J, et al. Seasonal variation of the essential oils of Salvia lavandulifolia: Antibacterial activity. *J Essent Oil Bear Plants.* 2012 Jan;15(20:195-203(9).
[8171] Zrira S, Menut C, Bessiere JM, et al. A study of the essential oil of Salvia lavandulifolia Vahl from Morocco. *J Essent Oil Bear Plants.* 2004;7(3):232-38.
[8172] Jirovetz L, Buchbauer G, Denkova Z, et al. Chemical composition, antimicrobial activities and odor descriptions of various Salvia sp. And Thuja sp. essential oils. *ERNÄHRUNG/NUTRITION.* 2006;30(4):152-59.
[8173] Porres-Martinez M, Gonzalez-Burgos E, Accame MEC, et al. Phytochemical composition, antioxidant and cytoprotective activities of essential oil of Salvia lavandulifolia Vahl. *Food Res Int.* 2013 Nov;54(1):523-31.
[8174] Khine H, Weiss D, Graber N, et al. A cluster of children with seizures caused by camphor poisoning. *Pediatrics.* 2009 May;123(5):1269-72.
[8175] Michiels EA, Mazor SS. Toddler with seizures due to ingesting camphor at an Indian celebration. *Pediatr Emerg Care.* 2010 Aug;26(8):574-75.
[8176] Koren G. Medications which can kill a toddler with one tablet or teaspoonful. *J toxicol Clin Toxicol.* 1993;31(3):407- 13.
[8177] Bar-Oz B, Levicheck Z, Koren G. Medications that can kill a toddler with one tablet or teaspoonfull – A 2004 update. *Paediatr Drugs.* 2004;6(2):123-6.
[8178] Craig JO. Poisoning by the volatile oils in childhood. *Arch Dis Child.* 1953;28:259-67.
[8179] Melis K. Bochner A, Janssens G. Accidental nasal eucalyptol and menthol instillation. *Eur J Pediatr.* 1989 Aug;148(8)786-7.
[8180] Day LM, Ozanne-Smith J, Parsons BJ, et al. Eucalyptus oil poisoning among young children: mechanisms of access and the potential prevention. *Aust N Z J Public Health.* 1997 Jun;21(3):297-302.
[8181] Chandar SD, Prashanti M, Kumar CL, et al. Eucalyptus Oil-Induced Seizures in Children: A Single-Center Prospective Study. *Cureus.* 2021 Mar 25;13(3):e14109.
[8182] Flaman Z, Pellechia-Clarke S, Bailey B, et al. Unintentional exposure of young children to camphor and eucalyptus oils. *Paediatr Child Health.* 2001 Feb;6(2):80-83.
[8183] Rabl W, Katzgraber F, Steinlechner M. Camphor ingestion for abortion (case report). *Forensic Sci Int.* 1997 Sep 19;89(1-2):137-40.
[8184] Pages N, Fourier G, Baduel C, et al. Sabinyl acetate, the main component of Juniperus sabina L'Herit. essential oil, is responsible for antiimplantation effect. *Phytother Res.* 1996 Aug;10(5):438-40.
[8185] Pages N, Fourier G, Velut V, et al. Potential teratogenicity in mice of the essential oil of Salvia lavandulifolia Vahl. study of a fraction rich in sabinyl acetate. *Phytother Res.* 2006;6(2):80-83.

[8186] Burkhard PR, Burkhardt K, Haenggeli CA, et al. Plant-induced seizures: reappearance of an old problem. *J Neurol.* 1999 Aug;246(8):667-70.
[8187] Culic M, Kekovic G, Grbic G, et al. Wavelet and fractal analysis of rat brain activity in seizures evoked by camphor essential oil and 1,8-cineole. *Gen Physiol Biophys.* 2009;Special Issue(28):33–40.
[8188] Mathew T, Kamath V, Kumar RS, et al. Eucalyptus oil inhalation–induced seizure: A novel, underrecognized, preventable cause of acute symptomatic seizure. *Epilepsia Open.* 2017 Sep;2(3):350–354.
[8189] Narayan S, Singh N. Camphor poisoning-An unusual cause of seizure. *Med J Armed Forces India.* 2012 Jul;68(3):252-53.
[8190] Chanaranaj KJ, G MV, S M. Camphor poisoning in a child. *Natl Med J India.* 2013 Jan-Feb;26(1):60.
[8191] Olowe SA, Ransome-Kuti O. The risk of jaundice in glucose-6-phosphate dehydrogenase deficient babies exposed to menthol. *Acta Paediatr Scand.* 1980 May;69(3):341-5.
[8192] Dillon Remy M, Manning Alleyne P, Bratt DE, et al. Neonatal jaundice at Port-of-Spain General Hospital abstract. *West Indian Med J.* 1987;36(Suppl):28.
[8193] Manoguerra AS, Erdman AR, Wax PM, et al. Camphor poisoning: an evidence-based practice guideline for out-of- hospital management. *Clin Toxicol (Phila).* 2006;44(4):357-70.
[8194] Gibson DE, Moore GP, Pfaff JA. Camphor ingestion. *Am J Emerg Med.* 1989 Jan;7(1):41-43.
[8195] Koppel C, Martends F, Schirop T, et al. Hemoperfusion in acute camphor poisoning. *Intensive Care Med.* 1988;14(4):431-33.
[8196] Jori A, Bianchetti A, Prestini PE, et al. Effect of eucalyptol (1,8-cineole) on the metabolism of other drugs in rats and in man. *Eur J Pharmacol.* 1970;9(3):362-66.
[8197] de Sousa DP, Raphael E, Brocksom U, et al. Sedative effect of monoterpene alcohols in mice: A preliminary screening. *Verlag der Zeitschrift fur Naturforschung.* 2007;62c:563-66.
[8198] Lamborn LL. Modern soaps, candles and glycerin: A practical manual of modern methods of utilization of fats and oils in the manufacture of soaps and candles, and of the recovery of glycerin. Library of the University of Wisconsin.
[8199] Oyen LP, Dung NX. Plant resources of South-East Asia. 1999. Backhyus, Leiden.
[8200] Kim NH, Hyun SH, Jin CH, et al. Pretreatment with 1,8-cineole potentiates thioacetamide-induced hepatotoxicity and immunosuppression. *Arch Pharm Res.* 2004 Jul;27(7):781-9.
[8201] Savelev S, Okello E, Perry NSL, et al. Synergistic and antagonistic interactions if anticholinesterase terpenoids in Salvia lavandulaefolia essential oil. *Pharmacol Biochem Behav.* 2003 Jun;75(3):661-68.
[8202] Perry NS, Houghton PJ, Sampson J, et al. In-vitro activity of S. lavandulaefolia (Spanish sage) relevant to treatment of Alzheimer's disease. *J Pharm Pharmacol.* 2001 Oct;53(10):1347-56.
[8203] Perry NS, Houghton PJ, Theobald A, et al. In-vitro inhibition of human erythrocyte acetylcholinesterase by salvia lavandulaefolia essential oil and constituent terpenes. *J Pharm Pharmacol.* 2000 Jul;52(7):895-902.
[8204] Miroddi M, Navarra M, Quattropani MC, et al. Systematic review of clinical trials assessing pharmacological properties of Salvia species on memory, cognitive impairment and Alzheimer's disease. *CNS Neurosci Ther.* 2014 Jun;20(6):485-95.
[8205] Kennedy DO, Scholey AB. The psychopharmacology of European herbs with cognition-enhancing properties. *Curr Pharm Des.* 2006;12(35):4613-23.
[8206] Tildesley NT, Kennedy DO, Perry EK, et al. Positive modulation of mood cognitive performance following administration of acute doses of Salvia lavandulaefolia essential oil to healthy young volunteers. *Physiol Behav.* 2005 Jan 17;83(5):699-709.
[8207] Perry NS, Bollen C, Perry EK, et al. Salvia for dementia therapy: review of pharmacological activity and pilot tolerability clinical trial. *Pharmacol Biochem Behav.* 2003 Jun;75(3):651-59.
[8208] Porres-Martinez M, Gonzalez-Burgos E, Carretero ME, et al. Protective properties of Salvia lavandulifolia Vahl. essential oil against oxidative stress-induced neuronal injury. *Food Chem Toxicol.* 2015 Mar;80:154-62.
[8209] Porres-Martinez M, Gonzalez-Burgos E, Carretero ME, et al. Major selected monoterpenes alpha-pinene and 1,8-cineole found in Salvia lavandulifolia (Spanish sage) essential oil as regulators of cellular redox balance. *Pharm Biol.* 2015 Jun;53(6):921-9.
[8210] Savelev S, Okello E, Perry NSL, et al. Synergistic and antagonistic interactions if anticholinesterase terpenoids in Salvia lavandulaefolia essential oil. *Pharmacol Biochem Behav.* 2003 Jun;75(3):661-68.
[8211] Perry NS, Houghton PJ, Sampson J, et al. In-vitro activity of S. lavandulaefolia (Spanish sage) relevant to treatment of Alzheimer's disease. *J Pharm Pharmacol.* 2001 Oct;53(10):1347-56.
[8212] Perry NS, Houghton PJ, Theobald A, et al. In-vitro inhibition of human erythrocyte acetylcholinesterase by salvia lavandulaefolia essential oil and constituent terpenes. *J Pharm Pharmacol.* 2000 Jul;52(7):895-902.
[8213] Perry NS, Bollen C, Perry EK, et al. Salvia for dementia therapy: review of pharmacological activity and pilot tolerability clinical trial. *Pharmacol Biochem Behav.* 2003 Jun;75(3):651-59.
[8214] Cutillas AB, Carrasco A, Martinez-Gutierrez R, et al. Composition and Antioxidant, Antienzymatic and Antimicrobial Activities of Volatile Molecules from Spanish Salvia lavandulifolia (Vahl) Essential Oils. *Molecules.* 2017 Aug 21;22(8).
[8215] Lee MJ, Park JH, Lee HS. Acaricidal toxicities and synergistic activities of Salvia lavandulifolia oil constituents against synanthropic mites. *Pest Manag Sci.* 2018 Nov;74(11):2468-2479.
[8216] Dinel AL, Lucas C, Guillemet D, et al. Chronic Supplementation With a Mix of Salvia officinalis and Salvia lavandulaefolia Improves Morris Water Maze Learning in Normal Adult C57Bl/6J Mice. *Nutrients.* 2020 Jun 15;12(6):E1777.
[8217] Govindarajan M, Sivakumar R, Rajeswari M, et al. Chemical composition and larvicidal activity of essential oil from Mentha spicata (Linn.) against three mosquito species. *Parasitol Res.* 2012 May;110(5):2023-32.
[8218] Chauhan SS, Prakash O, Padalia RC, et al. Chemical diversity in Mentha spicata: antioxidant and potato sprout inhibition activity of its essential oils. *Nat Prod Commun.* 2011 Sep;6(9):1373-8.
[8219] Koliopoulos G, Pitarokili D, Kioulos E, et al. Chemical composition and larvicidal evaluation of Mentha, Salvia, and Melissa essential oils against the West Nile virus mosquito Culex pipiens. *Parasitol Res.* 2010 Jul;107(2):327-55.
[8220] Sokovic MD, Vukojevic J, Marin PF, et al. Chemical composition of essential oils of Thymus and Mentha species and their antifungal activities. *Molecules.* 2009 Jan 7;14(1):238-49.
[8221] Chauhan RS, Kaul MK, Shahi AK, et al. Chemical composition of essential oils in Mentha spicata L. accession [IIIM(J)26] from North-West Himalayan region, India. *Ind Crops Prod.* 2009;29(2-3):654-56.
[8222] Chowdhury JU, Nandi NC, Uddin M, et al. Chemical constituents of essential oils from two types of spearmint (Mentha spicata L. and M, cardiac L.) introduced in Bangladesh. *Bangladesh J Sci Ind Res.* 2007;42(1):79-82.
[8223] Joshi RK. Pulegone and menthone chemotypes of Mentha spicata Linn. from Western Ghats Region of North West Karnataka, India. *Natl Acad Sci Lett.* 2013 May-Jun;36(3):349-52.
[8224] Padmini E, Valarmathi A, Usha Rani M. Comparative analysis of chemical composition and antibacterial activities of Mentha spicata and Camellia sinensis. *Asian J Exp Biol Sci.* 2012;1(4):772-81.
[8225] Joshi RK, Sharma AK. Cis-Ocimenone chemotype essential oil of green mint (Mentha viridis L.) from Western Ghats region of North West Karnataka, India. *Plant Sci Today.* 2014;1(1):10-12.
[8226] Telci I, Demirtas I, Bayram E, et al. Environmental variation on aroma components of pulegone/piperitone rich spearmint (Mentha spicata L.). *Ind Crops Prod.* 2010;32:588-92.
[8227] Sallam SMA, Abdelgaleil SAM, Buenol CS, et al. Effect of essential oils on ruminal fermentation, microbial population and methane emission in vitro. Available at: http://om.ciheam.org/om/pdf/a99/00801549.pdf.
[8228] Kokkini S, Vokou D. Mentha spicata (Lamiaceae) chemotypes growing wild in Greece. *Economic Botany.* 1989 Apr-Jun;43(2):192-202.
[8229] de Sousa DP, Lima TC, Steverding D, et al. Evaluation of Antiparasitc Activity of Mentha crispa Essential Oil, Its Major Constituent Rotundifolone and Analogues against Trypanosoma brucei. *Planta Med.* 2016 Oct;82(15):1346-1350.
[8230] Zhelijazkov VD, Cantrell CL, Astatkie T, er al. Productivity, Oil Content, and Composition of Two Spearmint Species in Mississippi. *Agronomy J.* 2010;102(1):129-33
[8231] Chowshury JU, Nandi NC, Uddin M, et al. Chemical Constituents of Essential Oils from Two Types of Spearmint (Mentha spicata L. and M. cardiaca L.) Introduced in Bangladesh. *Bangladesh J Sci Ind Res.* 2007;42(1):79-82.
[8232] Akdogan M, Gultekin F, Yontem M. Effect of Mentha piperita (Labiatae) and Mentha spicata (Labiatae) on iron absorption in rats. *Toxicol Ind Health.* 2004 Sep;20(6-10):119-22.
[8233] Bakerink JA, Gospe SM Jr, Dimand RJ, et al. Multiple organ failure after ingestion of pennyroyal oil from herbal tea in two infants. *Pediatrics.* 1996;98(5):944-47.
[8234] Sudekum M, Poppenga RH, Raju N, et al. Pennyroyal oil toxicosis in a dog. *J Am Vet Med Assoc.* 1992;200:817-8.
[8235] Anderson IB, Mullen WH, Meeker JE, et al. Pennyroyal toxicity: measurement of toxic metabolite levels in two cases and review of the literature. *Ann Intern Med.* 1996;124:726-34.
[8236] Seeff L, Stickel F, Navarro VJ. Hepatotoxicity of herbals and dietary supplements. In, Kaplowitz N, DeLeve LD, eds. Drug-induced liver disease. 3rd ed. Amsterdam: Elsevier, 2013, pp. 631-58.
[8237] Moolla A. A phytochemical and pharmacological investigation of indigenous Agathosma species. MSc Dissertation, University of the Witwatersrand. 2006.
[8238] Mullen W, Anderson I, Oishii S, et al. Accidental pennyroyal oil ingestion in a toddler with the first human serum metabolite detection. *Vet Hum Toxicol.* 1994;36:342.
[8239] Barnes J, Anderson LA, Philpson JD. Herbal Medicine: A Guide for Healthcare Professionals. London, UK: The Pharmaceutical Press, 1996.
[8240] Ciganda C, Laborde A. Herbal infusions used for induced abortion. *J Toxicol Clin Toxicol.* 2003;41(3):235-9.
[8241] Zimmerman HJ. Unconventional drugs. Miscellaneous drugs and diagnostic chemicals. In, Zimmerman, HJ. Hepatotoxicity: the adverse effects of drugs and other chemicals on the liver. 2nd ed. Philadelphia: Lippincott,1999: pp. 731-34.
[8242] Sudekum M, Poppenga RH, Raju N, et al. Pennyroyal oil toxicosis in a dog. *J Am Vet Med Assoc.* 1992;200:817-8.
[8243] Anderson IB, Mullen WH, Meeker JE, et al. Pennyroyal toxicity: measurement of toxic metabolite levels in two cases and review of the literature. *Ann Intern Med.* 1996;124:726-34.
[8244] Seeff L, Stickel F, Navarro VJ. Hepatotoxicity of herbals and dietary supplements. In, Kaplowitz N, DeLeve LD, eds. Drug-induced liver disease. 3rd ed. Amsterdam: Elsevier, 2013, pp. 631-58.
[8245] Lassila T, Mattila S, Turpeinen M, et al. Tandem mass spectrometric analysis of S- and N-linked glutathione conjugates of pulegone and menthofuran and identification of P450 enzymes mediating their formation. *Rapid Commun Mass Spectrom.* 2016 Apr 15;30(7):917-26.
[8246] Nelson SD, McClanahan RH, Thomassen D, et al. Investigations of mechanisms of reactive metabolite formation from (R)-(+)-pulegone. *Xenobiotica.* 1992 Sep-Oct;22(9-10):1157-64.
[8247] Moorthy B, Madyastha P, Madyastha KM. Metabolism of a monoterpene ketone, R-(+)-pulegone--a hepatotoxin in rat. *Xenobiotica.* 1989 Feb;19(2):217-24.
[8248] Madyastha KM, Raj CP. Effects of menthofuran, a monoterpene furan on rat liver microsomal enzymes, in vivo. *Toxicology.* 1994 Apr 18;89(2):119-25.
[8249] Nelson SD. Mechanisms of the formation and disposition of reactive metabolites that can cause acute liver injury. *Drug Metab Rev.* 1995;27(1-2):147-77.
[8250] Moorthy B, Madyastha P, Madyastha KM. Hepatotoxicity of pulegone in rats: its effects on microsomal enzymes, in vivo. *Toxicology.* 1989 May 15;55(3):327-37.
[8251] Madyastha KM, Raj CP. Effects of menthofuran, a monoterpene furan on rat liver microsomal enzymes, in vivo. *Toxicology.* 1994 Apr 18;89(2):119-25.

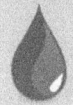

8252 Sullivan JB Jr, Rumack BH, Thomas H Jr, et al. Pennyroyal oil poisoning and hepatotoxicity. *JAMA*. 1979;242:2873-4.
8253 Sudekum M, Poppenga RH, Raju N, et al. Pennyroyal oil toxicosis in a dog. *J Am Vet Med Assoc*. 1992;200:817-8.
8254 Anderson IB, Mullen WH, Meeker JE, et al. Pennyroyal toxicity: measurement of toxic metabolite levels in two cases and review of the literature. *Ann Intern Med*. 1996;124:726-34.
8255 Zimmerman HJ. Unconventional drugs. Miscellaneous drugs and diagnostic chemicals. In, Zimmerman, HJ. Hepatotoxicity: the adverse effects of drugs and other chemicals on the liver. 2nd ed. Philadelphia: Lippincott,1999: pp. 731-34.
8256 Seeff L, Stickel F, Navarro VJ. Hepatotoxicity of herbals and dietary supplements. In, Kaplowitz N, DeLeve LD, eds. Drug-induced liver disease. 3rd ed. Amsterdam: Elsevier, 2013, pp. 631-58.
8257 Burkhard PR, Burkhardt K, Haenggeli CA, et al. Plant-induced seizures: reappearance of an old problem. *J Neurol*. 1999 Aug;246(8):667-70.
8258 Akdogan M, Gultekin F, Yontem M. Effect of Mentha piperita (Labiatae) and Mentha spicata (Labiatae) on iron absorption in rats. *Toxicol Ind Health*. 2004 Sep;20(6-10):119-22.
8259 Muruganathan U, Srinivasan S, Indumathi D. Antihyperglycemic effect of carvone: Effect on the levels of glycoprotein components in streptozotocin-induced diabetic rats. *J Acute Disease*. 2013;2(4):310-15.
8260 Souza FV, da Rocha MB, de Souza DP, et al. (-)-Carvone: antispasmodic effect and mode of action. *Fitoterapia*. 2013 Mar;85:20-24.
8261 Rajeshwari T, Raja B. Antihypertensive, antihyperlipidemicand antioxidantinfluence of D-carvone in L-NAME induced hypertensive rats. *Int J Pharmaceutical Biol Arch*. 2014;5(4):82-88.
8262 de Sousa DP, Farias Nobrega FF, de Almeida RN. Influence of the chirality of (R)-(-)- and (S)-(+)-carvone in the central nervous system: a comparative study. *Chirality*. 2007 May;19(4):264-268.
8263 Akdogan M, Gultekin F, Yontem M. Effect of Mentha piperita (Labiatae) and Mentha spicata (Labiatae) on iron absorption in rats. *Toxicol Ind Health*. 2004 Sep;20(6-10):119-22.
8264 Sessa R, Di Pietro M, De Santis F, et al. Effects of Mentha suaveolens essential oil on Chlamydia trachomatis. *Biomed Res Int*. 2015;2015:508071.
8265 Stringaro A, Vavala E, Colone M, et al. Effects of Mentha suaveolens Essential Oil Alone or in Combination with Other Drugs in Candida albicans. *Evid Based Complement Alternat Med*. 2014;2014:125904.
8266 Civitelli L, Panella S, Marcocci ME, et al. In vitro inhibition of herpes simplex virus type 1 replication by Mentha suaveolens essential oil and its main component piperitenone oxide. *Phytomedicine*. 2014 May 15;21(6):857-65.
8267 Akdogan M, Gultekin F, Yontem M. Effect of Mentha piperita (Labiatae) and Mentha spicata (Labiatae) on iron absorption in rats. *Toxicol Ind Health*. 2004 Sep;20(6-10):119-22.
8268 Cardoso NN, Alviano CS, Blank AF, et al. Synergism Effect of the Essential Oil from Ocimum basilicum var. Maria Bonita and Its Major Components with Fluconazole and Its Influence on Ergosterol Biosynthesis. *Evid Based Complement Alternat Med*. 2016;2016:5647182.
8269 Tayarani-Najaran Z, Talasaz-Firoozi E, Nasiri R, et al. Antiemetic activity of volatile oil from Mentha spicata and Mentha x piperita in chemotherapy-induced nausea and vomiting. *Ecancermedicalscience*. 2013;7:290.
8270 Hunt R, Dienemann J, Norton HJ, et al. Aromatherapy as treatment for postoperative nausea: a randomized trial. *Anesth Analg*. 2013 Sep;117(3):597-604.
8271 Rajeshwari T, Raja B. Antihypertensive, antihyperlipidemic and antioxidant influence of D-carvone in L-NAME induced hypertensive rats. *Int J Pharmaceutical Biol Arch*. 2014;5(4):82-88.
8272 Duarte MC, Figueira GM, Sartoratto A, et al. Anti-Candida activity of Brazilian medicinal plants. *J Ethnopharmacol*. 2005 Feb 28;97(2):305-11.
8273 Imai H, Osawa K, Yasuda H, et al. Inhibition by the essential oils of peppermint and spearmint of the growth of pathogenic bacteria. *Microbios*. 2001;106 Suppl 1;31-39.
8274 Soliman KM, Badeaa RI. Effect of oil extracted from some medicinal plants on different mycotoxigenic fungi. *Food Chem Toxciol*. 2002 Nov;40(11):1669-75.
8275 Sokovic MD, Vukojevic J, Marin PD, et al. Chemical composition of essential oils of Thymus and Mentha species and their antifungal activities. *Molecules*. 2009 Jan 7;14(1):238-49.
8276 Houicher A, Hechachna H, Teldji H, et al. In vitro study of the antifungal activity of essential oils obtained from Mentha spicata, Thymus vulgaris and Laurus nobilis. *Recent Pat Food Nutr Agric*. 2016;8(2):99-106.
8277 Rasooli I, Shayegh S, Astaneh S. The effect of Mentha spicata and Eucalyptus camaldulensis essential oil on dental biofilm. *Int J Dent Hyg*. 2009 Aug;7(3):196-203.
8278 Zhao CZ, Wang Y, Tang FD, et al. Effect of spearmint oil on inflammation, oxidative alteration and Nrf2 expression in lung tissue of COPD rats. *Zhejiang Da Xue Xue Bao Yi Xue Ban*. 2008 Jul;37(4):357-63.
8279 Rafii F, Shahverdi AR. Comparison of essential oils from three plants for enhancement of antimicrobial activity of nitrofurantoin against enterobacteria. *Chemotherapy*. 207;53(1):21-25.
8280 Jaradat NA, Al Zabadi H, Rahhal B, et al. The effect of inhalation of Citrus sinensis flowers and Mentha spicata leave essential oils on lung function and exercise performance: a quasi-experimental uncontrolled before-and-after study. *J Int Soc Sports Nutr*. 2016 Sep 22;13:36.
8281 Santana-Méridas O, González-Coloma A, Fe Andrés M, et al. Biocidal compounds from Mentha sp essential oils and their structure-activity relationships. *Chem Biodivers*. 2017 Mar;14(3).
8282 de Sousa DP, Lima TC, Steverding D, et al. Evaluation of Antiparasitc Activity of Mentha crispa Essential Oil, Its Major Constituent Rotundifolone and Analogues against Trypanosoma brucei. *Planta Med*. 2016 Oct;82(15):1346-1350.
8283 Mahboubi M. Mentha spicata as natural analgesia for treatment of pain in osteoarthritis patients. *Complement Ther Clin Pract*. 2017 Feb;26:1-4.
8284 Mogosan C, Vostinaru O, Oprean R, et al. A Comparative Analysis of the Chemical Composition, Anti-Inflammatory, and Antinociceptive Effects of the Essential Oils from Three Species of Mentha Cultivated in Romania. *Molecules*. 2017 Feb 10;22(2).
8285 Yones DA, Bakir HY, Bayoumi SA, et al. Chemical composition and efficacy of some selected plant oils against Pediculus humanus capitis in vitro. *Parasitol Res*. 2016 Aug;115(8):3209-18.
8286 Wiwattanaratanabut K, choonharuangdej S, Srithava T. In Vitro Anti-Cariogenic Plaque Effects of Essential Oils Extracted from Culinary Herbs. *J Clin Diagnostic Res*. 2017 Sep;11(9):DC30-5.
8287 Vetas D, Dimitropoulou E, Mitropoulou G, et al. Disinfection efficiencies of sage and spearmint essential oils against planktonic and biofilm Staphylococcus aureus cells in comparison with sodium hypochlorite. *Int J Food Microbiol*. 2017 Sep 18;257:19-25.
8288 Sadeghi Ataabadi M, Alaee S, Bagheri MJ, et al. Role of Essential Oil of Mentha Spicata (Spearmint) in Addressing Reverse Hormonal and Folliculogenesis Disturbances in a Polycystic Ovarian Syndrome in a Rat Model. *Adv Pharm Bull*. 2017 Dec;7(4):651-654.
8289 Bartoňková I, Dvořák Z. Essential oils of culinary herbs and spices display agonist and antagonist activities at human aryl hydrocarbon receptor AhR. *Food Chem Toxicol*. 2018 Jan;111:374-384.
8290 da Cruz Almeida ET, de Medeiros Barbosa I, Tavares JF, et al. Inactivation of Spoilage Yeasts by Mentha spicata L. and M. × villosa Huds. Essential Oils in Cashew, Guava, Mango, and Pineapple Juices. *Front Microbiol*. 2018 May 25;9:1111.
8291 Bardaweel SK, Bakchiche B, ALSalamat HA, et al. Chemical composition, antioxidant, antimicrobial and Antiproliferative activities of essential oil of Mentha spicata L. (Lamiaceae) from Algerian Saharan atlas. *BMC Complement Altern Med*. 2018 Jul 3;18(1):201.
8292 Turkez H, Tozlu OO, Lima TC, et al. A Comparative Evaluation of the Cytotoxic and Antioxidant Activity of Mentha crispa Essential Oil, Its Major Constituent Rotundifolone, and Analogues on Human Glioblastoma. *Oxid Med Cell Longev*. 2018 Jul 2;2018:2083923.
8293 Giatropoulos A, Kimbaris A, Michaelakis A, et al. Chemical composition and assessment of larvicidal and repellent capacity of 14 Lamiaceae essential oils against Aedes albopictus. *Parasitol Res*. 2018 Jun;117(6):1953-1964.
8294 Piras A, Porcedda S, Falconieri D, et al. Antifungal activity of essential oil from Mentha spicata L. and Mentha pulegium L. growing wild in Sardinia island (Italy). *Nat Prod Res*. 2019 Jul 19:1-7.
8295 Wu Z, Tan B, Liu Y, et al. Chemical Composition and Antioxidant Properties of Essential Oils from Peppermint, Native Spearmint and Scotch Spearmint. *Molecules*. 2019 Aug 2;24(15).
8296 Karaca N, Demirci B, Demirci F, et al. Evaluation of Lavandula stoechas L. subsp. stoechas L., Mentha spicata L. subsp. spicata L. essential oils and their main components against sinusitis pathogens. *Z Naturforsch C*. 2018 Sep 25;73(9-10):353-360.
8297 Wang H, Xie M, Charpin-El Hamri G, et al. Treatment of chronic pain by designer cells controlled by spearmint aromatherapy. *Nat Biomed Eng*. 2018 Feb;2(2):114-123.
8298 Ali-Shtayeh MS, Jamous RM, Abu-Zaitoun SY, et al. Biological Properties and Bioactive Components of Mentha spicata L. Essential Oil: Focus on Potential Benefits in the Treatment of Obesity, Alzheimer's Disease, Dermatophytosis, and Drug-Resistant Infections. *Evid Based Complement Alternat Med*. 2019;2019:3834265.
8299 Soutar O, Cohen F, Wall R. Essential oils as tick repellents on clothing. *Exp Appl Acarol*. 2019 Oct;79(2):209-219.
8300 Ekhtelat M, Borujeni FK, Siahposh A, et al. Chemical composition and antibacterial effects of some essential oils individually and in combination with sodium benzoate against methicillin-resistant Staphylococcus aureus and Yersinia enterocolitica. *Vet Res Forum*. Fall 2020;11(4):333-338.
8301 Santos AA, Wanderley-Teixeira V, Dos Santos Cruz G, et al. Essential oil toxicity on biological and reproductive parameters of Alabama argillacea (Hübner) (Lepidoptera: Erebidae). *Acta Histochem*. 2021 Apr 12;123(4):151714.
8302 Jayaram CS, Chauhan N, Dolma SK, et al. Chemical Composition and Insecticidal Activities of Essential Oils against the Pulse Beetle. *Molecules*. 2022 Jan 17;27(2):568.
8303 Yasir M, Nawaz A, Ghazanfar S, et al. Anti-bacterial activity of essential oils against multidrug-resistant foodborne pathogens isolated from raw milk. *Braz J Biol*. 2022 May 9;84:e259449.
8304 Fazal H, Akram M, Ahmad N, et al. Nutritionally rich biochemical profile in essential oil of various Mentha species and their antimicrobial activities. *Protoplasma*. 2022 Aug 9. Online ahead of print.
8305 Rasti F, Yousefpoor Y, Abdollahi A, et al. Antioxidative, anticancer, and antibacterial activities of a nanogel containing Mentha spicata L. essential oil and electrospun nanofibers of polycaprolactone-hydroxypropyl methylcellulose. *BMC Complement Med Ther*. 2022 Oct 7;22(1):261.
8306 Landeo-Villanueva GE, Salazar-Salvatierra ME, Ruiz-Quiroz JR, et al. Inhibitory Activity of Essential Oils of Mentha spicata and Eucalyptus globulus on Biofilms of Streptococcus mutans in an In Vitro Model. *Antibiotics (Basel)* . 2023 Feb 10;12(2):369.
8307 Salido S, Altarejos J, Nogueras M, et al. Chemical composition and seasonal variations of spike lavender oil from Southern Spain. *J Essential Oil Res*. 2004;16(3):206-10.
8308 Barazandeh MM. Essential oil composition of Lavandula latifolia Medik from Iran. *J Essent Oil Res*. 2002;14(2):103-04.
8309 Guillen MD, Cabo N, Burillo J. Characterisation of the essential oils of some cultivated aromatic plants of industrial interest. *J Sc Food Agric*. 1996 Mar;70(3):359-63.
8310 Khine H, Weiss D, Graber N, et al. A cluster of children with seizures caused by camphor poisoning. *Pediatrics*. 2009 May;123(5):1269-72.
8311 Michiels EA, Mazor SS. Toddler with seizures due to ingesting camphor at an Indian celebration. *Pediatr Emerg Care*. 2010 Aug;26(8):574-75.
8312 Koren G. Medications which can kill a toddler with one tablet or teaspoonful. *J toxicol Clin Toxicol*. 1993;31(3):407- 13.
8313 Bar-Oz B, Levicheck Z, Koren G. Medications that can kill a toddler with one tablet or teaspoonfull – A 2004 update. *Paediatr Drugs*. 2004;6(2):123-6.
8314 Craig JO. Poisoning by the volatile oils in childhood. *Arch Dis Child*. 1953;28:259-67.
8315 Melis K. Bochner A, Janssens G. Accidental nasal eucalyptol and menthol instillation. *Eur J Pediatr*. 1989 Aug;148(8)786-7.

8316 Day LM, Ozanne-Smith J, Parsons BJ, et al. Eucalyptus oil poisoning among young children: mechanisms of access and the potential prevention. *Aust N Z J Public Health.* 1997 Jun;21(3):297-302.

8317 Chandar SD, Prashanti M, Kumar CL, et al. Eucalyptus Oil-Induced Seizures in Children: A Single-Center Prospective Study. *Cureus.* 2021 Mar 25;13(3):e14109.

8318 Rabl W, Katzgraber F, Steinlechner M. Camphor ingestion for abortion (case report). *Forensic Sci Int.* 1997 Sep 19;89(1-2):137-40.

8319 Flaman Z, Pellechia-Clarke S, Bailey B, et al. Unintentional exposure of young children to camphor and eucalyptus oils. *Paediatr Child Health.* 2001 Feb;6(2):80-83.

8320 Day LM, Ozanne-Smith J, Parsons BJ, et al. Eucalyptus oil poisoning among young children: mechanisms of access and the potential prevention. *Aust N Z J Public Health.* 1997 Jun;21(3):297-302.

8321 Myott E. Case of eucalyptus poisoning. *Brit M J.* 1906;1:558.

8322 Hindle RC. Eucalyptus oil ingestion. *N Z Med J.* 1994 May 11;107(977)185-6.

8323 Tibballs J. Clinical effects and management of eucalyptus oil ingestion in infants and small children. *Med J Aust.* 1995 Aug;163(4):177-80.

8324 Waldman W, Barwina M, Sein Anand J. Accidental ontoxication with eucalyptus oil—a case report. *Przegl Lek.* 2011;68(8):555-6.

8325 Day LM, Ozanne-Smith J, Parsons BJ, et al. Eucalyptus oil poisoning among young children: mechanisms of access and the potential prevention. *Aust N Z J Public Health.* 1997 Jun;21(3):297-302.

8326 De Vincenzi M, Silano M, De Vincenzi A, et al. Constituents of aromatic plants: eucalyptol. *Fitoterapia.* 2002 Jun;73(3):269-75.

8327 Manoguerra AS, Erdman AR, Wax PM, et al. Camphor poisoning: an evidence-based practice guideline for out-of- hospital management. *Clin Toxicol (Phila).*2006;44(4):357-70.

8328 Gibson DE, Moore GP, Pfaff JA. Camphor ingestion. *Am J Emerg Med.* 1989 Jan;7(1):41-43.

8329 Koppel C, Martends F, Schirop T, et al. Hemoperfusion in acute camphor poisoning. *Intensive Care Med.* 1988;14(4):431-33.

8330 Sayyah M, Valizadeh J, Kamalinejad M. Anticonvulsant activity of the leaf oil of Laurus nobilis against pentylentetrazole- and maximal electroshock-induced seizure. *Phytomedicine.* 2002 Apr;9(3):212-16.

8331 Culic M, Kekovic G, Grbic G, et al. Wavelet and fractal analysis of rat brain activity in seizures evoked by camphor oil and 1,8-cineole. *Gen Physiol Biophys.* 2009;28 Sec No:33-40.

8332 Burkhard PR, Burkhardt K, Haenggeli CA, et al. Plant-induced seizures: reappearance of an old problem. *J Neurol.* 1999 Aug;246(8):667-70.

8333 Waldman N. Seizure caused by dermal application of over-the-counter eucalyptus oil head lice preparation. *Clin Toxicol (Phila).* 2011 Oct;49(8):750-1.

8334 Craig JO. Poisoning by the volatile oils in childhood. *Arch Dis Child.* 1953;28:259-67.

8335 Mathew T, Kamath V, Kumar RS, et al. Eucalyptus oil inhalation-induced seizure: A novel, underrecognized, preventable cause of acute symptomatic seizure. *Epilepsia Open.* 2017 Jul 4;2(3):350-354.

8336 Olowe SA, Ransome-Kuti O. The risk of jaundice in glucose-6-phosphate dehydrogenase deficient babies exposed to menthol. *Acta Paediatr Scand.* 1980 May;69(3):341-5.

8337 Dillon Remy M, Manning Alleyne P, Bratt DE, et al. Neonatal jaundice at Port-of-Spain General Hospital abstract. *West Indian Med J.* 1987;36(Suppl):28.

8338 Jori A, Bianchetti A, Prestini PE, et al. Effect of eucalyptol (1,8-cineole) on the metabolism of other drugs in rats and in man. *Eur J Pharmacol.* 1970;9(3):362-66.

8339 de Sousa DP, Raphael E, Brocksom U, et al. Sedative effect of monoterpene alcohols in mice: A preliminary screening. *Verlag der Zeitschrift fur Naturforschung.* 2007;62c:563-66.

8340 Lamborn LL. Modern soaps, candles and glycerin: A practical manual of modern methods of utilization of fats and oils in the manufacture of soaps and candles, and of the recovery of glycerin. Library of the University of Wisconsin.

8341 Oyen LP, Dung NX. Plant resources of South-East Asia. 1999. Backhyus, Leiden.

8342 Kim NH, Hyun SH, Jin CH, et al. Pretreatment with 1,8-cineole potentiates thioacetamide-induced hepatotoxicity and immunosuppression. *Arch Pharm Res.* 2004 Jul;27(7):781-9.

8343 Uc A, Bishop WP, Sanders KD. Camphor hepatotoxicity. *South Med J.* 2000;93:596-98.

8344 Roller S, Ernest N, Buckle J. The antimicrobial activity of high-necrodane and other lavender oils on methicillin-sensitive and -resistant Staphylococcus aureus (MSSA and MRSA). *J Altern Complement Med.* 2009 Mar;15(3):275-79.

8345 Rota C, Carraminana KK, Burillo J, et al. In vitro antimicrobial activity of essential oils from aromatic plants against selected foodborne pathogens. *J Food Prot.* 2004 Jun;67(6):1252-56.

8346 Charron JM. Use of Lavandula latifolia as an expectorant. *J Altern Complement Med.* 1997 Fall;3(3):211.

8347 Carrasco A, Martinez-Gutierrez R, Tomas V, et al. Lavandula angustifolia and Lavandula latifolia Essential Oils from Spain: Aromatic Profile and Bioactivities. *Planta Med.* 2016 Jan;82(1-2):163-70.

8348 Carrasco A, Martinez-Gutierrez R, Tomas V, et al. Lavandula angustifolia and Lavandula latifolia Essential Oils from Spain: Aromatic Profile and Bioactivities. *Planta Med.* 2016 Jan;82(1-2):163-70.

8349 Karaca N, Sener G, Demirci B, et al. Synergistic antibacterial combination of Lavandula latifolia Medik. essential oil with camphor. *Z Naturforsch C J Biosci.* 2020 Nov 2. Online ahead of print.

8350 Liu XC, Liu ZL. Evaluation of insecticidal activity of Nardostachys jatamansi essential oil against some grain storage insects. *J Entomol Zoolo Stud.* 2014;2(4):335-40.

8351 Paudyal MP, Rajbhandari M, Basnet P, et al. Quality assessment of the essential oils from Nardostachys jatamansi (D. Don) DC and Nardostachys chinensis batal obtained from Kathmandu valley market. *Sci World.* 2012 Jul;10(10):13- 16.

8352 Naquvi KJ, Ansari SH, Ali M, et al. Volatile constituents of Nardostachys Jatamansi DC., a critically endangered species. *Nat Prod: An Indian J.* 2013;9(3).

8353 Mahalwal VS, Ali M. Volatile constituents of the rhizomes of Nardostachys jatamansi DC. *J Essent Oil Bearing Plant.* 2002;5:83-89.

8354 Naquvi KJ, Ansari SH, Ali M. Composition of volatile oil of sambul-ut-teeb (Nardostachys jatamansi DC.), an endangered species. Anal Chem An Indian J 2013; 12:347-351.

8355 Mahalwal VS, Ali M. Volatile constituents of the rhizomes of Nardostachys jatamansi DC. *J Essent Oil Bearing Plants.* 2002;5:83-89.

8356 Satyal P, Chhetri B, Dosoky N, et al. Chemical Composition of Nardostachys grandiflora Rhizome Oil from Nepal – A Contribution to the Chemotaxonomy and Bioactivity of Nardostachys. *Nat Prod Commun.* 2015 Jun;10(6):1067-70.

8357 Satyal P, Chhetri B, Dosoky N, et al. Chemical Composition of Nardostachys grandiflora Rhizome Oil from Nepal – A Contribution to the Chemotaxonomy and Bioactivity of Nardostachys. *Nat Prod Commun.* 2015 Jun;10(6):1067-70.

8358 Maiwulanjiang M, Chen J, Xin G, et al. The volatile oil of Nardostachyos Radix et Rhizoma inhibits the oxidative stress-induced cell injury via reactive oxygen species scavenging and Akt activation in H9c2 cardiomyocyte. *J Ethnopharmacol.* 2014 Apr;153(2):491-98.

8359 Satyal P, Chhetri B, Dosoky N, et al. Chemical Composition of Nardostachys grandiflora Rhizome Oil from Nepal – A Contribution to the Chemotaxonomy and Bioactivity of Nardostachys. *Nat Prod Commun.* 2015 Jun;10(6):1067-70.

8360 Maiwulanjiang M, Bi CWC, Lee PSCL, et al. The volatile oil of Nardostachyos Radix et Rhizoma induces endothelial nitric oxide synthase activity in HUVEC cells. *PLoS One.* 2015 Feb 2;10(2):e0116761.

8361 Maiwulanjiang M, Chen J, Xin G, et al. The volatile oil of Nardostachyos Radix et Rhizoma inhibits the oxidative stress-induced cell injury via reactive oxygen species scavenging and Akt activation in H9c2 cardiomyocyte. J Ethnopharmacol. 2014 Apr;153(2):491-98.

8362 Han X, Beaumont C, Stevens N. Chemical composition analysis and in vitro biological activities of ten essential oils in human skin cells. *Biochim Open.* 2017 Apr 26;5:1-7.

8363 Feng YX, Wang Y, Geng ZF, et al. Contact Toxicity and Repellent Efficacy of Valerianaceae Spp. To Three Stored-Product Insects and Synergistic Interactions Between Two Major Compounds Camphene and Bornyl Acetate. *Ecotoxicol Environ Saf.* 2019 Dec;190:110106.

8364 Cornara L, Ambu G, Trombetta D, et al. Comparative and Functional Screening of Three Species Traditionally used as Antidepressants: Valeriana officinalis L., Valeriana jatamansi Jones ex Roxb. and Nardostachys jatamansi (D.Don) DC. *Plants (Basel).* 2020 Aug 5;9(8):E994.

8365 Garneau FX, Collin G, Gagnon H, et al. Chemical composition of the hydrosol and the essential oil of three different species of the Pinaceae family: Picea glauca (Moench) Voss., Picea mariana (Mill.) B.S.P., and Abies balsamea (L.) Mill. *J Essential Oil Bearing Plants.* 2012;15(2):227-36.

8366 Royer M, Houde R, Stevanovic T. Non-wood forest products based on extractives-A new opportunity for Canadian Forest Industry. Part 2-Softwood forest species. *J Food Res.* 2013;5(2):164-89.

8367 Hachey JM, Collin GJ, Simard S. Influence of sample preparation on the composition of the essential oil of the needles and twigs of Picea mariana (Mill.) B.S.P. *J Wood Chem Tech.* 1989;9(1):563-60.

8368 Kocak A, Kilic O. Identification of essential oil composition of four Picea Mill. (Pinaceae) species from Canada. *J Agric Sci Tech.*2014;b4:209-14.

8369 Chartier C. Red spruce, tradition and current use. *Phytoth Rapie.* 2009 Oct;7(5):251-54.

8370 Chao S, Young G, Oberg C, et al. Inhibition of methicillin-resistant Staphylococcus aureus (MRSA) by essential oils. *Flav Frag J.* 2008;23:444-49.

8371 Matsubara E, Fukagawa M, Okamoto T, et al. (-)-Bornyl acetate induces autonomic relaxation and reduces arousal level after visual display terminal work without any influences of task performance in low-dose condition. *Biomed Res.* 2011 Apr;32(2):151-57.

8372 Huang Y, Zhao J, Zhou L, et al. Antifungal Activity of the Essential Oil of Illicium verum Fruit and Its Main Component trans-Anethole. *Molecules.* 2010;15:7558-7569.

8373 Lee SOG, Park IK, Choi GJA, et al. Fumigant Activity of Essential Oils and Components of Illicium verum and Schizonepeta tenuifolia Against Botrytis cinerea and Colletotrichum gloeosporioides. *J Microbiol Biotechnol.* 2007;17(9):1568-1572.

8374 Gholivanda MB, Rahimi-Nasrabadiab M, Chalabib H. Determination of Essential Oil Components of Star Anise (Illicium verum) Using Simultaneous Hydrodistillation–Static Headspace Liquid-Phase Microextraction–Gas Chromatography Mass Spectrometry. *Analytical Letters.* 2009;42(10):1382-97.

8375 Ana D, Marina S, Mihalo R, et al. Chemical composition and antifungal activity of Illicium verum and Eugenia caryophyllata essential oils. *Chem Nat Constituents.* 2009 Mar;45(2):259-61.

8376 European Medicines Agency. Public statement on the use of herbal medicinal products containing estragole. Available at: http://www.ema.europa.eu/docs/en_GB/document_library/Scientific_guideline/2010/04/WC500089960.pdf.

8377 Turkyilmaz Z, Karabulut R, Sonmez K, et al. A striking and frequent cause of premature thelarche in children: Foeniculum vulgare. *J Pediatr Surg.* 2008 Nov;43(11):2109-11.

8378 Ostad SN, Khakinegard B, Sabzevari O. Evaluation of the teratogenicity of fennel essential oil (FEO) on the rat embryo limb buds culture. *Toxicol.* 2004 Oct;18(5):623-7.

8379 Tabanca N, Khan SI, Bedir E, et al. Estrogenic activity of isolated constituents and essential oils of Pimpinella species from Turkey, evaluated using a recombinant yeast screen. *Planta Med.* 2004 Aug;70(8):728-35.

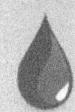

8380 Albert-Puleo M. Fennel and anise as estrogenic agents. *J Ethnopharmacol.* 1980 Dec;2(4):337-44.

8381 Malini T, Vanithakumari G, Megala N, et al. Effect of Foeniculum vulgare Mill. seed extract on the genital organs of male and female rats. *Indian J Physiol Pharmacol.* 1985 Jan-Mar;29(1):21-6.

8382 Dhar SK. Anti-fertility activity and hormonal profile of trans-anethole in rats. *Indian J Physiol Pharmacol.* 1995;39(1):63-67.

8383 Howes MJ, Houghton PJ, Barlow DJ, et al. Assessment of estrogenic activity in some common essential oil constituents. *J Pharm Pharmacol.* 2002 Nov;54(11):1521-28.

8384 Ostad SN, Soodi M, Shariffzadeh M, et al. The effect of fennel essential oil on uterine contraction as a model for dysmenorrhea, pharmacology and toxicology study. *J Ethnopharmacol.* 2001 Aug;76(3):299-304.

8385 Rosti L, Nardini A, Bettini ME, et al. Toxic effects of a herbal tea mixture in two newborns. *Acta Paediatrica.* 1994;83:683.

8386 Tognolini M, Barocelli E, Ballabeni V, et al. Comparative screening of plant essential oils; phenylpropanoid moiety as basic core for antiplatelet activity. *Life Sci.* 2006 Feb 23;78(13):1419-32.

8387 Yoshioka M, Tamada TT. Aromatic factors of anti-platelet aggregation in fennel oil. *Biogenic Amines.* 2005 Apr;19(2):89-96.

8388 Tognolini M, Ballabeni V, Bertoni S, et al. Protective effect of Foeniculum vulgare essential oil and anethole in an experimental model of theombosis. *Pharm Res.* 2007;56:254-60.

8389 Kreydiyyeh SI, Usta J, Knio K, et al. Aniseed oil increases glucose absorption and reduces urine output in the rat. *Life Sci.* 2003 Dec 19;74(5):663-73.

8390 Sheikh BA, Pari L, Rathinham A, et al. Trans-anethole, a terpenoid ameliorates hyperglycemia by regulating key enzymes of carbohydrate metabolism in streptozotocin induced diabetic rats. *Biochimie.* 2015 May;112:57-65.

8391 Pari L, Sheikh BA. Antihyperglycemic effect of trans-anethole in streptozotocin induced diabetic rats with special reference to glycoprotein components. *Int J Adv Res Biol Sci.* 2015;2(5):28-34.

8392 Kreydiyyeh SI, Usta J, Knio K, et al. Aniseed oil increases glucose absorption and reduces urine output in the rat. *Life Sci.* 2003 Dec 19;74(5):663-73.

8393 Samojlik I, Petković S, Stilinović N, et al. Pharmacokinetic Herb-Drug Interaction between Essential Oil of Aniseed (Pimpinella anisum L., Apiaceae) and Acetaminophen and Caffeine: A Potential Risk for Clinical Practice. *Phytother Res.* 2016 Feb;30(2):253-9.

8394 Samojlik I, Mijatović V, Petković S, et al. The influence of essential oil of aniseed (Pimpinella anisum, L.) on drug effects on the central nervous system. *Fitoterapia.* 2012 Dec;83(8):1466-73.

8395 Samojlik I, Mijatović V, Petković S, et al. The influence of essential oil of aniseed (Pimpinella anisum, L.) on drug effects on the central nervous system. *Fitoterapia.* 2012 Dec;83(8):1466-73.

8396 Wisniewski-Rebecca ES, Rocha BA, Wiirzler LA, et al. Synergistic effects of anethole and ibuprofen in acute inflammatory response. *Chem Biol Interact.* 2015 Dec 5;242:247-53.

8397 Samojlik I, Mijatović V, Petković S, et al. The influence of essential oil of aniseed (Pimpinella anisum, L.) on drug effects on the central nervous system. *Fitoterapia.* 2012 Dec;83(8):1466-73.

8398 Samojlik I, Mijatović V, Petković S, et al. The influence of essential oil of aniseed (Pimpinella anisum, L.) on drug effects on the central nervous system. *Fitoterapia.* 2012 Dec;83(8):1466-73.

8399 Howes MJ, Houghton PJ, Barlow DJ, et al. Assessment of estrogenic activity in some common essential oil constituents. *J Pharm Pharmacol.* 2002 Nov;54(11):1521-28.

8400 Chen CH, deGraffenreid LA. Anethole suppressed cell survival and induced apoptosis in human breast cancer cells independent of estrogen receptor status. *Phytomedicine.* 2012 Jun 15;19(8-9):763-7.

8401 Nessa MU, Beale P, Chan C, et al. Studies on combination of platinum drugs cisplatin and oxaliplatin with phytochemicals anethole and curcumin in ovarian tumor models. *Anticancer Res.* 2012 Nov;32(11):4843-50.

8402 Ostad SN, Soodi M, Shariffzadeh M, et al. The effect of fennel essential oil on uterine contraction as a model for dysmenorrhea, pharmacology and toxicology study. *J Ethnopharmacol.* 2001 Aug;76(3):299-304.

8403 Khorshidi N, Ostad SN, Mosaddegh M, et al. Clinical effects of fennel essential oil on primary dysmenorrhea. *Iran J Pharm Res.* 2003 Spring;2(2):89-93.

8404 Cao LX. Endometriosis as treated by traditional Chinese medicine. *J Am Coll Trad Chin Med.* 1983;1:54-57.

8405 Subehan UT, Iwata H, Kadota S, et al. Mechanism-based inhibition of CYP3A4 and CYP2D6 by Indonesian medicinal plants. *J Ethnopharmacol.* 2006 May;105(3):449-55.

8406 Subehan Z, Kadota SF, Tezuka Y. Inhibition on human liver cytochrome P450 3A4 by constituents of fennel (Foeniculum vulgare): Identification and characterization of a mechanism-based inactivator. *J Agric Food Chem.* 2007 Dec;55(25):10162-67.

8407 Yarnell E, Abascal K. Interaction of Herbal Constituents with Cytochrome P450 Enzymes. *Alt Complement Ther.* 2007 Nov;13(5):239-47.

8408 Sinitskaia ZF, Lashneva NV, Chichilanova GV, et al. [Effect of trans-anethole on liver monooxygenase system and its induction of polychlorinated diphenyls]. *Vopr Pitan.* 1994;(5):24-7.

8409 Rompelberg CJ, Verhagen H, van Bladeren PJ. Effects of the naturally occurring alkenylbenzenes eugenol and trans-anethole on drug-metabolizing enzymes in the rat liver. *Food Chem Toxicol.* 1993 Sep;31(9):637-45.

8410 Rompelberg CJ, Verhagen H, van Bladeren PJ. Effects of the naturally occurring alkenylbenzenes eugenol and trans-anethole on drug-metabolizing enzymes in the rat liver. *Food Chem Toxicol.* 1993 Sep;31(9):637-45.

8411 Tepe B, Akpulat HA, Sokmen M, et al. Screening of the antioxidative and antimicrobial properties of the essential oils of Pimpinella anisetum and Pimpinella flabellifolia from Turkey. *Food Chemistry.* 2006 Aug;99(4):719-24.

8412 Marin I, Sayas-Barberá E, Viuda-Martos M, et al. Chemical Composition, Antioxidant and Antimicrobial Activity of Essential Oils from Organic Fennel, Parsley, and Lavender from Spain. *Foods.* 2016 Mar 4;5(1).

8413 Shin EH, Song BG, Lee IH, et al. Repellency of cassia bark, eucalyptus, and star anise oils and their major constituents to Leptotrombidium pallidum (Acari: Trombiculidae). *J Med Entomol.* 2013 May;50(3):579-84.

8414 Sinthusiri J, Soonwera M. Oviposition deterrent and ovicidal activities of seven herbal essential oils against female adults of housefly, Musca domestica L. *Parasitol Res.* 2014 Aug;113(8):3015-22.

8415 Chaiyasit D, Choochote W, Rattanachanpichai E, et al. Essential oils as potential adulticides against two populations of Aedes aegypti, the laboratory and natural field strains, in Chiang Mai province, northern Thailand. *Parasitol Res.* 2006 Nov;99(6):715-21.

8416 Astani A1, Reichling J, Schnitzler P. Screening for antiviral activities of isolated constituents from essential oils. *Evid Based Complement Alternat Med.* 2011;2011:253643.

8417 Ritter AM1, Ames FQ1, Otani F, et al. Effects of anethole in nociception experimental models. *Evid Based Complement Alternat Med.* 2014;2014:345829.

8418 Kang P, Kim KY, Lee HS, et al. Anti-inflammatory effects of anethole in lipopolysaccharide-induced acute lung injury in mice. *Life Sci.* 2013 Dec 5;93(24):955-61.

8419 Domiciano TP1, Dalalio MM, Silva EL, et al. Inhibitory effect of anethole in nonimmune acute inflammation. *Naunyn Schmiedebergs Arch Pharmacol.* 2013 Apr;386(4):331-8.

8420 Ritter AM1, Domiciano TP, Verri WA Jr, et al. Antihypernociceptive activity of anethole in experimental inflammatory pain. *Inflammopharmacology.* 2013 Apr;21(2):187-97.

8421 Kim J, Jang M, Shin E, et al. Fumigant and contact toxicity of 22 wooden essential oils and their major components against Drosophila suzukii (Diptera: Drosophilidae). *Pestic Biochem Physiol.* 2016 Oct;133:35-43.

8422 Dwivedy AK, Singh VK, Prakash B, et al. Nanoencapsulated Illicium verum Hook.f. essential oil as an effective novel plant-based preservative against aflatoxin B1 production and free radical generation. *Food Chem Toxicol.* 2017 Nov 8;111:102-113.

8423 Bartoňková I, Dvořák Z. Essential oils of culinary herbs and spices display agonist and antagonist activities at human aryl hydrocarbon receptor AhR. *Food Chem Toxicol.* 2018 Jan;111:374-384.

8424 Zhang G, Yuan C, Sun Y, et al. Effect of Selective Encapsulation of Hydroxypropyl-β-cyclodextrin on Components and Antibacterial Properties of Star Anise Essential Oil. *Molecules.* 2018 May 9;23(5).

8425 Elmhalli F, Pålsson K, Örberg J, et al. Acaricidal properties of ylang-ylang oil and star anise oil against nymphs of Ixodes ricinus (Acari: Ixodidae). *Exp Appl Acarol.* 2018 Oct;76(2):209-220.

8426 Gomes da Rocha Voris D, Dos Santos Dias L, Alencar Lima J, et al. Evaluation of larvicidal, adulticidal, and anticholinesterase activities of essential oils of Illicium verum Hook. f., Pimenta dioica (L.) Merr., and Myristica fragrans Houtt. against Zika virus vectors. *Environ Sci Pollut Res Int.* 2018 Aug;25(23):22541-22551.

8427 Freitas JP, Raguel de Jesus IL, Karoline de Oliveira Chaves J, et al. Efficacy and residual effect of Illicium verum (star anise) and Pelargonium graveolens (rose geranium) essential oil on cat fleas Ctenocephalides felis felis. *Rev Bras Parasitol Vet.* 2021 Dec 10;30(4):e009321.

8428 Wu K, Zhang T, Chai X, et al. Preparation and antibacterial and antioxidant ability of β-cyclodextrin complexes of vaporized Illicium verum essential oil. *Food Sci Nutr.* 2022 Jul 26;10(11):4003-4018.

8429 Khalid KA. Essential Oil Constituents of Summer Savory Plants Propagated and Adapted under Egyptian Climate. *J Appl Sci.* 2016;16:54-57.

8430 Mohammadhosseini M, Beiranvand M. Chemical Composition of the Essential Oil from the Aerial Parts of Satureja hortensis As a Potent Medical Plant Using Traditional Hydrodistillation. *J Chem Health Risks.* 2013;3(4):43-54.

8431 Yazdanpanah L, Mohamadi N. Antifungal activity of Satureja hortensis L. essential oil against Alternaria citri. *Eur J Exp Biol.* 2014;4(1):399-403.

8432 Adiguzel A, Ozer H, Kilic H, et al. Screening of Antimicrobial Activity of Essential Oil and Methanol Extract of Satureja hortensis on foodborne Bacteria and Fungi. *Czech J Food Sci.* 2007 Jan;25(2):81-89.

8433 Mahboubi M, Kazempour N. Chemical composition and antimicrobial activity of Satureja hortensis and Trachyspermum copticum essential oil. *Iran J Microbiol.* 2011 Dec;3(4):194-200.

8434 Mihajilov-Krstev T, Radnovic D, Kitic D, et al. Antimicrobial activity of Satureja hortensis L. essential oil against pathogenic microbial strains. *Arch Biol Sci Belgrade.* 2010;62(1):159-66.

8435 Sefidkon F, Abbasi K, Khaniki GB. Influence of drying and extraction methods on yield and chemical composition of the essential oil of Satureja hortensis. *Food Chem.* 2006 Jan;99(1):19-23.

8436 Gormez A, Bozari S, Yanmis D, et al. Chemical Composition and Antibacterial Activity of Essential Oils of Two Species of Lamiaceae against Phytopathogenic Bacteria. *Polish J Micribiol.* 2015;64(2):121-27.

8437 Domaracky M, Rehak P, Juhas S, et al. Effects of selected plant essential oils on the growth and development of mouse preimplantation embryos in vivo. *Physiol Res.* 2007;56(1):97-104.

8438 Kohlert C, Schindler G, Marz RW, et al. Systemic availability and pharmacokinetics of thymol in humans. *J Clin Pharmacol.* 2002 Jul;42(7):731-7.

8439 Toxicology Data Network, National Library of Medicine. Thymol. Available at: http://toxnet.nlm.nih.gov/cgi-bin/sis/search/a?dbs+hsdb:@term+@DOCNO+866.

8440 Lemhadri A, Zeggwagh NA, Maghrani M, et al. Anti-hypoglycaemic activity of the aqueous extract of Origanum vulgare growing wild in Tafilalet region. *J Ethnopharmacol.* 2004 Jun;92(2-3):251-6.
8441 Mirazi N, Rezaei M, Mirhoseini M. Hypoglycemic effect of Satureja montanum L. hydroethanolic extract on diabetic rats. *J HerbMed Pharm.* 2016;5(1):17-22.
8442 Ezhumalai M, Radhiga T, Pugalendi KV. Antihyperglycemic effect of carvacrol in combination with rosiglitazone in high-fat diet-induced type 2 diabetic C57BL/6J mice. *Mol Cell Biochem.* 2014 Jan;385(1-2):23-31.
8443 Tognolini M, Barocelli E, Ballabeni V, et al. Comparative screening of plant essential oils; phenylpropanoid moiety as basic core for antiplatelet activity. *Life Sci.* 2006 Feb 23;78(13):1419-32.
8444 Tsai HH, Lin HW, Chen YL, et al. A review of potential harmful interactions between anticoagulant/antiplatelet agents and Chinese herbal medicines. *PLoS One.* 2013 May 9;8(5):e64255.
8445 Karkabounas S, Kostoula OK, Daskalou T, et al. Anticarcinogenic and antiplatelet effects of carvacrol. *Exp Oncol.* 2006 Jun;28(2):121-5.
8446 Langeveld WT, Veldhuizen EJ, Burt SA. Synergy between essential oil constituents and antibiotics. *Crit Rev Microbiol.* 2014 Feb;40(1);76-94.
8447 Jukic M, Politeo O, Maksimmovic M, et al. In vitro acetylcholinesterase inhibitory properties of thymol, carvacrol and their derivatives thymoquinone and thymohydroquinone. *Phytother Res.* 2007;21(3):259-61.
8448 Adiguzel A, Ozer H, Kilic H, et al. Screening of Antimicrobial Activity of Essential Oil and Methanol Extract of Satureja hortensis on foodborne Bacteria and Fungi. *Czech J Food Sci.* 2007 Jan;25(2):81-89.
8449 Mahboubi M, Kazempour N. Chemical composition and antimicrobial activity of Satureja hortensis and Trachyspermum copticum essential oil. *Iran J Microbiol.* 2011 Dec;3(4):194-200.
8450 Güllüce M, Sökmen M, Daferera D, et al. In vitro antibacterial, antifungal, and antioxidant activities of the essential oil and methanol extracts of herbal parts and callus cultures of Satureja hortensis L. *J Agric Food Chem.* 2003 Jul 2;51(14):3958-65.
8451 Cosentino S, Tuberoso CI, Pisano B, et al. In-vitro antimicrobial activity and chemical composition of Sardinian Thymus essential oils. *Lett Appl Microbiol.* 1999;29:130–135.
8452 Mihajilov-Krstev T, Radnovic D, Kitic D, et al. Antimicrobial activity of Satureja hortensis L. essential oil against pathogenic microbial strains. *Arch Biol Sci Belgrade.* 2010;62(1):159-66.
8453 Djenane D, Yangüela J, Amrouche T, et al. Chemical composition and antimicrobial effects of essential oils of Eucalyptus globulus, Myrtus communis and Satureja hortensis against Escherichia coli O157:H7 and Staphylococcus aureus in minced beef. *Food Sci Technol Int.* 2011 Dec;17(6):505-15.
8454 Alizadeh A, Zamani E, Sharaifi R, et al. Antifungal activity of some essential oils against toxigenic Aspergillus species. *Commun Agric Appl Biol Sci.* 2010;75(4):761-7.
8455 Shojaee-Aliabadi S, Hosseini H, Mohammadifar MA, et al. Characterization of antioxidant-antimicrobial κ-carrageenan films containing Satureja hortensis essential oil. *Int J Biol Macromol.* 2013 Jan;52:116-24.
8456 Saharkhiz MJ, Zomorodian K, Rezaei MR, et al. Influence of growth phase on the essential oil composition and antimicrobial activities of Satureja hortensis. Nat Prod Commun. 2011 Aug;6(8):1173-8.
8457 Dikbas N, Kotan R, Dadasoglu F, et al. Control of Aspergillus flavus with essential oil and methanol extract of Satureja hortensis. *Int J Food Microbiol.* 2008 May 31;124(2):179-82.
8458 Razzaghi-Abyaneh M, Shams-Ghahfarokhi M, Yoshinari T, Rezaee MB, et al. Inhibitory effects of Satureja hortensis L. essential oil on growth and aflatoxin production by Aspergillus parasiticus. *Int J Food Microbiol.* 2008 Apr 30;123(3):228-33.
8459 Anghel I, Grumezescu AM, Holban AM, et al. Biohybrid nanostructured iron oxide nanoparticles and Satureja hortensis to prevent fungal biofilm development. *Int J Mol Sci.* 2013 Sep 4;14(9):18110-23.
8460 Harmati M, Gyukity-Sebestyen E, Dobra G, et al. Binary mixture of Satureja hortensis and Origanum vulgare subsp. hirtum essential oils: in vivo therapeutic efficiency against Helicobacter pylori infection. *Helicobacter.* 2017 Apr;22(2).
8461 Samadi N, Masoum S, Mehrara B, et al. Application of linear multivariate calibration techniques to identify the peaks responsible for the antioxidant activity of Satureja hortensis L. and Oliveria decumbens Vent. essential oils by gas chromatography-mass spectrometry. *J Chromatogr B Analyt Technol Biomed Life Sci.* 2015 Sep 15;1001:75-81.
8462 Ceker S, Agar G, Alpsoy L, et al. Antagonistic effects of Satureja hortensis essential oil against AFB1 on human lymphocytes in vitro. *Tsitol Genet.* 2014 Sep-Oct;48(5):65-71.
8463 Mosaffa F, Behravan J, Karimi G, et al. Antigenotoxic effects of Satureja hortensis L. on rat lymphocytes exposed to oxidative stress. *Arch Pharm Res.* 2006 Feb;29(2):159-64.
8464 Najafian S, Zahedifar M. Antioxidant activity and essential oil composition of Satureja hortensis L. as influenced by sulfur fertilizer. *J Sci Food Agric.* 2015 Sep;95(12):2404-8.
8465 Dawidowicz AL, Olszowy M. Does antioxidant properties of the main component of essential oil reflect its antioxidant properties? The comparison of antioxidant properties of essential oils and their main components. *Nat Prod Res.* 2014;28(22):1952-63.
8466 Zeidán-Chuliá F, Keskin M, Könönen E, et al. Antibacterial and antigelatinolytic effects of Satureja hortensis L. essential oil on epithelial cells exposed to Fusobacterium nucleatum. *J Med Food.* 2015 Apr;18(4):503-6.
8467 Zeidán-Chuliá F, de Olivfeira B, Gursoy M, et al. MMP-REDOX/NO interplay in periodontitis and its inhibition with satureja hortensis L. Essential Oil. *Chem Biodiversity.* 2013 Apr;10(4):507-23.
8468 Gursoy UK, Gursoy M, Gursoy OV, et al. Anti-biofilm properties of Satureja hortensis L. essential oil against periodontal pathogens. *Anaerobe.* 2009 Aug;15(4):164-7.
8469 Sabzghabaee AM, Davoodi N, Ebadian B, et al. Clinical evaluation of the essential oil of "Satureja Hortensis" for the treatment of denture stomatitis. *Dent Res J (Isfahan).* 2012 Mar;9(2):198-202.
8470 Hajhashemi V, Zolfaghari B, Yousefi A. Antinociceptive and anti-inflammatory activities of Satureja hortensis seed essential oil, hydroalcoholic and polyphenolic extracts in animal models. *Med Princ Pract.* 2012;21(2):178-82.
8471 Hajhashemi V, Sadraei H, Ghannadi AR, et al. Antispasmodic and anti-diarrhoeal effect of Satureja hortensis L. essential oil. *J Ethnopharmacol.* 2000 Jul;71(1-2):187-92.
8472 Hajhashemi V, Sadraei H, Ghannadi AR, et al. Antispasmodic and anti-diarrhoeal effect of Satureja hortensis L. essential oil. *J Ethnopharmacol.* 2000 Jul;71(1-2):187-92.
8473 Yazdanpanah L, Mohamadi N. Antifungal activity of Satureja hortensis L. essential oil against Alternaria citri. *Eur J Exp Biol.* 2014;4(1):399-403.
8474 Gormez A, Bozari S, Yanmis D, et al. Chemical Composition and Antibacterial Activity of Essential Oils of Two Species of Lamiaceae against Phytopathogenic Bacteria. *Polish J Micribiol.* 2015;64(2):121-27.
8475 Kim JR, Haribalan P, Son BK, et al. Fumigant toxicity of plant essential oils against Camptomyia corticalis (Diptera: Cecidomyiidae). *J Econ Entomol.* 2012 Aug;105(4):1329-34.
8476 Sharifi A, Mohammadzadeh A, Zahraei Salehi T, et al. Antibacterial, antibiofilm and antiquorum sensing effects of Thymus daenensis and Satureja hortensis essential oils against Staphylococcus aureus isolates. *J Appl Microbiol.* 2018 Feb;124(2):379-388.
8477 Sharifi A, Ahmadi A, Mohammadzadeh A, et al. Streptococcus pneumoniae quorum sensing and biofilm formation are affected by Thymus daenensis, Satureja hortensis, and Origanum vulgare essential oils. *Acta Microbiol Immunol Hung.* 2018 Aug 1;65(3):345-359.
8478 Guo Y, Pizzol R, Gabbanini S, et al. Absolute Antioxidant Activity of Five Phenol-Rich Essential Oils. *Molecules.* 2021 Aug 29;26(17):5237.
8479 Štrbac F, Bosco A, Maurelli MP, et al. Anthelmintic Properties of Essential Oils to Control Gastrointestinal Nematodes in Sheep-In Vitro and In Vivo Studies. *Vet Sci.* 2022 Feb 19;9(2):93.
8480 Ghasemzadeh S, Messelink GJ, Avila GA, et al. Sublethal impacts of essential plant oils on biochemical and ecological parameters of the predatory mite Amblyseius swirskii. *Front Plant Sci.* 2022 Sep 16;13:923802.
8481 Sánchez-Quintero MJ, Delgado J, et al. Beneficial Effects of Essential Oils from the Mediterranean Diet on Gut Microbiota and Their Metabolites in Ischemic Heart Disease and Type-2 Diabetes Mellitus. *Nutrients.* 2022 Nov 3;14(21):4650.
8482 Mitic V, Stankov Jovanovic S, Ilic M, et al. Dittrichia graveolens (L.) Greuter Essential Oil: Chemical Composition, Multivariate Analysis, and Antimicrobial Activity. *Chem Biodiversity.* 2016 Jan;13(1):85-90.
8483 Aghel N, Mahmoudabadi AZ, Darvishi L. Volatile constituents and anti candida activity of the aerial parts essential oil of Dittrichia graveolens (L.) Greuter grown in Iran. *African J Pharm and Pharmacol.* 2011 Jun;5(6):772-75.
8484 Mahboubi M. Chemical composition, antimicrobial and antioxidant activities of Dittrichia graveolens (L.) Greuter essential oil. *Herba Polonica J.* 2011;57(3):20-31.
8485 Blanc MC, Muselli A, Bradesi P, et al. Chemical composition and variability of the essential oil of Inula graveolens from Corsica. *Flavour Frag J.* 2004 Jul-Aug;19(4):314-19.
8486 Ghosan MW, Chemali CB, Zaknoun FI, et al. Chemical Profile of the Dittrichia graveolens (Desf.) Greuter Essential Oil of Lebanese Origin. *J Essent Oil Res.* 2006 Jul-Aug;18:443-44.
8487 Beghidja N, Ikhlef F, Benayache S, et al. Composition of the essential oil of Inula graveolens Algerian origin species. *J Nat Prod Plant Resour.* 2014;4(1):1-3.
8488 Petropoulou A, Tzakou O, Verykokidou E. Volatile Constituents of Dittrichia graveolens (L.) Greuter from Greece. *J Essent Oil Res.* 2004;16(5):400-01.
8489 Kilic O. Chemical Composition of Two Inula sp. (Asteraceae) Species from Turkey. *Iğdır Univ J Inst Sci & Tech.* 2014;4(1):15-19.
8490 Craig JO. Poisoning by the volatile oils in childhood. *Arch Dis Child.* 1953;28:259-67.
8491 Melis K. Bochner A, Janssens G. Accidental nasal eucalyptol and menthol instillation. *Eur J Pediatr.* 1989 Aug;148(8)786-7.
8492 Day LM, Ozanne-Smith J, Parsons BJ, et al. Eucalyptus oil poisoning among young children: mechanisms of access and the potential prevention. *Aust N Z J Public Health.* 1997 Jun;21(3):297-302.
8493 Chandar SD, Prashanti M, Kumar CL, et al. Eucalyptus Oil-Induced Seizures in Children: A Single-Center Prospective Study. *Cureus.* 2021 Mar 25;13(3):e14109.
8494 Li YH, Sun XP, Zhang YQ, et al. The antithrombotic effect of borneol related to its anticoagulant property. *Am J Chin Med.* 2008;36(4):719-27.
8495 Sayyah M, Valizadeh J, Kamalinejad M. Anticonvulsant activity of the leaf oil of Laurus nobilis against pentylentetrazole- and maximal electroshock-induced seizure. *Phytomedicine.* 2002 Apr;9(3):212-16.
8496 Culic M, Kekovic G, Grbic G, et al. Wavelet and fractal analysis of rat brain activity in seizures evoked by camphor oil and 1,8-cineole. *Gen Physiol Biophys.* 2009;28 Sec No:33-40.
8497 Burkhard PR, Burkhardt K, Haenggeli CA, et al. Plant-induced seizures: reappearance of an old problem. *J Neurol.* 1999 Aug;246(8):667-70.
8498 Waldman N. Seizure caused by dermal application of over-the-counter eucalyptus oil head lice preparation. *Clin Toxicol (Phila).* 2011 Oct;49(8):750-1.
8499 Craig JO. Poisoning by the volatile oils in childhood. *Arch Dis Child.* 1953;28:259-67.
8500 Mathew T, Kamath V, Kumar RS, et al. Eucalyptus oil inhalation-induced seizure: A novel, underrecognized, preventable cause of acute symptomatic seizure. *Epilepsia Open.* 2017 Jul 4;2(3):350-354.
8501 Day LM, Ozanne-Smith J, Parsons BJ, et al. Eucalyptus oil poisoning among young children: mechanisms of access and the potential prevention. *Aust N Z J Public Health.* 1997 Jun;21(3):297-302.
8502 Myott E. Case of eucalyptus poisoning. *Brit M J.* 1906;1:558.
8503 Hindle RC. Eucalyptus oil ingestion. *N Z Med J.* 1994 May 11;107(977)185-6.

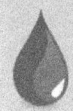

[8504] Tibballs J. Clinical effects and management of eucalyptus oil ingestion in infants and small children. *Med J Aust.* 1995 Aug;163(4):177-80.
[8505] Waldman W, Barwina M, Sein Anand J. Accidental ontoxication with eucalyptus oil—a case report. *Przeql Lek.* 2011;68(8):555-6.
[8506] Day LM, Ozanne-Smith J, Parsons BJ, et al. Eucalyptus oil poisoning among young children: mechanisms of access and the potential prevention. *Aust N Z J Public Health.* 1997 Jun;21(3):297-302.
[8507] De Vincenzi M, Silano M, De Vincenzi A, et al. Constituents of aromatic plants: eucalyptol. *Fitoterapia.* 2002 Jun;73(3):269-75.
[8508] Hiroi T, Miyazaki Y, Kobayashi Y, et al. Induction of hepatic P450s in rat by essential wood and leaf oils. *Xenobiotica.* 1995 May;25(5):457-67.
[8509] Chen JY, Wang JJ, Meng MR, et al. [Borneol is an inducer of rat hepatic CYP2D activity in vivo]. *Yao Xue Xue Bao.* 2015 Apr;50(4):459-63.
[8510] Zhang R1, Mi SQ, Wang NS. Effect of borneol on cytochrome P450 3A enzyme and midazolam pharmacokinetics in rats. *Eur J Drug Metab Pharmacokinet.* 2013 Sep;38(3):159-69.
[8511] Kim NH, Hyun SH, Jin CH, et al. Pretreatment with 1,8-cineole potentiates thioacetamide-induced hepatotoxicity and immunosuppression. *Arch Pharm Res.* 2004 Jul;27(7):781-9.
[8512] Chen JY, Huang XT, Wang JJ, et al. In vivo effect of borneol on rat hepatic CYP2B expression and activity. *Chem Biol Interact.* 2017 Jan 5;261:96-102.
[8513] Basak SS, Candan F. Effect of Laurus nobilis L. Essential Oil and its Main Components on α-glucosidase and Reactive Oxygen Species Scavenging Activity. *Iran J Pharm Res.* 2013 Spring;12(2):367-79.
[8514] Fathiazad F, Mazandarani M, Hamedeyazdan. Phytochemical analysis and antioxidant activity of Hyssopus officinalis L. from Iran. *Adv Pharm Bull.* 2011 Dec;1(2):63–67.
[8515] Miladinović DL, Ilić BS, Kocić BD, et al. In Vitro Trials of Dittrichia graveolens Essential Oil Combined with Antibiotics. *Nat Prod Commun.* 2016 Jun;11(6):865-8.
[8516] Jori A, Bianchetti A, Prestini PE, et al. Effect of eucalyptol (1,8-cineole) on the metabolism of other drugs in rats and in man. *Eur J Pharmacol.* 1970;9(3):362-66.
[8517] de Sousa DP, Raphael E, Brocksom U, et al. Sedative effect of monoterpene alcohols in mice: A preliminary screening. *Verlag der Zeitschrift fur Naturforschung.* 2007;62c:563-66.
[8518] Mitic V, Stankov Jovanovic S, Ilic M, et al. Dittrichia graveolens (L.) Greuter Essential Oil: Chemical Composition, Multivariate Analysis, and Antimicrobial Activity. *Chem Biodiversity.* 2016 Jan;13(1):85-90.
[8519] Guinoiseau E, Luciani A, Rossi PG, et al. Cellular effects induced by Inula graveolens and Santolina corsica essential oils on Staphylococcus aureus. *Eur J Clin Microbiol Infect Dis.* 2010 Jul;29(7):873-9.
[8520] Aghel N, Mahmoudabadi AZ, Darvishi L. Volatile constituents and anti candida activity of the aerial parts essential oil of Dittrichia graveolens (L.) Greuter grown in Iran. *African J Pharm and Pharmacol.* 2011 Jun;5(6):772-75.
[8521] Mahboubi M. Chemical composition, antimicrobial and antioxidant activities of Dittrichia graveolens (L.) Greuter essential oil. *Herba Polonica J.* 2011;57(3):20-31.
[8522] Miladinović DL, Ilić BS, Kocić BD, et al. In Vitro Trials of Dittrichia graveolens Essential Oil Combined with Antibiotics. *Nat Prod Commun.* 2016 Jun;11(6):865-8.
[8523] Mahboubi M. Chemical composition, antimicrobial and antioxidant activities of Dittrichia graveolens (L.) Greuter essential oil. *Herba Polonica J.* 2011;57(3):20-31.
[8524] Dohi S, Terasaki M, Makino M. Acetylcholinesterase inhibitory activity and chemical composition of commercial essential oils. *J Agric Food Chem.* 2009 May 27;57(10):4313-8.
[8525] Miladinović DL, Ilić BS, Kocić BD, et al. In Vitro Trials of Dittrichia graveolens Essential Oil Combined with Antibiotics. *Nat Prod Commun.* 2016 Jun;11(6):865-8.
[8526] Mitic V, Stankov Jovanovic V, et al. Dittrichia graveolens (L.) Greuter Essential Oil: Chemical Composition, Multivariate Analysis, and Antimicrobial Activity. *Chem Biodivers.* 2016 Jan;13(1):85-90.
[8527] Ben Mustapha M, Algethami FK, Elamin MR, et al. Chemical Composition, Toxicity and Repellency of Inula graveolens Essential Oils from Roots and Aerial Parts against Stored-Product Beetle Tribolium castaneum (Herbst). *Chem Biodivers.* 2023 Feb 19:e202200978.
[8528] El Bouzidi L, Abbad A, Hassani L, et al. Essential oil composition and antimicrobial activity of wild and cultivated Moroccan Achillea ageratum L.: a rare and threatened medicinal species. *Chem Biodivers.* 2012 Mar;9(3):598-605.
[8529] de la Puerta R, Saenz MT, Garcia MD. Antibacterial activity and composition of the volatile oil from Achillea ageratum L. *Phytother Res.* 1996;10:248-50.
[8530] Vavala E, Ragno R, Sivric S, et al. Antimycotic activity of Achillea ageratum L. essential oil. *Int J Essential Oil Ther.* 2009;3:101-05.
[8531] Burkhard PR, Burkhardt K, Haenggeli CA, et al. Plant-induced seizures: reappearance of an old problem. *J Neurol.* 1999 Aug;246(8):667-70.
[8532] Culic M, Kekovic G, Grbic G, et al. Wavelet and fractal analysis of rat brain activity in seizures evoked by
camphor essential oil and 1,8-cineole. *Gen Physiol Biophys.* 2009;Special Issue(28):33–40.
[8533] Mathew T, Kamath V, Kumar RS, et al. Eucalyptus oil inhalation–induced seizure: A novel, underrecognized, preventable cause of acute symptomatic seizure. *Epilepsia Open.* 2017 Sep;2(3):350–354.
[8534] Jori A, Bianchetti A, Prestini PE, et al. Effect of eucalyptol (1,8-cineole) on the metabolism of other drugs in rats and in man. *Eur J Pharmacol.* 1970;9(3):362-66.
[8535] de Sousa DP, Raphael E, Brocksom U, et al. Sedative effect of monoterpene alcohols in mice: A preliminary screening. *Verlag der Zeitschrift fur Naturforschung.* 2007;62c:563-66.
[8536] Lamborn LL. Modern soaps, candles and glycerin: A practical manual of modern methods of utilization of fats and oils in the manufacture of soaps and candles, and of the recovery of glycerin. Library of the University of Wisconsin.
[8537] Oyen LP, Dung NX. Plant resources of South-East Asia. 1999. Backhyus, Leiden.
[8538] Kim NH, Hyun SH, Jin CH, et al. Pretreatment with 1,8-cineole potentiates thioacetamide-induced hepatotoxicity and immunosuppression. *Arch Pharm Res.* 2004 Jul;27(7):781-9.
[8539] El Bouzidi L, Abbad A, Hassani L, et al. Essential oil composition and antimicrobial activity of wild and cultivated Moroccan Achillea ageratum L.: a rare and threatened medicinal species. *Chem Biodivers.* 2012 Mar;9(3):598-605.
[8540] de la Puerta R, Saenz MT, Garcia MD. Antibacterial activity and composition of the volatile oil from Achillea ageratum L. *Phytother Res.* 1996;10:248-50.
[8541] Vavala E, Ragno R, Sivric S, et al. Antimycotic activity of Achillea ageratum L. essential oil. *Int J Essential Oil Ther.* 2009;3:101-05.
[8542] de la Puerta R, Herrera MD. Spasmolytic action of the essential oil of Achillea ageratum L. in rats. *Phytother Res.* 1995;9:150-52.
[8543] Kasrati A, Alaoui Jamali C1, Bekkouche K, et al. Comparative evaluation of antioxidant and insecticidal properties of essential oils from five Moroccan aromatic herbs. *J Food Sci Technol.* 2015 Apr;52(4):2312-9.
[8544] Bilia AR, Santomauro F, Sacco C, et al. Essential Oil of Artemisia annua L.: An Extraordinary Component with Numerous Antimicrobial Properties. *Evid Based Complement Alternat Med.* 2014;2014:159819.
[8545] Mohammadreza V. Variation in the essential oil composition of Artemisia annua L. of different growth stages cultivated in Iran. *African J Plant Sci.* 2008 Feb;2(2):16-18.
[8546] Cavar S, Maksimovic M, Vidic D, et al. Chemical composition and antioxidant and antimicrobial activity of essential oil of Artemisia annua L. from Bosnia. *Industrial Crops Plants.* 2012 May;37(1):479-85.
[8547] Juteau F, Masotti V, Bessiere JM, et al. Antibacterial and antioxidant activities of Artemisia annua essential oil. *Fitoterapia.* 2002 Oct;73(6):532-35.
[8548] Tzenkova R, Kamenarska Z, Draganov A, et al. Composition of Artemisia Annua Essential Oil Obtained from Species Growing Wild in Bulgaria. *Biotechnology Biotechnological Equip.* 2010;24(2):1833-35.
[8549] Héthelyia EB, Csekoa IB, Grósza M, et al. Chemical Composition of the Artemisia annua Essential Oils from Hungary. *J Essent Oil Res.* 1995;7(1):45-48.
[8550] Cosge Senkal B, Kiralan M, Yaman C. The Effect of Different Harvest Stages on Chemical Composition and Antioxidant Capacity of Essential Oil from Artemisia annua L. *J Agric Sci.* 2015;21:71-77.
[8551] Radulović NS, Randjelović PJ, Stojanović NM, et al. Toxic essential oils—part II: chemical, toxicological, pharmacological and microbiological profiles of Artemisia annua L. volatiles. *Food Chem Toxicol.* 2013;58:37–49.
[8552] Verdian-Rizi MR, Sadat-Ebrahimi E, Hadjiakhoondi A, et al. Chemical composition and antimicrobial activity of Artemisia annua L. essential oil from Iran. *J Med Plants.* 2008;7(4):58–62.
[8553] Marinas IC, Oprea E, Chifiriuc MC, et al. Chemical Composition and Antipathogenic Activity of Artemisia annua Essential Oil from Romania. *Chem Biodivers.* 2015 Oct;12(10):1554-64.
[8554] Khine H, Weiss D, Graber N, et al. A cluster of children with seizures caused by camphor poisoning. *Pediatrics.* 2009 May;123(5):1269-72.
[8555] Michiels EA, Mazor SS. Toddler with seizures due to ingesting camphor at an Indian celebration. *Pediatr Emerg Care.* 2010 Aug;26(8):574-75.
[8556] Koren G. Medications which can kill a toddler with one tablet or teaspoonful. *J toxicol Clin toxicol.* 1993;31(3):407- 13.
[8557] Craig JO. Poisoning by the volatile oils in childhood. *Arch Dis Child.* 1953;28:259-67.
[8558] Melis K. Bochner A, Janssens G. Accidental nasal eucalyptol and menthol instillation. *Eur J Pediatr.* 1989 Aug;148(8)786-7.
[8559] Day LM, Ozanne-Smith J, Parsons BJ, et al. Eucalyptus oil poisoning among young children: mechanisms of access and the potential prevention. *Aust N Z J Public Health.* 1997 Jun;21(3):297-302.
[8560] Chandar SD, Prashanti M, Kumar CL, et al. Eucalyptus Oil-Induced Seizures in Children: A Single-Center Prospective Study. *Cureus.* 2021 Mar 25;13(3):e14109.
[8561] Rabl W, Katzgraber F, Steinlechner M. Camphor ingestion for abortion (case report). *Forensic Sci Int.* 1997 Sep 19;89(1-2):137-40.
[8562] Flaman Z, Pellechia-Clarke S, Bailey B, et al. Unintentional exposure of young children to camphor and eucalyptus oils. *Paediatr Child Health.* 2001 Feb;6(2):80-83.
[8563] Burkhard PR, Burkhardt K, Haenggeli CA, et al. Plant-induced seizures: reappearance of an old problem. *J Neurol.* 1999 Aug;246(8):667-70.
[8564] Narayan S, Singh N. Camphor poisoning-An unusual cause of seizure. *Med J Armed Forces India.* 2012 Jul;68(3):252-53.
[8565] Chanaranaj KJ, G MV, S M. Camphor poisoning in a child. *Natl Med J India.* 2013 Jan-Feb;26(1):60.
[8566] Manoguerra AS, Erdman AR, Wax PM, et al. Camphor poisoning: an evidence-based practice guideline for out-of- hospital management. *Clin Toxicol (Phila).*2006;44(4):357-70.
[8567] Gibson DE, Moore GP, Pfaff JA. Camphor ingestion. *Am J Emerg Med.* 1989 Jan;7(1):41-43.
[8568] Koppel C, Martends F, Schirop T, et al. Hemoperfusion in acute camphor poisoning. *Intensive Care Med.* 1988;14(4):431-33.
[8569] Perazzo FF, Carvalho JC, Carvalho JE, et al. Central properties of the essential oil and the crude ethanol extract from aerial parts of Artemisia annua L. *Pharmacol Res.* 2003 Nov;48(5):497-502.
[8570] Olowe SA, Ransome-Kuti O. The risk of jaundice in glucose-6-phosphate dehydrogenase deficient babies exposed to menthol. *Acta Paediatr Scand.* 1980 May;69(3):341-5.
[8571] Dillon Remy M, Manning Alleyne P, Bratt DE, et al. Neonatal jaundice at Port-of-Spain General Hospital abstract. *West Indian Med J.* 1987;36(Suppl):28.
[8572] Uc A, Bishop WP, Sanders KD. Camphor hepatotoxicity. *South Med J.* 2000;93:596-98.
[8573] Yu Z, Wang B, Yang F, et al. Chemical Composition and Anti-acetyl cholinesterase Activity of Flower Essential Oils of Artemisia annua at Different Flowering Stage. *Iran J Pharm Res.* 2011 Spring;10(2):265-71.
[8574] Perazzo FF, Carvalho JC, Carvalho JE, et al. Central properties of the essential oil and the crude ethanol extract from aerial parts of Artemisia annua L. *Pharmacol Res.* 2003 Nov;48(5):497-502.

8575 Covington TR, et al. Handbook of Nonprescription Drugs. 11th ed. Washington, D.C.: American Pharmaceutical Association. 1996.

8576 Li Y, Li MY, Wang L, et al. [Induction of apoptosis of cultured hepatocarcinoma cell by essential oil of Artemisia Annul L]. *Sichuan Da Xue Xue Bao Yi Xue Ban.* 2004 May;35(3):337-9.

8577 Bilia AR, Santomauro F, Sacco C, et al. Essential Oil of Artemisia annua L.: An Extraordinary Component with Numerous Antimicrobial Properties. *Evid Based Complement Alternat Med.* 2014;2014:159819.

8578 Cavar S, Maksimovic M, Vidic D, et al. Chemical composition and antioxidant and antimicrobial activity of essential oil of Artemisia annua L. from Bosnia. *Industrial Crops Plants.* 2012 May;37(1):479-85.

8579 Juteau F, Masotti V, Bessiere JM, et al. Antibacterial and antioxidant activities of Artemisia annua essential oil. *Fitoterapia.* 2002 Oct;73(6):532-35.

8580 Li Y, Hu HB, Zheng XD, et al. Composition and antimicrobial activity of essential oil from the aerial part of Artemisia annua. *J Med Plant Res.* 2011;5(16):3629–33.

8581 Verdian-Rizi MR, Sadat-Ebrahimi E, Hadjiakhoondi A, et al. Chemical composition and antimicrobial activity of Artemisia annua L. essential oil from Iran. *J Med Plants.* 2008;7(4):58–62.

8582 Massiha A, Majid M, Pahlaviani K, et al. Antibacterial activity of essential oils and plant extracts of artemisia (Artemisia annua L.) in vitro. *Zahedan J Res Med Sci.* 2013;15:14–18.

8583 Bedini S, Flamini G, Cosci F, et al. Artemisia spp. essential oils against the disease-carrying blowfly Calliphora vomitoria. *Parasit Vectors.* 2017 Feb 13;10(1):80.

8584 Viuda-Martos M, El Gendy AENGS, Sendra E, et al. Chemical composition and antioxidant and anti-Listeria activities of essential oils obtained from some Egyptian plants. *J Agric Food Chem.* 2010;58(16):9063–70.

8585 Marinas IC, Oprea E, Chifiriuc MC, et al. Chemical Composition and Antipathogenic Activity of Artemisia annua Essential Oil from Romania. *Chem Biodivers.* 2015 Oct;12(10):1554-64.

8586 Santomauro F, Donato R, Sacco C, et al. Vapour and Liquid-Phase Artemisia annua Essential Oil Activities against Several Clinical Strains of Candida. *Planta Med.* 2016;82(11-12):1016-20.

8587 Radulović NS, Randjelović PJ, Stojanović NM, et al. Toxic essential oils—part II: chemical, toxicological, pharmacological and microbiological profiles of Artemisia annua L. volatiles. *Food Chem Toxicol.* 2013;58:37–49.

8588 Radulović NS, Randjelović PJ, Stojanović NM, et al. Toxic essential oils—part II: chemical, toxicological, pharmacological and microbiological profiles of Artemisia annua L. volatiles. *Food Chem Toxicol.* 2013;58:37–49.

8589 Cavar S, Maksimovic M, Vidic D, et al. Chemical composition and antioxidant and antimicrobial activity of essential oil of Artemisia annua L. from Bosnia. *Industrial Crops Plants.* 2012 May;37(1):479-85.

8590 Juteau F, Masotti V, Bessiere JM, et al. Antibacterial and antioxidant activities of Artemisia annua essential oil. *Fitoterapia.* 2002 Oct;73(6):532-35.

8591 Viuda-Martos M, El Gendy AENGS, Sendra E, et al. Chemical composition and antioxidant and anti-Listeria activities of essential oils obtained from some Egyptian plants. *J Agric Food Chem.* 2010;58(16):9063–70.

8592 Islamuddin M, Chouhan G, Tyagi M, et al. Leishmanicidal activities of Artemisia annua leaf essential oil against Visceral Leishmaniasis. *Front Microbiol.* 2014 Nov 25;5:626.

8593 Yu Z, Wang B, Yang F, et al. Chemical Composition and Anti-acetyl cholinesterase Activity of Flower Essential Oils of Artemisia annua at Different Flowering Stage. *Iran J Pharm Res.* 2011 Spring;10(2):265-71.

8594 Zhang N, Tang L, Hu W, et al. Insecticidal, fumigant, and repellent activities of sweet wormwood oil and its individual components against red imported fire ant workers (Hymenoptera: Formicidae). *J Insect Sci.* 2014 Jan 1;14.

8595 Pirali-Kheirabadi Kh, Teixeira da Silva J. In-Vitro Assessment of the Acaricidal Properties of Artemisia annua and Zataria multiflora Essential Oils to Control Cattle Ticks. *Iran J Parasitol.* 2011 Mar;6(1):58-65.

8596 Palacios SM, Bertoni A, Rossi Y, et al. Insecticidal activity of essential oils from native medicinal plants of Central Argentina against the house fly, Musca domestica (L.). *Parasitol Res.* 2009 Dec;106(1):207-12.

8597 Bedini S, Flamini G, Cosci F, et al. Artemisia spp. essential oils against the disease-carrying blowfly Calliphora vomitoria. *Parasit Vectors.* 2017 Feb 13;10(1):80.

8598 Santomauro F, Donato R, Pini G, et al. Liquid and Vapor-Phase Activity of Artemisia annua Essential Oil against Pathogenic Malassezia spp. *Planta Med.* 2018 Feb;84(3):160-167.

8599 Zhigzhitzhapova SV, Dylenova EP, Gulyaev SM, et al. Composition and antioxidant activity of the essential oil of Artemisia annua L. *Nat Prod Res.* 2019 Jan 19:1-4.

8600 Liu H, Guo SS, Lu L, et al. Essential oil from Artemisia annua aerial parts: composition and repellent activity against two storage pests. *Nat Prod Res.* 2019 Apr 8:1-4.

8601 Das S, Voros-Horvath B, Bencsik T, et al. Antimicrobial Activity of Different Artemisia Essential Oil Formulations. *Molecules.* 2020 May 21;25(10):E2390.

8602 Golbarg H, Moghaddam MJM. Antibacterial Potency of Medicinal Plants including Artemisia annua and Oxalis corniculata against Multi-Drug Resistance E. coil. *Biomed Res Int.* 2021 Jun 1;2021:9981915.

8603 Mojarab-Mahboubkar M, Sendi JJ, Mahmoodi N. The sweet wormwood essential oil and its two major constituents are promising for a safe control measure against fall webworm. *Pestic Biochem Physiol.* 2022 Jun;184:105124.

8604 Chebbac K, Benziane Ouaritini Z, El Moussaoui A, et al. Antimicrobial and Antioxidant Properties of Chemically Analyzed Essential Oil of Artemisia annua L. (Asteraceae) Native to Mediterranean Area. *Life (Basel).* 2023 Mar 16;13(3):807.

8605 Moghaddam M, Omnidbiagi R, Sefidkon F. Chemical Composition of the Essential Oil of Tagetes minuta L. *J Essent Oil Res.* 2007 Jan;19(1):3-4.

8606 Héthélyi E, Dános B, Tétényi P, et al. GC-MS analysis of the essential oils of four tagetes species and the anti-microbial activity of Tagetes minuta. *Flavour Frag J.* 1986 Sep;1(4-5):169-73.

8607 Senatore F, Napolitano F, Mohamed M, et al. Antibacterial activity of Tagetes minuta L. (Asteraceae) essential oil with different chemical composition. *Flavour Frag J.* 2004 Nov;19(6):574-78.

8608 Moshen Taheri S, Gholami H, Kavoosi G, et al. Chemical composition, antioxidant, antimicrobial and cytotoxic activities of Tagetes minuta and Ocimum basilicum essential oils. *Food Sci Nutr.* 2014 Mar;2(2):146-55.

8609 Ali NA, Sharopov FS, Al-Kaf AG, et al. Composition of essential oil from Tagetes minuta and its cytotoxic, antioxidant and antimicrobial activities. *Nat Prod Commun.* 2014 Feb;9(2):265-8.

8610 Garcia MV, Matias J, Barros JC, et al. Chemical identification of Tagetes minuta Linnaeus (Asteraceae) essential oil and its acaricidal effect on ticks. *Rev Bras Parasitol Vet Jaboticabal.* 2012;21(4):405-11.

8611 Meshkataksadat MH, Safaei-Ghomi J, Moharramipour S, et al. Chemical characterization of volatile components of Tagetes minuta L. cultivated in South West of Iran by nano scale injection. *Digest J Nanomaterials Biostructures.* 2010 Mar;5(1):101-106.

8612 Scrivanti LR, Zunino MP, Zygadlo A. Tagetes minuta L. and Schinus arera L. essential oils as allelopathic agents. Available at: http://www.efn.uncor.edu/departamentos/divbioeco/divveg2/publicaciones/text%20fulltagetes%20minuta.pdf.

8613 Chamorro ER, Ballerini G, Sequeira AF, et al. Chemical composition of essential oil from Tagetes minuta L. leaves and flowers. *J Argentine Chem Soc.* 2008;96(1-2):80-86.

8614 Ruiz C, Cachay M, Dominguez M, et al. Chemical composition, Antioxidant and Mosquito larvicidal activities of essential oils from Tagetes filifolia, Tagetes minuta and Tagetes elliptica from Perú. *Planta Med.* 2011;77:PE30.

8615 Singh G, Singh OP, De Lampasona MP, et al. Studies on essential oils. Part 35: chemical and biocidal investigations on Tagetes erecta leaf volatile oil. *Flavour Frag J.* 2003 Jan;18(1):62-65.

8616 Sefidkon F, Salehyar S, Mirza M, et al. The essential oil of Tagetes erecta L. occurring in Iran. *Flavour Frag J.* 2004;19:579-81.

8617 Krishna A, Kumar S. Composition of the Essential Oils of the Leaves and Flowers of Tagetes erecta L. *J Essent Oil Res.* 2004 Nov-Dec;16:520-22.

8618 de Oliveira PF, Alves JM, Damasceno JL, et al. Cytotoxicity screening of essential oils in cancer cell lines. *Rev Bras Farmacog.* 2015 Mar-Apr;25(2):ISSN 1981-528X.

8619 Tripathi B, Bhatia R, Walia S, et al. Chemical composition and evaluation of tagetes erecta (var. Pusa narangi genda) essential oil for its antioxidant and antimicrobial activity. *Biopestic Int.* 2012 Dec;8(2):1-9.

8620 Armas K, Rojas J, Rojas L, et al. Comparative study of the chemical composition of essential oils of five Tagetes species collected in Venezuela. *Nat Prod Commun.* 2012 Sep;7(9):1225-6.

8621 Politi FA, de Souza-Moreira TM, Rodrigues ER, et al. Chemical characterization and acaricide potential of essential oil from aerial parts of Tagetes patula L. (Asteraceae) against engorged adult females of Rhipicephalus sanguineus (Latreille, 1806). *Parasitol Res.* 2013 Jun;112(6):2261-8.

8622 Romagnoli C1, Bruni R, Andreotti E, et al. Chemical characterization and antifungal activity of essential oil of capitula from wild Indian Tagetes patula L. *Protoplasma.* 2005 Apr;225(1-2):57-65.

8623 Dharmagadda VS, Naik SN, Mittal PK, et al. Larvicidal activity of Tagetes patula essential oil against three mosquito species. *Bioresour Technol.* 2005 Jul;96(11):1235-40.

8624 Marques MM, Morais SM, Vieira IG, et al. Larvicidal activity of Tagetes erecta against Aedes aegypti. *J Am Mosq Control Assoc.* 2011 Jun;27(2):156-8.

8625 Scientific Committee on Consumer Safety. Opinion on the fragrance ingredients Tagetes minuta and T. patula extracts and essential oils (phototoxicity only). Available at: http://ec.europa.eu/health/scientific_committees/consumer_safety/docs/sccs_o_172.pdf.

8626 Marin RH, Garcia DA, Martijena ID, et al. Anxiogenic-like effects of Tagetes minuta L essential oil on T-maze and tonic immobility behaviour in domestic chicks. *Fundam Clin Pharmacol.* 1998;12(4):426-32.

8627 García DA, Perillo MA, Zygadlo JA, et al. The essential oil from Tagetes minuta L. modulates the binding of [3H]flunitrazepam to crude membranes from chick brain. *Lipids.* 1995 Dec;30(12):1105-10.

8628 Shahverdi AR, Mirzaie S, Rafii F, et al. Monoterpenes as nitrofurantoin resistance modulating agents: minimal structural requirements, molecular dynamics simulations, and the effect of piperitone on the emergence of nitrofurantoin resistance in Enterobacteriaceae. *J Mol Model.* 2015 Aug;21(8):198.

8629 Shahverdi AR, Rafii F, Tavassoli F, et al. Piperitone from Mentha longifolia var. chorodictya Rech F. reduces the nitrofurantoin resistance of strains of enterobacteriaceae. *Phytother Res.* 2004 Nov;18(11):911-4.

8630 Nguyen LT, Mysliveckova Z, Szotakova B, et al. The inhibitory effects of β-caryophyllene, β-caryophyllene oxide and α-humulene on the activities of the main drug-metabolizing enzymes in rat and human liver in vitro. *Chem-Biol Interactoins.* 2017 Dec 25;278:123-8.

8631 Moshen Taheri S, Gholami H, Kavoosi G, et al. Chemical composition, antioxidant, antimicrobial and cytotoxic activities of Tagetes minuta and Ocimum basilicum essential oils. *Food Sci Nutr.* 2014 Mar;2(2):146-55.

8632 Ali NA, Sharopov FS, Al-Kaf AG, et al. Composition of essential oil from Tagetes minuta and its cytotoxic, antioxidant and antimicrobial activities. *Nat Prod Commun.* 2014 Feb;9(2):265-8.

8633 de Oliveira PF, Alves JM, Damasceno JL, et al. Cytotoxicity screening of essential oils in cancer cell lines. *Rev Bras Farmacog.* 2015 Mar-Apr;25(2):ISSN 1981-528X.

8634 Moshen Taheri S, Gholami H, Kavoosi G, et al. Chemical composition, antioxidant, antimicrobial and cytotoxic activities of Tagetes minuta and Ocimum basilicum essential oils. *Food Sci Nutr.* 2014 Mar;2(2):146-55.

8635 Ali NA, Sharopov FS, Al-Kaf AG, et al. Composition of essential oil from Tagetes minuta and its cytotoxic, antioxidant and antimicrobial activities. *Nat Prod Commun.* 2014 Feb;9(2):265-8.

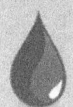

[8636] Ruiz C, Cachay M, Dominguez M, et al. Chemical composition, Antioxidant and Mosquito larvicidal activities of essential oils from Tagetes filifolia, Tagetes minuta and Tagetes elliptica from Perú. *Planta Med.* 2011;77:PE30.
[8637] Héthélyi E, Dános B, Tétényi P, et al. GC-MS analysis of the essential oils of four tagetes species and the anti-microbial activity of Tagetes minuta. *Flavour Frag J.* 1986 Sep;1(4-5):169-73.
[8638] Senatore F, Napolitano F, Mohamed M, et al. Antibacterial activity of Tagetes minuta L. (Asteraceae) essential oil with different chemical composition. *Flavour Frag J.* 2004 Nov;19(6):574-78.
[8639] Moshen Taheri S, Gholami H, Kavoosi G, et al. Chemical composition, antioxidant, antimicrobial and cytotoxic activities of Tagetes minuta and Ocimum basilicum essential oils. *Food Sci Nutr.* 2014 Mar;2(2):146-55.
[8640] Tripathi B, Bhatia R, Walia S, et al. Chemical composition and evaluation of tagetes erecta (var. Pusa narangi genda) essential oil for its antioxidant and antimicrobial activity. *Biopestic Int.* 2012 Dec;8(2):1-9.
[8641] Ali NA, Sharopov FS, Al-Kaf AG, et al. Composition of essential oil from Tagetes minuta and its cytotoxic, antioxidant and antimicrobial activities. *Nat Prod Commun.* 2014 Feb;9(2):265-8.
[8642] Singh G, Singh OP, De Lampasona MP, et al. Studies on essential oils. Part 35: chemical and biocidal investigations on Tagetes erecta leaf volatile oil. *Flavour Frag J.* 2003 Jan;18(1):62-65.
[8643] Tripathi B, Bhatia R, Walia S, et al. Chemical composition and evaluation of tagetes erecta (var. Pusa narangi genda) essential oil for its antioxidant and antimicrobial activity. *Biopestic Int.* 2012 Dec;8(2):1-9.
[8644] Bii CC, Siboe GM, Mibey RK. Plant essential oils with promising antifungal activity. *East Afr Med J.* 2000 Jun;77(6):319-22.
[8645] Romagnoli C1, Bruni R, Andreotti E, et al. Chemical characterization and antifungal activity of essential oil of capitula from wild Indian Tagetes patula L. *Protoplasma.* 2005 Apr;225(1-2):57-65.
[8646] Karimian P, Kavoosi G1, Amirghofran Z. Anti-oxidative and anti-inflammatory effects of Tagetes minuta essential oil in activated macrophages. *Asian Pac J Trop Biomed.* 2014 Mar;4(3):219-27.
[8647] Macedo IT, de Oliveira LM1, Camurça-Vasconcelos AL, et al. In vitro effects of Coriandrum sativum, Tagetes minuta, Alpinia zerumbet and Lantana camara essential oils on Haemonchus contortus. *Rev Bras Parasitol Vet.* 2013 Oct-Dec;22(4):463-9.
[8648] Garcia MV, Matias J, Barros JC, et al. Chemical identification of Tagetes minuta Linnaeus (Asteraceae) essential oil and its acaricidal effect on ticks. *Rev Bras Parasitol Vet Jaboticabal.* 2012;21(4):405-11.
[8649] Andreotti R, Garcia MV, Cunha RC, et al. Protective action of Tagetes minuta (Asteraceae) essential oil in the control of Rhipicephalus microplus (Canestrini, 1887) (Acari: Ixodidae) in a cattle pen trial. *Vet Parasitol.* 2013 Oct 18;197(1-2):341-5.
[8650] Ruiz C, Cachay M, Dominguez M, et al. Chemical composition, Antioxidant and Mosquito larvicidal activities of essential oils from Tagetes filifolia, Tagetes minuta and Tagetes elliptica from Perú. *Planta Med.* 2011;77:PE30.
[8651] Gillij YG, Gleiser RM, Zygadlo JA. Mosquito repellent activity of essential oils of aromatic plants growing in Argentina. *Bioresour Technol.* 2008 May;99(7):2507-15.
[8652] Singh G, Singh OP, De Lampasona MP, et al. Studies on essential oils. Part 35: chemical and biocidal investigations on Tagetes erecta leaf volatile oil. *Flavour Frag J.* 2003 Jan;18(1):62-65.
[8653] Chamorro ER, Ballerini G, Sequeira AF, et al. Chemical composition of essential oil from Tagetes minuta L. leaves and flowers. *J Argentine Chem Soc.* 2008;96(1-2):80-86.
[8654] Nchu F, Magano SR, Eloff JN. In vitro anti-tick properties of the essential oil of Tagetes minuta L. (Asteraceae) on Hyalomma rufipes (Acari: Ixodidae). *Onderstepoort J Vet Res.* 2012 Mar 30;79(1):E1-5.
[8655] Gillij YG, Gleiser RM, Zygadlo JA. Mosquito repellent activity of essential oils of aromatic plants growing in Argentina. *Bioresour Technol.* 2008 May;99(7):2507-15.
[8656] Gillij YG, Gleiser RM, Zygadlo JA. Mosquito repellent activity of essential oils of aromatic plants growing in Argentina. *Bioresour Technol.* 2008 May;99(7):2507-15.
[8657] Politi FA, de Souza-Moreira TM, Rodrigues ER, et al. Chemical characterization and acaricide potential of essential oil from aerial parts of Tagetes patula L. (Asteraceae) against engorged adult females of Rhipicephalus sanguineus (Latreille, 1806). *Parasitol Res.* 2013 Jun;112(6):2261-8.
[8658] Dharmagadda VS, Naik SN, Mittal PK, et al. Larvicidal activity of Tagetes patula essential oil against three mosquito species. *Bioresour Technol.* 2005 Jul;96(11):1235-40.
[8659] Marques MM, Morais SM, Vieira IG, et al. Larvicidal activity of Tagetes erecta against Aedes aegypti. *J Am Mosq Control Assoc.* 2011 Jun;27(2):156-8.
[8660] da Silva EM, Rodrigues VD, Jorge JO, et al. Efficacy of Tagetes minuta (Asteraceae) essential oil against Rhipicephalus sanguineus (Acari: Ixodidae) on infested dogs and in vitro. *Exp Appl Acarol.* 2016 Dec;70(4):483-489.
[8661] Politi FA, Nascimento JD, da Silva AA, et al. Insecticidal activity of an essential oil of Tagetes patula L. (Asteraceae) on common bed bug Cimex lectularius L. and molecular docking of major compounds at the catalytic site of ClAChE1. *Parasitol Res.* 2017;116:415-24.
[8662] Kimutai A, Ngeiywa M, Mulaa M, et al. Repellent effects of the essential oils of Cymbopogon citratus and Tagetes minuta on the sandfly, Phlebotomus duboscqi. *BMC Res Notes.* 2017;10:98.
[8663] Marin RH, Garcia DA, Martijena ID, et al. Anxiogenic-like effects of Tagetes minuta L essential oil on T-maze and tonic immobility behaviour in domestic chicks. *Fundam Clin Pharmacol.* 1998;12(4):426-32.
[8664] García DA, Perillo MA, Zygadlo JA, et al. The essential oil from Tagetes minuta L. modulates the binding of [3H]flunitrazepam to crude membranes from chick brain. *Lipids.* 1995 Dec;30(12):1105-10.
[8665] Politi FAS, Souza AA Júnior, Fantatto RR, et al. Chemical composition and in vitro anthelmintic activity of extracts of Tagetes patula against a multidrug-resistant isolate of Haemonchus contortus. *Chem Biodivers.* 2018 Feb;15(2).
[8666] Igwaran A, Iweriebor BC, Ofuzim Okoh S, et al. Chemical constituents, antibacterial and antioxidant properties of the essential oil flower of Tagetes minuta grown in Cala community Eastern Cape, South Africa. *BMC Complement Altern Med.* 2017 Jul 5;17(1):351.
[8667] Chaaban A, Santos VMCS, Martins CEN, et al. Tissue damage and cytotoxic effects of Tagetes minuta essential oil against Lucilia cuprina. *Exp Parasitol.* 2019 Mar;198:46-52.
[8668] Politi FAS, Fantatto RR, da Silva AA, et al. Evaluation of Tagetes patula (Asteraceae) as an ecological alternative in the search for natural control of the cattle tick Rhipicephalus (Boophilus) microplus (Acari: Ixodidae). *Exp Appl Acarol.* 2019 Apr;77(4):601-618.
[8669] Chaaban A, Carvalho Silva Santos VM, Nogueira Martins CE, et al. Effects of Tagetes minuta essencial oil on Lucilia cuprina third instar larvae. *Data Brief.* 2019 Jun 14;25:104008.
[8670] Cui G, Wei F, Wei M, et al. Modulatory effect of Tagetes erecta flowers essential oils via Nrf2/HO-1/NF-κB/p65 axis mediated suppression of N-methyl-N'nitro-N-nitroguanidine (MNNG) induced gastric cancer in rats. *Mol Cell Biochem.* 2021 Jan 4. Online ahead of print.
[8671] Czerniewicz P, Chrzanowski G. The Effect of Santolina chamaecyparissus and Tagetes patula Essential Oils on Biochemical Markers of Oxidative Stress in Aphids. *Insects.* 2021 Apr 17;12(4):360.
[8672] Birmann PT, Casaril AM, Zugno GP, et al. Flower essential oil of Tagetes minuta mitigates oxidative stress and restores BDNF-Akt/ERK2 signaling attenuating inflammation- and stress-induced depressive-like behavior in mice. *Brain Res.* 2022 Feb 24:147845.
[8673] Aati HY, Emam M, Al-Qahtani J, et al. Chemical Composition of Tagetes patula Flowers Essential Oil and Hepato-Therapeutic Effect against Carbon Tetrachloride-Induced Toxicity (In-Vivo). *Molecules.* 2022 Oct 25;27(21):7242.
[8674] Denett GO, Comelli NC, Rodriguez MR, et al. Chemical composition and insecticidal activity of essential oils from cultivated and native aromatic plants of Argentina against Carpophilus dimidiatus (Fabricius) (Nitidulidae) and Oryzaephilus mercator (L.) (Silvanidae). *Nat Prod Res.* 2023 Jan 9:1-5.
[8675] Mir SR, Ali M, Kapoor R. Chemical composition of essential oil of Cinnamomum tamala Nees et Eberm. Leaves. *Flavour Frag J.* 2004 Mar-Apr;19(2):112-14.
[8676] Ahmed A, Choudhary MI, Farooq A, et al. Essential oil constituents of the spice Cinnamomum tamala (HAM.) Nees & Eberm. *Flavour Frag J.* 2000;15:388-90.
[8677] Srivastava B, Sagar A, Dubey N. Evaluation of Cinnamomum tamala oil and its phenylpropanoid eugenol for their antifungal and antiaflatoxigenic activity. *Food Anal Methods.* 2011;4:347-56.
[8678] Joshi S, Padalia EC, Bisht DS, et al. Terpenoid diversity in the leaf essential oils of Himalayan Lauraceae species. *Chem & Biodiversity.* 2009 Sep;6(9):1364-73.
[8679] Rana VS, Langoljam RD, Verdeguer M, et al. Chemical variability in the essential oil Cinnamomum tamala leaves from India. *Nat Prod Res.* 2012 Jul;26(14):1335-57.
[8680] Kapoor IPS, Singh B, Singh G, et al. Chemistry, antimicrobial and antioxidant potentials of Cinnamomum tamala Nees & Eberm. (Tejpat) essential oil and oleoresins. *Nat Prod Radiance.* 2009;8(2):106-16.
[8681] Lohani H, Singh SK, Bhandari U, et al. Chemical polymorphism in Cinnamomum tamala (Buch.-Ham.) Nees. & Eberm. growing in Uttarakhand Himalaya (India). *J Chem Pharm Res.* 2015;7(8):67-71.
[8682] Chowdhury JU, Shaha GC, Begum F, et al. Essential oil composition from fresh and dried leaves of C. tamala. *Bangladesh J Sci Ind Res.* 2013;48(2):151-54.
[8683] Kumar S, Vasudeva N, Sharma S. Pharmacological and pharmacognostical aspects of Cinnamomum tamala Nees & Eberm. *J Pharm Res.* 2012;5(1):480-84.
[8684] Nath SC, Hazarika AK, Singh RS. Essential oil of leaves of Cinnamomum tamala Nees & Eberm. From North East India. *J Spices Aromatic Crops.* 1994;3(1):33-35.
[8685] Domaracky M, Rehak P, Juhas S, et al. Effects of selected plant essential oils on the growth and development of mouse preimplantation embryos in vivo. *Physiol Res.* 2007;56(1):97-104.
[8686] Forschmidt P. Teratogenic activity of flavor additives. *Teratology.* 1979;19:26A.
[8687] Mantovani A, Stazi AV, Macri C, et al. Pre-natal (segment II) toxicity study of cinnamic aldehyde in the Sprague- Dawley rat. *Food Chem Toxicol.* 1989;27:781-86.
[8688] Domaracky M, Rehak P, Juhas S, et al. Effects of selected plant essential oils on the growth and development of mouse preimplantation embryos in vivo. *Physiol Res.* 2007;56(1):97-104.
[8689] Vrskova D, Modra H. Evaluation of the developmental toxicity of 2-phenoxyethanol and clove oil anesthetics using the Frog Embryo Teratogenesis Assay: Xenopus (FETAX). *Veterinarami Medicina.* 2012;57(5):245-50.
[8690] Amini A, Cheraghi E, Safaee MR, et al. The role of eugenol in the reduction of teratogenic effects of retinoic acid on skeletal morphology of mice embryo. *Yakhteh Medical Journal.* 2003;4:195-200.
[8691] Chen R, Chen J, Cheng S, et al. Assessment of embryotoxicity of constituents in cosmetics by the embryonic stem cell tes. *Toxicol Mech Methods.* 2010 Mar;20(3):112-18.
[8692] Huang J, Wang S, Luo X, et al. Cinnamaldehyde reduction of platelet aggregation and thrombosis in rodents. *Thromb Res.* 2007;119(3):337-42.
[8693] Kim SY, Koo YK, Koo JY, et al. Platelet anti-aggregation activities of constituents from Cinnamomum cassia. *J Med Food.* 2010 Oct;13(5):1069-74.
[8694] Takenaga M, Hirai A, Terano T, et al. In vitro effect of cinnamic aldehyde, a main component of Cinnamomi Cortex, on human platelet aggregation and arachidonic acid metabolism. *J Pharmacobiodyn.* 1987 May;10(5):201-208.
[8695] Chen SJ, Wang MH, Chen IJ. Antiplatelet and calcium inhibitory properties of eugenol and sodium eugenol acetate. *Gen Pharmacol.* 1996 Jun;27(4):629-33.

8696 Tognolini M, Barocelli E, Ballabeni V, et al. Comparative screening of plant essential oils; phenylpropanoid moiety as basic core for antiplatelet activity. *Life Sci.* 2006 Feb 23;78(13):1419-32.

8697 Heck AM, DeWitt BA, Lukes AL. Potential interactions between alternative therapies and warfarin. *Am J Health Syst Pharm.* 2000;57(13):1221-1227.

8698 Saaeed SA, Gilani AH. Antithrombotic activity of clove oil. *J Pak Med Assoc.* 1994;44(5):112-15.

8699 Kamatou GP, Vermaak I, Viljoen AM. Eugenol—from the remote Maluku Islands to the international market place: A review of a remarkable and versatile molecule. *Molecules.* 2012;17:6953-81.

8700 Tao G, Irie Y, Li DJ, et al. Eugenol and its structural analogs inhibit monoamine oxidase A and exhibit antidepressant-like activity. *Bioorg Med Chem.* 2005 Aug 1;13(15):4777-88.

8701 Mack TS, Raner GM. Regulation of cytochrome P450 2A6 and phase II enzymes by unsaturated aldehydes. University of North Carolina at Greensboro. Available at: http://libres.uncg.edu/ir/uncg/listing.aspx?id=2343.

8702 Wickramasinghe RH, Muller G, Norpoth K. Spectral evidence of interaction of spice constituents with hepatic microsomal cytochrome P-450. *Cytobios.* 1980;29(113):25-27.

8703 Cochrane ML. Inhibition of Cytochrome P450 2C9 by essential oils. Available at: https://libres.uncg.edu/ir/uncg/listing.aspx?id=18102.

8704 Verspohl EJ, Bauer K, Neddermann E. Antidiabetic effect of cinnamomum cassia and cinamomum zeylanicum in vivo and in vitro. *Phytother Res.* 2005 Mar;19(3):203-06.

8705 Hua P, Guijun Z, Guixing R. Antidiabetic effects of cinnamon oil in diabetic KK-A mice. *Food Chem Toxicol.* 2010 Aug-Sep;48(8-9):2344-9.

8706 Sung HK, Sun HH, Choung SY. Anti-diabetic effect of cinnamon extract on blood glucose in db/db mice. *J Ethnopharmacol.* 2006 Mar 8;104(1-2):119-23.

8707 Babu PS, Prabuseenivasan S, Lgnacimuthu S. Cinnamaldehyde-A potential antidiabetic agent. *Phytomedicine.* 2007;14(1):15–22.

8708 Langeveld WT, Veldhuizen EJ, Burt SA. Synergy between essential oil constituents and antibiotics. *Crit Rev Microbiol.* 2014 Feb;40(1);76-94.

8709 Palaniappan K, Holley RA. Use of natural antimicrobials to increase antibiotic susceptibility of drug resistant bacteria. *In J Food Microbiol.* 2010 Jun 15;140(2-3):164-8.

8710 Langeveld WT, Veldhuizen EJ, Burt SA. Synergy between essential oil constituents and antibiotics. *Crit Rev Microbiol.* 2014 Feb;40(1);76-94.

8711 Dohi S, Terasaki M, Makino M. Acetylcholinesterase inhibitory activity and chemical composition of commercial essential oils. *J Agric Food Chem.* 2009 May 27;57(10):4313-8.

8712 Sarrami N, Pemberton MN, Thornhill MH, et al. Adverse reactions associated with the use of eugenol in dentistry. *British Dental J.* 2002;193:253-55.

8713 Tammannavar P, Pushpalatha C, Jain S, et al. An unexpected positive hypersensitive reaction to eugenol. *BMJ Case Rep.* 2013; 2013: bcr2013009464.

8714 National Toxicology Program. Cinnamaldehyde. 1989 Dec. Available at: https://ntp.niehs.nih.gov/ntp/htdocs/chem_background/exsumpdf/cinnamaldehyde_508.pdf

8715 National Toxicology Program. Cinnamaldehyde. 1989 Dec. Available at: https://ntp.niehs.nih.gov/ntp/htdocs/chem_background/exsumpdf/cinnamaldehyde_508.pdf

8716 Srivastava B, Sagar A, Dubey N. Evaluation of Cinnamomum tamala oil and its phenylpropanoid eugenol for their antifungal and antiaflatoxigenic activity. *Food Anal Methods.* 2011;4:347-56.

8717 Kapoor IPS, Singh B, Singh G, et al. Chemistry, antimicrobial and antioxidant potentials of Cinnamomum tamala Nees & Eberm. (Tejpat) essential oil and oleoresins. *Nat Prod Radiance.* 2009;8(2):106-16.

8718 Bisht D, Pal A, Chanotiya CS, et al. Terpenoid composition and antifungal activity of three commercially important essential oils against Aspergillus flavus and Aspergillus niger. *Nat Prod Res.* 2011 Dec;25(20):1993-8.

8719 Lohani H, Singh SK, Bhandari U, et al. Chemical polymorphism in Cinnamomum tamala (Buch.-Ham.) Nees. & Eberm. growing in Uttarakhand Himalaya (India). *J Chem Pharm Res.* 2015;7(8):67-71.

8720 Kumar S, Vasudeva N, Sharma S. GC-MS analysis and screening of antidiabetic, antioxidant and hypolipidemic potential of Cinnamomum tamala oil in streptozotocin induced diabetes mellitus in rats. *Cardiovasc Diabetol.* 2012 Aug 10;11:95.

8721 Lohani H, Singh SK, Bhandari U, et al. Chemical polymorphism in Cinnamomum tamala (Buch.-Ham.) Nees. & Eberm. growing in Uttarakhand Himalaya (India). *J Chem Pharm Res.* 2015;7(8):67-71.

8722 Kumar S, Vasudeva N, Sharma S. GC-MS analysis and screening of antidiabetic, antioxidant and hypolipidemic potential of Cinnamomum tamala oil in streptozotocin induced diabetes mellitus in rats. *Cardiovasc Diabetol.* 2012 Aug 10;11:95.

8723 Satyal P, Paudel P, Poudel A, et al. Bioactivities and compositional analyses of Cinnamomum essential oils from Nepal: C. camphora, C. tamala, and C. glaucescens. *Nat Prod Comm.* 2013 Sep;8(12):1777-84.

8724 Farisa Banu S, Rubini D, Rakshitaa S, et al. Antivirulent Properties of Underexplored Cinnamomum tamala Essential Oil and Its Synergistic Effects with DNase against Pseudomonas aeruginosa Biofilms - An In Vitro Study. *Front Microbiol.* 2017 Jun 26;8:1144.

8725 Rubini D, Banu SF, Nisha P, et al. Essential oils from unexplored aromatic plants quench biofilm formation and virulence of Methicillin resistant Staphylococcus aureus. *Microb Pathog.* 2018 Sep;122:162-173.

8726 Farisa Banu S, Rubini D, Shanmugavelan P, et al. Effects of patchouli and cinnamon essential oils on biofilm and hyphae formation by Candida species. *J Mycol Med.* 2018 Jun;28(2):332-339.

8727 Chakraborty A, Sankaran V, Murugan R, et al. Comparative spasmolytic effect between Cinnamomum tamala and Cinnamomum verum leaf essential oils and eugenol through in vitro and in silico approaches. *Z Naturforsch C J Biosci.* 2021 Apr 20. Online ahead of print.

8728 Chutia M, Deka Bhyan D, Pathak MG, et al. Antifungal and chemical composition of Citrus reticulata Blanco essential oil against phytopathogens from North East India. *LWT - Food Sci Tech.* 2009 Apr;42(3):777-80.

8729 Sultana HS, Ali M, Panda BP. Influence of volatile constituents of fruit peels of Citrus reticulata Blanco on clinically isolated pathogenic microorganisms under In-vitro. *Asian Pac J Trop Biomed.* 2012:S1299-S1302.

8730 Phi NTL, Sawamura M. Volatile constituents of Mandarin (Citrus reticulata Blanco) peel oil from Burundi. *J Essent Oil Res.* 2006;18(6):659-62.

8731 Njoroge SM, Koaze H, Mwaniki M. Essential oils of Kenyan citrus fruits: volatile components of two varieties of mandarins (Citrus reticulata) and a tangelo (C. paradisi X C. tangerina). *Flav Frag J.* 2005 Jan-Feb;20(10:74-79.

8732 Darjazi BB. Comparison of peel components of Dancy Tangerine (Citrus reticulata) obtained from cold-press and hydrodistillation method. *TI Journals.* 2015 Jan;5(1):21-26.

8733 Espina L, Somolinos M, Loran S, et al. Chemical composition of commercial citrus fruit essential oils and evaluation of their antimicrobial activity acting alone or in combined processes. *Food Control.* 2011 Jun;22(6):896-902.

8734 Ford RA, Api AM, Letizia C. Monographs on fragrance raw materials. *Food Chem Toxicol.* 1992;30(Suppl.):69S- 70S.

8735 International Fragrance Association. Citrus oils and other furocoumarins containing essential oils. Available at: http://www.ifraorg.org/view_document.aspx?docId=23169.

8736 Seo KA, Kim H, Ku HY, et al. The monoterpenoids citral and geraniol are moderate inhibitors of the CYP2B6 hydroxylase activity. *Chem Biol Interact.* 2008;174:141-46.

8737 Sheweita SA, Newairy AA, Mansour HA, et al. Effect of some hypoglycemic herbs on the activity of phase I and II drug-metabolizing enzymes in alloxan-induced diabetic rats. *Toxicology.* 2002 May 24;17(2):131-39.

8738 Raner GM, Vaz AD, Coon MJ. Metabolism of all-trans, 9-cis, and 13-cis isomers of retinal by purified isozymes of microsomal cytochrome P450 and mechanism-based inhibition of retinoid oxidation by citral. *Mol Pharmacol.* 1996;49(3):515-22.

8739 De Olivera AC, Ribeiro-Pinto LF, Paumgartten JR. In vitro inhibition of CYP2B1 monoxygenase by beta-myrcene and other monoterpenoid constituents. *Br J Nutr.* 1999;81:289-95.

8740 Williamson EA. Inhibition of cytochrome P450 2E1, cytochrome P450 3A6 and cytochrome P450 2A6 by citrus essential oils. University of North Carolina Thesis. Available at: http://libres.uncg.edu/ir/uncg/f/Williamson_uncg_0154M_10494.pdf.

8741 Modak T, Mukhopadhaya A. Effects of citral, a naturally occurring antiadipogenic molecule, on an energy-intense diet model of obesity. *Indian J Pharmacol.* 2011 May-Jun;43(3):300-05.

8742 Najafian M, Ebrahim-Habibi A, Yaghmaei P, et al. Citral as a potential antihyperlipidemic medicine in diabetes: a study on streptozotocin-induced diabetic rats. *J Diabetes Metabolic Disorders.* 2011;10(1):3.

8743 Choi JY, Damte D, Seung-Jin L, et al. Antimicrobial activity of lemongrass and oregano essential oil against standard antibiotic resistant Staphylococcus aureus and field isolates from chronic mastitis cow. *International Journal of Phytomedicine.* 2012;4(1):134-39.

8744 Kuhn GO, McCampbell P, Singmaster G, et al. Application of microencapsulation technology to improve the stability of citral in rodent diets. *Fundam Appl Toxicol.* 1991 Oct;17(3):635-40.

8745 De Mozzi P, Johnston GA. An outbreak of allergic contact dermatitis caused by citral in beauticians working in a health spa. *Contact Dermatitis.* 2014 Jun;70(6):377-9.

8746 Baylac S, Racine P. Inhibition of 5-lipoxygenase by essential oils and other natural fragrant extracts. *Int J Aromatherapy.* 2003;13(2-3):138-42.

8747 Singh P, Shukla R, Kumar A, et al. Effect of Citrus reticulata and Cymbopogon citratus essential oils on Aspergillus flavus growth and aflatoxin production on Asparagus racemosus. *Mycopathologia.* 2010 Sep;170(3):195-202.

8748 Sutthanot N, Choochote W, Tuetun B, et al. Chemical composition and larvicidal activity of edible plant-derived essential oils against the pyrethroid-susceptible and -resistant strains of Aedes aegypti (Diptera: Culicidae). *J Vector Ecol.* 2010 Jun;35(1):106-15.

8749 Zhou XM, Zhao Y, He CC, et al. Preventive effects of Citrus reticulata essential oil on bleomycin-induced pulmonary fibrosis in rats and the mechanism. *Zhong XI Yi Jie Xue Bao.* 212 Feb;10(2):200-09.

8750 Dyer J, Cleary L, McNeill S, et al. The use of aromasticks to help with sleep problems: A patient experience survey. Complement Ther Clin Pract. 2016 Feb;22:51-8.

8751 Johnson JR, Rivard RL, Griffin KH, et al. The effectiveness of nurse-delivered aromatherapy in an acute care setting. *Complement Ther Med.* 2016 Apr;25:164-9.

8752 Campolo O, Romeo FV, Algeri GM, et al. Larvicidal Effects of Four Citrus Peel Essential Oils Against the Arbovirus Vector Aedes albopictus (Diptera: Culicidae). *J Econ Entomol.* 2016 Feb;109(1):360-5.

8753 Badawy MEI, Taktak NEM, El-Aswad AF, et al. Chemical composition of the essential oils isolated from peel of three citrus species and their mosquitocidal activity against Culex pipiens. *Nat Prod Res.* 2018 Dec;32(23):2829-2834.

8754 Lu J. Effect of Citrus reticulata Blanco Essential Oil on Cryptolestes ferrugineus (Stephens) Adults. *J Food Prot.* 2017 Dec;80(12):2090-2093.

8755 Nair S A, Sr RK, Nair AS, et al. Citrus peels prevent cancer. *Phytomedicine.* 2018 Nov 15;50:231-237.

8756 Aumeeruddy-Elalfi Z, Lall N, et al. Selected essential oils inhibit key physiological enzymes and possess intracellular and extracellular antimelanogenic properties in vitro. *J Food Drug Anal.* 2018 Jan;26(1):232-243.

8757 Bedini S, Cosci F, Tani C, et al. Essential Oils as Post-Harvest Crop Protectants against the Fruit Fly Drosophila suzukii: Bioactivity and Organoleptic Profile. *Insects.* 2020 Aug 5;11(8):E508.

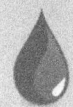

[8758] Ishfaq M, Akhtar B, Muhammad F, et al. Antioxidant and wound healing potential of essential oil from Citrus reticulata peel and its chemical characterization. Medicinal values of peels essential oil. *Curr Pharm Biotechnol.* 2020 Sep 17. Online ahead of print.

[8759] Feng K, Zhu X, Liu G, et al. Dietary citrus peel essential oil ameliorates hypercholesterolemia and hepatic steatosis by modulating lipid and cholesterol homeostasis. *Food Funct.* 2020 Aug 1;11(8):7217-7230.

[8760] Song X, Liu T, Wang L, et al. Antibacterial Effects and Mechanism of Mandarin (Citrus reticulata L.) Essential Oil against Staphylococcus aureus. *Molecules.* 2020 Oct 26;25(21):E4956.

[8761] Chandharakool S, Koomhin P, Sinlapasorn J, et al. Effects of Tangerine Essential Oil on Brain Waves, Moods, and Sleep Onset Latency. *Molecules.* 2020 Oct 21;25(20):4865.

[8762] Yabalak E, Eliuz EAE, Nazli MD. Evaluation of Citrus reticulata essential oil: Chemical composition and antibacterial effectiveness incorporated gelatin on E. coli and S. aureus. *Int J Environ Health Res.* 2021 Jan 11;1-10.

[8763] Denkova-Kostova R, Teneva D, Tomova T, et al. Chemical composition, antioxidant and antimicrobial activity of essential oils from tangerine ( Citrus reticulata L.), grapefruit ( Citrus paradisi L.), lemon ( Citrus lemon L.) and cinnamon ( Cinnamomum zeylanicum Blume). *Z Naturforsch C J Biosci.* 2020 Nov 23;76(5-6):175-185.

[8764] Lin X, Cao S, Sun J, et al. The Chemical Compositions, and Antibacterial and Antioxidant Activities of Four Types of Citrus Essential Oils. *Molecules.* 2021 Jun 4;26(11):3412.

[8765] Oliveira ACSD, Fernandes CC, Santos LS, et al. Chemical composition, in vitro larvicidal and antileishmanial activities of the essential oil from Citrus reticulata Blanco fruit peel. *Braz J Biol.* 2021 Jun 28;83:e247539.

[8766] Pasias IN, Ntakoulas DD, Raptopoulou K, et al. Chemical Composition of Essential Oils of Aromatic and Medicinal Herbs Cultivated in Greece-Benefits and Drawbacks. *Foods.* 2021 Oct 3;10(10):2354.

[8767] Bhandari DP, Poudel DK, Satyal P, et al. Volatile Compounds and Antioxidant and Antimicrobial Activities of Selected Citrus Essential Oils Originated from Nepal. *Molecules.* 2021 Nov 4;26(21):6683.

[8768] Tang M, Ai Y, Zhu S, et al. Antidepressant-like Effect and Mechanisms of Essential Oils From Citrus Reticulata in Reserpine-induced Depression Model Mice. 2021 Jul. Online ahead of print.

[8769] Infante V, Campos PM, Gaspar LR, et al. Safety and efficacy of combined essential oils for the skin barrier properties: in vitro, ex vivo and clinical studies. *Int J Cosmet Sci.* 2022 Jan 5. Online ahead of print.

[8770] Li C, Cai Q, Wu X, et al. Variation in compositions and biological activities of essential oils from four Citrus species: Citrus limon, Citrus sinensis, Citrus paradisi, and Citrus reticulata. *Chem Biodivers.* 2022 Feb 10. Online ahead of print.

[8771] Kwangjai J, Cheaha D, Manor R, et al. Modification of brain waves and sleep parameters by Citrus reticulata Blanco. cv. Sai-Nam-Phueng essential oil. *Biomed J.* 2021 Dec;44(6):727-738.

[8772] Li C, Zhu H, Zhao K, et al. Chemical constituents, biological activities and anti-rheumatoid arthritic properties of four citrus essential oils. *Phytother Res.* 2022 Jul;36(7):2908-2920.

[8773] Torshabi M, MoadabShoar Z, Negahban M. Preparation of Citrus reticulata peel nano-encapsulated essential oil and in vitro assessment of its biological properties. *Eur J Oral Sci.* 2023 Feb 16:e12924.

[8774] Haris A, Azeem M, Abbas MG, et al. Prolonged Repellent Activity of Plant Essential Oils against Dengue Vector, Aedes aegypti. *Molecules.* 2023 Jan 31;28(3):1351.

[8775] de la Cruz OA, Huerrero J, Podea R, et al. Composition of the essential oil from leaves of Palma Real (Tanacetum vulgare L.) from Peru. *Chem Bull POLITENICA Univ.* 2008;53(67):10–12.

[8776] Rohloff J, Mordal R, Dragland S. Chemotypical variation of tansy (Tanacetum vulgare L.) from 40 different location in Norway. *J Agric Chem.* 2004 Mar;52(6):1742–48.

[8777] de Pooter HL, Vermeesch J, Schamp NM. The essential oils of Tanacetum vulgare L. and Tanacetum parthenium (L.) Schultz-Bip. *J Essential Oil Res.* 1989 Jan;1(1):9–13.

[8778] Keskitalo M, Pehu E, Simon JE. Variation in volatile constituents from tansy (Tanacetum vulgare L.) related to genetic and morphological differences of genotypes. *Biochem Syst Ecology.* 2001;29:267–85.

[8779] da Silva Costa KC, Bezerra SB, Norte CM, et al. Medicinal plants with teratogenic potential: current considerations. *Braz J Pharm Sci.* 2012;48(3):427–33.

[8780] Brinker F. Herb Contraindications and Drug Interactions. 2nd ed. Sandy, OR. Eclectic Medical Publications. 1998.

[8781] European Medicines Agency. Public statement on the use of herbal medicinal products containing thujone. Available at: http://www.ema.europa.eu/docs/en_GB/document_library/Public_statement/2011/02/WC500102294.pdf.

[8782] Millet Y, Jouglard J, Steinmetz MD, et al. Toxicity of some essential plant oils. Clinical and experimental study. *Clin Toxicol.* 1981 Dec;18(12):1485–98.

[8783] Cristovao L, Carvalho F, Bastos MDL, et al. Hepatotoxicity of an essential oil of Salvia officinalis L.: an in vitro study using freshly isolated rat hepatocytes. *Congress Biomarkers.* 2001 Sep:165.

[8784] Perry NB, Anderson RE, Brennan NJ, et al. Essential oils from Dalmatian sage (Salvia officinalis L.) variations among individuals, plant parts, seasons, and sites. *J Agric Food Chem.* 1999;47:2048–54.

[8785] Pelkonen O, Abass K, Wiesner J. Thujone and thujone-containing herbal medicinal and botanical products: toxicological assessment. *Regul Toxicol Pharmacol.* 2013 Feb;65(1):100–07.

[8786] Godinho LS, Aleixo de Carvalho LS, Barbosa de Castro CC, et al. Anthelmintic activity of crude extract and essential oil of Tanacetum vulgare (Asteraceae against adult worms of Schistosoma mansoni). *ScientificWorldJournal.* 2014 Feb;2014:460342.

[8787] Palsson K, Jaenson TG, Baeckstrom P, Tick repellent substances in the essential oil of Tanacetum vulgare. *J Med Entomol.* 2008 Jan;45(1):88–93.

[8788] de la Cruz OA, Huerrero J, Podea R, et al. Composition of the essential oil from leaves of Palma Real (Tanacetum vulgare L.) from Peru. *Chem Bull POLITENICA Univ.* 2008;53(67):10–12.

[8789] Haliciglu O, Astarcioglu G, Yaprak I, et al. Toxicity of Salvia officinalis in a newborn and a child: an alarming report. *Pediatr Neurol.* 2011 Oct;45(4):259-60.

[8790] Lachenmeier DW, Walch SG. Epileptic seizure caused by accidental ingestion of sage (Salvia officinalis L.) oil in children: a rare, exceptional case or a threat to public health. *Pediatr Neurol.* 2012 Mar;46(3):201.

[8791] Stafstrom CE. Seizures in a 7-month-old child after exposure to the essential plant oil thuja. *Pediatr Neurol.* 2007 Dec;37(6):446-8.

[8792] Khine H, Weiss D, Graber N, et al. A cluster of children with seizures caused by camphor poisoning. *Pediatrics.* 2009 May;123(5):1269-72.

[8793] Michiels EA, Mazor SS. Toddler with seizures due to ingesting camphor at an Indian celebration. *Pediatr Emerg Care.* 2010 Aug;26(8):574-75.

[8794] Koren G. Medications which can kill a toddler with one tablet or teaspoonful. *J toxicol Clin Toxicol.* 1993;31(3):407- 13.

[8795] Bar-Oz B, Levicheck Z, Koren G. Medications that can kill a toddler with one tablet or teaspoonfull – A 2004 update. *Paediatr Drugs.* 2004;6(2):123-6.

[8796] Brinker F. Herb Contraindications and Drug Interactions. 2nd ed. Sandy, OR. Eclectic Medical Publications. 1998.

[8797] da Silva Costa KC, Bexerra SB, Norte CM, et al. Medicinal plants with teratogenic potential: current considerations. *Braz J Pharm Sci.* 2012;48(3):427-33.

[8798] Brinker F. Herb Contraindications and Drug Interactions. 2nd ed. Sandy, OR. Eclectic Medical Publications. 1998.

[8799] Rabl W, Katzgraber F, Steinlechner M. Camphor ingestion for abortion (case report). *Forensic Sci Int.* 1997 Sep 19;89(1-2):137-40.

[8800] Flaman Z, Pellechia-Clarke S, Bailey B, et al. Unintentional exposure of young children to camphor and eucalyptus oils. *Paediatr Child Health.* 2001 Feb;6(2):80-83.

[8801] Frohne D. Giftpflanzen: Cupressaceae. Stuttgart: Wissenschaftliche Verlagsgesellschaft mbH; 1997. pp. 153–6.

[8802] European Medicines Agency. Public statement on the use of herbal medicinal products containing thujone. Available at: http://www.ema.europa.eu/docs/en_GB/document_library/Public_statement/2011/02/WC500102294.pdf.

[8803] Millet Y, Jouglard J, Steinmetz MD, et al. Toxicity of some essential plant oils. Clinical and experimental study. *Clin Toxicol.* 1981 Dec;18(12):1485-98.

[8804] Cristovao L, Carvalho F, Bastos MDL, et al. Hepatotoxicity of an essential oil of Salvia officinalis L.: an in vitro study using freshly isolated rat hepatocytes. *Congress Biomarkers.* 2001 Sep:165.

[8805] Burkhard PR, Burkhardt K, Haenggeli CA, et al. Plant-induced seizures: reappearance of an old problem. *J Neurol.* 1999 Aug;246(8):667-70.

[8806] Burkhard PR, Burkhardt K, Haenggeli CA, et al. Plant-induced seizures: reappearance of an old problem. *J Neurol.* 1999 Aug;246(8):667-70.

[8807] Waldman N. Seizure caused by dermal application of over-the-counter eucalyptus oil head lice preparation. *Clin Toxicol (Phila).* 2011 Oct;49(8):750-1.

[8808] Craig JO. Poisoning by the volatile oils in childhood. *Arch Dis Child.* 1953;28:259-67.

[8809] Narayan S, Singh N. Camphor poisoning-An unusual cause of seizure. *Med J Armed Forces India.* 2012 Jul;68(3):252-53.

[8810] Chanaranaj KJ, G MV, S M. Camphor poisoning in a child. *Natl Med J India.* 2013 Jan-Feb;26(1):60.

[8811] Perry NB, Anderson RE, Brennan NJ, et al. Essential oils from dalmatian sage (Salvia officinalis L.) variations among individuals, plant parts, seasons, and sites. *J Agric Food Chem.* 1999;47:2048-54.

[8812] Millet Y, Jouglard J, Steinmetz MD, et al. Toxicity of some essential plant oils. Clinical and experimental study. *Clin Toxicol.* 1981 Dec;18(12):1485-98.

[8813] Olowe SA, Ransome-Kuti O. The risk of jaundice in glucose-6-phosphate dehydrogenase deficient babies exposed to menthol. *Acta Paediatr Scand.* 1980 May;69(3):341-5.

[8814] Dillon Remy M, Manning Alleyne P, Bratt DE, et al. Neonatal jaundice at Port-of-Spain General Hospital abstract. *West Indian Med J.* 1987;36(Suppl):28.

[8815] Uc A, Bishop WP, Sanders KD. Camphor hepatotoxicity. *South Med J.* 2000;93:596-98.

[8816] Frohne D. Giftpflanzen: Cupressaceae. Stuttgart: Wissenschaftliche Verlagsgesellschaft mbH; 1997. pp. 153–6.

[8817] Dolan LC, Matulka RA, Burdock GA. Naturally Occurring Food Toxins. *Toxins (Basel).* 2010 Sep;2(9):2289–2332.

[8818] United States National Toxicology Program (NTP). Alpha-Thujone. Dec 10, 1997. Available at: http://ntp.niehs.nih.gov/index.cfm?objectid=03DB8C36-E7A1-9889-3BDF8436F2A8C51F.

[8819] Schulz V, Hansel R, Tyler VE. Rational Phytotherapy: A Physician's Guide to Herbal Medicine. Terry C. Telger, transl. 3rd ed. Berlin, GER: Springer, 1998.

[8820] Godinho LS, Aleixo de Carvalho LS, Barbosa de Castro CC, et al. Anthelmintic activity of crude extract and essential oil of Tanacetum vulgare (Asteraceae against adult worms of Schistosoma mansoni). *ScientificWorldJournal.* 2014 Feb;2014:460342.

[8821] Palsson K, Jaenson TG, Baeckstrom P. Tick repellent substances in the essential oil of Tanacetum vulgare. *J Med Entomol.* 2008 Jan;45(1):88–93.

[8822] Coté H, Boucher MA, Pichette A, et al. Anti-Inflammatory, Antioxidant, Antibiotic, and Cytotoxic Activities of Tanacetum vulgare L. Essential Oil and Its Constituents. *Medicines (Basel).* 2017 May 25;4(2).

[8823] Devrnja N, Kostić I, Lazarević J, et al. Evaluation of tansy essential oil as a potential "green" alternative for gypsy moth control. *Environ Sci Pollut Res Int.* 2020 Apr;27(11):11958-11967.

[8824] Lazarević J, Kostić I, Milanović S, et al. Repellent activity of Tanacetum parthenium (L.) and Tanacetum vulgare (L.) essential oils against Leptinotarsa decemlineata (Say). *Bull Entomol Res.* 2020 Aug 11:1-10.

[8825] Korpinen RI, Valimaa AL, Liimatainen J, et al. Essential Oils and Supercritical CO 2 Extracts of Arctic Angelica ( Angelica archangelica L.), Marsh Labrador Tea ( Rhododendron tomentosum) and Common Tansy ( Tanacetum vulgare)-Chemical Compositions and Antimicrobial Activities. *Molecules.* 2021 Nov 25;26(23):7121.

8826 Kordali S, Kotan R, Mavi A, et al. Determination of the Chemical Composition and Antioxidant Activity of the Essential Oil of Artemisia dracunculus and of the Antifungal and Antibacterial Activities of Turkish Artemisia absinthium, A. dracunculus, Artemisia santonicum, and Artemisia spicigera Essential Oils. *J Agric Food Chem*. 2005;53(24):9452-58.

8827 Obistioiu D, Cristina RT, Schmerold I, et al. Chemical characterization by GC-MS and in vitro activity against Candida albicans of volatile fractions prepared from Artemisia dracunculus, Artemisia abrotanum, Artemisia absinthium and Artemisia vulgaris. *Chem Central J*. 2014;8(6):1-11.

8828 Fraternale D, Flamini G, Ricci D. Essential Oil Composition and Antigermination Activity of Artemisia dracunculus (Tarragon). *Nat Prod Commun*. 2015 Aug;10(8):1469-72.

8829 Obolskiy D, Pischel I, Feistel B, et al. Artemisia dracunculus L. (Tarragon): A Critical Review of Its Traditional 2 Use, Chemical Composition, Pharmacology, and Safety. *J Agric Food Chem*. 2011 Nov 9;59(21):11367-84.

8830 Obolskiy D, Pischel I, Feistel B, et al. Artemisia dracunculus L. (Tarragon): A Critical Review of Its Traditional 2 Use, Chemical Composition, Pharmacology, and Safety. *J Agric Food Chem*. 2011 Nov 9;59(21):11367-84.

8831 European Medicines Agency. Public statement on the use of herbal medicinal products containing estragole. Available at: http://www.ema.europa.eu/docs/en_GB/document_library/Scientific_guideline/2010/04/WC500089960.pdf.

8832 European Medicines Agency. Public statement on the use of herbal medicinal products containing estragole. Available at: http://www.ema.europa.eu/docs/en_GB/document_library/Scientific_guideline/2010/04/WC500089960.pdf.

8833 Ding W, Levy DD, Bishop ME, et al. In vivo genotoxicity of estragole in male F344 rats. *Environ Mol Mutagen*. 2015 May;56(4):356-65.

8834 Eisenmann SW, Poulev A, Struwe L, et al. Qualitative variation of anti-diabetic constituents in different tarragon (Artemisia dracunculus L.) cytotypes. *Fitoterapia*. 2011 Oct;82(7):1062–74.

8835 European Medicines Agency. Public statement on the use of herbal medicinal products containing estragole. Available at: http://www.ema.europa.eu/docs/en_GB/document_library/Scientific_guideline/2010/04/WC500089960.pdf.

8836 European Commission. Opinion of the Scientific Committee on Food on methyl eugenol (4-Allyl-1,2- dimethoxybenzene). Available at: http://ec.europa.eu/food/fs/sc/scf/out102_en.pdf.

8837 European Commission. Opinion of the Scientific Committee on Food on estragole (1-Allyl-4-methoxybenzene). Available at: http://ec.europa.eu/food/fs/sc/scf/out104_en.pdf.

8838 California Environmental Protection Agency. Evidence of the carcinogenicity of estragole. Available at: http://oehha.ca.gov/prop65/pdf/estragf.pdf.

8839 Drinkwater NR, Miller EC, Miller JA, et al. Hepatocarcinogenicity of estragole (1-allyl-4-methoxybenzene) and 1'-hydroxyestragole in the mouse and mutagenicity of 1'-acetoxyestragole in bacteria. *J Natl Cancer Inst*. 1976 Dec;57(6):1323-31.

8840 Zeller A, Horst K, Rychlik M. Study of the metabolism of estragole in humans consuming fennel tea. *Chem Res Toxicol*. 2009 Dec;22(12):1929-37.

8841 Tognolini M, Barocelli E, Ballabeni V, et al. Comparative screening of plant essential oils; phenylpropanoid moiety as basic core for antiplatelet activity. *Life Sci*. 2006 Feb 23;78(13):1419-32.

8842 Shahriyary L, Yazdanparast R. Tarragon (Artemisia d. has anti-platelet, anticoagulant activity. *J Ethnopharmacol*. 2007 Nov 1;114(2):194-8.

8843 Duric K, Kovac Besovic EE, Niksic H, et al. Anticoagulant activity of some Artemisia dracunculus leaf extracts. *Bosnian J Basic Med Sci*. 2015;15(2):9-14.

8844 Yazdanparast R, Shahriyary L. Comparative effects of Artemisia dracunculus, Satureja hortensis and Origanum majorana on inhibition of blood platelet adhesion, aggregation and secretion. *Vascul Pharmacol*. 2008 Jan;48(1):32-37.

8845 Lee HS. Anticoagulant properties of constituents derived from fennel (Foeniculum vulgare Gaertner) fruits. *Food Sci Biotech*. 2006 Oct;15(5):763-67.

8846 Khan MM. Masters Thesis: Inhibition of Cytochrome P450 2E1 and Cytochrome P450 2A6 by Essential Oils: Tarragon (Artemisia dracunculus) and Basil (Ocimum basilicum). 2014. Available at: https://libres.uncg.edu/ir/uncg/f/Khan_uncg_0154M_11587.pdf

8847 Dohi S, Terasaki M, Makino M. Acetylcholinesterase inhibitory activity and chemical composition of commercial essential oils. *J Agric Food Chem*. 2009 May 27;57(10):4313-8.

8848 Sayyah M, Nadjafnia L, Kamalinejad M. Anticonvulsant activity and chemical composition of Artemisia dracunculus L. essential oil. *J Ethnopharmacol*. 2004 Oct;94(2-3):283-7.

8849 Shin S, Pyun MS. Anti-Candida effects of estragole in combination with ketoconazole or amphotericin B. *Phytother Res*. 2004 Oct;18(10):827-30.

8850 Shin S. Essential oil compounds from Agastache rugosa as antifungal agents against Trichophyton species. *Arch Pharm Res*. 2004 Mar;27(3):295-9.

8851 Shin S, Kang CA. Antifungal activity of the essential oil of Agastache rugosa Kuntze and its synergism with ketoconazole. *Lett Appl Microbiol*. 2003;36(2):111-5.

8852 Maham M, Moslemzadeh H, Jalilzadeh-Amin G. Antinociceptive effect of the essential oil of tarragon (Artemisia dracunculus). *Pharm Biol*. 2014 Feb;52(2):208-12.

8853 Obistioiu D, Cristina RT, Schmerold I, et al. Chemical characterization by GC-MS and in vitro activity against Candida albicans of volatile fractions prepared from Artemisia dracunculus, Artemisia abrotanum, Artemisia absinthium and Artemisia vulgaris. *Chem Central J*. 2014;8(6):1-11.

8854 Raeisi M, Tajik H, Razavi RS, et al. Essential oil of tarragon (Artemisia dracunculus) antibacterial activity on Staphylococcus aureus and Escherichia coli in culture media and Iranian white cheese. *Iran J Microbiol*. 2012 Mar;4(1):30-4.

8855 Bedini S, Flamini G, Cosci F, et al. Artemisia spp. essential oils against the disease-carrying blowfly Calliphora vomitoria. *Parasit Vectors*. 2017 Feb 13;10(1):80.

8856 Dohi S, Terasaki M, Makino M. Acetylcholinesterase inhibitory activity and chemical composition of commercial essential oils. *J Agric Food Chem*. 2009 May 27;57(10):4313-8.

8857 Sayyah M, Nadjafnia L, Kamalinejad M. Anticonvulsant activity and chemical composition of Artemisia dracunculus L. essential oil. *J Ethnopharmacol*. 2004 Oct;94(2-3):283-7.

8858 Bedini S, Flamini G, Cosci F, et al. Artemisia spp. essential oils against the disease-carrying blowfly Calliphora vomitoria. *Parasit Vectors*. 2017 Feb 13;10(1):80.

8859 Bartoňková I, Dvořák Z. Essential oils of culinary herbs and spices display agonist and antagonist activities at human aryl hydrocarbon receptor AhR. *Food Chem Toxicol*. 2018 Jan;111:374-384.

8860 Pelarti SM, Zarehshuran LK, Babaeekhou L, et al. Antibacterial, antibiofilm and anti-quorum sensing activities of Artemisia dracunculus essential oil (EO): a study against Salmonella enterica serovar Typhimurium and Staphylococcus aureus. *Arch Microbiol*. 2021 Jan 5. Online ahead of print.

8861 Osanloo M, Ghaznavi G, Abdollahi A. Surveying the chemical composition and antibacterial activity of essential oils from selected medicinal plants against human pathogens. *Iran J Microbiol*. 2020 Dec;12(6):577-583.

8862 Azizkhani M, Kiasari FJ, Tooryan F, et al. Preparation and evaluation of food-grade nanoemulsion of tarragon ( Artemisia dracunculus L.) essential oil: antioxidant and antibacterial properties. *J Food Sci Technol*. 2021 Apr;58(4):1341-1348.

8863 Sahakyan N, Andreoletti P, Cherkaoui-Malki M, et al. Artemisia dracunculus L. essential oil phytochemical components trigger the activity of cellular antioxidant enzymes. *J Food Biochem*. 2021 Mar 10;e13691.

8864 Tomaś N, Myszka K, Wolko Ł. Black pepper and tarragon essential oils suppress the lipolytic potential and the type II secretion system of P. psychrophila KM02. *Sci Rep*. 2022 Mar 31;12(1):5487.

8865 Osanloo M, Firooziyan S, Abdollahi A, et al. Nanoemulsion and nanogel containing Artemisia dracunculus essential oil; larvicidal effect and antibacterial activity. *BMC Res Notes*. 2022 Aug 12;15(1):276.

8866 Lak F, Zandi-Sohani N, Ghodoum Parizipour MH, et al. Synergic effects of some plant-derived essential oils and Iranian isolates of entomopathogenic fungus Metarhizium anisopliae Sorokin to control Acanthoscelides obtectus (Say) (Coleoptera: Chrysomelidae). *Front Plant Sci*. 2022 Dec 9;13:1075761.

8867 Pereira TS, de Sant'anna JR, Silva EL, et al. In vitro genotoxicity of Melaleuca alternifolia essential oil in human lymphocytes. *J Ethnopharmacol*. 2014 Feb 3;151(2):852-57.

8868 Hammer KA, Carson CF, Riley TV, et al. Effects of Melaleuca alternifolia (Tea Tree) essential oil and the major monoterpene component terpinen-4-ol on the development of single- and multistep antibiotic resistance and antimicrobial susceptibility. *Antimicrobial Agents Chemo*. 2012 Feb;56(2):909-15.

8869 Gomez-Rincon C, Langa E, Murillo P, et al. Activity of tea tree (Melaleuca alternifolia) essential oil against L3 larvae of Anisakis simplex. *BioMed Res Int*. 2014;2014(2014):549510.

8870 World Health Organization. WHO Monographs on Selected Medicinal Plants. 2004. Available at: http://apps.who.int/medicinedocs/en/d/Js4927e/17.html.

8871 Carson CF, Hammer KA, Riley TV. Melaleuca alternifolia (tea tree) oil: A review of antimicrobial and other medicinal properties. *Clin Microbiol Rev*. 2006 Jan;19(1):50-62.

8872 Mertas A, Garbusińska A, Szliszka E, et al. The influence of tea tree oil (Melaleuca alternifolia) on fluconazole activity against fluconazole-resistant Candida albicans strains. *Biomed Res Int*. 2015;2015:590470.

8873 Valente JS, Fonseca AO1, Denardi LB, et al. In vitro activity of antifungals in combination with essential oils against the oomycete Pythium insidiosum. *J Appl Microbiol*. 2016 Oct;121(4):998-1003.

8874 Scazzocchio F, Garzoli S, Conti C, et al. Properties and limits of some essential oils: chemical characterisation, antimicrobial activity, interaction with antibiotics and cytotoxicity. *Nat Prod Res*. 2016 Sep;30(17):1909-18.

8875 Seawright, A. 1993. Tea tree oil poisoning. *Med. J. Aust*. 1993 Dec 6-20;159(11-12):830-31.

8876 Elliott C. Tea tree oil poisoning. *Med J Aust*. 1993 Dec;159(11-12):830-1.

8877 European Medicines Agency. Assessment report on Melaleuca alternifolia (Maiden and Betch) Cheel, M. linariifolia Smith, M. dissitiflora F. Mueller and/or other species of Melaleuca, aetheroleum. Available at: http://www.ema.europa.eu/docs/en_GB/document_library/Herbal_-_HMPC_assessment_report/2013/08/WC500148251.pdf.

8878 Jacobs MR, Hornfeldt CS. Melaleuca oil poisoning. *J Toxicol Clin Toxicol*. 1994:32(4):461-4.

8879 Del Beccaro MA. Melaleuca oil poisoning in a 17-month-old. *Vet Hum Toxicol*. 1995 Dec;37(6):557-8.

8880 Morris MC, Donoghue A, Markowitz JA, et al. Ingestion of tea tree oil (Melaleuca oil) by 4-year-old boy. *Pediatr Emerg Care*. 2003 Jun;19(3):169-71.

8881 Seawright, A. 1993. Tea tree oil poisoning. *Med. J. Aust*. 1993 Dec 6-20;159(11-12):830-31.

8882 Santamaria M Jr, Petermann KD, Vedovello SA, et al. Antimicrobial effect of Melaleuca alternifolia dental gel in orthodontic patients. *Am J Orthod Dentofacial Orthop*. 2014 Feb;145(2):198-202.

8883 Soukoulis S, Hirsch R. The effects of a tea tree oil-containing gel on plaque and chronic gingivitis. *Aust Dent J*. 2004 Jun;49(2):78-83.

8884 Santana-Méridas O, González-Coloma A, Fe Andrés M, et al. Biocidal compounds from Mentha sp essential oils and their structure-activity relationships. *Chem Biodivers*. 2017 Mar;14(3).

8885 Graziano TS, Calil CM, Sartoratto A, et al. In vitro effects of Melaleuca alternifolia essential oil on growth and production of volatile sulphur compounds by oral bacteria. *J Appl Oral Sci*. 2016 Nov-Dec;24(6):582-589.

8886 Catalan A, Pacheco JG, Martinez A. In vitro and in vivo activity of Melaleuca alternifolia mixed with tissue conditioner on Candida albicans. *Oral Surg Oral Med Oral Pathol Oral Radiol Endod*. 2008 Mar;105(3):327-32.

8887 Sharma S, Hedge V. Comparative Evaluation of Antifungal Activity of Melaleuca Oil and Fluconazole when Incorporated in Tissue Conditioner: An In Vitro Study. *J Prosthodontics*. 2014 Jan;23(5):367-73.

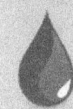

[8888] Iqbal Z, Zafar MS. Role of antifungal medicaments added to tissue conditioners: A systematic review. J Prosthodont Res. 2016 Oct;60(4):231-239.
[8889] Garozzo A, Timpanaro R, Stivala A, et al. Activity of Melaleuca alternifolia (tea tree) oil on Influenza virus A/PR/8: study on the mechanism of action. *Antiviral Res.* 2011 Jan;89(1):83-88.
[8890] Garozzo A, Timpanaro R, Bisignano B, et al. In vitro antiviral activity of Melaleuca alternifolia essential oil. *Lett Appl Microbiol.* 2009 Dec;49(6):806-08.
[8891] Ninomiya K, Maruyama N, Inoue S, et al. The essential oil of Melaleuca alternifolia (tea tree oil) and its main component, terpinen-4-ol protect mice from experimental oral candidiasis. *Biol Pharm Bull.* 212;35(6):861-65.
[8892] Pazyar N, Yaghoobi R. Tea tree oil as a novel antipsoriasis weapon. *Skin Pharmacol Physiol.* 2012;25(3):162-63.
[8893] Koh KJ, Pearce AL, Marshman G, et al. Tea tree reduces histamine-induced skin inflammation. *Br J Dermatol.* 2002 Dec;147(6):1212-17.
[8894] Khailil Z, Pearce AL, Satkunanathan N, et al. Regulation of wheal and flare by tea tree oil: complementary human and rodent studies. *J Invest Dermatol.* 2004 Oct;123(4):683-90.
[8895] Cuaron JA, Dulal S, Song Y, et al. Tea tree oil-induced transcriptional alterations in Staphylococcus aureus. *Phytother Res.* 2013 Mar;27(3):390-96.
[8896] Hammer KA, Carson CF, Riley TV. Antifungal effects of Melaleuca alternifolia (tea tree) oil and its components on Candida albicans, Candida glabrata and Saccharomyces cerevisiae. *J Antimicrob Chemother.* 2004 Jun;53(6):181-85.
[8897] Kwiecinski J, Eick S, Wojcik K. Effects of tea tree (Melaleuca alternifolia) oil on Staphylococcus aureus in biofilms and stationary growth phase. *Int J Microb Agents.* 2009 Apr;33(4):343-47.
[8898] Carson CF, Mee BJ, Riley TV. Mechanism of action of Melaleuca alternifolia (tea tree) oil on Staphylococcus aureus determined by time-kill, lysis, leakage, and salt tolerance assays and electron microscopy. *Antimicrob Agents Chemother.* 2002 Jun;46(6):1914-20.
[8899] Cox SD, Mann CM, Markham JL, et al. The mode of antimicrobial action of the essential oil of Melaleuca alternifolia (tea tree oil). *J Appl Microbiol.* 2000 Jan;88(1):170-75.
[8900] Cox SD, Gustafson JE, Mann CM, et al. Tea tree causes K+ leakage and inhibits respiration in Escherichia coli. *Lett Appl Microbiol.* 1998 May;26(5):355-58.
[8901] Rajkowska K, Kunicka-Styczyńska A, Maroszyńska M, et al. Selected Essential Oils as Antifungal Agents Against Antibiotic-Resistant Candida spp.: In Vitro Study on Clinical and Food-Borne Isolates. *Microb Drug Resist.* 2017 Jan;23(1):18-24.
[8902] Li WR, Li HL, Shi QS, et al. The dynamics and mechanism of the antimicrobial activity of tea tree oil against bacteria and fungi. *Appl Microbiol Biotechnol.* 2016 Oct;100(20):8865-75.
[8903] Li Y, Shao X, Xu J, et al. Effects and possible mechanism of tea tree oil against Botrytis cinerea and Penicillium expansum in vitro and in vivo test. *Can J Microbiol.* 2017 Mar;63(3):219-227.
[8904] Millar BC, Moore JE. Successful topical treatment of hand warts in a paediatric patient with tea tree oil (Melaleuca alternifolia). *Complement Ther Clin Pract.* 2008 Nov;14(4):225-27.
[8905] Gnatta JR, Pinto FM, Bruna CQ, et al. Comparison of hand hygiene antimicrobial efficacy: Melaleuca alternifolia essential oil versus triclosan. *Rev Lat Am Enfermagen.* 2013 Nov-Dec;21(6):1212-19.
[8906] Messager S, Hammer KA, Carson CF, et al. Effectiveness of hand-cleansing formulations containing tea tree oil assessed ex vivo on human skin and in vivo with volunteers using European standard EN 1499. *J Hosp Infect.* 2005 Mar;59(3):220-28.
[8907] Chin KB, Cordell B. The effect of tea tree oil (Melaleuca alternifolia) on wound healing using a dressing model. *J Altern Complement Med.* 213 Dec;19(12):942-45.
[8908] Low WL, Kenward K, Britland ST, et al. Essential oils and metal ions as alternative antimicrobial agents: a focus on tea tree oil and silver. *Int Wound J.* 2017 Apr;14(2):369-384.
[8909] Sherry E, Boeck H, Warnke PH. Percutaneous treatment of chronic MRSA osteomyelitis with a novel plant-derived antiseptic. *BMC Surgery.* 2001;1:1.
[8910] Tsao N, Kuo CF, Lei HY, et al. Inhibition of group A streptococcal infection by Melaleuca alternifolia (tea tree) oil concentrate in the murine model. *J Appl Microbiol.* 2010 Mar;108(3):936-44.
[8911] Hammer KA. Treatment of acne with tea tree oil (melaleuca) products: A review of efficacy, tolerability and potential modes of action. *Int J Antimicrob Agents.* 2015 Feb;45(2):106-10.
[8912] Bassett IB, Pannowitz DL, Barnetson RS. A comparative study of tea-tree oil versus benzoylperoxide in the treatment of acne. *Med J Aust.* 1990 Oct 15;153(8):455-58.
[8913] Enshaieh S, Jooya A, Siadat AH, et al. The efficacy of 5% topical ta tree gel in mild to moderate acne vulgaris: a randomized, double-blind placebo-controlled study. *Iranian J Dermatol Venereol Leprol.* 2007 Jan-Feb;73(1):22-25.
[8914] D'Arrigo M, Ginestra G, Mandalari G, et al. Synergism and postantibiotic effect of tobramycin and Melaleuca alternifolia (tea tree ) oil against Staphylococcus aureus and Escherichia coli. *Phytomedicine.* 2010 Apr;17(5):317-22.
[8915] Ferrini AM, Mannoni V, Aureli P, et al. Melaleuca alternifolia essential oil possesses potent anti-staphylococcal activity extended to strains resistant to antibiotics. *Int J Immunopathol Pharmacol.* 2006 Jul-Sep;19(3):539-44.
[8916] Furneri PM, Paolino D, Saija A, et al. In vitro antimycoplasmal activity of Melaleuca alternifolia essential oil. *J Antimicrob Chemother.* 2006 Sep;58(3):706-07.
[8917] F Souza C, Baldissera MD, A Vaucher R, et al. In vivo bactericidal effect of Melaleuca alternifolia essential oil against Aeromonas hydrophila: Silver catfish (Rhamdia quelen) as an experimental model. *Microb Pathog.* 2016 Jul 5;98:82-87.
[8918] Barker SC, Altman PM. A randomised, assessor blind, parallel group comparative efficacy trial of three products for the treatment of head lice in children—melaleuca oil and lavender oil, pyretrins and piperonyl butoxide, and a "suffocation" product. *BMC Dermatol.* 2010 Aug;10:6.
[8919] Barker SC, Altman PM. An ex vivo, assessor blind, randomised, parallel group, comparative efficacy trial of the ovicidal activity of three pediculicides after a single application--melaleuca oil and lavender oil, eucalyptus oil and lemon tea tree oil, and a "suffocation" pediculicide. *BMC Dermatol.* 2011 Aug 24;11:14.
[8920] Di Campli E, Di Bartolomeo S, Delli Pizzi P, et al. Activity of tea tree oil and nerolidol alone or in combination against Pediculus capitis (head lice) and its eggs. *Parasitol Res.* 2012 Nov;111(5):1985-92.
[8921] Tirabassi G, Giovannini L, Paggi F, et al. Possible efficacy of lavender and tea tree oils in the treatment of young women affected by mild idiopathic hirsutism. *J Endocrinol Invest.* 2013 Jan;36(1):50-54.
[8922] Kaur CD, Saraf S. In vitro sun protection factor determination of herbal oils used in cosmetics. *Pharmacognosy Res.* 2010 Jan;2(1):22-25.
[8923] Ireland DJ, Greay SJ, Hooper CM, et al. Topically applied Melaleuca alternifolia (tea tree) oil causes direct anticancer cytotoxicity in subcutaneous tumour bearing mice. *J Dermatol Sci.* 212 Aug;67(2):120-29.
[8924] Greay SJ, Ireland DJ, Kissick HT, et al. Inhibition of established subcutaneous murine tumour growth with topical Melaleuca alternifolia (tea tree) oil. *Cancer Chemother Pharmacol.* 2010 Nov;66(6):1095-102.
[8925] Bozzuto G, Colone M, Toccacieli L, et al. Tea tree oil might combat melanoma. *Planta Med.* 2011 Jan;77(1):54-6.
[8926] Calcabrini A, Stringaro A, Toccacieli L, et al. Terpinen-4-ol, the main component of Melaleuca alternifolia (tea tree) oil inhibits the in vitro growth of human melanoma cells. *J Invest Dermatol.* 2004 Feb;122(2):349-60.
[8927] Greay SJ, Ireland DJ, Kissick HT, et al. Induction of necrosis and cell cycle arrest in murine cancer cell lines by Melaleuca alternifolia (tea tree) oil and terpinen-4-ol. *Cancer Chemother Pharmacol.* 2010 Apr;65(5):877-88.
[8928] Kang HY, Na SS, Kim YK. Effects of oral care with essential oil on improvement in oral health status of hospice patients. *J Korean Acad Nurs.*2010 Aug;40(4):473-81.
[8929] De Campos Rasteiro VM, da Costa AC, Araujo CF, et al. Essential oil of Melaleuca alternifolia for the treatment of oral candidiasis induced in an immunosuppressed mouse model. *BMC Complement Altern Med.* 2014 Dec;14:489.
[8930] Sudjana AN, Carson CF, Carson KC, et al. Candida albicans adhesion to human epithelial cells and polystyrene and formation of biofilm is reduced by sub-inhibitory Melaleuca alternifolia (tea tree) essential oil. *Med Mycol.* 2012 Nov;50(8):863-70.
[8931] Hammer KA, Carson CF, Riley TV. Melaleuca alternifolia (tea tree) oil inhibits germ tube formation by Candida albicans. *Med Mycol.* 2000 Oct;38(5):355-62.
[8932] Nogueira MN, Aquino SG, Rossa Junior C, et al. Terpinen-4-ol and alpha-terpineol (tea tree oil components) inhibit the production of IL-1β, IL-6, and IL-10 on human macrophages. *Inflamm Res.* 2014 Sep;63(9):769-78.
[8933] Ninomiya K, Hayama K, Ishijima SA, et al. Suppression of inflammatory reactions by terpinen-4-ol, a main constituent of tea tree oil, in a murine model of oral candidiasis and its suppressive activity to cytokine production of macrophages in vitro. *Biol Pharm Bull.* 213;36(5):838-44.
[8934] Pazyar N, Yaghoobi R, Bagerani N, et al. A review of applications of tea tree oil in dermatology. *Int J Dermatol.* 2013 Jul;52(7):784-90.
[8935] Garozzo A, Timpanaro R, Bisignano B, et al. In vitro antiviral activity of Melaleuca alternifolia essential oil. *Lett Appl Microbiol.* 2009 Dec;49(6):806-08.
[8936] Papadopoulos CJ, Carson CF, Hammer KA, et al. Susceptibility of pseudomonas to Melaleuca alternifolia (tea tree) oil and components. *J Antimicrob Chemother.* 2006 Aug;58(2):449-51.
[8937] Caldefie-Chezet F, Fusillier C, Jarde T, et al. Potential anti-inflammatory effects of Melaleuca alternifolia essential oil on human peripheral blood leukocytes. *Phytother Res.* 2006 May;20(5):364-70.
[8938] Caldefie-Chezet F, Guerry M, Chalchat JC, et al. Anti-inflammatory effects of Melaleuca alternifolia essential oil on human polymorphonuclear neutrophils and monocytes. *Free Radic Res.* 2004 Aug;38(8):805-11.
[8939] Hart PH, Brand C, Carson CF, et al. Terpinen-4-ol, the main component of the essential oil of Melaleuca alternifolia (tea tree oil), suppressed inflammatory mediator production by activated by human monocytes. *Inflamm Res.* 2000 Nov;49(11):619-26.
[8940] Bagg J, Jackson MS, Petrina Sweeney M, et al. Susceptibility to Melaleuca alternifolia (tea tree) oil of yeasts isolated from the mouths of patients with advanced cancer. *Oral Oncol.* 2006 May;42(5):487-92.
[8941] Ramage G, Milligan S, Lappin DF, et al. Antifungal, cytotoxic, and immunomodulatory properties of tea tree oil and its derivative components: potential role in management of oral candidiasis in cancer patients. *Front Microbiol.* 2012 Jun 18;3:220.
[8942] Hammer KA, Dry L, Johnson M, et al. Susceptibility of oral bacteria to Melaleuca alternifolia (tea tree) oil in vitro. *Oral Microbiol Immunol.* 2003 Dec;18(6):389-92.
[8943] Kulik E, Lenkeit K, Meyer J. Antimicrobial effects of tea tree oil (Melaleuca alternifolia) on oral microorganisms. *Schweiz Monatsschr Zahnmed.* 2000;110(11):125-30.
[8944] Saxer UP, Stauble A, Szabo SH, et al. Effect of mouthwashing with tea tree oil on plaque and inflammation. *Schweiz Monatsschr Zahnmed.* 2003;113(9):985-96.
[8945] Farnan TB, McCallum J, Awa A, et al. Tea tree oil: in vitro efficacy in otitis externa. *J Laryngol Otol.* 2005 Mar;119(3):198-201.
[8946] Hammer KA, Carson CF, Riley TV. Antifungal activity of the components of Melaleuca alternifolia (tea tree) oil. *J Appl Microbiol.* 2003;95(4):853-60.
[8947] Oliva B, Piccirilli E, Ceddia T, et al. Antimycotic activity of Melaleuca alternifolia essential oil and its major components. *Lett Appl Microbiol.* 2003;37(2):185-87.
[8948] Ergin A, Arkan S. Comparison of microdilution and disc diffusion methods in assessing the in vitro activity of fluconazole and Melaleuca alternifolia (tea tree) oil against vaginal Candida isolates. *J Chemother.* 2002 Oct;14(5):465- 72.

8949 Hammer KA, Carson CF, Riley TV. In vitro activity of Melaleuca alternifolia (tea tree) oil against dermatophytes and other filamentous fungi. *J Antimicrob Chemother.* 2002 Aug;50(2):195-99.

8950 D'Auria FD, Laino L, Strippoli V, et al. In vitro activity of tea tree oil against Candida albicans myccelial conversion and other pathogenic fungi. *J Chemother.* 2001 Aug;13(4):377-83.

8951 Banes-Marshall L, Cawley P, Phillips CA. In vitro activity of Melaleuca alternifolia (tea tree) oil against bacterial and Candida spp. isolates from clinical specimens. *Br J Biomed Sci.* 2001;58(3):139-45.

8952 Hammer KA, Carson CF, Riley TV. In vitro activities of ketoconazole, econazole, micronazole, and Melaleuca alternifolia (tea tree) oil against Malassezia species. *Antimicrob Agents Chemother.* 2000 Feb;44(2):467-69.

8953 Hammer KA, Carson CF, Riley TV. In vitro susceptibility of Malassezia furfur to the essential oil of Melaleuca alternifolia. *J Med Vet Mycol.* 1997 Sep-Oct;35(5):375-77.

8954 Wallengren J. Tea tree oil attenuates experimental contact dermatitis. *Arch Dermatol Res.* 2011 Jul;303(5):333-38.

8955 Hammer KA, Carson CF, Riley TV. Susceptibility of transient and commercial skin flora to the essential oil of Melaleuca alternifolia (tea tree oil). *Am J Infect Control.* 1996 Jun;24(30:186-89.

8956 Sakkas H, Gousia P, Economou V, et al. In vitro antimicrobial activity of five essential oils on multidrug resistant Gram-negative clinical isolates. *J Intercult Ethnopharmacol.* 2016 Jun-Aug;5(3):212–18.

8957 Ziółkowska-Klinkosz M, Kedzia A, Meissner HO, et al. Evaluation of the tea tree oil activity to anaerobic bacteria—in vitro study. *Acta Pol Pharm.* 2016 Mar-Apr;73(2):389-94.

8958 Comin VM, Lopes LQ, Quatrin PM, et al. Influence of Melaleuca alternifolia oil nanoparticles on aspects of Pseudomonas aeruginosa biofilm. *Microb Pathog.* 2016 Apr;93:120-5.

8959 Syed TA, Qureshi ZA, Ali SM, et al. Treatment of toenail onychomycosis with 2% butenafine and 5% Melaleuca alternifolia (tea tree) oil in cream. *Trop Med Int Health.* 1999 Apr;4(4):284-87.

8960 Buck DS, Nidorf DM, Addino JG. Comparison of two topical preparations for the treatment of onychomycosis: Melaleuca alternifolia (tea tree) oil and clotrimazole. *J Fam Pract.* 1994 Jun;38(6):601-05.

8961 Satchell AC, Saurajen A, Bell C, et al. Treatment of interdigital tinea pedis with 25% and 50% tea tree oil solution: a randomized, placebo-controlled, blinded study. *Australas J Dermatol.* 202 Aug;43(3):175-78.

8962 Carson CF, Cookson BD, Farrelly HD, et al. Susceptibility of methicillin-resistant Staphylococcus aureus to the essential oil of Melaleuca alternifolia. *J Antimicrob Chemother.* 1995 Mar;35(3):421-24.

8963 Thompson G, Blackwood B, McMullan R, et al. A randomized controlled trial of tea tree oil (5%) body wash versus standard body wash to prevent colonization with methicillin-resistant Staphylococcus aureus (MRSA) in critically ill adults: research protocol. *BMC Infect Dis.* 2008 Nov 28;8:161.

8964 LaPlante KL. In vitro activity of lysostaphin, mupirocin, and tea tree oil against clinical methicillin-resistant Staphylococcus aureus. *Diagn Microbiol Infect Dis.* 2007 Apr;57(4):413-18.

8965 Brady A, Loughlin R, Gilpin D, et al. In vitro activity of tea tree oil against clinical skin isolates of methicillin-resistant and -sensitive Staphylococcus aureus and coagulase-negative staphylococci growing planktonically and as biofilms. *J Med Microbiol.* 2006 Oct;55(Pt 10):1375-80.

8966 Dryden MS, Dailly S, Crouch M. A randomized controlled trial of tea tree topical preparations versus a standard topical regimen for the clearance of MRSA colonization. *J Hosp Infect.* 2004 Apr;56(4):283-86.

8967 Bradley SF. MRSA colonisation (eradicating colonisation in people without active/invasive infection). *BMJ Clin Evid.* 2011 Jan 17;2011.

8968 Modello F, De Bernardis F, Girolamo A, et al. In vivo activity of terpinen-4-ol, the main bioactive component of Melaleuca alternifolia Cheel (tea tree) oil against azole-susceptible and -resistant human pathogenic Candida species. *BMC Infect Dis.* 2006 Nov 3;6:158.

8969 Mirza MA, Ahmad S, Mallick MN, et al. Development of a novel synergistic thermosensitive gel for vaginal candidiasis: an in vitro, in vivo evaluation. *Colloids Surf B Biointerfaces.* 2013 Mar;103:275-82.

8970 Azimi H, Fallah-Tafti M, Karimi-Darmiyan M, et al. A comprehensive review of vaginitis phytotherapy. *Pak J Biol Sci.* 2011 Nov 1;14(21):960-66.

8971 Joksimovic N, Spasovski G, Joksimovic V, et al. Efficacy and tolerability of hyaluronic acid, tea tree oil and methyl- sulfonyl-methane in a gel medical device for treatment of haemorrhoids in a double-blind, placebo-controlled clinical trial. *Updates Surg.* 2012 Sep;64(3):195-201.

8972 Markum E, Baillie J. Combination of essential oil of Melaleuca alternifolia and iodine in the treatment of molluscum contagiosum in children. *J Drugs Dermatol.* 2012 Mar;11(3):349-54.

8973 Gao YY, Xu DL, Huang IJ, et al. Treatment of ocular itching associated with ocular demodicosis by 5% tea tree oil ointment. *Cornea.* 2012 Jan;31(1):14-17.

8974 Schnitzler P, Reichling J. Efficacy of plant products against herpetic infections. *HNO.* 2011 Dec;59(12):1176-84.

8975 Pearce AL, Finlay-Jones JJ, Hart PH. Reduction of nickel-induced contact hypersensitivity reactions by topical tea tree oil in humans. *Inflamm Res.* 2005 Jan;54(1):22-30.

8976 Walton SF, McKinnon M, Pizzutto S, et al. Acaricidal activity of Melaleuca alternifolia (tea tree) oil: in vitro sensitivity of sarcoptes scabiei var hominis to terpinen-4-ol. *Arch Dermatol.* 204 May;140(5):563-66.

8977 Walton SF, Myerscough MR, Currie BJ. Studies In vitro on the relative efficacy of current acaricides for Sarcoptes scabiei var hominis. *Trans R Soc Trop Med Hyg.* 2000 Jan-Feb;94(1):92-96.

8978 Satchell AC, Aurajen A, Bell C, et al. Treatment of dandruff with 5% tea tree oil shampoo. *J Am Acad Dermatol.* 2002 Dec;47(6):852-55.

8979 Vazquez JA, Zawawii AA. Efficacy of alcohol-based and alcohol-free melaleuca oral solution for the treatment of fluconazole-refractory oropharyngeal candidiasis in patients with AIDS. *HIV Clin Trials.* 202 Sep-Oct;3(5):379-85.

8980 Budhiraja SS, Cullum ME, Sioutis SS, et al. Biological activity of Melaleuca alternifolia (Tea Tree) oil component, terpinen-4-ol, in human myelocytic cell line HL-60. *J Manipulative Ther.* 1999 Sep;22(7):447-53.

8981 Low P, Clark AM, Chou TC, et al. Immunomodulatory activity of Melaleuca alternifolia concentrate (MAC): Inhibition of LPS-induced NF-KB activation and cytokine production in myeloid cell lines. *Int Immunopharmacol.* 2015 May;26(1):257-64.

8982 Banjerdpongchai R, Khaw-On P. Terpinen-4-ol induces autophagic and apoptotic cell death in human leukemic HL-60 cells. *Asian Pac J Cancer Prev.* 2013;14(12):7537-42.

8983 Grando TH, Baldissera MD2, Gressler LT, et al. Melaleuca alternifolia anthelmintic activity in gerbils experimentally infected by Haemonchus contortus. *Exp Parasitol.* 2016 Nov;170:177-183.

8984 Plant J. Effects of essential oils on telomere length in human cells. *Med Aromat Plants.* 2016;5(2):1-6.

8985 Fang F, Candy K, Melloul E, et al. In vitro activity of ten essential oils against Sarcoptes scabiei. *Parasit Vectors.* 2016 Nov 22;9(1):594.

8986 Yim WT, Bhandari B, Jackson L, et al. Repellent effects of Melaleuca alternifolia (tea tree) oil against cattle tick larvae (Rhipicephalus australis) when formulated as emulsions and in β-cyclodextrin inclusion complexes. *Vet Parasitol.* 2016 Jul 30;225:99-103.

8987 Pazinatto Boito J, Santos RC, Vaucher RA, et al. Evaluation of tea tree oil for controlling Rhipicephalus microplus in dairy cows. *Vet Parasitol.* 2016 Jul 30;225:70-2.

8988 de Souza Silveira Valente J, de Oliveira da Silva Fonseca A, Denardi LB, et al. In Vitro Susceptibility of Pythium insidiosum to Melaleuca alternifolia, Mentha piperita and Origanum vulgare Essential Oils Combinations. *Mycopathologia.* 2016 Aug;181(7-8):617-22.

8989 Rajkowska K, Kunicka-Styczyńska A, Maroszyńska M, et al. Selected Essential Oils as Antifungal Agents Against Antibiotic-Resistant Candida spp.: In Vitro Study on Clinical and Food-Borne Isolates. *Microb Drug Resist.* 2017 Jan;23(1):18-24.

8990 Hadaś E, Derda M, Cholewiński M, et al. Evaluation of the effectiveness of tea tree oil in treatment of Acanthamoeba infection. *Parasitol Res.* 2017 Mar;116(3):997-1001.

8991 Nikolić MM, Jovanović KK, Marković TL, et al. Antimicrobial synergism and cytotoxic properties of Citrus limon L., Piper nigrum L. and Melaleuca alternifolia (Maiden and Betche) Cheel essential oils. *J Pharm Pharmacol.* 2017 Nov;69(11):1606-1614.

8992 Salvatori C, Barchi L, Guzzo F, et al. A comparative study of antibacterial and anti-inflammatory effects of mouthrinse containing tea tree oil. *Oral Implantol (Rome).* 2017 Apr 10;10(1):59-70.

8993 Xu J, Shao X, Wei Y, et al. iTRAQ Proteomic Analysis Reveals That Metabolic Pathways Involving Energy Metabolism Are Affected by Tea Tree Oil in Botrytis cinerea. *Front Microbiol.* 2017 Oct 12;8:1989.

8994 Monteiro DU, Azevedo MI, Weiblen C, et al. In vitro and ex vivo activity of Melaleuca alternifolia against protoscoleces of Echinococcus ortleppi. *Parasitology.* 2017 Feb;144(2):214-219.

8995 Lee SY, Chen PY, Lin JC, et al. Melaleuca alternifolia Induces Heme Oxygenase-1 Expression in Murine RAW264.7 Cells through Activation of the Nrf2-ARE Pathway. *Am J Chin Med.* 2017;45(8):1631-1648.

8996 Candy K, Nicolas P, Andriantsoanirina V, et al. In vitro efficacy of five essential oils against Pediculus humanus capitis. *Parasitol Res.* 2018 Feb;117(2):603-609.

8997 Zhang X, Guo Y, Guo L, et al. In Vitro Evaluation of Antioxidant and Antimicrobial Activities of Melaleuca alternifolia Essential Oil. *Biomed Res Int.* 2018 May 6;2018:2396109.

8998 Koseki Y, Tanaka R, Murata H. Development of antibacterial denture cleaner for brushing containing tea tree and lemongrass essential oils. *Dent Mater J.* 2018 Jul 29;37(4):659-666.

8999 Li M, Zhu L, Zhang T, et al. Pulmonary delivery of tea tree oil-β-cyclodextrin inclusion complexes for the treatment of fungal and bacterial pneumonia. *J Pharm Pharmacol.* 2017 Nov;69(11):1458-1467.

9000 Piekarz T, Mertas A, Wiatrak K, et al. The Influence of Toothpaste Containing Australian Melaleuca alternifolia Oil and Ethanolic Extract of Polish Propolis on Oral Hygiene and Microbiome in Patients Requiring Conservative Procedures. *Molecules.* 2017 Nov 13;22(11).

9001 Zhao X, Liu Z, Liu Z, et al. Phenotype and RNA-seq-Based transcriptome profiling of Staphylococcus aureus biofilms in response to tea tree oil. *Microb Pathog.* 2018 Jul 21;123:304-313.

9002 de Souza ME, Clerici DJ, Verdi CM, et al. Antimicrobial activity of Melaleuca alternifolia nanoparticles in polymicrobial biofilm in situ. *Microb Pathog.* 2017 Dec;113:432-437.

9003 Najafi-Taher R, Ghaemi B, Kharazi S, et al. Promising Antibacterial Effects of Silver Nanoparticle-Loaded Tea Tree Oil Nanoemulsion: a Synergistic Combination Against Resistance Threat. *AAPS PharmSciTech.* 2018 Apr;19(3):1133-1140.

9004 Vasireddy L, Bingle LEH, Davies MS. Antimicrobial activity of essential oils against multidrug-resistant clinical isolates of the Burkholderia cepacia complex. *PLoS One.* 2018 Aug 2;13(8):e0201835.

9005 Chohan TA, Chohan TA, Zhou L, et al. Repellency, Toxicity, Gene Expression Profiling and In Silico Studies to Explore Insecticidal Potential of Melaleuca alternifolia Essential Oil against Myzus persicae. *Toxins (Basel).* 2018 Oct 25;10(11).

9006 Noumi E, Merghni A, M Alreshidi M, et al. Chromobacterium violaceum and Pseudomonas aeruginosa PAO1: Models for Evaluating Anti-Quorum Sensing Activity of Melaleuca alternifolia Essential Oil and Its Main Component Terpinen-4-ol. *Molecules.* 2018 Oct 17;23(10).

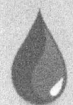

9007 Oliva A, Costantini S, De Angelis M, et al. High Potency of Melaleuca alternifolia Essential Oil against Multi-Drug Resistant Gram-Negative Bacteria and Methicillin-Resistant Staphylococcus aureus. *Molecules.* 2018 Oct 9;23(10).

9008 Assmann CE, Cadoná FC, Bonadiman BDSR, et al. Tea tree oil presents in vitro antitumor activity on breast cancer cells without cytotoxic effects on fibroblasts and on peripheral blood mononuclear cells. *Biomed Pharmacother.* 2018 Jul;103:1253-1261.

9009 Liao M, Yang QQ, Xiao JJ, et al. Toxicity of Melaleuca alternifolia essential oil to the mitochondrion and NAD+/NADH dehydrogenase in Tribolium confusum. *PeerJ.* 2018 Nov 13;6:e5693.

9010 Brun P, Bernabè G, Filippini R, et al. In Vitro Antimicrobial Activities of Commercially Available Tea Tree (Melaleuca alternifolia) Essential Oils. *Curr Microbiol.* 2019 Jan;76(1):108-116.

9011 Muchembled J, Deweer C, Sahmer K, et al. Gene expression responses of Listeria monocytogenes Scott A exposed to sub-lethal concentrations of natural antimicrobials. *Environ Sci Pollut Res Int.* 2018 Oct;25(30):29921-29928.

9012 Ramadan MA, Shawkey AE, Rabeh MA, et al. Expression of P53, BAX, and BCL-2 in human malignant melanoma and squamous cell carcinoma cells after tea tree oil treatment in vitro. *Cytotechnology.* 2019 Feb;71(1):461-473.

9013 Shi C, Zhang X, Guo N. The antimicrobial activities and action-mechanism of tea tree oil against food-borne bacteria in fresh cucumber juice. *Microb Pathog.* 2018 Dec;125:262-271.

9014 Agrawal SK, Dahal S, Bhumika TV, et al. Evaluating Sanitization of Toothbrushes Using Various Decontamination Methods: A Meta-Analysis. *J Nepal Health Res Counc.* 2019 Jan 27;16(41):364-371.

9015 Pereira Dos Santos E, Nicácio PHM, Coêlho Barbosa F, et al. Chitosan/Essential Oils Formulations for Potential Use as Wound Dressing: Physical and Antimicrobial Properties. *Materials (Basel).* 2019 Jul 10;12(14).

9016 Ergun SB, Saribas GS, Yarayici S, et al. Comparison of Efficacy and Safety of Two Tea Tree Oil-Based Formulations in Patients with Chronic Blepharitis: A Double-Blinded Randomized Clinical Trial. *Ocul Immunol Inflamm.* 2019 Aug 20:1-10.

9017 Karakurt Y, Zeytun E. Evaluation of the Efficacy of Tea Tree Oil On the Density of Demodex Mites (Acari: Demodicidae) and Ocular Symptoms In Patients With Demodectic Blepharitis. *J Parasitol.* 2018 Oct;104(5):473-478.

9018 Labib RM, Ayoub IM, Michel HE, et al. Appraisal on the wound healing potential of Melaleuca alternifolia and Rosmarinus officinalis L. essential oil-loaded chitosan topical preparations. *PLoS One.* 2019 Sep 16;14(9):e0219561.

9019 Tullio V, Roana J, Scalas D, et al. Enhanced Killing of Candida krusei by Polymorphonuclear Leucocytes in the Presence of Subinhibitory Concentrations of Melaleuca alternifolia and "Mentha of Pancalieri" Essential Oils. *Molecules.* 2019 Oct 23;24(21).

9020 Carmo PHF, Costa MC, Franco PH, et al. Essential Oils of Taxandria fragrans and Melaleuca alternifolia Have Effective Antidermatophytic Activities in vitro and in vivo That Are Antagonised by Ketoconazole and Potentiated in Gold Nanospheres. *Nat Prod Res.* 2020 Jan 2:1-4.

9021 Esmael A, Hassan MG, Amer MM, et al. Antimicrobial activity of certain natural-based plant oils against the antibiotic-resistant acne bacteria. *Saudi J Biol Sci.* 2020 Jan;27(1):448–455.

9022 Krzyśko-Lupicka T, Sokół S, Piekarska-Stachowiak A. Evaluation of Fungistatic Activity of Eight Selected Essential Oils on Four Heterogeneous Fusarium Isolates Obtained From Cereal Grains in Southern Poland. *Molecules.* 2020 Jan 10;25(2):292.

9023 Korona-Glowniak I, Glowniak-Lipa A, Ludwiczuk A, et al. The In Vitro Activity of Essential Oils Against Helicobacter Pylori Growth and Urease Activity. *Molecules.* 2020 Jan 29;25(3):586.

9024 Kamath NP, Tandon S, Nayak R, et al. The Effect of Aloe Vera and Tea Tree Oil Mouthwashes on the Oral Health of School Children. *Eur Arch Paediatr Dent.* 2020 Feb;21(1):61-66.

9025 Amorese V, Donadu M, Usai D, et al. In vitro activity of essential oils against Pseudomonas aeruginosa isolated from infected hip implants. *J Infect Dev Ctries.* 2018 Nov 30;12(11):996-1001.

9026 Dillmann JB, Cossetin LF, de Giacometi M. et al. Adulticidal Activity of Melaleuca alternifolia (Myrtales: Myrtaceae) Essential Oil With High 1,8-Cineole Content Against Stable Flies (Diptera: Muscidae). *J Econ Entomol.* 2020 Jun 9. [Online ahead of print]

9027 Francisconi RS, Huacho PMM, Tonon CC, et al. Antibiofilm Efficacy of Tea Tree Oil and of Its Main Component terpinen-4-ol Against Candida Albicans. *Braz Oral Res.* 2020 Jun 5;34:e050.

9028 Liu T, Wang J, Gong X, et al. Rosemary and Tea Tree Essential Oils Exert Antibiofilm Activities In Vitro Against Staphylococcus Aureus and Escherichia Coli. *J Food Prot.* 2020 Jul 1;83(7):1261-1267.

9029 Bedini S, Cosci F, Tani C, et al. Essential Oils as Post-Harvest Crop Protectants against the Fruit Fly Drosophila suzukii: Bioactivity and Organoleptic Profile. *Insects.* 2020 Aug 5;11(8):E508.

9030 de Assis KMA, da Silva Leite JM, de Melo DF, et al. Bicontinuous microemulsions containing Melaleuca alternifolia essential oil as a therapeutic agent for cutaneous wound healing. *Drug Deliv Transl Res.* 2020 Sep 13. Online ahead of print.

9031 Marcos-Tejedor F, Gonzalez-Garcia P, Mayordomo R. Solubilization in vitro of tea tree oil and first results of antifungal effect in onychomycosis. *Enferm Infecc Microbiol Clin.* 2020 Sep 7;S0213-005X(20)30245-7.

9032 Song YM, Zhou HY, Wu Y, et al. In Vitro Evaluation of the Antibacterial Properties of Tea Tree Oil on Planktonic and Biofilm-Forming Streptococcus mutans. *AAPS PharmSciTech.* 2020 Aug 6;21(6):227.

9033 Voros-Horvath B, Das S, Salem A, et al. Formulation of Tioconazole and Melaleuca alternifolia Essential Oil Pickering Emulsions for Onychomycosis Topical Treatment. *Molecules.* 2020 Nov 26;25(23):5544.

9034 Ossa-Tabares JC, Llanos CJ, Garcia AM, et al. Evaluation of tea tree oil physicochemical features and its antimicrobial activity against Cutibacterium acnes (Propionibacterium acnes) ATCC 6919. *Biomedica.* 2020 Dec 1;40(4):693-701.

9035 Kundu A, Dutta A, Mandal A, et al. A Comprehensive in vitro and in silico Analysis of Nematicidal Action of Essential Oils. *Front Plant Sci.* 2021 Jan 8;11:614143.

9036 Roana J, Mandras N, Scalas D, et al. Antifungal Activity of Melaleuca alternifolia Essential Oil (TTO) and Its Synergy with Itraconazole or Ketoconazole against Trichophyton rubrum. *Molecules.* 2021 Jan 17;26(2):461.

9037 Mohammadpour M, Maleki S, Khorrami-Nejad M. The effect of tea tree oil on dry eye treatment after phacoemulsification cataract surgery: A randomized clinical trial. *Eur J Ophthalmol.* 2020 Nov;30(6):1314-1319.

9038 Gnatta JR, Poveda VDB, Padoveze MC, et al. Melaleuca alternifolia essential oil soap: a potential alternative for hand hygiene. *Eur J Clin Microbiol Infect Dis.* 2021 Feb 26. Online ahead of print.

9039 Santos AA, Wanderley-Teixeira V, Dos Santos Cruz G, et al. Essential oil toxicity on biological and reproductive parameters of Alabama argillacea (Hübner) (Lepidoptera: Erebidae). *Acta Histochem.* 2021 Apr 12;123(4):151714.

9040 Melegari G, Iseppi R, Mariani M, et al. Keyboard Contamination in Intensive Care Unit: Is Cleaning Enough? Prospective Research of In Situ Effectiveness of a Tea Tree Oil (KTEO) Film. *Adv Exp Med Biol.* 2021;1323:91-102.

9041 Dudek-Wicher R, Paleczny J, Kowalska-Krochmal B, et al. Activity of Liquid and Volatile Fractions of Essential Oils against Biofilm Formed by Selected Reference Strains on Polystyrene and Hydroxyapatite Surfaces. *Pathogens.* 2021 Apr 23;10(5):515.

9042 Youn BH, Kim YS, Yoo S, et al. Antimicrobial and hand hygiene effects of Tea Tree Essential Oil disinfectant: A randomized control trial. *Int J Clin Pract.* 2021 May 5;e14206.

9043 Aryani R, Nurulhuda U, Dinarti, et al. Comparison of honey and natural ointment based on honey-tea tree oil on the healing of diabetic foot ulcer. *Enferm Clin.* 2020 Mar;30 Suppl 3:14-17.

9044 Puvaca N, Milenkovic J, Coghill TG, et al. Antimicrobial Activity of Selected Essential Oils against Selected Pathogenic Bacteria: In Vitro Study. *Antibiotics (Basel).* 2021 May 8;10(5):546.

9045 Ahmed Q, Agarwal M, Al-Obaidi R, et al. Evaluation of Aphicidal Effect of Essential Oils and Their Synergistic Effect against Myzus persicae (Sulzer) (Hemiptera: Aphididae). *Molecules.* 2021 May 20;26(10):3055.

9046 Martile MD, Garzoli S, Sabatino M, et al. Antitumor effect of Melaleuca alternifolia essential oil and its main component terpinen-4-ol in combination with target therapy in melanoma models. *Cell Death Discov.* 2021 May 31;7(1):127.

9047 Taalab MR, Mahmoud SA, Moslemany RME, et al. Intrapocket application of tea tree oil gel in the treatment of stage 2 periodontitis. *BMC Oral Health.* 2021 May 5;21(1):239.

9048 Marcos-Tejedor F, Gonzalez-Garcia P, Mayordomo R, et al. Solubilization in vitro of tea tree oil and first results of antifungal effect in onychomycosis. *Enferm Infecc Microbiol Clin (Engl Ed).* 2021 Jul 29;S2529-993X(21)00148-9.

9049 Wiatrak K, Morawiec T, Roj R, et al. Evaluation of Effectiveness of a Toothpaste Containing Tea Tree Oil and Ethanolic Extract of Propolis on the Improvement of Oral Health in Patients Using Removable Partial Dentures. *Molecules.* 2021 Jul 3;26(13):4071.

9050 Qi J, Gong M, Zhang R, et al. Evaluation of the antibacterial effect of tea tree oil on Enterococcus faecalis and biofilm in vitro. *J Ethnopharmacol.* 2021 Aug 24;281:114566.

9051 Manikandan S, Bhambal AM, Ratchambiga KS, et al. Comparative Evaluation of the Effect of 0.2% Chlorhexidine, 2% LemonGrass Oil, and 2% Tea Tree Oil Mouth rinse on Salivary pH: An In vivo Study. *J Pharm Bioallied Sci.* 2021 Jun;13(Suppl 1):S757-S760.

9052 Abrha S, Christenson JK, McEwen J, et al. Treatment of tungiasis using a tea tree oil-based gel formulation: protocol for a randomised controlled proof-of-principle trial. *BMJ Open.* 2021 Jul 29;11(7):e047380.

9053 Clark AM, Magawa C, Pliego-Zamora A, et al. Tea tree oil extract causes mitochondrial superoxide production and apoptosis as an anticancer agent, promoting tumor infiltrating neutrophils cytotoxic for breast cancer to induce tumor regression. *Biomed Pharmacother.* 2021 Aug;140:111790.

9054 Brozyna M, Paleczny J, Kozlowska W, et al. The Antimicrobial and Antibiofilm In Vitro Activity of Liquid and Vapour Phases of Selected Essential Oils against Staphylococcus aureus. *Pathogens.* 2021 Sep 17;10(9):1207.

9055 Haines RR, Putsathit P, Tai AS, et al. Antimicrobial effects of Melaleuca alternifolia (tea tree) essential oil against biofilm-forming multidrug-resistant cystic fibrosis-associated Pseudomonas aeruginosa as a single agent and in combination with commonly nebulized antibiotics. *Lett Appl Microbiol.* 2021 Oct 23. Online ahead of print.

9056 Yasin R, Younis A, Javed T, et al. River Tea Tree Oil: Composition, Antimicrobial and Antioxidant Activities, and Potential Applications in Agriculture. *Plants (Basel).* 2021 Oct 4;10(10):2105.

9057 Mergen B, Arici C, Yildiz-Tas A, et al. Swabs Containing Tea Tree Oil and Chamomile Oil Versus Baby Shampoo in Patients With Seborrheic Blepharitis: A Double-Blind Randomized Clinical Trial. *Eye Contact Lens.* 2021 Nov 1;47(11):604-610.

[9058] Melegari G, Iseppi R, Mariani N, et al. Keyboard Contamination in Intensive Care Unit: Is Cleaning Enough? Prospective Research of In Situ Effectiveness of a Tea Tree Oil (KTEO) Film. *Adv Exp Med Biol.* 2020 Sep 11. Online ahead of print.
[9059] Abrha S, Tesfaye W, Thomas J. Therapeutic Potential of Tea Tree Oil for Tungiasis. *Am J Trop Med Hyg.* 2021 Oct 26;105(5):1157-1162.
[9060] Wróblewska M, Szymańska E, Winnicka K. The Influence of Tea Tree Oil on Antifungal Activity and Pharmaceutical Characteristics of Pluronic ® F-127 Gel Formulations with Ketoconazole. *Int J Mol Sci.* 2021 Oct 20;22(21):11326.
[9061] Wei S, Zhao X, Yu J, et al. Characterization of tea tree oil nanoemulsion and its acute and subchronic toxicity. *Regul Toxicol Pharmacol.* 2021 Aug;124:104999.
[9062] Infante V, Campos PM, Gaspar LR, et al. Safety and efficacy of combined essential oils for the skin barrier properties: in vitro, ex vivo and clinical studies. *Int J Cosmet Sci.* 2022 Jan 5. Online ahead of print.
[9063] Chen L, Alrobaian M, Afzal O, et al. Crotamiton-loaded tea tree oil containing phospholipid-based microemulsion hydrogel for scabies treatment: in vitro, in vivo evaluation, and dermatokinetic studies. *Drug Deliv.* 2021 Dec;28(1):1972-1981.
[9064] Zarei-Ghanavati S, Nooghabi MJ, Zamani G. Comparison of the Effect of Tea Tree Oil Shampoo With Regular Eyelid Shampoo in Meibomian Gland Dysfunction Treatment. *Am J Ophthalmol.* 2021 Sep;229:45-51.
[9065] Arcella A, Sanchez M. Natural substances to potentiate canonical glioblastoma chemotherapy. *J Chemother.* 2021 Sep;33(5):276-287.
[9066] Borotová P, Galovičová L, Vukovic NL, et al. Chemical and Biological Characterization of Melaleuca alternifolia Essential Oil. *Plants (Basel).* 2022 Feb 20;11(4):558.
[9067] Aponso M, Patti A, Hearn MTW, et al. Anxiolytic effects of essential oils may involve anti-oxidant regulation of the pro-oxidant effects of ascorbate in the brain. *Neurochem Int.* 2021 Nov;150:105153.
[9068] Altun M, Yapici BM. Determination of chemical compositions and antibacterial effects of selected essential oils against human pathogenic strains. *An Acad Bras Cienc.* 2022 Mar 11;94(1):e20210074.
[9069] Man A, Mare AD, Mares M, et al. Antifungal and anti-virulence activity of six essential oils against important Candida species - a preliminary study. *Future Microbiol.* 2022 Jul;17:737-753.
[9070] Man A, Mare AD, Mares M, et al. Antifungal and anti-virulence activity of six essential oils against important Candida species - a preliminary study. *Future Microbiol.* 2022 Jul;17:737-753.
[9071] Yurekli A, Botsali A. The comparative in vitro killing activity of tea tree oil versus permethrin on Demodex folliculorum of rosacea patients. *J Cosmet Dermatol.* 2022 May;21(5):2268-2272.
[9072] Madia VN, Toscanelli W, De Vita D, et al. Ultrastructural Damages to H1N1 Influenza Virus Caused by Vapor Essential Oils. *Molecules.* 2022 Jun 9;27(12):3718.
[9073] Romeo A, Iacovelli F, Scagnolari C, et al. Potential Use of Tea Tree Oil as a Disinfectant Agent against Coronaviruses: A Combined Experimental and Simulation Study. *Molecules.* 2022 Jun 12;27(12):3786.
[9074] Brożyna M, Paleczny J, Kozłowska W, et al. Chemical Composition and Antibacterial Activity of Liquid and Volatile Phase of Essential Oils against Planktonic and Biofilm-Forming Cells of Pseudomonas aeruginosa. *Molecules.* 2022 Jun 25;27(13):4096.
[9075] Wei S, Tian Q, Zhao X, et al. Tea Tree Oil Nanoemulsion Potentiates Antibiotics against Multidrug-Resistant Escherichia coli. *ACS Infect Dis.* 2022 Jul 19. Online ahead of print.
[9076] BinShabaib MS, ALHarthi SS, Helaby BS, et al. Cɒmparison of the Anti-bacterial Efficacy of Saussurea costus and Melaleuca alternifolia Against Porphyromonas gingivalis, Streptococcus mutans, and Enterococcus faecalis: An in-vitro Study. *Front Oral Health.* 2022 Jun 27;3:950840.
[9077] Najafi-Taher R, Jafarzadeh Kohneloo A, Eslami Farsani V, et al. A topical gel of tea tree oil nanoemulsion containing adapalene versus adapalene marketed gel in patients with acne vulgaris: a randomized clinical trial. *Arch Dermatol Res.* 2022 Sep;314(7):673-679.
[9078] Gray BH, Green KJ, Haines RR, et al. Antibacterial interactions between two monofloral honeys and several topical antiseptics, including essential oils. *BMC Complement Med Ther.* 2022 Aug 26;22(1):228.
[9079] Fernandes L, Gonçalves B, Costa R, et al. Vapor-Phase of Essential Oils as a Promising Solution to Prevent Candida Vaginal Biofilms Caused by Antifungal Resistant Strains. *Healthcare (Basel).* 2022 Aug 29;10(9):1649.
[9080] Toschi A, Piva A, Grilli E. Phenol-Rich Botanicals Modulate Oxidative Stress and Epithelial Integrity in Intestinal Epithelial Cells. *Animals (Basel).* 2022 Aug 25;12(17):2188.
[9081] Kamel R, Afifi SM, Abdou AM, et al. Nanolipogel Loaded with Tea Tree Oil for the Management of Burn: GC-MS Analysis, In Vitro and In Vivo Evaluation. *Molecules.* 2022 Sep 20;27(19):6143.
[9082] Hu K, Jia E, Zhang Q, et al. Injectable carboxymethyl chitosan-genipin hydrogels encapsulating tea tree oil for wound healing. *Carbohydr Polym.* 2023 Feb 1;301(Pt B):120348.
[9083] Yürekli A. Adjunctive Agent for Treating Scabies: In vitro Killing Activity of Permethrin and Tea Tree Oil on Sarcoptes scabiei Collected from Patients. *Turkiye Parazitol Derg.* 2022 Nov 28;46(4):334-338.
[9084] Ibrahium SM, Wahba AA, Farghali AA, et al. Acaricidal Activity of Tea Tree and Lemon Oil Nanoemulsions against Rhipicephalus annulatus. *Pathogens.* 2022 Dec 9;11(12):1506.
[9085] Aquilano C, Baccari L, Caprari C, et al. Effects of EOs vs. Antibiotics on E. coli Strains Isolated from Drinking Waters of Grazing Animals in the Upper Molise Region, Italy. *Molecules.* 2022 Nov 24;27(23):8177.
[9086] Tullio V, Roana J, Cavallo L, et al. Immune Defences: A View from the Side of the Essential Oils. *Molecules.* 2023 Jan 3;28(1):435.
[9087] Bo R, Zhan Y, Wei S, et al. Tea tree oil nanoliposomes: optimization, characterization, and antibacterial activity against Escherichia coli in vitro and in vivo. *Poult Sci.* 2023 Jan;102(1):102238.
[9088] Iseppi R, Mariani M, Benvenuti S, et al. Effects of Melaleuca alternifolia Chell (Tea Tree) and Eucalyptus globulus Labill. Essential Oils on Antibiotic-Resistant Bacterial Biofilms. *Molecules.* 2023 Feb 9;28(4):1671.
[9089] Sathiyaseelan A, Zhang X, Wang MH. Enhancing the Antioxidant, Antibacterial, and Wound Healing Effects of Melaleuca alternifolia Oil by Microencapsulating It in Chitosan-Sodium Alginate Microspheres. *Nutrients.* 2023 Mar 7;15(6):1319.
[9090] Oran NT, Alan N, Akokay P, et al. The healing effect of topical tea tree oil on pressure ulcers in a rat model. *J Wound Care.* 2023 Mar 2;32(Sup3a):xiv-xxi.
[9091] Şahin E, Yildirim F, Büyükkayaci Duman N. Effect of Tea Tree Oil and Coconut Oil on Nipple Crack Formation in the Early Postpartum Period. *Breastfeed Med.* 2023 Mar;18(3):226-232.
[9092] Lawrence BM. Progress in essential oils. *Perfumer & Flavorist.* 1998;5:67-68.
[9093] Cedarwood Oil. Summary of data for chemical selection. Available at: https://ntp.niehs.nih.gov/ntp/htdocs/chem_background/exsumpdf/cedarwood_oil_508.pdf.
[9094] Barefut Essential Oils. Chromatogram Texas Cedarwood. Available at: http://barefut.com/dr-pappas/essential-oil-university/gc-ms-analysis-test/1510Texas-Cedarwood.pdf.
[9095] Jeong HU, Kwon SS, Kong TY, et al. Inhibitory effects of cedrol, β-cedrene, and thujopsene on cytochrome P450 enzyme activities in human liver microsomes. *J Toxicol Environ Health A.* 2014;77(22-24):1522-32.
[9096] Tumen I, Süntar I, Eller FJ, et al. Topical Wound-Healing Effects and Phytochemical Composition of Heartwood Essential Oils of Juniperus Virginiana L., Juniperus occidentalis Hook., and Juniperus ashei J. Buchholz. *J Med Food.* 2013 Jan;16(1):48-55.
[9097] Wanner J, Schmidt E, Bail S, et al. Chemical composition and antibacterial activity of selected essential oils and some of their main constituents. *Nat Prod Commun.* 2010 Sep;5(9):1359-64.
[9098] Szołyga1 B, Gniłka R, Szczepanik M, et al. Chemical composition and insecticidal activity of Thuja occidentalis and Tanacetum vulgare essential oils against larvae of the lesser mealworm, Alphitobius diaperinus. *Entonologia Experimentalis er Applicata.* 2014 Apr;151(1):1-10.
[9099] Simard S, Hachey JM, Collin GJ. The Variations of Essential Oil Composition During the Extraction Process. The Case of Thuja occidentalis L. and Abies balsamea (L.) Mill. *J Wood Chem Tech.* 1998;8(4):561-73.
[9100] Küpeli Akkol E, İlhan M, Ayşe Demirel M, et al. Thuja occidentalis L. and its active constituent, α-thujone: Promising effects in the treatment of polycystic ovary syndrome without inducing osteoporosis. *J Ethnopharmacol.* 2015 Jun 20;168:25-30.
[9101] Haliciglu O, Astarcioglu G, Yaprak I, et al. Toxicity of Salvia officinalis in a newborn and a child: an alarming report. *Pediatr Neurol.* 2011 Oct;45(4):259-60.
[9102] Lachenmeier DW, Walch SG. Epileptic seizure caused by accidental ingestion of sage (Salvia officinalis L.) oil in children: a rare, exceptional case or a threat to public health. *Pediatr Neurol.* 2012 Mar;46(3):201.
[9103] Stafstrom CE. Seizures in a 7-month-old child after exposure to the essential plant oil thuja. *Pediatr Neurol.* 2007 Dec;37(6):446-8.
[9104] Khine H, Weiss D, Graber N, et al. A cluster of children with seizures caused by camphor poisoning. *Pediatrics.* 2009 May;123(5):1269-72.
[9105] Michiels EA, Mazor SS. Toddler with seizures due to ingesting camphor at an Indian celebration. *Pediatr Emerg Care.* 2010 Aug;26(8):574-75.
[9106] Koren G. Medications which can kill a toddler with one tablet or teaspoonful. *J toxicol Clin toxicol.* 1993;31(3):407- 13.
[9107] Rabl W, Katzgraber F, Steinlechner M. Camphor ingestion for abortion (case report). *Forensic Sci Int.* 1997 Sep 19;89(1-2):137-40.
[9108] da Silva Costa KC, Bexerra SB, Norte CM, et al. Medicinal plants with teratogenic potential: current considerations. *Braz J Pharm Sci.* 2012;48(3):427-33.
[9109] Brinker F. Herb Contraindications and Drug Interactions. 2nd ed. Sandy, OR. Eclectic Medical Publications. 1998.
[9110] Flaman Z, Pellechia-Clarke S, Bailey B, et al. Unintentional exposure of young children to camphor and eucalyptus oils. *Paediatr Child Health.* 2001 Feb;6(2):80-83.
[9111] Frohne D. Giftpflanzen: Cupressaceae. Stuttgart: Wissenschaftliche Verlagsgesellschaft mbH; 1997. pp. 153–6.
[9112] European Medicines Agency. Public statement on the use of herbal medicinal products containing thujone. Available at: http://www.ema.europa.eu/docs/en_GB/document_library/Public_statement/2011/02/WC500102294.pdf.
[9113] Millet Y, Jouglard J, Steinmetz MD, et al. Toxicity of some essential plant oils. Clinical and experimental study. *Clin Toxicol.* 1981 Dec;18(12):1485-98.
[9114] Cristovao L, Carvalho F, Bastos MDL, et al. Hepatotoxicity of an essential oil of Salvia officinalis L.: an in vitro study using freshly isolated rat hepatocytes. *Congress Biomarkers.* 2001 Sep:165.
[9115] Millet Y, Jouglard J, Steinmetz MD, et al. Toxicity of some essential plant oils. Clinical and experimental study. *Clin Toxicol.* 1981 Dec;18(12):1485–98.
[9116] Burkhard PR, Burkhardt K, Haenggeli CA, et al. Plant-induced seizures: reappearance of an old problem. *J Neurol.* 1999 Aug;246(8):667–70.
[9117] Weisbord SD, Soule JB, Kimmel PL. Poison on line-acute renal failure caused by oil of wormwood purchased through the internet. *N Engl J Med.* 1997;337:825-7.
[9118] Arditti J, Faizende JJ, Bernard J, et al. Trois observations d'intoxication par des essences végétales convulsivantes. *Ann Med.* 1978;17:371-74.
[9119] Manoguerra AS, Erdman AR, Wax PM, et al. Camphor poisoning: an evidence-based practice guideline for out-of- hospital management. *Clin Toxicol (Phila).*2006;44(4):357-70.
[9120] Gibson DE, Moore GP, Pfaff JA. Camphor ingestion. *Am J Emerg Med.* 1989 Jan;7(1):41-43.
[9121] Koppel C, Martends F, Schirop T, et al. Hemoperfusion in acute camphor poisoning. *Intensive Care Med.* 1988;14(4):431-33.
[9122] Burkhard PR, Burkhardt K, Haenggeli CA, et al. Plant-induced seizures: reappearance of an old problem. *J Neurol.* 1999 Aug;246(8):667-70.
[9123] Narayan S, Singh N. Camphor poisoning-An unusual cause of seizure. *Med J Armed Forces India.* 2012 Jul;68(3):252-53.

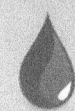

[9124] Chanaranaj KJ, G MV, S M. Camphor poisoning in a child. *Natl Med J India.* 2013 Jan-Feb;26(1):60.
[9125] Perry NB, Anderson RE, Brennan NJ, et al. Essential oils from dalmatian sage (Salvia officinalis L.) variations among individuals, plant parts, seasons, and sites. *J Agric Food Chem.* 1999;47:2048-54.
[9126] Millet Y, Jouglard J, Steinmetz MD, et al. Toxicity of some essential plant oils. Clinical and experimental study. *Clin Toxicol.* 1981 Dec;18(12):1485-98.
[9127] Abass K, Reponen P, Mattila S, et al. Metabolism of α-thujone in human hepatic preparations in vitro. *Xenobiotica.* 2011 Feb;41(2):101-11.
[9128] Olowe SA, Ransome-Kuti O. The risk of jaundice in glucose-6-phosphate dehydrogenase deficient babies exposed to menthol. *Acta Paediatr Scand.* 1980 May;69(3):341-5.
[9129] Dillon Remy M, Manning Alleyne P, Bratt DE, et al. Neonatal jaundice at Port-of-Spain General Hospital abstract. *West Indian Med J.* 1987;36(Suppl):28.
[9130] 2046 Uc A, Bishop WP, Sanders KD. Camphor hepatotoxicity. *South Med J.* 2000;93:596-98.
[9131] Dolan LC, Matulka RA, Burdock GA. Naturally Occurring Food Toxins. *Toxins (Basel).* 2010 Sep;2(9):2289–2332.
[9132] Küpeli Akkol E, İlhan M, Ayşe Demirel M, et al. Thuja occidentalis L. and its active constituent, α-thujone: Promising effects in the treatment of polycystic ovary syndrome without inducing osteoporosis. *J Ethnopharmacol.* 2015 Jun 20;168:25-30.
[9133] Thompson JD, Chalchat JC, Michet A, et al. Qualitative and quantitative variation in monoterpene co-occurrence and composition in the essential oil of Thymus vulgaris chemotypes. *J Chem Ecology.* 20003 Apr;29(4):859-80.
[9134] Sokovic MD, Vukojevic J, Marin PD, et al. Chemical composition of essential oils of Thymus and Mentha species and tier antifungal activities. *Molecules.* 209;14:238-49.
[9135] Kohlert C, Schindler G, Marz RW, et al. Systemic availability and pharmacokinetics of thymol in humans. *J Clin Pharmacol.* 2002 Jul;42(7):731-7.
[9136] Toxicology Data Network, National Library of Medicine. Thymol. Available at: http://toxnet.nlm.nih.gov/cgi-bin/sis/search/a?dbs+hsdb:@term+@DOCNO+866.
[9137] Sayyah M, Valizadeh J, Kamalinejad M. Anticonvulsant activity of the leaf oil of Laurus nobilis against pentylentetrazole- and maximal electroshock-induced seizure. *Phytomedicine.* 2002 Apr;9(3):212-16.
[9138] Culic M, Kekovic G, Grbic G, et al. Wavelet and fractal analysis of rat brain activity in seizures evoked by camphor oil and 1,8-cineole. *Gen Physiol Biophys.* 2009;28 Sec No:33-40.
[9139] Burkhard PR, Burkhardt K, Haenggeli CA, et al. Plant-induced seizures: reappearance of an old problem. *J Neurol.* 1999 Aug;246(8):667-70.
[9140] Waldman N. Seizure caused by dermal application of over-the-counter eucalyptus oil head lice preparation. *Clin Toxicol (Phila).* 2011 Oct;49(8):750-1.
[9141] Craig JO. Poisoning by the volatile oils in childhood. *Arch Dis Child.* 1953;28:259-67.
[9142] Mathew T, Kamath V, Kumar RS, et al. Eucalyptus oil inhalation-induced seizure: A novel, underrecognized, preventable cause of acute symptomatic seizure. *Epilepsia Open.* 2017 Jul 4;2(3):350-354.
[9143] Jukic M, Politeo O, Maksimmovic M, et al. In vitro acetylcholinesterase inhibitory properties of thymol, carvacrol and their derivatives thymoquinone and thymohydroquinone. *Phytother Res.* 2007;21(3):259-61.
[9144] Tognolini M, Barocelli E, Ballabeni V, et al. Comparative screening of plant essential oils; phenylpropanoid moiety as basic core for antiplatelet activity. *Life Sci.* 2006 Feb 23;78(13):1419-32.
[9145] Okazaki K, Kawazoe K, Takaishi Y. Human platelet aggregation inhibitors from thyme (Thymus vulgaris L.). *Phytother Res.* 2002 Jun;16(4):398-9.
[9146] Seo KA, Kim H, Ku HY, et al. The monoterpenoids citral and geraniol are moderate inhibitors of the CYP2B6 hydroxylase activity. *Chem Biol Interact.* 2008;174:141-46.
[9147] Ray S, Ghosal SK. Release and skin permeation studies of Naproxen from hydrophilic gels and effect of terpenes as enhancers on its skin. *Boll Chim Farm.* 2003;142(3):125-29.
[9148] Hofer R, Dong L, Ginglinger JF, et al. Geraniol hydroxylase and hydroxygeraniol oxidase activities of the CYP76 family of cytochrome P450 enzymes and potential for engineering the early steps of the (seco)iridoid pathway. *Metab Eng.* 2013 Nov;20:221-32.
[9149] Seo JY, Lim SS, Kim JR, et al. Nrf2-mediated induction of detoxifying enzymes by alantolactone present in Inula helenium. *Phytother Res.* 2008 Nov;22(11):1500-5.
[9150] Jukic M, Politeo O, Maksimmovic M, et al. In vitro acetylcholinesterase inhibitory properties of thymol, carvacrol and their derivatives thymoquinone and thymohydroquinone. *Phytother Res.* 2007;21(3):259-61.
[9151] Jukic M, Politeo O, Maksimovic M, et al. In vitro acetylcholinesterase inhibitory properties of thymol, carvacrol and their derivatives thymoquinone and thymohydroquinone. *Phytother Res.* 2007 Mar;21(3):259-61.
[9152] Langeveld WT, Veldhuizen EJ, Burt SA. Synergy between essential oil constituents and antibiotics. *Crit Rev Microbiol.* 2014 Feb;40(1);76-94.
[9153] Fadli M, Saad A, Sayadi S, et al. Antibacterial activity of Thymus maroccanus and Thymus broussonetii essential oils against nosocomial infection - bacteria and their synergistic potential with antibiotics. *Phytomedicine.* 2012 Mar 15;19(5):464-71.
[9154] Palaniappan K, Holley Ra. Use of natural antimicrobials to increase antibiotic susceptibility of drug resistant bacteria. *In J Food Microbiol.* 2010 Jun 15;140(2-3):164-8.
[9155] Ilic BS, Kocic BD, Ciric VM, et al. An in vitro synergistic interaction of combinations of Thymus glabrescens essential oil and its main constituents with chloramphenicol. *ScientificWorldJournal.* 2014 Jan 28;2014:826219.
[9156] Miladinovic DL, Ilic BS, Kocic BD, et al. Antibacterial investigation of thyme essential oil and its main constituents on combination with tetracycline. *J Med Food.* 2015 Aug;18(8):935-7.
[9157] Shin S, Lim S. Antifungal effects of herbal essential oils alone and in combination with ketoconazole against Trichophyton spp. *J Appl Micribiol.* 2004;97:1289-96.
[9158] Cardoso NN, Alviano CS, Blank AF, et al. Synergism Effect of the Essential Oil from Ocimum basilicum var. Maria Bonita and Its Major Components with Fluconazole and Its Influence on Ergosterol Biosynthesis. *Evid Based Complement Alternat Med.* 2016;2016:5647182.
[9159] Kissels W, Wu X, Santos RR, et al. Short communication: Interaction of the isomers carvacrol and thymol with the antibiotics doxycycline and tilmicosin: In vitro effects against pathogenic bacteria commonly found in the respiratory tract of calves. *J Dairy Sci.* 2017 Feb;100(2):970-974.
[9160] Hagvall L. Cytochrome P450-mediated activation of the fragrance constituent geraniol forms potent contact allergens. *Tox Appl Pharm.* 2008 Dec;233(2):308-13.
[9161] Ibrahim SM, El-Denshary ES, Abdallah DM. Geraniol, Alone and in Combination with Pioglitazone, Ameliorates Fructose-Induced Metabolic Syndrome in Rats via the Modulation of Both Inflammatory and Oxidative Stress Status. *PLoS One.* 2015 Feb 13;10(2):e0117516.
[9162] Srinivasan S, Muruganathan U. Antidiabetic efficacy of citronellol, a citrus monoterpene by ameliorating the hepatic key enzymes of carbohydrate metabolism in streptozotocin-induced diabetic rats. *Chem Biol Interact.* 2016 Apr 25;250:38-46.
[9163] Zu Y, Yu H, Liang L, et al. Activities of ten essential oils towards Propionibacterium acnes and PC-3, A-549 and MCF-7 cancer cells. *Molecules.* 2010;15:3200-10.
[9164] Sertel S, Eichhorn T, Polinkert PK, et al. Cytotoxicity of Thymus vulgaris essential oil towards human oral cavity squamous cell carcinoma. *Anticancer Res.* 2011 Jan;31(1):81-87.
[9165] Yin QH, Yan FX, Zu XY, et al. Anti-proliferative and pro-apoptotic effect of carvacrol on human hepatocellular carcinoma cell like HepG-2. *Cytotechnology.* 2012 jan;64(1):43-51.
[9166] Hsu SS, Lin KL, Chou CT, et al. Effect of thymol on Ca2+ homeostasis and viability in human glioblastoma cells. *Eur J Pharmacol.* 2011 Nov 16;670(1):85-91.
[9167] Fabio A, Cermelli C, Fabil G, et al. Screening of the antibacterial effects of a variety of essential oils on microorganisms responsible for respiratory infections. *Phytother Res.* 2007 Apr;21(4):374-77.
[9168] Inouye S, Yamaguchi H, Takizawa. Screening of the antibacterial effects of a variety of essential oils on respiratory tract pathogens, using a modified dilution assay method. *J Infect Chemother.* 201 Dec;7(4):251-54.
[9169] Sienkiewicz M, Lysakowska M, Denys P, et al. The Antimicrobial activity of thyme essential oil against multidrug resistant clinical bacterial strains. *Microb Drug Resist.* 2012 Apr;18(2):137-48.
[9170] Vázquez-Sánchez D, Cabo ML, Rodríguez-Herrera JJ, et al. Antimicrobial activity of essential oils against Staphylococcus aureus biofilms. *Food Sci Technol Int.* 2015 Dec;21(8):559-70.
[9171] Sakkas H, Gousia P1, Economou V, et al. In vitro antimicrobial activity of five essential oils on multidrug resistant Gram-negative clinical isolates. *J Intercult Ethnopharmacol.* 2016 May 30;5(3):212-8.
[9172] Seo HS, Beuchat LR, Kim H, et al. Development of an experimental apparatus and protocol for determining antimicrobial activities of gaseous plant essential oils. *Int J Food Microbiol.* 2015 Dec 23;215:95-100.
[9173] Vázquez-Sánchez D, Cabo ML, Rodríguez-Herrera JJ, et al. Antimicrobial activity of essential oils against Staphylococcus aureus biofilms. *Food Sci Technol Int.* 2015 Dec;21(8):559-70.
[9174] Kerekes EB, Vidács A, Török JJ, et al. Anti-listerial effect of selected essential oils and thymol. *Acta Biol Hung.* 2016 Sep;67(3):333-43.
[9175] Quesada J, Sendra E, Navarro C, et al. Antimicrobial Active Packaging including Chitosan Films with Thymus vulgaris L. Essential Oil for Ready-to-Eat Meat. *Foods.* 2016 Aug 29;5(3).
[9176] Possas A, Posada-Izquierdo GD, Pérez-Rodríguez F, et al. Application of predictive models to assess the influence of thyme essential oil on Salmonella Enteritidis behaviour during shelf life of ready-to-eat turkey products. *Int J Food Microbiol.* 2017 Jan 2;240:40-46.
[9177] Tohidpour A, Sattari M, Omnidbaigi R, et al. Antibacterial effect of essential oils from two medicinal plants against Methicillin-resistant Staphylococcus aureus (MRSA). *Phytomedicine.* 2010 Feb;17(2):142-45.
[9178] Mohsenzadeh M. Evaluation of antibacterial activity of selected Iranian essential oils against Staphylococcus aureus and Escherichia coli in nutrient broth medium. *Pak J Biol Sci.* 2007 Oct;10(20):3693-97.
[9179] Hili P, Evans CS, Veness RG. Antimicrobial action of essential oils: the effect of dimethylsulfoxide on the activity of cinnamon essential oil. *Lett Appl Microbiol.* 1997 Apr;24(4):269-75.
[9180] Rajkowska K, Kunicka-Styczyńska A, Maroszyńska M, et al. Selected Essential Oils as Antifungal Agents Against Antibiotic-Resistant Candida spp.: In Vitro Study on Clinical and Food-Borne Isolates. *Microb Drug Resist.* 2017 Jan;23(1):18-24.
[9181] Mandras N, Nostro A, Roana J, et al. Liquid and vapour-phase antifungal activities of essential oils against Candida albicans and non-albicans Candida. *BMC Complement Altern Med.* 2016 Aug 30;16(1):330.
[9182] Kovács JK, Horváth G, Kerényi M, et al. A modified bioautographic method for antibacterial component screening against anaerobic and microaerophilic bacteria. *J Microbiol Methods.* 2016 Apr;123:13-7.
[9183] Miladi H, Mili D, Ben Slama R, et al. Antibiofilm formation and anti-adhesive property of three mediterranean essential oils against a foodborne pathogen Salmonella strain. *Microb Pathog.* 2016 Apr;93:22-31.
[9184] Sakkas H, Gousia P, Economou V, et al. In vitro antimicrobial activity of five essential oils on multidrug resistant Gram-negative clinical isolates. *J Intercult Ethnopharmacol.* 2016 Jun-Aug;5(3):212–18.
[9185] Kulisic T, Krisko A, Dragovic-Uzelac V, et al. The effects of essential oils and aqueous tea infusions of oregano (Origanum vulgare L. spp hirtum), thyme (Thymus vulgaris L.) and wild thyme (Thymus serpyllum L.) on the copper- induced oxidation of human low-density lipoproteins. *Int J Food Sci Nutr.* 2007 Mar;58(2):87-93.

[9186] Meisinger C, Baumert J, Khuseyinova N, et al. Plasma oxidized low-density lipoprotein, a strong predictor for acute coronary heart disease events in apparently healthy, middle-aged med from the general population. *Circulation.* 2005 Aug 2;112(5):651-57.

[9187] Pérez-Rosés R, Risco E, Vila R, et al. Biological and Nonbiological Antioxidant Activity of Some Essential Oils. *J Agric Food Chem.* 2016 Jun 15;64(23):4716-24.

[9188] Zu Y, Yu H, Liang L, et al. Activities of ten essential oils towards Propionibacterium acnes and PC-3, A-549 and MCF-7 cancer cells. *Molecules.* 2010;15(5):3200-10.

[9189] Salmalian H, Saghebi R, Moghadamnia AA, et al. Comparative effects of thymus vulgaris and ibuprofen on primary dysmenorrhea: A triple-blind clinical study. *Caspian J Intern Med.* 2014 Spring;5(2):82-88.

[9190] Inouye S, Uchida K, Nishiyama Y, et al. Combined effect of heat, essential oils and salt on fungicidal activity against Trichophyton mentagrophytes in a foot bath. *Nihon Ishinjin Gakkai Zasshi.*2007;48(1):27-36.

[9191] Warnke PH, Becker ST, Podschun R, et al. The battle against multi-resistant strains: Renaissance of antimicrobial essential oils as a promising force to fight hospital-acquired infections. *J Craniomaxillofac Surg.* 2009 Oct;37(7):392- 97.

[9192] Pozzatti P, Scheid LA, Spader TB, et al. In vitro activity of essential oils extracted from plants used as spices against fluconazole-resistant and fluconazole-susceptible Candida spp. *Can J Microbiol.* 2008 Nov;54(11):950-56.

[9193] Giordani R, Regli P, Kaloustian J, et al. Antifungal effect of various essential oils against Candida albicans. Potentiation of antifungal action of amphotericin B by essential oil from Thymus vulgaris. *Phytother Res.* 2004 Dec;18(12):990-95.

[9194] Pina-Vaz C, Goncalves Rodriguez A, Pinto A, et al. Antifungal activity of Thymus oils and their major constituents. *J Eur Acad Dermatol Venereol.* 2004 Jan;18(1):73-78.

[9195] Rajkowska K, Kunicka-Styczyńska A, Maroszyńska M, et al. Selected Essential Oils as Antifungal Agents Against Antibiotic-Resistant Candida spp.: In Vitro Study on Clinical and Food-Borne Isolates. *Microb Drug Resist.* 2017 Jan;23(1):18-24.

[9196] Houicher A, Hechachna H, Teldji H, et al. In vitro study of the antifungal activity of essential oils obtained from Mentha spicata, Thymus vulgaris and Laurus nobilis. *Recent Pat Food Nutr Agric.* 2016;8(2):99-106.

[9197] Cisarová M, Tančinová D, Medo J, et al. The in vitro effect of selected essential oils on the growth and mycotoxin production of Aspergillus species. *J Environ Sci Health B.* 2016 Oct 2;51(10):668-674.

[9198] Kumar P, Mishra S, Kumar A, et al. Antifungal efficacy of plant essential oils against stored grain fungi of Fusarium spp. *J Food Sci Technol.* 2016 Oct;53(10):3725-3734.

[9199] Divband K, Shokri H, Khosravi AR, et al. Down-regulatory effect of Thymus vulgaris L. on growth and Tri4 gene expression in Fusarium oxysporum strains. *Microb Pathog.* 2017 Jan 3;104:1-5.

[9200] Koch C, Reichling J, Schneele J, et al. Inhibitory effect of essential oils against herpes simplex virus type 2. *Phytomedicine.* 2008 Jan;15(1-2):71-78.

[9201] Schnitzler P, Koch C, Reichling J. Susceptibility of drug-resistant clinical herpes simplex virus type 1 strain to essential oils of ginger, thyme, hyssop, and sandalwood. *Antimicrob Agents Chemother.* 2007 May;51(5):1859-62.

[9202] Hay IC, Jamieson M, Ormerod AD. Randomized trial of aromatherapy. Successful treatment for alopecia areata. *Arch Dermatol.* 1998 Nov;134(11):1349-52.

[9203] Muhlbauer RC, Lozano A, Palacio S, et al. Common herbs, essential oils, and monoterpenes potently modulate bone metabolism. *Bone.* 2003 Apr;32(4):372-80.

[9204] Inouye S, Takizawa T, Yamaguchi H. Antibacterial activity of essential oils and their major constituents against respiratory tract pathogens by gaseous contact. *J Antimicrobi Chemother.* 2001 May;47(5):565-73.

[9205] Sherry E, Boeck H, Warnke PH. Percutaneous treatment of chronic MRSA osteomyelitis with a novel plant-derived antiseptic. *BMC Surgery.* 2001;1:1.

[9206] Alinkina ES, Misharina TA, Fatkullina LD. Antiradical properties of oregano, thyme, and savory essential oils. *Prikl Biokhim Mikrobiol.* 2013 Jan-Feb;49(1):82-87.

[9207] Pérez-Rosés R, Risco E, Vila R, et al. Biological and Nonbiological Antioxidant Activity of Some Essential Oils. *J Agric Food Chem.* 2016 Jun 15;64(23):4716-24.

[9208] Saija A, Speciale A, Trombetta D, et al. Phytochemical, ecological and antioxidant evaluation of wild Sicilian thyme: Thymbra capitata (L.) Cav. *Chem Biodivers.* 2016 Dec;13(12):1641-1655.

[9209] Tohidi B, Rahimmalek M, Arzani A, et al. Essential oil composition, total phenolic, flavonoid contents, and antioxidant activity of Thymus species collected from different regions of Iran. *Food Chem.* 2017 Apr 1;220:153-161.

[9210] Santoro GF, das Gracas Cardoso M, Guimaraes LG, et al. Effect of oregano (Origanum vulgure L.) and thyme (Thymus culgaris L.) essential oil on Trypanosoma cruzi (Protozoa: Kinetoplastida) growth and ultrastructure. *Parasitol.* 2007 Mar;100(4):783-90.

[9211] Wei A, Shibamoto T. Antioxidant activities of essential oil mixtures toward skin lipid squalene oxidized by UV irradiation. *Cutan Ocul Toxicol.* 2007;26(3):227-33.

[9212] Kohiyama CY, Yamamoto Ribeiro MM, Mossini SA, et al. Antifungal properties and inhibitory effects upon aflatoxin production of Thymus vulgaris L. by Aspergillus flavus link. *Food Chem.*2015 Apr 15;173:1006-10.

[9213] Cisarová M, Tančinová D, Medo J, et al. The in vitro effect of selected essential oils on the growth and mycotoxin production of Aspergillus species. *J Environ Sci Health B.* 2016 Oct 2;51(10):668-674.

[9214] Khan MS, Ahmad I, Cameotra SS. Carum copticum and Thymus vulgaris oils inhibit virulence in Trichophyton rubrum and Aspergillus spp. *Braz J Microbiol.*2014 Aug;45(2):523-31.

[9215] Grespan R, Aguiar RP, Giubilei FN, et al. Hepatoprotective effect of pretreatment with Thymus vulgaris essential oil in experimental model of Acetaminophen-induced injury. *Evid Based Complement Altern Med.* 214;2014:954136.

[9216] Fachini-Queiroz FC, Kummer R, Estevao-Silva CF, et al. Effects of thymol and carvacrol, constituents of Thymus vulgaris L. essential oil, on the inflammatory response. *Evid Based Complement Alternat Med.* 2012;2012:657026.

[9217] Gholijani N, Gharagozloo M, Farjadian S, et al. Modulatory effects of thymol and carvacrol on inflammatory transcription factors in lipopolysaccharide-treated macrophages. *J Immunotoxicool.* 2016;13(2):157-64.

[9218] De Lira Mota KS, de Oliveira Pereira F, de Oliveira WA, et al. Antifungal activity of Thymus vulgaris L. essential oil and its constituent phytochemicals against Rhizopus oryzae: interaction with ergosterol. *Molecules.* 2012 Dec 5;17(12):14418-33.

[9219] Sienkiewicz M, Kalemba D, Wasiela M. Sensitivity assessment of thyme and lavender essential oils against clinical strains of Escherichia coli for their resistance. *Med Dosw Mikrobiol.* 2011;63(3):273-81.

[9220] Marino M, Bersani C, Comi G. Antimicrobial activity of the essential oil of Thymus vulgaris L. measured using a bioimpedometirc method. *J Food Prot.* 1999 Sep;62(9):1017-23.

[9221] Behnia M, Haghighi A, Komeylizadeh H, et al. Inhibitory effects of Iranian Thymus vulgaris extracts on in vitro growth of Entamoeba histolytica. *Korean J Parasitol.* 2008 Sep;46(3):153-56.

[9222] Sokovic M, Glamoclija J, Ciric A, et al. Antifungal activity of the essential oil of Thymus vulgaris L. and thymol on experimentally induced dermatomycoses. *Drug Dev Ind Pharm.* 2008 Dec;34(12):1388-93.

[9223] Jukic M, Politeo O, Maksimovic M, et al. In vitro acetylcholinesterase inhibitory properties of thymol, carvacrol and their derivatives thymoquinone and thymohydroquinone. *Phytother Res.* 2007 Mar;21(3):259-61.

[9224] Vigo E, Cepeda A, Gualillo O, et al. In-vitro and anti-inflammatory effect of Eucalyptus globulus and Thymus vulgaris: nitric oxide inhibition in J774A.1 murine macrophages. *J Pharm Pharmacol.* 2004 Feb;56(2):257-63.

[9225] Machado M, Dinis AM, Salquiero L, et al. Anti-giardia activity of phenolic-rich essential oils: effects of Thymbra capitata, Origanum virens, Thymus zygis subsp. Sylvestris, and Lippia graveolens on trophozoites growth, viability, adherence, and ultrastructure. *Parasitol Res.* 2010 Apr;106(5):1205-15.

[9226] Machado M, Sousa Mdo C, Salgueiro L, et al. Effects of essential oils on the growth of Giardia lamblia trophozoites. *Nat Prod Commun.* 2010 Jan;5(1):137-41.

[9227] Wechsler JB, HSU CL, Bryce PJ. IgE-mediated mast cell response are inhibited by thymol-mediated, activation- induced cell death in skin inflammation. *J Allergy Clin Immunol.* 2014 Jun;133(6):1735-43.

[9228] Hassan SB, Gali-Muhtasib H, Goransson H, et al. Alpha terpineol: a potential anticancer agent which acts through suppressing NF-kappaB signaling. *Anticancer Res.* 2010 Jun;30(6):1911-19.

[9229] Chaftar N, Girardot M, Labanowski J, et al. Comparative evaluation of the antimicrobial activity of 19 essential oils. *Adv Exp Med Biol.* 2016;901:1-15.

[9230] Yones DA, Bakir HY, Bayoumi SA. Chemical composition and efficacy of some selected plant oils against Pediculus humanus capitis in vitro. *Parasitol Res.* 2016 Aug;115(8):3209-18.

[9231] Gutiérrez MM, Werdin-González JO, et al. The potential application of plant essential oils to control Pediculus humanus capitis (Anoplura: Pediculidae). *Parasitol Res.* 2016 Feb;115(2):633-41.

[9232] Labib GS, Aldawsari H. Innovation of natural essential oil-loaded Orabase for local treatment of oral candidiasis. *Drug Des Devel Ther.* 2015 Jun 29;9:3349-59.

[9233] Azad MF, Schwiertz A, Jentsch HF. Adjunctive use of essential oils following scaling and root planing -a randomized clinical trial. *BMC Complement Altern Med.* 2016 Jun 7;16(1):171.

[9234] Labib GS, Aldawsari H. Innovation of natural essential oil-loaded Orabase for local treatment of oral candidiasis. *Drug Des Devel Ther.* 2015 Jun 29;9:3349-59.

[9235] Ozogul Y, Kuley E, Ucar Y, et al. Antimicrobial Impacts of Essential Oils on Food Borne-Pathogens. *Recent Pat Food Nutr Agric.* 2015;7(1):53-61.

[9236] D'Amato S, Mazzarrino G, Rossi C, et al. Thymus Vulgaris (Red Thyme) and Caryophyllus Aromaticus (Clove) Essential Oils to Control Spoilage Microorganisms in Pork Under Modified Atmosphere. *Ital J Food Saf.* 2016 Aug 3;5(3):5785.

[9237] Placha I, Chrastinova L, Laukova A, et al. Effect of thyme oil on small intestine integrity and antioxidant status, phagocytic activity and gastrointestinal microbiota in rabbits. *Acta Vet Hung.* 2013 Jun;61(2):197-208.

[9238] Seo YM, Jeong SH. [Effects of Blending Oil of Lavender and Thyme on Oxidative Stress, Immunity, and Skin Condition in Atopic Dermatitis Induced Mice]. *J Korean Acad Nurs.* 2015 Jun;45(3):367-77.

[9239] Hili P, Evans CS, Veness RG. Antimicrobial action of essential oils: the effect of dimethylsulfoxide on the activity of cinnamon essential oil. *Lett Appl Microbiol.* 1997 Apr;24(4):269-75.

[9240] Ferreira LE, Benincasa BI, Fachin AL, et al. Thymus vulgaris L. essential oil and its main component thymol: Anthelmintic effects against Haemonchus contortus from sheep. *Vet Parasitol.* 2016 Sep 15;228:70-76.

[9241] Plant J. Effects of essential oils on telomere length in human cells. *Med Aromat Plants.* 2016;5(2):1-6.

[9242] Seo YM, Jeong SH. [Effects of Blending Oil of Lavender and Thyme on Oxidative Stress, Immunity, and Skin Condition in Atopic Dermatitis Induced Mice]. *J Korean Acad Nurs.* 2015 Jun;45(3):367-77.

[9243] Placha I, Chrastinova L, Laukova A, et al. Effect of thyme oil on small intestine integrity and antioxidant status, phagocytic activity and gastrointestinal microbiota in rabbits. *Acta Vet Hung.* 2013 Jun;61(2):197-208.

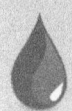

9244 Kim SW, Lee HR2, Jang MJ, et al. Fumigant Toxicity of Lamiaceae Plant Essential Oils and Blends of Their Constituents against Adult Rice Weevil Sitophilus oryzae. *Molecules*. 2016 Mar 16;21(3):361.

9245 Fani M, Kohanteb J. In Vitro Antimicrobial Activity of Thymus vulgaris Essential Oil Against Major Oral Pathogens. *J Evid Based Complementary Altern Med*. 2017 Oct;22(4):660-666.

9246 Rajkowska K, Kunicka-Styczyńska A, Maroszyńska M, et al. Selected Essential Oils as Antifungal Agents Against Antibiotic-Resistant Candida spp.: In Vitro Study on Clinical and Food-Borne Isolates. *Microb Drug Resist*. 2017 Jan;23(1):18-24.

9247 Basholli-Salihu M, Schuster R, Hajdari A, et al. Phytochemical composition, anti-inflammatory activity and cytotoxic effects of essential oils from three Pinus spp. *Pharm Biol*. 2017 Dec;55(1):1553-1560.

9248 Turchi B, Mancini S, Pistelli L, et al. Sub-inhibitory stress with essential oil affects enterotoxins production and essential oil susceptibility in Staphylococcus aureus. *Nat Prod Res*. 2017 Jun 8:1-7.

9249 Yones DA, Bakir HY, Bayoumi SA, et al. Chemical composition and efficacy of some selected plant oils against Pediculus humanus capitis in vitro. *Parasitol Res*. 2016 Aug;115(8):3209-18.

9250 Schött G, Liesegang S, Gaunitz F, et al. The chemical composition of the pharmacologically active Thymus species, its antibacterial activity against Streptococcus mutans and the antiadherent effects of T. vulgaris on the bacterial colonization of the in situ pellicle. *Fitoterapia*. 2017 Jul 10;121:118-128.

9251 Boskovic M, Djordjevic J, Ivanovic J, et al. Inhibition of Salmonella by thyme essential oil and its effect on microbiological and sensory properties of minced pork meat packaged under vacuum and modified atmosphere. *Int J Food Microbiol*. 2017 Oct 3;258:58-67.

9252 Gaire S, O'Connell M, Holguin FO, et al. Insecticidal Properties of Essential Oils and Some of Their Constituents on the Turkestan Cockroach (Blattodea: Blattidae). *J Econ Entomol*. 2017 Apr 1;110(2):584-592.

9253 Giordana F, Nicola M, Valentina C, et al. Chemical composition of essential oils from Thymus vulgaris, Cymbopogon citratus and Rosmarinus officinalis and their effects on the HIV-1 Tat protein function. *Chem Biodivers*. 2018 Feb;15(2).

9254 Grzesiak B, Kołodziej B, Głowacka A, et al. The Effect of Some Natural Essential Oils Against Bovine Mastitis Caused by Prototheca zopfii Isolates In Vitro. *Mycopathologia*. 2018 Jun;183(3):541-550.

9255 Singh P, Verma C, Mukhopadhyay S, et al. Preparation of thyme oil loaded κ-carrageenan-polyethylene glycol hydrogel membranes as wound care system. *Int J Pharm*. 2022 Apr 25;618:121661.

9256 Pellegrini M, Ricci A, Serio A, et al. Characterization of Essential Oils Obtained from Abruzzo Autochthonous Plants: Antioxidant and Antimicrobial Activities Assessment for Food Application. *Foods*. 2018 Feb 2;7(2).

9257 Tardugno R, Pellati F1, Iseppi R, et al. Phytochemical composition and in vitro screening of the antimicrobial activity of essential oils on oral pathogenic bacteria. *Nat Prod Res*. 2018 Mar;32(5):544-551.

9258 Scalas D, Mandras N, Roana J, et al. Use of Pinus sylvestris L. (Pinaceae), Origanum vulgare L. (Lamiaceae), and Thymus vulgaris L. (Lamiaceae) essential oils and their main components to enhance itraconazole activity against azole susceptible/not-susceptible Cryptococcus neoformans strains. *BMC Complement Altern Med*. 2018; 18: 143.

9259 Bartoňková I, Dvořák Z. Essential oils of culinary herbs and spices display agonist and antagonist activities at human aryl hydrocarbon receptor AhR. *Food Chem Toxicol*. 2018 Jan;111:374-384.

9260 Gucwa K, Milewski S, Dymerski T, et al. Investigation of the Antifungal Activity and Mode of Action of Thymus vulgaris, Citrus limonum, Pelargonium graveolens, Cinnamomum cassia, Ocimum basilicum, and Eugenia caryophyllus Essential Oils. *Molecules*. 2018 May 8;23(5).

9261 Polednik KM, Koch AC, Felzien LK. Effects of Essential Oil from Thymus vulgaris on Viability and Inflammation in Zebrafish Embryos. *Zebrafish*. 2018 Aug;15(4):361-371.

9262 Vinciguerra V, Rojas F, Tedesco V, et al. Chemical characterization and antifungal activity of Origanum vulgare, Thymus vulgaris essential oils and carvacrol against Malassezia furfur. *Nat Prod Res*. 2018 May 4:1-5.

9263 Benameur Q, Gervasi T, Pellizzeri V, et al. Antibacterial activity of Thymus vulgaris essential oil alone and in combination with cefotaxime against blaESBL producing multidrug resistant Enterobacteriaceae isolates. *Nat Prod Res*. 2018 May 4:1-8.

9264 Solarte AL, Astorga RJ, Aguiar F, et al. Combination of Antimicrobials and Essential Oils as an Alternative for the Control of Salmonella enterica Multiresistant Strains Related to Foodborne Disease. *Foodborne Pathog Dis*. 2017 Oct;14(10):558-563.

9265 Kot B, Wierzchowska K, Grużewska A, et al. The effects of selected phytochemicals on biofilm formed by five methicillin-resistant Staphylococcus aureus. *Nat Prod Res*. 2018 Jun;32(11):1299-1302.

9266 Perrin E, Maggini V, Maida I, et al. Antimicrobial activity of six essential oils against Burkholderia cepacia complex: insights into mechanism(s) of action. *Future Microbiol*. 2018 Jan;13:59-67.

9267 Ács K, Balázs VL, Kocsis B, et al. Antibacterial activity evaluation of selected essential oils in liquid and vapor phase on respiratory tract pathogens. *BMC Complement Altern Med*. 2018 Jul 27;18(1):227.

9268 Feng J, Shi W, Miklossy J, et al. Identification of Essential Oils with Strong Activity against Stationary Phase Borrelia burgdorferi. *Antibiotics (Basel)*. 2018 Oct 16;7(4).

9269 Abdolshahi A, Naybandi-Atashi S, Heydari-Majd M, et al. Antibacterial activity of some Lamiaceae species against Staphylococcus aureus in yoghurt-based drink (Doogh). *Cell Mol Biol (Noisy-le-grand)*. 2018 Jun 25;64(8):71-77.

9270 Mansouri N, Aoun L, Dalichaouche N, et al. Yields, chemical composition, and antimicrobial activity of two Algerian essential oils against 40 avian multidrug-resistant Escherichia coli strains. *Vet World*. 2018 Nov;11(11):1539-1550.

9271 Manconi M, Petretto G, D'hallewin G, et al. Thymus essential oil extraction, characterization and incorporation in phospholipid vesicles for the antioxidant/antibacterial treatment of oral cavity diseases. *Colloids Surf B Biointerfaces*. 2018 Nov 1;171:115-122.

9272 Muchembled J, Deweer C, Sahmer K, et al. Gene expression responses of Listeria monocytogenes Scott A exposed to sub-lethal concentrations of natural antimicrobials. *Environ Sci Pollut Res Int*. 2018 Oct;25(30):29921-29928.

9273 Braschi G, Serrazanetti DI, Siroli L, et al. Gene expression responses of Listeria monocytogenes Scott A exposed to sublethal concentrations of natural antimicrobials. *Int J Food Microbiol*. 2018;286:170-8.

9274 Kang J, Liu L, Wu X, et al. Effect of thyme essential oil against Bacillus cereus planktonic growth and biofilm formation. *Appl Microbiol Biotechnol*. 2018 Dec;102(23):10209-10218.

9275 Lorenzo-Leal AC, Palou E, López-Malo A. Evaluation of the efficiency of allspice, thyme and rosemary essential oils on two foodborne pathogens in in-vitro and on alfalfa seeds, and their effect on sensory characteristics of the sprouts. *Int J Food Microbiol*. 2019 Feb 12;295:19-24.

9276 Lagha R, Ben Abdallah F, Al-Sarhan BO, et al. Antibacterial and Biofilm Inhibitory Activity of Medicinal Plant Essential Oils Against Escherichia coli Isolated from UTI Patients. *Molecules*. 2019 Mar 23;24(6).

9277 Gedikoğlu A, Sökmen M, Çivit A, et al. Evaluation of Thymus vulgaris and Thymbra spicata essential oils and plant extracts for chemical composition, antioxidant, and antimicrobial properties. *Food Sci Nutr*. 2019 Apr 2;7(5):1704-1714.

9278 Namala BB, Hegde V. Comparative evaluation of the effect of plant extract, Thymus vulgaris and commercially available denture cleanser on the flexural strength and surface roughness of denture base resin. *J Indian Prosthodont Soc*. 2019 Jul-Sep;19(3):261-265.

9279 Boskovic M, Glisic M, Djordjevic J, et al. Antioxidative Activity of Thyme (Thymus vulgaris) and Oregano (Origanum vulgare) Essential Oils and Their Effect on Oxidative Stability of Minced Pork Packaged Under Vacuum and Modified Atmosphere. *J Food Sci*. 2019 Sep;84(9):2467-2474.

9280 Kubatka P, Uramova S, Kello M, et al. Anticancer Activities of Thymus vulgaris L. in Experimental Breast Carcinoma in Vivo and in Vitro. *Int J Mol Sci*. 2019 Apr 9;20(7).

9281 Uzair B, Niaz N, Bano A, et al. Essential oils showing in vitro anti MRSA and synergistic activity with penicillin group of antibiotics. *Pak J Pharm Sci*. 2017 Sep;30(5(Supplementary)):1997-2002.

9282 Kerekes EB, Vidács A, Takó M, et al. Antibiofilm Effect of Selected Essential Oils and Main Components on Mono- and Polymicrobic Bacterial Cultures. *Microorganisms*. 2019 Sep 12;7(9).

9283 Tian F, Lee SY, Chun HS. Comparison of the Antifungal and Antiaflatoxigenic Potential of Liquid and Vapor Phase of Thymus vulgaris Essential Oil Against Aspergillus flavus. *J food Prot*. 2019 Dec;82(12):2044-8.

9284 Kot B, Wierzchowska K, Piechota M, et al. Antimicrobial Activity of Five Essential Oils From Lamiaceae Against Multidrug-Resistant Staphylococcus aureus. *Nat Prod Res*. 2019 Dec;33(24):3587-3591.

9285 Kozics K, Buckova M, Puskarova A, et al. The Effect of Ten Essential Oils on Several Cutaneous Drug-Resistant Microorganisms and Their Cyto/Genotoxic and Antioxidant Properties. *Molecules*. 2019 Dec 13;24(24):24244570.

9286 Iseppi R, Sabia C, de Neiderhausern S, et al. Antibacterial Activity of Rosmarinus officinalis L. And Thymus vulgaris L. Essential Oils and Their Combination Against Food-Borne Pathogens and Spoilage Bacteria in Ready-To-Eat Vegetables. *Nat Prod Res*. 2019 Dec;33(24):3568-3572.

9287 Rajkowska K, Nowicka-Krawczyk P, Kunicka-Styczynska. Effect of Clove and Thyme Essential Oils on Candida Biofilm Formation and the Oil Distribution in Yeast Cells. *Molecules*. 2019 May 21;24(10):24101954.

9288 Krzyśko-Łupicka T, Sokół S, Piekarska-Stachowiak A. Evaluation of Fungistatic Activity of Eight Selected Essential Oils on Four Heterogeneous Fusarium Isolates Obtained From Cereal Grains in Southern Poland. *Molecules*. 2020 Jan 10;25(2):292.

9289 Stepanycheva E, Petrova M, Chermenskaya T, et al. Fumigant Effect of Essential Oils on Mortality and Fertility of Thrips Frankliniella Occidentalis Perg. *Environ Sci Pollut Res Int*. 2019 Oct;26(30):30885-30892.

9290 Al-Nabusi AA, Osali TM, Olaimat AN, et al. Inactivation of Salmonella Spp. In Tahini Using Plant Essential Oil Extracts. *Food Microbiol*. 2020 Apr;86:103338.

9291 Cho Y, Kim H, Beuchart LR, et al. Synergistic Activities of Gaseous Oregano and Thyme Thymol Essential Oils Against Listeria Monocytogenes on Surfaces of a Laboratory Medium and Radish Sprouts. *Food Microbiol*. 2020 Apr;86:103357.

9292 Korona-Glowniak I, Glowniak-Lipa A, Ludwiczuk A, et al. The In Vitro Activity of Essential Oils Against Helicobacter Pylori Growth and Urease Activity. *Molecules*. 2020 Jan 29;25(3):586.

9293 Jafri H, Ahmad I. Thymus Vulgaris Essential Oil and Thymol Inhibit Biofilms and Interact Synergistically With Antifungal Drugs Against Drug Resistant Strains of Candida Albicans and Candida Tropicalis. *J Mycol Med*. J Mycol Med. 2019 Nov 7:100911.

9294 Córdoba S, Vivot W, Szusz W, et al. Antifungal Activity of Essential Oils Against Candida Species Isolated from Clinical Samples. *Mycopathologia.* 2019 Oct;184(5):615-623.
9295 Xiao S, Cui P, Shi W, et al. Identification of essential oils with activity against stationary phase Staphylococcus aureus. *BMC Complement Med Ther.* 2020 Mar 24;20(1):99.
9296 Amorese V, Donadu M, Usai D, et al. In vitro activity of essential oils against Pseudomonas aeruginosa isolated from infected hip implants. *J Infect Dev Ctries.* 2018 Nov 30;12(11):996-1001.
9297 Alibi S, Ben Selma W, Ramos-Vivas J, et al. Anti-oxidant, antibacterial, antibiofilm, and anti-quorum sensing activities of four essential oils against multidrug-resistant bacterial clinical isolates. *Curr Res Transl Med.* 2020 Mar 16. [Epub ahead of print]
9298 El Euony OI, Elblehi SS, Abdel-Latif HM, et al. Modulatory role of dietary Thymus vulgaris essential oil and Bacillus subtilis against thiamethoxam-induced hepatorenal damage, oxidative stress, and immunotoxicity in African catfish (Clarias garipenus). *Environ Sci Pollut Res Int.* 2020 Apr 24. [Epub ahead of print]
9299 Oliveira RC, Carvajal-Moreno M, Correa B, et al. Cellular, physiological and molecular approaches to investigate the antifungal and anti-aflatoxigenic effects of thyme essential oil on Aspergillus flavus. *Food Chem.* 2020 Jun 15;315:126096.
9300 Sim JXF, Khazandi M, Chan WY, et al. Antimicrobial activity of thyme oil, oregano oil, thymol and carvacrol against sensitive and resistant microbial isolates from dogs with otitis externa. *Vet Dermatol.* 2019 Dec;30(6):524-e159.
9301 Kozics K, Buckova M, Puskarova A, et al. The Effect of Ten Essential Oils on Several Cutaneous Drug-Resistant Microorganisms and Their Cyto/Genotoxic and Antioxidant Properties. *Molecules.* 2019 Dec 13;24(24):4570.
9302 Mizan MFR, Ashrafudoulla M, Hossain MI, et al. Effect of Essential Oils on Pathogenic and Biofilm-Forming Vibrio parahaemolyticus Strains. *Biofouling.* 2020 Apr;36(4):467-478.
9303 Micucci M, Protti M, Aldini R,et al. Thymus vulgaris L. Essential Oil Solid Formulation: Chemical Profile and Spasmolytic and Antimicrobial Effects. *Biomolecules.* 2020 Jun 4;10(6):E860.
9304 Marinkovic J, Culafic DM, Nikolic B, et al. Antimicrobial potential of irrigants based on essential oils of Cymbopogon martinii and Thymus zygis towards in vitro multispecies biofilm cultured in ex vivo root canals. *Arch Oral Biol.* 2020 Jul 16;117:104842.
9305 Tardugno R, Serio A, Purgatorio C, et al. Thymus vulgaris L. essential oils from Emilia Romagna Apennines (Italy): phytochemical composition and antimicrobial activity on food-borne pathogens. *Nat Prod Res.* 2020 Jul 27;1-6.
9306 Rinaldi F, Oliva A, Sabatino M, et al. Antimicrobial Essential Oil Formulation: Chitosan Coated Nanoemulsions for Nose to Brain Delivery. *Pharmaceutics.* 2020 Jul 17;12(7):E678.
9307 Lazarevic J, Jevremovic S, Kostic I, et al. Toxic, Oviposition Deterrent and Oxidative Stress Effects of Thymus vulgaris Essential Oil against Acanthoscelides obtectus. *Insects.* 2020 Aug 24;11(9):E563.
9308 Csikos E, Cseko K, Ashraf AR, et al. Effects of Thymus vulgaris L., Cinnamomum verum J.Presl and Cymbopogon nardus (L.) Rendle Essential Oils in the Endotoxin-induced Acute Airway Inflammation Mouse Model. *Molecules.* 2020 Aug 4;25(15):3553.
9309 Salvaneschi S, Iriti M, Vitalini S, et al. Thymus vulgaris L. as a possible effective substitute for nitrates in meat products. *Ital J Food Saf.* 2020 Aug 19;9(2):7739.
9310 Pinto L, Bonifacio MA, Giglio ED, et al. Unravelling the Antifungal Effect of Red Thyme Oil ( Thymus vulgaris L.) Compounds in Vapor Phase. *Molecules.* 2020 Oct 16;25(20):4761.
9311 Abdallah FBm Lagha R, Gaber A. Biofilm Inhibition and Eradication Properties of Medicinal Plant Essential Oils against Methicillin-Resistant Staphylococcus aureus Clinical Isolates. *Pharmaceuticals (Basel).* 2020 Nov 6;13(11):369.
9312 Capatina L, Todirascu-Ciornea E, Napoli EM, et al. Thymus vulgaris Essential Oil Protects Zebrafish against Cognitive Dysfunction by Regulating Cholinergic and Antioxidants Systems. *Antioxidants (Basel).* 2020 Nov 4;9(11):1083.
9313 de Oliveira MA, da Vegian MR, Brighenti FL, et al. Antibiofilm effects of Thymus vulgaris and Hyptis spicigera essential oils on cariogenic bacteria. *Future Microbiol.* 2021 Feb 24. Online ahead of print.
9314 Netopilova M, Houdkova M, Urbanova K, et al. Validation of Qualitative Broth Volatilization Checkerboard Method for Testing of Essential Oils: Dual-Column GC-FID/MS Analysis and In Vitro Combinatory Antimicrobial Effect of Origanum vulgare and Thymus vulgaris against Staphylococcus aureus in Liquid and Vapor Phases. *Plants (Basel).* 2021 Feb 18;10(2):393.
9315 Kovacevic Z, Radinovic M, Cabarkapa I, et al. Natural Agents against Bovine Mastitis Pathogens. *Antibiotics (Basel).* 2021 Feb 19;10(2):205.
9316 Catella C, Camero M, Lucente MS, et al. Virucidal and antiviral effects of Thymus vulgaris essential oil on feline coronavirus. *Res Vet Sci.* 2021 Apr 22;137:44-47.
9317 Jaber H, Oubiji A, Ouryemchi I, et al. Chemical Composition and Antibacterial Activities of Eight Plant Essential Oils from Morocco against Escherichia coli Strains Isolated from Different Turkey Organs. *Biochem Res Int.* 2021 Mar 15;2021:6685800.
9318 Micucci M, Protti M, Aldini R, et al. Thymus vulgaris L. Essential Oil Solid Formulation: Chemical Profile and Spasmolytic and Antimicrobial Effects. *Biomolecules.* 2020 Jun 4;10(6):860.
9319 Horvath G, Horvath A, Reichert G, et al. Three chemotypes of thyme (Thymus vulgaris L.) essential oil and their main compounds affect differently the IL-6 and TNFα cytokine secretions of BV-2 microglia by modulating the NF-κB and C/EBPβ signalling pathways. *BMC Complement Med Ther.* 2021 May 22;21(1):148.
9320 Bagheri L, Khodaei N, Salmieri S, et al. Correlation between chemical composition and antimicrobial properties of essential oils against most common food pathogens and spoilers: In-vitro efficacy and predictive modelling. *Microb Pathog.* 2020 Oct;147:104212.
9321 Aebisher D, Cichonski J, Szpyrka E, et al. Essential Oils of Seven Lamiaceae Plants and Their Antioxidant Capacity. *Molecules.* 2021 Jun 22;26(13):3793.
9322 Niksic H, Becic F, Koric E, et al. Cytotoxicity screening of Thymus vulgaris L. essential oil in brine shrimp nauplii and cancer cell lines. *Sci Rep.* 2021 Jun 23;11(1):13178.
9323 Karpinski TM, Ozarowski M, Seremak-Mrozikiewicz A, et al. Plant Preparations and Compounds with Activities against Biofilms Formed by Candida spp. *J Fungi (Basel).* 2021 May 5;7(5):360.
9324 Proškovcová M, Čonková E, Váczi P, et al. Antibiofilm activity of selected plant essential oils from the Lamiaceae family against Candida albicans clinical isolates. *Ann Agric Environ Med.* 2021 Jun 14;28(2):260-266.
9325 Dos Santos LR, Alía A, Martin I, et al. Antimicrobial activity of essential oils and natural plant extracts against Listeria monocytogenes in a dry-cured ham-based model. *J Sci Food Agric.* 2021 Aug 11. Online ahead of print.
9326 Brozyna M, Paleczny J, Kozlowska W, et al. The Antimicrobial and Antibiofilm In Vitro Activity of Liquid and Vapour Phases of Selected Essential Oils against Staphylococcus aureus. *Pathogens.* 2021 Sep 17;10(9):1207.
9327 Galovičová L, Borotová P, Valková V, et al. Thymus vulgaris Essential Oil and Its Biological Activity. *Plants (Basel).* 2021 Sep 19;10(9):1959.
9328 Beicu R, Alexa E, Obistiou D, et al. Antimicrobial Potential and Phytochemical Profile of Wild and Cultivated Populations of Thyme (Thymus sp.) Growing in Western Romania. *Plants (Basel).* 2021 Sep 3;10(9):1833.
9329 Granata G, Stracquadanio S, Leonardi M, et al. Oregano and Thyme Essential Oils Encapsulated in Chitosan Nanoparticles as Effective Antimicrobial Agents against Foodborne Pathogens. *Molecules.* 2021 Jul 2;26(13):4055.
9330 Harčárová M, Čonková E, Proškovcová M, et al. Comparison of antifungal activity of selected essential oils against Fusarium graminearum in vitro. *Ann Agric Environ Med.* 2021 Sep 16;28(3):414-418.
9331 Omar HS, EL-Rahman SNA, AlGhannam SM, et al. Antifungal Evaluation and Molecular Docking Studies of Olea europaea Leaf Extract, Thymus vulgaris and Boswellia carteri Essential Oil as Prospective Fungal Inhibitor Candidates. *Molecules.* 2021 Oct 10;26(20):6118.
9332 Yan J, Wu H, Chen K, et al. Antifungal Activities and Mode of Action of Cymbopogon citratus, Thymus vulgraris, and Origanum heracleoticum Essential Oil Vapors against Botrytis cinerea and Their Potential Application to Control Postharvest Strawberry Gray Mold. *Foods.* 2021 Oct 15;10(10):2451.
9333 Michalczky A, Ostrowska P. Essential oils and their components in combating fungal pathogens of animal and human skin. *J Mycol Med.* 2021 Jun;31(2):101118.
9334 Milenkovic L, Ilic ZS, Sunic L, et al. Modification of light intensity influence essential oils content, composition and antioxidant activity of thyme, marjoram and oregano. *Saudi J Biol Sci.* 2021 Nov;28(11):6532-6543.
9335 Antih J, Houdkova M, Urbanova K, et al. Antibacterial Activity of Thymus vulgaris L. Essential Oil Vapours and Their GC/MS Analysis Using Solid-Phase Microextraction and Syringe Headspace Sampling Techniques. *Molecules.* 2021 Oct 29;26(21):6553.
9336 Guo Y, Pizzol R, Gabbanini S, et al. Absolute Antioxidant Activity of Five Phenol-Rich Essential Oils. *Molecules.* 2021 Aug 29;26(17):5237.
9337 Alshaikh NA, Perveen K. Susceptibility of Fluconazole-Resistant Candida albicans to Thyme Essential Oil. *Microorganisms.* 2021 Nov 28;9(12):2454.
9338 Martínez A, Manrique-Moreno M, Klaiss-Luna MC, et al. Effect of Essential Oils on Growth Inhibition, Biofilm Formation and Membrane Integrity of Escherichia coli and Staphylococcus aureus. *Antibiotics (Basel).* 2021 Nov 30;10(12):1474.
9339 de Aguiar FC, Solarte AL, Gómez-Gascón L, et al. Antimicrobial susceptibility of cinnamon and red and common thyme essential oils and their main constituent compounds against Streptococcus suis. *Lett Appl Microbiol.* 2022 Jan;74(1):63-72.
9340 Sardari S, Mobaien A, Ghassemifard L, et al. Therapeutic Effect of Thyme (Thymus Vulgaris) Essential Oil on Patients with COVID19: A Randomized Clinical Trial. *J Adv Med Biomed Res.* 2021;29(133):83-91.
9341 Radi FZ, Bouuhrin M, Mechchate H, et al. Phytochemical Analysis, Antimicrobial and Antioxidant Properties of Thymus zygis L. and Thymus willdenowii Boiss. Essential Oils. *Plants (Basel).* 2021 Dec 22;11(1):15.
9342 Mekkaoui M, Assaggaf H, Qasem A, et al. Ethnopharmacological Survey and Comparative Study of the Healing Activity of Moroccan Thyme Honey and Its Mixture with Selected Essential Oils on Two Types of Wounds on Albino Rabbits. *Foods.* 2021 Dec 23;11(1):28.
9343 Ismail HTH. The ameliorative efficacy of Thymus vulgaris essential oil against Escherichia coli O157:H7-induced hematological alterations, hepatorenal dysfunction and immune-inflammatory disturbances in experimentally infected rats. *Environ Sci Pollut Res Int.* 2022 Jan 28. Online ahead of print.
9344 Rodriguez Diaz C, Mith H, Bernard T, et al. In vitro study of antimicrobial activity of essential oils and their components against the main Clostridioides difficile PCR-ribotypes isolated in Belgium. *IAFP Eur Congress.* 2021.
9345 Štrbac F, Bosco A, Maurelli MP, et al. Anthelmintic Properties of Essential Oils to Control Gastrointestinal Nematodes in Sheep-In Vitro and In Vivo Studies. *Vet Sci.* 2022 Feb 19;9(2):93.
9346 Coimbra A, Miguel S, Ribeiro M, et al. Thymus zygis Essential Oil: Phytochemical Characterization, Bioactivity Evaluation and Synergistic Effect with Antibiotics against Staphylococcus aureus. *Antibiotics (Basel).* 2022 Jan 24;11(2):146.
9347 Romoli JCZ, Silva MV, Pante GC, et al. Anti-mycotoxigenic and antifungal activity of ginger, turmeric, thyme and rosemary essential oils in deoxynivalenol (DON) and zearalenone (ZEA) producing Fusarium graminearum. *Food Addit Contam Part A Chem Anal Control Expo Risk Assess.* 2022 Feb;39(2):362-372.
9348 Ahmed OM, Galaly SR, Mostafa MMA, et al. Thyme Oil and Thymol Counter Doxorubicin-Induced Hepatotoxicity via Modulation of Inflammation, Apoptosis, and Oxidative Stress. *Oxid Med Cell Longev.* 2022 Feb 7;2022:6702773.

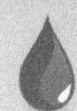

9349 El-Zehery HRA, Zaghloul RA, Abdel-Rahman HM, et al. Novel strategies of essential oils, chitosan, and nano- chitosan for inhibition of multi-drug resistant: E. coli O157:H7 and Listeria monocytogenes. *Saudi J Biol Sci*. 2022 Apr;29(4):2582-2590.
9350 Yasir M, Nawaz A, Ghazanfar S, et al. Anti-bacterial activity of essential oils against multidrug-resistant foodborne pathogens isolated from raw milk. *Braz J Biol*. 2022 May 9;84:e259449.
9351 Man A, Mare AD, Mares M, et al. Antifungal and anti-virulence activity of six essential oils against important Candida species - a preliminary study. *Future Microbiol*. 2022 Jul;17:737-753.
9352 Ebadollahi A, Naseri B, Abedi Z, et al. Chemical Profiles and Insecticidal Potential of Essential Oils Isolated from Four Thymus Species against Rhyzopertha dominica (F.). *Plants (Basel)*. 2022 Jun 14;11(12):1567.
9353 Ribeiro R, Fernandes L, Costa R, et al. Comparing the effect of Thymus spp. essential oils on Candida auris. *Ind Crops Prod*. 2022 Apr;178:114667.
9354 Akermi S, Smaoui S, Fourati M, et al. In-Depth Study of Thymus vulgaris Essential Oil: Towards Understanding the Antibacterial Target Mechanism and Toxicological and Pharmacological Aspects. *Biomed Res Int*. 2022 Jul 21;2022:3368883.
9355 Proškovcová M, Čonková E, Váczi P, et al. Efficacy of Lamiaceae essential oils with selected azoles against Candida albicans clinical isolates. *Pol J Vet Sci*. 2022 Jun;25(2):279-285.
9356 Alibi S, Selma WB, Mansour HB, et al. Activity of Essential Oils Against Multidrug-Resistant Salmonella enteritidis. *Curr Microbiol*. 2022 Jul 30;79(9):273.
9357 Abdelhamed FM, Abdeltawab NF, ElRakaiby MT, et al. Antibacterial and Anti-Inflammatory Activities of Thymus vulgaris Essential Oil Nanoemulsion on Acne Vulgaris. *Microorganisms*. 2022 Sep 19;10(9):1874.
9358 Toschi A, Piva A, Grilli E. Phenol-Rich Botanicals Modulate Oxidative Stress and Epithelial Integrity in Intestinal Epithelial Cells. *Animals (Basel)*. 2022 Aug 25;12(17):2188.
9359 El-Kased RF, El-Kersh DM. GC-MS Profiling of Naturally Extracted Essential Oils: Antimicrobial and Beverage Preservative Actions. *Life (Basel)*. 2022 Oct 12;12(10):1587.
9360 Bouymajane A, Filali FR, Ed-Dra A, et al. Chemical profile, antibacterial, antioxidant, and anisakicidal activities of Thymus zygis subsp. gracilis essential oil and its effect against Listeria monocytogenes. *Int J Food Microbiol*. 2022 Dec 16;383:109960.
9361 Alsakhawy SA, Baghdadi HH, El-Shenawy MA, et al.
9362 Goharrostami M, Sendi JJ, Hosseini R, et al. Effect of thyme essential oil and its two components on toxicity and some physiological parameters in mulberry pyralid Glyphodes pyloalis Walker. *Pestic Biochem Physiol*. 2022 Nov;188:105220.
9363 Zerkani H, Kharchoufa L, Tagnaout I, et al. Chemical Composition and Bioinsecticidal Effects of Thymus zygis L., Salvia officinalis L. and Mentha suaveolens Ehrh. Essential Oils on Medfly Ceratitis capitata and Tomato Leaf Miner Tuta absoluta. *Plants (Basel)*. 2022 Nov 14;11(22):3084.
9364 Naseri N, Kalantari Khandani A, Baherimoghadam T, et al. The Effect of Thymus Vulgaris Essential Oil and Chlorhexidine on Candida Albicans Accumulated on Removable Orthodontic Appliance: A Clinical Trial. *J Dent (Shiraz)*. 2022 Jun;23(1 Suppl):190-197.
9365 Sidiropoulou E, Marugán-Hernández V, Skoufos I, et al. In Vitro Antioxidant, Antimicrobial, Anticoccidial, and Anti-Inflammatory Study of Essential Oils of Oregano, Thyme, and Sage from Epirus, Greece. *Life (Basel)*. 2022 Nov 4;12(11):1783.
9366 Rostami R, Eslamifar Z, Nazemi S, et al. The Effect of Thyme Essential Oil on Liver Injuries Caused by Renal Ischemia-Reperfusion in Rats. *Biomed Res Int*. 2022 Oct 26;2022:2988334.
9367 Aquilano C, Baccari L, Caprari C, et al. Effects of EOs vs. Antibiotics on E. coli Strains Isolated from Drinking Waters of Grazing Animals in the Upper Molise Region, Italy. *Molecules*. 2022 Nov 24;27(23):8177.
9368 Zanotto AW, Kanemaru MYS, de Souza FG, et al. Enhanced antimicrobial and antioxidant capacity of Thymus vulgaris, Lippia sidoides, and Cymbopogon citratus emulsions when combined with mannosylerythritol a lipid biosurfactant. *Food Res Int*. 2023 Jan;163:112213.
9369 Ebani VV, Pieracci Y, Cagnoli G, et al. In Vitro Antimicrobial Activity of Thymus vulgaris, Origanum vulgare, Satureja montana and Their Mixture against Clinical Isolates Responsible for Canine Otitis Externa. *Vet Sci*. 2023 Jan 1;10(1):30.
9370 Luca SV, Zengin G, Sinan KI, et al. Post-Distillation By-Products of Aromatic Plants from Lamiaceae Family as Rich Sources of Antioxidants and Enzyme Inhibitors. *Antioxidants (Basel)*. 2023 Jan 16;12(1):210.
9371 Zanotto AW, Kanemaru MYS, de Souza FG, et al. Enhanced antimicrobial and antioxidant capacity of Thymus vulgaris, Lippia sidoides, and Cymbopogon citratus emulsions when combined with mannosylerythritol a lipid biosurfactant. *Food Res Int*. 2023 Jan;163:112213.
9372 Karpiński TM, Ożarowski M, Seremak-Mrozikiewicz A, et al. Anti-Candida and Antibiofilm Activity of Selected Lamiaceae Essential Oils. *Front Biosci (Landmark Ed)*. 2023 Feb 16;28(2):28.
9373 Bonetti A, Piva A, Grilli E. Botanicals as a zinc oxide alternative to protect intestinal cells from an Escherichia coli F4 infection in vitro by modulation of enterocyte inflammatory response and bacterial virulence. *Front Vet Sci*. 2023 Mar 9;10:1141561.
9374 Albuquerque KRS, Purgato GA, Piccolo MS, et al. Formulations of essential oils obtained from plants traditionally used as condiments or traditional medicine active against Staphylococcus aureus isolated from dairy cows with mastitis. *Lett Appl Microbiol*. 2023 Mar 1;76(3):ovad034.
9375 Bolatli G, Taş F, Alayunt NÖ. Effects of Thymus vulgaris Oil on Sodium Hypochlorite-Induced Damage in Rats. *Molecules*. 2023 Feb 25;28(5):2164.
9376 Galgano M, Capozza P, Pellegrini F, et al. Antimicrobial Activity of Essential Oils Evaluated In Vitro against Escherichia coli and Staphylococcus aureus. *Antibiotics (Basel)*. 2022 Jul 20;11(7):979.
9377 Pandur E, Micalizzi G, Mondello L, et al. Antioxidant and Anti-Inflammatory Effects of Thyme (Thymus vulgaris L.) Essential Oils Prepared at Different Plant Phenophases on Pseudomonas aeruginosa LPS-Activated THP-1 Macrophages. *Antioxidants (Basel)*. 2022 Jul 6;11(7):1330.
9378 Moyler DA. The flavor gum resins, their chemistry and uses. *Rivista Italiana EPPOS*. 2008;(Numero Speciale):351-60.
9379 National Library of Medicine. TOXNET. Benzyl acetate. Available at: https://toxnet.nlm.nih.gov/cgi-bin/sis/search/a?dbs+hsdb:@term+@DOCNO+2851.
9380 JECFA. Summary of evaluations performed by the Joint FAO/WHO Expert Committee on Food Additives. 2001. Available at: https://toxnet.nlm.nih.gov/cgi-bin/sis/search/a?dbs+hsdb:@term+@DOCNO+2851.
9381 Thyssen JP, Carlsen BC, Menne T, et al. Trends of contact allergy to fragrance mix I and Myroxylon pereirae among Danish eczema patients tested between 1985 and 2007. *Contact Dermatitis*. 2008 Oct;59(4):238-44.
9382 Sabroe RA, Holden CR, Gawkrodger DJ. Contact allergy to essential oils cannot always be predicted from allergy to fragrance markers in the baseline series. *Contact Dermatitis*. 2016 Apr;74(4):236-41.
9383 Boonchai W, Iamtharachai P, Sunthonpalin P. Prevalence of allergic contact dermatitis in Thailand. Dermatitis. 2008;19:142-45.
9384 Salam TN, Fowler JF Jr. Balsam-related systemic contact dermatitis. *J Am Acad Dermatol*. 2001 Sep;45(3):377-81.
9385 Machado TB, Leal ICR, Kuster M, et al. Brazilian phytopharmaceuticals-evaluation against hospital bacteria. *Phytother Res*. 2005;19(6):519-25.
9386 El-Shaer NS. Evaluation of some natural products and plant acids against UVB radiation (in vitro). *Alex J Pharm Sci*. 2006;20:7-11.
9387 Noudogbessi JP, Alitonou GA, Djenontin T, et al. Chemical Compositions and Physico-chemical Properties of Three Varieties Essential oils of Cymbopogon giganteus Growing to the Spontaneous State in Benin. *Oriental J Chem*. 2013;29(1):59-67.
9388 Ganjewala D. Cymbopogon essential oils: Chemical compositions and bioactivities. *Int J Essential Oil Ther*. 2009;3:56-65.
9389 Jirovetz L, Buchbauer G, Eller G, et al. Composition and Antimicrobial Activity of Cymbopogon Giganteus (Hochst.) Chiov. Essential Flower, Leaf and Stem Oils From Cameroon[Dagger]. *J Essent Oil Res*. 2007 Sep-Oct;12:207-12.
9390 Bassolé IH, Lamien-Meda A, Bayala B, et al. Chemical composition and antimicrobial activity of Cymbopogon citratus and Cymbopogon giganteus essential oils alone and in combination. *Phytomedicine*. 2011 Sep 15;18(12):1070-4.
9391 Rabehaja DJR, Raoelison G, Ihandriharison H, et al. Volatile Components from Cymbopogon giganteus (Hochst) Chiov var. madagascariensis (A. Camus). *J Essential Oil Bear Plants*. 2013 Mar;13(5):522-27.
9392 Alitonoua F, Avlessia DK, Sohuounhlouea H, et al. Investigations on the essential oil of Cymbopogon giganteus from Benin for its potential use as an anti-inflammatory agent. *Int J Aromather*. 2006;16:37-40.
9393 Sahouo BG, Tonzibo ZF, Boti B, et al. Antiinflammatory and analgesic activities: chemical constituents of essential oils of Ocimum gratissimum, Eucalyptus citriodora and Cymbopogon giganteus inhibited lipoxygenase L-1 and cyclooxygenase of PGHS. *Bull Chem Soc Ethiop*. 2003;17:191–97.
9394 Alitonoua F, Avlessia DK, Sohuounhlouea H, et al. Investigations on the essential oil of Cymbopogon giganteus from Benin for its potential use as an anti-inflammatory agent. *Int J Aromather*. 2006;16:37-40.
9395 Sahouo BG, Tonzibo ZF, Boti B, et al. Antiinflammatory and analgesic activities: chemical constituents of essential oils of Ocimum gratissimum, Eucalyptus citriodora and Cymbopogon giganteus inhibited lipoxygenase L-1 and cyclooxygenase of PGHS. *Bull Chem Soc Ethiop*. 2003;17:191–97.
9396 Jirovetz L, Buchbauer G, Eller G, et al. Composition and Antimicrobial Activity of Cymbopogon Giganteus (Hochst.) Chiov. Essential Flower, Leaf and Stem Oils From Cameroon[Dagger]. *J Essent Oil Res*. 2007 Sep-Oct;12:207-12.
9397 Bassolé IH, Lamien-Meda A, Bayala B, et al. Chemical composition and antimicrobial activity of Cymbopogon citratus and Cymbopogon giganteus essential oils alone and in combination. *Phytomedicine*. 2011 Sep 15;18(12):1070-4.
9398 Alitonoua F, Avlessia DK, Sohuounhlouea H, et al. Investigations on the essential oil of Cymbopogon giganteus from Benin for its potential use as an anti-inflammatory agent. *Int J Aromather*. 2006;16:37-40.
9399 Bayala B, Bassole IHN, Maqdasy S, et al. Cymbopogon citratus and Cymbopogon giganteus essential oils have cytotoxic effects on tumor cell cultures. Identification of citral as a new putative anti-proliferative molecule. Biochimie. 2018 Oct;153:162-170.
9400 Kilic O, Kocak A. Volatile constituents of Juniperus communis L., Taxus Canadensis Marshall. and Tsuga Canadensis (L.) Carr. From Canada. *J Agric Sci Tech*. 2014;B4:135-40.
9401 Aromatics International. Hemlock - Tsuga canadensis. Available at: http://www.aromaticsinternational.com/products/essential-oils/hemlock.
9402 Bernhart MW. Closely eluting bornyl and isobornyl acetates are chemotaxonomic markers in the Pinaceae by virtue of their unique mass spectra. *Am. J Essential Oils Nat Products*. 2016;4(2):41-46.
9403 Frank MB, Yang Q, Osban J, et al. Frankincense oil derived from Boswellia carterii induces tumor cell specific cytotoxicity. *BMC Complement Altern Med*. 2009;9:6.
9404 Ozogul Y, Kuley E, Ucar Y, et al. Antimicrobial Impacts of Essential Oils on Food Borne-Pathogens. Recent Pat Food Nutr Agric. 2015;7(1):53-61.
9405 Bagci E, Hayta S Dogan G. Chemical Composition of Essential Oils from Bark and Leaves of Pinus brutia Ten. from Turkey. *Asian J Chem*. 2011;23(6):2782-84.
9406 Ghosn MW, Saliba NA, Talhouk SY. Chemical Composition of the Needle-Twig Oils of Pinus brutia Ten. *J Essent Oil Res*. 2006 Jul-Aug;18:445-47.

9407 Ulukanli Z, Karaborklu S, Bozok F, et al. Chemical composition, antimicrobial, insecticidal, phytotoxic and antioxidant activities of Mediterranean Pinus brutia and Pinus pinea resin essential oils. *Chinese J Natural Med.* 2014;12(12):0901-10.
9408 Tumen I, Hafizoglu H, Kilic A, et al. Yields and Constituents of Essential Oil from Cones of Pinaceae spp. Natively Grown in Turkey. *Molecules.* 2010;15:5797-806.
9409 Loizzo M, Saab A, Tundis R, et al. Chemical composition and antimicrobial activity of essential oils from Pinus brutia (calabrian pine) growing in Lebanon. *Chem Nat Compounds.* 2008;44(6):784-86.
9410 Riahi L, Chograni H, Ziadi S, et al. Essential oil of Pinus brutia and Cupressus sempervirens from Tunisia: Chemical composition and antioxidant activity. *Revue Soc Sci Nat de Tunisie.* 2011-2012;38:55-60.
9411 Ustun O, Senol FS, Kurkcuoglu M, et al. Investigation on chemical composition, anticholinesterase and antioxidant activities of extracts and essential oils of Turkish Pinus species and pycnogenol [J]. *Ind Crop Prod.* 2012;38:115-23.
9412 Koutsaviti K, Giatropoulos A, Pitarokili D, et al. Greek Pinus essential oils: larvicidal activity and repellency against Aedes albopictus (Diptera: Culicidae). *Parasitol Res.* 2015 Feb;114(2):583-92.
9413 Ozogul Y, Kuley E, Ucar Y, et al. Antimicrobial Impacts of Essential Oils on Food Borne-Pathogens. Recent Pat Food Nutr Agric. 2015;7(1):53-61.
9414 Ulukanli Z, Karaborklu S, Bozok F, et al. Chemical composition, antimicrobial, insecticidal, phytotoxic and antioxidant activities of Mediterranean Pinus brutia and Pinus pinea resin essential oils. *Chinese J Natural Med.* 2014;12(12):0901-10.
9415 Loizzo M, Saab A, Tundis R, et al. Chemical composition and antimicrobial activity of essential oils from Pinus brutia (calabrian pine) growing in Lebanon. *Chem Nat Compounds.* 2008;44(6):784-86.
9416 Ulukanli Z, Karaborklu S, Bozok F, et al. Chemical composition, antimicrobial, insecticidal, phytotoxic and antioxidant activities of Mediterranean Pinus brutia and Pinus pinea resin essential oils. *Chinese J Natural Med.* 2014;12(12):0901-10.
9417 Ulukanli Z, Karaborklu S, Bozok F, et al. Chemical composition, antimicrobial, insecticidal, phytotoxic and antioxidant activities of Mediterranean Pinus brutia and Pinus pinea resin essential oils. *Chinese J Natural Med.* 2014;12(12):0901-10.
9418 Ustun O, Senol FS, Kurkcuoglu M, et al. Investigation on chemical composition, anticholinesterase and antioxidant activities of extracts and essential oils of Turkish Pinus species and pycnogenol [J]. *Ind Crop Prod.* 2012;38:115-23.
9419 Riahi L, Chograni H, Ziadi S, et al. Essential oil of Pinus brutia and Cupressus sempervirens from Tunisia: Chemical composition and antioxidant activity. *Revue Soc Sci Nat de Tunisie.* 2011-2012;38:55-60.
9420 Ustun O, Senol FS, Kurkcuoglu M, et al. Investigation on chemical composition, anticholinesterase and antioxidant activities of extracts and essential oils of Turkish Pinus species and pycnogenol [J]. *Ind Crop Prod.* 2012;38:115-23.
9421 Darvesh S, Hopkins DA, Geula C, Neurobiology of butyrylcholinesterase. *Nat Rev Neurosci.* 2003 Feb;4:131-38.
9422 Ulukanli Z, Karaborklu S, Bozok F, et al. Chemical composition, antimicrobial, insecticidal, phytotoxic and antioxidant activities of Mediterranean Pinus brutia and Pinus pinea resin essential oils. *Chinese J Natural Med.* 2014;12(12):0901-10.
9423 Lalthazuali, Mathew N. Mosquito repellent activity of volatile oils from selected aromatic plants. *Parasitol Res.* 2017 Feb;116(2):821-825.
9424 Liu VB, Jeena K, Kuttan R. An evaluation of antioxidant, anti-inflammatory, and antinociceptive activities of essential oil from Curcuma longa L. *Indian J Pharmacol.* 2011 Sep-Oct;43(5):526-31.
9425 Chowdhury JU, Nandi NC, Bhuiyan NI, et al. Essential oil constituents of the rhizomes of two types of Curcuma longa of Bangladesh. *Bangladesh J Sci Ind Res.* 2008;43(2):259-266.
9426 Singh G, Kapoor IP, Singh P, et al. Comparative study of chemical composition and antioxidant activity of fresh and dry rhizomes of turmeric (Curcuma longa Linn.). *Food Chem Toxicol.* 2010 Apr;48(4):1026-31.
9427 Singh S, Sankar B, Rajesh S, et al. Chemical composition of turmeric oil (Curcuma longa L. cv. Roma) and its antimicrobial activity against eye infecting pathogens. *J Essent Oil Res.* 2011 Nov-Dec;23:11-18.
9428 Ferreira FD, Mossini SAG, Ferreira FMD, et al. The inhibitory effects of Curcuma longa L. essential oil and curcumin on Aspergillus flavus link growth and morphology. *Sci World J.* 2013 Nov;2013(2013)343804.
9429 Raina VK, Srivastava SK. Rhizome and leaf oil composition of curcuma longa from the lower Himalayan region of Northern India. *J Essent Oil Res.* 2005 Sep-Oct;17:1-4.
9430 Sindhu S, Chempakam B, Leela NK, et al. Chemoprevention by essential oil of turmeric leaves (Curcuma longa L.) on the growth of Aspergillus flavus and aflatoxin production. *Food Chem toxicol.* 2011 May;49(5):1188-92.
9431 Mau JL, Lai EYC, Wang NP, et al. Composition and antioxidant activity of the essential oil from Curcuma zedoaria. *Food Chem.* 2003 Sep;82(4):583-91.
9432 Singh P, Singh S, Kapoor IPS, et al. Chemical composition and antioxidant activities of essential oil and oleoresins from Curcuma zedoaria
rhizomes, part-74. *Food Biosci.* 2013 Sep;3:42-48.
9433 Purkayastha J, Nath SC, Klinkby N. Essential Oil of the Rhizome of Curcuma zedoaria (Christm.) Rose. Native to Northeast India. *J Essent Oil Res.* 2006;18(2):154-55.
9434 Angel GR, Menon N, Vimala B, et al. Essential oil composition of eight starchy Curcuma species. *Ind Crops Products.* 2014;60:233-38.
9435 Kojima H, Yanai T, Toyota A. Essential oil constituents from Japanese and Indian Curcuma aromatica rhizomes. *Planta Med.* 1998 May;64(4):380-1.
9436 Zwaving JH, Bos R. Analysis of the Essential Oils of Five Curcuma Species. *Flavour Frag J.* 1992 Jan;7(1):19-22.
9437 Jarikasem S, Thubthimthed S, Chawananoraseth K, et al. Essential Oils from Three Curcuma Species Collected in Thailand. *Acta Hort.* 2005;677:37-41.
9438 Zhou L, Zhang K, Li J, et al. Inhibition of vascular endothelial growth factor-mediated angiogenesis involved in reproductive toxicity induced by sesquiterpenoids of Curcuma zedoaria in rats. *Reprod Toxicol.* 2013 Jun;37:62-9.
9439 Lai EY, Chyau CC, Mau JL, et al. Antimicrobial activity and cytotoxicity of the essential oil of Curcuma zedoaria. *Am J Chin Med.* 2004;32(2):281-90.
9440 Lee HS. Antiplatelet property of Cucuma longa L. rhizome-derived ar-turmerone. *Bioresource Tech.* 2006 Aug;97(12):1372-76.
9441 Kuroda M, Mimaki Y, Nishiyama T, et al. Hypoglycemic effects of turmeric (Curcuma longa L. Rhizomes) on genetically diabetic KK-$A^y$ mice. *Biol Pharm Bull.* 2005;28(5):937-39.
9442 Lekshmi PC, Arimboor R, Indulekha PS, et al. Turmeric (Curcuma longa L.) volatile oil inhibits key enzymes linked to type 2 diabetes. *Int J Food Sci Nutr.* 2012 Nov;63(7):832-34.
9443 Al-Jenoobi FI, Al-Thukair AA, Alam MA, et al. Effect of Curcuma longa on CYP2D6- and CYP3A4-mediated metabolism of dextromethorphan in human liver microsomes and healthy human subjects. *Eur J Drug Metab Pharm.* 2014 Feb:2107-0180.
9444 Zhou L, Zhang K, Li J, et al. Inhibition of vascular endothelial growth factor-mediated angiogenesis involved in reproductive toxicity induced by sesquiterpenoids of Curcuma zedoaria in rats. *Reprod Toxicol.* 2013 Jun;37:62-9.
9445 Khine H, Weiss D, Graber N, et al. A cluster of children with seizures caused by camphor poisoning. *Pediatrics.* 2009 May;123(5):1269-72.
9446 Michiels EA, Mazor SS. Toddler with seizures due to ingesting camphor at an Indian celebration. *Pediatr Emerg Care.* 2010 Aug;26(8):574-75.
9447 Koren G. Medications which can kill a toddler with one tablet or teaspoonful. *J toxicol Clin toxicol.* 1993;31(3):407- 13.
9448 Flaman Z, Pellechia-Clarke S, Bailey B, et al. Unintentional exposure of young children to camphor and eucalyptus oils. *Paediatr Child Health.* 2001 Feb;6(2):80-83.
9449 Rabl W, Katzgraber F, Steinlechner M. Camphor ingestion for abortion (case report). *Forensic Sci Int.* 1997 Sep 19;89(1-2):137-40.
9450 Flaman Z, Pellechia-Clarke S, Bailey B, et al. Unintentional exposure of young children to camphor and eucalyptus oils. *Paediatr Child Health.* 2001 Feb;6(2):80-83.
9451 Narayan S, Singh N. Camphor poisoning-An unusual cause of seizure. *Med J Armed Forces India.* 2012 Jul;68(3):252-53.
9452 Chanaranaj KJ, G MV, S M. Camphor poisoning in a child. *Natl Med J India.* 2013 Jan-Feb;26(1):60.
9453 Olowe SA, Ransome-Kuti O. The risk of jaundice in glucose-6-phosphate dehydrogenase deficient babies exposed to menthol. *Acta Paediatr Scand.* 1980 May;69(3):341-5.
9454 Dillon Remy M, Manning Alleyne P, Bratt DE, et al. Neonatal jaundice at Port-of-Spain General Hospital abstract. *West Indian Med J.* 1987;36(Suppl):28.
9455 Manoguerra AS, Erdman AR, Wax PM, et al. Camphor poisoning: an evidence-based practice guideline for out-of- hospital management. *Clin Toxicol (Phila).*2006;44(4):357-70.
9456 Gibson DE, Moore GP, Pfaff JA. Camphor ingestion. *Am J Emerg Med.* 1989 Jan;7(1):41-43.
9457 Koppel C, Martends F, Schirop T, et al. Hemoperfusion in acute camphor poisoning. *Intensive Care Med.* 1988;14(4):431-33.
9458 Noomhorm N, Chang CJ, Wen CS, et al. In vitro and in vivo effects of xanthorrhizol on human breast cancer MCF-7 cells treated with tamoxifen. *J Pharmacol Sci.* 2014;125(4):375-85.
9459 Kim MB, Kim C, Song Y, et al. Antihyperglycemic and Anti-Inflammatory Effects of Standardized Curcuma xanthorrhiza Roxb. Extract and Its Active Compound Xanthorrhizol in High-Fat Diet-Induced Obese Mice. *Evid Based Complement Alternat Med.* 2014;2014:205915.
9460 Zhou Y, Shen J, Xia L, et al. Curcuma zedoaria (Berg.) Rosc. essential oil and paclitaxel synergistically enhance the apoptosis of SKOV3 cells. *Mol Med Rep.* 2015 Jul;12(1):1253-7.
9461 Chen CC, Chen Y, Hsi YT, et al. Chemical constituents and anticancer activity of Curcuma zedoaria roscoe essential oil against non-small cell lung carcinoma cells in vitro and in vivo. *J Agric Food Chem.* 2013 Nov 27;61(47):11418-27.
9462 Chen W, Lu Y, Gao M, et al. Anti-angiogenesis effect of essential oil from Curcuma zedoaria in vitro and in vivo. *J Ethnopharmacol.* 2011 Jan 7;133(1):220-6.
9463 Lai EY, Chyau CC, Mau JL, et al. Antimicrobial activity and cytotoxicity of the essential oil of Curcuma zedoaria. *Am J Chin Med.* 2004;32(2):281-90.
9464 Li Y, Wo JM, Liu Q, et al. Chemoprotective effects of Curcuma aromatica on esophageal carcinogenesis. *Ann Surg Oncol.* 2009 Feb;16(2):515-23.
9465 Tawatsin A, Wratten SD, Scott RR, et al. Repellency of volatile oils from pants against three mosquito vectors. *J Vector Ecol.* 2001 Jun;26(1):76-82.
9466 Liju VB, Jeena K, Kuttan R. Gastroprotective activity of essential oils from turmeric and ginger. *J Basic Clin Physiol Pharmacol.* 2015 Jan;26(1):95-103.
9467 Lekshmi PC, Arimboor R, Indulekha PS, et al. Turmeric (Curcuma longa L.) volatile oil inhibits key enzymes linked to type 2 diabetes. *Int J Food Sci Nutr.* 2012 Nov;63(7):832-34.
9468 Honda S, Aoki F, Tanaka H, et al. Effects of ingested turmeric oleoresin on glucose and lipid metabolisms in obese diabetic mice: a DNA microarray study. *J Agric Food Chem.* 2006 Nov 29;54(24):9055-62.
9469 Funk JL, Frye JB, Oyarzo JN, et al. Anti-arthritic effects and toxicity of the essential oils of turmeric (Curcuma longa L.). *J Agric Food Chem.* 2010 Jan 27;58(2):842-49.
9470 Dohare P, Garg P, Sharma U, et al. Neuroprotective efficacy and therapeutic window of curcuma oil: in rat embolic stroke model. *BMC Complement Altern Med.* 2008 Sep 30;8:55.
9471 Dohare P, Varma S, Ray M. Curcuma oil modulates the nitric oxide system response to cerebral ischemia/reperfusion injury. *Nitric Oxide.* 2008 Aug;19(1):1-11.
9472 Rathore P, Dohare P, Varma S, et al. Curcuma oil: reduces early accumulation of oxidative product and is anti- apoptogenic in transient focal ischemia in rat brain. *Neurochem Res.* 2008 Sep;33(9):1672-82.
9473 Baylac S, Racine P. Inhibition of 5-lipoxygenase by essential oils and other natural fragrant extracts. *Int J Aromatherapy.* 2003;13(2-3):138-42.

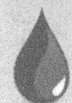

[9474] Jacob JN, Badyal DK. Biological studies of turmeric oil, part 3: anti-inflammatory and analgesic properties of turmeric oil and fish oil in comparison with aspirin. *Nat Prod Commun.* 2014 Feb;9(2):225-28.
[9475] Dias Ferreira F, Mossini SA, Dias Ferreira FM, et al. The inhibitory effects of Curcuma longa L. essential oil and curcumin on Aspergillus flavus link growth and morphology. *ScientificWorldJournal.* 2013 Dec 3;2013:343804.
[9476] Ferreira FD, Kemmelmeier C, Arroteia C, et al. Inhibitory effect of the essential oil of Curcuma longa L. and curcumin on aflatoxin production by Aspergillus flavus link. *Food Chem.* 213 Jan 15;136(2):789-93.
[9477] Hu Y, Zhang J, Kong W, et al. Mechanisms of antifungal and anti-aflatoxigenic properties of essential oil derived from turmeric (Curcuma longa L.) on Aspergillus flavus. *Food Chem.* 2017 Apr 1;220:1-8.
[9478] Singh V, Jain M, Misra A, et al. Curcuma oil ameliorates hyperlipidaemia and associated deleterious effects in golden Syrian hamsters. *Br. J Nutr.* 2013 Aug 28;110(3):437-46.
[9479] Lee KH, Kim BS, Keum KS, et al. Essential oil of Curcuma longa inhibits Streptococcus mutans biofilm formation. *J Food Sci.* 2011 Nov-Dec;76(9):H226-30.
[9480] Hassan W, Gul S, Rehman S, et al. Report - Gas chromatography coupled with mass spectrometric characterization of Curcuma longa: Protection against pathogenic microbes and lipid peroxidation in rat's tissue homogenate. *Pak J Pharm Sci.* 2016 Mar;29(2):615-21.
[9481] Jankasem M, Wuthi-Udomlert M, Gritsanapan W. Antidermatophytic properties of ar-turmerone, turmeric oil, and Curcuma longa preparations. *ISRN Dermatol.* 2013 Aug 26;2013:250597.
[9482] Hastak K, Lubri N, Jakhi SD, et al. Effect of turmeric oil and turmeric oleoresin on cytogenetic damage in patients suffering from oral submucous fibrosis. *Cancer Lett.* 1997 Jun 24;116(2):265-69.
[9483] Hans VM, Grover HS, Deswal H, et al. Antimicrobial Efficacy of Various Essential Oils at Varying Concentrations against Periopathogen Porphyromonas gingivalis. *J Clin Diagn Res.* 2016 Sep;10(9):ZC16-ZC19.
[9484] Aggarwal BB, Yuan W, Li S, et al. Curcumin-free turmeric exhibits anti-inflammatory and anticancer activities: Identification of novel components of turmeric. *Mol Nutr Food Res.* 2013 Sep;57(9):1529-42.
[9485] Sandur SK, Pandey MK, Sung B, et al. Curcumin, demethoxycurcumin, bisdemethoxycurcumin, tetrahydrocurcumin and turmerones differentially regulate anti-inflammatory and anti-proliferative responses through ROS-independent mechanism. *Carcinogenesis.* 2007;28:1765-73.
[9486] Murakami A, Furukawa I, Miyamoto S, et al. Curcumin combined with turmerones, essential oil components of turmeric, abolishes inflammation-associated mouse colon carcinogenesis. *Biofactors.* 2013 Mar-Apr;39(2):221-32.
[9487] Hong CH, Noh MS, Lee WY, et al. Inhibitory effects of natural sesquiterpenoids isolated from the rhizomes of Curcuma zedoaria on prostaglandin E2 and nitric oxide production. *Planta Med.* 2002;68:545-47.
[9488] Park SY, Kim YH, Kim Y, et al. Aromatic-turmerone attenuates invasion and expression of MMP-9 and COX-2 through inhibition of NF-kappaB activation in TPA-induced breast cancer cells. *J Cell Biochem.* 2012;113:3653-62.
[9489] Lee Y. Activation of apoptotic protein in U937 cells by a component of turmeric oil. *BMB Rep.* 2009,42:96-100.
[9490] Yue GG, Chan BC, Hon PM, et al. Evaluation of in vitro anti-proliferative and immunomodulatory activities of constituents isolated from Curcuma longa. *Food Chem Toxicol.* 2010;48:2011-20.
[9491] Cheng SB, Wu LC, Hsieh YC, et al. Super-critical carbon dioxide extraction of aromatic turmerone from Curcuma longa Linn. induces apoptosis through reactive oxygen species-triggered intrinsic and extrinsic pathways in human hepatocellular carcinoma HepG2 cells. *J Agric Food Chem.* 2012;60:9620-30.
[9492] Hucklenbroich J, Klein R, Neumaier B, et al. Aromatic-turmerone induces neural stem cell proliferation in vitro and in vivo. *Stem Cell Res Ther.* 2014 Sep;5:100.
[9493] Park SY, Jin ML, Kim YH, et al. Anti-inflammatory effects of aromatic turmerone through blocking of NF-KB, JNK, and p38 MAPK signaling pathways in amyloid β-stimulated microglia. *Int Immunopharmacol.* 2012 Sep;14(1):13- 20.
[9494] Lai EY, Chyau CC, Mau JL, et al. Antimicrobial activity and cytotoxicity of the essential oil of Curcuma zedoaria. *Am J Chin Med.* 2004;32(2):281-90.
[9495] Singh P, Singh S, Kapoor IPS, et al. Chemical composition and antioxidant activities of essential oil and oleoresins from Curcuma zedoaria rhizomes, part-74. *Food Biosci.* 2013 Sep;3:42-48.
[9496] Mau JL, Lai EYC, Wang NP, et al. Composition and antioxidant activity of the essential oil from Curcuma zedoaria. *Food Chem.* 2003 Sep;82(4):583-91.
[9497] Tsai HH, Lin HW, Chen YL, et al. A review of potential harmful interactions between anticoagulant/antiplatelet agents and Chinese herbal medicines. *PLoS One.* 2013 May 9;8(5):e64255.
[9498] Al-Reza SM1, Rahman A, Sattar MA, et al. Essential oil composition and antioxidant activities of Curcuma aromatica Salisb. *Food Chem Toxicol.* 2010 Jun;48(6):1757-60.
[9499] Phukerd U, Soonwera M. Repellency of essential oils extracted from Thai native plants against Aedes aegypti (Linn.) and Culex quinquefasciatus (Say). *Parasitol Res.* 2014 Sep;113(9):3333-40.
[9500] Phukerd U, Soonwera M. Larvicidal and pupicidal activities of essential oils from Zingiberaceae plants against Aedes aegypti (Linn.) and Culex quinquefasciatus say mosquitoes. *Southeast Asian J Trop Med Public Health.* 2013 Sep;44(5):761-71.
[9501] Pitasawat B, Champakaew D, Choochote W, et al. Aromatic plant-derived essential oil: an alternative larvicide for mosquito control. *Fitoterapia.* 2007 Apr;78(3):205-10.
[9502] Champakaew D, Choochote W, Pongpaibul Y, et al. Larvicidal efficacy and biological stability of a botanical natural product, zedoary oil-impregnated sand granules, against Aedes aegypti (Diptera, Culicidae). *Parasitol Res.* 2007 Mar;100(4):729-37.
[9503] Chaiyasit D, Choochote W, Rattanachanpichai E, et al. Essential oils as potential adulticides against two populations of Aedes aegypti, the laboratory and natural field strains, in Chiang Mai province, northern Thailand. *Parasitol Res.* 2006 Nov;99(6):715-21.
[9504] Suthisut D, Fields PG, Chandrapatya A. Contact toxicity, feeding reduction, and repellency of essential oils from three plants from the ginger family (Zingiberaceae) and their major components against Sitophilus zeamais and Tribolium castaneum. *J Econ Entomol.* 2011 Aug;104(4):1445-54.
[9505] Choochote W, Chaiyasit D, Kanjanapothi D, et al. Chemical composition and anti-mosquito potential of rhizome extract and volatile oil derived from Curcuma aromatica against Aedes aegypti (Diptera: Culicidae). *J Vector Ecol.* 2005 Dec;30(2):302-9.
[9506] Araújo LA, Araújo RG, Gomes FO, et al. Physicochemical/photophysical characterization and angiogenic properties of Curcuma longa essential oil. *An Acad Bras Cienc.* 2016;88(3 Suppl):1889-1897.
[9507] Chen M, Chang YY1, Huang S, et al. Aromatic-turmerone Attenuates LPS-Induced Neuroinflammation and Consequent Memory Impairment by Targeting TLR4-Dependent Signaling Pathway. *Mol Nutr Food Res.* 2018 Jan;62(2).
[9508] Zhang L, Yang Z, Chen D, et al. Variation on composition and bioactivity of essential oils of four common Curcuma herbs. *Chem Biodivers.* 2017 Nov;14(11).
[9509] Oyemitan IA, Elusiyan CA, Onifade AO, et al. Neuropharmacological profile and chemical analysis of fresh rhizome essential oil of Curcuma longa (turmeric) cultivated in Southwest Nigeria. *Toxicol Rep.* 2017 Jul 17;4:391-398.
[9510] Santos PASR, Avanco GB, Nerilo SB, et al. Assessment of Cytotoxic Activity of Rosemary (Rosmarinus officinalis L.), Turmeric (Curcuma longa L.), and Ginger (Zingiber officinale R.) Essential Oils in Cervical Cancer Cells (HeLa). *ScientificWorldJournal.* 2016; 2016: 9273078.
[9511] Kumar A, Agarwal K, Singh M, et al. Essential oil from waste leaves of Curcuma longa L. alleviates skin inflammation. *Inflammopharmacology.* 2018 Oct;26(5):1245-1255.
[9512] Bartoňková I, Dvořák Z. Essential oils of culinary herbs and spices display agonist and antagonist activities at human aryl hydrocarbon receptor AhR. *Food Chem Toxicol.* 2018 Jan;111:374-384.
[9513] Li YL, Du ZY, Li PH, et al. Aromatic-turmerone ameliorates imiquimod-induced psoriasis-like inflammation of BALB/c mice. *Int Immunopharmacol.* 2018 Sep 19;64:319-325.
[9514] Akinyemi AJ, Faboya OL, Paul AA, et al. Nephroprotective Effect of Essential Oils from Ginger (Zingiber officinale) and Turmeric (Curcuma longa) Rhizomes against Cadmium-induced Nephrotoxicity in Rats. *J Oleo Sci.* 2018;67(10):1339-1345.
[9515] Teles AM, Rosa TDDS, Mouchrek AN, et al. Cinnamomum zeylanicum, Origanum vulgare, and Curcuma longa Essential Oils: Chemical Composition, Antimicrobial and Antileishmanial Activity. *Evid Based Complement Alternat Med.* 2019 Jan 15;2019:2421695.
[9516] Chaaban A, Richardi VS, Carrer AR, et al. Insecticide activity of Curcuma longa (leaves) essential oil and its major compound α-phellandrene against Lucilia cuprina larvae (Diptera: Calliphoridae): Histological and ultrastructural biomarkers assessment. *Pestic Biochem Physiol.* 2019 Jan;153:17-27.
[9517] Mahmoudvand H, Pakravanan M, Aflatoonian MR, et al. Efficacy and safety of Curcuma longa essential oil to inactivate hydatid cyst protoscoleces. *BMC Complement Altern Med.* 2019 Jul 26;19(1):187.
[9518] Le TB, Beaufay C, Nghiem DT, et al. Evaluation of the Anti-Trypanosomal Activity of Vietnamese Essential Oils, with Emphasis on Curcuma longa L. and Its Components. Molecules. 2019 Mar 23;24(6).
[9519] Zheng Y, Pan C, Zhang Z, et al. Antiaging effect of Curcuma longa L. essential oil on ultraviolet-irradiated skin. *Michrochem J.* 2020 May;154:104608.
[9520] Wang S, Li Y, Li W, et al. Curcuma oil ameliorates benign prostatic hyperplasia through suppression of the nuclear factor-kappa B signaling pathway in rats. *J Ethnopharmacol.* 2020 Dec 16;113703.
[9521] Ogidi CO, Ojo AE, Ajayi-Moses OB, et al. Synergistic antifungal evaluation of over-the-counter antifungal creams with turmeric essential oil or Aloe vera gel against pathogenic fungi. *BMC Complement Med Ther.* 2021 Jan 28;21(1):47.
[9522] Qiang Y, Si R, Tan S, et al. Spatial variation of volatile organic compounds and antioxidant activity of turmeric ( Curcuma longa L.) essential oils harvested from four provinces of China. *Curr Res Food Sci.* 2021 Nov 29;4:882-890.
[9523] Li C, Zhang W, Wu X, et al. Aromatic-turmerone ameliorates DSS-induced ulcerative colitis via modulating gut microbiota in mice. *Inflammopharmacology.* 2022 Aug;30(4):1283-1294.
[9524] Sharma N, Gupta N, Orfali R, et al. Evaluation of the Antifungal, Antioxidant, and Anti-Diabetic Potential of the Essential Oil of Curcuma longa Leaves from the North-Western Himalayas by In Vitro and In Silico Analysis. *Molecules.* 2022 Nov 8;27(22):7664.
[9525] Zhang Y, Peng F, Yu C. Therapeutic potential of Curcuma oil and its terpenoids in gynecological cancers. *Biomed Pharmacother.* 2022 Nov 14;157:114016.
[9526] Albaqami JJ, Hamdi H, Narayanankutty A, et al. Chemical Composition and Biological Activities of the Leaf Essential Oils of Curcuma longa, Curcuma aromatica and Curcuma angustifolia. *Antibiotics (Basel).* 2022 Nov 3;11(11):1547.
[9527] Jugreet BS, Lall N, Anina Lambrechts I, et al. In Vitro and In Silico Pharmacological and Cosmeceutical Potential of Ten Essential Oils from Aromatic Medicinal Plants from the Mascarene Islands. *Molecules.* 2022 Dec 8;27(24):8705.
[9528] Tanveer M, Ejaz S, Zaka SM, et al. Toxicology of diatomaceous earth, phyto oils and their admixed emulsions against adults of Tribolium castaneum (Herbst). *Toxicol Rep.* 2022 May 16;9:1172-1179.

[9529] Guerrini A, Tacchini M, Chiocchio I, et al. A Comparative Study on Chemical Compositions and Biological Activities of Four Amazonian Ecuador Essential Oils: Curcuma longa L. (Zingiberaceae), Cymbopogon citratus (DC.) Stapf, (Poaceae), Ocimum campechianum Mill. (Lamiaceae), and Zingiber officinale Roscoe (Zingiberaceae). *Antibiotics (Basel)*. 2023 Jan 15;12(1):177.
[9530] Soonwera M, Wongnet O, Sittichok S. Ovicidal effect of essential oils from Zingiberaceae plants and Eucalytus globulus on eggs of head lice, Pediculus humanus capitis De Geer. *Phytomedicine*. 2018 Aug 1;47:93-104.
[9531] Raal A, Arak E. Variation in the Composition of the Essential Oil of Commercial Valeriana officinalis L. Roots from Different Countries. *J Essent Oil Res*. 2008 Dec;20(6):524-29.
[9532] Morteza E, Joorabloo. Evaluation of medicinal plant valerian (Valeriana officinalis L.) essential oil compositions cultivated at Garmsar Zone in Iran. *J Pharm Sci Innovation*. 2012 May-Jun;1(3):87-88.
[9533] Bos R, Woerdenbag H,J, Hendriks H, et al. Composition of the essential oil from underground parts of Valeriana officinalis L. s.l. and several closely related taxa. *Flavour Frag J*. 1997 Sep;12(5):359-70.
[9534] Raal A, Arak E. Variation in the Composition of the Essential Oil of Commercial Valeriana officinalis L. Roots from Different Countries. *J Essent Oil Res*. 2008 Dec;20(6):524-29.
[9535] Bos R, Woerdenbag HJ, van Putten FM, et al. Seasonal variation of the essential oil, valerenic acid and derivatives, and velopotriates in Valeriana officinalis roots and rhizomes, and the selection of plants suitable for phytomedicines. *Planta Med*. 1998 Mar;64(2):143-7.
[9536] Hadley S, Petry JJ. Valerian. *Am Fam Physician*. 2003 Apr 15;67(8):1755-8.
[9537] Albrecht M, Berger W, Laux P, et al. Psychotropic drugs and traffic safety. The influence of Euvegal-coated tablets on the ability to drive and combination effects with alcohol. *Z Allg Med*. 1995;71:1215-25.
[9538] Carrasco MC, Vallejo JR, Pardo-de-Santayana M, et al. Interactions of Valeriana officinalis L. and Passiflora incarnata L. in a patient treated with lorazepam. *Phytother Res*. 2009 Dec;23(12):1795-6.
[9539] Yuan CS, Mehendale S, Xiao Y, et al. The gamma-aminobutyric acidergic effects of valerian and valerenic acid on rat brainstem neuronal activity. *Anesth Analg*. 2004;98:353-8.
[9540] Letchamo W, Ward W, Heard B, et al. Essential oil of Valeriana officinalis L. cultivars and their antimicrobial activity as influenced by harvesting time under commercial organic cultivation. *J Agric Food Chem*. 2004 Jun 16;52(12):3915-9.
[9541] Chen JH, Chao YH, Lu SF, et al. The effectiveness of valerian acupressure on the sleep of ICU patients: a randomized clinical trial. *Int J Nurs Stud*. 2012 Aug;49(8):913-20.
[9542] Yuan CS, Mehendale S, Xiao Y, et al. The gamma-aminobutyric acidergic effects of valerian and valerenic acid on rat brainstem neuronal activity. *Anesth Analg*. 2004;98:353-8.
[9543] Feng YX, Wang Y, Geng ZF, et al. Contact Toxicity and Repellent Efficacy of Valerianaceae Spp. To Three Stored-Product Insects and Synergistic Interactions Between Two Major Compounds Camphene and Bornyl Acetate. *Ecotoxicol Environ Saf*. 2019 Dec;190:110106.
[9544] Feng YX, Wang Y, Geng ZF, et al. Contact toxicity and repellent efficacy of Valerianaceae spp. to three stored-product insects and synergistic interactions between two major compounds camphene and bornyl acetate. *Ecotoxicol Environ Saf*. 2020 Mar 1;190:110106.
[9545] Wang W, Wang Y, Guo Q, et al. Valerian essential oil for treating insomnia via the serotonergic synapse pathway. *Front Nutr*. 2022 Jul 28;9:927434.
[9546] Lee KB, Latif S, Kang YS. Differences in Neurotransmitters Level as Biomarker on Sleep Effects in Dementia Patients with Insomnia after Essential Oils Treatment. *Biomol Ther (Seoul)*. 2023 Mar 13. Online ahead of print.
[9547] Viljoen AM, Subramoney S, van Vuuren SF, et al. The composition, geographical variation and antimicrobial activity of Lippia javanica (Verbenaceae) leaf essential oils. *J Ethnopharmacol*. 2006;96:271-77.
[9548] Chagonda LS, Makanda CD, Chalchat JC. Essential Oils of Wild and Cultivated Lippia javanica (Spreng) and L. oatesii (Rolfe) from Zimbabwe. *J Essent Oil Res*. 2000 Jan/Feb;12:1-66.
[9549] Virijevic S. Antimicrobial and chemical properties of essential oils from indigenous South African Lippia species. *Tshwane University of Technology*. 2012 Jun.
[9550] Delgado IF, Carvalho RR, Nogueira, et al. Study on embryofetotoxicity of b-myrcene in the rat. *Food and Chemical Toxicology*. 1993;31(1):31-5.
[9551] De Olivera AC, Ribeiro-Pinto LF, Paumgartten JR. In vitro inhibition of CYP2B1 monoxygenase by beta-myrcene and other monoterpenoid constituents. *Br J Nutr*. 1999;81:289-95.
[9552] De-Oliveira AC1, Ribeiro-Pinto LF, Otto SS, et al. Induction of liver monooxygenases by beta-myrcene. *Toxicology*. 1997 Dec 26;124(2):135-40.
[9553] Freitas JC1, Presgrave OA, Fingola FF, et al. Effect of beta-myrcene on pentobarbital sleeping time. *Braz J Med Biol Res*. 1993 May;26(5):519-23.
[9554] Viljoen AM, Subramoney S, van Vuuren SF, et al. The composition, geographical variation and antimicrobial activity of Lippia javanica (Verbenaceae) leaf essential oils. *J Ethnopharmacol*. 2006;96:271-77.
[9555] Nzira L, Per M, Peter F, et al. Lippia javanica (Burm F) Spreng: its general constituents and bioactivity on mosquitoes. *Trop Biomed*. 2009 Apr;26(1):85-91.
[9556] Omolo MO, Okinyo D, Ndiege IO, et al. Repellency of essential oils of some Kenyan plants against Anopheles gambiae. *Phytochemistry*. 2004 Oct;65(20):2797-802.
[9557] Samie A, Housein A, Lall N, et al. Crude extracts of, and purified constituents from, Pterocarpus angolensis, and the essential oil of Lippia javanica: their in-vitro cytotoxicities and activities against selected bacteria and Entamoeba histolytica. *Ann Trop Med Parasitol*. 2009 Jul;103(5):427-39.
[9558] Manenzhe NJ, Potgieter N, van Ree T. Composition and antimicrobial activities of volatile components of Lippia javanica. *Phytochemistry*. 2004 Aug;65(16):2333-6.
[9559] Krzyśko-Łupicka T, Sokół S, Piekarska-Stachowiak A. Evaluation of Fungistatic Activity of Eight Selected Essential Oils on Four Heterogeneous Fusarium Isolates Obtained From Cereal Grains in Southern Poland. *Molecules*. 2020 Jan 10;25(2):292.
[9560] Kirici S, Inana M, Turk M, et al. To study of essential oil and agricultural properties of Vetiver (Vetiveria zizanioides) in the Southeastern of Mediterranean. *Adv Environ Biol*. 2011;5(2):447-51.
[9561] Champagnat P, Figueredo G, Chalchat JC, et al. A study of the composition of commercial Vetiveria zizanioides oils from different geographical origins. *J Essent Oil Res*. 2006;18(4):416-22.
[9562] Saraswathi KJT, Jayalakshmi NR, Vyshali P, et al. Comparative study on essential oil in natural and in vitro regenerated plants of Vetiveria zizanioides (Linn.) Nash. *America-Eurasian J Agric Environ Sci*. 2011;10(3):458-63.
[9563] Thubthimthed S, Thisayakorn K, Rerk-am U, et al. Vetiver oil and its sedative effect. *Thailand Institute of Scientific and Technological Research (TISTR, Bangkok, Thailand*. Available at: http://www.vetiver.com/ICV3-Proceedings/THAI_sedation.pdf.
[9564] Rotkittikhun P, Kruatrachue M, Pokethitiyook P, et al. Tolerance and accumulation of lead in Vetiveria zizanioides. *J Environ Biol*. 2010 May;31:329-34.
[9565] Adams RP, Habte M, Park S, et al. Preliminary comparison of vetiver root essential oils from cleansed (bacteria- and fungus-free) versus non-cleansed (normal) vetiver plants. *Biochem Syst Ecol*. 2004;32:1137-44.
[9566] Kadarohman A, Eko SR, Dwiyanti G, et al. Quality and chemical composition of organic and non-organic vetiver oil. *Indo J Chem*. 2014;14(1):43-50.
[9567] Peng HY, LaiCC, Lin CC, et al. Effect of Vetiveria zizanioides essential oil on melanogenesis in melanoma cells: downregulation of tyrosinase expression and suppression of oxidative stress. *ScientificWorldJournal*. 2014 Mar;2014:213013.
[9568] Kim HJ, Chen F, Wang X, et al. Evaluation of antioxidant activity of vetiver (Vetiveria zizanioides L.) oil and identification of its antioxidant constituents. *J Agric Food Chem*. 2005;53(20):7691-95.
[9569] Matsubara E, Shimizu K, Fukagawa M, et al. Volatiles emitted from the roots of Vetiveria zizanioides suppress the decline in attention during a visual display terminal task. Biomed Res. 2012;33(5):299-308.
[9570] Hammer KA, Carson CF, Riley TV. Antimicrobial activity of essential oils and other plant extracts. *J Appl Microbiol*. 1999 Jun;86(6):985-90.
[9571] Saiyudthong S, Pongmayteegul S, Marsden CA, et al. Anxiety-like behavior and c-fos expression in rats that inhaled vetiver essential oil. *Nat Prod Res*. 2015 Jan 2:1-4.
[9572] Saikia D, Parveen S, Gupta VK, et al. Anti-tuberculosis activity of Indian grass KHUS (Vetiveria zizanioides L. Nash). *Complement Ther Med*. 212 Dec;20(6):434-36.
[9573] Sathantriphop S, Achee NL, Sanguanpong U, et al. The effects of plant essential oils on escape response and mortality rate of Aedes aegypti and Anopheles minimus. *J Vector Ecol*. 2015 Dec;40(2):318-26.
[9574] Nararak J, Sathantriphop S, Chauhan K, et al. Avoidance Behavior to Essential Oils by Anopheles minimus, a Malaria Vector in Thailand. *J Am Mosq Control Assoc*. 2016 Mar;32(1):34-43.
[9575] Plant J. Effects of essential oils on telomere length in human cells. *Med Aromat Plants*. 2016;5(2):1-6.
[9576] Cheaha D, Issuriya A, Manor R, et al. Modification of sleep-waking and electroencephalogram induced by vetiver essential oil inhalation. *J Intercult Ethnopharmacol*. 2016 Feb 14;5(1):72-8.
[9577] Burger P, Landreau A, Watson M, et al. Vetiver Essential Oil in Cosmetics: What Is New? *Medicines (Basel)*. 2017 Jun 16;4(2).
[9578] Khater HF, Ali AM, Abouelella GA, et al. Toxicity and growth inhibition potential of vetiver, cinnamon, and lavender essential oils and their blends against larvae of the sheep blowfly, Lucilia sericata. *Int J Dermatol*. 2018 Apr;57(4):449-457.
[9579] Powers CN, Osier JL, McFeeters RL, et al. Antifungal and Cytotoxic Activities of Sixty Commercially-Available Essential Oils. *Molecules*. 2018 Jun 27;23(7).
[9580] Khater HF, Geden CJ. Potential of essential oils to prevent fly strike and their effects on the longevity of adult Lucilia sericata. *J Vector Ecol*. 2018 Dec;43(2):261-270.
[9581] Ramirez-Rueda RY, Marinho J, Salvador MJ. Bioguided identification of antimicrobial compounds from Chrysopogon zizaniodes (L.) Roberty root essential oil. *Future Microbiol*. 2019;14(14):1179-89.
[9582] Khater HF, Geden GJ. Efficacy and Repellency of Some Essential Oils and Their Blends Against Larval and Adult House Flies, Musca Domestica L. (Diptera: Muscidae). *J Vector Ecol*. 2019 Dec;44(2):256-63.
[9583] Sivakumar L, Chellappan DR, Sriramavaratharajan V, et al. Root essential oil of Chrysopogon zizanioides relaxes rat isolated thoracic aorta - an ex vivo approach. *Z Naturforsch C J Biosci*. 2020 Oct 14. Online ahead of print.
[9584] Kurrimboccus F, Orchard A, Danckwerts MP, et al. Antimicrobial Formulation of Chrysopogon zizanioides Essential Oil in an Emulsified Lotion for Acne. *Planta Med*. 2021 Dec 28. Online ahead of print.
[9585] Hanifa M, Wulandari R, Zulfin UM, et al. Different Cytotoxic Effects of Vetiver Oil on Three Types of Cancer Cells, Mainly Targeting CNR2 on TNBC. *Asian Pac J Cancer Prev*. 2022 Jan 1;23(1):241-251.
[9586] Nararak J, Giorgio CD, Thanispong K, et al. Behavioral avoidance and biological safety of vetiver oil and its constituents against Aedes aegypti (L.), Aedes albopictus (Skuse) and Culex quinquefasciatus Say. *Curr Res Insect Sci*. 2022 Aug 6;2:100044.
[9587] Pessoa Moreira AC, de Oliveira Lima E, Alves Wanderley P, et al. Chemical composition and antifungal activity of Hyptis suaveolens (L.) poit leaves essential oil against Aspergillus species. *Braz J Microbiol*. 2010 Jan-Mar;41(1):ISSN 1678-4405.
[9588] Azevedo NR, Campos IFP, Ferreira HD, et al. Chemical variability in the essential oil of Hyptis suaveolens. *Phytochemistry*. 2001;57:733-35.

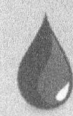

[9589] Peerzada N. Chemical Composition of the Essential Oil of Hyptis Suaveolens. *Molecules*. 1997;2(11):165-168.

[9590] Noudogbessi JP, Agbangnan CP, Yehoouenou B, et al. Chemical composition and physico-chemical characteristics of Hyptis suaveolens (L.) Poit. leaves essential oils from Benin. *Molecules*. 1997;2(11):165-168.

[9591] Nantitanon W, Chowwanapoonpohn S, Okonogi S. Antioxidant and antimicrobial activities of Hyptis suaveolens essential oil. *Sci Pharm*. 2007;75:35-46.

[9592] Grassi P, Nunez MJ, Varmuza K, et al. Chemical polymorphism of essential oils of Hyptis suaveolens from El Salvador. *Flavour Frag J*. 2005 May;20(2):131-35.

[9593] Eshilokun AO, Kasali AA, Giwa-Ajeniya O. Chemical composition of essential oils of tow Hyptis suaveolens (L.) Poit leaves from Nigeria. *Flavour Frag J*. 2005;20:528-30.

[9594] Chatri M, Bakitiar A, Mansyurdin, et al. Chemical Components of Essential Oils of the Leaves of Hyptis suaveolens (L.) Poit. from Indonesia. *Am J Res Commun*. 2014;2(10):30-38.

[9595] Flores SE, Medina JD. Estudio preliminar de los componentes del aceite esencial de Hyptis suaveolens (L.) Poit. *Acta Scientifica Venezolana*. 1970 Dec;21(4):161-162.

[9596] Noudogbessi JP, Agbangnan P, Yehouenou B, et al. Physico-chemical properties of Hyptis suaveloens essential oil. *Int J Med Arom Plants*. 2013 Jun;3(2):191-99.

[9597] Newall CA, Anderson LA, Phillipson JD. "Herbal Medicines: A Guide for Health-care Professionals." London: The Pharmaceutical Press, 1996, 108.

[9598] European Medicines Agency. Community herbal monograph on Eucalyptus globulus Labill., Eucalyptus polybractea R.T. Baker and/or Eucalyptus smithii R.T. Baker, aetheroleum. 2013 Jun. Available at: http://www.ema.europa.eu/docs/en_GB/document_library/Herbal_-_Community_herbal_monograph/2013/07/WC500147008.pdf

[9599] Fischer JH, Dethlefsen U. Efficacy of cineole in patients suffering from acute bronchitis: a placebo-controlled double-blind trial. *Cough*. 2013; 9: 25.

[9600] Worth W, Dethlefsen U. Patients with asthma benefit from concomitant therapy with cineole: a placebo-controlled, double-blind trial. *J Asthma*. 2012 Oct;49(8):849-53.

[9601] Day LM, Ozanne-Smith J, Parsons BJ, et al. Eucalyptus oil poisoning among young children: mechanisms of access and the potential prevention. *Aust N Z J Public Health*. 1997 Jun;21(3):297-302.

[9602] Myott E. Case of eucalyptus poisoning. *Brit M J*. 1906;1:558.

[9603] Hindle RC. Eucalyptus oil ingestion. *N Z Med J*. 1994 May 11;107(977)185-6.

[9604] Tibballs J. Clinical effects and management of eucalyptus oil ingestion in infants and small children. *Med J Aust*. 1995 Aug;163(4):177-80.

[9605] Waldman W, Barwina M, Sein Anand J. Accidental ontoxication with eucalyptus oil—a case report. *Przeql Lek*. 2011;68(8):555-6.

[9606] Day LM, Ozanne-Smith J, Parsons BJ, et al. Eucalyptus oil poisoning among young children: mechanisms of access and the potential prevention. *Aust N Z J Public Health*. 1997 Jun;21(3):297-302.

[9607] De Vincenzi M, Silano M, De Vincenzi A, et al. Constituents of aromatic plants: eucalyptol. *Fitoterapia*. 2002 Jun;73(3):269-75.

[9608] Burkhard PR, Burkhardt K, Haenggeli CA, et al. Plant-induced seizures: reappearance of an old problem. *J Neurol*. 1999 Aug;246(8):667-70.

[9609] Narayan S, Singh N. Camphor poisoning-An unusual cause of seizure. *Med J Armed Forces India*. 2012 Jul;68(3):252-53.

[9610] Chanaranaj KJ, G MV, S M. Camphor poisoning in a child. *Natl Med J India*. 2013 Jan-Feb;26(1):60.

[9611] Perry NB, Anderson RE, Brennan NJ, et al. Essential oils from dalmatian sage (Salvia officinalis L.) variations among individuals, plant parts, seasons, and sites. *J Agric Food Chem*. 1999;47:2048-54.

[9612] Millet Y, Jouglard J, Steinmetz MD, et al. Toxicity of some essential plant oils. Clinical and experimental study. *Clin Toxicol*. 1981 Dec;18(12):1485-98.

[9613] Lamborn LL. Modern soaps, candles and glycerin: A practical manual of modern methods of utilization of fats and oils in the manufacture of soaps and candles, and of the recovery of glycerin. Library of the University of Wisconsin.

[9614] Oyen LP, Dung NX. Plant resources of South-East Asia. 1999. Backhyus, Leiden.

[9615] Kim NH, Hyun SH, Jin CH, et al. Pretreatment with 1,8-cineole potentiates thioacetamide-induced hepatotoxicity and immunosuppression. *Arch Pharm Res*. 2004 Jul;27(7):781-9.

[9616] Nguyen LT, Mysliveckova Z, Szotakova B, et al. The inhibitory effects of β-caryophyllene, β-caryophyllene oxide and α-humulene on the activities of the main drug-metabolizing enzymes in rat and human liver in vitro. *Chem-Biol Interactoins*. 2017 Dec 25;278:123-8.

[9617] Lee HS. Anticoagulant properties of constituents derived from fennel (Foeniculum vulgare Gaertner) fruits. *Food Sci Biotech*. 2006 Oct;15(5):763-67.

[9618] Jori A, Bianchetti A, Prestini PE, et al. Effect of eucalyptol (1,8-cineole) on the metabolism of other drugs in rats and in man. *Eur J Pharmacol*. 1970;9(3):362-66.

[9619] de Sousa DP, Raphael E, Brocksom U, et al. Sedative effect of monoterpene alcohols in mice: A preliminary screening. *Verlag der Zeitschrift fur Naturforschung*. 2007;62c:563-66.

[9620] Nantitanon W, Chowwanapoonpohn S, Okonogi S. Antioxidant and antimicrobial activities of Hyptis suaveolens essential oil. *Sci Pharm*. 2007;75:35-46.

[9621] Xu DH, Huang YS, Jiang DQ, et al. The essential oils chemical compositions and antimicrobial, antioxidant activities and toxicity of three Hyptis species. *Pharm Biol*. 2013;51(9):1125–1130.

[9622] Abagli AZ, Alavo TB, Avlessi F, et al. Potential of the bush mint, Hyptis suaveolens essential oil for personal protection against mosquito biting. *J Am Mosq Control Assoc*. 2012 Mar;28(1):15-9.

[9623] Vongsombath C, Pålsson K, Björk L, et al. Mosquito (Diptera: Culicidae) repellency field tests of essential oils from plants traditionally used in Laos. *J Med Entomol*. 2012 Nov;49(6):1398-404.

[9624] Ashitani T, Garboui SS, Schubert F, et al. Activity studies of sesquiterpene oxides and sulfides from the plant Hyptis suaveolens (Lamiaceae) and its repellency on Ixodes ricinus (Acari: Ixodidae). *Exp Appl Acarol*. 2015 Dec;67(4):595-606.

[9625] Jaya, Singh P, Prakash B, et al. Insecticidal activity of Ageratum conyzoides L., Coleus aromaticus Benth. and Hyptis suaveolens (L.) Poit essential oils as fumigant against storage grain insect Tribolium castaneum Herbst. *J Food Sci Technol*. 2014 Sep;51(9):2210-5.

[9626] Conti B, Benelli G, Flamini G, et al. Larvicidal and repellent activity of Hyptis suaveolens (Lamiaceae) essential oil against the mosquito Aedes albopictus Skuse (Diptera: Culicidae). *Parasitol Res*. 2012 May;110(5):2013-21.

[9627] Soares SF, Borges LM, de Sousa Braga R, et al. Repellent activity of plant-derived constituents against Amblyomma cajennense (Acari: Ixodidae) nymphs. *Vet Parasitol*. 2010 Jan 20;167(1):67-73.

[9628] Benelli G, Flamini G, Canale A, et al. Repellence of Hyptis suaveolens whole essential oil and major constituents against adult granary weevil Sitophilus granarius. *Bulletin of Insectology*. 2012;65(2):177-183.

[9629] Moreira ACP, de Oliveria Lima E, Wanderley PA, et al. Chemical composition and antifunal activity of Hyptus suaveolens (L.) poit leaves essential oil against Aspergillus species. *Braz J Microbiol*. 2014;41:28-33.

[9630] Castro KNC, Canuto KM, Brito ES, et al. In vitro efficacy of essential oils with different concentrations of 1,8-cineole against Rhipicephalus (Boophilus) microplus. *Rev Bras Parasitol Vet*. 2018 Apr-Jun;27(2):203-210.

[9631] Bayla B, Nadembega C, Guenne S, et al. Chemical Composition, Antioxidant and Cytotoxic Activities of Hyptis suaveolens (L.) Poit. Essential Oil on Prostate and Cervical Cancers Cells. *Pak J Biol Sci*. 2020 Jan;23(9):1184-1192.

[9632] Peniche T, Duarte JL, Ferreira RMA, et al. Larvicidal Effect of Hyptis suaveolens (L.) Poit. Essential Oil Nanoemulsion on Culex quinquefasciatus (Diptera: Culicidae). *Molecules*. 2022 Dec 2;27(23):8433.

[9633] Lawrence BM. Progress in essential oils. *Perf Flavorist*. 1998;23(5):67-68.

[9634] Adams RP. Cedar wood oil – analyses and properties. *Essent Oils Waxes*. 1991;12:159-73.

[9635] Cedarwood Oil. Summary of data for chemical selection. Available at: https://ntp.niehs.nih.gov/ntp/htdocs/chem_background/exsumpdf/cedarwood_oil_508.pdf.

[9636] Dunford NT, Hiziroglu S, Holcomb R. Effect of age on the distribution of oil in Eastern redcedar tree segments. *Bioresour Technol*. 2007 Oct;98(14):2636-40.

[9637] Jeong HU, Kwon SS, Kong TY, et al. Inhibitory effects of cedrol, β-cedrene, and thujopsene on cytochrome P450 enzyme activities in human liver microsomes. *J Toxicol Environ Health A*. 2014;77(22-24):1522-32.

[9638] Tumen I, Süntar I, Eller FJ, et al. Topical Wound-Healing Effects and Phytochemical Composition of Heartwood Essential Oils of Juniperus Virginiana L., Juniperus occidentalis Hook., and Juniperus ashei J. Buchholz. *J Med Food*. 2013 Jan;16(1):48-55.

[9639] van Tol RW, Swarts HJ, van der Linden A, et al. Repellence of the red bud borer Resseliella oculiperda from grafted apple trees by impregnation of rubber budding strips with essential oils. *Pest Manag Sci*. 2007 May;63(5):483-90.

[9640] Eller FJ, Vander Meer RK, Behle RW, et al. Bioactivity of cedarwood oil and cedrol against arthropod pests. *Environ Entomol*. 2014 Jun;43(3):762-66.

[9641] Tumen I, Süntar I, Eller FJ, et al. Topical Wound-Healing Effects and Phytochemical Composition of Heartwood Essential Oils of Juniperus Virginiana L., Juniperus occidentalis Hook., and Juniperus ashei J. Buchholz. *J Med Food*. 2013 Jan;16(1):48-55.

[9642] Baylac S, Racine P. Inhibition of 5-lipoxygenase by essential oils and other natural fragrant extracts. *Int J Aromatherapy*. 2003;13(2-3):138-42.

[9643] Zhang K, Yao L. The anxiolytic effect of Juniperus virginiana L. essential oil and determination of its active constituents. *Physiol Behav*. 2018 May 15;189:50-58.

[9644] Zhang K, Lu J, Yao L. Involvement of the Dopamine D 1 Receptor System in the Anxiolytic Effect of Cedrol in the Elevated Plus Maze and Light-Dark Box Tests. *J Pharmacol Sci*. 2020 Jan;142(1):26-33.

[9645] Korona-Glowniak I, Glowniak-Lipa A, Ludwiczuk A, et al. The In Vitro Activity of Essential Oils Against Helicobacter Pylori Growth and Urease Activity. *Molecules*. 2020 Jan 29;25(3):586.

[9646] Santos AA, Wanderley-Teixeira V, Dos Santos Cruz G, et al. Essential oil toxicity on biological and reproductive parameters of Alabama argillacea (Hübner) (Lepidoptera: Erebidae). *Acta Histochem*. 2021 Apr 12;123(4):151714.

[9647] Dudek-Wicher R, Paleczny J, Kowalska-Krochmal B, et al. Activity of Liquid and Volatile Fractions of Essential Oils against Biofilm Formed by Selected Reference Strains on Polystyrene and Hydroxyapatite Surfaces. *Pathogens*. 2021 Apr 23;10(5):515.

[9648] Yohana R, Chisulumi PS, Kidima W, et al. Anti-mosquito properties of Pelargonium roseum (Geraniaceae) and Juniperus virginiana (Cupressaceae) essential oils against dominant malaria vectors in Africa. *Malar J*. 2022 Jul 14;21(1):219.

[9649] National Toxicology Program. Summary of data for chemical selection: Cedarwood oil. Available at: https://ntp.niehs.nih.gov/ntp/htdocs/chem_background/exsumpdf/cedarwood_oil_508.pdf.

[9650] Essential Oil Univeristy. Thuja plicata GC-MS report. Available at: https://www.facebook.com/EssentialOilUniversity/photos/a.10152083271143083.1073741825.82862428082/10152821671898083/?type=3&theater

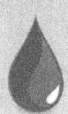
9651 Tsiri D, Graikou K, Poblocka-Olech L, et al. Chemosystematic Value of the Essential Oil Composition of Thuja species Cultivated in Poland—Antimicrobial Activity. Molecules. 2009;14:4707-15.

9652 Zusammensetzung C, Aktivitäten A, von Verschiedenen G. Chemical composition, antimicrobial activities and odor descriptions of various Salvia sp. and Thuja sp. essential oils. ERNÄHRUNG/NUTRITION. 2006;30:152-59.

9653 Northwest Aromatics. Giant arborvitae oil. Available at: http://www.nwaromatics.com/nwaproducts/documents/GAO_online.indd.pdf

9654 Haliciglu O, Astarcioglu G, Yaprak I, et al. Toxicity of Salvia officinalis in a newborn and a child: an alarming report. Pediatr Neurol. 2011 Oct;45(4):259-60.

9655 Lachenmeier DW, Walch SG. Epileptic seizure caused by accidental ingestion of sage (Salvia officinalis L.) oil in children: a rare, exceptional case or a threat to public health. Pediatr Neurol. 2012 Mar;46(3):201.

9656 Stafstrom CE. Seizures in a 7-month-old child after exposure to the essential plant oil thuja. Pediatr Neurol. 2007 Dec;37(6):446-8.

9657 da Silva Costa KC, Bexerra SB, Norte CM, et al. Medicinal plants with teratogenic potential: current considerations. Braz J Pharm Sci. 2012;48(3):427-33.

9658 Brinker F. Herb Contraindications and Drug Interactions. 2nd ed. Sandy, OR. Eclectic Medical Publications. 1998.

9659 European Medicines Agency. Public statement on the use of herbal medicinal products containing thujone. Available at: http://www.ema.europa.eu/docs/en_GB/document_library/Public_statement/2011/02/WC500102294.pdf.

9660 Millet Y, Jouglard J, Steinmetz MD, et al. Toxicity of some essential plant oils. Clinical and experimental study. Clin Toxicol. 1981 Dec;18(12):1485-98.

9661 Cristovao L, Carvalho F, Bastos MDL, et al. Hepatotoxicity of an essential oil of Salvia officinalis L.: an in vitro study using freshly isolated rat hepatocytes. Congress Biomarkers. 2001 Sep:165.

9662 Millet Y, Jouglard J, Steinmetz MD, et al. Toxicity of some essential plant oils. Clinical and experimental study. Clin Toxicol. 1981 Dec;18(12):1485-98.

9663 Burkhard PR, Burkhardt K, Haenggeli CA, et al. Plant-induced seizures: reappearance of an old problem. J Neurol. 1999 Aug;246(8):667-70.

9664 Burkhard PR, Burkhardt K, Haenggeli CA, et al. Plant-induced seizures: reappearance of an old problem. J Neurol. 1999 Aug;246(8):667-70.

9665 Narayan S, Singh N. Camphor poisoning-An unusual cause of seizure. Med J Armed Forces India. 2012 Jul;68(3):252-53.

9666 Chanaranaj KJ, G MV, S M. Camphor poisoning in a child. Natl Med J India. 2013 Jan-Feb;26(1):60.

9667 Perry NB, Anderson RE, Brennan NJ, et al. Essential oils from dalmatian sage (Salvia officinalis L.) variations among individuals, plant parts, seasons, and sites. J Agric Food Chem. 1999;47:2048-54.

9668 Millet Y, Jouglard J, Steinmetz MD, et al. Toxicity of some essential plant oils. Clinical and experimental study. Clin Toxicol. 1981 Dec;18(12):1485-98.

9669 Abass K, Reponen P, Mattila S, et al. Metabolism of α-thujone in human hepatic preparations in vitro. Xenobiotica. 2011 Feb;41(2):101-11.

9670 Uc A, Bishop WP, Sanders KD. Camphor hepatotoxicity. South Med J. 2000;93:596-98.

9671 Frohne D. Giftpflanzen: Cupressaceae. Stuttgart: Wissenschaftliche Verlagsgesellschaft mbH; 1997. pp. 153–6.

9672 Dolan LC, Matulka RA, Burdock GA. Naturally Occurring Food Toxins. Toxins (Basel). 2010 Sep;2(9):2289–2332.

9673 United States National Toxicology Program (NTP). Alpha-Thujone. Dec 10, 1997. Available at: http://ntp.niehs.nih.gov/index.cfm?objectid=03DB8C36-E7A1-9889-3BDF8436F2A8C51F.

9674 Zusammensetzung C, Aktivitäten A, von Verschiedenen G. Chemical composition, antimicrobial activities and odor descriptions of various Salvia sp. and Thuja sp. essential oils. ERNÄHRUNG/NUTRITION. 2006;30:152-59.

9675 Hudson J, Kuo M, Vimalanathan. The Antimicrobial Properties of Cedar Leaf (Thuja plicata) Oil; A Safe and Efficient Decontamination Agent for Buildings. Int J Environ Res Public Health. 2011 Dec;8(12):4477–4487.

9676 Han X, Parker TL, et al. Arborvitae (Thuja plicata) essential oil significantly inhibited critical inflammation- and tissue remodeling-related proteins and genes in human dermal fibroblasts. Biochim Open. 2017 Feb 20;4:56-60.

9677 McGregor RC, Parker KA, Hornby JM, et al. Microbial population dynamics under microdoses of the essential oil arborvitae. BMC Complement Altern Med. 2019;19:247.

9678 Kozics K, Buckova M, Puskarova A, et al. The Effect of Ten Essential Oils on Several Cutaneous Drug-Resistant Microorganisms and Their Cyto/Genotoxic and Antioxidant Properties. Molecules. 2019 Dec 13;24(24):24244570.

9679 Adams RP, Lanner RM, Kauffmann M. Taxonomy of intraspecific taxa of Abies concolor: Leaf essential oils of var. concolor and var. Iowiana. Phytologia. 2011 Apr;93(1):107-17.

9680 USDA Natural Resource Conservation Service. Available at: http://plants.usda.gov/core/profile?symbol=ABCO and http://plants.usda.gov/core/profile?symbol=abal3.

9681 Warren R, Johnson EW. A guide to firs (Abies spp.) of the Arnold Arboretum. Firs of the Arnold Arboretum. Available at: http://arnoldia.arboretum.harvard.edu/pdf/articles/730.pdf.

9682 Ulubelen A, Caldwell ME, Cole JR. Phytochemical Investigation of Abies concolor. J Pharm Sci. 1996 Nov;55(11): 1308-10.

9683 Kilic O, Kocak A. Essential Oil Composition of Six Pinus L. Taxa (Pinaceae) from Canada and Their Chemotaxonomy. J Aric Sci Tech B. 2014;4:67-73.

9684 Krauze-Baranowska M, Mardarowicz M, Wiwart M. Antifungal activity of the essential oils from some species of the genus Pinus. Zeitschrift fur Naturforschung C. 2002 May;57(5-6):478-82.

9685 von Rudloff E. The leaf oil terpene composition of eastern white pine, Pinus strobus L. Flavour Frag J. 1985 Nov;1(1):33-35.

9686 Koutsaviti K, Giatropoulos A, Pitarokili D, et al. Greek Pinus essential oils: larvicidal activity and repellency against Aedes albopictus (Diptera: Culicidae). Parasitol Res. 2015 Feb;114(2):583-92.

9687 Koutsaviti K, Giatropoulos A, Pitarokili D, et al. Greek Pinus essential oils: larvicidal activity and repellency against Aedes albopictus (Diptera: Culicidae). Parasitol Res. 2015 Feb;114(2):583-92.

9688 Krauze-Baranowska M, Mardarowicz M, Wiwart M. Antifungal activity of the essential oils from some species of the genus Pinus. Zeitschrift fur Naturforschung C. 2002 May;57(5-6):478-82.

9689 Ali A, Tabanca N, Demicri B, et al. Chemical Composition and Biological Activity of Four Salvia Essential Oils and Individual Constituents against Two Species of Mosquitoes. J Agric Food Chem. 2015;63(2):447-56.

9690 Takeoka GR, Hobbs C, Park BS. Volatile Constituents of the Aerial Parts of Salvia apiana Jepson. J Essent Oil Res. 2010 May-Jun;22:241-44.

9691 Borek TT, Hochrien JM, Irwin AN. Composition of the essential oil of white sage, Salvia apiana. Flavour Frag J. 2006;21:571-72.

9692 Craig JO. Poisoning by the volatile oils in childhood. Arch Dis Child. 1953;28:259-67.

9693 Melis K. Bochner A, Janssens G. Accidental nasal eucalyptol and menthol instillation. Eur J Pediatr. 1989 Aug;148(8)786-7.

9694 Day LM, Ozanne-Smith J, Parsons BJ, et al. Eucalyptus oil poisoning among young children: mechanisms of access and the potential prevention. Aust N Z J Public Health. 1997 Jun;21(3):297-302.

9695 Chandar SD, Prashanti M, Kumar CL, et al. Eucalyptus Oil-Induced Seizures in Children: A Single-Center Prospective Study. Cureus. 2021 Mar 25;13(3):e14109.

9696 Koren G. Medications which can kill a toddler with one tablet or teaspoonful. J toxicol Clin toxicol. 1993;31(3):407- 13.

9697 Flaman Z, Pellechia-Clarke S, Bailey B, et al. Unintentional exposure of young children to camphor and eucalyptus oils. Paediatr Child Health. 2001 Feb;6(2):80-83.

9698 Rabl W, Katzgraber F, Steinlechner M. Camphor ingestion for abortion (case report). Forensic Sci Int. 1997 Sep 19;89(1-2):137-40.

9699 Burkhard PR, Burkhardt K, Haenggeli CA, et al. Plant-induced seizures: reappearance of an old problem. J Neurol. 1999 Aug;246(8):667-70.

9700 Culic M, Kekovic G, Grbic G, et al. Wavelet and fractal analysis of rat brain activity in seizures evoked by camphor essential oil and 1,8-cineole. Gen Physiol Biophys. 2009;Special Issue(28):33–40.

9701 Mathew T, Kamath V, Kumar RS, et al. Eucalyptus oil inhalation-induced seizure: A novel, underrecognized, preventable cause of acute symptomatic seizure. Epilepsia Open. 2017 Sep;2(3):350–354.

9702 Olowe SA, Ransome-Kuti O. The risk of jaundice in glucose-6-phosphate dehydrogenase deficient babies exposed to menthol. Acta Paediatr Scand. 1980 May;69(3):341-5.

9703 Dillon Remy M, Manning Alleyne P, Bratt DE, et al. Neonatal jaundice at Port-of-Spain General Hospital abstract. West Indian Med J. 1987;36(Suppl):28.

9704 Newall CA, Anderson LA, Phillipson JD. "Herbal Medicines: A Guide for Health-care Professionals." London: The Pharmaceutical Press, 1996, 108.

9705 European Medicines Agency. Community herbal monograph on Eucalyptus globulus Labill., Eucalyptus polybractea R.T. Baker and/or Eucalyptus smithii R.T. Baker, aetheroleum. 2013 Jun. Available at: http://www.ema.europa.eu/docs/en_GB/document_library/Herbal_-_Community_herbal_monograph/2013/07/WC500147008.pdf

9706 Fischer JH, Dethlefsen U. Efficacy of cineole in patients suffering from acute bronchitis: a placebo-controlled double-blind trial. Cough. 2013; 9: 25.

9707 Worth W, Dethlefsen U. Patients with asthma benefit from concomitant therapy with cineole: a placebo-controlled, double-blind trial. J Asthma. 2012 Oct;49(8):849-53.

9708 Day LM, Ozanne-Smith J, Parsons BJ, et al. Eucalyptus oil poisoning among young children: mechanisms of access and the potential prevention. Aust N Z J Public Health. 1997 Jun;21(3):297-302.

9709 Myott E. Case of eucalyptus poisoning. Brit M J. 1906;1:558.

9710 Hindle RC. Eucalyptus oil ingestion. N Z Med J. 1994 May 11;107(977)185-6.

9711 Tibballs J. Clinical effects and management of eucalyptus oil ingestion in infants and small children. Med J Aust. 1995 Aug;163(4):177-80.

9712 Waldman W, Barwina M, Sein Anand J. Accidental ontoxication with eucalyptus oil—a case report. Przeql Lek. 2011;68(8):555-6.

9713 Day LM, Ozanne-Smith J, Parsons BJ, et al. Eucalyptus oil poisoning among young children: mechanisms of access and the potential prevention. Aust N Z J Public Health. 1997 Jun;21(3):297-302.

9714 De Vincenzi M, Silano M, De Vincenzi A, et al. Constituents of aromatic plants: eucalyptol. Fitoterapia. 2002 Jun;73(3):269-75.

9715 Manoguerra AS, Erdman AR, Wax PM, et al. Camphor poisoning: an evidence-based practice guideline for out-of- hospital management. Clin Toxicol (Phila).2006;44(4):357-70.

9716 Gibson DE, Moore GP, Pfaff JA. Camphor ingestion. Am J Emerg Med. 1989 Jan;7(1):41-43.

9717 Koppel C, Martends F, Schirop T, et al. Hemoperfusion in acute camphor poisoning. Intensive Care Med. 1988;14(4):431-33.

9718 Lamborn LL. Modern soaps, candles and glycerin: A practical manual of modern methods of utilization of fats and oils in the manufacture of soaps and candles, and of the recovery of glycerin. Library of the University of Wisconsin.

9719 Oyen LP, Dung NX. Plant resources of South-East Asia. 1999. Backhyus, Leiden.

9720 Kim NH, Hyun SH, Jin CH, et al. Pretreatment with 1,8-cineole potentiates thioacetamide-induced hepatotoxicity and immunosuppression. Arch Pharm Res. 2004 Jul;27(7):781-9.

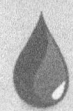

[9721] Gray AM, Flatt PR. Antihyperglycemic actions of Eucalyptus globulus (Eucalyptus) are associated with pancreatic and extra pancreatic effects in mice. *J Nutr.* 1998 Dec;128(12):2319–23.
[9722] Basak SS, Candan F. Effect of Laurus nobilis L. Essential Oil and its Main Components on α-glucosidase and Reactive Oxygen Species Scavenging Activity. *Iran J Pharm Res.* 2013 Spring;12(2):367-79.
[9723] Dey B. Chemo-profiling of eucalyptus and study of its hypoglycemic potential. *World J Diabetes.* 2013 Oct 15;4(5):170–76.
[9724] Tsai HH, Lin HW, Chen YL, et al. A review of potential harmful interactions between anticoagulant/antiplatelet agents and Chinese herbal medicines. *PLoS One.* 2013 May 9;8(5):e64255.
[9725] Moharam BA, Jantan I, bin Ahmad F, et al. Antiplatelet Aggregation and Platelet Activating Factor (PAF) Receptor Antagonistic Activities of the Essential Oils of Five Goniothalamus Species. *Molecules.* 2010;15:5124-38.
[9726] Jori A, Bianchetti A, Prestini PE, et al. Effect of eucalyptol (1,8-cineole) on the metabolism of other drugs in rats and in man. *Eur J Pharmacol.* 1970;9(3):362-66.
[9727] de Sousa DP, Raphael E, Brocksom U, et al. Sedative effect of monoterpene alcohols in mice: A preliminary screening. *Verlag der Zeitschrift fur Naturforschung.* 2007;62c:563-66.
[9728] Garneau FX, Collin G, Gagnon H, et al. Chemical Composition of the Hydrosol and the Essential Oil of Three Different Species of the Pinaceae Family: Picea glauca (Moench) Voss., Picea mariana (Mill.) B.S.P., and Abies balsamea (L.) Mill. *J Essent Oil-Bearing Plants.* 2013 Mar;15(2):227-36.
[9729] Kocak A, Kilic O. Identification of Essential Oil Composition of Four Picea Mill. (Pinaceae) Species from Canada. *J Agric Sci Tech.* 2014;b4:1939-1250.
[9730] Geron C, Rasmussen R, Arnts RR, et al. A review and synthesis of monoterpene speciation from forests in the United States. *Atmospheric Environ.* 2000;34(11):1761-81.
[9731] Hachey JM, Simard S. Extraction and Analysis of the Essential Oil of the Needles and Twigs of White Spruce Picea Glauca (Moench) Voss. *J Wood Chem Tech.* 1987;7(3):333-41.
[9732] Poaty B1, Lahlah J, Porqueres F, et al. Composition, antimicrobial and antioxidant activities of seven essential oils from the North American boreal forest. *World J Microbiol Biotechnol.* 2015 Jun;31(6):907-19.
[9733] von Rudloff E. Chemosytematic studies in the genus picea (Pinaceae) II. The leaf oil of Picea glauca and P. mariana. *Can J Botany.* 1967;45:1703-14.
[9734] von Ruloff E. Seasonal variation in the composition of the volatile oil of the leaves, buds, and twigs of white spruce (Picea glauca). *Can J Botany.* 1972;50:1595-1603.
[9735] Wilkinson RC, Hanover JW, Wright JW, et al. Genetic variation in the monoterpene composition of White Spruce. *Forest Sci.* 1971;17(1):83-90.
[9736] Aromatics International. White Spruce. Available at: https://www.aromatics.com/products/essential-oils/white-spruce.
[9737] Stillpoint Aromatics. White Spruce Essential Oil. Available at: http://www.stillpointaromatics.com/white-spruce-Picea-glauca-essential-oil-aromatherapy
[9738] Khine H, Weiss D, Graber N, et al. A cluster of children with seizures caused by camphor poisoning. *Pediatrics.* 2009 May;123(5):1269-72.
[9739] Michiels EA, Mazor SS. Toddler with seizures due to ingesting camphor at an Indian celebration. *Pediatr Emerg Care.* 2010 Aug;26(8):574-75.
[9740] Koren G. Medications which can kill a toddler with one tablet or teaspoonful. *J toxicol Clin Toxicol.* 1993;31(3):407- 13.
[9741] Bar-Oz B, Levicheck Z, Koren G. Medications that can kill a toddler with one tablet or teaspoonfull – A 2004 update. *Paediatr Drugs.* 2004;6(2):123-6.
[9742] Rabl W, Katzgraber F, Steinlechner M. Camphor ingestion for abortion (case report). *Forensic Sci Int.* 1997 Sep 19;89(1-2):137-40.
[9743] Flaman Z, Pellechia-Clarke S, Bailey B, et al. Unintentional exposure of young children to camphor and eucalyptus oils. *Paediatr Child Health.* 2001 Feb;6(2):80-83.
[9744] Manoguerra AS, Erdman AR, Wax PM, et al. Camphor poisoning: an evidence-based practice guideline for out-of- hospital management. *Clin Toxicol (Phila).*2006;44(4):357-70.
[9745] Gibson DE, Moore GP, Pfaff JA. Camphor ingestion. *Am J Emerg Med.* 1989 Jan;7(1):41-43.
[9746] Koppel C, Martends F, Schirop T, et al. Hemoperfusion in acute camphor poisoning. *Intensive Care Med.* 1988;14(4):431-33.
[9747] Uc A, Bishop WP, Sanders KD. Camphor hepatotoxicity. *South Med J.* 2000;93:596-98.
[9748] Burkhard PR, Burkhardt K, Haenggeli CA, et al. Plant-induced seizures: reappearance of an old problem. *J Neurol.* 1999 Aug;246(8):667-70.
[9749] Narayan S, Singh N. Camphor poisoning-An unusual cause of seizure. *Med J Armed Forces India.* 2012 Jul;68(3):252-53.
[9750] Chanaranaj KJ, G MV, S M. Camphor poisoning in a child. *Natl Med J India.* 2013 Jan-Feb;26(1):60.
[9751] Olowe SA, Ransome-Kuti O. The risk of jaundice in glucose-6-phosphate dehydrogenase deficient babies exposed to menthol. *Acta Paediatr Scand.* 1980 May;69(3):341-5.
[9752] Dillon Remy M, Manning Alleyne P, Bratt DE, et al. Neonatal jaundice at Port-of-Spain General Hospital abstract. *West Indian Med J.* 1987;36(Suppl):28.
[9753] Covington TR, et al. Handbook of Nonprescription Drugs. 11th ed. Washington, D.C.: American Pharmaceutical Association. 1996.
[9754] Poaty B1, Lahlah J, Porqueres F, et al. Composition, antimicrobial and antioxidant activities of seven essential oils from the North American boreal forest. *World J Microbiol Biotechnol.* 2015 Jun;31(6):907-19.
[9755] Glamoclija J, Sokovic M, Tesevic V, et al. Chemical characterization of Lippia alba essential oil: an alternative to control green molds. *Braz J Microbiology.* 2011 Oct-Dec;42(4): ISSN 1517-8382.
[9756] Lopez MA, Stashenko EE, Fuentes JL. Chemical composition and antigenotoxic properties of Lippia alba essential oils. *Genet Mol Biol.* 2011 Jul-Sep;34(3):479–488.
[9757] Mesa-Arango AC, Montiel-Ramos J, Zapata B, et al. Citral and carvone chemotypes from the essential oils of Colombian Lippia alba (Mill.) N.E. Brown: composition, cytotoxicity and antifungal activity. *Mem Inst Oswaldo Cruz, Rio de Janiero.* 2009 Sep;104(6):878-84.
[9758] Blank AF, Alves Camelo LD, Arrigoni-Blank MDF, et al. Chemical Diversity in Lippia alba (Mill.) N. E. Brown Germplasm. *Scientific World J.* 2015(2015):321924.
[9759] Hennebelle T, Sahpaz S, Dermont C, et al. The essential oil of Lippia alba: analysis of samples from French overseas departments and review of previous works. *Chem Biodivers.* 2006 Oct;3(10):1116-25.
[9760] Dellacassa E. Essential oils from Lippia alba (Mill.) N. E. Brown and Aloysia chamaedrifolia Cham. (verbenaceae) from Uruguay. *Flavour Frag J.* 1990 Jun;5(2):107-08.
[9761] Nogueira AC, Carvalho RR, Souza CA, et al. Study on the embryofeto-toxicity of citral in the rat. *Toxicology.* 1995;96(2):105-13.
[9762] Delgado IF, Carvalho RR, Nogueira, et al. Study on embryofetotoxicity of b-myrcene in the rat. *Food and Chemical Toxicology.* 1993;31(1):31-5.
[9763] Seo KA, Kim H, Ku HY, et al. The monoterpenoids citral and geraniol are moderate inhibitors of the CYP2B6 hydroxylase activity. *Chem Biol Interact.* 2008;174:141-46.
[9764] Sheweita SA, Newairy AA, Mansour HA, et al. Effect of some hypoglycemic herbs on the activity of phase I and II drug-metabolizing enzymes in alloxan-induced diabetic rats. *Toxicology.* 2002 May 24;17(2):131-39.
[9765] Raner GM, Vaz AD, Coon MJ. Metabolism of all-trans, 9-cis, and 13-cis isomers of retinal by purified isozymes of microsomal cytochrome P450 and mechanism-based inhibition of retinoid oxidation by citral. *Mol Pharmacol.* 1996;49(3):515-22.
[9766] De Olivera AC, Ribeiro-Pinto LF, Paumgartten JR. In vitro inhibition of CYP2B1 monoxygenase by beta-myrcene and other monoterpenoid constituents. *Br J Nutr.* 1999;81:289-95.
[9767] Modak T, Mukhopadhaya A. Effects of citral, a naturally occurring antiadipogenic molecule, on an energy-intense diet model of obesity. *Indian J Pharmacol.* 2011 May-Jun;43(3):300-05.
[9768] Najafian M, Ebrahim-Habibi A, Yaghmaei P, et al. Citral as a potential antihyperlipidemic medicine in diabetes: a study on streptozotocin-induced diabetic rats. *J Diabetes Metabolic Disorders.* 2011;10(1):3.
[9769] Jori A, Bianchetti A, Prestini PE, et al. Effect of eucalyptol (1,8-cineole) on the metabolism of other drugs in rats and in man. *Eur J Pharmacol.* 1970;9(3):362-66.
[9770] de Sousa DP, Raphael E, Brocksom U, et al. Sedative effect of monoterpene alcohols in mice: A preliminary screening. *Verlag der Zeitschrift fur Naturforschung.* 2007;62c:563-66.
[9771] do Vale TG, Furtado EC, Santos JG Jr, et al. Central effects of citral, myrcene and limonene, constituents of essential oil chemotypes from Lippia alba (Mill.) n.e. Brown. *Phytomedicine.* 2002 Dec;9(8):709-14.
[9772] Veras HN, Campos AR, Rodrigues FF, et al. Enhancement of the antibiotic activity of erythromycin by volatile constituents of Lippia alba (Mill.) N.E. Brown against Staphylococcus aureus. *Pharmacogn Mag.* 2011 Oct;7(28):334-7.
[9773] Zanini SF, Silva-Angulo AB, Rosenthal A, et al. Effect of citral and carvacrol on the susceptibility of Listeria monocytogenes and Listeria innocua to antibiotics. *Lett Appl Microbiol.* 2014 May;58(5):486-92.
[9774] Kuhn GO, McCampbell P, Singmaster G, et al. Application of microencapsulation technology to improve the stability of citral in rodent diets. *Fundam Appl Toxicol.* 1991 Oct;17(3):635-40.
[9775] De Mozzi P, Johnston GA. An outbreak of allergic contact dermatitis caused by citral in beauticians working in a health spa. *Contact Dermatitis.* 2014 Jun;70(6):377-9.
[9776] Souza FV, da Rocha MB, de Souza DP, et al. (-)-Carvone: antispasmodic effect and mode of action. *Fitoterapia.* 2013 Mar;85:20-24.
[9777] Rajeshwari T, Raja B. Antihypertensive, antihyperlipidemicand antioxidantinfluence of D-carvone in L-NAME induced hypertensive rats. *Int J Pharmaceutical Biol Arch.* 2014;5(4):82-88.
[9778] de Sousa DP, Farias Nobrega FF, de Almeida RN. Influence of the chirality of (R)-(-)- and (S)-(+)-carvone in the central nervous system: a comparative study. *Chirality.* 2007 May;19(4):264-268.
[9779] Muruganathan U, Srinivasan S, Indumathi D. Antihyperglycemic effect of carvone: Effect on the levels of glycoprotein components in streptozotocin-induced diabetic rats. *J Acute Disease.* 2013;2(4):310-15.
[9780] Cardoso NN, Alviano CS, Blank AF, et al. Synergism Effect of the Essential Oil from Ocimum basilicum var. Maria Bonita and Its Major Components with Fluconazole and Its Influence on Ergosterol Biosynthesis. *Evid Based Complement Alternat Med.* 2016;2016:5647182.
[9781] Khine H, Weiss D, Graber N, et al. A cluster of children with seizures caused by camphor poisoning. *Pediatrics.* 2009 May;123(5):1269-72.
[9782] Michiels EA, Mazor SS. Toddler with seizures due to ingesting camphor at an Indian celebration. *Pediatr Emerg Care.* 2010 Aug;26(8):574-75.
[9783] Koren G. Medications which can kill a toddler with one tablet or teaspoonful. *J toxicol Clin toxicol.* 1993;31(3):407- 13.
[9784] Craig JO. Poisoning by the volatile oils in childhood. *Arch Dis Child.* 1953;28:259-67.
[9785] Melis K. Bochner A, Janssens G. Accidental nasal eucalyptol and menthol instillation. *Eur J Pediatr.* 1989 Aug;148(8)786-7.
[9786] Day LM, Ozanne-Smith J, Parsons BJ, et al. Eucalyptus oil poisoning among young children: mechanisms of access and the potential prevention. *Aust N Z J Public Health.* 1997 Jun;21(3):297-302.
[9787] Chandar SD, Prashanti M, Kumar CL, et al. Eucalyptus Oil-Induced Seizures in Children: A Single-Center Prospective Study. *Cureus.* 2021 Mar 25;13(3):e14109.
[9788] Flaman Z, Pellechia-Clarke S, Bailey B, et al. Unintentional exposure of young children to camphor and eucalyptus oils. *Paediatr Child Health.* 2001 Feb;6(2):80-83.
[9789] Rabl W, Katzgraber F, Steinlechner M. Camphor ingestion for abortion (case report). *Forensic Sci Int.* 1997 Sep 19;89(1-2):137-40.
[9790] Burkhard PR, Burkhardt K, Haenggeli CA, et al. Plant-induced seizures: reappearance of an old problem. *J Neurol.* 1999 Aug;246(8):667-70.
[9791] Culic M, Kekovic G, Grbic G, et al. Wavelet and fractal analysis of rat brain activity in seizures evoked by camphor essential oil and 1,8-cineole. *Gen Physiol Biophys.* 2009;Special Issue(28):33–40.
[9792] Mathew T, Kamath V, Kumar RS, et al. Eucalyptus oil inhalation–induced seizure: A novel, underrecognized, preventable cause of acute symptomatic seizure. *Epilepsia Open.* 2017 Sep;2(3):350–354.
[9793] Narayan S, Singh N. Camphor poisoning-An unusual cause of seizure. *Med J Armed Forces India.* 2012 Jul;68(3):252-53.

9794 Chanaranaj KJ, G MV, S M. Camphor poisoning in a child. *Natl Med J India.* 2013 Jan-Feb;26(1):60.

9795 Uc A, Bishop WP, Sanders KD. Camphor hepatotoxicity. *South Med J.* 2000;93:596-98.

9796 Olowe SA, Ransome-Kuti O. The risk of jaundice in glucose-6-phosphate dehydrogenase deficient babies exposed to menthol. *Acta Paediatr Scand.* 1980 May;69(3):341-5.

9797 Dillon Remy M, Manning Alleyne P, Bratt DE, et al. Neonatal jaundice at Port-of-Spain General Hospital abstract. *West Indian Med J.* 1987;36(Suppl):28.

9798 Manoguerra AS, Erdman AR, Wax PM, et al. Camphor poisoning: an evidence-based practice guideline for out-of- hospital management. *Clin Toxicol (Phila).*2006;44(4):357-70.

9799 Gibson DE, Moore GP, Pfaff JA. Camphor ingestion. *Am J Emerg Med.* 1989 Jan;7(1):41-43.

9800 Koppel C, Martends F, Schirop T, et al. Hemoperfusion in acute camphor poisoning. *Intensive Care Med.* 1988;14(4):431-33.

9801 Jori A, Bianchetti A, Prestini PE, et al. Effect of eucalyptol (1,8-cineole) on the metabolism of other drugs in rats and in man. *Eur J Pharmacol.* 1970;9(3):362-66.

9802 de Sousa DP, Raphael E, Brocksom U, et al. Sedative effect of monoterpene alcohols in mice: A preliminary screening. *Verlag der Zeitschrift fur Naturforschung.* 2007;62c:563-66.

9803 Covington TR, et al. Handbook of Nonprescription Drugs. 11ᵗʰ ed. Washington, D.C.: American Pharmaceutical Association. 1996.

9804 Mesa-Arango AC, Montiel-Ramos J, Zapata B, et al. Citral and carvone chemotypes from the essential oils of Colombian Lippia alba (Mill.) N.E. Brown: composition, cytotoxicity and antifungal activity. *Mem Inst Oswaldo Cruz, Rio de Janiero.* 2009 Sep;104(6):878-84.

9805 Mesa-Arango AC, Montiel-Ramos J, Zapata B, et al. Citral and carvone chemotypes from the essential oils of Colombian Lippia alba (Mill.) N.E. Brown: composition, cytotoxicity and antifungal activity. *Mem Inst Oswaldo Cruz, Rio de Janiero.* 2009 Sep;104(6):878-84.

9806 Pandey AK, Sonker N, Singh P, et al. Efficacy of Some Essential Oils Against Aspergillus flavus with Special Reference to Lippia alba Oil an Inhibitor of Fungal Proliferation and Aflatoxin B1 Production in Green Gram Seeds during Storage. *J Food Sci.* 2016 Apr;81(4):M928-34.

9807 Shukla R, Kumar A, Singh P, et al. Efficacy of Lippia alba (Mill.) N.E. Brown essential oil and its monoterpene aldehyde constituents against fungi isolated from some edible legume seeds and aflatoxin B1 production. *Int J Food Microbiol.* 2009 Oct 31;135(2):165-70.

9808 Glamočlija J, Soković M, Tešević V, et al. Chemical characterization of Lippia alba essential oil: an alternative to control green molds. *Braz J Microbiol.* 2011 Oct;42(4):1537-46.

9809 Jarvis GE, Barbosa R1, Thompson AJ. Noncompetitive Inhibition of 5-HT3 Receptors by Citral, Linalool, and Eucalyptol Revealed by Nonlinear Mixed-Effects Modeling. *J Pharmacol Exp Ther.* 2016 Mar;356(3):549-62.

9810 Blanco MA, Colareda GA, van Baren C, et al. Antispasmodic effects and composition of the essential oils from two South American chemotypes of Lippia alba. *J Ethnopharmacol.* 2013 Oct 7;149(3):803-9.

9811 Sousa DG, Sousa SD1, Silva RE, et al. Essential oil of Lippia alba and its main constituent citral block the excitability of rat sciatic nerves. *Braz J Med Biol Res.* 2015 Aug;48(8):697-702.

9812 de Souza Chagas AC, de Sena Oliveira MC2, Giglioti R, et al. Efficacy of 11 Brazilian essential oils on lethality of the cattle tick Rhipicephalus (Boophilus) microplus. *Ticks Tick Borne Dis.* 2016 Apr;7(3):427-32.

9813 DA Silva Lima A, DE Carvalho JF1, Peixoto MG, et al. Assessment of the repellent effect of Lippia alba essential oil and major monoterpenes on the cattle tick Rhipicephalus microplus. *Med Vet Entomol.* 2016 Mar;30(1):73-7.

9814 Peixoto MG, Costa-Júnior LM, Blank AF, et al. Acaricidal activity of essential oils from Lippia alba genotypes and its major components carvone, limonene, and citral against Rhipicephalus microplus. *Vet Parasitol.* 2015 May 30;210(1-2):118-22.

9815 Santos IG, Scher R, Rott MB, et al. Amebicidal activity of the essential oils of Lippia spp. (Verbenaceae) against Acanthamoeba polyphaga trophozoites. *Parasitol Res.* 2016 Feb;115(2):535-40.

9816 Olivero-Verbel J, Barreto-Maya A1, Bertel-Sevilla A, et al. Composition, anti-quorum sensing and antimicrobial activity of essential oils from Lippia alba. *Braz J Microbiol.* 2014 Oct 9;45(3):759-67.

9817 Jaramillo-Colorado B, Olivero-Verbel J, Stashenko EE, et al. Anti-quorum sensing activity of essential oils from Colombian plants. *Nat Prod Res.* 2012;26(12):1075-86.

9818 Pino Alea JA, Ortega Luis AG, Rosado Perez A, et al. Composicion y propiedades antibacterianas del aceite esencial de Lippia alba (Mill.) N.E. Brown. *Revista Cubana de Farmacia.* 1996;30(1):ISSN 1561-2988.

9819 Hennebelle T, Sahpaz S, Joseph H, et al. Ethnopharmacology of Lippia alba. *J Ethnopharmacol.* 2008 Mar 5;116(2):211-22.

9820 Oliveira DR, Leitao GG, Santos SS, et al. Ethnopharmacological study of two Lippia species from Oriximina, Brazil. *J Ethnopharmacology.* 1996;108:103–108.

9821 Holetz FB, Pessini GL, Sanches NR, et al. Screening of some plants used in the brazilian folk medicine for the treatment of infectious diseases. *Memorias do Instituto Oswaldo Cruz.* 2002;97:1027–31.

9822 Hennebelle T, Sahpaz S, Joseph H, et al. Ethnopharmacology of Lippia alba. *J Ethnopharmacol.* 2008 Mar 5;116(2):211-22.

9823 Duarte MC, Figueira GM, Sartoratto A, et al. Anti-Candida activity of Brazilian medicinal plants. *J Ethnopharmacol.* 2005 Feb 28;97(2):305-11.

9824 Juiz PJ, Lucchese AM, Gambari R, et al. Essential oils and isolated constituents from Lippia alba leaves and flowers: antimicrobial activity and osteoclast apoptosis. *Int J Mol Med.* 2015 Jan;35(1):211-7.

9825 Vera SS, Zambrano DF, Méndez-Sanchez SC, et al. Essential oils with insecticidal activity against larvae of Aedes aegypti (Diptera: Culicidae). *Parasitol Res.* 2014 Jul;113(7):2647-54.

9826 Shukla R, Singh P, Prasad B, et al. Efficacy of essential oils of Lippia alba (Mill.) N.E. Brown and Callistemon lanceolatus (Sm.) Sweet and their major constituents on mortality, oviposition and feeding behaviour of pulse beetle, Callosobruchus chinensis L. *J Sci Food Agric.* 2011 Sep;91(12):2277-83.

9827 Caballero-Gallardo K, Olivero-Verbel J, Stashenko EE. Repellent activity of essential oils and some of their individual constituents against Tribolium castaneum herbst. *J Agric Food Chem.* 2011 Mar 9;59(5):1690-6.

9828 Gómez LA, Stashenko E, Ocazionez RE. Comparative study on in vitro activities of citral, limonene and essential oils from Lippia citriodora and L. alba on yellow fever virus. *Nat Prod Commun.* 2013 Feb;8(2):249-52.

9829 Meneses R, Ocazionez RE, Martinez JR, et al. Inhibitory effect of essential oils obtained from plants grown in Colombia on yellow fever virus replication in vitro. *Ann Clin Microbiol Antimicrob.* 2009 Mar 6;8:8.

9830 Ocazionez RE, Meneses R, Torres FA. Virucidal activity of Colombian Lippia essential oils on dengue virus replication in vitro. *Mem Inst Oswaldo Cruz.* 2010 May;105(3):ISSN 0074-0276.

9831 Costa DC, Vermelho AB, Almeida CA, et al. Inhibitory effect of linalool-rich essential oil from Lippia alba on the peptidase and keratinase activities of dermatophytes. *J Enzyme Inhib Med Chem.* 2014 Feb;29(1):12-7.

9832 Hatano VY, Torricelli AS, Giassi AC, et al. Anxiolytic effects of repeated treatment with an essential oil from Lippia alba and (R)-(-)-carvone in the elevated T-maze. *Braz J Med Biol Res.* 2012 Mar;45(3):238-43.

9833 Veras HN, Campos AR, Rodrigues FF, et al. Enhancement of the antibiotic activity of erythromycin by volatile constituents of Lippia alba (Mill.) N.E. Brown against Staphylococcus aureus. *Pharmacogn Mag.* 2011 Oct;7(28):334-7.

9834 Maynard LG, Santos KC, Cunha PS, et al. Chemical composition and vasorelaxant effect induced by the essential oil of Lippia alba (Mill.) N.E. Brown. (Verbenaceae) in rat mesenteric artery. *Indian J Pharmacol.* 2011 Nov;43(6):694-8.

9835 López MA, Stashenko EE, Fuentes JL. Chemical composition and antigenotoxic properties of Lippia alba essential oils. *Genet Mol Biol.* 2011 Jul;34(3):479-88.

9836 Shukla R, Kumar A, Singh P, et al. Efficacy of Lippia alba (Mill.) N.E. Brown essential oil and its monoterpene aldehyde constituents against fungi isolated from some edible legume seeds and aflatoxin B1 production. *Int J Food Microbiol.* 2009 Oct 31;135(2):165-70.

9837 Stashenko EE, Jaramillo BE, Martinez JR. Comparison of different extraction methods for the analysis of volatile secondary metabolites of Lippia alba (Mill.) N.E. Brown, grown in Colombia, and evaluation of its in vitro antioxidant activity. *J Chromatogr A.* 2004 Jan 30;1025(1):93-103.

9838 Vale TG, Matos FJ, de Lima TC, et al. Behavioral effects of essential oils from Lippia alba (Mill.) N.E. Brown chemotypes. *J Ethnopharmacol.* 1999 Nov 1;67(2):127-33.

9839 Neto AC, Netto JC, Pereira PS, et al. The role of polar phytocomplexes on anticonvulsant effects of leaf extracts of Lippia alba (Mill.) N.E. Brown chemotypes. *J Pharm Pharmacol.* 2009 Jul;61(7):933-9.

9840 Viana GS, do Vale TG, Silva CM, et al. Anticonvulsant activity of essential oils and active principles from chemotypes of Lippia alba (Mill.) N.E. Brown. *Biol Pharm Bull.* 2000 Nov;23(11):1314-7.

9841 Conde R, Corrêa VS, Carmona F, et al. Chemical composition and therapeutic effects of Lippia alba (Mill.) N. E. Brown leaves hydro-alcoholic extract in patients with migraine. *Phytomedicine.* 2011 Nov 15;18(14):1197-201.

9842 Tomazoni EZ, Pansera MR1, Pauletti GF, et al. In vitro antifungal activity of four chemotypes of Lippia alba (Verbenaceae) essential oils against Alternaria solani (Pleosporeaceae) isolates. *An Acad Bras Cienc.* 2016 May 31;88(2):999-1010.

9843 Montero-Villegas S, Polo M, Galle M, et al. Inhibition of Mevalonate Pathway and Synthesis of the Storage Lipids in Human Liver-Derived and Non-liver Cell Lines by Lippia alba Essential Oils. *Lipids.* 2017 Jan;52(1):37-49.

9844 Tofiño-Rivera A, Ortega-Cuadros M, Galvis-Pareja D, et al. Effect of Lippia alba and Cymbopogon citratus essential oils on biofilms of Streptococcus mutans and cytotoxicity in CHO cells. *J Ethnopharmacol.* 2016 Dec 24;194:749-754.

9845 Kumar P, Mishra S, Kumar A, et al. In vivo and in vitro control activity of plant essential oils against three strains of Aspergillus niger. *Environ Sci Pollut Res Int.* 2017 Sep;24(27):21948-21959.

9846 Porfirio EM, Melo HM, Pereira AMG, et al. In Vitro Antibacterial and Antibiofilm Activity of Lippia alba Essential Oil, Citral, and Carvone against Staphylococcus aureus. *ScientificWorldJournal.* 2017;2017:4962707.

9847 Santos NOD, Pascon RC, Vallim MA, et al. Cytotoxic and Antimicrobial Constituents from the Essential Oil of Lippia alba (Verbenaceae). *Medicines (Basel).* 2016 Aug 12;3(3).

9848 Carvalho PMM, Macedo CAF, Ribeiro TF, et al. Effect of the Lippia alba (Mill.) N.E. Brown essential oil and its main constituents, citral and limonene, on the tracheal smooth muscle of rats. *Biotechnol Rep (Amst).* 2018 Mar; 17: 31–34.

9849 Moreno ÉM, Leal SM, Stashenko EE, et al. Induction of programmed cell death in Trypanosoma cruzi by Lippia alba essential oils and their major and synergistic terpenes (citral, limonene and caryophyllene oxide). *BMC Complement Altern Med.* 2018 Jul 27;18(1):225.

9850 da Silva RER, de Morais LP, Silva AA, et al. Vasorelaxant effect of the Lippia alba essential oil and its major constituent, citral, on the contractility of isolated rat aorta. *Biomed Pharmacother.* 2018 Sep 22;108:792-798.

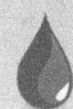

9851 Pereira-de-Morais L, Silva AA, da Silva RER, et al. Tocolytic activity of the Lippia alba essential oil and its major constituents, citral and limonene, on the isolated uterus of rats. *Chem Biol Interact.* 2018 Nov 14;297:155-159.
9852 Quintero Ruiz N, Córdoba Campo Y, Stashenko EE, et al. Antigenotoxic Effect Against Ultraviolet Radiation-induced DNA Damage of the Essential Oils from Lippia Species. *Photochem Photobiol.* 2017 Jul;93(4):1063-1072.
9853 Bonilla-Carvajal K, Stashenko EE, Moreno-Castellanos N. Essential Oil of Carvone Chemotype Lippia alba (Verbenaceae) Regulates Lipid Mobilization and Adipogenesis in Adipocytes. *Curr Issues Mol Biol.* 2022 Nov 18;44(11):5741-5755.
9854 Borges AS, Bastos CMS, Dantas DM, et al. Effect of Lippia alba (Mill.) N.E. Brown Essential Oil on the Human Umbilical Artery. *Plants (Basel).* 2022 Nov 7;11(21):3002.
9855 Santos Filho LGAD, Reis RBD, et al. Chemical composition and biological activities of the essential oils from Lippia alba and Lippia origanoides. *An Acad Bras Cienc.* 2023 Feb 10;95(1):e20220359.
9856 Zrira S, Menut C, Bessiere JM, et al. Chemical Composition of the Essential Oils of Moroccan Ormenis mixta (L.) Dumort. ssp. Multicaulis. *J Essent Oil Bear* Plants. 2007;10(5):278-85.
9857 Darriet F, Bendahou M, Costa J, et al. Chemical compositions of the essential oils of the aerial parts of Chamaemelum mixtum (L.) Alloni. *J Agric Food Chem.* 2012 Feb 15;60(6):1494-502.
9858 Elouaddari A, El Amrani A, Jamal Eddine J, et al. Yield and chemical composition of the essential oil of Moroccan chamomile [Cladanthus mixtus(L.) Chevall.] growing wild at different sites in Morocco. *Flavour Frag J.* 2013 Nov;28(6):360-66.
9859 Kim J, Kang JS, Kang KS, et al. Fumigant toxicity and acetylcholinesterase inhibitory activity of 4 Asteraceae plant essential oils and their constituents against Japanese termite (Reticulitermes speratus Kolbe). *Pesticide Biochem Physiol.* 2014 Jul;113:55-61.
9860 Satrani B, Ghanmi M, Farah A, et al. Composition chimique et activité antimicrobienne de l'huile essentielle de Cladanthus mixtus. *Bull Soc Pharm Bordeaux.* 2007;146:85–89.
9861 Elouaddari A, El Amrani A, JamalEddine J. Intraspecific variability of the essential oil of Cladanthus mixtus from Morocco. *Nat Prod Commun.* 2014 Jan;9(1):133-6.
9862 Darriet F, Bendahou M, Costa J, et al. Chemical compositions of the essential oils of the aerial parts of Chamaemelum mixtum (L.) Alloni. *J Agric Food Chem.* 2012 Feb 15;60(6):1494-502.
9863 Darriet F, Bendahou M, Costa J, et al. Chemical compositions of the essential oils of the aerial parts of Chamaemelum mixtum (L.) Alloni. *J Agric Food Chem.* 2012 Feb 15;60(6):1494-502.
9864 Satrani B, Ghanmi M, Farah A, et al. Composition chimique et activité antimicrobienne de l'huile essentielle de Cladanthus mixtus. *Bull Soc Pharm Bordeaux.* 2007;146:85–89.
9865 Kim J, Kang JS, Kang KS, et al. Fumigant toxicity and acetylcholinesterase inhibitory activity of 4 Asteraceae plant essential oils and their constituents against Japanese termite (Reticulitermes speratus Kolbe). *Pesticide Biochem Physiol.* 2014 Jul;113:55-61.
9866 Ouedrhiri W, Balouiri M, Bouhdid S, et al. Antioxidant and antibacterial activities of Pelargonium asperum and Ormenis mixta essential oils and their synergistic antibacterial effect. *Environ Sci Pollut Res Int.* 2018 Oct;25(30):29860-29867.
9867 Miguel G, Simoes M, Figueiredo AC, et al. Composition and antioxidant activities of the essential oils of Thymus caespititius, Thymus camphoratus and Thymus mastichina. *Food Chem.* 2004 Jun;86(2):183-88.
9868 Delgado T, Marinero P, Asensio-S-Manzanera M, et al. Antioxidant activity of twenty wild Spanish Thymus mastichina L. populations and its relation with their chemical composition. *Food Sci Tech.* 2014 Jul;57(1):412-18.
9869 Pina-Vaz C, Goncalves Rodrigues A, Pinto E, et al. Antifungal activity of Thymus oils and their major constituents. *JEADV.* 2004 Jan;18(1):73-78.
9870 Miguel MG, Guerrero C, Rodriguez H, et al. Main Components of the Essential Oils from Wild Portuguese Thymus mastichina (L.) L. ssp. Mastichina in Different Developmental Stages or Under Culture Conditions. *J Essent Oil Res.* 2004 Mar-Apr;16:111-14.
9871 Cutillas AB, Carrasco A, Martinez-Gutierrez R, et al. Thymus mastichina L. essential oils from Murcia (Spain): Composition and antioxidant, antienzymatic and antimicrobial bioactivities. *PLoS One.* 2018 Jan 5;13(1):e0190790.
9872 Craig JO. Poisoning by the volatile oils in childhood. *Arch Dis Child.* 1953;28:259-67.
9873 Melis K. Bochner A, Janssens G. Accidental nasal eucalyptol and menthol instillation. *Eur J Pediatr.* 1989 Aug;148(8)786-7.
9874 Day LM, Ozanne-Smith J, Parsons BJ, et al. Eucalyptus oil poisoning among young children: mechanisms of access and the potential prevention. *Aust N Z J Public Health.* 1997 Jun;21(3):297-302.
9875 Chandar SD, Prashanti M, Kumar CL, et al. Eucalyptus Oil-Induced Seizures in Children: A Single-Center Prospective Study. *Cureus.* 2021 Mar 25;13(3):e14109.
9876 Burkhard PR, Burkhardt K, Haenggeli CA, et al. Plant-induced seizures: reappearance of an old problem. *J Neurol.* 1999 Aug;246(8):667-70.
9877 Waldman N. Seizure caused by dermal application of over-the-counter eucalyptus oil head lice preparation. *Clin Toxicol (Phila).* 2011 Oct;49(8):750-1.
9878 Craig JO. Poisoning by the volatile oils in childhood. *Arch Dis Child.* 1953;28:259-67.
9879 Day LM, Ozanne-Smith J, Parsons BJ, et al. Eucalyptus oil poisoning among young children: mechanisms of access and the potential prevention. *Aust N Z J Public Health.* 1997 Jun;21(3):297-302.
9880 Myott E. Case of eucalyptus poisoning. *Brit M J.* 1906;1:558.
9881 Hindle RC. Eucalyptus oil ingestion. *N Z Med J.* 1994 May 11;107(977)185-6.
9882 Tibballs J. Clinical effects and management of eucalyptus oil ingestion in infants and small children. *Med J Aust.* 1995 Aug;163(4):177-80.
9883 Waldman W, Barwina M, Sein Anand J. Accidental ontoxication with eucalyptus oil—a case report. *Przeql Lek.* 2011;68(8):555-6.
9884 Day LM, Ozanne-Smith J, Parsons BJ, et al. Eucalyptus oil poisoning among young children: mechanisms of access and the potential prevention. *Aust N Z J Public Health.* 1997 Jun;21(3):297-302.
9885 De Vincenzi M, Silano M, De Vincenzi A, et al. Constituents of aromatic plants: eucalyptol. *Fitoterapia.* 2002 Jun;73(3):269-75.
9886 Jori A, Bianchetti A, Prestini PE, et al. Effect of eucalyptol (1,8-cineole) on the metabolism of other drugs in rats and in man. *Eur J Pharmacol.* 1970;9(3):362-66.
9887 Kim NH, Hyun SH, Jin CH, et al. Pretreatment with 1,8-cineole potentiates thioacetamide-induced hepatotoxicity and immunosuppression. *Arch Pharm Res.* 2004 Jul;27(7):781-9.
9888 Gray AM, Flatt PR. Antihyperglycemic actions of Eucalyptus globulus (Eucalyptus) are associated with pancreatic and extra pancreatic effects in mice. *J Nutr.* 1998 Dec;128(12):2319–23.
9889 Basak SS, Candan F. Effect of Laurus nobilis L. Essential Oil and its Main Components on α-glucosidase and Reactive Oxygen Species Scavenging Activity. *Iran J Pharm Res.* 2013 Spring;12(2):367-79.
9890 Dey B. Chemo-profiling of eucalyptus and study of its hypoglycemic potential. *World J Diabetes.* 2013 Oct 15;4(5):170–76.
9891 Jori A, Bianchetti A, Prestini PE, et al. Effect of eucalyptol (1,8-cineole) on the metabolism of other drugs in rats and in man. *Eur J Pharmacol.* 1970;9(3):362-66.
9892 de Sousa DP, Raphael E, Brocksom U, et al. Sedative effect of monoterpene alcohols in mice: A preliminary screening. *Verlag der Zeitschrift fur Naturforschung.* 2007;62c:563-66.
9893 Cutillas AB, Carrasco A, Martinez-Gutierrez R, et al. Thymus mastichina L. essential oils from Murcia (Spain): Composition and antioxidant, antienzymatic and antimicrobial bioactivities. *PLoS One.* 2018 Jan 5;13(1):e0190790.
9894 Cutillas AB, Carrasco A, Martinez-Gutierrez R, et al. Thymus mastichina L. essential oils from Murcia (Spain): Composition and antioxidant, antienzymatic and antimicrobial bioactivities. *PLoS One.* 2018 Jan 5;13(1):e0190790.
9895 Miguel G, Simoes M, Figueiredo AC, et al. Composition and antioxidant activities of the essential oils of Thymus caespititius, Thymus camphoratus and Thymus mastichina. *Food Chem.* 2004 Jun;86(2):183-88.
9896 Delgado T, Marinero P, Asensio-S-Manzanera M, et al. Antioxidant activity of twenty wild Spanish Thymus mastichina L. populations and its relation with their chemical composition. *Food Sci Tech.* 2014 Jul;57(1):412-18.
9897 Cutillas AB, Carrasco A, Martinez-Gutierrez R, et al. Thymus mastichina L. essential oils from Murcia (Spain): Composition and antioxidant, antienzymatic and antimicrobial bioactivities. *PLoS One.* 2018 Jan 5;13(1):e0190790.
9898 Peñalver P, Huerta B, Borge C, et al. Antimicrobial activity of five essential oils against origin strains of the Enterobacteriaceae family. *APMIS.* 2005 Jan;113(1):1-6.
9899 Faleiro ML, Miguel MG, Ladeiro F, et al. Antimicrobial activity of essential oils isolated from Portuguese endemic species of Thymus. *Lett Appl Microbiol.* 2003;36(1):35-40.
9900 Pina-Vaz C, Goncalves Rodrigues A, Pinto E, et al. Antifungal activity of Thymus oils and their major constituents. *JEADV.* 2004 Jan;18(1):73-78.
9901 Pavela R. Insecticidal activity of some essential oils against larvae of Spodoptera littoralis. *Fitoterapia.* 2005 Dec;76(7-8):691-6.
9902 Cutillas AB, Carrasco A, Martinez-Gutierrez R, et al. Thymus mastichina L. essential oils from Murcia (Spain): Composition and antioxidant, antienzymatic and antimicrobial bioactivities. *PLoS One.* 2018 Jan 5;13(1):e0190790.
9903 Arantes SM. Picarra A, Guerreiro M, et al. Toxicological and Pharmacological Properties of Essential Oils of Calamintha Nepeta, Origanum Virens and Thymus Mastichina of Alentejo (Portugal). *Food Chem Toxicol.* 2019 Nov;133:110747.
9904 Rodrigues M, Lopes AC, Vaz F, et al. Thymus mastichina: Composition and Biological Properties with a Focus on Antimicrobial Activity. *Pharmaceuticals (Basel).* 2020 Dec 19;13(12):479.
9905 Araujo ARTS, Périno S, Fernandez X, et al. Solvent-Free Microwave Extraction of Thymus mastichina Essential Oil: Influence on Their Chemical Composition and on the Antioxidant and Antimicrobial Activities. *Pharmaceuticals (Basel).* 2021 Jul 22;14(8):709.
9906 Vukovic NL, Vukic MD, Obradovic AD, et al. GC, GC/MS Analysis, and Biological Effects of Essential Oils from Thymus mastchina and Elettaria cardamomum. *Plants (Basel).* 2022 Nov 23;11(23):3213.
9907 Coimbra A, Miguel S, Ribeiro M, et al. Chemical composition, antioxidant, and antimicrobial activities of six commercial essential oils. *Lett Appl Microbiol.* 2023 Jan 23;76(1):ovac042.
9908 Nikolic M, Markovic T, Mojovic M, et al. Chemical composition and biological activity of Gaultheria procumbens L. essential oil. *Ind Crops Prod.* 2013 Aug;49:561-67.
9909 Baruh AKS, Bhagat SD. Oil of Indian wintergreen. *Indian J Pharm.* 1976;38:56-57.
9910 Ojha PK, Pudel DK, Dangol S, et al. Volatile Constituent Analysis of Wintergreen Essential Oil and Comparison with Synthetic Methyl Salicylate for Authentication. *Plants.* 2022;11:1090.
9911 National Institutes of Health, Medline Plus. Reye Syndrome. Available at: http://www.nlm.nih.gov/medlineplus/ency/article/001565.htm.
9912 Karabulut AK, Ulger H, Pratten MK. Protection by free oxygen radical scavenging enzymes against salicylate- induced embryonic malformation in vitro. *Toxicol In Vitro.* 2000 Aug;14(4):297-307.
9913 Overman DO, White JA. Comparative teratogenic effects of methyl salicylate applied orally or topically to hamsters. *Teratology.* 1983 Dec;28(3):421-6.
9914 Chan TY. Potential dangers from topical preparations containing methyl salicylate. *Hum Exp Toxicol.* 1996 Sep;15(9):747-5.
9915 Botma M, Colquhoun-Flannery W, Leighton S. Laryngeal oedema caused by accidental ingestion of Oil of Wintergreen. *Int J Pediatr Otorhinolaryngol.* 2001 May 11;58(3):229-32.
9916 Chyka PA. et al. Salicylate poisoning: an evidence-based consensus guideline for out-of-hospital management. *Clin Toxicol (Phila).* 2007;45(2):95-13.
9917 Johnson PN. Methyl salicylate/aspirin (salicylate) equivalence: who do you trust? *Vet Hum Toxicol.* 1984 Aug; 26(4):317-318.

[9918] Howrie DL, Moriarty R, Breit R. Candy flavoring as a source of salicylate poisoning. *Pediatrics.* 1985 May 1;75(5):869-71.
[9919] Tisserand R, Young R. *Essential Oil Safety* (Second Edition). 2014 Churchill Livingstone Elsevier.
[9920] Burkhard PR, Burkhardt K, Haenggeli CA, et al. Plant-induced seizures: reappearance of an old problem. *J Neurol.* 1999 Aug;246(8):667-70.
[9921] Tanen DA, Danish DC, Reardon JM, et al. Comparison of oral aspirin versus topical applied methyl salicylate for platelet inhibition. *Ann Pharmacother.* 2008 Oct;42(10):1396-401.
[9922] Le Bourhis B, Soenen AM. Recherches sur l'action psychotrope de quelques substances aromatiques utilisees en alimentation. *Food Cosmet Toxicol.* 1973;11:1-9.
[9923] Joss JD, LeBlond RF. Potentiation of warfarin anticoagulation associated with topical methyl salicylate. *Ann Pharmacother.* 2000 Jun;34(6):729-33.
[9924] Chan TY. Potential dangers from topical preparations containing methyl salicylate. *Hum Exp Toxicol.* 1996;15:747- 50.
[9925] Orra P, Bartle WR, Walker SE, et al. Serum concentrations of salicylic acid following topically applied salicylate derivatives. *Ann Pharmacother.* 1996 Sep;30(9):935-40.
[9926] Botma M, Colquhoun-Flannery W, Leighton S. Laryngeeal oedema caused by accidental ingestion of oil of wintergreen. *Int J Ped Otorhinolaryngology.* 2001 May;58(3):229-32.
[9927] Parker D, Martinez C, Stanley C, et al. The analysis of methyl salicylate and salicylic acid from Chinese herbal medicine ingestion. *J Analytical Tox.* 2004 Apr;28:214-16.
[9928] Zhang B, He XL, Ding Y, et al. Gaultherin, a natural salicylate derivative from Gaultheria yunnanensis. Towards a better non-steroidal anti-inflammatory drug. *Eur J Pharmacol.* 2006;530:166-171.
[9929] Zhang B, Li JB, Zhang DM, et al. Analgesic and anti-inflammatory activities of a fraction rich in gaultherin isolated from Gaultheria yunnanensis (FRANCH.) REHDER. *Biol Pharm Bull.* 2007 Mar;30(3):465-69.
[9930] Zhang D, Liu R, Sun L, et al. Anti-inflammatory activity of methyl salicylate glycosides isolated from Gaultheria yunnanensis (Franch.) Rehder. *Molecules.* 2011;16:3875-3884.
[9931] Xin W, Huang C, Zhang X, et al. Evaluation of the new anti-inflammatory constituent ethyl salicylate 2-O-β-D- glucoside and its possible mechanism of action. *Int Immunopharmacol.* 2013 Feb;15(2):303-08.
[9932] Zhang T, Sun L, Liu R, et al. A novel naturally occurring salicylic acid analogue acts as an anti-inflammatory agent by inhibiting nucleus factor-kappaB activity in RAW264.1 macrophages. *Mol Pharm.* 2012 Mar;9(3):671-77.
[9933] Logan CJ, Stewart JT. Treatment of post-electroconvulsive therapy headache with topical methyl salicylate. *J ECT.* 2012 Jun;28(2):e17-18.
[9934] Kim J, Jang M, Shin E, et al. Fumigant and contact toxicity of 22 wooden essential oils and their major components against Drosophila suzukii (Diptera: Drosophilidae). *Pestic Biochem Physiol.* 2016 Oct;133:35-43.
[9935] Pandey BP, Thapa R, Upreti A. Chemical composition, antioxidant and antibacterial activities of essential oil and methanol extract of Artemisia vulgaris and Gaultheria fragrantissima collected from Nepal. *Asian Pac J Tropical Med.* 2017 Oct;10(10):952-9.
[9936] Damos PT. An in vitro ULV olfactory bioassay method for testing the repellent activity of essential oils against moths. *MethodsX.* 2018 Apr 20;5:375-394.
[9937] Monzote L, Herrera I, Satyal P, et al. In-Vitro Evaluation of 52 Commercially-Available Essential Oils Against Leishmania amazonensis. Molecules. 2019 Mar 20;24(7):24071248.
[9938] Verdi CM, Machado VS, Machado AK, et al. Phytochemical characterization, genotoxicity, cytotoxicity, and antimicrobial activity of Gautheria procumbens essential oil. *Nat Prod Res.* 2020 Dec 28;1-5.
[9939] Jardim CM, Jham GN, Dhingra OD, et al. Composition and antifungal activity of the essential oil of the Brazilian Chenopodium ambrosioides L. *J Chem Ecology.* 2008;34:1213-18.
[9940] Cavalli JF, Tomi F, Bernardini AF, et al. Combined analysis of the essential oil of Chenopodium ambrosioides by GC, GC-MS and 13C-NMR spectroscopy: quantitative determination of ascaridole, a heat-sensitive constituent. *Phytochemical Analysis.* 2004;15:275-79.
[9941] Monzote L, Nance MR, Garcia M, et al. Comparative chemical, cytotoxicity and antileishmanial properties of essential oils from Chenopodium ambrosioides. *Nat Prod Commun.* 2011;6:281-86.
[9942] Owolabi MS, Lajide L, Oladimeji MO, et al. Volatile constituents and antibacterial screening of the essential oil of Chenopodium ambrosioides L. growing in Nigeria. *Nat Prod Commun.* 2009;4:989-92.
[9943] Gupta D, Charles R, Mehta VK, et al. Chemical examination of the essential oil of Chenopodium ambrosioides L. from the Southern Hills of India. *J Essent Oil Res.* 2002;14:93-94.
[9944] Chu SS, Hu JF, Liu ZL. Composition of essential oil of Chinese Chenopodium ambrosioides and insecticidal activity against maize weevil, Sitophilus zeamais. *Pest Management Sci.* 2011;67:714-18.
[9945] Lohani H, Chauhan NK, Haider KKSZ, et al. Comparative aroma profile of wild and cultivated Chenopodium ambrosioides L. from Uttarakhand. *J Essent Oil Bearing Plants.* 2012;15:657-661.
[9946] Al-kaf AG, Crouch RA, Denkert A, et al. Chemical composition and biological activity of essential oil of Chenopodium ambrosioides from Yemen. *Am J Essential Oils Nat Prod.* 2016;4(1):20-22.
[9947] Sa RD, Moraes Galvao MA, Assuncao Ferreira MR, et al. Chemical composition of the essential oil from leaves of Chenopodium ambrosioides L. grown in Recife-PE, Brazil. *Rev. Bras. Farm.* 2014;95(3):855–66.
[9948] Avila-Blanco ME, Rodriguez MG, Moreno Duque JL, et al. Amoebicidal Activity of Essential Oil of Dysphania ambrosioides (L.) Mosyakin & Clemants in an Amoebic Liver Abscess Hamster Model. *Evid Based Complement Alternat Med.* 2014;2014:930208.
[9949] Navaei MN, Mizra M. Chemical composition of the oil of Chenopodium ambrosioides L. from Iran. *Iranian J Pharm Res.* 2004 Autumn;3(S2):88.
[9950] de Andrade Santiago J, das Gracas Cardoso M, da Silva Figueiredo AC, et al. Chemical Characterization and Application of the Essential Oils from Chenopodium ambrosioides and Philodendron bipinnatifidum in the Control of Diabrotica speciosa (Coleoptera: Chrysomelidae). *Am J Plant Sci.* 2014;5:3994-4002.
[9951] Qi Bai C, Liu ZL, Liu QZ. Nematicidal Constituents from the Essential Oil of Chenopodium Ambrosioides Aerial Parts. *E-J Chem.* 2011;8(S1):S143-48.
[9952] MacDonald D, VanCrey K, Harrison P, et al. Ascaridole-less infusions of Chenopodium ambrosioides contain a nematocide(s) that is(are) not toxic to mammalian smooth muscle. *J Ethnopharmacol.* 2004 Jun;92(2-3):215-21.
[9953] Gadano AB, Gurni AA, Carballo MA. Argentine folk medicine: genotoxic effects of Chenopodiaceae family. *J Ethnopharmacol.* 2006 Jan 16;103(2):246-51.
[9954] European Medicines Agency. Assessment report on Peumus boldus Molina, folium. Available at: http://www.ema.europa.eu/docs/en_GB/document_library/Herbal_-_HMPC_assessment_report/2009/12/WC500018102.pdf.
[9955] Raintree Tropical Plant Database. Databse for Epazote (Chenopodium ambrosioides). Available at: http://www.rain-tree.com/epazote.htm#.V9BqjZgrKUk.
[9956] Potawale SE, Luniya KP, Mantri RA, et al. Chenopodium ambrosioides: An ethnopharmacological review. *Pharmacologyonline.* 2008;2:272-86.
[9957] Osol A, ed. The Dispensatory of the United States of America. 25th ed. Philadelphia, PA: Lippincott, 1955.
[9958] Piscaglia F, Leoni S, Venturi A, et al. Caution in the use of boldo in herbal laxatives: a case of hepatotoxicity. *Scand J Gastroenterol.* 2005;40:236-39.
[9959] Monzon S, Lezaun A, Saenz D, et al. Anaphylaxis to boldo infusion, a herbal remedy. *Allergy.* 2004;59:1019-20.
[9960] Msaada K, Salem N, Bachrouch O, et al. Chemical Composition and Antioxidant and Antimicrobial Activities of Wormwood (Artemisia absinthium L.) Essential Oils and Phenolics. *J Chem.* 2015;(2015):804658.
[9961] Sharopov FS, Sulaimonova VA, Setzer WN. Composition of the Essential oil of Artemisia absinthium from Tajikistan. *Rec Nat Prod.* 2012;6(2):127-34.
[9962] Orav A, Raal A, Arak E, et al. Composition of the essential oil of Artemisia absinthium L. of different geographical origin. *Proc Estonian Acad Sci Chem.* 2006;55(3):155-65.
[9963] Juteau F, Jerkovic I, Masotti V, et al. Composition and antimicrobial activity of the essential oil of Artemisia absinthium from Croatia and France. *Planta Med.* 2003;69:158-61.
[9964] Altunkaya A, Yildirim B, Ekici K, et al. Determining essential oil composition, antibacterial and antioxidant activity of water wormwood extracts. *GIDA.* 2014;39(1):17-24.
[9965] Judzentiene A, Tomi F, Casanova J. Analysis of essential oils of Artemisia absinthium L. from Lithuania by CC, GC(RI), GC-MS and 13C NMR. *Nat Prod Commun.* 2009 Aug;4(8):1113-8.
[9966] Mihajilov-Krstev T, Jovanović B, Jović J, et al. Antimicrobial, antioxidative, and insect repellent effects of Artemisia absinthium essential oil. *Planta Med.* 2014 Dec;80(18):1698-705.
[9967] Erel SB, Reznicek G, Senol SG, et al. Antimicrobial and antioxidant properties of Artemisia L. species from western Anatolia. *Turk J Biol.* 2012;36:75-84
[9968] Joshi RK. Volatile composition and antimicrobial activity of the essential oil of Artemisia absinthium growing in Western Ghats region of North West Karnataka, India. *Pharm Biol.* 2013 Jul;51(7):888-92.
[9969] Govindarajan M, Benelli G. Artemisia absinthium-borne compounds as novel larvicides: effectiveness against six mosquito vectors and acute toxicity on non-target aquatic organisms. *Parasitol Res.* 2016 Dec;115(12):4649-4661.
[9970] Haliciglu O, Astarcioglu G, Yaprak I, et al. Toxicity of Salvia officinalis in a newborn and a child: an alarming report. *Pediatr Neurol.* 2011 Oct;45(4):259-60.
[9971] Lachenmeier DW, Walch SG. Epileptic seizure caused by accidental ingestion of sage (Salvia officinalis L.) oil in children: a rare, exceptional case or a threat to public health. *Pediatr Neurol.* 2012 Mar;46(3):201.
[9972] Stafstrom CE. Seizures in a 7-month-old child after exposure to the essential plant oil thuja. *Pediatr Neurol.* 2007 Dec;37(6):446-8.
[9973] Casares R. Juniperus sabina. *Food Cosmet Toxicol.* 1964;2:680-81. Found in U.S. Food and Drug Administration. FDA Poisonous Plant Database. Available at: http://www.accessdata.fda.gov/scripts/plantox/detail.cfm?id=5133
[9974] Radulović NS, Mladenović MZ, Randjelovic PJ, et al. Toxic essential oils. Part IV: The essential oil of Achillea falcata L. as a source of biologically/pharmacologically active trans-sabinyl esters. *Food Chem Toxicol.* 2015 Jun;80:114-29.
[9975] Judzentiene A, Budiene J, Gircyte R, et al. Toxic activity and chemical composition of Lithuanian wormwood (Artemisia absinthium L.) essential oils. *Rec Nat Prod.* 2012;6(2):180-83.
[9976] da Silva Costa KC, Bexerra SB, Norte CM, et al. Medicinal plants with teratogenic potential: current considerations. *Braz J Pharm Sci.* 2012;48(3):427-33.
[9977] Brinker F. Herb Contraindications and Drug Interactions. 2nd ed. Sandy, OR. Eclectic Medical Publications. 1998.
[9978] Pages N, Fournier G, Chamorro G, et al. Teratological evaluation of Juniperus sabina essential oil in mice. *Planta Med.* 1989 Apr;55(2):144-46.
[9979] Pages N, Fournier G, Baudel C, et al. Sabinyl Acetate, the Main Component of Juniperus sabina L'Hérit. Essential Oil, is Responsible for Antiimplantation Effect. *Phytother Res.* 1996 Aug;10(5):438-440.
[9980] Pages N, Fournier G, Velut V, et al. Potential teratogenicity in mice of the essential oil of Salvia lavandulifolia Vahl. Study of a fraction rich in sabinyl acetate. *Phytother Res.* 1992 Mar;6(2):80-83.
[9981] Delgado IF, Carvalho RR, Nogueira, et al. Study on embryofetotoxicity of b-myrcene in the rat. *Food and Chemical Toxicology.* 1993;31(1):31-5.
[9982] Paumgartten FJ, De-Carvalho RR, Souza CA, et al. Study of the effects of beta-myrcene on rat fertility and general reproductive performance. *Braz J Med Biol Res.* 1998 Jul;31(7):955-65.
[9983] Frohne D. Giftpflanzen: Cupressaceae. Stuttgart: Wissenschaftliche Verlagsgesellschaft mbH; 1997. pp. 153–6.

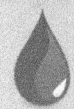

[9984] European Medicines Agency. Public statement on the use of herbal medicinal products containing thujone. Available at: http://www.ema.europa.eu/docs/en_GB/document_library/Public_statement/2011/02/WC500102294.pdf.
[9985] Millet Y, Jouglard J, Steinmetz MD, et al. Toxicity of some essential plant oils. Clinical and experimental study. *Clin Toxicol.* 1981 Dec;18(12):1485-98.
[9986] Cristovao L, Carvalho F, Bastos MDL, et al. Hepatotoxicity of an essential oil of Salvia officinalis L.: an in vitro study using freshly isolated rat hepatocytes. *Congress Biomarkers.* 2001 Sep:165.
[9987] Weisbord SD, Soule JB, Kimmel PL. Poison on line-acute renal failure caused by oil of wormwood purchased through the internet. *N Engl J Med.* 1997;337:825-7.
[9988] Millet Y, Jouglard J, Steinmetz MD, et al. Toxicity of some essential plant oils. Clinical and experimental study. *Clin Toxicol.* 1981 Dec;18(12):1485–98.
[9989] Burkhard PR, Burkhardt K, Haenggeli CA, et al. Plant-induced seizures: reappearance of an old problem. *J Neurol.* 1999 Aug;246(8):667–70.
[9990] Weisbord SD, Soule JB, Kimmel PL. Poison on line-acute renal failure caused by oil of wormwood purchased through the internet. *N Engl J Med.* 1997;337:825-7.
[9991] Arditti J, Faizende JJ, Bernard J, et al. Trois observations d'intoxication par des essences végétales convulsivantes. *Ann Med.* 1978;17:371-74.
[9992] Casares R. Juniperus sabina. *Food Cosmet Toxicol.* 1964;2:680-81. Found in U.S. Food and Drug Administration. FDA Poisonous Plant Database. Available at: http://www.accessdata.fda.gov/scripts/plantox/detail.cfm?id=5133
[9993] Abass K, Reponen P, Mattila S, et al. Metabolism of α-thujone in human hepatic preparations in vitro. *Xenobiotica.* 2011 Feb;41(2):101-11.
[9994] De-Oliveira AC1, Ribeiro-Pinto LF, Otto SS, et al. Induction of liver monooxygenases by beta-myrcene. *Toxicology.* 1997 Dec 26;124(2):135-40.
[9995] Burkhard PR, Burkhardt K, Haenggeli CA, et al. Plant-induced seizures: reappearance of an old problem. *J Neurol.* 1999 Aug;246(8):667-70.
[9996] Narayan S, Singh N. Camphor poisoning-An unusual cause of seizure. *Med J Armed Forces India.* 2012 Jul;68(3):252-53.
[9997] Chanaranaj KJ, G MV, S M. Camphor poisoning in a child. *Natl Med J India.* 2013 Jan-Feb;26(1):60.
[9998] Perry NB, Anderson RE, Brennan NJ, et al. Essential oils from dalmatian sage (Salvia officinalis L.) variations among individuals, plant parts, seasons, and sites. *J Agric Food Chem.* 1999;47:2048-54.
[9999] Millet Y, Jouglard J, Steinmetz MD, et al. Toxicity of some essential plant oils. Clinical and experimental study. *Clin Toxicol.* 1981 Dec;18(12):1485-98.
[10000] Uc A, Bishop WP, Sanders KD. Camphor hepatotoxicity. *South Med J.* 2000;93:596-98.
[10001] Frohne D. Giftpflanzen: Cupressaceae. Stuttgart: Wissenschaftliche Verlagsgesellschaft mbH; 1997. pp. 153–6.
[10002] Dolan LC, Matulka RA, Burdock GA. Naturally Occurring Food Toxins. *Toxins (Basel).* 2010 Sep;2(9):2289–2332.
[10003] Patoir A, Patoir G, Bedrine H. Note sur l'action de l'essence de rue sur l'organisme animal. *Computes Rendues Société Bologique.* 1938;127:1324-25.
[10004] United States National Toxicology Program (NTP). Alpha-Thujone. Dec 10, 1997. Available at: http://ntp.niehs.nih.gov/index.cfm?objectid=03DB8C36-E7A1-9889-3BDF8436F2A8C51F.
[10005] United States National Toxicology Program (NTP). Alpha-Thujone. Dec 10, 1997. Available at: http://ntp.niehs.nih.gov/index.cfm?objectid=03DB8C36-E7A1-9889-3BDF8436F2A8C51F.
[10006] Pages N, Fournier G, Chamorro G, et al. Teratological evaluation of Juniperus sabina essential oil in mice. *Planta Med.* 1989 Apr;55(2):144-46.
[10007] Radulović NS, Mladenović MZ, Randjelovic PJ, et al. Toxic essential oils. Part IV: The essential oil of Achillea falcata L. as a source of biologically/pharmacologically active trans-sabinyl esters. *Food Chem Toxicol.* 2015 Jun;80:114-29.
[10008] Judzentiene A, Budiene J, Gircyte R, et al. Toxic activity and chemical composition of Lithuanian wormwood (Artemisia absinthium L.) essential oils. *Rec Nat Prod.* 2012;6(2):180-83.
[10009] Freitas JC1, Presgrave OA, Fingola FF, et al. Effect of beta-myrcene on pentobarbital sleeping time. *Braz J Med Biol Res.* 1993 May;26(5):519-23.
[10010] Martínez-Díaz RA, Ibáñez-Escribano A, Burillo J, et al. Trypanocidal, trichomonacidal and cytotoxic components of cultivated Artemisia absinthium Linnaeus (Asteraceae) essential oil. *Mem Inst Oswaldo Cruz.* 2015 Aug;110(5):693-9.
[10011] Stanković N, Mihajilov-Krstev T, Zlatković B, et al. Comparative Study of Composition, Antioxidant, and Antimicrobial Activities of Essential Oils of Selected Aromatic Plants from Balkan Peninsula. *Planta Med.* 2016 May;82(7):650-61.
[10012] Martínez-Díaz RA, Ibáñez-Escribano A, Burillo J, et al. Trypanocidal, trichomonacidal and cytotoxic components of cultivated Artemisia absinthium Linnaeus (Asteraceae) essential oil. *Mem Inst Oswaldo Cruz.* 2015 Aug;110(5):693-9.
[10013] Monzote L, Piñón A, Sculli R, et al. Chemistry and leishmanicidal activity of the essential oil from Artemisia absinthium from Cuba. *Nat Prod Commun.* 2014 Dec;9(12):1799-804.
[10014] Tariku Y, Hymete A, Hailu A, et al. In vitro evaluation of antileishmanial activity and toxicity of essential oils of Artemisia absinthium and Echinops kebericho. *Chem Biodivers.* 2011 Apr;8(4):614-23.
[10015] Mihajilov-Krstev T, Jovanović B, Jović J, et al. Antimicrobial, antioxidative, and insect repellent effects of Artemisia absinthium essential oil. *Planta Med.* 2014 Dec;80(18):1698-705.
[10016] Erel SB, Reznicek G, Senol SG, et al. Antimicrobial and antioxidant properties of Artemisia L. species from western Anatolia. *Turk J Biol.* 2012;36:75-84.
[10017] Mohammadi A, Sani TA1, Ameri AA, et al. Seasonal variation in the chemical composition, antioxidant activity, and total phenolic content of Artemisia absinthium essential oils. *Pharmacognosy Res.* 2014 Oct-Dec;7(4):329-34.
[10018] Joshi RK. Volatile composition and antimicrobial activity of the essential oil of Artemisia absinthium growing in Western Ghats region of North West Karnataka, India. *Pharm Biol.* 2013 Jul;51(7):888-92.
[10019] Blagojević P, Radulović N, Palić R, et al. Chemical composition of the essential oils of Serbian wild-growing Artemisia absinthium and Artemisia vulgaris. *J Agric Food Chem.* 2006 Jun 28;54(13):4780-9.
[10020] Jaenson TG, Pålsson K, Borg-Karlson AK. Evaluation of extracts and oils of tick-repellent plants from Sweden. *Med Vet Entomol.* 2005 Dec;19(4):345-52.
[10021] Kordali S, Kotan R, Mavi A, et al. Determination of the chemical composition and antioxidant activity of the essential oil of Artemisia dracunculus and of the antifungal and antibacterial activities of Turkish Artemisia absinthium, A. dracunculus, Artemisia santonicum, and Artemisia spicigera essential oils. *J Agric Food Chem.* 2005 Nov 30;53(24):9452-8.
[10022] Kordali S, Cakir A, Mavi A, et al. Screening of chemical composition and antifungal and antioxidant activities of the essential oils from three Turkish artemisia species. *J Agric Food Chem.* 2005 Mar 9;53(5):1408-16.
[10023] Juteau F, Jerkovic I, Masotti V, et al. Composition and antimicrobial activity of the essential oil of Artemisia absinthium from Croatia and France. *Planta Med.* 2003;69:158-61.
[10024] Chiasson H, Bélanger A, Bostanian N, et al. Acaricidal properties of Artemisia absinthium and Tanacetum vulgare (Asteraceae) essential oils obtained by three methods of extraction. *J Econ Entomol.* 2001 Feb;94(1):167-71.
[10025] Govindarajan M, Benelli G. Artemisia absinthium-borne compounds as novel larvicides: effectiveness against six mosquito vectors and acute toxicity on non-target aquatic organisms. *Parasitol Res.* 2016 Dec;115(12):4649-4661.
[10026] Tamargo B, Monzote L, Piñón A, et al. In Vitro and In Vivo Evaluation of Essential Oil from Artemisia absinthium L. Formulated in Nanocochleates against Cutaneous Leishmaniasis. *Medicines (Basel).* 2017 Jun 9;4(2).
[10027] Raita MS, Iconaru SL, Groza A, et al. Multifunctional Hydroxyapatite Coated With Arthemisia absinthium Composites. *Molecules.* 2019 Jan 19;25(2):25020413.
[10028] Mathlouthi A, Saadaoui N, Pennacchietti E, et al. Essential oils from Artemisia species inhibit biofilm formation and the virulence of Escherichia coli EPEC 2348/69. *Biofouling.* 2021 Feb 15;1-11.
[10029] Mohammed HA. Phytochemical Analysis, Antioxidant Potential, and Cytotoxicity Evaluation of Traditionally Used Artemisia absinthium L. (Wormwood) Growing in the Central Region of Saudi Arabia. *Plants (Basel).* 2022 Apr 9;11(8):1028.
[10030] Khan FA, Khan NM, Ahmad S, et al. Phytochemical Profiling, Antioxidant, Antimicrobial and Cholinesterase Inhibitory Effects of Essential Oils Isolated from the Leaves of Artemisia scoparia and Artemisia absinthium. *Pharmaceuticals (Basel).* 2022 Oct 1;15(10):1221.
[10031] Tiwary M, Naik SN, Tewary DK, et al. Chemical composition and larvicidal activities of the essential oil of Zanthoxylum armatum DC (Rutaceae) against three mosquito vectors. *J Vector Borne Dis.* 2007 Sep;44(3):198-204.
[10032] Jain N, Srivastava S, Aggarwal K, et al. Essential oil composition of Zanthoxylum alatum seeds from northern India. *Flavour Frag J.* 2001;16(6)408-10.
[10033] Cardoso NN, Alviano CS, Blank AF, et al. Synergism Effect of the Essential Oil from Ocimum basilicum var. Maria Bonita and Its Major Components with Fluconazole and Its Influence on Ergosterol Biosynthesis. *Evid Based Complement Alternat Med.* 2016;2016:5647182.
[10034] Tiwary M, Naik SN, Tewary DK, et al. Chemical composition and larvicidal activities of the essential oil of Zanthoxylum armatum DC (Rutaceae) against three mosquito vectors. *J Vector Borne Dis.* 2007 Sep;44(3):198-204.
[10035] Wang CF1, Zhang WJ, You CX, et al. Insecticidal Constituents of Essential Oil Derived from Zanthoxylum armatum against Two Stored-Product Insects. *J Oleo Sci.* 2015;64(8):861-8.
[10036] Nadim MM, Malik AA, Ahmad J, et al. The Essential Oil Composition of Achillea millefolium L. Cultivated under Tropical Condition in India. *World J Agric Sci.* 2011;7(5):561-65.
[10037] Smelcerovic A, Lamshoeft M, Radulovic N, et al. LC-MS analysis of the essential oils of Achillea millefolium and Achillea crithmifolia. *Chromatographia.* 2010 Jun;71(1):113-16.
[10038] Suleimenov Y, Atazhanova GA, Ozek T, et al. Essential oil composition of three species of Achillea from Kazakhstan. *Chem Nat Constituents.* 2001 Sep;37(5):447-50.
[10039] Shawl AS, Srivastava SK, Syamasundar KV, et al. Essential oil composition of Achillea millefolium L. growing wild in Kashmir, India. *Flavour Frag J.* 2002;17:165-168.
[10040] Orav A, Arak E, Raal A. Phytochemical analysis of the essential oil of Achillea millefolium L. from various European Countries. *Nat Prod Res.* 2006 Nov;20(12):1082-88.
[10041] Tampe J, Parra L, Huaiquil K, et al. Repellent Effect and Metabolite Volatile Profile of the Essential Oilof Achillea millefolium Against Aegorhinus nodipennis (Hope)(Coleoptera: Curculionidae). *Neotrop Entomol.* 2015 Jun;44(3):1-7.
[10042] Haliciglu O, Astarcioglu G, Yaprak I, et al. Toxicity of Salvia officinalis in a newborn and a child: an alarming report. *Pediatr Neurol.* 2011 Oct;45(4):259-60.
[10043] Lachenmeier DW, Walch SG. Epileptic seizure caused by accidental ingestion of sage (Salvia officinalis L.) oil in children: a rare, exceptional case or a threat to public health. *Pediatr Neurol.* 2012 Mar;46(3):201.
[10044] Stafstrom CE. Seizures in a 7-month-old child after exposure to the essential plant oil thuja. *Pediatr Neurol.* 2007 Dec;37(6):446-8.
[10045] Casares R. Juniperus sabina. *Food Cosmet Toxicol.* 1964;2:680-81. Found in U.S. Food and Drug Administration. FDA Poisonous Plant Database. Available at: http://www.accessdata.fda.gov/scripts/plantox/detail.cfm?id=5133.
[10046] Radulović NS, Mladenović MZ, Randjelovic PJ, et al. Toxic essential oils. Part IV: The essential oil of Achillea falcata L. as a source of biologically/pharmacologically active trans-sabinyl esters. *Food Chem Toxicol.* 2015 Jun;80:114-29.
[10047] Judzentiene A, Budiene J, Gircyte R, et al. Toxic activity and chemical composition of Lithuanian wormwood (Artemisia absinthium L.) essential oils. *Rec Nat Prod.* 2012;6(2):180-83.
[10048] Khine H, Weiss D, Graber N, et al. A cluster of children with seizures caused by camphor poisoning. *Pediatrics.* 2009 May;123(5):1269-72.
[10049] Michiels EA, Mazor SS. Toddler with seizures due to ingesting camphor at an Indian celebration. *Pediatr Emerg Care.* 2010 Aug;26(8):574-75.

10050 Koren G. Medications which can kill a toddler with one tablet or teaspoonful. *J toxicol Clin toxicol.* 1993;31(3):407- 13.
10051 Millet Y, Jouglard J, Steinmetz MD, et al. Toxicity of some essential plant oils. Clinical and experimental study. *Clin Toxicol.* 1981 Dec;18(12):1485–98.
10052 Halicioglu O, Astarlioglu G, Yaprak I, et al. Toxicity of Salvia officinalis in a newborn and a child: an alarming report. *Pediatr Neurol.* 2011 Oct;45(4):259–60.
10053 Lachenmeier DW, Walch SG. Epileptic seizure caused by accidental ingestion of sage (Salvia officinalis L.) oil in children: a rare, exceptional case or a threat to public health. *Pediatr Neurol.* 2012 Mar;46(3):201.
10054 Khine H, Weiss D, Graber N, et al. A cluster of children with seizures caused by camphor poisoning. *Pediatrics.* 2009 May;123(5):1269–72.
10055 Michiels EA, Mazor SS. Toddler with seizures due to ingesting camphor at an Indian celebration. *Pediatr Emerg Care.* 2010 Aug;26(8):574–75.
10056 Craig JO. Poisoning by the volatile oils in childhobd. *Arch Dis Child.* 1953;28:259–67.
10057 Melis K. Bochner A, Janssens G. Accidental nasal eucalyptol and menthol instillation. *Eur J Pediatr.* 1989 Aug;148(8)786–7.
10058 Day LM, Ozanne-Smith J, Parsons BJ, et al. Eucalyptus oil poisoning among young children: mechanisms of access and the potential prevention. *Aust N Z J Public Health.* 1997 Jun;21(3):297–302.
10059 Burkhard PR, Burkhardt K, Haenggeli CA, et al. Plant-induced seizures: reappearance of an old problem. *J Neurol.* 1999 Aug;246(8):667–70.
10060 Waidyanatha S, Johnson JD, Hong SP, et al. Toxicokinetics of α-thujone following intravenous and gavage administration of α-thujone or α- and β-thujone mixture in male and female F344/N rats and B6C3F1 mice. *Toxicol Appl Pharmacol.* 2013 Sep;271(2):216–28.
10061 Albert-Puleo M. Van Gogh's vision: thujone intoxication. *JAMA.* 1981;246:42.
10062 Flaman Z, Pellechia-Clarke S, Bailey B, et al. Unintentional exposure of young children to camphor and eucalyptus oils. *Paediatr Child Health.* 2001 Feb;6(2):80-83.
10063 Blumenthal M, ed. The Complete German Commission E Monographs: Therapeutic Guide to Herbal Medicines. Trans. S. Klein. Boston, MA: American Botanical Council, 1998.
10064 da Silva Costa KC, Bezerra SB, Norte CM, et al. Medicinal plants with teratogenic potential: current considerations. *Braz J Pharm Sci.* 2012;48(3):427–33.
10065 Brinker F. Herb Contraindications and Drug Interactions. 2nd ed. Sandy, OR. Eclectic Medical Publications. 1998.
10066 Rabl W, Katzgraber F, Steinlechner M. Camphor ingestion for abortion (case report). *Forensic Sci Int.* 1997 Sep 19;89(1-2):137-40.
10067 Pages N, Fourier G, Baduel C, et al. Sabinyl acetate, the main component of Juniperus sabina L'Herit. essential oil, is responsible for antiimplantation effect. *Phytother Res.* 1996 Aug;10(5):438-40.
10068 Pages N, Fourier G, Velut V, et al. Potential teratogenicity in mice of the essential oil of Salvia lavandulifolia Vahl. study of a fraction rich in sabinyl acetate. *Phytother Res.* 2006;6(2):80-83.
10069 European Medicines Agency. Public statement on the use of herbal medicinal products containing thujone. Available at: http://www.ema.europa.eu/docs/en_GB/document_library/Public_statement/2011/02/WC500102294.pdf.
10070 Cristovao L, Carvalho F, Bastos MDL, et al. Hepatotoxicity of an essential oil of Salvia officinalis L.: an in vitro study using freshly isolated rat hepatocytes. *Congress Biomarkers.* 2001 Sep:165.
10071 Millet Y, Jouglard J, Steinmetz MD, et al. Toxicity of some essential plant oils. Clinical and experimental study. *Clin Toxicol.* 1981 Dec;18(12):1485–98.
10072 Casares R. Juniperus sabina. *Food Cosmet Toxicol.* 1964;2:680-81. Found in U.S. Food and Drug Administration. FDA Poisonous Plant Database. Available at: http://www.accessdata.fda.gov/scripts/plantox/detail.cfm?id=5133
10073 Manoguerra AS, Erdman AR, Wax PM, et al. Camphor poisoning: an evidence-based practice guideline for out-of- hospital management. *Clin Toxicol (Phila).*2006;44(4):357-70.
10074 Gibson DE, Moore GP, Pfaff JA. Camphor ingestion. *Am J Emerg Med.* 1989 Jan;7(1):41-43.
10075 Koppel C, Martends F, Schirop T, et al. Hemoperfusion in acute camphor poisoning. *Intensive Care Med.* 1988;14(4):431-33.
10076 Millet Y, Jouglard J, Steinmetz MD, et al. Toxicity of some essential plant oils. Clinical and experimental study. *Clin Toxicol.* 1981 Dec;18(12):1485–98.
10077 Burkhard PR, Burkhardt K, Haenggeli CA, et al. Plant-induced seizures: reappearance of an old problem. *J Neurol.* 1999 Aug;246(8):667–70.
10078 Weisbord SD, Soule JB, Kimmel PL. Poison on line-acute renal failure caused by oil of wormwood purchased through the internet. *N Engl J Med.* 1997;337:825-7.
10079 Arditti J, Faizende JJ, Bernard J, et al. Trois observations d'intoxication par des essences végétales convulsivantes. *Ann Med.* 1978;17:371-74.
10080 Burkhard PR, Burkhardt K, Haenggeli CA, et al. Plant-induced seizures: reappearance of an old problem. *J Neurol.* 1999 Aug;246(8):667-70.
10081 Millet Y, Jouglard J, Steinmetz MD, et al. Toxicity of some essential plant oils. Clinical and experimental study. *Clin Toxicol.* 1981 Dec;18(12):1485–98.
10082 Charanraj KJ, G MV, S M. Camphor poisoning in a child. *Natl Med J India.* 2013 Jan-Feb;26(1):60.
10083 Narayan S, Singh N. Camphor poisoning-An unusual cause of seizure. *Med J Armed Forces India.* 2012 Jul;68(3):252–53.
10084 Perry NB, Anderson RE, Brennan NJ, et al. Essential oils from Dalmatian sage (Salvia officinalis L.) variations among individuals, plant parts, seasons, and sites. *J Agric Food Chem.* 1999;47:2048–54.
10085 Olowe SA, Ransome-Kuti O. The risk of jaundice in glucose-6-phosphate dehydrogenase deficient babies exposed to menthol. *Acta Paediatr Scand.* 1980 May;69(3):341-5.
10086 Dillon Remy M, Manning Alleyne P, Bratt DE, et al. Neonatal jaundice at Port-of-Spain General Hospital abstract. *West Indian Med J.* 1987;36(Suppl):28.
10087 Jori A, Bianchetti A, Prestini PE, et al. Effect of eucalyptol (1,8-cineole) on the metabolism of other drugs in rats and in man. *Eur J Pharmacol.* 1970;9(3):362-66.
10088 de Sousa DP, Raphael E, Brocksom U, et al. Sedative effect of monoterpene alcohols in mice: A preliminary screening. *Verlag der Zeitschrift fur Naturforschung.* 2007;62c:563-66.
10089 Ganzera M, Schneider P, Stuppner H. Inhibitory effects of the essential oil of chamomile (Matricaria recutita L.) and its major constituents on human cytochrome P450 enzymes. *Life Sci.* 2006 Jan 18;78(8):856-61.
10090 Kim NH, Hyun SH, Jin CH, et al. Pretreatment with 1,8-cineole potentiates thioacetamide-induced hepatotoxicity and immunosuppression. *Arch Pharm Res.* 2004 Jul;27(7):781-9.
10091 Heck AM, DeWitt BA, Lukes AL. Potential interactions between alternative therapies and warfarin. *Am J Health Syst Pharm.* 2000;57(13):1221-1227.
10092 Tsai HH, Lin HW, Chen YL, et al. A review of potential harmful interactions between anticoagulant/antiplatelet agents and Chinese herbal medicines. *PLoS One.* 2013 May 9;8(5):e64255.
10093 Segal R, Pilote L. Warfarin interaction with Matricaria chamomilla. *CMAJ.* 2006;174:1281-82.
10094 Uc A, Bishop WP, Sanders KD. Camphor hepatotoxicity. *South Med J.* 2000;93:596-98.
10095 Frohne D. Giftpflanzen: Cupressaceae. Stuttgart: Wissenschaftliche Verlagsgesellschaft mbH; 1997. pp. 153–6.
10096 Dolan LC, Matulka RA, Burdock GA. Naturally Occurring Food Toxins. *Toxins (Basel).* 2010 Sep;2(9):2289–2332.
10097 United States National Toxicology Program (NTP). Alpha-Thujone. Dec 10, 1997. Available at: http://ntp.niehs.nih.gov/index.cfm?objectid=03DB8C36-E7A1-9889-3BDF8436F2A8C51F.
10098 Peng HY, Lin CC, Wang HY, et al. The melanogenesis alteration effects of Achillea millefolium L. essential oil and linalyl acetate: involvement of oxidative stress and the JNK and ERK signaling pathways in melanoma cells. *PLoS One.* 2014 Apr 17;9(4):e95186.
10099 Riley PA. Melanogenesis and melanoma. *Pigment Cell Res.* 2003 Oct;16(5):548-52.
10100 Song JE, Kim JM, Lee NH, et al. Acaricidal and Insecticidal Activities of Essential Oils against a Stored-Food Mite and Stored-Grain Insects. *J Food Prot.* 2016 Jan;79(1):174-8.
10101 Tampe J, Parra L, Huaiquil K, et al. Repellent Effect and Metabolite Volatile Profile of the Essential Oil of Achillea millefolium Against Aegorhinus nodipennis (Hope) (Coleoptera: Curculionidae). *Neotrop Entomol.* 2015 Jun;44(3):279-85.
10102 Benelli G, Bedini S, Flamini G, et al. Mediterranean essential oils as effective weapons against the West Nile vector Culex pipiens and the Echinostoma intermediate host Physella acuta: what happens around? An acute toxicity survey on non-target mayflies. *Parasitol Res.* 2015 Mar;114(3):1011-21.
10103 Conti B, Canale A, Bertoli A, et al. Essential oil composition and larvicidal activity of six Mediterranean aromatic plants against the mosquito Aedes albopictus (Diptera: Culicidae). *Parasitol Res.* 2010 Nov;107(6):1455-61.
10104 Jaenson TG, Pålsson K, Borg-Karlson AK. Evaluation of extracts and oils of mosquito (Diptera: Culicidae) repellent plants from Sweden and Guinea-Bissau. *J Med Entomol.* 2006 Jan;43(1):113-9.
10105 Chou ST, Peng HY, Hsu JC, et al. Achillea millefolium L. essential oil inhibits LPS-induced oxidative stress and nitric oxide production in RAW 264.7 Macrophages. *Int J Mol Sci.* 2013 Jun 24;14(7):12978-93.
10106 Falconieri D, Piras A, Porcedda S, et al. Chemical composition and biological activity of the volatile extracts of Achillea millefolium. *Nat Prod Commun.* 2011 Oct;6(10):1527-30.
10107 Santos AO, Santin AC, Yamaguchi MU, et al. Antileishmanial activity of an essential oil from the leaves and flowers of Achillea millefolium. *Ann Trop Med Parasitol.* 2010 Sep;104(6):475-83.
10108 de Sant'anna JR, Franco CC, Miyamoto CT, et al. Genotoxicity of Achillea millefolium essential oil in diploid cells of Aspergillus nidulans. *Phytother Res.* 2009 Feb;23(2):231-5.
10109 Santoro GF, Cardoso MG, Guimarães LG, et al. Trypanosoma cruzi: activity of essential oils from Achillea millefolium L., Syzygium aromaticum L. and Ocimum basilicum L. on epimastigotes and trypomastigotes. *Exp Parasitol.* 2007 Jul;116(3):283-90.
10110 Candan F, Unlu M, Tepe B, et al. Antioxidant and antimicrobial activity of the essential oil and methanol extracts of Achillea millefolium subsp. millefolium Afan. (Asteraceae). *J Ethnopharmacol.* 2003 Aug;87(2-3):215-20.
10111 Sharififard M, Safdari F, Siahpoush A, et al. Evaluation of Some Plant Essential Oils against the Brown-Banded Cockroach, Supella longipalpa (Blattaria: Ectobiidae): A Mechanical Vector of Human Pathogens. *J Arthropod Borne Dis.* 2016 Oct 4;10(4):528-537.
10112 El-Kalamouni C, Venskutonis PR, Zebib B, et al. Antioxidant and Antimicrobial Activities of the Essential Oil of Achillea millefolium L. Grown in France. *Medicines (Basel).* 2017 May 19;4(2).
10113 Guz L, Ziętek J, Puk K, et al. Inhibitory activities of essential oils against Babesia canis. *Pol J Vet Sci.* 2020 Mar;23(1):161-163.
10114 Mohamed ME, Elsayed SA, Madkor HR, et al. Yarrow oil ameliorates ulcerative colitis in mice model via regulating the NF-κB and PPAR-γ pathways. *Intest Res.* 2020 Aug 21. Online ahead of print.
10115 Acimovic M, Zoric M, Zheljazkov VD, et al. Chemical Characterization and Antibacterial Activity of Essential Oil of Medicinal Plants from Eastern Serbia. *Molecules.* 2020 Nov 23;25(22):5482.
10116 Guz L, Wawrzykowski J, Adaszek L. Anti-babesial potential and chemical composition of essential oil from yarrow Achillea millefolium. *Pol J Vet Sci.* 2021 Mar;24(1):79-84.
10117 Guz L, Zietek J, Puk K, et al. Inhibitory activities of essential oils against Babesia canis. *Pol J Vet Sci.* 2020 Mar;23(1):161-163.
10118 Mohamed ME, Elsayed SA, Madkor HR, et al. Yarrow oil ameliorates ulcerative colitis in mice model via regulating the NF-κB and PPAR-γ pathways. *Intest Res.* 2021 Apr;19(2):194–205.

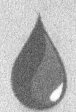

10119 Emtiazi H, Salari Sharif A, Hemati M, et al. Comparative Study of Nano-liposome and Nano-niosome for Delivery of Achillea Millefolium Essential Oils: Development, Optimization, Characterization and Their Cytotoxicity Effects on Cancer Cell Lines and Antibacterial Activity. *Chem Biodivers.* 2022 Sep 12:e202200397.

10120 Alomair MK, Alabduladheem LS, Almajed MA, et al. Achillea millefolium Essential Oil Mitigates Peptic Ulcer in Rats through Nrf2/HO-1 Pathway. *Molecules.* 2022 Nov 15;27(22):7908.

10121 Hadavi-Siahboomi M, Yegdaneh A, Talebi A, et al. Ulcer-Healing Effect of Hydroalcoholic Extract and Essential Oil of Achillea millefolium L. on Murine Model of Colitis. *Int J Prev Med.* 2022 Dec 26;13:155.

10122 Pickett LJ, Amiro M, Hawboldt C, et al. Common yarrow (Achillea millefolium) essential oil and main components as potential repellents and acaricides against Ixodes scapularis and Dermacentor variabilis (Acari: Ixodidae) ticks. *Exp Appl Acarol.* 2023 Mar 11. Online ahead of print.

10123 Brokl M, Fauconnier ML, Benini C, et al. Improvement of ylang-ylang essential oil characterization by GCXGC- TOFMS. *Molecules.* 2013;18:1783-97.

10124 Buccellato F. Ylang survey. *Perf Flav.* 1982;7:9-12.

10125 Stillpoint Aromatics. Ylang ylang complete essential oil. Available at: http://www.stillpointaromatics.com/ylang-ylang-complete-cananga-odorata-essential-oil-aromatherapy.

10126 Aromatics International. Ylang ylang (complete) - Cananga odorata Available at: http://www.aromaticsinternational.com/ylangylang106.

10127 Megawati, Saputra SWD. A combination of water-steam distillation and solvent extraction of Cananga odorata essential oil. *IOSR J Eng.* 2012 Oct;10(2):5-12.

10128 Gaydou EM, Randriamiharisoa R, Bianchini JP. Composition of the essential oil of Ylang-ylang (Cananga odorata Hook Fil. et Thomson forma genuina) from Madagascar. *J Agric Food Chem.* 1986;34(3):481-87.

10129 Kubeczka KH, Formacek V. Essential Oils Analysis by Capillary Gas Chromatography and Carbon-13 NMR Spectroscopy, 2nd, Completely Revised, Edition. 2002 May. John Wiley, Chichester.

10130 Kristiawan M, Sobolik V, Al Haddad M, et al. Effect of pressure-drop rate on the isolation of cananga oil using instantaneous controlled pressure-drop process. *Chem Engineering Processing.* 2008;47:66-75.

10131 Nguyen LT, Mysliveckova Z, Szotakova B, et al. The inhibitory effects of β-caryophyllene, β-caryophyllene oxide and α-humulene on the activities of the main drug-metabolizing enzymes in rat and human liver in vitro. *Chem-Biol Interactoins.* 2017 Dec 25;278:123-8.

10132 National Library of Medicine. TOXNET. Benzyl acetate. Available at: https://toxnet.nlm.nih.gov/cgi-bin/sis/search/a?dbs+hsdb:@term+@DOCNO+2851.

10133 JECFA. Summary of evaluations performed by the Joint FAO/WHO Expert Committee on Food Additives. 2001. Available at: https://toxnet.nlm.nih.gov/cgi-bin/sis/search/a?dbs+hsdb:@term+@DOCNO+2851.

10134 Cha JH, Lee SH, Too YS. Effects of aromatherapy on changes in the autonomic nervous system, aortic pulse wave velocity and aortic augmentation index in patients with essential hypertension. *J Korean Acad Nurs.* 2010 Oct;40(5):705-13.

10135 Hwang JH. The effects of the inhalation method using essential oils on blood pressure and stress responses of clients with essential hypertension. *Taehan Kanho Hakhoe Chi.* 2006 Dec;36(7):1123-34.

10136 Zhang N, Zhang L, Feng L, et al. The anxiolytic effect of essential oil of Cananga odorata exposure on mice and determination of its major active constituents. *Phytomedicine.* 2016 Dec 15;23(14):1727-1734.

10137 Kim IH, Kim C, Seong K, et al. Essential oil inhalation on blood pressure and salivary cortisol levels in prehypertensive and hypertensive subjects. *Evid Based Complement Alternat Med.* 2012;2012:984203.

10138 Soonwera M, Phasomkusolsil S. Efficacy of Thai herbal essential oils as green repellent against mosquito vectors. *Acta Trop.* 2015 Feb;142:127-30.

10139 Caballero-Gallardo K, Olivero-Verbel J, Stashenko EE. Repellent activity of essential oils and some of their individual constituents against Tribolium castaneum herbst. *J Agric Food Chem.* 211 Mar 9;59(5):1690-96.

10140 Bilcu M, Grumezescu AM, Oprea AE, et al. Efficiency of vanilla, patchouli and ylang ylang essential oils stabilized by iron oxide@C14 nanostructures against bacterial adherence and biofilms formed by Staphylococcus aureus and Klebsiella pneumoniae clinical strains. *Molecules.* 2014 Nov;49(11):17943-56.

10141 Gnatta JR, Piason PP, Lopes Cde L, et al. Aromatherapy with ylang ylang for anxiety and self-esteem: a pilot study. *Rev Esc Enferm USP.* 2014 Jun;48(3):492-99.

10142 Hongratanaworakit T, Buchbauer G. Relaxing effect of ylang ylang oil on humans after transdermal absorption. *Phytother Res.* 2006 Sep;20(9):758-63.

10143 Kim HJ, Yang HM, Kim DH, et al. Effects of ylang-ylang essential oil on the relaxation of rat bladder muscle in vitro and white rabbit bladder in vivo. *J Korean Med Sci.* 2003 Jun;18(3):409-14.

10144 Jantapan K, Poapolathep A, Imsilp K, et al. Inhibitory Effects of Thai Essential Oils on Potentially Aflatoxigenic Aspergillus parasiticus and Aspergillus flavus. *Biocontrol Sci.* 2017;22(1):31-40.

10145 Han X, Beaumont C, Stevens N. Chemical composition analysis and in vitro biological activities of ten essential oils in human skin cells. *Biochim Open.* 2017 Apr 26;5:1-7.

10146 Elmhalli F, Pålsson K, Örberg J, et al. Acaricidal properties of ylang-ylang oil and star anise oil against nymphs of Ixodes ricinus (Acari: Ixodidae). *Exp Appl Acarol.* 2018 Oct;76(2):209-220.

10147 Amadeo S, Nguyen NL, Teai T, et al. Supportive effect of body contact care with ylang ylang aromatherapy and mobile intervention team for suicide prevention: A pilot study. *J Int Med Res.* 2020 Sep;48(9):1:16.

10148 Upadhyay N, Singh VK, Dwivedy AK, et al. Assessment of nanoencapsulated Cananga odorata essential oil in chitosan nanopolymer as a green approach to boost the antifungal, antioxidant and in situ efficacy. *Int J Biol Macromol.* 2021 Jan 9;171:480-490.

10149 Upadhyay N, Singh VK, Dwivedy AK, et al. Assessment of nanoencapsulated Cananga odorata essential oil in chitosan nanopolymer as a green approach to boost the antifungal, antioxidant and in situ efficacy. *Int J Biol Macromol.* 2021 Feb 28;171:480-490.

10150 Lebanov L, Lam SC, Tedone L, et al. Radical scavenging activity and metabolomic profiling study of ylang-ylang essential oils based on high-performance thin-layer chromatography and multivariate statistical analysis. *J Chromatogr B Analyt Technol Biomed Life Sci.* 2021 Jul 15;1179:122861.

10151 Sukkanon C, Nararak J, Bangs MJ, et al. Cananga odorata (Magnoliales: Annonaceae) Essential Oil Produces Significant Avoidance Behavior in Mosquitoes. *J Med Entomol.* 2021 Sep 13;tjab143.

10152 Pavela R, Maggi F, Giordani C, et al. Insecticidal activity of two essential oils used in perfumery (ylang ylang and frankincense). *Nat Prod Res.* 2021 Nov;35(22):4746-4752.

10153 Lebanov L, Paull B. Comparison of chemometric assisted targeted and untargeted approaches for the prediction of radical scavenging activity of ylang-ylang essential oils. *J Chromatogr B Analyt Technol Biomed Life Sci.* 2021 Dec 29;1191:123093.

10154 Kurniasih DE, Erwanto R. The effectiveness differences of Cananga aromatherapy and Java Langgam music on blood pressure of the elderly with hypertension. *J Keperawatan Respati Yogyakarta.* 2021 Jamn;8(1):55-60.

10155 Tubachi SS, Rasal VP, Ugare SR, et al. Evaluation of Ylang Ylang essential oil on alcohol induced hepatotoxicity in rats. *Adv Trad Med.* 2022 Mar 4;191:1-14.

10156 Borgonetti V, López V, Galeotti N. Ylang-ylang (Cananga odorata (Lam.) Hook. f. & Thomson) essential oil reduced neuropathic-pain and associated anxiety symptoms in mice. *J Ethnopharmacol.* 2022 Aug 10;294:115362.

10157 de Freitas Junior RA, Lossavaro PKMB, Kassuya CAL, et al. Effect of Ylang-Ylang (Cananga odorata Hook. F. & Thomson) Essential Oil on Acute Inflammatory Response In Vitro and In Vivo. *Molecules.* 2022 Jun 7;27(12):3666.

10158 Sriboonlert J, Munkong W, Rintawut S, et al. Cananga odorata Aromatherapy Reduces Anxiety in Unexperienced Patients Hospitalized for Interventional Neuroradiology Procedures: A Randomized Control Trial. *J Evid Based Integr Med.* 2023 Jan-Dec;28:2515690X221150527.

10159 Zhang N, Wang ST, Yao L. Inhalation of Cananga odorata essential oil relieves anxiety behaviors in autism-like rats via regulation of serotonin and dopamine metabolism. *J Integr Med.* 2023 Feb. Online ahead of print.

10160 Swarma M, Lan-Phi NT. Chemical and aroma profiles of different cultivars of Yuzu (Citrus junos Sieb ex Tanaka) essential oils. *Kochi University.* Available at: https://home.zhaw.ch/yere/pdf/Teil108%20-%20Expression% 20of%20Multidisciplinary.pdf.

10161 Song HS, Sawamura M, Ito T, et al. Chemical compositions of the volatile part of yuzu (Citrus junos Tanaka) peel cold-pressed oils from Japan and Korea. *Flavour Frag J.* 1999;14:383-89.

10162 Akakabe Y, Sakamoto M, Ikeda Y, et al. Identification and characterization of volatile components of the Japanese sour citrus fruit Citrus nagato-yuzukichi Tanaka. *Biosci Biotechnol Biochem.* 2008 Jul;72(7):1965-8.

10163 Mauerman B, Ahmed N, Tambhar N, et al. Trends in Furanocoumarin Profiles Among Commerical-Scale Essential Oils. International Conference on the Science of Botanicals, Poster. Mar 2022.

10164 Sawarma M, Hasegawa K, Kashiwagi K, et al. Determination of bergapten in Japanese citrus essential oils. *Japanese J Aromatherapy.* 2009;9:30-7.

10165 Matsumoto T, Kimura T, Hayashi T. Aromatic effects of a Japanese citrus fruit-yuzu (Citrus junos Sieb. ex Tanaka)-on psychoemotional states and autonomic nervous system activity during the menstrual cycle: a single- blind randomized controlled crossover study. *Biopsychosoc Med.* 2016 Apr 21;10:11.

10166 Matsumoto T, Asakura H, Hayashi T. Effects of olfactory stimulation from the fragrance of the Japanese citrus fruit yuzu (Citrus junos Sieb. ex Tanaka) on mood states and salivary chromogranin A as an endocrinologic stress marker. *J Altern Complement Med.* 2014 Jun;20(6):500-6.

10167 Hirota R, Roger NN, Nakamura H, et al. Anti-inflammatory effects of limonene from yuzu (Citrus junos Tanaka) essential oil on eosinophils. *J Food Sci.* 2010 Apr;75(3):H87-92.

10168 Matsumoto T, Kimura T, Hayashi T, et al. Does Japanese Citrus Fruit Yuzu (Citrus junos Sieb. ex Tanaka) Fragrance Have Lavender-Like Therapeutic Effects That Alleviate Premenstrual Emotional Symptoms? A Single-Blind Randomized Crossover Study. *J Altern Complement Med.* 2017 Jun;23(6):461-470.

10169 Vitalini S, Iriti M, Vinciguerra V, Garzoli S. A Comparative Study of the Chemical Composition by SPME-GC/MS and Antiradical Activity of Less Common Citrus Species. *Molecules.* 2021 Sep 4;26(17):5378.

10170 Yang J, Lee SY, Jang SK, et al. Inhibition of Melanogenesis by Essential Oils from the Citrus Cultivars Peels. *Int J Mol Sci.* 2023 Feb 20;24(4):4207.

10171 Chalchat JC, Petrovic SD, Maksimovic ZA, et al. A comparative study on essential oils of Geranium macrorrhizum L. and Geranium phaeum L., Geraniaceae from Serbia. *J Essent Oil Res.* 2002 Sept-Oct;14:333-35.

10172 Radulovic NS, Dekic MS, Stojanovic-Radic ZZ, et al. Geranium macrorrhizum L. (Geraniaceae) Essential Oil: A Potent Agent Against Bacillus subtilis. *Chem Biodivers.* 2010;7:2783-2800.

10173 Sharopov F. Dissertation. Phytochemistry and bioactivities of selected plant species with volatile secondary metabolites. Available at: https://archiv.ub.uni-heidelberg.de/volltextserver/19495/1/Farukh%20Sharopov%20-%20Dissertation-HeidelberU,%202015.pdf.

10174 Pimkaew P1, Küblbeck J, Petsalo A, et al. Interactions of sesquiterpenes zederone and germacrone with the human cytochrome P450 system. *Toxicol In Vitro.* 2013 Sep;27(6):2005-12.

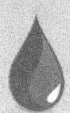
10175 Radulovic NS, Dekic MS, Stojanovic-Radic ZZ, et al. Geranium macrorrhizum L. (Geraniaceae) Essential Oil: A Potent Agent Against Bacillus subtilis. *Chem Biodivers*. 2010;7:2783-2800.

10176 American Institute of Stress. America's #1 Health Problem. Available at: http://www.stress.org/americas-1-health-problem/.

10177 Darben T, Cominos B, Lee CT. Topical eucalyptus oil poisoning. *Australas J Dermatol*. 1998 Nov;39(4):265-7.

10178 Myott E. Case of eucalyptus poisoning. *Brit M J*. 1906;1:558.

10179 Eikholt TH, Box RH. Toxicities of peppermint and Pycnanthemun albescens oils, Fam. Labiateae. *J Pharm Sci*. 1965;54:1071-72.

10180 Craig JO. Poisoning by the volatile oils in childhood. *Arch Dis Child*. 1953;28:259-67.

10181 Hindle RC. Eucalyptus oil ingestion. *N Z Med J*. 1994 May 11;107(977)185-6.

10182 Tibballs J. Clinical effects and management of eucalyptus oil ingestion in infants and small children. *Med J Aust*. 1995 Aug;163(4):177-80.

10183 Melis K. Bochner A, Janssens G. Accidental nasal eucalyptol and menthol instillation. *Eur J Pediatr*. 1989 Aug;148(8):786-7.

10184 Reynolds JEF. Martindale: The Extra Pharmacopoeia. *The Pharmaceutical Press, London*. 1993.

10185 No author listed. Monographs on the medicinal uses of plants. *Exeter: European Scientific Cooperative on Phytotherapy*. 1997.

10186 Javorka K, Tomori Z, Zavarska L. Protective and defensive airway reflexes in premature infants. *Physiol Bohemoslov*. 1980;29(1):29-35.

10187 Food and Drug Administration, HHS. Labeling for oral and rectal over-the-counter drug products containing aspirin and nonaspirin salicylates; Reye's Syndrome warning. Final rule. *Fed Regist*. 2003 Apr 17;68(74):18861-9.

10188 Kim HJ, Yang HM, Kim DH, et al. Effects of ylang-ylang essential oil on the relaxation of rat bladder muscle in vitro and white rabbit bladder in vivo. *J Korean Med Sci*. 2003 Jun;18(3):409-14.

10189 Kirsch F, Buettner A. Characterisation of the metabolites of 1,8-cineole transferred into human milk: concentrations and ratio of enantiomers. *Metabolites*. 2013 Jan 30;3(1):47-71.

10190 Kirsch F, Beauchamp J, Buettner A. Time-dependent aroma changes in breast milk after oral intake of a pharmacological preparation containing 1,8-cineole. *Clin Nutr*. 2012 Oct;31(5):682-92.

10191 Melli MS, Rashidi MR, Nokhoodchi A, et al. A randomized trial of peppermint gel, lanolin ointment, and placebo gel to prevent nipple crack primiparous breastfeeding women. *Med Sci Monit*. 2007 Sep;13(9):406-11.

10192 Ali Akbari SA, Alamolhoda SH, Baghban AA, et al. Effects of menthol essence and breast milk on the improvement of nipple fissures in breastfeeding women. *J Res Med Sci*. 2014 Jun;19(7):629-33.

10193 Melli MS, Rashidi MR, Delazar A, et al. Effect of peppermint water on prevention of nipple cracks in lactating primiparous women: a randomized controlled trial. *Int Breastfeed J*. 2007;2:7.

10194 Croker AK, Allan AL. Cancer stem cells: implications for the progression and treatment of metastatic disease. *J Cell Mol Med*. 2008;12:374-90.

10195 Mayo Clinic. Living with cancer blog: The high cost of cancer drugs. Available at: http://www.mayoclinic.org/diseases-conditions/cancer/expert-blog/high-cancer-drug-cost/bgp-20149406

10196 Mackillop WJ, Ward GK, O'Sullivan B. The use of expert surrogates to evalute clinical trials in non-small cell lung cancer. *Brit J Cancer*. 1986;54:661-67

10197 Tayarani-Najaran Z, Talasaz-Firoozi E, Nasiri R, et al. Antiemetic activity of volatile oil from Mentha spicata and Mentha x piperita in chemotherapy-induced nausea and vomiting. *Ecancermedicalscience*. 2013;7:290.

10198 Hwang JH. The effects of the inhalation method using essential oils on blood pressure and stress responses of clients with essential hypertension. *Taehan Kanho Hakhoe Chi*. 2006 Dec;36(7):1123-34.

10199 Kim IH, Kim C, Seong K, et al. Essential oil inhalation on blood pressure and salivary cortisol levels in prehypertensive and hypertensive subjects. *Evid Based Complement Alternat Med*. 2012;2012:984203.

10200 Sargolzaee MR, Faayyazi Bordbar MR, Shakiba M, et al. The comparison of the efficacy of Citrus Fragrance and Fluoxetine in the treatment of major depressive disorder. *J of Gonabad University of Med Sci and Health Sci*. 2004;10(3):43-48.

10201 Maignana Kumar R, Rukmani A, Saradha S, et al. Evaluation of antiepileptic activity of vetiveria zizanioides oil in mice. *Int J Pharm Sci Rev Res*. 2014 Mar-Apr;25(2):248-51.

10202 de Sousaa DP, Nóbregab FF, de Morais LC, et al. Evaluation of the Anticonvulsant Activity of Terpinen-4-ol. *Z Naturforsch C*. 2009 Jan-Feb;64(1-2):1-5.

10203 Lytle J, Mwatha C, Davis KK. Effect of lavender aromatherapy on vital signs and perceived quality of sleep in the intermediate care unit: a pilot study. *Am J Crit Care*. 2014 Jan;23(1):24-29.

10204 Maddocks-Jennings W, Wilkinson JM, Cavanagh HM, et al. Evaluating the effects of the essential oils Leptospermum scoparium (manuka) and Kunzea ericoides (kanuka) on radiotherapy induced mucositis: a randomized, placebo controlled feasibility study. *Eur J Oncol Nurs*. 2009 Apr;13(2):87-93.

10205 Johnson JR, Rivard RL, Griffin KH, et al. The effectiveness of nurse-delivered aromatherapy in an acute care setting. *Complement Ther Med*. 2016 Apr;25:164-9.

10206 Hasanzadeh F, Kashouk NM, Amini S, et al. The effect of cold application and lavender oil inhalation in cardiac surgery patients undergoing chest tube removal. *EXCLI J*. 2016 Jan 22;15:64-74.

10207 Tayarani-Najaran Z, Talasaz-Firoozi E, Jalali N, et al. Antiemetic activity of volatile oil from Mentha spicata and Mentha X piperita in chemotherapy-induced nausea and vomiting. *Ecancermedicalscience*. 2013;7:290.

10208 Lua PL, Salihah N, Mazlan N. Effects of inhaled ginger aromatherapy on chemotherapy-induced nausea and vomiting and health-related quality of life in women with breast cancer. *Complement Ther Med*. 2015 Jun;23(3):396-404.

10209 Kim MA, Sakong JK, Kim EJ, et al. Effect of aromatherapy massage for the relief of constipation in the elderly. *Taehan Kanho Hakhoe Chi*. 2005 Feb;35(1):56-64.

10210 Moss M, Cook J, Wesnes K, et al. Aromas of rosemary and lavender essential oils differentially affect cognition and mood in healthy adults. *Int J Neurosci*. 2003 Jan;113(1):15-38.

10211 Moss M, Oliver L. Plasma 1,8-cineole correlates with cognitive performance following exposure to rosemary essential oil aroma. *Ther Adv Psychopharmacol*. 2012 Jun;2(3):103-13.

10212 Khiewkhern S, Promthet S, Sukprasert A, et al. Effectiveness of aromatherapy with light Thai massage for cellular immunity improvement in colorectal cancer patients receiving chemotherapy. *Asian Pac J Cancer Prev*. 2013;14(6):3903-07.

10213 Johnson S. Supercritical Essential Oils. 2017. Scott A Johnson Professional Writing Services, LLC: Orem, Utah.

10214 Kim Y, Kim WJ, Cha EJ. Quercetin-induced Growth Inhibition in Human Bladder Cancer Cells Is Associated with an Increase in Ca2+-activated K+ Channels. *Korean J Physiol Pharmacol*. 2011 Oct; 15(5): 279–283.

10215 Wei L, Liu JJ, Cao J, et al. [Role of autophagy in quercetin-induced apoptosis in human bladder carcinoma BIU-87 cells]. *Zhonghua Zhong Liu Za Zhi*. 2012 Jun;34(6):414-8.

10216 Lee HP, Li TM, Tsao JY, et al. Curcumin induces cell apoptosis in human chondrosarcoma through extrinsic death receptor pathway. *Int Immunopharmacol*. 2012 Jun;13(2):163-9.

10217 Chang R, Sun L, Webster TJ, et al. Short communication: selective cytotoxicity of curcumin on osteosarcoma cells compared to healthy osteoblasts. *Int J Nanomedicine*. 2014;9:461-5.

10218 Shoba G, Joy D, Joseph T, et al. Influence of piperine on the pharmacokinetics of curcumin in animals and human volunteers. *Planta Med*. 1998 May;64(4):353-6.

10219 Yin H, Zhou Y, Wen C, et al. Curcumin sensitizes glioblastoma to temozolomide by simultaneously generating ROS and disrupting AKT/mTOR signaling. *Oncol Rep*. 2014 Oct;32(4):1610-6.

10220 Shoba G, Joy D, Joseph T, et al. Influence of piperine on the pharmacokinetics of curcumin in animals and human volunteers. *Planta Med*. 1998 May;64(4):353-6.

10221 Kirste S, Treier M, Wehrle SJ, et al. Boswellia serrata acts on cerebral edema in patients irradiated for brain tumors: a prospective, randomized, placebo-controlled, double-blind pilot trial. *Cancer*. 2011 Aug 15;117(16):3788-95.

10222 Wang DY, Yeh CC, Lee JH, et al. Berberine inhibited arylamine N-acetyltransferase activity and gene expression and DNA adduct formation in human malignant astrocytoma (G9T/VGH) and brain glioblastoma multiforms (GBM 8401) cells. *Neurochem Res*. 2002 Sep;27(9):883-9.

10223 Yin H, Zhou Y, Wen C, et al. Curcumin sensitizes glioblastoma to temozolomide by simultaneously generating ROS and disrupting AKT/mTOR signaling. *Oncol Rep*. 2014 Oct;32(4):1610-6.

10224 Shoba G, Joy D, Joseph T, et al. Influence of piperine on the pharmacokinetics of curcumin in animals and human volunteers. *Planta Med*. 1998 May;64(4):353-6.

10225 Kirste S, Treier M, Wehrle SJ, et al. Boswellia serrata acts on cerebral edema in patients irradiated for brain tumors: a prospective, randomized, placebo-controlled, double-blind pilot trial. *Cancer*. 2011 Aug 15;117(16):3788-95.

10226 Wang DY, Yeh CC, Lee JH, et al. Berberine inhibited arylamine N-acetyltransferase activity and gene expression and DNA adduct formation in human malignant astrocytoma (G9T/VGH) and brain glioblastoma multiforms (GBM 8401) cells. *Neurochem Res*. 2002 Sep;27(9):883-9

10227 Bayet-Robert M, Kwiatkowski F, Leheurteur M, et al. Phase I dose escalation trial of docetaxel plus curcumin in patients with advanced and metastatic breast cancer. *Cancer Biol Ther*. 2010 Jan;9(1):8-14.

10228 Bayet-Robert M, Kwiatkowski F, Leheurteur M, et al. Phase I dose escalation trial of docetaxel plus curcumin in patients with advanced and metastatic breast cancer. *Cancer Biol Ther*. 2010 Jan;9(1):8-14.

10229 Shang HS, Chang CH, Chou YR, et al. Curcumin causes DNA damage and affects associated protein expression in HeLa human cervical cancer cells. *Oncol Rep*. 2016 Oct;36(4):2207-15.

10230 Zhang X, Wang R, Chen G, et al. The Effects of Curcumin-based Constituents on Proliferation and Cell Death in Cervical Cancer Cells. *Anticancer Res*. 2015 Oct;35(10):5293-8.

10231 Shoba G, Joy D, Joseph T, et al. Influence of piperine on the pharmacokinetics of curcumin in animals and human volunteers. *Planta Med*. 1998 May;64(4):353-6.

10232 Ahn WS, Yoo J, Huh SW, et al. Protective effects of green tea extracts (polyphenon E and EGCG) on human cervical lesions. *Eur J Cancer Prev*. 2003 Oct;12(5):383-90.

10233 Basu P, Dutta S, Begum R, et al. Clearance of Cervical Human Papillomavirus Infection by Topical Application of Curcumin and Curcumin Containing Polyherbal Cream: A Phase II Randomized Controlled Study. *Asian Pac J Canc Prev*. 2013 Oct;14(10):5753-59.

10234 Maher DM, Bell MC, O'Donnell EA, et al. Curcumin suppresses human papillomavirus oncoproteins, restores p53, Rb, and PTPN13 proteins and inhibits benzo[a]pyrene-induced upregulation of HPV E7. *Mol Carcinog*. 2011 Jan;50(1):47-57.

10235 Verhoeven V, Renard N, Makar A, et al. Probiotics enhance the clearance of human papillomavirus-related cervical lesions: a prospective controlled pilot study. *Eur J Cancer Prev*. 2013 Jan;22(1):46-51.

10236 Cha MK, Lee DK, An HM, et al. Antiviral activity of Bifidobacterium adolescentisSPM1005-A on human papillomavirus type 16. *BMC Medicine*. 2012;10:17.

10237 Carroll RE, Benya RV, Turgeon DK, et al. Phase IIa clinical trial of curcumin for the prevention of colorectal neoplasia. *Cancer Prev Res (Phila)*. 2011;4:354-64.

10238 Patel KR, Brown VA, Jones DJ, et al. Clinical pharmacology of resveratrol and its metabolites in colorectal cancer patients. *Cancer Res*. 2010 Oct 1;70(19):7392-9.

10239 Citronberg J, Bostick R, Ahearn T, et al. Effects of ginger supplementation on cell-cycle biomarkers in the normal-appearing colonic mucosa of patients at increased risk for colorectal cancer: results from a pilot, randomized, and controlled trial. *Cancer Prev Res (Phila)*. 2013 Apr;6(4):271-81.

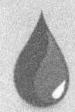

[10240] Zick SM, Turgeon DK, Vareed SK, et al. Phase II study of the effects of ginger root extract on eicosanoids in colon mucosa in people at normal risk for colorectal cancer. *Cancer Prev Res (Phila)*. 2011 Nov;4(11):1929-37.
[10241] Peiffer DS, Zimmerman NP1, Wang LS, et al. Chemoprevention of esophageal cancer with black raspberries, their component anthocyanins, and a major anthocyanin metabolite, protocatechuic acid. *Cancer Prev Res (Phila)*. 2014 Jun;7(6):574-84.
[10242] Medda R, Lyros O2, Schmidt JL, et al. Anti inflammatory and anti angiogenic effect of black raspberry extract on human esophageal and intestinal microvascular endothelial cells. *Microvasc Res*. 2015 Jan;97:167-80.
[10243] Subramaniam D, Ponnurangam S, Ramamoorthy P, et al. Curcumin induces cell death in esophageal cancer cells through modulating Notch signaling. *PLoS One*. 2012;7(2):e30590.
[10244] Shoba G, Joy D, Joseph T, et al. Influence of piperine on the pharmacokinetics of curcumin in animals and human volunteers. *Planta Med*. 1998 May;64(4):353-6.
[10245] Shrotriya S, Deep G, Gu M, et al. Generation of reactive oxygen species by grape seed extract causes irreparable DNA damage leading to G2/M arrest and apoptosis selectively in head and neck squamous cell carcinoma cells. *Carcinogenesis*. 2012 Apr;33(4):848-58.
[10246] Shrotriya S, Deep G, Lopert P, et al. Grape seed extract targets mitochondrial electron transport chain complex III and induces oxidative and metabolic stress leading to cytoprotective autophagy and apoptotic death in human head and neck cancer cells. *Mol Carcinog*. 2015 Dec;54(12):1734-47.
[10247] Tyagi A, Gu M, Takahata T, et al. Resveratrol selectively induces DNA Damage, independent of Smad4 expression, in its efficacy against human head and neck squamous cell carcinoma. *Clin Cancer Res*. 2011 Aug 15;17(16):5402-11.
[10248] Kodama N, Komuta K, Nanba H. Effect of Maitake (Grifola frondosa) D-Fraction on the activation of NK cells in cancer patients. *J Med Food*. 2003 Winter;6(4):371-7.
[10249] Kodama N, Komuta K, Nanba H. Can maitake MD-fraction aid cancer patients? *Altern Med Rev*. 2002 Jun;7(3):236-9.
[10250] Alexander B, Fishman AI, Eshghi M, et al. Induction of cell death in renal cell carcinoma with combination of D-fraction and vitamin C. *Integr Cancer Ther*. 2013 Sep;12(5):442-8.
[10251] Everett PC, Meyers JA, Makkinje A, et al. Preclinical assessment of curcumin as a potential therapy for B-CLL. *Am J Hematol*. 2007 Jan;82(1):23-30.
[10252] Shoba G, Joy D, Joseph T, et al. Influence of piperine on the pharmacokinetics of curcumin in animals and human volunteers. *Planta Med*. 1998 May;64(4):353-6.
[10253] Mingzhu M, Bangyuan Y. Progress in indirubin treatment of myelocytic leukemia. *J Tradit Chin Med*. 1983;3:245-248.
[10254] Xiao Z, Hao Y, Liu B, et al. Indirubin and meisoindigo in the treatment of chronic myelogenous leukemia in China. *Leuk Lymphoma*. 2002 Sep;43(9):1763-8.
[10255] Ghalaut VS, Sangwan L, Dahiya K, et al. Effect of imatinib therapy with and without turmeric powder on nitric oxide levels in chronic myeloid leukemia. *J Oncol Pharm Pract*. 2012 Jun;18(2):186-90.
[10256] Shoba G, Joy D, Joseph T, et al. Influence of piperine on the pharmacokinetics of curcumin in animals and human volunteers. *Planta Med*. 1998 May;64(4):353-6.
[10257] Xia L, Chen D, Han R, et al. Boswellic acid acetate induces apoptosis through caspase-mediated pathways in myeloid leukemia cells. *Mol Cancer Ther*. 2005 Mar;4(3):381-8.
[10258] Ghalaut VS, Sangwan L, Dahiya K, et al. Effect of imatinib therapy with and without turmeric powder on nitric oxide levels in chronic myeloid leukemia. *J Oncol Pharm Pract*. 2012 Jun;18(2):186-90.
[10259] Shoba G, Joy D, Joseph T, et al. Influence of piperine on the pharmacokinetics of curcumin in animals and human volunteers. *Planta Med*. 1998 May;64(4):353-6.
[10260] Xia L, Chen D, Han R, et al. Boswellic acid acetate induces apoptosis through caspase-mediated pathways in myeloid leukemia cells. *Mol Cancer Ther*. 2005 Mar;4(3):381-8.
[10261] Park SE, Park C, Kim SH, et al. Korean red ginseng extract induces apoptosis and decreases telomerase activity in human leukemia cells. *J Ethnopharmacol*. 2009 Jan 21;121(2):304-12.
[10262] Wang WH, Chiang IT, Ding K, et al. Curcumin-Induced Apoptosis in Human Hepatocellular Carcinoma J5 Cells: Critical Role of -Dependent Pathway. *Evidence-based Complement Altern Med*. 2012;2012:521907.
[10263] Hessien M, El-Gendy S, Donia T, et al. Growth inhibition of human non-small lung cancer cells h460 by green tea and ginger polyphenols. *Anticancer Agents Med Chem*. 2012 May;12(4):383-90.
[10264] Shoba G, Joy D, Joseph T, et al. Influence of piperine on the pharmacokinetics of curcumin in animals and human volunteers. *Planta Med*. 1998 May;64(4):353-6.
[10265] Zhu Y, Warin RF, Soroka DN, et al. Metabolites of ginger component [6]-shogaol remain bioactive in cancer cells and have low toxicity in normal cells: chemical synthesis and biological evaluation. *PLoS One*. 2013;8(1):e54677.
[10266] Kewitz S, Volkmer I, Staege MS. Curcuma Contra Cancer? Curcumin and Hodgkin's Lymphoma. *Cancer Growth Metastasis*. 2013; 6: 35–52.
[10267] Shoba G, Joy D, Joseph T, et al. Influence of piperine on the pharmacokinetics of curcumin in animals and human volunteers. *Planta Med*. 1998 May;64(4):353-6.
[10268] Wang HC, Pao J, Lin SY, Sheen LY. Molecular mechanisms of garlic-derived allyl sulfides in the inhibition of skin cancer progression. *Ann N Y Acad Sci*. 2012 Oct;1271:44-52.
[10269] Hakimzadeh H, Ghazanfari T, Rahmati B, et al. Cytotoxic effect of garlic extract and its fractions on Sk-mel3 melanoma cell line. *Immunopharmacol Immunotoxicol*. 2010 Sep;32(3):371-5.
[10270] Zhang YP, Li YQ2, Lv YT, et al. Effect of curcumin on the proliferation, apoptosis, migration, and invasion of human melanoma A375 cells. *Genet Mol Res*. 2015 Feb 6;14(1):1056-67.
[10271] Jiang AJ, Jiang G, Li LT, et al. Curcumin induces apoptosis through mitochondrial pathway and caspases activation in human melanoma cells. *Mol Biol Rep*. 2015 Jan;42(1):267-75.
[10272] Shoba G, Joy D, Joseph T, et al. Influence of piperine on the pharmacokinetics of curcumin in animals and human volunteers. *Planta Med*. 1998 May;64(4):353-6.
[10273] Miller JM, Thompson JK, MacPherson MB, et al. Curcumin: a double hit on malignant mesothelioma. *Cancer Prev Res (Phila)*. 2014 Mar;7(3):330-40.
[10274] Wang Y, Rishi AK, Wu W, et al. Curcumin suppresses growth of mesothelioma cells in vitro and in vivo, in part, by stimulating apoptosis. *Mol Cell Biochem*. 2011 Nov;357(1-2):83-94.
[10275] Shoba G, Joy D, Joseph T, et al. Influence of piperine on the pharmacokinetics of curcumin in animals and human volunteers. *Planta Med*. 1998 May;64(4):353-6.
[10276] Tyagi AK, Prasad S, Yuan W, et al. Identification of a novel compound (β-sesquiphellandrene) from turmeric (Curcuma longa) with anticancer potential: comparison with curcumin. *Invest New Drugs*. 2015 Dec;33(6):1175-86.
[10277] Sung B, Murakami A, Oyajobi BO, et al. Zerumbone abolishes RANKL-induced NF-kappaB activation, inhibits osteoclastogenesis, and suppresses human breast cancer-induced bone loss in athymic nude mice. *Cancer Res*. 2009 Feb 15;69(4):1477-84.
[10278] Bode AM, Dong Z. Herbal Medicine: Biomolecular and Clinical Aspects. 2nd edition. Chapter 7: The Amazing and Mighty Ginger. Available at: https://www.ncbi.nlm.nih.gov/books/NBK92775/.
[10279] Ghoneum M1, Gollapudi S. Synergistic apoptotic effect of arabinoxylan rice bran (MGN-3/Biobran) and curcumin (turmeric) on human multiple myeloma cell line U266 in vitro. *Neoplasma*. 2011;58(2):118-23.
[10280] Goel A, Aggarwal BB. Curcumin, the golden spice from Indian saffron, is a chemosensitizer and radiosensitizer for tumors and chemoprotector and radioprotector for normal organs. *Nutr Cancer*. 2010;62(7):919-30.
[10281] Shoba G, Joy D, Joseph T, et al. Influence of piperine on the pharmacokinetics of curcumin in animals and human volunteers. *Planta Med*. 1998 May;64(4):353-6.
[10282] Ghoneum M1, Gollapudi S. Synergistic apoptotic effect of arabinoxylan rice bran (MGN-3/Biobran) and curcumin (turmeric) on human multiple myeloma cell line U266 in vitro. *Neoplasma*. 2011;58(2):118-23.
[10283] Picone P, Nuzzo D, Caruana L, et al. Curcumin induces apoptosis in human neuroblastoma cells via inhibition of AKT and Foxo3a nuclear translocation. *Free Radic Res*. 2014 Dec;48(12):1397-408.
[10284] Shoba G, Joy D, Joseph T, et al. Influence of piperine on the pharmacokinetics of curcumin in animals and human volunteers. *Planta Med*. 1998 May;64(4):353-6.
[10285] Kirste S, Treier M, Wehrle SJ, et al. Boswellia serrata acts on cerebral edema in patients irradiated for brain tumors: a prospective, randomized, placebo-controlled, double-blind pilot trial. *Cancer*. 2011 Aug 15;117(16):3788-95.
[10286] Lee HP, Li TM, Tsao JY, et al. Curcumin induces cell apoptosis in human chondrosarcoma through extrinsic death receptor pathway. *Int Immunopharmacol*. 2012 Jun;13(2):163-9.
[10287] Chang R, Sun L, Webster TJ, et al. Short communication: selective cytotoxicity of curcumin on osteosarcoma cells compared to healthy osteoblasts. *Int J Nanomedicine*. 2014;9:461-5.
[10288] Shoba G, Joy D, Joseph T, et al. Influence of piperine on the pharmacokinetics of curcumin in animals and human volunteers. *Planta Med*. 1998 May;64(4):353-6.
[10289] Vallianou NG, Evangelopoulos A, Schizas N, et al. Potential anticancer properties and mechanisms of action of curcumin. *Anticancer Res*. 2015 Feb;35(2):645-51.
[10290] Terlikowska KM, Witkowska AM, Zujko ME, et al. Potential application of curcumin and its analogues in the treatment strategy of patients with primary epithelial ovarian cancer. *Int J Mol Sci*. 2014 Nov 25;15(12):21703-22.
[10291] Shoba G, Joy D, Joseph T, et al. Influence of piperine on the pharmacokinetics of curcumin in animals and human volunteers. *Planta Med*. 1998 May;64(4):353-6.
[10292] Rhode J, Fogoros S, Zick S, et al. Ginger inhibits cell growth and modulates angiogenic factors in ovarian cancer cells. *BMC Complement Altern Med*. 2007 Dec 20;7:44.
[10293] Vallianou NG, Evangelopoulos A, Schizas N, et al. Potential anticancer properties and mechanisms of action of curcumin. *Anticancer Res*. 2015 Feb;35(2):645-51.
[10294] Terlikowska KM, Witkowska AM, Zujko ME, et al. Potential application of curcumin and its analogues in the treatment strategy of patients with primary epithelial ovarian cancer. *Int J Mol Sci*. 2014 Nov 25;15(12):21703-22.
[10295] Shoba G, Joy D, Joseph T, et al. Influence of piperine on the pharmacokinetics of curcumin in animals and human volunteers. *Planta Med*. 1998 May;64(4):353-6.
[10296] Rhode J, Fogoros S, Zick S, et al. Ginger inhibits cell growth and modulates angiogenic factors in ovarian cancer cells. *BMC Complement Altern Med*. 2007 Dec 20;7:44.
[10297] Park B, Sung B, Yadav VR, et al. Acetyl-11-keto-β-boswellic acid suppresses invasion of pancreatic cancer cells through the downregulation of CXCR4 chemokine receptor expression. *Int J Cancer*. 2011 Jul 1;129(1):23-33.
[10298] Park B, Prasad S, Yadav V, et al. Boswellic acid suppresses growth and metastasis of human pancreatic tumors in an orthotopic nude mouse model through modulation of multiple targets. *PLoS One*. 2011;6(10):e26943.
[10299] Kanai M, Yoshimura K, Asada M, et al. A phase I/II study of gemcitabine-based chemotherapy plus curcumin for patients with gemcitabine-resistant pancreatic cancer. *Cancer Chemother Pharmacol*. 2011 Jul;68(1):157-64.
[10300] Dhillon N, Aggarwal BB, Newman RA, et al. Phase II trial of curcumin in patients with advanced pancreatic cancer. *Clin Cancer Res*. 2008 Jul 15;14(14):4491-9.
[10301] Shoba G, Joy D, Joseph T, et al. Influence of piperine on the pharmacokinetics of curcumin in animals and human volunteers. *Planta Med*. 1998 May;64(4):353-6.
[10302] Agarwal C, Sharma Y, Agarwal R. Anticarcinogenic effect of a polyphenolic fraction isolated from grape seeds in human prostate carcinoma DU145 cells: modulation of mitogenic signaling and cell-cycle regulators and induction of G1 arrest and apoptosis. *Mol Carcinog*. 2000;28:129-38.
[10303] Li J, Xiang S, Zhang Q, et al. Combination of curcumin and bicalutamide enhanced the growth inhibition of androgen-independent prostate cancer cells through SAPK/JNK and MEK/ERK1/2-mediated targeting NF-κB/p65 and MUC1-C. *J Exp Clin Cancer Res*. 2015 May 15;34:46.
[10304] Guo H, Xu Y, Fu Q, et al. Curcumin inhibits growth of prostate carcinoma via miR-208-mediated CDKN1A activation. *Tumour Biol*. 2015 Nov;36(11):8511-7.
[10305] Shoba G, Joy D, Joseph T, et al. Influence of piperine on the pharmacokinetics of curcumin in animals and human volunteers. *Planta Med*. 1998 May;64(4):353-6.

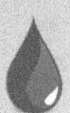
10306 Park SY, Lee YH, Choi KC, et al. Grape seed extract regulates androgen receptor-mediated transcription in prostate cancer cells through potent anti-histone acetyltransferase activity. *J Med Food.* 2011 Jan-Feb;14(1-2):9-16.

10307 Agarwal C, Sharma Y, Agarwal R. Anticarcinogenic effect of a polyphenolic fraction isolated from grape seeds in human prostate carcinoma DU145 cells: modulation of mitogenic signaling and cell-cycle regulators and induction of G1 arrest and apoptosis. *Mol Carcinog.* 2000;28:129-38.

10308 Zhou DY, Ding N, Du ZY, et al. Curcumin analogues with high activity for inhibiting human prostate cancer cell growth and androgen receptor activation. *Mol Med Rep.* 2014 Sep;10(3):1315-22.

10309 Shoba G, Joy D, Joseph T, et al. Influence of piperine on the pharmacokinetics of curcumin in animals and human volunteers. *Planta Med.* 1998 May;64(4):353-6.

10310 Zhang JY, Lin MT, Zhou MJ, et al. Combinational Treatment of Curcumin and Quercetin against Gastric Cancer MGC-803 Cells in vitro. *Molecules.* 2015;20:11524-34.

10311 Cheng AL, Hsu CH, Lin JK, et al. Phase I clinical trial of curcumin, a chemopreventive agent, in patients with high-risk or pre-malignant lesions. *Anticancer Res.* 2001 Jul-Aug;21(4B):2895-900.

10312 Liu X, Sun K, Chen H, et al. Curcumin inhibits proliferation of gastric cancer cells by impairing ATP-sensitive potassium channel opening. *World J Surg Oncology.* 2014;12:389.

10313 Shoba G, Joy D, Joseph T, et al. Influence of piperine on the pharmacokinetics of curcumin in animals and human volunteers. *Planta Med.* 1998 May;64(4):353-6.

10314 Zhou C, Zhao XM, Li XF, et al. Curcumin inhibits AP-2γ-induced apoptosis in the human malignant testicular germ cells in vitro. *Acta Pharmacol Sin.* 2013 Sep;34(9):1192-200.

10315 Shoba G, Joy D, Joseph T, et al. Influence of piperine on the pharmacokinetics of curcumin in animals and human volunteers. *Planta Med.* 1998 May;64(4):353-6.

10316 Zhang L, Cheng X2, Gao Y, et al. Induction of ROS-independent DNA damage by curcumin leads to G2/M cell cycle arrest and apoptosis in human papillary thyroid carcinoma BCPAP cells. *Food Funct.* 2016 Jan;7(1):315-25.

10317 Song F, Zhang L, Yu HX, et al. The mechanism underlying proliferation-inhibitory and apoptosis-inducing effects of curcumin on papillary thyroid cancer cells. *Food Chem.* 2012 May 1;132(1):43-50.

10318 Shoba G, Joy D, Joseph T, et al. Influence of piperine on the pharmacokinetics of curcumin in animals and human volunteers. *Planta Med.* 1998 May;64(4):353-6.

10319 Chen Q, Gao Q, Chen K, et al. Curcumin suppresses migration and invasion of human endometrial carcinoma cells. *Oncol Lett.* 2015 Sep;10(3):1297-1302.

10320 Feng W, Yang CX, Zhang L, et al. Curcumin promotes the apoptosis of human endometrial carcinoma cells by downregulating the expression of androgen receptor through Wnt signal pathway. *Eur J Gynaecol Oncol.* 2014;35(6):718-23.

10321 Shoba G, Joy D, Joseph T, et al. Influence of piperine on the pharmacokinetics of curcumin in animals and human volunteers. *Planta Med.* 1998 May;64(4):353-6.

10322 Lee A, Chui PT, Aun CST, et al. Possible interaction between sevoflurane and Aloe vera. *Ann Pharmacother.* 2004;38:1651-54.

10323 Blickstein D, Shaklai M, Inbal A. Warfarin antagonism by avocado. *Lancet.* 1991;337:914-15.

10324 Guivernau M, Meza N, Barja P, et al. Clinical and experimental study on the long-term effect of dietary gamma- linolenic acid on plasma lipids, platelet aggregation, thromboxane formation, and prostacyclin production. *Prostaglandins Leukot Essent Fatty Acids.* 1994;51:311-16.

10325 Asmis L, Tanner FC, Sudano I, et al. DMSO inhibits platelet activation through cyclooxygenase-1 inhibition. A novel agent for drug eluting stents? *Biochem Biophys Res Commun.* 2010 Jan;39(4):1629-33.

10326 Guivernau M, Meza N, Barja P, et al. Clinical and experimental study on the long-term effect of dietary gamma-linolenic acid on plasma lipids, platelet aggregation, thromboxane formation, and prostacyclin production. *Prostaglandins Leukot Essent Fatty Acids.* 1994;51:311-16.

10327 Chang WC, Hsu FL. Inhibition of platelet aggregation and arachidonate metabolism in platelets by procyanidins. *Prostaglandins Leukot Essent Fatty Acids.* 1989;38(3):181-88.

10328 de Lange DW, Scholman WL, Kraaijenhagen RJ, et al. Alcohol and polyphenolic grape extract inhibit platelet adhesion in flowing blood. *Eur J Clin Invest.* 2004;34(12):818-24.

10329 Petroni A, Blasevich M, Salami M, et al. Inhibition of platelet aggregation and eicosanoid production by phenolic components of olive oil. *Thromb Res.* 4-15-1995;78(2):151-160.

10330 Lee A, Chui PT, Aun CST, et al. Possible interaction between sevoflurane and Aloe vera. *Ann Pharmacother.* 2004;38:1651-54.

10331 Blickstein D, Shaklai M, Inbal A. Warfarin antagonism by avocado. *Lancet.* 1991;337:914-15.

10332 Guivernau M, Meza N, Barja P, et al. Clinical and experimental study on the long-term effect of dietary gamma- linolenic acid on plasma lipids, platelet aggregation, thromboxane formation, and prostacyclin production. *Prostaglandins Leukot Essent Fatty Acids.* 1994;51:311-16.

10333 Asmis L, Tanner FC, Sudano I, et al. DMSO inhibits platelet activation through cyclooxygenase-1 inhibition. A novel agent for drug eluting stents? *Biochem Biophys Res Commun.* 2010 Jan;39(4):1629-33.

10334 Guivernau M, Meza N, Barja P, et al. Clinical and experimental study on the long-term effect of dietary gamma- linolenic acid on plasma lipids, platelet aggregation, thromboxane formation, and prostacyclin production. *Prostaglandins Leukot Essent Fatty Acids.* 1994;51:311-16.

10335 Chang WC, Hsu FL. Inhibition of platelet aggregation and arachidonate metabolism in platelets by procyanidins. *Prostaglandins Leukot Essent Fatty Acids.* 1989;38(3):181-88.

10336 de Lange DW, Scholman WL, Kraaijenhagen RJ, et al. Alcohol and polyphenolic grape extract inhibit platelet adhesion in flowing blood. *Eur J Clin Invest.* 2004;34(12):818-24.

10337 Petroni A, Blasevich M, Salami M, et al. Inhibition of platelet aggregation and eicosanoid production by phenolic components of olive oil. *Thromb Res.* 4-15-1995;78(2):151-160.

10338 Lee A, Chui PT, Aun CST, et al. Possible interaction between sevoflurane and Aloe vera. *Ann Pharmacother.* 2004;38:1651-54.

10339 Blickstein D, Shaklai M, Inbal A. Warfarin antagonism by avocado. *Lancet.* 1991;337:914-15.

10340 Guivernau M, Meza N, Barja P, et al. Clinical and experimental study on the long-term effect of dietary gamma- linolenic acid on plasma lipids, platelet aggregation, thromboxane formation, and prostacyclin production. *Prostaglandins Leukot Essent Fatty Acids.* 1994;51:311-16.

10341 Asmis L, Tanner FC, Sudano I, et al. DMSO inhibits platelet activation through cyclooxygenase-1 inhibition. A novel agent for drug eluting stents? *Biochem Biophys Res Commun.* 2010 Jan;39(4):1629-33.

10342 Guivernau M, Meza N, Barja P, et al. Clinical and experimental study on the long-term effect of dietary gamma- linolenic acid on plasma lipids, platelet aggregation, thromboxane formation, and prostacyclin production. *Prostaglandins Leukot Essent Fatty Acids.* 1994;51:311-16.

10343 Chang WC, Hsu FL. Inhibition of platelet aggregation and arachidonate metabolism in platelets by procyanidins. *Prostaglandins Leukot Essent Fatty Acids.* 1989;38(3):181-88.

10344 de Lange DW, Scholman WL, Kraaijenhagen RJ, et al. Alcohol and polyphenolic grape extract inhibit platelet adhesion in flowing blood. *Eur J Clin Invest.* 2004;34(12):818-24.

10345 Petroni A, Blasevich M, Salami M, et al. Inhibition of platelet aggregation and eicosanoid production by phenolic components of olive oil. *Thromb Res.* 4-15-1995;78(2):151-160.

10346 Lee A, Chui PT, Aun CST, et al. Possible interaction between sevoflurane and Aloe vera. *Ann Pharmacother.* 2004;38:1651-54.

10347 Blickstein D, Shaklai M, Inbal A. Warfarin antagonism by avocado. *Lancet.* 1991;337:914-15.

10348 Guivernau M, Meza N, Barja P, et al. Clinical and experimental study on the long-term effect of dietary gamma- linolenic acid on plasma lipids, platelet aggregation, thromboxane formation, and prostacyclin production. *Prostaglandins Leukot Essent Fatty Acids.* 1994;51:311-16.

10349 Asmis L, Tanner FC, Sudano I, et al. DMSO inhibits platelet activation through cyclooxygenase-1 inhibition. A novel agent for drug eluting stents? *Biochem Biophys Res Commun.* 2010 Jan;39(4):1629-33.

10350 Guivernau M, Meza N, Barja P, et al. Clinical and experimental study on the long-term effect of dietary gamma-linolenic acid on plasma lipids, platelet aggregation, thromboxane formation, and prostacyclin production. *Prostaglandins Leukot Essent Fatty Acids.* 1994;51:311-16.

10351 Chang WC, Hsu FL. Inhibition of platelet aggregation and arachidonate metabolism in platelets by procyanidins. *Prostaglandins Leukot Essent Fatty Acids.* 1989;38(3):181-88.

10352 de Lange DW, Scholman WL, Kraaijenhagen RJ, et al. Alcohol and polyphenolic grape extract inhibit platelet adhesion in flowing blood. *Eur J Clin Invest.* 2004;34(12):818-24.

10353 Petroni A, Blasevich M, Salami M, et al. Inhibition of platelet aggregation and eicosanoid production by phenolic components of olive oil. *Thromb Res.* 4-15-1995;78(2):151-160.

10354 Ruiz-Gutierrez V, Muriana FJ, Guerrero A, et al. Plasma lipids, erythrocyte membrane lipids and blood pressure of hypertensive women after ingestion of dietary oleic acid from two different sources. *J Hypertens.* 1996;14:1483-90.

10355 Ferrara LA, Raimondi AS, d'Episcopo L, et al. Olive oil and reduced need for antihypertensive medications. *Arch Intern Med.* 2000;160:837-42.

10356 Brinker F. Herb Contraindications and Drug Interactions. 2nd ed. Sandy, OR: Eclectic Medical Publications, 1998.

10357 Brinker F. Herb Contraindications and Drug Interactions. 2nd ed. Sandy, OR: Eclectic Medical Publications, 1998.

10358 Brayton CF. Dimethyl sulfoxide (DMSO): a review. *Cornell Vet.* 1986;76:61-90.

10359 Jacob SW, Herschler R. Pharmacology of DMSO. *Cryobiology.* 1986;23:14-27.

10360 Cherif S, Rahal N, Haouala M, et al. [A clinical trial of a titrated Olea extract in the treatment of essential arterial hypertension]. *J Pharm Belg.* 1996;51:69-71.

10361 Ferrara LA, Raimondi AS, d'Episcopo L, et al. Olive oil and reduced need for antihypertensive medications. *Arch Intern Med.* 2000;160:837-42.

10362 Teotia S, Singh M. Hypoglycemic effect of Prunus amygdalus seeds in albino rabbits. *Indian J Exp Biol.* 1997;35(3):295-96.

10363 Vogler BK, Ernst E. Aloe vera: a systematic review of its clinical effectiveness. *Br J Gen Pract.* 1999;49:823-38.

10364 Huseini HF, Kianbakht S, Hajiaghaee R, et al. Anti-hyperglycemic and anti-hypercholesterolemic effects of Aloe vera leaf gel in hyperlipidemic type 2 diabetic patients: a randomized double-blind placebo-controlled clinical trial. *Planta Med.* 2012;78:311-16.

10365 Miller LG. Herbal medicinals: selected clinical considerations focusing on known or potential drug-herb interactions. *Arch Intern Med.* 1998;158(20):2200-11.

10366 Al-Khamees WA, Schwartz MN, Alrashdi D, et al. Status epilepticus associated with borage oil ingestion. *J Med Toxicol.* 2011 Jun;7(2):154-57.

10367 Miller LG. Herbal medicinals: selected clinical considerations focusing on known or potential drug-herb interactions. *Arch Intern Med.* 1998;158(20):2200-11.

10368 Falth-Magnusson K, Magnusson KE. Elevated levels of serum antibodies to the lectin wheat germ agglutinin in celiac children lend support to the gluten-lectin theory of celiac disease. *Pediatr Allergy Immunol.* 1995 May;6(2):98- 102.

10369 Sollid LM, Kolberg J, Scott H, et al. Antibodies to wheat germ agglutinin in coeliac disease. *Clin Exp Immunol.* 1986 Jan;63(1):95-100.

10370 Takwale A, Tan E, Agarwal S, et al. Efficacy and tolerability of borage oil in adults and children with atopic eczema: randomised, double blind, placebo controlled, parallel group trial. *BMJ.* 2003;327:1385.

10371 Gaylord Chemical Company. Dimethyl sulfoxide (DMSO) health and safety information. Available at: https://www.researchgate.net/file.PostFileLoader.html?id=547d95e4d2fd6436518b468c&assetKey=AS%3A273644578639890%401442253359624.

10372 The Review of Natural Products by Facts and Comparisons. St. Louis, MO: Wolters Kluwer Co., 1999.

10373 Duke JA. CRC Handbook of Medicinal Herbs. 1st ed. Boca Raton, FL: CRC Press, LLC, 1985.

10374 Miller LG. Herbal medicinals: selected clinical considerations focusing on known or potential drug-herb interactions. *Arch Intern Med.* 1998;158(20):2200-11.

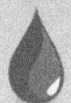

10375 Al-Khamees WA, Schwartz MN, Alrashdi D, et al. Status epilepticus associated with borage oil ingestion. *J Med Toxicol.* 2011 Jun;7(2):154-57.

10376 Miller LG. Herbal medicinals: selected clinical considerations focusing on known or potential drug-herb interactions. *Arch Intern Med.* 1998;158(20):2200-11.

10377 Newall CA, Anderson LA, Philpson JD. Herbal Medicine: A Guide for Healthcare Professionals. London, UK: The Pharmaceutical Press, 1996.

10378 Chojkier M. Hepatic sinusoidal-obstruction syndrome: toxicity of pyrrolizidine alkaloids. *J Hepatol.* 2003;39:437-46.

10379 Roeder E. Medicinal plants in Europe containing pyrrolizidine alkaloids. *Pharmazie.* 1995;50:83-98.

10380 Dove D, Johnson P. Oral evening primrose oil: its effect on length of pregnancy and selected intrapartum outcomes in low-risk nulliparous women. *J Nurse Midwifery.* 1999;44:320-24.

10381 Wedig KE, Whitsett JA. Down the primrose path: petechiae in a neonate exposed to herbal remedy for parturition. *J Pediatr.* 2008;152:140, 140.e1.

10382 Burfield T. The adulteration of essential oils – and consequences to aromatherapy and natural perfumery practice. 2003 Oct. Available at: http://www.users.globalnet.co.uk/~nodice/new/magazine/october/october.htm

10383 Quality assurance in spices and spice products; Modern of Analysis. 1999. Allied Publishers Pct. Ltd.

10384 American Herbal Pharmacopoeia Standards of Identity. Chaste tree fruit. Available at: http://www.herbal-ahp.org/documents/macroscopy/Chaste_Tree_macro.pdf.

10385 Lamborn LL. Modern soaps, candles and glycerin: A practical manual of modern methods of utilization of fats and oils in the manufacture of soaps and candles, and of the recovery of glycerin. Library of the University of Wisconsin.

10386 Oyen LP, Dung NX. Plant resources of South-East Asia. 1999. Backhyus, Leiden.

10387 Nhu-Trang TT1, Casabianca H, Grenier-Loustalot MF. Authenticity control of essential oils containing citronellal and citral by chiral and stable-isotope gas-chromatographic analysis. Anal Bioanal Chem. 2006 Dec;386(7-8):2141-52.

10388 Arctander S. Perfume and Flavor Materials of Natural Origin. 1990. Self-published, Elizabeth, New Jersey

10389 Kubeczka KH, Formacek V. Essential Oils Analysis by Capillary Gas Chromatography and Carbon-13 NMR Spectroscopy, 2nd, Completely Revised, Edition. 2002 May. John Wiley, Chichester.

10390 Singhal RS, Kulkarni PR, Rege DV. Handbook of indices of food quality and authenticity. Woodhead Publishing, Abington.

10391 Agarwood Indonesia. How to detect fake agarwood for both wood and oil. Available at: http://agarwoodindonesia.com/?p=121

10392 Vankar PS. Adulteration in rose oil. *Nat Prod Radiance.* 2003 Jul-Aug;2(4):180-181.

10393 Peter KV. Handbook of herbs and spices. 2001. Woodhead Publishing, Abington. Available at: https://babel.hathitrust.org/cgi/pt?id=mdp.39015000804453;view=1up;seq=98

10394 Radulović NS1, Blagojević PD, Miltojević AB. α-Linalool - a marker compound of forged/synthetic sweet basil (Ocimum basilicum L.) essential oils. *J Sci Food Agric.* 2013 Oct;93(13):3292-303.

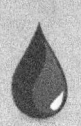

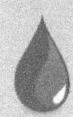

# INDEX

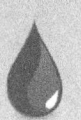

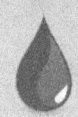

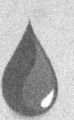

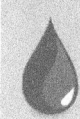

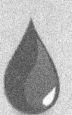

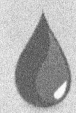

## M

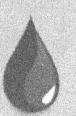

# N

# O

# P

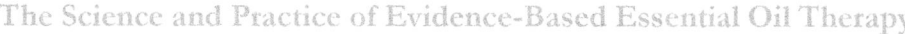
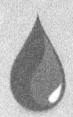

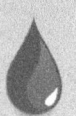

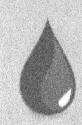